Mader's

REPTILE
AND
AMPHIBIAN
Medicine and Surgery

Mader's
REPTILE
AND
AMPHIBIAN
Medicine and Surgery

THIRD EDITION

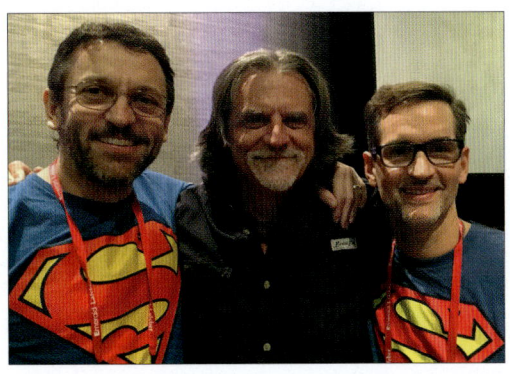

STEPHEN J. DIVERS
BVetMed, DZooMed, Dipl ECZM, (Herpetology and Zoo Health Management), DACZM, FRCVS

Royal College of Veterinary Surgeons Fellow and Recognized Specialist
in Zoo and Wildlife Medicine
European Veterinary Specialist in Zoo Health Management
Scientific Editor for the Journal of Herpetological Medicine & Surgery
Associate Editor for the Journal of Zoo and Wildlife Medicine
Professor of Zoological Medicine
Department of Small Animal Medicine and Surgery
College of Veterinary Medicine
University of Georgia
Athens, Georgia

SCOTT J. STAHL
DVM, Dipl ABVP (Avian)

Chief of Staff and Director
Stahl Exotic Animal Veterinary Services (SEAVS)
Fairfax, Virginia
Adjunct Professor
Virginia-Maryland College of Veterinary Medicine
Virginia Tech
Blacksburg, Virginia

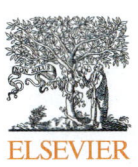

ELSEVIER

MADER'S REPTILE AND AMPHIBIAN MEDICINE AND SURGERY,
THIRD EDITION

ISBN: 978-0-323-48253-0

Previous editions copyrighted 2006 and 1996.

International Standard Book Number: 978-0-323-48253-0

Senior Content Strategist: Jennifer Flynn-Briggs
Senior Content Development Manager: Ellen Wurm-Cutter
Senior Content Development Specialist: Rebecca Leenhouts
Publishing Services Manager: Julie Eddy
Book Production Specialist: Clay S. Broeker
Design Direction: Renee Duenow

Printed in China

Last digit is the print number: 9   8   7   6   5   4   3   2   1

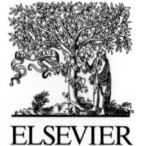

3251 Riverport Lane
St. Louis, Missouri 63043

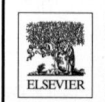

Working together
to grow libraries in
developing countries

www.elsevier.com • www.bookaid.org

This book is dedicated to our parents,
Alan and Christine Divers and Dale and Brenda Stahl.
Your unconditional love and support gave us
the opportunity to make this important contribution
to the health and welfare of these unique animals we love.
Thank you, mom and dad, for everything.

With love,
Steve and Scott

Sarah Alexander, BSc, BVMS, PGCert (Conservation Medicine), DVetMedSc, MANZCVS (Medicine of Zoo Animals)
Resident Veterinarian 2013-2016
New Zealand Centre for Conservation Medicine
Auckland Zoo
Auckland, New Zealand
Locum Veterinarian
Zoos Victoria, Zoos South Australia, and Taronga Western Plains Zoo
Australia
Tuatara Taxonomy, Anatomy, and Physiology
Tuatara

Kimberly M. Andrews, PhD, MS
Assistant Research Scientist
Odum School of Ecology
University of Georgia
Brunswick, Georgia
Working With Free-Ranging Amphibians and Reptiles

Frances M. Baines, MA, VetMB, MRCVS
Owner
UV Guide UK
Abergavenny, United Kingdom
Environmental Lighting

Stephen Barten, DVM
Partner
Vernon Hills Animal Hospital
Mundelein, Illinois
Program Coordinator
VMX Veterinary Meeting and Expo
Orlando, Florida
Lizard Taxonomy, Anatomy, and Physiology
Lizards
Differential Diagnoses by Clinical Signs—Lizards

James E. Bogan Jr., DVM, DABVP (Canine/Feline and Reptile/Amphibian), CertAqV
Chief Veterinary Officer
Veterinary Department
Central Florida Zoo & Botanical Gardens
Sanford, Florida
Chief of Staff and Owner
The Critter Fixer of Central Florida
Oviedo, Florida
Snake Taxonomy, Anatomy, and Physiology

Donal M. Boyer, BLA
Curator
Herpetology
Wildlife Conservation Society
Bronx Zoo
New York, New York
Tortoises, Freshwater Turtles, and Terrapins

Thomas H. Boyer, DVM, DABVP (Reptile and Amphibian Practice)
Owner
Small and Exotic Animal Medicine and Surgery
Pet Hospital of Penasquitos
Co-Founder and Editor-in-Chief (Emeritus)
Journal of Herpetological Medicine & Surgery
Association of Reptilian and Amphibian Veterinarians
San Diego, California
Chelonian Taxonomy, Anatomy, and Physiology
Tortoises, Freshwater Turtles, and Terrapins
Nutrition
Nutritional Diseases
Nutritional Therapy
Differential Diagnoses by Clinical Signs—Chelonians
Hypovitaminosis and Hypervitaminosis A
Nutritional Secondary Hyperparathyroidism

Teresa Bradley Bays, DVM, CVA, DABVP (ECM), CVMMP
Co-Owner, Medical Director, and Exotic Companion Mammal Specialist
Belton Animal Clinic and Exotic Care Center
Raymore Animal Clinic
Belton, Missouri
Clinical Behavioral Medicine
Mental Health Treatment (Psychopharmacology and Behavior Therapy)

Mary B. Brown, PhD
Professor
Infectious Diseases and Immunology
University of Florida
Gainesville, Florida
Otorhinolaryngology
Tortoise Mycoplasmosis

Melinda S. Camus, DVM, DACVP
Associate Professor
Pathology
College of Veterinary Medicine
University of Georgia
Athens, Georgia
Cytology

Brendan Carmel, BVSc, MVS, MANZCVS (Unusual Pets), GDipComp
Owner
Warranwood Veterinary Centre
Warranwood, Australia
Specialization

James W. Carpenter, MS, DVM, Dipl ACZM
Professor
Department of Clinical Sciences
College of Veterinary Medicine
Kansas State University
Manhattan, Kansas
Hematology and Biochemistry Tables
Reptile Formulary

Norin Chai, DVM, MSc, PhD, Dipl ECZM (Zoo Health Management)
Head Vet and Deputy Director
Ménagerie du Jardin des Plantes
Muséum National d'Histoire Naturelle
Paris, France
Amphibian Chytridiomycosis

Leigh Clayton, DVM
Vice President
Animal Care and Welfare
National Aquarium
Baltimore, Maryland
Differential Diagnoses by Clinical Signs—Amphibians

Jessica R. Comolli, DVM, LVT
Zoological Medicine Resident
Department of Small Animal Medicine and Surgery
College of Veterinary Medicine
University of Georgia
Athens, Georgia
Radiography—Snakes

Scott Connelly, PhD
Assistant Professor
Odum School of Ecology
University of Georgia
Athens, Georgia
Herpetofauna and Ecosystem Health

John E. Cooper, DTVM, FRCPath, FRSB, CBiol, FRCVS, RCVS Specialist in Veterinary Pathology, Dipl European College of Veterinary Pathologists, Dipl ECZM
Wildlife Health, Forensic and Comparative Pathology Services (UK)
Honorary Research Fellow
Durrell Institute for Conservation and Ecology (DICE)
University of Kent
Canterbury, United Kingdom
Forensics

Margaret E. Cooper, LLB, FLS, English Solicitor (Non-Practising)
Wildlife Health, Forensic and Comparative Pathology Services (UK)
Honorary Research Fellow
Durrell Institute for Conservation and Ecology (DICE)
University of Kent
Canterbury, United Kingdom
Laws and Regulations—International
Laws and Regulations—Europe
Forensics

Lara M. Cusack, DVM
Wildlife Veterinarian
Florida Fish and Wildlife Conservation Commission
Naples, Florida
Environmental Lighting
Photomodulation (Low-Level Laser Therapy)

Daniel Cutler, DVM
Zoological Medicine Resident
Department of Small Animal Medicine and Surgery
College of Veterinary Medicine
University of Georgia
Athens, Georgia
Esophagostomy Tube Placement
Hospitalization

Andre Daneault
Curator of Ectotherms
Animals, Science, and Environment
Disney's Animal Kingdom
Bay Lake, Florida
Behavioral Training and Enrichment of Reptiles

Leticia Mattos de Souza Dantas, DVM, MS, PhD, DACVB
Clinical Assistant Professor of Behavioral Medicine
Department of Veterinary Biosciences and Diagnostic Imaging
College of Veterinary Medicine
University of Georgia
Athens, Georgia
Clinical Behavioral Medicine
Mental Health Treatment (Psychopharmacology and Behavior Therapy)

Ryan De Voe, DVM, MSpVM, Dipl ACZM, Dipl ABVP (Reptiles and Amphibians)
Clinical Veterinarian
Animals, Science, and Environment
Disney's Animal Kingdom
EPCOT's The Seas with Nemo and Friends
Walt Disney's Parks and Resorts
Bay Lake, Florida
Gastroenterology—Oral Cavity, Esophagus, and Stomach
Gastrointestinal Tract
Stomatitis

Dale F. DeNardo, DVM, PhD
Associate Professor
School of Life Sciences
Arizona State University
Tempe, Arizona
Theriogenology

Geraldine Diethelm, DrVetMed
Chief of Staff
Marathon Veterinary Hospital
Marathon, Florida
Digit Abnormalities

Stephen J. Divers, BVetMed, DZooMed, Dipl ECZM (Herpetology and Zoo Health Management), DACZM, FRCVS
Royal College of Veterinary Surgeons Fellow and Recognized Specialist in Zoo and Wildlife
European Veterinary Specialist in Zoo Health Management
Scientific Editor for the Journal of Herpetological Medicine & Surgery
Associate Editor for the Journal of Zoo and Wildlife Medicine
Professor of Zoological Medicine
Department of Small Animal Medicine and Surgery
College of Veterinary Medicine
University of Georgia
Athens, Georgia
Specialization
Bacteriology
Mycology
Molecular Infectious Disease Diagnostics
Diagnostic Laboratory Listing
Medical History and Physical Examination
Diagnostic Techniques and Sample Collection
Catheter Placement
Esophagostomy Tube Placement
Hospitalization
Amphibian Anesthesia
Radiography—General Principles
Radiography—Lizards
Radiography—Snakes
Radiography—Chelonians
Diagnostic and Surgical Endoscopy Equipment
Endoscopy Practice Management (Fee Structures and Marketing)
Diagnostic Endoscopy
Endoscope-Assisted and Endoscopic Surgery
Urology
Hepatology
Otorhinolaryngology
Pulmonology
Surgical Equipment, Instrumentation, and General Principles
Ear
Rhinarium
Oral Cavity, Mandible, Maxilla, and Beak
Chelonian Prefemoral Coeliotomy
Chelonian Transplastron Coeliotomy
Lower Respiratory Tract
Urinary Tract
Photobiomodulation (Low-Level Laser Therapy)
Aural/Tympanic Abscessation
Hepatic Lipidosis
Pneumonia
Renal Disease
Tail Abnormalities

Andrew M. Durso, BS, MS, PhD
Postdoctoral Researcher
Institute of Global Health
University of Geneva
Geneva, Switzerland
Natural Behavior

Kevin Eatwell, BVSc (Hons), Dipl ZooMed (Reptilian), Dipl ECZM (Herpetology and Small Mammals), RCVS Recognized Specialist in Zoo and Wildlife Medicine, ECZM Recognized Veterinary Specialist in Herpetological Medicine, MRCVS
Senior Lecturer in Rabbit, Exotic Animal, and Wildlife Medicine and Surgery
Dick Vet Rabbit and Exotic Clinic
University of Edinburgh
Edinburgh, United Kingdom
Gastroenterology—Small Intestine, Exocrine Pancreas, and Large Intestine
Diarrhea
Lizard Cryptosporidiosis

Bruce Ferguson, MS, DVM
Instructor and Course Director
Tui-Na and Chinese Bodywork
Topographic Acupuncture
Chi Institute of Chinese Medicine
Reddick, Florida
Complementary and Integrative Veterinary Therapies

Shannon T. Ferrell, DVM, DACZM, DABVP (Avian)
Chief
Veterinary Services
Zoo de Granby
Granby, Canada
Conservation

Kevin T. Fitzgerald, PhD, DVM, DABVP
Staff Veterinarian
General Practice/Emergency/Exotics
VCA Alameda East Veterinary Hospital
Denver, Colorado
Toxicology
Acariasis
Spinal Osteopathy

Samuel P. Franklin, MS, DVM, PhD
Assistant Professor of Small Animal Orthopedic Surgery
Department of Small Animal Medicine and Surgery
College of Veterinary Medicine
University of Georgia
Athens, Georgia
Physical Therapy and Rehabilitation

Richard S. Funk, MA, DVM
Owner
Richard Funk Veterinary Services
Mesa, Arizona
Adjunct Professor
Midwestern University
College of Veterinary Medicine
Glendale, Arizona
Snake Taxonomy, Anatomy, and Physiology
Snakes
Venomoid Surgery
Snake Coeliotomy
Tail Amputation
Differential Diagnoses by Clinical Signs—Snakes
Tail Abnormalities
Vomiting and Regurgitation

Janos Gal, DVM, PhD, Dipl ECZM
Head of Department
Department of Exotic Animal and Wildlife Medicine
University of Veterinary Science
Budapest, Hungary
Salmonellosis
Zoonoses and Public Health

Paul M. Gibbons, DVM, MS, Dipl ABVP (Reptile/Amphibian)
Conservation Program Director
Behler Chelonian Center
Turtle Conservancy
Ojai, California
Associate Veterinarian
Avian and Exotic Veterinary Care
Portland, Oregon
Hematology and Biochemistry Tables
Reptile Formulary
Large Zoo and Private Collection Management

Simon Girling, BVMS (Hons), DZooMed, Dipl ECZM (ZHM), CBiol, FRSB, EurProBiol, FRCVS
Head of Veterinary Services
Veterinary Department, Living Collections
Royal Zoological Society of Scotland
Edinburgh, United Kingdom
Cardiology
Vascular, Hematopoietic, and Immune Systems

Nicole Gottdenker, DVM, MS, PhD, Dipl ACVP
Associate Professor
Department of Veterinary Pathology
College of Veterinary Medicine
University of Georgia
Athens, Georgia
Biopsy
Necropsy

Chris Griffin, DVM, DABVP (Avian)
Medical Director and Owner
Griffin Avian and Exotic Veterinary Hospital
Kannapolis, North Carolina
Breeders, Wholesalers, and Retailers

Craig A. Harms, DVM, PhD, Dipl ACZM
Professor
Clinical Sciences
College of Veterinary Medicine
North Carolina State University
Center for Marine Sciences and Technology
Morehead City, North Carolina
Sea Turtles

Tara M. Harrison, DVM, MPVM, Dipl ACZM, Dipl ACVPM, Dipl ECZM (ZHM), CVA
Assistant Professor
Department of Clinical Sciences
North Carolina State University College of Veterinary Medicine
Raleigh, North Carolina
Cancer Chemotherapy

J. Jill Heatley, DVM, MS
Associate Professor
Veterinary Small Animal Clinical Sciences
College of Veterinary Medicine and Biomedical Sciences
College Station, Texas
Hematology
Clinical Chemistry

Joanna Hedley, BVM&S, DZooMed (Reptilian), Dipl ECZM (Herpetology), MRCVS
Exotics Service
Royal Veterinary College
London, United Kingdom
Reference Resources for the Herpetological Clinician

Tom Hellebuyck, DVM, PhD, Dipl ECZM (Herpetology)
Head of Clinic
Division of Poultry, Exotic Companion Animals, Wildlife and Experimental Animals
Department of Pathology, Bacteriology and Avian Diseases
Faculty of Veterinary Medicine
Ghent University
Merelbeke, Belgium
Dermatology—Skin
Integument
Dysecdysis
Thermal Burns

Claudia Hochleithner, DVM
Managing Director
Tierklinik Strebersdorf Hochleithner GmbH
Tierklinik
Vienna, Austria
Ultrasonography

Shannon P. Holmes, DVM, MSc, Dipl ACVR
Founding Radiologist
AXIS—Animal Cross-Sectional Imaging Specialists
Athens, Georgia
Radiography—General Principles
Radiography—Lizards
Radiography—Chelonians
Magnetic Resonance Imaging

Elizabeth W. Howerth, DVM, PhD
Professor
Department of Veterinary Pathology
College of Veterinary Medicine
University of Georgia
Athens, Georgia
Immunopathology

Craig J-G. Hunt, BVetMed, CertSAM, DZooMed (Reptilian), MRCVS
RCVS Recognized Specialist in Zoo and Wildlife Medicine
Chine House Veterinary Hospital
Loughborough, United Kingdom
Stress and Welfare
Disinfection

Charles J. Innis, VMD, DABVP (Reptile and Amphibian Practice)
Director of Animal Health
New England Aquarium
Boston, Massachusetts
Chelonian Taxonomy, Anatomy, and Physiology
Urology
Medical Management and Rehabilitation of Sea Turtles

Robert Johnson, BVSc, MANZCVS, CertZooMed, BA
Zoologica Consulting
Mosman, Australia
Venomous Species
Tail Abnormalities

Cathy A. Johnson-Delaney, DVM
Special Projects Coordinator
Animal Facility
NW Zoological Supply
Everett, Washington
Consulting Veterinarian
Oregon Tiger Sanctuary
Eagle Point, Oregon
Consulting Veterinarian
Pacific Primate Sanctuary
Haiku, Hawaii
Contributing Author
Vetstream
Devon, United Kingdom
Salmonellosis
Zoonoses and Public Health

W. Michael Karlin, DVM, MS, Dipl ACVS SA and LA
Assistant Professor of Orthopedic Surgery
Cummings School of Veterinary Medicine
Tufts University
North Grafton, Massachusetts
Orthopedic Principles and External Coaptation
Fracture Fixation and Arthrodesis
Skull and Spinal Fracture Repair
Limb Amputation

Krista A. Keller, DVM, Dipl ACZM
Assistant Professor
Department of Veterinary Clinical Medicine
College of Veterinary Medicine
University of Illinois
Urbana, Illinois
Perinatology
Urolithiasis (Cystic Calculi and Cloacal Uroliths)

Marja J.L. Kik, DVM, PhD, Dipl ECZM (Herpetology), Dipl Pathology RNVA
Professor
Department of Pathobiology
Veterinary Pathological Diagnostic Center
Utrecht University
Utrecht, Netherlands
Bite Wounds and Prey-Induced Trauma

Michelle Kischinovsky, DVM, MRCVS
Head Veterinarian
Zoo Animal Health
Nordens Ark
Hunnebostrand, Sweden
Otorhinolaryngology
Ear
Rhinarium
Oral Cavity, Mandible, Maxilla, and Beak
Aural/Tympanic Abscessation

Eric Klaphake, DVM, Dipl ACZM, Dipl ABVP (Avian Practice), Dipl ABVP (Reptile/Amphibian Practice)
Associate Veterinarian
Cheyenne Mountain Zoo
Colorado Springs, Colorado
Hematology and Biochemistry Tables
Reptile Formulary

S. Emi Knafo, BS, DVM, DACZM
Zoological Medicine Specialist
Avian and Exotics Department
Red Bank Veterinary Hospital
Tinton Falls, New Jersey
Musculoskeletal System
Orthopedic Principles and External Coaptation
Fracture Fixation and Arthrodesis
Skull and Spinal Fracture Repair
Limb Amputation
Spinal Osteopathy

Zdenek Knotek, DVM, PhD, Dipl ECZM (Herpetological Medicine and Surgery)
Head
Avian and Exotic Animal Clinic
Faculty of Veterinary Medicine
University of Veterinary and Pharmaceutical Sciences Brno
Brno, Czech Republic
Pulmonology

Martin P.C. Lawton, BVetMed, CertVOphthal, CertLAS, CBiol, MRSB, DZooMed, FRSM, FRCVS
Lawton & Stoakes
Romford
Essex, United Kingdom
Ophthalmology
Eye
Jurisprudence, Expert Reports, Testimony, and Court Appearance

Daniel T. Lewbart, JD, MELP
Gerolamo, Divis, McNulty, & Lewbart
Philadelphia, Pennsylvania
Laws and Regulations—Americas

Gregory A. Lewbart, MS, VMD, Dipl ACZM and ECZM (Zoo Health Management)
Professor of Aquatic Animal Medicine
College of Veterinary Medicine
North Carolina State University
Raleigh, North Carolina
Laws and Regulations—Americas

Adolf Maas, DVM, DABVP (Reptile and Amphibian), CertAqV
Director
Research and Clinical Medicine
ZooVet Consulting, PLLC
Bothell, Washington
Developing a Successful Herpetological Veterinary Service

Ross A. Machin, DVM, MRCVS, GPCert (ExAP), PgC (EAS), RCVS
Advanced Practitioner in Zoological Medicine
Veterinary Surgeon
Exotics
MR Vet Ltd.
Leicester, United Kingdom
Gastroenterology—Cloaca
Cloacal Prolapse
Cloacal Prolapse

John C. Maerz, PhD, BSc
Josiah Meigs Distinguished Professor
Warnell School of Forestry and Natural Resources
University of Georgia
Athens, Georgia
Natural Behavior

Christoph Mans, DrMedVet
Clinical Assistant Professor of Zoological Medicine
Department of Surgical Sciences
School of Veterinary Medicine
University of Wisconsin-Madison
Madison, Wisconsin
General Anesthesia
Analgesia
Regional Anesthesia and Analgesia

Maud L. Marin, DMV, MSc, DACZM
Clinical Director
Veterinary Technician Program
Pima Medical Institute
Houston, Texas
Wound Management

Rachel E. Marschang, PD DrMedVet, Dipl ECZM (Herpetology), FTÄ Mikrobiologie, ZB Reptilien
Veterinarian
Microbiology
Laboklin GmbH & Co. KG
Bad Kissingen, Germany
Universität Hohenheim
Stuttgart, Germany
Virology
Antiviral Therapy

An Martel, DVM, MSc, PhD, Dipl ECZM (Wildlife Population Health)
Professor
Wildlife Health Ghent
Department of Pathology, Bacteriology, and Avian Diseases
Ghent University
Merelbeke, Belgium
Amphibian Taxonomy, Anatomy, and Physiology
Amphibians

Albert Martínez-Silvestre, DVM, MSc, PhD, Dipl ECZM (Herpetology), Acred AVEPA (Exotic Animals)
Scientific Director and Veterinarian
Catalonian Reptile and Amphibian Rescue Center (CRARC)
Masquefa, Spain
Advisory Board Member and Veterinarian
Turtle Conservancy
Los Angeles, California
Toxicology
Physical Therapy and Rehabilitation

Karina A. Mathes, DVM, Dipl ECZM (Herpetology), European Veterinary Specialist in Zoological Medicine (Herpetology), Certified Specialist in Reptiles (Fachtieraerztin für Reptilien), Certified Specialist in Reptiles and Amphibians (ZB Reptilien und Amphibien)
Head of the Department of Reptiles and Amphibians
Clinic for Small Mammals, Reptiles and Birds
University of Veterinary Medicine Hannover
Hannover, Germany
Neurological Disorders

Joerg Mayer, DVM, MSc, DABVP (SM), DECZM (SM), DACZM
Associate Professor
Department of Small Animal Medicine and Surgery
College of Veterinary Medicine
University of Georgia
Athens, Georgia
Oncology
Cancer Chemotherapy
Radiation Therapy
Allometric Scaling

Stuart McArthur, BVetMed
Veterinarian
The Animal Trust
Leeds, United Kingdom
Gastroenterology—Cloaca
Cloacal Prolapse
Cloacal Prolapse

Colin T. McDermott, VMD, CertAqV
Exotic and Aquatic Veterinarian
Exotics Department
Mount Laurel Animal Hospital
Mount Laurel, New Jersey
Hematology and Biochemistry Tables
Amphibian Formulary

Melinda Merck, DVM
Owner
Veterinary Forensics Consulting, LLC
Austin, Texas
Forensics

Jean Meyer, DrMedVet, FTA Kleintiere
Private Practice
Tierarztpraxis Voelkendorf
Villach, Austria
Lecturer
Department of Small Animal Medicine/Reptile Medicine
University of Veterinary Medicine
Vienna, Austria
Dermatology—Shell
Shell Surgery and Repair
Shell Abnormalities

Mark A. Mitchell, DVM, MS, PhD, DECZM (Herpetology)
Professor
Department of Veterinary Clinical Sciences
Louisiana State University
Hospital Director
Veterinary Teaching Hospital
Louisiana State University
Baton Rouge, Louisiana
The Importance of Herpetological Publication by Clinicians and
*   Academics*
Statistics for the Clinician Scientist
Therapeutic Overview and General Approach
Routes of Administration
Antibiotic Therapy
Antifungal Therapy
Antiinflammatory Therapy
Antiparasitic Therapy

Antony S. Moore, BVSc, MVSc, MANZCVS, Dipl ACVIM
(Oncology)
Co-Director
Veterinary Oncology Consultants
Wauchope, Australia
Oncology
Cancer Chemotherapy

Walter Mustin, MS, PhD
Chief Research Officer
Animal Programs
Cayman Turtle Farm
West Bay, Cayman Islands
Commercial Reptile Farming

Koichi Nagata, BVSc, DACVR (RO)
Radiation Oncology
Department of Veterinary Biosciences
College of Veterinary Medicine
University of Georgia
Athens, Georgia
Radiation Therapy

Giordano Nardini, DMV, PhD, Dipl ECZM (Herpetology)
Head of Hospital
Clinica Veterinaria Modena Sud
Spilamberto, Italy
Adjunct Professor
University of Teramo
Teramo, Italy
Hemoparasites

Javier G. Nevarez, DVM, PhD, DACZM, DECZM (Herpetology)
Professor
Veterinary Clinical Sciences
School of Veterinary Medicine
Louisiana State University
Baton Rouge, Louisiana
Crocodilian Taxonomy, Anatomy, and Physiology
Crocodilians
Euthanasia
Radiography—Crocodilians
Crocodilian Coeliotomy
Differential Diagnoses by Clinical Signs—Crocodilians
Commercial Reptile Farming

Terry M. Norton, DVM, Dipl ACZM
Director and Veterinarian
Rehabilitation, Education, and Research
Georgia Sea Turtle Center/Jekyll Island Authority
Jekyll Island, Georgia
Wildlife Veterinarian
St. Catherines Island Foundation
Midway, Georgia
Veterinarian
Turtle Hospital
Marathon, Florida
Vice President
St. Kitts Sea Turtle Monitoring Network
Basseterre, St. Kitts
Board Member and Wildlife Veterinarian
Osa Ecology
Osa Peninsula, Costa Rica
Adjunct Professor
College of Veterinary Medicine
University of Georgia
Athens, Georgia
North Carolina State University College of Veterinary Medicine
Raleigh, North Carolina
Lincoln Memorial University College of Veterinary Medicine
Harrogate, Tennessee
Cummings School of Veterinary Medicine at Tufts University
North Grafton, Massachusetts
Shell Surgery and Repair
Wound Management
Working With Free-Ranging Amphibians and Reptiles

Peter Nowlan, MVB, MSc, MRCVS, Cert LAS MA
Professor
Department of Zoology
Trinity College Dublin
Dublin, Ireland
Laboratory Management and Medicine

Dorcas P. O'Rourke, DVM, MS, DACLAM
Professor and Chair
Department of Comparative Medicine
The Brody School of Medicine
East Carolina University
Greenville, North Carolina
Laboratory Management and Medicine

Francesco C. Origgi, DVM, PhD, DACVM (Virology), DACVP, DECZM (Herpetology)
Centre for Fish and Wildlife Health (FIWI)
Vetsuisse Faculty
University of Bern
Bern, Switzerland
Inclusion Body Disease (Reptarenavirus)
Paramyxoviruses (Ferlaviruses)
Testudinid Herpesviruses

Jorge Orós, DVM, PhD, Dipl ECZM
Professor
Morphology
Veterinary Faculty
University of Las Palmas de Gran Canaria
Arucas, Spain
Gout
Pseudogout

Mariana A. Pardo, BVsc, MV
Emergency and Critical Care Resident
Department of Clinical Sciences
Cornell University
Ithaca, New York
Catheter Placement

Frank Pasmans, DVM, MSc, PhD, Dipl ECZM (Herpetology)
Professor
Wildlife Heath Ghent and Laboratory of Veterinary Bacteriology and
    Mycology
Ghent University
Merelbeke, Belgium
Amphibian Taxonomy, Anatomy, and Physiology
Amphibians

Michael Pees, Dipl ECZM (Avian and Herpetology)
Department for Birds and Reptiles
University Teaching Hospital
Leipzig, Germany
Thermal Burns

Sean M. Perry, DVM
Graduate Assistant
Department of Veterinary Clinical Sciences
Louisiana State University
Baton Rouge, Louisiana
The Importance of Herpetological Publication by Clinicians and
    Academics
Statistics for the Clinician Scientist
Therapeutic Overview and General Approach
Routes of Administration
Antibiotic Therapy
Antifungal Therapy

Olivia A. Petritz, DVM, DACZM
Assistant Professor
Department of Clinical Sciences
College of Veterinary Medicine
North Carolina State University
Raleigh, North Carolina
Emergency and Critical Care

Simon R. Platt, BVM&S, FRCVS, Dipl ACVIM (Neurology), Dipl ECVN
Professor of Neurology
Department of Small Animal Medicine and Surgery
College of Veterinary Medicine
University of Georgia
Athens, Georgia
Neurology
Neurological Disorders

Geoffrey W. Pye, BVSc, MSc, Dipl ACZM
Animal Health Director
Animals, Science, and Environment
Disney's Animal Kingdom
Bay Lake, Florida
Behavioral Training and Enrichment of Reptiles

Nathalie Rademacher, DrVetMed, DACVR, DECVDI
Associate Professor, Diagnostic Imaging
Veterinary Clinical Sciences
School of Veterinary Medicine
Louisiana State University
Baton Rouge, Louisiana
Radiography—Crocodilians

Paul Raiti, DVM, DABVP (Reptile and Amphibian Practice)
Owner
Beverlie Animal Hospital
Mount Vernon, New York
Endocrinology
Geriatric Medicine

Drury R. Reavill, DVM, DABVP (Avian and Reptile/Amphibian), DACVP
Owner
Zoo/Exotic Pathology Service
Carmichael, California
Breeders, Wholesalers, and Retailers

Leslie Retnam, BVetSc, MLAS, MRCVS
Director of Veterinary Services
Biological Resource Centre
Agency for Science, Technology and Research (A*STAR)
Singapore
Laboratory Management and Medicine

Jenna Richardson, BVM&S MRCVS
Lecturer and Clinician in Rabbit, Exotic Animal, and Wildlife
    Medicine and Surgery
Rabbit and Exotic Animal Department
University of Edinburgh
Edinburgh, United Kingdom
Gastroenterology—Small Intestine, Exocrine Pancreas, and Large
    Intestine
Diarrhea
Lizard Cryptosporidiosis

Sam Rivera, DVM, MS, DABVP (Avian), DACZM, DECZM (Zoo Health Management)
Senior Director of Animal Health
Zoo Atlanta
Atlanta, Georgia
Quarantine

Kelly Rockwell, DVM
Zoological Medicine Intern
Louisiana State University
Baton Rouge, Louisiana
Antiinflammatory Therapy
Antiparasitic Therapy

John V. Rossi, DVM MA
Private Practitioner
Riverside Animal Hospital
Jacksonville, Florida
General Husbandry and Management

Karen E. Russell, DVM, PhD, Dipl ACVP (Clinical Pathology)
Department of Veterinary Pathobiology
Texas A&M University
College Station, Texas
Hematology
Clinical Chemistry

T. Franciscus Scheelings, BVSc, MVSc, MANZCVSc (Wildlife Health), Dipl ECZM (Herpetology)
PhD Candidate
School of Biological Sciences
Monash University
Clayton, Australia
Dermatology—Skin
Integument
Bite Wounds and Prey-Induced Trauma
Dysecdysis

Lionel Schilliger, DVM, DECZM (Herpetology), DABVP (Reptile and Amphibian Practice)
Owner
Veterinary Clinic of Auteuil Village
Paris, France
Clinical Instructor
Exotics Medicine Service
Veterinary School of Alfort
Maisons-Alfort, France
Cardiology

Volker Schmidt, DrMedVet, Dipl ECZM (Avian and Herpetology)
Head of the Clinical Laboratory
Department for Birds and Reptiles, Veterinary Teaching Hospital
University of Leipzig
Leipzig, Germany
Specialization
Abscesses/Fibriscesses

Rodney W. Schnellbacher, DVM, Dipl ACZM
Staff Veterinarian
Animal Health
Dickerson Park Zoo
Springfield, Missouri
Sedation
Snake Coeliotomy
Miscellaneous Drug Therapy
Differential Diagnoses by Clinical Signs—Snakes
Snake Cryptosporidiosis

Juergen Schumacher, DrMedVet, Dipl ACZM
Professor and Head
Department of Small Animal Clinical Sciences
College of Veterinary Medicine
University of Tennessee
Knoxville, Tennessee
General Anesthesia

Peter W. Scott, MSc, BVSc, FRCVS
Director
Specialist Veterinary Services
Biotope
Winchester, United Kingdom
Nutrition
Nutritional Diseases
Nutritional Therapy
Nutritional Secondary Hyperparathyroidism

Paolo Selleri, DMV, PhD, SpecPACS, Dipl ECZM (Herpetology and Small Mammals)
Clinica per Animali Esotici
Centro Veterinario Specialistico
Rome, Italy
Dermatology—Shell
Shell Abnormalities

Ajay Sharma, BVSc, MVSc, DVM
Associate Professor, Diagnostic imaging
Veterinary Biosciences and Diagnostic Imaging
College of Veterinary Medicine
University of Georgia
Athens, Georgia
Ultrasonography
Computed Tomography

Molly Shepard, DVM, Dipl ACVAA, CCRP, cVMA
Anesthesiologist and Pain Management Specialist
MedVet
Chicago, Illinois
Sedation

Shane Simpson, BVSc (Hons), GCM (VP)
Partner
The Unusual Pet Vets
Frankston, Australia
Lizard Taxonomy, Anatomy, and Physiology
Lizards
Differential Diagnoses by Clinical Signs—Lizards

Michelle L. Skurski
Zoological Manager of Behavioral Husbandry
Animals, Science, and Environment
Disney's Animal Kingdom
Bay Lake, Florida
Behavioral Training and Enrichment of Reptiles

Izidora Sladakovic, BVSc (Hons I), MVS, DACZM
Director of Avian and Exotics Service
Northside Veterinary Specialists
Terrey Hills, Australia
Amphibian Anesthesia
Miscellaneous Drug Therapy

Kurt K. Sladky, MS, DVM, Dipl ACZM, Dipl ECZM
Professor
Zoological Medicine
Surgical Sciences
School of Veterinary Medicine
University of Wisconsin
Madison, Wisconsin
Hematology and Biochemistry Tables
General Anesthesia
Analgesia
Regional Anesthesia and Analgesia
Reptile Formulary

Lora L. Smith, MS, PhD
Scientist
Research
Joseph W. Jones Ecological Research Center
Newton, Georgia
Working With Free-Ranging Amphibians and Reptiles

Mauricio Solano, MV, DACVR
Assistant Professor
Clinical Sciences
Cummings School of Veterinary Medicine
Tufts University
North Grafton, Massachusetts
Scintigraphy

Tolina Tina Son, DVM, DACVECC, CVA
Director of Emergency and Critical Care
The Amanda Foundation
Beverly Hills, California
Emergency and Critical Care

Scott J. Stahl, DVM, Dipl ABVP (Avian)
Chief of Staff and Director
Stahl Exotic Animal Veterinary Services (SEAVS)
Fairfax, Virginia
Adjunct Professor
Virginia-Maryland College of Veterinary Medicine
Virginia Tech
Blacksburg, Virginia
Specialization
Snakes
Theriogenology
Lizard Coeliotomy
Reproductive Tract
Cloacal Scent Gland Adenitis
Dystocia and Follicular Stasis
Hyperglycemia
Periodontal Disease
Vomiting and Regurgitation

Paulo Steagall, DVM, MSc, PhD, Dipl ACVAA
Associate Professor of Veterinary Anesthesia and Pain Management
Department of Clinical Sciences
Faculty of Veterinary Medicine
Université de Montréal
Saint-Hyacinthe, Canada
Regional Anesthesia and Analgesia

Heather D.S. Walden, MS, PhD
Assistant Professor
Comparative, Diagnostic and Population Medicine
University of Florida College of Veterinary Medicine
Gainesville, Florida
Parasitology (Including Hemoparasites)

James F.X. Wellehan, DVM, MS, PhD, DACZM, DACVM (Virology and Bacteriology/Mycology)
Zoological Medical Service
College of Veterinary Medicine
University of Florida
Gainesville, Florida
Bacteriology
Mycology
Parasitology (Including Hemoparasites)
Molecular Infectious Disease Diagnostics

Lori D. Wendland, DVM, PhD
Veterinarian
Shelton Veterinary Clinic
Interlachen, Florida
Otorhinolaryngology
Tortoise Mycoplasmosis

Cynthia L. West, DVM, CVA, CVTP
Instructor
Traditional Chinese Veterinary Medicine
Chi Institute of Chinese Medicine
Reddick, Florida
Complementary and Integrative Veterinary Therapies

Brent R. Whitaker, MS, DVM
Research Associate Professor
Department of Marine Biology
Institute of Marine and Environmental Technology
University of Maryland
Baltimore, Maryland
Hematology and Biochemistry Tables
Amphibian Medicine
Amphibian Soft Tissue Surgery
Amphibian Formulary
Amphibian Chytridiomycosis

Stacey Leonatti Wilkinson, DVM, DABVP (Reptile and Amphibian)
Owner and Head Veterinarian
Avian and Exotic Animal Hospital of Georgia
Pooler, Georgia
Adjunct Assistant Professor
Companion Animal
North Carolina State University College of Veterinary Medicine
Raleigh, North Carolina
Understanding the Human-Herp Relationship

Elisa Wüst, DrMedVet
Certified Specialist in Poultry and Avian Medicine
Head of Clinical Department
Clinic for Birds, Reptiles, Amphibians, and Fish
Veterinary Department
Justus-Liebig University
Giessen, Germany
Chelonian Prefemoral Coeliotomy
Chelonian Transplastron Coeliotomy

Jeanette Wyneken, PhD
Professor
Department of Biological Sciences
Florida Atlantic University
Boca Raton, Florida
Sea Turtles
Computed Tomography
Magnetic Resonance Imaging

Wilson Yau, DVM, Dipl ACVP
Anatomic Pathologist
ANTECH Diagnostics
Fountain Valley, California
Biopsy
Necropsy

Taylor Yaw, DVM
Veterinary Intern
Animal Health
National Aquarium
Baltimore, Maryland
Zoological Resident
University of Wisconsin
Surgical Sciences
University of Wisconsin/Milwaukee County Zoo
Madison, Wisconsin
Differential Diagnoses by Clinical Signs—Amphibians

Corry K. Yeuroukis, DVM
Clinical Pathology Resident
Department of Veterinary Pathology
College of Veterinary Medicine
University of Georgia
Athens, Georgia
Cytology

FOREWORD

The art of reptile and amphibian medicine has progressed from knee-jerk reactions to basic signs and symptoms to advanced, pragmatic, evidenced-based medical care. Although there are still those that think a paramedian incision is the only way to enter a coelom or that Baytril is all you need to be a successful herp doctor, for the majority, the approach to diagnosis and treatment has finally started to catch up with real veterinary medicine. Of course, I am referring to the level practiced on dogs and cats.

As far as I can tell, the first published work on "Diseases of Reptiles" was authored by Dr. H. Spencer Glidden, an MD, *not* a DVM. The work was penned in 1936 and published by the Florida Reptile Institute, Silver Springs, Florida. The entire manuscript was a whopping *four* pages long. Dr. Glidden was an instructor in Pathology and Bacteriology at the Tufts College Medical School.

"Respiratory," "Mouth Rot," and "Bad Sheds" (which included retained eye-caps) were about the extent of the spectrum of reptilian diseases. For years, that was it.

Sick reptile treatments started with gentamicin and progressed to enrofloxacin. Now, dozens of pharmacodynamic studies exist to validate drugs and dosages. It is no longer "one dose fits all."

As a young herp doc, I was taught that anesthesia involved placing the lizard in the refrigerator for a few hours. Pain control? Not necessary—reptiles don't feel pain.

Fortunately, those antediluvian beliefs have gone the way of the dinosaurs.

Compared to Dr. Glidden's 4-page tome, the first edition of this series, *Reptile Medicine and Surgery,* had over 500 pages. This current edition has over 1500 pages of advanced medical knowledge.

Drs. Divers and Stahl have done an amazing job gathering and incorporating specialists in several disciplines into the production of this book. In addition, they have integrated experts from across the oceans, erasing the myopic tenet that only the United States' viewpoints were relevant. So much research has been done overseas that it is refreshing to see the valuable information being disseminated here.

Whether you are just a novice herp veterinarian, an ectoderm enthusiast, or someone studying for one of the specialty examinations, you need to have this book on your shelf—and you also need to read it!

I am so proud to pass the torch on to the next generation of brilliant herp medicine enthusiasts. It has been such a ride watching the evolution of herp care from simple antibiotics to advanced health care.

If you are going to talk the talk, you have to walk the walk.

Douglas R. Mader, MS, DVM
Diplomate, American Board of Veterinary Practitioners (Canine/Feline)
Diplomate, American Board of Veterinary Practitioners (Reptile/Amphibian)
Diplomate, European College of Zoological Medicine (Herpetology)
Fellow, Royal Society of Medicine

Welcome to the third edition of the quintessential veterinary reference on reptile and amphibian medicine and surgery. When Douglas Mader passed over the editorial reins of his book to us, we knew we had large shoes to fill. Doug remains a major contributor and pioneer in the field of herpetological medicine and surgery, and his contributions to the literature culminated in the first and subsequently greatly expanded second edition. The second edition represented the most comprehensive veterinary text on reptile medicine and surgery and quickly became established as *the* reference worldwide by private practitioners, specialists, and veterinary students. The second edition became standard reading for the veterinary specialty examinations of the American, European, and Australian specialty colleges and boards. Indeed, such was our reliance on this book that it quickly became a trusted resource or colleague, and basically everyone referred to the tome as *Mader*. It seemed only right and proper therefore that this sentiment be continued, and in honor of his numerous and ongoing contributions, this new edition bears the title of *Mader's Reptile and Amphibian Medicine and Surgery*.

The goal of the current editors was to continue the evolution of this specialty reference that Doug had started, and we have approached this challenging task in several ways. First, this third edition is 25% larger to accommodate our continued growth in knowledge of these animals, with each chapter undergoing a major review and rewrite. Some areas have expanded greatly, requiring the division of some topics into multiple chapters, while many chapters appear for the first time. A perusal of the table of contents will readily convey this expansion, including greater inclusion of amphibians with dedicated biology, husbandry, anesthesia, and surgery chapters. In addition, we have made great efforts to include many recognized specialists from around the world. This created obvious language challenges in some cases, and we are extremely grateful for the extra effort taken by authors, whether they were writing in a second language or providing additional editorial assistance to their international co-authors. However, the inclusion of such a varied assortment of international specialists has resulted in a truly global perspective that benefits us all. Second, we have tried to continue the evolution of our specialty away from anecdote and opinion and toward more evidence-based medicine through greater reliance on peer-reviewed science. To this end, the authors and editors have toiled to include only peer-reviewed journal and published book materials in their references. Non–peer reviewed and unavailable proceedings papers have not been utilized in the chapter bibliographies, so the reader is assured that any reference number refers to a peer-reviewed journal or published book chapter. This is particularly important in this edition because all references have been removed from the printed book and placed online. This proved necessary because of space constraints and is in keeping with other major texts like Ettinger's *Textbook of Veterinary Internal Medicine*.

Section 1 details practice management and development and has been expanded from 3 to 6 chapters, including specialization, the value of herpetological publication by clinicians and academics, and statistics for the clinician. Our specialty depends on continued informational growth, and we encourage everyone to be part of that development by submitting to the *Journal of Herpetological Medicine and Surgery*.

The previous biology and husbandry section has been separated into two separate sections and expanded. Section 2 covers anatomy, physiology, and taxonomy of all the major taxa and now includes tuatara and amphibians, as well as behavior, training, welfare, and stress. The husbandry Section 3 is updated for all reptile taxa and also includes tuatara and amphibians. There are also updated chapters on environmental lighting, disinfection, quarantine, and nutrition.

A new Section 4 details infectious diseases and laboratory sciences, while Section 5 focuses on clinical techniques and procedures. Our knowledge of anesthesia and analgesia has grown considerably in the last decade, and Section 6 includes dedicated chapters on sedation, general and regional anesthesia, analgesia, and amphibian anesthesia. Diagnostic imaging Section 7 has been expanded to include taxa-based radiography (for snakes, lizards, chelonians, and crocodilians), ultrasonography, CT, MRI, and scintigraphy. Section 8 details endoscopic equipment and diagnostic and surgical procedures. However, probably the greatest reorganization has occurred in the medicine and surgery sections, where we have tried to emulate domestic animal and human medical texts by organizing the material by major organ systems. Medicine Section 9 now includes dedicated chapters on urology, hepatology, cardiology, dermatology, ophthalmology, otorhinolaryngology, gastroenterology, pulmonology, neurology, oncology, endocrinology, theriogenology, musculoskeletal, vascular/hematopoietic/immunology, behavioral medicine, nutritional diseases, perinatology, geriatrics, emergency and critical care, toxicology, and amphibian medicine. The previous single surgery chapter has been expanded into a dedicated Section 9 and includes chapters focused on specific organs or systems, including eye, ear, rhinarium, oral cavity, integument, coeliotomy, respiratory tract, gastrointestinal tract, urinary tract, reproductive tract, cloaca, external coaptation, internal fracture fixation, spine, amputation, shell, and amphibian soft tissue surgery. Similarly, the previous single therapeutics chapter has been expanded into a 19-chapter Section 11, and in addition to updates of the usual drug classes also includes new chapters on mental health treatment, photobiomodulation, rehabilitation and physical therapy, and wound management. The clinically useful differential diagnosis Section 12 has been retained and updated to include a new amphibian chapter.

Another major area of change occurred with Section 13 on specific diseases and conditions. Much of the detailed information has been moved and incorporated into the aforementioned medicine and surgery sections. However, we recognized the value of retaining this section as a quick reference guide for busy practitioners needing a brief summary during a consultation. Therefore these clinical diseases and conditions have been condensed into a more abbreviated format to facilitate rapid review during a busy practice day, with cross-references to the major chapters for more in-depth information.

Section 14 is new and focused on population and public health, including zoonoses, free-ranging reptiles, management and rehabilitation of sea turtles, commercial reptile farming, large collection management, breeders/wholesale/retail, laboratory management, conservation, and ecosystem health. Section 15 on legal topics includes updated chapters on international, European, and American legislation, and there are new chapters on forensics and jurisprudence.

Our wives tell us that childbirth is one of the most painful but ultimately rewarding experiences. Pregnancy seems like an appropriate metaphor for this book, because after a 3-year gestation, months of labor, and a painful delivery, we can now, at last, lay back and bask in the glow of this wondrous creation. We invite you, our colleagues and friends, to peruse its contents. We hope it will become a valuable asset to your work, and we look forward to your feedback—just in case we are ever crazy enough to attempt a fourth edition. Welcome to the third edition of *Mader's*!

Stephen J. Divers
Scott J. Stahl

ACKNOWLEDGMENTS

First things first—thank you, Doug Mader. Thank you for being the driving force behind the first, second, and current therapy editions. Your dedication to the specialty has and continues to be an inspiration for all of us. It was the fall of 2015 when Penny Rudolph of Elsevier first approached Doug and myself about a third edition. Doug took a big gulp, staggered slightly, regained composure, and said he wanted to step down as editor. That's when I knew the editorial umbilicus had been cut and I was on my own! While quick to accept the challenge, I did so without any real thought to the monumental task that lay before me. Doug tried to convey this, but I was an enthusiastic and naive fool. However, in addition to maintaining the impeccable standards previously set by Doug, I knew that I wanted to see further progression away from anecdote and opinion, toward more evidence-based medicine and clinical science. I sent out an initial draft chapter outline to a series of close colleagues and trusted friends: Charles Innis, Steve Barten, Paul Gibbons, Mark Mitchell, Tom Boyer, Doug Mader, and Scott Stahl. Their positive feedback not only gave the vision structure but also highlighted the enormity of the task ahead and the need for additional help. Fortunately, I did not have to look far to locate an equally gullible and unwitting optimist, and Scott Stahl joined as co-editor.

Everyone has always referred to the first edition as *Mader*, then the second edition as *The New Mader*, so one thing was abundantly clear from the start—this book was going to be called *Mader*! Therefore, as homage to Doug, we elected to officially change the name of the text to *Mader's Reptile and Amphibian Medicine and Surgery*. In addition to Mader, it might also say Divers and Stahl on the front cover, but this was very much a community effort. They say it takes a village to raise a child; well, this big baby took 130 authors from around the world to produce what we believe is THE definitive text on reptile and amphibian medicine and surgery. The authors worked tirelessly, many in their second language, to ensure a truly international perspective.

None of us get rich writing textbooks. We do it out of passion for our colleagues and our specialty. Therefore, it was critically important to us as editors that the authors felt proud of their contributions and the final product. We hope you agree that the publishers have not disappointed. We are indebted to our *family* of contributors, not least because most, if not all, are close colleagues and personal friends. This is their book as much as ours. Our only sadness, and the one thing from the second edition that is sorely missing in the third, is Kevin Wright; however, Kevin is still in these pages in spirit and content, and his name remains as a co-author on the amphibian medicine and surgery chapters.

Penny Rudolph retired in 2017, and we thank her for her tireless support and wisdom over the years—we miss you. There was a dedicated group at Elsevier that stuck with us to the very end. Jennifer Flynn-Briggs (Senior Content Strategist) and Ellen Wurm-Cutter (Senior Content Development Manager) kept everyone's eyes on the goal, while Becky Leenhouts (Senior Content Development Specialist) endured a lot by being at the sharp interface between authors and editors. Clay Broeker (Book Production Specialist) also showed great professionalism in the face of numerous about-turns and changes during the proof stages, while Renee Duenow was responsible for book design and Madelene Hyde for Global Content.

There is no doubt that I am where I am today not because of any genetic talent but because of the environment and training I have been fortunate to experience. Professionally, I stand on the shoulders of those that gave me their time and shared their knowledge. Calvert Appleby, Oliphant Jackson, John Cooper, Martin Lawton, Neil Forbes, Peter Scott, Fred Frye, Phillip Lhermette, and Dermod Malley were mentors from my student and early post-graduate days in England. I remember fondly my friends and colleagues within the British Veterinary Zoological Society, and then, after I moved to the United States, within the Association of Reptilian and Amphibian Veterinarians (ARAV). The ARAV continues to play a critical role in my career, and I owe this group so much—not least for being the catalyst for the development of many close personal friendships, including Charles "Chuckles" Innis, Kevin "Lick" Wright, Mitchell "Elvis" Mitchell, and of course my co-editor, Scott "Baby Face" Stahl. Since I first met Scott in 1996, we have always been close friends, and I think of him as a brother. Although, over the years, he has been gracious enough to share his knowledge about reptiles and their medicine with me, my efforts at trying to educate him on the rules of cricket have been universally unsuccessful. I have enjoyed countless hours laughing with him (or at him) at conferences and working together on research projects and co-teaching wet-labs. I am especially grateful for his friendship, support, and the life lessons he has taught me. He is a gentleman and a scholar, and I am so thankful to be able to call him my friend.

I am particularly pleased that there are many contributions from my colleagues at the University of Georgia's (UGA) College of Veterinary Medicine (Departments of Small Animal Medicine and Surgery, Pathology, Veterinary Biosciences, and Diagnostic Imaging), Odum School of Ecology, and Warnell School of Forestry and Natural Resources. One area of nationally renowned expertise is Educational Resources at the College of Veterinary Medicine, with their award-winning medical illustrators. A look through these pages will reveal some incredible illustrations designed and drawn by a group of talented artists. Thanks to Kip Carter, Amanda Slade, Danielle VanBrabant, and Katelyn Snell for making the pages come alive. I am fortunate to work in an incredible state-of-the-art hospital with an amazing team of dedicated faculty, notably Joerg Mayer, and technicians, including Ashley McGaha, Nia Chau, and Danielle Stewart, within the zoological medicine service. Zoological medicine has become an integral part of the curriculum and clinical service at UGA, and many of the developments that can be found within these pages are due to the institutional support I have received from current (Spencer Johnston) and past department heads and the administration of the Veterinary Teaching Hospital. During the development of this text, zoological medicine interns/residents Emi Knafo, Rodney Schnellbacher, Lara Cusack, Izidora Sladakovic, Dan Cutler, Spencer Kehoe, and Jessica Comolli played crucial roles as authors and/or acquirers of clinical material. I am proud of their accomplishments to date and look forward to seeing their continued contributions to the field. Also deserving of special mention are Paul Gibbons, Eric Klaphake, Kurt Sladky, James Carpenter, Brent Whitaker, and Colin McDermott for enabling us to use their recently updated formularies and clinicopathology tables from the recently revised *Exotic Animal Formulary*.

There have been thousands of e-mails, telephone calls, text messages, meetings, and conference calls, not to mention the occasional sleepless night and sporadic (but essential) alcoholic drink. This undertaking consumed a lot of time, and my closest friends and family have endured much during this process. My parents, Alan and Christine, have always been completely dedicated and supportive of my education and career. They were visibly relieved when I elected veterinary medicine over human medicine, and I owe them everything. My wife, Leticia, whose lessons in compassion and forgiveness have helped me cope with missed deadlines and many other frustrations along the way, is my foundation and my rock, and her love and patience have given me the strength to finish what has at times seemed like a never-ending process. I was especially pleased to see her participate as an author. My 6-year-old son, John-Eduardo, on the other hand, was less patient than his mother, but his interruptions and insistence on regular breaks to build Lego rocket ships or duel with Star Wars lightsabers were equally essential to maintain my sanity and productivity. I look forward to spoiling them both now that this is finished.

Stephen J. Divers

As I began writing these acknowledgments, I assumed it would be a short and relatively easy endeavor. However, I quickly realized that this required just as much careful thought and attention as the rest of the book. There are so many people to thank for the opportunity to co-edit this contribution to the medical care of the beloved animals for which I have dedicated my career.

I am deeply grateful for Stephen J. Divers, my co-editor and dear friend of the last 20 years. My involvement in this project is the result of his belief in me and our mutual lifelong love for reptiles and amphibians (or maybe I was the only one who would agree to work with him). Since we met in 1996 at an Association of Reptilian and Amphibian Veterinary (ARAV) Conference in Tampa, Florida, we have been close.

I thank Steve for always encouraging me to grow and challenge myself professionally. We have traveled the world together, educating practitioners about exotic animal endoscopy. (Thank you for the support, Christopher Chamness and everyone at Karl Storz Veterinary Endoscopy). This opportunity has enriched my life with knowledge, adventure, and much laughter. Steve is an amazingly talented clinician, orator, and teacher. His willingness to share research ideas, techniques, studies, and publications with his students and colleagues is selfless. He truly is committed to the goal of improving our clinical knowledge and understanding of zoo and exotic animals. I am thankful he has allowed me to join him on numerous research endeavors, and although he left me out of his research trip to the Galapagos (he called me from the island to rub it in), I have since forgiven him. In hindsight, would I have wanted to be stuck on a small island with him for any great length of time anyway? I digress. However, because the completion of this book has sometimes felt never ending, I couldn't imagine collaborating with anyone else. Yes, I had to be the "voice of reason" at times and drag him off a few soapboxes, and there were a few spirited phone conversations, but we still like each other. Mate, thank you for this opportunity, and cheers to many more adventures together. I love you brother.

As Steve has mentioned in his acknowledgments, this book would not be possible without the monumental efforts of our veterinary colleagues and fellow herpetologists who have advanced this discipline. I would personally like to thank Frederick L. Frye for being the first of our clinical colleagues to put together a comprehensive surgical and medical book on reptiles (*Biomedical and Surgical Aspects of Captive Reptile Husbandry),* which was the catalyst for all subsequent books, including his even more comprehensive two-volume set years later. Fred had the foresight to recognize the need for clinical knowledge about these unique animals. I used to sleep with his books under my pillow as a pre-veterinary student (what a reptile geek). As a young veterinary student on a trip to California for a conference, Fred agreed to meet with me for a chat. He was gracious with his time and encouragement, and that meeting reinforced my commitment to herpetological medicine. Thanks, Fred, for your confidence in me and your friendship. Another personal hero and mentor of mine is Elliott R. Jacobson, who I fortuitously heard lecture on herpetological medicine in the early 1980s at a Virginia Herpetological Society meeting. At that time, I was an undergraduate studying biology at the University of Richmond. His dynamic presentation was an "a-ha" moment for me and skewed my original plan for a career in zoology (herpetology) to that of veterinary medicine. Elliott went on to become a legend in our field, recognizing the need for sound research and validation, especially regarding infectious diseases. I am grateful for his vast contribution to our field, his encouragement, and his friendship. And, of course, I thank Douglas R. Mader and echo Steve's sentiments that without Doug's tremendous effort, foresight, and dedication to the field of clinical herpetological medicine and surgery, we would not have this opportunity. I first met Doug when I attended a North American Veterinary Conference as a young veterinary graduate. Anyone who has attended one of Doug's lectures will confirm that his passion, charisma, and enthusiasm are contagious. Doug, thank you for your support, mentorship, and friendship over the years. I am delighted that we can honor you with this edition, appropriately entitled *Mader's Reptile and Amphibian Medicine and Surgery.*

I send love to all my colleagues in my ARAV family (many of whom made important contributions to this book) and thank them for their support and dedication to our field. I have enjoyed coming together annually to share ideas (okay, and drink beer and laugh till we cry), with the common goal of elevating our medical knowledge of these beloved animals. I don't have room to name everyone, but Charlie "Chuckles" Innis, Mark "Teddy Bear" Mitchell, Tom "Tommy-Boy" Boyer, and Steve "Shutterfly" Barten must be called out! It feels like we have grown up together professionally and we are family. You guys have always been an inspiration to me, and I'm so proud of your accomplishments.

Sadly, we lost one of our herpetological family members and one of my dearest friends, Kevin Michael Wright, in 2013. Kevin contributed so much to the field of herpetological medicine. He is present in this third edition because his previous work is so vital that he is the co-author of the amphibian medicine chapter along with his equally brilliant friend and colleague Brent Whitaker. I am thankful to have had Kevin in my life for nearly 30 years, as we met in 1984 at a Society for the Study of Amphibians and Reptiles meeting in Florida as undergraduates. It was an immediate bond because we seemed destined for the same goal, pursuing veterinary school to become herpetological veterinarians. I learned so much from Kevin over the years. He was an amazing human being. He was like a brother to me, and I cherish the time we shared together. Kevin lived life to the fullest, followed his interests and pursuits with passion, and looked for humor in any situation. What a valuable message for all of us. I know the professional goals I have accomplished and many of the opportunities I have pursued are because of his love, support, and friendship. I love you Kevin, and I miss you every day.

In our avian and exotic practice, we have many fourth-year veterinary students spending time learning from our team. I have always felt it is important to help train our future colleagues in this unique discipline. Over 350 students have trained at our clinic, including many international students. I gained a great deal of knowledge from this type of hands-on experience as a veterinary student, and I am grateful to my colleagues who taught me their craft, including Michael Cranfield, Richard Linnehan, Robert Wagner, Walt Rosskopf, Richard Woerpel, Jeff Jenkins, Tookie Meyers, H.J. Holshuh, Lois Roth, Larry Freeman, Michael Leib, Craig Thatcher, Phillip Sponenberg, Alan Adair, Cindy Adair, and many others I may have inadvertently omitted. I want to thank the Virginia-Maryland College of Veterinary Medicine (VMCVM) for allowing me to be a part of the veterinary class of 1989. During my veterinary school interview, I stated that I wanted to be a "snake doctor," and this was before cable television made exotic animal practice a popular choice of applicants today. My undergraduate research involved evaluating the reproductive cycle of the northern copperhead, *Agkistrodon contortrix,* with my mentor Joseph C. Mitchell at the University of Richmond, and this likely made me an unusual candidate. Thanks for taking a chance on me, VMCVM, and go Hokies!

I am indebted to Dr. Mitchell for taking me under his wing as an undergraduate to work in his herpetological ecology lab and help with research for his book, *The Reptiles of Virginia*. I know he was hoping that I would stay in the field of "true" herpetology rather than pursue veterinary medicine, but he supported my decision and taught me the value of research. Thank you also to the many science professors at the University of Richmond who supported my interest in reptiles and desire to pursue veterinary medicine.

I was known as the "reptile guy" during my years of vet school. Although the program was limited in organized instruction on avian and exotic animal medicine and surgery, the professors and staff were all supportive of me and encouraged my fascination. Thank you to my VMCVM professors for giving me the knowledge and tools to succeed in veterinary medicine and to my 1989 classmates for supporting my unique interests and making the 4 years fun (although, to date, no one has confessed to putting the green peanut M&Ms in Dr. Leib's gallbladder stone specimen jar). Special thanks to my dear friend and vet school roommate, board-certified veterinary surgeon Richard "Hogg" Suess, who had to share his apartment with many "creepy crawlies" over the years. I also want to note that as a veterinary student, I had the opportunity to work with Dr. Robin Andrews in her herpetology laboratory at Virginia Tech. She graciously allowed me to stay close to my herp passion by working with her research lizards and even giving me the opportunity to co-author a paper on reproduction in tropical anolis lizards.

In my first few years of clinical practice, I was lucky to be surrounded by an amazing and supportive group of colleagues who taught me so much about medicine, surgery, and how to be a caring professional. I thank you for the laughs, warm memories, and love Patrick Denny, John Schaff, Jody Clarke, Len Rice, Julia Finlayson, Kelli Rhymes, Andrew Voell, Daniel Morris, and Bill Tyrell (who encouraged me to follow my dream of starting my own specialty practice). Also, early in my career, I worked with numerous enthusiastic and brilliant veterinary associates and technicians. We learned a lot together, and I appreciated their insight. Thank you to Thomas Bankstahl, Carmine Bausone, Patty Bright, Jennifer Stampf, Janice Raab, Carol Canny, Meredith Davis, Ben Haas, Debbie Koth (RIP), Beth Steroitis, and Christopher Normand.

In 2003, I decided to start my own exclusive avian and exotic animal practice, Stahl Exotic Animal Veterinary Services (SEAVS). On opening day at SEAVS, I had one employee, my dear friend Jennifer Hutchins, LVT. Jennifer has been the glue that holds everything together in our practice and has been instrumental to its success. She is a highly skilled veterinary technician, and when she joined me in this adventure, she was coerced into being both business manager and technician. She had no interest in this managerial role, but 15 years later (now a 6-doctor practice, with more than 25 employees) she is still our fearless business manager. Let's face it, she is the real boss of the practice. It's a tough job, and I am so thankful for the sacrifices she has made and for dreaming big alongside me.

I would also like to thank our associates, ABVP avian residents, and interns over the last 15 years: David Crum (our first resident and associate), Lisa Carr, Scott Medlin, Greg Costanzo, Shoshana Sommer, Octavio Romo, Emily Nielsen, and Scott Hammer, for their hard work and dedication. They have all contributed so much and have been integral to the success of our practice. Although some of them have moved on, they will always be part of the SEAVS family. Grasshoppers, I am proud of you. The sky is the limit!

To Greg Costanzo, my previous resident and now senior associate, I'm grateful for your willingness to take on greater responsibilities over the last 3 years because of my abbreviated clinical schedule, which was necessary to allow me to focus on the monumental task of completing this book. Greg knew that contributing to the field of herpetological medicine by co-editing this book would fulfill a professional dream for me, and I am appreciative of his commitment to me and the team. You're a skilled clinician, a great human being, and so important to the success of SEAVS.

Thank you to my second family, the entire SEAVS team, for all your support over the years and especially the last few years during the completion of this book. I am so proud of you all. Your hard work and dedication have resulted in the creation of one of the largest exclusive avian and exotic animal practices in the world! I am especially grateful to my dedicated long-timers (10 years plus!) Alissa Hoklotubbe, Danya Mandery, Kathy Burrier, Anibal Armendaris, and Zach Romeo.

Away from work, my cycling coach and dear friend Jared Nieters helps me maintain some sanity and balance with the demands of life by routinely kicking my butt! Thanks coach.

Finally, my family has always been supportive of me, kept me grounded, and loved me unconditionally, which makes all this hard work and effort worthwhile. As mentioned in the dedication, I owe everything to my parents, Brenda and Dale "Buck" Stahl, who worked hard to provide every opportunity for their kids to pursue their dreams. My interest in reptiles and amphibians, which started at an early age while living on a farm in Maine, was always encouraged. Although I'm sure my parents had some concerns at times when, for example, a presumed male red-bellied snake produced a "surprise" litter of neonates ($n = 10$), an anolis lizard showed up in the mail from Florida (purchased for $1.99 from and ad in the back of a magazine), and numerous "live specimens" escaped in the house over the years! I am grateful to my sister Susie and brother Mark, who survived growing up with these animals around them but still supported me. I love you so much.

None of this would have been possible without the years of support and love from my wife, Stephanie. She has put up with this nonsense (the herps, not me, right?) since we first met when I was a veterinary student and she was an undergraduate at Virginia Tech. More than 25 years later, we still have a house full of reptiles! She has always supported my interest and fascination with these animals. She (and my daughters) have accepted that wherever we travel in the world, visiting zoos and reptile collections and herping in the wild are normal protocol. Being married to a veterinarian is challenging, and this is especially true with one obsessed with contributing to the scientific advancement of a group of animals. Long hours at the office along with writing, putting together lectures, and traveling to teach all reduce family time. Stephanie is the rock that keeps our family grounded, even while pursuing her own full-time career. Honestly, I don't know how she does it all, but I know the world of "content marketing" would be lacking without her input! I am proud of her and her amazing accomplishments in her field. As a writer and editor herself, she has been gracious with her time in helping me with many of my previous writing projects. For sanity reasons and the vastness of this project, I did not ask her to help with editing of this book (I am getting smarter with age); however, she has had to shoulder many responsibilities in the last several years due to my absence while working on this book. I greatly appreciate her making it possible for me to have the opportunity to make this contribution to my field. I love you, Stephanie!

My most important accomplishment of all is being the father to two amazing, smart, and beautiful daughters, Madeline and Macy. I am so proud of them and what they have already accomplished in life. To my loves, I say, "Chase your dreams. I will love and support you wherever life leads!" My co-editorship of this book and the success of Stahl Exotic Animal Veterinary Services is proof that hard work and determination can lead to the fulfillment of your dreams!

Scott J. Stahl

CONTENTS

Developing a Successful Herpetological Veterinary Service

Adolf Maas

Building a successful herpetological veterinary service is comprised of two important disciplines: the medicine practiced and the management of the business. Both are intrinsically necessary as one cannot succeed without the other.

The majority of veterinary medicine focuses on domestic species. However, the reptile clade is comprised of nearly 10,000 distinct species that occupy almost every biome on the planet. The evolutionary diversity is staggering; our own species has been present in multiple variants for a few hundred thousand years, while Emydidae (pond turtles) have been essentially unchanged for 45 million years. Furthermore, reptiles are incredibly diverse in their phylogenetic relationships to each other; chelonia are far more closely related to birds and crocodiles than to other reptiles, while geckos and bearded dragons are more distantly related to each other than humans are to rabbits. It is not difficult to understand why a reptile is not a "reptile" and that it is inappropriate to assume that one single therapy or treatment plan should apply to multiple, let alone all, species.

MEDICINE PRACTICED

The majority of herptile diseases have underlying husbandry etiologies; therefore having a strong knowledge of their natural history is essential and is a critical factor in practicing quality medicine. Without the ability to assess a patient's husbandry and determine if it is appropriate for that species, clinicians will have difficulty formulating an effective treatment plan.

The next most important factor for achieving success in herpetological medicine is to gain knowledge in the unique physiology and anatomy, disease syndromes, and therapies utilized in herptiles. This might seem counterintuitive, but, if husbandry and care are not appropriate and/or corrected, an accurate diagnoses and treatment protocol will not be successful.[1] It is not possible to separate natural history from disease management and therapeutics. Natural history and husbandry information can be found in other chapters throughout Sections 1 and 2 of this text, and the reader is encouraged to peruse this critical information.

Managing/Developing the Business

During the process of gaining an important knowledge base in herpetological medicine (an ongoing career process), clinicians must also focus on developing a business and facility that will support practicing this particular subset of medicine.[2] The following components are essential for a successful business:

(A) Attracting clients
(B) Proper organization
(C) Knowledgeable support staff
(D) Appropriate infrastructure
(E) Necessary equipment

(A) Attracting Clients.
Herptile-owning clients are not a particular anomaly, even if they are not the most common of pet owners. Zoological medicine and reptile/amphibian medicine are recognized specialties in veterinary medicine, and regardless of whom you ask, herpetological medicine is a small fraction (5%–20%) of their zoological case load. To date, there are no dedicated herptile-only veterinary practices in the United States, despite there being limited numbers of avian-exclusive, exotic companion mammal-exclusive, and even fish-exclusive practices.

However, a rewarding herpetological service can be built with similar approaches utilized to develop other successful services. Three strategies are important.

1. Marketing/advertising your herpetological service. Without a way to reach potential clients, there is no way to get them to consider your practice. Traditional print media has generally gone the way of the dinosaur and been replaced with the internet. One challenge with internet exposure/marketing is holding the attention of potential clients for more than a few seconds, and it becomes critical to "grab their attention" and differentiate your practice from others quickly. Even the practice name plays a role and needs to be focused and descriptive of the patients being targeted so potential clients can see the practice as uniquely filling their needs.

In today's internet age, the practice website has become a significant marketing tool. The website must be dynamic yet easy to use and intuitive. To hold the attention of the viewer, images of herptiles and procedures routinely performed on them can be displayed and discussed to reassure clients that the practice is comfortable with these species. The veterinarian(s)' and staff's credentials and experience can be listed along with continuing education attended. Also, the clinician's curriculum vitae can be posted on the site to show their active involvement in herpetological medicine through publications, lectures, and teaching. Nothing can build a client's confidence more than to see that the practice is contributing to the knowledge base of herpetological medicine. Additionally, the practice's memberships in important associations such as the Association of Reptilian and Amphibian Veterinarians (ARAV), as well as local, national, and international herpetological societies or associations, can be posted. As smartphones are one of the main tools for communication and internet connection, it is critical that websites are designed to be compatible with computers as well as mobile-based browsers.

Search-engine optimization is a skill in and of itself and is critical for more targeted internet placement. As with the development, maintenance, and management of a successful website, companies can be employed to improve the practice's website search-engine placement. This is a worthwhile investment, like the financial investment practices would make in the size and location of a telephone "Yellow Pages" advertisement in the past. This, as well as the inclusion of videos, blogs, regular updates, and changes, will dramatically increase the ever-important website presence.

Social media has become an intrinsic part of our culture and must be utilized to build a successful herpetological service. Facebook, Twitter, Instagram, Snapchat, and Flikr are all social media platforms (with more to follow) that have become popular and effective methods to gain exposure to and connect with potential clients.[3] Herpetological patients are considered interesting to the public, so posting pictures and videos of these animals on social platforms is a great way to promote your expertise as a herpetological veterinarian. A media release form should be utilized to allow the clinic to post pictures of client's animals on social media. Additionally, when their animal shows up on your social media page or in a post, the client will share that image and thus your practice, providing great exposure at a minimal cost.

If your practice has a media savvy employee who can be placed in charge of taking images and posting them regularly, this skill can be utilized. Posting frequently to blogs and social media will increase your standings on search engines; pictures rank higher than text, and videos rank higher than pictures. Use caution, however, as it is possible that too-frequent posting may result in a loss of followers, possibly due to overload.

These social media platforms are efficient, timely, and a preferred method to get information to clients about upcoming events, promotions, products, new employees, public service announcements (i.e., cautioning clients not to overheat pets in cars during summer travel), holiday business hour changes, and more. The timely nature of these social platforms is useful for situations such as emergency closure or other issues that may affect the practice hours.

Another successful form of promotion that is especially worthwhile in herpetological practice is direct exposure, going directly to the source of potential clients. Other than the time commitment, there is little cost. Opportunities abound, especially in urban environments, and attending/becoming a member and/or speaking/exhibiting is a great way to acquire new clients. Examples of such venues/organizations include the following:

- Herpetological societies and meetings
- General and order- or species-specific reptile rescues/shelters (focus on 501c3 organizations)
- Exotic animal shows/sales (may or may not be herptile-specific)
- Reptile subsets of animal rescue exhibits
- Pet shops that carry/sell herptile species
- Reptile hobbyist group (breeder and/or keeper) meetings
- Local/regional VMA groups/meetings

2. Establishing that your practice has herpetological expertise. Once you have reached these new clients, it is important that they perceive the value and expertise your practice can offer compared to others in your region. An excellent way to gain credibility in the herpetological community is by owning and successfully keeping the animals that you treat. Herptile keepers take great pride in their knowledge and often will not respect and/or trust a veterinarian that does not also keep herp species. In addition to gaining the confidence of clients, the knowledge gained by keeping and caring for these animals is invaluable.

Reaching out to and sharing information with owners that you hope to gain as clients is a great way to show your expertise. However, it is important not to diagnose or provide treatment to animals you have not examined. Providing discount services to pet stores and validated rescues (501c3 certification is important) not only allows you access to these cases but can also generate referrals.

3. Establishing yourself as a local expert. Although it can be challenging to find time during a busy practice day, personally taking calls from potential clients as well as from local veterinarians regarding cases will build your credibility in your region as a qualified and approachable herpetological veterinarian.[4] As mentioned above, it is important not to provide too much detailed information without seeing the case yourself. However, providing a list of possible differentials and diagnostic options can help these potential clients or referring veterinarians to see the value that your expertise and practice can offer. It is critical to show that there is more to treating herptiles than a home remedy or a dose of antibiotic. Obtaining a specialist qualification so that you can legitimately call yourself a "specialist" can have many advantages. Likewise, be careful not to give the impression of being a "specialist" if you do not hold a recognized qualification (e.g., DACZM, DABVP[R/A]) in the United States (see Chapter 4).

(B) Proper Organization: Client and Patient Processing

"You have only one chance to make a first impression." Every veterinary practice has standard procedures for addressing clients and their animals when they arrive for an appointment. Most canine/feline patients are socialized as well as socially accepted, and it would be considered an unusual event for another pet's owner to be startled or afraid by their presence. This is not always the case with herps. At a minimum, people that do not own herptiles may be surprised to see them in a practice lobby, and it is not uncommon to have the occasional client in terror. Furthermore, many herptile owners seek the attention associated with possessing an unusual pet and will carry them out in the open.

The reception staff is critical in instructing clients on the policies and procedures of the hospital. This communication must start when the client makes the appointment and be reinforced by the receptionists in person upon arrival. All herptile patients should arrive at the hospital in an appropriate carrying container or cage. During cool weather, owners should be instructed to consider insulated containers and advised that exposure to low temperatures can be damaging to the patient's health, as well as hinder an accurate veterinary evaluation. If there are specific clades or species that the clinician is not willing to take on as patients (i.e., crocodilians, venomous snakes) it should be stated clearly to potential clients at first contact. It would also be advisable for the clinician to research the local jurisdictional regulations regarding potentially dangerous and illegal species and determine the role the veterinarian should play if such species are presented.[5]

Technology can be utilized to easily alleviate potential issues. When the owner is making the initial appointment, along with obtaining the name and phone number of the client, the staff should obtain their e-mail address to send them hospital information and new patient forms. An added benefit of electronic communication is that the "no-show" occurrence rate decreases significantly because of the added communication and increased disclosure. Another system utilized is texting appointment reminders. Once you have the owner's cell phone number, it can be used as a brief reminder to owners regarding upcoming appointments and can even be programmed in advance. The dental profession has been utilizing this system and has had remarkable success, both with helping people keep appointments and encouraging rescheduling an appointment rather than simply not showing up.

Forms sent to the new client should include a summary of clinic policies and procedures, the basic consultation fee, and information regarding restraint and caging of their pet at the appointment, as well as patient health and husbandry questionnaires. To increase efficiency, new client forms are sent to the owner to read/fill out in advance. Compliance in completely filling out these forms is necessary, and reception staff must review them for completeness at the time of intake.

With the advent of camera phones, owners are encouraged to bring photographs of their enclosures, setups, and supplies. This way, it is easy for the clinician to assess husbandry almost as if they were making an onsite visit. The new client should understand that the more information provided at the first visit, the more accurate the assessment, diagnosis, and treatment plan can be.

The health and husbandry questionnaire can be utilized to help the owner summarize the husbandry and care of the animal they are presenting, as well as increase the efficiency of the technical staff and doctor. Table 1.1 is a condensed general outline of a typical form. While each practice should tailor the questionnaire form to their needs, it is important that the queries are kept simple and brief. The primary goal is to identify general issues rather than specific ones, allowing the clinician to easily investigate potential problems.

Other policies should be determined and documented at the hospital prior to first presentation. As many herptile owners often have multiple animals, a decision should be reached about how additional animals at a visit will be charged. Additionally, charges for large collections (i.e., breeders) might be best based on time and not the number of animals.

Reptiles and amphibians have lower requirements for after-hours emergency care than mammals and birds, but plans should be made in advance regarding where emergent cases should be sent, as well as for times when a herptile-skilled doctor (or specialist) is not on duty. Overnight care plans must be made in advance, as there will be cases that require a higher level of treatment than outpatient care can provide. Having a plan in place for these situations is important to prevent client/staff frustrations and avoid legal liability.

(C) Knowledgeable Support Staff

"You are only as good as those helping you." Recently a t-shirt was seen that said, "Behind every successful veterinarian is an exhausted technician." Not only is that true, but "technician" should also be replaced intermittently with "assistant," "receptionist," and "manager."

Staff are not generally trained in how to process, inquire, and assist a herptile veterinarian, nor is there much coursework available even in accredited technician programs. Although staff education is still primarily the responsibility of the herpetological clinician, there is now specialization through the National Association of Veterinary Technicians in America in "exotic companion animals" or "zoological medicine." Also, many veterinary conferences that incorporate material on herpetological medicine offer continuing education for technicians. There is a veterinary technician group within the Association of Reptilian and Amphibian Veterinarians (ARAV).

Similarly, just as policies need to be established and followed for the herptile-owning client, appropriate guidelines for staff must be in place to ensure each appointment and treatment plan works smoothly and efficiently.

The basic policies involving the front desk staff include those listed earlier, such as providing new clients with forms and hospital procedures in advance. Additional recommendations might include placing reptile-owning clients into exam rooms as quickly as possible (to avoid distressing other clients) and having receptionists learn from teaching tools such as flash cards about the more common species seen in the practice so that basic knowledge and familiarity can be demonstrated to owners. This familiarity builds confidence in the client.

Fear of herptiles is one factor that must be considered when selecting staff that will be encountering these patients. It is critical that all staff are able to approach nondangerous herptile patients (perhaps even be comfortable handling them) when they present in the office. The damage done by an owner seeing a staff member recoil in revulsion is irreparable.

Managers also need to understand the unique issues presented with herpetological medicine. An informal survey of exclusively exotic animal practices in the United States concluded that technical labor needs were nearly 50% higher than domestic animal practices because of the increased time the staff spent working directly with the patients (K. Wright, personal communication). Additional resources were required for these exclusive exotic animal practices, including a commitment to stock specialty medications and unique supplies and equipment. Other important requirements include providing special housing and husbandry materials and unique food resources (insects and rodents), along with additional training of staff. Doctors need to be scheduled appropriately for these patients because more time will be taken to get a complete anamnesis as well as samples for diagnostic testing. Management and accounting must charge appropriately for the increased resources applied to each case.[6]

As stated above, there is usually little instruction available for technical staff to learn to work with herpetological patients until they take a position in such a practice. There are good texts available, continuing education, and internet sources, but the best resource is the experienced herpetological veterinarian(s) in the practice. By taking the time to personally train and educate the technicians and the assistants, the doctor can have them perform the necessary duties as expected by the practice. This also provides a support mechanism for team members to be quizzed, challenged, and have their skills confirmed/corrected. This method of instruction will help them to complete tasks more effectively but also gives them an environment that encourages them to continually advance and improve their skills.

(D) Appropriate Infrastructure

"Better facilities make for smoother operations." Unique infrastructure is necessary to be able to provide quality care to herptiles. These provisions are necessary to accommodate the unique anatomy and physiology that these animals have and will make the practice both easier and more effective.

The lobby requires little more than what is found in any other small animal practice. The entry door should be large enough to facilitate the admission of larger carriers, tubs, and even carts carrying multiple units. Seating is best when there are distinct separate areas, allowing clients with herps to sit away from, or at least out of direct vision of, other clients that might be disturbed by their presence. As with all areas of the hospital, good thermal control is important to avoid exposing these patients to inappropriately hot or cold temperatures.

Making the entrance/lobby appealing to owners is a great way to connect with these clients as soon as they enter your facility. Having decorations that show your interest in these species facilitates comfort, and having reading material, brochures, diets, and other information available communicates to these clients that you take their nontraditional pets seriously (Fig. 1.1).

An exam room needs to have a large work area, both to accommodate larger patients as well as to put the carrying cases or enclosures in which the animals were transported (Fig. 1.2). A sink with running water is essential for the ability to clean off both the patient and the doctor and/or technician. Drawers and cabinets should all close completely and securely, and there should be no gaps or spaces around, under, or behind fixed furniture that might allow a smaller patient an opportunity to hide or escape. For that same reason, the sink should have a permanently mounted mesh drain strainer. Doors entering the exam room work best with automatic closers and should have no more than a 1 cm gap between the bottom of the door and the floor. Any vents or wall perforations should have covers or have only small gaps (<1 cm) to

TABLE 1.1   Reptile History Form

Date: _____

Referring veterinarian: _____

First and last name: _____

Pet's name: _____

Species:_____ Age/DOB: _____

Sex: _____ Male _____ Female _____ Unknown _____

Where did you obtain your reptile? _____

How long have you had your reptile? _____ Is your reptile: Wild caught? ___ Captive bred? ___

Housing

What type of enclosure does your reptile live in? _____

What are the dimensions? H _____ W _____ L _____

Do you use a hygrometer (humidity meter)? YES _____ NO _____ If yes, what is the humidity? _____

How is the enclosure heated (e.g., light, heating pad, heat rock)?_____

What is the temperature? Day: _____ Night: _____ Basking site: _____

Do you use thermometers? YES _____ NO _____

Where are they located? _____

Do you use a full-spectrum UVB bulb? YES _____ NO _____ UNKNOWN _____

What kind of bulb is it? _____

How often is it replaced and when was the last time? _____

How long are the lights on/off? Day: _____ Night: _____

Does your pet spend time outside of the enclosure? If yes, explain: _____

What is the substrate (bedding)? _____

What is the water source? _____

Are there plants, branches, or other climbing structures? _____

Is there a hiding area? If so, what kind? _____

Are there any other reptiles in the same enclosure? YES _____ NO ___ If so, what species?_____

For Aquatic Species:

How often do you change the water completely? _____Partially?_____

Do you use a water heater? _____ YES _____ NO _____ Water temperature: _____

Does the aquarium have a filter? YES _____ NO _____ Do you test water quality? YES _____ NO _____

Diet

Please fill in the percentage of the total diet and types of food in each category that your pet actually eats:

Leafy greens: _____ Legumes/beans: _____ Fruits: _____ Other vegetables: _____

Insects/small rodents: (circle one: live/dead) Pellets: _____ Other (including treats): _____

How often do you offer food? _____

Where do you feed your reptile? _____

Do you add vitamin or calcium supplements to the food? YES _____ NO_____

How often? _____ What kind? _____

If insects are fed, are they gut loaded? _____ YES _____ NO _____ UNKNOWN

Miscellaneous

Do you soak or bathe your reptile? YES ___ NO _____ How often? _____

Do they have any seasonal behavior changes? _____

Medical History

Has your reptile ever been checked for intestinal parasites? _____

Has your reptile ever laid eggs? YES _____ NO _____ UNKNOWN _____

How often does your reptile defecate? _____

How often does your reptile shed? _____When was the last shed? _____Any problems?_____

Check any boxes that apply to your pet:

_____ mites	_____ wounds	_____ weight loss	_____ weight gain	_____ not defecating
_____ anorexia	_____ diarrhea	_____ shedding problems	_____ difficulty breathing	
_____ lethargy	_____ inactivity	_____ increased appetite	_____ decreased appetite	
_____ limping	_____ vomiting	_____ deformed limbs	_____ swollen eyes	

Is there anything else you would like us to know today? _____

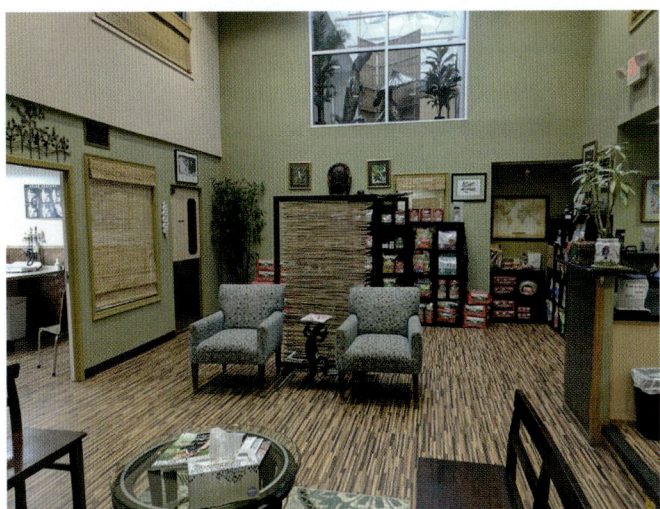

FIG 1.1 A reasonable amount of space in the waiting room is an excellent investment to promote nontraditional species care and husbandry but also showcase your herpetological and exotic species practice. (Courtesy of Scott J. Stahl, Stahl Exotic Animal Veterinary Services.)

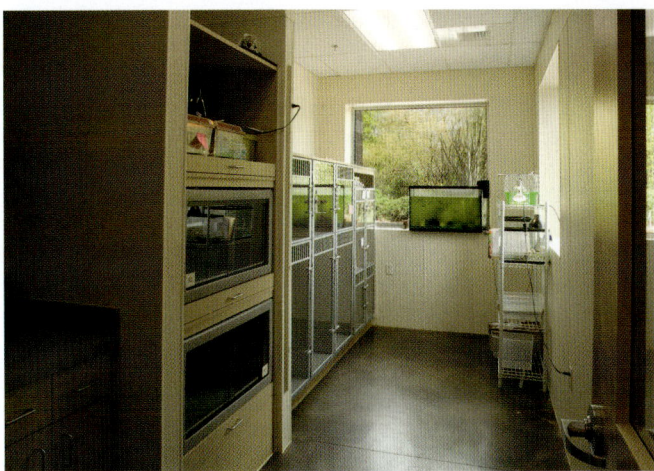

FIG 1.3 To provide quality reptile and amphibian medicine, an appropriate hospital room must be part of the practice. This room provides controlled heat and ventilation, with multiple enclosures available depending on the size and husbandry of the patient. Additionally, this room is well insulated, blocking sounds that might disturb exotic species.

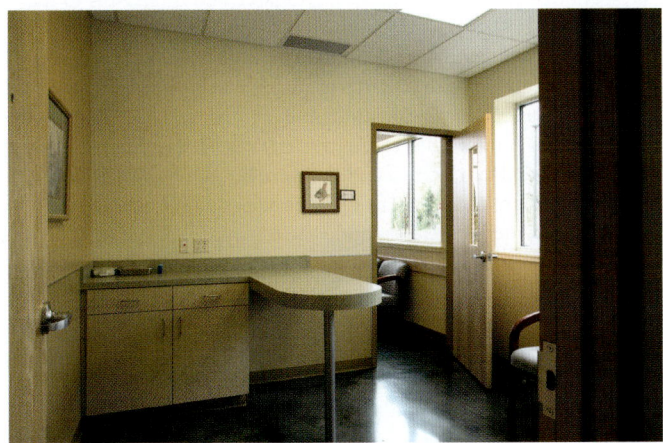

FIG 1.2 It is critical to have at least one room designed to accommodate herpetological patients. LED lighting, small-size screens over any wall and ceiling perforations, and no inaccessible openings to cabinets or chairs are critical considerations. All surfaces that might come in contact with patients must be solid and easily cleaned.

prevent the escape of small patients. All surfaces (floor, walls, tables, etc.) must be of nonporous, smooth material and easily cleaned, with supplies present.

Lighting is critical for an effective examination but also needs to have the patient in mind when selected. Traditionally, incandescent bulbs were selected to provide both light and heat, but, because they are no longer available, halogen or very high-frequency or constant-light LED bulbs should be utilized. Many species of herptiles have broader spectral ranges of vision than mammals, so the quality of light produced is as important as the quantity. Further information on the LED lights should be obtained from the manufacturer to ensure that they provide a balanced spectrum. Fluorescent lights (CFL included) should be avoided due to the limited spectrum produced (due to the types of phosphors present), as well as the potential strobe effect that they may generate. These lighting concerns should be applied to the exam room, as well as any boarding and/or hospital spaces.

There will need to be hospital space in a designated ward for reptiles and amphibians (Fig. 1.3). The concerns above apply to this space as well (controllable heat, lighting, security, sanitation), along with the ability to isolate patients from each other to minimize intimidation, predation, and disease transmission and to provide optimal husbandry for each patient. Mesh or wire-fronted cages are not appropriate in most cases, so close-tolerance clear plastic or tempered glass doors are advisable. This style also has the added benefit of being able to control heat and humidity so that cages can be optimized for the health of the individual patient. When selecting cage design and materials, consider their ability to have heat sources installed within each unit, their resistance to heat damage and moisture, and ease of disinfection (see Chapter 46).

In the treatment area and critical care ward, it is important to have open floor space with clear lighting. At least one dedicated treatment table with an overhead focused beam exam light (individually controlled) will allow for basic procedures with most animals, whereas the floor will make for an easy exam area for very large individual patients. A large sink or a wet table is necessary for washing, soaking, and even holding some animals, but a clean bathtub will work. Avian/reptile incubators can be an excellent addition to the critical care ward, but they are not all equal. Each model should be considered prior to purchase for oxygen concentration abilities, thermostat accuracy, ventilation, security (e.g., escape proof), and the ability to be easily and completely cleaned and sanitized between uses (see Chapter 46).

(E) Necessary Equipment

"No good carpenter blames his tools." Appropriate materials and equipment kept in the treatment areas are a necessity, and if you have poor-quality tools, you will have poor-quality results. Specific medical equipment is necessary for examinations. Ophthalmoscopes and otoscopes found in any basic practice work well for examining most eyes, ears, and oral cavities; a Doppler monitor is necessary for assessing heart rate and quality; a gram (to the nearest 1 gram or better still 0.1 gram) scale for small reptiles and a cat/baby scale for most others is adequate for getting accurate weights; and a set of sexing probes to determine gender is required. Wooden-stick, cotton-tipped applicators and tongue depressors work well for opening mouths for examination; the soft wood works well for encouraging them to open without damaging sensitive gingiva or teeth. A cordless rotary tool (e.g.,

Dremel) with a diamond grinder bit is preferred for trimming and rounding nails.

Appropriate diagnostic equipment is also imperative to provide quality herpetological veterinary services (Fig. 1.4). Table 1.2 provides a list of recommended equipment needed in different areas of the hospital.

Medical supplies required in a herpetological service are like those required in most veterinary practices. Anti-inflammatories, antibiotics, antifungals, and other medications should be stocked based on current research and known safety data and selected for each patient based on all available information, including patient specificities such as species, condition, husbandry, plasma biochemistries, and culture and sensitivity results. Just as in domestic animal medicine, there is no "one-size-fits-all" medical therapy, and a diversity of therapies must be immediately available. Access to a compounding pharmacy is important.

Table 1.3 provides a short list of some (not necessarily complete) of the most essential medications and drug products necessary for a herptile veterinary service.

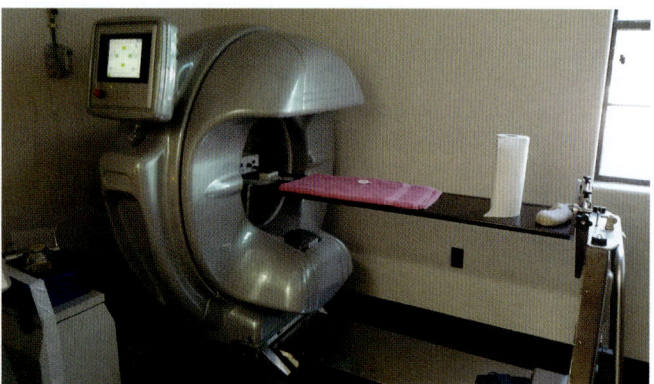

FIG 1.4 An example of a compact, affordable CT scanner (Vimago HDCT, Epica Medical Innovations) now available for private practices, providing advanced resolution and data for the herpetological practitioner.

APPROACH AND ATTITUDE

"A Clear Statement of Our Ignorance Does More to Advance Science Than Does an Assumption of Knowledge."

Probably the single most important aspect of building a successful reptile practice is the approach and attitude the doctor takes in each case managed. The correct approach builds a doctor's reputation, is a measure for success, and can be the inspiration to guide their career. Specifically, the proper approach involves the ability to differentiate what one knows versus what one does not and the ability to build on each. For example, clinicians need to understand that some clients may know more about a specific species than they do. Many owners report disappointment when a veterinarian pretends to have knowledge about a particular species but actually does not. This can be a fatal error in relating to clients and damages the reputation of the clinician. However, clinicians must also be prepared for clients who have spent time on the internet gathering selective "wisdom"; this misinformation spreads through herp-related sites and is presented as absolute certainty, often with no evidence or validation to support the claims. Obviously, clinicians cannot be expected to know all there is about every species and case presented. However, clinicians are obligated to seek out the best (often peer-reviewed journal) information available and utilize this to make evidence-based treatment decisions.

To avoid mismanagement of these cases, as described above, clinicians should complete as much research as possible in advance and never be embarrassed to admit they are not familiar with a species. Additionally, they should willingly defer to the owner's knowledge unless they can readily validate their difference of opinion. In the case of an error, it is best to admit ignorance of a fact or mistake and take action to follow up with the owner after researching the topic.

In this information age, there is constant availability and a never-ending supply of material on almost any subject. A recent Google search for "causes of iguana diarrhea" produced over 130,000 website hits in less than a second. This exemplifies the need to specifically focus such searches and utilize only reliable sources that involve peer-reviewed research. Google Scholar (https://www.scholar.google.com), PubMed

TABLE 1.2 Critical Areas and Basic Equipment Needs for a Practice Seeing Reptiles and Amphibians		
Treatment/Lab Area	**Hospitalization/Critical Care**	**Operating Room**
Microscope	Oxygen cage/oxygen concentrator	Radiosurgical unit or laser
Centrifuge capable of processing hematocrit tubes, blood tubes, and fecal samples	Programmable incubator(s)	Ventilator (oxygen and room air), programmable for small volume and low tidal pressure
Bacterial and fungal culture supplies	Syringe pump	Endotracheal tube size 1–12 mm
Acid-fast stain kit	Esophagostomy tubes	Doppler
Wright's stain kit	IO and cut-down IV supplies	Surgical loupes or magnification
Gram's stain kit	Blood transfusion supplies	Endoscopy
Radiology, preferably digital, and including horizontal beam capability	Bandaging materials	Bone and external fixator supplies plating supplies
Ultrasonography	Fluid bags and warmer	Microsurgery instrumentation
In-house biochemistry analyzer (or access to a commercial lab)	Blood transfusion supplies	Surgical heaters
Hemocytometer, diluents, and stains for in-house hematology (or access to a commercial lab)		Gas anesthesia
Heparin and EDTA blood tubes		Hemoclips/Ligasure
Digital in–out thermometer		Retractors such as Lone Star retractor
PCR testing supplies, formalin jars		

EDTA, Ethylene diamine tetra acetate; *PCR,* polymerase chain reaction.

TABLE 1.3   Drugs and Other Therapeutic Products Commonly Used in Herpetological Practice

Antibiotics/Antifungals	Antiparasitics	Anesthetic/Analgesic/Anti-Inflammatory	Other	Nutritional
Ceftazidime	Metronidazole	Meloxicam	Furosemide	Vitamin A
Amoxicillin/clavulanate	Fenbendazole	Ketoprofen	Plasmalyte, LRS, or equivalent	Calcium gluconate
TMP-SMZ	Ponazuril	Butorphanol	Dexamethasone	Vitamin E
Enrofloxacin	Ivermectin	Hydromorphone or morphine, tramadol	Lactulose	Vitamin D
Ceftiofur	Fipronil spray	Lidocaine	Heparin	Vitamin C
Doxycycline	TMP-SMZ	Bupivicaine	Sodium citrate	
Metronidazole	Praziquantel	Isoflurane	Iohexol	
Azithromycin	Permethrin (Provent-a-mite)	Propofol	Barium	
Florfenicol		Alfaxalone	Epinephrine	
Itraconazole		Midazolam	Glycopyrrolate	
Voraconazole		Flumazenil	Allopurinol	
		Ketamine		
		(Dex)medetomidine		
		Atipamezole		

TMP-SMZ, Trimethoprim/sulfamethoxazole.

(https://www.ncbi.nlm.nih.gov/pubmed), and BioOne (http://www.bioone.org) are all excellent search engines for research publications. There are many textbooks and journals (including *Journal of Herpetological Medicine and Surgery, Journal of Herpetology, Journal of Zoo and Wildlife Medicine,* and the *Journal of Wildlife Diseases*) available. In general, peer-reviewed clinical trials, studies, and case series are among the strongest and most reliable sources, followed by case reports, roundtable discussions/reports, and conference proceedings. (See Chapter 2 for herpetological reference resources.)

Once information has been researched and reviewed, clinicians must attempt to incorporate substantiated and updated information into the management of the case at hand. If clinical questions can be answered with substantiated information such as research and published material, a specific treatment may be able to be initiated. However, in herpetological medicine, answers are often unclear, and application of evidence-based veterinary medicine, although always the goal, may not always be entirely possible. In these situations clinicians still have an obligation to provide treatment for these unique patients. Subsequently, it is important for the clinician to utilize the *best* available information in managing a case.

REFERENCES

See www.expertconsult.com for a complete list of references.

2

Reference Resources for the Herpetological Clinician

Joanna Hedley

Finding reference resources has historically been a challenge for the reptile clinician. Despite published recommendations, reptile medicine has not been well-represented in the core curriculum of the majority of veterinary schools.[1] Thus, in comparison to the more traditional companion animals, there has been a lack of resources available for veterinary students wanting to learn about reptile medicine and surgery. Early literature was based primarily on personal experience, from both clinicians and experienced reptile keepers. Currently, however, as the field of herpetological medicine has developed, there are many more resources available, ranging from textbooks to peer-reviewed research articles. Additionally, a large amount of nonveterinary herpetological literature, including information on taxonomy, anatomy, physiology, ecology, nutrition, and behavior, is available and is relevant to reptiles treated in veterinary practice. Likewise, literature published in other languages should not be overlooked.

With the widespread use of the internet, more resources are available online and even on mobile devices, making access to information easy. Obtaining reliable information, however, can still be problematic and requires the clinician to critically evaluate the quality of reference resources. The advantages and disadvantages of each type of resource will be examined in more detail below.

ASSOCIATIONS AND SOCIETIES

First, for any clinician with a keen interest in reptile medicine, membership in a specialist veterinary association is highly recommended. Membership usually allows access to various resources, including publications, conference proceedings, and an opportunity to network and collaborate with other veterinarians in the field.

The largest association is the Association of Reptilian and Amphibian Veterinarians (ARAV) (http://www.arav.org), which, although primarily based in North America, does have active international involvement and considers itself an international organization. Regular conferences are held in North America and Europe, and members have access to the peer-reviewed *Journal of Herpetological Medicine and Surgery* (JHMS).

Other useful organizations, depending on location, include the American Association of Zoo Veterinarians (AAZV) (http://www.aazv.org) and the European Association of Zoo and Wildlife Veterinarians (http://www.eazwv.org). Many countries also have their own local reptile or zoological veterinary organizations.

Herpetological societies can also be an extremely helpful source of information. The North American–based Society for the Study of Amphibians and Reptiles (http://www.ssarherps.org) is the largest international herpetological society. Other useful societies in North America include The American Society of Ichthyologists and Herpetologists (http://www.asih.org) and The Herpetologists League (http://www.herpetologistsleague.org). Other large international and national organizations include Societas Europaea Herpetologica (http://www.seh-herpetology.org) in Europe, and Australian Society of Herpetologists (http://www.australiansocietyofherpetologists.org), but many countries will also have multiple regional organizations, which can be good sources of information on local herpetofauna.

BOOKS

Textbooks have previously been the standard starting point for those looking for information, and, although they are now often available as online resources, many clinicians still prefer to keep at least some hard copies available for quick reference. Books can provide a good general overview of a topic but may not always be well-referenced or have undergone rigorous review. The reader will therefore need to evaluate the information carefully to decide whether it is based primarily on the author's personal opinion (and whether that author is a recognized specialist in the field) or backed up by references (to material other than previous textbooks).

Many standard veterinary textbooks or exotic pet textbooks contain a section on reptiles, but more reptile-specific literature is now available. Aside from this book (and previous volumes), some useful titles are listed below. This list is limited to the last 20 years because older titles can be harder to obtain. However, the older titles should not be completely disregarded; although some information is outdated, many still contain useful reference material found nowhere else. A classic example would be *Biomedical and Surgical Aspects of Captive Reptile Husbandry*, volumes 1 and 2 (Frye), which contains a wealth of information and high-quality color photographs.

Identification and Husbandry

- Bartlett RD, Bartlett P (2010) *Reptiles, Amphibians and Invertebrates: An Identification and Care Guide* (Reptile Keepers Guide), New York, Barron's Educational series—this basic husbandry manual covers more than 250 commonly kept species, with excellent photographs for identification
- Behler JL, King FW (2013) *National Audubon Society Field Guide to North American Reptiles and Amphibians*, New York, Alfred A. Knopf—this field guide describes all the native and introduced reptiles and amphibians found in North America, with full-color photographs for identification
- Huchzermeyer FW (2003) *Crocodiles. Biology, Husbandry and Diseases*, Cambridge, CABI—a review of the crocodilian species, in particular their biology and captive management

Anatomy and Physiology

- O'Malley B (2005) *Clinical Anatomy and Physiology of Exotic Species*, Philadelphia, Elsevier—a concise, easily read summary of clinically relevant reptile and amphibian anatomy and physiology
- *Biology of the Reptilia*—a 22-volume collection of information, which provides the most comprehensive review of this topic to date; useful for more in-depth reading on a specific topic and now also available for free online at http://www.carlgans.org/biology-reptilia-online

Pathology

- Campbell TW (2015) *Exotic Animal Hematology and Cytology*, 4th edition, Oxford, Wiley Blackwell—an excellent reference guide with good-quality pictures, especially for those routinely performing their own in-house laboratory work
- Fudge AM (2000) *Laboratory Medicine: Avian and Exotic Pets*, Philadelphia, WB Saunders—although some information has now been superseded by newer publications, the reptile chapters provide a useful background in reptile clinical pathology
- Jacobson E (2007) *Infectious Diseases and Pathology of Reptiles: Color Atlas and Text*, Boca Raton, CRC Press—an incredibly detailed reference guide with many useful pictures and further references for the reptile clinician

Clinical Medicine

- Fowler ME, Miller RE (2012) *Zoo and Wild Animal Medicine, Current Therapy*, 7th edition, St. Louis, WB Saunders—the reptile section provides a thorough review of selected topics. The previous six editions also contain sections on different reptile-related topics
- Fowler ME, Miller, RE (2015) *Zoo and Wild Animal Medicine* (vol. 8), St Louis, Elsevier Health Sciences—this revised edition provides an up-to-date overview of reptile and amphibian medicine, including biology, anatomy, and husbandry
- Girling SJ, Raiti P (2004) *Manual of Reptiles*, 2nd edition, Quedgeley, British Small Animal Veterinary Association—this book provides information in an easy-to-use format for the busy clinician
- Jacobson ER (2003) *Biology, Husbandry and Medicine of the Green Iguana*, Malabar, Krieger Publishing—although not as up-to-date as some of the more recent texts, this book is still a valuable source of information, particularly about the biology of the green iguana
- Krautwald-Junghanns ME, Pees M, Reese S, Tully T (2011) *Diagnostic Imaging of Exotic Pets*, Hannover, Schlütersche—a helpful atlas including both normal and abnormal images of a variety of reptile species
- Longley L (2008) *Anaesthesia of Exotic Pets*, Edinburgh, Saunders—the reptile and amphibian sections provide a practical and detailed guide to anesthesia
- McArthur S, Wilkinson R, Meyer J (2004) *Medicine and Surgery of Tortoises and Turtles*, Oxford, Blackwell—a well-illustrated, extremely practical guide for the reptile clinician
- Schneller P, Pantchev N (2008) *Parasitology in Snakes, Lizards and Chelonians*, Edition Chimaira, Frankfurt am Main—a useful reference source for those performing in-house parasitology
- Wright KM, Whitaker BR (2001) *Amphibian Medicine and Captive Husbandry*, Malabar, FL, Krieger Publishing Company—a comprehensive guide to amphibian biology, nutrition, husbandry, and medicine
- Zug GR, Vitt LJ, Caldwell JP (2001) *Herpetology: An Introductory Biology of Amphibians and Reptiles*, 2nd edition, San Diego, Academic Press—a detailed herpetology text
- *Veterinary Clinics of North America* (Exotic Animal Practice)—published three times per year, this journal reviews a different topic with each issue, with contributions from multiple international authors

In addition to the larger textbooks, specific exotic pet formularies are also available, which can provide a quick reference guide for the clinician. These include the *Exotic Animal Formulary*, 5th edition (Carpenter and Marion), and the *BSAVA Small Animal Formulary*, 9th edition, Part B: Exotic Pets (Meredith). In addition to drug doses and some normal blood reference ranges, both of these are well-referenced, so clinicians can assess the evidence (whether based on pharmacokinetic studies or personal communications) before selecting their dosage.

JOURNALS

Both veterinary journals and herpetological journals can be useful sources of information. Peer-reviewed original research articles should provide the most reliable evidence base for reptile medicine. However, articles need to be critically evaluated by the reptile clinician to assess their validity and relevance to clinical cases. Case reports and review articles can also provide valuable clinically relevant information.

The main reptile veterinary journal is the *Journal of Herpetological Medicine and Surgery* (JHMS), published by ARAV and available online for members. However, other veterinary journals are now beginning to include more herpetological articles. These include zoological or exotic animal–based publications, such as the following:

- *Journal of Wildlife Diseases*
- *Journal of Zoo and Wildlife Medicine*
- *Journal of Exotic Pet Medicine* (previously *Seminars in Avian and Exotic Pet Medicine*)
- *Zoo Biology*

Herpetological research and case reports are also now being featured more frequently in mainstream veterinary journals, such as *Journal of American Veterinary Medical Association*, *American Journal of Veterinary Research*, *Veterinary Record*, *Veterinary Journal*, and *Journal of Small Animal Practice*. Publications on more specific reptile topics can even be found in discipline-specific journals such as *Veterinary Radiology and Ultrasound*, *Veterinary Ophthalmology*, *Veterinary Anaesthesia and Analgesia*, *Journal of Veterinary Diagnostic Investigation*, *Veterinary Pathology*, and *Veterinary Parasitology*.

Herpetological journals of interest may include:

- *Journal of Herpetology* (Society for the Study of Amphibians and Reptiles)
- *Herpetological Review* (Society for the Study of Amphibians and Reptiles)
- *Copeia* (The American Society of Ichthyologists and Herpetologists)
- *Herpetologica* (The Herpetologists League)
- *Amphibia-Reptilia* (Societas Europaea Herpetologica)
- *Chelonian Conservation and Biology* (Chelonian Research Foundation)
- *Herpetological Conservation & Biology* (open-access online journal)

It may not be economically feasible to subscribe to all of these journals, and although more journals are now moving toward an open-access online format, many still require substantial subscription fees. In most cases, electronic reprints of articles can be provided for a fee, or alternatively, journals may be accessed via libraries of veterinary colleges or other academic institutions.

ONLINE RESOURCES

As more resources become available online, determining which of these are actually reliable sources of information will be a challenge for the reptile clinician. Searching with a standard search engine such as http://www.google.com provides a basic overview of the information available. Because most websites, wikis, and blogs can be set up or edited by anyone, quality is highly variable. However, these websites can be a helpful insight into the information (often confusing and conflicting) available to clients attempting to research their pet's needs or medical conditions.

For a more focussed search, there are a number of free literature database search engines available. Pubmed (http://www.ncbi.nlm.nih.gov/pubmed) covers primarily biomedical literature and is easy to navigate, whereas others such as Bioone (http://www.bioone.org) include a number of natural history publications that are not available on Pubmed. Google Scholar (http://www.scholar.google.com) covers a wider range of literature types including books, which can result in a more extended search. However, it has the advantage of providing links to other articles that cite the original, which can be helpful when searching for more current research. Whichever type of search is conducted, it is important to critically assess the information retrieved. This applies whether the resources are books, journal articles, websites, wikis, blogs, or any other format.

Some useful websites for veterinary information and husbandry advice are listed below, although website addresses are subject to change.

- Veterinary Information Network (VIN): http://www.vin.com—a membership fee is charged, but this is an extremely useful resource. Members can access a wide range of information, such as journal abstracts (including several, such as JHMS, that are not listed on Pubmed), conference proceedings, drug formularies, and forums moderated by experienced reptile consultants.
- LaFeber has a website specifically designed for exotic animal veterinarians at http://lafeber.com/vet that provides reviews of many reptile-specific topics in addition to step-by-step guides and videos of procedures
- Reptile Database: http://www.reptile-database.org—this database (originally the EMBL Database) covers current reptile classification and taxonomy for all living species of reptiles and is updated several times per year
- http://www.kingsnake.com—a comprehensive information portal for reptile and amphibian keeping. It contains several hundred links, including breeders, dealers, stores, classified ads, forums specific to various species, organizations, events, care sheets, frequently asked questions (FAQs), and products.
- http://www.anapsid.org—this site contains hundreds of articles on the care of most herpetological species seen in the pet trade, with an exhaustive section on green iguanas. It also lists information on herpetological societies and veterinarians, literature, supplies, and links to other important sites.
- http://www.reptilesmagazine.com—this site provides current news, information, and care sheets on many commonly kept species of reptiles and amphibians.
- World Chelonia Trust: http://www.chelonia.org—dedicated to the conservation and species survival of turtles and tortoises, this website also has many care sheets and images to facilitate species identification.
- Tortoise Trust: http://www.tortoisetrust.org—an easy-to-navigate website containing numerous useful articles on chelonian care, breeding, and conservation
- USDA Nutrient Database: https://ndb.nal.usda.gov—a useful online resource providing complete nutritional information on any human food type
- http://www.herplit.com—a website that offers out-of-print and hard-to-find herpetological literature for sale

As demand for instant access to information has increased, so too has application software (apps) available for mobile devices. These apps can provide quick, concise reference resources, particularly for clinicians working between multiple sites or on the move. Examples include apps such as Merck Veterinary Manual, Veterinary Care of Exotic Pets, and Exotic Pet Vet. Several formularies are also now available as apps, including The Veterinary Formulary, which lists information on drugs and doses for a variety of exotic species. Alternatively, PDF versions of formularies or textbooks may be downloaded onto mobile devices for easy access.

Finally, online veterinary forums such as those run by VIN or Exotic DVM (http://www.exoticdvm.com) can provide clinicians with an opportunity to discuss cases, exchange ideas about topics, and advance their understanding of reptile medicine. Alternatively, more specialist forums are also available, such as the European College of Zoological Medicine (ECZM) forum, although access is restricted to European Diplomates (https://www.eczm.eu).

CONFERENCES

Attendance at conferences is one of the main ways of keeping up to date with advances in the field of reptile medicine. ARAV hosts an annual conference running over several days, concentrating solely on herpetological medicine, although this is often in collaboration with other exotic pet or zoological associations. This conference includes both basic and advanced lecture sessions and wet labs and so provides a helpful learning experience for clinicians at any stage in their career. Other conferences to consider in North America include the North American Veterinary Conference (http://www.navc.com), which usually runs a reptile lecture stream, and the Western Veterinary Conference (http://www.wvc.org). Both conferences take place annually.

In Europe, the International Conference on Avian heRpetological and Exotic mammal medicine (ICARE) runs every other year in various locations around Europe and hosts a reptile stream (including lecture sessions and wet labs) in collaboration with ARAV. The World Congress of Herpetology (http://www.worldcongressofherpetology.org) meets every 3 to 5 years in various locations around the world. Topics include reptile and amphibian biology, ecology, reproduction, and behavior. There are also smaller conferences run by the reptile or zoological veterinary and herpetological associations for each country that may be more accessible for many clinicians and can still provide a good source of continuing education.

REFERENCES

See www.expertconsult.com for a complete list of references.

3

Understanding the Human-Herp Relationship

Stacey Leonatti Wilkinson

Reptile ownership represents the fastest-growing population of pets in the United States, and amphibians are becoming more popular as well.[1] At one time, buying a new reptile or amphibian was cheaper than taking an ill animal to the veterinarian, and there was a lack of veterinarians experienced in herpetological medicine. This is simply no longer the case. With the rapid advance in veterinary medical knowledge in exotic pets and the strengthening of the human-animal bond, herp owners are now seeking health care once not even considered an option. Services only available for canine and feline patients are now offered routinely for reptile and amphibian patients.

Veterinarians no longer enter the profession to avoid working with people. In fact, it is well understood that the "people part" of a clinician's job may be the most important. Veterinarians who have poor bedside manner lose out on both the financial and personal satisfaction aspects of this special profession. Preparation for work with owners and caretakers of nontraditional pets takes extra training—training that generally does not come from a classroom. The veterinarian gains this knowledge either in the field through trial and error or from an experienced mentor. This chapter offers veterinary clinicians and technicians a scaffold for building a better understanding of the concerns of these clients and their unique relationships with their nontraditional patients.

THE HUMAN-ANIMAL BOND

Who gets attached to a pet and why? The many answers to this question probably equal the number of clients in a practice. In general, people are attracted to pets for companionship, a sense of security they may provide, unconditional love (free of criticism and judgment), or because of a biological fascination with the species. For many people, experiencing consistent positive feelings with animals is easier than it is with people. Relationships with animals do not take as much emotional work to maintain.

Much truth can be found in the previous statements, even with herps as pets. Depending on the reptile or amphibian in consideration, many owners claim that their pets show reciprocal affection (Fig. 3.1). This affection is a matter of interpretation, and one person's definition likely differs from the next. However, regardless of how the veterinarian rationalizes a particular animal's ability to relate, the owner's emotional interplay is what matters. There is no doubt that certain herps recognize their owners, and many species tolerate handling and interaction very well.

The first step to take with a client and animal, in any situation, is to assume that some degree of emotional investment exists. This emotional investment could be in the form of "my lizard Iggy is deathly ill, and I may lose him" or "my lizard breeder number 14 is sick, and I could be out several hundred dollars." Regardless of the connection, whether an obvious true emotional dependence or a financial dependence,

some type of emotion almost always plays a part in the decision making. Three general categories of the human-herp bond are considered in this chapter: the "pet" reptile/amphibian, the "commercial" reptile/amphibian, and the "large collection" group.

THE PET REPTILE OR AMPHIBIAN

To take the position of "pet," the animal generally assumes and fills some niche in a person's life. The relationship may be as simple as the owner dropping some crickets in the animal's cage every morning. Alternatively, it may be more complex, with the owner considering the animal a true part of the family; this may include routine conversations with the pet and even Christmas presents purchased in the animal's name. This bond can affect the owner's relationship with the herp veterinarian. The type and quality of medicine and care offered should not be dictated by the perceived bond between the client and animal. Recommendations should be made based on what is best for the animal, and it is up to the client to decide what they can afford and are willing to pursue. Often one might be surprised by which clients are willing to do whatever is needed for their pet. Part of establishing a trusting relationship with a client is not judging them or their relationship with their animal.

There are some owners who have one or more reptiles or amphibians that are considered members of the family (Fig. 3.2). The pets are typically out of their enclosures, held frequently, and even watch TV with their owners in a similar fashion to how owners spend time with a dog or cat. Owners may buy treats and presents for them and provide intensive detailed care for them such as changing the cage daily. When questioned by clinicians they can often recite their exact environmental temperatures, cage dimensions, type of lighting, food, supplements, and more provided to their cherished pet. These pets are often referred to by people as their "child" or their "best friend," and veterinary recommendations are eagerly accepted, and economics are not of concern. The author often sees this type of bond with green iguanas (*Iguana iguana*), bearded dragons (*Pogona vitticeps*), and large tortoises, among others. The bond between the owner and their herp pets can be profound (Fig. 3.3).

There are also owners who really enjoy their herp pet, love it, and take good care of it but are not as involved with it on a daily basis. They usually do everything correctly in regards to husbandry, but there may be some areas to improve on. When it comes to veterinary care, they are often willing to spend some money but may not commit to expensive diagnostic tests, hospitalization, or surgery without significant thought. They love their pet but may have limits. A common example of this is the college student with a bearded dragon.

Some pets have a more ornamental or decorative value. Reptiles are often used to enhance an image, such as the outlaw biker with the pet

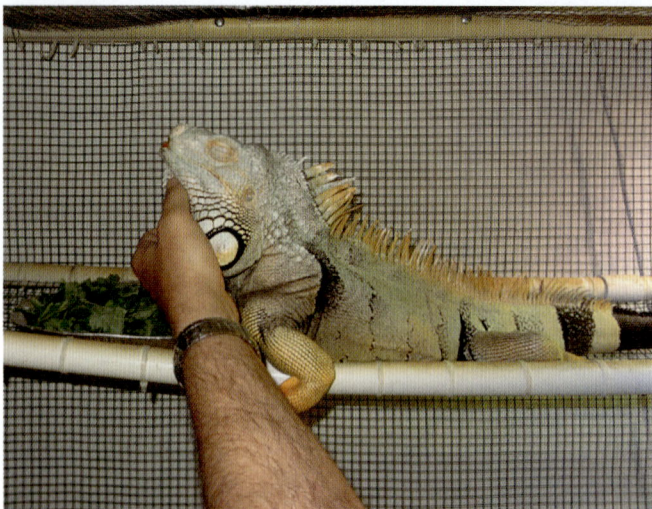

FIG 3.1 A green iguana (*Iguana iguana*) who appears to be enjoying human attention. Closing the eyes can be a defense mechanism (ignoring their surroundings), but in this case the lizard was leaning into the hand as if he is enjoying the attention. (Courtesy of Stacey Leonatti Wilkinson.)

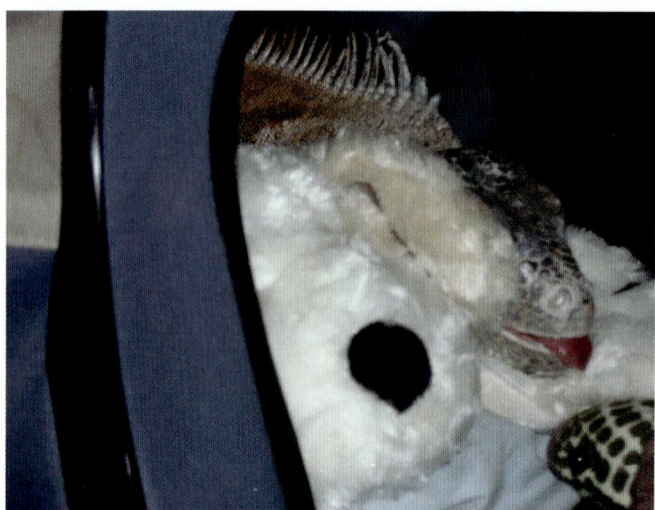

FIG 3.2 A green iguana (*Iguana iguana*) sleeping on blankets with a stuffed animal. (Courtesy of Nanette Gunn.)

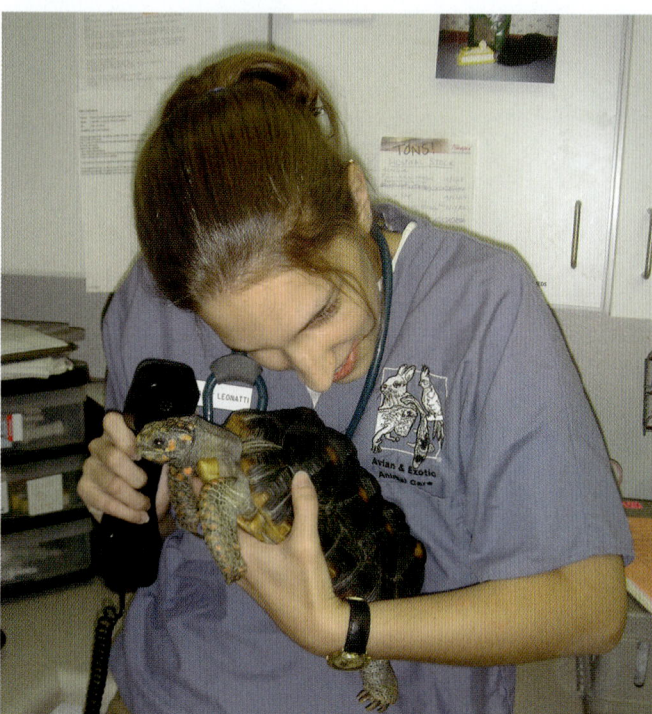

FIG 3.3 A hospitalized red-footed tortoise (*Chelonoidis carbonaria*) being held by the veterinarian so that the owner can speak to it over the phone. (Courtesy of Dan Johnson.)

rattlesnake, the dancer with the python, or the surfer kid with the pet iguana. These reptiles, although important facets in the lives of these individuals, likely do not take on the same significance as the herp pet considered to be a part of the family.

Veterinarians will also encounter parents of children with pet reptiles or amphibians. Often the child really wanted the animal and the parent agreed, neither understanding the commitment they were making nor the level of care required. Once realizing the care may be challenging, some parents do research on the care required, help their child, and bond with the animal just as much or more than the child; these relationships are often rewarding. However, some parents are discouraged with the extensive care required and may resent the pet. They are not interested in continuing to care for an animal that their child fails to be responsible for or loses interest in. They also resent having to bring it to a veterinarian or spend any money on it at all. They often would prefer to euthanize rather than treat but may do the bare minimum treatment to appease their child. Of course there are variations between these two extremes,

and some parents are often responsible and actively involved in the care of the pet from the beginning.

Along with the child/parent impulse purchasers, there are adults who purchase reptiles or amphibians with no forethought either, but rather because it "looks cool" or "my friend has one." They do little to no research, buy what a pet store tells them or they find online, and often end up with a sick animal. Many times these owners feel extremely guilty when they realize they have done something wrong and will do whatever it takes to save the animal. If it is beyond saving, they may request humane euthanasia but are willing to learn what they need to do should they get another herp in the future. Although these cases can be frustrating, it is important not to make these clients feel guilty as they are at least seeking veterinary care when realizing there is a problem. Along these same lines, giving a herp pet as a surprise gift is never recommended. These "gifted" pets are often given to people who are not prepared to own a herp and are not aware of the commitment involved. Often the animal is the least expensive part of the purchase; the cage, lighting, heating, food, and more cost significantly more.

THE COMMERCIAL ANIMAL

The commercial animal refers to a reptile or amphibian that is part of a breeding collection (Fig. 3.4). Some professional herpetoculturists have thousands of breeding animals. Breeders with large collections will often vary in their approach to veterinary care depending on the worth of the individual animal and their previous experience with veterinarians. If an individual animal has valuable genetics, they will often be willing to spend money on it, especially if there is a problem that could affect the entire collection. If there is a disease outbreak, they are often willing to sacrifice a critically ill animal for a necropsy in order to obtain a diagnosis. The financial investment generally far outweighs the emotional attachment.

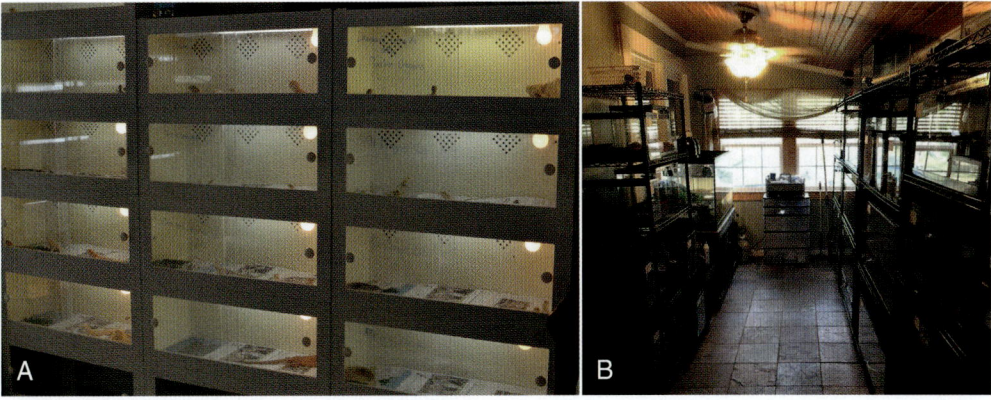

FIG 3.4 An example of commercial animals/large collections. Part of a breeding colony of bearded dragons. In large collections, animals are often kept in rack systems or uniform cages for ease of care and visualization of all the animals daily. (Courtesy of David Freeman.)

Often these clients have been keeping herps for many years, sometimes before there were knowledgeable herp veterinarians available. They often perform their own medical care on their animals. They may still trust other keepers more than veterinarians. The herp veterinarian may have to work hard to prove to this client that they are knowledgeable and offer what is best for the animal. These keepers are often quite experienced, especially with specific species of reptiles or amphibians, and it is important to respect their knowledge while sharing clinical information with them. Often if this is done correctly, a mutually beneficial, respectful relationship can be formed.

LARGE COLLECTIONS

The last general category is the large collection. Examples include animals on display, such as zoo animals or animals in a research colony. In this last category, the bond between caretaker (not an owner but someone assigned to provide daily care for the animals) and the animal often may be just as strong as that between an owner and the pet reptile or amphibian. Caretakers may be asked to spend a significant part of their lives attending to these captive animals. Emotional attachment is not uncommon when one of the animals becomes ill or has to be euthanized, such as in the case of a research setting.

END-OF-LIFE CONSIDERATIONS

Palliative, end-of-life, or hospice care can be a valuable service to offer reptile and amphibian clients. In many cases these animals are as important to a client as a dog or cat may be, and the same standards of care should be offered. Often owners need time to understand or come to accept their pet's diagnosis, and there are frequently palliative measures that can be used to maintain a good quality of life. Often owners will ask if their pet is "in pain" or "suffering," and this can be more difficult to interpret in herps. Although they are not as demonstrative as other species, the same indicators can be used to assess their quality of life, including lethargy, lack of appetite, unwillingness to ambulate, and increased aggression. Remember the owner generally knows their animal best; often what is seen in an exam room is different from what is occuring at home.

Hospice care for reptiles and amphibians usually starts with optimizing husbandry: keep the animal in its preferred optimum temperature zone; provide appropriate lighting; modify the enclosure and furnishings to make it easier for them to move around; provide excellent water quality for amphibians; and generally provide a nutritious, highly digestible diet or modify the diet as needed for the condition being treated. Supportive care may be needed, such as additional soaking, fluid therapy, or syringe or tube feeding for an animal that is not eating. Many times there are medications that can be used to manage conditions being treated, and pain management can be incorporated if necessary.

For the emotionally attached client, regardless of the category, the decision to euthanize a cherished animal is agonizing and heart wrenching. Some people withdraw into a state of denial that gives relief from the psychological pain of a beloved animal in declining health. Many different conflicts and questions must be addressed in each category. An experienced veterinarian (and staff) is a great help to the client in making these difficult decisions.

With pets, regardless of the type of animal, the dilemma is always "treat or don't treat" or "euthanize and replace." Some reptile pets have extended life expectancies. Some of the smaller lizards may only live a few years, but some of the larger snakes and lizards may live much longer, and some tortoises may live more than 100 years. Longevity has an obvious impact on the decision for treatment or euthanasia.

The client who wants heroic efforts made at all costs to keep the terminal animal alive can create resentment in veterinarians and staff members who feel the animal is suffering. Practitioners also may disagree with clients who, in their opinion, prematurely or inappropriately choose euthanasia rather than attempt to treat an apparently correctable health problem. The owner has the right to make the decision to euthanize a pet, and veterinarians have the right to refuse continued therapy if euthanasia is indicated on humane grounds. Owners who feel they are discouraged from or coerced into a euthanasia decision may leave the office feeling misunderstood and manipulated. Euthanasia of a beloved pet can be the single event by which a pet owner judges the veterinary service; one should always be sensitive to an owner's needs in these situations.

In a commercial situation, the decision to treat or euthanize may not be emotional but intellectual and financial (i.e., if the cost of treatment can be recuperated with production profits) or scientific/diagnostic. If an animal is ill and a risk for infectious disease (or other colony danger) exists, then sacrifice of an ill or dying individual for the benefit of the colony is often wise. Even in these situations, a veterinarian should be cognizant of the owner's emotions, because the inherent loss of any animal, commercial or not, may have an emotional impact.

The animals in the large collection category present their own concerns regarding the human-herp bond. The caretaker, and even the general public, develops bonds with certain display animals. The decision to euthanize a charismatic zoo animal requires careful planning and media announcements to prevent public discourse. In a research setting, the value of an animal to a caretaker/scientist takes on different meanings. Again, caretakers commonly form bonds with long-term research specimens. When one of these animals dies or is sacrificed, an emotional toll may result on the caretaker. From a more objective perspective, if a colony animal is ill and is in imminent danger of dying or may have to be sacrificed, the associated loss of scientific worth (i.e., lost data and future potential data) also brings some consternation. In many cases, the decision for euthanasia or treatment may be a financial one and completely out of the control of the caretaker, which can have a serious effect on their emotions.

COMPASSIONATE EUTHANASIA GUIDELINES

Reptilian euthanasia can be a technically difficult procedure and should not be learned through trial and error in the presence of a client. See Chapter 47 for procedures to follow. Learn the techniques on either non–client owned animals or on patients with clients who do not want to be present.

From beginning to end, all cases of euthanasia should be handled with the utmost sensitivity and compassion. Acknowledge to the client the difficulty of saying goodbye. If possible, reminisce with the client about the animal. Offer at-home euthanasia or a referral for that service.

Give the client the option to be with the animal during the procedure. Many people need to feel that they were at the animal's side until the end. If a practice is not comfortable with this, a referral should be made to a practice where clients can be present during the pet's euthanasia. Many clients appreciate honoring their feelings about being present and remain loyal to the practice in the future.

Take time to educate the client. Talk about the process of euthanasia: the solutions that are used and how they work on the body; the length of time for an animal to die; that twitching, writhing, and elimination can occur; and that animals may die with their eyes open. Because a herp's metabolism is slow, and they can have continued electrical activity in the heart after death, it can take hours for the heart to stop after the euthanasia solution is given. Warn owners about this, and if they wish to take the pet's body home for burial it may be best to return the next day for pickup. Owners who want to be present for euthanasia may wish to stay while the animal is sedated and the euthanasia solution given but then leave once the animal is unaware of their surroundings, as the entire process can take hours. If possible, handle financial matters beforehand. If the client is billed, consider a phrase like "special services" rather than "euthanasia" on the billing statement. Schedule euthanasia when people are not feeling rushed between other client appointments. Some veterinarians worry about crying in front of a client. Getting teary-eyed on occasion is normal. Keep in mind, though, that you have a job to do, so tell yourself that you will take some private time to feel and express emotion after the procedure is completed. Clients appreciate sensitivity and can feel especially supported when the veterinary staff shares in the emotional climate of a particular event or experience.

Once the animal is deceased, allow the client to see the veterinarian check for a heartbeat (using a Doppler monitor in herps). This can be reassuring to some clients who may not be convinced that their animal has actually died. Some clients might appreciate a private moment to say goodbye to their pet. Ask clients who are upset to have someone drive them home, or keep them at your practice until they seem calm enough to drive. One can show support by making a referral to a local pet loss support group or hotline by simply handing the client a brochure telling them that they might be interested in these services because other clients have found them helpful.

Handle the body of a deceased animal with respect and gentleness. Disposal of remains should be discussed with the owner beforehand.

If the owner wishes to have the body for burial, use plain boxes or boxes designed for this purpose; do not reuse shipping boxes or those with logos on them. Cremation services should be offered, and many of these services will offer additional mementos such as clay paw prints, poems, or other keepsakes. A sympathy card signed by the employees of the practice should be sent to every owner who loses a pet. Sometimes it is appropriate to send a gift to a client who is very special to the practice, such as one who has been coming there for many years with their pet or recently had a long protracted illness. A plant that the owner can keep in memory of their pet is often much appreciated. Alternatively, a donation can be made in their name to an animal rescue group or animal conservation and research organization.

Update the client's records to reflect the death of the animal so reminders of future examinations, parasite checks, and more, are not sent. If the case was referred, remember to inform the primary practice that the animal was euthanized. It is embarrassing for a well-meaning primary care veterinarian to call the owner to discover what has happened at the referral practice. If applicable, note what examination room was used for the euthanasia and then refrain from using that room for that client who may bring other pets. Providing a photo of the pet to add to a memorial board in the waiting room or web page may give them the courage to return to that practice due to their compassionate care.

COMMON CONCERNS FOR THE CLINICIAN AND THE CLIENT REGARDING ANIMAL LOSS

There are many concerns that both the clinician and the client may have regarding end-of-life care and euthanasia. Delivering bad news is an unpleasant part of the job but is a skill that can be learned. Use a gentle tone of voice, and starting the conversation with a phrase like "I'm afraid I have some bad news" will help prepare the client for what is about to come. Sometimes the client will react with anger, especially if their pet has died unexpectedly. Listen to their concerns and be empathetic and truthful about what happened. It is acceptable to express shock as well. Given time, many clients will be understanding, while some will never be satisfied. Contain feelings of defensiveness when speaking with the client, and document all conversations.

When the decision for euthanasia or not is necessary, often clients will ask the veterinarian "What would you do if you were me?" No perfect answer exists, but one should be careful about answering this question and swaying the client one way or the other; they need to make their own decision for their pet. Review everything that has been done and be honest about the animal's prognosis. Encourage people to think about a definition for a good quality of life; are they still seeing those behaviors? The clinician can often be more objective than the client. Many times people will feel guilty about this choice, feeling they "gave up" too soon or that they waited too long to euthanize their pet. Reassure them that all we can do when faced with tough choices is to make decisions based on the information we have at the time.

Many clients feel unsure about how to talk to their child about the loss of a pet. They may ask you to lie for them because they do not want their child to suffer, but try to avoid this. If you are comfortable you can coach parents about how to talk to their kids, or you can suggest a book on the topic of children and pet loss. Children can benefit from memorializing a beloved pet in their own personal way or by holding a memorial service in which everyone participates.

Older clients often have concerns about what will happen to their pet if something happens to them, particularly when long-lived species are involved. Think about all the people (e.g., friends, relatives, their veterinarian) who would be willing to adopt the animal in case of the owner's death or at least provide short-term care if the owner needs to be in the hospital for a time. Other possibilities include an animal sanctuary or an arrangement with an informed attorney. Some veterinary schools have programs that provide arrangements for the lifetime care of pets of deceased owners.

CONCLUSION

The profession of veterinary medicine is full of trials, tribulations, and triumphs. It can be demanding when, within the same day, you find yourself sharing the excitement of a client's new pet only to enter the next examination room to deliver bad news about the beloved pet of a familiar client. Euthanasia of animals you have come to know and like also takes its toll on your emotional well-being. Given the emotional challenges you face as a veterinary professional, you need to take care of yourself so that you can maintain patience and a sense of compassion for your clients. Stay current with your medical skills, have confidence in your interpersonal skills, and take good care of yourself physically and emotionally. Many veterinary schools now require self-care classes and more training in client communication in an effort to prepare future veterinarians for some of the challenges of private practice

(Kenwright M, http://veterinarynews.dvm360.com/university-tennessee-requires-self-health-classes-veterinary-students).

If you find that you are feeling impatient or you are reacting to people in a cold fashion, you could be experiencing some symptoms of burnout or compassion fatigue. Instead of focusing on the complaints you have about work, think about possible solutions to what you have identified as problems. Do what you can to make constructive changes and accept the aspects of your job you feel you cannot change. If you definitely cannot accept certain things, maybe a different strategy or a new path should be considered.

Working in the veterinary field, especially in a unique discipline such as herpetological medicine, can be a most rewarding experience. Because of the compassion you show, the job is one in which you can truly make a difference in the lives of many animals and the people who love them. Take good care of yourself so you can maintain compassion in all the work you do.

REFERENCES

See www.expertconsult.com for a complete list of references.

4

Specialization

Volker Schmidt, Brendan Carmel, Scott J. Stahl, and Stephen J. Divers

Often within any profession there is a drive to "take things to another level," to achieve a higher level of expertise, perhaps with the goal of developing a niche within the profession. Part of this drive is for personal growth; in other cases, it may be more financially driven to develop a "product" for the practice that allows the practice to offer a service not otherwise available within the community. Legally and ethically there are guidelines as to how one may advertise such a product. For example, an American Board of Veterinary Practitioners (ABVP) (avian) specialist cannot advertise as a specialist in reptiles/amphibians and vice versa. While beyond the scope of this chapter, the American Veterinary Medical Association's website (http://www.avma.org) and the European Board for Veterinary Specialization (EBVS) (http://www.ebvs.eu), as well as the Australasian Veterinary Boards Council Inc. (AVBC) (http://www.avbc.asn.au), provides such guidelines for the United States and the European Union, as well as for Australia and New Zealand. Communicating directly with the state veterinary board can also provide guidance as to how to advertise such skills. Ultimately, however, the term *specialist* is considered the gold standard for indicating the highest level of expertise. Because this chapter resides within a herpetological book, the discussion will be directed toward different opportunities for specialization in reptiles and amphibians. The process of specialization will vary depending on which part of the world a veterinarian is eligible to work in, although there are efforts in many areas (unfortunately zoological/herpetological medicine is not one of them) to establish global criteria and reciprocation. A veterinary specialist is a registered veterinarian with an exceptionally high level of skills well above those of a general practitioner in the same discipline. An entry-level specialist must have undergone extensive advanced supervised training, culminating in the passing of a rigorous set of examinations. The specialty must be a branch of veterinary practice having sufficient depth and breadth to allow one to spend a significant time practicing within the specialty. The roles of the American Board of Veterinary Specialization (ABVS), EBVS, and AVBC are simply to maintain the standards established by each specialty. Veterinarians who are eligible to work in the United States have the opportunity to become a Diplomate of the American Board of Veterinary Practitioners with specialization in reptile and amphibian medicine (ABVP R/A) or a Diplomate of the American College of Zoological Medicine (ACZM), which includes reptile and amphibian medicine.[1]

Although many countries offered veterinary specialization, veterinary specialization was not standardized in the European Union until the advent of the EBVS. Standardization on a European level is a central aim of the EBVS. European colleges of different veterinary specialties are established on the European level, for example, a Diplomate of the European College of Zoological Medicine (ECZM) in the subspecialty herpetology would hold the title "European Veterinary Specialist in Herpetology."

The Australian and New Zealand College of Veterinary Scientists (ANZCVS) fellowship is one of the most common pathways for veterinary specialist registration in Australia and New Zealand. The subject *Medicine and Surgery of Unusual Pets* includes native and exotic reptile species legally kept as pets in Australia and New Zealand. *Medicine of Zoo Animals* membership includes reptiles commonly encountered in zoos and so is applicable for veterinarians working in zoos. Membership in the discipline *Medicine of Australasian Wildlife Species* has reptiles included in its learning outcomes. However, the AVBC lists certifying bodies that set the standards acceptable for specialist registration, besides the fellowship, which includes ABVS, EBVS, and The Royal College of Veterinary Surgeons (RCVS), thus a veterinarian who holds a specialist registration from one of these bodies may be registered as a specialist in Australia or New Zealand without having to undergo further examinations. Such reciprocity is generally lacking in Europe and the United States, although some colleges have moved in this direction by allowing diplomates to train residents of either US or EU colleges. In addition, although the ACZM is accepted as a specialist qualification in Europe (e.g., RCVS in the UK) and Australia/New Zealand, the AVBC and ECZM qualifications are not recognized by the ABVS in the United States.

ADVICE TO CANDIDATES SEEKING SPECIALIST REGISTRATION

Before an examination can be taken, a period of 2 or up to 11 years of training is required, depending on whether the training was completed through a structured residency program or an alternative practitioner program. Training programs typically consist of a 1-year internship followed by a 2-year (EU, ABVP) to 3-year (ACZM) residency or 2 to 6 years of comparable general practice experience. Mentors often have the job of motivating residents to undertake research, publish, and study, but mentors and their programs also benefit by having more of their residents take and eventually pass boards. Candidates may be apprehensive about preparation for the specialist examinations. A good course of action is to work on and complete the credentialing process and then focus on studying. Achieving approval to sit for the examination strongly motivates the candidate to focus on study and preparation to pass the exam. For credentialing, some may prefer to work through one case report or submit one publication at a time, whereas others may find it more efficient to work on several simultaneously. Having an online study group to review publications, discuss cases, and test each other can be extremely helpful. The main regulatory bodies offer advice and often provide dedicated short courses to aid candidates in examination preparation. The pass rate for the examinations varies between the examination bodies. Check the relevant organization to access the most current information regarding timelines, credentialing, and recredentialing requirements, and examination structure and content (Table 4.1).

TABLE 4.1	Specialty Colleges and Boards			
	ACZM (American College of Zoological Medicine)	**ABVP-Reptile/Amphibian Medicine (American Board of Veterinary Practitioners)**	**ECZM (Herpetology) (European College of Zoological Medicine)**	**ANZCVS (Australian and New Zealand College of Veterinary Scientists)**
Definition	Zoological—A broad spectrum of disciplines involved with the medical problems of invertebrates, fish, amphibians, reptiles, birds, and mammals. Includes all exotic or nondomesticated species, including exotic pets, wildlife, and zoo/aquaria species.	Specialty recognition in the specific animal taxa reptile/amphibian	Herpetology—the veterinary treatment, health care, and preventative medicine of all reptilian and amphibian species Zoo Health Management—veterinary medicine as applied in zoological collections	Membership (MANZCVS) and fellowship (FANZVCS) Fellowship is the college qualification required by those seeking veterinary specialist registration. There are currently no subjects with significant reptile content at fellowship level. It is envisaged that the Unusual Pets Chapter of the ANZCVS, which currently provides a membership level qualification, will consider the introduction of a fellowship level in the future
Foundation	Founded in response to National Academy of Science Committee on Veterinary Medical Research and Education, and the comprehensive PEW report of veterinary education. The majority of diplomates work in institutions (e.g., zoo, universities, state, federal and international commissions and panels). As of May 2017, there are currently 186 diplomates (all examined), with the vast majority (>90%) working in clinical practice.	ABVP recognized a specialty in avian medicine and with strong support and interest, later followed with an exotic mammal specialty. The establishment of these specialties supported the development of the reptile/amphibian specialty, which had its first examination in 2010. As of May 2017, there are 11 reptile/amphibian diplomates (all examined) out of a total of 817 ABVP diplomates.	European Veterinary Specialist College formed under the auspices of the European Board of Specialisation (https://www.ebvs.eu). The ECZM evolved from the European College of Avian Medicine and Surgery (ECAMS), itself a veterinary specialist organization founded in 1993. Herpetology was added in 2009 and zoo health management in 2012. As of May 2017 there are 26 and 41 herpetology and zoo health management diplomates, respectively. The vast majority are de facto (not examined).	Formed in 1971 through the Australian Veterinary Association, it seeks to serve the veterinary profession and reward excellence. College membership signifies that a veterinarian has expertise and competence in a nominated subject area. College fellowship is associated with scholarly and technical excellence in a particular subject. Standards required for training and examination in fellowship subjects meet or exceed the prerequisites for registration as a veterinary specialist in Australia and/or New Zealand.
Official website	http://www.aczm.org	http://www.abvp.com	http://www.eczm.eu	http://www.anzcvs.org.au
Examined areas	Avian Reptiles and amphibians Mammals Fish and aquatic mammals Wildlife	Reptiles and amphibians	Reptile and amphibians	Subjects with a significant component of reptile content: Medicine and surgery of unusual pets Medicine of zoo animals Medicine of Australasian wildlife species
Required training	3-year ACZM-approved residency (100% time allocation) OR 6 years of 100% exotic/zoo/wildlife practice experience	1 year in small animal practice or small animal internship and 2- or 3-year ABVP-approved residency (10+ cases per week) OR 5 years in practice for credentialing application, 6 years prior to sitting for exam. First year may be nonspecialty specific, as with the residency option. There is no % time requirement, but an emphasis on reptile/amphibian medicine with a biannual self-reporting form, including detailed case logs listing, procedures, diagnoses, and diseases seen.	1 year companion animal or zoological species clinical sciences internship in a recognized institution that provides a broad range of clinical assignments or two years in clinical practice, and 2.5 to 3 years approved postgraduate training program (min. 24 hrs per week or 60% time allocation) under supervision of an ECZM diplomate.	Membership: at least 4 years in a full-time veterinary activity between graduation and taking the examination Fellowship: a minimum of 96 weeks of full-time, directly supervised training, or its equivalent At least 25 hours per week working in the clinical and technical aspects of the discipline Specialist registration requires 3 years of work in the appropriate discipline. This is a requirement of the ACRVS, not of the college

Continued

TABLE 4.1   Specialty Colleges and Boards—cont'd

	ACZM (American College of Zoological Medicine)	ABVP-Reptile/Amphibian Medicine (American Board of Veterinary Practitioners)	ECZM (Herpetology) (European College of Zoological Medicine)	ANZCVS (Australian and New Zealand College of Veterinary Scientists)
Publications and research	3 first-author, peer-reviewed journal papers, including at least one full manuscript on original research	2 (unpublished) case reports must be submitted OR 1 first-author publication (within 5 years of January 15 credentialing year) in an ABVP-approved scientific journal and 1 (unpublished) case report Must present two 1-hr seminars every year	Herpetology: 2 first-author papers of which at least 1 must be original research (the second can be a case report or case series). Zoo health management: 3 papers, of which 2 must be first author and include at least 1 investigative research project. Resident as first author must have the work accepted for publication in a peer-reviewed, well-established, internationally refereed scientific journal (i.e., mentioned in the Science Citation Index or in the reading list relevant to their own specialty) prior to sitting the examination, second manuscript as first author should also be accepted for publication and can be original scientific research, a case series, or a single case report	Membership: no formal requirements Fellowship: all fellowship candidates as a minimum requirement must submit a total of 2 original, first-author, scientific, peer-reviewed publications in peer-reviewed journals and evidence of presenting at one national or international scientific conference
Examination	Day 1 (qualifying exam, 375 points): 375 multiple-choice on avian, mammals, reptiles and amphibians, fish and aquatics, wildlife. Timed multiple-choice exams, each question has 5 possible answers. Must pass by 65% overall to continue. Day 2 (certifying exam, 300 points): slide (85 points), multiple-choice (75 points), and essays (140 points) in one of the following areas (all of which include herps); Zoological companion animals General zoo Aquatics Wildlife	Day 1 (core examination): 300 multiple-choice on preclinical and basic veterinary sciences 300 multiple-choice questions on reptile/amphibian medicine Day 2 (practical examination): 50–100 multiple-choice questions based on images. May also contain short-answer and essay questions. Timed multiple-choice exams, each question has 3 possible answers.	1-day examination for a total of 370 points, consisting of 100 timed multiple-choice questions, with one correct answer and four distractors, and a practical/written section of the exam is designed to test interpretive skills. Candidates must pass the examination within 8 years of being notified that they have satisfied the credentials process and may sit the examination on 4 occasions only.	College membership: Written paper 1 (2 hours): basic concepts and principles relevant to the subject Written paper 2 (2 hours): the practice and clinical applications of the subject Practical/oral: For most disciplines there is a 45–60 min oral exam A pass will be awarded if the candidate achieves at least 55% in one component (written or oral) AND at least 70% in the other component (written or oral) of the examination, AND achieves an overall average mark of at least 70% College fellowship: Written paper 1 (minimum 3 hours): basic science and principles of the subject. Written paper 2 (minimum 3 hours): practice and clinical applications of the subject. Practical (minimum 1 hour): case presentations, multimedia, problem solving, and theory, for which written answers will be required. Oral examination (minimum 1 hour) Pass mark (70%) in all four components

TABLE 4.1	Specialty Colleges and Boards—cont'd			
	ACZM (American College of Zoological Medicine)	**ABVP-Reptile/Amphibian Medicine** (American Board of Veterinary Practitioners)	**ECZM (Herpetology)** (European College of Zoological Medicine)	**ANZCVS** (Australian and New Zealand College of Veterinary Scientists)
Recognition and role (as outlined in published board information)	ACZM diplomates advance competency and scientific progress in zoological medicine, including birds, reptiles/amphibians, mammals, aquatics, wildlife; establish standards for post-doctoral training and experience and to certify veterinarians as specialists in zoological medicine through comprehensive examination; encourage research on the medical, surgical, and management problems of nondomestic species; disseminate information relative to zoological medicine to the veterinary profession DACZM is recognized as a specialist in zoological medicine (including birds, reptiles, mammals, amphibians, fish/aquatics, wildlife)	The DABVP (R/A) advances the quality of veterinary medicine through certification of veterinarians who demonstrate excellence in reptile and amphibian clinical practice	DECZM (herpetology) and DECZM (zoo health management) work primarily as clinicians and can function in academic and research institutions, as well as industry/zoos. The primary objectives of diplomates are to advance the specialties in Europe and increase the competency of those who practice in this field by: (a) Establishing guidelines for postgraduate training; (b) examining and authenticating veterinarians as specialists; and (c) encouraging research and other contributions to knowledge relating to the subspecialties of zoological medicine. A registered specialist shall spend at least 50% (i.e., >20 hours/week) of the time working at the specialist level.	Membership of the ANZCVS is not considered sufficient for application of specialist registration in Australia or New Zealand. Membership candidates are expected to demonstrate a high level of interest and competence in a given area of veterinary activity, which would make the person suitable to give professional advice to veterinary colleagues not similarly qualified on problems or procedures often encountered or used in general practice, in the relevant area of veterinary endeavor. A fellowship level herpetological qualification with reptiles as a significant component does not currently exist but may be available in the future.

REQUIREMENTS FOR CONTINUING EDUCATION IN THE CHOSEN SPECIALTY

Recertification of Diplomate status is required every 5 years in the ECZM and every 10 years in the ACZM and ABVP. Recertification is based on a standardized point system to quantify continued activity within the specialty. These include points awarded for publications and presentations, continuing education, training of residents, active involvement in committees, and annual general meetings of the colleges, as well as preparing questions for the specialty examination.

SPECIALTY BOARDS

The American College of Zoological Medicine

The ACZM website is http://www.aczm.org. In 1983 the ABVS for the formation of the American College of Zoological Medicine (ACZM) was provisionally approved and ratified by the AVMA House of Delegates. The initiating constitution approved by the ABVS stated that the ACZM would be the parent body for three or more sub-groups: (a) Captive Wild Animals, (b) Free-Living Wild Animals, (c) Fish and Aquatic Animals, and (d) such others as might be appropriate in the future. Deliberations between the ABVS and the ACZM organizing committee established that the ACZM would be developed by charter diplomates. An invitation for experienced zoological veterinarians with 10 years or more of experience was made at the October 1983 conference of the AAZV. The ABVS appointed an ad hoc committee to assist in establishing the ACZM. The original organizing committee prevailed upon the ABVS

ad hoc committee to determine the number of charter diplomates and to select them from the 22 curricula vitae submitted in response to the call for candidates. The ABVS ad hoc committee chose to limit the charter diplomates to eight and selected Drs. Mitchell Bush, William Boever, Martin Dinnes, Murray Fowler, George Kollias, Kay Mehren, Richard Montali, and Phillip Robinson as ACZM Charter Diplomates. This recommendation was ratified by the ABVS.

ACZM is an international specialty organization for certification of veterinarians with special expertise in zoological medicine. Of note, zoological medicine includes all exotic species, so a Diplomate is not restricted to being just a reptile/amphibian specialist. Six individuals sat for the first examination in 1984. ACZM became a stand-alone college in 1988. As of May 2017, there were 186 active Diplomates in the college (all certified by examination). ACZM is responsible for establishing training requirements, evaluating and accrediting training programs, and examining and certifying veterinarians in the veterinary specialty of zoological medicine. ACZM Diplomates foster high-quality medical care for nondomestic animals and are actively involved in the discovery of new knowledge in the discipline and the dissemination of this knowledge to the veterinary profession and public.[2]

Eligibility for examination can occur either by practicing 100% in the specialty for at least 6 years (or 50% for 12 years, or some combination thereof) or completing an ACZM-approved residency program (minimum of 3 years, 100% dedicated to zoological medicine).

For credentialing the applicant must have at least three senior-authored (first author), peer-reviewed journal publications, and at least one must be original research (hypothesis driven, experimental, prospective or retrospective). Papers must be fully accepted by the journal(s) before the application deadline—a letter from the editor indicating this may be sufficient proof if a paper is *in press*. Papers must make a meaningful contribution to the literature. Book chapters, review papers, and proceedings papers *are not* acceptable. The ACZM examination occurs over 2 full days, and the total point allocation is 675 points. On Day 1, all candidates take five sections of the test: avian, herpetofauna, terrestrial mammal, wildlife, and aquatics (fish and invertebrates). Continuation to Day 2 is contingent on passing all five Day 1 sections with a score of 65% or higher overall. There are 75 multiple-choice questions for each of the five Day 1 components, and each question has one right answer and four distractors (five options). There are still some encouraging rewards if three or four of the sections are passed. On returning the next year, examinees only need to pass the remaining one or two sections to continue on to Day 2. However, failure to pass those final one or two components will cause the examinee to have to repeat all five sections of the Day 1 examination the next year. The Day 2 examination for ACZM is based on one of four options of a subspecialty—general zoo, zoological companion animal ("exotic pets"), aquatics, or wildlife. Obviously, reptiles and amphibians are a component of each of these four disciplines; however, many examinees choose one of the first two options. Each option has three sections: an essay examination (140 points), a slide examination (85 points), and an advanced multiple choice examination (75 questions). One must pass with 65% or greater. If examinees do not pass Day 2 on the first try, they return the following year for one last try. Failure on the second try for Day 2 requires the examinee to start completely over with passing Day 1, all sections, again.

The American Board of Veterinary Practitioners

The ABVP website is http://www.abvp.com. This specialty is focused more on the private practitioner, although other opportunities are available. Certification provides professional and public recognition of advanced knowledge, skills, and competency in a species category. The organization began in 1978, and the first examination was given in 1981. In 2010 the first reptile/amphibian specialty examination was administered, and five individuals successfully passed the inaugural test. As of May 2017, 11 out of 817 ABVP Diplomates are in the reptile and amphibian medicine specialty. There are no specified % time allocations to be an ABVP specialist or in a residency program, but according to their website the typical caseload is 10 or more herp cases per week.

Two paths are available to qualify an individual for credentialing. One is to practice a minimum of 5 years (6 years prior to sitting for the examination) in any combination of practice that allows the minimal amount of professional exposure and caseload of reptiles and amphibians as required (see table). The first year does not have to be in the recognized veterinary specialty (RVS), but for the subsequent 5 years it is required. The second is to complete a 2- or 3-year ABVP R/A–approved residency program. This often involves a 1-year internship that does not have to be in the RVS, followed by 2 years in the RVS specifically. The applicant should contact the current ABVP R/A regent for up-to-date requirements at the time of application (see Table 4.1). As of 2017 the credentialing process timeline starts with a straightforward first-time application form and fee due by September 1 of each year. The more complex credentials packet, which is described later, is due by January 15 of the earliest year a candidate hopes to sit for the examination. The final evaluation of the credentials packet is completed and notification of acceptance or rejection (complete or partial) of that packet is provided to the candidate by June 1 of the same year. Accepted candidates must decide by September 1 if they will register for that year's examination or wait an additional year. One of the most challenging components of the credentials packet is the case report. An applicant may submit one unpublished case report and a publication or two unpublished case reports. To demonstrate excellence in reptile and amphibian medicine and surgery, it behooves the candidate to show some breadth of expertise in these case reports. Each case report's species should be different. The topic and species of each case should be different from each other. Generally, it is recommended to avoid obscure, new, or uncommon diseases; instead, show expertise at thoroughly working up a standard case. Case reports must have been personally seen and investigated by the applicant within the past 5 years. Applicants should demonstrate their thought processes in the case report: significant presenting signs, diagnostic characteristics, problem lists, pathophysiology, differential diagnoses, treatments, and management options. Additionally, if certain diagnostic or therapeutic steps are not pursued, an explanation for why they were not performed and how they could have been useful in the case must be discussed.

More specific guidelines and example case reports are available on the website (also see Table 4.1). The most common reason for failing to credential is inadequate case reports. It is highly advisable that applicants begin writing their case reports *before* submitting the application and application fee. Study groups and mentors are available through the ABVP and can help with case report guidelines, review, and specialty examination preparation.

For the refereed (peer-reviewed) publication, the applicant must be the first author. The topic of publication must make a meaningful contribution to the literature of the species specialty and must be different from that of the case report. The publication must have been published no more than 5 years before the January 15 deadline in a refereed, ABVP-approved scientific journal. Conference proceedings, online publications, clinical vignettes, short/brief communications, serial features, and review articles will *not* be accepted. Acceptance for publication in a refereed scientific journal does not guarantee that the manuscript will be admissible in lieu of an ABVP-style case report.

The ABVP examination is offered every year in October and is a two-day examination. Day one is broken into two parts; both are timed multiple-choice examinations. The morning is a core examination with 300 questions on preclinical and basic veterinary sciences. The afternoon is a specialty examination on reptile/amphibian medicine. Day two involves a practical examination in the morning with 50 to 100 questions primarily based on slide images. This exam may also include short-answer and essay questions. Multiple-choice questions for both days have one correct answer and two distractors (three options) and are timed examinations. A standard passing score for the ABVP examination is a 70% raw score.

The European College of Zoological Medicine

The ECZM is a European Veterinary Specialist College formed under the auspices of the European Board of Specialization (http://www.eczm.eu). The ECZM evolved from the European College of Avian Medicine and Surgery (ECAMS), itself a veterinary specialist organization founded in 1993. ECAMS was an initiative of the European Committee of the Association of Avian Veterinarians in response to a growing demand for better avian medical and surgical services for birds through specialization and a need to harmonize certification in this area. ECAMS became recognized as a fully functional college in 2005.[3] In 2007 an initiative was commenced to broaden the membership and areas of specialty of ECAMS. The aims were to strengthen the college by increasing membership, provide the opportunity for those working at a specialist level within allied zoological fields to gain recognition, and facilitate greater recognition of the clinical area by the profession within veterinary academia, by governments and by the public. The result was that ECAMS changed to ECZM, and herpetology was added in April 2009. As of April 2016 and according to the ECZM website, there were 26 ECZM (herpetology) diplomates, including five members from the United States and one member from Australia. In 2012 the zoo health management specialty within ECZM was created and currently has 41 diplomates. As of May 2017 the ECZM (herpetology) and ECZM (zoo health management) qualifications are not currently accepted by the ABVS as a specialist qualification in the United States.

The herpetology specialty encompasses the veterinary treatment, healthcare, and preventative medicine of all reptilian and amphibian species (captive or wild). The zoo health management specialty also includes reptiles and amphibians within institutional and zoological collections. The ECZM website provides detailed information about the ECZM, including the constitution, bylaws, and information brochures on all specialties, including herpetology and zoo health management. The latter contains information about requirements for admission to the college, a profile of the specialties, and application and examination procedures. To become a European specialist in zoological medicine the training period is split into (a) internship (minimum 1 year) in companion animal or zoological species clinical sciences in a recognized institution that provides a broad range of clinical assignments or 2 years in clinical practice; and (b) residency (minimum of 2.5 years, minimum 60% time dedicated to the specialty) program under the supervision of a ECZM Diplomate (i.e., an ECZM resident can spend significant time outside of their specialty). Alternatively, the candidate must have followed a preapproved alternative program, with a minimum of 2 years in general practice (first phase) and 4 years in specialty practice (60% minimum time allocation to the specialty). For the alternate residency route the credentials committee evaluates the suitability of the practice at which the alternative internship period (2 years) was undertaken. The alternative route is intended for clinicians for whom a standard residency would be impossible (e.g., moving to another country). If an alternative residency is proposed, a program must be suggested that is appropriate for the resident, such that they achieve the required standard by the time of completion. All programs must be considered and approved by the ECZM Education and Residency Committee. The alternative training residency must, at the discretion of the Education and Residency Committee, be equivalent to a standard residency. An alternative residency, as with any other, must be approved prior to commencement. At least 20% of the resident's program must be off clinical duty. During this time, residents must fulfil their requirements for research, publications (two journal papers), and presentation engagements. Besides a sufficient case, continuing education, and postmortem log, the resident must complete an investigative project that contributes to the advancement of medicine and surgery of reptiles and amphibians. The resident, as first author, must have the work accepted for publication in a peer-reviewed journal prior to sitting the examination. A second first-author paper should also be accepted for publication and can be original scientific research, a case series, or a single case report. The current ECZM examination structure is composed of only a 1-day examination for a total of 370 points and is the smallest examination of any European specialty college (see Table 4.1).

Veterinary Specialization in Australia and New Zealand

The Advisory Committee on the Registration of Veterinary Specialists (ACRVS) is a standing committee of the AVBC and handles the assessment of applications. The purpose of the ACRVS is to establish uniformity between the registering authorities in terms of the standards applied to assessment of applications for specialist registration. Veterinary registration authorities normally send applications to the ACRVS for assessment, and the ACRVS advises the authority if the application meets the criteria accepted by the AVBC. Eligibility for specialist registration is listed in the AVBC specialist registration information booklet: Section 5 of the AVBC booklet sets out the minimum standards as part of the requirements for registration as a veterinary specialist in Australia and New Zealand, including details of approval of training programs and examinations and selection and roles of supervisors and fees.

College membership of the ANZCVS signifies that a veterinarian demonstrates a high level of interest and competence in a given area of veterinary activity. To become a member of the college, a candidate must have at least 4 years post-graduate experience as a full-time veterinarian and have successfully completed both written and oral/practical examinations in one of the diverse range of subjects offered (see Table 4.1). College fellowship is associated with scholarly and technical excellence in a particular subject. Standards required for training and examination in fellowship subjects meet or exceed the prerequisites for registration as a veterinary specialist in Australia and/or New Zealand. ANZCVS fellowship is one of the most common pathways for veterinary specialist registration in Australia and New Zealand. It is envisaged that the Unusual Pets Chapter of the ANZCVS, which currently provides a membership level qualification, will consider the introduction of a fellowship level in the future for consideration by the AVBC.

SPECIALTY COLLEGES AND BOARDS WEB PAGES

The American College of Zoological Medicine: http://www.aczm.org
The American Board of Veterinary Practitioners: http://www.abvp.com
The European College of Zoological Medicine: http://www.eczm.eu
Australian and New Zealand College of Veterinary Scientists: http://www.anzcvs.org.au

REFERENCES

See www.expertconsult.com for a complete list of references.

5

The Importance of Herpetological Publication by Clinicians and Academics

Mark A. Mitchell and Sean M. Perry

The majority of the veterinarians or veterinary nurses reading this chapter received minimal exposure to herpetological medicine in their curricula. In the three institutions that the authors have attended or taught at, representing approximately 10% of US veterinary colleges, the herpetological curricula were limited to 1 to 2 elective or graduate courses, consisting of 1 to 3 credit hours, or lectures within a zoological medicine course. Overall, the herpetological medicine course offerings at these institutions represented <2% of the overall curriculum. When compared with the amount of a curriculum that is devoted to two species of small mammals or a few more species of food or farm animals, it is quite obvious that most of us are provided minimal exposure to the >10,000 species of reptiles or >7500 species of amphibians that exist in the world.[1,2] For those that routinely see exotic or zoological medicine cases, this is no new revelation. Veterinary medicine, unlike human medicine, remains a generalists' profession. In human medicine, subspecialization occurs within a specialty and is limited to a single species, whereas in veterinary medicine specialization remains more broad for more than one species (e.g., disciplines such as pathology and zoological medicine) or more restricted to certain species and body systems (e.g., cardiology, dermatology, ophthalmology). The only way for us to move toward greater specialization is to generate evidence-based knowledge that provides insight into the medical and surgical needs of these animals. It is also important to recognize that because of this limitation, we should approach these cases as clinician scientists rather than practitioners (see Chapter 6) to ensure we are generating new questions and problem solving rather than simply moving from case to case without using the knowledge gained to grow the profession.

WHAT IS "HERPETOLOGICAL LITERATURE"?

Herpetological literature includes all written (paper and digital) documentation that encompasses reptiles and amphibians. This can include taxonomy, physiology, husbandry, medicine, surgery, or any topic related to these species. For practical purposes, this chapter will focus on the medical and surgical herpetological literature. When considering herpetological literature, it is generally divided into lay literature, conference proceedings, scientific abstracts, book chapters, and peer-reviewed articles. Each of these will be addressed.

Lay Literature

The lay literature represents an important component to the overall literature. This type of literature is typically associated with husbandry-related information, although examples of medically relevant information are also available.[3] The information provided in these articles is really intended for herpetoculturists and other lay individuals looking to hear the opinion of a specific author on a topic. This type of literature is rarely peer reviewed and thus represents the opinion (good, bad, or indifferent) of the author. The level of review for these types of articles is primarily limited to copyediting, editorial assistants, or an editor; however, these individuals are generally more interested in format than content and may not have a high level of experience with the topic covered. These types of articles have been important in disseminating author experiences on issues such as husbandry and nutrition and will likely continue to do so in the future. They also serve as an important method of educating herpetoculturists on the health and welfare of the animals in their care. These types of articles tend to have wide distribution. Unfortunately, the lack of peer review can lead to the dissemination of misinformation. Thus it is important for veterinarians to remain vigilant when reviewing these types of articles and responding through editorial feedback to ensure best practices. However, the importance of this information cannot be overstated. Much of what we know in our peer-review literature is based on discussions being initiated in the lay literature (e.g., nutrition) and clinician scientists rigorously testing specific hypotheses generated through these writings/discussions.

Conference Proceedings

Conference proceedings are similar to lay articles in their review process but represent a more specific veterinary perspective. Conference proceedings are provided as a supplement to the lectures given to veterinarians and veterinary nurses at continuing education programs; the information gained at these meetings is intended to meet specific continuing education guidelines for state boards. These types of herpetological literature represent the opinions of the author and are rarely peer reviewed; instead, they are copyedited for format. Because there is an expectation that all licensed individuals must obtain continuing education, this type of information is one of the primary mechanisms veterinarians and veterinary nurses use to expand their knowledge. However, a limitation of this "new knowledge" is that it represents the opinion of the author and has not been rigorously tested. In many cases, the information provided is a review of the literature, although it is disseminated through the interpretation of the author/presenter. It is important for veterinarians and veterinary nurses to follow up on the information derived through conference proceedings by delving into the peer-reviewed literature to review and confirm the message being shared. Veterinarians presenting this type of material should, at a minimum, attempt to have this type of material converted to a review paper for publication after peer or editorial review. It is important to convert proceedings material for three reasons: (1) It strengthens the value of the material, (2) there is an increased distribution to members of the profession, and (3) it expands the quantity and quality of literature available for clinician scientists to apply. Indeed, it is for the reasons outlined above that conference proceedings have been essentially removed from the bibliographies of the chapters in this textbook. The editors hope that such a move will help encourage veterinarians to seek journal publication and rely less on proceedings as we have done in the past.

Scientific Abstracts

Scientific abstracts typically represent the first attempt at sharing evidence-based information. These abstracts may include case reports, case series, or hypothesis-driven research. The primary limitations of these types of literature is (1) the length of the material and (2) that it is seldom freely available to those that did not attend the conference (most herpetological abstracts are not printed in journals or available electronically). Most scientific abstracts are limited to 250 words. There are professional organizations that do not limit the word count; however, this is not recommended. The word count limit was primarily established to ensure that the scientific material shared in these settings could still be submitted for publication in the peer-reviewed literature. When word counts are not limited, peer-reviewed journals are less likely to publish the material. The restrictive word count does minimize how much information can be shared with the reader, especially when it comes to study design, analysis, and the conclusions of the author(s); however, the scientific abstract is not intended to serve as the final publication of the material, and thus this should be less of a concern. Another limitation of scientific abstracts is associated with the review process. In some organizations, the scientific abstracts are peer reviewed, whereas in others they are reviewed by the proceedings editor(s). Although these both represent a step up from conference proceedings, there are limitations as to how detailed the review can be because of the limited amount of information provided in the scientific abstract. Ultimately, all clinician scientists who are working with reptiles and amphibians should be contributing at this level. In this book, as an example, such research abstracts published in proceedings have been permitted where they represent very recent information (within the last 1–2 years) but have again been largely avoided because of their limited availability.

Book Chapters

Veterinary textbooks, such as the one you are reading here, remain an important method for disseminating herpetological literature; however, much like the other offering discussed earlier, the information obtained in book chapters is limited to review of the literature and is typically editorially and not rigorously peer reviewed. This by no means limits the value of the material but should remind each of us to delve into the peer-reviewed literature being covered in the book chapter to confirm its value and validity. The authors always review the references or literature cited to determine the source of the information used to generate the book chapter. A it is not uncommon for scientific abstracts to serve as a primary constituent of the references, we are seeing an increase in the number of peer-reviewed papers. It is becoming more routine for some texts to not include any reference that is not from a peer-reviewed journal, and this certainly helps to highlight deficiencies within the peer-reviewed literature. As we noted earlier, all literature has value; it is knowing how much weight each provides that is important. If we take a narrower view of the literature, then books, such as this one, might also be considered nothing more than the opinions of the author(s) without ample peer review to affirm its value. However, textbooks remain an important, readily available source of information for busy clinicians that will continue to serve as an important source of knowledge. Although the authors always recommend searching the literature for peer-reviewed articles relevant to a topic of interest, there are times when a quick answer is needed and a book chapter serves that purpose. Book chapters serve as a continuation of the method in which many of us learned veterinary medicine. A lecturer would review and compile the literature and present it to us as students. Book chapters serve the same function, with the author replacing the lecturer. For many of us, our lecturers "knew everything" and were the source of our knowledge. This type

of unconscious acceptance that book chapters are all we need to be successful can be dangerous and lead to some instability in the foundation of our knowledge, especially as books are typically 1 to 2 years out of date by the time of publication. Thus, as with the other sources of herpetological literature available to us, we should understand the limitations of the book chapter and always seek peer-reviewed literature when available.

Peer-Reviewed Literature

Peer-reviewed literature serves as the foundation for the evidence we use to practice medicine. The premise behind the peer-review process is that literature is evaluated by individuals within the field to ensure that the hypothesis(es), design, analyses, and conclusions drawn by an author(s) are legitimate based on current knowledge, or what is currently in the peer-reviewed literature. The authors routinely hear colleagues note that peer-reviewed literature is a gold standard; however, although it is true to say that it represents the most reliable source of information, it is important to appreciate that it may not be infallible and should be interpreted using a critical eye. A review of the peer-reviewed literature will show that many studies have flaws and still pass peer review.[4-18] Many authors will acknowledge flaws in their discussion, and that in itself does not negate publication; however, the unappreciated and unacknowledged flaws are more dangerous and can be associated with unanswered hypotheses, poor study design, a lack of or the use of incorrect statistics, and erroneous conclusions drawn based on these shortcomings. Peer review at its core is subjective. It is based on the opinions of the reviewers, experience of the reviewer (i.e., are they an expert on the material and how current are they with the literature?), and state of the literature (i.e., has something been previously published on the subject, and if so, does it have shortcomings?). There are many examples that could be used to show this, but the authors have selected an early publication of the lead editor to reinforce this point.[19] In this article, blood samples were collected from 10 green iguanas (*Iguana iguana*), 7 male and 3 female. Back in 1996, the authors used the term "normal range" throughout the article to describe the results. Of course, the limited sample size and a lack of any statistical analysis of the results beyond descriptive statistics would not be considered acceptable as a reference range by today's standards because the criteria for the establishment of reference intervals were published 16 years later in 2012.[20] However, that was cutting edge for the day. Veterinarians working with reptiles were looking for any help from the literature to better manage their green iguana patients. Interestingly, this article has been cited 58 times, including by articles being published at the time this chapter is being written.[21] What the authors want the readership of this chapter, and scientists in general, to appreciate is that these types of articles, much needed when they were written because there was nothing else, are often dated and flawed by modern standards. Although study design, sample size determinants, and statistical methods were well known in 1996 when this article was published, there were no published standards for normal reference range determination, and therefore the peer-review process was limited. Nowadays, similar "reference range" papers are still being submitted but should not make it through the review process because of established and published guidelines.[20] If they are allowed through to publication, then this represents a failure of the peer-review process. The subjectivity comes in when the reviewers, including the associate editor and editor, allow for these flaws to be published. This remains an issue today because herpetological medical literature is still being produced by a limited number of individuals, the science remains clinical and basic, and many serving as peer-reviewers have limited understanding of study design and statistics. How do we rectify this? (1) By ensuring that recognized system specialists (e.g., clinical pathologists, pathologists, virologists, anesthesiologists, etc.) are paired with herpetological specialists for peer review, and (2) by having this discussion—it is important for us to challenge ourselves to not believe we are just "practitioners." Instead we must see ourselves as clinician scientists and be prepared to challenge ourselves to learn about these different review processes.

Once we can understand that peer-reviewers can have some inherent flaws, it is important to consciously correct for them and celebrate the value of peer-reviewed literature. We need to take the experiences we gain from working in herpetological medicine and share them with the entire profession. This can take many forms, from case reports and case series to cross-sectional studies, longitudinal prospective studies, and experimental studies. There are experts in our field who can assist with helping guide prospective authors with their work. The Association of Reptile and Amphibian Veterinarians (ARAV) is an excellent resource, and the *Journal of Herpetological Medicine and Surgery* is an excellent medium for peer-reviewed publication.

NEGATIVE RESULTS DON'T EXIST...ONLY HYPOTHESES THAT NEED TO BE TESTED

Negative results are publishable. Unfortunately, there has been some cultural bias against the publication of negative results that has been promoted through the scientific community and also touches herpetological medicine. It is unfortunate that some who are supposed to be objective believe this statement. Evidence-based medicine should be based on hypothesis-driven research. For every hypothesis identified, a null and alternative hypothesis should be generated. A null hypothesis is generally derived by thinking that there will be "no difference" between what is being analyzed, while the alternative hypothesis is the exact opposite; that a difference will exist. An example of null and alternative hypotheses is: Ho (null): there will be no difference in the hounsfield units (generated on computed tomography) of the mandibles of bearded dragons fed a standard non-gut-loaded cricket diet and a commercial diet specifically developed for bearded dragons. The alternative hypothesis is that there will be a difference. This alternative difference can be one-tailed or two-tailed. If the investigators believe that the hounsfield units for one group will be higher than the other, than a one-way directional hypothesis can be used. The benefit of a directional hypothesis is that a smaller sample size can be used. If the authors are unsure of which group will have higher or lower hounsfield units, then the hypothesis should be two-tailed. Regardless of which hypothesis is ultimately accepted, the research answers the hypothesis. The results are not "negative" if there is no difference between the groups; they just reinforce that that the null hypothesis was accepted. It is as important to publish that something is not different as it is when a difference exists, because research is hypothesis-driven, not result driven. In addition, when resources for pursuing research are limited, as they are in the field of herpetological medicine, it is important that we do not repeat research simply because results were not published. This should be a familiar approach to clinicians because it is similar to how we pursue our clinical cases. A "negative" radiograph does not represent a waste of financial resources, instead it serves to rule out a number of potential diseases such as organomegaly, foreign bodies, ascites, etc.

PEER-REVIEWED HERPETOLOGICAL MEDICINE PUBLICATIONS

There are several journals that serve as excellent repositories for herpetological medicine research. The journal that is specific to herpetological medicine is the *Journal of Herpetological Medicine and Surgery* (JHMS). This is the official journal of the ARAV. The journal publishes a variety of editorially reviewed and peer-reviewed articles. Peer-reviewed articles include brief communications, "what's your diagnosis?" reports, case reports/case series, cross-sectional studies, cohort studies, case-control studies, and experimental studies. Brief communications and "what's your diagnosis?" articles are the most basic publications and represent examples of articles that all practicing veterinarians can contribute to. Although these articles are peer reviewed, they are not always accepted by credentialing boards; all of the other articles noted previously are universally accepted. As the authors have stated previously, all clinicians practicing herpetological medicine should feel a professional obligation to share their knowledge and experiences with the profession through peer-reviewed journals (rather than conference proceedings). Additional benefits of the JHMS is that there is no charge to publish, and all images are in color at no additional charge.

The *Journal of Exotic Pet Medicine* (JEPM) is another peer-reviewed journal that routinely publishes peer-reviewed herpetological medicine articles, in addition to exotic small mammal and bird articles. The JEPM accepts the same types of articles noted for the JHMS, has no publishing charge, and has color images at no additional cost. The *Journal of Zoo and Wildlife Medicine* (JZWM) is the official journal of the American Association of Zoo Veterinarians. This journal also accepts the same types of articles but does have a publication charge and does not publish color images. Of course, there are a broad range of journals that will accept herpetological medicine research (e.g., *Journal of the American Veterinary Medical Association*, *American Journal of Veterinary Research*, and *Veterinary Record*) and may be considered by those looking to publish their work.

When selecting a journal to publish in, the authors believe it is important to consider the target audience. Too many times, the impact factor of a journal is considered to be the most important. Impact factors are an objective method of assigning weight to a journal based on its audience size. The audience for the field of herpetological medicine is small. We will never have a high impact value. For that matter, veterinary medicine is a small field and has journals of low impact compared with other scientific fields. The Scimago Journal Rank (http://www .scimagojr.com/journalrank.php?area=3400) for 2016 ranked the *Annual Review of Animal Biosciences* as the highest ranking veterinary journal with a score of 2.4533. Journals 2 to 50 had rank scores of 1.956 to 0.613. The highest ranked journal in the Scimago review is *CA: A Cancer Journal for Clinicians* with a score of 39.285. The previously mentioned top veterinary journal's rank in the overall list is 877/28,606. These findings should reinforce that directing published research to a specific audience is more important than a rank score. These ranks should have no impact on clinician scientists working outside of academia; however, we have had a number of colleagues question publication in certain journals because of either (1) their impact score or (2) their slower review and turnaround times. Science should remain an unbiased and hypothesis-driven endeavor, and those publishing their findings should be focused on distributing it to the audience that will most benefit from it.

BEING AN ACTIVE PARTICIPANT IN PEER REVIEW

For the peer-review process to work, each of us has to contribute. A common problem encountered by the senior author in his role as an editor is getting individuals to accept invitations to review manuscripts and perform the review in a timely manner. In a small field such as herpetological medicine, it is important that everyone feel a sense of responsibility to serve in this role. The peer-review process is at its best when a diverse number of specialists are involved (including those from other specialties such as pathology, anesthesiology, surgery, diagnostic imaging, dermatology, cardiology, and so on). Each specialist brings a unique perspective to the review process based on our understanding of the literature and the experiences we have gained seeing cases or performing research in the field of herpetological medicine. Manuscript review is typically done using at least two peer-reviewers, and it is the job of the associate editor and editor to pair up reviewers on manuscripts with different backgrounds to ensure a complete review of a manuscript. It is not uncommon for manuscripts reviewed in the JHMS to have a specialist with minimal reptile knowledge but great depth in the specialty (e.g., cardiology, anesthesia, ophthalmology) to be paired with a clinician scientist who has great depth in the field of herpetological medicine and an understanding of the specialty. During the review process it is important for the reviewers to let the editors know of any deficiencies, such as their understanding of statistics or some other aspect of the review. This will ensure that the editors will know of any shortcomings and be sure to obtain additional coverage if needed. Remember, the herpetological literature will only expand if we each contribute to making it so.

CONCLUSION

So in the end what is the point of all this? If you are actively receiving reptile and amphibian cases at your veterinary hospital or teaching institution, you are responsible, nay we say obligated, to contribute to the herpetological literature. The growth of the profession depends on all of its members, especially the recognized specialists. All information, from a brief communication to a well-designed experimental study, has the potential to grow and expand the evidence we use to manage these animals and ensure their conservation. Additionally, each specialist can contribute by reviewing scientific abstracts or peer-reviewed manuscripts when asked. They say knowledge is power. We need to move our profession forward from being the 98-pound weakling to being muscled and fit like editors Steve Divers and Scott Stahl.

REFERENCES

See www.expertconsult.com for a complete list of references.

6

Statistics for the Clinician Scientist

Mark A. Mitchell and Sean M. Perry

"Fear not the statistics!" is the primary objective in the syllabus of a graduate biostatistics course taught by one of the authors (M.A.M.). The course is started with this note because the authors have always found it comical that veterinarians, a highly ambitious and intellectual group of individuals, find the idea of learning about statistics or applying them to their research or clinical work a difficult task. However, as it is with all things we learn, if we take the time to understand how and why something is done, it is possible for us to capture and own that knowledge.

There are many things that we need to change in our profession if we ever hope to meet our potential as veterinarians. Because of the limited space available in this chapter, we will focus on two of these needs as they are relevant to the chapter topic. First, we must stop limiting ourselves by identifying simply as "practitioners." Instead, we need to accept that we are clinician scientists. You "practice" some procedure and use it because it works or stop using it because it fails. A scientist is willing to formally test hypotheses and search for new knowledge as to why something works or doesn't. For the scientist, success is met with validation by further review, while failure is met with additional testing to identify why it failed and how to correct it. If we are not providing our clients and patients the latter, we fail them and our profession. The second is using and welcoming rigorous evidence-based science to dictate how we perform our duties as clinician scientists. A large part of this second recommendation is understating the value of statistics in interpreting evidence-based results. There is a general assumption that once a manuscript passes peer-review it is correct and infallible; however, because of this "fear of statistics" I noted earlier, many peer-reviewers are unsure of how to interpret the statistics used to analyze the results of a manuscript they are reviewing. If the associate editor and/or editor are also unsure of what is appropriate, and there is no official statistical review of the manuscript by a trained statistician, then what becomes published may be flawed. This is more common than most of us recognize. It is well documented within the medical literature that statistical errors are common. Study design, data analysis, data reporting, data presentation, and interpretation of data are all areas where errors are commonly made when preparing manuscripts.[1–8] Sometimes these mistakes can result in serious clinical consequences.[9–15] Ultimately, the knowledge each of us gains through reading, listening to lectures, and gaining real-time clinical experience is filtered through our effort to evaluate the truth behind each of these. If we accept them on face value, we may be laying an unstable foundation to our collective knowledge. As it is the focus of this chapter, we will discuss how embracing a basic understanding of statistics can help ensure that when we constructively review a paper we can be sure the statistics were done in an appropriate manner.

HYPOTHESES

Successful research starts with well-defined hypotheses. However, it is only now becoming common for scientists to include the specific hypotheses for their study in their published articles. The reason we see the publication of the hypotheses as important is because they can give us guidance as to the direction of the research, regarding the biological relevance of the work, as well as guide the selection of the statistical tests required to analyze the data. Specific and detailed hypotheses provide insight into the type of data to be collected, which is the first real guide to selecting statistical tests. It is important to recognize that the same basic hypothesis can be answered using categorical, ordinal, or continuous data; however, the level of detail in the answer provided depends on the robustness of the type of data, with continuous data being more robust than ordinal and categorical data, and ordinal data being more robust than categorical data. The concept of using hypotheses to test our scientific opinions regarding our clinical cases is something else we should be doing. The more we think like a clinician scientist, the more likely we are to be more thorough and complete with our cases. For example, every time we submit a diagnostic test to evaluate our hypothesis regarding a specific problem/differential, we are also testing a hypothesis regarding the test method used. When we submit a plasma biochemistry analysis for a tortoise case, we hypothesize what the results are for each analyte measured. If the result for an analyte is what we hypothesized, then we can have more confidence in the direction we are taking the case. However, if the result for an analyte is different from what we expected, then we need to determine whether we are on the right track or if there is some other reason for this difference (e.g., failure of analyzer to correctly perform assay?). A "practitioner" would assume they are wrong and redirect how they are managing the case, such as run another test, whereas a clinician scientist could see that it is possible that they are on the wrong path or that there could be a deficiency in the assay, how the sample was handled, or some other issue. In this latter case, the clinician scientist will reset their hypotheses and do some further investigation.

DATA

When preparing to do a study or interpret the results of a study, it is important to define the type of data used. There are three primary types of data: categorical, ordinal, and continuous. Categorical, or nominal, data represent the most basic data. These data are simply characterized into categories. Many times these data are reported in a binary fashion: yes/no; infected/not infected; present/absent. Ordinal data are assigned a numerical rank, but the assigned numbers have no

TABLE 6.1 Regression Tests Used for Different Types of Data

Data Type	Types of Regression Analysis
Nominal/dichotomous measure of data	Logistic regression
Ordinal/ranked measure of data	Ordinal regression
Continuous/interval measure of data	Linear regression

specific numerical quantity. Examples of this type of data might include a ranking of pathologic lesions from none (1), minimal (2), moderate (3), to severe (4). Each data point represents a qualitative difference, but there is no quantitative value to the difference. Finally, continuous data represents the most robust style of data. It includes data that can be found on a continuous scale, including many of the different types of objective data we use as clinicians to assess our patients, including body temperature, heart rate, body weight, and clinical pathology data (e.g., plasma biochemistry data). These data provide us with quantitative results that can be used for comparison, such as comparing a green iguana (*Iguana iguana*) patient's calcium concentration to a reference interval for captive green iguanas.

It is important to recognize that these three types of data can be used interchangeably to test the same hypotheses (Table 6.1). However, our ability to explain some phenomena improves based on the type of data used. For example, if we are testing a hypothesis that electroejaculation can be used to collect semen from chameleons, we could test the hypothesis by collecting categorical, ordinal, or continuous data. The categorical data would represent a binary outcome: semen yes/no; the ordinal data would include general ranks of data: 0: no semen; 1: <10 sperm/high dry field (hdf); 2: 10 to 100 sperm/hdf; 3: >100 sperm/hdf; and continuous data would count actual numbers of sperm collected in the sample. While the continuous data would provide the most information, with a small sample size and a high degree of variability, it would be difficult to interpret the data. In this example, showing that the technique would produce semen was sufficient to provide proof of concept and serve as a foundation to pursue additional resources (e.g., animals and research grants) for a study where more robust continuous data could be collected. The more robust continuous data could then be collected using a larger sample size to characterize semen concentrations. Those results could then be used to identify the most productive animals for breeding programs.

DISTRIBUTION

The reporting of data can have a significant impact on how we use it as clinician scientists. When reporting continuous data, it is commonplace to report the data by a mean to define the central tendency and the standard deviation to define the variability in the data. However, while these descriptive statistics are considered the "best methods" for presenting continuous data, they are only appropriate when the data is normally distributed. Therefore it is important to always evaluate the distribution of data to determine the best method for reporting it. This is also important for selecting the most appropriate statistical tests for analyzing the data, as parametric statistical testing requires that data be normally distributed. There are a number of different methods for evaluating the distribution of data, much like there are many different methods for treating the same disease; therefore, the authors find it best to identify those tests that provide a consistent result, similar to how we select clinical treatments. The most common methods used by the authors

to evaluate the distribution of the data include the Shapiro-Wilk test, skewness, kurtosis, and Q-Q plots. The Shapiro-Wilk test is one of several statistical tests that can be used to determine whether continuous data collected from a group of study subjects meet the assumption of normality. The null hypothesis associated with this test is that the data come from a normal distribution. A test statistic (W) is calculated for this test and a P-value generated. If the $P < 0.05$, the null is rejected and the distribution is not normal. Skewness is a measure that evaluates the distribution of the data; it is affected by outliers. A statistic is generated for the distribution that can be positive or negative. The more positive the skewness, the larger the number of outliers to the right of the distribution, while the more negative the skewness, the more outliers to the left of the distribution. Kurtosis describes the shape of the distribution. A normal distribution, or classic bell-shaped curve, has a mesokurtic shape, while a flat shape or peaked shape, both representing nonnormal distributions, are termed platykurtic and leptokurtic, respectively. The platykurtic and leptokurtic distributions are associated with highly negative or highly positive kurtotic values. Q-Q plots represent a visual method of looking at data without a numerical inference. This method is preferred by some for its simplicity but is subject to some personal interpretation. The combination of all four factors in a parallel method ensures the greatest confidence for the authors.

Once the distribution of the data is determined, this information can be used to confirm how the data should be reported. For normally distributed data, the mean (weighted average), median (middle value), and mode (most frequent value) are similar, and it is commonplace to report the mean; however, when the data isn't normally distributed, the median represents the best estimate of central tendency. In addition to reporting the central tendency, it is also important to report the variability of the data. For normally distributed data, the standard deviation serves this purpose; however, when the data isn't normally distributed, this statistic can be confusing to interpret. The authors prefer to use percentiles to describe the variability in the data when the distribution is not normal. In most cases, 25% to 75% or 10% to 90% are used; these represent where 50% or 80% of the data fall. It is now finally becoming common for data to be reported using these methods, although some journals still report these data incorrectly.

SAMPLE SIZE

One of the struggles that clinician scientists face when designing a study or interpreting an article is determining the sample size required to ensure success and minimize the potential for introducing error. This is another reason that the authors believe that hypotheses should be incorporated into an article. By knowing what the specific hypothesis(es) is/are, it is possible to identify the type of data needed and thus the sample size needed. Ultimately, sample size can help determine the risk for introducing Type I or Type II errors into a study. Type I error occurs when a null hypothesis is rejected, when it is true. These types of error are tied to the alpha (or P-value). This type of error is less common because the scientific community routinely accepts an alpha or P-value of 0.05. In cases where this value is decreased, the likelihood for a Type I error increases; however, this is less common in clinical studies. Type II error is more common in veterinary studies and is the error that we are most concerned about. Type II error occurs when a null hypothesis is accepted, stating there is no difference, when it is false. Because most clinical studies are designed to prove the alternative hypothesis, this can lead to accepting that something isn't significant when it indeed is significant. This type of error is often attributed to small sample sizes; thus, it can be limited or minimized by determining an appropriate sample size before starting the study. As we now understand the importance of preemptive analgesia for controlling pain postoperatively, preemptively setting a sample size for a study can control poststudy issues. There are a number of different methods available for calculating sample sizes for a study, and to cover them is beyond the scope of this chapter. Instead, the authors recommend that readers of this chapter use available commercial software (MedCalc Software bvba, Ostend, Belgium; http://www.medcalc.org; 2017) or sample size calculators available on the internet. To do so does require some *a priori* information. The *a priori* information is used to estimate sample size. The source of this *a priori* information may come from pilot data, previously published results, or experts in the field. In cases where none of this is available, the authors select values that would have real-world relevance. To start, alpha and beta (1-power [0.8]) values are needed. The standard values for these two parameters are 0.05 and 0.20, respectively. However, if you are concerned about a Type I or II error, you can alter these values to reduce the likelihood of erroneous results. The additional *a priori* information needed will depend on the study. For experimental studies that have a hypothesis that will compare two means, the additional information required includes the "expected difference between the means" and the "expected standard deviations" for each group (e.g., control group and treatment group). In a recent study being conducted by one of the authors (M.A.M) evaluating the impact of ultraviolet B radiation on the plasma 25-hydroxyvitamin D concentrations of leopard geckos *(Eublepharis macularius)*, the authors used the following *a priori* information to determine sample size: an alpha = 0.05, a power = 0.8 (beta = 0.2), an expected difference in the 25-hydroxyvitamin D concentrations of the UVB exposed and non-UVB exposed gecko of 25 nmol/L, and expected standard deviations for each group of 15 nmol/L. The sample size required to detect a difference of at least as big as outlined above is 14 animals, 7 UVB exposed and 7 controls. The authors used pilot data and previously published data in other species of reptiles to generate the *a priori* information. While the authors find estimating a study's sample size *a priori* an excellent way to prepare for a study, it is also important to recognize that many granting agencies now expect researchers to show how they determined their study sample size in order to be given full consideration. As noted earlier, the methods outlined for this study example only represent one study type. Different *a priori* information is needed, other than alpha and beta values, to estimate the sample size for other study types; however, this becomes self-explanatory when using a sample size calculator for a specific study type.

THE *P*-VALUE

The *P*-value is a statistical term known by all but understood by few. The probability of an event occurring, or the *P*-value, is used by scientists to ultimately determine whether or not to accept a null hypothesis. Unfortunately, to most clinician scientists, the *P*-value is a fixed value, .05, and represents a hard line in determining the significance associated with an event. This dogma unfortunately leads us to create evidence-based knowledge that is flawed. The *P*-value selected for a particular hypothesis should not be set at 0.05 for convenience but instead based on the sample size of the study (i.e., is it a small sample size because of resource [animal number, financial] constraints?), the number of comparisons being made in the hypothesis(es), the types of variables being tested, and the risks for Type I and Type II errors, among other factors. Ultimately, the 0.05 value being used suggests that an event occurring would be unlikely to occur no more than 5% or 1 out of 20 times by chance alone. While the authors do find it to be a reasonable value, it is how hard the line is that gives me pause. During peer-review, it is not uncommon for the authors to have reviewers or editors question the significance of a *P*-value that includes 0.05 (e.g., 0.05–0.055). In these cases, individuals have argued that the value is >0.05 and is thus

not significant. Is there really that great of a difference in the likelihood of an event happening no more than 4.9% or 0.98 out of 20 times versus 5.1% or 1.02 times out of 20 times? These are the cases where knowledge of what a Type II error represents is important, as well as the power and sample size. Because many of the studies done in herpetological medicine are limited to smaller sample sizes, not addressing these concerns may lead to accepting a null hypothesis and reporting no difference, when indeed there is a difference. One of the ways to officially acknowledge this in a manuscript is to perform a post-hoc power analysis. The authors routinely include a post-hoc power analysis for *P*-values = 0.06 to 0.10. By including post-hoc power and acknowledging the risk of a Type II error in these studies, it guides the reader to consider the limitation associated with the results.

PARAMETRIC VERSUS NONPARAMETRIC STATISTICAL TESTS

Selecting a statistical test to evaluate a hypothesis is no different, and thus should be no scarier to a clinician scientist, than selecting diagnostic tests to rule in/out a disease. While there are entire texts written not only on statistics, but also on select topics in statistics (e.g., logistic regression), it is beyond the scope of this chapter to do anything more than provide a cursory introduction into statistical test selection. However, for the majority, if not all, of the readers of this text, it is not necessary to become an expert in statistics. Instead, we should work to become expert clinician scientists in our field and understand statistics as one of the many tools at our disposal.

The first step in selecting statistical tests is to determine which group of statistics to use. For simplicity, we will divide the statistics into two categories: parametric and nonparametric statistics. Certain assumptions must be met in the study design to properly perform and utilize a statistical test. Two of the most common assumptions, which are needed in both parametric and nonparametric tests, are: (1) data collected for analysis should be obtained from study subjects randomly selected from the population represented in the study, and (2) the individuals and their data should be independent of one another. These represent basic tenets to follow regardless of the statistics used. Note other assumptions must be met for each specific statistical test; the experimental design should reflect these assumptions. A major difference between the two types of statistics is related to the distribution of the data; parametric statistics should only be used on data that meet the assumption of normality, while nonparametric statistics do not have this restriction. Thus, if we simplify this to the types of data, it is obvious that categorical and ordinal data must always be analyzed using nonparametric statistics and that continuous data that doesn't meet the assumption of normality must also be analyzed using nonparametric statistics. The only data type that we would use parametric statistics for are those that meet the assumption of normality. Now, it is important to point out that continuous data that do not meet the assumption of normality can be transformed (e.g., log transformed) to potentially normalize the data. If this transformation is successful, then the more robust parametric statistics could be used to analyze the data; however, it would still be important to report the data by their median and percentiles because the transformed data would not be clinically relevant.

Because veterinarians tend to rely on visual learning aids, we have included Figs. 6.1 through 6.3 as flowcharts that allow us to follow the same hypothetical-deductive reasoning we use to investigate clinical cases. The figures are divided into the three different types of data that we typically use: categorical (Fig. 6.1), ordinal (Fig. 6.2), and continuous (Fig. 6.3). Please note that the flow through each chart is similar and that the only real difference in the type of tests used is based on number of variables. As a refresher, an outcome or dependent variable represents

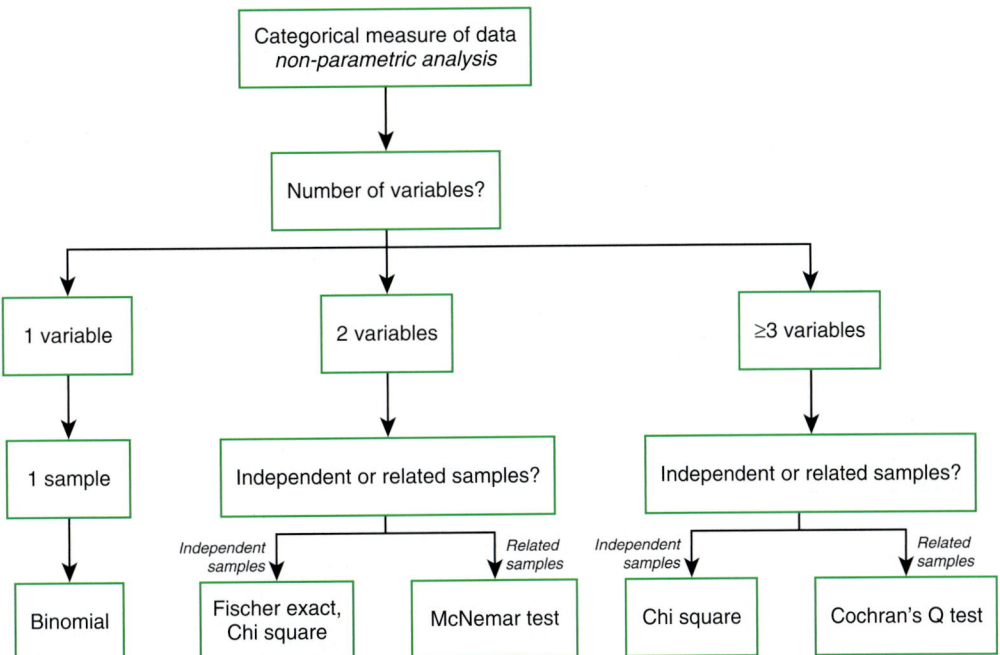

FIG 6.1 Statistical flowchart for categorical data. Independent samples represent the independent variable or predictors, and the related samples represent outcome or dependent variables. These examples are used only to simplify the process, as there are additional tests that can be put into each category; however, the goal of this example is to show commonly used statistical tests and not to overwhelm the reader.

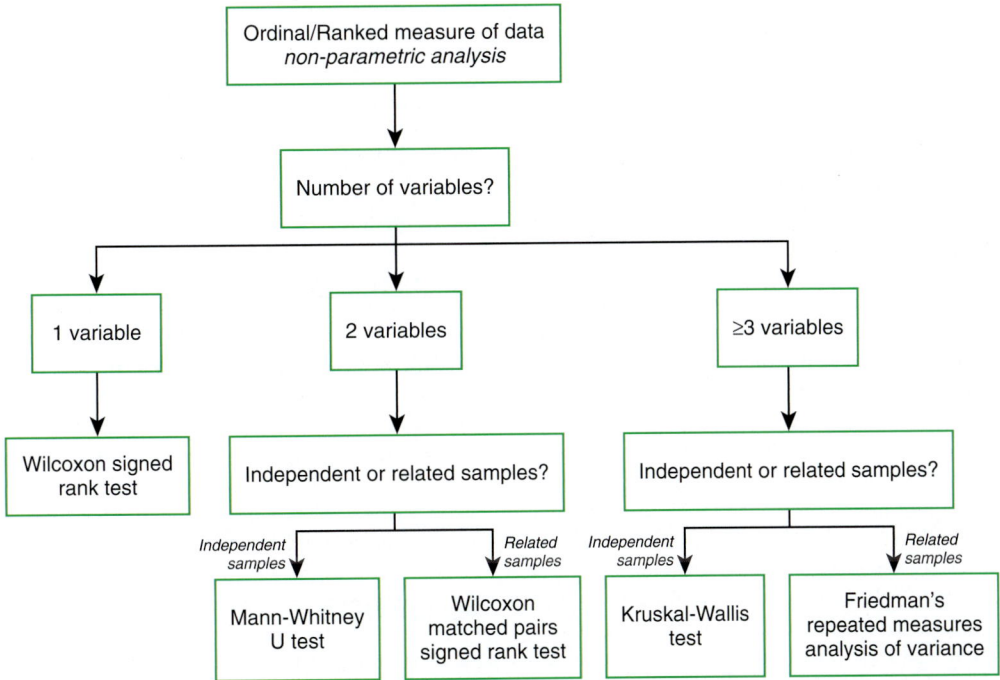

FIG 6.2 Statistical flowchart for ordinal data. Independent samples represent the independent variable or predictors, and the related samples represent outcome or dependent variables. These examples are used only to simplify the process, as there are additional tests that can be put into each category; however, the goal of this example is to show commonly used statistical tests and not to overwhelm the reader.

the data we are measuring, while the independent variable represents the data that may predict or influence the dependent variable. When using the flowcharts, the "related samples" are for those cases where there are two (paired) or three or more (serial) data points for the same outcome variable. For example, if you are measuring 25-hydroxyvitamin D concentrations in leopard geckos (*Eublepharis macularius*) over time and collect a baseline value and a final concentration 30 days later, you have paired data. If you collected samples on baseline (day 0), day 15, and day 30 to evaluate additional samples over time, you have serial data. Paired and serial sampling are excellent methods for reducing

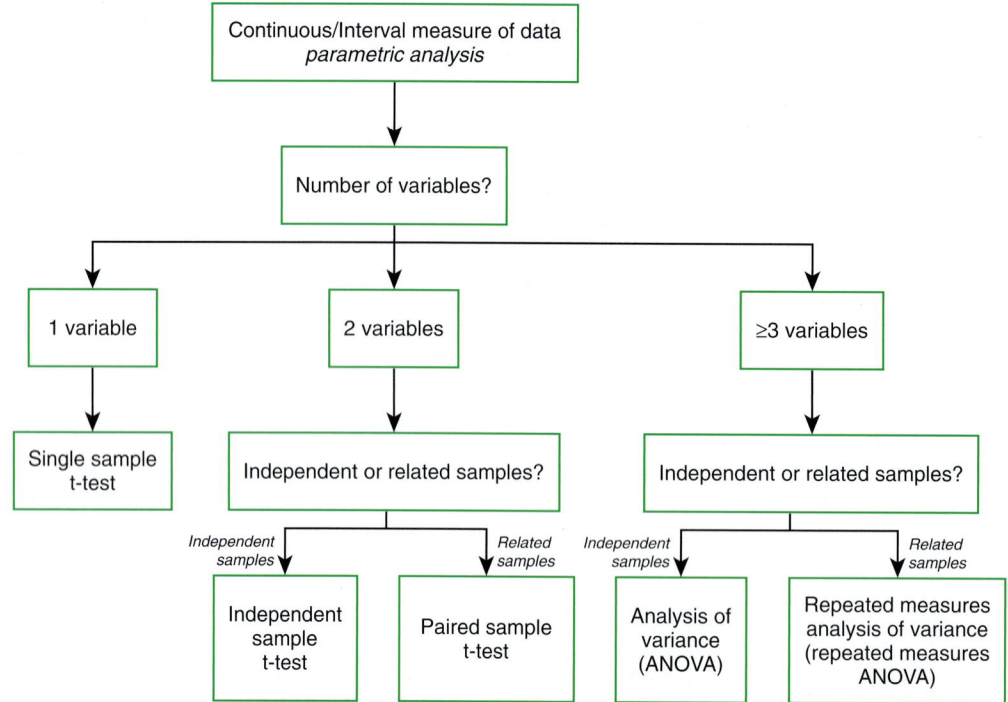

FIG 6.3 Statistical flowchart for continuous data. Independent samples represent the independent variable or predictors, and the related samples represent outcome or dependent variables. These examples are used only to simplify the process, as there are additional tests that can be put into each category; however, the goal of this example is to show commonly used statistical tests and not to overwhelm the reader.

within subject bias and making your analysis more robust. For those looking for an excellent statistical text to pursue additional statistical expertise, the authors recommend *The Handbook of Parametric and Nonparametric Statistical Procedures* by David J. Sheskin.[16]

STATISTICAL SOFTWARE

Statistical software is available that has simplified the process for analyzing data. These software programs come in a variety of packages, from those that require programming to those that don't require programming. The programs that require programming tend to be more robust in what they can accomplish. Examples of these types of programs include SAS (SAS Institute Inc., Cary, NC) and R (https://www.r-project.org/). R is free. MedCalc and SPSS (current version 24.0; IBM Statistics, Armonk, NY) do not require programming, although programming can be done with SPSS when more involved statistical methods are required. The authors use a combination of these programs. For those running very basic statistics, such as chi squared and Fisher exact tests, free calculators are available on the internet. The Centers for Disease Control and Prevention also have a free software program, EpiInfo

(https://www.cdc.gov/epiinfo/index.html). Regardless of the software being used, it is important to understand when to select a test (Figs. 6.1 through 6.3) to ensure the analysis is correct, because these software programs will generate results for whatever test is selected, even if it is the wrong test.

CONCLUSION

The field of herpetological medicine is in its infancy, and maturation requires evidence-based knowledge to expand our understanding of these magnificent animals. Evidence-based knowledge requires hypothesis-generated research that is validated using appropriate study design and statistical analysis. Every member of our profession can and should feel an obligation to contribute to the generation of evidence-based science. For it is only through this new knowledge that we can achieve our potential as a true specialty.

REFERENCES

See www.expertconsult.com for a complete list of references.

Chelonian Taxonomy, Anatomy, and Physiology

Thomas H. Boyer and Charles J. Innis

Chelonians (turtles, tortoises, and terrapins) were traditionally thought of as primitive basal reptiles because of their anapsid skull (without temporal fennestra). Recent morphologic and molecular studies have discarded this notion; chelonians are now thought of as diapsids (having two temporal fennestra) that have secondarily evolved into anapsids.[1–4] As such, chelonians are a sister clade to the Archosaurs (crocodilians, birds, and extinct dinosaurs) and less closely related to the living Lepidosaurs (lizards, snakes, amphisbaenids, and tuataras). Chelonians are the most ancient reptiles, evolving before the dinosaurs over 300 million years ago.[4,5] They survived multiple mass extinctions with little change to their basic body plan; their armored shell served them well until man evolved. Pursuit by man for food, traditional medicine, and pets, as well as introduced invasive species, diseases, anthropogenic trauma, fisheries interactions, habitat degradation, and fragmentation have resulted in population declines for many chelonian species. Chelonians are under siege on a global basis and are the most threatened of any major group of vertebrates—more than mammals, birds, or amphibians.[5] More than half of freshwater turtles worldwide, and 75% of the Asian species, are threatened with extinction. Due to the magnitude of this crisis, concerned organizations and individuals have been developing strategies to conserve chelonians through better education, enforcement, legislation, and international cooperation. Zoos and private individuals can play a role in preserving assurance colonies of threatened species before they are gone. The Turtle Survival Alliance (http://www.turtlesurvival.org) has been effective in prioritizing and coordinating conservation action.

Turtles are near the top in the number and proportion of species that have been known to live more than 50 years in captivity.[6] All species of chelonians can potentially live half a century or more, certain species may exceed 100 years, and fortunate individuals have been known to exceed 150 years.[7] However, in the Anthropocene, death by man is more likely to result in mortality than old age. Anyone who obtains chelonians is encouraged to act responsibly and observe all regulations set forth by the Convention on the International Trade in Endangered Species of Fauna and Flora, in addition to other applicable state, local, and federal wildlife laws. Asking questions about chelonian origin and verification of legal importation are important. Seek captive-born animals.

TAXONOMY

Turtles, tortoises, and terrapins are the only living representatives of the order variously referred to as Testudines, Testudinata, or Chelonia. The two suborders of chelonians are the Cryptodira (hidden-neck turtles) (Fig. 7.1) and the Pleurodira (side-neck turtles) (Fig. 7.2). Cryptodiran turtles can, by a vertical cobralike bending of the neck vertebrae, retract the head and neck straight back into the shell, thereby hiding the neck.[8] Although sea turtles are Cryptodirans, they are anatomically unable to retract their heads into their shells. Pleurodirans are not able to fully retract the neck inside the shell and must fold it sideways hence the common name of side-necks. Currently, approximately 14 families, 97 genera, and 327 species encompass the Chelonia (Tables 7.1 and 7.2), including seven species of sea turtles.[9]

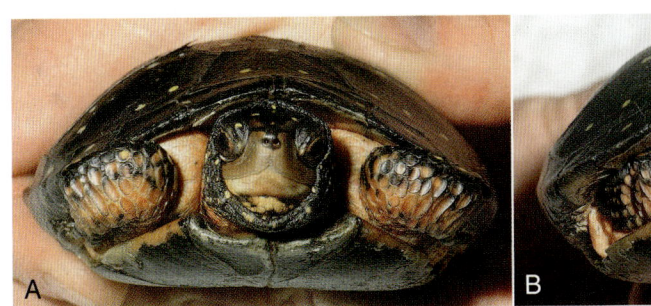
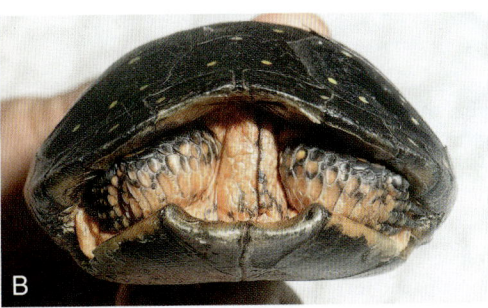

FIG 7.1 (A) Cryptodiran turtles are able to retract the neck straight back into the shell, cobralike, thereby hiding the neck, such as this extreme example (B) in a spotted turtle (Clemmys guttata). (Courtesy of Thomas H. Boyer.)

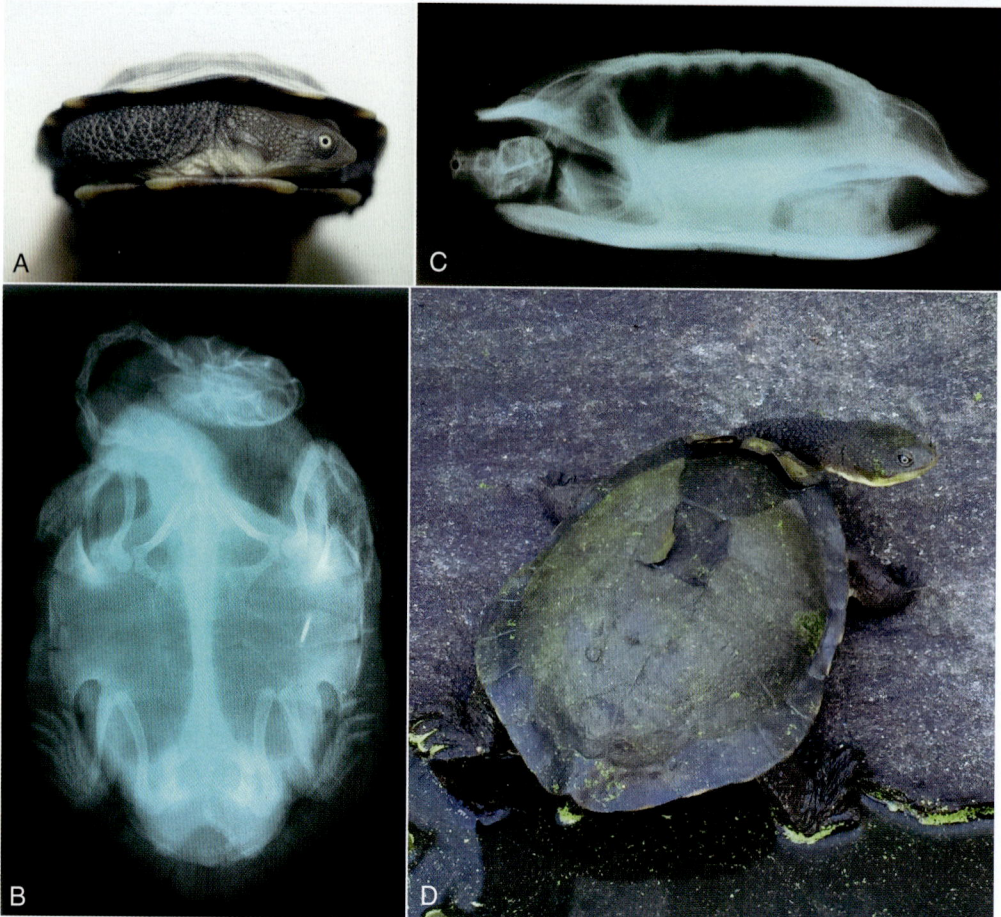

FIG 7.2 (A) Pleurodiran turtles are not able to retract the neck and must fold it up sideways; hence, the common name of side-necks, such as this common snake-necked turtle (*Chelodina longicollis*) with (B) lateral and (C) dorsoventral radiographs. (D) Note the start of annual scute shedding. (Courtesy of Thomas H. Boyer.)

TABLE 7.1   The Suborder Pleurodira Consists of 3 Families, 16 Genera, and Over 80 Species[9]

Family	Common Names	Example Species
Chelidae (Fig. 7.2 and 7.3)	Austro-American side-necked and snake-necked turtles	Common snake-neck turtle (*Chelodina longicollis*) Mata mata, (*Chelys fimbriata*)
Pelomedusidae (Fig. 7.4)	Afro-American side-neck turtles	African helmeted turtle (*Pelomedusa subrufa*)
Podocnemididae (Fig. 7.5)	Madagascar big-headed turtles, big-headed Amazon river turtles, South American side-neck river turtles	Madagascar big-headed turtles (*Erymnochelys madagascariensis*)

The common names of chelonians vary throughout the world and change from language to language.[10] Tortoise usually refers to terrestrial species, such as members of the family Testudinidae. Australians, however, refer to all but one of their turtles as tortoises, despite the fact that no Testudinidae exist there and all of their chelonians are aquatic. In the United Kingdom, terrapin refers to freshwater/brackish chelonians, turtle refers to marine chelonians, and tortoise refers to terrestrial chelonians. In South Africa, fresh water turtles are also referred to as terrapins. North Americans restrict the use of terrapin to a single species, the diamondback terrapin (*Malaclemys terrapin*), a brackish water species, while all other aquatic turtles are called turtles. Vernacular names such as sliders, sawbacks, or cooters may also be used. The Spanish language refers to chelonians as tortugas, tortugas de tierra (land tortoises), tortugas de aqua (water turtles), and tortugas de mar (sea turtles). One can appreciate scientific names that are the same from language to language. The Turtle Taxonomy Working Group has standardized English common names with generic names by compiling a checklist of turtles of the world, their distribution, and conservation status.[9]

TABLE 7.2 The Suborder Cryptodira Consists of 11 Families, 74 Genera, and Over 250 Species[9]

Family	Common name	Examples
Carettochelyidae (Fig. 7.6)	Pig-nosed turtle	Pig-nosed, or Fly River, turtle (*Carettochelys insculpta*)
Cheloniidae (Fig. 7.7)	Hard-shelled sea turtles	Green sea turtle (*Chelonia mydas*), loggerhead sea turtle (*Caretta caretta*)
Chelydridae (Fig. 7.8)	Snapping turtles	Alligator snapping turtle (*Macrochelys temminckii*)
Dermatemydidae (Fig. 7.9)	Central American river turtles	Central American river turtle (*Dermatemys mawii*)
Dermochelyidae (Fig. 7.10)	Leatherback sea turtle	Leatherback sea turtle (*Dermochelys coriacea*)
Emydidae (Fig. 7.11)	Box turtles, pond turtles, map turtles, wood turtles, terrapins, sliders, cooters	Red-eared slider (*Trachemys scripta elegans*), Eastern box turtle (*Terrapene carolina carolina*), European pond turtle (*Emys orbicularis*)
Geoemydidae (Fig. 7.12)	Asian river, leaf, roofed, or Asian box turtles	Malayan box turtle (*Cuora amboinensis*), yellow-margined box turtle (*Cuora flavomarginata*)
Kinosternidae (Fig. 7.13)	Mud and musk turtles	Stinkpot (*Sternotherus odoratus*)
Platysternidae (Fig. 7.14)	Big-headed turtle	Big headed turtle (*Platysternon megacephalum*)
Testudinidae (Fig. 7.15)	Land tortoises	Mojave desert tortoise (*Gopherus agassizii*)
Trionychidae (Fig. 7.16)	Softshell turtles	Spiny softshell (*Apalone spinifera*)

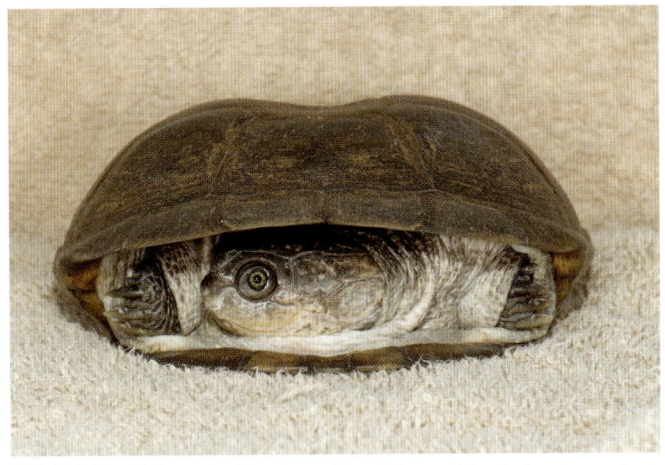

FIG 7.4 The Pelomedusidae is another side-neck turtle family, such as this *Pelomedusa* spp. (Courtesy of Stephen Barten.)

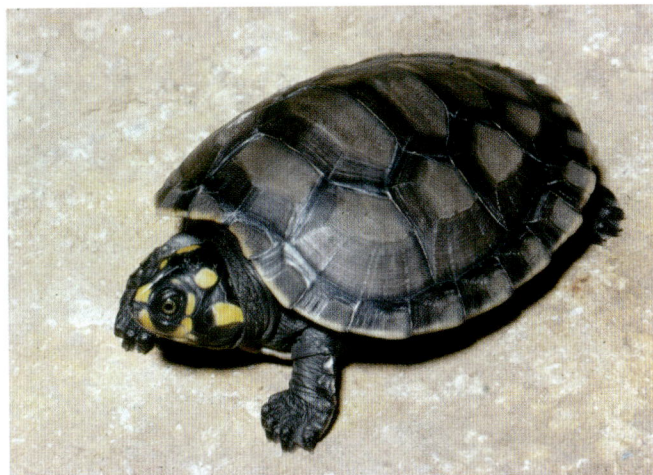

FIG 7.5 The yellow-spotted Amazon River turtle (*Podocnemis unifilis*) is a large member of the Podocnemididae. (Courtesy of John Tashjian.)

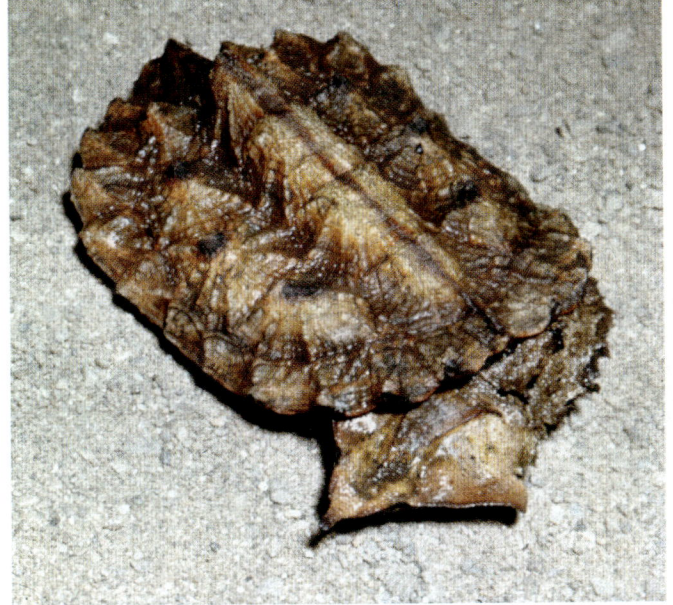

FIG 7.3 The mata mata (*Chelus fimbriata*) is a South American side-neck Chelidae and blends beautifully with its flooded forest floor habitat. (Courtesy of John Tashjian.)

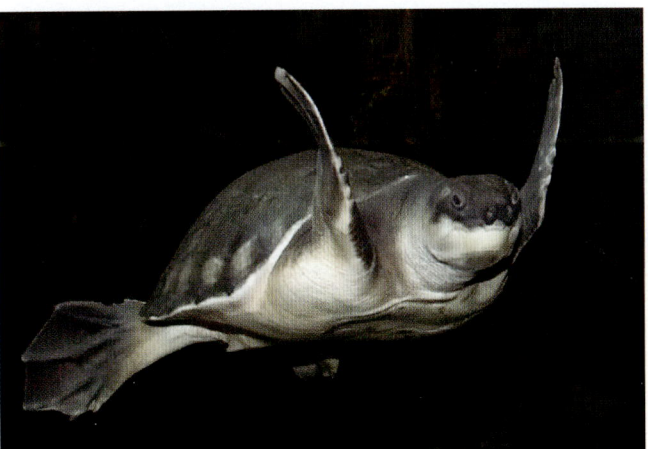

FIG 7.6 The Fly River turtle (*Carettochelys insculpta*) is the only chelonian that is not a sea turtle with flippers and can fly through the water. (Courtesy of Stephen Barten.)

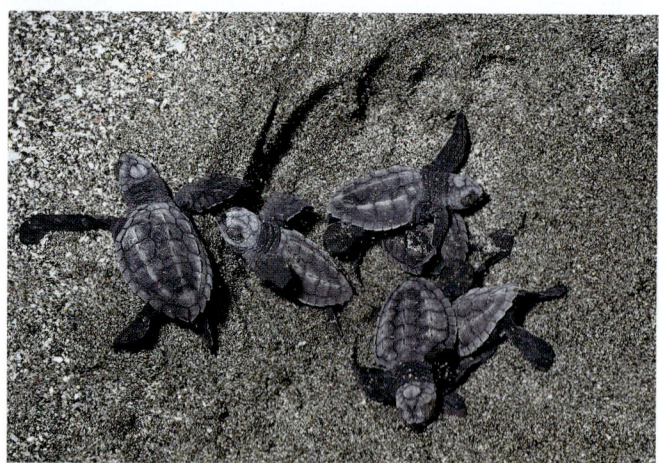

FIG 7.7 Olive ridley sea turtles (*Lepidochelys olivacea*) hatching at night on Playa Naranjo, Guanacaste, Costa Rica. Olive ridleys are one of seven sea turtle species, six species being within this family, Cheloniidae. (Courtesy of Donal M. Boyer.)

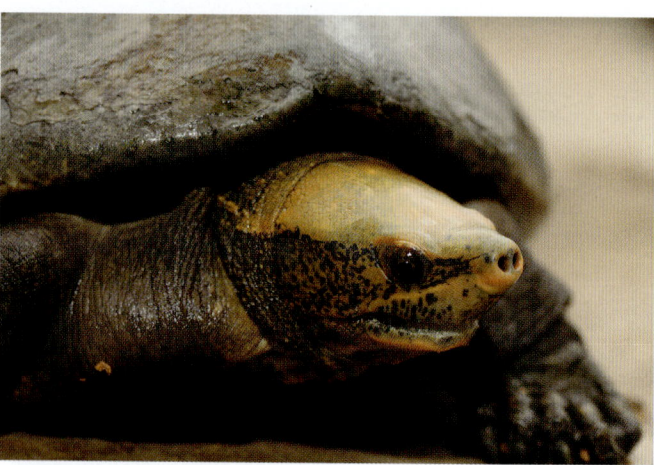

FIG 7.9 The Central American river turtle (*Dermatemys mawii*) is the sole representative of Dermatemydidae, entirely aquatic, herbivorous, and nocturnal. It has been intensively harvested for meat, eggs, and shell and is critically endangered. (Courtesy of Sam Rivera.)

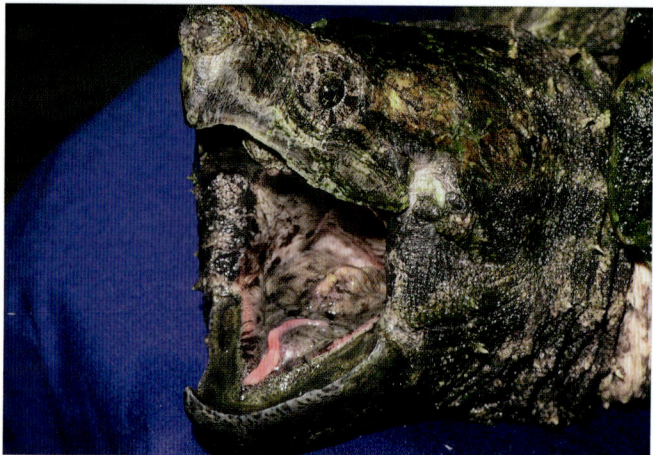

FIG 7.8 The alligator snapping turtle (*Macrochelys temminckii*) is one of the heaviest freshwater species and has a lingual vermiform appendage that it uses to lure fish. (Courtesy of Donal M. Boyer.)

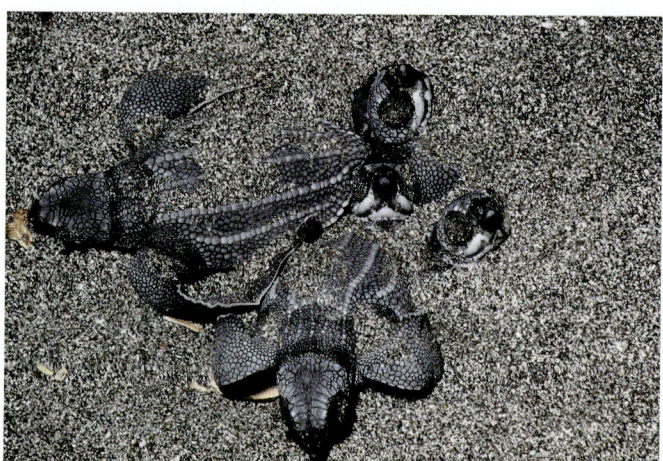

FIG 7.10 The leatherback sea turtle (*Dermochelys coriacea*) grows to be the largest, fastest, and deepest diving of all living turtles. Leatherbacks are endothermic; core body temperatures can be 18°C (32°F) above water temperature. (Courtesy of Donal M. Boyer.)

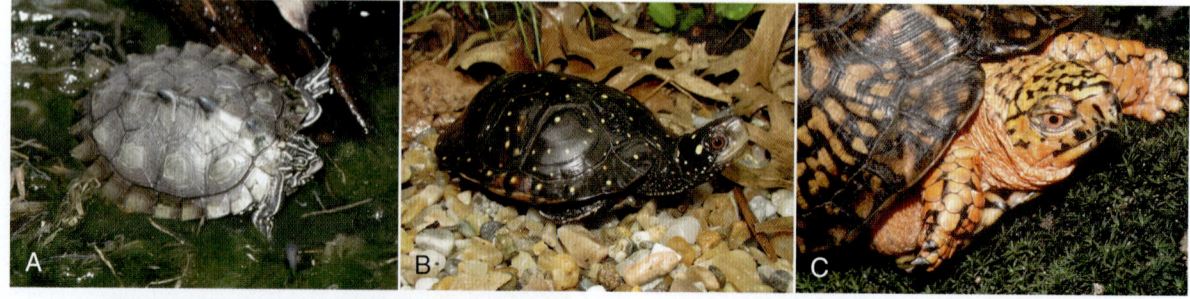

FIG 7.11 Emydidae is the largest and most diverse turtle family, accounting for almost a third of all species and distributed around the world. Emydids are primarily freshwater turtles, some are semiaquatic to terrestrial, represented here by the (A) black-knobbed map turtle or sawback (*Graptemys nigrinoda*), (B) spotted turtle (*Clemmys guttata*), and (C) eastern box turtle (*Terrapene carolina carolina*). (A and C, Courtesy of Stephen Barten; B, courtesy of Donal M. Boyer.)

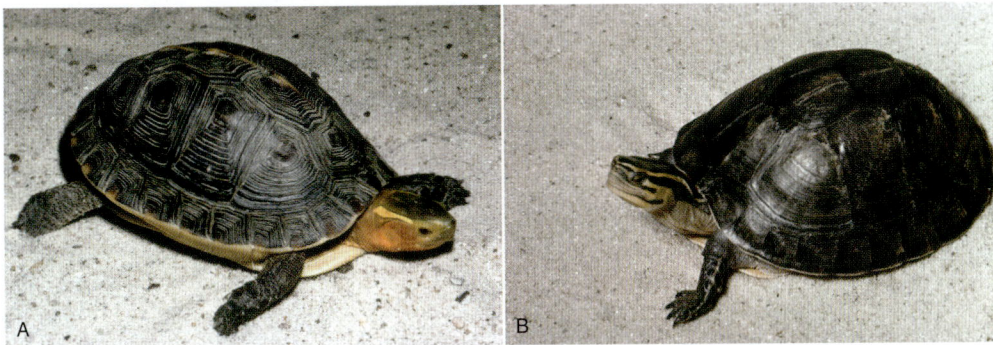

FIG 7.12 (A) The yellow-margined box turtle (*Cuora flavomarginata*) and (B) the southeast Asian box turtle (*Cuora ambionensis*) were both once ubiquitous in the pet trade but are now rare. (Courtesy of John Tashjian.)

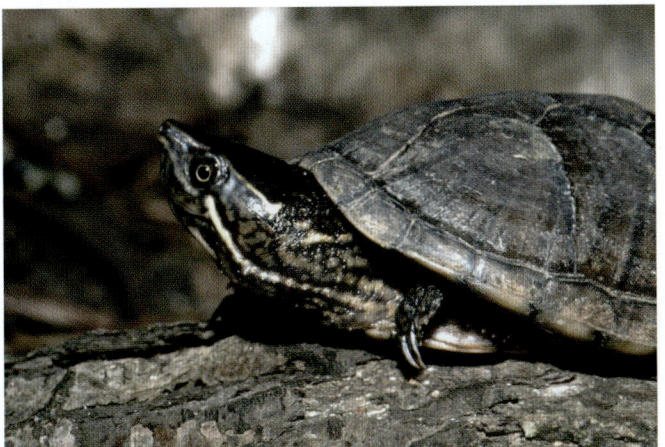

FIG 7.13 The mud and musk turtles, Kinosternidae, are a large group of New World aquatic turtles. This stinkpot (*Sternotherus odoratus*) has musk glands along the bridge that are a predator deterrent. (Courtesy of Stephen Barten.)

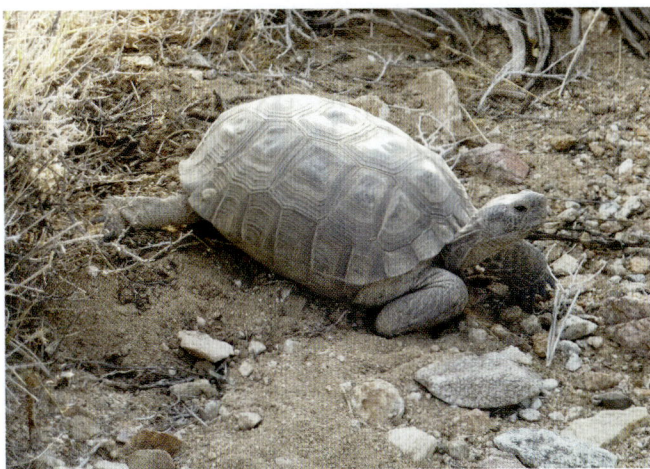

FIG 7.15 The desert tortoise (*Gopherus agassizii*) has recently been split into several species and is the most common reptile in the senior author's veterinary practice. (Courtesy of Donal M. Boyer.)

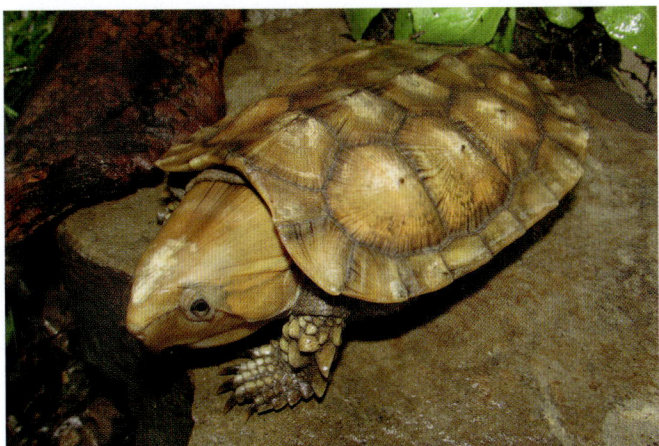

FIG 7.14 The monotypic big-headed turtle (*Platysternon megacephalum*) lives in cool, fast-moving rivers and streams in Southeast Asia and is an excellent climber. Human consumption is rapidly removing it from the wild. (Courtesy of John Tashjian.)

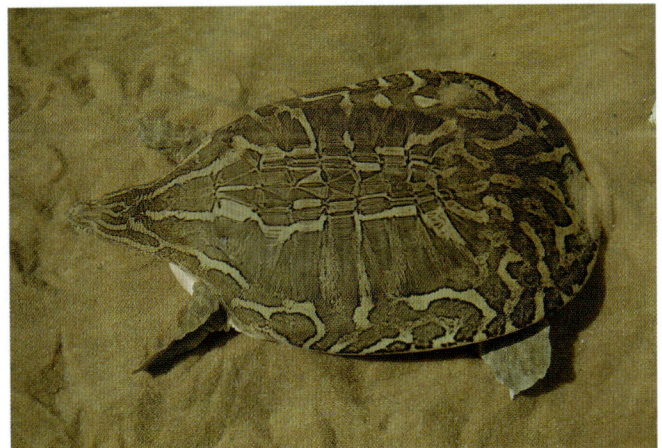

FIG 7.16 Softshell turtles (Trionychidae) are the largest freshwater turtle species, such as this Indian narrow-headed softshell turtle (*Chitra indica*), which has cervical vertebrae at the carapacial junction that can flip 180 degrees. (Courtesy of Donal M. Boyer.)

ANATOMY AND PHYSIOLOGY

Chelonians are vertebrates, but they possess several unique aspects to their anatomy and physiology. Figs. 7.17 through 7.23 illustrate the gross anatomy of the chelonian.

Musculoskeletal System

Chelonians are immediately recognizable by their shell. The shell consists of an upper carapace and lower plastron connected laterally by bony bridges. The carapace consists of some 50 bones derived from ribs, vertebrae, and dermal elements of the skin; the plastron has 9 bones evolved from the clavicles, coracoids, interclavicles, and gastralia (abdominal ribs).

The bony shell is covered by a superficial layer of keratin shields, called scutes (Fig. 7.23). Scutes are staggered so that the seams between them are not directly over bone sutures. Turtles produce new scutes with each major growth period and retain (terrestrial chelonians) or shed (aquatic to semiaquatic chelonians) the scutes from the preceding growth period.[11] Scutes grow outward from their central nucleus, or areola. Each year, a new scute forms beneath the previous year's scute and, if it is larger, its outer edge shows around the perimeter of the older scute in the form of a growth ring (an annulus). If nutrition is compromised, instead of expanding level with the shell surface, the annuli will invert, which is abnormal, but a good indicator of chronic nutritional inadequacy (Fig. 7.24). In some species, annuli can be used to estimate age, similar to growth rings in a tree. This requires considerable expertise and is reliable only when a distinct growth period is present, as in wild temperate turtles.[11] The difficulty of estimating age from annuli is complicated by continuous growth in captivity, without distinct annuli; annuli that are worn off with age, wear, or shedding scutes; or multiple annuli per year. Therefore, contrary to popular belief, the age of most turtles cannot be determined accurately by counting annuli.[12] Scutes and underlying bone are capable of incredible regeneration (Fig. 7.25), such that necrotic bones and scutes are shed, or can be debrided, and eventually replaced by underlying new shell with both bones and scutes.[13] Scute nomenclature is useful to veterinarians to describe shell lesions and surgical sites and to identify species.[11] Scutes are named for their adjacent body portion (see Fig. 7.23).

Shell modifications are numerous. The bones in the shells of leatherback sea turtles (*Dermochelys coriacea*), softshell turtles (Trionychidae), and Fly River turtles (*Carettochelys insculpta*) have been reduced and the scutes replaced with tough leathery skin with α keratin, but no β keratin. All other turtles have both α and β keratin, the latter is hard and brittle.[14] Most hatchling tortoises have fontanelles or fenestrae (openings) between carapacial bones that fuse as the tortoise ages (provided bone growth is normal). Some species, such as pancake tortoises (*Malacochersus torneiri*), adult male and immature giant Asian river turtles (*Batagur* spp.),[15] and softshell turtles retain these fenestrae.

Many chelonians have connective tissue hinges in their shell. These include plastronal hinges in box turtles (*Terrapene* spp., *Cuora* spp.), spider tortoises (*Pyxis* spp.), and mud turtles (*Kinosternon* spp.); a caudal carapacial hinge in hinged-back tortoises (*Kinixys* spp.); and slight caudal plastron mobility in female Mediterranean tortoises (*Testudo* spp.).

Chelonians are the only extant vertebrates in which pectoral and pelvic girdles are within the rib cage, an early evolutionary change first apparent 260 million years ago.[7] The vertical orientation of the pectoral and pelvic girdles buttresses the shell and provides strong ventral anchors for the humerus and femur. With few exceptions, the appendicular bones are typical of other vertebrates. The tripartite rectilinear pectoral girdle consists of a dorsoventral scapula, ventromedial acromium process and ventrocaudal coracoid (procoracoid), which resembles the mammalian scapula, especially on dorsoventral radiographs. Marine species and one freshwater species, the Fly River turtle, have elongated metacarpals and phalanges that form elaborate forelimb flippers so that they can "fly" through water (Fig. 7.26; also see Fig. 7.6).

Chelonians have 8 cervical, 10 trunk, and variable numbers of up to 33 caudal vertebrae. Chelonians have well-developed musculature associated with retraction of the head and neck and the limb girdles and limbs, but because of the shell, they have reduced trunk musculature.[16,17] Appreciating the boundaries of the pectoral and pelvic muscles is important when plastron celiotomy is contemplated.

Integumentary System

The skin of chelonians varies from smooth and scaleless to thickly scaled. A tendency toward thicker scales is seen among the Testudinidae. Injections should be given through finely scaled areas, avoiding the larger, thicker scales that may have osteoderms, which are difficult to penetrate. As with all reptiles, skin is shed periodically, although in a much more piecemeal fashion than in squamates. This is particularly noticeable in aquatic turtles, often misinterpreted by laypersons as a fungal infection.

Text continued on p. 41

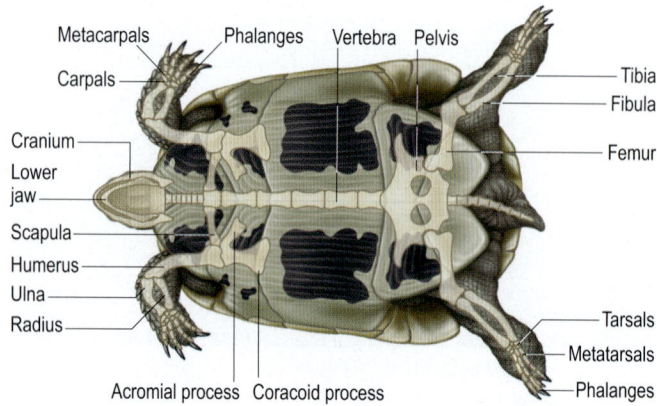

FIG 7.17 Ventral view, with the plastron removed, of the axial and appendicular skeleton of a Greek tortoise (*Testudo graeca*).

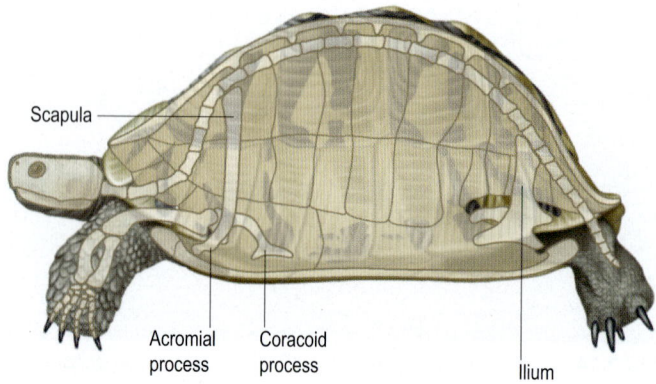

FIG 7.18 Saggital view of the axial and appendicular skeleton of a Greek tortoise (*Testudo graeca*).

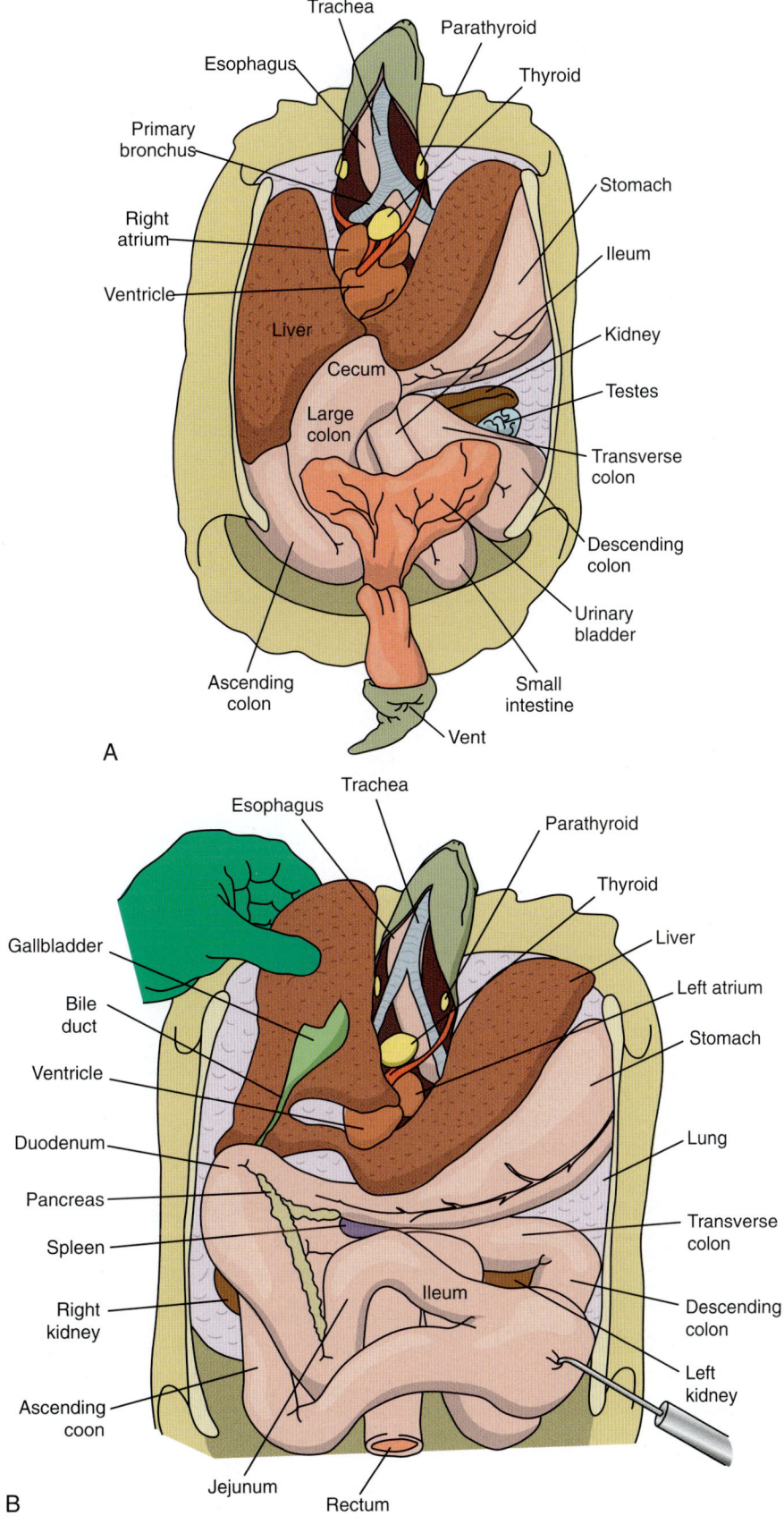

FIG 7.19 (A) Gross anatomy of the tortoise, ventral view; the plastron has been removed. (B) Ventral view. The bladder has been removed to permit visualization of the intestinal tract. The right lobe of the liver is reflected to expose the gallbladder. *Continued*

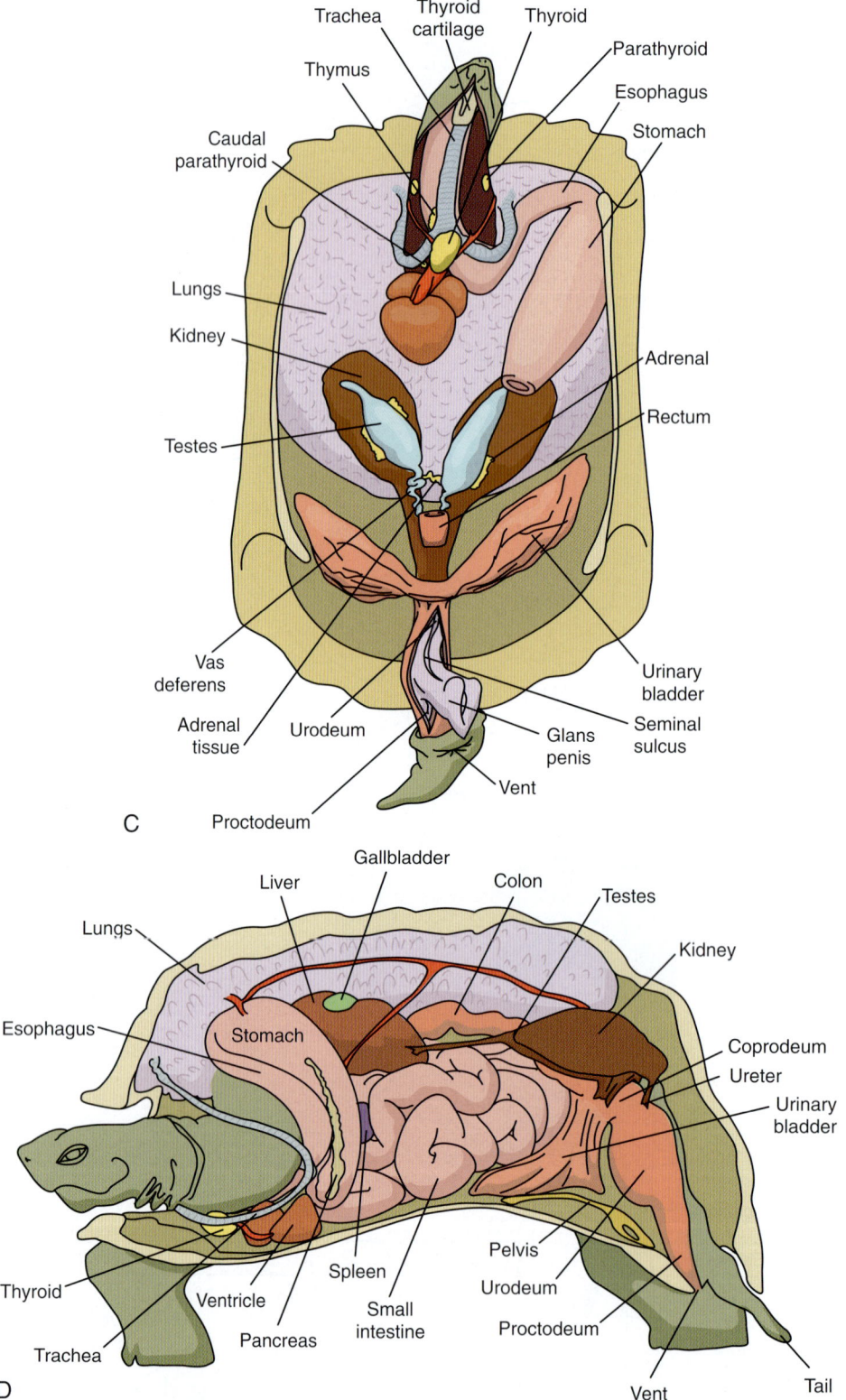

FIG 7.19, cont'd (C) Ventral view. The liver and intestinal tract have been removed. In this male, the testicles are attached to the ventral aspect of the kidneys. (D) Midsagittal view of the gross anatomy of the tortoise.

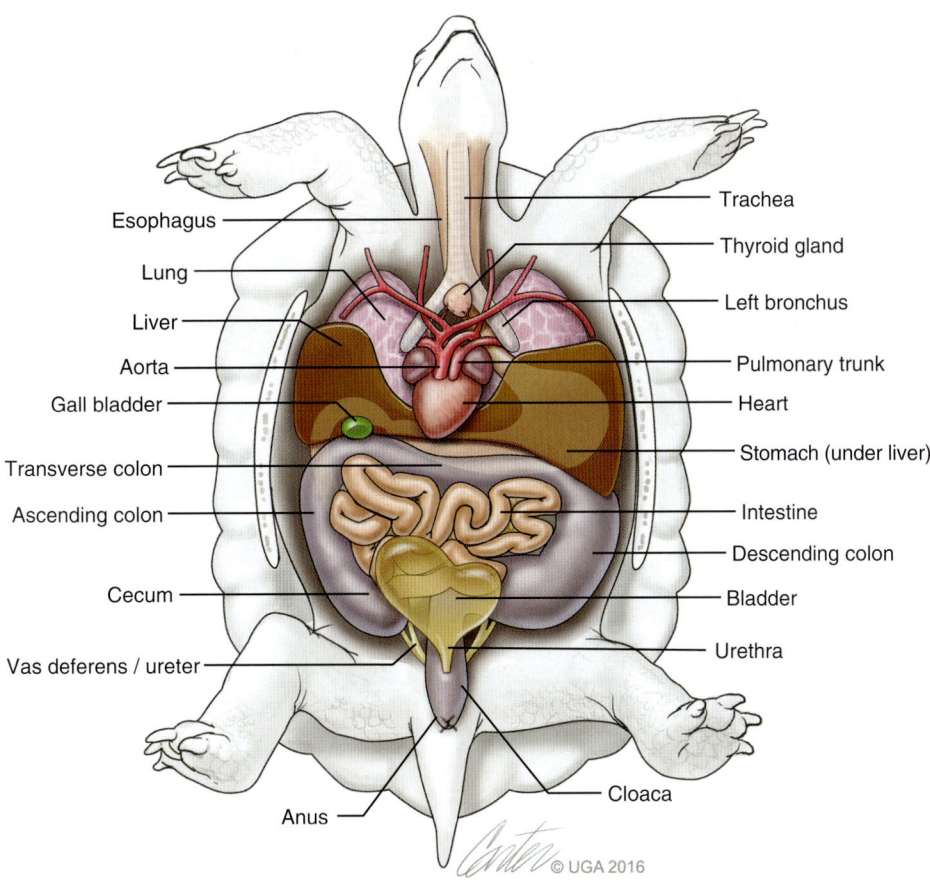

FIG 7.20 Ventral view of the desert tortoise (*Gopherus agassizii*), with plastron removed after Meyer. (Redrawn from McArthur S, Wilkinson R, Meyer J, et al. *Medicine and Surgery of Tortoises and Turtles.* Oxford, UK: Blackwell Publishing Ltd.; 2004.)

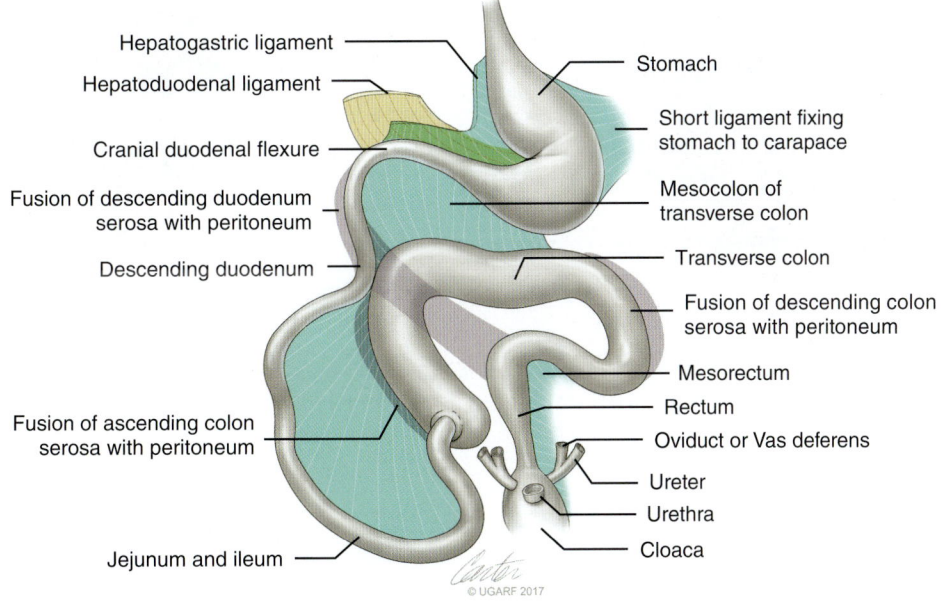

FIG 7.21 Ventral view of the attachments and mesenteries of the intestinal tract of a desert tortoise (*Gopherus agassizii*) after Meyer. (Redrawn from McArthur S, Wilkinson R, Meyer J, et al. *Medicine and Surgery of Tortoises and Turtles.* Oxford, UK: Blackwell Publishing Ltd.; 2004.)

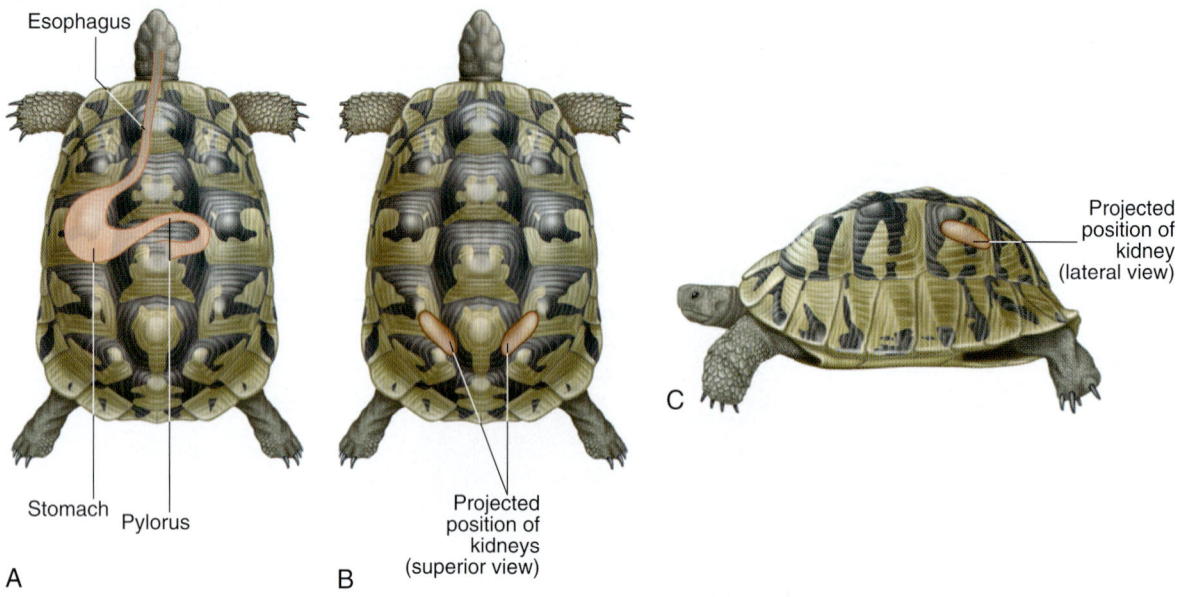

FIG 7.22 Dorsal view of the stomach (A) and kidneys (B) and lateral view of the kidneys (C) in a Greek tortoise (*Testudo graeca*).

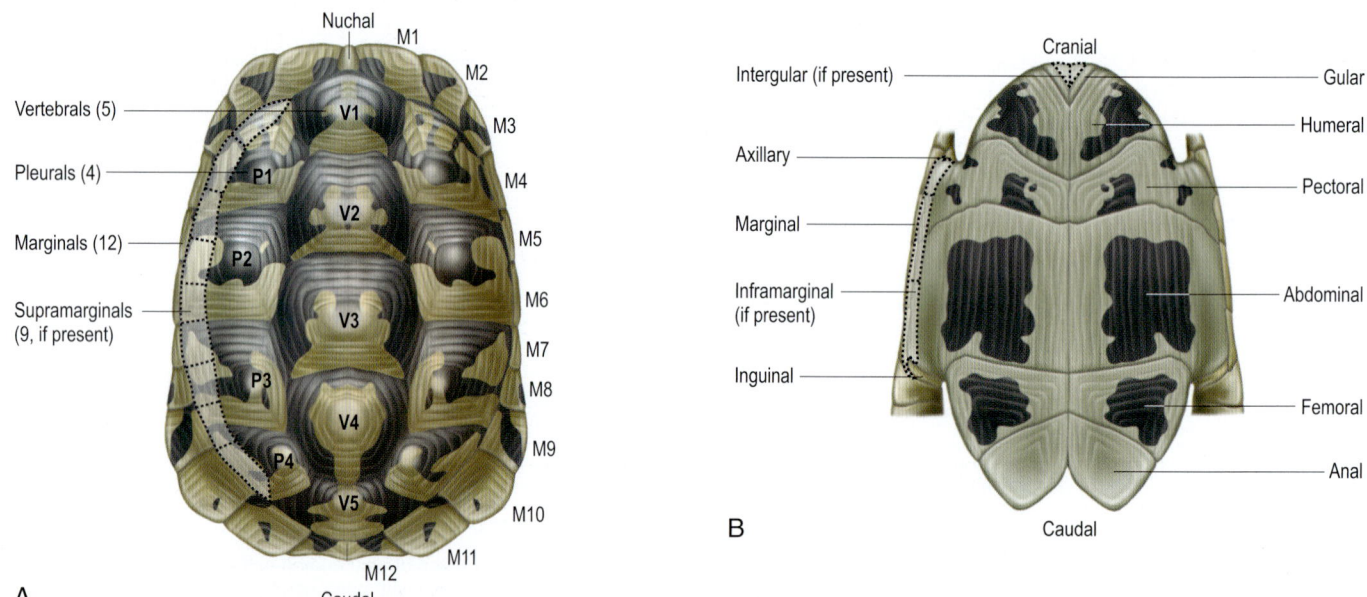

FIG 7.23 Nomenclature of carapacial (A) and plastronal (B) scutes of a Greek tortoise (*Testudo graeco*).

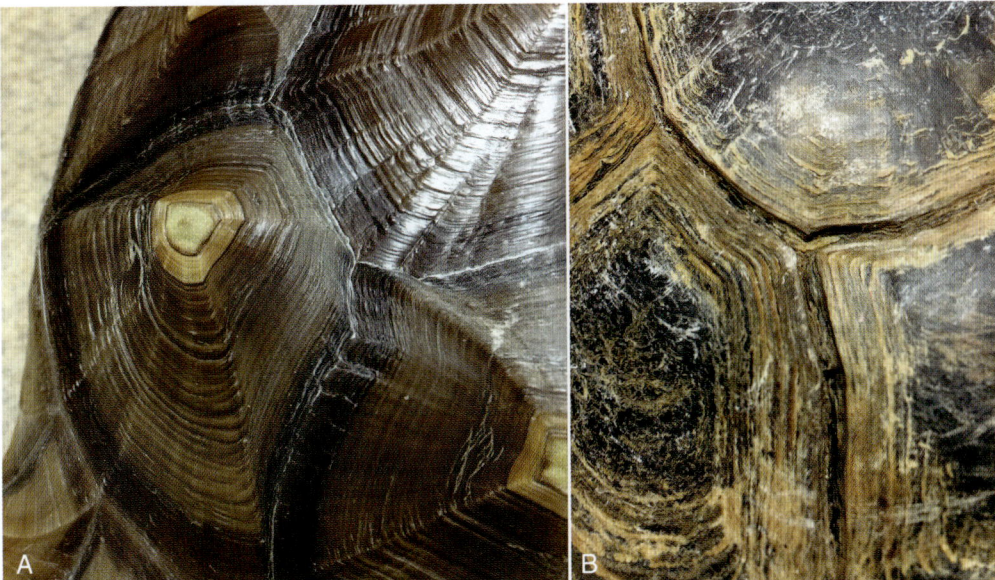

FIG 7.24 If nutrition is compromised, instead of expanding level with the shell surface (A), the annuli (growth rings) will invert; this abnormality (B) indicates chronic nutritional issues. (Courtesy of Thomas H. Boyer.)

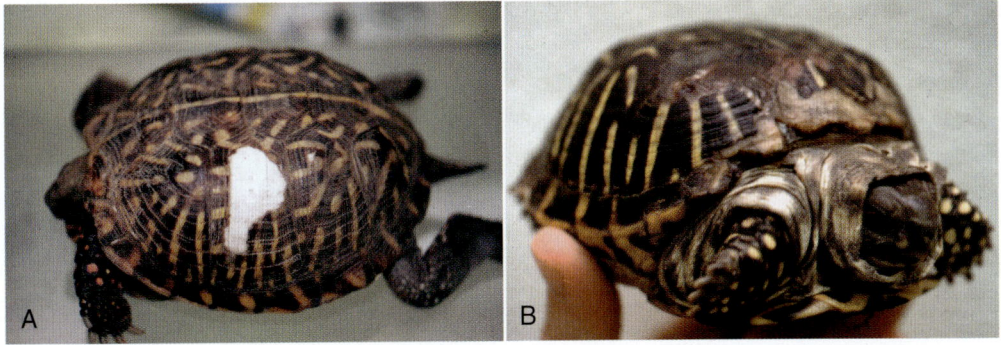

FIG 7.25 Scutes and underlying bone are capable of regeneration, such that dead bone and scutes are shed or can be debrided and eventually replaced by underlying new shell with both bone and scutes. If there is no odor, discharge, or active inflammation, as in these ornate box turtles *(Terrapene ornata ornata)* (A and B), no treatment is indicated. (Courtesy of Thomas H. Boyer.)

Respiratory System

The rigid shell makes respiration much different for chelonians compared with other vertebrates with expandable chests. Chelonians are obligate nasal breathers; mouth breathing is abnormal and often indicates airway pathology. Air from the external nares passes over the partial hard palate (there is no soft palate) into the much larger nasal sinus (Fig. 7.27), separated into halves by the internasal septum, then opens into choanae (the internal nares) in the dorsal oral cavity. The nasal sinus is lined with dorsal olfactory and ventral, mucous producing epithelium. The glottis is located at the base of the tongue, and the tracheal rings are complete. In cryptodiran turtles, the trachea is relatively short and bifurcates midcervically into two main-stem, unbranched bronchi that open directly into the entire dorsal surface of the paired lungs. The cranial bifurcation and complete tracheal rings of the trachea enables chelonians to breathe unimpeded when the neck is withdrawn[18] but can also be a hazard if endotracheal intubation is too deep. The dorsal lungs are adherent to the carapace and ventrally separated and weighted by the septum horizontale, which is attached to the liver, stomach, and intestinal tract. No true diaphragm separates the lungs from other internal organs, thus there is a pleuroperitoneal or coelomic cavity. Grossly, the lungs are large, multicameral (partitioned), saccular structures reminiscent of hollow porous sponges. Lungs are divided into 3 to 11 chambers dependent on the family.[19] The lung surface is reticular and interspersed with bands of smooth muscle and connective tissue. Although lung volume is large, respiratory surface area is only 10% to 20% of a comparably sized mammal but adequate for animals with a metabolic rate that is only 10% to 30% of that of mammals.[6,17] Large lung volume provides an obvious advantage as a hydrostatic organ for aquatic turtles.[19] In three-toed box turtles *(Terrapene carolina triunguis)*, researchers found relatively small tidal volumes (2.2 ± 1.4 mL/breath) coupled with high respiratory rates (36.6 ± 26.4 breaths/min).[20]

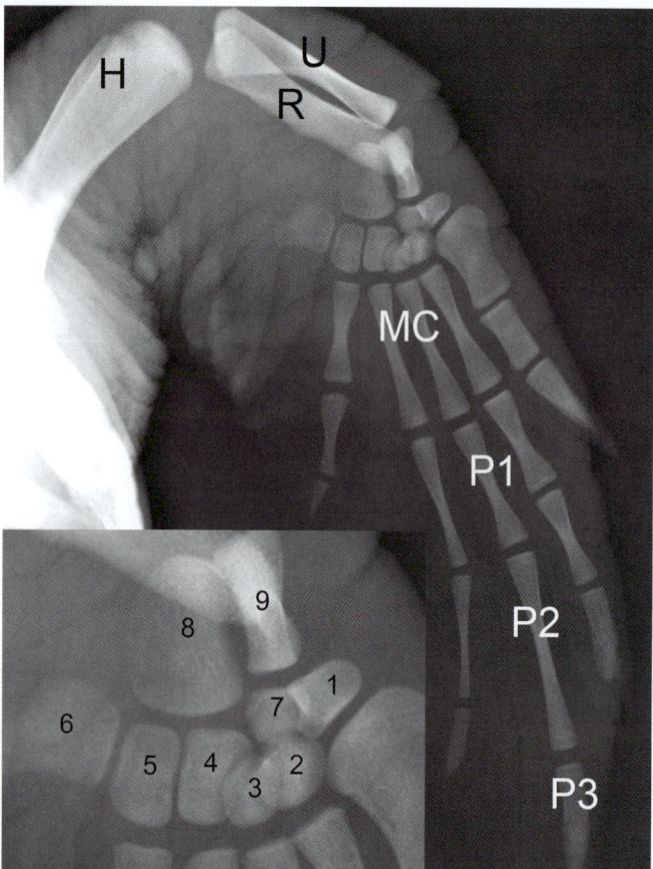

FIG 7.26 Radiograph of the front flipper of a loggerhead turtle (*Caretta caretta*), showing the elongated metacarpal and phalangeal bones that form the majority of the length of the flipper. There are five metacarpals, one for each digit. The first and fifth digits have two phalanges, while digits 2–4 have three phalanges. Inset shows close-up of the carpal bones. H, Humerus; U, ulna; R, radius; MC, metacarpal; P1, P2, and P3, first, second, and third phalanges; 1-5, distal carpal bones 1-5; 6, pisiform; 7, centrale; 8, radiale; 9, ulnare. (Courtesy of Charles J. Innis.)

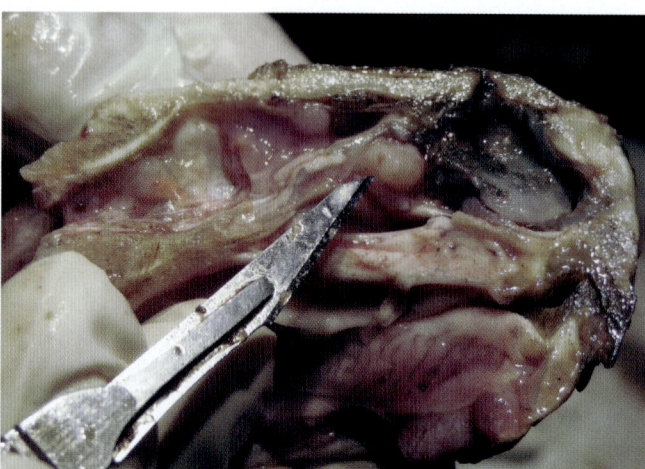

FIG 7.27 Saggital section of the skull of a leopard tortoise (*Stigmochelys pardalis*); note the large olfactory lobes (scapel tip) and anterior nasal sinus. (Courtesy of Brian Horne.)

Intrapulmonary pressure varies from slightly negative to 5 cm H_2O.[19] Peak airway pressures during anesthesia are recommended to be less than 10 cm H_2O.[21]

Antagonistic pairs of muscles essentially decrease or increase lung and visceral volume.[22] This action may or may not be supplemented with limb and head movements and anatomically varies considerably among chelonians. Amphibians and monitors breathe, in part, through positive pressure gular pumping. Turtles are capable of gular pumping, but this assists olfaction, not ventilation (except in some aquatic species that do have gular respiration).[22] In the submerged snapping turtle, inspiration is active and expiration passive because of hydrostatic pressure that affects visceral volume. On land, the opposite is true; inspiration is passive, and expiration is active.[11] Some aquatic turtles have supplemental cloacal, buccopharyngeal, or cutaneous respiration to enable them to remain submerged longer. The Fitzroy River turtle (*Rheodytes leukops*) can extract from 40% (adults) to 73% (juveniles) of their oxygen requirement via highly modified cloacal fimbriated bursae[23] and can pump water in and out of their cloaca 15 to 60 times per minute.[24] Underwater respiration may sustain aquatic turtles during periods of low activity, but when they are active, they still need to surface for air (bimodal respiration).[7] Chelonians are capable of long periods of apnea that makes induction of gas anesthesia by chamber or mask more difficult, especially in cryptodirans, without injectable preanesthetics. Open fractures of the shell, exposing the lung, typically do not result in obvious respiratory distress. Many factors make removing secretions or foreign bodies from the lungs difficult for chelonians. These include termination of the mucociliary elevator outside the glottis, poor drainage through the dorsally located bronchi, compartmentalization of the lungs, large potential space within the lungs, and lack of a complete muscular diaphragm to facilitate coughing.[25] Consequently, pneumonia can be difficult to manage and life threatening in chelonians.

Digestive System

Chelonians have large, fleshy tongues that are not able to distend from the mouth as in squamates. As a general rule, most terrestrial species are herbivorous, whereas aquatic species are carnivorous or omnivorous; however, numerous exceptions exist.[12] Chelonians lack teeth and depend on the scissorlike actions of their horny beak, or rhamphotheca, for biting off pieces of food that are swallowed whole. In captivity, chronic nutritional disease may produce deformity of the rhamphotheca (Fig. 7.28). Salivary glands produce mucus devoid of enzymes to enable swallowing of bite-sized pieces,[24] especially in tortoises. Aquatic turtles eat under water. The ciliated esophagus courses along the neck. Sea turtles have large esophageal papillae to entrap ingested food while expelling sea water (Fig. 7.29). Passing a stomach tube with the neck extended, rather than retracted, is easier. However, in large chelonians, the mouth is easier to open with the head retracted, and it is possible to pass a flexible stomach tube. The stomach lies along the ventral left side, caudal to the liver, and has a gastroesophageal sphincter on the left and pyloric sphincter centrally, as well as greater and lesser curvatures (see Figs. 7.19, 7.20, and 7.21) (Edwards, Proc AAZV, 1991, pp 139–143). The small intestine is relatively short (compared with mammals), mildly convoluted, and absorbs nutrients and water.[27] The stomach, small intestine, and pancreas produce digestive enzymes, while the liver and gallbladder produce and store bile. The pale orange-pink pancreas empties into the proximal duodenum via a short duct or ducts and has functions similar to other vertebrates. The pancreas is in direct contact with the spleen (cryptodirans) or separate in the mesentery along the duodenum (among examined pleurodirans).[17] Tissue amylase and lipase levels have been found to be highest in pancreatic tissue in loggerhead (*Caretta caretta*) and Kemp's ridley (*Lepidochelys kempii*) sea turtles and low in all other tissues.[28,29]

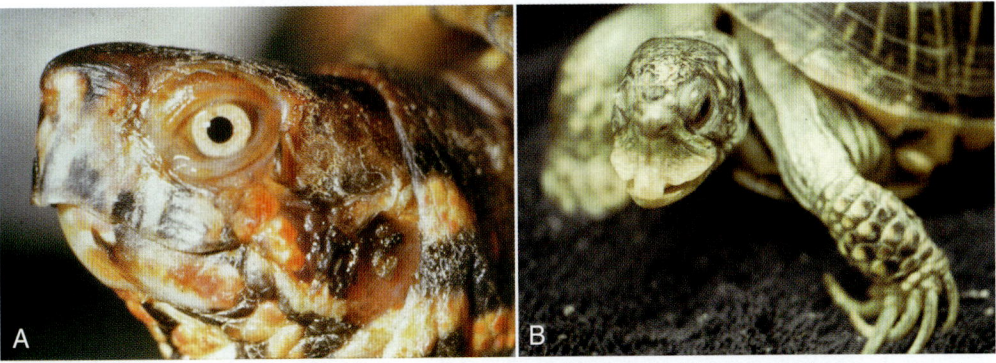

FIG 7.28 The normal rhamphotheca (A) of a box turtle should be vertical. Nutritional disease may produce deformity of the rhamphotheca (B). (Courtesy of Thomas H. Boyer.)

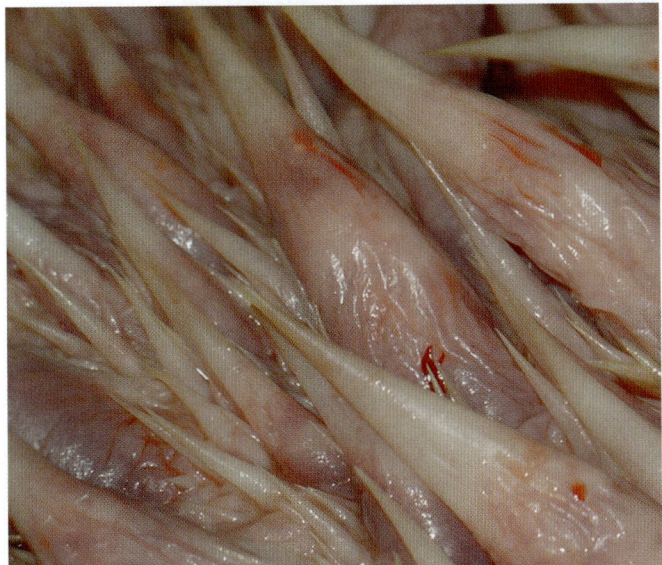

FIG 7.29 Necropsy specimen of a Kemp's Ridley sea turtle (*Lepidochelys kempii*) showing the large keratinized esophageal papillae that are found in all sea turtle species. (Courtesy of Charles J. Innis.)

The liver is a large, ventral, saddle-shaped organ that spreads from side to side under the lungs. It has two major lobes, envelops the gallbladder on the right, and has indentations for the heart and stomach. The liver is dark red to brown, similar to other animals; some chelonian livers may be normally pigmented with melanin (melanomacrophages).[18] Pale yellow to tan color to the liver can be abnormal and an indication of hepatic lipidosis (Fig. 7.30); however, this color change can also be associated with vitellogenesis in females (see Chapter 67). Chelonian bile acids differ somewhat structurally from those typically found in other vertebrates, but 3α hydroxybile acid, the most common clinicopathologic analyte, is conserved. Little is known about the diagnostic use of plasma bile acid concentrations in chelonians, but one study did not detect a postprandial increase in red-eared sliders.[30,31]

The small intestine joins the large intestine at the ileocolic valve. The large intestine, the primary site of microbial fermentation in herbivorous tortoises, includes the cecum, ascending colon, transverse colon, and descending colon (see Figs. 7.19 and 7.20). The cecum is not well developed and not especially distinct; it is more of an expansion of the proximal colon and, fortuitously for the surgeon, lacks mesentric attachments. The ascending and descending colons have short dorsal mesenteric attachments, whereas the transverse colon has a wider mesenteric attachment to the stomach, giving it more dorsoventral mobility.[32] Because of this, heavy ingested material (rocks, sand, metal foreign bodies) sink ventrally in the transverse colon, become entrapped,[32] and accumulate at the descending colon (Fig. 7.31; also see Fig. 7.21). Foreign body removal is facilitated by milking material anterograde into the cecum (which is easiest to exteriorize) from the descending, transverse, and ascending colon, then exteriorizing the cecum for enterotomy and extraction of foreign bodies. The colon terminates in the coprodeum of the cloaca. Gastrointestinal (GI) transit time is affected by many factors, including temperature, species, feeding frequency, food particle size, and water or fiber content of food. GI transit time is shortest in omnivores (e.g., *Trachemys* spp), longer in carnivores, and longest in herbivores (such as tortoises).[32] No digestion takes place below 7°C (45°F), intestinal peristalsis decreases below 10°C (50°F), and extremely slow digestion occurs between 10° to 15°C (50°–59°F).[32] Captive diets generally move faster through the GI tract than natural diets, especially in tortoises. For example, GI transit times for spur-thighed tortoises (*Testudo graeca*), kept at 28°C, varied from 3 to 8 days when fed *ad libitum* lettuce but increased to 16 to 28 days when fed thistles, grasses, and dog food.[33] In Hermann's tortoises (*Testudo hermanni*), diatrizoate (Gastrograffin, 100 mg sodium amidotrizoate [sodium diatrizoate] and 660 mg meglumine amidotrizoate [meglumine diatrizoate]/ml, Bayer, Berkshire, UK) mean total transit time was 2.6 hours at 30.6°C (87°F), 6.6 hours at 21.5°C (70°F), and 17.3 hours at 15.2°C (60°F).[34] In loggerhead sea turtles (*Caretta caretta*), radiographic contrast studies documented transit times of 2 to 3 weeks.[35,36] Metoclopramide, cisapride, and erythromycin did not significantly reduce GI transit time compared with water in desert tortoises (*Gopherus agassizii*).[37]

Genitourinary Systems

The retrocoelomic kidneys of chelonians are located deep to the caudodorsal carapace and posterior to the acetabulum, except in marine turtles in which they are usually anterior to the acetabulum (see Figs. 7.22B and C).[18] The kidneys are metanephric. Reptiles cannot concentrate urine above that of plasma because of the absence of the loop of Henle.[27] Urine is not sterile, and, in chelonians, the urinary tract is not easily accessible. Soluble urinary nitrogenous wastes, such as ammonia and urea, require relatively large amounts of water for excretion. This is only practical for aquatic and semiaquatic chelonians. Marine and highly aquatic freshwater turtles (such as *Trachemys*) excrete more ammonia and urea than uric acid (amino-ureotelic); semiaquatic turtles excrete two to four times as much urea as ammonia or uric acid (ureo-uricotelic).[32] Terrestrial chelonians produce more insoluble uric acid and urates that can be passed from the body in a

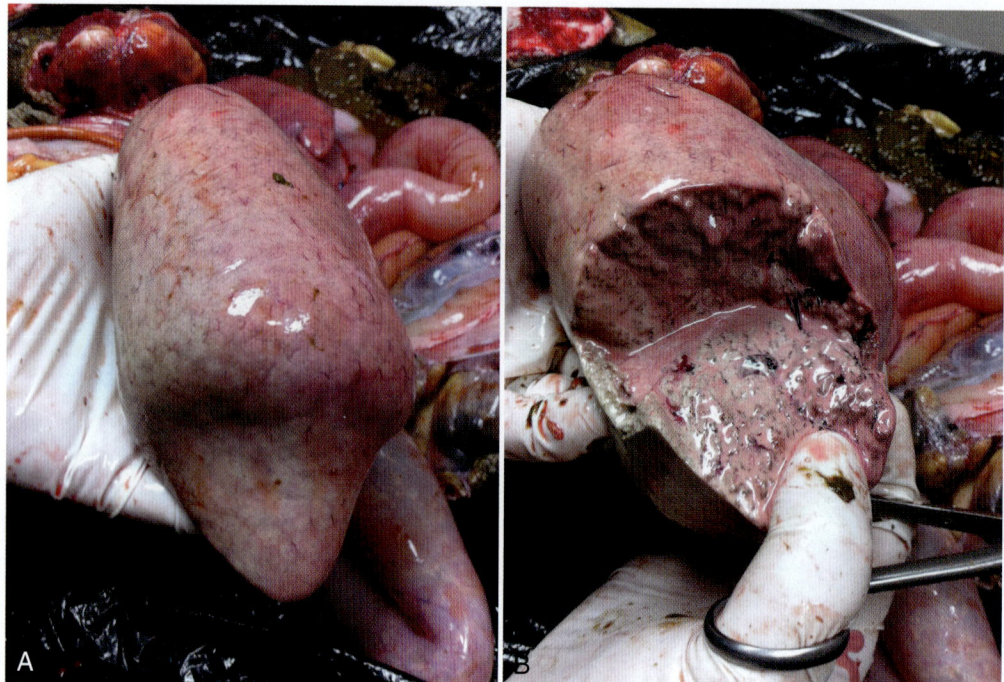

FIG 7.30 Hepatic lipidosis is common in tortoises; notice the swollen rounded liver edges, pale color, and cut surface oozing fatty liquid. (Courtesy of Thomas H. Boyer.)

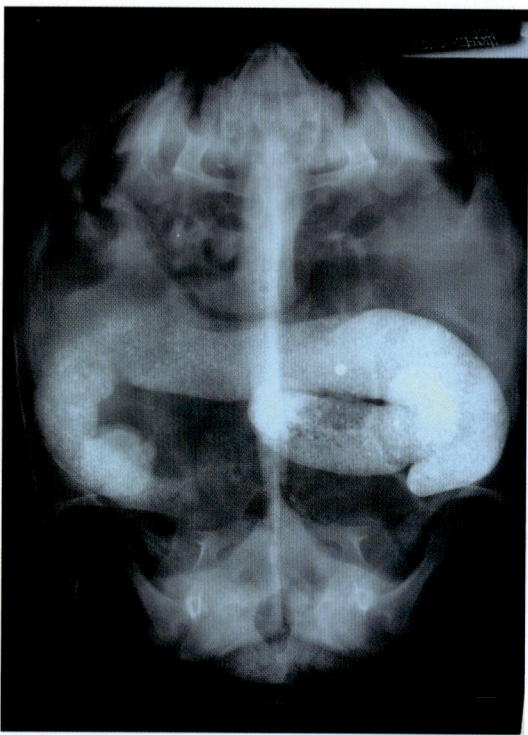

FIG 7.31 Radiograph of sand in transverse colon and descending colon; both act as foreign body traps because they are more ventrally dependent. There is also urocystolith in the left limb of the bladder. (Courtesy of Thomas H. Boyer.)

semisolid state, requiring much less water (ureo-uricotelic to urico-telic).[27] These differences make detection of kidney disease on the basis of mammalian markers, such as blood urea nitrogen (BUN) and creatinine, more difficult in chelonians. Healthy carnivorous sea turtles maintain very high plasma BUN blood urea nitrogen (BUN) concentrations in comparison to most other vertebrates and other chelonians (e.g., often >100 mg/dL), perhaps to aid in osmoregulation in a hypertonic environment as seen in elasmobranchs. Healthy herbivorous tortoises have basic urine, while tortoises in a catabolic state may have acidic urine, but again, this is not specific to renal disease. Urine pH of two healthy captive hawksbill turtles (14 urine samples) was 5.9 to 6.2, as expected for a carnivore.[38]

The urinary bladder opens into the urodeum of the cloaca. A fold separates the coprodeum from the urodeum, which has openings to the ureters, oviducts or vas deferens, the bladder, and, if present, accessory urinary bladders. Terrestrial chelonians have the largest urinary bladders of all chelonians; the bladder is bilobed with a thin, membranous, distensible, ciliated, mucus secreting wall and used for water storage and potassium/sodium ion exchange during drought.[17,18] Aquatic turtles have smaller bladders with thicker walls.[17] The cloaca, colon, and urinary bladder can reabsorb urinary water across a concentration gradient, which can increase urine osmolality but still not above that of plasma.[27] Bladder prolapses are not uncommon with uroliths or colonic foreign bodies and can be reduced endoscopically, if acute.

The paired gonads are located anterior to the kidney. Fertilization is internal in chelonians. Sexual maturity is reached by 15 years in the wild and often much sooner under captive conditions, probably more a function of size than age. Reproductive physiology has been closely studied in *Gopherus* spp. Seasonal patterns for testosterone, estrogen, and progesterone, summarized here, are similar to those reported in other species.[39,40] Spermatogenesis is temperature- and testosterone-dependent, all rising in the spring/summer and falling in the fall/winter. However, spermatazoa may be retained through the winter in the epididymis and released during the following spring's mating season. In temperate and subtropical species, ovulation occurs in the spring following emergence. Sperm are stored, for months to years, by the female in the albumin gland region within the isthmus of the oviduct, where fertilization occurs. Following fertilization, this same area produces membranes and albumin layers around the developing ovum. Further down the widening oviduct, the shell gland produces shell membranes and the eggshell; the eggs are held here as new eggs are added bilaterally until oviposition.

Each ovary has a hierarchy of follicles at different stages of development.[17] Small white previtellogenic follicles secrete estradiol in response to pituitary gonadotropin. Estradiol stimulates the liver to secrete vitellogenic protein, which is taken up by the maturing enlarging yellow follicles, typically in the fall, sometimes in the spring. Nesting female sea turtles have higher concentrations of total protein, albumin, globulin, calcium, phosphorus, triglycerides, and cholesterol.[41] Testosterone appears to regulate seasonal reproduction in both males and females. Follicular testosterone production increases as the follicles mature and increase in size. In females, there is a biphasic increase in testosterone associated with spring and fall mating. As testosterone falls after ovulation, females become nonreceptive to breeding and avoid males. Ovulation occurs after courtship and mating, then again within days of nesting, associated with luteinizing hormone and progesterone surges. Chelonians may produce single or multiple clutches of eggs in a given breeding season depending on the species. Sea turtles generally migrate to nesting beaches and produce multiple clutches over a several-week period, separated by 2 or more years of nonreproductive activity. Arginine vasotocin peaks during the first oviposition, returning to baseline within an hour. After nesting season, any fully mature follicles that haven't ovulated

undergo atresia. Atresia is a process of yolk resorption, and as the follicle reduces in size it eventually becomes a corpora albicans. Repeated folliculogenesis and atresia without production of eggs may lead to egg yolk coelomitis. In temperate species, thyroxine (T_4) levels peak in both sexes following hibernation emergence; males undergo a second peak in late summer as male combat and spermatogenesis return.

Male chelonians possess a single, large, smooth, dark-colored, expansile, spade-shaped phallus (Fig. 7.32). When not erect, the phallus lies in the ventral floor of the proctodeum and is not used for urine transport (no urethra). Females have a much smaller clitoris in the same area. When engorged, the muscular phallus extends from the cloaca and can reach as much as half the length of the shell, with a seminal groove for transport of sperm. Laypersons understandably often mistake an engorged phallus for another organ prolapse. No inversion of the phallus occurs as it does in squamates.[27] The distal proctodeum can entrap uroliths or eggs, which can be broken down and accessed per cloacal manipulation.

Male chelonians often vocalize during copulation or masturbation, causing uninformed owners to suspect that something is wrong with their tortoise. Intermittent cloacal hemorrhage resulting from phallus lacerations associated with breeding or masturbation may require surgical intervention. Under general anesthesia, the phallus is often the last area of the turtle body to be desensitized unless intrathecal local anesthesia is utilized.

Chelonians are oviparous, with either soft flexible eggshells, or, more commonly, hard-shelled eggs. Depending on species, clutches may consist of single or multiple eggs, with some very large species producing dozens of eggs per clutch. Temperature-dependent sex determination occurs in most chelonians, which typically produces females at higher

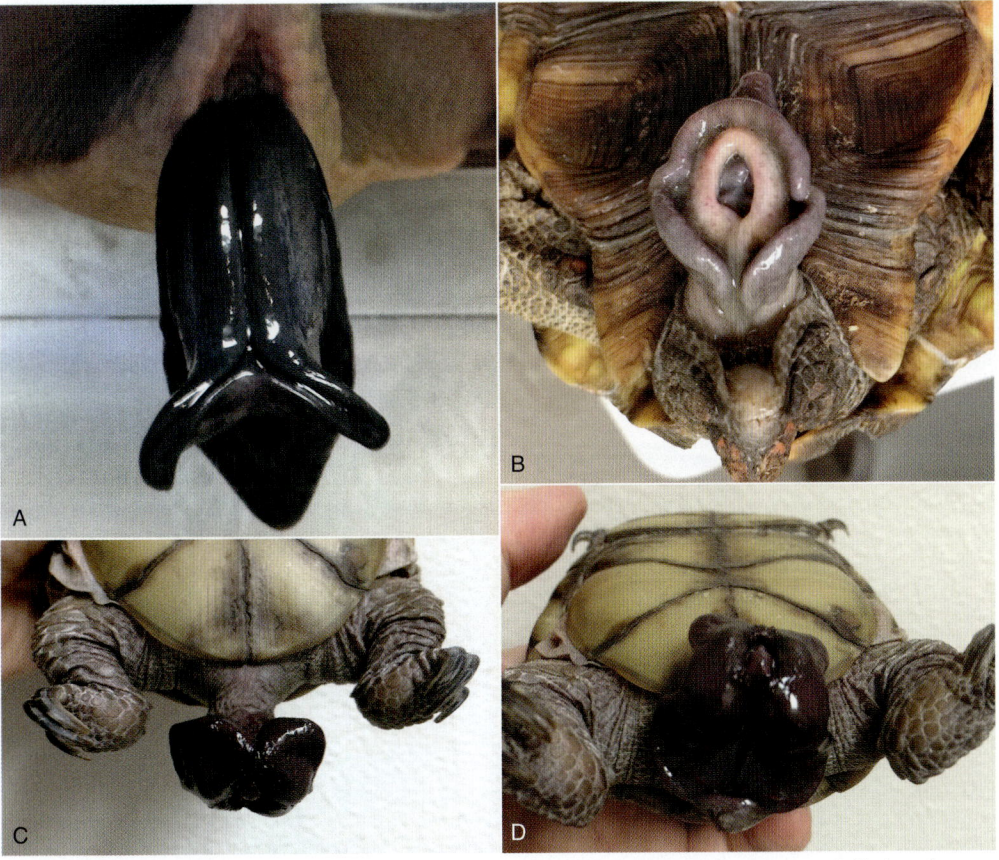

FIG 7.32 Chelonians have large phalluses (A–D) that, when fully engorged, can span half the plastron. (Courtesy of Thomas H. Boyer.)

temperatures and males at lower temperatures (pattern Ia) during early to mid incubation. However, other species produce females at both high and low temperatures and males at intermediate temperatures (pattern II). With temperature-dependent sex determination the smaller gender typically occurs at cooler temperatures, males for pattern Ia and females for pattern II.[42] Some turtles have genetic sex determination, such as the common snake-necked turtle (*Chelodina longicollis*) and the wood turtle (*Glyptemys insculpta*).[32,42] To produce both sexes, pivotal species-dependent temperatures are somewhere between 27° to 31°C (81°–88°F).

Sexual Dimorphism

Sexual dimorphism is known to occur in most postpubertal chelonians. Where present, differences can be seen in coloration, tail or claw length, size, and shell shape. Perhaps the most obvious form of sexual dimorphism is tail length and shell shape (Fig. 7.33). In many species, to facilitate intromission, mature males have longer, thicker tails, a more distal vent, a curved or concave plastron, and, if present, an anal notch on the plastron that is narrower and deeper than that of the female (Fig. 7.34). In contrast, females have shorter tails that abruptly taper

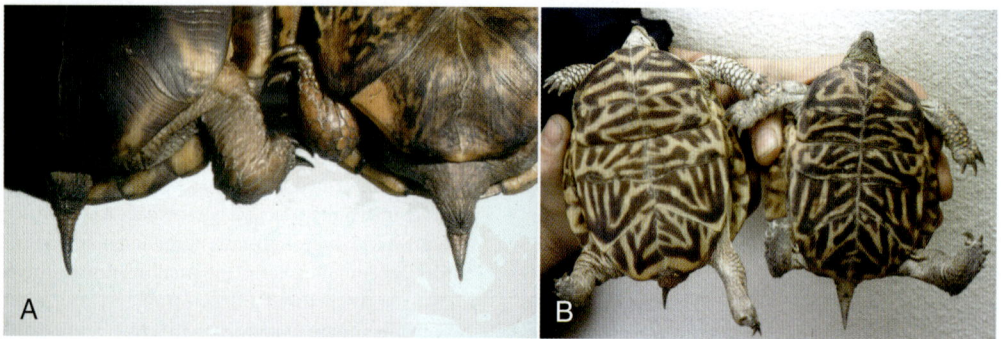

FIG 7.33 One of the most consistent distinguishing characteristics between mature male and female chelonians is the length of the tail. (A) The male (on the right in both photographs) box turtle *(Terrapene carolina)* has a longer broader tail, and the cloacal opening is beyond the margin of the carapace. (B) The female (on the left in both photographs) ornate box turtle *(Terrapene ornata ornata)* has a cloacal opening within the margin of the carapace. These differences are not apparent in juveniles. (Courtesy of Thomas H. Boyer.)

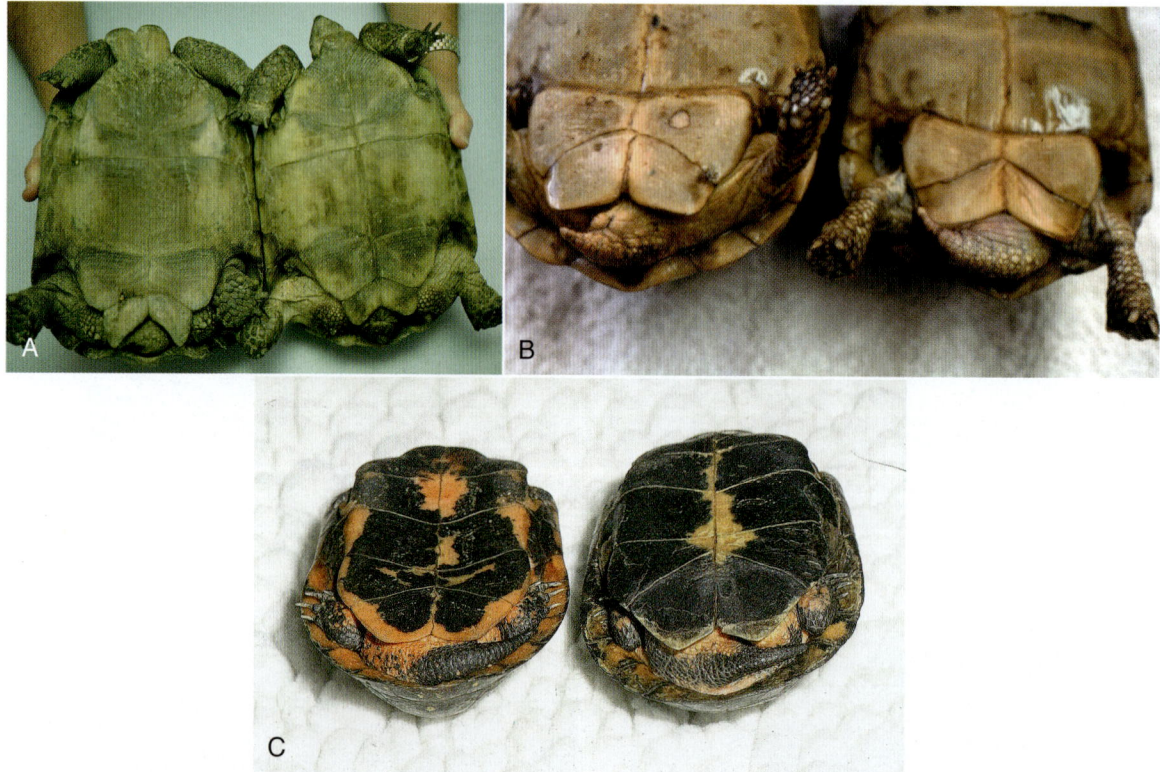

FIG 7.34 (A) In *Gopherus* species, the male (left) has a large epiplaston projection, a deeper V to the anal notch, and a concave plastron. (B) The male Egyptian tortoise *(Testudo kleinmanni*, on right) has a longer thicker tail. (C) Both spotted turtles *(Clemmys guttata)* have long tails, but notice the male's tail touches the rear leg while the female's does not, and the male has a concavity to his plastron (on left). (Courtesy of Thomas H. Boyer.)

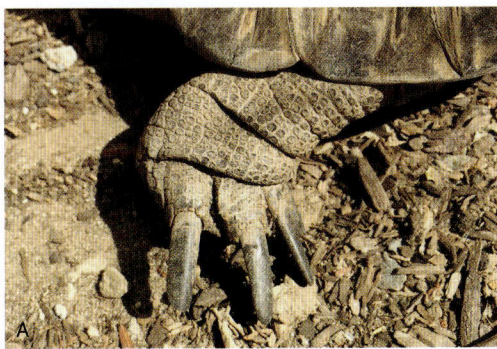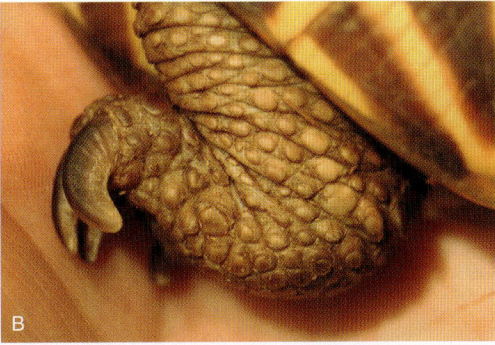

FIG 7.35 (A) Sexually mature female leopard tortoises (*Stigmochelys pardalis*) have elongated rear claws, perhaps as an aid to nest digging, and males do not. These claws should not be trimmed. (B) The inner rear claw of the male three-toed box turtle (*Terapene c. triunguis*) is thickened and curved inward to aid clasping the female's shell during intromission. (Courtesy of Thomas H. Boyer.)

posterior to the vent, the vent is cranial to the carapace margin, plastron is usually flat, and the anal notch wider and shallower, perhaps as an aid to oviposition (see Fig. 7.34). With the onset of sexual maturity, these differences may allow for easy sex identification, especially with both sexes present. Often these differences are subtle, and sex identification is very difficult prior to sexual maturity; however, endoscopic sex identification is possible. Males sometimes evert their phallus during defecation or cloacal manipulation.

A difference in size between the sexes is common among cryptodiran turtles. In 70% of 50 taxa examined by Fitch,[43] females were significantly larger, especially in highly aquatic species. Males were larger in 22% of the taxa, and in the remaining 8%, the sexes were equal in size. In general, females are typically larger in smaller-sized species and males are larger in larger-sized species and in terrestrial forms.[32,43]

Many male aquatic turtles have elongated foreclaws that they use to court females. Forelimb claw length is dimorphic in *Trachemys*, *Pseudemys*, *Chrysemys*, and *Graptemys*. Male three-toed box turtles (*Terapene c. triunguis*) have a thickened, curved inner rear claw (Fig. 7.35), and males of some marine species have a hooked claw on the front flipper. These claws allow the male to hold onto the female during copulation. Sexually mature female leopard tortoises (*Stigmochelys pardalis*) have elongated rear claws, perhaps as an aid for nest digging (see Fig. 7.35). Chin (or mental) glands, unique to *Gopherus*, are more developed in males than females, vary seasonally under testosterone influence, and are largest during the fall breeding season (Fig. 7.36). Chin glands ooze long chain fatty acids, which are thought to identify conspecifics and establish rank and territory during courtship and mating.[44]

Sexual dichromatism is especially common among the emydid and geomydid turtles. Mature males and females may differ in coloration of the head, iris, chin, or markings on the head. A well-known example in the box turtle is the bright red iris of males compared with the yellow to reddish brown iris of females (Fig. 7.37). Some of these differences are observable only in males during the breeding season; for example, breeding male bataguids have much more colorful heads than females (Fig. 7.38).

Cardiovascular System

Chelonians have four-chambered hearts[45,46] consisting of one sinus venosus, two atria, and one ventricle with three subchambers (cavas), which effectively segregate oxygenated and deoxygenated blood. Heart location moves caudally with neck retraction. The heart is situated on midline except in Trionychidae, which have a more flattened carapace,

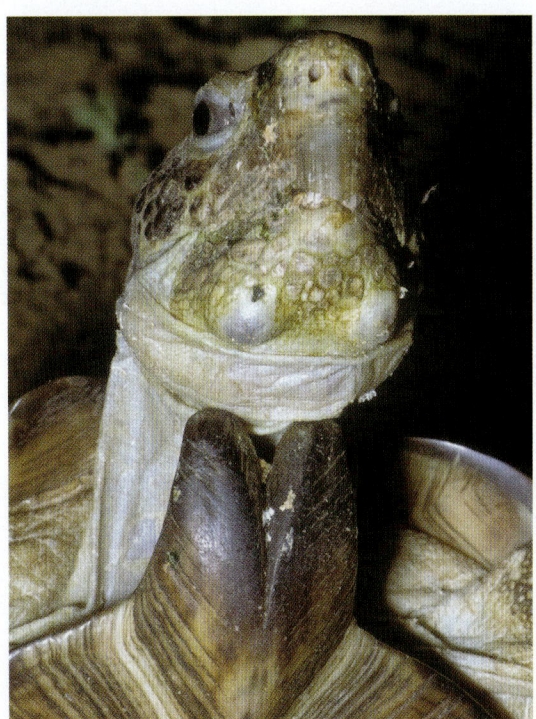

FIG 7.36 Chin, or mental glands, are more prominent in male *Gopherus* spp., enlarge during the breeding season under the influence of testosterone, and are used to identify conspecifics and mark territory. (Courtesy of Thomas H. Boyer.)

and, perhaps to make more room for neck retraction, the heart and liver are displaced to the right with the stomach on the left.[45] The heart is bathed in clear colorless to slightly yellow pericardial fluid within the pericardial sac and bordered laterally by the acromium and coracoid processes.[46] Comparatively there is more pericardial fluid than one sees in mammals. A ligamentous gubernaculum cordis attaches from the ventricular apex to the posterior pericardial sac and serves as the anchor for the ventricle.[45,46] The pericardial sac is contiguous ventrally with the coelomic membrane. Surgeons should be aware that a ventral midline, anterioposterior, coelomic membrane incision can inadvertently enlarge into the pericardial sac, which can be repaired or avoided. Deoxygenated blood returns to the dorsally located, thin-walled, but muscular, sinus

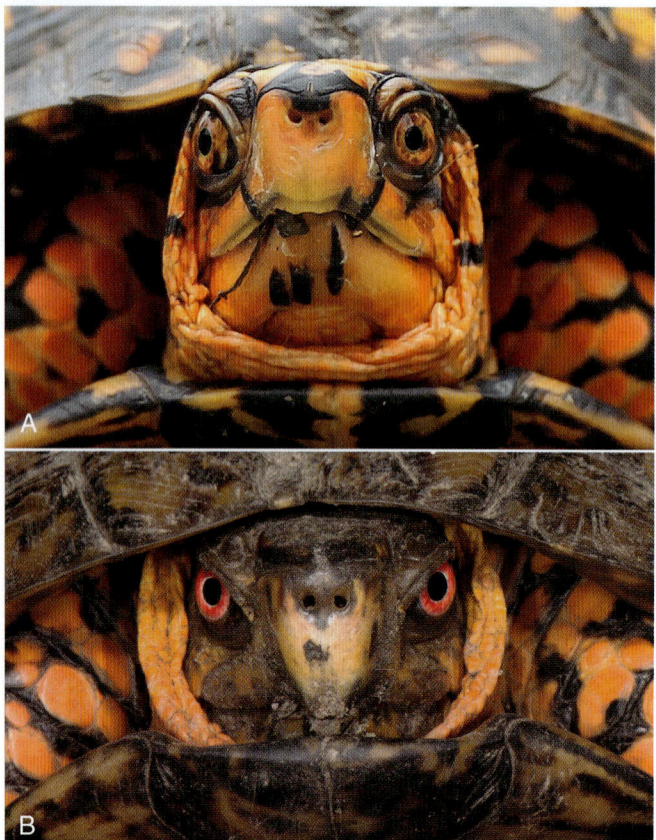

FIG 7.37 Female box turtles have yellow, yellow-brown, or red-brown irises (A), compared to the bright red irises of the male (B). (Courtesy of Stephen Barten.)

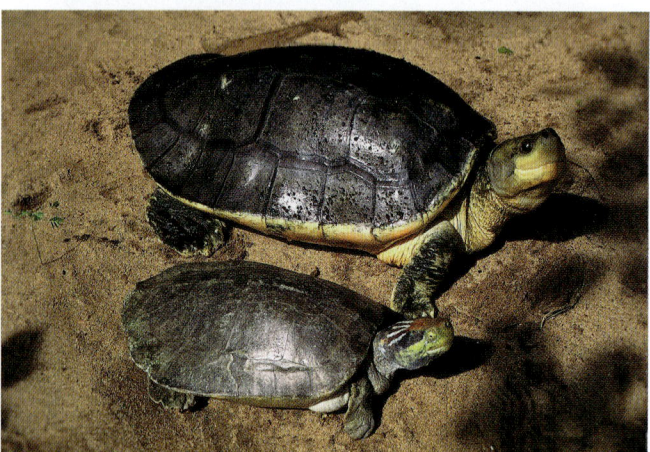

FIG 7.38 Male Batagurs are sexually dichromatic during the breeding season. Notice the brightly colored head of this male Indian red-crowned roof turtle (*Batagur kachuga*) compared to the larger female. (Courtesy of Donal M. Boyer.)

venosus, which receives blood from the right and left cranial vena cavas, caudal vena cava, and the left hepatic vein.[47] The sinus venosus has cardiac muscle that acts as a cardiac pacemaker, and size varies considerably between genera.[45] The right atrium is considerably larger than the left atrium and neither has auricles. Three great vessels arise from the

ventricle, including two aortas and the common pulmonary artery or trunk. The left-most trunk is the pulmonary artery, which splits into pulmonary arteries to each lung. The middle trunk, the left aorta, supplies blood to the viscera. The third, the right aorta, is obscured ventrally at its base by a brachiocephalic artery or trunk that immediately arises from it. The brachiocephalic trunk, or artery, supplies blood to the head and limbs and bifurcates into the large subclavian arteries, which are good landmarks for the thyroid gland located between them, just anterior to the heart.[46,47] The left and right aortae curve posteriodorsally to rejoin caudal to the heart and form the dorsal aorta.

Chelonians are capable of remarkable apnea (see neurology and pulmonology). During apnea of diving, the heart rate and pulmonary blood flow decrease by 50% and 80%, respectively, with a 150% increase in pulmonary resistance, resulting in a 50% or more intracardiac R-to-L shunt. During air breathing, heart rate and pulmonary blood flow increase two- and three-fold, respectively, which results in a net L-to-R shunt.[48] Baseline mean arterial and systolic pressures, ± SD, of six gopher tortoises (*Gopherus polyphemus*) were 56 ± 10 mmHg and 65 ± 11 mmHg, respectively.[49]

Renal portal systems exist in chelonians, as in other reptiles (see nephrology). The clinical significance of this is debatable; however, drugs are often given in the front half of the body to avoid the potential for renal toxicity or accelerated clearance of drugs excreted by tubular secretion.

Nervous System

Like other vertebrates, turtles have a central nervous system (CNS) consisting of the brain and spinal cord and a peripheral nervous system, which transmits signals between the CNS and the remainder of the body (see neurology). The turtle brain includes the typical vertebrate components, including the olfactory bulb, cerebral cortex, thalamus, hypothalamus, pituitary, optic lobes, cerebellum, and medulla.[50] While in most reptiles the neocortex is lacking, in chelonians, there is some evidence that the dorsal cortex is homologous to the neocortex of mammals.[51] The brain is well protected within the osseous brain case, which is surrounded by the more superficial but very dense bones of the skull. Accessing the brain during postmortem investigation can be challenging, especially in very large individuals. The spinal cord is surrounded by vertebrae as in other species, including the mobile cervical and coccygeal vertebrae, as well as the fixed vertebrae that are incorporated into the carapace. As a result, traumatic midline carapace injuries may affect the spinal cord. The brain and spinal cord are surrounded by two meningeal layers, including the inner leptomeninx and the outer dura mater. Cerebrospinal fluid (CSF) fills the space between these meninges, and this is the space that is targeted for intrathecal injections of analgesics or anesthetics, as well as cerebrospinal fluid collection. Reptiles lack a subarachnoid space. The epidural space is generally rich in vascular supply but does not contain CSF.[50] The brains of some turtle species have evolved a suite of physiological mechanisms to be extremely tolerant of hypoxia or even anoxia.[52] For example, one study found that painted turtles (*Chrysemys picta*) submerged in hypoxic water at 3°C survived for an average of 126 days, with some surviving as long as 177 days.[53]

Chelonians have the typical 12 cranial nerves as seen in other vertebrates, and some authors also include the nervous terminalis, or nerve 0, in the list of reptilian cranial nerves.[50] The cranial nerves are involved with olfaction, vision, taste, hearing, balance, and movement of the eye, facial muscles, tongue, pharynx, glottis, neck, and shoulders. In addition, nerve X, the vagus, has its typical role in regulation of the heart and viscera. Cranial nerve examination and general neurologic examination methods[54–58] are effective for chelonians, although some responses (e.g., olfaction) may be difficult to determine.[55]

Nonreproductive Endocrine System

The thyroid gland is unpaired and located just anterior to the heart. Anterior to the thyroid gland is the thymus. The thymus does not involute as in mammals and is not part of the endocrine system. Chelonians have two pairs of parathyroid glands, one pair within the thymus, one pair near the aortic arch. Parathyroid hormones regulate calcium and phosphorus metabolism. Also found with the caudal parathyroid glands are miniscule paired ultimobranchial bodies, which are homologous with the thyroid parafollicular cells of mammals that secrete calcitonin.[17] The adrenal glands are located retrocoelomically just cranial to the kidneys and produce catecholamines, glucocorticoids, and mineralocorticoids. Increased corticosterone concentrations have been documented in chelonians under physical or physiological stress.[59] The pituitary gland produces nine hormones and is found just below the optic chiasma in the sella tursica of the sphenoid bone.[17] The chelonian pancreas serves the typical vertebrate endocrine functions of insulin and glucagon production.

Special Senses and Salt Glands

Chelonians lack a parietal eye, but do have a pineal gland that may affect behavior, gonadal activity, and thermoregulation.[17] The sense of smell is well developed; terrestrial chelonians have large olfactory bulbs and a modified Jacobson's organ. Chelonians have excellent hearing, especially freshwater emydid species, even though they have no external ears.[7] Chelonians respond to low tones ranging from 100 to 700 Hz,[51] good for sensing ground vibrations and predator approach. Sea turtles appear to be most sensitive to underwater acoustic stimuli below 1000 Hz, suggesting that sea turtles are able to detect much of the low-frequency and high-intensity anthropogenic sound in the ocean, including shipping, pile driving, low-frequency active sonar, and oil and gas exploration and extraction.[60] Chelonians have a large middle and internal ear beneath the tympanic membrane, just caudal to the angle of the jaw, with a large bony case surrounding them. Sound reception involves the tympanic membrane, the attached extracolumella cartilaginous footplate, and the thin osseous columella, which connects to the inner ear. The Eustachian, or auditory tube, connects the inner ear to the oropharynx.

Freshwater turtles are more far-sighted than terrestrial species, and both react more to movement than shape. Cones are the predominant photoreceptors, typical for predominantly day-active animals. Color vision is especially good for red, yellow, and orange wavelengths, which may partially explain chelonian attraction to colorful foods.[7,32] The retina is avascular but does have a vascular projection from the optic nerve, the conus papillaris. Chelonians have upper and lower eyelids, a nictitating membrane (greatly reduced in Carettochelys) and scleral ossicles surround the globe. The iris is composed of skeletal muscle. Red-eared sliders possess slow pupillary light reflexes (PLRs). Direct pupil diameter decreased by 31% from 36 to 72 seconds, and consensual pupil diameter

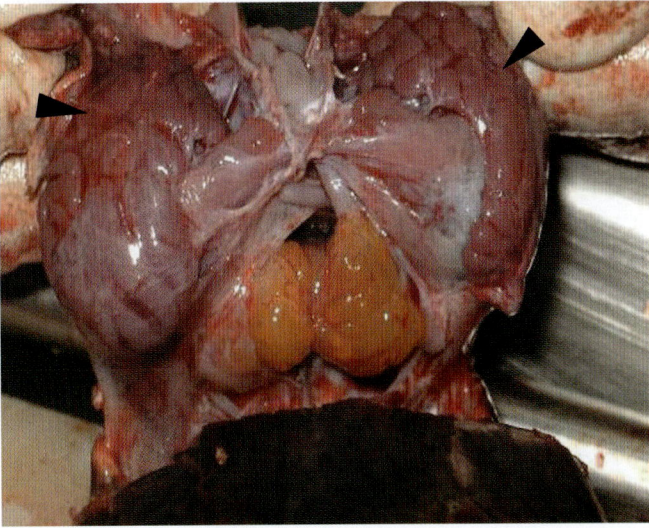

FIG 7.39 Necropsy of a Kemp's Ridley sea turtle (*Lepidochelys kempii*) in which the anterior portion of the skull has been removed to expose the large periocular salt glands (arrowheads). (Courtesy of Charles J. Innis.)

decreased by 11% from 85 to 120 seconds.[61] Given the small size of chelonian eyes, without specialized testing equipment, PLRs can be difficult to observe. Intraoccular pressure has been measured in several species (see ophthalmology). The craniomedial Harderian and caudomedial lacrimal glands produce the tear film. These glands and ducts are prone to obstruction and cystic enlargement in carnivorous and some omnivorous chelonians with hypovitaminosis A. Herbivorous chelonians can synthesize vitamin A endogenously. Chelonians have no nasolacrimal ducts, so tears spill over lid margins, which is especially pronounced in sea turtles and red-footed (*Chelonoidis carbonaria*) and yellow-footed tortoises (*Chelonoidis denticulata*). Tears are also lost by evaporation or conjunctival tissue absorption.[17]

In sea turtles and diamondback terrapins, the lacrimal gland has evolved into a salt-excreting gland (Fig. 7.39). These glands function along with the kidneys to regulate plasma electrolytes in the presence of a hypertonic environment. Plasma osmolality and concentrations of sodium, chloride, potassium, and magnesium can be influenced by salt gland function.[62]

REFERENCES

See www.expertconsult.com for a complete list of references.

8

Snake Taxonomy, Anatomy, and Physiology

Richard S. Funk and James E. Bogan, Jr.

Of the approximately 3400 species of living snakes (see http://www.reptile -database.org/), relatively few are well known in nature, and some are threatened with extinction. For example, the unique Round Island burrowing boa (*Bolyeria multocarinata*) has become extinct in recent times due to soil erosion and general habitat decline.[1] Snake species seen by practicing veterinarians are mainly from three families, the Boidae, Pythonidae, and Colubridae (Fig. 8.1). We cannot assume the anatomy and physiology is the same for all these species, and we must keep in mind that we are extrapolating drug dosages and clinical therapies based on research from relatively few species.

Snakes and lizards are related and classified together in the order Squamata. Snakes are subgrouped into the clade Ophidia, which contains a dozen clades of extinct, prehistoric snakes, as well as the suborder Serpentes, which includes modern snakes.[2] Among the more than 70 anatomical features shared by lizards and snakes are the paired copulatory organs, the hemipenes, located in the base of the tail. Limb reduction has occurred in at least 25 lineages among the Squamata.[3] In pythons the presence of more than 300 precloacal vertebrae, limb loss, body elongation, and loss of axial regionalization are a result of the expression of Hox (homeobox) genes; the Hox genes for thoracic development are expressed but those programming for forelimb development are not.[4,5]

Snakes are limbless with a rigid braincase that has the frontal and parietal bones articulating with the sphenoid bones and a kinetic skull with a joint between the frontals and the nasal region. They lack external ear openings and a tympanum. The ophthalmic branch of the trigeminal nerve enters the orbit via the optic foramen, whereas in other squamates it enters the orbit posteriorly. They have many precloacal vertebrae, from 120 to more than 400, with no regional differentiation posterior to the atlas and axis. Snake eyes have no scleral ossicles and no muscle in the ciliary body, and the eye is covered with a transparent spectacle or reduced and covered with a scale. They have no dermal osteoderms.[5–7] Within a snake's elongated body, paired organs are also elongated and tend to be staggered with one cranial to the other.

Among the snakes are species that mature at less than 10 cm (4 inches) in total length, and those that attain huge proportions of several meters and consume large prey. Much discussion and publicity centers around the so-called giant snakes. Many of the records of truly huge snakes remain dubious and unsubstantiated, because they are poorly documented. A review of the literature on giant snakes lists the four species that probably exceed 6 m (20 ft) in total length: the anaconda (*Eunectes murinus*) of South America, the Burmese python (*Python bivittatus*) of Southeast Asia, the reticulated python (*Malayopython reticulatus*) of Southeast Asia, and the African Rock Python (*Python sebae*) of Africa.[8,9] The two largest species are the anaconda and the reticulated Python, both of which approach 9 m (30 ft), but no valid records are seen of either beyond that length. An anaconda has a greater girth and mass than a reticulated python of the same length.

In captivity many snakes can live for over 20 years, with the record being a 47.5-year-old ball python (*Python regius*) at the Philadelphia Zoo.[10]

This discussion of snake biology focuses on the clinically significant aspects of their lives for an appreciation of their uniqueness and diversity. Few disease conditions are mentioned in this discussion because they are covered elsewhere in this volume.

TAXONOMY

Snake systematics is constantly changing. Difficulties occur when trying to arrange snakes into a meaningful higher classification because of a poor fossil record. Additionally, because snakes have evolved an elongated body adapted to a crawling mode of existence, they have relatively few external features, thus systematists have relied heavily on features of internal morphology. More recently, molecular data have been analyzed to elucidate the relationships among the living snakes.

Snakes are characterized by features that are shared with lizards. Recent trends in phylogenetics, considering both morphologic and molecular data, place the lizards, snakes, and tuataras in the clade Lepidosauria, as a sister taxon to the Archosauria, which includes chelonians, crocodilians, and birds.[5,11–14]

The classification listed here differs dramatically from that presented in the second edition of this text, particularly in recognizing new families and subfamilies. Molecular analyses of snakes reveal major departures from previous phylogenies that were based primarily upon morphology. The most recent and thorough phylogeny is based upon analyzing nuclear and mitochondrial DNA of 4161 squamate species, including all known families and subfamilies of snakes,[11] and appears to be the most accurate reflection of relationships of extant snakes. Table 8.1 summarizes this classification.

A brief listing of the content and some characteristics of the higher snake taxa may be useful in appreciating the diversity of living species. Brief listings are also given of their geographical distributions. The * indicates families most often seen in herpetoculture (Figs. 8.2 to 8.16).

Infraorder Scolecophidia: The Blind Snakes

These snakes have blunt heads, short tails, vestigial eyes with only rods, and a multilobed liver, and the lower jaws are attached to each other anteriorly. They are fossorial and oviparous, have smooth scales with no enlarged ventral scales, and eat invertebrates, especially ants and termites.

Family Anomalepididae: Dawn blind snakes. Four genera, 15 species, Central and South America. These may prove to be a sister taxon to all other living snakes and not be scolecophidians.

Family Leptotyphlopidae: Thread snakes. Four genera, 50+ species. Southwest United Sates through South America, Africa, and Southwest Asia. Unique among vertebrates in having a mandibular mechanism used to rake food into the mouth.

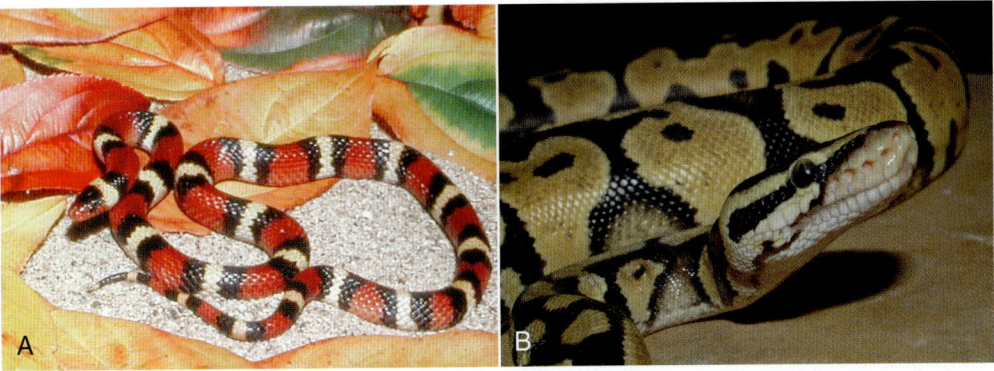

FIG 8.1 The two most common groups of snakes seen by veterinarians in clinical practice are colubrids, such as (A) the scarlet king snake (*Lampropeltis elapsoides*) and boids, such as (B) the ball python (*Python regius*).

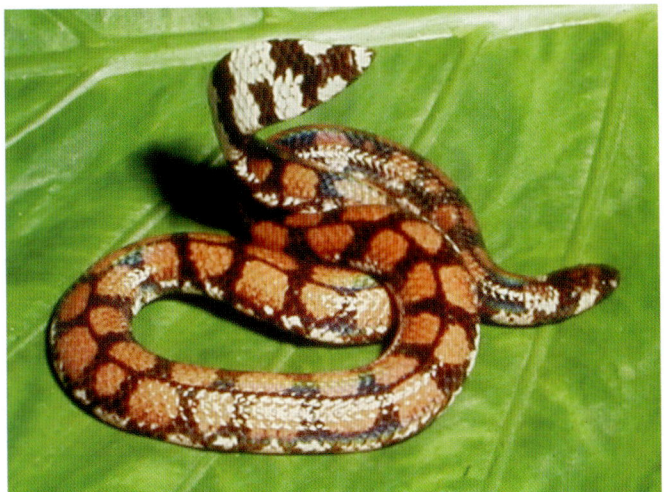

FIG 8.2 This adult Sri Lankan pipe snake (*Cylindrophis maculatus*) of the family Cylindrophidae exhibits automimicry with a flattened, elevated tail that is slowly moved in a side-to-side fashion. These viviparous snakes eat relatively large, elongated prey.

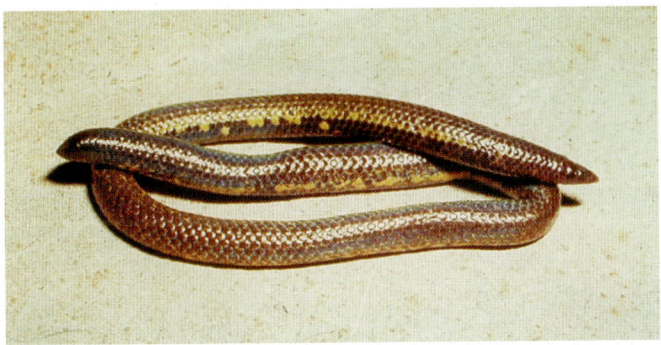

FIG 8.3 Sri Lankan shield-tail snake (*Uropeltis phillipsi*) of the family Uropeltidae. The head is the small pointed end. The soil adheres to the robust tail and helps block the burrow from behind.

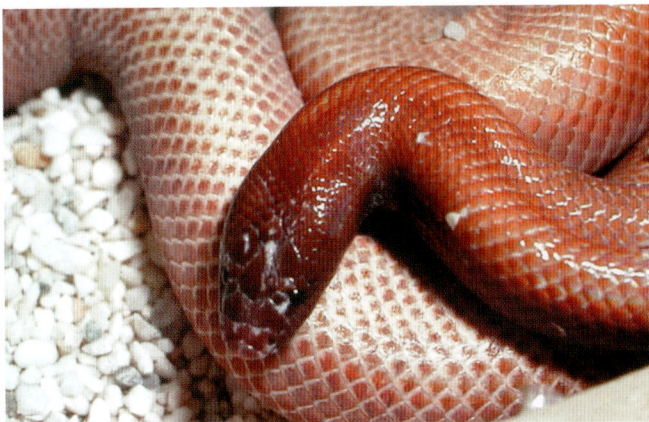

FIG 8.4 Neotropical sunbeam snake (*Loxocemus bicolor*) was formerly called the "new world python." This oviparous and fossorial snake feeds on lizards, reptile eggs, and rodents.

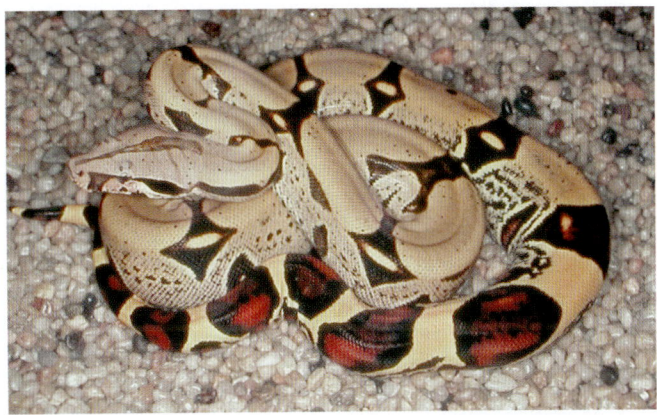

FIG 8.5 Boa constrictor (*Boa constrictor*), a common pet snake, is generally considered docile. It is now available in a number of colors and patterns. Although these snakes can attain lengths of more than 3 m (10 ft), most do not grow that large.

Family Gerrhopilidae: Blind snakes. One genus, 15 species. Indonesia, New Guinea, Southeast Asia, India.

Family Xenotyphlopidae: Malagasy blind snakes. One genus, Madagascar.

Family Typhlopidae: Cosmopolitan blind snakes. Ten genera, more than 250 species. Worldwide in tropical climes. One parthenogenetic species also becoming worldwide.

Infraorder Alethinophidia

Now defined to include all of the living snakes except the blind snakes. These snakes have a kinetic skull and share other important details of morphology. A diverse variety of sizes and habitats.

Family Aniliidae: South American or red and black pipe snakes. One species. Northern South America.

TABLE 8.1 Higher Classification of Living Snakes (Suborder Serpentes)

Infraorder Scolecophidia
Family Anomalepididae
Family Leptotyphlopidae
Family Gerrhopilidae
Family Xenotyphlopidae
Family Typhlopidae

Infraorder Alethinophidia
Family Aniliidae
Family Tropidophiidae
Family Xenophidiidae
Family Bolyeriidae
Family Calabariidae
Family Boidae*
    Subfamily Sanziniinae
    Subfamily Ungaliophiinae
    Subfamily Candoiinae
    Subfamily Erycinae
    Subfamily Boinae
Family Anomochilidae
Family Cylindrophiidae
Family Uropeltidae
Family Xenopeltidae*
Family Loxocemidae
Family Pythonidae*
Family Acrochordidae
Family Xenodermatidae
Family Pareatidae
Family Viperidae*
    Subfamily Viperinae
    Subfamily Azemiopinae
    Subfamily Crotalinae
Family Homalopsidae
Family Lamprophiidae*
    Subfamily Prosymniinae
    Subfamily Psammophiinae
    Subfamily Atractaspidinae
    Subfamily Aparallactinae
    Subfamily Pseudaspidinae
    Subfamily Lamprophiinae
    Subfamily Psuedoxyrhophiinae
Family Elapidae*
Family Colubridae*
    Subfamily Calamariinae
    Subfamily Pseudoxenodontinae
    Subfamily Sibynophiinae
    Subfamily Grayiinae
    Subfamily Colubrinae
    Subfamily Natricinae
    Subfamily Dipsadinae

*Indicates families most often seen in herpetoculture.

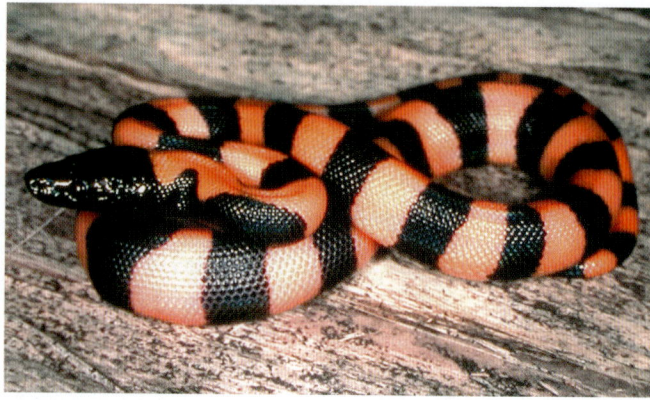

FIG 8.6 Juvenile ringed python (*Bothrochilus boa*) from the Bismarck Archipelago. An active species in which adults are brown ringed with black or uniformly brown, with high iridescence.

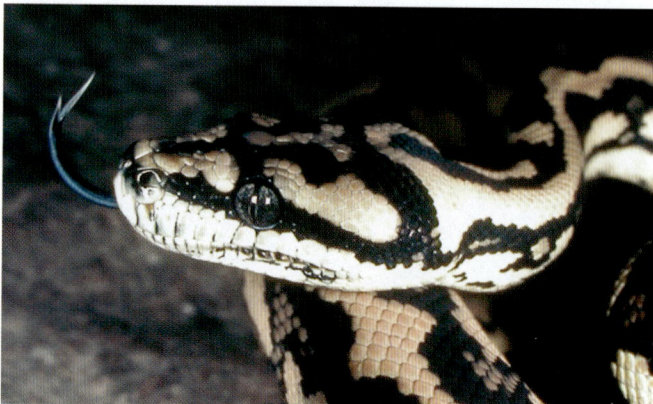

FIG 8.7 The popular carpet python (*Morelia spilotus variegatus*) is from Australia. This photo shows the typical forked tongue and also, in this case, the labial heat pits. This python typically reaches lengths of 2 m (6–7 ft).

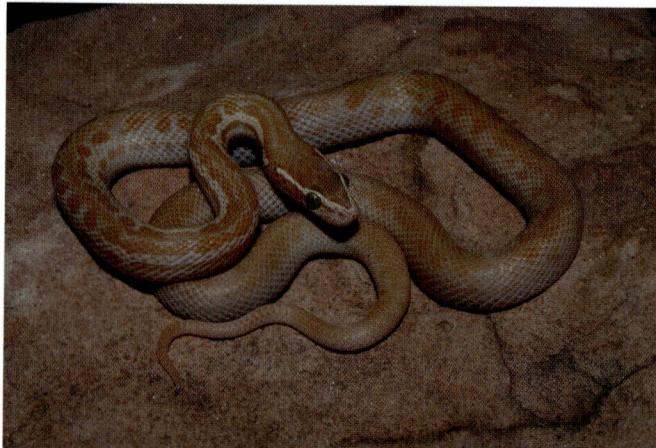

FIG 8.8 Albino house snake, *Lamprophis fuliginosis*, Lamprophiidae. A nonvenomous African snake that is hardy in captivity, producing multiple clutches per season.

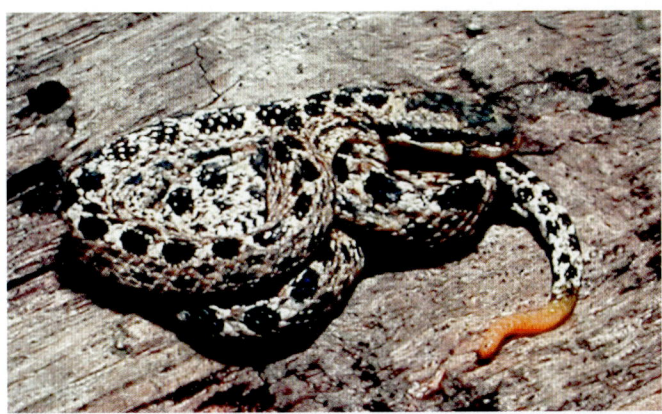

FIG 8.9 The dwarf boa (*Tropidophis canus curtus*) of the family Tropidophiidae is a live-bearing snake. Species in this genus have a defensive behavior involving flushing blood across the subspectacular space and out the mouth onto a predator (or human handler). This species possesses a yellowish tail tip that functions as a caudal lure for its prey of frogs and lizards.

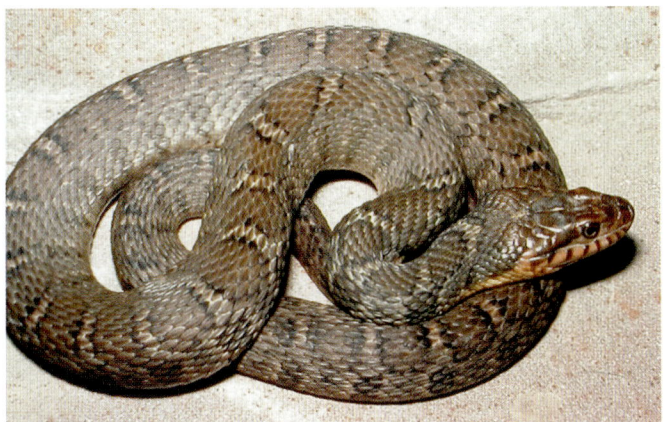

FIG 8.10 The yellow-bellied water snake (*Nerodia erythrogaster flavigaster*) is a representative of a group called Natricines, which are mostly associated with aquatic habitats. North American natricines are viviparous, but most old-world species are oviparous.

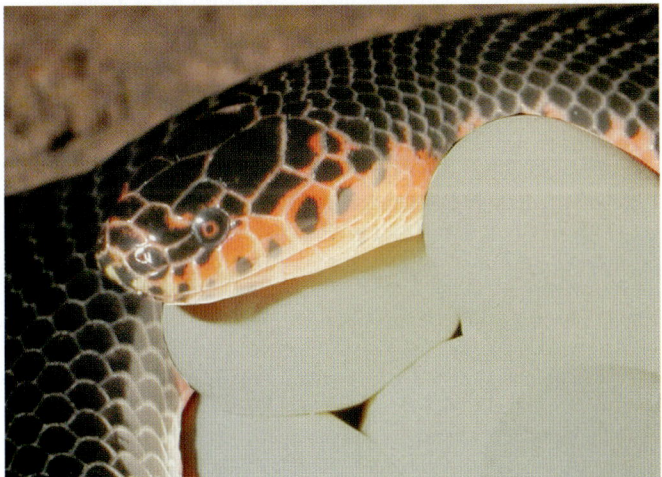

FIG 8.11 This adult mud snake (*Farancia abacura reinwardti*) is exhibiting parental care, coiling around her clutch of eggs until they hatch. This type of parental care is also seen in some pit vipers and notoriously among pythons, the latter of which thermoregulate to control their clutch's incubation temperature.

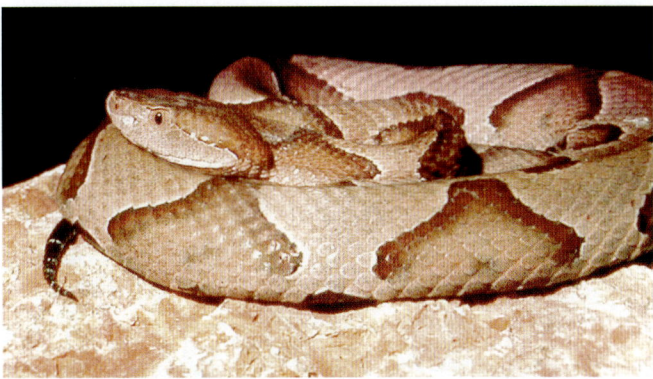

FIG 8.12 The copperhead (*Agkistrodon contortrix contortrix*) is a terrestrial pit viper from eastern United States, with a pattern that is cryptic among leaves on the ground.

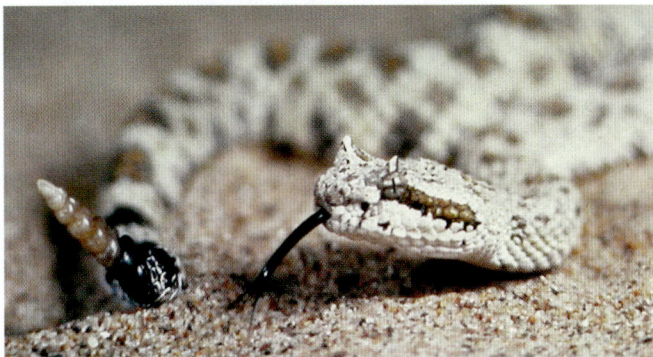

FIG 8.13 The sidewinder (*Crotalus cerastes laterorepens*) is a species of rattlesnake from the deserts of the southwestern United States. Shown are the rattle on the tail tip, facial heat pit, forked tongue, and supraocular horns that may function to keep blowing sand off the eyes. Rattlesnakes occur only in the New World, and all species are viviparous. A new rattle segment is added with each shed, and rattles may break off. Certain African vipers that sidewind also have supraocular horns.

Family Tropidophiidae: Caribbean wood snakes. Two genera, 25 to 30 species. West Indies and Central and South America. Viviparous small constrictors, most with pelvic vestiges. A unique defensive mechanism starts with ocular (subspectacular) hemorrhage that progresses to oral hemorrhage, the function of which is conjectural. Once placed within the Boidae.

Family Xenophidiidae: Spine-jaw snakes. Two species, Malaysia. They have a large anterior caninelike tooth on their dentary bone.

Family Bolyeriidae: Round Island boas. Two monotypic genera. *Bolyeria* became extinct about 1975. Unique among tetrapod vertebrates in having divided (hinged) maxillary bones. *Casarea* is oviparous. Formerly placed with the Boidae.

Family Calabariidae: Calabar ground boa. One monotypic genus. Central and West Africa. A cylindrical, mostly fossorial, oviparous constrictor with tiny eyes.

*Family Boidae: The boas. Eight genera and about 40 species. Viviparous except two oviparous species of *Eryx*. New World and Madagascar, Africa to southern Asia, and Southwest Pacific Islands. Most have infrared labial receptors. All are constrictors. Cloacal spurs present.

Subfamily Sanziniinae: Madagascan tree boas. One genus and species, Madagascar.

Subfamily Ungaliophiinae: Dwarf boas. Four genera and 5 species, now defined to include the rubber boas *Charina* and the rosy

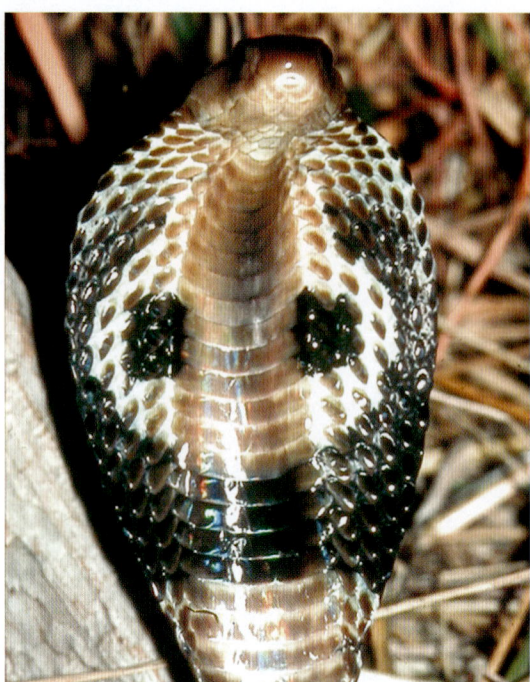

FIG 8.14 This spectacled cobra (*Naja naja*) is showing the "hood," an extended portion of the neck that can spread by expanding neck ribs laterally. Cobras are highly venomous elapids, and some species can even spit venom at a predator's (or human's) face or eyes. Cobras account for many human deaths and also figure widely in religion and folktales.

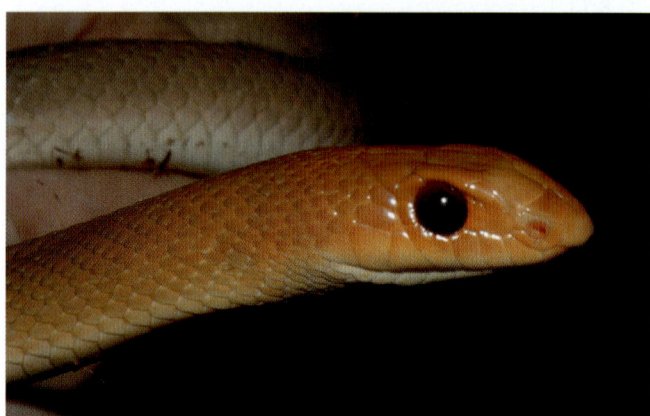

FIG 8.15 Western beaked snake (*Rhamphiopus oxyrhynchus*) Lamprophiidae. A mildly venomous terrestrial and burrowing African snake. (Courtesy of Richard S. Funk.)

boas *Lichanura* of western North America. From the United States southward to Colombia.

Subfamily Candoiinae: Pacific boas. One genus, 3 to 4 species. Southwest Pacific Islands. One is quite viperlike in habitus.

Subfamily Erycinae: Sand boas. One genus, 8 species. Central Africa through Asia to China. Viviparous with two oviparous species.

Subfamily Boinae: The boas. Central and South America, West Indies. Includes the anaconda and boa constrictor. Most with labial infrared receptors.

Family Anomochilidae: Dwarf pipe snakes. Sumatra, Bornea, Malaysia. Two species known from less than a dozen specimens. Oviparous. Have yellow or white spots and a red tail band.

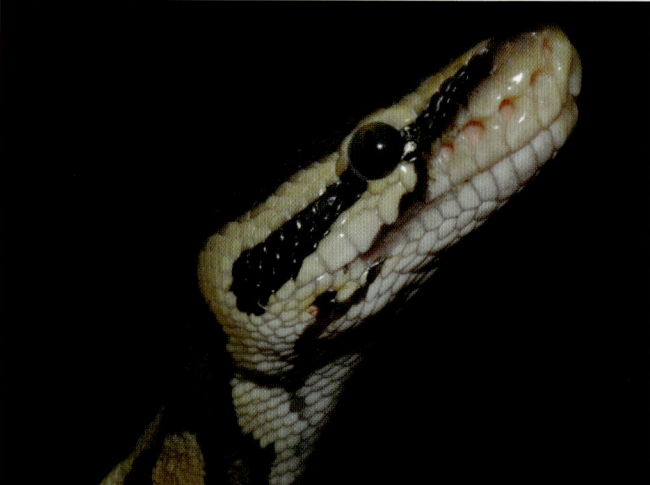

FIG 8.16 Adult ball python (*Python regius*) showing the row of facial sensory pits in the upper lip scales. (Courtesy of Richard S. Funk.)

Family Cylindrophidae: (Asian) Pipe snakes. One genus, 8 species. Sri Lanka, Southwest Asia, Indoaustralian Archipelago. Fossorial, viviparous, utilize caudal automimicry.

Family Uropeltidae: Shieldtail snakes. India and Sri Lanka. Eight genera and 50 species. Specialized burrowers with blunt tails and a unique locomotion with the skin in contact with, and pushing off of, the walls of the burrow, while the inner body is moving along relative to the skin.

*Family Xenopeltidae: Sunbeam snakes. One genus with 2 species. Southeast Asia, Burma to the Philippines. Highly iridescent fossorial snakes, constrictors, no pelvic vestiges, oviparous; hinged teeth that change ontogenetically reflecting dietary shifts, bicuspid in juveniles.

Family Loxocemidae: Neotropical sunbeam snake (called New World Python in older literature). One monotypic genus, originating from Mexico to Costa Rica. Similar to Xenopeltidae, they are also iridescent and fossorial/terrestrial constrictors with no pelvic vestiges and oviparous.

*Family Pythonidae: Pythons. Eight genera, 25 species. Africa, South Asia, Indoaustralia, and Australia. Oviparous with maternal care of the eggs. Includes several of the largest known living snakes.

Family Acrochordidae: Wart snakes or elephant trunk snakes. One genus with 3 species. India to northern Australia and Solomon Islands. Aquatic, mainly marine and brackish waters. Scales small and strongly keeled that gives them a sandpaper-like texture, with loose skin; can catch fish with body folds and skin. One species known to be parthenogenetic.

Family Xenodermatidae: Dragon snakes, tubercle snakes. Six genera, 17 species. Southern India, Indochina to Japan, Malaysia to Java, Borneo, and Sumatra. Have small eyes, over 20 maxillary teeth, and are oviparous.

Family Pareatidae: Slug-eating snakes. Three genera, 15 species. Southeast Asia to Borneo, Java, Mindanao. Oviparous slender arboreal snakes with a blunt snout, no teeth on anterior maxillary; able to pull snails from their shells with elongated mandibles and sharp teeth.

*Family Viperidae: The vipers and pit vipers. About 25 genera with 240 species. Basically, worldwide except Australia, New Guinea, and the Pacific oceanic islands. All are venomous, some highly dangerous. Solenoglyph dentition, with fang erection in a posterior-anterior direction. Includes the true vipers, pit vipers, rattlesnakes, moccasins, and their allies. Many habitats and lifestyles, both oviparous and viviparous species, including some rattlesnakes with parental care.

Subfamily Viperinae: Vipers. Thirteen genera and 90 species. Europe, Africa, and Asia. All less than 2 m in length, both oviparous and viviparous species, no loreal pit.

Subfamily Azemiopinae: Fea's viper. One monotypic genus. China, Vietnam, and Burma. Oviparous, no loreal pit.

Subfamily Crotalinae: Pit vipers. Twenty-three genera, 220 species. Southwest and southern Asia and the New World. Have a well-developed loreal pit that is infrared receptive. Both oviparous and viviparous species, some with parental care of eggs or neonates. Bushmasters (*Lachesis*, 3 species) of Central and northern South America are the longest venomous snakes and may reach 3.75 m in length.

Family Homalopsidae: Asian water snakes. Eleven genera with 40 species. South Asia southward to northern Australia. Aquatic with dorsal valvular nostrils and dorsally oriented eyes and tightly fitting labials. Viviparous and venomous with 2 to 3 grooved posterior maxillary teeth.

*Family Lamprophiidae: Stiletto snakes and mole vipers, keeled snakes. About 300 species. Subsaharan Africa and Madagascar. Diverse sizes and habitats, oviparous. Sister group to elapids.

Subfamily Prosymninae: Shovelsnout snakes. One genus, 16 species. Subsaharan Africa. Oviparous, with a diet mainly of lizard and snake eggs.

Subfamily Psamophiinae: Grass snakes. Seven genera, 50 species. Africa, South Asia, southern Europe, and the Middle East. Oviparous. Fast diurnal predators mainly of lizards, and one species purported to be the fastest snake.

Subfamily Atractaspidinae: Stiletto snakes (formerly called mole vipers). Two genera, 21 species. Subsaharan Africa, Israel, and Arabian Peninsula. Highly venomous, envenomate with a lateral and posterior jab; cannot be safely handheld.

Subfamily Aparallactinae: Centipede-eaters. Subsaharan Africa. Two genera with 50 species. Oviparous and viviparous with opisthoglyphic or proteroglyphic teeth.

Subfamily Pseudaspidinae: Mole snakes or mole vipers. Two monotypic genera. Africa, Southeast Asia, Malaysia. Viviparous.

Subfamily Lamprophiinae: House snakes, et al. Eleven genera, 70 species. Subsaharan Africa. Grouping defined mainly by molecular data. Oviparous.

Subfamily Pseudoxyrhophiinae: Malagasy brown snakes, brook snakes. Sixteen genera, 50 species. Subsaharan Africa, Madagascar, Yemen. Oviparous. Includes *Langaha* and *Lioheterodon*.

*Family Elapidae: the elapids, including cobras, kraits, taipans, death adders, mambas, coral snakes, and sea snakes. Sixty-two genera with 350 species. North, Central, and South America; Africa; southern Asia to Australia; Pacific and Indian Oceans. Proteroglyph dentition. All venomous, some not dangerous to humans but some among the deadliest. Most oviparous.

*Family Colubridae: "Common" colubrid snakes. Over 100 genera and 1800 species. Most of the world except Antarctica, Greenland, Iceland, and Ireland. Previous concepts of this family proved to be a polyphyletic assemblage of snakes. As now perceived it is a somewhat smaller but still widespread and diverse grouping. Aside from the boas and pythons, colubrids include most of the nonvenomous snakes we see in herpetoculture, such as king snakes, rat snakes, racers, garter snakes, and gopher snakes. Oviparous and viviparous.

Subfamily Calamariinae: Reed snakes. Six genera, 90 species. India, Southeast Asia, South China, Japan, and Malaysia through Indonesia and the Philippines. Fossorial.

Subfamily Pseudoxenodontinae: Bamboo snakes. Three genera, 13 species. Southeast Asia, Tibet, Taiwan, Indonesia, often at high elevations.

Subfamily Sibynophiinae: Collared or black-headed Snakes. One genus, 6 to 8 species. Southeast Asia, Malaysia, Taiwan. So-called "goo-eaters" feeding on slugs and snails. Oviparous.

Subfamily Grayiinae: African water snakes. One genus, 4 species. Subsaharan Africa, mainly aquatic, oviparous.

Subfamily Colubrinae: Common or colubrid Snakes. One hundred genera, 650 species. Worldwide as for the family. Diverse sizes and habitats, generalists and specialists, oviparous and viviparous. Includes king snakes, rat snakes, racers, and gopher snakes.

Subfamily Natricinae: Water snakes. Thirty-eight genera, 215 species. North and Central America, Africa, Eurasia, East Indies. Many are aquatic. Old World members are oviparous, New World ones viviparous. Includes *Natrix* and *Nerodia*.

Subfamily Dipsadinae: Dipsadine snakes. Ninety-seven genera, 740 species. Most of the New World. Mostly oviparous, diverse in sizes and habitats. Includes several familiar North American snakes, including *Diadophis*, *Farancia*, and *Heterodon*. Mostly oviparous.

ANATOMY AND PHYSIOLOGY

The following sections refer to Fig. 8.17.

Integument

Snake scales are essentially made of folds of the epidermis and dermis, but the scales themselves are epidermal in origin. Except for the head, they typically overlap each other. A variety of pits, ridges, keels, and tubercles, mostly of unknown function, are present on snake scales. Regional differences occur, with enlarged head shields, a series of rows of small dorsal scales covering the body and tail dorsally and laterally, as well as larger and wider ventral scales that provide support and protection ventrally. Scolecophidians and some sea snakes lack enlarged ventral scales. Most snakes have an enlarged scale or pair of scales that cover the cloacal opening. Dorsal scales are usually in odd numbers or rows, with a maximum number near midbody and fewer rows near the head and cloaca. The keratinized scales and skin protect the snake from abrasions and dehydration.

Almost no skin glands are present in snakes, but paired scent glands are characteristic (Fig. 8.18). These glands are a pair of organs located within the base of the tail, dorsal to the hemipenes in males, and they open into the posterior margin of the cloacal opening. Their unpleasant odor plays a part in defense and may also carry social signals. In captivity, they may become enlarged, impacted, or abscessed. (See Chapters 80 and 171.)

Shedding, or ecdysis, is a complex event histologically.[5,6,15–19] With hormonal input from the thyroid gland, during shedding, a synchronous proliferation of the epithelial cells from the stratum germinativum occurs. This forms a new epithelial generation between the stratum germinativum and the older outer epidermal layer. This younger epidermal layer keratinizes and comes to resemble the (older) outer layer. During separation of these two generations of epithelium, anaerobic glycolysis assists in separating the outer layer, and acid phosphatase helps break down the cementing material. The snake has a dull "blue" look to it as a thin fluid forms between the two layers (Fig. 8.19).

Herpetoculturists call their snakes "blue" or "opaque" at this time. A snake will go blue for several days, then clear up as the fluid is resorbed, and then proceed to shed its entire skin. Healthy snakes shed the entire outer layer as one event, but the older outer layer may tear during shedding especially in larger snakes. The epithelium covering the spectacles (the eye caps) are also shed together with the rest of the skin (Fig. 8.20). During this shed cycle, many snakes refuse food and seek

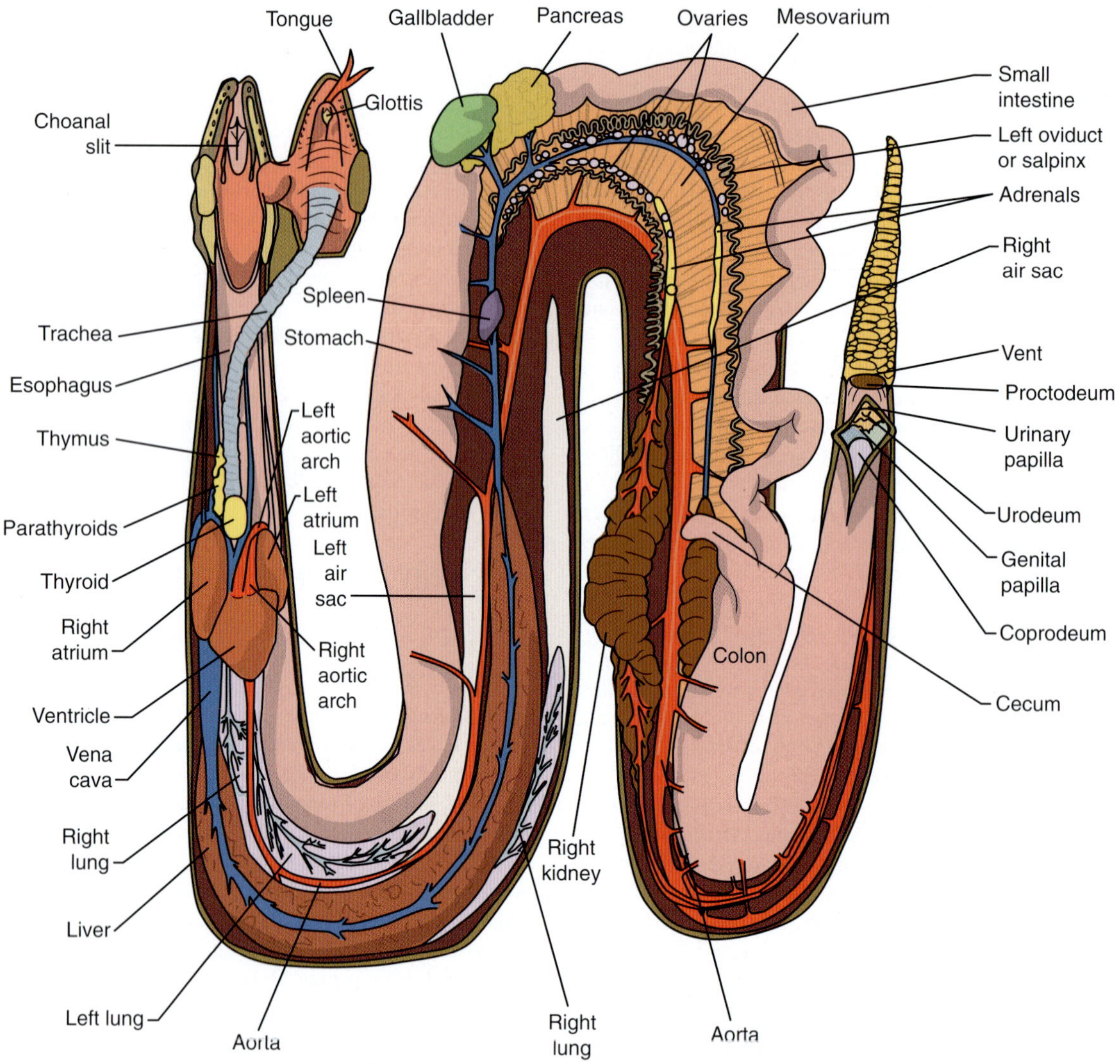

Tongue

Gallbladder

Pancreas

Ovaries   Mesovarium

Choanal slit

Glottis

Small intestine

Left oviduct or salpinx

Adrenals

Right air sac

Trachea

Spleen

Stomach

Esophagus

Thymus

Left aortic arch

Left atrium

Parathyroids

Left air sac

Thyroid

Right atrium

Right aortic arch

Ventricle

Vena cava

Right lung

Liver

Left lung

Aorta

Right kidney

Right lung

Colon

Aorta

Vent

Proctodeum

Urinary papilla

Urodeum

Genital papilla

Coprodeum

Cecum

FIG 8.17 Gross anatomy of the snake, ventral view.

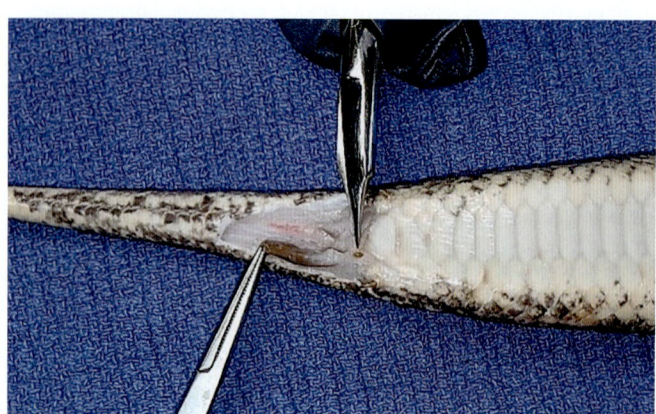

FIG 8.18 Almost no skin glands occur in snakes, but cloacal scent glands are characteristic. A prosection of a female ball python (*Python regius*) showing the location of the paired cloacal scent glands in the tail base. The caudal vent rim and some subcaudal scales have been removed to show the location of the left scent gland (grasped by hemostats) and the opening of the scent gland with scent gland material evident (at the tip of the scissors). (Courtesy of Greg Costanzo, Stahl Exotic Animal Veterinary Services).

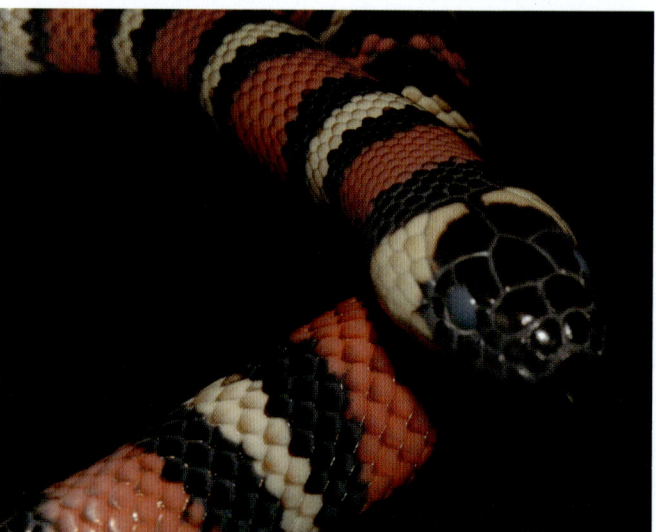

FIG 8.19 A shedding snake has a dull blue look to it as fluid forms between old and new layers of skin. Herpetoculturists call their snakes blue or opaque during this time. A snake "goes blue" for several days, clears, and then sheds. Arizona mountain king snake (*Lampropeltis pyromelana*) nearing shedding, showing dulled coloration and bluish coloration of the eyes. (Courtesy of Richard S. Funk.)

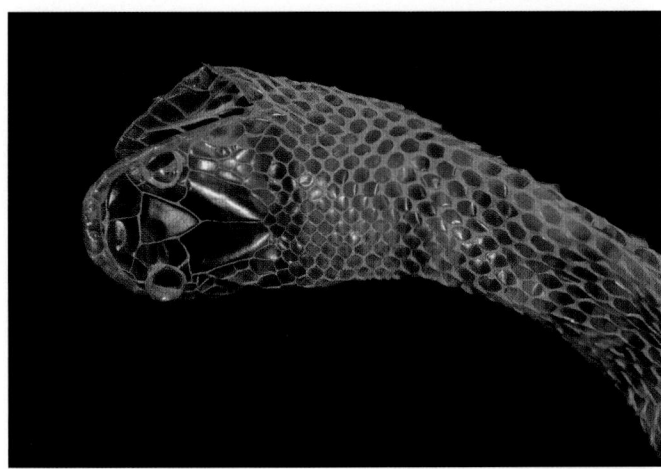

FIG 8.20 Shed head and neck skin of a variable king snake (*Lampropeltis leonis*). Note that the skin has also been shed over each eye (eye caps). (Courtesy of Richard S. Funk.)

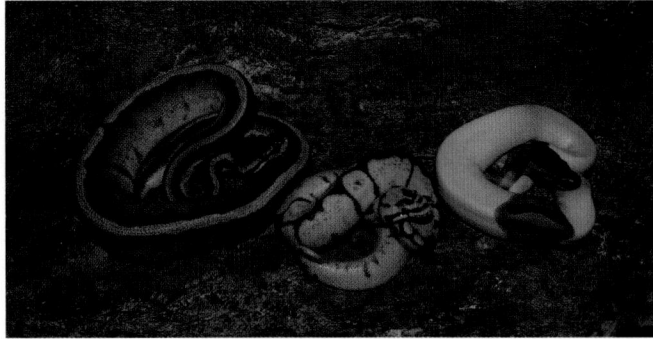

FIG 8.21 Captive propagation has produced a variety of genetic mutations, including partial albinos and leucistic individuals, and many pattern types, and has contributed to marketing of designer snakes or cultivars. Three neonate ball pythons (*Python regius*) illustrating some of the phenotypic variation being selectively produced in captivity. (Courtesy of Richard S. Funk.)

shelter, often in a moist or humid site. They will often resume feeding immediately after ecdysis.

Dysecdysis is the term for improper shedding and may be caused by incorrect humidity, lack of a proper substrate, improper handling, malnutrition, dermatopathy including ectoparasites, or trauma.

Pigment cells within the skin create the skin coloration and pattern, but microscopic surface structures can yield an iridescence. Ontogenetic color and/or pattern changes occur in some species. Some species, especially in juveniles, have brightly colored tails that are used as caudal lures to attract prey. Coloration may also vary geographically. Polymorphism is unusual, but for example the Turk's Island boa (*Chilabothrus chrysogaster*) and California king snake (*Lampropeltis californiae*) have both striped and blotched or banded individuals within the same populations. Many boas are darker during the day and lighter or paler at night.

In recent years there has been great success in the captive propagation of a variety of snake species with a wide variety of color and pattern mutations. Albinos, leucistics, hypomelanistic, patternless, and even scaleless varieties have become popular. For example, well over 100 "morphs" of the ball python are currently available in the pet trade in the United States.[20] These new mutations are often marketed under unusual names, often coined by the first breeder to produce the morph, for example, the "bumblebee," "clown" and "GHI" (got to have it) ball python morphs (Fig. 8.21). Of course, price varies with pattern and coloration. Such color mutant production often unfortunately necessitates significant inbreeding.

Cardiovascular System

Snakes have traditionally been thought to have a three-chambered heart, but with recent study the sinus venosus has been determined to function as a true chamber, and now many experts consider snakes to have a four-chambered heart. The four chambers include the sinus venosus, a right and left atrium, and a ventricle (see Chapter 68). Although communication exists between the ventricular halves, considerable functional separation exists between the oxygenated and unoxygenated circuits leaving the heart. The heart becomes functionally five-chambered, with the two systemic arches and the pulmonary artery all exiting the ventricle. Further, right-to-left and left-to-right shunting is also possible between the oxygen-rich and the oxygen-poor circuits, under control of several mechanisms.[21] Details of this are complex and beyond the scope of this brief introduction (see Chapter 68). Burmese pythons

have been shown to have the remarkable ability to increase the ventricular mass of their hearts by 40% within 2 days of feeding by synthesizing new protein.[22] Once the digestive process has been completed, the cardiac hypertrophy resolves, and the heart returns to its previous size.[23] These findings, however, are often inconsistent and not always reproducible,[23] and the hypertrophy may instead reflect stressed conditions.[24]

The position of the heart within a snake's body varies somewhat with its ecological niche; arboreal snakes' hearts are more cranial, and fully aquatic snakes tend to have a more centrally located heart.[21] The long axis of the heart is oriented craniocaudally with the atria located cranially. With no diaphragm, the heart is somewhat mobile within the rib cage, perhaps facilitating the passage of relatively large prey past it. Two aortae are present, with the right aorta exiting the left side of the ventricle and the left aorta exiting the right side; they fuse caudal to the heart and form the abdominal aorta. The left systemic arch is larger than the right, which is the opposite of most tetrapods. Paired carotid arteries and jugular veins are located anterior to the heart near the trachea. The jugulars may be easily cannulated via a simple cut-down for placement of an intravenous catheter for obtaining samples or administering fluids or medications.

Snakes have been shown to be able to control arterial pressure reflexively, but this control is reduced when the snake's body temperature is higher or lower than preferred.[21,25] Additionally, oxygen dissociation curves of snake blood may also be influenced by temperature.[25] This has not been shown to be true in ball pythons, however.[26]

Snakes have both renal and hepatic portal circulations. For this reason, it has been recommended to administer parenteral medications eliminated from the body via the renal system, in the front half of the body, to avoid potential nephrotoxicity and first pass effects. However, studies have indicated that clearance of drugs via the renal portal system may rely more on how the kidneys clear a drug with tubular excretion affected more than glomerular filtration[27,28] (see Chapter 66 for a thorough discussion of the renal portal system). A ventral coelomic vein courses through much of the coelom, and it should be avoided when making a surgical approach to the coelomic cavity by entering at the edge of the rib cage between the second and third dorsal (lateral) scale rows.

The primary sites for obtaining blood samples in snakes include a ventral coccygeal vein and cardiocentesis. An alternative venipuncture site not commonly used is the jugular vein. The jugular vein is typically located 1/3 to 1/2 the distance between the base of the heart and the base of the skull. A blood sample can be collected by blindly inserting

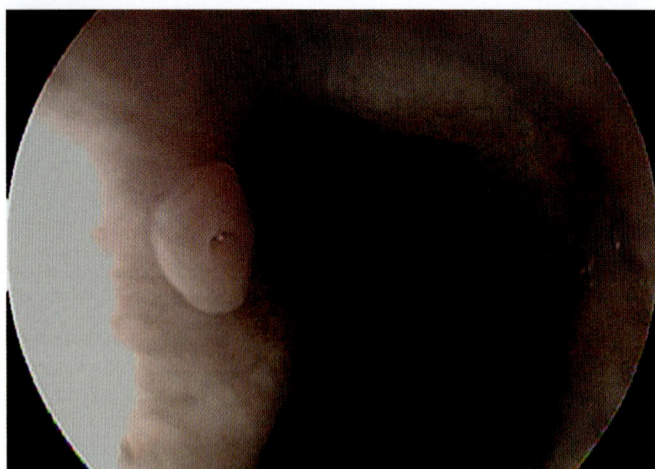

FIG 8.22 Endoscopic view of esophageal tonsil in an eastern indigo snake (*Drymarchon couperi*). (Courtesy of James E. Bogan.)

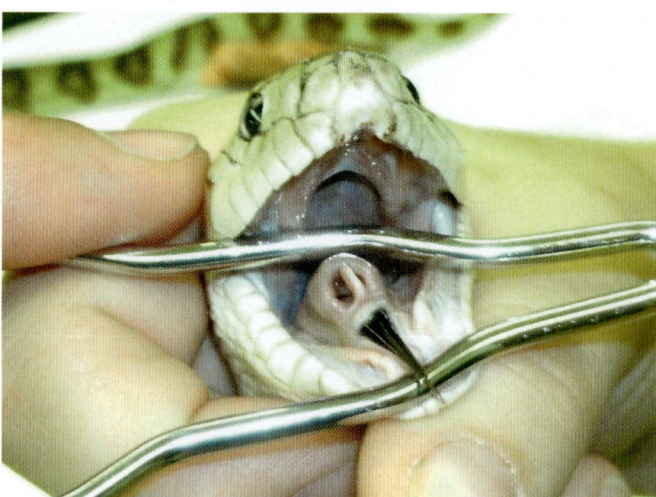

FIG 8.23 Epiglottal cartilage in a Florida pine snake (*Pituophis melanoleucus mugitus*). This enlarged cartilage will vibrate during exhalation, producing a dramatically louder hissing sound than snakes that lack this unique anatomical feature. (Courtesy of James E. Bogan.)

the needle along the medial rib margins.[29] A cannulated jugular vein may also be used. Venipuncture of the dorsal palatine vein is frequently referenced; however, it is difficult to utilize without sedation and may result in a difficult to manage hematoma at the venipuncture site.

The normal hematocrit (packed cell volume) of snakes is about 20% to 30%. Based on a study in the black rat snake (*Pantherophis obsoletus*), the blood volume is equivalent to about 6% of the animal's body weight.[30] All circulating blood cells are nucleated, and the presence of occasional mitotic figures in the peripheral blood is normal. Azurophils are unique granulocytes that are seen in snakes and other reptiles. Although many snakes seem to lack eosinophils,[31,32] they have been documented in several species, including the king cobra (*Ophiophagus hannah*), puff-faced water snakes (*Homalopsis buccata*), grass snakes (*Natrix natrix*), and Asian vine snakes (*Ahaetulla prasina*)[32–37] (see Chapter 33). Snakes have lymphoid tissue associated with the gastrointestinal tract, and in boas, pythons, and a few colubrids there are tonsil-like structures in the esophagus;[38] these may have clinical significance in the identification of viral infections (Fig. 8.22).

Respiratory System

Although squamates typically have two lungs, in most snakes the left lung is greatly reduced, never more than 85% of the size of the right lung, or absent.[7,39] In boas and pythons the left lung is moderately large. The right lung generally courses from near the heart to just cranial to the right kidney. The cranial portion of a lung is vascularized, functioning in gas exchange, and the caudal portion functions mainly as an air sac (see Chapter 76); these can be termed the vascular lung and the saccular lung, respectively. Air is drawn into the nostrils and delivered to the choana medial to the maxillae, where the epiglottis fits when the mouth is closed.

The trachea has incomplete cartilaginous rings, with the ventral portion being rigid and the dorsal fourth being membranous. In many snakes, the vascular portion of the lung extends cranially into the trachea, with expansion of this dorsal membrane into a "tracheal lung"; in extreme cases the most functional portion of the lung is tracheal.[7,39,40] The wall of the vascular lung is comprised of honeycombed units called faveoli, through which gas exchange occurs; these are not homologous to mammalian alveoli. The Acrochordidae have tracheal air sacs, and in some aquatic snakes the lung extends posteriorly nearly to the cloaca as a hydrostatic adaptation. Variations in lung and tracheal morphology are useful taxonomic characteristics. Snakes lack a diaphragm, and

inspiration occurs by muscular expansion of the rib cage to create negative pressure.

The glottis opens in the floor of the mouth caudodorsal to the tongue and is generally easily visualized, making intubation for anesthesia relatively straightforward. When consuming large prey, the glottis is quite mobile and can extend cranial and/or lateral as necessary to facilitate breathing during protracted ingestion. The epiglottal cartilage is quite enlarged and modified to facilitate defensive hissing in bull, gopher, and pine snakes (*Pituophis* spp.) (Fig. 8.23).

Digestive System

The digestive tract is essentially a linear duct from the oral cavity to the cloaca, which also receives products from the urinary and reproductive systems (see Chapters 73 through 75 on gastroenterology). The palatine, lingual, sublingual, and labial mucus-secreting glands in the oral cavity moisten the mouth and lubricate prey. Venom glands are modified labial glands and have evolved independently in several snake lineages. Snake venoms are extremely complex and used mainly for obtaining prey.

Six rows of teeth are generally present in snakes found in the pet trade, with one row on each of the lower mandibular bones and two on each maxillary region. Teeth are generally not regionally differentiated except for modified fangs in some species or in species with specialized feeding habits (none have molars, incisors, etc.). The dentigerous bones include the mandibles, maxillae, palatines, pterygoids, and sometimes the premaxillae. The teeth, including fangs, continue to be replaced throughout life. Usually a membranous flap covers the fangs when not in use. In vipers and pit vipers, the fangs fold caudodorsally and lie sheathed when the mouth is closed. But in elapids and others including colubrids with fangs, the fangs remain erect and cannot fold.

Snake teeth are basically elongated, slender, pointed, and slightly curved posteriorly. Snake teeth are modified pleurodont teeth with a rudimentary socket and are attached to the side of the bone.[41] More primitive snakes have all the teeth the same (homodont), whereas in the more advanced snakes, some teeth may be modified into grooved and hollow fangs. Historically, variations in the maxillary teeth have been classified as follows[41]:

Aglyphous: having homodont maxillary teeth.
Opisthoglyphous: "rear-fanged" with enlarged teeth on the posterior maxilla.

Proteroglyphous: a solitary enlarged fang on the long maxillary bone that does not allow for erection of the fang (elapid type).

Solenoglyphous: the only tooth is a hollow fang on the short maxilla that can be erected by maxillary rotation on the prefrontal bone (viper type).

Many variations occur among these types. In elapids and vipers, the anterior fangs are hollow with a distinctive venom canal. These fangs are shed periodically. It is not uncommon to observe a functional fang and an adjacent replacement fang (destined to replace the currently functional one when it is shed) during examination of the oral cavity. The fangs may be lost as the prey is bitten and pass through the snake relatively undigested and appear in the feces.

Venom glands are modified labial glands, located in the upper jaw below the orbit, and have evolved independently in several snake lineages. The size and shape of the gland varies with the species. Rarely, the venom glands extend far caudally into the body even to the level of the heart (*Causus*, Viperidae; *Atractaspis*, Lamprophiidae; *Maticoura*, Elapidae). Venoms are extremely complex, containing toxic proteins varying from a few amino acids to much higher molecular weight that are used mainly for subduing prey. These toxins have been characterized by their activities: neurotoxins acting at neuromuscular junctions and synapses; hemorrhagins act to destroy blood vessels; and myotoxins act on skeletal muscle. Among the venom toxins are RNAses, DNAses, phospholipases, proteolytic enzymes, thrombinlike enzymes, hyaluronidases, lactic dehydrogenases, acetylcholinerases, L-amino acid oxidases, and others.[42] At least 10 enzymes are found in nearly all snake venoms, and a venom may contain more than two dozen proteins. A particular venom may have a number of receptor sites, and venoms can also have digestive properties. In fact, snake venoms are theorized to have evolved from digestive enzymes.[43] Older classifications of venoms as hemotoxic or neurotoxic are oversimplifications and inaccurate, and some venoms contain mixtures of both. The relative abundance of venom components in a particular species can vary geographically, seasonally, or with age.

Many colubrid and lamprophiid snakes have been reported to have elicited toxic reactions in humans. These reports need to be carefully evaluated; some species, lacking venom glands, may have oral secretions that can elicit an inflammatory reaction when a person is bitten. However, several colubrids are venomous and capable of serious and even fatal human envenomation.[18,44,45] Many colubrids have venoms that are toxic to their prey but not to humans. Individual human reactions can depend on many variables, such as the general health status of the person, the species involved, nature of the bite, the amount of venom injected, the site of the bite, the depth of the bite, and the activity of the venom. A full discussion of human snakebites is beyond the scope of this chapter. Nevertheless, understanding the risks involved is essential before seeing venomous snakes (see Chapter 22). Many jurisdictions have restrictions regarding the possession of venomous reptiles, and legal restrictions must be appreciated. Not all local human hospitals have the appropriate experience or antivenom on hand to treat bites particularly from exotic species. Proper identification of an exotic snake may be difficult. Prevention of snakebite is always preferred to treatment of a bite.

The tongue has a forked tip and lies within a sheath beneath the epiglottis and functions in olfaction, delivering particulate odors to the vomeronasal organs located in the roof of the mouth. Snakes that lose their tongues to trauma or infection may cease feeding.

The esophagus is distensible, and about half its length is largely amuscular. Snakes generally use their axial musculature and skeleton to help transport food to the stomach. Snakes do not masticate food items; rather, they swallow their prey intact. Snakes lack a well-defined cardiac (gastroesophageal) sphincter.

The stomach is muscular and distensible. The process of prey digestion begins in the stomach. The small intestines are relatively uncoiled and straight (compared with mammals, birds, and even lizards). The pancreas is generally located in a triad together with the gall bladder and spleen, distal to the posterior tip of the elongated, spindle-shaped liver. Some species have a splenopancreas.

The small intestine empties into the colon, which in turn empties into the cloaca. The cloaca has three regions and from cranial to caudal the order is coprodeum, urodeum, and proctodeum, and it receives products from the digestive, urinary, and reproductive systems. Urates and feces may be temporarily stored within the colon and cloaca. In boas and pythons a small cecum is present at the proximal colon. The intestines and cloaca play important roles in water conservation.

Fat bodies are present within the coelom, a row on each side of the body cavity and a smaller group cranial to the heart; these may be huge in an obese snake and tiny in an emaciated one.

Reproductive and Urinary Systems

The paired kidneys are located in the dorsocaudal coelom, approximately the last 25% of the snout-to-vent length, with the right kidney situated cranial to the left, far forward from the cloaca (see Chapter 66 Nephrology chapter). The kidneys are lobulated and elongated and arranged in a craniocaudal orientation. The ureters empty into the urodeum. Snakes lack a urinary bladder. Male snakes possess a sexual segment, consisting of distal convoluted renal tubules that hypertrophy during the reproductive season to produce a contribution to seminal fluid (Fig. 8.24). Affected kidneys may appear abnormal because of their increased size and paler coloration, and to the untrained eye, these kidneys may appear diseased (see Chapter 80). Uric acid is the primary nitrogenous waste and appears as whitish to yellowish urates, often voided with the feces. Snake kidneys are unable to excrete urine at a higher concentration than that of plasma.[25]

Male snakes have two paired intromittent organs that are invaginated within pouches in the ventral tail base. Each is called a hemipenis (plural, hemipenes). Hemipenial morphology has proven to be a valuable taxonomic character. During copulation, a hemipenis evaginates into the cloaca of the receptive female. The functional surface of the hemipenis facing her cloacal wall, when not in use, lines the lumen of the cavity in the male's proximal tail. Because of the presence of the hemipenes,

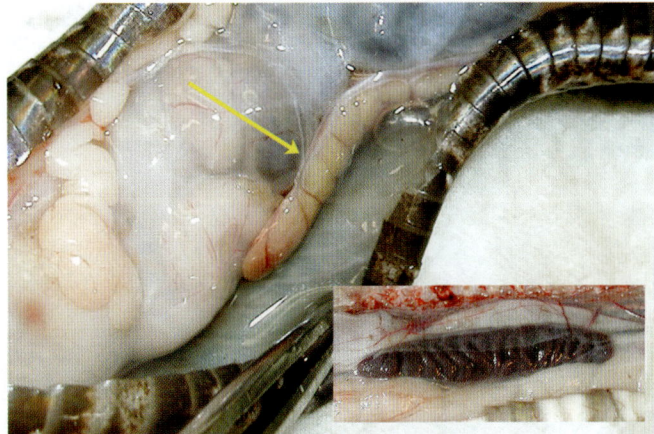

FIG 8.24 Male snakes have a "sexual segment" in their kidneys (yellow arrow), consisting of the distal renal tubules that enlarge during the reproductive season to produce a contribution to the seminal fluid. During this seasonal period, the kidneys appear abnormal because of dramatic size and color change, and this should not be misinterpreted as pathology. Insert shows a normal kidney during the nonreproductive season. (Courtesy of Douglas R. Mader.)

a smooth lubricated (water-soluble) blunt-tipped probe may be carefully inserted into the base of the tail of a snake and into the lumen of the hemipenis to accurately identify gender. The male probes relatively deeply compared with the conspecific female. In many snakes, the tail base of a male is wider and straighter than a female's due to the presence of the hemipenes. With practice, probing is relatively safe and easy, and the authors recommend probing most snakes to ascertain their sex as part of the clinical physical examination.

In males and females, the gonads are situated cranial to the kidneys, with the right one more cranial than the left. The ovaries are located nearer the pancreas. The developing eggs or fetuses in the right uterus are carried cranial to those on the left side. Each oviduct has a separate opening into the cloaca at the urodeum. A few fossorial species have lost one ovary and oviduct. The fusiform testes are intracoelomic, situated between the pancreatic triad and the kidneys, and they enlarge and regress in size as the season changes (Fig. 8.25). Sperm is carried in the Wolffian ducts (vasa defferentia) into the urodeum and to the base of the hemipenis during copulation and travels up the sulcus spermaticus on the outside of the erected hemipenis into the female's cloaca (see Chapter 80).

Some snakes are oviparous (egg-laying) and others are viviparous (live-bearing). Very few snakes (notoriously the king cobra, *Ophiophagus*

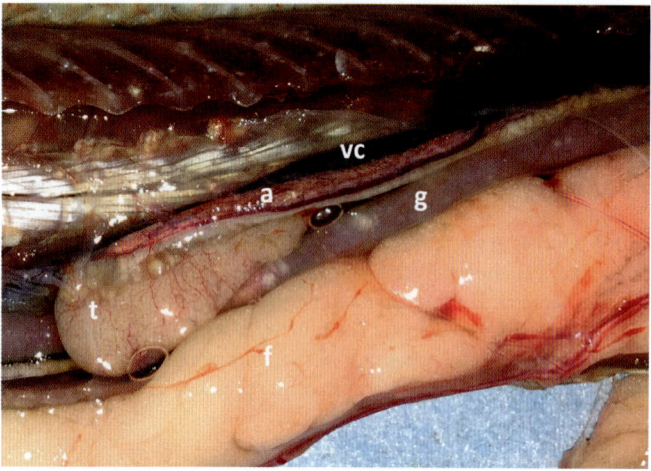

FIG 8.25 Fusiform testes are seen cranial to the kidneys, with the right being more cranial than the left. During breeding season, testes undergo recrudescence, often doubling in size. The pink adrenal gland can be seen in the gonadal mesentery. Cranial is to the left. a, Adrenal gland; f, fat body; g, gastrointestinal tract; t, testicles; vc, vena cava. (Courtesy of James E. Bogan.)

hannah) build a nest for egg incubation. Egg-brooding has evolved in several lineages (pythons; *Farancia* in the Colubridae; some *Trimeresurus* in the Viperidae); these females coil around their eggs until hatching (see Fig. 8.11). Some rattlesnakes (*Crotalus*) in the southwestern United States are known to exhibit some parental care and remain with their newborn until after they have shed.

No temperature-dependent sex determination has yet been documented in snakes, although it is known to occur in crocodilians, chelonians, and lizards. Where studied, snakes have genetic sex determination, and in advanced snakes the female is heterogametic (ZW) and the male is homogametic (ZZ).[46,47] In more primitive snakes, such as boids and pythonids, the male is heterogametic (XY) and the female is homogametic (XX).[47,48] Sexual dimorphism in coloration or morphology except for size differences is rare in snakes, but in the leaf-nosed snakes of Madagascar (*Langaha* spp.), there is sexual dimorphism in their nasal protuberances. In most species, female snakes attain larger sizes than males.

Most snakes reproduce sexually, although the blind snake *Indotyphlops* (formerly *Rhamphotyphlops*) *braminus* and the file snake (*Acrochordus arafurae*) are parthenogenetic (no males). Rare parthenogenesis has also been reported in several North American snakes and one python; further investigation will prove interesting and likely identify more species with this ability.[26,49]

Musculoskeletal System

Snakes show great modifications in their musculoskeletal systems from their lizardlike ancestry. The braincase is solid. However, the skull is kinetic, with the quadrate bones articulating with the lower jaw and the palatomaxillary arch. This facilitates, along with the elasticity in lacking a mandibular symphysis, the ingestion of prey items that are larger than the head or the diameter of the body. The ribs are not joined ventrally, and the body may expand to accommodate prey items that are larger than the diameter of the body. Caudal autotomy, widespread in lizards, is known in only a few snakes and occurs between caudal vertebrae rather than within the vertebral body, and no regeneration occurs (see Chapter 168). Many snakes feed by grasping the prey and ingesting it; others by ingesting it first; and others kill their prey by constriction, suffocating, and/or blocking blood flow to the brain.[22]

Endothermic prey tend to die faster than ectothermic prey when constricted. Snakes do not have thoracic limbs, but a few do have pelvic vestiges, including external spurs, that may be used during courtship, particularly in the boas and pythons (Fig. 8.26).

Locomotion centers around an axial skeletal system of precloacal vertebrae numbering from 120 to more than 400, most of which have ribs, plus axial skeletal muscles with multiple attachments. The ribs and vertebrae lack marked regional differentiation. Snake locomotion has been found to be relatively low in energy expenditure: a garter

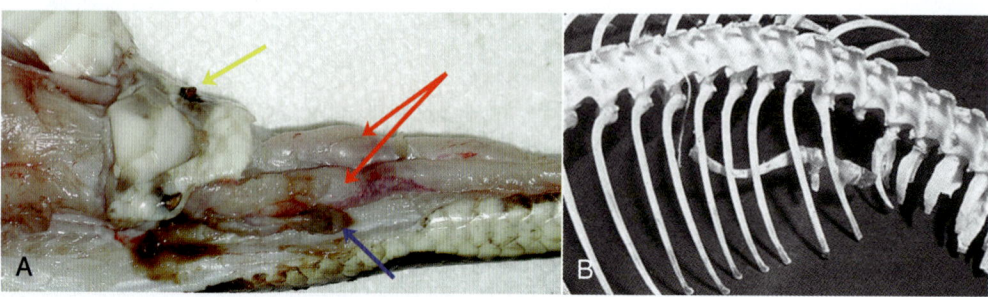

FIG 8.26 (A) Male boids have vestigial pelvic appendages. The yellow arrow points to the "spurs," red arrows highlight paired hemipenes, and the blue arrow points to the scent gland. (B) Skeleton shows relationship of the "spur" to the vestigial pelvis. The tail is to the right in both A and B. (A, Courtesy of Douglas R. Mader; B, courtesy of Richard S. Funk.)

snake expends only about 13% as much energy in locomotion as does a lizard of comparable size.[25] The diversity of snake locomotory types has been classified as follows, although a snake can switch from one form of locomotion to another as it changes habitat, substrate, or activity.[6,25]

Lateral undulation: involves bending the vertebral column laterally, where contractions occur on opposite sides of the body; this is characteristic of most tetrapods. The fastest terrestrial snakes utilize this method.

Rectilinear locomotion: a "caterpillar crawling" in which muscle contractions are bilaterally symmetrical in waves, with the body contacting the substrate at intervals and the progression occurring essentially in a straight line. Common in boas, pythons, and stocky vipers and pit vipers.

Concertina locomotion: the body moves forward by making a purchase and then moving a portion of the body forward to gain a new purchase. Common in arboreal and fossorial snakes; the most energy-expensive method of snake locomotion.

Sidewinding: a difficult mode to describe, much more easily understood when observed; used by snakes on smooth surfaces such as sand or mud; the body essentially contacts the substrate at two points and creates a series of separate parallel straight lines as it progresses. *Crotalus cerastes* and *Cerastes cerastes* are textbook examples.

Nervous System and Special Senses

Snakes have a typical reptilian brain with 11 to 12 pairs of cranial nerves, depending on whether you count cranial nerve 0 (nervus terminalis).[50] Researchers have not yet been able to identify cranial nerve XI in snakes.[51] Snakes have no external auditory opening, tympanic membrane, or middle ear cavity. For years, snakes were presumed to be unable to hear sounds, merely substrate vibrations. However, snakes have been shown electrophysiologically to be sensitive to airborne sound in a low frequency range of 150 to 600 Hz.[52–54]

The eyes of snakes are unique among vertebrates in lacking ciliary bodies. Accommodation occurs by moving the lens toward or away from the retina by means of iris muscle movements. In contrast, other vertebrates use ciliary body muscles to change the shape of the lens.[5,25,55] The eyelids fuse embryologically to form a transparent spectacle that is keratinized, covers the eye, and is continuous with the epidermis. The outer portion of the spectacle is shed during ecdysis, along with the rest of the integument. When a snake is near shedding, the spectacle may appear cloudy or "blue." Lacrimal secretions flow through the subspectacular space between the cornea and the spectacle and drain into the oral cavity at the distal aspect of the medial maxillae. The shape of the pupil varies with habitat and activity. Some fossorial snakes have reduced eyes covered by a scale without a spectacle. Additional details of eye anatomy, clinical examination, and diseases are discussed in Chapter 71.

Independent evolution of specialized infrared receptors has occurred in the heat pits of pit vipers and the labial pits of different groups of boas and pythons[56,57]; they do not appear to be homologous.[58] In pit vipers, one organ occurs on each side of the head slightly ventral to a line drawn between the nostril and the orbit. In boas and pythons these organs occur in labial or rostral scales or both, but the location, arrangement, and number vary with the species. Innervation is via branches of the trigeminal nerve. Pit viper facial pits (also sometimes termed loreal pits or heat pits) have a thin membrane stretched over an air-filled inner cavity. The pit organs are extremely sensitive to infrared radiation changes as small as 0.002°C.[58] These pits provide not only infrared information but also direction and distance, and because these pits are integrated in the brain within the optic region, they provide the snake with both infrared and visual imaging, apparently superimposed.[59,60]

Research shows that many snakes without pits can also detect infrared radiation with other nerve endings in their head. It is theorized that some and possibly many snakes may be able to "see" their environment as well with this infrared system as they can optically.[56,58–62] Snake keepers are commonly bitten when they are feeding cool (e.g., frozen and thawed to room temperature) rodents to snakes because the snakes may smell prey but orient toward the heat source (in this case radiant heat from the "live" keeper's hand).

Snakes have a specialized pair of vomeronasal organs (also called the Jacobson's organs) in the roof of the mouth, which are spherical and separate from the nose, containing a thick sensory epithelium, and are innervated by part of the olfactory nerve. The lacrimal duct enters the duct of the vomeronasal organ. These organs have an olfactory function, and particulate odors are relayed to it by the forks of the tongue.[63,64]

Central nervous system diseases are poorly understood in snakes (see Chapter 77). Boas and pythons with inclusion body disease (arenavirus) show varying degrees of CNS signs, including ataxia and opisthotonos[18] (see Chapter 30).

Endocrine System

The single or paired thyroid glands lie just cranial to the heart (Fig. 8.27). Thyroid function is involved in controlling growth and the shedding cycle. Issues with the skin such as dysecdysis, continual shedding cycles, dermatitis, etc., have suggested links with dysfunction of the thyroid gland. The thymus does not involute in adult snakes as it does in mammals but may be difficult to find in the adipose tissue just cranial to the thyroid(s). Parathyroid glands are paired and often imbedded in the thymus cranial to the heart and thyroid(s) and play a role in calcium metabolism. The adrenal glands are usually located within the gonadal mesentery (see Fig. 8.25). The pituitary gland appears to function as a master gland much as it does in mammals. Melatonin is secreted by the pineal gland. The clinical significance of endocrine function and dysfunction are poorly understood in snakes (see Chapter 79).

BEHAVIOR

Being ectothermic, snakes depend on behaviorally regulating their temperatures by interfacing with their environment. Different species have different preferred body temperatures. Snakes that are ill, gravid, or digesting prey may seek out warmer temperatures. Facultative endothermy is exhibited by brooding females of many python species that are able to maintain their temperatures several degrees warmer than the ambient temperature.[25,65] Both the clinician and the client must understand the thermal physiology of reptiles to ensure success

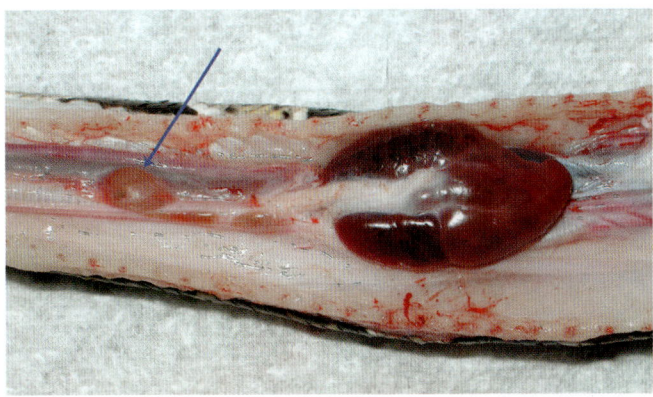

FIG 8.27 Single or paired thyroid gland is found just cranial to the heart.

in captivity. Each species needs to reach its selected (or preferred) body temperature (T_S or T_P), which occurs within the range of physiologically tolerated temperatures or the thermal neutral zone. Herpetoculturists find that their captives thrive better when provided with a thermal gradient that incorporates the T_S for species being maintained. Summary discussions of research on thermoregulation are available.[66–76] Brumation is the term for winter dormancy in reptiles (as opposed to true hibernation).[77,78]

Other snake behaviors, including defense, aggression, courtship, and death-feigning, are covered in behavior-related Chapters 13, 80, 83, and 121.

REFERENCES

See www.expertconsult.com for a complete list of references.

9

Lizard Taxonomy, Anatomy, and Physiology

Stephen Barten and Shane Simpson

Ranging in size from the tiny Mount d'Ambre leaf chameleon (*Brookesia tuberculate*) to the giant Komodo dragon (*Varanus komodoensis*) (Fig. 9.1), lizards are arguably the most diverse group of reptiles. They demonstrate a wide range of morphologic, physiological, and behavioral adaptations that have allowed them to colonize an array of environments on every continent except Antarctica.

With such diversity and distribution, it is not surprising that of the over 10,000 known living reptile species, nearly 6200 of them are lizards.[1]

From private reptile keepers to zoo collections alike, lizards offer considerable choice as to what can be kept in captivity. Many species adapt well and can be handled with ease. Similarly, many species have been bred in captivity with great success, and there is no better example of these traits than the most popular pet reptile, the central or inland bearded dragon (*Pogona vitticeps*).

TAXONOMY

Living reptiles, or as they are more correctly referred to, sauropsids, can be divided into three clades. The first reptilian clade is the chelonians (turtles and tortoises), the second is the archosaurs (crocodiles and birds), and the third clade is the lepidosaurs, which consists of lizards, snakes, amphisbaenians, and tuataras (Fig. 9.2).

Common nomenclature recognizes lizards and snakes as two different groups of reptiles. This is not true, however, when classificatory labels are used. Snakes and lizards are collectively known as squamates and have more than 50 shared-derived features that demonstrate their close affiliation with each other. These include skeletal features such as a single fused premaxillary bone and soft tissue features such as males having well-developed, paired copulatory organs known as hemipenes. It should be appreciated that snakes are actually lizards with either reduced limbs or no limbs.[2] Because of this relationship, it is taxonomically incorrect to refer to lizards without also including snakes. Nethertheless, this is exactly the group that this chapter discusses. It is, however, difficult to describe the taxonomy of lizards because there is no clear consensus among taxonomists. The following outline therefore is based on historical thinking in combination with current cladistic theories (Table 9.1).

The first branch of the squamate cladogram divides them into the Iguania and all the others, which collectively are called the Scleroglossa.

Historically Iguania has contained three groups: the Iguanidae, the Agamidae, and the Chamaeleonidae. The family Iguanidae or Iguanids is the dominant group of lizards in the new world and differs from the other two by having pleurodont dentition (teeth attached to the medial side of the jaws without sockets that are regularly shed and replaced) and fracture planes in the caudal vertebrae. There are at least 12 families in this group, and examples include the green iguana (*Iguana iguana*) (Fig. 9.3), green anole (*Anolis carolinensis*), basilisks (*Basiliscus* spp.),

horned lizards (*Phrynosoma* spp.), spiny lizards (*Sceloporus* spp.), and West Indian rock iguanas (*Cyclura* spp.).

Together the Agamidae and Chamaeleonidae make up the Acrodonta because of their acrodont dentition (teeth attached to the biting edge of the jaw without sockets that are not shed and replaced). This group also lacks caudal vertebral fracture planes; exceptions include some *Uromastyx*. Because of these similar features, the Agamidae and the Chamaeleonidae are considered to be more closely related to each other than either of them are to the Iguanidae. Members of the family Agamidae are the dominant family of lizards in the old world. Examples include the central or inland bearded dragon (*Pogona vitticeps*), agama (*Agama agama*), frilled lizard (*Chlamydosaurus kingii*) (Fig. 9.4), Chinese water dragon (*Physignathus cocincinus*), Egyptian spiny-tailed lizard (*Uromastyx aegyptius*), and Philippine sail-fin lizard (*Hydrosaurus pustulatus*). The family Chamaeleonidae consists of the old-world, or true, chameleons. Examples include the veiled chameleon (*Chamaeleo calyptratus*), the panther chameleon (*Furcifer pardalis*), and the Parson's chameleon (*Calumma* parsonii).

The relationships between the remaining squamate groups in the Scleroglossa are less certain and are where the greatest amount of conjecture occurs. The following structure is just one proposal and will no doubt raise debate among those with a penchant for taxonomy.

The first main group, the Nyctisaura, contains the Gekkonidae, the Xantusiidae, the Dibamidae, and the Amphisbaenidae.

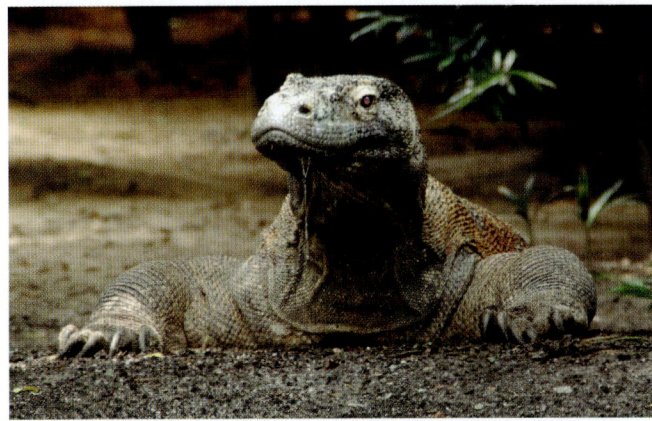

FIG 9.1 Komodo dragon (*Varanus komodoensis*). The largest living species of lizard, these animals can reach 3 meters in length and weigh up to 70 kilograms. Found only on five Indonesian islands, they hunt and ambush prey such as deer and water buffalo. Human fatalities from Komodo dragon attacks have been reported. (Courtesy of Shane Simpson.)

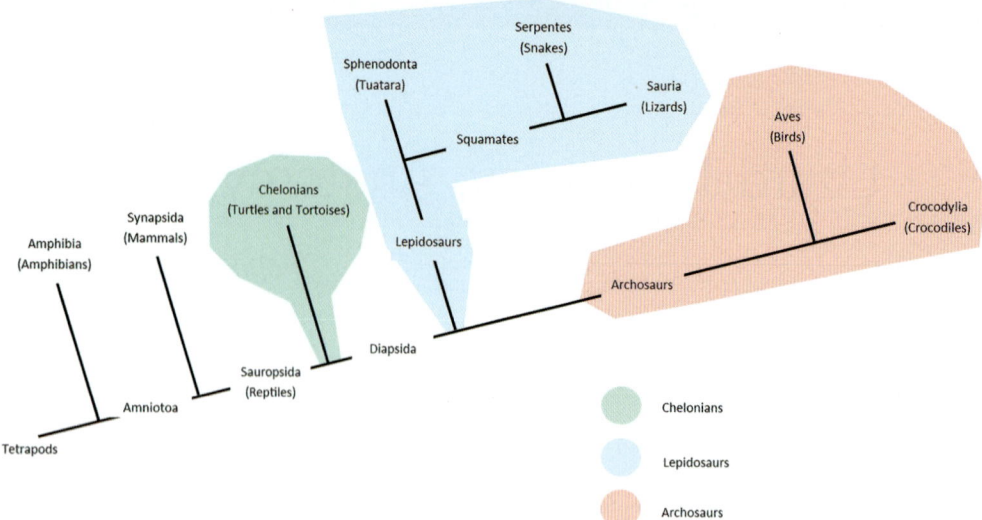

FIG 9.2 A simplified cladogram showing the three extant reptilian clades. There is still much conjecture among taxonomists as to the exact relationships among the reptile groups. Table 9.1 provides an overview of the assorted lizard families.

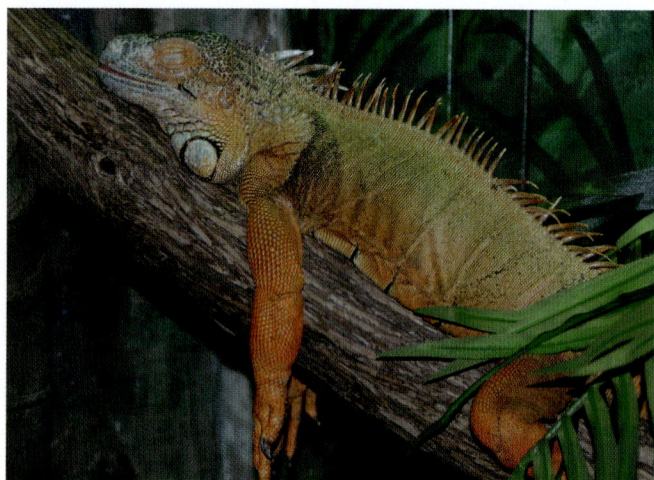

FIG 9.3 Green iguana (*Iguana iguana*). Dominant males of this species take on an orange coloration as seen in this sleeping specimen. Males also show more developed dorsal spines, larger dewlaps, and larger operculum scales than females. (Courtesy of Shane Simpson.)

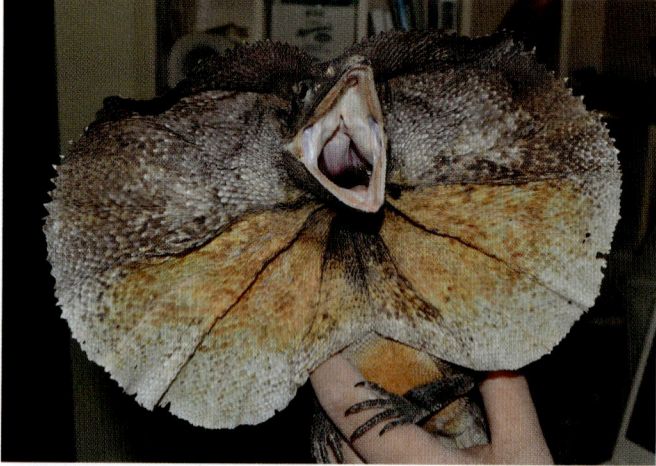

FIG 9.4 Frilled lizard (*Chlamydosaurus kingii*). When threatened and during courtship, this predominantly arboreal species will gape its mouth and expand the large ruff of skin that is normally folded back on the neck and head. (Courtesy of Shane Simpson.)

The Gekkonidae family is comprised of the Eublepharidae geckos with movable eyelids and include the leopard gecko (*Eublepahris macularius*); the Diplodactylidae, otherwise known as Austral geckos,[3] of which examples include the three-lined, knob-tailed gecko (*Nephrurus levis*) and the crested geckos (*Correlophus [Rhacodactylus] spp.*); the Gekkoninae, which are the typical geckos including the tokay gecko (*Gekko gecko*) and leaf-tailed geckos (*Uroplatus* spp.); the Phyllodactylidae or leaf-toed geckos; the Sphaerodactylidae or dwarf geckos; and finally the Pygopodinae, which are snakelike without forelimbs and with their hind limbs reduced to flaps of skin containing a few phalanges, such as seen with the common scaly-foot (*Pygopus lepidopodus*) and Burton's snake-lizard (*Lialis burtonis*). The Xantusiidae contain the night lizards (*Xantusia* spp.). The Dibamidae, or blind lizards (*Dibamus* and *Anelytropsis* spp.), also are snakelike lizards with no forelimbs and flaplike hind limbs. The Amphisbaenidae, or worm lizards, are legless, covered with wormlike annular rings made of scales, and all species are fossorial, including the red worm lizard (*Amphisbaena alba*).

The remaining squamates, the Antarchoglossa, contain two diverse subgroups. The subgroup Lacertoiformes includes three families. First is the Lacertidae, or wall and rock lizards. Some examples are the jeweled lizard (*Timon lepida*), rock lizard (*Lacerta saxicola*), and viviparous lizard (*Zootoca vivipara*). Second is the Teiidae, which are the new-world equivalent of the Lacertidae and include the whiptails and racerunners (*Aspidoscelis* and *Cnemidophorus* spp.), jungle runners (*Ameiva* spp.), and tegus (*Salvator* and *Tupinambis* spp.). The final family is the Gymnophthalmidae or spectacled lizards. The other subgroup is the Diploglossa, which contains the remaining lizard groups. One is the family Scincidae or true skinks, familiar species of which include the blue-tongued skink (*Tiliqua* spp.), prehensile-tailed skink (*Corucia zebrata*), five-lined skink (*Plestiodon [Eumeces] fasciatus*), and the

TABLE 9.1 Lizard Taxonomy

Iguania
Agamidae [Agamas]
Chamaeleonidae [Chameleons]
Iguanidae [Iguanas]
    Corytophaninae [Casquehead Lizards]
    Crotaphytidae [Collared and Leopard Lizards]
    Dactyloidae [Anoles]
    Hoplocercinae [Wood lizards and Clubtails]
    Iguaninae [Iguanas and Spinytail Iguanas]
    Leiocephalidae [Curly-tailed Lizards]
    Leiosauridae
    Liolaemidae [Liolaemids]
    Oplurinae [Madagascar Iguanids]
    Phyrynosomatinae [Earless, Spiny, Tree, Side-blotched, and Horned
      Lizards]
    Polychrotinae [Bush Anoles]
    Tropidurinae [Neotropical Ground Lizards]

Scleroglossa
Nyctisaura
    Gekkonidae [Geckos and Pygopods]
    Diplodactylidae [Austral Geckos]
    Eublepharidae [Eyelid Geckos]
    Gekkoninae [Typical Geckoes]
    Phyllodactylidae [Leaf-toed Geckos]
    Pygopodinae [Legless Lizards]
    Sphaerodactylidae [Dwarf Geckos]
    Xantusiidae [Night Lizards]
    Dibamidae [Blind Lizards]
    Amphisbaenidae [Worm Lizards]
Antarchoglossa
    Lacertoiformes
      Gymnophthalmidae [Spectacled Lizards]
      Lacertidae [Wall and Rock Lizards]
      Teiidae [Whiptails, Racerunners, Jungle Runners, and Tegus]
    Diploglossa
      Cordylidae [Girdle-tailed or Spinytail Lizards]
      Gerrhosauridae [Plated Lizards]
    Scincidae [Skinks]
    Anguimorpha
      Xenosauridae [Knob-scaled Lizards]
      Shinisauridae [Chinese Crocodile-Tailed Lizards]
      Anguidae [Alligator Lizards, Glass Lizards, and Legless Lizards]
      Varanoidae
        Helodermatidae [Gila Monsters]
        Varanidae [Monitors]
        Lanthanotidae [Earless Monitor Lizards]

crocodile skinks (*Tribolonotus* spp.). Two others are the Cordylidae or girdle-tailed lizards (*Cordylus* spp. and others) and Gerrhosauridae or plated lizards (*Gerrhosaurus* spp. and others). The Diploglossid group also incorporates a lesser subgroup, Anguimorpha, which contains several families. The Xenosauridae or knob-scaled lizards include the new world viviparous xenosaurs (*Xenosaurus* spp.), and the Shinisauridae contains only the Chinese crocodile-tailed lizard (*Shinisaurus crocodilurus*). The family Anguidae are long and snakelike in form. They include the alligator lizards (*Elgaria* spp.), glass lizards (*Ophisaurus* spp.), legless lizards (*Anniella* spp.), the sheltopusik or European glass lizard (*Pseudopus*

apodus), and the galliwasps (*Diploglossus* ssp. and *Celestus* ssp.). The final three families in the Anguimorpha are members of the Varanoidae group. The Helodermatidae contain only two species, the gila monster (*Heloderma suspectum*) and the Mexican beaded lizard (*Heloderma horridum*). The family Varanidae consists of the monitor lizards. Australian monitor lizards and certain species from Southeast Asia are often referred to as goannas. Familiar examples include the savannah monitor (*Varanus exanthematicus*), the Nile Monitor (*Varanus niloticus*), and the perentie (*Varanus giganteus*). Lanthanotidae has a single species, the Bornean earless lizard (*Lanthanotus borneensis*).[1–3]

ANATOMY AND PHYSIOLOGY

The following sections refer extensively to Figs. 9.5 through 9.7.

Integument

Lizards have relatively thick, keratinized skin with ectodermal scales formed by folding of the epidermis and outer dermal layers.[4] Epidermal growth is cyclic, and lizards undergo regular periods of shedding or ecdysis, during which the skin comes off in pieces in most lizards rather than in one piece as seen in snakes. Some species eat their sloughed skin. Normal shedding is one indication of good health. The frequency of ecdysis varies with species, size, temperature, humidity, state of nutrition, age, gender, rate of growth, skin damage including surgically induced, state of health, and endocrine factors.[5] Rapidly growing juveniles may shed every 2 weeks, whereas adults may shed three to four times a year.[6] Wounds and skin infections cause more frequent shed cycles.

The skin contains few glands. Many lizards, notably iguanas and many agamids, have femoral pores in a single row on the ventral aspect of the thigh (Fig. 9.8). Many geckos and agamids also have precloacal pores arranged in a V-shaped row anterior to the cloaca. These are not true glands but rather are invaginations of the skin that produce a waxy secretion for territorial marking and social communication.[7] They can be used as a method for sex identification as they tend to be larger and more developed in mature males.

The skin color patterns seen in lizards, like all reptiles, is due to presence of multiple types of pigment cells referred to collectively as chromatophores. These cells are located in the dermis of the skin. Many species of lizards, such *Chamaeleo* spp. and *Anolis* spp., are able to undergo rapid color changes due to hormonal and neurologic control mechanisms of the chromatophores to alter their size and positioning within the dermis.

Osteoderms are dermal bones that support the epidermal scales. They are present in the Heliodermata, some skinks (such as the shingle-back lizard, *Tiliqua rugosa*) (Fig. 9.9), legless lizards, and girdle-tailed lizards. These are usually confined to the back and sides where they have a protective role. Dewlaps, spines, crests, and horns may be present and often are secondary sex characteristics, being more prominent in males. These all may play a role in defense, protection, and dominance behaviors. The integument can also have a role in locomotion in some species of lizards. Of particular note are the anatomical features of the feet of many gecko species that allow them to seemingly defy gravity. Adhesive setae on the feet of these animals enable them to adhere to smooth vertical and horizontal surfaces.[8]

The integument of lizards not only functions to protect from desiccation and predation but is also innately involved in the synthesis of vitamin D_3. UVB light of the appropriate wavelength striking the skin converts cholesterol to the inactive form of vitamin D as part of the pathway to the ultimate formation of 1,25-dihydroxycholecalciferol.[9] Without such a chemical conversion susceptible lizards may develop secondary nutritional hyperparathyroidism. For further details, see Chapter 69.

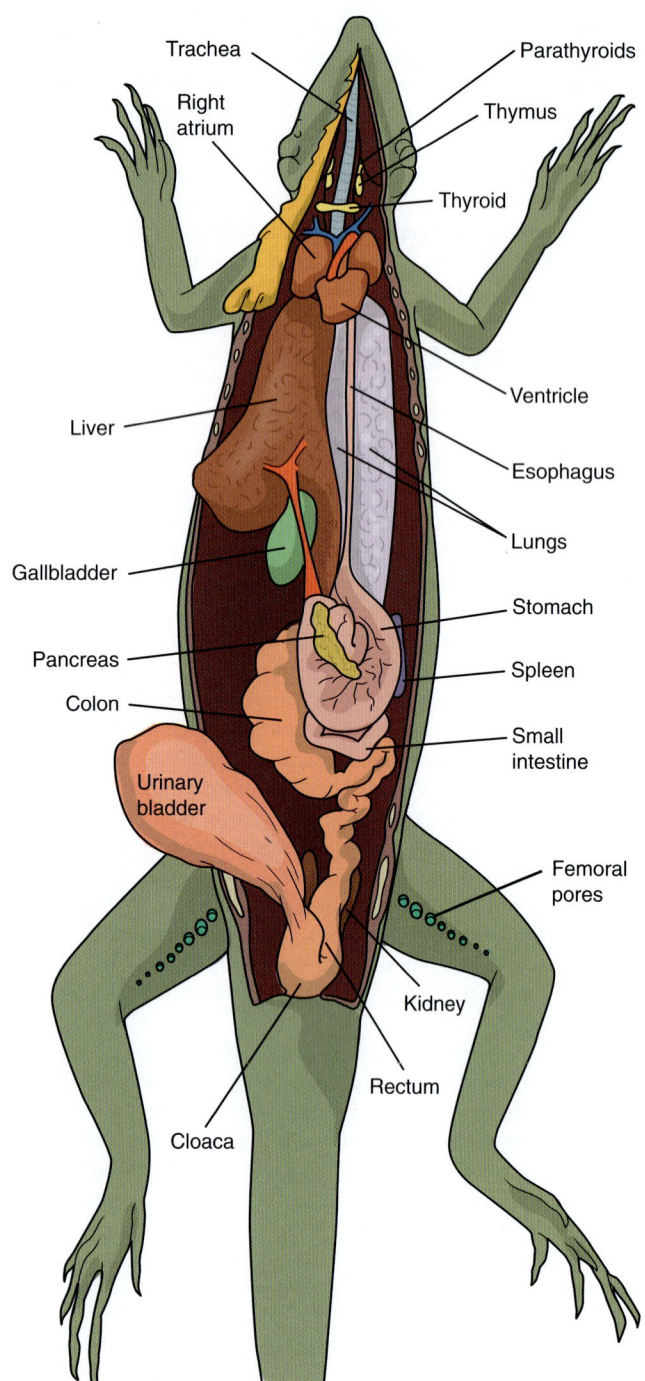

FIG 9.5 Ventral view of a green iguana (*Iguana iguana*). Note the anterior location of the heart between the shoulder joints. Also, note the caudal position of the kidneys within the pelvic canal.

Cardiovascular System

In lizards, the heart is three chambered, with left and right atria and a single ventricle. The ventricle is divided into three chambers: the cavum arteriosum, cavum venosum, and cavum pulmonale.[10] The cavum venosum receives deoxygenated venous blood from the right atrium, and the cavum arteriosum receives oxygenated blood from the left atrium. Blood leaves the heart through the pulmonary artery arising from the cavum pulmonale and the two aortic arches arising from the

cavum venosum. All three cava communicate, but a muscular flap and two-stage ventricular contraction minimizes mixing among the three cava. Deoxygenated blood flows from the cavum venosum into the cavum pulmonale. An atrioventricular valve prevents mixing of this blood with the oxygen-rich blood in the cavum arteriosum. Next the ventricle contracts, forcing the deoxygenated blood in the cavum pulmonale into the pulmonary artery. The atrioventricular valve then closes, allowing oxygenated blood to flow from the cavum arteriosum into the cavum venosum and out the aortic arches. Thus the three-chambered squamate heart function is similar to that of a four-chambered heart.[10]

In all lizards the heart lies within the pectoral girdle except for the monitors (*Varanus* spp.) and tegus (*Salvator* and *Tupinambis* spp.), where it is located more caudally in the coelomic cavity. For further details, see Chapter 68.

The renal portal system of reptiles is well documented in the literature for its parenteral therapeutic implications.[10–13] Although the anatomy of the blood vessels varies somewhat from group to group, venous circulation from the tail, and little from the hind limbs, routes directly to the kidneys via the renal portal system.[12] The injection of drugs (that are cleared via tubular secretion) into the caudal half of the body could result in lower than anticipated serum concentrations because of their first-pass excretion from the kidneys before entering the systemic circulation. This practice could also result in increased renal toxicity in the case of nephrotoxic drugs, such as aminoglycosides. Only limited pharmacokinetic studies on the effect of the renal portal system on serum drug concentrations have been done, but the results suggest that the renal portal system has less effect on drug uptake and distribution than was once thought. Moreover, shunts exist that carry blood directly from the renal portal system to the postcava, bypassing the renal parenchyma. For more details, see Chapter 66.

Venous blood from the hind limbs and tail in reptiles drains to the ventral abdominal vein (Fig. 9.10), which connects to the hepatic portal vein and enters the liver.[10] This is in contrast to what occurs in mammals and birds, in which blood drains into the caudal vena cava then to the heart, thus bypassing the liver. Consequently, drugs administered in the caudal half of the reptilian body enter the liver first and are subject to a hepatic first-pass effect. Those drugs that undergo hepatic metabolism or excretion may therefore be rendered ineffective and should not be administered in the caudal half of the body. Given the presence of both renal and hepatic portal systems in reptiles, it would seem prudent to avoid administering drugs in the caudal half of the body to avoid any potential metabolism or excretion effects.

Maintaining adequate blood pressure is important for ensuring appropriate tissue perfusion. Baroreceptor control of blood pressure has been identified in a number of lizard species.[14,15] The level of baroreceptor control in response to hypotension may not be influenced by temperature and is still maintained through periods of reduced metabolic activity such as brumation.[14]

Respiratory System

Nasal salt glands are present in herbivorous iguanid lizards such as the green iguana. Solutions with high concentrations of sodium and potassium can be excreted by these glands, and their importance in osmoregulation in some species is greater than that of the kidneys and is vital for the animal's survival.[10] Generally, lizards sneeze and expel a clear fluid that dries to a fine white powder consisting of sodium and potassium salts. This mechanism allows water conservation and should not be mistaken for an upper respiratory infection. The paired internal nares are anterior in the roof of the mouth and are a common site for discharges to accumulate and a good site for bacteriologic sampling when respiratory infection is present.

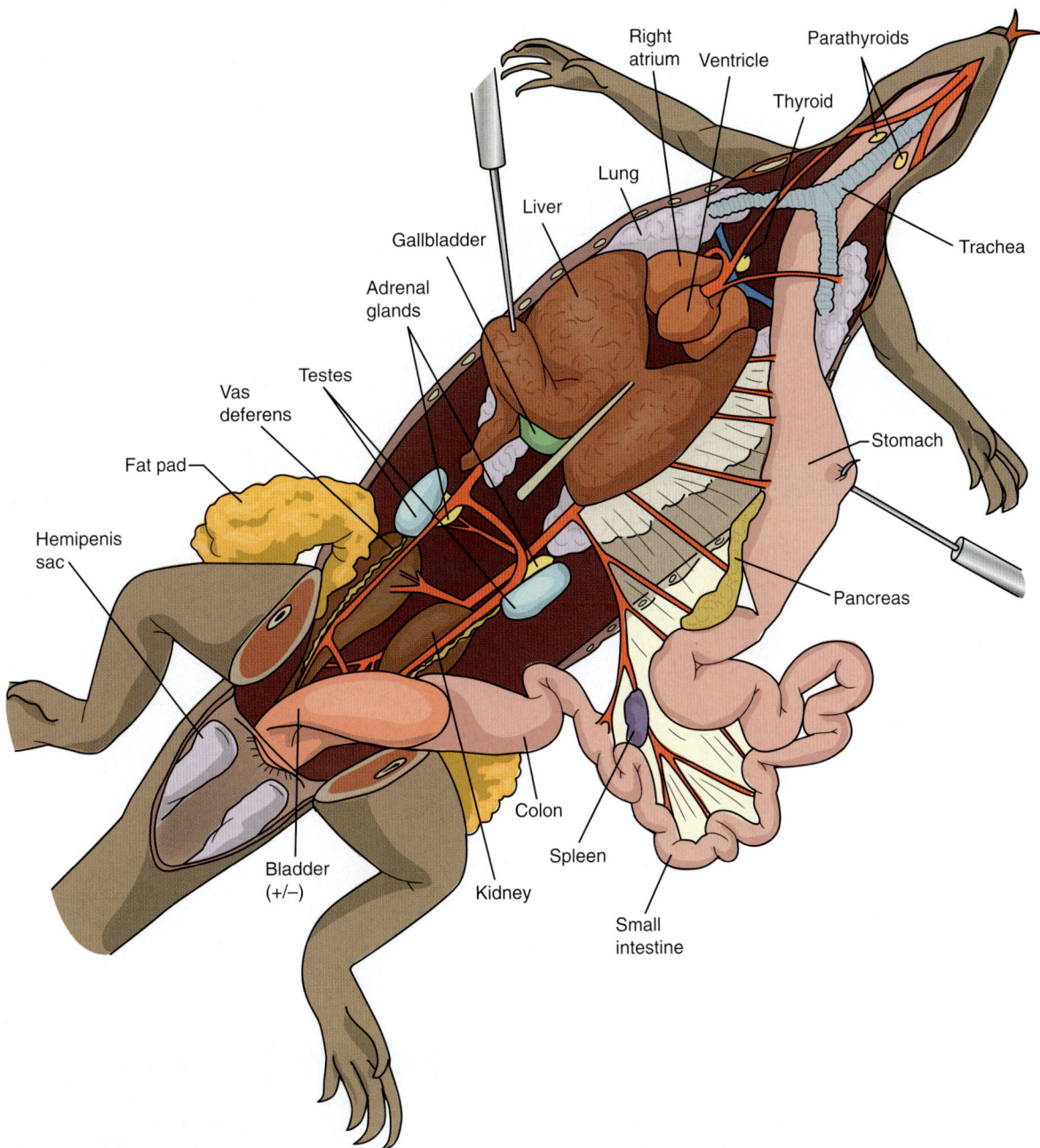

FIG 9.6 Ventral view of a savannah monitor (*Varanus exanthematicus*). Note the more typical location of the heart compared to the green iguana (*Iguana iguana*). Likewise, although the caudal portions of the kidneys extend into the pelvic canal, the cranial portions are within the coelomic cavity, unlike in the green iguana.

The location of the glottis is variable. In some species such as monitors (*Varanus* spp.) it is found rostrally; however, in agamids it is located caudally, behind the tongue. The glottis is normally closed except during inspiration and expiration. Vocal cords are occasionally present, most notably in some geckos, which can produce loud vocalizations. The trachea is composed of incomplete tracheal rings and bifurcates near the level of the heart.[4]

Primitive lizards (e.g., the European green lizard, *Lacerta viridis*) possess so-called unicameral lungs that consist of a hollow single chamber lined with faveoli (small sacs) that are more spongelike than saclike to increase surface area for gas exchange. Some species, particularly skinks (Scincidae), may have large, caudal nonrespiratory sacs that are thin-walled and poorly vascularized.[4,10] In more advanced lizards (e.g., Chamaeleonidae), the lungs are further divided into interconnected chambers by a few large septae, and there is a membrane that connects to the pericardium. Chameleons specifically have hollow, smooth-sided, fingerlike projections on the margins of their lungs that must be identified and avoided during coelomic surgery. These are not used in gas exchange but rather to inflate the body and intimidate would-be predators. Some chameleons also have an accessory lung lobe that projects from the anterior trachea cranial to their forelimbs. This may fill with secretions with infection, resulting in swelling of the ventral neck. Monitors' lungs are multichambered with bronchi that continue to divide until small tertiary bronchi extend toward the pleural surface to form hexagonal

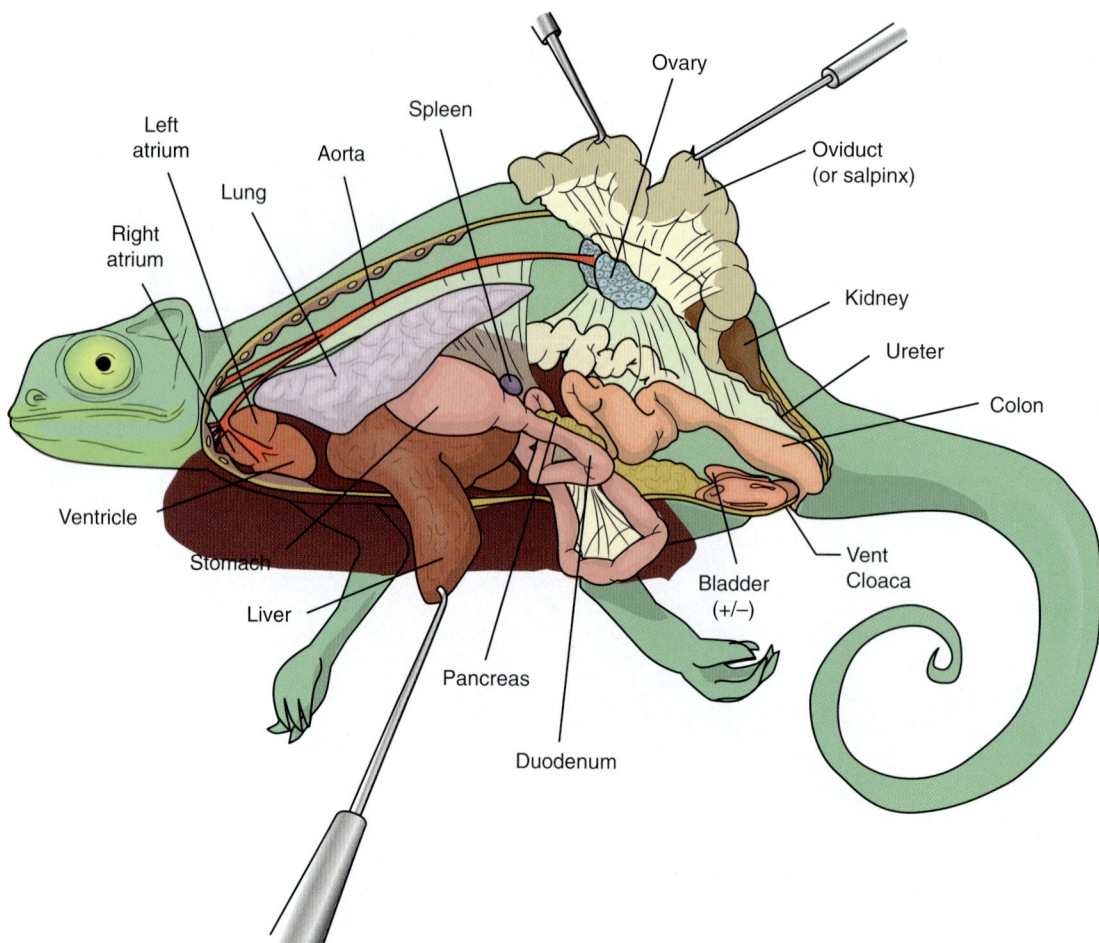

FIG 9.7 Lateral, midsagittal view of a female chameleon. Serosal surfaces in the coelom of many chameleons are starkly melanotic.

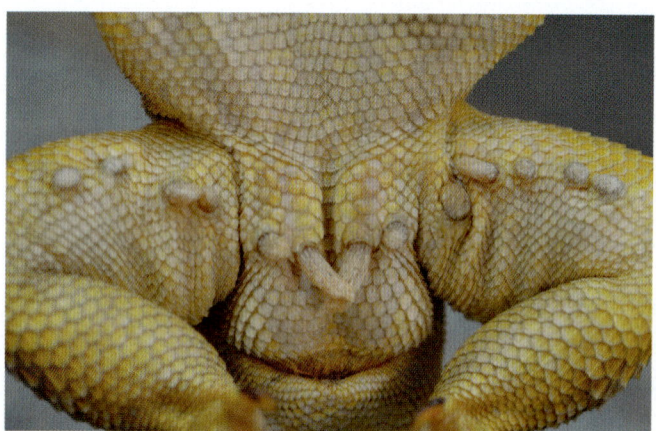

FIG 9.8 The femoral and precloacal pores on the ventral aspect of the thighs of this central bearded dragon (*Pogona vitticeps*) indicate that this is a male. Femoral pores of adult male dragons like this one are larger than those in females, although this specimen has an accumulation of secretions in the pores. (Courtesy of Shane Simpson.)

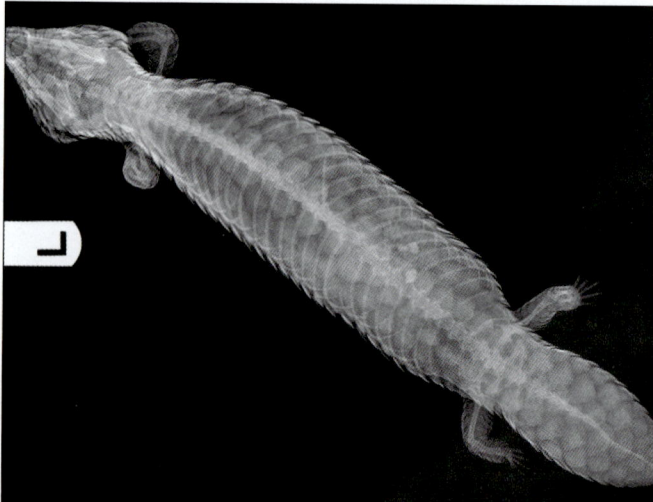

FIG 9.9 The shingleback lizards (*Tiliqua rugosa* sp.) are one of a number of species of lizard that possess bony plates or osteoderms within their scales. Normally confined to the dorsum and sides, they are clearly visible in this radiograph. Notice the vertebral lysis and rib loss in the left mid-body area secondary to neoplasia. (Courtesy of Shane Simpson.)

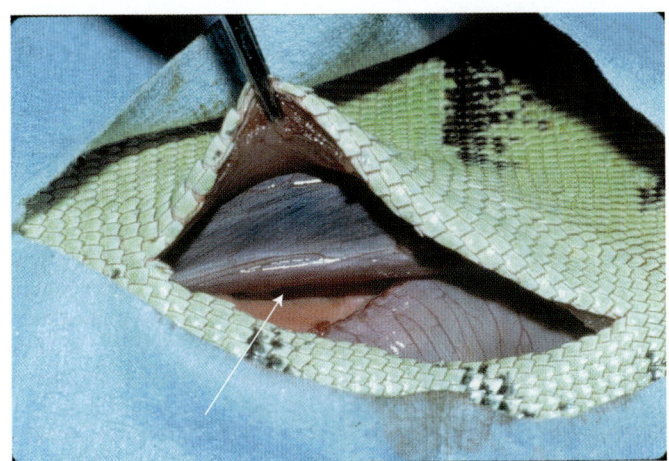

FIG 9.10 Paramedian coeliotomy incision in a green iguana (*Iguana iguana*). The medial body wall has been elevated to show the large ventral vein as it hangs in its suspensory ligament from the medial aspect of the linea alba. This vessel is best avoided during coeliotomy incisions. (Courtesy of Stephen Barten.)

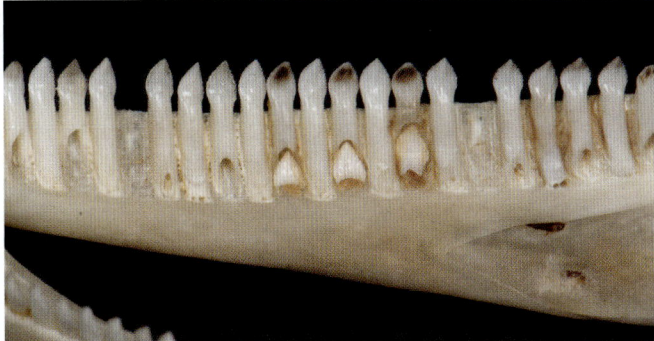

FIG 9.11 Mandible of a green iguana (*Iguana iguana*) showing pleurodont dentition. Teeth are attached to the medial side of the jaw without sockets. Note that alternate teeth have shortened roots with buds of new teeth below them. Teeth are shed and replaced throughout life. Rostral is to the right. (Courtesy of Stephen Barten.)

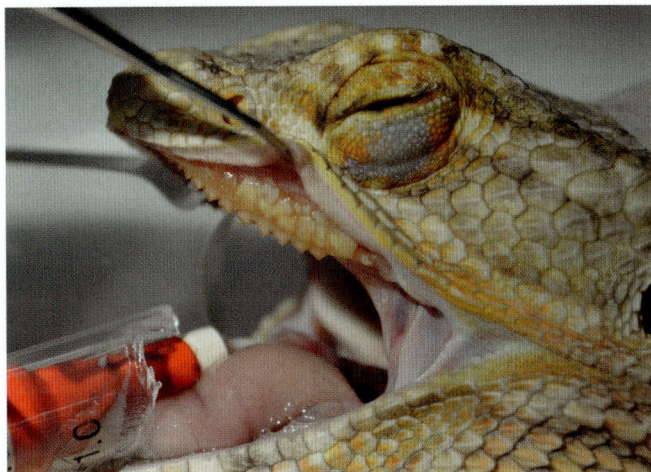

FIG 9.12 Periodontal disease of the left maxillary arcade of a central bearded dragon (*Pogona vitticeps*). Captive lizards with acrodont dentition such as this are prone to periodontal disease. An improper diet with excessive fruits and lack of abrasive items is thought to be a contributing factor. (Courtesy of Shane Simpson.)

faveolar parenchyma for gas exchange.[10,16] These lungs most closely resemble the lungs of primitive mammals.

Lizards lack a diaphragm and rely on the expansion and contraction of the ribs using the intercostal muscles, aided by the skeletal muscles of the coelomic wall to move air through the lungs. Given that these muscles are under voluntary control, this has implications when lizards are anesthetized as they will require artificial ventilation. The monitors and gila monsters have an incomplete, post-pulmonary, fascialike septum that divides the coelomic cavity but does not aid respiratory movements.[17] Monitors have been shown to have unidirectional pulmonary airflow similar to that seen in birds and crocodilians.[16] The fluttering of the ventral throat does not result in significant respiration but probably ventilates the oropharynx for olfaction and may play a role in cooling.

Some lizards can revert to anaerobic metabolism during prolonged periods of apnea and will switch to anaerobic metabolism quite quickly with sustained activity due to their limited capacity for aerobic respiration.[4,10]

Control of respiration in lizards is similar to that in other reptile species. CO_2 chemoreceptors and O_2 receptors have been found in the periphery. The dominant drive to breathe in reptiles is an increasing CO_2 concentration in the blood rather than a decreasing O_2 level. In addition, pulmonary stretch receptors act to suppress inspiration and enhance expiration when stimulated. Clinically these methods of control are important to understand, because overventilation with highly oxygenated gas during and after anesthesia can result in apnea and delayed recovery. For further details, see Chapter 76.

Digestive System

The lips of lizards are composed of flexible skin but are not moveable. The teeth of lizards fall into two types. Pleurodont dentition is characterized by teeth attached to the lingual sides of the mandible without sockets and is the most common type of dentition as seen in iguanids and varanids (Fig. 9.11). Pleurodont teeth are regularly shed and replaced. The odd-numbered teeth are shed in one cycle, and the even-numbered teeth in the next, so that a tooth being shed has a functional tooth on either side allowing normal mastication. Agamidae and Chamaeleonidae possess acrodont dentition, where the teeth are attached to the biting edges of the jaws without sockets. Acrodont teeth are not replaced except in very young specimens, although new teeth may be added to the posterior end of the tooth row as the lizard grows. Some agamids

have a few caninelike pleurodont teeth on the anterior jaws, along with the normal acrodont teeth. Care should be taken to avoid damaging the irreplaceable acrodont teeth in agamids and chameleons when opening the mouth with a rigid speculum during physical examination. Peridontal disease has been reported in species with acrodont dentition but not pleurodont dentition (Fig. 9.12).[18] Lizard teeth generally grasp, pierce, or break up food, and, unlike snakes and chelonians, they will chew their food before swallowing. In many monitors, the teeth slice and cut. Mollusc-eating caiman lizards (*Dracaena guianensis*) and adult Nile monitors (*Varanus niloticus*) have broad rounded cheek teeth for crushing shells.

The tongue of the lizard varies with the species. In general, it is mobile and protrusible, being attached to the hyoid apparatus at its base. Taste buds are abundant in species with fleshy tongues, and in these species the tongue has both mechanical and chemosensory function. Taste buds also are found in the lining of the pharynx. In monitors and tegus, the tongue is highly keratinized and has minimal taste buds. Lizards with deeply forked tongues protrude it to bring scent particles to the vomeronasal (Jacobson's) organ for olfaction. The tongue is a projectile for food gathering in chameleons (*Chamaeleo* spp.). In green iguanas and many Agamids, the tip of the tongue is darker in color and should not be mistaken for a lesion. The paired vomeronasal (Jacobson's) organs have tiny openings in the anterior roof of the mouth, just cranial to the openings to the paired internal nares. Lizards have well developed multicellular mucous glands that line the oral cavity and produce saliva. The saliva lubricates food, allowing it to pass down the esophagus with greater ease.[10,19]

The gila monster and Mexican beaded lizard were considered to be the only venomous extant lizards for many years. These species have grooved rather than hollow teeth, which have no direct connection to the venom glands. The venom glands are sublingual rather than temporal as seen in snakes. Venom flows from the glands along the dental grooves and is injected with the chewing action. Symptoms of envenomation include pain, hypotension, tachycardia, nausea, and vomiting. Work with various varanid and iguanid lizards has since revealed they too possess venom that can have potent effects on blood pressure and clotting ability.[20,21]

The esophagus in lizards is short, thin-walled, and enters the stomach on the left side of the coelom. The stomach of lizards is simple, C-shaped, and not gizzard-like. The stomach can be divided into the fundic (corpus) and parspylorica regions. Some lizard species have prominent cardia regions, and rugae may or may not be present.[19] The swallowing of stones to assist digestion is not a normal behavior in lizards.

The length and complexity of the intestine of lizards depends greatly on the type of diet the animal consumes. In general, herbivores have the longest intestine and carnivores the shortest. In herbivores the distinction between the small and large intestines is often obvious but this is less so in carnivores. A number of vegetarian species have a colon that is divided into sacculations to facilitate hindgut fermentation for more complete digestion. Lizards in this group include the green iguana, prehensile-tailed skink, Egyptian spiny-tailed lizard, and chuckwalla (*Sauromalus ater*).[22]

A cloaca is present and is divided into three parts: the coprodeum, which collects feces; the urodeum, which collects urinary waste and receives the sexual structures (vas deferens/oviducts); and the proctodeum, which is the final chamber before the vent.[23] The cloacocolonic region has an important role in the reabsorption of electrolytes and fluids from the excreted wastes. The vent or cloacal slit is transverse in lizards.

The liver is an encapsulated, bilobed organ in lizards. The right lobe is the larger of the two lobes and usually has the gall bladder closely associated with it. Its exact location in the body cavity can vary in the cranial-caudal direction.[23,24]

The gall bladder of lizards has an important role in digestion, particularly of fats, by acting as a storage organ for bile. Bile emulsifies fat and allows it to be absorbed in the intestine. In most lizards it is attached to the liver, though in some species it may be located some distance from the liver, similar to snakes.[10,23]

The pancreas of lizards is an elongated structure that lies along the mesenteric border of the duodenum.[19,24] For further details see Chapters 73, 74, and 75.

Reproductive System

Lizards have breeding seasons determined by cycles of photoperiod, temperature, rainfall, and availability of food. In males, a corresponding fluctuation is seen in testicular size. Male iguanas and other lizards are often noted to be more territorial and aggressive during their breeding season.

Gender identification can be a challenge in lizards, particularly in juvenile animals. Some species may show sexual dimorphism as they mature. Mature male iguanas have taller dorsal spines, larger dewlaps, and larger operculum scales than do females. They also have bilateral hemipenal bulges at the base of the tail. Male chameleons often have

elaborate head ornamentation in the form of horns, crests, and plates that are lacking in females. Many other male lizards have larger heads, bigger crests, brighter colors, erectable dewlaps, or may have a larger body size than females. In addition, males may possess greatly enlarged femoral and precloacal pores. Sexing probes to determine the depth of the hemipenal sac (if present) can be used but is less definitive than is seen in snakes. Female lizards often have hemiclitoral structures that result in similar probing depths as are seen in males. The hemipenes of some species may be temporarily everted with application of gentle pressure to the base of the tail, just caudal to the cloaca. This should not be attempted in species that undergo tail autotomy, such as geckos. Transillumination of the tail base with a strong light source may allow visualization of the hemipenal structures in small or lightly colored species of lizard. The hemipenes of mature male monitor lizards of many species may show calcification of an internal skeleton, termed a hemibaculum, and are demonstrable on radiographs (Fig. 9.13 and Table 9.2).[25,26] The introduction of radio-opaque solutions into the hemipenal sac has been shown to be a useful method of sex identification in eastern blue-tongue lizards (*Tiliqua scincoides* scincoides) (pers. comm., Steven Mallet, 2016). Endoscopy to visualize the gonads may be used to identify gender.[27] Ultrasonography of the gonads or the presence or absence of hemipenes in the proximal tail also may be used to identify the gender of a lizard.[28] See Chapter 80 for more details.

Male lizards have paired testes, epididymides, and vasa deferentia. The testes are located anterior to the kidney, with the right testis positioned more anteriorly than the left in most lizards.[10] The male has paired hemipenes that are saclike and lack erectile tissue; these are an invagination from the cloacal wall and are stored in an inverted position in a pocket in the base of the tail. They may produce noticeable bulges in the ventral proximal tail. There may be considerable morphologic differences in the structure of the hemipenes between different lizard species, with some varanids in particular having very elaborate hemipenal structures. During mating the male aligns his cloaca with that of the female, and one hemipenis everts and penetrates the female cloaca. Sperm runs from the cloaca down a groove in the wall of the hemipenis,

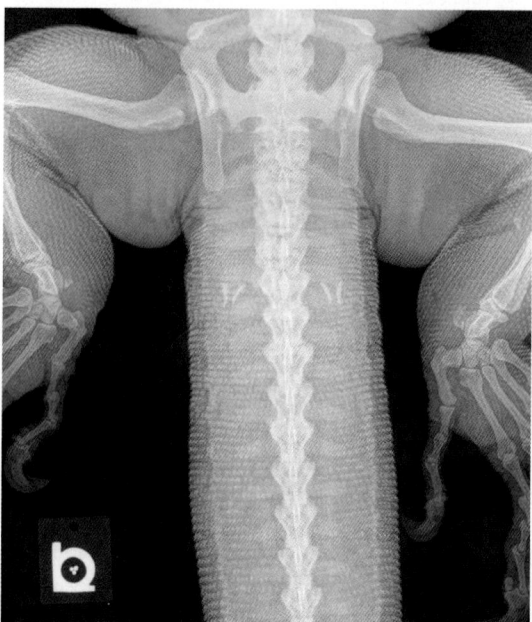

FIG 9.13 Mature male monitors of several species like this lace monitor (*Varanus varius*) can develop ossification of the hemibaculae within the hemipenes. This can be used as a method of identifying the sex of an individual. (Courtesy of Stephen Barten.)

TABLE 9.2 Species of Monitors (*Varanus* spp.) in Which Mineralized Hemibacula Are Present within Hemipenes and the Basic Hemibacula Shape[27]

Mineralization Present

Hemipenal Category	Species	Basic Hemibacula Shape
A	black tree monitor (*Varanus beccari*) emerald tree monitor (*V. prasinus*)	Single, short, parallel sides
B	pygmy desert monitor (*V. eremius*)	Long curved, spike-shaped horn
C	Perentie (*V. giganteus*) Gould's monitor (*V. gouldii*) mangrove monitor (*V. indicus*) yellow-spotted monitor (*V. panoptes*) lace monitor (*V. varius*) peach-throat monitor (*V. karlschmidti*) Komodo dragon (*V. komodensis*) crocodile monitor (*V. salvadori*) Merten's water monitor (*V. mertensi*)	Two components, equal sized, concave centrally
D	ridge-tailed monitor (*V. acanthurus*) striped-tailed monitor (*V. caudolineatus*) Gillen's monitor (*V. gilleni*) Storr's monitor (*V. storri*) black-headed monitor *(V. tristis)* spotted tree monitor (*V. scalaris*)	Two or three components, slightly different sizes, concave at the distal (tail) end
E	Gray's monitor (*V. olivaceous*)	Two components, lateral component much larger

Mineralization Absent

Bengal monitor (*V. bengalensis*)
Dumeril's montitor (*V. dumereli*)
savannah monitor (*V. examthematicus*)
desert monitor (*V. griseus*)
Nile monitor (*V. niloticus*)
roughneck monitor (*V. rudicollis*)
water monitor (*V. salvator*)
Timor monitor (*V. timorensis*)

the sulcus spermaticus, into the female, resulting in internal fertilization. There is no urethral structure. A retractor hemipenis muscle retracts the hemipenis after mating.[25,29]

Female lizards have paired ovaries and oviducts supported by mesenteries, which terminate at the urodeum of the cloaca. In lizards at least, the caudal pole of each ovary is attached to the peritoneum along the ventromedial surface of each kidney. In some lizards with highly modified lungs, such as chameleons, the ovary may extend cranially between the two lungs. The ovaries and oviducts can vary dramatically in terms of size and composition depending on age and time of year in relation to breeding season.[29]

Parthenogenesis is defined as reproduction without fertilization and occurs when the female gamete develops into a new individual without being fertilized by a male gamete. This is the sole method of reproduction in several all-female lizard species, including at least eight *Lacerta* spp.,[30] a number of *Aspidoscelis* spp., and assorted gecko species (e.g., Bynoe's gecko, *Heteronotia binoei*) among others, and is an incidental and anomalous observation in other lizards including the Komodo dragon.[31]

The storage of sperm in the female reproductive tract has been well documented in many vertebrates, and lizards are no exception.[32] Sperm storage has several functions including supporting the sperm to aid in increased fertility, sustaining female fertility duration, and allowing for the choice of the strongest sperm.

Lizards may be oviparous (i.e., egg-laying) or viviparous (i.e., live-bearing). In older literature a third term, ovoviviparous, is referred to and is used to describe the method of reproduction where the eggs are retained within the female until birth of live young. Current studies indicate that even in these species there is nutrient transfer from mother to young, and the appropriate term is viviparous. Some genera of lizards contain both oviparous and viviparous species (e.g., *Phrynosoma, Sceloporus, Rhacodactylus*).[27] See Chapter 80 for more details.

Urinary System

The kidneys are metanephric, paired, symmetric, elongated, slightly lobulated, and flattened dorsoventrally except in chameleons where they are flattened laterally. Depending on the species of lizard, the kidneys may be located deep in the pelvic canal (such as in Agamidae) or in the dorsal coelomic area (as in chameleons and varanids), but as in all reptiles the kidneys are located retrocoelomically.[33] In those species with intrapelvic kidneys, nephromegaly from any cause can result in obstruction of the colon as it passes between the kidneys within the pelvic canal. The posterior segment of the kidney in some male geckos, skinks, and members of the iguana family is sexually dimorphic. This area is called the sexual segment and represents hypertrophy of the distal convoluted tubules. It becomes swollen during the breeding season and contributes to the seminal fluid. The color of the sexual segment may change dramatically during the breeding season and may be misinterpreted as pathology by the untrained eye.

Reptiles can excrete nitrogenous waste as uric acid, urea, or ammonia.[10] Reptile kidneys have fewer nephrons than mammals, lack a renal pelvis, and also lack the loop of Henle and thus are unable to concentrate urine above that of plasma. However, water may be resorbed from the bladder across an osmotic gradient, resulting in the postrenal modification of urine. The excretion of ammonia or urea results in significant water loss, and the excretion of insoluble uric acid allows water conservation. Thus ammonia and urea are excreted in significant amounts only in aquatic and semiaquatic species (Table 9.3).

A thin-walled bladder is present in most species of lizard; however, several species either lack a bladder or develop a vestigial bladder including some agamids (including *Pogona* spp., some varanids, some *Crotophytus* spp., *Scleroporus* spp, teids, and a few geckos). When absent, urine is stored in the distal colon. In some instances, this urate may become desiccated and lead to constipation (Fig. 9.14). Because urinary waste flows from the kidney through the ureter into the urodeum of the cloaca before entering the bladder (or colon in species that lack a bladder), it is not sterile. Urine cannot be concentrated above that of plasma and may change within the bladder, so urinalysis and specific gravity results may not indicate renal function as in mammals.[27] Cystic calculi occur and may be caused in part by water deprivation and diets containing excessive levels of protein. The calculi tend to be singular, smooth-surfaced, layered, and quite large when discovered. For more information, see Chapter 66.

Musculoskeletal System

The skull of lizards is kinetic, resulting in a wide gape and mechanical advantages when closing their jaws. Unlike snakes, the mandibular

TABLE 9.3 Nitrogenous End-Products Produced by Lizards

Species	% TOTAL NITROGEN[a]		
	Ammonia	**Urea (BUN)**	**Uric acid**
Cuban rock iguana	<1	1	98–99
Cyclura nubila			
Carolina anole	13	13	73
Anolis carolinensis			
Sandfish skink	3	0	93
Scincus scincus			

BUN, Blood urea nitrogen.

[a]Calculated as % sum of the ammonia, urea, and uric acid when total nitrogen data was not available. Molecular weights of 18, 60.1, and 168.1 and percentages of 83%, 46.7%, and 33.3% were used respectively, in calculations.

Source: Campbell JW: Excretary nitrogen metabolism in reptiles and birds. In Walsh PJ, Wright P, editors: *Nitrogen Metabolism and Excretion.* London: CRC Press; 1995;147–170.

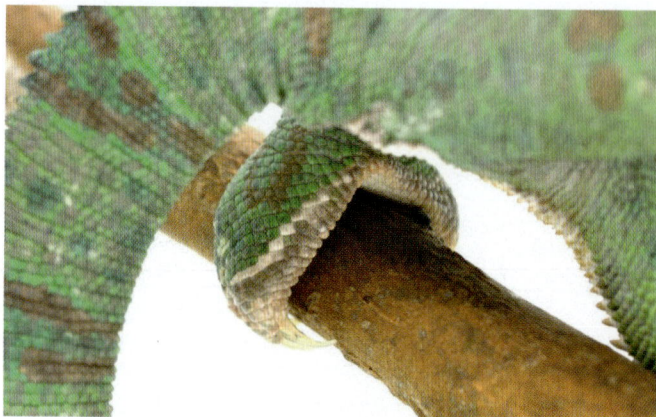

FIG 9.15 Chameleons have pincerlike zygodactyl feet with the first through third digits opposing the fourth and fifth in the front feet, and the first and second digits opposing the third through fifth in the hind feet. This veiled chameleon (*Chamaeleo calyptratus*) demonstrates their ability to grasp onto branches as they walk. (Courtesy of Shane Simpson.)

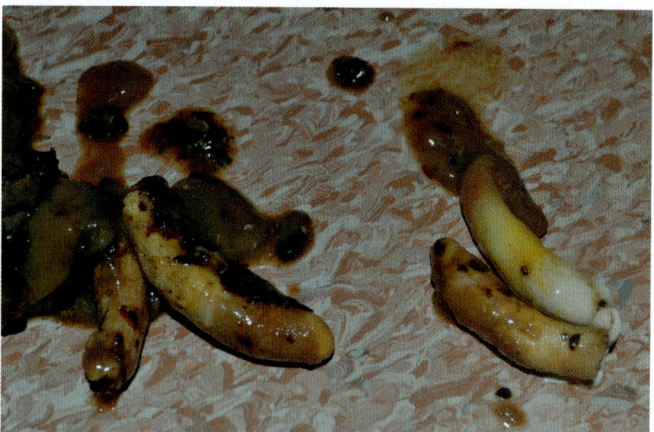

FIG 9.14 A large amount of hardened urates and fecal matter passed by a central bearded dragon (*Pogona vitticeps*). Lizards without a bladder store urate in the distal colon prior to passing it. In cases of dehydration this urate may become hardened and lead to constipation. (Courtesy of Shane Simpson.)

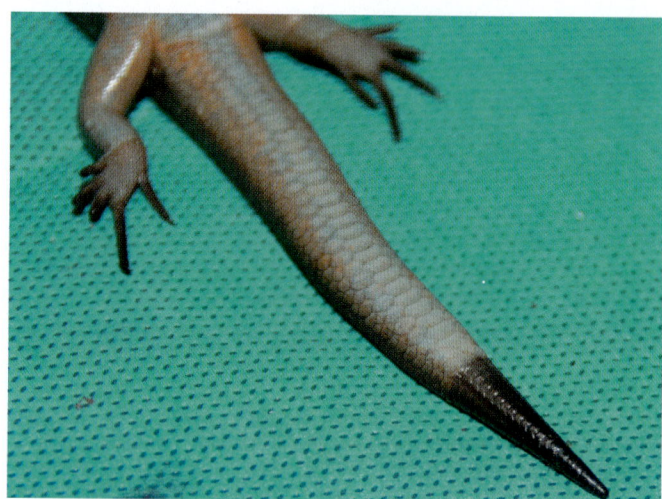

FIG 9.16 Tail autonomy and regeneration is a common trait amongst many lizard species, including the Guthega skink (*Liopholis guthega*). The newly grown tail is normally shorter and darker in appearance than the original one. (Courtesy of Shane Simpson.)

symphysis is fused in lizards. The arrangement of the musculature of the skull results in most lizards having the ability to rapidly and powerfully close the jaws. The backbone of lizards is very mobile and flexible. With the exception of cervical and coccygeal regions, all the vertebrae bear ribs that either join the sternum, the opposite member, or end free in the body wall.[4] The pectoral girdle consists of the scapulae, coracoid bones, and clavicles. The forelimb is composed of a short humerus and the radius/ulna. The hind limb is made up of a short femur and the tibia and fibula along with a patella. The pelvic girdle is comprised of the ilia, ischia, and pubes bones that are firmly braced against the sacrum. Legless lizards have lost the long bones but still retain their pectoral and pelvic girdles. The forefeet and hind feet are usually pentadactyl. The typical phalangeal formula is 2-3-4-5-3 in the forefoot and 2-3-4-5-4 in the hind foot.[2] Chameleons have pincerlike zygodactyl feet with the first through third digits opposing the fourth and fifth in the front feet, and the first and second digits opposing the third through fifth in the hind feet (Fig. 9.15). Bipedal locomotion is seen in some lizards, such as the basilisk and the collared lizard (*Crotaphytus collaris*), and results in great speed.

Many lizards are capable of tail autotomy, or loss of the tail. The advantage of autotomy is to escape from or distract predators when grabbed by the tail. Tails are often brightly colored to attract the attention of predators and wiggle extensively for a few minutes when they detach. Those species that undergo autotomy possess a vertical fracture plane through the body and part of the neural arch of each caudal vertebra. This is a plate of cartilage or connective tissue that develops after ossification. Fracture planes are absent in the cranial part of the tail to protect the hemipenes, fat deposits, and other structures. In iguanas, the fracture plane is replaced by bone during maturation, resulting in a more stable tail in adults. The lost tail is regenerated with a cartilaginous rod for support rather than vertebrae. It generally has smaller darker scales in a more irregular pattern than the original tail and may be shorter and blunter (Fig. 9.16).

Most iguanid lizards, anguids, and many skink genera can undergo autotomy, but most agamids do not. Likewise, the monitors and true chameleons (*Chamaeleo* spp.) do not have fragile tails. Those species with strong tails usually cannot regenerate a complete tail if the original is lost. For more information, see Chapter 81.

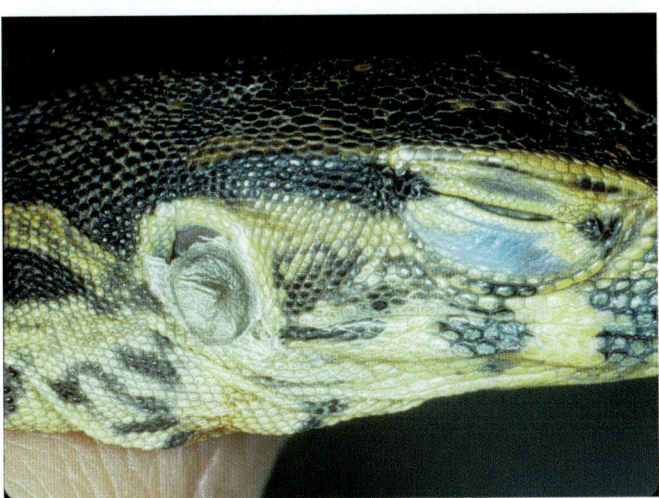

FIG 9.17 A monitor lizard (*Varanus* spp.) undergoing ecdysis sheds the outer layer of transparent skin that covers the tympanic membrane. (Courtesy of Stephen Barten.)

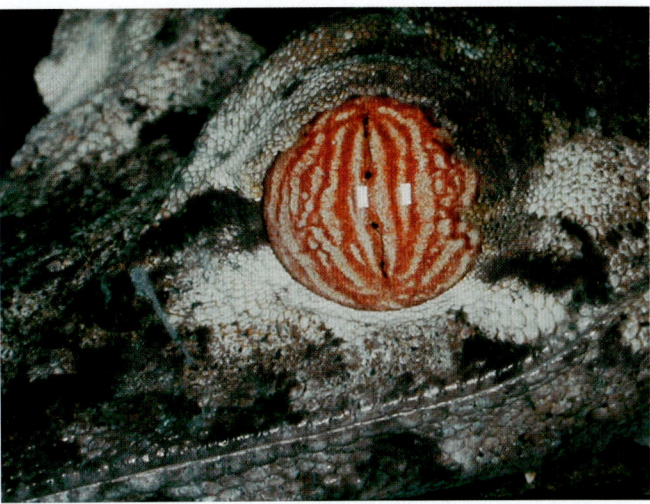

FIG 9.18 Madagascar leaf-tailed gecko (*Uroplatus fimbriatus*). The serrated vertical pupil is completely closed in the bright light used for photography, resulting in a series of pinholes (seen as a vertical line of tiny black dots in the center of the highly ornamented iris). These allow acute vision. (Courtesy of Stephen Barten.)

Nervous System

Like all vertebrates, the reptilian brain consists of the forebrain and the hindbrain. The reptile brain is more advanced, with a larger cerebrum and cerebellum than that of amphibians or fishes. Still, the brain is small, not exceeding 1% of the body mass in its tubular structure. Nevertheless, lizards should not be considered unintelligent; they are capable of learning and benefit from environmental enrichment in captivity. Reptiles are the earliest group of vertebrates with 12 pairs of cranial nerves. The spinal cord differs from that of mammals in that it extends to the tail tip. A subarachnoid space is not present, and as such myelography cannot be performed.

Neurologic disorders are poorly understood and documented in reptiles, but basic neurologic reflexes should be examined during any evaluation. Nutritional requirements and history must also be evaluated, because unbalanced diets may result in neurologic symptoms, such as hypocalcemic tetany. For more information, see chapter 77, Neurology.

Special Senses

Hearing. The ear has both auditory and vestibular functions. The tympanic membrane is generally visible within a shallow depression on the side of the head. It is covered with thin transparent skin, the outer layer of which is shed during ecdysis (Fig. 9.17). In some lizards, such as the lesser earless lizard (*Holbrookia maculata*) and horned lizards, the tympanic membrane is covered with scaly skin. Although mammals have three auditory ossicles, lizards only have two: the slender columnar stapes and its cartilaginous tip, the extracolumella, which are suspended within an air-filled cavity. Airborne vibrations are detected by the tympanic membrane and transmitted via these auditory ossicles across the middle ear to the inner ear. Geckos have the best hearing of all lizards. The inner ear consists of two sacs joined by a broad passage. The dorsal component or utriculus has three semicircular canals arranged perpendicular to each other. This arrangement allows for the detection of movement in three different planes and provides information for the sense of balance.[2,10] Some burrowing lizards have no external or middle ear but transmit sound via bone conduction in a manner the same as snakes. The eustachian tubes connect the middle ear cavities to the dorsolateral pharynx.

Vision. The structure of the reptile eye is similar to that of other vertebrates. The iris contains striated, not smooth, musculature, and

common mydriatics therefore have no effect. The lizard pupil is usually round and relatively immobile in diurnal species and is usually vertically slitlike in nocturnal species. Many geckos have a serrated pupillary opening that results in a series of small holes when the pupil is completely closed (Fig. 9.18). The images that pass through these holes are superimposed on the retina, resulting in acute vision even in dim light. The lens does not move for accommodation, but rather muscles in the ciliary body change the lens shape for this purpose. Consensual pupillary light reflex is absent. The cornea does not contain Descemet's membrane. A ring of bony scleral ossicles is present in most species. Eyelids are usually present, except for some geckos and the oscellated skink (*Ablepharus* sp.), which have snakelike spectacle scales. The lower lid is more movable and moves upward to close the eye. In some lizards, the lower lid may be transparent, allowing vision when the lids are closed and the eyes protected. The nictitating membrane is usually present.

The retina is relatively avascular but contains a conus papillaris, a large vascular body that protrudes into the vitreous. The fovea centralis, a depression in the retina responsible for acute vision, is often present in diurnal species. Lizards have good color vision but only a narrow binocular field. This is why they often cock their heads to the side to get the best monocular vision.[4]

A well-developed parietal eye is found on the dorsal midline of the head in some lizards, particularly the Iguanidae (Fig. 9.19). It is a degenerate eye that contains a lens and retina and connects neurologically to the pineal body and is thought to play an important role in regulating circadian rhythms. It does not form images.[10]

Endocrine System

The endocrine system is comprised of numerous glands scattered throughout the body. The gonads produce gametes, but they are also responsible for producing sex hormones. Photoperiod, temperature, and seasonal cycles influence the levels and production of these reproductive hormones. The pituitary gland functions in much the same way as in other vertebrates by producing hormones, such as adrenocorticotropin, prolactin, and follicle-stimulating hormone. These hormones along with others produced by the pituitary gland control such things as growth, water balance, and reproduction.[10]

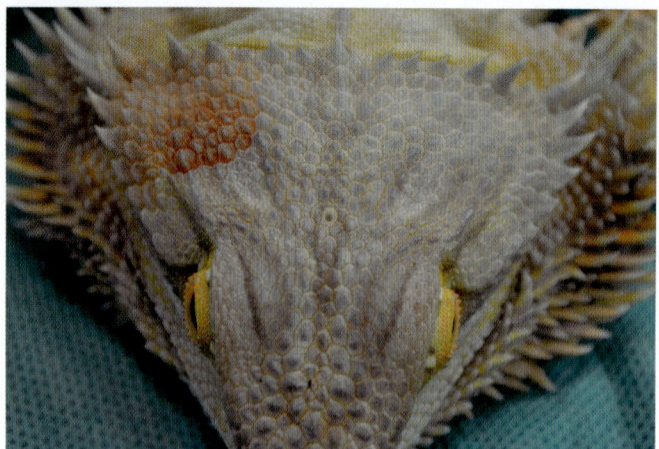

FIG 9.19 A well-developed parietal eye, like that seen in the center of this central bearded dragon's (*Pogona vitticeps*) head is a degenerate eye that contains a lens and retina. It connects to the pineal body and plays an important role in regulating circadian rhythms. (Courtesy of Shane Simpson.)

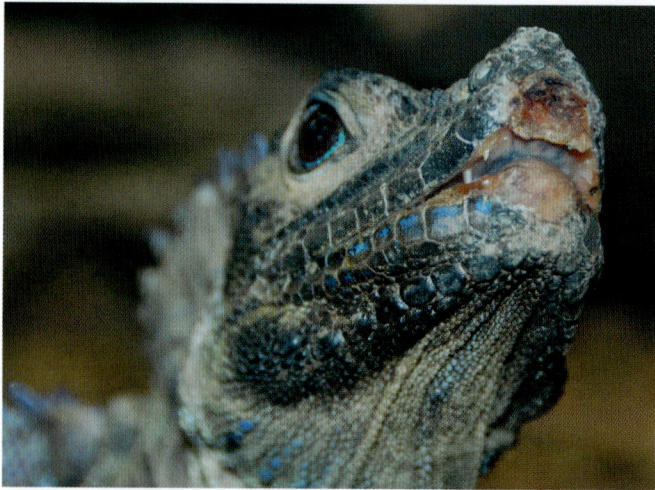

FIG 9.20 A male Philippines sail-fin lizard (*Hydrosaurus pustulatus*) with severe rostral abrasion. High-stress species like this can inflict serious damage to themselves with their constant rubbing on the glass walls of the enclosure. (Courtesy of Shane Simpson.)

The pineal body or complex detects the presence and absence of light and as a glandular structure produces the hormone melatonin. This hormone plays a vital role in both daily cycles (or circadian rhythms) and seasonal cycles. It is therefore intrinsically linked with the reproductive cycles of the lizard.[10]

The thyroid gland varies with the species and may be single, bilobed, or paired. The thyroid controls normal ecdysis. Lizards have paired parathyroid glands that control plasma calcium and phosphorus levels. Secondary nutritional and renal hyperparathyroidism are among the most commonly diagnosed diseases in captive reptiles.[4,10] Adrenal glands are suspended in the mesorchium or mesovarium and must be avoided during surgery for neutering.[10] The reptile pancreas has both exocrine and endocrine functions. The beta cells produce insulin, but primary diabetic changes are rare and often are associated with widespread disease. Insulin and glucagon have the same functions in controlling blood sugar levels as they do in other vertebrates.[10]

Despite all the advances in reptile medicine, endocrine disorders are poorly documented and are probably underdiagnosed in these species. See Chapter 79 for more details.

BEHAVIOR

Lizards tend to be alert and responsive, almost inquisitive. Captive-born lizards tend to be tame, docile, and tolerate handling. Wild-caught lizards tend to be shy and wary. They frantically try to escape at the slightest disturbance. Iguanas, monitors, and other lizards may exhibit defensive aggression when threatened. They stand sideways to the threat, swallow air to increase their size, stand high off the ground to look bigger, and lash out at the threat with their tails. Some may gape and threaten to bite if provoked. Some other "normal" behaviors include sneezing in those species with nasal salt glands, color and body size changes in basking animals, and sleeping underwater for semiaquatic reptiles.[34] Many lizards exhibit head bobbing and push-ups when another lizard or human invades their territory. Cage-mate aggression is common in central bearded dragons, and as such they should be kept separate. Offensive aggression is rare and usually involves sexually mature male iguanas during the breeding season. They may attack anyone entering their territory and attempt to bite. These lizards must be confined to their cage during these times.

Iguanas, some geckos, and others frequently defecate in the same spot. If paper is put in that spot, the lizard may become litter-trained. Iguanas loose in the house frequently defecate in the bathtub, which is easy to clean.

A common behavioral problem is rostral nose rubbing. This is most often seen in some of the more "high-stress" species of lizards such as water dragons (*Intellagama lesuerii, Physignathus cocincinus*) and Philippines sail-fin lizards (Fig. 9.20). It can be a frustrating condition to overcome. See Chapter 13 for more details.

LONGEVITY

Owners often question their veterinarian about how long their pet is expected to live. An appreciation of expected lifespans of the various commonly kept lizard species can therefore be useful in answering this question and determining if the patient is nearing its normal end of life.

This can be difficult though because specific and accurate longevity data on assorted species is lacking. Adding to the difficulty is the fact that it can be challenging to estimate the age of reptiles. Reptiles show little outward signs of aging. Body size is not an accurate method due to variations in food amounts and quality that can result in stunting or an increased rate of growth.

In general, it is considered that captive animals are longer-lived than wild relatives due to less exposure to potential dangers

Lizards are relatively long-lived animals when compared to mammals but not when compared with some of the other reptilian groups such as tortoises and crocodilians.

Bearded dragons live 10 to 12 years, with older specimens reaching 14 years. Green iguanas are reported as living 10 to 15 years, but some have been known to live to 20 years of age.[35] Owners should be educated about the difference between record lifespans, which are usually reported in common references, and average lifespans, which often are considerably less than the record for a given species.

REFERENCES

See www.expertconsult.com for a complete list of references.

10

Crocodilian Taxonomy, Anatomy, and Physiology

Javier G. Nevarez

Crocodilians are some of the largest reptiles in the world. They can be found through the Americas, Africa, Asia, and Australia in approximately 90 countries. They mostly inhabit tropical and subtropical regions. Crocodilians range in length from 1.5 m for smaller caiman and crocodile species to over 6 meters and over 450 kg for the saltwater crocodile (*Crocodylus porosus*). Most are also long-lived species, although there is no way to determine their true age in the wild. In general, smaller species such as caimans have a lifespan of 20 to 40 years, whereas crocodiles can live 60+ years. As such they require a large enclosure and people committed to their care in captivity. Crocodilians are displayed in zoological institutions, and there are even crocodilian-specific parks that house a majority of the species. Many species are also raised in commercial operations for their meat and hides (see Chapter 177). While they are legal as pets in some states/countries, their large size precludes most individual private owners from providing an adequate environment that is safe for animals and humans alike. Crocodilians have unique anatomy and physiology that separates them from other reptilian groups. Knowledge of these unique features is essential for their proper care in captivity.

TAXONOMY

All living crocodilians belong to the clade Archosauria, which also includes birds and extinct dinosaurs. Crocodilian taxonomy is varied depending on the source and interpretation. The information presented in this chapter is based on currently accepted classification, especially as it pertains to recognition by the International Union for the Conservation of Nature (IUCN) and Convention on International Trade in Endangered Species (CITES), which have important implications for the commercial trade and conservation of crocodilians. Based on this parameter, there are 24 recognized species of crocodilians divided into three families: Alligatoridae, Crocodylidae, and Gavialidae (Table 10.1). Some classifications will include subspecies, but these are not universally accepted. In the future, additional species may be added because recent work suggests *Osteolaemus tetraspis* should be divided into *O. tetraspis*, *O. osborni*, and *O. sp. nov.*[1,2] It is also proposed that *Mecistops cataphractus* (*Crocodylus cataphractus*) be divided into Central and West African subspecies,[2,3] but this has not been universally accepted. *Tomistoma schlegelii*, formerly known as the false gharial, was formerly included in the family Gavialidae, but now it is recognized under Crocodylidae, and the common name Tomistoma is more widely accepted. These taxonomic variations can have important implications for the conservation of the species in their native habitat and selection of animals for captive breeding programs.

ANATOMY AND PHYSIOLOGY

Integument

The skin of crocodilians, like that of other reptiles, is comprised of β- and α-keratin. The outer scales are made up of the rigid β-keratin, whereas the hinge regions are comprised of the more flexible α-keratin. These layers are arranged in alternating lateral distribution as opposed to an alternating vertical arrangement found in squamates and tuataras.[4] This lateral arrangement is responsible for shedding in a gradual, exfoliation pattern more similar to mammals than that of other reptile groups.[4] Despite belief to the contrary, crocodilians do shed their skin, but it is not easily observed grossly as in other reptile species. Crocodilians also have a higher distribution of dermal bones known as osteoderms. The arrangement and number of scales and osteoderms in the dorsal neck region can be used for species identification.[5] The skin over the skull is tightly adhered without a subcutaneous space. While the majority of osteoderms are found in the dorsal skin, some caiman and alligator species have them in the ventral skin, making them less ideal for the skin trade. The tail has a double row of triangular scales that merge into a single row midway along the length.

The skin coloration varies with age. Hatchlings and juveniles often have well-defined bands or spots that will fade as they grow. Adult skin coloration ranges from black-gray to light brown or off-green depending on the species. The ventral and lateral skin tends to be lighter than the back and head.

The skin of all crocodilians possesses intradermal sensory organs (ISO). The distribution of ISOs varies across species. In Alligatoridae, they are strictly found on the head region (Fig. 10.1), whereas in Crocodylidae and Gavilaidae they are found throughout the whole body but are more prominently noted on the ventral skin (Fig. 10.1).[6] These structures have highly sensitive free nerve endings similar to the lateral line system of fish. The function of ISO includes detection of water movement and tactile discrimination.[6] Leitch and Catania report that ISO have a mechanical sensitivity exceeding that of primate fingertips.[6] This is an important consideration when handling crocodilians as it implies their skin is capable of very minute tactile receptivity.

Crocodilians have paired gular and paracloacal glands (Fig. 10.2). The compounds secreted by these glands vary between glands and sexes. Their true function is not fully elucidated but may include mating, defense, and communication.[7]

Cardiovascular System

The cardiovascular system of crocodilians is perhaps the most complex in the animal kingdom due to anatomic features that allow right-to-left

TABLE 10.1   Taxonomy, Geographic Location, and Size of Crocodilians

Taxonomy	Common Name	Location	Average Adult Length
Family Alligatoridae			
Alligator mississippiensis	American alligator	Southeastern United States	4.5 m
Alligator sinensis	Chinese alligator	Eastern China, lower Yangzi river	2 m
Caiman crocodilus	Spectacled caiman	Central and South America	1.5–2 m
Caiman latirostris	Broad-snouted caiman	Argentina, Bolivia, Brazil, Paraguay, Uruguay	2 m
Caiman yacare	Yacare caiman	Argentina, Bolivia, Brazil, Paraguay	2.5 m
Melanosuchus niger	Black caiman	Bolivia, Brazil, Colombia, Ecuador, French Guiana, Guyana, Peru	4 m
Palaeosuchus palpebrosus	Cuvier's dwarf caiman	Bolivia, Brazil, Colombia, Ecuador, French Guiana, Guyana, Paraguay, Peru, Surinam, Venezuela	1.5 m
Palaeosuchus trigonatus	Schneider's smooth-fronted caiman	Bolivia, Brazil, Colombia, Ecuador, French Guiana, Guyana, Peru, Surinam, Venezuela	2 m
Family Crocodylidae			
Crocodylus acutus	American crocodile	Belize, Colombia, Costa Rica, Cuba, Dominican Republic, Ecuador, El Salvador, Guatemala, Haiti, Honduras, Jamaica, Mexico, Mexico, Nicaragua, Panama, Peru, United States, Venezuela	5 m
Crocodylus cataphractus	African slender-snouted crocodile	Central and West Africa	2.5 m
Crocodylus intermedius	Orinoco crocodile	Colombia, Venezuela	4–5 m
Crocodylus johnstoni	Australian freshwater crocodile	Northern Australia	2–2.5 m
Crocodylus mindorensis	Philippine crocodile	Philippines (Busuanga, Luzon, Masbate, Mindanao, Mindoro, Negros, Samar islands)	2–3 m
Crocodylus moreletii	Morelet's crocodile	Belize, Guatemala, Mexico	3 m
Crocodylus niloticus	Nile crocodile	Central-Southern Africa	5 m
Crocodylus suchus	West African crocodile	West Africa	5 m
Crocodylus novaeguineae	New Guinea freshwater crocodile	Indonesia, Papua New Guinea	2–3 m
Crocodylus palustris	Mugger crocodile	Iran, India, Nepal, Pakistan, Sri Lanka	4–5 m
Crocodylus porosus	Saltwater crocodile	Australia, Bangladesh, Brunei, Myanmar, Timor Leste (East Timor), India (incl. Andaman & Nicobar islands), Indonesia, Malaysia, Palau, Papua New Guinea (incl. Bismarck archipelago and other island chains), Philippines, Sri Lanka, Solomon Islands	3 m (females) 5 m (males)
Crocodylus rhombifer	Cuban crocodile	Cuba	3.5 m
Crocodylus siamensis	Siamese crocodile	Cambodia, Indonesia (including Borneo and possibly Java), Laos, Malaysia, Thailand, Vietnam	3 m
Osteolaemus tetraspis	Dwarf crocodile	West and West-central Africa	1–1.5 m
Tomistoma schlegelii	Tomistoma	Indonesia (Sumatra, Kalimantan, Java), Malaysia (Sarawak, Sabah, Peninsular Malaysia)	5 m
Family Gavialidae			
Gavialis gangeticus	Gharial	Northern India subcontinent: Bangladesh, Bhutan, Burma, India, Nepal, Pakistan	5 m

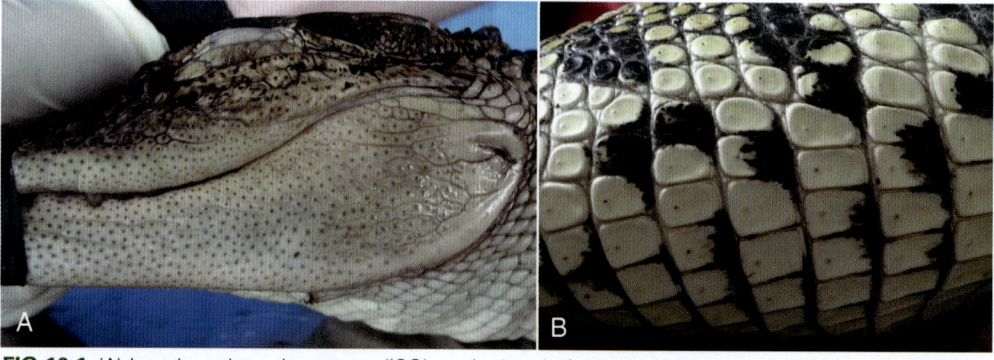

FIG 10.1 (A) Intradermal sensing organs (ISO) on the head of *A. mississippiensis*. (B) ISO on the flank of a crocodile. (Courtesy of Javier G. Nevarez.)

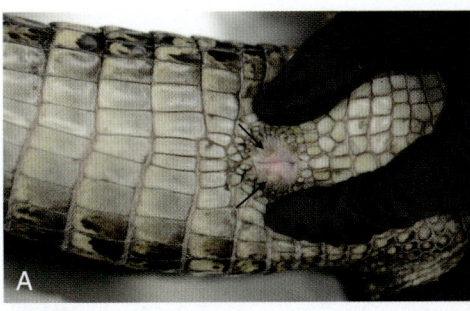
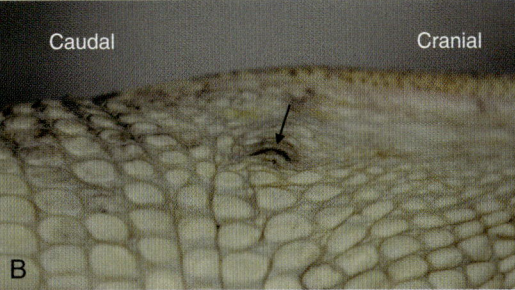

FIG 10.2 (A) Opening of the paracloacal glands (black arrow). (B) Opening of the right gular gland (black arrows) on the ventral mandibular vaspect of *A. mississippiensis*. (Courtesy of Javier G. Nevarez.)

shunting in a way not found in any other taxa. Crocodilians are the only reptiles with a true four-chamber heart. There is a prominent pericardial sac that often contains a large amount of fluid compared to similarly sized mammals (Fig. 10.3). The significance of this fluid volume is unknown. There is a prominent sinus venosus on the right side associated with the right atria. Salient features of the crocodilian heart include a foramen of Panizza, a left aorta originating from the right ventricle, anastomosis between left and right aortas, and cog-teeth-like valves in the right ventricle.[8] The foramen of Panizza is a high septal opening anterior to the aortic valves that connects the right and left aortas. A critical function is the perfusion of the coronary vessels and brain during blood shunting.[8] Because the left aorta originates from the right ventricle, it also plays a significant role in shunting, specifically as it relates to digestion.[9] The anastomosis between left and right aortas lies dorsal to the lungs. Past this anastomosis, the left aorta becomes the celiac artery, and the right becomes the dorsal aorta. The cog-teeth-like valves in the pulmonary outflow of the right ventricle, proximal to the bicuspid valve, help control shunting. These three features combined play a role in right-to-left shunting in crocodilians.[8,10] Shunting occurs as a result of complex anatomical and physiological factors including changes in ventricular pressures, pulmonary pressure, and systemic resistance. The shunting process cannot be predicted or controlled; therefore gas anesthesia alone is not recommended because, if shunting occurs, it can lead to unpredictable levels of anesthesia.

An important role of the shunting process is to allow crocodilians to stay submerged for prolonged periods of time. During diving, an increase in the pulmonary pressure leads to an increase in central pressure due to reduced blood flow from the pulmonary artery. This in turn leads to blood flow through the foramen of Panizza to the left aorta and to the systemic circulation allowing both conservation of oxygen and perfusion of organs.

Respiratory System

The nostrils of all crocodilians are located on a raised area at the end of their dorsal snouts and can be closed with muscular flaps when the animal submerges. Crocodilians lack a choanal slit; instead there is a complete hard palate creating a true division between the oral and pharyngeal cavities (Fig. 10.4). A highly vascular sinus system allows the nasal passage to seal out water when vessels are engorged so that animals do not drown under water. The nasal passage is divided into a vestibulum, nasal cavity (cavum), and nasopharyngeal duct. The nasal cavity has conchae and gives rise to a complex system of nasal sinuses. The internal nostrils open at the level of the glottis in the pharynx.

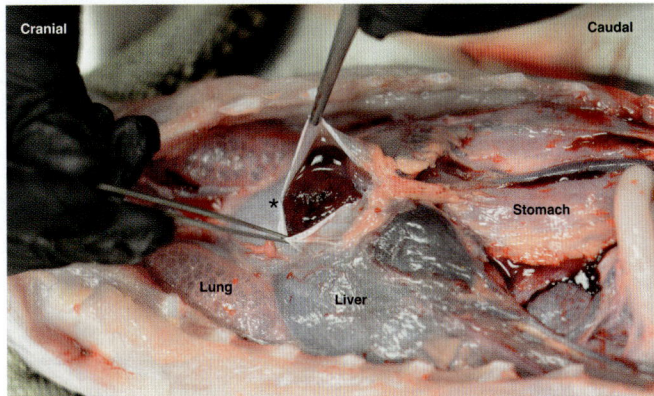

FIG 10.3 Incised pericardial sac (*) of *A. mississippiensis* revealing normal amount of fluid surrounding the heart. It is normal to find a large amount of pericardial fluid and sometimes free coelomic fluid as well, especially in free-ranging alligators. (Courtesy of Javier G. Nevarez.)

There is a gular valve composed of the velum palati dorsally and the gular fold ventrally (Fig. 10.4).[11] The velum palati is a soft tissue extension of the dorsal palate. The gular fold is a cartilaginous extension of the basihyoid cartilage.[11] Together they create a tight seal separating the oral and pharyngeal cavity (Fig. 10.4), which allows crocodilians to grab and hold prey underwater without drowning. Water that is taken into the mouth can be swallowed without being inhaled. They can open-mouth breath in cases of trauma to the nasal passages. Crocodilians have complete tracheal rings and multicameral lungs with a single left and right lung lobe. There is an extensive bronchial tree. The lungs are in direct contact with the liver and extend dorsocaudally within the coelomic cavity. On radiographs, the lungs normally encompass one-third to one-half of the coelomic cavity. Framer et al. have described the airflow through the lungs of crocodilians.[12] Despite the absence of air sacs, there is a unidirectional flow of air similar to birds.[12] Respiration is an active process by the intercostal muscles and the diaphragmaticus muscle, also known as the post-hepatic septum. The diaphragmaticus originates from the ischia and last gastralia and inserts on connective tissue on the caudal aspect of the liver (Fig. 10.5).[13] It is incomplete and more horizontally oriented so it does not create a true separation of the cavity. It is a thin muscle that has often been associated with respiration but also plays an active role in buoyancy.[13,14] Uriona et al. revealed that transection of the diaphragmaticus muscle can lead to decreased submersion times in *Alligator mississippiensis*.[15]

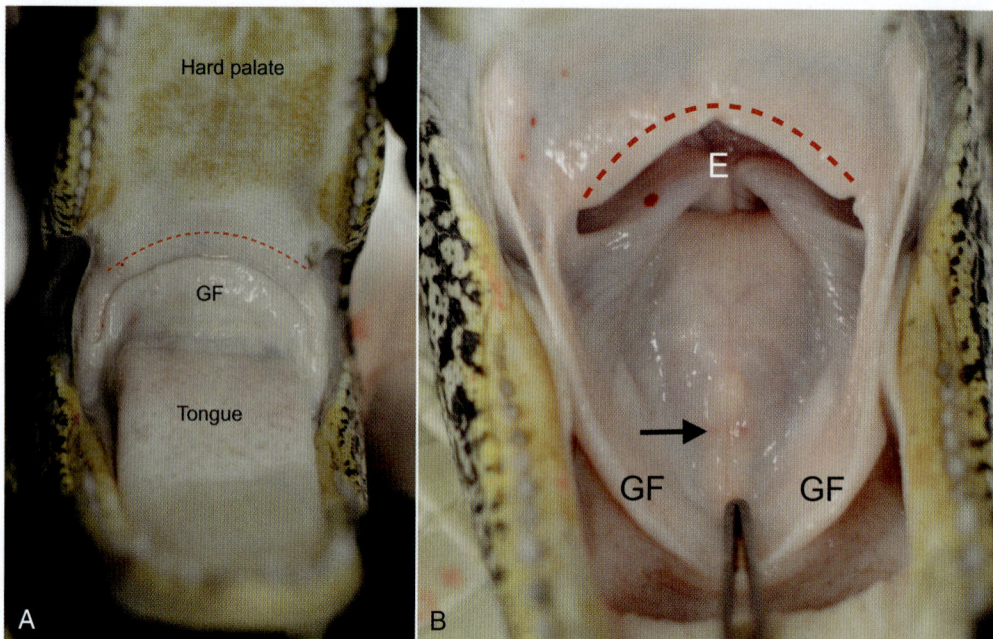

FIG 10.4 (A) Oral cavity of *A. mississippiensis* revealing the gular valve composed of the velum palati dorsally (red dotted line) and the gular fold ventrally (GF). (B) The gular fold (GF) retracted cranioventral to reveal the pharyngeal cavity. The larynx (black arrow) and esophageal opening (E) can be observed. The velum palti is dorsal (red dotted line). (Courtesy of Javier G. Nevarez.)

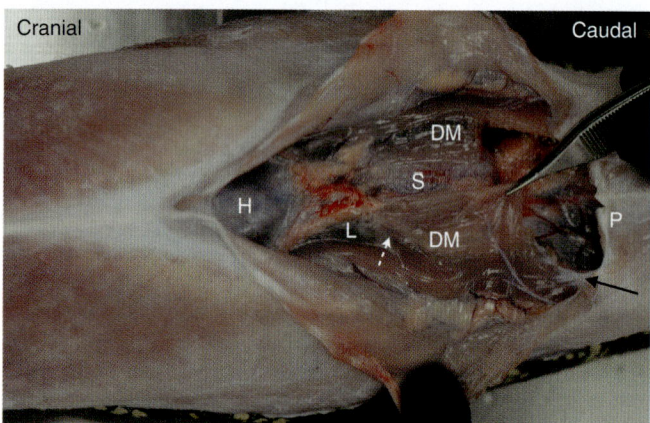

FIG 10.5 Exposed coelomic cavity of *A. mississippiensis*. The diaphragmaticus muscle (DM) has been partially resected during dissection from its origin on the ischia and last gastralia (black arrow) and insertion on connective tissue on the caudal aspect of the liver (white dotted arrow) are intact. H = heart; S = stomach; L = liver. (Courtesy of Javier G. Nevarez.)

Digestive System

Crocodilians are polyphyodonts with thecodont dentition. As such they have continually replaced teeth that live in a socket. Their teeth are conical, hollow, and without any roots. Estimates are that crocodilians can replace their teeth up to 50 times in their lifespan. Older animals may be missing teeth due to old age bind/or damage that has affected tooth growth. There is varied conformation of their tooth arrangement,

and some dental formulas have been proposed by Grigg and Kishner.[16] These formulas divide the teeth into premaxillary and maxillary rather than traditional mammalian formulas. Dental disease is usually of low clinical significance in crocodilians.

The tongue is attached to the floor of the mouth along the entire ventral surface, thereby preventing any protrusion of the organ. The crocodilian stomach is divided into two distinct regions, the corpus and the pars pylorica (Fig. 10.6). The corpus or cardiac region is the first compartment and glandular portion of the stomach. Gastroliths and other foreign bodies can sometimes be found in the corpus, leading some to compare it to the ventriculus of birds. However, gross and histologic structure differ from the avian ventriculus. Past the corpus there is a sphincter that opens into a small dilatation, the pars pylorica (Fig. 10.6), before a thick sphincter leads into the duodenum. There is rarely any ingesta observed within the pars pylorica, and its function is largely unknown. The stomach's high acidic secretion is partially controlled by shunting of deoxygenated blood after ingestion of a meal.[9] Crocodilians have shifts in plasma pH levels on a frequent basis.[17] Because of the high production of concentrated hydrochloric acid in the stomach, a shift of chloride ions from plasma leaves a large amount of sodium to react with plasma carbonic acid.[17] This results in large amounts of sodium bicarbonate causing an alkaline tide.[17] Thus a profound plasma alkalemia in crocodilians is associated with food ingestion. The most efficient temperatures for ingestion and digestion are between 25°C and 35°C (77°F–95°F).

The duodenum is thick and U-shaped (Fig. 10.6). The pancreas is closely adhered to the duodenum and runs its entire length (Fig. 10.6). The small intestines have a rather thick wall compared to in other animals, and the mucosa commonly displays a crosshatch pattern. Gut-associated lymphoid tissue is found throughout the intestines. These can sometimes be observed grossly, especially in cases of enteritis. The large intestine is short, thin walled, and with a diameter of approximately twice the

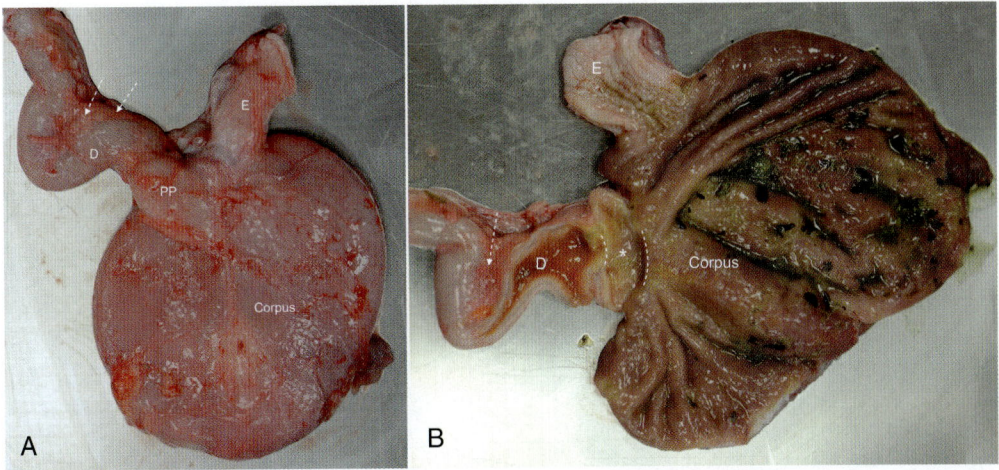

FIG 10.6 (A) The distal esophagus (E), corpus and pars pylorica (PP) of the stomach, duodenum (D), and pancreas (white dotted arrows) of *A. mississippiensis*. (B) Exposed mucosa of the esophagus (E), corpus, pars pylorica (*), and proximal loop of the duodenum (D). The dotted white lines mark the sphincters separating the pars pylorica from the corpus and duodenum. The pancreas (white dotted arrows) is located between the loops of the duodenum. (Courtesy of Javier G. Nevarez.)

small intestines. Urine and fluids are often found within the colon. There are prominent ileocolic and colon sphincters. The small and large intestines are enveloped by an extensive mesentery that creates a true separation between the lungs, liver, stomach, and the rest of the organs. This mesentery in essence creates a bag that encases and/or incorporates the small and large intestines, spleen, kidneys, and gonads (Fig. 10.7).

There are two liver lobes, with the right being larger. A gallbladder is present within the right lobe. A prominent triangular fat pad can normally be found caudal to the right liver lobe. A small fat pad may be indicative of chronic anorexia, particularly in captive animals. The liver lobes are concave medially to accommodate the shape of the heart. On cut surface, the liver tissue is dark brown-red in color. Unlike most reptiles and birds, crocodilians produce bilirubin. The author has observed icterus, elevated bilirubin levels, and liver fibrosis in cases of aflatoxicosis (Fig. 10.8).

Reproductive System

All crocodilians are oviparous. The time of year and length of various stages of the reproductive cycle are somewhat variable depending on the species, habitat, and hemisphere of location, but overall they share common anatomy and reproductive cycles. The testes and ovaries are located ventrally on the craniomedial aspect of the kidneys. Both gonads increase in size during the reproductive season. The reproductive cycle and follicular development of alligators has been described and can be monitored with ultrasonography.[18,19] During vitellogenesis, higher amounts of lipids, phosphorus, calcium, and vitamin E are found in the blood.[20] Blood plasma collected from female alligators at this time of year has a characteristic white appearance as a result of the increased circulating lipids.[19,20] After ovulation, the plasma loses the white appearance and is similar to that of males and nonreproductive females. In the alligator, a hierarchy of follicle groups develops, with each group representing a clutch. The clutch to be fertilized may contain as few as 20 or as many as 80 follicles, with an average of 40 eggs laid per clutch. Alligators and most of the crocodilian species go through a refractory period after ovulation. An exception to this is the Indian mugger crocodile (*Crocodylus palustris*), which produces two clutches per year under natural conditions.

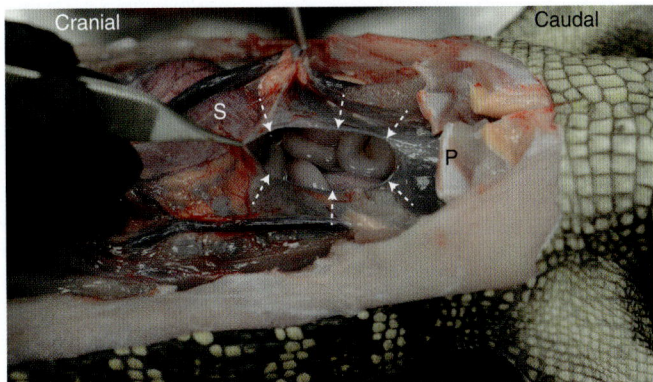

FIG 10.7 View of incision through the mesentery (white arrows) in *A. mississippiensis* revealing intestinal loops. While the intestinal loops come in contact with the stomach (S), they do not contact the lungs or heart. The pubis (P) has been cut for easier visualization. (Courtesy of Javier G. Nevarez.)

Sexing can be performed by examination of the cloaca. Males have a phallus that can be easily everted from the cloaca. The phallus is located on the ventroposterior surface of the cloaca near the cranial opening of the vent, and the dorsal surface has a single open groove that serves for conduction of spermatozoa. Two thick fibrous plates, the crus penis, are located at the base of the phallus. The groove is the result of the fusion of the crus penis. The phallus is primarily cartilaginous and has little erectile tissue. Females have a clitoris that is similar in appearance to the phallus but smaller and will not evert from the cloaca. Therefore when sexing crocodilians, palpating the cloaca is not accurate enough. It is important to attempt to evert the phallus to confirm it is a male, particularly in small animals because the well-developed clitoris is easily confused with a phallus.

Crocodilian gender is a result of temperature-dependent sex determination (TDSD) with an incubation temperature range of 29°C to 34°C (84°F–93°F) being reported as ideal for embryo viability and

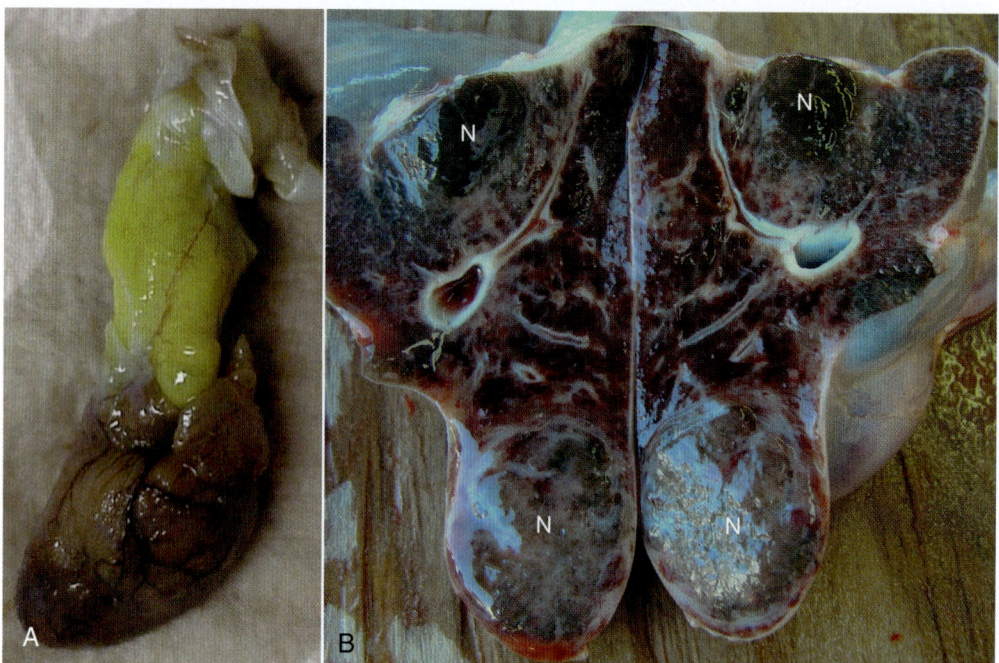

FIG 10.8 (A) Icteric cardiac vessels of *A. mississippiensis* diagnosed with aflatoxicosis. (B) Liver from the same animal revealing fibrosis and necrosis (N), replacing the more normal red-colored hepatic tissue. Affected animals were found to have higher bilirubin levels than healthy animals. (Courtesy of Javier G. Nevarez.)

hatching.[21,22] In all species, low incubation temperatures (29°C–30°C; 84°F–86°F) result in all females, and temperatures above 34°C (93°F) result in a high proportion of malformations or embryonic deaths.[22,23] However, the data on mid-range and high-range temperatures vary among studies. While it was proposed that *A. mississippiensis* and *C. crocodilus* followed a female-male pattern (FM) at low and high temperatures respectively,[22,23] Lang and Andrews found a female-male-female (FMF) pattern similar to other crocodilians.[22] In the FMF pattern, females are produced at low and high temperatures while males predominate at intermediate temperatures. It was determined that in *A. mississippiensis*, 100% males are produced at the narrow range of 31.5°C to 31.8°C (88.7°F–89.2°F), which appears to be unique in crocodilians.[22] At 33°C (91.4°F) there is again a shift toward a more-even distribution of male and females, and beyond 33.5°C (92.3°F), females predominate.[22] Based on their results, Lang and Andrews proposed an FMF pattern for *A. mississippiensis, C. crocodilus, C. palustris, C. moreletii, C. siamensis, C. porosus, C. johnstoni, C. niloticus,* and *G. gangeticus.* The period of temperature sensitivity at which sex is determined is proposed to be during stages 21 to 24 of the third quarter of embryonic development, which is the period of gonadal development.[21,22] In addition to incubation temperatures, there also appears to be a clutch effect that influences sex ratios.[22]

Urinary System

Crocodilians are both ammoniotelic and uricotelic, with ammonia excretion being predominant.[24] There is no urinary bladder, but urine is often stored in the urodeum and coprodeum.[25] Urine collection via catheter insertion into these chambers has been reported.[25] All crocodilians possess salt-excretory lingual glands, but these are less developed in species that live primarily in freshwater habitats.[26,27] Periodic submergence in water is necessary for all crocodilians to counteract water loss. Water intake consists of incidental drinking (and drinking when feeding. Water may also be absorbed through the skin. Small crocodilians

such as hatchlings and juveniles may lose up to 20% of body weight per day through insensible losses. Daily movement between land and water is necessary to maintain the correct osmoregulation. Loss of sodium in fresh water is fairly low, and the main route of sodium loss is through the skin. Evaporative water loss occurs from the respiratory tract, the oral cavity, and the skin. The kidney and cloaca are the primary route for the excretion of nitrogenous waste but not for salt excretion. Some salt and water absorption is reported to occur in the cloaca.

Musculoskeletal System

The crocodilian skull is elongated and composed of 30 fused bones. All species of crocodilians have long, flattened, tooth-lined skulls of various sizes and shapes. Both upper and lower jaws have teeth that are set in sockets via connective tissue. The upper and lower jaws articulate at the posterior aspect of the skull, which allows the wide opening of the jaws. The one to two muscle pairs that open the jaw are quite weak, and therefore the jaws can be held closed with a minimal amount of effort.[16] The five to six muscle pairs that close the jaws are very strong, creating an extreme bite force, the highest measured in animals.[16] In adult animals, attempting to open the mouth can be dangerous because of this strength. If one opens the mouth of an adult that has recently died, a point comes where the muscles are stimulated to close with tremendous force. The stimulatory effect may occur up to 24 hours after death.

The approximately 55 to 67 vertebrae consist of 8 to 9 cervical, 15 to 16 dorsal (thoracolumbar), 2 sacral, and 30 to 40 caudal.[16] Crocodilians, like most reptiles, have procoelous vertebrae, which are concave anteriorly and convex posteriorly. This is in contrast to the acoelous vertebrae of mammals, which are flattened on both ends. Exceptions in crocodilians include the atlas and axis, the two sacral, and the first caudal vertebrae, which are all acoelous.[16] There are eight pairs of ribs and an additional eight pairs of gastralia or floating ribs (Fig. 10.9). Gastralia are embedded in the ventral body wall superficial to the rectus abdominis muscles. The so-called sacral ribs are heavy bones that articulate with the transverse

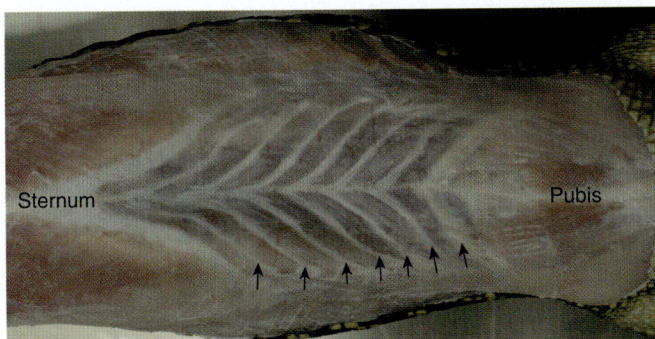

FIG 10.9 Ventral coelom of *A. mississippiensis* with the skin removed to reveal the gastralia (black arrows) and sternum. The eighth gastralia is not visible in the image as it lies within the soft tissues in the caudal coelom. (Courtesy of Javier G. Nevarez.)

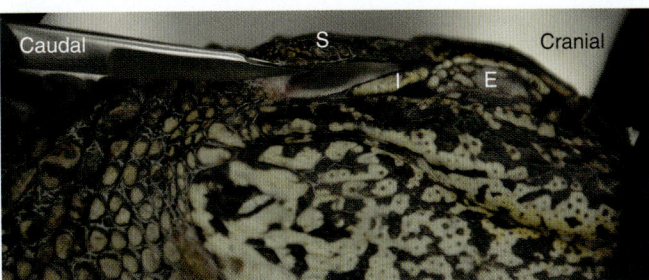

FIG 10.10 External auditory meatus of *A. Mississippiensis* showing the large superior (S) and smaller inferior (I) flaps that protect the tympanic membrane. The ear is located caudal to the eye (E). (Courtesy of Javier G. Nevarez.)

processes of the sacral vertebrae. A difference of opinion exists as to whether these are true ribs or merely thickened transverse processes. They are not fused to the vertebrae and so are frequently referred to as ribs. The pelvic girdle has a short ilium, a narrow but elongated pubis, and a short wide ischium. The front and hind limbs are anatomically similar to those of mammals and attach in an analogous fashion. The femur is longer than the humerus and holds the posterior portion of the body higher than the anterior. The front limbs have five digits with claws on the medial three digits, and the webbed hind limbs have four digits that are longer than the front limbs and also have claws on the medial three digits.

Nervous System

Crocodilians have features of the brain and nervous system that distinguish them from other reptiles. They have a cerebral cortex albeit small in size, lack a pineal body, and have a larger cerebellum than other reptiles.[28] They have small brains that account for 0.004% of their total body weight; however, they are still known to have good cognitive and learning capacity.[28] There are 12 pairs of cranial nerves, with a salient feature being enlargement of the trigeminal nerves. It is proposed that this serves the increased sensory function of skin on the face and head, along with the ISO.[28] The dorsal roots of the first two spinal nerves, are absent but do occur on the remaining spinal nerves. The spinal cord of crocodilians extends almost to the tip of the tail. The dorsal and ventral caudal nerves leave the spinal cord in the same way as the body trunk nerves due to the lack of a cauda equina.[29]

Species Senses

Vision. Crocodilians are visually oriented and have eyes that are well suited for both day and night. Because they are located high and lateral on the head, the eyes, like the nostrils, can remain above the surface of the water when the animal is partially submerged. The eyes of caimans and alligators are more prominent than those of crocodiles. The bony orbits of the skull surround the eyes, and if the eyes are pressed, they sink into the orbit. In crocodilians the upper eyelid provides most the movement for closing the eye. The upper lid may also contain a bony structure, or tarsus, which is absent from the lower lid.[30] There is a nictitating membrane with a cartilaginous edge. The third eyelid arises ventral and cranial and moves in a dorso-caudal direction when closing. The nictitans is transparent to translucent in most species. A harderian gland is present and described as discharging on the inner aspect of the nictitans.[30] A lachrymal gland is present on the medial aspect of the orbit.[30] There is a vertical slitlike pupil that dilates in a medial-lateral direction. The pupil position remains vertical with the horizon, even

when the head is raised or lowered. It is postulated that when the animal is turned over on its back, it becomes disoriented because of this particular eye configuration. Scleral ossicles are absent, but there is a cuplike scleral cartilage that extends more cranially.[28,30] There is a predominance of rods over cones, an adaptation for night vision. A tapetum lucidum is well developed and located on the dorsal aspect of the retina. This makes it easy to locate the animals at night when a spotlight is used.

The muscles of the eye (the superior rectus, inferior rectus, the internal rectus, and the inferior oblique) serve to allow retraction of the eye into the orbit when the animal is threatened. Almost all crocodilians use vision to capture prey that is out of the water, but such vision under the water is limited, and other senses are used. The lateral placement of the eyes means that the anterior binocular vision is not well developed. In the American alligator, the eyes are oriented to permit 25 degrees of binocular vision and a field of view of approximately 260 degrees.[28] When working with large crocodilians, an approach directly from the front or from behind is advisable and somewhat safer whenever feasible. The poor binocular vision means that the defensive mechanism for the animal is better adapted to lateral approaches. When approached from the side, the rapid defensive movement of the head and tail is directed in the same direction, with an attempt to strike the individual with the head, tail, or both.

Hearing. The external auditory meatus are slitlike openings that are closed by a large superior and smaller inferior flap and are protected by a dorsal shelf of bone (Fig. 10.10).[28] The fibrous flaps serve to close the external opening when the animal submerges. The middle ear is separated from the external ear by a tympanic membrane. Crocodilians have a well-developed hearing mechanism. They have good auditory acuity across a wide range of frequencies from approximately 20 to 2000 Hz.[28] A variety of sounds are used by crocodilians, such as grunts by hatchlings and hissing or snarling sounds when threatened. A characteristic bellowing sound is used during the mating season. Evidence of this is found in their behavior when strange sounds occur and in their ability to respond to vocalizations at specific times, such as during the breeding season or when hatchlings are in the nest. It is not unusual for females to become disturbed when hatchlings are stimulated to make grunting sounds.

BEHAVIOR

Parental care at hatching and post hatching are universal traits in the wild. In captivity, however, some species such as *A. mississippiensis* become accustomed to repeated approaches to the nest and do not display protective behavior. *C. porosus* is reported to aggressively defend the nest at all times.

Thermophile or heat seeking occurs in all crocodilians after feeding. This increase in body temperature apparently benefits the animal by increasing the rate of digestion and absorption. Even though environmental temperature has an influence on their body temperature, crocodilians select behavior that enhances their activity in relation to the environment. Evidence also shows that the particular temperature of incubation of an embryo may have an effect on selected body temperature later in life.[22] Lang has reported that when *A. mississippiensis* are fed, they select the warmer area in the enclosure.[31] When not fed, the same animals move to a cooler area. Coulson and Hernandez[17] reported that digestion and absorption took twice as long at 20°C as they did at 28°C in *A. mississippiensis*. Diefenbach also reported that passage of food through the digestive system was three times faster at 30°C than at 15°C in *Caiman crocodilus*.[32] This selection in body temperature differential appears to occur in captive *A. mississippiensis* hatchlings and juveniles when given the opportunity. Adults living in the wild or in outside captive facilities also display this selection process. They come out of the water to bask in the sun. At this time, they may lie with their jaws open in an effort to obtain evaporative cooling of the head. Heating and cooling are accomplished by entering and leaving the water.

The requirement for heat is greater in hatchlings and juveniles than in adults. An experimental infection reported by Lang caused an increase in selected body temperature within a short time and returned to normal by day 4.[31] Increases in body temperature ranged from +1.68°C to +7.88°C (35°–46°F). None of the animals showed ill effects in growth or behavior as a result.

In another study, Glassman and Bennett reported that *A. mississippiensis* subjected to an induced infection and held at constant temperatures responded to the infection with increased white blood cells.[33] The animals were maintained at 25°C (77°F), 30°C (86°F), and 35°C (95°F). The animals held at 30°C (86°F) displayed the greatest hematologic response and recovered. Infected animals held at 35°C (95°F) succumbed within 3 weeks, which was attributed to the stress of high temperature and an ineffective immune response.

Behavioral fever, which has been reported in other reptile species, appears to be an important factor in survival. However, an adequate thermal gradient must be available for the optimum immune response, which is temperature dependent.[34] When temperatures are maintained at a constant, the stress combined with a reduced antibody response can lead to stunted growth or a high mortality in the group.

REFERENCES

See www.expertconsult.com for a complete list of references.

11

Tuatara Taxonomy, Anatomy, and Physiology

Sarah Alexander

Tuatara (*Sphenodon punctatus*) are unique reptiles endemic to New Zealand and are the only extant members of the order Rhynchocephalia, a once widespread and moderately diverse group. The name "tuatara" is derived from the Maori language, where "tua" means back or far side, and "tara" means spike or spine. This is translated as "peaks on the back," a reference to the tuatara's spiny dorsal crest. The scientific name *Sphenodon* is derived from the Greek words for wedge (sphen) and tooth (odous), describing the wedge-shaped acrodont teeth of tuatara. The species name *punctatus* refers to the large number of spots on the tuatara's body. Tuatara were once widespread throughout New Zealand but effectively disappeared from the mainland following the arrival of Polynesians in AD 1250 to 1300 due to associated land use modification and the introduction of Pacific rats (*Rattus exulans*).[1] The arrival of Europeans and associated predators in the 1840s sounded the death knell for mainland tuatara populations, and today they survive on about 32 offshore islands and several mainland sanctuaries, approximating 0.5% of their former range.[2] The tuatara population today is estimated to number approximately 50,000 animals, and they are listed on CITES Appendix 1.

Tuatara are long-lived reptiles thought to survive for 80 years or more in the wild,[1] although there are several animals in captive institutions estimated to be more than 100 years of age. Adult tuatara exhibit sexual dimorphism. Males are larger than females, have a proportionally larger head, and have more prominent nuchal and dorsal crests and spines. Juveniles may exhibit this to a lesser degree but are more accurately sexed by coelioscopy.[3] Adult tuatara weigh between 200 and 1100 g, with a snout-vent length of 170 to 280 mm. Size varies with geographic location, with animals on larger islands consistently being bigger than their counterparts in more size-restricted habitats, presumably due to differences in food availability.[1] Tuatara are considered nocturnal, though they often emerge during the day in suitable weather, primarily to bask.[4]

TAXONOMY

Tuatara are members of the superorder Lepidosauria, which includes modern lizards and snakes. While tuatara bear a superficial resemblance to lizards, their ancestors are thought to have diverged from snakes and lizards in the early Triassic, an estimated 240 to 250 million years ago (Fig. 11.1).[5] *Sphenodon punctatus* is currently the only recognized species of tuatara, although the Brothers Island subpopulation was briefly classified as a separate species (*S. guntheri*) in the 1990s on the basis of variation in blood proteins.[6] Subsequent molecular studies have confirmed these animals all belong to the single species *S. punctatus*,[7] and they are currently managed as a single species with distinct geographic variants.

ANATOMY AND PHYSIOLOGY

The body shape of tuatara superficially resembles that of terrestrial lizards, but unique anatomic and physiological features set them apart from other squamates.

Integument

The dorsal scales of tuatara are small, granular, and usually an olive-brown color, though green, orange, and gray variants exist. Juveniles often exhibit brighter coloration than adults, and this fades with age (Fig. 11.2). The dorsal surface of the animal is covered in white-yellow spots of varying size, and there is a spiny crest that runs along the dorsal surface of the head and back. The ventral scales are larger than the dorsal scales and are pale gray to white in color. Tuatara slough in a ragged, fragmentary fashion similar to that of lizards, a process that can take up to 1 month and usually takes place once a year in late summer, although it can occur more frequently in juveniles and in captive animals.

Cardiovascular System

Tuatara have a heart structure similar to lizards, with two atria and a single ventricle. The ventricle has a poorly developed vertical septum and muscular ridge; however, functionally there is considerable separation of pulmonary and systemic blood flow, as seen in other squamates.[8] Tuatara have the largest erythrocytes and granular leukocytes of any reptile studied.[9] As in most other reptiles, tuatara lack lymph nodes[10] but have an extensive network of perivascular lymph vessels running throughout the body.

Respiratory System

The trachea of tuatara divides into two very short bronchi, each ending in a thin-walled, single-chambered lung.[11] The surface area for respiration is low compared with similar-sized reptiles, likely a function of the tuatara's low metabolic rate and oxygen demand.[12] Similar to many lizards, tuatara have a biphasic breathing pattern. After inspiration there is a small, incomplete exhalation, followed by a pause, and then active expiration, followed immediately by the next inspiration.[13] Tuatara have limited vocalizations but will make a croaking noise when disturbed or distressed.

Digestive System: Dentition

Tuatara have acrodont dentition, with two upper rows of teeth—a complete outer row attached to the maxilla, and a shorter inner row attached to the lateral edge of the palatine bone (Fig. 11.3). A single lower row of teeth fits into the gap between the two upper rows and moves rostrally relative to the upper jaw, producing a painful crushing bite with a saw-like motion.[14] Tuatara also have a pair of large incisor-like

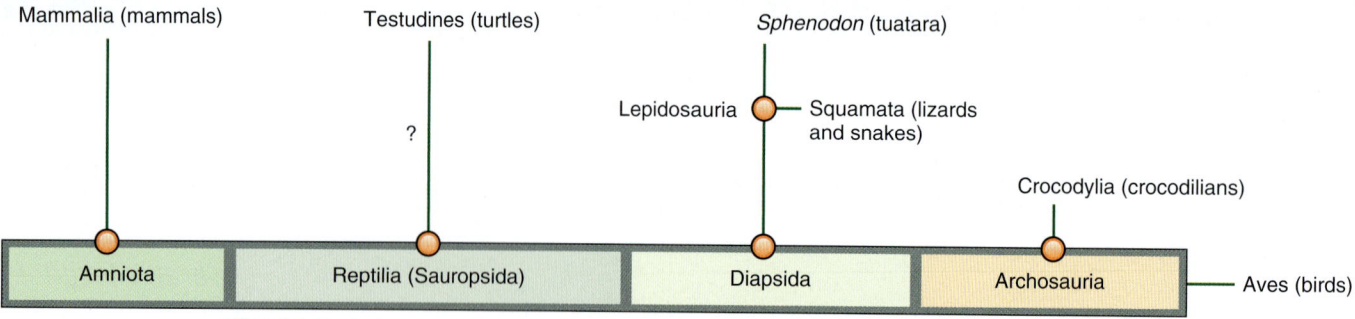

FIG 11.1 Evolutionary relationship of tuatara to other vertebrates. (Modified from Cree A, 2014.)[1]

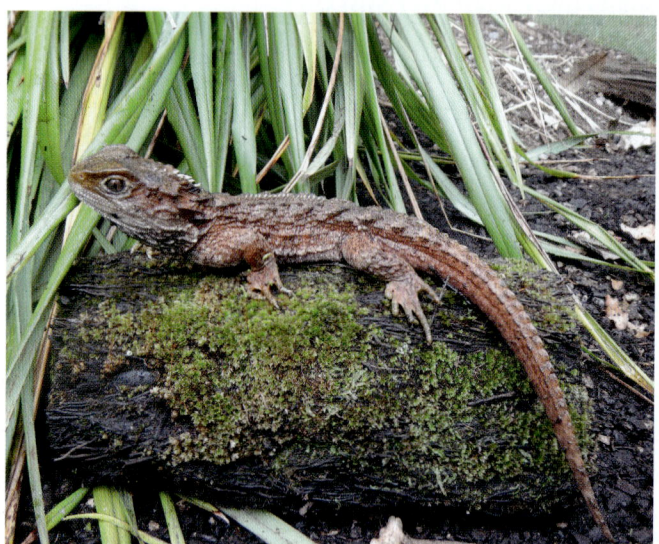

FIG 11.2 A juvenile tuatara *(Sphenodon punctatus)* with bright red coloring; this will fade with age. (Courtesy of Auckland Zoo.)

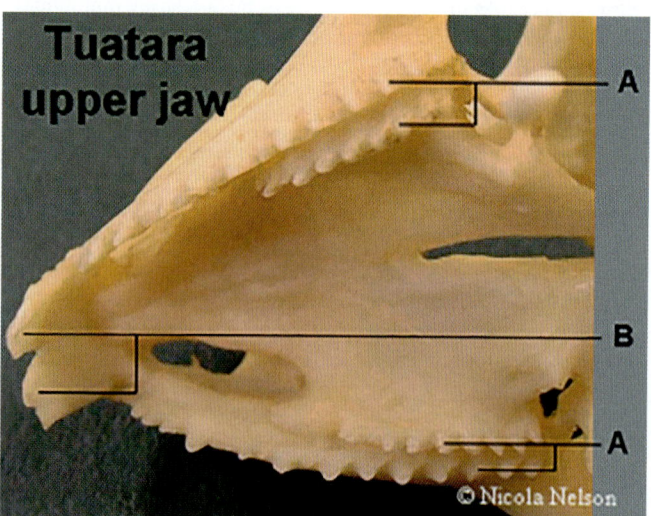

FIG 11.3 Tuatara *(Sphenodon punctatus)* have two rows of teeth in the upper dental arcade: A, wedge-shaped teeth attached to maxilla and palatine bone; B, incisor-like teeth attached to premaxilla. (Courtesy of Nicola Nelson.)

teeth at the front of the upper jaw, attached to the premaxilla. Additional teeth are added caudally as the animal grows.[15]

Liver

The tuatara liver is large, bilobed, and a typical dark red-brown color, extending from the heart to the posterior half of the abdominal cavity. There is a small gall bladder, and hepatocytes produce several types of bile acids, predominantly varanic acid.[16]

Pancreas and Spleen

The tuatara pancreas is pink and bilobed and histologically contains islets of Langerhans and exocrine glands.[10] The spleen is small and elongated with white and red pulp and is the only organ in adult tuatara with discernible lymphoid characteristics.[11]

Gastrointestinal System

Tuatara have a large, fleshy tongue that aids in capturing small prey. The J-shaped stomach contains both fundic and pyloric glands and has several internal longitudinal folds near the pyloric region.[11] The small intestine is longer and narrower than the large intestine,[17] and no cecum has been reported.

Reproductive System

Tuatara reach sexual maturity at 9 to 16 years of age[18–20] and are confirmed to breed into their sixties,[21] although there are anecdotal reports of tuatara reproducing far beyond this age. Male tuatara have paired testes that are closely apposed to the adrenal glands in the middle of the coelom. The testes are not associated with the kidneys, and, unlike squamates, there is no renal sex segment.[22] There is little seasonal variation in testicular size, although testosterone peaks substantially in mating season (March–December, southern hemisphere summer).[23] Spermatozoa are thin and threadlike and are transported from the testes via the epididymis and vas deferens to the urogenital papilla in the cloaca.[24] Male tuatara possess no intromittent organ, and copulation is achieved via cloacal apposition.[25]

Female tuatara have paired ovaries located in the posterior coelom. Vitellogenesis is protracted and can be spread over several years,[26] and eggs are present in the oviduct for 6 to 8 months.[23] Wild tuatara lay eggs every 2 to 5 years,[27] though annual reproduction has been reported in several captive institutions. Females gain a significant amount of weight in late gravidity, and this should not be confused with obesity. Tuatara exhibit temperature-dependent sex determination within a narrow range, with artificially incubated eggs producing all-female clutches below 21.2°C and all male clutches above 22.2°C.[28] Tuatara usually lay between 1 and 18 eggs per nesting event[21]; however, a female at Auckland Zoo has laid 25 eggs in a single clutch. Incubation time is

10 to 16 months in wild populations, the longest of any known reptile,[29] although eggs incubated artificially at 24°C hatched in just over 5 months.[30] Eggs are softshelled and ovoid, and tuatara emerge from them with the aid of a horny shell-breaker, similar to that seen in crocodile and turtle hatchlings.[31]

Male tuatara become increasingly territorial and aggressive during breeding season. In the presence of an intruding male, the resident male will elevate his body off the substrate, inflate the trunk and gular region, and erect the nuchal and dorsal crests.[25] He will then approach the intruder, sometimes swaying the head and neck from side to side, occasionally escalating to jaw snapping and fighting. A similar display is made when courting a female. After making himself look larger, the male will approach and circle the female in a stiff, exaggerated walk known as the *stoltzer Gang*.[32] Mating can last between 15 seconds and 2 hours.[32,33] Multiple paternity has been reported infrequently in both captive and wild tuatara clutches.[34]

Urinary System

Tuatara have two irregularly lobed kidneys located within the pelvis that are grossly and histologically similar to those of other reptiles.[17] A urinary bladder is present, which opens into the urodeum and has no direct connection with the ureters, which transport nitrogenous waste from the kidneys to the cloaca. Tuatara produce uric acid, urea, and ammonia in varying quantities depending on their hydration status.[35] As with other reptiles, tuatara do not possess a loop of Henle and are incapable of concentrating their urine.[11]

Musculoskeletal System

Tuatara share the same basic body plan as lizards, with several distinguishing features. The skull is diapsid with a fixed quadrate bone, contributing to their powerful but relatively slow bite.[36] Like crocodilians, tuatara possess abdominal ribs (gastralia), which are not true ribs but develop within the dermis, probably to provide protection and support for the abdominal organs.[1] Tuatara can autotomize their tails during instances of stress or aggression, though less readily than many lizards. The gait of the tuatara is a diagonal couplet type seen in many vertebrates and has the appearance of a ground-hugging crawl. Tuatara generally move in a fast, jerky stop-start pattern over short distances, presumably tiring quickly as they become anaerobic.[1]

Nervous System and Special Senses

The nervous system of the tuatara is very similar to that of lizards. Tuatara possess a parietal ("third") eye on the midline of the top of their head,[37] which is part of the pineal complex. It is sometimes visible in hatchlings as a dark spot covered by a translucent skin layer. The parietal eye has a lens and retina that contains what appear to be photoreceptive cells and is thought to have a role in regulating basking behavior.[38] Tuatara have two laterally positioned eyes with upper and lower eyelids, as well as a nictitating membrane.[17] The iris is often brightly colored in juveniles but fades with age. Tuatara have good visual acuity and track objects using head and eye movement.[39] Similarly to snakes, tuatara do not have an external ear opening or functional tympanic membrane, and the middle ear cavity is filled with connective and adipose tissue.[40] The inner ear, however, is well developed, and tuatara appear very responsive to sound.

Endocrine System

Apart from male and female reproductive cycles, the physiology of the tuatara's endocrine system is not well studied. The primary androgen is testosterone, which increases during the mating season in both males and females.[23] The roles of estradiol, progesterone, prostaglandin, and arginine vasotocin in female tuatara reproductive cycles have been elucidated,[23,26,41] and oxytocin has been used successfully to induce oviposition. The adrenal glands produce adrenaline and noradrenaline and are anatomically in close association with the gonads.[42] The thyroid is single, transversely elongate, and situated just anterior to the heart, not to be confused with the more cranial, bilobed thymus.[11] There are four parathyroid glands situated in the neck region. The endocrine functions of the pancreas have not been investigated but based on histology are presumed to be similar to other reptiles.[11]

Thermal Physiology and Metabolic Rate

Tuatara are renowned among reptiles for their low metabolic rate and relatively high activity level in cold temperatures. Wild tuatara have been observed to be nocturnally active when their body temperatures are between 5.5° and 20.5°C, and this can increase to 30°C when basking.[1] Sustained body temperatures over 28°C can cause signs of heat stress, and loss of locomotion occurs at 3.5°C.[43,44] The metabolic rate of tuatara at 13°C is similar to that of lizards and some turtles at the same temperature, the difference being that tuatara are active at these temperatures while many other reptiles are not.[45,46] Tuatara can undergo short periods of torpor in cold weather but still emerge periodically to eat and bask in appropriate conditions.[1]

ACKNOWLEDGMENTS

I am indebted to Peter Johnston for providing anatomic interpretation and illustrations, to Auckland Museum for the provision of tuatara specimens, and to Richard Jakob-Hoff and Richard Gibson for their support in preparation of this manuscript.

REFERENCES

See www.expertconsult.com for a complete list of references.

12

Amphibian Taxonomy, Anatomy, and Physiology

Frank Pasmans and An Martel

With currently some 7867 described species (Amphibian Species of the World; http://research.amnh.org/vz/herpetology/amphibia/), the number of amphibians known to science has increased by approximately five times compared with the year 1900 and is still steeply increasing.[1] Amphibians inhabit all continents except for Antarctica, the main requirement for their presence being sufficient moisture. The class Amphibia is highly diverse, ranging in size from the tiny frog *Paedophryne amauensis*, the smallest known vertebrate at 7.7 mm in length, to the Chinese giant salamander (*Andrias davidianus*), which reaches a length of 180 cm. Their small size, often attractive colors, and behavior render many amphibians and especially frogs and toads popular terrarium animals. Provided with proper husbandry and nutrition, many amphibians easily live for 10 to 20 years in captivity. Amphibians are being mass bred and collected for human consumption, mainly frogs (the best know example is the American bullfrog *Lithobathes catesbeianus*) but also salamanders (for example the Chinese giant salamander, which is farm bred in China). Due to the global amphibian declines and extinction of more than 200 species, amphibians are emblematic for the current sixth mass extinction event, and amphibian conservation is a hot topic. Amphibians have become the focus of many biodiversity conservation efforts involving zoos, research institutions, and authorities.[2]

TAXONOMY

The class of Amphibia is divided into three orders. With 66829 species described species, the tailless, four-legged frogs and toads (Anura) constitute the vast majority of known amphibian species and occur on all continents except Antarctica. Although species with more terrestrial habitats, drier skin, and a more stocky appearance are generally referred to as toads, there is no scientific delineation between frogs and toads. The Anura comprises 56 families, ranging from being species-rich (e.g., the tree frogs, Hylidae, with 710 species) to families containing a single taxon (the strange Indian frog *Nasikabatrachus sahyadrensis*). Most species kept in captivity belong to the families of the European and Asian fire-bellied toads (Bombinatoridae), the globally distributed true toads (Bufonidae), the South American horned frogs (Ceratophryidae), the neotropical poison frogs (Dendrobatidae), tree frogs (Hylidae), African reed frogs (Hyperoliidae), the Malagasy Mantellidae, the Asian toads (Megophryidae), the narrow-mouthed frogs (Microhylidae), the African and neotropical tongueless frogs (Pipidae), the Afro-Asian tree frogs (Rhacophoridae), and the true frogs (Ranidae).

The 720 species of salamanders and newts (Caudata) are tailed amphibians, mostly with four legs (except for the sirens, Sirenidae, with only two front legs), and are distributed in the Americas, Europe, Asia, and North Africa. With 473 species, the lungless salamanders (Plethodontidae) constitute the most species-rich family, occurring mainly in the Americas, with a limited number of species in Europe and Asia.

Most species kept in captivity, such as the "fire-bellied newts" (actually comprising newts of the genera *Cynops, Paramesotriton,* and *Pachytriton*) belong to the true salamanders (Salamandridae) or mole salamanders (Ambystomatidae, to which the famous axolotl *Ambystoma mexicanum* belongs) and to a lesser extent to the lungless salamanders, Asian salamanders (Hynobiidae), and sirens (Sirenidae).

The least-known amphibian order is that of the caecilians (Gymnophiona), with 10 families and 7867 species distributed across the (sub)tropical regions of the Americas, Africa, and Asia. Caecilians are aquatic or terrestrial wormlike amphibians that range in size from 10 cm to more than 1 m. Only very few species are being kept in captivity, notably some aquatic species (Typhlonectidae) and terrestrial neotropical and west African species (Herpelidae, Dermophiidae).

ANATOMY AND PHYSIOLOGY

For an in-depth review on amphibian biology and ecology, readers are directed to reference textbooks.[3,4] An overview of the position of the organs inside the coelomic cavity is provided in Figs. 12.1 and 12.2.

Integument

The skin of frogs and toads, salamanders, newts, and caecilians has a thin outer layer (epidermis) that is not covered by keratinized structures such as scales, hair, or feathers. Few layers of epidermal cells overlay the epidermal basement membrane. A thin stratum corneum covers the epidermis and is shed and eaten periodically. The presence of shed skin (dysecdysis) should be regarded as an anomaly, which is one of the hallmarks of chytridiomycosis. The dermis of salamanders and newts is firmly connected with the underlying tissue, rendering subcutaneous administration of compounds impossible. In anurans, large lymphatic spaces lie under the dorsal skin, with the result that "subcutaneous" injections should rather be considered intralymphatic. Caecilians are the only amphibians with scales in the deeper layer of the skin (the dermis). The amphibian skin is rich in glands, which can be roughly divided into mucous and serous or granular glands. The epidermis can be covered by mucous secretions or can be dry, which is species and often life-stage specific. Assessing skin texture is one of the key parameters for assessing an amphibian's health. The holocrine serous glands secrete a myriad of bioactive molecules, such as antimicrobial peptides, biogenic amines, steroids, alkaloids, and hormonelike peptides. The impressive arsenal of antimicrobial peptides controls microbial populations on the amphibian skin. Many amphibians secrete highly potent and potentially lethal toxins, such as tetrodotoxin,[5] as a defense against predators, notably some widely kept species such as poison frogs (species of the family Dendrobatidae with aposematic coloration; Fig. 12.3) or some newts (*Notophthalmus, Taricha, Cynops* sp.). Often, the presence of strong toxins is clearly advertised by amphibians with bright, aposematic colors. In many species such as poison frogs but also Malagasy

Mantella species, these toxins are largely derived from prey items, the lack of which in captivity results in marked loss of toxicity.[6] The amphibian skin is of vital importance for respiration and fluid balance. In many salamander and newt species, gas exchange even takes place entirely through the skin and mucous membranes. Most amphibians never drink through their mouths but absorb water via their skin, in frogs and toads often via a highly permeable region of the skin at the caudoventral coelomic region called the pelvic or drinking patch. Damage or disruption of the skin and its critical functions from diseases such as chytridiomycosis results in loss of homeostasis and death. The

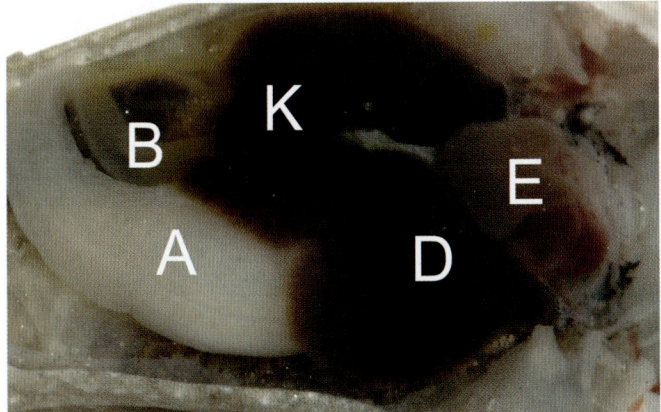

FIG 12.1 Abdominal anatomy of a frog (*Discoglossus pictus*) with skin, muscles, and coelomic membrane removed. A: stomach, B: small intestine, D: liver, E: heart, K: gall bladder. (Courtesy of Frank Pasmans.)

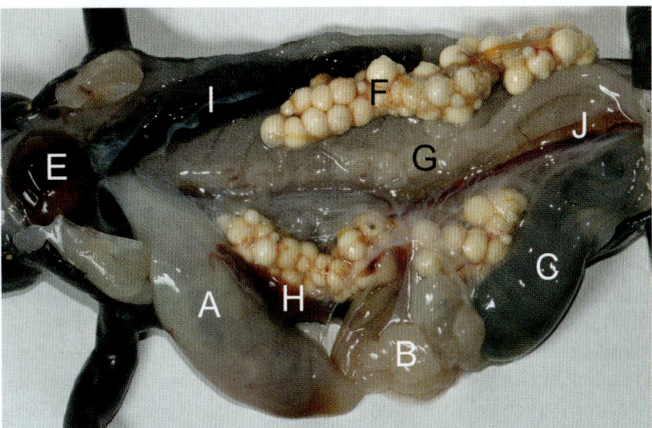

FIG 12.2 Coelomic cavity anatomy of a salamander (*Salamandra infraimmaculata*) with liver removed. A: stomach, B: small intestine, C: colon, E: heart, F: ovary, G: oviduct, H: spleen, I: lung, J: kidney. (Courtesy of Frank Pasmans.)

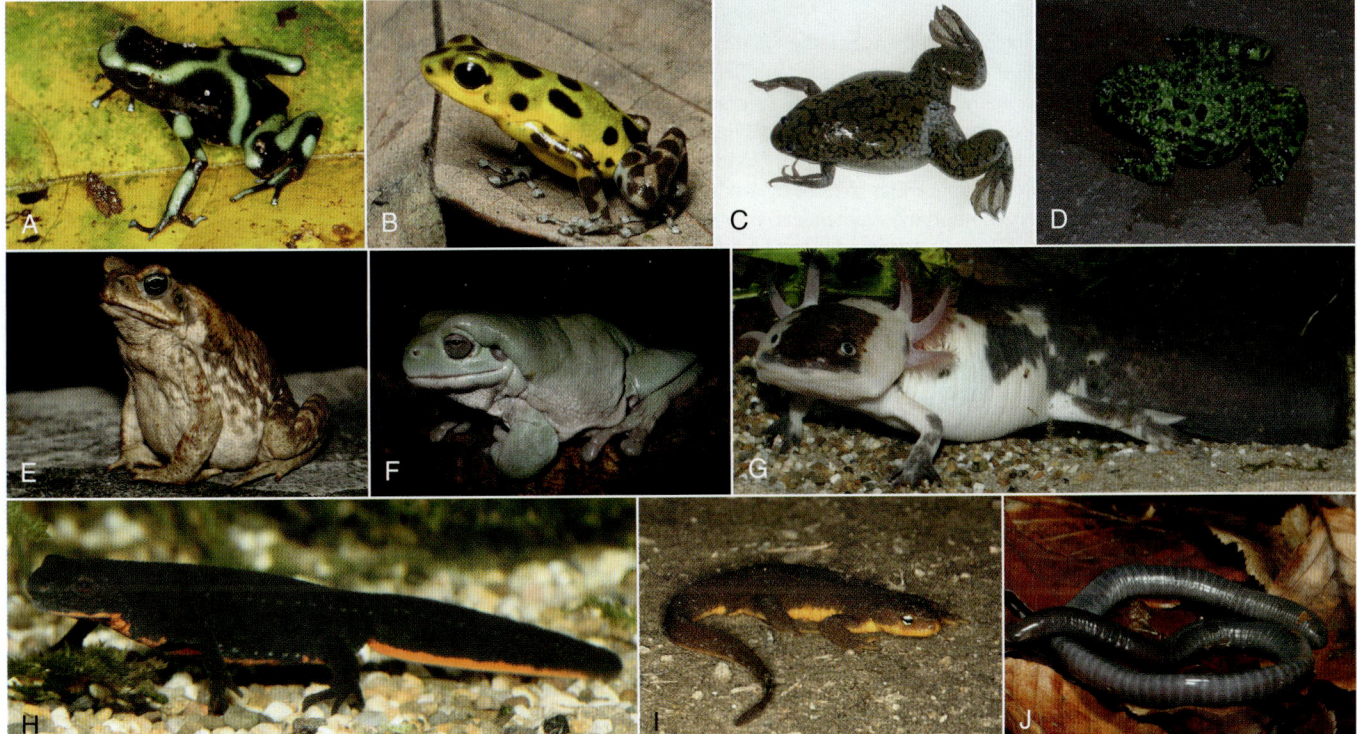

FIG 12.3 Amphibians frequently kept in captivity. (A) Green poison frog (*Dendrobates auratus*) showing aposematic colors as a warning for their feed-derived skin toxins. (B) Strawberry frogs (*Oophaga pumilio*) exhibit maternal care. (C) African clawed frogs (*Xenopus laevis*) are widely used laboratory animals and often carrier of chytrid infections. (D) Oriental fire-bellied toads (*Bombina orientalis*) are traded in large numbers as pets. (E) The introduction of cane toads (*Rhinella marina*) for insect pest control has resulted in the establishment of invasive colonies in many countries. (F) Green tree frogs (*Litoria caerulea*) are popular pets. (G) The axolotl (*Ambystoma mexicanum*) is a widely kept paedomorphic salamander. (H) The most widely traded "fire-bellied newt" is *Cynops orientalis*. (I) Several popular amphibian pet species such as this rough-skinned newt (*Taricha granulosa*) are highly toxic. (J) Little is known regarding most caecilians such as this *Herpele squalostoma*. (Courtesy of Frank Pasmans.)

disadvantage of a naked, semipermeable skin is that amphibians become susceptible to desiccation, toxins, and metabolites including nitrogen metabolites (ammonia, nitrite) absorbed from the environment. However, although amphibians are thought to be more susceptible to environmental changes such as pollution or to be useful as early bio-indicators ("canaries in the coal mine"), there are actually few indications that amphibians are any more susceptible to environmental toxins than other vertebrates. Amphibians even seem to adapt to the presence of toxins, and associations between the use of agricultural pesticides and amphibian declines are not clear.[7,8]

Cardiovascular System

Whereas larval amphibians have a two-chambered heart, postmetamorphic amphibians have one ventricle and two atria. Both hepatic and renal portal vein systems are present; the veins of the hind limb and tail combine to form the paired Jacobson's veins, which pass anteriorly on the dorsolateral surface of the kidney. In anurans, the subcutaneous space is largely occupied by an extensive system of lymphatic sacs, which provides an ability to administer medications intravascularly. Lymph fluid is actively circulated through lymph hearts. This also implies that subcutaneous administration in anurans is virtually impossible in practice. The number of accessible blood vessels for venipuncture is limited. A midline abdominal vein is present in most amphibians. In urodeles, a caudal tail vein is present, which is situated ventral to the caudal vertebrae. In anurans, the femoral vein is often used for obtaining blood samples.

Respiratory System

Depending on the species and life stage, amphibians breathe via their skin, mucous membranes, gills, and/or lungs to a varying extent. Skin breathing (gas exchange through the highly vascularized dermis) plays a major role in all species but is of particular importance for those living in the water (aquatic) and obviously for lungless salamanders living on land. Gills are branched structures that are either covered by a skin pouch (most anuran tadpoles, some paedomorphic salamanders) or not (most early-stage anuran tadpoles, all aquatic salamander larvae, and some paedomorphic salamanders). Lungs are present in the majority of amphibians after metamorphosis (but in the minority of salamander species) and present as relatively simple, thin-walled, saclike structures with folding to increase the surface for gas exchange. Most terrestrial amphibians breathe through the nares. Many aquatic amphibians take air in through the mouth. A diaphragm is lacking. Air is forced in the lungs through a force-pump mechanism of the floor of the buccal cavity.

Digestive System

All postmetamorphosis amphibians and larval salamanders, newts, and caecilians are carnivores whose diet consists primarily on live prey items. Although specialist feeders exist (e.g., termites, ants), most amphibians are not picky and will ingest any vertebrate or invertebrate prey that fits into their mouth. Some caecilians (*Typhlonectes* spp.) are known to feed on carrion. In contrast, the diet of larval anurans is extremely variable and ranges from species filtering debris from the water surface, predatory tadpoles, tadpoles that are being fed unfertilized eggs by their mother, or tadpoles that scrape organic substances from surfaces using specialized keratinized mouthparts. In some caecilians, the offspring are fed by scraping off the adult's differentiated skin.[9]

Prey may be caught by grabbing with the jaws, projecting a sticky-ended tongue, or in aquatic species, by sucking the prey into the oral cavity. Teeth are not used for chewing but mainly serve to prevent prey animals from escaping. An epiglottis is lacking. Oral cavity, esophagus, stomach, and duodenum are all separated by sphincters. However, these sphincters can easily be overcome, and the relatively short and broad,

cilia-lined esophagus makes the insertion of a gastric tube (for force feeding and gastric flushes) relatively simple to perform. The intestine is relatively short and receives bile from the gall bladder and pancreatic secretions. Since all postmetamorphic amphibians are carnivorous, the intestinal microbiome is likely to be of minor importance. The liver is generally large, bilobate in anurans and elongate in urodeles, contains a gall bladder, and, as in other vertebrates, is dark red/brown in color. The amphibian liver typically contains melano-macrophages (pigment-containing cells), which are thought to increase in size and/or frequency with age, chronic inflammation, and environmental stress.

Reproductive System

The paired testes are either lobed (many urodeles) or not (anurans) and attached to the kidneys by the mesorchium. The paired ovaries are suspended by the mesovarium from the kidneys. Ovulation results in the thin sheath of connective tissue surrounding the follicles, the ovisac, rupturing to release the ova into the coelom. The coelom, with its ciliated epithelium, moves the ova anteriorly to the opening of the oviduct. The gonads are closely associated with the fat bodies, which are suspended from the dorsal wall (anurans) or the gonadal mesentery (urodeles). Copulatory organs are present only in male caecilians and a small number of Anura and Caudata.

The reproduction of amphibians is driven by environmental determinants (temperature and/or humidity). During the mating season, the males will respond to visual, auditive, and/or olfactory cues from females. Only male anurans are able to attract females by means of advertisement calls that are often amplified by one or two vocal sacs. Many amphibian species are sexually dimorphic (Fig. 12.4). In anurans, males are often (but not always) smaller than females; in salamanders and newts males often have a more swollen cloaca region and often show sex-specific coloration and patterns. Males of many amphibian species develop marked secondary sexual characteristics during the breeding season, the most constant being the development of keratinized, darkly colored patches on the skin (nuptial pads) in anurans and a markedly swollen cloaca in salamanders and newts.

Mating can involve either physical contact (e.g., amplexus in many species, actual copulation in caecilians) or not (many species of salamanders and newts). In most anurans and some salamanders and newts, fertilization of the eggs takes place externally. In most salamanders and newts and all caecilians, fertilization is internal. Most amphibians produce eggs that are either deposited on land or in water where larvae or already metamorphosed juveniles hatch. Larvae then pass through an aquatic life stage, whereas metamorphosed juveniles are already adapted for a terrestrial life. Anurans especially have a huge repertoire of reproductive strategies. Parental care is common in salamanders but rare in anurans. The widely kept poison frogs (Dendrobatidae) guard their eggs and transfer the hatchlings to water reservoirs for further development. In some species such as the strawberry frog (*Oophaga pumilio*), the female feeds the aquatic larvae with unfertilized eggs (see Fig. 12.3). A small number of anurans, a large number of caecilians, and several salamanders give birth to a few larvae in an advanced stage of development (ovoviviparity) or even fully metamorphosed young (vivipary).

Neoteny or paedomorphosis describes a phenomenon of incomplete metamorphosis of animals that retain larval characteristics even though they become sexually mature. The best known example for this is the axolotl (*Ambystoma mexicanum*) in which metamorphosis can only be induced artificially by administering thyroid hormones (see Fig. 12.3).

Urinary System

In adult amphibians the paired, mesonephric kidneys are located dorsocaudally in the coelom. The bladder is a ventral outgrowth of the cloaca and is inconspicuous in many urodelans. Most amphibian larvae

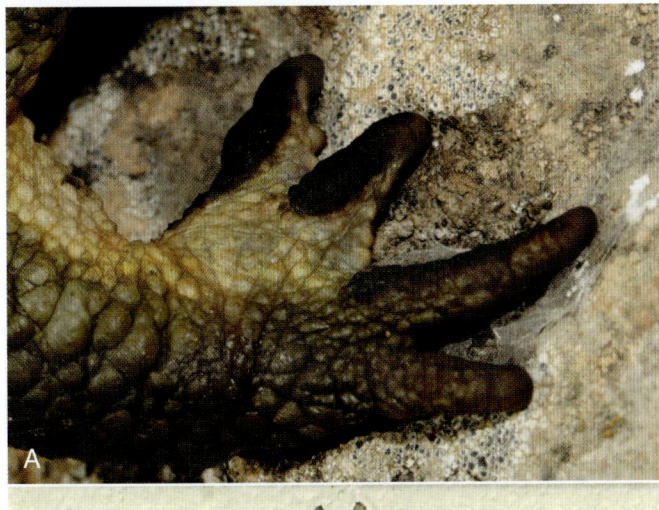

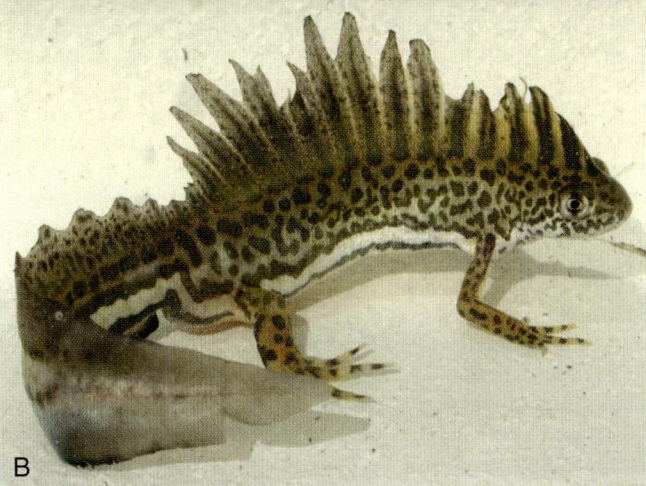

FIG 12.4 Sexual dimorphism in amphibians. (A) The presence of keratinized nuptial pads on the fingers of a male European common toad (*Bufo bufo*). (B) A markedly swollen cloaca and the presence of a crest in the southern-banded newt (*Ommatotriton vittatus*). (Courtesy of Frank Pasmans.)

and aquatic amphibians excrete nitrogen as ammonia through urine and gills. Terrestrial species excrete mainly urea. Some arboreal frogs even excrete uric acid, which requires much less water for excretion.

Musculoskeletal System

Amphibians have a skeletal system that is structurally homologous to other tetrapods, though with a number of variations. They all have four limbs except for the legless caecilians and a few species of salamander have reduced or no limbs. The bones are hollow and lightweight but fully ossified. In anurans, the ilium of the well-developed pelvic girdle is attached to the spine by a pair of sacral ribs, and the caudal vertebrae are fused and constitute a single bony structure, the urostyle.

Nervous System

The brain consists of equal parts: cerebrum, midbrain, and cerebellum. Various parts of the cerebrum process sensory input, such as smell in the olfactory lobe and sight in the optic lobe, and it is additionally the center of behavior and learning. The cerebellum is the center of muscular coordination, and the medulla oblongata controls some organ functions, including heartbeat and respiration. The pineal body is involved in hibernation and aestivation in amphibians. Amphibians have 10 cranial nerves, lacking XI and XII. Amphibians can feel pain.

Species Senses

Prey is located by means of scent, vision, and/or touch. The sense of touch can be developed as a lateral line organ in larvae and aquatic amphibians that, like fish, will respond to movements in the surroundings or as the sensitive fingertips of aquatic frogs of the Pipidae. A unique feature of caecilians is the presence of a tentacle below the eye. Most terrestrial amphibians use vision for locating prey and to a lesser extent their sense of smell. Feeding is mainly evoked by moving prey.

Endocrine System

Many amphibians pass through two different free-living life stages, beginning with an aquatic larval stage. Metamorphosis is the transformation from larval form to adult life stage, which involves fundamental anatomical and physiological modifications largely controlled by the thyroid gland.[10] The thyroid glands play a crucial role in amphibian metamorphosis through the production of T_3 and T_4. In Anuran tadpoles, first the hind legs become visible, then the front legs. The tail is resorbed, lungs replace gills, the mostly spiral-shaped intestinal tract of the tadpoles is modified to process prey items, and the jaw and tongue and the mature immune systems develop. Tailed amphibians first grow their front legs and then the hind limbs. During metamorphosis, their external gills disappear and they develop eyelids. In caecilians with a larval stage, metamorphosis includes the loss of the lateral line organ. Overall, metamorphosis is a life stage of increased susceptibility for amphibians with losses from drowning or infectious diseases such as chytridiomycosis. Amphibian declines related to chytridiomycosis are often associated with mass mortality shortly after metamorphosis.[11]

BEHAVIOR

All amphibians are ectothermic. Due to the majority of amphibians being nocturnal, these animals are less exposed to direct solar radiation than diurnal reptiles. Active thermoregulation by basking is observed in many diurnal anurans. In salamanders and newts, it is unclear to what degree they actively thermoregulate. Preferred thermal ranges of amphibians are highly species specific, and for anurans no general rule can be provided. Generally speaking, newts and salamanders prefer relatively low ambient temperatures in a range of 10°C to 20°C. Caecilians generally require much higher temperatures around 25°C.

If ambient temperatures decrease, amphibians from temperate regions will enter a state of dormancy (hibernation). Some amphibian species are well known for their ability to tolerate freezing, even for long periods of times. To survive freezing, these species use antifreeze molecules like glucose or glycerol that prevent the intracellular fluid from freezing.

REFERENCES

See www.expertconsult.com for a complete list of references.

13

Natural Behavior

Andrew M. Durso and John C. Maerz

The more than 17,750 species of extant reptiles and amphibians have a wide variety of behaviors that allow them to escape notice, defend themselves, reproduce, obtain food, maintain homeostasis, and otherwise interact with their environment. This chapter is meant to serve as an introduction to the general patterns of behavior seen in reptiles and amphibians. Many behaviors that are normal for a particular species but unfamiliar to hobbyists or clinicians may be misinterpreted as signs of disease or trauma. Unfortunately examples of all these behaviors cannot be presented in a single chapter, and research into the biology and natural history of many species is ongoing. Comprehensive scholarly reviews are available on the behavior of both reptiles and amphibians.[1–3] Throughout this chapter we address general patterns among these two diverse taxonomic groups while highlighting some widespread or special examples. We focus predominantly on anurans (frogs), salamanders, crocodilians, chelonians, lizards, and snakes. Because far less is known about the natural history and behavior of caecilians and tuataras,[4] their coverage here is limited.

The key to understanding amphibian and reptile behavior lies in their reliance on ectothermy and their associated reliance on anaerobic metabolism to produce energy. Pough[5,6] synthesized this understanding in his description of amphibians and reptiles as "low-energy systems." Reptiles and amphibians differ from many mammals and birds in that (1) their metabolic rates are flexible and their resting metabolic rates are nearly an order of magnitude lower than those of birds and mammals;[5,6] (2) as a result, they do not necessarily need food as often as we might assume; (3) the majority of their energy comes from anaerobic metabolism,[5] which leads to rapid exhaustion when active; (4) they spend a lot of their time doing nothing (or appearing to do nothing), with punctuated bursts of activity; and (5) much of their behavior is proximately motivated by regulating temperature or moisture. Frequent and extended periods of immobility or inactivity should not necessarily be taken as a sign that something is medically wrong with an amphibian or reptile.

ECTOTHERMY

As with birds and mammals, amphibians and reptiles operate at body temperatures elevated above the ambient conditions of their environment. The key difference is that amphibians and reptiles do this by absorbing heat from their environment. Therefore behavioral thermoregulation is, arguably, the key activity of all amphibians and reptiles. Behavioral thermoregulation is widely recognized in reptiles but is also demonstrated among amphibians.[5] However, because elevated temperatures accelerate evaporative water loss, many amphibians may be more constrained in their ability to thermoregulate and will choose areas of high moisture over warmer temperatures if both are not available together.[7] As a result of behavioral thermoregulation, many reptiles and some amphibians have relatively stable body temperatures.[5] It is important to recognize

that there are no optimal temperatures for an amphibian or reptile species. Rather, amphibians and reptiles need gradients of temperature and the ability to regulate their body temperature behaviorally by moving along that gradient. The inability to behaviorally thermoregulate can cause stress or death, and the absence of behavioral thermoregulation may be an indication of disease or illness.

Because they use ectothermy to elevate their body temperatures, amphibians and reptiles have dramatically lower metabolic energetic demand and higher assimilation efficiencies compared to birds and mammals.[6] Low metabolic demands allow amphibians and reptiles to feed on small, less energetically profitable prey and to take meals less frequently or fast for extended periods when food is unavailable or weather conditions favor estivation or hibernation. A consequence of ectothermy in amphibians and reptiles (and cutaneous gas exchange in some amphibians) is limited aerobic energy production and a reliance on anaerobic metabolism to sustain high activity. Amphibians and reptiles exhaust rapidly and can require hours to recover from only a few minutes of strenuous activity.[5] As a result, most amphibians and reptiles engage in infrequent, short bouts of activity with extended periods of limited activity. During periods of inactivity, amphibians and reptiles will often retreat to cooler areas, and body temperatures often reduce to near ambient temperatures, which reduces energetic demands and improves metabolic efficiency.[5,8] Among amphibians and reptiles there is considerable variation around these generalities. Some larger, often predatory reptiles have higher aerobic capacities that can sustain longer periods of activity, and reptile species that are passive or cruising foragers tend to operate at lower body temperatures for longer periods of time, whereas species that are intensive foragers tend to operate at higher body temperatures for more punctuated periods of time.[6] Body size differences between juvenile and adult amphibians and reptiles often exceed several orders of magnitude. This affects energetics and performance, which in turn affects behavior. Some amphibians (e.g., toads) that are particularly small at metamorphosis are diurnal until they achieve sufficient size to become nocturnal. Among reptiles, juveniles exhaust more quickly after short bouts of activity, and activity endurance tends to increase linearly with size. This phenomenon appears to drive ontogenetic changes in reptile diets. For example, because they can become exhausted when attempting to handle large, live prey, juvenile snakes often take prey that are smaller relative to their body size.

WATER CONSERVATION AND OSMOTIC BALANCE

Both reptiles and amphibians must balance their gain and loss of water and salts. Amphibians absorb water by soaking or extracting it from moist substrates. Through the use of hormones and specialized tissues, amphibians are capable of absorbing water from remarkably dry soils (e.g., water tension below 2 atm), but absorbing water from soils often takes far longer than from standing water.[9] Reptiles gain water by drinking. Both amphibians and reptiles acquire water from their food and by chemically producing it as a by-product of metabolism. Most reptiles and some amphibians excrete uric acid, and those species are able to retain more of their metabolic water than animals that excrete urea (mammals, terrestrial chelonians, and many amphibians) or ammonia (fishes, crocodilians, aquatic chelonians, most aquatic amphibians). Reptiles and amphibians lose water through urine, feces, evaporation, and their salt glands. Evaporation is the major route of water loss for terrestrial amphibians and reptiles.[2,3] Comparatively, amphibians are more prone to evaporative water loss, but some reptiles are sensitive to evaporative water loss,[10] and water stress can constrain activity.

Amphibians and reptiles generally deal with short-term avoidance of evaporative water loss through altered activity patterns and microhabitat selection. They will be more active during cooler parts of the day or select cooler or wetter microhabitats.[2,7] Many amphibians will concentrate activity around rain events. During periods of inactivity, amphibians will move under cover objects where conditions are typically cooler, moister, and there is reduced exposure to air movement that facilitates water loss. They will assume water conserving postures where bodies are pressed against the substrate, limbs are typically pulled in close to or under the body, the head may be tucked ventrally, and the eyes are typically closed (Fig. 13.1). This reduces their exposed surface area and protects more sensitive tissues from evaporative water loss. Amphibians resting on dry soils may establish a "wetting front," which limits water loss to dry soils.[7,9,11] As water is initially lost from the amphibian to the drier soil, water accumulates between the animal and the soil. When a locally steep gradient of water is formed between a wet region (the amphibian and soil immediately beneath it) and a dry

region (the rest of the soil), no water can move from wetter to drier soils. Thus the initial loss of water to establish a wetting front prevents additional, continuous water loss to the soil provided the animal does not move (or is not forced to move by a predator or person).

To deal with more protracted dehydrating environments, amphibians and reptiles may concentrate their activities seasonally or spend extended periods in deeper refugia.[12] Because of their greater reliance on anaerobic metabolism and lower dependence on aerobic metabolism, amphibians and reptiles are capable of burrowing deep in sand and soils where oxygen concentrations are reduced.[5] Body temperatures will cool to near ambient, and metabolic rates are reduced, allowing the animals to remain underground for months or years. Some aquatic and terrestrial amphibians will form cocoons from shed skin to remain moist during protracted droughts.[13]

Marine reptiles, many herbivorous or invertebrate-eating reptiles, and some invertebrate-eating amphibians must excrete excess ions from their diet. Marine reptiles, including sea snakes, sea turtles, marine iguanas, and saltwater crocodiles, dehydrate in sea water and must drink fresh water to survive.[14] They excrete salt through a variety of specialized glands in the eyes, nose, or mouth.[15] Salt glands are about seven times more water-efficient than kidneys at excreting excess salt, although they require more energy for active transport. Species that inhabit hypersaline environments may limit ingestion of high saline water and ingest high amounts of hyposaline water when available. For example, fresh rain water is less dense than hypersaline water and will temporarily form a surface layer. Diamondback terrapins (*Malaclemys terrapin*), which inhabit brackish tidal marshes, will float at the surface during a rain event and drink copious amounts of fresh rain water.[16] Sea snakes exhibit a similar behavior.[17] Freshwater is typically not limited for most temperate and tropical reptiles. Many desert reptiles harvest dew, rain, sleet, and snow off of the ground, plants, or their own bodies.[18,19] For some desert reptiles, such as Gila monsters (*Heloderma suspectum*) and desert tortoises (*Gopherus agassizii*), dietary and metabolic water are sufficient, and these animals rely on seasonal rainfall and inactivity in subterranean burrows to maintain water balance.[20] Some desert reptiles have special morphologic features and associated behaviors that aid in collecting moisture. For example, some lizards (e.g., *Moloch horridus*, *Phrynosoma cornutum*) have a network of channels between their scales to aid in the collection and transport of dew to their mouth.[21]

SENSORY ADAPTATIONS

Most reptiles and amphibians have good eyesight, hearing, tactile, and chemosensory abilities and exhibit notable sensory exploration behaviors and responses to information. The majority of surface-dwelling species have color vision, and vision plays an important role in amphibian and reptile behavior. Several lineages of snakes have evolved infrared sensory organs that reside in anterior facial pits. The nerves from these organs join the nerves from the eyes before reaching the brain and therefore enhance the detail of objects or allow snakes to see objects outside the field of view of their lateral eyes.[22] Amphibians and reptiles also have extra-optic photoreception for sensing light and dark, and these organs can be important in regulating endogenous biorhythms, physiology, and behaviors.[23–25] Some burrowing, cave-dwelling, or aquatic species that live in murky water have lost much or all of their vision but may still exhibit phototaxis based on extraoptic photoreception. Most amphibians appear to have an optimum level of ambient illumination above which an animal becomes negatively phototaxic and below which the animal becomes positively phototaxic.[26] For many nocturnal species, this manifests as an avoidance of high light environments, and species that occupy caves or burrows often emerge during twilight to forage. Color vision plays an important role in social communication, including

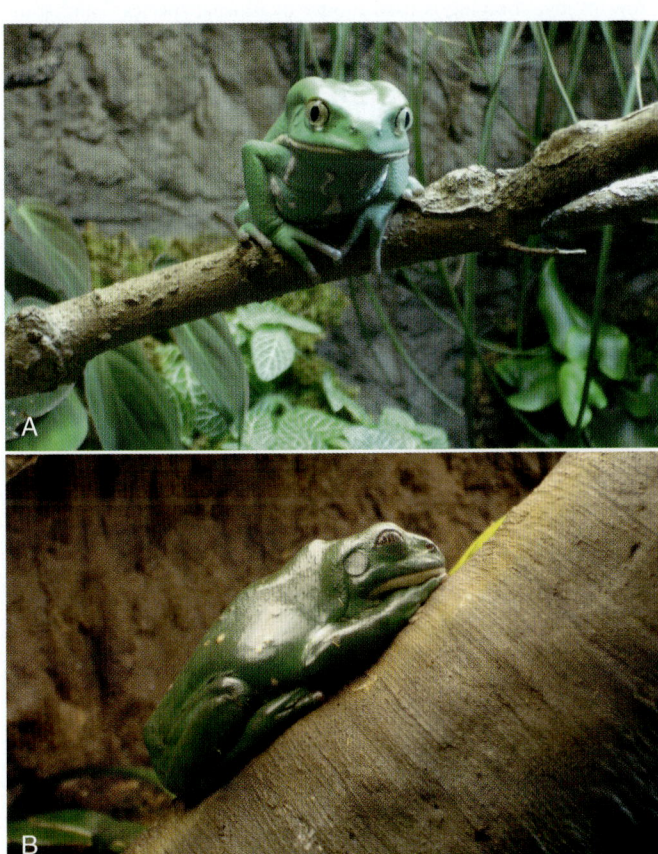

FIG 13.1 Active (A) and moisture-conserving (B) postures in a waxy monkey treefrog (*Phyllomedusa sauvagii*). (Courtesy of John C. Maerz.)

mate assessment,[27–29] location and identification of prey,[30] microhabitat selection,[31] and, for some species, color changing associated with camouflage or social interactions.[23,32]

Hearing is also relatively well developed in reptiles[33] and amphibians,[34,35] though perhaps more variable in capacity and importance than vision. Anurans are widely recognized for their derived ear structure and strong reliance on auditory communication for advertising to mates or rivals, individual recognition, despotic spacing, and release and alarm calls.[2,36] Reptiles also use their hearing for a variety of purposes.[37] Some lizards eavesdrop on the alarm calls of birds.[38] Some geckos use acoustic communication at night.[39] Contrary to popular belief, behavioral, neurological, and physiological experiments have shown that salamanders and snakes can hear both airborne and ground-borne sounds, even though they lack external ear openings.[35,40] Snakes can hear louder and lower frequency sounds more easily; their optimal range is 80 to 600 Hz (compared with 20–20,000 Hz for humans). Saharan sand vipers (genus *Cerastes*) ambush lizards and rodents from a position partially or completely buried in sand and probably rely heavily on hearing or feeling vibration to hunt.[41] Anurans and salamanders are particularly sensitive to seismic vibrations and can use them in communication.[35,42,43] Anurans and salamanders have a peculiar anatomy in which the operculum is attached by a muscle to the suprascapula. In a normal resting position with the forelimbs erect, this anatomy allows the efficient "hearing" of seismic vibrations.[43,44] The lower jaw may also be used in hearing; many reptiles and amphibians press their chin to the ground to amplify ground-borne sounds, and some aquatic amphibians can also sense motion via a lateral line system like that of fishes (e.g., *Amphiuma*). Tortoises have good tactile abilities in their shells.[45]

Along with vision, chemoreception is a dominant sense among amphibians and reptiles. Chemosensing is well developed in almost all reptiles and amphibians and is used extensively in communication and mating, movement, prey location, and predator identification and risk assessment. Salamanders have well-developed vomeronasal tissues and a relatively large portion of the brain dedicated to olfactory stimuli. Salamander species in the family Plethodontidae, which includes approximately two thirds of all salamander species, have unique nasal-labial grooves that carry chemical cues from protrusions on the upper lip to the nares via capillary action.[46] Plethodontid and ambystomatid salamanders frequently engage in nose-tapping behaviors as part of chemosensory exploration.[47,48] Chemoreception in salamanders and other amphibians is important in prey location and recognition,[49] conspecific and heterospecific recognition,[50] recognition of predators,[51,52] homing,[48,53] identifying territories,[48,54] and mate assessment.[55,56] Similar importance of the vomeronasal system and chemical cues are known among reptiles.[57–60] Aquatic turtles rely more on chemosensory cues than semiaquatic or terrestrial species.[61] Snakes and some lizards are well known for their deeply forked tongues and tongue-flicking behavior, which is used to determine directionality when following chemical cues.[62] Scent-trailing is a common behavior for many snakes and other reptiles for both locating mates and prey. Among naïve juvenile snakes, chemicals may be the only cues that can elicit prey-attacking behaviors,[63] although some species can be conditioned to respond to chemical cues of novel prey.[64] Because of the strong effect of chemical cues on amphibian and reptile risk perception and behavior, caution should be taken to minimize stress by limiting exposure to chemical cues associated with predators or rivals and to maintain individual chemical cues when cleaning or changing housing.

FORAGING AND PREDATION

Most reptiles and amphibians are carnivores, and many are ambush foragers. As a result, they can be foraging at almost any time that weather

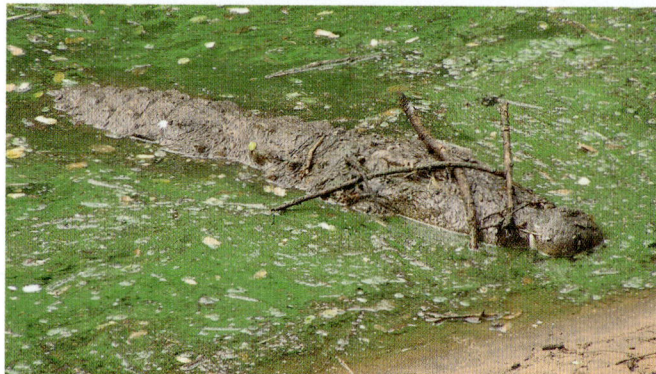

FIG 13.2 A mugger crocodile (*Crocodylus palustris*) luring birds with stick-displaying behavior. (Courtesy of Vladimir Dinets.)

conditions permit, although their energetic requirements are sufficiently low that they do not necessarily spend significant time foraging.[5] Many species (e.g., chameleons, plethodontid salamanders) use projectile tongues in prey capture.[65,66] Many heavy-bodied snakes make use of habitual ambush sites, which they select using chemical cues from their prey.[67] For most amphibians and reptiles, prey strikes are triggered by particular prey movements[68]; however, chemical cues can trigger instinctive or learned strikes, and striking a prey item can induce chemosensory searching behavior in both snakes[69] and lizards.[70] Herbivorous reptiles use both visual and chemical cues to locate and select fruits, flowers, and other parts of plants.[71] Amphibians and most reptiles swallow their prey whole. Many snakes use venom or constriction to subdue large prey.[72] Active foraging is used mostly by diurnal species,[73] and some reptiles and amphibians use additional behaviors to lure prey. Wood Turtles (*Glyptemys insculpta*) stomp their feet to create vibrations in the soil similar to those caused by rain, which lures earthworms to the surface to avoid drowning.[74] Some chameleons use chemical substances derived from their insect prey to lure their food to ambush sites.[75] Several species of frogs (e.g., Argentine horned frogs, *Ceratophrys calcarata* and *C. ornata*), as well as alligator snapping turtles (*Macrochelys temminckii*) and many species of snakes that prey on vertebrates or large predatory invertebrates have specialized toes (amphibians[76]), tongues (snapping turtle[77] and snakes[78]), or tails (snakes[79]) that are wiggled to lure their prey. Some crocodilians appear to use sticks as hunting lures during the nest-building season of their avian prey (Fig. 13.2).[80]

SLEEP AND OTHER ENDOGENOUS RHYTHMS

Sleep appears to be present in all amphibians and reptiles.[81] Periods of rest or quiescence associated with electroencephalogram (EEG) changes similar to those seen in mammalian sleep are clearly present in amphibians, turtles, and crocodilians, but EEG data suggest that they do not exhibit rapid-eye movement (REM or "deep") sleep. Some experiments have found REM-like sleep in lizards,[82] whereas others have not. In experiments where lizards, turtles, and crocodilians were subjected to continuous arousal for 24 to 48 hours, they appeared to get tired, sleeping more afterward and producing more high-voltage EEG spikes. Some reptiles sometimes seem to exhibit sleeplike brain activity when they are awake, perhaps because of sleeplike behavior induced by cold in ectotherms. Crocodilians may sleep one hemisphere of the brain at a time.[83] The single study of a snake[84] reported that an African rock python (*Python sebae*) produced sleeplike brain waves almost 16 hours a day, increasing to over 20 hours following feeding, and that these brainwaves corresponded with slower breathing and heart rate, some muscle relaxation, and perhaps a lowered behavioral response threshold. There was no evidence for REM sleep in this snake.

COLOR CHANGE

Some reptiles and amphibians can change color for camouflage, thermoregulation, or social communication. Chameleons are well known for their ability to change color, although many lizards can do this. Contrary to conventional wisdom, chameleons and other lizards use their colors primarily for communication, rather than for camouflage, with brighter coloration signaling dominance.[85] Color change is also present in a few snakes,[86] where it seems to be used mostly to aid thermoregulation. Rapid color change is not known from turtles or crocodilians. Color changing in amphibians appears largely related to camouflage and plays an important role in temperature regulation and reducing evaporative water loss. Generally, amphibian color changing occurs more slowly than in reptiles and invertebrates (e.g., octopus); therefore it is unlikely that color changing functions as a rapid antipredator response. Rather, color changing when at rest likely reduces detection of animals and can be used to alter heat absorption, the latter of which facilitates increased control of water loss and more flexible metabolic rates matched to activity.[2] Although some amphibians may use color cues in mate assessment, there is no evidence that color changing in amphibians is used in social interactions.

DEFENSE

Predator Avoidance and Immobility

In the wild, most reptiles and amphibians rely on immobility and cryptic coloration as their primary defense from predators.[87,88] Immobility and cryptic coloration may be accompanied by a reduction in respiration rate to conceal movement associated with ventilation,[89] the selection of substrates that improve camouflage,[2] or positioning themselves partially concealed and where they can quickly retreat to a more secure location. Reducing detection through immobility and crypsis is likely the primary defense of amphibians and reptiles because of their limited endurance for fight-or-flight defenses. Many amphibians also show behavioral responses to chemical cues of their predators or injured conspecifics that clearly function to reduce predatory encounters.[2] Behavioral responses to chemical alarm cues include avoiding substrates containing alarm cues,[51,90–93] increasing use of or delaying emergence from refugia,[93,94] and reducing movement rates.[52]

When predator avoidance has failed and amphibians and reptiles perceive an attack is eminent or they have been attacked, the first line of defense is nearly always an attempt to escape.[1,95] Among amphibians, frogs generally rely on their superior jumping ability to avoid attack. Plethodontid salamanders will jerk violently, causing them to spring away from the predator. Several large lizards[96] (e.g., *Sauromalus ater*, *Uromastyx aegyptia*, Cordylidae) and pancake tortoises[97] (*Malacochersus tornieri*) retreat to rock crevices where they wedge themselves in with their legs, sometimes inflating their lungs or using their tails to block access to their bodies. However, if escape is impossible or if the animal is seized, it may resort to one or more of the following tactics.

Defensive Postures and Displays

Many reptiles and amphibians assume stereotypical defensive display postures when confronted by a predator.[1,2] These postures range from inflating or elevating the body on four limbs to appear larger to displays (e.g., pushups) that signal alertness to the predator and likelihood of escape.[98,99] Some reptile defensive displays include expanding frills or hoods around the head[100] or generating noises by hissing, tail-rattling, growling, scale rubbing, and cloacal popping.[101] Many amphibians also

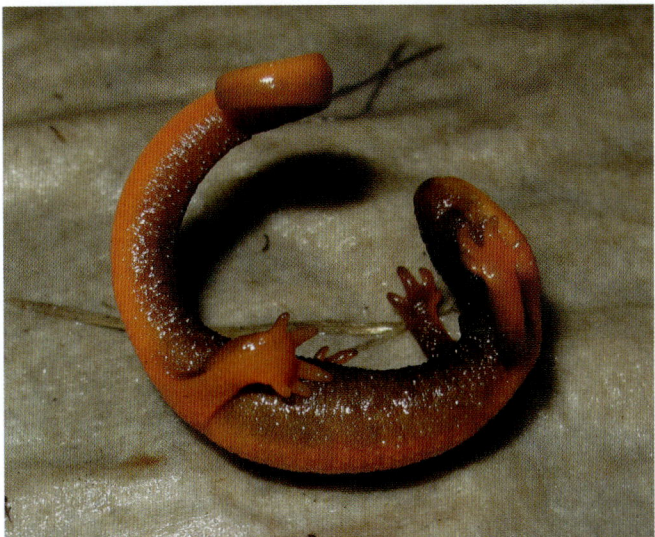

FIG 13.3 Unken behavior in a rough-skinned newt (*Taricha granulosa*). (Courtesy of Andrew M. Durso.)

use defensive calls, the exact function of which is debated.[102] Some amphibian and reptile postures may expose or emphasize expendable or durable body parts such as tails, spines, aposematically colored areas,[103] or glands where mucous or chemical defenses are stored, all of which function to deter attack or minimize its impact. Some snakes have specialized nuchal glands on the back of the neck, which they present to predators. The glands contain sequestered toxic compounds from their amphibian prey.[104] Reptiles capable of counter-attacking may turn to face their enemy gaping their mouths.

The most stereotypical display postures of amphibians are collectively known as the "unken" reflex (Fig. 13.3). Many noxious or mildly poisonous amphibians are generally cryptically patterned with concealed aposematic coloration. More potently poisonous species are often fully aposematic. When disturbed by a predator, amphibians will raise their head, limbs, and tail (for salamanders only) dorsally to expose or accentuate their aposematic coloration. Occasionally salamanders will wiggle their tail as part of their defensive display, which may serve as an additional warning or to direct an attack toward the tail and away from the head or trunk. Most toxic amphibians and some nontoxic species will contract the body with the limbs kept bent and close to the body, eyes usually open, and the head tucked ventrally potentially to present concentrated areas of poison glands positioned dorsally at the base of the head (e.g., toads and ambystomatid salamanders).[2,105,106]

If seized by a predator, many reptiles and amphibians struggle, hiss, urinate, defecate, or discharge their anal/cloacal glands.[1] Salamanders often writhe and coil around predators when seized, which often covers the predator in adhesive or irritating secretions and increases the likelihood of escape.[107,108] Vipers that are eaten by kingsnakes (*Lampropeltis*) use specific defensive postures when exposed to kingsnakes or their scent, including body bridging (a laterally raised loop of the trunk region, with the head and tail held low), inflation, and body flips and jerks, which presumably make them harder to swallow.[109] Colubrid snakes do not exhibit body bridging.[110] A number of lizards and snakes exhibit "death-feigning" behavior (thanatosis), where they flip on their back, the eyes usually remain open, and limbs (if present) remain limp and away from the body.[105] Sometimes death-feigning includes gaping the mouth with the tongue out and defecating, vomiting, or musking on themselves (Fig. 13.4). Although tests in the wild are limited,[111] the function of death-feigning seems to be to deter predator interest or

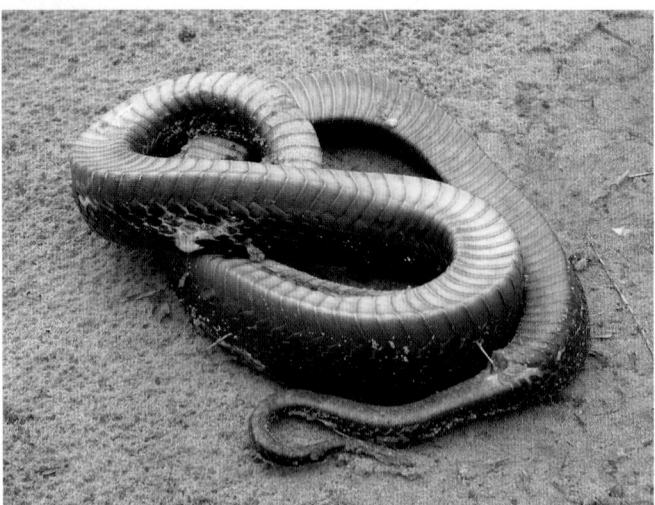

FIG 13.4 Death-feigning behavior in an Eastern hog-nosed snake (*Heterodon platirhinos*). (Courtesy of Andrew M. Durso.)

inhibit a predator's attack behavior, which allows the prey to slip away unnoticed when the predator's attention decreases.[112] It is often noted that death-feigning in species such as hog-nosed snakes (*Heterodon*) is common in the wild but wanes in captivity, potentially through habituation.

Tail Displays and Tail Autotomy

With the exception of adult anurans, most reptiles and amphibians have tails. Tails are important for balance, gait, and fat storage and are often used in displays with various functions, including luring prey[113] and signaling to predators[114] and conspecifics.[115] Because the loss or damage of a tail is normally not lethal, some reptiles and amphibians use their tails in defense.

Turtles and most snakes do not use their tails in defense, but crocodilians and some large lizards, such as green iguanas (*Iguana iguana*) and mace-tailed lizards (*Uromastyx*), will use their tails to whip or strike their enemies. Most salamanders, lizards, and some snakes can autotomize their tails.[116,117] Tail autotomy is a convergent adaptation among amphibians (salamanders) and reptiles (squamates). Salamander tail autotomy is achieved by a weakness in the skin and musculature between caudal vertebrae, whereas reptiles have fracture planes within each caudal vertebra. Some salamander species only autotomize the entire tail, whereas other salamander species and reptiles can break the tail off at any length. Ease of tail autotomy can vary among species and populations, is often correlated with local predation risk, and can differ between males and females and between previously unbroken and regenerated tails. Tail autotomy is clearly demonstrated to result in higher survival rates among amphibians and reptiles. Although the tail can regrow, there are often nutritional, social, and locomotory consequences to losing a tail.[118] Not all lizards recover well from autotomizing their tails. For example, the consequences of tail loss for leopard geckos (*Eublepharis macularius*) and other fat-tailed geckos, which store more water and fat in their tails than other lizards, can be severe and require more treatment than thin-tailed species such as anoles (*Anolis*) and grass lizards (*Takydromus*). Several groups of salamanders and lizards cannot autotomize their tails, many of which use them for some other purpose (e.g., locomotion, grasping; Table 13.1).[119,120] Many snakes, some amphisbaenians, and some salamanders will conspicuously display their tails when threatened.[108,121] Among reptiles, these species normally have short tails with blunt tips, often with contrasting colors, which probably

TABLE 13.1 Presence or Absence of Tail Breakage in Lepidosaurs

Squamate Family or Group	Common Name	Tail Autotomy Present?
Agamidae	Dragons and relatives	Some*[118–120]
Amphisbaenia	Worm lizards	Some[114,118,119,202]
Anguidae	Slowworms, glass lizards, alligator lizards, and relatives	Some*[118–120,201]
Chamaeleonidae	Chameleons	No[118–120,201]
Cordylidae	Girdled lizards	Yes*[118,119,201]
Corytophanidae	Basilisks and casquehead lizards	Some*[119,120,201]
Crotaphytidae	Collared and leopard lizards	Some*[118–120,201]
Dactyloidae	Anoles	Yes[118,119]
Dibamidae	Blind skinks	Yes[119]
Gekkota	Geckos	Almost all*†[118–120,201]
Gerrhosauridae	Plated lizards	Yes[118]
Gymnophthalmidae	Microteiids	Yes[118–120,201]
Helodermatidae	Gila monster and beaded lizard	No[118–120,201]
Hoplocercidae	Clubtails and wood lizards	Some*‡[119,120,201]
Iguanidae	Iguanas	Some*[118–120,201]
Lacertidae	Wall lizards and relatives	Yes[118–120,201]
Lanthanotidae	Earless monitors	No[118–120]
Leiocephalidae	Curly-tailed lizards	Yes*[115,118]
Leiosauridae	South American tree and ground lizards	No[119]
Liolaemidae	Tree iguanas, snow swifts, and relatives	Yes[118–120]
Opluridae	Madagascan iguanas	Yes*[201]
Phrynosomatidae	Sand and spiny lizards	Some*[118–120,201]
Polychrotidae	Bush anoles	Some[118–120,201]
Scincidae	Skinks	Some*[118–120,201]
Serpentes	Snakes	Few[3,119]
Shinisauridae	Chinese crocodile lizard	Yes*[119]
Sphenodontidae	Tuataras	Yes*[201]
Teiidae	Whiptails, tegus, and relatives	Some*[118–120,201]
Tropiduridae	Lava lizards	Some[118–120,201]
Varanidae	Monitor lizards and goannas	No[118–120,201]
Xantusiidae	Night lizards	Yes[118,119,201]
Xenosauridae	Knob-scaled lizards	No[119,120,201]

*Indicates groups for which tail loss has a significant consequence.
†Of more than 675 species, only one gecko, *Nephrurus asper*, is known to lack vertebral fracture planes.
‡Fracture planes are present in young *Enyalioides* but are lost as they age.
Data from references 3, 114, 115, 118–120, 201, and 202.

aid in misdirecting the attacks of predators or in sending aposematic or mimetic signals.[114]

Counter-Attack

Many amphibians and reptiles use counter-attacks, usually biting, as a last resort defense. For humans and large predators, the bites of most species are incapable of inflicting any significant damage, but some amphibians and reptiles are capable of delivering significant bites. Many reptiles and salamanders will bite and seize a predator to prevent

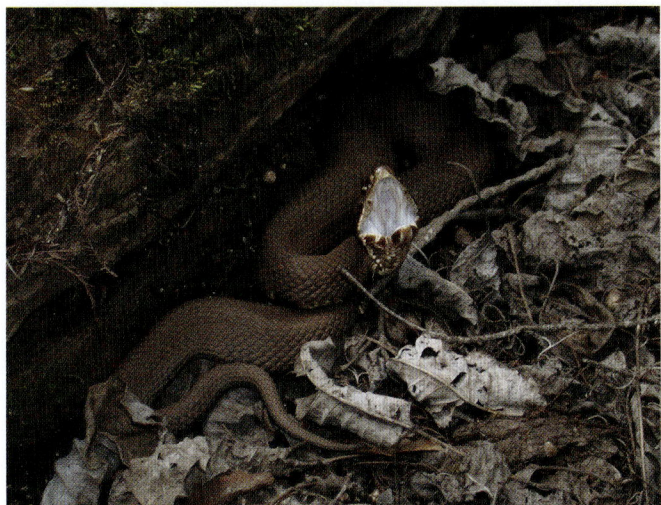

FIG 13.5 Mouth-gaping defensive behavior in a cottonmouth (*Agkistrodon piscivorus*). (Courtesy of John D. Wilson.)

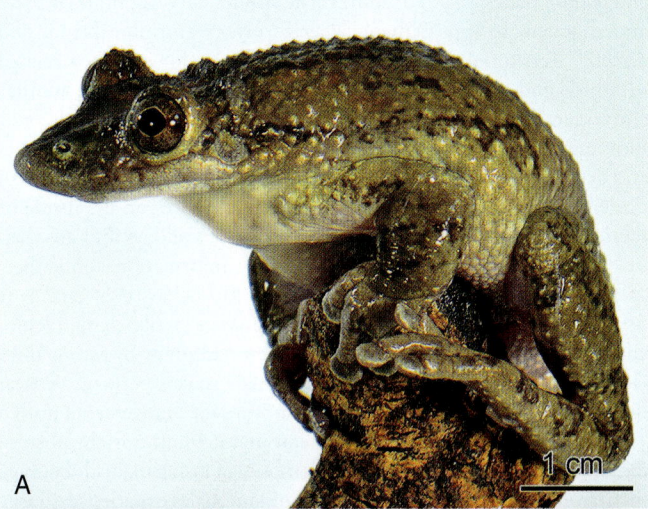

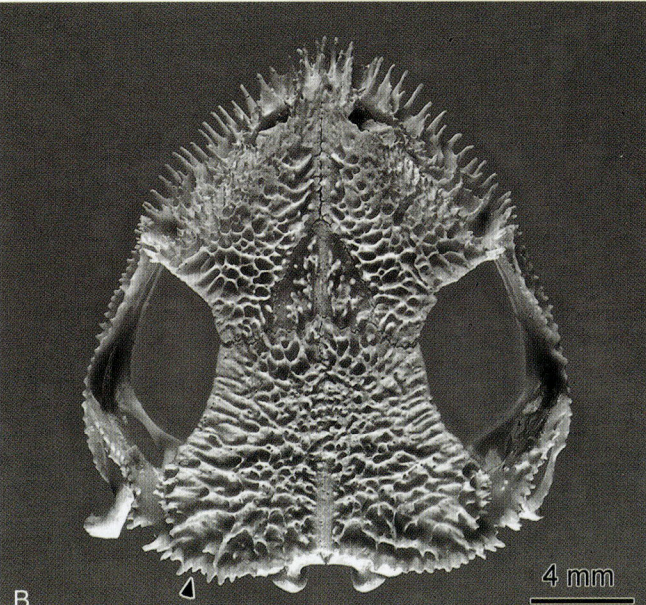

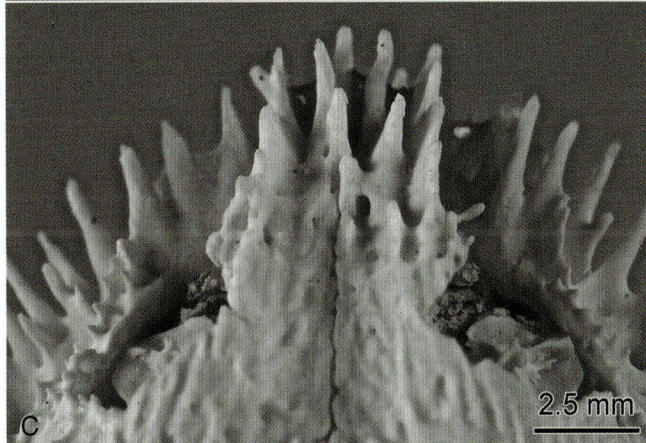

FIG 13.6 (A) The Greening's frog *(Corythomantis greeningi)*. (B and C) Head spines of the Greening's frog. (From Jared C., Mailho-Fontana PL, Antoniazzi MM, et al. Venomous frogs use heads as weapons. *Curr Biol.* 2015;25:2166-2170.)

ingestion.[1,2,107] The predator may have to release the animal, which creates an opportunity for escape.

Reptile venom evolved to accelerate prey digestion and enhance prey capture and therefore functions only indirectly in defense. Venom is energetically expensive to produce, and some venomous snakes do not always elect to use their venom in their own defense.[122] Nonetheless, some species have evolved to advertise their venomous nature through aposematic coloration, tail rattles, or visual displays such as mouth gaping (e.g., cottonmouths, *Agkistrodon piscivorous*; Fig. 13.5). Some reptiles and amphibians can spray their venom (e.g., spitting cobras, *Hemachatus*, and some *Naja*)[123] or poison (e.g., some toads)[124] at an enemy. Northwestern salamanders (*Ambystoma gracile*) have concentrations of poison glands along their tail ridge and will lash their tails to fling or slap irritating toxins into the eyes of a potential predator.[106] Some amphibian species are capable of injecting poisons as a defense.[125,126] Salamanders in the genera *Pleurodeles*, *Salamandrina*, and *Tylototriton* have long, spear-shaped ribs that can penetrate through the animal's skin when it assumes a defensive posture, facilitating the injection of toxic skin secretions into a predator that seizes the salamander.[126,127] Similarly, Greening's frogs (*Corythomantis greeningi*) and Bruno's casque-headed frogs (*Aparasphenodon brunoi*) have bony spines on the skull that penetrate the skin (Fig. 13.6) and can presumably facilitate envenomation of potently poisonous skin secretions.[125]

SOCIAL & REPRODUCTIVE ADAPTATIONS

Courtship

Reptiles and amphibians exhibit a remarkable diversity of courtship behaviors that are beyond the capabilities of this chapter to explore fully.[1,2,60] In many species, male courtship behaviors take the form of ritualized male-male combat or visual or vocal displays intended to advertise mate quality or entice females to breed. Chemical communication is an integral part of courtship for many reptiles and amphibians, and some have evolved elaborate courtship pheromones.

Male crocodilians establish a dominance hierarchy during courtship, and dominant males court females by vocalizing and blowing bubbles at them.[128] Courtship in turtles primarily involves visual and chemical cues. Males of some species turn brighter colors when they are ready to mate.[129] Species that live in murky water, such as mud and musk turtles (family Kinosternidae), rely mostly on pheromonal cues to find and choose mates. Males of some turtle species have elaborate displays aimed at female appeasement, whereas others are more brutal and direct.[130] Territorial defense and courtship behavior are often related in lizards and tuataras.[4] Males advertise their quality to one another and to females using bright colors and stereotyped body positions or movements, such as head-bobs, arm-waving, push-ups, tail-flagging, and dewlap displays.[131] Many male lizards also secrete nonvolatile, high protein-content chemical signals from femoral pores on the inside of their upper legs, which probably persist for several days and are used to mark their territories and communicate information about their species, social, and sexual status.[132] Courtship behavior of snakes is usually initiated by males and has three phases: tactile-chase, tactile-alignment, and coitus. Females indicate their receptivity by gaping their cloaca, and intromission follows. Many male snakes perform vertical displays in pairs punctuated by periodic "topping" movements until a "winner" is established. Snakes that can maintain an upright posture for longer are more dominant. The hormones of losing males discourage them from further courtship, while dominant males experience a surge of testosterone following combat that aids them in courting females.[133,134] Male Madagascan boas (*Sanzinia madagascariensis*) use their spurs in combat.[135] Because sperm competition is a major component of sexual selection,[136] males of many species of lizards and some snakes engage in mate-guarding behavior (Fig. 13.7).[137-140]

Wells[2] provides a thorough review of amphibian courtship and mating behaviors. Like reptiles, amphibians use visual, vocal, tactile, and chemical cues in courtship, but the relative importance of those modes differs among major lineages. Male anurans rely strongly on calls to attract females, and females have evolved to prefer very specific call patterns in order to mate. In addition to auditory calls, some male anurans use vibrations transmitted through substrates to communicate and court. Some anurans, especially those from naturally noisy environments such as fast-flowing streams have replaced or enhanced their calls with visual displays, such as waving of limbs in the "Dancing Frogs "of India (*Micrixalus* spp.), Brazilian torrent frogs (*Hylodes* spp.), and Panamanian golden frogs (*Atelopus zeteki*). Visual courtship displays are less commonly

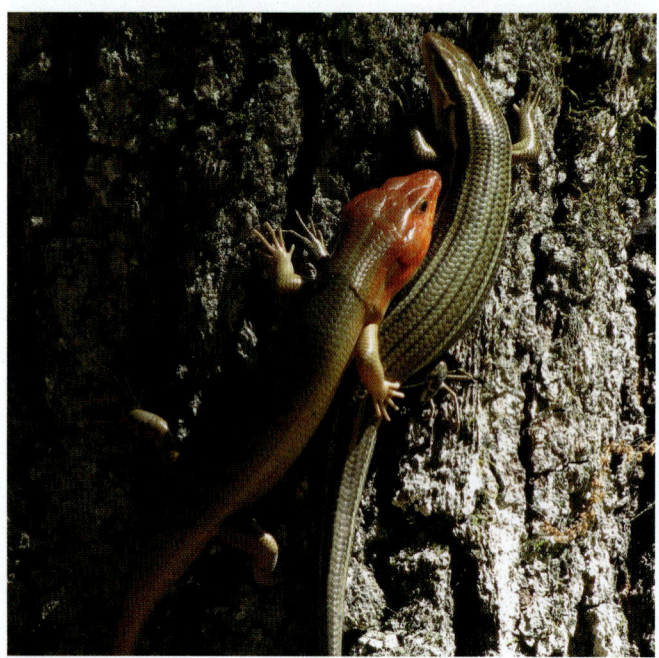

FIG 13.7 A male (left) broad-headed skink (*Plestiodon laticeps*) guarding a female (right). (Courtesy of Sandy Durso.)

known among salamanders except within particular lineages. Males of some species of salamanders such as crested newts (*Triturus cristatus*) have elaborate secondary sexual characters including bold body patterning and enlarged dorsal crests or tail fins that are used in visual displays to attract females. Waving of the tail in aquatic species may also involve the directional dispersal of a chemical pheromone that increases female receptivity.

Tactile and chemical signals are very important in the courtship of all salamanders. Ritualized tactile displays occur among a diversity of salamander lineages and involve using the tail to touch the female while delivering a pheromone, touching or bumping the male's head to the female's body, or tail straddle walking, where males position their tail under the female's body, her chin on the base of his tail, and the tail is undulated until the male perceives the female is receptive to mating. Chemical cues are important in locating and recognizing mates. Male newts (Salamandridae) and males of many species in the family Plethodontidae have glands on the head that produce a courtship pheromone. Because these salamanders have external sperm transfer but internal fertilization, these pheromones increase female receptivity to mating and increase the likelihood that she will complete the mating process. Male Eastern newts (*Notophthalmus viridescens*) court females by seizing the female around the neck with their hind legs and placing the glands in their cheek directly against a female's nares. The male uses his tail to create a current that concentrates pheromones near the female's head. Male plethodontids such as those in the genera *Desmognathus* and *Plethodon* have mental-"hedonic" glands in the chin. These species engage in "snapping" behavior that involves scraping or biting the female with their teeth to facilitate application of the pheromone to the female's bloodstream. Some large eastern *Plethodon* species will rub or slap the gland to the female's nares to deliver the courtship pheromone into the vomeronasal cavity. Beyond direct courtship, males of some amphibian species may acquire mates through defense of key resources such as oviposition sites or areas rich in prey resources, and males of many species will engage in direct combat with rivals for mates or key resources. In many species, male combat is enhanced by special morphologic adaptations such as enlarged thumbs, forearms, or specialized teeth or "tusks."

Female amphibians will also engage in courtship or mate assessment behaviors. Beyond selection of male courtship cues, females of some species will directly compete with other females for access to males. For example, male Majorcan midwife toads (*Alytes muletensis*) provide parental care, and females will interfere with matings between a male and another female in an attempt to secure the male for herself. Female Eastern red-backed salamanders (*Plethodon cinereus*) will smash open fecal pellets of conspecifics.[141] Although this behavior appears to function to track prey resources,[56] females may also use the quality of prey in male fecal pellets in mate assessment.[55]

Mating

Fertilization in reptiles and amphibians is either internal or external. Almost all male reptiles have intromittent organs that they use to transfer their sperm directly to individual females. Male turtles and crocodilians have a single phallus, whereas snakes and lizards have two hemipenes, although they only use one at a time. Male tuataras do not have an intromittent organ; sperm transfer is accomplished by "cloacal kissing," as in birds. Amphibians have an enormous diversity of reproductive modes.[2,142] All anurans and salamanders have external sperm transfer, but caecilians have a phallic structure for internal sperm transfer.[143] The vast majority of anurans, as well as salamanders in the families Cryptobranchidae and Hynobiidae, have external fertilization. The vast majority of salamanders have external sperm transfer but internal fertilization. Only a dozen species of anuran are known to have internal

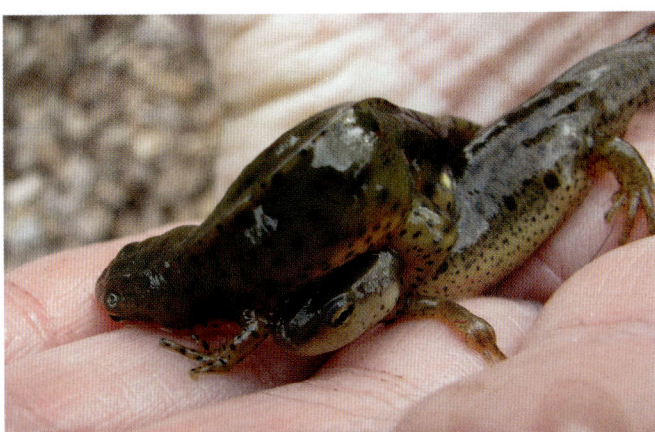

FIG 13.8 Cephalic amplexus in a pair of Eastern newts (*Notophthalmus viridescens*). (Courtesy of Sandy Durso.)

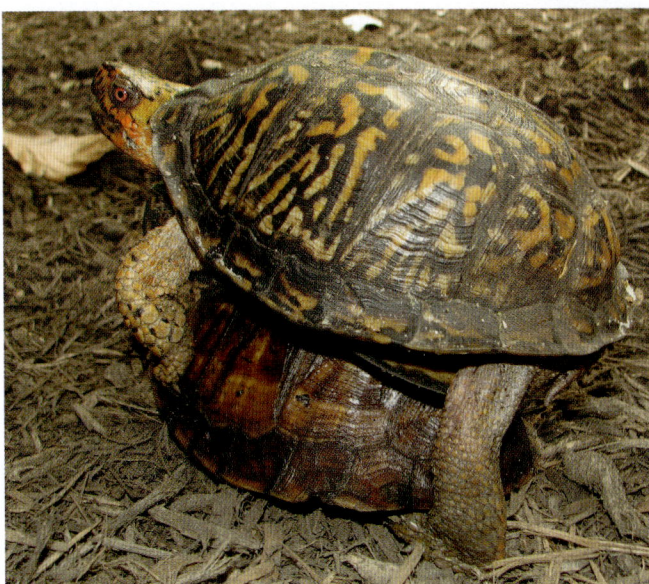

FIG 13.9 Mating in eastern box turtles (*Terrapene carolina*). (Courtesy of Kerry Wixted.)

fertilization.[144] For species with external fertilization, males generally engage in amplexus, where they seize the female from behind using the forearms around the female's waist (inguinal), under the forearms (axillary), or around the neck (cephalic; Fig. 13.8). Other males or females may try to dislodge amplexing males, so grip is often aided with adhesive pores along the male's arms or on enlarged pads on the male's thumbs. External sperm transfer with internal fertilization is accomplished through the deposition of a spermatophore (a sperm packet on a proteinaceous stalk). Male salamanders that deposit a spermatophore will guide females to pick up the sperm packet by tail straddle walking or nudging, and males may continue to use courtship pheromones to sustain female progression through mating.[2] Long-term sperm storage allows many female reptiles and amphibians to become gravid many months or even years after mating[145–147] and to dissociate mating from reproduction, which is useful in highly seasonal or unpredictable climates.

Most male reptiles are aggressive toward other males, and sometimes even toward females, during the mating season. Male crocodilians and many male lizards establish and defend territories around females. Male snakes follow the scent trails of receptive females[148] or scramble to mate with them upon emerging from hibernation.[149] Many male snakes and lizards guard their mates.[150] Actual mating behavior is quite variable. Some species mate very quickly, whereas mating in others takes hours. Most aquatic turtles mate in the water and most terrestrial turtles mate on land. Male box turtles (*Terrapene*) wedge their hind feet into the space between the female's carapace and plastron to prevent her closing her shell on his phallus when it is inserted (Fig. 13.9). Many lizards mate quickly, since their courtship displays make them conspicuous to predators. Overall, the courtship behaviors of most species of snakes are poorly known.[72] Many snakes lay side-by-side, intertwining their bodies, as the male inserts one of his hemipenes into the female's cloaca. Some male pythons use their spurs to titillate the female during mating,[151] and some male colubrid snakes bite the female during mating. Many male vipers exhibit a jerky "tapping" behavior with their chins on the female's back.

Gestation

Female behavior during gestation involves a trade-off between minimizing predation risk and maintaining optimal developmental temperature. Females of some species aggregate in the vicinity of habitat features that offer optimal protection from predators and thermoregulation opportunities.[152] Female reptiles and amphibians are generally less active during gestation than at other times. Many female snakes do not feed during gestation, because there is not enough room for their digestive tract to expand to accommodate a large meal. In temperate regions, they may alternate between feeding in one year and reproducing in the subsequent year.[153] Many female pythons brood their eggs, coiling tightly around them for up to 2 months, and some species can increase the temperature of their clutch by >7°C using muscle contractions ("shivering").[154] The brooding instinct in mother pythons is very strong—lab experiments have shown that they will brood the eggs of other pythons, as well as rocks that are roughly the right size.[155] Female king cobras (*Ophiophagus hannah*) use their coils to build a nest measuring up to 4 feet in diameter out of sticks and bamboo leaves and guard their eggs for 2 to 3 months.[156] Less sophisticated maternal attendance of eggs is widespread in lizards and snakes.[157] Nest-building during or at the end of gestation is also ubiquitous in turtles and crocodilians.

Gestation is not a common focus of behavioral research in amphibians because it appears to be a less important component of their reproductive natural history. Most aquatic-breeding amphibians lay small eggs that expand dramatically when laid, and gravid females may cease foraging shortly before breeding and during migrations to breeding sites. Terrestrial breeding species often have smaller clutch sizes of proportionately larger eggs; therefore females of some terrestrial breeding species may have more prolonged periods where they do not forage while they accommodate their clutches. Live bearing is rare among anurans and salamanders, but the majority of caecilians likely retain eggs for some portion of larval development.[158] Some African toad species (Bufonidae) and *Eleutherodactylus jasper* retain eggs in the oviducts and birth either tadpoles or developed froglets. Some newts (*Salamandra* spp. and *Mertensia* spp.) retain eggs in the oviducts and birth larvae or fully metamorphosed offspring. No special behaviors have been described associated with gestation in these amphibian species. A number of other anuran species have evolved specialized mechanisms for retaining and caring for developing eggs and larvae that are analogous to gestation. Male midwife toads (*Alytes* spp.) carry their eggs wrapped around the male's legs until the tadpoles hatch. Females of several South American anuran species in the family Hemiphractidae carry their fertilized eggs on their back (*Stefania* spp., *Cryptobatrachus* spp., and *Hemiphractus* spp.) or in special dorsal skin pouches (e.g., *Gastrotheca* spp.) until they hatch directly as developed frogs or the tadpoles are deposited in water.

Some pipid species, such as Surinam toads (*Pipa pipa*), also roll their eggs onto the female's back where they are carried in cavities in her skin until the tadpoles hatch.[159] Two of the most exceptional forms of gestation known among amphibians occur among males of the two species of Darwin's frogs (*Rhinoderma* spp.) and females of the two Australian Gastric Brooding Frogs (*Rheobatrachus* spp.), the latter of which are now extinct. After fertilizing the eggs, male Darwin frogs remain with the fertilized eggs until the tadpoles hatch. The male will gather the tadpoles and hold them in thick secretions in his vocal sac where the tadpoles are provisioned by skin secretions for two months until they metamorphose.[160] Female Gastric Brooding Frogs swallowed their eggs after external fertilization and brooded their developing tadpoles in their stomachs.[161] Digestion in the stomach, including the production of stomach acids, shut down and females did not feed for 1 to 2 months. The young would eventually emerge from the mother via the mouth, after which time feeding and digestive processes resumed.

Parental Care

In general, reptiles and amphibians do not exhibit parental care that is as prolonged and intricate as that of many mammals and most birds. However, parental care is found in every major group of reptiles and amphibians,[157,162] has probably evolved multiple times in most groups, is prevalent within specific lineages, and in some groups can be prolonged and intricate.

Crocodilians have particularly well-developed parental care, a trait they share with their closest living relatives (birds), as well as possibly with some dinosaurs. Most chelonians abandon their nests after burying them, although there are exceptions.[163] Hatchling crocodilians and some turtles vocalize from within their eggs to coordinate hatching with their clutch-mates and sometimes with their parents.[164,165] Some lizards guard their eggs against predators,[166] and Australian scincid lizards of the genus *Egernia* live in large aggregations of closely-related individuals and exhibit long-term monogamy and group stability, with up to three annual cohorts of full-sibling offspring living with their biological parents.[167] Parental care is also widespread within certain groups of snakes, such as pythons[168] and vipers,[169] particularly pit vipers, which may remain with their young for several days after they are born. Young pit vipers also seem to follow the scent-trails of their adult relatives to locate preferred hibernation sites[170] and may obtain thermoregulatory[171] and other[172] benefits from aggregating.

Parental care is highly variable within and among amphibian lineages and includes uniparental male or female care and biparental care.[2,173,174] Compared to anurans, which do not generally exhibit parental care, parental care is more common among caecilians and salamanders, particularly among the Plethodontidae. Generally, parental care is most common among terrestrial breeding and direct developing species that have few, large eggs, or among species that have specific constraints on completing their life cycle that require a parent to facilitate. Whether a species will exhibit male versus female parental care is best predicted by fertilization mode; external fertilization is often associated with male parental care and internal fertilization with female parental care.[173,174] Therefore, among anurans that exhibit parental care, males commonly provide the care (though females will as well), and male parental care occurs among external fertilizing salamander species such as hellbenders (*Cryptobranchus alleganiensis*). Among the majority of salamanders and all caecilians, females provide parental care.

Amphibian parental care is most commonly related to egg attendance and defense or egg or tadpole transport.[174] Among terrestrial breeding salamanders (e.g., *Plethodon* spp.), females will remain coiled around their eggs for 2 months or longer, seldom breaking contact with the clutch and often rubbing against and moving eggs around (Fig. 13.10). Egg attendance in these species is known to reduce desiccation and

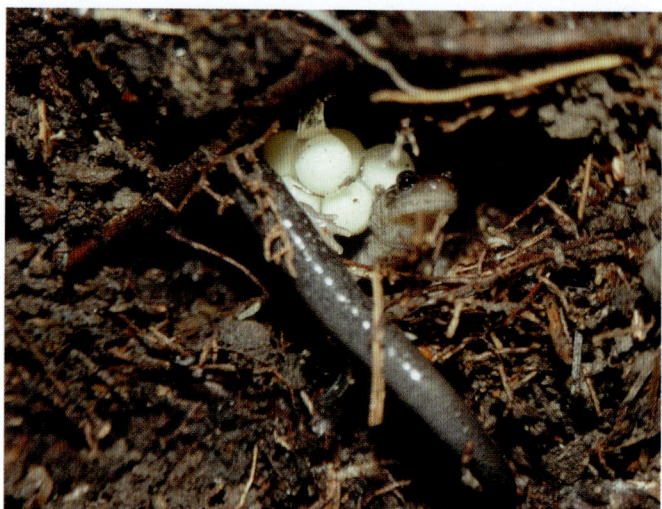

FIG 13.10 Red-backed salamander (*Plethodon cinereus*) female coiled around her clutch of eggs. (Courtesy of John C. Maerz.)

predation risk,[174–177] and females will often consume dead or infected eggs to prevent the spread of fungi to other embryos.[175] It is also hypothesized that female contact with eggs may facilitate the transfer of beneficial microbes that inhibit fungal colonization.[178,179] Upon hatching, young salamanders will remain in contact with their mother for up to 2 weeks, often positioning themselves under her chin or on her back, and juveniles may remain within their parent's territory for several years. Chemical communication between developing embryos and the parent and after hatching has been demonstrated to be important in facilitating parental care behaviors among these species.[180,181]

Beyond the examples of gastric or vocal sac brooding described previously, there are other examples of elaborate parental care in anurans. Tadpole and juvenile transport is documented among several anuran families. Generally, fertilization occurs out of water and males wait with fertilized eggs, or males or females hold eggs on their back or in specialized pouches until the tadpoles hatch, at which time the parent will transport the tadpoles to water. In several species, tadpoles climb on to the parent's back (e.g., *Sooglossus* spp., *Colostethus* spp.) or into skin pouches (e.g., *Assa darlingtoni*) where they will complete their larval development without feeding or ever being deposited in water. Several species of anuran also attend their developing tadpoles. Some species aerate tadpoles by kicking the water around the tadpoles, and some species may facilitate the movement of their tadpoles out of nests or among water bodies by digging channels for the tadpoles to swim between pools.[182] Arguably one of the most advanced forms of active parental care in anurans has evolved in several lineages that breed in or transport tadpoles to small water bodies (e.g., tree holes or bromeliads) where food resources may be limited or competition high. For example, several species of dart frogs (Dendrobatidae) distribute their tadpoles among multiple bromeliads.[183] Males and females will regularly visit the bromeliads to check on their tadpoles, and tadpoles may signal hunger by touching the parent. Females will deposit unfertilized eggs for their tadpoles to consume, and males have been observed signaling females to provide eggs to developing tadpoles. Arguably, this form of parental care is highly derived among amphibians and rivals the complexity often observed in birds and mammals. Finally, arguably the strangest form of amphibian parental care is the discovery of skin feeding in the caecilian *Boulengerula taitana*.[184] Young caecilians were observed feeding directly on the skin of adult females as a means to provision them with nutrients.

NONREPRODUCTIVE SOCIAL BEHAVIOR

Although reptiles and amphibians are generally thought of as nonsocial, many are highly social, even outside of mating. Play behavior has been documented in a number of reptiles and amphibians,[185,186] often in captive settings. All crocodilians are highly social,[128] with a social hierarchy and males that defend territories, females, and juveniles. Although most male turtles are not territorial, they may engage in combat if they encounter one another, even outside the breeding season. Sometimes male and female turtles, such as wood turtles[187] and gopher tortoises,[188] spend time together outside of the breeding season. It has been suggested that tortoises can learn by watching each other.[189] Male lizards are territorial toward one another in general,[190] but some species spend considerable time with females outside of the breeding season (e.g., sleepy lizards, *Tiliqua rugosa*).[191] Great desert skinks (*Liopholis kintorei*) build and maintain elaborate subterranean burrow systems, where they live in cooperative multigenerational family groups.[192] The few other lizard species that form family groups live in rock crevices that require no maintenance.[193] Snakes are generally not social,[194] but rattlesnakes may aggregate outside of the breeding season,[195] and they can use their chemosensory abilities to communicate information about foraging sites even when they are physically distant from one another.[196]

Similarly, social behavior of amphibians outside the context of mating and parental is not widely documented.[2,197] Most species are presumed solitary outside the breeding season, though some species may aggregate for specific purposes such as thermoregulation.[2] A number of amphibian species have been observed huddled during dry conditions, which presumably functions to reduce surface area to volume ratio and evaporative water loss. Many terrestrial salamanders (e.g., *Plethodon* spp., *Aneides* spp.) can be highly territorial in relation to refugia and food resources.[198] The species often engage in scent marking of territories and have visual threat (dominance) and submission displays that are used in territorial encounters. Fights are common among these species, particularly among adults of the same sex and outside breeding seasons, and can result in significant injuries including scarring to the face and the loss of the tail. Female salamanders may also routinely inspect the fecal pellets of other adults as a means to track resource availability.[56]

BEHAVIORS PARTICULAR TO CAPTIVITY

If captive reptiles and amphibians are prevented from thermoregulating or maintaining water balance or are exposed to cues associated with threats, they often exhibit behavioral signs of distress, such as refusing food, difficulty shedding, or weight loss. Some animals engage in "edging" behaviors where they continually push against the walls of their enclosure. This can cause significant lesions, particularly if some aspect of their care is inadequate. Some animals defecate very infrequently, sometimes as little as once per year,[199] but frequent defecation can be induced in captive animals by frequent cleaning of their cages.[200] Some important behaviors may also require stimulation or enrichment in captivity, which is now expected as part of quality husbandry. For example, some species are gregarious when they bask and will not engage in basking when housed individually, and some species or individuals may require live prey to stimulate feeding (which is illegal in some countries). Awareness of important behaviors and the factors that can either result in behavioral displacement or that are needed to stimulate healthy behaviors are important for maintaining animal welfare.

ACKNOWLEDGMENTS

In addition to the numerous references in this chapter, this review is largely possible due to the tremendous review texts produced and edited by F. Harvey Pough et al., Carl Gans, and Kentwood D. Wells, which we have cited throughout this chapter. Their contributions to synthesizing our understanding of amphibian and reptile behaviors cannot be understated. Thanks to P. Zani for reviewing Table 13.1.

REFERENCES

See www.expertconsult.com for a complete list of references.

14

Behavioral Training and Enrichment of Reptiles

Michelle L. Skurski, Gregory J. Fleming,[†] Andre Daneault, and Geoffrey W. Pye

Reptiles have historically carried the stigma of being unintelligent, uncharismatic, and easy to care for with minimal husbandry needs. Nothing could be further from the truth. Animal caretakers now recognize a need for all animals, including reptiles, to be able to perform biologically appropriate behaviors. The environment provided should be determined by the animals' natural and individual histories. Training and enrichment are great ways to provide reptiles opportunities to display their natural behaviors, to allow for people who keep reptiles to interact with these animals and observe their behavior close at hand, and to have the reptiles participate in their own veterinary medical care.[1-3]

Animal enrichment and training have become standard practice in most zoological and aquarium facilities and can also be implemented in private homes. The concepts of training and enrichment are interrelated. In recent years, many professional animal care facilities have seen improvements in the health and well-being of reptiles by providing an environment in which reptiles can make choices. For example, natural behaviors such as foraging, climbing, digging, or swimming cannot take place if animals are housed in a barren plastic box. With a small amount of effort, private owners can successfully encourage natural behaviors such as these in their reptiles.

ENRICHMENT

Enrichment is more than just placing a new branch or a plant in a reptile's environment. Although there are many different definitions of enrichment, for the sake of consistency we will follow the definition used by the Association of Zoos and Aquariums (AZA) Behavior Scientific Advisory Group:

> Enrichment is a dynamic process for enhancing animal environments within the context of the animal's behavioral biology and natural history. Environmental changes are made with the goal of increasing the animal's behavioral choices and drawing out their species-appropriate behaviors, thus enhancing animal welfare.

In practice, enrichment means encouraging species-appropriate behaviors and providing the animal with choices in every aspect of reptile husbandry, from food presentation to housing. The diversity of reptile habitats, microhabitats, and ecosystems, as well as the range and complexity of their behaviors, can actually increase the opportunities for enrichment to enhance the animals' lives.

Based on the aforementioned definition, there are three main goals for enrichment:
1. To promote species-appropriate behaviors
2. To provide behavioral opportunities
3. To provide animals with choices or control over their environment

All three of these goals require a clear understanding of the animal's natural and individual histories. This information is critical to making the enrichment successful. Useful natural history information includes how the reptile thermoregulates; the optimum body temperature range for the species; normal activity levels for the reptile; diel cycle (i.e., is the reptile diurnal or nocturnal?); natural diet and foraging style; and whether the reptile is arboreal, terrestrial, aquatic, or semiaquatic. This information will help to prepare clients to properly care for a reptile. Based on the natural history, each enrichment initiative should have a behavioral goal. One benefit of setting behavioral goals for enrichment is that it offers a way to measure success. For example, a client may want to encourage an overweight arboreal snake to climb and utilize more of the enclosure. The question the client may ask is, "Did the addition of branches into the snake enclosure encourage the snake to climb and utilize the enclosure?" If the answer is yes, the behavioral goal was achieved. If the answer is no, then other options such as platforms, heat sources, or even different types of branches may be explored to encourage the snake to climb (Fig. 14.1).

Another behavioral goal may be to encourage an animal to forage. One approach might be to utilize natural scents resulting from dragging a prey item through the enclosure to leave a scent trail that can stimulate the reptile to forage. In some cases the scent just needs to be novel to engage the reptile. Animal keepers have successfully utilized a cinnamon scent trail scattered throughout an enclosure to encourage foraging in a Komodo dragon (*Varanus komodoensis*).

Choice of housing, enclosure furnishings, and behavioral opportunity depend on whether the reptile is arboreal, terrestrial, aquatic, or semiaquatic. Something as simple as providing different levels in an enclosure can encourage exploration and foraging. Many species of monitor lizard are known to stand bipedal to forage in the wild. This behavior can be recreated through minor alterations of an enclosure and delivery of food to the animal (Fig. 14.2). Although animals in the wild seem to exhibit this behavior without much effort, a monitor lizard while in human care may need to be encouraged to stand through small and successive approximations of gradually increasing the height at which food is placed. Captive lizards are likely novices at standing bipedal and will need to develop the skills and physical ability to accomplish some behavioral goals.

The way in which food is presented can also provide behavioral opportunity. Multiple behaviors can be encouraged by varying the size of the food item, the placement or location of the food, and the time of day of the feeding. For example, tree pythons are nocturnal; as such, their activity level typically increases at night. During the more active periods, foraging and hunting behaviors will be displayed. Therefore feeding during these periods could encourage active behaviors that stimulate and exercise the snake.

Providing complexity and choices to an environment can be achieved through addition of, or changes to, rocks, branches, plants, light, and

---

[†]Deceased.

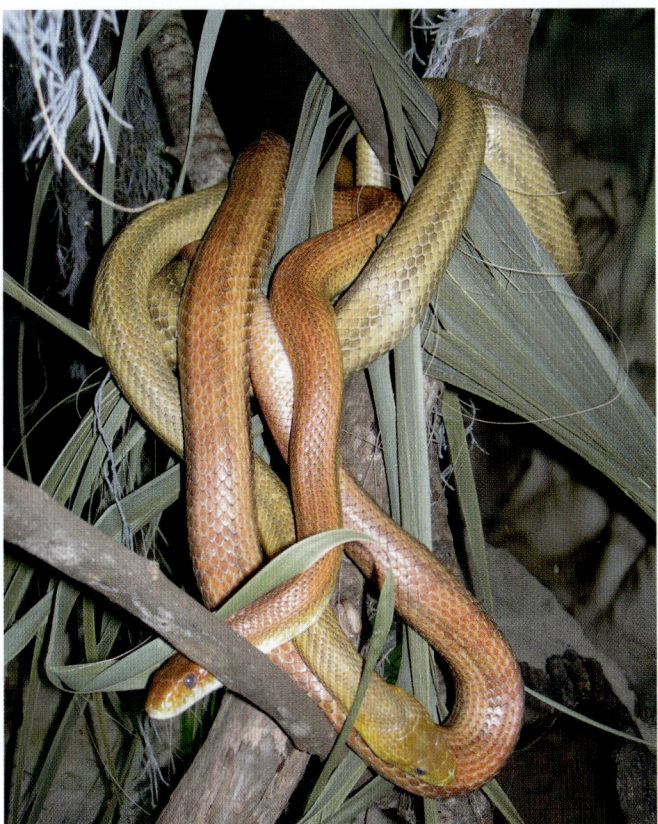

FIG 14.1 Everglades ratsnake (*Pantherophis obsoleta rossalleni*) utilizing natural climbing materials.

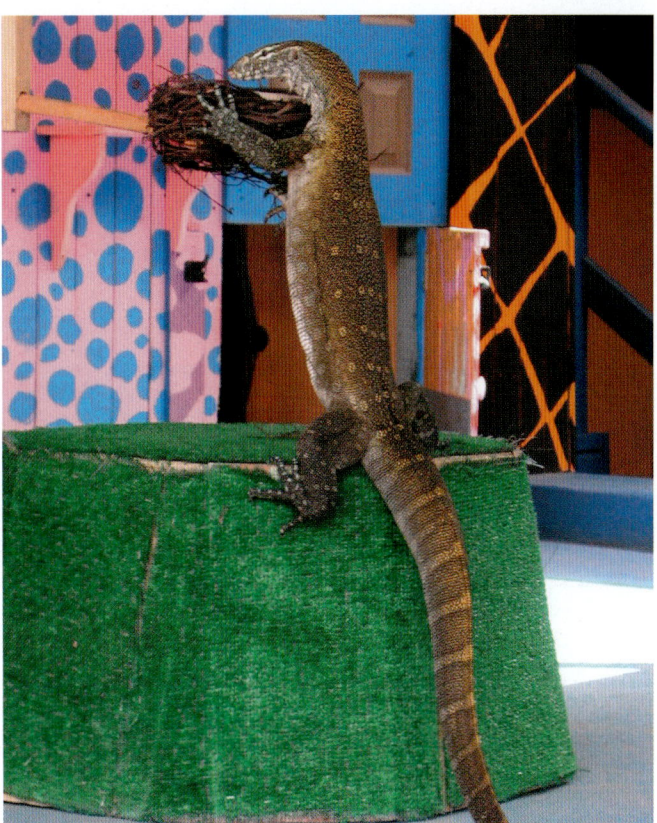

FIG 14.2 A Nile monitor (*Varanus niloticus*) standing bipedal to acquire a food item.

substrate within an enclosure. Providing choices for and control over thermoregulation opportunities is vital for the reptiles. Opportunities for thermoregulation can be provided with the use of lights, under-cage heat pads, water of variable temperatures, and heat-emitting ceramic bulbs. Recently, improvements in technology allow changes in the temperature and humidity of enclosures by the minute. Environmental temperature and humidity may be altered throughout the day, allowing for natural changes in the animal's environment that mimic a natural sunrise or an afternoon rainstorm.

Offering different levels in an enclosure provides reptiles an opportunity to utilize heat and light sources to varying degrees. Understanding the general environment for the reptile in the wild is not enough; a caretaker must dig deeper into the natural history and behavior of the animal to meet its needs. For instance, the animal could come from the desert but spend the majority of its day burrowed underground, escaping from the sun and heat. In this case, the assumption that the animal would need a very warm, barren environment would take into account only a part of its natural history. Providing a way to escape the heat would also be vital to this animal's well-being. Appropriate lighting is essential not only for health but also for enriching a reptile's life.

Encouraging clients to study the natural and individual history of the species they care for will be the first step in the creation of a successful enrichment program for their reptiles. Enrichment done appropriately will improve the health of the animal, enhance their welfare, and assist in facilitating their care. To find some additional examples of enrichment ideas, see Disney's Animal Programs' enrichment website at http://www.animalenrichment.org.[3]

TRAINING

Since the early 1990s, there has been a dramatic increase in the use of operant conditioning techniques to train exotic animals for husbandry and medical purposes. These animal training techniques can assist in facilitating day-to-day care, routine medical procedures, and management of reptiles. The act of training can be enriching for both the animal and its caretaker as they interact. Any reptile brought into clinics, such as bearded dragons (*Pogona vitticeps*), green iguanas (*Iguana iguana*), monitor lizards, boas and pythons, and turtles and tortoises, can be trained to calmly and voluntarily enter a crate instead of being physically restrained for crating. Reptiles can also be trained to accept various veterinary procedures such as ultrasonography, nail clipping, venipuncture, or even being medicated. Reptiles with chronic conditions requiring regular visits and/or treatments can be trained to cooperate for many procedures. This kind of training allows for treatment with reduced stress to the animals and client.

To create a well-thought-out behavioral plan for a reptile, many zoo and aquarium facilities use the "SPIDER" framework[4] taught in several courses given by the Association of Zoos and Aquariums. The SPIDER framework includes **S**etting goals, **P**lanning, **I**mplementing, **D**ocumenting, **E**valuating, and **R**eadjusting (Table 14.1). More information on this process can be found at http://www.animaltraining.org.[5]

The first step *(S)* in the SPIDER process is setting goals. It is beneficial to start a training program by determining the overall behavioral goals (i.e., detailing the specific behaviors to be trained). During this goal-development process, it is important to include all parties involved with the management of the animals. Goals should

TABLE 14.1   SPIDER Framework

Step	SPIDER Framework Details	Example
Setting Goals	Detail the specific behaviors to be trained.	Train the monitor lizard to enter a crate voluntarily and be calm and comfortable in the crate.
Planning	Create a series of steps for shaping the behavior. Plan who will be training the animal, when the animal will be trained, and any equipment or tool needed to achieve the training plan.	Wait for the lizard to move toward the crate; use crickets to reinforce. Continue to reinforce movements toward the crate until the lizard enters the crate. Reinforce calm behavior inside the crate by continuing to provide crickets. Close the door to the crate and continue to provide crickets for calm behavior.
Implementing	Train the behavior over many sessions, advancing only when the animal is ready. Ensure clear communication among participants regarding training steps and timelines.	The lizard's two owners will each train crating for two sessions per week. They will review each other's notes before each session. The crate will not be lifted with the lizard inside until the lizard has successfully entered the crate and remained inside calmly with the door closed for 10 minutes.
Documenting	Create a historical document that tracks the progress of the animal and shows trends in behavior.	Each of the owners will take notes on their training sessions, including a rating of the session and comments on the lizard's progress.
Evaluating	Review the documentation and training plan.	After 3 weeks, the lizard has not yet completely entered the crate.
Readjusting	Make any changes necessary to achieve the behavioral goals.	The owners decide to adjust the plan and begin placing a few crickets at the back of the crate to encourage the lizard to enter completely. Once this occurs, they will continue to provide crickets if the lizard remains calmly in the crate.

be based on the joint needs of owners, veterinary staff, and the reptile. For example, if the monitor lizard can shift into a crate for transport to the veterinarian, the lizard is more easily crated and less distressed when in the crate. This outcome facilitates a better veterinary evaluation. The goals in this case would then be to train the monitor lizard to enter a crate voluntarily and be calm and comfortable in the crate.

The next step (*P*) is planning. This is when a training plan is created for the behavior. The training plan is a series of steps for shaping the behavior. The plan is meant to be a way for the trainer to think through the process before beginning to train an animal. If crate training is used as the example, the first step is to reinforce being comfortable with the presence of the crate itself. This process starts with providing positive reinforcement when the animal merely approaches the crate and then slowly encouraging the animal to enter the crate. The reinforcer or reward for learning to enter the crate could be small bits of a highly desirable food that are delivered as soon as the reptile approaches and/or moves closer to the entry of the crate.

The third step (*I*) is implementing. The behavior should be trained over a number of sessions, and training should advance only when the animal is ready. If more than one trainer is involved, having clearly laid out plans, assignments, and timelines helps to facilitate a smooth process. Defining roles and creating clear avenues of communication among all participants is also important.

Before the training is implemented, a decision should be made regarding how the training sessions will be documented (*D*). Video recording sessions are an easy way to document and track progress of training. Taking notes, including session ratings and comments, is another useful way to document and track training outcomes. The goals of documenting are to create a historical record that can be used to track the progress of the animal, look for trends in behavior, and facilitate training new animals in the future.

The last two steps of the SPIDER process, evaluating (*E*) and readjusting (*R*), require reviewing the documentation and training plan and making any changes necessary to achieve the behavioral goals. Often these two steps are occurring throughout the shaping of a behavior. For more information on how to apply this process, visit Disney's Animal Programs website or http://www.animalenrichment.org[6] or http://www.animaltraining.org.[5]

PRACTICAL EXAMPLES OF TRAINING AND ENRICHMENT

Nile Monitor (*Varanus niloticus*)

Providing a pool with cascading water to a Nile monitor's habitat for enrichment will enhance the complexity of the environment. The keeper controls the water level, temperature, and flow rate of the water. Food items such as live fish, crustaceans, invertebrates, cut meat, and deceased whole prey items may also be presented in the pool. This encourages the animal to exhibit natural behaviors, including swimming, soaking, thermoregulation, foraging, and interacting with the cascading water (Fig. 14.3).

Training a Nile monitor to enter a crate on cue may be a safer alternative to physically restraining the reptile. It is certainly less stressful for both the caretaker and the lizard. A Nile monitor can be trained to enter a crate voluntarily for transport (Fig. 14.4). This trained behavior also allows the keepers to clean the enclosure safely.

Komodo Dragon (*Varanus komodoensis*)

A Komodo dragon crate is not only designed for transport but also to facilitate medical examinations and sampling of the animals. Historically, hands-on medical examinations for large Komodo dragons involved the animals being anesthetized. Today, with a solid training program and appropriate crate design, the animal can voluntarily enter the crate to be transferred to the hospital (Fig. 14.5). While at the hospital and during the exams, the animal remains calmly within the crate for multiple procedures. The animal can be asked to move into specific positions in the crate as needed. These exams include evaluation of overall body condition, obtaining weights and body measurements, radiography, ultrasonography, coelomic palpation, and wound evaluation and care (Fig. 14.6). The crate is designed with removable portions to gain safe access to the tail and hind area of the animal for cloacal swabs, nail trims, venipuncture, and hind limb evaluation. Once the examination is complete, the crate and animal are secured and returned to the holding area where the animal is safely released into its enclosure.

Crocodilians

The creation of a training and enrichment program for large crocodilians is an invaluable tool for the animal husbandry and veterinary staff. The

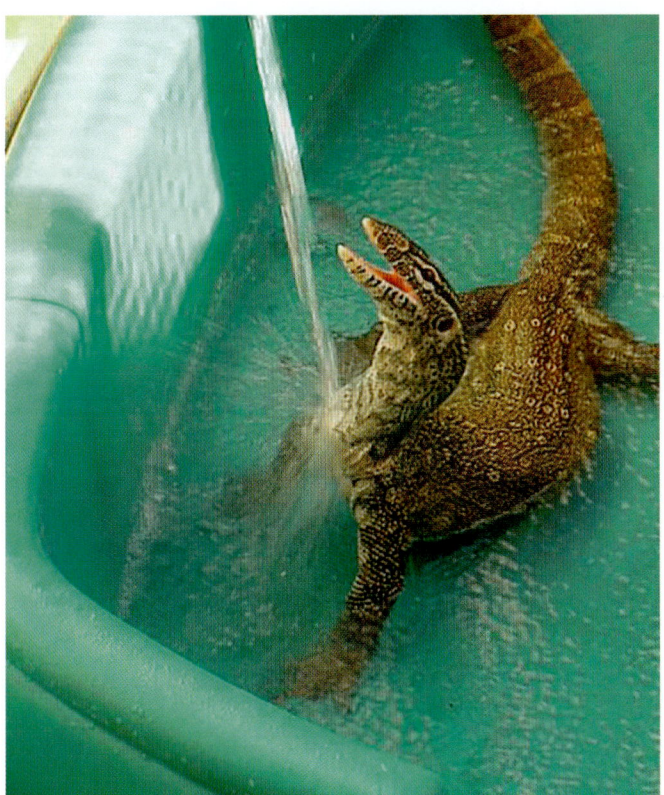

FIG 14.3 A Nile monitor (*Varanus niloticus*) interacting with a water element.

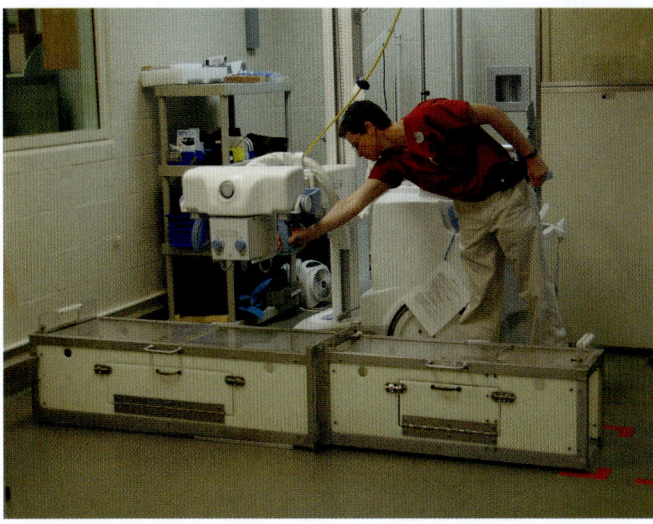

FIG 14.5 A Komodo dragon (*Varanus komodoensis*) in a crate at a veterinary hospital.

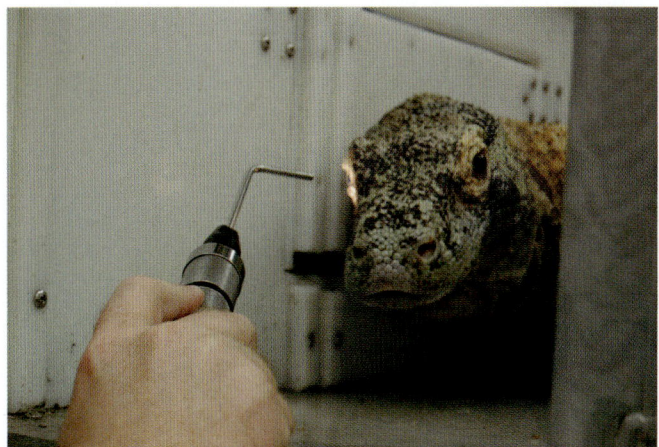

FIG 14.6 A Komodo dragon (*Varanus komodoensis*) in a crate having an eye exam.

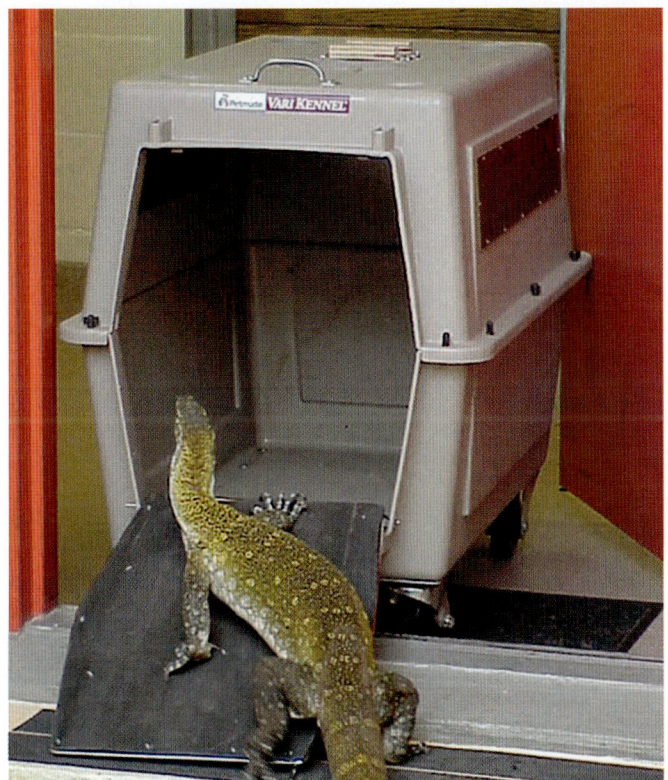

FIG 14.4 A Nile monitor (*Varanus niloticus*) being cued to move into a transport crate.

program can facilitate a safe working environment for the staff and animals while providing great care and medical opportunities that would normally not be possible. Traditionally crocodilians were manually restrained and/or chemically immobilized for medical procedures and transport. Crocodiles are trained to shift off exhibit into holding areas where pools and specially designed crates are located. The shift training of the crocodiles facilitates opportunities for the keepers to provide enrichment, opportunities that would not be feasible with the animals being present in the exhibit. Keepers can strategically place enrichment items within the exhibit, manipulate the environment, and control how many animals are in the exhibit at any given time. The act of shifting the crocodiles is enriching as it allows the animals to move and explore other areas and increase activity levels. While in the off-exhibit area the crocodiles can be asked to voluntarily enter crates for medical procedures and examinations that could include transport, obtaining weights and body measurements, venipuncture, radiography, safe injection administration of medications, and wound evaluation and care (Fig. 14.7) (Fig. 14.8). Once the examination and medical procedures have been completed, the crocodile can be safely released back into their holding pool(s) and shifted back into their habitat.

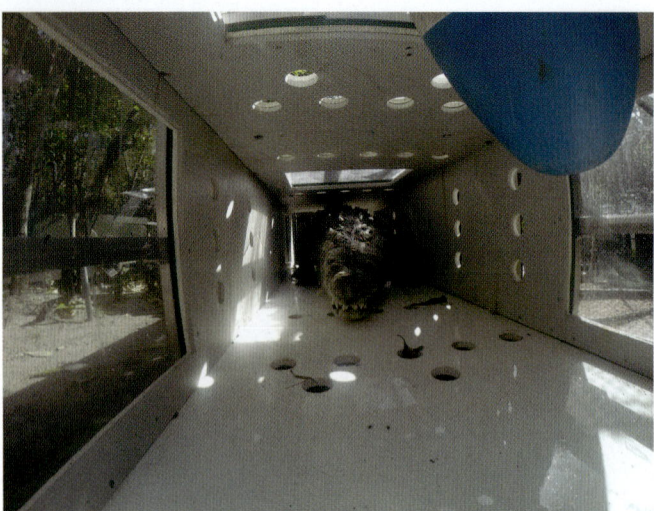

FIG 14.7 An American crocodile (*Crocodylus acutus*) entering a training crate.

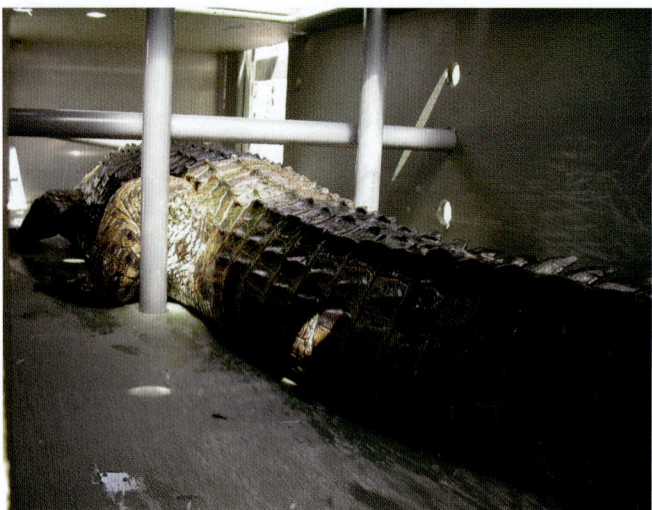

FIG 14.8 A Nile crocodile (*Crocodylus niloticus*) inside a training crate. Once crocodile is in place, pvc poles can be used to minimize movement for procedures. (From Miller RE, Fowler ME. *Fowler's Zoo and Animal Medicine*. Vol. 7. St. Louis: Elsevier; 2012;215. Used with permission.)

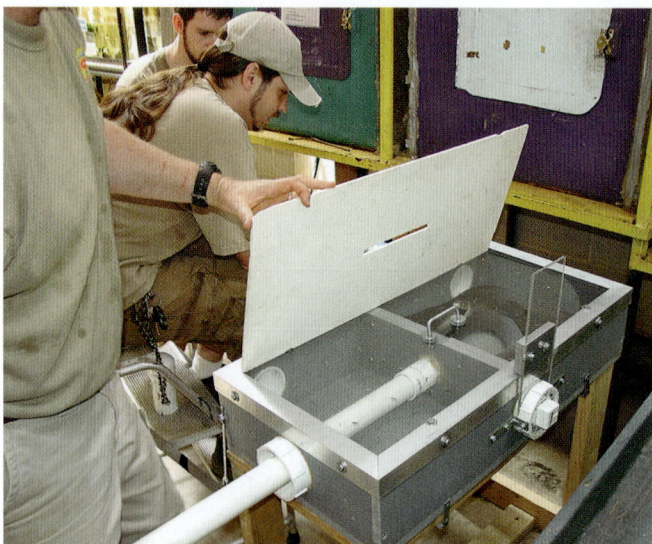

FIG 14.9 A Black mamba (*Dendroaspis polylepis*) has shifted from his enclosure to the holding box. A handling tube is attached to the side of the box. Once this is attached, the door will open and the snake will move into the tube. (Courtesy of Brad Lock.)

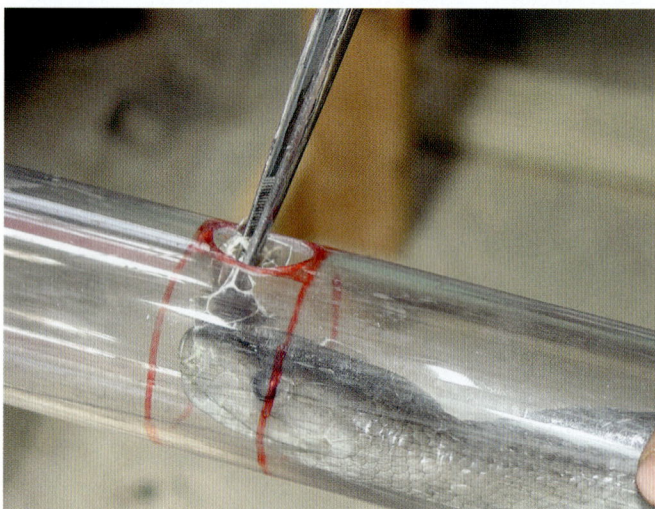

FIG 14.10 Once the snake is in the handling tube, the veterinarian can remove the retained eye cap without sedation. (Courtesy of Brad Lock.)

Venomous Snakes

Training snakes to shift into a box is helpful, particularly when dealing with venomous species (Fig. 14.9). Once the snake is safely in the holding box, a handling tube can be attached to the box, and the snake can enter the tube. The husbandry staff then detaches the tube from the box with the snake gently restrained by the tube. Using this technique allows safe and humane examination or treatment (Fig. 14.10). The snake does not come into direct contact with the handlers, making the entire procedure safer and less stressful for both the snake and the handlers.

CONCLUSION

The key to creating a successful training and enrichment program with a reptile is to develop the knowledge of the reptile's natural history.

This is critical for understanding the needs and capabilities of the reptile and, ultimately, improves the reptile's welfare. Consulting with a veterinarian can be helpful in deciding on proper enrichment objectives and appropriate behaviors to train for daily activity and medical procedures. In any case, training and enrichment can benefit both the owner and the reptile by providing a closer relationship and a fuller enriching life for both participants.

REFERENCES

See www.expertconsult.com for a complete list of references.

15

Stress and Welfare

Craig J-G. Hunt

Stress may be defined as any physical, chemical, or emotional force that disturbs or threatens homeostasis and the accompanying adaptive responses (the stress response) that attempts to restore homeostasis.[1] When stress results in mental or physical damage the welfare of the animal becomes compromised, thus stress and welfare are inextricably linked.

A stimulus that evokes a stress response is called a *stressor*. Broadly, stressors can be divided into two categories.[2] Physiological stressors affect the animal's ability to maintain homeostasis necessitating physiological changes to cope with such conditions. Contrarily, psychological stressors do not pose a direct challenge to body physiology but rather may be indicative of imminent physiological challenge and can induce a stress response without actual physiological insult. Examples of common stressors are provided in Box 15.1.

Physical and mental well-being are intricately related; any physical injury or dysfunction has the potential to impact behavior, causing mental stress that, in turn, often negatively impacts physical health such as immune function, reproduction, and growth. Maintenance of animals in good condition requires not only an assessment of physiological health but also psychological health.[3]

PHYSIOLOGY OF THE STRESS RESPONSE

The normal stress response is a result of the response of the sympathetic nervous system and the hypothalamic-pituitary-adrenal axis with subsequent release of norepinephrine (sympathetic nervous system) and epinephrine (adrenal medulla), preparing the body for fight or flight.[1] The hypothalamus releases corticotrophin-releasing factor, which triggers the release of adrenocorticotropic hormone from the pituitary gland, which then stimulates the release of glucocorticoids from the adrenal cortex. Several other hormones, including prolactin, glucagon, thyroid hormones, and vasopressin, are secreted from other endocrine organs. The overall effect of these two systems is to increase the immediate availability of energy; increase oxygen intake; decrease blood flow to areas not critical for movement; and inhibit digestion, growth, immune function, reproduction, and pain perception. This system works well when responding to discrete short-term stresses.[1]

If the system is chronically activated, the stress response persists and eventually becomes dysregulated. Chronic stress develops when an animal is unable to adapt to a particular stressor that does not go away. Cardiovascular, metabolic, reproductive, digestive, immune, and anabolic processes can be pathologically affected, subsequently leading to myopathy, fatigue, hypertension, decreased growth rates, gastrointestinal distress, and suppressed immune function.[1]

The predominant glucocorticoid in reptiles is corticosterone,[4] and an elevated serum corticosterone level is often used as an indicator that an animal has experienced stress. Increased corticosterone levels influence whole-body physiology and behavior by acting on numerous target organs. Glucocorticoids potentiate their effect by altering the circulating levels of sex steroid[5–8] and other hormones.[9] Combined, the direct and indirect effect of the sympathetic nervous system, epinephrine, and corticosterone rapidly induces substantial changes in physiological conditions that can be long lasting.

EFFECTS OF STRESS ON THE VARIOUS BODY SYSTEMS

As stated earlier, the role of the stress response is to maximize energy availability to vital body systems. Therefore the stress response stimulates lypolysis and gluconeogenesis[10] and alters cardiovascular function.[11] In addition, the stress response is a potent inhibitor of systems that are nonessential. Specifically, growth[12] and reproduction[13] are oftentimes dramatically inhibited during times of stress since the release of catabolic stress hormones (catecholamines and glucocorticoids) is incompatible with the release of anabolic hormones (growth hormone and gonadal hormones).[14] Although these processes are critical to long-term survival and fitness, they are nonessential for day-to-day survival. The effect of the stress response on the immune system is complex; however, typically the inflammatory response and antibody production are inhibited.[10] Such changes minimize energy utilization and enhance immediate performance, but immune suppression also increases the incidence of disease.

The stress response also has a substantial effect on behavior. Behaviors that are energy demanding such as aggression are usually drastically inhibited; however, behavioral changes can be complex. Corticosterone inhibits reproductive behaviors that consume substantial amounts of energy, such as aggression[7,8] and territory maintenance,[15] yet copulation itself is unaffected.[8] For males, copulation is a relatively low-energy behavior with high fitness value, so with copulatory behavior maintained, stressed males remain able to produce offspring during challenging times. However, without the supportive behaviors associated with male-male competition, such opportunities for reproduction are likely to be reduced.

The role of corticosterone in female reproduction appears complicated. Captivity-induced stress inhibits estrogen and therefore inhibits the production of vitellogenin.[16] However, corticosterone levels are frequently elevated during at least some stages of reproduction in wild female reptiles,[17-19] and this elevation is positively correlated with

BOX 15.1   Common Stressors of Captive Reptiles and Amphibians

Psychological Stressors	Physiological Stressors
Social dominance	Inadequate or excessive environmental temperature, humidity, or photoperiod
Overcrowding	
Confinement	
Novel environments	Thirst and dehydration
Human-reptile interactions	Hunger and undernutrition
Lack of appropriate seclusion	Inappropriate diet (malnutrition)
Excessive differences in the size of cage mates	Oxygen deprivation
	Disease
Poorly matched social dominance or sexually established territories	Trauma
	Courtship including male-male combat, production of sperm, eggs, or embryos.

reproductive output.[19] In fact, treatment with exogenous corticosterone implants increases reproductive output.[20] Therefore corticosterone likely plays a constructive role in female reproduction rather than simply reflecting the stressful nature of reproduction.

WHEN DOES THE STRESS RESPONSE BECOME NONADAPTIVE?

Although the stress response is clearly an adaptive process, it also can lead to disease and ultimately the death of an individual. Exposure to stressors is a common occurrence, and the stress response adjusts an individual's physiology to cope with a given situation in the short term. The dramatic physiological effects of the stress response provide a state in which the individual can overcome the stimuli or distance itself from it in a relatively short time frame. However, the extreme mobilization of energy and inhibition of other body systems cannot be supported for a lengthy period without detrimental effects. Repeated exposure to a stimulus leads to long-term adjustments in body physiology and/or perception, and thus tolerance may evolve to a stimulus previously recognized as a stressor.

THE STRESS OF CAPTIVITY

Reptiles live in a vast array of habitats throughout the world, and each species has evolved behavioral and physiological mechanisms that enable them to use the environment to meet both short-term and long-term needs. In captivity, reptiles and amphibians are entirely dependent on their keeper for all of their needs, including provision of shelter, water, food, and access to appropriate environmental parameters. Failure to provide such needs is the cause of a significant percentage of health problems in reptiles and amphibians.[21]

Cowan[22] described a maladaptation syndrome in reptiles and amphibians, which typically results in nonspecific degenerative conditions and diseases attributable to adaptational failures in the captive environment and has been reported to be responsible for an outbreak of salmonellosis in a colony of lizards that were subclinical carriers of *Salmonella*.[23] Signs of stress in reptiles and amphibians may initially be subtle and are often vague and nonspecific and may include ill-thrift, weight loss, increased parasite burdens, inactivity or hyperactivity, and a failure to thermoregulate. There is variation in how individuals perceive a given environmental stimulus or cope with the same environmental change;

thus the same environment may cause a greater stress response in one animal compared with another.[1] It is likely that captive breeding over several generations selects individuals that are more adapted to captivity and therefore less likely to suffer stress. Even when reptiles are held in conditions that properly provide for physiological needs, captivity can potentially be stressful. Escape behaviors, foraging activity, and mate-searching activity are all potentially altered by captivity therefore confinement in itself can be stressful.[24,25] However, this effect can be eliminated as the animal acclimates to the confinement.[26]

Another potential stressor that is unavoidable in captivity is handling. In nature, direct restraint is usually closely tied to consumption by a predator, so handling as a stressor of reptiles is not surprising. Handling leads to increases in both corticosterone[27,28] and adrenal catecholamines[29] even in some reptiles that are habituated to humans,[30] although, some can acclimate to handling.[31]

Routine management and cleaning of a reptile's or amphibian's enclosure may cause stress due to the frequent need to handle the animal and by removing important chemical cues.[32] Snakes have been shown to use pheromone on newspaper bedding in order to mark territory,[33] and removal of feces and cage cleaning has been shown to disrupt reproduction in the red-backed salamander (*Plethodon cinereus*).[34,35] Naturalistic enclosures with bioactive substrate may reduce stress by increasing the potential to provide microclimates and natural foraging behaviors; additionally such enclosures require less cleaning resulting in less disturbance. Reptiles in naturalistic environments were shown to be the least stressed when compared with those in more clinical environments,[32] but, if poorly done, there is the potential to increase pathogen and disease exposure.[36] Even in naturalistic enclosures, transparent barriers present a potential stressor as fear responses in snakes and turtles (and probabaly lizards) may be triggered with only visual stimuli.[32]

Psychological stress can also be induced by inappropriate social housing (Fig. 15.1); when kept together in captivity, many solitary or noncolonial animals display some degree of social dominance and territoriality, which may lead to stress.[37] Most reptile and amphibian species are not considered to be social, but there are numerous exceptions, and many exhibit a more social lifestyle at certain stages of life. Some animals come together in large numbers during certain events but remain solitary for the rest of the year, for example, garter snakes (*Thamnophis spp.*) during mating and Komodo dragons (*Varanus komodoensis*) feeding on a large carcass. Australian black rock skinks (*Egernia saxatilis*) exhibit long-term monogamy, stable social grouping, and evidence of nuclear family systems.[38] Group housing in some species such as the red-bellied cooter (*Pseudemys nelsoni*)[39] results in greater food consumption; in others such as hatchling chameleons (*Chamaeleo spp.*),[40] some crocodiles,[41] and snapping turtles (*Chelydra serpentina*),[42] dominance hierarchy discourages some individuals from feeding and limits access to food. Aggression and competition at basking sites has been demonstrated in some species such as the North American painted turtle (*Chrysemys picta*),[43] and dominant male iguanas (*Iguana iguana*) have been shown to grow more rapidly and use supplementary heat sources twice as often as subordinate males.[44] It has been demonstrated that in crocodilians and iguanas isolation from their peers may be stressful in their first year,[45] which suggests that such animals may be best group-housed (with suitable room) as juveniles but kept solitarily when subadults/adults.

Psychological and behavioral compromise due to constraints of a captive environment may result in frequent or constant attempts to escape or in inappropriate prolonged and repetitive locomotory behaviors that often result in self-induced trauma.[37] Reptiles appear unable to perceive the presence of glass as a barrier and may repeatedly rub against or crash into it causing physical injury.[46] Pica, the deliberate ingestion

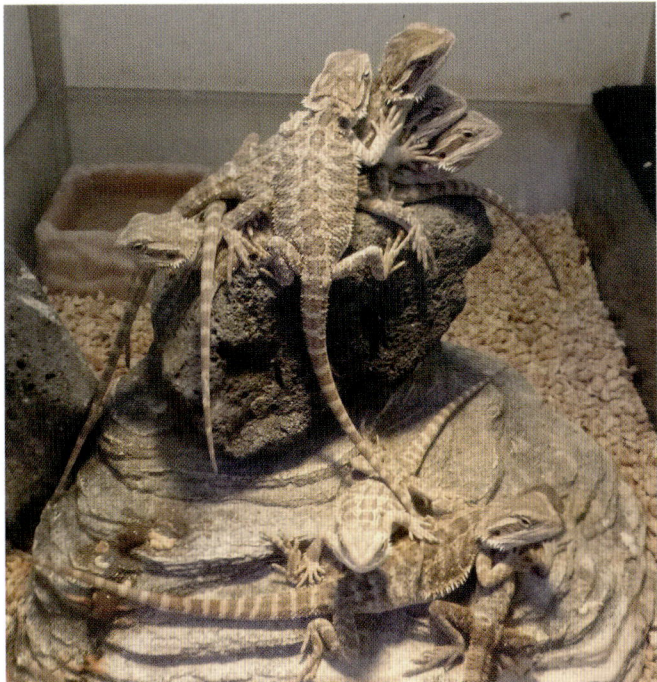

FIG 15.1 An overcrowded group of juvenile bearded dragons (*Pogona vitticeps*) housed in a barren enclosure with a single basking area. Such conditions are likely to cause psychological stress due to lack of individual space and refuge and physical stress due to an inability of all animals to bask appropriately. (Courtesy of Craig J-G. Hunt.)

of nonfood items, appears common especially in chelonia and may be caused by a lack of, or inappropriate, stimulation.[37]

HOW IS STRESS IMPORTANT TO REPTILE MEDICINE?

Because the stress response leads to a wide range of dramatic physiological changes, veterinarians must understand and consider the role of stress relative to the patient's condition. A thorough understanding of stress and the physiological changes associated with stress is vital for client education and patient treatment. Treatment regimes must incorporate both the immediate treatment of the disease and the reduction or elimination of any stressors in the animal's home environment. Without consideration of both, long-term improvement in the animal's condition is unlikely.

In addition to recognizing the role of stress in the etiology of a patient's condition, veterinarians must recognize the potential for stress associated with medical care. Diagnostic procedures and medical treatment can provide great benefits to an ill reptile, but they also unavoidably include many potentially stressful stimuli. All manipulations associated with both diagnosis and treatment must be evaluated in terms of their potential for inducing stress versus their potential medical benefit, being mindful that physiological changes induced by the stress response can be catastrophic to an already compromised animal.

Proper preparation minimizes the duration of stress associated with handling. All instruments and equipment necessary for physical examination and possible treatments should be ready before an animal is handled. Examination of reptile and amphibian patients in a dedicated room that has been properly sanitized since the last patient is optimal to reduce the potential stress of sounds and odors from other species such as dogs, cats, and ferrets.

ASSESSING WELFARE NEEDS

Animal welfare has been defined as being about how an animal feels about its world.[47,48] The husbandry of captive reptiles and amphibians has a major potential impact on the animals' physical and mental well-being and therefore its welfare in captivity. Appropriate husbandry is the most important factor in keeping captive reptiles and amphibians healthy both physically and mentally, and failure to provide appropriate husbandry is the number one cause of illness in captive reptiles.

In the United Kingdom "The Five Freedoms" were devised as a means by which the welfare needs of farm animals could be assessed; though originally designed for farm animals, their application has been accepted as a guideline for many other species, including those kept in laboratories, zoos, and as pets.[49] In the United States, San Diego Zoo Global developed a five-point animal welfare assessment guideline titled "Opportunities to Thrive" (Proc AAZV 2014, p 18-24), which was derived from and expands on the five freedoms: (1) freedom from hunger, thirst, and malnutrition; (2) freedom from thermal and physical discomfort; (3) freedom from fear and distress; (4) freedom from pain, injury, and disease; and (5) freedom to express normal patterns of behavior. Reptile welfare is protected by law in many countries (see Chapters 184 through 186).

RECOGNIZING STRESS AND ITS IMPACTS ON WELFARE

As previously discussed the causes and types of stress experienced by captive reptiles and amphibians are varied and not always easy to recognize, especially by the inexperienced.

Reptiles and amphibians have evolved mechanisms to mask signs of disease, which in extreme cases can result in an apparently healthy animal showing no signs of illness or distress dying acutely. Such cases are perhaps more likely where animals are kept in "clinical" conditions where the display of the normal repertoire of activities and behaviors is prevented.[50]

Some signs suggestive of stress may be quite obvious and include skin color changes; open mouth; hissing/spitting; coiling; inflating the body, neck, or throat; flattening the body against the ground; broadside posturing; standing more erect; biting; striking; tail whipping; spraying/voiding feces, urine, musk, blood, or stomach contents; retraction into shell; feigning death; tail autotomy; and attempts to escape. Other signs of stress may be much more subtle and/or may mimic other behaviors. Social stress for example may be subtle and is commonly observed when two juvenile reptiles are housed and raised together; in many instances one of the pairs will develop and grow more slowly with a resultant obvious disparity in their adult size. The eventual disparity in size is obvious, but the underlying stress often goes unrecognized (Fig. 15.2).

Hypoactivity with or without seeking out cooler temperatures such as normally occurs during hibernation, aestivation, and brumation is a biological shut-down strategy to avoid the rigors of a hostile environment that in some circumstances can be a sign of stress.[50] Prolonged bathing or basking may occur naturally at certain times of need such as posthibernation and gravidity, respectively; at other times such behavior may indicate stress.

Pain is a significant cause of stress and poor welfare in reptiles and amphians. Signs of acute pain in reptiles and amphibians include flinching, muscle contractions, aversive movements away from the

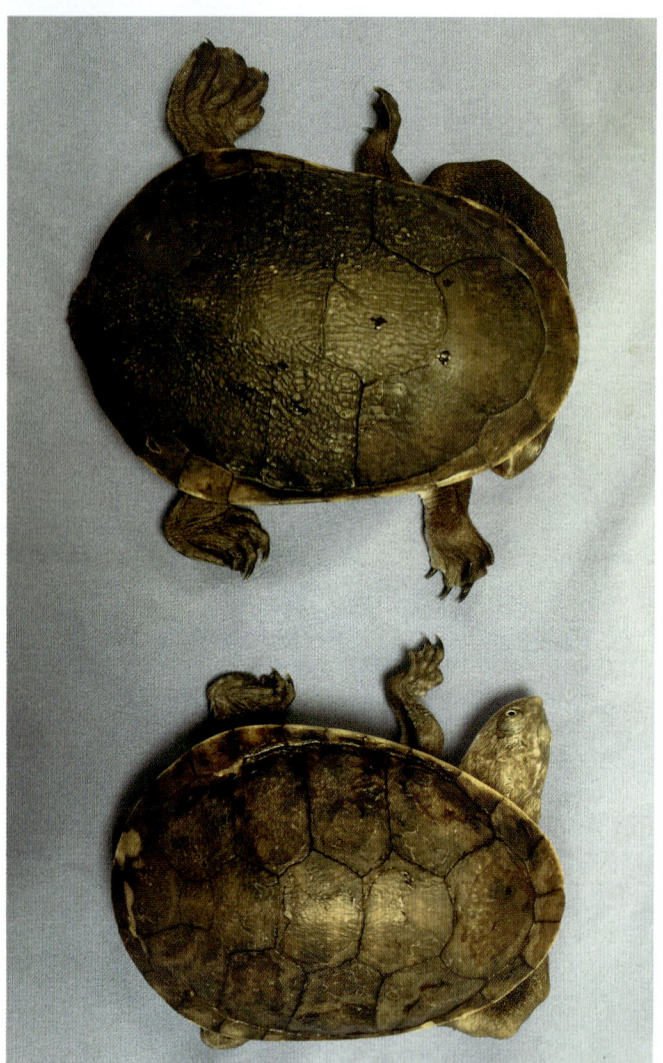

FIG 15.2 A pair of side-necked turtles (*Macrochelodina rugosa*) reared together in an inadequately sized enclosure with poor water quality. The larger specimen appeared healthy whilst the smaller was undersized and anorexic with poor body condition score (1/5). The potential reason(s) for the smaller specimen's condition are numerous; however, psychological stress due to overcrowding and social stress is likely, in addition to the physical stress from poor environmental conditions. (Courtesy of Craig J-G. Hunt.)

unpleasant stimulus, and attempts to bite. Chronic and persistent pain may be associated with nonspecific signs of inappetance lethargy and weight loss.[51]

CONCLUSION

Although the stress response is an adaptive response that maximizes immediate survival, it jeopardizes long-term survival, especially of compromised individuals. Critical to optimal veterinary care to reptiles is an understanding of the physiology of stress and the potential of seemingly innocuous stimuli to induce a stress response and compromise welfare.

ACKNOWLEDGMENTS

The author would like to thank Dr. Dale DeNardo, DVM, whose chapter in the second edition of *Reptile Medicine and Surgery* formed the framework for this chapter.

REFERENCES

See www.expertconsult.com for a complete list of references.

16

General Husbandry and Management

John V. Rossi

Reptile medicine is a challenging discipline. These unique animals require more than just a diagnosis and treatment to achieve successful medical management. For years experienced reptile clinicians have been aware of the importance of the "third rail" of reptile medicine. This additional evaluation requires establishing the correct physical and biological captive environment for our patients. Indeed, the paradigm of western medicine with regard to the treatment of infectious disease by using antimicrobials alone is being challenged. Questioning these concepts is even more critical in the reptile patient because stimulating a reptile's immune response depends so much on external factors. So what does this mean for the treatment of captive reptiles? Essentially, it means that we need to take a holistic approach to our reptile patients. Providing the correct captive husbandry is the most important factor in encouraging a healthy immune system. Keep in mind that the correct captive environment includes both physical and biological components. Physical factors include temperature, humidity, caging size and materials, substrate, lighting (both quality and quantity), ventilation, water provision, and water quality. Biological factors (or stressors) include competitors, predators, and infectious organisms, with the latter including metazoan, protozoan, bacterial, fungal, and viral diseases. Biological factors also may include symbiotic organisms, such as bacteria that assist in digestion or that may compete with pathogenic bacteria elsewhere on/in the body of a captive reptile.

Along with establishing the proper captive environment, providing the correct diet is critical to maintaining the health of a captive reptile and supporting successful reproduction. The correct diet includes the proper levels of proteins, fats, and carbohydrates, as well as vitamins, minerals, and micronutrients. These lesser minerals often serve as components of enzymes or coenzymes necessary for the immune response, and in many cases, these are deficient in the diet of captive reptiles. Water is also a critical component of the diet, and since many reptiles do not drink readily from standing water sources, the water content of the diet may become an important factor as well. For more detail on nutrition see Chapter 27.

Because there is such a strong correlation between the successful maintenance and reproduction of reptiles in captivity and providing the correct environment and diet, clients must be educated about such requirements and encouraged to research and correct any deficiencies. Reptile clinicians may think of this relationship in terms of a simple equation: $S_R = CE^2$, where *success with reptiles* in captivity (S_R) = both the *correct environment* and *client education* (CE^2). Even with years of

research in attempting to understand and gain knowledge in the keeping and breeding of reptiles in captivity, incorrect husbandry and diet are the number one reason for illness in captive reptiles. Therefore clinicians need to be aware of basic reptile biology and husbandry to properly diagnose and treat this group of animals.

Additionally clinicians need to provide their reptile clients with important guidance concerning quarantine, disinfection, regular examination, fecal examinations, and deworming.

In reptile collections disease transmission is an important concern. Reptile keepers often create multi-individual or multispecies enclosures, which increase the likelihood of contagious issues.

There has been a recent shift away from simple enclosures to those that are more environmentally enriched. More complex environments traditionally were considered more difficult to maintain and were not often utilized. However, the benefits of enriched enclosures have become increasingly obvious in recent years (Fig. 16.1). These benefits appear to be both behavioral and physiological. Increased environmental complexity leads to increased activity, which appears to result in leaner, more reproductively active animals. The physiological benefits of microclimates within the enclosure enables the reptile to regulate body temperature and cutaneous water losses accurately (Fig. 16.2). These benefits may prevent illness and allow a reptile to live to an age approximating genetic potential. Another recent advance in herpetoculture involves the use of bioactive substrates in reptile enclosures. Bioactive substrates are believed to encourage the growth of bacteria and fungi that compete with pathogenic bacteria and fungi, thereby protecting the captive reptile from infection. This is discussed in more detail later in this chapter, but examples would include thick layers of natural substrates like cypress mulch or coconut chips. These layers maintain moisture gradients that allow for the growth of beneficial organisms.

The purpose of this chapter will be to associate biology with basic husbandry. Biology will be summarized to help build a foundation for understanding the basic husbandry techniques discussed in more detail in later chapters of this section. The reader is also referred to the Current Therapy chapter on recent updates in herpetologic equipment by Barten and Fleming.[1]

BIOLOGY

More than 10,000 species of reptiles have been divided into three major orders and one minor order. The species vary widely in terms of size,

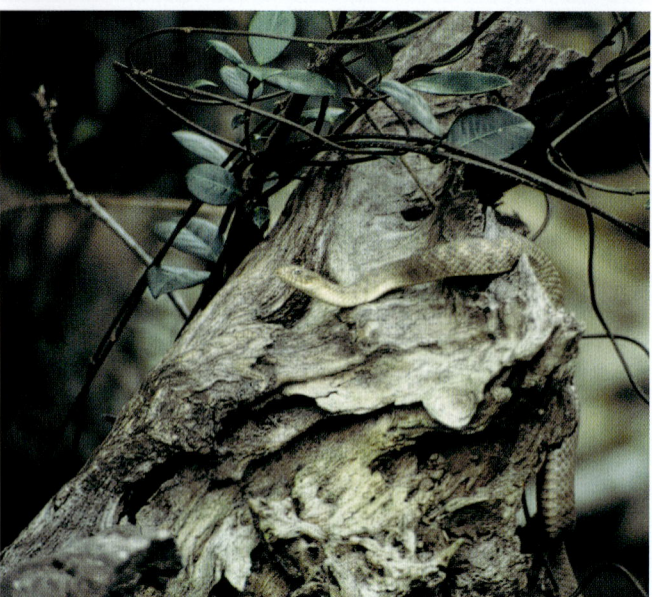

FIG 16.1 A Brazos water snake (*Nerodia harteri*) in a natural enclosure is more wary and maintains a leaner appearance than those housed in a typical aquarium-style cage. This snake also grows at a rate similar to those found in the wild and maintains oral bacterial flora more similar to a wild snake than one housed in an indoor aquarium-style enclosure.

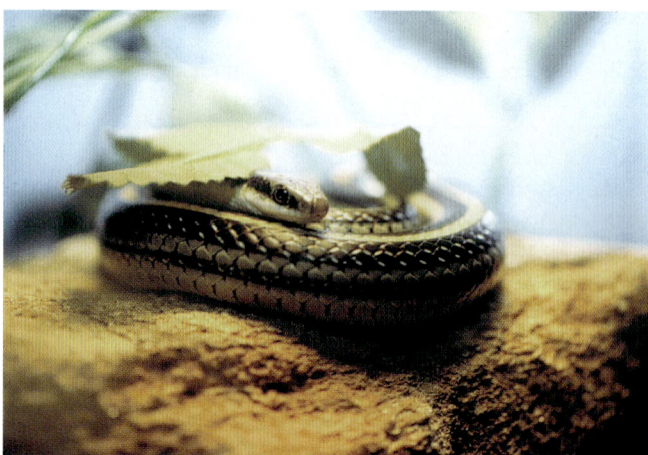

FIG 16.2 Texas patch-nose snake (*Salvadora grahamiae*) basks on a rock in its cage. Ability to thermoregulate is critical for long-term successful maintenance and reproduction of captive reptiles.

shape, physiology, behavior, and diet. Their captive requirements may vary just as widely. Providing every detail for each of these species is beyond the scope of this chapter. But details of the biology of each group are presented in the previous section, and the husbandry of each group is discussed in more detail in the chapters of this section. However, a basic understanding of the biology of the reptiles a clinician is working with is important when giving guidance on designing an enclosure or attempting to treat a captive reptile. The most important factor is that most reptiles are ectothermic, which means they derive the vast majority of their body heat from outside heat sources. Some reptiles are considered stenothermal, accurately controlling body temperature within a narrow range, and others are eurythermal, allowing body temperature to vary

widely according to external temperatures. In general, terrestrial reptiles are more stenothermal than arboreal or aquatic reptiles. There are exceptions, however; large sea turtles, for example, leatherbacks (*Dermochelys coriacea*) are extremely stenothermal because they are primarily endothermic. That means they derive the majority of body heat from metabolic and muscular functions and conserve that heat with a variety of physiological means, including countercurrent multipliers within their peripheral circulatory system. This extremely tight control of internal body temperature is also referred to as homeothermy, which is seen in many birds and mammals. However, all reptiles are believed to thermoregulate to some extent, making use of thermal gradients within their environment. Most aspects of their physiology are intimately tied to body temperatures, and hence, so is their behavior and ultimately their health. The preferred body temperature range of reptiles is referred to as the preferred optimum temperature range or zone (POTR or POTZ); this range is known for most wild reptiles (Table 16.1).

Ambient lighting and photoperiod (both quantity and quality) are important for health and reproduction in reptiles. Knowledge of the light exposure reptiles receive in their natural habitat will be important in providing proper captive lighting. Seasonal reproduction is often strongly influenced by seasonal changes in photoperiod. Some reptiles (e.g., many iguanid lizards and the tuatara, *Sphenodon punctatus*) actually have a light receptor on top of their head called the parietal eye. It is now believed that provision of a light gradient to captive reptiles may be as important as temperature and humidity gradients.

The use of herpetological field studies that describe the natural environment of a species can be helpful for determining captive conditions for that reptile patient. Botanists and gardeners have done this for years. In fact, in the absence of specific information on a species in question, one may refer to maps of solar insolation (hours of sunshine per day or kWh/m²/day) and temperature zone maps (average minimum and maximum temperatures) for the geographical area that encompasses the natural range of that species. Other maps that indicate average rainfall, elevation, and predominant plant cover may also be used to help determine the environmental preferences of a species. Use of these maps does not take into account the microhabitat selection of a species, but may provide information on appropriate physical parameters to recreate in the enclosure. Lighting is discussed in more detail in the husbandry section of this chapter and in Chapter 17.

Water regulation of reptiles also varies dramatically from one group of reptiles to another and even between species. Generally speaking, reptiles from dry environments are uricotelic, essentially producing the large, relatively insoluble molecules of uric acid in an effort to conserve water at the renal tubule level. Reptiles from aquatic environments generally produce the smaller, more soluble urea, or in some cases ammonia, to eliminate nitrogenous wastes (Fig. 16.3). Many reptiles use various combinations of nitrogenous waste likely related to taxonomy, as well as current environmental factors of the species in question. All reptiles have insensitive cutaneous and respiratory water loss, which may be minimized with microhabitat selection such as seeking an environment with higher humidity. This is properly termed hydroregulation, and all reptiles appear to engage in microhabitat selection and possibly hydroregulation to some extent. The ability to reduce these minute water losses is considered important for long-term health and for reducing the likelihood of developing degenerative renal disease. These microenvironments may also harbor beneficial bacteria and fungi that compete with pathogenic bacteria and fungi, thereby providing other benefits to the reptile. See the subsequent discussion on bioactive substrates.

Behavior is an extremely important factor that is intricately associated with and controls (and/or is controlled by) the physiology of this diverse group of animals (see Chapters 13 and 14). As primarily ectothermic

TABLE 16.1	Preferred Optimum Temperature Ranges for Commonly Housed Captive Reptiles				
	PREFERRED OPTIMUM TEMPERATURE RANGE °C (°F)				
Common Name (Scientific Name)	**Day**	**Night**	**Winter Cooling***	**Underfloor Heat Source**	**Radiant Heat Source**
Snakes					
Boa constrictor (Boa constrictor)	27–32 (80–90)	21–27 (70–80)	21–24 (70–75)	Yes	Optional
Rosy boa (Lichanura trivirgata)	27–29 (80–85)	21–24 (70–75)	14–16 (58–60)	Yes	Optional
Ball python (Python regius)	27–32 (80-90)	21–27 (70–80)	16–21 (60–70)	Yes	Optional
Burmese python (Python bivittatus)	27–32 (80-90)	21–27 (70–80)	16–21 (60–70)	Yes	Optional
Green tree python (Morelia viridis)	24–28 (75–82)	21–24 (70–75)	16–18 (60–64)	Optional	Yes
Carpet python (Morelia spilota)	27–29 (80–85)	21–24 (70–75)	16–18 (60–64)	Yes	Optional
Corn snake (Pantherophis guttatus)	25–29 (78–84)	19–24 (67–75)	13–16 (55–60)	Yes	Optional
Yellow rat snake (Pantherophis obsolete)	25–29 (78–84)	19–24 (67–75)	13–16 (55–60)	Yes	Optional
Gopher/bull snake (Pituophis catenifer)	25–29 (78–84)	19–23 (67–74)	10–16 (50–60)	Yes	Optional
Common king snake (Lampropeltis getula)	25–29 (78–84)	20–23 (68–74)	13–16 (55–60)	Yes	Optional
Mountain king snake (Lampropeltis zonata)	25–29 (78–84)	19–23 (66–74)	13–16 (55–60)	Yes	Optional
Gray-banded king snake (Lampropeltis alterna)	25–29 (79–84)	21–24 (70–75)	14–16 (58–60)	Yes	Optional
Garter snakes (Thamnophis)	24–27 (75–80)	18–22 (65–72)	12–15 (54–59)	Yes	Optional
Lizards					
Green iguana (Iguana iguana)	29–32 (84–90)	19–25 (67–77)	18–21 (64–69)	Optional	Yes
Basilisks (Basiliscus)	28–31 (82–87)	24–25 (75–77)	20–21 (68–70)	Optional	Yes
Leopard gecko (Eublepharis macularius)	25–29 (77–85)	18–24 (65–75)	None	Yes	Yes
African fat-tailed gecko (Hemitheconyx caudicinctus)	25–29 (78–85)	19–24 (67–75)	None	Yes	Yes
Day geckos (Phelsuma)	27–29 (80-85)	24–25 (75-78)	None	Optional	Yes
Leaf-tailed geckos (Uroplatus)	27–29 (81–84)	22–25 (72–78)	None	Optional	Yes
Chameleons, montane (Chamaeleo)	25–29 (77–84)	13–19 (55–67)	None	Optional	Yes
Chameleons, lowland (Chamaeleo)	27–29 (80–84)	21–24 (70-75)	None	Optional	Yes
Bearded dragons (Pogona)	29–31 (84–88)	20–23 (68–74)	17–21 (62–69)	Optional	Yes
Blue-tongued skinks (Tiliqua)	27–29 (80–85)	19–24 (67–75)	16–18 (60–65)	Optional	Yes
Monitor lizards (Varanus)	29–31 (84–88)	23–25 (74–78)	19–21 (66–70)	Optional	Yes
Tegus (Tupinambis)	27–30 (80–86)	21–25 (70–78)	16–21 (60–70)	Optional	Yes
Chelonians					
Temperate freshwater turtles (Emydidae)	27–29 (80–84)	18–21 (65–70)	Optional	Optional	Yes
Tropical freshwater turtles, most species	28–30 (82–86)	23–27 (74–80)	Optional	Optional	Yes
Temperate tortoises, box turtles (Testudo, Terrapene)	25–32 (78–89)	21–24 (70-75)	10–18 (50–65)	Yes	Yes
Tropical tortoises, most species (Testudinidae)	28–31 (82–88)	21–24 (70–76)	None	Yes	Yes

*Following fasting and with an empty gastrointestinal tract.
Most species probably benefit from the provision of natural sunlight and outdoor enclosures when local climatic conditions permit.

animals, their selection of, and precise control of, body temperatures using primarily exogenous heat sources is absolutely critical for nearly every biochemical reaction. Digestion, reproduction, and immunity are just three of the many functions that are affected by temperature selections. However, reptiles are also behaviorally regulating a myriad of other factors including not just those mentioned above (hydroregulation and lighting selection) but also the biological factors within the environment. Hence, normal behavior should be researched and understood when possible. Often changes in that behavior will provide important indicators of potential problems.

Behavioral changes in captivity fall into three major categories. These are seasonal/hormonal, learned, and medical/pathological. Seasonal/hormonal changes are those normal changes in behavior that occur each year and are associated with the season and/or reproductive behavior.

This would include anorexia in males prior to mating or in females after mating. Learned behaviors are random behaviors that are rewarded directly or indirectly and are therefore repeated. This would include such things as approaching an owner for food or making use of another temporary food resource. Medical/pathological changes are those changes in behavior associated with disease, and they are of concern to veterinarians. In reptiles, the most common behaviors associated with disease are excessive wandering and anorexia, followed by inactivity and anorexia. Hence, excessive wandering and anorexia that occurs during nonreproductive times of the year should be viewed with concern. The same is true for inactivity and anorexia that occurs during nonhibernation/nonestivation times of the year. This can make medical problems more difficult to detect at certain times of the year, and it is important to monitor the reptile's weight. Significant weight loss is often pathological,

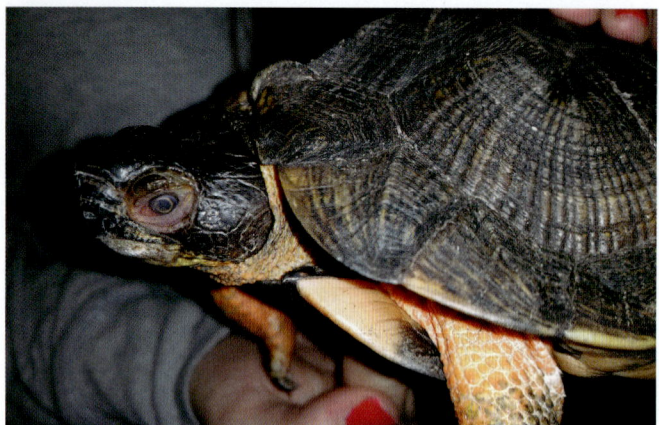

FIG 16.3 Wood turtle (*Glyptemys insculpta*) is a semiaquatic turtle that is more likely to produce urea as a primary nitrogenous waste product; squamates produce primarily uric acid. This particular turtle is demonstrating corneal edema and conjunctivitis after being placed in chlorinated water. Letting water sit for 24 hours or treating with dechlorinating agents may be helpful for many aquatic turtles.

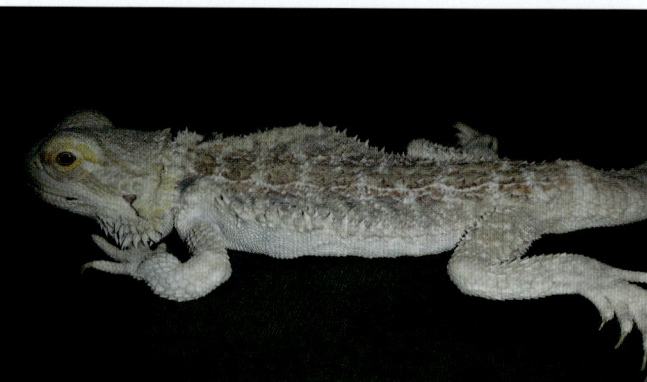

FIG 16.4 The classic juvenile form of nutritional secondary hyperparathyroidism in a bearded dragon (*Pogona vitticeps*) receiving insufficient calcium in the diet and/or a lack of UVB light. Note the deformed skull shape (an indication of poorly mineralized maxillary and mandibular bones), scoliosis of the spine, pathological fractures, and sternal recumbency.

while normal hibernation/estivation weight loss rarely exceeds 10% of body mass in captive reptiles. In wild reptiles, weight loss may exceed this mark and is usually related to dehydration. Biologists have noted that dehydration is the leading cause of death in hibernating reptiles, not starvation or cold. Hence, behavioral observation and regular weighing and record-keeping are essential as an early warning system for captive reptiles. A common medical reason for behavioral change is parasitism, especially in wild-caught reptiles. The author has observed numerous wild snakes that appeared sluggish or exceptionally docile that were heavily parasitized with ticks or mites. Captive snakes that are normally nocturnal that suddenly displayed more diurnal behavior have been diagnosed with coccidiosis.

The immune response of reptiles appears to vary dramatically on a seasonal basis and is also intricately tied to the temperature range available to the reptile in question. Maximum immune response appears to occur in most reptiles when they are held in or near their POTR. This range needs to be researched for the species in question. Both the humoral and cellular immune responses appear to be measurably lower in winter months, and thus reptiles may be more vulnerable to infection during this time. In fact, it appears that one of the most dangerous times for captive reptiles is at the end of hibernation, or early spring, as they emerge from hibernation. Sudden death of reptiles is common at this time, and it is hypothesized that as they warm up, infectious agents and parasites increase exponentially, while their immune response increases arithmetically. This may leave them with a "posthibernation immunity gap," and susceptibility to infectious agents and possibly death. Hence, clinicians should recommend physical exams, fecal exams, and parasite control prior to hibernation and immediately upon emergence from hibernation.

Certainly, the subject of stress and its relationship to disease in captive reptiles has been discussed in detail by a number of authors. Perhaps the most interesting and detailed report on the subject is that of Cowan.[2] To summarize their discussion, the amount of stress may be directly related to differences between the captive environment and the wild environment. Therefore captive environments that lack suitable temperature, lighting and humidity clines, and secure hiding places or have inappropriate photoperiods are more likely to result in diseased reptiles than those that have these key factors addressed (Fig. 16.4). See Chapter 15 for more details on stress.

BASIC HUSBANDRY REQUIREMENTS

Requirements for captive reptiles are based on their needs in nature. Requirements are summarized in this chapter and in more detail in subsequent chapters in this husbandry section. Unlike domestic animals, most reptiles have not been bred for generations to survive in "human habitations." A reptile's unique dietary requirements and ectothermic nature must be understood and addressed by keepers and clinicians to successfully maintain their health in captivity.

Temporary Housing or Hospitalization

Because the reptile patient has unique requirements, providing temporary housing or hospitalization is often challenging. Clinicians may be forced to provide these patients with just the bare necessities of a thermal gradient and a clean, usually dry, cage. For example a hospital cage may have a heat source, newspaper substrate, a water bowl, and a hiding place. A stable perch, such as a stick or a plastic rod, may be securely wedged into a temporary cage for an arboreal reptile. For species requiring high humidity a humid retreat may be provided if the cage is large enough and well ventilated.

While not ideal, the average veterinary hospital can temporarily house most reptiles for short periods in large plastic bins with secure, ventilated lids, as long as they are maintained in a climate-controlled area or provided with additional heat. For larger reptiles, stainless steel dog cages or runs may be adapted by adding hiding areas and the appropriate substrate for the reptile in question.

Ultimately for most reptiles, making a diagnosis, initiating treatment, and releasing the patient to the owner as soon as possible is beneficial. This reduces stress by allowing a rapid return to their permanent cage. Husbandry issues should have been reviewed and environmental corrections instituted by the owner while the reptile is hospitalized. Some animals must be hospitalized for longer periods of time requiring daily maintenance, such as cage cleaning and soaking or spraying a patient. Chapter 46 includes a more detailed discussion on hospitalization.

The staff may need additional training to care for hospitalized reptiles. A review of handling techniques to prevent injury to staff, clients, and reptiles is important (Fig. 16.5). Many reptiles may be easily injured if dropped, and staff may be bitten or scratched if they handle reptiles carelessly. In addition, cage security is critical. Snakes and lizards are especially good at escaping, and this is unacceptable in a veterinary hospital. In addition to a client's outrage and surprise of being informed

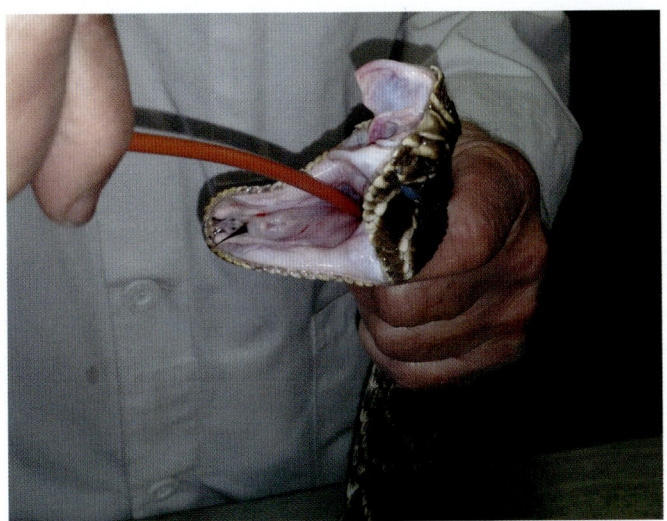

FIG 16.5 Handling reptiles requires additional training in order to avoid injury to the staff or patient. Handling venomous reptiles safely may require sedation or additional equipment. This eastern diamondback rattlesnake (*Crotalus adamanteus*) has been sedated in order to administer medication via a stomach tube.

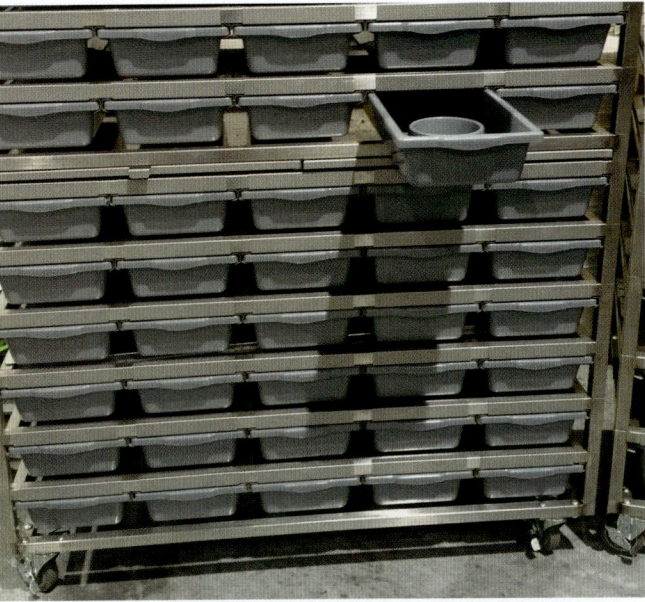

FIG 16.6 Reptile housing rack system (freedombreeder.com). These mobile units have lightweight, easily cleaned, and heated drawers that can house many reptiles in a relatively small space. A separate rack may be used for quarantine purposes and ideally should be in a separate room.

about the absence of the reptile left in the hospital's care, there are risks that large snakes or lizards may ingest an endothermic patient or frighten clients at the time of reappearance. It is the clinician's responsibility to take every precaution needed to secure reptile patients in proper cages.

Clinics that hospitalize many reptiles should invest in a rack-style system, where small to medium reptiles may be housed in plastic drawers in a rack (Fig. 16.6). These racks are often on wheels and can be conveniently moved from place to place with some degree of ease, and they may be ordered with heat tape included. Unfortunately, this style of cage makes providing a light source difficult, but most reptiles seem to tolerate this for short periods of time. Recently drawer systems (lizard racks, pmherps.com) have been designed with deeper tubs and screen tops to allow lighting for reptiles that require it in a similar space-efficient design (Fig. 16.7). Another company, Freedom Breeder, produces excellent racks for housing snakes (https://www.Freedombreeder.com, Turlock, California).

Ideally one should have separate rooms or at least separate racks for long-term healthy reptiles and those that have been recently captured or been in another collection. This allows a limited hospital quarantine, which is extremely important for reptiles.

An introduction to quarantine, as well as cleaning and disinfection, is found later in this chapter. See Chapters 18 and 19 for a more thorough discussion.

Remember that wild reptiles often show no outward signs of infection or parasitism at the time of capture. In some cases, reptiles may not show signs of a viral disease contracted for up to 6 months.[3,4] Therefore precautions must be taken when handling reptiles of unknown origin. With large numbers of hospitalized reptiles, wearing gloves to handle or examine new reptiles may be beneficial. Temporary identification of hospitalized reptiles with tape or other marking methods is also important and discussed in more detail in Chapter 46.

The handling and hospitalization of venomous reptiles requires strictly followed procedures and protocols; these are discussed in more detail in Chapter 22. This author requires that all venomous reptiles be dropped off in clearly marked, locked boxes with the key handed to the doctor in charge of the case. The reptile is also to be bagged inside of the box.

At the time of treatment, the box is unlocked and opened with a pair of snake tongs. The bag is then removed with tongs and placed in an anesthesia chamber. Upon loss of the righting response, the venomous reptile is removed from the bag, again using tongs to lift the bag and slide the venomous reptile out and back into the anesthesia chamber, where it may be further anesthetized or removed for treatment. This discourages handling accidents. Once samples are taken and treatment is administered, the venomous reptile is placed back in the bag, which is knotted, and then placed back in the box, which is then locked. The animal remains in the box until it is discharged at the end of the day. Admittedly, this protocol is extremely weighted toward providing safety for the veterinarian and staff and not on comforts for the venomous reptile while it is hospitalized. But unless the clinician is an experienced venomous snake handler, this protocol is advisable. There is no safe way to house venomous reptiles in the average veterinary hospital, due to the need for additional security measures such as locking cages with detachable shift boxes and preferably a separate locked room. Additionally a highly trained staff, a strict venomous reptile protocol, and warning labels and signs are imperative. See Chapter 22 for more detailed information on working with venomous reptiles.

Temperature

A useable thermal gradient should be provided to every captive reptile. In addition, daily temperature fluctuations and seasonal temperature fluctuations should be provided. Various lamps, heating pads, and heat tapes usually provide a useable thermal gradient for most terrestrial reptiles (Fig. 16.8). These same devices, however, do not provide a useable thermal gradient for aquatic or arboreal reptiles. For aquatic reptiles, a submersible water heater may be necessary, and for arboreal reptiles, a radiant heat source is often necessary to create a hot spot somewhere among the branches in which they reside. There are now radiant heat panels created specifically to provide broad areas of heat to arboreal reptiles (Pro-Heat, Pro-products.com) (Fig. 16.9). Basking areas are considered important for most reptiles, which includes many

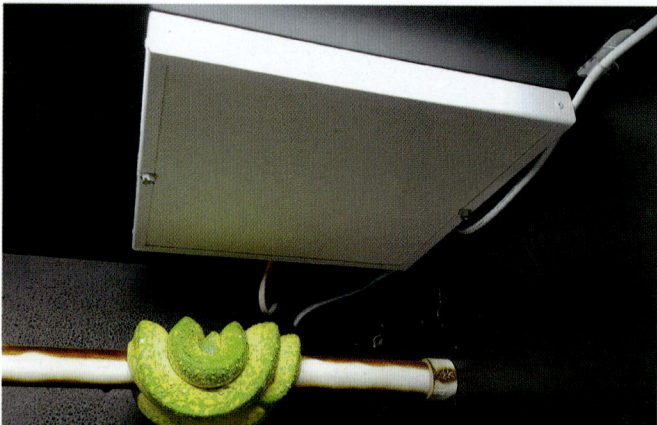

FIG 16.9 Radiant heat panel (pro-products.com/pro-heat/). These devices generate a broad area of gentle heat from above without any light. This is beneficial for arboreal reptiles.

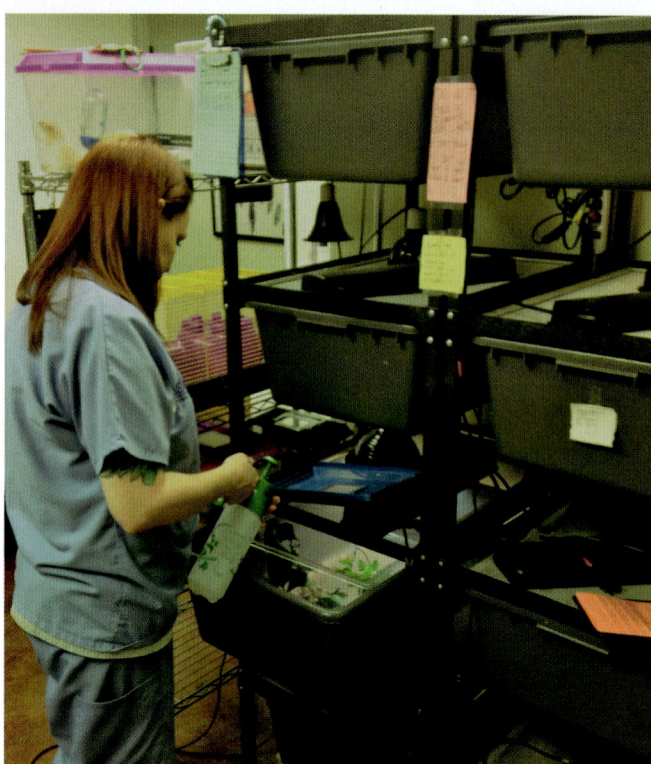

FIG 16.7 Lizard/chelonian rack systems (pmherps.com) provide a compact rack concept for efficiently housing reptiles that require overhead lighting and radiant heat sources. (Courtesy of Scott J. Stahl, Stahl Exotic Animal Veterinary Services.)

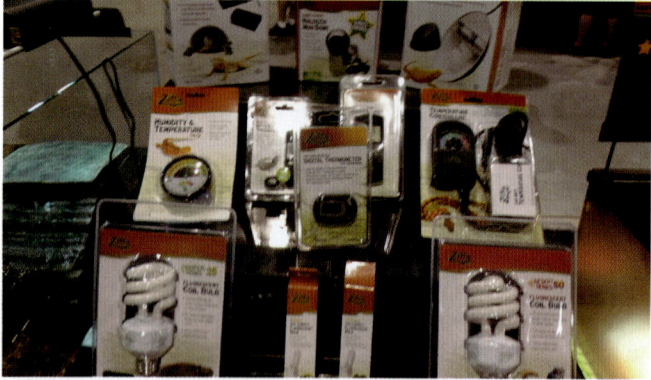

FIG 16.8 A wide variety of heat sources, vaporizers, temperature and humidity gauges, thermostats, and other tools are now available to help maintain reptiles in their preferred optimum temperature range (POTR) and preferred optimum humidity range (POHR). Thermostats are important because heat lamps/heat sources commonly cause reptile burns. Keepers tend to underestimate the amount of heat they produce and thus fail to provide a proper heat gradient.

aquatic reptiles. The preferred temperature ranges of many commonly kept reptiles are listed in Table 16.1. A simple rule of thumb is to maintain a hot spot in the cage that is near the upper end of the POTR. Then reptiles can achieve the highest temperatures that they would normally seek in nature but also can choose lower temperatures, including those that may be outside the POTR. McKeown[5] defines a primary heat source as that which is used to maintain an appropriate background

temperature in the enclosure. For most, this is the central heating unit in their house. Secondary heat sources are those used to create additional heat in some areas of the enclosure to provide a thermal gradient.[5] If either is insufficient or unusable to the reptile, disease is a likely.

Hot rocks, a source of artificial heat, are commonly used by reptile keepers. These generally provide very focal heat, directed from the ground upward, and generally are not useable except by the smallest reptiles. They often become progressively hotter with age, and larger reptiles frequently burn themselves by coming in contact with focal "hot spots" on the surface, likely trying to reach an optimal temperature. This can be minimized by covering and insulating these heaters, but generally these are not recommended for larger reptiles. Better heat sources include adjustable heating pads placed under the cage and incandescent bulbs placed at various heights above the cage. Ceramic heaters have become more popular because they produce radiant heat with no light emission. However sick reptiles often do not thermoregulate properly, so the background heat must be controlled carefully for these animals. Another group of reptiles at risk are male snakes during breeding season. Male boas and pythons commonly seek out the coolest area of the cage at this time, often staying too cool for extended periods of time resulting in illness. This may be avoided with careful control of the background temperature.

A general guideline for daytime air temperatures to provide for most diurnal reptiles is 80° to 90°F (27°–32°C) with a basking area of 90° to 100°F (32°–38°C). Diurnal desert lizards such as Uromastyx seem to prefer basking areas of 120° to 130°F (49°–54.5°C) for short periods of time. Nocturnal or montane reptiles often do well with daytime air temperatures of 70° to 80°F (21°–27°C) but still seem to benefit by having a warmer area of 90° to 95°F (32°–35°C) present in the enclosure. Field research on the habitat of montane rattlesnakes in southeastern Arizona showed that even though air temperatures in the early morning were barely exceeding 21°C (70°F), the snakes were found basking in areas where the sun had created hot spots of 32° to 35°C (90°–95°F).[6] Nighttime air temperatures for most reptiles should not drop below a temperature of 21°C (70°F) during the active season, although temperate zone reptiles can usually tolerate temperatures lower than this for short periods with access to a heat source. Experience shows that maintaining most reptiles for prolonged periods at temperatures ranging from 60° to 70°F (15°–21°C) is potentially harmful. This temperature range appears to be too cold to allow normal digestion or immune system response and too warm to allow for normal brumation (hibernation). Without any supplemental heat or the absence of a daytime temperature that rises sharply into the 90° to 95°F (32°–35°C) range, many reptiles kept consistently in this 60° to 70°F temperature range often become ill (Fig. 16.10). In fact, this has been such a common problem in practice that the author has referred to this temperature range as "reptile thermal limbo" for clients so that they can easily remember to keep their reptiles out of this temperature range for any length of time. It commonly occurs when reptiles are housed in air-conditioned rooms at ground level or during the winter when insufficient heat sources are provided.

Brumation (hibernation) temperatures for temperate zone reptiles generally may be maintained between 35° to 59°F (3.8°–15°C) for a minimum of 10 weeks. Montane reptiles or those from temperate climates may need brumation (hibernation) temperatures at the lower end of this range and possibly for a longer period of time. Of course, no feeding should occur at this time (Fig. 16.11). Subtropical reptiles can be brumated (hibernated) at similar temperatures but should have access to some heat source at all times. Tropical reptiles should not be brumated (hibernated) but instead may be exposed to nighttime lows that are lower than those to which they are exposed in the summer, and daytime highs remain similar to those that are provided during the summer. Typically, nighttime low temperatures for tropical reptiles should not drop below 21°C (70°F). Python and boa breeders often attempt to cycle their snakes by dropping the temperatures below this level at night during the late fall and winter to induce breeding behavior and ovulation. This is not necessary for most snakes and is also potentially dangerous, often resulting in respiratory infections. The photoperiod can safely be shortened during this time as discussed below.

Modern thermostats are capable of providing both temperature gradients and daily temperature fluctuations (i.e., diurnal and nocturnal temperatures).

Photoperiod and Light Quality (Lighting)

The amount of light received per day, or photoperiod, is important to reptiles. In general, day length and temperature should be decreased during the winter months for subtropical and temperate species. Failure to do so often results in reproductive failure or disease. Inappropriate photoperiod and temperature fluctuations have been correlated with repeated reproductive failure. Poor reproductive success has been related to abnormal vitellogenesis, chronic resorption of yolk, ovarian cysts, and ultimately ovarian granulomas or tumors (Fig. 16.12).

Obesity is another possible sequela to abnormal photoperiod. Reptiles that are normally inactive and anorectic during the winter months may continue eating when exposed to a consistent photoperiod, even though their metabolism is lower due to a reduction in ambient temperature. In most cases with temperate zone or subtropical zone reptiles, the artificial photoperiod may mimic that which is naturally occurring outside. Modifications may be made depending on the latitude of the reptile's origin and the latitude where the reptile is being housed. For example, seasonal changes can be manipulated appropriately by increasing the day length slightly for tropical reptiles housed in a subtropical area or more so if housed in a temperate zone area. Alternatively, decreasing the day length would be appropriate if housing a northern temperate zone reptile in a subtropical area.

Electric timers are inexpensive and widely available, and lights may be set to mimic the naturally occurring photoperiod or to adjust it in either direction. Not surprisingly, reptiles housed with access to the natural light cycles (i.e., a window or skylight) respond more strongly to the natural light than to an artificial light source. This must be taken into consideration when cycling reptiles for breeding purposes. A general

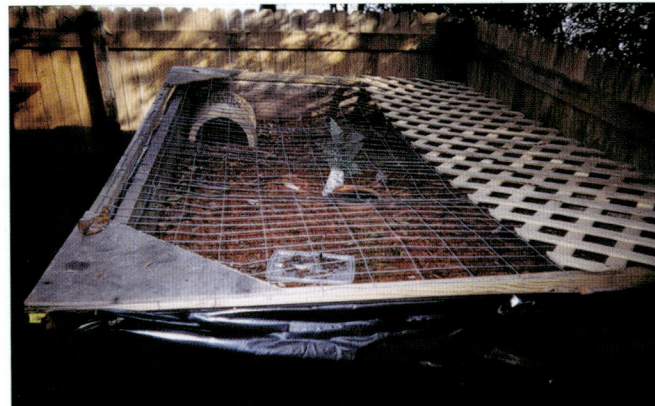

FIG 16.11 This outside turtle enclosure has thick mulch and a plastic barrier as insulation against cold for turtles overwintering. They may not eat for up to 6 months during brumation (hibernation). Such outside enclosures are excellent for housing small and medium-sized chelonians throughout the year but need to be kept covered with wire or hardware cloth to protect the inhabitants against predation.

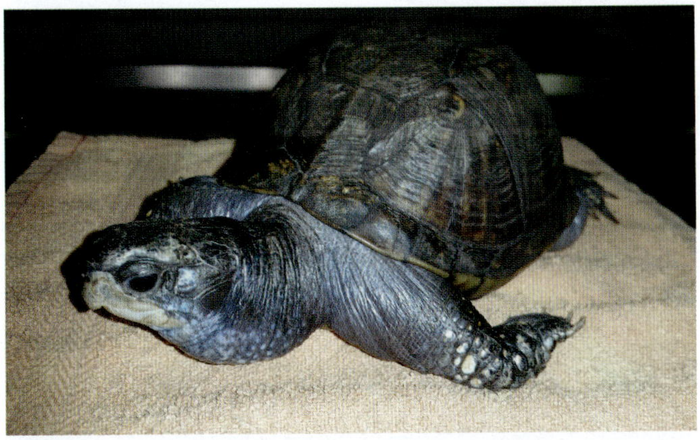

FIG 16.10 Box turtle (*Terrapene* sp.) with edema secondary to a cardiac abscess. This turtle was maintained at room temperature with little or no access to a usable secondary heat source. Constant exposure to these "middle temperatures" often results in various manifestations of disease.

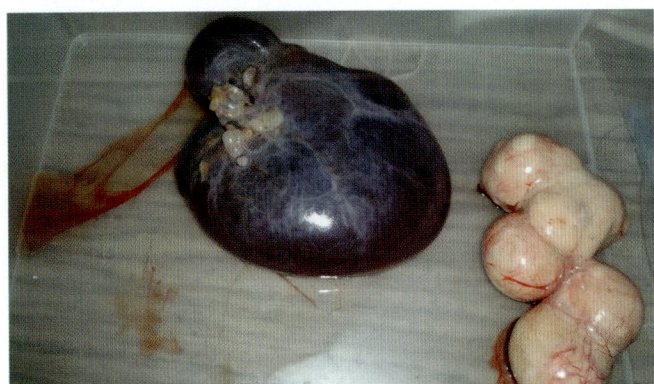

FIG 16.12 Large ovarian cyst (approximately 500 grams) and necrotic eggs surgically removed from an argus monitor (*Varanus panoptes*). These cysts often progress to neoplasms and are not uncommon in intact, long-term captive reptiles that are not cycled and bred regularly.

guideline relating to photoperiod is to provide about 14 hours of light in the summer and 12 hours of light in the winter. Another author suggested that temperate zone reptiles be exposed to 15 hours of light during the summer, 12 hours during spring and fall, and 9 hours during the winter, with tropical reptiles exposed to 13 hours of light during the summer and 11 hours of light during the winter.[7]

The quality of light is also important, and as with temperature and humidity, a gradient should be created in the enclosure. Some ultraviolet (UVB) light is necessary for most reptiles to manufacture vitamin D_3. Vitamin D_3 is necessary for the absorption of calcium from the intestinal tract. A deficiency of UVB light (290–320 nm) often results in nutritional secondary hyperparathyroidism (NSHP). UVA light, or light in the 320 to 400 nm range, does not assist in converting vitamin D into an active molecule but may have some beneficial effects in terms of behavior (i.e., improved visualization of prey or mates). Infared light is also critical for many reptiles because it provides much of the heat they require as ectotherms. Most curators and experienced herpetoculturists believe that natural lighting is the best light and may even be mandatory for success with some captive reptiles. One study with Hermann's tortoises showed a significant difference in measurable Vitamin D_3 in tortoises exposed to natural light versus two kinds of artificial UV lights, with those in the natural light having higher levels.[8] However, keep in mind that some species have adapted to lower light levels and shorter photoperiods, and for these species, too much or an increased intensity of light may be detrimental. For example, forest-dwelling tortoises, such as red- or yellow-footed tortoises (*Chelonoidis*), box turtles (*Terrapene* sp.), Blanding's turtles (*Emys blandingii*), and wood turtles (*Glyptemys insculpta*), may become anorectic if exposed to high levels of artificial UV light or natural lighting that exceeds what they have adapted to.[9]

As mentioned above, both natural and artificial lighting may be beneficial for these animals. However, two kinds of artificial lights are commonly used. Incandescent bulbs, which are generally bulblike, provide both heat and light. Fluorescent bulbs, which can be tubular or compact, provide a wider spectrum of light but little heat. Popular and widely available fluorescent bulbs that produce light in the proper spectrum are ZooMed's Reptisun lights (http://www.zoomed.com). Diurnal lizards, diurnal snakes, small crocodilians, and basking species of turtles and tortoises do well with the Reptisun 5.0 or 7.0, and amphibians and many temperate zone snakes do well with the Reptisun 2.0. For many diurnal desert reptiles, the Reptisun 10.0 is recommended. Providing both kinds of light (incandescent and fluorescent) for most reptiles is advisable, unless a combination light is used. Mercury halide lamps that are capable of providing both high-intensity light and heat are becoming more popular (e.g., Zoomed Powersun and UV Heat bulbs). There are a wide variety of excellent lights available, and the author does not wish to imply that these are the only useful lights. However, at this time these bulbs are readily available and have been safely utilized. Clinicians also need to be aware that the UV light production from these lights is often very low compared to natural sunlight and decreases over time even though the light still appears to be working. Therefore it is recommended that most lights be replaced at least every six months, whereas Mercury halide lamps may be replaced every 12 months.

Additionally, LED lights (both UVB and non-UVB) are becoming more readily available and popular. More research is needed to determine their effectiveness.

See Chapter 17 on lighting for more types of lights and details on the provision of light, light gradients, light combinations, and measurement of light intensity.

Generally speaking, however, no substitute exists for natural light for many reptiles. It is perhaps one of the most powerful health resources/treatments known in captive reptile management and is a strong argument for maintaining reptiles in outdoor enclosures when weather conditions permit. It is also a potent appetite stimulant for many reptiles and may have many other unknown beneficial effects. However, one must be extremely cautious when utilizing natural lighting. Reptiles should not be placed outside in direct sunlight in glass-sided enclosures. The greenhouse effect has resulted in the deaths of many captive reptiles, and this can occur in minutes! Reptile keepers should consider the construction of outdoor enclosures specifically designed for the reptiles in question. See the discussion on outdoor enclosures in this chapter.

Humidity and Ventilation

Providing a high humidity retreat or a humidity gradient may be difficult. One must remember that the higher humidity areas in the cage must not be created at the expense of total cage ventilation because humidity and ventilation are inversely related to each other. If ventilation is severely restricted (and it often is in many molded fiberglass cages or plastic rack systems), stagnant air often contributes to the growth of bacterial or fungal pathogens. Instead, high humidity zones within otherwise well-ventilated cages should be created. This may be done in confined areas, such as plastic boxes of varying sizes, or with moisture-containing substrates in different parts of the cage. The most commonly used method of providing a high humidity retreat for some reptiles is the use of the humidity box, in which a plastic box is filled with a moisture-containing substrate, such as sphagnum moss or peat moss (Fig. 16.13). A small hole is created in the cover (top) of such a box for snakes, or in the side for lizards and tortoises, to allow the reptile to enter or exit the structure. These boxes often show visible condensation within and provide the moisture needed to aid in ecdysis, or egg deposition, and to prevent chronic dehydration via cutaneous and respiratory water loss. Humidity boxes are now produced commercially in more aesthetically pleasing, naturalistic appearing shapes, such as artificial rocks or logs.

Many reptile keepers use vaporizers, humidifiers, automatic misters, or small fountains to humidify the enclosure directly or indirectly. This is acceptable because it does not interfere with ventilation. Chameleon keepers have been known to place intravenous (IV) drip–type systems or ice above a screen lid to allow water to drip into the environment. A number of keepers of both lizards and snakes simply maintain moistened sphagnum moss at the bottom of the cage. For some strictly arboreal reptiles, the bottom of the cage may be filled with several inches of water. In a well-ventilated cage, this maintains a high and constant humidity. Chameleons and arboreal snakes, such as emerald tree boas

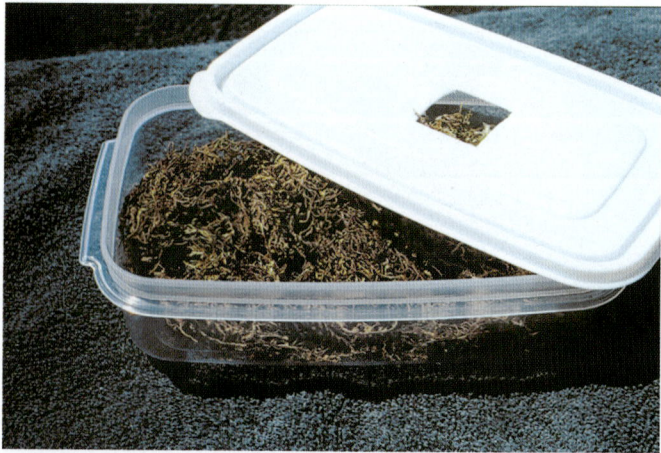

FIG 16.13 A humidity box is a plastic box containing substrate that holds some moisture. The most commonly used substrate for this purpose is sphagnum moss. More naturalistic appearing humidity boxes are now produced commercially.

(*Corallus caninus*) and green tree pythons (*Morelia viridis*) are now successfully maintained in tall, well-ventilated cages with mister systems maintaining the humidity. (Fig. 16.14). These cages and others may also gain increased ventilation via the use of axial fans, where necessary.

Substrate

Perhaps the next most important physical factor in determining the success or failure of a captive reptile is the substrate used. Both artificial and natural substrates may be used to achieve a level of humidity, physical support, and psychological security. Shredded newspaper, butcher's paper, and artificial turf have been popular with many herpetoculturists because of their availability and low price. However, although these materials are satisfactory and readily cleanable substrates for many reptiles, they are not aesthetically pleasing and do not appear to provide microenvironments similar to those found in nature. Certain kinds of wood chips, such as cypress or coconut chips, appear to provide a substrate with all of the features previously listed and an aesthetic appearance. Large, smooth stones have been successfully used as a substrate for many lizards and snakes; small stones and gravel, however, may be ingested. One of the more recent substrates that appears to have worked well is shredded coconut shells, called ReptiChips, and indeed they may prove to be superior to many other substrates for

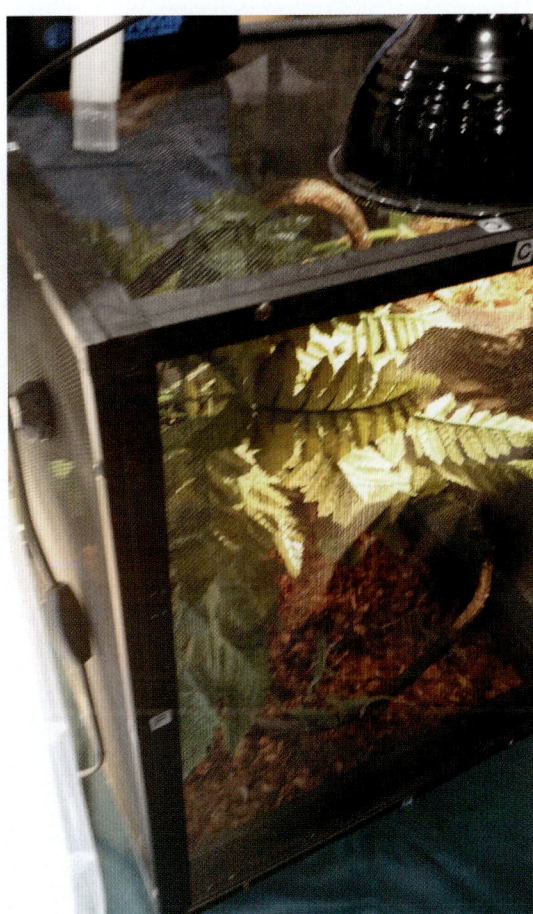

FIG 16.14 A small plastic mesh cage is ideal for many species of arboreal reptiles, because they are tall, light, and well ventilated. However, with excellent ventilation comes the challenge of maintaining proper humidity. Note the vaporizer as well as the UV lights on top of the cage. Chameleons, emerald tree boas (*Corallus caninus*), and green tree pythons (*Morelia viridis*), among others, are often housed in this manner, although mesh cages are usually replaced by tall glass cages for arboreal snakes.

reasons discussed below. Many species of snakes, lizards, and tortoises can be maintained on a variety of substrates; however, refer to herpetocultural sources for specific recommendations on the species in question. Substrates that are too basic, too acidic, too dry, too moist, or dirty may contribute to dermatologic or respiratory conditions in captive reptiles. Substrates that contain irritating aromatic compounds, such as cedar, eucalyptus, or pine shavings, may also result in skin or respiratory irritation and possible secondary infection. Natural substrates that absorb moisture, such as wood chips of any kind, are likely to harbor heavy growth of potentially pathogenic bacteria or fungi if placed in a poorly ventilated cage. Thus wood chip substrates should not be used in plastic shoe box or drawer style cages, unless good (top)ventilation is present. With regard to ventilation, it appears that top ventilation is the most critical factor in determining the usage of natural substrates. Remember that warm (often moist) air rises and is replaced by cooler (often drier) air. Without excellent top ventilation, and often regardless of excellent side ventilation, moisture is often trapped in an enclosure to the degree that natural substrates cannot be used. This ventilation issue may be improved if fans are utilized.

Many tortoises do well on a substrate of rabbit pellets, but occasionally loose footing may lead to splay leg in young tortoises. Also, tortoises such as Burmese mountain tortoises (*Manouria emys*) that need higher moisture substrates do not do well on this substrate. Semimoist cypress mulch or coconut chips work better for these species. It is often placed over cork bark to provide more solid footing and reduce the likelihood of splay leg. In addition, rabbit pellets may also contribute to respiratory disease if the pellets get wet and moldy. Most larger snakes commonly kept as pets do well on shredded newspaper, indoor/outdoor carpet, and wood chips, such as cypress or aspen. Smaller species of snakes generally do not do well on newspaper but may thrive when cypress or coconut mulch is used. Lizards often do well on dry, loose sand or indoor/outdoor carpet. Crushed pecan or walnut shells have been associated with many intestinal impactions in smaller lizards and are best avoided unless they are extremely finely ground. However, crushed pecan or walnut shells have been used successfully with many snakes and larger lizards. Keep in mind however that these substrates often increase exposure to fungal organisms such as *Aspergillis* sp. so if used must be kept clean. Sand may also be ingested and has been associated with impactions in smaller lizards, so it must be used with care. In addition, sand in poorly ventilated cages (i.e., those that lack top ventilation) may retain a large amount of water, which may lead to contact dermatitis. However, loose, dry sands (commercially available children's play sand, calcium-based sands, or Reptisand) have been successfully used as substrates in well-ventilated cages. Commercially available fine color-dyed sand is not recommended because it may become embedded in and color-stain the reptile's skin. This fine "talcum powder style" sand is not a natural type substrate. One must often provide some sand-free areas, such as large flat rocks, on which to feed.

Water itself may be considered a specialized substrate for some reptiles. However, tap water is often a poor substitute for the naturally occurring acidic bacteria-laden water from which many of our freshwater reptiles are derived. Tap water is also not usable for brackish or saltwater reptiles. Aquatic reptiles placed in cages where water is available frequently spend a great deal of time in that medium. However, these reptiles often have skin lesions develop under these circumstances. The neutral tap water is often contaminated with reptile feces, resulting in a suitable medium for opportunistic pathogens such as bacteria and fungi. This water is often devoid of the bacterial milieu and not in the appropriate temperature range found in the reptile's natural habitat, resulting in superficial infections and ultimately in sepsis. The warm acidic bacteria-laden water found in many natural situations is believed to form a bioactive substrate, which interferes with the growth of pathogens on many of the animals that have evolved to live there (see the discussion on bioactive substrates in this chapter). Attempting to recreate this bioactive milieu by acidifying the water and providing organic material to maintain acid-loving bacteria may be indicated. Some authors have used dilute mixtures of tea; others have added peat to filters, and some have just used swamp mud and live plants.[5,7,8] Commercially available acidifying buffers for tropical fish have also been used successfully for aquatic reptiles. Interestingly, an alternative that seems to help fresh water reptiles avoid skin lesions is the addition of some salt to the water. The addition of 1 cup (approximately 300 grams) of table salt per 20 gallons (approximately 80 L) of water often provides a brackish water solution that reduces the likelihood of infection but does not result in dehydration. This is particularly true if the water temperature is maintained at a warmer temperature than is generally recommended, such as a minimum of 82° to 85°F (28°–29.5°C) with drying/basking areas available in which the reptile can raise its body temperature to more than 90°F (32°C) during the daytime. In some cases, merely a diurnal rise in the water temperature is suitable, and this can be achieved with incandescent lights placed over the water during the daytime. Indeed, this mimics what occurs in nature as the sun warms up the top 4 inches (10 cm) of water in smaller bodies of water during the daytime over much of the earth's surface. Full-strength seawater may be created by purchasing one of the commercially available seawater mixes (e.g., Instant Ocean, http://www.aquariumsystems.com) and following the directions. However, this is only necessary for marine reptiles.

Keep in mind that some reptiles do not follow these general guidelines, and the reader is referred to one of the many references listed for specific information on the species in question.[10–30]

Measuring and Monitoring

In the words of Lord Kelvin, creator of the Kelvin temperature scale, "You don't know what you are talking about unless you count it." This is especially true when creating and maintaining captive environments for reptiles. Not only must one research the physical parameters of the wild habitat of said reptiles, but one must also strive to recreate them as accurately as possible. Aiding in this effort are some of the newer, very accurate digital meters that can measure temperature, humidity, and light levels in different areas of the enclosure and monitor them over time. Remember that the goal is to provide gradients of temperature, humidity, and light and allow the reptile to choose the level required for the particular function required. Data Loggers (Omega model OM-62, Omega.com, works well but there are multiple manufacturers) are typically small devices that can be placed in any area of a cage and record temperature, humidity, or pressure ranges over time (Fig. 16.15). External digital thermostats (Spyderrobotics.com or Vivariumelectronics.com) can also be used with small sensors placed in multiple areas of the cage (Fig. 16.16A and 16.16B). These monitors are also recording humidity. UV light meters (Solartech Inc., Solarmeter.com) are now widely available as well (Fig. 16.17). A detailed description of the available thermostats and their differences is available in Barten and Fleming.[1]

Cage Size and Construction

In general, the larger the enclosure for any captive reptile, the better the reptile fares, with the caveats that a larger cage must be successfully heated to avoid cold areas, humidity must be maintained in the proper range, and that the captive reptile can locate (and in some cases, capture) food and water sources. Larger cages are associated with fewer self-inflicted injuries and better body condition. Captive reproduction is also more likely to occur when larger cages or enclosures are used. One exception is hatchling or juvenile reptiles, which often do not thrive when provided with large enclosures. This is thought to be related to

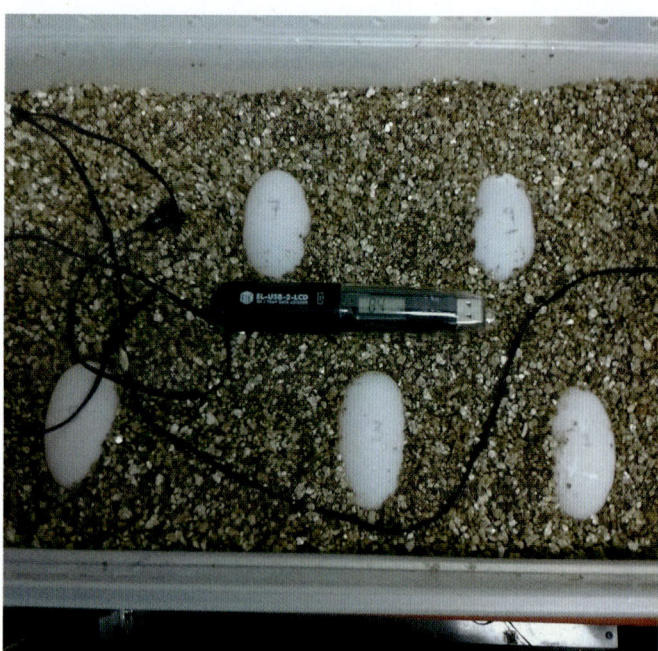

FIG 16.15 A data logger, used here to monitor eggs in an incubator. These small devices can be placed in various locations in reptile enclosures and can measure and record temperature and humidity changes over time.

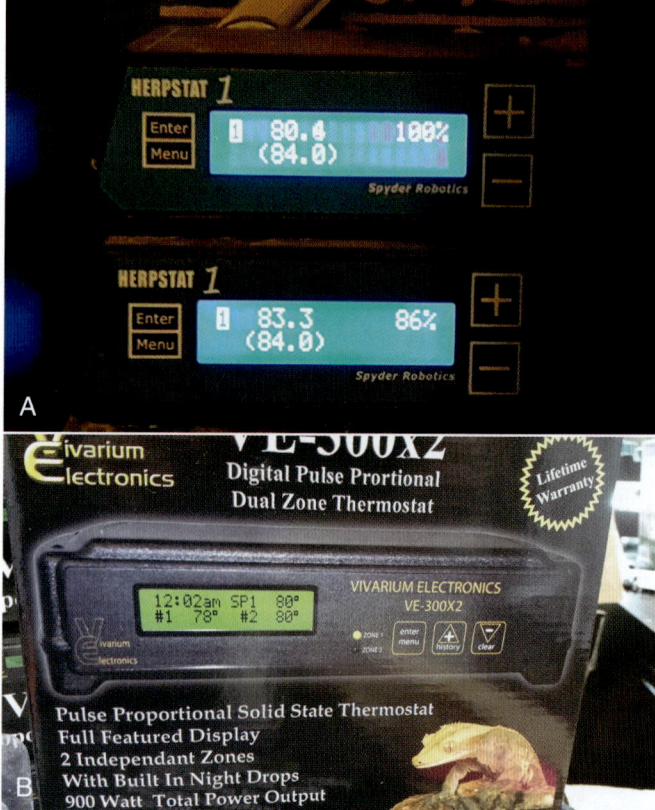

FIG 16.16 (A) A digital thermostat mounted to the outside of the enclosure. These devices take the guesswork out of setting up the thermal and humidity gradients required for different reptiles. (B) Another thermostat commonly used by herpetoculturists that allows for daily, gradual increases and decreases of temperature, as well as thermal gradients.

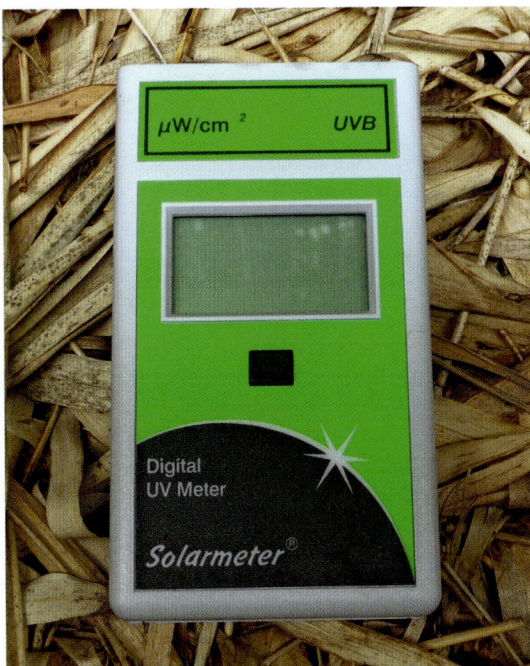

FIG 16.17 Solar meter. These devices may be used to determine the UVB intensity provided to a reptile.

Table 16.2 Successful Maintenance Areas (SMA) and Ideal Maintenance Areas (IMA) for Reptiles Based on Total Body Length (BL)

BL m (inches)	SNAKES SMA/IMA (m²)	LIZARDS SMA/IMA (m²)	TERRESTRIAL CHELONIANS SMA/IMA (m²)
0.1 (4)	0.04/0.12	0.12/0.25–0.50	0.4/1
0.2 (8)	0.08/0.24	0.24/0.50–1.0	0.8/2
0.3 (12)	0.12/0.36	0.36/0.75–1.5	1.2/3
0.4 (16)	0.16/0.48	0.48/1.0–2.0	1.6/4
0.5 (20)	0.20/0.60	0.60/1.25–2.5	2.0/5
0.6 (24)	0.24/0.72	0.72/1.50–3.0	2.4/6
0.7 (28)	0.28/0.84	0.84/1.75–3.5	2.8/7
0.8 (31)	0.32/0.96	0.96/2.00–4.0	3.2/8
0.9 (35)	0.36/1.08	1.08/2.25–4.5	3.6/9
1.0 (39)	0.40/1.20	1.20/2.50–5.0	4.0/10
2.0 (79)	0.80/2.40	2.40/5.00–10.0	8.0/20
3.0 (118)	1.20/3.60	3.60/7.50–15.0	
4.0 (157)	1.60/4.80		
5.0 (197)	2.00/6.00		
6.0 (236)	2.40/7.20		

Multiply m × 39.4 to obtain inches.
Multiply m² × 35.3 to obtain cubic feet.

an inability to properly thermoregulate and/or find food and water in these larger enclosures early in life.

With regard to the actual amount of recommended space per captive reptile, one is referred to species-specific references in the following chapters in this section of this book. However, formulas for minimum cage sizes for reptiles are presented here.

Many herpetoculturists follow anecdotal cage floor space recommendations put forth by Kaplan (Kaplan M, tank sizes available at http://www.anapsid.org/resources/tanksize.html). These cage size lengths and widths may be determined by using the following formulas: snakes: .75x BL × .33 BL; lizards: 2 to 3x BL × 1 to 1.5 BL, turtles and tortoises 4 to 5x BL × 2 to 3x carapace length, where BL is body length (total length, which equals STL or snout tail length). Cage height recommendations range from 1.5 to 2 × BL. Kaplan stresses that at least 30% to 40% of the cage should be open floor space for the reptile to feed, move about, and defecate. Furthermore, if a naturalistic habitat is used, more space is required to maintain that amount of floor space. For each additional reptile, an additional one-half the amount of floor space is recommended, and even more space is recommended for territorial reptiles. Although these recommendations have been largely successful, it is our goal to enrich the environment, increase more normal activity, and reduce stress, so an analysis of floor space area as determined by the Kaplan formulas was performed.

Assuming that the relationship of area required by a reptile is based on the size of the reptile and that this is a linear positive correlation, one may generate a floor space area required by simply multiplying the BL (body length) of a reptile by a factor that varies with each group of reptile. These factors, as determined by analysis of success by various herpetoculturists, are as follows, where meters squared is represented by (m²): snakes: .4 m²/1 m BL; lizards: 1.2 m²/1 m BL; turtles and tortoises: 4 m²/1 m BL (in this case, carapace length). These low-end factors, hence referred to as the successful maintenance factor (SMF) for each group, when multiplied by body length (in meters) results in what might be considered a "successful maintenance area" (SMA)

(Table 16.2). However, larger areas have been proposed by some herpetoculturists and veterinarians, and at least one peer-reviewed journal publication exists (Table 16.3).[32] They are as follows: snakes: 1.2 m²/1 m BL; lizards: 2.5 to 5.0 m²/1 m BL; turtles and tortoises: 10 m²/1 m BL (actually carapace length). These high end factors, hence referred to as the ideal maintenance factor (IMF) for each group, when multiplied by the body length results in what might be termed the "ideal maintenance area" (IMA). Using these factors results in a linear graph of usable areas by the captive reptile (Graphs 16.1, 16.2, and 16.3). Furthermore, any area between the SMA and the IMA will likely be successful for that group of reptiles. Hence, one might refer to areas in this range as the "successful maintenance area range" (SMAR). However, using these factors results in a linear graph of usable areas for reptiles of varying sizes but does not intuitively provide a length, width, or height of the cage. These cage lengths and widths may be approximated by using BL formulas similar to Kaplan's above, which have been calculated to result in an area lying close to or within the SMAR. Using the SMARs for the various groups, the formulas for cage size would be increased over the Kaplan formulas as follows: snakes: 1.25 to 1.5 BL by .5 to .75 BL; lizards: 3 to 10 × BL by 2 to 5 BL; turtles and tortoises: 6 to 12 × carapace length by 3 to 4 × carapace length. Note however that these formulas, like the Kaplan formulas, result in curvilinear (exponential growth) graphs, which may be used to approximate the minimum and maximum areas of a cage within the SMAR. These curvilinear graphs reveal several things. Firstly, that the Kaplan recommendations match fairly well for lizards and turtles, but that snakes require more space. Secondly, that the low-end formulas fail to produce an area that enters the SMAR or even reaches the SMA for medium-sized and small reptiles. Hence, to provide the same usable area for a small reptile, one needs to use a formula of BL toward the top end of the new recommendations. Furthermore, one must remember that the amount of usable area produced by multiplying length times width of the cage is not always

Table 16.3   Recommended Space Requirements for Reptiles[32]

Taxa	Minimum Floor Area or Volume Requirements[a]	Recommended Floor Area or Volume Requirements for Indoor Enclosures[b]
Boas and pythons	0.6 m² per m snake	1.2 m² per m snake
Kingsnakes, cornsnakes	0.6 m² per m snake	1.2 m² per m snake
Whipsnakes, racers	1.0 m² per m snake	2.0 m² per m snake
Arboreal snakes	0.6 m³ per m snake	1.2 m³ per m snake
Terrestrial lizards	0.2 m² per 0.1 m lizard	0.5 m² per 0.1 m lizard
Arboreal lizards	0.2 m³ per 0.1 m lizard	0.5 m³ per 0.1 m lizard
Tortoises and semi-aquatic turtles	0.2 m² per 0.1 m chelonian	0.5 m² per 0.1 m chelonian
Purely aquatic turtles	0.2 m³ per 0.1 m chelonian	0.5 m³ per 0.1 m chelonian

Snake example: A 1.2-m (47″) ball python (*Python regius*) requires at least 0.72 m² (7.7 feet²), which could be provided by an enclosure measuring 1.5 m (59″) long × 0.48 m (19″) wide. However, the recommended area is 1.44 m² (15.5 feet²), which could be provided by an enclosure measuring 2 m (79″) long × 0.72 m (28″) wide.

Lizard example: A 15-cm (6″) veiled chameleon *(Chamaeleo calyptratus)* requires at least 0.3 m³ (10.6 feet³), which could be provided by an enclosure measuring 0.55 m (22″) square × 1 m (39″) high. However, the recommended space is 0.75 m³ (26.5 feet³), which could be provided by an enclosure measuring 0.75 m (30″) square × 1.34 m (53″) high.

Chelonian example: A 30-cm (12″) Greek tortoise *(Testudo graeca)* requires at least 0.6 m² (6.5 feet²), which could be provided by an enclosure measuring 1.5 m (59″) long × 0.4 m (16″) wide. However, the recommended area is 1.5 m² (16.1 feet²), which could be provided by an enclosure measuring 2 m (79″) long × 0.75 m (30″) wide.

Quoted animal lengths are total length including tail.

Increasing occupancy does not necessitate multiplying these space requirements by the number of animals as space can be shared; however, increasing enclosure size and resources is important if multiple animals are maintained in the same enclosure.

[a]These minimum space requirements are geared towards wholesalers and retailers.

[b]These recommended space requirements are geared towards private pet ownership; however, in general, the largest enclosure possible should be provided, and larger outdoor enclosures are preferred.

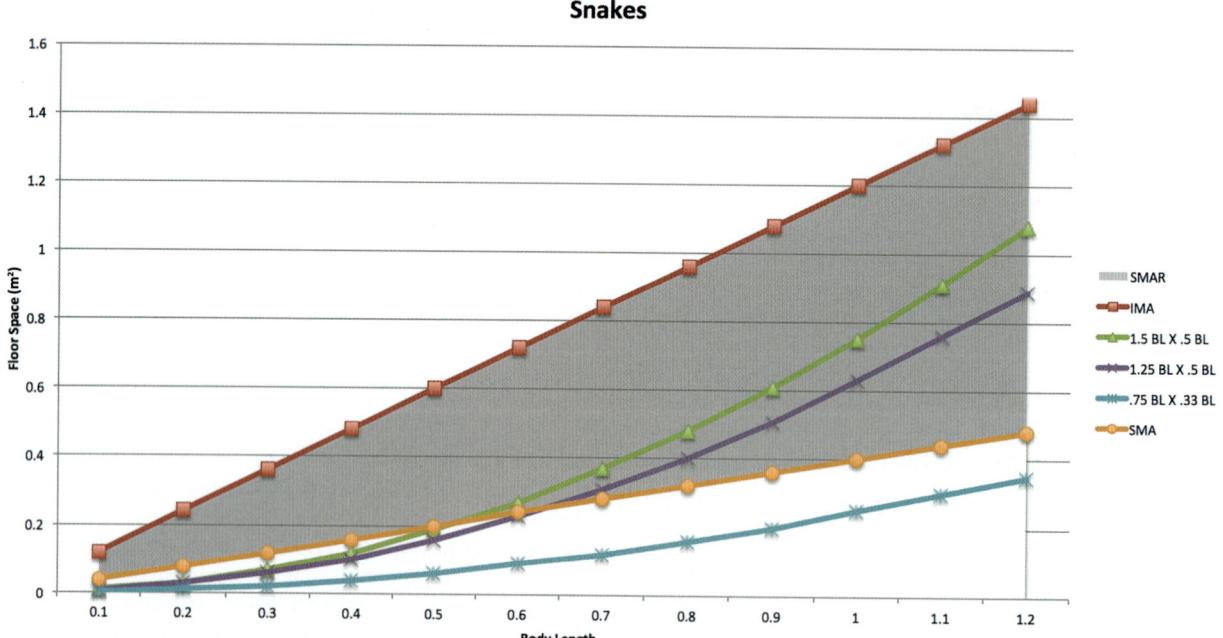

Graph 16.1 Floor space area graph (in meters² [m²]) of successful maintenance area (SMA) vs. ideal maintenance area (IMA) compared to common formulas for cage size in snakes. SMAR = successful maintenance area range. BL = body length = STL (snout total length) in meters.

Lizards

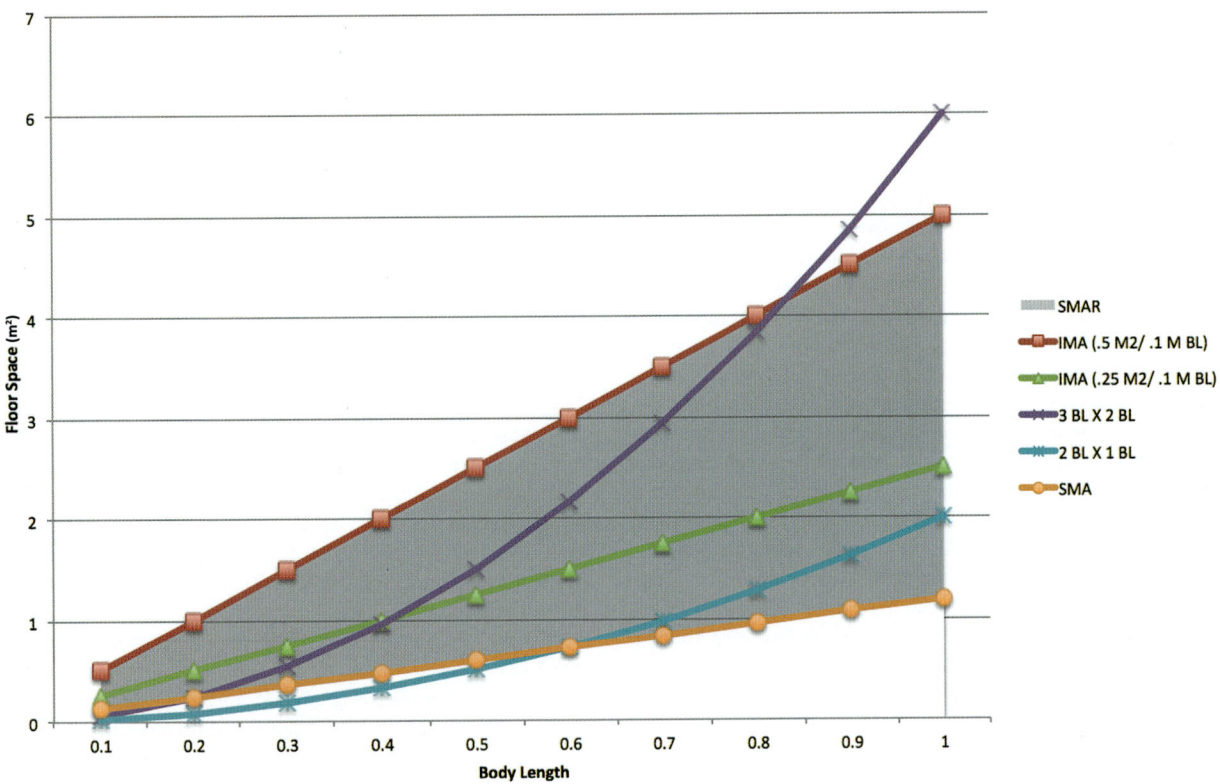

Graph 16.2 Floor space area graph (in meters^2 [m^2]) of successful maintenance area (SMA) vs. ideal maintenance area (IMA) compared to common formulas for cage size in lizards. SMAR = successful maintenance area range. BL = body length = STL (snout total length) in meters.

Turtles and Tortoises

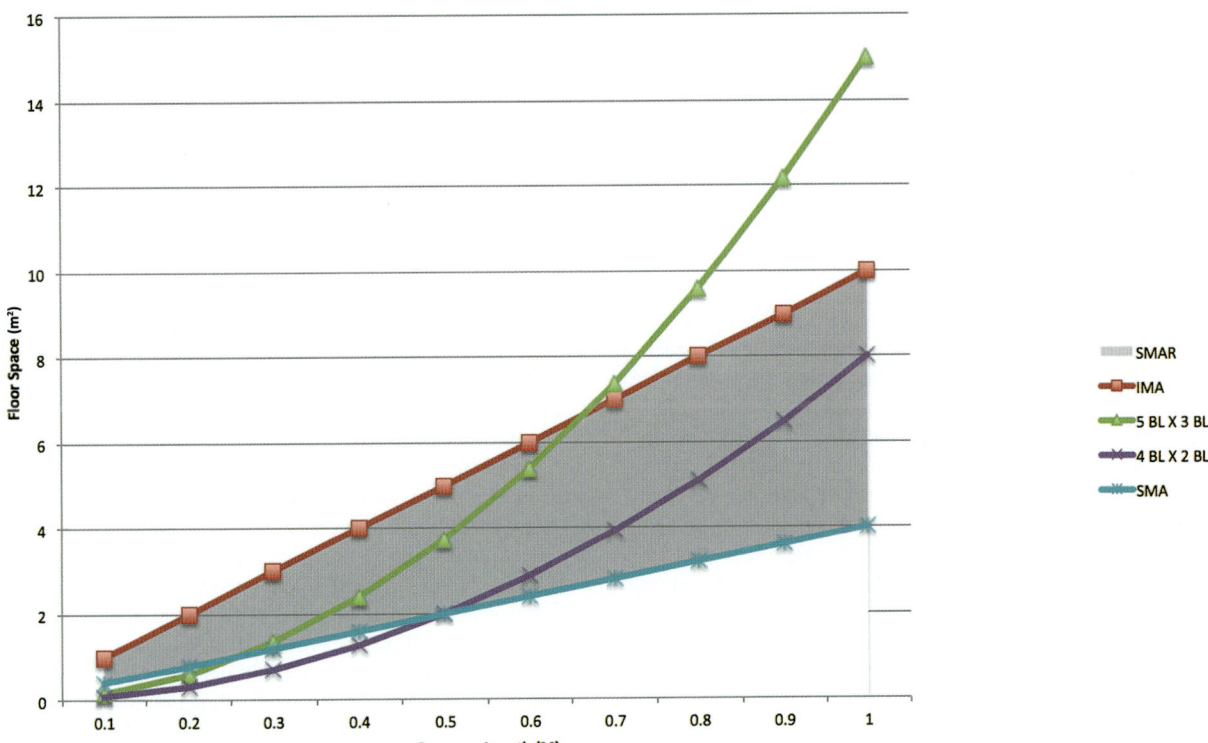

Graph 16.3 Floor space area graph (in meters^2 [m^2]) of successful maintenance area (SMA) vs. ideal maintenance area (IMA) compared to common formulas for cage size in tortoises. SMAR = successful maintenance area range. BL = carapace length in meters.

intuitive. For example, if one increases the length of a cage by 10% and decreases the width by 10%, one would think that the area is the same. This is not the case. For example, a tortoise pen that is 10 times the carapace length by 4 times the carapace length of a .1 m tortoise provides a floor space of .4 m². A pen that is 9 times the carapace length by 5 times the carapace length is .45 m², 8 × 6 provides .48 m², and 7 × 7 (a square) provides the maximum floor space of .49 m² for a tortoise with a carapace length of .1 m.

Indeed, it is hard to produce a formula for minimum cage size when comparing primarily fossorial skinks or earth snakes to active widely ranging monitor lizards or whip snakes respectively. Although our ultimate goal is to provide for the maximum comfort and welfare of the animals in question, we must be wary of recommending minimum cage sizes that governmental agencies will use to prohibit the average person from maintaining reptiles. Furthermore, the quality of a captive environment is based on more than just the cage size. It includes the environmental enrichment within the enclosure. The author does not mean to malign the Kaplan recommendations. They are an excellent starting point, and they actually align well with the successful maintenance areas. Finally, even though the snake recommendations are slightly lower than the SMA graph for snakes (see Graph 16.1), an interesting observation about juvenile snakes is that they often become anorectic when placed in cages too large. This suggests that the Kaplan recommendations for snakes may actually work very well for small snakes, even though they are mathematically below the newly recommended cage sizes.

As might be expected, some of the recommendations for aquatic chelonians and arboreal snakes are volumetric in nature, with recommendations for aquatic chelonians at 0.75 m³/0.1 M and for arboreal snakes at 1.6 m³/1 M of body length. Divers adds the same caveat as above, that active individuals may require more space, while less active reptiles may require less.[32] Be aware that many municipalities and other governmental entities have regulations dictating the minimum cage size for captive reptiles, depending on the length of the reptile and the number to be housed together. The cage sizes recommended above, even successful maintenance numbers for area (SMAs), exceed those minimum recommendations (see Graphs 16.1, 16.2, and 16.3). Hence, a clinician may simply use an SMF to approximate a cage size. For reference, a 5-gallon aquarium has a floor space of .08 M², a 10-gallon aquarium has a floor space of .12 m², a 20 gallon aquarium has a floor space of .23 M², a 40-gallon aquarium has a floor space of .41 m², a 75-gallon aquarium has a floor space of .56 m², a 125-gallon aquarium has a floor space of .83 m², and a 180-gallon aquarium has 1.11 m² of floor space. (Note that gallons here and elsewhere in this chapter are US gallons.)

The material from which cages are constructed is also important. Cages should be made of smooth, nonabrasive, and nonabsorbent materials. Examples of such materials are glass, plastic, plexiglass, and stainless steel. One of the most ideal recent materials to be utilized is HDP (high-density polyethylene). This material is extremely smooth, strong, light, and nonporous. All of these materials are less likely to result in rostral abrasions as are rougher materials, and they are easily cleaned and disinfected. Bare wood has notoriously been a problem material used in the construction of large reptile cages. It is abrasive, difficult to clean, and nearly impossible to disinfect. Additionally, eliminating mites from wooden cages is difficult and often requires that the cage be destroyed or at minimum repainted. Melamine-coated, wooden cages do provide a smooth, nonabrasive, cleanable, and disinfectable surface; however, mites may still be difficult to eliminate from such cages.

The most common cage shape used in herpetoculture is the rectangle. These cages are structurally sound hund readily available, and they minimize the angles into which a reptile might collide. Unusual shapes such as pentagons, hexagons, octagons, and others often provide less usable space and are associated with more injuries than simple rectangular cages. As mentioned above, a square cage would actually provide the most floor space, but rectangular cages have been far more commonly used and are much easier to produce gradients within. The height of a cage is also an important parameter. For terrestrial reptiles, the "foot space" is more important than the vertical height of the enclosure; however, the top of the cage must not be so low as to allow the reptile to reach it easily and traumatize itself or facilitate an easy escape. For arboreal reptiles, the opposite is true; a cage with increased height provides more usable habitat than a cage with increased foot space. Tall, plastic mesh cages are now available for arboreal reptiles, such as chameleons (e.g., ZooMed Naturalistic Terrarium), and they come in various sizes, including 12 × 12 × 18 in. (30 × 30 × 46 cm = .04 m³), 18 × 18 × 24 in. (46 × 46 × 61 cm), and 18 × 18 × 36 in. (46 × 46 × 91 cm = .19 m³) with the latter numbers referring to the height of the cage. Mass-produced aquariums, which are commonly converted to reptile terrariums, use terminology that may be helpful to the herpetoculturist and veterinarian. Aquariums with the maximum floor space are referred to as "long" aquariums, and those of the same volume with a smaller foot space are referred to as "high" aquariums. High aquariums are more suitable for arboreal reptiles because they can use this vertical space.

The use of aquariums for reptile maintenance has been attacked by some well-respected herpetoculturists, stating poor ventilation, poor insulation, and greater exposure. However, the successful use of these structures for years cannot be ignored. With regard to ventilation, they provide nearly perfect top ventilation when utilized with screens instead of the typical light hoods. This is in stark contrast to some of the newer molded plexiglass cages, which have restricted top ventilation, or many of the rack-style cages, which have extremely poor top ventilation. Excellent top ventilation is absolutely critical (see humidity and ventilation discussed earlier in this chapter) when natural substrates are used, as they tend to retain moisture. These substrates provide numerous benefits, including physical support, and even visual security as the reptiles often burrow in them. The fact that they are constructed of clear material, namely glass, has advantages as well as disadvantages. For reptiles that prefer bright habitats, supplemented by natural lighting, this material has a major advantage over many of the more opaque substances. Poor insulation may be a problem compared with some of the newer materials; however, this may be an advantage when primary heat sources (room temperature controls) are utilized to allow the development of a heat cycle for a large number of cages for treatment or hibernation purposes. For reptiles that prefer a high level of visual security and require excellent insulation for narrowly controlled temperature gradients, aquariums may not be the best option. Additionally glass is heavy compared to plastic enclosures, making them more cumbersome and difficult to clean.

On the opposite end of the reptile enclosure maintenance spectrum, compared with the well-decorated terrarium/aquarium, are the popular reptile rack systems or drawer-style enclosures. The newer rack-style cages are constructed of HDP (high-density polyethylene), reasonably ventilated, often wired to provide a thermal gradient, and frequently have molded places to prevent water bowls from tipping over. They are often filled with a satisfactory substrate, such as newspaper or aspen bedding, and by their nature provide good visual security. The individual cages/drawers are light, strong, smooth, and easily cleaned and disinfected. In short, they are very effective at providing the requirements necessary for snakes and many other reptiles. The size of individual cages in such a rack varies from a "shoe box" size, 19 × 8 × 3.5 in (48 × 20 × 9 cm) or approximately .1 m² of floor space, to the "boa box" size, which is 51 × 25 × 8 in (130 × 64 × 20 cm) or approximately .8 m² of floor space.

Note that the cage size numbers are listed as length by width by height and that there is very little height to these cages. However, the low height issue does not appear to be a problem for the successful maintenance of most species of snakes commonly kept by herpetoculturists at this time. In fact, multiple generations of many species have been maintained and bred in such enclosures. In spite of the success of these rack-style cages, the author is intuitively "dissatisfied" with this style of caging as a permanent, final enclosure for a captive snake. It is not aesthetically pleasing to see a snake housed in an opaque "box." Hence, this explains the encouragement of the more enriched, well-decorated aquarium/terrarium-type enclosure. However, there is no scientific evidence at this time that snakes or other reptiles require more intellectual stimulation than what they receive in these "boxes," and indeed many snakes commonly maintained are semifossorial, or are nocturnal/crepuscular, and thereby may be comfortable and secure in dark, relatively small spaces.

Quarantine

Isolating reptiles from each other during their initial entry into a collection is critical. Often parasitic or infectious diseases have been introduced into a collection because of a lack of proper quarantine. A recommended period of 3 months is advisable for most reptiles. Some experts have suggested that reptiles be quarantined for up to 6 months because of the risk of viruses.[2,3] Isolation should theoretically be accomplished in separate rooms that do not exchange air with each other. However, this is not often practical or possible with hospitalized reptiles. Under these circumstances, prevention of direct contact or fomite spread is often what can be achieved. Animals that will enter a reptile hospital area or bank of cages should be carefully examined first for any evidence of external parasitism. Snake mites and lizard mites may rapidly travel from cage to cage in a rack-style arrangement. Snakes with mites are not housed in the same room as other reptiles. After the newly arrived reptile has been placed in its new enclosure, the bag or box used to transport that reptile should either be disinfected or discarded.

Also, reptiles from different areas of the world should never be housed together because organisms that may be commensals for reptiles from one area may be pathogens for reptiles from other areas. Healthy animals, or long-term hospital patients, should be serviced and treated first, and new arrivals, or quarantined animals, last. In some cases, reptiles of the same species, captured in the same area and shipped at the same time, can be quarantined in a communal cage. However, this should only be attempted if the species in question is not cannibalistic and all of the previous conditions are met. Reptiles housed together may compete with each other for food and basking sites, so care should be exercised when housing communally. See Chapter 19 for a thorough discussion of quarantine procedures.

Cleaning and Disinfection

Disease is often considered an opportunistic event. A potential pathogen is given the "opportunity" to invade an organism, and it enters and reproduces. Microbiologists have turned this possibility into an equation, $D = V \times E \div I$, where D is disease; V is virulence of the invading organism; E is Exposure, or how many potential pathogens are involved; and I is the immunity of the organism invaded. There is generally little that the clinician can do to change the virulence of the invading organism. Immunity however, is increased by providing the correct environment and diet as discussed. Increased immunity, of course, reduces the risk of disease. But it is exposure that we are attempting to control with disinfectants. Heat and certain kinds of UV light (especially in the UVC range) may act as disinfectants, but generally, the word disinfectant refers to a group of chemicals known for their ability to kill pathogenic

organisms. There are several groups of disinfectants, including the halogens (bleach and povidone iodine), phenols or coal tar derivatives (such as Lysol, Pine Sol, and Amphyl), and quaternary ammonium compounds (e.g., Roccal and DiQuat). Of these groups, the halogens and quaternary ammonium compounds are generally the most effective and safest for reptile enclosure disinfection. No disinfectant should be used in a soiled cage (i.e., cages should be cleaned with soap and water prior to disinfection). See Chapter 18 for a detailed discussion on disinfectants.

Use of disposable paper towels instead of a single cleaning sponge/cloth is imperative when cleaning from cage to cage. Keep in mind that no disinfectant is 100% effective against all pathogens; therefore one should dispose of towels after use in a single cage. Only clean paper towels are dipped into the chosen disinfectant bucket. In this manner, the disinfectant solution itself does not become contaminated. Hands should also be washed between cages with a suitable antibacterial soap or perhaps some of the disinfectant solution in a separate container from that used to disinfect the cages. A common, inexpensive, and effective disinfectant is household bleach (sodium hypochlorite), which can be diluted to a concentration of one part bleach to 30 parts water (30 mL per liter of water or $\frac{1}{2}$ cup per gallon). Full-strength bleach is not necessary and has been associated with the destruction of respiratory epithelium and death of reptiles when used in their cages. A 5% ammonia solution is effective against coccidia and cryptosporidia, but remember that bleach and ammonia when mixed produce toxic fumes.

Another commonly used and effective disinfectant is Roccal-D. This is a quaternary ammonium compound that has a broad spectrum of activity against common reptile pathogens. McKeown[5] recommends a dilution with water of 1:200 to 1:400 for reptile cages and bowls.[5] Remembering that disinfection cannot occur without first physically removing the organic debris. Cleaning is defined as the removal of organic material from the cage or pen. Thus, the clinician should advise herpetoculturists, zookeepers, and technicians to thoroughly clean a cage first and then disinfect it. Cleaning should occur daily unless a bioactive substrate is being used, in which case, nonpathogenic bacteria breaks down the fecal matter. See the discussion on bioactive substrates. It is also important to remember that most disinfectants work best above 20°C (68°F).

Ideally, hospitals that treat reptiles benefit by having foot pump water faucets and soap dispensers. This helps prevent cross contamination of hands and cages and cage accessories at the sink/faucet level. An important point to remember about cleaning these cage accessories, including water bowls, hide boxes, and artificial plants, is to avoid placing them together in the same water-filled sink. Even when soap and a disinfectant are added, certain infectious agents may not be eliminated and instead spread from dish to dish within the ineffective soapy solution. For example, if one placed a water bowl contaminated with coccidia in a sink filled with bleach water, all other dishes in that sink may be contaminated with coccidia because sodium hypochlorite is an ineffective disinfectant against coccidia. See Chapter 18 for a more detailed discussion on disinfectants and disinfection.

Examinations

Careful examination of reptiles entering a facility where other reptiles are housed is critically important in protecting that collection. (See Chapter 42 for a more detailed discussion on performing a physical examination.) Any signs of illness, including nasal or ocular discharges; excessive sneezing or wheezing; loose, mucous, or bloody stools; neurological signs; or skin lesions should alert the clinician to isolate such an animal immediately. It is not uncommon for large stable collections to have drastic losses after a new "unquarantined" animal was introduced.

A collection of reptiles that does not admit new animals is referred to as a closed collection.

A fecal examination is advisable for all reptiles immediately after acquisition and again 3 months later. Annual or semiannual fecal examinations are advisable after that.

Hematology and blood chemistry may also be helpful in determining the apparent health of a reptile. Often a reptile appears healthy outwardly but has a disorder that is only revealed with a complete blood cell count (CBC) or chemistry (see Chapters 33 and 34). A blood smear evaluation may reveal parasites in wild-caught reptiles (see Chapter 32). Normal blood values for numerous species of reptiles have now been published and are readily accessible (see Chapter 35).[33,34]

Parasite Control

Parasites and commensal organisms are extremely common in captive reptiles. Problems associated with parasites include diarrhea, constipation, obstruction, colitis, perforation of the intestine, peritonitis, bloating, bleeding from the cloaca, anorexia, cachexia, anemia, and death. Commensal organisms are organisms that live in or on a reptile but do not result in any damage. Symbiotic organisms may also be present, and these may actually help reptiles digest their food or possibly compete with potential pathogens. When performing a fecal exam it is often difficult to distinguish pathogens from symbiotic organisms, particularly in herbivorous reptiles. Hence, evaluating fecal exams and determining a treatment protocol must include evaluating the overall health of the reptile in question. A moderate amount of protozoans in an otherwise healthy herbivorous reptile may be normal, whereas any protozoans in an anorectic snake or carnivorous lizard should be viewed as potential pathogens, and the clinician must consider treatment to reduce or eliminate these organisms. In spite of the difficulty determining the pathogenicity of organisms discovered on a fecal exam, all recently captured reptiles or reptiles that are new to a collection should be suspected of parasitism. Repeated fecal examinations should be performed during the first several months in captivity and then regularly thereafter. The eggs of many parasites may not appear immediately in the first fecal examination performed on a recently captured reptile; they often appear on fecal examinations performed 3 to 6 months later. This was observed in numerous species of North American snakes after their capture.[6] The cause of this is not known. Presumably, the parasite infections are present at the time of capture, but either they are not yet reproductive and need time to mature and produce ova or the stress of captivity may suppress the immune response of the captive reptile and allow the parasites to increase in numbers. Thus, fecal examinations performed on reptiles after recent capture or importation are important screens to evaluate for a heavy parasite load but not as definitive tests to rule out parasitism. Fecal analyses should be performed both at the beginning and the end of the quarantine period.

Once parasitism is diagnosed, appropriate parasiticides should be administered at the doses recommended elsewhere in this book (see Chapters 32 and 120). Some authors recommend a routine deworming be performed even in the absence of positive fecal examination results. Furthermore, those parasites with direct life cycles are particularly difficult to eliminate, even in a single animal enclosure, so a regular deworming schedule may be indicated even for some long-term captives. Examples of parasites that are extremely difficult to eliminate are cryptosporidia in many species of snakes and lizards and coccidia in bearded dragons. Grazing tortoises present a unique problem in reptile parasite control. Following a deworming, grazing reintroduces parasites (as well as commensals and symbionts) back into the gut. Hence, their parasite control may be considered similar to that of other grazing animals such as horses and cattle, in which regular deworming in combination with rotational grazing is recommended.

Parasites and other infectious agents may be brought into a collection by wild rodents, birds, insects, and other arthropods. Mosquitoes are well-known vectors for certain blood parasites, and flies can serve as mechanical vectors for many pathogenic bacteria. Thus, a simple but extremely effective method of disease control is to maintain insect screens over and between all cages. Flies, mosquitoes, and roaches are not able to move easily from cage to cage with this protection. Unfortunately, most insect screens do not inhibit movement of fruit flies, gnats, or mites, and other methods are necessary for the control of these pests.

Snake mites (*Ophionyssus*) and lizard mites (*Hirtstiella*) are frustrating parasites for herpetoculturists to manage. Once in a collection, they are extremely difficult to eliminate, so major efforts should be made to prevent their entry into a collection. Usually all new reptiles should be quarantined for at least 3 months and probably longer to visualize a potential infection. If the newly acquired animal is found to have these ectoparasites, treating this individual is far easier than treating an entire collection. Food items and humans (such as caretakers, especially those working around other groups of reptiles) may also serve as vectors for mites.

Food items such as live mice have also been incriminated in transferring snake mites into collections. Pet shops often maintain rodent cages near snake cages, and when the snakes have mites, they often get into the rodent cages. Thus, an unsuspecting owner may carry home mites with a live prey item. The clinician should warn owners of this potential risk. This problem may be eliminated by purchasing rodents from clean reputable sources where reptiles are not housed near rodents or by purchasing frozen rodents. Freezing prekilled rodents appears to eliminate snake mites; however, freezing is not effective for eliminating pathogenic bacteria or protozoans. Keep in mind that feeding live prey items is illegal in some countries, states, provinces, or municipalities. Hence, purchasing humanely euthanized, frozen rodents will eliminate the risk of mites from this source. See Chapters 32 and 120 for more details on parasite identification and control.

As mentioned previously, insects, including prey insects, may also serve as vectors for the transmission of parasites or other pathogenic organisms. Prey insects arriving from a supplier with flies, maggots, or the larvae of other insects should be suspect, and one might want to consider recommending a different supplier.

Lastly, keep in mind that a substrate intended for use in the bottom of an enclosure may harbor mites as well, particularly if purchased from a vendor that also carries reptiles. A simple solution is to freeze the substrate for several days (or, if nonflammable, oven bake for a short time) prior to using.

Control of Disease Transmission in Closed Collections

A closed collection is a group of reptiles where new specimens are not permitted to enter. This arrangement has tremendous advantages in the prevention of disease. The only reason to allow a new animal into a closed breeding colony is to add more genetic diversity to the group. This reduces the likelihood of inbreeding and associated diseases.

Multi-Individual and Multispecies Enclosures

Recently, herpetoculturists have made efforts to house reptiles in naturalistic enclosures that mimic not only the naturally occurring physical environment but also the biological environment of the animals. Numerous species of plants and animals that coexist with the species may be considered for the captive environment, if the cage is suitably sized and complex enough to provide the proper habitat for all species considered. However, if two or more species are to be considered for cohabitation, the relationship to each other must be determined. Will they compete with each other for food and habitat? Will they prey on each other? Do they carry any diseases or parasites that may negatively affect each other? What is a suitable population density for the species? Are the species being considered somewhat social in nature or entirely independent from each other and potentially cannibalistic? These and other questions need to be answered to safely house different species of reptiles together. For many years, we have correctly advised clients to house reptiles alone when they are using small cages. Only in this way can feeding be monitored and competition for food reduced. Larger, more complex cages may house more than one individual of the same species, but they must be monitored closely. Clients frequently misinterpret reptiles maintaining close proximity to each other under basking lights as a positive social indicator. A frequent comment is that "they are buddies because they hang out on each other." To which the author responds, "so do people in a lifeboat." Indeed, there is a great risk for two or more individuals of the same species to compete heavily for limited basking sites, food, water, and even hiding areas. The stress of such competition may be detrimental to both the submissive and dominant reptile over time. Usually this competition manifests itself first in the submissive individual. Unable to bask effectively, limited in feeding, the submissive individual begins to lose size and body condition relative to the dominant individual. As the size difference increases the dominance of one individual over another appears to increase, and often the submissive individual ends up with an infection from opportunistic pathogens. Typically, it will succumb in exactly the same environment, and consuming the same diet, where the dominant reptile is thriving. This has been referred to as "big reptile, little reptile syndrome," and it is extremely common (see Fig. 16.18). It has been observed in captive squamates (both snakes and lizards), chelonians, and crocodilians. Indeed, this may be one of the best demonstrations of the effects of biological stress on an individual, given that all physical factors in the environment and the diet offered are the same for both reptiles involved. The best way to avoid this "syndrome" is to either house reptiles separately or increase the size and complexity of the cage, such that there are multiple basking areas, feeding areas, and hiding areas. Tortoise keepers have been known to create a feeding stall arrangement so that tortoises in the same enclosure can eat without disturbance from other tortoises yet gain the benefit of social contact. See the discussion on stress in this chapter and in Chapter 15.

Generally, reptiles from different geographic areas should not be maintained together because of the risk of introducing disease into a susceptible (immunologically naive) population. Hence, clinicians should strongly advise their clients against this practice. As mentioned above, two individual rodent-eating snakes maintained in a small enclosure or two groups of rodent-eating snakes in a large enclosure may not be compatible. Similarly, two species of tortoises that feed on the same food at the same time of the day may compete directly or indirectly. Also, chelonians and crocodilians appear to naturally carry a number of commensal protozoans that may be pathogenic for some snakes and lizards (e.g., Entamoeba). Thus, chelonians and terrestrial snakes should not be housed together in small enclosures. Crocodilians, of course, are likely to eat snakes and small chelonians, thereby making their cohabitation ill-advised.

In a large, outdoor enclosure maintained by the author, six species of snakes were maintained. These included water snakes (*Nerodia harteri harteri*), queen snakes (*Regina septemvittata*), hog-nosed snakes (*Heterodon simus*), rough green snakes (*Opheodrys aestivus*), fox snakes (*Pantherophis vulpinus*), and ribbon snakes (*Thamnophis proximus*) (Fig. 16.19). Theoretically, these snakes should have been able to cohabitate on the basis of their differing food preferences. Their preferred foods included, respectively, fish, crayfish, toads, insects, rodents, and small amphibians. However, the ribbon snakes also preyed on small fish, effectively competing with young water snakes. The fox snakes and green snakes contracted amoebiasis, presumably from drinking water contaminated by the heavy population of water snakes and queen snakes, for which the amoeba appeared to be nonpathogenic commensals. The hog-nosed snakes were preyed on by large local birds. Thus, it became evident how difficult it can be to maintain health in these multiple species enclosures. Even when predation was controlled, the water snakes increased rapidly to such a number that parasitism, fungal disease, and even cannibalism became significant factors for these snakes housed outdoors.[35,36] See the discussion on outdoor enclosures to follow.

Environmental Enhancement and Outdoor Enclosures

As a small boy visiting the large cat enclosure at a zoo in the early 1960s, I was struck by the constant activity level of the caged cats. In small concrete-bottomed bare cages, they appeared to pace back and forth incessantly. Reptiles caged in similarly stark cages appear to show similar

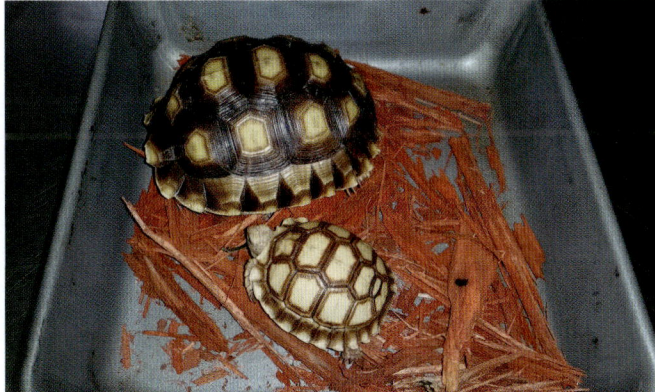

FIG 16.18 Measuring stress in a captive reptile is difficult but important as stress plays a major role in survival, longevity, and reproductive success. These two tortoises were raised together in exactly the same environment and offered the same diet. Their size difference is likely a manifestation of stress, probably from competition for food or thermal resources. This is referred to as "big reptile, little reptile syndrome."

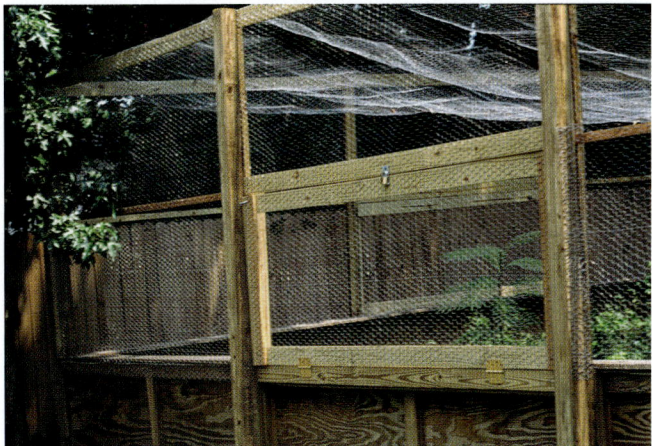

FIG 16.19 A large outdoor enclosure allows reptiles to establish territories, forage, and avoid confrontations with cage mates. These behaviors are not often observed in those reptiles housed indoors.

stereotypic behaviors, and generally, reptiles that pace are more likely to have health problems in captivity. A direct observation that may be associated with pacing is rostral abrasion, which often leads to stomatitis, anorexia, and rapid decline. However, a constantly pacing reptile likely is under stress and all the sequelae of that stress, including immune system suppression and ultimately disease. Ideally, one should observe that a captive reptile finds certain areas within its enclosure and stays in one of those areas for periods of time, rather than constantly wandering.

Numerous hiding, resting, and activity areas should be provided. Activities might include foraging for food or water, seeking mates, thermoregulating, or seeking more suitable shelter. Admittedly, some energy may be directed toward escaping from an enclosure, but in a large well-designed enclosure, this activity should be minimized. In open outdoor enclosures, some reptiles establish territories and defend them. They may exhibit normal escape reactions when approached and normal defensive actions when approached closely or picked up (e.g., they may bite, flail wildly, or defecate on the keeper). In short, they may live like and behave much more like wild reptiles than captive ones.[35] All of those factors that affect them in nature may affect them in a large outdoor enclosure (i.e., competition, predation, parasitism, disease, starvation, dehydration, cold exposure). However, these animals are not wild but rather captive reptiles in elaborate naturalistic cages. They may become more heavily parasitized than their wild counterparts, because they are confined to much smaller areas, thereby increasing exposure to parasites. They may become obese because of reduced activity associated with confinement. And they may exhibit unusual behaviors not seen in wild reptiles of the same species. But in spite of all of the potential problems, it is interesting to note that in the study with snakes conducted by the author mentioned above, snakes housed in a large outdoor enclosure were anatomically and physiologically more similar to their siblings released back into the wild in a number of measurable parameters than those raised in aquariums. These parameters included length, weight, defensive behavior, and oral bacterial cultures (see Figs. 16.1 and 16.19). Large outdoor enclosures have been used successfully for years with crocodilians and tortoises; only recently have they become more popular for lizards and snakes.

Bioactive Substrates

Some advances in herpetoculture may seem counterintuitive regarding the way we keep reptiles in captivity and think about their captive requirements. DeVosjoli[37] discusses in detail the use of bioactive substrate systems (BSS).[37] The basic theory behind these substrates is that they provide an environment where beneficial bacteria compete with pathogenic bacteria and fungi to support a healthy microhabitat for the captive. Stirring the substrate is apparently the key. Stirring mixes the competitive bacteria in lower layers with fecal bacteria and others at the surface, thereby inhibiting their growth. Successful creation of the bioactive substrate, according to DeVosjoli, requires that the substrate is at least 6.5 cm (2.5 in) deep and that it allows for good oxygenation and moisture retention. If the substrate dries out, it does not work. This system has been tested primarily on snakes, but theoretically it is useful for many captive reptiles.

The moisture-containing substrate mentioned previously probably has other benefits as well. Lillywhite[38] and others have recently commented on cutaneous water loss that captive snakes endure when they are placed in completely dry cages. This chronic water loss is suspected of being a major factor leading to the premature demise of captive snakes; by contributing to renal damage. Thus, a moist substrate may create a microhabitat that protects a captive reptile from both dehydration and infection. Indeed, the author has seen many small species of snakes do well in moist substrates or where moist substrates are offered as one of the choices available. An example of a bioactive substrate is a thick layer of cypress mulch, which has been regularly misted with water and stirred occasionally. Typically, this will result in layering of humidity within the substrate, with the driest areas on top and the moister areas near the bottom. Beneficial bacteria are encouraged within this acidic medium, and these appear to compete with pathogens in a well-ventilated cage. The author has successfully used this substrate for over 5 million snake hours (hours in which over 90 species of captive snakes have been housed in this substrate).

Other substrates successfully utilized are finely shredded coconut husks (coir), sphagnum or peat moss of varying particle size, and natural soil (baked or not). Each one of these substrates has potential for being successfully used as a natural (and bioactive) substrate. However, each substrate has its unique qualities of pH, moisture retention, air pocket size, compressibility, and the amount of physical support it provides to the reptile in question. Those substrates that are naturally less compressible will retain more air and less moisture (e.g., aspen bedding) will also tend to stay looser and provide less physical support. While this may be ideal for larger terrestrial reptiles, it is not a good substrate for smaller, semifossorial reptiles. Indeed, it appears that recommendations for substrate particle size may be correlated (loosely), with the size of the reptile in question. For example, larger reptiles generally do well on larger particle size substrates, which are less compressible and retain less moisture. Whereas smaller reptiles generally do well on smaller particle substrates that are more compressible and more moisture retentive. Any time a natural substrate is used, it is critical that enough top ventilation is provided or moist stagnant air will lead to the development of an unhealthy, fungal-laden environment.

Regarding the use of natural soil, some have questioned the value or necessity of baking the soil first before using. Some argue that baking the soil before use kills the naturally occurring bacteria and reduces its quality as a bioactive substrate. Others argue this is not the case. Indeed, natural soil may contain a variety of potentially symbiotic bacteria. However, there is also a risk that it may contain pathogens, including soil arthropods, nematodes, fungi, bacteria, and viruses that may opportunistically invade a reptile in close contact for an extended period of time, and thus baking is advisable.

Water

Water should be available at all times for most reptiles. However, exceptions do exist. The constant presence of water in poorly ventilated cages often becomes a health hazard for many reptiles. Unable to escape the excessively humid air in such a cage, these animals become susceptible to dermatitis or respiratory disease. The situation may be aggravated by excessive substrate moisture. However, with suitable conditions in a well-ventilated cage, the presence of a clean reliable source of water is extremely important to most captive reptiles. As mentioned previously, definite cutaneous and respiratory water losses must be compensated for or the captive reptile suffers either acute or chronic dehydration. This concept of chronic dehydration, and possibly associated kidney disease, has captured the interest of some physiologists and zookeepers recently.[38] Some have suggested that merely providing sufficient drinking water cannot prevent chronic dehydration and kidney disease if the reptile does not have access to a suitable microenvironment that reduces cutaneous and respiratory water loss. See the discussion on basic husbandry requirements.

How water is provided is also important. An arboreal reptile, such as a vine snake, a tree boa, or a chameleon, may rarely come to the ground level. Therefore a water bowl on the floor of the cage may be futile as a method of providing drinking water. However, misting the branches on a regular basis or providing a tree-mounted water bowl may be effective. Modern herpetoculturists have responded to this requirement by creating naturalistic water bowls and hiding areas that can be mounted high in the enclosure with the use of magnets. Desert reptiles may also benefit from misting rocks in their enclosure on a regular basis, as they often lap water from these rocks but may not always use a water bowl. Conversely, some may sit in their water bowls for excessively long periods of time if these are provided, sometimes resulting in associated dermatitis. Many tortoises seem to need a daily rain to thrive, but the substrate should not stay excessively moist on a continual basis. Water intake may also be increased significantly by soaking or misting food prior to feeding it to captive reptiles.

The size and shape of a container is another factor that should be considered. Steep-sided water containers may prevent easy entry or exit by many chelonians, resulting in dehydration or drowning. Terrestrial chelonians and even some aquatic species are not strong swimmers and may easily drown if the water is deeper than their legs are long, and thus chelonians should not be put in water deeper than this. Even the most aquatic of reptiles, including crocodilians, chelonians, and certain snakes, need a resting area or "haul out" where they can climb out to bask or rest. In many cases, they must be able to raise their body temperatures significantly and dry the skin completely during the basking process or dermatitis may occur.

Be aware that daily soakings are an important maintenance requirement for many terrestrial chelonians. It is recommended to soak hospitalized tortoises for at least one half hour daily in shallow water. The tortoises may drink at this time, but often the soaking merely facilitates defecation and appears to encourage activity and alertness. Furthermore, bathing and the manual scrubbing or removal of debris or old skin may be healthful (Fig. 16.20).

Additives to reptile water have been the subject of many discussions during the last 10 years. Several commercial vitamin and mineral formulations are presently available, but the values of these products are largely unknown. The dosing of such products is purely empirical. Some authors have recommended the use of dilute bleach in the drinking water to control bacteria. At 1 to 5 mL per gallon (4 L), this addition is both safe for the reptile and efficacious against some bacteria. This addition is probably unnecessary for most captive reptiles; however, it may be helpful in cases where a particular bacterial organism may be thought to be spreading through a group of reptiles in the same cage. Conversely, chlorinated water may be a problem for aquatic turtles because it may cause conjunctivitis, so dechlorinating additives may be used or the water should be allowed to sit for 24 hours prior to use (see Fig. 16.3).

Feeding

Poor nutrition is as common as an inadequate environment for causing disease in captive reptiles (see Chapter 27). Together, these factors are likely responsible directly or indirectly for more than 80% of illness in captive reptiles.

Both the quantity and quality of food is important. Feed reptiles the highest quality food items possible. When possible, feeding fresh food items is ideal. "Old" food items or those that have been stored improperly may be contaminated with various fungi or bacteria.

Items that have been frozen for more than 6 months often lose nutritive value. Nevertheless, short-term freezing of most food items is an economical and convenient way to store food. Freezing may actually increase the digestibility of certain plant materials by rupturing the cell wall and thereby making the cell contents more accessible at an earlier stage in the digestive process. Unfortunately, the freezing process has also been associated with a reduced thiamin content in certain species of fish (see Chapter 27).

Cooking some vegetables accomplishes the same function of breaking down cell walls as freezing but does not reduce the thiamin content, and this process may be helpful in softening hard vegetables, such as sweet potatoes. Recently steaming and canning insects and other foods for reptiles has become popular. The preservation of nutritive value with this process appears to be excellent and provides a reliable food source, if accepted by reptiles. (Fig. 16.21) Under normal circumstances, however, most herbivorous reptiles should be fed uncooked green leafy vegetables. Mustard greens, collard greens, turnip greens, dandelion greens, escarole, endive, and watercress are all excellent foods. Other nutritious vegetables to offer include squash, snap peas, and carrot tops. Vegetables to avoid in large quantities include cabbage, Brussels sprouts, cauliflower, broccoli, kale, bok choy, and radish because they contain goitrogenic substances (i.e., iodine-binding agents); however, these vegetables are safe when fed in moderation. Another group, including spinach, beets, and celery stalks, contain oxalic acid in a sufficient quantity to interfere with normal calcium uptake and metabolism but again can be safely fed in moderation. Many fruits are nutritious but are low in

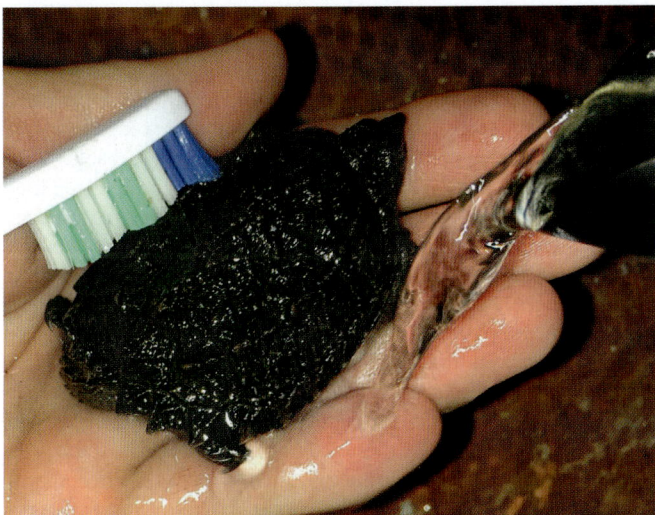

FIG 16.20 Hospitalized tortoises should be soaked in shallow water at least every other day. This author recommends soaking every hospitalized tortoise for at least a half hour every day. Bathing tortoises and turtles is also advisable as needed to help remove debris or old skin. Here a technician uses a soft bristle toothbrush to remove old skin from a juvenile snapping turtle (*Chelydra serpentina*).

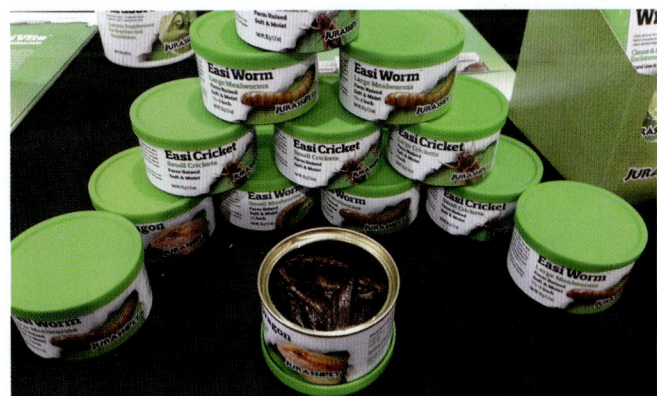

FIG 16.21 A wide variety of commercially prepared reptile foods are now available. Canning insects stabilizes the nutrient value and provides a reliable food source.

calcium or have a poor calcium to phosphorus ratio or both. Bananas and grapes also contain tannins, which can interfere with protein metabolism in reptiles. As with birds, avocados are generally considered toxic to reptiles, although it is not uncommon to see wild iguanas eating avocados that have fallen from trees. Rhubarb and eggplant are also believed by some to be toxic for reptiles. If concern exists over the safety of a food item, it is best left out of the captive diet.

Some flowers are considered safe and nutritious. The most notable and common among these are dandelions, hibiscus, and roses. Flowers that are toxic and extremely dangerous are azaleas, oleander, daffodils, and tulips. Marijuana is also toxic to reptiles (see Chapter 88 for more information on toxins).

The use of live prey food has been discouraged in the last few years, only utilized if necessary, and remains illegal in many countries. Reasons for this include the increased risk of injury to the captive reptile and the inhumanity associated with placing a frightened prey animal in with one of its predators. The latter observation notwithstanding, some benefits may exist to feeding live prey. First, the energy spent hunting and subduing food in a large enclosure represents a significant percentage of total energy expenditure for some reptiles. Second, the act of hunting may represent a series of necessary intellectual stimuli for the maintenance of normal behavior. Certainly, it is a survival skill that is needed if a reptile is to be released back into the wild. The combination of physical activity and intellectual stimulation helps to maintain a predatory reptile in "better fitness" than a stationary, stagnant, and stimulus-free environment. The same may be said for herbivorous reptiles, although the hunting behavior is limited to finding suitable forage.

Food may also serve as a vector or fomite for parasites, bacteria, fungi, or viruses. Clients must be advised to avoid wild-caught food and not to transfer food items from one cage to another.

The preferred foods of many reptiles are discussed in Chapter 27 and in detail in many references.[6,13,20,33,34,39] Generally, however, all snakes are carnivores, with foods ranging in size from insects, slugs, and earthworms to mammals the size of capybaras, deer, and antelope. Most snakes seen in practice are rodent or rabbit eaters, but a small percentage eat birds, fish, or other vertebrates (see Chapters 20, 22, and 27). Many lizards and turtles are also carnivorous, with foods ranging from insects to large rodents, birds, fish, and small deer. The entire family Varanidae (monitors), with a few rare exceptions, are carnivorous. The most commonly seen captive species (e.g., savannah, water, and Nile monitors) all are primarily small vertebrate feeders. The family Teiidae, commonly known as whiptails and tegus, occupy the same niche in the western hemisphere as the monitors do in the eastern hemisphere and eat primarily insects and small vertebrates. Certainly most members of the five other lizard families are insectivorous, namely the Scincidae (skinks), Chamaeleonidae (chameleons), Iguanidae (new world anoles, fence lizards, swifts, chuckwallas, and iguanas), Agamidae (old world lizards occupying the same niche as the new world iguanids [e.g., agamas, water dragons]), and Gekkonidae (geckos). Other species of lizards are herbivorous or omnivorous, including many of the species commonly kept as pets (e.g., green iguanas, bearded dragons) (see Chapters 21 and 27; for tuataras, see Chapter 26).

Most tortoises and turtles are herbivorous, but many are omnivorous and a few are primarily carnivorous. Box turtles (*Terrapene* sp. and *Cuora* sp.) and hingeback tortoises (*Kinyxis* sp.) are examples of chelonians that are primarily carnivorous. Among aquatic turtles, carnivorous or scavenging species include mud turtles (family Kinosternidae), chicken turtles (*Deirochelys reticularia*), and snapping turtles (*Chelydra serpentina* and *Macroclemmys temmincki*) (see Chapters 23, 24, and 27).

Crocodilians are all carnivorous, with adults preferred prey varying from fish in some species to mammals and birds in others. The young

of all species of crocodilians may consume some insects but rapidly switch to vertebrate prey, which has a higher calcium content (see Chapters 25 and 27).

Knowledge of these basic diets is helpful in establishing guidelines for captive and hospitalized reptiles. In an emergency situation, leafy greens or a high-quality pelletized rodent food may be used for herbivorous reptiles, a (quality) canned dog food may be used for an omnivorous reptile, and a (quality) canned cat food may be used for a carnivorous reptile. The latter two options, however, may be too high in protein for long-term use in many reptiles. Gout or renal disease can result from such diets. Better nutrition for hospitalized reptiles can be provided by utilizing diets prepared specifically for this purpose. These include the Critical Care Diets (Oxbow Pet Products) or Emeraid Critical Care Diets (LaFeberVet).

Be aware that concentrated pelletized diets, if used as the primary diet of a reptile, even those marketed as "balanced" diets, may lead to nutritional disorders. A variety of foods that may include some pellets is always preferable to any monotypic diet.

Fruits may have limited nutritional value but are often added to diets to stimulate consumption for herbivorous reptiles. Reptiles are capable of seeing color. Brightly colored fruits such as strawberries, tomatoes, bananas, and melons often attract the attention of many herbivorous lizards and tortoises and invite consumption. These are particularly valuable in many cases to entice recently captured or ill animals to eat, and they contain large quantities of water. Yellow (summer) squash and cooked sweet potato are also brightly colored and can be valuable additions to the diet of many herbivorous reptiles. Some lizards, such as *Uromastyx*, consume significant quantities of seeds in the wild, so a variety of seeds should be included as part of the captive diet.

Monoculture insects raised in captivity are also often of questionable value as a balanced diet. Captive raised crickets and mealworms often have a low calcium content and must be "fortified" to improve nutrition. Perhaps the most widely accepted method of raising the calcium content is to "dust" these food items with calcium powder; however, feeding the insects a high calcium diet for 24 hours or more before feeding them to a reptile has been shown to be more efficient at providing the needed calcium to the reptile.[40] This is referred to as "gut loading" in the herpetological vernacular. Current recommendations are to gut load and dust to provide maximum levels of calcium (see Chapter 27).

Regarding gut-loading diets, there are several commercially available. However, all gut-loading diets are not the same. Many feature powdered calcium in the metallic form, mixed with a food source (e.g., oatmeal). Only a small percentage of calcium in this form is absorbable by the reptile, whereas calcium in the chelated form, as found in green leafy vegetables, is highly absorbable. Hence, gut-loading insects with shredded turnip greens (7/1 calcium to phosphorus ratio), collard greens (3/1 calcium to phosphorus ratio), or other greens is preferable to a powdered gut-load diet. Furthermore, the cubed (gel) calcium supplements are not by themselves a satisfactory gut-load meal. In one study performed by the author, hatchling insectivorous snakes (ground snakes, *Sonora semiannulata*) were fed crickets gut loaded with turnip greens or calcium gel cubes. Those that were fed crickets gut loaded with turnip greens developed normally, while those fed crickets gut loaded solely with calcium gel cubes developed multiple kinks in the spine. In addition, numerous juvenile lizards have been presented to the author in practice with signs of nutritional secondary hyperparathyroidism, where the history included being fed crickets gut loaded solely with these cubes.

Mice and rats raised in captivity are usually considered to be a good quality food source. However, the nutritional quality of these rodents is affected by what they have been fed. Rodents fed a diet exclusively of dog food have a tendency to be fat and "greasy," and snakes and monitors that have eaten rodents fed this way also have a tendency to become obese. Many rat and corn snakes (*Pantherophis*) that develop lipomas have a common history of primarily feeding on a diet of ex-breeder mice or mice fed primarily a dog food diet. Feeding reptiles young lean mice that have been fed a high-quality, plant-based rodent chow provides a healthier diet. Additionally a high-quality food should be available to the rodents until the time they are fed to the reptile. These gut contents probably contain valuable nutrients and roughage, and thus, multivitamin and mineral supplementation for rodent feeders is usually not considered necessary, because properly fed rodents represent a complete diet (entire rodent ingested). In fact, one study showed no significant difference in size, weight, or bone density in two groups of hatchling corn snakes fed supplemented and nonsupplemented mice (Backner B, personal communication, 1991).

Herbivorous reptiles need a quality vitamin and mineral supplement. However, the vitamin and mineral requirements for most reptiles have not been determined, and most recommendations are anecdotal. Oversupplementation has occurred when vitamins, especially fat-soluble vitamins, are administered too frequently or in large quantities. Also, oversupplementation does not always balance an otherwise deficient diet (i.e., appropriate vitamin and mineral intake in the absence of sufficient roughage may still result in an unhealthy reptile). As in mammals, sometimes oversupplementation of one nutrient may result in a deficiency of another. In most cases, calcium dusting should occur with every meal, while multivitamin and mineral supplementation once weekly or every other week is usually sufficient (see Chapter 27).

Stress

Stress is an important factor for captive reptiles (see Chapter 15). Stress is difficult to define but may be thought of as the increased energy required for a reptile to maintain itself, compared with that which is required in the normal habitat (see Fig. 16.19). Reptiles generally can survive for prolonged periods in captivity and may reproduce if they are maintained in low-stress environments. Clean adequately sized cages with the proper substrate, thermal gradients, light quality and photoperiod, ventilation, and humidity are considered important physical requirements to reduce stress in the captive environment. Predators, competitors, parasites, and pathogens are biological factors that must be controlled to reduce stress, but these factors act independently to increase the morbidity and mortality of captive reptiles in high-stress environments.

Constantly changing cages, substrates, cage accessories, or cage mates adds stress to the life of a captive reptile. Adding or interacting with a cage mate is likely the most stressful factor in a confined captive reptile's environment. See the discussion on "big reptile, little reptile syndrome" in the section on multi-individual and multispecies enclosures. Even a change of keepers may add stress. However, many reptiles, once they adjust to a certain routine, adapt well to captive maintenance.

Other factors that may contribute to stress include handling or disruption. In addition, placing a cage in a high traffic area with associated vibration can be stressful. We often advise our clients not to handle any anorexic reptile until the animals have adapted and are feeding regularly.

CONCLUSION

Reptile clinicians should be aware that reptiles are not domestic pets. Even though some species are bred extensively in captivity, millions of years of evolution cannot be erased in a few generations of captive propagation. As wild animals in captivity, they need a recreation of many of the physical and biological features of their natural habitat. Successful management of reptiles in a contrived environment requires

veterinarians to become familiar with the habitat (particularly the substrate likely to be found where the reptile lives), diet, and preferred temperature range of the species in question. We need to approximate those parameters as close as possible in the captive setting. The same is true for biological factors. Will competition with other animals negatively impact them or stimulate normal activity? Are the animals in question social in nature or asocial (i.e., only interacting with the same species during mating season)? If there is any doubt, it may be safer to house reptiles alone.

Some reptile species appear to be more adaptable than others. Those which occupy large geographic ranges in nature with a broad diet may be considered more adaptable. Many of these adaptable species have the ability to tolerate a wide range of captive habitats. As clinicians we need to be aware of ideal temperature, lighting, and humidity range for our patients so that we can guide our clients. For all captive reptiles, whether the natural history is well known or not, the safest and best way to prevent problems is to provide environmental gradients. Not only should a thermal gradient be provided but also a humidity and lighting gradient. In this manner, the reptile may choose the microenvironment that best suits it for the function at hand, such as digestion, reproduction, or immune system stimulation.

Finally veterinarians and herpetoculturists must strive to go beyond just providing the correct environment. Attempts should be made to provide an enriched environment.[41] In recent years, herpetoculturists have developed a variety of inventions to help reduce stress in captive reptiles by enriching the captive environment. Some of those recent innovations are illustrated in these figures (Figs. 16.22, 16.23, and 16.24). Ultimately reptile enclosures should be large and enriched to allow the reptile to have "needs fulfilled" and practical enough for the keeper to be able to keep that reptile "healthy" (see Fig. 16.25).

Inappropriately housed reptiles may survive but not thrive. This difference between ideal and a deficient captive environment can result in stress, and chronic stress leads to reproductive failure, disease, and death.[42]

To summarize, the first step in successfully treating reptiles is the examination of the captive environment and the second step is educating the client on how to correct errors in the captive environment. Thus, as mentioned early in this chapter, success with maintaining captive reptiles involves both client education and correcting the environment ($S_R = CE^2$).

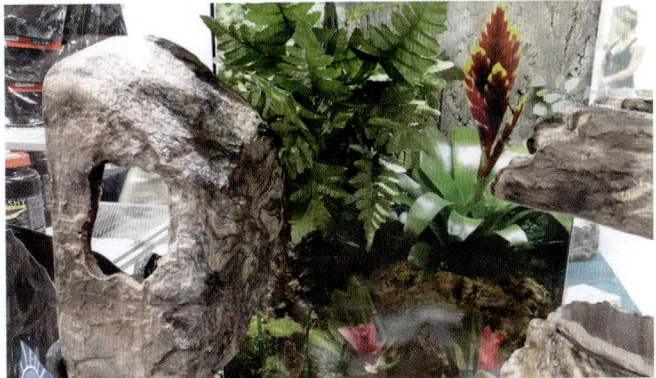

FIG 16.22 Magnetized devices are available that allow ledges, hiding areas, and water sources to be placed at elevated locations in aquariums for arboreal reptiles.

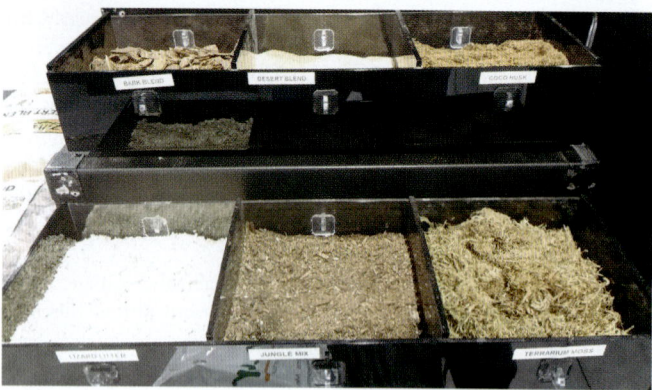

FIG 16.23 The substrate or bottom material is an important component of the captive reptile environment. Herpetoculturists may select from a wide variety of naturalistic substrates, which vary in texture, particle size, absorbency, and the physical support that they provide to a reptile. Many substrates also provide additional hiding areas, which can reduce captive stress.

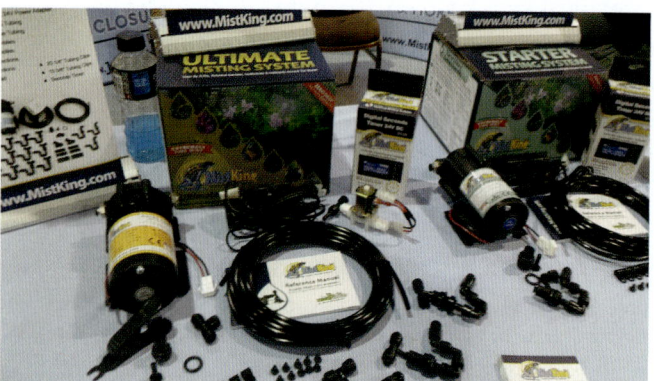

FIG 16.24 Misting devices have become increasingly popular and are adaptable to a variety of cage sizes.

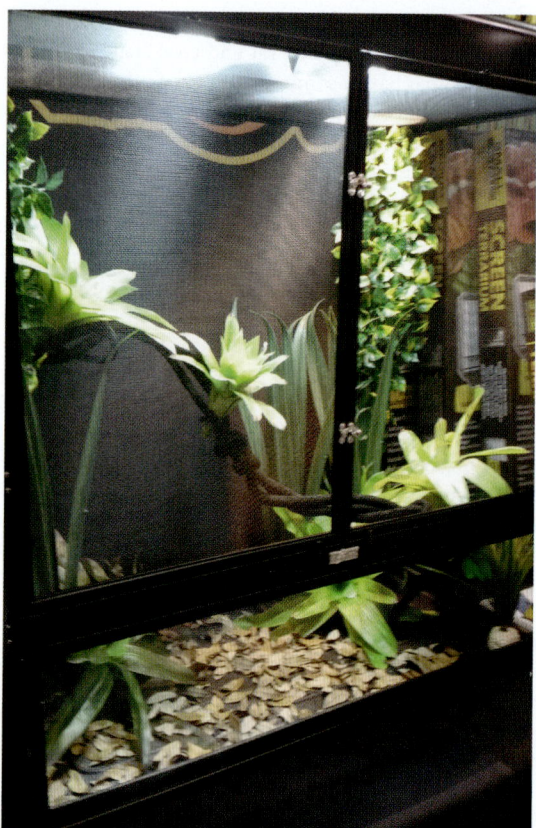

FIG 16.25 The "ideal" reptile enclosure provides all of the requirements discussed, including correct size, excellent ventilation, lighting, temperature and humidity control (and gradients), a naturalistic substrate suitable for the species in question, and environmental enrichment.

ACKNOWLEDGMENTS

I would like to thank the late Sean McKeown for setting the standard for this chapter in the first edition and all of his guidance in so many areas of herpetoculture. I would also like to thank Brian R. Eisele, senior reptile curator at the Jacksonville Zoological Garden, as well as Chris Lechowicz, director of wildlife habitat management at the Sanibel-Captiva Conservation Foundation, for sharing their experiences. Vic Morgan and Michael Pilch, experienced herpetoculturists, also provided me with some excellent suggestions. In addition, I would like to extend thanks to the staff of Riverside Animal Hospital in Jacksonville, Florida, for their suggestions on practical solutions to common reptile problems.

REFERENCES

See www.expertconsult.com for a complete list of references.

17

Environmental Lighting

Frances M. Baines and Lara M. Cusack

In nature, sunlight interacts with features of a reptile's environment, creating a microhabitat with superimposed gradients of heat, light, and ultraviolet (UV), extending from full sun into full shade. Reptiles utilize these gradients for thermoregulation and, at least in some cases, for UV photoregulation[1,2]; they do so by self-regulating their exposure to solar radiation. Deviations from the optimal range are likely to act as stressors, with negative repercussions on health. Providing a suitable photo-microhabitat in captivity is, however, challenging. To date, very few field studies have recorded the daily light and UV exposure of wild reptiles of any species; this work has been pioneered by Drs. Gary Ferguson and William Gehrmann and colleagues at Texas Christian University.[3,4] Natural sunlight varies constantly, its spectrum and radiance determined by the solar altitude (the height of the sun in the sky) and the degree of cloud cover, as well as the degree of shading from features within the landscape. In a typical vivarium, a lamp is either on or off, and its spectrum and radiance vary little, if at all, over the course of a day. However, it is possible to utilize combinations of lamps to create full spectrum gradients from ultraviolet to infrared. Although artificial lighting cannot replicate natural sunlight it can, when used properly, make a huge contribution to reptile husbandry.

NATURAL SUNLIGHT

Free-living reptiles, even crepuscular and nocturnal species, utilize every part of the solar spectrum from ultraviolet to infrared (Fig. 17.1). Their exposure levels are determined by their microhabitat and their daily activity patterns. Sunlight includes short-wavelength infrared (IR-A), so-called visible light (visible to humans) and ultraviolet (UV), subdivided into UVA and UVB from around 290 to 295 nm (depending on solar altitude). Earth's atmosphere blocks hazardous shorter wavelengths (UVB below 290 nm and UVC) from reaching the surface.

Infrared

Short-wavelength infrared (IR-A) is responsible for the warming effect of sunlight. Sunlight reaching the earth's surface passes through water vapor, which absorbs certain infrared wavelengths. This "water-filtered IR-A" passes through the epidermis, reaching the internal organs of small-bodied reptiles, without excessively heating water molecules in the tissues.[5,6] IR-A also warms the surface of the earth, which reradiates in longer wavelengths (IR-B and IR-C). Long-wavelength infrared does not penetrate the epidermis, but transfers all of its energy as heat,[7] which is conducted or carried by convection in bodily fluids to deeper tissues. Infrared is invisible to humans and most reptiles, although some snakes can perceive the longer wavelengths (above 3000 nm) through their facial pit organs.

Visible Light and UVA

Most reptiles have full color vision, in which UVA is a vital component, with wavelengths from 350 nm (within the UVA band) to those at the boundary with infrared being visible. The presence of UVA-reflective markings on many animals and plants aids in the recognition of conspecifics and food. Some nocturnal reptiles even have good color vision in dim moonlight, in which humans see no color at all.

In addition to enabling conscious vision, sunlight reaches nonvisual photoreceptors in the reptile retina, pineal body, and parietal eye (when present), and even deep brain photoreceptors that respond to light filtering through the skull.[8] Information is relayed to a complex neuroendocrine network controlling daily and seasonal behaviors, including activity levels, thermoregulation, the immune system, and the reproductive cycle, and which is mediated via hormones secreted by the pituitary (Fig. 17.1).

UVB

The amount of UVB in sunlight depends on the solar altitude, because the earth's atmosphere absorbs and scatters UV light, affecting the shortest wavelengths most strongly. When the sun is low in the sky, near dawn or sunset, the sun's rays have a longer path through the atmosphere, so more filtering occurs, leaving only traces of UVB in the spectrum. As the sun rises, the total UVB rises, reaching a maximum with the sun directly overhead. The dose of UVB received by a reptile therefore depends on the time of day when sun exposure occurs. A wild reptile's photo-microhabitat may bear little resemblance to solar data collected by meteorological stations; climate data is rarely indicative.

UVB and warmth are required for cutaneous vitamin D3 synthesis in reptiles. A cholesterol in the epidermis, 7-dehydroxycholesterol (7DHC), is converted to previtamin D_3 when exposed to short-wavelength UVB (range 290 nm–315 nm). This undergoes a temperature-dependent isomerization into vitamin D_3, which enters the bloodstream. This process has been demonstrated in both diurnal and crepuscular lizards and snakes. The vital vitamin D pathways (endocrine, autocrine, and paracrine)[9] are summarized in Fig. 17.1. For more details, see Chapters 27, 79, and 84. Overproduction of vitamin D_3 is prevented by the conversion of excess previtamin D_3 and vitamin D_3 in the skin into inert photoproducts by UVB and short-wavelength UVA (range 290 nm–335 nm). UVB in sunlight also has direct effects on the skin: it acts as an effective disinfectant, modulates the immune system, improves skin barrier functions, and upregulates melanin synthesis.

Utilizing Natural Sunlight

Many reptiles, especially basking species, benefit from outdoor enclosures where they can experience natural sunlight. Ambient temperatures must

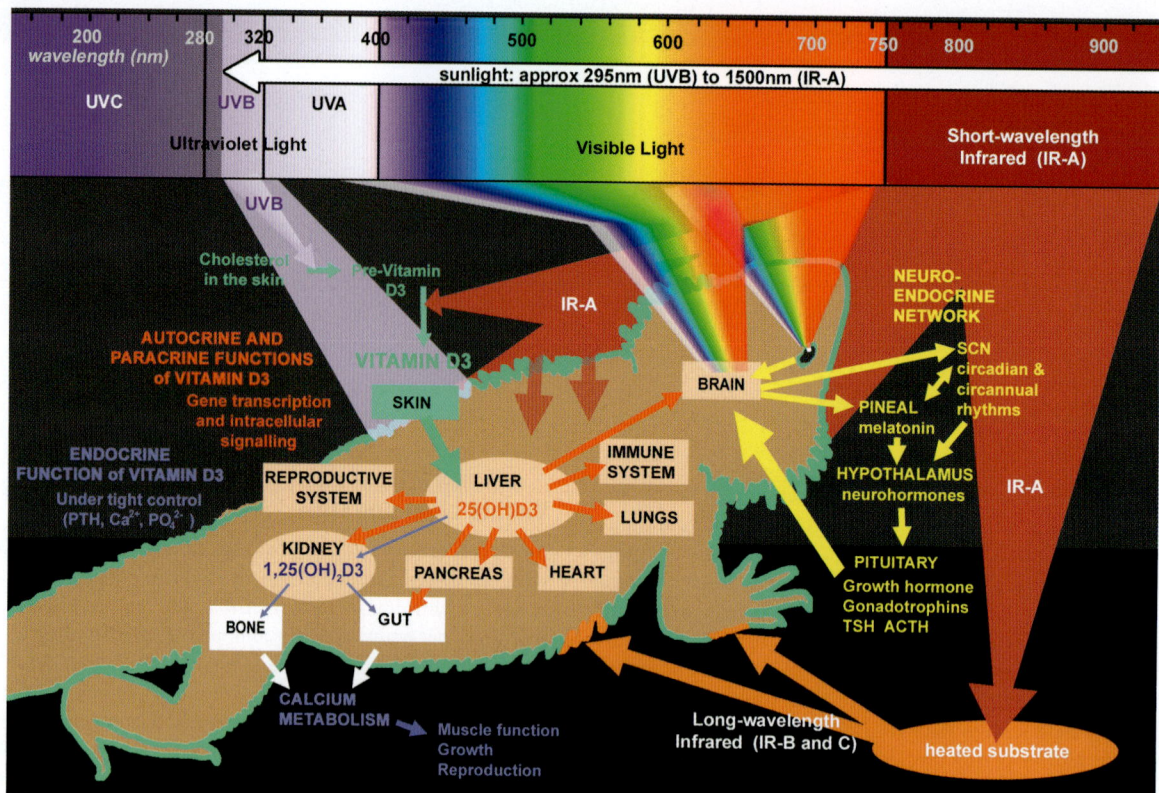

FIG 17.1 Reptiles utilize every part of the solar spectrum. (Courtesy of Frances M. Baines.)

be suitable, and the amount of direct sunlight required will depend on the species. All enclosures must provide areas of full shade and shelter. "Greenhouse"-type shelters may be glazed with special UV-transmitting acrylic sheets ("sunbed acrylics"), allowing up to 80% transmission of UVB, or low iron glass, which may allow 50% transmission. Horticultural UV-transmitting plastic sheeting, with up to 65% UVB transmission, can be used to create covers for more temporary outdoor shelters and polytunnels. Care must be taken to avoid excess heat buildup caused by direct sunlight through glass or plastics into restricted airspaces. Glass tanks and vivariums should never be placed in direct sunlight as lethal temperatures can swiftly develop. Natural sunlight can rarely be utilized inside unmodified buildings. Ordinary window glass and most plastics block all UVB and some UVA.

ELECTROMAGNETIC RADIATION

To be successful, vivarium lighting must create superimposed heat, visible light, and UV gradients similar to those found in nature. Sun-basking species will require a basking zone with a gradient into full shade, allowing the reptile to self-regulate its exposure. It is virtually impossible to simulate sunlight using just one type of lamp, but combining simple incandescent bulbs ("basking lamps"), lamps emitting additional visible light, and specialist UV-emitting products can be very effective.

Infrared
Ceramic Heaters, Panel Heaters, and Heat Mats. These emit only long-wavelength infrared (IR-B and IR-C), which can put an excessive heat load on the upper epidermis and increase the risk of thermal burns. They make excellent background or nighttime heaters but are not suitable for basking zones. The absence of a visible light output is

also a significant disadvantage, as many reptiles use light as a cue for locating a basking area.

Incandescent Lamps. Basic tungsten or halogen lamps are widely used to create basking zones. Their spectrum contains no UVB and very little blue or UVA. Orange and red visible light and short-wavelength infrared (IR-A) predominate, but this IR-A includes the wavelengths removed from natural sunlight by atmospheric moisture. They also emit longer-wavelength IR-B and some IR-C. Intense exposure may overheat the skin surface and water molecules in the epidermis before deeper structures reach optimum temperatures. To minimize the risk of thermal burns, the basking zone must cover an area at least as large as the whole body of the animal, and the radiation must be evenly distributed, with no focal hot spots. "Flood" bulbs (with beam angles of 30 degrees or more) are essential. Basking zones for large reptiles are best created with a cluster of several lower-wattage bulbs rather than with one high-wattage lamp.

Thermal imaging (Fig. 17.2A and B) demonstrates the contrast between the uniform body temperature of a reptile basking in natural sunlight and the extremely localized heating provided by a "spot" basking lamp. The head and limbs of the animal may remain at ambient (air) temperature. Such abnormal heating of a tortoise carapace may contribute to localized dehydration and development of pyramiding deformities in captive tortoises.[10] A reptile may remain under such a lamp long enough for serious burns to occur, typically over the shoulders and cranial coelomic spine (Fig. 17.2C). For further details, see Chapters 69 and 169.

Incandescent lamps should be controlled using dimming thermostats. Surface temperatures underneath basking lamps need to be measured directly, as they are very different from ambient (air) temperatures. Noncontact infrared thermometers (so-called "temperature guns") are ideal for this purpose.

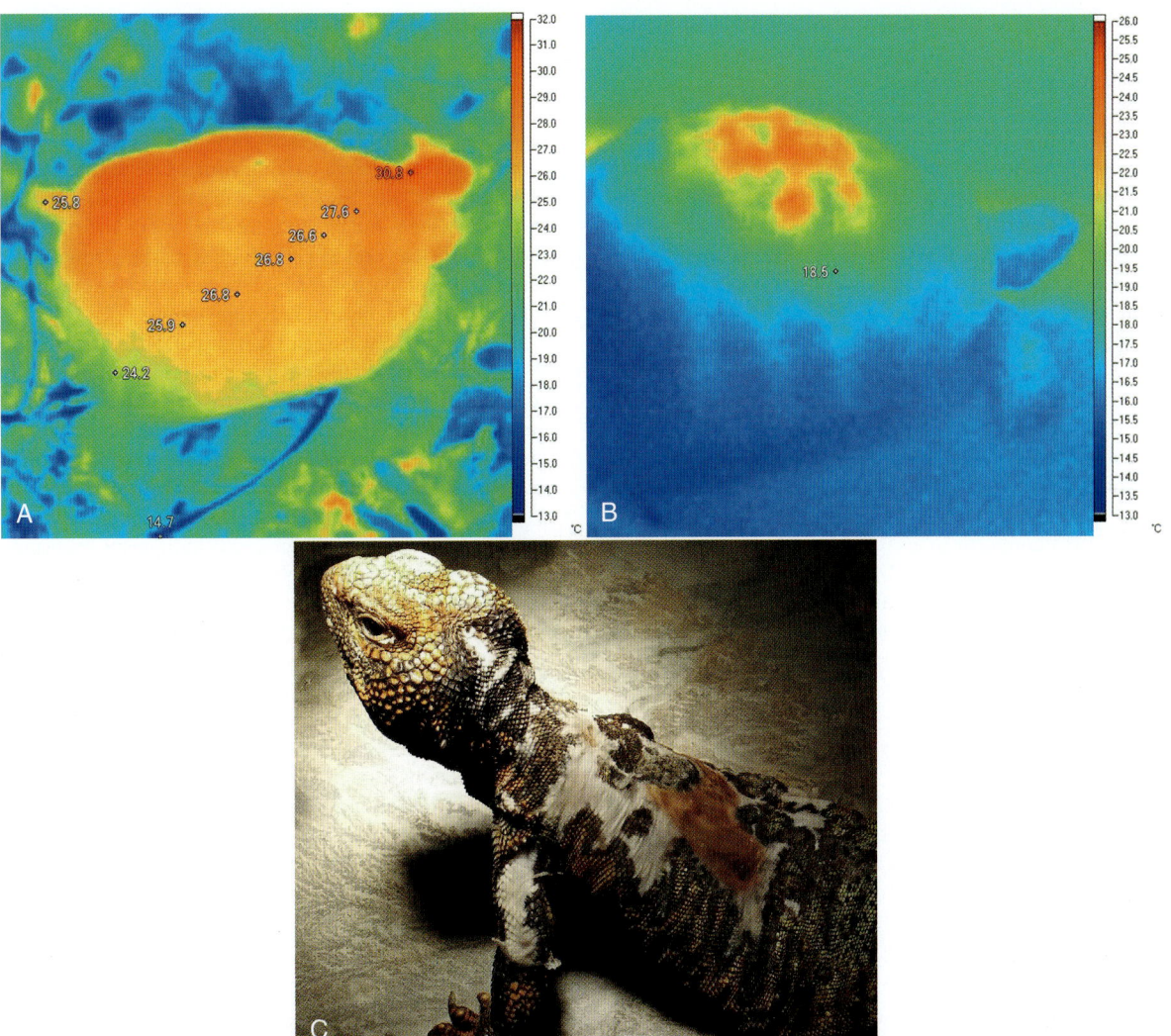

FIG 17.2 (A) Thermal image: Wild *Testudo graeca*, basking in natural sunlight, Murcia, Spain. (B) Thermal image: *Testudo graeca* in captivity, basking under a 100-watt "spot" lamp. (C) Moroccan Uromastyx (*Uromastyx acanthinuris*) recovering from severe thermal burns from inappropriate "spot" basking lamp. Note typical location of burned skin. (A and B, Courtesy of A.C. Highfield; C, courtesy of D. Chatham.)

Visible Light

"Daylight" Fluorescent Tubes and Compact Lamps. Sometimes misleadingly called "full-spectrum," these emit no UVB and very little UVA but can be useful for improving general light levels in cooler areas of a vivarium.

Metal Halides. High-quality "daylight" metal halide lamps, such as those used for freshwater aquaria and display lighting in store windows, can reproduce the full brilliance of sunlight, including UVA (but no UVB) and significant infrared. These are high-intensity discharge (HID) lamps requiring external ballasts and cannot be used with a proportional/dimming thermostat. Positioning them directly above the vivarium is crucial because ocular damage can occur if they are placed in an animal's direct line of sight.

LED Lighting. There are two types of LED currently available:
(1) "White" LEDs, which use a blue LED and a phosphor to simulate white light. The spectrum of these contains no UVA or UVB and is deficient in cyan and red.
(2) LEDs that emit just one color, in a very narrow band of wavelengths. "White" is created using a combination of red, blue, and green LEDs in a single bulb. However, this light will not appear white to any reptile, owing to their different visual range from humans. Neither type of LED should be the primary light source in a vivarium. However, they may be suitable for supplementary lighting or for enhancing plant growth.

In the near future lamps may be developed that utilize multiple LEDs covering a wide range of wavelengths from UVB to infrared, creating a more sunlike spectrum. A recent trial of a prototype

UVB-emitting LED lamp by one of the current authors (L.M.C.) has shown promising results with regard to cutaneous vitamin D_3 synthesis in bearded dragons (*Pogona vitticeps*).[11]

Colored Lamps. These should be avoided, since reptiles need full-spectrum, white light during the day for normal color vision and nonvisual perception. Neodymium coatings do not improve the spectrum of an incandescent bulb; they merely absorb some yellow wavelengths so that the light appears more "blue" to a human observer. The use of red and blue lamps at night is also extremely unnatural as reptiles can see both colors. Reptiles should not be illuminated at night; their circadian rhythms require regular periods of darkness and daylight.

Ultraviolet

There are five main types of UVB-emitting lamps that are commonly available, all of which also emit significant UVA and visible light (Fig. 17.3).

Regular T8 UVB fluorescent tubes (diameter 25 mm) have a low, well-diffused output (Figs. 17.3A and 17.4A). T5-high output (T5-HO) UVB fluorescent tubes (diameter 16 mm) can have a much higher output, especially when used with a reflector (Figs. 17.3A and 17.4B) Very wide UVB coverage can be obtained for large vivaria and zoo enclosures using multiple T5-HO tubes in reflective fixtures.

Compact fluorescent UVB lamps (Figs. 17.3B and 17.4C) have a well-diffused but very steep UV gradient and limited range. They are only suitable for use in small vivaria.

Mercury vapor UVB lamps (Fig. 17.3C) are self-ballasted HID lamps, which do not require a ballast. They can have a high UV output, but all have a poor visible spectrum. Lamps with clear front glass produce very narrow beams, creating "hot spots" of either UV or infrared; these must be avoided in favor of those with coatings diffusing and widening the beam.

UVB-emitting metal halides, a relatively new development (Figs. 17.3D and 17.4D), produce intense visible light, UVA and UVB. Many brands have fairly narrow beams, however; wide flood versions should be chosen to create large basking zones. Like all metal halides, these need external ballasts; "kits" are available that include a lamp, a matching ballast, and a lamp-holder. Both mercury vapor and metal halide bulbs produce sufficient heat to contribute to basking zones but cannot be controlled by a proportional/dimming thermostat, so previously discussed cautions regarding infrared radiation apply.

Brands vary widely in their UVB output. High-quality products from well-known brands should be chosen to ensure suitable spectra, output, and longevity although even these will show some individual variability. Manufacturers' recommended distances should be carefully observed. Independent test results for a range of lamps are available on the internet (e.g., http://www.uvguide.co.uk) but only provide rough guides, since UV at the level of the reptile is affected by external factors such as the presence of reflectors, which can greatly increase the irradiance beneath a lamp, or mesh screens, which physically block 30% to 50% of visible light and UV. The effect of aluminum reflectors and a typical mesh "vivarium screen top" on the output of a T5-HO UVB fluorescent tube is shown in Fig. 17.5. Lamp output also declines with use, mainly due to solarization of the glass: most lamps show a sharp initial fall in UVB output over the first few days of use (the "burning-in period") followed by a much slower loss over weeks and months. Ideally, owners should purchase a UV meter and test their lamps *in situ* at the closest lamp-to-reptile distance, repeating the tests monthly to monitor decay. Some veterinarians offer a lamp testing service, but care must be taken not to expose staff to a UV-radiation hazard. The most suitable meter currently available is the Solarmeter 6.5 UV Index Meter (Solartech Inc., Glenside, PA), also sold

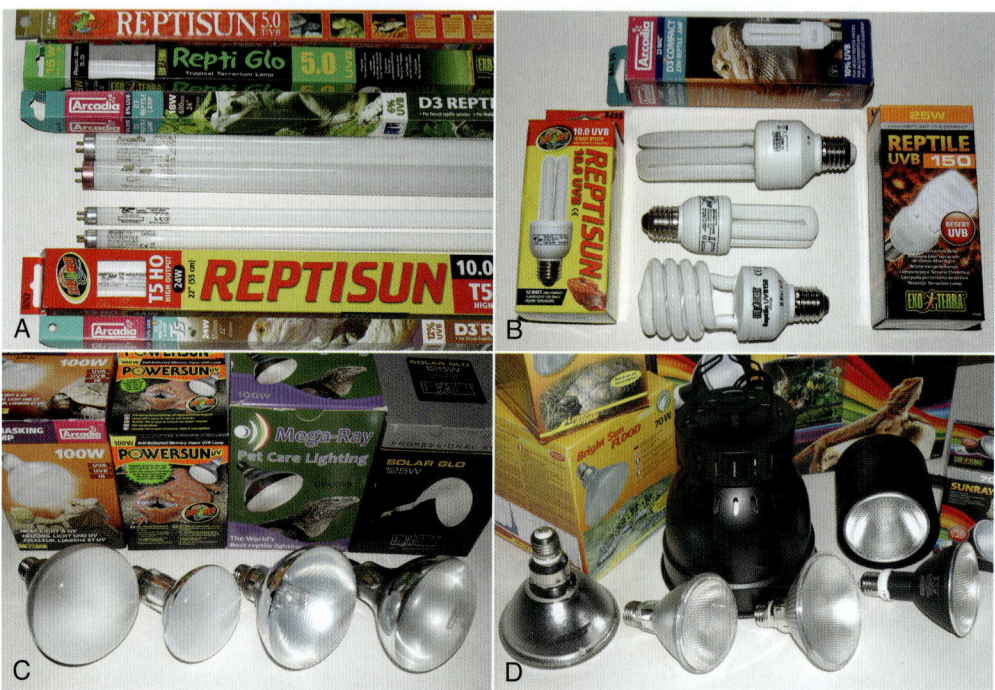

FIG 17.3 Examples of specialist UVB-emitting lamps used in reptile husbandry. (A) Fluorescent tubes: regular T8 (2.5 cm diameter) and high-output T5-HO (16 mm diameter). (B) Compact fluorescent lamps, available as coil- or bar-type lamps in a range of styles. (C) Self-ballasted mercury vapor lamps. (D) Metal halide lamps, sold with matching external ballasts and lamp-holders. (Courtesy of Frances M. Baines.)

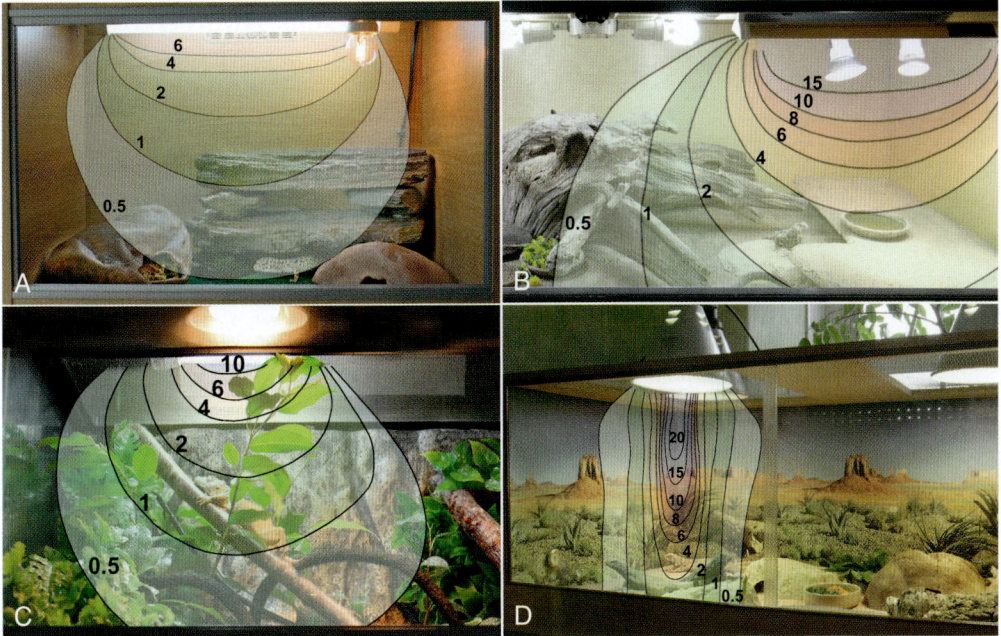

FIG 17.4 Creating UV, light, and heat gradients. Overlaid iso-irradiance charts visualize the UV index gradients. (A) Shade method using regular T8 5% UVB fluorescent tube and diffuse halogen lighting for leopard gecko (*Eublepharis macularius*) vivarium. (B) Sunbeam method using T5-HO 12% UVB fluorescent tube with aluminum reflector, twin halogen floodlamps, and non-UVB compact fluorescent lamps for *Uromastyx yemenensis* vivarium. (C) Shade method using 6% UVB compact fluorescent lamp and halogen reflector, both above mesh, for gargoyle gecko (*Rhacodactylus auriculatus*) vivarium. (D) Sunbeam method using 150W PAR38 flood UVB metal halide with PAR38 halogen floodlamp and non-UVB metal halide for chuckwalla (*Sauromalus ater*) vivarium. (A, C, and D, Courtesy of Frances M. Baines; B, courtesy of M.J. Versweyveld and Frances M. Baines.)

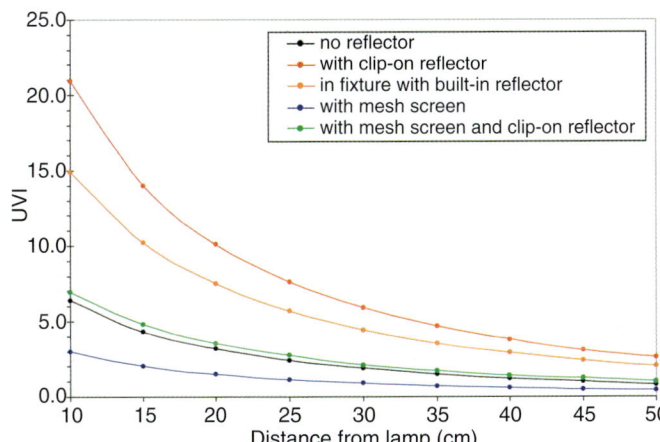

FIG 17.5 The effect of reflectors and mesh upon UV irradiance in the vivarium. UV index recordings made at increasing distances directly beneath the midpoint of a T5-HO UVB fluorescent tube (Arcadia T5 D3+ 12%UVB 24 watt lamp; Arcadia Products plc., Redhill, UK). When the tube was fitted with a clip-on aluminum reflector (Arcadia T5 Reflector; Arcadia Products plc., Redhill, UK) readings increased by 218%. Mounting the tube in a fixture with an integral aluminum reflector (Sunblaster T5 fixture; FHD Europe, Tyne & Wear, UK) increased readings by 138%. Placing a thick flyscreen mesh vivarium screen (Komodo screen top cover; Happy Pet Products Ltd., Syston, UK) under the tube reduced output by 52%. However, use of the clip-on reflector counteracted the effect of the screen. (Courtesy of Frances M. Baines and Lara M. Cusack.)

under the brand name ZooMed Digital UV Index Radiometer (ZooMed Laboratories Inc., San Luis Obispo, CA). The sensitivity response of this meter follows the action spectrum for vitamin D_3 synthesis fairly closely, making this meter suitable for estimating UV from both sunlight and lamps. Cheap "sun-smart" UV index meters should not be used; typically they do not register short wavelength UVB and are unable to give accurate readings with reptile lamps.

The Solarmeter 6.2 UVB meter is another handheld meter that has been popular for many years. This gives a readout in microwatts per square centimeter ($\mu W/cm^2$) and measures the total UVB output (from 280 nm–320 nm). However, this is a less helpful measurement when comparing the output of reptile lamps with each other and with natural sunlight, because the photobiological activity of UV is wavelength-dependent. Short-wavelength UVB is far more effective than long-wavelength UVB in enabling vitamin D synthesis—and in causing cellular damage. So if a lamp has a greater proportion of its UVB output in the shorter wavelengths, then less total UVB will be needed to have the same biologic effect as another lamp (or sunlight), which has a greater proportion of its output in the longer wavelengths. Most reptile lamps do have a significantly higher proportion of short-wavelength UVB than sunlight; total UVB readings from sunlight cannot therefore be used as a guide to suitable UVB levels from reptile lamps, because overirradiation may result.

However, the Solarmeter 6.5 has a sensitivity response weighted toward the shorter wavelengths. If any UVB lamp gives a reading of UVI 3.0, for example, with a Solarmeter 6.5 then its "strength" is likely to be similar to sunlight of UVI 3.0 regardless of the total UVB recorded.

TABLE 17.1   Meter Readings: UV Index, Total UVB, and Visible Light

Distance From Lamp (cm)	UV INDEX				TOTAL UVB (µW/cm²)				ILLUMINANCE (lux)			
	20	30	40	50	20	30	40	50	20	30	40	50
T8 Fluorescent Tubes (610 mm 18–20 watt)												
ZooMed Reptisun 10.0 T8	1.5	0.9	0.6	0.4	50	31	20	15	748	448	302	222
Arcadia D3+ 12% Reptile UVB T8	1.5	0.9	0.6	0.4	45	28	18	13	631	383	263	186
Arcadia D3+ 12% Reptile UVB T8 with reflector	3.2	2.0	1.3	0.9	100	61	40	29	1710	1035	692	494
T5 High Output Fluorescent Tubes (550 mm 24 watt)												
ZooMed Reptisun 10.0 T5-HO	3.2	1.9	1.3	0.9	103	62	41	28	1220	738	485	343
Arcadia D3+ Reptile 12% UVB T5	3.1	1.8	1.2	0.8	109	65	42	30	1420	831	545	384
Arcadia D3+ Dragon 14% UVB T5	4.6	2.7	1.8	1.2	131	79	52	36	1460	882	586	418
Arcadia D3+ Dragon 14% UVB T5 with reflector	(13.1)	7.8	5.0	3.5	381	225	146	103	4250	2590	1680	1206
Compact Fluorescent Lamps (20–26 watt)												
ExoTerra Reptile UVB 200	1.8	0.9	0.5	0.3	46	23	13	9	1050	580	374	276
Arcadia D3+ 10%UVB Compact Reptile Lamp	1.4	0.6	0.4	0.2	48	23	13	9	1107	535	323	223
ZooMed ReptiSun 10.0 Compact Lamp	1.8	0.9	0.4	0.3	55	26	15	10	1520	761	441	299
Metal Halide Lamps												
Lucky Reptile Bright Sun UV Desert 70 watt	(14.8)	6.8	3.6	2.1	446	202	108	67	(>200,000)	94,200	51,500	32,500
Lucky Reptile Bright Sun Flood Jungle 150 watt	(14.1)	6.3	3.5	2.1	499	225	120	72	(>200,000)	(>200,000)	(142,900)	84,400
ExoTerra SunRay 35 watt PAR30	(26.2)	(10.3)	5.4	3.3	670	264	139	84	72,200	29,400	15,200	9060
ExoTerra SunRay 70 watt PAR30	(17.3)	7.4	4.0	2.4	615	262	141	85	(>200,000)	84,500	45,300	28,200
Mercury Vapor Lamps												
ExoTerra Solar Glo 160 watt	1.7	1.0	0.5	0.4	33	19	11	8	15,900	8070	5140	3500
ZooMed Powersun 160 watt	8.5	4.7	2.9	2.0	157	83	52	36	11,500	6020	3730	2600
Arcadia D3 Basking Lamp 160 watt	(13.0)	6.4	3.8	2.5	245	122	72	48	12,700	6300	3900	2670
Natural Tropical Sunlight: October 4th 2006 Kakadu, NT, Australia. Latitude 12°39′ S												
09:00h Solar altitude 40°		3.5				175				117,300		
10:00h Solar altitude 50°		7.6				312				128,000		
12:30h Solar altitude 80°		13.5				457				130,400		

UV index (Solarmeter 6.5), total UVB (Solarmeter 6.2), and lux motor (SkyTronic LX101-600.620) readings from individual samples of reptile lamps and natural tropical sunlight. (Numbers in brackets: UV Index/lux too high–lamp is unsuitable at this distance.) Lamps all in use for 100 hours before testing; measurements taken after 30 minutes warm-up. No mesh, glass, or plastic between lamp and meter; no reflectors used except where indicated.
Source: Frances M. Baines (unpublished data).

Table 17.1 gives examples of UVI, total UVB, and visible light (lux) meter readings from a range of lamps on sale at the time of writing, with solar readings for comparison.

Estimating the UV Requirement: the Ferguson Zone Concept. Ferguson and colleagues recorded the daily UV exposure of 15 reptile species and placed these into four sun exposure ranges or "zones," since designated as "UVB zones" or "Ferguson zones" (Fig. 17.6).[3,4] They suggested that knowledge of any species' microhabitat and basking behavior enables an estimate of its range of UV exposure, with the average daily exposure used as a suitable "midbackground" level of UV and the recorded maximum UVI used as the upper acceptable limit for the UV gradient in captivity. This concept has been used to develop a living document estimating suitable UV ranges for more than 250 species of reptiles and amphibians.[12]

Two methods of providing UVB are described. A "shade method" provides low-level "background" UV over a large proportion of the animal's enclosure, with a gradient to zero in shade (Fig. 17.4A and C). This would be suitable for shade-dwelling reptiles and occasional baskers, that is, those in Zones 1 and 2. Provision of UVI up to approximately 1.0 would seem appropriate. Fluorescent T8 UV tubes may be used if the animals will be close to the lamps; other sources may be suitable if positioned at greater distances.

A "sunbeam method" provides a higher level of UV for species known to bask (Fig. 17.4B and D). The aim is to provide UV similar to that which the animal would experience when in direct sunlight *during a typical early to midmorning period* when most reptiles bask. This higher level needs to be restricted to the basking zone ("like a sunbeam") with a gradient to zero in shade. T5-HO UV tubes fitted with an aluminum reflector, UV metal halide, and mercury vapor lamps can be used. This method would seem appropriate for reptiles in Zones 3 and 4; a maximum of UVI 7.0 at reptile level is suggested. Zone 2 (occasional baskers) in larger enclosures that can accommodate a high-output lamp would probably utilize this type of UV gradient as well, with a maximum UVI around 3.0.

Excessive UV Exposure/Nonterrestrial UVB and UVC

All guidelines to date are still very experimental. It is vital to watch the animals' responses and adjust the UV levels immediately if problems are seen. Albino and hypomelanistic animals may be at increased risk of UV-induced skin damage and cancer and likely need much lower UV levels than normally-pigmented conspecifics.

Zone	1	2	3	4	Suggested method of UVB provision
Characteristics	**Crepuscular or shade dweller**	**Partial sun or occasional basker**	**Open or partial sun basker**	**'Mid-day' open sun basker**	
Species in original study (Ferguson et al. 2010)	**Cottonmouth water moccasin** (*Agkistrodon piscivorus*) **Texas rat snake** (*Elaphe obsoleta*) **Jamaican brown anole** (*Anolis lineotopus*) **Broad-banded water snake** (*Nerodia fasciata*)	**Western ribbon snake** (*Thamnophis proximus*) **Green anole** (*Anolis carolinensis*) **Jamaican blue-pants anole** (*Anolis grahami*) **Yellow-bellied water snake** (*Nerodia erythrogaster*)	**Desert side-blotched lizard** (*Uta stansburiana stejnegeri*) **Eastern fence lizard** (*Sceloporus undulatus hyacinthinus*) **Cuban brown anole** (*Anolis sagrei*) **Texas spiny lizard** (*Sceloporus olivaceous*)	**Lesser earless lizard** (*Holbrookia maculata*) **Sagebrush lizard** (*Sceloporus graciosus*) **Northern prairie lizard** (*Sceloporus undulatus garmani*)	
UVI Zone range (all-day average)	**0 - 0.7**	**0.7 - 1.0**	1.0 - 2.6	2.6 - 3.5	**Shade Method** (Fluorescent UVB) **UV Index up to approx 1.0**
Maximum UVI recorded (one-off maximum)	0.6 - 1.4	**1.1 - 3.0***	**2.9 - 7.4**	**4.5 - 9.5**	**Sunbeam Method** (Mercury vapour, metal halide or T5-HO Fluorescent UVB) **UV Index up to approx. 7.0**
Species typical of Zone commonly held in captivity	**Leopard gecko** (*Eublepharis macularius*) **Crested gecko** (*Correlophus cilliatus*) **Corn snake** (*Pantherophis guttatus guttatus*) **Burmese python** (*Python bivittatus*)	**Redfooted tortoise** (*Geochelone carbonaria*) **Monkey-tailed skink** (*Corucia zebrata*) **Chinese water dragon** (*Physignathus cocincinus*) **Boa constrictor** (*Boa constrictor*)	**Bearded dragon** (*Pogona vitticeps*) **Spur-thighed tortoise** (*Testudo graeca*) **Red-eared slider** (*Trachemys scripta elegans*) **Standing's Day Gecko** (*Phelsuma standingi*)	**Saharan Uromastyx** (*Uromastyx geyri*) **Chuckwalla** (*Sauromalus ater*) **Rhinoceros iguana** (*Cyclura comuta cornuta*) **(NB: shade is vital even for these)**	***** Zone 2 reptiles in a larger enclosure would probably utilise gentle "sunbeam" UVB up to approx. UVI 3.0

FIG 17.6 UV index estimates based on the Ferguson zones. The original 15 species of reptiles studied in their natural habitat in Jamaica and south and west United States were allocated to one of four zones according to their basking behavior and recorded UV range. Other species, such as the examples given, may also be assigned to these zones based upon their known basking behavior, and this also acts as a guide as to choice of shade or sunbeam methods of UV provision. (Modified from Baines et al., 2016.)[12]

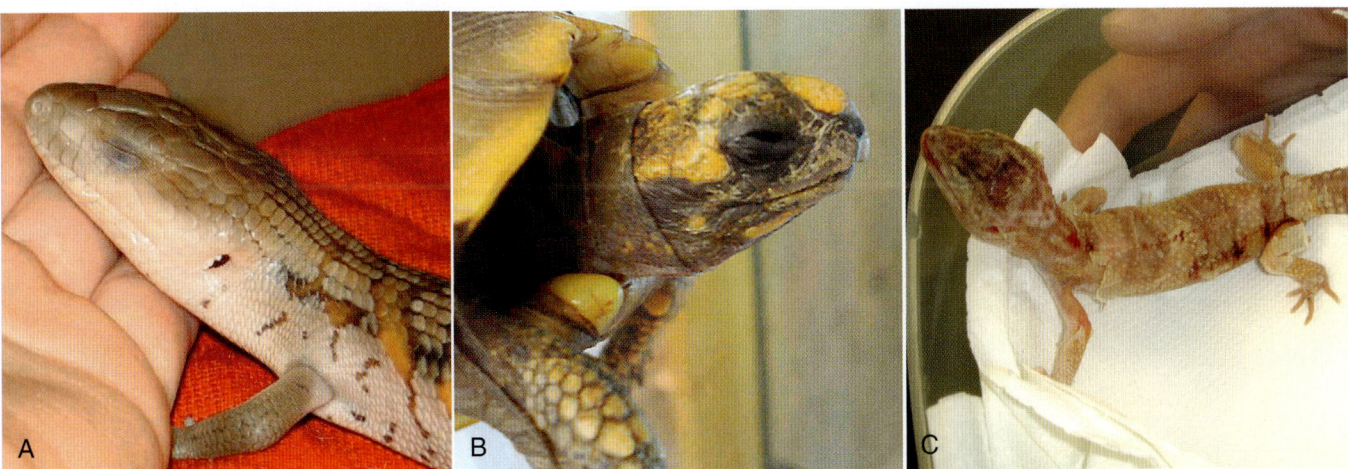

FIG 17.7 Effects of hazardous, abnormally short-wavelength UVB from "problem" UV lamps marketed in 2006 to 2007. (A) Juvenile blue-tongue skink (*Tiliqua scincoides intermedia*) with photo-kerato-conjunctivitis. (Courtesy of A. Murphree.) (B) Yellow-footed tortoise (*Chelonoidis denticulata*) with photo-kerato-conjunctivitis. (Courtesy of M. Buono.) (C) Leopard gecko (*Eublepharis macularius*) hatchling with very severe UV "burns," which proved fatal. (Courtesy of M. Buono.)

A few brands of reptile lamps, found to emit hazardous, very short wavelength UVB and UVC, have caused photo-kerato-conjunctivitis, severe photo-dermatitis, burns, and death in a significant number of cases[13] (Fig. 17.7). These were withdrawn from sale but similar products may inadvertently be marketed. In mild cases, recovery is spontaneous following removal of the lamp.

Excessive doses of "solar" UVB and UVA can also result in eye and skin damage and, in mammals, can lead to the formation of skin cancers. Squamous cell carcinomas have been reported in captive reptiles, but their association with use of artificial UV lighting is, as yet, undetermined.[14]

REFERENCES

See www.expertconsult.com for a complete list of references.

18

Disinfection

Craig J-G. Hunt

Disinfection is an essential tool to help provide a healthy environment for amphibians and reptiles in the home environment and veterinary clinic by helping to reduce pathogen loads, disease transmission, and postoperative infections. Although often used interchangeably, cleaning, disinfecting, and sterilizing are not the same. Cleaning refers to the physical act of removing organic matter and solid debris (dirt, grease, feces, body fluids, etc.) and must always precede disinfection and sterilization in order to eliminate infectious microorganisms.[1] Disinfection reduces the pathogen load but does not eliminate it; a properly disinfected surface may still harbor a low level of potentially pathogenic bacteria, fungi, and viruses, but the pathogen level is usually so low as to not cause problems for otherwise healthy inhabitants.[2] Sterilization, as opposed to simple cleaning or disinfecting, kills all life (bacteria, fungi, and viruses). Exposure to steam at high pressures and certain chemicals such as ethylene oxide gas, peroxide, or formalin may be used. These methods require special equipment and safety considerations.

TECHNIQUES AND PRODUCTS

Disinfection techniques differ depending on specific needs. Maintenance of hygiene in a single, private-home cage versus a large breeding colony, pet store, or quarantine facility can vary dramatically. Veterinarians must properly advise clients with specific instructions for specific needs. Many disinfectants are on the market, and choosing the right one can be confusing. One must take the time to read labels to choose the right disinfectant and to use appropriate personal protection equipment such as gloves, aprons, and masks. In choosing a disinfectant, one should keep in mind that it should be safe, easy to use and effective against target pathogens, be fast acting, and have predictable risk to animals in the vivarium and not leave toxic residues. More than one disinfectant may be needed to kill all target organsisms.

Good housekeeping is the best ally against disease. Cleaning and disinfecting on a scheduled basis prevents the buildup of potential pathogens and reduces the spread of disease. Few disinfectants work effectively in the presence of organic debris (blood, feces, and urine), therefore thorough cleaning with a mild detergent followed by a thorough rinse in hot water before disinfection is essential. Dish soaps work well because they are easily rinsed and generally effective against grease. Washing should be performed in a dedicated area away from food preparation areas, and disposable gloves should be worn as a minumim.

Disinfectants should be mixed following the manufacturer's directions. Too dilute a concentration is ineffective, and too strong may be toxic, hard to rinse, and expensive.

Some disinfectants may not be compatible when mixed; ammonia and bleach for example can produce toxic, potentially lethal fumes.

Some plastics and rubber may retain chemicals such as disinfectants, and if they are not thoroughly rinsed and soaked, can leech out back into an animal's environment, water, or substrate with potentially toxic effects. Stoskopf[3] reported a case of iodine toxicity, resulting in the death of several individuals in a group of red and black poison arrow frogs (*Dendrobates histrionicus sylvaticus*), which had been temporarily housed in styrene plastic containers previously disinfected with povidone iodine solution.

There may be individual variation in tolerance to disinfectants and particular care should be exercised when using disinfectants in different species. For example, two red-bellied short-necked turtles (*Emydura subglobosa*) developed partial flaccid paralysis and death when bathed for 45 minutes in a 0.024% clorhexidine solution.[4] In one study a 0.75% chlorhexidine solution used as presurgical skin preparation in African clawed frogs (*Xenopus laevis*) was associated with erythema, skin ulceration, and death in some individuals, whereas 0.5% povidone-iodine was associated with minimal reaction.[5]

Ammonia and bleach are both excellent, inexpensive, and readily available disinfectants. Ammonia can be used undiluted (full strength), and bleach should be diluted to a working concentration of 1% to 5% (1:50 to 1:10 dilution).[6] Both of these solutions are adequate to kill most common pathogens. Contact time is the key to effectiveness, and items should be soaked for a minimum of 5 to 30 minutes depending on the pathogen(s) of concern and which disinfectant is used (Table 18.1). Placement of disinfectants in spray bottles is an excellent way to disperse the material. Some disinfectatants should be rinsed following application to prevent toxicity and/or damage to treated surfaces and should subsequently be allowed to air dry. Ammonia can be rinsed with water, and chlorine bleach can be neutralized with the addition of a dechlorinator to the rinse water or with placement of the items in direct sunlight for a few hours, which deactivates the chlorine. Other disinfectants may have residual activity and are preferably not rinsed for optimal effect.

Extra bowls and cages allow rotation of items through this cleaning process, with minimal stress to the occupants. Substrates that cannot be effectively cleaned, such as paper towel, aspen, soil, and coco bedding, should be replaced when soiled. Porous items such as wood may be impossible to disinfect and may be best discarded, preferably by incineration, in quarantine facilities or in the event of a disease outbreak.

Nine broad categories of disinfectants exist. Each has a different spectrum of activity, advantages, and disadvantages, and each is used for a variety of applications (see Table 18.1).

In addition to disinfection of enclosures, food bowls, and furnishings, good hand hygiene is extremely important in preventing spread of potential pathogens between animals and between animals and humans (see also Chapter 19). In one study, less than half of the respondents

TABLE 18.1   Characteristics of Common Disinfectants

Type	Examples	Dilutions	Spectrum of Activity	Comments	Common Uses	Contact Time	Mode of Action
Iodophore solutions	Betadine Povidine-iodine Pevidine Tamodine	10%–100% solution	B+/-, (s), tb, m, (f), ev, nev	Inactivated by organic debris and alcohol. Stains skin and porous material.	Wound antiseptic, preoperative scrubs	1–5 min depending on concentration used.	Denature proteins and disrupt nucleic acids
Chlorines	Sodium hypochlorite Bleach	2%–10% solution	B+/-, (s), tb, m, (f), ev, nev	Corrosive, irritant, fumes irritant to mucous membranes. Must be rinsed well. Inactivated by organic debris, high water ph, and UV light. Inactivated by some soaps.	Hard surfaces	10 min	Denature proteins
Chlorhexidine	Nolvasan Chlorhexiderm Hibitane Savlon Virosan	0.5%–2% solution	B+(-), m, (f), (ev), (nev) (not effective vs. Pseudomonas spp.)	Not inhibited by organic matter or alcohol. May be affected by alkaline ph. Generally safe when in contact with animal but potentially toxic in baths, especially to amphibians.	Instruments, cages, and all hard surfaces. Preoperative scrub; may not be suitable for amphibians	10 min	Alter cell membrane permeability
Quaternary ammonium compounds	Roccal-d Parvosol Disintegrator Ark-klens Anistel F10 (combined with a biguanide) Benzalkonium chloride	0.5%–1%	B+/-, (s), (tb), (m), (f), (ev), (nev) (may not be effective vs. Pseudomonas spp.)	Inhibited by organic matter. Inactivated by soaps. Poor activity in hard water. Can be toxic to amphibians. F10 has been used in some amphibians and appears safe in those species.[9,10,11]	Instruments, rubber equipment, and hard surfaces. Used as bath and aerosol in some species to treat environment with animals in situ	5–10 min	Denature proteins, disrupt cell membrane, inactivate enzymes
Alcohols	Ethyl alcohol Isopropyl alcohol	70%–90%	B+/-, (s), tb, (f), ev, (nev)	Good skin antiseptic. Inactivated by organic matter. Fumes may be irritating.	Instruments and skin	20 min	Cell lysis, precipitates proteins, and denatures lipids
Phenolic compounds	Lysol Synphenol-3	Follow data sheet	B+(-), tb, f, (ev), (nev)	Not inactivated by organic material. Irritating and corrosive to skin; must be rinsed well. Potentially toxic to reptiles and amphibians.	Hard surfaces, floors, foot baths, laundry rinse.	10 min	Alter cell membrane permeability and denature proteins
Aldehydes: glutaraldehyde, formaldehyde	(Formula h)	Follow data sheet	B+/-, s, (tb), m, f, ev, nev	Not inactivated by organic material. Corrosive, toxic, and irritating to the eyes, skin, and respiratory tract. Toxic to humans/animals.	Endoscopy equipment, empty cages, and furnishings. A fixative for electron microscopy.	20 min	Denature proteins and alkylate nucleic acids
Peroxide	Hydrogen peroxide, peroxygen compounds	3%–6%	B+/-, (s), tb, (f), ev, nev	Toxic gases form when in contact with chlorine and bi-sulfites. Dilute always by adding acid to water. Stable and effective when used on inanimate surfaces. Breaks down very quickly when contaminated with impurities.	Endoscopy equipment instruments and used to fog rooms	10–30 mins	Denature protein and lipids

B = bacteria, s = bacterial spores, tb = mycobacteria, m= mycoplasma, f=fungi, ev = enveloped viruses, nev = nonenveloped viruses; parentheses indicate partial effectiveness. Data from references 1, 2, 8, and 12.

(76 of 182 [41.7%]) reported washing their hands regularly between handling patients.[7] Environmental contamination is known to be an important factor in the transmission of hospital-borne infections and surfaces with regular hand contact are most at risk of contamination.[6] Alcohol-based hand rubs remain the initial choice for hand hygiene in human medicine, unless the hands are visibly contaminated with dirt and organic material, in which case liquid soap and water is recommended.[8]

Glutaraldehyde-based disinfectants are commonly used to sterilize instruments such as endoscopes that may not be easily or safely sterilized using heat or steam-based protocols; a 2% solution used for a maximum of 30 minutes is recommended.

REFERENCES

See www.expertconsult.com for a complete list of references.

19

Quarantine

Sam Rivera

Quarantine is defined as the period in which a new arrival to a collection is kept isolated for observation, habituation to its new environment, disease testing, and subsequent treatment or relocation if required. The inadvertent introduction of an infectious pathogen into an established reptile collection can have devastating consequences, both emotional and financial due to associated animal disease and loss. The goals of quarantine are to prevent the introduction of infectious diseases into an established collection, provide a recovery period from shipment, and allow an animal the opportunity to adapt to new husbandry procedures and protocols with minimal stress. Additionally, it has been well-documented that transport and exposure to a novel environment can be stressful and may result in animals being both more susceptible to, and more likely to, shed infectious agents. Therefore it is important to separate newly acquired animals from the established collection during this quarantine period to mitigate disease transmission.[1,2]

Traditionally quarantine has been defined as a period of time to isolate a newly acquired animal from an established collection. The parameters of this quarantine period were based on the origin of the animal (captive-born vs wild-caught) and/or resources available at each individual facility. The current concept of quarantine has evolved, however, and the principles of disease risk assessment and management are now specifically tailored for both the species involved and the individual institution. The inherent goals are to optimize the resources available to properly isolate new animals while minimizing risk to the established collection.[3,4]

Disease risk assessment requires having an intimate knowledge of the new arrival's previous environment and health history, as well as that of the collection of origin. In many cases, performing a thorough disease risk assessment may allow for modifications in the quarantine period, resulting in reduced labor cost and ease of transition.[4] Compared with a traditional quarantine, the disease risk assessment approach can be more efficient and effective. With this approach, if a new animal originates from an institution that can provide detailed medical records for review prior to acquisition then modifications to a traditional quarantine may be permissible.[3] In contrast, when acquiring animals with an unknown health history, a traditional quarantine becomes an important tool to protect the health of the individual animal and the collection animals at the receiving institution.

DISEASE RISK ASSESSMENT

The goals of disease risk assessment are to estimate presence, exposure, and consequences of introducing an infectious disease of concern.[5–7] Reviewing medical and pathology records from both the sending and receiving institutions is a crucial part of assessing the risk of disease presence and potential for exposure. A disease risk assessment is a method by which the likelihood and consequences of an adverse effect are calculated.[5,6] In the case of quarantine, the most devastating consequences would involve the introduction of an infectious disease agent with high morbidity/mortality to a naive or healthy population.

A proper disease risk assessment involves reviewing current knowledge about the diseases of concern, reviewing medical records from the sending institution regarding both the animal in question and the relevant collection, reviewing pertinent historical data of both the animal and collections involved, and finally reviewing important natural history information.

To complete such a disease risk assessment, four interconnected steps must be considered and performed. These include (1) hazard identification, (2) risk assessment, (3) risk management, and (4) risk communication.[5–7] For hazard identification, diseases of concern must be identified. This is accomplished by performing a thorough review of the medical history of the individual animal to be acquired and the original collection/source. In many zoological collections, comprehensive preventive medicine and pathology programs can provide essential information about the presence of diseases of concern. This identification of hazards, or diseases of concern, should start with consideration of the species involved and the diseases to which those species may be particularly susceptible. Table 19.1 lists important diseases per taxa that should be considered when performing the disease risk assessment. This list is dynamic, and recent literature should be reviewed on a regular basis to stay current on the ever-increasing body of knowledge regarding infectious diseases in reptiles and amphibians. It is also important to review the animal's history regarding temperament, nutrition, and enclosure requirements to identify potential noninfectious hazards prior to acquiring the animal.

Risk management helps to develop and implement policies and procedures that decrease the likelihood of specific diseases being introduced into an established collection. These actions may include refusal to accept an animal, extending the quarantine time period, additional disease testing, euthanasia of an animal based on results or necessity, or acceptance of an animal if the disease in question is already present in the collection. It is arguable that the risk management step is the most important component of the disease risk assessment process, because it integrates the identification of a specific pathogen with the actions needed to minimize its introduction into a naive collection.[6,7] Risk communication involves keeping all relevant individuals and departments informed and updated on the progress of the disease risk assessment and the plans and outcomes of the actions taken.

QUARANTINE DURATION

The results of the disease risk assessment are then utilized to determine the length of the quarantine period and requirements for specific infectious disease testing. An animal with no exposure to a disease of concern could potentially bypass a lengthy quarantine period and enter the collection after a shorter acclimation and observation period. The

TABLE 19.1 Selected Group of Diseases/Infectious Agents That Should Be Considered When Performing a Disease Risk Assessment

Amphibians	Chelonians	Crocodilians	Lizards	Snakes
Chlamydiosis	Amoebiasis	Chlamydiosis	Acariasis	Acariasis
Chytridomycosis	Helminthiasis	Helminthiasis	Adenovirus	Amoebiasis
Helminthiasis	Herpesvirus	Mycoplasmosis	Cryptosporidiosis	Arenavirus
Ranavirus	Intranuclear coccidiosis	Pox virus	Fungal dermatitis	Cryptosporidiosis
	Mycoplasmosis	West Nile Virus	Helminthiasis	Helminthiasis
	Ticks		Ticks	Nidovirus
				Paramyxovirus
				Snake fungal disease
				Ticks

length of the quarantine period can be difficult to determine when the health history is unknown. Currently, at Zoo Atlanta, reptiles originating from unknown sources and/or suspected to be wild caught are quarantined for a minimum of 90 days. This period overlaps with or exceeds the incubation period of the majority of pathogens of concern, although there are an ever-increasing number of novel pathogens being identified for which we have little or no epidemiological information. Reptiles arriving from known institutions with well-documented health history and without hazards identified during the disease risk assessment may have a quarantine period as short as 14 days.

During quarantine, there are some important principles to be followed. The space allocated for quarantine should be separate from the established collection, ideally in a separate building with a separate air-handling system. The greater the distance, the less likely a disease agent may be transmitted or transported by fomites. Quarantine care and husbandry routines must be completed in a manner that minimizes cross-contamination within the established collection. In the ideal world, the person taking care of quarantined animals is not the same person taking care of the established collection, but this may not always be possible. Alternatives may include providing hands-on care on alternate days or caring for quarantined animals after working with the animals in the established collection.

Animals in quarantine must be housed in an enclosure that meets their husbandry needs with regard to size, thermal gradient, hiding areas, and climbing structures balanced with ease of cleaning and disinfection (Fig. 19.1). Setting up a quarantine enclosure, which is based on a good understanding of the animal's natural history, minimizes stress and eases the transition period. Paper makes an ideal substrate for quarantine purposes because it can be easily replaced, is relatively inexpensive, and allows for observation and collection of fecal samples for analysis. Porous surfaces should be avoided, because they are difficult to clean and disinfect, but if they are used they should be disposable. Dedicated tools and equipment should be designated for quarantine use only and should be cleaned and disinfected on a regular basis during the quarantine period (Fig. 19.2). Adequate disinfection of quarantine space, tools, and equipment is paramount to minimize disease transmission (see Chapter 18).

QUARANTINE EVALUATION

When an animal arrives into quarantine a thorough physical examination should be performed as soon as possible. Record the entry weight, body condition score, and any distinguishing external characteristics (i.e., scars, missing digits, shell notches). If not already present, some form of permanent identification, such as microchip placement, should be established. Photographs of individuals are an easy and convenient way

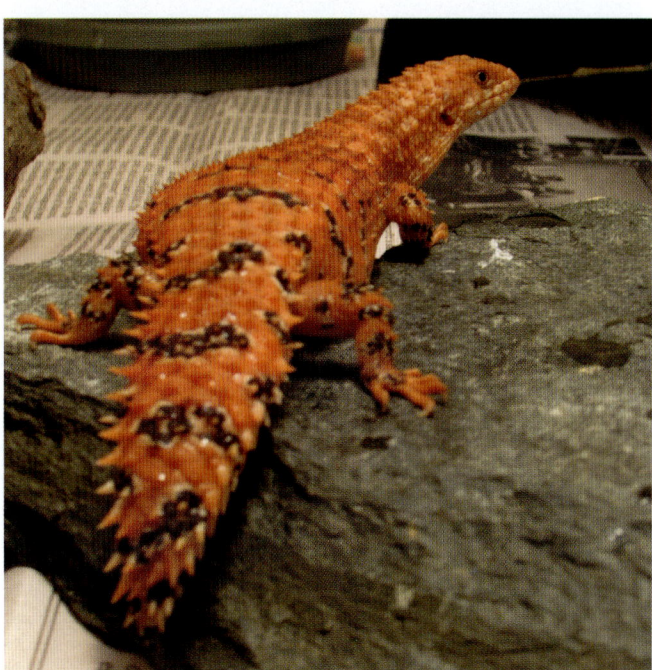

FIG 19.1 A newly arrived spiny-tailed skink (*Egernia epsisolus*). The animal is housed in an enclosure adequate for its size. Note that all cage furniture is disposable or easily disinfected, and newspaper is used as a substrate during this quarantine period. (Courtesy of Stephanie Earhart, Zoo Atlanta.)

to identify animals when dealing with large groups. Chelonians can be temporarily identified by painting a number on the shell.

During quarantine note the animal's behavior and demeanor, appetite, defecation frequency, and fecal consistency. Any deviation from these normal baseline observations may be an indication of illness and may require further diagnostic investigation. Abnormal clinical signs that should alert the clinician that something is wrong include vomiting/regurgitation, diarrhea, anorexia, weight loss, dysecdysis, lethargy, lameness or abnormal locomotion, and dehydration. If problems are identified during quarantine, quarantine duration may need to be extended to accommodate for treatments or diagnostics to be performed and results obtained.

Screening for infectious agents, especially if the health history is unknown, is critical to the goals of quarantine.[1] Intestinal parasites, while common in some species, must be monitored and controlled in many cases. Certain parasites such as oxyurids and *Nyctotherus* sp. can be commensal organisms and under normal circumstances

Furthermore, cross-reactivity among closely related strains may limit their usefulness. Molecular assays, such as PCR, may be helpful but are of limited value when screening healthy animals that may not be shedding the infectious agent's nucleic acid at the time of sample collection.

All animals coming into a new collection should be screened for ectoparasites, particularly if the animal's origin is unknown. Ectoparasites such as snake mites (*Ophionyssus natricis*) can be easily missed during quarantine if the infestation is mild. Multiple attempts should be made to identify mites on both the animal and in the enclosure before the animal is released from quarantine. Ticks are common in reptiles, especially in wild-caught animals, and can pose a risk as reservoirs of infectious agents.[8,11] The African tortoise tick (*Amblyomma marmoreum*) was identified in Florida outside importation facilities where it had become established.[9] Further investigations found that at least eight premises in Florida had been infested with this tick, including reptile importation facilities, reptile breeding operations, zoos, and wildlife theme parks.[10] Studies confirmed that *A. marmoreum* was a vector of heartwater, an acute rickettsial disease of domestic and wild ruminants.[11] At Zoo Atlanta's quarantine facility, we have identified tick species found on illegally imported tortoises that were from the tortoises' countries of origin.

It is often difficult, unrealistic, or impractical to screen for every potential pathogen. In some cases, there are unknown or emerging pathogens that pose great danger to an established collection. As an example, a confiscated group of Sulawesi tortoises (*Indotestudo forstenii*) illegally imported into the United States exhibited a high mortality rate, and subsequent studies revealed a novel adenovirus.[12] These animals had been screened for the majority of commonly recognized pathogens of tortoises, and the results were negative. These tortoises either died or became severely ill shortly after being placed into quarantine, thus demonstrating the importance of establishing and adhering to a quarantine period as an effective tool to identify signs of illness and take appropriate action.

Ideally, once an animal enters quarantine, no other animals should be allowed into quarantine until these specific animals leave quarantine. However, this is not always feasible. Some institutions have an all in/all out policy where animals from different institutions are brought into quarantine around the same time and complete their quarantine period simultaneously. In cases where animals are brought into an occupied quarantine space, it is ideal to extend the quarantine period on the basis of the time the last animals arrived.

Quarantine serves a vital role in preventing the introduction of a potentially fatal infectious agent into an established collection. There is value, however, in rethinking the traditional concept of quarantine by utilizing a disease risk assessment. Such an assessment can help to design and implement an optimum plan that is tailored for each new acquisition with the benefit of maximizing resources and minimizing risk to a collection.

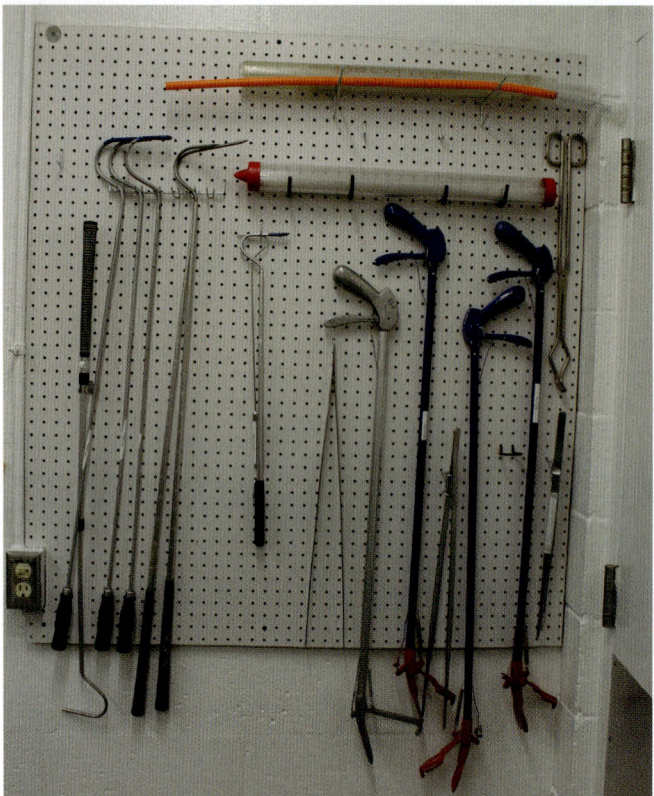

FIG 19.2 The quarantine area should have a dedicated set of tools that are easily disinfected and kept separate from the tools used for the established animal collection. (Courtesy of Stephanie Earhart, Zoo Atlanta.)

are nonpathogenic. On the other hand, direct life-cycle ascarids and strongyles can be pathogenic, and an attempt should be made to eliminate infestation or keep the parasite load as low as possible. Keep in mind that reptiles kept on the same substrate, especially when housed in naturalistic exhibits, will have an increased exposure to higher parasite concentrations in their environment that can be extremely detrimental to their health. Other parasitic infections such as cryptosporidiosis, intranuclear coccidiosis, and amoebiasis must be kept from entering the collection. Screening for these agents requires molecular techniques such as a polymerase chain reaction (PCR) test (*Cryptosporidium* sp. and intranuclear coccidiosis) or frequent fecal examinations and special stains (amoeba). The decision to test for a specific parasite is largely based on the results of the disease risk assessment.

Serology screening for infectious diseases can be challenging due to the limited availability and poor reliability. Serologic assays are available to screen for ophidian paramyxovirus in snakes and *Mycoplasma agassizii* and *Mycoplasma testudineum* in chelonians. These assays if positive are indicative of infection by the pathogen, but a negative result does not exclude exposure or early infection, and the test may need to be repeated.

REFERENCES

See www.expertconsult.com for a complete list of references.

20

Snakes

Richard S. Funk and Scott J. Stahl

Snakes are among the most fascinating, beautiful, and wonderful animals inhabiting our planet. During the past 3 decades, they have steadily increased in popularity in the pet trade. An increasing variety of species is becoming available every year. The most commonly kept species include the boas, pythons, and colubrids, many of which adapt well and will readily reproduce in captivity.

In choosing a snake, clients should closely examine the individual for alertness, good body strength and muscle tone, body weight and conformation, any open wounds or scars, oral lesions, signs of respiratory disease, stool quality, and evidence of external parasites. Captive-bred animals are preferred because they originate in captivity, are generally well established and feeding, usually lack parasites, and are less likely to have the poor adaptation issues commonly associated with wild-caught snakes. Additionally, captive-breeding reduces pressures on wild populations. Many snakes are purchased through Internet sales, and, although most are healthy, the health status of some may be misrepresented, and buyers must be cautious. Legislation concerning reptile ownership exists in many jurisdictions and is constantly changing, and this may prohibit the ownership of certain species in some areas, such as large constrictors, native or endangered species, and venomous snakes. Both the keeper and the clinician must be aware of applicable regulations. See Section 15.

Newly acquired snakes should always be quarantined away from other captives in the home or facility. Ideally, a separate room or even a separate building should be used. During quarantine, the new snake is observed for normal activity, feeding, shedding, stool quality, and general health. Medical problems are identified and addressed during quarantine. A quarantined snake should be managed only after the resident snakes have been cared for, and equipment used in quarantine should be carefully disinfected and remain with the quarantined animal. See Chapter 19 for more information on quarantine.

RESTRAINT

Venomous snakes should only be handled by trained, experienced individuals using appropriate equipment (e.g., tongs, snake hooks, plastic tubes, large transparent viewing containers). The remaining discussion focuses on nonvenomous snakes (see Chapter 22 for details on handling venomous species).

The head of an aggressive snake or snake of unknown disposition should be identified and restrained before opening the transportation bag and removing the animal. In general, the head is held behind the occiput using the thumb and middle finger to support the lateral aspects of the cranium. The index finger is placed on top of the head. The other hand is used to support the serpentine body. By restraining the snake's head in this manner greater support can be given to the cranium-cervical junction, which, having only a single occiput, is more prone to dislocation with rough or inappropriate handling. Upon removal from the transportation bag, the snake should be supported using one or two hands depending upon size. The largest pythons and anacondas can exceed 5 m and 80 kg and are powerful and potentially dangerous. When dealing with large, even docile, boas and pythons, an additional handler is recommended for each meter of snake. An assessment of demeanor can usually be quickly done. A healthy individual that is permitted to wrap a coil around the handler's wrist while the head is allowed to hang down should be able to raise its head to the level of the tail. Nervous or aggressive (nonvenomous) snakes can be restrained using plexiglass tubes or in clear plastic viewing containers.

SPECIFIC HOUSING REQUIREMENTS

Snakes are quite adept at escaping from enclosures, so the first consideration for any vivarium or cage is security; it must be escape-proof when properly closed. Cages may be plastic shoe boxes, sweater boxes, modified aquaria, or homemade from wood. Commercially manufactured cages now can be purchased specifically for snakes and are typically made of fiberglass or acrylonitrate-butadiene-styrene (ABS) plastic (Fig. 20.1). Cages can be solitary or part of a rack system, where multiple plastic tubs slide in and out of openings; many professional breeders utilize rack systems (Fig. 20.2A and B). Table 20.1 lists the minimum requirements for snake caging. See Chapter 16 for more detailed information on appropriate cage sizing.

Lighting requirements for captive snakes are not as well understood as they are for lizards. However, attention to the photoperiod promotes good health and successful reproduction in snakes. Many successful breeders provide only subdued artificial lighting for their snakes and have excellent results. UVB lighting is not documented to be necessary for successful husbandry and breeding, but keepers who provide diurnal snakes access to UVB lighting report these snakes will exhibit some degree of increased activity and basking behavior.

One concern for cages kept in dim light is that snakes may not be cleaned as routinely or as thoroughly because excrement is not as easily observed. Fresh water should always be available and changed frequently. Some keepers use disposable plastic cups that fit into premolded holders in the tubs of rack systems to improve sanitation and cleaning efficiency (Fig. 20.3). Arboreal species may appreciate an elevated water bowl. Water bowls should be cleaned and disinfected at least once weekly.

Humidity varies geographically and seasonally. During the winter, when forced air heat is utilized to maintain appropriate temperatures, the drying effect (with reduced humidity) may cause problems such as dysecdysis and respiratory disease. Alternatively, too much humidity may be harmful to a desert-adapted species. Many snakes do well if the humidity is between 50% and 70%, but this must be maintained while still providing adequate ventilation, or the humidity inside a cage will rise dramatically and air quality will be adversely affected. Desert or xeric-adapted species should be maintained with less humidity than riparian or semiaquatic species. Snakes kept in aquaria or plastic sweater boxes, with only substrate, a water bowl, and a hide, may have the essentials but are being housed more like laboratory animals rather than pets (see Fig. 20.2A and B). A recent trend is to use larger cages or *vivaria* with cage furnishings such as plants, rocks, and tree branches. Most clients feel that their snakes are more fulfilled in these environments, even though more maintenance may be necessary (Fig. 20.4). This type of vivarium provides the snake with environmental enrichment, which may help to minimize captive stress and provide more enjoyment in maintaining snakes for the keeper as well.[1]

The authors prefer a newspaper or paper substrate for hospitalized patients unless their needs dictate otherwise, such as with fossorial or aquatic species (see Fig. 20.2A and B). For clients, simple (spartan or barren) cages may also work well. But many species, especially fossorial or more sensitive species, need more attention to cage setup, including

some attempt to duplicate more natural conditions. Woodland burrowers generally will not thrive in dry sand and vice versa for desert burrowing snakes. Among the most popular substrates utilized are aspen shavings or chips; they are relatively dust free, may be spot-cleaned, are inexpensive, and allow snakes traction and some burrowing ability. Aspen is a popular substrate used in rack systems. Newspaper is inexpensive but does wrinkle and fold and is less absorbent. Nonprinted paper with varying absorption abilities and specifically cut (for cage size and if desired with a cut-out for molded water cup holders) for certain rack systems are commercially available and help with efficiency and sanitation in large collections of snakes (Fig. 20.5). Pelleted and shredded paper products are available and are more absorbent than flat paper. Well thought out vivaria with naturalistic setups may utilize sand, gravel, soil, or mixtures and may include living plants.

Briefly, several different styles of caging for snakes are as follows:[2]

- *Basic enclosure setup:* One type of substrate, with a water bowl, a hide box, and perhaps with a plant or tree branch added.
- *Wet-dry enclosure setup:* Like the basic, but this type has one or two types of substrate, with a moist area and a dry area, providing a horizontal moisture gradient.

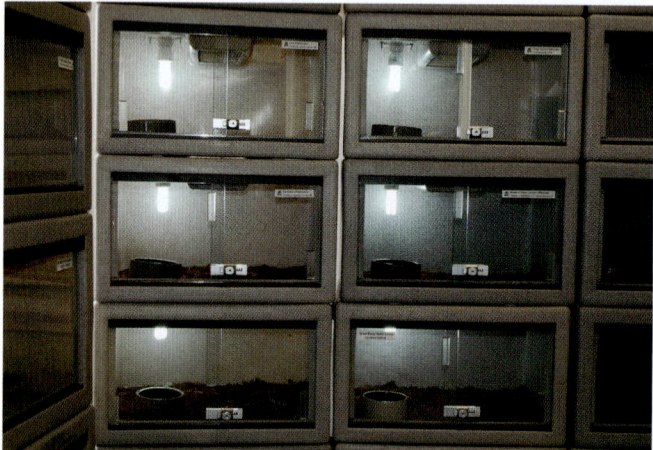

FIG 20.1 Commercially manufactured modular, stackable cages made of ABS plastic with locks placed on the horizontally sliding glass doors. Individual lighting is present within each cage. This is a private collection of rattlesnakes (*Crotalus* spp.). (Courtesy of Richard S. Funk.)

TABLE 20.1   **Minimal Requirements for Snake Caging**
Escape-proof with latch or lock
Easy access for cleaning, feeding, and monitoring occupant
Avoid design/materials that allow for ectoparasites or uneaten prey to hide
Easy to clean and disinfect
Appropriate substrate both for snake's needs and for serviceability
Hide box or shelter(s)
Constructed to prevent water or feces absorption
Appropriate lighting, ventilation, and humidity
Large enough to accommodate the snake and allow some activity
With multiple captives, uniform or modular cages are conducive to good husbandry (see Figs. 20.1 and 20.2A and B)

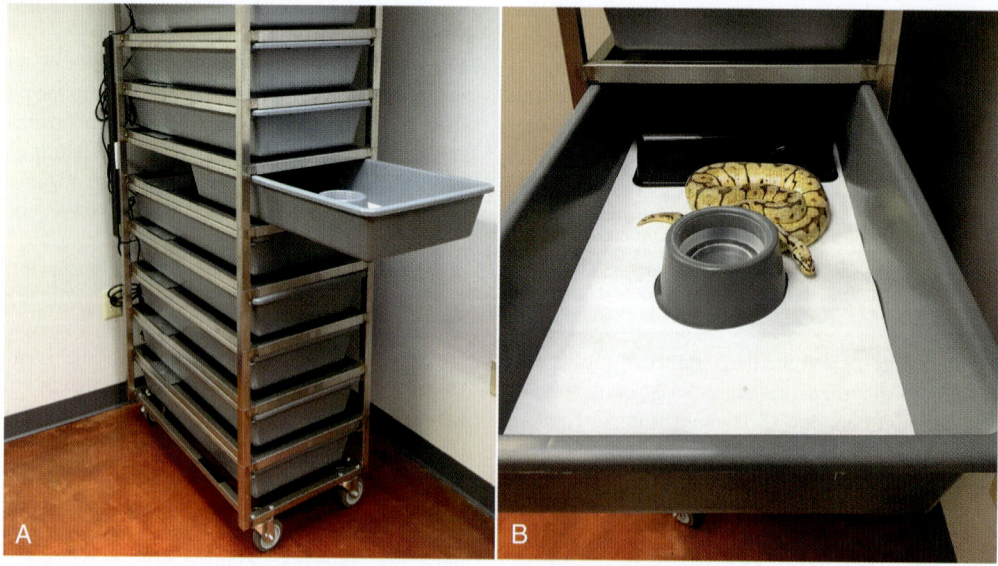

FIG 20.2 (A) Commercially produced rack systems are available for housing snakes efficiently utilizing multiple plastic tubs that slide in and out of tight openings that do not require tops (https://www.freedombreeder.com). Heat tape controlled by a thermostat is then utilized along the back of the tub system to establish a temperature gradient for the snakes. This rack is on wheels to allow mobility of the entire system. (B) A "bumblebee" color morph ball python (*Python regius*) is housed in one of the tubs showing the molded water holders and a plastic hide box provided over the heated area. (Courtesy of Scott J. Stahl, Stahl Exotic Animal Veterinary Services.)

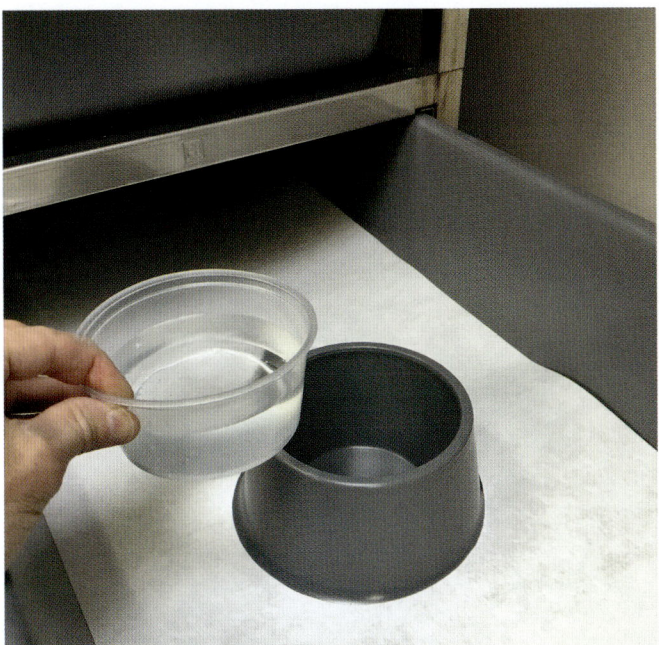

FIG 20.3 Some keepers use disposable plastic cups that fit into pre-molded holders in the tubs of rack systems to improve sanitation and cleaning efficiency. (Courtesy of Scott J. Stahl, Stahl Exotic Animal Veterinary Services.)

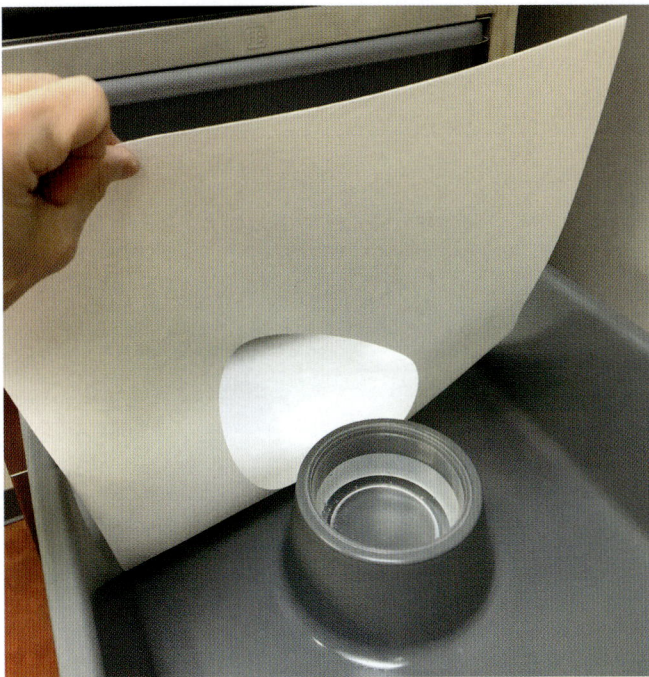

FIG 20.5 Nonprinted paper with varying absorption abilities and specifically pre-cut (for cage size and if desired with a cut-out for molded water cup holders) for certain rack systems are commercially available and help with efficiency and sanitation in large snake collections. (Courtesy of Scott J. Stahl, Stahl Exotic Animal Veterinary Services.)

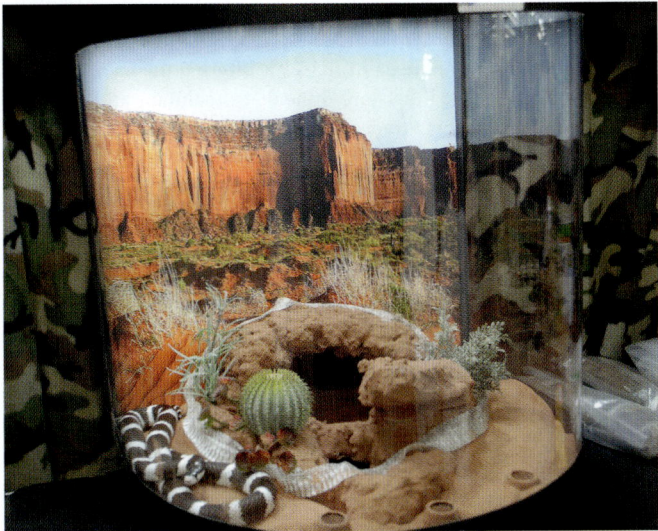

FIG 20.4 Commercially manufactured, vivarium-type cage, housing a single snake. The cage is decorated for esthetics and to provide environmental enrichment for the inhabitant. (Courtesy of Richard S. Funk.)

- *Three-layer enclosure setup:* Three layers of substrate are used; from bottom upward they are gravel, sand, and then mulch. The gravel can be moistened, and a vertical moisture gradient achieved.
- *Desert enclosure setup:* Basically, a thick layer of sand for the substrate. Small water bowl, good ventilation, and in some situations, depending on species housed, occasional moisture in a small focal area.
- *Swamp tea setup:* Rarely used, primarily for swamp snakes, with a dilute solution of tea for the water environment.
- *Natural setups and outdoor enclosures:* Indoor vivaria are often naturalistic and esthetically pleasing, but they must also be functional.

Unfortunately, difficulty in maintaining these enclosures often relates to their degree of complexity.

Outdoor enclosures can be rewarding, as they allow the snake to experience a true natural environment, but the environment must be similar to their native environment. However, being housed outside has inherent risks that must be avoided. The enclosure must be escape-, vermin-, and vandal-proof, and meeting these requirements can be challenging. See Section 3 for more information on cage setups.

THERMOREGULATION

Snakes, like other reptiles, are ectotherms. In a captive setting, providing a thermal gradient to allow the snake to move in and out of preferred temperature zones (similar to the temperatures they would experience in the wild) will allow proper thermoregulation. A variety of commercially available products exist to give the herpetoculturist an opportunity to provide such a regimen. Heat tapes are popular and effective and may be used with thermostats (Fig. 20.6). Light bulbs and hot rocks are inefficient and dangerous heat sources that and are not recommended; they may lead to thermal burns if a snake has prolonged contact. Shine provides a discussion of behavioral thermoregulation in wild diamond pythons (*Morelia s. spilotes*), describing variations in their activity based on seasonal and gender differences.[3] Both the clinician and the client must understand the thermal biology of reptiles (Fig. 20.7). Each species needs to reach its selected (or preferred) body temperature (T_s or T_p), which occurs within the range of physiologically tolerated temperatures or the thermal neutral zone (TNZ). Snakes that are ill, gravid, or digesting food often seek out

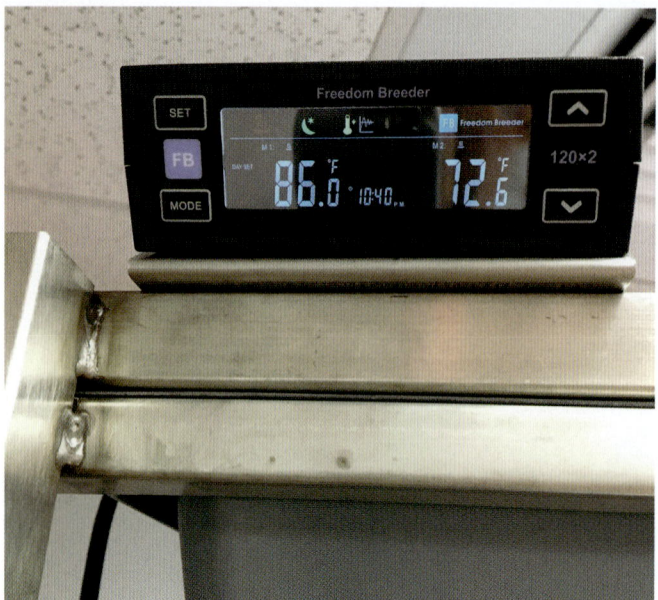

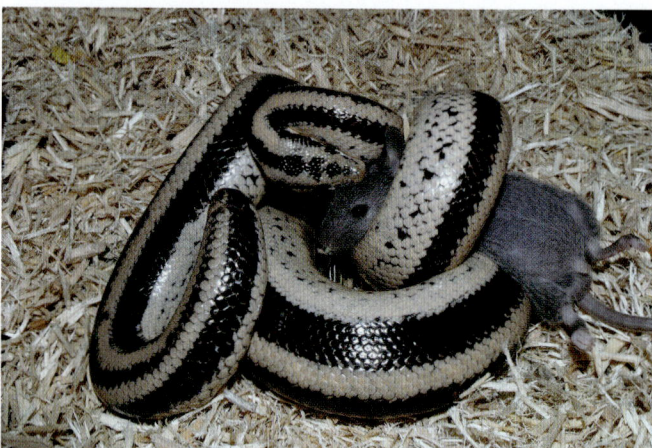

FIG 20.8 Adult rosy boa (*Lichanura trivirgata*) constricting its prey even though the mouse was offered already dead. (Courtesy of Richard S. Funk.)

FIG 20.6 Snakes, like other reptiles, are ectotherms. In a captive setting, providing a thermal gradient to allow the snake to move in and out of preferred temperature zones (similar to the temperatures they would experience in the wild) will allow proper thermoregulation. Sophisticated thermostats to control heat tape are available (https://www.freedom-breeder.com), with multiple features including day and night temperature control and alarm systems to warn keepers if temperatures are out of a preset temperature range. (Courtesy of Scott J. Stahl, Stahl Exotic Animal Veterinary Services.)

FEEDING AND NUTRITION

All snakes are carnivorous. Some species may eat a wide variety of prey, some primarily endothermic prey, some only invertebrates, and some have specialized diets (e.g., slugs, eggs, frogs, fish, eggs, termites). Therefore it is critical for both the clinician and the client to understand the appropriate diet for a snake species (Table 20.2). One of the most common reasons for anorexia in snakes is offering the incorrect prey. Species with specialized diets are difficult to maintain and require a dedicated owner. Most pet trade species feed on captive-reared rodents, which are whole (dietarily complete) animals, therefore nutritional problems are not often seen in feeding snakes. However, rodents must be fed a nutritionally complete commercial rodent diet to be a balanced diet for snakes. Similarly, if a client is feeding insects or fish to a snake, these prey items should be fed a nutritionally sound food to improve their dietary quality before feeding them to the snake. It is preferred to feed dead rodents to snakes to avoid possible bite wounds and injury to the snake but also for humane considerations for the rodents (Fig. 20.8). Rodents can be offered fresh-killed or purchased frozen and then thawed and rewarmed just before offering to the snake. Dead prey items should be placed in the enclosure or if simulated movement is necessary, offered from long forceps or tongs instead of by hand. The "live" human hand tends to radiate more heat than the warmed prey item, and keepers are frequently bitten when feeding snakes by hand, as the snake is confused where to strike. If a snake is not feeding, the natural history and husbandry for that species should be reviewed and changes made to provide a diet, timing, and strategy for feeding that more closely resembles that in the wild. Snakes may become anorexic if appropriate environmental temperatures are not provided for the species. Additionally, it is normal for most snakes not to feed during an active shed cycle. Underlying illness could also be a cause of anorexia, and a health evaluation should be performed if other etiologies are ruled out. Frequency of meals varies with the age and species of snake. Many juvenile and adult rodent-feeding species thrive and grow well with once-weekly feedings, but babies may need two feedings per week. Very active species may need more frequent feedings. For example, garter snakes (*Thamnophis* spp.) fed primarily fish do poorly if fed only once weekly and must be fed more frequently. Most keepers increase the feedings for female snakes as the breeding season approaches. Many gravid female

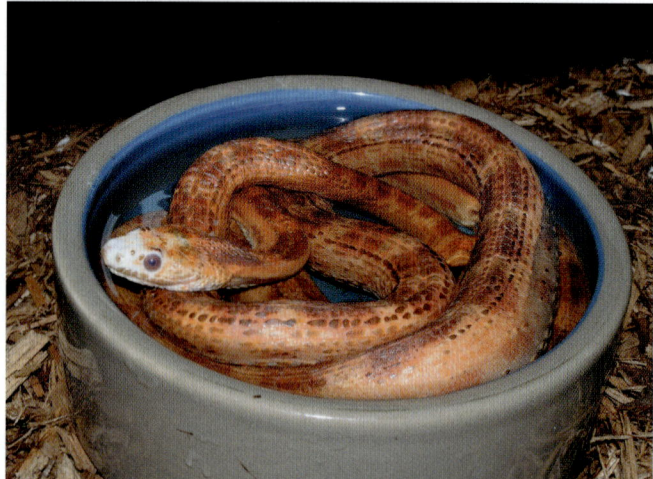

FIG 20.7 Adult partially scaleless corn snake (*Pantherophis guttatus*) soaking in her water bowl after the cage temperature had increased to an uncomfortable level. (Courtesy of Richard S. Funk.)

situations that allow them to achieve a slightly elevated body temperature. Captives thrive better when provided with a thermal gradient that incorporates the T_s for each species. Summary discussions of research on thermoregulation in snakes have been published.[4–6] Also, see Section 3 for more information on captive thermal considerations in snakes.

TABLE 20.2 Suggested Diets for Snakes

Snake Group	Example	PRIMARY FOOD PREFERENCES Adults	Young
Scolecophidia	Blind snakes	A	
Tropidophiidae	Wood snakes (*Troidophis* spp.)	Am, L, M	
Calabariidae	Calabar ground boa (*Calabaria*)	M	
Boidae	Anacondas, *Eunctes* spp.	F, M, B	
	Boa constrictor (*Boa constrictor*), Dumeril's (*Acrantophis dumerili*)	M, B	
	Pacific/Solomon Island (*Candoia* spp.)	L, M, B	
	Rubber (*Charina bottae*)	L, M	
	Amazon, Emerald, Annulated (*Corallus* spp.)	M, B	L, M
	Rainbow/Caribbean (*Chilabothrus* spp., *Epicrates cnchria*)	M, B	Am, L, M
	Sand boas (*Eryx* spp.)	M	
	Rosy (*Lichanura trivirgata*)	M	
Xenopeltidae	Asian sunbeam snake (*Xenopeltis unicolor*)	M	L
Loxocemidae	Neotropical Sunbeam Snakes (*Loxocemus bicolor*)	M	
Pythonidae	Burmese, Indian, black-headed, woma, carpet, diamond, reticulated, ball, African Rock, blood, short-tailed (*Aspidites*, *Malayopython*, *Morelia*, and *Python* spp.)	M, B	
	Green Tree (*Morelia viridis*)	M, B	L, M
	Indoaustralian (*Liasis*, *Leiopython* spp.)	M, B	L, M
Acrochordidae	Elephant trunk snake (*Acrochordus* spp.)	F	
Viperidae	Copperheads and Asian relatives (*Agkistrodon, Calloselasma, Deinagkistrodon, Gloydius, Hypnale, Protobothrops, Trimeresurus* spp.)	M, B, L	Am, L, M
	Cottonmouth (*Agkistrodon piscivorus*)	F, A, L, M	Am, F, M
	Rattlesnakes (*Crotalus* and *Sistrurus* spp.)	M, L, B	L, M
	Most other pit vipers (*Bothrops* spp., *Lachesis* spp.)	M, B	Am, L, M
	Sawscale vipers (*Echis* spp.)	A, M	I, L, M
	Horned sand vipers (*Cerastes* spp.)	L, M	
	Most other vipers (*Vipera* spp.)	M, B	L, M
Lamprophiidae	House snakes (*Lamprophis* spp.)	M	L, M
	Madagascan hog-nosed (*Liohetrodon* spp.)	M, B	
Elapidae	King cobra (*Ophiophagus hannah*)	S, M, B	
	Most other cobras (*Naja* spp.)	M, B	
	Kraits (*Bungarus* spp.)	M, B	
	Coral snakes (*Micrurus* spp.)	S, M, L	
Colubridae	Brown, red-bellied (*Storeria* spp.)	OI	
	Garter and ribbon (*Thamnophis* spp.)	F, Am, M	
	Glossy (*Arizona elegans*)	L, M	
	Bull, gopher, pine (*Pituophis* spp.)	M, B	
	Green (*Opheodrys* spp.)	A, L	
	Hog-nosed (*Heterodon* spp.)	Am, M	
	Indigo, cribo (*Drymarchon* spp.)	S, M, B	Am, L, M
	King snake (*Lampropeltis* spp.)	M, L	L, M
	Long-nosed (*Rhiinocheilus lecontei*)	L, M	L
	Milk snake (*Lampropeltis triangulum* complex)	M	L, M
	Patchnosed (*Salvadora* spp.)	L, M	
	Racers (*Coluber, Drymobius, Masticophis* spp.)	M, B	L, M
	Rat snakes, new world (*Bogertophis, Elaphe, Senticolis, Spilotes* spp.)	M, B	Am, L,
	Rat snakes, old world (*Coelognathus, Elaphe, Eupreplophus, Gonyosoma, Oreocryptophis, Orthriophis, Ptyas* spp.)	M, B, L	M, L
	Ringneck (*Diadophis* spp.)	OI, Am, S	

A, Arthropods; *Am*, amphibians; *B*, birds; *F*, fish; *L*, lizards; *M*, mammals; *OI*, other invertebrates; *S*, snakes.

snakes will not feed during gestation, and actively breeding males may also have reduced appetites. See Chapter 27 for a thorough discussion of nutrition in snakes.

BEHAVIOR

If the cage is opened primarily for feeding, the snake is likely to exhibit a feeding response every time the cage is opened. Sometimes snakes can be conditioned to a "feeding" experience if the keeper repeats an action at feeding time. For example, tapping on the enclosure with metal forceps (recommended to feed snakes) before feeding can train the snake that a prey item is soon to be presented. If the snake is large and potentially dangerous to the keeper, feeding it outside the cage (within another enclosure) may be safer. Many social behaviors observed in captive snakes are related to reproductive activities, and these courtship-related interactions can be quite dramatic and variable among species. Pheromones along with visual and tactile cues are often involved in these complex behaviors. During the mating season, the behavior of some snakes is completely different, sometimes becoming aggressive, and courtship, mating, and combat can occasionally result in injuries. Most clients can recognize behavioral changes in snakes as the mating season arrives, and they can track when a female is ready to oviposit or give birth. See Chapter 80 for more information on reproduction in snakes. In most circumstances, housing captive snakes singly is preferable. If housed in groups, they must be monitored closely, especially during feeding times or during the breeding season to avoid injuries or even cannibalism. For example, if two snakes attempt to swallow the same prey item, a larger snake may eventually ingest both the prey and the other snake (Fig. 20.9A and B). Before interacting with a snake, hands should be washed, especially after handling prey species such as rats and mice, or after handling predator species such as cats, ferrets, or king snakes. Otherwise, the snake may become confused and react to these odors by biting the hand in a feeding or defensive response. Having an ophiophagus (snake-eating) snake, such as a king snake (*Lampropeltis getula* or *L.californiae*), housed in an adjacent cage, or having just treated one on the same examination table, can affect the behavior of another snake likely in response to pheromone production.

BRUMATION

Brumation is the proper term for winter dormancy in reptiles (as opposed to true hibernation).[7–9] Many temperate zone snakes must be brumated to induce successful reproduction. For successful, safe brumation snakes are fed well during the summer and fall, then feeding is stopped, and the snakes can pass stool (empty the gastrointestinal tract) before the cooling cycle. The cage temperature is slowly dropped over a period of several weeks. Dropping the temperature 2.8°C (5°F) every few days for a total drop of 10°C to 14°C (20°F–25°F) "conditions" the snakes to enter the brumation period. They are maintained in the dark with water available but no food for about 3 months, then slowly the temperatures are increased again. Feeding may begin 2 to 3 weeks later. Unlike temperate colubrids, most tropical boas and pythons do not require as drastic a temperature drop. Usually a 5°C (10°F) temperature reduction suffices, and often this may only need to occur at night, and total darkness is not required. These tropical snakes are prone to respiratory or neurologic disease if kept too cool. Neonate temperate zone snakes that are not yet feeding, if in good physical condition, can be brumated, which may induce them to feed after the brumation period. No snake, regardless of age, should be brumated if it is not in good physical condition or if it is showing evidence of illness.

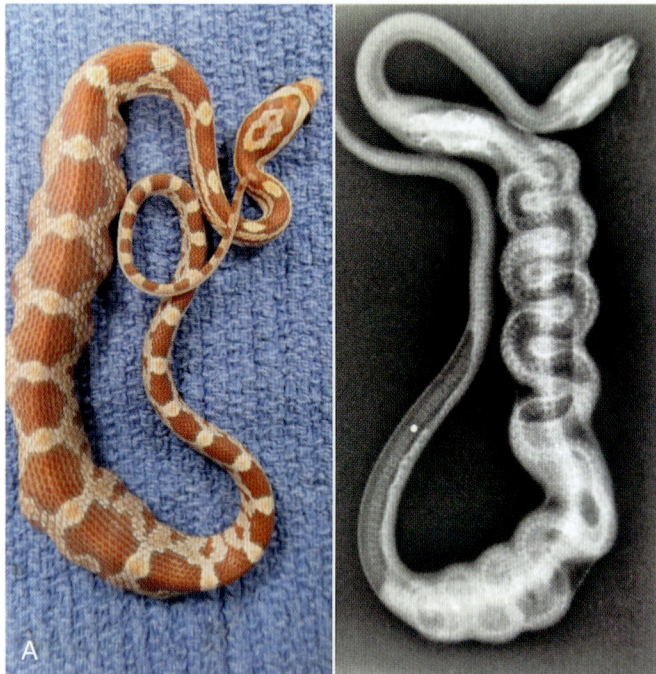
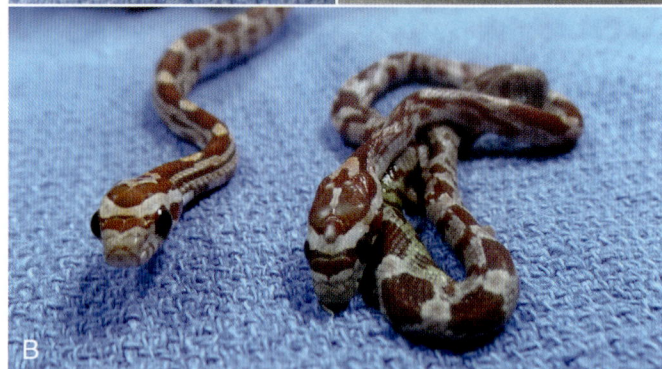

FIG 20.9 (A) It is recommended to feed snakes separately if they are housed together, as cannibalism may occur. A juvenile corn snake (*Pantherophis guttatus*) was presented for ingesting its cage mate (another juvenile corn snake) after prey items were offered in the same enclosure. Radiographs identified the cage mate was ingested tail first. (B) The ingested snakes head was visualized in the cranial esophagus and gently pulled out, but the ingested snake was no longer alive. Pictured here is the patient and its extracted cage mate "meal." (Courtesy of Scott J. Stahl, Stahl Exotic Animal Veterinary Services.)

LONGEVITY

Clients frequently ask about the life expectancy of their snakes. A ball python (*Python regius*) set the longevity record at 47.5 years in the Philadelphia Zoo.[10] Table 20.3 lists longevity records for a number of commonly kept snakes, showing many snakes can potentially live a long life in captivity. Little is known about longevity in nature, but experts doubt that many snakes reach these ages in the wild. Many herpetoculturists believe that female snakes, bred repeatedly for high production, may have a shorter lifespan because of reproductive activity.

TABLE 20.3 Longevity in Years of Some Selected Snakes in Captvity

Boidae

Dumeril's boa, *Acrantophis dumerili*	26
Boa constrictor, *Boa c. constrictor*	40
Solomon Island ground boa, *Candoia carinata paulsoni*	16
Rubber boa, *Charina bottae*	26
Emerald tree boa, *Corallus caninus*	19
Colombian rainbow boa, *Epicrates cenchria maurus*	31
Smooth sand boa, *Eryx johni*	24
Anaconda, *Eunectes murinus*	31
Rosy boa, *Lichanura trivirgata*	31

Xenopeltidae

Asian sunbeam snake, *Xenopeltis unicolor*	12

Loxocemidae

Neotropical sunbeam snake, *Loxocemus bicolor*	32

Pythonidae

Children's python, *Antaresia childreni*	24
Black-headed python, *Aspidites melanocephalus*	22
Woma, *Aspidites ramsayi*	16
Brown water python, *Liasis mackloti fuscus*	26
Reticulated python, *Malayopython reticulatus*	29
Carpet python, *Morelia s. spilotes*	19
Green tree python, *Morelia viridis*	20
Short-tailed python, *Python curtus*	27
Burmese python, *Python bivittatus*	28
Indian python, *Python m. molurus*	34
Ball python, *Python regius**	47.5
African rock python, *Python sebae*	27

Viperidae, Crotalinae

Northern copperhead, *Agkistrodon contortrix*	29
Western cottonmouth, *Agkistrodon piscivorous leucostoma*	26
Jumping pit viper, *Atropoides nummifer*	19
Eyelash palm pit viper, *Bothriechis schlegeli*	19
Terciopelo, *Bothrops asper*	20
Eastern diamondback rattlesnake, *Crotalus adamanteus*	22
Western diamondback rattlesnake, *Crotalus atrox*	27
South American rattlesnake, *Crotalus durissus terrificus*	17
Timber rattlesnake, *Crotalus h. horridus*	30
Banded rock rattlesnake, *Crotalus lepidus klauberi*	33
Southern Pacific rattlesnake, *Crotalus oreganus helleri*	24

Central American bushmaster, *Lachesis stenophrys*	24
Western Massasauga, *Sistrurus catenatus tergeminus*	20
Pope's pit viper, *Trimeresurus popeorum*	13

Viperidae, Viperinae

Puff adder, *Bitis arietans*	15
Gaboon viper, *Bitis gabonica*	18
Horned sand viper, *Cerastes cerastes*	18
Russell's viper, *Daboia russelli*	15
Carpet viper, *Echis coloratus*	28
Common adder, *Vipera berus* spp.	19

Lamprophiidae

House snake, *Lamprophis fuliginosus*	9

Elapidae

Black mamba, *Dendroaspis polylepis*	21
Texas coral snake, *Micrurus tenere*	19
Monocled cobra, *Naja kaouthia*	32
Black Forest cobra, *Naja melanoleuca*	29
Cape cobra, *Naja nivea*	26
King cobra, *Ophiophagus hannah*	22
Taipan, *Oxyuranus scutellatus*	15

Colubridae

Trans-Pecos rat snake, *Bogertophis subocularis*	23
Eastern Indigo snake, *Drymarchon couperi*	25
Black rat snake, *Pantherophis obsoletus*	22
Western mud snake, *Farancia abacura reinwardti*	18
Plains hog-nosed snake, *Heterodon nasicus*	19
False water cobra, *Hydrodynastes gigas*	16
Grey-banded king sake, *Lampropeltis alterna*	19
California king snake, *Lampropeltis californiae*	44
Prairie king snake, *Lampropeltis c. calligaster*	23
Arizona mountain king snake, *Lampropeltis p. pyromelana*	22
Scarlet king snake, *Lampropeltis triangulum elapsoides*	23
Coastal mountain king snake, *Lampropeltis zonata multicincta*	28
Grass snake, *Natrix natrix*	20
Blotched water snake, *Nerodia erythrogster transversa*	14
Corn snake, *Pantherophis guttatus*	32
Great Basin gopher snake, *Pituophis catenifer deserticola*	33
Northern pine snake, *Pituophis m. melanoleucus*	20
Northwestern garter snake, *Thamnophis ordinoides*	15

*Conant R. The oldest snake. *Bull Chicago Herpetol Soc.* 1993;28(4):77.
Data from Slavens FL, 1999.[11]

REFERENCES

See www.expertconsult.com for a complete list of references.

21

Lizards

Stephen Barten and Shane Simpson

Great advances have been made in the captive care of lizards, in part from our increased knowledge of their ecology and natural history but also due to the global dissemination of information through internet-based resources. Unfortunately, this information is not always accurate and must be critically interpreted. Keepers acquiring a new lizard species should be familiar with the natural history and any special husbandry requirements necessary for that species. Thorough research should include speaking with people who keep or have kept the species; reading reference material from as many different, reliable sources as possible; and speaking with a reptile veterinarian. Unfortunately, many acquire the lizard first and do research later, often to the detriment of the animal.

Despite advancements in the captive management of lizards, veterinarians are still frequently presented with animals suffering from medical conditions related to poor husbandry.

RESTRAINT

Lizards may need to be restrained for a number of reasons including environmental management, examination, diagnostic procedures, or therapeutic delivery. No matter the reason, the method of restraint should always be performed with care to avoid injury to both the animal and the handler. Never assume that because someone owns an animal they know how to handle it safely.

Although many captive reptiles seem calm and relaxed when handled, they are not domesticated. Therefore restraint methods should allow appropriate control with minimal stress and handling time.[1]

Small lizards may simply be caught and held in bare hands. If needed towels and blankets should be available. These can be placed over the head and/or body of the lizard to avoid being bitten or scratched, as well as to provide some comfort for the animal. Covering the head reduces light and visual stimulation, and most lizards will relax and become motionless when this is performed. In short-bodied species such as skinks, a thick sock can be used over the body to restrain the animal to allow for examination of the head and oral cavity (Fig. 21.1). Equipment such as catching poles and tongs may be required in larger, faster species, although care should be taken to avoid injury to the animal.[2] In fieldwork circumstances a fine noose has proven to be an effective method to capture lizards and could be used in a captive situation if deemed necessary and appropriate. If a large, uncooperative lizard needs to be restrained for accurate morphologic measurements, the construction of a restraining tray using Velcro straps and a plastic base may be considered.[3] Clear, plastic tubes that are more known for the handling of venomous snakes are very effective in restraining lizards for procedures such as radiology (Fig. 21.2). For the short-term restraint of small lizards, a clear ziplock bag can be used.[4] Some species, such as the eastern water dragons (*Intellagama lesuerrii* spp.), can be placed in a hypnotic-like trance when positioned on their backs, with their throat and ventral coelomic area gently stroked. This relaxed state allows for minimal procedures such radiology and ultrasonography to be performed. Once placed back in normal recumbency they return to their normal state.

The use of the ocular vasovagal response has been reported as an effective short-term method of restraint for iguanids,[5] monitors, and other large, hyperactive lizards. This method requires applying gentle pressure on the eyes (through closed eyelids) to stimulate the vagal nerve and cause a reduction in the heart rate and, through vasodilation, a subsequent drop in blood pressure. This can be achieved using digital pressure or, alternatively, soft gauze placed over the eyes and held in place with self-adherent bandage material. Pressure is applied for 30 seconds to 2 minutes to achieve the effect. Unfortunately, not all patients respond, and the technique may only allow for several minutes of restraint. If there are excessive external stimulants, such as noise and movement, this method is less successful. It can be repeated but is often less effective on subsequent applications unless a suitable time interval is allowed. The simple process of covering the eyes may also calm the animal due to a reduction of external stimuli.

In some cases, the use of physical restraint can actually be avoided all together. When radiographing small lizards, they can simply be placed in a radiolucent box for images to be taken. This is considerably less stressful for the animal and is often adequate to obtain satisfactory diagnostic images.

Another method for reducing the need to restrain and handle lizards is training (see Chapter 14). While once thought impossible, several successful training outcomes with reptiles, including lizards, have been reported.[6] Target training and visual and auditory cues can all be utilized to aid the handler.

Utilizing the ectothermic nature of reptiles may also aid in the restraint of lizards. Allowing a lizard to cool to below its preferred optimum body temperature will result in a less active animal and one that may be easier to handle. This can be achieved by handling animals in the cooler parts of the day or simply not providing any supplemental heat for a period. Animals should not be actively cooled by artificial means (e.g., placing in the refrigerator) to achieve this. Different species have particular defensive behaviors of which handlers should be aware. Iguanas and monitors are proficient at tail whipping and can deliver a nasty blow if the tail is left unrestrained. If a single person is holding such an animal the tail can be pinned gently between the holder's hip and a table while the head and body are restrained. Probably the most common defensive behavior is biting. Large lizards can cause serious

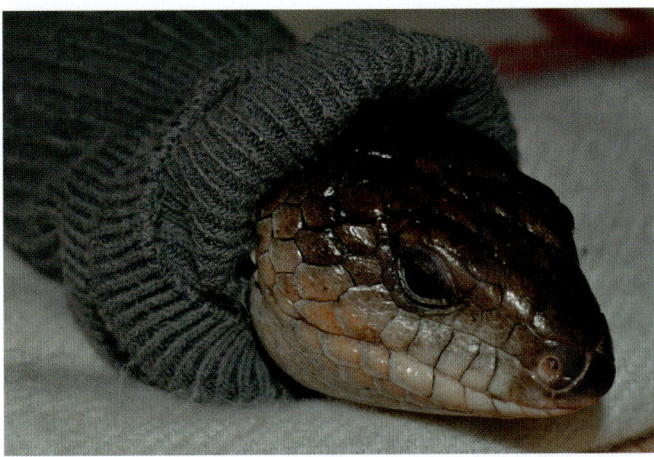

FIG 21.1 Large skinks such as eastern blue-tongue skinks (*Tiliqua scincoides*) can be well restrained in a thick sock. This is particularly useful for allowing radiographs to be taken and for examination of the head and mouth structures. (Courtesy of Shane Simpson.)

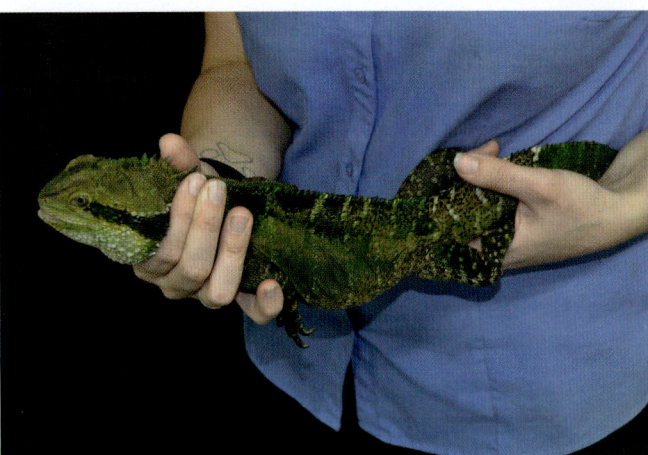

FIG 21.3 Larger lizards, such as this eastern water dragon (*Intellagama lesueurii lesueurii*), may be adequately restrained by grasping behind the head to reduce the chances of being bitten. The pelvis and hind legs are supported in the other hand while the tail is pinned against the handler's body to prevent being whipped. (Courtesy of Shane Simpson.)

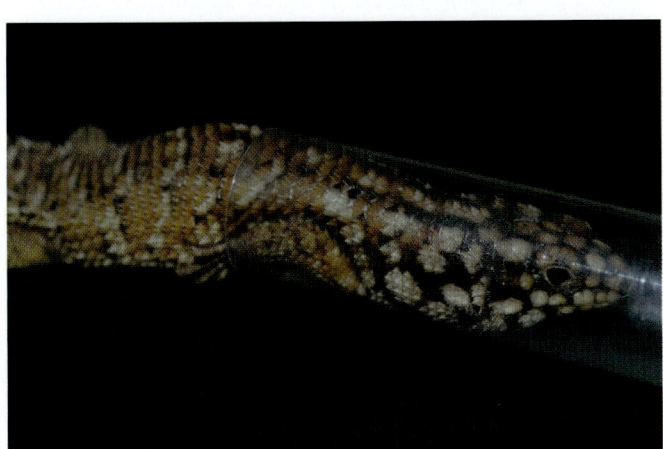

FIG 21.2 Clear plastic tubes normally used for restraining snakes can be used just as effectively to immobilize lizards, particularly small, flighty species such as this Hosmer's skink (*Egernia hosmeri*), for procedures such as radiography. (Courtesy of Shane Simpson.)

damage, so it is vital that the method of restraint minimizes this risk. The head can be controlled by holding it firmly behind the mandible with the thumb and index finger. The front feet can be controlled by holding them against the body with the remaining fingers. The rear legs can be grasped with the other hand and held against the lizard's body or tail just below the pelvis (Fig. 21.3).[7] Never reach over an iguana or other large lizard that is not being restrained, because they may bite and claw. This is particularly so in arboreal species, and it may be prudent to clip nails prior to an examination or procedure to minimize the risk of injury to the handler. Lizards do not tolerate leashes well. They do not walk to follow an owner. When the leash is tugged, the lizard usually spins becoming tangled in the leash, which often results in injury.

Care must be taken to prevent tail autotomy in species that possess this ability. These include most iguanids, skinks, geckos, and anguids but not monitors, chameleons, or agamids (refer to Chapter 9). They

must never be grasped by the tail, and it is advisable to inform owners that there is a risk of tail autotomy prior to any restraint or procedure. Small geckos, such as *Phelsuma* spp., have delicate skin that can tear during handling and may best be captured with a soft net. Other geckos of the *Strophurus* genus possess a series of tail glands that can exude a sticky amber fluid. The secretion is quite pungent and can be an irritant to the eyes and mucous membranes of the handler. Some species are able to explosively eject this fluid up to 50 cm.[8] Special considerations should be taken when handling the two species of venomous lizards that are dangerous to humans, gila monsters (*Heloderma suspectum*) and beaded lizards (*Heloderma horridum*).

Regardless of the method of restraint used, lizards are best controlled with a light touch. The more pressure that is exerted, the more lizards tend to struggle. When necessary, lizards can be chemically sedated or anesthetized (see Chapters 48 and 49).

IDENTIFICATION

In both zoological collections and with private keepers, individual animals may need to be permanently identified. The appropriate method of identification will depend on many factors, including the species involved, size and temperament of the lizards, the length of time identification is required, the actual reason for the identification, and whether the lizard is in a captive situation or wild.

Photo-identification of lizards is a method of identifying animals based on their natural markings and other features present on one or more parts of the body. It is an excellent noninvasive method of identification that has become more accessible with digital cameras and imaging software. High-resolution, standardized photographs of predefined regions of the lizard can be taken and stored for future comparisons. Disadvantages for this method include excessive handling to obtain adequate photos, accuracy issues in those species in which natural markings change over time, and limited use in species that lack distinguishing marks.

A simple, cheap, and fast method of identification that is particularly useful for field situations is to use a felt-tip permanent marker or paint pen to write a number or other mark on the lizard's side. These identification markers can be seen from a distance, especially with binoculars, thus minimizing stress to the animals. The amount of marking should

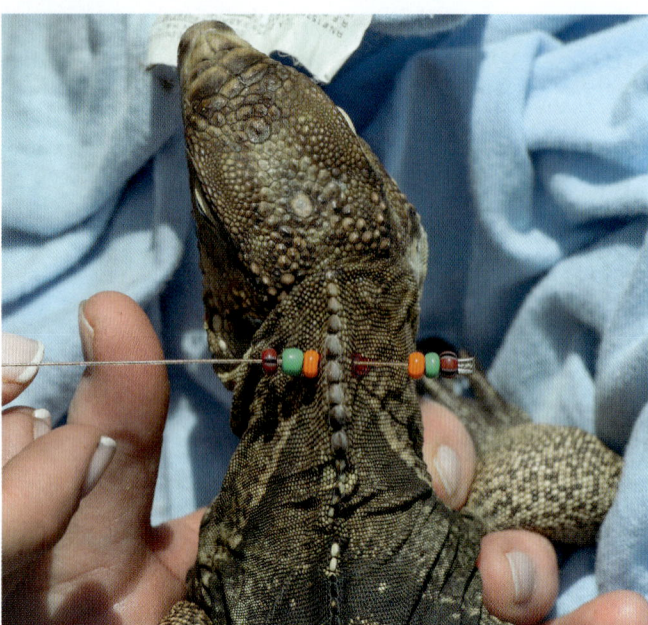

FIG 21.4 Colored beads threaded onto wire that is inserted through the nuchal crest of lizards can be used as a means of identification. By using different color combinations and repeating this on both sides of the animal, it can be easily identified from any angle, such as in this Sister Islands iguana (*Cyclura nubila caymanensis*) from Cayman Brac. (Courtesy of Stephen Barten.)

TABLE 21.1 Microchip Implant Sites in Lizards	
WSAVA Guidelines[12]	
Lizards >12.5 cm snout to vent length	Subcutaneously in the left inguinal region
Lizards <12.5 cm snout to vent length	Intracoelomic
British Veterinary Zoological Society[13]	
Lateral aspect of the left femoral area, over the quadriceps muscle, or subcutaneous on the caudal half of the left flank if too small or legs too skinny or absent	

WSAVA, World Small Animal Veterinary Association.

be kept to a minimum to avoid an increase in mortality from predation. Unfortunately, markings will only last until the lizard sheds its skin. Spray paint can also be used and is a great tool for mark-recapture studies estimating population size over time. If lizards are seen on subsequent days, researchers can mark them with different colored paint each day. The nontoxic, water-based paint is applied as minimally as possible but in a manner that allows the animal to be identified from any angle. Using a spray device means the animal may not have to be captured for the paint to be applied.[9] Different colored nail polishes and highly reflective paints applied to the animal's body and/or its nails have also been utilized.

The use of colored beads provides a more permanent method of marking and identification. Colored beads can be sutured into the tail musculature or crests of the neck using thin wire or nylon suture (Fig. 21.4).[10] A combination of colors and patterns can be used to create a unique code. When the neck is used, it is common for the same bead combination to be placed on either side to allow the animal to be identified from any direction. This method is more stressful for the animal, and some practice is required to perform the "beading" quickly.

Visible implant elastomers (VIE) are biologically inert solids that can be injected just beneath areas of translucent skin where they remain externally visible. Available in multiple colors, including some that fluoresce under ultraviolet light, they can be injected into different positions on the body to create an inordinate number of unique combinations. Unfortunately, these implants are not visible from a distance and so the animal must be restrained to allow accurate identification.

Visible implant alpha tags (VI Alpha Tags) are biologically inert, implantable tags with a letter and number combination printed on a fluorescent background color. When implanted under translucent skin the combination is visible when the animal is restrained.

For times when identification is only required for a short period of time the use of bee tags has been reported.[11] These cardboard tags come in 5 colors and are numbered 1–99. Used for the identification of queen bees in a hive, the tags can easily be glued to a small lizard in appropriate locations.

The most common method of animal identification known to veterinarians is the microchip. More correctly referred to as passive integrated transponder (PIT) tags or passive radio frequency identification (RFID) tags, these small devices are used extensively for permanent identification in dogs, cats, and other animals. PIT tags can also be used to identify lizards, whether in captive or wild populations. Standardization of microchip implantation sites is essential for integrity of the system, and recommended sites have been developed (Table 21.1).

Another classic method of identification for small vertebrates is toe clipping. By clipping toes in different combinations on different limbs lizards can be identified. Although toe clipping is a permanent identification method for lizards, there is a high prevalence of lost toes in wild populations. Thus this method could lead to errors and misidentification of lizards. Loss of toes in captive populations is less likely; however, toe clipping is invasive, and in some species of lizards the procedure has had a negative impact on survivability.[14,15] In addition there is always public concern for the humane treatment of animals in research, and toe clipping is a contentious issue.[16] Other methods of lizard identification involving permanent modification of body parts include tail notching and clipping of dorsal body spines. Researchers using identification techniques that involve alteration or removal of body parts must keep the animals' welfare in mind and consider alternatives when possible. In general toe/spine clipping and notching should only be performed under a research license and cannot be recommended for clinical practice.

Other temporary identification methods used by field researchers that can be utilized in captive lizards include colored cloth tape around the tail, aluminum leg rings around the upper thigh, collars, and subcutaneous tattooing with ultraviolet fluorescent tattoo ink.[17]

SPECIFIC HOUSING REQUIREMENTS

Design of captive lizard enclosures basically can be split into two broad categories. Reptiles were once considered quite basic animals, and so traditionally spartan, easily cleaned cages were recommended and popular. Bare cages with newspaper substrate, a single branch if needed, and a water bowl were considered adequate. The advantage was ease of maintenance at the cost of stimulation and enrichment for the cage inhabitants. The other category, naturalistic, is one that has become more popular over recent years, particularly with keepers taking on

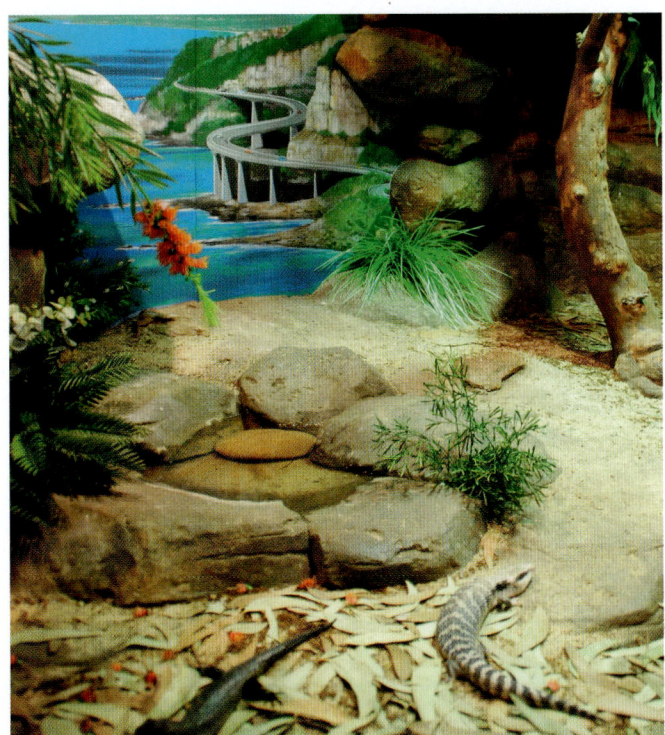

FIG 21.5 Zoos, wildlife parks, and other establishments with reptiles on display need to have animals presented in naturalistic settings. Such enclosures need to be well planned with respect to providing the animals with all their requirements, as well as being suitable for the viewing public. (Courtesy of Shane Simpson.)

lizards as pets. These keepers want more lush, complex, naturalistic vivaria to show off their animals and provide them with a more realistic setting in which to live. Many of these enclosures become part of the decor in the home and become a talking point among friends and family. Keepers will literally spend thousands of dollars on creating mini-landscapes for their animals to enjoy. They often take great pride in not only having a healthy animal but one that is living as it would in the wild (or as close to that as possible). Naturalistic enclosures are a must for display systems at zoos and wildlife parks (Fig. 21.5). The visiting public like and demand to see animals represented as if they were taken directly out of the wild. These facilities often need to balance the wants and needs of the animal with the need for the paying public to see the animal. Although these vivaria are more aesthetically pleasing for both the owner or member of the public and the pet, they do not come without cost. Such cages are labor intensive to maintain, and, if inadequately done, bacteria and fungi build up to levels that result in illness for the cage inhabitants. Few but the most dedicated and experienced hobbyists do an adequate job of maintaining hygiene in such complex cages. If a keeper cannot properly maintain a complex vivarium, then a simpler setup is a better choice.

Cage Size and Orientation

In general, lizards need large cages to accommodate their active behavior. As another generality, most keepers provide cages that are too small or of inappropriate dimensions for the species being kept. Not all space is created equally when it comes to the highly diverse lizard group. An enclosure that is perfectly suitable for an arboreal lizard is likely to be

totally unsuitable for a terrestrial one. Keepers need to keep this in mind when deciding what species they wish to keep so that appropriate space can be planned for and allocated. It has been recommended that for lizards the cage length should equal 1.5 to 2 times the total length of the lizard housed within and the cage width at least half that length.[18] These dimensions are very conservative, and others have suggested even more space, quantifying requirements as 0.2 m² cage space per 0.1 m total length for terrestrial lizards and 0.4 m³ cage space per 0.1 m total length for arboreal lizards.[19] That equals a cage two times as long and one time as wide as a terrestrial lizard is long or two times as long, two times as high, and one time as wide as an arboreal lizard is long. For example, a 1 m–long iguana should have a cage measuring 2 m long, 2 m high, and 0.5 to 1 m wide, and a 2 m long one needs a cage measuring 4 m long, 2 m high, and 1 m wide, almost the size of a whole room. Few commercial cages exceed 1.2 m in length, so once a lizard reaches a length of 0.8 m, it needs a custom-built or room-sized cage. This is only one example why green iguanas (*Iguana iguana*) are not the most ideal pet for most reptile keepers. Aquariums often sold for juvenile iguanas and monitors are rarely adequate for more than a year. Chameleons need proportionately even more space, and cages varying from 1 m × 0.5 m × 0.6 m high for dwarf species to 1.3 m × 0.6 m × 1.3 m high for large species are minimum standards.[20] All these measurements are purely minimums, and attention needs to be given to how the cage furniture is arranged to make appropriate use of the space for species being housed. Additionally, the larger an enclosure the more microhabitats can be created using temperature, light, and humidity.

Terrestrial lizards need a horizontally oriented enclosure. Enclosure height is not a priority for these species, although they often use rocks and branches for climbing. These also are essential to allow the lizard to move closer to and further away from overhead heat and light sources. Arboreal lizards need height in their enclosures, and many species fail to thrive if denied the opportunity to climb at will. To achieve this, the enclosure should be fitted throughout with both vertical and horizontal climbing structures of varying widths and textures that are securely anchored to prevent falling and causing injury to the cage inhabitant. This will allow the animal to access all the environmental zones.

All lizards should be housed within a suitable enclosure, because lizards allowed to roam free in the house are subject to hypothermia, trauma, ingestion of foreign material (Fig. 21.6), and escape.

Construction Materials

A multitude of materials are available. Glass, acrylic, timber, assorted plastics, fiberglass, and wire may all be utilized. Each has its pros and cons, and the correct material is used to meet the unique husbandry needs of the species.

Keepers must be aware of these needs for each species of lizard being housed. An enclosure for a larger chameleon should be constructed of plastic-coated, wire mesh with timber or metal framing. The mesh should be no smaller than 10 mm × 10 mm square, because this provides good ventilation and protection yet is still a physical barrier. Aluminum window mesh should be avoided because there is a risk of trapping and removing toes and claws. Medium to large chameleons should not be housed in glass or plastic aquariums. First, the lizard's reflection in the glass may cause stress for these solitary animals. Second, this type of enclosure is also not ventilated well enough to provide adequate air exchange and can lead to eye, skin, and respiratory infections.[21] Semiaquatic lizards such as caiman lizards (*Dracaena* sp.) need a large bathing area that allows them to fully submerge and swim. A simple bowl of water is not sufficient for these species. As such the enclosure base needs to be constructed of glass or plastic to accommodate water and handle the humidity associated with it. Wire mesh for the enclosure walls should be avoided when housing highly stressed or active animals

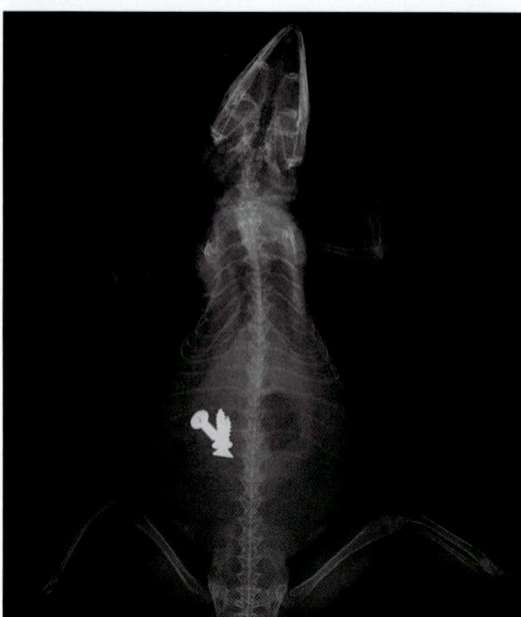

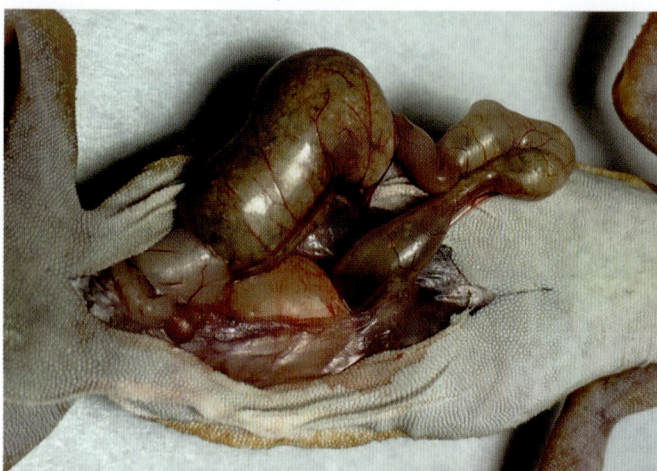

FIG 21.7 A smooth knob-tailed gecko (*Nephrurus levis levis*) necropsy showing severe sand impaction in the lower regions of the intestinal tract. (Courtesy of Shane Simpson.)

FIG 21.6 Lizards should not be allowed to roam freely outside of their enclosure. They can be inquisitive animals and will use their tongue to sample their surroundings. This can often lead to the ingestion of inappropriate items such as screws, as seen in this radiograph of an eastern water dragon (*Intellagama lesueurii lesueurii*). (Courtesy of Shane Simpson.)

like basilisks (*Basiliscus* spp.) and water dragons (*Physignathus* spp., *Intellagama* spp.). These animals often rub their noses on the walls of their enclosures in an attempt to escape. The wire mesh acts like coarse sandpaper and can inflict severe damage to the rostral area. Ideally these animals should be housed in enclosures with opaque walls and a smooth surface to minimize damage. Geckos with adhesive lamellae on their feet prefer solid surfaces to screening. Glass provides poor visual security and is a poor insulator. Many reptiles are escape artists and can squeeze through narrow cracks; thus cages must be secure, with tight-fitting lids.

Substrates

There is possibly no single subject that creates more debate amongst reptile keepers than that of substrates. With such diversity in the lizard group and with animals coming from such a broad range of habitats and lifestyles, it is not unexpected that there is controversy. As herpetoculture has grown, so has the boundless number of different substrates available in the market place. Keepers must balance the natural history requirements of their animals with the ability to adequately maintain hygiene and minimize other risks associated with using particular substrates. An ideal substrate is one that is inexpensive, aesthetically pleasing, easily cleaned, absorbent, and digestible or easily passed if swallowed. Examples of commonly used substrates include newspaper, unprinted paper sheets, outdoor or marine carpet, bark chips, assorted mulches and commercially available wood shavings, soil, ground coconut fiber (coir), vermiculite, recycled paper, and compressed wooden pellets. Like construction materials, each substrate has its good and bad qualities. Newspaper is easy to keep clean and is cheap to obtain but is not aesthetically pleasing. Carpets require regular washing and replacement. Bark made from redwood and cedar should not be used because there are anecdotal reports of the toxic aromatic oils in them causing respiratory

and dermatological issues. Soils containing fertilizers should be avoided in case of accidental ingestion. Recycled paper pellets are a popular substrate because they are absorbent, contain minimal dust, and if swallowed are digestible. Additionally, from an environmental standpoint many of these products, with the exception of carpet, are compostable. Sand or a mixture of soil and sand may be used for desert species. However, color-dyed fine desert sand made for reptiles often results in discoloration of the skin.

Of greatest concern with most lizards kept on particulate substrates is the risk of accidental ingestion and gastrointestinal impaction. Cases of this have been reported in animals kept on fine bark chips, crushed corn cob, clay kitty litter, crushed walnut shell, shredded coconut husk, and calcium carbonate sands marketed as digestible among others (Fig. 21.7).[22] There are anecdotal stories of obstructions occurring in lizards housed on other sands (e.g., washed play sand and sand sold as "red desert sand"), but actual documented reports in the literature are scarce. Regardless of the particulate substrate used, there is always a risk of ingestion, especially at feeding time, or associated with pica due to mineral-deficient diets. The risk of ingestion can be minimized by feeding an appropriate, balanced diet from a large, flat food bowl or feeding the animal in a separate enclosure free from particulate substrates. Chameleons are best kept in an enclosure free of substrate or a non-particulate substrate such as outdoor or marine carpet. This will minimize the risk of ingestion of foreign material should the chameleon's tongue miss a prey item at feeding time.

Some fossorial species prefer substrates that hold their moisture and allow burrows to be made, whereas others such as sand skinks (*Scincus scincus*) prefer a looser sand mix that they can "swim" through.

Both public and private displays sometimes use natural-appearing, artificial rock substrates and walls made of concrete or gunite. These surfaces can be excessively rough and result in open sores and granulomas on the ventral surfaces of the body and feet of inhabitant lizards. If such lesions occur, case management must include smoothing out the surfaces, for instance, using an epoxy-based top coat.

Cage Furniture

The extent and type of enclosure furnishings used for lizards should keep the natural history of the species in mind. Some keepers prefer minimalistic setups that allow easy cleaning and visibility of the animal.

Others like a more naturalistic approach that provides environmental enrichment for the animal and encourages natural behavior.

There is a vast array of natural and artificial products that can be used in enclosures. These include hides, branches, backgrounds, and plants. What and how these products are utilized will be dependent on budget, the species being kept, and the imagination of the keeper.

Many species such as the frilled lizard (*Chlamydosaurus kingii*), helmeted iguana (*Corytophanes cristatus*), and Boyd's forest dragon (*Hypsilurus boydii*) need vertical or strongly inclined branches on which to perch and become stressed and anorectic if these are not available.[23]

Live, nontoxic plants that lack spines and slick surfaces and are big enough to bear the weight of the lizard are recommended. Live plants should be potted to facilitate cleaning and easy replacement if needed. Plants with small, easily swallowed pieces should be avoided. Plants, whether live or artificial, act as cage furniture, provide shelter, and visually enhance an enclosure. Live plants have the additional benefits of adding humidity and providing egg-laying sites. An array of realistic-looking artificial plants is also commercially available.

The provision of at least one hide area and preferably two is essential to ensure ongoing health. Lizards may become stressed if they are unable to seek refuge from heat, light, and other stimulation outside the enclosure. Hide boxes can be made from a cardboard box, terra cotta pottery, cardboard tubes, PVC tubes, corrugated black plastic drainage tubes, sheets of cork bark, or the saucer that fits under a flowerpot. The latter is inverted, and a hole is cut through the top or side to allow access. Arboreal species should be provided with real or artificial plants in which to hide. Many animals may refuse to eat and become stressed if they lack a secure hiding place. If a lizard does not use a particular hiding place, a different size or shape should be tried.

An additional benefit of providing a hide box is that they can be used to create a humid microclimate within the enclosure. Certain species may benefit from this when undergoing ecdysis.

An alternative to a hide box is a Retes stack. This multilayered type of hide allows the lizard to hide and thermoregulate at the same time, as the lizard can move from the lower layers to upper (near the heat source) layers of the hide.

OUTDOOOR ENCLOSURES

Where climatic conditions allow, many lizard keepers use outdoor enclosures to take advantage of natural sunshine, humidity, and weather. Escape and exposure to potential predators is prevented by the use of wire mesh walls and ceiling, or, for some species, smooth, nonclimbable walls made of corrugated tin or similar material. These should be buried deep enough to prevent the lizard from tunneling to freedom. Nontoxic plants, climbing branches, and a water source should be utilized. A shelter to provide refuge from direct sun and inclement weather is essential.

Thermoregulation

Reptiles are ectothermic and need supplemental heat in captivity. The preferred body temperature (T_p) is a behavioral choice and is the temperature range a reptile selects when placed in a thermal gradient. The optimal body temperature (T_o) is a physiological constant that represents the temperature at which performance is maximized. T_o is necessary to optimize metabolic processes, including digestion, growth, healing, reproduction, and immune system function. T_p and T_o usually overlap.

Keepers should be aware of the difference between overhead and substrate heat sources. Radiant heat sources are the preferred method for heating most species of lizard. Overhead radiant heat sources include spot lamps (such as incandescent, mercury vapor, metal halide, and dichroic), ceramic heaters, and radiant heat panels. When radiant heat sources are used, direct contact must be prevented to avoid burns. This can be achieved through the use of wire guards. Examples of substrate heat sources include heat cables and heat mats. These must be used in accordance with the manufacturer's instructions to avoid potential fire hazards.

Heat sources should be used in conjunction with a thermostat so that the temperature in the cage can be precisely controlled. A number of models designed for use with reptile heating systems are commercially available. The simplest form is the on/off thermostat. This type simply turns off the supply of electricity when the temperature in the enclosure reaches a set point. Similarly, the electricity is turned on if the temperature gets too low. These types of thermostats have a degree of swing in the temperature since the enclosure needs to cool below the set point for the heater to be turned back on. Proportional thermostats allow much finer control over the temperature; rather than shutting off the electricity completely they adjust the flow based on the temperature at the probe. The thermostat or its probe should be positioned in close proximity to the basking area within the enclosure to control what will be the hottest area. This reduces the risk of overheating. As a consequence of this, thermostats that are able to register higher temperatures are more useful. If they cannot, then they will need to be positioned further from the basking site.

Even with a thermostat in use, temperatures within the cage must be monitored with a thermometer. Digital and analogue thermometers are available as are infrared temperature "guns." These should be positioned and used to monitor the temperatures at both the basking site and cooler end of the enclosure to gain an appreciation of the thermal gradient present.

Thermal gradients must be provided. In nature, the environment consists of multiple microenvironments with varying temperatures and humidity levels. Reptiles in the wild control their core body temperature to within a few degrees of their T_o via thermoregulation—they move all or parts of their bodies into or out of direct sunlight. A thermally complex environment is recommended for captive reptiles to allow them to adjust their body temperature behaviorally as they would in the wild. A thermal gradient on both a horizontal and vertical axis is ideal. This can be created by providing a focal hot spot on one side of the cage with a combination of substrate and radiant heat. This area should reach the T_o for the species being housed. A captive lizard can heat up in the morning by sitting in the focal hot spot and move out of the hot spot when it exceeds its T_o. Having the entire cage maintained at a uniform temperature is unnatural.

Diurnal temperature fluctuations occur between day and night in the wild, so heat sources should not be left on 24 hours a day. Daily fluctuations in temperature seem to be important for lizards. Timers can be used to turn the heaters off at night. Should temperatures drop too low at night, supplemental heat should be provided by using non-light-emitting radiant sources such as ceramic heat emitters or heat mats. The particular needs of a given species should be researched, because some require hotter or cooler temperatures (Table 21.2).

Stressed, sick, or injured reptiles need to reach their T_o to optimize immune system function. Drug uptake and distribution is influenced by temperature, and reptiles should be maintained at their T_o when receiving medications or anesthetics.

Once commonly used as a heat source, so-called "hot rocks" are inappropriate because most lizard species derive external heat from basking in the sun (radiant heat) and not from lying on rocks heated by the sun (conductive heat). Hot rocks also do not heat the air adequately to increase the ambient temperature. Hot rocks can also be dangerous because they allow direct contact with the heat source. They also have the ability to short circuit and can progressively get hotter with age,

TABLE 21.2   Preferred Optimum Temperature Ranges for Common Captive Lizards

| Common Name | Scientific Name | PREFERRED OPTIMUM TEMPERATURE RANGE (°C/°F) | | Basking Site Temperature (°C/°F) |
		Day	Night	
Bearded dragons	*Pogona* sp.	29–31/84–88	17–20/63–68	35–40/95–104
Green iguanas	*Iguana iguana*	29–32/84–90	19–25/66–77	35–37/95–99
Leopard geckos	*Euphapharis macularius*	25–29/77–84	18–24/64–75	31–32/88–90
Crested geckos	*Correlophus ciliatus*	26–28/79–82	21–23/70–73	Not required
Chameleons (montane)	*Chamaeleo* sp.	25–29/77–84	13–19/55–66	28–29/82–84
Chameleons (lowland)	*Chamaeleo* sp.	27–29/81–84	21/70	29–35/84–95
Blue-tongue skinks	*Tiliqua* sp.	27–29/81–84	19–24/66–75	32–35/90–95
Monitors	*Varanus* sp	29–31/84–88	23–26/73–79	40–45/104–113
Tegus	*Tupinambis* sp.	27–30/27–86	21–26/70–79	39–42/102–108

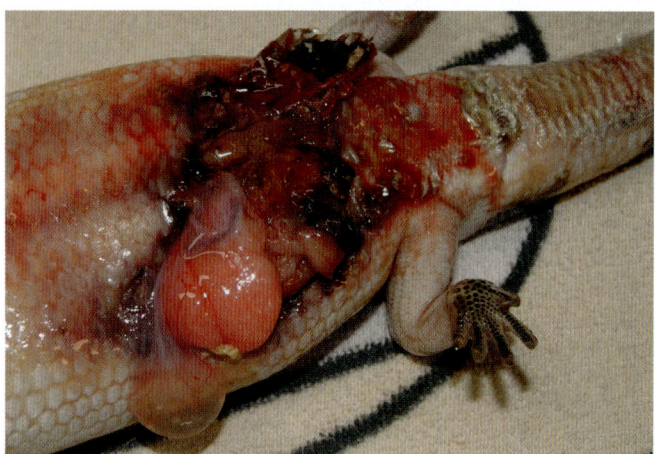

FIG 21.8 The surface of a hot rock can become extremely hot and lead to serious burns as seen in this western blue-tongue lizard (*Tiliqua occipitalis*). (Courtesy of James Haberfield.)

resulting in dangerous surface temperatures. This can lead to severe burns when lizards come in contact with these hot spots (Fig. 21.8) (see Chapter 16).

Lighting

The full spectrum of natural light, specifically the ultraviolet wavelengths (UV), is important for vitamin D synthesis and calcium metabolism in diurnal lizards that do not eat vertebrate prey (see Chapter 17).

No artificial UV source matches the sun, but certain precautions must be taken before exposing captive lizards to direct sunlight. First, window glass filters out UV rays, so sunlight through a window is of no benefit. A reptile in a glass cage should never be placed in direct sunlight, or overheating and death may occur. Reptiles should be in a screen or mesh cage to allow sunlight to enter, but at the same time prevent the escape of the lizard. Part of this enclosure must be shaded with an overhang or plants to allow the animal to get out of direct sun. Basking outside should not be allowed if the ambient temperature is excessively high or low. Even 15 to 30 minutes of direct sunlight a week can be quite beneficial.

A number of artificial UVB light sources for reptiles are commercially available. Traditionally, fluorescent tubes have been used but other lamps such as mercury vapor and metal halide bulbs that provide UVB and heat in a single bulb are excellent alternatives in the right enclosure. These latter lamps get very hot and must be used with caution and only with larger lizards.

There should never be glass or plastic between a UV light source and the reptile because it will filter out the beneficial UV rays. Follow manufacturer recommendations for distance between the lamp and the reptile and how frequently to replace the bulb.

Caution should be taken to avoid human exposure or eye contact with the UV rays because these have been associated with skin cancer and cataract formation.[24,25] Artificial UV light sources should mimic natural photoperiods and be turned off at night.

Artificial light sources cannot replace natural sunlight, and reptiles with access to the sun in outdoor enclosures, even on a screen porch or patio, invariably have better growth, health, behavior, reproduction, and longevity than those kept exclusively indoors.

With advances in technology, LED (light-emitting diode) products made for the reptile hobby are entering the market. These LED lights can provide an energy-efficient and economical method of providing visible light in an enclosure. They do not provide any additional heat. At the time of this writing, few if any provide UV light, and they should not be relied upon as a UVB source. However, as the technology advances and costs come down, UVB-emitting LEDs are likely to become available in the future.

WATER PROVISION, HUMIDITY, AND OSMOREGULATION

Pseudomonas spp. bacteria grow rapidly in water bowls, so bowls should be changed and disinfected or washed in hot soapy water daily.[26] Alternatively, using disposable plastic water bowls is another way of maintaining hygiene in large collections. Arboreal species, such as Old World chameleons, geckos, and anoles, only lap dew from leaves. These species need daily misting of the cage or a drip system.

Tap water usually is adequate, but filtered or bottled water might be used where the tap water quality is in question. Aging the water for dechlorination is generally not necessary.

Humidity is an important but often overlooked factor when keeping lizards. In general, tropical species need higher humidity and desert species lower humidity. Most species do well at humidity levels around 50%.

Low humidity levels result in skin issues such as dysecdysis, because the shed skin dries back onto the animal before it has had the opportunity to be shed. Dysecdysis is most common in winter months when humidity

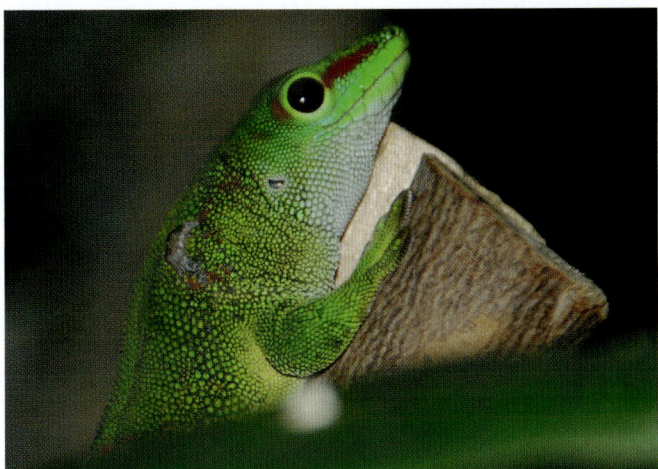

FIG 21.9 A Madagascar day gecko (*Phelsuma grandis*) with a tear in its skin over the right shoulder area. These lizards have very fragile skin, and handling them should be avoided. (Courtesy of Shane Simpson.)

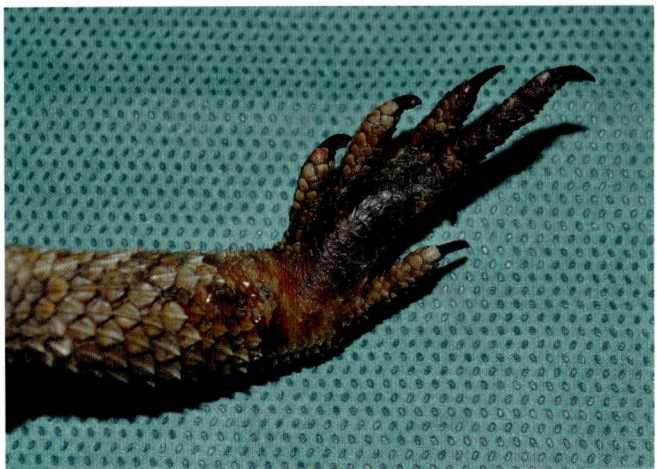

FIG 21.10 Many species of lizard, such as central/inland bearded dragons (*Pogona vitticeps*), are territorial and should not be kept together. They tend to fight often, resulting in injuries to the legs and feet. Avascular necrosis often develops from these crush injuries, necessitating the amputation of the foot, leg, or tail. (Courtesy of Shane Simpson.)

in the average home can get as low as 10%. Low humidity can be corrected by placing damp sponges or clean cloths in the hide boxes or by using a so-called humidity box. This is made by cutting an access hole in the side or top of a plastic storage container and partially filling it with damp but not soaked sphagnum moss. Frequent spraying with a plant mister is also effective to maintain a higher level of humidity but is more labor intensive. Commercial fogging and misting machines for reptile enclosures are increasingly available in the pet trade. Fogging machines are best used in small enclosures, whereas misting systems are generally preferred for larger ones. Manufacturer recommendations for use should be followed. These machines can be controlled by timers. For more precise control, higher end thermostats are available that contain a channel to be used with a hygrometer probe; this triggers the mister whenever the humidity level drops below a preset level. Some misting system models can be directly plumbed into the building water supply. Room humidifiers or vaporizers may be more efficient for controlling humidity in collections with numerous cages; however, care should be taken to ensure hot steam is not directed at housed lizards. All these misting and humidity systems must be monitored for bacterial growth and should be periodically cleaned and disinfected. Decreasing ventilation to maintain humidity is inappropriate. Without adequate ventilation, high humidity and temperature can result in rapid growth of bacteria and mold. Adequate drainage must be provided to avoid flooding of enclosures.

COMMUNAL HOUSING AND HANDLING

Pet stores often display lizards for sale in crowded community enclosures, suggesting these are social animals. Additionally, dealers and breeders may encourage customers to purchase multiple animals. However, many lizard species, especially males, are highly territorial and are stressed by the presence of conspecifics.[27,28] Hormone fluctuations, and thus territoriality, are seasonal and are manifested most acutely during the breeding season.[29] Chameleons are especially territorial, and when two or more are kept together, the larger or more aggressive individual may physically attack and inflict serious wounds on the subordinate one (Fig. 21.9). Often the signs of chronic social stress are subtler where subordinate lizards are merely denied free access to food, heat sources, and hides. This results in "failure to thrive syndrome" for these subordinate cage mates. Symptoms include slow growth, emaciation, poor

muscle tone, lethargy, poor coloring, and susceptibility to opportunistic infectious agents. Keepers often interpret lizards lying together as a compatible behavior; however, in nonsocial lizard species, stress is likely present, even in the absence of overt aggression. Separating the lizards to individual enclosures often solves these issues.

If providing each lizard with its own cage is not possible, then at least housing same-sized members of the same species together, with adequate resources, is acceptable. However, placing males together should always be avoided.

For these communal cages a large cage is necessary, with enough spatial complexity that lizards are able to stay out of sight of one another while still having access to heat, UV light, water, and food.

Human nature is to be enthused with pet lizards, especially newly acquired ones, and to handle them frequently. However, unless a pet lizard is tame and acclimated to captivity, this practice may cause stress and lead to anorexia.[30] In general, the relatively large species, such as iguanas and monitors, tolerate handling and are less prone to panic and flight behavior. Bearded dragons (*Pogona* spp.) and plated lizards (*Gerrhosaurus* spp.) are especially docile and easily handled. Small, high-strung species and juvenile lizards of any species are readily startled and stressed with handling. They are commonly injured by jumping and frantically trying to escape. Day geckos (*Phelsuma* spp.) have fragile skin that is torn even with gentle restraint and should not be handled (Fig. 21.10). Generally, excessive handling of lizards should be avoided. One should strive for a balance, with enough contact to train the lizard to tolerate gentle handling without stress, but not so much as to induce stress. For instance, a monitor that is never handled can become a wild, aggressive animal. Another factor to consider is that during handling, the lizard is at room temperature and humidity, away from its basking sites. Because lizards may be carriers of zoonotic diseases. Handlers should wash their hands thoroughly after interaction.

FEEDING AND NUTRITION

No other group of reptiles shows the diversity of diet that lizards do. Although some species have quite specific dietary requirements, others show more flexibility in what they will eat. Nutrition of reptiles is a complex and ever-changing topic. The guidelines listed below are only very basic recommendations, but please refer to Chapter 27 for more detailed information. Many keepers provide a diet based on what the lizard prefers, but, as with humans, this has no relationship to nutritional value. Diets appropriate to the biology of the species in question must be used.

Herbivores

Green iguanas are herbivorous for their entire lives and in the wild feed almost entirely on leaves of trees and vines.[31] They do not have gizzard-like stomachs and do not need grit or gravel to help digest their food. In fact, intestinal obstruction with gravel is a common problem when iguanas are kept on this substrate. Iguanas, like most herbivores, use microbial fermentation in the hindgut to digest high-fiber diets as efficiently as ruminants. However, this requires suitable environmental temperatures. Newly hatched iguanas lack the microbes necessary for hindgut fermentation and obtain them in the wild by eating the feces of adult iguanas.[32] Other species of herbivorous lizards, such as the Caicos rock iguana (*Cyclura carinata*) and Gray's monitor lizard (*Varanus olivaceus*), do undergo an ontogenetic change from a carnivorous diet as juveniles to an herbivorous diet as adults. Ground iguanas (*Cyclura* spp.), the prehensile-tailed skink (*Corucia zebrata*), spiny-tailed iguanas (*Ctenosaura* spp.), spiny-tailed lizards (*Uromastyx* spp.), and chuckwallas (*Sauromalus* spp.) are herbivores with hindgut fermentation like green iguanas and, in general, do well with similar nutritional provisions.

In captivity, herbivorous lizard diets should be based on a variety of chopped, dark green, leafy vegetables. The use of greens that contain high levels of oxalates, like spinach, or goitrogens, like kale, is controversial, but such items can be fed in moderation. Fruit should be minimized, not because it is toxic but because it dilutes the beneficial nutrients of the other ingredients. Commercial iguana diets can be used as part of a varied diet but vary in quality and palatability.[31, 33] We can approximate a nutritious diet, but most formulations are based on anecdote, experience, and speculation rather than scientific feeding trials. See Chapter 27 for more details.

Insectivores

Crickets (*Acheta domestica*), like those that are readily available in pet stores, are in general overused in lizard diets. Crickets by themselves are low in protein and calcium.[34] Many pet stores do not feed the crickets before sale to reduce mess and clean up, but this practice results in less nutritional value. Commercial cricket foods are available and should be fed to the crickets for at least 4 days before their use as prey items to improve nutritional value (gut loading).[35] Nevertheless, crickets should not be more than 50% of the diet. The remainder of the diet can consist of a variety of wild-caught and captive-raised insects and other prey items, including but not limited to mealworms (*Tenebrio molitor*), king or super mealworms (*Zophobas morio*), wax worms (*Achroia grisella, Galleria mellonella*), earthworms, butterworms (*Chilecomadia moorei*), horn worms (*Manduca sexta*), phoenix worms or soldier fly larvae (*Hermetia illucens*), silk worms (*Bombyx mori*), cockroaches (including Dubia [*Blaptica dubia*], hissing [*Gromphadorhina portentosa*], and speckled [*Nauphoeta cinereal*]), flies, cicadas, grasshoppers/locusts, field crickets, stick insects, caterpillars (smooth-skinned, lacking any hairlike covering that can be irritating), and newborn pinkie mice. "Sweepings" are obtained by sweeping a butterfly net through a grassy field to collect a variety of insect life. Porch lights attract a variety of nocturnal insects. Certain insect species such as fruit fly (*Drosophila melanogaster*) and springtails (*Collembola*) can be cultured to feed to tiny or hatchling insectivorous lizards.

However, fireflies or lightning bugs (family *Lampyridae*) and some butterflies can be potentially toxic, and lizard deaths have resulted from the ingestion of a single firefly.[36] Many caterpillars with bushy, hairlike, or spikey appendages are toxic or irritating.

Multivitamin and calcium supplements may be applied to the insect prey with a salt shaker or by shaking the insects in a plastic bag with a small amount of supplement powder. Supplement particle size affects the bioavailability with smaller particle size resulting in higher blood levels. Insects groom themselves and remove this powder, so they should be offered immediately to the lizard. Young growing lizards should receive vitamin supplements once or twice a week and calcium supplements daily, and adults should receive vitamins every other week and calcium two to three times a week. Insects should be presented in a controlled manner such as a plastic tub so that the appetite can be monitored and insects are not wasted. In addition, insects such as crickets may begin to feed on the lizards themselves if left in an enclosure.

When possible, chameleons should be hand-fed. The insect may be held in front of the chameleon or may be placed in a smooth-sided bowl suspended in the climbing branches. Juvenile chameleons must be fed several times a day, and a single daily feeding suffices for adults.

Commercially prepared insectivore diets are available in a number of forms, including pelleted, powdered, dried, frozen, and canned. The formulations of the pelleted diets vary with respect to ingredients used and nutrient levels available. There is little to no regulation to control their production, ingredients, and the claims of being complete and balanced nutrition. The powdered diets are most often mixed with boiling water and allowed to set as a gel before feeding. Because data is lacking on the exact nutritional requirements for individual species of lizards, these diets may be deficient in essential nutrients and as such should be incorporated into a varied diet rather than being fed exclusively. Similarly, dried, frozen, and canned insects can be used as part of the diet should they be accepted by the animal.

Many species of lizards, particularly the agamids and skinks, are omnivorous in food preferences. These animals will readily take insects, fruit, vegetables, and meat if presented.

Many keepers are falsely led to believe that central/inland bearded dragons are predominantly insectivores as juveniles and change to predominantly herbivores as they reach adulthood. Adults should be considered as dietary generalists and opportunistic predators. Although recent research shows that free-ranging adult bearded dragons do maintain a high level of insect intake as adults, in captivity a much less active adult diet should include plant material to reduce the common occurrence of obesity and hepatic lipidosis.[37] Because of their acrodont dentition, central/inland bearded dragons, similar to other agamids and to old world chameleons, are predisposed to the development of periodontal disease (see Chapter 161). Feeding proportionally more hard-bodied insects such as cockroaches and locusts along with fibrous vegetables such as pumpkin, sweet potato, and green-leafed vegetables aids in keeping the teeth clean and avoids periodontal disease. Diets with higher fruit content increase the risk of developing periodontal disease and as such should be minimized.[38]

Carnivores

Carnivorous lizards should be fed prekilled whole prey (either thawed or fresh killed). Rodents are preferable to chicks, and chicks are preferable to fish due to more balanced nutrition and firmer stools produced. Live rodents should never be offered as a food source. Not only does this prevent rodent bites to the lizard, but it is also more humane for the prey. In many jurisdictions, it is also illegal to feed live rodents to predators. Appropriate-sized prey should be offered to prevent trauma during swallowing or subsequent impaction or regurgitation. Juveniles should be fed once or twice a week, and adults every week or two. Obesity is common in adults, and these animals should be fed smaller amounts and/or less frequently. Alternatively, the amount of rodents fed can be reduced and replaced with cockroaches and stick insects.

If whole rodents and chicks make up the bulk of the diet, vitamin and mineral supplementation is not necessary. Newborn pinkie mice have less total calcium than do adult mice, and calcium should be supplemented if these are used.

Other items may be offered to help reduce feeding costs, but these are less optimal than whole prey items and should always be less than 50% of the diet. These include chicken parts, ground beef, dog food, cat food, and trout food. It should be noted that none of these are designed or formulated for reptiles and should be considered nutritionally inadequate.

Nectivore

Once considered rare in captivity, nectar-eating lizard species such as the crested gecko (*Correlophus [Rhacodactylus] ciliatus*), gargoyle gecko (*Rhacodactylus auriculatus*), and New Caledonian giant gecko (*Rhacodactylus leachianus*) have exploded in popularity. Much of this stems from the fact they can be easily fed using commercially available powdered nectar and fruit diets such as Crested Gecko MRP (Repashy Ventures, Oceanside, California) and Pangea Fruit Mix With Insects (Pangea Reptile LLC, Hudsonvile, Michigan). Although insects can be supplemented into the diet, these lizards can be fed exclusively on these products.

DISINFECTION

Cages and bowls must be cleaned frequently. It is important to remove all organic waste using something such as hot, soapy water. The cage and its furniture must be rinsed thoroughly before returning a lizard to the cage. Solutions of bleach or one of many commercial disinfectants can be used periodically, after treating a sick lizard and before a new lizard is placed in a cage previously occupied by a different lizard. Keepers must wash their hands thoroughly after cleaning each cage and not transfer water bowls, uneaten food, or climbing branches between cages without disinfecting them first (see Chapter 18).

QUARANTINE

New reptiles to a collection must be kept in a separate area from the main collection until they can be appropriately monitored and screened for health problems. New arrivals should have physical examinations, recorded body weights, fecal examinations, parasite treatment, and monitoring for appetite, normal behavior, and symptoms of illness. At the very least, the owner should inspect new arrivals. The main collection should be fed and cleaned first and the quarantined animals second, with no transfer of animals, cages, food and water bowls, uneaten food items, or cage furniture between the two. Keepers must wash their hands and consider clothing changes after working with either collection to prevent the inadvertent transfer of pathogens. Ideally, different keepers should care for the two collections. The farther apart the two collections are physically, the less likely an epizootic will occur. No transfer of air should occur between the two groups. When multiple animals are quarantined, they should enter and leave the quarantine area as a group (see Chapter 19).

REFERENCES

See www.expertconsult.com for a complete list of references.

22

Venomous Species

Robert Johnson

Approximately 450 species of venomous snakes and two species of venomous lizards exist, many of which are kept in captivity. The effects of venom are sometimes categorized as neurotoxic, myotoxic, and coagulopathic, with each victim having a unique clinical picture because of the wide range of effects produced by the various venom components.[1] Venomous reptiles are kept at most zoos, at a few aquariums, and by some hobbyists. Although bites from captive animals are rare, developing, implementing, and following appropriate emergency protocols can help to minimize the likelihood of permanent disability or mortality from an accidental envenomation.

Globally, snake bites are an important public health problem in rural and developing communities, particularly in poor, tropical, and subtropical areas.[2] As many as 4.5 to 5 million snake bites occur every year, causing 2.5 million envenomations, 125,000 deaths, and perhaps three times that number of permanent disabilities.[3] In the United States in a study of calls to poison control centers on animal bites from 2001 to 2005, an annual average of 6803 calls were reportedly due to snake bites.[4] An average of five deaths occur from reptile bites each year in the United States.[5] Three families of venomous snakes are native to Australia, including Colubridae, Homalopsidae, and Elapidae. Nearly all clinically significant bites are from elapids. There are around 2000 bites each year in Australia, and an average of two deaths per annum according to Commonwealth Serum Laboratories (CSL) data (Morgan, unpublished data). The most common snakes to cause severe clinical signs and death are the Eastern brown snake (*Pseudonaja textilis* [Fig. 22.1]), Coastal taipan (*O. scutellatus*) and Mainland tiger snake (*Notechis scutatus*).

DEVELOPMENT OF EMERGENCY PROTOCOLS FOR THE MANAGEMENT OF VENOMOUS ANIMAL BITES[6]

Emergency protocols for handling venomous reptiles should be developed and implemented before the acquisition of a venomous animal or before deciding to provide veterinary services for venomous animals (Fig. 22.2). These protocols include specific plans for venomous animal escape/recovery, venomous animal bite, first-aid procedures for a venomous animal bite, and medical treatment protocols. Sources of information that may be useful in the development of these protocols include direct contact with other zoos or aquariums and the American Association of Zoos and Aquariums Resource Center (http://www.aza.org), where emergency plans developed by several zoos have been published. In addition, the Antivenom Index published and updated periodically by the American Zoo and Aquarium Association and the American Association of Poison Control Centers (https://www.aza.org/antivenom-index) lists the amount and location of available antivenom for most venomous species.

In the United States, venomous reptiles are classified as Code 1 and Code 2 animals (Table 22.1). The venom of a Code 1 animal is capable of causing death, long-term illness, or permanent disability, and the venom of a Code 2 animal is unlikely to have severe or long-lasting effects. The protocols developed must be specific for the type and number of venomous reptiles in the collection. For each protocol, contact information for responsible staff and outside consultants must be readily available. It should be emphasized that the guidelines in this chapter may not be applicable, economical, or practical for all facilities. It is recommended that a physician knowledgeable in the treatment of venomous reptile bites be consulted in the development of protocols for venomous animal bites. Once developed, these protocols should be given to authorities at the medical facility that will be responsible for treating an envenomation.

CLASSIFICATION OF VENOMOUS REPTILES

Venomous snakes occur in the following families: Viperidae, Elapidae, Lamprophiidae, Homalopsidae, and Colubridae. A revised phylogenetic classification of squamate reptiles at the family and subfamily level has been suggested.[7] There are two species of venomous lizards (Gila monster, *Heloderma suspectum,* and the beaded lizard, *H. horridum*), with no recorded human deaths occurring from bites. The multilobed venom glands are located on the lower jaws, whereas in venomous snakes the glands are in the maxillary region. Studies have also reported the presence of venom toxins in two additional lizard lineages, monitor lizards and iguanids.[8,9]

VENOMS

Venoms are key evolutionary innovations in the animal kingdom that have evolved independently in multiple taxa.[10] Venoms allow predators such as snakes, with their lack of limbs, to feed on a far wider range of prey items than would otherwise be possible. Venom is also an effective defense for an otherwise vulnerable animal. The favored terminology is "venom gland" for the venom glands of viperids, elapids, and atractaspidids, and "Duvernoy's gland" for the venom glands of all other colubrids.[11] There is strong developmental evidence that both originate from dental glands, which are present in most squamates.[12] Snake venoms are chemically complex mixtures of proteins, including peptides, polypeptides, enzymes, and glycoproteins, which together produce a variety of pharmacological activities in prey animals. Ranging from a molecular mass of 6 to 100 kD,[13] venoms may contain 30 to 100 protein toxins, with no two venoms identical.[14] Many of these proteins have enzymatic properties. The peptides in venom appear to bind to multiple receptor sites in the prey. For example, components of pit-viper venom affect almost every organ system; therefore some sources claim it is

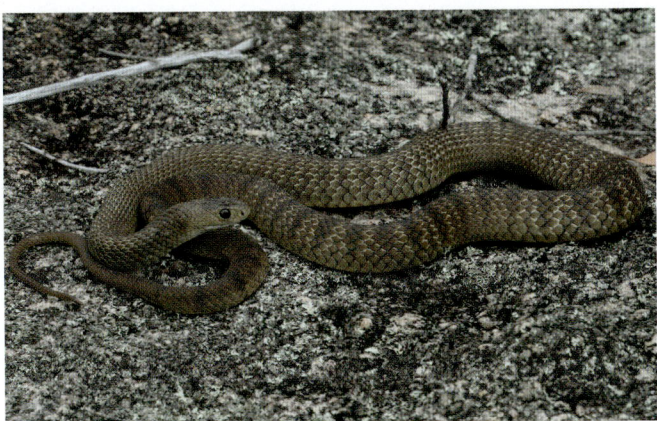

FIG 22.1 The Eastern brown snake, *Pseudonaja textilis*, is responsible for the greatest number of deaths from snakebite in Australia. (Courtesy of M. McFadden.)

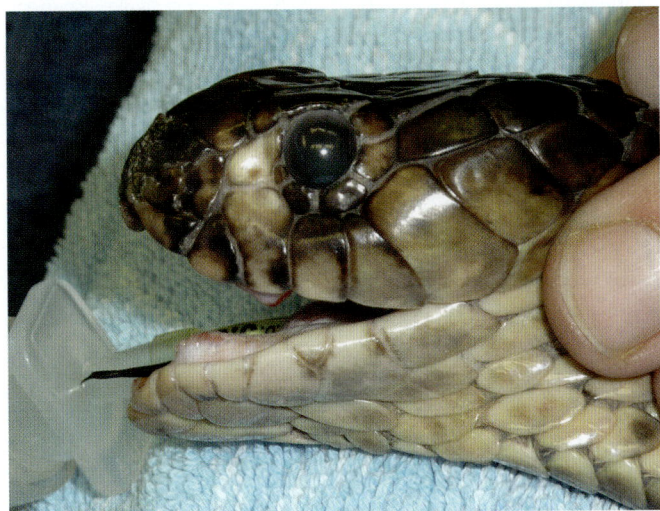

FIG 22.2 Emergency protocols must be prepared when handling or treating venomous snakes such as this Egyptian cobra (*Naja haje*). (Courtesy of L. Vogelnest.)

TABLE 22.1 Classification of Venomous Reptiles in the United States

Family	Code 1	Code 2
Viperidae (Crotalinae: pit vipers)	Rattlesnake, cottonmouth, copperhead, lance-headed pit viper, Fer-de-lance, bushmaster, and Asiatic pit viper	
Viperidae (Viperinae: true vipers)	African, European, and Middle Eastern vipers	
Elapidae	Cobras, mambas, kraits, coral snakes, and most venomous snakes of Australia	
Hydrophiidae	True sea snakes	
Colubridae	Boomslang, bird or twig snake, and red-necked keelback	Brown vine snake, Amazonian vine snake, and cat-eyed snake
Laticaudidae	Sea kraits	
Atractaspididae	African and Middle East mole vipers	
Helodermatidae	Gila monster and Mexican beaded lizard	

inaccurate to label a venom according to the body system affected, that is, as a neurotoxin, hemotoxin, cardiotoxin, or myotoxin. Accordingly, the most deleterious effects are seen in the cardiovascular, hematologic, respiratory, and nervous systems.[15] Recent studies have used molecular techniques of high throughput proteomics and transcriptomics, aiming to characterize further the components of snake venom.[16]

Hemotoxic Effects

Venoms may interfere with blood clotting, either by procoagulant or anticoagulant activity. Procoagulants (prothrombin-activating enzymes, serine proteases, and PLA_2) produce disseminated intravascular coagulation (DIC) defibrination and bleeding. Anticoagulants produce anticoagulation without fibrin depletion. Bleeding may occur from the nose and gums, skin (petechiae and echymoses), intravenous catheter sites, urinary tract, gastrointestinal tract, and the intracerebral space. Thrombotic microangiopathy is a more recently recognized condition that is always associated with a venom-induced consumption coagulopathy (VICC) and is characterized by thrombocytopenia, microangiopathic hemolytic anemia, with fragmented red blood cells, and acute renal

impairment.[17] Analysis of blood films reveals fragmented red blood cells (microangiopathic hemolytic anemia) and a thrombocytopenia, accompanied by a rising creatinine level (>120 mmol/L), which may lead to renal impairment or even acute renal failure requiring dialysis.

Neurotoxic Effects

Both pre- and postsynaptic neurotoxins exist. Postsynaptic neurotoxins (neurotoxic peptides "3 finger toxins") bind competitively to acetylcholine receptors. They are readily reversed by antivenom and may be reversed by physostigmine. The venom of the death adder (*Acanthophis antarcticus*) is mainly postsynaptic. Presynaptic neurotoxins (neurotoxic PLA_2) cause structural damage to nerve terminals either at the level of the cell membrane or synaptic vesicle. They respond poorly to antivenom and are found to a variable degree in all Australian elapids. The venom of the coastal taipan, *Oxyuranus scutellatus*, is mostly presynaptic (Fig. 22.3). Symptoms include a descending flaccid paralysis that initially involves the eye muscles (ptosis, diplopia, and blurred vision), followed by bulbar muscles, respiratory muscle paralysis, and limb paralysis.[17]

Myotoxic Effects

Phospholipases (PLA_2) produce rhabdomyolysis and only affect striated skeletal muscle. Symptoms include generalized muscle pain and tenderness; muscle weakness and edema; myoglobinuria, hyperkalemia, and renal failure; and local pain and tissue destruction. For example, common and abundant components of *Bothrops* spp. (Central and South American vipers) venoms are myotoxic phospholipases A2 (PLA_2) and play a major role in the pathogenesis of local tissue damage. These myotoxins are responsible for local myonecrosis, inflammation, and pain.[18]

LD_{50}

The lethal dose of venom required to kill 50% of mice injected is termed the LD_{50}. For example, the inland taipan, *Oxyuranus microlepidotus* (0.025 mg/kg), and the eastern brown snake, *P. textilis* (0.053 mg/kg),

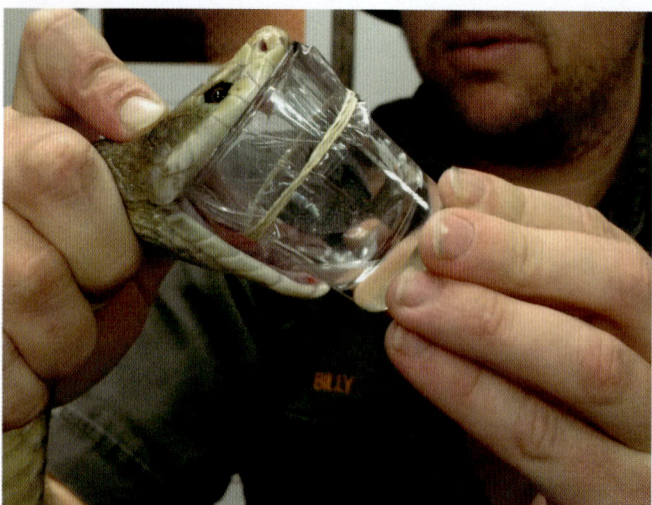

FIG 22.3 Venom collection in a Coastal taipan (*Oxyuranus scutellatus*) yields a large volume compared with many other elapids. (Courtesy of Robert Johnson.)

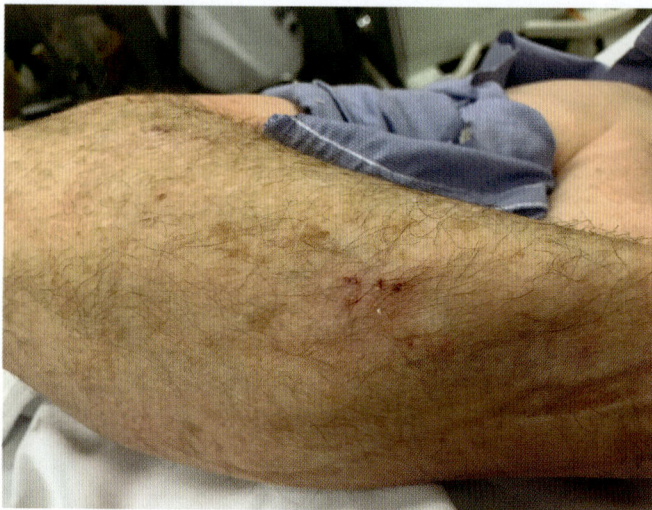

FIG 22.4 Snakebite on the arm of a veterinarian from an eastern brown snake (*Pseudonaja textilis*). Only a small volume of venom is delivered by the bite of this small-fanged but highly venomous snake. (Courtesy of Robert Johnson.)

deliver a much smaller volume to achieve the LD_{50} compared with the king cobra, *Ophiophagus hannah* (1.8 mg/kg), and the eastern diamond-backed rattlesnake, *Crotalus adamanteus* (11.4 mg/kg) (Australian Venom Research Unit: http://biomedicalsciences.unimelb.edu.au/departments/pharmacology/engage/avru). However, grading venomous snakes by comparing the LD_{50} is not of great benefit because many other factors determine whether a snake is termed "dangerous," for example, the volume and manner in which the venom is delivered, the fang size, and the behavior of the snake.

MEDICAL MANAGEMENT OF SNAKEBITE

Every bite is unique and depends on human factors: age, weight, sex, preexisting conditions, bite site, and first aid (time and quality); and snake factors: species, degree and number of bites, and the age and size of the snake (Fig. 22.4). Not all patients bitten will have been envenomated, and antivenom is not needed in every case. Each patient presented for treatment for a suspected snakebite should be rapidly triaged, with management of any cardiovascular or respiratory impairment taking priority. It should not be assumed that medical or nursing staff are familiar with assessing snakebite victims or recognizing symptoms. Consequently, treating staff should be instructed to monitor specific signs such as ptosis, dysarthria, weakness, diplopia, persistent bleeding from a bite site or venipuncture wound, or dark or discolored urine (myoglobinuria, hematuria).[19]

In summary, the treatment of snakebite may be divided into two components: management of tissue damage and supportive care and neutralization of the venom using antivenom. The time to onset of symptoms depends on the size and species of the snake, the number of bites, the size and health of the victim, the activity of the victim after the bite, and whether adequate first aid was administered in a timely manner (Morgan, observation). Symptoms usually develop over hours, and deaths usually occur after 24 hours. Common nonspecific symptoms are headache, abdominal pain, back pain, nausea, vomiting, and dizziness.

Snake Venom Detection Kit (SVDK)

The Snake Venom Detection Kit (SVDK; CSL, Commonwealth Serum Laboratories, Parkville, Melbourne, Australia), based on the immunoassay

of venom enzymes, may assist in regions of Australia when the identification of a snake is not known and where the range of possible snakes is too broad to allow the use of monovalent antivenoms.[17] The optimal sample is a swab from the bite or urine. Blood yields unreliable results in the SVDK.

Antivenom

Any venomous snakebite should be considered a medical emergency, and antivenom is the only effective antidote for a venomous snakebite; however, in some cases antivenom administration can cause anaphylaxis and delayed serum sickness. For these reasons antivenom use is usually reserved for cases that decompensate or deteriorate despite supportive measures. Dry bites may occur, wherein no venom is injected.

Antivenoms can be classified as monovalent (when they are effective against the venom of a single species) or polyvalent (when they are effective against a range of species or several different species at the same time). Antivenom is a hyperimmune serum containing antibodies (immunoglobulin G) that bind to the venom molecules, rendering them inactive. The IgG molecule is divided into two main fragment types; the Fc is involved in mounting a cellular response to antigens and in complement fixation and two antigen-binding fragments, Fabs, which recognize and bind to foreign substances.[20] Currently in North America, the most widely used antivenom in humans is CroFab Crotalidae Polyvalent Immune Fab (Ovine) (BTG International, Inc., http://www.crofab.com). In Australia, species-specific equine IgG antivenoms are available for black snakes, tiger snakes, taipans, death adders, brown snakes, sea snakes, or polyvalent snakes. The World Health Organization maintains a list of antivenoms available on the world market (http://www.who.int/bloodproducts/snake_antivenoms/en/).

HANDLING AND TREATING VENOMOUS SNAKES IN THE VETERINARY HOSPITAL[21]

Venomous snakes should be expertly restrained for the physical examination, preferably by the keeper, wildlife rescuer, or owner and not the veterinarian or veterinary technician, leaving them free to treat the patient. It is recommended that only experienced reptile veterinarians examine and treat venomous species and that they are fully aware of the legalities involved (Box 22.1). Veterinarians are liable for any injuries that occur under their supervision. Equipment required for the safe handling of venomous snakes includes the following: jiggers, hooks, pinning sticks, hoop bags with sewn corners, clear plastic tubes (Fig. 22.5), pads (foam rubber), secure containers, and holding facilities. If possible, it is preferable to treat venomous snakes on site or as outpatients. If hospitalization is necessary, ensure that a locked, labeled enclosure is available in a secured room. Access should be restricted to authorized and fully trained staff only. Snake hooks, jiggers, and tubes should be easily accessible. Protective eyewear and gloves should be worn when handling anesthetized or dead snakes, as envenomation may still occur. Care should be taken when dissecting the venom gland. To minimize the chance of envenomation it is often safer to decapitate the dead snake or encase the head in a crush-proof container before commencing the postmortem examination (Fig. 22.6). Place the head directly into decalcifying formalin solution.[21]

> ### BOX 22.1 Legal Issues for Consideration When Treating Venomous Snakes[21]
>
> - Legal responsibilities of the veterinarian should be considered when handling venomous snakes.
> - Who is responsible in the event of a bite—rescuer, handler, staff, or veterinarian?
> - Does the veterinary hospital have a protocol for the handling of venomous snakes?
> - Has the insurer been informed that venomous snakes are handled at the veterinary hospital?
> - Veterinarians treating venomous snakes should have a good understanding of the legal and licensing issues of owning or keeping exotic venomous reptiles in private collections.
> - Understand and consider the legal requirements involved in possessing a venomous reptile.
> - Understand and have a commitment to maintaining a safe work environment. Ensure that there is a plan for emergencies and access to a local hospital and antivenoms.
> - There should be a written protocol in place for handling and for emergency snakebite.

Venomoid Snakes

Venomoid snakes are snakes that have undergone surgery involving the sectioning of the venom duct or ablation of the venom gland. This practice is viewed by most reptile veterinarians and herpetologists as a disfiguring surgery and, in many countries, is illegal and considered professional malpractice. Venomoid snakes can never be guaranteed as "de-venomed." Concerns include an incomplete, or incorrectly performed (often by nonveterinarians), surgery. It is apparent that there are considerable legal and liability issues associated with this practice. In addition, there is the subsequent risk of people being bitten by apparently venomoid snakes that may still have remnants of venom gland tissue and/or patent venom ducts. Venomoid snakes should always be regarded as venomous.

VENOMOUS ANIMAL BITE PLAN (UNITED STATES)[6]

In the United States, venomous reptiles are classified as Code 1 or Code 2. Example protocols are provided for the response to Code 1 (Box 22.2) and 2 (Box 22.3) venomous animal bites. Routine emergency drills are important to ensure that personnel are prepared and alarms are working properly. Appropriate antivenoms, if available, must be acquired, properly stored, and replaced when expired.

VENOMOUS ANIMAL ESCAPE PLAN[6]

Every facility that holds venomous reptiles must have a plan for recapturing escaped animals (Box 22.4). A well-developed plan is critical for management of escape. The plan must include procedures for managing an escape into both public and contained areas and a course of action if the animal cannot be located.

FIRST-AID PROCEDURES

Veterinarians treat venomous snakes at their own discretion and should be acutely aware of the risks involved. These notes are meant as a guide only, and the advice contained within may change with time. Veterinarians are also advised to familiarize themselves with snake identification and make their own enquiries. Veterinary hospitals should ensure that there is always a fully trained first aider in attendance when venomous snakes are being handled or treated.

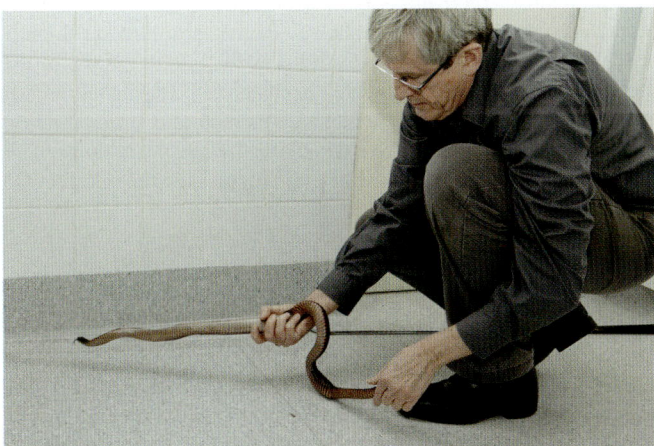

FIG 22.5 Tubing a red-bellied black snake (*Pseudechis porphyriacus*) is usually a gentle and stress-free procedure for the snake and safe for the handler and veterinarian. (Courtesy of M. Wilson.)

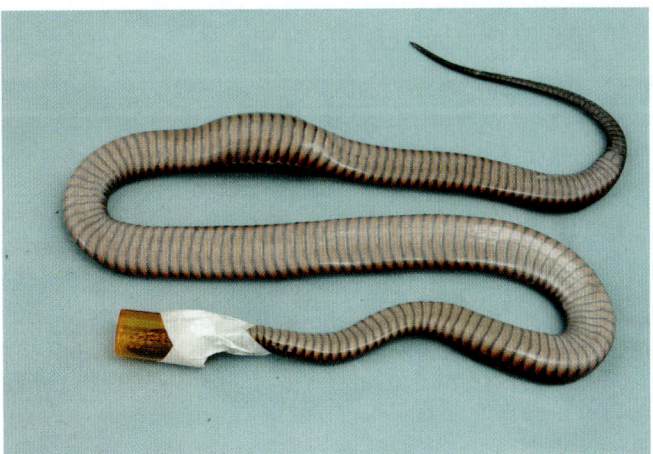

FIG 22.6 Enclosing the head of a venomous snake in a crush-proof receptacle prior to necropsy or disposal is a safe alternative to decapitation. (Courtesy of M. Wilson.)

> **BOX 22.2** **Protocols for Code 1 Venomous Animal Bites**
>
> **Victim**
> Leave area
> Secure area to prevent animal escape
> Activate emergency bite alarm
> Notify others in area of the bite, type of animal, and whether the animal is secured
> Remain calm; remove all jewelry to prevent further injury from swelling
>
> **First Assistant**
> Call 911; report that a venomous animal bite has occurred and give address
> Call for further assistance
> Ensure jewelry has been removed and keep victim calm
> Administer first aid
> When help arrives, ensure that the antivenom, Antivenom Index, and other reference documents accompany victim to hospital
>
> **Second Assistant**
> Enlist trained staff to recapture venomous animal, if necessary
> Gather antivenom, AZA Antivenom Index, and other documents needed to accompany victim to hospital

> **BOX 22.3** **Protocols for Code 2 Venomous Animal Bites**
>
> **Victim**
> Recapture and secure animal if easily done
> Leave area and close door
> Request assistance from staff
> Remove all jewelry to prevent swelling-associated injuries
> Begin first aid
>
> **Assistant**
> Treat as a Code 1 venomous animal bite if victim is in severe pain or shows signs of shock or other systemic effects
> If available, request an emergency medical technician; otherwise, take victim directly to a medical facility for treatment
> Notify appropriate staff of injury

> **BOX 22.4** **Example Protocols for the Recapture of Venomous Animals**
>
> **Contained Escape (i.e., in a secured area)**
> Alert appropriate staff of the escape, including the type of animal and its location, via radio, pager, or telephone
> Alert any personnel in the immediate vicinity of an animal escape
> For Code 1 animals, secure the area and wait until a minimum of two trained staff members arrive before recapture is attempted
> Code 2 animals may be recaptured by one trained staff person
> If alone or untrained in the capture of venomous reptiles, secure the area and monitor the animal from a distance until trained staff arrives
> Recapture and secure animal
> Report incident to appropriate staff
>
> **Public Area Escape**
> Report escape to appropriate staff, including the type of animal and its location, via radio, pager, or telephone
> If members of the public are present, evacuate them from area
> Secure area. This may include:
>   Closing doors, windows, or other escape routes
>   Shutting off escalators and elevators
> Recapture and secure animal
> Maintain communication with appropriate staff, such as the head of visitor services, security, and other departments that need to ensure public and staff safety
>
> **Missing Venomous Animal**
> Report to appropriate staff that an animal is missing; include the type of animal and location of escape
> Once the animal has been confirmed missing, appropriate actions are determined by:
>   The species of animal
>   The area involved
>   The potential risk to visitors or staff

FIRST-AID PROCEDURES FOR A VENOMOUS REPTILE BITE (UNITED STATES)[6]

First aid for bites by a Code 1 animal should be administered immediately after activating the venom alarm and calling 911 (see Boxes 22.2, 22.3, and 22.5). Do not activate the venom alarm or call 911 for Code 2 animal bites unless the victim is in severe pain or shock. Previously, the Sawyer Extractor was recommended to aid in the extraction of venom from viperid and crotalid bites. The effectiveness of this device has not been proven, and its use in North America is no longer recommended, although these kits are still readily available. Apart from being ineffective there is also evidence that these devices can aggravate or facilitate tissue damage at the bite site.[22] The technique of lancing bites and sucking out venom is ineffective and may result in greater tissue damage and possible infection. The use of a tourniquet or an ice pack is contraindicated.[22] Pressure bandages are not recommended if the venom has proteolytic properties, which cause tissue necrosis. A pressure wrap is recommended for bites by sea snakes, sea kraits, or other animals with venom that has primarily cardiotoxic or neurotoxic effects. Many types of venom may cause respiratory failure; therefore maintenance of an airway is a top priority.

ELAPID SNAKEBITE (AUSTRALIA)

In regions where pressure immobilization is indicated to slow uptake of neurotoxins/hemotoxins, appropriate measures should be used.[1] A pressure bandage should be applied as soon as possible over the bite site and then around the limb from below the bite to the top of the limb (except in the case of rattlesnake or viper bites). The limb is splinted and placed in a sling if appropriate. Both pressure and immobilization must be used to reduce the rate of venom absorption and movement from the bite site. Do not wash, clean, cut, or suck the bite site. Do NOT use a tourniquet (Box 22.6).

PRESSURE/IMMOBILIZATION

Other than those from Australasia and North America and all viper species, the use of measures to reduce local venom uptake in elapid snakes is not formally agreed upon, and first aid measures used vary widely. Pressure/immobilization (PI) should be considered for envenomation by any lethally potent coagulopathic or neurotoxic species. However, pending further research, it should not be used for species known to cause serious local tissue injury.[1] A review of the treatment of snakebite in Australia has shown that PI is safe for Australasian elapid

---

BOX 22.5 Snakebite First Aid (United States)

What to Do if You Are Bitten by a Snake

- Keep still and calm; do not panic.
- Call the poison center immediately by dialing the national, free Poison Help number at 1 (800) 222-1222. If the person who was bitten is having trouble breathing or losing consciousness, call 911 immediately.
- If you are in a remote location and do not have mobile phone service, ask someone to drive you to the nearest emergency medical facility. Only drive yourself as a last resort.
- Keep the part of your body that was bitten straight and at heart-level unless told otherwise by the specialist at the poison center.
- Remove all jewelry and tight clothing.
- Wash the bite with soap and water and cover the bite with a clean, dry dressing, if available, and if doing so does not cause delay.

- Being able to describe the snake to medical professionals can help them decide on the best treatment for you. Only take a photograph of the snake if you can do so from a safe distance.
- Note the time the bite happened.

What Not to Do

- DO NOT pick up, attempt to trap, or kill the snake.
- DO NOT apply a tourniquet or attempt to restrict blood flow to the affected area.
- DO NOT cut the wound.
- DO NOT attempt to suck out the venom.
- DO NOT apply heat, cold, electricity, or any substances to the wound.
- DO NOT drink alcohol or caffeinated beverages or take any drugs or medicines.

From American Association of Poison Control Centers. https://aapcc.s3.amazonaws.com/pdfs/releases/2016_AAPCC_BTG_Press_Release_Updated_with_PH.pdf. Accessed June 30, 2017.

BOX 22.6 Snakebite First Aid (Australia)

What to Do

1. Follow DRSABCD, which stands for:
   a) **D**anger—always check the danger to you, any bystanders, and then the injured or ill person. Make sure you do not put yourself in danger when going to the assistance of another person.
   b) **R**esponse—is the person conscious? Do they respond when you talk to them, touch their hands, or squeeze their shoulder?
   c) **S**end for help—call triple zero (000). Don't forget to answer the questions asked by the operator.
   d) **A**irway—is the person's airway clear? Is the person breathing?
   e) **B**reathing—check for breathing by looking for chest movements (up and down). Listen by putting your ear near to their mouth and nose. Feel for breathing by putting your hand on the lower part of their chest. If the person is unconscious but breathing, turn them onto their side, carefully ensuring that you keep their head, neck, and spine in alignment. Monitor their breathing until you hand over to the ambulance officers.
   f) **C**PR (cardiopulmonary resuscitation)
   g) **D**efibrillator—for unconscious adults who are not breathing, apply an automated external defibrillator (AED) if one is available. Some AEDs may not be suitable for children.
2. Reassure the patient and ask them not to move.
3. Apply a broad crepe bandage over the bite site as soon as possible.
4. Apply a pressure bandage (heavy crepe or elasticized roller bandage) starting just above the fingers or toes of the bitten limb and move upward on the limb as far as can be reached (include the snake bite). Apply firmly without stopping blood supply to the limb.

5. Immobilize the bandaged limb with splints.
6. Ensure the patient does not move.
7. Write down the time of the bite and when the bandage was applied. Stay with the patient.
8. Regularly check circulation in fingers or toes.
9. Manage for shock.
10. Ensure an ambulance has been called.

What Not to Do

DO NOT wash venom off the skin.
DO NOT cut the bitten area.
DO NOT try to suck venom out of wound.
DO NOT use a tourniquet.
DO NOT try to catch the snake.

Signs and Symptoms

Signs are not always visible but may be puncture marks, bleeding, or scratches. Symptoms developing within an hour may include headache, impaired vision, nausea, vomiting, diarrhea, breathing difficulties, drowsiness, faintness, problems speaking or swallowing.

Disclaimer

St John Ambulance Australia first aid protocols are for the Australian market only. All care has been taken in preparing the information but St John takes no responsibility for its use by other parties or individuals.

From St John Ambulance. http://stjohn.org.au/assets/uploads/fact%20sheets/english/ FS_snakebite.pdf. Accessed June 30, 2017.

---

snakebite; however, PI is still not used correctly in the majority of snakebites in Australia.[23] Immobilization is critical in addition to pressure bandaging. It is not known to what extent PI retards venom absorption in the snakebite patient. The timing of PI application appears critical, especially for bites involving species such as the brown snake (*Pseudonaja* sp.), where venom may be absorbed rapidly via the capillary venous system.

MEDICAL TREATMENT

In the event of a venomous snakebite the patient should be referred immediately to the nearest hospital with appropriate facilities for the treatment of snakebite. It is not within the scope of this chapter to expand further upon the current medical treatment of snakebites in humans.

ACKNOWLEDGMENTS

The author acknowledges the work of Drs. Whitaker and Gold in the previous edition and thanks Dr. Richard Funk for his input in the production of this chapter.

REFERENCES

See www.expertconsult.com for a complete list of references.

23

Tortoises, Freshwater Turtles, and Terrapins

Thomas H. Boyer and Donal M. Boyer

HANDLING

Temperament varies considerably among the chelonians. As an over-generalization, terrestrial forms rarely bite, whereas aquatic forms typically will. Handle chelonians by their shell, not their appendages or tail. The main hazards are from bites and scratches, although being urinated, defecated, or musked on can be unpleasant. Large species may require several people to safely handle. In large tortoises the rear limb can withdraw, trap, and crush an unwary handler's finger in the prefemoral fossa. Avoid this risk when moving large species (Fig. 23.1). Some turtles can inflict a serious bite with a surprisingly fast and long reach. The head may be blocked, with a thick folded cloth towel, and the turtle held posterior to the bridge of the shell. Placing a tongue depressor in front of the head of smaller turtles allows safe front limb access.

LIGHTING

Chelonians require ultraviolet light (UVB, 290–315 nm); natural sunlight is the best source (see Chapter 17 for more information). There should be no light at night and a photoperiod of 12 hours light for tropical chelonians year round. For temperate chelonians an annual photoperiod should be followed.[1] All lighting should be controlled by timers for consistant photoperiod regulation and adjustment.

TEMPERATURE

Most chelonians are heliotherms; they obtain radiant heat by basking in the sun. The nonlethal temperature range for all chelonians is 8°C (46°F) to 45°C (113°F). The optimal for terrestrial species is 28°C (84°F) with a range of 22° to 30°C (72°–86°F),[2,3] with exceptions. At temperatures less than 15°C (59°F), chelonians are inactive and anorexic; at less than 10°C (50°F), chelonians are hibernating.[2] Sudden freezes, especially in late winter or early spring, are a major cause of mass mortalities in box turtles (*Terrepene*), even though box turtles are the largest freeze-tolerant taxa.[4] Some montane species, such as impressed tortoises (*Manouria impressa*), do poorly above 30°C (86°F). Above 35°C (95°F) chelonians actively seek cooler areas, such as burrows or burrowing in the mud, and may aestivate.[2] Temperatures of 39° to 43°C (102°–109°F) are within the lethal or critical thermal maximum for most chelonians; 45°C (113°F) is rapidly lethal for all species.[2,5] A drop in temperature at night is beneficial and may help lessen pyramidal shell growth.[6] Larger chelonians have much more thermal inertia than small chelonians. Small chelonians are more prone to temperature fluctuations because of their high ratio of surface area to volume. Perhaps this is one reason pneumonia is much more common in young turtles.[7]

In captivity, a temperature gradient within the preferred optimal temperature zone or range (POTZ, POTR) is best so that the chelonian can regulate its own body temperature. Basking areas can be created under various incandescent light bulbs, infrared heat lamps or porcelain heating elements, or self-ballasted mercury vapor flood lamps with reflector hoods. In addition, one can place a heating pad underneath the cage in the basking area, or even better, a radiant heat panel overhead (see the tortoise barn discussion later in this chapter). Chelonians should not be within the 18-inch focal heating range of infrared fixtures or severe burns could occur. Chelonians need not stay within their POTZ; a nighttime drop in temperature preserves natural circadian rhythms. Ambient temperatures should be regularly monitored with minimum-maximum thermometers. Indoor-outdoor varieties allow ambient and basking temperature monitoring. Noncontact temperature measurement guns (Raytek Ranger ST, Total Temperature Instrumentation Inc, Williston, VT) are also useful to spot check temperatures throughout enclosures.

HIBERNATION

Hibernation (or brumation) is part of the normal physiology for many temperate chelonians. It precedes reproduction, utilizes stored glycogen and fat, and can be an essential component of husbandry. With colder temperatures thyroid values plummet, and most hibernating species become anorectic. All temperate chelonians should be hibernated if in good health. Most *Gopherus* and *Testudo* tortoises hibernate, with the exception of African *Testudo* tortoises (Greek tortoise spp. *T. graeca graeca* and the Egyptian tortoise *T. kleinmanni*). In contrast, none of the tropical tortoises (e.g., leopard, African spurred, red-footed, yellow-footed, star, radiated) hibernate. Most temperate zone terrestrial and freshwater turtles hibernate. Of the North American box turtles, all hibernate except for the Gulf Coast (*Terrepene c. major*) and Florida box turtles (*Terrapene c. bauri*). Some other commonly kept species that should hibernate are wood turtles (*Glyptemys insculpta*), spotted turtles (*Clemmys guttata*), common snapping turtles (*Chelydra serpentina serpentina*), northernly distributed eastern mud turtles (*Kinosternon subrubrum*), stinkpots (*Sternotherus odoratus*), red-eared sliders (*Trachemys scripta elegans*), and painted turtles (*Chrysemy picta*).

Hibernation onset is primarily governed by falling temperatures, which inhibits appetite. In the wild, this drives chelonians toward their hibernaculi. Hibernaculi are areas that are slightly warmer than the surrounding environment to avoid freezing and provide some moisture to protect against dessication.[3] Glycogen and fat stores in the liver and body are the main energy source during hibernation. Metabolism slows down considerably as temperature and thyroid levels plumet, resulting in reduced energy expenditure.[3] Emergence is triggered by rising temperatures, not photoperiod.[3]

Only healthy chelonians should hibernate, which means they have been eating and are in good body condition. Sick, convalescing, or underweight turtles should not hibernate. A physical examination, weight-to-length ratio, complete blood count, plasma chemistry panel,

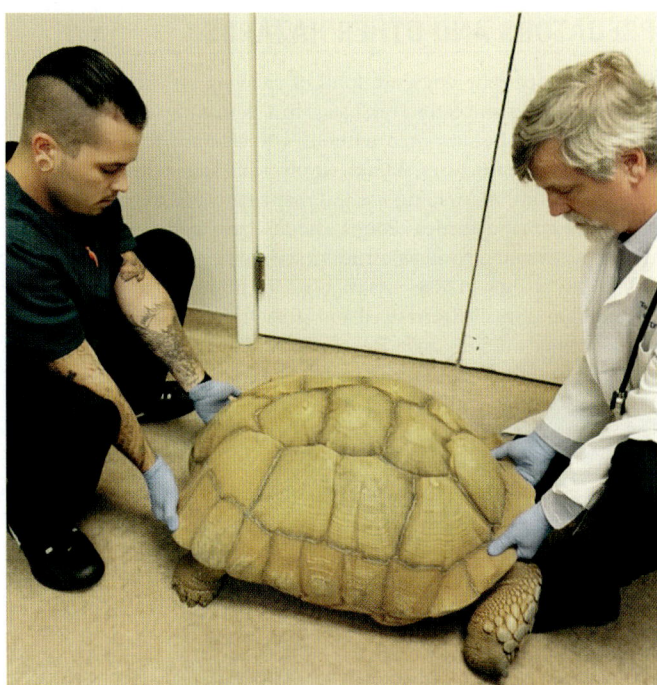

FIG 23.1 When handling large tortoises, be sure your finger doesn't get drawn into and crushed in the prefemoral fossa.

and, if possible, survey radiographs are recommended in late summer to early fall, before hibernation. Low body condition, weight loss, edema, hypoalbuminemia, hypocalcemia, hyperuricemia, anemia, diarrhea, or other signs of illness, such as nasal discharge or hepatic lipidosis, are some of the indications not to hibernate. If the chelonian does not have sufficient body reserves, it will catabolize its own tissues and may die. There is no one clinical parameter regarding hibernation; clinical acumen and keeper judgment are needed.

Body condition scores have been described for desert tortoises,[8] with 1 to 3 being poor or in undercondition, 4 to 6 in good condition, and 7 to 9 obese or in overcondition. Jackson's ratio[9] compares body weight with midline, straight carapace length and is a simple partial estimation of normal or healthy body condition for *Testudo graeca* and *T. hermanni* (but not applicable to other *Testudo*). Sick tortoises often exhibit a reduced body condition (low weight for a given length), while obese tortoises are well above normal weight for a given length. However, the presence of uroliths, coelomic exudates, or intestinal gravel can elevate body weight of ill tortoises.[10] Mader and Stoutenberg (Mader et al, Proc ARAV, 1998, p 103) charted maximum carapace length, width, and height (volume) against weight, as another estimation of the health status of desert tortoises. More charts should be produced for other species of chelonians, along with some already available on the internet or in research papers.[12–14]

Supplemental food should be discontinued several weeks prior to hibernation; larger animals may require 3 or 4 weeks, smaller turtles 1 or 2 weeks. Backyard grasses, weeds, or leaves can still be consumed. Water should be available, and soaking prior to hibernation is recommended. Most chelonians enter hibernation in the fall/autumn when nighttime temperatures drop to 8° to 21°C (40°–60°F), and the days are cooler. However, there is great individual variation in the timing and duration of hibernation. Onset of hibernation in northeastern Mojave desert tortoises is from late October to early November, and they emerge 4 to 5 months later in mid-February to late April. Mean temperatures of hibernaculi were 11° to 16°C (52°–61°F), with minimum temperatures of 7° to 10°C (45°–50°F).[15] Hibernaculi often maintained

higher temperatures than the surrounding open environment, with less temperature variation.

Hibernaculi can be indoors or outdoors, with outdoors preferred for species that naturally hibernate in a given geographic area. Outdoor hibernation is not advisable in areas with severe winters or in areas outside the species' normal geographical distribution. For desert tortoises, an outdoor burrow, or tortoise barn, works well. Temperatures should be between 7° to 15°C (45°–59°F), ideally around 13°C (55°F), and always above freezing. Ensure that burrows can't flood during winter rains because wet and cold conditions are dangerous. Indoors, tortoises can be hibernated in cool areas, such as an unheated garage, storeroom, closet, or even in modified refrigerators.[1] A Styrofoam box, or a cardboard box insulated with thick layers of newspaper, within a larger cardboard, plastic, or wooden box can be used. The box should be large enough for the tortoise to turn around in, lined with newspaper and filled with shredded newspaper, or humid substrate, covered with blankets and kept dark. Do not put the box directly on cold concrete, unless it is too warm. Insulation minimizes temperature swings. Indoors low humidity can dehydrate tortoises; juveniles should be soaked every 2 to 3 weeks and adults every 4 to 6 weeks. Soak for 15 to 30 minutes in shallow lukewarm water during the day and allow the tortoise to dry before returning to the hibernaculum. Contrary to popular belief, disturbing turtles during hibernation is not harmful.[16] Low humidity is generally not a problem outdoors, but turtles should still be encouraged to drink if active on warmer days. During warm periods tortoises may be active only to return to hibernation as it cools again. As overnight temperatures stay above 18°C (65°F), and days warm, the tortoise will start to move around and can emerge from hibernation. Soak the tortoise and watch to see if it urinates. Healthy tortoises will start eating and urinating within a week of emergence; make sure they stay above 18°C (65°F) at night.

Box turtles (*Terrapene* spp.) and *Testudo* tortoises can tolerate much colder hibernation temperatures, ideally from 2° to 9°C (36°–48°F).[1] They generally dig into outdoor substrates but do not use burrows, except for ornate box turtles (*Terrapene ornata*) and Russian tortoises (*Agrionemys horsfeldii*). Eastern box turtles (*Terrapene carolina carolina*), hibernate near the surface, whereas ornate box turtles dig down into the soil.[4] A simple outdoor hibernaculum can be constructed in an area sheltered from the wind, near a foundation or wall. Excavate an area 2.5 ft by 4 ft, about 2 ft deep, and line it with stacked masonry blocks to about 6 inches above ground level, with several openings that turtles can enter through. Spread a mixture of mulch and soil, with a leaf layer on top, to the top of the block wall. Place marine-grade plywood on top of the hibernaculum, bury the entire structure in soil, and clear tunnels into the openings. Once the turtle enters in the fall, after a week or so, the entrance can be sealed shut with masonry blocks until the following spring. Compost piles are not suitable for hibernation. Some box turtles and Russian tortoises can survive freezing, but it is not recommended and can result in blindness, damage to extremities, or even death.[1]

Postemergence turtles and tortoises are often dehydrated, immuno-compromised, and vulnerable to disease. Suboptimal nutrition, as well as suboptimal hibernation conditions, can result in a dehydrated, malnourished chelonian with major organ system failure upon emergence. Tortoises should lose no more than 6% to 7% of their body weight over hibernation.[17] Under ideal conditions *Testudo* spp. lose less than 1% body weight.[1]

Aquatic turtles housed outdoors that hibernate will cease feeding in late fall/autumn if they have no supplemental heat. Aquatic turtles can hibernate under water, in terrestrial environments, or both. If hibernating indoors one can use a stock tank in a garage or unheated room. Multiple turtles can be hibernated together if they are compatible species. Reduce feeding in preparation for hibernation so that when temperatures are 15°C (59°F) feeding has ceased. Water level depth should cover shell by about 6 inches. A few blocks or rocks can be added to allow the turtle easy access to the surface but not allow them to emerge from the water. A filter should be run to help keep the tank clean, circulate water, and keep it oxygenated. Allow water temperature to fall into the 4.4° to 10°C (40°–50°F) range and provide reduced lighting, less than 10 hours per day, or no lighting. Turtles may still move about, but they should not be disturbed. A more controlled hibernation is possible with refrigeration units or incubators that can be programmed to cool. Feeding can be started again as it warms in the spring. Watch for signs of pneumonia such as asymmetric lateral floating, inability to submerge, discharge from the nostrils or mouth, or closed eyes. If any signs of illness are present during hibernation, warm the turtle up to 27°C (80°F) over 24 to 48 hours and perform diagnostic testing, including culture and sensitivity, before beginning antibiotic treatment.

PREDATORS AND OTHER HAZARDS

Predators, especially dogs, are fond of chewing on chelonians' shells and appendages and can wreak havoc in a short time (Fig. 23.2). Small chelonians can be devoured without a trace. Small carnivores (e.g., raccoons, opossums, foxes, skunks, coyotes) and large birds (e.g., raptors, ravens, sea gulls, and wading species) may enter yards to prey on turtles, especially aquatic turtles. Ponds should have sufficient depth and underwater shelters to allow turtles to seek cover and prevent predators from easily wading in. Rats can chew on the limbs and heads of turtles, even indoors. Smaller terrestrial and aquatic chelonians should always have screened outdoor cages.[18] Fire ants (*Solenopis* spp.) and Argentine ants (*Linepithema humile*) can attack and kill small chelonians. Eggs should always be removed for incubation to avoid predation by an even larger suite of predators.

Tortoises will eat anything that falls into their enclosure. Enclosures must be regularly screened for trash (Fig. 23.3). Produce is often bound

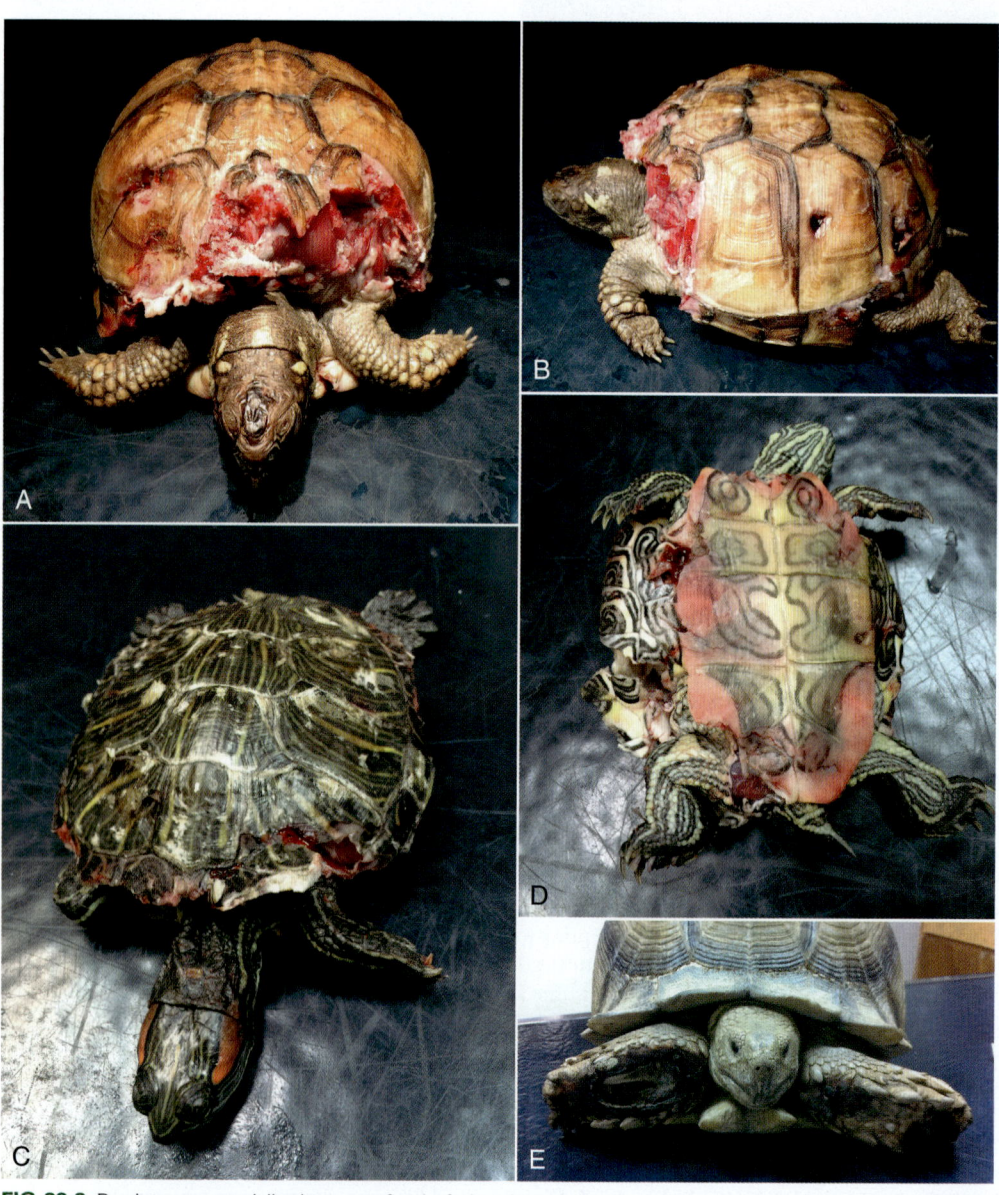

FIG 23.2 Predators, especially dogs, are fond of chewing on turtles and can cause a tremendous amount of damage (A–E) in a short time. Raccoons can smell aquatic turtles and will travel large distances to prey on them at night.

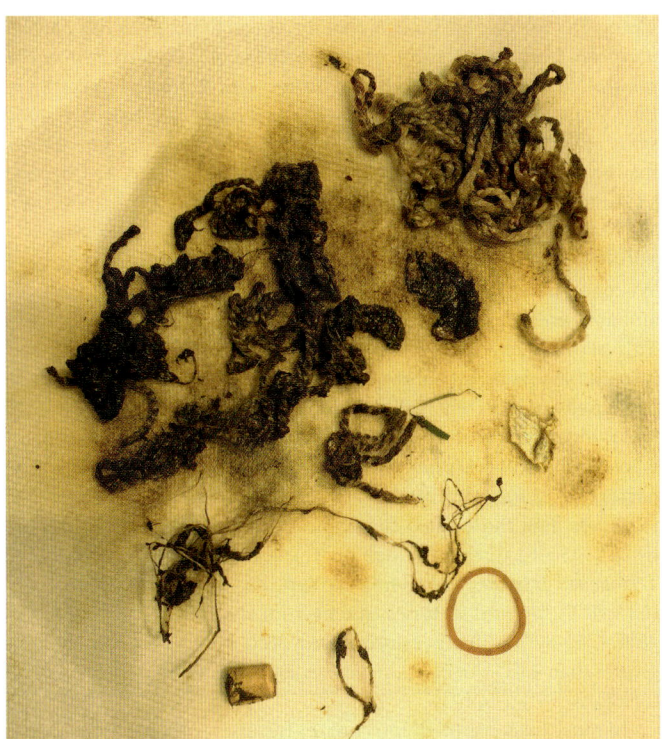

FIG 23.3 Chelonians will eat anything in their enclosure. This tortoise ate carpet, rubber bands, rubber erasers, twist ties, string, and metal foil, which resulted in several colonic prolapses before resolution.

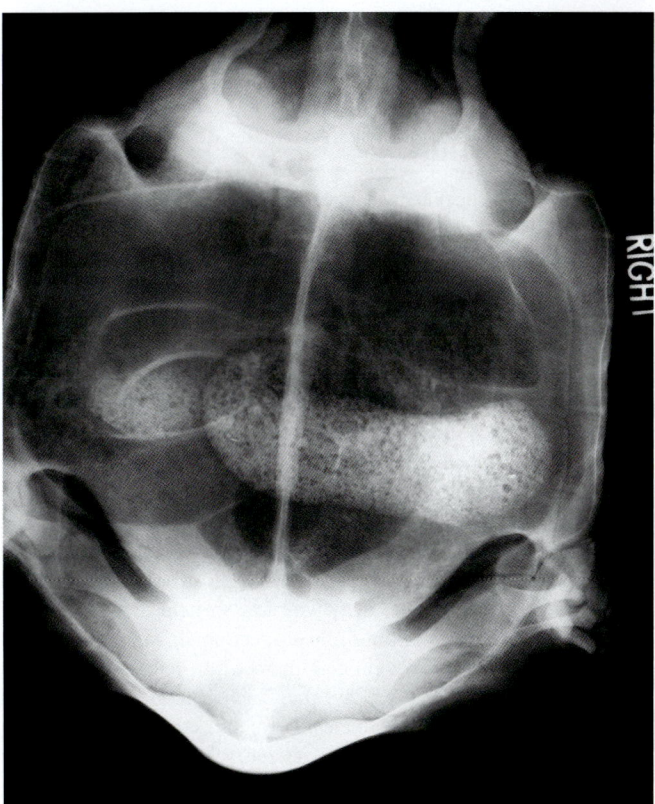

FIG 23.4 Large amounts of ingested sand or gravel can cause colonic impactions, chelonians should not be housed on dry sand or gravel.

with wire ties or rubber bands, so be sure to remove these from salad mixtures or they may be eaten (see Fig. 23.3). Tortoises will also consume small rocks, gravel, decomposed granite, pumice, pebbles (perhaps if they don't have enough calcium in their diet), and sand. These are rarely cause for concern unless large quantities are consumed. Large amounts of ingested sand or gravel can cause intestinal impactions (Fig. 23.4). Another potential hazard is pesticide spraying; do not spray tortoise enclosures with pesticides. Theft is an unfortunate reality as well.

ANNUAL EXAMINATIONS

Annual examinations are important to discuss overall care and feeding, educate owners, compare weight to species' normals, and screen for parasites and diseases. After a year, review of husbandry is again indicated, to get back to healthy habits. Reliance on diagnostics, especially hematology chemistry panels, fecal analysis (both direct and fecal flotation), and three-view survey radiographs are vital for the early detection of abnormalities. If an owner thinks something is wrong with the chelonian, there generally is. Do not delay diagnostic investigation; often the chelonian has been sick for weeks to months and adopting a wait-and-see attitude is often catastrophic.

IDENTIFICATION

Microchips are an accurate, permanent way to identify turtles and tortoises. The chip should be scanned first to ensure it is working and then injected subcutaneously in the skin fold over the left dorsal femur. All CITES Appendix I chelonians over 6 cm need to be microchipped as part of registration for a CITES Transaction or Specimen Specific Certificate, which allows them to be sold. Another method of identification is by using 5-minute epoxy to apply the patient's name, address,

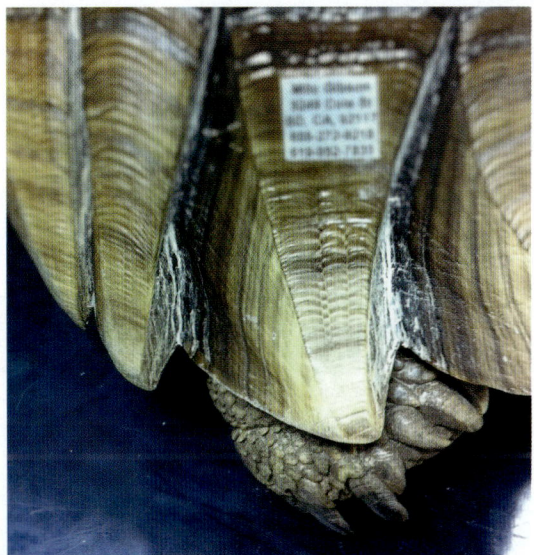

FIG 23.5 Microchipping is a permanent identification method; however, most chelonians are lost and found locally but not scanned for a microchip. Applying a tiny identification tag to a caudal central costal scute, covered with 5-minute epoxy, may help get the chelonian back to its home.

and phone number, in 8-point print, in the center of a costal scute, not overlapping a seam—a service most tortoise owners appreciate (Fig. 23.5). Most tortoises are lost locally and often not scanned for microchips; visible identification makes it easier to find the owner. Wildlife biologists will often notch marginal scutes to provide a unique number identifier.

While this system is appropriate for fieldwork when performed appropriately, it is not recommended for captive-owned pets. Inappropriate notching can result in damage to the sensitive underlying bone.

ACCLIMATIZATION

Wild-caught adult chelonians adapt poorly to captivity, and their purchase should be actively discouraged. Wild-caught temperate chelonians should be established in spring or early summer; late summer and fall does not allow them time to acclimate and feed enough prior to hibernation. Prior to obtaining chelonians, review the natural history and pertinent literature on captive care. All new arrivals should be quarantined away from the main collection to allow for veterinary diagnostics, parasite treatment, and establishment of a feeding regimen for 3 to 6 months. This basic safeguard should not be overlooked because diseases are easy to introduce into a collection but difficult and costly to eliminate. If healthy, new arrivals should be set up in as large a cage as possible or placed outdoors if the weather is favorable. Most chelonians are naturally secretive animals, and frequent handling or disturbance deters them from settling into captivity. Try to minimize disturbance and provide the turtles with plenty of security with low shelters they can retreat under, with proper cage substrates, broad-spectrum lighting, and basking areas. For finicky eaters try enticing them with preferred foods. For carnivorous species this means live prey, such as insects, worms, fish, or pink mice (taking into account legislative restrictions on feeding live vertebrate prey). For herbivorous species, red, yellow, or orange-colored foods, and fresh dark leafy greens, such as dandelions, are often favored (refer to Chapter 27). Rainstorms often increase activity; thus spraying the enclosure can stimulate appetite. Never release tortoises back into the wild; it is illegal, they rarely if ever survive, and more importantly they are likely to pose a serious health threat to the endemic chelonian populations.

TORTOISE AND BOX TURTLE CARE

Tortoises and box turtles are popular backyard pets. Many of these species are commonly treated by veterinarians, including Mojave desert tortoises (*Gopherus agassizii*), Sonoran desert tortoises (*G. morafkai*), Texas tortoises, (*G. berlandieri*), Greek tortoises, (*Testudo graeca spp.*), Hermann's tortoise (*Testudo hermanni*), Russian tortoises (*Agronemys horsfieldii*), and the African spurred tortoise or sulcata (*Centrochelys sulcata*). Several subspecies of box turtles were common, especially in the U.S. pet trade, including the Eastern box turtles (*Terrapene carolina spp.*), and the ornate box turtles (*Terrapene ornata spp.*). Some species may be controlled by international or national legislation (see Chapters 183 and 184 on legislation).

Outdoor Housing

Whenever possible, house tortoises and box turtles outdoors, in as large an enclosure as possible, even if only for a small portion of the year. This allows them space to exercise, graze, and bask. Hatchling and juveniles should be kept above 21°C (70°F). Adult tropical tortoises can be housed outdoors when morning temperatures are above 18°C (65°F) and midday temperatures exceed 24°C (75°F). Bring them in at night when temperatures are below 18°C (65°F) or provide a heated tortoise barn (Fig. 23.6). Adult temperate species tolerate temperatures 3°C (5°F) less than those listed for tropical species provided it warms up to 24°C (75°F) during the day or if a heated barn is present. Many *Terrapene*, *Testudo*, and *Gopherus* spp. do well from 20° to 32°C (68°–90°F); tropical tortoises benefit from less variability, from 22° to 28°C (72°–82°F).[1] Temperatures above 38°C (100°F) are too hot, and greater than 43°C (110°F) is critically dangerous for all box turtles and tortoises.

In most areas it is often too cold for tortoises without supplemental heat, especially at night. All tortoises benefit from heated shelters (e.g., the tortoise barn, Fig. 23.6), which can be constructed of plywood with a hinged, sloped, insulated, slightly overhanging, and heated inner roof. The floor is open to the dirt to boost humidity and ease cleaning or can be floored in colder areas. Hinging the roof makes it easier to clean; waterproofing the plywood will extend its lifespan. A 12-inch by 36-inch Kane pig blanket (Kane MKG, Inc., Des Moines, IA) or waterproof radiant heat panel, suspended loosely from the solid inner roof insulation, provides heat, and temperature can be controlled with a rheostat or thermostat. A dusk-to-dawn timer will keep heat on at night and off on warmer days, or it can be run continuously. The doorway should be just large enough for tortoises to fit through and left open to provide an avenue to escape heat should the timer fail. The doorway opening can be covered with heavy gauge clear vinyl strips, which allows for

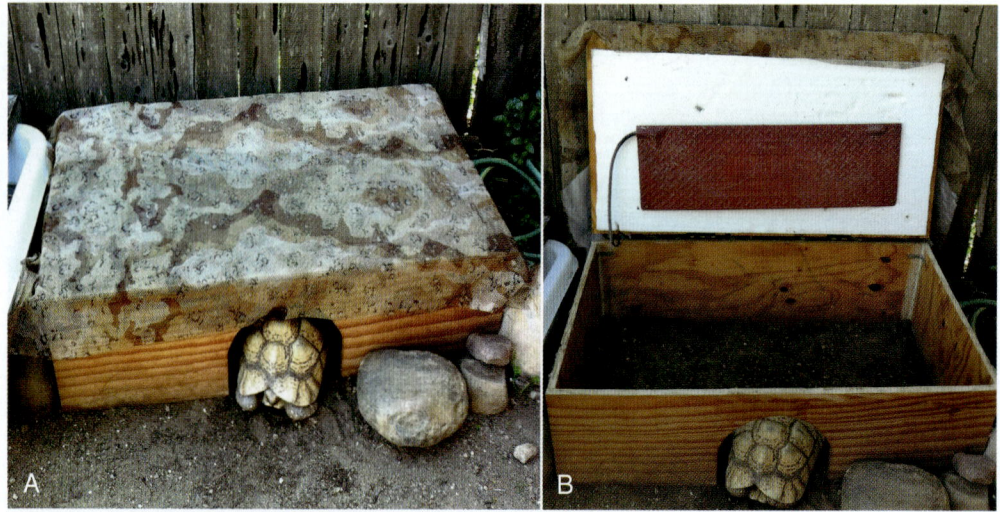

FIG 23.6 A heated waterproof insulated tortoise barn (A, B) is advantageous for tortoises. The insulated roof reflects heat down from the heat pad. Hinging the roof makes cleaning easier, and a dusk-to-dawn timer turns on heat at night and off on hot days.

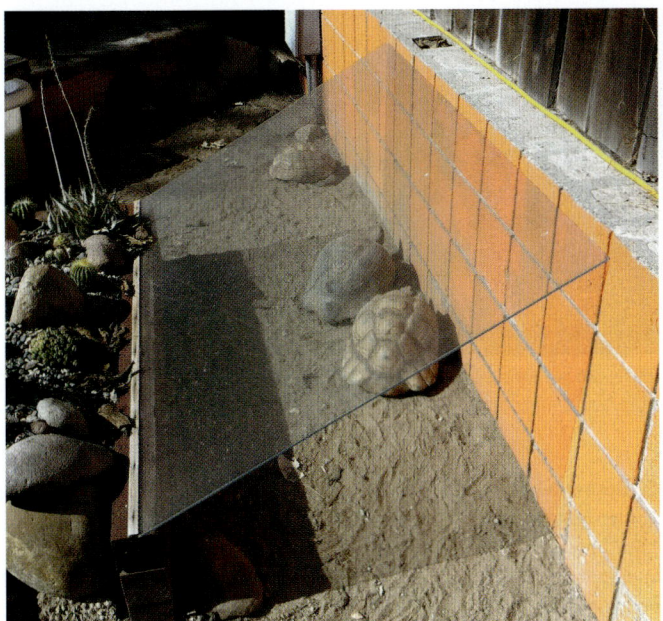

FIG 23.7 Tortoise solariums boost ambient heat to provide a basking area so the tortoise can better thermoregulate.

easy tortoise access but traps heat. On really cold nights a waterproof wrap or space blanket can increase heat retention.

Another way to boost heat and allow better thermoregulation is to make a solarium, with 1/4-inch safety glass, leaned up at a 45-degree angle against a sun-facing wall and secured on the other side by quarter round on top of two or more stacked 4-inch by 4-inch landscape timbers, drilled through and secured to the ground with rebar spikes. Leave this structure open at both ends (Fig. 23.7).

Burrowing species (e.g., desert tortoises, African spurred, Russians, ornate box turtles) may excavate a burrow to escape cold or hot temperatures. Be sure the opening cannot flood during heavy rains, either by berming around the entrance or providing drainage away from the entrance. Artificial burrows can also be constructed (see the Arizona Game and Fish Department website).[19] Do not allow African spurred tortoises to burrow near foundations; they can do extensive damage.

When planning outdoor enclosures, several factors should be considered to suit the needs of species. An understanding of the species microhabitat use and environment will be useful in designing the enclosure. Desert species can tolerate higher temperatures and drier enclosures than can tropical rainforest species. For grassland or desert species, such as *Gopherus*, *Testudo*, sulcatas, leopard tortoises (*Stigmochelys pardalis*), Indian star tortoises (*Geochelone elegans*), and ornate box turtles (*Terrapene ornata* spp.), enclosures can be more sparsely planted with shrubs and grasses. For tropical forest forms, such as red- and yellow-footed (*Chelonoidis carbonaria* and *C. denticulata*), Burmese tortoises (*Manouria spp.*), hingeback tortoises (*Kinixys* spp.), *Indotestudo* spp., Eastern box turtles (*Terrapene carolina* sspp.), provide densely planted enclosures with shelters they can retreat under and shallow pools they can cool off in. Loose mulch piles in shaded areas will allow additional refuge to burrow under. All enclosures should have sun areas, as well as shade. The strategic use of rocks, boulders, hollow logs, branches, and varied topography can provide a more complex and enriched environment.

Outdoor enclosures must have secure, solid perimeters. Tortoises pace perimeters and constantly try to get through perimeters they can see through. If there is a way over, under, or through, the turtle or tortoise will find it. Solid barriers, such as wooden fencing, block walls, or smooth concrete, are far more preferable to open fencing. Open fencing should be small, or large, enough that turtles or tortoises cannot entrap and cut an appendage. Materials will vary in size from hardware cloth to welded wire, depending on species size. Small tortoise species can climb chain link. Fencing should be buried 12 inches to 24 inches and be at least two to three times the carapace length in height. Large powerful species, such as African spurred, Aldabra, and Galapagos tortoises, or giant yellow foots, require more substantial containment barriers of welded pipe or concrete/block construction. Tethering a tortoise by a leg, or through a hole in the shell, is unacceptable, inhumane, and potentially disastrous if a leg gets entrapped.

Indoor Housing

Indoor housing is usually required for a good portion of the year, except in subtropical to tropical areas. The combined shell size of all turtles/ tortoises present should not exceed a quarter of the floor surface area available to the tortoises (Mader et al, Proc ARAV, 1998, p 103), or at minimum, 0.4 m² per 0.1 m carapace length and recommended is 1.0 m² per 0.1 m carapace length.[12] Provide as much space as possible. Aquariums, plastic or metal livestock troughs, or plastic containers can be used for small turtles/tortoises. Large commercially available plastic tubs are waterproof, easy to clean, and much more suitable for larger tortoises than aquariums (Vision Products, Tubs, Canoga Park, CA, or Waterlandtubs). Cages can also be constructed out of plywood for larger tortoises. The inner cage surfaces should be caulked and sealed with several coats of polyurethane, which facilitates cleaning. Allow the cage to dry out thoroughly and any varnish smell to completely dissipate before placing any tortoises inside. To prevent chilling, the cage bottom should not be in direct contact with cold concrete; a gap of several inches is advisable, such as resting on 2 inch by 4 inch (5 cm × 10 cm) wood blocks. Ambient indoor temperature should be 24° to 32°C (75°–90°F) depending on the species. Rooms can be heated with thermostatically controlled space heaters, radiant heat panels, and basking lights to provide a thermogradiant.

Substrates

Tortoises vary in environmental requirements from desert to tropical forest. More xeric-adapted tortoise species can be maintained indoors on alfalfa pellets or newspaper. As they graduate to larger cages, a mixture of medium to large rice hulls, newspaper, indoor-outdoor carpeting (be sure to avoid frayed edges), or corrugated cardboard can be used. Forest tortoises and box turtles will fair better on humid substrates such as a mixture of conifer bark nuggets and peat moss, coconut coir, or soil (which is a good source of cellulolytic bacteria). Remove fecal material from the enclosure several times per week and replace the substrate several times per year. Avoid sand, gravel, cat litter, crushed corncob, or walnut shells.

Water

Water should be regularly available for indoor and outdoor chelonians (Fig. 23.8). Shallow plastic plant saucers work well for most tortoises, with the exception of desert tortoises. Chelonians often defecate in their water; thus water bowls should be changed frequently and whenever visibly soiled. Desert tortoises, and other species outdoors, will also drink from standing water. An alternative to the water bowl is to soak the desert or xeric species in chin-deep water every 1 to 2 weeks.

Feeding

What to feed tortoises is an evolving empirical science and fraught with misconceptions (Box 23.1, Tortoise Diet; see also Chapter 27).[16,18,20] Most desert tortoises in the backyards of southern California suffer from chronic protein and fiber deficiency, as well as carbohydrate

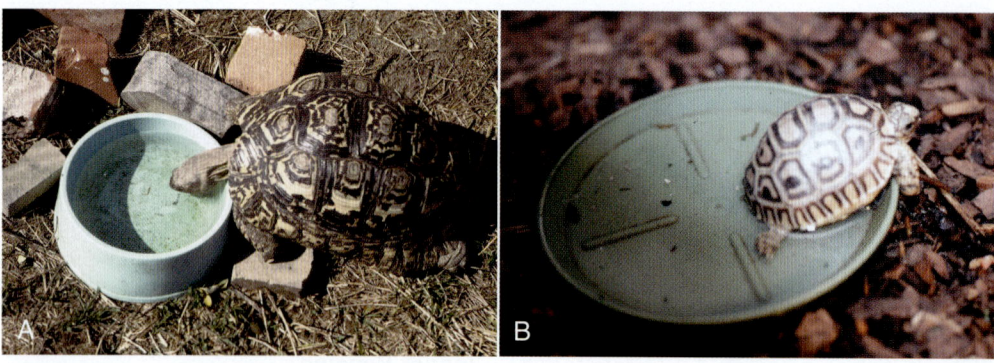

FIG 23.8 Water should always be available for chelonians, such as these leopard tortoises *(Stigmochelys pardalis)*, either by water bowls (A) or soaking (B).

BOX 23.1   Tortoise Diet[18,20]

Adults should be fed three times per week, and hatchlings fed daily. If pelleted commercial tortoise foods are used, calcium and multivitamin supplementation isn't needed. If not feeding pellets (not recommended) every feeding, dust food with calcium lactate, carbonate, citrate, or gluconate and multivitamins once or twice a month.

Majority—50% to 80% good quality commercial pelleted tortoise diets and grass hays (Bermuda, timothy, buffalo, brome, tall fescue, orchard grass but not alfalfa hay or Kentucky bluegrass). See Chapter 27 for more information.

Minority—20% to 50% native plants consumed by tortoises in the wild: backyard weeds (especially dandelions, clover, burclovers, purslane, spurges, crabgrass, cheese weed, creeping wood sorrel, and others), spineless prickly pear cactus pads and fruits *(Opuntia ficus-indica)*, dark leafy greens (collards, mustards, turnip tops, bok choy, kale, spinach, cabbage, endive, Romaine lettuce), flowers (roses, nasturtiums, hibiscus, carnations, geraniums, primroses, ice plant, and cactus flowers), leaves (mulberry, grape, hibiscus, squash) can also be fed. Very little to no fruit should be fed.

---

excess, and many have calcium deficiencies. The same is likely true in other areas.

Most wild tortoises consume a wide variety of plants (over 200 for *Gopherus morafkai*), switching diet species to obtain the freshest plants until only dry senescent plants are available.[21] Commercial tortoise diets, grasses, and grass hays tend to have better calcium levels and nutrient profiles similar to what tortoises naturally consume. Getting tortoises to eat hay and commercial foods can be a challenge. Much like a dog content with table food, a tortoise will eat pellets and hay once hungry enough, but not if better tasting or more familiar foods are available. Use good quality hays, not stems or stalks that smell stale or moldy. Chopping the hay with scissors, or a food processor, and sprinkling or spraying the hay with water to moisten it helps, or it can be soaked in water for several minutes. Soaking too long will leach out nutrients. Mixing the normal food in or under the hay also helps. Pellets can be soaked in water until just soft and mixed into the greens. Be patient and persistent, and tortoises will switch over to hay and commercial pellets, as fruits and vegetables are gradually reduced. Feeding less or less often will encourage turtles and tortoises to try new foods. For information on native plant species naturally consumed by desert tortoises, see the websites of AZ Game and Fish Department[22] and the CA Turtle and Tortoise Society.[23] Similar resources probably exist in other countries.

Be aware of several persistent widespread misconceptions. Members of the vegetable family Brassica (cabbages, kale, mustard greens, broccoli, cauliflower, Brussels sprouts) do not cause thyroid problems (goiter) and are completely harmless in moderation as part of a balanced diet. Foods rich in oxalic acid, such as spinach, beet greens, collards, Swiss chard, Brussels sprouts, prickly pear cactus, and purslane, do not contribute to calcium oxalate uroliths. The adverse effects of oxalates must be considered in terms of the oxalate:Ca ratio of food (see Chapter 27). Diets low in Ca and high in oxalates are not recommended, but occasional consumption of high oxalate foods as part of a nutritious diet does not pose any particular health problem. Tortoises commonly form uric acid stones but very rarely calcium oxalate stones, which were considered an incidental finding in wild desert tortoises.[24,25] Plant poisoning is rare in tortoises. Tortoises either avoid poisonous plants or are more resistant to their effects, unless no other forage is available. Some toxic plant exceptions include rhododendrons (grayanotoxins cause flaccid paresis), oleanders, chinaberry trees, tree tobacco, and poisonous mushrooms. Tortoises love fruits and will consume them preferentially over more nutritious foods; however, most species are not frugivorous. Red and yellow-footed tortoises are more frugivorous than other tortoises and can be offered more fruit, but no more than 20% of the entire balanced ration. Fruits, in general, are mineral poor, yet high in sugars and can disrupt the normal gut flora and may lead to hepatic lipidosis. Limit fruits to a small portion of the diet, more of an occasional treat than a staple, or do not feed them at all.

Tortoises should be fed on a flat board, metal or plastic trays, or newspaper. Wash, or dispose of, these after use. Do not feed tortoises on loose substrate or they will incidentally ingest it. Feed as much variety as possible! The majority of the diet should be commercial tortoise chows, hay, grasses, weeds, and flowers (see Box 23.1, Tortoise Diet). Adults should be fed a minimum of three times per week and hatchlings daily. If the diet consists largely of commercial pellets, then supplemental calcium and multivitamins are not needed. It is easier to achieve proper shell growth with commercial pellets than a fresh vegetable diet (Fig. 23.9). If not using commercial pellets or natural foods, every feeding should be lightly dusted with calcium carbonate, lactate, citrate, or gluconate for juveniles, and weekly for adults. If vitamin-fortified tortoise foods are not being consumed, twice a month lightly dust food with multivitamins. If the tortoises are exposed to unfiltered sunlight or indoor ultraviolet (UVB) lights, vitamin D supplements are not needed or desired.

Box turtles are quite predatory, eating whatever they can catch, consequently, moving prey appeals to them.[4] Box turtles are opportunistic omnivores that consume a wide variety of invertebrate and small vertebrate prey along with a diversity of plants. See Box Turtle Diet (Box 23.2)[20,26] and Chapter 27 for information on captive feeding.

Reproduction

Males of bowsprit tortoises (*Chersina angulata*), chaco Tortoises (*C. chilensis*), African spurred tortoises, and *Gopherus* spp. will fight relentlessly, may kill one another, and should be housed singly. Females may be housed together separate from males. It is no longer recommended to breed desert or African spurred tortoises as there is an overabundance of them in captivity. Celioscopic-assisted prefemoral oophorectomy,[27] or orchiectomy,[28] or phallectomy is recommended to reduce unwanted numbers of these tortoises. Orchiectomy is difficult as the testicles are deep in the coelom. Phallectomy will not change the male's belligerent mating behavior.

Courtship behavior and breeding season varies. Posthibernation rising temperatures and increasing daylength stimulate temperate chelonians to breed. Tropical species may respond to the onset of the rainy season. Storms and associated changes in barometric pressure seem to stimulate breeding activity in many species. Courtship behavior involves visual, tactile, and olfactory cues including trailing, smelling, biting, ramming, male/male combat, female copulatory posture (presentation), and male vocalization.[29] Female tortoises must be in prime condition before egg production, including a well-balanced diet with adequate calcium. Additional calcium should be provided for females that produce large or multiple clutches. Chelonians are known to be able to store sperm up to 4 years.[30] Gravid females feel heavier than normal and tend to be more active, often pacing in the enclosure. Eggs can be palpated in the prefemoral fossa and can be readily demonstrated by radiography and ultrasonography. Some females may excavate several nests before actually laying eggs. Eggs should be carefully excavated and removed for incubation. Fertile eggs, when candled, develop a dorsal chalk spot, or band, that slowly spreads ventrally as the extraembryonic membranes develop, and blood vessels may be visible, whereas infertile eggs have neither (Fig. 23.10).

Neonatal Care

Once the neonate has pipped the eggshell with its caruncle, or eggtooth, it emerges from the shell within 1 to 4 days. During this time, the neonate's shell begins to unfold, facilitating yolk absorption. As the neonate's shell straightens and the tortoise begins to move, the eggshell

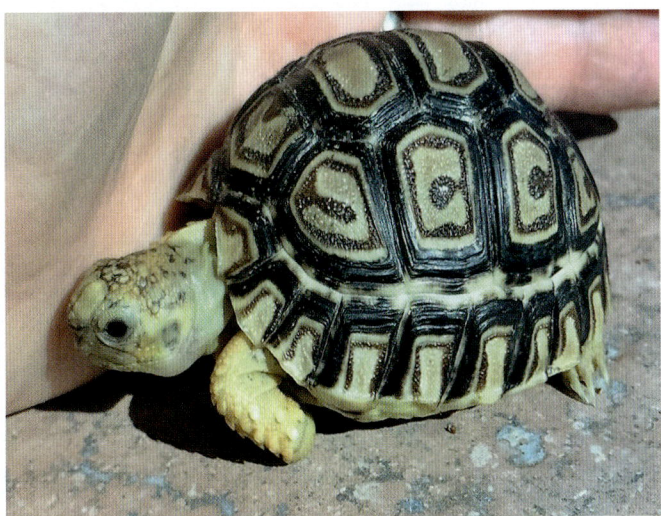

FIG 23.9 Juvenile leopard tortoise (*Stigmochelys pardalis*), raised primarily on commercial pellets, dark leafy greens, weeds, flowers, and no fruit. A nighttime drop in temperature, and humid substrate or hidebox, may also help prevent pyramidal shell growth.

BOX 23.2 Box Turtle Diet[20,26]

Items listed in italics often entice anorexic animals to eat. Adults should be fed three or more times per week in the morning, and juveniles fed daily. Juveniles tend to be much more carnivorous than adults. If pelleted foods are not a large part of the diet, lightly dust food with calcium lactate, carbonate, citrate, or gluconate every feeding and give multivitamins twice monthly. Provide variety.

>50% Pellets or animals—commercial good quality box turtle or aquatic turtle pellets (see Chapter 27 for more information), earthworms, crickets, grasshoppers, slugs, snails, pill bugs, cicadas, whole-skinned chopped mice, baby mice (pinkies), mealworms, waxworms, silk moth larvae, and other insects.

<50% Plants—25% fruits and 75% vegetables

25% Fruits: tomatoes, strawberries, raspberries, blackberries, mulberries, blueberries, apples, grapes, cherries, peaches, pears, plums, nectarines, figs, melons.

75% Vegetables: mushrooms; dark leafy greens (mustard, collard, radish, beet and turnip greens or tops, kale, cabbage, dandelion leaves, stems or flowers, spinach, bok choy, pak choi, broccoli rabe); red leaf or romaine lettuce (be careful not to overfeed lettuces); Swiss chard; steamed chopped squashes; sweet potatoes; shredded (not chopped) carrots; thawed frozen mixed vegetables (peas, corn, carrots, green beans, lima beans); alfalfa, radish, clover, or bean sprouts; soaked alfalfa pellets; bell peppers; broccoli; green beans; peas in the pod; okra; and prickly pear (*Opuntia* spp.) cactus pads (be sure to shave off spines).

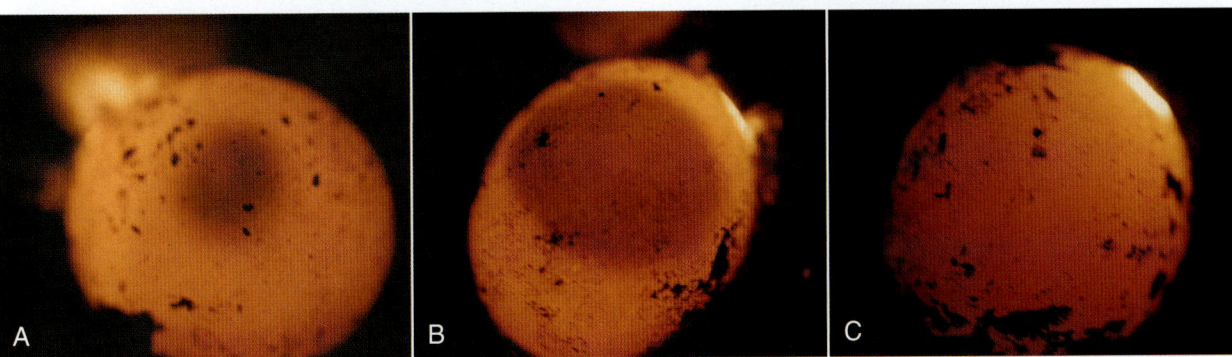

FIG 23.10 Fertile eggs, when candled, have a dorsal chalk line (A) that spreads slowly ventrally during development (B), whereas infertile eggs do not (C).

breaks further. Once out of the egg, the neonate may still have a considerable yolk sac (Fig. 23.11). The hatchling should be carefully rinsed off and transferred to a small plastic container, and kept on clean moist paper towels at the same temperature as the incubator. Replace and remoisten towels as the yolk sac slowly absorbs over the next few days (Fig. 23.12). Once the yolk sac is fully absorbed and the umbilicus sealed, the neonate can be transferred to a cage with previously mentioned substrates.

Hatchlings usually begin feeding within 1 to 14 days of leaving the egg. Hatchlings are prone to dehydration; therefore shallow water bowls should constantly be available (see Fig. 23.8B). An alternative is to soak neonates in shallow water several times a week. A drop in ambient temperature at night,[6] provision of humid substrate,[31] or humidity box,

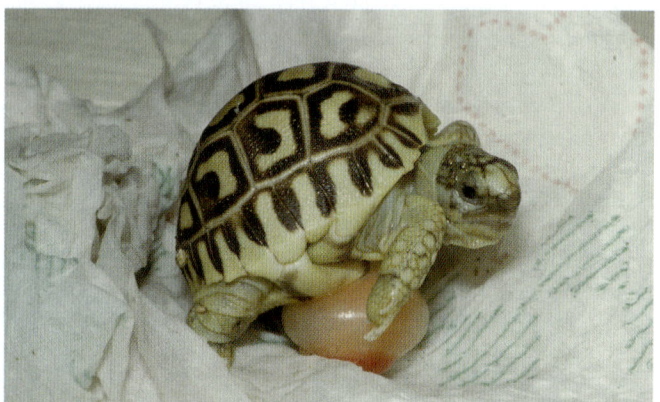

FIG 23.11 Once out of the egg, neonatal chelonians, such as this leopard tortoise *(Stigmochelys pardalis),* may still have considerable yolk sac. The hatchling should be carefully rinsed off and transferred to a small plastic container and kept on clean moist paper towels, at the same temperature as the incubator, until the yolk is absorbed.

and feeding pelleted commercial pellets seems to reduce pyramidal shell growth. Ambient temperature should gradually warm to 30°C (85°F) during the day, with a thermal gradient. Hatchlings should develop a firm shell in the first year.

AQUATIC TURTLES

Aquatic turtles are popular pets, yet among the most labor intensive of all reptiles to maintain properly.[32] Improper husbandry often results in health problems, such as skin and shell infections, pneumonia, hypovitaminosis A, and shell deformities. An understanding of proper captive care helps to avoid these issues. Keep in mind that there are many species-specific differences, and no substitute exists for knowledge of natural history to direct captive care. The most common aquatic turtle seen by veterinarians is the red-eared slider or terrapin (*Trachemys scripta elegans*).

Housing

Housing requirements vary according to the size of the turtle and the number being kept. A variety of enclosures can be used from glass aquaria, plastic tubs, livestock watering tanks, and pond liners to elaborate outdoor ponds. Waterland Tubs, ZooMed, and Vision Cages all make commercially available turtle enclosures (Fig. 23.13). Outdoor enclosures should have some shade available. Never place a plastic or glass aquarium in full sun because it could easily overheat. A rule of thumb, for minimum cage size, is the combined shell size of all residents should not exceed 25% of the cage's accessible space for turtles,[33] or 0.25 m^3 per 0.1 m carapace length and 0.75 m^3 per 0.1 m carapace length is recommended.[34]

Temperature

Water and air must be warm; 24° to 28°C (75°–82°F) are recommended for most species. A combination heat and broad-spectrum lighting (including UVB), with reflector, directed toward the basking area creates

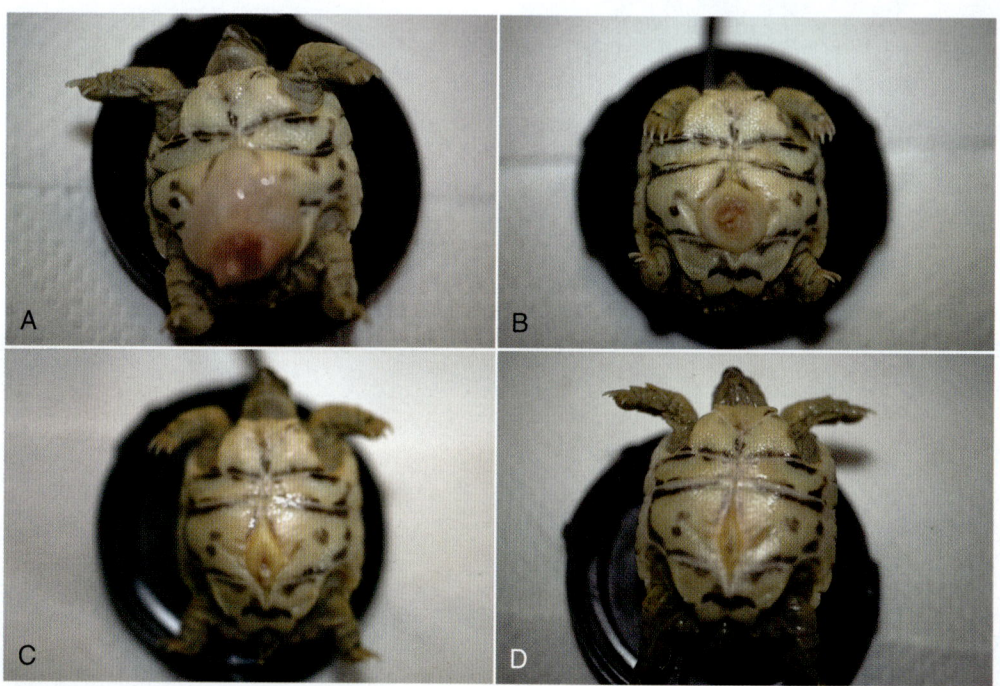

FIG 23.12 Leopard tortoise (*Stigmochelys pardalis*) hatchling on days 1 (A), 3 (B), 5(C), and 8(D) as it rapidly resorbs its yolk sac and the umbilicus closes.

a hot spot for basking. Submersible aquarium heaters (Eheim Jager, Deizisau, Germany, makes good, durable ones) will keep the water warm; this is especially important for hatchlings. Provide barriers around submersible heaters to prevent contact burns on the turtle. In larger setups, an inline heater can be plumbed to the filtration system. Alternatively, one can keep the room temperature within this range, without heating the water. Some species such as mud and musk turtles, common snapping turtles (not alligator snapping turtles), and big-headed turtles (*Platysternon megacephalum*) prefer it cooler; the latter may need an aquarium chiller to cool the water.

Water Quality

Clean water is crucial to prevent skin and shell infections in turtles. Warm water promotes bacterial, fungal, and parasitic growth. Water laden with bacteria, feces, and urine is malodorous; clean water should have little to no odor. Likewise, turtles should have no odor, unless they are overly excited and express their musk glands. Water should be kept clean by frequent water changes and/or sufficient filtration.

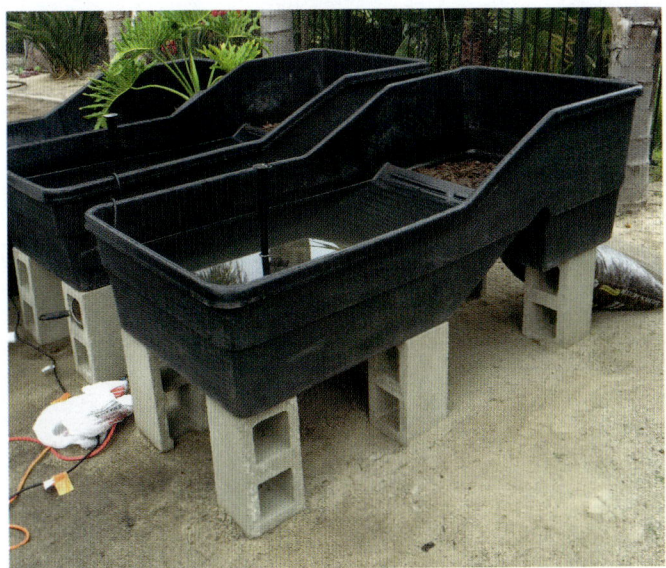

FIG 23.13 A variety of commercial aquatic turtle enclosures are available, such as this Waterland Tub.

Small aquatic turtles can be kept in simple, small, closed water systems that afford more freedom from water conditioning because reptiles are not dependent on ultraclean water for respiratory needs as for fish.[35] The bacterial nitrification cycle that converts ammonia in urine to nitrites, then to less toxic nitrates, is much more important for delicate fish gills. Being less sensitive, full water changes (as opposed to partial water changes) are regularly needed to keep bacterial levels low, unless filtration is profound and well maintained. Dechlorination of water is also not normally necessary for turtles; however, it should be performed if biologic filtration is used or fish are present. A common misconception of inexperienced turtle owners is that the mechanical and biologic filtration recommended for specific water volumes for fish will keep a similarly sized turtle tank clean. However, the much greater biomass of turtles in the same volume necessitates considerably greater filtration.

How often the water needs to be changed depends on several factors, including stocking density, water volume, temperature, feeding frequency, and available filtration. One can keep the water cleaner by feeding in a separate container, because most foods foul the water quickly and promote bacterial growth, but this is not essential. Initially some turtles may be reluctant to feed in the separate container but can be acclimated to this over time. Using the same water from the home container helps.

Full water changes are easier if no substrates, or easily removable substrates, are present. Sand and gravel are harder to clean, and aquatic turtles can ingest gravel, which can cause intestinal obstruction (Fig. 23.14). Some species (e.g., soft shells, Trionychidae), however, like to burrow into sand and gravel. Keep in mind that cleaning areas are a potential source of zoonosis, such as Salmonella. Avoid food preparation, or infant bathing areas, when cleaning turtle cages.

For larger enclosures, too heavy to move, make it as easy as possible to dump and fill water. By far the easiest way to drain a tank is to install a PVC bulkhead fitting (http://pentairaes.com) and valve that attaches to a hose. Use a hole drill bit to cut through plastic and a diamond hole saw (http://www.grainger.com) to cut through glass, or buy a predrilled aquarium before installing a PVC bulkhead fitting. The next easiest method of drainage is portable electric submersible pumps (e.g., Little Giant Water Wizard model 50500 5-MSP, http://www.lilgiantpump-products.com). Be sure to purchase a bottom suction pump, not a side suction pump. When in use, make sure a turtle doesn't get caught in the pump's suction, panic, and drown. Alternatively, one can use a siphon to drain the water into a toilet, floor drain, or outdoors to water plants. Siphons take longer than pumps. After draining, the empty tank

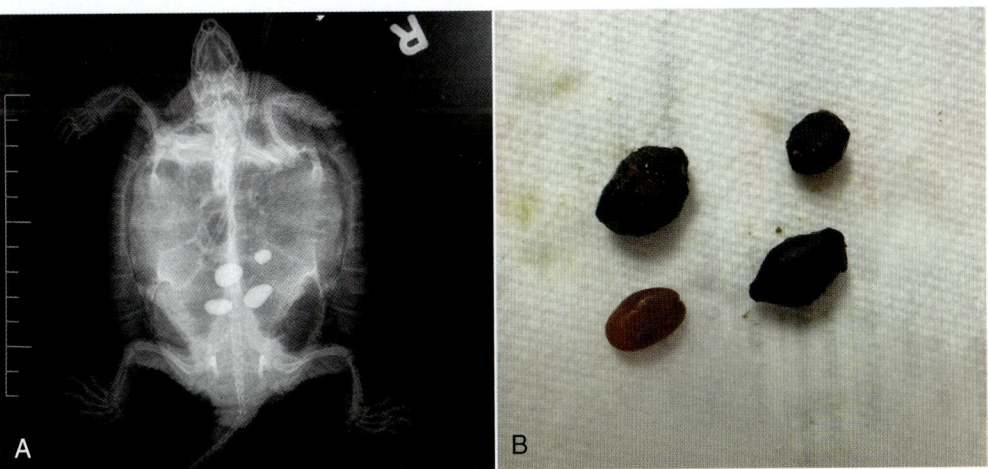

FIG 23.14 Aquatic turtles can ingest small pebbles and gravel, this anorectic red-eared slider (A) responded to food and fluids through an esophagostomy tube and was able to pass these stones (B).

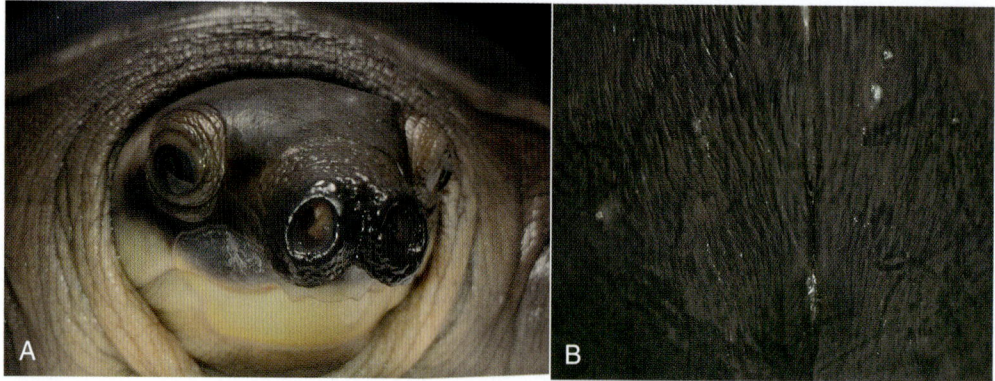

FIG 23.15 Multiple acid-fast granulomas in the nostril (A) and on the shell (B) of a Fly River turtle (*Carettochelys inscuplta*) that resolved after adding a simple external canister filter with ultraviolet disinfection designed to eliminate algae.

can be rinsed out, and occasionally even scrubbed out, but need not be disinfected. When refilling be aware that abrupt changes in water temperature can kill turtles, especially hot water; make sure the water temperature refilling the tank is similar to what it was prior to cleaning. Thermometers facilitate this; with experience, one can gauge this by hand.

Proper filtration makes aquatic turtle care easier. The best filters for turtles are large external canister filters, such as those designed for Koi, or rapid sand filters. A weir tank, fed from the holding enclosure, increases water volumes and can allow for prefiltering of the water through a floss pad. Sterilizing ultraviolet (UV, 254 nm) filters irradiates pathogens and is an easy way to eliminate algae and as an adjunct to managing infectious disease (Fig. 23.15). Ozone is even better at water disinfection but much more expensive and has the potential for harm if not accurately monitored and controlled. Aeration of water is important to support aerobic bacterial growth in biological filters. Under-gravel filters need a deep gravel bed, 7.5 cm or more, or the turtle may dig and expose the filter plate.[16] Once exposed, water will bypass the gravel as it follows the path of least resistance, and the benefits of biological filtration will be decreased. For small enclosures with low biological load, internal submersible filters are gaining in popularity but need to be cleaned frequently. Foam rubber filters are generally inadequate as a sole method of keeping water clean.

Water should be at least as deep as the width of the turtle's shell at the widest point so that if overturned the turtle will be able to right itself and avoid drowning. For the most part, turtles can be maintained in water with neutral pH, except for some South American blackwater species, such as red-headed river turtles (*Podocnemis erythocephala*), snake-necked turtle (*Hydromedusa tectifera*), red side-neck turtle (*Phyrnops rufipes*), and other *Phyrnops* spp., which need more acidic conditions.[16] There are numerous aquarist buffer systems available to maintain such conditions. Diamondback terrapins live in brackish water and require the addition of two tablespoons of aquarium salt and mineral mix per gallon of water (5 g per L).

Haul Out and/or Nesting Area

A dry haul out or nesting area should be present so that turtles can crawl out of the water, dry off, and bask. A broad spectrum (including UVB) basking light that provides heat should be directed toward the basking area to create a hot spot (<35°C, 95°F). Basking areas can be as simple as a flat rock resting on submerged bricks, a cinder block, or fixed pieces of cork, hardwood driftwood, or plastic platforms. More elaborate platforms can be built above water level with access via a plastic or wooden ramp or branch (Fig. 23.16). Snapping turtles (*Chelydra*

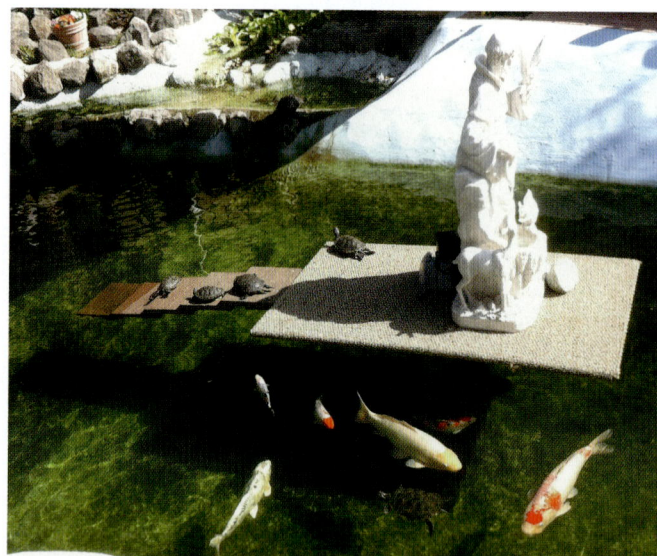

FIG 23.16 A haul out area is important for aquatic turtles to dry off, bask, thermoregulate, and for vitamin D synthesis via ultraviolet light.

and *Malaclemys* spp.), matamatas (*Chelus fimbriata*), and Fly River turtles (*Carettochelys insculpta*) do not need basking areas.

Nesting areas, which double as a basking area, should be provided for adult females, even if males are not present. If sufficient nest area is provided, dystocia may be avoided and oviposition stimulated. Temporarily rigging a nesting area, or shifting a gravid female to a cage with a nesting area, is far less successful than keeping a nesting area present year round.[36] The nest area should be approximately four to five times larger than the female, and twice as deep as the carapace length. Nest medium should be a mixture of 50% moist sand mixed with potting soil or peat moss. Nest area containers can be made from a variety of plastic tote containers, with wet sand weighing down the bottom, which prevents the nest area from floating and tipping over. Some aquatic turtle enclosures, such as those from Waterland Tubs and Zoo Med, have built in basking/nest areas, with a ramp coming up out of the water (see Fig. 23.13).

Feeding

The majority of the diet should consist of soaked, softened, commercial fish-based aquatic turtle pellets (Box 23.2). Patience and persistence is

---

BOX 23.3 Aquatic Turtle Diet[20,26]

Feed adults one to three times per week, and hatchlings daily. Feed as much variety as possible. If a balanced commercial pellet is provided, multivitamin and mineral supplementation is not required.

Majority of the diet—Commercial, good-quality, soaked, fish-based aquatic turtle pellets (see Chapter 27 for more information), or whole animals (mice, rats, earthworms, tubifex worms, slugs, snails, fresh whole shrimp [with shells, not freeze dried], thawed frozen guppies, trout, bait fish, freshwater (not saltwater) smelt.

Minority of the diet—Insects (crickets, wax worms, mealworms, flies, moths, and grasshoppers), in moderation, if properly gut loaded with calcium-enriched diet (>8% calcium). Desiccated insects are nutritionally inadequate and should not be fed.

In older omnivorous species (many sliders and pond turtles), gradually increase dark leafy greens (kale, spinach, dandelion greens, romaine lettuce, cabbage, watercress, endive, bok choy, escarole), yams, carrots, duckweed, water lettuce, and algae.

---

required with commercial diets because acceptance can take several weeks. See Box 23.2 for other options. Whole fish are better than gutted fish and can be fed chopped or whole. Ideally, fish should be well fed prior to being fed to turtles. Freezing for more than three days may eliminate transfer of some, but not all, parasites. Wild-caught sticklebacks, mosquito fish, and goldfish should not be fed because they are natural vectors for several serious parasites[37] and mycobacteria. Most aquatic turtles will readily consume mice, from pinkies to chopped, skinned adults. Mice and rats are skinned to reduce indigestible keratin. Older mice have more mineralized bone, which is preferable for shell growth, whereas mouse liver is an excellent source of vitamin A. A variety of gut-loaded insects can also be fed as a minority of the diet (Box 23.3). Mineral or antibiotic blocks in the water do not help nutritionally, or medically, and should be discouraged.

Commercial gel diets are also available. Cut gelatin into bite-sized pieces or strips. The strips can be tightly wrapped in plastic wrap, placed in self-sealing polyethylene plastic bags, and frozen for up to a month. Remove as much air as possible before freezing to minimize freezer burn. Do not refreeze the ration once thawed. Refrigerated gel diet should be discarded after a week.

Neonatal Care

Hatchling aquatic turtles can be a challenge to raise, and overcrowding must be avoided. Hatchlings may be shy and scramble for cover at your approach and can be reluctant to feed. Provide hatchlings with cover to retreat under such as floating pieces of cork, clay flower-pot pieces, plastic leaves (large enough that they cannot be ingested), or a board or flat rock over bricks. Be certain that cage props are stable so that they do not shift and trap young turtles underwater and drown them. Live plants such as cuttings of pothos (*Epipremnum aureum*) or java moss (*Vesiclaria duyana*) work well for cover and can thrive in shallow water. The tank can be tilted by placing a small block of wood under one end, providing a gradual taper from shallow to deep. Nontransparent plastic containers are easy to clean and may offer additional security.

To coerce young turtles to feed, try feeder guppies (taking into account national welfare legislation); small live insects such as two-week-old crickets, mealworms, wax worms, chopped pink mice or earthworms; frozen krill; or soaked, softened, pelleted fish-based diets. Live small worm species such as black worms (*Lumbriculus variegatus*) or tubifex (*Tubifex tubifex*) often initiate feeding. As the hatchlings begin to feed with more vigor, try a wider variety of foods. Broad spectrum (including UVB) lights, proper temperature, and a wide variety of foods are important to prevent nutritional disease, improper growth, and imprinting on a single food.

Species Interactions

Some turtle species, such as snapping turtles, large softshell turtles, mud and musk turtles (*Kinosternon* and *Sternotherus* spp.), big-headed turtles, and Hamilton's pond turtles (*Geoclemys hamiltonii*) are aggressive toward other turtles, and cannibalism is known to occur. They can cause severe trauma and even kill other species, and should only be kept with others of the same species and size. When establishing groups of turtles watch for evidence of aggression, including bite marks along rear shell margins, neck, or tail, and be ready to separate if necessary. If a turtle refuses to enter the water, aggression from another turtle may be the cause. Many turtles can be carriers of *Entamoeba invadens*, which can cause serious gastrointestinal disease in chelonians and other reptiles.[38]

ACKNOWLEDGMENTS

Portions of this chapter have been previously published and reviewed by Stephen Barten, DVM; Jim Jarchow, DVM; Jeffrey Jenkins, DVM, DABVP; Douglas Mader, MS, DVM, DABVP; Roger Klingenburg, DVM; Chuck Smith; Scott Stahl, DVM, DABVP; and Brett Stearns.

REFERENCES

See www.expertconsult.com for a complete list of references.

24

Sea Turtles

Craig A. Harms and Jeanette Wyneken

Seven species of sea turtles are found worldwide (Table 24.1). All are listed in Appendix I of the Convention on International Trade in Endangered Species of Wild Fauna and Flora (CITES; https://cites.org/eng/app/appendices.php), signifying the species' risk of decline and extinction, with international trade permitted only in exceptional circumstances. Six species are listed in whole or as subpopulations with designated status by the International Union for the Conservation of Nature and Natural Resources (IUCN; http://www.iucnredlist.org) red list of threatened species. Status identifies those with too little information to rank (data deficient: the flatback [*Natator depressus*]) and those designated as vulnerable to critically endangered: leatherback (*Dermochelys coriacea*), Kemp's and olive ridley (*Lepidochelys kempii* and *L. olivacea*), hawksbill (*Eretmochelys imbricata*), loggerhead (*Caretta caretta*), and green turtle (*Chelonia mydas*). Those same six species are listed in whole or in distinct populations segments (DPS) as threatened or endangered under the US Endangered Species Act (ESA; https://www.fws.gov/endangered/), and the flatback is listed as vulnerable by the Australian Department of Environment and Energy (https://www.environment.gov.au/biodiversity/threatened/publications/flatback-turtle-natator-depressus-2008). Generally, listings agree, yet there is also some divergence. For instance, leatherbacks are listed as endangered, wherever found, under the ESA, but some subpopulations are designated of least concern and others as critically endangered by IUCN. It is, however, safest to assume that some level of regulatory protection applies when working with any sea turtle species.

Pressures from interactions with humans (industry and recreation), poaching, predation, habitat encroachment and degradation, and infectious and noninfectious diseases together contribute to the worldwide decline in sea turtle populations. Veterinarians working along coastal regions may be presented with opportunities to provide veterinary care to these animals. Sea turtles also are popular exhibit animals and can convey a powerful conservation message to visitors (Fig. 24.1). Because of the legal implications of working with protected species, which vary greatly from location to location, veterinarians must communicate with federal and local authorities regarding medical intervention with these animals.

This chapter is intended to give the veterinary professional a working background for understanding basic sea turtle biology and species identification, as well as husbandry and management in human care. Assessing medical problems and providing treatment are covered in Chapter 176.

SEA TURTLE SPECIES AND IDENTIFICATION

Sea turtles are taxonomically separated into the leathery-shelled (dermochelyid) and the hard-shelled (cheloniid) species. The key characteristics include the presence or absence of complete longitudinal ridges along the carapace versus a hard-keratinous shell (Dermochelyidae versus Cheloniidae, respectively). The family Dermochelyidae is represented by just one extant species. Within the Cheloniidae, the six species can be distinguished by the number and patterns of specific scales on the head (prefrontals), jaw form, the number of claws, and the numbers and patterns of the plates or scutes on the shell. The plastron also has distinct scute patterns, but these scutes are used most often as landmarks for internal structures rather than for species identification. Inframarginal (bridge) scutes are found between the

TABLE 24.1	Conservation Status and Distribution of Sea Turtles		
Common Name	**Scientific Name**	**Distribution**	**ESA Status (IUCN)**
Loggerhead	*Caretta caretta*	Tropical and subtropical Atlantic, Pacific, and Indian Oceans; Mediterranean Sea	T/E (LC to CE)
Green turtle	*Chelonia mydas*	Tropical and subtropical Atlantic, Pacific, and Indian Oceans	T/E (E [LC Hawaii population])
Hawksbill	*Eretmochelys imbricata*	Tropical Atlantic, Pacific, and Indian Oceans; Black Sea	E (CE)
Kemp's ridley	*Lepidochelys kempii*	Western Atlantic, Nova Scotia south to Mexico	E (CE)
Olive ridley	*Lepidochelys olivacea*	Tropical and subtropical Atlantic, Pacific, and Indian Oceans	T/E (V)
Leatherback	*Dermochelys coriacea*	Atlantic, Pacific, and Indian Oceans; north to Alaska and south to Australia; Mediterranean Sea; Great Britain to South Africa	E (LC to CE, and two DD)
Flatback	*Natator depressa*	Tropical and subtropical Australian waters	[V] (DD)

Conservation status as listed under the United States Endangered Species Act (ESA) and in parentheses, by the International Union for Conservation of Nature (IUCN). Some species are divided into distinct population segments (ESA) or subpopulations (IUCN) with different conservation status assignments. CE = critically endangered, DD = data deficient for determination, E = endangered, T = threatened, LC = least concern, V = vulnerable. The flatback turtle has no listing under the ESA but is listed as Vulnerable by the Australian Government, Department of the Environment and Energy.

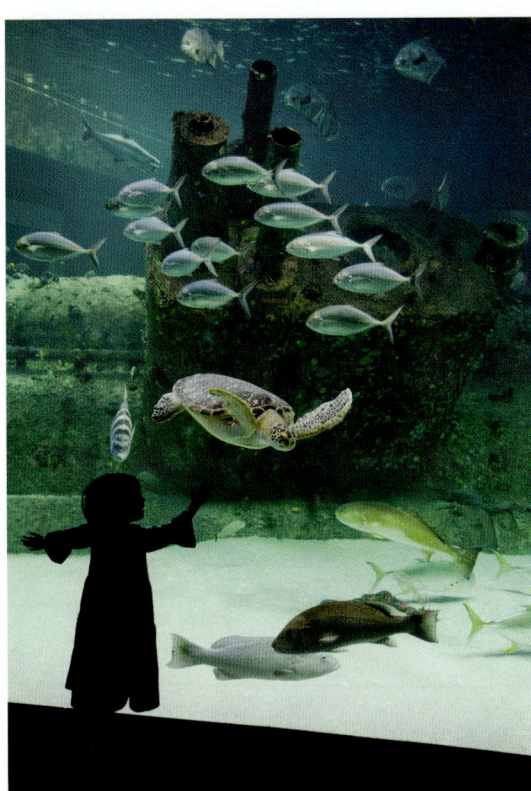

FIG 24.1 Green turtle (*Chelonia mydas*) in a large multispecies exhibit tank at a public aquarium. (Courtesy of North Carolina Aquarium at Pine Knoll Shores.)

carapace and plastron.[1] Inframarginal counts usually range from three to four but can be highly variable and hence are of limited use as diagnostic characters.

Scutes of the carapace are the marginals, laterals (= costals), and vertebrals (= centrals). The first marginal caudal to the neck is the nuchal. The most posterior marginal scutes on each side are termed supracaudals (= postcentrals). The paired scutes of the plastron (listed cranial to caudal) are the gular, humeral, pectoral, abdominal, femoral, and anal; unpaired intergular and interanal scutes sometimes are not present (Fig. 24.2). Supernumerary scutes are common in species that incubate under very warm or very dry conditions.

Leatherbacks lack distinct head scales as adults, lack claws, and have a thin keratin covering on the jaws. The cheloniid sea turtles are characterized and distinguished from one another by the prefrontal scales on the head, carapace shape and scute pattern, inframarginal scute characteristics, the numbers of claws on the flippers, and details of the robust keratinous covering of the jaws (rhamphotheca). Most species have two claws associated with digits I and II. The claw I on digit I is usually larger than claw II; in adult males, claw I is enlarged and strongly curved ventrally. The number of claws on the front and hind limbs is the same. Fig. 24.3 compares the distinguishing features of all seven species.

The hard-shelled sea turtles have keratinous scales on the dorsal and lateral head that are used in identification of species. The prefrontal scales are a key characteristic. They occur in pairs on the snout. Green turtles and flatbacks have one pair of prefrontal scales. The other species all have two pairs and may have one or more supernumerary scales along the midline that separate the pairs. Other head scales are not diagnostic.

The rhamphotheca may be used for species identification. Most species have sharp cutting edges or crushing plates. In green turtles, the rhamphotheca has serrated edges for cropping sea grasses (Fig. 24.4).

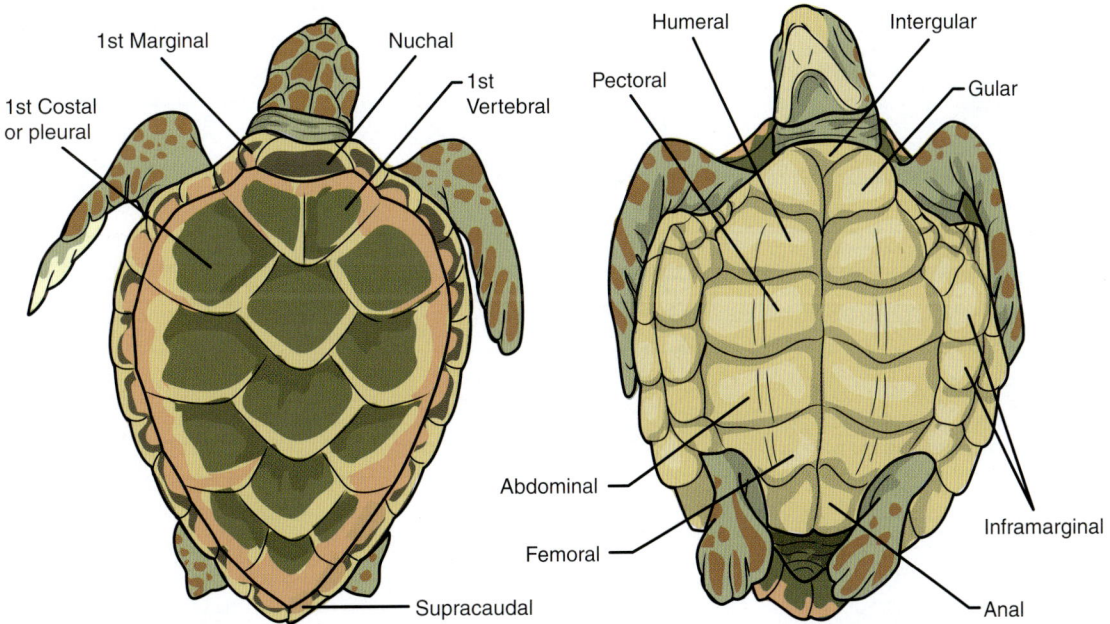

FIG 24.2 The scutes of the carapace and plastron are keratinous. Their pattern and number can be diagnostic in determination of species. Scutes in different parts of the carapace, bridge, or plastron are named here. (With permission of Jeanette Wyneken, 2001, "Guide to the Anatomy of Sea Turtles," NMFS Tech. Publication NOAA Tech., Memo NMFS-SEFSC-470.)

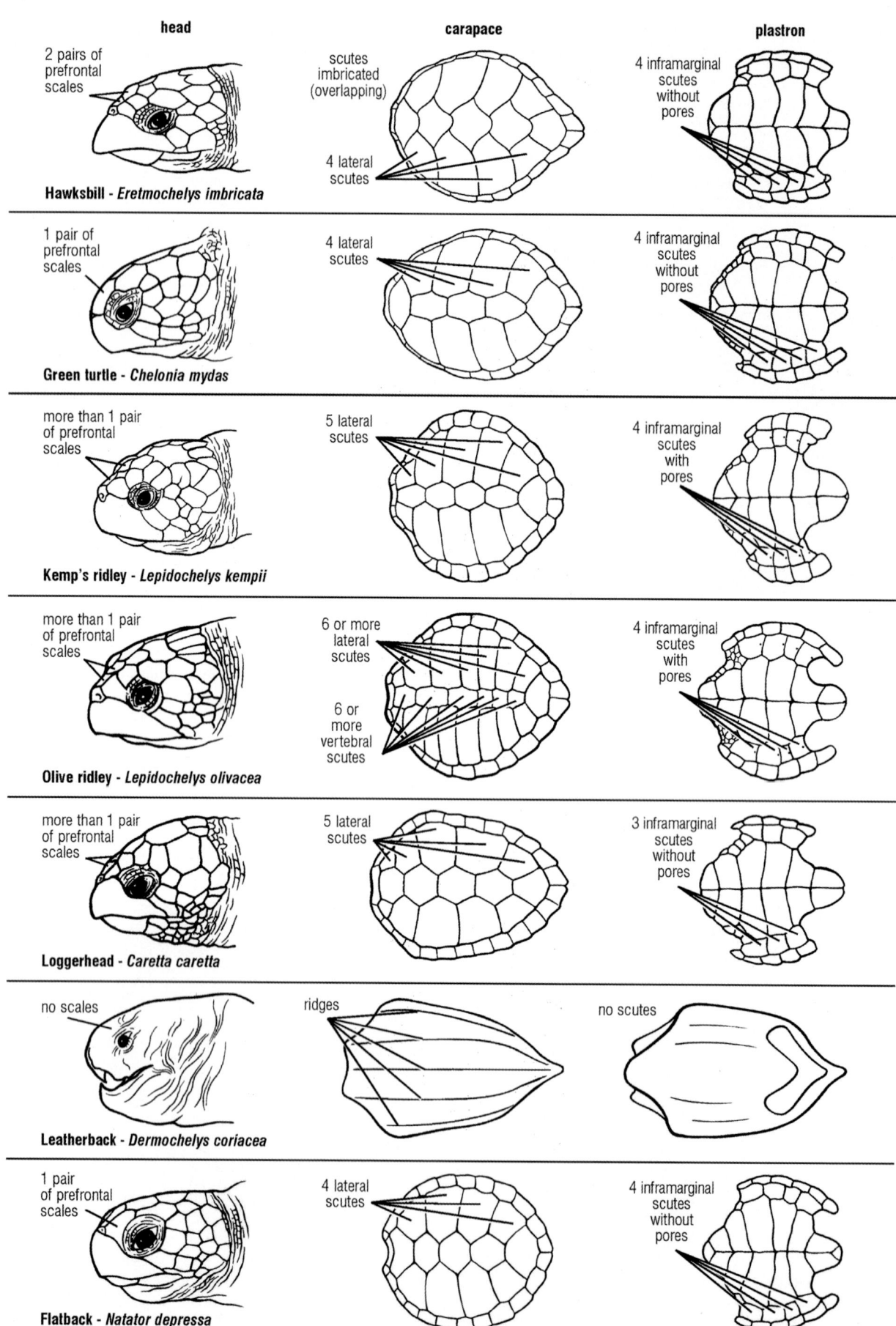

head   **carapace**   **plastron**

2 pairs of prefrontal scales

scutes imbricated (overlapping)

4 inframarginal scutes without pores

4 lateral scutes

Hawksbill - *Eretmochelys imbricata*

1 pair of prefrontal scales

4 lateral scutes

4 inframarginal scutes without pores

Green turtle - *Chelonia mydas*

more than 1 pair of prefrontal scales

5 lateral scutes

4 inframarginal scutes with pores

Kemp's ridley - *Lepidochelys kempii*

more than 1 pair of prefrontal scales

6 or more lateral scutes

6 or more vertebral scutes

4 inframarginal scutes with pores

Olive ridley - *Lepidochelys olivacea*

more than 1 pair of prefrontal scales

5 lateral scutes

3 inframarginal scutes without pores

Loggerhead - *Caretta caretta*

no scales

ridges

no scutes

Leatherback - *Dermochelys coriacea*

1 pair of prefrontal scales

4 lateral scutes

4 inframarginal scutes without pores

Flatback - *Natator depressa*

FIG 24.3 Key to sea turtle species. (Modified from Jeanette Wyneken, 2001, "Guide to the Anatomy of Sea Turtles," NMFS Tech. Publication NOAA Tech., Memo NMFS-SEFSC-470.)

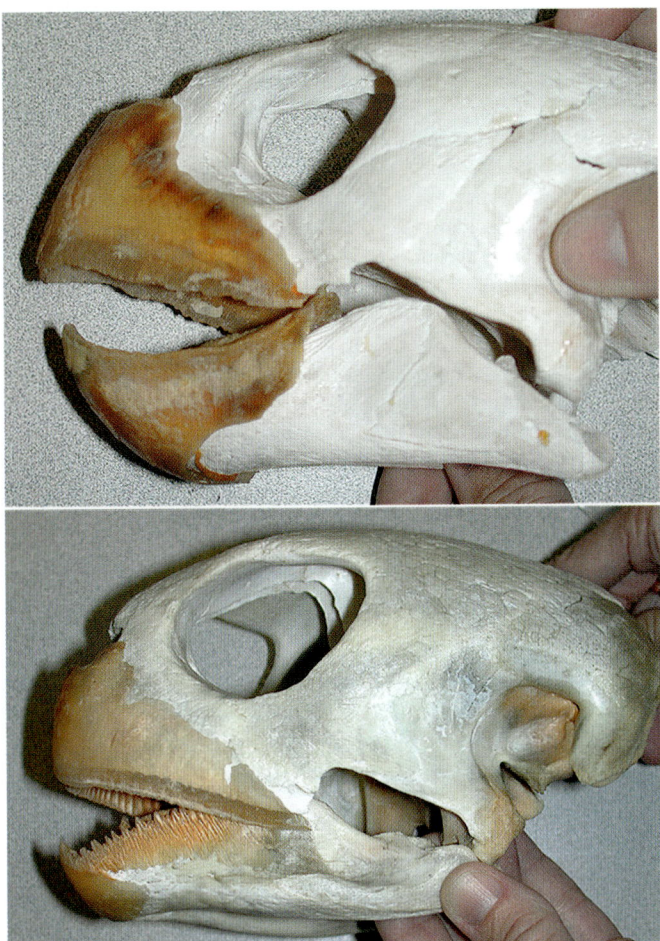

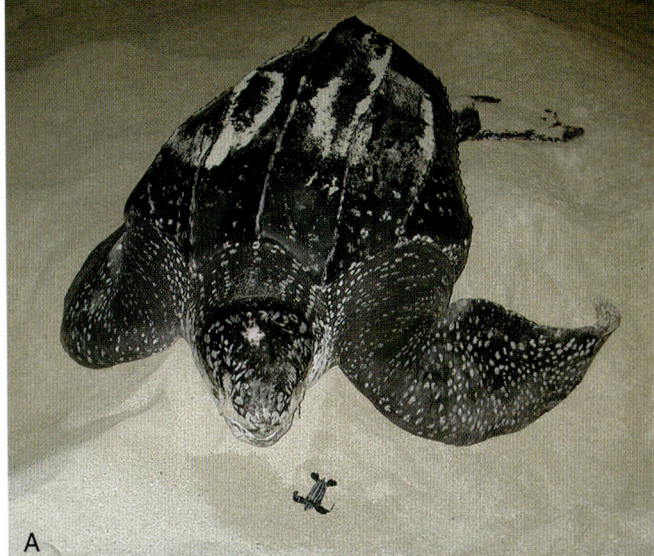

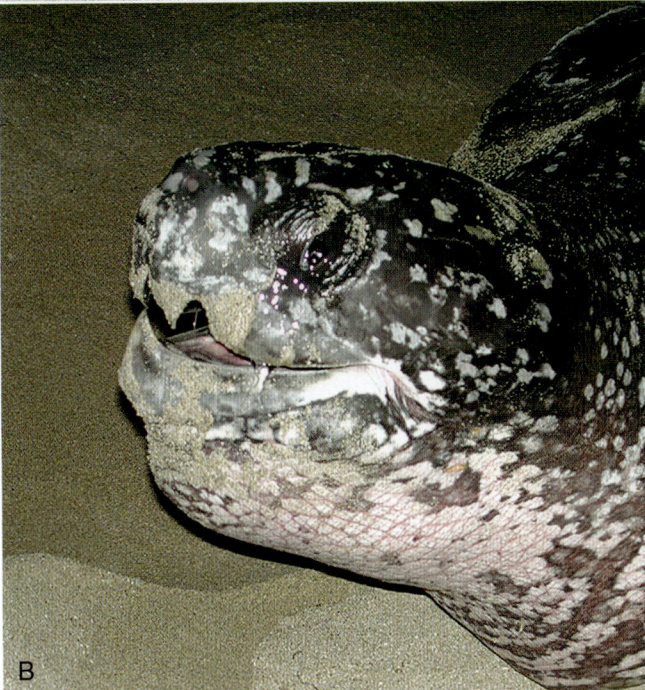

FIG 24.4 Sea turtles lack teeth, as do other turtle species. The upper and lower jaws are covered by keratinous rhamphothecae. Most species have sharp, cutting edges on crushing plates (top); however, the herbivorous green turtles (*C. mydas*) (bottom) have serrated edges on the rhamphothecae. (Courtesy of Jeanette Wyneken.)

FIG 24.5 A The leatherback (*D. coriacea*) is the largest of all the sea turtles and is black with white stripes (young) or white spots (juveniles and adults). The hatchlings have scales that are lost in the juveniles. The carapace has five longitudinal ridges running its length. (B) The jaws have little keratin, and a characteristic notch is seen in each side. (Courtesy of Jeanette Wyneken.)

Just one dermochelyid species exists: the leatherback (Fig. 24.5). It is black with white speckling. Five dorsal ridges run the length of the carapace, two ridges form the margins, and ventral ridges are seen in hatchlings but are usually not obvious in adults. The upper jaws have a notch in each side. The flippers and hind feet lack claws.

The six cheloniid species can be distinguished geographically in some cases (see Table 24.1).[2] The flatback is endemic to Australia; Kemp's ridley (both described subsequently) is restricted to the North Atlantic. All can be distinguished from one another with external characteristics, starting with the prefrontal scales and the carapacial scutes (see Fig. 24.3).

The green turtle and the flatback each have one pair of prefrontal scales. The green turtle has a smooth carapace that lacks keels and four pairs of lateral scutes (Fig. 24.6). Carapace color changes with age. It is black in hatchlings and then turns brown and tan in juveniles; in adults it is olive or gray-green, sometimes with speckles of yellow and brown. The plastron is white in hatchlings. It turns creamy yellow, sometimes pink or gray in juveniles, depending on the population. Adult green turtles have a creamy yellow plastron except in more melanistic Pacific green turtles (referred to as black turtles) that have a gray plastron. The green turtle has one claw on each limb.

The flatback is distinct from other cheloniid species (Fig. 24.7). Flatback hatchlings are light gray, and each carapacial scute is rimmed with dark gray. The marginal scutes caudal to the flippers form a serrated edge. As flatbacks grow, the carapace becomes solid gray; the carapacial scutes are thin and appear softer than in other cheloniids and feel waxy. The body is not as tall as in other cheloniids; however, the carapace is not flat as the name implies. The lateral margins of the carapace curl slightly upward. The plastron is white or pale yellow. The flippers and hind feet typically have one claw.

The remaining cheloniid species (*C. caretta, L. olivacea, L. kempii,* and *E. imbricata*) each have two pairs of prefrontal scales, and, as young, they have keels (ridges) on their shells. All have two claws on each flipper or foot. The loggerhead (Fig. 24.8) has a large head and brown

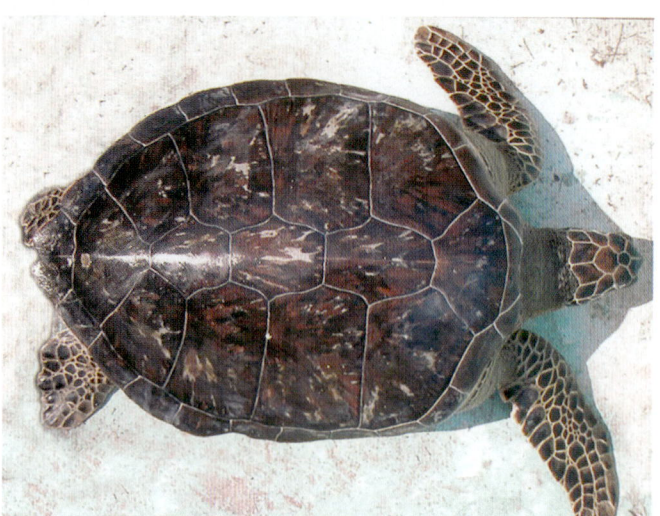

FIG 24.6 The green turtle (*C. mydas*) lacks keels on its smooth shell. This species changes colors dramatically from hatchling (black carapace with white ventral surfaces) to adult (brown, tan, or olive gray). (Courtesy of Douglas R. Mader.)

carapace with five (sometimes four) lateral scutes. The nuchal scute (the marginal just dorsal to the neck) is in contact with the first lateral scute on each side. In hatchlings, the carapace is brown with various shades of dark gray (see Fig. 24.8). The plastron of hatchlings is light tan to brown. In juveniles and adults, it is cream to tan. The carapaces of juveniles often develop streaks of yellow and tan, and sometimes the scutes slightly overlap at their caudal margins. In adults, no overlap of scutes is seen. The carapace is primarily brown, with occasional individuals retaining some tans or even black. The shells of juvenile and adult loggerheads often host large epibiont communities. Loggerheads have two claws on each limb.

Hawksbill hatchlings have carapace and plastron colors that range from medium to dark brown. The head of the hawksbill soon elongates, so that, even in turtles as small as 15 cm SCL, the head is nearly twice as long as it is wide, and the rhamphothecae form a long, narrow, distinctive beak (Fig. 24.9). The carapaces of juveniles and adults have distinctive patterns of yellow, black, tan, and brown radiating through scutes that overlap at their margins (Fig. 24.10). This color persists through adulthood. The nuchal scute does not articulate with the first lateral scute in hawksbills. The plastron of adults is light tan. Each plastral scute may retain a spot of dark color in juveniles.

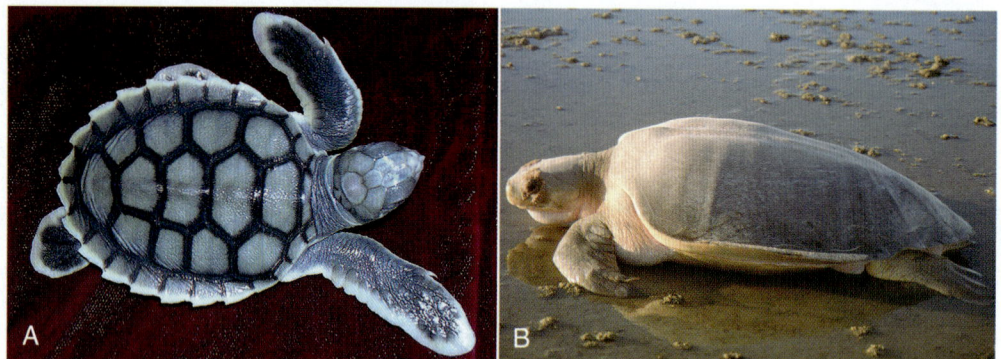

FIG 24.7 Flatback sea turtles (*N. depressa*) are endemic to Australia. (A) This species has dark pigment around each scute in hatchlings. (B) As a juvenile or an adult, it is primarily gray or gray and tan dorsally and white or light tan ventrally. The carapace of the adult flatback has upturned lateral edges. This species has thin keratinous scutes and scales, so the skin is pliable and the carapacial scute pattern is not easily discerned. The flippers retain more flexibility in the digits than many other cheloniids. The flatback has powerful jaws and can have a contrary disposition. (A, Courtesy of Jeanette Wyneken; B, courtesy of K. Pendoley.)

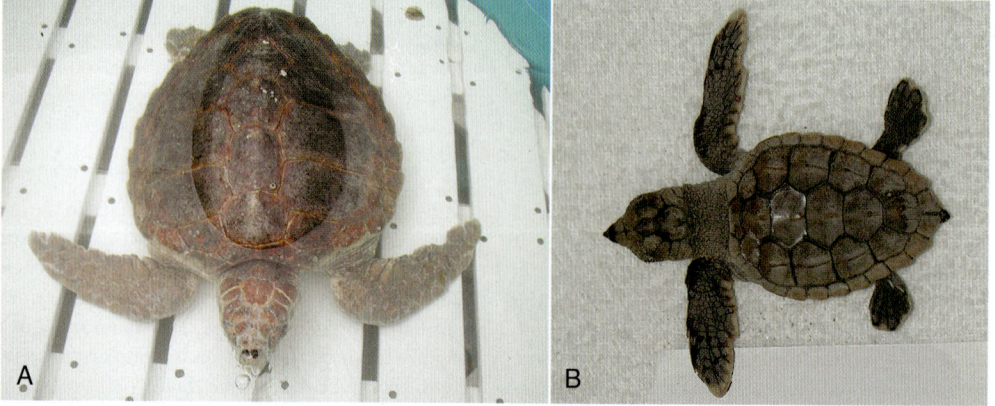

FIG 24.8 (A) The loggerhead (*Caretta caretta*) is a brown turtle with an obviously proportionately larger head than the other cheloniid species. It has two pairs of prefrontal scales and two claws on its limbs. (B) Hatchlings, juveniles, and adults are mostly brown with gray and tan coloration. (A, Courtesy of Douglas R. Mader; B, courtesy of Jeanette Wyneken.)

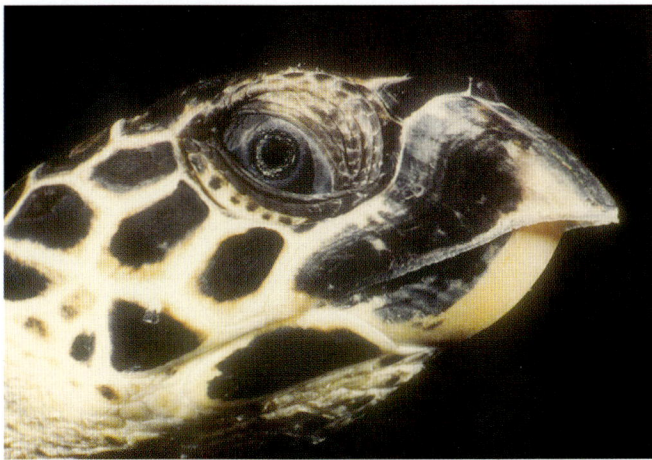

FIG 24.9 The head of the hawksbill (*E. imbricata*) is elongated so that, even in turtles as small juveniles, the head is nearly twice as long as it is wide, and the rhamphothecae form a long narrow distinctive beak. (Courtesy of Douglas R. Mader.)

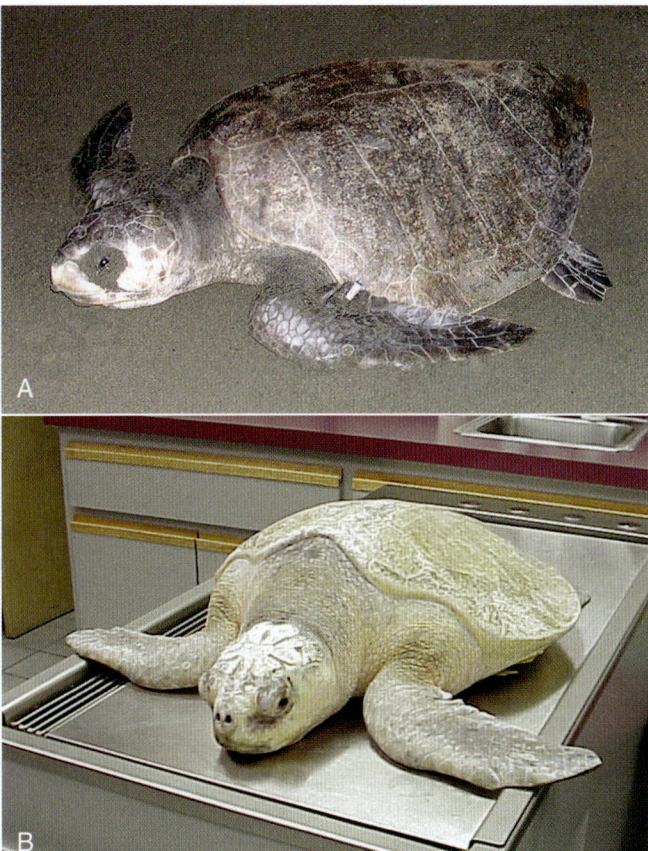

FIG 24.11 Both species of the ridleys are primarily gray, and the carapace is nearly round in outline. (A) The olive ridley (*Lepidochelys olivacea*) has many more vertebral and lateral scutes than the Kemp's ridley (*L. kempii*). (B) Kemp's ridleys have four or five lateral scutes and just five vertebrals. (A, Courtesy of Jeanette Wyneken; B, courtesy of Douglas R. Mader.)

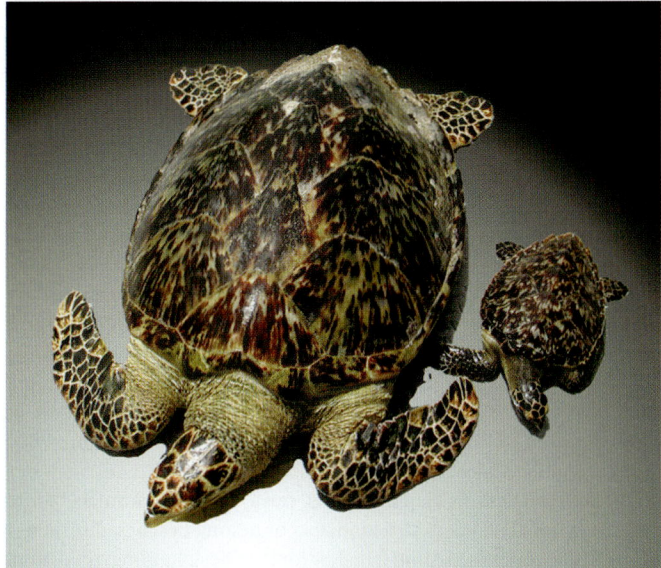

FIG 24.10 Hawksbills (*E. imbricata*) have overlapping scutes at most life stages. The beautiful epidermal scutes on the carapace and plastron are the source of the "Tortoiseshell" used in jewelry. These colors differ little between juvenile and adult stages. (Courtesy of Jeanette Wyneken.)

NATURAL HISTORY

Sea turtles are long-lived and late maturing. In most species, longevity records are limited and often are best estimates. Life spans are estimated to be in the range of 50 to 75 years, based on long-term mark-and-recapture studies and captive records.

The sexes can be differentiated from one another by external characteristics only at puberty, which, depending on species, ranges in age from 8 to 20 or more years. Mature males have long, prehensile tails that extend well beyond the carapace margins (Fig. 24.13), and the cloacal opening is closer to the tail tip than to the most caudal part of the plastron. The tails of mature females (and immature turtles) are short and seldom extend beyond the carapace except in adult leatherbacks. The cloacal opening is close to the plastron in females.

The age to maturity is becoming better understood in several species through skeletochronological approaches using lines of arrested growth (LAGs) in the humerus or scleral ossicles on histologic sections, although considerable variability probably exists. Age estimates in adult females may also be independently assessed using DNA fingerprinting and mark-and-recapture techniques. Age to maturity within the same species may vary by the ocean basin in which it lives. Maturity in cheloniid species have estimates of roughly 25 to 50 years, with the younger estimates primarily coming from Atlantic populations and the older estimates from Pacific populations.[3,4] Kemp's ridleys appear to mature

The remaining two species of sea turtles that occur in U.S. waters are both members of the genus *Lepidochelys* (Fig. 24.11). Both are primarily gray. The Kemp's ridley occurs in the Gulf of Mexico and East Coast waters. The olive ridley occurs in Pacific and South Atlantic waters (but occasionally strays into North Atlantic regions). The hatchlings of both species are gray-brown. The carapace grows more rapidly in width than length for some periods so that both species are nearly round in dorso-ventral silhouette. Much of the width increase is due to growth in the marginal scutes, which become wide. Olive ridleys typically have more than six normally aligned lateral scutes, six or more normally aligned vertebral scutes, and many supraoccular scales on the head. Kemp's ridleys, in contrast, have four (sometimes five) lateral scutes and just five vertebrals. In both ridley species, often four (sometimes three) inframarginal scutes characteristically each have a pore (Fig. 24.12).

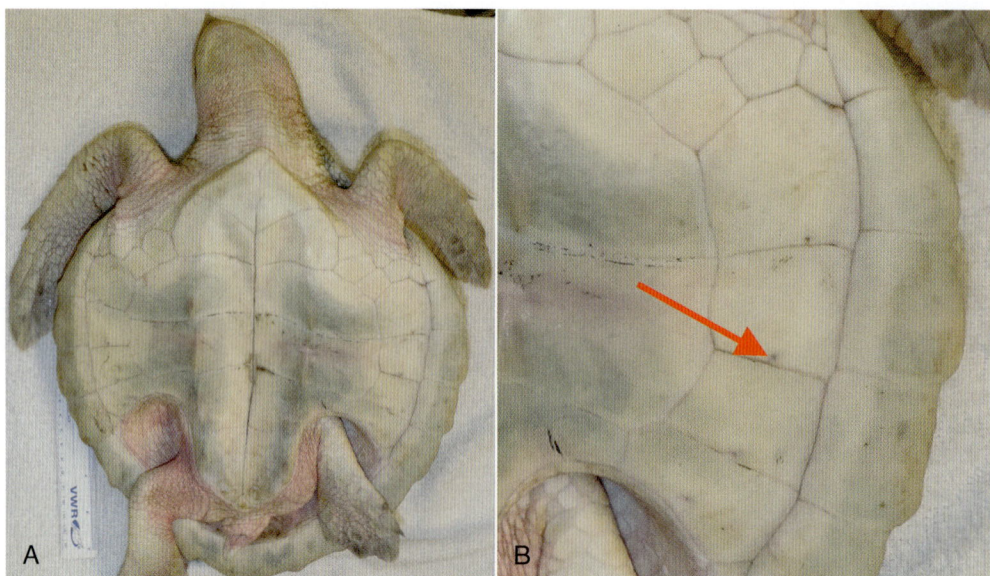

FIG 24.12 (A) This ventral view of a Kemp's ridley (*Lepidochelys kempii*) shows the almost round outline of the shell, the wide marginal scutes, and the pores (B, arrow) in the inframarginal scutes that are characteristic of this genus. (Courtesy of Craig A. Harms.)

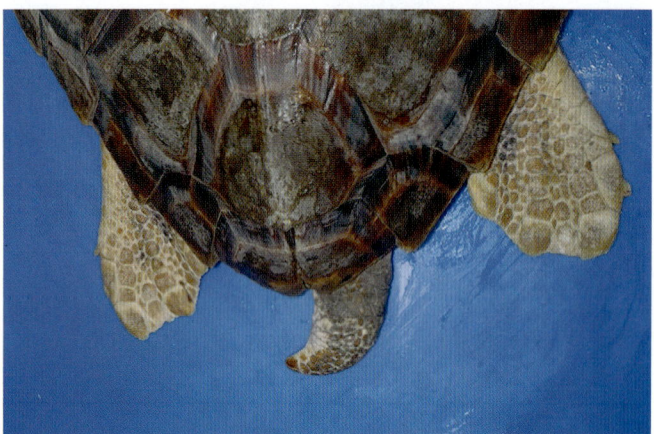

FIG 24.13 Dorsal view of an adult male loggerhead (*Caretta caretta*) shows the tail extending well beyond the carapace margin. (Courtesy of Craig A. Harms.)

at younger ages, around 10 to 12 years.[5] There is some disagreement in the literature regarding age at maturity in leatherbacks, with early estimates at 13 to 14 years[6] and later estimates of 20 to 25 years.[7] Adult body weights vary by species and within species by location. Table 24.2 lists approximate adult size and weights.

Members of the genus *Lepidochelys* exhibit a coordinated nesting event known as an "arribada." Kemp's ridleys and some populations of olive ridleys mass nest for several months of the year. This occurs mainly at night for olive ridleys and during the night and day for Kemp's ridleys. Solitary nesters occur as well. The synchronous emergence of 100 to 10,000 females to oviposit occurs over a 1-to-3-day period and repeats approximately every 30 days for the season.[8] Decades of egg and turtle harvesting during these events combined with heavy incidental mortality in fisheries and other industry-associated threats have taken a toll on the Kemp's ridley population, which has improved over decades but remains endangered.

For centuries, sea turtles have been exploited for meat, oils, leather, and shell for jewelry. Green turtles and hawksbills, with their beautiful shells, were killed for curios. The sea turtle industry has been banned in the United States and other countries. In many places, possession or trade in sea turtle artifacts is illegal. Illegal harvest still occurs in many countries, and legal harvest (particularly for indigenous peoples) or even farming occurs in some countries (see Chapter 177). Current threats to sea turtles include accidental capture by fishing nets and long lines and entanglement in fishing, lobster, or crab trap lines. Trauma from boats, personal watercraft, fishing gear, and dredging equipment accounts for many of the calls to rehabilitation facilities. Environmental pollution (chemical, agricultural run-off) may debilitate, and in-water pollution (plastics, plastic bags, other trash) may kill animals before they are found. Habitat destruction, loss of nesting beaches, disorientations of hatchlings or nesting females from artificial lighting, predation, and natural disease take a toll on sea turtles.

PERMIT CONDITIONS FOR SEA TURTLE CAPTIVE CARE AND REHABILITATION

Permit conditions for captive care and rehabilitation of sea turtles vary by country. In the United States, permits are issued by the US Fish and Wildlife Service (US FWS).[9] These directives cover a wide range of topics related to husbandry and management of sea turtles, including transportation conditions, tank size and depth, public display and educational messaging, water quality, lighting, temperature, quarantine and biosecurity, environmental enrichment, nutrition, veterinary care and release determination, among others. They allow a certain degree of latitude based on the medical judgment of the attending veterinarian to meet the needs of turtles undergoing treatment and rehabilitation, and for specific research needs. Although US FWS permit conditions are specific to the United States, general principles are applicable to sea turtle captive care anywhere. Major points are included below, but direct reference to country-specific permit conditions is recommended, and as more information is learned about sea behavior and habitats, adjustments may need to be considered.

Species	SCL Hatchling	SCL Adult	Weight Range*	Natural Diets
Loggerhead (*Caretta caretta*)	38–55 mm	70–125 cm	170–182 kg	Omnivorous-carnivorous: mollusks, crustaceans, algae and sea grass
Green turtle (*Chelonia mydas*)	45–57 mm	59–117 cm	96–186 kg	Hatchlings omnivorous; juveniles and adults herbivorous: sponges, jellyfish, algae, and sea grass
Hawksbill (*Eretmochelys imbricata*)	39–50 mm	63–94 cm	78–91 kg	Hatchlings omnivorous; adults omnivorous or spongivorous
Kemp's ridley (*Lepidochelys kempii*)	38–46 mm	58–75 cm	32–49 kg	Omnivorous: vegetation, crustaceans, and mollusks
Olive ridley (*Lepidochelys olivacea*)	40–50 mm	56–78 cm	35–45 kg	Omnivorous: vegetation, crustaceans, tunicates, and jellyfish
Leatherback (*Dermochelys coriacea*)	56–63 mm	114–176 cm CCL	200–916 kg	Gelatinivorous: jellyfish, cnidarians, and tunicates
Flatback (*Natator depressa*)	56–66 mm	81–97 cm	80–90 kg	Omnivorous: echinoderms, crustaceans, and sea grass

TABLE 24.2 Size, Weight, and Diet of Sea Turtles

*Adult female.

CCL, Curved carapace length; *SCL,* straight carapace length.

From Bjordal KA. Foraging ecology and nutrition of sea turtles. In Lutz PL, Musick JA, editors. *The Biology of Sea Turtles.* Boca Raton, FL: CRC Press; 1997; 199–231; Ernst CH, Barbour RW. *Turtles of the World.* Washington, DC: Smithsonian Institute Press; 1989; Hirth HF: Synopsis of the biological data on the green turtle *Chelonia mydas* (Linnaeus 1758). *Biological Report* 97(1), Fish and Wildlife Service, U.S. Department of the Interior, 120 pp, 1997; Witzell WN: Synopsis of biological data on the hawksbill turtle, *Eretmochelys imbricata* (Linnaeus, 1766). *FAO Fisheries Synopsis* 137, 78 pp, 1983.

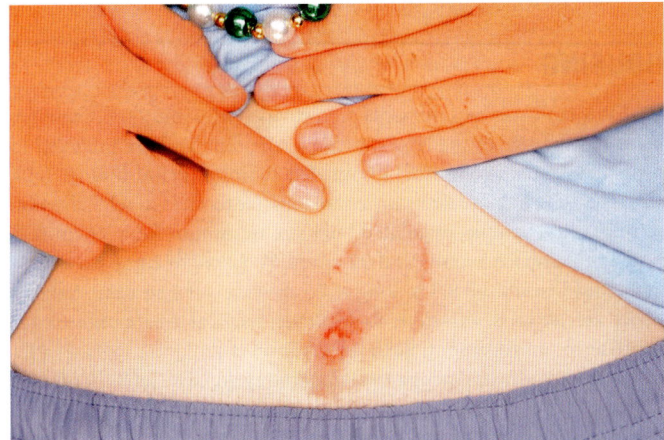

FIG 24.14 Beak-shaped bruise from a loggerhead (*Caretta caretta*) bite that could have been much worse. The turtle was inappropriately picked up by a single person from the front and was too heavy to maintain with arms extended away from the carrier's body. (Courtesy of Craig A. Harms.)

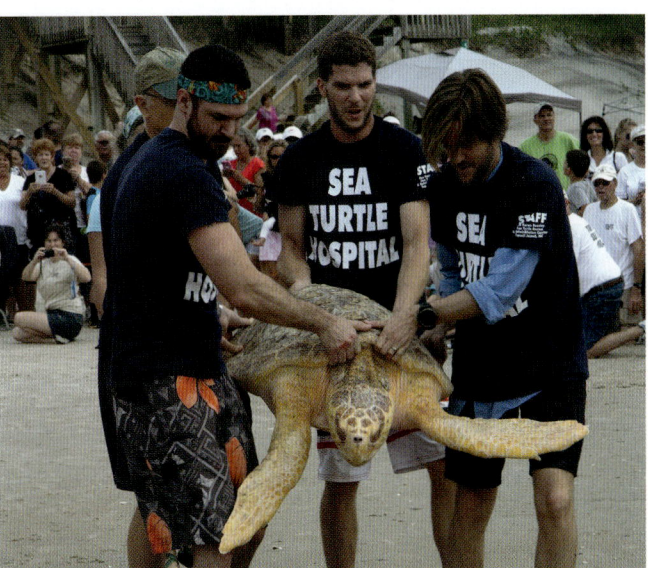

FIG 24.15 Rehabilitated loggerhead (*Caretta caretta*) being carried down the beach for release by four individuals gripping the carapace and lifting from the side. (Courtesy of Craig A. Harms.)

HANDLING AND TRANSPORTATION

Sea turtle handling is usually straightforward, constrained mainly by the size and strength of larger individuals, however, hazards to personnel must be considered. Sea turtles typically are not actively aggressive and have a limited range of motion with their heads, but with extremely powerful jaws capable of crushing shellfish, they have the capacity to inflict serious injury if mishandled (Fig. 24.14). Forelimbs (flippers) can slap forcefully enough to bruise restrainers, and claws can scrape exposed skin. Handlers must always be aware of their position relative to the turtle's mouth and should lift sea turtles from the sides. In most cases, lifting adults and large juveniles requires more than two people. The edges of the carapace at the neck and near the rear flippers provide convenient and secure grasping sites for safely lifting the turtle with less risk of joint damage than lifting by the limbs (Fig. 24.15). Sea turtles with shell fractures may be lifted and transported by sliding a strong tarp or board underneath the plastron and lifting that instead of the shell. A custom-made turtle stretcher with Velcro straps

(http://wmblanchardco.com/custom-sewing/) can be useful for lifting and carrying larger injured or refractory turtles (Fig. 24.16). Humeral fractures and glenohumeral luxations can occur if foreflippers are restrained improperly with either too much force on the joint or by immobilizing the distal flipper while allowing proximal flipper movement.

Sea turtles are surprisingly responsive to tactile stimulation through their carapace, and many respond by becoming calm when scratched or patted. Covering the eyes with a dry towel may also calm some sea turtles, although patting the carapace or covering the eyes occasionally agitates rather than calms a turtle. Resting the plastron on a tire or other padded elevated surface where flippers cannot gain traction provides convenient nonrestrictive restraint for examinations and minor procedures (Fig. 24.17).

Sea turtles must be protected from heat and cold and kept moist during transport, ideally between 21° to 27°C (70°–81°F). One exception is cold-stunned turtles, which should be kept near the temperature at which they stranded or started on a very slow rewarming en route to a rehabilitation facility.[9] Moisture can be provided by covering with a wet towel at temperatures above 24°C (75°F) or with a thin layer of water-based, water-soluble lubricant at lower temperatures. Eyes can be protected with ophthalmic gel for longer transports. Use rigid, covered crates with padding, ventilation holes, and sufficient room for normal flipper and head positioning. Transporting more than one turtle per container is sometimes unavoidable but adds risks of bite wounds. Face the turtles in the direction of motion to reduce agitation from abnormal acceleration backward or sideways. A container with moist sand substrate is recommended for transporting hatchlings, which mimics the beach environment, keeps them from dehydrating, and avoids initiating the swimming frenzy. Hatchling turtles typically undergo a period of hyperactive swimming that distances them from the shore. Hatchlings that are placed in a pool or bucket of water usually cease vigorous swimming prematurely, may fail to reach offshore nursery areas, and deplete yolk reserves.[9] Sand can cause irritation, particularly to the eyes and umbilicus, during the jostling of transportation, so some facilities prefer transporting hatchlings and post-hatchlings on a damp cloth instead. If transporting a turtle by air, follow International Air Transport Association (IATA) Live Animals Regulations (http://www.iata.org/publications/store/Pages/live-animals-regulation.aspx).

HOUSING

US FWS tank size requirements are provided in Table 24.3. These are based on the size of the largest turtle in the tank and are intended to provide adequate room for unimpeded swimming and diving. Tank size requirements for larger turtles are difficult to meet in rehabilitation settings. For example, calculated tank size minimum for a 99 cm SCL (straight carapace length) and 77 cm SCW (straight carapace width) loggerhead would be 8.9 m long × 1.5 m wide × 1.2 m deep. Smaller tanks are allowed, however, to facilitate medical treatments or for short-term management, such as while arranging for release after complete recovery or during mass stranding events. The intent for turtles undergoing rehabilitation is that once medically cleared, they should be released within 2 weeks, so that the duration of holding in smaller tanks is brief. Tank sizes should increase when holding more than one turtle, but permit conditions do not allow for housing hatchlings together, and, even when permitted, caution is warranted to prevent trauma from tank-mate aggression (Fig. 24.18). Green turtles are generally, though not always, more amenable to short-term cohabitation than loggerheads and Kemp's ridleys, although dominance hierarchies develop, and biting increases with time in all species, particularly in the absence of abundant space and hiding places afforded by some large exhibit

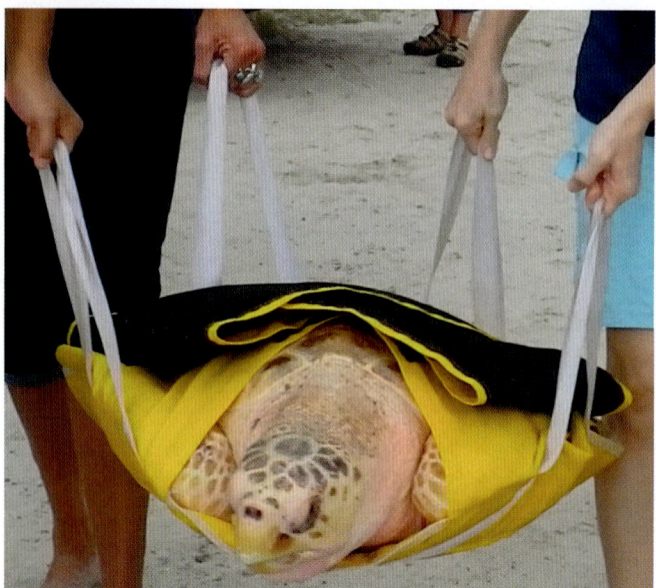

FIG 24.16 Restraint stretcher useful for carrying large injured sea turtles. Time of complete physical restraint in the stretcher should be minimized. (Courtesy of Craig A. Harms.)

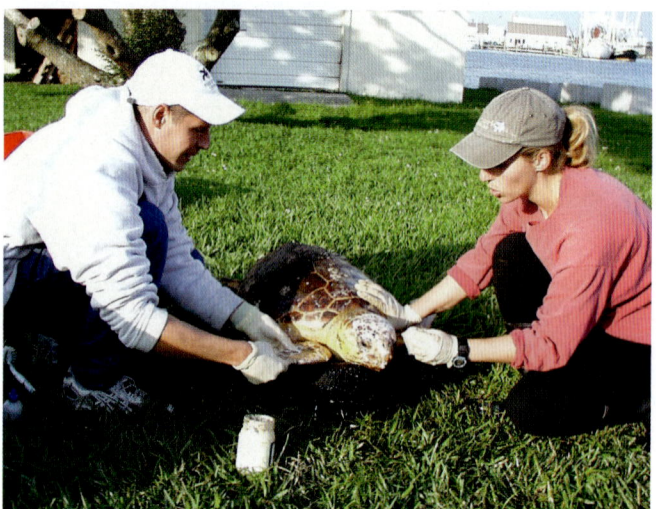

FIG 24.17 Loggerhead (*Caretta caretta*) restrained on a tire while mayonnaise is used to remove adhered tar. (Courtesy of Craig A. Harms.)

TABLE 24.3 **Tank Size Requirements (US Fish and Wildlife Service 2013)**[9]			
Turtle Size (SCL)	**Minimum Surface Area**	**Minimum Width**	**Minimum Depth cm (ft)**
Hatchlings and post-hatchlings up to 6 cm	5x SCL by 2x SCW	>2x SCW	30.5 (1)
6–50 cm	7x SCL by 2x SCW (increase by 50% for each additional turtle)	>2x SCW (>2x the sum of SCW for more than one turtle)	76 (2.5)
50–65 cm	7x SCL by 2x SCW (increase by 50% for each additional turtle)	>2x SCW (>2x the sum of SCW for more than one turtle)	91.5 (3)
>65 cm	9x SCL by 2x SCW (increase by 100% for each additional turtle)	>2x SCW (>2x the sum of SCW for more than one turtle)	122 (4)

Exceptions include allowing smaller tanks to facilitate treatments and short-term management situations. Hatchlings and post-hatchling must not be housed together. Pairings and groupings of larger turtles need to be monitored for compatibility in order to avoid trauma from aggression. *SCL,* Straight carapace length; *SCW,* straight carapace width.

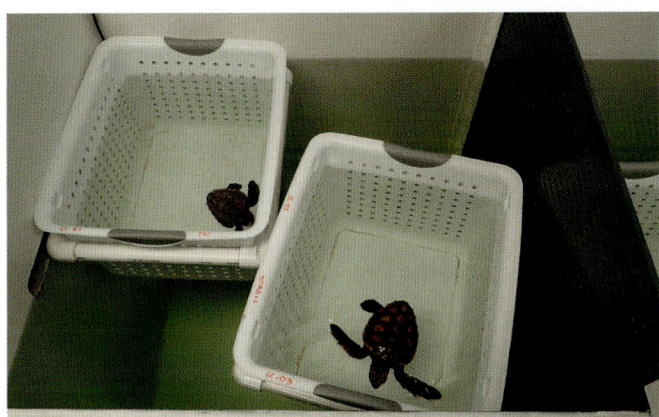

FIG 24.18 Floating plastic baskets are used to keep loggerhead (*Caretta caretta*) post-hatchlings separate to avoid intraspecific aggression, while taking advantage of the stability and water quality management of a larger tank system.

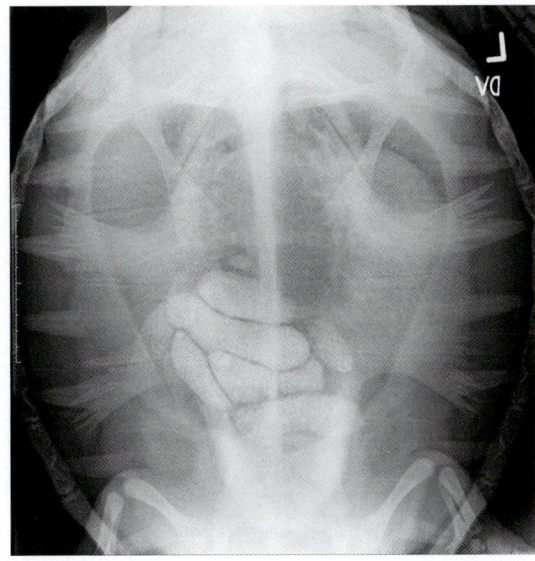

FIG 24.20 Sand in the intestines of a loggerhead (*Caretta caretta*). This turtle was managed with mineral oil in food items to help clear the sand from the intestines and changing the tank substrate to eliminate the ingestion hazard. (Courtesy of Craig A. Harms.)

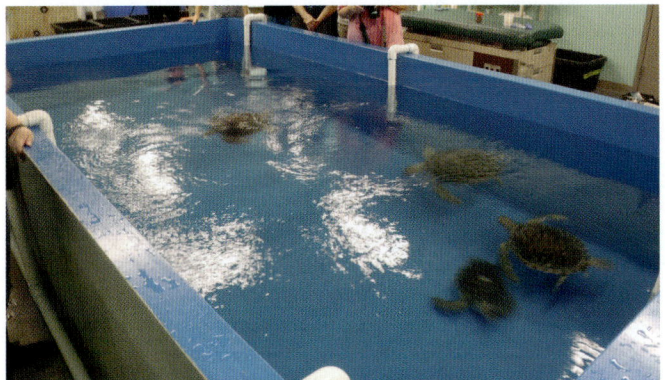

FIG 24.19 Large pool with multidirectional jetted currents used to stimulate swimming for physical therapy. Small green turtles (*Chelonia mydas*) can swim together under observation with relatively low risk of conspecific aggression, and grouping them together also promotes increased activity. (Courtesy of Craig A. Harms.)

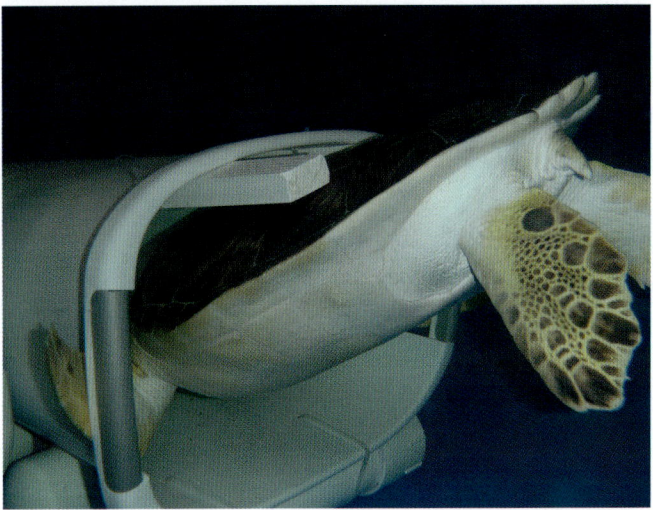

FIG 24.21 A weighted plastic clothes hamper modified by an extension to expand a ledge, and removing the bottom to allow swim-through, provides a mechanism for a positively buoyant green turtle (*Chelonia mydas*) to remain comfortably submerged. (Courtesy of Craig A. Harms.)

tanks. A tank with directed or haphazard currents (e.g., a commercial jetted lap pool or custom-designed currents) can maximize swimming within limited space (Fig. 24.19).

Besides size minimums, additional conditions of tanks should include smooth surfaces that will not abrade turtle skin; nontoxic coatings; use of only finished concrete; and avoiding foreign body ingestion hazards (Fig. 24.20), entangling material, and potential entrapment hazards that could prevent surfacing to breathe. Additionally, using barriers to prevent the public from reaching into tanks is important.

Weak, debilitated, or seriously injured turtles may require dry-docking or shallow wet-docking (water level below the nares) temporarily. Provide padding and keep the turtle moist with wet towels or a sprinkler system when they are not allowed to immerse. Even shallow water can help with hydration, provide some buoyant support, and reduce pressure on the plastron. If wounds are above water, cover the enclosure with insect netting and dress the wounds to protect the turtle from myiasis. Sea turtles need to be submerged for normal voluntary feeding, so ultimately water depth needs to be increased to facilitate adequate nutrition for convalescence and wound healing. After an initial phase of healing, wounds can tolerate water exposure well, as long as good water quality is maintained, and in conjunction with continued topical

and systemic treatment. A false bottom made of mesh or a fenestrated platform that can be raised or lowered within a fixed volume intensive care tank can be used gradually to adjust the water depth a turtle can manage, and to raise the turtle with minimal handling for wound treatments.[10]

Environmental enrichment is encouraged to facilitate normal swimming, feeding, and resting behaviors. Ledgelike items are used for submerged resting and back scratching to remove epibiota and loose keratin scutes[11] and are particularly useful to help positively buoyant turtles to remain submerged (Fig. 24.21), although they should not be a risk for entrapment. Enrichment devices including various configurations of PVC pipes (Fig. 24.22), water cooler jugs, jugs and PVC pipes containing food items to simulate foraging (Fig. 24.23), and falling

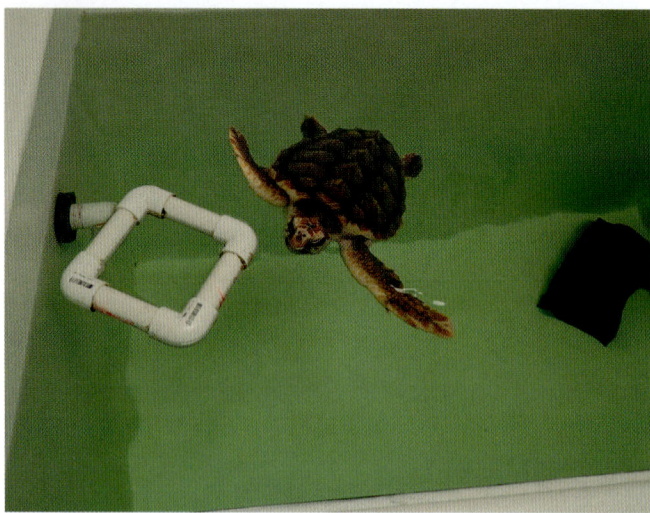

FIG 24.22 Floating PVC-pipe square and submerged half-pipe ledge provide basic enrichment in a tank for a small loggerhead (*Caretta caretta*). (Courtesy of Craig A. Harms.)

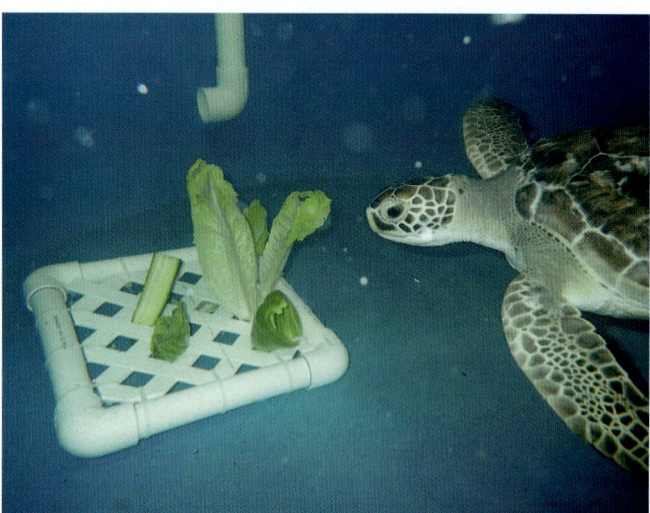

FIG 24.23 Green turtle (*Chelonia mydas*) feeding on fresh cucumber, green pepper, and romaine lettuce anchored in a custom-made weighted PVC-pipe-framed feeding tray. (Courtesy of Craig A. Harms.)

TABLE 24.4	**Acceptable Water Quality Parameters for Systems Housing Sea Turtles (US Fish and Wildlife Service 2013)[9]**
Water Quality Parameter	**Acceptable Range**
Salinity	20–35 ppt (or g/L)
pH	7.2–8.5
Temperature	20–30°C (68-86°F)
Chlorine	<1.0 ppm
Redox potential (ozonated system)	<400 mV
Coliform bacteria	<1000 MPN (most probable number)/100 ml

Exceptions include lower salinity under veterinary supervision for rehydration and for epibiota removal and lower temperatures being raised gradually for cold-stunned turtles.

wounds. Recommended water quality parameters are listed in Table 24.4. Use these recommendations in conjunction with knowledge of the species, life stage, and habitat from which a turtle is rescued and make adjustments gradually. Additionally, water clarity must be adequate for easy viewing of sea turtles. Freshwater or reduced salinity water can be used therapeutically short-term for rehydration and epibiota/ectoparasite removal, but caution and monitoring of behavior and plasma electrolytes are warranted to prevent hyponatremia, particularly in smaller turtles. Nitrogenous waste products (ammonia, nitrite, nitrate) are more of a concern for fish and are important to monitor if fish are kept in a mixed species exhibit with sea turtles but are not specifically addressed for sea turtle permit conditions. Ammonia and combinations with halogen disinfectants (chlorine, bromine) can be irritating to mucous membranes, however, so maintaining low concentrations of nitrogenous wastes is advisable, even if systems contain only sea turtles. Similarly dissolved oxygen and total dissolved gas tension are of greater concern for fish cohabiting with sea turtles, but adequate dissolved oxygen is necessary for biofilter function (minimum of 5–6 mg/L), and there are anecdotal reports of gas emboli in sea turtles from inhabiting gas supersaturated water.

When sampling for water quality testing, be consistent in timing and locations to ensure reproducible results for monitoring changes, and be strategic about sampling to obtain desired information. For instance, sampling from filtration outflow into the tank provides an indication of filter function, while sampling from mid-water column of the tank shortly after feeding provides an indication of what may be the least optimal water quality the turtle experiences in a 24-hour period.

Water quality is maintained by filtration or water turnover, or a combination of the two. Recirculating systems with filtration, flow-through systems with variable degrees of filtration, and periodic complete water change (dump and fill) systems all can provide either excellent or substandard water quality conditions, depending on rates of filtration or water turnover and properly functioning filters. Water quality being equal, however, dump-and-fill systems, in which all water is removed and replaced at one time and left static between water changes, are discouraged except on a short term, such as in managing a higher number of cases than usual or during power outages.[9]

Filtration includes four basic functions—mechanical, biological, chemical, and disinfection—and multiple filter types are commonly used together.[11,13] A single filter can perform more than one function. Mechanical filters remove suspended particles based on size and type of filter media and include sand, canister, and bag filters. The surface area of mechanical filtration media supports a biofilm that contributes

water (e.g., from a hose) are important to provide. (However, some turtles ingest bubbles and may develop positive buoyancy if the water flow produces a stream containing bubbles.) Enrichment devices increase random swimming and focused behavior while decreasing resting and pattern swimming in captive sea turtles, indicating that effective environmental enrichment can be provided for sea turtles similarly as with other animals in human care.[12] Feeding seafood or vegetables in ice blocks is another way to simulate more active foraging behavior and to help prevent rhamphothecal overgrowth. Conch or whelk shells also stimulate biting activity and promote tomial wear if suitably sized, that is, small enough to serve as a source of calcium and roughage without causing obstruction or large enough to prevent ingestion. Sea turtles also are amenable to basic behavioral training for such things as positioning for weighing and examination and separation from mix-species tank mates for focused feedings.

Appropriate water quality and composition are important for maintaining skin and ocular health and avoiding infection of healing to biologic filtration. Foam fractionators and skimmers remove a film of organic waste from the surface of the water (skimming) or bubbles (foam), along with some particulates and hydrophobic chemicals, so these filters can be considered mechanical and chemical filtration. Biologic filters combine large surface areas and aeration to promote growth of bacteria that convert ammonia to nitrite and nitrite to nitrate. Activated carbon is used to remove a wide range of chemicals from the water and some suspended particulates.

Disinfection using ozone, UVC light, or chlorine can reduce microbial loads (including pathogens) in the water column, but true sterilization is not feasible or desirable for tanks holding living animals. Ozone and UV light are applied to water flowing through chambers separate from the holding tank, whereas chlorine is applied to the whole system, including the inhabitants. All filtration and disinfection systems require regular monitoring and maintenance, cleaning, or replacement to remain effective. Water should be changed daily in dump-and-fill systems. Feeding 1 to 2 hours before water change and cleaning minimizes the time turtles spend in fouled water, because sea turtles often defecate soon after a new meal. Physical removal of feces and uneaten food with a dip net is labor intensive but dramatically reduces the burden on the filtration system, limits bacterial proliferation, and slows deterioration of water quality in static systems.

Wastewater disposal must follow local, state, and federal regulations. Water discharged from sea turtle facilities may contain a high nutrient load (nitrogen and phosphorous compounds), microbes, drugs and their metabolites, and high salt content. Municipal sewer systems may be an option, but local rules apply. Tertiary wastewater treatment systems can effectively reduce bacterial and nutrient loads, but drugs may pass through unaltered, and some systems may not tolerate high volumes of salt water, necessitating limits on discharge volumes. If discharge directly back into the environment is allowed, some pretreatment is advisable to destroy pathogens (e.g., ozonation, chlorination/dechlorination with sodium thiosulfate), break down or absorb drugs (e.g., ozonation, carbon filtration), or absorb nutrients (e.g., designed wetlands).

Lighting must be adequate for easy viewing of sea turtles in all areas of the tank, with a seasonally appropriate photoperiod. Shaded areas must be provided to give turtles the option of choosing light levels and degree of visual exposure and for outdoor tanks to prevent water from overheating and to allow behavioral thermoregulation. If artificial lighting is the primary light source, full-spectrum UVB bulbs have been mandated for vitamin D production and calcium metabolism.[9] Exposure of sea turtle tanks to adequate UVB by artificial lighting is challenging.[14] The close proximity needed is at odds with electrical appliance splash safety, tank access, and keeping the light (or light guard) surface free of spray and salt caking that can interfere with light transmission. Because of the close proximity of the lights to water, all fixtures should be wired with ground-fault circuit interrupters (GFCIs). Bulb variability, and diminished performance over time, make monitoring UVB exposure important. A commercially available UV radiometer can be used to ensure lighting at the water surface is adequate. The need for UVB lighting to maintain normal vitamin D and calcium metabolism in sea turtles is not entirely clear. Plasma 25-hydroxyvitamin D concentrations decreased over 4 to 5 months in green turtles housed indoors without natural sunlight and continued to decline over a 6 to 8 year period, although clinical signs of vitamin D deficiency were not evident.[15] No significant differences in plasma 25-hydroxyvitamin D concentrations were found between green turtles housed at least 75 days in a rehabilitation facility lacking a UVB source and a wild cohort from the same region.[16] Despite the lack of a clear demonstration of UVB requirement in these limited studies, replicating a complete natural diet in managed care is challenging, and UVB may compensate for dietary deficiencies and imbalances in vitamin D, calcium, and phosphorus. Therefore

provision of UVB light by some means is advisable, especially for hatchlings and juveniles that have requirements for growth. Smaller turtles are also easily moved, and rotating them outside periodically for brief exposure to natural sunlight under favorable weather conditions is likely to be more effective than artificial lighting.

Water temperature should be maintained between 20° to 30°C (68°–86°F),[9] although 25° to 30°C (77°–86°F) may be more suitable for maintaining appetite and promoting healing and immune response. Cooler temperatures are required initially for rehabilitating cold-stunned turtles (see Chapter 176). Rapid temperature changes should be avoided, preferably no more than 2° to 3°C over 24 hours.

Hatchlings intended for immediate release from shore should not be kept in water, because they will undergo a swimming frenzy that is essential to propel them to offshore currents and floating vegetation, depleting their energy reserves. Once hatchlings end their frenzy, it will not resume, and they will require a boat ride for release to favorable currents. Hatchlings should instead be kept moist in a quiet, low-light container. If they are held for treatment (e.g., dehydration, superficial wounds from failed predation attempts), keeping them in water is necessary, but they will need to be released offshore in suitable habitat, because they will lack the energy reserves for the swim from shore. Post-hatchlings that have washed back to shore require similar release considerations after rehabilitation.

Mixing of adult male and female turtles is prohibited under USFWS permit conditions to prevent breeding, and if an adult female deposits eggs in the tank, consultation with USFWS within 24 hours is required to discuss the best course of action for the turtle and her eggs.[9] Special considerations for housing and treating leatherbacks are addressed in Chapter 176.

QUARANTINE AND BIOSECURITY

Biosecurity for a facility keeping sea turtles comprises all measures taken to prevent the spread of infectious agents among sea turtles within the facility, to wild turtles from released or translocated turtles, to wildlife from discharge water, and to personnel. Biosecurity measures (including quarantine) can be effective in minimizing transmission of known and, perhaps even more importantly, unknown pathogens. Water supply can be a source of pathogen introduction into a facility, so incoming water should undergo some level of filtration (e.g., particulate, ozone, UVC). Using sea salt mixtures with municipal or well water minimizes the risk of environmental pathogen introduction, though at greater expense than natural seawater. If discharge into adjacent surface waters is allowed, intake pipes should be separated from discharge as much as possible. Indirect transfer of pathogens can occur in water (tanks on the same system, splashes from tanks, and drips from carried seawater), in aerosols, in improperly handled food, and on fomites (e.g., feeding utensils, scrub brushes, towels, enrichment items, clothing, unwashed hands). Physical separation of tanks and water handling systems provides an important barrier against waterborne pathogen transfer. Quarantine is an important measure to prevent introduction of disease to turtles already under care. Sea turtles admitted to a rehabilitation facility are in some state of debilitation and so are more likely to be shedding infectious agents, as well as more susceptible to infection. Quarantine tanks should be on separate water systems from those holding turtles under long-term care and ideally in separate rooms with dedicated air handling, cleaning, and feeding utensils. Minimize personnel traffic in the quarantine area. If staffing levels permit, have individuals dedicated only to quarantine, or if not, service the quarantine area after the nonquarantine areas. Any duration of quarantine can reduce the risk of pathogen introduction; the US FWS specifies a 60-day quarantine period for juvenile and adult turtles.[9] Completion of a quarantine period is not a prerequisite to release from the rehabilitation facility. During mass stranding events such as cold stunning or oil spills, space limitations may make adherence to the all-in-all-out principle of quarantine difficult or impossible, but some batching may be possible as groups progress through quarantine. Releasing turtles promptly after they are medically cleared minimizes overlap of healthy recovered turtles with compromised recent admissions and alleviates overcrowding that can foster cross-contamination.

After a turtle has vacated a tank, the tank should be cleaned, disinfected (e.g., bleach, quaternary ammonium compound), and well rinsed before occupancy by another turtle. If a turtle dies, following postmortem examination to ascertain likely cause of death, the carcass should be incinerated/cremated or buried deeply to avoid transfer of drug residues or pathogens to scavengers and the environment.

Preventing zoonotic disease transmission to staff is a priority. Sea turtles are not particularly high-risk animals from a zoonotic perspective in husbandry and rehabilitation settings, but they do harbor many gram-negative and gram-positive bacteria that have been documented in infections of humans, including *Vibrio* spp., *Enterococcus* spp., and others. Some of these bacteria may be resistant to multiple antibiotics even before selection by antimicrobial therapy in rehabilitation,[17,18] which could complicate treatment in the event of a human infection. Reasonable hygienic and personal protection measures are warranted when working with sea turtles as with any animal. These include, but are not limited to, nonsterile examination gloves, hand washing, eye protection when irrigating wounds, not immersing cuts or open sores in tank water, changing soiled clothes, and showering after working with sea turtles.

NUTRITION

Food should ideally replicate or mimic the natural diet for species and life stage (see Table 24.2), although this can be difficult to achieve for herbivorous green turtles, gelatinovorous leatherbacks, and spongivorous hawksbills. Animal-based feed is easier and more economical to provide to green turtles and is readily accepted, but it is not suitable for long-term maintenance. Green turtles can be adequately maintained with a mix of calcium-rich greens, even though terrestrial-source vegetation does not match the nutritional profile of sea grasses they normally consume. Even for omnivorous-carnivorous loggerheads and ridleys, fish and shellfish available commercially in economical quantities may be higher in fat (e.g., herring, mackerel) and deficient in calcium (e.g., squid) compared with their natural diets, risking obesity, hepatic lipidosis, or calcium/phosphorus imbalance. Food must be high quality, uncontaminated, and unspoiled (Fig. 24.24). To minimize nutrient loss and bacterial growth, frozen food should be thawed under refrigeration, finishing thaw shortly before feeding, and should never be refrozen.[19] Live food has the advantages of freshness and being stimulating to the appetite but can also transmit parasites and be more active and effectively defensive than a debilitated turtle can manage, and it is better reserved for prerelease conditioning. A floating pellet diet for fish has long been used with good success in a sea turtle–rearing facility and mimics pelagic-phase feeding,[20] but it may not be readily accepted by sea turtles in rehabilitation. A homemade gel diet listed in Table 24.5 can be modified based on available ingredients and monitoring turtle growth and plasma biochemistry values and used as a vehicle for delivery of oral medications.[21] A commercial gel diet for sea turtles is also available (http://www.mazuri.com/seaturtle-aquatic.aspx). Without gelatin (i.e., meal diet for the commercial product), these may also be used as a tube-feeding formula for anorexic turtles. Feeding rates vary by life stage, with younger, faster growing turtles requiring a greater amount. Good growth rates using a dry feed have been achieved starting at ~2%

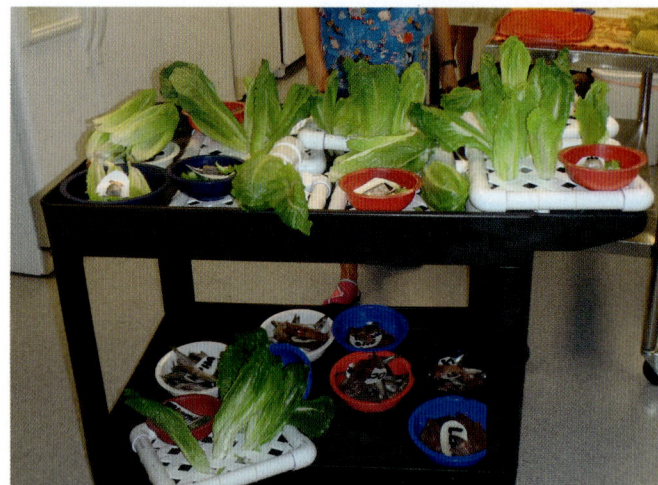

FIG 24.24 Food preparation cart with fresh greens for green turtles (*Chelonia mydas*) and fresh fish and shellfish for loggerheads (*Caretta caretta*) and Kemp's ridleys (*Lepidochelys kempii*) measured out in individual sanitized dishes and feeding trays. (Courtesy of Craig A. Harms.)

TABLE 24.5	**Gelatin Diet for Sea Turtles**	
Ingredient	**Weight (g)**	**Percent of Diet**
Staple diet		
Trout chow	425	8
Fish, various species	565	10.6
Squid (viscera removed)	282	5.3
Peeled shrimp	282	5.3
Carrots (fresh, washed)	142	2.7
Spinach (fresh or frozen)	142	2.7
Gelatin (unflavored)	450	8.5
Water	2800 mL	53
Supplements		
Sea tabs (Pacific Research Labs, Inc, El Cajon, Ca) #4	500 mg tabs	0.04
Amino acid complex 1000 #4	500 mg tabs	0.04
Spirolina (Lightforce, Santa Cruz, Calif)	50 mL powder (28 g)	0.5
Rep-Cal (Rep-Cal Research Labs, Los Gatos, Calif)	200 mL powder (180 g)	3.4

Diet can be modified based on available ingredients and can be used as a vehicle for oral medications.
Modified from Whitaker BR, Krum H. Medical management of sea turtles in aquaria. In Fowler ME, Miller RE, editors. *Zoo and Wild Animal Medicine 4*. Philadelphia: WB Saunders; 1999:217–231.[21]

body weight per day, scaling down to 1.2%.[20] Wet gel foods would be about five times that amount by weight.[20] For maintenance in a healthy subadult to adult turtle, feeding rate could be as low as 1% wet feed per week.[20] Regular weighing of sea turtles is required to assess and adjust feeding rate.

Restoring a positive plane of nutrition is essential for adequate wound healing and immune response. For weak debilitated turtles, feeding rate must start slow to avoid impaction and to prime the gastrointestinal system, which may have developed ileus during prolonged inanition. After verifying digestive function and defecation, the above rates can be increased to allow normal maintenance or growth and recovery of body condition. Rehydration and correcting electrolyte imbalances also helps ensure digestive system function. Softer highly palatable foods (e.g., fish fillets, debeaked squid) are appropriate in early stages of rehabilitation to provide essential protein and calories and reduce chances of impaction. However, once a turtle is feeding well, transition to a more balanced whole food diet for carnivores and to a primarily plant-based diet for green turtles is recommended. Debilitated turtles may require some level of assisted feeding initially. This can range from tong feeding to gently lifting the beak and placing food in the oral cavity or pharynx (with tongs) to tube feeding. Overly aggressive assisted feeding may lead to impactions. Tube feeding is a stressful procedure but in some cases is unavoidable. Tube-feeding formula is easily regurgitated by sea turtles, so they must be tilted head up during tube feeding and for a period afterward. The volume for tube feeding may start at 0.5% of body weight and gradually increase to 3%, once or twice daily. Continue trying to transition to less aggressive forms of feeding in between tube-feeding sessions. If a turtle is too weak to remain in water continuously, it may still be placed in water supervised for short periods to encourage voluntary feeding. Once a turtle no longer requires assisted feeding, cease hand or tong feeding as quickly as possible and transition to broadcast or bottom feeding to discourage habituation and promote natural feeding. Parenteral nutrition has been used successfully in recent years during the initial recovery phase for emaciated, debilitated sea turtles that are not amenable to enteral assisted feeding.[22]

CONCLUSION

The ability of sea turtles to recover from major injuries and serious medical conditions, given adequate time and supportive care, make them incredibly rewarding patients to treat. The population-level impact of rehabilitating sick and injured sea turtles is unclear, even considering their threatened or endangered status,[23] but the opportunities afforded

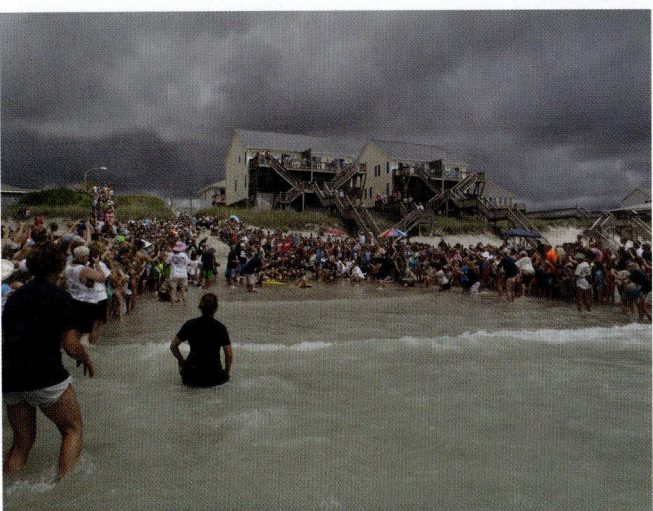

FIG 24.25 A crowd gathered for the shore-based release of several rehabilitated sea turtles. Such events are celebrations and an opportunity to inspire people to conserve and protect sea turtles and their environment. (Courtesy of Craig A. Harms.)

for education, research, and environmental advocacy are invaluable. Release of a successfully rehabilitated sea turtle is a celebration with potential to inspire greater stewardship of the entire marine environment (Fig. 24.25).

REFERENCES

See www.expertconsult.com for a complete list of references.

25

Crocodilians

Javier G. Nevarez

Crocodilians are among the largest reptiles in the world. They range in length from 1.5 meters for smaller caiman and crocodile species to over 6 meters and more than 450 kg for the saltwater crocodile (*Crocodylus porosus*). Most are also long-lived species, but there is no easy way to determine their true age in the wild. A general rule is that smaller species such as caimans will live a shorter life (20–40 years) than the larger crocodiles (60+ years). Therefore, with their size and longevity, they require large enclosures and people committed to their long-term care in captivity. Crocodilians can be found in zoos, aquariums, commercial farms/ranches, breeding facilities, and under private ownership. Commercial farming/ranching is discussed in Chapter 177. While it is certainly possible for some private individuals to properly maintain crocodilians in captivity, the large size and aggressive nature of some species makes them less suited for this scenario. In addition, not all states or countries allow private ownership of crocodilians. Crocodilian exhibits help educate the public about both the importance of protecting these reptiles and the dangers of not respecting them in their natural environment. In general, crocodilians are fairly low-maintenance animals with respect to need for frequent veterinary care; however, when required it can be daunting for all involved. Proper habitat design can help provide ease of capture, allow separation of sick animals, and make it easier to perform daily observations. As a group, crocodilians have unique husbandry and management requirements that are key for the safety and well-being of both crocodilian and personnel alike.

RESTRAINT

The methods and requirements for handling and restraint vary, depending on the size, species, and the procedure to be accomplished. Crocodilians are powerful animals, and their physical capture and restraint should always be performed by experienced personnel. Contrary to popular belief, crocodilians are quite astute and very observant of their surroundings. They will quickly be aware of a change in routine, leading them to be on high alert. Alligators and most caimans tend to be more defensive in nature whereas crocodiles are more aggressive and can take an offensive stance when threatened. Therefore capture and restraint plans must be carried out in a careful but swift manner. Crocodilians will lunge forward and can move their heads quickly side to side but are not very fast crawling backward. They can, however, turn around very quickly. Approaching a crocodilian is best performed from behind the animal, never from the front or the sides. It is also important that all personnel are committed to follow through in synchrony once contact has been made with the animal, otherwise a small number of individuals will quickly be overpowered, which increases the risk of injury.

A minimum of one person is required for every meter of body length (tip of snout to tip of tail) for animals up to 2 m. Beyond 2 m, there should be two persons for every additional meter. Manual restraint can be safely performed for crocodilians up to 3.5 m in length. Physical restraint of animals larger than 3.5 m should be reserved for only the most experienced of crews. In the absence of such a crew, or when dealing with aggressive animals, chemical immobilization is the only safe option (see Chapters 48 and 49). Large crocodiles of any species are extremely dangerous to handle (more so than alligators). They are faster and more aggressive than alligators or caimans.

The first goal of manual restraint is to control the head, followed by the tail and limbs. The muscles used to open the mouth are relatively weak, so the mouth can be easily held closed. Care must be taken when working around the head, because the teeth that are exposed even when the jaws are closed can cause injury to the handler (Fig. 25.1). The tail must be controlled at all times to prevent vigorous lashing that can cause injury. The limbs must be controlled to prevent them from rolling and attempting to escape. Staying as close as possible to the animal will minimize the risk of injury, because the tail cannot travel as far, thereby minimizing the damage of a tail strike. When collecting diagnostic samples, one should work in line with the long axis of the animal and avoid working beside them to avoid injury from the head or tail. Hands should be kept as far away from the mouth as possible (Fig. 25.2). Applying pressure over the eyes helps decrease visual stimulation and also induces vagal tone to help calm the animal (Fig. 25.3).

Hatchlings and juveniles up to 1 m can be physically restrained with one hand to hold the mouth closed and the other hand to control the lower body and tail. Once the mouth is taped, control can be maintained by grasping the cervical area and supporting the tail (Fig. 25.4). An effective grasp for animals up to 1 m is to bring their body close to the handler, support their neck, and simultaneously hold the rear limb facing away from the person's body at the base of the tail. By holding the limb and tail, the animals are less likely to attempt rolling.

Animals between 1 and 3 m can be caught by hand or with the aid of a catchpole or snare. The metal cable of the snare should be encased in plastic to prevent injury to the animal. Again the animal should be approached from behind, and the handlers must commit to reaching out to grab the animal. Any hesitation can provide the animal enough time to turn around, possibly causing injury to the personnel. Their nature is to roll or twirl once the snare is around the neck. One must be prepared to rotate the snare to prevent injury or strangulation of the animal. The tail should be grasped as soon as possible because this serves to immobilize the animal to some extent until the mouth can be securely closed. However, one must remember they are capable of turning around, and holding the tail does not guarantee personal safety. The head can be swiftly moved from side to side even with a snare around the neck. One can then pin the head manually and secure the mouth with tape. Placing a towel, rag, or taping over the eyes tends to help keep the animal calmer (Fig. 25.5). This can be done before or after restraining the head.

For animals over 3.5 m, physical capture and restraint can be as simple as all crew members forming a single line to approach the animal

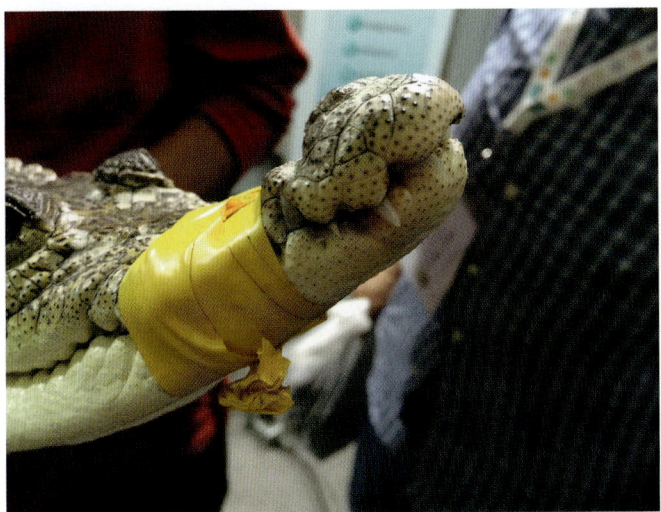

FIG 25.1 Morelet's crocodile (*Crocodylus moreletii*) with tape around the mouth and still revealing prominent mandibular and maxillary teeth. These teeth are very sharp and can cut a handler's hand. (Courtesy of Javier G. Nevarez.)

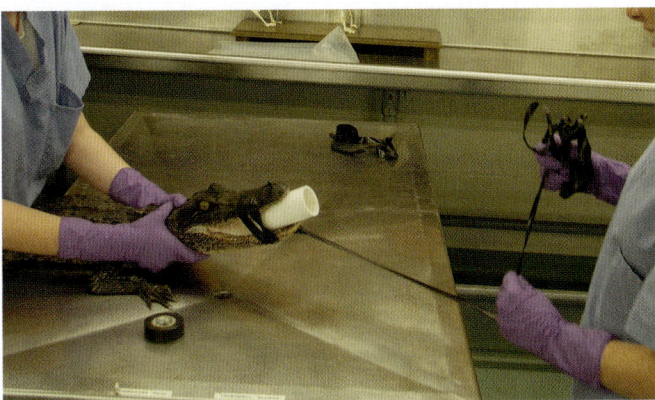

FIG 25.2 Removal of tape that was securing the mouth of an American alligator (*Alligator mississippiensis*). Notice the handler is leaning over the animal to secure the rear limbs and tail while holding the neck of the animal. The person removing the tape is working directly in front of the alligator and taking advantage of slack in the tape to remain a safe distance from the head. (Courtesy of Javier G. Nevarez.)

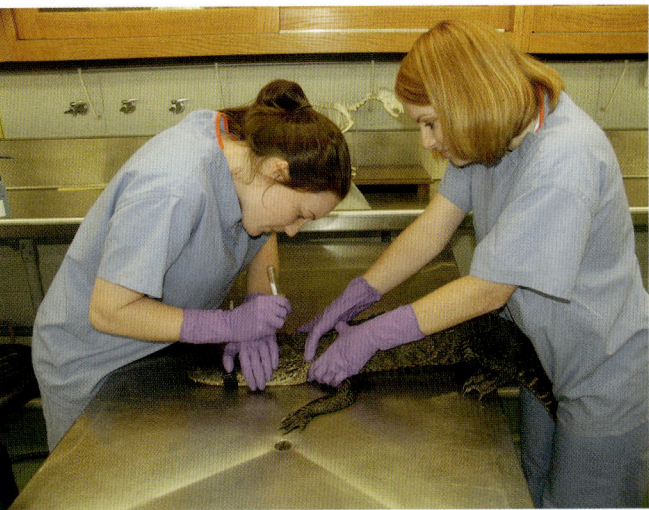

FIG 25.3 Restraint for supravertebral venipuncture in an American alligator (*Alligator mississippiensis*). Notice the eyes are being covered by the handler's hand to decrease visual stimulation and elicit vagal tone to calm the animal. The person holding the animal has a firm hold on the neck while putting slight downward pressure. The tail is controlled between the handler's legs; however, the rear limbs of the alligator are on the table, which would provide leverage if it attempted to roll. It would be better to have the limbs off the table for added safety. (Courtesy of Javier G. Nevarez.)

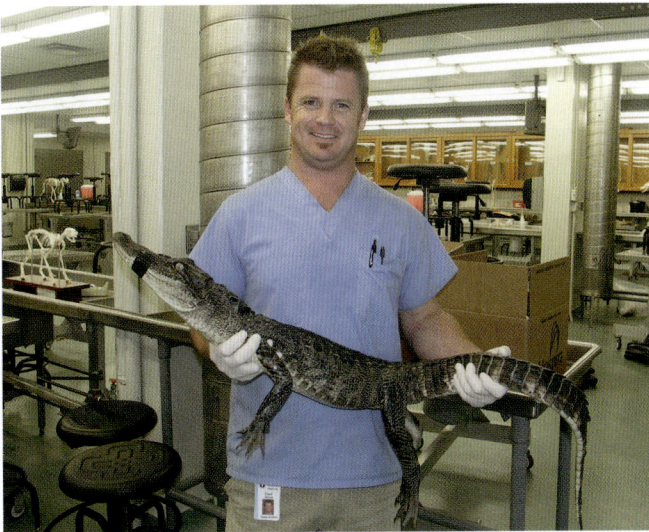

FIG 25.4 Restraint of an American alligator (*Alligator mississippiensis*) after its mouth has been taped. The neck and tail are held in order to both control and support the animal. The animal is kept close to the handler's body. Aggressive species (e.g., crocodiles) would require a more secure grip. (Courtesy of Javier G. Nevarez.)

from behind and then quickly landing on top of the animal in synchrony. For larger and more aggressive animals, special nets and ropes should be used to secure them before any attempt is made to tape the mouth. For large crocodiles, roping the jaws shut and then taping is advisable. Multiple ropes can be used to restrain the head, tail, and limbs before any hands-on contact with the animal. A pole snare or ropes around the neck and another around the jaw plus control of the tail and feet are necessary before tape can be applied to the jaws. The selection of technique will vary with individual and species demeanor, animal accessibility (enclosure design, animal in vs out of the water), personal experience, animal's activity level, and more. Regardless of the technique, the head, tail, and hind limbs must be controlled. If the animal must be transported or restrained for a period of time, both the front and hind feet may be secured to the body by tying over the back (see Fig. 25.5), or the animal can be tied/taped to a wooden board. Care must be taken to ensure the limbs are not tied too tight or for long periods of time to avoid injury to the animal.

Transportation of these animals can be accomplished in either burlap sacks, custom crates, or cages, depending on the size and circumstances.

One must use caution because overheating is possible, especially if the animals continue to thrash about with the mouth closed. Removal of the tape from the eyes or mouth can also be dangerous. The usual procedure is to place a tie or rope around the tape on the ventral side of the jaws between the mandibles. A quick pull from a distance, after the other restraints have been removed, allows the animal to move away. Occasionally an animal escapes after all the restraints except the mouth tape are removed. In these instances, the animal must be recaptured to remove the tape to prevent starvation. Recapture is usually much more difficult.

Operant conditioning is also recommended to train crocodilians to perform various procedures, including moving within the enclosure,

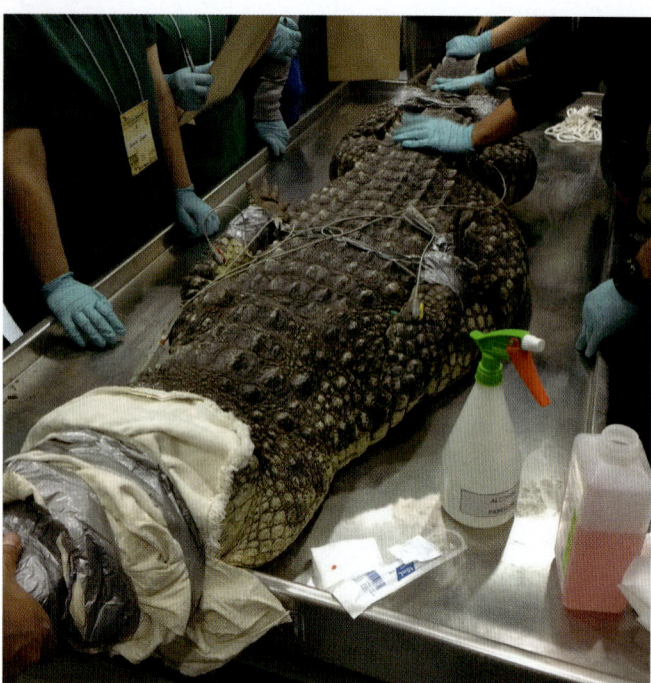

FIG 25.5 Anesthetized *Crocodylus niloticus* with a rag taped around the head and eyes, and the limbs taped across on the dorsum. Notice the head and tail as still being held by personnel to ensure the safety of all present. (Courtesy of Javier G. Nevarez.)

getting into a crate, tail access for venipuncture, and more. Engaging enthusiastic personnel in this repetitive activity is key to ensure successful training.

Finally, electrical stunning has been used in commercial crocodile farms in Australia and South Africa to safely immobilize and transport *Crocodylus porosus* and *C. niloticus*.[1,2] In *C. porosus*, the stunned animals had a lower stress response versus restraint with ropes. Stunned animals had no increase in corticosterone or glucose levels.[1] In *C. niloticus*, blood lactate levels were significantly higher in animals captured with a noose versus those captured via stunning.[2] The author has evaluated electrical stunning in alligators with similar results. These data suggest that electrical stunning could be a useful technique to reduce the stress of restraint and improve safety for both animals and personnel.

IDENTIFICATION

Identification of individual animals in a group of captive crocodilians is frequently advantageous. The use of collars, bands, or tattoos is considered unsatisfactory in most instances because collars and bands are frequently lost during normal animal activity. Tattoos are often difficult to read and fade away. Tags and transponders are better alternatives.

Metal swine ear tags can be used as toe tags for crocodilians. These tags can be placed on the web of the feet (Fig. 25.6). These are not permanent identification but could last for over a year in small animals. Placing tags bilaterally also increases the possibility of longer-term identification. The use of plastic cattle or swine ear tags has been accomplished in the dorsal area of the mid-tail of larger animals. Although animals can be identified, they must be out of the water to do so. The tags can also be lost or bitten off by other animals.

Another method that has been successfully used in some facilities is the placement of a tag on the head (see Fig. 25.6). The numbered half of a common swine tag can be attached to the head by passing a stainless steel surgical wire around the jugal bone midway between the

eye and the auditory meatus. The jugal bones are elongated bones that form the lateral borders of the orbits. Each forms a part of the postorbital bar that separates the orbit from the lateral temporal fossa. The advantage of this method is that the tags are inexpensive, easily attached, and visible from a distance of up to 20 ft (6 m). The variety of tag colors allows the left or right side of the head to be used, depending on parameters of gender, clutch group, or age. The disadvantage of the head-tagging method is that the wire must be securely fastened or the tags come off. Also, if the wire is too tight, the jugal bone is weakened and scarred. Identification methods using exposed tags may not be not ideal for animals in zoological institutions, as they are readily visible to the public.

A more permanent identification method is the use of implanted passive integrated transponder (PIT) microchips, commonly known as PIT tags. These are cost effective and are available from a number of manufacturers. The main disadvantage of the smaller (approximately 8×2 mm) full duplex PIT tags is that the scanner must be within a few centimeters of the microchip; however, larger (approximately 23×4 mm) half-duplex PIT tags provide greater range. PIT tags can be implanted in just about any muscle, but placement posterior to the dorsal plate of the head or in the tail provides easier access for reading (see Fig. 25.6). These sites also have a decreased subcutaneous space, which limits migration of the transponder. When possible, the entry point of the needle should be closed with surgical glue or suture to decrease the risks of infection and the transponder migrating out of the animal.

Finally, a permanent identification method is the use of tail notches. The distal tip of the tail scutes are cartilaginous and do not contain any bone. There is blood supply, but bleeding is minimal after notching. Both the paired lateral and single dorsal scutes of the tail can be used to create a numbering system (see Fig. 25.6). In young animals, the scutes are easily cut using a scalpel blade or sharp knife. In older/adult animals, the tissue is more fibrotic; hence, notching takes slightly more effort, but it is still plausible. In either case, no more than 50% of the scute should be notched. This prevents cutting deeper into the tissue, which is likely to be more painful. Tail notching is commonly performed in farmed American alligators before being released to the wild. They appear to tolerate this well, and there are no reported cases of detrimental effects associated with tail notching. However, this technique may be more acceptable for farmed or research animals rather than exhibit animals.

SPECIFIC HOUSING REQUIREMENTS

In a zoological institution, the facilities are aimed at exhibiting the animals in the most appropriate artificial environment possible. While having a naturalistic enclosure is ideal, this may not always be possible. Priorities include water quality, appropriate diet, and enough space to accommodate the growth and number of animals. A rear holding area should also be considered. The size of the enclosure will largely depend on the species of crocodilian and their purpose in captivity. One should have a general understanding of their biology and natural behavior in order to design an appropriate enclosure for display versus breeding. If in doubt, you should contact an institution housing the species for advice on what has or has not worked for them.

When designing an enclosure, first consider the species of interest. Some species grow larger than others and may be more territorial, necessitating a larger enclosure. Also consider how many animals will be kept in the enclosure and their gender. Both males and females can become aggressive during the reproductive season, and keeping them separated should be a consideration if enough space is not available in the primary enclosure. This is often not taken into account, and many crocodilian exhibits do not have any separations or back holding areas. The lack of separate holding areas makes management of aggressive and ill crocodiles challenging.

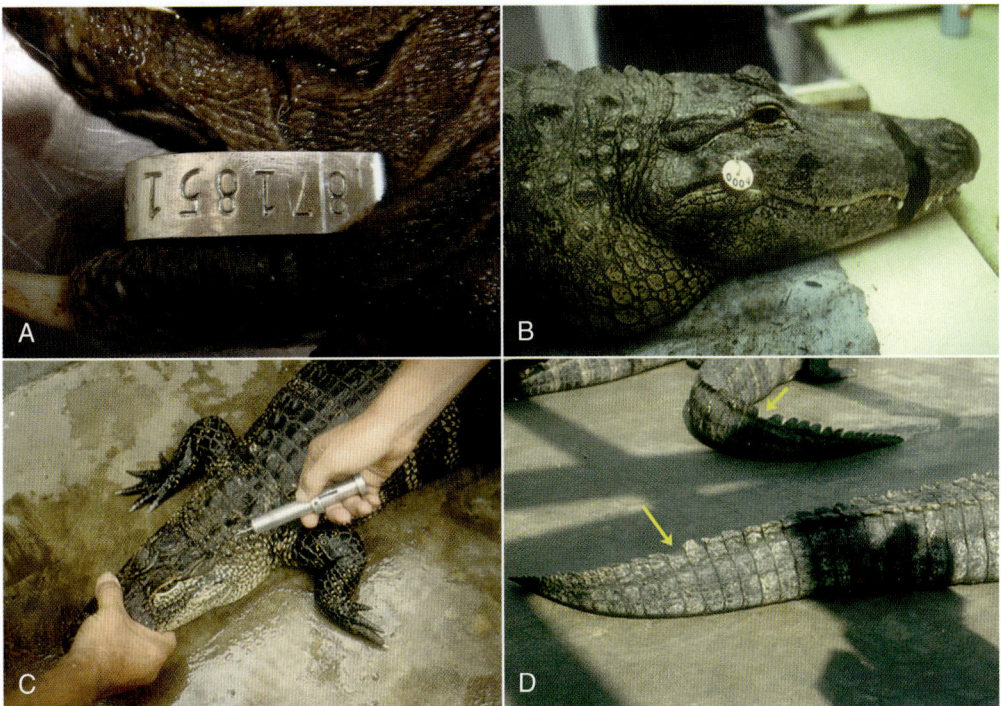

FIG 25.6 Crocodilian identification methods. (A) Metal ear tag used to identify a crocodilian by placing it in the webbing of the feet. Tags with the same number can be placed on multiple feet to create redundancy in case a tag is lost. (B) A head tag placed by passing stainless steel surgical wire around the jugal bone midway between the eye and the auditory meatus. (C) Location for implantation of microchip on the neck region. (D) Tail notching (*arrows*) is a permanent method but cannot be easily visualized when animals are in water.

Exhibits can be outdoors, indoors, or a combination thereof. Outdoor exhibits will likely mimic the natural environment more closely, but also present their own challenges for maintaining water quality and enclosure hygiene. Geographic location will also play a role in the value of outdoor exhibits, because not all species of crocodilians can tolerate cold weather. Finally, some species can create large burrows or tunnels and may escape an exhibit that does not have suitably deep footings. Crocodilians are also adept at climbing; therefore chain-link and horizontal fencing must be avoided.

The temperature and humidity requirements for crocodilians vary with species. As a general rule, 25°C to 32°C is optimal for the growth and well-being of most species. Animals maintained constantly at higher temperatures (e.g., indoor farmed crocodilians) may be more susceptible to certain diseases that are normally restricted to mammals (e.g., West Nile virus). In an enclosure, the water temperature can be maintained via heating elements contained within concrete slab or in-line water heaters and a recirculating system. The water temperature must also be maintained during the wash and refilling period to avoid a drastic temperature change that could lead to cold shock. Relative air humidity should be approximately 40% to 60%. The provision of circadian variations of both environmental temperature and light cycle to mimic the natural environment is recommended.

The UVB requirement for crocodilians is unknown. As true carnivores it might be expected that they can thrive with minimal exposure to UVB as long as they are offered whole prey or a commercial diet supplemented with vitamin D_3. Studies with 5-month-old broad-snouted caimans (*Caiman latirostris*) identified immune activity alterations and genotoxic effects after exposure to 30% UVA 5% UVB Sylvannia Reptistar lights.[3,4] These are the first studies to evaluate the deleterious aspects of ultraviolet radiation (UVR) in reptiles and conclude that provision of UVR must be carefully planned.[3,4] However, natural

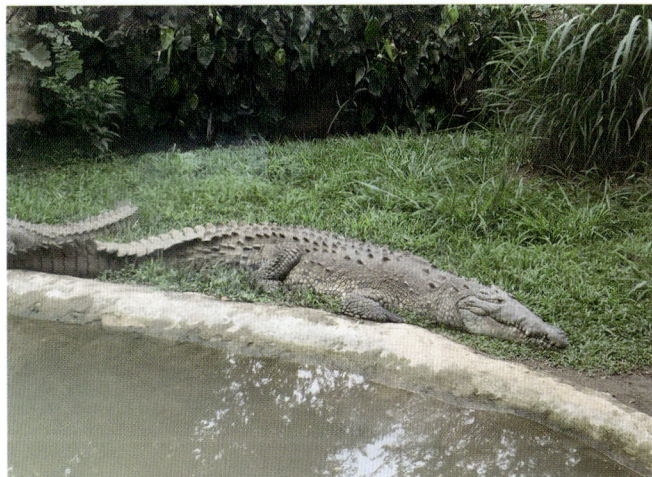

FIG 25.7 Outdoor enclosure for *Crocodylus acutus*. An artificial pond with sloped concrete leads to a natural soil and grass area. Notice the condition of the tall grass indicating little use of this area of the enclosure.

photoperiods of natural sunlight were associated with greater growth than any artificial lighting regime or darkness.[3] The clinical implications of these findings are not clear at this time. Most captive crocodilians are not offered artificial UVR within large enclosures. For young animals exposed to artificial UVR, a gradient must be provided to allow them to hide from the light as needed. Provision of natural sunlight must be done concurrently with the provision of shaded areas so the animals can seek shelter from the sun.

The two main areas in a crocodilian exhibit will be water and land. Soil, grass, sand, and concrete can be used for land surfaces (Fig. 25.7).

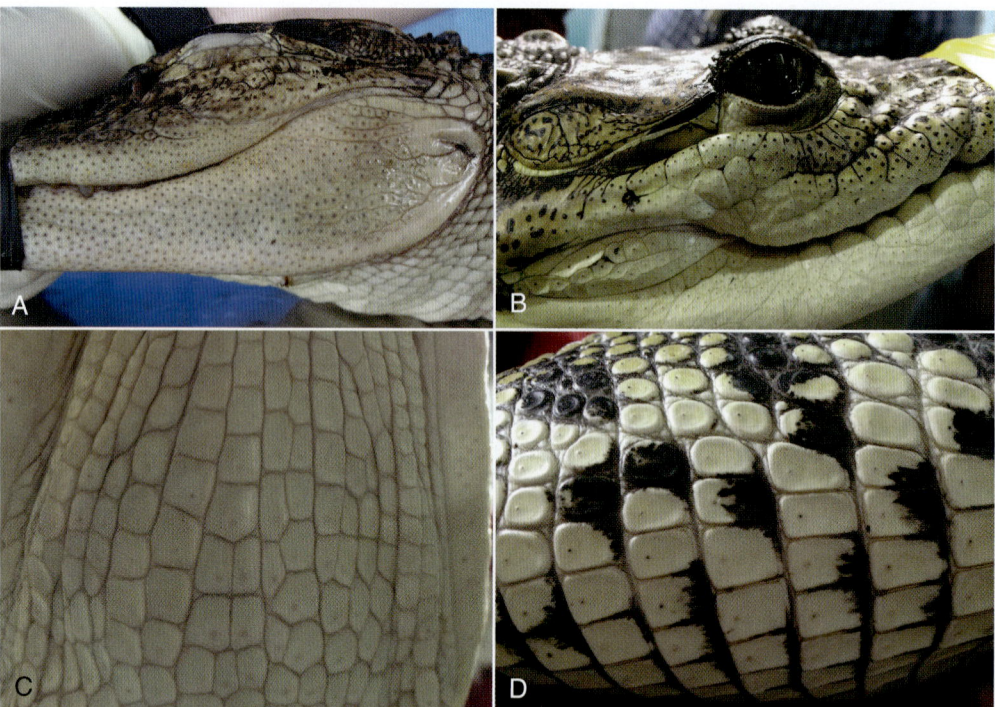

FIG 25.8 Intradermal sensing organs (ISO) (*gray dots*) on the lateral aspect of the head of an alligator (A), crocodile (B), the ventral mandible of a crocodile (C), and the lateral and ventral skin of a crocodile (D). These ISO allow crocodilians to sense water movement and prey proximity, allowing them to hunt even in murky water. (Courtesy of Javier G. Nevarez.)

All-concrete flooring is the least ideal because it can lead to pressure sores and irritation of the skin on the feet and legs. Concrete ramps leading in and out of the water should slope over a distance of 1 to 2 m to minimize haul-out efforts and reduce the risk of skin abrasions. An important consideration for the design of water features is the presence of intradermal sensory organs (ISO) (see Chapter 10), which are highly sensitive free nerve endings similar to the lateral line system of fish (Fig. 25.8). ISO are reported to have mechanical sensitivity exceeding that of primate fingertips.[5] For these reasons, waterfalls and other features creating surface water movement may serve as a source of overstimulation and stress in species that naturally inhabit calm waters. The behavior of animals in these enclosures must be monitored closely to determine if they appear to avoid areas of high water movement. Currently no studies have evaluated this as a potential stressor for captive crocodilians.

FEEDING AND NUTRITION

As true carnivores, crocodilians require a high-protein, high-fat diet that is low in fiber. Their feeding habits in the wild vary with age and food availability. The diet of juvenile animals is often comprised of small invertebrates, amphibians, and reptiles. As they grow, they pursue larger prey of the same type and may add fish and birds to their diet.

As adults, they will usually prey on mammals as well. There are various commercial feeds available for captive alligators. A variety of whole prey foods, such as chicken, nutria, and fish, may also be used as part of an overall nutritional plan. Lead toxicosis has been reported in alligators fed nutria killed with lead shot.[6] Lead ingestion was also suspected to affect reproduction in captive alligators.[7] Similar effects have not been observed in *C. porosus* after ingestion of lead shot,[8] suggesting there may be species-specific sensitivity to the toxic effects of lead. If feeding frozen fish, thiamine supplementation may be needed to prevent thiamine deficiency because thiaminases are released from the fish tissues upon thawing. Obesity is a common problem of captive crocodilians due to overfeeding combined with a sedentary lifestyle. Feeding amounts and frequency should be tailored to the age, size, and activity level of the species. Young crocodilians may require feeding three to four times per week whereas adults may only have to be fed once weekly to maintain their body condition. Gastrointestinal foreign bodies can be a common problem, and it is important to prevent the public from throwing coins and trash into exhibits. Hoses, buckets, and other tools must also be stored securely outside of exhibit areas.

REFERENCES

See www.expertconsult.com for a complete list of references.

26

Tuatara

Sarah Alexander

Tuatara (*Sphenodon punctatus*) are widely held in captivity in New Zealand and have historically contributed to reintroduction programs. At the time of writing there are six institutions outside New Zealand that house tuatara for display and education purposes. Tuatara superficially resemble lizards, their husbandry is accordingly similar, with a few significant exceptions, and many of the restraint and identification methods used in lizards are also applicable to tuatara.

RESTRAINT

Physical restraint of tuatara is best accomplished by one person. Tuatara are most at ease when lightly restrained horizontally and will often sit comfortably on a handler's forearm with the tail partially wrapped around the arm for security (Fig. 26.1). Vertical restraint may be required for physical examination or blood sampling; in these situations the tuatara is held firmly behind the head with one hand, and the pelvis is supported with the other hand, as in medium-sized lizards. We have found this to be the best method for restraint of captive animals for blood collection from the ventral tail vein, although other methods involving a single operator have been described.[1] A head bandage can be utilized to reduce visual stimulation and induce a vasovagal response, although we have found this method to be of varying success in tuatara. Tuatara can inflict painful bites and may be reluctant to release their grip, in which case placing the tuatara on the ground may encourage it to let go. Their sharp claws can also result in scratches and damaged gloves. Although Salmonella has been infrequently detected in tuatara,[2,3] gloves and appropriate disinfection protocols should be routinely utilized. Tuatara have the ability to autotomize their tails, and this can be caused by tail trauma or improper restraint during handling. This is not a common occurrence, even in conscious animals, when properly handled.

Chemical restraint of tuatara has similarities with other reptiles, but special consideration is given to the tuatara's low metabolic rate, which can result in prolonged recovery times when injectable anesthesia is used. Ketamine hydrochloride should be avoided in tuatara, because prolonged apnea and recoveries ranging from 3 to 12 hours have been documented with doses from 4.5 to 70 mg/kg IM. Alfaxalone (Alfaxan, Jurox NZ Ltd., Auckland, New Zealand) administered IM or IV at 5 mg/kg did not produce appreciable sedation but did prolong recovery from subsequent inhalational anesthesia, whereas at 10 mg/kg IM or IV it produced deep sedation to light anesthesia, with recoveries taking up to 2 hours. The anesthesia agents of choice at Auckland Zoo are isoflurane (Isoflurane-Vet, Merial NZ Ltd., Auckland, New Zealand) and sevoflurane (Sevorane, Abbott, Botany, New South Wales, Australia). Tuatara often breath-hold when administered isoflurane, but this can be reduced by using a tight-fitting facemask to allow partial ventilation, using medical air rather than oxygen on induction, increasing the isoflurane concentration slowly, and gently compressing the cranial coelom or squeezing a toe to encourage ventilation. Similar problems have been experienced with sevoflurane induction, although often to a lesser degree. Several animals have been successfully induced with sevoflurane, with the aid of a darkened induction chamber. After anesthetic induction, the tuatara is intubated in the same manner as a lizard and maintained on the preferred inhalational anesthetic in oxygen. Intermittent positive pressure ventilation (IPPV), typically at 1 to 6 breaths/min, is frequently needed to supplement respirations and maintain anesthesia. Heart rate is easily monitored by use of a Doppler probe placed on the cranioventral coelomic area over the heart. Changing from oxygen to medical air before the end of the procedure may speed return to spontaneous ventilation and anesthetic recovery. Using this protocol, recovery times of 10 to 30 minutes can be expected.

IDENTIFICATION

Adult tuatara are reliably identified by microchip, implanted subcutaneously in the left inguinal region. However, at Auckland Zoo several juvenile tuatara (<2 years of age) have expelled their microchips when implanted in this region or over the lateral coelomic wall, despite appropriate placement and closure of the resulting wound with tissue adhesive. Juvenile tuatara can be visually identified by the placement of beads on nonabsorbable monofilament suture material that is threaded through the nuchal crest (Fig. 26.2) or temporarily by permanent marker or correction fluid on the dorsum. Photographic identification can be sufficient in small groups of animals. Toe clipping is still used as a means of identification in juveniles in field situations if other methods are not available or practical, but it should be avoided in captivity where less-invasive options are available.

SPECIFIC HOUSING REQUIREMENTS

Tuatara are cold-adapted reptiles and should be housed in conditions that mimic those in their natural environment as closely as possible. Temperatures should be carefully monitored and not be above 25°C (77°F) or below 4°C (39°F) for prolonged periods. It has been recommended that ambient air temperature be kept between 4°C (39°F) and 15°C (59°F) in winter and 10°C (50°F) and 25°C (77°F) in summer,[1] with the provision of an artificial heat source for basking in indoor enclosures. In the absence of access to direct sunlight, appropriate UVB supplementation should be provided. Recommended levels are as for other native New Zealand reptiles and are 50–200 uw/cm² of UVB 290–315 nm or UV index 1–4 (Gibson R, 2016, personal communication). At Auckland Zoo artificial UVB lighting is provided using Reptisun 10.0 UVB T5 lamps, with output measured regularly using a UVB meter. Humidity levels should be maintained above 60% in the enclosure and above 80% in burrows with the aid of misting if required. Temperature, humidity, photoperiod, and UVB supplementation should be varied seasonally in indoor enclosures to match natural conditions, and adequate ventilation should be provided to achieve good air exchange.

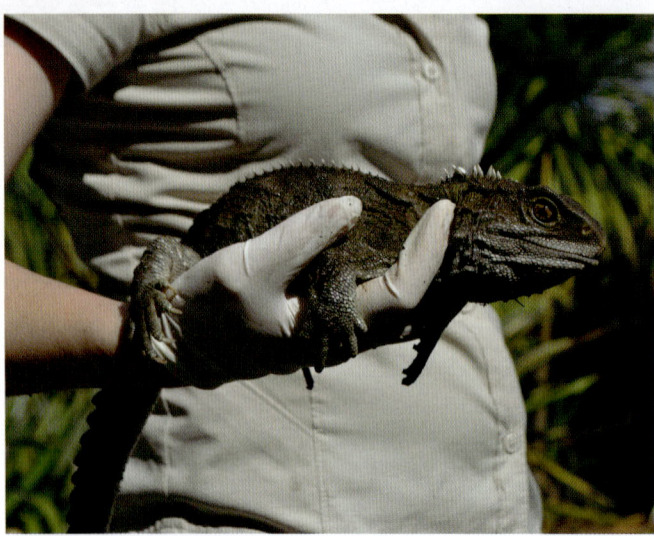

FIG 26.1 Comfortable restraint of an adult tuatara *(Sphenodon punctatus)*. (Courtesy of Auckland Zoo.)

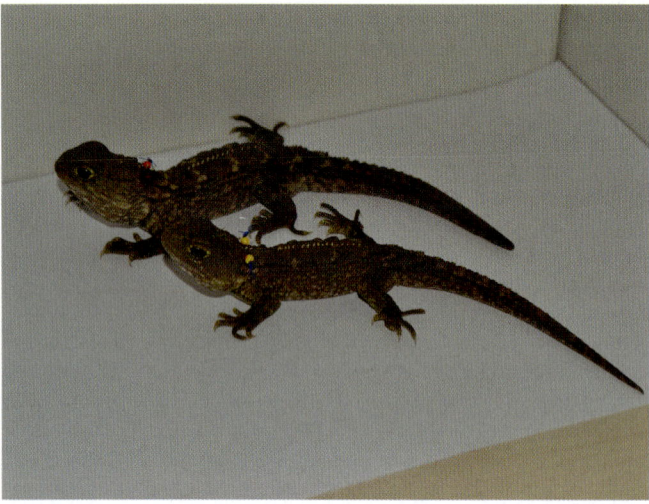

FIG 26.2 Identification of juvenile tuatara *(Sphenodon punctatus)* using beads on suture material placed through the nuchal crest. (Courtesy of Auckland Zoo.)

Enclosures should have a minimum of 3 m² of floor space for each adult animal if housed alone and at least 5 m² if housed in a group situation (Gibson R, 2016, personal communication). Enclosure substrate should drain freely and be deep enough to allow tuatara to dig their own burrows and nests for egg-laying. Leaf litter is an ideal surface layer, with the remaining substrate comprising soil with the addition of coarse sand or fine pumice for drainage. Substrate should be replaced as necessary to prevent the build-up of waste products. Artificial burrows should also be provided; these can be in the form of partially buried hollow logs, appropriately sized plastic pipes, or purpose-built wooden boxes with hinged lids to allow inspection and capture of their inhabitants (Fig. 26.3). Cage furniture such as low-growing shrubs and rocks provide shade and visual screens between animals. A shallow water dish provides a water source and aids in preventing dysecdysis; tuatara will also often pass urates and feces in water. Like many reptiles, tuatara can develop rostral abrasions by rubbing their noses on the walls of enclosures; this can be prevented by ensuring enclosures have smooth, nonabrasive walls and sufficient space for all animals. Tuatara are vulnerable to

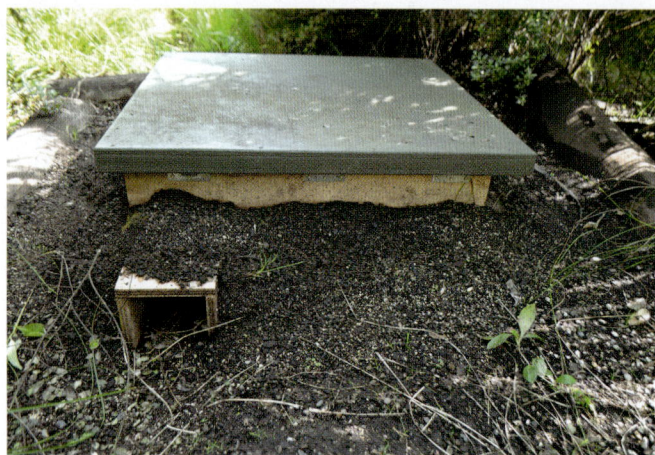

FIG 26.3 A partially buried artificial burrow that allows inspection of its inhabitants (Courtesy of Auckland Zoo.)

predation, and off-display areas should be fully enclosed with wire mesh or similar.

Young tuatara should be housed separately from adults to prevent predation. Newly hatched animals can be housed in large groups, but from 6 months of age juveniles can become territorial, so incompatible animals should be separated.[1] At 12 months of age, juveniles can be moved to enclosures that are similar to but smaller than those housing adult tuatara.

FEEDING AND NUTRITION

Tuatara are primarily insectivorous, and wild tuatara subsist primarily on a variety of invertebrates, including darkling beetles (*Mimopeus* sp), weevils, spiders, earthworms, adult moths, and tree weta.[4] Wild adult tuatara also occasionally consume vertebrate prey, most commonly fairy prion (*Pachyptila turtur*) chicks, seabird eggs, reptiles including juvenile tuatara, and crustaceans if available.[4] Tuatara rarely intentionally consume plant material, but they do appear to have a preference for ripe kawakawa (*Macropiper excelsum*) berries.[5] The captive diet of tuatara should mimic the nutrient composition of the wild diet as much as possible[6] and should include a variety of invertebrates and appropriate vitamin and mineral supplementation. At Auckland Zoo, tuatara are primarily fed live field crickets (*Teleogryllus commodus*) and locusts (*Locusta migratoria*) dusted with a vitamin and mineral supplement (Calcium Plus, Repashy Superfoods). They are also offered woodlice (*Porcellio scaber*), mealworm beetles (*Tenebrio* sp.), and cockroaches (*Celatoblatta* spp. and *Drymaplaneta semivitta*) when available and forage for other invertebrates in their naturalistic enclosures. Kawakawa berries are offered when in season. Captive tuatara can become obese, and careful attention should be paid to weight and body condition relative to similar-sized wild counterparts. Secondary nutritional hyperparathyroidism has been diagnosed in captive tuatara and is caused by insufficient UVB and/or inadequate calcium provision,[7] as in other reptiles.

ACKNOWLEDGMENTS

Many thanks to Richard Gibson and Richard Jakob-Hoff for their contributions to these chapters and to Wayne Boardman and Barbara Blanchard for their previous work on this subject.

REFERENCES

See www.expertconsult.com for a complete list of references.

27

Nutrition

Thomas H. Boyer and Peter W. Scott

Inadequate nutrition is a leading cause of morbidity and mortality in herpetological medicine because owners, as well as most veterinarians, are often not well educated about the nutrition needs of these animals. Much less is known about herpetological nutrition compared with domestic animal nutrition. Therefore veterinarians must be a dependable source of information for reptile and amphibian owners, otherwise, they will seek advice from the internet, pet stores, or outdated literature, usually with highly variable, and sometimes dangerous, results.

Always evaluate the reptile patient's diet as part of any detailed medical history. Never assume the owner has good nutritional knowledge, regardless of their experience. Keeping a reptile alive for years is no guarantee that it is healthy. Chronic nutritional disease, often with environmental components, remain common, including nutritional secondary hyperparathyroidism (NSHP), hepatic lipidosis, protein deficiency, hypovitaminosis A, hypervitaminosis A, pyramidal shell growth, renal disease, urocystoliths, thiamine deficiency, vitamin E/selenium deficiency, steatitis, corneal lipidosis, obesity, loose stools, and starvation (see Chapter 84).

As veterinarians we need to take a proactive approach to reptile and amphibian nutrition rather than treating an endless stream of nutritional disease. The goal of this chapter is to educate veterinarians so they are competent and confident in evaluating, reformulating, and implementing herpetological diets.

WATER

Water is the most important of all nutrients. All animals need water, it is the most essential nutrient, and there is enormous diversity in methods utilized to obtain it. Mammals can survive loss of most fat and glycogen reserves, and half of their bodies' protein, but a 10% to 15% water loss is life threatening. Water remains of critical importance to reptiles, even desert species, which can withstand greater losses but still require water.

Three sources of water are available to animals: dietary water (in food), metabolic water (formed from cellular metabolism), and environmental water. Few animals are able to survive without environmental water, and those that do are generally herbivores consuming plants with a high water content. Their dependence on, or independence from, environmental water is not well understood.[1] Many desert species can behaviorally conserve water by retreating to a humid underground burrow, but this may not be available in a cage or yard with low relative humidity. In captivity, it is safest to assume all reptiles depend on environmental water. Some reptiles are not adept at drinking from water bowls. Many terrestrial species (e.g., desert tortoises, *Gopherus agassizii* and *G. morfakai*; bearded dragons, *Pogona* spp.; spiny-tailed lizards, *Uromastyx* spp.) seem to prefer to walk into shallow water to drink or to have water dripped on their head; while arboreal species (e.g., anoles, *Anolis* spp.; chameleons, Chamaeleonidae; day geckos,

Phelsuma spp.; arboreal vipers, *Atheris*, *Bothrops*, *Bothriechis*, *Trimeresurus* spp.; boids, *Corallus* spp., *Morelia viridis*; green and ribbon snakes, *Thamnophis*, *Opheodrys* spp.) imbibe water droplets from foliage or their skin. The thorny dragon or devil (*Moloch horridus*) is an Australian lizard with hydroscopic channels within its skin that channel water (from dew condensation at night or rainfall) via capillary action from all over its body to its mouth. This same system, first reported by Gans et al.,[2] has now been shown in a number of agamid and iguanid lizards.[3] All these species need water, whether misted, sprayed, dripped, or provided as free-standing water. Some need water provision several times daily (e.g., misting), while others may only need water to be provided a few times each week.

COMPLETE MANUFACTURED DIETS

The goal is to feed captive reptiles a balanced diet, although in the wild state reptiles likely balance their diet over long periods of time. A balanced diet is one that leads to no net gain, or loss, of nutrients from the body, allowing the body to maintain a state of metabolic equilibrium. The important factors are nutrient content, energy content, digestibility, and the species-specific requirements, which may change with age, gender, season, and reproductive status.

Major differences in mammalian nutritional requirements have been identified, for superficially similar species, or even the same species, such as humans. We simply do not have the same body of knowledge for any reptile species that we have for the more familiar domesticated animals. Nevertheless, manufactured diets are available, and while some have reasonably long-term feeding data, most do not. Much more work is needed in this area, especially in relation to the many reptile species being kept.

The main advantage of appropriately processed or manufactured diets is they can contain all of the nutrients for a given species, assuming we know what they are. The disadvantages are that if any nutrients are omitted or included at inappropriate levels, the consequences can be substantial.[4] The data and research to formulate complete herp diets are not currently available; however, companies may falsely claim to have data. No regulatory agencies oversee reptile diets or advertising claims, so veterinarians should be cognizant of a wide variation in quality and be prepared to evaluate the diets themselves before making recommendations. In general, manufactured foods use the National Research Council (NRC) guidelines for some species (such as laboratory rats and domestic carnivores) as a starting point, or known nutritional studies from herps, where they are available. Some complete diets are from feed manufacturers with PhD nutritionists, or veterinarians, on staff to provide professional input, while others are from pet suppliers with little training or expertise in diet formulation. Meats used may be human grade in Europe, but not in the United States. Routinely offals are used. National guidelines exist in different countries for declarations and layouts on labels, although these may be limited to the familiar domesticated species.

Reading a Product Label

Protein is the most costly component, and therefore manufactured diets will often use less expensive plant proteins in combination with smaller quantities of mammalian or fish proteins. Examining ingredient lists may help estimate digestibility since plant materials are generally less digestible by carnivores. Reviews of how to "read" labels are available.[5]

The best way to read a product label is to start with the guaranteed analysis. If ingredients are listed without a guaranteed analysis, then readers are advised to be skeptical of nutritional adequacy. The more nutritional information provided, the better. The water content of foods varies, so for direct comparison, diets are compared on a dry matter basis (DMB), with water removed, and not by the nutrient levels on the label (which are as fed, or AF). For example, suppose three foods (frozen, canned, and pellets) had a label guaranteed analysis of 15% protein as fed. Do they have the same protein content? The moisture content is 80% for the frozen food, 75% for the canned food, and 12% for the pelleted food. On a DMB the frozen food contains 75% protein, the canned food 60% protein, and the pelleted food 18% protein. So no, the protein content is not the same on a DMB, but they look the same on the label, or on an AF basis. By removing water, diets can be more accurately compared to one another. See Box 27.1 for an explanation on how to calculate the DMB of a food. See Tables 27.1 through 27.3 for nutritional information for various herbivorous foods, and Tables 27.4 through 27.7 for tortoise, iguana, box turtle, aquatic turtle, and bearded dragon manufactured diets.

Metabolizable Energy

Another way to look at foods is by metabolizable energy (ME) or kcal ME per unit volume (e.g., cup) or weight. For carnivores, which consume variably energydense foods, ME estimates can be useful. ME estimates are calculated using Atwater calculations. In cats and dogs, estimated digestibility coefficients determined in humans overestimated ME in pet foods, so modified Atwater calculations are preferred.[9] Using guaranteed analysis data from four current commercial diets, the calculations allow some comparisons (Table 27.8). In general, juvenile reptiles require higher dietary ME than adults.

Protein

Overall growth rate in animals is protein driven, although food intake can be controlled somewhat by energy intake. As animals mature, active growth slows and less protein is needed in relation to energy. The consumption of excess calories resulting in a maximal growth rate is not compatible with optimal skeletal development and may result in skeletal deformities in juvenile reptiles.

A protein:energy ratio (P:E ratio) can also be calculated for a diet; this is not something that directly relates to an established "need" but is a useful "descriptor" of the nutritional quality of a diet. It represents the proportional contribution of dietary protein to total dietary energy. In general, the P:E ratio needed by an animal changes throughout its life, with a higher proportion of protein to energy needed as animals are growing. It also varies depending on activity and reproductive status.

BOX 27.1 Converting a Nutrient Analysis From "as Fed" to "Dry Matter" (DM)

To calculate DM, first determine the percentages of protein, fat, fiber, moisture, ash, and carbohydrate listed as fed, fresh-weight basis, or as sold (all the same). Carbohydrate is not included in the guaranteed analysis but is equal to 100 − (% protein + % fat + % moisture + % ash). Note that fiber is not included because it is a carbohydrate. Next, remove the moisture or water content to give the % total dry matter (TDM). Then divide each nutrient % by % TDM and multiply by 100 (DM = 100 [% nutrient/% TDM]).

For example, the guaranteed analysis lists:

Protein 15%, fat 3%, fiber 18%, moisture 12.5%, ash 8%, Ca 1.2%, P 0.65% AF

The carbohydrate content would be 100 − (15+3+12.5+8) = 38.5%

Next, remove water, TDM = 100 − 12.5% (moisture) = 87.5%

For DM basis protein, 100(15/87.5) = 17% protein

DM basis for the others are: 3% fat, 21% fiber, 44% carbohydrate, 1.4% Ca, 0.74% P

TABLE 27.1 Nutritional Composition (% DM) of Commonly Fed Greens Compared to Nutrient Profile of Desert Tortoises (*Gopherus agassizii* and *G. morafakai*)[6,7] and Suggested Nutrient Profile for Green Iguanas (*Iguana iguana*)[4]

Food	Protein	Fat	Fiber	CHO	Ca	P	Ca : P
Iceberg lettuce	25	0	11	59	0.4	0.5	0.8 : 1
Endive	26	3	11	60	1.17	0.78	1.5 : 1
Cabbage	17	2	11	71	0.64	0.38	1.7 : 1
Kale	35	5	8	52	1.4	0.6	2.7 : 1
Romaine lettuce	36	7	11	50	1.1	0.4	2.8 : 1
Spinach	36	3	7	50	1.1	0.4	2.8 : 1
Beet greens	24	3	14	51	1.31	0.44	3.0 : 1
Collards	33	5	6	51	1.70	0.56	3.0 : 1
Dandelions	18	5	11	61	1.3	0.4	3.3 : 1
Mustards	29	5	11	53	1.74	0.48	3.6 : 1
Desert tortoise natural diet[6]	9–15.4	<3	18.7–34.0	45.5–52.3	NL	NL	3.2–5.8 : 1
Suggested green iguana diet[4]	26[Juveniles] ≥22[Subadults] 15–17[Adults]	3	6–10	NL	1.1	0.6	1.8 : 1

NL, Not listed.

TABLE 27.2 Nutritional Composition (% DM) of Commonly Fed Fruits and Vegetables Compared to Nutrient Profile of Desert Tortoises (*Gopherus agassizii* and *G. morafakai*)[6,7] and Suggested Nutrient Profile for Green Iguanas (*Iguana iguana*)[4]

Food	Protein	Fat	Fiber	CHO	Ca	P	Ca : P
Banana	4	2	2	86	0.02	0.07	0.3:1
Cantaloupe	8	2	4	79	0.1	0.2	0.5:1
Tomatoes	15	3	9	66	0.18	0.38	0.5:1
Watermelon	6.8	2.5	8.1	86	0.09	0.14	0.6:1
Apples	1	2	4	86	0.04	0.06	0.7:1
Blueberries	4	2	12	80	0.1	0.1	1:1
Strawberries	6	4	6	77	0.2	0.2	1:1
Corn	7	2	12	45	0.006	0.22	0.03:1
Zucchini	23	1	9	67	0.51	0.54	0.9:1
Frozen mixed	28	1	13	51	0.2	0.2	1:1
Carrots	8.4	1.5	8.5	73.1	0.28	0.27	1:1
Squash	17	2	3	65	0.4	0.4	1:1
Green beans	19	2	14	72	0.57	0.44	1.3:1
Broccoli floret	33	3	12	54	0.94	0.72	1.3:1
Prickly pear (wild)	7	3.1	9.3	60.4	6.29	0.8	78.7:1
Prickly pear (store)	4.8	2	14	69	9.6	0.1	96:1
Desert tortoise natural diet[6,7]	**9–15.4**	**<3**	**18.7–34.0**	**45.5–52.3**	**NL**	**NL**	**3.2–5.8:1**
Suggested green iguana diet[4]	**26**[Juveniles] **≥22**[Subadults] **15–17**[Adults]	**3**	**6–10**	**NL**	**1.1**	**0.6**	**1.8:1**

NL, Not listed.

TABLE 27.3 Nutritional Composition (% DM) of Commonly Fed Grasses, Hays, and Clover, Compared to Nutrient Profile of Desert Tortoises (*Gopherus agassizii* and *G. morafakai*)[6-8]

Forage	Protein	Fat	Fiber	CHO	Ca	P	Ca : P
Kentucky bluegrass	5.2	2	8.1	75	0.1	0.1	1:1
Orchard grass hay	8.4–15	3	31	41	0.4	0.4	1:1
Fescue	9.5–12.4	NL					
Timothy hay	7.8–17	3	28	45	0.5	0.2	2.5:1
Ryegrass	16.3	4.2	21.8	42	0.64	0.41	2:1
Bermuda grass hay	8–16	2.0	29.6	52.8	0.46	0.22	2.3:1
Bermuda grass	11.6	2.1	25.9	50.0	0.53	0.22	2.4:1
Clover	19	1	23	47	1.7	0.4	4.3:1
Alfalfa hay	17–23	2.1	31.4	45	1.64	0.26	6.3:1
Desert tortoise natural diet[6-8]	**9–15.4**	**<3**	**18.7–34.0**	**45.5–52.3**	**NL**	**NL**	**3.2–5.8:1**

NL, Not listed.

TABLE 27.4 Nutritional Composition (%DM) of Commonly Fed Commercial Tortoise Pellets Compared to Nutrient Profile of the Most Frequently Consumed Plant Species Reported From Studies of Free-Ranging Desert Tortoises (*Gopherus agassizii* and *G. morafakai*)[6,7]

Commercial Diet	Protein (min)	Fat (min)	Fiber (max)	CHO (est)	Ca (min max)	P (min)	Ca : P (ratio)
Desert tortoise natural diet	9–15.4	<3	18.7–34.0	45.5–52.3	NL	NL	3.2–5.8:1
Score = 4							
ZooMed Gourmet Tortoise	9	2	25	NC	0.9–1.4	0.3	3–4.7:1
Agrobs Pre Alpin Testudo Baby	11	2	28	79	1.03	0.32	3.2:1
Score = 3							
Zoo Med (ZM)	10	2	30	66	1.0–1.5	0.5	2.0–3.0:1
Natural Grassland Tortoise ZM Forest Tortoise	15	2	26	62	1.0–1.5	0.5	2.0–3.0:1
Agrobs Pre Alpin Testudo Fibre	9	3	31	80	0.67	0.28	2.4:1
ExoTerra European Tortoise Juvenile Soft Pellets	12.6	2.3	27.6	73	1.5	0.5	3:1

Continued

TABLE 27.4 Nutritional Composition (%DM) of Commonly Fed Commercial Tortoise Pellets Compared to Nutrient Profile of the Most Frequently Consumed Plant Species Reported From Studies of Free-Ranging Desert Tortoises (*Gopherus agassizii* and *G. morafakai*)[6,7]—cont'd

Commercial Diet	Protein (min)	Fat (min)	Fiber (max)	CHO (est)	Ca (min max)	P (min)	Ca : P (ratio)
ExoTerra European Tortoise Adult Soft Pellets	10.3	2.3	29.9	76	1.5	0.5	3:1
Exoterra Forest Tortoise Adult Soft Pellets	14.9	2.3	26.4	71	1.5	0.5	3:1
Score = 2							
Agrobs Pre Alpin Testudo Original	8	2	32	65	0.62	0.27	2.3:1
Agrobs Pre Alpin Testudo Herbs	8	3	33	82	0.58	0.27	2.1:1
Mazuri Tortoise LS Diet	14	5	25	72	1.4	0.72	1.9:1
Mazuri Tortoise or NutraZu Tortoise (same)	17	3	21	71	1.4	0.74	1.9:1
Repashey Superfoods Grassland Grazer Tortoise Gel Premix	16	3	33	71	1.6	NL	NL
Exoterra Forest Tortoise Juvenile Soft Pellets	18.4	2.3	24.1	68	1.5	0.5	3:1
Pretty Pets Small Tortoise or Large Tortoise (same)	9	3	14	76	NL	NL	2:1
Rep-Cal Tortoise	22	2	20	NC	NL	NL	NL
Score = 1							
Ziegler Monster	14	6	10	74	NL	NL	NL
Nature Zone Bites Tortoise	5	2	10	NL	NL	NL	NL
Score = 0							
Zilla Land Tortoise and Turtle Food	16	5	11	66	NL	NL	NL
Marion Zoological Mozaic Reptile Food	22	7	12	63	1.0	0.8	1.4:1
Mazuri Small Tortoise Diet LS	23	5	16	60	1.99–2.56	1.1	1.8–2.3:1
Dietex Intl. Mazuri Zoo Foods Exotic Leaf Eater	26	4	13	62	1.3	0.9	1.4:1
Nature Zone Natural Bites Tortoise	3	10	9	NL	NL	NL	NL

Scores were assigned based on whether the diet met the free-ranging nutrient profiles in references, with 4 being the best score. Not all diets had Ca or P listed, which was reflected in their lower scores; scores listed from highest to lowest.
NL, Not listed.

TABLE 27.5 Nutritional Composition (% DM) of Commonly Fed Commercial Iguana Diets Compared to Suggested Nutrient Profile for Green Iguanas (*Iguana iguana*)[4]

Commercial Diet	Protein% (min)	Fat% (min)	Crude Fiber% (max)	Ca% (min-max)	P% (min)	Ca : P (ratio)
Suggested green iguana diet[4]	26[Juveniles] ≥22[Subadults] 15–17[Adults]	3	6–10	1.1	0.6	1.8:1
Score = 5						
Exoterra Iguana Juvenile Soft Pellets	27.5	2.9	17.2	1.4	0.6	2.3:1
Exoterra Iguana Adult Soft Pellets	16.1	2.9	17.2	1.4	0.6	2.3:1
Score = 4						
ZooMed Natural Iguana Food Adult Formula	15	2	21	0.9–1.4	0.5	1.8–2.8:1
Score = 3						
ZooMed Natural Iguana Food Juvenile Formula	28	3	15	0.9–1.4	0.6	1.5–2.3:1
Mazuri Herbivorous Reptile LS Diet-Small	24	5	17	1.99–2.60	1.1	1.8–2.4:1
Rep-Cal Adult Iguana Food	18	1	20	NL	NL	NC
Zilla Juvenile Iguana	22	3	11	NA	NL	NC
Pretty Pets Juvenile Iguana Food	13	3	10	NL	NL	2:1
Score = 2						
Rep-Cal Juvenile Iguana Food	27	1	18	NL	NL	NC
Marion Zoological Mozaic Reptile Iguana	22	7	12	1.1	0.8	1.4:1
Zeigler Monster Diets Adult Iguana	14	3	14	NL	NL	NC
Zilla Adult Iguana	14	3	14	NL	NL	NC
Score = 1						
Zeigler Monster Diets Juvenile Iguana	29	8	10	NL	NL	NC
Zilla Fortified Food Juvenile Iguana	21.6	3.4	11.4	NL	NL	NL
Zilla Fortified Food Adult Iguana	14.2	3.4	13.6	NL	NL	NL
Nature's Zone Bites Iguana	11.4	2.1	5.7	NL	NL	NL

Scores were assigned based on whether the diet met the suggested nutrient profile. Not all diets had Ca or P listed, which was reflected in their lower scores; scores listed from highest (5) to lowest (1).
NL, Not listed.

TABLE 27.6 Nutritional Composition (% DM) of Commonly Fed Commercial Aquatic Turtle (AT) and Box Turtle (BT) Foods, Listed Alphabetically

Diet	Protein	Fat	Ash	CHO	Fiber	Ca	P	Ca : P
API AT Pellets	47.2	6.7	NL	NL	3.4	NL	NL	NL
ExoTerra Floating Pellet Hatchling AT Food	49.4	11.5	11.5	27.6	1.1	2.5	1.1	2.3
ExoTerra Floating Pellet Juvenile AT Food	40.2	5.7	11.5	42.5	3.8	2.5	1.1	2.3
ExoTerra Floating Pellet Adult AT Food	28.7	5.7	11.0	54.0	9.2	2.5	1.1	2.3
Fluker's Buffet Blend AT Formula	42.3	8.7	14.3	34.9	2.6	4.8	1.1	4.4
Mazuri AT	45.5	11.4	10.8	32.4	5.7	2.4	1.1	2.2
Monster Diets AT	45.5	11.4	11.4	31.8	2.3	NL	NL	NL
Nature Zone Bites AT	30.0	10.0	NL	NL	8.8	NL	NL	NL
Saki-Hikari Turtle	45.0	4.4	15.6	34.0	2.2	2.2	1.1	2
Rep-Cal AT Food	37.5	6.8	NL	NL	9.1	NL	NL	NL
Tetra Fauna Reptotreat Suprema Krill Enriched Food Sticks	51.6	7.7	NL	NL	4.4	NL	1.0	NL
Tetra ReptoMin Floating Food Sticks, (Baby, Jumbo) and Mini Pellets	46.2	9.2	NL	NL	2.2	2.2	2.0	1.1
Tetra ReptoMin Floating Food Sticks, Plus	48.9	9.2	NL	NL	2.2	2.2	1.7	1.3
Tetra ReptoMin Select A Food	42.9	4.9	NL	NL	2.2	NL	1.3	NL
Wardley Reptile Sticks	41.8	4.4	NL	NL	3.3	NL	NL	NL
Wardley Turtle Delight	56.8	1.7	NL	NL	4.5	NL	NL	NL
Wardley Turtle Treat	22.2	4.4–8.9	NL	NL	2.2	NL	NL	NL
Zilla Clam Turtle Chasers AT Treats	66.6	1.1	NL	NL	3.3	NL	NL	NL
Zilla Fortified AT Food	39.8	11.4	NL	NL	5.7	NL	NL	NL
Zilla Shrimp Turtle Chasers AT Treats	37.5	5.7	NL	NL	13.6	NL	NL	NL
Zoo Med BT Canned	13.6	2.3	NL	NL	4.5	NL	NL	NL
Zoo Med Gourmet BT	9.1	4.5	NL	NL	20.4	NL	NL	NL
Zoo Med Natural AT Food Hatchling Form	48.3	11.2	11.5	29.0	3.4	2.2	1.7	1.3
Zoo Med Natural AT Food Growth Form	39.3	5.6	9.0	46.0	5.6	1.3	1.3	1.0
Zoo Med Natural AT Food Maintenance Form	28.1	5.6	10.7	55.6	9.0	1.3	1.3	1.0
Zoo Med Natural BT Food	27.5	2.9	9.7	59.8	14.9	1.2	0.8	1.5
Zoo Med Repti Sticks	40.4	6.7	NL	NL	3.4	2.0	0.9	2.2
Zoo Med Sinking Mud & Musk Turtle Food	39.3	5.6	11.0	44.0	5.6	1.5	1.3	1.2

NL, Not listed.

TABLE 27.7 Nutritional Composition (%DM) of Commonly Fed Commercial Bearded Dragon (BD) Foods, Listed Alphabetically

Diet	Protein	Fat	Ash	CHO	Fiber	Ca	P	Ca : P
Exoterra BD Juvenile Soft Pellets	34.5	4.6	11.5	49.4	13.8	1.1	0.6	1.8
Exoterra BD Adult Soft Pellets	20.5	4.5	12.5	62.5	13.6	1.1	0.6	1.8
Fluker's Buffet Blend Juvenile BD	35	8.2	11.5	45	7.1	2.5	2.2	1.1
Fluker's BD Diet For Juveniles	35.5	13.3	4.4	47.0	7.8	NL	NL	NL
Fluker's BD Diet For Adults	26.7	8.9	10.0	54.4	3.9	NL	NL	NL
Monster Diets Adult BD	29.3	9.8	12.3	48.8	11.0	NL	NL	NL
Nature's Zone BD Bites Reptile Food	13.3	2.7	NL	NL	8.0	NL	NL	NL
Repashey Veggie Burger	38.0	8.7	9.8	43.5	9.8	1.3	NL	NL
Rep-Cal Maintenance Formula Adult BD Food	27.0	2.3	NL	NL	14.7	NL	NL	NL
Rep-Cal Maintenance Formula Juvenile BD Food	28.2	4.7	8.2	58.8	12.9	NL	NL	NL
T-Rex BD Gourmet Food Blend	21.6	6.7	5.9	65.9	8.9	0.3	NL	NL
Zilla Fortified Food BD	27.8	6.7	NL	NL	6.7	NL	NL	NL
Zilla Reptile Munchies Omnivore Mix with Ca	18.9	6.7	NL	NL	6.7	2.2	NL	NL
Zilla Reptile Munchies Vegetable Mix with Ca	8.8	0.8	NL	NL	6.7	2.2	NL	NL
ZooMed Gourmet BD Food	10.3	2.3			29.9	1.1	0.5	2.2
ZooMed Juvenile BD Food	27.5	3.4	9.7	59.1	14.9	1.2	0.8	1.5
ZooMed Adult BD Food	18.4	3.0	10.1	68.6	18.4	1.1	0.6	1.8

NL, Not listed.

TABLE 27.8   Metabolizable Energy (ME) and Protein Requirements Can Change as Reptiles Age, So One Diet Does Not Always Work for All Age Groups

	Juvenile Iguana	Adult Iguana	Juvenile Bearded Dragon	Adult Bearded Dragon
Crude protein (min)	24	13	24	16
Crude fat (min)	2.5	2	3	2.5
Crude fiber (max)	13	18	13	16
Moisture (max)	13	13	13	13
Ash (max)	11	11	10	10
Calcium (min)	0.8	0.8	0.8	0.8
Calcium (max)	1.2	1.2	1.2	1.2
Phosphorus (min)	0.4	0.4	0.4	0.4
Ca : P	2–3:1	2–3:1	2–3:1	2–3:1
Calculated carbohydrate	36.5	43	37	42.5
ME/100 g using modified Atwater	233	213	239	226
Protein/energy	0.10	0.06	0.10	0.07

Currently we have no in-depth knowledge of the actual needs of herps, but we can assess effects clinically. Animals short of energy will use protein as an energy source, whereas a physiological excess of protein tends to be stored as fats. The metabolism of excess protein in this way can lead to excess nitrogenous waste excretion. Looking at levels of declared calcium (Ca) and phosphorus (P) is also useful. The diets listed in Table 27.8 provide close to "ideal" vertebrate ratios of Ca:P if nothing else is fed. If live foods or greens are used in addition, then the ratio may become inadequate without additional calcium supplementation.

MULTIVITAMINS AND CALCIUM SUPPLEMENTS

Multivitamins

Multivitamins marketed for reptiles and amphibians can be broken down into multivitamins with and without Ca (Tables 27.9 and 27.10). Ca supplements are typically used on a daily or regular basis. Some argue that multivitamins with Ca should not be used as a daily Ca source, because they may not contain sufficient Ca to prevent NSHP (thus giving owners a false sense of adequate Ca supplementation), and long-term inclusion of fat-soluble vitamins (particularly A and D) or trace minerals (such as copper, iron, or zinc) may lead to oversupplementation; however, taking calcium supplements with iron or zinc compromises the absorption of these minerals. Others believe that properly formulated supplements containing multivitamins (including low level D_3) and calcium are required daily. Such opinions and controversies probably stem from the variable quality, availability, and experience of using supplements and are unlikely to be resolved until definitive research is published.

For most animals, the presumed maximal safe levels of vitamins A and D_3 for long-term feeding (>60 days) is 4 to 10 times the recognized dietary requirement.[10] Unfortunately for herps, we still do not know their dietary requirements for either A or D, nor any other vitamins. In green iguanas (*Iguana iguana*), the risk of oversupplementation of vitamin A was thought to be especially great in supplements with vitamin A levels >1100 IU/gm.[4] The estimated daily vitamin A requirements of green iguanas was 56 IU/kg, and long-term intake of vitamin A 2 to 3

times the recommended dietary level of 8000 IU/kg feed could produce hypervitaminosis A.[4] Using human-formulated products should be done with great care, as it may be impossible to subdivide a tablet into small enough portions for safe dosing.[4] If multivitamins are used, the amount provided should be restricted to that amount that supplies the daily requirement for vitamin A, but at this level many supplements are poor sources of other vitamins and trace minerals.[4] One author (Boyer) has had empirical success recommending multivitamins once or twice a month for diets lacking vitamin A, and no multivitamins if commercial gut-loading diets, or dry, formulated feeds with vitamin A, are used. Vitamin deficiencies typically arise from a total lack of the vitamin in the diet; small amounts of the vitamin, with a balanced diet, generally avoid deficiencies.

Multivitamins without Ca should be evaluated to see if they are true multivitamins (all vitamins A, B, C, D, E, and K, as well as trace minerals). Insectivores, such as chameleons (Chamaeleonidae), leopard geckos (*Eublepharis macularius*), toads, and some frogs (Anura), need vitamin A in their diet because of poor conversion of β-carotene precursors into vitamin A. All herbivores seem capable of vitamin A synthesis. Carnivores typically avoid vitamin A deficiency because liver in whole animal diets is an excellent source of vitamin A. Emydid turtles, such as box turtles (*Terrapene* spp.) and sliders (*Trachemys*), cooters (*Pseudemys*), and painted turtles (*Chrysemys*) often develop hypovitaminosis A; however, it is not clear if this is from a dietary deficiency or if they are poor converters of β-carotene precursors. An informal survey of popular reptile multivitamins showed that about a third contained no vitamin A but instead list β-carotene, and half are not true multivitamins (see Table 27.9). This could be an issue for insectivores if not fed properly gut-loaded insects, or for emydid turtles, if their diet were vitamin A deficient. The ratio of A:D:E should be roughly 100:10:1. Essential amino acid supplementation should not be necessary if insects, whole animals, or a nutritionally complete commercial diet are fed, as these foods all have adequate essential amino acids.

The vitamin D content must also be considered; vitamin D enhances Ca absorption. As we have discussed, Ca is often used on a daily or regular basis. Vitamin D is a fat-soluble vitamin or hormone, and excess may be retained in fat. Large doses of vitamin D can be toxic (hence, its widespread usage as a rodenticide), although these doses far exceed levels used in most supplements. Not all reptiles (especially *Iguana* and *Cyclura* spp.) seem to be able to efficiently utilize dietary vitamin D.[4,11] If adequate UVB light exposure is available, there is less need for dietary vitamin D_3 in Ca supplements, especially if multivitamins or fortified foods containing vitamin D_3 are already in use. It is important to note that reptiles are thought to only utilize D_3, many human products use D_2 but "mathematically convert" the D_2 into the equivalent D_3 for their label information using the known rate of human conversion. Reptiles cannot convert D_2 to D_3. The important point is that clinicians evaluate the vitamin label (see Table 27.9 or online resources) to make sure the product is appropriate.

Calcium Supplements

Ca supplements are listed in Table 27.10. Ca supplementation is needed on a regular basis (daily to every other day) for all growing herps not consuming whole vertebrates regularly. Once adults have fully formed skeletons, Ca demands decrease, but there is still a need, especially in reproductive females. Most calcium salts are better absorbed with food and help to competitively inhibit P absorption. Ideally, Ca supplements should be independent of multivitamins (other than vitamin D) and contain little to no P. Most insects have a 1:10 Ca:P ratio, therefore a Ca supplement with a 2:1 Ca:P ratio (common with bone meal products) will never achieve a positive Ca:P ratio until the mass of the supplement is greater than the mass of the insect. Also heavily dusting salads adds

TABLE 27.9   Alphabetical Listing by Manufacturer of Multivitamins Marketed for Reptiles and Amphibians

Manufacturer, Name	Vitamin A Present?	All Multivitamins Present?	Ingredients
Dendrocare, Vitamin/ Mineral Powder	Yes	No	Vitamin A (450,000 IU/kg), Vitamin D_3 (120,000 IU/kg), Vitamin E (10,200 mg/kg), Vitamin B_1, Vitamin B_2, Pantothenic acid, Niacin, Vitamin B_6, Copper, Iodine, Iron, Manganese, Zinc, Cobalt, Sodium, Magnesium, Potassium, Calcium 22%, Phosphorus 8.8%
Exo Terra, Multi-vitamin Supplement	No	No	Seaweed Meal, Yeast, Oyster Shell Flour, Dextrose, Beta-Carotene (8980 IU/kg), Menadione Sodium Bisulfite Complex (Source of Vitamin K Activity), Biotin, Inositol, Choline Chloride, Salt, Calcium Phosphate, Calcium Carbonate, Potassium Chloride, Manganese Oxide, Ferrous Fumarate, Calcium Sulfate, Manganous Oxide, Zinc Oxide, Copper Sulfate, Potassium Iodate. Calcium (4.4%–4.6%), Vitamin D_3 (21,954 IU/kg), Vitamin E (100 IU/kg)
Fluker's, Liquid Vitamin Electrolyte Spray	No	No	Vitamins: Niacin, DI-Alpha Tocopheryl Acetate, Vitamin D_3, Calcium Pantothenate, Ascorbic Acid, Riboflavin, Menadione Sodium Bisulfite Complex, Pyridoxine Hydrochloride, Thiamine Mononitrate, D-Biotin, Folic Acid, Vitamin B_{12}. Minerals: Sodium Bicarbonate, Potassium Chloride, Magnesium Sulfate, Manganese Sulfate, Zinc Sulfate, Copper Sulfate, Ethylene Diamine Dihydriodide. Amino Acids: L-Glutamic Acid, L-Aspartic Acid, L-Leucine, L-Valine, L-Serine, L-Lysine, L-Alanine, L-Phenylalanine, L-Arginine, L-Isoleucine, L-Threonine, L-Tyrosine, L-Proline, DI-Methionine, Glycine, L-Cystine, L-Histidine, L-Tryptophan.
Fluker's, Repta Boost Insectivore/Carnivore High Amp Boost Reptile Supplement	Yes	Yes	Egg Product, Wheat Flour, Starch, Isolated Soy Flour, Corn Oil, Brewers Yeast, Kelp, Calcium Carbonate, Dicalcium Phosphate, Pollen, Dextrose, Sodium Chloride, Potassium Sorbate, DI-Methionine, Lecithin, Choline Chloride, Potassium Chloride, Spirulina, Manganese Sulfate, Mixed Natural Tocopherols, Zinc Sulfate, Magnesium Oxide, Ascorbic Acid, Beta Carotene Supplement, Niacin, Vitamin E Supplement, Copper Sulfate, Vitamin B_{12} Supplement, Vitamin A Acetate, Calcium Pantothenate, Vitamin D_3, Pyridoxine HCl, Menadione Sodium Bisulfite Complex, Riboflavin, Thiamine Mononitrate, Ethylene Diamine Dihydriodide, Biotin Supplement, Folic Acid, Sodium Selenite.
Fluker's, Reptile Vitamin with Beta Carotene Reptile Supplement	Yes	Yes	Dibasic Calcium Phosphate, Kelp Flour, Oyster Shell Flour, Calcium Carbonate, Bone Ash, L-Glutamic Acid, L-Aspartic Acid, L-Leucine, Iron Sulfate, Beta Carotene, L-Valine, L-Sarine, Choline Chloride, L-Lysine, L-Alanine, L-Phenyfalanine, L-Arginine, L-Isoleucine, Canthaxanthin, L-thereoline, L-Tyrosine, L-Proline, L-Methionine, Glycine, L-Cystine, Niacin, L-Histindine, Potassium Chlorine, Ascorbic Acid, Inositol, L-Tryptophan, Manganese Sulfate, Sodium Chloride, Zinc Sulfate, Thiamine Mononitrate, Para-Aminobenzoic Acid, Pyridoxine Hydrochloride, Apo-Carotenal, Rutin, Vitamin B_{12}, Magnesium Oxide, Copper Sulfate, Riboflavin, Calcium Pantothenate, DI-Alpha Tocopherol Acetate, Vitamin A Acetate, Sulfur, Calcium Iodate, Folic Acid, Hesperidin, Vitamin D_3, D-Biotin, Menadione Dimethylpyrimidinol Bisulfite.
National Geographic, Reptile Multivitamin Supplement Powder	Yes	Yes	Dicalcium Phosphate, Soy Protein Isolate, Calcium Carbonate (Ca 21%–25%, P 9%), Oyster Shell Flour, Calcaxanthin, Choline Chloride, Beta Carotene, Ferrous Sulfate, Kelp, Niacin, Potassium Chloride, Ascorbic Acid, Inositol, Vegetable Oil, DL-Methionine, Manganese Sulfate, Salt, Zinc Sulfate, Thiamine Mononitrate, Para–Aminobenzoic Acid, Pyridoxine HCl, Mixed Tocopherals, Rosemary Extract, Citric Acid, Magnesium Oxide, Riboflavin, Copper Sulfate, d–Calcium Pantothenate, Vitamin B_{12}, Vitamin E, Vitamin A (23,129 IU/kg), Vitamin D_3 (5,124 IU/kg), Vitamin E (49 IU/kg), Sulfur, Ethylenediamine Dihydriodide, Folic Acid, Natural and Artificial Flavoring, Neohespiridin Dihydrochalcone, Biotin, Menadione Sodium Bisulfite Complex Biotin, Vitamin B_{12}, Ascorbic Acid, Inositol
Nekton-Rep, Vitamin Mineral Supplement for Reptiles	Yes	No	Dextrose, Calcium Carbonate, Silicic Acid, Vitamin A (6,600,000 IU/kg), Vitamin D_3 (10,000 IU/kg), Vitamin E (6600 mg), Vitamin B_1, Vitamin B_2, Pantothenic acid, Nicotinamide, Vitamin B_6, Folic acid, Vitamin B_{12}, Vitamin C, Vitamin K_3, Menandione sodium bisulfate, Iron Zinc, Manganese, Copper, Iodine
Nekton, Multi-Rep	Yes	Yes	Dicalcium phosphate, Dextrose, Calcium Carbonate, Magnesium Carbonate, (Ca 21.3%, Phosphorus 7%), Vitamin A (200,000 IU/kg), Vitamin D_3 (40,000 IU/kg), Vitamin E (2,000 mg/kg), Vitamin B_1, Vitamin B_2, Pantothenic Acid (calcium-D pantothenate), Nicotinamide, Vitamin B_6, Folic Acid, Vitamin B_{12}, Biotin, Vitamin C, Selenium, Carnitine, Taurine, Choline Chloride, Iron, Zinc, Manganese, Copper, Iodine

Continued

TABLE 27.9 Alphabetical Listing by Manufacturer of Multivitamins Marketed for Reptiles and Amphibians—cont'd

Manufacturer, Name	Vitamin A Present?	All Multivitamins Present?	Ingredients
Repashey Superfood, Vitamin A Plus	Yes	No—Not listed as multivitamin	Calcium Carbonate, Kelp, Brewer's Yeast, Rose Hips, Calendula Flower, Marigold Flower, Paprika, Hibiscus Flower, Algae Meal, Turmeric, Rosemary Extract, Natural Fruit Flavor, Magnesium Amino Acid Chelate, Zinc Methionine Hydroxy Analogue Chelate, Manganese Methionine Hydroxy Analogue Chelate, Copper Methionine Hydroxy Analogue Chelate, Selenium, Yeast, Vitamin A Acetate (440,000 IU/kg), Vitamin D_3 (44,000 IU/kg), Calcium L-Ascorbyl-2-Monophosphate, Vitamin E (4400 IU/kg), Niacin, Beta Carotene, Pantothenic Acid, Riboflavin, Pyridoxine Hydrochloride, Thiamine Mononitrate, Menadione Sodium Bisulfite Complex, Folic Acid, Biotin, Vitamin B_{12}
Repashey Superfood, Vitamin A Plus LoD	Yes	Yes	Calcium Carbonate, Dried Kelp, Brewer's Yeast, RoseHips, Calendula Flower, Marigold Flower, Paprika, Hibiscus Flower, Algae Meal, Turmeric, Rosemary Extract, Natural Fruit Flavor, Magnesium Amino Acid Chelate, Zinc Methionine Hydroxy Analogue Chelate, Manganese Methionine Hydroxy Analogue Chelate, Copper Methionine Hydroxy Analogue Chelate, Selenium, Yeast, Potassium Iodide. Vitamin A (176,000 IU/kg), Vitamin D_3 (17,600 IU/kg), Calcium L-Ascorbyl-2-Monophosphate, Vitamin E (1760 IU/kg), Niacin, Beta Carotene, Pantothenic Acid, Riboflavin, Pyridoxine Hydrochloride, Thiamine Mononitrate, Menadione Sodium Bisulfite Complex, Folic Acid, Biotin, Vitamin B_{12}
Repashey Superfood, Vitamin A Plus HyD	Yes	Yes	Calcium Carbonate, Dried Kelp, Brewer's Yeast, RoseHips, Calendula Flower, Marigold Flower, Paprika, Hibiscus Flower, Algae Meal, Turmeric, Rosemary Extract, Natural Fruit Flavor, Magnesium Amino Acid Chelate, Zinc Methionine Hydroxy Analogue Chelate, Manganese Methionine Hydroxy Analogue Chelate, Copper Methionine Hydroxy Analogue Chelate, Selenium, Yeast, Potassium Iodide. Vitamin A (880,000 IU/kg), Vitamin D_3 (88,000 IU/kg), Calcium L-Ascorbyl-2-Monophosphate, Vitamin E (8800 IU/kg), Niacin, Beta Carotene, Pantothenic Acid, Riboflavin, Pyridoxine Hydrochloride, Thiamine Mononitrate, Menadione Sodium Bisulfite Complex, Folic Acid, Biotin, Vitamin B_{12}
Repashey Superfood, SuperVite	Yes	Yes	Cellulose Powder, Calcium Carbonate, Vitamin C, Vitamin A (440,000 IU/kg), Vitamin D_3 (44,000 IU/kg), Vitamin E (4400 IU/kg), Niacin, Beta Carotene (1100 IU/kg), Pantothenic Acid, Riboflavin, Pyridoxine Hydrochloride, Thiamine Mononitrate, Menadione Sodium Bisulfite Complex, Folic Acid, Biotin, Vitamin B_{12}, Vitamin K (Metadione), Choline
Rep-Cal's, Herptivite with Beta-carotene Multivitamins for All Reptiles and Amphibians	No	No	Glutamic Acid, Aspartic Acid, Leucine, Valine, Serine, Lysine, Alanine, Phenylalanine, Arginine, Isoleucine, Threonine, Tyrosine, Methionine, Proline, Glycine, Cysteine, Histidine, Alfalfa, Kelp, Calcium Carbonate, Dicalcium Phosphate, Ascorbic Acid, Potassium Chloride, Riboflavin Supplement, Thiamine Mononitrate, Pyridoxide Hydrochloride, Manganous Oxide, Sulfur, Zinc Oxide, Vitamin B_{12}, Copper Oxide, d-Calcium Pantothenate, Magnesium Oxide, Menadione Sodium Bisulfite Complex (source of Vitamin K activity), Biotin, Folic Acid
Vetark Professional, ACE-High	Yes	No—Not listed as a multivitamin	Vitamins A, Vitamin C, Vitamin E, Vitamin K, Vitamin B_1, Vitamin B_2, Vitamin B_6, Vitamin B_{12}, Folic, Nicotinic and Pantothenic Acids, Biotin, Choline, Niacin, Calcium, Phosporus, Sodium, Iron, Cobalt, Iodine, Magnesium, Zinc, Selenium, Copper
Vetark Professional, BSP Vitamin Drops	Yes	Yes	Vitamins A (retinyl acetate) 6,000,000 IU/L, Vitamin C, Vitamin E 9000 IU/L, Vitamin D_3 1,000,000 IU/L, Vitamin B_1, Vitamin B_2, Vitamin B_6, Vitamin B_{12}, Biotin, Folic Acid, Nicotinic Acid, Pantothenic Acid, Vitamin K_3
Vetark Professional, Nutrobal	Yes	Yes	Calcium Carbonate, Vitamin D3 (150,000 IU/kg), Vitamins A, C, E, K, B_1, B_2, B_6, B_{12}, Folic, Nicotinic & Pantothenic Acids, Biotin, Choline, Niacin, Phosporus, Sodium, Iron, Cobalt, Iodine, Magnesium, Zinc, Selenium, Copper
Zilla, Food Spray Vitamin Supplement	No	No	Water, Ascorbic Acid, Riboflavin, Calcium (60 ppm = 0.006%), Pantothenate, Pyridoxine Hydrochloride, Thiamine, Folic Acid, Vitamin D_3 (5 mg/kg), Beta Carotene (4 mg/kg), Niacin, Vitamin B_{12} Supplement, Potassium Iodide, Biotin
Zoo Med, Reptivite Reptile Vitamins with D_3	Yes/No (older versions did not have vitamin A)	No	Dicalcium Phosphate, Precipitated Calcium Carbonate, Maltodextrins, Salt, Potassium Chloride, Choline Bitartrate, Magnesium Oxide, L-Leucine, Manganese Sulfate, Ascorbic Acid, L-Arginine, L-Lysine Monohydrochloride, A-Tocopherol Acetate, L-Valine, L-Isoleucine, L-Threonine, L-Glutamine, L-Alanine, L-Glutamic Acid, Calcium Pantothenate, L-Phenylalanine, Dried Kelp, L-Tyrosine, Lecithin, Ferrous Fumarate, L-Cystine, L-Histidine, Glycine, DL-Methionine, L-Serine, L-Aspartic Acid, Niacin, Copper Sulfate, Zinc Oxide, Vitamin A Acetate, (220,264 IU/kg), Riboflavin, Vitamin D_3 (10,390 IU/kg), Thiamine Hydrochloride, Folic Acid, Pyridoxine Hydrochloride, Menadione Sodium Bisulfite Complex, Biotin, Vitamin B_{12}

"All multivitamins present" refers to 13 essential vitamins (vitamins A,C, D, E, and K, as well as vitamins B_1 thiamine, B_2 riboflavin, B_3 niacin, B_5 pantothenic acid, B_6 pyridoxine, B_7 biotin, B_9 folate/folic acid, and B_{12} cyanocobalamine).

TABLE 27.10 Calcium Supplements for Reptiles and Amphibians Listed Alphabetically By Manufacturer

Manufacturer, Calcium Supplement	Phosphorus Present?	Other Vitamins Besides Vitamin D₃ Present?	Ingredients
Aristopet, Repti-Cal	No	No	Calcium Carbonate, Vitamin D₃ (70,000 IU/kg)
Exo Terra Liquid Calcium-Magnesium Supplement	No	No	Water, Calcium Chloride, Magnesium Chloride, Calcium Lactate, 8%–8.5% Calcium
Exo Terra Calcium D₃	No	No	Calcium Carbonate, Oyster Shell Flour, Dextrose, Vitamin D3 (6,700 IU/kg)
Exo Terra Calcium	No	No	Calcium Carbonate, Oyster Shell Flour, Salt, Calcium Sulfate, Potassium Chloride, Ferrous Fumarate, Magnesium Oxide, Zinc Oxide, Manganous Oxide, Copper Sulfate
Flukers Repta-Calcium Dietary Supplement With Or Without Vitamin D₃	No	No	Limestone Flour, Flavor, Vitamin D₃ Or Limestone Flour, Flavor
Flukers Liquid Calcium Supplement For All Reptiles	No	No	Water, Calcium Chloride, Calcium Lactate. Calcium is 560 ppm = 0.06% Calcium Not Less Than 6%
Fluker's Calcium: Phosphorus	Yes	No	Dicalcium Phosphate, Limestone Flour, Vitamin D₃
Jurassipet Jurassical Reptile & Amphibian Dry Calcium Supplement	No	No	Calcium Carbonate
Lloyd Osteoform SA	Yes	Yes	Dicalcium Phosphate, Tricalcium Phosphate, Calcium Carbonate, (Ca 27%–32%, P 16.5%), Polysorbate 80, Citric Acid, Ascorbic Acid, Vitamin A Palmitate (328,571 IU/kg), Cholecalciferol (32,857 IU/kg)
Repashey Superfoods Ca Plus	No	No	Calcium Carbonate, Kelp, Brewer's Yeast, Rosehips, Calendula Flower, Marigold Flower, Paprika, Hibiscus Flower, Algae Meal, Turmeric, Rosemary Extract, Natural Fruit Flavor, Magnesium Amino Acid Chelate, Zinc Methionine Hydroxy Analogue Chelate, Manganese Methionine Hydroxy Analogue Chelate, Copper, Methionine Hydroxy Analogue Chelate, Selenium, Yeast Vitamins: Vitamin A, Vitamin D₃, Calcium L-Ascorbyl-2-Monophosphate, Vitamin E, Niacin, Beta Carotene, Pantothenic Acid, Riboflavin, Pyridoxine HCl, Thiamine Mononitrate, Menadione Sodium Bisulfite Complex, Folic Acid, Biotin, Vitamin B₁₂
Repashy Superfoods Supercal NoD	No	No	Calcium Carbonate, no Vitamin D
Repashy Superfoods Supercal LoD	No	No	Calcium Carbonate, Vitamin D₃ (4,545 IU/kg)
Repashy Superfoods Supercal MeD	No	No	Calcium Carbonate, Vitamin D₃ (11,354 IU/kg)
Repashy Superfoods Supercal HyD	No	No	Calcium Carbonate, Vitamin D₃ (22, 727 IU/kg)
Repashy Superfoods Rescuecal+ Liquid Calcium Supplement	No	No	Calcium Lactate Gluconate, Magnesium Lactate, Sucrose, Potassium Citrate, Malic Acid, Sodium Chloride, Potassium Sorbate Analysis (when mixed to 30% solution with water): Sucrose 40 mg/mL, Calcium 25 mg/mL, Magnesium 2.5 mg/mL, Sodium 1 mg/mL, Potassium 0.7 mg/mL, Chloride 0.1 mg /mL
Rep-Cal Original or Ultrafine Calcium powder with Vitamin D₃	No	No	Calcium Carbonate, Vitamin D₃
Rep-Cal Calcium without Vitamin D₃	No	No	Calcium Carbonate
TerraFauna, ReptoCal	Yes	Yes	Dicalcium Phosphate, Bone Meal, Calcium Carbonate, Oyster Shell Flour, Brewer's Yeast, Alfalfa Leaf Concentrate, Desiccated Liver, Vitamin D₃
T-Rex Bone Aid Liquid	No	No	Distilled Water, Calcium, Magnesium, Nature Identical Cricket Flavor, Potassium Sorbate, Sodium Benzoate
T-Rex 2:1 Calcium to Phosphorus Powdered Supplement with Vitamins	Yes	Yes	Dicalcium Phosphate, Bone Ash, Calcium Carbonate, Soy Flour, Bone Meal, Ascorbic Acid, Vitamin A Acetate, Vitamin D₃, Vitamin C, Stabilizers
T-Rex 2:0 Calcium/No Phosphorus Powdered Supplement with Vitamins	No	Yes	Calcium, no Phosphorus, Ascorbic Acid, Vitamin A Acetate, Vitamin D₃, Vitamin C, Stabilizers
Vetark Professional Calci-Dust	No	No	Calcium Carbonate
Vetark Professional Calcium Lactate	No	No	Calcium Lactate
Vetark Professionals Zolcal D	No	No	Calcium Borogluconate, Vitamin D, Magnesium

Continued

TABLE 27.10 Calcium Supplements for Reptiles and Amphibians Listed Alphabetically By Manufacturer—cont'd

Manufacturer, Calcium Supplement	Phosphorus Present?	Other Vitamins Besides Vitamin D₃ Present?	Ingredients
Zilla Food Spray Calcium Supplement	No	No	Water, Calcium Gluconate, Calcium Carbonate, Calcium Chloride, Potassium Sorbate, Sodium Benzoate, Xantham Gum
ZooMed, Repti Calcium with or without D3	No	No	Calcium Carbonate, Vitamin D₃ or Calcium Carbonate
Zoo Med Tortoise Calcium Block	Yes	Yes	Calcium Sulfate, Nopales (Spineless Opuntia Cactus), Carrot, Alfalfa, Dicalcium Phosphate, Niacin, Vitamin C, Thiamine HCl, D-Calcium Pantothenate, Pyridoxine Hydrochloride, Biotin, Beta-Carotene, Artificial Tropical Fruit Flavor, Yellow 5, Blue 1, Calcium 23.0%–28.0%

TABLE 27.11 Type of Calcium Can Be Important as not All are Absorbed Equally; Calcium Carbonate and Calcium Citrate are Best Absorbed

Ca Salt (1 gram)	Elemental Calcium (mg)	Percent Calcium Salt Absorbed or Elemental Ca Available
Ca carbonate	400	40%
Ca citrate	211	21%
Ca lactate	130	13%
Ca gluconate	93	9.3%
Ca glubionate	66	6.6%

a mildly salty, sour, or chalky taste (for humans), which may reduce palatability for herps. Therefore any herp Ca supplement should be P free or have a very high Ca:P ratio (>20:1). Furthermore, there are a number of similar-sounding products that make distinguishing Ca powders more confusing. For example, Rep-Cal (Rep-Cal Research Labs, Los Gatos, CA), ReptaCalcium (Flukers, Monroe, LA), and Repti-Calcium (Zoo Med, San Louis Obispo, CA), all have P-free Ca with and without vitamin D. Reptical (Aristopet, Brisbane, Australia) is a P-free Ca supplement with vitamin D, and ReptoCal (TetraFauna, Blacksburg, VA) has dicalcium phosphate with vitamin D (phosphate is a source of P). Note that one of these products has Ca and P, the other four do not. It is often difficult to distinguish among these products, therefore owners should bring supplements with their animal to the veterinarian's office and compare them to Tables 27.9 and 27.10.

The type of Ca used is also important as different kinds of Ca salts have different amounts of elemental Ca available for absorption and utilization. One gram of Ca carbonate has 40%, or 400 mg elemental Ca, available for absorption, followed by 1 gram of Ca citrate with 211 mg (Table 27.11). You would have to use almost three times as much Ca lactate to equal Ca carbonate in elemental Ca. Fortunately, Ca carbonate is the most commonly used Ca salt in Ca powders.

How well the product adheres to the insect depends on electrostatic properties and the fineness of grind. Finer particles adhere better than coarser particles. Companies manufacturing these supplements regard component particle sizes as commercially sensitive, but often the ingredients other than the calcium will be larger and will adhere for a much shorter time. Particle sizes can be appreciated on gross examination of most supplements.

NUTRITIONAL BIOLOGY

Although some particularly interesting exceptions exist, caecilians generally feed on earthworms and other invertebrates; frogs, toads, and salamanders feed almost exclusively on insects (at least as adults, tadpoles are detritivores); crocodilians feed largely on other vertebrates; turtles feed on a combination of plants and animals; and squamates feed largely on invertebrates or vertebrates.[12] Herbivory is uncommon, generally the exception within groups rather than the rule, except for Testudinidae, Iguanidae, and Leiolepidinae (Butterfly agamids).[12] Adult amphibians and reptiles do not necessarily eat the same prey as larvae or juveniles; ontogenetic shifts in diet are probably common but not well studied.[12] On a very simplistic level, reptile and amphibian diets can be categorized as insectivores, carnivores, herbivores, or omnivores. These can all be regarded as simply a means of obtaining the necessary amino acids, fatty acids, carbohydrate components, and more that make up a diet. Many reptiles have specialized dietary needs that require extensive appreciation of natural history. Some will have needs for certain components not yet identified. The following information serves as a foundation for most common species in captivity.

Insectivores

This group includes many lizards, most amphibians, some turtles, and a few snakes. Many obligate carnivorous adults may be insectivores as growing juveniles. Insectivory is a broad term that also includes consumption of arachnids, annelids, and crustaceans.[13] Nutrient levels of insects are listed in Table 27.12. Nutritional requirements of most insectivorous reptiles are unknown, so nutritionists often extrapolate from better-known species, such as the rat, or other carnivores, that have known NRC requirements.[14,15] Although these comparisons are unlikely to be appropriate for all insectivores, they do provide a basis for comparison. Deficiencies by nutrient (percentage of samples deficient vs. NRC rat growth requirements on a DMB) for fasted adult and nymphal house crickets (*Acheta domesticus*), superworms (*Zophobas morio* larvae), larval and adult mealworms (*Tenebrio molitor*), giant mealworms (*Tenebrio molitor* mealworm larvae treated with juvenile hormone to prevent them from molting into adults), waxworm larvae (*Galleria mellonella*), silkworm larvae (*Bombyx mori*), and earthworms (*Lumbricus terresstris*), were as follows: calcium (100%), vitamin D₃ (100%), vitamin A (89%), vitamin B₁₂ (75%), thiamin (63%), vitamin E (50%), iodine (44%), manganese (22%), methionine-cystine (22%), and sodium (11%).[15] Simply put, as dietary items, insects are Ca and multivitamin deficient. All invertebrates are a good source of protein and meet or exceed NRC requirements for growth in rats.[15] It is true that some of the protein nitrogen may be chitin, which forms the cuticle (exoskeleton) of invertebrates and may not be nutritionally available. However, some insectivores have chitinases, while others rely on gut bacterial chitinases.[13] Invertebrates contain little or no carbohydrates except silkworms fed a high (60%) carbohydrate diet.[15] Larval insects (except silkworm larvae) have high fat content (35%–60% DMB), especially mealworms, wax-worms, and butterworms (*Chilecomadia moorei*).[22] If these larvae constitute a substantial portion of the diet, this may lead to disproportion-ally high fat content.[13] Earthworms, silkworms, false katydids (Phaner-opterinae), adult fruit flies (*Drosophila*), wood louse (Oniscidea), termites (Isoptera), and krill (Euphausiacea) have lower fat content.[23] Insects contain significant quantities of fiber, highest in mealworms and lowest in silkworms and earthworms.[15] Invertebrates appear to be a good source of essential amino acids (except for superworms and waxworms, which are limited only in methionine and cysteine)[15] and adequate sources of trace minerals copper, iron, manganese, and zinc.[14]

Calcium and vitamin A and D levels of insects are below the NRC requirements for rat growth[15,22] and carnivores.[14] Consequently Ca and vitamin A deficiencies are the most common nutritional diseases of both reptiles and amphibians. One study found that juvenile veiled chameleons (*Chamaeleo calyptratus*) fed locusts (*Locusta migratoria*) with adequate artificial UVB developed symptoms of NSHP (if no supplemental Ca, vitamin A, or vitamin D_3 was provided to locusts) within 152 to 186 days, and even faster if no UVB was present (within 110 to 146 days).[24] When Ca, vitamin A, and UVB were supplemented, chameleons did not develop NSHP, and the best results were in cha-meleons supplied with Ca, vitamins A and D, and UVB. Healthy Ca to P ratios for most vertebrates are generally 2:1 to 3:1 but may be higher for growing herps. For example, rapidly growing juvenile saltwater crocodiles (*Crocodylus porosus*) eat insects, amphibians, crustaceans, small reptiles, fish, and rats, with an overall Ca:P ratio of 6.7 to 1, primarily because of the calcium-rich crustacean shells. Adult saltwater crocodiles consume more mammals and fish but fewer crabs and shrimp, and consequently the Ca to P ratio of their diet drops to 1.85 to 1.[25] Ca:P ratios of commonly fed insects are as follow: 0.2 crickets, 0.1 mealworms and waxworms, and 0.06 super mealworms. All analyzed insects are Ca deficient, with few exceptions. Cocooning eastern tent moths (*Malacosoma americanum*), stone flies (Plecoptera), and black soldier fly larvae (*Hermetia illucens*, sold as Phoenix worms) all have a higher Ca content,[14,18] but only the last is commercially available. When fed to mountain chicken frogs (*Leptodactylus fallax*) the calcium digest-ibility of whole soldier fly larvae was only 44%, compared with 88% for soldier fly larvae that had been "mashed" to expose calcium in mineralized exoskeletons.[18,26]

So, for client discussions, it is appropriate to say all insects are severely Ca deficient (Fig. 27.1). Earthworms, night crawlers (*Lumbricus terrestris*), and terrestrial crustaceans (Isopods), such as the wood louse (*Porcellio scaber*) and pill bugs, or roly-polies (*Armadillidium* spp.), all have positive Ca:P ratios.[15,22] Crustacean shells are good sources of amorphous calcium carbonate, which is reported to have higher bioavailability than crystalline calcium carbonate.[23]

All analyzed insects are vitamin A deficient with the exception of false katydids (e.g., greater angle-wing katydid, *Microcentrum rhombi-folium*), migratory locust (*Locusta migratoria*), termites (*Nasutitermes* spp.), silkworms, and four other wild-caught species of lepidopteran larvae, which may be able to convert β-carotene to vitamin A.[15,22] Insects are also vitamin D deficient,[15] which is not a problem because most insectivores are kept under UVB lights and should also receive Ca dusted and gut-loaded prey (discussed later). Interestingly, nocturnal geckos, such as the leopard gecko, have the ability to utilize UVB light but also appear to thrive utilizing only dietary vitamin D.

Compared to NRC requirements for growing rats, most invertebrates contain sufficient vitamin E (except mealworms and superworms) and trace minerals, except superworms, giant mealworm larvae, waxworms,

and silkworms, which are deficient in iodine.[15] Vitamin B_{12} is below the NRC requirements for growing rats for all larval insects. Thiamine is below the NRC requirements for growing rats in crickets, superworms, and giant and adult mealworm larvae.[15]

From this discussion it is obvious that commercially available invertebrates and annelids are nutritionally incomplete.[15] Feeding herps store-bought crickets and mealworms without supplementation will result in calcium or vitamin A deficiencies and may induce obesity and hepatic lipidosis. Improving insectivore nutrition is a simple triad of feeding a nutritionally complete, calcium-rich diet to insects, dusting insects with calcium (and, less frequently, multivitamins), and feeding a wide variety of insects, crustaceans, annelids, and rodent pups. Both gut loading and dusting are recommended to provide more balanced nutrition and boost Ca. One case of hypovitaminosis A in a panther chameleon (*Furcifer pardalis*) resulted from refusal of the chameleon to eat multivitamin-dusted insects until 2 hours after they had been offered, enough time for the insects to groom off the multivitamins (Boyer, personal observation). Providing a gut-loading diet resolved the problem.

Gut-Loading Insects. Originally, feeding a Ca-rich diet to improve the insect's Ca content was called gut loading.[27] Early studies in feeder insects demonstrated that feeding high Ca diets (≥8% Ca DM) increased the Ca content and developed a positive Ca:P ratio after 24 hours (mealworms), 48 hours (crickets), or 72 hours (waxworms).[27-29] Higher Ca levels (12%) result in poor viability of mealworms, and Ca levels begin to decline after a week of high-Ca diets.[30] Unfortunately, over time, the term gut loading has lost its original meaning and degenerated into just feeding crickets, often with foods rich in β-carotene (even though crickets and some insectivores do not convert β-carotene to vitamin A). For instance, feeding mealworms and crickets a 3% Ca DM diet with a 2.8 Ca:P ratio for 72 hours resulted in a mean Ca:P ratio of 0.19 for mealworms and 0.26 for crickets (i.e., negative Ca:P ratios).[30] Not all cricket diets designed to boost Ca content are equal. In one study, three out of four commercial calcium-fortified dry diets designed for feeder crickets contained no more calcium than unfortified diets.[31] Despite claims on their labels, only one diet actually increased the calcium content of the crickets (T-Rex Calcium Plus Food for Crickets).[31] Calcium-fortified, high-moisture cricket waters or high-moisture foods (gel water cubes) are also ineffective at increasing calcium content.[32] A typical cube has 600 ppm Ca or 0.06% Ca, about twice the content of tap water. One study noted that as fed, gel water cube labels claimed 0.1% to 0.12% Ca but when analyzed were found to have only 0.01% Ca and caused some mealworms to asphyxiate. Another problem with gel water cubes is that insects, as well as reptiles, will consume them preferentially over high-Ca diets. Instead of gel water cubes, offer water, such as a water-soaked cotton ball in a bottle cap (for crickets and roaches) or damp paper towel (for mealworms or superworms) (Fig. 27.2). One of the reasons cubes became popular is that insects drown in standing water. The same study found that by day 3 mealworms on a Ca-fortified insect diet and offered either apple slices or gel water cubes had a mean negative Ca:P ratio of 0.62 and 0.91, respectively. Presumably, the mealworms ate more apples and gel cubes and less Ca-fortified diet (see Fig. 27.2). Therefore do not offer fruit, vegetables, or gel water cubes as a water source to feeder insects. Additionally, fruit and vegetables tend to mold and may result in aflatoxin ingestion by the insects and accumulation by herps. Assume store-bought insects are nutritionally inadequate at purchase. Mealworms are typically shipped and sold in 100% wheat bran, with 0.14% Ca and a Ca:P ratio of 0.12, or even worse, inedible saw dust. Only mealworms and superworms fed a high-calcium cricket feed met NRC dietary calcium recommendations for nonlactating rats; those fed wheat millings, avian hand-feeding formula, or organic avian mash diet

TABLE 27.12 Nutrient Levels of Insects

	Typical Body Mass (g)	Water (%)	DM (%)	Crude Protein %	Crude Fat %	Total Nitrogen (% DM)	CHITIN BOUND ADF-N (% DM)	NDF (% DM)	Ash (% DM)	ME (kcal/g)	Ca (%)	P (%)
Traditional "Feeder Insects"												
Mealworm (*Tenebrio molitor*)	0.126	61.9	38.1	49.1	35	-	6.6	15	2.4	5.395	0.0444	0.748
	0.136	63.7	36.3	65.3	14.9	-	20.4	31.7	3.3	3.796	0.0636	0.763
Giant mealworm	0.304	61	39	47.2	43.1	-	6.4	7.4	3.1	5.774	0.0472	0.697
Superworm (*Zophobas morio*)	0.61	57.9	42.1	46.8	42	-	6.3	9.3	2.4	5.755	0.042	0.5629
Moth Larvae												
Silkworm (*Bombyx mori*)	1.04	82.7	17.3	53.8	8.1	-	6.4	6.4	6.4	3.896	0.102	1.37
Hornworm (*Manduca* spp., probably *sexta*)				60	17-21.5				7.68-8.4			
Butterworm/trevo/tebo (*Chilecomadia moorei*)	0.392	60.2	39.8	38.9	73.9	-	3.5	6.6	1.9	7.479	0.0314	0.565
Waxworm (*Galleria mellonella*)	0.314	58.5	41.5	34	60	-	8.1	19.2	1.4	6.6	0.059	0.47
Commercial Cricket (*Acheta domestica*)												
Pinhead/juvenile	<0.01	66.8±9.8	33.2	55*	9.8±1.4	8.8±0.5	0.6±0.1	16.4±5.6	9.1±6.7	-	1.29±2.26	0.79±0.19
Adults	0.2	73.2±1.9	26.8	64.38*	22.8±1.5	10.3±0.4	0.7±0.1	19.1±2.5	5.1±1.4	-	0.21±0.03	0.78±0.08
Fly Larvae												
Soldier fly larvae (*Hermetia illucens*)	0.082	61.2	38.8	45.1	36.1	-	7.6	9.7	9	5.139	2.407	0.917
Housefly pupae (*Musca domestica*)	<0.01	67.1±3.5	32.9	56.25*	17.9±3	9±0.1	1±0.3	16.2±1.5	5.2±0.7		0.14±0.22	1.1±0.05
Fruit fly (*Drosophila melanogaster*) adult	-	74.8	25.2	78.2	7.5	-	11.5	14.4	6.8	3.644	0.304	1.476
Turkestan/Rusty Red Roaches (*Blatta lateralis*)	0.153	69.1	30.9	61.5	32.4	-	7	8.9	3.9	5.183	0.125	0.569
Earthworms												
Earthworm (*Lumbricus terrestris*) "wild"	1.1±0.7	74.5±2	25.5	32.5*	12.6±1	5.2±1.1	0.2±0.1	51.2±6.3	45.7±6.6	-	0.97±0.28	0.79±0.13
Commercial	2.9±1.1	75.8±4.8	24.2	50.6*	10.6±1.7	8.1±1.5	0.3±0.1	20.9±13.2	24.9±11.4	-	1.21±0.03	0.86±0.15
Red wrigglers/ brandlings (*Eisenia fetida*)	204	83.6	16.4	64	9.8	-	0.6	-	3.7	4.32	0.27	0.97
Aquatic Invertebrates												
Tubifex spp.	-	88.2	11.8	46.1	15.1	-	-	-	6.9		0.19	0.73
Northern crayfish (*Orconectes virilis*)	-	74.31±4.16	25.69	54.1±4.14	2.96±1.47	-	13.7±0.66	17.27±0.95	35.69±4.42	-	12±1.79	1.16±0.04
Freshwater prawn (*Macrobrachium rosenbergii*) (cultured)	43–138	77.1	22.9	74.85	9.15	-	-	-	10.14		-	-

**= Calculated from values in Finke 2002.[15]

GE = Gross energy, determined in the lab rather than calculated using Atwater.

Crude protein (marked *) has been calculated by total nitrogen x 6.

ADF-N is considered to be chitin-bound nitrogen and so is unavailable to many species; crude protein (adjusted) may be more accurately calculated by deducting ADF-N from total nitrogen.

Insect exoskeletons contain not just chitin but also sclerotized protein, fat, and other compounds. Some species have chitinases.

Thiaminase has been reported in a wide range of genera, freshwater and marine, vertebrate and invertebrate. It has been demonstrated to vary through the year.

Mg (%)	Cu (mg/kg)	Fe (mg/kg)	Zn (mg/kg)	Mn (mg/kg)	Vitamin A (IU/kg)	Vitamin D3 (IU/kg)	Vitamin E (IU/kg)	Carotenoid (mg/kg)	Presence of Thiaminase	Source
0.21	16	54.1	136.5	13.6	811±324	-	30±3	-	-	14, Finke, unpublished data
0.167	20.6	60.1	127.3	11	-	-	-	-	-	14, Finke, unpublished data
0.2215	16.4	55.1	114.1	9.2	-	-	-	-	-	14, Finke, unpublished data
0.118	8.6	39.2	72.9	10.2	972±570	-	32±6	-	-	14, Finke, unpublished data
0.29	20.8	95.4	177.5	24.9	9133	<1479**	51.4	<1.16**	Yes (low)	Finke, unpublished data, 15, 16, 17
0.0698	7.4	35.2	89.7	1.8	-	399.5	48.7	1.4	-	Finke, unpublished data
0.076	9.2	50.4	61.2	3.2	150±160	-	509±232	-	-	14, Finke, unpublished data
0.16±0.04	9.61±1.74	196.8±79.75	159.06±14.97	52.76±17.83	471±585	-	71±42	-	-	14
0.08±0.01	8.5±1.01	112.33±58.1	186.36±16.48	29.65±4.54	811±849	-	81±41	-	-	14
0.4485	10.3	171.6	144.8	159.3	-	257	23.7	-	-	Finke, unpublished data
0.13±0.02	8.66±3.98	454.22±50.91	146.95±71.05	16.09±2.68	ND	-	23±13	-	-	14
0.319	51.2	496	340.5	105.6	-	395.6	175.4	-		
0.0809	25.7	47.9	105.8	8.5	-	624.6			-	Finke, unpublished data, 18
0.31±0.03	32.86±17.88	11087.45±2938.07	270.8±88.94	199.4±44.86	2400±279	-	70±12	-	-	14
0.19±0.03	8.09±1.66	5801.76±2323.5	231.15±55.54	113.13±51.04	328±171	-	229±82	-	-	14
0.083	9.4	307.3	107.9	7.9	-	-	-	-	-	Finke, unpublished data
0.09	108	1702	190	30	-	-	-	-	-	13
0.4±0.06	107.44±12.19	133.78±53.6	87.78±6.04	108.44±101.15	1619.26±237.06	-	478.24±220.34	54.67±16.88	-	13
-	-	-	-	-	-	-	-	-	Yes	19, 20

To convert a nutrient analysis from "as fed" to "dry matter," see Box 27.1

Thiaminase has been reported in a wide range of genera, freshwater and marine, vertebrate and invertebrate. It has been demonstrated to vary through the year.

- 1 mg alpha tocopherol = 1.1 IU, and 0.3 µg retinol = 1 IU vitamin A activity
  mg/kg = µg/g
- Gross energy (GE) calculated by adding the product of % crude protein x 5.43 kcal/g to the product of % crude fat x 9.11 kcal/g.[4,21]

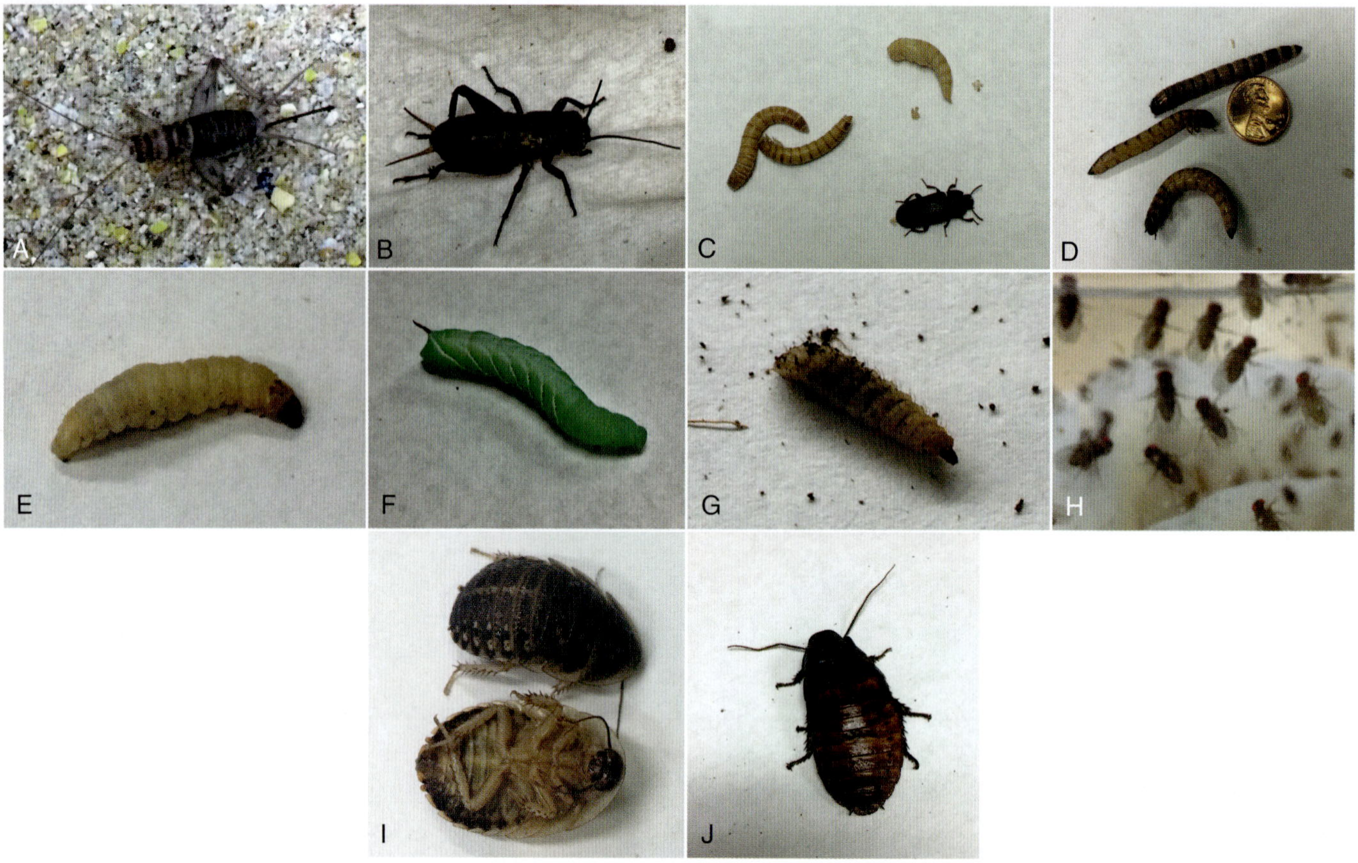

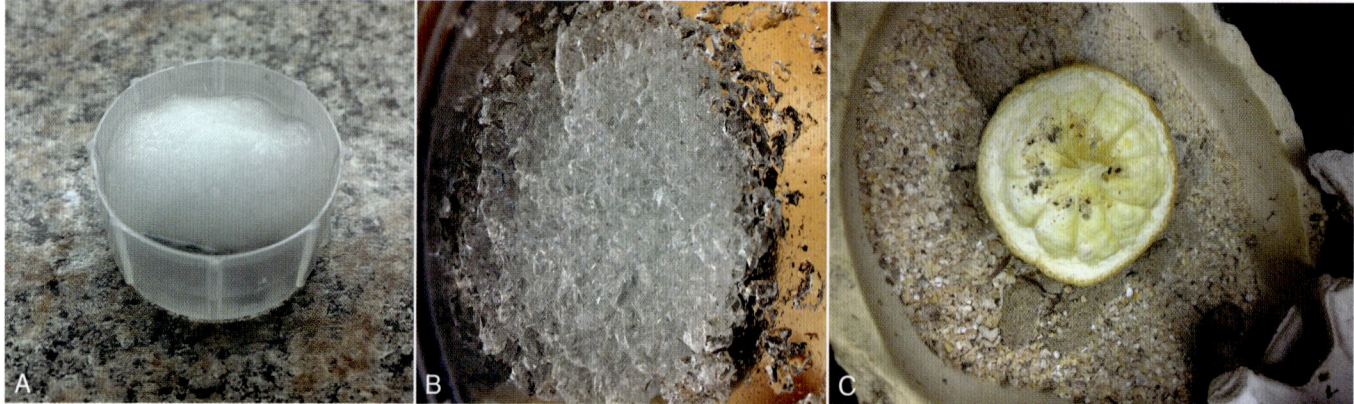

FIG 27.1 Practically speaking, almost all insects are calcium deficient (approximately 1 Ca:5 to 10 P for most insects) and must be fed a diet greater than 8% Ca to develop a positive Ca:P ratio. Note that gut loading does not mean mere feeding; it entails providing a diet fortified with high levels of calcium, as well as multivitamins and trace minerals. Common feeder insects include (A) house or gray crickets (*Acheta domesticus*); (B) black field crickets (*Gryllus bimaculatus*); (C) mealworms (*Tenebrio molitor*), larvae, instar, and beetle; (D) superworms (*Zophobas morio* larvae); (E) waxworm larvae (*Galleria mellonella*); (F) tobacco hornworms or goliath worms (*Manduca sexta*); (G) black soldier fly larvae or Phoenix worms (*Hermetia ilucens*); (H) fruitflies (*Drosophila melanogaster* or *D. hydei*) and cockroaches; (I) dubias (*Blaptica dubia*); and (J) hissing cockroaches (*Gromphadorhina portentosa*).

FIG 27.2 (A) All insects need water; a cotton ball in a bottle cap works for crickets and cockroaches, a damp paper towel on the surface of the gut-loading diet works for mealworms and superworms. (B) Cubes are not recommended because they are consumed preferentially over gut-loading diets, do not change the nutritional profile of the insect, and some insects can choke on them. (C) When gut-loading insects, offer only water (not cubes) and the gut-loading diet, nothing else. Good gut-loading diets have a high Ca content and probably reduced palatability. If better-tasting foods are available, such as fruits or vegetables, the insects will eat them, avoiding the gut-loading diet.

did not.[33] Owners should purchase a high-quality, gut-loading diet (such as Mazuri Hi Calcium Gut Loading Diet) or veterinarians should buy, stock, and supply such products. Food products should be appropriately stored in a cool dry area, refrigerator (4°C, 39°F), or freezer (−20°C, −4°F) and discarded after expiration dates (varies with manufacturer but typically 6–12 months).[27] Crickets, mealworms, superworms, and Dubia cockroaches (*Blaptica dubia*) can be maintained on cricket high-Ca (≥8% Ca DM) diets, even though these diets are not intended as maintenance diets, and Ca content of feeders declines after a week. Newer commercial gut-loading diets can produce a positive Ca:P ratio as quickly as 12 hours, compared with experimental diets that required several days. Be sure to use a Ca-enriched diet (such as Mazuri Hi Calcium Gut Loading Diet, 8%–9% Ca) and not a maintenance diet (such as Mazuri Cricket Diet, 1% Ca). Remember, water is the most essential nutrient, and insects will die rapidly without it. Feeder insects should not be refrigerated; they should be maintained at their preferred optimum temperature zone, when in doubt, around 27°C (80°F). Refrigeration merely extends shelf life without essential nutritional supplementation. Feeding starved insects will result in a malnourished reptile, even though the reptile is still eating. For crickets, a temperature range of 26°C to 34°C (79°F to 93°F), with a vertical temperature gradient from top to bottom is desirable (easily provided with egg flats or other cage furniture), and a relative humidity of 20% to 50%.[34,35]

Many of the gut-loading studies produced variable results on final nutrient content (especially Ca:P) because of variations in insect age (crickets do not feed readily in the last week of life), food or insect size (smaller insects cannot consume larger food particles, gut capacity is slightly higher relative to body weight for nymphal stage vs adult crickets), or developmental stage (where the insect is in its instar; see later), temperature (higher or lower temperatures may adversely affect food intake; optimum temperature maximizes food intake and growth), sex (female crickets develop faster than males), water sources or lack of water (water cubes, produce, or fruit decreases consumption of gut-loading diets, as does a lack of water), humidity, and, of course, palatability.[34,35] Perhaps the most important is developmental stage. All insects grow through various life stages by shedding their exoskeleton. The time between sheds is called an instar, or growth period. Crickets begin feeding about 6 hours after shedding, then feed well until about mid-instar, at which point they have filled their exoskeleton and reached their critical weight to get through molting. At this stage, they reduce feeding until after the next molt. Instars can last days (at 35°C or 95°F) to weeks (at 28°C or 82°F), last longer in older crickets, and have obvious implications on how well the insect can be gut loaded.[34,35] Practically the best way to minimize these variables is to gut load all insects, with the hope that short-term deficiencies will be corrected over the long term. Additionally, it is important to consistently dust insects and provide a variety of different species. If insects are left in the cage for more than a few hours, a gut-loading diet and water should always be available.

Dusting Insects.

An additional essential method of improving Ca, or vitamin content, is dusting insects with calcium or multivitamins (Fig. 27.3). To dust, insects and the Ca, or multivitamin powder, are placed in a plastic bag, or deep plastic cup, and lightly shaken or swirled, until the insects are coated. This method can produce variable results depending on the type of calcium or multivitamin used (e.g., particle size and electrostatic properties). One study found crickets would groom off 50% of either multivitamin/mineral or calcium/vitamin D powder within 90 seconds of dusting.[36] A larger study involving two cricket species (*Gryllus bimaculatus* and *G. assimilis*), and multiple life stages, found dusting with Ca boosted Ca:P ratio above 1:1 for 5.5 hours (endpoint of study).[37] There were no statistically significant differences between the dusting powders, but there were differences between cricket

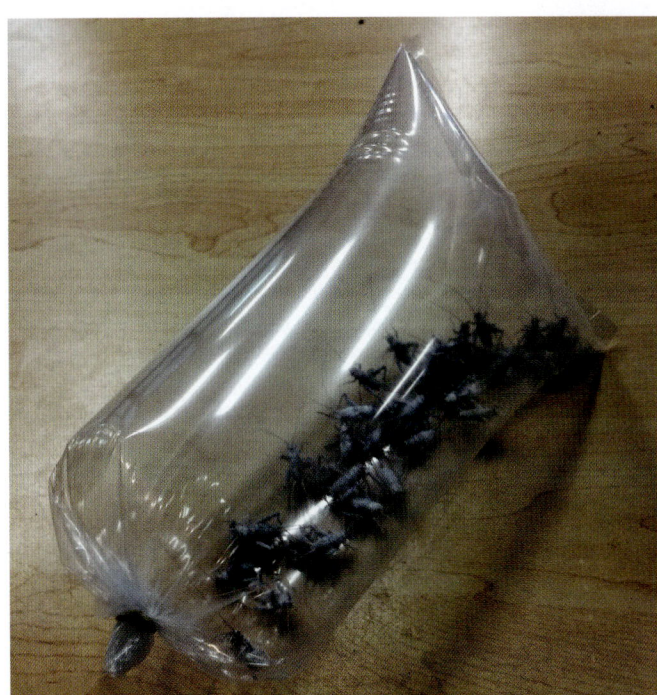

FIG 27.3 Dusting insects with Ca is recommended every feeding, in addition to gut loading, to further boost Ca content. Insects can be dusted with multivitamins once or twice per month. Some insectivores will avoid multivitamin dusted insects for several hours until the insects have groomed off the multivitamins, thus gut loading is also important.

species and life stages. Overall, adult black field crickets (*Gryllus bimaculatus*) were the least effective at delivering calcium, with Ca:P ratio barely exceeding 2:1 immediately after dusting and eventually declining to just below 1:1, whereas hatchlings of both species were the most effective, with Ca:P ratios remaining above 4:1 for at least 5.5 hrs. Other instars of both species were intermediate.[37]

Dusting insects in environments with high humidity is less effective and generally ineffective for aquatic insectivores unless they take insects off the water surface.[38] Multivitamins do not contain enough Ca to prevent NSHP, regardless of what the label claims. Calcium carbonate has the most elemental Ca (see Ca discussion earlier) and is most useful. Little to no P should be present in the Ca supplement as insects are already high in P; vitamin D is generally not required if appropriate UVB is present. Dusting can be effective in raising calcium; however, unless the other component vitamins in the product are of equal size and electrostatic charge, they may not adhere to the insects for long.

Insect Variety.

The third vital aspect of feeding insectivores, in addition to gut loading and dusting, is to offer a wide variety of insects (see Fig. 27.1). Senegalese chameleons (*Chamaeleo senegalensis*) maintained on grasshoppers (*Scuderia* spp.) developed a statistically significant preference for crickets (*Acheta domestica*).[39] Jamaican anoles (*Anolis lineatopus*) experienced significantly higher growth rates when they ate a variety of insect larvae species compared to just a monoculture diet.[40] Insectivores naturally consume a diverse diet. Individual chameleons that steadfastly refuse crickets may immediately take a novel insect. Store-bought insects such as crickets, waxworms, mealworms, super mealworms, and Dubia cockroaches should be supplemented with commercially available silkworms, black soldier fly larvae (Phoenix worms), tobacco or tomato horn worms (*Manduca sexta* and *M. quinquemaculata*), bean beetles (*Callosobruchus maculates*), fruit flies, springtails (Collembolands), and wood lice (e.g., European wood lice, *Porcellio scaber*; dwarf tropical wood lice, *Trichorhina tomentosa*), as well as wild-caught, seasonally available insects such as moths, cicadas, flies, grasshoppers, bees (remove stingers), cockroaches, and crustaceans. Insects are easily collected at night around lights, with funnel traps or by children, and pill bugs accumulate in damp soil under a piece of shaded plywood. Owners often are overly concerned about pesticide hazards, but this is rarely ever a problem. Fireflies (*Photinus* sp.) contain toxic lucibufagins, and deaths have been reported in bearded dragons (*Pogona vitticeps*), a panther chameleon (*Furcifer pardalis*), Derjugin's lizard (*Darevskia derjugini*) and a White's tree frog (*Litoria caerulea*) following ingestion.[41] Many insectivores can be trained, or naturally take, baby mice and annelids, which are excellent dietary supplements. It is recommended that owners feed as wide a variety of invertebrates as possible, not just two or three varieties.

In summary, veterinarians should advise insectivore owners that almost all insects are deficient in Ca and vitamins A and D, and larval insects can have inappropriately high fat levels if fed exclusively. Broad-spectrum lighting including UVB is recommended for all insectivores. Gut-loading insects (i.e., feeding a nutrient-dense diet with ≥8% Ca DM, for 12 hours to 5 days, but no longer than 7 days) is essential. Proactive veterinary involvement, such as stocking a good gut-loading product, may be required to ensure compliance. Calcium dusting of insects is a good way to boost Ca and is recommended to augment gut loading.[35] Multivitamins must have, but are also limited by, their vitamin A content. Multivitamins are regularly needed for all reptiles (especially insectivores) not eating dry formulated feeds or whole vertebrates. A wide variety of foods is necessary to keep insectivores healthy.

Carnivores

This group includes all snakes, crocodilians, adult amphibians, and most aquatic turtles and lizards. Carnivores require high levels of protein (25%–60%) and fat (30%–60%) and low levels of carbohydrates (<10% DM).[8,42]

Snakes. One reason snakes remain popular is that rodents are a completely balanced diet and are easily procured. Therefore snakes are easier to provide a healthy, well-balanced diet for, and nutritional diseases are uncommon. See Table 27.13 for nutrient levels of whole vertebrates. Nutritionists consider whole vertebrate animals nutritionally complete foods that do not require supplementation.[43,50] Most pet stores, as well as numerous online vendors, sell frozen mice and rats, in all sizes. Veterinarians should be aware of different rodent life stages as owners often ask what size rodent to feed (Fig. 27.4). Pinkies are neonatal rodents (*Mus musculus* and *Rattus norvegicus*) without fur and have been found to have an almost even Ca:P ratio (slightly negative to slightly positive). After 5 to 9 days mice develop fur to become fuzzies, and from then on have a positive Ca to P ratio. After 2 to 2.5 weeks, mice open their eyes and are known as hoppers (because of their propensity to jump when startled). By 21 to 25 days they wean and are known as weanlings or small adults, then on to large and extra-large adults. Rodents and other whole animal prey should be frozen in moisture-impermeable plastic or vacuum packed to reduce dehydration during storage.[43] Frozen whole animals should be completely thawed and warmed before feeding to prevent a bacterial bloom in the prey's gut. This also occurs commonly if rodents are allowed to thaw over several hours at room temperature. Feeding cold or partly frozen prey is not recommended, as it can cause gastrointestinal dysfunction and slow digestion. For the die-hard reptile breeder still producing their own rodents, it is recommended to feed commercial pelleted rodent diets, not seed mixes or dog food (which can pass on nutritional deficiencies to the predator). Feeding live prey, although legal in the United

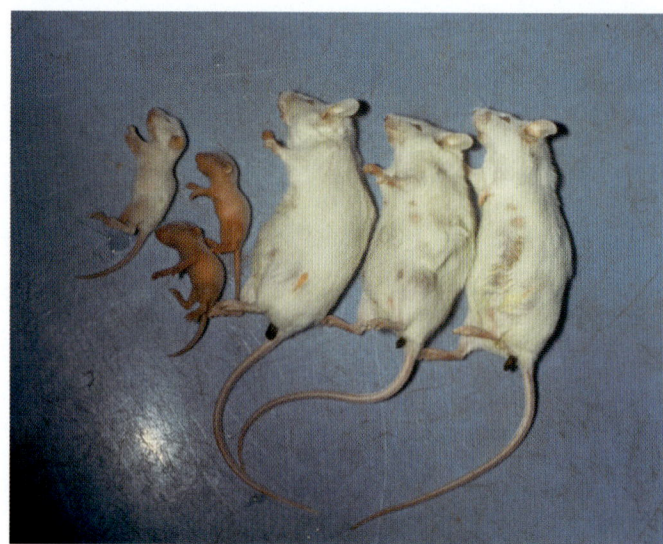

FIG 27.4 Rodents come in a variety of sizes from pinkies, fuzzies, hoppers, and small and large adults and can be purchased frozen from most pet stores. From left to right, fuzzies, pinkies, and small adult mice. (Courtesy of Don Boyer).

States, is ethically unacceptable in most countries and should be avoided. The feeding of live prey has been the subject of much discussion; see Cooper[51] for the welfare and ethics of feeding live prey. Prey should be killed (cervical dislocation or gassed with CO_2) prior to feeding.[52] Serious trauma can be inflicted by a live rodent on a reptile (Fig. 27.5). Given the choice, boids and colubrids may prefer thawed mice over freshly killed ones.[53] Rabbits, hamsters, gerbils, chicks, lizards, snakes, frogs, toads, or fish are also appropriate food items. It is important for owners to appreciate the natural history of the species to identify food preferences. Muscle meat and viscera lack bone and therefore have little Ca. For example, Ca:P ratios of chicken meat (0.08:1), hamburger (0.06:1), chicken liver (0.14:1), and gizzards (0.1:1) are all inadequate for bone growth or maintenance.

An interesting digestive strategy has been noted in pythons.[54] As digestion of a meal begins, the snake's metabolic rate rises dramatically as a result of the energy requirements of digestion, known as the specific dynamic action (SDA). The python selectively digests the protein components first, releasing amino acids for oxidation (even if the prey has been through a blender). These amino acids provide the immediate needs of the SDA, with digestion of lipids occurring more slowly. Previously, it was assumed that the needs of the SDA were met from endogenous stores. The fatty acids released are then stored and used as an energy source during times of the prolonged fasting, which is common in these ambush predators.

Hatchling snakes often refuse pinkies, and several sequential tricks can be used to induce feeding. Handling should be curtailed, and at least one hide box should be present in the enclosure. A pink mouse can be left in the cage overnight. Washing, to remove all rodent scent, and/or then scenting a pink mouse with the preferred natural prey (such as lizards for king snakes and milk snakes [*Lampropeltis* spp.]; toads for hognoses [*Heterodon* spp.]; or fish for garter, ribbon, [*Thamnophis* spp] or water snakes [*Nerodia* spp]). Scenting involves rubbing, or attaching a small amount of skin, or limb, from the preferred prey onto the pink mouse, especially around the head. "Braining" also works well, even in snakes that have steadfastly refused pinkies. Brain material is forced out the pink mouse's nostrils or through a skull incision, onto

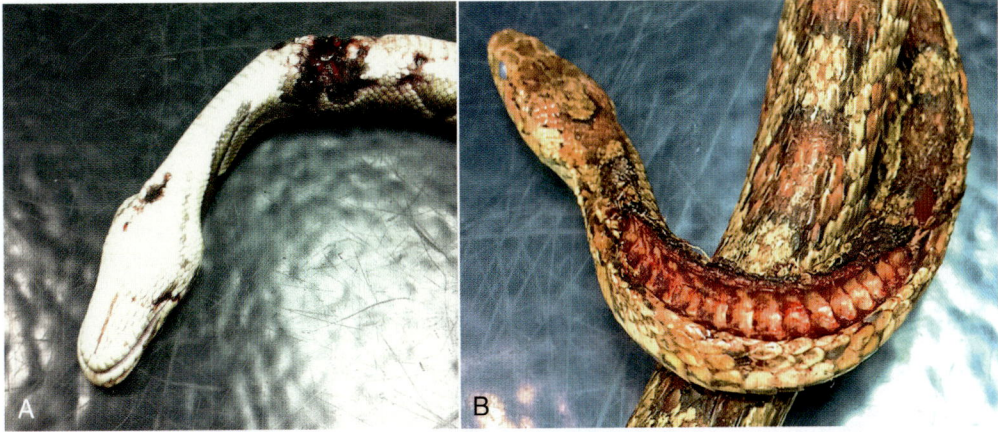

FIG 27.5 (A, B) Live prey should be humanely killed by cervical dislocation or gassed with CO_2, prior to feeding. Alternatively, rodents can be purchased frozen and thawed completely before feeding. Feeding live prey can result in serious injury to reptiles.

the snout, and presented close to the snake, or left in the cage overnight. Tongue flicking by the snake of the pinky brain seems to be a super optimal stimulus releaser for feeding.

Fish is often used as a food for snakes, turtles, and crocodilians. Whole fish are relatively good sources of most nutrients except for thiamine and vitamin E.[48] Thiaminases, enzymes that destroy or inactivate thiamin, are present in many marine animals, such as clams, herring, smelt, and mackerel.[48] The recommended supplementation is 25 mg to 30 mg thiamine per kg of wet fish. Trout and most freshwater fish do not contain thiaminases and do not require thiamin supplementation. Vitamin E is abundant in fresh fish, but oxidation of fish lipids while frozen can deplete vitamin E content.[50] Much of the vitamin E can be destroyed after a few weeks of freezing, and frozen fish should be used within 4 to 6 months.[48] The recommended level of supplementation is 100 IU of vitamin E per kg of wet fish. Many freshwater reptiles will not eat saltwater fish. The types of fish fed should be varied, and many piscivores will also eat rodents, snails, slugs, earthworms, shrimp, krill (frozen, not freeze dried), or pelleted commercial diets. Aquatic turtles do well on fish-based aquatic turtle pellets (see Table 27.6), earthworms, waxworms, mealworms, crickets, whole fish (freshly killed guppies or minnows, chopped trout, and freshwater smelt [Fig. 27.6], whole shrimp, and pinkies or chopped skinned mice. Goldfish are not recommended due to frequent infection with *Mycobacteria*. Many sliders and cooters will take dark leafy greens as they get older.

Crocodilians. Nutritional studies of saltwater crocodiles (*Crocodylus porusus*) reveal average diets to be 70% water, 13% to 15% protein, 3% to 4% fat, and with a Ca:P ratio of 2–7:1, which are similar to other crocodilians.[55,56] Crocodilians are generalist opportunistic carnivores, which eat a wide variety of prey. Gharials (*Gavialis gangeticus*) are the singular exception, being largely fish specialists. Hatchlings feed mostly on small prey items such as insects, spiders, crustaceans, fish, and amphibians; adults feed mainly on larger prey (fish, crustaceans, mammals, reptiles, and birds). Small crocodilians typically stay in shallow, warmer water. Hatchling American alligators (*Alligator missippiensis*) have metabolic rates 25 times that of large adult males. Consequently, they need about 25 times more food per unit of body weight, have faster digesta transit times, and higher food conversion rates.[56] Food is not chewed by crocodilians but swallowed whole or as large chunks;

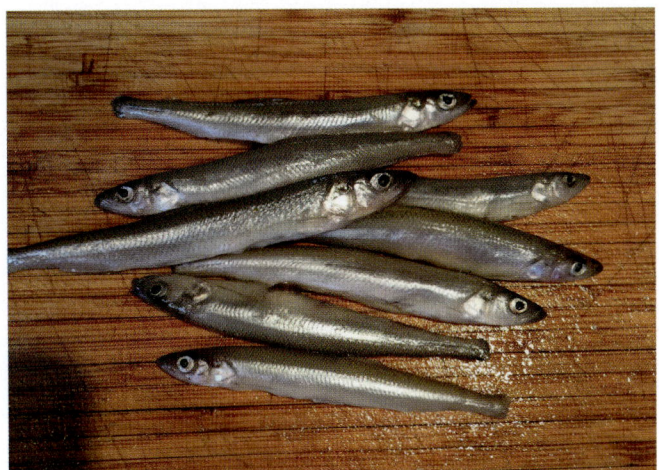

FIG 27.6 Freshwater smelt (not saltwater smelt), and chopped, skinned whole mice, can be fed to aquatic turtles that will not consume aquatic turtle pellets.

however, food may be crushed by the powerful jaws. If the prey or food item is too large to be swallowed or attached to a large dead animal, the crocodile bites and rolls its body in an attempt to tear off smaller pieces. Crocodiles are ambush predators and active scavengers (but will not take putrid prey), can be cannibalistic, and some occasionally even feed on fruits.[56] Small captive crocodilians can be fed gut-loaded insects, rodents, and whole fish or shrimp. Larger crocodilians can be fed larger prey, such as crustaceans, fish, rodents, rabbits, chickens, pigs, nutria, cats, dogs, and sheep. Crocodilian farms often utilize waste food, or byproducts, unfit for human consumption, which works if animals are culled young, but can be lethal to long-term zoo captives.[55] Rancid fish, or fish high in polyunsaturated fatty acids, can cause steatitis (see Chapter 84). As a general rule, juveniles should be offered food 2 to 3 times/week, subadults 1 to 2 times/week, and adults 1 time/week to every 2 weeks.[55] In the wild, juveniles eat 3% to 4% of their body weight/week, while adults consume 0.5% to 1% body weight/week. Farms encourage

TABLE 27.13 Nutrient Levels of Whole Vertebrates (ALL Values Expressed on a Dry Matter Basis)

Species	Typical Body Mass (g)	Water (%)	DM (%)	Crude Protein (%)	Crude Fat (%)	Ash (%)	GE (kcal/g)	Ca (%)	P (%)	Mg (%)
Hamster, Syrian	100–150	69.7	30.3	49.8	34.7	7.5	5.98	2.51	2.03	0.12
Mouse (range of ages)										
Pinkie 1–2 d	1.7±0.5	82±1.8	18	64.2±6.4	15.2±9.6	9.7±2.1	-	1.17±0.17	-	0.11±0.01
Fuzzy 4–13 d	3.8±1.1	70.8±4.3	29.2	41.8±2.8	46.7±4.3	8.4 ±1.6	-	1.47±0.18	-	0.09±0.01
Crawler 14–21 d	6.5±1.3	69±2.9	31	46.6±5.4	46.6±3	8.5±2.1	-	-	-	-
Small 21–23 d	7.4 ±1	71.3±2.8	28.7	55.8±4.3	23.4±2.4	13.4 ±4.6	-	2±0.43	-	0.12±0.01
Medium 4–6 wk	14.8±3	69.7±2	30.3	58.6±4.1	17±4.3	17±4.3	-	2.62±0.62	-	0.13±0.01
Large 2–10 m	36.2±8.8	62.9±5.6	37.1	45±9	13.6±4	13.6±4	-	1.73±0.25	-	0.09±0.01
Mouse, neonate	<3g	80.9	19.1	64.2	17	9.7	4.87	1.17	-	0.11
Mouse, juvenile	3–10g	81.8	18.2	44.2	30.1	8.5	6.65	1.47	-	0.09
Mouse, adult	>10g	67.3	32.7	55.8	23.6	11.8	5.25	2.98	1.72	0.16
Rat (range of sizes)										
Pinkie 14 days	10±3.6	79.2±1.9	20.8	57.9±3.6	23.7±7.4	12.2±1.2	-	1.85±0.36	-	0.14±0.02
Fuzzy 5–13 d	15.5±2.1	-	-	-	-	-	-	2.08±0.19	-	0.13±0.01
Crawler 2–3 wk	21.3±2.3	-	-	-	-	-	-	2.05±0.52	-	0.11±0.01
Small 4 wk	54.1±9.9	70±3.5	30	56.1±5.8	27.5±7.9	14.8±5.3	-	1.96±0.67	-	0.14±0.01
Medium 5–6 wk	117.2±4.5	69.8±1.1	30.2	60.1±4.3	24±1.5	15.9±8.5	-	3.34±1.32	-	0.18±0.01
Large 7–8 wk	256.9±39	65.2±3.8	34.8	45±9	35.1±9	8.8±3.6	-	3±1.12	-	0.15±0.02
Rat, neonate	<10	79.2	20.8	57.9	23.7	12.2	5.3	1.85	-	0.14
Rat, juvenile	10–50	70	30	56.1	27.5	14.8	5.55	2.07	-	0.12
Rat, adult	>50	66.1	33.9	61.8	32.6	9.8	6.37	2.62	1.48	0.08
Guinea pig, neonate	60–120	70.9	29.1	51.2	34.7	14.1	5.95	-	-	-
Guinea pig, 10 wk	500–550	68.7	31.3	51.4	46.1	9.2	6.99	3.02	-	0.07
Rabbit, neonate	50–80	84.6	15.4	72.1	13	14.9	5.06	-	-	-
Rabbit, dressed carcass	-	73.8	26.2	65.2	15.8	3.4	5.3	5.93	3.43	0.18
Chick, day old	40	74.4	25.6	64.9	22.4	6.4	5.8	1.69	1.22	0.05
Chicken	-	67.5	32.5	42.3	37.8	9.4	5.9	2.22	1.4	0.5
Quail	90–100	65.4	34.6	71.5	31.9	9.9	6.79	3.43	-	0.06
Lizard, anolis, adult	2.65±0.16	70.56	29.44±0.33	67.36±0.64	9	15.2	4.8	5.54	2.88	0.15
Bearded dragon neonate	2.55±0.25	82.01	17.99±0.53	61.07±1.11	-	-	-	3.6±0.25	2.31±0.13	0.185
11 day	3.19±0.32	81.65	18.35±0.63	66.13±1.22	-	-	-	3.52±0.3	2.4±0.16	0.143
17 day	3.13±0.29	82.55	17.45±0.57	63.88±1.22	-	-	-	3.42±0.27	2.36±0.14	0.147
Toad, Southern	-	71.8	28.2	61.07±1.11	14		4.25	2.94	1.79	0.06
Frog, green	-	77.5	22.5	71.2	10.2		4.8	42.9	1.89	2.47
Atlantic herring	-	79.4	20.6–28.6	44.2–70.2	2–22.8	11.1–16.5	5.12–5.33	1.56–1.85	1–2.13	0.1–0.24
Whitebait	-	79.6	20.4–25.4	67.7	10	12.3	4.94	2.32	1.95	0.18
Atlantic smelt	-	79.6	20.4–25.4	63.6–65.2	17–19.3	9–9.4	5.36–5.77	1.74–2.81	1.57–1.71	0.11–0.15
Atlantic mackerel	-	68.8	31.2–36.9	41.8–50.1	42.3–48.4	6.2–6.4	6.43–6.84	0.73–1.16	1.09–1.23	0.1–0.14
Pacific mackerel	-	76.3	23.7–33.4	43.4–79.2	3.7–37.5	7–13.8	4.46–5.94	1.55–3.08	1.21–2.65	0.09–0.23
Goldfish	-	80.6	19.4	58.8	8.5	23	4.15	6.99	4.36	0.17
Rainbow trout	-	72.3	27.7–30.7	54.7–68.5	27.2–33.9	7–9.2	5.68–6.15	1.54–1.82	1.54–1.78	0.1–0.11
Freshwater/rainbow smelt (*O. mordax*)	-	79.6	20.4–25.4	63.6–65.2	17–19.3	9–9.4	5.36–5.77	1.64–2.56	1.62–2.01	0.1–0.15

There are many sources of these figures that differ in detail; it is useful to recognize trends and ideally work with one set.

Often sources are regionally varied, dependent on food source and sampled in small numbers, so using the data requires some caution.

Some of these analyses do not show corresponding Ca and P; there is a basic assumption that these are present in healthy vertebrates in a classic ratio of approximately 1.5–2.0:1

Diet of the prey species has some variable effects on nutrients.[46]

• Pinkies, fuzzies, and crawlers have only fed on milk from the mother; other sizes receive commercial rodent diets.

• Vitamin E as alpha tocopherol, and A as retinol.

Na (%)	K (%)	Cu (mg/kg)	Fe (mg/kg)	Zn (mg/kg)	Mn (mg/kg)	Se (mg/kg)	Vitamin A (IU/kg)	Vitamin D3 (IU/kg)	Vitamin E (IU/kg)	Reported to Contain Thiaminase	Source
0.46	0.88	12	237	94	-	-	26,666	-	12.4	-	43
-	-	19.2±4.9	181.3±22.2	-	-	-	20,033–51,033	-	35.04±12.38	-	44, 45
-	-	14.8±7	113.4±27.9	-	-	-	7333–26,533	-	36.26±12.86	-	44, 45
-	-	-	-	-	-	-	11,766–21,567	-	43.26±6.5	-	44, 45
-	-	13.4±1.4	153.6±7.8	-	-	-	54,133–63,933	-	36.34±7.26	-	44, 45
-	-	10.5±1.2	169±9.9	-	-	-	87,066–182,800	-	35.74±9.51	-	44, 45
-	-	7.9±1.7	171.6±17.5	-	-	-	11,046–463,600	-	50.02±15.36	-	44, 45
-	-	19.2	181.3	82.5	-	-	17,000–35,500	-	7–52.7	-	43
-	-	13.4	153.6	75.4	13.1	-	-	-	-	-	43
-	-	6.7	137.9	67.5	-	-	130,000–578,272	—	6–100	-	43
-	-	60.6±37.5	275.8±86.9	-	-	-	13,500–29,167	-	426.35±143.83	-	44, 45
-	-	11.7±2.5	155±31.4	-	-	-	-	-	-	-	45
-	-	10.9±2	111.3±9.3	-	-	-	-	-	-	-	45
-	-	12.4±3	208.2±59.8	-	-	-	30,967–60,300	-	128.54±71.41	-	44, 47
-	-	10.8±0.8	332.6±27.4	-	-	-	28,900–20,443	-	106.54± 49.15	-	44, 47
-	-	15.9±2	280±37.6	-	-	-	31,470–35,590	-	137.63±61.12	-	44, 47
-	-	60.6	275.8	113.6	-	-	-	-	-	-	43
-	-	11.3	133.2	81.9	2.6	-	-	-	-	-	43
-	-	148	62.1	11	-	-	-	-	-	-	43
-	-	-	-	-	-	-	-	-	-	-	43
-	-	5.6	56.4	46.4	-	-	16,506	-	24.2	-	43
-	-	-	-	-	-	-	-	-	-	-	43
0.26	0.72	4.6	100	84	2.4	1.18	6200	-	60	-	43
0.71	0.8	5.2	119.5	97.4	-	-	-	-	-	-	43
-	-	3.6	122.2	116.1	-	-	35,600	-	51.3	-	43
-	-	2.6	74.9	53	-	-	32,988–155,222	-	34.9–115.3	-	43, 46
0.33	0.73	5	127.8	142.5	-	-	4880±1960	-	11.9–44.8	-	47
0.6	1.03	7.63	438	99.4	-	-	29,650±3540	-	115.6±6.8	-	47
0.7	1.15	8.28	196	155	-	-	48,950±5780	-	68.5±11.1	-	47
0.69	1.19	11.28	145	154.7	-	-	42,280±1960	-	88.8±7.9	-	47
0.36–0.63	-	117,4	286	662.9	4.7		38,261	-	369	-	43
0.55	-	11.28	102.6	100.3	11.5		25,110	-	82.2	-	43
0.35–0.85	0.94–1.94	4–6	64–132	44–80	3–7	0.93–4.48	10,704–31,864	7593	25–129	Yes	48, 49
0.46	1.47	4–6	112	75	10	0.8	14,706	2510	25	Yes	48, 49
0.36–0.63	0.93–1.42	2–3	29–36	80–94	7–14	0.55–1	17,717–25,980	476	39–49	Yes	48, 49
0.38–0.48	0.77–1.03	5–10	63–100	39–46	2–3	2.09–2.67	59,108	16,800	33	Possibly	48, 49
0.35–1.17	0.75–1.6	4–8	153–184	41–82	0–2	2.9–4.67	-	-	-	Yes	48, 49
0.65	1.22	14	307	225	64	1.22	-	-	-	Yes	48, 49
0.22–0.27	1.33–1.6	5–9	41–62	96–130	0–1	0.69–1.03	-	-	-	No	48, 49
0.24–0.58	0.95–1.41	2–8	26–87	78–113	4–19	0.73–1.29	9287–75,091	633	85–282	Yes	48

To convert a nutrient analysis from "as fed" to "dry matter," see Box 27.1.
Thiaminase has been reported in a wide range of genera, freshwater and marine, vertebrate and invertebrate. It has been demonstrated to vary through the year.

- 1 mg alpha tocopherol = 1.1 IU, and 0.3 µg retinol = 1 IU vitamin A activity
  mg/kg = µg/g
- Gross energy (GE) calculated by adding the product of % crude protein x 5.43 kcal/g to the product of % crude fat x 9.11 kcal/g.[4,21]

growth by feeding juveniles and subadults 20% of their body weight/ week. All crocodilians can be fed commercial crocodilian extruded biscuits, such as Small or Large Crocodilian Diet or Crocodilian Gel Diet (Mazuri, PMI Nutrition International, LLC, St. Louis, MO). See Chapter 25 and Britton reference for more information.[55]

Herbivores

Herbivores average dietary composition is 15% to 35% protein, less than 10% fat, and 50% to 75% carbohydrates, of which 15% to 40% is crude fiber (DM).[8,42] Herbivores are the greatest challenge to feed correctly. Extant herbivorous reptiles are found in the Cheloniidae, Testudinae, and some Agamidae and Iguanidae. Only three other herbivorous lizard species exist outside the latter two families, including the Solomon Island prehensile-tailed skink (*Corucia zebrata*). Thus herbivory in lizards is limited to only about 50 species, and folivory is unique to the green iguana.[4,57,58] However, herbivorous species are popular and a large portion of the reptile veterinarian's caseload. Herbivores are typically generalized grazers and browsers. Some species are only herbivorous as adults and insectivores, carnivores or omnivores as juveniles, such as the bearded dragon and Emydid turtles, including *Chrysemys*, *Pseudemys*, *Trachemys*, and *Terrapene*.[59] All herbivores require UVB light. Green iguanas and rock iguanas (*Cyclura*) seem to utilize dietary vitamin D relatively inefficiently and are far more dependent on UVB radiation.[4,11] Herbivorous reptiles are hindgut fermenters with an enlarged cecum or colon, particularly well developed and partitioned in herbivorous iguanids and agamids but not in chelonians. The hindgut contains symbiotic microbes (bacteria, protozoa, and fungi) that anaerobically ferment plant material to produce proteins, vitamins, and volatile fatty acids.[57] A common misconception is that herbivores will select a balanced diet from the foods offered. While this may be true for free-ranging herbivores, this is not the case in captivity. Complex natural diets of herbivores are only slowly beginning to be appreciated. For example, Sonoran desert tortoises (*Gopherus morafkai*) consume well over 200 plant species, and this dietary diversity is probably true of many species.[60] Plants vary seasonally, annually (dependent on rainfall), phenologically (freshest plants eaten first, dry senescent plants last), and ecologically. Consumed plants in Arizona upland habitat included 55% forbs (herbaceous flowering nongrasses), 22% woody plants (especially desert vine, *Janusia gracilis*), 18% grasses, and 5% succulents (*Opuntia* cactus). In contrast, in more xeric habitats, tortoises consumed 50% to 90% woody plants, 3% to 29% forbs, and 13% to 19% grasses.[61] Dietary overlap between two desert tortoise species (*G. agassizii* and *G. morafkai*) was less than 25% of diet plants found in both the Mojave and Sonoran deserts. Thus there is much intraspecies and interspecies variability, even between closely related species. One researcher commented that the abundance and diversity of annual plants varied so much from year to year and site to site that it was difficult, if not misleading, to characterize an average desert tortoise diet.[62] Nonetheless, captive desert tortoise diets should attempt to emulate the nutrient composition of wild diets, with a goal of ≤15% crude protein, 2% to 4% fat, and 25% to 30% fiber (% DM).[6,62] Captive herbivore nutrition is more of an art than a science, primarily because of the scarcity of nutritional information. Nutritional studies are difficult and tedious. Consider, for example, studying the green iguana. Green iguanas are tough to observe in the field because they are arboreal folivores and wary of humans. They are also inactive 90% of the time[63] and spend little time foraging (0.6% of total observation time in one study).[59] Once you observe them foraging, arboreal plants consumed must be collected and nutritionally analyzed. However, one must be careful to collect exactly what they consumed. In another study, iguanas never ate mature leaves with ≤20% DM crude protein content but always selected younger leaves with higher crude protein contents of ≥25% DM.[64] It is therefore

understandable that we still know so little about the nutrient composition of wild iguana diets. Nutritionists, working on captive propagation of green iguanas for decades, have produced some valuable estimates.[4] For green iguanas, the recommended DM nutrient levels are 26% gross protein for hatchlings to 6 months, 22% gross protein after 6 months, 15% to 17% gross protein for nonreproductive adults, as well as 3% fat, 6% to 10% crude fiber, and a 2:1 Ca:P ratio (% DM).

Salad-type diets are problematic in that commercial fruits and vegetables produced for humans typically are too low in Ca, fiber, trace minerals, and some vitamins; too high or too low in protein; and too high in simple carbohydrates for herbivorous reptiles (see Tables 27.1 and 27.2).[4] It is no surprise that captive herbivores commonly present with calcium deficiencies, difficulty laying eggs, cystic calculi, renal diseases, and loose stools. In southern California, chronic nutritional disease is endemic in tortoises fed backyard grasses, weeds, and grocery store fruits and vegetables. Most suffer from chronic protein, calcium, and fiber deficiencies and simple carbohydrate excess, with many dying from hepatic lipidosis. Captive iguanas typically die from calcium deficiency, hypovitaminosis D, or renal failure. Nutritional analysis of the most frequently consumed plant species reported from four studies of free-ranging desert tortoises,[6,7] and a recommended nutrient profile for green iguanas,[4] are compared to commonly fed greens (see Table 27.1) and fruits and vegetables (see Table 27.2). It is difficult to provide a balanced range of necessary nutrients with greens, vegetables, and fruits. That is not to say that they have no place in herbivorous reptile diets, but, by themselves, are often poor alternatives to wild foods.[4] Another problem with salads is that animals can be selective in favor of fruit and other food items that are nutritionally incomplete. The USDA nutrient database (https://ndb.nal.usda.gov/ndb/) is an online, searchable database that enables veterinarians to obtain complete nutritional information on any human food item.

Attempts to compensate for nutritional inadequacies in salad diets by supplementing with vitamin-mineral supplements is difficult without knowing what they need, how much they need, and how much they are consuming, and does not correct nutritional excesses. This also applies to natural foods planted for browse in the herbivores exhibit. In the wild, they consume dozens to hundreds of species, although they may concentrate on a few. Most backyards or exhibits simply are too space limited to support a wide variety of plant species, and herbivores often overgraze whatever is in their exhibit. This is not to say that native palatable species should not be offered, but rather that it is hard to provide a nutritionally complete diet in such a manner.

There is a difficult trade-off to be made between trying to mimic a reasonably normal diet while accepting that the actual components are nothing like those encountered in the wild, against using a totally abnormal commercial diet based on in-house extrapolation with little to no validation. The former presumably fills more of the nonnutritional behavioral needs of the animal, which will not be experienced by eating uniform pellets. Some prefer to attempt to simulate normality in the types of food items presented often with the choices dependent on availability of suitable natural or commercial foodstuffs. Others believe providing a high-quality commercial pelleted diet as a large portion of the diet probably offers a superior dietary alternative to what the typical owner can accomplish.

Most grasses and hays (except for Kentucky bluegrass and alfalfa) approach or meet the nutrient profile for desert tortoises, except some are low in Ca (see Table 27.3).[6,65] Clover (*Trifolium* spp.) and alfalfa (*Medicago sativa*) have more Ca but are also higher in protein. Alfalfa is a nitrogen-fixing legume hay that has higher crude protein than grass hays. Early season vegetative alfalfa has a 23% crude protein content that drops to 17% crude protein by full bloom,[65] all levels above what desert tortoises naturally consume and therefore may be excessive.

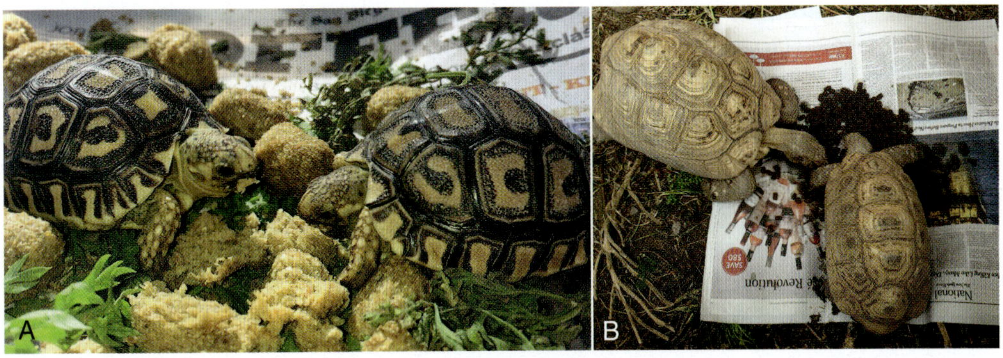

FIG 27.7 Chronic nutritional deficiency, such as anemia, hypoalbuminemia, and hepatic lipidosis is prevalent in backyard tortoises fed grasses, weeds, flowers, and grocery store produce. Better alternatives include commercial pelleted mixes, grasses, grass hays, and plant species normally consumed in the wild. Converting reptiles to pellets and hay is much like getting a dog off table scraps and onto dog food; patience, persistence, and feeding less often will eventually convert them.

Commercial diets are also compared to nutritional analysis of the most frequently consumed plant species reported from free-ranging desert tortoises[6,7] in Table 27.4 and recommended nutrient levels for green iguanas[4] in Table 27.5. On a DM basis, there is a great deal of variation in these diets, and some are better than others in approaching free-ranging nutrient profiles. Overall, they appear better than greens, fruits, or vegetables. However, a diet for juvenile iguanas with a 13% protein DM is not only inappropriate for juveniles but for adult iguanas as well. Only two of the tortoise diets had the recommended 3.2 to 5.8 Ca:P ratio, so additional Ca supplementation may be needed, and all tortoise diets were high in carbohydrates. Scores were assigned based on whether the diet met the free-ranging nutrient profiles (for tortoises, protein, fat, fiber, carbohydrates, and Ca:P; for iguanas, the same, except carbohydrates were not listed by Allen and Oftendal[4]). Not all diets had Ca or P listed, which was reflected in their lower scores. The diets in Tables 27.4 and 27.5 are listed from highest to lowest scores.

Getting tortoises to eat hay and commercial foods can be difficult (Fig. 27.7). Much like a dog content with table food, a tortoise will eat pellets and hay once hungry enough, but not if better-tasting foods are available. Feeding less frequently will often encourage the reptile to try new foods. Use good-quality hays, not stems or stalks, and ensure it is not stale or moldy. Chopping the hay with scissors, or a food processor, and sprinkling, spraying, or briefly soaking the hay with water improves palatability. Soaking too long will leach out nutrients. Short hay segments may decrease colonic obstructions. Mixing greens in or under the hay also helps with acceptance. Pellets can be soaked in just enough water to be absorbed and soften and then mixed into the greens. Be patient and persistent, tortoises and iguanas will switch over to commercial pellets, or hay (for tortoises), once hungry enough. African spurred tortoises (*Centrochelys sulcata*), as well as other giant tortoise species, grow so large and eat so much that reliance on grass hays often becomes a practical necessity.

Diluting commercial diets with natural foods and creating an unbalanced ration should be avoided. By definition, complete diets are intended as sole diets, unless the feeding instructions specify they are formulated to be fed with natural foodstuffs. Some manufacturers have anticipated this, and Mazuri recommends feeding their pelleted tortoise diets with good quality grass hay, and, if desired, up to 5% fruit and 20% vegetables by total diet weight.

Misconceptions. Be aware of several persistent and widespread misconceptions. Members of the Brassica family (cabbages, kale, mustard greens, broccoli, cauliflower, Brussels sprouts, bok choy) are thought, but not proven, to cause thyroid problems (goiter) if fed exclusively long term but are harmless in moderation as part of a balanced diet. Goiters appear exceedingly rarely in tortoises, and goiter association with feeding Brassicas has never been validated in tortoises. Galapagos and Aldabra tortoises may have enlarged thymuses in their ventral neck, but these should not be confused with goiter. Massively enlarged thyroid glands are generally tumors, not goiter (see Chapter 79).

Many greens contain oxalates, which can bind Ca in the intestinal tract and decrease calcium absorption. The adverse effects of oxalates must be considered in terms of oxalate:Ca molar ratio of food.[66] Spinach, beet greens, sorrels (*Oxalis* and *Rumex spp.*), and purslane (*Portulaca spp.*) have oxalate:Ca ratios >2, therefore they have no utilizable Ca and possess excess oxalate, which can bind Ca in other foods eaten at the same time. They are not good sources of Ca despite their apparently high Ca levels.[66] Other foods, such as prickly pear cactus (*Opuntia ficus indica*), collards, Swiss chard, dandelions, kale, turnip greens, Brussels sprouts, and parsley, have oxalate:Ca ratios <2, indicating that they are good sources of Ca. Diets low in Ca and high in oxalates are not recommended, but occasional consumption of high-oxalate foods, as part of a nutritious diet, does not pose any particular health problem.[66] Indeed, it is recommended to feed these greens, just not exclusively. Cattle and sheep, as well as humans, possess a bacterium, *Oxalobacter formigenes*, that can metabolize oxalic acid, and perhaps herbivorous reptiles do as well.[66] Another unfounded concern with oxalates is that they can cause urocystoliths, probably because they may contribute to renoliths in humans. Reptiles form urate stones, not Ca oxalate stones. There are only two reports of Ca oxalate stones in tortoises, one in a Moorish tortoise (*Testudo graeca graeca*, the cystourolith was only 20% calcium oxalate)[67] and one in a deceased wild desert tortoise with renoliths.[68] The latter study concluded that oxalates in desert tortoises were an incidental finding and nonpathogenic.[68] In contrast, humans do get Ca oxalate stones, yet oxalate-rich foods are still widely and safely consumed and only restricted in people predisposed to Ca oxalate stone formation.

Plant poisoning is extremely rare in tortoises. Leopard tortoises (*Stigmochelys pardalis*) and tent tortoises (*Psammobates oculifer*) regularly eat the invasive African species, goat's head (*Tribulus terrestris*), which causes staggers (limb paresis) and death in livestock.[69,70] Leopard tortoises are known to consume more than six plant species suspected to contain toxic substances, including oxalates.[69] Most of the plants consumed by Russian tortoises (*Agrionemys horsfeildii*) are notorious for their toxicity to herbivorous mammals.[71] More than 10% of plant species regularly consumed by Hermann's tortoises (*Testudo hermanni*) contained toxic alkaloids.[72] Tortoises will typically avoid poisonous plants, dilute their effects with other foods, or are resistant to their effects. Some exceptions include rhododendrons (*Rhododendron* spp., grayanotoxins cause flaccid paresis), oleanders (*Nerium oleander*), chinaberry trees (*Melia azedarach*), tree tobacco (*Nicotiana glauca*), and toadstools (Agaricomycetes).

Given the previous discussion, it is apparent that making recommendations for an appropriate herbivorous reptile diet can be challenging. However, some important points for guidance are summarized here. All herbivores require UVB light to assist with Ca requirements, and it must be routinely provided with either exposure to unfiltered sunlight or appropriate lighting. Regarding diet for both tortoises and iguanas, it is important to concentrate more on dietary variety than limiting foods. For tortoises, grasses, grass hays, native plants and good-quality commercial tortoise diets should make up at least 80% of the diet. The remaining 20% can be dark leafy greens, Mulberry tree leaves, grape leaves, backyard weeds, and nonstarchy vegetables, as well as calcium-rich flowers (roses, *Rosa* spp., nasturtiums, *Tropaeolum* spp., carnations, *Dianthus caryophyllus*, cactus flowers). For iguanas, produce should be no more than 50% of the diet, on an AF basis, with the remainder being a rationally formulated commercial diet.[4] Produce should be limited to dark leafy greens and nonstarchy vegetables. Commercial fruits and starchy vegetables should be avoided.[6] Additional multivitamins are not needed for iguanas or tortoises, as long as they consume commercial foods formulated for them but ensure that Ca levels are acceptable, or additional supplementation should be used. If the commercial diet is supplemented with produce, or grass, then additional calcium supplementation may again be required.

Omnivores

Omnivores' average dietary composition consists of 15% to 40% protein, 5% to 40% fat, and 20% to 75% carbohydrates.[42] Many aquatic turtles, box turtles, wood turtles, forest tortoises, sea turtles, and lizards consume both plant and animal material. Many omnivores consume more animals as juveniles to fuel increased demands for protein and fat than as adults.[8]

Box Turtles. Box turtles are more carnivorous than initially thought, and they eat whatever stimulates them and whatever they can catch; moving prey especially appeals to them.[73] Box turtles are opportunistic omnivores that consume beetles, insect larvae (caterpillars, grubs, maggots), cicadas, crickets, cockroaches, flies, grasshoppers, termites, millipedes, centipedes, land snails, slugs, earthworms, spiders, dragonfly larvae, sowbugs or pillbugs, crayfish, carrion, fish, frogs, tadpoles, toads, small mammals, birds, salamanders, lizards, snakes, smaller turtles, and all types of carrion, as well as plant material, such as mushrooms (even poisonous ones), strawberries, raspberries, blackberries, blueberries, elderberries, mulberries, persimmons, sea grapes, tomatoes, apples, grasses, leaves, shoots, buds, roots, mosses and Opuntia fruits, pads, and flowers.[73] Again fruits should be limited, and good-quality commercial diets designed for box turtle or aquatic turtles should make up a large portion of the diet (see Table 27.6).

Bearded Dragons. One study of the stomach contents of 10 bearded dragons found a wide variety of arthropods (9 orders, 80% Isopterans [termites]) but a larger volume of plant matter. The diets were high in crude protein (41%–50% DM), and fatty acid content was 14%–27% of the DM intake. Mealworms most closely resembled the nutritional profile of termites, and the authors concluded a diet with a variety of insects and dark leafy greens would closely resemble the natural diet.[74] Another study showed adult bearded dragons consumed 90% plant material, whereas juveniles consumed 50% plant material and 50% animal material.[75] Bearded dragons are also lizard eaters and cannibalistic if size disparity is present. Suitable vegetables include calcium-dusted dark leafy greens (kale, collards, mustards, turnip or beet tops, spinach, dandelions, cabbage, bok choy, broccoli rape, and lettuces such as romaine, red leaf, green leaf, or boston lettuces but not iceberg lettuce), carrots, squash, zucchini, peas, and beans. Flowers such as roses, nasturtiums, carnations, and hibiscus are also good. Dragons should be fed a wide variety of insects, including mealworms, crickets, super worms, waxworms, Dubia cockroaches, black soldier fly larvae, locusts, silkworms, butter worms, grasshoppers, and tomato hornworms. Insects should be gut loaded and dusted before becoming prey. Commercial pelleted (not cubed) bearded dragon foods can also be fed (see Table 27.7). Baby mice can be offered several times per month. Even though bearded dragons enjoy fruits, they are not recommended. Overfeeding and obesity are major problems in captivity. Growing juveniles can be fed daily, while adults should be fed 2 to 3 times weekly. Growing dragons need more calcium than adults. Calcium is provided in calcium-rich insect gut-loading diets, dusted on insects or sprinkled on plant food. If multivitamins are not included in the gut-loading, dusting preparation, or fortified foods, multivitamins can be given twice a month.

Sea Turtles. Sea turtles can be carnivorous, herbivorous, or omnivorous, and most undergo a change in diet as they age.[12] Adult leatherbacks (*Dermochelys coriacea*) are gelatinovores; their diet consists of jellyfish, tunicates, and sea squirts. Sea turtles have large caudally directed papillae in their oropharynx and esophagus to help them swallow soft food (see Fig. 7.29). Their fondness for jellyfish can also lead to fatal consumption of plastic bags. Adult hawksbills (*Eretmochelys imbricate*) eat sponges primarily but also feed on soft corals, tunicates, shrimp, and squid. Kemp's ridley sea turtles (*Lepidochelys kempii*) are also carnivores that eat crab, fish, jellyfish, shrimp, and mollusks. Green sea turtle hatchlings (*Chelonia mydas*) are carnivorous until juveniles, when they switch to eating sea grasses, especially turtle grass (*Thalassia testudinum*) in the Caribbean, as well as red, green, and brown algae, jellyfish, mollusk eggs, and sponges. Near the coast of Peru, invertebrates are much more common in green sea turtle diets, and some fish are taken.[12] Adult loggerheads (*Caretta caretta*) are carnivorous, eating crabs (especially horseshoe crabs) and mollusks, while hatchings are omnivores. Olive ridley sea turtles (*Lepidochelys olivacea*) are omnivores, eating crabs, shrimp, lobster, urchins, jellies, algae, and fish. Flatbacks (*Natator depressus*) are also omnivores, eating sea cucumbers, jellyfish, soft corals, shrimp, crabs, mollusks, cuttlefish, fish, and seaweed. In captivity, all sea turtles can be maintained on a carnivorous diet. Mazuri (PMI Nutrition International, LLC, St. Louis, MO) makes a meal form product (Sea Turtle Meal Diet for Carnivorous Turtles) that may be fed via gavage, as well as a gel diet (Sea Turtle Gel Diet for Carnivorous Turtles). See Chapter 24 for more information.

Freshwater Turtles. Many large emydid turtles, including *Chrysemys*, *Graptemys*, *Pseudemys*, and *Trachemys* spp. undergo an ontogenetic shift in diet as they mature.[76] The red-eared slider (*Trachemys scripta elegans*) starts out predominantly carnivorous when juvenile, inhabiting shallower warmer waters that are rich in invertebrate and animal prey (the latter are good sources of protein and Ca). As they get older and larger, they cannot maneuver in shallow water and move into deeper, cooler water (typically 5°–6°C lower) where prey is more dispersed, and so they shift to eating more plant material (with lower protein content), such as duckweed (*Spirodela polyrhiza*) and hydrilla (*Hydrilla verticillata*).[76] See Table 27.6 for an alphabetical list of freshwater turtle manufactured diets.

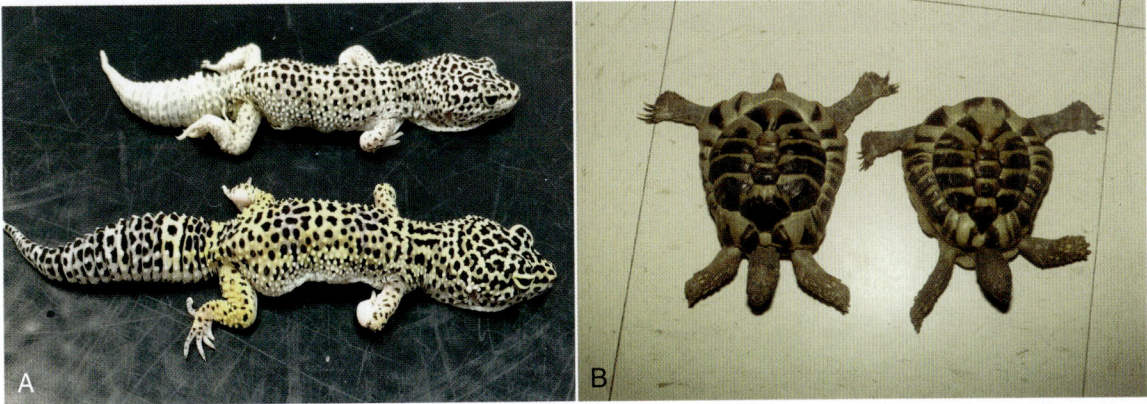

FIG 27.8 Always consult with your reptile and amphibian owners (from novice to breeder) about nutrition. As their veterinarian, you are their best knowledgeable source for this vital information. If you do not provide it, they may acquire the information from questionable sources, often leading to disastrous results, as illustrated here in these stunted and nutritionally unsound reptile patients (A) leopard geckos *(Eublepharis macularius)* and (B) tortoises *(Testudo),* that can be completely preventable.

CONCLUSION

Veterinarians have been trained in animal nutrition. The herp veterinarian must evaluate dietary history on a regular basis to keep their reptile and amphibian patients healthy. Information within this chapter covers the majority of reptiles and amphibians seen by veterinarians in private and zoological veterinary practice. With basic information and as vocal advocates for good nutrition, veterinarians can have a tremendous impact on the health of captive herps (Fig. 27.8).

REFERENCES

See www.expertconsult.com for a complete list of references.

Amphibians

Frank Pasmans and An Martel

Captive propagation of amphibians has gained increased attention due to the global amphibian crisis, which renders amphibians the most severely threatened vertebrate class on earth.[1] Indeed, ex situ captive breeding programs are far from ideal; however, they may prove to be the only available measure to prevent extinction of amphibian species from global threats such as chytridiomycosis (Fig. 28.1).[2,3] Although amphibians are currently being kept in fairly large numbers in different settings (e.g., zoos and aquaria, research laboratories, private collections), principles for keeping these animals healthy in a sustained way are widely applicable. For example, avoiding pathogen pollution and the establishment of invasive alien species, securing amphibian welfare and conservation, and avoiding negative effects on public health all apply within these settings. Because issues with infectious diseases are especially prominent in amphibian conservation and relevant in most aspects of amphibian captive management, veterinarians play a key role in the sustainability of captive amphibians.

RESTRAINT

Restraining amphibians should be kept to the absolute minimum, for example, for collecting blood or cloacal samples or administering therapeutics. In general, the smaller the amphibian, the less it will tolerate prolonged periods of contact with the warm and relatively salty human skin. Manipulation can result in severe signs of (heat) stress and even death. Signs of distress are excessive production of skin secretions, cramps, and in some urodelan species caudal autotomy (tail loss). Many critically important clinical parameters can be assessed visually in amphibians without the need for manipulation (posture, skin texture, presence of dysecdysis, body condition, appetite). Parasitologic examination is preferably done on fresh feces instead of cloacal lavage.

Wearing vinyl (nonpowdered) gloves is highly recommended when manipulating amphibians. The use of latex gloves is discouraged, given the potential adverse reactions of amphibians, especially after repeated manipulation.[4] Changing gloves between animals is advised, not only to prevent disease transmission but also to prevent intoxication by skin secretions that adhere to the glove. Frogs and toads can be restrained by grasping the animal firmly just cranial to the hind legs (Fig. 28.2). Most salamanders and newts can be carried easily on the open palm of the hand. For restraining these animals, the same techniques as for lizards can be used. Amphibians with particularly slippery skin may be restrained by using a wet towel, tissue, or a dip net. Some amphibians (for example, large and slippery salamanders or caecilians) can only be properly manipulated with sedation. Most amphibians will not attempt to bite when grasped, with very few exceptions, such as some large anurans (notably horned frogs, *Ceratophrys* sp., *Lepidobatrachus* sp., and African bullfrogs [*Pyxicephalus* sp.]) and some, mostly very large

salamanders (large sirens, amphiumas, and giant salamanders but also some smaller species like *Aneides lugubris*). All amphibians should be considered to contain several skin toxins that may cause irritation or (in very rare cases and invariably after ingestion) intoxication. Notoriously toxic taxa include the popular pet species like poison dart frogs (family Dendrobatidae) or Malagasy poison frogs (genus *Mantella*) but also many urodelans (e.g., the genus *Taricha*), many of which are aposematically colored (with warning colors) and secrete defensive alkaloids. However, at least in anurans, much of this toxicity is commonly derived from prey items,[5–7] which are generally not available in captivity and, hence, toxicity of these species is reduced over time in captivity. Intoxication by amphibian skin secretions can be easily avoided by wearing gloves. A very small number of amphibians such as the frequently kept frogs of the genus *Trachycephalus* may cause mucosal irritation even without contact[8] (Fig. 28.3) or by active spraying of poison from skin glands (*Salamandra*).

Alternatives to oral and parenteral application should be preferentially used where applicable, for example, by percutaneous drug administration, which is possible for several frequently used antiparasitic drugs (metronidazole, levamisole). Only in rare cases do these authors utilize force feeding. Opening an amphibian's mouth can be done by gently forcing a nontraumatic device (e.g., credit card, double-folded piece of paper) in the mouth.

IDENTIFICATION

Identifying individual amphibians for research or legislation purposes (e.g., CITES) may pose some challenges given the small size of many species. Methods to identify individuals include toe-clipping (amputation of one or several toes), branding, tattooing, implantable polymers, pattern mapping, and transponders.[9] For reasons of animal welfare and technique reliability, only the use of polymers, pattern mapping, and transponders will be discussed. Passive integrated transponder tags (PIT tags or microchips) are widely used and provide long-term, unambiguous identification. The only limitation is the size of the animals, the minimum size for frogs and toads being some 4 cm and the minimal snout-vent length for salamanders and newts being approximately 5 cm (but depending on the animal's girth) when using 1.4 mm × 9 mm transponders. In anurans, transponders can be placed either in the coelomic cavity or in the dorsal lymphatic sac (Fig. 28.4). In salamanders and newts, transponders can be placed in the coelomic cavity or, in very large species, intramuscularly in the tail. For some species that are difficult to handle, sedation is recommended to prevent trauma from the PIT tag applicator. Potential complications are the loss of transponders (often reported but actually, when performed secundum artem, loss of transponders is very limited) and the potential of causing trauma in

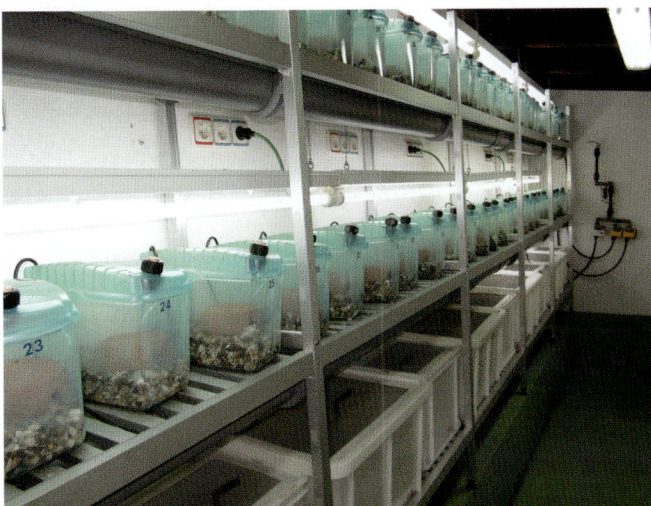

FIG 28.1 Ex situ breeding of midwife toads (*Alytes obstetricans*) in Spain (Peñalara National Park), where the species suffers from massive chytridiomycosis-driven declines (Courtesy of Frank Pasmans.)

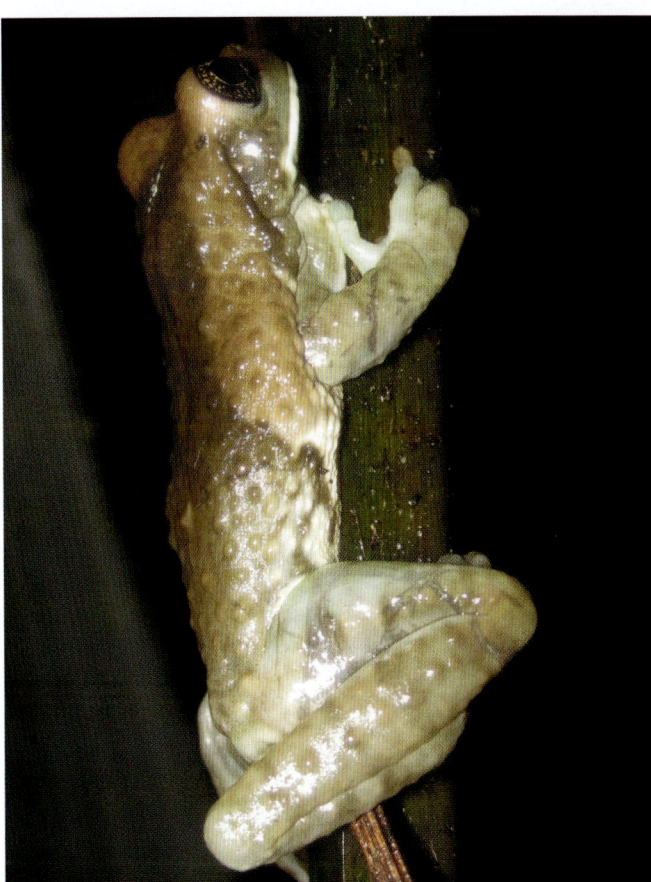

FIG 28.3 The commonly kept frogs of the genus *Trachycephalus* (here *T. typhonius*) secrete toxic skin substances that may irritate even without direct contact (Courtesy of Frank Pasmans.)

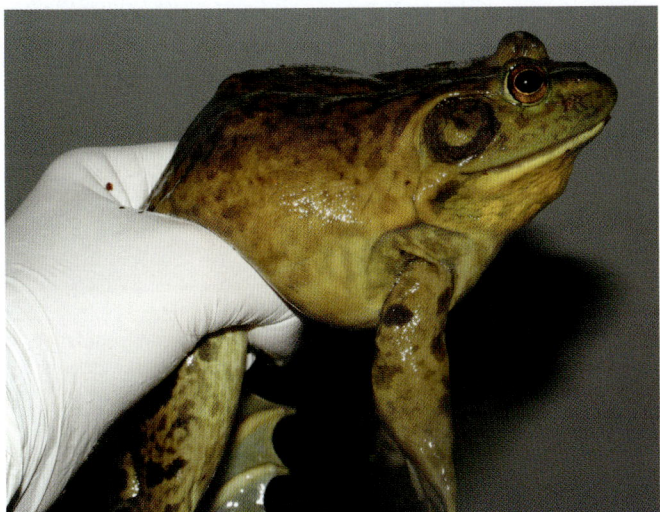

FIG 28.2 Restraining many anurans can be done by grasping the animal in front of the hind legs (Courtesy of Frank Pasmans.)

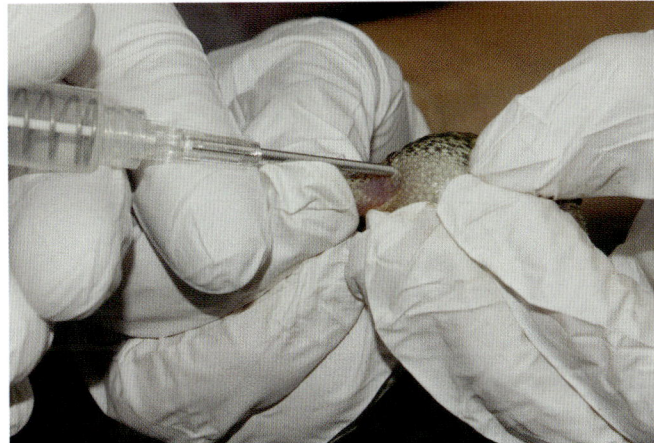

FIG 28.4 Intracoelomic injection of a PIT tag in a midwife toad (*Alytes obstetricans*) for a capture-mark-recapture study (Courtesy of Sergé Bogaerts.)

small animals. PIT tags should be applied by trained persons only. The insertion site should be gently wiped clean with a sterile gauze or cotton-tipped applicator. These authors prefer not to disinfect the insertion site to avoid possible irritation or even intoxication.

High-quality detailed photographs of amphibians against a contrasting background and with indication of size can be used for pattern mapping in species with unique patterns that remain stable with age. For several amphibian species, software has been developed for quick matching of a given pattern with a pattern database. Finally, colored or fluorescent polymers (e.g., elastomers) are widely used in amphibians, mainly in field studies. These are injected subcutaneously. The technique is cheap, allows a large number of individual identifications (by alternating dyes and application sites), and is applicable to very small amphibians, including tadpoles. Disadvantages are loss of visibility of the tags and the lack of unique code combinations, rendering this technique limited for CITES and other legal purposes.

SPECIFIC HOUSING REQUIREMENTS

Before acquiring any amphibian, the relevant literature should be consulted to identify the species husbandry and nutritional needs. Indeed, given the often highly species-specific requirements, it is impossible to provide general instructions that meet all species' needs. Ample literature is easily available,[10,11] and a wealth of high-quality monograph booklets have been published on most of the commonly kept species. Most amphibian enclosures are constructed from glass or plastics. Only glues and sealants, such as silicone-based or two-component epoxy glues, that are safe for use in fish aquaria should be used. Newly glued materials should be thoroughly dried and rinsed with water. All amphibians need moisture in at least part of their terrarium to maintain their fluid balance. Amphibians typically do not drink, but rather absorb fluid through their skin (such as the drinking patch on the ventral coelom of many anurans). Depending on their life history, amphibians should be kept in aquaria or terraria, the latter containing an aquatic part, the size of which depends on the amphibian species. It is of vital importance to keep the water quality in any amphibian enclosure optimal (see below) to avoid intoxication. Most amphibians can easily overcome the glass sides of their enclosure and should be prevented from escaping by securing a tightly fitting lid covered with fine mesh. For many salamanders and newts a frame of overhanging strips of at least 5 cm will prevent the inmates from escaping, although some species, notably plethodontid salamanders, are capable of walking around on glass sheets upside down (Fig. 28.5). An abundance of shelters, provided by PVC tubes, piles of flat stones, bark, or similar should be available.

Fully aquatic species can be housed in escape-proof aquaria (Fig. 28.6) that can be otherwise designed similar to aquaria used for ornamental fish. A water level of 15–20 cm will be sufficient in most instances, and potable tap water will be fine for most of the commonly kept amphibians, as long as chlorine levels are low or absent, acidity (pH) is between 6–8, and overall hardness of the water is moderate to high (8°dH–18°dH, 2.9–6.5 meq/L). The pH values below 4 or above 11 are lethal and must be avoided. Water hardness, expressed in degrees of German hardness (°dH), reflects levels of dissolved calcium and magnesium and is an indirect measure of the alkalinity of the water, that is, the amounts of dissolved carbonates and bicarbonates. The lower the hardness, the lower its capacity for buffering, with the potential of severe pH fluctuations. Chlorine can be removed from tap water by leaving the water in a bucket for at least 24 hours, preferably with aeration. The use of chloramine-treated water for amphibians is discouraged. Chloramine is more stable and requires the use of dechlorinators for removal. Only a limited number of amphibian species require a more specific water quality. One of the most crucial parameters that should

be monitored is the level of nitrogen metabolites and especially ammonia, nitrite, and nitrate. Total ammonia nitrogen consists of NH_3 and ionized NH_4^+. The latter is far less toxic. The rate NH_3/NH_4^+ increases with increasing pH and temperature. The maximum levels for these metabolites are for ammonia: 0.02 mg/L, nitrite: 0.1 mg/L, and nitrate: 50 mg/L, but for ammonia and nitrite, values should be zero.[12,13] Ammonia is continuously being produced by aquatic amphibians but also by decaying organic matter, such as leftover feed items. In a well-conditioned aquarium, ammonia is quickly metabolized to nitrite and further to nitrate by bacteria. When these bacteria are lacking (typically in newly installed tanks or following inappropriate antibiotic use in the environment) or do not have the capacity to break down ammonium and nitrite, buildup of these metabolites causes overt disease and death (Fig. 28.7).[14] This "new tank syndrome" is an often overlooked but very frequent cause of death in captive amphibians. Accumulation of nitrates

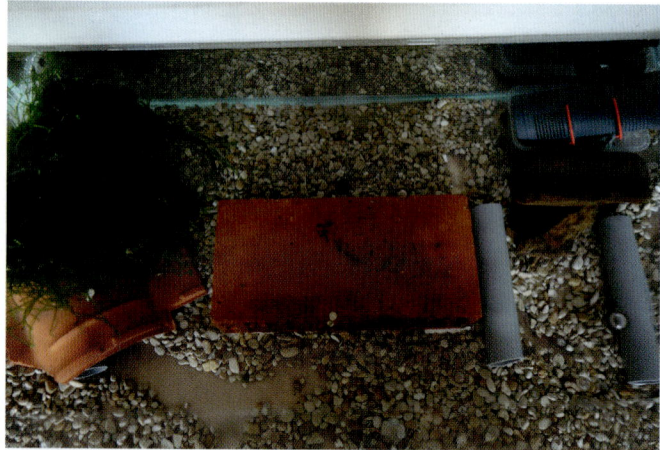

FIG 28.6 Aquarium for a pair of stream-dwelling salamanders (*Necturus lodingi*). The substrate consists of coarse gravel, aquatic vegetation of cold-tolerant Java moss, and hiding places of PVC tubes. Water is circulated, aerated, and filtered by a submersible filter. (Courtesy of Frank Pasmans.)

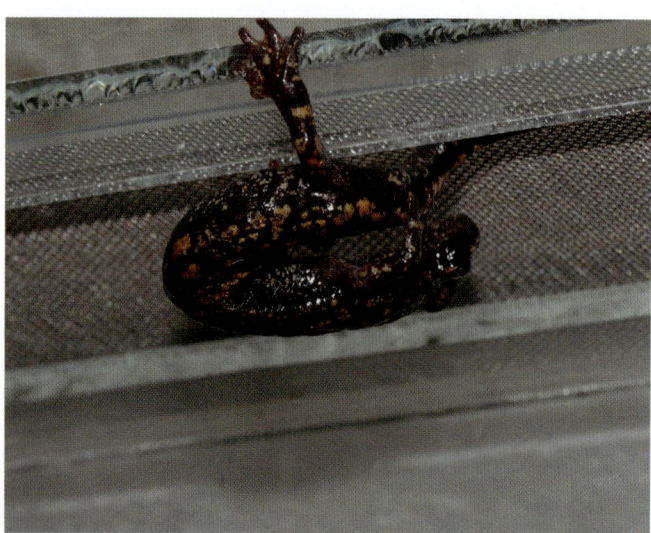

FIG 28.5 Cave salamander (*Speleomantes strinatii*) clinging to the glass ceiling of the terrarium (Courtesy of Frank Pasmans.)

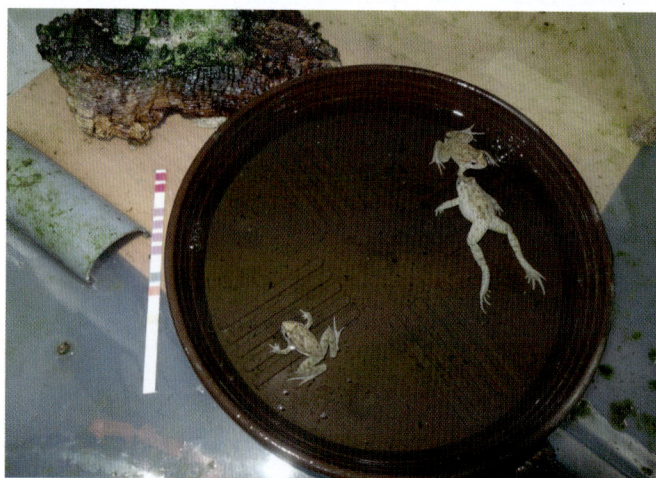

FIG 28.7 Mortality in a colony of painted frogs (*Discoglossus pictus*) due to elevated nitrite concentrations in the water container, despite the water looking rather clean to the naked eye. The dark pink coloration on the test strip demonstrates the very high levels of nitrogen metabolites. (Courtesy of Frank Pasmans.)

causes more subtle clinical symptoms such as anorexia. Buildup of toxic nitrogen metabolites is an important cause of disease and death in both larval and adult amphibians. It is important not only in aquatic settings but also in terrestrial species kept on substrates with a poor capacity to metabolize waste products (e.g., tissue paper), and a water-quality check should be part of any routine veterinary evaluation. A weekly water-quality check by the owner using commercially available testing kits is highly recommended. Optimal water quality can be maintained by proper water filtration to eliminate ammonium and nitrite, combined with regular, partial water changes to remove excessive nitrates. Anaerobic filters and resins to remove nitrate from the water are commercially available. Charcoal or activated carbon can reduce the amount of toxins or chemicals. Thus, when medication is applied to an aquarium, charcoal should be removed from the filter. The surface for nitrogen converting bacteria should be maximized, for example, by including special substrates (e.g., ceramic tubes, filter foam) in the filter compartment and by providing an aquarium substrate of sand or gravel. Likewise, a proper substrate increases the surface for bacterial growth. Generally, sand (which does not contain sharp particles) or gravel is used as substrate. Sand generally allows the roots of aquatic plants to anchor easily but has the disadvantage of easily accumulating large amounts of detritus. Gravel must be preferably smooth and of such a size that, if ingested, it will not cause foreign body impaction. Small- to medium-sized gravel generally works well. Aquatic plants not only add to the aquarium's aesthetics but create environmental enrichment for the inmates, spawning substrate, produce oxygen during the day and remove metabolic waste products such as nitrate from the water. A newly set up aquarium should be left to establish an efficient nitrogen cycle before the amphibians are added. This process takes at least 6 weeks but can be shortened by adding substrate and/or filter material from a mature aquarium to the new tank. Living aquatic plants use nitrate as fertilizer and help keep nitrate levels low. A sufficiently high concentration of dissolved oxygen in the water is particularly important for amphibian species or life stages that breathe mainly via gills and the skin but also for the proliferation of aerobic bacteria that metabolize amphibian waste products. The amount of dissolved oxygen in the water should be at least 5 mg/L (ppm). However, oversaturating the water with oxygen may cause "gas bubble disease" (Fig. 28.8).[15] The oxygen content of the water may be raised by creating a water current and, during the daytime, by the presence of aquatic plants. Even though most stream-dwelling amphibians prefer at least some water current, this does not mean that they prefer to be exposed to strong currents continuously. In fact, many stream-dwelling amphibians inhabit stream sections with weak currents.

The majority of terrestrial amphibians are best kept in well-structured terraria with a moisture gradient and a water container, the size and depth of which depend on the life history of the species kept. The shape of the terrarium should reflect the species' behavioral preferences; for example, most arboreal species appreciate climbing opportunities in a terrarium as high as possible. Easy access into and exit out of the water container is vital to prevent drowning, especially in metamorphing juveniles but also many adult terrestrial amphibians that are poor swimmers. For these aquatic sections, the same requirements with regard to water quality apply as discussed above, especially with small water containers, which are prone to pollution with feces and drowned feeder insects. A constantly wet substrate without the opportunity to retreat to drier places is detrimental to the skin of many terrestrial species. A drainage layer below the actual substrate, for example, from expanded clay balls or foam mats, can prevent stagnant moisture. Comparable to the importance of a heat gradient in reptile enclosures to facilitate thermoregulation, a moisture gradient in the amphibian terrarium is necessary. This can be accomplished by stacking layers of bark on the substrate or by keeping only part of the substrate moist by regular misting. The substrate used must be nontoxic and easy to keep clean. When using inert substrates (e.g., paper toweling), these must be regularly exchanged to avoid buildup of toxic metabolites. The use of bleached paper towels is under debate, but actual evidence of resulting health problems is lacking. Organic substrates that allow the development of metabolite-degrading bacterial communities (e.g., loam, forest soil) can be used as well. However, regular cleaning (removal of feces, dead prey items), removal, and replacement are recommended to prevent buildup of metabolites and parasites. Commercial topsoils should be avoided because many contain fertilizers or chemical additions that might prove toxic for amphibians. Live moss is esthetically pleasing but is often not long-lived in the terrarium environment and must be frequently replaced. Mulch can be used as well, if not derived from trees that produce toxic or irritating substances (pine trees, cedar). Peat can be used for species that tolerate acid soil. We discourage the use of tree fern substrate in terraria since this is often not harvested in a sustainable way. Nontoxic foam (e.g., filter mats for garden ponds) can be used but should also be regularly cleaned. Fossorial species require a substrate similar to that in their natural habitat. Notably for fossorial species, which often defecate below the surface, the substrate should be replaced regularly and a drainage layer (filter mat or clay balls) used to avoid the buildup of excessive moisture and prevent anaerobiosis of the substrate (with the production of H_2S). The use of dead leaves (we prefer oak or beech leaves, which are less prone to fungal overgrowth) on the substrate provides additional hiding places and moisture gradients. When materials are being used from amphibian-rich forests, prior decontamination (heating for 30 minutes at 80°C) will kill most potential pathogens, such as ranaviruses, Batrachochytrium sp., many bacteria, and trombiculid mites.[16–18] For all amphibians, it is vital that proper shelters are provided, with at least one shelter per animal. The type of shelter depends on the species' requirements: many arboreal species rest on or between leaves or branches. Many terrestrial species seek shelters that fit their body dimensions and prefer contact of the roof of the shelter with their back to feel secure. Shelters can include bark, PVC pipes, shells from clay pots, roof tiles, and more. Some "sit and wait" predators that rely on camouflage (e.g., Ceratophrys sp.) partially dig in the substrate to blend with their environment and should be given the opportunity to do so. When heavy objects are used in the terrarium (rocks, branches, water bowls), they must be securely attached to avoid trauma to amphibians that may try to dig underneath. Adding plants to the terrarium offers additional niches for the inmates. Many

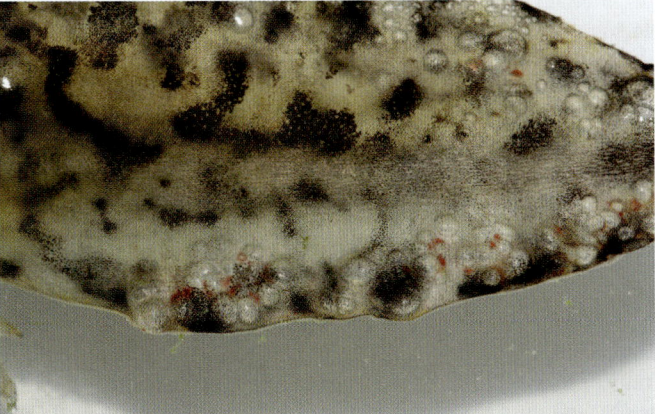

FIG 28.8 Gas bubble disease in a salamander (*Ambystoma andersonii*), visible as gas bubbles in the tissue of the tail. (Courtesy of Frank Pasmans.)

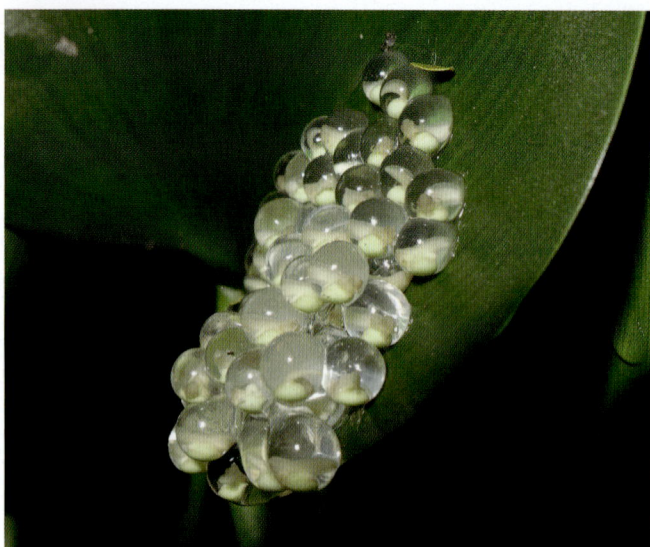

FIG 28.9 Live or plastic plants are important cage enrichment for many amphibians, for example, providing opportunities to lay eggs for these tree frogs (*Agalychnis annae*). Eggs are deposited on leaves overhanging water, and when the tadpoles hatch, they fall in the water beneath. (Courtesy of Frank Pasmans.)

arboreal species appreciate the opportunity to rest on leaves, and many species (e.g., many poison dart frogs) breed in the axils of plants, such as bromeliads, or deposit eggs on leaves overhanging water (e.g., *Agalychnis* sp., Fig. 28.9). Alternatives to these axils can be provided using dark-walled, nontoxic canisters, for example, film containers (although increasingly hard to come by) or amber plastic pill pots. When living plants are used, their leaves should not have sharp edges or spines. The relative humidity of the air should, in general, be kept high, at least at 80%. This can be achieved by regular misting using manual or automated misting systems. Either rainwater or demineralized water should be used to prevent mineral depositions. Variations in moisture should reflect seasonal moisture variations of the species concerned and are important to cycle reproductive behavior. For example, in many species, mimicking the onset of the wet season by increased misting of water or transferring the animals to a rain chamber will trigger reproduction. A limited number of species (e.g., certain *Phyllomedusa* sp.) do not tolerate a continuously high relative humidity.

Temperature

The endothermic amphibians require a taxon-specific temperature range in which they function optimally. In the case of species undergoing marked seasonal temperature differences in nature, captive conditions should reflect these thermal needs, for example, by providing a period of hibernation where appropriate. Providing these natural seasonal fluctuations is an important key to inducing amphibian reproduction. In contrast to reptiles, most amphibians do not require the presence of a thermal gradient for active thermoregulation. Providing a temperature within the range that is consistent with the species' thermal preference and taking natural day/night fluctuations into account often suffices. However, species that exhibit basking behavior such as many diurnal anurans (e.g., the widely kept fire-bellied toad, *Bombina orientalis*) or tree frogs, do benefit from access to a basking area, which can be provided by a low-power spotlight or ceramic heater. The use of high-power heat mats in amphibian enclosures to create basking areas is not recommended because accidents resulting in quick desiccation of the terrarium and inmates can occur. Providing general temperature

recommendations is not possible, and we recommend looking up thermal requirements of a given species in the relevant literature. Many species such as poison dart frogs appreciate a circadian thermal regime, with cooler nights (Table 28.1). One important temperature-related consideration is that the majority of the urodeles require temperatures that are cooler than those in most modern households. Many urodelan species do not tolerate temperatures higher than 20°C, and when kept at these higher temperatures tend to develop secondary infections including chlamydiosis.[19] A limited number of widely available species (e.g., *Tylototriton shanjing*, *Cynops ensicauda*) are notable exceptions. Cooling and heating devices are readily available commercially.

Lighting

Lighting is less of an issue for keeping healthy amphibians healthy than is the case for reptiles. A preference for a high light intensity is only appreciated by a limited number of diurnal amphibians that voluntarily expose themselves to sunlight. Although not as well understood in amphibians as in reptiles, these (partially) diurnal species likely benefit from UVB radiation for calcium metabolism to prevent secondary nutritional hyperparathyroidism, and also for color rendition.[20] Most amphibians have been bred successfully over generations without providing any UVB radiation. For nocturnal species, lighting serves the purposes of stimulating plant growth, and many species prefer dim light conditions—some are even markedly photophobic. Care must be taken not to use light sources that emit heat, which could result in overheating; fluorescent bulbs or LED lights are often recommended. Likewise, amphibian terraria should be kept from direct insolation to prevent overheating. Illumination of the terrarium should follow a photoperiod experienced by the free-ranging species. The seasonal variation in photoperiod (when appropriate) is an important reproductive stimulus in many species. Mimicking the natural photoperiod can be done stepwise, for example, with 1 hour increases or decreases of light every 2 weeks.

Outdoor Enclosures

When kept in a climate similar to that of their region of origin, many amphibians do well in outdoor enclosures, especially when provided with a pond and underground retreats to escape from heat, drought, and frost. Captive breeding of species in their home range in outdoor enclosures (e.g., for conservation purposes) mimicking the species' habitat is often successful and is far less time-consuming than breeding attempts indoors (Fig. 28.10). Such outdoor enclosures must be well fenced to prevent entry of predators (rats, cats, birds, rodents, mustelids, etc.) but also to prevent escapes. One major drawback is that outdoor enclosures for amphibians render regular health checks difficult, and major health issues, including mass mortality, can go unnoticed. Escape and direct or indirect contact of captive amphibians with native amphibians should be avoided to prevent pathogen pollution of the environment (or the inverse: infection of inmates from wild amphibians) or establishment of invasive alien species. Unless strict biosecurity can be enforced, the housing of exotic pet amphibians in outdoor enclosures should be discouraged.

QUARANTINE AND DISINFECTION PROCEDURES

Often overlooked, proper quarantine procedures are mandatory to minimize the risk of introducing infectious diseases by newly acquired amphibians (see also Chapter 19).[21,22] Independent of the source, all amphibians should be kept in quarantine for a period of at least 6 weeks, and until they appear to be healthy (or are euthanized). This determination includes no anomalies upon clinical examination (including parasitological examination of feces), normal appetite and behavior,

TABLE 28.1	**Key Husbandry Requirements of Frequently Kept Amphibian Species**				
Scientific Name/ Common Name	**Total Length/ Sexual Dimorphism**	**Life History/ Terrarium/ Temperature (Day/Night)**	**Breeding Induction**	**Reproduction**	**Suitability/Remarks**
Anura					
Ceratophrys ornata/ Bell's horned frog	10–12 cm/Male smaller, with darker throat and nuptial pads on fingers	Sit and wait predator buried in leaf litter, nocturnal/ forest floor terrarium/25°C–28°C/20°C–22°C	Drier and cooler (20°C) period followed by wet and warm period (rain chamber).	Spawn up to 2000 eggs, tadpoles carnivorous and cannibalistic	High/bred in large numbers, often carrier of *B. dendrobatidis*
Dendrobates auratus/ green poison frog	25–60 mm/Finger disks in males larger	Ground dweller, diurnal, lowland to premontane rain forest/forest floor terrarium/24°C–27°C/19°C–20°C	Breeds throughout year, alternating drier periods provides a resting period and stimulates breeding	Clutch of 6–10 eggs on land, tadpoles are carried on the male's back to the water and should be raised individually or in large containers	High/bred in large numbers in several color morphs, frequent carrier of *B. dendrobatidis*
*Dendrobates tinctorius/*dyeing poison frog	34–60 mm/Finger disks in males larger	Ground dweller, diurnal, lowland rainforest/forest floor terrarium, due to intraspecific aggression, pairwise keeping recommended/24°C–27°C/19°C–20°C	Breeds throughout year, alternating drier and wetter periods stimulates breeding	Clutch of 2–16 eggs on land, tadpoles are carried on the male's back to the water and should be raised individually or in large containers	High/bred in large numbers in several color morphs, frequent carrier of *B. dendrobatidis*
Phyllobates vittatus/ Golfo Dulce poison dart frog	26–31 mm/Females larger	Ground dweller, diurnal, lowland rainforest near brooks/forest floor terrarium, can be kept in groups/25°C–27°C/19°C–20°C	Breeds throughout year	Clutch of 7–21 eggs on land, tadpoles are carried on the male's back to the water and can be raised in groups	High
Oophaga pumilio/ strawberry poison frog	17.5–24 mm/Males of some populations have darker throats	Ground dweller, climbs regularly, diurnal, lowland rainforest/forest floor terrarium with sufficient height (>60 cm) for climbing. males very territorial/25°C–27°C/19°C–20°C	Breeds throughout year, drier period provides resting period.	Clutch of 3–10 eggs on land, tadpoles are carried on the female's back to bromeliad axils and fed with unfertilized eggs	Intermediate/extreme, locality-dependent color and pattern variation
*Litoria caerulea/*green tree frog	10–12 cm/Male with darker, wrinkled skin on throat	Nocturnal, forests, cultivated landscapes/large and high terrarium with ample climbing opportunities/23°C–28°C/20°C	Breeding induced in rain chamber after a drier period	Eggs deposited in small clumps, in total up to 2000 eggs	High
*Rhinella marina/*cane toad	To 24 cm/male smaller with nuptial pads on fingers	Nocturnal, forests, highly adaptive/very large surface terrarium/21°C–28°C/20°C	Breeding can be induced using hormones	Eggs in long jelly strings, up to 36,000 eggs	High/highly invasive species
Bombina orientalis/ oriental fire-bellied toad	To 6 cm/male with extensive foot webbing and nuptial pads on fingers	Diurnal and nocturnal, near shallow parts of brooks/ terrarium with large and shallow water part/20°C–25°C/15°C–20°C	Hibernation at 5°C; with increasing temperature in spring, animals come in breeding condition	Eggs in clutches up to 100 eggs	High/most specimens available as wild-caught animals from mass importations, frequent carrier of *B. dendrobatidis* infection
Xenopus laevis/ African clawed frog	4.5–15 cm/Male smaller, with nuptial pads, female with skin fold above cloaca	Nocturnal, in all kinds of water bodies/ aquarium/18°C–22°C	Cool period at 7°C–14°C; with increasing temperature, animals come in breeding condition.	Up to 17,000 eggs deposited singly or in small groups, tadpoles are filter feeders	High/common laboratory animal, highly invasive species, many breeding colonies infected by *B. dendrobatidis* and/or mycobacteria

Continued

TABLE 28.1	**Key Husbandry Requirements of Frequently Kept Amphibian Species—cont'd**				
Scientific Name/ Common Name	Total Length/ Sexual Dimorphism	Life History/ Terrarium/ Temperature (Day/Night)	Breeding Induction	Reproduction	Suitability/Remarks
Hymenochirus boettgeri/Zaire dwarf clawed frog	32–41 mm/Male smaller, with whitish to pinkish spot in the post axillar region	Nocturnal, rainforest ponds/ aquarium/22°C–27°C	Breeds throughout year	Up to 1000 eggs, tadpoles are predators	High/commonly sold for tropical aquaria
Dyscophus guineti/ tomato frog	60–95 mm/Males yellowish, females orange-red, Males smaller	Nocturnal, lowland rainforest ground dweller/Forest floor terrarium, Burrows in soil/23°C–28°C/20°C–22°C	After a drier period, breeding can be induced in a rain chamber	Up to 15,000 eggs per clutch, tadpoles are filter feeders	High
Mantella aurantiaca/ golden Mantella	19–31 mm/Males smaller	Diurnal, rainforest, ground dweller in swampy areas/ forest floor terrarium, especially froglets are extremely sensitive to stress/18°C–22°C/12°C–14°C	After a cooler and drier period, breeding can be induced by increasing temperature and humidity	Up to 60 eggs produced, eggs laid on land, tadpoles are flushed to water by rain	Low/critically endangered in its native range in Madagascar
Urodela					
Cynops orientalis/ Chinese fire-bellied newt	Up to 9 cm/males smaller with shorter tail and cloaca more pronounced	Nocturnal on land, nocturnal and diurnal in water, pond dweller/can be housed fully aquatic in aquarium or in an aquaterrarium/15°C–25°C	After a hibernation period (2°C–5°C), breeding starts with increasing temperatures	Up to 100 eggs folded between leaves of aquatic vegetation	High/mass imports from China, potential carrier of *B. salamandrivorans*
Paramesotriton chinensis/Chinese warty newt	Up to 18.5 cm/male smaller, with more pronounced cloaca and with silver-white stripe on tail during breeding season	Nocturnal, stream dweller, in captivity fully aquatic/ stream aquarium, males highly territorial/15°C–20°C	After a hibernation period (7°C–10°C), newts come in breeding condition with increasing temperature	Eggs are deposited singly between leaves of aquatic plants	Low/mass imports from China despite local protection, potential carrier of *B. salamandrivorans*
Ambystoma mexicanum/axolotl	Up to 30 cm/male with more pronounced cloaca	Nocturnal, fully aquatic, originally from canal system/aquarium/15°C–22°C	Sudden cooling the water to 10°C for a few days with subsequent gradual increase in temperature	Up to 1000 eggs deposited in small clumps among vegetation	High/paedomorphic species, most widely used urodelan species in research, near extinct in the wild but bred at large scale, several color morphs available
Ambystoma tigrinum/ tiger salamander	Up to 30 cm/male with more pronounced cloaca	Nocturnal, fossorial, terrestrial but breeds in ponds/terrarium for burrowing species, aquaterrarium or aquarium during breeding season/15°C–20°C	Depending on the origin of the animals, mostly start breeding after hibernation	Up to 800 eggs deposited in small clumps among vegetation	High, but produces large amounts of waste
Salamandra salamandra/fire salamander	Up to 28 cm/male with more pronounced cloaca	Nocturnal, terrestrial ground dweller in cool forests with streams/forest floor terrarium, males can be territorial/10°C–20°C	Courtship mostly in autumn, deposition of larvae in spring	Up to 75 larvae are deposited in streams or ponds	Intermediate
Tylototriton shanjing/ Mandarin salamander	Up to 17 cm/male with somewhat more pronounced cloaca	Nocturnal, terrestrial ground dweller in forests, breeds in ponds/forest floor terrarium/15°C–25°C	After a cooler and drier period in winter, increased temperatures and humidity induces breeding	Up to 291 eggs are deposited singly in or near water	High when captive bred/ several species of *Tylototriton* are being imported from China despite local protection, potential carrier of *B. salamandrivorans* and ranaviruses

TABLE 28.1 Key Husbandry Requirements of Frequently Kept Amphibian Species—cont'd

Scientific Name/ Common Name	Total Length/ Sexual Dimorphism	Life History/ Terrarium/ Temperature (Day/Night)	Breeding Induction	Reproduction	Suitability/Remarks
Pleurodeles waltl/ ribbed newt	Up to 30 cm/male with longer tail and nuptial pads on upper arm	Nocturnal, terrestrial salamander, aquatic during breeding season/can be kept fully aquatic in an aquarium/15°C–20°C	Often starts breeding when temperature drops in autumn	Up to 1300 eggs deposited singly or in clusters among aquatic vegetation	High
Taricha granulosa/ rough-skinned newt	Up to 22 cm/males with longer tail, smoother skin, and nuptial pads on toe tips during breeding	Terrestrial but reproduces in all types of water, flowing and standing/can be kept fully aquatic in an aquarium/18°C–20°C	Often starts breeding after hibernation at 10°C	Up to 160 eggs singly among aquatic vegetation	Intermediate/one of the most toxic newts, the skin containing tetradotoxin
Necturus maculosus/ mudpuppy	Up to 50 cm/males with papillae on the cloaca	Fully aquatic, rivers and lakes/aquarium/15°C–20°C	Winter temperature between 5°C–10°C, mates in autumn or winter, eggs deposited in spring	Up to 193 eggs laid on the roof of a nesting site and guarded by the female	Low/wild specimens still caught in large numbers and sold a.o. as fish bait or laboratory animals
Gymnophiona					
Typhlonectes compressicauda/ rubber eel	Up to 45 cm/larger white spot in the cloacal region of the male	Fully aquatic/aquarium/23°C–27°C	Appears to mate mainly in autumn	Viviparous with up to 11 young born	High

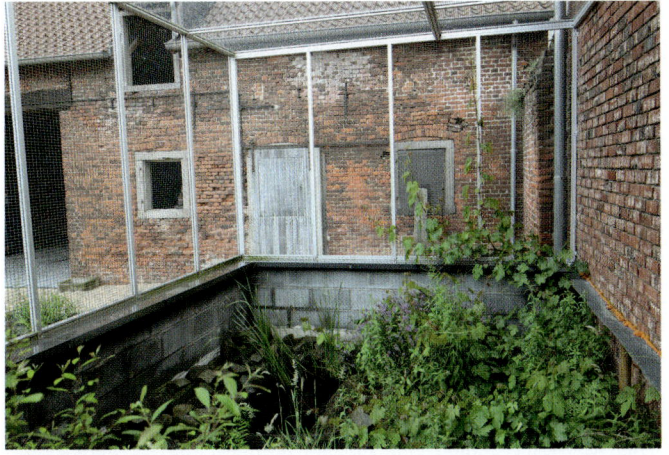

FIG 28.10 Outdoor enclosure for European anurans (midwife toads, *Alytes obstetricians*, and spadefoot toads, *Pelobates fuscus*) protected against predators by the fence and against escape of the inmates by overhanging cover stones. When properly built, such enclosures provide excellent opportunities for mass propagation of species within their geographical range. (Courtesy of Frank Pasmans.)

and completion of any required veterinary treatment, for example, against parasitic or bacterial infections. Effective treatment against enteric flagellate and/or enteric or respiratory nematode infections can make the difference between successfully establishing a captive colony or mass mortality.

Quarantine enclosures (similar enclosures can be used for amphibian patient hospitalization) for amphibians should meet all of their needs (temperature, light, humidity, proper nutrition), with an emphasis on hygiene and creating a stress-free environment. A hygienic environment that meets these demands can be created by using moist paper toweling as a substrate when possible (e.g., not for burrowing species), providing proper, easy to inspect and clean hiding places (e.g., PVC tubes), and a water bowl of appropriate size for the species. The use of paper towels facilitates inspection and collection of feces for coprologic examination. The production of feces is a good indication of the animal's appetite, with a lack suggesting anorexia. During quarantine, amphibians are preferably kept in isolation. Disturbance and handling of the animals should be kept to an absolute minimum. For nervous species, making transparent sides visible (e.g., by taping colored paper to the enclosure) avoids the development of rostral ulcerations (Fig. 28.11). The size of the container for anurans should preferably be at least the length of the frog's leap to avoid trauma. Climbing species will appreciate the presence of a variety of elevated surfaces (e.g., PVC pipes, branches, plastic plants). We prefer not to use living plants in quarantine enclosures since these cannot be properly decontaminated between uses.

Any animal that dies during quarantine should be subjected to a full necropsy examination. When possible, diagnostics should not be limited to the relatively few known amphibian pathogens but should include gross pathology and thorough histopathology including viral, bacterial, fungal, and parasitic evaluations of tissues. For all quarantined animals, testing for the most common diseases during this period (ranaviruses, *Batrachochytrium dendrobatidis*, and *B. salamandrivorans*) is mandatory. Whereas this is reliable for chytrid infections, noninvasive sampling for ranaviruses using skin swabs is less reliable, and so negative results do not invariably mean that animals are free from ranaviruses. There is no reliable method to examine the presence of many other common amphibian pathogens in clinically healthy amphibians, for example, Chlamydiales or mycobacteria. When the absence of these pathogens is a requirement (for example, in laboratory colonies or for conservation breeding programs), and where appropriate, a proportion

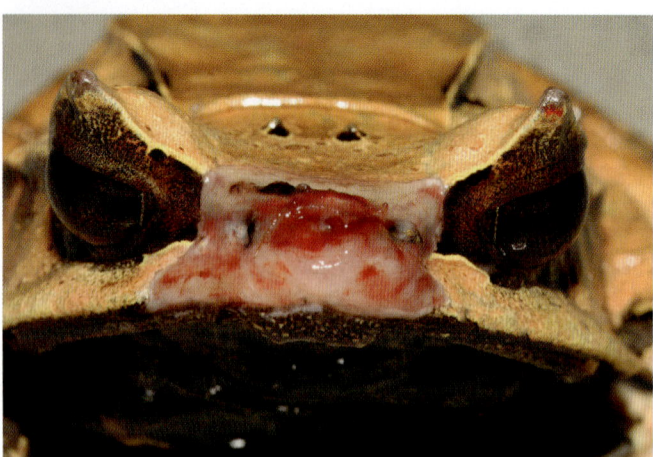

FIG 28.11 Snout ulceration in a frog (*Megophrys nasuta*) by leaping against the glass windows of the terrarium. (Courtesy of Frank Pasmans.)

of these animals could be euthanized and thoroughly examined. However, depending on pathogen prevalence, even such radical entry control is not guaranteed to prevent pathogen introduction. Although it is not clear to which extent most pathogens can be vertically transmitted, it is safe to assume that establishing captive colonies starting from eggs reduces the likelihood of introducing infectious diseases.

Given the risk of pathogen pollution, all materials, including water that has come into contact with captive amphibians, should be disinfected before disposal. Decontamination can be done using chemical compounds (often recommended are sodium hypochlorite or Virkon S) or by heat treatment. All materials should be thoroughly rinsed after disinfection. Disinfectants with residual activity (e.g., phenolics such as chloroxylenol-containing products) can be toxic and should not be used around amphibians. See Chapter 18 for more details.

ENVIRONMENTAL TOXINS

Zinc and copper from galvanized copper tubes are a source of possible intoxication and should be avoided. Instead, tubes should be of polyethylene, polypropylene, or nylon construction. Lead intoxication may occur as a consequence of using lead piping, or lead may be introduced in the aquarium as weights, attached to aquatic plants. Plastic softeners may release dioxinlike PCBs (polychlorinated biphenyls) in phenol and acrylic plastics or phthalate esters.[23] Only products specifically produced for aquaria or used for human food/water storage should be used. Nongloved handling of amphibians by smokers may result in acute nicotine intoxication.[24] The use of insect repellents, especially those based on DEET, is generally contraindicated when handling amphibians, although toxicity studies for amphibians are largely lacking.

TRANSPORTATION OF AMPHIBIANS

The transportation of amphibians may be subject to legal limitations for conservation or sanitary reasons (e.g., due to the emergence of *B. salamandrivorans*, the transportation of many urodelan species to and within the United States and Switzerland has been temporarily banned). International animal transportation requires fulfilling all legal and administrative obligations and following guidelines set for animal transportation. Sending amphibians by mail is illegal in most countries. When transporting amphibians, this should preferably be done in individual containers. Cohousing specimens, even from the same species,

during transportation may result in mass mortality due to massive secretion of amphibian toxins when the animals are stressed. Containers should be lined with a substrate that prevents trauma when the container is rocked (e.g., foam rubber, rehydrate sphagnum), should contain ample ventilation (use caution when drilling ventilation holes as they can result in sharp edges) and provide sufficient moisture (for example, wet paper toweling or sphagnum). For short-term transportation, providing food is not advisable. Temperatures should be kept as constant as possible during transportation and at a temperature within the species' preferred thermal range. Enclosures containing animals can be put in styrofoam boxes that should comply with all relevant legislation and cushioned with newspaper or other padding. Transportation boxes should never be exposed to sunlight, because this quickly results in overheating. Aquatic species or larvae can be either transported on a wet substrate (e.g., many aquatic, nonpaedomorphic urodelans) or in plastic bags used for the transportation of live fish. These bags must be filled with water for $\frac{1}{3}$ of the total volume. Silicon or breathable bags for fish transportation that allow gas exchange must be filled completely, which prevents the contained animals from being shaken too much. These bags even allow for the transportation of very sensitive tadpoles from stream-breeding frogs.

SUITABILITY OF SPECIES

Most species of amphibians can be kept and bred successfully in captivity. Important factors for success include acquiring healthy animals, a knowledgeable keeper, providing proper husbandry and nutrition, and use of expert veterinary care when needed. Some species have requirements that can be difficult to provide, such as some of the larger species for giant salamanders (*Andrias* sp.). Additionally, species with specific husbandry demands can be more challenging (e.g., aquatic species from cool caves or high mountain streams, species with specific dietary requirements such as ants). Overall, many species are currently being bred in sufficient numbers, and in general, acquisition of captive-bred offspring is recommended. Wild-caught animals should be avoided. The latter pose a significant risk of introducing exotic diseases not only into the captive collection but also to populations of wild indigenous species, as recently demonstrated by the emergence of *B. salamandrivorans* in Europe.[25] This fungus has likely been vectored into Europe through the pet trade in Asiatic urodelans and is currently decimating salamander populations. Introduction of wild-caught amphibians into the pet trade is stressful for the animals and often results in high mortality. Collection of wild caught amphibians often occurs when large numbers congregate, such as during breeding. Often these wild-caught animals end up in poor condition with heavy parasitic infections, secondary and often lethal bacterial skin infections, and viral or fungal diseases (Fig. 28.12).[26] Unsustainable harvesting of amphibians is one of the causes of the current global amphibian declines.[27]

STOCKING DENSITY

Generally adults of many amphibian species and most juveniles tolerate relatively high densities. However, males (primarily) of many species, especially dart frogs and urodeles, do exhibit or aggressive behavior. For these species, only a single male with one to several females should be kept in the same enclosure. Otherwise overt or cryptic aggression will result in the suppressed animal(s) becoming stressed, showing loss of appetite and behavioral anomalies, and becoming more susceptible to secondary infections. In general, only amphibians of similar size should be cohoused, because cannibalism is common. Although many amphibian larvae live in dense communities in nature, others (e.g., many species of poison dart frogs and urodeles) are highly cannibalistic

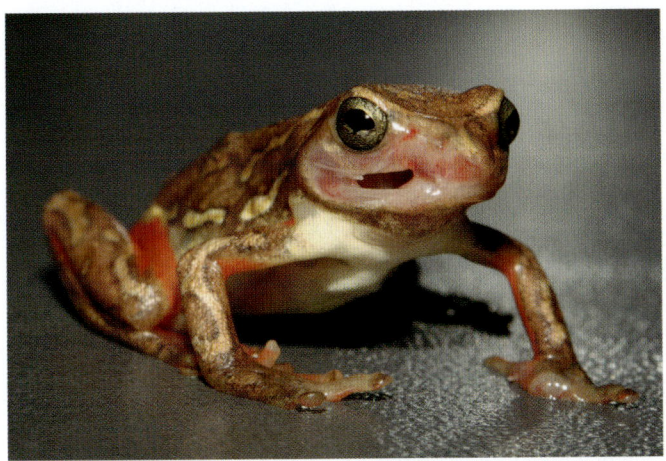

FIG 28.12 Wild-caught tree frog (*Afrixalus* sp.) with severe snout ulceration due to secondary bacterial infection following recent importation. (Courtesy of Frank Pasmans.)

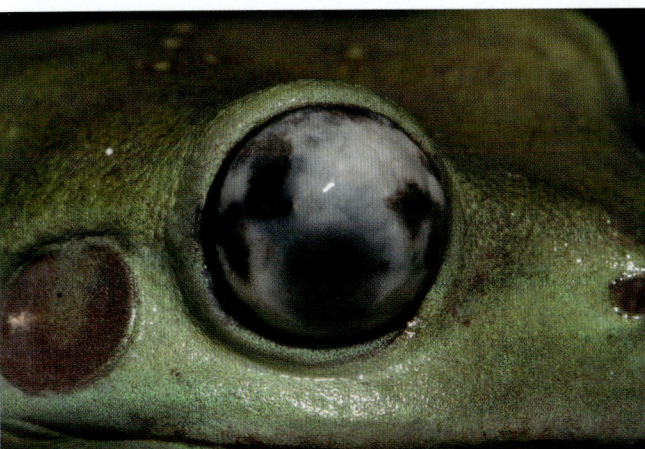

FIG 28.13 Corneal lipidosis in a tree frog (*Litoria caerulea*), which is associated with hypercholesteremia. (Courtesy of Frank Pasmans.)

and must be raised in small groups consisting of similarly sized individuals or even in isolation.

FEEDING AND NUTRITION

Most amphibians post-metamorphosis feed on living, mostly invertebrate prey items. In captivity, many species, mainly aquatic, can be conditioned to accept substitutes like commercial pellets produced for turtles, fish, or aquatic amphibians. The advantage of feeding pellets is that these can be supplemented with minerals (calcium) and vitamins (e.g., vitamin A) that may be largely lacking when feeding live invertebrate prey. Leftovers must be removed within one hour after feeding to prevent deterioration of water quality. Other dead food items may be offered occasionally such as raw meat. However, this should not be used routinely because nutritional deficiencies, including nutritional secondary hyperparathyroidism (NSHP), can occur. Although pellets are commonly used to sustain amphibians over generations, we recommend offering a variety of food items, not only for dietary needs but also as enrichment, allowing the amphibian to display natural predatory behavior.

Amphibians not accepting pellets should be fed live prey, mostly invertebrates. For large amphibians, depending on the species, vertebrates such as fish and rodents can also be offered; however, the feeding of live vertebrates may be illegal in some areas. In principle, invertebrate prey items discussed in the section on reptile nutrition can be used. Most amphibians are not picky eaters and will consume whatever fits in their mouth. The most common commercially bred food items are crickets (Gryliidae), buffalo worms or mealworms (*Alphitobius laevigatus* or *Tenebrio molitor*), fruit flies (*Drosophila* sp.), springtails (Collembola), woodlice (Oniscidea), and annelid worms (Lumbricidae, Tubificidae, Enchytraeidae) for terrestrial amphibians. Good-quality commercial feeder animals can provide an excellent staple diet for most terrestrial amphibians. However, these invertebrates must be properly fed themselves and enriched at least with calcium and vitamin A (see below). A varied diet reduces chances of nutritional disorders (Fig. 28.13). With regard to feeding nematodes, many amphibians do not accept the commonly sold worm bait species belonging to the genera *Dendrobaena* or *Eisenia*, because these worms excrete a foul-smelling substance. Aquatic amphibians can be fed crustaceans (*Daphnia* sp.), arthropod larvae ("bloodworm," *Chironomus* larvae), nematodes (*Tubifex*, several species of terrestrial worms) or, if legally permissible, aquatic vertebrates (small fish, tadpoles). When feeding vertebrate prey to amphibians, care must

be taken not to introduce parasites or infectious diseases. Hence (and also for legal and ethical aspects), these prey items should always be captive bred, and the source should be free of the most common infectious amphibian diseases (at least chytrid fungi, ranaviruses, mycobacteria). Some fish and anuran species are indeed easily bred in large numbers, for example, guppies or frogs from the genus *Discoglossus* (Pasmans et al., in press). When feeding commercial aquatic live prey like bloodworms (*Tubifex*), these should first be thoroughly rinsed to remove dead animals. Quality of these feed items often is poor and may be a source of heavy metals.[28] Use caution with quantity offered because massive die-offs of these prey items in the aquarium may quickly pollute the water. Although crustaceans like *Artemia* sp. are readily available and constitute a suitable food item, they have a short life span in fresh water, quickly die, and can pollute the water.

In general, feeding live prey items to amphibians can result in the same nutritional problems described for reptiles. Insects must be enriched with at least calcium (and vitamin D_3) and vitamin A using gut-loading of the feeder insects or dusting of the insects with a mineral- and vitamin-containing powder before feeding them to the amphibians. NSHP and hypovitaminosis A are both common nutritional disorders of amphibians. In aquatic amphibians, SNHP signs may be less obvious, given that body weight is largely supported by the water. In terrestrial amphibians, NSHP problems are often obvious, resulting in bone deformations, often of the skull and spine (Fig. 28.14). A calcium/phosphorous ratio of 1.5:1 in prey items should be attempted (combining gut-loading and dusting of feeder insects). There are no established guidelines for the recommended daily intake of vitamin A by amphibians but hypovitaminosis A (often noted as "short tongue disease") is common in captives.[29] It is likely that amphibians are not capable of processing beta-carotene in significant amounts to make vitamin A physiologically available. Thus preformed vitamin A should be provided in the diet. Excess supplementation should be avoided since hypervitaminosis A is of equal concern as it is in reptiles (see relevant chapters on nutrition, hypo-, and hypervitaminosis A). Adding vitamin D_3 to the feeder insects may likewise be beneficial, especially if diurnal amphibians do not have access to UVB radiation. As in reptiles, predation of amphibians by feeder insects occasionally occurs. This can be avoided by providing the feeder insects with food in the amphibian terrarium (e.g., a dog pellet) by not overfeeding (minimizing the number of live insects in the environment at a time) and by respecting predator–prey size relationships. Notable losses to prey can occur in amphibian larvae-fed predatory

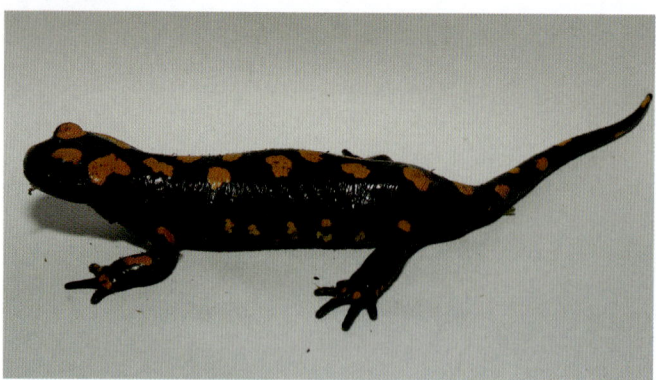

FIG 28.14 Nutritional secondary hyperparathyroidism in a salamander (*Salamandra infraimmaculata*), with severe spinal deformation. (Courtesy of Frank Pasmans.)

species of *Cyclops*. A final problem with live prey items is poor adaption of prey (e.g., crickets) to the cooler temperatures required for keeping many urodelans, resulting in prey death and contribution to rapid fungal growth of the substrate. Dead prey items must be removed promptly.

Aquatic amphibian larvae should receive a more species-specific diet. Urodelan larvae predate on small live prey (rule of thumb: prey items smaller than the eye). Anuran tadpoles, however, have highly divergent feeding habits. These range from herbivorous to omnivorous species, with some that scrape algae and detritus from surfaces to specialized amphibian egg feeders and predatory tadpoles. For many anuran species, feed composed of fish flakes, turtle pellets, frozen and thawed vegetables such as lettuce, and *Spirulina* cyanobacteria, enriched with yeast and a vitamin/mineral mixture provides a suitable diet. Feeding oxalate-containing plants such as spinach or kale should be avoided to prevent renal oxalosis. When feeding tadpoles, frequently feeding smaller amounts reduces deterioration of water quality. Many species exhibit direct development in ovo on land and when they hatch, can be fed small prey items. During metamorphosis, most amphibians refuse feeding.

Feeding frequency depends on the species and on the life stage. Feeding several smaller-sized prey items instead of a few large ones is recommended. For many adult amphibians, feeding once or twice weekly is sufficient. Very active amphibians with higher metabolic rates (e.g., poison dart frogs, *Mantella* sp.) and adults during the breeding period require more intensive feeding. Larval or juvenile amphibians benefit from a near-constant food supply.

A common problem when raising larvae, especially those with bright red markings, is poor color development. Although this apparently does not affect the animal's health, this can be remedied by providing carotenoid-containing prey items such as crustaceans. Carotenoids may be artificially added to the amphibian feed, for example, by feeding carotenoids to crickets. Mixed carotenoids appear to have a more beneficial effect on reddish coloration than mere beta-carotene.[30]

REFERENCES

See www.expertconsult.com for a complete list of references.

Bacteriology

James F.X. Wellehan and Stephen J. Divers

REPTILES AS MICROBIAL ECOSYSTEMS

Reptile patients are often approached as a collection of eukaryotic cells organized into organ systems. This is highly misleading; most of the cells in a vertebrate are prokaryotic. Bacteria are especially critical for digestion and immune function, and maintenance of healthy bacterial flora is essential. Although birds nest in the middle of the reptile family tree, making them clearly reptiles, for the purposes of this chapter, only the bacteriology of paraphyletic nonavian reptiles is emphasized.

Clinicians are also often misled by Koch's postulates; by fulfilling or not fulfilling these requirements in a controlled experiment, a microbe is often then considered dichotomously as a pathogen or not a pathogen. This is far from the case; in the real world, numerous host, pathogen, and environmental factors (including coinfections, temperature, nutrition, handling stress, crowding, and others) play significant roles in whether a pathogen manifests as disease. There are numerous documented asymptomatic Ebola virus infections in humans, and *Lactobacillus acidophilus,* which is usually thought of as a probiotic in yogurt, has caused fatal sepsis.[1,2] When infectious disease is more properly considered as ecology, it is obvious that a typical disease scenario involves several infectious agents in concert with other environmental factors. Coinfection with both *Austwickia chelonae* and ranavirus has been found in skin lesions in bearded dragons (*Pogona vitticeps*), and coinfection with *Paranannizziopsis guarroi* and *Devriesea agamarum* has been seen in skin lesions in other bearded dragons.[3,4] Like all vertebrates, reptile patients are complex ecosystems, and we are still in the early stages of learning about the complex ecological interactions between the eukaryotic components of a reptile patient and the diverse prokaryotic components. Rather than thinking of a war on bacteria, clinicians should have the goal of improving ecosystem health within a reptile patient.

Evolution is an essential concept in biology; when one considers definitions for life, perhaps the simplest and most elegant definition is that life consists of things that evolve. Clinically, this is most immediately apparent with infectious disease. Because of short generation times, evolution of bacteria occurs in a time frame impacting clinical management of a patient. To compensate, the most rapidly evolving genes in vertebrates are immune-related. A bacterium does not "want" to cause disease or not cause disease. All life on earth has been selected for billions of years to reproduce successfully, and this is all that matters from an evolutionary standpoint. If pathogenic traits provide an evolutionary advantage in a given situation, they will be selected for. If they provide a disadvantage, they will be selected against.

There are a number of important selective pressures impacting microbes in a reptile host, including nutrition, temperature, the need to transfer to a new host, competition with other microbes, and the host immune system. A reptile host is a nutrient-rich environment for bacteria. However, some nutrients may be sequestered; one example is iron, which is a limiting factor for the growth of many bacteria. Significant resources are spent by the host synthesizing transferrin, lactoferrin, and ferritin to make iron unavailable. Many bacterial virulence pathways have evolved to access this sequestered iron.[5,6] Iron storage disease or clinical administration of iron may rapidly favor bacteria with these pathways. Nutrition also plays a major and long-lasting role in the host immune response. In southern grass skinks (*Pseudemoia entrecasteauxii*), maternal carotenoid intake has been shown to have a significant effect on the immune response of offspring by providing lipopolysaccharide (LPS), which is important in developing an immunogenic bacterial cell wall component.[7]

Ectothermic hosts require bacterial flora to have the ability to survive at different temperatures. Infectious disease manifestation may be highly temperature dependent in ectotherms.[8] In reptiles, temperature manipulation is often the most significant therapeutic approach. Further investigation of the role of temperature in disease manifestation in reptiles is strongly indicated, especially with populations of many species critically declining and likely to be impacted by anthropogenic climate change.[9,10]

The need to transfer to a new host creates significant selective pressure. This often involves secretion of large amounts of bacteria via respiratory discharge or diarrhea, but other routes occur, such as use of insect vectors. There are three fundamental strategies that can be utilized to deal with limited host lifespans. First, bacteria may adapt to a balance with the host environment, creating a selective pressure to keep the host alive. Second, bacteria may survive well in the environment, decreasing selective pressure to keep the host alive. Finally, bacteria may move quickly to a new host, also decreasing selective pressure to keep the host alive; high host density favors this, and increased stocking density creates environments selecting for pathogenicity.

Microbial competition is also a major selective pressure in a reptile; many organisms want to live in such a nutrient-rich environment. The majority of antimicrobials are derived from products secreted by other microbes that help them compete for ecologic niches. Animal guts are some of the most diverse and rich ecosystems to be found anywhere. Many organisms that have evolved in such a competitive environment have resistance to many antimicrobials, with *Enterococcus* sp. being a classic example.

There are far more bacterial cells than eukaryotic cells in a healthy reptile. Traditional approaches to examining bacterial diversity have depended on culture; this is a poor way of assaying diversity. Culture-independent methods, such as 16S PCR and cloning, or high-throughput sequencing methods, have revealed that standard culture-based methods will detect between 1% and 10% of bacterial species present in most ecologic niches. A vertebrate is a complex ecosystem.[11] This system may be very dynamic. The gut flora of Burmese pythons (*Python bivittatus*) changes significantly in response to feeding.[12] Postprandially, bacteria in the phylum Firmicutes (the "classic" gram positives, containing organisms such as *Clostridium*, *Lactobacillus*, and *Peptostreptococcus*) increase dramatically, whereas those in the phylum Bacteroidetes (primarily containing anaerobic gram negatives such as *Bacteroides* and *Prevotella*) make up a greater percentage of the fewer species present after fasting. The gut flora did not significantly share species with prey mice, with the exception of the temporary postprandial establishment of *Lactobacillus* sp.

Microbial ecologic disturbance may have significant negative impacts on many aspects of health. Damage to healthy gut flora by antibiotic use provides opportunity for invasive species; recent treatment with antibiotics markedly increases host susceptibility to *Salmonella*.[13] A 5-day course of ciprofloxacin will change human gut flora diversity and composition for several weeks, and the original composition may never reestablish.[14] In many ways, the use of broad-spectrum antibiotics for a bacterial infection in a vertebrate is analogous to starting a forest fire to get rid of coyotes. The ideal treatment for a bacterial pathogen would be as narrow-spectrum as possible, minimally disturbing the rest of the host ecosystem. Fidoxamicin, which targets only *Clostridium difficile* and a few very closely related species, and does not even significantly impact many other *Clostridium* sp., is an excellent example. Unfortunately, current market forces have resulted in pharmaceutical companies markedly cutting antibiotic development; the few antibiotics developed in recent years have as broad a spectrum as possible, and narrow spectrum antibiotics are generally not put through further development and clinical trials.

Antibiotic use without consideration of microbial ecology and evolution rapidly leads to failure. Back in the 1980s, gentamicin was promoted for eradication of *Salmonella* from turtles.[15] Over the next few years, the *Salmonella* isolates from farmed turtles acquired a high rate of aminoglycoside resistance, and therefore posed a greater risk to human health than they had previously.[16] Several studies have suggested that wild turtles may have a lower carriage rate for *Salmonella*.[17,18] The only realistic way to reduce the risk of *Salmonella* in farmed turtles over the long term is to alter the ecologic niche that it inhabits. Keeping farmed animals in high population densities increases contact rates, pathogen loads, and stress, lowering barriers to transmission. Increased ease of transmission reduces the selective pressure to keep the host alive, selecting toward virulence.[19] The stress of close confinement also has significant negative impacts on numerous health parameters.[20] The only realistic way to reduce the risk of *Salmonella* in hatchling turtles is to alter the ecology, getting rid of high-density turtle farming, as well as farming at lower densities.[21]

Other routine husbandry practices in the reptile pet trade also create strong evolutionary selective pressures toward bacterial pathogenicity. It is also common to select for color mutants. This usually involves some degree of inbreeding to select for what are often recessive traits. A major driving force for the evolution of sex is acquisition of genetic diversity for immune function. Inbreeding results in selection for greater disease.[22] Finally, reptile species from all over the world, stressed with capture, holding, and transport, are brought to large dealers and placed in the same facility. This is an ideal situation for pathogens to host jump, often resulting in dramatic disease outbreaks.[23]

To reduce significant selective pressures toward highly pathogenic bacterial diseases, major changes in the reptile industry are indicated. Genetic diversity in populations needs to be valued and monitored through appropriate use of studbooks and cooperative rather than competitive interactions with breeders. Breeding for mutations needs to be discouraged. Proper biosecurity practices must be understood and implemented. Housing needs to be revised, with larger enclosures for individual animals designed so that feeding and cleaning is accomplished without cross-contamination. Importation of wild animals for pets needs to be strongly discouraged. Facilities should focus on single species and have smaller numbers of animals at lower densities.

The routine use of antibiotics implies a low level of expertise on the part of the clinician. The use of antibiotics should be limited to cases where there are specific indications of bacterial disease. Empirical use of antibiotics should be limited to cases where a delay in therapy is likely to have a significant negative impact on the health of the patient, and diagnostic samples should be collected before starting therapy. Antibiotic therapy should always be done in conjunction with concurrent therapies and husbandry changes, addressing the patient's ability to fight infection. Antibiotic use should be based on sound pharmacokinetic data whenever possible. Allometric scaling is not reliable and should not be used for drug calculations.[24] The half life of cefovecin in dogs is 133 hours; in green iguanas, it is less than 4 hours.[25,26] If pharmacokinetic data were lacking, empirical use of cefovecin extrapolating from dog doses would result in subtherapeutic levels in iguanas. Alternate scenarios could result in toxicosis. Subtherapeutic antibiotic levels may have significant negative impacts on patient health and also have significant public health implications.[27] Subtherapeutic antibiotic use often significantly increases resistance to entirely different classes of antibiotics, due to gene linkage.[28] Development of resistance is much lower with administration of appropriate therapeutic doses.[29] Within the constraints of available knowledge, drug selection should emphasize the most narrow-spectrum, first-line antibiotic for which knowledge of therapeutic dosing is available. In keeping with numerous recommendations regarding antimicrobial stewardship, advanced cephalosporins and fluroquinolones should be reserved for resistant cases.[30]

BACTERIAL DIAGNOSTICS

In order to make a diagnosis of bacterial disease, a thorough understanding of the microbial ecology of the patient is necessary. A history and physical examination is a good starting point, with the recognition that husbandry has played a major role in almost any disease process for which a captive reptile is presented, and husbandry improvements will need to be part of the therapeutic approach. When visible lesions are present, cytology or histology is often a good next step. It is important to develop reasonable in-house cytology skills; rapid evaluation of a dif-quik, gram stain (Box 29.1), and acid-fast staining (Box 29.2) is important for further test selection; this should later be confirmed with a board-certified veterinary clinical pathologist. A complete blood count to look for evidence of infection/inflammation and a plasma biochemistry to narrow concerns to specific organ systems are often helpful. Ultrasonography, endoscopy, or other diagnostic imaging may be helpful to identify internal lesions and guide sample collection. Once the results of initial diagnostic tests are in hand, appropriate diagnostic testing for bacteria can be selected.

There are two major approaches to testing for bacterial disease. These tests are based on either the animal's acquired immune response to an agent or the presence of the agent. Acquired immune responses can be further subdivided into two categories. Tests that evaluate antibody production against specific bacteria assess the reptile's humoral immune response. The most commonly used tests for acquired immune response

BOX 29.1 Gram Stain

Materials required:
Clean glass slides
Inoculating loop or sterile Q-tips or sterile microbrushes
Bunsen burner or similar
Distilled water
Crystal violet (primary stain)
Grams iodine (mordant)
95% Ethyl alcohol or ethanol (decolorizer)
Safranin (secondary stain)
Bibulous or absorbent paper
Microscope with x1000 oil immersion

Procedure:
1. Use a flamed inoculating loop, sterile Q-tip, or microbrush to apply a thin layer of clinical material to the cleaned surface of a glass slide.
2. Air dry and heat fix.
3. Gently flood smear with crystal violet and let stand for 1 minute.
4. Tilt the slide and gently rinse with distilled water.
5. Gently flood the smear with Gram's iodine and let stand for 1 minute.
6. Tilt the slide and gently rinse with distilled water.
7. Decolorize using 95% ethyl alcohol or acetone. Tilt the slide and apply the alcohol drop by drop for 5–10 seconds until the alcohol runs almost clear. Be careful not to overdecolorize.
8. Immediately rinse with distilled water.
9. Gently flood with safranin to counterstain and let stand for 45 seconds.
10. Tilt the slide and gently rinse with distilled water.
11. Blot dry the slide with bibulous paper, or quickly air dry.
12. View the smear using a light-microscope under oil-immersion x1000.

Gram-positive bacteria appear blue, and gram-negative bacteria pink.

BOX 29.2 Acid-Fast Stain

Materials required:
Clean glass slides
Inoculating loop or sterile Q-tips or sterile microbrushes
Bunsen burner or similar
Beaker with water in tripod stand
Tweezers
Distilled water
Carbol fuschin (primary stain)
25% sulfuric acid (decolorizer)
Methylene blue (secondary stain)
Bibulous or absorbent paper
Microscope with x1000 oil immersion

Procedure:
1. Use a flamed inoculating loop, sterile Q-tip, or microbrush to apply a thin layer of clinical material to the cleaned surface of a glass slide.
2. Air dry and heat fix.
3. Cover the bacterial smear with a piece of absorbent paper cut to fit the smear and slide.
4. Place the slide over a container of boiling water.
5. Saturate the paper with carbol fuschin and steam for 5 minutes. Keep the paper moist by adding more stain as required.
6. Remove the absorbent paper using tweezers; wash the excess stain with distilled water, and allow the slide to cool.
7. Decolorize the slide with 25% sulfuric acid.
8. Rinse the slide with distilled water.
9. Counterstain the cells with methylene blue stain for 45 seconds.
10. Wash the slide with distilled water and blot dry the slide.
11. View the smear using a light-microscope under oil-immersion x1000.

Acid-fast bacteria are stained pink.

---

to bacteria in reptiles are western blots and ELISAs for *Mycoplasma agassizii* in *Gopherus* sp. tortoises. Tests that evaluate the presence of cellular immunity, which is centered around the T-cell receptor, are unfortunately not commonly available; assays that are used in human medicine include T-cell proliferation assays. It is important when assaying humoral immunity to consider that it is only part of the acquired immune response and generally the less important aspect for defense against intracellular pathogens.

Commonly used assays for the presence of bacteria include culture and PCR based techniques; these should be targeted as much as possible. Diverse normal flora are present on the external surfaces and in the gastrointestinal tract of reptiles; untargeted cultures of these without significant corollary data are clinically uninterpretable. If cytology indicates a morphology and gram or acid fast staining result, this should be communicated to the laboratory. An appropriate differential diagnoses list should be formulated based on the initial diagnostic findings, and it should be decided whether culture is likely to be the most practical route to diagnosis, or whether other methods such as PCR should be used.

Specimens for bacterial testing are collected before beginning antimicrobial therapy. All specimens should be transported in clean, tightly sealed, leak-proof containers according to postal regulations. Biopsies or aspirates of lesions are preferable to swabs when possible due to a lesser degree of contamination. Selection of appropriate transport media is essential for useful culture results. Hardier organisms, such as pseudomonads and enterobacteria, can be expected to survive overnight transport at room temperature on a standard collection swab in a transport medium, such as Amies with charcoal. Anaerobic samples should be placed immediately into anaerobic transport media such as thioglycollate agar; nonspore-forming obligate anaerobes rapidly die when exposed to room air, and rapid placement into media and minimizing transport time are critical. More fastidious organisms require specific transport media and should be discussed with the laboratory in advance. Molecular diagnostic testing is discussed in Chapter 36. Another important consideration when deciding on a diagnostic approach is additional testing that may be needed; sensitivity testing (diffusion disc or minimum inhibitory concentrations) is currently only economically feasible for cultured isolates.

A blood culture is indicated when an animal is suspected of being bacteremic. The spleen of reptiles is less efficient than that of mammals; bacteremia is more common in reptiles than in mammals. Blood culture can be useful for identification of organisms, especially in difficult sites to sample, such as a case of vertebral osteomyelitis.[31] However, interpretation needs to be taken in context; anaerobic spore-forming bacteria, such as *Clostridium* spp., are not uncommonly found in blood cultures of apparently healthy reptiles.[32] For blood culture, the skin at the venipuncture site should be aseptically prepared. The needle should be changed and the bottle wiped with alcohol before placing the sample in the blood culture bottle. Pediatric blood culture bottles are available and require smaller samples. Although it

TABLE 29.1   Medically Important Bacterial Phyla

Phylum	Example Genera	Morphology	Diagnostic Testing	Comments
Firmicutes	Streptococcus Staphylococcus Enterococcus Erysipelothrix Clostridium Listeria	Gram-positive rods and cocci	Grow relatively well in culture compared with other phyla, although some taxa are fastidious	The "classic" gram-positive bacteria, some taxa are spore-producing, a dominant phyla in gut flora, often obesity associated
Proteobacteria	Salmonella Pseudomonas Providencia Morganella Helicobacter Neisseria Anaplasma	Gram-negative rods and cocci, may be spiral shaped	Grow relatively well in culture compared with other phyla, although some taxa are fastidious	The "classic" gram-negative bacteria, often associated with increased inflammation in GI tracts
Actinobacteria	Mycobacterium Nocardia Austwickia Devriesea Corynebacterium Actinomyces	Many are gram positive or acid fast, often filamentous	Often difficult to culture, often slow growing, poorly identified by biochemical testing. PCR may be a reasonable option.	Variable antibiotic susceptibility makes profile important, often require multidrug therapy for long courses, often associated with granulomatous inflammation
Bacteroidetes	Bacteroides Capnocytophaga Elizabethkingia Myroides	Gram negative, many anaerobes	Often difficult to culture	A dominant phyla in gut flora, often associated with reduced inflammation and decreased obesity
Chlamydiae	Chlamydia Parachlamydia Simkania	Gram negative, obligate intracellular cocci	Very difficult to culture, PCR diagnostics	Often associated with granulomatous inflammation
Tenericutes	Mycoplasma Acholeplasma	Gram negative, cell-associated cocci	Often difficult to culture, require specialized media	Lack cell wall, will not respond to beta-lactam drugs, osmotically sensitive
Spirochaetes	Borrelia Leptospira	Spiral-shaped gram-negative rods, axial filament	Very difficult to culture, PCR diagnostics	Dark field microscopy may aid with diagnosis
Fusobacteria	Fusobacterium Streptobacillus	Gram negative, anaerobes	Often challenging to culture	Large fraction of gut microbiota in alligators
Cyanobacteria	Microcystis Lyngbya	Gram negative, often filamentous	Testing typically focuses on toxin identification	Blue-green algae, pathology is related to toxin ingestion rather than colonization of reptile

is ideal to sample the volume recommended by the manufacturer of the culture bottle, collecting such a volume may be contraindicated by the size of smaller patients, and the relatively higher loads seen in bacteremia in reptiles make it much more probable to have a colony-forming unit in a smaller volume.

Many bacteria found in reptiles grow best at lower temperatures than do those of mammals, so samples may need to be incubated at different temperatures (25°C and 37°C are commonly used, but further study is needed). Additionally, many if not all biochemical identification protocols for laboratories are developed around organisms likely to be found in mammals or birds. If an identification appears unusual, it is appropriate to question the result with a microbiologist.

AN OVERVIEW OF BACTERIAL TAXA

When working on an exotic animal, it is helpful to know what taxa you are dealing with; the clinical approach to a tortoise is different from the approach to a rodent. Unfortunately, bacteria are commonly taught as a list of genera and species, giving no higher level context. Although they may be described as gram-positive or gram-negative, these are not true clades; just as birds, bats, and dragonflies are all "animals with

wings" but not closely related to each other, gram-positive or gram-negative bacteria are not necessarily groups most closely related to each other. When dealing with bacteria, the phylum level is a clinically useful starting point (Table 29.1). A useful source for the clinician to find higher-level classification of a given bacterial isolate is the National Center for Biotechnology Information's Taxonomy Browser (https://www.ncbi.nlm.nih.gov/Taxonomy/Browser/wwwtax.cgi).

FIRMICUTES

The phylum Firmicutes are the "classic" gram-positive bacteria. They comprise a large part of normal gut flora, and an increase in their proportion in gut flora is often associated with obesity and increased inflammation in humans.[33] In pythons, there is a massive postprandial shift in gut flora composition toward the Firmicutes.[12] Significant increase in oxidative damage is seen postprandially in snakes.[34] As a whole, Firmicutes are more likely to be cultivable using standard culture methods.

Streptococcus. The genus *Streptococcus*, firmicutes in the order Lactobacillales, are chain-forming gram-positive cocci. They were the second most common cause of vertebral osteomyelitis in snakes in one study, although species were not identified.[31] *Streptococcus agalactiae* is the species most commonly associated with disease in reptiles, with reports of mortality events in green tree monitors (*Varanus prasinus*) and necrotizing fasciitis in saltwater crocodiles (*Crocodylus porosus*).[35,36] Both of these reports involved juvenile animals. Group B streptococci, containing *S. agalactiae,* are typically susceptible to penicillin, making it a good empirical choice while sensitivity results are pending.

A probiotic containing a mixture of bacteria including *Streptococcus thermophilus* was associated with increased intestinal villous height and increased mucosal thickness in yellow-bellied sliders (*Trachemys scripta scripta*) and common musk turtles (*Sternotherus odoratus*), which was interpreted as a positive difference for health.[37]

Enterococcus.

Enterococcus. The genus *Enterococcus,* firmicutes in the order Lactobacillales, are chain-forming gram-positive cocci. They have a long evolutionary association with the vertebrate gastrointestinal tract, dating back approximately 500 million years ago.[38] This led to the development of a hardened cell wall, osmotic resistance, and resistance to antimicrobial compounds made by other gut flora and now appropriated by humans for use as antibiotics. These traits make clinical treatment of enterococcal infections challenging, and *Enterococcus fecalis* has emerged as a significant nosocomial pathogen in humans.

Enterococcus spp. were identified as a significant cause of infection in 17% of cold-stunned Kemp's ridley turtles (*Lepidochelys kempii*) over a 6-year period.[39] This likely represents translocation of gut flora in immunosuppressed animals. Blood, bone, joint, and respiratory tract cultures were identified as *E. fecalis* (36 cases), unidentified *Enterococcus* sp. (13 cases), and *Enterococcus faecium* (1 case), although sequence-based methods were not reported to be done. Findings of significant coevolution among *Enterococcus* spp. And their hosts suggest that species found in sea turtles may likely be divergent from those found in humans.[38]

A novel *Enterococcus* sp. most closely related to *E. faecium* has been reported in a blue-tailed skink (*Cryptoblepharus egeriae*) and several gecko species in a captive breeding facility.[40] This isolate was not successfully cultured and was identified by next-generation sequencing. These lizards had thickly encapsulated gram-positive cocci effacing many tissues including bone, lung, liver, and kidney. Unfortunately, any investigation of the presence of this organism in normal gut was not reported, and the only viral diagnostic reported was attempted viral culture of pooled tissues.

When enterococcal disease is identified in a patient, it is important to identify the cofactors that have led to the establishment of clinical disease by these normal gastrointestinal flora. Factors resulting in immunosuppression, such as thermal stress, nutritional stress, toxins, and coinfections, should be evaluated and, if possible, addressed. A history of cephalosporin use is associated with enterococcal disease, likely due to microbial ecological perturbation.[41] In humans, outcome of *E. fecalis* infection is associated with patient comorbidities and not with virulence genes.[42] Many enterococci are susceptible to an ampicillin/aminoglycoside combination, making this a reasonable empirical choice while sensitivity results are pending and predisposing conditions are being addressed.

A probiotic containing a mixture of bacteria including *Enterococcus faecium* was associated with increased intestinal villous height and increased mucosal thickness in yellow-bellied sliders (*Trachemys scripta scripta*) and common musk turtles (*Sternotherus odoratus*), which was interpreted as a positive difference for health.[37]

Staphylococcus.

Staphylococcus. The genus *Staphylococcus,* firmicutes in the order Bacillales, are cluster-forming gram-positive cocci. They appear to be relatively uncommon as causes of disease in reptiles, in contrast to mammals. The emergence of multidrug resistance in this genus is of major public health concern. There are case reports of a methicillin-resistant *S. aureus* (MRSA) subspectacular abscess in a Burmese python (*Python bivittatus*) and MRSA-associated dermatitis in a turtle (species not given); these were most likely of anthropogenic origin.[43,44] Use of topical antibiotics has been shown to shift human skin flora, reducing competitors and increasing *S. aureus* loads more than 100-fold.[45]

Listeria.

Listeria. The genus *Listeria,* firmicutes in the order Bacillales, are small gram-positive rods. *Listeria* are common components of gut flora. There are two case reports of *Listeria monocytogenes* disease in reptiles, both in bearded dragons; one presented as meningitis and septicemia and the other as a myocardial abscess.[46,47] *Listeria* are cold-tolerant and will grow at 4°C in a refrigerator. Whereas disease often progresses so rapidly that waiting for culture results is not feasible. *Listeria* are susceptible to a wide array of antibiotics; first- or second-generation cephalosporins, penicillin, and trimethoprim-sulfamethoxazole are reasonable empirical choices.

Clostridium.

Clostridium. The genus *Clostridium,* firmicutes in the order Clostridiales, are anaerobic spore-forming gram-positive rods. The ability to form spores makes them highly stable in the environment. *Clostridium* are commonly found in blood cultures of apparently healthy reptiles.[32] Clostridial abscesses or gangrene may arise in a variety of species when an anaerobic site is created through loss of blood supply; closing a contaminated wound with poor blood supply creates ideal conditions. Enteric clostridial disease is also commonly seen following use of antibiotics, due to ecological perturbation of the flora. Species reported from disease in reptiles include *C. perfringens, C. glycolicum,* and *C. novyi.*[48,49]

Initial diagnostics when clostridial disease is suspected include a fecal gram stain; large numbers of large spore-forming gram-positive rods are seen, often with inflammatory cells. Anaerobic cultures may be helpful, although some species, such as *C. dificile,* are more fastidious. Toxin immunoassays may support a diagnosis, although many clostridial toxins degrade rapidly, so false-negative rates may increase within hours after collection. PCR for toxin genes may also be utilized.

Many *Clostridium* spp. are susceptible to metronidazole, making it a reasonable empirical choice while predisposing conditions are being addressed; other antibiotics should be discontinued if not otherwise contraindicated. Transfaunation is perhaps the most effective therapy for enteric clostridial disease.

In pythons, there is a massive postprandial shift in gut flora composition toward *Clostridium* spp.[12] Significant increase in oxidative damage is seen postprandially in snakes.[34] A probiotic containing a mixture of bacteria that did not include *Clostridium* spp. was associated with decreased intestinal *Clostridium perfringens* counts and increased intestinal villous height in turtles, which was interpreted as a positive difference for health.[37]

Erysipelothrix.

Erysipelothrix. The genus *Erysipelothrix,* firmicutes in the order Erysipelotrichales, are small gram-positive rods. *E. rhusiopathiae* is the species associated with disease in a wide variety of vertebrates. It is not uncommonly found in fish, and there is greater diversity of strains found in marine environments.[50] Disease often involves rapid sepsis with thrombus formation, known in pigs and marine mammals as diamond skin disease. Disease has been seen in crocodilians.[51] *E. rhusiopathiae* represents a significant zoonotic risk to the veterinarian and direct contact with suspect infected tissues should be avoided. Very small colonies are seen on culture, which may be overgrown if a mixed infection is present. Penicillin is a reasonable empirical choice.

PROTEOBACTERIA

The phylum Proteobacteria are the "classic" gram-negative bacteria. They typically comprise a smaller part of normal gut flora than Firmicutes or Bacteroidetes, and an increase in their proportion in gut flora is often associated with increased inflammation and obesity in humans.[52] As a whole, Proteobacteria are more likely to be cultivable using standard culture methods. They are divided into several classes, of which the Alphaproteobacteria, Betaproteobacteria, Gammaproteobacteria, and Epsilonproteobacteria are most relevant in reptile medicine.

α-Proteobacteria

The class Alphaproteobacteria have many members adapted for life inside eukaryotic cells, including members involved in nitrogen fixation for plants. They tend to be more fastidious than other members of the Proteobacteria, and PCR methods are often preferable to culture for diagnostics.

Bartonella. The genus *Bartonella,* proteobacteria in the order Rhizobiales, are small gram-negative rods that are primarily intracellular. They are often vectored by arthropods. Human diseases associated with *Bartonella* sp. include cat scratch fever, trench fever, and Carrion's disease. They are difficult to culture and require specialized media. PCR-based diagnostics are more practical. PCR and sequencing of blood samples from loggerhead sea turtles (*Caretta caretta*) found that two species were present; one was *B. henselae*-like and one was *B. vinsonii*-like.[53] Unfortunately, these sequences are not available in public databases. It is very probable that *Bartonella* spp. are medically relevant for reptiles, but the diagnostic challenges have resulted in limited investigation to date.

Rickettsia. The genus *Rickettsia,* proteobacteria in the order Rickettsiales, are small gram-negative pleomorphic bacteria that are primarily intracellular. They are often vectored by arthropods. *R. honei, R. bellii, R. tamurae,* and unnamed species have been found in ticks on reptiles.[54–59] There has been little investigation of the reptiles on which these ticks were found. It is very probable that *Rickettsia* spp. are medically relevant for reptiles, but diagnostic challenges have resulted in limited investigation to date.

Ehrlichia. The genus *Ehrlichia,* proteobacteria in the order Rickettsiales, are small gram-negative pleomorphic bacteria that are primarily intracellular. They are often vectored by arthropods. *E. ruminantium,* the causative agent of heartwater in cattle, has been found in ticks on African tortoises imported into Florida.[60] A possible *Ehrlichia* sp. was reported in three *Bitis* sp. vipers that presented with neurological signs, pneumonia, and mottled kidneys.[61] When liver was cultured with viper heart cells and bovine endothelial cells, cytopathic effects were seen. PCR for *E. ruminantium* was done, but no sequencing results were reported. There were no reported diagnostics for Ferlaviruses performed, which is most consistent with the clinical findings. It is very probable that *Ehrlichia* spp. are medically relevant for reptiles, but diagnostic challenges have resulted in limited investigation to date.

Anaplasma. The genus *Anaplasma,* proteobacteria in the order Rickettsiales, are small gram-negative pleomorphic bacteria that are primarily intracellular. They are often vectored by arthropods. *A. phagocytophilum,* an agent of granulocytic anaplasmosis, was found in approximately 10% of wild squamates in a survey in northern California, but disease was not investigated.[62] An *Anaplasma* has been identified by PCR and sequencing in 13% of sand lizard (*Lacerta agilis*) skin samples from Poland.[63] Again, disease in the reptiles was not investigated. This *Anaplasma* was highly divergent and is closest to sequences found

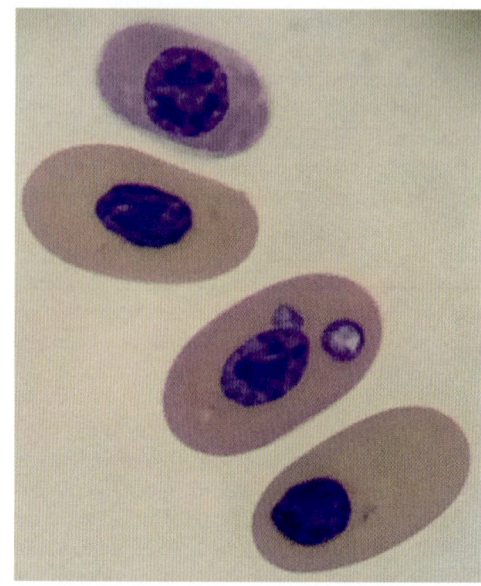

FIG 29.1 A novel *Anaplasma* in an erythrocyte of an anemic gopher tortoise (*Gopherus polyphemus*). Modified Wright's Giemsa, ×1000.

in ticks in Tunisia, Morocco, China, Korea, and California; it has been proposed that this may represent a new genus, provisionally called *Cryptoplasma californiense.*[64]

In anemic gopher tortoises (*Gopherus polyphemus*), a novel *Anaplasma* has been identified in erythrocytes (Fig. 29.1) (Wellehan et al, Proc WDA, 2016). PCR and sequencing identified it as a novel species, basal to the erythrocytic clade containing *A. marginale* and *A. ovis,* which cause anemia in ruminants. The organism was also found in gopher tortoise ticks (*Amblyomma tuberculatum*), and qPCR surveillance of tortoises found a negative correlation with packed cell volume. Treatment with doxycycline resulted in clinical resolution of anemia.

β-Proteobacteria

The class Betaproteobacteria are metabolically diverse and adapted to utilize a wide variety of nutritional substrates. They tend to be more easily cultured than average clades of bacteria.

Burkholderia. The genus *Burkholderia,* proteobacteria in the order Burkholderiales, are gram-negative rods that typically live in soil. *B. pseudomallei* is the causative agent of melioidosis. It presents significant risk of human mortality and is classified by the US government as a tier 1 select agent. Humans with diabetes are at especially high risk. It is not endemic in the United States and Europe. It has been identified in abscesses of green iguanas (*Iguana iguana*) in the United States and the Czech Republic.[65,66] Strain typing found they were consistent with strains of Central American origin. All iguanas had been in captivity with their owners for over a year. *B. pseudomallei* has also been cultured from the granulomatous liver of an elephant trunk snake (*Acrochordus javanicus*).[67] Biochemical identification of *B. pseudomallei* cultures may result in misidentification as *Chromobacterium violaceum* or *B. cepacia,* and this should be discussed with the laboratory if these are reported from abscesses. *B. pseudomallei* often has extensive resistance profiles. If the clinician encounters this organism, public health authorities should be contacted immediately.

Neisseria. The genus *Neisseria,* proteobacteria in the order Neisseriales, are gram-negative cocci typically found in oral flora. Septicemia and abscesses have been seen in iguanas (*Cyclura cornuta* and *Iguana iguana*) associated with *N. iguanae*. It is closely related to *N. meningitidis,* the agent of meningococcal encephalitis in humans.[68,69] Bite wounds should be considered as a probable source when *Neisseria* is cultured from reptiles. Penicillin is a reasonable empirical choice.

Chromobacterium. The genus *Chromobacterium,* proteobacteria in the order Neisseriales, are gram-negative cocci that typically are found in water. Although *Chromobacterium* are not known to be clinically relevant for reptiles, biochemical identification of *Burkholderia pseudomallei* cultures may result in misidentification as *C. violaceum,* and this should be discussed with the laboratory if *C. violaceum* is reported from abscesses.

γ-Proteobacteria

The Gammaproteobacteria are the largest class of Proteobacteria. They tend to be more easily cultured than average clades of bacteria.

Pseudomonadales: *Pseudomonas aeruginosa* and *Acinetobacter baumanii.*

The Pseudomonadales are an order of Gammaproteobacteria. The most relevant species for reptile medicine are *Pseudomonas aeruginosa* and *Acinetobacter baumanii.* They are gram-negative rods that are often found in water or soil. They tend to have extensive resistance profiles and are opportunists. When one of the Pseudomonadales is found in a lesion on a patient, it should provoke a search for factors causing the reptile to be compromised. The Pseudomonadales and underlying cause(s) need to be addressed. It is critical when dealing with these organisms to get a sensitivity profile. While sensitivity results are pending, aminoglycosides are reasonable empirical choices. Third-generation cephalosporins or fluoroquinolones may be required following sensitivity results.

Aeromonadales: *Aeromonas hydrophila.*

The Aeromonadales are an order of Gammaproteobacteria. The most relevant species for reptile and amphibian medicine is *Aeromonas hydrophila.* They are gram-negative rods that are often found in water. They tend to have extensive resistance profiles and are opportunists. When one of the Aeromonadales is found in a lesion on a patient, it should provoke a search for factors causing the reptile to be compromised. The Aeromonadales and underlying cause(s) both need to be addressed. It is critical when dealing with these organisms to get a sensitivity profile. Standard biochemical methods may result in misidentification of *Elizabethkingia meningoseptica* as *Aeromonas salmonicida,* and this should be discussed with the laboratory if *A. salmonicida* is reported.[70] While sensitivity results are pending, aminoglycosides are reasonable empirical choices.

Xanthomonadales: *Stenotrophomonas maltophila.*

The Xanthomonadales are an order of Gammaproteobacteria. The relevant species for reptile and amphibian medicine is *Stenotrophomonas maltophila.* They are gram-negative rods that are often found in soil and water. They tend to have extensive resistance profiles and are opportunists. When *S. maltophila* is found in a lesion on a patient, it should provoke a search for factors, causing the reptile to be compromised. *S. maltophila* and the underlying cause(s) both need to be addressed. It is critical when dealing with this organism to get a sensitivity profile. While sensitivity results are pending, trimethoprim-sulfamethoxazole is a reasonable empirical choice.

Enterobacteriales.

The Enterobacteriales are an order of Gammaproteobacteria. They are gram-negative rods that are often found in vertebrate intestines. While often opportunists, for several taxa, such as *Salmonella, Providencia,* and *Morganella,* the opportunity can be minimal. The emergence of multidrug resistance in this order is of major public health concern. Other Enterobacteriales not discussed below that may be seen in association with disease in reptiles include *Citrobacter, Serratia, Klebsiella, Enterobacter, Escherichia,* and *Proteus.* A probiotic containing a mixture of bacteria that did not include Enterobacteriales was associated with decreased intestinal Enterobacteriacae counts and increased intestinal villous height and increased mucosal thickness in turtles, which was interpreted as a positive difference for health.[37]

Salmonella. The genus *Salmonella* represents the reptile bacteria best known by the public. *Salmonella* infection in reptiles typically begins enterically and then translocates across the gut. Hematogenous spread to other organs then occurs. Lesions often include necrotizing enteritis, granulomatous hepatitis, and proliferative osteomyelitis. *Salmonella* was the most common cause of vertebral osteomyelitis in snakes in one study, although types were not identified.[31]

Salmonella contains two species: *S. bongori* and *S. enterica. S. enterica* is subdivided into six subspecies. They are further subdivided into over 2500 serotypes, and isolates are often referred to by serotype name rather than species or subspecies name. Of the six *S. enterica* subspecies, subspecies IIIa (arizonae) and IIIb (diarizonae) are most commonly associated with both wild and captive reptiles. Human disease due to these subspecies tends to occur in young children, geriatrics, and the immunosuppressed. *S. enterica* subspecies IIIa is most strongly associated with disease in reptiles, and *S. enterica* subspecies IIIa with flagellar antigens z4 and z23 has been documented to cause loss of multiple snakes at more than one facility.[71,72] Significant disease associated with z4/z23+ strains has been reported from children with reptiles in the household.[73]

S. enterica subspecies I (enterica), especially serovars Poona, Java, Pomona, Newport, Saintpaul, and Muenchen, are also associated with captive reptiles. Studies of wild reptiles suggest that infection in wild reptiles may be less frequent, although more data are needed. *S. enterica* subspecies I is most strongly associated with disease in humans, but the serovars most pathogenic in humans, such as Typhimurium and Enteritidis, are often food-associated and are not usually reptile-associated.

Other animal sources of *Salmonella,* such as feral cat colonies, are not as appreciated by the public, with one report finding 51% of group-housed cats shedding *Salmonella,* a much higher figure than is seen in individual pet cats.[74] Nonetheless, the level of concern regarding salmonellosis in reptiles is not inappropriate. Parallel to cat colonies, the high stocking density and poor sanitation standards of animals in the pet reptile trade, especially in species housed in aquatic environments, has led to much higher carriage than what is seen in wild reptile populations (see previous section Reptiles as Microbial Ecosystems). The ban on selling aquatic turtles under 4 inches (10 cm) in length has been an enormous public health success, with a 77% reduction in frequency of turtle-associated serotypes in humans during the 6 years after passage.[75]

Owners may want their animals tested to find them *Salmonella*-free. Because no test is 100% sensitive, the possibility of a false-negative result is significant. To declare an animal *Salmonella*-free opens up a clinician to litigation, especially in the event of the death of a child. Clients should be educated on good hygiene and biosecurity techniques, and appropriate husbandry will minimize the risk.

Salmonella will grow on standard bacterial media. Since reptiles with clinical salmonellosis are often septic, blood cultures are often useful. If fecal cultures are taken, selective enrichment media should be used. Serotyping of the organism should be done to assess clinical significance, potential sources, and extent of zoonotic potential; flagellar antigen typing should be emphasized. In some countries, *Salmonella* isolation is reportable to the authorities.

Salmonella are often present in the feces of normal animals. A positive culture of *Salmonella* from feces does not necessarily mean that it is causing disease; it needs to be correlated with other findings. Eradication from an animal through antibiotic use is not feasible. Antibiotic use in a normal animal may favor antibiotic resistance and induction of disease through disruption of normal competitive flora.[76]

In cases of clinical salmonellosis, empirical therapy using aminoglycosides is a reasonable first-line drug. However, due to antibiotic overuse, there are now strains that are resistant to aminoglycosides and may not be easily treatable.[16,77] Surgical therapy to remove granulomas may be helpful. In cases of vertebral osteomyelitis in snakes, surgical therapy is not feasible, and the prognosis is poor.

Morganella. *Morganella* is a genus in the order Enterobacteriales. *M. morganii* is the species of concern in reptiles. *Morganella* infection in reptiles typically begins enterically and then translocates across the gut. Hematogenous spread to other organs then occurs. Lesions often include necrotizing enteritis, soft tissue granulomas, and sepsis.[78–80] It is clinically similar to salmonellosis but is less commonly associated with osteomyelitis. *M. morganii* often have extensive resistance profiles that require advanced antimicrobials after sensitivity results.

Providencia. *Providencia* is a genus in the order Enterobacteriales. *P. rettgeri* is the species of concern in reptiles. Although all reptiles are affected, it is of greatest concern in crocodilians, where large epizootics with high mortality rates are seen.[81–83] Lesions often include sepsis, pneumonia, meningoencephalitis, splenitis, and hepatitis. *P. rettgeri* often have extensive resistance profiles that require advanced antimicrobials after sensitivity results, but rapid progression of disease in crocodilians may limit therapeutic response.

Coxiella burnetti. The Legionellales are an order of Gammaproteobacteria. They are gram-negative rods that are often found intracellularly in eukaryotes. They tend to be more fastidious than other members of the Proteobacteria, and PCR methods are preferable to culture for diagnostics. The known species of concern in reptiles is *Coxiella burnetti*, the agent of Q fever; it is a listed bioterrorism agent in the United States. *C. burnetti* has been isolated from Indian pythons (*Python molurus*), roofed turtles (*Batagur* or *Pangshura* spp.) and mangrove monitors (*Varanus indicus*) in India.[84] This report was before use of DNA sequence identification for bacteria identification. More diverse *Coxiella* sp. have recently been found in birds, and it is likely they are also present in reptiles.[85] Cases of splenomegaly especially merit further investigation. It is very probable that *Coxiella* spp. are medically relevant for reptiles, but diagnostic challenges have resulted in limited investigation to date. Doxycycline is the treatment of choice. If the clinician encounters *C. burnetti*, public health authorities should be contacted immediately.

Pasteurella testudinis and **Chelonobacter oris.** The Pasteurellales are an order of Gammaproteobacteria. They are gram-negative rods that are typically found in the nose and mouth of terrestrial vertebrates. They tend to be less stable in the environment than other members of the Proteobacteria, often do not survive transport well, and often require specialized media. *Pasteurella testudinis* was described from California desert tortoises (*Gopherus agassizii*) with rhinitis.[86] Later work showed a major role for *Mycoplasma agassizii* in rhinitis in this species, but *Pasteurella testudinis* may play a role as well. *Chelonobacter oris* has recently been described from Hermann's tortoises (*Testudo hermanni*) with upper respiratory disease, and the phylogenetic analysis showed that *P. testudinis* should be moved to this genus as well.[87] Again, the role of the bacterium in disease remains to be investigated. Given the significance the Pasteurellales play in disease in birds and mammals, it

is likely they are significant in reptiles as well. Empirical antibiotic treatment is not recommended.

Vibrio spp. The Vibrionales are an order of Gammaproteobacteria. They are gram-negative rods that are associated with marine environments. Although all reptiles may be affected, they are of greatest concern in sea turtles. In stranded sea turtles with concurrent fibropapillomatosis, *Vibrio* spp. were the most common isolate from the blood.[88] Species commonly isolated from septic sea turtles include *V. parahaemolyticus*, *V. harveyi*, and *V. alginolyticus*. Trimethoprim-sulfas, amoxycillin-clavulanic acid, and 1st generation fluoroquinolones are reasonable choices pending sensitivity testing.

ε-Proteobacteria

The class Epsilonproteobacteria are often curved or spiral-shaped gram-negative rods. Many inhabit vertebrate gastrointestinal tracts. They tend to require specialized media for culture.

Campylobacter. The genus *Campylobacter*, in the order Campylobacterales, are gram-negative curved rods that are typically found in gastrointestinal tracts. *Campylobacter iguaniorum*, most closely related to *C. fetus*, is not uncommonly found in the gastrointestinal tract of reptiles; one study found it in 10% of turtles and 3% of squamates.[89] There is genetic segregation between *C. fetus* strains of mammal origin and *C. iguaniorum* of reptile origin, but *C. iguaniorum* have been shown to cause disease in humans.[90] Most investigation has focused on risks to human health rather than on reptile health; *C. iguaniorum* has been isolated from a leopard tortoise (*Stigmochelys pardalis*) with lethargy and anorexia that responded to therapy with enrofloxacin.[91]

A second species (*Campylobacter geochelonis*) from Hermann's tortoises has also been described, but there are no data on disease or zoonotic potential.[92] *C. jejeuni*, a known human pathogen, has also been reported by qPCR identification from lizards; further strain typing may reveal whether this is actually *C. jejeuni* or a distinct reptile species.[93]

Campylobacter spp. require specific media for growth and grow under microaerophilic conditions. Samples should not be refrigerated, because *Campylobacter* is not tolerant of cooling. Antibiotic therapy is not indicated for mild cases; in a more severe case, erythromycin and potentiated sulfas are reasonable empirical choices while sensitivity results are pending.

A probiotic containing a mixture of bacteria that did not include *Campylobacter* spp. was associated with decreased intestinal *Campylobacter* counts and increased intestinal villous height and increased mucosal thickness in turtles, which was interpreted as a positive difference for health.[37]

Helicobacter. The genus *Helicobacter*, proteobacteria in the order Campylobacterales, are gram-negative spiral-shaped rods that are typically found in gastrointestinal tracts. Sepsis with a novel *Helicobacter* species was seen in a pancake tortoise (*Malacochersus tornieri*) that had concurrent cryptosporidiosis.[39] Enteritis may have led to gut translocation and sepsis. In surveillance, *Helicobacter* sp. were detected by PCR in 57% of tortoises and 29% of squamates.[94] A sequence from a Greek tortoise (*Testudo graeca*) was closely related to the pancake tortoise species. Several sequences from diverse lizards formed a separate clade. Nasal cytology from two gopher tortoises with rhinitis and weight loss, presenting 2 years apart, showed large numbers of spiral-shaped bacteria (Fig. 29.2). Neither tortoise responded to ceftazidime treatment and both died. PCR and sequencing identified the same *Helicobacter* in both tortoises, which was related to but distinct from the pancake tortoise and Greek tortoise *Helicobacter* spp. (Wellehan et al, Proc WDA, 2016). *Helicobacter* require specific media

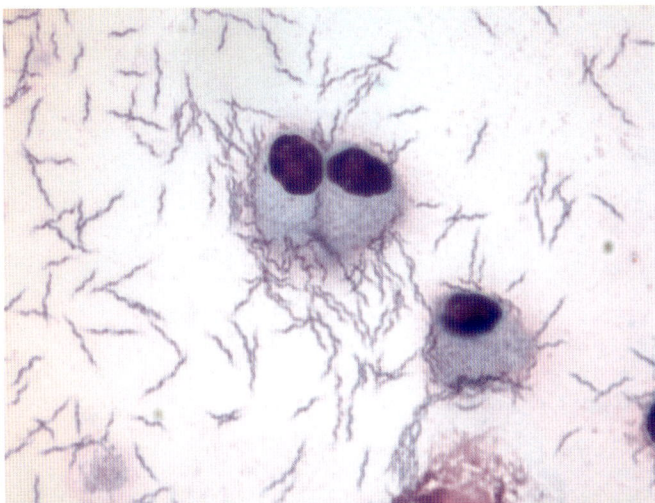

FIG 29.2 Nasal cytology from a gopher tortoise (*Gopherus polyphemus*) with rhinitis. Note the large numbers of spiral-shaped bacteria that were subsequently identified as *Helicobacter* by PCR. DiffQuik, ×1000.

for growth and grow under microaerophilic conditions. Empirical treatment is not recommended without diagnosis, but if confirmed, a clarithromycin, amoxicillin, and metronidazole combination is appropriate.[95]

ACTINOBACTERIA

The phylum Actinobacteria may stain gram-positive or may stain acid fast. Members of this phylum have thick cell walls, and many produce filaments; some can produce spores. They comprise a small part of normal gut flora and play a large role in soil ecology. They often have large immunomodulatory effects on the host. As a whole, Actinobacteria are often slow growing and poorly identified by traditional biochemical means.

***Actinomyces, Arcanobacterium,* and *Trueperella*.** *Actinomyces*, *Arcanobacterium*, and *Trueperella* are genera of arcanobacteria in the family Actinomycetaceae. They are gram-positive rods and do not stain acid fast. *T. pyogenes* has been reported in the intestine of an unidentified gecko species and the lung of a bearded dragon.[96] These grow well on standard cultures, but standard biochemical identification has a high error rate, and DNA sequence ID may be preferable. Penicillins have been demonstrated to be effective and are reasonable empirical choices while sensitivity results are pending.

Rhodococcus. *Rhodococcus* is a genus of arcanobacteria in the family Corynebacteriales. They are gram-positive short rods that normally live in soil. *R. equi*, an important pathogen of horses, has been reported to cause sepsis in crocodilians.[97]

Corynebacterium. *Corynebacterium* is a large genus of arcanobacteria in the family Corynebacteriales. They are gram-positive, club-shaped rods that are common in soil and skin flora. Although there are reports of *Corynebacterium* infections in reptiles, they are typically considered contaminants and not clinically relevant.[98,99]

Nocardia. *Nocardia* is a genus of arcanobacteria in the family Corynebacteriales. They are weakly gram-positive bacteria that stain partially acid fast and form branching filaments. They normally live in soil. They are often slow growing and poorly identified by

traditional biochemical means; molecular identification is indicated. They have primarily been reported in osteomyelitis in sea turtles.[100,101] Trimethoprim-sulfamethoxazole is a reasonable empirical choice while sensitivity results are pending.

Mycobacterium. *Mycobacterium* is a genus of arcanobacteria in the family Corynebacteriales. They do not take up gram stain and are often seen as unstained "ghost cells." They stain acid fast. Many mycobacterial species are found in biofilms in aquatic environments; they are usually found in large numbers in shower heads.[102] A large number of mycobacterial species have been identified in reptile disease, including *M. agri*, *M. avium*, *M. chelonae*, *M. confluentis*, *M. fortuitum*, *M. haemophilum*, *M. hiberniae*, *M. intracellulare*, *M. kansasii*, *M. marinum*, *M. neoaurum*, *M. nonchromogenicum*, *M. phlei*, *M. smegmatis*, *M. szulgai*, and *M. ulcerans*. There are significant differences in drug susceptibility and zoonotic risk, and any identified mycobacterial infection should be speciated. The most common lesions are granulomas; one study found that mycobacteria could be found in 14.6% of reptiles with granulomatous inflammation by acid-fast staining and 25.6% by PCR.[103] However, other lesions may also be seen less commonly, including disseminated intravascular coagulation.[104] Neurotropism has been seen with *M. haemophilum* in leatherback turtles, a close relative of *M. leprae;* leprosy is also neurotropic.[105]

Mycobacterial or actinomycete cultures are often most successful from unfixed biopsy samples. Concurrent histology with acid-fast staining is recommended if mycobacterial disease is suspected. Many granulomatous infections are paucibacterial, and it may be necessary to cut in multiple sections to see organisms. Tissue samples may be sent directly to the laboratory in a sterile sealed container. Mycobacteria are very slow growing, and culture results may take as long as several months, but culture is needed for a susceptibility profile. They are poorly identified by traditional biochemical means; molecular identification is indicated. Because culture is often slow, and knowledge of species provides important information about culture conditions, zoonotic risk, and typical susceptibility profile, submission of concurrent direct molecular diagnostic testing is recommended. Using *Mycobacterium tuberculosis* as a model, antibody response is not likely to be diagnostically useful; the World Health Organization has a position statement against the use of serological testing for *M. tuberculosis*.[106]

Before treatment is initiated, the organism should be speciated to determine zoonotic potential and probable drug susceptibility. Euthanasia should be considered for mycobacterial species of significant zoonotic concern. Any husbandry deficiencies should be addressed and corrected. Zoonotic risks need to be discussed with the owner, and the clinician needs to determine that the owner understands the risks and expense and is committed to the long-term therapy necessary. If not, euthanasia should be recommended. Antibiotic therapy will need to involve multiple drugs over a course of at least 6 months to 1 year. Single drug therapy or shorter courses are likely to result in treatment failure and antibiotic resistance. Biopsies of affected tissues should be taken and hematology repeated after 6 months to 1 year to determine whether therapy needs to be continued. Hematology should be checked every 3 months for several years to look for leukocytosis, which may be a sign of recurrence. With appropriate therapy, mycobacteriosis is a treatable disease (Wilkinson et al, Proc NAVC, 2016, pp 1302–1304).

Austwickia. *Austwickia* is a genus of arcanobacteria in the family Micrococcales. They stain gram positive, have a characteristic branching, filamentous structure, and the ability to produce motile cocci called zoospores. Formerly known as *Dermatophilus chelonae*, *Austwickia chelonae* is the sole member of the genus.[3] Histologically, although it does form filaments, they do not typically have the "train track"

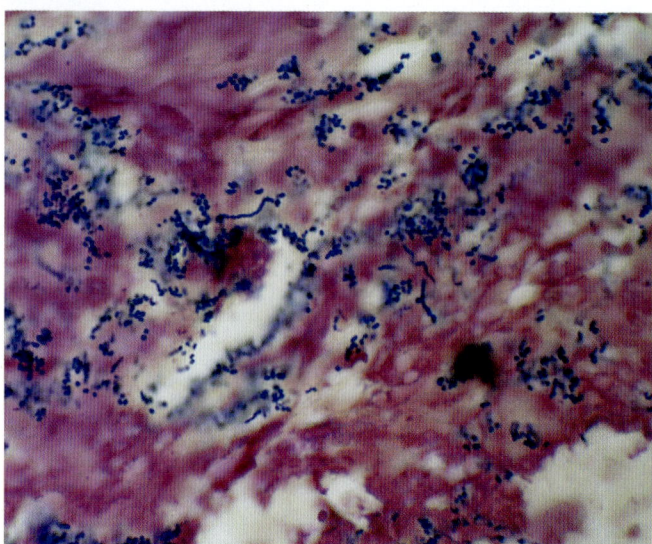

FIG 29.3 *Austwickia chelonae* (formerly known as *Dermatophilus chelonae*) form gram-positive staining rods with characteristic branching, filamentous structure. Gram stain, ×1000.

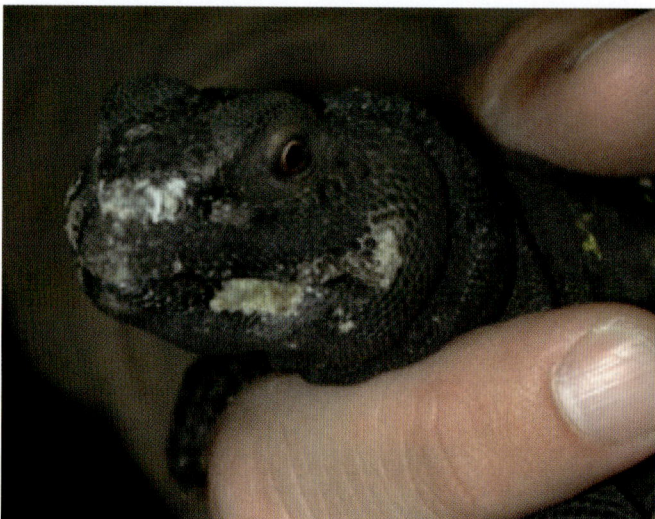

FIG 29.4 *Devriesea* cheilitis in a spiny-tailed lizards (*Uromastyx* sp.).

appearance seen with *Dermatophilus congolensis* (Fig. 29.3). *A. chelonae* is associated with granulomatous disease in reptiles. It was first isolated from turtles but has also been identified in squamates.[3,107,108] Infection typically starts in the skin and invades deeper tissues, resulting in granulomas. Coinfection with ranavirus has been documented.[3]

The clinician should communicate in advance with the microbiology laboratory when *A. chelonae* is suspected, and the microbiology laboratory should be prepared to look for actinomycete-like colonies. *A. chelonae* grows faster at 27°C than 37°C. They are poorly identified by traditional biochemical means; molecular identification is indicated. It is likely that extensive protocols comparable to mycobacterial treatment protocols may be needed. Antibiotic therapy may need to involve multiple drugs over a course of 6 months to 1 year. Single drug therapy or shorter courses seem likely to result in treatment failure.

Devriesea. *Devriesea* is a genus of arcanobacteria in the family Micrococcales. They are small, gram-positive rods. It initially presents as cheilitis and is most commonly seen in *Uromastyx* sp. (Fig. 29.4) and often leads to sepsis.[109] It has been found in association with disease in diverse agamids and iguanids, as well as a single isolate from the oral cavity of a leopard gecko without reported clinical signs.[110] It was demonstrated to cause dermatitis in inland bearded dragons by experimental infection, but this species is not usually clinically affected and is considered a carrier.[109] Despite not forming spores, it is very stable in the environment; disinfectants labeled with activity against *Mycobacterium* should be used.[111] Use of a killed vaccine on bearded dragons prevented sepsis but not dermatitis in experimental infections and elicited an antibody response; species in which disease is seen naturally were not studied.[112] Using *Mycobacterium tuberculosis* as a model, it is likely that antibody response will be less predictive of protection than cellular immunity. First-line drugs erythromycin and tetracyclines are often effective, while the third-generation cephalosporin, ceftiofur, has also demonstrated efficacy. Fluoroquinolones are often ineffective.[113]

BACTEROIDETES

The phylum Bacteroidetes stain gram negative. Many of them are anaerobic. They comprise a large part of normal gut flora, and an increase in their proportion in gut flora is often associated with decreased

obesity and reduced inflammation in humans.[33] In pythons, there is a massive postprandial shift in gut flora composition away from the Bacteroidetes.[12] Significant increase in oxidative damage is seen postprandially in snakes.[34] A probiotic containing a mixture of bacteria that were mostly in the phylum Firmicutes and did not include any Bacteroidetes was associated with decreased intestinal *Bacteroides* and *Prevotella* sp. counts in turtles; this may be a negative change for health.[37]

In their usual context, most of the Bacteroidetes are commensal. In compromised patients, normal gut flora such as *Bacteroides* sp. or *Prevotella* sp. may function as opportunistic pathogens. The notable exception, in reptile medicine, is *Elizabethkingia*.

Elizabethkingia. *Elizabethkingia* is a genus of bacteroides in the family Flavobacteriales. They are small gram-negative rods that are found in aquatic environments. *E. meningoseptica* can invade intracellularly and is the species known to cause disease in reptiles. It also affects a wide variety of other vertebrates, including humans.[114,115] Former names for *E. meningoseptica* include *Chryseobacterium meningosepticum* and *Flavobacterium meningosepticum*. Little molecular identification has been done on *Elizabethkingia* in reptiles, and *E. anophelis* and *E. miricola* have also recently been recognized as human pathogens.[116] Clinical signs in reptiles typically consist of depression, anorexia, and edema shortly followed by death. Blood cultures are good antemortem samples. Standard biochemical methods may result in misidentification as *Aeromonas salmonicida*, and this should be discussed with the laboratory if *A. salmonicida* is reported.[70] *Elizabethkingia* often have extensive resistance profiles, and do not respond to many drugs commonly used for Proteobacteria, such as third-generation cephalosporins. A trimethoprim-sulfamethoxazole combination is a reasonable empirical choice, but rapid progression of disease may limit therapeutic response.[116]

CHLAMYDIAE

Chlamydia, Neochlamydia, Parachlamydia,* and *Simkania. The phylum Chlamydiae are gram-negative, obligate, intracellular bacteria that have a biphasic developmental cycle consisting of the infectious elementary body and the noninfectious replicating reticulate body. They are not known to serve commensal roles. A number of species in the phylum Chlamydiae have been identified in reptiles. The most common appears to be *Chlamydia pneumoniae*, but *C. abortus*, *C. felis*, *C. psittaci*, *C. muridarum*, unnamed *Chlamydia* sp., *Neochlamydia* sp., *Parachlamydia* sp., and *Simkania* sp. have also been identified from reptiles.[103,117] They are very prevalent in captive reptiles; this is likely an artifact of the poor biosecurity and high stocking density standard in the reptile trade. A recent study in asymptomatic snakes found a prevalence of *Chlamydia* sp. ranging between 5% to 33% in six snake collections in Europe.[118]

Chlamydiae are challenging to culture and poorly identified by traditional biochemical means; PCR is the standard for identification. Occasionally, Chlamydiae can be seen in circulating leukocytes on a blood smear, but this is not reliable. The most common lesions in reptiles are granulomas. One study found that Chlamydiales could be found in 5.6% of reptiles with granulomatous information by immunohistochemistry, and 64.4% by PCR, underscoring both the high prevalence and the much greater sensitivity of PCR to identify the organism.[103] They are often disseminated in many tissues, although infection of a novel *Chlamydia* sp. in false gharials (*Tomistoma schlegleii*) lesions was confined to the central nervous system.[119] Nasal lavage of tortoises with nasal discharge found that 10% were PCR positive for a novel *Chlamydia*.[120]

When known granulomas are accessible at biopsy or necropsy, these are the best samples for testing. When this is not accessible, PCR of choanal and cloacal swabs has been most commonly used, but data on sensitivity, or comparison to other samples such as buffy coats, nasal lavage, or conjunctival swabs, needs to be studied.

Treatment of Chlamydiales consists of surgical removal of any known granulomas, and a 45 to 60-day course of tetracyclines or macrolides. Repeat PCR testing and hematology should be performed at 6 months and 1 year after treatment to look for evidence of treatment failure.

TENERICUTES

Mycoplasma, Ureaplasma, and *Acholeplasma*. The phylum Tenericutes are gram–negative, obligate cell-associated bacteria that have lost their cell walls and many biochemical pathways, becoming highly dependent on their host cells. Medically relevant genera include *Mycoplasma, Ureaplasma,* and *Acholeplasma. Mycoplasma* sp. has been found in all vertebrates that have been significantly investigated, including reptiles. Infection appears to be much more common than significant disease for most *Mycoplasma* sp. in most species.

In turtles, *Mycoplasma agassizii* has been shown to be one cause of significant upper respiratory tract disease (URTD) in California desert tortoises (*Gopherus agassizii*) and Florida gopher tortoises (*Gopherus polyphemus*).[121,122] It is not uncommon to find asymptomatic tortoises; temperature is one cofactor indicated to play a role in this. There has been an association between *M. agassizii* URTD in desert tortoises and colder winters.[123] Gopher tortoises with severe URTD have been found to move longer distances over short time periods than unaffected tortoises; they also have higher body temperatures, and increased activity may be heat seeking for a behavioral fever.[124] Other factors such as reproductive status and nutrition are likely to play significant roles in manifestation of disease. Coinfection, especially with agents such as Chlamydiales, Pasteurellales, and viruses, needs further investigation.

A different species in the upper respiratory tract of California desert tortoises, *M. testudineum*, may be associated with URTD, although a causal relationship with URTD has not definitively been shown. *M. testudinis,* isolated from the cloaca of Greek tortoises (*Testudo graeca*), has not been associated with disease and is not currently considered a pathogen.

A different *Mycoplasma* sp., yet unnamed, has been found in association with URTD, first in eastern box turtles (*Terrapene carolina carolina*) and then in other North American emydid turtles.[125] This organism may cross-react serologically with *M. agassizii* and *M. testudineum*, complicating serodiagnostics.[126]

In squamates, *Mycoplasma* is not uncommonly seen in pythons, often in association with tracheitis and pneumonia.[127] This organism is closely related to but distinct from *M. agassizii* and *M. testudineum*.[128] It is commonly seen as a coinfection with python nidoviruses, and study of the interactions of these agents is indicated. *M. iguanae,* isolated from a green iguana (*Iguana iguana*), did not cause lesions in experimentally infected green iguanas.[129] *M. insons* is also likely normal flora in green iguanas.[130] An unnamed *Mycoplasma* sp. related to *M. iguanae* has been identified from the lungs of a bearded dragon with Helodermatid adenovirus 2-associated pneumonia.[130a]

In crocodilians, *M. crocodyli* is associated with polyarthritis in Nile crocodiles (*Crocodylus niloticus*).[131] *M. alligatoris* has been shown to cause pneumonia, polyserositis, and polyarthritis in American alligators (*Alligator mississippiensis*) and broad-nosed caiman (*Caiman latirostris*) but did not cause disease in Siamese crocodiles (*Crocodylus siamensis*).[132]

There is likely significant tenericute diversity in reptiles still to be determined, and a large amount of work has to be done to understand their clinical implications in different reptile species. There are no known zoonotic concerns for any of the reptile-associated mycoplasmas. Most *Mycoplasma* sp. appear to be somewhat host specific.

Tenericutes require special media for culture. Because mycoplasmas lack cell walls, they are highly susceptible to desiccation, and samples should immediately be placed into a mycoplasma culture broth such as SP4 or Frey's. If the sample is taken with a swab, chances for successful culture are greatly improved by premoistening swabs in sterile mycoplasma broth. Media typically contains a cell wall inhibitor, such as ampicillin, to inhibit the growth of other bacteria. Many mycoplasmas are slow growing, and it may take up to several weeks to obtain culture results. They are poorly identified by traditional biochemical means; PCR with sequence identification is the standard for diagnosis, whether done from cultures or directly from clinical samples.

The goal of therapy is treatment of disease. Eradication of the organism is a second goal, but *Mycoplasma* sp. are difficult to completely eradicate, and the possibility of having an asymptomatic carrier after treatment is significant. Because of the lack of a cell wall, antibiotics targeting the cell wall, such as penicillins or cephalosporins, will not be effective. Fluoroquinolones are likely to result in temporary success and relapse, and tetracyclines are recommended as a first-line choice. There is pharmacokinetic data on azithromycin in ball pythons (*Python regius*), clarithromycin in California desert tortoises (*Gopherus agassizii*), tulathromycin in desert tortoises, and oxytetracycline in American alligators (*Alligator mississippiensis*) and loggerhead sea turtles (*Caretta caretta*).[133–137] In the absence of further data, treatment should be for at least 45 to 60 days.

SPIROCHAETES

The phylum Spirochaetes are gram-negative bacteria with a double membrane and a spiral shape. They have central flagella that are between the membrane layers. Spirochaetes are difficult to grow and require special media for culture.

Borrelia. *Borrelia* is a genus of spirochaetes in the family Borreliaceae. They are gram-negative spiral-shaped rods that are usually transmitted by ticks. Most investigation has focused on ticks rather than their reptile hosts; *Borrelia* sp. have been identified in ticks from diverse reptile hosts. *B. turcica* was cultured from seven of eight (88%) *Testudo* sp. tortoises being imported into Japan, and a novel *Borrelia* sp. was cultured from five of seven (71%) leopard tortoises (*Stigmocheys pardalis*).[138] These *Borrelia* were also seen in *Amblyomma* sp. ticks. When these *Borrelia* were inoculated into juvenile African spur-thighed tortoises

(*Centrochelys sulcata*), the leopard tortoise *Borrelia* but not *B. turcica* was isolated from the African spur-thighed tortoises when the animals were sacrificed after 4 weeks. The African spur-thighed tortoises were not reported to show clinical signs, but histopathology was not performed. When *B. turcica* and the leopard tortoise *Borrelia* were inoculated into mice, no culture-positive samples were found when the mice were sacrificed after 4 weeks, suggesting that mammals may not be competent hosts.[138]

Borrelia lusitaniae, found in skin lesions of humans, was present in 19% of green lizards (*Lacerta viridis*), suggesting they may be a significant reservoir.[139] In contrast, western fence lizards (*Sceloporus occidentalis*) and southern alligator lizards (*Elgaria multicarinata*) are not competent hosts for *B. burgdorferi*, the agent of Lyme disease, and their plasma has been shown to be borreliacidal through activation of complement.[140]

Given the high prevalence in reptiles and the nebulous clinical signs and chronic nature of disease seen in mammals, it is very probable that *Borrelia* spp. are medically relevant for reptiles, but diagnostic challenges have resulted in limited investigation to date.

Skin appears to be a good sample to test, followed by blood.[138] *Borrelia* are challenging to culture; Barbour-Stoenner-Kelly (BSK) media is commonly used. PCR diagnostics may be a more practical option. A reasonable approach to treatment of *Borrelia* is a 45- to 60-day course of tetracyclines. PCR testing of a skin biopsy should be taken at 6 months and 1 year after treatment to look for evidence of treatment failure.

Leptospira. *Leptospira* is a genus of spirochaetes in the family Leptospiraceae. They are gram-negative spiral-shaped rods that are found in aquatic habitats. They are associated with renal disease in diverse species and are typically transmitted through urine. Serologic data have suggested that antibodies against *Leptospira* sp. are present in reptiles. However, validation of serologic assays has been very limited. Gastric and cloacal contents of Geoffroy's side-necked turtles (*Phrynops geoffroanus*) were found to be PCR positive for *Leptospira* sp., although sequencing identification of PCR products was not done.[141] There was no correlation of PCR results with serologic status; 5 of 25 (20%) samples from seropositive turtles were PCR positive, and 6 of 30 (20%) samples from seronegative turtles were PCR positive.

Leptospira interrogans and an unnamed *Leptospira* sp. have been identified by sequencing PCR products from the kidneys of a herald snake (*Crotaphopeltis hotamboeia*), a Jararaca viper (*Bothrops pauloensis*), and two Brazilian lancehead vipers (*Bothrops moojeni*).[142,143]

Given the presence of *Leptospira* sp. in reptiles, the challenges of leptospiral and renal diagnostics in reptiles, and the disease seen in mammals, it is very probable that *Leptospira* spp. are medically relevant for reptiles, but diagnostic challenges have resulted in limited investigation to date.

Renal samples appear to be the best tissue samples for *Leptospira* PCR.[142] Gastric washes and cloacal washes have been used as minimally invasive samples.[141] *Leptospira* are challenging to culture; specialized media is needed. PCR diagnostics may be a more practical option. Darkfield microscopy of urine to look for spirilliform bacteria may be helpful as a rapid initial test. A reasonable approach to treatment of *Leptospira* is a 45- to 60-day course of a tetracycline (e.g., doxycycline) or macrolide (e.g., erythromycin). PCR testing should be repeated after treatment to look for evidence of treatment failure.

FUSOBACTERIA

Fusobacterium necrophorum. The phylum Fusobacteria are gram-negative nonspore-forming obligate anaerobes. In most vertebrates that have been studied, they may be found in oral flora but are a very small component of gut flora (<1%). The known exception is alligators, where the flora in the colon of both wild and farmed American alligators was typically composed of more than 50% Fusobacteria.[144] The most clinically relevant species in reptiles is *Fusobacterium necrophorum*, which has been reported in clinical lesions from squamates and turtles.[145] When *F. necrophorum* is found in a lesion on a patient, it should provoke a search for factors, causing the reptile to be compromised. *F. necrophorum* needs to be addressed, but the underlying cause also needs to be addressed. Metronidazole is a reasonable empirical therapy.

CYANOBACTERIA

The phylum Cyanobacteria includes photosynthetic bacteria that are often referred to as "blue-green algae," although they are not eukaryotes. They are common in diverse habitats, especially aquatic and marine environments. They were critical in oxygenation of the early atmosphere. In reptiles, they are not typically seen as part of internal flora but are common epibiota on aquatic and marine turtles. Their clinical relevance is not from infection of animals but from toxin production.[146] In freshwater environments, *Microcystis* is one genus commonly associated with toxin production; in marine environments, *Lyngbya* is a common toxic genus. Lesions seen include vacuolar myelinopathy.[147] However, deaths without lesions may be seen. Measurement of microcystin or *Lyngbya* toxins may be helpful with diagnosis. Management includes careful monitoring of water systems and maintenance of water quality with low nitrogen and phosphate loads to avoid cyanobacterial overgrowth.[148] Antibiotic therapy is not likely to be useful.

REFERENCES

See www.expertconsult.com for a complete list of references.

30

Virology

Rachel E. Marschang

Reptile virology has undergone rapid development over the past few decades. The use of next-generation sequencing (NGS) techniques has led to a rapid increase in the number of viruses described in reptiles. Additionally, transmission studies proving the role of specific viruses in disease processes have been carried out for a number of viral infections in various reptile species. Despite many advances, the factors involved in the development of viral disease in reptiles are, in many cases, unclear. Both host and viral factors are involved. Environmental factors, particularly temperature, have long been known to influence the immune system of reptiles. Increasing evidence suggests that other factors can play an important role in the outcome of viral infections in reptiles, including various pollutants and other infectious agents. Concurrent infections with several infectious agents, including multiple viruses, may occur, and the interactions and effects of these concurrent infections are not yet understood. This makes clinical evaluation of individual test results difficult and reinforces the need to consider multiple pathogens and critically evaluate results in these individual cases. It is critical to differentiate between infection and clinical disease caused by true viral pathogens in our reptile patients.

Many different methods are available for the diagnosis of viral infections in reptiles. These include methods for the detection of viruses, viral proteins, or viral genomes and serologic methods for the detection of an immune response to viral infection (generally restricted to antibody detection). Which method should be used in a specific situation depends on many different factors. These include the host species, clinical observations, time since infection, virus species, reason for testing, and test availability. Unfortunately, some of these factors such as virus species involved or time since infection are often unknown. None of the test systems available for reptile virology are fully standardized in that repeatability and reproducibility are not consistently studied. In addition, cross-reactivity and relationships between reptile viruses are not fully understood, and the specificity of some tests may therefore be lower than expected in some cases, or may be too high, and only a subset of related viruses may be detected using some assays. It is recommended to contact your laboratory before submitting samples (Table 30.1).

The viruses in this review are presented according to taxonomic position, with double-stranded (ds) DNA viruses (adenoviruses, including atadenoviruses, siadenoviruses, and "testadenoviruses"; herpesviruses; iridoviruses, including ranaviruses, invertebrate iridoviruses, and erythrocytic viruses; papillomaviruses; poxviruses) presented first, followed by single-stranded (ss) DNA viruses (circoviruses and a "tornovirus," parvoviruses), reverse transcribing DNA and RNA viruses (hepadnaviruses, retroviruses), dsRNA viruses (reoviruses), negative sense ssRNA viruses (members of the order *Mononegavirales*, including bornaviruses, paramyxoviruses [ferlaviruses], sunviruses, rhabdoviruses; arenaviruses; bunyaviruses), and positive sense ssRNA viruses (members of the order *Nidovirales* [corona- or toroviruses], members of the genus *Picornavirales* [picornaviruses], caliciviruses, flaviviruses, togaviruses) (Table 30.2).

ADENOVIRIDAE

Adenoviruses (AdVs) are the viruses most commonly identified in many squamate species, particularly bearded dragons (*Pogona* spp.), although they have also been detected in various chelonians and crocodilians. AdVs have a relatively high resistance to inactivation and can be difficult to disinfect. Current taxonomy of the family *Adenoviridae* suggests a coevolutionary lineage of the viruses with their hosts and additional host switches. Atadenoviruses have been hypothesized to have coevolved with squamate reptiles, while a new genus ("Testadenovirus") has been proposed to have coevolved with chelonian hosts.[1] This can be important in understanding the pathogenicity of the viruses, because viruses that have coevolved with their hosts may not cause disease or may only cause disease in immune-suppressed animals or in conjunction with other infectious agents or other factors, whereas switching of hosts may lead to severe disease and death. AdVs from crocodilians have not yet been characterized.

Adenoviruses in Squamates

AdVs appear to occur worldwide in captive populations, and antibodies to AdVs have been detected in wild boa constrictors (*Boa constrictor*) from Costa Rica (Marschang et al, Proc 6th Int Cong Vet Virol, 2003, p 152) and in wild-caught rattlesnakes from the United States.[3] All of the AdVs detected in squamates so far have belonged to the genus *Atadenovirus*. Clinical signs most commonly associated with AdV infection in squamates are gastrointestinal and neurologic, including anorexia, lethargy, wasting, head tilt, opisthotonus, and circling (Fig. 30.1) In individual cases, stomatitis, dermatitis, and pneumonia have also been described.[4] AdVs have also been detected in animals with no clinical signs of disease. Koch's postulates have been fulfilled for an AdV-induced hepatic necrosis in a boa constrictor.[5] Gross pathologic examination of animals that die with AdV infection can involve only the liver, which may be enlarged and have petechiae or pale areas scattered throughout. Histologically, these animals generally have hepatic necrosis. The intestine is also frequently affected, and documented changes include dilatation of the duodenum and hyperemia of the mucosa. Basophilic intranuclear inclusions are often seen in hepatocytes and enterocytes (Fig. 30.2), as well as in myocardial endothelial cells, renal epithelial cells, endocardium, epithelial cells of the lung, and glial and endothelial cells in the brain.[4]

An important observation in many squamate AdVs is their relative species specificity: specific lizard AdVs are mostly found in a single host species, most notably Agamid AdV-1 in bearded dragons. However,

TABLE 30.1   Laboratories to Contact for Additional Information and Reptile Virus Testing

Name	Website	Address for Submissions	Contact Person	Email Contact
North America				
UF Diagnostic Laboratories, College of Veterinary Medicine	labs.vetmed.ufl.edu/sample-requirements/zoo-med-infections/	April Childress, University of Florida, 2015 SW 16th Ave., Building 1017, Room V2-186, Gainesville, FL 32608	April Childress or James F.X. Wellehan	childressa@ufl.edu
Wildlife Epidemiology Lab, University of Illinois, College of Veterinary Medicine	vetmed.illinois.edu/wel	2001 S. Lincoln Ave., Urbana, IL 61802	Matt Allender	WildlifeEpi@vetmed.illinois.edu
Europe				
Laboklin	laboklin.com/?lang=en	Steubenstr. 4, 97688 Bad, Kissingen, Germany	Rachel E. Marschang	marschang@laboklin.com
Wildlife Diagnostic Service	fiwi.vetsuisse.unibe.ch/	Länggassstrasse 122, 3001 Bern, Switzerland	Francesco Origgi	francesco.origgi@vetsuisse.unibe.ch
Center for Fish and Wildlife Medicine, Department of Infectious Diseases and Pathobiology, College of Veterinary Medicine, Vetsuisse Faculty, University of Bern				
Chemisches- und Veterinäruntersuchungsamt Ostwestfalen-Lippe (CVUA-OWL) AöR	cvua-owl.de	Westerfeldstraße 1, 32758 Detmold, Germany	Silvia Blahak	silvia.blahak@cvua-owl.de
Australia				
The Hyndman Reptile Pathogen Lab	profiles.murdoch.edu.au/myprofile/tim-hyndman/	School of Veterinary & Life Sciences, South Street, Murdoch University, Western Australia 6150	Tim Hyndman	T.Hyndman@murdoch.edu.au
Asia				
Laboratory of Veterinary Pathology, School of Veterinary Medicine, Azabu University	www.azabu-u.ac.jp/english/laboratories/	1-17-71 Fuchinobe, Chuo-ku, Sagamihara, Kanagawa 252-5201, Japan	Yumi Une	une@azabu-u.ac.jp

This table includes only laboratories that offer qualified consultations, regularly publish their methods in peer-reviewed publications, and are known to the author. There are many other labs available that offer qualified testing, but it is important that the practitioner understands what each test offered detects.

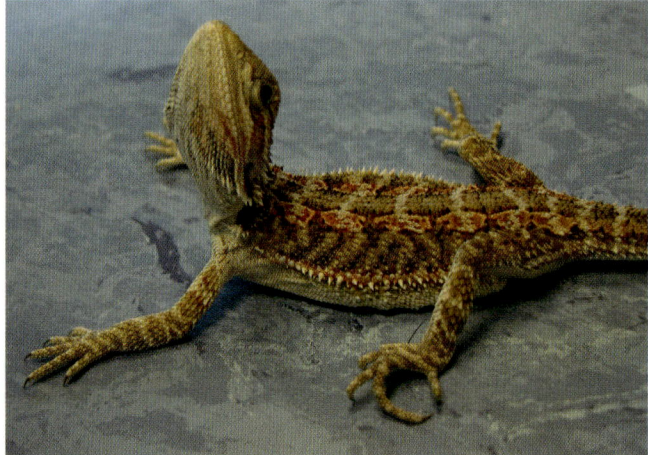

FIG 30.1 Bearded dragon (*Pogona vitticeps*) infected with an adenovirus. This lizard showed neurological signs including opisthotonus. (Courtesy of Jutta Wiechert.)

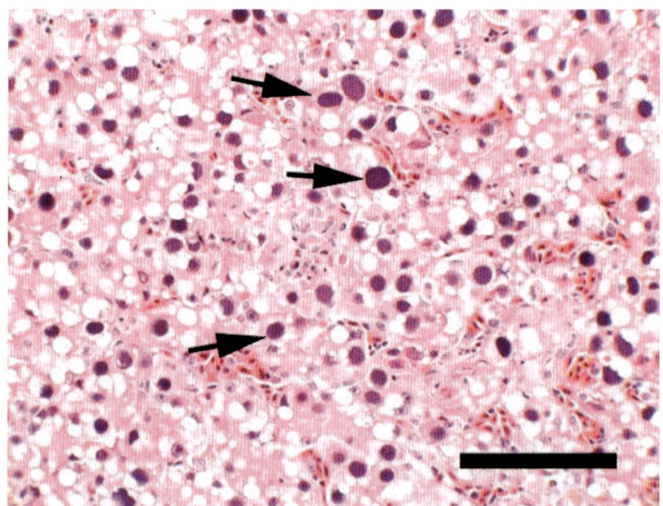

FIG 30.2 Liver of a bearded dragon (*Pogona vitticeps*). Note the large numbers of hepatocytes with large intranuclear basophilic or amphophilic inclusions (arrows). The hepatocytes also have moderate lipidosis. Hematoxylin and eosin; bar = 250 μm. (Courtesy of Michael M. Garner, Northwest ZooPath.)

TABLE 30.2 Virus Families Described in Select Groups of Reptiles (Including Endogenous Viruses)

Virus Family	Chelonians Ch1	Ch2	Ch3	Ch4	Ch5	Squamates S1	S2	S3	Crocodiles
Adenoviridae	X	X				X	X	X	X
Herpesviridae	X	X	X		X	X	X	X	X
Iridoviridae	X	X		X		X	X	X	
Papillomaviridae	X		X		X	X		X	
Poxviridae	X						X	X	X
Circoviridae		X	X			X			
Parvoviridae						X	X		
Hepadnaviridae		X		X		X			X
Retroviridae		X	X			X	X	X	X
Reoviridae	X					X	X	X	
Bornaviridae						X			
Paramyxoviridae	X					X	X	X	?
Sunviridae						X			
Rhabdoviridae		X		X		X		X	
Orthomyxoviridae									?
Arenaviridae						X			
Bunyaviridae				X				X	
Coronaviridae						X			?
Picornaviridae	X					X			
Caliciviridae						X			
Flaviviridae	X	X		X		X	X	X	X
Togaviridae	X	X		X		X	X	X	X

Ch1, Tortoises; *Ch2*, pond, box, and freshwater turtles; *Ch3*, sea turtles; *Ch4*, other Cryptodira; *Ch5*, side-necked turtles; *S1*, snakes; *S2*, Iguania (e.g., agamas, iguanas, chameleons); *S3*, other squamates; *?*, Some evidence of infection with these viruses in this group of reptiles.

there are a number of exceptions to this apparent rule, including the detection of a Helodermatid AdV-2-like virus in liver tissue of a western bearded dragon (*Pogona minor*) in Australia.[6] Serologic studies have also indicated that many different squamate reptiles can be infected with a variety of atadenoviruses.[3] AdV infections in squamates are also frequently found in conjunction with multiple other infections, including infections with parvo, reo, iridoviruses, coccidia, and microsporidia.

Adenoviruses in Chelonians

AdVs have only relatively recently been detected in several species of chelonians. In Travancore (Sulawesi) tortoises (*Indotestudo forstenii*), as well as in other tortoises in contact with the Travancore tortoises, infection was associated with severe systemic disease and a very high mortality rate (82%). Pathological findings in infected tortoises were multifocal hepatic necrosis, amphophilic to basophilic intranuclear inclusions and diffuse hepatic lipidosis, myeloid necrosis in bone marrow, and severe necrotizing enterocolitis. The virus detected in these tortoises differed distinctly from the AdVs characterized from squamates so far and was determined to belong in the *Siadenovirus* genus.[7] A single case of AdV infection has been reported in a leopard tortoise (*Stigmochelys pardalis*) that was also infected with a herpesvirus. This animal had biliverdinuria, wasting, and episodes of hemorrhages.[8] In Hungary, an AdV was detected in a box turtle with degeneration of liver cells, pronounced vacuolization of the cytoplasm, pyknosis of nuclei, and inclusion bodies in some hepatocytes.[9] Similar viruses have since been detected in a wider range of turtle and tortoise species in the United States and in Europe, including both healthy and diseased individuals. It has been proposed to classify these viruses in a new genus in the family *Adenoviridae*, "Testadenovirus."[1] There is some evidence that this lineage may have coevolved with chelonian hosts.

Adenoviruses in Crocodilians

Adenoviruses have been described in crocodilians, where they are mostly associated with liver disease in juvenile animals. The intestines, pancreas, and lungs are less commonly affected. Clinical signs that have been reported in infected animals have generally been limited to lethargy and anorexia. In chronically infected animals, hepatitis may lead to runting. Gross pathology may show swelling of the liver. Intestines may also be affected and show swelling. Histologically, intranuclear inclusions have been described mainly in hepatocytes and enterocytes.[10]

Identification of Adenovirus Infections

Virus Detection. A PCR targeting the DNA polymerase gene[11] has been frequently used to detect various AdVs in reptiles (Tables 30.3 and 30.4). It has been used on a wide range of samples and can detect AdVs described in squamates and chelonians. The PCR products should be sequenced, because this PCR can also detect AdVs of prey animals.[12] Recommended samples for the detection of AdVs in lizards and snakes are cloacal swabs (Fig. 30.3), liver, and intestine. Specific PCRs for the detection of reptilian AdVs have also been described. A real-time PCR has been developed for the detection of Agamid AdV-1.[13] This method will not detect other AdVs found in reptiles.

A number of AdVs from reptiles have been isolated in cell culture, which has facilitated further characterization of individual viruses. Snake AdVs have been isolated in several cases.[4] In lizards, AdVs have been isolated from helodermatid lizards,[12] and Agamid AdV-1 has been isolated on cells from bearded dragon embryos.[14]

Serology. Virus neutralization testing was first used for the detection of antibodies against a snake AdV (SAdV-1) (Marschang et al, Proc 6th Int Cong Vet Virol, 2003, p 152), demonstrating the presence of anti-AdV

TABLE 30.3 Select Viruses of Chelonians and Common Methods for Virus and Antibody Detection

Virus Family and Virus Genus	Virus Species or Strain	Host Species	Clinical Signs and/or Pathologic Changes Described in Infected Animals[1]	Diagnostic Samples in Order from Least to Most Invasive (if known, priority samples in bold)[2]	Virus Detection	Serology
Adenoviridae						
Siadenovirus[7]		Sulawesi tortoise (Indotestudo forsteni), Burmese star tortoise (Geochelone platynota)	Systemic disease, hepatic necrosis, necrotizing enterocolitis	Cloacal swabs, choanal swabs, **nasal flush**, oral/nasal mucosal tissue, plasma, **liver**, other tissues	PCR*	n.d.
"Testadenovirus"[1,9]		Various testudinid and emydid species	Hepatic and gastrointestinal lesions	Cloacal swabs, liver, intestine	PCR*	n.d.
Herpesviridae						
Scutavirus[33,54]	Lung, eye, and trachea disease (LETD) virus	Green sea turtles (Chelonia mydas)	Respiratory signs, buoyancy abnormalities, caseated material on the eyes, around the glottis, and in the trachea	Lung and trachea	PCR*, virus isolation	ELISA
Scutavirus[105]	Chelonid alphaherpesvirus 5 (ChHV5), fibropapilloma-associated turtle HV (FPTHV)	Green sea turtles, loggerhead sea turtles, hawksbill turtles (Eretmochelys imbricate), Olive Ridley (Lepidochelys olivacea)	External and internal fibropapillomas	Fibropapillomas	PCR*	ELISA
Scutavirus-like[36]	LGRV	Loggerhead sea turtles (Caretta caretta)	Ulcers in the trachea, around the cloaca, and on the base of the phallus	Material from lesions	PCR*	n.d.
Scutavirus-like[36]	LOCV	Loggerhead sea turtles	Ulcers in the oral cavity, cutaneous plaques, pneumonia	Material from lesions	PCR*	n.d.
Scutavirus-like[39,41,60]	Testudinid HV1 (TeHV1)	Russian tortoise (Testudo horsfieldii), other testudinid spp.	Stomatitis, glossitis, rhinitis	**Oral swabs, tongue,** liver, brain, other tissues	PCR*, virus isolation	NT*, ELISA
Scutavirus-like[40,56]	TeHV2	Desert tortoise (Gopherus agassizii)	Stomatitis, glossitis	**Tongue,** liver, other tissues	PCR*, rtPCR	ELISA
Scutavirus-like[41,60]	TeHV3	Many different species of Testudinidae	Stomatitis, glossitis, rhinitis, paralysis, incoordination	**Oral swabs, tongue,** liver, brain, other tissues	PCR*, virus isolation	NT*, ELISA
Scutavirus-like[42,43]	TeHV4	Bowsprit tortoise (Chersina angulata), leopard tortoise (Stigmochelys pardalis)	No clinical signs detected in first description, respiratory signs	Oral swab	PCR*	n.d.
Scutavirus-like[47,48]	Emydid HV 1	Eastern river cooter (Pseudemys concinna concinna), northern map turtle (Graptemys geographica), painted turtle (Chrysemys picta)	Hepatic necrosis, nasal discharge, pneumonia	Choanal/cloacal swabs, liver	PCR*	n.d.
Scutavirus-like[49]	Emydid HV 2	Spotted turtle (Clemmys guttata), bog turtle (Glyptemys muhlenbergii)	No disease detected	Choanal/cloacal swabs	PCR*	n.d.
Scutavirus-like[49]	Glyptemys HV1	Bog turtle (Glyptemys muhlenbergii)	No disease detected	Choanal/cloacal swabs	PCR*	n.d.
Scutavirus-like[49]	Glyptemys HV2	Wood turtle (Glyptemys insculpta)	No disease detected	Choanal/cloacal swabs	PCR*	n.d.

Virus	Virus name	Host species	Disease[1]	Tissue samples[2]	Method	Serology
Scutavirus-like[50]	Terrapene HV1	Eastern box turtle (Terrapene carolina carolina)	Stomatitis, rhinitis, esophagitis, tracheobronchitis, pneumonia, gastritis, enterocolitis, splenic vasculitis, hepatitis, interstitial nephritis,	Oropharyngeal swabs, pharyngeal, and nasal mucosa	PCR*	n.d.
Scutavirus-like[51,57]	Terrapene HV2	Eastern box turtle (Terrapene carolina carolina)	Papillomas	Skin lesions	PCR*, rtPCR	n.d.
Scutavirus-like[53]	Pelomedusid HV 1	West African mud turtle (Pelusios castaneus)	No disease detected	Oral and cloacal swabs	PCR*	n.d.
Iridoviridae						
Ranavirus[67,76,77]	FV3-like, CMTV-like	Many different species of turtles and tortoises	Lethargy, anorexia, nasal discharge, conjunctivitis, subcutaneous cervical edema, ulcerative stomatitis, hepatitis, enteritis, pneumonia	Cloacal swabs, oral swabs, blood, liver, gastrointestinal tract	PCR*, rtPCR virus isolation	ELISA
Reoviridae						
Orthoreovirus[125,137]	Unnamed	Spur-thighed tortoise (Testudo graeca)	Stomatitis	Oral swabs, tongue	PCR*, virus isolation	NT
Paramyxoviridae						
Ferlavirus[146,153,154]		Spur-thighed tortoise (Testudo graeca), hermann's tortoise (Testudo hermanni), leopard tortoise (Stigmochelys pardalis)	Pneumonia, dermatitis	**Lung**, other tissues	RT-PCR*, virus isolation	HI*
Picornaviridae						
Torchivirus[139,179,184]	Called virus "x"	Many different species of Testudinae, most often spur-thighed tortoises (Testudo graeca)	Softening of the carapace, stomatitis, rhinitis, conjunctivitis, ascites, tubular vacuolization in the kidneys	**Oral swabs**, tongue, trachea, **intestine**, other tissues	RT-PCR*, virus isolation	NT
"Rafivirus"[180]		Travancore (Sulawesi) tortoise (Indotestudo forstenii)	Found together with a siadenovirus during an outbreak of severe systemic disease	Liver, kidney	RT-PCR	n.d.

*Method most commonly commercially available.

[1]A causative relationship between infection and disease has not always been proven and, in some cases, viruses may also have been detected in animals with no overt clinical signs of disease.

[2]In general, tissues with lesions should be included in diagnostic testing in sick animals.

CMTV, Common midwife toad virus; ELISA, enzyme-linked immunosorbent assay; FV3, frog virus 3; HI, hemagglutination inhibition test; HV, herpesvirus; LETD, lung, eye, and trachea disease; LGRV, loggerhead genital-respiratory HV; LOCV, loggerhead orocutaneous HV; n.d., not described; NT, neutralization test; PCR, polymerase chain reaction; rtPCR, real-time PCR; RT-PCR, reverse-transcriptase PCR; TeHV, testudinid herpesvirus.

TABLE 30.4 Select Viruses of Squamate Reptiles and Common Methods for Virus and Antibody Detection

Virus Family and Virus Genus	Virus Species or Strain	Host Species	Clinical Signs and/or Pathologic Changes Described in Infected Animals[1]	Diagnostic Samples in Order from Least to Most Invasive (if known, priority samples in bold)[2]	Virus Detection	Serology
Adenoviridae *Atadenovirus*[3,11,13]	Multiple including *Snake atadenovirus A*, Agamid AdV-1	Many different species	Gastrointestinal and neurological signs (including anorexia, wasting, head tilt), hepatic necrosis, stomatitis, dermatitis, pneumonia	**Cloacal swabs, liver, intestine**, other tissues	PCR,* virus isolation; Agamid AdV 1: rtPCR*	NT
Herpesviridae Unclassified[23,26]		Various snake and lizard species	Oral lesions, skin lesions (papilloma-like), hepatic necrosis, necrosis of endothelial cells, reduced venom production	Material from lesions, liver, intestine	PCR*	n.d.
Iridoviridae *Ranavirus*[64,65]	FV3-like, BIV-like, others	Various snake and lizard species	Oral lesions, hepatic necrosis, skin lesions	Oral/cloacal swabs, blood, skin, liver	PCR,* rtPCR, virus isolation	n.d.
Iridovirus (invertebrate iridoviruses, IIV)[95]	IIV6-like	Various lizard species, including agamid, chameleonid, and iguanid lizards	Skin lesions, anorexia, emaciation	Skin, kidney, liver	rtPCR,* PCR, virus isolation	n.d.
Unclassified: erythrocytic viruses[80,86,88]		Numerous species including bearded dragons (*Pogona vitticeps*), Iberian rock lizards (*Iberolacerta monticola*), and ribbon snakes (*Thamnophis sauritus sackenii*)	Anemia, oral lesions, blepharospasm	Erythrocytes	PCR (generally diagnosed by histological examination and EM)	n.d.
Papillomaviridae Unclassified[90]		Various snakes and lizards	Papillomas	Skin lesions	PCR	n.d.
Parvoviridae *Dependoparvovirus*[110]	*Squamate dependoparvovirus 1*, others	Various snake and lizard spp.	Mostly found together with adenovirus infections, gastrointestinal, neurologic, and respiratory signs	**Intestine**, other tissues	PCR, cell culture	n.d.
Reoviridae *Orthoreovirus*[125]		Many different species	Pneumonia, enteropathy, hepatopathy, CNS signs, skin lesions	Oral and cloacal swabs, liver, kidney, intestine, lung, spleen, brain	RT-PCR,* virus isolation	NT

Family / Virus	Host / Species	Disease	Specimens / Tissues	Method	Serology
Bornaviridae					
Bornavirus (Hyndman T, personal communication, 2016)[141,142] / *Elapid 1 bornavirus*, others	Gaboon viper (*Bitis gabonica*), African garter snake (*Elapsoidea loveridgei*), various python spp.	Neurologic disease	**Oral-cloacal swabs**, blood, venom glands, **brain**, various other tissues	RT-PCR, NGS	n.d.
Paramyxoviridae					
Ferlavirus[146,149,151,15]	Many different snake and lizard species; most commonly viperid snakes	Pneumonia, CNS signs	Oral and cloacal swabs, **tracheal washes**, **lung**, brain, kidney, and other tissue	RT-PCR,* virus isolation	HI*
Sunviridae					
Sunshinevirus[160]	Australian pythons (including black-headed python [*Aspidites melanocephalus*], woma python [*A. ramsayi*], spotted python [*Aspidites maculosa*], and carpet python [*Morelia spilota* spp. and *M bredli*]), ball python (*Python regius*)	CNS signs, pneumonia	Oral-cloacal swabs, liver, kidney, lung, **brain**	RT-PCR, virus isolation	n.d.
Arenaviridae					
Reptarenavirus[166,167]	Multiple species	Inclusion body disease	Oral-esophageal swabs, blood, esophageal tonsils, **liver**, kidney, pancreas, **brain**, other tissues	RT-PCR,* virus isolation	n.d.
Nidovirales: Coronaviridae					
Unassigned[175] / *Ball python nidovirus 1*	Ball python (*Python regius*), Indian rock python (*Python molurus*), green tree python (*Morelia viridis*), carpet python (*Morelia spilota* spp.), boa constrictors (*Boa constrictor*)	Pneumonia, stomatitis/pharyngitis	**Oral swabs, tracheal washes,** blood, liver, **lung,** trachea, esophagus, spleen, heart, brain	RT-PCR*	n.d.

*Method most commonly commercially available.

†A causative relationship between infection and disease has not always been proven and in some cases, viruses may also have been detected in animals with no overt clinical signs of disease.

‡In general, tissues with lesions should be included in diagnostic testing in sick animals.

BIV, Bohle iridovirus; *EM*, electron microscopy; *FV3*, frog virus 3; *HI*, hemagglutination inhibition test; *IBD*, inclusion body disease; *n.d.*, not described; *NT*, neutralization test; *PCR*, polymerase chain reaction; *rtPCR*, real-time PCR; *RT-PCR*, reverse-transcriptase PCR.

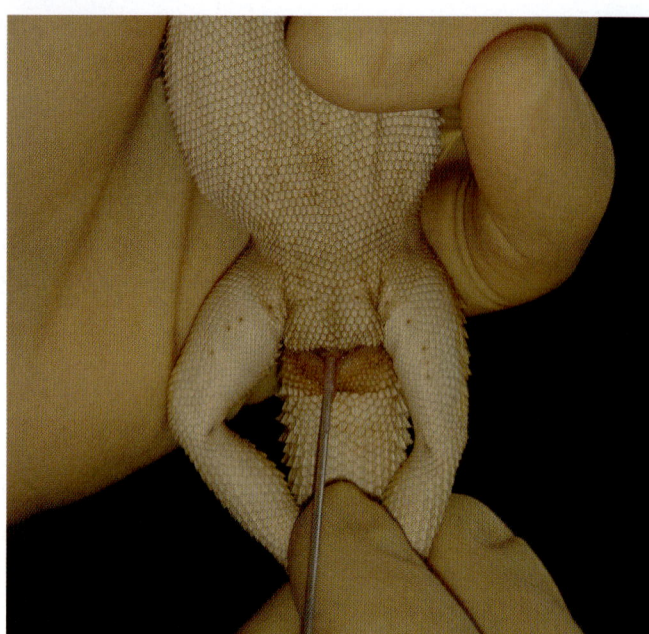

FIG 30.3 Bearded dragon (*Pogona vitticeps*). Cloacal swabs are recommended for the diagnosis of adenovirus infections in live animals.

antibodies in wild-caught snakes in Central America. In a study using Agamid AdV-1, Helodermatid AdV-1 and -2, and Snake AdV-1 and -2 in neutralization tests, antibodies against Agamid AdV-1 were most commonly found in agamid lizards, as well as in viperid and pythonid snakes, while antibodies against Helodermatid AdV-1 were most commonly found in iguanid lizards, and antibodies against Helodermatid AdV-2 were most commonly detected in helodermatid lizards.[3]

HERPESVIRIDAE

All of the reptilian HVs described so far appear to belong to the subfamily *Alphaherpesvirinae*. The genus *Scutavirus* has been created with the type species *Chelonid alphaherpesvirus 5* (chHV), also known as chelonid fibropapilloma-associated herpesvirus,[15] and herpesviruses from other chelonians have been shown to cluster with this genus.[16] It is considered probable that all vertebrates carry multiple HV species. In most cases, severe infection is only observed in very young or immunosuppressed animals or following infection of an alternative host.

Herpesviruses are relatively susceptible to disinfectants and are therefore easy to inactivate in the environment with the use of standard virucidal disinfectants. Studies on viral persistence in soil have shown that they are inactivated within about 2 weeks in the summer but may persist for longer at lower temperatures.[17] It is important to remember, though, that HV cause latent infections. Thus an HV-infected animal that survives initial infection must be considered a lifelong carrier.

In reptiles, HVs have been detected in lizards, snakes, chelonians, and crocodylians.[18] Infections are most often detected in various chelonian species, while detections in other species have been sporadic. In many, but not all, cases, infections have been associated with severe disease.

Herpesviruses in Squamates

In snakes, HVs have been detected in venom glands of various species, in some cases associated with decreased venom production,[19] and in a group of juvenile boa constrictors that died with hepatic necrosis.[20] In a disease outbreak among captive adult horned vipers (*Vipera ammodytes*

ammodytes), all 71 horned vipers in the collection died within 2 weeks of developing lethargy, anorexia, and dyspnea. Common European vipers (*Vipera berus*) in the same collection were unaffected. Gross lesions in necropsied animals included petechiae and serosanguinous effusion throughout the body. Histology showed multiple foci of severe coagulative necrosis and necrosis of sinusoidal endothelial cells in the livers, myocardium, fat bodies, and spleens. Large acidophilic inclusion bodies were observed in the nuclei of endothelial cells in the liver.[21]

In lizards, a number of different HVs have been detected. HV-like particles, as well as particles resembling papova- and reoviruses, were detected by electron microscopy in papillomas of green lizards (*Lacerta viridis*).[22] Herpesviral DNA has also been detected by PCR in tissues from papillomas from green lizards.[23] A number of cases have been documented in which lizard HVs were associated with oral lesions in infected animals. Varanid HV 1 was detected in the oral mucosa and brain of emerald tree monitor lizards (*Varanus prasinus*) with proliferative stomatitis.[24] Three distinct HVs (gerrhosaurid HVs 1-3) were detected in Sudan plated lizards (*Gerrhosaurus major*) and a black-lined plated lizard (*Gerrhosaurus nigrolineatus*) with stomatitis.[25]

A few reports are available of HVs in lizards associated with lesions in the liver. Hepatitis and enteritis were diagnosed in juvenile monitor lizards that died acutely in the United States. Intranuclear inclusions were found in hepatocytes and enterocytes, and electron microscopy confirmed the presence of herpesvirus-like particles. The virus was shown to be closely related to Varanid herpesvirus 2 (GenBank accession No. AB189433), found in a monitor lizard in Japan (unpublished).[26]

Iguanid HV1 is the only lizard HV that has been isolated in cell culture from cell cultures derived from an infected green iguana (*Iguana iguana*). Transmission of the isolate to other lizards did not lead to the development of clinical signs.[27] In another case with a green iguana, HV-like particles were detected by electron microscopy in a lizard with hepatitis.[28]

Herpesviruses in Crocodilians

Several HVs have been reported in crocodilians. The first report was of the detection of HV-like particles in the skin of saltwater crocodiles (*Crocodylius porosus*) in Australia with a crust on the abdominal skin.[29] However, a direct link between the lesions and the HV detected could not be drawn, as the animals with lesions were shown to also have a poxvirus infection, as well as bacterial infections precipitated by biting. In the United States, an HV was detected in American alligators (*Alligator mississippiensis*) with lesions in the cloaca.[30] The virus was found to be very closely related to testudinid HV3, and the authors have suggested that it might have been a contaminant (GenBank accession number AY913769.1). Three different herpesviruses (Crocodyline HV1–3) were detected in saltwater and freshwater crocodiles from two large farms in Australia. The viruses were isolated in cell culture during an investigation into disease syndromes associated with conjunctivitis and pharyngitis, systemic lymphoid proliferation and encephalitis, and lymphonodular skin infiltrates in saltwater crocodiles and systemic lymphoid proliferation in freshwater crocodiles.[31]

Herpesviruses in Chelonians

Of the reptilian HVs, the chelonian HVs are most common and have been best characterized. HVs have been detected in members of the families Cheloniidae (sea turtles), Testudinidae (tortoises), Emydidae (pond turtles, box and freshwater turtles), Chelidae (Austro-American sideneck turtles), and Pelomedusidae (Afro-American sideneck turtles) so far.

In sea turtles, HV infections have been associated with skin lesions (gray patch disease); fibropapillomatosis; lung, eye, and trachea disease (LETD); loggerhead genital–respiratory HV (LGRV)-associated disease;

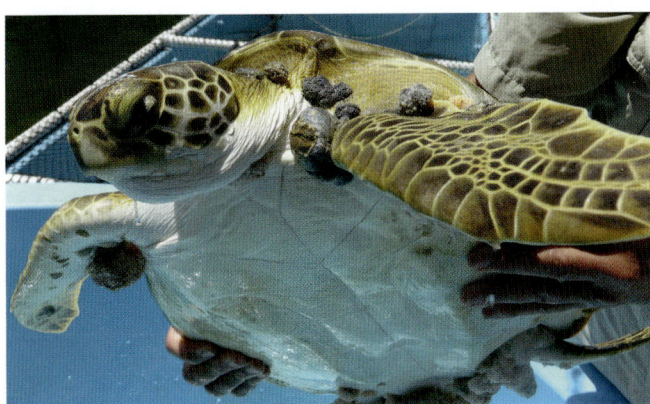

FIG 30.4 Green turtle (*Chelonia mydas*) with fibropapillomas.

and loggerhead orocutaneous HV (LOCV)-associated disease. Gray patch disease virus was one of the first HVs to be described in chelonians. It infects green sea turtles (*Chelonia mydas*). Aquaculture-reared, 2- to 3-month-old turtles appear to be most commonly affected. The virus was described by electron microscopy.[32]

Lung, eye, and trachea disease (LETD) has also been described in green sea turtles. Clinical signs associated with infection are gasping; harsh respiratory sounds; buoyancy abnormalities; inability to dive properly; and the presence of caseated material on the eyes, around the glottis, and within the trachea. Some of the infected turtles died after several weeks, while others became chronically ill. An HV (LETV) was isolated from diseased turtles in green sea turtle kidney cells.[33]

In sea turtles, fibropapillomatosis (Fig. 30.4) has been associated with HV infection and has been described in many different species of marine turtles, including green, loggerhead (*Caretta caretta*), Hawksbill (*Eretmochelys imbricata*), and olive ridley (*Lepidochelys olivacea*) sea turtles around the world. Infected turtles develop fibropapillomas, and individual or multiple tumors can occur externally all over the body. Internal tumors are also possible. The viral etiology has been tested by tumor transmission using cell-free tumor extracts.[34] The fibropapillomatosis HV has never been isolated in cell culture. Fibropapilloma-associated turtle HV (FPTHV) (also known as ChHV5) is considered the type species of the genus *Scutavirus*.[15] A study of geographically and genetically diverse FPTHVs indicated that these can be divided into groups, which cluster according to geographic origin, not host species.[35] Fibropapillomatosis has been treated by surgical removal of external fibropapillomas. These may recur, and the prognosis is poor in animals with extensive internal lesions or severely weakened animals.

Two HV-associated disease syndromes have been described in wild-caught loggerhead sea turtles, LGRV- and LOCV-associated disease. LGRV was associated with ulcers in the trachea, around the cloaca, and on the base of the phallus, while LOCV was associated with ulcers in the oral cavity and cutaneous plaques, which were covered with exudate and had an erythematous border, as well as with pneumonia.[36]

HV infections have been reported in many different species of tortoises. Clinical signs commonly associated with infections include rhinitis, conjunctivitis, stomatitis, and glossitis, which frequently develop into a diphtheroid-necrotizing stomatitis and glossitis (Fig. 30.5), with diphtheroid membranes covering parts of the oral cavity and extending down into the trachea and esophagus. Edema of the neck is a common sign. Affected animals are generally anorexic and lethargic. Animals that survive acute HV infection may develop central nervous system disorders, including paralysis or incoordination.[37] Hepatitis has also been described in affected animals. In a transmission study, spur-thighed tortoises inoculated with a tortoise HV either intramuscularly or intranasally developed disease signs consistent with HV infection.[38]

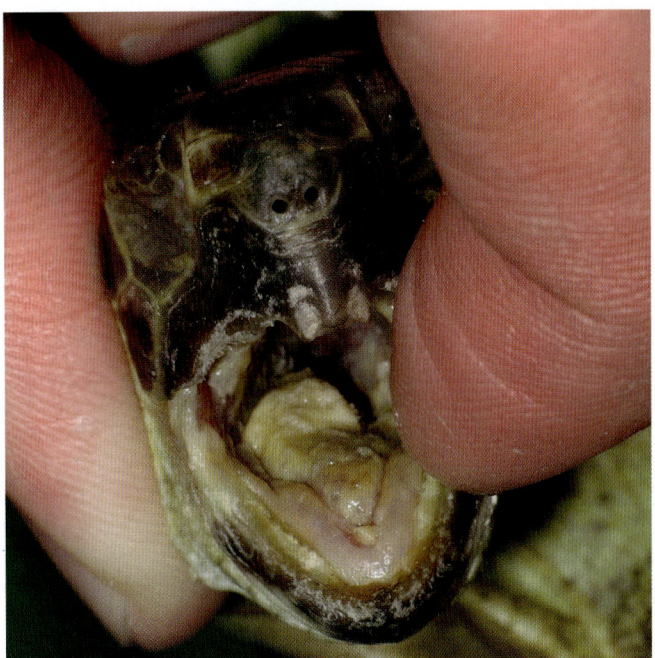

FIG 30.5 Russian tortoise (*Agrionemys horsfieldii*) with herpesvirus infection. Severe stomatitis with diphtheroid plaques visible throughout the oral cavity. (Courtesy of Volker Schmidt, Universität Leipzig, Leipzig, Germany.)

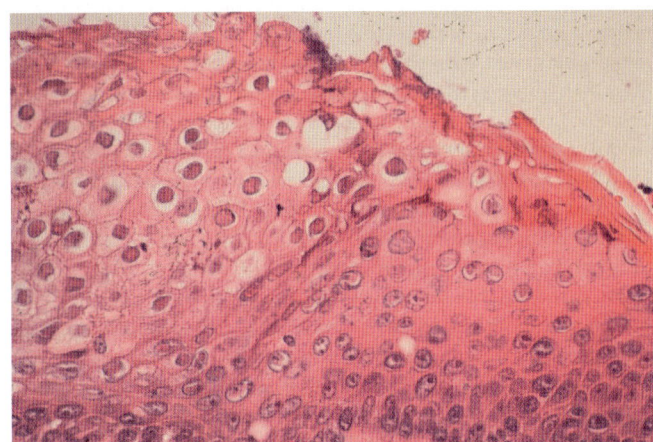

FIG 30.6 Herpesvirus infection in a tortoise (*Testudo hermanni*). Photomicrograph of the epithelium of the tongue. Ballooning degeneration is evident in numerous epithelial cells. Large intranuclear inclusions are also visible in several cells. H&E stain, ×400. (Courtesy of Horst Posthaus, Universität Bern, Berne, Switzerland.)

Development of disease and prognosis appear to depend both on the host species and on the virus involved.[37]

Histologically, HV infections in tortoises may be associated with eosinophilic or amphophilic intranuclear inclusions in infected tissues, most frequently in epithelial cells of the tongue, oral mucosa, and upper respiratory tract, as well as in the gastrointestinal tract (Fig. 30.6). Occasionally, inclusions can also be found in epithelial cells of the urinary tract, brain, liver, and spleen.[37]

There are currently four different HVs that have been shown to infect tortoises. They have been named testudinid HV1 to 4 (TeHV1 to 4).[18] TeHV1 was first detected in Russian tortoises (*Testudo horsfieldii*) and pancake tortoises (*Malacochersus tornieri*) in Japan.[39] Similar viruses have also been found in tortoises in Europe. Although they have been detected in several different species, many cases so far have had direct contact with Russian tortoises. TeHV1 is associated with stomatitis in infected animals but does not appear to cause high morbidity or mortality. TeHV2 was described in a California desert tortoise (*Gopherus agassizii*) in the United States. The animal exhibited anorexia, lethargy, and yellow-white caseous plaques on the tongue and palate.[40] TeHV3 has been most frequently described in Mediterranean tortoises (Hermann's [*T. hermanni*], spur-thighed [*T. graeca*] and marginated [*T. marginata*] tortoises) and Russian tortoises in Europe. It has also been detected in tortoises in the United States and in northern Africa. This virus is associated with severe disease and high morbidity and mortality, particularly in Hermann's and Russian tortoises. Spur-thighed tortoises develop disease less frequently and appear to be able to survive and carry the infection.[41] TeHV4 was detected in a clinically healthy bowsprit tortoise (*Chersina angulata*) in a zoo in the United States.[42] A similar virus has since been detected in a leopard tortoise with respiratory disease that was co-infected with a mycoplasma in Europe.[43] Studies of the genomes of several distinct TeHV3 isolates have shown genetic differences between isolates, including deletions, which appear to influence the ability of the viruses to invade the brain and may therefore influence the virulence of individual strains.[16]

A number of reports are available on HV infection in water turtles. These were first described based on histological changes in Pacific pond turtles (*Actinemys* (*Clemmys*) *marmorata*), painted turtles (*Chrysemys picta*), and map turtles (*Graptemys* spp.). Clinical signs reported in affected animals include lethargy, anorexia, and subcutaneous edema. Characteristic necropsy findings include hepatomegaly and pulmonary edema. Areas of hepatic necrosis with the presence of intranuclear inclusion bodies in hepatocytes were reported. Inclusions have also been demonstrated in the spleen, lungs, kidneys, and pancreas.[44–46] More recent descriptions have included data on the genomes of the viruses detected. In all cases the detected viruses have clustered with other chelonian alphaherpesviruses. In one case in a captive freshwater turtle (*Pseudemys concinna concinna*) the animal died with no previous clinical signs. Histologic examination showed hepatic lipidosis with intranuclear inclusion bodies in hepatocytes.[47] A similar virus was also found in a northern map turtle (*Graptemys geographica*). The turtle had shown weakness and nasal discharge prior to death. Postmortem examination showed pneumonia, as well as hepatocellular and splenic necrosis, all associated with intranuclear inclusion bodies.[48] In a study screening wild bog turtles (*Glyptemys muhlenbergii*), wood turtles (*G. insculpta*), and spotted turtles (*Clemmy guttata*) in the northeastern United States, three different HVs were detected; 51.5% of the bog turtles sampled were HV positive. None of the animals in that study were clinically ill.[49] Herpesviruses have also been described in box turtles in the United States in association with stomatitis and papillomas.[50,51]

A single report is available of an HV infection in an Australian sideneck turtle, a captive Krefft's river turtle (*Emydura macquarii kreffti*). The animal showed ulcerative lesions of the skin and shell, and histopathology showed orthokeratotic hyperkeratosis with intranuclear inclusions in keratinocytes.[52] A single report also exists of an HV infection in African sideneck turtles (West African mud turtles [*Pelusios castaneus*]). The animals were imported into Germany from a farm in West Africa. A herpesvirus was detected in oral and cloacal swabs from clinically healthy animals by PCR.[53]

Identification of Herpesvirus Infections

Virus Detection. Detection of viral DNA by PCR is the most commonly used method for detecting HVs in infected reptiles (Tables 30.3 to 30.5). A PCR using degenerate primers in a nested format targeting a highly conserved portion of the DNA polymerase gene has been used to detect HVs in chelonians, squamates, and crocodylians.[54] Results from this

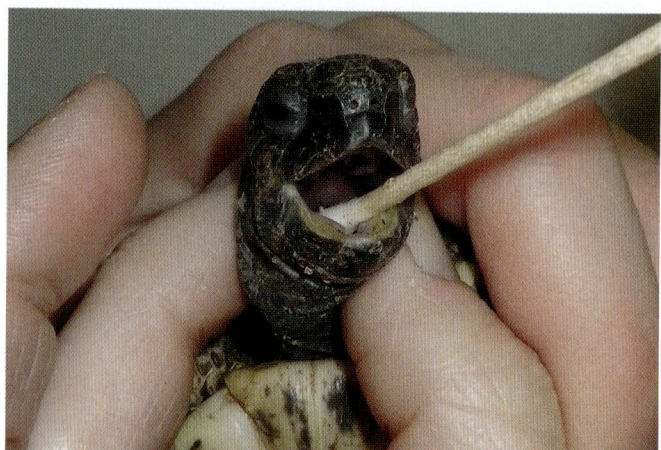

FIG 30.7 Hermann's tortoise (*Testudo hermanni*). Oral swabs can be used to diagnose several different viral infections in live tortoises, particularly herpes, picorna, and ranavirus infections.

PCR must be confirmed (e.g., by sequencing). Other PCRs have been described targeting specific TeHVs (e.g., only TeHV1 or only TeHV3).[41] A PCR for the differentiation of TeHV3 strains has been suggested.[55] A duplex PCR has been designed for the detection of CrHVs 1, 2, and 3 in formalin-fixed tissues from infected crocodiles.[31] Real-time, quantitative PCRs have also been developed for the detection of specific viruses in specific animal species, including TeHV2 in desert tortoises[56] and Terrapene HV1 in box turtles.[57] Virus isolation in cell culture has been used to detect LETV, TeHV1, and TeHV3. Samples for HV detection in chelonians should generally include tissues with lesions. For fibropapillomatosis, viral DNA can be detected in fibropapillomas removed from live or dead animals. In tortoises, HV DNA has been detected in oral swabs from live animals. Swabs should be taken from the base of the tongue and should include cellular material (Fig. 30.7). In dead tortoises, the tongue is generally considered the best tissue for virus detection. Esophagus, stomach, intestine, trachea, liver, and brain can also be helpful in virus detection. In water turtles, HV detection has most often been reported from the liver in dead animals. In crocodylians, CrHVs have been detected in conjunctiva, skin, liver, kidney, and mixed tissues of infected animals.

Serology. Detection of antibodies against HVs is particularly important because HVs cause latent infections, therefore, any animal found to be serologically positive for HVs must be considered a lifelong carrier, even if the animal appears healthy. Serologic tests have been described for the detection of antibodies against FPTHV and LETV in sea turtles and against TeHV1 and TeHV3 in tortoises.[58–61] High seroprevalences were found in wild green sea turtles in Florida and in loggerhead turtles with an ELISA used for the detection of antibodies against glycoprotein H of an FPTHV.[58] Seropositivity did not correlate with clinical disease. However, testing for antibodies against this virus is not widely available. An ELISA has also been described for the detection of antibodies against LETV.[59]

Virus neutralization tests and ELISAs have been described for the detection of antibodies against TeHV1 and against TeHV3.[60,61] Virus neutralization testing with both TeHV1 and TeHV3 has shown that these viruses do not cross-react serologically; thus testing for antibodies against both is recommended in Europe. Detection of antibodies against these two viruses has been shown to depend on the tortoise species involved. Hermann's tortoises, which are particularly susceptible to HV infection and disease, do not often develop neutralizing antibodies after

TABLE 30.5 **Select Viruses of Crocodilians and Common Methods for Virus and Antibody Detection**

Virus Family and Virus Genus	Virus Species or Strain	Host Species	Clinical Signs and/or Pathologic Changes Described in Infected Animals[1]	Diagnostic Samples in Order from Least to Most Invasive (if known, priority samples in bold)[2]	Virus Detection	Serology
Herpesviridae[31]	Crocodyline HV 1–3	Saltwater crocodile (*Crocodylus porosus*), freshwater crocodile (*Crocodylus johnsoni*)	Conjunctivitis, pharyngitis, systemic lymphoid proliferation, encephalitis, lymphonodular skin infiltration	Conjunctiva, pharynx, skin, fat body, liver, kidney, lung, spleen, pancreas, intestine, thymus, heart, eye, brain	PCR, virus isolation	n.d.
Poxviridae						
Unclassified[96,97]	Caiman pox virus	Common caiman (*Caiman crocodilus*)	Gray-white papular skin lesions	Skin lesions	Histology and EM	n.d.
Crocodylidpoxvirus[101]	Nile crocodilepox virus (CRV) and others	*Crocodylus* spp.	Brownish wartlike skin lesions, in some cases, deeply penetrating skin lesions	Skin lesions	Histology and EM, PCR	n.d.
Flaviviridae						
Flavivirus[196,198,203,204]	*West Nile virus*	*Alligator mississippiensis*, *Crocodylus niloticus*	Neurologic signs (e.g. tremors, disorientation, opisthotonus), stomatitis, lymphohistiocytic proliferative cutaneous lesions	Cloacal swabs, **blood**, serum, **liver**, lung	RT-PCR*, virus isolation	NT, ELISA

*Method most commonly commercially available.

[1]A causative relationship between infection and disease has not always been proven, and, in some cases, viruses may also have been detected in animals with no overt clinical signs of disease.

[2]In general, tissues with lesions should be included in diagnostic testing in sick animals.

ELISA, Enzyme-linked immunosorbent assay; *n.d.*, not described; *NT*, neutralization test; *PCR*, polymerase chain reaction; *RT-PCR*, reverse-transcriptase PCR.

infection. In contrast, antibodies are frequently detected in spur-thighed tortoises that have been infected. An ELISA originally developed for the detection of antibodies against TeHV3 has also been adapted to detect antibodies against TeHV2 in California desert tortoises on the basis of putative serologic cross-reactivity between TeHV2 and 3.[40,62]

IRIDOVIRIDAE

Iridoviruses belonging to two (or three) genera have been detected in reptiles—ranaviruses, invertebrate iridoviruses and a putative additional genus in the family consisting of erythrocytic viruses. Although iridoviruses are enveloped, some viruses in this family (notably the ranaviruses) do not require their envelopes to be infectious. This makes them somewhat more resistant to disinfection (especially by organic solvents) than other enveloped viruses. Studies have shown that iridoviruses may be quite resistant to inactivation in water and soil at cool temperatures and may be able to survive over winter in regions with a temperate climate.[63] There is, however, evidence that ranaviruses can be inactivated in soil in the summer (at relatively high temperatures) within several weeks.[17] Under clean conditions, iridoviruses can be disinfected using standard virucidal disinfectants.

RANAVIRUSES

Ranaviruses have been increasingly shown to be important pathogens of ectothermic animals and are one of the major causes of global amphibian declines. Both phylogenetic studies and transmission studies indicate that some ranaviruses can be transmitted between reptiles, amphibians, and fish. Analysis of whole and partial genomes from reptilian ranaviruses indicates that several different species of amphibian ranaviruses, including viruses closely related to *Frog virus 3* (FV3), the type species of the genus *Ranavirus*, as well as *Bohle iridovirus* (BIV)-like, *common midwife toad virus* (CMTV)-like, and *European catfish virus* (ECV)-like viruses can infect reptiles.[64,65] Development of disease in infected animals is dependent on the virus strain, on the host species, and on environmental factors, particularly temperature. Some animals can become inapparent carriers, while in others, infection leads to severe disease and death.

Chelonians

In chelonians, ranaviral infection has been associated with lethargy, anorexia, nasal discharge, conjunctivitis, severe subcutaneous cervical

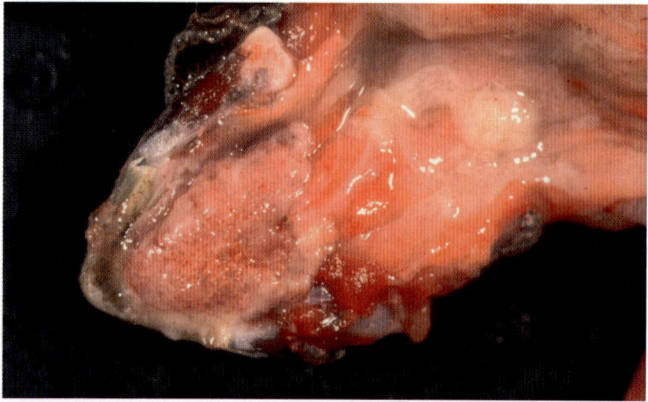

FIG 30.8 Hermann's tortoise (*Testudo hermanni*) infected with a ranavirus. Severe stomatitis. (Courtesy of Dr. Horst Posthaus, Universität Bern, Berne, Switzerland.)

edema, ulcerative stomatitis, and "red-neck disease" (Fig. 30.8). Infection induces an inflammatory response, and detection of an acute-phase protein response has been described.[66] Histologically, infected animals have been found to have hepatitis, enteritis, and pneumonia. Basophilic intracytoplasmic inclusions have in some cases been described in epithelial cells of the gastrointestinal tract and hepatocytes of infected animals, although inclusion bodies are not always detected. In a transmission study with box turtles (*Terrapene ornata ornata*) and red-eared sliders (*Trachemys scripta elegans*), intramuscular injection of a ranavirus led to disease, including lethargy, anorexia, ocular discharge, conjunctivitis, oral plaques, and death in some animals.[67] Studies on turtles that have survived ranavirus outbreaks have suggested that some animals may become persistently infected.[68] Other transmission studies have shown that environmental temperature can affect the development of clinical disease and death in infected turtles, with a higher mortality rate documented in infected red-eared sliders kept at 22°C than at 28°C.[69]

Squamates

In the first description of infection in squamates, infected green tree pythons (*Morelia [Chondropython] viridis*) showed ulceration of the nasal mucosa, hepatic necrosis, and severe necrotizing inflammation of the pharyngeal submucosa.[70] In a giant leaf-tailed gecko (*Uroplatus fimbriatus*), infection was associated with granulomatous lesions in the tail and liver. In an Iberian mountain lizard (*Iberolacerta (Lacerta) monticola*), no overt disease was documented. That lizard was also infected with erythrocytic virus. In recent descriptions of ranavirus infections in various lizard species, variable skin lesions have been the most common lesion observed (Fig. 30.9). In many cases, infected lizards were from the international pet trade and had multiple other infections.[71–73]

Transmission. There is evidence that ranaviruses can be transmitted to reptiles by several different routes, including direct contact between animals, contact with contaminated water or pond sediment, and ingestion of infectious material, for example, from dead amphibians. In transmission studies, injection of virus into susceptible species has been successful,[67] but transmission via water has also been demonstrated.[74] Transmission by mosquitoes has also been proposed for FV3 in terrestrial turtles.[75]

Identification of Ranavirus Infections

Virus Detection. Molecular methods, including both conventional and real-time PCR, have been frequently used for the detection of ranaviruses in reptiles (see Tables 30.3 and 30.4). The gene most frequently targeted is the major capsid protein (MCP) gene.[76] A real-time PCR has been described for the detection of ranaviruses in eastern box turtles in the United States.[77] However, real-time PCRs can be very strain specific, and methods described so far in reptiles have generally only been able to detect FV3, not other ranavirus strains found in reptiles, thus the use of these methods could lead to false-negative results. Ranaviruses also grow well in cell culture and can be grown on a wide range of cell lines from reptiles, fish, mammals, and birds if the cells are kept at appropriate temperatures (below 32°C).

Samples for the detection of ranaviruses in chelonians should include liver and gastrointestinal tract. Spleen and kidney may also be virus positive.[67] In a transmission study viral DNA was detected in oral and cloacal swabs from intramuscularly infected red-eared sliders as early as 5 days postinoculation (p.i.) and until 26 days p.i. or until the animals died or were euthanized.[67] Oral and cloacal swabs and blood have all been used to detect ranavirus in naturally infected chelonians.[78,79]

Samples for ranavirus detection in squamates should include liver tissue and skin. A ranavirus has been detected in the blood of a live

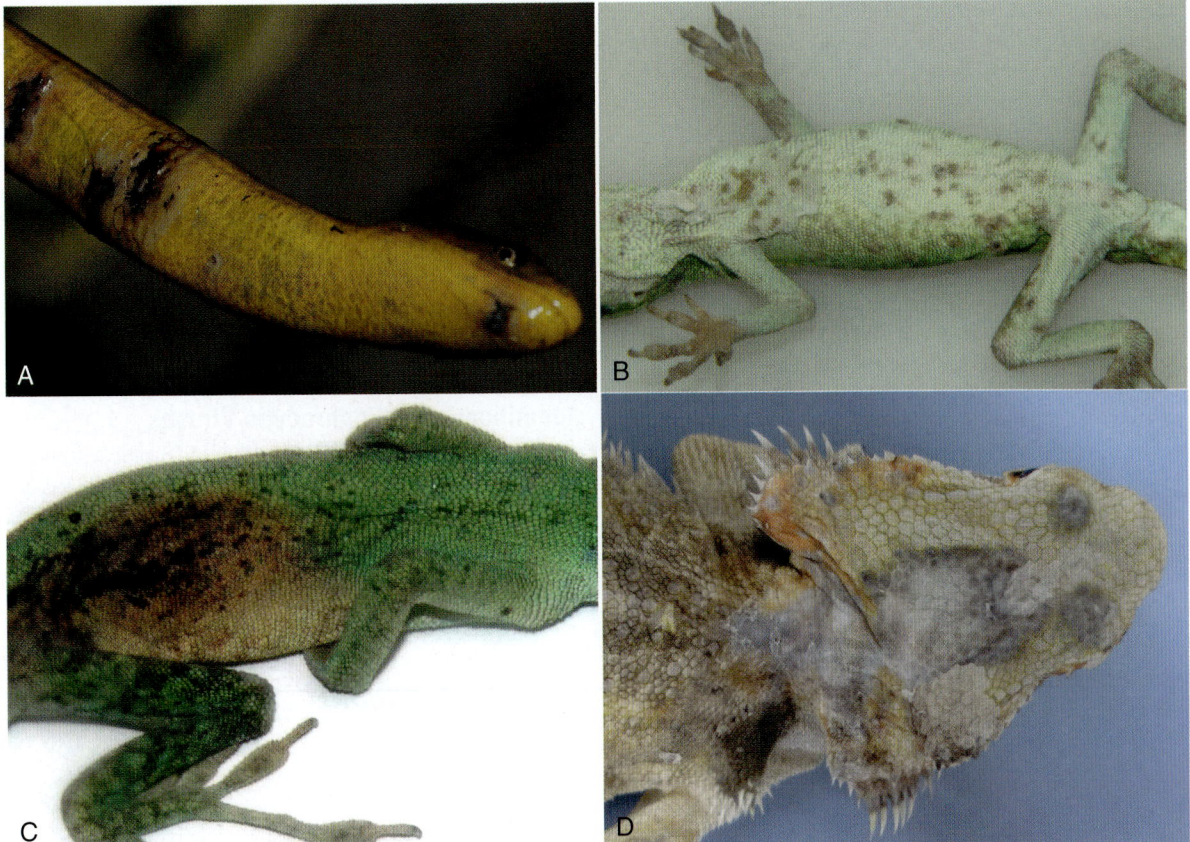

FIG 30.9 (A) Ranavirus-infected Asian glass lizard (*Dopasia gracilis*). Skin lesions on the ventral surface of the body. An invertebrate iridovirus was also found in the skin of this animal. (B and C) Skin alterations observed in ranavirus-infected green anoles (*Anolis carolinensis*). An invertebrate iridovirus was also detected in these animals. (B) Multiple ulcera on the ventral abdominal surface. (C) Beige gray discoloration of the skin at the lateral abdomen. (D) Skin lesions in a ranavirus-infected central bearded dragon (*Pogona vitticeps*). (From Stöhr et al, 2013.)[72]

Iberian mountain lizard.[80] The optimal sample for the detection of ranaviruses in live squamates is unknown, but testing of mixed oral/cloacal swabs and blood is recommended. Skin biopsies can also be tested in cases with dermatologic signs.

Serology. An ELISA for the detection of anti-ranavirus antibodies in Burmese star tortoises, gopher tortoises (*Gopherus polyphemus*), and eastern box turtles has been developed.[81] Testing of various species with and without previous histories of ranaviral infection showed a low prevalence of anti-ranavirus antibodies in all cases.[81] This ELISA has also been adapted for the detection of anti-ranavirus antibodies in *Testudo* spp. in Europe.[78]

INVERTEBRATE IRIDOVIRUSES (IIV)

Until recently, viruses of the genus *Iridovirus* had only been described in invertebrates, in which they can cause lethal infections in a wide range of host species. These viruses have been repeatedly detected in various species of crickets sold as feed animals in the pet trade in Europe. Infected crickets show hypertrophy and bluish iridescence of the affected fat body cells.[82] In reptiles, IIVs have been isolated from the lung, liver, kidney, and intestine of two bearded dragons (*Pogona*

vitticeps) and a chameleon (*Trioceros* (*Chamaeleo*) *quadricornis*) and from the skin of a frilled lizard (*Chlamydosaurus kingii*). The frilled lizard showed poxlike skin lesions, and one of the bearded dragons had pneumonia. The other lizards had died with nonspecific signs. A host-switch of this virus from prey insects to the predator lizards was postulated.[83] An IIV was isolated from several tissues of a high-casqued chameleon (*Trioceros* [*Chamaeleo*] *hoehnelii*) and successfully used to infect crickets of the species *Gryllus bimaculatus*.[84] IIV-like viruses have also been detected in multiple other lizards from various owners, as well as from crickets,[85] and in multiple lizards with skin lesions in which other viruses (e.g., ranaviruses) were detected (Fig. 30.9A–C).[71,72] The clinical significance of IIV infection in lizards is not always clear, because virus has been detected in clinically healthy animals, as well as in animals that were emaciated, had skin lesions, or died acutely.

Identification of IIV Infections

IIVs have been detected by virus isolation, conventional, and real-time PCRs (see Table 30.4). All of the methods used to detect IIVs in samples from reptiles can also be used to detect these viruses in feed insects.[85] IIVs grow on multiple cell lines from insects, reptiles, and mammals at 28°C. Because feed insects are often infected with IIVs, samples from the gastrointestinal tract, including oral and cloacal swabs in live animals, should not be used for IIV detection in reptiles. Skin biopsies have been used for virus detection in live animals with skin lesions, and various internal tissues including liver have been successfully used in dead animals. IIVs are often detected together with other infectious agents, particularly adenoviruses (AdVs) in agamids.

ERYTHROCYTIC VIRUSES

Viral erythrocytic infections have been described in fish and amphibians as well as lizards, snakes, and turtles. These viruses have been preliminarily classified as iridoviruses, and recent studies based on partial sequences of the DNA polymerase gene have shown that erythrocytic viruses (also called erythrocytic necrosis viruses) of reptiles and fish probably belong to a new genus in the family *Iridoviridae*.[80,86,87] They have been hypothesized to be transmitted by invertebrates. These viruses are associated with inclusions in erythrocytes of infected animals (Fig. 30.10), and

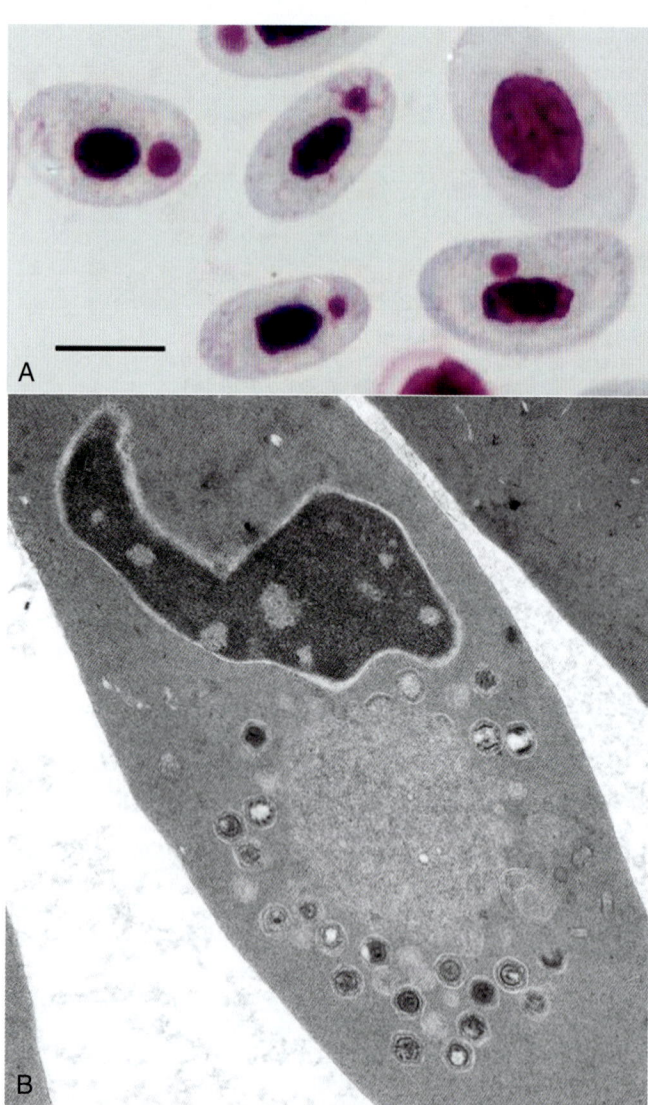

FIG 30.10 Iberian rock lizard (*Iberolacerta monticola*) erythrocytes with erythrocytic virus infection. (A) Erythrocytic necrosis virus has caused intracytoplasmic inclusions in multiple erythrocytes. H&E stain. (B) Transmission electron photomicrograph of the inclusion in an erythrocyte. The inclusions consist of viral precursors and viral particles in a crystalline array. (Courtesy of Antonio Pedro Alves de Matos, Curry Cabral Hospital, Lisbon, Portugal.)

inclusions were originally believed to be parasites (*Toddia* and *Pirhemocyton* sp.). Clinical signs in infected animals range from apparently healthy to severe systemic disease and death. Lethargy and weight loss associated with anemia have been reported. In a study of an outbreak in bearded dragons, infection was associated with lesions on the tongue, reduced appetite and weight loss, lethargy, and blepharospasmus in several infected animals.[88] Morphological changes in infected erythrocytes, including anisocytosis and polychromasia, as well as hepatic necrosis have been documented in reptiles with erythrocytic necrosis virus infections. A transmission study conducted with the lizards *Iberolacerta* (*Lacerta*) *monticola* and *Lacerta schreiberi* showed that infection with these agents can become systemic and may lead to death if the animals are kept at suboptimal temperatures.[89]

Identification of Erythrocytic Viruses

Erythrocytic viruses have generally been diagnosed by detection of inclusions in erythrocytes in blood smears, followed by electron microscope confirmation of their etiology. Following partial characterization of the genomes of erythrocytic viruses from fish and reptiles, several PCRs have been published and may prove usefull for diagnostics.[87,88] Sampling for these viruses should always include peripheral blood as well as liver in dead animals.

PAPILLOMAVIRIDAE

Papilloma-like lesions (Fig. 30.11) have been repeatedly described in various reptiles. Their cause is not always known, and various viruses have been associated with such lesions. Papillomaviruses have only been associated with them in select cases. The papillomaviruses are highly host specific and tissue restricted. They generally cause benign tumors (warts, papillomas) in their natural host. Papillomaviruses are highly resistant to inactivation and can persist in the environment for long periods of time.

Papillomaviruses in Squamates

The first description of a papilloma-like virus (papovavirus) in reptiles was in wartlike skin lesions in a European green lizard. The virus was identified by electron microscopy based on morphologic characteristics. Herpeslike and reolike viruses were also identified in the lesions.[22] A papillomavirus has also been detected in a diamond python (*Morelia spilota spilota*) with multiple small black papillated and pedunculated skin proliferations, approximately 3 mm in diameter, as well as signs of respiratory disease.[90] The skin lesions were found to be a papilloma-like

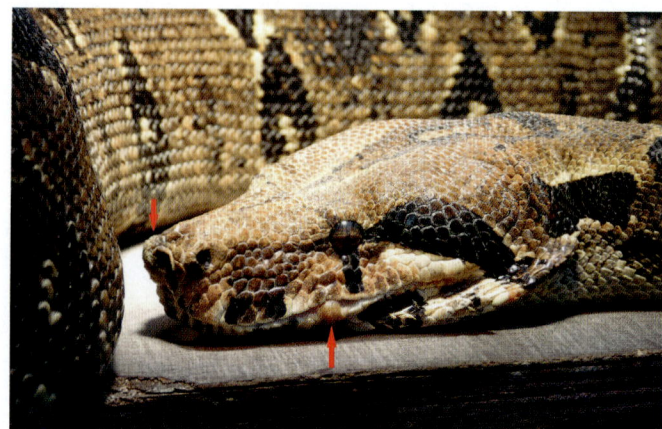

FIG 30.11 Wart-like lesions on the mouth and nares of a boa constrictor (*Boa constrictor*). This animal had inclusion body disease (IBD).

neoplasia, and inclusion bodies were found in some of the papillomas. A papillomavirus was identified in skin biopsies from this animal by PCR.[90]

Papillomaviruses in Chelonians

In chelonians, papillomaviruses have been described in Bolivian side-neck turtles (*Platemys platycephala*) with circular papular skin lesions that in some cases progressed to areas of necrosis. Viral particles were detected by electron microscopy in skin biopsies.[91] Papillomavirus-like particles were detected in a lung wash (but not in oral scrapings) by electron microscopy in a Russian tortoise with a history of stomatitis.[92] Lesions similar to those described in the Bolivian side-neck turtles were found in a loggerhead turtle and a green sea turtle.[93] The lesions resolved after several months. These two viruses (CcPV-1 and CmPV-1) were shown to be distinct from one another and from previously described papillomaviruses.[93]

Identification of Papillomavirus Infections

Diagnosis of papillomavirus infections has been mostly by detection of viral particles in infected tissues via electron microscopy. The complete sequences of CcPV-1 and CmPV-1 have been determined as has the complete sequence of a snake papillomavirus, so future development of diagnostic PCRs is possible.[94,95] However, these viruses are phylogenetically quite distant from one another, and nothing is known about genetic diversity of most reptilian papillomaviruses. Tissues for analysis should include affected skin.

POXVIRIDAE

Although poxviruses are enveloped, they are much more resistant to inactivation in the environment than other enveloped viruses and can remain infectious at ambient temperatures for months, especially when protected by cellular material (e.g., sloughed skin cells or blood). They are, however, inactivated by standard virucidal disinfection protocols.

The first report of poxvirus-associated disease in a reptile was in captive caimans (*Caiman crocodilus*) in the United States.[96] Similar cases have since been reported from caimans throughout the world.[97,98] Affected animals develop gray-white skin lesions on various parts of the body (Fig. 30.12).

Poxviruses have also been detected in Nile crocodiles (*Crocodylus niloticus*), as well as saltwater crocodiles (*Crocodylus porosus*) and freshwater crocodiles (*Crocodylus johnsoni*) in Australia.[99] Infected animals develop brownish wartlike skin lesions that can occur over the entire body (Fig. 30.13). Infection is associated with high morbidity but low mortality. A recent study of farmed saltwater crocodiles in Australia found that 40% to 45% of the examined animals were affected with mild cutaneous poxvirus infections.[100] An atypical form of crocodile pox has also been observed in Nile crocodiles. This virus was associated with deeply penetrating skin lesions in farmed crocodiles in Africa. A PCR was developed and used to amplify a portion of the genome of the virus associated with these lesions. Analysis of the PCR product showed that this virus was related to, but not identical with, crocodilepox virus (CRV).[101] Transmission is likely by contaminated water, possibly from infected wild animals as well as direct contact between animals. Infection by arthropod vectors as described for poxviruses of other animals may be possible.

Poxvirus infections have been detected in individual cases in other reptiles by electron microscopy. Papular skin lesions around the eyes of a Hermann's tortoise were found to contain poxlike viruses.[102] A flap-necked chameleon (*Chamaeleo dilepis*) in Tanzania was found to have two different types of intracytoplasmic inclusions in circulating monocytes. The inclusions were found to be caused by a chlamydialike organism and a poxlike virus.[103] A poxvirus infection in a tegu lizard was associated with brown papules on various parts of the body.[104]

Identification of Poxvirus Infections

Poxvirus infection in crocodilians has generally been diagnosed on the basis of the detection of intracytoplasmic inclusions in hypertrophic epithelial cells followed by electron microscopic demonstration of viral particles within these inclusions or by electron microscopic detection of viral particles in unfixed scrapings from lesions.[101,105] A PCR for the detection of CRV in scrapings from fresh lesions has also been described (see Table 30.5).[101]

CIRCOVIRIDAE AND TORNOVIRUS

Circoviruses are very resistant to inactivation in the environment and are very difficult to disinfect. A single circolike virus has been reported in macrophages of a painted turtle (*Chrysemys* sp.), with multifocal areas of necrosis in the spleen and liver. The virus was identified based on electron microscopy.[105] Studies of the genomes of snakes have shown that sequences of endogenous circoviruses can be found in these animals.[106]

A novel ssDNA virus with a circular genome (named sea turtle tornovirus 1, STTV1) was detected in two green sea turtles with fibropapillomatosis using metagenomics. Part of the genome was found

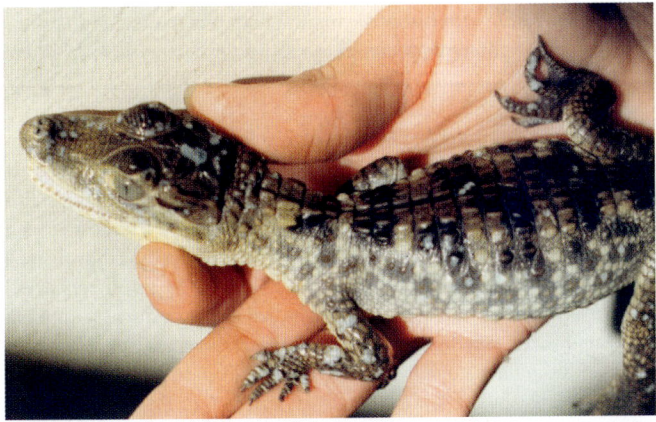

FIG 30.12 Caiman (*Caiman crocodilus*) with poxvirus infection. The skin lesions are covered with a white-gray crust. (Courtesy of Fritz W. Huchzermeyer, University of Pretoria, Onderstepoort, South Africa.)

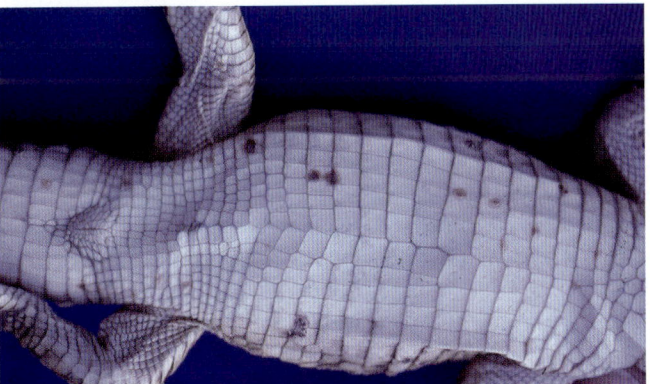

FIG 30.13 Nile crocodile (*Crocodylus niloticus*) infected with crocodile pox virus. Brownish lesions are seen on the abdominal skin. (Courtesy of Fritz W. Huchzermeyer, University of Pretoria, Onderstepoort, South Africa.)

to be distantly related to the circovirus *Chicken anemia virus*. Both of the infected turtles were severely afflicted with fibropapillomatosis. STTV1 was detected in the fibropapillomas, as well as in external swabs from the conjunctiva, oral cavity, cloaca, unaffected skin, and numerous internal tissues. The herpesvirus FPTHV was also detected in the fibropapillomas, but not in other tissues. STTV1 was also detected in leeches collected from one of the green sea turtles. It was hypothesized that STTV1 might affect the immune system of infected sea turtles or that it might be an opportunistic pathogen.[107]

PARVOVIRIDAE

The parvoviruses are highly resistant to inactivation in the environment and are therefore difficult to disinfect. They are particularly resistant to heat. The only classified reptile parvovirus, *Squamate dependoparvovirus 1*, is a species within the genus *Dependoparvovirus*.[108] Dependoparvoviruses are generally associated with a helper virus (adeno- or herpesviruses). In reptiles, parvolike viruses were first described by electron microscopy in the duodenum of a four-lined rat snake (*Elaphe quatuorlineata*) and of an Aesculapian snake (*Zamenis* [*Elaphe*] *longissimus*), both with gastrointestinal disease. Adenolike viruses were also detected in the duodenums of both and herpes- and picornalike viruses in the duodenum of one snake.[109] Co-infections of adenovirus- and parvoviruslike viruses have been described repeatedly from both snakes and lizards, with clinical signs including gastrointestinal disease, as well as neurologic signs and pneumonia.[18] A parvovirus but no helper virus was detected in a bearded dragon with malfunctioning ovaries and aberrant yolk formation, indicating that this virus is capable of independent replication.[110] Parvoviruses isolated in cell culture from a boa constrictor and a ball python (*Python regius*) were identical and were given the name serpentine adeno-associated virus (SAAV) or *Squamate dependoparvovirus 1*. It is unclear whether SAAV can replicate without a helper virus, as both isolates were obtained together with adenoviruses.[111]

Diagnosis of parvoviruses in reptiles has been by isolation in cell culture in various reptilian cell lines and, more recently, by PCR detection of viral DNA using degenerate primers targeting a portion of the genome of dependoparvoviruses.[110] Tissues from the intestinal tract have most often been used for virus detection, although mixed samples from various internal tissues have also tested positive in some cases.

HEPADNAVIRIDAE

Hepadnaviruses are enveloped viruses that include *Hepatitis B virus* (HBV). Integration of viral DNA into the host genome is rare but possible. Hepadnaviruses generally have narrow host specificity, although studies of virus evolution indicate frequent, recent host-switching, with incongruencies between host and virus phylogenies.[106] They are hepatotropic, and infection may be transient or persistent. Endogenous hepadnavirus sequences have been detected in the genomes of avian species and in rattlesnakes (*Crotalus mitchellii*) and the king cobra (*Ophiophagus hannah*).[106] In a transmission study, HBV-positive human serum was inoculated intramuscularly into yellow pond turtles (*Mauremys* [*Clemmys*] *mutica*) and Reeves' turtles (*Mauremys* [*Geoclemys*] *reevesii*). Viral antigene and antibodies against HBV were detected in most of the inoculated animals over a period of several weeks, and viral antigen and viral DNA were detectable in cultured liver cells from the inoculated animals. No signs of acute hepatitis were noted in the animals, although edematous changes in hepatocytes and minor cellular infiltration were reported and attributed to an inflammatory response.[112] HBV DNA has also been detected in a cloacal swab from a bearded dragon. The animal was from a reptile rescue in Germany and appeared clinically healthy at the time of sampling (Ball et al, Proc 9th Int Cong Vet Virol, 2012, p 60).

RETROVIRIDAE

Historically, retrovirus nomenclature was based on electron microscopy and classified members of the genera *Alpharetrovirus* and *Gammaretrovirus* as C-type viruses (assembly of immature capsids at the plasma membrane) and members of the genus *Betaretrovirus* as A-type particles (immature capsids) in the cytoplasm. A-type particles then budded with either B- or D-type morphology.[114] Retroviruses are widely distributed among vertebrates as exogenous infectious agents. Endogenous proviruses resulting from infection of germline cells also occur widely. Various retrovirus-like particles have been described in healthy snakes and in snakes with neoplasms.[18] Retroviral sequences have been detected in the genomes of many different reptiles. Systematic searches for sequences of murine leukemia–related retroviruses have shown that related viruses can be found in a wide range of animals, including reptiles, amphibians, birds, and mammals. In reptiles these viral sequences have been detected in the genomes of a number of chelonians, squamates, and in tuatara (*Sphenodon punctatus*).[115–117] A study on endogenous retroviral sequences from crocodilians showed that the genomes of several different species from different families in the order Crocodylia contain retrovirus sequences that are related to one another but highly divergent from other members of the *Retroviridae*, some of which appear to be species specific.[118] Retroviruses have been repeatedly isolated from boid snakes with inclusion body disease (IBD),[119,120] although IBD is now believed to be caused by arenaviruses. A retrovirus was isolated from an Indian rock python (*Python molurus*) that was kept together with IBD-positive pythons. Further study indicated that this is a highly expressed endogenous virus of pythons that is not associated with IBD. A similar virus was also identified in blood pythons (*Python curtus*).[121]

REOVIRIDAE

The family *Reoviridae* consists of non-enveloped viruses that are very stable in the environment. Reoviruses of reptiles that have been characterized so far have been classified in the genus *Orthoreovirus*. Viruses in this genus infect only vertebrates and are spread by the respiratory or fecal-oral route. Many orthoreovirus infections may cause no clinical signs of disease, or only mild upper respiratory tract illness and/or enteritis, while other species have been shown to cause significant and often fatal disease in avian and mammalian hosts. Five species have been classified in the genus *Orthoreovirus*, including *Reptilian orthoreovirus*. All but the *Mammalian orthoreovirus* isolates are fusogenic in cell culture.[122] Full genome sequencing of several reptilian othoreoviruses has shown that these may have originated from a common ancestor with fusogenic mammalian reoviruses and that they likely represent different species in the genus *Orthoreovirus*.[123,124] There is also evidence that individual reptilian reovirus strains are not host species specific.[125]

Reovirus infections have been relatively frequently described in reptiles. In lizards, reoviruses have been described by electron microscopy associated with papillomas in green lizards.[22] Other viruses were also detected in those lesions. Isolation of reoviruses from lizards has been described from green iguanas that died with no specific clinical signs in Germany[126] and from a spiny-tailed lizard (*Saara* [*Uromastyx*] *hardwickii*) in the United Kingdom that died during a disease outbreak associated with pneumonia.[127] An outbreak of reovirus-associated enteropathy and hepatopathy was described in leopard geckos (*Eublepharis macularius*) in the United States (Garner et al, Proc ARAV, 2009, p 82). Serologic tests have provided evidence of reovirus infections among other lizards as well, including wild-caught lizards in Central America.[129,130]

In snakes, reoviruses have been isolated from Chinese vipers (*Azemiops feae*) with enteritis, from ball pythons, emerald tree boas, and Aesculapian snakes.[18] Virus was isolated from the brain of a prairie rattlesnake (*Crotalus viridis*) with signs of central nervous system (CNS) disease, including incoordination, loss of proprioception, and convulsions.[131] A reovirus was detected in rough green snakes (*Opheodrys aestivus*) in the United States with a necrotizing hepatitis.[132] Rough green snakes imported into Hungary from the United States were also found to be infected with an orthoreovirus (Gál et al, Proc 8th Int Cong Vet Virol, 2009, p 228). Reoviruses were isolated from Moellendorff's rat snakes (*Orthriophis* [*Elaphe*] *moellendorffi*) and beauty snakes (*Orthriophis* [*Elaphe*] *taeniuris*) with fatal respiratory disease. The virus isolated from that outbreak was inoculated intratracheally, orally, and nasally into a black rat snake (*Pantherophis* [*Elaphe*] *obsoletus*). That snake died with pneumonia 26 days p.i. A reovirus was reisolated from the lungs of the dead snake.[134] Reoviruses were isolated from three boa constrictors with IBD in Germany, and a transmission study was carried out using one of these isolates. No specific disease or pathology was observed in the infected animals, although the virus was reisolated from the infected snakes up to 18 weeks p.i.[135] A reovirus was also detected repeatedly in a collection of corn snakes with increased mortality, as well as reported dyspnea, vomitus, and cachexia. A ferlavirus and an adenovirus were also detected in the same collection.[136]

Reovirus infections have been much less frequently described in tortoises. In one case a reovirus was isolated from a captive spur-thighed tortoise in Switzerland. The tortoise was cachectic and had a necrosis of the epithelium of the tongue.[137] A disease outbreak in spur-thighed tortoises in Germany with sudden softening of the carapax in juvenile animals, as well as an increased mortality rate, was associated with nematode, picornavirus, and reovirus infections in multiple animals (Blahak et al, Proc 33 Tagung der DVG Fachgruppe AVID 2014, pp 59-60).

Identification of Reovirus Infections

Virus Detection. Reoviruses of squamates are relatively easily isolated in cell culture (VH2 and IgH2), in which they cause the formation of giant syncytia. Virus has been isolated from oral and cloacal swabs from live snakes[136] and from liver, kidney, spleen, intestine, brain, and lung of dead animals. An RT-PCR has been described and used to detect and characterize reoviruses from various reptiles[125] but appears to be less sensitive than virus isolation in cell culture (see Tables 30.3 and 30.4).[136]

Serology. Virus neutralization tests have been used to detect antibodies against reoviruses in wild-caught green iguanas, Utila iguanas (*Ctenosaura bakeri*), spiny-tailed iguanas (*C. similis*), and knob-scaled lizards (*Xenosaurus grandis*).[129,130] In a study surveying wild-caught spur-thighed tortoises in Turkey, 4.9% of the animals tested had antibodies against a tortoise reovirus.[139] A study of the serologic cross-reactivity of six different reovirus isolates from lizards showed that at least three different serogroups exist; thus results of testing for antibodies using a virus neutralization test will depend on the virus used.[126]

BORNAVIRIDAE

Bornaviruses are neurotropic and do not cause the death of infected cells. Transmission may be direct or indirect, although bornaviruses of mammals do not appear to be readily transmissible between hosts. Bornaviruses are easily disinfected. In infected animals, virus persists in the host-cell nucleus. Endogenous bornalike elements (EBL) that have been integrated into the host genome have been found in the genomes of multiple species.[140] Both exogenous and endogenous bornaviruses have been detected in various reptile species in recent years. EBLs have been detected in the genomes of snakes, including speckled rattlesnakes (*Crotalus mitchellii*) and Burmese pythons (*Python bivittatus*).[106] Bornavirus N- and X/P-like sequences have been described in the venom glands (but not the genomic DNA) of a Gaboon viper (*Bitis gabonica*),[141] indicating that this is an exogenous virus, although no information about the clinical relevance of that virus (preliminarily named reptile bornavirus) is available. The full genome of a bornavirus, named Loveridge's garter snake virus 1, was sequenced from tissues of a museum specimen of an African garter snake (*Elapsoidea loveridgei*). It is unknown if any disease was associated with infection in that animal.[142] Recently, novel bornaviruses have been detected in pythons with neurologic disease in Australia. Virus detection by PCR has been successful in live animals from oral-cloacal swabs and whole blood, and from a range of tissues from dead animals. An oral-cloacal swab appears to be the priority sample from a live animal, and the brain appears to be the priority sample from a dead animal. Further research on these viruses and their clinical significance is ongoing, but preliminary results indicate that snakes can be persistently infected, and the correlation between clinical signs, histologic findings, and the presence of virus are not strong (Hyndman T, personal communication, 2016). These findings are not inconsistent with other bornaviruses known to be pathogenic.

PARAMYXOVIRIDAE: FERLAVIRUS

Paramyxoviruses (PMVs) are easily inactivated in the environment and by standard disinfectants. Some, but not all, members of this family have hemagglutinating and neuraminidase activity. The PMVs documented in reptiles belong to the genus *Ferlavirus*, which contains PMVs detected in snakes, lizards, and chelonians. These viruses have also been referred to as ophidian PMVs or reptilian PMVs. The genus *Ferlavirus* is named after the first PMV isolated from a snake, Fer-de-Lance virus (FDLV),[143] which is considered the type species of the genus.[108] All ferlaviruses hemagglutinate chicken red blood cells and hemagglutination inhibition assays have been used for serologic comparisons between isolates, as well as for diagnostic testing. Serologic studies have, however, shown that several ferlavirus strains can be distinguished from one another.[144,145] Isolates from squamates have been divided into three different genotypes (A, B, and C). A fourth genotype ("tortoise") has been isolated from a tortoise.[136,146] These genotypes do not appear to be host-species specific, and types A and B viruses have been found in a wide range of squamate hosts, as well as in chelonian hosts in individual cases.

Ferlaviruses in Squamates

The first PMV outbreak in snakes was described in 1976 in a serpentarium in Switzerland. During that outbreak, 87% of the snakes in one room died with dyspnea, opisthotonus, and apathy, followed by abnormal activity, mydriasis, and terminal convulsions.[147] Transmission appeared to be possible via aerosol, as well as via direct contact between snakes and fomites. Since that outbreak, ferlavirus outbreaks have been documented in numerous snake collections in North and South America and Europe, and the virus has been detected in wild-caught snakes from South America. Common clinical signs described in infected snakes include abnormal posturing, regurgitation, anorexia, head tremors, abnormal respiratory sounds, and exudate in the oral cavity (Fig. 30.14). In many cases, no clinical signs may be noticed, and infected animals may be found dead in their enclosures.[147,148] Severe disease has mostly been described in viperid snakes, but ferlaviruses have also been found in snakes from the families Colubridae, Elapidae, Boidae, and Pythonidae.[149] Koch's postulates have been fulfilled for pulmonary lesions associated with ferlavirus infection in Aruba Island rattlesnakes (*Crotalus durissus*

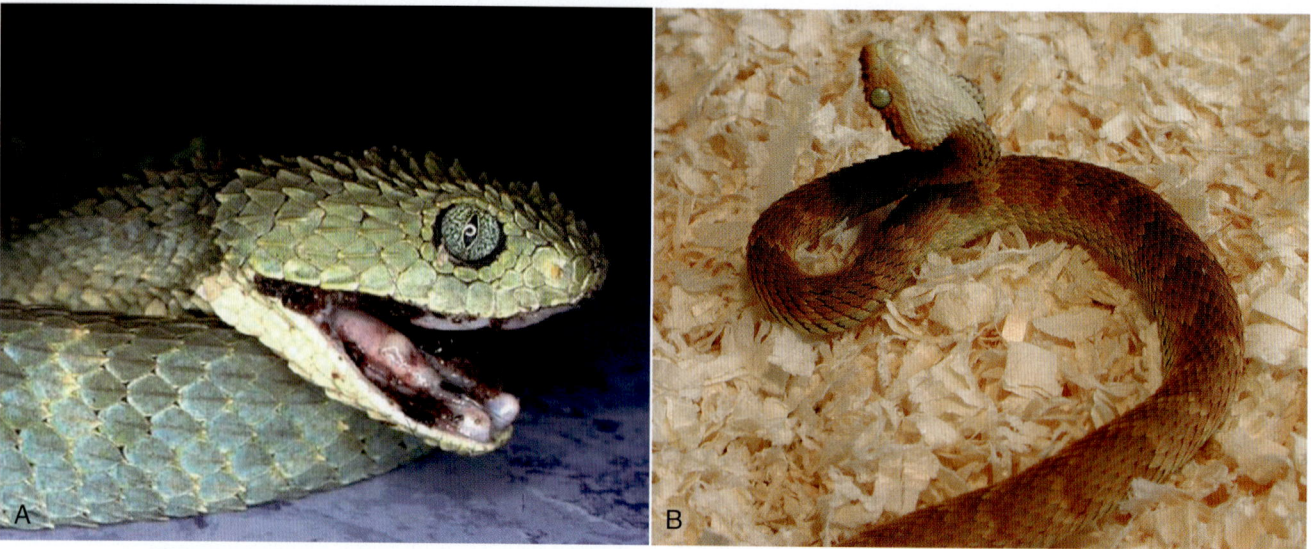

FIG 30.14 Bush vipers (*Atheris squamigera*) infected with ferlaviruses. (A) Dyspnea and bloody secretions in the oral cavity. (B) Opisthotonus. (Courtesy of Jutta Wiechert.)

unicolor). A ferlavirus isolated from several tissues of an Aruba Island rattlesnake that died of the infection was inoculated intratracheally into four Aruba Island rattlesnakes. Several snakes developed pulmonary signs, including blood in the lungs, trachea, and oral cavity. The two animals that were not euthanized earlier died 19 and 22 days p.i.[150] In another transmission study, genotypes A, B, and C ferlaviruses were inoculated intratracheally in corn snakes. That study demonstrated clear differences in pathogenicity between the three isolates used, with the type B virus causing the greatest pathology, with the lungs most severely affected.[151]

Gross abnormalities are most consistently found in the lungs of infected snakes. Changes include congestion and hemorrhage. Histologic findings often show proliferative interstitial pulmonary disease with proliferation and vacuolation of epithelial cells lining the faveoli. In rare cases, intracytoplasmic inclusions can be seen in lining epithelial cells.[148,150]

Although ferlaviruses are most commonly described in snakes, these viruses have also been detected in several species of lizard, including a spotted false monitor (*Callopistes maculatus*), an emerald tree monitor, a flathead knob-scaled lizard (*Xenosaurus platyceps*), and a group of Caiman lizards (*Dracaena guianensis*).[149] Ferlavirus infections in lizards have been associated primarily with pneumonia, although virus infections in clinically healthy lizards have been documented. The viruses do not appear to be host specific, and transmission between different species of snakes and lizards, as well as chelonians may be possible.

Ferlaviruses in Chelonians

Descriptions of ferlavirus infections in chelonians are rare. These infections have been associated with dermatitis (Zangger et al, Proc 4th Int Coll Path Med Rept Amphib, 1991, pp 25-29) and pneumonia.[146,153] In a single case, a PMV was isolated from a Hermann's tortoise with pneumonia. That virus was further characterized and found to be related to but distinct from the described ferlaviruses from snakes and lizards so far.[146] In another case, two distinct squamate ferlaviruses were detected in a leopard tortoise with pneumonia (Fig. 30.15). The detected viruses were each most closely related to ferlaviruses from snakes. However, it was unclear whether the virus was a causative agent, because no virus was detected in the lungs of the diseased animal.[153] Antibodies against ferlaviruses have been detected in several tortoise species.[154]

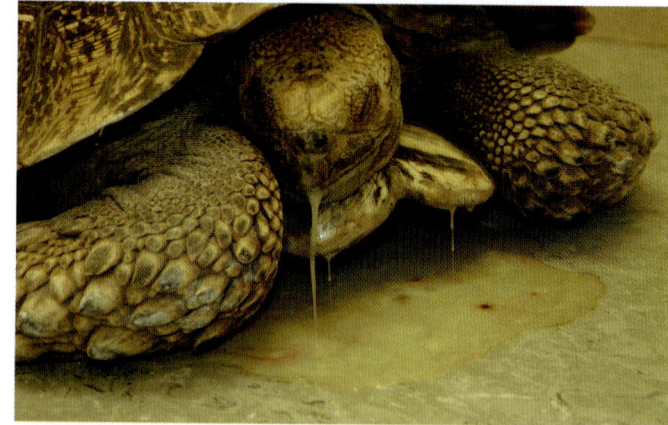

FIG 30.15 Leopard tortoise (*Stigmochelys pardalis*) with severe pneumonia. A ferlavirus was detected in this animal. (From Papp T, Seybold J, Marschang RE. Paramyxovirus infection in a leopard tortoise [*Geochelone pardalis babcocki*] with respiratory disease. *J Herp Med Surg* 2010;20:64–68. With permission.)

Identification of Ferlavirus Infections

Virus Detection. Ferlaviruses were first diagnosed in snakes by isolation in cell culture.[143] Virus isolation has since been used in many cases to detect these viruses in clinical samples from snakes and lizards. A number of RT-PCRs have also been described for the detection of ferlaviruses in reptiles. An RT-PCR targeting the conserved large polymerase (L) gene has been used to detect all of the ferlavirus genotypes detected to date.[146,155] In live animals, oral and cloacal swabs, as well as transtracheal washes, can be used as diagnostic samples. Oral and cloacal shedding can be inconsistent, and tracheal washes (Fig. 30.16) were found to be the most sensitive sample for ferlavirus detection in snakes during a transmission study, although virus was inoculated intratracheally in that study.[151] In dead animals, the highest viral load is found in the lung, and this tissue is recommended for testing (see Tables 30.3 and 30.4).[145,151] In addition, virus was frequently detected in intestine, pancreas, and brain.[151] The RT-PCR is not highly specific for ferlaviruses, and

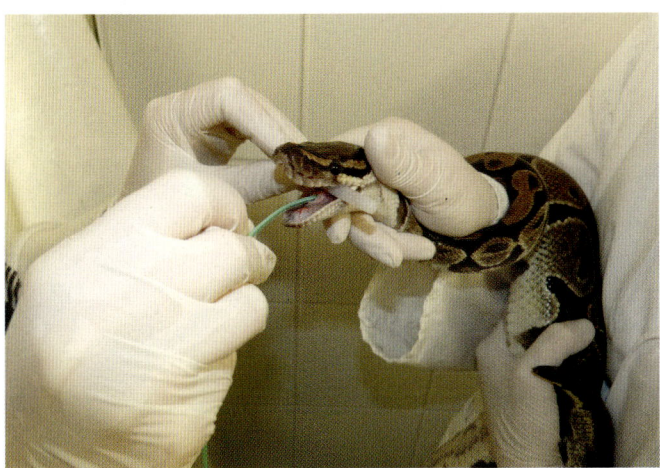

FIG 30.16 Collection of a tracheal wash from a ball python (*Python regius*). Tracheal washes are the preferred sample for ferlavirus testing.

false-positive reactions have been shown to occur. For this reason, PCR products of the expected size (566 base pairs) should be sequenced. A direct comparison of virus isolation and virus detection by PCR showed that the PCR was more sensitive, although the highest sensitivity was achieved using a combination of both methods.[151]

Serology. Antibodies against ferlaviruses can be detected by hemagglutination inhibition (HI) assays using chicken red blood cells (see Tables 30.3 and 30.4). HI testing has been used repeatedly to detect exposure to ferlaviruses in squamates, including wild-caught snakes and lizards.[129,130,148] Serologic cross-reactivity among ferlaviruses and between ferlaviruses and other PMVs is not fully understood, and some (but not all) ferlaviruses have been shown to serologically cross-react with some avian PMVs.[145] Although serologic cross-reactivity exists between ferlaviruses, there is some indication that testing with different virus isolates will lead to different results. In a study comparing results of HI testing of plasma from eastern massasaugas (*Sistrurus catenatus catenatus*) from three different laboratories, different results were obtained from each; thus interpretation of results may be difficult.[156] Following transmission studies with three different ferlavirus genotypes (A, B, and C), clear differences were documented in the antibody titers detected against each virus, with lower or no titers detected in the group in which the highest pathogenicity was documented (infected with a genotype B virus), so that viral factors and pathogenicity may also play a role in development, titers, and persistence of antibodies.[157] Detection of anti-PMV antibodies indicates that an animal has been exposed to ferlaviruses or serologically related viruses. Persistence of ferlavirus infection in reptiles has not been recorded, but there is clinical evidence that this may occur. It is not known how long virus replication and shedding may persist after the development of HI antibodies.

SUNVIRIDAE: SUNSHINEVIRUS

A virus that is distantly related to the PMVs but differs distinctly from the ferlaviruses has been described in snakes in Australia. The virus has been named *Sunshinevirus* for the geographic location of the first isolation on the Sunshine coast of Australia. It has now been placed in a new family *Sunvirdae* in the order *Mononegavirales*. This virus was associated with neurorespiratory disease in Australian pythons and has been detected in black-headed pythons (*Aspidites melanocephalus*), woma pythons (*A. ramsayi*), spotted pythons (*Antaresia maculosa*), and carpet pythons (*Morelia spilota* spp. and *M. bredli*).[158] A single report exists of

Sunshinevirus detection outside of Australia, in a ball python in Germany (Marschang et al, Proc ARAV, 2013, p 15). Clinical signs associated with infection may be similar to those reported for ferlavirus infections or be nonspecific (e.g., lethargy, inappetance). Histologically, the hindbrain white matter often exhibits spongiosis and gliosis. Neuronal necrosis has been described in severe cases. Some snakes may develop bronchointerstitial pneumonia.[160] Transmission is assumed to occur horizontally from oral and cloacal secretions, and there is evidence that the virus can also be transmitted vertically, although it may lead to the death of infected embryos.[161]

Sunshinevirus was originally detected by isolation in VH2 from diseased and contact snakes. A PCR has been described for the detection of this virus and appears to be more sensitive than isolation in cell culture. Virus detection has been carried out from oral and cloacal swabs in live animals. In dead animals, the virus is most often detected in the brain (see Table 30.4).[160]

RHABDOVIRIDAE

In reptiles, rhabdovirus infections have been documented based on both serology and virus detection. Little is known about the importance of rhabdoviruses in reptiles, but the rhabdoviruses detected in reptiles so far all appear to be arboviruses, some of which are also capable of infecting mammals. Antibodies against a vesicular stomatitis virus and Bahia Grande virus have been detected in wild-caught reptiles in Texas, while Charleville virus and Almpiwar virus have been isolated from lizards in Australia. Marco, Timbo, Chaco, and Sena Madureira viruses have been isolated from teiid lizards in South America as has another rhabdovirus from Caiman lizards.[162] Transmission studies with the rhabdovirus viral hemorrhagic septicemia virus (VHSV) and snapping turtles (*Chelydra serpentina*) and red-eared sliders have shown that aquatic turtles may be a vector for VHSV and that this virus may be able to infect turtles.[163] No clinical disease has been reported in association with these viruses in reptiles.

ARENAVIRIDAE

The family *Arenaviridae* has recently been divided into two genera, *Mammarenavirus* and *Reptarenavirus*. The genus *Reptarenavirus* was created to include arenaviruses detected in snakes and associated with IBD. These viruses have only been detected in snakes (no mammalian host), and their proteins differ from those of mammalian arenaviruses in several aspects.[164] Reptarenaviruses have been shown to be a genetically diverse group of viruses, including multiple species. It is even possible that arenaviruses of snakes may represent more than one genus.[165] Sequencing of full or partial genomes from a number of infected snakes has also shown that infection with multiple genotypes is common in captive infected snakes and that recombination and reassortment are common occurences.[166] Diversity is unequal between the genomic segments, with more L genotypes detected in infected animals than S genotypes. It has been hypothesized that human activity has led to an increased rate of viral evolution and that mixing of infected animals in captivity is a factor in virus diversity and in disease development.[165,166] The prevalence of reptarenaviruses in snakes in captivity, the existence of a possible reservoir hosts other than boid and/or pythonid snakes, and the genetic diversity of arenaviruses in the wild are not yet known.

INCLUSION BODY DISEASE (IBD)

IBD is a disease of snakes of the families Boidae and Pythonidae that has been described worldwide in captive snakes. The disease is characterized by the formation of intracytoplasmic inclusions in neurons and

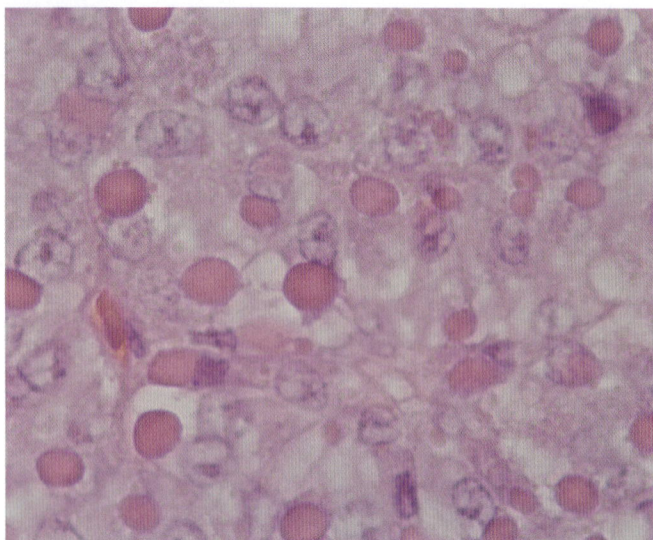

FIG 30.17 Multiple eosinophilic intracytoplasmic inclusion bodies in the pancreas of a *Boa constrictor* with IBD. H&E stain, 1000x. (Courtesy of Kim Heckers.)

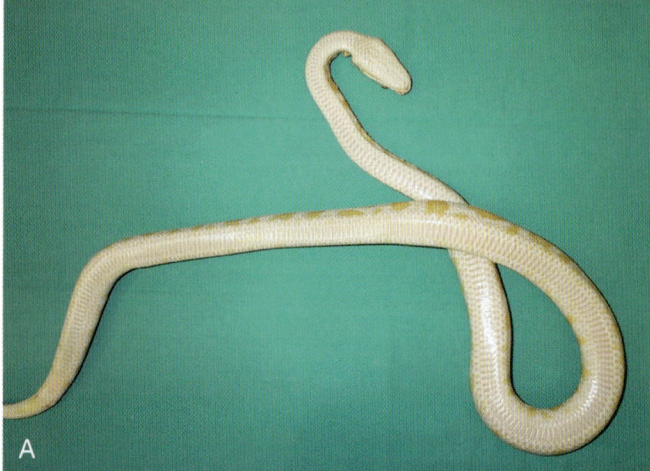

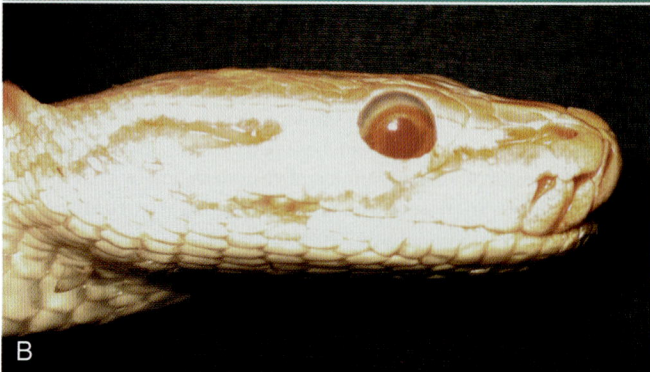

FIG 30.18 (A) Juvenile Burmese python (*Python molurus*) presented with acute onset of neurologic signs, including loss of the righting reflex and disorientation. (B) The same snake with mydriasis. (Courtesy of Jürgen Schumacher.)

in epithelial cells of various organs (Fig. 30.17). The etiology of IBD was long unknown, and various viruses have been proposed as possible causes of this disease over time.[119,120] Reptarenaviruses are now believed to be the cause of IBD.[167–169] In the first study describing the detection of these viruses, genetically variable arenaviruses were detected in 6 of 8 tested IBD-positive snakes and in none of 18 IBD-negative snakes by metagenomics and RT-PCR.[167] The inclusions are made up of a unique protein (inclusion body disease protein, IBDP), which appears to correspond to the reptarenaviral nucleoprotein.[167,168]

IBD was originally most commonly detected in Burmese pythons but is now most commonly diagnosed in boa constrictors.[105] Anecdotally, pythons tend to develop clinical diseases more quickly, while boas may remain inclusion-body positive but clinically healthy (or low morbidity, chronically diseased) for extended periods of time. The host range of IBD also includes the green anaconda (*Eunectes murinus*), yellow anaconda (*Eunectes notaeus*), rainbow boa (*Epicrates cenchria*), Haitian boa (*Chilabothrus [Epicrates] striatus*), Madagascan boa (*Acrantophis madagascariensis*), annulated tree boa (*Corallus annulatus*), Indian rock python, reticulated python (*Malayopython [Python] reticulatus*), ball python, and carpet python.[167,170] Similar inclusions have also been reported in palm vipers (*Bothriechis marchi*) and an eastern king snake (*Lampropeltis getula*),[105,171] although it is not known if these were caused by the same virus. Clinical signs associated with IBD are variable and can range from subclinical carriers to severe neurologic disease and death. IBD is believed to cause immune suppression in affected animals, and many diverse clinical signs may result. Common signs in infected snakes include torticollis, disequilibrium, opisthotonus, inability to right itself, regurgitation, and flaccid paralysis (Fig. 30.18). Other signs that may also be observed include stomatitis and pneumonia. Skin lesions of various types have also been regularly observed in affected snakes. Lymphoproliferative disorders and round cell tumors have been described in infected snakes. Some snakes with IBD may die within weeks, but others may survive for extended periods of time. In some cases, boa constrictors have been described with inclusions but no apparent signs of clinical disease.

Studies on reptarenavirus-infected snakes with IBD have shown that infections with multiple genetically distinct viruses are very common.[165,166] As these viruses are believed to be immune suppressive, it has been hypothesized that reptarenaviruses may establish chronic infections in

snakes, possibly leading to acquired immunosuppression. Co- or superinfection of such snakes with another reptarenavirus could then result in amplified replication, with disease developing due to immunosuppression induced by the chronically infecting virus.[165]

Transmission of reptarenaviruses and development of IBD are not yet fully understood. Transmission from one animal to another appears to involve close contact over time, and cohabitation over a period of weeks or months has been demonstrated to lead to virus transmission.[166] Mites have been implicated as a possible vector,[170] and studies showing that a reptarenavirus can replicate in tick cells at 30°C support the hypothesis that these viruses may be transmitted by arthropod hosts and may even be arboviruses capable of replicating in arthropod and vertebrate hosts.[165] Transmission via biting among snakes and via aerosole have also been discussed. Vertical transmission appears to be possible, and reptarenaviruses have been detected in offspring from IBD-positive parents.[172]

Identification of IBD and Reptarenaviruses

Because IBD is defined by the presence of inclusion bodies in cells of affected snakes, cytology and histology remain important tools for IBD diagnostics. Typical eosinophilic to amphophilic intracytoplasmic inclusions in hematoxylin and eosin–stained tissue sections can be found in various tissues. The distribution of inclusions in tissues appears to depend on the host species. In pythons, inclusions are most commonly found in neurons within the central nervous system. In boa constrictors, they can also be found in glial cells, as well as in cells in the "esophageal tonsils" (Fig. 30.19), hepatocytes, pancreatic acinar cells, renal tubular

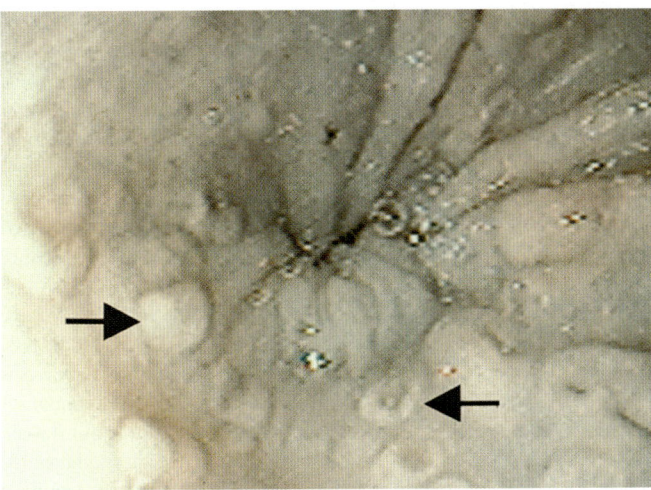

FIG 30.19 Endoscopic demonstration of prominent esophageal tonsils (arrows) in the distal esophagus of a boa constrictor (*Boa constrictor*) with inclusion body disease. (Courtesy of Jürgen Schumacher.)

epithelial cells, and epithelial cells lining the gastrointestinal and respiratory tracts.[170] In live boid snakes, inclusions can be detected in biopsies of the "esophageal tonsils," liver, and kidney. They can also be found in peripheral blood cells. Detection of inclusion bodies in live animals is much more common in boas than in pythons.

Virus detection via PCR has also become an important tool in the detection of infected animals and may be more sensitive than detection of inclusion bodies in many cases. A PCR targeting a portion of the glycoprotein gene has been described[166,167] and used for the detection of reptarenaviruses in live and dead snakes.[172] The glycoprotein gene is found on the S segment, in which less diversity has been detected than on the L segment, and this PCR has been shown to be able to detect diverse reptarenaviruses.[166] Samples used for virus detection in live snakes have included esophageal swabs/biopsies of esophageal tonsils, kidney, liver, gastric mucosa, and whole blood. In dead animals, brain is most often positive in pythons, while virus may be detectable in a wide range of tissues in boas (see Table 30.4). In some cases, animals that are arenavirus positive may not develop IBD. Persistence of virus in the brains of apparently clinically healthy animals has also been described.[172] Reptarenaviruses have also been isolated in cell culture in several cases, mostly in cell lines derived from boa constrictor kidney cells.[167,168]

BUNYAVIRIDAE

Bunyaviruses found in reptiles have all been arboviruses. A bunyavirus was isolated from the blood of a Texas soft-shelled turtle (*Apalone* [*Trionyx*] *spinifer emoryi*), which was wild-caught in Texas. The virus was isolated in suckling mice by intracerebral inoculation and caused 100% mortality in the mice. The virus was not further characterized but was found to serologically cross-react with Cache Valley and Tensaw viruses, both mosquito-borne viruses of the genus *Orthobunyavirus*.[173] Kowanyama virus, an unassigned member of the family *Bunyaviridae*, has been isolated from both mosquitoes and a skink (*Cryptoblepharus* [*Ablepharus*] *virgatus*) in Australia.[174] No disease has been described in association with bunyavirus infections in reptiles.

NIDOVIRALES: CORONAVIRIDAE

The order *Nidovirales* contains enveloped, positive-strand RNA viruses with the largest known RNA genomes. These viruses are relatively easily inactivated by chemical disinfectants. Nidoviruses have been identified in snakes, and these viruses appear to be most closely related to viruses in the family *Coronaviridae*, subfamily *Torovirinae*, and may represent a new genus in this subfamily.[175–177] Coronaviruses generally target the epithelia and are mostly associated with respiratory and gastrointestinal disease. A number of recent emerging viruses belong in this family.

In reptiles, nidoviruses have been found in snakes, particularly ball pythons in the United States and in Europe.[175,176] Nidoviruses have also been detected in Indian rock pythons, green tree pythons, a carpet python, and boa constrictors.[176,178] The most common manifestations of disease appear to be an interstitial proliferative pneumonia, but infected snakes have also been reported with a mild-to-severe tracheitis, mild-to-severe sinusitis/rhinitis, mild-to-moderate stomatitis/pharyngitis, esophagitis, mucous or caseous material in air passageways, and pulmonary hemorrhage.[175,176] Changes in other organ systems have also been detected in individual cases, including encephalitis, nephritis, nephrosis, multifocal dermatitis, salpingitis, hepatic lipidosis, conjunctivitis, and pancreatic necrosis. It is unknown if changes in tissues outside the respiratory tract were related to the nidovirus infection.[175,176] Viruslike particles consisting of circular and elongated rod-shaped nucleocapsids were observed within pneumocytes of individual affected snakes by electron microscopy. Metagenomic sequencing was carried out on tissues from affected snakes, leading to detection of novel nidoviruses. No similar viruses were detected in nonaffected snakes.[175] Real-time and conventional PCRs have been used to detect nidoviruses in infected snakes. In live snakes, virus has most frequently been detected in oral swabs, although blood has also tested positive.[178] Tracheal washes may also be a sensitive sample for virus detection. Lung tissue has most often tested positive for nidoviruses, and the highest viral loads are detectable in respiratory tissues,[175] but virus has also been detected in the trachea, esophagus, liver, spleen, heart, and brain (see Table 30.4).[175,176]

PICORNAVIRIDAE

Two genetically distinct picornaviruses from reptiles have been characterized so far, both found in chelonians. They have been named torchiviruses (originally called topiviruses) and rafiviruses.[179,180] As unenveloped viruses, picornaviruses can be moderately difficult to disinfect. Studies of environmental persistence of torchiviruses show that these can persist for extended periods of time in water at cold temperatures, and inactivation at 37°C can take weeks. Inactivation in soil can take 3 weeks or more in the summer but significantly longer at lower temperatures.[17]

The first report of picornalike viruses in reptiles was based on the detection of 20- to 27-nm large viral particles in duodenal and splenic cells in a boa constrictor and in duodenal cells in an Aesculapian snake. Both snakes showed signs of gastrointestinal disease. An adenolike virus was also found in the duodenum and spleen of the boa constrictor, while parvo-, adeno-, and herpeslike viruses were detected in the duodenum of the Aesculapian snake.[109]

Picornalike viruses have been detected repeatedly by isolation in cell culture in a number of different tortoise species (Marschang et al, Proc ARAV, 2002, p 102). These viruses have been called Virus "X." They have most frequently been isolated from spur-thighed tortoises but have also been found in marginated tortoises, Hermann's tortoises, leopard tortoises, Egyptian tortoises (*Testudo kleinmanni*), and spider tortoises (*Pyxis arachnoides*). They have been associated with various signs of disease in infected animals, including softening of the carapace in young animals, diphtheroid-necrotizing stomatitis, rhinitis, conjunctivitis, and ascites (Fig. 30.20) but have also been isolated from clinically healthy animals.[137,182] There are no typical histologic lesions associated with infection. In numerous cases, tortoises infected with Virus "X"

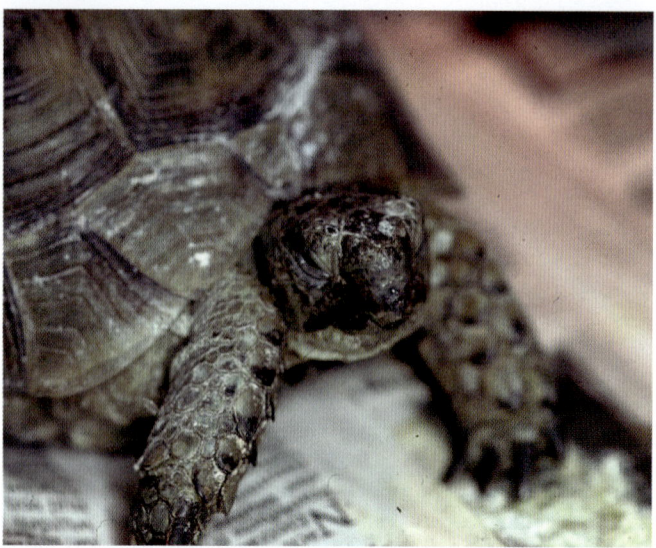

FIG 30.20 Spur-thighed tortoise (*Testudo graeca*) with rhinitis. This animal was infected with a picornavirus (topivirus, "virus X"), as well as with a herpesvirus and *Mycoplasma*.

have also been shown to be infected with other pathogens, especially herpesviruses and *Mycoplasma* spp.[18] Sequencing of a large part of the genomes of isolates obtained from tortoises in Germany and Hungary over several years showed that all isolates were related to one another and belonged to the family *Picornaviridae*. They clearly form a new genus that has now been named "Torchivirus."[179] A transmission study in which juvenile spur-thighed and Hermann's tortoises were inoculated with a torchivirus isolate led to a decrease in bone density and tubular vacuolization in the kidneys (Paries et al, Proc iCARE 2015, p 351).

A genetically distinct picornavirus was detected in the spleen of a Travancore (Sulawesi) tortoise. The animal was from a group that died during a severe disease outbreak in which an adenovirus (Sulawesi tortoise adenovirus 1) was considered the causative agent.[7] The genus name "Rafivirus" was proposed for this new virus. The role of the detected picornavirus in the disease outbreak was unknown.[180]

Identification of Picornavirus Infections in Tortoises

Virus Detection. The detection of torchiviruses in tortoises has most often been described via isolation in cell culture. Virus can be isolated on TH-1 (*Terrapene* heart cells, ATCC CCL-50). An RT-PCR for the detection of viral RNA has also been developed.[184] The best samples for virus detection in live animals are oral swabs. In dead animals, samples from the entire gastrointestinal tract (tongue to cloaca) can all be used for virus detection. Virus is frequently also found in other tissues (including liver, kidney, heart, brain, and lung) (see Table 30.3).

Rafiviruses have not been isolated in cell culture. A PCR for their detection in tissues from affected animals has been described.[180] It has been successfully used to detect virus in liver and kidney samples from animals in the original disease outbreak.

Serology. Serological detection of antibodies against torchiviruses can be carried out using virus neutralization methods. Antibodies against this virus are frequently found in tortoises in Europe, and low titers have also been detected in wild-caught tortoises in Turkey.[139] It is unknown how closely related all torchivirus isolates are to one another, so cross-reactivity among these viruses and between these viruses and other picornaviruses is not yet understood.

CALICIVIRIDAE

Caliciviruses (CVs) infect a broad range of animals, and most individual CV species exhibit a natural host restriction. However, the vesicular exanthema of swine virus (VESV) is an exception, with a broad host range. Transmission is generally via contaminated food, water, fomites, and sometimes via aerosolization.[185] Caliciviruses can be inactivated using standard virucidal disinfectants (e.g., bleach and acid-based disinfectants) very quickly and are generally inactivated by alcohol formulations used for hand disinfection.

In reptiles, CVs closely related to the San Miguel sea lion CV have been isolated from four different snake species—Aruba island rattlesnakes, a rock rattlesnake (*Crotalus lepidus*), and an eyelash viper (*Bothriechis* [*Bothrops*] *schlegeli*)—as well as from Bell's horned frogs (*Ceratophrys ornata*) in a single collection in the United States.[186] Some, but not all, of the animals from which virus was isolated had enteritis and hepatitis. A transmission study with prairie rattlesnakes showed that these animals could be infected and the virus could be reisolated (in one out of two snakes inoculated), but no pathognomonic disease was observed in the infected snake. Transmission of the virus to pigs led to seroconversion but not disease.[186] A PCR for the detection of reptile calicivirus, as well as other vesiviruses, has been described,[187] but no information is available on the prevalence of this virus in reptiles.

FLAVIVIRIDAE

All of the flaviviruses described in reptiles belong to the genus *Flavivirus*, which contains viruses that are transmitted by hematophagous arthropods (arboviruses). Some flaviviruses are able to infect and replicate in a wide variety of vertebrate hosts (including mammals, birds, and reptiles). The focus of much interest in flaviviruses of reptiles has been the role of these animals as reservoirs for human disease.

Antibodies against various flaviviruses, including St. Louis encephalitis virus, Powassan virus, Japanese encephalitis virus, and West Nile virus (WNV), have been found in chelonians, snakes, and crocodilians in various parts of the world.[18,188] Japanese encephalitis virus has been isolated from Chinese rat snakes in Korea.[189] Transmission studies with Japanese encephalitis virus have shown that lizards can be infected with this virus both by parenteral inoculation and, in some species, by feeding on infected mosquitoes. Infected animals develop viremia, and the development of viremia is temperature dependent.[190] No clinical signs of disease were reported in the lizards. A flaviviruslike virus was isolated from a leopard tortoise with epistaxis, cloacal hemorrhage, biliverdinuria, and anemia. Herpes and adenoviruses were isolated from other animals in the same collection, and intraerythrocytic inclusions of unknown etiology were also described in these tortoises.[8,191] The most commonly described flavivirus in reptiles is West Nile virus.

WEST NILE VIRUS (WNV)

WNV is a flavivirus that primarily cycles between mosquitoes and birds. It is zoonotic, and care should be taken when dealing with suspected cases (especially in crocodilians). A number of transmission studies have been carried out with WNV and various reptile species. In one transmission study iguanas, snakes, and frogs became infected, and the iguanas and frogs both developed low-level viremias. No disease was reported in any of the infected animals.[192] Viremia was induced by subcutaneous inoculation into common garter snakes (*Thamnophis sirtalis*).[193] Another transmission study was able to induce a moderate viremia in four western fence lizards following inoculation with WNV.[194]

WNV has been shown to be pathogenic for crocodilians and causes high-titer viremias in these animals. Antibodies against WNV have been detected in crocodilians in many different countries, including crocodiles at a commercial farm in Israel,[195] wild alligators in Florida,[196] and farmed and wild crocodiles in Mexico.[188,197] In the United States, WNV has been detected in disease outbreaks in American alligators in a number of different states, including Georgia,[198] Florida,[196] and Louisiana.[199] Infection of crocodilians can occur by bite from infected mosquitoes, orally by consumption of contaminated meat (e.g., infected horses), and by contact with viremic tankmates.[198,200] The development and duration of viremia are dependent on ambient temperature.[200] The highest mortalities have been found in young animals. Neurologic signs have included anorexia, tremors, swimming on their sides, spinning in the water, and opisthotonus. Oral lesions (stomatitis) have also been noted. Death may occur 24 to 48 hours after the appearance of clinical signs. The highest viral loads were detected in the livers of affected animals.[196,198] WNV has also been associated with lymphohistiocytic proliferative cutaneous lesions in American alligators. Round to ovoid lesions were described in the superficial dermis of infected alligators. No virus was detectable in the lesions, but animals with lesions consistently tested positive for antibodies against WNV and 97.5% tested positive for WNV RNA in pooled skin and liver-brain samples.[201] In a transmission study with alligators, viremia developed in all alligators infected by subcutaneous injection, with the time to development and duration of viremia dependent on temperature (32°C or 27°C), with longer duration of viremia at 27°C, while only tankmates of infected alligators kept at 32°C became infected. Viremia also developed after oral infection and also led to the infection of tankmates. Viral titers in serum of infected animals were sufficiently high to infect mosquitoes (*Culex quinquefasciatus*), and high virus loads were also documented in the cloaca.[200] WNV has been detected in mosquitoes associated with alligator farms.[202]

Identification of WNV Infections

Detection of WNV can be performed with the use of serum or whole blood in infected crocodilians. Viremic alligators have also been shown to shed virus via the cloaca.[200] In dead animals, virus can be detected in a number of tissues, including liver, lung, and blood. Liver has been shown to have the highest titers and yield the most positive results in American alligators (see Table 30.5).[196,198] Virus detection has been carried out by isolation in cell culture (e.g., Vero cells) or by detection of viral RNA using RT-PCR. A number of RT-PCR protocols have been described for the detection of WNV RNA in various animals. WNV is currently grouped into five different lineages, and the choice of RT-PCR will affect which lineages can be detected. Lineage 1 is found in North America, southern Europe, Asia, and Africa, whereas lineage 2 is found in southern Africa and has recently also been found in Europe. Real-time quantitative PCRs have been described for the combined detection of both lineages but have not been tested with crocodilian samples.[203]

Antibodies against WNV can be detected in tthe serum of infected crocodilians. In a transmission study with American alligators, antibodies were detected within 25 days of virus detection in infected animals. Methods used for the detection of anti-WNV antibodies have included a plaque reduction assay for the detection of neutralizing antibodies and an ELISA. The plaque reduction assay requires live virus and must therefore be carried out in a biosafety level 3 laboratory. An ELISA has been developed for the specific detection of antibodies against WNV in alligators.[204] Antibodies against WNV can cross-react with antibodies against other related flaviviruses.

TOGAVIRIDAE

The togaviruses detected in reptiles to date have all belonged to the genus *Alphavirus*, which contains viruses that have the ability to replicate in and be transmitted horizontally by mosquitoes. Most alphaviruses can infect a wide range of vertebrates, mostly birds and mammals, but several have also been reported in reptiles. Studies on alphaviruses in reptiles have mostly focused on the possible role of these animals for the transmission of alphaviruses to humans and livestock. This has led to a focus on persistence of alphaviruses in reptiles, particularly viral persistence over winter in temperate regions in the absence of mosquito activity.[205] Detection of alphavirus infection in reptiles has been carried out by detection of virus in blood or detection of antibodies. Eastern equine encephalitis virus (EEEV), Western equine encephalitis virus (WEEV), and antibodies against these viruses have been found in various chelonians, lizards, and snakes, including a number of wild-caught reptiles in the United States.[105] Antibodies against Venezuelan equine encephalitis virus (VEEV) have been found in free-ranging caimans in Brazil.[206] In a serosurvey of various frogs, turtles, lizards, and snakes in Alabama for antibodies against EEEV, seropositivity was detected most often in various snake species,[207] and repeated cycles of viremia were documented in garter snakes. EEEV RNA was detected in serum of wild-caught copperheads (*Agkistrodon contortrix*) and cottonmouths (*Agkistrodon piscivorus*) in Alabama.[208] Experimental transmission of WEEV and EEEV to garter snakes has shown that these animals can develop sufficiently high viremias to infect mosquitoes following hibernation.[18,209] Transmission studies with EEEV and WEEV in spotted turtles (*Clemmys guttata*) and Texas tortoises (*Gopherus berlandieri*) both led to viremia in injected animals.[210,211] Viremia was longer at lower temperatures than at high environmental temperatures. None of the transmission studies described any signs of clinical disease in infected reptiles.

REFERENCES

See www.expertconsult.com for a complete list of references.

31

Mycology

James F.X. Wellehan and Stephen J. Divers

REPTILE-FUNGAL ECOLOGY

Reptile patients are often approached as a collection of vertebrate cells organized into organ systems. This is highly misleading; most of the cells in a vertebrate are microbial. Microbes are especially critical for digestion and immune function, and maintenance of healthy flora is essential to the health of a reptile patient.

Clinicians are also often misled by Koch's postulates; by fulfilling or not fulfilling these requirements in a controlled experiment, a microbe is then considered dichotomously as a pathogen or not a pathogen. This is far from the case; in the real world, numerous host, pathogen, and environmental factors (including coinfections, temperature, nutrition, handling stress, crowding, and others) play significant roles in whether a pathogen manifests as disease. When infectious disease is properly considered as ecology, it becomes obvious that a typical disease scenario involves several infectious agents in concert with other environmental factors. Coinfection with both *Nannizziopsis guarroi* and *Devriesea agamarum* has been seen in skin lesions in inland bearded dragons (*Pogona vitticeps*),[1] and coinfection with *Encephalitozoon pogonae*, coccidia, and Agamid adenovirus 1 has been reported in other bearded dragons.[2] Like all vertebrates, reptile patients are complex ecosystems, and we are still in the early stages of learning about the complex ecological interactions between the microbial components of a reptile patient. Rather than thinking of a war on fungi, clinicians should have the goal of improving ecosystem health within a reptile patient.

Evolution is an essential concept in biology; when one considers definitions for life, perhaps the simplest and most elegant definition is that life consists of things that evolve. Clinically, this is most immediately apparent with infectious disease. Because of short generation times, evolution of microbes occurs in a time frame impacting clinical management of a patient. To compensate, the most rapidly evolving genes in vertebrates are immune related. A fungus does not "want" to cause disease or not cause disease. All life on earth has been selected for billions of years to reproduce successfully, and this is all that matters from an evolutionary standpoint. If pathogenic traits provide an evolutionary advantage in a given situation, they will be selected for. If they provide a disadvantage, they will be selected against.

There are a number of important selective pressures impacting microbes in a reptile host, including nutrition, temperature, the need to transfer to a new host, competition with other microbes, and the host immune system. A reptile host is a nutrient-rich environment for fungi. However, some nutrients may be sequestered; one example is iron, which is a limiting factor for the growth of many fungi. Significant resources are spent by the host synthesizing transferrin, lactoferrin, and ferritin to make iron unavailable. Many fungal virulence pathways have evolved to access this sequestered iron.[3] Iron storage disease or clinical administration of iron may rapidly favor fungi with these pathways.

Ectothermic hosts require microbial gut flora to have the ability to survive at different temperatures. Infectious disease manifestation may be highly temperature dependent in ectotherms.[4] In reptiles, temperature manipulation is often a significant therapeutic approach. Further investigation of the role of temperature in disease manifestation in reptiles is strongly indicated, especially with populations of many species critically declining and likely to be impacted by anthropogenic climate change.[5,6]

The need to transfer to a new host creates significant selective pressure. Most fungi may survive well in the environment, decreasing selective pressure to keep the host alive. High host density also favors virulence, and increased stocking density creates environments selecting for pathogenicity.

Microbial competition is also a major selective pressure in a reptile; many organisms want to live in such a nutrient-rich environment. The majority of antimicrobials are derived from products secreted by other microbes that help them compete for ecologic niches. Animal guts are some of the most diverse and rich ecosystems to be found anywhere. Microbial ecologic disturbance may have significant negative impacts on many aspects of health. Damage to healthy flora by antimicrobial use provides opportunity for invasive species; recent treatment with antibiotics markedly increases host susceptibility to *Candida*,[7] and previous treatment with itraconazole makes frogs more susceptible to *Batrachochytrium*.[8] A 5-day course of ciprofloxacin will change human gut flora diversity and composition for several weeks, and the original composition may never reestablish.[9] Reduction in antibiotic use should result in reduction in fungal disease.

Other routine husbandry practices in the reptile pet trade also create strong evolutionary selective pressures toward fungal pathogenicity. It is common in the pet reptile trade to select for color mutants. This usually involves some degree of inbreeding to select for what are often recessive traits. A major driving force for the evolution of sex is acquisition of genetic diversity for immune function. Inbreeding results in selection for greater disease.[10]

ISSUES IN MYCOLOGY

Mycology is a field with serious flaws. Bacteriology and virology long ago abandoned morphology as a definitive method for identification; it is still commonly used in mycology. Because microbes have relatively few morphologic characteristics on which to base identification, it is not unexpected to find a high error rate. This has led to serious errors, such as the misidentification of multiple significant reptile pathogens as "*Chrysosporium* anamorph of *Nannizziopsis vriesii*." Information on morphologic ID of fungi is interspersed throughout the literature, and it has become an arcane field. A paper on a snake fungal infection indicated "The identification of the fungus can cause some difficulties to the nonskilled mycologist…. The final diagnosis can be performed only by a skilled specialist."[11] Ironically, this was later shown by molecular methods to be a different species.[12] A good mycologist should not have complete confidence in morphologic identification.

Mycologists have also used a nomenclature inconsistent with the rest of biology. With other clades of organisms, such as coccidia, cestodes, or cnidaria, life stages with very different morphology had not been recognized as the same species and had been named as separate organisms. However, as soon as they were recognized as the same organism, they were merged under one name. In mycology, separate taxonomic systems for asexual anamorph stages and sexual teleomorph stages of the same organism were deliberately kept, resulting in multiple species names and paraphyletic taxa. The anamorph species *Blastomyces dermatitidis* and *Histoplasma capsulatum* are in different genera, but their teleomorphs *Ajellomyces dermatitidis* and *Ajellomyces capsulatus* are congeneric. The availability of sexual structures meant that teleomorph classification was somewhat more accurate. In 2011 it was decided by the Nomenclature Section meeting of the International Botanical Congress that teleomorph names should be used.[13] This is very problematic for clinicians, because nearly all names of systemic fungi routinely used in medicine are anamorph names (e.g., *Cryptococcus*, *Blastomyces*, *Histoplasma*, etc.).

There is a significant need for major revision of fungal nomenclature.

FUNGAL DIAGNOSTICS

Diagnosis of fungal disease needs to be done with an understanding of the microbial ecology of the patient. A history and physical examination is a good starting point, with the recognition that husbandry has played a major role in almost any disease process for which a captive reptile is presented to a veterinarian, and husbandry improvements will need to be part of the therapeutic approach. When visible lesions are present, cytology or histology is often a good next step. A complete blood count to look for evidence of infection/inflammation and a plasma biochemistry to narrow concerns to organ systems are often helpful. Ultrasonography, endoscopy, or other diagnostic imaging may be helpful to identify internal lesions and guide sample collection. Once the results of initial diagnostic tests are in hand, appropriate diagnostic testing for fungi can be selected.

There are two major approaches to testing for infectious diseases. These tests are based on either the animal's acquired immune response to an agent or the presence of the agent. There is a lack of availability of validated immunological testing for fungi in reptiles, and currently available testing for fungal disease looks directly for the fungus.

Commonly used assays for the presence of fungi include culture and polymerase chain reaction (PCR)–based techniques; these should be targeted as much as possible. Diverse normal flora are present on the external surfaces and in the gastrointestinal tract of reptiles; untargeted cultures of these without significant corollary data are clinically uninterpretable. If cytology or histology indicates the presence of and morphologic information on fungi, this should be communicated to the laboratory. An appropriate differential diagnoses list should be formulated based on the initial diagnostic findings, and it should be decided whether culture is likely to be the most practical route to diagnosis or other methods such as PCR should be used.

Whenever possible, specimens for fungal testing are collected before antifungal therapy is begun. All specimens should be transported in clean, tightly sealed, leak-proof containers. Biopsies of lesions are preferable to swabs whenever possible. Once a laboratory has cultured and isolated a fungus, the most common method of identification is morphologic identification. As might be expected for a microbe, the error rate for morphologic identification is high, and it is strongly recommended that molecular diagnostic testing be considered for any serious fungal disease. Molecular diagnostic testing is discussed in Chapter 36. If corollary diagnostics suggest fungal infection and there does not appear to be multiple species present, it may be possible and more rapid to proceed directly to molecular diagnostic testing on uncultured samples. However, an important consideration when deciding on diagnostic approach is additional testing that may be needed; sensitivity testing is currently only economically feasible for cultured isolates. If an identification appears unusual, it is appropriate to question the result with a microbiologist.

PHARMACOLOGIC ANTIFUNGAL THERAPY

As members of the eukaryote clade Opisthokonta, the fungi are among the closest relatives of metazoan animals.[14] A lizard and a mushroom are more closely related to each other than either one is to an oak tree or a coccidian. Antimicrobial drug therapy targets differences between microbe and host; there are significantly fewer differences between animals and fungi than there are between animals and bacteria. Although we have a number of different targets for antibacterial drug therapy, antifungal drugs have comparatively few targets, with most targeting ergosterol. Antifungal drugs also tend to have more toxic side effects. Treatment of fungal disease often needs drug courses of months or years. Intermittent therapy may be more likely to lead to drug resistance and is not advised.

Polyene drugs bind to ergosterol in the fungal cell membrane. Commonly used polyenes include nystatin, natamycin, and amphotericin B. They are generally not well-absorbed enterically and require parenteral administration for systemic use. Nystatin is commonly given orally to achieve high levels in the gastrointestinal tract without significant systemic levels.

Azole drugs inhibit ergosterol synthesis via lanosterol 14α-demethylase. They are generally well-absorbed enterically. Fluconazole and ketoconazole have fairly limited spectra, significantly limiting their utility. Ketoconazole also disrupts host steroid synthesis more significantly, causing greater toxicosis. Itraconazole tends to have a broader spectrum than fluconazole and ketoconazole, and although expensive, is significantly less costly than voriconazole, posaconazole, or ravuconazole. However, there are fungal taxa that tend to be itraconazole resistant, with the most problematic for reptile clinicians being *Nannizziopsis guarroi*. Voriconazole, posaconazole, and ravuconazole all have significantly broader spectra but are very expensive.

Allylamines inhibit ergosterol synthesis via squalene epoxidase. The most commonly used allylamine is terbinafine. It is generally well-absorbed enterically. It is often synergistic with azoles and is relatively nontoxic and inexpensive. Combination therapy with terbinafine and an azole is often a reasonable empirical choice.

Echinocandins inhibit glucan synthesis in fungal cell walls via β-1-3-glucan synthase. They were primarily developed for use against non–*albicans Candida*, which tend to be highly resistant to other drug classes. Commonly used echinocandins include caspofungin, anidulafungin, and mycofungin. They are generally not well absorbed enterically and require parenteral administration for systemic use. They are expensive, and data on their use in reptiles is lacking.

AN OVERVIEW OF FUNGAL TAXA

When working on an exotic animal, it is helpful to know what taxa you are dealing with; the clinical approach to a tortoise is different from the approach to a rodent. Unfortunately, fungi are commonly taught as a list of genera and species, giving no higher-level context. When dealing with fungi, the phylum level is a clinically useful starting point (Table 31.1). A useful source for the clinician to find higher-level classification of a given fungal isolate is the National Center for Biotechnology

TABLE 31.1   Medically Important Fungal Taxa

Taxonomy (SK, P, O, F, G)	Morphology	Diagnostic Testing	Typical Lesions	Comments

Microsporidia (P)
  Encephalitozoon (G)
  Enterocytozoon (G)
  Heterosporis (G)
	Oval or pyriform spores	Histology/cytology, PCR/sequencing	Disseminated	Periodic acid–Schiff positive, gram positive, acid-fast positive spores

Chytridiomycota (P) Batrachochytrium (G)	Flask-shaped sporangia in epithelium	Histology/cytology, PCR/sequencing, probe hybridization qPCR, skin cytology	Keratinized skin, electrolyte imbalance	Major amphibian pathogens, not reptile pathogens
Zoopagomycota (P) Schizangiella (G)	Primarily seen in vivo as yeast	Histology/cytology, culture, PCR/sequencing for definitive diagnosis	Fungal granulomas	Some previous reports of *Basidiobolus* in amphibian deaths may have been chytrids
Mucormycota (P) Mucor (G)	Hyphae	Histology/cytology, cultures well, PCR/sequencing for definitive diagnosis	Dermatitis	Opportunists, extensive drug resistance
Dikarya (SK)	Life stage with two nuclei			Largest extant fungal clade

Basidiomycota (P)
  Tremellales (O)
  Cryptococcus (G)
	Yeast with thick capsule	Histology/cytology, cultures infectious, PCR/sequencing or probe hybridization qPCR	Pulmonary granulomas	Significant human pathogen, contagious if cultured; notify diagnostic laboratory if suspected.

Trichosporonales (O) Cutaneotrichosporon (G)	Yeast	Histology/cytology, culture, PCR/sequencing for definitive diagnosis	Dermatitis	
Ascomycota (P) Onygenales (O)				

Onygenaceae (F)
  Ophidiomyces (G)
  Coccidioides (G)
  Aphanoascella (G)
	Ophidiomyces form hyphae in tissues, *Coccidioides* form characteristic spherules	Histology/cytology, culture, PCR/sequencing of ITS2 for definitive diagnosis, qPCR available for *Coccidioides*, *Ophidiomyces*	*Coccidioides:* pneumonia
			Ophidiomyces, Aphanoascella: dermatitis
				Coccidioides is a significant human pathogen, contagious if cultured; notify diagnostic laboratory if suspected; *Ophidiomyces* having population-level effects

Nanniziopsiaceae (F)
  Nannizziopsis (G)
  Paranannizziopsis (G)
	Hyphae in tissues		Dermatitis	Significant diversity with differing temperature tolerance; major reptile pathogens

Chaetothyriales (O)
  Exophiala (G)
  Veronaea (G)
	Pigmented yeast		Disseminated fungal granulomas	*Exophila equina* in Galapagos tortoises

Hypocreales (O)
  Ophiocordycipitaceae (F)
  Purpureocillium (G)
	Hyphae in tissues		Pneumonia, dermatitis	Extensive drug resistance

Cordycipitaceae (F)
  Beauveria (G)
  Lecanicillium (G)
			Beauveria: pneumonia
			Lecanicillium: dermatitis, disseminated granulomas
				Used as insect biocontrol agents

Clavicipitaceae (F) Metarhizium (G)			Pneumonia, dermatitis, glossitis, disseminated granulomas	Used as insect biocontrol agents, some species have extensive drug resistance
Nectriaceae (F) Fusarium (G)		Histology/cytology, culture, PCR/sequencing of EF-1α for definitive diagnosis, ITS2 not definitive	Pneumonia, dermatitis, glossitis, disseminated granulomas	Opportunists, extensive drug resistance
Saccharomycetales (O) Candida (G)	Yeast	Histology/cytology, culture, PCR/sequencing for definitive diagnosis	Enteritis, pneumonia, disseminated granulomas	Clinical disease typically secondary to antibiotic use; non-*albicans* species have extensive drug resistance

SK, Sub kingdom; *P,* phylum; *O,* order; *F,* family; *G,* genera.

Information's Taxonomy Browser (https://www.ncbi.nlm.nih.gov/Taxonomy/Browser/wwwtax.cgi). The earliest divisions within the fungi, the microsporidia and chytrids, have atypical morphology.[15] The remaining taxa generally have a hyphal morphology, making them more recognizable as fungi. There are several primitive groups of fungi that branch off next. Formerly known as zygomycetes, these primitive hyphal fungi are not more closely related to each other than to the Dikarya and should be considered as several independent clades rather than a single group. The most speciose group of fungi is the subkingdom Dikarya, which are further divided into the phyla Basidiomycetes and Ascomycetes.[16]

Microsporidia

Members of the phylum Microsporidia do not have typical fungal morphology. They are obligate animal parasites and lack mitochondria. They have two life stages, spore and meront. Spore morphology is typically oval or pyriform and includes a chitin coat and a polar filament. The polar filament is attached to one end of the spore, coils around the spore contents, and ends near the posterior vacuole at the other end of the spore. It has morphologic similarity to stinging cells of jellyfish. The spore injects the sporoplasm into the host cell via the polar filament, and development of the meront occurs inside the host cell.

In reptile hosts, microsporidiosis was first reported in lizards and tuatara (Sphenodon punctatus), and most reports are from squamates.[17,18] The first molecular characterization of a microsporidian in a reptile host was Encephalitozoon pogonae in inland bearded dragons.[19] Closely related to E. cuniculi from rabbits (Oryctolagus cuniculus), E. pogonae is most commonly associated with nonspecific signs in bearded dragons such as lethargy, anorexia, weight loss, and polydipsia. It develops within macrophages in granulomas in multiple tissues, especially kidneys, but also including intestine, liver, ovary, spleen, lungs, vascular endothelium, and ventricular ependymal cells in the brain. Prevalence appears to be fairly high in captive inland bearded dragons outside Australia. Fecal shedding occurs, and it is likely that fecal-oral is the primary route of transmission. Coinfection with Agamid adenovirus 1 and coccidia has been reported, and it is probable that coinfection exacerbates disease.[2] Also seen in squamates is Heterosporis anguillarum, described by DNA sequence identification from eels (Anguilliformes) before it was found in a garter snake (Thamnophis) and sea snakes (Hydrophiinae).[20,21] Granulomas are seen in the muscle of the body wall.

Enterocytozoon bieneusi has also been identified by DNA sequence from the feces of two snake species, Indian cobra (Naja naja) and Oriental rat snakes (Ptyas mucosus).[22] Enterocytozoon bieneusi is known to use diverse amniotes as hosts and is of zoonotic concern. Although lesions were not investigated in the snakes, in other hosts, E. bieneusi causes enteritis.

Encephalitozoon hellem has been identified by DNA sequence from a juvenile freshwater crocodile (Crocodylus johnstoni) in Australia.[23] The animal was found dead with no previously identified signs of illness. Kupffer cells in the liver contained large numbers of E. hellem, and it was attributed as the primary cause of death.

Microsporidia have been described morphologically in four Hermann's tortoises (Testudo hermanni) from Germany.[24] The primary lesion seen histologically was granulomatous hepatitis, with organisms also seen in lung, heart, intestine, and kidney. The microsporidian was not identified.

Diagnosis. Specific diagnosis of microsporidiosis is best accomplished by histopathology in combination with PCR and sequencing of affected tissue. Encephalitozoon and Enterocytozoon are often shed per cloaca and may be an acceptable sample for testing, although data on sensitivity in reptiles are lacking.

Treatment. Treatment of microsporidiosis is challenging; they do not respond to traditional antifungal drugs.[25] Benzimidazoles such as oxfendazole, fenbendazole, and albendazole have some activity against microsporidia in vitro. However, the effects on the host can be significant, with bone marrow suppression and enterocyte necrosis seen particularly with fenbendazole.[26] It remains to be determined whether benzimidazole therapy of microsporidia in reptiles is beneficial or deleterious. Fumagillin is efficacious against microsporidia but bone marrow suppression is a significant potential side effect,[27] and data in reptiles is lacking.

Chytridiomycota

Members of the phylum Chytridiomycota do not have typical fungal morphology. Most are parasites of plants, algae, or oomycetes. Only two species are known vertebrate pathogens; Batrachochytrium dendrobatidis and B. salamandrivorans, both causing significant disease in amphibians. Neither appears to be a reptile pathogen. Batrachochytrium dendrobatidis has been associated with significant population declines in amphibians worldwide; to date, B. salamandrivorans has only been found in salamanders in Europe and Asia. They have two life stages; flask-shaped zoosporangia and uniflagellated motile zoospores. Zoosporangia are found in squamous epithelium of amphibians and also in gastrointestinal tracts of crayfish.[28] Amphibian skin is crucial for respiration and osmoregulation, and chytridiomycosis causes fatal electrolyte imbalances.[29] Maintenance of healthy skin flora is important for disease resistance; normal bacterial skin flora significantly inhibit Batrachochytrium spp.[30] Fungal skin flora are likely also important; previous treatment with itraconazole makes frogs more susceptible to Batrachochytrium.[8]

Diagnosis. Skin of the ventrum, especially the thighs and caudal abdomen, is generally the best diagnostic sample. Infected frogs often show a higher shed rate. Thalli containing zoosporangia may be seen in epithelium on cytologic examination of skin (Fig. 31.1), although the orientation of the thalli is usually such that the narrower "flask-shaped" portion is not visible, as is often seen histologically. Definitive disease diagnosis may be made through use of histopathology/cytology and PCR and sequencing or validated probe hybridization quantitative PCR (qPCR) (see Chapter 36).

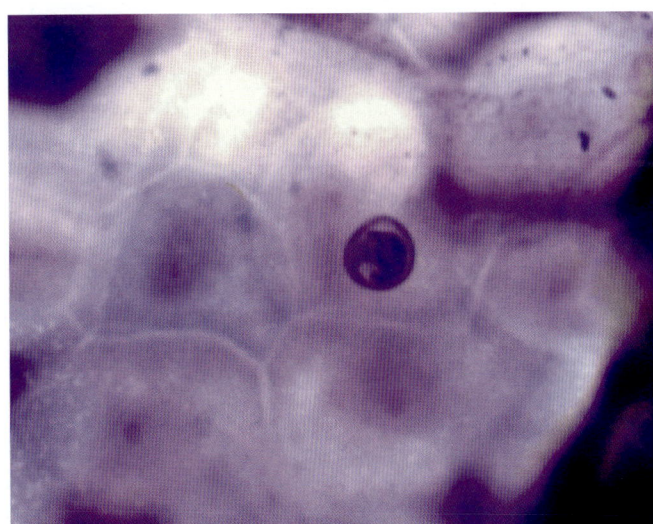

FIG 31.1 Cytological appearance of Batrachochytrium dendrobatidis in a White's tree frog (Litoria caerulea). (Courtesy of Jennifer L. Owen.)

Treatment. For amphibian species tolerant of higher temperatures, temperature manipulation may be the best therapeutic approach. Housing frogs at 37°C for 16 hours was found to clear frogs of *B. dendrobatidis.*[31] Housing frogs at 30°C for 10 days has also been found to clear frogs of *B. dendrobatidis.*[32] This may be at least partially due to alteration of bacterial skin flora.[33]

Pharmacologic therapy of *Batrachochytrium* is also possible. Itraconazole treatment in 0.01% baths has been shown to be effective in reducing *B. dendrobatidis* beyond detectable levels, but follow-up testing often found that infection was still present several months later.[34] Itraconazole also has significant toxic effects with negative effects on growth and weight gain, with fatal side effects seen, and some trials have found that a lower dose of 0.0025% itraconazole for 5 minutes/day for 6 days may be more efficacious.[35] Terbinafine, amphotericin B, voriconazole, and chloramphenicol all have activity against *B. dendrobatidis*, and further study is indicated.[36] Study of terbinafine/azole combinations is especially merited.

Batrachochytrium salamandrivorans tends to be more drug resistant than *B. dendrobatidis.* Combinations of voriconazole, polymyxin E, and temperature therapy were found to clear infection in infected fire salamanders (*Salamandra salamandra*), although follow-up testing was only done for 3 weeks.[37]

Zoopagomycota

The fungi formerly grouped as the now-defunct zygomycetes have been shown to be paraphyletic, with Zoopagomycota a more basal branch than Mucoromycota.[38] Zoopagomycota have more recognizable hyphal fungal morphology than microsporidians or chytrids. Most are pathogens or commensals of invertebrates, other fungi, or amoeba. The Zoopagomycota that are known potential vertebrate pathogens are in the subphylum Entomophthoromycotina, which are primarily known as arthropod pathogens.

Basidiobolus ranarum. *Basidiobolus ranarum*, in the class Basidiobolomycetes, order Basidiobolaceae, is commonly found as commensal intestinal flora in reptiles and amphibians. While it has been reported as a cause of fatal skin disease in anurans, these reports all date before the discovery of *Batrachochytrium dendrobatidis*. Histologic images from at least one report of *Basidiobolus ranarum* infection in anurans show what appear to be *Batrachochytrium dendrobatidis* thalli.[39] *Basidiobolus ranarum* is much more easily cultured than *Batrachochytrium dendrobatidis*, and, in hindsight, many reports of basidioboliasis in anurans may have been misattributed chytridiomycosis cases.

Schizangiella serpentis. *Schizangiella serpentis*, also in the class Basidiobolomycetes, order Basidiobolaceae, has been reported from an esophageal granuloma in an eastern rat snake (*Pantherophis alleghaniensis*).[40] Growth is yeastlike. Definitive diagnosis may be made through use of PCR and sequencing; susceptibility and treatment response has not been reported.

Mucormycota

The fungi formerly grouped as the now-defunct zygomycetes have been shown to be paraphyletic, with Mucoromycota being more closely related to Dikarya than Zoopagomycota.[15,38] Mucoromycota have more recognizable hyphal fungal morphology than microsporidians or chytrids. Most are associated with plants as commensals or decomposers.

Mucor. *Mucor* spp. have been reported from skin lesions in Florida softshell turtles (*Apalone ferox*).[41] Five of 30 recently captured wild Marlborough green geckos (*Naultinus manukanus*) developed skin lesions, from two of which *Mucor ramosissimus* was cultured, and both died.[42] It is probable that capture stress and husbandry played significant roles in disease. *Mucor* are relatively easy to culture and are not uncommon in the environment. Colonies are fluffy and white to gray, with wide hyphae and terminal round, spore-filled sporangia. Once infection is established, pharmacologic therapy is difficult. *Mucor* are often susceptible to amphotericin B and posaconazole, with limited susceptibility to other azoles and resistance to echinocandins.[43] Terbinafine is usually synergistic in combination.[44]

Dikarya

Dikarya is a subkingdom containing the largest extant clade of fungi. They do not have any flagellated life stages. Their name comes from dikaryons, a life stage containing two genetically distinct nuclei. They are divided into two phyla, Basidiomycota and Ascomycota.

Basidiomycota. Basidiomycota is a phylum in the Dikarya. Members of the phylum Basidiomycota have typical fungal morphology, with diploid zygotes called basidiospores. They often have large fruiting bodies; mushrooms are basidiomycetes. Most are associated with plants as decomposers or pathogens. Typically, animals eat mushrooms and mushrooms do not eat animals; the most major exception is *Cryptococcus/Filobasidiella.*

Cryptococcus/Filobasidiella. Although best known by the anamorph name *Cryptococcus*, the medically relevant members of the genus are technically more correctly called by the teleomorph name *Filobasidiella.*[13] It remains to be seen whether this will ever be generally accepted by the medical field. There are other members of the anamorph genus associated with several other teleomorph genera, but only two species, *C. neoformans* and *C. gattii*, are significant pathogens, and both are *Filobasidiella*. *Cryptococcus/Filobasidiella* is in the subphylum Agaricomycotina, class Tremellomycetes, order Tremellales. They cause pneumonia and encephalitis in a variety of animals, including humans. In animals, it is seen as a yeast with a distinctive thick capsule. This capsule helps avoid phagocytosis. The yeast form that grows in the animal is not the infective stage, and direct contact with a *Cryptococcus*-infected animal does not present undue zoonotic risk. The infective stage is environmental and has strong geographical and plant associations. It is strongly associated with trees, especially Douglas firs (*Pseudotsuga menziesii*) in Pacific northwestern North America, *Eucalyptus* trees in Australia, and carob (*Ceratonia siliqua*) and olive trees (*Olea europaea*) in the Mediterranean.

In reptiles, *Cryptococcus* has been reported in a captive green anaconda (*Eunectes murinus*) with ataxia, weight loss, and lethargy.[45] Interestingly, it had been raised in captivity in a region of the United States where *Cryptococcus/Filobasidiella* is not endemic. Granulomatous pneumonia and meningoencephalitis with intralesional yeast were seen histologically. It was identified by immunohistochemistry as *C. neoformans*, although this was before the recognition of *C. neoformans* and *C. gattii* as separate species. Cryptococcosis has also been reported in a captive eastern water skink (*Eulamprus quoyii*) in Australia.[46]

Diagnosis. Although standard radiography is insensitive for diagnosis of pneumonia in reptiles, computed tomography or endoscopy may be of more use. Histology or cytology may reveal the presence of yeast with thick capsules. If there is strong suspicion of *Cryptococcus*, culture should only be done by a referral laboratory; cultures will have the infective stage and are a biosafety level 3 risk to laboratory personnel. Direct testing of infected tissue without culture may be preferable. Definitive identification may be made through use of PCR and sequencing or validated probe hybridization qPCR (see Chapter 36).

Treatment. Whenever feasible, infected tissue should be excised surgically. An azole/terbinafine combination is a reasonable therapeutic approach.

Cutaneotrichosporon. *Cutaneotrichosporon* are Basidiomycetes in the class Tremellomycetes, order Trichosporonales. *Cutaneotrichosporon* were formerly known as *Trichosporon*.[47] They are yeasts, and sexual reproduction is not known. *Cutaneotrichosporon jiroveci* has been reported from ulcerative skin lesions on a Hermann's tortoise.[48] The author is aware of additional cases in emydid turtles and snakes. Although *C. mucoides* is a human pathogen that may have systemic effects, *C. jiroveci* does not grow above 36°C and is not considered a significant zoonotic risk.[49]

Diagnosis. Skin biopsies are indicated to diagnose cutaneotrichosporonosis. Histologically, 14- to 16-μm round yeasts and pseudohyphae are seen. On culture, colonies are white and waxy and frequently have a wrinkled appearance. Biochemical methods of identification frequently result in errors.[50] Confirmation of identity should be based on molecular identification. Sequencing of the ITS2 region of the ribosomal RNA genes is commonly used.

Treatment. The Hermann's tortoise reported with cutaneotrichosporonosis responded to surgical debridement and topical iodine therapy.[48] Pharmacologic antifungal therapy may not be needed. If indicated, clinical *C. jiroveci* isolates from humans are resistant to amphotericin B and susceptible to itraconazole and voriconazole.[50]

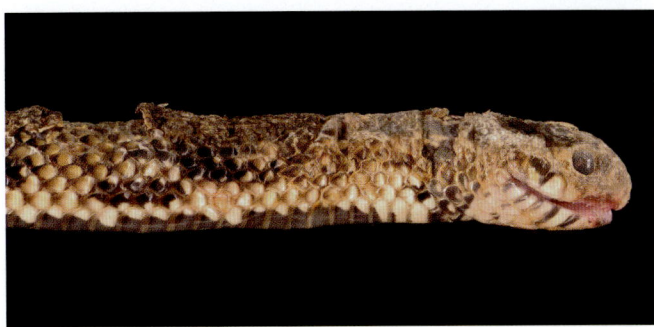

FIG 31.2 *Ophidiomyces ophiodiicola* dermatitis in an eastern king snake (*Lampropeltis getula*). (Courtesy of Rob Ossiboff.)

Ascomycota

Ascomycota is a phylum in the Dikarya. Members of the phylum Ascomycota have typical fungal morphology, with diploid zygotes called ascospores. They are often called sac fungi. They are the largest extant fungal phylum.

Pezizomycotina—Eurotiomycetes: Onygenales. Within the ascomycete order Onygenales (subphylum Pezizomycotina, class Eurotiomycetes), the majority of the fungal pathogens most significant for immunocompetent vertebrates are found, including *Blastomyces*, *Histoplasma*, *Coccidioides*, *Microsporum*, *Trichophyton*, *Lacazia*, *Paracoccidioides*, *Nannizziopsis*, *Paranannizziopsis*, and *Ophidiomyces*. The Onygenales have been shown to have reduced numbers of plant cell wall–degrading enzymes and tend to have increased numbers of proteases, especially keratinases, which may be adaptations for living on animal hosts.[51]

The anamorph name *Chrysosporium* is used widely for diverse anamorphs found widely across the order Onygenales and contains organisms in diverse teleomorph genera, including *Amaurascopsis*, *Amauroascus*, *Aphanoascus*, *Arthroderma*, *Bettsia*, *Ctenomyces*, *Neogymnomyces*, *Pectinotrichum*, *Renispora*, *Uncinocarpus*, *Ophidiomyces*, and *Nannizziopsis*.[52] There are significant differences in appropriate clinical approaches to king cobras (*Ophiophagus hannah*), Oustalet's chameleons (*Furcifer oustaleti*), and Mexican blind lizards (*Anelytropsis papillosus*), all in the order Squamata. Similarly, the wide distribution of the genus *Chrysosporium* across an entire diverse order renders it a relatively clinically useless name, and teleomorph names should be used.[13] Older reports may have misidentified members of the Onygenales as *Geotrichum*, *Trichophyton*, or *Microsporum*.

Ophidiomyces. *Ophidomyces ophiodiicola*, in the order Onygenales, family Onygenaceae, has recently been recognized as a major concern in North American snakes. The clinical presentation of the organism is commonly uncreatively called "snake fungal disease," although ophidiomycosis is a better term. Initially misidentified in reports as "*Chrysosporium* anamorph of *Nannizziopsis vriesii*,"[53] *O. ophiodiicola* is more closely related to *Coccidioides immitis* than it is to *Nannizziopsis* spp.[12,54] It was first characterized in 2009 from a black rat snake (*Pantherophis obsoletus*).[55] Reports of cases consistent with ophidiomycosis date to significantly earlier.[56,57] Snakes present with crusting dermatitis, often distributed around the head (Fig. 31.2). Invasion of deeper tissues is possible. It is capable of causing population-level impacts; it appears to be the primary cause for the near-extinction of the timber rattlesnake (*Crotalus horridus*) in New Hampshire.[58] Most reports have involved snakes in eastern North America, where most investigations have focused, but distinct strains of the organism have been reported in Europe.[59] Taxa most commonly affected are viperids and colubrids. Normal

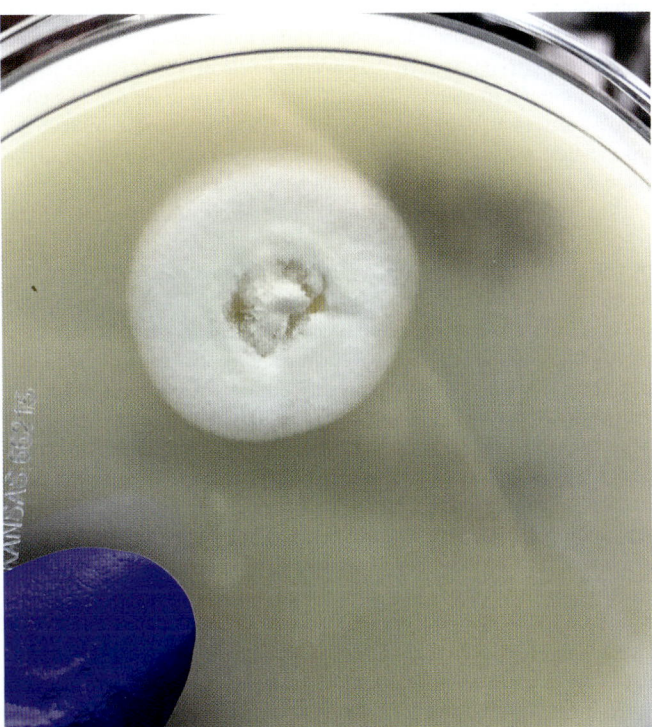

FIG 31.3 *Ophidiomyces ophiodiicola* colony. (Courtesy of Rebecca Richardson.)

cutaneous flora inhibit the growth of *O. ophiodiicola*, so antibiotic use may predispose animals to ophidiomycosis.[60]

Diagnosis. Histological examination of affected skin reveals 2 to 6 μm wide, parallel-walled, septate, rarely branching hyphae. Arthroconidia may be seen. Culture of *Ophidiomyces* cases commonly results in growth mixed with other more rapidly growing fungi, such as *Cladosporium* sp., and overgrowth by nontarget fungi can delay diagnosis. *Ophidiomyces* colonies are white and powdery on potato dextrose agar (Fig. 31.3). Narrow, cylindrical-to-slightly clavate conidia are seen. Confirmation of identity should be based on molecular identification. Sequencing of the ITS2 region of the ribosomal RNA genes is commonly used. There are also validated probe hybridization quantitative PCR assays for diagnosis of *O. ophiodiicola*.[61,62]

Treatment. Initial data on susceptibility of *O. ophiodiicola* suggests it is relatively drug resistant. The minimal inhibitory concentration (MIC) of itraconazole for two *O. ophiodiicola* isolates was 0.5 to 1 μg/mL.[63] Another member of the Onygenales, *Blastomyces dermatitidis*, has an itraconazole MIC <0.016 μg/mL, and the EUCAST breakpoint for *Aspergillus fumigatus* susceptibility is ≤1 μg/mL,[64,65] suggesting that a small shift in susceptibility would result in resistance. Administration of itraconazole at 10 mg/kg per cloaca also did not result in expected therapeutic levels.[63]

The MIC of voriconazole for two *O. ophiodiicola* isolates was 0.25 μg/mL (*B. dermatitidis* MIC 0.063 μg/mL, EUCAST *A. fumigatus* breakpoint ≤1 μg/mL), and the MIC of posaconazole for two *O. ophiodiicola* isolates was 0.5 μg/mL (*B. dermatitidis* MIC 0.016 μg/mL, EUCAST *A. fumigatus* breakpoint ≤0.125 μg/mL), suggesting voriconazole may be effective, and posaconazole is unlikely to be effective.[63–65] Voriconazole and itraconazole have been found to kill *O. ophiodiicola* in vitro.[63] There are significant concerns with safety; injection of voriconazole at 5 mg/kg subcutaneously resulted in the death of 3 of 6 cottonmouths (*Agkistrodon piscivorus*) within 12 hours.[63] Use of implantable osmotic pumps for voriconazole did not result in consistent therapeutic levels.[63] Clinical ophidiomycosis lesions on timber rattlesnakes resolved when given 10 mg/kg voriconazole per cloaca 3 times per week for 4 weeks, with no adverse effects detected.[54] However, levels of voriconazole in the snakes were not measured. The MIC of clotrimazole for two *O. ophiodiicola* isolates was <0.03 μg/mL, and the MIC of miconazole was 0.06 μg/mL.[63] These are low values, suggesting likely efficacy; further study of these drugs for *O. ophiodiicola* treatment is indicated.

The MIC of terbinafine for two *O. ophiodiicola* isolates was 0.015 μg/mL, suggesting this drug is likely to be effective.[63] Terbinafine administered by nebulization or subcutaneous implant resulted in levels expected to be therapeutic.[66] Terbinafine is often synergistic with azoles, and study of combination therapy is merited; clotrimazole/terbinafine nebulization may be effective. Bleach and 70% ethanol are effective for environmental disinfection of *O. ophiodiicola* on cleaned nonporous surfaces.[67]

Coccidioides. *Coccidioides,* in the order Onygenales, family Onygenaceae, contains the species *C. immitis* and *C. posadasii*, which are both significant pathogens in a variety of vertebrates. These two species are not morphologically distinguishable and were only recognized as separate species in 2002. Both species like arid environments with alkaline soil, with *C. immitis* endemic in California and *C. posadasii* endemic in the rest of the southwestern United States and northern Mexico, Guatemala and Honduras, eastern Brazil, and eastern Bolivia/Paraguay to central Argentina. There is no corresponding teleomorph name. Disease in humans is primarily pulmonary and is known as valley fever. In reptiles, natural coccidioidomycosis has been documented in snakes, and experimental infection in other toxicoferan squamates.[68–70] Of these, only one report has attempted molecular identification; in this case, although DNA from other fungi were amplified and sequenced from formalin-fixed paraffin-embedded tissues, *Coccidioides* spp. could not be detected by PCR.[70] A report of histological identification of coccidioidomycosis in a reticulated python (*Malayopython reticulatus*) from Dhaka Zoo in Bangladesh is surprising; neither the location of the zoo nor the endemic range of reticulated pythons are within known range of *Coccidioides* sp.[69] Soil in this area is also acidic. There are sporadic reports of human coccidioidomycosis in nonendemic areas, and further investigation is indicated.[71]

Diagnosis. Although standard radiography is insensitive for diagnosis of pneumonia in reptiles, computed tomography and/or endoscopy can be more useful. Pulmonary lavage or endoscopic biopsy are viable sampling techniques in snakes with potential coccidioidomydosis. Histological examination of affected tissue reveals 10 to 100 μm diameter spherules containing 2 to 5 μm endospores.[72] There is significant cross-reactivity of *Coccidioides* enzyme immunoassays with other endemic mycoses.[72] Although not considered directly infectious from contact with an infected animal, cultures of *C. immitis* or *C. posadasii* are biosafety level 3 (BSL3) agents in the United States, presenting significant risk to laboratory personnel. If a patient is suspected to have coccidioidomycosis, the laboratory should be informed of this when diagnostic

samples are submitted. *Coccidioides* colonies produce white cottony mycelia on potato dextrose agar. Confirmation of identity should be based on molecular identification. Sequencing of the ITS2 region of the ribosomal RNA genes is commonly used; specific probe hybridization qPCR is also available.[73]

Treatment. In humans, pharmacological treatment of coccidioidomycosis is only recommended in symptomatic patients.[72] *C. immitis* and *C. posadasii* are not highly antifungal resistant; only 1% of isolates are resistant to itraconazole.[73a] Surgical debridement may be an important component of therapy when possible.[72]

Aphanoascella. *Aphanoascella galapagosensis,* in the order Onygenales, family Onygenaceae, has been isolated from carapacial keratitis lesions on a Galapagos tortoise (*Chelonoidis nigra*).[74] Data on susceptibility and treatment of this organism is lacking. *Aphanoascella* colonies are white and cottony. Arthroconidia are cylindrical to slightly barrel-shaped. Confirmation of identity should be based on molecular identification. Sequencing of the ITS2 region of the ribosomal RNA genes is appropriate.

Nannizziopsis. *Nannizziopsis* spp., in the order Onygenales, family Nannizziopsiaceae, have been recognized as a major concern in squamates. They are commonly known by reptile hobbyists as "yellow fungus disease," although nannizziomycosis is a better term. Patients initially present with crusting dermatitis, but invasion of deeper tissues is common and fatality rates are high. Initially misidentified in reports as "*Chrysosporium* anamorph of *Nannizziopsis vriesii* (CANV)," much of the literature unfortunately is incorrect on which fungal species is actually found, resulting in significant confusion. The term CANV should not be used.

Nannizziopsis dermatitidis was first reported in 1999 from chameleons.[12,75] *N. dermatitidis* has also been reported from leopard geckos (*Eublepharis macularius*) and day geckos (*Phelsuma*).[12] The name *N. arthrosporioides* may have also been used with an isolate of this organism from a water dragon (*Physignathus* sp.), and this characterization involved a more robust gene set.[76] It remains to be determined which name will be accepted. It is the *Nannizziopsis* species most closely related to *N. vriesii*. It does not typically grow at temperatures greater than 30°C, and temperature manipulation may be therapeutically useful.

The best-studied and most clinically common species is *Nannizziopsis guarroi*. It was first characterized in 2010.[77] The genetic distance between *N. guarroi* and *N. vriesii* is similar to that between *Blastomyces dematitidis* and *Histoplasma capsulatum*, implying that similar differences in clinical management are probable.[54] *N. guarroi* is widespread in captive inland bearded dragons and green iguanas (*Iguana iguana*) in North America and Europe and has been reported in green iguanas in South Korea.[78] Growth is more rapid at 35°C than at 30°C, and temperature manipulation is unlikely to be therapeutically useful for most patients.

Nannizziopsis chlamydospora was identified in inland bearded dragons from the United States.[76] It is most closely related to *N. guarroi* and *N. draconii*. Unlike *N. guarroi* and *N. draconii*, it will grow on Sabouraud's dextrose agar with 3% NaCl.[76] It grows at temperatures up to 40°C, even higher than *N. guarroi*, and temperature manipulation is unlikely to be therapeutically useful.

Nannizziopsis draconii was identified in an inland bearded dragon from Spain.[76] It is most closely related to *N. guarroi* and *N. chlamydospora*. It grows at 25°C but not at 40°C, and further study is needed to determine whether temperature manipulation is likely to be therapeutically useful.

Nannizziopsis pluriseptata was identified in a five-lined skink (*Plestiodon inexpectatus*) from the United States.[76] It is divergent from other known *Nannizziopsis* species, making extrapolation from other species more tenuous. It grows at temperatures up to 40°C, even higher than *N. guarroi,* and temperature manipulation is unlikely to be therapeutically useful.

Nannizziopsis barbata was identified in captive and wild coastal bearded dragons (*Pogona barbata*) in southwest Australia.[79] It has not yet been reported outside of Australia. It is most closely related to *N. crocodili*, from Australian crocodiles.[12] It does not grow at temperatures greater than 30°C, and temperature manipulation may be therapeutically useful.

Nannizziopsis crocodili has been associated with fatalities in farmed saltwater crocodiles *(Crocodylus porosus)* in Australia and is the first species identified from lesions in nonsquamate reptiles.[80] It is most closely related to *N. barbata,* possibly representing an Australian clade.[12] Forty-eight hatchlings died in two outbreaks, suggesting a possible age predisposition. It grows at 25°C, more slowly at 35°C, and not at 37°C, so temperature manipulation may be therapeutically useful.

Nannizziopsis infrequens, N. obscura, and *N. hominis* have only been identified in human patients. They are all very close relatives of *N. guarroi,* raising concerns of zoonosis by the more thermophilic *Nannizziopsis* spp.[12] There is debate as to whether an isolate termed UTHSC R-4317 from a human represents *N. guarroi* or *N. hominis*.[12,76]

Diagnosis. Histologic examination of affected skin reveals 2 to 12 μm wide, parallel-walled, septate, occasionally branching hyphae.[81] Arthroconidia may be seen. *Nannizziopsis* colonies are white and powdery on potato dextrose agar and grossly resemble *Ophidiomyces*. Morphologic identification is not reliable, and confirmation of identity should be based on molecular identification. Sequencing of the ITS2 region of the ribosomal RNA genes is commonly used.

Treatment. There is a significant lack of antifungal susceptibility data for *Nannizziopsis* spp.; it consists largely of uncontrolled case reports of treatment. This is confounded by lack of proper identification; most reports lack proper fungal species identification. A report of susceptibility of "CANV" isolates from inland bearded dragons in Belgium says that sequence data matched *Nannizziopsis vriesii* 100%, but the GenBank accession number given was for *Aphanoascus fulvescens* (*Chrysosporium keratinophilum*).[82] There are significant differences in antifungal susceptibility profiles between different species in the same genus for other fungi, and it is probable that this will be found in *Nannizziopsis* sp.[65]

There is only a single report of *N. dermatitidis/arthrosporioides* therapy. In one of two infected chameleons treated with itraconazole therapy, clinical resolution was seen.[75] There are more reports of *N. guarroi* treatment. In one report, one of three infected inland bearded dragons responded to itraconazole therapy; the other two died.[83] Combination therapy with terbinafine and ketoconazole resulted in clinical resolution in two green iguanas.[84] Treatment of an infected inland bearded dragon with oral voriconazole for 14 days resulted in initial improvement, but the animal recrudesced and was euthanized.[85]

Treatment of inland bearded dragons infected with *N. chlamydospora* has been attempted with either oral voriconazole or oral itraconazole; disease recrudesced in all animals and the animals were euthanized.[85] Treatment of *N. barbata* has been attempted with oral itraconazole, topical nystatin, and topical iodine.[79] All attempted treatments were unsuccessful, resulting in progression of disease and euthanasia.

In summary, there are currently no consistently effective therapy recommendations for any *Nannizziopsis* sp., and the available data are concerning. Clinically it is crucial to determine which species is present in a patient. For some species, environmental temperature manipulation may be an important part of therapy. Surgical debridement may be an important component of therapy when possible. Susceptibility to antifungal drugs should be determined when possible. While susceptibility panels are waiting, a combination of terbinafine and voriconazole is a reasonable empirical therapy, and it is expected that therapy will need to be continued for at least several months. There are concerns about possible itraconazole toxicosis in bearded dragons; in one case series,

5 of 7 inland bearded dragons died when given 5 mg/kg PO q24h for 4 weeks.[82] The cost of long-term voriconazole justifies the cost of drug susceptibility testing.

Paranannizziopsis. *Paranannizziopsis* spp., in the order Onygenales, family Nannizziopsiaceae, have been recognized as a significant clinical concern in squamates and tuatara. Patients initially present with crusting dermatitis, but invasion of deeper tissues is common and fatality rates may be high. Initially misidentified in reports as "*Chrysosporium* anamorph of *Nannizziopsis vriesii* (CANV)," much of the literature unfortunately is incorrect on which fungal species is actually found, resulting in significant confusion. The term CANV should not be used.

Paranannizziopsis crustacea has been identified in an unidentified skink with multifocal dermatitis and in tentacled snakes (*Erpeton tentaculum*).[12,76] The name *Chrysosporium longisporum* has also been used with this organism.[76]

Paranannizziopsis australasiensis has been identified in file snakes (*Acrocordus* sp.), a coastal bearded dragon, and tuatara.[12,86] There appear to be significant differences in susceptibility between species; all cases in tuatara resolved with or without therapy, whereas the coastal bearded dragon was euthanized due to disease progression despite itraconazole treatment.[86] Rapid fatal disease was also seen in file snakes.[12] It is possible that the lower normal temperatures of tuatara may have played a role in case outcomes, and there may be host differences in immune response.

P. californiensis, reported from a tentacled snake isolate, is a very close relative of *P. australasiensis*.[12] Several snakes died in the outbreak.

Diagnosis. Histologic examination of affected skin reveals 2 to 3 μm wide, parallel-walled, septate, branching hyphae.[86] Arthroconidia may be seen. *Paranannizziopsis* colonies are white and powdery on potato dextrose agar and grossly resemble *Nannizziopsis* or *Ophidiomyces*. Morphologic identification is not reliable, and confirmation of identity should be based on molecular identification. Sequencing of the ITS2 region of the ribosomal RNA genes is commonly used.[87]

Treatment. There is a significant lack of antifungal susceptibility data for *Paranannizziopsis* spp. Treatment of a coastal bearded dragon with itraconazole for *P. australasiensis* was ineffective.[86] For some species, environmental temperature manipulation may be an important part of therapy. Surgical debridement may be an important component of therapy when possible. Susceptibility to antifungal drugs should be determined when possible.

Pezizomycotina—Eurotiomycetes: Chaetothyriales.
Within the ascomycete order Chaetothyriales (subphylum Pezizomycotina, class Eurotiomycetes), a variety of darkly pigmented fungi may be found, which may cause chromomycosis or phaeohyphomycosis.

Exophiala and Veronaea. The genera *Exophiala* and *Veronaea*, in the order Chaetothyriales, family Herpotrichiellaceae, are significant reptile pathogens. *Exophiala* is a large, paraphyletic genus, and *Veronaea* nests within it.[52] Teleomorphs of *Exophiala* sp have been named *Capronia* sp., but this name is not used significantly in the medical literature. These organisms appear to be most significant in chelonians. *Exophiala equina* was first reported from a Galapagos tortoise.[88] This organism seems to be a specific problem for Galapagos tortoises, and the author is aware of at least three additional cases of *E. equina* in this species. Lesions may be disseminated, and common sites include lungs and bone (Fig. 31.4). Carapacial phaeohyphomycosis due to *E. oligosperma* has been reported in an Aldabra tortoise (*Aldabrachelys gigantica*).[89] An *Exophiala* sp. was reported from a wild eastern box turtle (*Terrapene carolina*) with an extensive granulomatous lesion of the right hind leg.[90] Although the organism was thought to be *E. jeanselmei* based on morphology, there was no molecular characterization done, and organisms with *E. jeanselmei*-like morphology have been shown to be

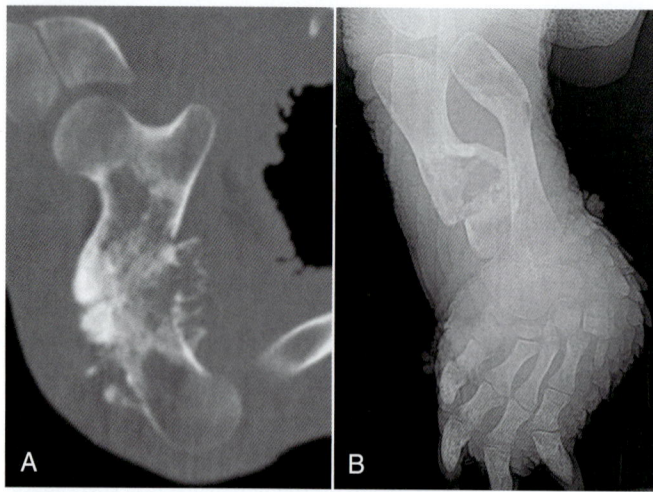

FIG 31.4 (A) Computed tomography of *Exophiala equina* osteomyelitis in the femur of a Galapagos tortoise (*Chelonoidis nigra*). (B) Radiograph of *Exophiala equina* osteomyelitis in the tibia of a Galapagos tortoise. (Courtesy of James F.X. Wellehan.)

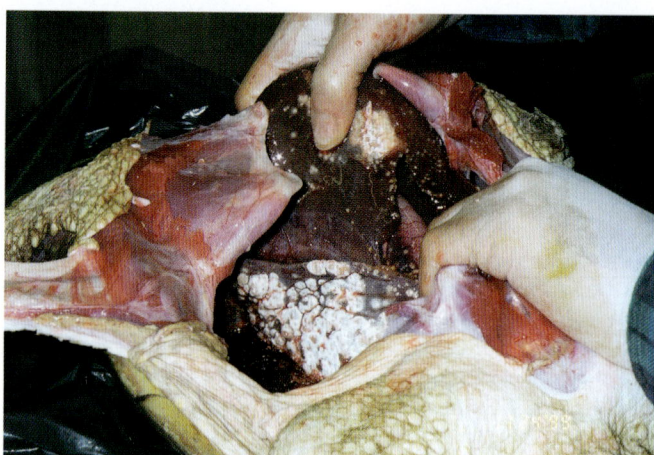

FIG 31.5 Disseminated *Beauveria bassiana* in a common snapping turtle (*Chelydra serpentina*). (Courtesy of James F.X. Wellehan.)

phylogenetically diverse.[91] Obstructive tracheitis due to *Veronaea botryosa* has been reported in green turtles (*Chelonia mydas*).[92]

Diagnosis. Infection with *Exophiala* or *Veronaea* typically causes destructive granulomatous lesions. If present in bone, they may be seen radiographically. Whereas standard radiography is insensitive for diagnosis of respiratory disease in reptiles, computed tomography and/or endoscopy may be more useful (see Fig. 31.4). When tissues are examined histologically, pigmented fungi in granulomatous lesions may be seen. In culture, colonies are dark on potato dextrose agar. Early growth shows yeast; older colonies may show hyphae with clusters of oval conidia. Morphological identification is not reliable, and confirmation of identity should be based on molecular identification. Sequencing of the ITS2 region of the ribosomal RNA genes is commonly used.

Treatment. *E. equina* isolates are susceptible to itraconazole and posaconazole but resistant to fluconazole and voriconazole.[93] *E. oligosperma* is also most susceptible to itraconazole and posaconazole, as well as amphotericin B.[94] Terbinafine also shows activity against many *Exophiala* isolates and may be synergistic in combination with azoles.[94] Susceptibility to antifungal drugs should be determined when possible. Surgical debridement may be an important component of therapy when possible.

Pezizomycotina—Sordariomycetes: Hypocreales. The ascomycete order Hypocreales (subphylum Pezizomycotina, class Sordariomycetes) contains a number of significant reptile pathogens. This order contains many significant arthropod pathogens, and some members are used for biological control of arthropod pests.

Purpureocillium. *Purpureocillium lilacinum*, in the order Hypocreales, family Ophiocordycipitaceae, was originally classified in the genus *Penicillium*, then *Paecilomyces*, before being classified as *Purpureocillium*. Clinical disease typically presents as pneumonia, although disseminated infection may be seen.[95–97] Turtles in the Trionychia are also prone to skin lesions.[98–99]

Diagnosis. Whereas standard radiography is insensitive for diagnosis of pneumonia in reptiles, computed tomography or endoscopy may be more useful. Pulmonary lavage or endoscopic biopsy are viable sampling techniques in reptiles with potential *Purpureocillium* infection. Histologically, fungal granulomas with hyphae are seen. Colonies are initially white but take on a reddish-purple color. Morphology is similar to

Penicillium, with bowling pin–shaped phialides supporting chains of oval conidia. Confirmation of identity should be based on molecular identification. Sequencing of the ITS2 region of the ribosomal RNA genes is commonly used.

Treatment. *Purpureocillium lilacinum* isolates tend to be resistant to amphotericin B and itraconazole but susceptible to voriconazole, posaconazole, and terbinafine. A combination of posaconazole and terbinafine is the best empirical choice for treating *P. lilacinum* infection.[100] Topical malachite green has also been used for cutaneous lesions.[98] Susceptibility to antifungal drugs should be determined when possible. Surgical debridement may be an important component of therapy when possible.

Beauveria and Lecanicillium. *Beauveria bassiana*, in the order Hypocreales, family Cordycipitaceae, is best known as an insect pathogen. It is also a significant reptile pathogen. The teleomorph name has been *Cordyceps bassiana*. Commercial use of *B. bassiana* as an insect biocontrol agent is widespread and has implications for wild reptile populations. Whereas there has been significant study of virulence mechanisms in insect hosts, these studies have primarily been focused on how to increase virulence.[101] Lesions in reptiles are typically pulmonary and have been reported in alligators, tortoises, and emydid turtles (Fig. 31.5).[102–104]

Lecanicillium, like *Beauveria*, are in the order Hypocreales, family Cordycipitaceae. They are also known as arthopod pathogens and are used commercially for insect control, which may have implications for wild reptiles. Members of the genus were formerly known as *Verticillium* before being moved to *Lecanicillium*. A *Lecanicillium* most closely related to *L. attenuatum* and *L. muscarium* caused systemic mycosis in captive Guthega skinks (*Liopholis guthega*).[105] Lesions were first seen as necrotic dermatitis which progressed to myositis, hepatitis, and pneumonia.

Diagnosis. Whereas standard radiography is insensitive for diagnosis of pneumonia in reptiles, computed tomography and/or endoscopy may be more useful. Pulmonary lavage or endoscopic biopsy are viable sampling techniques in reptiles with potential *B. bassiana* infection. Histologically, fungal granulomas with hyphae are seen. Birefringent calcium oxalate crystals may be seen.[103] *B. bassiana* and *Lecanicillium* spp. colonies are typically white to yellow in color. *Beauveria* have flask-shaped structures supporting small numbers of small oval conidia. *Lecanicillium* have elongate pointed phialides with single conidia. Confirmation of identity should be based on molecular identification. Sequencing of the ITS2 region of the ribosomal RNA genes is commonly used.

Treatment. *B. bassiana* isolates tend to be comparatively susceptible to itraconazole, less so to voriconazole, and resistant to fluconazole.[106,107] Data on *Lecanicillium* spp. susceptibility is not yet published, but skinks treated with a regime including oral voriconazole showed clinical resolution.[105] Susceptibility to antifungal drugs should be determined when possible.

Metarhizium. *Metarhizium* spp., in the order Hypocreales, family Clavicipitaceae, are best known as insect pathogens. Characterized teleomorph names are in the genus *Metacordyceps*. *M. anisopliae* is used commercially for insect control, which has implications for wild reptiles. In experimental challenges, fringe-toed lizards (*Acanthodactylus dumerili*) exposed to *M. anisopliae* either by ingestion or inhalation showed decreased activity compared with controls, with mycotic pneumonia seen at necropsy in some animals.[108] Pneumonia caused by *M. anisopliae* has also been reported in alligators.[109]

Metarhizium granulomatis, previously described as *Chamaeleomyces granulomatis* and *Paecilomyces viridis*, has been associated with dermatitis, glossitis, and disseminated granulomatous mycosis. Veiled chameleons (*Chamaeleo calyptratus*) are the most commonly affected species, with disease in an inland bearded dragon and a panther chameleon (*Furcifer pardalis*) also reported.[110] There are distinct genotypes of *M. granulomatis*, with genotype A more associated with dermatitis, and genotypes B to E more associated with glossitis.[110] *M. granulomatis* has been found in environmental soil samples, and it is probable that this is its usual habitat.

Metarhizium viride, previously described as *Chamaeleomyces viridis* and *Paecilomyces viridis*, has been associated with dermatitis, pharyngitis, glossitis, and disseminated granulomatous mycosis.[111] *M. viride* appears to have a broader host range than *M. granulomatis*; there is a distribution of reported hosts, including veiled chameleons, inland bearded dragons, panther chameleons, and carpet chameleons (*Furcifer lateralis*); the bias toward veiled chameleons seen with *M. granulomatis* is not seen with *M. viride*.

Diagnosis. Glossitis or dermatitis lesions due to *M. granulomatis* or *M. viride* are fairly easily accessible. Whereas standard radiography is insensitive for diagnosis of *M. anisopliae* pneumonia in reptiles, computed tomography and endoscopy may be more useful.[109] Pulmonary lavage or endoscopic biopsy are viable sampling techniques in reptiles with potential *M. anisopliae* infection. Histologically, fungal granulomas with hyphae are seen. Birefringent calcium oxalate crystals may be seen.[109] *Metarhizium* colonies are typically olive green in color. They have cylindrical conidia produced in long chains from branched, subcylindrical phialides. Confirmation of identity should be based on molecular identification. Sequencing of the ITS2 region of the ribosomal RNA genes is commonly used.

Treatment. *M. anisopliae* isolates tend to be susceptible to itraconazole and voriconazole but highly resistant to fluconazole and amphotericin B.[112] *M. granulomatis* isolates were found to be resistant to all doses of itraconazole and ketoconazole tested, and inhibitory concentrations of terbinafine, clotrimazole, voriconazole, posaconazole, and amphotericin B were high enough that clinical therapy with these drugs as a single therapy is unlikely to be susceptible.[110] Treatment of chameleons with *M. granulomatis* using terbinafine and nystatin resulted in continued disease progression and death.[110] Further studies on synergy of posaconazole and terbinafine against *M. granulomatis* are indicated. *M. viride* showed high resistance to voriconazole, fluconazole, clotrimazole, nystatin, posaconazole, nystatin, and amphotericin B, and treatment appears problematic.[111] Whenever feasible, infected tissue should be excised surgically.

Fusarium. *Fusarium* spp. are in the order Hypocreales, family Nectriaceae. It is a large genus with at least 200 species divided into 20 complexes, and many members are common in soil in association with plants and in marine environments. A number of them are plant pathogens. Although *Fusarium* infections are typically not primary pathogens, once they have become established as secondary infections, they are typically very drug resistant and difficult to treat. Cutaneous and respiratory infections are most common in reptiles.

Most infections in reptiles are from members of the *F. solani* complex, which contains at least 18 species associated with disease in animals.[113] Juvenile sea turtles and eggs are commonly affected; loggerhead turtle (*Caretta caretta*) eggs exposed to *F. solani* complex had an 83.3% mortality rate in comparison to 8.3% mortality in control eggs.[114]

Fusarium incarnatum, formerly known as *F. semitectum*, is a member of the *F. incarnatum-equiseti* species complex. It has been associated with scute lesions in Texas tortoises (*Gopherus berlandieri*).[115] *Fusarium proliferatum*, a member of the *F. fujikuroi* species complex, has been associated with dermatitis in 9 of 40 (22.5%) wild fringe-toed lizards (*Acanthodactylus nilsoni*).[116] Lesions were distributed on the front digits and the back of the neck, which may be consistent with combat and mating bite wounds providing a route for infection. The *F. fujikuroi* species complex has also been associated with pneumonia in an alligator.[117] A member of the *F. oxysporum* complex caused disseminated granulomatous infection in a red-bellied black snake (*Pseudechis porphyriacus*).[118] Treatment with itraconazole was unsuccessful.

Diagnosis. Dermatitis lesions due to *Fusarium* spp. are easily accessible. Whereas standard radiography is insensitive for diagnosis of *Fusarium* pneumonia in reptiles, computed tomography and/or endoscopy may be more useful. Pulmonary lavage or endoscopic biopsy are viable sampling techniques. Histologically, fungal granulomas with hyphae are seen. *Fusarium* colonies are white to cream initially but may develop purple to peach coloration as they mature. They have both larger canoe-shaped septate conidiophores and smaller single oval conidiophores. Confirmation of identity should be based on molecular identification. The ITS2 region of the ribosomal RNA genes, commonly used in other fungal taxa, is not sufficient for species identification in *Fusarium* spp. Sequencing of the *ef-1α* and *rbp2* genes is indicated.[119]

Treatment. Treatment of fusariomycosis is very challenging. They are usually multidrug (including itraconazole) resistant. Empirically, a combination of terbinafine with either posaconazole or voriconazole may be used while identification, speciation, and sensitivity results are pending. Whenever feasible, infected tissue should be excised surgically.[120]

Pezizomycotina—Eurotiomycetes: Eurotiales

Aspergillus. *Aspergillus* spp. are in the order Eurotiales, family Aspergillaceae. They are widespread and extremely common in decaying plant matter. Although common pathogens of birds and mammals, they are surprisingly uncommon as pathogens in reptiles. There is only one report of aspergillosis in reptiles with molecular sequence identification; a case of granulomatous pneumonia and hepatitis in a Siamese crocodile (*Crocodylus siamensis*) due to *A. fumigatus*.[121] Unfortunately, details on PCR or sequencing were not given, and sequence data were not placed in a public database.

Saccharomycotina—Saccharomycetes: Saccharomycetales

Candida. *Candida* is a genus in the order Saccharomycetales, which are ascomycete yeasts. They are common in vertebrate gastrointestinal tracts, including reptiles.[122] They are typically benign and form a normal part of gut flora. A major risk factor for development of clinical disease due to *Candida* spp. is the use of antibiotics, disrupting normal bacterial flora.[7] Cephalosporin use, β-lactam–β-lactamase inhibitor combination use, and fluoroquinolone use are especially inked with candidiasis.[7,123] Clinical candidiasis is more common in chelonians than in other reptiles.

Candida albicans has been reported to cause disseminated disease in an elongated tortoise (*Indotestudo elongata*).[124] The animal had recently been treated with enrofloxacin for a wound and subsequently developed fatal candidiasis. *C. albicans* pneumonia has been reported in a Greek tortoise (*Testudo graeca*).[125]

Several reports of clinical candidiasis in reptiles lack identification of which species of *Candida* was present. From healthy tortoises, *C. tropicalis*, *C. famata*, *C. albicans*, *C. guillermondi*, *C. intermedia*, and *C. parapsilosis* were identified in oral and cloacal swabs from *Testudo* and *Chelonoidis* tortoises.[126,127] In healthy sea turtles, *C. parapsilosis*, *C. guillermondi*, *C. tropicalis*, *C. albicans*, and *C. intermedia* were identified.[127] Prevalence is high in healthy chelonians, with 67% of healthy *Chelonoidis* tortoises colonized.[127]

Diagnosis. A history of recent broad-spectrum antibiotic use in chelonians increases the concern for candidiasis. Light-colored plaques are often present with severe overgrowth, and cytology of affected mucosa will reveal large numbers of yeast. Histologically, 2- to 12-μm round yeasts and pseudohyphae are seen. *C. albicans* tends to be at the larger end of the range, whereas other species tend to be smaller. In disseminated cases, blood culture may be useful. On culture, colonies are cream colored and waxy. Confirmation of identity should be based on molecular identification. Sequencing of the ITS2 region of the ribosomal RNA genes is commonly used.

Treatment. Although *C. albicans* are frequently susceptible to azoles, non–*albicans Candida* spp. are frequently significantly more drug resistant. Susceptibility to antifungal drugs should be determined when possible. When mucosal surfaces are affected, nystatin may be effective. Pneumonia due to *C. albicans* in a Greek tortoise (*Testudo graeca*) was successfully treated with intrapulmonary amphotericin B delivered via a transcarapacial pulmonary catheter.[125]

REFERENCES

See www.expertconsult.com for a complete list of references.

32

Parasitology (Including Hemoparasites)

James F.X. Wellehan and Heather D.S. Walden

REPTILE-PARASITE ECOLOGY

Parasites are organisms that live in or on other host organisms and benefit by deriving nutrients at the host's expense. In common medical jargon, and for the purposes of this chapter, only nonfungal eukaryotic parasites will be considered. Reptile patients are often approached as a collection of vertebrate cells organized into organ systems. This is highly misleading; most of the cells in a vertebrate are microbial. Microbes are especially critical for digestion and immune function, and maintenance of healthy flora is essential to the health of a reptile patient.

Clinicians are also often misled by Koch's postulates; by fulfilling or not fulfilling these requirements in a controlled experiment, an organism is often considered dichotomously as a pathogen or not a pathogen. This is far from the case; in the real world, numerous host, pathogen, and environmental factors (including coinfections, temperature, nutrition, handling stress, crowding, and others) play significant roles in whether a pathogen manifests as disease. When infectious disease is more properly considered as ecology, it is obvious that a typical disease scenario involves several infectious agents in concert with environmental factors. It is critical to determine whether an organism is acting as a parasite in a given context. Bullfrog tadpoles (*Rana catesbeiana*) that have the pinworm *Gyrinicola batrachiensis* develop more quickly and have better gut fermentation than controls without pinworms, indicating a mutualistic rather than parasitic relationship.[1] Vertebrates have more than likely had gut helminths over most of their evolution.[2] The vertebrate immune system has adapted to living with gut helminths; eradication of gut helminths is associated with a significant increase in autoimmune and allergic disease.[3] Rather than thinking of a war on parasites, clinicians should have the goal of improving ecosystem health within a reptile patient.

Evolution is an essential concept in biology; when one considers definitions for life, perhaps the simplest and most elegant definition is that life consists of things that evolve. Clinically, this is most immediately apparent with infectious disease. Because of short generation times, evolution of parasites occurs in a time frame impacting clinical management of a patient. To compensate, the most rapidly evolving genes in vertebrates are immune related. A parasite does not "want" to cause disease or not cause disease. All life on earth has been selected for billions of years to reproduce successfully, and this is all that matters from an evolutionary standpoint. If pathogenic traits provide an evolutionary advantage in a given situation, they will be selected for. If they provide a disadvantage, they will be selected against.

The need to transfer to a new host creates significant selective pressure. Some parasites, such as *Rhabdias* spp., with both homogonic and heterogonic life cycles, may survive and reproduce well without their hosts, decreasing selective pressure to keep the host alive. High host density also favors virulence by increasing access to new hosts, and increased stocking density creates environments selecting for pathogenicity.

Other routine husbandry practices in the reptile pet trade also create strong evolutionary selective pressures toward pathogenicity. It is common in the pet reptile trade to select for color mutants. This usually involves some degree of inbreeding to select for what are often recessive traits. A major driving force for the evolution of sex is acquisition of genetic diversity for immune function. Inbreeding results in selection for greater disease.[4]

Understanding life cycles is crucial for parasite control. Parasites with direct life cycles complete their life cycles using one host. Keeping that host alive maintains their habitat and is advantageous for the parasite. Parasites with indirect life cycles utilize more than one host and include intermediate hosts. It is often advantageous for the parasite to cause disease in intermediate hosts that will result in death or illness of that host and allow completion of the life cycle. If a rodent with *Baylisascaris procyonis* is mentally impaired by neural larval migrans, that rodent is more likely to be predated upon by a raccoon, completing the life cycle. Clinical parasitic disease is typically much more significant for intermediate hosts than definitive hosts.

DIAGNOSTIC CONFIRMATION

Diagnosis of parasitic disease needs to be done with an understanding of the ecology of the patient and parasite. A history and physical examination is a good starting point, with the recognition that husbandry has played a major role in almost any disease process for which a captive reptile is presented to a veterinarian, and husbandry improvements will need to be part of the therapeutic approach. Wild-caught animals are more likely to have parasitic disease than captive-bred animals, and parasites with direct life cycles are much more likely to persist in captive populations than those with indirect life cycles.

Diagnosis of parasites in their definitive hosts, where ova, oocysts, cysts, or larvae are produced, is much easier than diagnosis of parasites in intermediate hosts. Many of these parasite diagnostic stages are shed in feces. Fecal flotation is very useful for diagnosis of enteric coccidia, as well as many nematodes, cestodes (if eggs have been released from proglottids), and sometimes pentastomids. Different flotation media are used; some are concentrated salts, and others are sugars. Some parasites are best identified using specific solutions. The specific gravities of these solutions are important, as are the specific gravities of the diagnostic stages of the parasites in question. Using a centrifuge for fecal flotations, in addition to a solution with higher specific gravity, increases the ability to detect these diagnostic stages, especially when sample sizes are small, as many reptile samples are, and when there are few ova, oocysts, cysts, or larvae present in the samples. Some enteric parasite diagnostic stages have a high specific gravity, including ova of trematodes, acanthocephalans, and some nematodes and pentastomids, and fecal sedimentation is preferred. The salt or sugar flotation solutions can sometimes distort the morphologic characteristics of larvae recovered in feces, so a sedimentation can also be used to preserve these characteristics and allow identification. Quantification of parasite egg counts using modified McMaster techniques or larval counts using modified Baermann techniques can also provide valuable information on parasite burden and response to therapy. This can be especially important when formulating strategic anthelmintic strategies for reptiles kept outside.

Direct microscopic examination of feces by direct fecal smear in saline is the best way to detect motile enteric protozoa. Feces need to be fresh and at room temperature to observe motility of trophozoites, including flagellates, ciliates, and amoeba, because these organisms are susceptible to desiccation and cold or hot temperatures. Fresh feces can also be fixed in zinc polyvinyl alcohol (Zinc-PVA) and stained with a trichrome or iron hematoxylin stain to show the internal characteristics of the protozoans. The trichrome stain method is preferred for identification of amoeboid cysts and trophozoites. Hemoparasites can be detected with blood smears stained with Wright's or Giemsa stain or a combination. Some blood parasites are intracellular, and some are extracellular. Additional blood samples should be stored frozen for molecular identification.

Pseudoparasites are parasites found during patient or fecal examinations of a reptile, but the parasite is actually from another host. For example, if reptiles are fed mice, four helminth eggs might appear in fecal examinations that are parasites of the mice (prey) and not the reptile (Figs. 32.1 through 32.4). Pseudoparasites are common and can be easily confused with true parasites, an important distinction because the former do not require treatment.

For the diagnosis of gastric *Cryptosporidium*, gastric biopsies are the gold standard. For intestinal species, the biopsy should be from the intestines. If animals in a collection are dying, necropsy and histopathologic examination of gastric and intestinal tissue are helpful in determination of the cause.

Reptiles fed mice may have false-positive fecal examination results because mice harbor their own *Cryptosporidium* species, and these cause problems for diagnosis based on lack of morphologic differences from those that are parasites of reptiles (Fig. 32.5).

Diagnosis of parasites in intermediate hosts, where parasites are more typically encysted in tissues, waiting to be ingested by the definitive host, is more challenging. Physical examination or imaging may identify potential sites of encysted parasites, and excisional biopsy may be needed to acquire samples. Samples of parasites are best kept in 70% ethanol or at −80°C; formalin fixation damages DNA, preventing molecular diagnostics, and can hinder gross identification. Further detail on parasite preservation may be found in Sepulveda and Kinsella.[5]

SINGLE-CELLED PARASITES

Identification of single-celled parasites is more challenging. They generally are not visible without magnification and lack sufficient morphologic

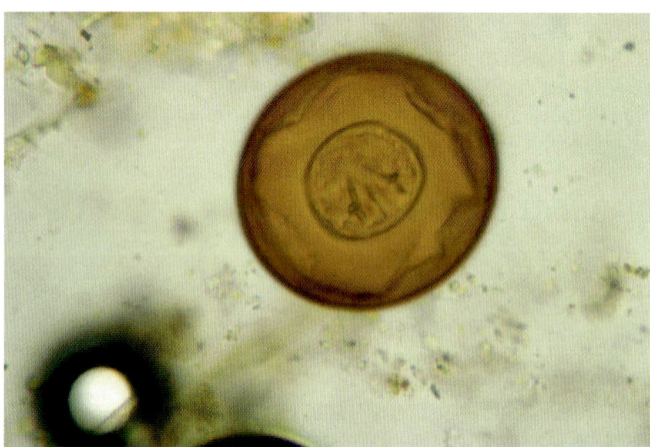

FIG 32.1 *Hymenolepis diminuta*, pseudoparasite. Photomicrograph magnification, 400×.

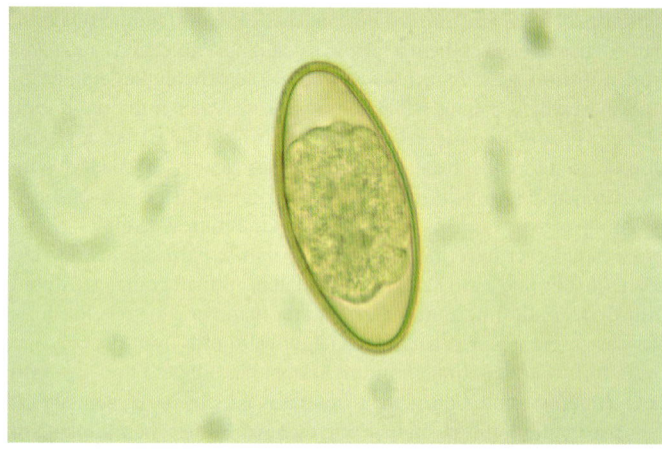

FIG 32.3 *Aspicularis tetraptera*, pseudoparasite. Photomicrograph magnification, 400×.

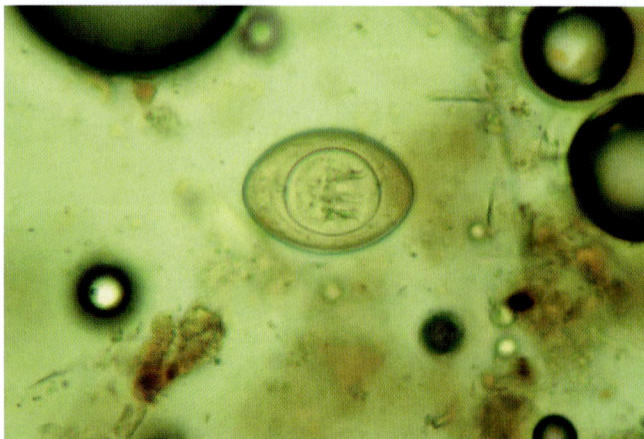

FIG 32.2 *Hymenolepis nana*, pseudoparasite. Photomicrograph magnification, 400×.

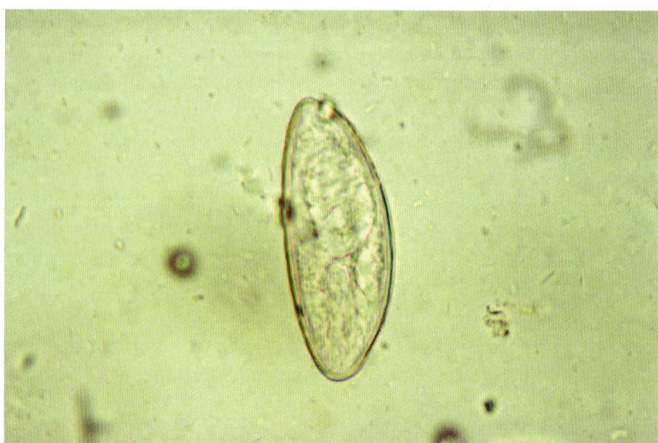

FIG 32.4 *Syphacia muris*, pseudoparasite. Photomicrograph magnification, 400×.

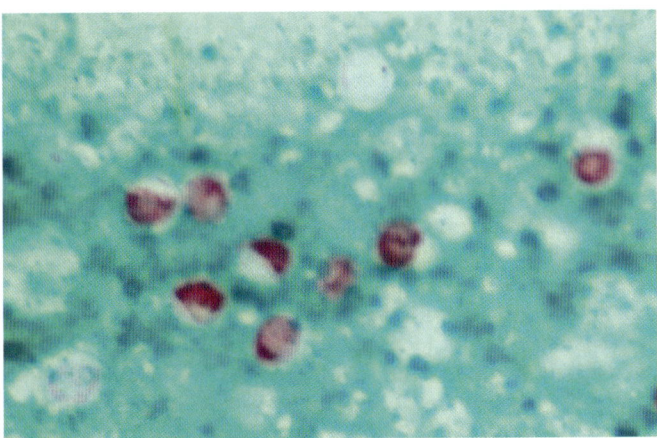

FIG 32.5 *Cryptosporidium muris* from a corn snake (*Pantherophis* sp.), pseudoparasite. Photomicrograph magnification, 400×.

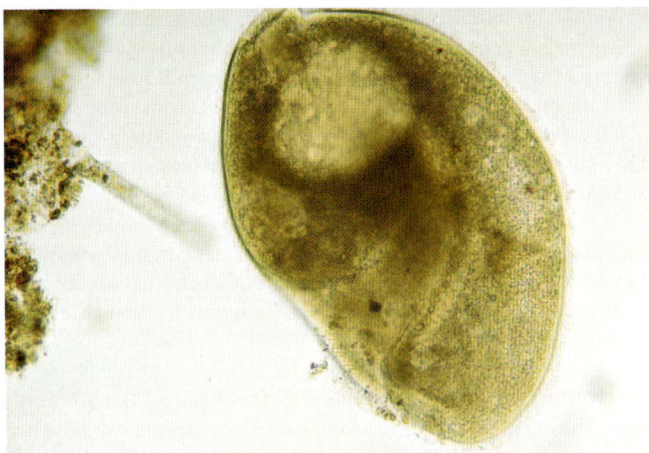

FIG 32.6 Ciliate trophozoite from a star tortoise (*Geochelone elegans*). Photomicrograph magnification, 160×.

features to make morphologic identification reliable. There is also significantly more diversity present. Multicellular parasites are found in one clade, the Metazoa, or animals; unicellular parasites are found across the Eukaryota. Morphologic groupings, such as flagellates or amoeba, are widespread across diverse taxa and do not imply relatedness. There is a life stage of humans and reptiles that is a flagellate, and phagocytic immune cells are amoeboid. Molecular sequence may be necessary for accurate identification, and, for PCR-based methods, it is necessary to have primers that amplify primer but not host. Because flagellates are widespread across eukaryotes, primers that would amplify DNA from all eukaryotes would also amplify DNA from animal hosts. It is therefore necessary to target PCR assays more narrowly toward specific clades. Techniques such as next-generation sequencing (NGS), which involve obtaining large numbers of nontargeted nucleic acid sequences from a given sample and then identifying the resultant sequences, may hold promise for the future. However, although costs have dropped dramatically, NGS is still too expensive for routine diagnostic use, and the lack of reference sequence, especially in nondomestic animals and their parasites, is a major impediment to interpretation of data.

Alveolata

The Alveolata are a clade of eukaryotes that have cortical alveoli, which are vesicles underlying the cell membrane. There are a number of phyla within the alveolates, of which the Ciliophora and Apicomplexa are the most relevant for reptile parasitology.

Ciliophora (*Balantidium, Nyctotherus*).

Ciliophora is a phylum of aveolates that have short hairlike cilia that move in an undulating pattern (Fig. 32.6). Although common in gastrointestinal tracts of vertebrates, there is limited data on their pathogenicity. There is a single case report of ciliate-associated enteritis in a puff adder (*Bitis arietans*) kept at inappropriate temperatures.[6] A collection of snakes with enteritis had ciliates morphologically consistent with *Balantidium* sp. present, as well as bacteria morphologically consistent with *Clostridium,* and improved after treatment with metronidazole.[7] Overall, ciliates do not appear to be highly pathogenic in reptiles, and high numbers are more indicative of gut dysbiosis. Cysts of the genus *Nyctotherus* strongly resemble trematode ova; one way to differentiate them is that *Nyctotherus* cysts will be commonly found on a fecal flotation, whereas trematode ova usually will not (Fig. 32.7). However, there are occasions where trematode ova are detectable on a fecal flotation, so this should not be used as a sole method of differentiation.

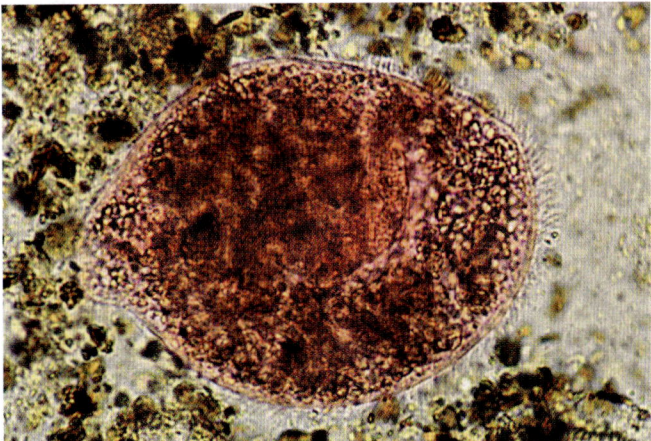

FIG 32.7 *Nyctotherus* (merthiolate stain). (Courtesy of F.L. Frye.)

Apicomplexa.

Apicomplexa is a phylum of alveolates that have apicoplasts, unique organelles that have their own genomes and are involved in important cellular functions, much like mitochondria or chloroplasts. They typically do not have cilia, flagella, or pseudopods, and they move using gliding motility. This phylum contains many of the most clinically significant reptile parasites. They are divided into the classes Aconoidasida, containing the orders Haemosporidia and Piroplasmida, and Conoidasida, containing the subclasses Coccidia and Gregarinasina.

Haemosporidia (*Plasmodium, Haemoproteus, Haemocystidium*).

The order Haemosporidia are intraerythrocytic parasites in the class Aconoidasida with indirect life cycles, typically transmitted by invertebrates. Important genera infecting reptiles in this group include *Plasmodium, Haemoproteus,* and *Haemocystidium.* All are insect vectored and target erythrocytes. Molecular sequence data have shown that the *Plasmodium* of reptiles are paraphyletic.[8] Although haemosporidians are generally considered to have high host fidelity, *Haemoproteus anatolicum* has been found to infect both Horsfield's tortoises (*Agrionemys horsfieldii*) and Greek tortoises (*Testudo graeca*).[9] Much work needs to be done to determine the diversity of haemosporidians using nonavian reptile hosts and their clinical significance. *Plasmodium falciparum* caused 212 million cases of malaria in humans, resulting in 429,000 deaths from the infection in 2015.[10] The significance of malarial parasites in mammals suggests that they are likely significant in reptiles as well. Their indirect life cycles tend to make them less significant in captivity, where life cycles may be interrupted by separation from vectors. Drugs used for treatment of human malaria include mefloquine, primaquine, chloroquine, doxycycline, and atovaquone; data on these drugs in reptiles are lacking.

Coccidia. The subclass Coccidia are intracellular parasites in the class Conoidasida, phylum Aveolata. The order Eucoccidiorida contains the vertebrate parasites and is divided into the suborders Adeleorina and Eimeriorina.

Adeleorina (*Hepatozoon, Hemolivia, Haemogregarina, Karyolysus*). The suborder Adelorina are intracellular coccidian parasites. They have indirect life cycles and may be transmitted by hematophagous insects, ticks, or leeches. They are most commonly found in aquatic reptiles. Disease appears to be most strongly associated with aberrant hosts.[11] Diagnosis is commonly made through examination of blood smears or through histopathology. Specific identification of organisms may be done though nucleic acid sequencing. There is a lack of data on safety or efficacy of pharmacologic treatment of adelorine parasites in reptiles; in dogs, *Hepatozoon americanum* is most commonly treated with decoquinate or ponazuril.[12] Limited data found a decrease in hemogregarine loads in lizards treated with atovaquone.[13]

Eimeriorina (*Cryptosporidium, Isospora, Sarcocystis, Eimeria, Caryospora, Schellackia, Choleoeimeria,* Intranuclear Coccidium of Tortoises). The suborder Eimeriorina are intracellular coccidian parasites. There are three families that are relevant for reptile medicine: Cryptosporidiidae, Eimeriidae, and Sarcocystidae. Sexual reproduction is typically in the intestine of the definitive host, followed by fecal shedding. In many cases in which coccidian oocysts are seen in the feces, whether disease or simply infection exists is unknown, and additional clinical data such as histopathology are needed. Cryptosporidiidae and Eimeriidae typically have direct life cycles, utilizing a single host, with oocysts passed in the feces. Sarcocystidae typically have obligate two-host cycles, although exceptions exist, and oocysts are passed in the feces of the definitive host (Figs. 32.8 to 32.11). To date, vertical transmission of coccidia has not been shown in reptiles.

Coccidian oocysts generally need time to sporulate after they are shed before they are infective; *Cryptosporidium* and some species of *Sarcocystis* are exceptions. In general, once the sporulated oocyst is ingested, the sporozoites leave the oocyst and penetrate epithelial cells that line gastrointestinal mucosa. Development is intracellular, and with each phase of the cycle, more host cells are killed as the parasites exit the host cells in which they were produced and enter other cells.

Set numbers of asexual generations exist within one life cycle, and then the sexual phase ensues and produces gametes and zygotes. A wall is produced by the parasite around the zygote that is now an oocyst. It is expelled from the host cell and passes in the feces.

Whether disease is caused by the developing coccidian depends on the number of oocysts initially ingested, the ability of the host to replace the cells killed quickly enough to preclude clinical disease, the genetics of the parasite itself, and the host immune status. Coccidia that infect cells beyond the gastrointestinal tract are often associated with more significant pathology. Enteric coccidiosis is most commonly a disease of young animals, where stunting or slowing of growth and maturation may be evident. See Table 32.1 for generic oocyst morphology.

Cryptosporidiidae. Cryptosporidiidae contains a single genus, *Cryptosporidium.* Cryptosporidian parasites are epicytoplasmic in host cells rather than intracytoplasmic, unlike most other coccidia. All *Cryptosporidium* species have direct life cycles. Oocysts are less than 8 μm in diameter and stain acid-fast (see Fig. 32.5). It should be noted that *Cryptosporidium* only stains acid-fast on fresh smears and not in

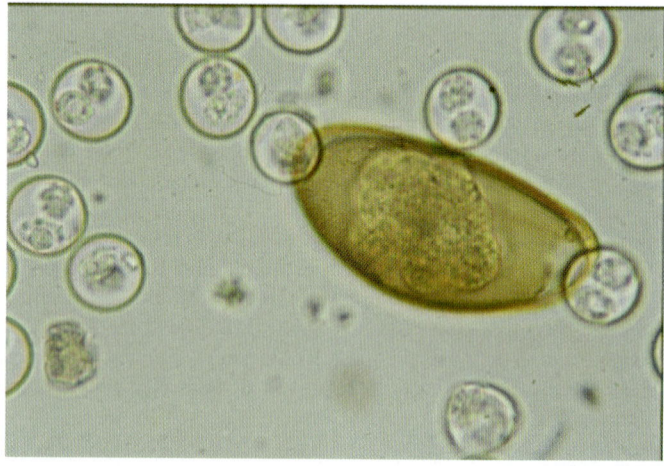

FIG 32.8 *Isospora amphiboluri* from a bearded dragon (*Pogona vitticeps*). A pinworm egg is also pictured in the center (larger, yellow color). Photomicrograph magnification, 400×. (Courtesy of Ellis Greiner.)

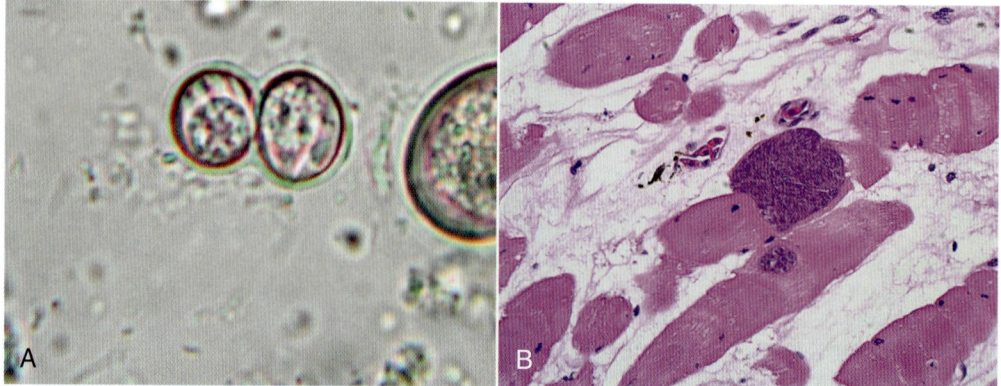

FIG 32.9 (A) *Sarcocystis* sp. sporocyst. Photomicrograph magnification, 400×. (B) *Sarcocystis* sarcocysts in the muscle of a pancake tortoise (*Malacochersus tornieri*). Photomicrograph magnification, 600×. (A, Courtesy of Heather Walden; B, courtesy of Ellis Greiner.)

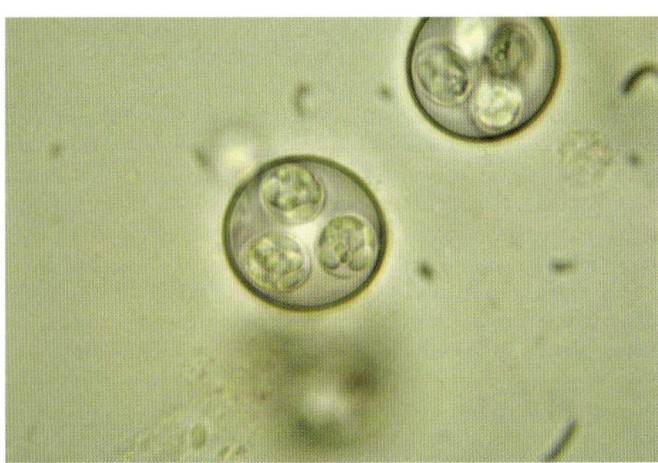

FIG 32.10 *Eimeria tokayae* from a tokay gecko (*Gekko gecko*). Photomicrograph magnification, 1000×.

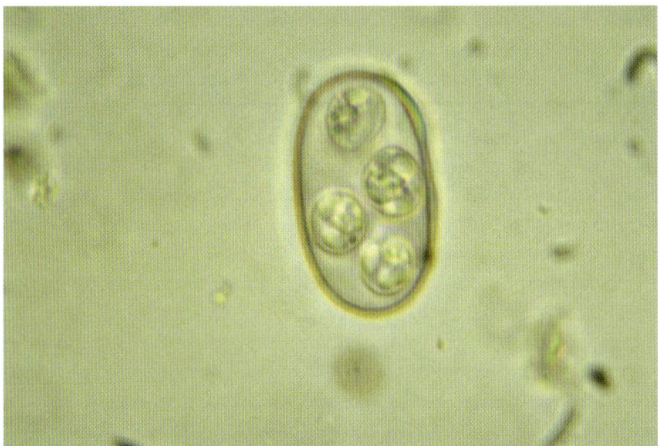

FIG 32.11 *Eimeria* sp. from a bearded dragon (*Pogona vitticeps*). Photomicrograph magnification, 1000×.

TABLE 32.1	**Generic Oocyst Morphology**	
	Sporocyst No.	**Sporozoites/Sporocyst No.**
Cryptosporidium	0	4/oocyst
Caryospora	1	8
Isospora	2	4
Sarcocystis	2	4[a]
Eimeria	4	2

[a]Oocysts of Sarcocystis rupture while passing through the gut; thus, one typically sees sporulated sporocyst.

formalin-fixed tissues. Oocysts are sporulated and infective when feces is passed. Morphologic species identification is not reliable, and sequence-based techniques are needed to differentiate species.[14] Differentiation of species is especially important because prey items may have *Cryptosporidium* sp. that do not infect reptiles but may pass intact through the gastrointestinal tract and be seen in feces; *C. muris* is commonly seen in rodent-eating reptiles and has no clinical significance for reptiles. Some studies have found *C. muris* to have a higher prevalence in snakes than *C. serpentis*.[15] *Cryptosporidium* sp. vary significantly in their host specificity; some are highly tropic for one host taxon, whereas others have a broad host range.

There are two major clades of *Cryptosporidium;* one is tropic for the stomach and the other is tropic for the intestines. In squamates, the most common gastric species is *C. serpentis*. In chelonians, the most common gastric species is *C. testudinis.*[16] *Cryptosporidium testudinis* has also been reported in ball python (*Python regius*) feces, indicating that squamates may also be susceptible.[16] Neither is known to be zoonotic, although *C. serpentis* has been found in cattle.[17] Gastric cryptosporidiosis often presents with regurgitation. In snakes, gastric thickening may be externally visible.

In squamates, the most common intestinal species is *C. varanii*. This species has also been incorrectly reported in the literature as *C. saurophilum.*[18] In chelonians, the most common intestinal species is *C. ducismarci.*[16] There is comparatively more diversity among intestinal *Cryptosporidium,* with several additional species possibly present.[19] Intestinal cryptosporidiosis often presents as poor growth or weight loss.

An uncharacterized *Cryptosporidium* has been seen in the ears of green iguanas (*Iguana iguana*), and *Cryptosporidium* avian genotype V has been seen in urinary bladders of the same species.[20,21]

Advanced cryptosporidiosis is typically fatal in reptiles, although subclinical infections may persist without clinical signs. Coinfections with agents such as adenoviruses appear to increase the likelihood of disease manifestation.

Diagnostic samples vary depending on site of infection. For gastric species, gastric biopsies or washes are better samples than feces. For intestinal species, biopsy or feces are preferred. Histopathologic evidence of disease is ideal, and endoscopic biopsies are a good way of obtaining antemortem samples. Organisms may be seen on the apical surface of enterocytes. There are significant gaps in knowledge of antigen cross-reactivity with antibody-based assays, making them unreliable. PCR with sequencing is the current best approach for identification of the etiologic agent.

There are no known effective treatments for cryptosporidiosis in reptiles. Drugs such as paromomycin or nitazoxanide have been used and do not consistently clear infection. Maintenance of a closed group, testing of populations, strict quarantine, and stringent biosecurity practices are the most effective means of prevention. *Cryptosporidium* oocysts are exceptionally stable in the environment; they are not susceptible to ultraviolet disinfection, and even 6% bleach with a 2-hour contact time only resulted in 92.7% reduction. Chloro-m-cresol was more effective.[22]

Eimeriidae. Eimeriidae are intracellular coccidian parasites. They tend to have direct life cycles and are typically transmitted by fecal-oral routes. Important members of this group include *Isospora, Eimeria, Caryospora, Schellackia, Choleoeimeria,* and the intranuclear coccidium of tortoises. Eimeriidae with extraintestinal life stages tend to be associated with more significant disease. Although initial morphologic identification was based on sporulation patterns, use of this has led to errors. Molecular sequence data has shown conclusively that what was formerly considered to be *Isospora,* based on sporulation patterns, consisted of two evolutionarily distinct groups. The presence or absence of Stieda bodies, the use of paratenic hosts, and reptilian or mammalian host specificity, are more phylogenetically informative than number of sporocysts or sporozoites for these genera.[23] The use of sporulation patterns has resulted in paraphyletic definitions of *Caryospora* and *Eimeria* that are widespread across the Eimeriidae.[24]

Caryospora are an eimeriid genus with both direct and indirect life cycles, containing more than 25 species. Oocysts have a single sporocyst with eight sporozoites. Carnivorous birds and other carnivorous reptiles serve as definitive hosts, where *Caryospora* sp. replicate in the intestines. Known intermediate hosts are typically prey mammals, where extraintestinal tissue cysts may be in the skin. Clinical signs in carnivorous reptiles center around enteritis, weight loss, and diarrhea. Management centers around excluding *Caryospora* sp. from collections through quarantine surveillance, disinfection of contaminated areas, and breaking the life cycle by obtaining food animals that are free of *Caryospora*. *Caryospora* have recently been recognized as significant pathogens associated with mortality events in sea turtles.[24]

Eimeria is a diverse eimeriid genus with direct life cycles. Oocysts have four sporocysts, which each contain two sporozoites. Most species replicate in intestinal epithelium. Management centers around excluding *Eimeria* sp. from collections through quarantine surveillance and disinfection of contaminated areas. *Eimeria* tend to be very host specific, and host-jumping between distantly related reptile taxa is rare. However, there are potential concerns for transmission between more closely related taxa. Coinfections with agents such as adenoviruses may play significant roles in disease manifestation. Infections in otherwise healthy adult animals are often subclinical.

Isospora is a diverse eimeriid genus with direct life cycles. Oocysts have two sporocysts, which each contain four sporozoites. However, molecular sequence data have shown conclusively that what was formerly considered to be *Isospora*, based on sporulation patterns, consisted of two evolutionarily distinct groups. All former *Isospora* of mammals are members of the Sarcocystinae, and not the Eimeriidae, and were moved into the new genus *Cystoisospora*. All true *Isospora* utilize reptilian hosts, including the Dinosauria (birds). *Isospora amphibolouri* (see Fig. 32.8) is the most common coccidian found in bearded dragons (*Pogona vitticeps*); it is not known to have extraintestinal stages but can cause significant enteritis in young animals.

Schellackia are a group of eimeriid coccidia that have indirect life cycles and infect squamates. Oocysts contain eight naked sporozoites. After undergoing sexual reproduction in the intestine, sporozoites are released into the bloodstream rather than the intestinal lumen, where they infect erythrocytes or lymphocytes. They are then transmitted by hematophagous invertebrates. Because they are not shed in feces, they will not be seen on fecal examination and may be found on blood smears. Because of their indirect life cycle, they are uncommon in captive-bred animals. They are closely related to the sea turtle *Caryospora* and to *Eimeria gruis,* an extraintestinal coccidian of cranes.[24]

Choleoeimeria are eimeriid coccidia that are similar to *Eimeria*, but endogenous development occurs in biliary epithelium rather than intestinal epithelium. *Choleoeimeria hirbayah* is a significant pathogen of veiled chameleons (*Chamaeleo calyptratus*).[25]

The still-unnamed intranuclear coccidium of tortoises (TINC) is a major tortoise pathogen, especially in Old World tortoises such as radiated tortoises (*Astrochelys radiata*) and leopard tortoises (*Stigmochelys pardalis*), although red-footed tortoises (*Chelonoidis carbonaria*) have also been infected.[26] Detections thus far have been restricted to hosts in the superfamily Testudinoidea, with most reports in the family Testudinidae (tortoises). TINC has also been identified in the members of the families Emydidae (Eastern box turtle [*Terrapene carolina*]) and Geoemydidae (Arakan forest turtle [*Heosemys depressa*]).[27]

TINC is often multisystemic, infecting epithelial cells, and can be associated with lymphoplasmacytic, or mixed inflammation, and variable necrosis and epithelial hyperplasia. Clinical findings in TINC-infected tortoises are nonspecific and may include anorexia, lethargy, weight loss, emaciation, weakness, diarrhea, ocular and nasal discharge, ulcers of the oral or gastrointestinal mucosa, respiratory distress, swollen erythematous vent, and ascites. The course of disease is often very rapid, and mortality rates are high.

The life cycle of TINC is not fully understood. Oocysts have yet to be identified. The organism may be shed cloacally in large amounts in Old World tortoises, but this was not seen in red-footed tortoises.[26]

Surprisingly, the organism was found by qPCR in the blood of affected red-footed tortoises but was not found in cloacal swabs, which is the opposite of what is seen in Old World tortoises.

Antemortem diagnosis of TINC was first achieved through PCR of nasal lavages from Sulawesi tortoises (*Indotestudo forstenii*) with rhinosinusitis.[28] A quantitative polymerase chain reaction assay (qPCR) targeting a unique region from the TINC 18S rRNA gene was developed to be specific for TINC and can detect as few as 10 copies of target DNA.[27]

Treatment of intranuclear coccidiosis with ponazuril is possible. The clinical signs of treated animals often improve with ponazuril, but follow-up testing often reveals shedding of the organism. This may be because ponazuril is more active against actively dividing parasites and may not affect encysted latent organisms. Pharmacokinetic data show low oral bioavailability but a very long half-life of ponazuril in red-footed tortoises.[29]

Two additional unnamed coccidia in the Eimeriidae have been found in the adrenal glands of leatherback sea turtles (*Dermochelys coriacea*) in the Atlantic.[30] They were associated with lesions in the adrenal glands of 100% of 17 adult and subadult turtles, although none of the four juvenile turtles had lesions or parasites detected.

Sarcocystidae. Sarcocystidae contains several different genera, not all of which have proven to be valid when further examined. The clinically relevant genera in reptile hosts include *Sarcocystis*, *Besnoitia*, and *Toxoplasma*. Sarcocystidae typically have obligate indirect life cycles, although some species may be facultatively direct in their definitive hosts. Reptiles may be intermediate, definitive, or both hosts, depending on the parasite. Host fidelity is typically higher, and pathology is less significant in definitive hosts.

Sarcocystis are a sarcocystid genus containing more than 120 known species. Oocysts have two sporocysts with four sporozoites (see Fig. 32.9A), similar to *Isospora* in the Eimeriidae. Carnivorous or omnivorous vertebrates serve as definitive hosts, where *Sarcocystis* sp. replicate in the intestines. Clinical disease in definitive hosts centers around enteritis, with weight loss and diarrhea the most common signs. Definitive host ranges tend to be more limited than intermediate host ranges. Intermediate hosts are prey animals, where initial stages replicate in blood vessels, followed by development of sarcocysts in tissues, commonly muscle (see Fig. 32.9B). Sarcocysts are often grossly visible and may appear as white streaks in muscle. The most significant disease is seen in intermediate hosts, where signs may include depression and sudden death. Induction of disease in intermediate hosts may make predation more likely, completing the parasite's life cycle. There is zoonotic potential for humans to serve as intermediate hosts for *Sarcocystis* sp., with snakes as definitive hosts.[31] Management centers around excluding *Sarcocystis* sp. from collections through separation of definitive hosts and their feces from intermediate hosts and, for carnivorous/omnivorous reptiles, exclusion of potential other intermediate hosts that may be ingested.

Besnoitia is a sarcocystid genus with a facultatively indirect life cycle. In intermediate hosts, meronts develop in mesenchymal cells forming cysts. Various squamate species have been reported to serve as intermediate hosts, although further characterization to species has not been done.[32]

Toxoplasma is a sarcocystid genus with a facultatively indirect life cycle, containing one species, *T. gondii*. Cats are the definitive hosts. *Toxoplasma gondii* has very little specificity for intermediate hosts and is a zoonotic disease. All amniote species should be considered susceptible intermediate hosts; those that ingest other intermediate hosts or cat feces are at greater risk, and infection has been best characterized in vipers and cobras from areas with higher temperatures.[33] Management centers around excluding *T. gondii* from collections through exclusion of cats and cat feces and, for carnivorous/omnivorous reptiles, exclusion of potential other intermediate hosts that may be ingested.

Excavata

The Excavata are a clade of eukaryotes that are often flagellated, may lack mitochondria, and often have a ventral feeding groove. Within the Excavata, the superclass Fornicata, superclass Parabasalea, and phylum Euglenozoa contain the most relevant reptile parasites.

Fornicata (*Giardia, Hexamita*).
The excavate superclass Fornicata contains the Diplomonadida, which contains the family Hexamitinae. The Hexamitinae are flagellates that have two nuclei and lack true mitochondria, although they may have homologous mitosomes that do not synthesize ATP. The most clinically relevant organisms within the Hexamitinae are the genera *Giardia*, *Spironucleus*, and *Hexamita*.

All parasites in this group have direct life cycles. Although *Giardia* are significant enteric pathogens in mammals, their pathological role in reptiles, including the birds, is not as well established. The mammal pathogen *G. duodenalis* was found in 16% of wild lizards in Europe; although disease associated with this organism has not been reported in lizards, it is of significant zoonotic concern.[34] *Giardia* is a graceful swimmer, and on a direct smear as it rolls over, one can see the concave sucking disc (Fig. 32.12).

The genus *Hexamita* contains significant but poorly understood reptile pathogens. Reported clinical disease caused by *Hexamita* sp. is typically tubulointerstitial nephritis, leading to renal failure and death.[35] Disease is most commonly seen in chelonians but also occurs in squamates. They are thought to have direct life cycles, and renal infection is thought to ascend from the cloaca.

Diagnosis of hexamitiasis is challenging; there is a lack of clinically applicable molecular diagnostic assays for these agents. *Hexamita* is smaller than other flagellates, usually less than 8 microns in length, and quickly swims directly out of the field of view at high magnifications (Fig. 32.13). Current disease reports have been based on morphological diagnosis of binucleate flagellates lacking the disc structure seen with *Giardia* or *Spironucleus*. Controlled studies on treatment of hexamitiasis in reptiles are lacking; metronidazole has been found to be effective for treatment of *H. salmonis* in rainbow trout.[36]

Parabasalea (*Monocercomonas*).
The excavate superclass Parabasalea are flagellates, often associated with animal gut flora. They have single nuclei, are anaerobic, and lack mitochondria and a feeding groove. The best studied reptile pathogen in this clade is *Monocercomonas colubrorum*,

in the order Tritrichomonadida. However, it is probable that there is significant diversity still to be identified.

Monocercomonas has a stiff axostyle running its length, three anterior flagella, and a single trailing flagellum. *Monocercomonas colubrorum* is a significant disease in squamates, where it causes enteritis.[37] Large numbers of flagellates are seen on a fresh fecal wet mount in saline. Morphological identification led to significant misclassification of the Parabasalea, especially the family Monocercomonadidae, and sequence data is more reliable.[38] An in situ hybridization (ISH) assay has been developed for diagnosis of *M. colubrorum*, and it was found in 34 of 182 (19%) snakes with enteritis, a greater proportion than was found for *Cryptosporidium* (4%) or *Entamoeba* (7%).[39]

Controlled data on treatment of *M. colubrorum* is lacking, but Tritrichomonadida tend to be responsive to metronidazole.[40] Pharmacokinetic data is available in squamates.[41]

Euglenozoa (*Trypanosoma, Leishmania*).
The excavate superclass Euglenozoa are flagellates. The medically significant members are in the order Kinetoplastida. Kinetoplastida have a kinetoplast, a large mitochondrion near the flagellar basal body. Within the Kinetoplastida, the family Trypanosomatidae contains the genera *Trypanosoma* and *Leishmania*, which both contain significant human hemoparasitic pathogens that are primarily insect-vectored.

The genus *Trypanosoma* have a single flagellum. They cause significant human diseases, including African sleeping sickness and Chagas disease. They typically have an indirect life cycle, utilizing insects as intermediate hosts, although some *Trypanosoma* sp. found in aquatic reptiles are vectored.[42] However, *T. equiperdum*, the agent of dourine in horses, is primarily transmitted through direct contact, usually sexual.

Trypanosoma brucei, the causative agent of African sleeping sickness and a close relative of *T. equiperdum*,[43] has been found to successfully infect Nile monitors (*Varanus niloticus*), and there is serologic evidence wild monitors may be infected.[44] The vectors for *T. brucei* are tsetse flies (*Glossina* sp.), and *G. fuscipes* was found in one study to take up to 27% of its blood meals from Nile monitors.[45] The import of wild-caught Nile monitors is still common, and the potential for zoonotic disease should be considered. Although tsetse flies are not yet endemic outside of Africa, veterinarians may be at higher risk for contact with blood.

There are very limited data on pathology of *Trypanosoma* sp. in reptiles. *T. therezieni*, found in short-horned chameleons (*Calumma brevicorne*), was experimentally inoculated into carpet chameleons (*Furcifer lateralis*). Infected carpet chameleons died within 11 to 18 days with high levels of parasitemia.[46] It is probable that trypansomes

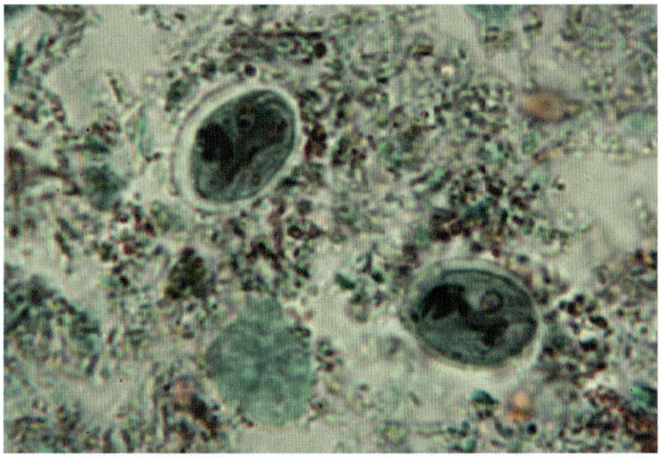

FIG 32.12 *Giardia lamblia.* (Courtesy of F.L. Frye.)

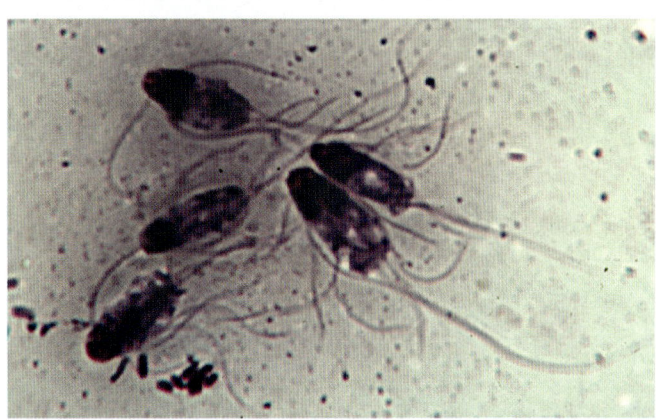

FIG 32.13 *Hexamita* from *Clemmys marmorata.* (Courtesy of F.L. Frye.)

will be most pathogenic in nonendemic hosts that are closely enough related to their adapted endemic hosts for trypanosomes to infect but have not yet had selection on their populations by the given parasite. Diagnosis of trypanosomiasis in reptiles is currently based on visualization of trypomastigotes in stained blood smears. Molecular identification by PCR and sequencing is needed for species identification.

Data on treatment of trypanosomiasis in reptiles are lacking. Antitrypanosomal drugs tend to be toxic, and different drugs are used in humans for African sleeping sickness and Chagas disease. In one author's experience, use of eflornithine in an African side-necked turtle (*Pelusios* sp.) was rapidly followed by death, consistent with toxicosis.

Leishmania is a genus in the family Trypanosomatidae with indirect life cycles that are transmitted by sandflies. The motile promastigote stage develops in the sandfly vector, and amastigotes, lacking flagella, reproduce in the vertebrate host. In reptiles, reproduction typically occurs in erythrocytes. Although organisms from reptile hosts were formerly considered as a separate genus, *Sauroleishmania,* sequence data has shown this to be incorrect. A *Leishmania* isolated from a plated lizard has been shown to cause cutaneous leishmaniasis in mice.[47] There has been a long relationship between *Leishmania* and reptiles; nucleated red cells in the gut of sandflies in early Cretaceous amber contain organisms morphologically consistent with *Leishmania.*[48] Despite the fact that leishmaniasis causes 20,000 to 40,000 human deaths per year,[49] there has been no published investigation of disease in reptiles.

Amoebozoa (*Entamoeba*)

The Amoebozoa are a clade of eukaryotes with trophozoites that primarily move by extension of pseudopods and whose primary mode of nutrition is phagocytosis. They are not the only clade with these characteristics (e.g., *Naegleria* is not in the Amoebozoa), and some members do have flagellar motion. They appear to be the closest relatives of the Opisthokonta, the clade containing fungi and animals. Diverse members of the Amoebozoa are found in association with reptile gastro-intestinal tracts, including *Rhizomastix, Hartmannella, Echinamoeba,* and *Acanthamoeba.*

Entamoeba Invadens. The taxon most strongly associated with disease in reptiles is *Entamoeba,* and *E. invadens* is the best-characterized reptile pathogen in the genus. This organism has a direct life cycle, and transmission is through fecal-oral route. Disease due to *E. invadens* presents as necrotic enteritis and hepatitis. Signs include lethargy, depression, hematochezia, and death. The life cycle of *E. invadens* consists of a motile trophozoite and a more environmentally stable cyst (Fig. 32.14).

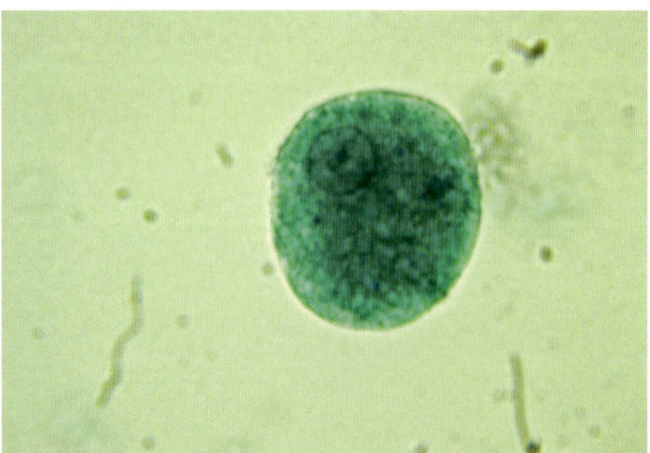

FIG 32.14 Amoeba, *Entamoeba invadens* trophozoite. Photomicrograph magnification, 1000×.

Although disease often presents more dramatically in squamates than in chelonians or crocodilians, chelonians are certainly susceptible to disease, and all nonavian reptiles should be considered at risk.

Diagnosis is often made based on trichrome staining and morphologic characterization; however, many species can potentially be present and, combined with poor sample quality, may hinder identification. Molecular sequencing has also found *E. terrapinae, E. insolita, E. barreti, E. testudinis,* and *E. ranarum* in reptiles.[50] Unfortunately, the sensitivity of currently described PCR techniques is rather poor, and improved methods are needed. Amplification of nonspecific products is common with available methods, and all PCR products should be identified by sequencing.

The most important component of therapy for *E. invadens* is temperature manipulation. In experimentally inoculated snakes, snakes that were maintained at 13°C, 33°C, and 35°C did not develop clinical disease. However, snakes kept at 25°C consistently died with clinical disease.[51,52] Metronidazole is also commonly used for treatment of *E. invadens.*[41] For species with appropriate thermal tolerances, the author treats *E. invadens* by raising enclosure temperatures to a minimum of 33°C for 60 days and administering metronidazole at 20 mg/kg PO daily.

METAZOAN PARASITES

The Metazoa are multicellular animals. They cluster with fungi in the clade Opisthokonta. Reptile parasites are largely found in the Bilateria, animals with bilateral symmetry. Within the Bilateria, reptiles and other vertebrates fall within the Deuterostomia, and metazoan parasites of reptiles fall within the Protostomia. In the Protostomia, the important reptile parasites are found within the Platythelminthes, Annelida, Lophotrochozoa, and Ecdysozoa.

Platyhelminthes

The Platyhelminthes are acoelomate flatworms, with no specialized circulatory or respiratory organs and a single opening into the digestive cavity. Platyhelminth parasites of reptiles are found in the Trematoda, Cestoda, and Monogenea.

Trematoda (Flukes). The Trematoda are composed of the Digenea and the Aspidogastrea. Trematodes have obligate indirect life cycles, although aspidogastrans do not asexually reproduce as larvae in intermediate hosts.

Aspidogastrean trematodes have the ventral surface subdivided as a holdfast organ. Most of these are parasites of molluscs, but a few species are gastrointestinal parasites of turtles. They are not usually associated with significant pathology.

Digeneans are commonly found in all groups of reptiles, and some are extremely pathogenic. They are the most diverse group of trematodes (Figs. 32.15 through 32.21). All digeneans require at least one intermediate host to complete their cycles, and some require two or more. These live in nearly every soft tissue organ in the body of their reptilian hosts, although most reside in the gastrointestinal tract. They all have the potential to alternate between generations of sexual and asexual reproduction. The former occurs in the definitive host, and the latter occurs in the first intermediate host, which is normally a mollusc. Some use terrestrial gastropods for their intermediate hosts and are therefore not tied to an aquatic habitat.

Other digenetic trematodes need aquatic snails for their first intermediate host, and thus flukes have different potentials to be found in captive reptilian collections kept in natural settings. Many digenetic trematodes are associated with little or no pathology in definitive hosts. The presence of trematodes attached to the oral mucosa and esophagus may be more of an esthetic concern than a medical problem. These

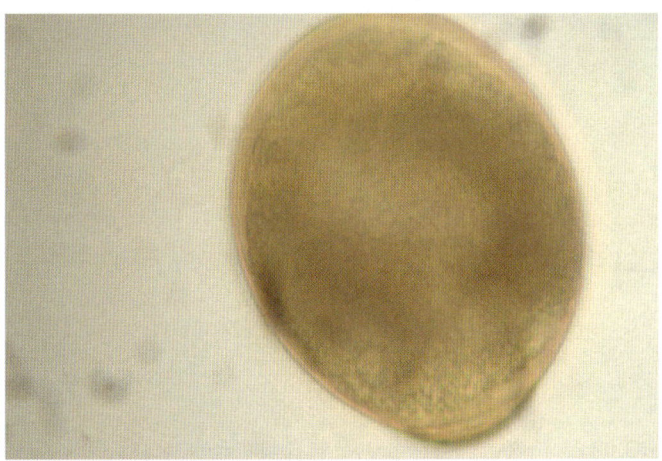

FIG 32.15 *Nematophila* sp. egg from a yellow-footed tortoise (*Chelonoidis denticulata*). Photomicrograph magnification, 400×.

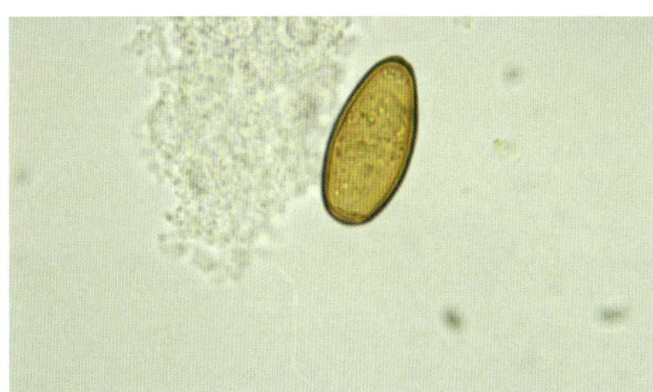

FIG 32.18 *Enodiotrema* sp. from a loggerhead sea turtle (*Caretta caretta*). Photomicrograph magnification, 400×.

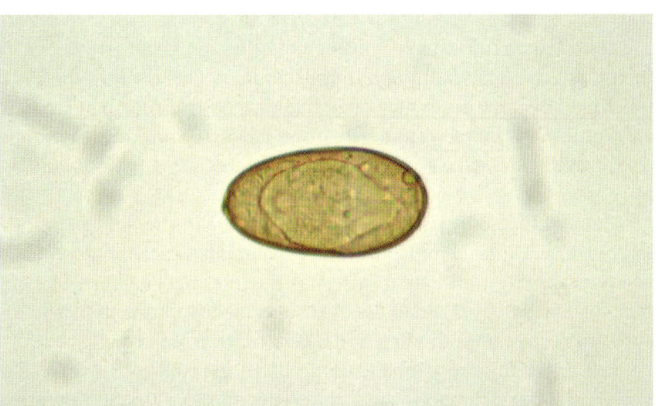

FIG 32.16 *Euparadistomum* sp. from a green-eyed gecko (*Gekko smithii*). Photomicrograph magnification, 400×.

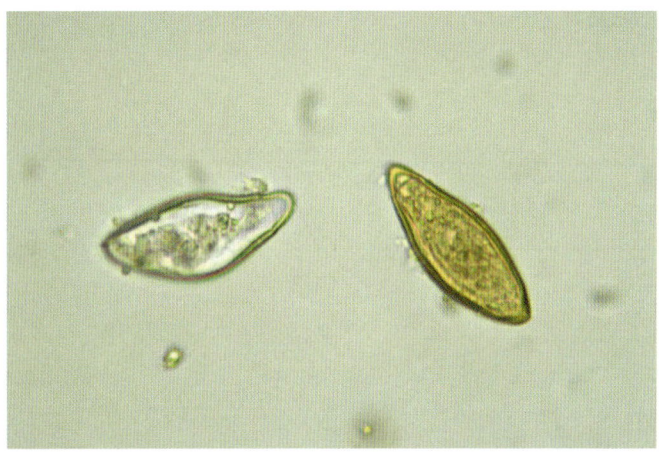

FIG 32.19 *Pachypsolus irroratus* from a loggerhead sea turtle (*Caretta caretta*). Photomicrograph magnification, 400×.

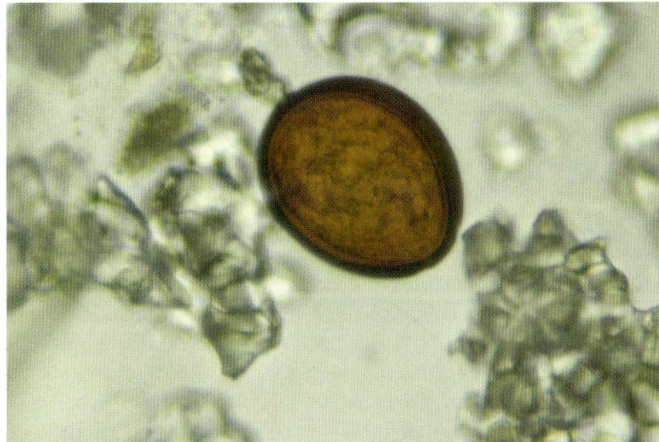

FIG 32.17 *Orchidasma amphiorchis* from a loggerhead sea turtle (*Caretta caretta*). Photomicrograph magnification, 400×.

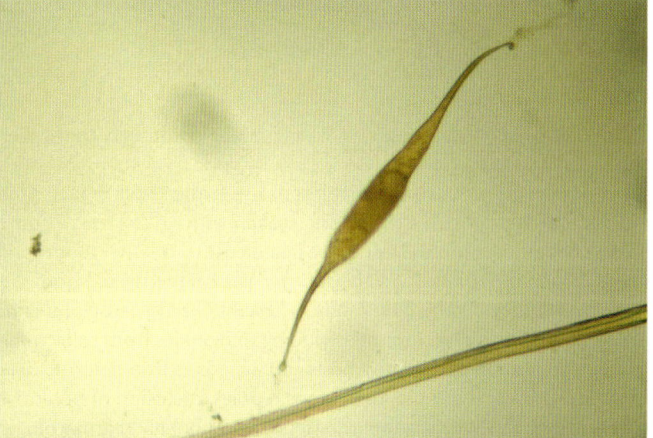

FIG 32.20 *Hapalotrema loossi* from a loggerhead sea turtle (*Caretta caretta*). Photomicrograph magnification, 400×.

flukes include *Haplometroides, Ochetosoma, Pneumatophilus, Stomatrema,* and *Zeugorchis.* They are acquired by eating a vertebrate second intermediate host containing encysted metacercariae.

Spirorchiidae, a family of flukes whose adults live in blood vessels and the heart, are pathogenic. To disseminate eggs from the blood, the eggs are trapped in capillary beds and then worked passively through the host tissue into the gut, where they are then shed in the feces. Adults or eggs may be numerous enough to block smaller vessels (capillaries), causing ischemia and tissue damage. Eggs that leave the gut may also be trapped by the host and form granulomas. These can be found in most soft tissues of the body, and the more of these that develop in an organ, the less functional that organ becomes.[53] Marine turtles are most

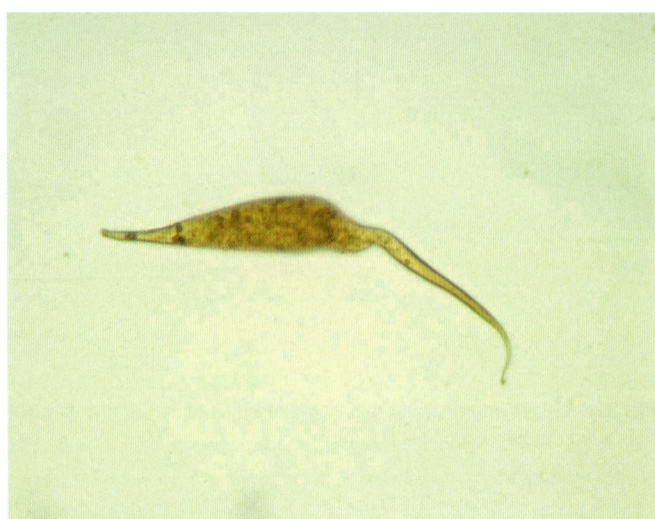

FIG 32.21 *Learedius learedi* from a green sea turtle (*Chelonia mydas*). Photomicrograph magnification, 400×.

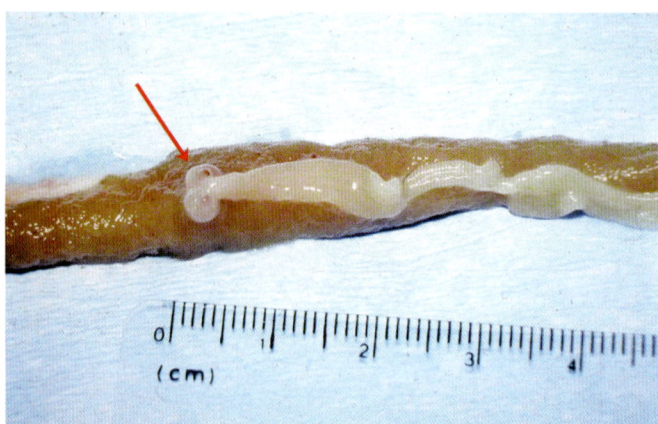

FIG 32.23 *Bothridium* sp. tapeworm in the intestine of a ball python (*Python regius*). Note the scolex on the left side of the photograph (arrow). (Courtesy of Stephen Barten.)

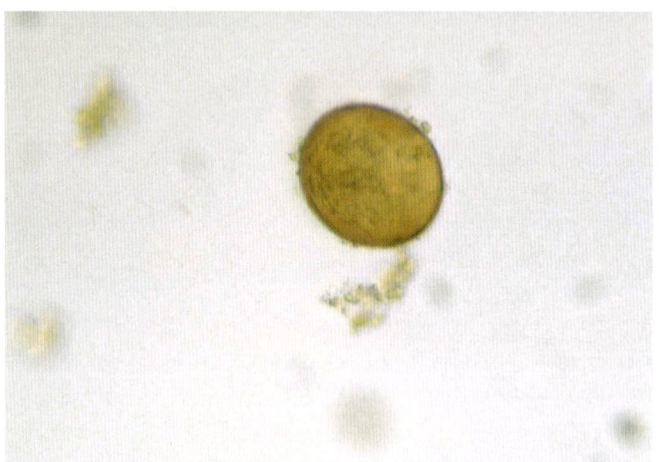

FIG 32.22 *Neospirorchis* sp. from a loggerhead sea turtle (*Caretta caretta*). Photomicrograph magnification, 400×.

commonly affected by these flukes (Fig. 32.22), although freshwater turtles may also be affected.[54]

Other flukes, such as *Styphlodora* spp., live in the urinary tract. This is a common parasite in free-ranging snakes, with up to 66% of some snake populations infected. A captive boa died after about 6 months of anorexia, and the adults of *Styphlodora horrida* were recovered from the preserved kidneys.[55] The flukes were believed to be the cause of death.

Management centers around excluding trematodes from collections through separation of definitive hosts and their feces from intermediate hosts and, for carnivorous/omnivorous reptiles, exclusion of potential other intermediate hosts that may be ingested. Although pharmacologic therapy with praziquantel is possible, especially with trematodes in viscera such as with spirorchids, the inflammatory response to large numbers of dead trematodes in tissues has the potential to be fatal.

Cestoda (Tapeworms).

Cestodes are platyhelminths with obligate indirect life cycles. They have a scolex (holdfast organ) and a chain of proglottids (repetitive reproductive sections). Each proglottid increases in maturity as they move farther from the scolex with budding of new sections. The adults reside in the small intestine of their definitive host (Fig. 32.23). Tapeworms parasitize all groups of reptiles.

Cestodes are not usually considered to be significant pathogens in their definitive hosts, although they can outcompete the host for basic nutrients, and heavy loads may cause intestinal obstruction. In intermediate reptile hosts, larval cestodes are often subcutaneous, causing bumps or ridges in the skin, and make a reptile less attractive for display purposes.

Many of the adult tapeworms of reptiles are in the families Anoplocephalidae, Diphyllobothriidae, and Proteocephalidae. Anoplocephalidae typically use a mite or an insect as the intermediate host. The life cycle of Diphyllobothriidae uses two intermediate hosts, typically an aquatic crustacean as the first and a vertebrate as the second.

The eggs of Proteocephalidae are eaten by copepods, where the procercoid larva develops, and these are infective to the definitive host, where they develop into plerocercoids. These develop in the solid organs, such as the liver. The parasite then wanders through the host, and if it reaches the lumen of the intestine, it attaches and matures. Adult tapeworms may be diagnosed with fecal flotation if the eggs are released from the proglottids or with visualization of free proglottids in the feces and a search for eggs in normal saline solution. All tapeworm eggs (except species of the Diphyllobothriidae) from reptile feces should contain a fully formed oncosphere with six hooks (Figs. 32.24 through 32.30).

Larval tapeworms of *Spirometra* (spargana) may be found in the viscera or subcutaneously in snakes and lizards, and the same is true for the tetrathyridia of *Mesocestoides*. The latter should contain an inverted scolex with four suckers, but this is not always obvious.

Management centers around excluding cestodes from collections through separation of definitive hosts and their feces from intermediate hosts and, for carnivorous/omnivorous reptiles, exclusion of potential other intermediate hosts that may be ingested. Although pharmacologic therapy with praziquantel is possible, especially with larval cestodes in intermediate hosts, the inflammatory response to large numbers of dead cestodes in tissues has the potential to be fatal, and surgical removal may be preferred.

Monogenea. Formerly classified in the Trematoda, the Monogenea are now recognized as phylogenetically distinct platyhelminths. They have direct life cycles and can build to high levels in captivity. Although most are parasites of fish, the family Polystomatidae often utilize aquatic turtles as hosts. Host fidelity is not particularly high, and host-switching from red-eared sliders (*Trachemys scripta*) to Mediterranean pond turtles (*Mauremys leprosa*) has been documented.[56] Adult parasites may be found in the urinary bladder, cloaca, pharynx, and conjunctival sacs of

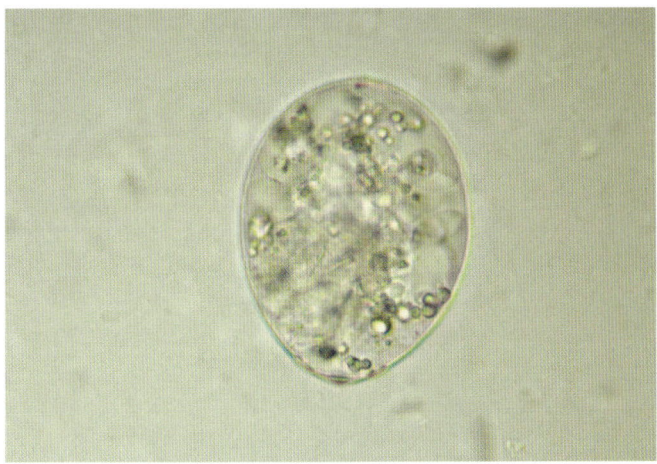

FIG 32.24 Cestode eggs as passed in feces from a python (*Python* sp.). Photomicrograph magnification, 400×.

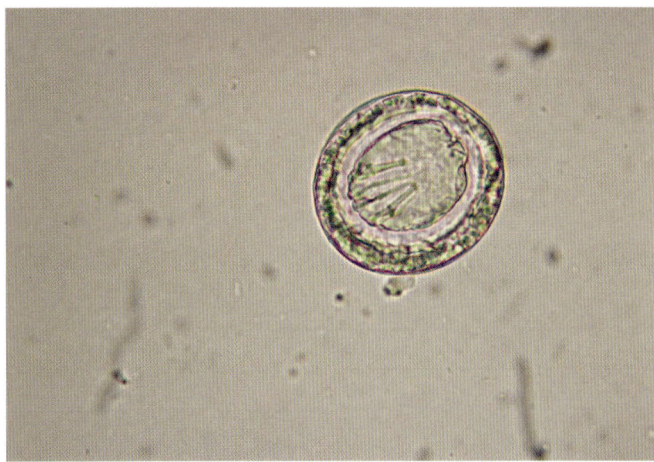

FIG 32.27 Unknown tapeworm egg from a rhinocerous iguana (*Cyclura cyclura*). Photomicrograph magnification, 400×.

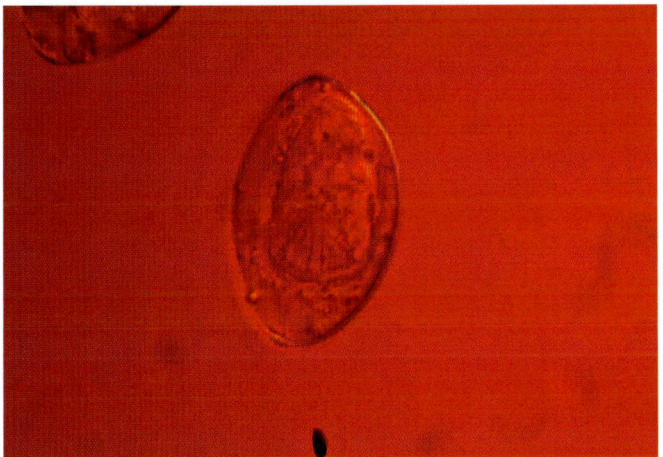

FIG 32.25 Cestode larva from a python (*Python* sp.). Photomicrograph magnification, 400×.

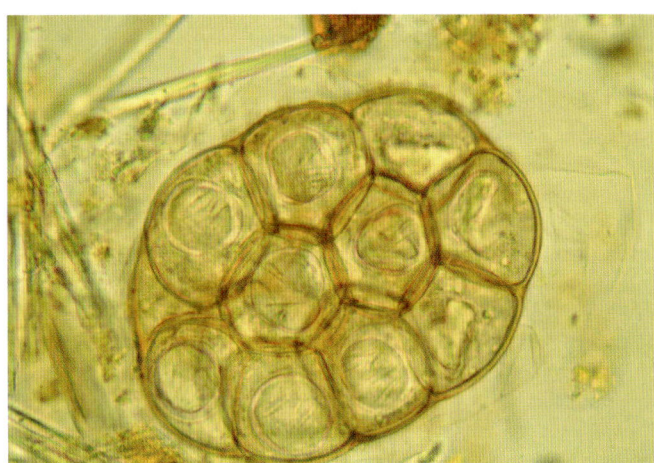

FIG 32.28 Unknown tapeworm egg from a boa *(Boa)*. Photomicrograph magnification, 400×.

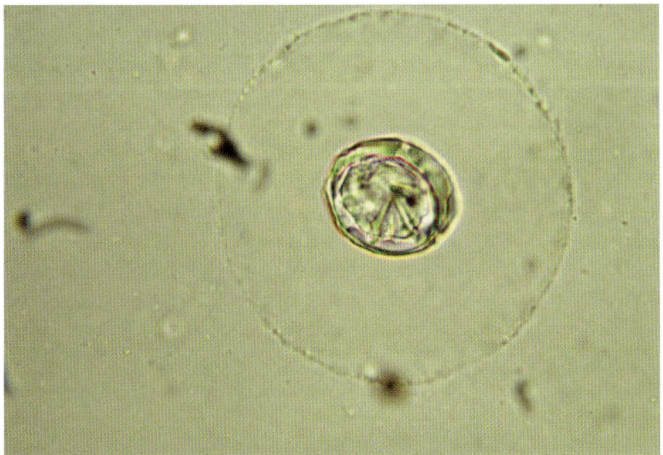

FIG 32.26 *Oochoristica* from a tokay gecko (*Gekko gecko*). Photomicrograph magnification, 400×.

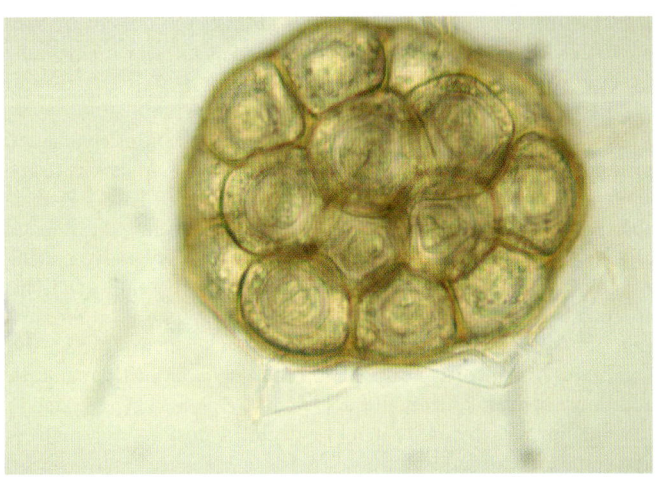

FIG 32.29 Unknown tapeworm egg from a green tree python (*Morelia viridis*). Photomicrograph magnification, 400×.

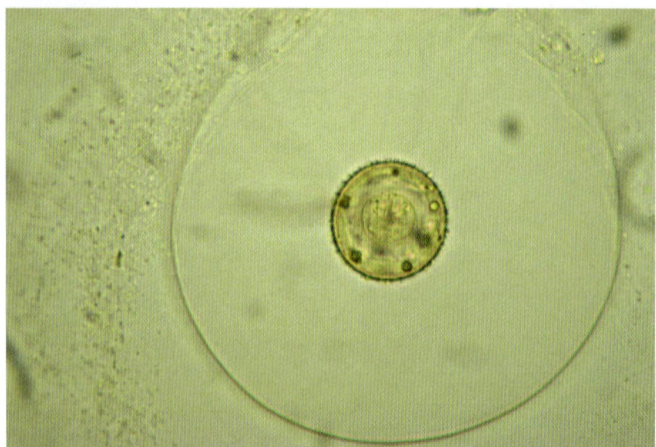

FIG 32.30 Unknown tapeworm egg from a python (*Python* sp.). Photomicrograph magnification, 400×.

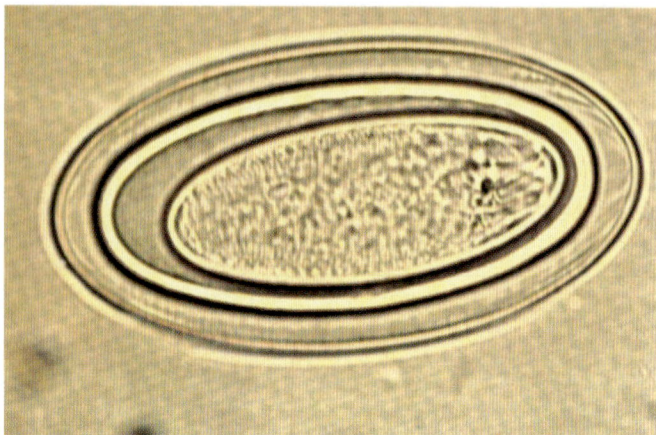

FIG 32.31 Acanthocephalan egg from a monitor lizard *(Varanus)*. Note the multiple layers enclosing the acanthor larva (Courtesy of F.L. Frye.)

fresh-water turtles. Treatment by manual removal is often possible, and use of praziquantel may also be effective. Environmental decontamination is essential, because free swimming oncomiracidia can build to high levels.

Lophotrochozoa

The Lophotrochozoa are a clade in the Protostomia containing molluscs, annelids, rotifers, and acanthocephalans. They are a sister group to the platyhelminths.

Annelida (Leeches). Annelids are a phylum in the Lophotrochozoa and are commonly known as segmented worms. Most annelids are free-living organisms, but the subclass Hirudinea, the leeches, has a number of parasitic members. These hematophagous annelids are found on aquatic reptiles such as turtles and crocodilians. The leeches on American alligators (*A. mississippiensis*) are *Placobdella multilineata* and *P. papillifera*.[57,58] They are able to transmit hemogregarines, such as *Haemogregarina crocodilinorum*.[59] Infestations of large numbers of leeches have been reported to cause anemia in young crocodilians.

When leeches feed on aquatic animals, the resultant lesion may allow secondary bacteria to invade and establish infections. Marine leeches (*Ozobranchus margoi*) can be found in massive numbers on green sea turtles (*Chelonia mydas*), Atlantic hawksbill (*Eretomochelys imbricata*), loggerhead sea turtles (*Caretta caretta*), and Atlantic ridleys (*Lepidochelys kempi*). High populations of this leech usually are seen on severely emaciated turtles. Treatment by manual removal is typically the best way to deal with leech infestations.

Acanthocephala (Thorny-Headed Worms). Acanthocephala is a phylum in the Lophotrochozoa. They are most closely related to the rotifers. Adults live within the small intestines. They have a retractable proboscis armed with spines that is inserted into the mucosa as a holdfast. They have separate sexes and lack a digestive system. Acanthocephalans have indirect life cycles. The eggs of acanthocephalans are usually complex, with multiple layers enclosing the acanthor larva (Fig. 32.31). The first intermediate host is usually an arthropod, and within this intermediate host it matures to a cystacanth. There may be additional paratenic hosts, and cystacanth larvae may be encysted in the abdominal cavity until eaten by a definitive host, when it matures and embeds in the gut wall.

Eggs of some acanthocephalan species may rise on fecal flotation, but most must be detected with a sedimentation procedure. *Neoechi-*

norhychus sp. are seen in emydid turtles; *Bolbosoma* sp. and *Rhadinorhynchus* sp. have been reported in sea turtles; and *Acanthocephalus* sp., *Centrorhynchus* sp., *Corynosoma* sp., *Oligacanthorhynchus* sp., *Oncicola* sp., *Pseudoacanthocephalus* sp., and *Sphaerirostris* sp. have been reported in squamates. The proboscis often embeds deeply into the gut wall, causing significant pathology.

Management centers around excluding acanthocephalans from collections through separation of definitive hosts and their feces from intermediate hosts and, for carnivorous/omnivorous reptiles, exclusion of potential other intermediate hosts that may be ingested. Acanthocephalans do not typically respond well to most anthelminthic drugs. Loperamide, normally thought of as an antidiarrheal drug, has shown activity at high doses against acanthocephalans in pigs and ray-finned fish and may have application for treatment of acanthocephalans in reptiles.[60,61] Surgical removal is also an option.

Ecdysozoa

The Ecdysozoa are a clade of Protostomes whose members all grow by ecdysis, shedding their exoskeletons. Important reptile parasite groups in the Ecdysozoa include nematodes, arthropods, and pentastomids.

Nematoda. The phylum Nematoda has more than 25,000 described species, with much more undescribed diversity likely present. They are commonly called roundworms. More than half of known species are parasitic, and hosts include all orders of reptiles. They may have either direct or indirect life cycles. They have separate sexes and complete digestive systems. The two classes within the phylum are the Chromadorea and the Enoplea.

The effects of most nematodes are unknown, and many could be neutral or even beneficial in their influence on their hosts, depending on context. Nematodes are the most diverse group of helminths that infect reptiles. Some produce eggs, some release first stage (L1) larvae, and some produce microfilariae that are motile embryos. Those that produce eggs shed in feces are diagnosed with fecal flotation, and those that release larvae into the gastrointestinal tract are easily diagnosed with a Baermann funnel or fecal sedimentation. These larvae do float but may be greatly distorted by the flotation medium. Nematodes that produce microfilariae can be seen in the blood by direct smear or Modified Knott's.

Pharmacologic treatment of nematodes typically uses four classes of drugs: avermectins, benzimidazoles, pyrantel, or octadepsipeptides. Avermectins, such as ivermectin or selamectin, kill the worm by binding to glutamate receptors; the drugs are normally excluded from receptors in the brain by the blood-brain barrier. However, in turtles and crocodilians, the blood-brain barrier is less effective at excluding avermectins, and there is a greater risk of toxicity. Benzimidazoles work by binding to tubulin, interfering with cytoskeletal structure. For the host, this has greatest implications for rapidly dividing cells, and some benzimidazoles may have significant effects on bone marrow and gut epithelium; heterophil numbers drop quickly after high doses.[62] Pyrantel and octodepsipeptides hold promise, but controlled studies in reptiles are lacking.

Strongyloidoidea. The family Rhabdiasidae is in the order Strongyloidoidea, class Chromadorea, and includes the genera *Rhabdias*, *Serpentirhabdias*, *Pneumonema*, and *Entomelas* (Fig. 32.32).[63] Larvae typically hatch in feces and are seen on fecal examination rather than eggs. Molecular sequence data are usually needed to differentiate species within these genera. All of these genera alternate generationally between the host and a free-living phase, known as heterogony. The genus *Serpentirhabdias* may also have multiple generations of parthenogenetic females in the host, known as homogony.[63] The ability to survive as free-living worms without a host reduces the selective pressure to keep the host alive. Environmental removal is an essential part of addressing *Rhabdias* in a patient. Infective stages can penetrate intact skin and usually move to the lungs, although *Entomelas* may move to the esophagus. Clinical signs often include great quantities of mucus production, pneumonia, and gasping for air. The eggs are larvated when shed by the females, and these may hatch as they exit the host.

The family Strongylidae is in the order Strongyloidoidea, class Chromadorea, and includes the genus *Strongyloides* (Fig. 32.33). These should not be confused with the similarly named hookworm suborder Strongylida, which is not closely related. *Strongyloides* alternate generationally between the host and a free-living phase. The ability to survive as free-living worms without a host reduces the selective pressure to keep the host alive. Environmental removal is an essential part of addressing *Strongyloides* in a patient. Infective stages can penetrate intact skin and usually move to the intestine, where they embed in the mucosa. Either larvae or larvated eggs may be seen on fecal examination. Significant enteritis was seen in colubrid snakes (*Liophis miliaris*) experimentally infected with *S. ophidiae*, with resultant mortalities.[64] Four of five experimentally infected snakes died. Interestingly, three of three snakes treated with ivermectin died, whereas only one of two untreated snakes died. Further studies are needed, but it is possible that the inflammatory response to a large burden of dead worms contributed to mortality.

Rhabditida. The suborder Strongylida is in the order Rhabditida, class Chromadorea. The Rhabditida should not be confused with the similarly named family Rhabdiasidae, which is not closely related. Similarly, Strongylida should not be confused with the order Strongyloidoidea, another confusingly similar unrelated group. Life cycles have not been elucidated for most species, but in general, they are direct, with hosts ingesting infective larvae. *Kalicephalus,* found in snakes, can cause significant pathology (Fig. 32.34). They normally reside in the small intestine but have been reported from the mouth and esophagus of snakes (Fig. 32.35). The oral cavity is distinctive (Fig. 32.36), and the males have a prominent copulatory bursa (Fig. 32.37). *Oswaldocruzia* and *Bakeria* are other significant genera in squamates. *Chapiniella* is a genus of strongylids found in New World tortoises (Fig. 32.38).[65] Management of strongylids involves removal of organic substrates that may sustain infective larvae, as well as pharmacologic therapy.

Spirurida. The order Spirurida are in the class Chromadorea. They have indirect life cycles, typically utilizing arthropod intermediate hosts, sometimes with additional vertebrate intermediate hosts. Reptiles may be either definitive or intermediate hosts. Ova, when present, are larvated.

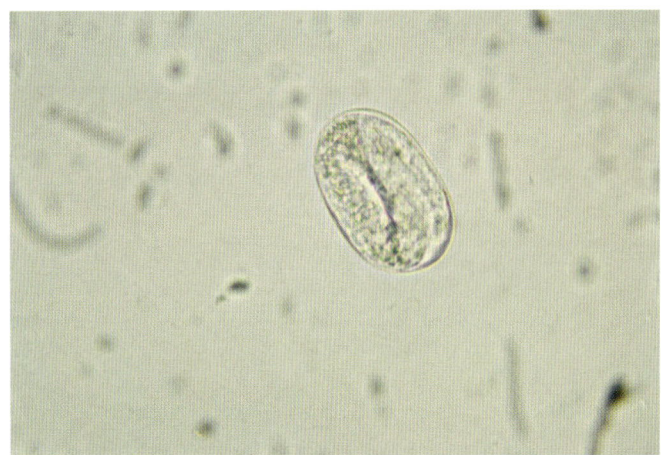

FIG 32.33 Nematode egg from a blue-tailed monitor (*Varanus doreanus*). Photomicrograph magnification, 400×.

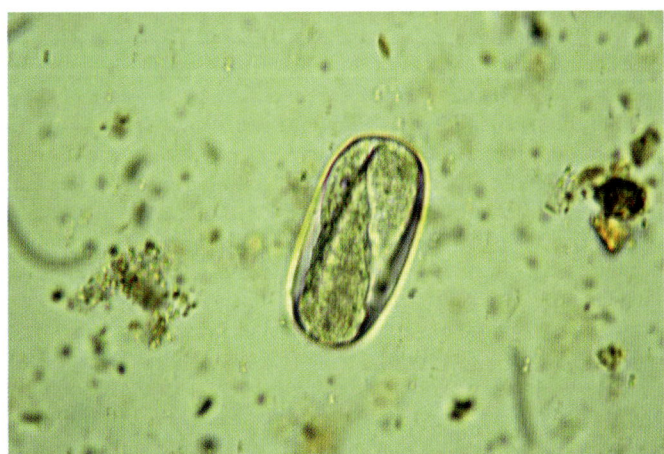

FIG 32.32 Nematode egg (*Rhabdias* sp.) from a corn snake (*Pantherophis guttata*). Photomicrograph magnification, 400×.

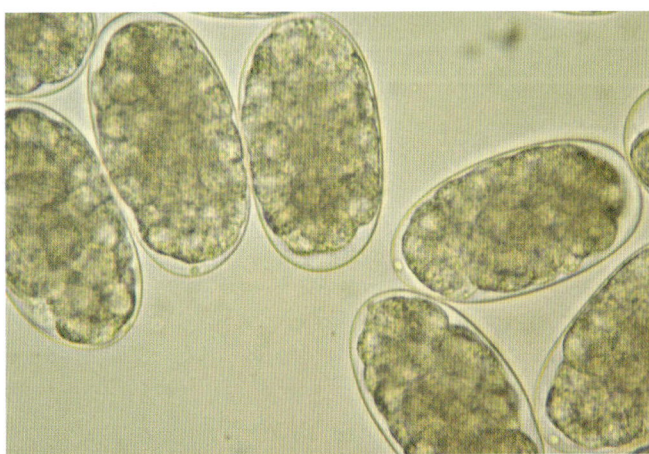

FIG 32.34 *Kalicephalus* sp. eggs from a black racer (*Coluber constrictor*). Photomicrograph magnification, 400×.

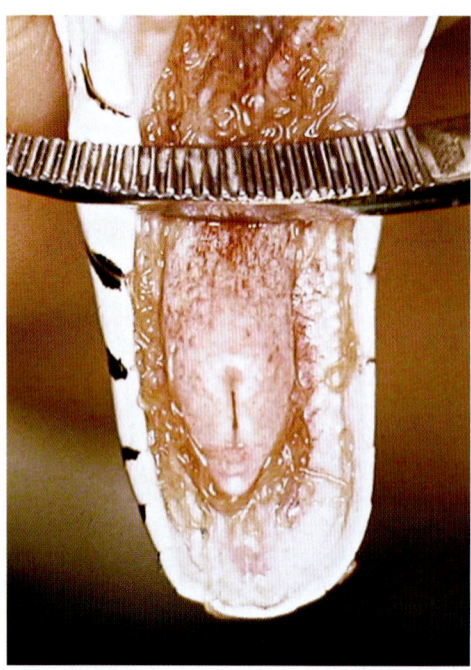

FIG 32.35 *Kalicephalus* sp. larva in the oral cavity of a snake. (Courtesy of Douglas R. Mader.)

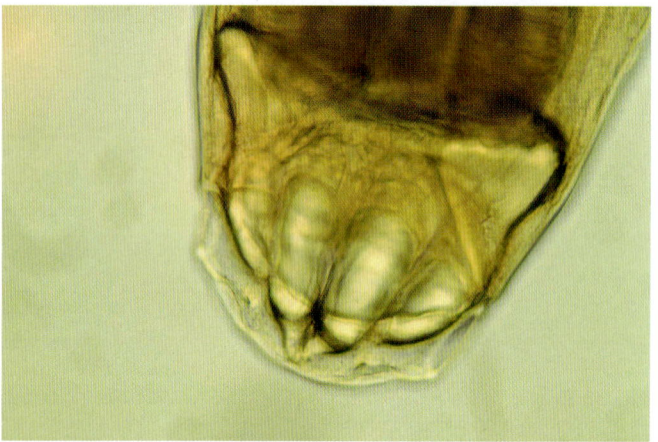

FIG 32.36 *Kalicephalus* sp. anterior end shows the distinctive oral cavity (from *Bothrops* sp.). Photomicrograph magnification, 160×.

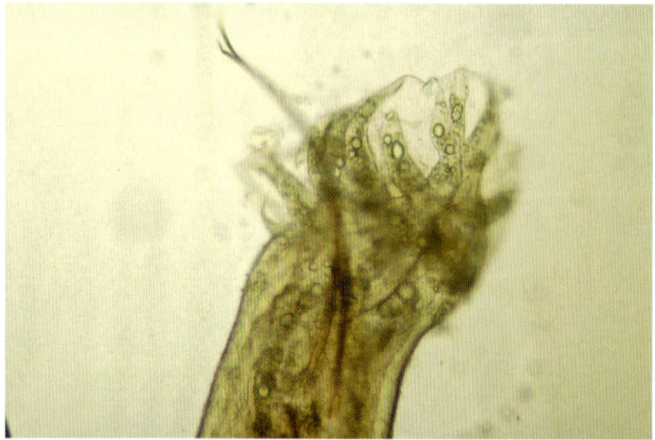

FIG 32.37 *Kalicephalus* sp. prominent copulatory bursa from a black racer (*Coluber constrictor*). Photomicrograph magnification, 100×.

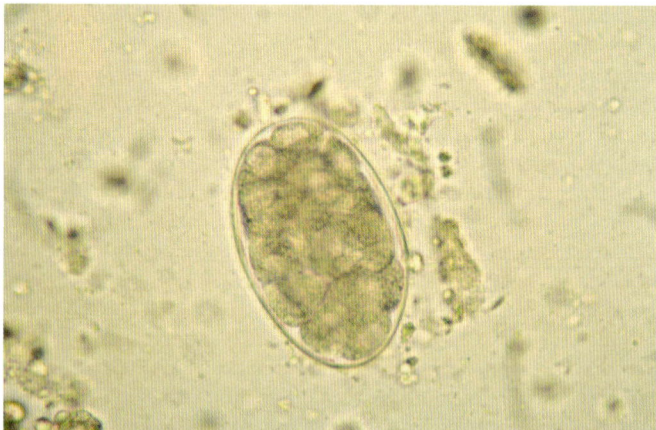

FIG 32.38 *Chapiniella* sp. egg from an ornate box turtle (*Terrapene ornata*). Photomicrograph magnification, 400×.

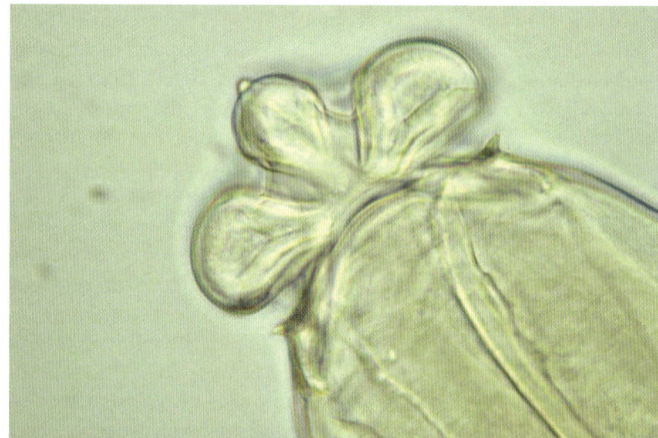

FIG 32.39 Distinctive mouth parts of *Spiroxis* sp. from a freshwater turtle. Photomicrograph magnification, 400×.

The genus *Abbreviata* in the family Physalopteridae and the genus *Tanqua* in the family Gnathostomatidae are commonly found in monitor lizards (*Varanus* sp.), where gastric lesions are seen in definitive hosts.[66,67] It is also common to see encysted larvae in squamates acting as paratenic hosts. *Spiroxys,* in the family Gnathostomatidae, lives in the stomachs of freshwater turtles, where it may cause severe granulomatous lesions (Fig. 32.39).[68] *Serpinema*, in the family Camallanidae, is also common in freshwater turtles and has been associated with pancreatitis due to migrating worms (Fig. 32.40).[69] Management of nonfilarial spirurids centers around excluding them from collections through separation of definitive hosts and their feces from intermediate hosts, and exclusion of arthropod intermediate hosts that may be ingested. Due to their indirect life cycle, they are more typically a problem of wild-caught animals. Although spirurids may be significant pathogens, the presence of potentially large numbers of worms in tissues complicates treatment of intermediate hosts; use of anthelminthics may result in a massive inflammatory response to dead worms. When possible, coelioscopic inspection and removal is advisable before pharmaceutical therapy.

Within the order Spirurida, the superfamily Filarioidea are distinct in that they have larvae that circulate in blood and are vectored by hematophagous arthropods. Adult worms may be in blood vessels, connective tissue, or subcutaneous, and larvae are found circulating in blood. Microfilariae will precipitate to the level of the buffy coat when a microhematocrit tube is spun, and their motion can be seen when

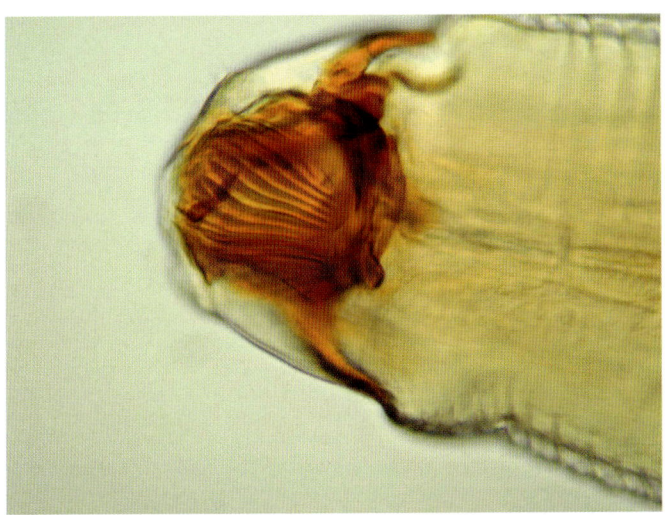

FIG 32.40 *Serpinema* sp. common spirurid from a freshwater turtle. Note the distinctive buccal capsule. Photomicrograph magnification, 160×.

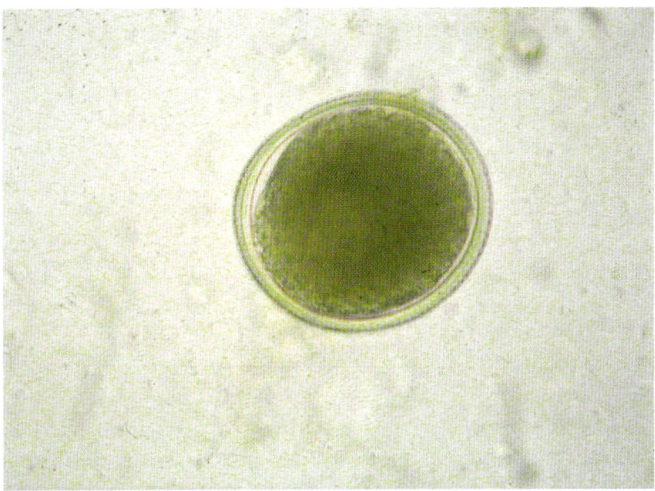

FIG 32.42 *Polydelphis* sp. from a reticulated python (*Malayopython reticulatus*). Photomicrograph magnification, 400×.

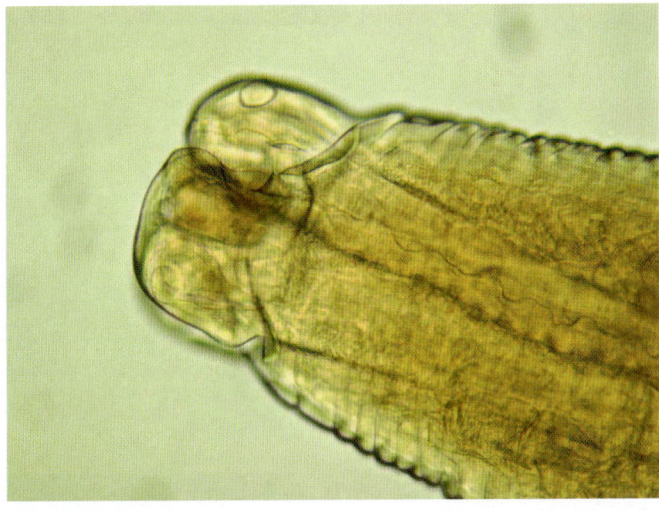

FIG 32.41 Prominent lips on the mouthpart of an ascarid nematode. Photomicrograph magnification, 100×.

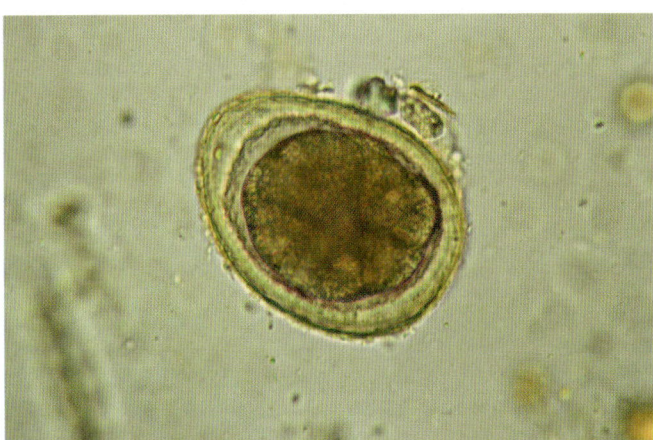

FIG 32.43 *Dujardinascaris* sp. from an American alligator (*Alligator mississippiensis*). Photomicrograph magnification, 400×.

the tube is examined under a microscope. Some genera that use reptile hosts include *Foleyella*, *Macdonaldius*, *Madathamugadia*, and *Oswaldofilaria*. Studies in frilled lizards (*Chlamydosaurus kingii*) found that the presence of *Oswaldofilaria chlamydosauri* was not associated with changes in hematocrit, body condition, or oxygen consumption.[70] A necrotic muscle lesion was attributed to occluded arteries caused by *Macdonaldius*.[71] *Foleyella* adults are often subcutaneous, and surgical removal may be a reasonable option.[72] A chameleon treated with ivermectin for *Foleyella* died, and lesions seen were consistent with an inflammatory response to dead worms.[73] Management of filarial spirurids centers around excluding them from collections through exclusion of hematophagous arthropod intermediate hosts. Due to their indirect life cycle, they are more typically a problem of wild-caught animals. The presence of potentially large numbers of worms in tissues complicates treatment of intermediate hosts; use of anthelminthics may result in a massive inflammatory response to dead worms. When possible, coelioscopic inspection and removal is advisable before pharmaceutical therapy.

Ascaridida. The order Ascaridida in the class Chromadorea contains very large worms that have three prominent lips (Fig. 32.41) and have indirect life cycles. The eggs are large and have pitted or roughened shells. Typically, they may initially utilize a wide range of invertebrate or vertebrate hosts, then are eaten by vertebrates, where they mature in the coelom. If in their definitive host, they then migrate to the gastrointestinal tract.[74] There are exceptions to this; *Cyrtosomum penneri*, in the family Atractidae, is transmitted between lizards venereally.[75] Primates have experimentally been found to be suitable intermediate hosts for *Hexametra*, raising zoonotic concerns.[76] Ascarids may cause significant enteritis in their definitive reptile hosts.[77] The genera *Hexametra*, *Amplicaecum*, *Ophidascaris*, and *Polydelphis* utilize squamates as definitive hosts (Fig. 32.42) and lack sequence data for appropriate phylogenetic classification. *Dujardinascaris* and *Ortleppascaris* in the family Heterocheilidae utilize crocodilians as definitive hosts (Fig. 32.43).[78,79] *Ortleppascaris* can cause significant gastric pathology.[80]

Krefftascaris, also in the Heterocheilidae, utilizes side-necked turtles as definitive hosts.[81] *Sulcascaris sulcata*, in the family Anisakidae, utilizes loggerhead sea turtles as definitive hosts and oysters as intermediate hosts (Figs. 32.44 and 32.45). Loggerhead sea turtles have also been found to be intermediate hosts for *Anisakis* spp.[82] *Angusticaecum* spp. utilize tortoises as definitive hosts, where they are associated with disease.[83]

Management centers around excluding ascarids from collections through separation of definitive hosts and their feces from intermediate

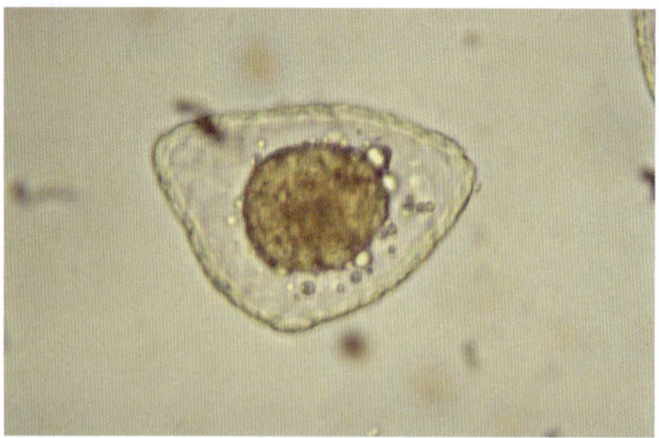

FIG 32.44 *Sulcascaris sulcata* from a loggerhead sea turtle (*Caretta caretta*). Photomicrograph magnification, 400×.

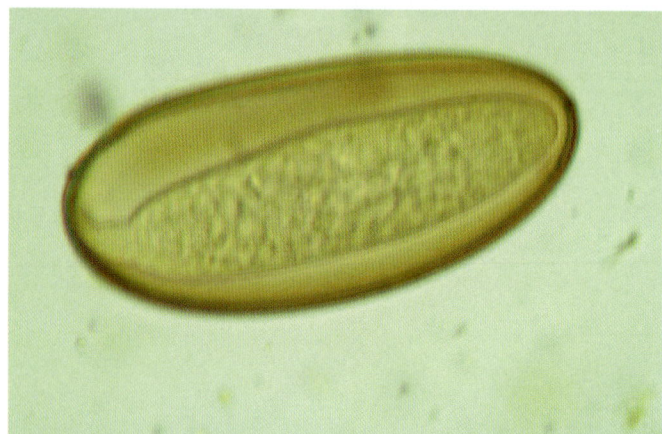

FIG 32.46 *Ozolaimus* sp. from a green iguana (*Iguana iguana*). Photomicrograph magnification, 400×.

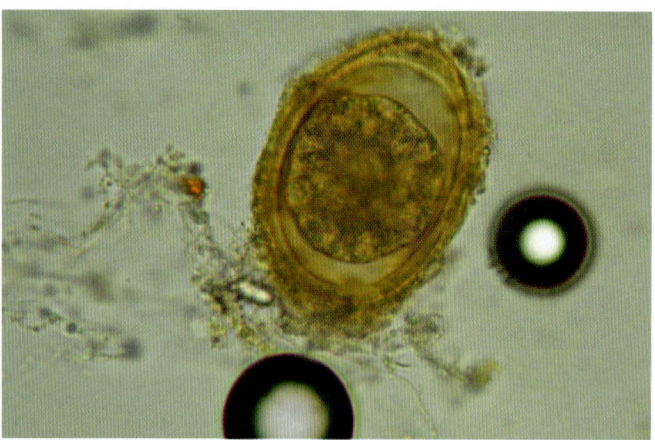

FIG 32.45 *Sulcascaris sulcata* from a loggerhead sea turtle (*Caretta caretta*). Photomicrograph magnification, 400×.

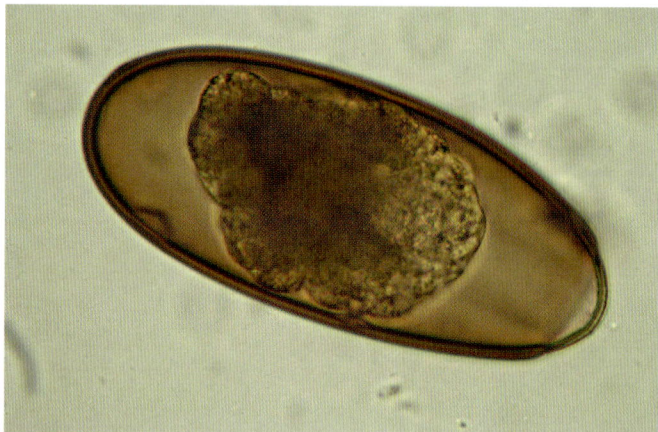

FIG 32.47 Unknown pinworm from a spur-thighed (Greek) tortoise (*Testudo graeca*). Photomicrograph magnification, 400×.

hosts and, for carnivorous/omnivorous reptiles, exclusion of potential intermediate hosts that may be ingested. Due to their indirect life cycle, they are more typically a problem of wild-caught animals. Although ascarids are significant pathogens, the presence of potentially large numbers of worms in the coelomic cavity complicates treatment; use of anthelminthics may result in a massive inflammatory response to dead worms. When possible, coelioscopic inspection and removal is advisable before pharmaceutical therapy.

Oxyurida. The order Oxyurida, in the class Chromadorea, contains pinworms. They have direct life cycles and, because of this, are the most common helminths seen in captive-breeding facilities. There are many genera that infect reptiles, and they tend to be host-specific. Eggs are smooth and elongate, with a straight side and a lens-shaped plug at one end (Figs. 32.46 to 32.48). It is important to differentiate oxyurid ova from strongyle ova, as the clinical approach to these two groups is markedly different. Pinworms have an esophageal bulb, and the females have a long tapering tail that gives them their name. Tortoises often have a community of multiple species of these short worms (Fig. 32.49). The male posterior ends are all-important in identification, and two such tails are illustrated: *Ozolaimus* lateral view (Fig. 32.50) and *Aleuris* sp. ventral view (Fig. 32.51). They live in the lumen of the large intestine (Fig. 32.52). Normally these worms pose little pathologic significance, and may even potentially be beneficial, and could therefore be commensals and not parasites. Bullfrog tadpoles (*Rana catesbeiana*) that

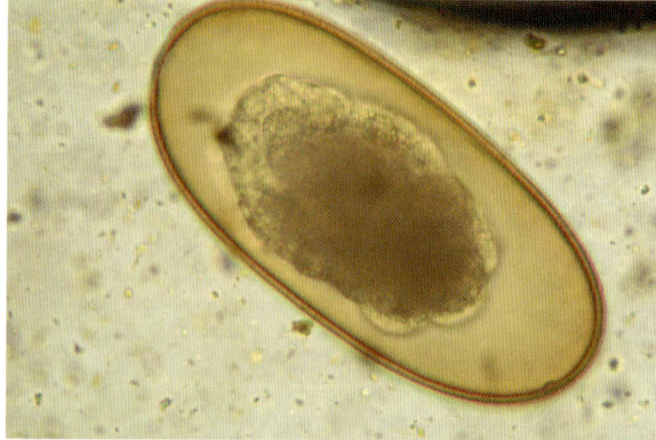

FIG 32.48 Unknown pinworm from a spur-thighed (Greek) tortoise (*Testudo graeca*). Photomicrograph magnification, 400×.

have the pinworm *Gyrinicola batrachiensis* develop more quickly and have better gut fermentation than controls without pinworms, indicating a mutualistic rather than parasitic relationship.[84] Unlike ascarids, oxyurids are not associated with disease in tortoises.[83] Under extremely poor husbandry, very high worm burdens may accumulate; captive reptiles

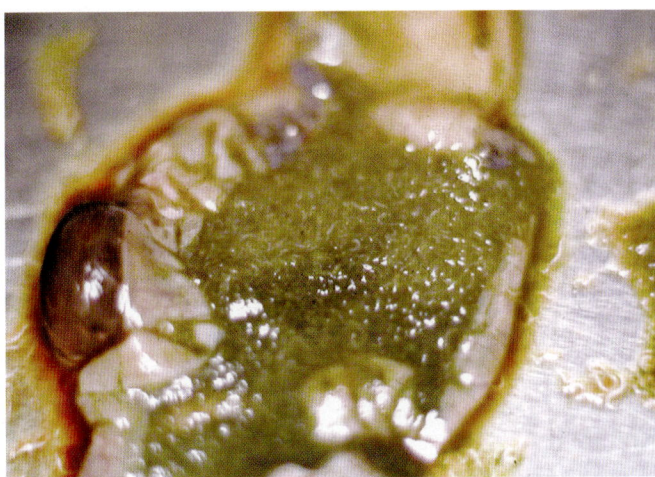

FIG 32.49 Large colon from a desert tortoise (*Gopherus agassizii*) impacted with oxyurid larva. (Courtesy of Douglas R. Mader.)

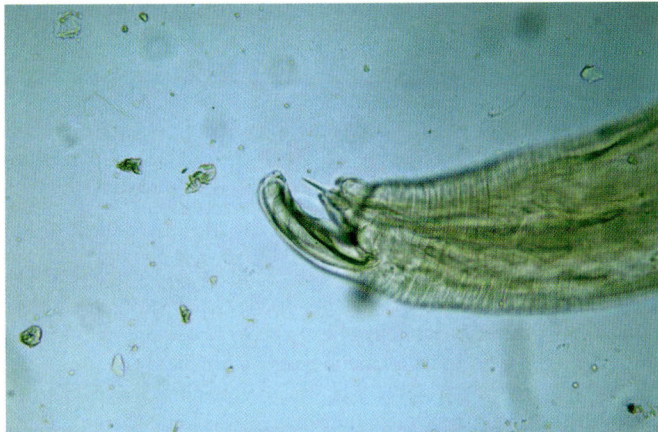

FIG 32.50 Posterior end of male *Ozolaimus* sp., lateral view. This is an important distinction for identification of different species of pinworms.

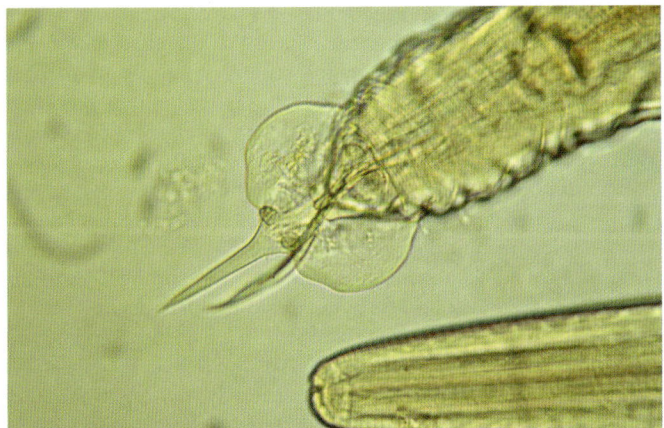

FIG 32.51 Posterior end of a male *Aleuris* sp., ventral view.

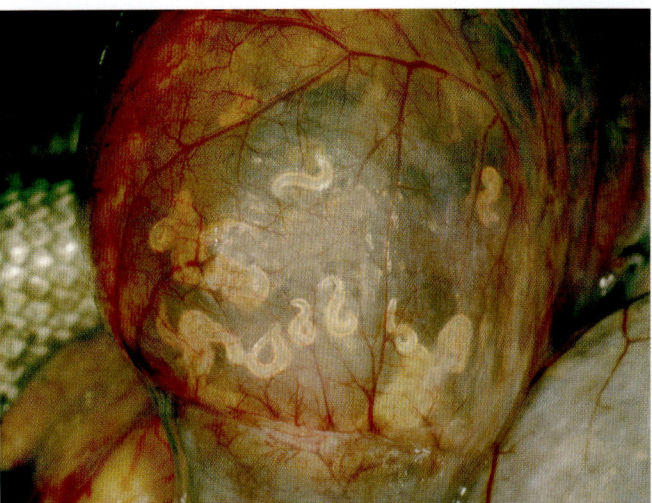

FIG 32.52 Oxyurids in the distended colon of a green iguana (*Iguana iguana*). (Courtesy of Stephen Barten).

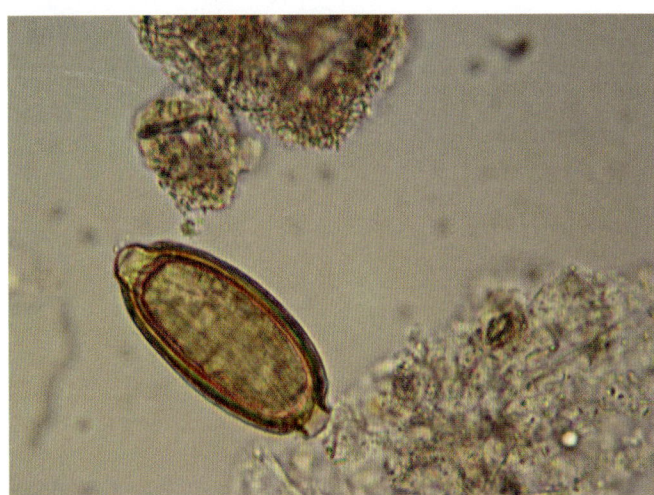

FIG 32.53 *Capillaria* sp. egg from a green tree python (*Morelia viridis*). Photomicrograph magnification, 400×.

Capillaria spp., in the family Capillariidae, are primarily found in the GI tract and have bipolar eggs like whipworms (*Trichuris* spp.) (Figs. 32.53 through 32.56).[85] Life cycles are thought to be direct. *Paratrichosoma* spp., in the family Trichosomoididae, live under the skin of crocodilians and leave dark tracks in the skin as they migrate, damaging leather quality.[86] Low rainfall is associated with higher *Paratrichosoma* worm burdens.[86]

Dioctophymatida. The order Dioctophymatida is in the class Enoplea. This class difference is most significant during treatment; they tend not to respond as well to most anthelminthics as the Chromeadorea do. *Eustrongylides* sp., in the family Dioctophymatidae, have indirect life cycles involving at least two intermediate hosts. Reptiles are usually intermediate hosts, but crocodiles have rarely been found to be definitive hosts.[87] Severe granulomatous lesions may be seen in reptiles acting as intermediate hosts.[88]

Management centers around excluding *Eustrongylides* from collections through separation of definitive hosts and their feces from intermediate hosts and, for carnivorous/omnivorous reptiles, exclusion of potential intermediate hosts that may be ingested. Due to their indirect life cycle, they are more typically a problem of wild-caught animals. Although

can always benefit from husbandry improvements. The risk/benefit ratio of pharmacologic therapy is poor, and it is not indicated.

Trichinellida. The order Trichinellida is in the class Enoplea. This class difference is most significant during treatment; they tend not to respond as well to most anthelminthics as the Chromeadorea do.

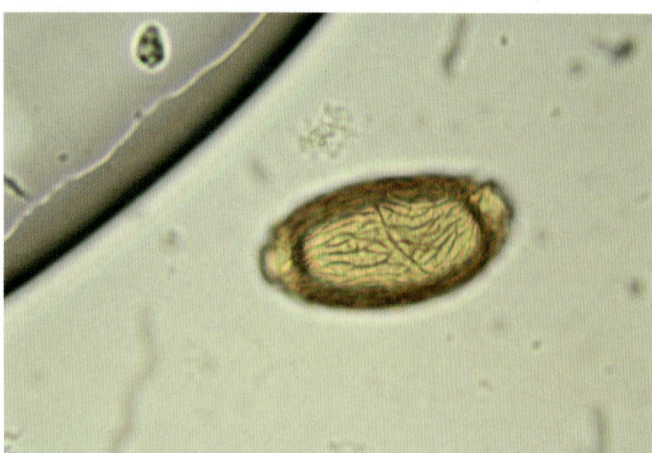

FIG 32.54 *Capillaria* sp. egg from a green tree python (*Morelia viridis*) (same egg as in Fig. 32.53—focus is on the shell surface). Photomicrograph magnification, 400×.

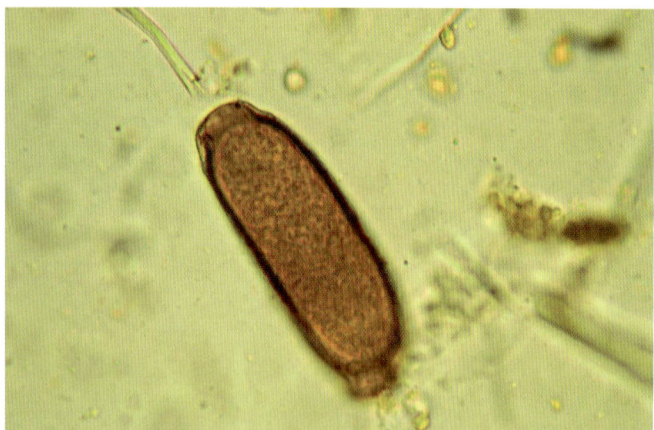

FIG 32.55 *Capillaria* sp. egg from a boa. Photomicrograph magnification, 400×.

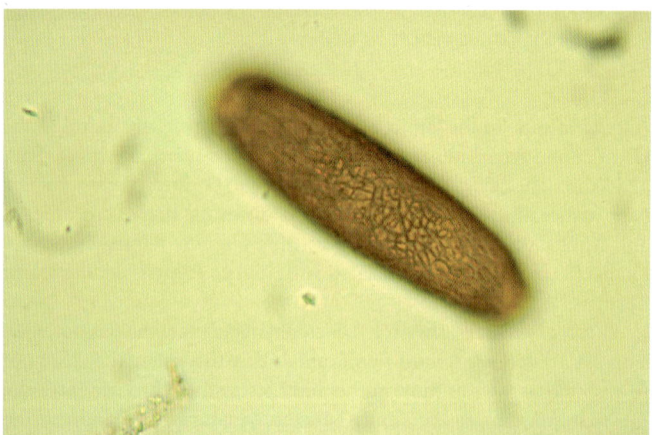

FIG 32.56 *Capillaria* sp. egg from a boa (same egg as in Fig. 32.55—focus is on the shell surface). Photomicrograph magnification, 400×.

Eustrongylides are significant pathogens, the presence of potentially large numbers of worms in the coelomic cavity complicates treatment; use of anthelminthics may result in a massive inflammatory response to dead worms. When possible, coelioscopic inspection and removal is advisable before pharmaceutical therapy.

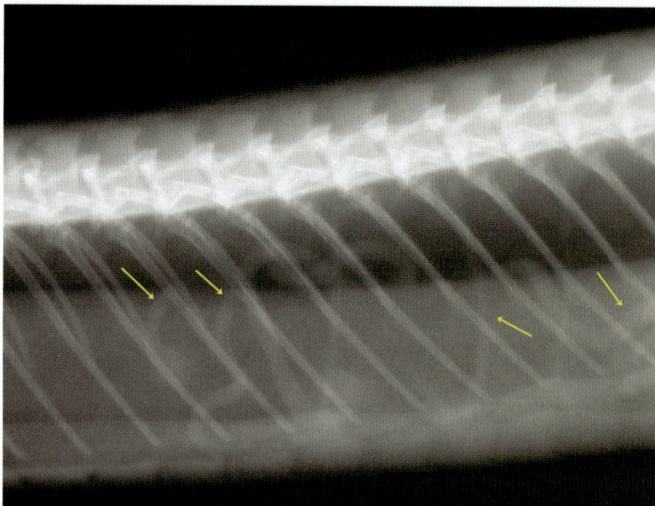

FIG 32.57 Radiograph of a wild indigo snake (*Drymarchon couperi*). Note the radiodense serpiginous pattern within the lungs (*yellow arrows*). These are internal pentastomid parasites. (Courtesy of Douglas R. Mader.)

Arthropoda. The phylum Arthropoda have chitinous exoskeletons with jointed appendages. The most clinically relevant taxa that parasitize reptiles are the subclass Pentastomida, the class Arachnida, and the class Insecta.

Pentastomida. The subclass Pentastomida is a member of the subphylum Crustacea in the ecdysozoan phylum Arthropoda. Their closest known relatives are branchiuran fish lice, such as *Argulus*.[89] They have indirect life cycles, typically utilizing vertebrate hosts. Many species use reptiles as definitive hosts, and adults are typically found in the lungs. Eggs are then coughed up, swallowed, and excreted in feces. Especially in squamates, where the lumen of the lung is large and the diameter of the trachea may be smaller than the pentastomid, there is a risk of respiratory obstruction by adult pentastomes, but the greatest pathology is seen in intermediate hosts, where they may be embedded in diverse tissues. There are two orders, the Cephalobaenida and the Porocephalida. The Porocephalida present a greater zoonotic risk. The porocephalan *Armillifer armillatus*, which typically utilizes *Bitis* spp. vipers as definitive hosts, is not uncommonly found in humans in endemic regions and may cause fatal lesions in the brain.[90] Feces from wild-caught *Bitis* sp. should be handled with appropriate protection. The porocephalan *Porocephalus crotali* utilizes North American vipers as definitive hosts and has caused fatal infection in dogs.[91] The porocephalan *Kiricephalus coarctatus* is common in North American colubrids; due to its close relationship to *Porocephalus* and *Armillifer*, feces from positive snakes should be handled with caution. The porocephalan genus *Sebekia*, in the family Sebekidae, utilizes crocodilians as definitive hosts. Greater inflammatory response was seen in experimentally infected rodent paratenic hosts than in turtles.[92] *Alofia* sp., also in the Sebekidae, utilize chelonian definitive hosts. The genus in the Cephalobaenida most commonly seen by practitioners is *Raillietiella*, which utilizes squamate hosts and is not uncommon in wild-caught geckos.

Evidence of the adult worms living in the lungs on survey radiographs is not uncommon (Fig. 32.57). Eggs may be seen on fecal flotation. A pulmonary wash is an even better sample. Eggs contain larvae and have four leg-like appendages; it is not uncommon to see hatched larva and empty eggshells (Figs. 32.58 through 32.61). Specific diagnosis may be done via morphologic characterization of adults or DNA sequencing.[93]

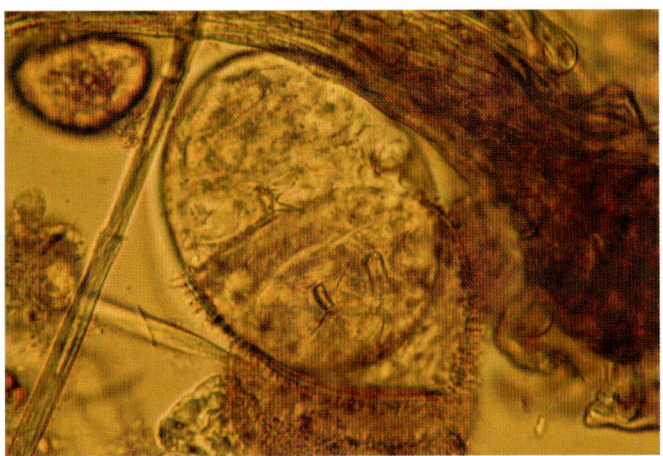

FIG 32.58 Pentastome eggs are characteristically thin walled and can measure up to 130 μm in diameter. Larvae with four hooklets are typically seen within eggs. This is an unidentified pentastome from a water monitor (*Varanus* sp.).

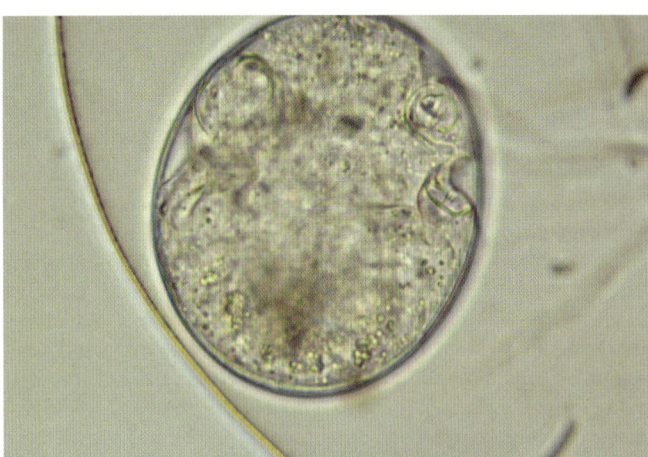

FIG 32.61 Unknown pentastome from a narrow-head softshell turtle (*Chitra indica*). Photomicrograph magnification, 400×.

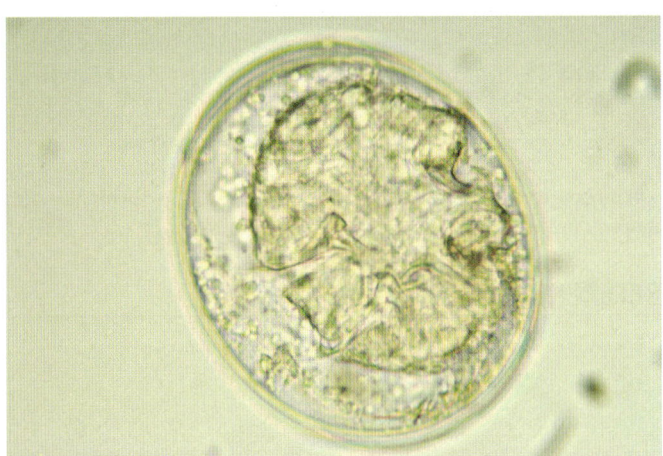

FIG 32.59 *Railietiella frenatus* from a Tokay gecko (*Gekko gecko*). Photomicrograph magnification, 400×.

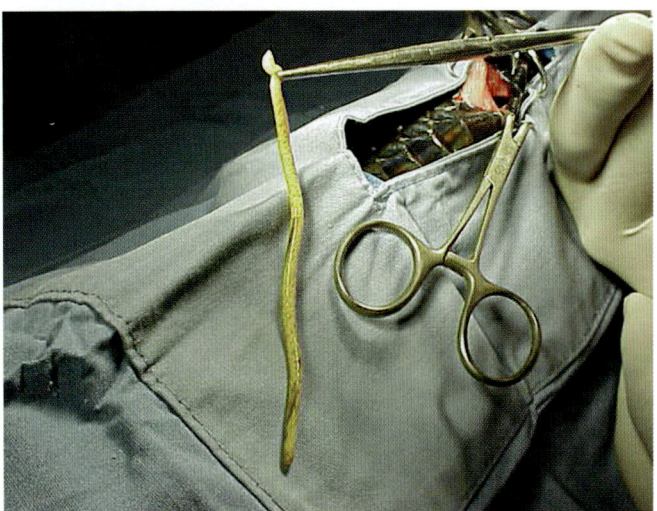

FIG 32.62 Extracted adult pentastomid from the lung of an indigo snake (*Drymarchon couperi*). Endoscopy allows simple, safe extraction of the typically low worm burden. (Courtesy of Douglas R. Mader.)

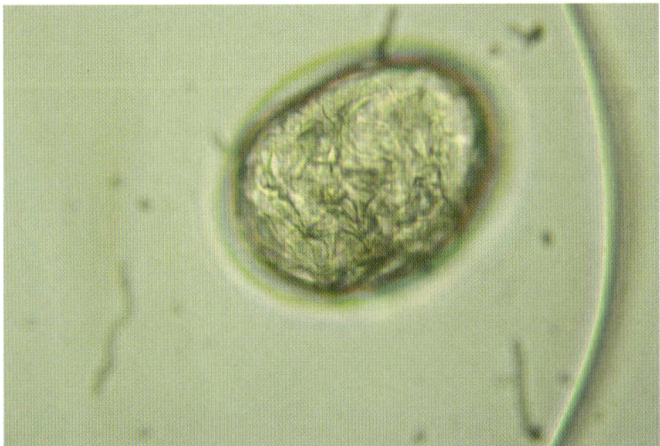

FIG 32.60 *Sebekia* sp. from a softshell turtle (*Apalone* sp.). Photomicrograph magnification, 400×.

Management centers around excluding pentastomids from collections through separation of definitive hosts and their feces from intermediate hosts and, for carnivorous/omnivorous reptiles, exclusion of potential intermediate hosts that may be ingested. Due to their indirect life cycle, they are more typically a problem of wild-caught animals. There are no effective anthelminthics for treatment of pentastomids, although there are reports of high doses of ivermectin arresting ova shedding. Pulmonoscopy and removal of adult pentastomes is the best therapeutic approach (Fig. 32.62).[93]

Arachnida. The class Arachnida is a member of the subphylum Chelicerata in the ecdysozoan phylum Arthropoda. They have eight legs as adults. The subclass Acari contains mites and ticks, which are both significant ectoparasites of reptiles.

The order Ixodida contains ticks, hematophagous arthropods. The two major groups of ticks are the hard ticks (Ixodidae) and the soft ticks (Argasidae). Most ticks seen on reptiles are ixodids. Some of the tick genera that feed on reptiles include *Amblyomma*, *Aponomma*, *Haemophysalis*, *Hyalomma*, and *Ixodes*. *Aponomma* is the genus most commonly seen on squamates. *Amblyomma* is the most common genus seen on tortoises and are known vectors for *Ehrlichia ruminantium,* the agent causing heartwater in ruminants. Although *E. ruminantium* has not been found to infect tortoises, it has been found in *Amblyomma* sp. on tortoises, and imports of tortoises from heartwater-endemic regions represent an agricultural risk. *Amblyomma tuberculatum,* the gopher tortoise tick, also carries an *Anaplasma* sp. that causes anemia in tortoises. The best therapeutic approach to ticks is manual removal. See Chapter 120 for more therapeutic options.

The order Mesostigmata are parasitic mites. The mite most commonly seen causing concerns in captive reptiles is *Ophionyssus natricis,* found on squamates (Fig. 32.63). The life cycle of *O. natricis* is egg > larva > protonymph > deutonymph >adult. Only the protonymph and adult feed on the blood of the squamate host; other stages are off the host and in the environment. Although it has been proposed as a potential vector of reptarenaviruses, this remains to be proven. It is a small black mite that may often be found in the gular fold, at the margins of the spectacles, or in water bowls. Diagnosis is by identification of adult mites. Environmental cleanup is an essential part of management. Pyrethrins are commonly used to treat infested squamates. Predatory mites have also been used to control *O. natricis.*[94] Maintenance of environments at temperatures over 42°C together with removal of water sources for several days will eliminate stages off the reptiles, provided they do not have access to cooler areas. See Chapter 120 for additional therapeutic options.

The order Trombidiiformes are a diverse order of mites. The family Cloacaridae contains the genera *Cloacarus* and *Caminacarus,* which live in the cloaca of turtles.[95] The impacts of Cloacaridae on reptile health has not yet been studied.

Insecta. The class Insecta is a member of the subphylum Hexapoda in the ecdysozoan phylum Arthropoda. They have six legs as adults. The order Diptera contains flies, which can be significant ectoparasites of reptiles. Hematophagous flies may be important disease vectors. The most significant dipteran parasite of North American reptiles is *Cistudinomyia cistudinis.*[96] This fly will lay eggs on box turtles (*Terrapene* sp.), most commonly beneath the carapace dorsal to the head. Larva

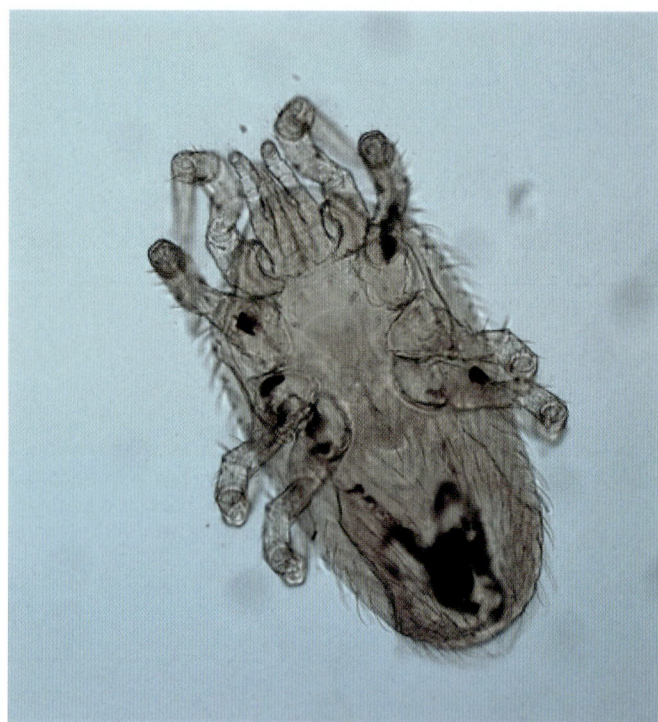

FIG 32.63 The snake mite, *Ophionyssus natricis.* Photomicrograph magnification, 200x. (Courtesy of Heather Walden.)

will burrow in and eat underlying tissue, causing large defects. Surgical removal of the larva is the most effective treatment.

REFERENCES

See www.expertconsult.com for a complete list of references.

33

Hematology

J. Jill Heatley and Karen E. Russell

This chapter strives to provide a clinically useful guide for veterinarians and other biologists on sample collection, sample handling and clinical interpretation of hematology results from reptile and amphibian species. This detailed summary will focus on hematologic principles and knowledge specific to reptiles and amphibians commonly presented in clinical practice. Although most information in this chapter will be based on more commonly seen species, other esoteric species may have been studied in more detail and may be included when necessary to illustrate general and expected findings (venomous species, tuatara crocodilians, etc). Should the reader require more specifics for zoo or wildlife species beyond this chapter, a review of primary literature is highly recommended.

Indications for hematologic assessment in reptiles and amphibians are numerous and are similar to those of companion mammals (Table 33.1). However, based on numerous factors including lack of baseline clinicopathologic data and normal physiology of ectotherms, results may be less accurate or specific for diagnosis than in traditional species. Most hematology information available for amphibians and reptiles, although valuable and peer reviewed, does not conform to the current ASVCP guidelines for reference range creation.[1] Finally, initial hematologic assessment generally provides nonspecific results to support (or refute) the clinician's working diagnosis based on historical and physical examination findings.[1] Additionally, more specific diagnostic testing (serology, PCR, histopathology, culture, etc) may be necessary to arrive at a definitive diagnosis. Though expensive and sometimes challenging to obtain in clinical practice, these additional steps maybe particularly necessary in the case of herpetological patients wherein few standard clinicopathologic tests have been rigorously investigated or validated. This chapter has three major sections: (1) sample collection, handling, and storage, (2) brief review of selected analyte methodologies as it pertains to analyte choice, and (3) analyte choice and evaluation, which have been carefully edited to provide information deemed essential for the clinician. For more in depth information regarding analyte or sample collection methodology, review of the primary literature and basic clinical pathology texts is recommended.

SAMPLE COLLECTION AND PRESERVATION

Choice of materials for blood collection from reptiles and amphibians is dependent on a number of factors, including species, patient size, anatomy, temperament, sample desired, sample collection conditions, equipment availability, and practitioner skill. A sample collection plan should be determined and materials prepared before sample collection for best results.

Restraint and Site Preparation

Sedation or anesthesia for routine diagnostic sampling is seldom necessary in reptile species commonly maintained as exotic pets but may be necessary for larger or potentially dangerous species. Excellent resources for reptile and amphibian sedation anesthesia and immobilization are available (see Chapters 48 and 49).[2] For amphibians, submersion or gas anesthesia may be necessary for best results. Should topical local anesthetics (lidocaine or benzocaine creams or gels) be used to facilitate amphibian venipuncture, avoid overzealous application, as overdose may results in anesthesia or death.[3] Cleaning and disinfecting the venipuncture site is highly recommended in reptiles, and small synthetic bristle (tooth, nail or scrub) brushes may be required for adequate surface cleaning of the heavily scaled skin of some species. However, application of alcohol alone is seldom advantageous in reptiles with thick, scaled, and opaque skin. Conversely in amphibians, topical antiseptic use is not advised.[4]

Venipuncture Equipment

For most reptiles and amphibians 27- to 22-gauge needle ranges and 0.3- to 3-mL syringes are sufficient. However, sampling of large lizards, snakes, or tortoises may require longer (1.5- to 2-inch) needles. The low blood pressure, slow heart rate, and large but relatively sturdy osmotic nature of blood cells in some reptile and amphibian species supports the preference of a larger-gauge needle but smaller-size syringe than one might choose in similarly sized birds or mammals (Table 33.2).[5,6] These syringe-needle combinations allows blood to flow slowly into the smaller syringe while minimizing aspiration pressure to preserve cell integrity and lessening the concern of thrombocyte activation and microclot formation. Furthermore, in amphibians, use of smaller than 25-gauge needles in species with relatively large RBCs may result in hemolysis.[3] Butterfly administration sets may also be useful when the sample size is sufficient to lose the 0.05 mL, which may coat the tubing. Use of syringes or needles precoated with heparin or other anticoagulant is unnecessary, and avoidance precludes dilutional and cellular staining artifact.[7-9] However, in amphibians relatively decreased clotting times may necessitate use of syringes or needles precoated or flushed with heparin.[3]

Anticoagulant

Whole anticoagulated blood, without lymphatic or cerebrospinal fluid dilution, is the preferred sample for routine hematology. Choice of anticoagulant and blood collection equipment is based on similar factors as detailed under equipment, but species, sample collection conditions, availability, and postcollection sample use are also primary concerns. All anticoagulants can affect cell morphology and staining characteristics (Figs. 33.1 and 33.2). Although lithium heparin is commonly used, EDTA has been shown to be superior for assessment of leukocyte count and morphology and other parameters in lizards and snakes but can cause hemolysis in chelonians.[8,10] However, lithium heparin provides the added possible benefit of obtaining both whole blood for hematology (complete blood count [CBC], packed cell volume [PCV], total solids) and plasma for biochemical analyte determination from the same sample. Sodium citrate has received minimum study in reptiles but resulted in hemolysis of samples from Burmese pythons (*Python bivittatus*).[11] An overview of current knowledge regarding anticoagulant choice for hematology is provided in Table 33.3. Lithium or ammonium heparin is the preferred anticoagulant for amphibian blood, unless the blood is intended for bacterial culture.[3]

Acceptable blood collection tubes include microtainer, pediatric, or larger sizes based on sample requirements. Microtainer plastic tubes coated with freeze-dried anticoagulant are preferred for blood storage before diagnostic testing to avoid sample dilution and allow small sample

collection. Heparinized microhematocrit tubes (75 mm) may be used for blood collection from very small species, but sample recovery compared with microtainer tubes appears somewhat less and is challenging without specialized sample expulsion bulbs.[3] Furthermore, diagnostic assays available from this method are limited based on the relatively small sample size collected.

Two to three smears of blood not exposed to anticoagulant should be created for each blood sample collected.[4] Blood smears may be made on cover slips or slides. The best blood smear technique is one that provides for the best creation of a monolayer of cells and the fewest damaged cells. Technique options include cover slip to slide, slide to slide (wedge), and cover slip to cover slip. A single study that evaluated these methods for use in reptiles found the slide-to-slide method preferred for use in green iguanas (*Iguana iguana*).[9] The small fragile nature of cover slips is generally prohibited from use as the primary mode for assessing reptile and hematology based on their small fragile nature, which makes shipping, review, and storage challenging. In addition, cover slips are generally incompatible with automated slide stainers. Blood smears should be actively and quickly air dried to reduce drying artifact. Blood films are best fixed in methanol within 1 to 4 hours of preparation.[12] Based on current methodologies available in veterinary diagnostic laboratories, assessment of CBC is highly dependent on the quality of the blood smear provided. Samples for hematology and cytology should never be shipped in the same container as those containing biopsied tissues in formalin; formalin fumes will markedly

TABLE 33.1	Indications for Clinicopathologic Assessment of Reptiles
Health assessment	Entry or exit of collection, baseline determination, presurgical assessment, pre- or posthibernation assessment
Diagnosis	Clinical suspicion of inflammation or organ dysfunction
Therapeutic assessment	Assessment of treatment plan as for renal or liver dysfunction, sepsis, chemotherapy, other chronic diseases
Prognosis	Assessment of seriousness of infection, inflammation, blood loss, etc

TABLE 33.2	Comparative Osmotic Fragility of Select Reptilian and Mammalian Erythrocytes[5]	
Common Name	**Scientific Name**	**Solution %***
Green iguana	*Iguana iguana*	15–70
Bengal monitor, common Indian monitor	*Varanus bengalensis*	15–55
Gold or golden tegu, common tegu, black tegu, Colombian tegu, tiger lizard	*Tupinambis teguixin*	20–60
Broad-snouted caiman, Yacare caiman	*Caiman latirostris, Caiman jacare*	20–40
Nile crocodile	*Crocodylus nilotocus*	20–70
Common agama, red-headed rock agama, rainbow agama	*Agama agama*	10–60
Camel	*Camelus* spp.	21–30
Rabbit	*Oryctolagus* spp.	30–50
Human	*Homo sapiens*	35–50

*Range of buffered saline solution percentages at which cells maintained their integrity (i.e., did not undergo lysis).

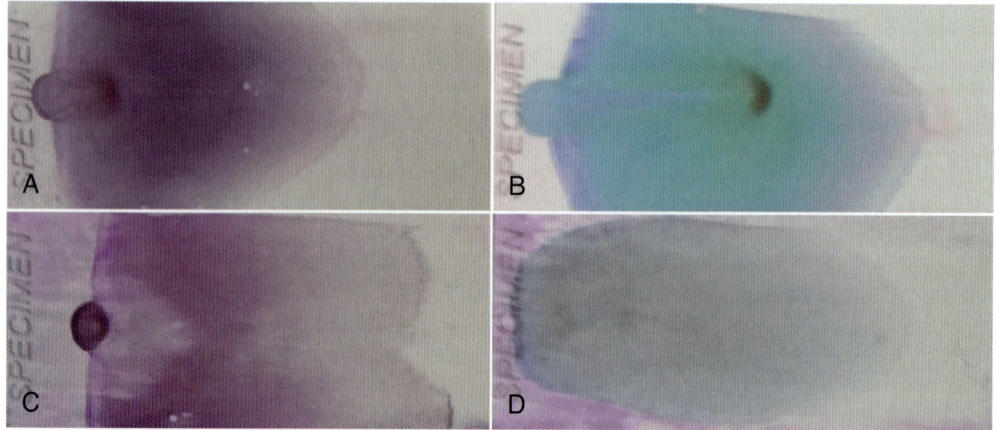

FIG 33.1 Gross appearance of multiple blood smears without anticoagulant from a red-footed tortoise (*Chelonoidis carbonaria*) based on stain and formalin exposure. (A) Methanol-based rapid stain. (B) Methanol-based rapid stain after formalin exposure. (C) Modified Wright's stain. (D) Modified Wright's stain after formalin exposure. (Courtesy of J. Jill Heatley and Karen E. Russell.)

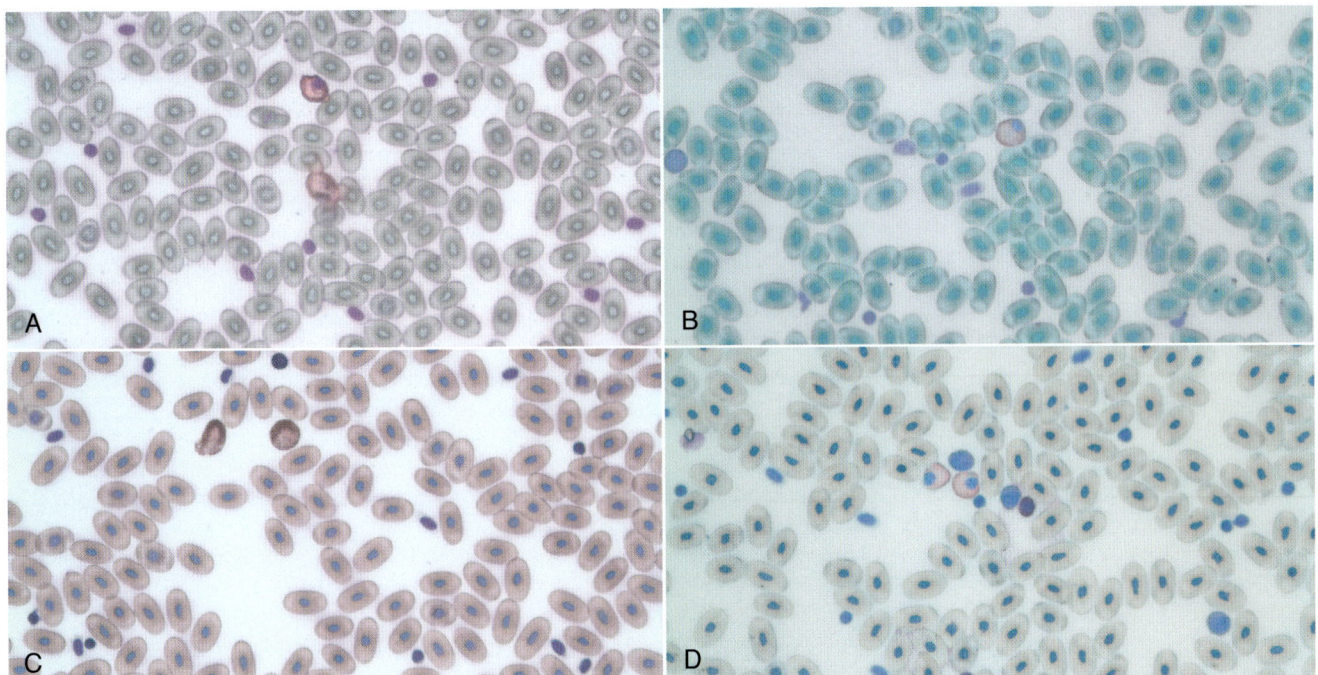

FIG 33.2 Microscopic appearance (400× magnification) of multiple blood smears without anticoagulant from a red-footed tortoise (*Chelonoidis carbonaria*) based on stain and formalin exposure. (A) Methanol-based rapid stain. (B) Methanol-based rapid stain after formalin exposure. (C) Modified Wright's stain. (D) Modified Wright's stain after formalin exposure. (Courtesy of J. Jill Heatley and Karen E. Russell.)

TABLE 33.3 Impactful Studies for Anticoagulant Choice in Reptiles: Exceptions to and Support for the Rule of Green

Anticoagulant(s)	Species	Parameter Changes
CPDA-1, ACD	American alligator (*Alligator mississippiensis*)	Comparable; blood may be stored up to 35 days based on PCV, methemoglobin, osmotic fragility, and morphologic evaluation[67]
K₂- or Na₂-EDTA, Heparin	Puff adder (*Bitis arientans*)	All PCV similar[65]
EDTA	Burmese python (*Python bivitattus*)	No hematologic differences[11]
Lithium heparin		
K₃-EDTA	**Hermann's tortoises (Testudo hermanni)**	**Lysis in EDTA at 6 hours; no lysis in lithium heparin[64]**
Lithium heparin		
EDTA	**Spiny softshell turtle (Apalone spinifera)**	**All EDTA samples hemolyzed[10]**
Lithium heparin		
EDTA	*American alligator (Alligator mississippiensis)*	*Used for hematologic parameter determination without apparent problems[68]*
EDTA	*Green iguana (Iguana iguana)*	*Thrombocytes, WBC, heterophils, and monocytes of EDTA sample had best agreement with differential of fresh blood smear[8]*
EDTA	*Yellow-blotched map turtle (Graptemys flavimaculata)*	*EDTA preferred[66]*
Lithium heparin		
EDTA	*Yellow rat snake (Pantherophis obsoleta quadrivittatta)*	*Acceptable results with EDTA for cellular morphology[56]*
Ca-EDTA	*Chinese water dragon (Physignathus cocincinus)*	*Morphologic features of distortion and leukergy (WBC clumping) in LiHep samples; EDTA preferred[69]*
Lithium heparin		

Studies in which heparin was a preferred anticoagulant are boldface, while those in which EDTA was preferred are italic. Equivocal studies or those with different anticoagulants are neither.

When confronted with a reptile or amphibian for which anticoagulants have not been studied, generally one should choose lithium heparin as the anticoagulant of choice.

ACD, acid-citrate-dextrose; *CPDA-1*, citrate-phosphate-dextrose-adenine; *EDTA*, Ethylenediaminetetraacetic acid; *PCV*, packed cell volume; *WBC*, white blood cells.

TABLE 33.4 Effects of Venipuncture Site and Lymphatic* Contamination Upon Reptile Cellular Components and Total Solids

Species	Sampling Sites	Differences Found in Samples with Lymphatic Contamination (LC)* or Associated With Venipuncture Site (VS)
Desert tortoise (Gopherus agasizzi)	Jugular vein Occipital plexus	VS: PCV, RBC count, WBC count, and hemoglobin were lower in samples from the occipital sinus;[70] VS: PCV, RBC count, WBC count, and hemoglobin were lower in samples from the occipital sinus[70]
Marginated tortoise (Testudo marginata)	Coccygeal vein Brachial vein	VS: RBC, Hct, and Hb were greater in brachial vein samples compared with coccygeal vein samples;[71] VS: RBC, Hct, and Hb were greater in brachial vein samples compared with coccygeal vein samples[71]
Northern map turtle (Graptemys geographica)	Coccygeal vein Subcarapacial vein	LC: Visual hemodilution noted in 16% of coccygeal samples but 75% of subcarapacial samples;[72] LC: Visual hemodilution noted in 16% of coccygeal samples but 75% of subcarapacial samples[72]
Red-eared slider (Trachemys scripta elegans)	Coccygeal vein Occipital vein	VS: Total WBC count, total plasma protein lower in samples from the dorsal coccygeal vein;[73] VS: Total WBC count, total plasma protein lower in samples from the dorsal coccygeal vein[73]
Leatherback sea turtle (Dermochelys coriacea)	Occipital vein Interdigital vein	VS: PCV, total solids, WBC count, heterophils, lymphocyte, monocyte, eosinophil, basophil from each site were comparable;[74] VS: PCV, total solids, WBC count, heterophils, lymphocyte, monocyte, eosinophil, basophil from each site were comparable[74]
African spurred tortoise (Centrochelys sulcata)	Coccygeal vein Subcarapacial vein	VS: Total solids had increased concentrations in samples from the tail versus the subcarapacial sampling site[18]
Common chameleon (Chameleo chameleon)	Jugular vein Tail vein	VS: No difference in WBC, RBC. Jugular venipuncture preferred based on likelihood of obtaining sample and darkening of the tail;[75] VS: No difference in WBC, RBC. Jugular venipuncture preferred based on likelihood of obtaining sample and darkening of the tail[75]
Hydrophiine sea snakes (Hydrophis spp.)	Tail vein	LC: Samples with observed lymphatic contamination had increased azurophils, total WBC count, and decreased PCV and total solids;[76] LC: Samples with observed lymphatic contamination had increased azurophils, total WBC count, and decreased PCV and total solids[76]

*Although previously identified as lymphatic contamination, venipuncture sites close to the cervical or coccygeal spine may be contaminated with cerebrospinal fluid.

Hb, Hemoglobin; *Hct*, hematocrit; *PCV*, packed cell volume; *RBC*, red blood cells; *WBC*, white blood cells.

affect cellular staining properties and render the sample unacceptable for microscopic evaluation (formalin fog)[12] (see Figs. 33.1 and 33.2).

Lymphatic dilution may occur from any venipuncture site in reptiles but is least likely to occur when samples are obtained from the jugular vein or heart.[13] Contamination of samples with CSF may be more likely to occur from venipuncture sites near the vertebral column (subcarapacial, supravertebral, coccygeal veins) (Divers S, personal observations). Thus the venipuncture site may affect multiple hematologic analytes based on lymphatic or CSF dilution or other factors. Lymphatic or CSF dilution should be suspected based on the rapid filling of the syringe with clear to light transparent light yellow fluid, which may be followed by blood. With cardiocentesis, clear fluid obtained should be differentiated from pericardial fluid. In humans, expected cell count, glucose and protein concentrations, and LDH activities of pericardial fluid are known; for reptiles these values have yet to be investigated. In mammals, most pericardial fluid samples are blood tinged and may have mesothelial cells not present in peripheral blood. Rather than discarding lymphatic samples, the authors recommend they be used for assessment of serology, PCR, or select plasma chemistries. Expected hematologic differences associated with lymph/CSF contamination of the blood sample include decreased PCV and RBC. In addition, increased lymphocytes may be seen with lymph-contaminated samples. When lymph is obtained during venipuncture we recommend drawing a reasonable sample for serology and/or plasma chemistries, or until a slight tinge of blood is seen, which may signal the collapse of local lymphatics. Use of a new needle and syringe in an approach along the same route will often provide a blood sample without lymphatic contamination. Both venipuncture site and lymph/CSF contamination may affect analyte results in reptiles.[14] Unfortunately, the effects of such contamination, venipuncture site,

and associated changes in hematological analytes have been studied in relatively few species (Table 33.4).

Venipuncture Sites

Choice of the best sample site depends on many factors, including vascular anatomy, patient temperament, and practitioner skill. Consultation of taxa-specific reviews are recommended should training via a skilled and experienced veterinarian not be available (see also Chapter 43).[3,15–17] An overview of multiple options for vascular access based on reptile class and common site usage are provided in Table 33.5; however, other sites may be appropriate and preferred based on practitioner experience and knowledge. Sample site alone or in conjunction with lymph/CSF dilution may affect multiple hematologic parameters (see Table 33.4).[14] Clinically and for experimental purposes one should always document the venipuncture site used for each sample obtained. Further, for serial sampling, when possible, the same sample site should be used to facilitate direct comparisons. Samples obtained from more craniad sites may be more valid for interpretation of health or experimental outcomes in some reptiles.[14,18]

Sample Storage and Expected Analyte Changes

Few studies have focused on best or acceptable storage methodologies for reptilian blood samples bound for hematological analysis. The effect of delay upon hematology values has been studied in relatively few reptilian and amphibian species. Thus testing within 24 hours of sample collection is recommended for most hematologic analytes, and the sooner a sample can be analyzed, the better. However, amphibian blood samples diluted with Natt and Herrick's solution shortly after collection and refrigerated can maintain integrity for up to 2 years, and cell counts

TABLE 33.5 Venipuncture Site Options in Reptiles and Amphibians

Reptile Class	Preferred	Other Options
Snakes	Caudal (ventral coccygeal) vein, cardiocentesis	Jugular vein
Lizards	Caudal (ventral coccygeal) vein, jugular vein	Ventral abdominal vein, casque vein
Chelonians	Jugular vein	Brachial vein, subcarapacial sinus, caudal (dorsal and ventral coccygeal) veins, postoccipital venous sinus
Crocodilians	Supraoccipital sinus, tail vein	Ventral abdominal vein
Amphibians	Caudal (ventral coccygeal) vein, ventral abdominal vein, maxillary (facial) vein	Lingual vein, femoral vein

TABLE 33.6 Common Analytes Provided in the Reptile and Amphibian Complete Blood Count

Analyte	Measurement, Abbreviation, Units	Methodology Gold Standard	Other Methods	
Erythrocytes	PCV, %	Packed cell volume, centrifugation	Hematocrit calculation from hemoglobin and cell dimension often invalid/inappropriate	Derivation from impedance (iSTAT) requires validation/correction factor for the species
Leukocytes	WBC, 10^9/L or 10^3/mm^3 or /μL	Natt and Herrick's stain, cell counting chamber	Phloxine stain, cell-counting chamber	Slide estimate
		Total WBC count, manual, direct	Total WBC count, manual, indirect	Total WBC count, slide estimate
Heterophil	Absolute 10^9/L or 10^3/mm^3 or /μL,%	Differential leukocyte counts based upon % from blood smear × TWBC	Direct count of phloxine-stained eosinophils + heterophils	Estimate, %
Lymphocyte	Absolute 10^9/L or 10^3/mm^3 or /μL,%		Indirect calculation	Estimate, %
Monocyte	Absolute 10^9/L or 10^3/mm^3 or /μL,%		Indirect calculation	Estimate, %
Azurophil*	Absolute 10^9/L or 10^3/mm^3 or /μL,%		Indirect calculation	Estimate, %
Basophil	Absolute 10^9/L or 10^3/mm^3 or /μL,%		Indirect calculation	Estimate, %
Eosinophil	Absolute 10^9/L or 10^3/mm^3 or /μL,%		Direct count of phloxine stained eosinophils + heterophils	Estimate, %
Thrombocytes	Cells/μL		Slide estimation (low, adequate, high)	Estimate, %
Plasma Protein	Total solids (TS) or total protein (TP) g/dL or g/L**	Protein electrophoresis (EPH)	Refractometry	BCG binding, Biuret

*Many laboratories may include azurophils as or within monocytes for the count of percentage. Consultation with your laboratory and clinical pathologist is recommended to determine your lab's methodology
**Total solids may or may not be equivalent to total protein; for more information, see Chapter 34.

may be performed days to weeks after collection without compromise of result quality.[3] Older amphibian blood samples stored in this way suffer from loss of differential staining properties, thrombocyte-lymphocyte confusion, and leukocyte aggregation or clumping (Leukergy) resulting in decreased WBC counts.[3] In heparinized blood samples of loggerhead sea turtles (*Caretta caretta*) in which cells remained in contact with plasma and were refrigerated for up to 96 hours, minimal hemolysis occurred by 24 hours but moderate hemolysis occurred at 48 and 96 hours. Samples from Burmese pythons collected into heparin-coated syringes and transferred to containers with multiple anticoagulants and bovine serum albumin were evaluated for cellular changes over time.[11] Python blood samples anticoagulated with lithium heparin or K3-EDTA and refrigerated at 4°C for up to 24 hours had similar hematologic results to those immediately processed and were therefore preferred, whereas the addition of bovine serum albumin failed to provide any advantage for the analytes assessed.[19]

THE HEMATOLOGY REPORT

Complete Blood Count (CBC)

The parameters provided in a hematology report (often referred to as a complete blood count or CBC for other species) from commercial and university reference laboratories are more limited compared with those provided for mammals. These differences are based on a lack of automation for cell counts and the necessity of performing many tests manually, which increases the cost and time needed. Common evaluated parameters provided for the herpetological hematology report (complete blood count [CBC]) include PCV and total solid concentration (also referred to as plasma protein or total protein), thrombocyte estimate (low, adequate, high, clumped), leukocyte count and differential, evaluation of leukocyte and erythrocyte morphology, and examination for cell inclusions and hemoparasites (Table 33.6). Reptile and amphibian veterinarians are urged to choose a laboratory that provides a cell count based on hemocytometer rather than slide estimation for more accurate and precise results. No peer-reviewed, database publication in reptile or amphibian medicine has suggested that a WBC (slide) estimate provides results comparable to that of a hemocytometer-based WBC count. However, in both cases results are highly dependent on the quality of the blood smear, which is best made at the time of sampling. Although determination of the leukocyte count and differential may be beyond the time constrains of a practitioner, it is highly recommended that at least a PCV, total solids concentration (refractometric), and a slide review be performed in house to obtain actionable clinico-pathologic data until results from the reference laboratory are available. This method, along with slide storage, provides an insurance policy against shipment loss, slide breakage, and cellular change/artifact that may occur based on storage, transport, and shipping to a reference laboratory.

Multiple methodologies may be used to determine the CBC, which may lead to confusion regarding clinical interpretation. Commonly used methods are not interchangeable and rarely agree. Manual leukocyte counts remain the preferred method for amphibian and reptilian blood samples but have an inherent error of approximately 20% despite use of experienced personnel.[3,20] Methodologies commonly used to determine the total and differential WBC count and differential include slide estimates (estimated WBC) and hemocytometer counts using Phloxine staining (indirect total WBC; e.g., Leukopet, Vetlab Supply, Palmetto Bay, FL) or Natt and Herrick's staining (direct total WBC; e.g., Natt and Herrick's stain, Vetlab Supply); these methods are listed in order of increasing accuracy, cost, time, and training necessary for correct performance. As most reptiles are predominantly lymphocytic, Phloxine techniques, which are based on granulocyte counts, may easily underestimate lymphocytes. Staining choices for determination of cell counts may also influence results. In general, eosin stains are recommended to provide more accurate counts from species that have leukograms predominated by heterophils and eosinophils, whereas Natt & Herrick's solution may be more appropriate for cell counts of lymphocytic reptile and amphibian species. Further, the preferred method of leukocyte counting (Natt and Herrick's staining, hemocytometry of all cells) is often not what is most commonly provided for reptiles and amphibians in commercial reference laboratories (likely based on cost, time, and technical difficulty prohibitions). Estimating the total WBC count based upon blood smear evaluation is seldom accurate except to subjectively judge whether leukocyte numbers appear low, adequate, or high. However, the differential percentages are generated from the blood smear in all cases; therefore, the quality of the slide and smear can greatly affect the differential and the relative WBC counts derived therefrom. Commonly provided hematologic parameters and methodologies are provided in Table 33.6, and examples are provided in Figs. 33.3 through 33.5. See Box 33.1 for specific instructions and methodologies used for determination of the total and differential WBC counts in reptiles and amphibians.

For the clinician, review and banking of the fixed blood smear is just as important as the receipt and interpretation of CBC results. Observing the blood smear in house, one may make several important clinical conclusions that may benefit the patient without a 24- to 48-hour

REPTILIAN PROFILE #3	AVIAN/EXOTIC CBC AND PLASMA PROTEIN			
Test	Result	Reference Range	Flag	
WBC-EST	7.5	THOUS 1.2-25.6 (7.97)		
WBC	7.5	K/uL		
WBC ESTIMATE				
HCT	26.0	% 9.48 (28)		
HETEROPHILS	70	%		
HETEROPHIL BANDS	0.0	%		
% NEUTROPHIL	0.0	%		
% LYMPHOCYTE	24.0	%		
% MONOCYTE	1.0	%		
AZUROPHIL	0.0	%		
% EOSINOPHIL	5.0	%		
% BASOPHIL	0.0	%		
THROMBOCYTES	ADEQUATE			
BLOOD PARASITES	NO PARASITES SEEN			
REMARKS				
SLIDE REVIEWED MICROSCOPICALLY. INCREASED NUMBERS OF LYSED CELLS NOTED MAY CAUSE ERRONEOUS DIFFERENTIAL COUNTS.				
ABSOLUTE HETEROPHIL	5250	/uL		
ABSOLUTE HETEROPHIL BAND	0	/uL		
NEUTROPHIL	0	/uL		
LYMPHOCYTE	1800	/uL		
MONOCYTE	75	/uL		
ABSOLUTE AZUROPHIL	0	/uL		
EOSINOPHIL	375	/uL		
BASOPHIL	0	/uL		

FIG 33.3 Hematology report of a subadult sulcata tortoise (*Centrochelys sulcata*) with a necrotic and infected rear limb in need of amputation. Note (1) the lack of reference ranges provided, which is appropriate and typical for many laboratories; (2) the WBC count has been estimated (EST), likely from the slide; and (3) that the venipuncture site is not provided. The referral veterinarian's attempt to assess this animal is provided by the handwritten notes, which resulted in the assessment of anemia. However, the most striking hematologic abnormality of this animal is the heterophilia, as evidenced by a ratio approximately 3 heterophils per 1 lymphocyte in this normally lymphocytic species. (Courtesy of J. Jill Heatley and Karen E. Russell.)

Pertinent History:
anorexia 3 weeks, emaciated

Test Name	Result	Flag	Reference	Unit
Manual WBC	47.8			
Packed Cell Volume	spun 21			%
Plasma Protein	2.7			TS-g/dl
Heterophil	66			%
Absolute Heterophil	31548			
Band Heterophil				%
Absolute Band Heterophil				
Lymphocytes	2			%
Absolute Lymphocyte	956			
Monocytes	31			%
Absolute Monocyte	14818			
Azurophils				%
Absolute Azurophils				
Eosinophil				%
Absolute Eosinophil				
Basophil	1			%
Absolute Basophil	478			
Other				
Absolute Other				

Panel Name	Interpretation Name	Result
RBC Morphology	Polychromasia	rare to occ
Platelets	Thrombocytes	adeq
Neutrophil Morphology	Toxic Change	few to mod

Approximately 2% of the herterophils have a large nucleus with increased N:C ratios, increased basophilia of the cytoplasm, decreased granularity, and the presence of dark purple granules. These findings are consistent with immature heterophils and therefore a left shift.

Addendum: Occasionally, monocytes contain blue to green to yellow to rarely black, refractile, granular to globular material. Monocytes in the peripheral blood of reptiles often exhibit phagocytic activity and erythrophagia and leukocytophagia in the peripheral blood of reptiles can be associated with anemia and infectious diseases. Additionally, the cells with black material may represent melanophages, a type of macrophage common in lower vertebrates, which can be found in blood smears of reptiles with inflammatory diseases. Overall, this finding is most likely associated with a systemic inflammatory process given the inflammatory leukogram, and no overt cause for the inflammation is noted within the blood smear. Continued monitoring of CBCs to assess the inflammatory process as well as the presence of these cells is recommended if clinically warranted.

FIG 33.4 Adult female leopard tortoise (*Stigmochelys pardalis*) presented moribund despite previous treatment with systemic parenteral antibiotics and fluids. The WBC count was provided by hemocytometry, and the packed cell volume was provided by centrifuge rather than by calculation (Hct). Note the profound leukocytosis, heterophilia with left shift and toxic changes, and monocytosis suggestive of chronic, severe inflammation/infection. (Courtesy of J. Jill Heatley and Karen E. Russell.)

delay. Major tasks for review of the blood smear include differentiation of cell types, assessment of cell morphology and observation of morphological cell abnormalities, and observation of cellular inclusions or extracellular abnormalities such as hemoparasites. Cellular morphology based on systemic inflammation, infection, etc., has been minimally investigated in reptiles. However, toxic change associated with whole body toxins affecting the bone marrow and left shift associated with acute severe inflammation have been anecdotally reported (Figs. 33.9 through 33.11). Increased glucocorticoid levels are associated with degranulation of the granulocytes (heterophils and eosinophils) in some species.[21] Detection of these cellular morphologic changes may be vitally important for practitioners to detect life-threatening conditions in patients that show minimal signs of ill health yet may lack a leukocytosis or overt leukopenia.

Leukogram (White Blood Cell Count and Differential)

Most reptiles and amphibians are lymphocytic. Table 33.7 provides examples of species, which in contrast to most other reptiles, have a leukogram predominated by a cell type other than lymphocytes in the apparently healthy state.

Clinical interpretation of the leukogram is made challenging by numerous factors. First, rigorous reference ranges, including total WBC and expected cell percentages, are seldom available for healthy reptiles. Additionally, species' cellular percentages and total count ranges vary widely even within healthy members of each class of reptile. Second, as primarily ectothermic species, numerous normal physiological factors may greatly affect the leukogram such as season, temperature, sex and reproductive status, and age, among others. Third, the expected leukocyte effects of specific conditions such as fungal, bacterial, viral, or parasitical infection or stress have been minimally investigated in these species. Few studies have attempted to induce increased or decreased numbers of specific cell types within the WBC differential. Additionally, many classical cellular changes associated with stress, toxic change, parasitism, and more, have only been anecdotally reported as supportive of an existing condition rather than prospectively induced by said condition. Therefore we are left with anecdotal reports of cellular numbers and morphologic changes observed in association with diseases or conditions. In the future, meta-analysis of the literature might be worthwhile to further investigate leukogram values and their association with inflammatory disease. Currently, clinicians must coordinate case clinical pathology

Test	Results		Adult Reference Range	
CBC (Avian and Exotics)				
WBC Estimate	9.2 1000/uL		3-8	HIGH
HCT	22 %		23-35	LOW
RBC Morphology	Normal			
Blood Parasites	None Seen		NONE SEEN	
Differential	**Absolute**	**%**		
Heterophils	7,452 /uL	81		
Toxic Changes	None Seen	0-1		
Differential	**Absolute**	**%**		
Bands	0 /uL	0		
Lymphocytes	1,656 /uL	18		
Monocytes	0 /uL	0		
Eosinophils	0 /uL	0		
Basophils	92 /uL	1		
Azurophilic Monocytes	0	0		
Thrombocyte Estimate	Adequate		ADEQUATE	

FIG 33.5 Hematology report of a juvenile sulcata tortoise (*Centrochelys sulcata*) with a cloacolith blockage. WBC count is provided by slide estimate and leukocytosis was determined. However, based on the likely minimum 20% expected variability of the estimated count, and the few reference ranges available for this species, this conclusion is debatable. Anemia is also identified and would be more acceptable if the jugular vein was used for venipuncture (avoiding lymphatic contamination), and this was not a 100-g (juvenile) animal. Heterophilia is present (4:1 ratio), but the young age of this animal may be contributory. Toxic changes may or may not be present. (Courtesy of J. Jill Heatley and Karen E. Russell.)

TABLE 33.7 Exemplar Reptiles and Amphibians in Which Lymphocytes Are Not the Predominant Leukocyte

Predominant Leukocyte	Species
Basophil	Common snapping turtle, *Chelydra serpentina*[59]
	Juvenile Northern red-bellied cooter, *Pseudemys rubriventris*[61]
	Pascagoula map turtle, *Graptemys gibbonsi*[77]
	Painted turtles, *Chrysemys picta*[78]
	Chinese and yellow pond turtles, *Mauremys mutica, M reevessii*[79]
	Japanese newt, *Cynops pyrrhogaster*[3]
	African clawed frog, *Xenopus laevis*[3]
	Sapito de jardin, little garden toad, *Bufo fernandezae*[3]
Azurophil	Eastern indigo snakes, *Drymarchon couperi*[80]
	Massasauga rattle snakes, *Sistrurus catenatus catenatus*[81]
Heterophil	Southeast Asian box turtle, *Cuora amboinensis*[77]
	Yellow-headed temple turtle, *Heosemys annandalii*[82]
	Yellow-marginated box turtle, *Cuora flavomarginata*[77]
	Asian yellow pond turtle, *Ocadia sinensis*[83]
	Basilisk, *Basiliscus plumifrons*[84]
	Spiny-tailed lizard, *Uromastyx* spp.[85]
	Desert tortoise, *Gopherus agassizii*[86]
	Radiated tortoise, *Geochelone radiate*[24,87]
	Mediterranean pond turtles, *Mauremys leprosa*[88]
Neutrophil	American bullfrog, *Rana catesbeiana*
	African tropical clawed frog, *Xenopus tropicalis*

results with pathology and microbiology results retrospectively. Reporting this information remains critical for the advancement of herpetologic clinical pathology and health care.

Stress may account for increased WBC and differential derangements, but the extent of these changes has not been extensively investigated in reptiles. Increased glucocorticoid levels are associated with heterophilia, lymphopenia, and degranulation of the granulocytes (heterophils and eosinophils) in some species.[21] Free living box turtles affected by clear-cutting of their home range suffered increased total WBC counts.[22] In *Uromastyx aegyptius*, heat stress is associated with increased WBC counts.[23] With few exceptions, we lack fundamental knowledge regarding the timing of inflammation and the associated cellular responses in reptiles. Based on the author's experience, in many species, inflammation, as caused by infection, trauma, neoplasia, and so on, may be more likely to cause a shift in leukocyte percentages rather than an increased total leukocyte count. Thus leukocytosis, although reported in reptiles, may occur less commonly in reptiles than in birds or mammals. Consequently, leukopenia in reptiles, possibly even more so than in birds and mammals, may be cause for clinical concern and a guarded prognosis. However, many natural reptile processes may be associated with a relative decrease in WBC count.

Red Blood Cells

Erythrocytes of reptiles and amphibians are nucleated ellipsoidal disks. Comparative erythrocyte size and volume generally proceeds from the smallest in some lizards, to snakes, crocodilians, chelonians, and the largest in amphibians. This spectrum of increasing red cell size is accompanied by decreasing red cell number, resulting in similar PCVs among these groups.[24] However, multiple species diverge from this generality (Table 33.8). In general, despite great variability in the total number of red blood cells (RBC), the mean cell volume (MCV) and mean cell hemoglobin (MCH), the hemoglobin level (Hb), PCV, and mean cell hemoglobin concentration (MCHC) are relatively constant but lower in reptiles compared with birds and mammals.[25] Thus oxygen carrying capacity also tends to be relatively lower in exothermic species.[25]

RBC, MCV, MCHC, MCH, Hb, and the attendant calculations are rarely determined for reptiles based on current analyzer methodologic limitations and incompatibility with the analysis of nucleated nonround cells. Some methods require sophisticated cell analysis techniques or lysis of cells to remove the nuclei.[26] However, these values have been determined for some species experimentally.[24,27,28] Beware of calculated

---

BOX 33.1 **Methods for Determining Total and Differential White Blood Cell Counts in Reptiles and Amphibians**

1. Slide estimate
   a. Materials needed: Slides with well-executed blood smears, cellular differentiating stain, microscope with at least ×400 magnification, ×1000 magnification preferred. Microscopist trained in differentiation of reptile or amphibian leukocytes.
   b. Time investment
      i. Differential 20 minutes
      ii. WBC estimate 10 minutes
   c. Technique
      i. 100 WBCs are counted and differentiated to create a percentage of cells = differential
      ii. At 400 magnification (high-dry, 40×), WBCs are counted in 10 separate fields in the monolayer, in which RBC are just barely touching. Sources vary as to the multiplier best used to provide an estimate of the total white blood count, which is generally from 1500 to 2500.
   d. Advantages: Minimum expense, small volume requirement (1 drop)
   e. Disadvantages: Time consuming for clinical practice, requires a well-trained eye, results likely very inaccurate, it is an estimate
2. Indirect phloxine stain technique (indirect method)
   a. Description: In the indirect method, acidophilic granulocytes (heterophils and eosinophils) are stained with phloxine solution and counted in a hemacytometer. Additionally, a differential cell count is performed on a blood film stained with Romanowsky-type stains (e.g., Wright-Giemsa).
   b. Materials needed: Slides with well-executed blood smears; cellular differentiating stain; aliquoted eosinophil stain; pipettor; anticoagulated blood; Neubauer improved hemocytometer; microscope with ×10, ×20, ×40, and ×100 objectives preferred. Microscopist trained in differentiation of reptile/amphibian leukocytes on blood smears and able to count granulocytes within the hemocytometer.
   c. Time investment
      i.   Differential 20 minutes
      ii. Granulocyte count 30 minutes
      iii. Calculations 10 minutes
   d. Technique
      i.   Mix 25 µL blood with 0.775 µL mL phloxine stain. Mix and stand for 10-15 mins.
      ii. Charge both sides of the Neubauer improved hemocytometer (Fig. 33.6, 33.7)
      iii. Place in humidity chamber for 10 minutes to allow cell settling
      iv. Count all granulocytes (pink dots) in large corner squares from one side = X
         1. Should any quaker be less than 50% of another square, cells were not distributed evenly; start count on other side of hemocytometer or return to (ii) with new hemocytometer.
      v.   The total WBC (×10⁹/L) = (average number of stained heterophils + eosinophils in 9 squares of hematocytometer × 1.1 × 16 × 0.1), divided by the percentage of heterophils + eosinophils in the differential. Multiply by 1000 for TWBC/µL.

   e. Advantages: Faster than Natt and Herrick's, more accurate than an estimate
   f. Disadvantages: Requires specialized equipment and reagents. Indirect method may underestimate total cell count in species that have nongranulocytic cells as the predominant inflammatory cell. This technique is heavily reliant on a quality blood smear to produce an accurate differential; a damaged or poorly fixed blood smear will cause erroneous results. When heteropenia exists the total leukocyte count may be falsely elevated.
3. Direct Natt and Herrick's stain technique
   a. Materials needed: Slides with well-executed blood smears; cellular differentiating stain; aliquoted Natt and Herrick's stain; pipetter; anticoagulated blood; Neubauer improved hemocytometer; microscope with ×10, ×20, ×40, and ×100 objectives preferred. Microscopist trained in differentiation of reptile/amphibian leukocytes in both Natt and Herrick's stain and within blood smears.
   b. Time investment
      i.   Differential 20 minutes (not necessary for numbers, but slide review of morphology and platelet estimate should be performed)
      ii. Cellular counts 60 to 90 minutes
      iii. Calculation 5 minutes
   c. Technique: Dilute whole anticoagulated blood 1:200 with Natt and Herrick's solution. Allow the diluted blood to mix for a minute or two before discharging into the hemocytometer counting chamber. Allow the hemocytometer contents to settle for approximately 3 minutes.
      i. Performing the total erythrocyte count using the high dry (40×) objective of the microscope; count the total number of RBCs (easily recognizable by their nuclei) in the four corners and central squares of the central large square of the counting chamber. Count all cells that overlap the top and left border. Do not count any cells that overlap the bottom or right borders. Multiply the total number of cells counted by 0.01 to obtain TRBC ×10¹²/L. Multiply total number of counted cells by 10,000 to obtain TRBC/µL.
      ii. WBCs tend to stain dark blue to purple and may exhibit some granularity. The total leukocyte count is obtained by counting all leukocytes present in the nine large ruled squares of both sides of the hemacytometer, and calculating the average of the two. Count all cells that overlap the top and left border. Do not count any cells that overlap the bottom or right borders (Fig. 33.8). The computation for total leukocyte count is: Total WBC × 10⁹/L = total leukocytes counted in 9 squares (average of both sides) × 1.1 × 0.2. For total WBC/µL ×1000.
   d. Advantages allow for direct counting of both erythrocytes and leukocytes in amphibian and reptilian species. As the same dilution is used for both red and white cells, a total leukocyte and a total erythrocyte count can be obtained simultaneously from the same charged hemacytometer.
   e. Disadvantages: Because many more cells are there for the counting, this method can be very time consuming. Differentiating WBC from thrombocytes may be difficult; thrombocytosis could result in an erroneously high WBC.

---

hematocrits in reptiles, which, based on cellular size and shape, may or may not be reflective of a centrifuge-determined PCV (the gold standard). Similarly, RBC count by automated cell counters may be suspect when species-specific standards are not provided. Calculated or other methodologies for determination of HCT are seldom validated for use in reptiles. Manual methods for manual determination of RBC necessitate use of dilution pipettes, hemocytometers, and Natt and Herrick's or other specialized cell stains, as well as a trained and proficient hematology technician.[24]

Packed Cell Volume

Clinical evaluation of the reptilian and amphibian RBC parameters is often best provided by PCV determination (Tables 33.8 and 33.9). Causes for relatively increased or decreased PCV of reptiles are numerous and

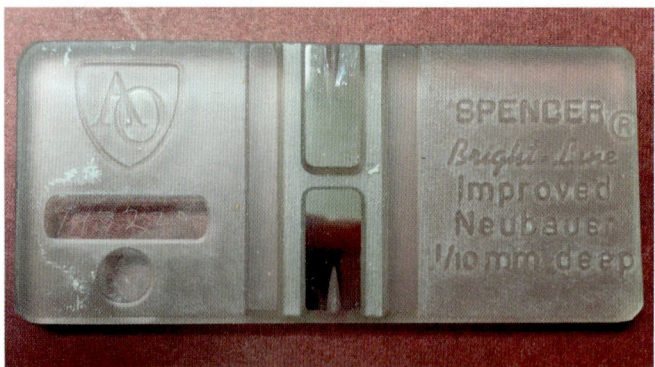

FIG 33.6 Glass Neubauer cell counter, which can be used for hemocytometry. These antiques may be used for prolonged periods, but as glass they are fragile, must be carefully cleaned and dried between counts, and require a new cover slip for each count. For more detail, see Fig. 33.8. (Courtesy of J. Jill Heatley and Karen E. Russell.)

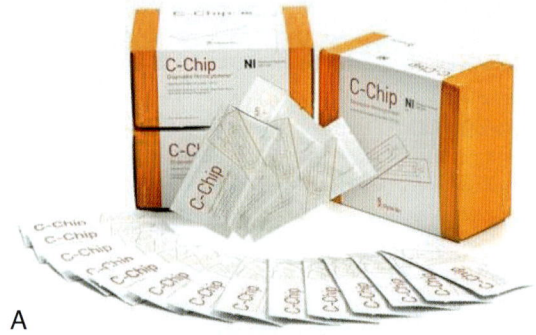

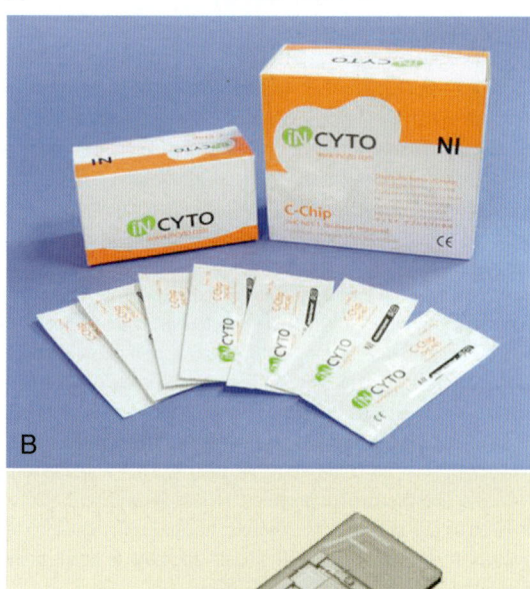

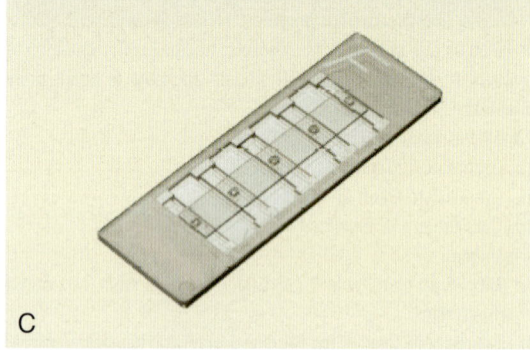

FIG 33.7 (A–C) Disposable hemocytometer examples. These hemocytometers are plastic and relatively inexpensive but must be bought in batches of 50 from standard laboratory supply companies. Four- rather than two-chamber disposable counters are also available (C, four-chip Neubauer improved plastic cell counting chamber, bulldog-bio.com). (Courtesy of J. Jill Heatley and Karen E. Russell.)

include both normal physiological and disease-based origins. Causes for increased or decreased PCV in ill or injured reptiles parallel those of companion mammals. For example, chronic lower gastrointestinal tract strictures of green sea turtles *Chelonia mydas* have been associated with a persistent anemia.[29] Table 33.10 provides etiologies of PCV change in reptiles.

Causes for physiological change in RBC parameters for reptiles are numerous. As reptiles age, MCV, MCHC, MCH, RBC, PCV, and Hb tend to increase.[30–32] In general, one might expect increased RBC and PCV posthibernation compared with prehibernation, as well as during active periods compared with hibernation or less active periods.[33] Similarly, posthibernation reptiles can have a marked regenerative erythroid response accompanied by basophilic stippling.[26] However, many exceptions exist; for example, the captive South American rattlesnake (*Crotalus durissus terrificus*) had significantly higher RBC, PCV, Hb, MCV, MCH, and MCHC in winter than in summer.[31] Relatively increased Hb, PCV, and/or RBC mass occur in some male chelonia compared with females, but many reptile species do not adhere to this expectation.[34] For example, captive female green iguanas had higher PCV and MCHC values than males.[33]

Pathologic changes in PCV or other RBC parameters can be characterized as anemia or polycythemia. True polycythemia has not been reported in reptiles; however, hyperviscosity syndrome may occur in association with rapid temperature change or envenomation.[13] Increased PCV and RBC count have been reported in terrapins subjected to hyperosmotic stress.[21] Polycythemia may be considered when PCV exceeds 40% but is rare and more commonly caused by dehydration.[13]

Anemia, a decreased PCV and/or RBC count, may be classified as regenerative or nonregenerative. Clinicopathologic markers of regenerative anemia of reptiles include cytoplasmic basophilic stippling, polychromasia, binucleation, increased anisocytosis and anisokaryosis, and an increased number of mitotic figures and/or early erythroid precursors.[33] A regenerative response in reptiles is also typically associated with a decrease in MCV and MCHC.[33] As in other vertebrates common differentials for regenerative anemia include acute blood loss from trauma or parasitism, hemolytic diseases (including oxidative damage from zinc toxicosis), hemoparasites or other infectious disease, microangiopathic disease, and marked hypophosphatemia. Hemoparasitism or heavy metal toxicity may result in hemolytic anemia.[26] However, hemoparasitism does not dictate hemolytic anemia, and this sign likely depends on a number of factors including the species of hemoparasite, host adaptation, and the primarily affected cell type. In the teiid lizard

(*Ameiva ameiva*), hematozoon parasitism causes a monocytosis and ultrastructural changes in infected monocytes but does not affect erythrocyte parameters.[35]

Nonregenerative anemias are characterized by a lack of cytologically appreciable response; however, normal reptile regenerative response times have not been characterized and are likely slower than mammals, based on their expected RBC lifespan of 600 to 800 days.[36] Reptiles with iron-deficiency anemia may have hypochromic erythrocyte with decreased MCH and MCHC. Causes for iron deficiency in reptiles are similar to other vertebrates and include chronic inflammatory disease, iron-deficient diets, and malabsorption due to gastrointestinal disease. Anemia of chronic disease is likely the most common cause of nonregenerative anemia in reptiles and includes a multitude of etiologies:[33]

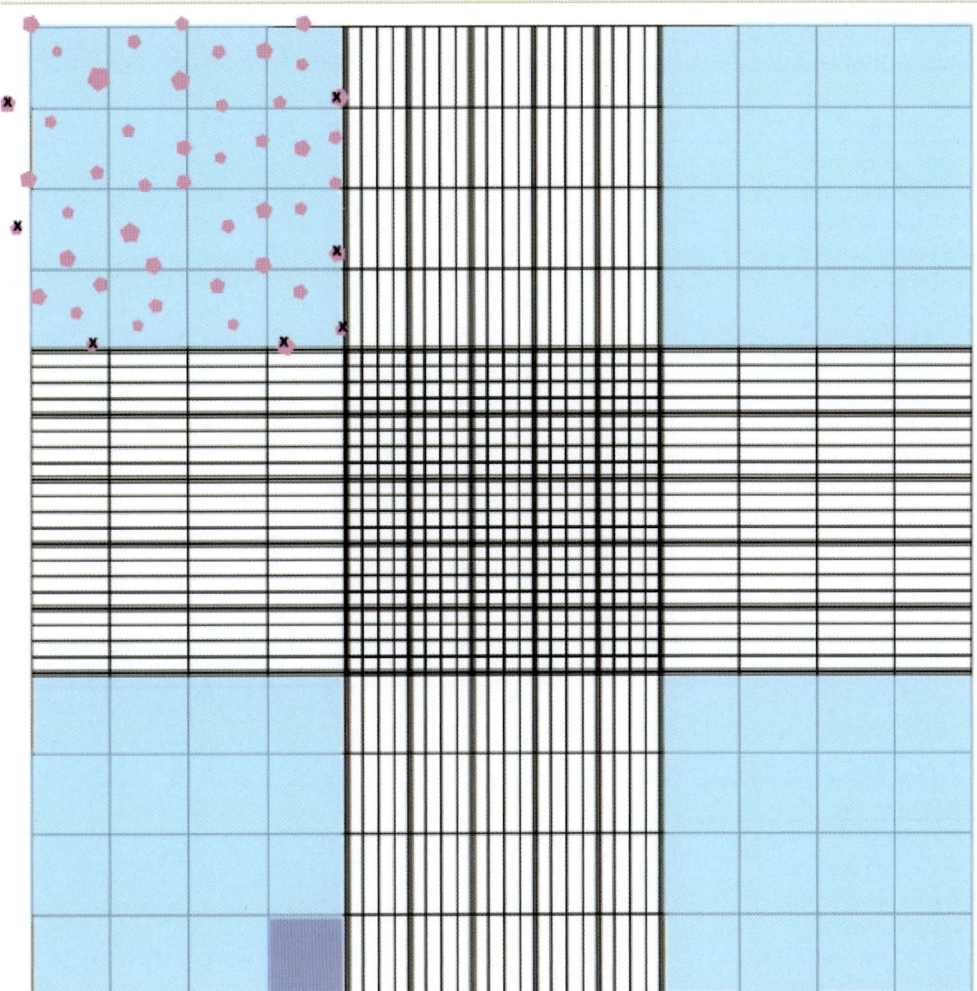

FIG 33.8 Microscopic grid of a Neubauer cell counter. The small purple square is 0.25 × 0.25 mm, whereas squares created by the bold lines (area filled in light blue) are 1 × 1 mm. Areas filled with light blue are used for counting granulocytes in the indirect eosinophil stain method. In the upper left square, an example of the counting method is demonstrated. Cells (pink pentagons) outside the grid or, by convention, those on the inner or lower lines (bottom and right, X) are not counted whereas those on the upper and outer lines (top and left) are counted. (Courtesy of J. Jill Heatley and Karen E. Russell.)

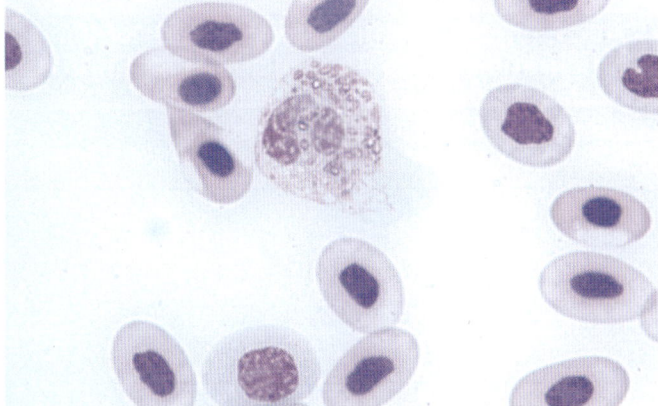

FIG 33.9 Blood smear from a green iguana (*Iguana iguana*), 1000× magnification, Modified Wright Giemsa stain. Foamy cytoplasm and poor granulation of this heterophil are suggestive of toxic change. (Courtesy of J. Jill Heatley and Karen E. Russell.)

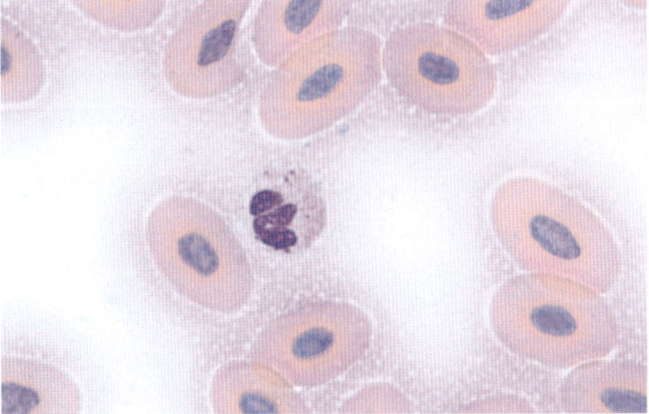

FIG 33.10 Blood smear from a bearded dragon (*Pogona vitticeps*), 1000× magnification, Modified Wright Giemsa stain. Foamy cytoplasm, poor granulation, and purple granules of this heterophil are suggestive of toxic change. (Courtesy of J. Jill Heatley and Karen E. Russell.)

TABLE 33.8   Comparative Mean Corpuscular Volume, Erythrocyte Count, and Packed Cell Volume of Select Reptiles and Amphibians

Class	Species	MCV (fl)	RBC x 10^{12}/L (x10^6/µL)	PCV %
Snake[89]	Grass snake, male	190 ± 7	1.545 ± 0.33	29.4 ± 6
	Natrix natrix natrix, female	191 ± 8	1.748 ± 0.32	36.3 ± 6
Lizard[90]	Prehensile-tailed skink	263 (152–600)	1.5 (0.8–1.4)	35 (24–60)
	Corucia zebrata			
Lizard[35]	Tegu	264 ± 57	1.36 ± 0.24	35 ± 3
	Ameiva ameiva			
Crocodilian[91]	Nile crocodiles	312 ± 60	0.59 ± 0.12 0.35–1.00	17.9 ± 2.0 14–22
	Crocodylus niloticus	200–465		
Lizard[32]	Green iguana	346 ± 60	1.04 ± 0.16	35 ± 5
	Iguana iguana			
Tortoise[92]	Mediterranean spur-thighed Tortoise	383 ± 37	0.758 ± 0.147	28 ± 4
	Testudo graeca			
Turtle[93]	Red-eared slider	401 ± 22	0.45 ± 0.08	18 ± 4
	Trachemys scripta elegans			
Crocodilian[94]	Broad-snouted caiman	404 ± 16	0.727 ± 0.05	28.6 ±1.2
	Caiman latirostris			
Crocodilian[68]	American alligator	430–446	0.476–0.697	24.5–32.0
	Alligator mississippiensis			
Snake[95]	Indian rat snake, captive	434 ± 55	0.88 ± 0.10	34 ± 2
	Ptyas mucosa			
Tortoise[92]	*Testudo hermanni*	435 ± 95	0.649 ± 0.09	27 ± 5
Snake[95]	Indian rat snake, wild rescued	444 ± 37	0.89 ± 0.10	36 ± 1
	Ptyas mucosa			
Anuran	Argentine horned frog	450		
	Ceratophrys ornata			
Anuran[96]	American bull frog	714		22 ± 5
	Rana catesbeiana			
Anuran[97]	Oriental fire-bellied toad	607–750	Males 0.34; females 0.29	19.5
	Bombina orientalis			
Urodele[98]	Eastern newt	2204		21–28
	Notophthlamus viridescens			
Urodele[99,100]	Hellbender	No value given		27–57
	Cryptobranchus alliganiensis			
Urodele[101]	Mudpuppy	No value given	0.007–0.063	
	Necturus maculosis			

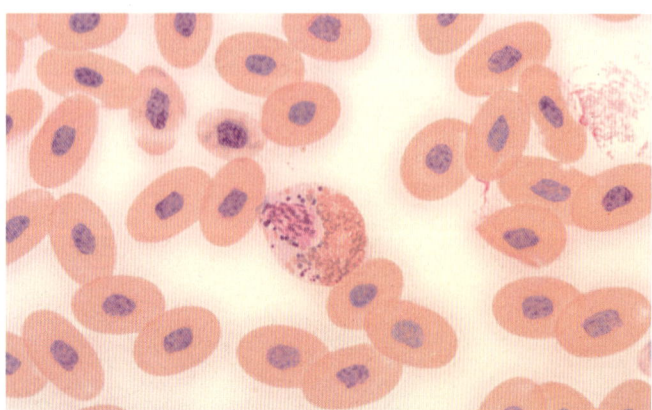

FIG 33.11 Blood smear from a savannah monitor lizard (*Varanus exanthematicus*), 1000× magnification, Modified Wright Giemsa stain. This central granulocyte shows evidence of toxic granulation. (Courtesy of J. Jill Heatley and Karen E. Russell.)

TABLE 33.9   Erythrocyte Variables of a Comparative Study That Included 33 Reptile Species From the Orders Testudines, Crocodylia, Sauria, and Serpentes[25]

Variable	Mean SD	Observed Range
RBC (×10^{12}/L)	0.75 ± 0.32	0.24–1.57
MCV (fL)	398 ± 121.4	214.3–707.4
MCH (pg)	125.5 ± 46.8	60.2–270.8
Hb (g/dL)	8.5 ± 1.9	5.1–12.0
PCV (%)	25.7 ± 6.5	15.0–38.8
MCHC (g/dL)	31.1 ± 4.0	22.5–39.3

Hb, Hemoglobin; *MCH*, mean cell hemoglobin; *MCHC*, mean cell hemoglobin concentration; *MCV*, mean cell volume; *PCV*, packed cell volume; *RBC*, red blood cells.

TABLE 33.10   Etiologies of Packed Cell Volume (PCV) Changes in Reptiles[22,24,26]

	Factor	Comments
Increased PCV		
Physiological	**Male**	Reproductive activity and hydration status
	Pre-hibernation [brumation]	Activity increased need for blood cells
	Favorable environmental conditions	Summer, increased temperature, geographic variation
Disease	Dehydration	Husbandry, renal disease, gastrointestinal disease
Decreased PCV		
Physiological	**Female**	Reproductive activity and hydration status
	Juvenile	Hatchling to year one
	Posthibernation [brumation]	Inactivity reduced need for blood cells
	Unfavorable environmental conditions	Winter, decreased temperature, other unfavorable climatic conditions, lack of food, clear cutting, poor husbandry
Disease	**Systemic chronic inflammation or degenerative disease**	Coagulation disorders, thrombocytopenia*
		Neoplasia, infection
	Blood loss	Trauma to include surgery, gastrointestinal tract ulcers, hemoparasitism, hematophagous ectoparasitism
	Pollution	Lead, zinc, other environmental toxins
Artifactual	**Collection technique**	Lymphatic or cerebrospinal fluid contamination
		Hemolysis from inappropriate choice of handling, storage, venipuncture technique, anticoagulant

Italic factors are commonly regenerative. Boldface factors are commonly nonregenerative.
*May be regenerative in early stages until iron stores are depleted. Reptilian regenerative and nonregenerative anemias have not been well characterized and are assumed to follow the same general trends as mammals. However, time until visualization of regenerative cytological signs may be relatively prolonged in these ectothermic species.

- Systemic infectious disease
- Chronic degenerative or inflammatory diseases of the liver, kidney, spleen, or lungs
- Gastrointestinal disease
- Inappropriate husbandry/starvation
- Hematopoietic neoplasia
- Multifactorial from above

Assessment of anemia relies heavily upon evaluation of cellular morphology to identify a regenerative response. Polychromatophilic cells are often assessed as synonymous with reticulocytes, which are generally <1% to 2.5% in healthy reptiles. Increased polychromasia may have also been associated with ecdysis and young age (Fig. 33.12). Similarly, anisocytosis, variation in cell size, is mild to minimal in healthy reptiles and amphibians. A highly regenerative response is associated with polychromasia as well as binucleated erythrocytes, a few mitotic figures, and even younger erythroid precursors such as rubricytes and prorubricytes. However, similar regenerative responses (binucleated RBC, anisokaryosis, mitosis) have, in reptiles, been associated with hibernation emergence, severe inflammation, malnutrition, starvation, and in amphibians with increased lactate or changes in oxygen and carbon dioxide tension of polluted water.[37] Basophilic stippling of reptilian erythrocytes is rare but associated with lead toxicity, iron deficiency, or regenerative responses.[26] An increased number of fusiform or teardrop-shaped erythrocytes has been associated with septicemia or chronic infectious disease; however, these cell shapes are commonly found in the circulation of healthy amphibians.[3,33]

LEUKOCYTE MORPHOLOGY, FUNCTION, AND INTERPRETATION

Leukocytes of amphibians and reptiles are thought to have similar function as those of other vertebrates, but few functional studies have

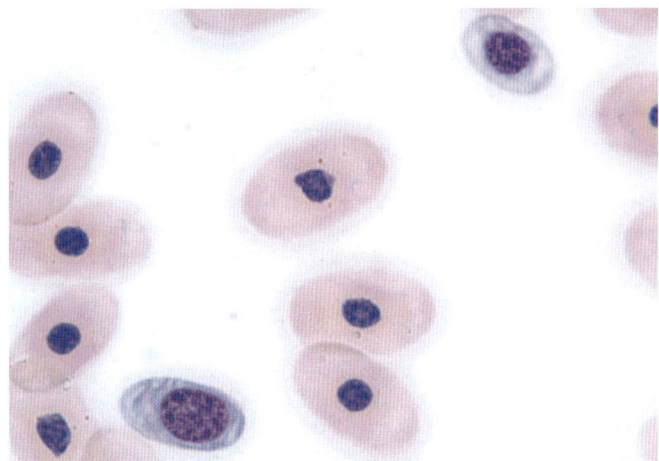

FIG 33.12 Blood smear from a red-eared slider (*Trachemys scripta elegans*), 1000× magnification, Modified Wright Giemsa stain. Polychromatophils (immature bluish RBCs, upper right, lower left) starkly contrast the adult erythrocytes and support a regenerative response to anemia in this patient, which was infected by hemogregarines. (Courtesy of J. Jill Heatley and Karen E. Russell.)

been performed.[3] As reptiles age, WBC counts tend to decrease.[30,31] The agranulocytes consist of lymphocytes, monocytes, and azurophils. The granulocytes include the heterophil, eosinophil, and basophil. Cell differentiation may be complicated by species variety.

Lymphocyte

Reptilian and amphibian lymphocytes and monocytes have similar morphology and likely similar function to those of mammals.

TABLE 33.11	**Clinical Differentiation of Reptile and Amphibian Mononuclear Cells With Immune Function**		
Factors	Monocyte	Lymphocyte	Thrombocyte
Shape	Round-oval	Round	Inactivated: Elongate oval similar to erythrocyte Activated: Round sometimes with small pseudopodia
Cytoplasm	Abundant pale blue-gray, vacuoles variably present Vacuoles may contain: melanin, nucleoproteinaceous debris, lipid, erythrocytes, hemosiderin	No granules, thin, blue	Clear to very light purple or blue, small pink granules
Nucleus	Round, oval, reniform, or multilobed Smooth to slightly clumped chromatin	Eccentric, round dark blue-purple, chromatin clumping, or nucleoli may be seen	Centric, very dark purple, often indented, no internal structures visible
N:C	1:3	4:1	1:1
Activity	Clumping uncommon	Clumping uncommon but may be induced by some anticoagulants	Rafting (clumps) common
Size (μm)	8–25	5–15	8–16 × 5–9

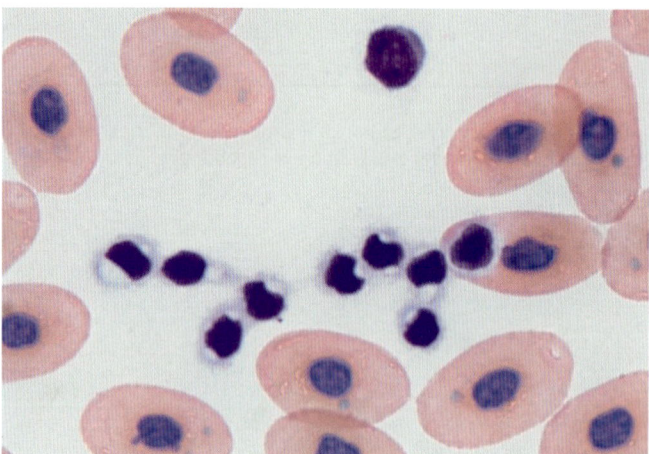

FIG 33.13 Blood smear from a box turtle (*Terrapene carolina*), 1000× magnification, Modified Wright Giemsa stain. Thrombocytes (central) and lymphocyte (upper). (Courtesy of J. Jill Heatley and Karen E. Russell.)

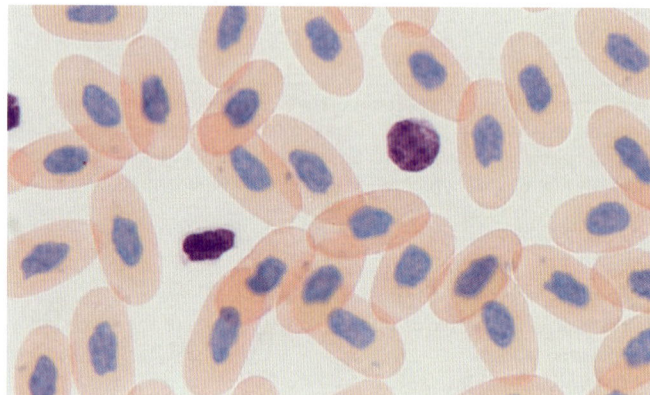

FIG 33.14 Blood smear from a red tegu (*Tupinambus rufescens*), 1000× magnification, Modified Wright Giemsa stain. Thrombocyte (left) and lymphocyte (right). (Courtesy of J. Jill Heatley and Karen E. Russell.)

Lymphocytes are the most common leukocyte, accounting for up to 80% of the differential of most healthy reptiles, although exceptions to this general rule exist (see Table 33.7).[33] The thrombocyte may be challenging to differentiate from small lymphocytes, resulting in erroneously high lymphocyte counts within differentials (see Table 33.11 and Figs. 33.13 and 33.14). Immune stimulation based on inflammatory or infectious disease has been associated with the peripheral circulation of large lymphocytes, reactive lymphocytes, lymphoblasts, plasmacytoid lymphocytes, granular lymphocytes, and rarely, plasma cells.[33] Plasma cells are larger than the normal lymphocyte with a deep blue cytoplasm, a round eccentric nucleus with chromatin clumping, and a perinuclear halo created by the golgi apparatus. Etiologies of lymphocytosis include subacute causes of inflammation associated with infection, wound healing, parasitism, and viral disease.[33] Clinicopathologic etiologies of lymphopenia should include exogenous testosterone administration, endogenous or exogenous steroid exposure, acute bacterial infection, and other causes of immunosuppression (including poor husbandry and malnutrition).[38] Reptile B lymphocyte and T lymphocyte functions include immunoglobulin production and cell-mediated immune responses.[33]

Monocyte

Reptilian and amphibian monocytes have similar morphology and likely similar functions to those of mammals (Figs. 33.15 through 33.17). Monocytes may comprise up to 10% of the leukocytes in a healthy reptile.[33] Physiological causes of relative monocytosis include (pre)hibernation in free-ranging gopher and desert tortoises; however, similar findings were not apparent in pre- and posthibernation captive vipers.[39–41] Otherwise, and in comparison to other leukocytes of reptiles, monocyte counts change minimally between seasons. Absolute monocytosis may occur due to chronic antigenic stimulation or chronic inflammation associated with bacterial and parasitical diseases, dystocia, and leukemic neoplasia.[33,42] Circulating monocytes may phagocytose erythrocytes, hemosiderin, melanin, and other cellular components. Differential etiologies of these cells in circulation include postsurgical or other trauma, wound healing, sepsis, infectious disease, delayed sample processing, and immune-mediated disease.[33,43–45] Differentiation between large lymphocytes and monocytes may also be challenging during the cell counting process if Natt and Herrick's solution is used. In the teiid lizard *Ameiva ameiva*, hematozoon parasitism causes ultrastructural changes in infected monocytes, monocytosis and leukocytosis.[35]

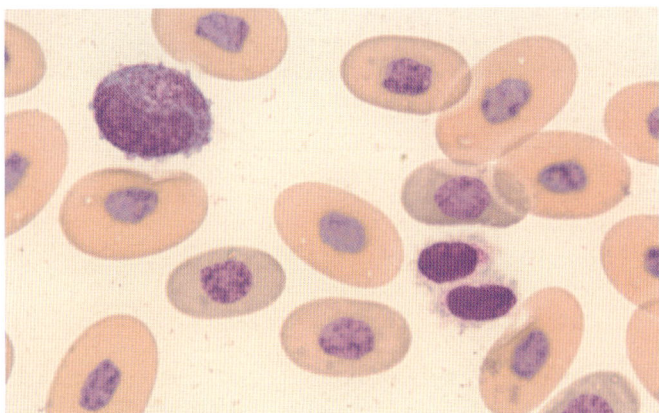

FIG 33.15 Blood smear from a Panther chameleon (*Furcifer pardalis*), 1000× magnification, Modified Wright Giemsa stain. An azurophilic monocyte (upper left) and two activated thrombocytes (lower right) are shown. (Courtesy of J. Jill Heatley and Karen E. Russell.)

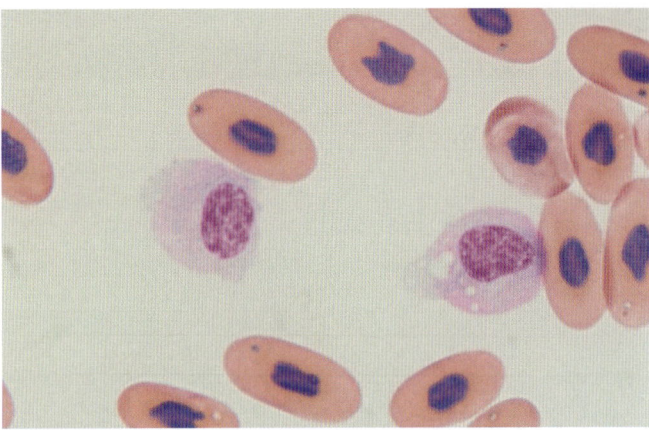

FIG 33.17 Blood smear from a ball python (*Python regius*), 1000× magnification, Modified Wright Giemsa stain, monocytes. (Courtesy of J. Jill Heatley and Karen E. Russell.)

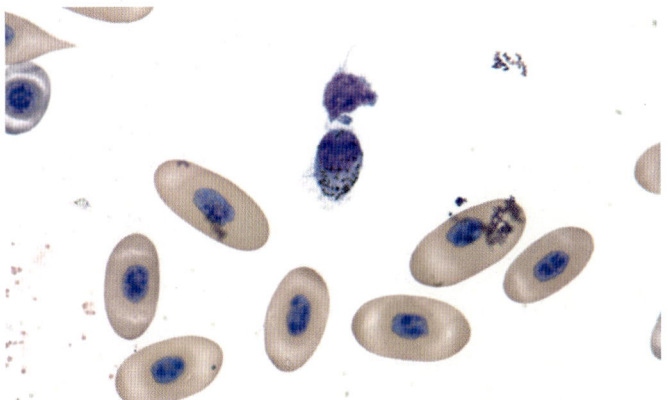

FIG 33.16 Blood smear from a long-nosed horned frog (*Megaphrys nasuta*), 1000× magnification, Modified Wright Giemsa stain, melanomacrophage.

Azurophil

The azurophil is a relatively large mononuclear cell that appears unique to the monocyte line of reptiles and amphibians. This cell is similar in size to the monocyte but has a fine dusting of small azurophilic granules that may impart a darker blue (azure) appearance. These cells occur commonly in snakes and may account for up to 35% of the WBC differential in healthy specimens.[33] These cells also occur on lizards, crocodilians, and least commonly chelonians[33] (see Fig. 33.15). The azurophil may function differently based on the species. Cytochemical staining of snake azurophils indicates a function similar to mammalian neutrophils, whereas those of lizards may function more like mammalian monocytes.[33] Thus in snakes, azurophilia has been associated with acute stages of inflammation and infectious disease, whereas in other reptiles increased number of azurophils may more likely signal chronic inflammation.[33,46,47] Although the exact function of the azurophil remains unknown, functions likely include those similar to the monocyte including phagocytosis. Azurophils have been tentatively identified in amphibians.[48,49] Based on the variable presence and likely function of this cell in reptiles and amphibians, the clinician must be familiar with the cell-counting procedures of their reference laboratory because azurophils may or may not be counted separately from monocytes. The

resultant differential, especially in snakes, could vary markedly depending on the laboratory classification of these cells.

Heterophil

Heterophils are commonly the most numerous granulocytes followed by eosinophils and basophils (Table 33.12). Heterophils are a granular leukocyte characterized by granules that have variable sizes and staining characteristics. As such, the term heterophil is most often used to describe the granulocyte (and second-most common leukocyte) with rod or variably shaped granules that may fail to uptake stain (appear clear) or appear pale pink, bright orange, or even green-blue (see Figs. 33.9 through 33.11). In some crocodilians and chelonians, heterophils may account for greater than 50% of the differential in the healthy animal.[33] Heterophils are believed to function similarly to that of mammalian neutrophils; they can phagocytize bacteria and other foreign materials. As primary responders for the innate immune system, increased heterophils in the peripheral blood may occur based on a variety of inflammatory stimuli. The term heterophil has been used for the primary amphibian granulocyte, but based on cytochemical staining and enzyme contents, neutrophil is now preferred.[3]

Heterophil number changes have been reported based on numerous physiological factors. In general, relative increases are often associated with adult males, juveniles, summer season (compared with hibernation), and free-living states (compared with captivity).[33] Etiologies of pathologic heterophilia are presumed similar to those of other vertebrates, including acute, active inflammatory conditions, such as infectious diseases (bacterial, parasitical), tissue injury, necrosis, gravidity, exogenous or endogenous glucocorticoids, and neoplasia, including granulocytic leukemia.[33] Severe, acute inflammation may result in heteropenia with a left shift or toxic changes.[47] Heteropenia may occur due to acute toxicity (e.g., fenbendazole administration) or severe, acute inflammatory disease, such as overwhelming sepsis (which may also be accompanied by left shift and/or toxic changes).[68]

Eosinophils

Eosinophil morphology of reptiles and amphibians is similar to that of mammals (see Table 33.12 and Figs. 33.18 and 33.19). An important exception to this rule is the "green" eosinophil of some iguanid, teiid, and agamid lizards, so named based on their pale blue-green granules (Fig. 33.20). Eosinophils are rare to absent in most snakes but have been documented in the king cobra (*Ophiophagus hannah*), Burmese

TABLE 33.12 Differential Morphology of Reptile Granulocytes Based on Modified Wright Stain

Cell	Cytoplasm	Granules	Nucleus	Size (μm)
Heterophil	Clear	Distinct fusiform (crocodilians, chelonians) Angular pleomorphic, densely packed (squamates) Orange-pink	Round to oval (snakes, chelonians, crocodilians) Bilobed or multilobed (lizards) Eccentric	10–23 (Figs. 33.5 and 33.6)
Eosinophil	Clear	Round and pink Exceptions: blue-green in iguanas, tegu, rainbow lizard	Eccentric, round to oval elongated or bilobed	9–20 (Figs. 33.9, 33.15, and 33.17)
Basophil	Pale purple	Numerous, small round, deep purple (metachromic)	Round eccentric, often obscured by granules	7–12 (Figs. 33.7 and 33.9)

Cells are listed in decreasing order of appearance in most reptilian species.[47,52]

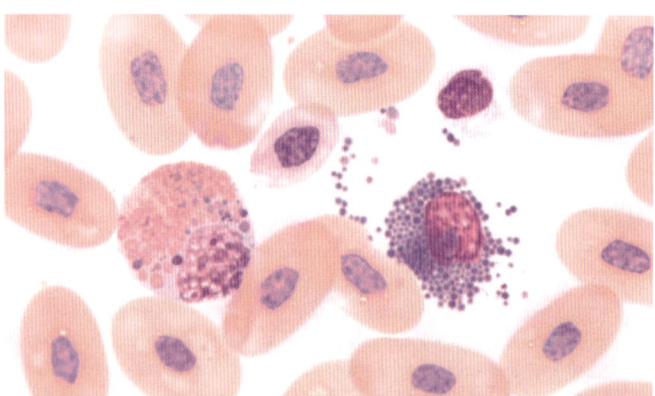

FIG 33.18 Blood smear from a savannah monitor (*Varanus exanthematicus*), 1000× magnification, Modified Wright Giemsa stain. Two granulocytes are present: An eosinophil is shown on the left and a fractured basophil with free granules is on the right. (Courtesy of J. Jill Heatley and Karen E. Russell.)

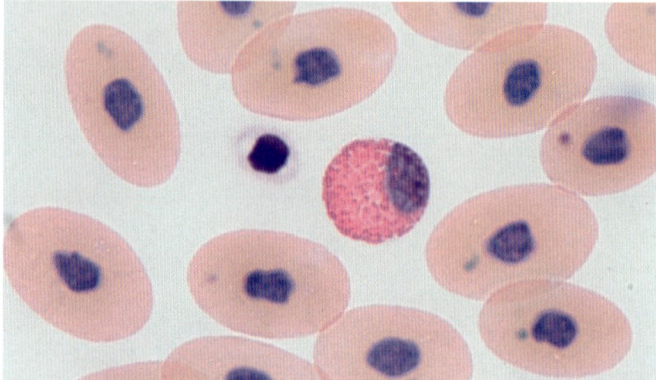

FIG 33.19 Blood smear from a box turtle (*Terrapene carolina*), 1000× magnification, Modified Wright Giemsa stain. Eosinophil (center) and a thrombocyte to the left. (Courtesy of J. Jill Heatley and Karen E. Russell.)

python, reticulated python (*Malayopython reticulatus*), African rock python (*Python sebae*), green tree python (*Morelia viridis*), and boa constrictor (*Boa constrictor*).[50,51,52,53] Eosinophils may represent a second heterophil type in snakes.[54,52,55,56] In healthy reptiles, eosinophils range from 7% to 20% of the WBC differential, with relatively fewer cells in lizards and increased numbers in chelonia. The functions of reptile and amphibian eosinophils remain minimally studied, but increased numbers have been associated with parasitic disease.[33,57] Reptile eosinophils can phagocytose immune complexes and bacteria and have microbicidal properties.[33]

Basophils

Basophils, the small "cluster of grapes" cell, are usually easily differentiated from other reptile and amphibian granulocytes (Table 33.11 and Figs. 33.18 and 33.21). However, basophils may degranulate to expose their eccentric nucleus, pale purple cytoplasm, and the remaining clear distinct cytoplasmic vacuoles. Occasionally, nearby granules may be observed or, even more rarely, the act of granule expulsion may be evident.[48] Basophil degranulation may occur because of a number of external factors including methanol quick-based stains (e.g., DiffQuik) and inappropriate sample collection, handling, slide preparation, or delayed processing.[33,48] Lack of metachromatic staining of basophil granules may also occur with use of aqueous-based stains.[58] Despite documented possession and release of histamine and expression of immunoglobulin, the function of the reptile basophil remains poorly understood.[59,60]

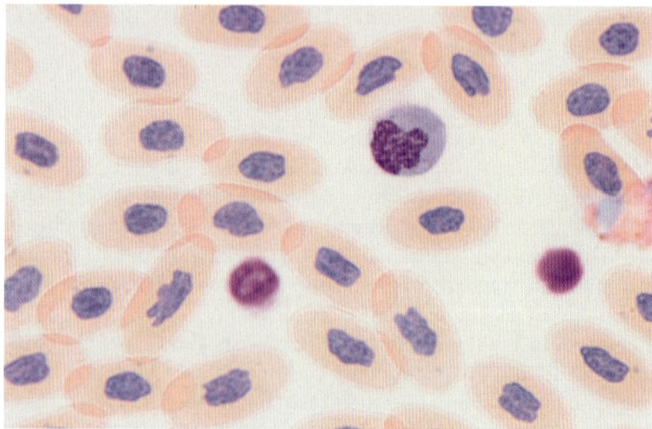

FIG 33.20 Blood smear from a red tegu (*Tupinambus rufescens*), 1000× magnification, Modified Wright Giemsa stain. "Green" eosinophil. (Courtesy of J. Jill Heatley and Karen E. Russell.)

Basophils appear more commonly in chelonians with up to 40% to 65% reported in some healthy species.[59,61] In some amphibians, basophils can be the predominant leukocyte (see Table 33.7).[3] Likely based on the predominance of basophils in some chelonia, reports of relatively increased numbers of these cells based on physiological factors so far appear limited to these species. In chelonia, one might expect increased

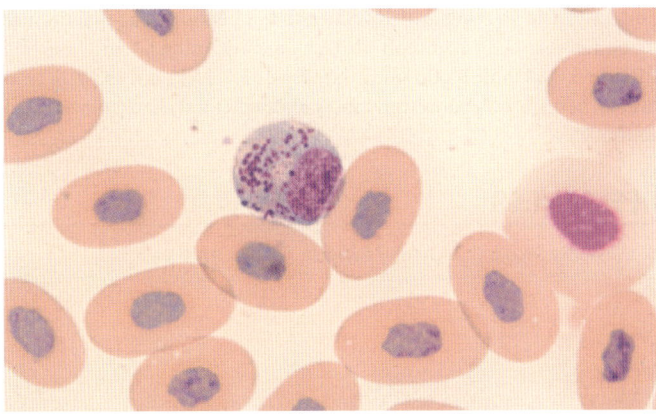

FIG 33.21 Blood smear from a Panther chameleon (*Furcifer pardalis*), 1000× magnification, Modified Wright Giemsa stain. Minimal granulation in a basophil, which allows the eccentric nonlobulated nucleus to be observed. (Courtesy of J. Jill Heatley and Karen E. Russell.)

basophil numbers in spring versus summer or during active periods versus hibernation.[33] Pathologically increased numbers of basophils have been associated with hemic infections, including hemoparasites and iridovirus.[33]

Thrombocytes

Thrombocytes are ovoid cells with pale cytoplasma but transform to round cells when activated (see Figs. 33.13, 33.14, and 33.19). Fig. 33.2A depicts multiple small lymphocytes as well as multiple inactivated thrombocytes. The thrombocyte may be challenging to differentiate from the small lymphocyte, resulting in erroneously high lymphocyte counts within differentials. Table 33.11 provides figures and explanations to differentiate these cells. Best methods for accurate determination of thrombocyte counts remain to be demonstrated in reptiles.[62] Comparison among the many differing methodologies makes meaningful clinical interpretation of the extant literature challenging. Platelet estimation from the blood smear is most commonly reported as reduced, adequate, increased or clumped. Direct thrombocyte counting techniques are hampered by numerous, similarly stained, shaped, and sized mononucleated cells, most notably small lymphocytes. Despite these challenges, the reptile thrombocyte is an important part of the clotting response and is also thought to have phagocytic properties. Currently, use of thrombocyte counts as a significant prognostic or diagnostic tool is unreliable.[62] The hematology report should include thrombocyte numbers if direct (Natt and Herrick's) hemocytometry methods were used. Otherwise, these cells could have been mistaken for lymphocytes, resulting in an erroneously high lymphocyte count.[3] As reptiles age, thrombocyte counts tend to decrease.[32,30,31]

Hemoparasites and Cellular Inclusions

Hemoparasites are not uncommonly encountered in the blood smears of wild-caught or free-living reptiles. Specific treatment is seldom pursued unless clinical disease is evident; supportive care and removal of intermediate hosts from the environment are generally sufficient. Hemoparasites include: *Hemogregarina* spp. (Fig. 33.22), *Karyolysus* spp., *Trypansoma* spp., and microfilaria of *Filarid* spp. (Fig. 33.23). For a more detailed description of the numerous species and host interactions and morphology of hemoparasites of reptiles a complete text is available.[63] Cellular inclusions of multiple types are not uncommon in reptiles and may signal a variety of conditions, ranging from benign to life threatening. Differentials include reptarenavirus (Fig. 33.24) iridovirus, poxvirus, *Chlamydia*, degenerate organelles (see Figs. 33.23

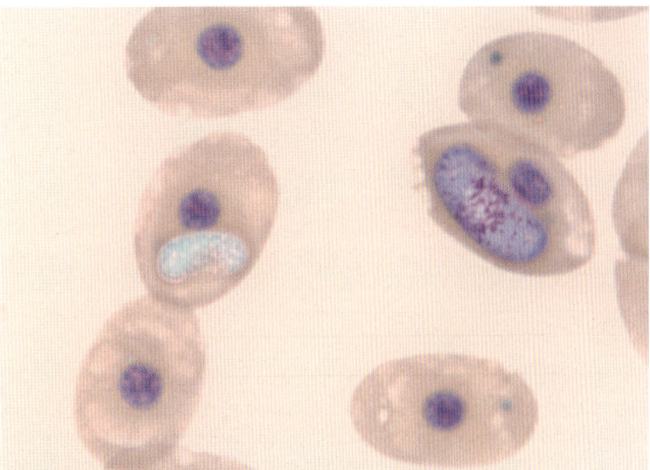

FIG 33.22 Blood smear from a common snapping turtle (*Chelydra serpentine*), 1000× magnification, Modified Wright Giemsa stain. Two forms of the hemogregarine parasite are observed within erythrocytes. Also note multiple clear areas within several RBCs that likely represent drying artifact. (Courtesy of J. Jill Heatley and Karen E. Russell.)

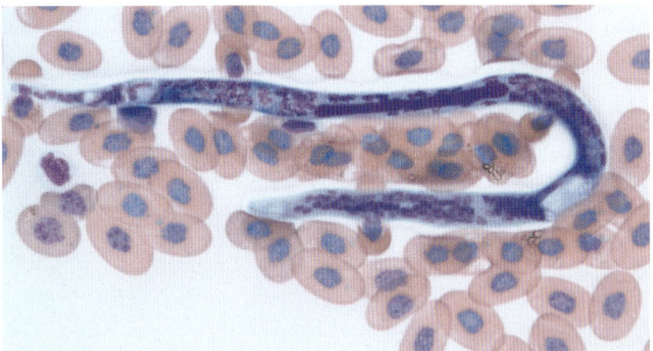

FIG 33.23 Blood smear from an adult male box turtle (*Terrapene carolina*), 600× magnification, Modified Wright Giemsa stain, Microfilariasis (spp. unknown). Punctate blue inclusions in multiple erythrocytes are considered degenerate organelles but lack clinical importance. (Courtesy of J. Jill Heatley and Karen E. Russell.)

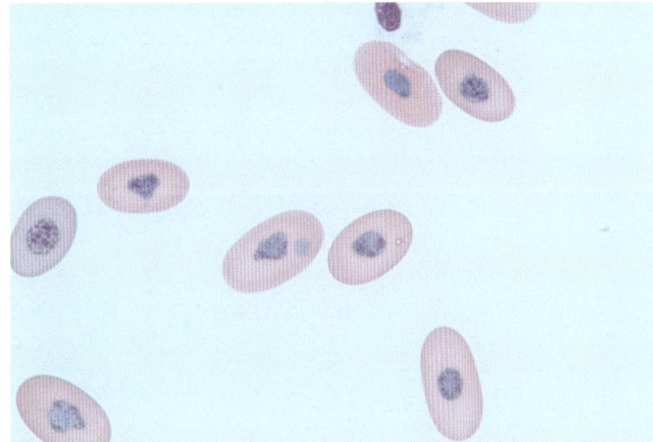

FIG 33.24 Blood smear from a reticulated python (*Malayopython reticulatus*) suffering regurgitation and dehydration, 1000× magnification, Modified Wright Giemsa stain. Note the blue-tinged cytoplasmic inclusion body in the central erythrocyte. This animal had classical histopathologic lesions of inclusion body disease and was PCR positive for Reptarenavirus. (Courtesy of J. Jill Heatley and Karen E. Russell.)

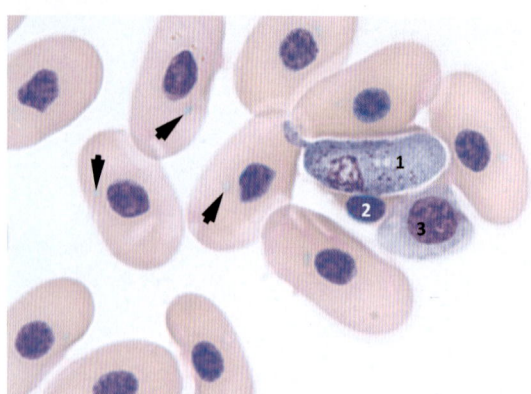

FIG 33.25 Blood smear from a red-eared slider (*Trachemys scripta elegans*), 1000× magnification, Modified Wright Giemsa stain. The hemogregarine (1) that displaces the nucleus and deforms the host erythrocyte (2) is seen above the erythroblast (3). The small, intracytoplasmic, light green-blue structures (arrows) are artifacts commonly observed in reptile blood smears that likely represent degenerate organelles. (Courtesy of J. Jill Heatley and Karen E. Russell.)

and 33.25), and drying artifacts. Therefore it behooves the practitioner to be familiar with common artifacts and inclusions, which may be found on the reptile blood smear (see Figs. 33.1, 33.3, and 33.4). In teiid lizards, hematozoon parasitism causes ultrastructural changes in infected monocytes.[35]

REFERENCES

See www.expertconsult.com for a complete list of references.

34

Clinical Chemistry

J. Jill Heatley and Karen E. Russell

This chapter strives to provide a clinically useful guide for veterinarians and biologists of indications and methodologies for collection, handling, storage, and clinical interpretation of bodily fluid samples (plasma, serum, coelomic effusions, and cerebrospinal fluids). Although most information in this chapter will be based on more commonly seen species, other esoteric species may have been studied in more detail and may be included when necessary to illustrate general and expected findings. Should the reader require more specifics, a review of primary literature is recommended. Indications for clinical chemistry assessment in reptiles and amphibians are numerous and are similar to those of companion mammals (Table 34.1). However, based on numerous factors, including lack of baseline data, clinical chemistry data, and variable physiology of ectotherms, results may be less accurate and/or specific for diagnostic purposes compared with more domesticated species. Additionally, more specific diagnostic testing (serology, PCR, histopathology, culture, etc.) may be necessary to arrive at a definitive diagnosis. This chapter has two major sections: (1) sample collection, handling, and preservation and (2) laboratory tests/techniques and clinical interpretation. For more in-depth information on this material, a review of the primary literature and veterinary clinical pathology texts is recommended.[1]

VENIPUNCTURE

Choice of materials for blood collection from reptiles and amphibians is dependent on a number of factors, including species, patient size/weight, anatomy, temperament, sample desired, sample collection conditions, equipment availability, and practitioner skill. A sample collection plan should be determined and materials prepared beforehand. Sedation or anesthesia for routine diagnostic sampling is seldom necessary in companion reptile species but may be necessary for larger or potentially dangerous species. Operant conditioning for voluntary blood draws has been performed in reptiles.[2] Cleaning and disinfecting of the venipuncture site is recommended, and small brushes (such as a toothbrush or surgical scrub brush) may be required in cases of thick or heavily keeled scalation. Application of alcohol alone to the intended sampling site often provides little benefit, as contact time necessary for disinfection is seldom achieved, and the keratinized skin of reptiles does not usually allow better visualization of vessels. Alcohol is contraindicated for use in amphibians. An overview of sample site options preferred to provide the volume and sample integrity necessary for biochemical and hematological analysis is provided in Chapter 33. However, additional sites may prove acceptable for sampling volumes for genetic and other analyses as sample requirements become smaller, and less reliant on cellular integrity.[3] The clinician and biologist are advised to choose the least invasive sample and sample collection techniques that still provide adequately viable results.

For most animals, 21- to 26-gauge needles and 1 to 3 mL syringes are sufficient. However, sampling of large reptiles may require longer or larger-gauge (3–6 cm, 1.5–2 inch) needles. Butterfly administration sets may also be useful when the sample size is sufficient to lose the 0.05 mL that may coat the tubing. Use of syringes or needles precoated with heparin or other anticoagulant is unnecessary and avoidance precludes dilutional and cellular staining artifacts. Acceptable blood collection tubes include microtainer, pediatric, or larger sizes based on desired sample volume. The low blood pressure, slow heart rate, and large but relatively osmotically robust nature of the herpetological erythrocyte supports the preference of a larger-gauge needle and smaller syringe than one might choose for similarly sized birds or mammals.[4–6] This syringe–needle combination allows blood to flow slowly into the smaller syringe while minimizing aspiration pressure to preserve cell integrity.

GROSS PLASMA EVALUATION

Plasma is generally the sample of choice for determination of biochemistry profiles. Factors for this choice include the lower harvest expected from serum and the (variable and prolonged) time for complete clot formation, which may result in serum analyte changes, associated with increased clot contact time.[7,8] However, in some cases lymph may be an acceptable sample for select biochemistries and may be particularly suitable for serological or PCR-based assays (Table 34.2). Gross color, opacity/ transparency, and turbidity should be subjectively evaluated and recorded for plasma samples to facilitate quality control and as a diagnostic assessment. Amphibian plasma may be clear to yellow or even blue, as in the case of the Japanese giant salamander (*Andrias japonicas*) and the white-lipped tree frog (*Litoria infrafrenata*).[1] Common abnormalities of plasma that deserve attention consideration include lipemia, biliverdinemia, lymphatic or cerebrospinal fluid dilution, and hemolysis. Green plasma in reptiles and amphibians has been associated with biliverdinemia, which may be associated with active hemic or hepatic disease. However, in some lizard species, biliverdinemia is physiologically normal (Figure 34.1).[8a] Interference and other effects of many of these gross abnormalities upon analytes are often inferred from other species and have yet to be adequately investigated for many reptiles and amphibians. The effect of biliverdinemia upon analytes in reptilian and amphibian blood remains uninvestigated.

Lipemia

The expected gross plasma findings for lipemia are a white opaque milky layer that may float to the top of the sample (Figs. 34.2 and 34.3). The most common physiologic causes of lipemic plasma in reptiles are lack of adequate fasting before sample collection or reproductive activity.[9] In other species, measurements of many metabolite activities (including alanine aminotransferase [ALT], aspartate aminotransferase [AST], and glucose) and most electrolyte concentrations are known to be falsely decreased by lipemia.[10] Analyte differences caused by lipemia may also vary based on the analyzer.[10] In most cases, lipemia can be removed and measurement can be done from a "cleared" sample without interferences based on ultracentrifugation at the reference laboratory or extraction with nonpolar solvents or polymer binding for precipitation. However, polymer-binding treatment (Lipoclear) may also result in low recovery of cardiac troponins, gamma-glutamyl transferase (GGT), and some isoforms of creatine kinase (CK).[10]

Lymphatic and Cerebrospinal Fluid Dilution

Lymphatic dilution may occur from any venipuncture site in reptiles, whereas cerebrospinal fluid (CSF) contamination is more likely from blood collection sites close to the vertebral column (e.g., subcarapacial, supravertebral, coccygeal), and pericardial fluid may contaminate cardiocentesis samples. Blood dilution seems least likely when sampling from the jugular vein, followed by the heart.[11] Lymphatic or CSF dilution is recognized by a rapid filling of the syringe with clear to lightly

transparent yellow-colored fluid, often followed by blood. The appearance of lymphatic dilution in plasma may be difficult to detect grossly, but a lighter color than that encountered in pure plasma would be expected. In the case of cardiocentesis, clear fluid obtained should be differentiated from pericardial fluid. In humans, expected cell count, glucose and protein concentrations, and LDH activities of pericardial fluid are known. However, for amphibians and reptiles, these values have yet to be

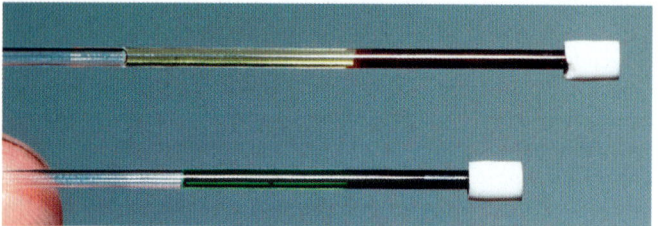

FIG 34.1 Green plasma from a skink (*Prasinohaema*). Biliverdinemia is normal for this species. (Courtesy of Christopher C. Austin.)

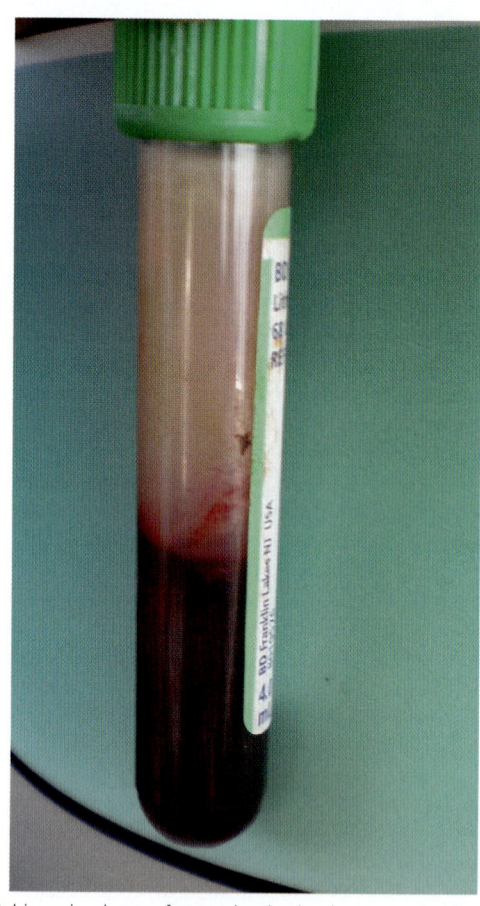

FIG 34.2 Lipemic plasma from a leatherback sea turtle (*Dermochelys coriacea*). Note the use of the green top lithium heparin tube (Becton, Dickinson and Company, Franklin Lakes, NJ) as the most appropriate anticoagulant for this species. (Courtesy of Charles J. Innis.)

TABLE 34.1	Indications for Clinicopathologic Assessment of Reptiles
General health assessment	Entry or exit from collection, baseline determination, presurgical assessment, pre- or posthibernation assessment
Diagnosis	Clinical suspicion of organ dysfunction or abnormal fluid accumulation
Therapeutic assessment	Assessment of treatment plan for renal, liver, or other organ dysfunction, chemotherapy, other chronic diseases, response to treatment
Prognosis	Assessment of seriousness or etiology of organ dysfunction or fluid accumulation

TABLE 34.2 Impactful Studies for Anticoagulant Choice in Reptiles Based on Biochemical Changes		
Anticoagulant	**Species**	**Parameter Changes**
EDTA Lithium heparin	Burmese python (*Python bivitattus*)	Glucose concentration decreased; potassium concentration increased over time in heparinized blood samples[34]
Citrate- phosphate-dextrose-adenine (CPDA-1), acid-citrate-dextrose (ACD)	American alligator (*Alligator mississippiensis*)	Comparable, blood may be stored up to 35 days based on blood culture, blood gas analysis, methemoglobin, osmotic fragility[154]
Lithium heparin	Hermann's tortoises (*Testudo hermanni*), spur-thighed tortoises (*Testudo graeca*), and Horsfield tortoises (*Agrionemys horsfieldii*)	Ionized Ca: no significant differences between heparinized plasma samples stored for 48 hr at 5°C (23°F) and fresh heparinized whole blood. Sodium and potassium: significantly lower sodium and higher potassium in the stored heparinized whole blood compared to the fresh heparinized whole blood.[139]
Sodium heparin, sodium citrate, and citrate-phosphate-dextrose-adenine (CPDA-1).	Loggerhead sea turtle (*Caretta caretta*)	No change in total solids (TS) over 24 hours Electrolytes, glucose, and venous blood gas analytes all change over time[31]

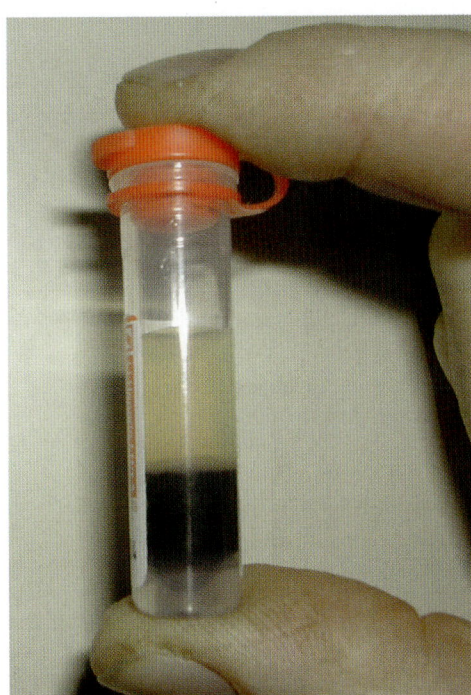

FIG 34.3 Lipemic plasma from a bearded dragon (*Pogona vitticeps*). Note the use of the lithium heparin tube, which is orange in the EU (Sarstedt AG & Co. KG, Nümbrecht, Germany) (Courtesy of Lionel Schilliger.)

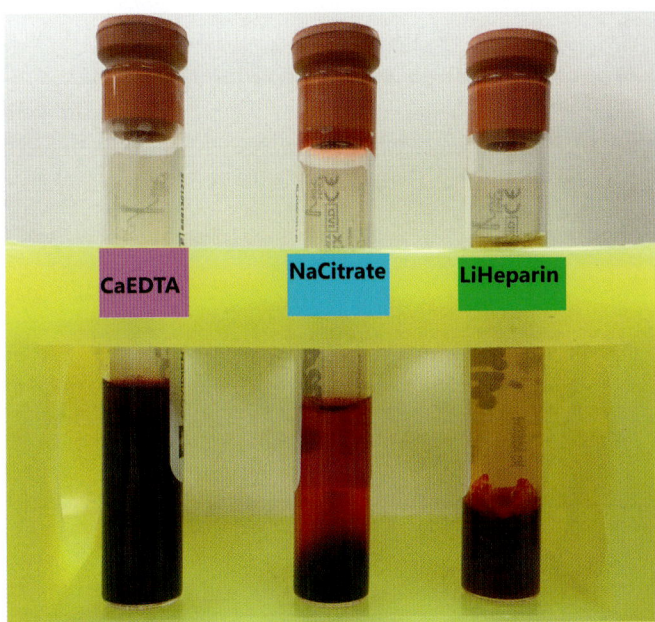

FIG 34.4 Plasma and packed cells from placement of chelonian blood (*Gopherus berlandieri*) in EDTA (hemolyzed), lithium heparin, and sodium citrate.

investigated. Both venipuncture site and lymphatic/CSF contamination may affect analytes results in reptiles.[12] Unfortunately the effects of lymphatic/CSF contamination, venipuncture site comparisons, and their associated effects on biochemistry analytes have been studied in only a few reptilian species. Rather than discarding lymphatic samples the authors recommend they be considered for serology or PCR. Select analytes of lymph that are similar to plasma chemistries obtained from blood are presented in Table 34.3.

Hemolysis

Hemolysis may impart an orange, red, or pink hue to plasma. The specific effects of hemolysis upon biochemical constituents of reptilian and amphibian blood remain minimally investigated. Because the internal biochemical constituents of the erythrocytes of many of these species are also unknown, expected effects of hemolysis also remain obscure. In samples from iguanas (*Iguana iguana*) and red-eared sliders (*Trachemys scripta* elegans), the samples with hemolysis had altered protein electrophoretic profiles, which may reflect species differences in hemoglobin structure.[13] In the green iguana, hemolysis did not affect concentrations of sodium, calcium, uric acid, or CK but did increase potassium, phosphorus, total protein, albumin, and aspartate aminotransferase.[14]

ANTICOAGULANTS, PRESERVATION, AND VENIPUNCTURE SITES

Anticoagulants

Choice of anticoagulant and blood collection equipment is based on similar factors as detailed in Chapter 33 and above under venipuncture, but species, sample collection conditions, availability, and sample use are also primary concerns. All anticoagulants can damage cell architecture and affect biochemical parameters. An overview of current knowledge regarding anticoagulant choice for biochemistry in reptiles is provided

in Table 34.2. Microtainer, plastic tubes coated with freeze-dried anticoagulant, are preferred to avoid sample dilution and allow small volume collection. Hematocrit tubes may be used for blood collection from very small species, but the authors find that sample recovery (when compared with microtainer tubes) is less effective as well as challenging without specialized sample expulsion bulbs. Appropriate anticoagulants for use with cerebrospinal, joint, or coelomic fluids have not been investigated for amphibians or reptiles. However, based on extant literature review, anticoagulation may be unnecessary for these fluids and red-top tubes, without additive, may be suitable.[15–24] For biochemical determinations, plasma, rather than serum, remains the sample of choice based on prolonged or unpredictable clotting times.

Lithium heparin is the most commonly used anticoagulant, may be accompanied by plasma separator gel, and appears less likely to cause hemolysis of reptile blood, particularly in chelonians (Figure 34.4). However, investigation of other anticoagulants with reptile blood remains minimally studied.[25–28] Blood collection into heparin also yields more heparinized plasma than the volume of serum from clotting of whole blood.[29]

Heparin-gel separator tubes are convenient and facilitate plasma separation from cells. However, gel may only prevent migration of some analytes (notably potassium, phosphate, and glucose) between plasma and cells for only a few hours.[30] Further, inadequate centrifugation may result in a cell layer remaining on top of the gel, which could cause further change in the resultant concentration of some plasma analytes with this method of storage.[30] Lastly, many instrument companies discourage use of tubes with separator gels because the gel can affect tubing and other instrument parts, causing malfunction.

A recent comparison of total solids (TS), electrolytes, glucose, and venous blood gas analytes over a 24 hr storage from 8 loggerhead sea turtles (*Caretta caretta*) was performed for the anticoagulants sodium heparin, sodium citrate, and citrate-phosphate-dextrose-adenine (CPDA-1) with whole blood.[31] Blood was stored at 4°C to 8°C (39°F–46°F) for up to 24 hours before analysis. Total solids, evaluated at 0, 3, 6, 12, and 24 hours, did not change significantly, independent of the anticoagulant chosen. However, pink plasma was observed in 62.5%

TABLE 34.3   Effects of Venipuncture Site (VS) and Lymphatic Contamination (LC)* Upon Reptile Biochemical Analytes[12]

Species	Sampling Sites	Differences Found in Samples with Lymphatic Contamination (LC) or Site Based (VS)
Gopherus agasizzi[155]	Jugular, occipital plexus	For samples obtained from the occipital sinus, most values were relatively lower: Glu, K, UA, Ca, P, TP, Alb, Glob, ALP, AST, ALT, and total Chol. Cl was relatively increased
Chelonia mydas[156]	Jugular, coccycgeal, subcarapacial	Analytes of clear fluid obtained from the jugular vein area were similar to values of blood plasma for the same species based on biochemical analysis
Testudo marginata[157]	Coccygeal, brachial	TP, UA, AST, ALT, LDH, ALKP, Ca, and P greater in brachial vein samples than from coccygeal vein samples
Graptemys geographica[158]	Coccygeal, subcarapacial	Visual hemodilution noted in 16% of coccygeal samples and 75% of subcarapacial samples
Apalone spinifera[159]	Coccygeal, subcarapacial	Glu and K concentrations increased in samples from the subcarapacial vein
Trachemys scripta[160]	Coccygeal, occipital	Total protein lower in samples from the dorsal coccygeal vein
Dermochelys coriacea[161]	Occipital, interdigital	Values for Alb, Ca, Glob, Glu, P, K, Na, TP, TS, and UA from each site comparable; AST and CK activities higher in samples obtained from cervical sinus
Centrochelys sulcata[37]	Coccygeal, subcarapacial	Total solids, TP, P, and Glob had increased concentrations in samples from the coccygeal versus the subcarapacial
Chameleo chameleon[162]	Jugular, tail	No difference in TP, UA; jugular venipuncture preferred based on likelihood of obtaining sample and darkening of the tail
Hydrophis spp.[36]	Tail	Observed lymph contamination; increased Na, decreased TS, Alb, ALP, Ca, Chol, Glob, and protein
Mauremys leprosa[12]	Jugular, subcarapacial, coccygeal	Subcarapacial samples had lower Alb, TP, Glu, Chol, Trig, UA, BUN, Ca, P, iron, and ALP than those of jugular blood; corticosterone, Alb, TP, Glu, Chol, Trig, UA, Ca, P, ALP higher in samples from more cranial sites than those from caudal sites
Trachemys scripta elegans[163] N = 36	Multiple	Blood-lymph mixtures had lower concentrations of TP and K but values for Glu, BUN, Ca, P, ALP, CK, LDH, AST, and Na were comparable; although not significantly different, chloride concentrations of blood-lymph samples were lower than in pure plasma
Centrochelys sulcata[37] N = 60	Dorsal coccygeal (tail), subcarapacial v.p., based on body size	TS, TP, P, Glob were higher values in samples from the tail versus the subcarapacial sampling site; reading of Glob failed in over 50% of samples from the subcarapacial site

*When sampling close to the spinal cord (e.g., subcarapacial, coccygeal), cerebrospinal fluid contamination is likely and may be confused with lymphatic contamination.

Alb, Albumin; *ALT*, alanine transaminase; *ALP*, alkaline phosphatase; *AMS*, amylase; *AST*, aspartate transaminase; *BA*, bile acids; *BUN*, blood urea nitrogen; *Ca*, calcium/total calcium; *Chol*, cholesterol; *CK*, creatine kinase; *Cl*, chloride; *Cort*, corticosterone; *Fib*, fibrinogen; *GGT*, glutamyltransferase; *Glob*, globulin; *Glu*, glucose; *GMD*, glutamate dehydrogenase; *HDL*, high-density lipoproteins; *iCa*, ionized calcium; *K*, potassium; *Lact*, lactate; *LDH*, lactate dehydrogenase; *LDL*, low-density lipoproteins; *Lip*, lipase; *Mg*, magnesium; *Na*, sodium; *NH₃*, ammonia; *OSM*, osmolality; *P*, phosphorus; *SDH*, sorbitol dehydrogenase; *Trig*, triglycerides; *TP*, total protein; *TS*, total solids; *UA*, uric acid; *VLDL*, very low–density lipoproteins;

(5/8) of CPDA-1 and 12.5% (1/8) of citrate specimens at 24 hours. Specimens in CPDA-1 and citrate had increased potassium concentrations at 24 hours. Specimens stored in heparin and citrate had relatively decreased pH and increased P_{CO_2} at 24 hours postcollection. Sodium values decreased over time in citrate and CPDA-1 specimens. Thus in these sea turtles as in many other chelonian species, based on the assay of multiple biochemical constituents and short-term storage, heparin remains the preferred anticoagulant.

Sample Preservation

Few studies have focused on acceptable storage methodologies for reptilian blood or bodily fluid samples. Thus testing within 24 hours of sample collection is recommended for most analytes, and the sooner a sample can be analyzed, the better. Plasma should be separated immediately after centrifugation and kept refrigerated or frozen until processed or shipped to a diagnostic laboratory.[1] Proteins, enzymes and electrolytes are the most sensitive biochemical analytes, and the most likely to be affected by storage.[32]

For chelonia, studies of the effect of time on plasma analytes are limited to those of tortoises and sea turtles. In heparinized blood samples from loggerhead sea turtles (*Caretta caretta*), plasma in contact with cells and refrigerated for up to 96 hours had relatively few biochemical changes. Minimal hemolysis occurred by 24 hours, but moderate hemolysis was present at 48 and 96 hours. Of the 17 analytes measured (alkaline phosphatase [ALP], AST, GGT, CK, sodium, chloride, potassium, magnesium, calcium, phosphorus, cholesterol, glucose, blood urea nitrogen [BUN], uric acid, total protein, albumin, and calculated globulin) no significant changes (compared with time 0) were detected at 4 hours postcollection for any analyte. At 24 hours postcollection, only GGT had a significant difference in mean activity compared with activity at 0 hours. This decrease persisted throughout the time period of the study. At 24 to 96 hours of storage, glucose concentrations and GGT activities were decreased compared with fresh samples. At 96 hours, AST increased by 2%, GGT decreased by 25%, glucose increased by 7%, and uric acid increased by 25%. Storage also affected phosphorous and cholesterol.[32] In Aldabra tortoises (*Aldabrachelys gigantea*) storage time and temperature (4°C and 25°C) did not affect potassium concentrations, but decreases in sodium concentration occurred over time regardless of storage temperature.[8] In Burmese mountain tortoises (*Manouria emys*) potassium concentrations increased over time, although increases were less at 4°C than at 25°C and sodium concentrations decreased over time at both temperatures.[8]

For squamates, studies on the effect of time upon plasma biochemical analytes is limited to a single lizard and large constricting snake species. In the green iguana, hemolysis did not affect concentrations of sodium, calcium, uric acid, or CK but did increase potassium, phosphorus, total protein, albumin, and aspartate aminotransferase.[14] Blood samples of free-living anacondas (*Eunectes murinus*) processed after cold storage for 1 to 2 days had relatively decreased concentrations of glucose, total CO_2, total bilirubin, and iron, and increased concentrations of lactate and lactate dehydrogenase activities compared with samples processed within 12 hrs of collection.[33] Blood samples from Burmese pythons (*Python bivittatus*) were collected into heparin-coated syringes and transferred to containers with the anticoagulants lithium heparin, K3-EDTA, or sodium citrate and/ or bovine serum albumin. These samples were evaluated for biochemical and cellular changes based on time and anticoagulant.[46] Samples anticoagulated with lithium heparin and refrigerated at 4°C for up to 24 hours had potassium concentrations that increased and glucose concentrations that decreased over time compared with those anticoagulated with K3-EDTA.[34]

Protein analytes may also be affected by sample storage. Protein electrophoresis of samples from loggerhead sea turtles showed that storage temperature and duration affected albumin, β-globulin, and A/G ratio but not total protein concentrations. Albumin percentage was decreased with 2 and 7 days of storage +4°C or −20°C whereas β-globulins were increased after 2 days at −20°C and after 7 days at both storage temperatures, which resulted in a reduced AG ratio. Thus for plasma protein determination, plasma should not be refrigerated for >48 hrs before analysis.[35] Comparison of samples obtained from healthy sea snakes (*Hydrophis* spp.) for protein with standard methods versus reconstitution from freeze-dried samples resulted in lower values (~10 g/L or 1.0 g/dL less) for frozen samples, suggesting this method of storage is unsatisfactory.[36]

Venipuncture Sites

Choice of the best sample site depends on many factors, including vascular anatomy, patient temperament, and practitioner skill. An overview of multiple options for vascular access based on taxa is provided in Table 33.5. However, other sites may be appropriate and preferred based on practitioner experience and knowledge. Sample site alone or in conjunction with lymphatic or CSF dilution may affect multiple hematologic, biochemical, metabolite, and enzyme parameters (see Tables 33.2 and 34.3).[12] Clinically and for experimental purposes one should always document the venipuncture site used for each sample obtained. Further, for serial sampling, when possible, the same sample site should be used to facilitate analyte comparison and health evaluation. Samples obtained from more craniad sites may be more valid for interpretation of health or experimental outcomes in some reptiles.[12,37]

BLOOD CHEMISTRY

Review of commonly available plasma biochemical panels available to private practitioners reveals a diversity of analytes, some of which may or may not be appropriate for diagnostic use (Table 34.4). The lack of other apparently useful analytes, based upon literature review, is also notable. Significant interspecies variation in many analytes occurs. Blood biochemistry can be affected by seasonal variation and by disease. In a comprehensive study of the Hermann's tortoise (*Testudo hermanni*) no less than 13 parameters showed distinct seasonal variation.[38] For amphibians, a recent review of amphibian clinical pathology perfectly summarized our current understanding and interpretation of enzymes for use in these species: "Almost nothing is known of the diagnostic significance of hepatic, pancreatic, muscular, or cardiac enzymes in amphibian blood."[1]

As we progress in the age of data, we will likely continue to discover appropriate enzymes and biochemical combinations to allow better discrimination of health (including life stage and seasonal changes) and disease (Table 34.5). For example, a recent study of captive Balkan whip snakes (*Hierophis gemonensis*) reviewed biochemical parameters during different periods of the biological cycle, including pre- and posthibernation, hibernation, sexual activity, and normal activity. Use of values for urea, glucose, and LDH simultaneously could discriminate between the various physiological conditions during the biological cycle for this species. Thus these parameters may also be useful in clinical assessment of snakes.

Enzyme Activities

Choice and clinical interpretation of enzyme activities remains minimally studied in reptiles, in comparison to companion mammals such as dogs and cats. Most commonly used or recommended analytes were designed for humans, with assays run at 37°C. Studies of analytes determined by in-house analyzers with those of reference labs show that values obtained are seldom directly comparable.[39] Most of these assays have not been validated for reptiles or amphibians. Practitioners are encouraged to compare clinicopathologic results with anatomical pathology and report their findings to improve our knowledge base. Foundational studies of tissue enzyme activities in reptiles are summarized in Table 34.6. To our knowledge, half-lives of commonly used enzymes for reptiles have not been determined. The assumption that half-lives of reptile enzymes are similar or even relative to those of mammals or humans should be viewed with circumspection.

Creatine kinase or phosphokinase (CK or CPK) and AST are commonly evaluated and generally attributed to muscle injury (skeletal myocytes, cardiac myocytes, smooth muscle myocytes), but significant CK activity also occurs in the brain (~10% that of skeletal muscle).[40–47]

TABLE 34.4	Commercially Available Plasma Biochemical Panels for Use in Reptile Species	
Laboratory	**Specific Panel or Rotor**	**Analytes Available**
Abaxis VS2 (in house)	Rotor: Avian /Reptilian Profile Plus	Alb, AST, BA, Ca, CK, Glob, K, Na, P, TP, UA
Comparative Path Laboratory Miami	Advanced Reptile Chemistry Panel	ALP, AMS, anion gap, AST, BUN, CK, Ca, Chol, Cl, CO_2, GGT, Glu, K, Lip, Mg, Na, osmolality, P, TP, Trig, UA
IDEXX Reference laboratories	Reptile Profile 5	Alb, AST, BUN, Ca, Cl, Chol, CK, Glu, P, K, Na, Trig, TP, UA
IDEXX Reference laboratories	Reptile Profile 2 with Bile Acids	Alb, AST, BUN, Ca, CK, Glu, LDH, P, TP, BUN, UA, BA
Avian & Exotic Clin Path Lab	Complete reptile	TP, AST, total bilirubin, UA, glucose, CK, Ca, P

For a full list of abbreviations, see Table 34.3.

TABLE 34.5 **Recommended Biochemical Analytes for Health Assessment of Major Groups of Reptiles and Amphibians***

Class	Enzymes	Ions, Glucose, Blood Gases	Proteins, Lipids	Other
Squamates *Lizard*	CK, AMS, LDH, AST, SDH, LDH	Glu, Na, K, Cl, Ca, iCa, P, OSM	Chol (HDL, LDL, VLDL) Trig, Alb,* Glob, TP	BA, UA
Squamates *Snake*	LDH, AST, ALT, CK	Glu, Na, K, Cl, Ca, iCa, P, OSM	Alb,* Glob, TP	UA
Terrestrial chelonian *Tortoises*	AST, CK, ALT, ALP	Glu, Na, K, Cl, Ca, iCa, P, OSM	Alb,* Glob, TP Fib	BA, BUN, UA
Aquatic chelonian *Sea turtle*	AST, CK, LDH, AMS, Lip, ALP, ALT, ALP, GGT	pH, PO_2, Pco_2, Lact, Glu, Na, K, Cl, Ca, iCa, P, OSM	Alb,* Glob, TP, Fib	BA, BUN, UA, NH_3 (creatinine)
Crocodilian	CK, LDH, ALT, AST	Na, K, Ca, iCa, P, Mg, Cl, OSM	Chol (HDL, LDL, VLDL) Trig, Alb,* Glob, TP, Fib	UA, NH_3
Amphibian	CK, LDH, ALT, AST, GGT, ALP, Lip	Glu, glycerol Na, K, Cl, pH, iCa, Ca, P, OSM	Chol (HDL, LDL, VLDL) Trig, Alb,* Glob, TP, Fib	Aquatic, NH_3; adult terrestrial, BUN; some tree frogs, UA

*Albumin measurements are often inaccurate by bromocresol green methods; protein electrophoresis is preferred.
For a full list of abbreviations, see Table 34.3.

TABLE 34.6 **Foundational Studies of Reptile and Amphibian Tissue and Plasma Enzymes**[42–47]

Species	Tissues Examined	Enzymes Examined	Useful Enzyme Activities	Useless Enzymes
Green iguana (*Iguana iguana*)	Liver, kidney, epaxial muscle, heart, lung, spleen, small intestine, pancreas from 6 juveniles	ALP, LDH, AST, ALT, GGT, CK, GMD, AMS	High CK confined to epaxial muscle, heart. AMS activity confined to pancreas. Moderate LDH and AST activities in all tissues. Low ALT and ALP activities in many tissues.	Plasma, tissue activities of GGT, GMD low to undetected.
Loggerhead sea turtle (*Caretta caretta*)	30 tissues of 5 stranded turtles	AMS, Lip, CK, GGT, ALP, LDH, AST, ALT	High CK activity confined to epaxial and heart muscle. AMS activity confined to pancreas. Moderate LDH and AST activities in all tissues. Low ALT and ALP activities in many tissues.	Plasma, tissue activities of GGT, GMD low to undetected
Yellow rat snake (*Pantherophis obsoleta quadrivitatta*)	Liver, kidney, skeletal muscle, heart, intestine, lung, pancreas, free-living snakes	ALP, LD, AST, ALT, GGT, CK	Major enzyme activities of liver were LD and AST. Kidney had moderate activities of LDH, AST, ALT, and CK. Skeletal muscle and heart had high CK activity. Intestine, lung, and pancreas had low activities for most enzymes. Serum enzyme activities of CK were increased in rat snakes compared with other reptiles.	Little to no GGT in serum or tissues
Kemp's ridley turtles (*Lepidochelys kempii*)	Liver, kidney, skeletal muscle, cardiac muscle, pancreas, lung, small intestine, and spleen from 13 juvenile strandings	ALT, ALP, AST, CK, GGT, LDH, lipase	AST, CK, and LDH highest in cardiac and skeletal muscle but found in all other tissues. AMS and Lip highest in the pancreas, low in other tissues. ALP highest in lung. ALT highest in liver, kidney, and cardiac muscle. GGT highest in kidney.	ALT, GGT low in all tissues
Cuban tree frogs (*Osteopilus septentrionalis*)	Liver, cardiac muscle, lung, kidney, skeletal muscle, gonad, and pancreas	Amylase, lipase, ALP, ALT, AST, LDH, CK, GGT	CK, LDH mainly from skeletal and cardiac muscles; ALT mainly from kidney and liver; AST mainly from liver, kidney, and skeletal and cardiac muscles; GGT mainly from kidney; ALP mainly from kidney and cardiac muscle; Lip mainly from liver.	AMS highest in the plasma, lacked other tissue specificity
American alligator (*Alligator mississippiensis*)	Liver, cardiac muscle, lung, kidney, skeletal muscle, and mid–small intestine	ALP, ALT, AST, LDH, CK, GGT	CK and LDH mainly in skeletal and cardiac muscle; ALT mainly in kidney and skeletal muscle tissue; AST mainly in liver and skeletal muscle.	GGT, ALP of little diagnostic value in sampled tissues

For a full list of abbreviations, see Table 34.3.

In comparison, increased AST may derive in large quantities from muscle, liver, or other tissues. Although plasma CK activities may increase based on capture stress of reptiles,[48] intramuscular injections have yet to be documented to increase CK activities in reptiles and amphibians. Increased AST in the absence of increased CK is often considered indicative of liver damage but could be based on other tissue damage as well (as this enzyme is fairly widespread in body tissues, despite relatively high concentrations occurring in the liver). Loggerhead sea turtles suffering illness may have relatively increased AST and decreased ALT (alanine aminotransferase) plasma activities. However, in another study of the same species, AST activity was lower in turtles with serious illness compared with those in good health.[49] This finding may serve as an example of end-stage disease wherein a lack of hepatocytes result in relatively "normal" liver enzyme activities. Rat snakes (*Patherophis obsoleta*) appear to have relatively high CK plasma activities whereas the yellow-marginated box turtle (*Cuora flavomarginata*) has lower ALT activities compared with other chelonians.[41,50] Additionally, in juvenile alligators (*Alligator mississippiensis*) body condition index, AST, and CK were correlated.[51] Of interest, a study of 43 wild-caught southwest carpet pythons (*Morelia spilota imbricate*) failed to reveal any effects of intrinsic or extrinsic factors (season, locale, sex, presence of hemoparasites, surgical transmitter replacement, or anesthetic state) upon CK or AST plasma activities.[52] These findings suggest that although CK and AST may be more specific to serious disease processes than physiological changes, they may also be less sensitive for detection of organ disease in this species. Based on a few extant studies in reptiles, GGT and glutamate dehydrogenase (GLDH, GDH) are less useful diagnostically based on their pan organ distribution, low analyte activities, and/or lack of detection in the tissues assayed.[42,43,45-47]

Enzyme activity interpretation for health assessment of reptiles may be further complicated by changes based on season, sex, age class, and species, as well as inadequate reference ranges. In alligators, LDH activities of muscle were greater in winter compared with summer, and although mitochondrial enzyme activity was relatively increased in males, LDH activity did not differ between sexes.[53,54] In plasma of male Herman's tortoises, ALT, bile acids, LDH and GLDH, and in both sexes ALP were relatively increased by midsummer. Similar seasonal variations occur in both captive and free-living reptile species.[55-57] In apparently healthy adult hawksbill turtles (*Eretmochelys imbricate*), ALP, AST, bilirubin, LDH, CK, and amylase were increased and ALT was decreased during nesting compared with the foraging season, which the authors attributed to reproductive output.[58] In male radiated tortoises (*Astrochelys radiata*), LDH activity was decreased during winter; LDH and CK activities similarly increased in summer, compared with females.[59] Feeding and activity may also affect multiple analytes. In 2-hour postprandial green sea turtles (*Chelonia mydas*), but not Kemp's ridley turtles (*Lepidochelys kempii*), plasma activities of ALP, AST, ALT, and amylase were significantly increased.[9] In captive mugger crocodiles (*Crocodylus palustris*), the effect of age was studied. Subadults had lower mean ALP activities than juveniles, but adults had the lowest AST and ALT activities. Subadult LDH activities were lower than for juveniles and adults.[60] In the yellow-marginated box turtle, marked seasonal variations of ALP, AST, and CK were attributed to the gender, reproduction, and seasonal temperature changes.[50] Additionally, in summer, captive female panther chameleons (*Furcifer pardalis*) have increased ALT and AST compared with winter.[61] In summer, gravid females had increased ALT activity whereas males had higher CK activities in winter.[61] Experimentally induced toxic hepatopathy in green iguanas has demonstrated ×40 increases in AST, ×4 increases in ALT, ×15 increases in sobital dehydrogenase (SDH), and 100× increases in LDH (Schnellbacher et al, Proc ARAV, 2014, pp 127–128).

Biliverdin and Bilirubin

Heme pigment metabolism in reptiles and amphibians remains poorly understood. In some species (green lizard, *Lacerta viridis*, and common frog, *Rana temporaria*) bilirubin is not produced in appreciable amounts due to the lack of the biliverdin reductase and bilirubin conjugation enzyme (uridyl diphosphate glucuronyltransferase, UDPG).[62] Therefore unconjugated biliverdin is the main product excreted in the bile of these species. Bilirubin does occur in the bile of alligators (*Alligator missisipiensis*) but not in eastern racers (*Coluber constrictor*).[63] Some reptiles, such as the indigo snake (*Drymarchon corais*), anaconda (*Eunectes*), and green iguana (and likely other squamates), have significant plasma bilirubin and may therefore develop hyperbilirubinemia (jaundice or icterus).[33,64] Activity of UDPG is less in some snakes than in mammals. The indigo snake serves as a model of hyperbilirubinemia, having 10 times more unconjugated plasma bilirubin than other snake species.[65] Therefore we know that for this species, hepatic uptake of injected bilirubin is relatively slow (compared with mammals) and that plasma clearance of bilirubin and sulfobromophthalien in indigo snakes is slower than in rat snakes. In the anaconda, blood samples processed within 12 hours of collection had higher total bilirubin levels than samples processed after cold storage (on ice in a cooler or refrigerated) for 1 to 2 days, suggesting that this analyte is best measured in snakes within <12 hours of sampling.[33] In amphibians, bilirubin may be present in appreciable quantities, but this analyte's diagnostic value remains unproven.

Biliverdin is present in the green plasma of skinks (*Prasinohaema*), some arboreal snakes, monitor lizards (*Varanus*), and the Cambodian frog (*Chiromantis samkosensis*).[66] Biliverdinemia may represent an ecological or physiological adaptation. Green blood that imparts a green body color occurs nearly exclusively in species inhabiting green vegetation, and accumulation of biliverdin might also deter *Plasmodium* spp. hemoparasitism.[67,68] Despite the short half-life of biliverdin, as the end product of heme synthesis in reptiles and other lower vertebrates, the lack of a commercially available biliverdin assay continues to confound diagnosis of liver disease in these species. Interestingly, an assay of total bile pigments (to include biliverdin) was reported in 1966, and multiple assays for biliverdin have been developed, including a more recent high throughput assay via infrared fluorescence.[66,69,70]

Bile Acids

Bile acids (3α-hydroxy bile acids) have been scientifically evaluated for clinical use in relatively few reptile species (see Table 67.1).[71] Nonetheless they are commonly assayed and used as an indicator of hepatic dysfunction when fasted values are >60 μmol/L (>24.5 μg/mL) (see Chapter 67). Bile acids assess function whereas liver enzyme activities are associated with hepatocellular damage. As in other species, postprandial effects have been demonstrated and so obtaining both fasted and postprandial samples for bile acids are more diagnostically valuable. Bile acid stimulation procedures for use in reptiles are provided in Box 67.1. Bile acids of the Hermann's tortoise were increased midsummer.[38] Mean plasma bile acid concentration in plasma samples from healthy 24-hr fasted green iguanas was 15.89 ± 15.61 μmol/L (6.49 ± 6.38 μg/mL) and 48-hr fasted was 9.56 ± 8.52 μmol/L (3.91 ± 3.48 μg/mL). Bile acids increase in plasma of green iguanas with chronic liver diseases with the highest concentrations (>70 μmol/L; >28.6 μg/mL) present in patients suffering from liver cirrhosis, liver lipidosis, and liver neoplasms.[72-74] Plasma appears to be the preferred sample for determination of bile acids based on increased values obtained from serum samples.[7] The validity, sensitivity, and specificity of bile acids as a diagnostic for liver disease in some reptiles remains suspect as demonstrated by a recent case report of suspected hepatic encephalopathy in a boa (*Boa constrictor*) with a plasma bile acid concentration of less than 35 μmol/L (<14.3 μg/mL).[75]

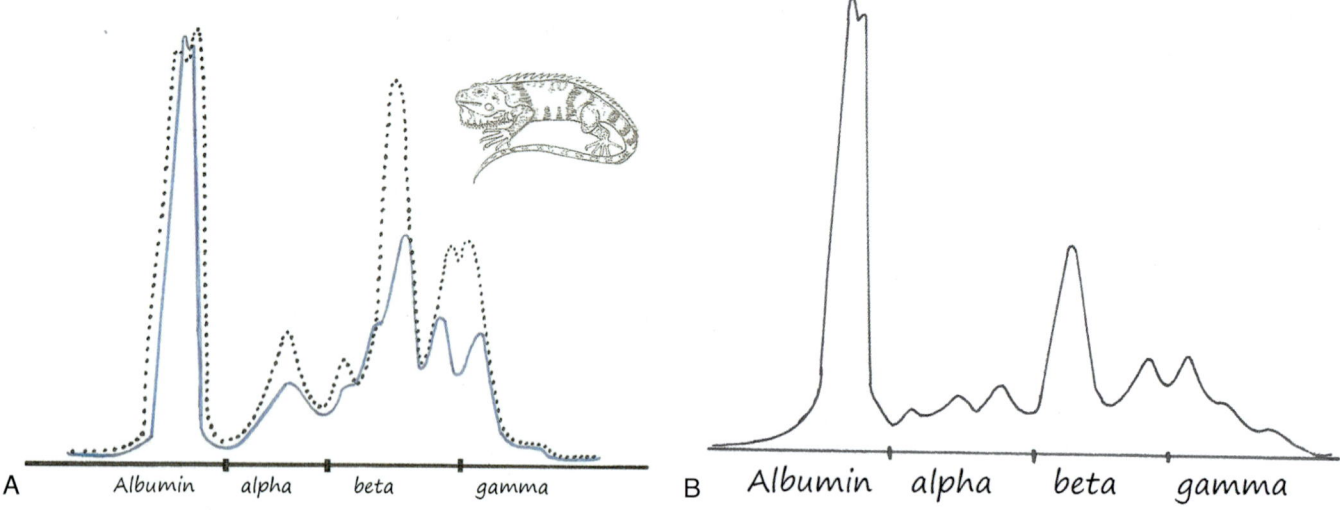

FIG 34.5 Diagrammatic representations of reptile electrophoretograms. Albumin, alpha-globulins (alpha), beta-globulins (beta), and gamma-globulins (gamma) are demarcated horizontally along the x axis. Overall, species, seasonal and protein charge, and size variation from that of mammals make accurate diagnostic interpretation of results from this assay challenging. (A) Agar gel electrophoretogram (AGE) of different iguanas *(Iguana iguana)*. Overlying diagrams show the wide acceptability of variation within healthy animals and bisalbuminemia (dotted line), which occurs in approximately 40% of healthy iguanas.[13,86] (B) Cellulose acetate electrophoretogram (CAE) of the same iguana in (A) (blue solid line), which demonstrates the lack of interchangeability of the two techniques.[13] (Redrawn from cited source by Sylvia Hester.)

Proteins and Acute Phase Reactants

Plasma and serum proteins are commonly evaluated in reptiles based on the myriad of systems in which they may reflect health and disease. Common causes of relatively increased total protein include dehydration and active reproductive processes (vitellogenesis) in females.[58,76] Plasma and serum proteins may change due to inflammation, hydration status, liver, kidney, and gastrointestinal function.

Proteins may also be affected by a variety of factors that are more specific to reptiles, including venipuncture site, gender and reproductive status, season, age, fasting or feeding status, sample type, and assay used (Figures 34.5 through 34.10).[55,77] Two distinct albumins occur in red-eared slider plasma and may also occur in other reptiles.[78] In healthy loggerhead sea turtles, albumin concentrations in juvenile and subadult turtles are lower compared with adults, and total protein concentrations are lower in subadults compared with adults.[49] Gravid females tend to have greater concentrations of albumin and therefore total protein.[50,61] Seasonal variation also occurs with increased total protein and albumin expected in the summer for some species.[50,61] In green sea turtles, albumin and consequently total protein were increased 2 hrs after feeding compared with a preprandial samples.[9]

The methods commonly used to determine plasma protein in reptiles, in order of increasing specificity/accuracy but also cost, include refractometry, dry or wet analyzers (dye binding/biuret), and electrophoresis.[79] Although protein electrophoresis is the gold standard for protein determination in reptiles, few studies have compared techniques, and comparison to other protein determination techniques have shown mixed results.[13,80–82] Comparisons between protein electrophoresis (EPH) and bromocresol green dye-binding (BCG) methods for determination of proteins indicated poor agreement between healthy and especially ill turtles of multiple species. Recent work at the University of Georgia has also demonstrated inaccuracies between albumin measurements by bromocresol green when compared with electrophoresis in the bearded dragon *(Pogona vitticeps)* (Comolli et al, Proc ICARE, 2017, pp 575–576).

Plasma EPH may also be the most appropriate assay to measure albumin and globulins in amphibians.[83] However, EPH of plasma rather

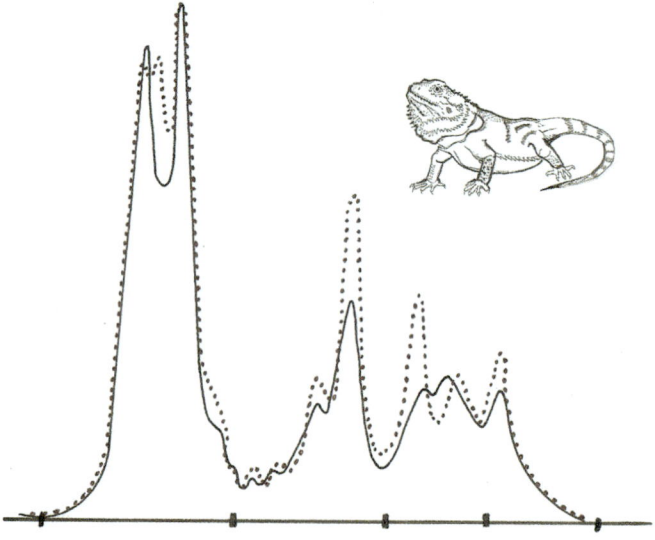

FIG 34.6 Diagrammatic representation of plasma electrophoretogram of two apparently healthy bearded dragons *(Pogona vitticeps)* that illustrates the inherent variability of this diagnostic assay, which may result in difficulty of interpretation or diagnosis of health or disease in reptiles.[168] (Redrawn from cited source by Sylvia Hester.)

than serum may yield heparin and/or fibrinogen bands or spikes. The validity of changes in amphibian proteins determined by EPH, such as acute phase proteins, reduced or increased albumin:globulin ratios, or monoclonal gammopathies, remains unknown.

Studies conflict regarding agreement of BCG and EPH methods in reptiles. For diseased Hermann's tortoises, protein values for BCG were increased compared with EPH.[79,84,85] Evaluation of protein electrophoretic profiles is further confounded because of inherent differences within commonly available EPH assays and the lack of comparability of results.[13] Electrophoretic protein patterns must be interpreted based on the method

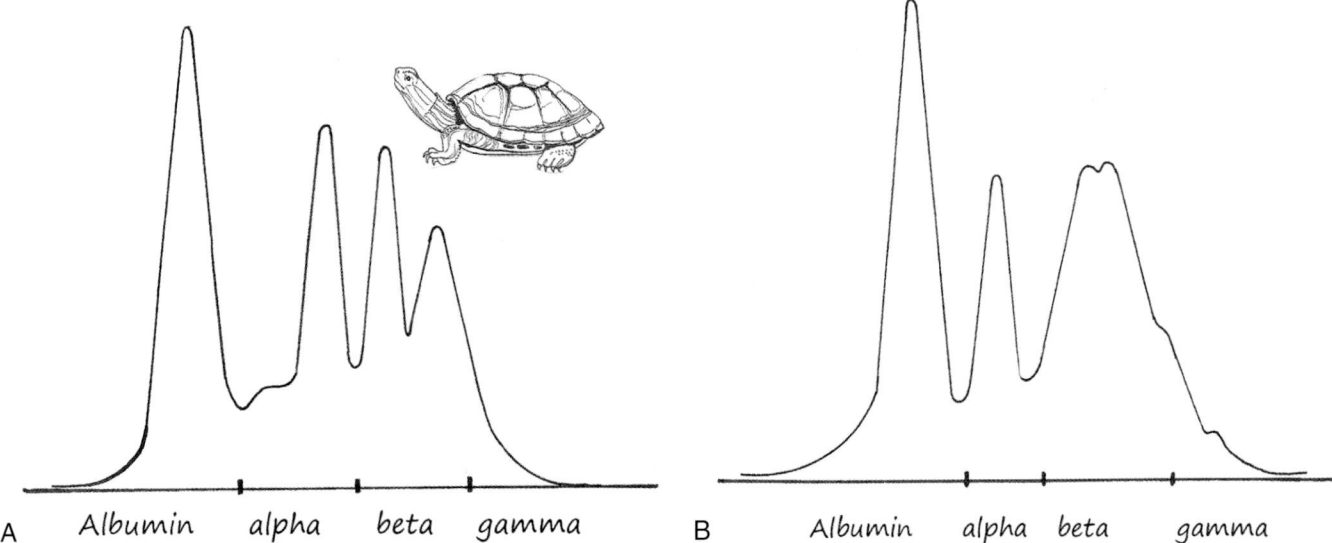

FIG 34.7 Diagrammatic representation of plasma electrophoretogram of a red-eared slider (*Trachemys scripta elegans*). The variability between the two methods: (A) Agarose gel (AGE) and (B) cellulose acetate (CAE) is illustrated.[13] (Redrawn from cited source by Sylvia Hester.)

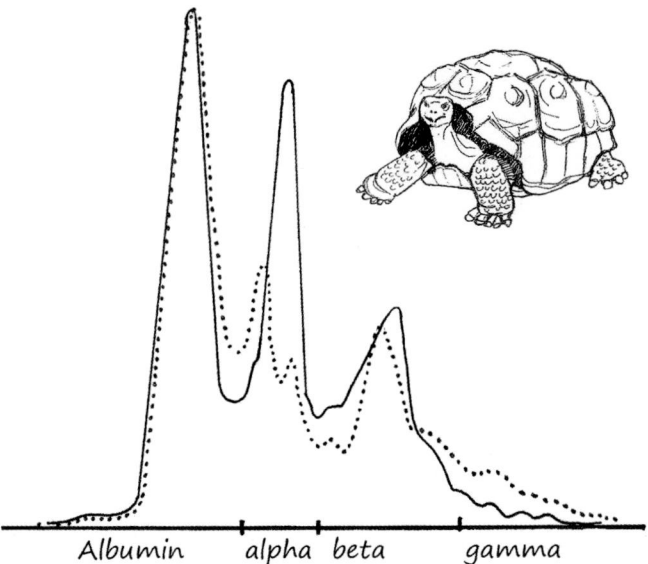

FIG 34.8 Diagrammatic representation of comparative seasonal plasma protein electrophoretogram of the Hermann's tortoise (*Testudo hermanni*) based on the agarose gel method. Summer (July) is denoted by the black line whereas fall (September) is shown via the dotted line.[84] (Redrawn from cited source by Sylvia Hester.)

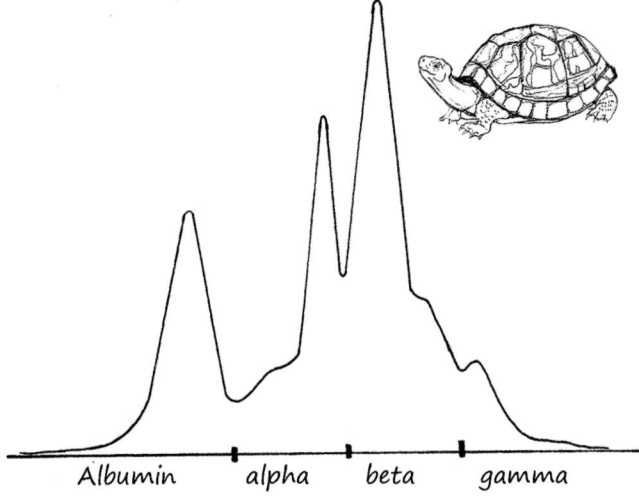

FIG 34.9 Diagrammatic representation of plasma electrophoretogram of an apparently healthy Eastern box turtle (*Terrapene carolina*).[82] (Redrawn from cited source by Sylvia Hester.)

used, the species analyzed, the sex and season, and the quality of the plasma sample, as each of these factors may affect the resultant pattern (see Figs. 34.5 through 34.9).[13,55,84,86] In box turtles (*Terrapene carolina*), EPH fractions were affected by variables such as age, sex, season, and location.[82] Total protein concentrations were similar in male and female radiated tortoises (*Astrochelys radiata*); however, female tortoises had higher concentrations of alpha1- and beta-globulins compared with males.[59] In wild-caught carpet pythons (*Morelia spilota imbricate*), no intrinsic or extrinsic factors appeared to influence total protein, but albumin and therefore albumin:globulin ratios were increased in summer.[52] In captive panther chameleons, albumin and therefore total protein plasma concentrations were lower in the summer compared

with winter for both sexes, and males tended to have higher values than females, independent of season.[61]

Determination of total serum solids via refractometry in the Arrau turtle (*Podocnemis expansa*) and Geoffroy's toadhead side-necked turtle (*Phrynops geoffroanus*) agreed with the biuret method of protein determination. This finding suggests that for clinical application in some reptiles, refractometry may be an acceptable substitute for determination of total solids.[87] In juvenile green sea turtles, the formula for conversion of refractive index (Y, total solids) to total plasma proteins (X, biuret method for total protein) was $Y = 1.34 + 0.00217(X)$.[88] The albumin to globulin ratio (A:G) in most reptiles is inverted (compared with mammals), with higher globulins than albumins often encountered in apparently healthy reptiles.[82,88] Healthy gravid female iguanas have lower A:G than males or nongravid females.[76]

Potential etiologies for decreased total protein or albumin include kidney, liver or gut dysfunction, secondary protein loss (e.g., severe

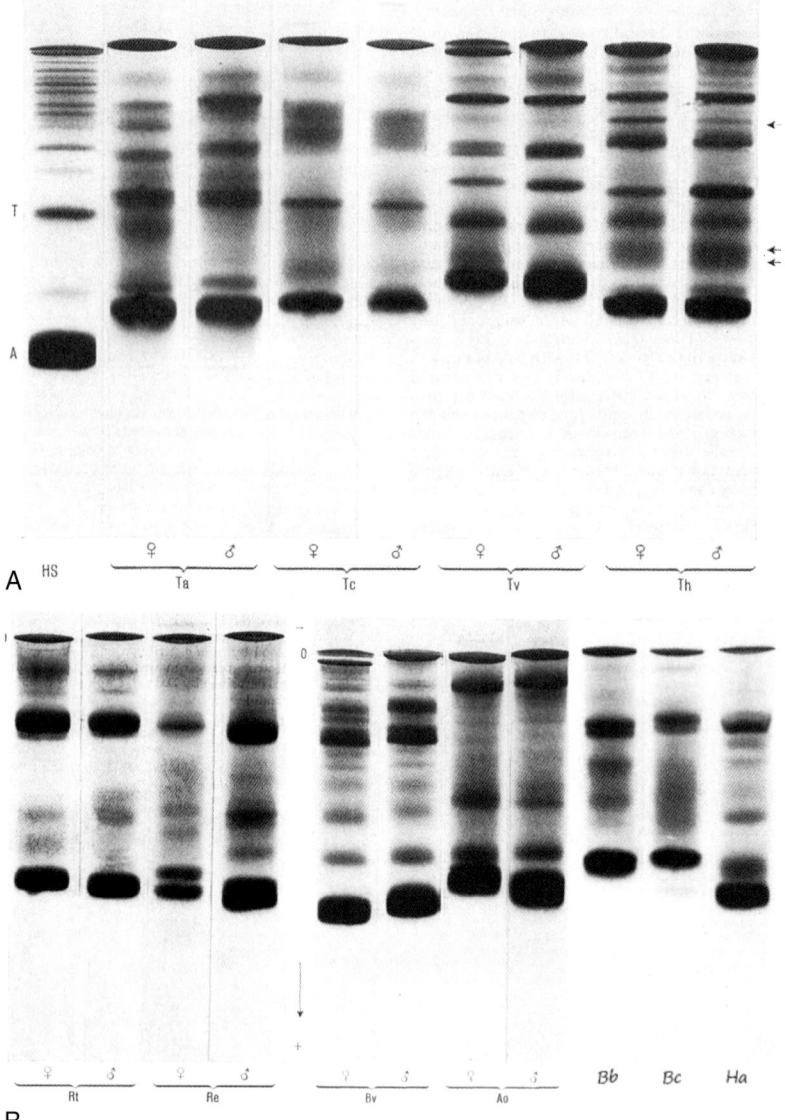

FIG 34.10 Comparative polyacrylamide gels of serum proteins of multiple amphibians, illustrating normal species and class diversity of proteins. All samples were collected during the breeding season.[169] (A) Electrophoretic separation of human serum (HS) and serum proteins of *Triturus alpestris* (Ta), *T. cristayus* (Tc), *T. vulgaris* (Tv), and *T. helveticus* (Th) in polyacrylamide gels. *A*, Albumin; *T*, transferrin. (B) Electrophoretic patterns of serum proteins of multiple anurans illustrative of natural species diversity among proteins: *Rana temporaria* (Rt) and *R. esculenta* (Re); *Bombina variegata* (Bv) and *Alytes obstetricans* (Ao); *Bufo bufo* (Bb), *B. calamita*, (Bc) and *Hyla arbores* (Ha) (all males). The largest band on the bottom is presumed albumin; the male Re shows bisalbuminemia.

burns), or extreme and prolonged inanition leading to catabolism and loss of total body protein stores. Lower gastrointestinal tract strictures of green sea turtles have been associated with a persistent hypoproteinemia and hypoalbuminemia.[89] Ill loggerhead sea turtles had lower total protein and albumin concentrations than subjects in good health.[49] Upper gastrointestinal obstruction and vomiting in a red-footed tortoise (*Chelonoidis carbonaria*) was associated with hyperproteinemia attributable to dehydration.[77]

Acute Phase Proteins

Acute phase reactants (APR) or acute phase proteins (APP) have been studied in a few reptiles, mainly chelonia.[90,91] These nonspecific components of the innate immune system provide restoration of homeostasis in response to inflammation and infection. Thus APR may be more sensitive to detect early and/or continuing acute inflammation than assessment of cellular counts or protein ratios. However, APR increases are nonspecific and may be caused by infection, surgery, trauma, autoimmune responses, toxin exposure, neoplasia, and stress (including transport) and affected by dehydration. Preliminary investigations suggest that fibrinogen, serum amyloid (SAA), complement (C3), and cathepsin-L may serve as positive acute phase reactants in reptiles, and albumin may serve as a negative acute phase protein.[92] However, expression of these molecules were only assessed via PCR of liver; plasma concentrations were not determined. Fibrinogen has received more attention, but preliminary results are not readily comparable based on the variety of methodologies and anticoagulants used. Fibrinogen's clinical usefulness

TABLE 34.7 Acute Phase Reactant Data for Apparently Healthy Reptiles

Species	Units	Method	Data	Acute Phase Reactant	Data Format
Box turtle[91] (*Terrapene carolina*)	mg/dL	Modified clauss	97.9–117	Fibrinogen	95% CI
Box turtle[82] (*Terrapene carolina*)	mg/mL	Haptoglobin	0.27–0.38	hemoglobin binding protein ([HBP], haptoglobin)	95% CI
Spiny-tailed lizard[90] (*Uromastyx* spp.)	g/L	Heat precipitation	1.80 ± 0.13 (0.0–6.0)	Fibrinogen	Mean ± SEM (min-max)
Red-eared slider[93] (*Trachemys scripta elegans*)	mg/mL	Jacobsson	1.68–6.71	Fibrinogen	RI
Brown tree snakes[164] (*Boiga irregularis*)	mg/dL	Heat precipitation	150 ± 92.7 [0–500]	Fibrinogen	Mean ± SD [min-max]

is further hindered by gender and reproduction (e.g., female red-eared sliders have higher concentrations than males).[93] Alligator serum contains a protein antigenically similar and with nearly identical molecular weights as human complement protein C3.[94,95] A complement-facilitated humoral immune response analogous to that of mammals is present in alligator serum, partially based on the presence of this protein.[94,95] Reference data for circulating APR in apparently healthy and unhealthy reptiles is provided in Table 34.7.

Reptile Glucose

In reptiles, blood glucose concentrations tend to be lower than that of mammals and birds. Blood glucose may vary with metabolic rate, environmental adaptations or influence, and physiological changes. Thus season, gender, health, temperature, and many other factors may affect blood glucose concentrations. Examples of expected physiological changes include increased glucose with increased body length in Galapagos marine iguanas (*Amblyrhynchus cristatus*) and maturity in mugger crocodiles.[60,96] Increased glucose concentrations are evident in nesting versus foraging hawksbill turtles.[58] A relative increase in glucose in warmer or summer months have been documented in the Hermann's and yellow-marginated box turtle.[38,50] In captive panther chameleons, blood glucose concentrations varied based on gender and season.[61] Males tended toward higher glucose concentrations than females, independent of season, and both sexes tended toward lower blood sugar concentrations in summer.[53,54,61]

Hypoglycemia. Normal low blood glucose states (prolonged physiological hypoglycemia) may occur during hibernation or brumation in some species. For example, hibernation is associated with an approximately 60% decrease in mean blood glucose in the desert monitor (*Varanus griseus*).[97,98] However, in the common water snake (*Nerodia sipedon*), experimental fasting for 15 days had no effect on blood glucose.[99] Serious, profound, and/or prolonged hypoglycemia has been associated with a number of serious abnormalities in reptiles. Profound hypoglycemia is commonly associated with sea turtle strandings and may be more severe or prolonged based on the degree of debilitation (52.80 ± 43.01 mg/dL; 2.93 ± 2.39 mmol/L) or disease processes such as intestinal and cloacal strictures, enterococcal infection, or phaeohyphomycosal obstructive tracheitis (18 mg/dL; 1 mmol/L).[89,100–102] In other species, hypoglycemia associated with specific disease processes has rarely been documented. Mycobacterial cholecystitis of a Pacific gopher snake (*Pituophis catenifer*) was associated with a blood glucose of 28 mg/dL (1.55 mmol/L).[103] Experimental application of the organochlorine endosulfan to the garden lizard (*Calotes versicolor*) resulted in a decrease of blood glucose from ~114 mg/dL (6.33 mmol/L) in controls to ~75 mg/dL (4.16 mmol/L) 120 hrs postadministration.[104] Hypoglycemia associated with the neurological signs of mydriasis, altered mentation, and/or opisthotonus has been described in crocodilians.[15]

Hyperglycemia. Hyperglycemia in reptiles is rarely confirmed as a consistent or specific indicator of any disease, including diabetes mellitus.[105] Stress-associated hyperglycemia has been reported in a number of species, including freshwater and sea turtles, crocodilians, and snakes. Upper ranges for blood glucose levels due to stress often vary between species from 100 to 175 mg/dL (5.56–9.71 mmol/L).[48,105–111] Physiologically increased blood glucose has also been noted postprandially (particularly following starvation), seasonally during emergence from hibernation, as a cryoprotective mechanism, during the breeding season of temperate reptiles, and upon diving or forced submergence in turtles.[105,112,113] Vomiting and gastrointestinal obstruction in reptiles may be accompanied by hyperglycemia and hypochloremic metabolic alkalosis.[77,114] Experimental hyperglycemia has been induced in multiple species after injections of glucose or epinephrine (lizards, snakes, tortoises, caiman) and pancreatectomy (tegus, snakes).[115–118]

For the more than 20 cases of reptile hyperglycemia reported, affected taxa appears limited to snakes, lizards, turtles, and tortoises.[73,105,119,120] Pancreatic disease, liver disease (often hepatic lipidosis), or renal disease often occur in association with changes in blood glucose.[105] Neoplasia, of a variety of types, deriving from the liver, pancreas, gastrointestinal tract, or undifferentiated tissues, is often reported in these cases.[105] Gastric neuroendocrine carcinoma appears to be the most common cause of hyperglycemia in bearded dragons (*Pogona vitticeps*).[119,121] In a single free-living timber rattlesnake (*Crotalus horridus*) affected by *Ophidiomyces ophiodiicola* dermatitis that died during biopsy, hyperglycemia (220 mg/dL, 12.21 mmol/L) could not be attributed to any histopathologic lesions.[122] Mild hyperglycemia (257 mg/dL; 14.26 mg/dL) has been documented in a single case of atherosclerosis and pericardial effusion in a male bearded dragon.[123] Intracoelomic administration of 5% dextrose + 0.9% Na Cl solutions 1:1 to rehabilitating sea turtles resulted in approximately 100 mg/dL (5.55 mmol/L) higher concentrations of blood glucose compared with other fluid combinations.[100]

Amphibian Glucose

Freeze-tolerant overwintering amphibians such as wood frogs (*Lithobates sylvaticus*), spring peepers (*Pseudacris crucifer*), and western chorus frogs (*Pseudacris triseriata*) accumulate glucose or glycerol in tissues (including blood) for cryoprotection.[124] Thus a physiological hyperglycemia is present if animals are sampled soon after hibernation or during hibernation. Blood glucose concentrations of wood frogs 1 hour post hibernation can reach > 400 mmol/L (>7000 mg/dL), while blood glucose of those that have not withstood freezing temperatures is ~1.5 mmol/L (27 mg/dL). In the gray tree frog (*Hyla versicolor*), this cryoprotective response is dependent on age. Glucose concentrations of adults remain unchanged during freezing, while glycerol concentrations increase from 6.8 to 423 mmol/L (122.5–7621.6 mg/dL). However, immature gray tree frogs have a mild increase in both glycerol (0.1–16.3 mmol/L; 0.09–150.1 mg/dL) and glucose (1.46– 25.9 mmol/L; 26.3–25.9 mg/dL).

Lipids and Lipoproteins

Hypercholesterolemia can be associated with excessive production or decreased excretion (e.g., extrahepatic biliary obstruction). Normal female reptiles undergoing vitellogenesis often exhibit increases in cholesterol and triglycerides; however, sustained elevations or elevations in males may be associated with hepatic lipidosis. In addition to cholesterol and triglycerides, some commercial laboratories offer lipoprotein profiles. Plasma triglyceride concentrations are reasonable indicators of long term feed intake but may be slow to rise due to slow rates of digestion. For example, at 2 hours post feeding of green sea turtles, plasma cholesterol increased significantly.[9] In Hermann's tortoises, plasma triglycerides and cholesterol were significantly higher in females.[38] As postprandial effects on triglyceride and cholesterol concentrations remain minimally studied, fasting before sampling is recommended.

Extrinsic factors that may affect lipids and lipoproteins in reptiles include age and season. Decreased cholesterol occurs with increased age in the male iguanid, *Tropidurus torquatos,* possibly based on the change from omnivory to herbivory as the animal matures.[36] Similarly, differences in cholesterol and fatty acids have been documented between captive and free-living tuatara (*Sphenodon*).[125,126] In the captive mugger crocodile, cholesterol and triglycerides vary based on age class.[60] Cholesterol concentrations were relatively increased for subadults and juveniles compared with adults, while triglyceride concentrations were relatively decreased for subadults and highest for juveniles. Cholesterol concentrations were also relatively increased in juvenile males compared with juvenile females. Free-ranging Moreletti's crocodiles (*Crocodylus moreletii*) had decreased plasma cholesterol concentrations compared to those of the captive animals.[127] Marked seasonal variation in triglycerides has been documented in the yellow-marginated box turtle.[50]

Concentrations of cholesterol and triglycerides tend to decrease due to stress.[48] In the Indian spiny-tailed lizard (*Uromastix hardwickii*), plasma cholesterol concentrations and HDL:LDL ratios are affected by emergence from hibernation, activity periods, prehibernation preparation, and hibernation states (Table 34.8).[98,128] Similar changes are expected during vitellogenesis. Female radiated tortoises had higher triglyceride concentrations in winter (presumably during early vitellogenesis), and lower cholesterol and triglyceride concentrations in summer (presumable after laying), compared with males.[59] Hypercholesterolemia (cholesterol 937 mg/dL; 24.27 mmol/L) has been documented in a single case of atherosclerosis and pericardial effusion in a male bearded dragon.[123] Xanthomatosis in lizards has been associated with mild (20.1 and 22.4 mmol/L; 776–865 mg/dL) to marked increases (35.46 mmol/L, 1369 mg/dL) in plasma cholesterol.[129,130]

Captive anurans (especially tree frogs) are prone to obesity and other lipid disorders such as xanthomatosis and corneal lipidosis.[131] These diseases are associated with an increased plasma cholesterol of captive specimens (27.5 mmol/L, 1062 mg/dL) compared with their free-living counterparts, unaffected by lipidosis (3.86 (0–8.26, 95% CI) mmol/L or 149 (0–319, 95% CI) mg/dL). However, despite multiple publications, the overall number of amphibians investigated for these diseases based on plasma assessment of blood lipids and lipoproteins remains low at less than 75 individuals.[131]

Calcium, Phosphorus, and Magnesium

Calcium and phosphorous remain important analytes in the reptile and amphibian biochemical panel. Seasonal plasma increases of total calcium and phosphorous in free-living and captive females during vitellogenesis occurs in all major reptile taxa.[38,59,61,132 52] A similar trend of relatively increased serum or plasma calcium in females, compared with males, has been reported for eastern hellbenders (*Cryptobranchus alleganiensis*), African clawed frogs (*Xenopus laevis*), and American bull frogs (*Lithobates catesbeianus*).[1] In some amphibians, calcium metabolism changes with season and life stage.[1] Amphibian plasma calcium increases in spring and summer as larvae approach metamorphosis, but decreases in winter.[133] In nesting loggerhead sea turtles, a positive correlation between plasma phosphorous and successful hatching was observed, however nesting turtles were more likely to have lower plasma calcium concentrations than those that false crawled.[134] Differentiation of seasonal changes and reproduction from disease is not straightforward. Seasonal changes of calcium and phosphorous in the apparent absence of reproductive activity also occurs in reptiles.[50,61] In captive panther chameleons, winter values of Ca and P for both sexes were significantly higher than in summer. But within summer, gravid females had significantly higher Ca and P than nonreproductive females Ca (5.3 ± 3.5 vs. 2.9 ± 2.9 mmol/L), P (2.6 ± 1.1 vs. 1.9 ± 0.6 mmol/L).[61] Finally, species differences in total calcium and phosphorous values may be dramatic. Normal physiological hypercalcemia and hyperphosphatemia and relative hypervitaminosis D of indigo snakes has been documented and could be based on their specific diet, UVB exposure, or possibly PTH levels.[135]

To avoid seasonal, gender, and species related complexities of calcium analyte interpretation, the practitioner is encouraged to assess ionized (or free) calcium concentrations (iCa) as well as the total calcium provided by standard biochemical panels. As the biologically active form of calcium, iCa concentrations are relatively conserved across reptile taxa with expected values from healthy reptiles and amphibians being approximately 1.4-1.9 mmol/L.[136-139] Pathological derangements in calcium or phosphorous include nutritional/renal secondary hyperparathyroidism, primary hyperparathyroidism, osteolytic bone disease and pseudohyperparathyroidism.[138] Muscle tremors, fasiculations, and seizures may be caused by hypocalcemia, which most commonly occurs in herbivorous or omnivorous reptiles.[15] Lower gastrointestinal tract strictures of green sea turtles have been associated with persistent hypocalcemia.[89]

If magnesium is the forgotten analyte in mammals, then it remains doubly so in reptiles and amphibians. While one study of reproductive female alligators associated an increase in plasma magnesium with vitellogenesis, a similar study of cobras failed to provide similar results.[132,140] Magnesium toxicosis in leopard geckos (*Eublepharis macularius*) based on ingestion of vermiculite has been reported; however, blood concentrations of the offending ion were not confirmed.[141]

Osmolality, Sodium, Potassium, Chloride, and Bicarbonate

The evaluation of electrolytes from reptiles is made challenging because of widely differing physiology. As an example, Galápagos marine iguanas exhibit some of the highest known blood sodium concentrations, (~ 178 mEq/L = mmol/L), among reptiles.[96] Similarly, increased plasma sodium, chloride, and potassium concentrations have been reported

TABLE 34.8 Cholesterol Values for a Seasonally Active Reptile *Uromastix hardwickii*[128]		
Activity State	**Cholesterol (mg/dL, mmol/L)**	**Mean HDL:LDL**
Hibernation	250 ± 110, 6.47 ± 2.85	70.9: 29.1
Arousal	226 ± 104, 5.85 ± 2.69	73.5: 26.5
Activity	348 ± 117, 9.01 ± 3.03	72.3: 27.7
		(Max in May: 85.7:14.3)
Prehibernation	457 ± 134, 11.84 ± 3.47	57.1: 42.9

in sliders subjected to hyperosmotic stress.[142] In aquatic Chinese soft shelled turtles (*Pelodiscus sinensis*), exposed to 15% salt water, plasma osmolality and concentrations of Na, Cl and BUN increased.[143] Similarly, sea turtles tend to have relatively increased reference intervals for plasma electrolytes compared with other land or freshwater reptiles.[48] Many reptiles have the ability to modulate electrolyte balance using multiple organs: salt gland, kidney, adrenal gland, and the gastrointestinal tract. Dysfunction in these organs may be assumed, but is seldom proven, to have the same effects that one would classically encounter in a mammal. Vomiting and gastrointestinal obstruction may result in hyperglycemia, hypochloremia, and metabolic alkalosis.[77,114] Low potassium has occurred in sea turtles in association with debilitation, nesting, diarrhea, and inanition. In nesting loggerhead sea turtles, those that actually nested had lower potassium concentrations than those that false crawled.[134]

Relative electrolyte concentrations may also be affected by species or size. For example, in postprandial green sea turtles (but not Kemps' ridleys), plasma chloride was relatively decreased.[9] In the Galápagos marine iguana, body length positively correlated with increased HCO_3 and glucose. Electrolyte values may also be affected by season, activity, and sex.[132] For example, male radiated tortoises had increased sodium concentrations during winter compared with females.[59] In captive mugger crocodiles, potassium concentrations were significantly greater in juvenile males than in juvenile females, and subadult animals also had a comparatively lower potassium concentration than other age classes.[60] Prolonged storage of heparinized whole blood may result in relatively increased potassium and decreased sodium concentrations of plasma. The clinician should separate plasma from the cellular components of blood before overnight shipment for analysis.[34,139]

Plasma osmolality, an indicator of hydration state and electrolyte status, has been determined for a number of reptiles. As the concentration of active particles in an aqueous solution, osmolality is best measured directly by an analyzer. Freezing point depression osmometers are more common and more accurate than vapor pressure depression osmometers.[40] However, in the absence of measured osmolality, for some species, calculations may allow the practitioner to calculate an estimate of osmolality. Measured osmolality ranges for select reptiles and amphibians as well as associated recommended osmolality estimate calculations are provided in Table 34.9. Amphibians and reptiles appear tolerant of relatively wide ranges of osmolality, which are likely affected by environmental and physiological conditions.[1] Overwintering frogs and salamanders purposefully dehydrate; thus a healthy hibernating or near-hibernating amphibian should have relatively increased plasma osmolalities,[1] whereas plasma osmolality of active toads from arid areas remain similar throughout the year.[144] Chytridiomycosis, infection with *Batrachochytrid dendobatidis*, is associated with reduced plasma osmolality and decreased sodium, potassium, magnesium, and chloride in affected frogs (green [White's] tree frogs, mountain yellow-legged frogs [*Rana muscosa*]).[1]

Blood Gases and Acid-Base Balance

Few clinically relevant studies of acid–base status and blood gas values have been performed in reptiles or amphibians. However, electrolyte and acid–base status as well as venous blood gas values hold promise as indicators of function and integrity in organs such as kidney, lung, and gastrointestinal tract. For these organs many standard mammalian biomarkers remain inapplicable, poorly sensitive, nonspecific, or irrelevant. However, reptile and amphibian physiology may also allow a relatively wide variation in many acid–base, electrolyte, and blood gas values compared with mammals. Thus, values that would be considered diagnostic of disease in mammals may be within normal physiologic ranges for highly adapted and evolved reptiles or amphibians.[96,145] At present, evaluation of these analytes is mainly relegated to research purposes wherein arterial samples may be obtained. Within the genre of sea turtle stranding, however, determination of values from venous blood has proven useful for determination of prognosis and continued case management.[100,146,147] In anurans, an overly acidic habitat substrate (pH ≤ 4–5) may interfere with the integumental sodium–potassium pump, resulting in hyponatremia, often accompanied by subcutaneous edema.[1] Wild-caught mountain yellow-legged frogs infected with *B. dendrobatidis* retained apparently normal acid–base balance and blood gas values despite electrolyte imbalance.[148]

Uric Acid, Urea, and Ammonia

Evaluation of renal disease in reptiles and amphibians based on plasma markers remains challenging based on a number of factors including the diversity of species and physiological adaptations for nitrogenous waste excretion. For a review of urinalysis in reptiles, please see Chapter 66. Nitrogenous end-products vary in reptiles (see Table 66.2) and amphibians. Quantification of blood urea nitrogen (BUN) and ammonia is recommended for chelonians and crocodilians (see Table 66.2.) but is expected to change due to hydration, postprandial effects, hepatobiliary function, and renal impairment. Uric acid (UA) is most commonly assessed in lizards and snakes but is neither sensitive nor specific for renal disease and may increase in association with profound dehydration, a recent carnivorous meal, or decreased temperature. UA may decrease due to anorexia, fasting, or possibly severe hepatopathy.[9,149] Analysis of blood samples from 43 wild-caught southwest carpet pythons failed to reveal intrinsic or extrinsic factors that influenced UA in apparently healthy snakes.[52] Published cases in which hyperuricemia is linked to primary renal disease are actually relatively few. Hyperuricemia has been reported in a green iguana with small intestinal obstruction and volvulus, which was suspected to be secondary to vomiting and dehydration.[114] In tortoises, increased BUN may indicate renal disease or dehydration. However, ammonia is a major nitrogenous waste product excreted by crocodilians and some aquatic chelonians. Increased plasma or serum BUN concentrations may be associated with normal physiological processes in some desert species or following emergence from hibernation.[150] Multiple changes in plasma analytes are often seen in conjunction with azotemia and hyperosmolality, including hypercholesterolemia, hypophosphatemia, increased AST, and to a lesser extent, hyperchloremia, hypocalcemia, and anemia.[150–152] Thus renal assessment via plasma is best performed in the fasted, normothermic reptile, before and after fluid therapy.

TABLE 34.9	Plasma Osmolalities of Select Reptiles and Amphibians				
Species		**n**	**Osmolality (mOsm/Kg)**	**Data Format**	**Recommended Calculation**
Corn snakes, *Pantherophis guttatus guttatus*[165]		12	344.5 (304.5–373.0)	Mean (Range)	$2 \times [Na^+ + K^+] + ([Glu$ in mg/dL]/18)
Bearded dragons, *Pogona vitticeps*[166]		11	295.4 ± 9.35	Mean ± SD	$1.85 (Na^+ + K^+)$
American alligators, *Alligator mississippiensis*[167]		46	267.7–270.9; 269.3 ± 10.8	95% CI; Mean ± SD	$1.79 \times Na^+ + 0.05 \times [Glu$ in mg/dL]
European green toad, *Bufo viridis*[144]		47	377 ± 5	Mean ± SEM	Not determined

UA and other renal biomarkers may be affected by a number of extrinsic factors. In captive mugger crocodiles, multiple analytes associated with renal function were affected by age and gender. BUN was lower for subadults than for adults or juveniles, whereas UA concentrations were higher in juvenile (than for subadult and adult) females (compared with males). In healthy loggerhead sea turtles, lower plasma creatinine and BUN concentrations occurred in juvenile and subadult turtles, compared with adults.[49] Free-ranging Morelet's crocodiles had greater UA values than captive crocodiles.[127]

Season may also affect renal markers in apparently healthy reptiles, whether free-living or captive. In plasma of the yellow-marginated box turtles, marked seasonal variations occur with BUN, UA, and creatinine.[50] In captive panther chameleons, summer and winter UA values differed based on gender, with relatively increased plasma uric acid concentrations in gravid females.[61] Seasonal effects have also been reported in Hermann's tortoise with UA increased during midsummer.[38] In captive radiated tortoises, UA, BUN, and chloride values were higher in summer than in winter and were higher in males than in females. These changes were attributed to increased activity and seasonal dehydration, which may be normal in males of this arid species.[59]

Evaluation of renal disease in amphibians based on biochemical constituents of plasma is challenging due to the variety of nitrogenous end products and variable, environmentally adapted physiology. Many amphibians have a tolerance for relatively high plasma BUN concentrations to facilitate water uptake via the skin.[1] The appropriate nitrogenous end product to measure varies with species. In the ammonotelic aquatic adults and larvae (*Xenopus* spp., tadpoles) ammonia is the most appropriate analyte to determine. Examples of obligatory ammonotelics are Kuhl's creek frog (*Limnonectes kuhlii*), the fork-tongued frogs (Dicroglossidae), the striped stream, spotted stream, or Matang frog (*Pulchrana signata*), as well as Schlegel's, the brown stream, copper-cheeked, or white-lipped frog (*H. chalconota*).[153] Adult terrestrial amphibians, like most toads, are ureotelic and BUN should be measured. Some tree frogs (waxy tree frogs, *Phyllomedusa* spp.; painted-belly monkey frogs, *Phyllomedusa sauvagii*; leaf frogs, *Phyllomedusa tarsius;* and some species of foam-nesting tree frogs, *Chiromantis* spp.) are uricotelic. These frogs produce UA even when ample water is available and are prone to urate cystic calculi.[153] Thus UA would be the most appropriate nitrogenous end-product analyte to evaluate for these species.[1] In anurans, edema and renal disease are associated with hypoproteinemia (due to renal losses) and hyponatremia (due to lack of tubular resorption).[1]

REFERENCES

See www.expertconsult.com for a complete list of references.

35

Hematology and Biochemistry Tables

Paul M. Gibbons, Brent R. Whitaker, James W. Carpenter,
Colin T. McDermott, Eric Klaphake, and Kurt K. Sladky

The following clinicopathology tables are in US units only. For conversion to SI, see http://www.amamanualofstyle.com/page/si-conversion-calculator.

TABLE 35.1 Hematologic and Serum Biochemical Values of Reptiles[a]

Measurement	Boa Constrictor (*Boa constrictor*)[1,2,3,4]	Emerald Boa (*Corallus caninus*)[2,4]	Rainbow Boa (*Epicrates cenchria*)[2,4]
Hematology			
PCV (%)	29 (12–40)	26 (7–44)	29 (15–44)
RBC (10^6/μL)	0.71 (0.16–1.4)	2.16 (0.54–5.05)	0.87 (0.23–1.74)
Hgb (g/dL)	8.2 (3.1–13.2)	8.2 (6.1–11.4)	10.6 (8–13.1)
MCV (fL)	395 (122–669)	237 (37–360)	314 (45–619)
MCH (pg)	117 (51–184)	120 (113–128)	160
MCHC (g/dL)	31 (21–40)	34 (30–36)	36 (33–40)
WBC (10^3/μL)	7.37 (1.47–19.6)	4.87 (0.48–11.1)	7.64 (1–21.23)
Heterophils (10^3/μL)	1.93 (0.20–6.50)	1.25 (0.18–3.64)	1.07 (0.03–3.67)
Lymphocytes (10^3/μL)	2.89 (0.34–11.9)	1.92 (0.14–5.68)	4.71 (0.1–14.1)
Monocytes (10^3/μL)	0.27 (0.03–2.38)	0.17 (0.02–1.11)	0.9 (0.03–3.06)
Azurophils (10^3/μL)	0.84 (0–4.74)	0.23 (0–3.22)	0.60 (0–2.47)
Eosinophils (10^3/μL)	0.13 (0–0.60)	0.07 (0.06–0.08)	0.11 (0.04–0.22)
Basophils (10^3/μL)	0.21 (0.03–1.01)	0.06 (0.03–0.21)	0.1 (0.02–0.27)
Chemistries			
ALP (U/L)	189 (46–652)	87 (0–236)	27 (14–37)
ALT (U/L)	11 (0–30)	7 (0–27)	4 (1–6)
Amylase (U/L)	14 (0–76)	371 (61–847)	—
AST (U/L)	15 (2–64)	23 (2–61)	18 (3–54)
Bilirubin, total (mg/dL)	0.2 (0–0.6)	0.2 (0.2–0.3)	0.4 (0–0.8)
BUN (mg/dL)	2 (0–8)	2 (1–4)	2 (1–3)
Calcium (mg/dL)	15.3 (10–20)	12.8 (8.1–17.5)	13.8 (10.2–17.5)
Chloride (mEq/L)	125 (108–138)	131 (112–149)	129 (94–158)
Cholesterol (mg/dL)	120 (46–289)	304 (77–614)	206 (140–314)
Creatine kinase (U/L)	489 (57–2099)	454 (41–1445)	95 (0–347)
Creatinine (mg/dL)	0.2 (0–0.5)	0.6 (0.4–0.9)	0.4 (0.1–0.7)
GGT (U/L)	4 (0–23)	2 (1–2)	5
Glucose (mg/dL)	34 (7–74)	27 (5–64)	36 (2–80)
Iron (μg/dL)	113 (103–122)	—	—
LDH (U/L)	149 (0–452)	128 (14–754)	401 (141–661)
Lipase (U/L)	2730	—	—
Magnesium (mEq/L)	2.95 (2.9–3)	—	—
Osmolarity (mOsm/L)	306	—	—
Phosphorus (mg/dL)	4.3 (2.4–8.6)	4.1 (1.8–8)	4.3 (1.6–7.1)
Potassium (mEq/L)	4.7 (3.1–7.3)	5 (3–8.7)	4.8 (2.4–6.7)
Protein, total (g/dL)	7.0 (4.0–10.3)	4.5 (2.6–7.2)	6.8 (4.7–8.9)
Albumin (g/dL)[b]	2.9 (1.6–4.3)	2.6 (2–3.6)	2.4 (1.1–3.6)
Globulin (g/dL)[b]	3.9 (2.0–6.8)	2.8 (1.8–3.6)	4.2 (1.9–6.5)
Sodium (mEq/L)	159 (143–173)	157 (148–167)	162 (142–181)
Triglyceride (mg/dL) Uric acid	103 (3–457)	24 (10–49)	72 (64–90)
(mg/dL)	4.0 (0.3–15.0)	4.7 (1.4–19.2)	3.6 (1.1–9.7)

Continued

TABLE 35.1	Hematologic and Serum Biochemical Values of Reptiles—cont'd		
Measurement	**Rosy Boa** (*Lichanura trivirgata*)[2,4]	**Ball Python** (*Python regius*)[4,5]	**Blood Python** (*Python curtus*)[2]
Hematology			
PCV (%)	37 (20–54)	24 (10–33)	25 (15–49)
RBC (10^6/μL)	—	0.74 (0.31–1.16)	0.65
Hgb (g/dL)	—	7.8 (4.5–11.1)	—
MCV (fL)	—	328 (131–524)	340
MCH (pg)	—	102 (28–175)	—
MCHC (g/dL)	—	32 (24–40)	—
WBC (10^3/μL)	4.65 (0.57–8.73)	7.46 (2.22–21.6)	11.7 (1.13–42.5)
Heterophils (10^3/μL)	1.67 (0.39–4.13)	1.78 (0.32–6.17)	1.82 (0.31–3.99)
Lymphocytes (10^3/μL)	1.74 (0.18–4.92)	3.21 (0.35–13.8)	6.71 (0.34–33.6)
Monocytes (10^3/μL)	0.10 (0.03–0.65)	0.73 (0.01–3.26)	0.62 (0.13–2.12)
Azurophils (10^3/μL)	0.40 (0–1.68)	0.65 (0.01–4.12)	2.82 (0.27–6.8)
Eosinophils (10^3/μL)	—	0.10 (0.02–0.53)	0.08
Basophils (10^3/μL)	—	0.22 (0.04–1.08)	0.93 (0.32–1.83)
Chemistries			
ALP (U/L)	—	37 (11–98)	44 (8–56)
ALT (U/L)	—	9 (1–25)	10 (3–17)
Amylase (U/L)	—	1647 (383–2911)	—
AST (U/L)	20 (1–107)	25 (4–97)	56 (6–209)
Bilirubin, total (mg/dL)	—	0.1 (0–0.2)	0.3 (0.2–0.5)
BUN (mg/dL)	—	2 (0–7)	1 (0–2)
Calcium (mg/dL)	13.1 (9.4–17.4)	14.7 (10.4–19.3)	14.7 (13.5–16.2)
Chloride (mEq/L)	—	121 (107–134)	131 (123–138)
Cholesterol (mg/dL)	—	111 (15–232)	214 (76–445)
Creatine kinase (U/L)	—	526 (55–2136)	668 (327–1009)
Creatinine (mg/dL)	—	0.2 (0–0.7)	0.9 (0.5–1.3)
GGT (U/L)	—	—	8 (0–16)
Glucose (mg/dL)	37 (3–73)	25 (8–53)	30 (13–74)
LDH (U/L)	—	122 (4–376)	207 (49–364)
Phosphorus (mg/dL)	2.9 (0.8–6.1)	3.0 (1.4–7.3)	3.7 (3.1–4.5)
Potassium (mEq/L)	5.9 (3.7–10.3)	5.5 (2.4–10.0)	6.3 (3.3–11.2)
Protein, total (g/dL)	5.8 (3.7–8.3)	6.8 (3.6–9.0)	6.2 (3.6–8.1)
Albumin (g/dL)[b]	2.1 (1.2–2.9)	2.1 (1.1–3.6)	2.3 (1.6–2.8)
Globulin (g/dL)[b]	3.7 (2.3–4.8)	4.5 (2.1–6.5)	4.1 (3.1–4.9)
Sodium (mEq/L)	155 (115–174)	153 (137–171)	160 (155–164)
Triglyceride (mg/dL)	—	—	16 (13–22)
Uric acid (mg/dL)	6.4 (1.9–19.0)	3.0 (0.8–8.3)	4.3 (2.1–7.1)
Measurement	**Burmese Python** (*Python bivittatus*)[2,4]	**Reticulated Python** (*Malayopython reticulatus*)[2,4]	**Green Tree Python** (*Morelia viridis*)[2,4]
Hematology			
PCV (%)	28 (13–38)	26 (13–39)	25.3 (13–38)
RBC (10^6/μL)	0.83 (0.13–1.54)	0.72 (0.41–1.25)	0.85 (0.4–1.3)
Hgb (g/dL)	9.0 (4–11)	10.7 (5.2–30)	5.9 (4–7)
MCV (fL)	319 (84–554)	343 (176–429)	229 (208–250)
MCH (pg)	98 (32–143)	138 (60–186)	100
MCHC (g/dL)	32 (18–44)	37 (29–45)	36 (33–40)
WBC (10^3/μL)	7.6 (2.19–24.2)	7.48 (1.32–15.8)	7.28 (1.2–18.7)
Heterophils (10^3/μL)	2.25 (0.31–5.76)	1.92 (0.08–4.83)	1.59 (0.24–3.49)
Lymphocytes (10^3/μL)	3.73 (0.46–17.4)	2.24 (0.12–7.47)	3.46 (0.07–11.8)
Monocytes (10^3/μL)	0.17 (0.02–2.13)	1.22 (0.02–5.50)	0.61 (0.02–2.86)
Azurophils (10^3/μL)	0.27 (0.01–5.89)	0.10 (0.01–4.30)	0.72 (0.00–3.17)
Eosinophils (10^3/μL)	0.45 (0.10–1.4)	0.68 (0.04–1.95)	0.16 (0.1–0.22)
Basophils (10^3/μL)	0.12 (0.03–0.33)	0.06 (0.06–0.7)	0.17 (0.04–0.70)

TABLE 35.1 Hematologic and Serum Biochemical Values of Reptiles—cont'd

Measurement	Burmese Python (*Python bivittatus*)[2,4]	Reticulated Python (*Malayopython reticulatus*)[2,4]	Green Tree Python (*Morelia viridis*)[2,4]
Chemistries			
ALP (U/L)	58 (4–230)	61 (4–211)	177 (43–425)
ALT (U/L)	7 (0–26)	16 (0–51)	18 (0–52)
Amylase (U/L)	3255	1690 (416–2963)	902 (564–1240)
AST (U/L)	14 (3–65)	12 (2–34)	18 (1–63)
Bilirubin, total (mg/dL)	0.6 (0–2)	0.3	0.2
BUN (mg/dL)	2 (1–5)	2 (1–7)	2 (0–2)
Calcium (mg/dL)	16.1 (7.2–25.0)	16.3 (10.9–26.6)	13.8 (9.8–17.9)
Chloride (mEq/L)	118 (104–132)	118 (92–141)	124 (90–153)
Cholesterol (mg/dL)	264 (120–479)	285 (81–531)	251 (72–561)
Creatine kinase (U/L)	381 (39–1577)	351 (24–2338)	606 (21–1843)
Creatinine (mg/dL)	0.3 (0–1.6)	0.2 (0.1–0.4)	0.2 (0.2–0.5)
GGT (U/L)	25 (4–51)	22	—
Glucose (mg/dL)	24 (1–83)	31 (1–77)	37 (1–76)
LDH (U/L)	144 (12–807)	313 (43–1048)	206
Phosphorus (mg/dL)	4.4 (2.3–9.2)	5.6 (2.4–13.0)	5.1 (2.3–10.2)
Potassium (mEq/L)	4.8 (2.6–7.0)	5.0 (3.4–8.1)	5.5 (3.6–7.9)
Protein, total (g/dL)	7.2 (4.4–11.1)	7.8 (4.8–10.7)	7.2 (3.6–10.9)
Albumin (g/dL)[b]	2.3 (1.2–3.4)	2.1 (0.8–3.9)	2.0 (0.4–3.7)
Globulin (g/dL)[b]	4.9 (1.9–7.8)	5.0 (0.8–9.0)	4.9 (3.2–8.1)
Sodium (mEq/L)	158 (145–172)	160 (142–178)	161 (142–179)
Triglyceride (mg/dL)	114 (16–532)	45	—
Uric acid (mg/dL)	4.3 (0.4–10.1)	7.8 (3.5–17.4)	3.6 (0–11.0)

Measurement	Carpet Python (*Morelia spilota* ssp.)[2,4,6]	Gopher Snake (*Pituophis catenifer*)[2,4,7]	Indigo Snake (*Drymarchon corais*)[2,4,8]
Hematology			
PCV (%)	24 (16–32)	35 (13–49)	32 (23–45)
RBC (10^6/μL)	0.89 (0.32–1.45)	0.67 (0.14–1.4)	0.62 (0.43–0.76)
Hgb (g/dL)	7.9 (4.9–9.7)	9.7 (4.3–12.3)	9.2 (7.3–11.1)
MCV (fL)	327 (260–386)	578 (246–1571)	369 (221–558)
MCH (pg)	111 (86–170)	111 (81–132)	258
MCHC (g/dL)	34 (29–39)	33 (27.5–36)	40 (33–46)
WBC (10^3/μL)	13.4 (2.7–24.8)	7.31 (1.66–24.0)	16.3 (4–46)
Heterophils (10^3/μL)	7.13 (1.79–16.8)	1.58 (0.33–5.99)	3.09 (0.32–7.82)
Lymphocytes (10^3/μL)	2.59 (0.60–6.91)	4.06 (0.21–13.2)	5.29 (0.65–13.5)
Monocytes (10^3/μL)	0.67 (0.03–2.67)	0.14 (0.01–0.86)	—
Azurophils (10^3/μL)	1.09 (0.01–5.72)	0.58 (0.01–3.23)	6.92 (1.79–12.1)
Basophils (10^3/μL)	0.16 (0–1.01)	0.14 (0.01–0.44)	0.32 (0.16–2.12)
Chemistries			
ALP (U/L)	36 (10–81)	61 (15–128)	123 (6–547)
ALT (U/L)	17 (6–78)	15 (1–70)	30 (10–259)
Amylase (U/L)	—	711 (107–1315)	1107 (532–3887)[i]
AST (U/L)	17 (2–45)	20 (5–103)	47 (3–215)
Bilirubin, total (mg/dL)	0.5	0.4 (0.3–0.6)	2.1 (0.6–3.5)
BUN (mg/dL)	3 (2–3)	2.2 (1–5)	2.3 (1–5)[i]
Calcium (mg/dL)	14.3 (10.9–20.5)	15.5 (11.0–20.0)	50 (13.6–116)[c]
Ionized Ca (mmol/L)	—	—	1.89 (1.39–2.39)
Chloride (mEq/L)	118 (102–131)	120 (103–138)	121 (104–138)
Cholesterol (mg/dL)	318 (126–630)	368 (118–630)	255 (138–423)
Creatine kinase (U/L)	349 (3–1230)	330 (34–1702)	378 (27–1607)
Creatinine (mg/dL)	1.3 (0.3–3.7)	0.3 (0.1–0.6)	0.49 (0.1–2.8)
GGT (U/L)	32 (9–55)	10 (0–34)	8.7 (6–12)
Glucose (mg/dL)	30 (3–57)	57 (23–99)	102 (42–247)[i]
LDH (U/L)	201 (11–728)	112 (1–405)	1005 (100–2809)
Magnesium (mEq/L)	330 (48–547)	76 (20–191)	313 (13–1055)

Continued

TABLE 35.1   Hematologic and Serum Biochemical Values of Reptiles—cont'd

Measurement	Carpet Python (*Morelia spilota* ssp.)[2,4,6]	Gopher Snake (*Pituophis catenifer*)[2,4,7]	Indigo Snake (*Drymarchon corais*)[2,4,8]
Phosphorus (mg/dL)	4.1 (0.8–7.9)	3.6 (1.7–7.9)	9.4 (5.8–16.6)[c]
Potassium (mEq/L)	4.9 (3.0–7.1)	4.8 (2.2–7.4)	4.4 (3.2–6.1)[i]
Protein, total (g/dL)	7.2 (5.4–10.3)	6.0 (3.7–8.8)	7.6 (5.2–12.1)[i]
Albumin (g/dL)[b]	2.1 (1.6–2.9)	2.0 (1.1–3.0)	2.4 (1.0–4.3)
Albumin (PEP; g/dL)[b]	—	—	2.3 (1.40–3.27)
Globulin (g/dL)[b]	5.1 (3.7–7.6)	4.0 (1.7–6.3)	—
α-1 (PEP; g/dL)[b]	—	—	0.8 (0.37–1.5)
α-2 (PEP; g/dL)[b]	—	—	1.32 (0.4–2.16)
β (PEP; g/dL)[b]	—	—	1.89 (1.1–3.7)
γ (PEP; g/dL)[b]	—	—	1.09 (0.23–3.73)
A/G Ratio	—	—	0.49 (0.24–0.74)[i]
Sodium (mEq/L)	156 (140–172)	163 (146–180)	167 (158–180)[i]
Triglyceride (mg/dL)	30	27 (16–37)	154 (12–552)[i]
Uric acid (mg/dL)	4.1 (0–9.3)	4.6 (1.9–12.6)	6.7 (1.5–18.3)

Measurement	Corn Snake (*Pantherophis guttata*)[2,4]	Common King Snake (*Lampropeltis getula*)[2,4]	Rat Snake (*Pantherophis obsoleta*)[2,4,9]
Hematology			
PCV (%)	30 (13–50)	31 (9–47)	30 (12–46)
RBC (10^6/μL)	0.88 (0.40–1.60)	0.77 (0.10–1.88)	0.83 (0.23–1.43)
Hgb (g/dL)	11.5 (9.7–13.5)	—	9.8 (2.8–16.2)
MCV (fL)	307 (67–546)	311 (28–618)	354 (73–636)
MCH (pg)	127 (110–143)	—	121 (90–175)
MCHC (g/dL)	35 (32–40)	—	31 (18–45)
WBC (10^3/μL)	5.93 (1.12–16.9)	7.45 (1.55–27.7)	7.83 (1.02–25.2)
Heterophils (10^3/μL)	1.24 (0.23–5.08)	1.01 (0.16–5.50)	1.20 (0.10–3.89)
Lymphocytes (10^3/μL)	2.92 (0.29–11.8)	3.92 (0.35–20.9)	3.89 (0.41–16.1)
Monocytes (10^3/μL)	0.31 (0.03–1.78)	1.98 (0.05–5.83)	0.48 (0.02–2.52)
Azurophils (10^3/μL)	0.42 (0.01–3.29)	0.24 (0–4.77)	0.41 (0–3.50)
Eosinophils (10^3/μL)	0.09 (0.03–0.48)	0.08 (0.02–0.37)	0.11 (0.01–0.55)
Basophils (10^3/μL)	0.19 (0.04–1.04)	0.27 (0.04–1.08)	0.18 (0.01–0.72)
Chemistries			
ALP (U/L)	35 (0–85)	41 (13–102)	70 (11–212)
ALT (U/L)	19 (1–57)	11 (0–50)	10 (0–32)
Amylase (U/L)	540 (255–2225)	1268 (371–2671)	1337 (630–2626)
AST (U/L)	25 (4–149)	20 (4–107)	19 (3–75)
Bilirubin, total (mg/dL)	0.3 (0–1.0)	0.4 (0.1–0.7)	0.2 (0–0.8)
BUN (mg/dL)	3 (1–6)	2 (1–10)	2 (1–12)
Calcium (mg/dL)	15.6 (11.9–19.9)	14.9 (9.1–22.2)	15.3 (10.6–21.0)
Chloride (mEq/L)	122 (105–139)	119 (97–141)	121 (96–146)
Cholesterol (mg/dL)	473 (267–678)	294 (75–513)	340 (92–588)
Creatine kinase (U/L)	270 (31–967)	406 (59–1909)	228 (41–1049)
Creatinine (mg/dL)	0.6 (0.2–2)	0.6 (0–1.6)	0.3 (0–0.8)
GGT (U/L)	9 (0–25)	9	9 (1–35)
Glucose (mg/dL)	49 (17–92)	38 (8–92)	62 (11–121)
Iron (μg/dL)	—	190 (30–488)	—
LDH (U/L)	178 (10–585)	126 (15–417)	175 (4–452)
Lipase (U/L)	—	—	4 (3–4)
Magnesium (mg/dL)	—	—	2.5
Phosphorus (mg/dL)	3.7 (1.8–8.0)	3.8 (1.7–11.3)	3.8 (1.5–9.3)
Potassium (mEq/L)	4.9 (1.8–9.1)	4.6 (2.3–9.2)	5.0 (1.2–8.7)
Protein, total (g/dL)	7.0 (3.3–10.7)	6.4 (3.8–10.3)	6.3 (3.8–10.7)
Albumin (g/dL)[b]	2.1 (1.0–3.4)	1.8 (0.8–2.9)	2.3 (1.4–3.6)
Globulin (g/dL)[b]	4.7 (2.6–7.4)	4.4 (2.1–7.2)	4.0 (1.5–6.6)
Sodium (mEq/L)	162 (149–181)	161 (140–180)	164 (148–180)
Triglyceride (mg/dL)	331 (47–1118)	—	195 (21–1017)
Uric acid (mg/dL)	4.4 (1.0–13.6)	4.6 (1.4–16.0)	4.1 (0.9–14.0)

TABLE 35.1　Hematologic and Serum Biochemical Values of Reptiles—cont'd

Measurement	Milk Snake (*Lampropeltis triangulum*)[2,4]	Prehensile-Tailed Skink (*Corucia zebrata*)[4,10]	Blue-Tongued Skink (*Tiliqua scincoides*)[2,4]
Hematology			
PCV (%)	30 (10–43)	32 (21–43)	28 (16–39)
RBC (10^6/μL)	0.88 (0.36–1.45)	1.59 (0.91–2.28)	0.89 (0.30–2.00)
Hgb (g/dL)	10.4 (6.9–11.9)	9.3 (5.7–12.0)	10.4 (6–13)
MCV (fL)	354 (135–615)	213 (126–311)	297 (34–441)
MCH (pg)	119 (89–164)	61 (35–91)	98 (44–173)
MCHC (g/dL)	34 (29–45)	28 (19–35)	33 (16–57)
WBC (10^3/μL)	7.33 (1.66–23.8)	11.5 (3.4–31.2)	5.93 (2.00–17.7)
Heterophils (10^3/μL)	1.29 (0.09–5.32)	3.66 (0.70–10.6)	2.24 (0.43–6.64)
Lymphocytes (10^3/μL)	3.55 (0.61–10.33)	3.87 (0.50–16.2)	1.93 (0.31–7.31)
Monocytes (10^3/μL)	0.12 (0.03–1.19)	0.68 (0.07–4.55)	0.16 (0.03–1.03)
Azurophils (10^3/μL)	0.76 (0.02–6.13)	0.11 (0.02–4.28)	0.16 (0.01–1.93)
Eosinophils (10^3/μL)	—	0.45 (0.05–1.48)	0.37 (0.02–1.50)
Basophils (10^3/μL)	0.24 (0.02–0.67)	1.26 (0.10–5.30)	0.67 (0.03–2.27)
Chemistries			
ALP (U/L)	115 (27–338)	118 (33–344)	80 (25–159)
ALT (U/L)	8 (3–17)	6 (1–20)	20 (5–34)
Amylase (U/L)	665	792 (255–1971)	—
AST (U/L)	19 (1–74)	14 (3–54)	20 (5–80)
Bilirubin, total (mg/dL)	0.4 (0.1–0.9)	0.2 (0–0.5)	—
BUN (mg/dL)	2 (1–14)	1 (0–4)	2 (1–27)
Calcium (mg/dL)	14.9 (11.0–18.9)	11.8 (8.9–15.2)	12.7 (10.0–15.9)
Chloride (mEq/L)	122 (106–137)	124 (107–138)	116 (100–132)
Cholesterol (mg/dL)	446 (51–631)	97 (39–265)	207 (49–601)
Creatine kinase (U/L)	157 (7–566)	234 (26–1319)	629 (59–5570)
Creatinine (mg/dL)	0.5 (0.3–1.1)	0.3 (0–0.6)	0.3 (0.1–0.6)
GGT (U/L)	8 (3–13)	2 (0–11)	8
Glucose (mg/dL)	52 (12–128)	107 (35–171)	127 (72–202)
LDH (U/L)	816 (18–2807)	183 (28–625)	735 (364–1106)
Lipase (U/L)	—	25 (8–63)	364
Phosphorus (mg/dL)	3.5 (1.0–7.3)	4.3 (2.3–9.8)	4.4 (2.3–10.8)
Potassium (mEq/L)	4.6 (2.2–8.1)	5.0 (2.9–8.1)	5.1 (3.3–7.9)
Protein, total (g/dL)	6.5 (3.9–10.0)	5.8 (4.1–8.3)	6.1 (3.7–8.5)
Albumin (g/dL)[b]	2.0 (0.8–3.2)	2.3 (1.4–3.4)	2.1 (1.1–3.1)
Globulin (g/dL)[b]	4.6 (2.4–6.8)	3.5 (2.3–5.0)	3.9 (2.4–5.8)
Sodium (mEq/L)	164 (148–180)	160 (145–177)	151 (139–175)
Triglyceride (mg/dL)	428 (68–1620)	48 (12–309)	—
Uric acid (mg/dL)	4.9 (1.3–15.0)	1.8 (0.3–5.0)	2.7 (0.6–9.5)

Measurement	Panther Chameleon (*Furcifur pardalis*)[2,4,11]	Veiled Chameleon (*Chameleo calyptratus*)[2,4]	Spiny-Tailed Lizard (*Uromastyx* spp.)[2,12]
Hematology			
PCV (%)[i]	Nov-51	24 (12–37)	29 (4.9–44.5)
RBC (10^6/μL)	4.5–16.7	—	0.78 (0.33–4.1)
Hgb (g/dL)	—	—	9.9 (3.3–17.4)
MCV (fL)	330 (200–418)	—	415 (119–614)
MCH (pg)	—	—	133 (1.2–203)
MCHC (g/dL)	—	—	33 (22–41)
Thrombocytes (10^3/μL)	—	—	958 (290–2290)
WBC (10^3/μL)[i]	0.3–21.3	6.30 (1.20–21.0)	3.1 (1–8.1)
Heterophils (10^3/μL)	2.68 (0.09–6.64)	2.35 (0.50–8.32)	2 (0.59–5.36)
Lymphocytes (10^3/μL)	5.98 (0.21–16.8)	2.18 (0.07–10.8)	0.99 (0.27–4.05)
Monocytes (10^3/μL)	—	—	0.04 (0–0.5)
Azurophils (10^3/μL)	0.46 (0–2.29)	0.50 (0–2.75)	—
Eosinophils (10^3/μL)	—	—	0.04 (0–0.2)
Basophils (10^3/μL)	0.13 (0.03–0.92)	—	0.03 (0–0.33)

Continued

TABLE 35.1   Hematologic and Serum Biochemical Values of Reptiles—cont'd

Measurement	Panther Chameleon (*Furcifur pardalis*)[2,4,11]	Veiled Chameleon (*Chameleo calyptratus*)[2,4]	Spiny-Tailed Lizard (*Uromastyx* spp.)[2,12]
Chemistries			
ALP (U/L)	32 (1–109)	—	31 (5.9–139)
ALT (U/L)[i,j]	0–19.2	—	11 (2.4–35)
Amylase (U/L)	—	—	134
AST (U/L)[i,j]	0–104.5	397 (93–967)	73 (29–172)
Bilirubin, total (mg/dL)	—	—	0.3 (0.1–0.7)
BUN (mg/dL)	0–3.9	—	0.56 (0–3)
Calcium (mg/dL)	10.9 (7.1–14.6)	11.9 (8.7–14.5)	9.9 (7.2–13.2)
Chloride (mEq/L)	—	—	126 (111–135)
Cholesterol (mg/dL)	—	—	161 (64–295)
Creatine kinase (U/L)[j]	0–836	1873 (5–8905)	1778 (141–10k)
Creatinine (mg/dL)	—	—	0.4 (0.1–3)
GGT (U/L)	—	—	0.8 (0–5.0)
Glucose (mg/dL)[i,j]	50.7–395.5	270 (125–444)	200 (68–356)
LDH (U/L)[i]	0–670.7	—	209 (22–899)
Magnesium (mg/dL)	—	—	3.48 (2.1–10.2)
Phosphorus (mg/dL)	9.8 (2.1–17.5)	8.4 (4.4–16.1)	4.5 (1.3–10)
Potassium (mEq/L)	5.5 (1.1–10.0)	6.5 (3.5–12.0)	3.7 (3–4.6)
Protein, total (g/dL)[i,j]	2.6–7.0	6.4 (4.4–10.9)	4 (2.6–7.4)
Albumin (g/dL)[b,i,j]	0.5–3.3	3.1 (1.4–4.2)	2 (1.2–3.1)
Globulin (g/dL)[b]	3.2 (2.0–4.4)	3.3 (2.0–5.9)	2.9 (2.2–4.6)
Sodium (mEq/L)	143 (127–159)	144 (132–169)	173 ± 4
Triglyceride (mg/dL)	—	—	175 (111–238)
Uric acid (mg/dL)[i,j]	0–21.2	5.6 (0–21.9)	2.94 (0.3–7.3)

Measurement	Bearded Dragon (*Pogona vitticeps*)[2,13]	Gila Monster (*Heloderma suspectum*)[14]	Green Iguana (*Iguana iguana*)[4,15,16,17,18,] (Nevarez et al, Proc ARAV, 2002, pp 87–91)
Hematology			
PCV (%)	30 (17–45)	37 (22–50)	25–38
RBC (10⁶/µL)	1 (0.40–1.60)	0.50 (0.22–0.67)	1–1.9
Hgb (g/dL)	9.3 (4.7–14)	7.4 (6.0–9.5)	12-Aug
MCV (fL)	292 (77–506)	812 (415–1773)	165–305
MCH (pg)	90 (16–163)	—	65–105
MCHC (g/dL)	32 (19–46)	21 (14–36)	20–38
WBC (10³/µL)	6.21 (1.45–19.0)	4.72 (3.30–6.40)	10-Mar
Heterophils (10³/µL)	2.09 (0.24–7.77)	2.17 (1.35–3.31)	0.35–5.2
Lymphocytes (10³/µL)	2.77 (0.29–11.3)	1.54 (0.58–3.39)	0.5–5.5
Monocytes (10³/µL)	0.25 (0.03–1.39)	0.07 (0–0.19)	0–0.1
Azurophils (10³/µL)	0.11 (0.01–1.98)	0.38 (0–1.14)	0–1.7
Eosinophils (10³/µL)	0.12 (0.01–0.37)	—	0–1
Basophils (10³/µL)	0.26 (0.04–1.28)	0.57 (0.23–1.05)	0–0.5
Fibrinogen (mg/dL)	180 (0–300)	—	0–300
Chemistries			
ALP (U/L)	133 (21–569)	—	40 (4–170)
ALT (U/L)	9 (0–33)	—	21 (0–97)
Amylase (U/L)	1670 (497–3430)	—	1815 (996–2988)
AST (U/L)	20 (2–90)	42 (20–66)	52 (2–100)
Bile acids (rest; µmol/L)	—	16.2 (2.6–55.1)	7.5 (2.6–30.3)
Bile acids (7.5h; µmol/L)	—	—	32.5 (15.2–44.1)
Bilirubin, total (mg/dL)	0.4 (0–1.4)	—	0.3 (0–4.9)
BUN (mg/dL)	2 (1–5)	15 (6–30)	2 (0–10)
Calcium (mg/dL)	11.9 (8.6–18)	12.2 (10.2–13.4)	12 (6–18)[d]
Ionized Ca⁺⁺ (mmol/L)	—	1.26 (1.09–1.50)	1.01–1.62
Chloride (mEq/L)	120 (94–149)	—	117 (102–130)
Cholesterol (mg/dL)	271 (79–606)	—	104–333[d]

TABLE 35.1 Hematologic and Serum Biochemical Values of Reptiles—cont'd

Measurement	Bearded Dragon (*Pogona vitticeps*)[2,13]	Gila Monster (*Heloderma suspectum*)[14]	Green Iguana (*Iguana iguana*)[4,15,16,17,18,] (Nevarez et al, Proc ARAV, 2002, pp 87–91)
Creatine kinase (U/L)	563 (33–4042)	600 (144–1812)	1876 (174–8768)[d]
Creatinine (mg/dL)	0.2 (0–0.7)	—	0.5 (0.2–1.3)
GGT (U/L)	1 (0–21)	—	3 (0–10)
Glucose (mg/dL)	202 (108–333)	48 (4–109)	169–288
Iron (µg/dL)	—	—	88–133
LDH (U/L)	347 (25–1906)	—	617 (36–7424)[d]
Lipase (U/L)	—	—	21 (17–24)
Magnesium (mEq/L)	—	—	2.4–4
Phosphorus (mg/dL)	4.4 (2.1–10.6)	3.4 (1.1–8.6)	5 (2.5–21)[d]
Potassium (mEq/L)	4.0 (1.5–7.1)	3.9 (2.8–4.6)	1.3–3
Protein, total (g/dL)	5.0 (3.0–8.1)	6.3 (5.4–6.9)	5.4 (4.1–7.4)[d]
Albumin (g/dL)[b]	2.5 (1.2–4.0)		2.1–2.8
Albumin (PEP; g/dL)[b]	—	2.61 (2.14–3.23)	1.8 (1.4–3.1)
Globulin (g/dL)[b]	2.5 (1.1–4.5)	—	2.5–4.3[d]
α-1 (PEP; g/dL)[b]	—	2.09 (1.48–2.60)	0.9 (0.4–1.2)
α-2 (PEP; g/dL)[b]	—	0.59 (0.44–0.76)	—
β (PEP; g/dL)[b]	—	0.58 (0.41–0.77)	2.2 (1.6–3.8)[d]
γ (PEP; g/dL)[b]	—	0.33 (0.18–0.68)	0.3 (0.1–0.4)
A/G Ratio	—	—	0.5 (0.41–0.78)
Sodium (mEq/L)	157 (140–179)	144 (140–151)	158–183
Triglyceride (mg/dL)	261 (93–437)	—	383 (7–1323)[d]
Uric acid (mg/dL)	3.1 (0.5–9.8)	16.8 (9.8–24.7)	2.6 (0–8.2)[d]
Vitamin D_3 (25-OH; nmol/L)	—	—	51–393[d]

Measurement	Green Iguana (*Iguana iguana*), Male[e,19,20]	Green Iguana (*Iguana iguana*), Female[e,19,20]	Green Iguana (*Iguana iguana*), Juvenile[e,19]
Hematology			
PCV (%)	34 (29–39)	38 (33–44)	38 (30–47)
RBC (10^6/µL)	1.3 (1–1.7)	1.4 (1.2–1.8)	1.4 (1.3–1.6)
Hgb (g/dL)	8.6 (6.7–10.2)	10.6 (9.1–12.2)	9.6 (9.2–10.1)
MCV (fL)	266 (228–303)	270 (235–331)	—
MCHC (g/dL)	25 (23–28)	28 (25–31)	—
WBC (10^3/µL)	15 (11–25)	15 (8–25)	16 (8–22)
Heterophils (10^3/µL)	3.6 (1–5.4)	3.2 (0.6–6.4)	2.2 (1–3.8)
Lymphocytes (10^3/µL)	9.7 (5–16.5)	9.9 (5.2–14.4)	12.9 (6.2–17.2)
Monocytes (10^3/µL)	1.3 (0.2–2.7)	1.2 (0.4–2.3)	0.4 (0.3–0.6)
Eosinophils (10^3/µL)	0.1 (0–0.3)	0.1 (0–0.2)	0.3 (0–0.4)
Basophils (10^3/µL)	0.4 (0.1–1)	0.5 (0.2–1.2)	0.5 (0.1–0.7)
Fibrinogen (mg/dL)	100 (100–200)	100 (100–300)	100 (100–300)
Chemistries			
ALP (U/L)	39 (14–65)	59 (22–90)	—
ALT (U/L)	32 (4–76)	45 (5–96)	—
Anion gap (mEq/L)	22 (12–30)	29 (19–41)	—
AST (U/L)	33 (19–65)	40 (7–102)	41 (13–72)
Bilirubin, total (mg/dL)	0.8 (0.1–1.4)	1.5 (0.3–3.1)	—
Calcium (mg/dL)	11.3 (8.6–14.1)	12.5 (10.8–14)	14.3 (12.1–23.2)
Chloride (mEq/L)	119 (115–124)	121 (113–129)	—
Cholesterol (mg/dL)	161 (82–214)	255 (204–347)	—
CO_2 (mEq/L)	19.9 (15.2–24.7)	19 (16–23)	—
Estradiol (pg/mL)	79 (36–162)	270 (81–512)	—
Glucose (mg/dL)	166 (70–244)	170 (105–258)	273 (131–335)
Phosphorus (mg/dL)	5.3 (3.2–7.6)	6.3 (2.8–9.3)	7.7 (4.3–9)
Potassium (mEq/L)	4 (2.8–6.1)	3.6 (2–5.8)	—

Continued

TABLE 35.1 Hematologic and Serum Biochemical Values of Reptiles—cont'd

Measurement	Green Iguana (*Iguana iguana*), Male[e,19,20]	Green Iguana (*Iguana iguana*), Female[e,19,20]	Green Iguana (*Iguana iguana*), Juvenile[e,19]
Protein, total (g/dL)	5.4 (4.4–6.5)	6.1 (4.9–7.6)	5 (4.2–6.1)
Albumin (g/dL)[b]	2 (1.3–3)	2.4 (1.5–3)	2.3 (2–2.8)
Globulin (g/dL)[b]	3.5 (2.5–4.4)	3.8 (2.8–5.2)	2.7 (2.2–3)
A:G (ratio)	0.6 (0.4–0.9)	0.7 (0.3–1)	0.8 (0.7–0.9)
Sodium (mEq/L)	157 (152–162)	163 (156–172)	—
Testosterone (ng/mL)	10.2 (2.2–15.7)	0.26 (0.07–0.35)	—
Uric acid (mg/dL)	2.7 (1.5–5.8)	3.6 (0.9–6.7)	3.3 (0.7–5.7)

Measurement	Chinese (Asian) Water Dragon (*Physignathus cocincinus*)[21]	Crested Gecko (*Correlophus ciliatus*), Male[22]	Crested Gecko (*Correlophus ciliatus*), Female[22]
Hematology			
PCV (%)	35 (32–40)	36 (23–45)	31 (24–43)
WBC (10³/µL)	13.5 (11.7–18.2)	15.4 (3.5–38.9)	15.4 (3.5–38.9)
Heterophils (10³/µL)	5.1 (3.9–6.9)	1.5 (0.6–4.2)	1.5 (0.6–4.2)
Lymphocytes (10³/µL)	7.2 (5.6–9.5)	10.7 (2.2–24.9)	10.7 (2.2–24.9)
Monocytes (10³/µL)	1.1 (0.4–1.9)	1.9 (0.8–5.1)	1.9 (0.8–5.1)
Azurophils (10³/µL)	0 (0–0.6)	—	—
Eosinophils (10³/µL)	0.2 (0.1–0.3)	0 (0–0.2)	0 (0–0.2)
Basophils (10³/µL)	0.5 (0.2–0.8)	0.3 (0–0.8)	0.3 (0–0.8)
Chemistries			
AST (U/L)	16.5 (8–52)	30 (12–84)	30 (12–84)
Bile acids (µmol/L)	—	43 (<35–89)	43 (<35–89)
Calcium (mg/dL)	12.4 (11.6–13.3)	12.5 (11.8–13.9)	>20 (15.6–20.0)
Creatine kinase (U/L)	1747 (19–6630)	489 (89–2104)	489 (89–2104)
Glucose (mg/dL)	157 (112–243)	107 (56–180)	107 (56–180)
Phosphorus (mg/dL)	5.7 (3.4–8.2)	4.0 (2.6–6.2)	9.6 (3.8–18.8)
Potassium (mEq/L)	4.2 (3.8–4.5)	2.6 (1.5–4.5)	2.6 (1.5–4.5)
Protein, total (g/dL)	7 (6.6–7.5)	6.0 (4.9–7.7)	6.6 (5.2–8.0)
Albumin (g/dL)[b]	2.2 (2.1–2.3)	2.7 (2.3–3.2)	2.9 (2.4–3.4)
Globulin (g/dL)[b]	4.7 (4.5–5.3)	3.5 (2.6–5.2)	3.5 (2.6–5.2)
Sodium (mEq/L)	150 (147–153)	143 (136–148)	143 (136–148)
Uric acid (mg/dL)	2.3 (1.9–2.7)	2.6 (0.9–6.0)	2.6 (0.9–6.0)

Measurement	Savannah Monitor (*Varanus exanthematicus*)[2,4]	Water Monitor (*Varanus salvator*)[2,4]	Tegu Lizard (*Tupinambus* spp.)[f,2,23]
Hematology			
PCV (%)	34 (16–51)	34 (20–47)	25 ± 2.6
RBC (10⁶/µL)	1.23 (0.63–1.58)	0.98 (0.42–1.42)	0.96 ± 0.14
Hgb (g/dL)	10.5 (6.2–13.2)	10.5 (9.8–11.5)	11.4 ± 1.6
MCV (fL)	284 (229–382)	335 (227–595)	261 ± 23
MCH (pg)	94 (89–99)	140 (104–177)	119 ± 12.5
MCHC (g/dL)	32 (26–38)	33 (30–40)	45.6 ± 3.4
WBC (10³/µL)	4.67 (0.10–10.9)	9.49 (2.9–18.8)	16.8 ± 2.5
Heterophils (10³/µL)	1.58 (0.03–4.55)	4.30 (0.16–8.44)	2.2 ± 0.45
Lymphocytes (10³/µL)	1.87 (0.06–4.88)	2.84 (0.3–7.98)	7.5 ± 0.58
Monocytes (10³/µL)	0.42 (0.01–2.32)	0.81 (0.06–3.38)	1 ± 0.41
Azurophils (10³/µL)	0.02 (0–0.69)	0.75 (0.01–3.72)	1.8 ± 0.56
Eosinophils (10³/µL)	—	—	4.1 ± 0.11
Basophils (10³/µL)	0.15 (0.07–0.28)	0.11 (0.06–0.14)	0.4 ± 0.01
Fibrinogen (mg/dL)	156 (100–300)	500 (200–700)	133 (0–200)
Chemistries			
ALP (U/L)	20 (4–101)	176 (14–405)	160 ± 85
ALT (U/L)	70 (7–374)	19 (1–93)	33 ± 24
Amylase (U/L)	—	1021 (265–1868)	—

TABLE 35.1　Hematologic and Serum Biochemical Values of Reptiles—cont'd

Measurement	Savannah Monitor (*Varanus exanthematicus*)[2,4]	Water Monitor (*Varanus salvator*)[2,4]	Tegu Lizard (*Tupinambus spp.*)[f,2,23]
AST (U/L)	26 (5–80)	24 (2–58)	18 ± 14
Bilirubin, total (mg/dL)	0.1 (0–0.3)	0.1 (0–0.3)	0.3 ± 0.2
BUN (mg/dL)	1 (0–5)	2 (1–5)	1 ± 1
Calcium (mg/dL)	13.6 (10.8–16.5)	14.0 (9.8–18.2)	12.2 ± 0.8
Chloride (mEq/L)	115 (93–133)	111 (97–124)	121 ± 7
Cholesterol (mg/dL)	116 (49–231)	78 (22–126)	206 ± 67
Creatine kinase (U/L)	1529 (7–6624)	772 (176–1818)	641 ± 568
Creatinine (mg/dL)	8.7 (0–67)	0.5 (0–1)	0.3 ± 0.1
GGT (U/L)	7 (1–11)	24 (7–48)	7
Glucose (mg/dL)	108 (54–163)	98 (29–170)	128 ± 30
Iron (μg/dL)	—	242 (111–429)	—
LDH (U/L)	427 (29–3699)	157 (34–1288)	540 ± 537
Magnesium (mEq/L)	3.1	2.5 (2.2–2.7)	
Osmolarity (mOsm/L)	332 (319–345)	—	—
Phosphorus (mg/dL)	4.2 (0.8–7.7)	5.2 (2.9–8.9)	5.6 ± 2.1
Potassium (mEq/L)	4.9 (3.0–6.9)	4.6 (3.5–6.1)	2.4 ± 1.4
Protein, total (g/dL)	6.6 (3.4–9.8)	7.0 (5.1–9.8)	6.6 ± 1.3
Albumin (g/dL)[b]	2.0 (0.6–3.3)	2.4 (1.4–3.4)	3.6 ± 0.7
Albumin (PEP; g/dL)[b]	3.2 (3.1–3.3)	3.1 (3–3.2)	—
Globulin (g/dL)[b]	4.6 (1.4–7.9)	4.7 (2.0–7.3)	2.9 ± 1.2
α-1 (PEP; g/dL)[b]	—	0.1	—
α-2 (PEP; g/dL)[b]	—	0.9 (0.8–1)	—
β (PEP; g/dL)[b]	—	0.9	—
γ (PEP; g/dL)[b]	—	4.7 (2.6–6.8)	—
Sodium (mEq/L)	156 (142–169)	156 (143–170)	159 ± 4
Triglyceride (mg/dL)	135 (17–476)	35 (6–78)	31
Uric acid (mg/dL)	6.5 (2.0–14.6)	4.7 (1–12.2)	3.2 ± 2

Measurement	Broad-Snouted Caimen (*Caiman latirostris*)[24]	Nile Crocodile (*Crocodylus niloticus*)[25]	Freshwater Crocodile (*Crocodylus johnsoni*)[26]
Hematology			
PCV (%)	26.0–31.2	18 (14–22)	23 (18–32)
RBC (10^6/μL)	6.1–8.5	0.59 (0.35–1.00)	—
Hgb (g/dL)	7.5–9.5	7.1 (4.7–9.5)	—
MCV (fL)	404 (335–479)	312 (200–465)	—
MCH (pg)	120 (97–153)	123 (84–221)	—
MCHC (g/dL)	30 (27–32)	40 (29–48)	—
WBC (10^3/μL)	12.0–21.0	11.3 (3.75–26.2)	8.0 (2.2–17.5)
Heterophils (10^3/μL)	6.27 (2.41–8.80)[g]	2.09 (0.45–3.66)	1.3 (0.1–6.8)
Lymphocytes (10^3/μL)	16.1 (12.8–20.9)[g]	7.20 (1.65–17.8)	5.1 (1.4–9.8)
Monocytes (10^3/μL)	1.28 (0.31–2.39)[g]	0.09 (0.0–0.79)	1.0 (0.0–2.7)
Azurophils (10^3/μL)	—	0.60 (0.0–3.93)	—
Eosinophils (10^3/μL)	0.90 (0.33–1.60)[g]	0.53 (0.0–2.14)	0.7 (0.0–1.6)
Basophils (10^3/μL)	1.09 (0.23–2.56)[g]	0.69 (0.0–2.90)	0.0 (0.0–0.6)
Chemistries			
ALP (U/L)	21–30	21 (3–72)	—
ALT (U/L)	55–84	44 (15–63)	—
Amylase (U/L)	—	—	—
AST (U/L)	94–138	67 (14–211)	37 (19–74)
BUN (mg/dL)	3-Feb	—	—
Calcium (mg/dL)	—	10.92 (9.36–12.6)	9.2 (4.0–11.6)
Ionized Ca++ (mmol/L)	—	1.35 (1.08–1.61)	—
Chloride (mEq/L)	—	120 (97–135)	—
Cholesterol (mg/dL)	—	212 (0–381)	—
Creatine kinase (U/L)	1975–6450	—	1086 (109–4448)

Continued

TABLE 35.1   Hematologic and Serum Biochemical Values of Reptiles—cont'd

Measurement	Broad-Snouted Caimen (*Caiman latirostris*)[24]	Nile Crocodile (*Crocodylus niloticus*)[25]	Freshwater Crocodile (*Crocodylus johnsoni*)[26]
Creatinine (mg/dL)	0.3–0.5	0.38 (0.19–0.63)	—
GGT (U/L)	—	—	—
Glucose (mg/dL)	110–140	68 (32–86)	65 (36–112)
LDH (U/L)	763–1434	—	—
Lipase (U/L)	—	—	—
Magnesium (mq/dL)	—	2.79 (1.58–4.18)	—
Phosphorus (mg/dL)	—	—	3.71 (1.55–5.88)
Potassium (mEq/L)	—	4.88 (3.30–7.65)	3.7 (2.3–5.3)
Protein, total (g/dL)	4.5–5.0	4.12 (2.89–5.71)	3.96 (1.50–7.0)
Albumin (g/dL)[b]	2.3–2.5	1.47 (1.11–1.94)	0.77 (0–1.5)
Globulin (g/dL)[b]	2.2–2.6	2.65 (1.65–4.26)	1.58 (0–5.5)
Sodium (mEq/L)	—	148 (122–164)	139 (111–154)
Triglyceride (mg/dL)	12–18.5	—	—
Uric acid (mg/dL)	2.5–4.8	2.02 (0.67–5.04)	1.2 (0.45–1.9)

Measurement	Radiated Tortoise (*Astrochelys radiata*)[4,27,28]	Red-Footed Tortoise (*Chelonoidis carbonaria*)[2,4]	Indian Star Tortoise (*Geochelone elegans*)[2,4]
Hematology			
PCV (%)	Oct-51	25 (6–38)	23 (14–38)
RBC (10[6]/μL)	0.3–1.1	0.46 (0.14–1.15)	0.37 (0.24–0.55)
Hgb (g/dL)	5.6 (4–8)	7.5 (7–7.9)	7.9 (6.9–8.5)
MCV (fL)	454 (319–571)	482 (22–940)	—
MCH (pg)	108 (82–133)	136 (123–149)	—
MCHC (g/dL)	28 (26–33)	31 (29–32)	27 (26–28)
WBC (10[3]/μL)	2.5–14	6.51 (1.15–20.0)	6.71 (1.35–27.9)
Heterophils (10[3]/μL)	0.7–8	1.67 (0.16–7.26)	2.56 (0.24–10.9)
Lymphocytes (10[3]/μL)	0.4–5.8	1.89 (0.12–9.10)	2.83 (0.20–15.4)
Monocytes (10[3]/μL)	0.02–0.5	0.16 (0.02–0.58)	0.20 (0.02–0.75)
Azurophils (10[3]/μL)	0–0.82	0.05 (0–0.87)	0.05 (0.01–0.87)
Eosinophils (10[3]/μL)	0.03–0.82	0.17 (0.02–0.80)	0.26 (0.03–1.51)
Basophils (10[3]/μL)	0.1–2.5	0.92 (0.03–3.48)	0.49 (0.09–1.79)
Fibrinogen (mg/dL)	117 (100–200)	—	—
Chemistries			
ALP (U/L)	72–392	60 (6–145)	72 (20–164)
ALT (U/L)	0–17	7 (0–18)	4 (0–14)
Amylase (U/L)	—	—	1235
AST (U/L)	25–348	130 (20–406)	54 (14–152)
Bile acids (μmol/L)	0.3–31.3	—	—
Bilirubin, total (mg/dL)	0–0.5	0.5 (0.1–1.1)	0.2 (0–0.5)
BUN (mg/dL)	Feb-34	14 (1–34)	3 (0–9)
Calcium (mg/dL)	8.6–18	12.2 (7.1–24.1)	11.7 (7.6–21.2)
Chloride (mEq/L)	91–112	99 (81–111)	100 (88–112)
Cholesterol (mg/dL)	56–154	121 (10–257)	115 (15–255)
Creatine kinase (U/L)	33–5666	695 (54–3593)	374 (22–2644)
Creatinine (mg/dL)	0.1–0.5	0.4 (0.2–1.3)	0.3 (0.2–0.5)
GGT (U/L)	5 (0–11)	28 (7–130)	4 (0–5)
Glucose (mg/dL)	21–93	67 (13–154)	76 (37–186)
Iron (μg/dL)	60	107	—
LDH (U/L)	213–6444	638 (118–1644)	438 (12–863)
Lipase (U/L)	May-50	—	5
Phosphorus (mg/dL)	2.5–7	3.5 (1.0–8.3)	3.6 (1.4–9.4)
Potassium (mEq/L)	3.1–5.8	5.5 (2.8–9.4)	4.8 (2.0–7.7)
Protein, total (g/dL)	3–6.6	4.7 (1.9–7.4)	4.7 (2.2–7.6)
Albumin (g/dL)[b]	0.6–2.4	1.6 (0–3.0)	1.7 (0.4–3.0)
Albumin (PEP; g/dL)[b]	0.9–2.4	—	—

TABLE 35.1   Hematologic and Serum Biochemical Values of Reptiles—cont'd

Measurement	Radiated Tortoise (*Astrochelys radiata*)[4,27,28]	Red-Footed Tortoise (*Chelonoidis carbonaria*)[2,4]	Indian Star Tortoise (*Geochelone elegans*)[2,4]
Globulin (g/dL)[b]	1.4–3.2	3.1 (0.2–4.8)	2.9 (1.3–4.6)
α-1 Glob (PEP; g/dL)[b]	0.1–0.5	—	—
α-2 Glob (PEP; g/dL)[b]	0.6–1.9	—	—
β Glob (PEP; g/dL)[b]	0.6–1.5	—	—
γ Glob (PEP; g/dL)[b]	0.4–0.9	—	—
Sodium (mEq/L)	121–146	130 (117–143)	127 (117–137)
Triglyceride (mg/dL)	26–303	246 (28–480)	60 (27–110)
Uric acid (mg/dL)	0.3 (0–0.6)	0.6 (0.1–2.1)	3.3 (0.2–7.9)

Measurement	Desert Tortoise (*Gopherus agassizii*)[29,30,31,32]	Gopher Tortoise (*Gopherus polyphemus*)[33]	Russian Tortoise (*Agrionemys horsfieldii*)[34,35]
Hematology			
PCV (%)	15–39	23 (15–30)	23 (22–34)
RBC (10⁶/μL)	0.28–1.34	0.54 (0.24–0.91)	—
Hgb (g/dL)	3.6–10.3	6.4 (4.2–8.6)	—
MCV (fL)	197–688	—	—
MCH (pg)	39–189	—	—
MCHC (g/dL)	19–35	—	—
WBC (10³/μL)	0.97–10.9	15.7 (10–22)	8.5 (5–12.5)
Heterophils (10³/μL)	0.49–7.3	4.7 (1–12.5)[g]	3.7 (1.3–4.6)
Lymphocytes (10³/μL)	0–3.8	8.9 (3.2–17.4)[g]	4.7 (3.6–7.6)
Monocytes (10³/μL)	0–0.57	1.1 (0.3–2.9)[g]	0.01 (0–0.02)
Azurophils (10³/μL)	0–0.9	—	0.05 (0.03–0.12)
Eosinophils (10³/μL)	0–0.95	—	0.05 (0.02–0.06)
Basophils (10³/μL)	0–4.3	0.94 (0.2–2.4)[g]	0.05 (0.02–0.08)
Chemistries			
ALP (U/L)	43–176	39 (11–71)	498 (181–1188)
ALT (U/L)	21 (0–66)	15 (2–57)	1 (0–2)
AST (U/L)	41–106	136 (57–392)	20 (12–32)
Bile acids (μmol/L)	0–5.4	—	—
Bilirubin, total (mg/dL)	0–0.9	0.02 (0–0.1)	0.015 (0–0.09)
BUN (mg/dL)	0–4	30 (1–130)	12 (4–17)
Calcium (total; mg/dL)	9.3–14.7	12 (10–14)	13.2 (9.9–19.5)
Ionized calcium (mmol/L)	—	—	1.28 (1–1.6)
Chloride (mEq/L)	94–112	102 (35–128)	—
Cholesterol (mg/dL)	56–233	76 (19–150)	109 (25–210)
Creatine kinase (U/L)	2262 (944–3880)	160 (32–628)	123 (6–344)
Creatinine (mg/dL)	0.11–0.37	0.3 (0.1–0.4)	—
GLDH (U/L)	—	—	1 (0.6–1.5)
Glucose (mg/dL)	92–165	75 (55–128)	59 (40–86)
LDH (U/L)	25–250	273 (18–909)	—
Magnesium (mEq/L)	2.1 (1.8–2.4)	4.1 (3.3–4.8)	—
Phosphorus (mg/dL)	1–6.3	2.1 (1–3.1)	2.6 (1.3–3.9)
Potassium (mEq/L)	3.5–4.7	5 (2.9–7)	5.3 (1.9–7.2)
Protein, total (g/dL)	3–4.6	3.1 (1.3–4.6)	3 (2.5–4.6)
Albumin (g/dL)[b]	1.2–2.2	1.5 (0.5–2.6)	1.6 (1.2–2.3)
Albumin (PEP; g/dL)[b]	—	—	—
Globulin (g/dL)[b]	1.2–2.6	—	1.4 (1.3–2.3)
α-1 Glob (PEP; g/dL)[b]	1	—	—
α-2 Glob (PEP; g/dL)[b]	1	—	—
β Glob (PEP; g/dL)[b]	0.6	—	—
γ Glob (PEP; g/dL)[b]	—	—	—
Sodium (mEq/L)	122–139	138 (127–148)	138 (131–149)
Triglyceride (mg/dL)	0–425	—	—
Uric acid (mg/dL)	2.7–7.2	3.5 (0.9–8.5)	1.2 (0.8–3.9)
Vitamin A (μg/mL)	0.2–0.6	—	—
Zinc (ppm)	0.4–3.7	—	—

Continued

TABLE 35.1 Hematologic and Serum Biochemical Values of Reptiles—cont'd

Measurement	African Spurred Tortoise (*Centrochelys sulcata*)[2,4,36]	Leopard Tortoise (*Stigmochelys pardalis*)[2,4]	Galapagos Tortoise (*Chelonoidis nigra*)[4]
Hematology			
PCV (%)	14–28	23 (8–37)	18 (7–29)
RBC (10^6/µL)	0.61 (0.08–1.15)	0.52 (0.15–1.06)	0.40 (0.16–0.63)
Hgb (g/dL)	7.7 (2.4–13.1)	16.1 (8.8–28)	5.5 (3.3–8.9)
MCV (fL)	418 (156–678)	488 (179–833)	535 (266–769)
MCH (pg)	116 (2.1–193)	83	160 (100–239)
MCHC (g/dL)	30 (20–40)	44 (42–46)	31 (24–38)
WBC (10^3/µL)	4.41 (0.87–13.23)	4.24 (0.6–10.0)	4.57 (0.71–17.5)
Heterophils (10^3/µL)	1.92 (0.23–7.43)	1.92 (0.11–4.87)	1.57 (0.10–6.76)
Lymphocytes (10^3/µL)	1.41 (0.17–6.06)	1.61 (0.05–4.74)	1.45 (0.04–6.56)
Monocytes (10^3/µL)	0.01 (0.01–0.37)	0.08 (0.02–0.62)	0.08 (0.02–0.33)
Azurophils (10^3/µL)	0.04 (0–0.84)	0.02 (0–0.51)	0.03 (0–0.52)
Eosinophils (10^3/µL)	0.10 (0.01–0.43)	0.15 (0.02–0.37)	0.09 (0.02–0.40)
Basophils (10^3/µL)	0.12 (0.01–0.36)	0.11 (0.01–0.34)	0.34 (0.03–1.38)
Chemistries			
ALP (U/L)	36 (10–70)	107 (21–278)	77 (27–235)
ALT (U/L)	9 (0–33)	8	3 (0–18)
Amylase (U/L)	1359 (399–2240)	—	22 (3–41)
AST (U/L)	34–151	54 (5–119)	40 (16–122)
Bile acids	<35	—	—
Bilirubin, total (mg/dL)	0.1 (0–0.7)	0.1	0.3 (0–0.8)
BUN (mg/dL)	3 (1–6)	12 (1–36)	12 (3–35)
Calcium (mg/dL)	9.6–14.7	11.8 (6.5–18.3)	10.4 (6.6–17.8)
Chloride (mEq/L)	109 (93–124)	104 (90–119)	98 (83–112)
Cholesterol (mg/dL)	129 (36–283)	111 (9–239)	172 (42–450)
Creatine kinase (U/L)	191–3727	359 (223–704)	592 (35–2378)
Creatinine (mg/dL)	0.3 (0.1–0.4)	0.6	0.2 (0–0.4)
GGT (U/L)	14 (3–19)	—	4 (0–11)
Glucose (mg/dL)	63–155	75 (10–152)	98 (35–312)
Iron (µg/dL)	81 (80–82)	—	73 (8–593)
LDH (U/L)	977 (140–3264)	446 (346–546)	469 (71–1212)
Phosphorus (mg/dL)	3.8 (1.5–6.5)	2.7 (1.1–5.2)	3.7 (2.0–8.0)
Potassium (mEq/L)	5.8–9.7	5.4 (2.3–8.8)	4.8 (3.4–7.2)
Protein, total (g/dL)	3.8 (1.2–6.3)	3.3 (1.9–6.2)	4.7 (1.8–7.9)
Albumin (g/dL)[b]	0.3–2.7	1.6 (0.3–2.9)	1.6 (0.4–2.7)
Globulin (g/dL)[b]	2.3 (0.4–3.8)	2.6 (0.6–4.6)	3.1 (1.1–5.5)
Sodium (mEq/L)	125–139	132 (115–148)	130 (119–140)
α-tocopherol (µg/dL)	—	—	2 (1–2)
Triglyceride (mg/dL)	163 (53–388)	—	271 (29–1345)
Free T_3	—	—	29
Uric acid (mg/dL)	1.5–5.1	2.5 (0.5–6.6)	1.7 (0.1–4.0)

Measurement	Hermann's Tortoise (*Testudo hermanni*)[37]	Yellow-Marginated Box Turtle (*Cuora flavomarginata*)[38]	Golden Coin Turtle (*Cuora trifasciata*)[39]
Hematology			
PCV (%)	23 (11–40)	(23–44)[i,j]	20–40
RBC (10^6/µL)	—	(0.38–1.47)[i,j]	—
Hgb (g/dL)	8.4 (4.1–13.5)	(3.9–10.5)[i,j]	—
MCV (fL)	—	(204–620)[i]	—
MCH (pg)	—	(53–160)	—
MCHC (g/dL)	—	(17–31)[i,j]	—
WBC (10^3/µL)	—	(0.60–10.4)	—
Heterophils (10^3/µL)	—	(0.58–7.17)	—
Lymphocytes (10^3/µL)	—	(0–3.11)	—
Monocytes (10^3/µL)	0	(0–0.76)[i,j]	—

TABLE 35.1 Hematologic and Serum Biochemical Values of Reptiles—cont'd

Measurement	Hermann's Tortoise (*Testudo hermanni*)[37]	Yellow-Marginated Box Turtle (*Cuora flavomarginata*)[38]	Golden Coin Turtle (*Cuora trifasciata*)[39]
Azurophils (10^3/μL)	—		—
Eosinophils (10^3/μL)	—	(0–0.43)[i]	—
Basophils (10^3/μL)	—	(0–1.82)	—
Chemistries			
ALP (U/L)	122–606	(15–98)[i,j]	—
ALT (U/L)	1–12.5	(0–2)	—
Amylase (U/L)	—	—	234–706[i]
AST (U/L)	0–359	(46–299)[i,j]	42–198
Bile acids	—	—	<35
Bilirubin, total (mg/dL)	—	—	
BUN (mg/dL)	0–11.1	(2–48)[i,j]	—
Calcium (mg/dL)	4.8–20.5	(8.9–29.9)[i]	8.9–24.9
Chloride (mEq/L)	92–111	—	74–375[i]
Cholesterol (mg/dL)	—	(48–420)[i]	46–517
Creatine kinase (U/L)	0–732	(61–2156)[i,j]	—
Creatinine (mg/dL)	0.03–0.27	(0.1–0.4)[i]	4.9–24.7[i]
GGT (U/L)	—	—	43–95
Glucose (mg/dL)	15–120	(28–182)[i,j]	1355–9296[i]
LDH (U/L)	0–800	—	2.7–6.8[i]
Phosphorus (mg/dL)	0.6–5.5	(1.8–12.3)[i,j]	2.8–7.0
Potassium (mEq/L)	3.5–7.7	—	3.0–7.1
Protein, total (g/dL)	2.4–6.1	(3.9–9.1)[i]	1.1–2.9
Albumin (g/dL)[b]	0.8–2.6	(1.3–3.2)[i]	—
Albumin (PEP; g/dL)[b]	1.36 (0.69–1.94)	—	0–4.8
Globulin (g/dL)[b]	—	—	—
α-1 Glob (PEP; g/dL)[b]	1.29 (0.7–1.62)	—	—
β Glob (PEP; g/dL)[b]	0.91 (0.38–1.53)	—	—
γ Glob (PEP; g/dL)[b]	0.26 (0.04–0.55)	—	111–139
Sodium (mEq/L)	116–143	—	31–1195[i]
Triglycerides (mg/dL)	—	(30–1708)[i,j]	0.4–3.8[i]
Uric acid (mg/dL)	0–5.2	(0.4–3.1)[i,j]	

Measurement	Eastern Box Turtle (*Terrapene carolina*)[4,40,41,42]	Ornate Box Turtle (*Terrapene ornata*)[2,4,43]	Wood Turtle (*Glyptemys insculpta*)[4]
Hematology			
PCV (%)	24 (8–37)	23 (10–37)	25 (9–41)
RBC (10^6/μL)	0.56 (0.08–1.03)	0.62 (0.46–0.8)	—
Hgb (g/dL)	6.8 (2.6–11.0)	7.2 (6–9)	—
MCV (fL)	396 (117–750)	408 (350–463)	—
MCH (pg)	110 (30–207)	122 (108–136)	—
MCHC (g/dL)	29 (14–43)	33 (31–33)	—
WBC (10^3/μL)	5.48 (1.34–15.9)	5.76 (1.2–13.4)	5.20 (0.8–20.0)
Heterophils (10^3/μL)	1.61 (0.15–6.4)	2.01 (0.10–5.9)	—
Lymphocytes (10^3/μL)	1.61 (0.15–9.82)	2.19 (0.10–7.60)	3.15 (0.59–13.0)
Monocytes (10^3/μL)	0.19 (0.18–0.80)	0.13 (0.02–0.74)	—
Azurophils (10^3/μL)	0.03 (0–0.80)	0.03 (0–0.13)	0.08 (0–1.11)
Eosinophils (10^3/μL)	0.47 (0.42–3.01)	0.23 (0.03–1.32)	—
Basophils (10^3/μL)	0.55 (0.4–2.14)	0.25 (0.02–0.92)	—
Fibrinogen (mg/dL)	277 (195–360)		
Chemistries			
ALP (U/L)	77 (20–225)	61 (14–139)	71 (21–268)
ALT (U/L)	6 (0–20)	30 (25–33)	—
Amylase (U/L)	1033 (87–2526)	691 (2–1893)	—
AST (U/L)	64 (14–191)	61 (11–141)	79 (14–212)

Continued

TABLE 35.1   Hematologic and Serum Biochemical Values of Reptiles—cont'd

Measurement	Eastern Box Turtle (*Terrapene carolina*)[4,40,41,42]	Ornate Box Turtle (*Terrapene ornata*)[2,4,43]	Wood Turtle (*Glyptemys insculpta*)[4]
Bilirubin, total (mg/dL)	0.1 (0.1–0.4)	0.3 (0.1–0.4)	—
BUN (mg/dL)	52 (6–121)	60 (4–154)	—
Calcium (mg/dL)	10.5 (6.8–23.2)[d]	78 (14–140 +)	11.8 (6.3–29.4)
Ionized Ca (mmol/L)	—	1.3 (0.8–1.8)	—
Chloride (mEq/L)	106 (89–121)	103 (89–114)	—
Cholesterol (mg/dL)	205 (42–483)	201 (20–469)	—
Creatine kinase (U/L)	153 (23–747)	196 (0–777)	—
Creatinine (mg/dL)	0.2 (0–0.5)	1 (0.2–2.4)	—
Glucose (mg/dL)	48 (23–114)	65 (22–154)	53 (13–108)
LDH (U/L)	307 (20–1032)	362 (300–424)	—
Phosphorus (mg/dL)	3.5 (1.7–7.5)	3.3 (1.9–5.8)	3.2 (1.6–10)
Potassium (mEq/L)	4.7 (3.1–9.4)	4.7 (2.4–8.2)	—
Protein, total (g/dL)	3.20 (3.10–3.90)	3.6 (2.0–5.7)	4.7 (1.5–6.5)
Protein, total (male; g/dL)	3.00 (1.80–5.20)	—	—
Protein, total (female; g/dL)	4.00 (2.20–6.20)	—	—
Haptoglobin	0.25 (0.27–0.38)	—	—
Albumin (g/dL)[b]	2.2 (1.2–3.2)	1.5 (0.2–2.8)	—
Prealb (PEP; g/dL)[b]	0 (0–0.002)	—	—
Albumin (PEP; g/dL)[b]	0.71–0.85	—	—
Globulin (g/dL)[b]	3.4 (2.5–4.7)	2.4 (0.6–4.3)	—
α-1 Glob (PEP; g/dL)[b]	0.25–0.30	—	—
α-2 Glob (PEP; g/dL)[b]	0.76–0.92	—	—
β Glob (PEP; g/dL)[b]	1.27–1.55	—	—
γ Glob (PEP; g/dL)[b]	0.27–0.32	—	—
A:G ratio	0.27–0.31	—	—
Sodium (mEq/L)	139 (120–155)	134 (125–143)	—
Uric acid (mg/dL)	0.7 (0.1–2.9)	0.6 (0–1.9)	1.0 (0–4.1)

Measurement	Pacific Pond Turtle (*Actinemys marmorata*)[4]	Sliders (*Trachemys scripta* ssp.)[2,4,44]	Painted Turtle (*Chrysemys picta*)[2,4]
Hematology			
PCV (%)	24 (7–42)	26 (8–44)	25 (6–43)
RBC (10[6]/μL)	0.69 (0.24–1.20)	0.84 (0.33–2.21)	0.57 (0.41–0.68)
Hgb (g/dL)	7.6 (3.0–12.6)	11.1 (10–12.2)	11.2 (10.7–11.7)
MCV (fL)	377 (200–634)	409 (179–697)	271 (183–365)
MCH (pg)	107 (19–186)	108	—
MCHC (g/dL)	27 (18–42)	30	—
WBC (10[3]/μL)	5.94 (1.02–17.0)	6.73 (1.0–19.4)	9.49 (0.40–23.2)
Heterophils (10[3]/μL)	1.83 (0.14–5.52)	2.33 (0.18–5.86)	2.30 (0.17–8.39)
Lymphocytes (10[3]/μL)	2.46 (0.22–8.48)	2.28 (0.03–6.90)	2.60 (0.01–7.07)
Monocytes (10[3]/μL)	—	0.18 (0.04–0.65)	—
Azurophils (10[3]/μL)	0.04 (0–0.43)	0.05 (0–0.48)	0.05 (0–0.26)
Eosinophils (10[3]/μL)	0.37 (0.02–1.81)	0.52 (0.01–3.06)	—
Basophils (10[3]/μL)	0.62 (0.05–2.09)	1.07 (0.01–3.56)	1.95 (0.04–5.91)
Chemistries			
ALP (U/L)	—	113 (30–372)	208
ALT (U/L)	—	14 (1–66)	—
Amylase (U/L)	—	493 (411–535)	—
AST (U/L)	105 (26–228)	141 (44–358)	132 (45–284)
Bilirubin, total (mg/dL)	—	0.2 (0.1–0.5)	0.1
BUN (mg/dL)	—	23 (2–64)	37
Calcium (mg/dL)	10.0 (7.0–14.5)	12.6 (6.5–22.6)	11.7 (5.5–19.1)
Chloride (mEq/L)	—	98 (88–112)	96 (73–109)
Cholesterol (mg/dL)	—	162 (106–227)	—
Creatine kinase (U/L)	242 (63–747)	516 (108–2125)	352 (35–1608)
Creatinine (mg/dL)	—	0.3 (0.2–0.5)	—

TABLE 35.1 Hematologic and Serum Biochemical Values of Reptiles—cont'd

Measurement	Pacific Pond Turtle (*Actinemys marmorata*)[4]	Sliders (*Trachemys scripta* ssp.)[2,4,44]	Painted Turtle (*Chrysemys picta*)[2,4]
GGT (U/L)	—	7 (0–21)	—
Glucose (mg/dL)	53 (4–113)	54 (21–143)	63 (10–133)
Iron (µg/dL)	—	—	—
LDH (U/L)	—	1713 (371–5763)	412
Lipase (U/L)	—	6 (1–15)	—
Magnesium (mEq/L)	—	2.2	4.8
Phosphorus (mg/dL)	3.6 (1.9–6.6)	4.0 (1.8–8.8)	3.6 (1.7–7.2)
Potassium (mEq/L)	4.3 (2.3–7.1)	3.8 (2.4–7.5)	3.6 (2.2–11.6)
Protein, total (g/dL)	4.4 (1.8–7.0)	4.8 (1.1–8.8)	4.4 (1.8–7.7)
Albumin (g/dL)[b]	1.7 (0.7–2.7)	1.8 (0.6–3.3)	1.3 (0–2.7)
Globulin (g/dL)[b]	2.8 (1.0–4.6)	3.2 (1.1–5.9)	3.0 (0.1–5.9)
Sodium (mEq/L)	135 (123–147)	134 (123–147)	137 (119–146)
Triglyceride (mg/dL)	—	304 (30–664)	—
Uric acid (mg/dL)	0.9 (0–3.1)	0.8 (0.1–1.9)	0.7 (0.1–1.8)

Measurement	Loggerhead Sea Turtle (*Caretta caretta*)[4,45]	Green Sea Turtle (*Chelonia mydas*)[4,46,47]	Hawksbill Sea Turtle (*Eretmochelys imbricata*)[h,4,48,49]
Hematology			
PCV (%)	32 (18–40)	33 (23–45)	13–41
RBC (10⁶/µL)	0.52 (0.22–1.22)	0.52 (0.21–0.97)	—
Hgb (g/dL)	10.7	10.7	—
MCV (fL)	416 (82–1027)	717 (320–1429)	—
MCH (pg)	55	55	—
MCHC (g/dL)	36	36	—
WBC (10³/µL)	9.00 (5.00–12.50)	9.98 (3.76–21.7)	—
Heterophils (10³/µL)	3.67 (0.35–7.16)	6.69 (1.57–15.7)	—
Lymphocytes (10³/µL)	2.72 (0.30–4.83)	2.14 (0.94–4.34)	—
Monocytes (10³/µL)	0.96 (0.22–1.84)	0.91 (0.23–1.81)	—
Azurophils (10³/µL)	—	—	—
Eosinophils (10³/µL)	1.15 (0.45–2.10)	0.12 (0–0.48)	—
Basophils (10³/µL)	—	0.13 (0–1.94)	—
Chemistries			
ALP (U/L)	64 (11–254)	Jun-67	Jul-80
ALT (U/L)	—	32 (3–241)	23-Jan
Amylase (U/L)	—	534	1614 (1266–1782)
AST (U/L)	154 (10–480)	74–245	74–245
Bilirubin, total (mg/dL)	—	0.03–0.2	0–10
BUN (mg/dL)	105 (19–162)	64 (13.9–173)	Jul-34
Calcium (mg/dL)	6.9 (2.2–11.5)	8–8.8	2.6–11.6
Ionized Ca (mmol/L)	—	—	1.09 (0.94–1.32)
Chloride (mEq/L)	118 (103–137)	101–121	106–134
Cholesterol (mg/dL)	—	221 (142–354)	—
Creatine kinase (U/L)	899 (258–3586)	326–2729	14–6008
Creatinine (mg/dL)	—	0.25 (0.1–1.6)	0.29 (0.12–0.68)
GGT (U/L)	—	6 (0–21)	—
Glucose (mg/dL)	120 (66–177)	67–178	79–162
Iron (µg/dL)	—	362 (117–600)	Jun-67
LDH (U/L)	—	75–477	—
Lipase (U/L)	—	—	—
Magnesium (mEq/L)	—	4.8–12.2	3.4–7.1
Phosphorus (mg/dL)	9.3 (3.7–14.0)	4.9–11.1	1.9–8.7
Potassium (mEq/L)	3.9 (2.7–5.1)	3–7.1	3.0–5.3
Protein, total (g/dL)	3.3 (1.2–6.9)	2.1–6.2	1.3–5.1
Albumin (g/dL)[b]	1.5 (0.7–2.6)	0.7–1.8	0.3–1.4
Globulin (g/dL)[b]	2.2 (0.2–4.9)	1.5–4.7	0.8–4.8

Continued

TABLE 35.1 Hematologic and Serum Biochemical Values of Reptiles—cont'd

Measurement	Loggerhead Sea Turtle (*Caretta caretta*)[4,45]	Green Sea Turtle (*Chelonia mydas*)[4,46,47]	Hawksbill Sea Turtle (*Eretmochelys imbricata*)[h,4,48,49]
Sodium (mEq/L)	153 (142–164)	139–158	146–159
Triglyceride (mg/dL)	—	492 (124–932)	—
Uric acid (mg/dL)	0.5 (0–1.2)	1.1 (0–2.7)	0.6 (0–1.8)

[a]Listed values are median followed by either min-max or a confidence interval in parentheses depending on reported methods and the authors' judgment from the available evidence, unless there is a single value indicating n = 1, a range enclosed in parentheses indicating min-max, or a range that is not enclosed in parentheses indicating a reported reference interval.

[b]Albumin is measured by colorimetry (e.g., bromocresol green), and globulin value is calculated unless otherwise indicated "PEP" (protein electrophoresis).

[c]Remarkably high reference ranges for Ca (mean, 159 mg/dL; range, 30–337 mg/dL) and P (mean, 35 mg/dL; range, 8–69) have also been reported.[50]

[d]Can be elevated in gravid females.[19]

[e]These data were obtained from iguanas housed outdoors with unfiltered sunlight.

[f]Adults.

[g]Calculated from data.

[h]Juveniles.

[i]Varies between sexes.

[j]Varies between summer and winter.

TABLE 35.2 Hematologic and Serum Biochemical Values of Amphibians[a,b]

Measurement	African Clawed Frog (*Xenopus laevis*)[51,52*]	American Bullfrog (*Lithobates catesbeiana*)[52,53*]	Leopard Frog (*Lithobates pipiens*)[52] ♂	Leopard Frog (*Lithobates pipiens*)[52] ♀	Edible Frog (*Rana esculenta*)[52]	Grass Frog (*Rana temporaria*)[52]
BW (g)	—	—	25–42	25–46	—	—
Blood volume (mL/100 g BW)	—	3.1–3.6	—	—	—	—
Hematology[a]						
PCV (%)	23.3–47.0	19.3–40.9	19–52	16–51	—	—
RBC (10⁶/µL)	0.80–1.48	0–1.82	0.23–0.77	0.17–0.70	0.31	0.46
Hgb (g/dL)	6.06–15.19	3.84–9.76	3.8–14.6	2.7–14	9.7	14.34
MCV (fL)	31.6–62.8	—	722–916	730–916	—	—
MCH (pg)	6.9–22.1	—	182–221	182–238	—	—
MCHC (g/dL)	19.3–32.3	—	22.7–26.8	19.9–27.7	—	—
WBC[b] (10³/µL)	0.64–9.56	11.3–29.7	3.1–22.2	2.8–25.9	6.1	14.4
Early stages[b] (%)	—	—	—	—	1	1.5
Neutrophils[b] (%)	8 ± 1.1	36.1–85.7	—	—	8.8 ± 2.1	6.5 ± 1
Lymphocytes[b] (%)	65.3 ± 2.7	17–36.6	—	—	52 ± 3.3	68.5 ± 2.9
Monocytes[b] (%)	0.5	0.7–5.1	—	—	1.3	0.8
Eosinophils[b] (%)	—	2.6–9	—	—	19.4 ± 1.3	14.5 ± 2.9
Basophils[b] (%)	8.5 ± 1.4	1.1–5.9	—	—	16.6 ± 1.3	24.2 ± 2.2
Plasmocytes[b] (%)	0.2	—	—	—	1	0.4
Thrombocytes (10³/µL)	17.1	—	—	—	16.3	20.8
Chemistries						
ALP (U/L)	59–282	155.1–158.9	—	—	—	—
ALT (U/L)	10–39	10.52–14.28	—	—	—	—
AST (U/L)	27–1774	—	—	—	—	—
Bilirubin, total (mg/dL)	0.01–0.26	—	—	—	—	—
BUN (mg/dL)	2–10	—	—	—	—	—
Calcium (mg/dL)	5.2–12.3	6.89–9.73	—	—	—	—
Chloride (mEq/L)	72.7–92.7	96–121.2	—	—	—	—
Cholesterol (mg/dL)	56–563	34.0–89.6	—	—	—	—
Creatine kinase (U/L)	10–5400	262–602	—	—	—	—
Creatinine (mg/dL)	0.1–1.1	0.24–0.73	—	—	—	—
GGT (U/L)	1–19	—	—	—	—	—
Glucose (mg/dL)	18–111	25.8–74.0	—	—	—	—
LDH (U/L)	21–240	73–161	—	—	—	—

TABLE 35.2 Hematologic and Serum Biochemical Values of Amphibians—cont'd

Measurement	African Clawed Frog (*Xenopus laevis*)[51,52]*	American Bullfrog (*Lithobates catesbeiana*)[52,53]*	Leopard Frog (*Lithobates pipiens*)[52] ♂	♀	Edible Frog (*Rana esculenta*)[52]	Grass Frog (*Rana temporaria*)[52]
Phosphorus (mg/dL)	3.5–11.6	5.23–12.41	—	—	—	—
Potassium (mEq/L)	2.3–7.3	2.5–2.9	—	—	—	—
Protein, total (g/dL)	2.0–4.6	3.02–5.66	—	—	—	—
Albumin (g/dL)	0.1–2.3	0.92–2.24	—	—	—	—
Globulin (g/dL)	1.1–4.1	—	—	—	—	—
Sodium (mEq/L)	111–134	108.7–111.4	—	—	—	—
Triglyceride (mg/dL)	57–555	23–67.9	—	—	—	—
Uric acid (mg/dL)	0.1–0.4	0–7.1	—	—	—	—

Measurement	Wood Frog (*Rana sylvatica*)[53,*]	Australian Common Green Frog (*Litoria caerulea*)[54,*]	Australian White-Lipped Tree Frog (*Litoria infrafrenata*)[54,*]	Cuban Tree Frog (*Osteopilus septentrionalis*)[52,55,*,**]	Himalayan Tree Frog (*Polypedates maculatus*)[56,**] ♂	♀
BW (g)	—	—	—	28–35	—	—
Blood volume (mL/100 g BW)	—	—	—	7.2–7.8	—	—
Hematology[a]						
PCV (%)	18.6–40.5	34–40.8	26.0–34.0	20–24	28.6 ± 7.8	23.8 ± 6.5
RBC (10⁶/μL)	0.25–0.57	0.62–0.82	0.63–0.82	—	0.48	0.57
Hgb (g/dL)	—	8.0–10.6	6.1–8.2	5.6–6.8	—	—
MCV (fL)	—	461–602	374–486	—	582 ± 10.7	419.56 ± 40.1
MCH (pg)	—	111–148	84–115	—	137.5 ± 11.4	135.8 ± 13.9
MCHC (g/dL)	—	236–268	210–250	25–31	—	—
WBC[b] (10³/μL)	2.2–13.1	12.4–22.1	14.2–29.1	—	14.6 ± 1.3	16.6 ± 2.1
Early stages[b] (%)	—	—	—	—	—	—
Neutrophils[b] (%)	0.4–13.3	14–27	15.0–32.0	—	27.4 ± 1.7	22.0 ± 1.6
Lymphocytes[b] (%)	63.7–90.0	—	57.0–78.3	—	49.7 ± 6.1	50.3 ± 4.4
Monocytes[b] (%)	0–3.4	5.0–10.0	4.0–8.0	—	7.6 ± 1.4	7.4 ± 1.3
Eosinophils[b] (%)	0–4.5	1.0–5.0	0–1.3	—	12.6 ± 21.3	12.7 ± 2.0
Basophils[b] (%)	5.9–14.8	0	0–1.0	—	2.7 ± 0.6	3.7 ± 0.8
Plasmocytes[b] (%)	—	—	—	—	—	—
Thrombocytes (10³/μL)	1.3–5.2	23.2–33.5	25.8–38.8	—	—	—
Chemistries						
ALP (U/L)	—	—	—	18.5 ± 16.1	—	—
ALT (U/L)	—	—	—	132 ± 14.9	—	—
AST (U/L)	—	66–122	41–119	494.2 ± 59.9	—	—
Bilirubin, total (mg/dL)	—	—	—	—	—	—
BUN (mg/dL)	—	—	—	—	—	—
Calcium (mg/dL)	—	10.6–13.1	8.6–11.3	—	—	—
Chloride (mEq/L)	—	—	—	—	—	—
Cholesterol (mg/dL)	—	—	—	—	—	—
Creatine kinase (U/L)	—	347–705	233–722	1292 ± 959.3	—	—
Creatinine (mg/dL)	—	—	—	—	—	—
GGT (U/L)	—	—	—	1.5±0–18.7	—	—
Glucose (mg/dL)	—	55–78	45–81	—	—	—
LDH (U/L)	—	—	—	2907.7 ± 610.9[c]	—	—
Phosphorus (mg/dL)	—	3.3–5.0	3.2–4.9	—	—	—
Potassium (mEq/L)	—	4.9–7.7	3.2–4.7	—	—	—
Protein, total (g/dL)	—	5.5–6.8	3.0–4.1	—	—	—
Albumin (g/dL)	—	—	—	—	—	—
Globulin (g/dL)	—	—	—	—	—	—
Sodium (mEq/L)	—	107–114	104–108	—	—	—
Triglyceride (mg/dL)	—	—	—	—	—	—
Uric acid (mg/dL)	—	0.2–0.7	0.1–0.2	—	—	—

Continued

TABLE 35.2   Hematologic and Serum Biochemical Values of Amphibians—cont'd

Measurement	Dubois's Tree Frog (*Polypedates teraiensis*)[57,**] ♂	♀	Eastern Hellbender (*Cryptobranchus alleganiensis*)[58,**] ♂	♀	Ozark Hellbender (*Cryptobranchus alleganiensis*)[58,**] ♂	♀	Mexican Axolotl (*Ambystoma mexicanum*)[59,*]	Tiger Salamander (*Ambystoma tigrinum*)[52]
BW (g)	—	—	372 ± 58	511 ± 140	605 ± 196	440 ± 90	42.1–77.1	35
Blood volume (mL/100 g BW)	—	—	—	—	—	—	—	—
Hematology[a]								
PCV (%)	50.62 ± 1.1	51.6 ± 0.95	38 ± 5	33 ± 7	45 ± 6	42 ± 15	28–32.7	40
RBC (10⁶/μL)	0.59 ± 0.01	0.62 ± 0.01	—	—	—	—	—	1.66
Hgb (g/dL)	—	—	—	—	—	—	—	9.4
MCV (fL)	851.3 ±27.1	822.4 ±13.3	—	—	—	—	—	—
MCH (pg)	100.1 ± 3.7	96.7 ± 6.9	—	—	—	—	—	—
MCHC (g/dL)	—	—	—	—	—	—	—	—
WBC[b] (10³/μL)	12.1 ± 0.3	12.2 ± 0.7	—	—	—	—	—	4.6
Early stages[b] (%)	—	—	—	—	—	—	—	—
Neutrophils[b] (%)	23.5 ± 1.3	26.7 ± 1.2	32 ± 17	34 ± 9	54 ± 21	33 ± 14	—	—
Lymphocytes[b] (%)	55.5 ± 2.0	54.9 ± 0.5	51 ± 18	48 ± 13	28 ± 21	47 ± 22	—	—
Monocytes[b] (%)	6.4 ± 0.5	5.7 ± 0.5	0.7 ± 1.1	0.8 ± 0.8	0.4 ± 0.7	0.7 ± 0.8	—	—
Eosinophils[b] (%)	11.0 ± 1.1	10.0 ± 0.2	11 ± 6	12 ± 7	13 ± 10	15 ± 14	—	—
Basophils[b] (%)	3.5 ± 0.2	2.8 ± 1.1	4.4 ± 3.9	5.8 ± 5.4	4.2 ± 4.2	4.1 ± 3.2	—	—
Plasmocytes[b] (%)	—	—	—	—	—	—	—	—
Thrombocytes (10³/μL)	—	—	—	—	—	—	—	—
Chemistries								
ALP (U/L)	—	—	—	—	—	—	452.1–561.3	—
ALT (U/L)	—	—	—	—	—	—	14.9–20.6	—
AST (U/L)	—	—	136 ± 73	113 ± 59	205 ± 152	95 ± 41	201.3–263.8	—
Bilirubin, total (mg/dL)	—	—	—	—	—	—	—	—
BUN (mg/dL)	—	—	2.4 ± 0.6	2.5 ± 0.7	4.1 ± 3.7	4.1 ± 3.8	9.9–14.5	—
Calcium (mg/dL)	—	—	8.4 ± 1.1	13 ± 2	8.7 ± 2.2	11 ± 2	7.3–8.2	—
Chloride (mEq/L)	—	—	80 ± 9	76 ± 2	77 ±17	76 ± 3	78.1–80.3	—
Cholesterol (mg/dL)	—	—	—	—	—	—	—	—
Creatine kinase (U/L)	—	—	—	—	—	—	—	—
Creatinine (mg/dL)	—	—	—	—	—	—	0.25–0.37	—
GGT (U/L)	—	—	—	—	—	—	—	—
Glucose (mg/dL)	—	—	22 ± 14	18 ± 8	25 ± 14	23 ± 12	26.9–32.1	—
LDH (U/L)	—	—	—	—	—	—	—	—
Phosphorus (mg/dL)	—	—	8.4 ± 2.9	7 ± 2	14.5 ± 16.5	11 ± 2	3.4–3.9	—
Potassium (mEq/L)	—	—	4.0 ± 1.3	3.2 ± 1.3	11.4 ± 15.7	4.0 ± 1.2	2.0–4.6	—
Protein, total (g/dL)	—	—	3.4 ± 0.8	3.8 ± 0.6	4.6 ± 3.0	2.8 ± 0.6	1.2–2.8	—
Albumin (g/dL)	—	—	1.0 ± 0.4	1.4 ± 0.2	1.9 ± 1.7	1.0 ± 0.5	0.44–0.51	—
Globulin (g/dL)	—	—	2.3 ± 0.6	2.5 ± 0.4	2.7 ± 1.9	1.8 ± 0.4	1.34–1.55	—
Sodium (mEq/L)	—	—	113 ± 15	107 ± 4	101 ± 28	105 ± 8	102–119	—
Triglyceride (mg/dL)	—	—	—	—	—	—	—	—
Uric acid (mg/dL)	—	—	0.7 ± 0.3	1.0 ± 0.6	4.1 ± 7.9	0.5 ± .04	—	—

*Reference interval = 95% CI
**Mean ± SD
[a]Hematology is presently of limited diagnostic value because of the lack of normal data and the wide variation in hematologic and biochemical values according to sex, season, and state of hydration.
[b]For leukocyte totals and percentages for various species, refer to the wildlife leukocytes website at wildlifehematology.uga.edu.
[c]Median ± 25% to 75%
BW, Body weight; *Hb*, hemoglobin; *MCH*, mean corpuscular hemoglobin; *MCV*, mean cell volume; *PCV*, packed cell volume; *RBC*, red blood cell; *WBC*, white blood cell

REFERENCES

See www.expertconsult.com for a complete list of references.

36

Molecular Infectious Disease Diagnostics

James F.X. Wellehan and Stephen J. Divers

Molecular techniques have resulted in rapid advances in both our understanding of the diversity of infectious agents in reptiles and amphibians and our ability to specifically and sensitively diagnose these agents. This has brought a more nuanced understanding of the complex interactions between host, pathogen, coinfections, and environment in causing disease. Conversely, these techniques may not be well understood by the practitioner, leading to misinterpretation of results and bad clinical decisions. It is important for clinicians to understand the basics of molecular diagnostic testing and the potential problems, common errors, and clinical implications of results.

SEROLOGY OR CULTURE COMPARED WITH MOLECULAR TECHNIQUES

When testing for infectious agents, it is first important to determine what information is being sought. Are you looking for a pathogen, such as a virus or bacterium, or are you looking for a reaction to a pathogen, such as an antibody response? The molecular testing emphasized in this chapter tests directly for the presence of a pathogen. Immunologic testing gives evidence that an animal has had an immune response to a pathogen, but does not give information whether the pathogen is currently present. Looking at changes in immune response over time is typically needed to determine the current relevance of an immune response; this requires assaying immune response at more than one time point (e.g., paired rising titers).

For immunologic testing, it is also important to consider whether the patient has had time to develop an immune response to a pathogen. This may take several weeks in reptiles.[1] In acute infections, a specific immune response may not be present. There are large seasonal and temperature effects on the immune response of reptiles, as well as species differences.[2-4] Other factors, including reproductive status and exogenous corticosteroid administration, may also affect development of a measurable immune response.[5,6]

When testing immune response, it is also important to consider what aspect of the acquired immune system is being measured. There are two branches of the acquired immune system, cellular immunity and humoral immunity. A humoral immune response primarily produces antibodies to fight specific pathogens extracellularly. A cellular immune response centers around T-cell receptor recognition of a specific intracellular pathogen presented by a major histocompatibility complex, which are present on all host cells. Cellular and humoral immune responses are often found together but not always. An animal may have a cellular immune response without a significant humoral immune response and vice versa. Most common assays measure humoral immunity. A cellular immune response is typically most protective for intracellular pathogens such as viruses. Many intracellular pathogens elicit a relatively poor humoral immune response. A study of tortoise herpesvirus 3 (TeHV3) in *Testudo graeca* found that only three of four experimentally infected animals developed detectable humoral immune responses, and the responses in the three that did react were relatively transient.[7]

Especially in reptile species, whose pathogen diversity has not been well studied, there is concern of nonspecific cross-reactivity of antibodies against as-yet unstudied but antigenically related species. Although antibody cross-reactivity does correlate with genetic distance,[8] small genetic distances may be clinically significant. For example, *Testudinid herpesvirus 2* (TeHV2) (endemic in California desert tortoises, *Gopherus agassizii*) is distinct from TeHV3 (endemic in Greek tortoises) at a level greater than that seen between *human herpesvirus 1* (causing cold sores in humans, rapidly fatal in marmosets) and *Macacine herpesvirus 1* (causing cold sores in rhesus macaques; rapidly fatal herpes B in humans). It is probable that the clinical significance of the different tortoise herpesviruses in different species is comparable.

Before the diversity of tortoise herpesviruses was understood, a serosurvey of California desert tortoises using what was later shown to be TeHV3 as an antigen found that a number of California desert tortoises were seropositive; this was almost certainly cross-reactivity of antibodies to TeHV2 with TeHV3.[9] Treating diverse herpesviruses as a single entity may lead to inappropriate management decisions. From a population management perspective, it is crucial to know which viruses are endemic in a host species and the pathogenic implications of these viruses in other potential contact species.

Similarly, hemagglutination inhibition assays for ophidian paramyxoviruses in the genus *Ferlavirus* show poor concordance between different assays using different isolates.[10] There has recently been work done expanding the known diversity of the genus *Ferlavirus,* and at least three distinct clades are known.[11] The seroreactivity of samples from different snakes to different paramyxovirus strains differs significantly (Wellehan et al., unpublished data), and this may account at least in part for the lack of concordance seen. Overall, there are few pathogen clades whose diversity in reptiles is well enough understood to be confident of the specificity of a detected antibody. This limits the current utility of serological diagnostics in reptile medicine.

Culture of a pathogen from a diseased reptile has traditionally been utilized for direct identification of infectious agents. Although culture is still important, for some highly significant reptile pathogens such as *Chlamydia pneumoniae* or *Mycoplasma agassizii,* standard culture conditions will not support growth. Successful culture conditions have yet to be determined for the vast majority of microbes. Typically, around 10% of bacterial species can be cultured in a given ecologic niche,[12] and success at culturing viruses or protozoa is even lower.

Even if an agent has been cultured, it is still necessary to identify it. Biochemical methods for bacterial identification have been the standard for the past century. These methods have been best developed for two phyla of bacteria: Proteobacteria, the "typical" gram negatives, and Firmicutes, the "typical" gram positives. However, some of the most medically significant phyla in reptiles, such as Actinobacterium (containing *Mycobacterium, Devriesea,* and *Austwickia,* and others) and Chlamydiae (containing *Chlamydia* and others) are poorly identified by standard biochemical methods. Molecular methods involving nucleic acid sequencing are superior for identification.[13] The contrast is even more stark in molecular versus classical fungal identification, where identification has been morphologic, missing significant cryptic diversity. The most significant fungal pathogens of reptiles are *Ophidiomyces ophiodiicola* and *Nannizziopsis guarroi.* Although these were commonly called anamorphs of *Nannizziopsis vriesii,* there was no support for this when sequence data from these isolates were examined.[14,15] Sequence-based identification methods should be used to identify any agent where there is reason to question identification by conventional means.

POLYMERASE CHAIN REACTION (PCR)

Polymerase chain reaction (PCR) directly tests for the presence of a specific nucleic acid, in this context from an infectious agent (pathogen). Like other pathogen isolation techniques, this requires that the clinician submit an appropriate sample that contains the actual pathogen. A negative test does not mean that the pathogen is not present elsewhere in the patient. Unlike pathogen isolation, with PCR, the suspected agent does not need to be viable, but nucleic acid needs to be intact. Formalin degrades nucleic acids significantly.[16] The first step in sample processing is nucleic acid extraction. If an RNA template (typically an RNA virus) is to be amplified, the RNA will have to be transcribed into DNA, a process known as reverse transcription.

DNA is composed of two complementary strands oriented in opposite directions (Fig. 36.1A). Primers (short single-stranded segments of DNA) are designed to match the sequence of the two strands of pathogen DNA in a manner such that they face one another. Validation of primers is critical, and labs should provide a peer-reviewed publication on validation of a given primer set for diagnostic use to clinicians for evaluation (required for accreditation by the AAVLD, American

Association of Veterinary Laboratory Diagnosticians). The DNA is heated so that the two strands separate (see Fig. 36.1B). The temperature is then decreased to an appropriate temperature for the primers to anneal (bind) with the DNA (see Fig. 36.1C). If the primers do not match with the DNA sequence, they will not anneal, and no product will be formed. The temperature is then increased to an appropriate temperature for thermostable DNA polymerase to extend the primer, making a matching strand for the DNA (see Fig. 36.1D). The amount of DNA between the primers present is thus doubled. The cycle starts over again as the DNA is reheated to separate the strands. The cycle is repeated many times, and the amount of DNA increases geometrically.

The PCR product must then be validated, meaning that it must be determined to be the appropriate product and not an accidental binding of the primers to an unexpected site on a different DNA template. Formerly, older validation methods were limited to measurement of the size of the product by gel electrophoresis or restriction fragment length polymorphism (RFLP). These methods are significantly less accurate than modern methods, such as sequencing or probe hybridization, and should no longer be considered acceptable.

The most definitive way to determine the identity of the PCR product is to sequence it. Whereas this was once expensive, with the rapid improvements in sequencing technology that have taken place in the past decade, costs are now minimal. This provides not only the possibility of identifying known organisms but also characterization of novel organisms by comparison to reference sequences and subsequent phylogenetic analysis. Although capable of identifying novel organisms, it is slower and more labor intensive than probe hybridization quantitative (qPCR).

Alternatively, a labeled piece of DNA containing part of the target sequence may be used to probe the PCR product. The probe must be designed to a sequence unique to the pathogen found within the PCR product. When done under the appropriate conditions, binding of the probe to the PCR product indicates that the PCR product is correct. Some protocols, such as probe hybridization qPCR, have the probe incorporated as the PCR is running, and this is discussed in the following section.

PROBE HYBRIDIZATION QUANTITATIVE PCR

Probe hybridization quantitative PCR (qPCR), also known as real-time PCR, is a PCR variant. Similar to standard PCR, primers (short single-stranded segments of DNA) are designed to match the sequence of the two strands of pathogen DNA in a manner such that they face one another. The difference is the addition of a dye-labeled probe that matches and binds to sequences between the two primers. Two dyes, a reporter dye, to be detected by a spectrophotomer during the reaction, and a quencher dye, which absorbs the spectrum emitted by the reporter dye, are bound to the probe (Fig. 36.2A). As before, the DNA is heated so that the two strands separate (see Fig. 36.2B). The temperature is then decreased to an appropriate temperature for the primers and probe to anneal (bind) with the DNA (see Fig. 36.2C). If the primers do not match with the DNA sequence, they will not anneal and no product will be formed. The temperature is then increased to an appropriate temperature for thermostable DNA polymerase to extend the primer, making a matching strand for the DNA (see Fig. 36.2D). DNA polymerase, in addition to extending the primer to match the template DNA, also has exonuclease activity, which means that it will chew up any DNA in front of it that gets in the way as it is extending the primer. If the probe is bound to the template in front of the primer, the polymerase will chew through the probe, releasing the labeled dye. This separates the reporter dye from the quencher dye, and the released reporter dye can be measured with a spectrophotometer.

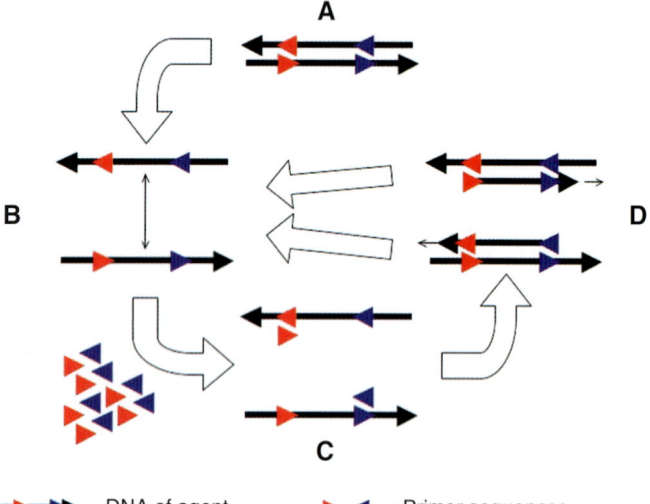

➤➤➤ = DNA of agent ▶ ◀ = Primer sequences

FIG 36.1 (A) DNA is composed of two complementary strands oriented in opposite directions. (B) The DNA is heated so that the two strands separate. (C) The temperature is then decreased for the primers to anneal (bind) with the DNA. (D) The temperature is then increased for thermostable DNA polymerase to extend the primer, making a matching strand for the DNA. The amount of DNA between the primers present is thus doubled. The cycle starts over again as the DNA is reheated to separate the strands. The cycle is repeated many times, and the amount of DNA increases geometrically. (Courtesy of James F.X. Wellehan.)

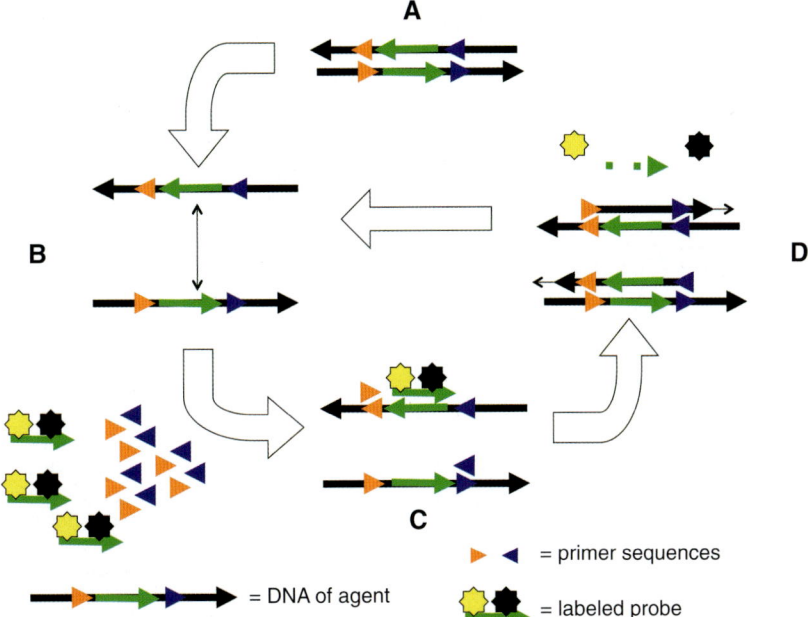

FIG 36.2 (A) Probe hybridization quantitative PCR (qPCR), also known as real-time PCR, is a PCR variant. Similar to standard PCR, primers are designed to match the sequence of the two strands of pathogen DNA in a manner such that they face one another. The difference is the addition of a dye-labeled probe that matches and binds to sequences between the two primers. (B) Two dyes, a reporter dye, to be detected by a spectrophotomer during the reaction, and a quencher dye, which absorbs the spectrum emitted by the reporter dye, are bound to the probe. As before, the DNA is heated so that the two strands separate. (C) The temperature is then decreased to an appropriate temperature for the primers and probe to anneal (bind) with the DNA. If the primers do not match with the DNA sequence, they will not anneal and no product will be formed. (D) The temperature is then increased to an appropriate temperature for thermostable DNA polymerase to extend the primer, making a matching strand for the DNA. DNA polymerase, in addition to extending the primer to match the template DNA, also has exonuclease activity, which means that it will chew up any DNA in front of it that gets in the way as it is extending the primer. (Courtesy of James F.X. Wellehan.)

This has two distinct advantages. First, the validation of the PCR product is rapid. Validation in probe hybridization qPCR is done during the reaction, data output is simple, and no further steps are necessary. Second, the release of dye depends on the amount of template present, providing quantitative information. In Fig. 36.3, a qPCR standard curve is shown. The horizontal axis is number of cycles, and the vertical axis is fluorescence. The arrows drawn on the figure indicate the number of template copies present in the initial reaction. When there are only 10 copies initially present, it takes approximately 37 cycles for the reaction to release enough dye to cross the threshold (green) line. When there are 1,000,000 copies initially present, the threshold is crossed after approximately 19 cycles. This provides a standard to compare samples to and also provides a control to ensure that reactions are working well and efficiently. Quantitative information can be clinically useful to determine whether loads are sufficient to consider as a disease etiology and to follow trends over time to assess response to therapy. A well-designed qPCR is a highly useful tool for specific identification of a known agent. When well designed and properly validated to ensure the assay specifically identifies only the target DNA, probe hybridization qPCR can be a sensitive, specific, rapid, quantitative, and relatively inexpensive test. Proper validation is critical, and labs should provide a peer-reviewed publication on validation of a given probe hybridization qPCR assay for diagnostic use to clinicians for evaluation. There are established guidelines for validation of a qPCR assay.[17]

It is important to realize that there are other assays commonly called real-time PCR that do not involve validation by probe hybridization. The most common of these utilizes SYBR green dye, which is incorporated into DNA as it is synthesized. This methodology does not provide any data on the size or sequence of the PCR amplicon, making it even more prone to false positives than gel electrophoresis. Especially when dealing with diverse host species, as is commonly done in reptile medicine, this methodology should not be utilized.

CONSENSUS PCR TECHNIQUES

Before primers can be designed, the nucleic acid sequence must be known. Some nucleic acid sequences are specific to a given species or even strain. Other nucleic acid sequences have stayed the same through evolution and are found across groups of related organisms. These are known as consensus sequences. Genes that are conserved throughout evolution are typically essential for function of the organism, such as ribosomal RNAs (rRNA) or viral polymerases. Gene choice is critical and depends on the level of taxonomic resolution needed. Within adenoviruses, the polymerase is the most conserved gene, and primers have been designed that will amplify any adenovirus.[18] However, when looking specifically at Agamid adenovirus 1 in bearded dragons, all polymerase sequences obtained to date show minimal variation, and it was necessary to obtain sequence from the hexon gene to differentiate strains.[19] Once consensus sequences have been identified, PCR primers

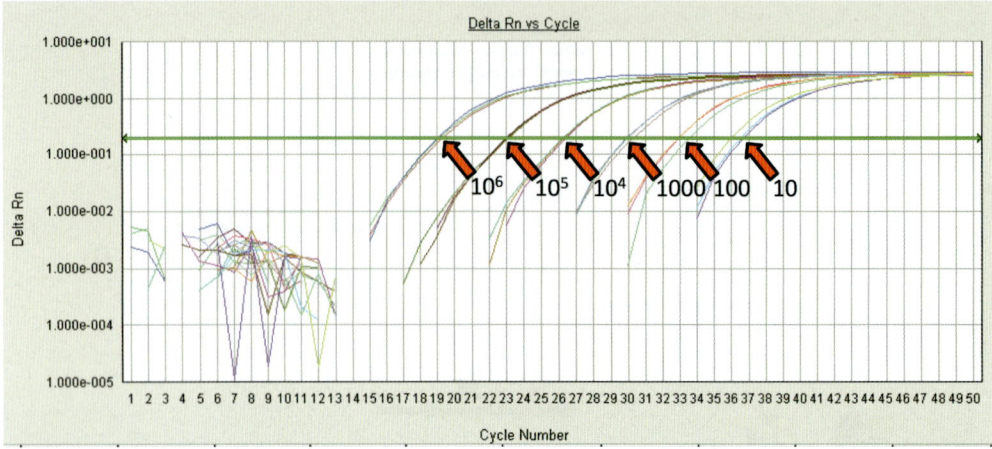

FIG 36.3 A qPCR standard curve is shown. The horizontal axis is number of cycles, and the vertical axis is fluorescence. The arrows drawn on the figure indicate the number of template copies present in the initial reaction. When there are only 10 copies initially present, it takes approximately 37 cycles for the reaction to release enough dye to cross the threshold (green) line. When there are 1,000,000 copies initially present, the threshold is crossed after approximately 19 cycles. (Courtesy of James F.X. Wellehan.)

can be designed in these conserved regions and used to amplify the more variable region between the consensus primers. In reptile medicine, many pathogens remain to be identified. If primers designed to conserved sequences are used in a PCR, the PCR will amplify all organisms containing the conserved sequence, providing the ability to identify novel pathogens in a known clade. Diverse published assays are available for a wide variety of taxonomic levels, ranging from the entire domain of prokaryotes,[20] the class Coccidia,[21] the family Adenoviridae,[18] and the genus *Orthoreovirus*,[22] to allow even more specificity. However, caution is needed. When more than one member of a clade is present in a sample, direct Sanger sequencing of a PCR product will result in mixed sequence that is unreadable. Protocols such as pan-bacterial or pan-fungal PCR are useful for identification of isolated bacteria or fungi, respectively, when ID by conventional methods is questionable. However, application of these methods directly to clinical samples that are likely to have diverse bacterial or fungal flora present, such as oral samples or fecal samples, it is unlikely to result in a product that can be directly sequenced and interpreted. More narrowly targeted assays should therefore be used on such samples (e.g., genus *Mycobacterium*-specific PCR, if that is an important differential) to detect more specific agents of possible concern.

Although consensus sequence PCR is useful for amplification of sequence from novel pathogens, the amplification of novel sequences does not lend itself to specific probe design, eliminating qPCR as an option for this application. Consensus PCR should always be accompanied by sequencing of the PCR product.

ROLLING CIRCLE AMPLIFICATION

Rolling circle amplification (RCA) is a technique for amplification of small circular DNA genomes, as are found in several families of viruses, including papillomaviruses, polyomaviruses, anelloviruses, circoviruses, and tornoviruses. It does not require knowledge of any sequence from the agent. The technique involves a polymerase that moves around the circle as it synthesizes a complementary strand. When the beginning of the circle is reached, the polymerase continues around again, and the new strand is a long series of repeated copies of the circle. This strand is then cut with a restriction enzyme, which recognized specific

short 4 to 6 base pair sequences. Since these sequences will be in the same place every time the circle is repeated, the restriction enzymes cut the circle into a set of pieces of specific size. These pieces can then be cloned and used as sequencing template. Because it does not require any known sequence, RCA has proven useful for obtaining sequence templates of divergent agents, such as tornoviruses in sea turtles.[23] However, this technique requires a significant amount of cloning and sequencing and is therefore highly labor intensive, raising costs.

HIGH THROUGHPUT SEQUENCING

Recent years have seen amazing advances in sequencing technology. Costs have been reduced several orders of magnitude. New techniques, including pyrosequencing, Illumina sequencing, PacBio, and SOLiD sequencing are capable of producing millions of sequences in a single run. This has enabled the development of metagenomics, in which nucleic acid representing an entire sample is sequenced, rather than targeted amplification of a specific region. This enables an understanding of the diversity of complex and diverse environments such as the reptile GI tract.[24] The ability to obtain such data sets is a double-edged sword; although it provides the ability to obtain sequences from previously unknown and divergent pathogens, it requires the ability to recognize and sift these sequences out of literally millions of nontarget sequences. This is a major bioinformatics challenge but has already resulted in significant advances in our knowledge of reptile/amphibian infectious disease. Recent discoveries of important reptile pathogens, such as sunshine virus, reptarenaviruses, and ball python nidovirus, have all been based on next-generation sequencing techniques.[25–27] Although costs for metagenomic methods are still considerable, they are decreasing rapidly, and what was a $100,000 project a couple of years ago is a $1000 project now. It is only a matter of time before these techniques become clinically affordable.

SAMPLE COLLECTION FOR NUCLEIC ACID–BASED DIAGNOSTICS

The first thing the practitioner needs to do is open a dialogue with the diagnostic laboratory. It is important first to understand what methodologies are offered, and ideally, peer-reviewed references describing testing methodologies should be provided to the clinician. Common problems and pitfalls should be discussed in advance, as well as limitations of diagnostic testing.

Histologic evaluation of a necropsy is often one indication that an agent requiring molecular testing is present. As such, although it is critical to collect a complete set of tissues in formalin for histologic evaluation, it is also important to save and freeze another set for further diagnostics if indicated by histology. Frozen tissues should be routinely kept until histologic results are back, and there is no indication for further diagnostics.

Sample choice is critical for nucleic-acid based diagnostics; the agent must be in the sample. This requires an understanding of the common distribution of the agent in the animal. Although plasma has historically been a common sample collected for infectious disease diagnostics (due to the use of serodiagnostics), relatively few infectious agents are themselves commonly found in plasma, making it a suboptimal sample choice for testing for most reptile pathogens. A laboratory with significant clinical experience with a given reptile pathogen may be able to advise on sample choice.

PCR is a highly sensitive technique, and the potential for false-positive results from slight contamination anywhere from collection to laboratory is high. As such, it is critically important that measures are taken to avoid contamination during sample collection and transport and that appropriate controls are run.

Transport is also crucial and needs to be discussed with the laboratory in advance. Agents such as RNA viruses, especially enveloped ones, tend to be significantly less environmentally stable. Media such as RNAlater can be used to preserve viability of nucleic acids. Shipping on ice or even dry ice is often preferable. When same-day transport is not available, overnight shipping is indicated. The laboratory should be notified in advance so that potential problems can be identified and brought up with the shipping service on the same day if a delivery does not arrive.

It is an exciting time in herpetological medicine. Molecular techniques are enabling us to begin to unravel the diversity of pathogens in reptiles and amphibians and detect them in a clinically applicable fashion. An understanding of molecular diagnostic options and their clinical interpretation are essential in modern reptile practice.

HOW TO CHOOSE A LABORATORY

It is important for the clinician to be able to assess the quality of results from the laboratory. The American Association of Veterinary Laboratory Diagnosticians accredits public laboratories, and AAVLD accredited laboratories should be preferred. Any project receiving US federal funding has to use a laboratory meeting GLP (Good Laboratory Practice) standards, but this is not required of private diagnostic submissions. There is no useful accreditation organization for private veterinary diagnostic laboratories in the United States. Important questions that practitioners should ask laboratories include:

1. What protocols are used? Are they from peer-reviewed literature? If so, are they used as in the literature or modified? Practitioners should obtain copies of peer-reviewed literature on protocols used.
2. What controls are used? Nucleic-acid-based testing should have both extraction controls and reaction controls.
3. If PCR-based testing, how are products validated? Acceptable methods include sequencing of products and validated probe hybridization (such as TaqMan). Older, less-specific methods, such as size of a band on electrophoresis, restriction digest fragment size or SYBR green dye incorporation should be avoided. It is important that probe hybridization protocols are properly validated; this should be published in a peer-reviewed journal.

REFERENCES

See www.expertconsult.com for a complete list of references.

37

Immunopathology

Elizabeth W. Howerth

Reptiles have a functional and complex immune system that includes innate, humoral, and cell-mediated components. However, the efficiency of the immune system is influenced by a variety of factors, such as health, nutritional status, age, and stress. In addition, environmental temperature, brumation (hibernation) or estivation, and seasonal changes also affect the efficiency of the immune system. Because reptiles are ectothermic, the immune system is dependent on the ability of the animal to maintain adequate core body temperature.

CELLS AND TISSUES OF THE IMMUNE SYSTEM

The tissue components of the reptile immune system include bone marrow, thymus, and spleen, as well as gastrointestinal-, respiratory-, and urogenital-associated lymphoid tissue. In some cases lymph node–like organs are present.[1] Reptiles, unlike mammals, do not have usual lymph nodes and do not form germinal centers, which is where B-cell and helper T-cell interaction, B-cell proliferation, isotype switching, and affinity maturation associated with an adaptive immune response occur in mammals.[1,2] In the reptile, the spleen is thought to be critical for reptilian immune function, assuming the functional role of lymph nodes.[3] Reptiles also do not have a bursa, but a bursalike lymphoid organ is found in the cloacal wall in some reptiles.[4]

The reptilian bone marrow produces both red and white cells, including lymphocytes, and is found in medullary bone throughout the body. In turtles and tortoises this includes the carapace and plastron of the shell.

In general, the thymus of reptiles is bilateral and composed of a variable number of lobulated or nonlobulated glandlike nodules or lobes. Frequently the thymus of each side consists of two small white lobes that are separate from each other. The thymus is located in the cervical region and may be contiguous with or immediately adjacent to the parathyroid glands and next to the ultimobranchial bodies and great arterial vessels and often extends to the base of the heart. It may be embedded in fatty tissue in well-nourished animals and be difficult to identify.

In lizards and tuatara, the thymus is described as nonlobulated, whereas chelonians and crocodilians have distinct thymic lobules.[4,5] Snakes have a spherical, single-lobed, double-lobed thymus immediately anterior to the heart between the thyroid gland and lateral fat body on each side.[5] The sea turtle thymus is an elongated gland on each side of the body, usually within fat, which may be thin and diffuse in chronically ill animals.[6] Crocodiles and alligators have a thymus more like a bird, which is elongated and may be embedded in fat and traverse the length of the neck on both sides of the trachea and into the thorax to the base of the heart.[5,7] In young crocodilians, there may be posterior enlargement of the right and left sides that may meet over the thyroid.[5]

Histologically, the thymus is delimited by a capsule, and the parenchyma is subdivided into a cortex and medulla composed of predominantly small- and medium-sized lymphocytes and a stroma of epithelial cells (Fig. 37.1). Hassall's corpuscles may be present, as well as other cell types such as myoid cells and secretory-like cells.[8]

The spleen produces red and white cells and in most reptiles is spherical, oval, or elongated triangularly and is histologically similar to higher vertebrates being composed of red and white pulp. In some reptiles, the spleen is contiguous with the pancreas, and there may be some admixture of both splenic and pancreatic tissue. This is entirely normal in many chelonians and some snakes, where it is referred to as splenopancreas (Fig. 37.2); in other reptiles the two organs are entirely separate.[4]

The reptilian thymus and white pulp of the spleen exhibit seasonal changes, involuting during the winter and becoming well developed again by the spring (Fig. 37.3).[1] It has been noted in snakes that cortex and medulla of the thymus are poorly defined during winter.[8] Splenic lymphocytolysis may lead to impaired immune function in the winter in some species.[9] Seasonal variation in GALT also has been noted but appears to be species specific.[1]

Lymphoid aggregations composed of lymphocytes and plasma cells occur in the gastrointestinal tract (gut associated lymphoid tissue [GALT]).[8] GALT occurs throughout the intestine, but the most important sites are esophagus, ileum, ileo-cecal junction, colon, and cloaca. These are small nonencapsulated aggregates mainly in the lamina propria, but they may extend deeper in the submucosa. These may reach a large size in certain sites of various reptiles. The lymphoid cloaca complex described in some reptiles may not be related to the bursa of Fabricius

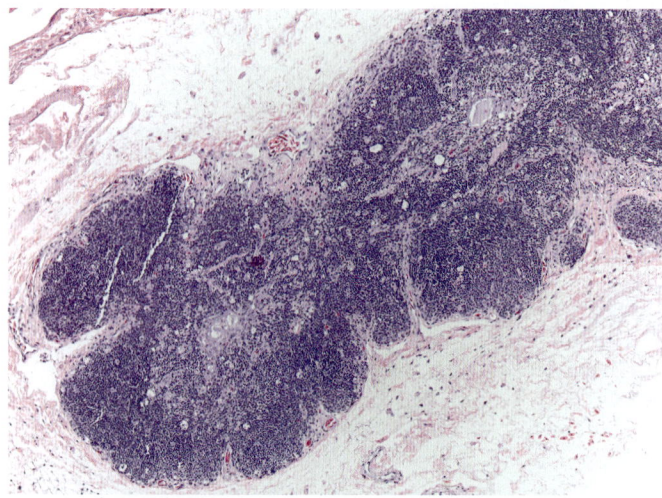

FIG 37.1 Normal lobulated thymus from an alligator (*Alligator mississippiensis*). (H&E, ×10). (Courtesy of Elizabeth Howerth, University of Georgia.)

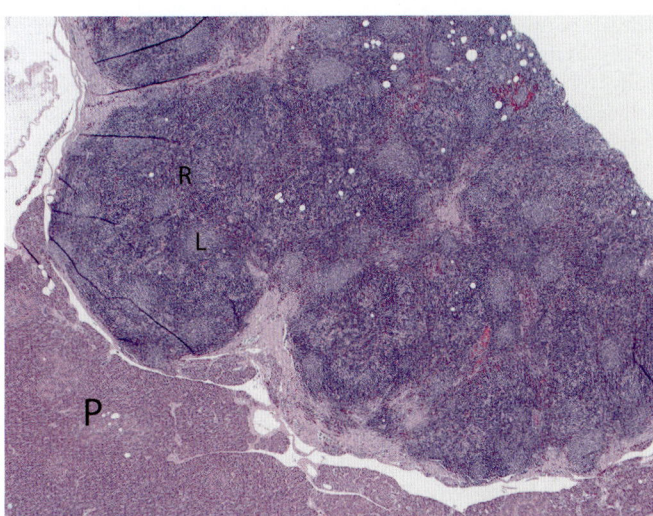

FIG 37.2 Normal splenopancreas from a corn snake (*Pantherophis guttatus*). The spleen is similar to a mammal with red (R) and white (L) pulp. P = pancreas (H&E, ×4). (Courtesy of Elizabeth Howerth, University of Georgia.)

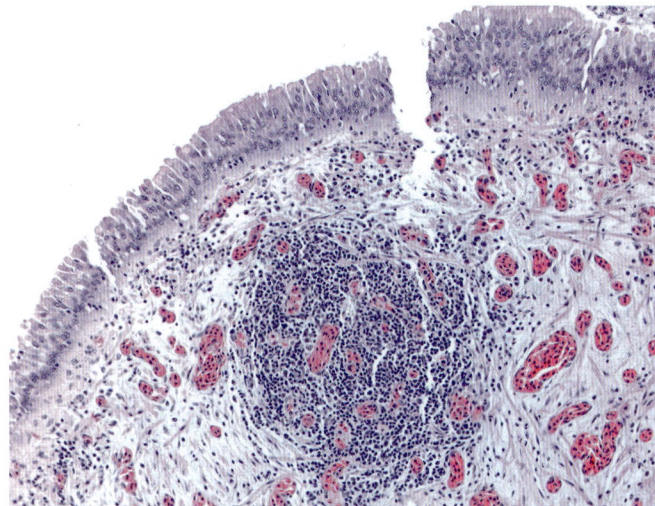

FIG 37.4 Normal urinary bladder from a turtle with typical sub-epithelial lymphoid aggregate. Similar aggregates occur throughout the gastrointestinal and respiratory tracts (H&E, ×20). (Courtesy of Elizabeth Howerth, University of Georgia.)

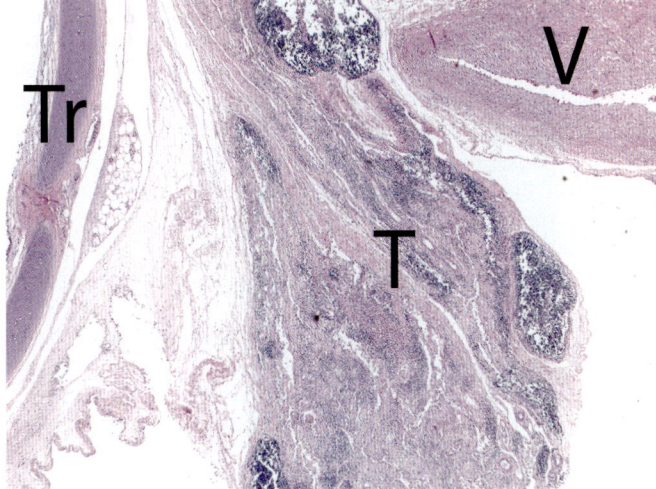

FIG 37.3 Thymic involution in a tortoise. Involution or atrophy can occur for a variety of reasons, including a normal seasonal response, but can also be driven by such things as exposure to estrogenic compounds, high levels of testosterone, or endocrine-disrupting chemicals. T = lymphoid depleted thymus; Tr = trachea; V = cervical vessel (H&E, ×4). (Courtesy of Elizabeth Howerth, University of Georgia.)

of birds because the histology is different. Lymphoid aggregates also occur in the lung, pancreas, urinary bladder, testes, and axillary and inguinal regions (Fig. 37.4). The esophagus of boid snakes has raised ovoid structures with a central cleft referred to as esophageal tonsils. Histologically these are submucosal lymphoid aggregates covered by mucosal epithelium and are important sites for the detection of viral inclusion bodies in boid snakes with arenavirus inclusion body disease.[10] Similar esophageal submucosal nodules have been described in other species of snakes.[11] In some species, small organs similar to lymph nodes have been found in axillary and inguinal areas.[8]

INNATE IMMUNITY

Innate immunity is the first line of defense against pathogens and has a critical role in the activation and regulation of adaptive immunity.

The concept of innate immunity being nonspecific to an antigen and lacking memory has evolved into one of a more specific immunity based on pattern recognition receptor molecules (PRRs) and even memory development.[12] In the reptile, the major components include intact epithelial barriers (e.g., skin, gastrointestinal, respiratory, urinary), physiological parameters (e.g., stomach pH, body temperature), and humoral and cellular effector components.[12]

Humoral innate immunity in reptiles includes lysozyme, antimicrobial peptides, acute phase proteins, complement, and certain cytokines.[12] Antimicrobial peptides are known in three of the four orders of reptiles, the testudines, crocodilians, and the squamata, and include members of the cathelicidin and defensin families unlike birds, reptiles also express hepcidins.[13] Reptile heterophils have granules that contain both cathelicidin-like peptides, as well as β-defensin. The β-defensin-like peptides and lysozyme are also found in reptile eggs. The few reptilian antimicrobial peptides that have been isolated and studied demonstrate broad-spectrum antimicrobial and antifungal activity. Expression of these peptides has also been found in wounds, such as when lizards lose their tails.[13]

The acute phase response is an early defense system activated by infection, injury, and inflammation, which results in changes in the concentration of many plasma proteins, known as acute phase proteins (APP), mostly produced by the liver. In reptiles, described APPs are serum amyloid A and fibrinogen.[12] The complement system is composed of serum proteins that react against pathogens through a molecular cascade; however, the molecular makeup of the reptilian complement system remains poorly defined, and only complement protein C3 has been identified.[12] Likewise, information on cytokines in reptiles is sparse, but they appear to have certain cytokines that are well-conserved among vertebrates, such as type II interferons, certain interleukins, and TGF-β.[12]

Cell-mediated innate immunity in reptiles includes intraepithelial T lymphocytes in the intestinal epithelium, phagocytic cells (monocytes-macrophages, heterophils, and dendritic cells), basophils, eosinophils, possibly nonspecific cytotoxic cells, and phagocytic B cells.[12,14] In reptiles, phagocytosis plays an important role in immune response, because it is less influenced by temperature than adaptive immune mechanisms.[12] However, the phagocytic response appears to have seasonal variation.[15,16]

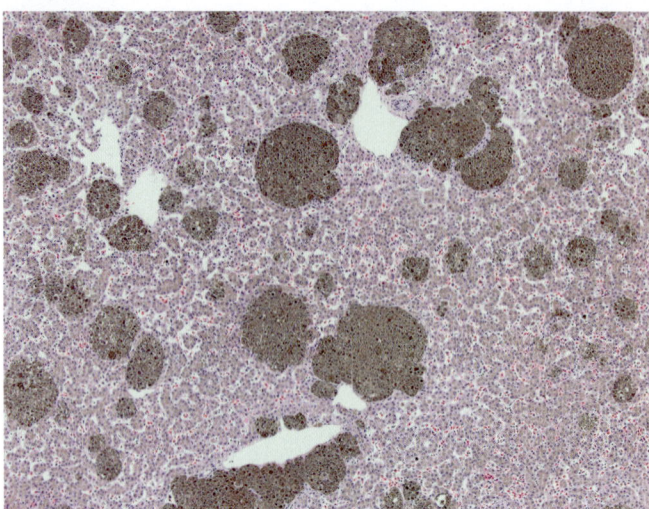

FIG 37.5 Liver from an emaciated Indian star tortoise (*Geochelone elegans*) that had severe pseudogout with an increased number and size of melanomacrophage systems (H&E, ×10). (Courtesy of Elizabeth Howerth, University of Georgia.)

Natural killer cells are an important subset of lymphocytes with the innate ability to kill infected cells without being primed and activated. Although NK cells have not been specifically identified in reptiles, there is evidence of the existence of specific cell types or a functionally similar group of cells in reptiles.[15–18] Reptiles also have circulating monocytes called azurophils due to their azurophilic-staining granules that appear to function similar to mammalian monocytes.[19]

In vertebrates, the "professional phagocytes" recognize senescent cells and microbes by pattern-recognizing receptors (PRRs), including Toll-like receptors and C-type lectin receptors. However, as important as these receptors are and how well-studied they are in other vertebrates, knowledge of PRRs in reptiles is scarce.[20]

The reptilian heterophil is functionally similar to birds, and phagocytosis is its primary function.[21] They are morphologically variable among species but contain two, possibly three, types of granules that contain cationic proteins, lysozyme, acid phosphatases, and acid hydrolases but lack myeloperoxidase, catalase, and alkaline phosphatase. Therefore heterophils depend on a nonoxidative method of killing and do not form pus. Heterophils also contain B-defensins, which have a broad spectrum of activity against infectious agents.[19]

Although eosinophils likely play a role in parasitic infections, little is known about their function.[1] Reptilian basophils are likely to be important in inflammation as they degranulate and release histamine when triggered by an antigen; the release is dependent on antigen concentration and temperature.[1] Aggregates of melanin-containing macrophages (melanomacrophages) normally occur in the liver of reptiles, and with systemic inflammation they can proliferate and even develop in other sites, such as the spleen (Fig. 37.5).[22] In the yellow mud turtle, and most likely in all reptiles, liver aggregations increase in number and size with age.[23] These cells contain melanin granules and also hemosiderin and lipofuscin and are phagocytic. The melanin granules are thought to produce free radicals and therefore may be involved in bacterial killing.[22,23]

ADAPTIVE IMMUNITY

Adaptive immunity occurs following the innate immune response. Current knowledge regarding the function of the reptilian adaptive immune system is poor, although T-cells and B-cells are recognized.

The site of origin of reptilian B-cells is unknown, but sites of lymphopoiesis likely include bone marrow, spleen, and other locations in the body.[21] There is evidence that reptilian B-cells possess phagocytic activity.[24] T-cells probably arise from lymphocytes in the bone marrow that colonize the thymus and differentiate into T-cells.[21]

Antibodies in reptiles are considered to be IgM, IgY, IgA, and IgD.[25,26] IgM is probably present in all reptiles as it is conserved across vertebrates, but there is variability among species as to which other classes are present, and in some species more than one form of certain immunoglobulin classes may be present (e.g., sea turtles have three forms of IgM and two of IgY).[27] Immunoglobulins are poorly studied in reptiles, but, in general, the structure of the reptile immunoglobulin is thought to be similar to mammals, although reptile immunoglobulins apparently do not have a hinge.[28] IgM is highest in blood and spleen but is also present in lung and intestine and so may play a role in mucosal immunity.[26] IgY is often considered the functional equivalent to IgG of mammals and expressed in liver and spleen in a T-cell-dependent manner when present.[26] Turtle IgY binds to protein G in contrast to IgY of birds, which does not, so reptile IgY might be more similar to mammalian IgG.[27] IgD may play a role in mucosal protection too.[26] An IgA-like gene is present in some species but lost in others. In gecko and crocodiles, it is expressed in high levels in the intestines and may have a role in mucosal immunity.[26] Reptile immunoglobulins undergo class switch recombination similar to mammals and function similarly to mammals in regard to agglutination, precipitation, and virus neutralization.[26]

Lymphocyte production is affected by stress, temperature, and season (decreased during fall and winter). Both cold and prolonged high temperature can affect antibody production.[29] Pregnancy in viviparous lizards may impair the immune response and is associated with splenic involution.[30] Environmental temperature can affect both antibodies and leukocytes.[26]

Measurement of the humoral immune response in reptiles has typically been measured with an indirect enzyme-linked immunosorbent assay (ELISA).

A variety of cell-mediated immune phenomena similar to mammals are present in a wide range of reptiles, including cutaneous delayed hypersensitivity reaction to tuberculin and alloantigens, allogeneic and xenogeneic graft rejection, phagocytosis, the two-way mixed lymphocyte reaction, and graft-versus-host phenomena.[31] Similar to mammals, the cell-mediated immune response in reptiles can be measured by in vitro cell proliferation assays using whole blood or peripheral blood mononuclear cells cultured with phytohemagglutinin, concanavalin A, or soluble chicken egg white lysozyme.[32]

RESPONSES AND DISORDERS

Sex Hormone–Induced Immunopathology

Physiologically, sex hormones modulate immune function, with both estrogens and androgens impacting immunocompetence. Reptiles, including lizards and turtles, demonstrate immune-related pathologies after estrogen administration. For example, 17β-estradiol (E2) exposure induced thymic atrophy and inhibited thymocyte proliferation in *Hemidactylus flaviviridis*, and injection of 17α-ethinylestradiol, an environmental estrogen often present in sewage-treatment plant effluent, decreased peripheral blood leukocyte and total splenocyte levels in *Sceloporus occidentalis*.[33,34] Testosterone induces lymphopenia in turtles,[35] and high levels of testosterone have been associated with decreased immune function and thymic degeneration in some reptiles.[3]

Endocrine-Disrupting Chemicals

Estrogenic endocrine-disrupting chemicals (EDC), for example, DDT metabolites and PCBs, which may structurally resemble estrogens or act similarly, can disrupt normal immune homeostasis. Estrogenic EDCs may induce autoimmune susceptibility by way of an overstimulated immune response, while at the same time promoting infection and disease development through specific immune deficiencies. Exposure to environmental estrogens by altering testosterone levels (or the estrogen:testosterone ratio) might result in the mobilization of lymphocytes and an increase in thymic hematopoiesis. This could shift the immune response toward a proinflammatory response, which could enhance responses to self-antigen or even downregulate other immune pathways.[36,37] Exposure to these environmental contaminants appears to result in damage to lymphoid tissue and may be seen as decreased thymic ratio (medulla:cortex) and decreased size of malpighian bodies and lymphocyte sheaths in spleen.[3,38]

Response to Infectious Agents

The typical response to infectious agents, such as bacteria, fungus, and parasites, in reptiles is granulomatous, seen as either a heterophilic granuloma (heterophils accumulate and degranulate and elicit a macrophage response) or histiocytic granulomas (composed mostly of macrophages).[39]

In mycobacterosis, there is a granulomatous lesion often with multinucleated giant cells and variable numbers of other inflammatory cells, heterophils, lymphocytes, and plasma cells. Granulomas range from nodules of viable and degenerate heterophils or nodules with a central core of necrosis surrounded by epithelioid macrophages, multinucleated giant cells (MGCs), and a variable mantel of mixed inflammation to older lesions composed primarily of epithelioid cells and MGCs (Fig. 37.6). These lesions rarely mineralize but will become walled off with fibrous tissue.[40,41]

The response to mycoplasmas, which typically colonize ciliated epithelial mucosa, is somewhat different as these organisms typically cause epithelial hyperplasia with infiltration of heterophils and histiocytes and lymphoid hyperplasia, the latter often being a trigger that a mycoplasma is present (Fig. 37.7).[42]

The response to non-mycobacterial bacteria and fungi is also typically a heterophilic granuloma. For example, lesions in *Ophidiomyces ophidiicola* infection, which is a fungus, are characterized by central necrosis surrounded by degenerate heterophils, macrophages, and MGCs.[43,44]

Even though reptiles have eosinophils, an eosinophilic response to parasites is rare, and more typically the response is granulomatous.

Immune Complex-Associated Glomerulonephritis

Glomerulonephritis occurs fairly frequently in reptiles and may range from acute to chronic with glomerular tuft sclerosis (Fig. 37.8).[45] Histologically there may be changes suggestive of immune complex glomerulonephritis, including thickening of capillary membranes due to deposition of hyaline periodic acid Schiff reactive-positive material.[42,45] However, these cases have yet to have been investigated beyond the light microscopic level.

Splendore-Hoeppli Reaction

The Splendore-Hoeppli reaction, characterized by eosinophilic clublike material radiating around an infectious agent, is reported commonly in mammals but only rarely seen in reptiles. Such a response was reported in *Neisseria* sp. infection in two species of iguana.[46]

Hypersensitivity

Except for a type IV hypersensitivity reaction to mycobacteria, there is little evidence to suggest that reptiles have a hypersensitivity response.

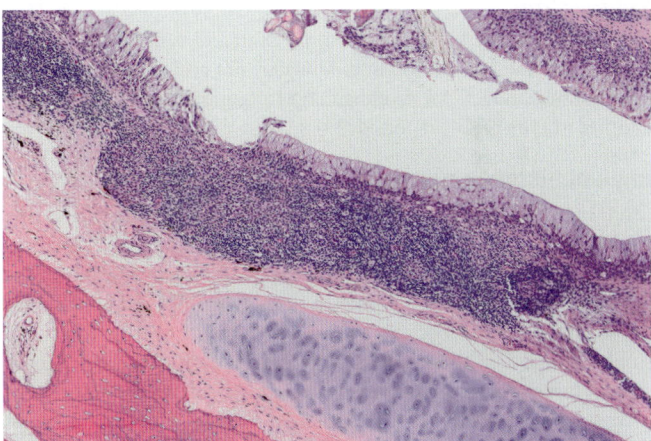

FIG 37.7 Lymphoid proliferation is a common response with mycoplasmosis, as seen in the nasal mucosa of this tortoise (H&E, ×20). (Courtesy of Elizabeth Howerth, University of Georgia.)

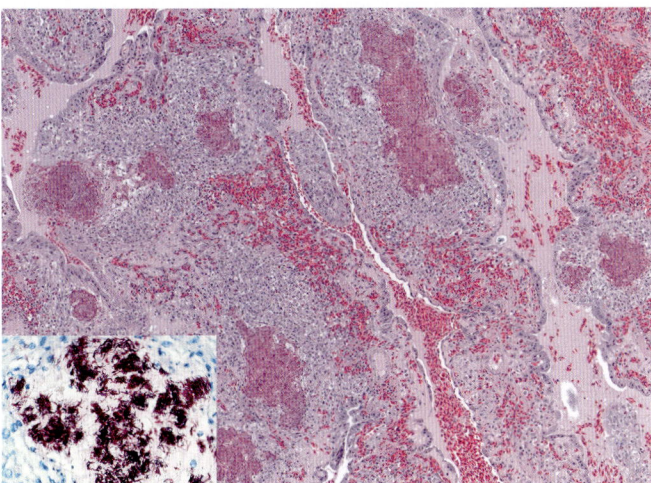

FIG 37.6 Coalescing granulomatous inflammation in the lung of a reticulated python (*Malayopython reticulatus*) with disseminated mycobacteriosis (H&E, ×10). (*Inset*) Acid-fast stain with myriad acid-fast bacilli (Ziehl-Neelson acid fast stain, ×100). (Courtesy of Elizabeth Howerth, University of Georgia.)

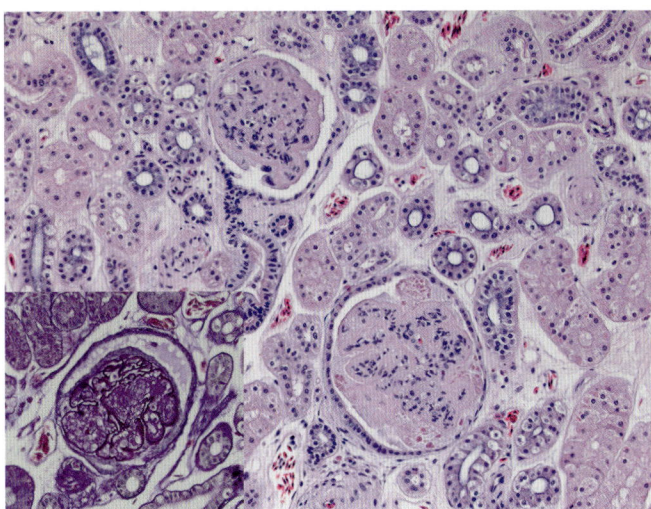

FIG 37.8 Glomerulopathy in an approximately 12-yr-old red diamond rattlesnake (*Crotalus ruber*). Glomeruli are obliterated by a hyaline matrix (H&E, ×20). (*Inset*) The matrix stains purple with a Masson's Trichrome/PAS stain, which is similar to mammals with glomerulosclerosis (×20). (Courtesy of Elizabeth Howerth, University of Georgia.)

However, delayed type hypersensitivity has been used to assess immune function.[47] Although not substantiated, acute hypersensitivity reaction in lungs of *Terrapene carolina* has been reported.[8]

Amyloidosis

In animals, the most common form of amyloidosis is associated with chronic infection and deposits derived from the acute-phase protein serum AA. Although common in mammals and birds, reports of amyloidosis or amyloidlike material in reptiles are few.[45,48,49] Why amyloid deposition is rare in reptiles is unknown. Information about the acute phase reaction and the production of serum amyloid A (SAA) is limited in reptiles, although it has been shown to exist in some reptilian species, for example, the Chinese soft-shelled turtle (*Trionyx sinensis*).[50] Amyloid-like plaques, similar to senile plaques in humans, have been reported in brains of reptiles exhibiting severe neurologic signs.[4]

Neoplasia of the Immune System

Lymphoma, plasmacytoma, and leukemia have been reported multiple times in many families and species of reptiles.[8]

Vaccination

Immunization studies indicate that the humeral response is slow in reptiles, and antigen-specific antibodies may not peak until 6 to 9 weeks postimmunization.[26,51] A prolonged IgM response before switching to another isotype is also reported.[26]

Immunohistochemistry

Immunohistochemistry is widely used in veterinary medicine, mostly in mammalian species, for the identification of tumors. Numerous commercially available antibodies are used for this purpose, but these antibodies are usually against human or mouse antigens, and their use in other mammalian species is based on their ability to cross-react with similar antigens in these species. Immunohistochemistry can also be helpful in determining tumor type in reptiles, but the ability of commercially available antibodies to cross-react in reptiles is often unknown and may vary between reptile species. Vimentin expression was shown in a snapping turtle fibroma (cutaneous fibroma in a snapping turtle, *Chelydra serpentina*),[52] but in other reports vimentin antibodies did not cross-react. Failure to cross-react could be related to species, but it could also be related to the specific vimentin antibody used. Certain cytokeratin antibodies, specifically the pancytokeratin antibodies AE1/AE3 and Lu-5, appear to cross-react in some reptiles and were used to help characterize an undifferentiated ovarian tumor in a corn snake and an esophageal adenocarcinoma in a matamata turtle (*Chelus fimbriata*).[53,54] However, in other reports (referenced in Petterino et al) other specific cytokeratin antibodies were not apparently cross-reactive.[53] While there have been variable results with anti-desmin antibodies, anti-actin antibodies seem more likely to cross-react in reptiles.[53] A variety of antibodies that might be used to differentiate neuroendocrine tumors, including protein gene product 9.5, synaptophysin, gastrin, glucagon, chromogranin, insulin neuron-specific enolase, endorphin, somatostatin, vasoactive intestinal peptide, pancreatic peptide, neurofibromin, have been shown to cross-react, at least in bearded dragons (*Pogona vitticeps*) where they have been used to identify gastric neuroendocrine carcinomas.[55] Melan A was also shown to cross-react in crocodile lizards so might be useful in identifying melanomas in reptiles.[22] Lymphoid tumors have been reported in many species and have sometimes been immunophenotyped. Antibodies to CD3 (T-cell marker) work well in most reptile species,[56] but the common B-cell markers CD79A and CD20 do not seem to be cross-reactive in reptiles (Howerth EW, personal communication, 2017). However, PAX-5 appears to be cross-reactive, at least in snapping turtles, and may hold promise in other species.[56] Cross-reactivity with human factor VIII–related antigen was demonstrated in a cardiac hemangiosarcoma in a Madagascar giant hognose snake (*Leioheterodon madagascariensis*).[57] In conclusion, antibody and species are both important considerations in using immunohistochemistry for tumor identification in reptiles, and a positive control of the same species should always be used.

REFERENCES

See www.expertconsult.com for a complete list of references.

38

Cytology

Melinda S. Camus and Corry K. Yeuroukis

Cytology is literally defined as the "study of cells." Cytologic examinations can be performed on body fluids (e.g., blood, urine, synovial fluid, effusions) or on material that is aspirated, scraped, or washed from a solid tissue. Cytology is often preferred to biopsy, at least as an initial diagnostic step, because it is typically less expensive, less invasive, requires less equipment, and has a more rapid turnaround time. Although cytologic examinations can be performed by general practitioners, microscopic interpretation can be challenging and is often best accomplished by a board-certified clinical pathologist. Submission of nondiagnostic samples results in loss of information, difficulties associated with resampling, and ultimately client dissatisfaction. Preanalytic factors including sample acquisition, handling, and submission are critical for optimizing chances of an accurate cytologic diagnosis.

SAMPLE ACQUISITION

Cytologic samples can be collected in a variety of ways, based on the sample location. Collection methods include aspiration, tissue impression, scraping, and swabbing. Regardless of sample type, the desired outcome is acquisition of enough intact cells with minimal contamination to allow for accurate interpretation. Broken cells often become unrecognizable or morphologically altered, which can yield incorrect conclusions. Samples diluted with iatrogenic blood contamination from sample collection contain leukocytes (white blood cells) from the peripheral blood that confound cytologic evaluation. Minimizing cell breakage and sample contamination should be a priority when collecting cytological samples using all methods but should not prevent collection of an adequate number of cells for interpretation. Use of the biggest possible needle while minimizing discomfort and hemorrhage is recommended.

Aspirates

This technique is used for collecting samples from masses, subcutaneous tissues, and internal organs. It is also commonly used in the acquisition of fluid samples. This method can be done in a number of ways. Typically, minimal cleansing preparation to the surface overlying the area of aspiration is desired. For large lesions where central necrosis is suspected, aspiration of the marginal areas may provide a higher diagnostic yield. If a sample is acquired via ultrasound guidance, care should be taken to avoid aspiration through ultrasound gel, as the gel can obscure microscopic evaluation of cells.

The most common aspiration technique involves stabilization of the structure to be aspirated with one hand, while a needle with an attached syringe is inserted into the structure with the other hand (Fig. 38.1). The length of the needle and the size of the syringe should be selected based on lesion size, depth, and character (e.g., hard versus fluctuant). For example, a 1-inch-long, 22-gauge needle attached to a 3-mL syringe should be adequate to aspirate a small, fluctuant subcutaneous mass, with minimal patient discomfort and iatrogenic hemorrhage. Once the needle is inserted firmly into the structure, negative pressure is applied by repeatedly pulling back on the syringe plunger. The needle tip can be redirected within the lesion or multiple aspirates can be performed in an attempt to sample several representative areas. The negative pressure should be released before removing the needle from the lesion to minimize tissue damage and avoid aspirating cells far into the syringe barrel, where they are difficult to retrieve.[1] Once the needle is withdrawn from the aspirated structure, the needle should be removed carefully from the syringe, and the syringe should then be filled with air. The needle is then replaced and the plunger rapidly depressed to disperse all collected sample onto one or more microscope slides. Once the sample is on a slide, an attempt should be made to distribute the cells gently and uniformly before they dry, typically with the weight of a clean "pusher" slide either held horizontally at a right angle to the sample slide or as done when making a blood smear (Fig. 38.2). Diagnostic sample may adhere to the "pusher" slide, which should also be submitted to the laboratory.

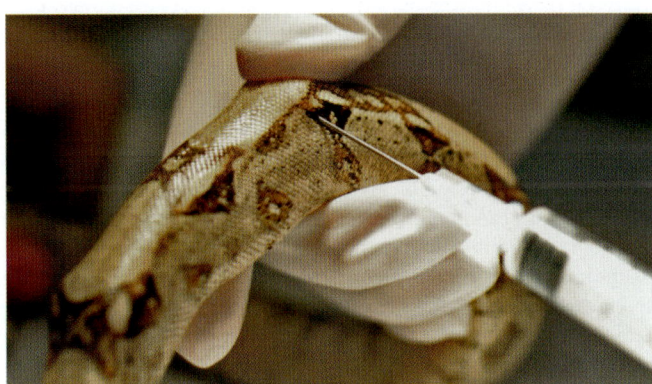

FIG 38.1 Aspiration technique. Adequate and appropriate restraint should be used to ensure patient and staff safety. Prepare and isolate the structure to be aspirated. Insert the needle into the lesion with the syringe plunger depressed. Once the needle is seated in the lesion, pull back on the syringe multiple times while directing and redirecting the needle. Make sure the syringe plunger is depressed when removing the needle to avoid aspirating sample contents into the syringe itself. (Courtesy of Stephen J. Divers.)

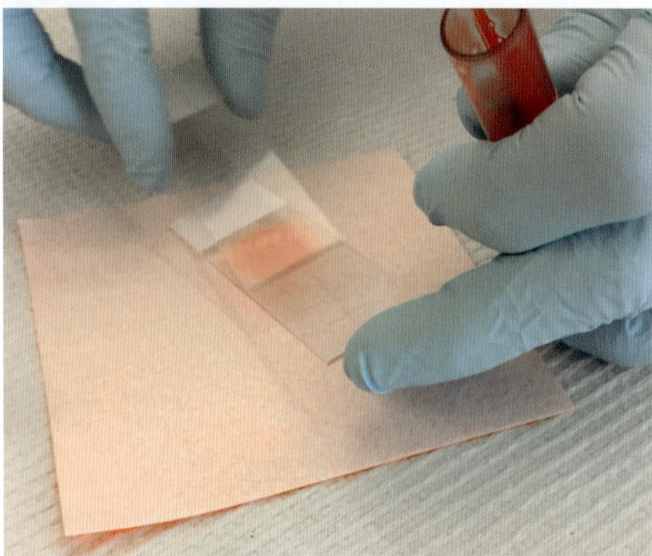

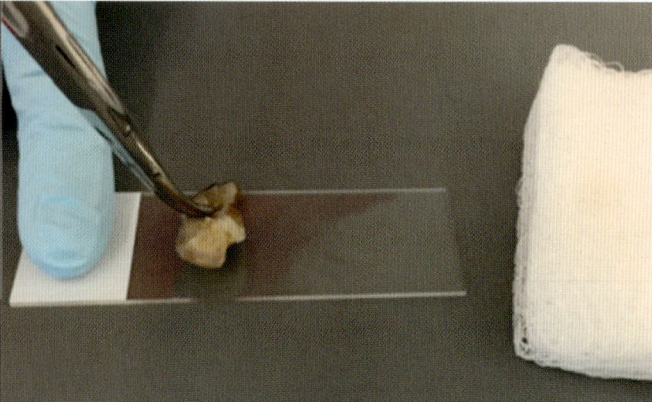

FIG 38.3 Impression smear. Blot the cut surface of the tissue on clean gauze until tacky and relatively free of blood. Touch the cut surface multiple times along the length of a clean slide. (Courtesy of Melinda S. Camus and Corry K. Yeuroukis.)

FIG 38.2 Smear preparation. The technique used to prepare well-distributed blood smears may also be utilized for fluid samples. A well-distributed fluid smear will have a curved shape and occupy approximately ¾ of the slide length. (Courtesy of Melinda S. Camus and Corry K. Yeuroukis.)

Another "aspiration" technique is the "pin prick" method or "stab technique."[1] This method involves using the needle, with or without an attached syringe, and rapidly moving the needle up and down in a vertical motion along the same needle tract in an attempt to "cut" the tissue and loosen the cells. After the sample is collected, an air-filled syringe is attached (if not already present), which is used to rapidly expel cells onto slides, as with the aspiration method. The "pin prick" method works well for vascular samples (e.g., spleen) because it minimizes bleeding and reduces blood contamination that can interfere with interpretation.[2]

Impression Smears

Impression smears are utilized when a solid piece of tissue is blotted onto a slide. This is typically done with (1) biopsy specimens that have been surgically collected and then pressed directly onto a slide to allow for rapid diagnosis; (2) skin lesions that have an ulcerated surface against which a slide can be pressed (Fig. 38.3); or (3) fresh necropsy tissues where a rapid provisional diagnosis may be possible while awaiting definitive histologic results. With all samples, it is essential to blot away any visible blood prior to making the impressions, because blood contamination can obscure the cells, which can make interpretation challenging. Additionally, it is important to realize that only the cells on the imprinted surface are transferred to the slide. Biopsy and necropsy specimens should be transected to allow for imprinting of the cut surface. Limitations of sampling only the surface, rather than deeper tissues, within a skin lesion must be recognized.

Scrapes

Tissue scrapings are often utilized with skin lesions and other surfaces in an attempt to minimize the superficial contamination obtained with the impression technique. A sterile scalpel blade coated in mineral oil is rubbed rapidly against the area to be sampled in an attempt to loosen cells that can be transferred onto a slide for microscopic evaluation. This can be more difficult in reptiles than in other animals due to their tough, keratinized integument. This is most frequently done to obtain tissue cells that would not otherwise exfoliate well.

Swabs

Sterile cotton-tipped applicators can be used to collect tissues and tissue discharges easily and with minimal disruption. Adding a drop of sterile saline prior to gently rolling the swab on or in the sample collection area minimizes tissue trauma and prevents contamination of the slide with cotton fibers. Collected cells are transferred onto a clean slide by gently rolling the swab across the slide's surface. Care must be taken not to press too hard, in an attempt to minimize cell breakage.

SAMPLE HANDLING

Sample handling is a critical component to achieving accurate cytologic diagnoses. Properly collected samples should be handled with care and packaged appropriately for transport to the laboratory to minimize cell deterioration and breakage. Fluid samples and slides have different handling requirements, and any questions regarding best practices for sample handling should be directly addressed to the laboratory prior to collection.

All samples should be labeled with the patient's identifying information and sample location immediately after collection. Slides with a frosted edge allow for easy labeling and are designed for use with a standard number 2 pencil. Slides without a frosted edge should be labeled near one end in an attempt to avoid covering potentially diagnostic material. Identifying information should be written directly on the slide and should not be placed on tape, which can fall off or obscure diagnostic material. Slides should never be labeled with permanent marker, which will wash off during many staining processes. A specific laboratory marker should be utilized to ensure that slides remain properly identified after processing.

Once a cytologic sample has been placed on a slide, a single slide should be stained using a standard Romanowsky-type stain (e.g., Diff-Quik), if possible. Heat fixing slides before staining is unnecessary and may compromise the integrity of the cells. The stained slide should then be examined to ensure that there is adequate cellularity for evaluation. In the event that no cells are seen or all cells are broken or deteriorated beyond recognition, additional samples can be obtained prior to incurring costs and delays associated with sending nondiagnostic

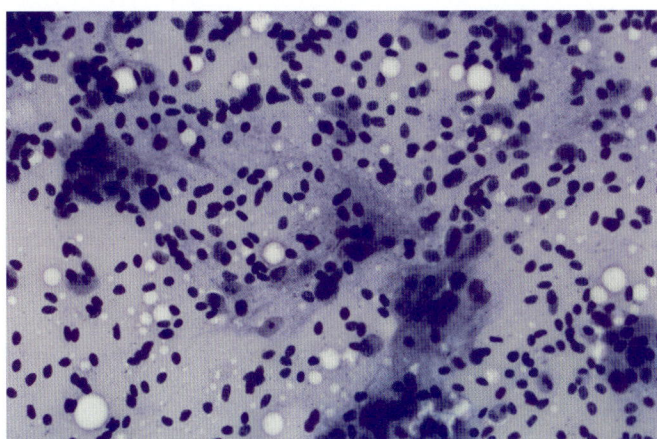

FIG 38.4 Slide examination. Prior to slide submission, stain a representative slide and examine it for sample quality. This slide (a liver aspirate from an iguana taken at 50x magnification and stained with modified Wright's stain) is of poor quality, consisting primarily of numerous free nuclei from ruptured cells in the background, with no microscopic evidence for cytoplasmic borders. The few cells with remaining cytoplasm have indistinct borders and swollen nuclei, which are additional features of ruptured cells. (Courtesy of Melinda S. Camus and Corry K. Yeuroukis.)

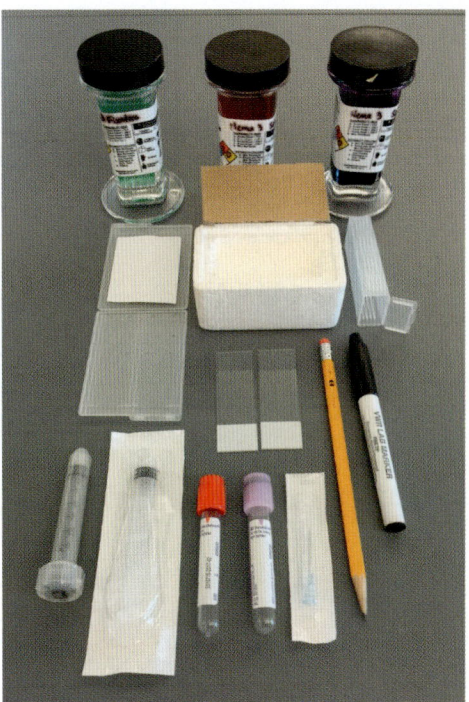

FIG 38.5 Recommended items for effective collection of specimens for sample submission and cytologic examination. The use of plastic slide containers for sample transport is ideal to minimize slide breakage. (Courtesy of Melinda S. Camus and Corry K. Yeuroukis.)

slides to the laboratory (Fig. 38.4). All additional slides for submission should remain untouched, with no fixation, including heat, methanol, or formalin. Specifically, extra care must be taken with cytology samples if they are to be used in conjunction with surgical biopsy or necropsy to establish a diagnosis, because formalin cross-links proteins. Exposure of unstained slides to formalin fumes, even when packaged within the same box for shipping, results in poor tinctorial properties due to protein cross-linking and typically precludes an accurate cytologic diagnosis. Submitting unstained slides allows for application of special stains at the discretion of the pathologist, in the event that it is necessary (e.g., for additional characterization of bacterial microorganisms in advance of culture results). All slides (both stained and unstained) should be packaged in a protective container for transport to the laboratory (Fig. 38.5). Many laboratories recycle slide containers and provide them free of charge for laboratory clients on request.

Fluid samples for cytology should be placed into sterile collection tubes. Although a no additive (red top) tube is most desirable to minimize dilutional effects, submission in species-appropriate anticoagulant is occasionally required to prevent sample clotting when large amounts of blood are obtained during sample collection. If culture is desired, or the need is even anticipated, a small amount of fluid should be collected into a separate no additive tube (or culturette with transport medium) at the time of sample collection. All fluid samples should be analyzed as soon as possible, because cellular detail diminishes in fluid suspension. Because even a small delay in time to sample analysis is inevitable, making a direct smear of a fluid sample at the time of sample collection is strongly encouraged. Preparation of the direct smear can be performed with the same technique used to create a blood film, stopping 1/4 inch from the end of the slide to prevent loss of potentially diagnostic samples off the end of the slides. Preparation of a direct smear for diagnostic fluid samples helps preserve cell morphology and may aid the pathologist in interpretation.

SAMPLE SUBMISSION

All laboratory submission forms should be filled out completely and concisely. As context accounts for the majority of interpretation, providing the pathologist with all pertinent medical history and a thorough description of the lesion helps with diagnostic accuracy (Fig. 38.6).[3] A good history includes answers to the questions: (1) Why was the sample acquired?; (2) what are the objective clinical findings (e.g., condition of the patient, duration and severity of the problem, appearance of the tissue, previous treatment or lab results)?; (3) what are differential diagnoses?; and (4) what exactly was sampled? Forms should be typed or written legibly in pen, and all patient information must match exactly what is written on the sample slides themselves. Abbreviations on the form should be limited to those that are standard and well recognized and should be reviewed prior to submission. Highlighting on submission forms should be avoided, because it often blurs text when copied or scanned.

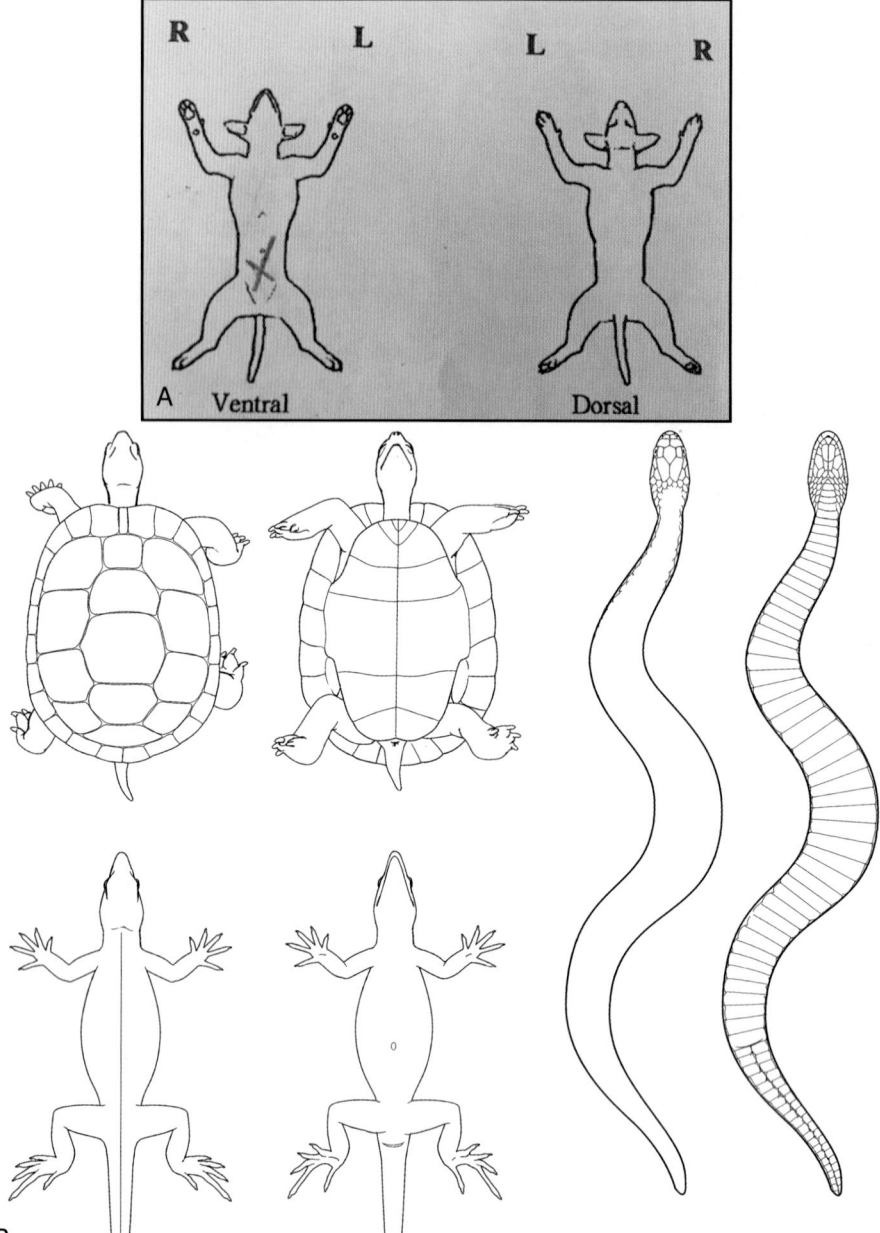

FIG 38.6 (A) Most laboratory submission forms show a picture of a canine patient. This can be utilized or a reptile-specific diagram (see B) can be attached. A visible "X" can be placed on the diagram to indicate the location of the sampled lesion. A thorough description of size, color, texture, and location of the lesion must also be included on the submission form to receive the most complete interpretation possible from the pathologist. The "X" in this image, without an accompanying history, could represent a skin lesion, a bladder aspiration, or a sample of an intra-abdominal structure. (B) Reptile-specific submission form diagram. These figures can be copied and attached to laboratory requests to indicate the location of the sampled lesion. (Courtesy of Educational Resources, University of Georgia.)

REFERENCES

See www.expertconsult.com for a complete list of references.

39

Biopsy

Nicole Gottdenker and Wilson Yau

Diagnostic biopsy samples provide clinically relevant information that helps with treatment and management at both individual and population levels. Obtaining and submitting a biopsy that results in a nondiagnostic report can be frustrating. Table 39.1 lists common errors associated with non-diagnostic samples, and steps to optimize sample collection. Fig. 39.1 illustrates some useful biopsy sampling supplies.

A complete medical history, including a summary of supportive diagnostic information such as clinical pathology, specific infectious disease testing (e.g., PCR, ELISA), and diagnostic imaging results, significantly helps the pathologist in providing meaningful diagnoses, comments, and feedback. In addition to patient signalment, pertinent information should include clinical signs and duration, husbandry conditions, and any recent changes or additions, treatments administered, and number of animals affected. In particular, husbandry specifics include type of cage and substrate, temperature, humidity, photoperiod, diets, and nutritional supplementation. Detailed descriptions of the submitted sample should include size, gross appearance, tissues involved and location on the body (Fig. 39.2), and whether the entire lesion has been submitted (incisional versus excisional biopsy).

When infectious or toxic etiologies are suspected, collecting paired samples (fresh and formalin-fixed) is recommended. Although formalin-fixed tissues allow for histopathology and immunohistochemistry, fresh tissues and swabs can be submitted for a wide variety of ancillary testing, such as bacterial and fungal cultures, fluorescent antibody testing, PCR, mineral analysis, and liquid chromatography-mass spectrometry. Fresh tissues stored in Whirl-Pak Bags can be frozen, held, and, if histopathology results indicate, subjected to ancillary testing later. Because some ancillary tests are specific to reptiles and are not widely available, it is important to identify and become familiar with diagnostic laboratories that offer such tests and the associated sample requirements, shipping guidelines, and turnaround times.

Recommended guidelines for submission for veterinary surgical pathology have been published.[1] In brief, most types of biopsy samples should be placed in 10% neutral buffered formalin as soon as possible to minimize tissue artifacts. To ensure adequate fixation, the volume of the formalin should be at least 10 times that of the tissue (10:1 ratio). If surgical margins are of interest, application of surgical ink or placement of sutures is helpful. Ink must dry completely prior to placing the tissue in formalin, which can take up to 10 minutes, and the designated margins should be clearly labeled on the submission form. Use the end of a cotton-tip applicator to minimize the amount of ink applied to the tissue.

Making tissue imprints often allows for quick identification of neoplastic populations and infectious etiologic agents, especially when a mass is identified during surgical exploration or necropsy. If tissue imprints are to be made, the procedure and slides should be made far away from formalin fumes, because the latter can introduce significant artifacts in the resulting imprints. Cut the tissue into a small block, such that forceps can hold onto opposite sides of the block while allowing for the downward-facing surface to be used for imprinting. Blot the surface onto clean absorbent material (such as paper towels) until no wet imprints are left, because excess blood and tissue fluids prevent cells and organisms from sticking onto the glass slide. After the surface is blotted dry, gently press the surface onto a clean glass slide. Depending on the size of the surface, often times multiple imprints

TABLE 39.1 "Dos and Don'ts" That Apply to Procurement and Submission of Biopsies

Do	Don't
Use 10% neutral buffered formalin, 10:1 ratio	Mix samples from multiple sites in the same container without labeling
Handle biopsy sample at margins	Grasp body of biopsy with forceps
Obtain more than one biopsy if possible	Submit the biopsy sample previously used for tissue imprints
Use scalpel or forceps to collect sample	Cauterize the tissue submitted for biopsy
Collect paired samples (fresh and formalin fixed)	Neglect to collect fresh tissues with suspected infectious or toxic etiologies
Double-pack samples & use absorbent liner	Use glass containers or zipper storage bags

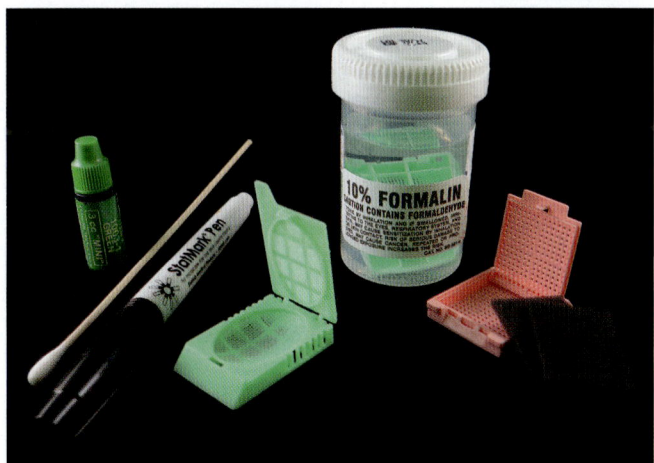

FIG 39.1 Useful biopsy sampling supplies, including formalin-filled jar with screw-top lid, cassette with sponge pads, Vortex cassette, StatMark pen, tissue ink, and cotton-tip applicator. (Courtesy of Wilson Yau.)

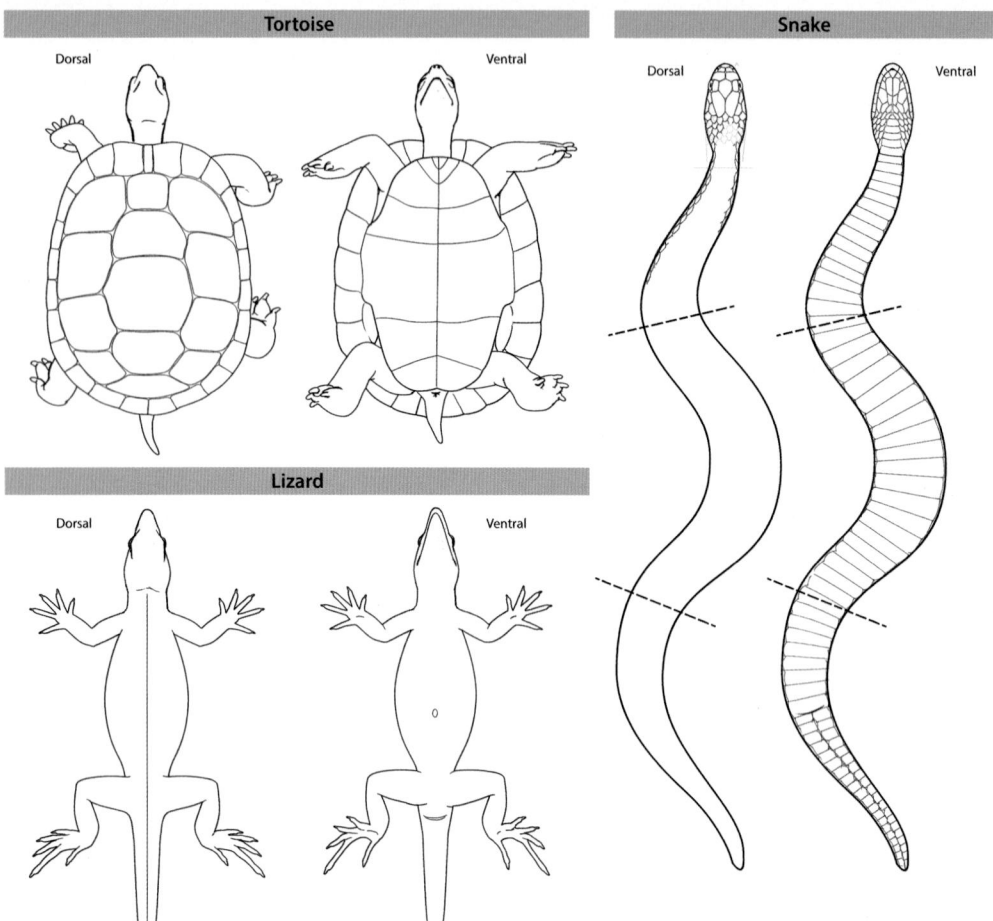

FIG 39.2 Reptile-specific submission form diagram. These figures can be copied and attached to laboratory requests to indicate the location of sampled lesions. (Courtesy of Educational Resources, University of Georgia.)

can be made onto the same slide in a row. Do not drag the tissue along the glass slide, because cells can rupture easily. Allow the glass slide to air dry before staining it with Diff-Quik or another Romanowsky-type stain. Consider making multiple duplicates of unstained glass slides, especially if infectious agents are suspected, in case special stains are indicated. The process of making imprints can distort tissue architecture (especially with kidney, liver, and gut mucosa), such that submission of other pieces of tissue not subjected to imprints is preferred. Endoscopic biopsies have been validated and produce clinically relevant results in lizards, chelonians, and snakes.[2,3] Refer to Chapters 63 and 64 for obtaining endoscopic biopsies. Similar small samples should be placed in screen cassettes and sandwiched between two sponge pads, which helps reduce sample movement and minimize the chance of sample loss or omission. Alternatively, Vortex cassettes eliminate the need for sponge pads. Do not use needles to immobilize tissues, which pose an unnecessary safety hazard to laboratory personnel handling the specimens. When multiple anatomic sites are sampled (e.g., proximal vs distal intestines), it is recommended to use separate cassettes. The cassettes should be labeled with pencils or StatMark pens. Do not use ballpoint pens or other ink markers, because the ink often smudges.

Small, soft tissue biopsy specimens are best obtained using a scalpel or biopsy forceps (crush technique). In contrast, radiosurgery, laser, and cautery techniques can cause extensive coagulation artifacts, which

can significantly impede microscopic interpretation at the margins. Because some biopsy sites, such as the oral or nasal cavity, can bleed profusely, the use of hemostatic devices may be required to control bleeding after the biopsy has been obtained. One should avoid the use of tissue forceps directly on the biopsy specimen, because this can cause microscopic crush artifact and impede interpretation. These principles also apply to core biopsies.

Disease processes are generally dynamic, and lesions or parts of lesions may be in different stages of formation or regression. For this reason, obtaining more than one biopsy from different parts of a lesion or from different sites of the same disease process is recommended. This is particularly applicable for multicentric skin lesions and core biopsies of large or nonresectable masses.

Bone biopsies often pose a significant challenge, because the reactive hyperostosis associated with many underlying bone lesions can be more prominent than the primary lesion, and obtaining representative biopsies becomes difficult, particularly with core biopsy techniques.

Because formalin is a hazardous substance that is irritating to the skin and mucous membranes, shipping the samples securely is important to ensure personnel safety. The samples should be placed in formalin-filled, plastic, and leak-proof containers, preferably with wide necks and screw-on lids. Parafilm-M can be used at the bottle neck to further minimize the chance of formalin leakage. The container should then be placed in a sealed plastic bag, surrounded by absorbent packing material, and shipped in accordance with postal regulations.

GROSS PHOTOGRAPHY

Photographs of gross lesions are extremely valuable, especially to pathologists correlating gross and histologic findings in both biopsy and necropsy cases.

The lesion should be of a magnification that occupies about 70% to 80% of the field, but an attempt should be made to include a margin of surrounding normal tissue to aid in viewer orientation. Including both low- and high-magnification images helps fully illustrate the location and gross features of the lesion. One should obtain more than one image at each magnification, adjusting for each to obtain the best contrast and focus.

For in situ and ex situ lesion photography, framing the lesion in the center of the image is important. For ex situ photography, a black or dark blue background is best to aid in tissue contrast, such as a flat, black rubber mat or a piece of clear glass placed over blue or black cloth. Many backgrounds can be distracting, such as newspaper, paper towels, wooden cutting boards, cage grates, or tile flooring. Fluid seepage and subsequent glare should be minimized by blotting the tissues before final positioning. A ruler is a useful size guide, especially for ex situ tissue photography; however, the ruler should not occupy more than 10% of the image and should not overlap the tissue of interest.

REFERENCES

See www.expertconsult.com for a complete list of references.

40

Necropsy

Nicole Gottdenker and Wilson Yau

Necropsies provide valuable information for diagnostic and educational purposes and often provide insight into population health management. A carcass can be submitted for necropsy with or without histopathology at a diagnostic laboratory. On the other hand, costs incurred and logistics of transferring whole carcasses can become prohibitive, and in-house necropsies are often performed. In addition, shipping intervals can contribute to autolytic change, postmortem bacterial overgrowth, and pseudomelanosis, which can significantly impede diagnostic evaluation. This chapter describes techniques to effectively perform a gross necropsy, including obtaining fresh and formalin-fixed samples for ancillary testing. Fig. 40.1 shows supplies useful for performing a necropsy.

Consultation with the pathologist regarding the animal's case history before shipping an entire carcass for a diagnostic lab necropsy or shipping formalin-fixed and fresh tissues from an in-house necropsy prevents many errors that arise from inadequate communications. This is particularly important with legal cases or cases that are being shipped on weekends or holidays. To prevent excessive autolysis, carcasses should be submitted with cold packs using the most expedient form of transport possible. Ideally, the carcasses should be necropsied as soon as possible after death. Carcasses waiting to be shipped or necropsied should be placed in a cooler (4°C) to slow autolysis. Avoid freezing carcasses directly, as freezing and thawing introduces tissue artifacts.

Gross pathology alone may not be sufficient to reach a specific diagnosis in many cases, and histopathology is indicated. At the minimum, formalin-fixed tissues of the brain, heart, lung, liver, spleen, kidney, reproductive organs, skeletal muscle, and a long bone should be collected.

Tissues should be fixed in 10% neutral-buffered formalin. To ensure adequate fixation, the volume of the formalin should be at least 10 times that of the tissue. Tissue thickness should not exceed 1 cm because formalin takes a considerable time to penetrate into the center of the tissue, and thick sections may not have adequate fixation, leading to autolytic change. Specific tissues may benefit from other types of fixatives. For example, eyes can be fixed in Davidson's solution, whereas tissues affected by gout should be fixed in ethanol instead, as formalin dissolves uric acid crystals. For cases where electron microscopy is anticipated, small vials containing 3% glutaraldehyde jars are ideal. Table 40.1 describes the dos and don'ts of submitting samples for necropsy.

When infectious or toxic etiologies are suspected, collecting paired samples (fresh and formalin-fixed) is highly recommended. Although formalin-fixed tissues allow for histopathology, immunohistochemistry, and in situ polymerase chain reaction (PCR), fresh tissues and swabs can be submitted for ancillary testing, such as aerobic and fungal cultures, fluorescent antibody testing, PCR, mineral analysis, and liquid chromatography–mass spectrometry. In cases suspected of toxins, save large quantities of liver, coelomic fat, kidney, and stomach contents, as certain toxicology tests require substantial amounts of sample to run. Fresh tissues stored in Whirl-Pak Bags can be frozen at −20°C or −80°C, held, and, if histopathology results indicate, subjected to ancillary testing. As some ancillary tests are specific to reptiles and are

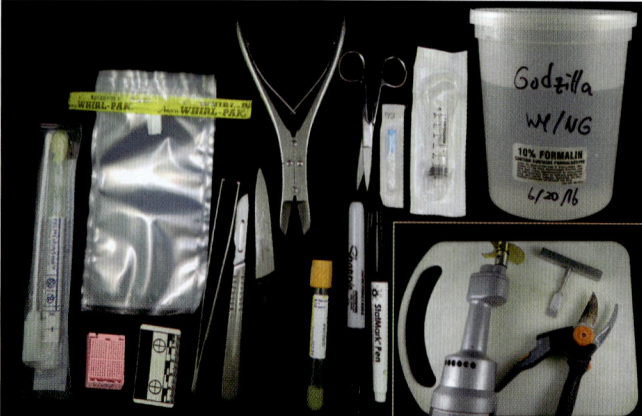

FIG 40.1 Useful necropsy instruments and sampling supplies. Formalin-filled container, syringe and needle, scissors, bone rongeur, Whirl-Pak Bag, culturette swab, tissue cassette, ruler, tissue forceps, scalpel blade, knife, blood tube, permanent marker (for labeling bags and containers), StatMark pen (for labeling cassettes), cutting board, Stryker saw, T-bar, and garden shears. (Courtesy of Wilson Yau.)

TABLE 40.1 "Dos and Don'ts" That Apply to Procurement and Submission of Necropsy Samples

Do	Don't
Use 10% neutral buffered formalin, 10:1 ratio	Overfill container with tissues
Ensure tissues are less than 1 cm thick for formalin fixation	Immerse entire carcasses in formalin without incising the coelom to allow for infusion
Use and label tissue cassettes for very small samples	Overfill a cassette and create "waffle" indentations on the tissue
Obtain multiple representative pieces of lung and liver for fixation	Submit only a single small piece of lung or liver
Call laboratory before sending fresh carcass/tissue	Send fresh tissue and carcasses without calling or on weekend/holiday
Keep extra set of formalin-fixed tissues	Discard tissues before biopsy/necropsy results are known
Collect paired samples (fresh and formalin-fixed)	Neglect to collect fresh tissues for cases with suspected infectious or toxic etiologies

not widely available, it is important to identify and become familiar with diagnostic laboratories that offer such tests, as well as their associated sample requirements, shipping guidelines, and turnaround times.

Although collecting fresh samples using aseptic techniques is ideal, it may not be practical in many situations. Nonsterile equipment can be dipped in alcohol, and the alcohol burned off with a Bunsen burner or lighter. In addition, diagnostic labs often have the ability to sanitize samples to minimize bacterial contamination. Any fresh tissues collected must not touch formalin, as formalin inactivates and destroys microorganisms and cross-links surface proteins, which drastically reduces the value of many ancillary tests.

Making tissue imprints often allows for quick identification of neoplastic populations and infectious etiologic agents, especially when a mass is identified during exploratory or necropsy. If tissue imprints are to be made, the procedure and slides should be made far away from formalin fumes, as the latter can introduce significant artifacts in the resulting imprints. Cut the tissue into a small block, such that forceps can hold onto opposite sides of the block while allowing for the downward-facing surface to be used for imprinting. Blot the surface onto clean absorbent material (such as paper towels) until no wet imprints are left, as excess blood and tissue fluids prevent cells and organisms from sticking onto the glass slide. After the surface is blotted dry, gently press the surface onto a clean glass slide. Depending on the size of the surface, often times multiple imprints can be made onto the same slide in a row. Do not drag the tissue along the glass slide, as cells can rupture easily. Allow the glass slide to air dry before staining it with Diff-Quik. Consider making multiple duplicates of unstained glass slides, especially if infectious agents are suspected, in case special stains are indicated. The process of making imprints can distort tissue architecture (especially with kidney, liver, and gut mucosa), such that submission of other pieces of tissue not subjected to imprints is preferred.

Table 40.2 lists reagents, instruments, and sampling supplies useful to perform a necropsy. Most necropsy equipment can be purchased at the local hardware store, but some equipment, such as dissecting scissors, forceps, and T-bars, may be purchased from medical suppliers (see Fig. 40.1).

Personal protective equipment should be used, as reptiles can carry multiple zoonoses, including salmonellosis, aeromoniasis, campylobacteriosis, mycobacteriosis, and zygomycoses. At minimum, personnel should wear dedicated protective clothing, footwear, and disposable gloves. Other equipment to consider includes safety goggles and facemasks, especially when using power tools (e.g., bone saws to separate turtle plastron and carapace) and high-pressure hoses. In addition, extra care should be exercised when handling venomous species, such as taping the mouth shut prior to handling the head to prevent accidental contact with fangs and subsequent envenomation.

NECROPSY PROCEDURES

Before starting a necropsy, ensure that the animal is indeed deceased (see Chapter 47 for proper euthanasia methods). Euthanasia by prolonged exposure to CO_2 alone often is not sufficient to ensure death of a reptile, such that application of a secondary lethal procedure may be indicated.[1] On the other hand, excessive injectable euthanasia solution, including intracoelomic or intravenous, creates extensive tissue artifacts resembling coagulative necrosis, which can obscure findings.

A necropsy examination must be methodical and complete, because, unlike a clinical physical examination, it cannot be repeated. Table 40.3 is a sample necropsy form that includes a tissue checklist, which should accompany all histopathologic submissions to help the pathologist put findings in context. A necropsy can be broken down into six steps:

1. Obtain signalment and medical history
2. External examination, including body weight
3. Open the body and examine body systems "in situ"
4. Remove and set aside the organs
5. Examine and sample the organs
6. Write the report

1. Obtain Medical History

A complete medical history significantly helps the pathologist in providing meaningful diagnoses and comments. In addition to patient signalment, pertinent information should include clinical signs and duration, husbandry conditions, and any recent changes, treatments administered, number of animals affected, whether the animal died or was euthanized, and any recent additions to the population. In particular, husbandry specifics include diet, type of cage and substrate, temperature, humidity, and photoperiod.

If multiple animals are affected in a die-off, do not necropsy just one carcass. Lesions present at different stages may be present in different individuals in a population, such that performing a necropsy on multiple affected individuals increases the likelihood of reaching a diagnosis. Attached clinical data, including hematology, biochemistry, culture and sensitivity, infectious disease testing (e.g., PCR, ELISA), and diagnostic imaging information, are often tremendously helpful.

2. External Examination

Record the body weight, snout-to-vent length, and total length. Observe for ocular, nasal, vent/cloacal discharge, discoloration, trauma, retained shedding of the skin (dysecdysis), and ectoparasites. In forensic necropsies, imaging techniques are invaluable, especially in detecting the presence of fractures, dislocations, bullets, or pellets that can be easily missed in cases without externally apparent wounds.[2]

Integument and Musculoskeletal System. Skin conditions are common in reptiles, especially trauma, burns, and infectious dermatopathies. A magnifying glass or dissection scope can help with examining small carcasses. Any cutaneous abnormalities or asymmetrical discoloration should be noted and collected in formalin. Photographs should also be taken of any suspected lesions and provided to the diagnostic pathologist (this applies to internal and external lesions). Fresh tissue should also be collected if infectious etiologies are suspected. Distribution and size of the abnormality should be succinctly noted on the necropsy

TABLE 40.2	**Equipment Needed for Performing a Gross Necropsy**		
Reagents and Supplies	**Safety Equipment**	**Instruments**	**Sampling Supplies**
Disinfectant detergent	Protective clothing	Knives, scalpel holders and blades, cutting board	Whirl-Pak Bags, culturette swabs
Neutral buffered 10% formalin solution	Nitrile or latex gloves	Bone rongeur, pruning shears, T-bar, Stryker saw or hacksaw	Needles and syringes, blood tubes
90% ethyl alcohol solution	Goggles, surgical face mask, face shield	Tissue forceps and scissors	Glass slides for imprints
		Ruler, permanent marker, StatMark pen	
		Camera, gram scale, dissecting scope or magnifying glass	

TABLE 40.3   Necropsy Form and Tissue Checklist

Prosector: _____   Date of necropsy: _____

Animal ID: _____   Species: _____

Age: _____   Sex: _____

Body weight: _____   Date of death: _____

Type of death (spontaneous/euthanized/unknown): _____

Clinical history and data: _____

Clinical diagnoses: _____

Gross photos taken (yes/no): _____

Samples submitted for ancillary testing (specify tissue and test): _____

Total body length (cm): _____

Snout-to-vent length (cm): _____

Body condition (emaciated/thin/moderate/stout/obese): _____

Postmortem autolysis (minimal/mild/moderate/marked/severe): _____

Body System	Tissue	Formalin-Fixed (Check if Collected)	Fresh Tissue (Check if Collected)	Abnormal Findings
Integument and Musculoskeletal	Skin	☐	☐	_____
	Skeletal muscle, peripheral nerve*	☐	☐	_____
	Coelomic fat	☐	☐	_____
	Bone, shell*	☐	☐	_____
	Joints	☐	☐	_____
Hematopoietic	Spleen*	☐	☐	_____
	Bone marrow	☐	☐	_____
	Thymus	☐	☐	_____
Endocrine	Pancreas	☐	☐	_____
	Adrenal	☐	☐	_____
	Thyroid, parathyroid	☐	☐	_____
Cardiovascular	Heart*	☐	☐	_____
	Great vessels	☐	☐	_____
Respiratory	Trachea	☐	☐	_____
	Lung*†	☐	☐	_____
	Pseudodiaphragm	☐	☐	_____
Urogenital	Kidney*†	☐	☐	_____
	Urinary bladder	☐	☐	_____
	Ovary, testes*	☐	☐	_____
	Uterus, phallus, hemipenes*	☐	☐	_____
Gastrointestinal	Liver, gallbladder*†	☐	☐	_____
	Tongue, teeth, gingiva	☐	☐	_____
	Esophagus	☐	☐	_____
	Stomach*	☐	☐	_____
	Small intestines*	☐	☐	_____
	Cecum, large intestines*	☐	☐	_____
	Cloaca	☐	☐	_____
Nervous	Brain*	☐	☐	_____
	Spinal cord	☐	☐	_____
	Eye	☐	☐	_____
Other (Specify)				

_____

_____

_____

*Formalin-fixed tissue should be collected.
†Fresh tissue should be collected.

form (i.e., "random on the back and legs," "confined to ventral aspects of body [or legs]," "tip of nose [or tail]"). For chelonians, this information also applies to the carapace, plastron, and bridges.

The musculoskeletal system provides useful information regarding current and past nutritional status, which can be affected by traumatic, degenerative, and infectious conditions. Palpate the appendicular skeleton for signs of fracture or unusual softness (metabolic bone disease). For carcasses too large to submit whole, an effort should be made to submit the head, a segment of vertebral column, and at least one long bone with the articular surface, such as the femur, tibia, humerus, or radius, especially if degenerative joint diseases or osteomyelitis are suspected. Postmortem radiographs may also be helpful for diagnostic and legal purposes. Peripheral nerves are often incorporated when collecting large muscles. Processing of bone most often requires decalcification, which can add days to weeks of processing time, depending on the thickness of the bone submitted and decalcification reagents used.

Snakes: All snakes possess secretory sacs at the base of the tail (scent glands). They may enlarge as inspissated secretions accumulate.

Crocodiles: Two pairs of musk-producing glands are present, one nuchal and the other cloacal.

Lizards: A single row of femoral pores are present on the ventral aspect of the thighs in many lizards, such as iguanas. Geckos can have both femoral and precloacal pores. Mature males tend to have larger femoral pores. Lizards such as geckos have paired endolymphatic sacs in the ventrolateral cervical region. These sacs often contain chalk-white liquid when normal.

3. Open the Body Cavity

Although many variations among reptile anatomy exist, a general necropsy approach can be applied to all, with modifications made for specific orders and species (Figs. 40.2–40.9). In particular, specific and detailed protocols on groups of reptiles are published, such as sea turtles.[3] Most animals should be placed in dorsal recumbency, while chameleons and other laterally compressed lizards may be better placed in lateral recumbency.

Many reptile specimens are small, which makes necropsy relatively easy. For animals less than 10 cm in length, use scissors to cut through the skin and coelomic wall from cloaca to the intermandibular symphysis,

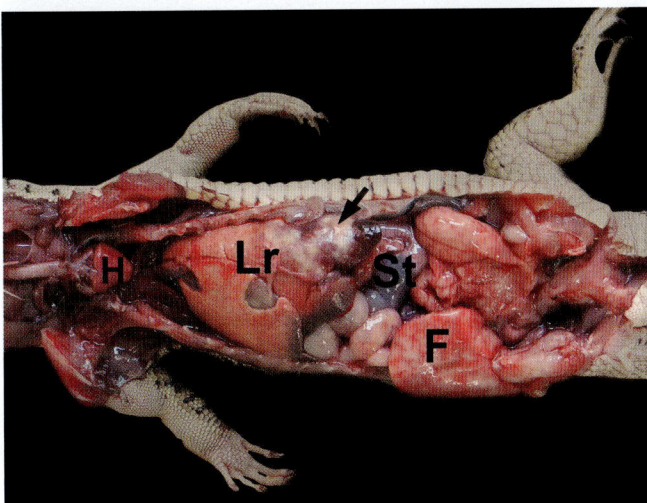

FIG 40.2 Ocellated lizard *(Timon lepidus)* necropsy. The ventrum and ribcage have been removed to reveal coelomic contents. Note the heart (H), liver (Lr), stomach (St), and coelomic fat pad (F). A large granuloma is present on the caudoventral aspect of the liver (arrow). (Courtesy of Wilson Yau.)

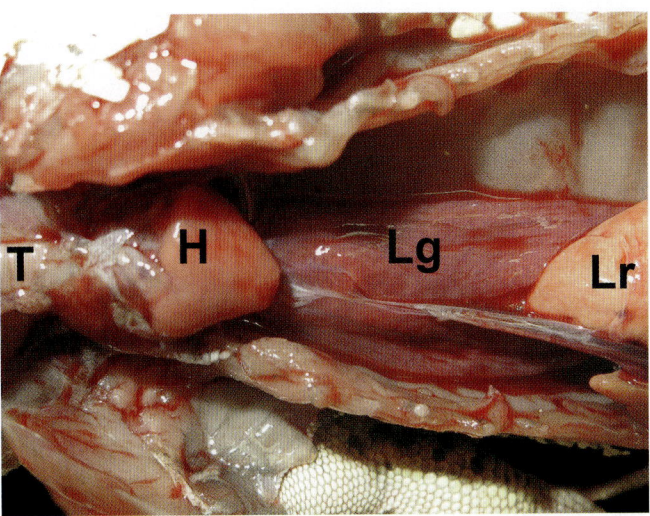

FIG 40.3 Ocellated lizard *(Timon lepidus)* necropsy. Higher magnification of the cranial coelom. Note the trachea (T), heart (H), lung (Lg), and liver (Lr). (Courtesy of Wilson Yau.)

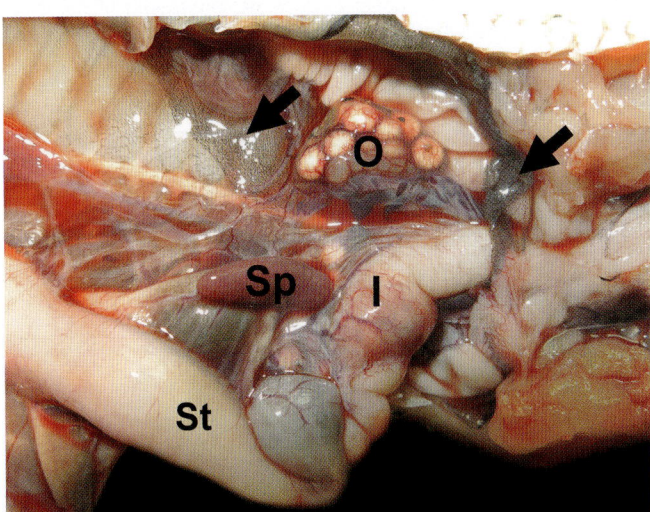

FIG 40.4 Ocellated lizard *(Timon lepidus)* necropsy. Higher magnification of the caudal coelom. Note the normal melanin pigmentation throughout the serosa (arrows), spleen (Sp), stomach (St), intestines (I), and ovary (O). (Courtesy of Wilson Yau.)

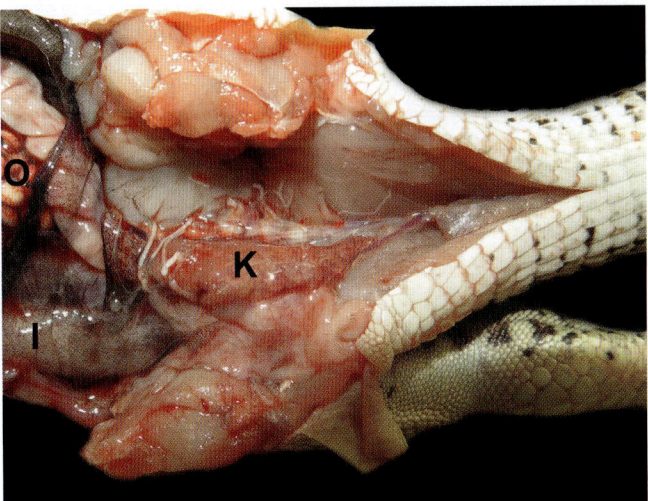

FIG 40.5 Ocellated lizard *(Timon lepidus)* necropsy. The pelvic symphysis has been split to reveal the left kidney (K). Note how caudal the kidney is compared to the ovary (O) and intestine (I). (Courtesy of Wilson Yau.)

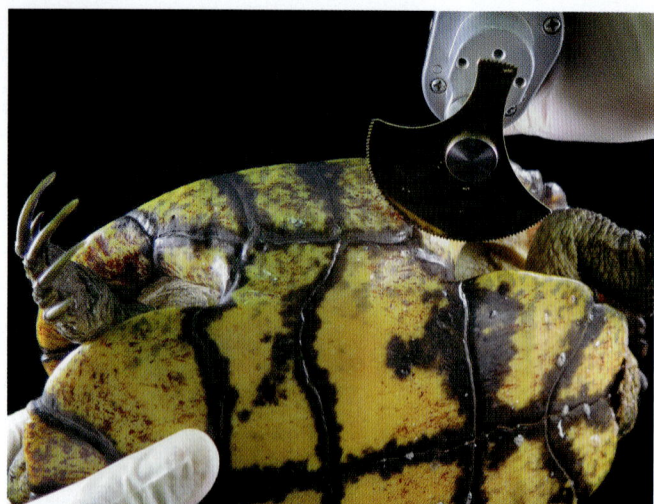

FIG 40.6 Chelonian necropsy. Incising the shell bridge with a Stryker saw. The carcass is inverted and angled at approximately 45 degrees. The initial cut is at the extreme caudal or cranial bridge junction, and a straight cut is made to the opposing end. The contralateral bridge is cut in the same manner. Alternatively, a hacksaw may be used if a Stryker saw is not available. (Courtesy of Wilson Yau.)

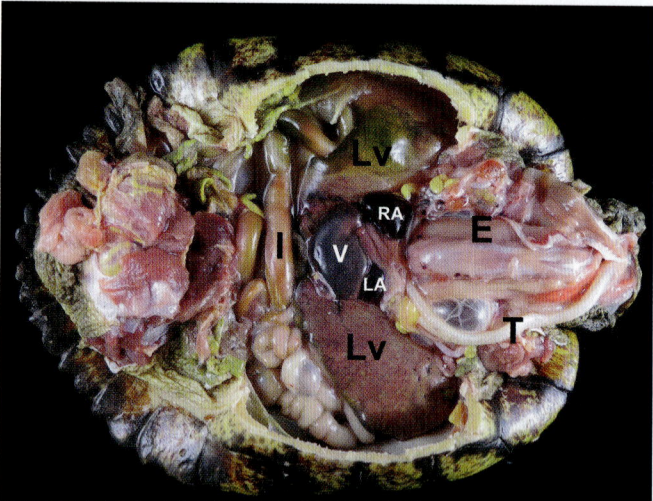

FIG 40.8 Chelonian necropsy. The pectoral and pelvic musculature, ventral coelomic wall, and pericardium have been removed to reveal the left atrium (LA), right atrium (RA), ventricle (V) of the heart, liver (Lv) with bile imbibition of the right lobe clearly visible, intestines (I), esophagus (E), and trachea (T). (Courtesy of Wilson Yau.)

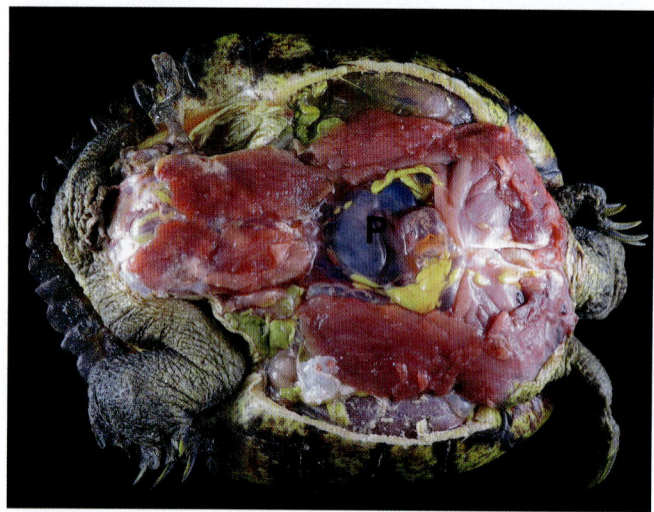

FIG 40.7 Chelonian necropsy. The plastron has been removed to reveal the pectoral and pelvic musculature and pericardium (P). (Courtesy of Wilson Yau.)

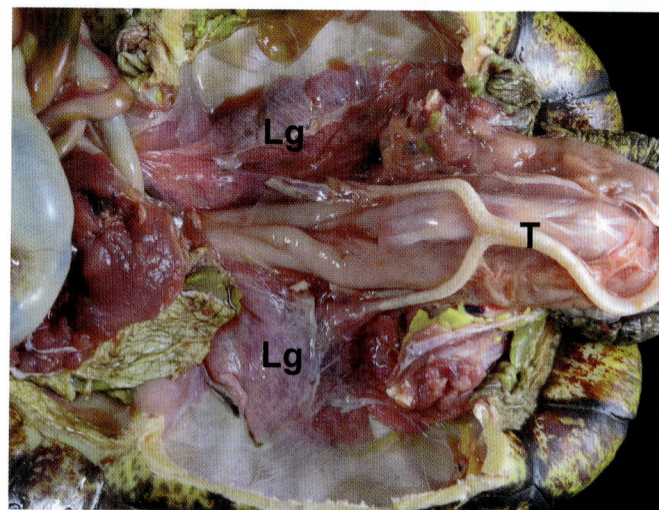

FIG 40.9 Chelonian necropsy. The liver and intestines are removed to reveal the bifurcating trachea (T) and lungs (Lg). The lungs are tightly attached to the ventral aspect of the carapace. (Courtesy of Wilson Yau.)

avoiding the ventral midline vein. Collect fresh tissues and swabs for ancillary testing (refer to the upcoming Step 5). Incise the skin and musculature over the cranium, and expose part of the calvarium using rongeurs, such that formalin can permeate the brain effectively. The entire carcass can then be submerged in 10% neutral buffered formalin. The formalin-to-tissue ratio should exceed 10:1 to ensure thorough fixation.

Larger snakes and lizards: The skin and body wall are gently parted with fingers, forceps, or scissors. When the body is opened, evaluate body condition, evident by the amount of coelomic fat present, and, in some cases, subcutaneous fat (e.g., tail fat storage in leopard geckos). Lizards generally have two paired intracoelomic fat bodies initiating ventrally near the pelvis and growing cranially and laterally as they enlarge with stored fat. Crocodilians have a single intracoelomic fat body on the right side of the coelom caudally. Note the degree of postmortem autolysis, including bile imbibition and pseudomelanosis. Note any effusions present within the coelom or pericardium, including volume, color, and consistency. Observe the visceral arrangement and any apparent displacement of organs. Observe the serosal surfaces for deposition of any abnormal material (such as visceral gout or yolk peritonitis). Some lizards, particularly chameleons and bearded dragons, normally have extensive melanin pigmentation in the mesentery and inner surfaces of the body wall and coelomic fat bodies, and this pigmentation should not be interpreted as a pathologic condition (see Fig. 40.4).

In cases with a high index of suspicion for infectious etiologies, fresh samples should be taken at this point from the lung, liver, and kidney using sterile instruments.

Chelonians: Several methods are used to remove the plastron. In young chelonians or those with significant loss of shell bone, the shells can be separated at the bridge with stout scissors. For larger animals, separation of the shells with a Stryker saw or hacksaw may be necessary (see Fig. 40.6). In all cases, the chelonian is placed on its back, then tilted laterally to a 45-degree angle. This angle allows gravity to shift the viscera downward, so they are not inadvertently incised during the sawing procedure. This is especially important for obtaining sterile cultures of the viscera and for avoiding a full urinary bladder. With care taken not to go too deeply with the saw, the shell is cut at the junction between the plastron and carapace without damaging the underlying soft tissues. Both bridges are sawed through in this manner. With the animal still in dorsal recumbency, scissors are used to cut through the skin at the front and rear attachments to the plastron. The soft tissue attachments are bluntly dissected from the top of the plastron, from rear to front, exposing the intact coelomic wall. For cultures, a small incision can be made in the coelomic wall to allow access to viscera. This provides access to the liver but not the lungs. The lungs are adhered to the ventral surface of the carapace, extend the full length of the carapace, and can be difficult to dissect from the dorsal body wall.

If sterile access to lungs is indicated in a particular case, then the carapace should also be removed. Use scissors to cut the skin at the junction of the carapace (chelonian still in dorsal recumbency), front and rear. A thick screwdriver, wedge, or T-bar is used to disarticulate the tail vertebrae and the cervical (neck) vertebrae from their attachments to the ventral aspect of the carapace. The chelonian is carefully turned over, and gravity is allowed to pull down on the viscera. The tissues are digitally dissected away from the inside aspect of the carapace, starting from the back and moving forward. The large skeletal muscle bundles in the shoulder and pelvic regions may need to be cut with scissors. The carcass is placed in sternal recumbency on the necropsy table, which allows for sterile access to the lung fields by an incision through the wall. This technique is modified for the giant land tortoises and large sea turtles that are too heavy to suspend during dissection of the carcass away from the carapace.

4. Remove and Set Aside the Organs

After examining the organs in situ, including relatively small frequently overlooked organs such as the thyroid glands, thymus, pancreas, adrenal glands, and spleen, isolate "the pluck" from the body wall to thoroughly examine the organs. The pluck incorporates the tongue and the gastrointestinal tract, heart, respiratory tract, and the cloaca. Some prosectors prefer to remove and set aside the spleen before removing the pluck, as this important organ is often small and difficult to locate after the organs have been manipulated. See below for discussion on hematopoietic organs.

Remove the pluck by cutting the tongue away from its attachments and pulling it through the ventral intermandibular space. While applying caudal traction to the tongue, use scissors or fingers to dissect the soft tissue attachments to the dorsal body wall. This procedure may be difficult in large crocodilians and chelonians, and the tissue collection and inspection may need to be done in situ. For better exposure, some prosectors prefer to incise around the perimeters of the ventral body wall on large lizards and crocodilians (with pruning shears to cut through the ribs), rather than on the ventral midline.

5. Examine and Sample the Organs

To minimize cross-contamination when taking fresh samples, start from the cleanest organs and end with the dirtiest organs. In other words, start with lymphoid tissue (spleen, thymus) and then proceed to brain, lungs and heart, kidneys, reproductive tract, liver, and finally the gastrointestinal tract.

Note any abnormalities in each, including distribution of lesions, color, size, shape, consistency, and the presence of any exudates. Examine both the capsular surface, as well as the cut surfaces. Make serial cuts of the liver, lung, and kidney to check for any focal lesions. Crushing should be avoided when using forceps to take samples. Using a sharp blade and a hard surface (cutting board) can minimize artifacts. When sampling mucosal surfaces, avoid rubbing the mucosa vigorously with fingers or instruments. If particular organs appear enlarged or small, obtain a weight of the organ to calculate percentage body weight (%BW) as an objective measurement.

In-house cytology performed on intestinal contents, masses, and granulomas is inexpensive and can sometimes offer quick insights into infectious or neoplastic etiologies. If tissue imprints are to be made, the procedure and slides should be made far away from formalin fumes, as the latter can introduce significant artifacts in the resulting imprints. The process of making imprints can distort tissue architecture (especially with kidney, liver, and gut mucosa), such that submission of other pieces of tissue not subjected to imprints is preferred (see Chapter 38).

Hematopoietic and Lymphoid Tissues (Spleen, Thymus, Bone Marrow, Peripheral Blood). Most reptiles lack discrete lymph nodes, although extensive lymphatic networks are present. Examination of these tissues provides clues to immune status, anemia, and various infectious and nutritional problems. Evaluation of overall lymphoid cellularity can give a crude estimation of immune status and can also provide evidence of exposure to stress.

The spleen is generally a small ovoid brown/red or tan structure located in the mesentery, off the greater curvature of the stomach, and often close to the gallbladder and pancreas (see Fig. 40.3). The association of these three organs is often referred to as the triad in snakes and is useful in helping to find the organs during imaging, surgery, or necropsy. The spleen can be difficult to find but is important to examine for the presence of infectious disease processes. The thymus is a lobulated structure and variable in location and may be found from the base of the heart to the neck.

Bone marrow can be collected from the medullary cavity of long bones. Crack open a long bone to ensure the presence of bone marrow, and then the whole bone can be placed in formalin. For larger species, bone marrow can be scooped out and placed in a cassette to be fixed in formalin.

Snakes and chelonians: In many species the spleen is fused with the pancreas (splenopancreas). Snapping turtles have lymphoid follicles present in the cloaca. The bone marrow is "trabecular" in nature and may be difficult to collect separately.

Lizards: The bone marrow is normally gelatinous.

Endocrine Organs (Adrenal, Pancreas, Thyroid, Parathyroid, Ultimobranchial, Pituitary, Pineal Glands). The adrenal gland is paired in reptiles but varies considerably in shape and location. Generally, it is a tubular-shaped or an ovoid structure closely associated with the kidneys and gonads. Microscopic changes in the adrenal gland can indicate stress, which can be difficult to evaluate by external observation.

The thyroid is a single structure (except variations in lizards) located at the base of the heart or at the bifurcation of the greater vessels. It is amber and appears multilobulated on cut surfaces. It can be mistaken for an abnormal mass. Examination of the thyroid for evidence of goiter or neoplasia is important. Thyroid size may vary from seasonal changes in follicular diameter, so mild enlargement may be a physiological rather than pathologic event. Also in the region of the thyroid are small lobulated structures that represent the thymus, parathyroid, and ultimobranchial bodies. Normally, ultimobranchial bodies are difficult to locate on gross examination.

The pancreas has both exocrine (digestive) and endocrine functions. Pancreatic examination is important because it develops microscopic changes indicative of nutritional status. Some infectious disease processes have a tropism for the pancreas, such as paramyxovirus and monocercomoniasis in snakes. It is important to be aware of the location of the islet cell tissue in the pancreas of the reptile patient, as much variability exists. It may be best to submit the entire pancreas for histopathology to allow thorough evaluation of endocrine and exocrine tissue.

The pituitary and pineal glands are extremely small structures that are rarely diseased. If examination is warranted, it is recommended to submit the entire head of a necropsy specimen and request their examinations explicitly on the submission form. The head will then be decalcified and serial sectioned to look for these organs.

Snakes and chelonians: The pancreas is often fused with the spleen (splenopancreas) and located in the mesentery next to the gut and gallbladder.

Snakes and lizards: The adrenals are incorporated into the mesorchium of the male and mesovarium of the female.

Crocodilians: The adrenal gland is retroperitoneal, lying dorsolateral to the genital ducts.

Cardiovascular System (Heart, Great Vessels).

A broad array of disease processes affects the cardiovascular system, such as atherosclerosis, bacterial endocarditis, endocardiosis, degenerative cardiomyopathy, thrombosis of the greater vessels and their main branches, and mineralization of the greater vessels. If cardiac pathology is of concern in a case, avoid intracardiac injections of euthanasia solution, as this can introduce significant histologic artifacts to the myocardium and vasculature.

Other than crocodilians, all reptiles possess a three-chambered heart, with muscular ridges partitioning the single ventricle. A fibrous attachment is sometimes present, connecting the pericardial sac to the apex of the ventricle (gubernaculum cordis), which is normal. For microscopic examination, routine submission of the entire heart of small reptiles (minus any fresh tissue for cultures) is recommended. For larger reptiles, full-thickness sections of the ventricle, both atria, and sections of the valves of larger reptiles is recommended. Opening the heart during dissection to allow for formalin perfusion is helpful for adequate fixation and may reveal lesions worthy of culture before formalin submersion. If the size of the heart permits, open the heart at the vena cava with blunt-tipped scissors at its insertion in the right atrium, extend the incision through the wall of the ventricle toward the apex, and then back up the left side to the aortic outflow. Reflecting the ventricles after this procedure exposes the valves for visual examination.

Visual identification of the aorta and major branches, and full-length examination of the luminal surfaces, is also recommended, especially if the animal has a history suggestive of thrombosis or vasculitis. A short length of cardiac outflow vessels (greater vessels) should routinely be submitted.

Blood films on slides can be made from heart blood at necropsy, provided the blood is not clotted. Blood collected in blood tubes can be centrifuged, and the resulting serum can be frozen and held for specific tests, such as electrolyte measurements.

Respiratory System (Trachea, Bronchi, Lung, Pseudodiaphragm).

Numerous disease processes affect the respiratory tract, especially infectious diseases and mineralization from metabolic or nutritional disorders. Submission of the entire head ensures microscopic examination of the nasal cavity and larynx. Representative sections of the trachea and lung should always be submitted. In reptiles, the lung is a hollow sac with a honeycomb appearance on the inner surface. The anterior portion often has a thick, vascularized wall for respiratory function. The posterior portions are often thin-walled in nature. If size permits,

open the trachea in its entirety and extend the incisions into the bronchi to look for parasites, effusions, or reddening of the mucosa. Palpate all lobes, if present, of the lungs for firmness (granulomas or neoplasia). The nasal cavity can be exposed by rongeurs to examine the nasal turbinates. Reptiles do not possess a muscular diaphragm, although tuataras, monitors, and crocodiles have a pseudodiaphragm.

Snakes: In nonboids, the right lung is well developed, while the left lung is generally reduced in size or absent. The lungs continue posteriorly as an air sac and can extend to the most caudal aspects of the coelomic cavity.

Lizards: The tracheal rings are incomplete. Geckos have chambered lungs, while iguanas and chameleons have transitional lungs with a large septum dividing a single chamber. The monitor and beaded lizards have multichambered lungs.

Chelonians: Complete cartilaginous rings are present. In sea turtles, the central bronchus extends throughout the length of the lungs. The lungs are attached to the ventral surface of the carapace, which consists of large, multichambered structures separated by septa (see Fig. 40.9). These can be difficult to dissect and remove from the carapace.

Crocodilians: The extrapulmonary bronchi can be extensive.

Urogenital System (Kidney, Urinary Bladder, Ovary, Uterus, Testes, Phallus/Hemipenes).

Common disease conditions in reptiles that involve the urinary tract include chronic renal disease (especially iguanas), gout, urolithiasis (often large stones), nephrocalcinosis, bacterial and parasitic infections, and neoplasia.[4] The kidneys are paired and are generally located in the caudal coelomic cavity. Routine collection of reproductive tissues is important. Common reproductive problems in reptiles and amphibians include bacterial infections, neoplasia, and preovulatory and postovulatory follicular stasis; uterine/oviductal/cloacal disease; and mineralization, impaction, or prolapse of the hemipenes.[4] The urogenital system is similar in most reptiles. Gonads are paired. Females have paired oviducts (salpinx), and males have a paired epididymides and vasa deferentia. Identification of the kidneys, gonads, and adrenals in situ is important so that they are not lost or inadvertently overlooked during prosection. When present, the urinary bladder should be opened to look for cystic calculi, eggs, and parasites.

Lizards: The kidneys are especially caudal and can be missed at necropsy (see Fig. 40.5). The urinary bladder is absent in certain lizards. Lizards possess hemipenes tucked inside the base of the tail. Hemipenal appearance varies in size, shape, and external appearance among species.

Snakes: The kidneys are lobulated, elongated, and resemble an oblique stack of coins. During breeding season, male snakes (and some male lizards) can undergo a renal change and develop a "sexual segment," resulting in a more swollen and pale appearance to the kidney. The urinary bladder is absent, such that ureters directly enter the urodeum. The right gonad is cranial to that of the left. The testes are elongated, lightly colored, and are located between the pancreas and the kidneys. On the other hand, the ovaries are often nearer the pancreas. Snakes possess hemipenes inside the base of the tail, which vary in size, shape, and external appearance among different species.

Chelonians: Similar to lizards, the kidneys are especially caudal, and removal of pelvic bones ventrally is recommended to access and visualize them. Chelonians possess a phallus, while the tuatara do not have any specialized intromittent organ.

Crocodilians: The urinary bladder is absent. Crocodiles possess a phallus.

Liver.

The liver is the largest organ in the coelomic cavity (see Figs. 40.2 and 40.8). It is generally bilobed, and all species have a gallbladder. The gallbladder is intimately associated with the right liver lobe in most lizards and chelonians. Hepatic diseases include infectious processes, neoplasia, toxicosis, lipidosis, cirrhosis, and melanosis.[4] Observe all the lobes for any uneven coloration and palpate for any evidence of friability or firmness. Although the normal liver is brown, abundant melanin can turn it black. A pale yellow to white and fatty liver can be associated with not only overfeeding and obesity but also impaired metabolism, anoxia, and toxins. However, seasonal, metabolic, and often associated reproductive activity can result in normal lipid movement into the liver of females, and this must be differentiated from true pathology (see Chapters 67 and 151). If sections of liver float in 10% neutral buffered formalin, consistent with lipidosis, then this should be noted. The gallbladder should be incised to examine the mucosal surface and look for any choleliths or parasites that may be present.

Snakes: The gallbladder is separated from, and caudal to, the liver, located close to the spleen and pancreas. There is a cystic duct that connects the gall bladder to the duodenum.

Nervous System (Brain, Spinal Cord). Diseases of the nervous system are commonly seen in reptiles and amphibians and are usually manifestations of other visceral disorders, such as gout, neoplasia, intoxication, or infectious disease. For small reptiles, the brain and cord are best examined when the entire head and vertebrae are submitted. For those animals too large for submission of an entire head and vertebral column, prosection of the spinal cord and brain is necessary. Using a knife or scalpel blade, the skin and musculature overlying the atlanto-occipital junction is incised, while moving the head up and down to facilitate separation without having to cut through bone. Exposure of the dorsocaudal aspect of the calvarium is achieved by removing the overlying soft tissue. The skull is removed piecemeal using rongeurs, starting at the foramen magnum and working rostrally, paying attention not to damage the brain underneath. Larger heads may require a Stryker saw or handsaw to cut through the calvarium. The top of the vertebral body (spinal process and lamina) can be removed for access to the spinal cord.

Extra care should be exercised when examining venomous snakes. The mouth should be taped shut so fingers are not impaled on fangs, and the top of the skull should be removed with a Stryker saw or bone rongeur for exposure to the brain. With submission of the head from venomous reptiles, labeling the containers "venomous" is important. Taping the mouth shut is useful when removing the brain, but fixation of the tissues may be impeded if the entire head is placed in formalin.

Gastrointestinal Tract. Disease conditions of the alimentary tract are especially common in reptiles, including a wide variety of bacterial, fungal, viral, and parasitic diseases.[4] Obstruction, plication, or ulceration from luminal passage of foreign bodies, intussusception (telescoping), stasis, and rectal/cloacal prolapse also are occasionally seen. Preferably, the pathologist should examine microscopically all segments of the alimentary tract, including the oral cavity (included with the head), esophagus, stomach, small intestine (duodenum, jejunum, and ileum regions), colon, rectum, and cloaca. Identifying particular segments of the intestines can be difficult histologically, especially when compounded by autolysis. Placing segments of intestines in separate and labeled cassettes can be helpful for the pathologist. If anaerobic etiological agents are suspected, segments of intestines should be tied off (if size permits) before placing into Whirl-Pak Bags. This allows for anaerobic culture of the intestinal contents, which would otherwise be compromised if the lumen is exposed to air. If ingestion of heavy metal is suspected, radiographs can be useful to demonstrate metal within the gastrointestinal tract that can easily be missed on the gross necropsy.

Snakes: Most snakes do not possess a cecum but have cloacal glands that exit at the caudolateral vent margins.

Lizards: Green iguanas (*Iguana iguana*) normally have a darkened tongue tip. They also have a sacculated large intestine.

Chelonians: Turtles lack teeth. Sea turtles have prominent spines associated with the esophageal mucosa, which should normally be directed caudally toward the stomach and are rigid. The intestinal tract is relatively short in carnivores and longer in herbivores.

6. Write the Report

Although formalin-fixed and frozen tissues can be stored for long periods of time, the written report and photographs are the only legal documents and physical evidence that remain once a gross necropsy is completed. Therefore it is critical that the thorough and succinct report includes high-quality photographs and is based on the contemporaneous notes taken during the necropsy examination. Table 40.3 is a sample necropsy form that includes a tissue checklist, which should accompany all histopathologic submissions to help the pathologist put findings in context.

The report should include at least the following information:

- Animal signalment: species, breed, age, sex
- Clinical history
- Died or euthanized, nutritional status
- Findings organized by organ system: external findings and musculoskeletal, lymphoid, respiratory, digestive, urogenital, and nervous systems

AFTER THE NECROPSY

Carcasses should be disposed of according to federal, state, and county regulations. Saved formalin-fixed tissues and Whirl-Pak Bags should be properly labeled and stored. If large amounts of fixed tissues need to be shipped, it may be preferable to thoroughly fix the tissues in formalin (at least 48 hours) and then pour off the formalin and wrap the fixed tissues in formalin-soaked power towels or gauze to be shipped. This avoids the need to ship large jars of formalin. However, proper infrastructure to handle formalin disposal and fumes is required.

ACKNOWLEDGMENTS

We would like to thank Dr. Mike Garner for his work on the previous edition of this textbook chapter, and Dr. Rita McManamon and Dr. Stephen Divers for collecting carcasses to be photographed. Several necropsy protocols, both specific to reptiles and modified from mammals, have been referenced as well.[4-8]

REFERENCES

See www.expertconsult.com for a complete list of references.

41

Diagnostic Laboratory Listing

Stephen J. Divers

Below is a list of diagnostic laboratories that have been fully or provisionally accredited through the American Association of Veterinary Laboratory Diagnosticians (AAVLD) (North America). This list is regularly updated and readers are advised to check current listings at http://www.aavld.org/accredited-laboratories.

Additional laboratories that are not accredited through the AAVLD have been included by recommendations from members of the Association of Reptilian and Amphibian Veterinarians, American Association of Zoo Veterinarians, American College of Zoological Medicine, and the European College of Zoological Medicine. It is the responsibility of those wishing to use these labs to ensure that they are satisfied with laboratory quality control and methodology validations.

NORTH AMERICA (ACCREDITED LABORATORIES)

Alabama

Thompson-Bishop Sparks State Diagnostic Laboratory
890 Simms Road
PO Box 2209
Auburn, AL 36832
Director: Dr. David G. Pugh
Ph: 334-844-7207
Fax: 334-844-7206
Email: dgp0003@auburn.edu
http://labs.alabama.gov

Arizona

Arizona Veterinary Diagnostic Laboratory
2831 N. Freeway
Tucson, AZ 85705
Interim Director: Dr. Sharon Dial
Phone: 520-621-2356 Ex 16
Fax: 520-626-8696
Email: sdial@email.arizona.edu
http://www.cals.arizona.edu/vdl

California
Main Laboratory
CA Animal Health & Food Safety Laboratory System
University of California
Davis Shipping Address:
620 W. Health Science Dr.
Davis, CA 95616
Mailing Address:
PO Box 1770
Davis, CA 95617-1770

Director: Dr. Pam Hullinger
Phone: 530-752-8709
Fax: 530-752-5680
Email: phullinger@ucdavis.edu
www.cahfs.ucdavis.edu

Branch Laboratories

CAHFS, San Bernardino Laboratory
105 W. Central Avenue
San Bernardino, CA
92408-2113
Branch Chief: Dr. Francisco Uzal
Phone: 909-383-4287
Fax: 909-884-5980
Email: sanbernardinocahfs@ucdavis.edu

CAHFS, Turlock Laboratory
1550 North Soderquist Rd.
Turlock, CA 95380
Branch Chief: Dr. Simone Stoute
Phone: 209-634-5837
Fax: 209-667-4261
Email: turlockcahfs@ucdavis.edu

CAHFS, Tulare Laboratory
18830 Road 112
Tulare, CA
93274-9042
Branch Chief: Dr. John Adaska
Phone: 559-688-7543
Fax: 559-686-4231
Email: tularecahfs@ucdavis.edu

Colorado
Main Laboratory
Veterinary Diagnostic Laboratory
Colorado State University
Shipping Address:
300 West Drake Road
Fort Collins, CO 80523
Mailing Address:
200 West Lake Street 1644 Campus Delivery
Fort Collins, CO 80523-1644
Director: Dr. Barbara Powers
Phone: 970-297-1281
Fax: 970-297-0320

Email: CVMBSEmaildlab@colostate.edu
http://www.dlab.colostate.edu

Branch Laboratories
Rocky Ford Veterinary Diagnostic Laboratory
27847 Road 21
Rocky Ford, CO 81067
Director: Dr. Gene Niles
Phone: 719-254-6382
Email: gene.niles@colostate.edu

Western Slope Veterinary Diagnostic Laboratory
425 29 Road
Grand Junction, CO 81504
Director: Dr. Don Kitchen
Phone: 970-243-0673
Email: vdl_western_slope@colostate.edu

Connecticut
Connecticut Veterinary Medical Diagnostic Laboratory
University of Connecticut
Department of Pathobiology & Veterinary Science
Shipping Address:
61 N. Eagleville Road, Unit 3089
Storrs, CT 06269-3089
Mailing Address:
61 N. Eagleville Road, Unit 3089
Storrs, CT 06269-3089
Director: Dr. Joan Smyth
Phone: 860-486-3738
Fax: 860-486-2794
Email: joan.smyth@uconn.edu
http://www.patho.uconn.edu

Florida
Bronson Animal Disease Diagnostic Laboratory
Florida Dept. of Agriculture & Consumer Services
Shipping Address:
2700 N. John Young Parkway
Kissimmee, FL 34741
Mailing Address:
2700 N. John Young Parkway
Kissimmee, FL 34741
Director: Dr. Y. Reddy Bommineni
Phone: 321-697-1400
Fax: 321-697-1467
Email: reddy.bommineni@freshfromflorida.com
www.freshfromflorida.com/baddl

Georgia
Athens Veterinary Diagnostic Laboratory
University of Georgia
College of Veterinary Medicine
501 W. Brooks Drive
Athens, GA 30602-7383
Director: Dr. Jeremiah Saliki
Phone: 706-542-5568
Fax: 706-542-5977
Email: jsaliki@uga.edu
http://www.vet.uga.edu/dlab

Tifton Veterinary Diagnostic and Investigation Laboratory
University of Georgia
Shipping Address:
43 Brighton Road
Tifton, GA 31793
Mailing Address:
PO Box 1389
Tifton, GA 31793
Director: Dr. Murray E. Hines II
Phone: 229-386-3340
Fax: 229-386-7128
Email: mhinesii@uga.edu
http://www.vet.uga.edu/dlab

Illinois
Animal Disease Laboratory, Illinois Department of Agriculture
Mailing Address:
2100 S. Lake Storey Road
Galesburg, IL 61401
Director: Dr. Dale M Webb
Phone: 309-344-2451
Fax: 309-344-7358
Email: dale.webb@illinois.gov
www.agr.state.il.us

Veterinary Diagnostic Laboratory
University of Illinois
Shipping Address:
2001 South Lincoln Avenue, Room 1224
Urbana, IL 61802
Mailing Address:
PO Box U
Urbana, IL 61802
Director: Dr. Richard Fredrickson
Phone: 217-333-1620
Fax: 217-244-2439
Email: vdldirectoroffice@vetmed.illinois.edu
http://www.cvm.uiuc.edu/vdl

Indiana
Main Laboratory
Animal Disease Diagnostic Laboratory
Purdue University
406 South University Street
West Lafayette, IN 47907
Director: Dr. Steven Lenz
Phone: 765-494-7440
Fax: 765-494-9181
Email: slenz@purdue.edu
http://www.addl.purdue.edu

Branch Laboratory
Heeke Animal Disease Diagnostic Laboratory (Southern Indiana)
11367 E. Purdue Farm Road
Dubois, IN 47527-9666
Director: Dr. Grant Burcham
Phone: 812-678-3401
Fax: 812-678-3412
gburcham@purdue.edu

Iowa

Veterinary Diagnostic Laboratory, College of Veterinary Medicine
Iowa State University
1600 S. 16th Street
Ames, IA 50011
Director: Dr. Rodger Main
Phone: 515-294-1950
Fax: 515-294-3564
Email: rmain@iastate.edu
http://www.vdpam.iastate.edu

Kentucky

Breathitt Veterinary Center
Murray State University
Shipping Address:
715 North Drive
Hopkinsville, KY 42240
Mailing Address:
PO Box 2000
Hopkinsville, KY 42241-2000
Director: Dr. Debbie Reed
Phone: 270-886-3959
Fax: 270-886-4295
Email: dreed@murraystate.edu
https://breathitt.murraystate.edu/

Veterinary Diagnostic Laboratory—Lexington
Shipping Address:
1490 Bull Lea Road
Lexington, KY 40511
Mailing Address:
PO Box 14125
Lexington, KY 40512
Director: Dr. Craig Carter
Phone: 859-257-8283
Fax: 859-255-1624
Email: craig.carter@uky.edu
http://www.vdl.uky.edu/

Louisiana

LA Animal Disease Diagnostic Laboratory
Shipping Address:
River Road, Room 1043
Baton Rouge, LA 70803
Mailing Address:
River Road, Room 1043
Baton Rouge, LA 70803
Director: Dr. Daniel Paulsen
Phone: 225-578-9777
Fax: 225-578-9784
Email: dpauls1@lsu.edu
http://laddl.lsu.edu

Michigan

Michigan State University Veterinary Diagnostic Laboratory (MSU VDL)
Shipping Address:
4125 Beaumont Road, Room 122
Lansing, MI 48910-8104
Mailing Address:
PO Box 30076
Lansing, MI 48909-7576

Director: Dr. Rachel Reams
Phone: 517-353-0635
Fax: 517-353-5096
Email: reamsrac@dcpah.msu.edu
http://www.animalhealth.msu.edu

Minnesota

Veterinary Diagnostic Laboratory
University of Minnesota
1333 Gortner Avenue
St. Paul, MN 55108-1098
Director: Dr. Jerry Torrison
Phone: 612-624-0497
Fax: 612-624-8707
Email: torri001@umn.edu
http://www.vdl.umn.edu

Mississippi

Main Laboratory

Mississippi Veterinary Research and Diagnostic Laboratory System
Mississippi State University
Shipping Address:
3137 Highway 468 West
Pearl, MS 39208
Mailing Address:
PO Box 97813
Pearl, MS 39288
Executive Director: Dr. Lanny Pace
Phone: 601-420-4700
Fax: 601-420-4719
Email: lpace@mvrdl.msstate.edu
http://www.cvm.msstate.edu

Branch Laboratories

Poultry Research & Diagnostic Laboratory
PRDL College of Veterinary Medicine
3137 Highway 468 West
Pearl, MS 39208
Phone: 601-420-4700
Fax: 601-420-4719
Director: Dr. Danny Pagee
Phone: 601-420-4700
Fax: 601-420-4719

The College of Veterinary Medicine Diagnostic Laboratory Services (CVM-DLS)
Full service, all species
Veterinary Specialty Center
1207 Highway 182 W, Suite D
Starkville, MS 39759
Phone: 662-325-7339
Fax: 662-325-3436

The Aquatic Research and Diagnostic Laboratory - ARDL
Thad Cochran National Warmwater Aquaculture Center
Stoneville, MS 38776
Phone: 662-686-3302

Missouri

Veterinary Medical Diagnostic Laboratory
University of Missouri
Shipping Address:

1600 East Rollins Road
Columbia, MO 65211
Mailing Address:
PO Box 6023
Columbia, MO 65205
Director: Dr. Shuping Zhang
Phone: 573-882-6811
Fax: 573-882-1411
Email: zhangshup@missouri.edu
http://www.cvm.missouri.edu/vmdl

Montana

Montana Department of Livestock
Montana Veterinary Diagnostic Laboratory
Shipping Address:
South 19th and Lincoln
Bozeman, MT 59718
Mailing Address:
PO Box 997
Bozeman, MT 59771
Director: Dr. A.W. Layton
Phone: 406-994-4885
Fax: 406-994-6344
Email: blayton@mt.gov
http://www.discoveringmontana.com/liv/lab/index.asp

Nebraska

Veterinary Diagnostic Center
Shipping Address:
PO Box 82646
Fair Street, E. Campus Loop
Lincoln, NE 68501-2646
Mailing Address:
PO Box 830907
Lincoln, NE 68583-0907
Director: Dr. Al Doster
Phone: 402-472-1434
Fax: 402-472-3094
Email: adoster@unl.edu
http://vbms.unl.edu/nvdls.shtml

New York
Main Laboratory
Animal Health Diagnostic Center
College of Veterinary Medicine Cornell University
Shipping Address:
240 Farrier Road
Ithaca, NY 14853
Mailing Address:
PO Box 5786
Ithaca, NY 14852
Director: Francois Elvinger
Phone: 607-253-3900
Fax: 607-253-3943
Email: fe65@cornell.edu
http://diaglab.vet.cornell.edu

Branch Laboratories
AHDC Quality Milk Production Service
4530 Millennium Drive
Geneseo, NY 14454
Director: Dr. Rick Waters

Phone: 585-243-1780
rdw34@cornell.edu

AHDC Quality Milk Production Service
34 Cornell Drive
Canton, NY 13617
Phone: 315-379-3930
jgs385@cornell.edu

AHDC Quality Milk Production Service
111 Schene Ctady
Cobelskill, NY 12043
Phone: 518-255-5681
mjz6@cornell.edu

North Carolina
Main Laboratory
North Carolina Department of Agriculture & Consumer Services
Rollins Laboratory
Shipping Address:
2101 Blue Ridge Road
Raleigh, NC 27607
Mailing Address:
1031 Mail Service Center
Raleigh, NC 27699-1031
Interim Director: Dr. James Trybus
Phone: 919-733-3986
Fax: 919-733-0454
Email: james.trybus@ncagr.gov
http://www.ncagr.gov/vet/ncvdl

Branch Laboratories
Western Animal Disease Diagnostic Laboratory
Arden Laboratory
785 Airport Road
Fletcher, NC 28732
Director: Dr. Richard C. Oliver
Phone: 828-684-8188
Fax: 828-687-3574

Northwestern Animal Disease Diagnostic Laboratory
Elkin Laboratory
1689 N. Bridge Street
Elkin, NC 28621
Director: Dr. Brad Barlow
Phone: 336-526-2499
Fax: 336-526-2603

Hoyle C. Griffin Animal Disease Diagnostic Laboratory
Griffin Laboratory
401 Quarry Road
Monroe, N.C. 28112
Director: Dr. Kim Hagans
Phone: 704-289-6448
Fax: 704-283-9660

North Dakota

Veterinary Diagnostic Laboratory
North Dakota State University
Shipping Address:
Veterinary Diagnostic Laboratory, Van Es Hall

1523 Centennial Boulevard
Fargo, ND 58105
Mailing Address:
NDSU Dept 7691
PO Box 6050
Fargo, ND 58108-6050
Director: Dr. Neil Dyer
Phone: 701-231-8307
Fax: 701-231-7514
Email: neil.dyer@ndsu.edu
http://www.vdl.ndsu.edu

Ohio

Animal Disease Diagnostic Laboratory
8995 E. Main Street, Building 6
Reynoldsburg, OH 43068
Director: Dr. Beverly Byrum
Phone: 614-728-6220
Fax: 614-728-6310
Email: byrum@agri.ohio.gov
http://www.ohioagriculture.gov/addl

Oklahoma

Oklahoma Animal Disease Diagnostic Laboratory
Oklahoma State University
Shipping Address:
Center for Veterinary Health Sciences
Farm and Ridge Road
Stillwater, OK 74078
Mailing Address:
PO Box 7001
Stillwater, OK 740767001
Director: Dr. Keith Bailey
Phone: 405-744-6623
Fax: 405-744-8612
Email: keith.bailey@okstate.edu
http://www.cvm.okstate.edu

Oregon

Veterinary Diagnostic Laboratory
Oregon State University
Magruder Hall, Room 134
Shipping Address:
30th and Washington Way
Corvallis, OR 97331
Mailing Address:
134 Magruder Hall
Corvallis OR 97331
Interim Director: Rob Bildfell
Phone: 541-737-3261
Fax: 541-737-6817
Email: bildfelr@oregonstate.edu
http://vetmed.oregonstate.edu/diagnostic

Pennsylvania

Department of Agriculture Pennsylvania Veterinary Laboratory
2305 N. Cameron Street
Harrisburg, PA 17110-9408
Director: Dr. Deepanker Tewari
Phone: 717-787-8808
Fax: 717-772-3895

Email: dtewari@pa.gov
http://www.padls.org

Pennsylvania State University
PADLS—Penn State Animal Diagnostic Laboratory
Orchard Road
University Park, PA 16802-1110
Resident Director: Dr. Bhushan Jayarao
Phone: 814-863-0837
Fax: 814-865-3907
Email: bmj3@psu.edu
http://www.padls.org

University of Pennsylvania
PADLS
382 West Street Road
Kennett Square, PA 19348
Director: Dr. Lisa Murphy
Phone: 610-444-5800
Fax: 610-925-8106
Email: murphylp@vet.upenn.edu
http://www.padls.org

South Dakota

Animal Disease Research and Diagnostic Laboratory
South Dakota State University
Shipping Address:
Animal Disease Research Building
North Campus Drive
Brookings, SD 57007-1396
Mailing Address:
Box 2175, North Campus Drive
Brookings, SD 57007-1396
Director: Dr. Jane Christopher-Hennings
Phone: 605-688-5171
Fax: 605-688-6003
Email: jane.hennings@sdstate.edu
http://vetsci.sdstate.edu

Tennessee

CE Kord Animal Health Diagnostic Laboratory
Ellington Agriculture Center
Shipping Address:
440 Hogan Road, Porter Building
Nashville, TN 37220
Mailing Address:
PO Box 40627
Nashville, TN 37204
Director: Dr. Bruce G. McLaughlin
Phone: 847-714-2753
Fax: 615-837-5250
Email: bruce.mclaughlin@tn.gov
http://www.state.tn.us/agriculture/regulate/labs/kordlab.html

Texas

Main Laboratory
Texas A&M Veterinary Medical Diagnostic Laboratory (TVMDL)
TVMDL—College Station
Shipping Address:
1 Sippel Road
College Station, TX 77843

Mailing Address:
PO Drawer 3040
College Station, TX 77841-3040
Director: Dr. Bruce Akey
Phone: 979-845-3414
Fax: 979-845-1794
Email: bakey@tvmdl.tamu.edu
http://tvmdl.tamu.edu

Branch Laboratories

TVMDL—Amarillo
Shipping Address:
6610 Amarillo Blvd., West
Amarillo, TX 79106
Mailing Address:
PO Box 3200
Amarillo, TX 79116-3200
Resident Director: Dr. Gayman Helman
Phone: 806-353-7478
Fax: 806-359-0636
Email: ghelman@tvmdl.tamu.edu
http://tvmdl.tamu.edu

TVMDL - Gonzales
Shipping Address:
1162 East Sarah DeWitt Drive
Gonzales, TX 78629
Mailing Address:
PO Box 84
Gonzales, TX 78629
Resident Director: Dr. Martin Ficken
Phone: 830-672-2834
Fax: 830-672-2835
Email: mficken@tvmdl.tamu.edu
http://tvmdl.tamu.edu

TVMDL - Center
Shipping/Mailing Address:
635 Malone Drive
Center, TX 79535
Resident Director: Dr. Randle Moore
Phone: 936-598-4451
Fax: 936-598-2741
Email: rmoore@tamu.edu
http://tvmdl.tamu.edu

Utah
Main Laboratory
Utah Veterinary Diagnostic Laboratory
Utah State University
950 East 1400 North
Logan, UT 84341
Director: Dr. Thomas Baldwin
Phone: 435-797-1885
Fax: 435-797-2805
Email: tom.baldwin@usu.edu

Virginia

Virginia Maryland College
Virginia Tech Animal Laboratory Services
Virginia Maryland
College of Veterinary Medicine

Blacksburg, VA
Shipping/Mailing Address:
245 Duckpond Drive
Blacksburg, VA 24061
Director: Dr. Tanya LeRoth
Phone: 540-231-4320
Email: tleroith@vt.edu

Branch Laboratory

Central Utah Branch Laboratory
1451 South Main
Nephi, UT 84648
Director: Dr. Thomas Baldwin
Phone: 435-623-1402
Fax: 435-623-1548
www.usu.edu/uvdl

Washington
Main Laboratory
**Washington Animal Disease Diagnostic
    Laboratory**
Washington State University
Shipping Address:
Hall Room 155N
Pullman, WA 99164-7034
Mailing Address:
PO Box 647034
Pullman, WA 99164-7034
Executive Director: Dr. Tim Baszler
Phone: 509-335-6047
Fax: 509-335-7424
Email: baszlert@vetmed.wsu.edu
http://www.vetmed.wsu.edu/depts_waddl

Branch Laboratory

**WADDL-Puyallup, Avian Health Food Safety
    Laboratory**
Washington State University
2607 W Pioneer
Puyallup, WA 98371-4990
Phone: 253-445-4537
Email: http://waddl.vetmed.wsu.edu/avian

Wisconsin
Main Laboratory
Wisconsin Veterinary Diagnostic Laboratory
University of Wisconsin
445 Easterday Lane
Madison, WI 53706
Director: Dr. Philip Bochsler
Phone: 608-262-5432
Fax: 847-574-8085
Email: Phil.bochsler@wvdl.wisc.edu or info@wvdl.wisc.edu
http://www.wvdl.wisc.edu

Branch Laboratory

Wisconsin Veterinary Diagnostic Laboratory
1521 E. Guy Avenue
Barron, WI 54812
Phone: 715-637-3151
Toll Free: 800-771-8387
Fax: 715-637-9220

Wyoming

Wyoming State Veterinary Laboratory
1174 Snowy Range Road
Laramie, WY 82070
Director: Dr. Will Laegreid
Phone: 307-766-9925
Direct line: 307-766-9929
Fax: 307-721-2051
Email: vetrec@uwyo.edu or wlaegrei@uwyo.edu

Canada

Animal Health Laboratory
University of Guelph
Shipping Address:
419 Gordon Street
NW Corner Gordon/McGilvray
Guelph, Ontario N1G 2W1
Mailing Address:
PO Box 3612, Guelph
Ontario N1H 6R8
Director: Dr. Grant Maxie
Phone: 519-824-4120, ext. 54530
Fax: 519-827-0961
Email: gmaxie@lsd.uoguelph.ca
http://ahl.uoguelph.ca

The Animal Health Centre
1767 Angus Campbell Road
Abbotsford, BC V3G 2M3 Canada
Director: Dr. Jane Pritchard
Phone: 604-556-3003
Fax: 604-556-3010
Email: jane.pritchard@gov.bc.ca
http://www.agf.gov.bc.ca/ahc/

University of Montreal
Diagnostic Services
Faculte de medecine veterinaire
Shipping Address:
3200 rue Sicotte
Saint-Hyacinthe, Quebec
Canada J2S 2M2
Mailing Address:
C. P. 5000 Saint-Hyacinthe
Quebec, J2S 7C6
Director: Dr. Estela Cornaglia, DMV, PhD
Phone: 450-773-8521
Fax: 450-778-8107
Email: estela.cornaglia@umontreal.ca
http://servicediagnostic.com

NORTH AMERICA (LABS WITH PROVISIONAL ACCREDITATION)

Kansas

Kansas State Veterinary Diagnostic Laboratory
Kansas State University
1800 Denison Avenue
Moiser Hall Manhattan, KS 66506
Interim Director: Dr. Jamie Henningson
Phone: 785-532-5650

Fax: 785-532-4481
Email: Heningsn@vet.k-state.edu
http://www.ksvdl.org

NORTH AMERICA (NONACCREDITED LABORATORIES)

California

Zoo/Exotic Pathology Service
6020 Rutland Drive #14
Carmichael, CA. 95608
Director: Dr. Drury Reavill
Phone: 800-457-7981
Fax: 916-725-6155
zooexotic@icloud.com
http://zooexotic.com
Histology, cytology, and necropsy services

Amphibian Disease Laboratory
15600 San Pasqual Valley Road
Escondido, CA 92027
Director: Dr. Josephine Braun
Phone: 760-291-5471
Fax: 760-291-5427
Email: amphibianlab@sandiegozoo.org
http://institute.sandiegozoo.org/resources/amphibian-disease
 -laboratory

Zoologix
9811 Owensmouth Avenue, Suite 4
Chatsworth CA 91311
Phone: 818-717-8880
Email: info@zoologix.com
http://zoologix.com
PCR infectious disease testing for amphibians and other species

Florida

Aquatic, Amphibian, and Reptile Pathology Program
University of Florida
2015 SW 16th Avenue, Room VS-50
Gainesville, FL 32610
Director: Dr. Salvatore Frasca
Phone: 352-294-4726
Fax: 352-392-2938
Email: sfrasca@ufl.edu
http://labs.vetmed.ufl.edu/services/aqarpath/
Histology, cytology, necropsy, molecular disease investigation, and in
 situ hybridization

Avian & Wildlife Laboratory
University of Miami
1600 NW 10th Avenue, RSMB 7101A
Miami FL 33136
Phone: 800-596-7390 or 305-243-6700
Fax: 305-243-5662
http://www.cpl.med.miami.edu

Georgia

Infectious Disease Laboratory, UGA
University of Georgia
College of Veterinary Medicine
501 W. Brooks Drive

Athens, GA 30602-7383
Molecular diagnostics and C/S

Illinois

Wildlife Epidemiology Laboratory
2001 S. Lincoln Avenue
Urbana, IL 61802
Phone: 217-333-1620
Email: WildlifeEpi@vetmed.illinois.edu
http://vetmed.illinois.edu/wel/
Quantitative and qualitative PCR and ancillary testing

Ohio

Avian & Exotic Animal Clin Path Labs
2712 N. US Highway 68
Wilmington, OH 45177
Phone: 800-350-1122
Fax: 937-383-3667
Email: aeacpl@yahoo.com
http://avianexoticlab.com
Exclusively dedicated to avian, reptilian (amphibian), and exotic small mammals; full-service diagnostic laboratory

Veterinary Molecular Diagnostics, Inc. (VMD)
5989 Meijer Drive, Suite 5
Milford, OH 45150
Owner/Director: Dr. Bob Dahlhausen
Phone: 513-576-1808
Fax: 513-576-6177
http://vmdlabs.com
DNA-based testing services for veterinary medicine; opened in 2003

Utah

Animal Reference Pathology, LLC
Exotic Companion Animal, Zoo Animal, & Wildlife Pathology Section
525 East 4500, South Suite F200
Salt Lake City, UT 84107
Phone: 800-426-2099
Fax: 801-584-5104
http://animalreferencepathology.com
Histology, cytology, and necropsy services only

Washington

Northwest ZooPath
654 West Main Street
Monroe, WA 98272
Phone: 360-794-0630
Fax: 360-794-4312
Email: Zoopath1@gmail.com
Histology, cytology, and necropsy only

Sound Diagnostics LLC
4909 236th Place SE
Woodinville, WA 98072
Phone: 206-363-0787
Fax: 425-482-9292
http://www.sounddiagnosticsllc.com
Rabbit/rodent serology

EUROPE

Germany

Clinic for Birds, Reptiles, Amphibians and Fish
Frankfurter Strasse 91
35392 Giessen, Germany
Laboratory Director: Prof. Dr. Michael Lierz
Phone: + 49-641-9938450
Fax: + 49-641-9938439
email: labor-kvraf@vetmed.uni-giessen.de
http://www.uni-giessen.de/fbz/fb10/institute_klinikum/klinikum/kvraf
Exclusively for nonmammal exotic animals; molecular biology, virology, parasitology, bacteriology, and necropsy

Chemical and Veterinary Investigation Office Ostwestfalen-Lippe (CVUA-OWL)
Westerfeldstraße 1
D-32758 Detmold
Laboratory Director: Herr Dr. Stolz
Phone: + 49-5231911-9
Fax + 49 5231911-503 (head office or +49 5231911-641 (pathology))
https://cvua-owl.de/tiergesundheit/allgemein

Laboklin GmbH & Co. KG
Steubenstr. 4
D-97688 Bad Kissingen
Laboratory Director: Frau Dr. Elisabeth Müller
Contact for reptile diagnostics: Rachel E. Marschang
Email: info@laboklin.com or marschang@laboklin.com
Phone: + 49-971-72020
Fax: + 49-971-68546
www.laboklin.com
Accredited according to DIN EN ISO/IEC 17025:2005

Spain

Catalonian Reptile and Amphibian Rescue Center
Maresme Avenue, 45
08783 Masquefa, Barcelona, Spain
Laboratory Director: Dr. Albert Martínez-Silvestre
Phone: 0034-937726396
Fax: 0034-937725311
Email: crarc@amasquefa.com
http://www.crarc-comam.net
Exclusively dedicated to reptile and amphibian pathology, necropsy, cytology, and histology

United Kingdom

Carmichael Torrance Diagnostic Services (CTDS) 2015 Ltd.
Blacksmiths Forge, Brookfield Court
Selby Road, Garforth, Leeds
LS25 1NB
Tel: + 44 113 2870175
https://www.ctdslab.co.uk

Australia

The Hyndman Reptile Pathogen (HRP) Laboratory
Murdoch University, Perth, Western Australia
Contact: Tim Hyndman
Email: t.hyndman@murdoch.edu.au

Tel: + 61 (08) 9360-7348
Molecular testing of reptile samples for pathogens

ASIA

Hong Kong

Asia Veterinary Diagnostics
Room 2106, 2101-2, 21st Floor
9 Wing Hong Street
Cheung Sha Wan
Kowloon
Hong Kong
Director of Pathology: Emeritus Professor Michael J. Day
Phone: (852) 2371 0080

Fax: (852) 2371 3183
Email: info@asiaveterinarydiagnostics.com
http://vetdiagnosticcentre.com.hk

Singapore

Asia Veterinary Diagnostics
466 Serangoon Road
03-01
Singapore
218 225
Director of Pathology: Emeritus Prof. Michael J. Day
Phone: (65) 6291 5412
Email: info@asiaveterinarydiagnostics.com
website: http://vetdiagnosticcentre.com.hk

Medical History and Physical Examination

Stephen J. Divers

The successful diagnosis and treatment of reptile disease requires an ability to properly restrain, examine, and perform a variety of clinical techniques. The principles are similar to those used in domestic companion animal medicine. The ability to perform a thorough physical examination, which depends on adequate restraint, is considered a cornerstone of clinical practice. However, there are herp-specific peculiarities that must be appreciated to avoid potentially serious errors or injuries. The following descriptions include clinical techniques employed for the purposes of diagnosis in pet, zoo, and free-ranging reptiles. Some descriptions are general and apply to most if not all species within a group, while others may be more taxa or even species specific. It is vital that the species is identified prior to clinical interaction so that potential dangers can be appreciated and avoided. Strikes, bites, scratches, crushing injuries, envenomation, and zoonoses are some of the common dangers facing the clinician.

Clinical evaluation starts with a detailed history, and inexperienced clinicians are advised to consult a history form to ensure that no items are overlooked (Table 42.1). The aim of the physical examination is to identify and document any lesions or clinical signs to an organ system or systems and formulate a list of differential diagnoses (Table 42.2). It may be possible to observe calm specimens unrestrained, permitting an assessment of demeanor, locomotion, and obvious neurologic disorders such as lameness, paralysis, paresis, and head tilt.[1] Observation while the animal is in its normal enclosure is particularly valuable, and clients should be encouraged to share smartphone videos whenever possible. Nervous or aggressive species are best restrained at all times using towels, snake hooks, clear plastic containers, restraint tubes, and for larger animals, ropes and snares. Gloves and gauntlets severely reduce the clinician's tactile sensation but may be required when dealing with large pugnacious lizards or small-to-medium aggressive crocodilians.

A systematic examination from rostrum to tail tip is always indicated, whether the reptile is being presented for a postpurchase exam, yearly health exam, presurgical assessment, or because it is clinically unwell.[2–4] The clinicians' senses of sight, sound, smell, and touch are all utilized to examine all accessible areas for abnormalities. When taking the first tentative steps into reptile medicine, it can be invaluable to seek the help of individuals from a local herpetological society or herpetocultural-ist for the purposes of examining clinically healthy animals.

A common stress response of many species to handling is the voiding of feces, urine, and urates during the clinical examination (Fig. 42.1). In many cases, material will be deposited on the table or on the clinician.

Any veterinarian blessed with an abundance of clinically valuable material should consider immediate collection for possible laboratory investigation, including urine dipstick, fecal wet preparation, and flotation. Microbiologic results must be interpreted with caution when dealing with material collected in such an unsterile manner.

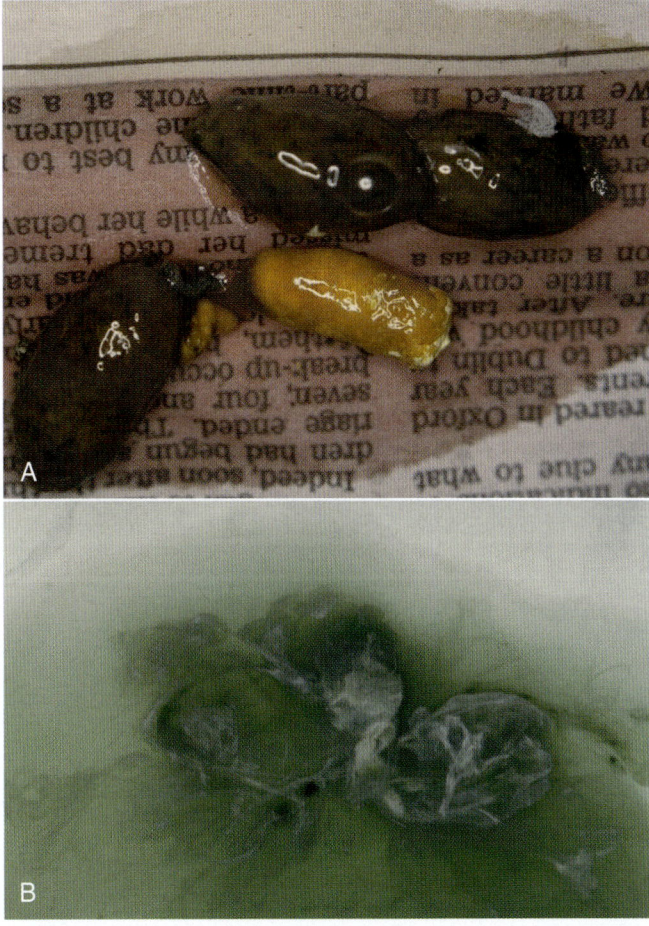

FIG 42.1 (A) Normal feces, urates, and urine from a snake. (B) Biliverdinuria and green urates from a tortoise with severe hepatobiliary disease. (Courtesy of Stephen J. Divers.)

SPECIAL CONSIDERATIONS

Reception and Preparation

Reception staff should ideally be knowledgeable of common species, and many of the best staff have direct experience of keeping reptiles themselves. If the practice also sees domesticated dogs and cats, then consideration should be given to seeing herps at specific times, often at the end of surgery hours when the waiting room is quieter.

Although little specific equipment is required, technicians should prepare examination areas ahead of time, especially with regard to availability of clean towels, mouth speculums, syringes, needles, and specimen containers (see Chapter 1).

Transportation

Herps should be transported in insulated containers, but careful thought should be given to whether supplemental heating is necessary—overheating is more acutely fatal than cooling. No reptile should be unsecured and free-handled in the public waiting area.

Large Dangerous or Venomous Reptiles

Careful consideration should be given to the safety of veterinary staff, curatorial staff, and private owners when dealing with potentially dangerous animals. Some species may be covered by legislation restricting their ownership (see Chapters 183, 184, and 185 on legislation). Venomous snakes (especially front-fanged species), venomous lizards (*Heloderma* spp), crocodilians, and large aquatic turtles can be aggressive and dangerous. Examination of such animals should only be performed by experienced, recognized specialists with due regard to required equipment, practice facilities, and trained staff, as well as legal and liability issues.

Chemical Restraint

In many cases the judicious use of chemical agents can expedite procedures and reduce risks to both herp and human considerably, particularly when dealing with dangerous or venomous animals. Given the improvements in sedation and anesthesia, even reasonably manageable "pet" species may be preferentially sedated or anesthetized for clinical

---

TABLE 42.1   Reptile and Amphibian History Form

A detailed history is essential to provide the most appropriate veterinary care for your animal. Please complete this form as accurately as possible. If there is anything you are unsure about, you can discuss it in more depth with the veterinary staff during your appointment.

Animal Details

Animal's name or identification: _____   Common or scientific species name: _____

Date of birth: _____   Age: _____   Sex: M □ F □   Unknown □   Neutered/spayed □   Origin: captive bred □   wild-caught import □   unknown □

How long have you had this animal? _____

From where did you obtain this animal? _____

Does your reptile have any history of breeding or laying eggs? N □ Y □ Please give details: _____
_____

When did your reptile last shed? _____   How often has your reptile been shedding? _____

Do you have any other reptiles or pets? N □ Y □ Please give details: _____
_____

Have you or your reptile had any contact with other reptiles in the last 90 days? N □ Y □ Please give details: _____
_____

When was the last reptile added to your collection? _____
_____

Reason for Presentation Today

What is the primary complaint or what signs have you noticed? How long have these problems been present?
_____
_____

What health problems has your reptile had previously? _____
_____

When & why did you last see a veterinarian? _____
_____

Has your reptile received any treatment in the last 30 days? N □ Y □ Please give details (what was used, dosage, how often, duration?): _____
_____

Have you noticed any change in your reptile's behavior? N □ Y □ Please give details: _____
_____

Have any other animals or persons in the household had any illness in the last 30 days? _____
_____

TABLE 42.1   Reptile and Amphibian History Form—cont'd

Cage Environment

What type of cage is used? arboreal (tall, climbing) □ terrestrial □ aquatic □ Cage size: _____

_____

What is the cage made of? plastic/fiberglass □ wooden □ metal □ glass □ other: _____

_____

What is the floor substrate? paper □ corn cob □ sand □ astroturf □ bark □ other: _____

_____

What décor and furnishings are present? _____

Is there additional ventilation (grills or mesh)? N □ Y □ Please give size/details: _____

_____

Are bathing facilities provided? N □ Y □ Please give details: _____

How often is the cage cleaned? _____

What cleaning/disinfectant agents are used? _____

What heating equipment is used?

Ceramic/infrared □, power _____ W   thermostat control: N □ Y □

Spot light/bulb □, power _____ W   thermostat control: N □ Y □

Heat mat □, size: _____   under cage □ or inside cage □   thermostat control: N □ Y □

Aquarium water heater □, power _____ W   thermostat control: N □ Y □

Other heaters, please give details: _____

Are the heat sources screened from the animals? N □ Y □ Please give details: _____

_____

Can the animal(s) touch or access the heat source? N □ Y □ Please give details: _____

_____

Is additional lighting provided inside the cage? N □ Y □

If yes, what type of light is used? Light bulb □ Fluorescent strip light □

What is the model and manufacturer? _____

When was the light last replaced? _____

Are the lights screened from the animals? N □ Y □ Please give details: _____

Can the animal(s) touch or access the lights? N □ Y □ Please give details: _____

How many hours of light are provided each day? _____

Is there ever access to direct sunlight (not through glass or plastic)? N □ Y □

If yes, how many hours per day or per week? _____

Do you measure the humidity in the cage? N □ Y □ If yes, what is the humidity level? _____

_____

What are the day time temperatures? Hottest area, basking area = _____ Coolest area = _____

What are the night time temperatures? Hottest area, basking area = _____ Coolest area = _____

Are these temperatures measured using a thermometer? Y □ N □

Does anyone in the household smoke? N □ Y □   Do you use any aerosolized products? N □ Y □

Have there been changes in the reptile's environment in the last 3 months? N □ Y □ Please give details: _____

_____

Continued

TABLE 42.1	**Reptile and Amphibian History Form—cont'd**

Diet

How often do you feed your animal? _____

Indicate which foods are eaten and in what amounts (by number, weight, or approx volume):

Fresh vegetables ☐ type and amount per feed: _____

Frozen/thawed or processed vegetables ☐ fresh ☐ other ☐ _____

Flowers ☐ type and amount per feed: _____

Fresh fruits ☐ type and amount per feed: _____   Frozen/thawed ☐ fresh ☐ other ☐

Frozen/thawed or processed fruits ☐ fresh ☐ other ☐ _____

Insects: crickets ☐   locusts ☐   mealworms ☐   waxworms ☐   earthworms ☐   other ☐ _____

Mice ☐ type and number per feed: _____   Freshly killed ☐

Rats ☐ type and number per feed: _____   Frozen/thawed ☐

Birds or fish, please give details: _____   Live prey ☐

Do you feed any wild animals to your animal? N ☐ Y ☐, please give details: _____

Any other food items fed? Please give details: _____

Do you use any nutritional supplements? N ☐ Y ☐, if yes what, how much, and how often: _____

What water supply do you provide? tap water ☐ bottled water ☐ rain/river water ☐

How is water provided? bowl ☐ dripper system ☐ spray ☐, how often: _____

How often is the water changed? _____

Do you use any water supplements? N ☐ Y ☐ Please give details: _____

Have you noticed any changes in feeding or drinking behavior? Please give details: _____

Have you noticed any changes in droppings (fecal material, urine and urates)? Please give details: _____

Any other comments or information: _____

_____

_____

procedures that would otherwise take longer to accomplish and cause unnecessary stress or discomfort (see Chapters 48 and 49). When dealing with venomous snakes and other dangerous reptiles, anesthesia should be routinely considered before examination.[5] Potential effects of sedation or anesthesia on clinicopathologic results, especially hematology and biochemistry, should be appreciated even if they cannot be avoided.

Operant Conditioning and Training

An overlooked facet of reptile examination has been the value of operant conditioning and training. Several zoos have instigated such behavioral programs, which can greatly improve the ability to perform physical examinations and collect diagnostic samples from large tortoises, lizards, and crocodilians (see Chapter 14).[6] Even in private practice, this approach deserves further consideration with clients encouraged to desensitize their animals to transportation containers, physical restraint, mouth opening, coelomic palpation, and more.

Zoonoses

Reptiles, like all other animal groups, can be a source of disease in humans. The risks of reptile-borne zoonoses are probably no greater than for other animal groups, and basic personal hygiene after handling patients will reduce these risks to an acceptable, minimal level. The major zoonoses of potential concern include *Salmonella* sp, *Pseudomonas* sp, *Mycobacteria* sp, *Cryptosporidia* sp, *Rickettsia* sp, and pentastomids (arachnid lung parasites). Major public concern centers on the commensal reptile salmonellas, and clinicians are advised to obtain a copy of the statement policy and client brochure on this subject produced by the Association of Reptile and Amphibian Veterinarians (see Chapter 174).

Weight, Length, and Body Condition Score

Every animal must be accurately weighed, because deaths associated with drug overdose, particularly anesthetics and aminoglycosides, are avoidable. Serial weight measurements permit an appraisal of growth and captive management, response to treatment, and disease progression. Relating body weight to length to give an assessment of body condition is valuable but takes practice and experience to master; however, it does promote differentiation between the acutely sick (less common) and terminal presentation of chronic disease (more common). A calculated ratio of weight:length (snout to vent length in lizards and snakes, straight carapace length in chelonians) provides a numerical body condition index, and there are published charts that utilize this ratio for several common species.[7–10] In addition, body condition scoring can be useful, albeit more subjective, and a system from 1 to 5 is practical (1 emaciated, 2 underweight, 3 normal, 4 overweight, 5 obese). Loss of bodily reserves

TABLE 42.2 Zoologic Medicine: Medical History and Physical Examination Form

Medical History (in addition, complete husbandry form with management details)

_____

_____

_____

_____

Resp rate: _____/min   **Heart rate**: _____/min   **Temp**: _____°F/°C   **Weight**: _____g/kg

General (demeanor, posture, neurologic status)

_____

_____

_____

_____

_____

_____

Head

_____

_____

_____

_____

_____

_____

Neck

_____

_____

_____

_____

_____

_____

Body

_____

_____

_____

_____

_____

_____

Pectoral Limbs

_____

_____

_____

_____

_____

_____

_____

Continued

TABLE 42.2 Zoologic Medicine: Medical History and Physical Examination Form—cont'd

Pelvic Limbs

Tail

Problem List and Differential Diagnoses

Initial Plan (use to create estimate/consent form)

are usually most obvious around the tail, pelvic, and hind limb areas in lizards and crocodilians. Some species, such as the leopard gecko (*Eublepharis macularius*), store most of their fat reserves within a bulbous tail, and therefore tail size and shape in this species is a good means of assessing body condition. In snakes, the fat reserves tend to be more diffuse throughout the elongated coelomic fat bodies, nevertheless weight loss leads to loose skin folds with pronounced spine and ribs. Obese snakes will often exhibit soft, fatty swellings just cranial to the vent. The snout-vent length of a snake is important to note as organ position and growth can be calculated as a result. Chelonians present more of a problem. The musculature of the limbs and subcutaneous fat stores can be palpated, but the best estimation of body condition relies on relating total weight to carapace length or body volume.

Cloacal Temperature

It may seem a paradox to recommend taking a cloacal temperature from an ectotherm, but in certain situations it can be rewarding. Obviously, small reptiles maintained out of their heated enclosures for prolonged periods will experience changes in core temperature. However, larger reptiles (especially large tortoises, crocodilians, and snakes) that are examined in their home environment or soon after leaving their normal enclosure will not demonstrate dramatic changes in their core temperature if they are transported in an insulated container. Consequently, cloacal temperature may provide an indication of the thermal environment from which the reptile came.

Transillumination

Transillumination of the coelom using a cold light source can be beneficial for visualizing the internal structures of small lizards and snakes and is particularly useful for confirming suspected impactions and foreign bodies in the examination room. The light can be held against the body of a small herp, or lubricated and inserted into the esophagus or cloaca of a sedated animal. Transillumination in a darkened room enables coelomic masses to be identified, and the cardiac shadow can be located for cardiocentesis.

Auscultation

Auscultation is certainly possible, but the use of a standard diaphragm stethoscope does require an absolutely silent consulting room and is often unrewarding. The adventitious sounds produced between the shell or scales and the stethoscope diaphragm may be reduced by placing a dampened swab or towel between the stethoscope and the reptilian integument. More recently, the use of electronic stethoscopes has improved the appreciation of heart and respiratory sounds, although Doppler devices are favored for recording heart rates. In general, auscultation is of limited value.

SNAKES

The head of an aggressive snake or a snake of unknown disposition should be identified and restrained before opening the transportation bag and removing the animal. Venomous snakes should be placed in clear plastic tubes or anesthetic induction chambers and anesthetized using an inhalant prior to examination. In general, the head of the snake is held behind the occiput using the thumb and middle finger to support the lateral aspects of the cranium. The index finger is placed on top of the head. The other hand is used to support the serpentine body (Fig. 42.2A). By restraining the snake's head in this manner, greater support can be given to the cranium-cervical junction, which, having only a single occiput, is more prone to dislocation with rough or inappropriate handling. The largest pythons and anacondas can exceed 5 m and 80 kg and are powerful and potentially dangerous. When dealing

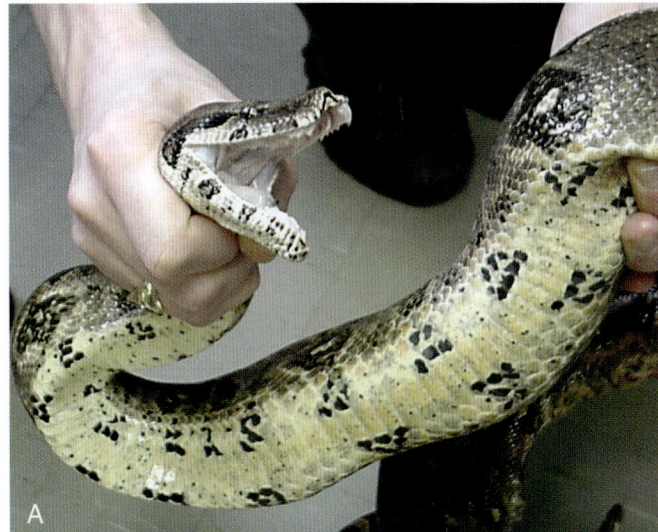
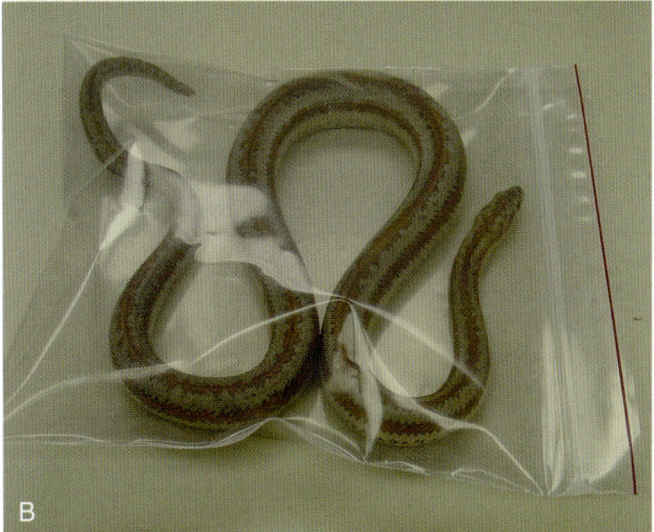

FIG 42.2 (A) Restrained snakes must have their head and body supported. Aggressive snakes like this boa constrictor (*Boa constrictor*) cannot harm the handler when their heads have been securely grasped and controlled. (B) Nonvenomous snakes that are too nervous to examine properly, such as the rosy boa (*Lichanura trivirgata*), can be sedated by placing them in a clear plastic bag with 5% isoflurane or 8% sevoflurane in oxygen. Once righting reflexes have been lost (typically 5–30 mins) the snake can be removed for examination and will recover within 10 mins. (Courtesy of Stephen J. Divers.)

with large, even docile boids, an additional handler is recommended for each meter of snake.

Nonvenomous species should be removed from their cloth bag and supported using one or two hands depending on size. An assessment of demeanor can usually be quickly determined. Nervous or aggressive (nonvenomous) snakes can be restrained using clear plastic bags and/ or sedated prior to examination (Fig. 42.2B). The docile snake should be permitted to roam over the hands and arms, thereby enabling the clinician to gauge muscle tone, proprioception, and mobility. Proprioception can be assessed by placing the snake in dorsal recumbency and monitoring the effort and ability of the snake to right itself (Fig. 42.3). Systemically ill serpents will often be limp, weak, and less mobile. The healthy serpent will impart a sense of strength and be active during handling. A healthy individual that is permitted to wrap a coil around

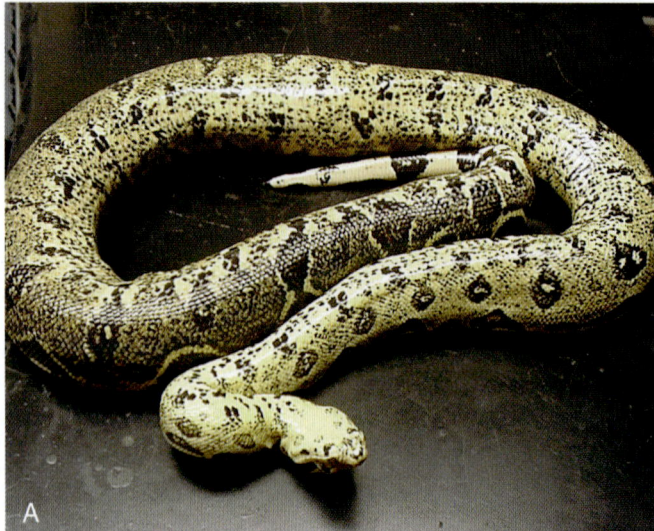

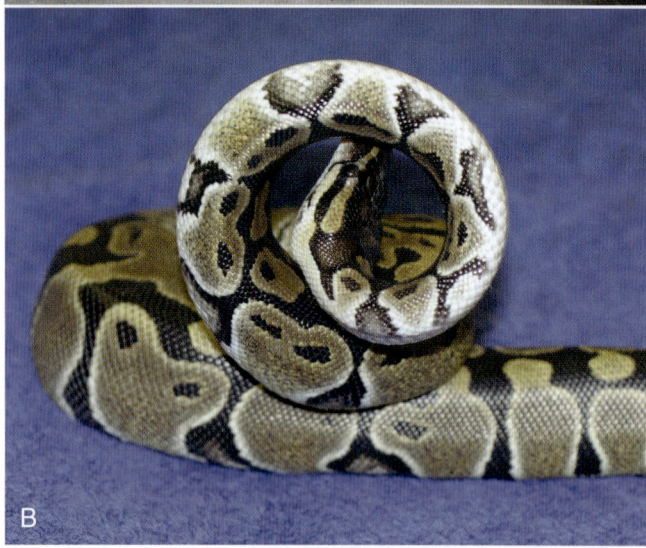

FIG 42.3 (A) Complete lack of righting reflex in a *Boa constrictor* suffering from arenavirus (boid inclusion body) disease (IBD). (B) Loss of righting reflex and opisthotonus in a ball python (*Python regius*). (Courtesy of Stephen J. Divers.)

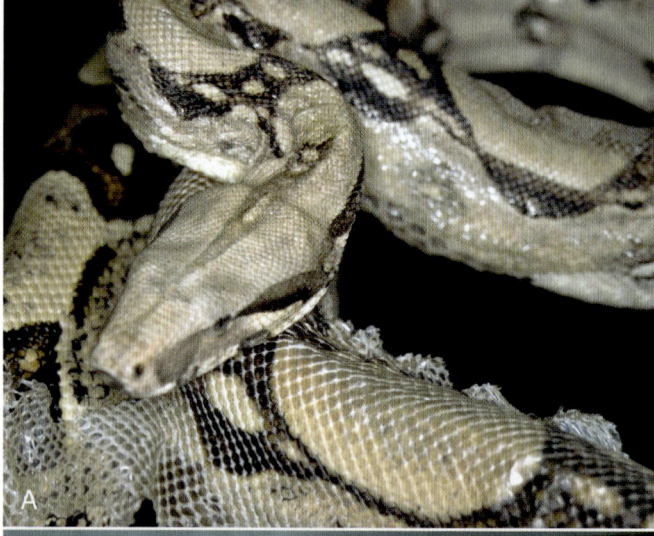

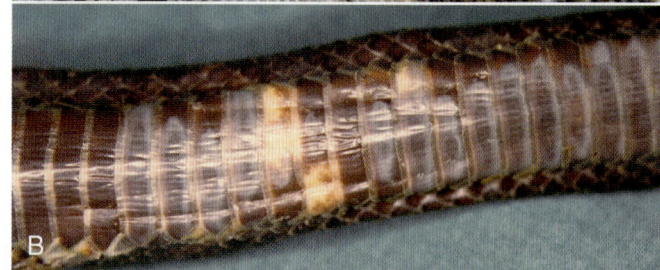

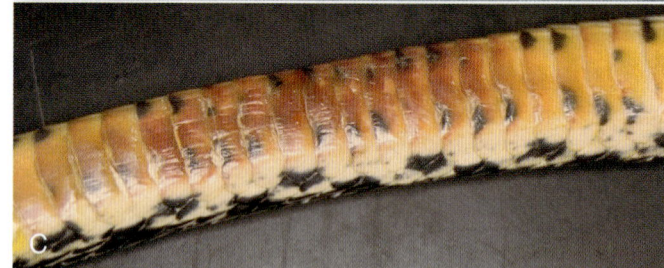

FIG 42.4 (A) Dysecdysis in a *Boa constrictor*. (B) Blister disease associated with the ventrum of a colubrid snake caused by constant dampness within the vivarium. (C) Thermal burn on the ventrum of a kingsnake (*Lampropeltis* sp), caused by a poorly controlled heat mat. (Courtesy of Stephen J. Divers.)

the handler's wrist while the head is allowed to hang down should be able to raise its head to the level of the tail. Head carriage, body posture, cloacal tone, proprioception, skin pinch, withdrawal, and ocular and righting reflexes can be used to assess neurologic function.

The entire integument, particularly the head and ventral scales, should be thoroughly examined for evidence of dysecdysis (poor shedding), trauma, parasitism (especially the common snake mite, *Ophionyssus natricis*, and ticks), and microbiologic infection (Fig. 42.4). If available, the recently shed skin should also be examined for evidence of retained spectacles. Skin tenting and ridges may indicate cachexia or dehydration, whereas ticks and mites may congregate in skin folds, infraorbital pits, nostrils, and perispectacular rims. The infraorbital pits (where present) and the nostrils should be free from discharge or retained skin. The eyes should be clear, unless ecdysis is imminent. In preparation for shedding, snakes produce a lymphlike fluid that creates a white to bluish haze to the eyes. It is this fluid that creates the cleavage zone and facilitates the lifting of the old skin. The spectacles covering the eyes should be smooth, as any wrinkles usually indicate the presence of a retained spectacle. The spectacle represents the transparent fused eyelids, and

therefore the cornea is not normally exposed. The subspectacular fluid drains through paired ducts, close to the vomeronasal openings in the maxilla. When blocked, the buildup of fluid causes a subspectacular swelling that often becomes infected, resulting in a subspectacular abscess. Damage to the underlying cornea can result in panophthalmitis and ocular swelling, while retrobulbar abscessation will result in protrusion of a normal-sized globe. Other ocular pathologies can include uveitis, corneal lipidosis, and spectacular foreign bodies, including slivers of wood chip or other vivarium materials (see Chapter 71).

Examination of the oral cavity is often left until the end of the examination, as many snakes object to such manipulation. However, even before the mouth is opened, the tongue should be seen flicking in and out of the philtrum with regularity. The mouth can be gently opened using a plastic/wooden spatula or wood portion of cotton-tip applicators to permit an assessment of mucous membrane color and buccal examination for evidence of mucosal edema, ptyalism, hemorrhage, necrosis, and inspissated exudates (Fig. 42.5). The presence of white deposits may indicate uric acid deposition due to visceral gout.

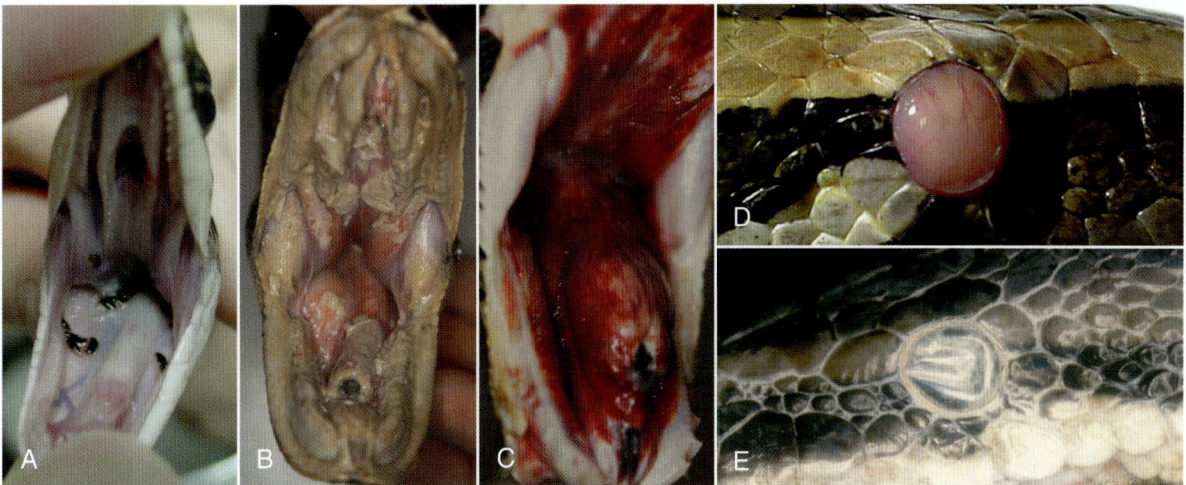

FIG 42.5 (A) Digenic trematodes (*Renifer*) in the oral cavity of a free-ranging black racer (*Coluber constrictor*). (B) Severe bacterial stomatitis in a *Boa constrictor*. (C) Severe buccal erythema and petechiation associated with stomatitis in a boid snake. (D) Subspectacular abscess in a Burmese python (*Python bivittatus*). (E) Retained spectacle in a ball python (*Python regius*). (Courtesy of Stephen J. Divers.)

The pharynx, choana, and larynx should be examined for hemorrhage, foreign bodies, and discharges. It is important to observe the larynx during respiration to differentiate between discharges originating from the respiratory or gastrointestinal tracts. Unfortunately, due to the stress of examination, respiratory rates are often elevated in normal reptiles, and therefore tachypnea may not be considered a definitive indicator of respiratory disease unless observed in the undisturbed snake. However, open mouth breathing is a reliable indicator of severe respiratory compromise. During the oral examination the patency of the internal nares and the state of the polyphyodontic teeth should be noted.

Working from cranial to caudal, the head and body are palpated for abnormal swellings, wounds, and other abnormalities. The position of any internal anomalies, noted as a distance from the snout and interpreted as a percentage of snout-vent length (SVL), will enable an assessment of possible organ involvement (Fig. 42.6).[11] Depending on the musculature, feeding habits, and fat reserves of the snake, it may be possible to palpate the normal heart, stomach, liver, active ovaries, eggs, kidneys, and fecal material. Recently fed snakes will have a midbody swelling associated with the prey within the stomach, and postprandial handling can lead to regurgitation. The clinical examination should differentiate between coelomic (internal) and extracoelomic (subcutaneous) masses. The majority of subcutaneous masses are usually abscesses, but parasitic cysts, blisters, and neoplasia are occasionally seen. Internal masses may represent abscesses, neoplasia, granulomas, obstipation, organ hypertrophy, retained eggs, or ova (Fig. 42.7). The cloaca should have muscle tone, not be gaping, and be free from fecal staining, discharge, and prolapse (Fig. 42.8). Just distal and slightly lateral to the cloaca the paired cloacal scent glands are palpable and should be soft and bilaterally symmetrical. Nervous snakes, especially colubrids, will often expel the contents of these cloacal glands in a defensive reaction to a perceived threat. This foul-smelling material does not represent infection but merely an annoyance, as the smell is difficult to eradicate from clothing. Examination of the cloaca can be carried out using a dedicated otoscope or rigid endoscope. Digital palpation is often overlooked but is a useful technique. In medium-to-large snakes a latex-gloved, lubricated finger can be passed into the cloaca and may allow palpation of eggs, cloacoliths, fecoliths, or abscesses. In the giant constrictors it is possible to insert a lubricated, gloved arm and perform an internal cloacal and even colonic examination. Care is required not to force the colonic examination, because the lower intestinal wall is thin and prone to laceration. Internal palpation often induces defecation and urination and can be useful to aid the collection of samples. Examination of tail length or probing of the hemipenes should confirm gender (Fig. 42.9). The tail length (and the number of subcaudal scales) is always shorter (less) in females than in males; however, this method requires access to published information on tail length and scale counts (which is not available for all species) or the presence of both sexes for simultaneous examination, and thus is a less reliable technique. The hemipenes are entered by directing a blunt, water-soluble lubricated probe, caudally, on either side of midline. In males the probe passes to a depth of 6 to 14 subcaudal scales, whereas in females the probe enters a cloacal gland to a depth of only 2 to 6 subcaudal scales. Some species of snakes such as short-tailed or blood pythons (*Python curtis*) can be difficult to sex with probing, as the probing depths are so similar for males and females (see Chapter 80 for more information on gender identification).

LIZARDS

Lizards vary considerably in size, strength, and temperament, and therefore a variety of handling techniques are required to cover most examination scenarios. The tegus (Teiidae) and monitors (Varanidae) are renowned for their powerful bites, whereas other species, particularly the green iguana (*Iguana iguana*), are much more likely to use their claws and tail to painful effect. The main problem when handling small lizards is restraining them before they flee from an open bag or container. In all cases, the lizard should be transported in a securely tied cloth bag so that the position of the lizard can be identified and held before the bag is even opened. Large lizards are best restrained with the forelimbs held laterally against their cranial coelom and the hind limbs held laterally against the tail base (Fig. 42.10). The limbs should not be held over the spine, as fractures and dislocations may occur. Smaller lizards can be restrained around the pectoral girdle, holding the forelimbs against the cranial coelom, although care is required not to impair respiratory movements. Restricting the vision of these animals is often the simplest way to facilitate handling, and a towel or sock placed over the head will often facilitate examination of the rest of

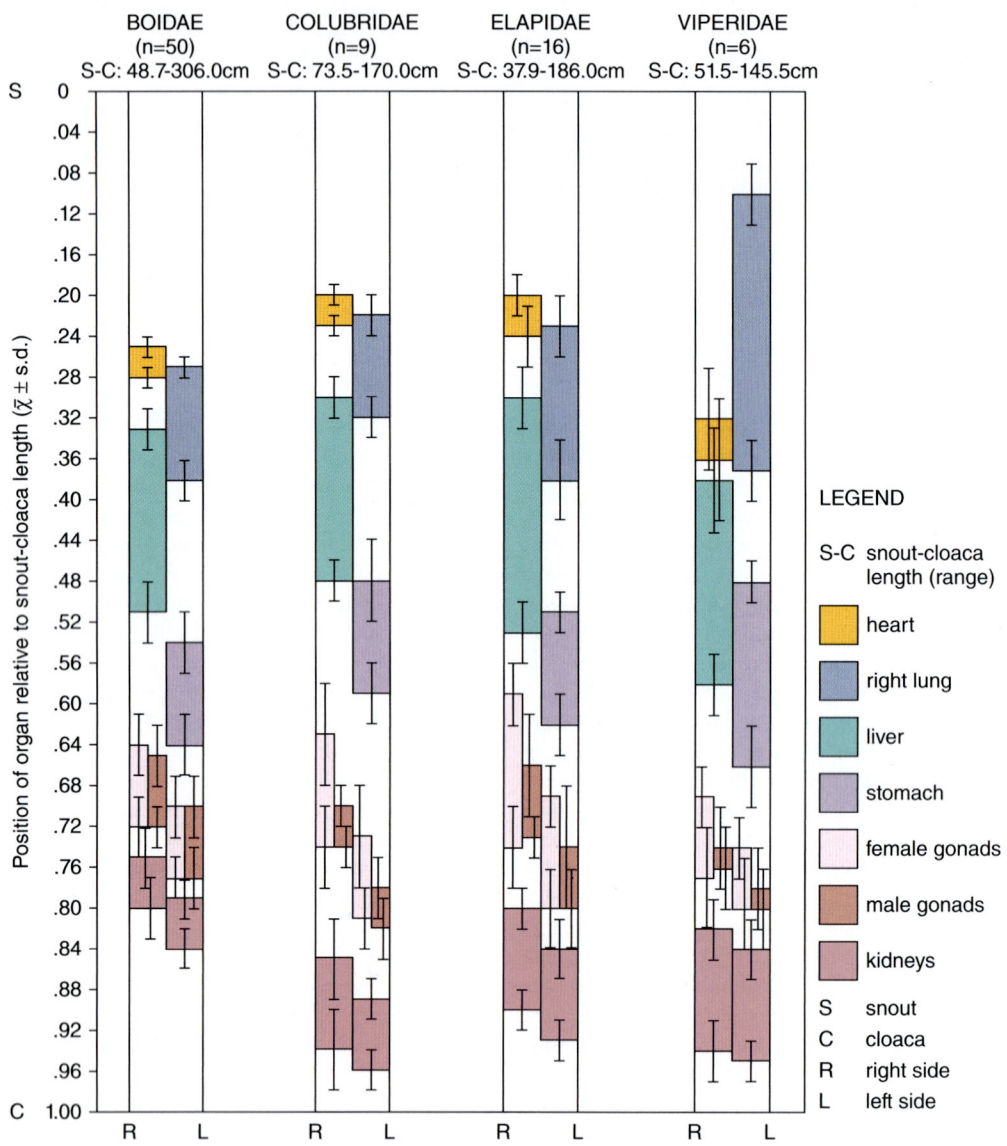

FIG 42.6 Positions of internal organs relative to body length in snakes. (Original Figure 31.3 from McCracken HE. Organ location in snakes for diagnostic and surgical evaluation. In Fowler ME, Miller RE, editors: *Zoo and wild animal medicine current therapy.* Vol. 4. St. Louis: Elsevier; 1999:247.)

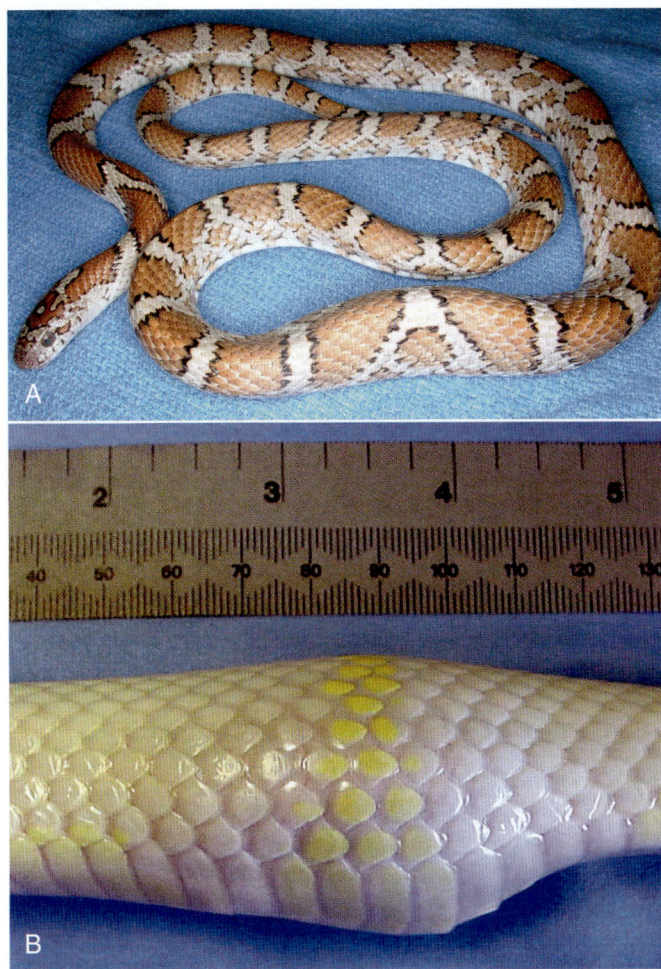

FIG 42.7 (A) Midbody swelling in a corn snake (*Pantherophis guttata*) associated with gastric cryptosporidiosis. (B) Intracoelomic mass in a kingsnake (*Lampropeltis* sp.). This mass was located approximately 90% from snout-vent and was subsequently confirmed as a renal carcinoma. (A, Courtesy of Scott J. Stahl, Stahl Exotic Animal Veterinary Services; B, courtesy of Stephen J. Divers.)

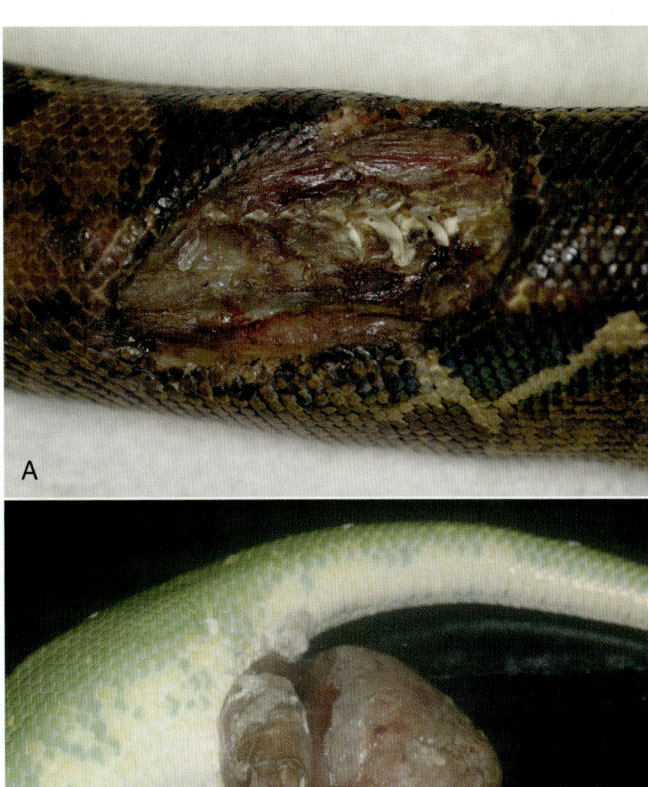

FIG 42.8 (A) Severe rat-induced trauma in a *Boa constrictor*. (B) Cloaco-colonic prolapse in a green tree python (*Morelia viridis*). (Courtesy of Stephen J. Divers.)

the body and limbs. Particularly nervous lizards can be wrapped in a towel to aid restraint (Fig. 42.11). A useful restraint technique for iguanid lizards utilizes the vasovagal response: gentle digital pressure is applied to both orbits, and in many cases the lizard will enter a state of stupor for up to 30 minutes or until a painful or noisy stimulus is applied. This technique can be used to calm nervous iguanids and monitors and enables the mouth to be gently opened without the need for excessive force.

If possible the lizard should be observed unrestrained to appreciate any neurologic problems or lameness (Fig. 42.12). Calm lizards may be permitted to walk around the examination table or on the floor. However, if in any doubt, the lizard should be placed in a large plastic enclosure to prevent escape during the observation period. Never grasp a lizard by the tail, because many species can perform autotomy and drop their tails in an attempt to evade a predator.

The integument should be examined for parasites (mites and ticks) and evidence of trauma due to fighting, mating, burns, or repeated escape attempts (Fig. 42.13). Most lizards tend to shed their skin in stages, and therefore retained skin (often dry and brown) must be differentiated from normal piecemeal ecdysis (flexible and transparent). Classically, dysecdysis and skin retention occurs around the digits and

tail, causing ischemic necrosis. Extensive skin folding and tenting are indicators of cachexia and possible dehydration.

The head should be examined for abnormal conformation (Fig. 42.14). The mouth can be opened using a blunt spatula or by gently applying pressure to the dewlap. Thorough buccal examination for evidence of trauma, infection, neoplasia, and edema, especially pharyngeal edema, and examination of the choana and larynx are considered routine (Fig. 42.15). In addition, the internal extent of any rostral abrasions can be evaluated. The nostrils, eyes, and tympanic scales should be clear and free from swelling and discharge (Fig. 42.16). The presence of white dried material around the nostrils of some iguanid lizards is normal, as some species excrete salt through specialized nasal glands. The head, body, and limbs must be palpated for masses, swellings, and fractures. Focal soft tissue masses are usually abscesses, whereas more diffuse swellings around the long bones or mandible are likely to be related to metabolic bone diseases. Lizards suffering from severe hypocalcemia and hyperphosphatemia due to nutritional or renal secondary hyperparathyroidism exhibit periodic tremors and muscle fasiculations. The coelomic body cavity of most lizards can be gently palpated. In the normal animal food and fecal material within the gastrointestinal tract, fat bodies, liver, ova, and eggs are usually appreciable. Cystic calculi, fecoliths, enlarged kidneys, impactions, retained eggs or ova, large fat bodies, and unusual coelomic masses are abnormal (Fig. 42.17). An appreciation of species, gender, age, body size, and weight will permit

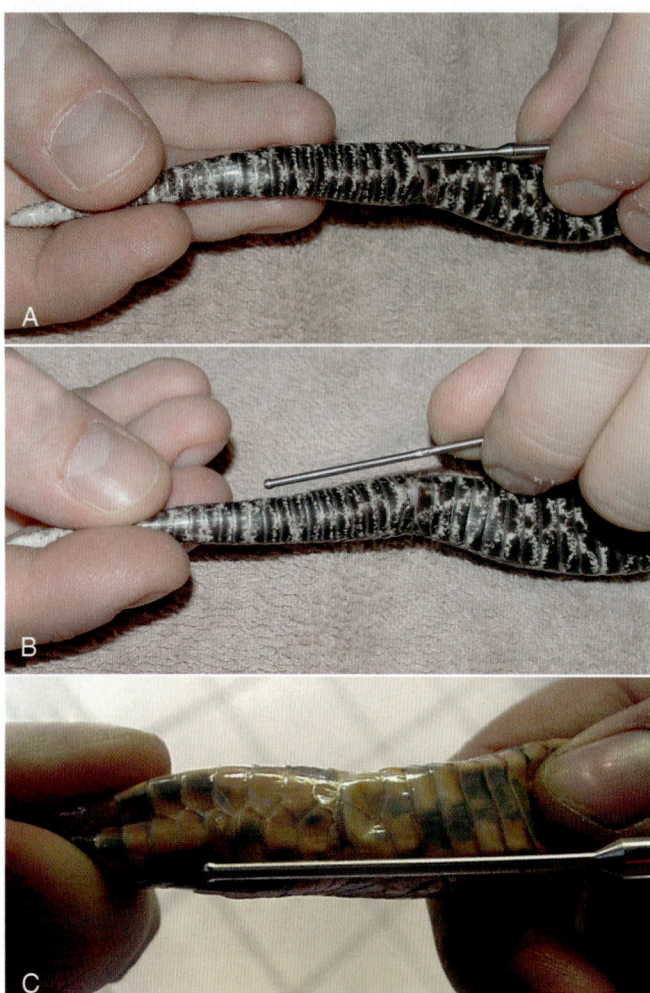

FIG 42.9 Gender identification of snakes: (A) a lubricated blunt sexing probe is inserted into the vent and advanced caudad; (B) the probe penetrates to a level of 6 to 14 subcaudal scales in males; (C) the probe penetrates to a level of only 2 to 4 subcaudal scales in females. (Courtesy of Stephen J. Divers.)

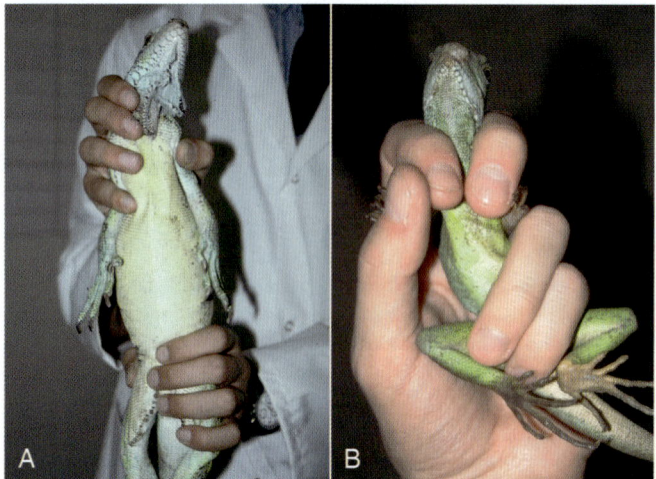

FIG 42.10 (A) Physical restraint of a large lizard such as this green iguana (*Iguana iguana*) should include holding the forelimbs against the body and the hind limbs against the tail base, as shown. (B) Single-handed restraint of small lizards such as this Asian water dragon (*Physignathus cocincinus*) must not inhibit coelomic breathing movements. (Courtesy of Stephen J. Divers.)

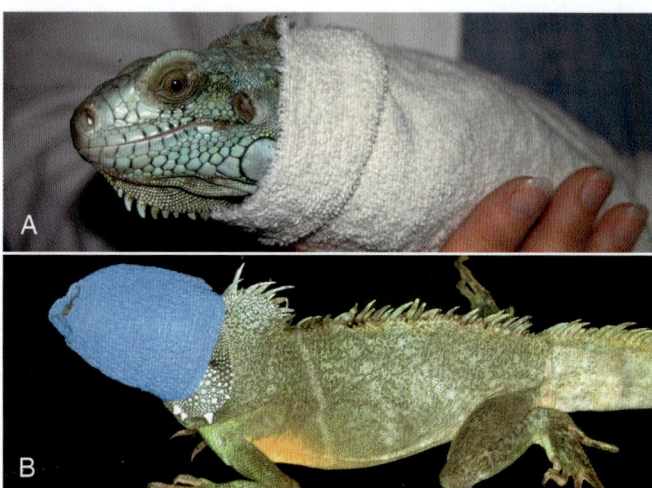

FIG 42.11 (A) Restraint of a green iguana (*Iguana iguana*) using a towel wrap technique. (B) Wrapping cotton wool and self-adherent tape over the closed eyes of an Asian water dragon (*Physignathus cocincinus*) to induce a vasovagal response. (Courtesy of Stephen J. Divers.)

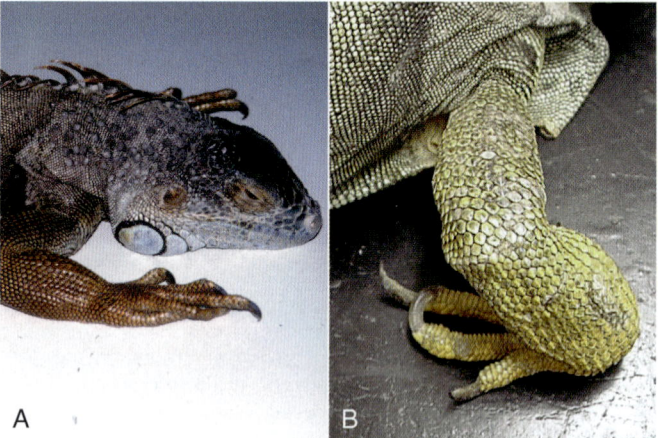

FIG 42.12 Neurologic assessment. (A) Moribund green iguana (*Iguana iguana*). Depression is most often associated with severe sepsis or metabolic derangements. (B) Propioceptive (placement) deficit in a green iguana with localized cervical spinal cord compression. Similar presentations can occur with limb fractures. (Courtesy of Stephen J. Divers.)

an assessment of growth and body condition. Auscultation of the heart using Doppler ultrasound is possible, whereas lungs are more challenging.

The cloaca should be free from fecal staining with visual and digital palpation considered routine in larger lizards where enlarged kidneys may be appreciated. The high incidence of dystocia necessitates a need to identify gender in the examination room. Many species of lizards are sexually dimorphic, although sexing juveniles can be difficult. Adult males tend to be generally larger with specifically larger heads; have more well-developed integumental appendages such as tubercules, spines, jowls, and dewlaps; are more colorful; exhibit more courting (head bobbing) and territorial behaviors; and possess paired hemipenal bulges at the tail base and more developed femoral or preanal pores (Fig. 42.18). Hemipenal eversion and probing are techniques that can be used but are generally more difficult to master than in snakes (see Chapter 80 for more information on gender identification lizards).

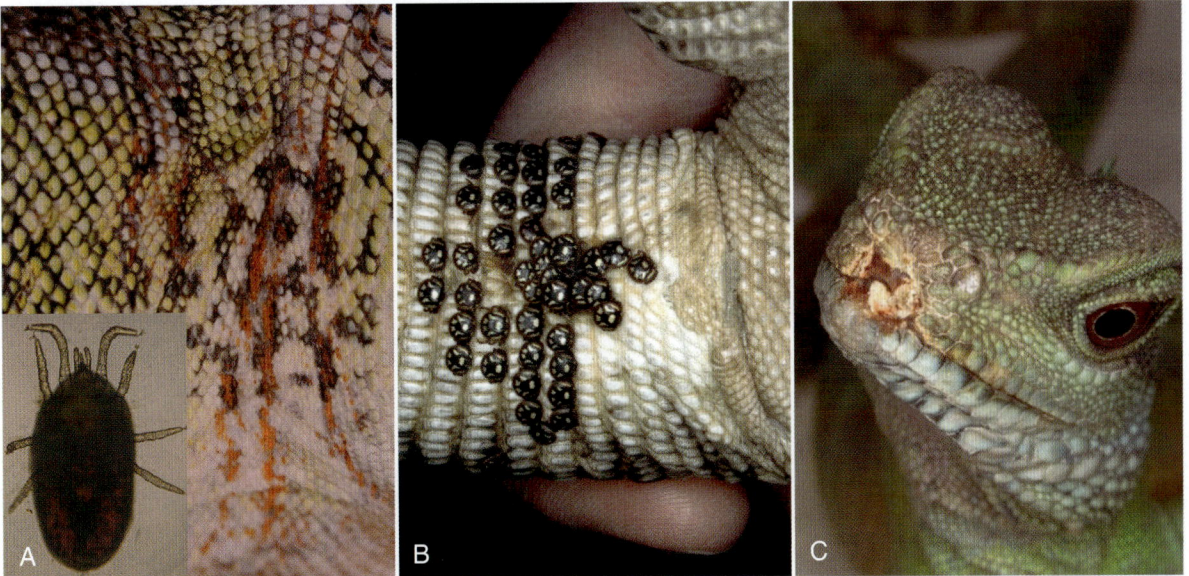

FIG 42.13 (A) *Hirstiella* mites are commonly found around skin folds. Inset, microscopic appearance of the mite. (B) Ticks located along the ventral tail base of an imported savannah monitor (*Varanus exanthematicus*). (C) Rostral abrasions are common in many lizards, like this Asian water dragon (*Physignathus cocincinus*), that fail to recognize and avoid glass barriers. (Courtesy of Stephen J. Divers.)

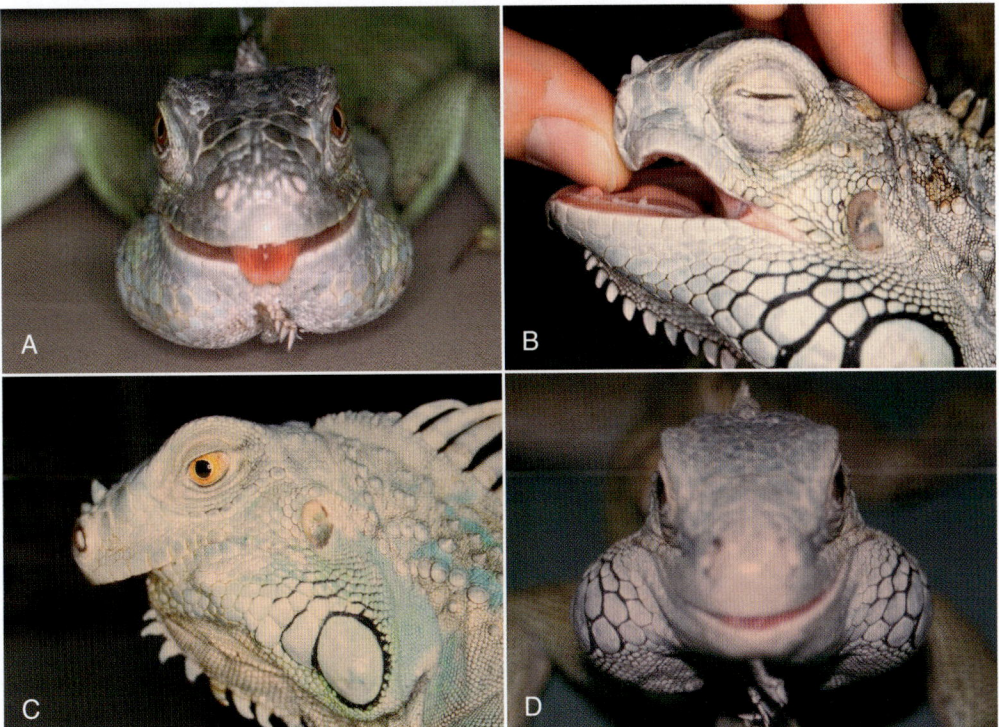

FIG 42.14 Abnormal head conformations in the green iguana (*Iguana iguana*). (A) Bilateral submandibular swellings associated with nutritional secondary hyperparathyroidism. (B) Softening and compressibility of the maxilla associated with renal secondary hyperparathyroidism. (C) Acquired agnathia caused by nutritional secondary hyperparathyroidism and the continual forces of the glossopharyngeal musculature on the softening mandible. (D) Bilateral submandibular fibromas or osteomas (not associated with classic nutritional secondary hyperparathyroidism although their cause remains unclear). (Courtesy of Stephen J. Divers.)

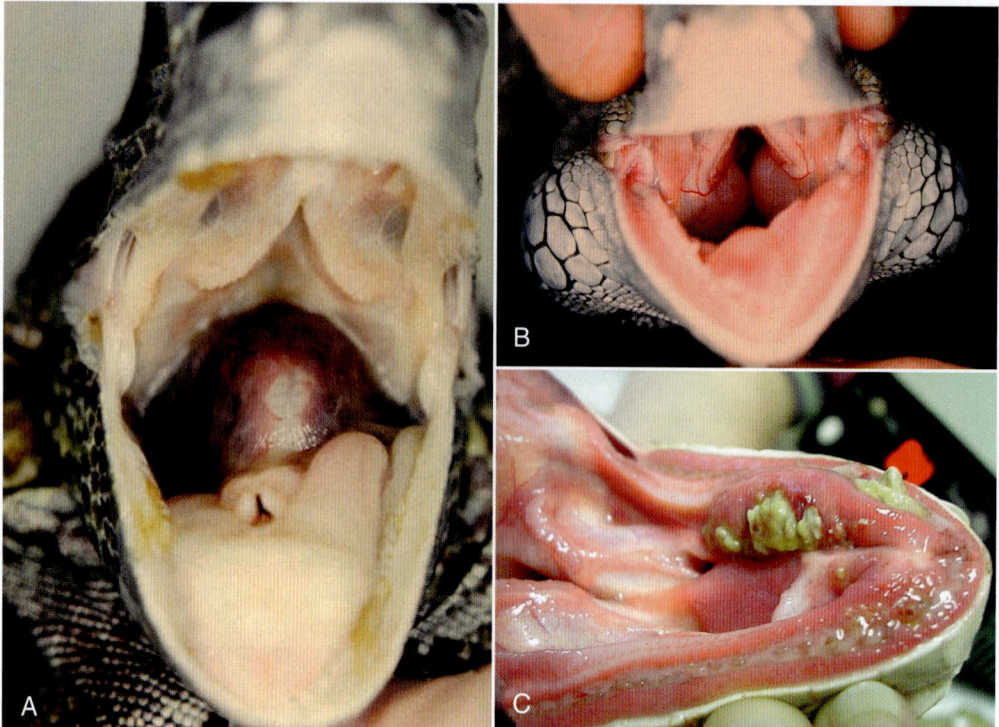

FIG 42.15 Oral abnormalities in lizards. (A) Pharyngeal edema due to chronic renal disease. (B) Intraoral appearance of bilateral fibroma/osteoma as they impinge within the dorsal pharynx. (C) Oral abscess. (Courtesy of Stephen J. Divers.)

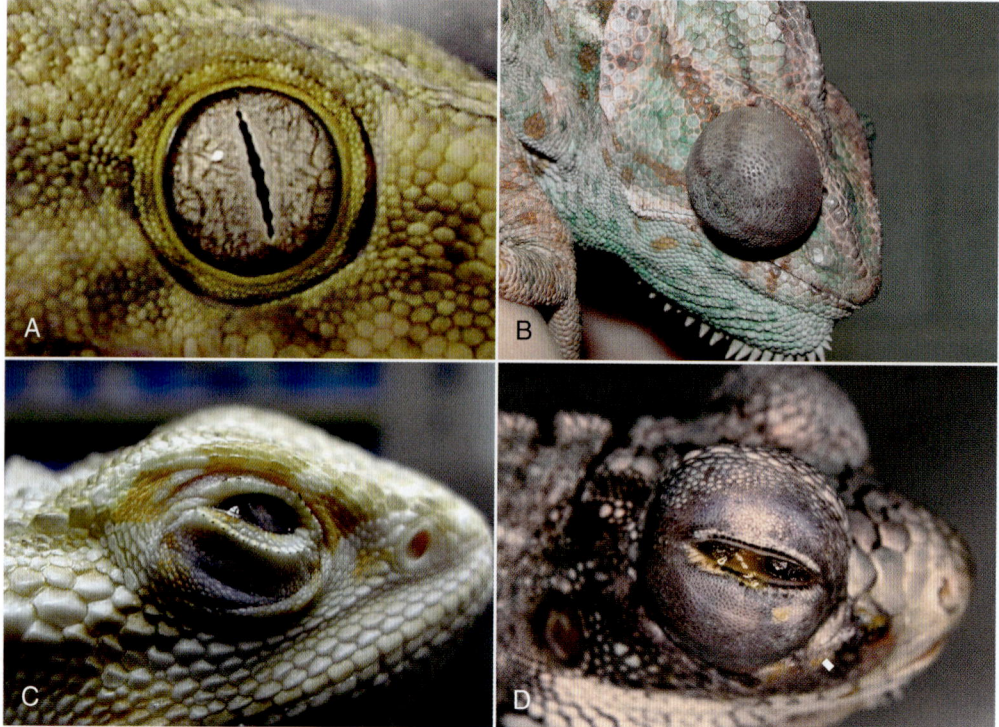

FIG 42.16 Lizard eyes. (A) Normal spectacled eye of the gecko, *Rhacodactylus leachianus*. (B) Acute swelling associated with trauma and engorgement of the retrobulbar venous plexus in a veiled chameleon (*Chameleo calyptraptus*). (C) Blepharospasm and conjunctivitis in a bearded dragon (*Pogona vitticeps*) associated with corneal ulceration tend sand in the conjunctival sac. (D) Gross distension of the eye in a green iguana (*Iguana iguana*) due to panopthalmitis and retrobulbar abscessation. (Courtesy of Stephen J. Divers.)

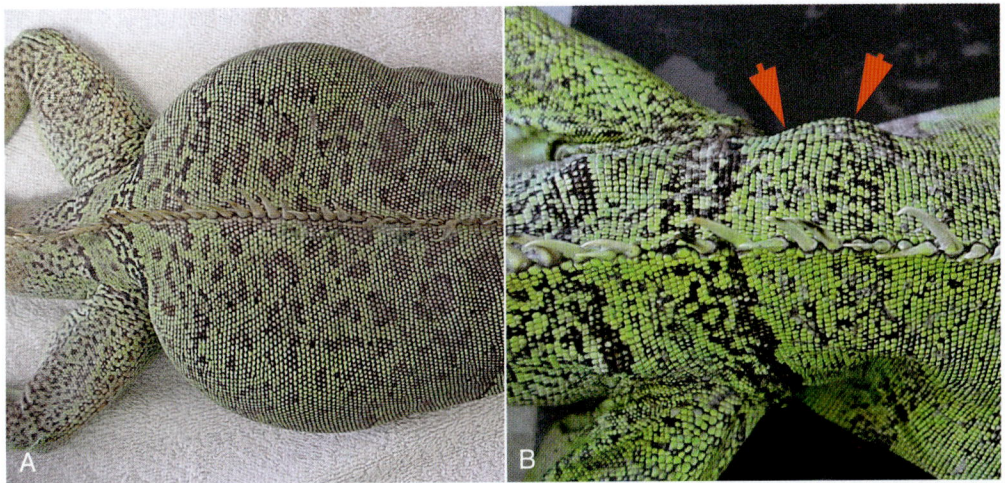

FIG 42.17 Coelomic distension in a lizard may be due to ascites, reproductive activity, organomegaly, neoplasia, or abscess. (B) Enlarged kidney (arrow) in a green iguana (*Iguana iguana*). (Courtesy of Stephen J. Divers.)

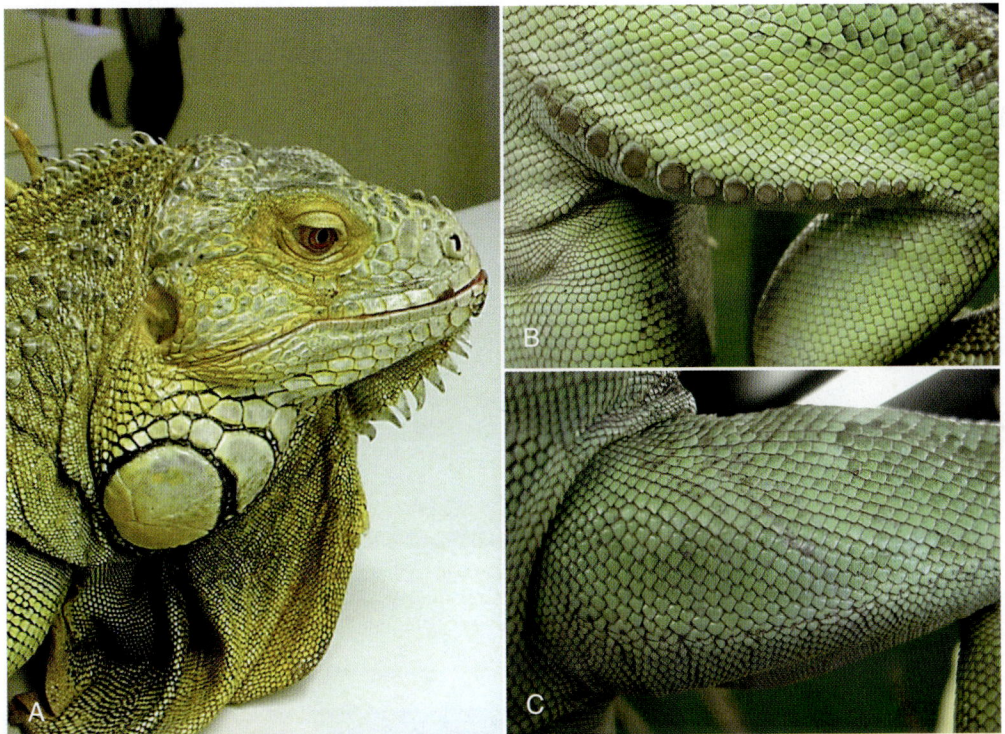

FIG 42.18 Secondary sexual characteristics of lizards, depicted in these figures in green iguanas (*Iguana iguana*). (A) Mature males often have larger, broader heads with more developed crests, dewlaps, or jowls. (B) Mature males have more developed preanal or femoral pores. (C) Female lizards tend to have reduced or absent preanal or femoral pores. (Courtesy of Stephen J. Divers.)

CHELONIANS

Aquatic species tend to have a formidable bite that may belie an apparently gentle disposition. The major biologic peculiarity of all chelonia is the presence of the shell. The plastron and carapace not only give this group their characteristic structure but also doubles as a barrier to physical examination. Nevertheless, much can still be achieved in the consulting room before resorting to imaging techniques. Small-to-medium tortoises are not difficult to handle, although their strength and uncooperative

nature can hinder the examination and cause frustration. A little patience while holding the tortoise head down will often persuade a shy individual to protrude the head from the shell, allowing the thumb and middle finger to then be placed behind the occipital condyles to prevent retraction of the head back into the shell. Alternatively, a long 18- to 20-g hypodermic needle with the terminal 3 mm bent at a 60-degree angle can be inserted into the mouth of a retracted head and used to engage the buccal surface of the upper beak. Sustained traction is often successful at extracting the head from the shell. In the larger species (e.g.,

Centrochelys, Stigmochelys, Geochelone) it may be physically impossible to overpower an individual, and reliance on sedation is often necessary.

Applying steady distractive pressure to the maxilla and mandible can open the mouth, and once open the index finger (in small, gentle specimens) or a mouth gag (in larger or aggressive specimens) can be inserted to prevent closure. This method enables the handler to keep the mouth open using one hand, leaving the other free to examine the head and take samples for laboratory investigation. In aggressive species, open-mouth threat displays provide a good opportunity to examine the buccal cavity with minimal handling. The buccal cavity must always be examined, particularly for evidence of inflammation, infection, gout, and foreign bodies (Fig. 42.19). Stomatitis can quickly lead to a generalized esophagitis, and examination down the pharynx and into the esophagus using a rigid endoscope is advisable. Mucous membrane coloration should be noted and is normally pale pink. Hyperemic membranes may be associated with septicemia or toxemia. Icterus is rare but may occur with biliverdinemia due to severe liver disease. Pale membranes are often observed in cases of true anemia. Pale deposits within the oral membranes may represent infection or urate tophi

associated with visceral gout. The larynx may be difficult to visualize, being positioned at the back of the fleshy tongue; however, it is important to check for any inflammation and glottal discharges that may be consistent with respiratory disease. Examination of the head should include the nostrils for any discharge and the beak for damage and overgrowth (Fig. 42.20). The eyelids should be open and not obviously distended or inflamed, and the eyes should be clear and bright. Conjunctivitis, corneal ulceration, and opacities are frequent presentations (Fig. 42.21). The retina can often suffer from degeneration as a consequence of freezing during hibernation, and ophthalmic examination is warranted in every animal. The tympanic scales should be examined for signs of swelling associated with aural abscessation (Fig. 42.22). Verification of a tympanic abscess can often be made by observing exudate emanating from the eustachian tube openings at the lateral walls of the pharynx.

The withdrawn limbs can also be extended from the shell of small-to-medium chelonians by applying steady traction. The coelomic space within the shell is restricted, and therefore gently forcing the hind limbs into the shell will often lead to partial protrusion of the forelimbs and head and vice versa. The more aggressive aquatic species should be held

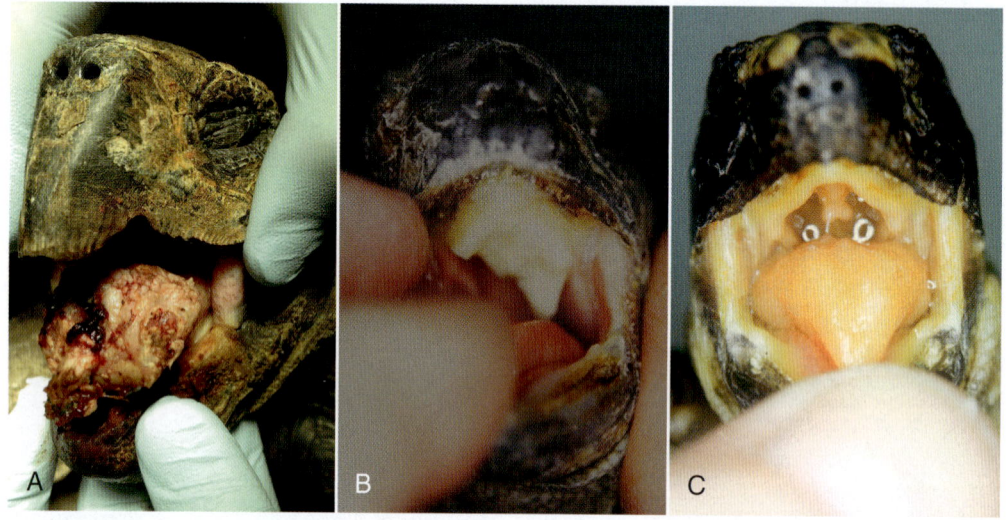

FIG 42.19 Oral abnormalities in chelonians. (A) Mycotic glossitis in a Galapagos tortoise (*Geochelone nigra*). (B) Hard palate stomatitis due to *Candida* in a Greek tortoise (*Testudo graeca*). (C) Pronounced icterus in a tortoise (*Testudo*) due to hepatobiliary disease. (Courtesy of Stephen J. Divers.)

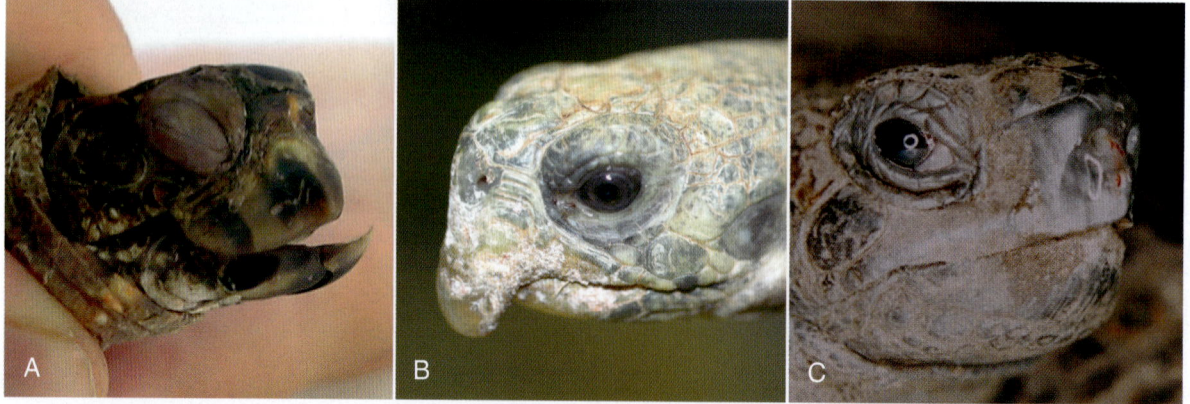

FIG 42.20 (A) Overgrown maxillary and mandibular beak in a *Testudo* tortoise. (B) Overgown maxillary beak in a bell's hinge-back tortoise (*Kinixys belliana*). (C) Serosanguinous nasal discharge from a tortoise (*Testudo*). (Courtesy of Stephen J. Divers.)

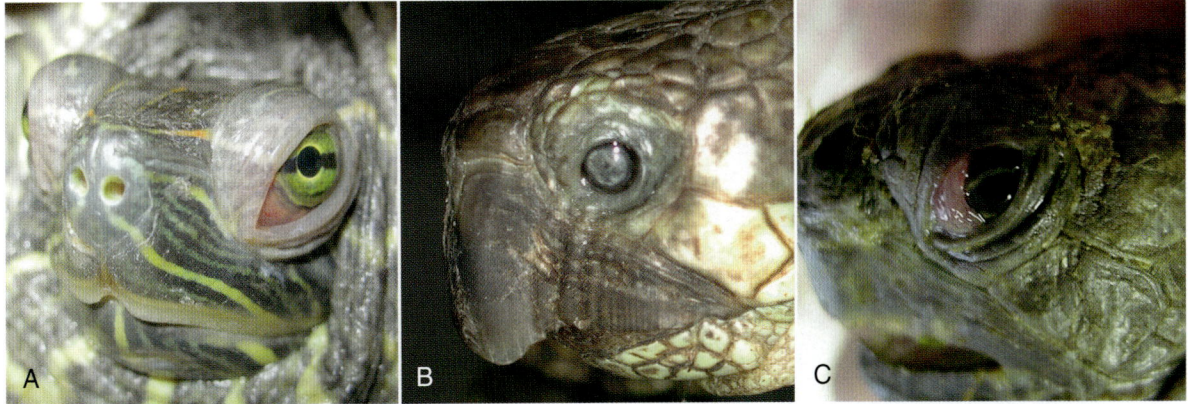

FIG 42.21 (A) Bilateral blepharitis and conjunctivitis in a red-eared slider (*Trachemys scripta elegans*). (B) Large hypermature cataract in a *Testudo* tortoise following freeze damage. (C) Protrusion of the nictitating membrane in a Hermann's tortoise (*Testudo hermanni*) with bacterial conjunctivitis. (Courtesy of Stephen J. Divers.)

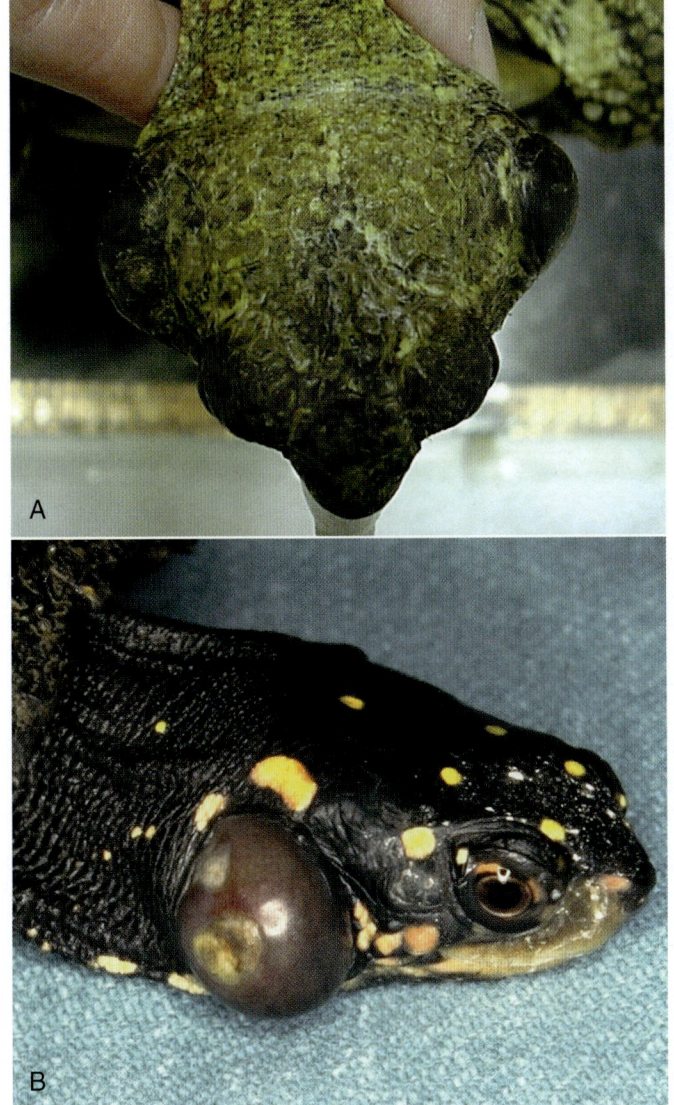

FIG 42.22 (A) Bilateral aural abscesses in a tortoise (*Testudo*). (B) Right aural abscess in a spotted turtle (*Clemmys guttata*). (Courtesy of Stephen J. Divers.)

at the rear of the carapace. Some species (e.g., common snapping turtle, *Chelydra serpentina*) can deliver a rapid and extremely powerful bite, and so great care is required at all times. Certain species also possess functional hinges at the front and/or back of the plastron, and care should be taken not to allow a finger to become trapped. A wedge or mouth gag can be used to prevent complete closure of a hinge, and chelonians will not close a hinge on their own extended appendage. The integument should be examined for parasites, particularly ticks and flies, dysecdysis, trauma, and infection resulting from rodent, raccoon, or small carnivore attacks. Aggressive conflicts and courting trauma must also be considered in the communal environment. Limb fractures are less commonly reported in chelonians than in lizards but are often caused by rough handling and falls, with a greater incidence possible in those individuals suffering from nutritional secondary hyperparathyroidism. The integument should be free of damage and subcutaneous swellings, which if present are often abscesses, myiasis (if housed outdoors), or neoplasia, which is less frequent (Fig. 42.23). Aquatic species appear more susceptible to superficial and deep mycotic dermatitis, especially around the head, neck, and limbs. Grossly swollen joints or limbs are more often cases of fracture, osteomyelitis, septic arthritis, or rarely neoplasia.

The prefemoral fossae should be palpated with the chelonian held head-up. Gently rocking the animal may then enable the clinician to appreciate eggs, cystic calculi, or other coelomic masses. The shell should be examined for hardness, conformation, trauma, and infection (Fig. 42.24). Soft, poorly mineralized shells of juveniles are usually a result of nutritional secondary hyperparathyroidism resulting from dietary deficiencies of calcium, excess phosphorus, or a lack of full-spectrum lighting. Pyramiding of the shell has been linked to reduced environmental humidity and high nocturnal temperatures, although it is likely multifactorial. Shell infection may present as loosening and softening of the scutes with erythema, petechiae, purulent, or caseous discharge and a foul odor. Deep infections usually involve the bones of the shell with resulting osteomyelitis.

Prolapses through the vent are obvious, but it is necessary to determine the structure(s) involved. Prolapses may include cloacal tissue, shell gland, colon, bladder, or phallus (Fig. 42.25). Internal examination using digital palpation or an endoscope is recommended. Male chelonians can be differentiated from females by their longer tails and a more distal position of their vent past the caudal edge of the carapace (Fig. 42.26). Other sexually dimorphism characteristics may also be obvious,

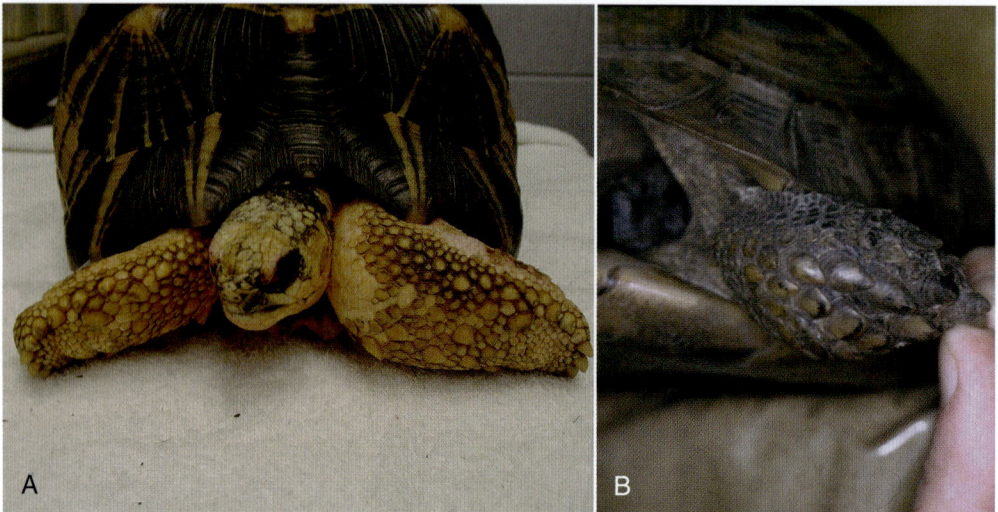

FIG 42.23 (A) Grossly enlarged left forelimb in a radiated tortoise (*Astrochelys radiata*) due to an undifferentiated sarcoma. (B) Grossly swollen left forelimb of a tortoise (*Testudo*) due to osteomyelitis. (Courtesy of Stephen J. Divers.)

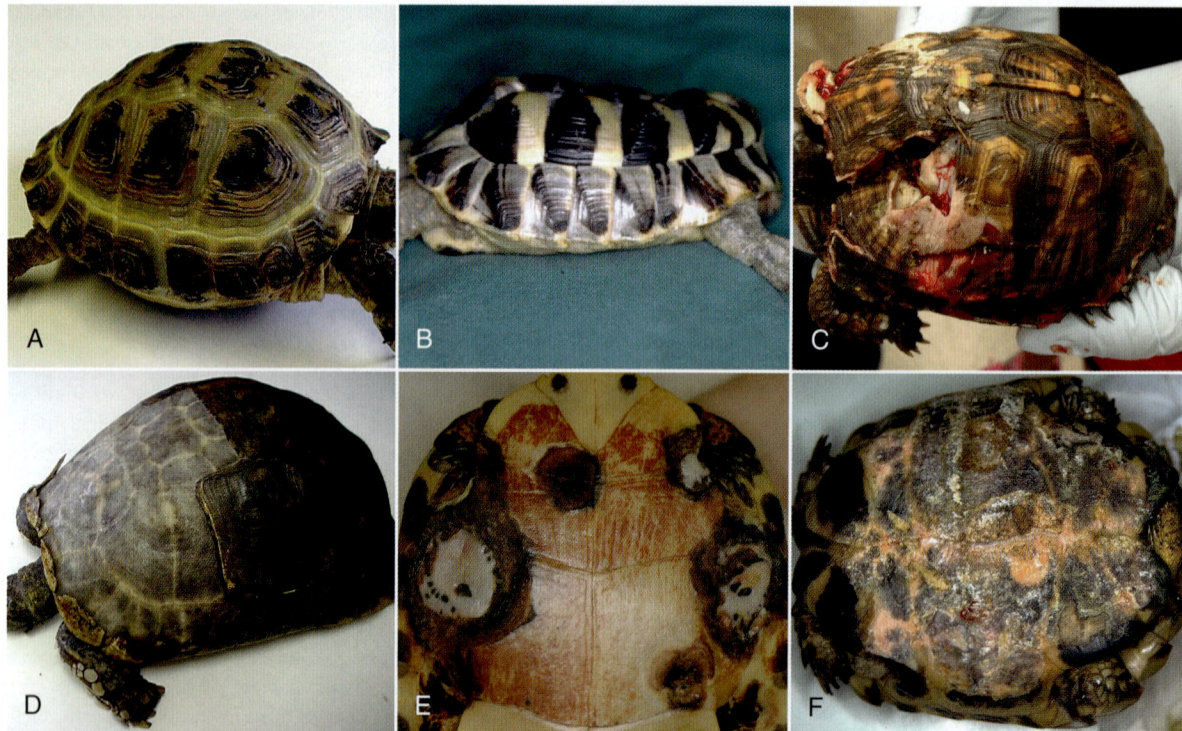

FIG 42.24 (A) Excessive growth in a juvenile tortoise (*Agrionemys*) indicated by broad growth lines between the scutes. (B) Carapacial concavity associated with nutritional secondary hyperparathyroidism in a tortoise (*Testudo*). (C) Shell fractures in a box turtle (*Terrapene*). (D) Fire trauma in a Greek tortoise (*Testudo graeca*). (E) Multifocal osteomyelitis from a mixed bacterial and mycotic infection in a map turtle (*Graptemys*). (F) Bacterial osteomyelitis of the plastron in a tortoise (*Testudo*) due to underfloor heating, excessive humidity, and poor cage hygiene. (Courtesy of Stephen J. Divers.)

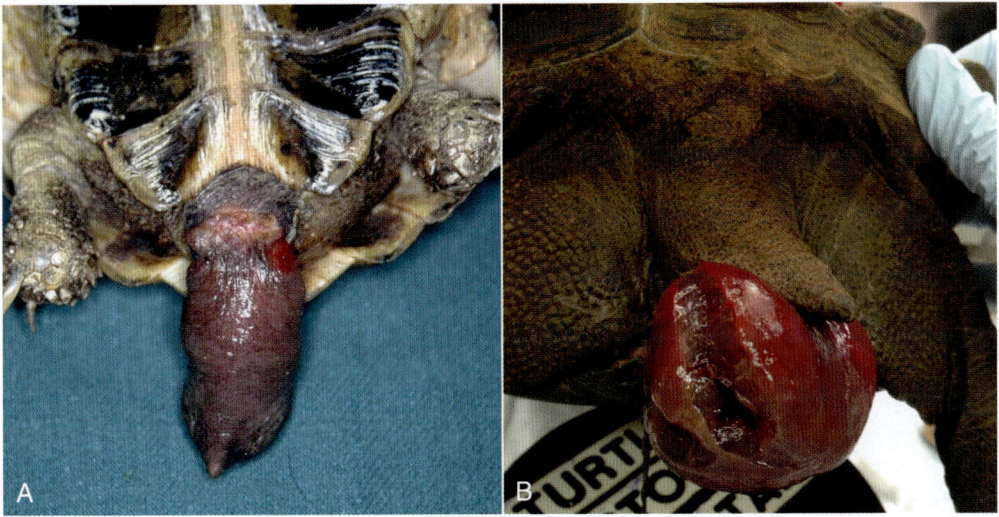

FIG 42.25 (A) Phallus prolapse in a tortoise (*Testudo*). (B) Cloacocolonic prolapse in an Aldabra tortoise (*Aldabrachelys gigantea*). (Courtesy of Stephen J. Divers.)

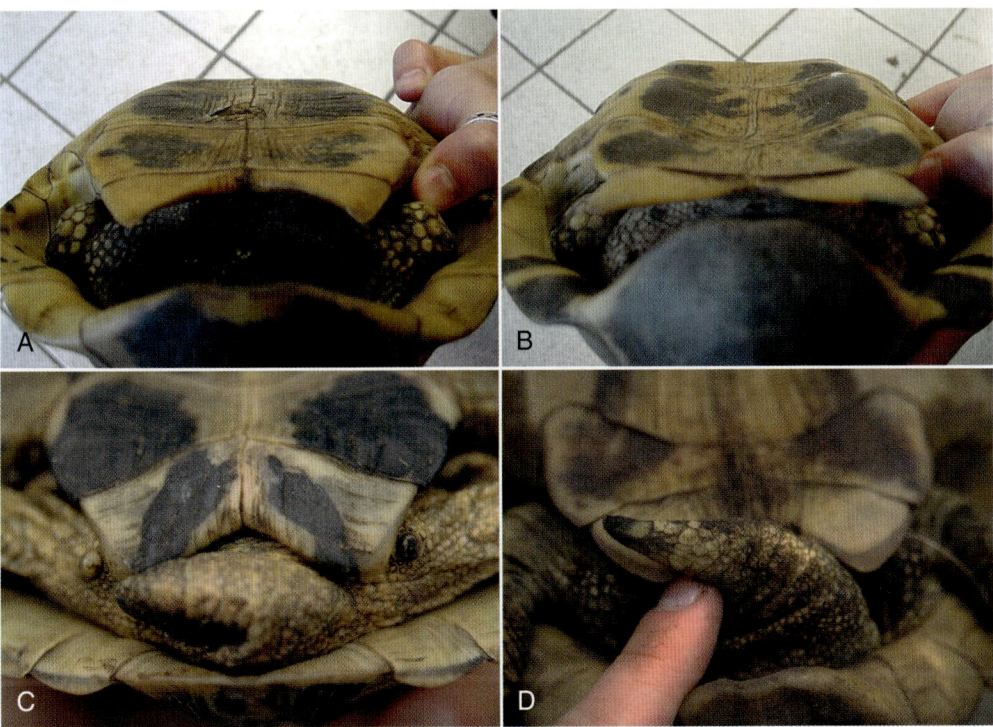

FIG 42.26 Gender identification in chelonians. (A) Female red-footed tortoise (*Chelonoidis carbonaria*) with flat plastron. (B) Male red-footed tortoise (*Chelonoidis carbonaria*) with more concave plastron. (C) Female Greek tortoise (*Testudo graeca*) with shorter tail. (D) Male hermann's tortoise (*Testudo hermanni*) with longer tail. (Courtesy of Stephen J. Divers.)

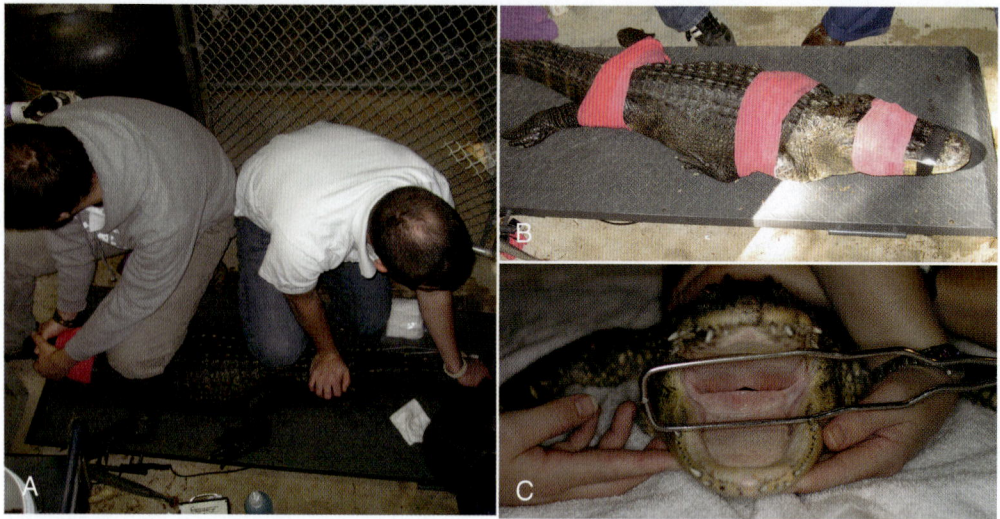

FIG 42.27 (A) Physical restraint of medium-to-larger crocodilians requires a well-trained team to control the head and tail. (B) Improved restraint can be achieved by taping the mouth and eyes closed and securing the limbs against the body and tail base. (C) Always use a sturdy mouth gag when performing an oral examination—even in an anesthetized crocodilian. (Courtesy of Stephen J. Divers.)

including the concavity of the male plastron in many species and the longer forelimb claws of some male freshwater species. (See Chapter 80 for a thorough review of sex determination.)

CROCODILIANS

Individuals under 2 m in total length can often be handled conscious, albeit with extreme caution. Even the small crocodilians can use both tail and jaw to cause injury. Examination of large crocodilians requires the coordinated efforts of an experienced team, and the mouth should always be taped shut and the tail firmly restrained (Fig. 42.27). A vasovagal-induced torpor can be elicited by gently taping the eyes closed. Examination of the eyes and mouth are carried out at the very end of the examination process, just before the animal is released. Animals may be strapped to a wooden plank to improve physical restraint, but when dealing with animals more than 2 m in length, serious consideration should be given to the routine use of chemical restraint. The physical examination of crocodilians follows a similar pattern to that used for large saurians, as their body patterns are similar. The clinician should pay particular attention to the extremities and integument, which are often traumatized by conspecifics or interactions with poorly designed environments.

REFERENCES

See www.expertconsult.com for a complete list of references.

43

Diagnostic Techniques and Sample Collection

Stephen J. Divers

The successful diagnosis and treatment of herpetologic disease requires an ability to properly restrain, examine, and perform a variety of clinical techniques. The principles of such techniques are similar to those employed in domestic companion animal medicine. The following descriptions include clinical techniques that the author has employed for the purposes of disease diagnosis in pets, zoo animals, and wildlife. Some descriptions are general and apply to most if not all species within a group, while others may be more specific. Careful consideration should be given to the context of disease investigation, and zoological veterinarians need to be able to switch perspectives from individual animal (i.e., extensive antemortem diagnostic testing is appropriate) to population health (i.e., when elective necropsy of an affected animal may be more efficient and cost-effective). Definitive diagnosis of nontraumatic issues requires demonstration of both a pathologic response by the animal and etiologic agent. Pathologic responses can be documented by histopathology (often considered the gold standard), cytology (less favored due to loss of tissue architecture), and paired rising antibody titers (of which the few that are available take 6–12 weeks to develop and are more retrospective in value). Demonstration of the etiologic cause typically requires microbiology (culture, PCR), parasitology, toxicology, or again, paired rising titers. As zoological clinicians we need to get past disease diagnosis at the organ level (i.e., kidney disease) and strive for an antemortem definitive diagnosis at a histologic level (e.g., glomerulonephritis due to *E. coli*). The advent of various clinical techniques (especially endoscopic biopsy) have enabled antemortem diagnosis, where previously necropsy was the only means of achieving a definitive answer.[1–7]

DIAGNOSTIC SAMPLE COLLECTION

Blood and Hemopoietic System

Venipuncture and Blood Collection. The ability to collect quality blood samples is essential in any animal class. Complete or selective hematologic and biochemical evaluations are possible, but the accuracy of results is often adversely affected by poor venipuncture, handling, or laboratory skills. The production of poor quality blood data can be useless or, even worse, misleading to the clinician. Likewise, the ability to administer intravenous medications especially anesthetics, or place intravenous catheters also relies on proficient venous access. Venipuncture is generally a blind technique in reptiles. The jugular vein of certain tortoises may be visible particularly following temporary caudal occlusion of the vessel or by positioning the animal in a head-down position; however, anatomic knowledge of the position of reptile veins is vital. It is wise to aseptically prepare the venipuncture site, as infection and abscessation following venous access is a potential complication. Despite a continuous trickle of published blood ranges, there is still a paucity of hematologic or biochemical data for reptiles compared to domesticated animals. The issue is further complicated by variations, often dramatic, associated with species, environment, nutrition, age, gender, breeding status, hibernation, and disease status. Consequently, few, if any, of these published ranges can claim to satisfy the American Society of Veterinary Clinical Pathologists guidelines for reference range production and therefore should be described as observed ranges.[8] Given this variability, published ranges are often of limited value, and clinicians should develop a healthy distrust of such data, which becomes clear when you start comparing clinicopathology to histopathology findings. Greater value should be placed on (i) establishing a healthy individual's observed range by annual or biennial sampling, which should form the basis of identifying abnormalities, and (ii) monitoring the progress of hematologic and biochemical changes during disease rather than relying on a single result. The following descriptions indicate the most humane and practical venipuncture sites. Others have been indicated for completeness but may have reduced clinical application due to increased risk, poor quality sample, or significant welfare and ethical concerns. For example, the use of a toenail clip to obtain blood may result in fecal or urate contamination, elevated tissue enzymes, abnormal hemogram, and electrolyte changes due to the peripheral nature of the sample and the crushing artifact of collection. Of even greater concern are the ethical and welfare issues that surround a procedure that causes more pain and carries a greater risk of post-sampling sepsis.

Approximately 0.4 to 0.8 mL blood per 100 g body weight may be safely collected from healthy reptiles, but when dealing with compromised animals, restricting collection to 0.4 to 0.5 mL/100 g on any occasion is sensible. The established dogma that lithium heparin is the preferred anticoagulant for reptile hematology is simply false. EDTA has been shown to be superior for most, if not all, squamates and even some chelonians.[9–11] Only in the Chelonia are there examples of species-specific, EDTA-induced erythrocyte lysis necessitating the use of lithium heparin.[12] When blood-sampling chelonians of unknown EDTA sensitivity, it is wise to submit both heparin and EDTA whole blood samples and to measure the PCV of both. Only if the PCV of the EDTA sample is lower should the heparin sample be used in preference. When dealing with small chelonians of unknown EDTA sensitivity (where only a single hematology sample is possible), heparin should be submitted. Another misconception is the value of manually preheparinized syringes to prevent clotting and improve sample quality. The use of preheparinized syringes results in significant and inconsistent blood dilution with reductions in PCV and total solids and is not recommended.[13]

Snakes. The two common sites for venipuncture in snakes are the caudal (ventral tail) vein and the heart (Fig. 43.1). The caudal (tail) vein is accessed caudal to the cloaca, between 25% and 50% down the tail. It is wise to avoid the paired hemipenes of males (that may extend up to 14–16 subcaudal scales down the tail), and the paired cloacal musk glands in both sexes (that may extend up to 6 subcaudal scales).

The needle is angled at 45 to 60 degrees and positioned in the ventral midline. The needle is advanced in a craniodorsal direction, while maintaining slight negative pressure. If the needle touches a vertebral body, it is withdrawn slightly and redirected more craniad or caudad. Gravity can be utilized to help with venous blood flow by "hanging" the tail down prior to and during blood collection. This vessel is most easily entered in larger snakes and lymphatic or cerebrospinal fluid contamination is possible.

With the snake restrained in dorsal recumbency, the heart is located approximately 22% to 33% from snout to vent. The heart is palpated and immobilized. The needle is advanced at 45 degrees in a craniodorsal direction into the apex of the beating ventricle. Blood often enters the syringe with each heartbeat. If an initial attempt does not result in blood entering the syringe, the needle should be withdrawn and a new needle and attempt should be made. Do not move the needle laterally "searching" for blood flow as laceration to the ventricle or pericardium

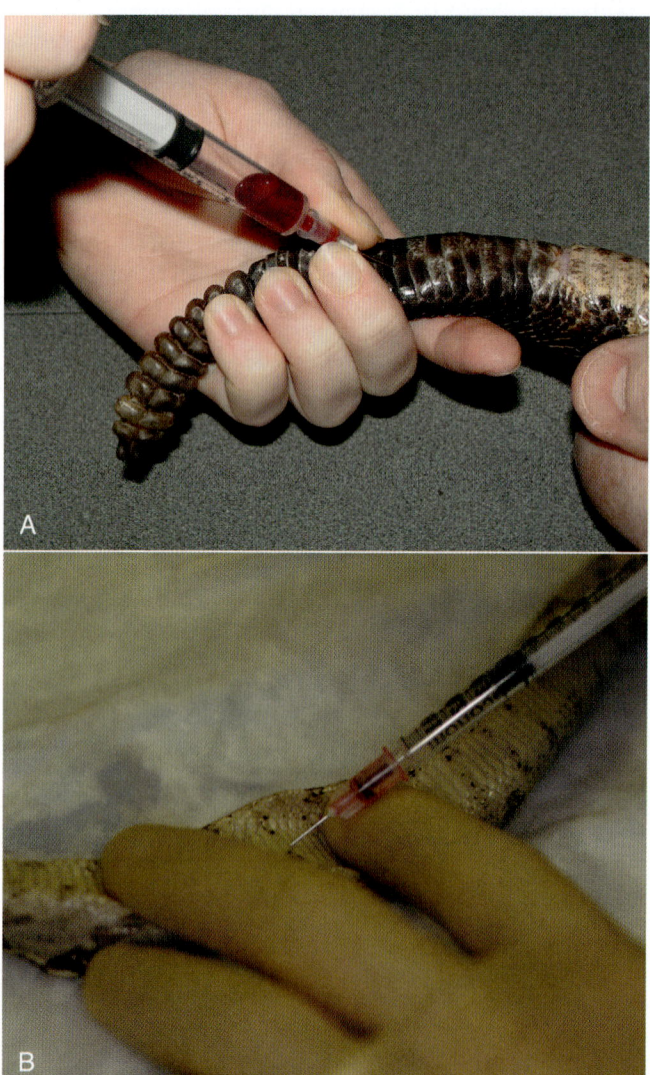

FIG 43.1 (A) Blood collection from the caudal (tail) vein of a rattlesnake (*Crotalinae*). Note the position of the needle caudal to the cloacal. (B) Blood collection by cardiocentesis in a juvenile *Boa constrictor*. The heart is digitally immobilized prior to introducing the needle. (Courtesy of Stephen J. Divers.)

may occur and result in severe damage and hemorrhage. It is wise to maintain digital pressure for 30 to 60 seconds following this technique. This technique appears to be safe in snakes of all sizes, although pericardial hemorrhage has been appreciated by the author at necropsy following this technique. Lymphatic or pericardial contamination appears uncommon but pericardial fluid, and it has been used in snakes ranging from 10 g neonates to 100 kg constrictors. Nevertheless, excellent restraint is essential if significant cardiac trauma is to be avoided, and this technique should be reserved for animals that are moribund, anesthetized, or where tail venipuncture failed. The palatine-pterygoid veins are easily visualized in the dorsal aspect of the oral cavity of large snakes; however, difficulties concerning physical restraint, appropriate access, and the prevention of a large hematoma make this technique less acceptable.

Lizards. The most clinically useful vessel is the caudal (tail) vein (Fig. 43.2). The needle is positioned in the ventral midline between 20% to 80% down the tail and advanced at 45 to 60 degrees in a craniodorsal direction while maintaining slight negative pressure. If a coccygeal vertebra is encountered, the needle is withdrawn slightly and redirected either further craniad or caudad. An alternative approach that is particularly useful for the larger species is to insert the needle from the lateral midline. The needle is advanced at 45 to 60 degrees in a craniomedial direction, aiming just ventral to the lateral processes of the coccygeal vertebrae. Lymphatic contamination appears more likely with the lateral approach.

Lizards possess a large ventral abdominal vein that runs within a suspensory ligament just below the linea alba. This vessel is most easily entered in the midcoelomic region. The needle is positioned in the ventral midline and advanced in a craniodorsal direction. Apart from the risks of puncturing the gastrointestinal tract or bladder, it is difficult to apply pressure to this vessel, making postvenipuncture hemorrhage a potential complication.

Jugular vein venipuncture is also practical, especially in larger lizards. The jugular veins lie lateral and deep and are seldom visible even when caudally occluded by digital pressure. For most species, the tympanum is a useful anatomic landmark. The lizard is restrained in lateral recumbency, and the clinician should insert the needle in a caudal direction behind the tympanum.

Cardiocentesis in lizards is not as acceptable as it is in snakes, because the heart cannot be stabilized. Other potential sites include the axillary plexus, orbital sinus, and toenail clip. but their use is more problematic, clinically unwarranted, and ethically less acceptable.

Tortoises, turtles, and terrapins. The left and right external jugular veins (also referred to as the left and right dorsal cervical sinuses) are preferred because of the greatly reduced risk of lymphatic or cerebrospinal fluid contamination (Fig. 43.3). The regional anatomy varies with species, but the vessel is generally located laterally and may even be visible by occluding the vessel at the base of the neck or restraining the animal in a 30-degree head-down position. The needle is positioned caudal to the tympanum and directed in a caudal direction. Following venipuncture, the chelonian should be held in a head-up position with pressure applied to the jugular to prevent hematoma formation.

There are variable, species-specific ventral, lateral, and dorsal coccygeal vessels that can be utilized in many chelonia. The dorsal coccygeal vein is probably the most commonly used of the tail veins (Fig. 43.4A). The needle is angled at 45 to 90 degrees and placed, as craniad as possible, in the dorsal midline of the tail. The needle is advanced in a cranioventral direction while maintaining slight negative pressure. If the needle encounters a vertebra, it is withdrawn slightly and redirected more craniad or caudad. The exact position, size, and even presence of this vessel may vary between species, and there is a significant risk of lymphatic or cerebrospinal fluid contamination.

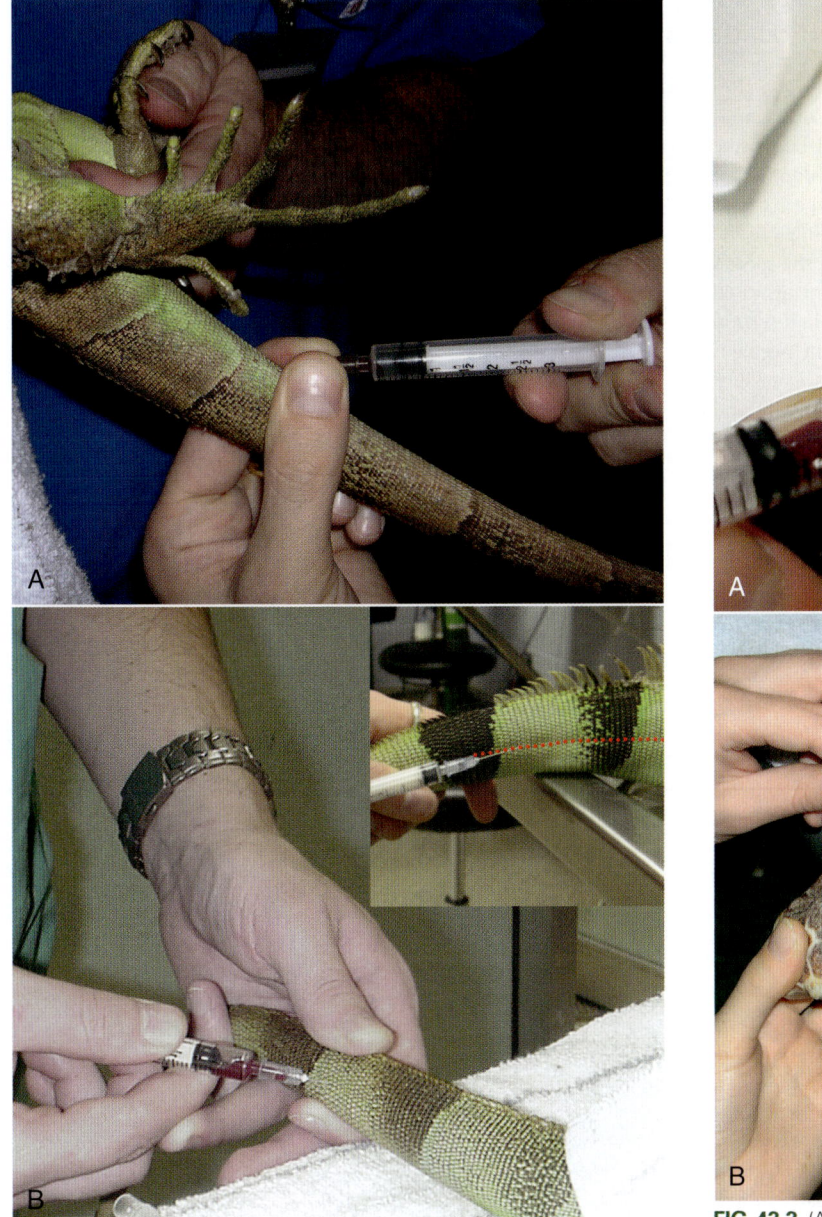

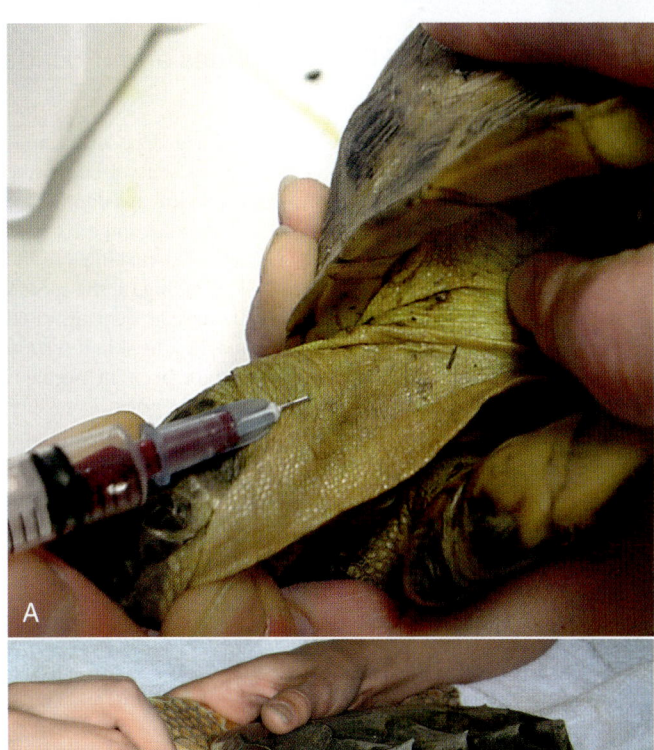

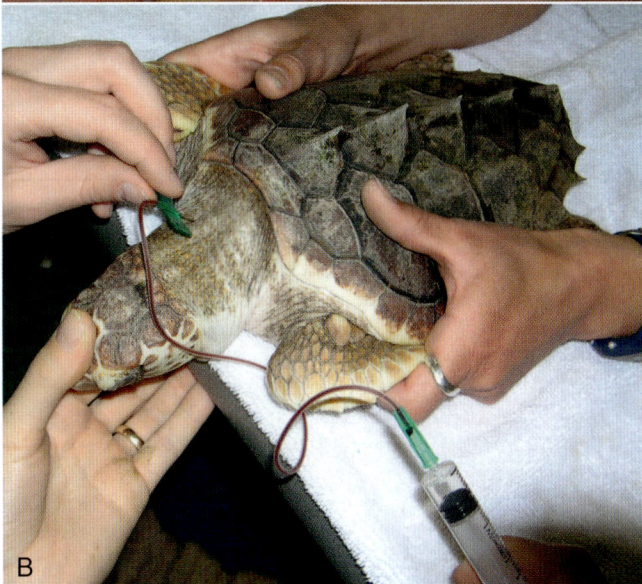

FIG 43.2 Ventral (A) and lateral (B) approaches to the caudal (tail) vein of lizards. (Courtesy of Stephen J. Divers.)

FIG 43.3 (A) Blood collection from the jugular vein of a Greek tortoise (*Testudo graeca*). Note how the assistant is restraining the forelimbs and occluding the vein at the caudolateral region of the neck. (B) Blood collection from the external jugular vein (also called the dorsal cervical sinus) of a juvenile loggerhead sea turtle (*Caretta caretta*). (Courtesy of Stephen J. Divers.)

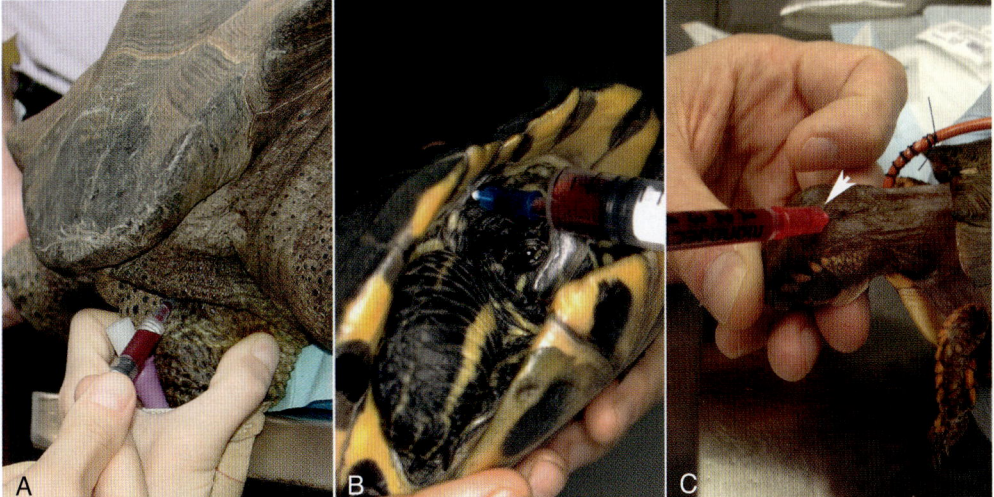

FIG 43.4 (A) Blood collection from the dorsal coccygeal vein of an adult Aldabran tortoise (*Dipsochelys elephantina*). (B) Blood collection from the subcarapacial venous sinus (junction of the last caudal anastomosis of the caudal external jugular veins and the cranial intercostal veins) from a red-eared slider (*Trachemys scripta elegans*). (C) Blood collection from the postoccipital sinus in a box turtle (*Terrapene* sp.). (Courtesy of Stephen J. Divers.)

A subcarapacial site is also available and formed by the venous communication between the most craniad intercostal vessels arising from the paired azygous veins and the caudal cervical anastomosis of the left and right jugular veins (Fig. 43.4B). This sinus can be accessed with the chelonian's head either extended or retracted, making it useful for uncooperative or aggressive individuals. Depending on the species and conformation of the carapace, the needle may be bent up to 60 degrees and positioned in the midline just caudal to the skin insertion on the ventral aspect of the cranial rim of the carapace. The needle is advanced in a caudodorsal direction, maintaining slight negative pressure. If a vertebra is encountered, the needle is withdrawn slightly and redirected further craniad or caudad. Lymph, or more commonly cerebrospinal fluid, contamination can occur.

There is a significant postoccipital vessel that lies in the midline, dorsal to the vertebral column. This vessel can be accessed just behind the head (Fig. 43.4C). The needle is inserted from the parietal notch, lateral to the supraoccipital crest, directed at 45 degrees to the midline and advanced in a caudomedial direction. The lateromedial advancement of the needle reduces the chances of trauma to the spinal cord. If unsuccessful, the needle can be inserted in the dorsal midline and aimed ventrally (much like access to the supravertebral sinus of crocodilians); however, excessive penetration can more easily damage the spinal cord, and therefore excellent restraint is necessary. In general, this dorsdal midline approach is reserved for anesthetized or moribund animals where there is a critical need for blood collection and other techniques have failed.

Cardiocentesis is rarely indicated (unless other approaches have failed) or practical due to the obstruction caused by the plastron. In those chelonians with soft shells (e.g., soft-shelled turtles [*Apalone* spp], neonates of most species, and individuals with severe secondary nutritional hyperparathyroidism) a needle can be inserted through the soft plastron directly into the heart. The exact position of the heart varies with species but is generally located just dorsal to the plastron, in the midline at the intersection of the abdominal and pectoral scutes. In hard-shelled animals, a temporary osteotomy over the cardiac point of the plastron also permits access to the heart. Alternatively, the heart may be approached from a soft tissue approach. The chelonian is held in dorsal recumbency and on the right side a point is located midway between the plastron and carapace vertically and between the base of the neck and the shoulder joint horizontally. The needle is inserted at this point and directed toward the junction of the humeral and pectoral scutes.[14]

There are a variety of other venipuncture sites, including the brachial and femoral veins and plexuses, orbital sinus, and toenail clips. Brachial and femoral approaches may be clinically useful in large tortoises, but lymphatic contamination is a concern. Orbital sinus and toenail clips are inappropriate clinically but may have legitimate research applications.

Crocodilians. The most appropriate venipuncture sites are the caudal (tail) vein in small-to-medium crocodilians and supravertebral vein/sinus in medium-to-large specimens (Fig. 43.5). The supravertebral vein is approached with the needle positioned in the dorsal midline, just caudal to the occiput and perpendicular to the surface of the skin. The needle is slowly advanced while maintaining slight negative pressure. Excessive penetration may lead to spinal trauma, but this appears rare in larger animals. The technique for caudal (tail) vein access is as described for lizards. The heart is located on the ventral midline, approximately 11 scale rows caudal to the forelimbs. Cardiocentesis in crocodilians is not as safe as it is in snakes because the heart cannot be stabilized.

Bone Marrow. On occasions it may be necessary to submit bone marrow to permit a more detailed hematologic evaluation. The technique for bone marrow collection depends on the size and nature of the

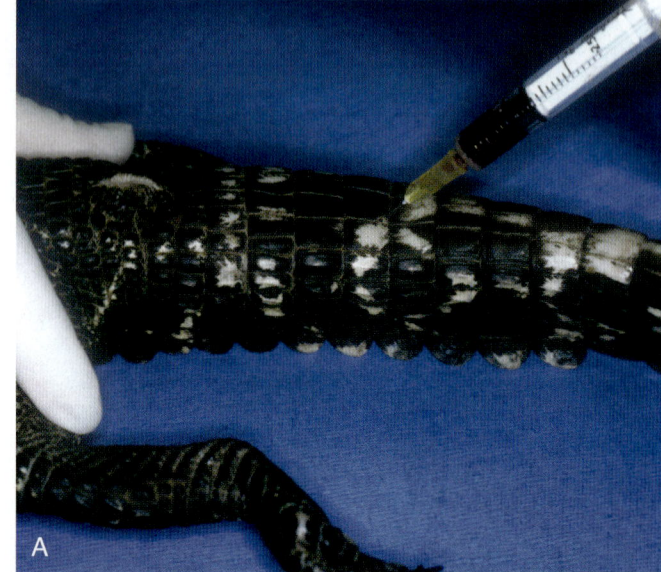
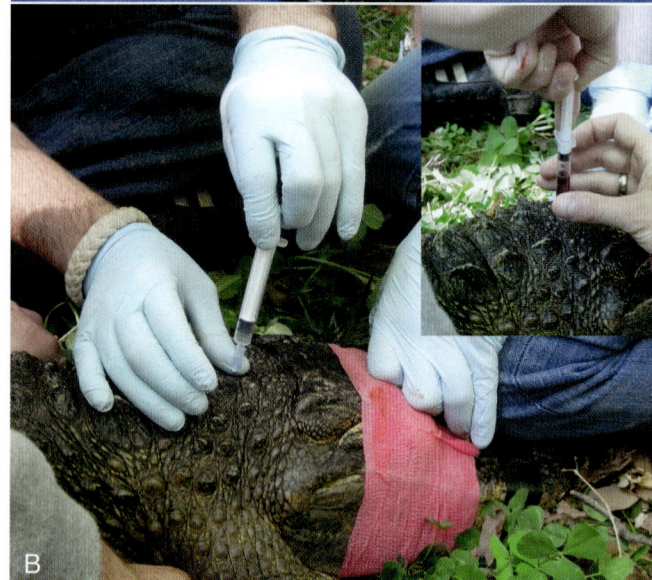

FIG 43.5 (A) Blood collection from the caudal (ventral tail) vein of a West African dwarf crocodile (*Osteolaemus tetraspis*). (B) Blood collection from the supravertebral venous sinus of an American alligator (*Alligator mississippiensis*). (Courtesy of Stephen J. Divers.)

reptile. Diagnostic samples can be collected from the femoral or tibial medullary cavities of most lizards, crocodilians, and large chelonians (although chelonians often have more solid bones and less medullary cavity) (Fig. 43.6A). In these reptiles, a suitably sized spinal needle (or hypodermic needle in very small individuals) can be placed into the medullary cavity of the bone, and gentle-to-moderate aspiration is used to obtain a sample. An alternative site in chelonia is the plastrocarapacial bridge that laterally connects the plastron and carapace, but again the medullary tissue is often limited (Fig. 43.6B). It is generally necessary to drill through the outer layer of keratin and bone and gain access to the medullary cavity and marrow beneath.

In snakes it is often necessary to surgically remove and submit a rib for marrow evaluation. A large midbody rib should be selected. A dorsoventral incision is made in the dorsolateral aspect of the body directly over a rib. The rib is palpated and located before cutting as far dorsad as possible, close to the epaxial musculature. The lateral muscular

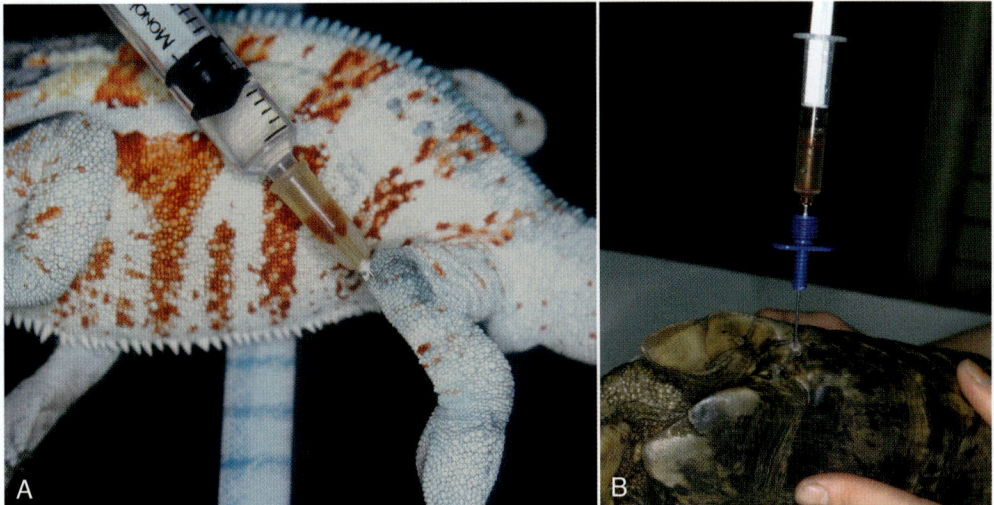

FIG 43.6 (A) Bone marrow aspiration from the tibia of a panther chameleon (*Furcifer pardalis*) using a hypodermic needle. (B) Bone marrow aspiration from the plastrocarapacial bridge of a tortoise (*Testudo sp*). (Courtesy of Stephen J. Divers.)

attachments are dissected free in a dorsoventral direction using scissors. The rib is dissected free and elevated through the skin incision. Hemorrhage has not been a complication, but any damaged intercostal vessels can be sealed using radiosurgery. Depending on the size of the rib and preferences of the histopathologist and hematologist, the entire rib or aspirated marrow may be submitted.

Spleen. The spleen has been cited as an important organ in regard to hemopoietic and lymphopoietic roles, and therefore biopsies or aspirates may be required for further evaluation of hematologic disorders. The spleen varies in size and shape but is usually closely associated with the stomach and pancreas within the dorsal mesentery. In snakes the spleen and pancreas may be combined into a single splenopancreas organ located approximately 60% to 65% from snout-vent. The spleen can be approached and biopsied in two ways: open surgery and endoscopy. Open surgical biopsy requires a standard coeliotomy approach, whereas endoscopic visualization and biopsy is less invasive and quicker to accomplish. Postbiopsy hemorrhage rarely requires intervention but can be controlled with the use of transendoscopic radiosurgery, laser, or a hemostatic sponge.

Cardiovascular Function. There are several means of assessing the cardiovascular system in the exam including the use of visual appearance, palpation, and sensitive electrical stethoscopes. The detection of abnormal rhythm or rate, as well as cardiac murmurs, may be appreciated. Further investigation using electrocardiography, diagnostic ultrasonography, and radiology, are necessary and are dealt with elsewhere (see Chapter 68).

Integument

Dermatologic disease is a frequent presentation, and there are various levels at which the clinician can intervene and collect biological samples. Shed skin, skin scrapes, impression smears, fine needle aspiration, and scale and skin biopsies can all be utilized in the pursuit of a diagnosis (Fig. 43.7A). The skin and associated structures are perhaps the easiest to sample for laboratory analysis due to their accessibility. However, they can also be the most demanding to interpret, as contamination and secondary changes often mask the underlying primary complaint. For example, impression smear cytology and bacterial culture may

diagnose *Pseudomonas* sp. dermatitis but miss the underlying burn that caused the initial skin damage and facilitated infection. Alternatively, normal and diseased skin often becomes contaminated from fecal Enterobactereace. It is therefore vital to sample correctly and interpret findings with caution.

Ectoparasites. Various ectoparasites may be clearly seen on the surface of the skin, around nostrils, eyes, and skin folds.[3,7] Mites, ticks, lice, maggots, and flies can often be physically removed and submitted in specimen containers for taxonomic identification. The shed skin of reptiles can be a valuable asset and should be inspected for evidence of parasitism (Fig. 43.7B). Suspected mites can be collected directly using a wet cotton-tipped applicator and transferred to a microscope slide for closer inspection and identification.

Skin Scrapes and Impression Smears. Skin lesions are frequently contaminated, and therefore superficial sampling may not demonstrate the primary cause or agent by the time the reptile is presented. Skin lesions are best cleaned and partially debrided using aseptic techniques prior to the collection of clinical samples.[3,7] Microbiologic swabs should be taken from the periphery of the lesion but deep to any exposed areas. Impression smears can be taken after the lesion has been cleaned with sterile saline and gently dabbed dry with sterile gauze. Skin scrapes may be useful, especially when dealing with drier, more proliferative lesions. Samples may be prepared for immediate microscopy or submitted to an external laboratory.

Scale and Skin Biopsies. Where the clinician requires a skin biopsy, the removal of a single scale may be all that is required, as scales contain both epidermal and dermal elements. A small volume (0.02–0.1 mL) of local anesthetic (e.g., 2% lidocaine) is injected subcutaneously in the area(s) of interest. Using aseptic techniques, a single scale is then elevated and cut close to its insertion using a scalpel blade. If a larger sample is required then a combination of local, regional, or general anesthesia and sharp excision or a skin punch biopsy instrument is effective (Fig. 43.8). A single suture closes the deficit. Biopsy of the chelonian shell requires general anesthesia and cortical biopsy devices (see the sections Bone and Shell Biopsy as well as Musculoskeletal System in this chapter).

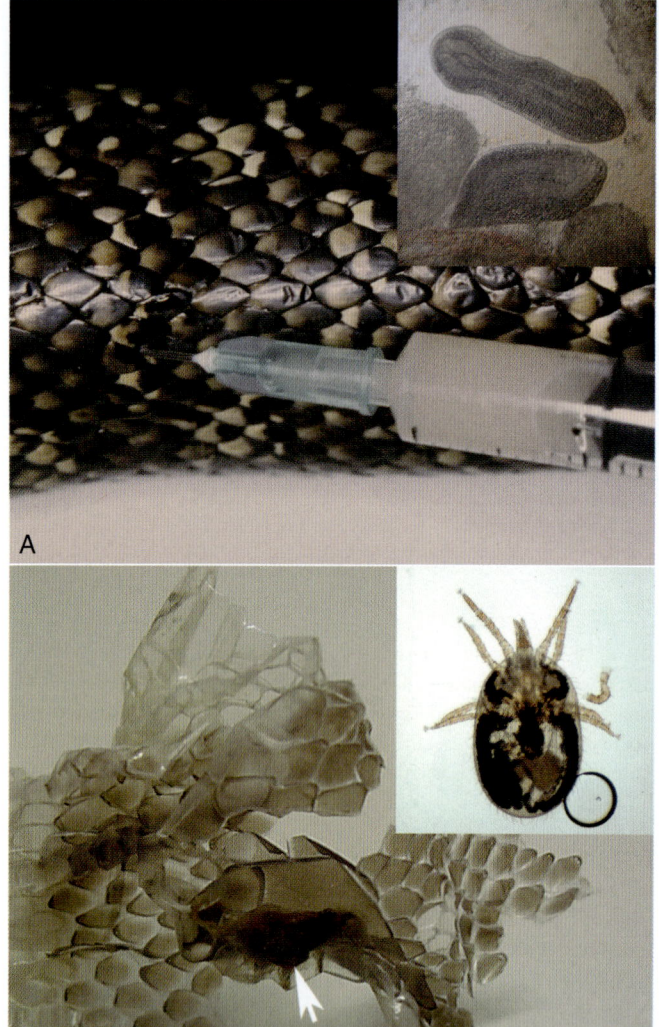

FIG 43.7 (A) Fine needle aspiration of a fluctuant cutaneous lesion in a Florida kingsnake (*Lampropeltis getula*). *(Inset)* Microscopic examination revealed numerous flukes. (B) Shed skin from a snake that was suffering from severe mite infestation and self-inflicted wounds from intense pruritis. One of these lesions can be appreciated from the abnormal slough (arrow). *(Inset)* The common snake mite, *Ophionyssus natricis*, was recovered from the shed skin. (Courtesy of Stephen J. Divers.)

Respiratory System

The respiratory system can be conveniently divided into upper and lower respiratory tracts. The upper respiratory tract consists of the nares, buccal cavity, larynx, and trachea, while the lower respiratory tract consists of the bronchus/bronchi, lung(s), and, where present, air-sac(s). There is very little in the way of tubular subdivision into secondary bronchi, bronchioles, and alveoli, as in mammals. The reptilian lung is more reticulated with a large central cavity, although chelonia are an exception because they possess a more three-dimensional, spongelike lung.

Abnormal respiration is a common presentation, and some of these are due to true disease, but many are associated with poor environments that resolve with husbandry improvements. The ability to diagnose pathologic changes within the respiratory system is relatively straightforward if

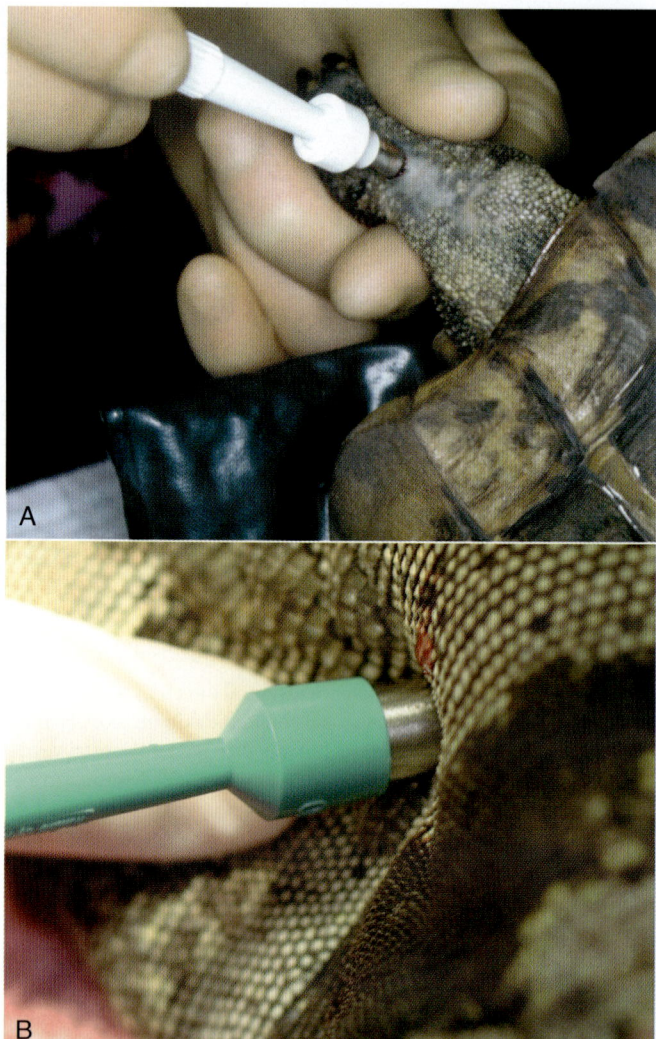

FIG 43.8 Skin punch biopsies being collected from the limb of a tortoise (A) and flank of a lizard (B). (Courtesy of Stephen J. Divers.)

reliance is placed upon the use of lung lavage for the collection of cytologic and microbiologic samples.[3,7] The collection of tissue biopsies requires anesthesia and surgical or endoscopic techniques.

Nares, Larynx and Cranial Trachea. The upper respiratory tract, including the nares, buccal cavity, larynx, and cranial trachea, can be visualized and often sampled directly without a surgical plane of anesthesia. Small-diameter swabs permit the collection of samples, although the greatest concern comes from bacterial contamination by oral commensals. Swabs can be submitted for microbiology or rolled onto glass slides for staining and cytologic evaluation.

Caudal Trachea and Lung Lavage. The simplest method of obtaining a representative sample from the lower respiratory tract is by lavage (Fig. 43.9). Although a lung wash or lavage can be carried out in the conscious reptile, the discomfort of such a procedure warrants sedation or light anesthesia. A sterile catheter of appropriate size is placed through the glottis, taking great care not to touch the oral membranes. The catheter is advanced down the trachea and into the lungs. In snakes the catheter is advanced caudal to the heart (>30% snout-vent), but in large specimens it may not be possible to reach the lung(s), and a tracheal lavage is performed. In lizards the catheter is advanced to a

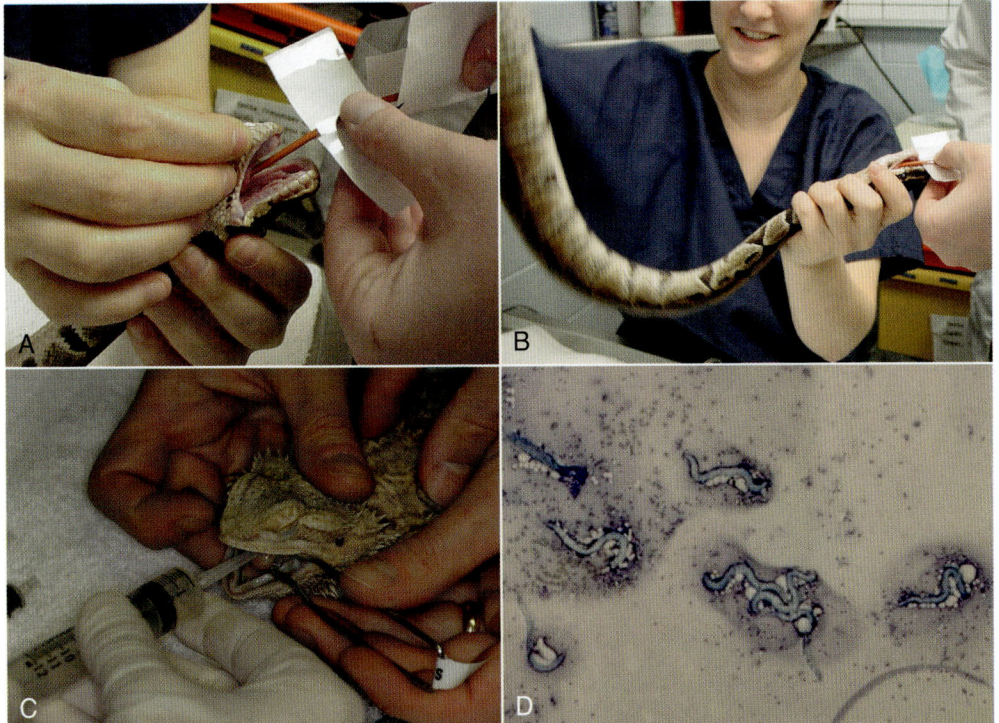

FIG 43.9 (A, B) Aseptic insertion of a sterile catheter through the glottis, down the trachea, and into the cranial lung of a sedated ball python (*Python regius*). Gentle rolling and rocking often improves the diagnostic quality of the aspirated sample. (C) Lung lavage of an anesthetized bearded dragon (*Pogona vitticeps*). (D) Microscopic view of a lung lavage sample from a snake indicating multiple, unidentified nematode larvae. (Courtesy of Stephen J. Divers.)

point just caudal to the forelimbs, whereas in chelonia a central position appears most appropriate. In lizards and chelonia the catheter can be preferentially directed into either the left or right lung by inserting a sterile metal stylet down the catheter prior to introduction. The catheter and stylet is then given a gentle bend to facilitate introduction into the left or right lung. Proper positioning of the stylet and catheter can be confirmed by radiography (Fig. 43.10A). Once in place, 0.5 to 1.0 mL of sterile saline per 100 g body weight can be infused. Sample recovery is often aided by rotating the animal and repeatedly aspirating, although in larger reptiles the use of dedicated bronchoalveolar lavage systems that utilize house vacuums are often most rewarding (Fig. 43.10B). In snakes, lifting the head and tail will also help accumulate fluid at the dependent area, near the catheter tip. In chelonia, a unilateral lung wash can also be obtained via a long fine hypodermic needle. The needle is positioned in the dorsocranial area of the prefemoral fossa and directed dorsomedially. Aspiration of air confirms entry into the lung prior to lavage. Similar techniques are possible in lizards and snakes, but anesthesia and lung inflation are usually required. Dependent upon the volume and quality of the sample obtained, material should be divided and submitted as requested by the laboratory. The submission of fresh and fixed material, multiple air-dried smears, and a microbiologic swab permits detailed investigation.

Lung Biopsy. Lavage samples do not permit an appreciation of lung architecture. For this, and many other pathological evaluations, tissue biopsies are preferred. Surgical access to the lung can be achieved using a standard coeliotomy, as there is no functional diaphragm or concern regarding the maintenance of pleural negative pressure in most squamates.[3,7] In snakes, the respiratory active anterior part of the lung is typically located between 35% to 45% snout-vent (i.e., just caudal to

the heart). However, there is great species variation with regard to lung anatomy, including the presence of a tracheal lung in some elapids and viperids, both left and right lungs in boids, and only a right lung in most other snakes. Surgical biopsy of the anterior lung commonly results in hemorrhage unless appropriate hemostatic measures are taken. Biopsy of the thinner posterior lung (or air sac) is not complicated by hemorrhage, although closing the thin pulmonary membrane without tearing can be challenging. In lizards the anterior lung is also more highly vascularized than the posterior areas. A cranial coeliotomy, close to the xiphoid process of the sternum, may permit sufficient exposure; otherwise, a lateral approach between ribs may offer better exposure for biopsy of the anterior lung. The tuatara, varanids, and crocodilians possess a significant post-pulmonary membrane that should be respected and, if surgically breached, sutured closed prior to closure of the coelom. In chelonia, the lungs are protected by the carapace, making surgical access more difficult. Creation of a 4- to 5-mm temporary osteotomy in the carapace, over the lung area of interest, does not give sufficient exposure for an excisional biopsy but does permit the collection of a tru-cut biopsy (Fig. 43.11).[15] The osteotomy can then be closed using acrylic or epoxy. Alternatively, an intrapneumonic catheter can be secured in the osteotomy site to permit continued local therapy.[15] A ventral coeliotomy is not recommended in chelonia because the septum horizontale (post-pulmonary membrane) is deep to the coelomic viscera and again should be repaired if surgically incised or penetrated in any way.

Endoscopic Biopsy. The use of small rigid telescopes and fine flexible endoscopes permits access to, and biopsy of, lung tissue in most reptiles. The use of 3- to 5-Fr biopsy instruments permits the collection of tissue samples from reptiles as small as 150 g without deleterious effects. Small biopsies are best submitted in histology filters to avoid loss during

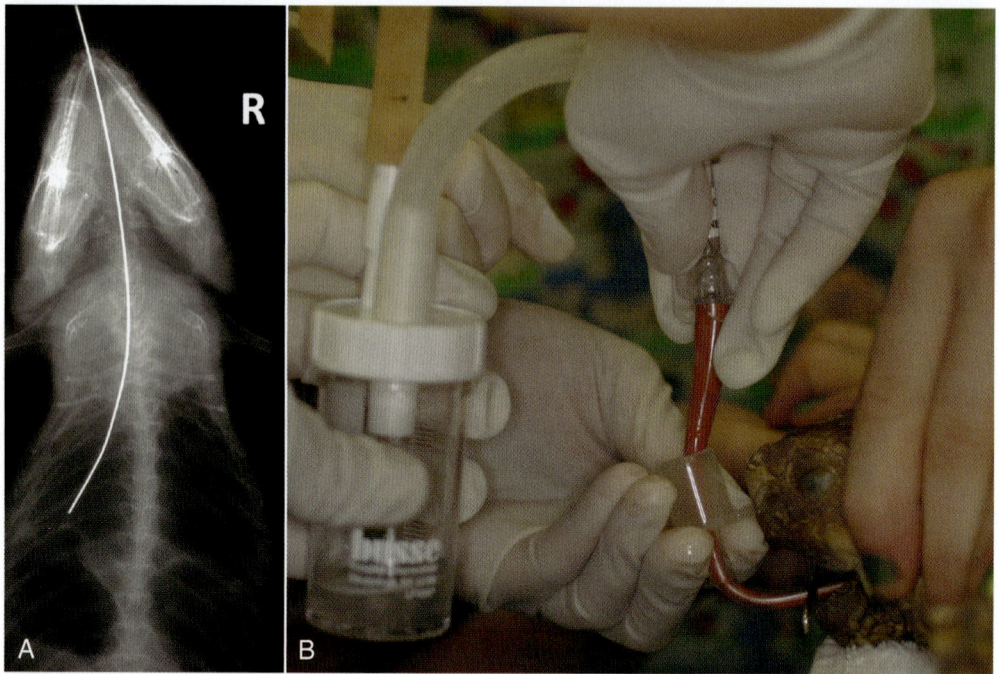

FIG 43.10 (A) By using a curved metal stylet it is relatively easy to ensure unilateral placement of a lung catheter into a specific lung—in this case the left lung of a bearded dragon (*Pogona vitticeps*). (B) For larger reptiles, like this large tortoise, the use of dedicated bronchoalveolar lavage supplies and house vacuums generally provide the most efficient means of sample collection. (Courtesy of Stephen J. Divers.)

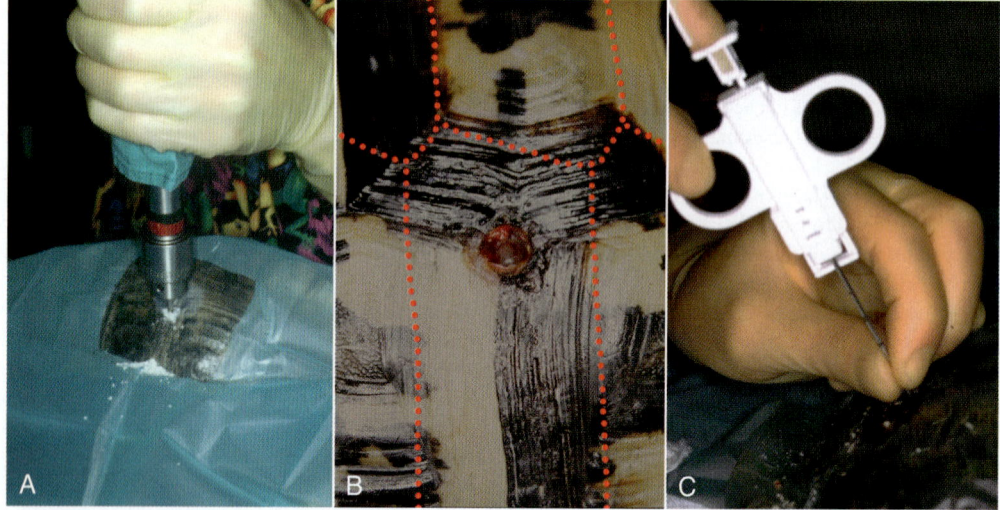

FIG 43.11 Lung biopsy of a tortoise. (A) Drilling a temporary osteotomy in the carapace to gain access to a diseased lung. (B) The general area of interest is determined by radiography or CT, but the osteotomy site should ideally be through a bone plate at the intersection of the keratin scutes and not through the peripheral growth plates (outlined by red dotted line). (C) Needle biopsy via the osteotomy hole. (Courtesy of Stephen J. Divers.)

transportation and processing. The submission of (digitally captured endoscopy) images of the lesion with the biopsies greatly assists the pathologist in histologic interpretation. There are also a variety of other sampling devices available including brush biopsy instruments and remote aspiration needles that can also be used deep within the respiratory system to obtain diagnostic material.

In snakes it may be impossible to reach the lung using a small-diameter bronchoscope via a laryngeal approach. In larger constrictors, a flexible bronchoscope or gastroscope can be inserted via a surgical approach to the lung and passed craniad and caudad to examine the entire lung. The use of a rigid endoscope via a surgical approach to the lungs of boids has also been widely advocated (Fig. 43.12).[7,16] In some lizards, the lungs can be reached via the larynx because the bronchi are often short and easily negotiated. However, in most chelonia the short trachea and long narrow bronchi make access to the chelonian lung extremely difficult via a laryngeal approach, although it is possible in large animals when using fine-diameter flexible bronchoscopes. Endoscopic entry to the lungs can also be achieved via a carapacial osteotomy

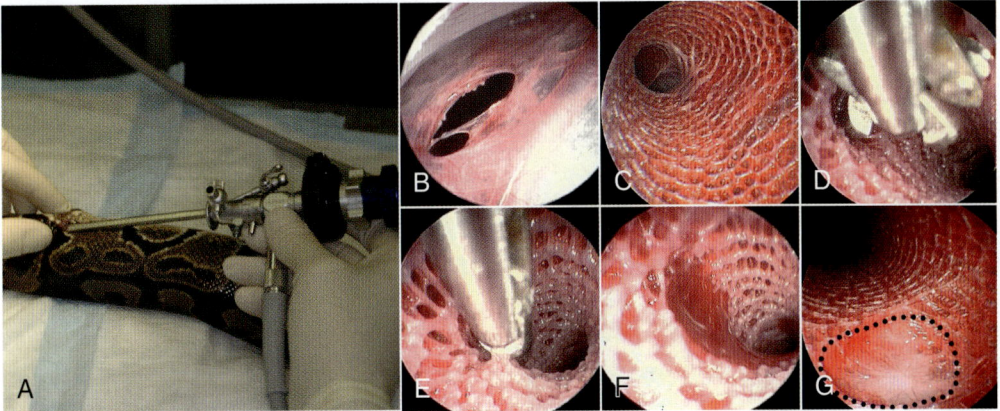

FIG 43.12 (A) Transcutaneous pulmonoscopy in a ball python (*Python regius*). The drape has been removed to facilitate photography. (B) Endoscopic appearance of the perforation into the lung. (C) Endoscopic view of the healthy cranial (faveolar) lung. (D, E, F) Endoscopic lung biopsy. (G) Endoscopic view of a previous lung biopsy site 12 months later (outlined in black dotted line). Note the minimal scarring. (Courtesy of Stephen J. Divers.)

(as described for chelonian lung biopsy) or a prefemoral approach (see Chapter 64). The prefemoral approach to the lungs requires a small incision in the craniodorsal aspect of the prefemoral fossa and identification of the septum horizontale (the membrane that divides the lungs from the remaining viscera). Retaining sutures are placed through this membrane to elevate it close to the skin incision. A small incision in this membrane permits the entry of the endo scope and examination of the lung as far cranially as the bronchial opening. It is important to close the septum horizontale following biopsy to prevent pneumocoelom and emphysema.

Gastrointestinal System

In cases of severe diarrhea or regurgitation, material for laboratory submission will be forthcoming and may be collected and presented along with the animal by well-educated owners or keepers. In addition, many reptiles will spontaneously defecate and urinate when handled during the examination process. It is important to appreciate that, like birds, the stools of reptiles are composed of fecal, urate, and urine components and that the cloaca is a common chamber for the gastrointestinal, urinary, and reproductive systems. For example, watery stools due to polyuria must be differentiated from true diarrhea, and cloacal bleeding may be intestinal, reproductive, or urinary in origin. Fecal material can be submitted for a variety of parasitologic, cytologic, and microbiologic tests. The submission of only fecal material in appropriate sterile containers will prevent further mixing and contamination by urates and urine during transportation and processing. Microbiologic results from deposited feces should be interpreted with caution because contamination from other organ systems can occur in the cloaca prior to elimination, while environmental contamination invariably occurs after elimination. The fresher the material, the more meaningful the laboratory results, although some parasitological investigations (e.g., helminth egg examination) can be performed on refrigerated material up to 4 weeks or more after elimination.

Oral Biopsy. Stomatitis is common, and sampling prior to initiating treatment is important because bacterial, fungal, parasitic, and viral causes are known (Fig. 43.13). Culture of superficial lesions frequently results in culturing commensal gram-negative bacteria and as deeper samples are required, biopsy is preferred. It is critical to submit material for histopathology (or cytology) in addition to microbiology to attribute pathogenicity to any cultured organisms.

Cloacocolonic Lavage. Unfortunately, the slow intestinal transit times of most reptiles often necessitates a more direct approach to obtain material. A cloacocolonic lavage can be performed on most conscious reptiles and provides the clinician with a diagnostic sample (Fig. 43.14A). A sterile lubricated round-tipped catheter is inserted into the cloaca and cranially toward the colon. A relatively large catheter should be used, as this helps prevent kinking of the tube and perforation of the thin intestinal wall. It is important not to force the catheter. Once in place, 0.5 to 1.0 mL sterile saline per 100 g body weight should be gently infused through the catheter and repeatedly aspirated until a sample is obtained. It is possible to infuse an additional 1.0 mL/100 g if no sample is forthcoming. It is surprisingly easy to catheterize the bladder and obtain a feces-free sample. The direct collection of fecal material from the distal colon using a lubricated, gloved hand offers another practical option in giant reptiles.

Gastric Lavage. A similar technique to cloacocolonic lavage can be used to collect samples from the stomach. A relatively large, round-tipped catheter can be inserted into the stomach of most conscious or sedated reptiles. In crocodilians, lizards, and chelonia, it is wise to use a mouth gag to prevent damage to the tube (Fig. 43.14B). The catheter should pass to the midcoelomic region before instilling 0.5 to 1.0 mL sterile saline per 100 g body weight. In large snakes it may not be possible to reach the stomach, in which case esophageal lavage is a more appropriate term. Such samples can be examined as a fresh wet preparation for parasites or stained to demonstrate microorganisms. Microbiological cultures are often worthy, but care is required in their interpretation, as contamination from the respiratory system and oral cavity is possible.

Gastroscopy and Biopsy. For the collection of gastric or intestinal biopsies, standard coeliotomy and excisional biopsies can be undertaken, but endoscopy is much less invasive. In lizards and chelonia endoscopic access to the stomach is straightforward but negotiating the pylorus and entering the duodenum is more difficult (Fig. 43.15). In snakes the small intestine can be readily entered via the gastric pylorus. It is unwise to endoscopically biopsy the large bowel because the intestinal wall is often thin and easily perforated. Even excisional biopsies of the large intestine can be challenging to ensure adequate closure and the prevention of leakage.

Liver Biopsy. Blood biochemistry, diagnostic imaging, and endoscopy may suggest hepatopathy, but they seldom provide the definitive diagnosis.

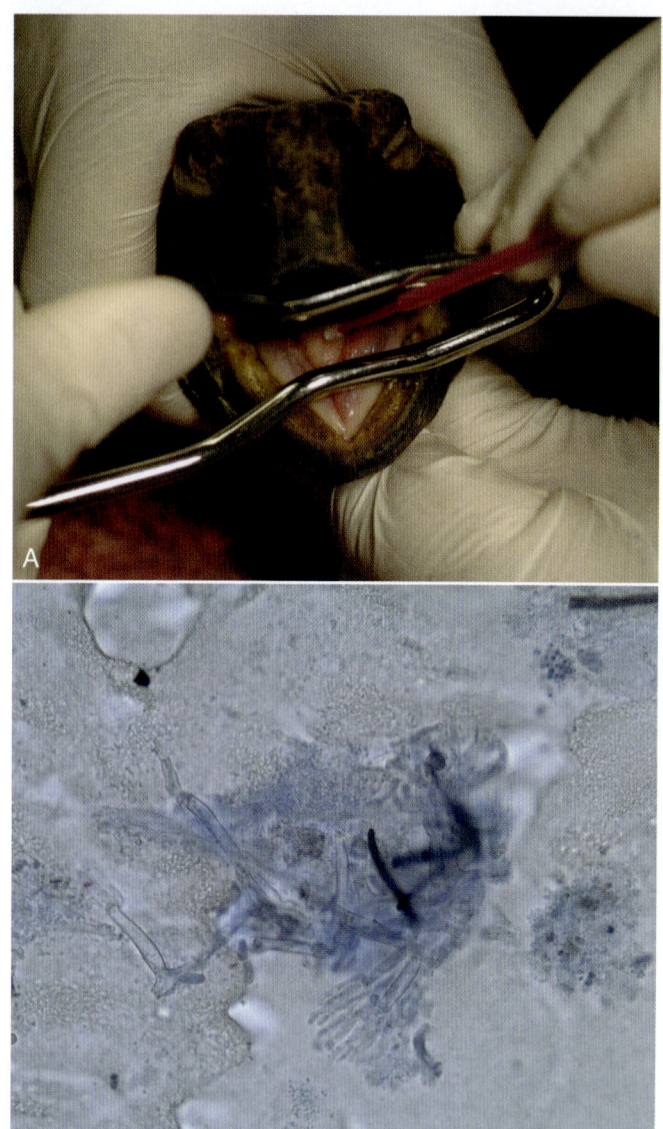

FIG 43.13 (A) Examination of and sampling from the oral cavity of a large tortoise. (B) Microscopy indicating budding fungal elements from the oral swab. (Courtesy of Stephen J. Divers.)

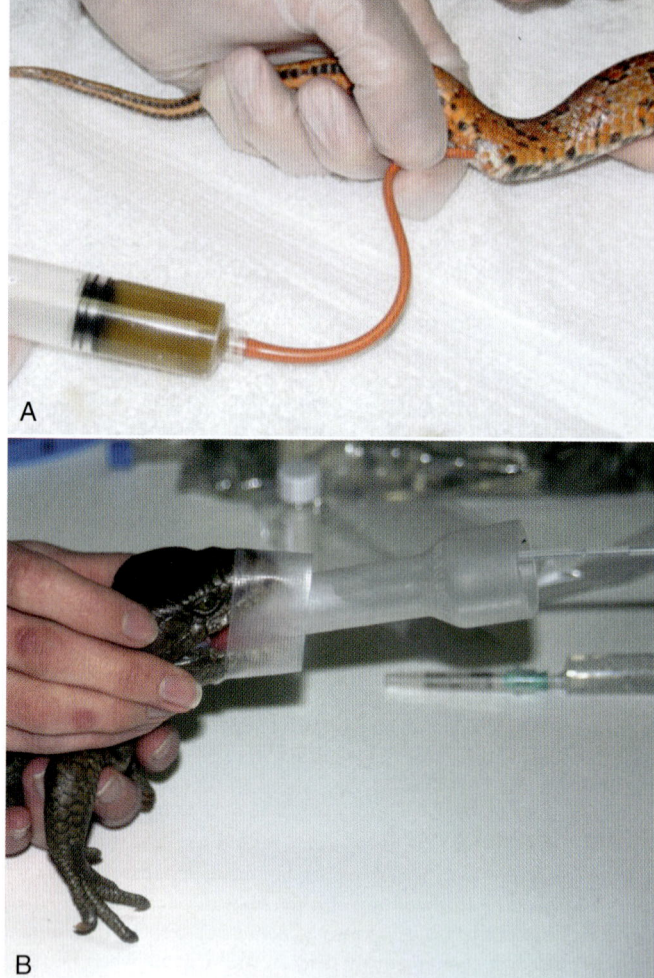

FIG 43.14 (A) Cloacocolonic lavage of a corn snake (*Pantherophis guttatus*) using a flexible catheter. (B) Gastric lavage of a Solomon Island skink (*Corucia zebrata*). The cut-off syringe casing acts as a mouth gag and protects the lavage catheter. (Courtesy of Stephen J. Divers.)

Liver biopsy remains the most effective tool for conclusively reaching a diagnosis, indicating specific therapies and providing a more accurate prognosis. Correlation between biochemical tests and histopathology are generally lacking, but serial blood sampling and biopsy currently offers the best diagnostic and monitoring approach to hepatic disease.

Biopsies may be collected for histopathology and microbiology. Liver samples may be collected percutaneously (with or without ultrasound guidance), surgically, or endoscopically. Surgical approaches generally rely on a standard coeliotomy approach to the liver, which in snakes usually results in only a small part of the organ being visible and available for biopsy (Fig. 43.16). Biopsies are best collected using large tru-cut needles or biopsy punches, with the defect packed with hemostatic foam to prevent post-biopsy hemorrhage. Wedge techniques can be used for sampling from the periphery in lizards and chelonians. Endoscopic techniques are typically less invasive, permit closer examination of more of the organ, and enable the collection of multiple biopsies

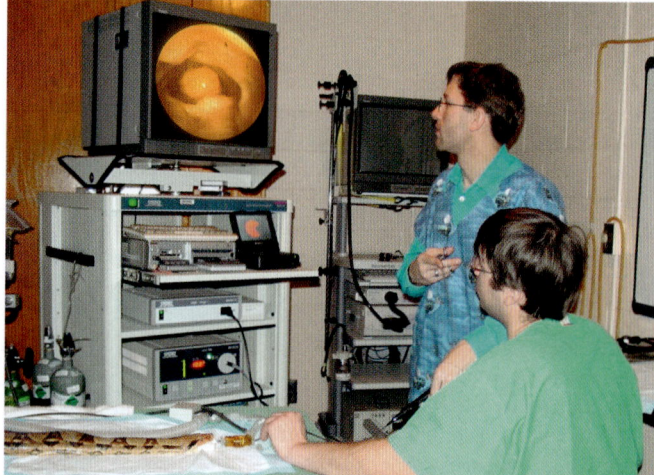

FIG 43.15 Gastroscopy of a *Boa constrictor*. (Courtesy of Stephen J. Divers.)

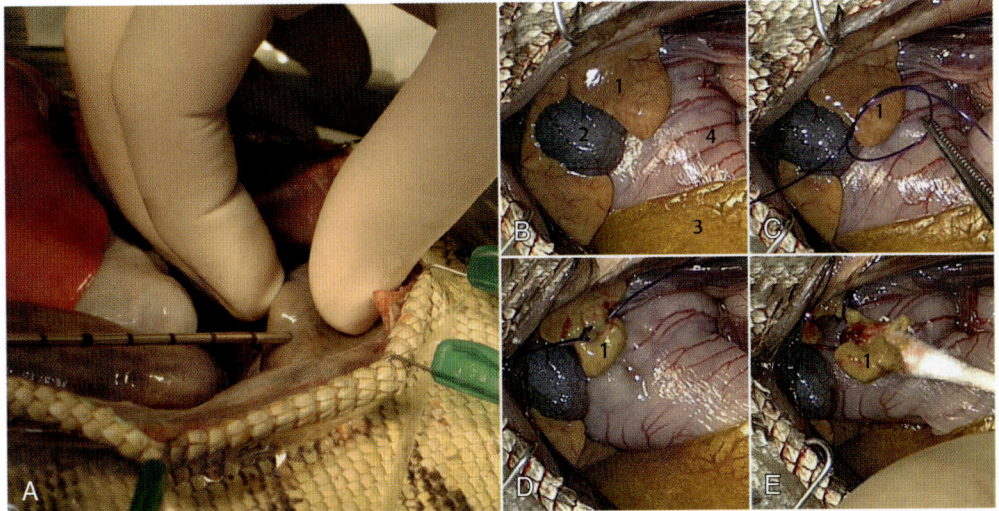

FIG 43.16 (A) Needle biopsy of an iguanid liver during coeliotomy. (B–E) Liver biopsy using a wedge technique in a juvenile bearded dragon by operating microscopy (1, liver; 2, gall bladder; 3, fat body; 4, stomach). (Courtesy of Stephen J. Divers.)

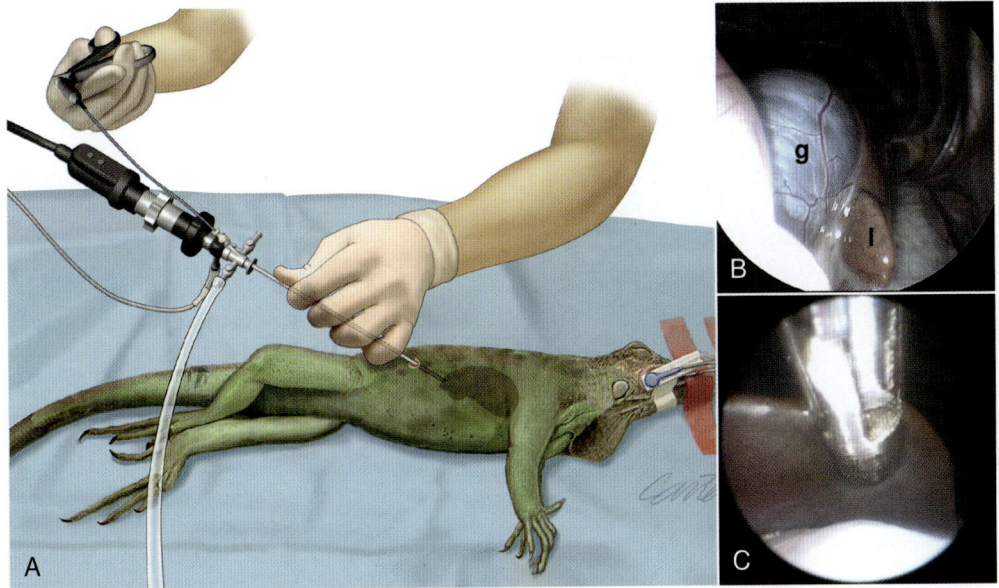

FIG 43.17 (A) Endoscopic examination and biopsy of the iguanid liver. (B) View of the liver (l) and gallbladder (g) from a right lateral approach. (C) Endoscopic liver biopsy of an iguanid liver. (Courtesy of Stephen J. Divers.)

(Fig. 43.17).[2,6] Ultrasound-guided biopsies in snakes and lizards have resulted in serious complications, including gastrointestinal perforation and fatal hemorrhage, and cannot be recommended for most reptiles.[17,18]

Pancreatic Biopsy. Blood glucose values can vary dramatically due to many factors, including stress, metabolic disease, systemic disease, neoplasia, and other extrinsic variables (see Chapters 79 and 155). However, pancreatic disease does exist, and a diagnosis should rely on the histopathologic demonstration of disease following endoscopic pancreatic evaluation and biopsy. Likewise, elevations of blood amylase levels may not be specific for pancreatic disease and should also be viewed cautiously unless disease can be confirmed histopathologically.

Musculoskeletal System

Despite major clinical interest in osteomyelitis and secondary nutritional hyperparathyroidism, there are a variety of other skeletal abnormalities that can affect reptiles. The ability to obtain bone material for histologic and microbiologic interpretation greatly aids our understanding and ability to advise on appropriate treatments for these conditions.

Bone and Shell Biopsy. Proliferative and lytic lesions affecting the axial and appendicular skeleton are not uncommon. The radiographic interpretation seldom provides a definitive pathologic diagnosis. The use of cortical bone biopsy instruments designed for humans can also be used in reptiles. Care is required not to cause excessive damage and risk fracture, but generally excellent samples can be obtained with only minor surgical exposure (Fig. 43.18A). In very small specimens a hypodermic needle can be used to obtain a core of bone. This bone core can then be expelled from the needle by inserting wire through the needle hub. In cases of vertebral osteomyelitis, where biopsy may be contraindicated due to the proximity of the spinal cord, blood cultures are often useful for identifying the bacterial cause.[19] Septic arthritis is

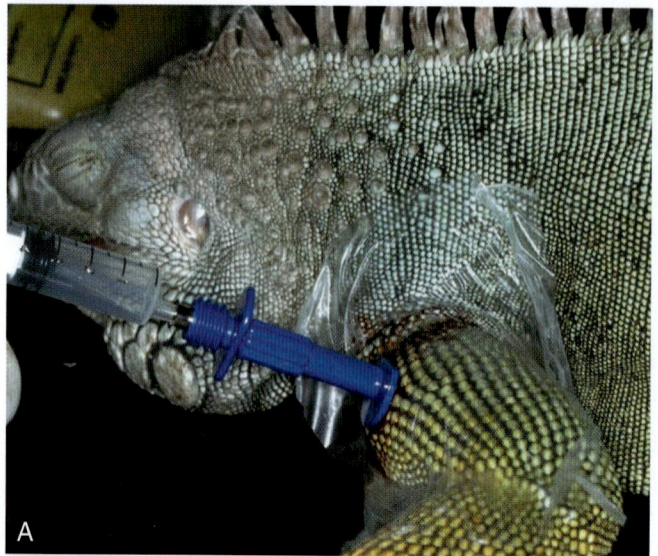

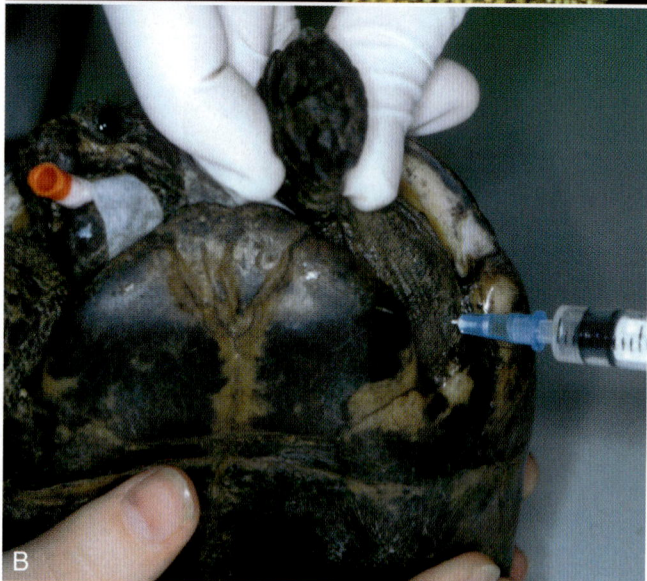

FIG 43.18 (A) Cortical bone biopsy in a green iguana (*Iguana iguana*). (B) Scapulohumeral joint aspiration of a *Testudo* tortoise. (Courtesy of Stephen J. Divers.)

commonly reported following bite wounds to the joints of lizards and tortoises. Following aseptic preparation of the area, fine-needle aspiration will permit the collection of samples for microbiologic and cytologic diagnosis (Fig. 43.18B).

Shell disease of chelonians is also common, and a Michele trephine has been shown to produce diagnostic samples (Fig. 43.19).[20] Diseased bone is often softer and easier to biopsy compared with healthy shell. Care is required to ensure that only a small length of the instrument is exposed so that overly deep penetration into the coelom does not occur. Acrylic or epoxy can be used to seal the biopsy site unless obvious infection is present.

Muscle Biopsy. Most cases of muscle wastage or weakness are related to nutrition or debilitating disease, but, if warranted, muscle biopsies may be collected for histopathologic investigations. The largest affected muscle masses should be selected because many reptiles, especially chameleons and other small lizards, have limited musculature. Surgical exposure of the muscle and longitudinal separation of a number of

fibers permits ligation using fine absorbable material at the proximal and distal margins of the biopsy. Sharp excision permits removal of the biopsy. Hemostasis by ligation is preferred over radiosurgery or laser because of the coagulation artifacts that are produced.

Urinary System

Diseases of the urinary system can include the kidneys, ureters, bladder, urethra, and cloaca. In addition to the kidneys, the bladder, cloaca, posterior colon, and remote salt glands can all play important roles in osmoregulation and should be considered part of the osmoregulatory system of reptiles. The clinician may assess the osmoregulatory system by sampling urine and biopsies from the kidney, bladder, and cloaca. Ancillary structures such as salt glands are seldom biopsied, although their secretions can often be collected from the reptile's nares or the glass surfaces of enclosures.

Urine. Urinalysis is less helpful in reptiles than mammals. The reptilian kidney cannot concentrate urine, and so urine-specific gravity is of limited use in the assessment of renal function. Furthermore, renal urine passes through the urodeum of the cloaca before entering the bladder (or posterior colon in those species that lack a bladder). Bladder urine is therefore not necessarily sterile. The clinical picture is further complicated by the fact that electrolyte and water changes can occur across the bladder or cloacocolonic mucosa. Despite these biochemical drawbacks, urine samples are useful for cytologic assessments of inflammation, infection, and for the identification of renal casts (see Chapter 66).

Voided urine. The urinary, genital, and intestinal tracts empty into a common cloaca, and therefore any samples voided from the cloaca may represent material derived from, or contaminated by, any of these systems. Voided urine and urates, although useful for cytology, must be critically evaluated whenever a culture is obtained. Urine microbiology must be even more critically judged if the sample was collected from the floor of the enclosure or the examination table. Fresher urine and urate samples can be collected as a free catch. Many reptiles will spontaneously void urine and urates (often with fecal material) when handled. More stoic individuals may be encouraged to urinate by gentle digital stimulation of the cloaca.

Cystocentesis. A more representative and less contaminated sample may be collected by cystocentesis in chelonia and those lizards that possess a bladder (Fig. 43.20A). However, given the thin, fragile nature of the reptilian bladder, the potential danger of postsampling leakage of unsterile urine into the coelom exists. Given the passage of urine through the cloaca, and the electrolyte and water changes that can occur in the bladder, urine collected by cystocentesis may not be representative of renal urine with respect to electrolyte composition and osmolarity. Such samples are often unsterile, although a heavy, pure microbiological growth should alert the clinician to potential infection.

Catheterization. One means of obtaining bladder urine without puncturing the bladder is by the placement, blind or preferably with the assistance of an endoscope, of a urethral catheter (Fig. 43.20B and C). This procedure has been performed in sedated and anesthetized tortoises and lizards that possess a bladder. Care must be taken not to damage the thin bladder wall. The indwelling catheter can be used to empty the bladder and may then be used to collect fresh urine (Fig. 43.2C). Collection of bladder urine that has not resided within the bladder for a prolonged period may be more representative of renal urine (i.e., before major post-renal electrolyte changes have occurred across the bladder membrane).

Renal Biopsy. A variety of infectious, degenerative, and neoplastic renal diseases have been reported in reptiles, particularly snakes and

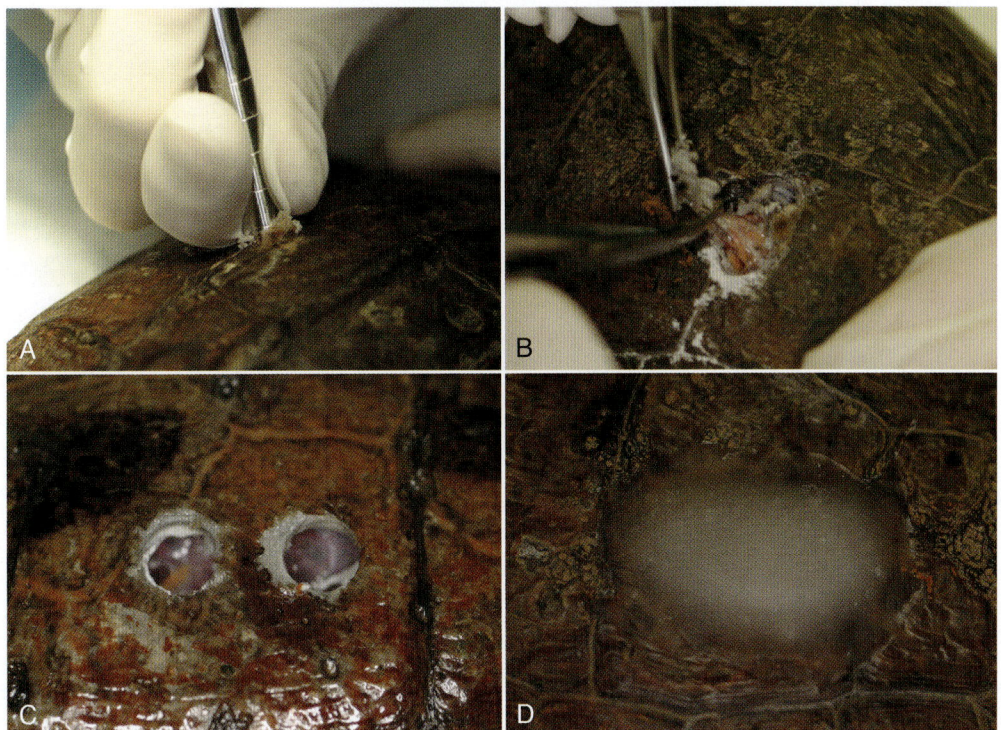

FIG 43.19 (A) Full thickness shell biopsy using a Michele trephine in a map turtle (*Graptemys* sp.). (B) Sharp incision to free the shell biopsy from its underlying attachments. (C) View of the double biopsy site. Note that the unpenetrated lung can be seen below the surface of the carapace. (D) Closure of the biopsy site using methylacrylate. (Courtesy of Stephen J. Divers.)

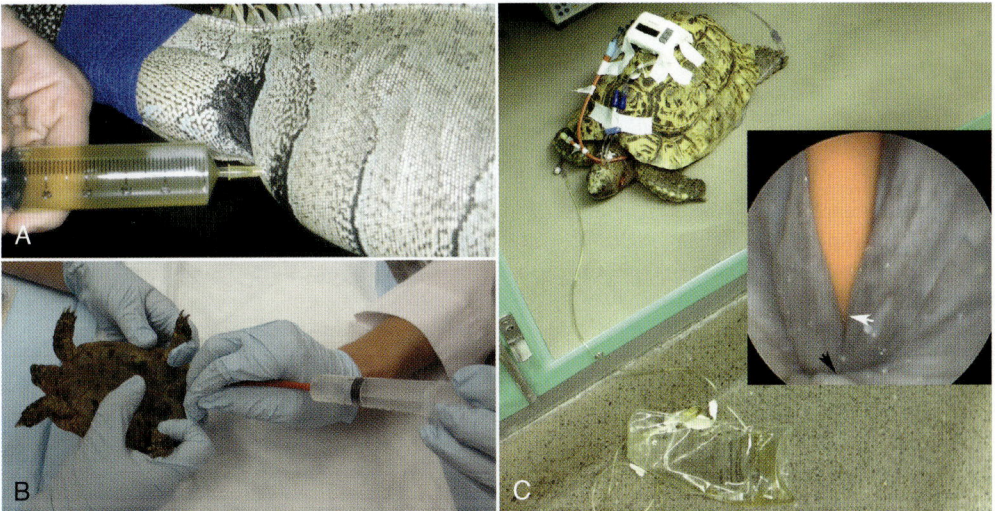

FIG 43.20 (A) Cystocentesis in a large green iguana (*Iguana iguana*). (B) Bladder catheterization in a tortoise. Care is required to direct the catheter dorsally in the cloaca to minimize the chances of colonic catheterization. (C) Indwelling bladder catheter in a leopard tortoise (*Stigmochelys pardalis*). Note the collected urine within the fluid bag. Inset: endoscopic urinary catheter placement through the urodeum and into the bladder. The animal is in dorsal recumbency and the red rubber catheter has been placed through the urodeal opening into the urethra (white arrow), avoiding the coprodeal opening to the colon (black arrow). (Courtesy of Stephen J. Divers.)

lizards. The poor regenerative capabilities of the kidney make early diagnosis essential. The relatively poor diagnostic value of urinalysis and the late detection of renal disease by blood biochemistry further exemplify the importance of renal biopsy early in the diagnostic process. The cranial tail cut-down and minimally invasive coeliotomy biopsy techniques permit unilateral access to a single kidney. In these cases, cloacal and coelomic palpation, diagnostic imaging (including

intravenous urography) can be used to determine whether a left or right approach is most appropriate. Major coeliotomy, ultrasound-guided, and endoscopic biopsy procedures can usually examine and biopsy either or both kidneys.

Coeliotomy biopsy. Where renomegaly is obvious, a coelomic entry and biopsy can be undertaken (Fig. 43.21A and B). A standard midline or paramedian coeliotomy enables both kidneys to be assessed in lizards,

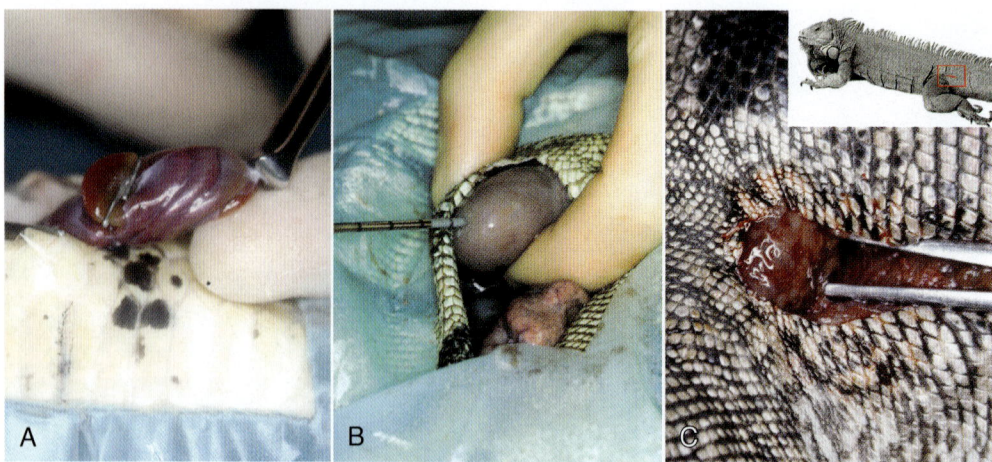

FIG 43.21 (A) Renal biopsy of a *Boa constrictor* following a standard coeliotomy. In this case vascular clips have been used to isolate a small kidney lobule prior to sharp excision. (B) Needle biopsy of an enlarged iguanid kidney during coeliotomy. (C) Cranial tail cut-down procedure to biopsy the caudal pole of an iguanid kidney. Inset: the incision is marked by the red line. (Courtesy of Stephen J. Divers.)

and excisional or tru-cut biopsies can be collected. In snakes, the elongated left and right kidneys overlap for a short distance, and coeliotomy and renal biopsy are readily accomplished. If an enlarged kidney can be palpated it can usually be immobilized just under the skin, permitting the use of a tru-cut needle biopsy or minimally invasive coeliotomy incision directly over the organ. This technique is best suited to the detection of diffuse renal disease, as focal diseases may be missed.

Cranial tail cut-down biopsy. A relatively simple technique for biopsy of the intrapelvic kidneys of iguanas requires a cranial tail cut-down under local or general anesthesia. A small longitudinal incision is made in the lateral midline just below the lateral processes of the coccygeal vertebrae. The incision extends for 1 to 3 cm caudad, starting just behind the hind limb. Blunt dissection between the dorsal and ventral coccygeal muscles permits exposure of the caudolateral aspect of the kidney that can then be sampled (Fig. 43.21C). Hemorrhage depends on the size of the biopsy, but the temporary application of hemostatic dressings or radiosurgery is effective. This technique is particularly valuable when the kidneys are not enlarged, coelomic approaches to the intrapelvic kidneys are more difficult, or shorter anesthesia time is a major advantage. It is limited to unilateral biopsy unless bilateral cut-down procedures are undertaken. Furthermore, as only a small area of kidney can be visualized and sampled from, this technique is best suited for the investigation of diffuse renal disease.

Ultrasound-guided biopsy. Ultrasound-guided biopsies have been performed in dogs and humans but are higher risk for smaller animals, including most reptiles. While ultrasound imaging permits the identification of gross lesions and aids biopsy needle guidance, there are still dangers associated with the voluminous bladder, gastrointestinal tract, dorsal aorta, and renal arteries and veins that must be appreciated and avoided. Depending on the quality of the equipment and skill of the ultrasonographer, multifocal or focal lesions may be missed. Indeed, given the complications encountered with ultrasound-guided biopsies of larger and more accessible organs like the liver, such ultrasound-guided renal sampling is not recommended for most reptiles.

Endoscopic biopsy. The endoscope permits evaluation of the size, color, and shape of both coelomic kidneys via a single surgical entry but is less able to examine intrapelvic tissue. The use of endoscopic scissors and biopsy forceps under direct visual control permits the incision of the renal capsule and collection of quality samples with less risk to surrounding structures (Fig. 43.22). The optics of the telescope also permits an assessment of diffuse, focal, and multifocal disease and the selection of appropriate biopsies that may otherwise be difficult to ascertain without a real-life, color, magnified image.[1-3]

Bladder Biopsy. The bladder performs important osmoregulatory functions in many reptiles and biopsy may rarely be required for an overall assessment of osmoregulation function. Proliferative masses of the bladder can also be biopsied to aid identification and direct treatment plans.

Endoscopic biopsy. Endoscopic entry into the bladder of larger lizards and chelonia has been accomplished with practice. However, endoscopic biopsy of the bladder is not recommended for anything other than grossly proliferative lesions, because there are major risks associated with perforation and leakage of unsterile urine and urates into the coelom.

Excisional biopsy. Surgical excisional biopsy is preferred in most cases due to the importance of preventing postbiopsy leakage. There are no ureteral connections to the bladder, and so bladder biopsies can be collected from almost any site. However, care should be taken to maintain the neural and vascular supplies and avoid the urethra. The technique is similar to that used in mammals, although a double-layer closure can be more difficult due to the very thin nature of the bladder wall. To ensure a waterproof seal the incision should be closed using an approximating continuous or simple interrupted pattern, followed by a second inverting pattern.

Cloacocolonic Biopsy. Biopsies of the cloacocolonic region may rarely be required for a complete assessment of osmoregulatory function, especially in those species that lack a bladder. Due to the intrapelvic position of the coprodeum and urodeum in most reptiles, endoscopic examination and mucosal biopsy is preferred. The cloacal wall tends to be relatively thick and perforation less likely compared to the bladder. Nevertheless, care must be taken not to biopsy or damage the urogenital papillae within the urodeum. Endoscopic biopsy of the colon is not recommended, as the intestinal wall is often thin and prone to perforation.

Reproductive System

Antemortem pathologic assessment of the reproductive system has not been undertaken to a large degree. However, the advent of minimally invasive endoscopic techniques has brought about an increase in obstetric evaluation and sampling.

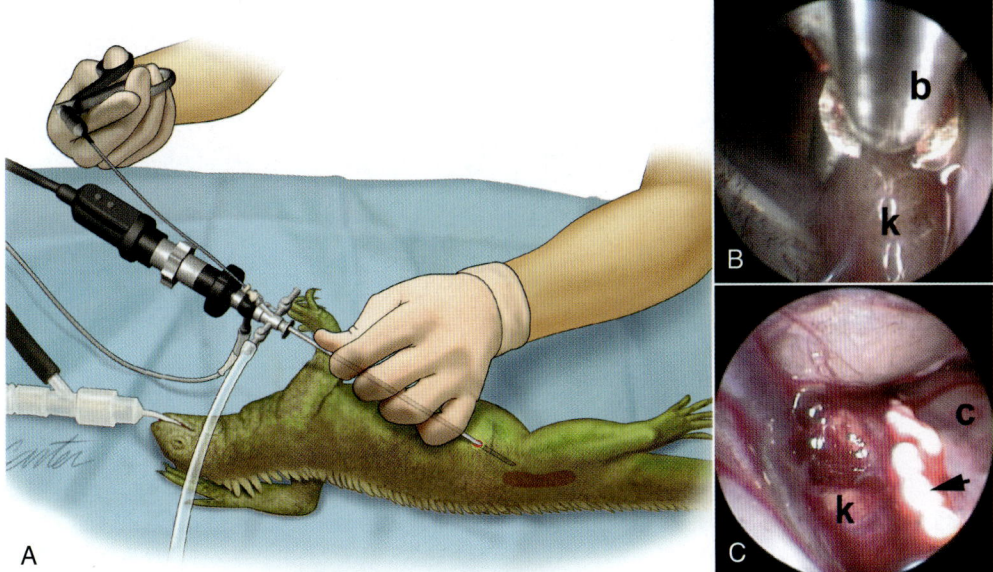

FIG 43.22 (A) Endoscopic evaluation and biopsy of the iguanid kidney. (B) Endoscopic view of an iguanid kidney (k) about to be sampled using 1.7 mm biopsy forceps (b). (C) Postbiopsy view of the same kidney (k) with the intact vas deferens (arrow) and colon (c). (Courtesy of Stephen J. Divers.)

Phallus and Hemipenes. The phallus of chelonians and crocodilians and the hemipenes of squamates may become infected or traumatized. Paraphimosis is not uncommon, and impression smear cytology and culture may indicate primary or secondary infectious causes that need to be addressed once the organ has been replaced. Where the hemipenes are retracted a small sterile lubricated catheter can be inserted into the hemipenal sulcus, and aspiration or lavage procedures can provide material for cytology and cultures. In some cases, there can be such an accumulation of cellular debris that a hemipenal "plug" forms that can be removed from the sulcus using forceps. The cytologic evaluation of hemipenal material may aid the investigation of male infertility by evaluating for the presence of spermatozoa and petroleum-based spermicidal lubricants, which may have been previously used for gender identification by probing.

Cloacal (Musk) Glands. The cloacal or musk glands of snakes connect to the cloaca and may on occasion become impacted and infected (see Chapter 171). Material can often be expressed from these areas manually in the conscious snake, or swabs and lavage techniques can be used for the collection of diagnostic samples.

Oviducts and Vas Deferens. A detailed knowledge of cloacal anatomy and expert proficiency in endoscopic techniques can permit examination of the oviduct. It may also be possible to catheterize the vas deferens, which may aid the investigation of male infertility.

Gonads. The gonads of reptiles can be approached surgically or with endoscopy. The endoscopic identification of gonads has been used as an aid to control reproduction and breeding (see Chapter 64). Testicular biopsy has been used as an aid in the assessment of male infertility in lizards and chelonia. Biopsy of the active ovary is not recommended because of the dangers of yolk leakage and coelomitis. Biopsies have been taken from inactive and diseased ovaries without incident.

Nervous System and Special Senses

The increasing interest in neurological diseases has led to the pursuit of improvements in neurological assessment and antemortem sampling techniques. Previously, cytologic and histopathologic assessment of the nervous system was only possible with necropsy, although investigations in the live reptile are still quite limited.

Cerebrospinal Fluid. Reptiles lack a subarachnoid space, but cerebrospinal fluid (CSF) can be collected from an intrathecal site. Cervical and lumbar tap techniques to obtain CSF samples have been performed in a limited number of cases.[13] It is obviously important to be aware of the potential misidentification and misinterpretation of lymph as cerebrospinal fluid.

The technique is essentially similar to that employed in mammals, with emphasis on proper positioning and accurate anatomic knowledge. The anesthetized lizard is placed in sternal recumbency with the head and neck maximally flexed. Following aseptic preparation of the dorsal neck and lateral retraction of the dorsal crest, the spinal processes of the cervical vertebrae can be palpated. Careful advancement of the needle between C1 and C2 permits the collection of a small volume of CSF. CSF, often blood contaminated, has been collected from the cervical region of lizards, snakes, and chelonians and from the lumbar region of lizards (Fig. 43.23). Strict asepsis is essential, and it is important that either the fluid is permitted to flow from the needle or only very minor negative pressure is applied. The greatest complication with this technique is blood contamination, and concurrent hematologic assessment of blood samples can be helpful in assessing CSF blood contamination and artifact. Cytologic and microbiologic evaluations of CSF would appear to be of value in the assessment of CNS disease.

Eyes. Subspectacular infections in snakes and some lizards occur with some frequency. Surgical wedge resection of the spectacle permits the collection of exudate for cytologic and microbiologic tests (Fig. 43.24A).[3,7] Likewise, proliferative corneal lesions can be carefully scraped and retrobulbar swellings aspirated for further investigation (Fig. 43.24B). Occasionally, eyelid lesions may be seen that can be biopsied using magnification with fine biopsy forceps.

Ears. Tympanic abscessation in chelonians is common, and surgical access to evacuate the inspissated contents also allows the collection of

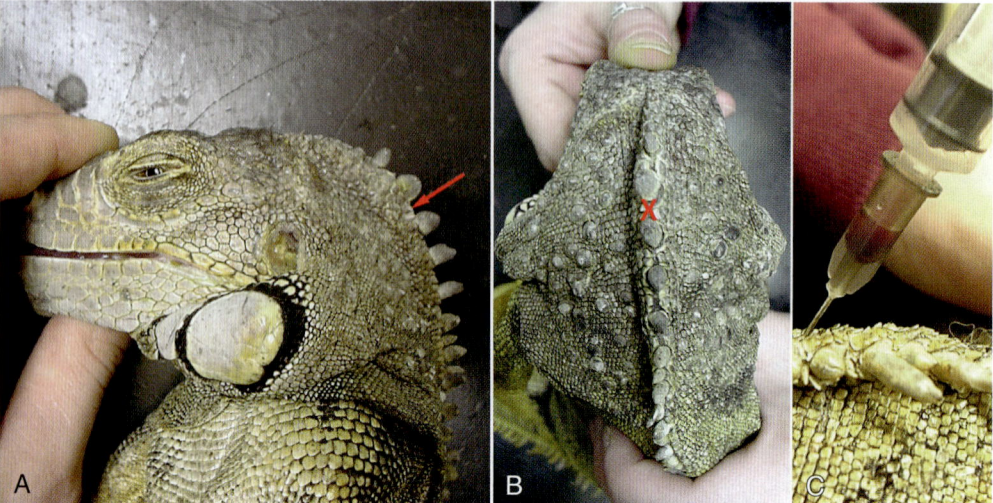

FIG 43.23 Positioning for cerebrospinal fluid tap in an iguana (*Iguana iguana*). (A, B) The head and neck are maximally flexed to improve dorsal access to the spinal canal. The needle is advanced in the dorsal midline; retracting the crest laterally and palpating the dorsal spinal processes aids proper needle placement (red cross and arrow). (C) Note that blood contamination is a common complication. A more caudal approach can also be attempted cranial to the pelvis or along the tail; however, reptiles do not possess a cauda equina, and therefore the potential for spinal damage remains. (Courtesy of Stephen J. Divers.)

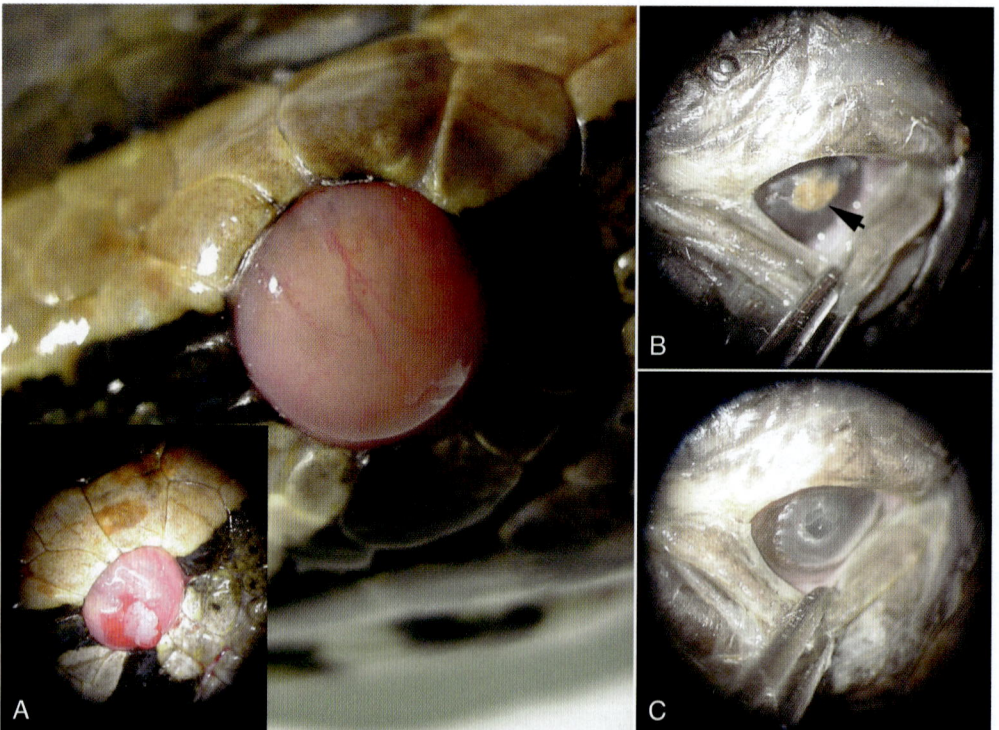

FIG 43.24 (A) Wedge resection of a python's spectacle to allow drainage and collection of subspectacular exudates for cytologic and microbiologic investigations. (B) Corneal lesion (arrow) of a *Testudo* tortoise as seen at 6x magnification. (C) The lesion has been carefully removed from the cornea for cytology, leaving the debrided ulcer for further medical therapy. (Courtesy of Stephen J. Divers.)

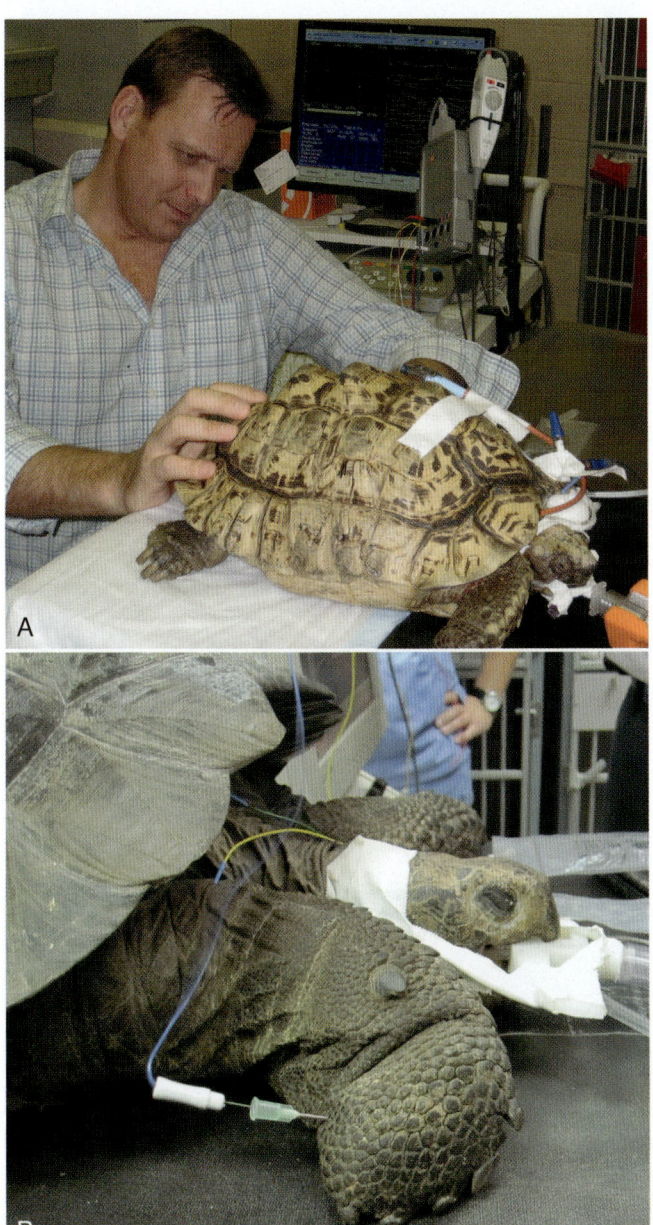

FIG 43.25 (A and B) Dr. Simon Platt (world-famous neurologist) performing electromyography in two anesthetized tortoises. (Courtesy of Stephen J. Divers.)

appropriate samples. In lizards, tympanic disease appears to be less common, but a variety of infectious causes, including *Cryptosporidia* sp have been identified and may not be appreciated without the collection of aspirates or biopsies. The removal of 25% to 50% of the tympanum facilitates both collection of samples and evacuation of exudates. This procedure does not damage the ear and the tympanum will heal by second intention.

Peripheral Nerve Evaluation and Biopsy. Peripheral neuropathies are seldom reported, but similar techniques to those used in mammals can be employed. Electromyography can be used to evaluate for potential neuromuscular diseases (Fig. 43.25). In most cases gastrointestinal or muscle biopsies often contain neural tissue.

REFERENCES

See www.expertconsult.com for a complete list of references.

44

Catheter Placement

Mariana A. Pardo and Stephen J. Divers

Vascular access in reptiles can present unique challenges for clinicians due to their intrinsic and particular anatomy. Peripheral vessels are not readily visualized, with the exception of the dorsal buccal vein in snakes. Because of this, additional visualization techniques such as surgical exposure and ultrasonography have been used to improve vascular access. A combination of appropriate patient restraint, technique, and technical expertise can facilitate venous access. Although vascular catheterization is not required for blood collection or fluid and drug administration, it is considered standard of care when treating critically ill patients. Often these critical reptiles require repeated or continuous drug administration or serial blood sampling. Additionally intravenous (IV) administration of medications are more rapid and reliable and may decrease variables that influence pharmacokinetics when medications and fluids are given through alternate routes to critically ill patients (Fig. 44.1).[1,2]

PERIPHERAL VENOUS CATHETERIZATION

Catheter Types

There are a variety of commercially available catheters. The selection of the appropriate gauge and length of the catheter is dependent on the species and size of the animal, the condition and availability of veins, and the needs of the patient. The maximum flow rate of a catheter is determined by the radius and the length of the catheter. A rapid delivery of large volumes of fluid will require a short, large-gauge catheter. If a slower rate is acceptable, then smaller-gauge catheters may be appropriate.

- Over-the-needle catheter: This is the most commonly used catheter type. They are easy to place and inexpensive. They are available in a variety of sizes and are composed of several materials. The point of the needle is beveled and extends a few millimeters past the catheter tip.
- Through-the-needle catheter: This type of catheter is passed through the lumen of the needle. They are much longer (8–12 inches, 20–30 cm) in comparison to over-the-needle catheters and also come in a variety of diameters. The catheter is covered by a plastic sheath to prevent catheter contamination during placement. Once the catheter is fed through the needle, the needle is withdrawn and removed completely or covered with a needle guard to prevent laceration or damage to the catheter lumen (Fig. 44.2).

Catheter Insertion Sites (Table 44.1)

- Cephalic vein: This is a common site of insertion in lizards and is located running from medial to lateral in a proximal to distal direction across the antebrachium (Fig. 44.3). Using sterile techniques, a superficial transverse cut down, starting from the midmedial antebrachium to lateral, is performed. The vein is superficial; hence, an aggressive skin incision may easily damage the vessel. Blunt dissection may be

used to further expose the vein. An appropriately sized catheter can then be placed and secured. An ultrasound-guided technique has been used in turtles under 15 kg.[3] This technique requires ultrasonographic visualization of the cephalic vein and is then used to guide the catheter insertion. Due to skin thickness, this technique may not be adequate in turtles more than 15 kg without previously performing a surgical cut down.[3]

- Ventral coccygeal vein: This is a common site of insertion in lizards, snakes, and crocodilians (Fig. 44.4). Using sterile technique, the transverse vertebral processes are palpated, and the tail is bent laterally. The catheter is inserted horizontally just below the level of the transverse vertebral processes in a proximal direction and then directed toward midline ventral to the vertebral body.[4] Alternatively, the catheter may be placed through the ventral midline approach

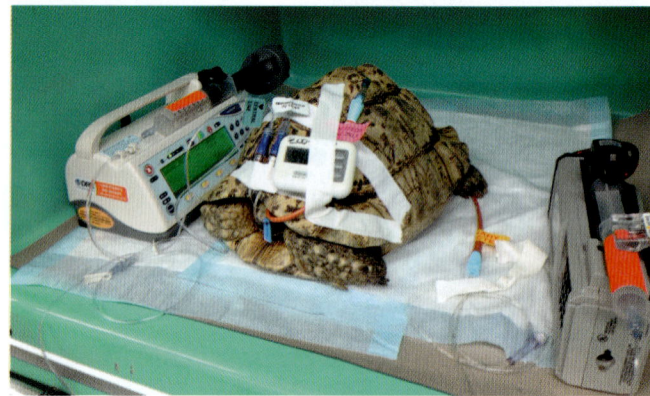

FIG 44.1 A critically ill leopard tortoise (*Stigmochelys pardalis*) with dual lumen jugular central line for receiving two intravenous medications, an esophagostomy feeding tube, and an indwelling bladder catheter for urine collection. (Courtesy of Stephen J. Divers.)

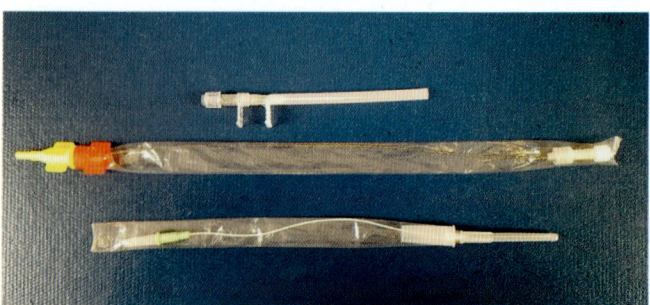

FIG 44.2 Through-the-needle catheters. Top: 18 G x 32 cm Cavafix MT Jugular Catheter (Braun, Germany); bottom: 19 G x 30.5 cm BD Intracath (BD, Sandy, UT). (Courtesy of Mariana A. Pardo.)

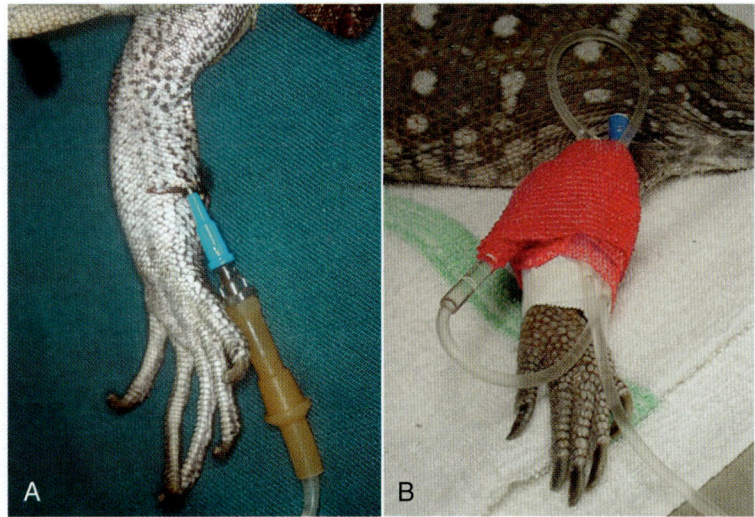

FIG 44.3 Lizard cephalic venous catheters. (A) Placement of the catheter in an iguanid lizard; note the transverse skin incision to permit better exposure to locate the vein. (B) Bandaged cephalic catheter in a monitor lizard. (Courtesy of Stephen J. Divers.)

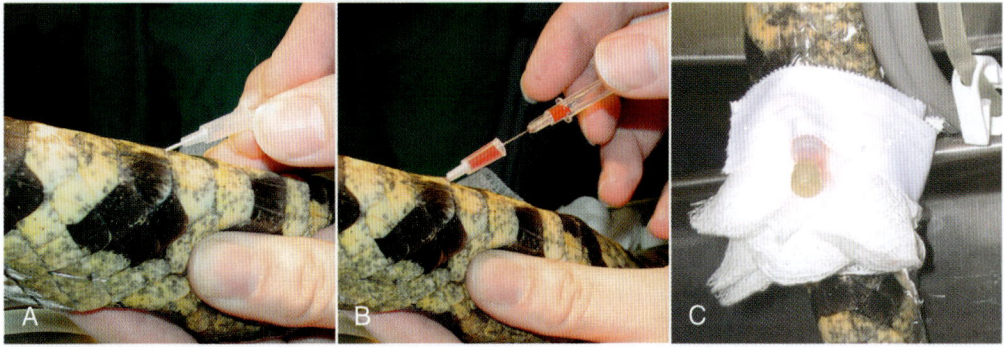

FIG 44.4 (A, B) Ventral coccygeal venous catheter placement in a snake. (C) While bandaging in place helps maintain patency, such catheters are difficult to impossible to maintain in active snakes. (Courtesy of Stephen J. Divers.)

TABLE 44.1 Available Intravenous and Intraosseous Catheter Sites for Reptiles

Species	Catheter Site	Comment
Chelonian	Jugular vein	Right jugular larger than left
	Cephalic vein	<15 kg, requires ultrasound guidance
	Plastrocarapacial bridge	Requires a drilled pilot hole, less effective than long bones
	Humerus/femur	Similar principle to small animals
Crocodilian	Ventral coccygeal vein	Similar principle to blood sampling
	Humerus/femur/tibia	Similar principle to small animals
Lizard	Cephalic vein	Requires a cut down
	Ventral coccygeal vein	Similar principle to blood sampling
	Femur/humerus/tibia	Similar principle to small animals
Snake	Jugular vein	Right jugular larger than left
	Heart	Only for emergency situations in moribund or anesthetized animals

in anesthetized reptiles. This has the advantage of being less likely affected by lateral tail movement or position but cannot be easily maintained in a conscious animal in sternal orientation.

- Dorsal coccygeal vein: This approach can be used in chelonians but is prone to lymphatic or cerebrospinal fluid contamination, is more difficult to maintain, and is therefore restricted to nonmobile or anesthetized animals where other routes prove unsuccessful. Using sterile technique, the transverse vertebral processes are palpated, and the tail is bent ventrally. The catheter is inserted vertically in the dorsal midline, between the spinous processes of the coccygeal vertebrae (Fig. 44.5).
- Jugular Vein: This is a common site of insertion in chelonians and snakes but can also be used in lizards (Fig. 44.6). The right jugular vein may be larger than the left; however, both sides may be used. The vein is located by drawing an imaginary line between the tympanic membrane and the carapace, under which the vein normally runs its path.[5] Ultrasonographic guidance can also aid in locating the vein.[3] A small cut down and blunt dissection is made at least one third of the way back from the tympanum down the neck. The further caudal the catheterization entry site, the more difficult it is to place, but the less likely it will be dislodged by the animal. An

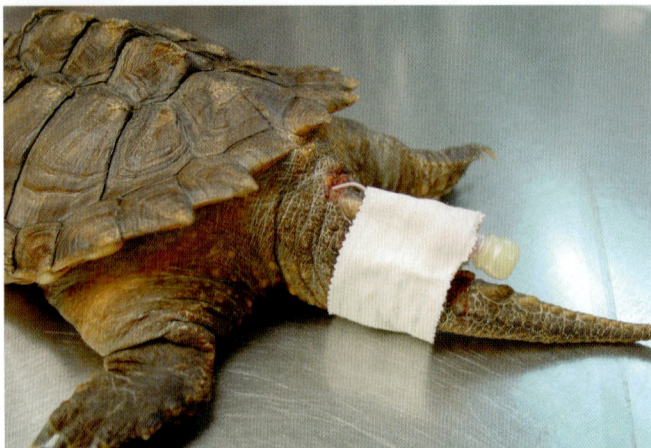

FIG 44.5 Dorsal coccygeal venous catheter in a turtle. Such catheters are difficult to impossible to maintain in active animals. (Courtesy of Stephen J. Divers.)

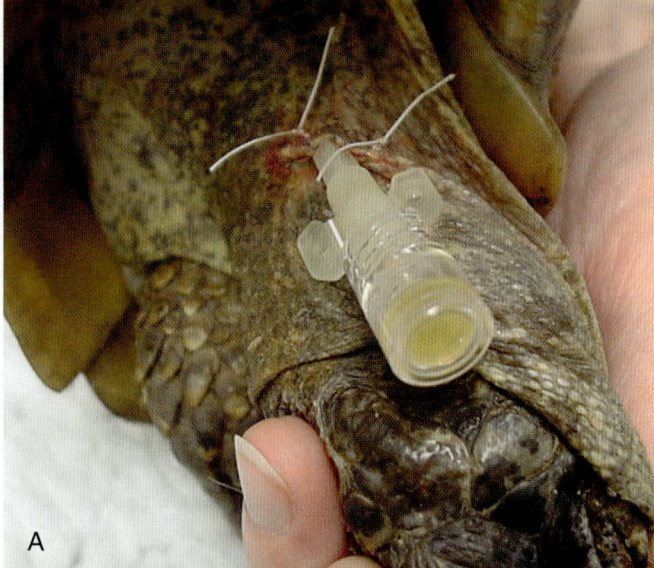

A

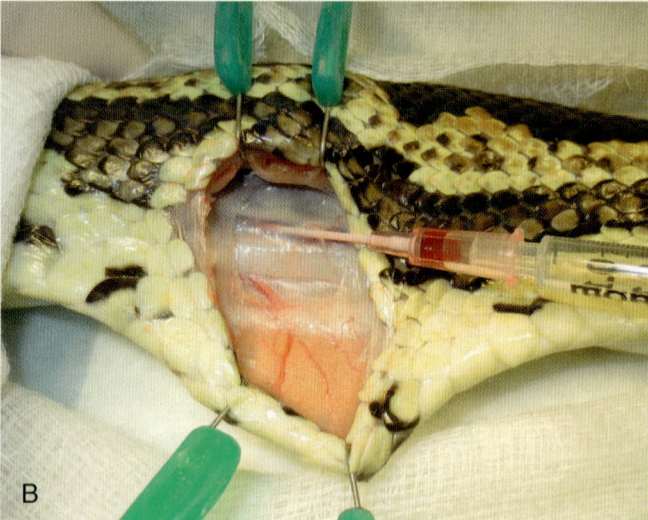

B

FIG 44.6 (A) Jugular venous catheter sutured in place in a chelonian. (B) Placement of a jugular venous catheter in a snake following a small coeliotomy cranial to the heart. (Courtesy of Stephen J. Divers.)

appropriately sized catheter is placed and secured. Longer catheters can flex when the neck is retracted and produce catheter failure; hence, central venous catheters may be considered instead (see the section Central Venous Catheterization). These catheters are more easily maintained in active animals.

- As in chelonians, the right jugular vein is typically preferred in snakes for placement of an indwelling catheter. The patient is placed in dorsal recumbency, and the heart is located by watching for the beating ventral scutes. Using a sterile technique, a small incision is made 10 scutes cranial to the heart and should be 3 scutes long at the margin of the scutes and the first row of lateral body scales. Using blunt dissection, the jugular vein is exposed; it is superficial and runs medial and parallel to the free margins of the ribs. An appropriately sized catheter is then inserted and directed toward the heart. Sutures will be needed to secure the catheter in place.

INTRAOSSEOUS CATHETERIZATION

Intravenous access can be difficult in dehydrated or hypotensive reptiles, and therefore intraosseous catheters may be placed in lizards, crocodilians, and chelonians. Intraosseous (IO) catheters should occupy between 33% to 67% of the marrow cavity at the thinnest portion. Intraosseous catheters should not be kept in place for more than 72 hours, and they should be replaced by IV catheters when possible. Intraosseous fluid delivery has been shown to be significantly slower than IV administration. The location of the IO catheter can influence delivery, and in desert tortoises, uptake from the shell was significantly lower than for the humerus and femur.[6] Due to the nonexpansive nature of the IO route, administration rates may be limited, with higher rates likely to result in patient discomfort. Contraindications for IO catheters include fractures, neoplasia, osteopenia, burns, and infection of the access site. Complications associated with IO catheters in human patients are <1% but include local cellulitis, osteomyelitis, fracture, IO needle bending, and occlusion. Additionally, extravasation of fluids or medications from an improperly placed catheter or due to the use of excessive force during bolus administration may occur.[7]

Catheter Types

A variety of human commercial intraosseous needles are available, including the Jamshidi needle (Baxter Health Care Corp., McGraw Park, IL) and the Sur-Fast Intraosseous needle (Cook, Bloomington, IN). These may be used in larger reptiles. More frequently, spinal needles are used for intraosseous catheters; however, if not available, hypodermic needles can also be used in small reptiles or amphibians, although they are more likely to become blocked with a bone plug during placement.

Catheter Insertion Sites

Intraosseous catheters should ideally be placed with analgesia and, in some cases, anesthesia depending on the patient's condition. Local anesthesia with 2% lidocaine over the placement site may be adequate to reduce pain associated with catheter placement. The site should be aseptically prepared.

- Proximal tibia: This is the most common IO site used in lizards (Fig. 44.7). The tibial crest is localized, and the catheter is introduced at the insertion of the patellar ligament. Penetration into the joint should be avoided. With the proximal tibia firmly grasped, the stifle is flexed while the needle is advanced through the skin and tibial crest while gently rotating the needle, until a subtle give is felt. Care is needed to keep the needle straight. The needle is then advanced within the marrow cavity. Depending on the angle at which the

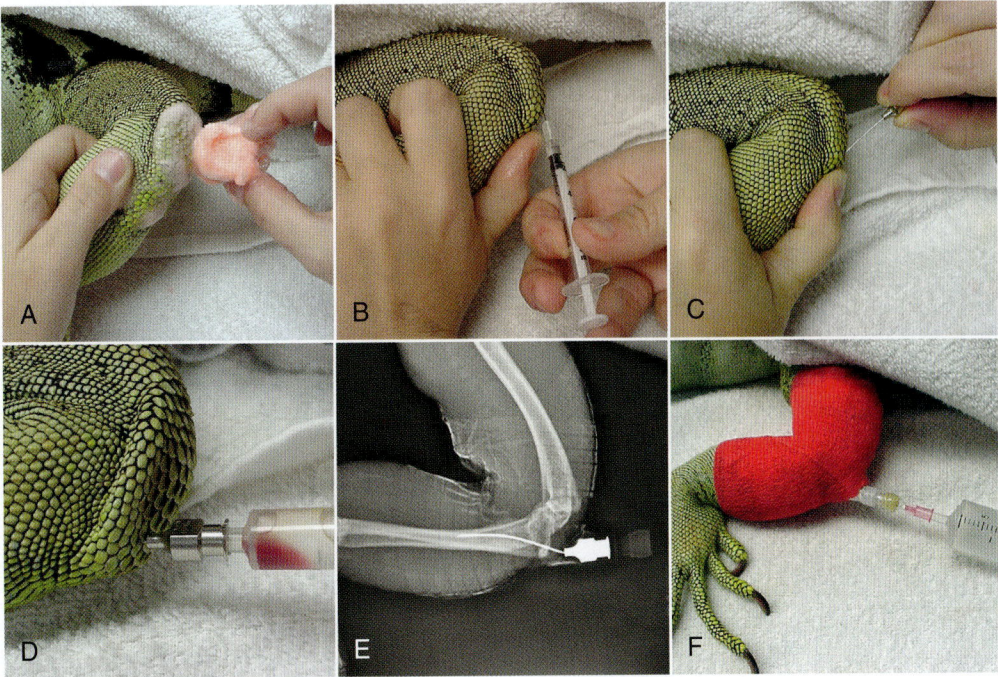

FIG 44.7 Intraosseous catheterization in a green iguana *(Iguana iguana)*. (A) Aseptic preparation of the right proximal tibia. (B) Injection of lidocaine subcutaneously. (C) Insertion of a 22 g 1-inch (2.5-cm) spinal needle. (D) Aspiration of bone marrow confirming correct placement. (E) Radiographic confirmation of intramedullary placement. (F) The catheter has been securely taped using a self-adhesive bandage, and a slow bolus of intravenous fluids is being given. (Courtesy of Stephen J. Divers.)

needle was bored, the catheter can be advanced to its full length in the case of catheters placed parallel to the long axis of the bone. In catheters placed at an angle, the needle is advanced until the tip of the catheter encounters resistance, indicating the opposite bone cortex. Care must be taken not to advance the catheter past this point of resistance because this can lead to penetration through the opposite cortex and extravasation of fluids into soft tissues.[7]

- Proximal humerus/femur: This technique can be used in chelonians, lizards, and crocodilians. The humerus and the femur can be catheterized by grasping the bone and firmly placing one finger along its long axis to indicate the direction of the bone. The needle is then introduced distally by use of a combination of a rotational movement and gentle pressure on the needle. Once the needle passes through the cortex into the medullary canal, a sudden loss of resistance will be detected.[8]

- Plastrocarapacial junction: In chelonians this technique can be used by locating the widest cranial aspect of the most dorsal-lateral scute of the bridge. A small pilot hole is created with a wire driver drill and sterile wire in a parallel plane to the shell in a cranial–caudal direction.[6] The wire is then removed, and the catheter is inserted by hand. Care should be taken to avoid celomic placement, and delivery at this site is less effective than the humerus and femur (Fig. 44.8).

INTRACARDIAC CATHETERIZATION

In emergency situations where a jugular catheter is unsuccessful, an intracardiac catheter may be placed in snakes (Fig. 44.9). Using sterile techniques, place the patient in dorsal recumbency in the usual manner used to identify cardiac beat. Using an appropriately sized catheter, direct the catheter through the ventral skin between scutes toward the heart. The heart beat will be felt against the catheter. Once a flash is observed,

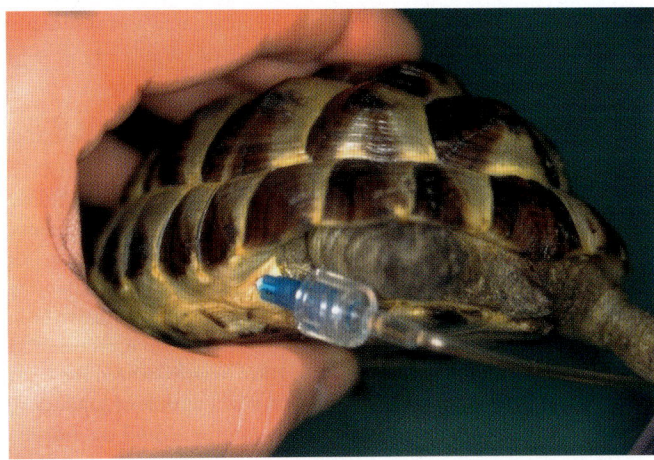

FIG 44.8 Intraosseous fluid administration via a plastrocarapacial bridge catheter in a chelonian. (Courtesy of Stephen J. Divers.)

remove the stylet, advance the catheter, and secure appropriately.[5] This technique is generally restricted to anesthetized or moribund snakes due to the difficulties of maintenance in an active animal.

ARTERIAL CATHETERIZATION

Arterial catheterization is important for the evaluation of invasive arterial blood pressure and serial arterial blood gas analysis. Unfortunately, arterial catheterization is invasive and challenging and tends to be restricted to research studies. Femoral artery and carotid catheterization has been successfully performed in iguanas,[9,10] and the vertebral

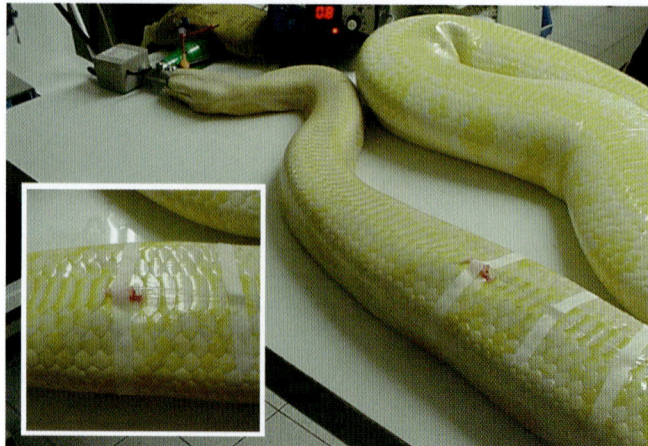

FIG 44.9 Intracardiac catheterization and intraoperative fluid administration in an anesthetized albino Burmese python *(Python bivittatus)*. (Courtesy of Stephen J. Divers.)

artery has been used in rattlesnakes.[11,12] In snakes, the vertebral artery is accessed by making a ventrolateral incision approximately 3 cm cranial to the heart. The tip of the catheter is then advanced toward the right aortic arch and secured in place with sutures.[11] The left carotid artery has been successfully catheterized in iguanas and used for evaluation of invasive arterial blood pressure.[13] The skin over the lateral neck is aseptically prepared, and the left carotid artery is surgically exposed. The carotid artery is ligated cranially with 5–0 nonabsorbable sutures, and the artery is occluded proximally with a sterile cotton-tipped applicator. An arterial catheter can then be inserted with the tip of the catheter positioned near the aortic arch and sutured in place (Fig. 44.10).

CENTRAL VENOUS CATHETERIZATION

Long-term IV access can be difficult to obtain and maintain; however, it may be critically important for administration of medications, fluids, blood products, and repeated blood sampling in hospitalized patients. Jugular catheterization provides the most rapid and secure route for vascular access, but catheters can be difficult to place, and maintaining catheter patency can be challenging. Central venous catheters have been shown to provide flexibility and sampling access while minimizing catheter displacement in chelonians.[14] Jugular veins have been the most commonly catheterized vessel; however. any vessel capable of supporting the diameter and length of these catheters may be a good candidate.

Catheter Types

Central venous catheters are available in a variety of gauges and lengths and with multiple lumens through Mila International (Florence, KY) and Arrow International (Reading, PA). This selection should be based on vessel diameter and length of catheter required.

- Single lumen catheter: These catheters may be appropriate when there is only one purpose for the central venous catheter, such as serial blood draws or fluid therapy.
- Multilumen catheter: These catheters may have up to four lumens. They are useful in critical care settings; incompatible drugs and fluids can be delivered simultaneously, they serve as a blood sampling line, and assessments such as central venous pressures can be performed. (Fig. 44.11). Dual-lumen catheters have been most commonly used by the authors, with one line for dedicated blood collection and the second for fluid/drug administration.

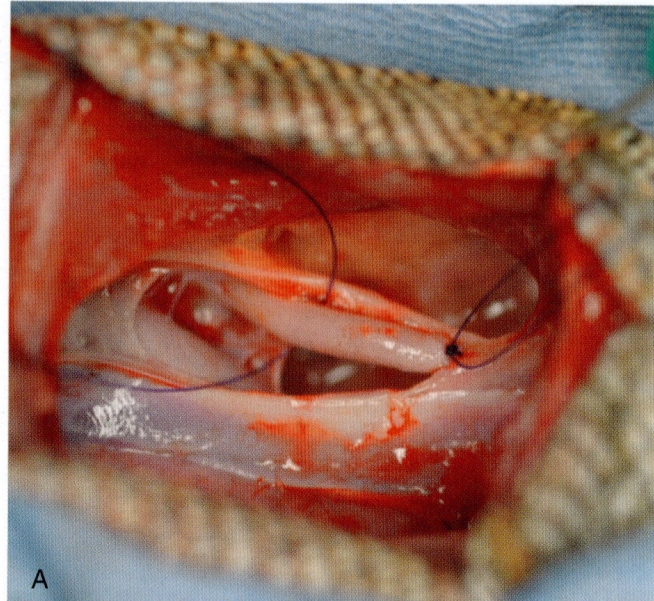

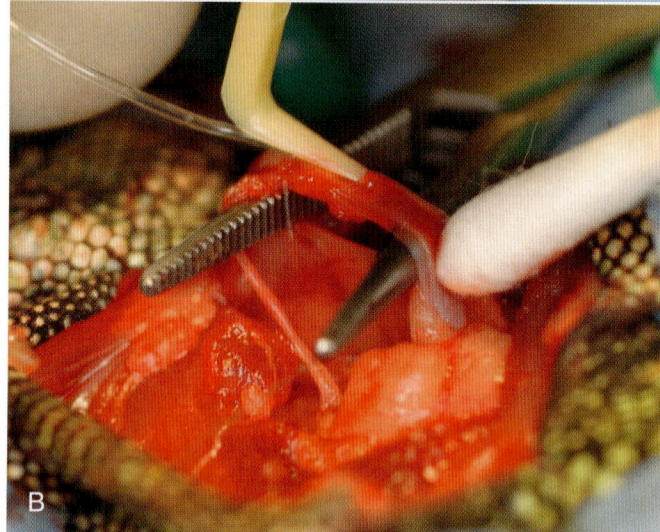

FIG 44.10 Intra-arterial catheterization in an iguanid lizard. (A) After surgical exposure of the lateral cervical region, the carotid artery has been isolated using stay sutures. (B) After small arteriotomy and while occluding the artery proximally, a catheter is being placed into the carotid artery. (Courtesy of Mariana A. Pardo.)

Seldinger Technique

This technique has been previously described in tortoises and sea turtles.[14,15,16] Under anesthesia or sedation, the jugular site is surgically prepared and draped in a standard fashion, and the patient is placed in sternal recumbency in a 20- to 30-degree head-down position. Ultrasound-guided placement and surgical cut downs have been used to improve success of catheterization.[3] The jugular vein is exposed through blunt dissection and then catheterized with an over-the-needle introducing catheter in a caudal direction. The J-tipped wire is introduced through the catheter, taking care to advance to the level of the proximal humeral plastron scutes and not to the level of the heart. Once the guidewire is placed, the introducing catheter and wire introducer are then carefully removed while keeping the wire in place. The vein dilator is then threaded over the wire and introduced a couple of centimeters into the vein while applying firm torsion. The dilator is removed and digital pressure is applied to prevent blood leakage. The central venous catheter is then threaded over the guide wire and introduced caudally. The guidewire will then appear through the uncapped distal lumen. Care must be taken to not lose sight of the guidewire as the catheter is introduced. As the catheter is threaded

over the wire and into the patient caudally, the wire is slowly removed in the opposite direction. The catheter should be introduced to the desired depth. Air entrapped in the catheter should be removed and then primed with sterile saline. The catheter is then sutured in place; a spacing clamp fastener may or may not be needed depending on patient size (Fig. 44.12).

Verification of Placement

Correct placement should be confirmed radiographically; the tip of the catheter should lie anterior to the heart. If the catheter is placed too far into the heart or past it, it should be backed up an appropriate distance until it is located in the desired area.

Rewiring of Catheters

Central venous catheters that are no longer patent or problematic can be replaced through an exchange technique. Catheters should be rewired only when there is no evidence of infection and the insertion site is clean and does not appear inflamed. Sterile techniques should be used as previously indicated. The Seldinger technique is again used by passing the guidewire through the existing catheter and then removing the catheter while keeping the guidewire in place. The replacement catheter is the threaded over the wire and into the vein as previously described.

Catheter Maintenance

Catheter maintenance involves twice daily flushing of the catheter port with sterile saline or heparinized saline if the ports are not being currently used with a continuous infusion. Monitoring of the insertion site for signs

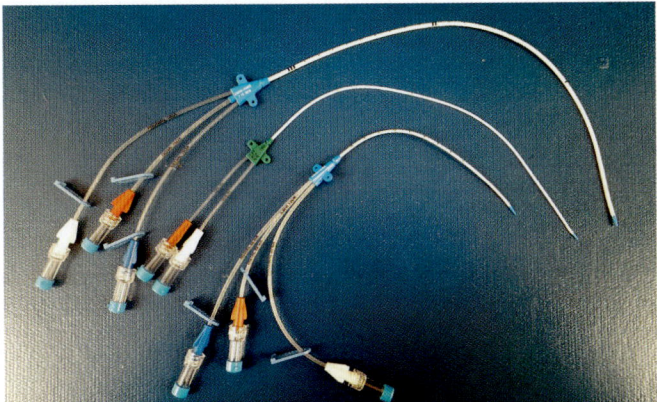

FIG 44.11 Multilumen central venous catheters. Top: triple lumen 7Fr 30 cm central venous catheter (Arrow International, Reading, PA); middle: double lumen 5Fr. 25 cm central venous catheter (Mila International, Florence, KY); bottom: triple lumen 5.5Fr 13 cm central venous catheter (Arrow International, Reading, PA). (Courtesy of Mariana A. Pardo.)

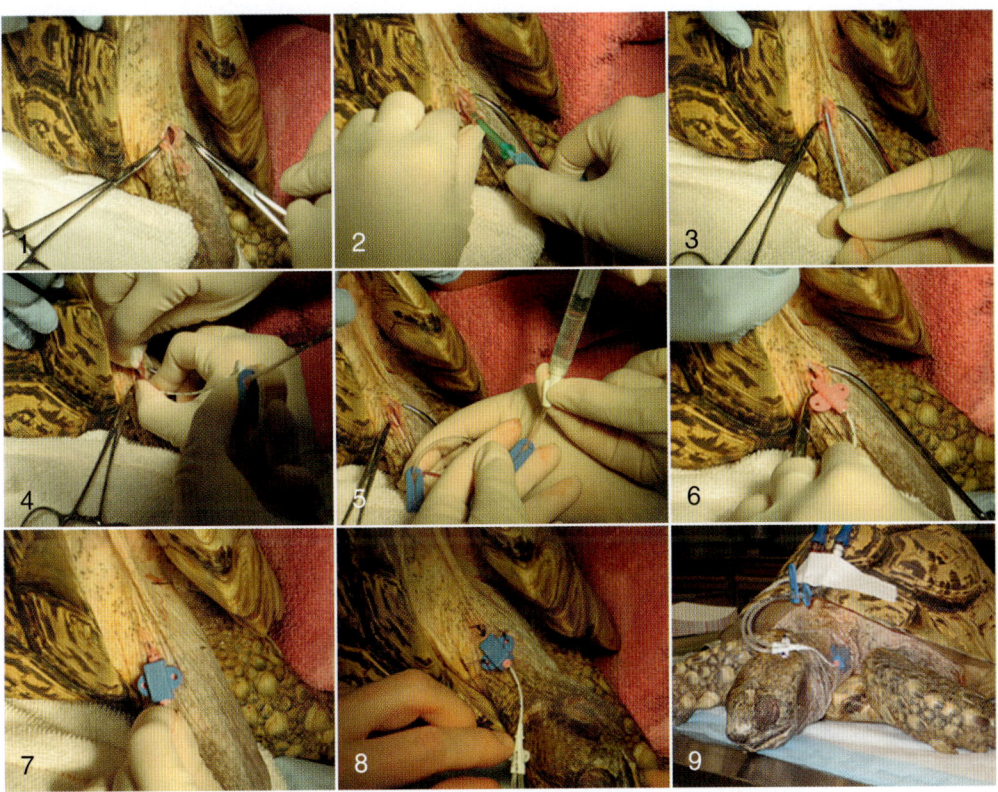

FIG 44.12 (1) Surgical cut down in preparation for jugular catheterization in a chelonian with an over-the-needle catheter. (2) Placement of J-tipped wire through the catheter. (3) Vein dilator placed over the wire. (4) Placement of central venous catheter over the wire. (5) Removal of air from catheter and priming with saline. (6) Placement of soft clamp directly onto the catheter. (7) Placement of hard fastener on top of the soft clamp. (8) Suturing of the catheter clamp and fastener. (9) Catheter in place with ports taped on carapace. (Courtesy of Mariana A. Pardo and Stephen J. Divers.)

of infection, thrombosis, and phlebitis should be performed daily. Catheter sites should be gently cleaned of any obvious organic material daily.

VASCULAR ACCESS PORTS

Vascular access ports may be placed in reptiles that require serial blood sampling.[17] The technique has been previously described in iguanas, where arterial blood gases were evaluated.[18] Using sterile techniques, blunt dissection ventral to the external jugular vein is performed to expose the internal and external carotid arteries near their bifurcation. The catheter was inserted into the internal carotid artery and then guided to the common carotid artery. The opposite end of the vascular access port is then tunneled under the skin to a dorsal location near the scapula. Maintenance of the port included flushing twice a week with heparinized saline. Placement of a cardiac port in tortoises has also been described: a hole is drilled at the cardiac level in the plastron, and once the heart is visualized a sterile rubber is custom fitted and sealed in place with epoxy.[19] Myocardial fibrosis was seen in some of these subjects.[18]

CATHETER MAINTENANCE

Regardless of the catheter insertion site, inspection of the catheter site should be performed daily and examined for signs of pain, phlebitis, infection, thrombosis, and subcutaneous infiltration of fluids. Catheters should be removed if any of these signs are observed (Box 44.1).

BOX 44.1   Complications Associated With Catheterization

- Dislodgement
- Mechanical (phlebitis, hematoma, laceration)
- Subcutaneous extravasation
- Infection
- Thrombosis

CONCLUSION

Unhindered access to the vascular compartment of reptiles has huge implications for serial clinicopathologic evaluations and therapy. Just as they have become an essential and integral aspect of human and domesticated animal critical care, they should be utilized in herpetological medicine. In particular, given the slow response of many reptiles, central line catheters have provided a mechanism for serial sampling and IV drug administration over periods of weeks to months. This has revolutionized our management of these cases from inpatient to outpatient, in much the same way that esophagostomy feeding tubes have.

REFERENCES

See www.expertconsult.com for a complete list of references.

45

Esophagostomy Tube Placement

Daniel Cutler and Stephen J. Divers

Compared with other veterinary patients, the debilitated reptile often requires an extended period of supportive care and treatment. For this reason the esophagostomy tube has proven especially useful as a method for delivering oral fluid therapy, nutrition, and medications, both in the hospital and on an outpatient basis.

Correction and maintenance of proper hydration is imperative in any sick patient.[1,2] Intravenous, subcutaneous, and intracoelomic routes for providing fluid therapy are utilized in hospitalized patients and particularly in those with dysfunctional gastrointestinal tracts or abnormal body temperatures.[3] However, long-term hospitalization may not be practical or financially viable, and these hydration techniques may not be possible by the caretaker.[1]

Ensuring proper nutrition and caloric intake should not be ignored and is vital to recovery. In addition to nutritional support, various medical therapies may need to be given for an extended period. Therapeutic drugs can be given via intramuscular or subcutaneous routes; however, the owner may not be able to give injections, and drugs that require multiple dosing throughout the day may be stressful to the patient. Depending on the species, oral medications may be easily administered by the owner with minimal stress. Most lizard and snake species are good candidates for oral dosing. Caretakers of such species can be trained to give both oral medications and nutritional supplementation via syringe or gavage needle. However, larger lizards such as monitors or iguanas may not allow repeated restraint and oral administration without putting the caretaker in unnecessary danger, in addition to being stressful to the patient.[4] Also, concurrent pathology of the oral cavity such as severe stomatitis or mandibular fractures may contraindicate giving treatments via the oral route.[2,5] Chelonian's anatomic adaptations make oral medicating and assist-feeding more challenging, if not impossible.

A solution to these challenges is placement of an esophagostomy tube.[4] An esophagostomy tube (E-tube) allows a long-term route for enteral treatments to be given. The E-tube is well tolerated by most reptiles and can be left in place when the patient is discharged from the hospital. Also, the patient is able to eat and swallow with the tube in place. This allows the animal to transition back to eating unaided while weaning off nutritional support. Caretakers can be trained on proper use and maintenance of the E-tube, allowing it to be used and kept in place for weeks to months. Placement of the E-tube is easily performed with sedation and local anesthesia to light anesthesia, and this is virtually identical to methods used in domestic small animal medicine. Removal of the E-tube rarely requires sedation. When the E-tube is removed, the esophagus is allowed to heal by second intention, and the skin typically does not require sutures. Due to the ease in placing and removing E-tubes, when sedating for other diagnostics/procedures, the reptile clinician should consider whether an E-tube may be necessary for ongoing case management.

PROCEDURE

See Table 45.1 for a list of materials needed for E-tube placement. Once the patient is adequately sedated/anesthetized, the tube entry site is aseptically prepared. The location of the tube should allow normal movement of the head (e.g., retraction of the head into the shell) but should not be placed too far forward to allow the front limbs to dislodge the tube. In general, the caudolateral neck is preferred, taking care to avoid the carotid and jugular vessels. The tube should be premeasured so that the end is at the level of the stomach (Fig. 45.1) and marked (with a permanent marker) where the tube would exit the neck. Curved hemostats are directed into the oral cavity and down the esophagus (Fig. 45.2A). The tips of the hemostats are pressed against the wall of the lateral esophagus to tent the skin at the preferred location. The hemostat tip (and ultimately, the tube) should be approximately halfway between the dorsum and ventrum of the neck (i.e., lateral at the 3 or 9 o'clock position) to best avoid any major vasculature. Applying firm pressure of the hemostats against the esophagus and skin helps to create an incision window with the least amount of tissue dissection and minimizes the risk of vascular laceration.

TABLE 45.1 Recommended Materials for E-Tube Placement

- Surgical scrub (e.g. chlorhexidine/povidone iodine and alcohol)
- #15 scalpel blade and handle
- Esophagostomy tube—A soft rubber or feeding tube should be chosen with the appropriate length to reach the stomach as well as adequate lumen diameter to prevent clogging.
- Christmas tree adapter and injection port
- Permanent marker
- Curved hemostats—It is important to ensure that the hemostats selected are long enough to reach the E-tube site and also long enough to direct the tube beyond the E-tube site and down the esophagus. In giant tortoise species, a large, curved Doyen clamp can be used.
- Nonabsorbable suture material (e.g., nylon)
- Needle drivers
- Suture scissors
- Materials for securing tube
  - Chelonians—White tape or duct tape can be used to affix the tube to the shell.
  - Squamates—White tape can be used to make a butterfly bandage and affix the tube to the skin with nonabsorbable suture material.
  - Antimicrobial ointment—Topical antibiotic or antiseptic treatment should be applied at least once daily after cleaning to deter local infection.

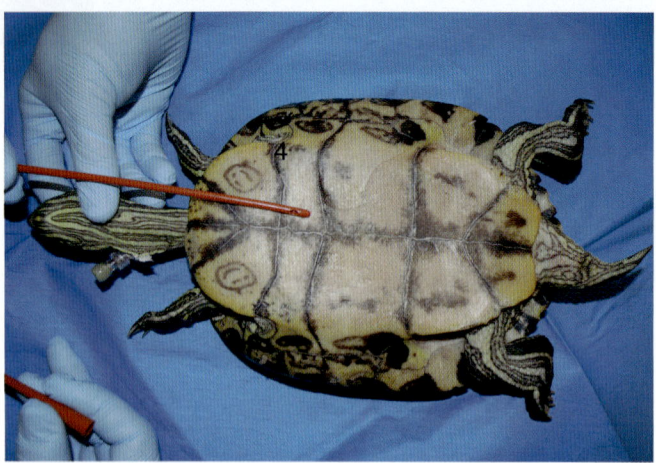

FIG 45.1 Prior to placement, the esophagostomy tube should be premeasured to the level of the stomach and marked at the point where it will leave the neck. In chelonians, the tube can be measured to the level of the pectoral scutes. (Courtesy of Daniel Cutler and Stephen J. Divers.)

Once the hemostats are properly placed, a #15 scalpel blade is used to make a small incision directly over the hemostats (Fig. 45.2B). Continual lateral pressure of the hemostat tips should be applied to cause the hemostat tips to protrude through the incision as soon as it is wide enough. A small incision provides a better seal around the tube and leaves a smaller incision to heal when the tube is removed. With the hemostat tips protruding, an appropriately sized E-tube is placed between the jaws of the hemostats and firmly grasped (Fig. 45.2C). The hemostat and E-tube tip is then pulled into the esophagus and out of the oral cavity (Fig. 45.2D). This step is crucial to prevent subcutaneous placement. The end of the tube is grasped with hemostats; the tip of the tube should be in the same direction as the hemostat tips. The hemostat and tube are then directed into the mouth and down the esophagus (Fig. 45.2E). The hemostat and tube should be pressed against the opposite side of the esophagus as they are directed caudally. This helps ensure that the tube is not directed into the esophageal defect created during the procedure. As the tube approaches and passes the location where the tube enters the neck, it is often helpful to retract and then feed the tube so as not to introduce any kinks. Once the

FIG 45.2 While the anatomy is different between species of reptiles, the steps are similar to those performed on this red-eared slider *(Trachemys scripta elegans)*. (A) Hemostats are inserted into the esophagus and pressed against the lateral side of the caudal neck. (B) An incision is made over the tips of the hemostats. (C) The hemostats are forced through the incision and used to grasp the tube and (D) pull the tube out of the mouth. (E) The tube is then redirected down the esophagus with the hemostats until (F) the premeasured mark is reached. (G) The tube is then secured with a purse-string and finger-trap suture techniques. (H) Following placement, the tube should be secured to allow normal movement but prevent contamination or removal by the patient. In chelonians, this is easily achieved by taping the tube to the carapace. (Courtesy of Daniel Cutler and Stephen J. Divers.)

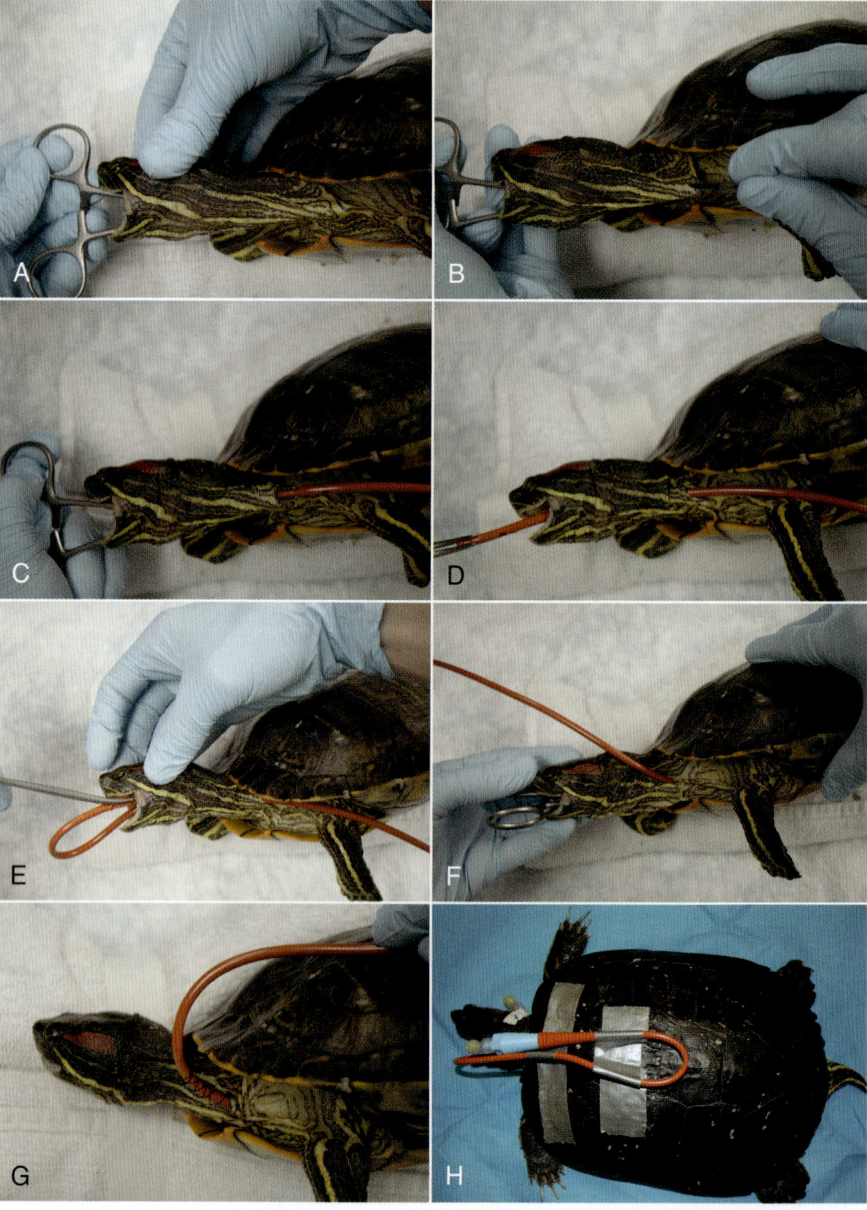

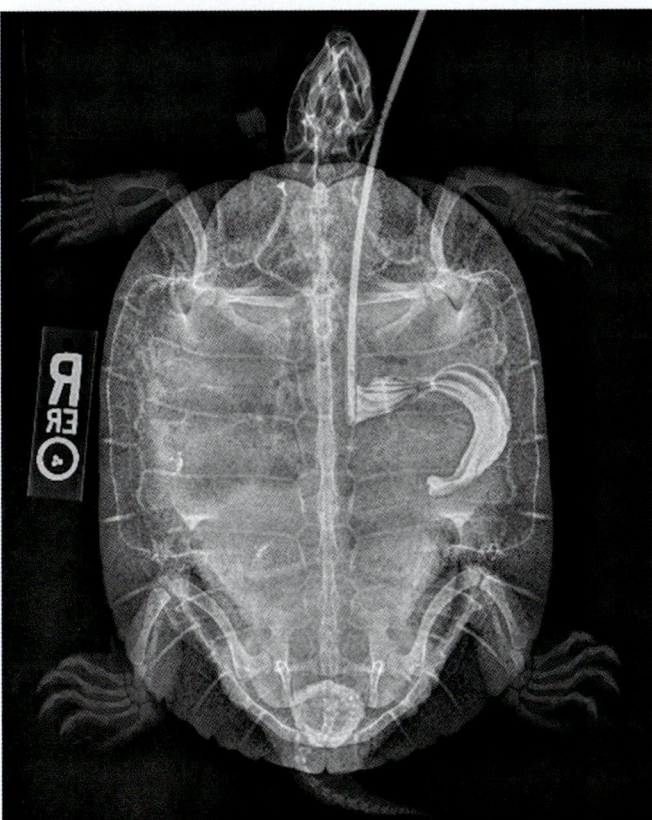

FIG 45.3 Placement should always be checked prior to giving any fluids via the tube. Contrast material can be given to assist in confirmation of proper placement in the distal esophagus or stomach. (Courtesy of Daniel Cutler and Stephen J. Divers.)

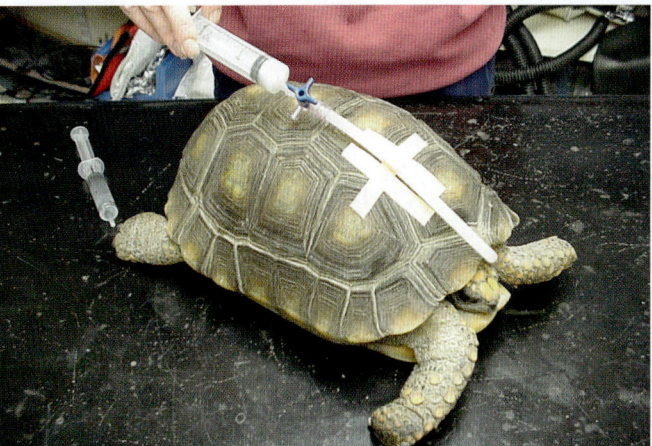

FIG 45.4 Delivering medication via an esophgostomy tube in a yellow foot tortoise *(Chelonoidis denticulata)* with minimal restraint. Note the syringe of water on the table, ready to flush the tube. (Courtesy of Stephen J. Divers.)

hemostats reach the extent of their reach, their grasp can be disengaged, the hemostats are removed, and the tube is fed until the proper location is reached (Fig. 45.2F). The tube may be palpated through the skin and stabilized to help direct it toward the stomach.

Once the tube has reached the premeasured location, the tube is secured using a purse-string and finger-trap suture pattern with nonabsorbable sutures (Fig. 45.2G). The tube should be checked to ensure that it will not easily move in or out of the neck incision. The tube end is secured with either butterfly sutures or tape, depending on the species (Fig. 45.2H). The end of the tube should be kept closed (e.g., Christmas tree adapter and injection port) when not in use.

Before food, medication, or water is administered through the tube, proper placement should be verified. Radiographic imaging with contrast or endoscopy can quickly verify proper tube placement (Fig. 45.3).

MAINTENANCE AND USE

While in place, the tube entry site should be cleaned with an antiseptic daily and a topical antibiotic ointment applied to the incision site to prevent local infection. Generally, before and after giving medications or food, and at least once per day, the tube should be flushed with a volume of water at least equal to the volume of the tube (Fig. 45.4). Flushing of the tube helps prevent clogging, which may necessitate

replacement. Any nutritional support delivered via the tube should be of an appropriate consistency to allow easy passage without excessive force.

Possible complications include secondary infection, blockage of tube, perforation/ulceration of gastrointestinal tract, and removal of the tube by the patient. Most of these can be prevented using the proper technique described above. The latter is the most common complication, especially in tortoises because of the large protective scales on the front limbs. Placing the tube more caudally and wrapping the "keratinized scales" on the front limbs of tortoises with vet wrap or tape can minimize these scales hooking the tube and pulling it out.

REMOVAL

Removal of the tube is a simple procedure and rarely requires sedation, unless the patient is fractious, dangerous, or uncooperative. Once the purse-string suture is cut, the tube can be pulled. The wound is generally left open to heal by second intention. Food can be offered to the patient the day after the procedure.

CONCLUSION

The E-tube is an important tool for the rehabilitation and treatment of sick and debilitated reptiles. The placement is minimally invasive and allows long-term, reliable delivery of fluids, nutrition, and medications. Use of the tube is not complicated and can easily be taught to the client to decrease hospitalization periods. Placement of an esophagostomy tube should always be considered for the sick, debilitated reptile that is likely to require prolonged, oral treatments.

REFERENCES

See www.expertconsult.com for a complete list of references.

46

Hospitalization

Daniel Cutler and Stephen J. Divers

The decision to hospitalize a reptile patient can be made for multiple reasons and are influenced by the medical goals and the patient's condition. The great variability in natural histories and physical attributes among reptile taxa makes finding a "one-size-fits-all" solution for hospitalization difficult. It is important to recognize the basic, daily requirements that must be met for each individual patient, along with addressing the reason(s) for hospitalization.[1] Improper hospitalization can exacerbate presenting pathology and patient stress or even create new problems, which can complicate the clinical picture and disrupt therapy.

INDICATIONS FOR HOSPITALIZATION

Proper requirements for hospitalization can vary based on the length of time the reptile patient will be staying.

Short-term hospitalization: A patient may be housed until a diagnostic or elective surgical procedure can be performed within the next 1 to 3 days. Such animals may only require basic amenities to address temperature, humidity, lighting, and security. Several days of stabilization and monitoring are often required for ill or unstable patients. In these cases, ensuring and monitoring the appropriate humidity, photoperiod, weight changes, appetite/caloric intake, and defecation/urination becomes more important.

Long-term hospitalization: If necessary, reptiles may need to be hospitalized for weeks to months. These reptile patients are usually chronically debilitated and require intensive daily care that the owner is unable to perform. Such hospitalization is far less common due to expense, and usually efforts are made to treat such cases on an outpatient basis using esophagostomy tubes and central line catheters. Fullspectrum lighting (including UVB) should be utilized for these long-term patients to prevent secondary nutritional hyperparathyroidism, as well as facilitate normal behaviors and color recognition. It is also increasingly important to ensure that the diet given to long-term inpatients meets all nutritional requirements (not just calories). Acknowledging these components of husbandry and addressing them proactively will allow the presenting complaint to be treated without management-induced complications.

ENCLOSURES AND SECURITY

Besides meeting requirements for proper medical care, hospital enclosures must also be safe and escape proof. Escaped patients can pose significant dangers to themselves, other patients, and staff, notwithstanding the embarrassment and liability if the animal cannot be recovered. For larger reptiles, walk-in kennels used for dogs may be appropriate (Fig. 46.1). Some designs incorporate sloped flooring to provide aquatic areas. Many reptiles are adept climbers, so the cage must be completely enclosed. Such large kennels are more difficult to heat or maintain

humidity unless they have dedicated thermostats, heat sources, and humidifiers.

Enclosures and incubators designed specifically for reptiles provide the most security, particularly for smaller species. Purpose-built caging offers the ability for custom designs and sizes for small areas and, although expensive, can create easily controllable and cleanable environments (Figs. 46.2 and 46.3). In general, the ability to divide or combine cage spaces provides more versatility, as does having both terrestrial and arboreal options (Figs. 46.4 and 46.5).

It is advisable to have locking mechanisms for cages because some (especially snakes) are escape artists, whereas others may be especially valuable or dangerous (e.g., venomous snakes). Venomous snake enclosures must be lockable and require special shift boxes integrated into their design (Fig. 46.6) that can be easily disconnected and moved to connect to practice anesthesia machines. It is beneficial to be able to view all enclosures, especially those that contain venomous species, from outside the reptile room. It is also useful for such windows to have integrated blinds to improve animal seclusion. If housing venomous snakes, the veterinarian should review any local, regional, and federal requirements. In addition, protocols for escapes and envenomation incidents should be developed, clearly posted, and periodically reviewed.

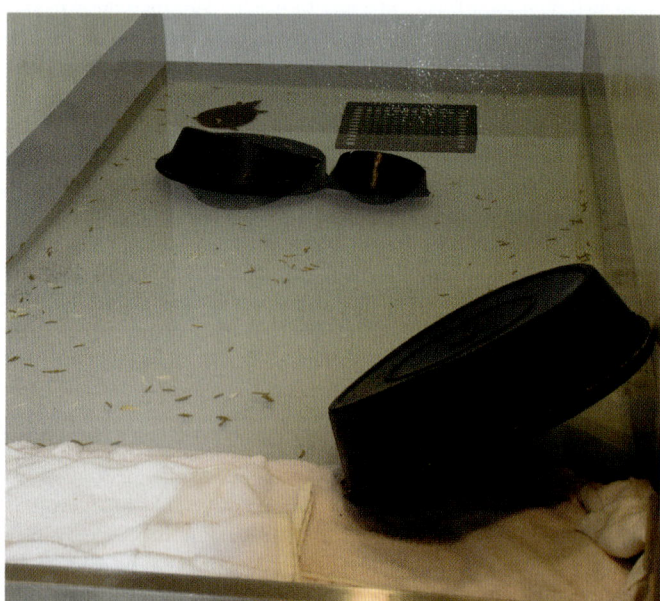

FIG 46.1 Dog kennels or runs can be used for reptiles such as large tortoises, lizards, or crocodilians. This walk-in cage was designed with a large drain and sloping floor so that larger turtles could be housed. (Courtesy of Stephen J. Divers and Daniel Cutler.)

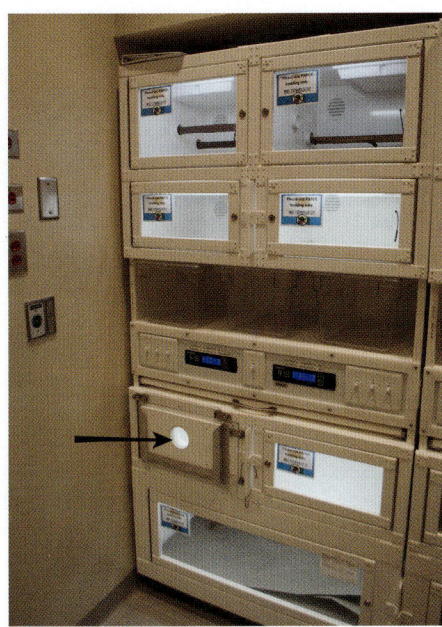

FIG 46.2 Custom reptile enclosures like this unit by Habitat Systems Ltd allow more comprehensive and automated control of environmental conditions, including temperature, humidity, and light cycle. Note the arboreal cages at the top with resin branches that can be sterilized. Each cage also has a lock and a separate temperature probe. The large enclosure at the bottom has a divider enabling it to be connected to the adjacent enclosure for large constrictors. There is also a shift box connector for moving venomous snakes (arrow). (Courtesy of Stephen J. Divers and Daniel Cutler.)

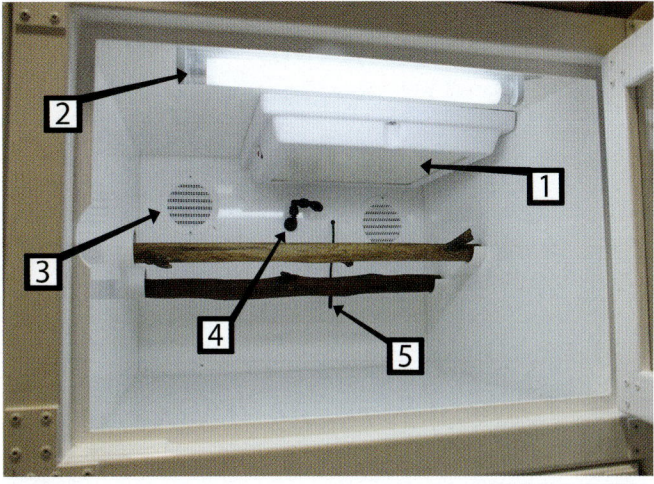

FIG 46.4 Arboreal reptiles, such as chameleons and some snakes, benefit from having suitable perching available. The perches are made of resin and can be easily cleaned and disinfected. Notice also the (1) heating element, (2) light, (3) ventilation panels, (4) sprinkler output, and (5) temperature probe. (Courtesy of Stephen J. Divers and Daniel Cutler.)

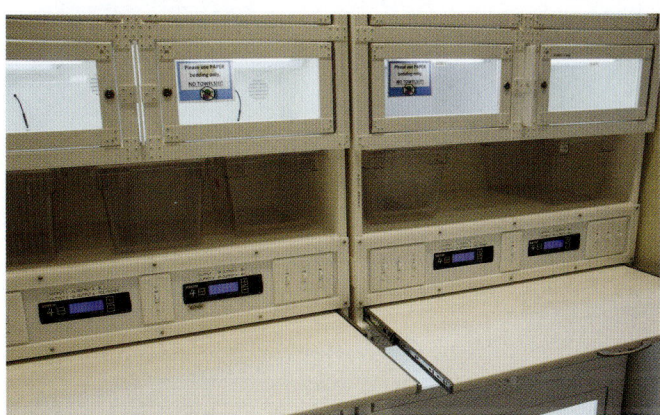

FIG 46.3 Reptile enclosures can also have customized furnishings, such as slide-out tables, to allow more convenient cage side treatment. Plastic bins can be incorporated into reptile housing units to provide temporary holding. These bins can easily be removed for disinfection. (Courtesy of Stephen J. Divers and Daniel Cutler.)

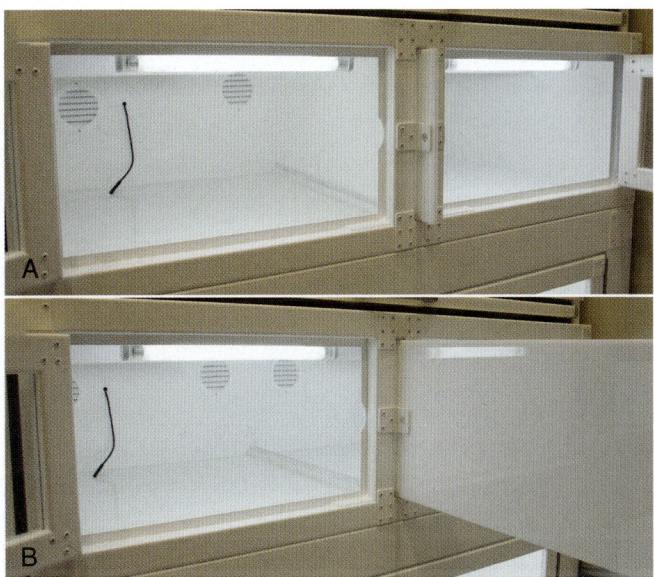

FIG 46.5 Caging units with dividers give the clinician more options in providing appropriately sized enclosures for patients (A and B). The access between separate units allows different temperature ranges to be accessible to the patient. (Courtesy of Stephen J. Divers and Daniel Cutler.)

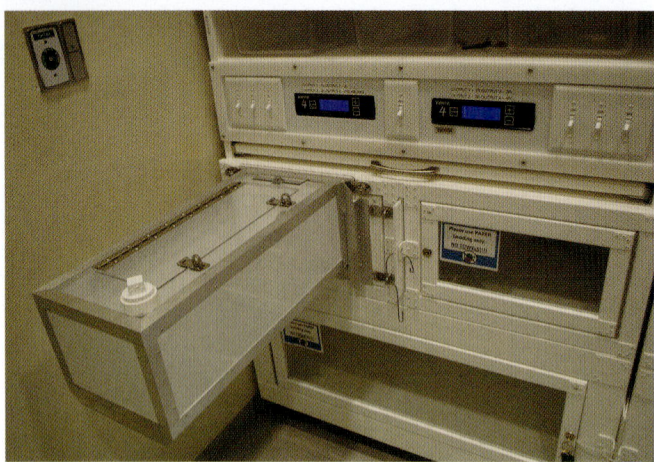

FIG 46.6 Venomous snakes should only be handled by trained individuals following established standard operating protocols. Enclosures with incorporated shift boxes can minimize the risk to veterinary personnel. (Courtesy of Stephen J. Divers and Daniel Cutler.)

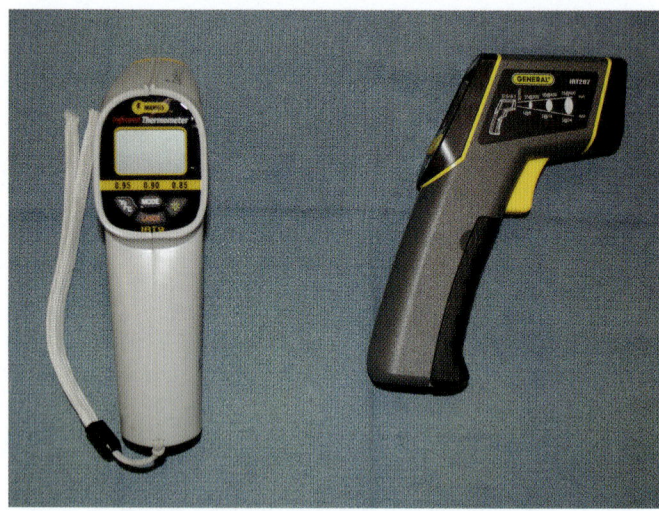

FIG 46.7 Infrared temperature guns are useful in determining the external temperature of a reptile, in addition to specific areas of the enclosure. (Courtesy of Stephen J. Divers and Daniel Cutler.)

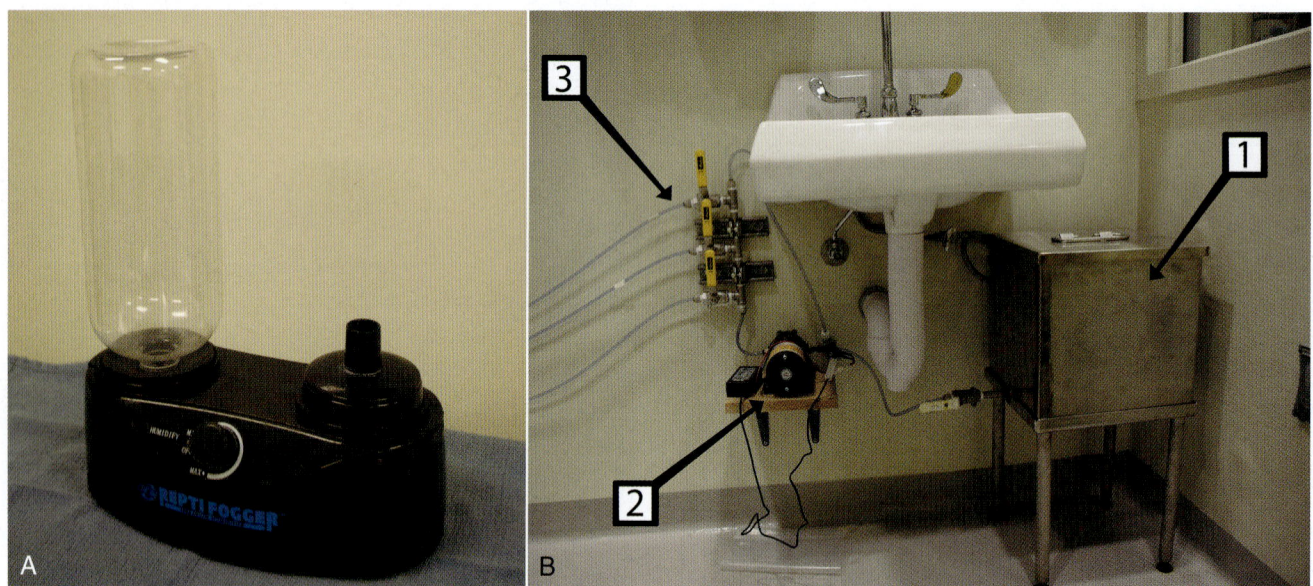

FIG 46.8 (A) Low-cost fogging equipment can be easily purchased from pet supply stores and provides a reliable method of increasing enclosure humidity. (B) Sprinkler/humidity system incorporating a (1) water reservoir, (2) pump, controlled by a detailed timer schedule (e.g., activate pump and sprinklers for 15 seconds at 9 AM, 11 AM, 1 PM, and 3 PM), and (3) water feed lines to separate cages. (Courtesy of Stephen J. Divers and Daniel Cutler.)

Temperature

As discussed elsewhere (see Section 2), maintaining appropriate temperatures and temperature gradients are imperative for healthy reptiles, with specific temperatures varying from species to species and dependent on natural history.[2] A sick reptile may be unable to ambulate and select an appropriate temperature within a gradient. Therefore moribund or nonambulatory reptiles should be provided with a steady temperature at the upper end of the preferred optimum temperature zone. Failure to provide an appropriate temperature will adversely affect drug absorption, distribution, and elimination. Temperature should be checked with digital instrumentation (not "dial" thermometers). For chelonians, a thermometer can be taped to the carapace to measure the animal's external temperature. An infrared laser thermometer is a convenient tool to measure both enclosure and external body temperatures (Fig. 46.7). Thermal support should be automated using reliable thermostats to ensure consistency, even on weekends. Dimming or proportional thermostats reduce temperature cycling. On-off thermostats cannot be used with lights. For larger chelonians and crocodilians, the general air temperature can be controlled in a small room with dedicated thermostat control (background heating), which is supplemented with a heat lamp suspended inside a large enclosure (basking area). Regardless of the methods used, providing safe, consistent, appropriate, and monitored thermal support is vital.[3]

Humidity

Hospital systems for maintaining appropriate environmental humidity can be simple or complex. Periodic misting of an enclosure can often provide short-term humidity for small enclosures. The humidity of larger rooms can be raised by providing larger water areas and/or allowing water to continually drip. Humidity boxes can also be placed in enclosures and provide microclimates for reptiles to selectively choose to enter. Fogging and misting systems can also be used to greatly elevate the amount of water in the air. These systems can be relatively inexpensive, with no automation, or can be built into an enclosure and controlled via hygrometers and timers (see Figs. 46.2 and 46.8). It is important to periodically disinfect or replace tubing on these fogging, misting, and drip systems, because hydrophilic bacterial growth can result overtime.

Enclosure Substrate

In contrast to the aesthetics of the normal enclosure, the main objectives during hospitalization are monitoring and hygiene. Compared to particulate materials, paper provides an inexpensive, easily replaceable floor cover that allows monitoring for urination, defecation, and vomiting/regurgitation, and reduces the chances of wound contamination. In some cases, particulate substrate may be necessary to promote natural behaviors such as egg laying. Also, aquatic and semiaquatic animals require a water-filled area of the enclosure. Enclosures made of glass or plastics can easily accommodate water. It is important that any substrates can be easily replaced and the enclosure and any utensils cleaned and disinfected. Perches and enclosures made of porous material (e.g., wood) should be avoided or discarded after use.

Nutrition

Appropriate food should be provided based on the medical history and natural history. Foods should be recognizable and presented in accordance with usual husbandry practices. Using dishes and food sources from the animal's home enclosure may be beneficial to a reptile housed in a foreign environment. If a reptile is to be fasted for medical or surgical procedures, then this should be clearly indicated on the cage door and in the medical record.

Some reptiles may require more intensive and calorically dense nutrient sources, especially when debilitated. A liquid diet is a good option as it can be delivered to an anorectic patient via feeding tube or gavage (see Chapter 45). Commercial powdered diets are available and are formulated for herbivorous, omnivorous, and carnivorous animals. When using such products, it is important to ensure that portion size and total daily amount is appropriate for the stomach size of the animal and also meets the daily caloric requirements. Cachectic reptiles that have been rehydrated should initially be fed very small quantities (approximately 10% of metabolic requirements) that are increased slowly over 2 to 4 weeks (see Chapter 122).

Staff

Staff directly involved with animal care and hospitalization must be appropriately trained and supervised, and qualified veterinary technicians and nurses are preferred. When dealing with potentially dangerous species (e.g., venomous snakes, crocodilians, large constrictors), staff must receive specific training, adhere to standard operating protocols, and never work alone. An incident log should be created for recording any mishaps, whether or not they are associated with injury to the patient or staff.

Monitoring

Any hospitalized reptile should receive at least daily examinations, and all observations and treatments must be accurately and contemporaneously recorded (Fig. 46.9). Changes in the environment, if not monitored, recorded, and addressed, can hamper recovery. Reptiles typically exhibit slower and more subtle changes, either positive or negative, which can easily be missed day to day. By regularly monitoring and maintaining a thorough record, changes in the patient's status can be more readily recognized and addressed. At a minimum, a patient's weight, demeanor, appetite, eliminations, environmental temperature, and environmental humidity should be recorded at least once if not twice daily. For more critical or postsurgical patients, more frequent monitoring and recording should be performed. Patient monitoring values can be recorded along with treatments given and case notes (Fig. 46.10).

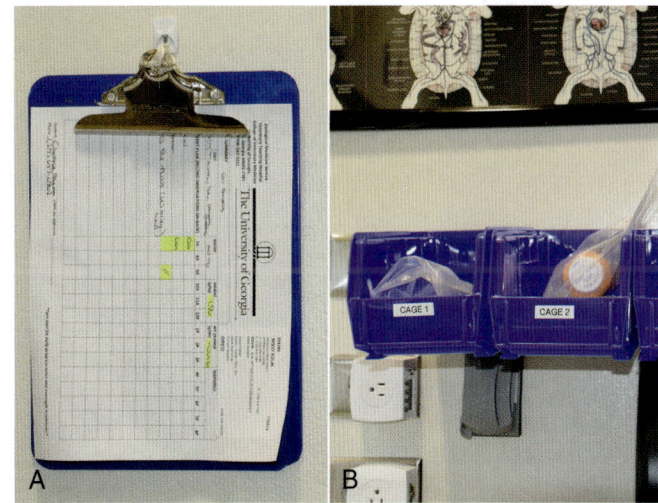

FIG 46.9 In a busy reptile practice, ensuring accurate and up-to-date records is essential to avoid medical errors. (A) Hanging records adjacent to caging and (B) labeled bins with medications and other supplies decreases the likelihood of confusion between patients. (Courtesy of Stephen J. Divers and Daniel Cutler.)

[Clinic Info]   [Patient Info]

Clinical Summary													
Date	Cage #	Diet	Water		Weight (g/kg)		Wt Change (q24)		WARNINGS				
TREATMENT PLAN RECORD OBSERVATIONS ON BACK			7A	8A	9A	10A	11A	12P	1P	2P	3P	4P	5P	6P	7P	8P

Technician_____ Clinician_____

Page____ of ____

Name		Case Number		Species		Weight					
Clinical Summary				WARNING							
TREATMENT PLAN RECORD OBSERVATIONS ON BOTTOM		9P	10P	11P	12A	1A	2A	3A	4A	5A	6A

Notes/Comments/Observations:

Technician_____ Clinician_____

Page____ of ____

FIG 46.10 Contemporaneous recording of patient vital parameters, medications, and procedures is a legal requirement and greatly enhanced by using dedicated treatment sheets. (Courtesy of Stephen J. Divers and Daniel Cutler.)

REFERENCES

See www.expertconsult.com for a complete list of references.

47

Euthanasia

Javier G. Nevarez

The word *euthanasia* originates from two Greek words, *Eu* meaning good and *Thanatosis* meaning death. Hence, its literal translation is "Good death." In contemporary terms, euthanasia is defined as ending the life of an individual animal in a way that minimizes or eliminates pain and distress.[1] Within this context, the American Veterinary Medical Association Guidelines for the Euthanasia of Animals (AVMA Guidelines) states that veterinarians carrying out euthanasia have two primary responsibilities: "his or her humane disposition to induce death in a manner that is in accord with an animal's interest and/or because it is a matter of welfare, and the use of humane techniques to induce the most rapid and painless and distress-free death possible."[1] It is further stated, "These conditions, while separate, are not mutually exclusive and are codependent."[1] Whereas in the United Sates the term euthanasia is widely accepted, in some parts of the world, the term killing of animals rather than euthanasia is often used. In these countries, killing of animals is an accepted term regardless of the context within which the life of the animal is terminated (pets, food, etc.). Although the use of the term killing may connote a more negative emotion, it is a literal interpretation of what is effectively being done, which is to terminate a life. As such, the euthanasia of animals carries significant professional, moral, and ethical responsibilities for veterinarians. In veterinary medicine, euthanasia is a tool available to ease the pain and suffering of animals, as well as a necessary part of management of animals for food and textiles. In all instances it must be conducted in the most humane manner possible. Veterinarians must also be sensitive to local customs and perceptions toward this act and perform euthanasia in a manner that conforms to accepted cultural, religious, and societal norms within their country. The human-animal bond should also be a consideration, even when working with herpetological species.

The AVMA Guidelines have long been regarded as the most important reference for euthanasia methods in the United States, and similar recommendations have been published by other veterinary bodies internationally (e.g., British Veterinary Association, Universities Federation for Animal Welfare). Nonetheless, the information contained with respect to reptiles and amphibians has been limited due to the low amount of research on euthanasia of these species. Anatomic and physiological differences of herpetological species add to the difficulties in providing objective data specific to the euthanasia of these animals.

There has been an ongoing debate about whether reptiles and amphibians feel pain and suffer in the same manner as mammals do or if a simple nociceptive response with no central processing in the brain is involved. This debate is a strong point of contention among biologists and veterinarians alike. In the United Kingdom, protection of animals, including reptile and amphibian welfare, has been legally defined and defended by veterinarians since 1911. However, in the United States, it was not until 2011 that the US veterinarians' oath was changed to reflect the need to prioritize animal welfare, and even today, herpetological species remain excluded from the US Animal Welfare Act. As such it is indeed our responsibility as veterinarians to practice under the premise that reptiles and amphibians do feel pain and therefore should be treated with the same humane standards as other species, including providing them with proper analgesics. Sladky and Mans provide a review of clinical analgesia in reptiles.[2]

Concerning euthanasia, the AVMA Guidelines state: "it is often difficult to ascertain that an amphibian or reptile is, in fact, dead."[1] Although this statement has become a paradigm when dealing with euthanasia of herpetological species, the truth is there are methods to ensure reptiles and amphibians are indeed dead, and it is our responsibility as veterinarians to educate ourselves and apply those methods in a manner that respects their welfare.

The AVMA has recently acknowledged the need for establishing separate guidelines that address the euthanasia of animals destined for food. As a result, the AVMA Guidelines for the Slaughter of Animals (AVMA Slaughter Guidelines) was published in 2016.[3] A third AVMA document addressing depopulation is also planned.[3] The AVMA Slaughter Guidelines include recommendations for hoof stock, poultry, fish, alligators, and rabbits. In 2013, the Swiss Federal Veterinary Office (Swiss FVO) published the analysis on humane killing methods for reptiles in the skin trade.[4] This Swiss FVO document aims to establish international standards for the humane slaughter of reptiles. Both of these documents represent the first time that governments have established reptile-specific guidelines and are pivotal in the advancement of the welfare of reptiles. In addition to these guidelines, other resources for information on euthanasia of reptiles include various textbooks and studies, most notably, Cooper's monograph on Euthanasia of Amphibians and Reptiles, which has been considered a gold standard since it was first published.[5-8]

For clarity purposes, the term euthanasia will be used when referring to reptiles and amphibians maintained as pets, zoological specimens, laboratory animals, and more. The term slaughter will be strictly used for animals in the commercial food and textile trade. Anyone performing euthanasia or slaughter has the responsibility to stay up to date on the current methods and recommendations to ensure they are using the most humane techniques available.

EUTHANASIA TECHNIQUES

Regardless of whether dealing with a pet, zoo animal, or laboratory subject, euthanasia should always provide a humane death in the fastest way possible with the least amount of distress to the animal. The first decision to be made is whether a one-step or two-step euthanasia method will be applied (Table 47.1). One-step euthanasia is ideally performed when there is adequate venous access and the animal can be safely restrained without causing additional stress. Injection of euthanasia solution via the intracoelomic route and cardiac puncture

TABLE 47.1	Review of Euthanasia Methods With Routes and Techniques for Their Application		
Single Methods	**Route/Technique**	**Species**	**Comment**
Injectable Agents			
Sodium pentobarbital (60–100 mg/kg)	IV	R, A	
MS 222 (>500 mg/L)	IV, ICe, Bath	A	While advocated in reptiles by some, its humaneness is not proven.
Benzocaine hydrochloride (>250 mg/L)	Bath, topical, ice	A	
Physical Methods			
Penetrating captive bolt	Placed over brain	R, A	Due to the force exerted, it will obliterate the head of any species smaller than crocodilians.
Nonpenetrating captive bolt	Placed over brain	R, A	Due to the force exerted, it will obliterate the head of any species smaller than crocodilians.
Firearm	Aim for the brain	R, A	Shot placement is critical for this procedure to be humane.
Blunt force trauma to the head	Aim for the brain	R, A	An adjunct method, such as decapitation or pithing, must be promptly applied to ensure death.
Adjunct Methods			
Decapitation	Atlanto-occipital joint	R, A	Must use sharp instruments and perform in a single swift motion. Facilitated by single occipital condyle.
Pithing	Needle or rod	R, A	Select the largest needle or metal rod possible.
Unacceptable Methods			
Hypothermia		R, A	
Inhalants		R	Because reptiles can hold their breath for an extended period of time, this can prolong death.

A, Amphibian; *ICe*, intracoelomic; *IV*, intravenous; *R*, reptile.

BOX 47.1 Three-Step Approach to Euthanasia of Reptiles to Ensure Death

Step 1
Inject Telazol (Fort Dodge, Inc, Fort Dodge, Iowa), 50 mg/kg IM, SQ, or ketamine HCl, 100 mg/kg IM, SQ.

Step 2
Option A. Once anesthetized, inject pentobarbital 0.5–1 ml/kg IV, IO, intracardiac, intrahepatic, or intracoelomic.
Option B. Once anesthetized, apply a physical method of euthanasia (see Table 47.1).

Step 3
Confirm lack of corneal reflex +/- fixed and dilated pupils. Then perform pithing, decapitation, or freezing.

(in snakes and lizards) is often advocated; however, one must wonder how much pain and discomfort a fully awake and aware reptile experiences with these procedures. In addition, in cases where postmortem evaluation and histopathology will be performed, cardiac puncture may result in mechanical or chemical damage to heart tissue and thus is not ideal. For these reasons, whenever possible, it is strongly suggested that one-step injectable euthanasia should be performed via the intravenous route. When venous access is not easily obtained, or if dealing with large, potentially dangerous, or unrestrainable animals, a two-step euthanasia should be performed. In two-step euthanasia the first step leads to a deep anesthetic plane while the second step results in death (Box 47.1). The authors recommend starting with anesthetics such as Telazol (Fort Dodge, Inc, Fort Dodge, Iowa), 50 mg/ kg intramuscularly (IM) or subcutaneously (SQ), or ketamine HCl, 100 mg/kg IM or SQ. At these high dosages, approximately 10 to 20 minutes are needed for the drugs to take effect when the patient is at

room temperature (see Box 47.1). Both of these drugs can be administered intramuscularly or subcutaneously, thereby facilitating delivery to a fractious or dehydrated patient or a patient with inaccessible peripheral veins. After the patient has been anesthetized, the second step of the euthanasia procedure can proceed. At this time, an intravenous, intracardiac, intracranial, intrahepatic, or intracoelomic injection of euthanasia solution can be administered (see Box 47.1). Alternatively, a physical method of euthanasia can be applied (see Table 47.1).

Even when performing two-step euthanasia, assessment of whether a reptile is, in fact, deceased can be difficult. This is important because occasionally a client takes the remains home for burial, taxidermy, and so forth. It would behoove the practitioner to make absolutely, positively sure that the pet is deceased before it is released to the owner. The situation can be embarrassing if owners call wanting to know why the animal they just paid to have euthanized is walking around. To prevent this type of medicolegal catastrophe, a third step in the euthanasia process can be performed.

Fixed, dilated pupils combined with lack of corneal reflex are good indicators that the animal is at least unconscious if not dead. After confirming a lack of corneal reflexes, pithing can be performed to ensure the brain tissue is destroyed. This technique also creates minimal external damage that may otherwise be unpleasant for an owner to visualize. Pithing is a technique by which a rigid tool or rod is inserted through the foramen magnum to the level of the brain. Once in the brain cavity, the rod can be rotated in circles 4 to 6 times to ensure destruction of the brain and, hence, death. For pet reptiles, the author utilizes a 14 to 16 g needle. In larger reptiles, a metal rod with a sharp tip can be used. For pithing to be successful, veterinarians must be familiar with the skull anatomy and location of the brain (Figs. 47.1 and 47.2). Pithing should only be performed as part of a two- or three-step euthanasia after an animal has been injected with euthanasia solution and there is a lack of corneal reflexes. In cases where the use of euthanasia solution may affect examination or testing

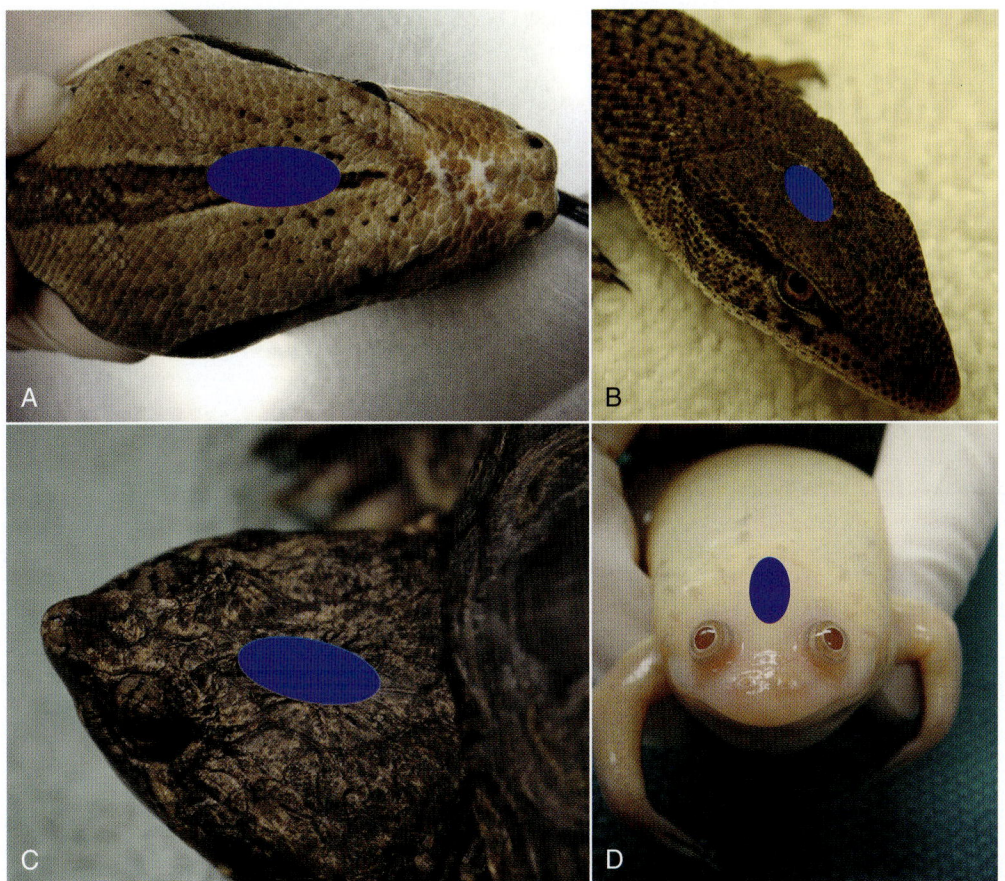

FIG 47.1 Approximate location of the brain (blue oval) in reptiles and amphibians. Proper localization of the brain is essential when applying physical methods of euthanasia to ensure the procedure is effective and humane. (Courtesy of Javier G. Nevarez.)

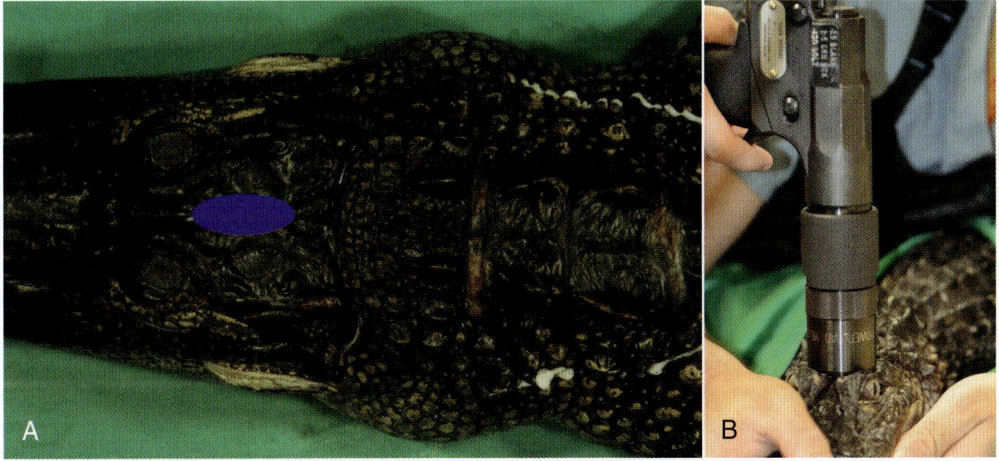

FIG 47.2 (A) Location of the brain (blue oval) in an American alligator. (B) Placement of a nonpenetrating captive bolt on the skull of an American alligator *(Alligator mississippiensis)*, directly over the brain location. (Courtesy of Javier G. Nevarez.)

of tissues (e.g., histopathology), pithing should only be performed in a reptile that is in a deep/surgical level of anesthesia.

An alternative to pithing is decapitation. Decapitation is visually unpleasant and therefore not ideal for reptiles that an owner wants to take home. Also it must be noted that decapitation by itself is not an effective euthanasia technique and must only be performed following complete unconsciousness with absent reflexes. Finally, freezing (only after rendering complete unconsciousness with no intact reflexes) for

at least 24 hours before the carcass is released to the owner is another alternative to ensure death.

Assessment of heart rate by electrocardiogram or Doppler blood flow analysis does not provide an accurate determination of death because the heart occasionally continues to beat, even hours after the apparent euthanasia. Movement of the limbs and head should also be interpreted cautiously because this is often normal even after pithing and decapitation. This is due to inherent differences in the nervous system of reptiles and amphibians, including the presence of spinal ganglia. Nonetheless if movement is present, a thorough assessment of the patient must be performed to ensure it is deceased.

In summary, euthanasia of reptiles is best performed as a two- or three-step procedure (see Box 47.1). First the reptile is sedated or anesthetized; this is then followed with an injection of euthanasia solution. Potassium chloride may also be injected intracardially in fully anesthetized animals.[1] As an added assurance of death or when sending a patient home with the owners, pithing or freezing can be performed. By following a stepwise, two- to three-step (see Box 47.1) approach to the euthanasia of reptiles, death can indeed be confirmed and performed in a humane manner.

EUTHANASIA OF FIELD-COLLECTED ANIMALS

The collection of specimens is an essential part of the advancement of science. This often creates the need for euthanasia of reptiles and amphibians in field situations away from laboratories and under the care of nonveterinarians. Although anesthetics are often not available, in the United States it is possible in some instances to obtain special licenses to possess certain euthanasia solutions. When this is not possible (e.g., working in foreign countries), scientists must utilize physical methods in the most humane manner possible when a veterinarian is not available. Nevertheless, a veterinarian should be consulted during the development of any such scientific study.

SLAUGHTER

A number of reptile species, most notably chelonians and crocodilians, are raised for food and textiles throughout the world (see Chapter 177). The AVMA Slaughter Guidelines provide recommendations for the slaughter of alligators based on the most current scientific information for this species.[3,9] The FVO Analysis on the humane killing of reptiles includes slaughter recommendations that can be applied to various reptile species.[4] The species, size, age of the animals, and personnel safety and training should all be considered before selecting a method of slaughter to ensure it is applied in the most humane manner possible. Specific slaughter recommendations can be found in Table 47.2.

In the United States, reptiles do not fall under the regulation of the Humane Slaughter Act; therefore it is up to the individual states and industries to establish their own regulations. Such legislation often exists elsewhere, including Europe. In alligators, spinal cord severance followed by pithing of the brain and application of a penetrating or nonpenetrating captive bolt is more humane and effective for inducing death, whereas spinal cord severance alone was determined to be inappropriate.[9] In 2016, the Louisiana Department of Wildlife and Fisheries established a regulation that requires all alligator ranchers and farmers to slaughter the animals according to established guidelines by the AVMA and Swiss FVO. Specifically, it includes the use of penetrating or nonpenetrating captive bolt (Fig. 47.2) and spinal cord severance followed immediately by pithing. This regulation had the full support of the Louisiana Alligators Farmers and Ranchers Association and represents the first instance of regulatory governing of slaughter methods for a commercial reptile species in the United States. These guidelines and regulations also acknowledge that methods may be refined as more research becomes available and strongly encourage consultation with veterinarians to ensure that the methods being used are the most humane possible for each species and circumstances.

AMPHIBIANS

The same basic considerations for the euthanasia of reptiles apply to amphibians; however, because of their skin permeability, there are some methods that are unique to this group of animals. External or topical

TABLE 47.2 Acceptable Methods of Slaughter for Reptile Species

Method	Comment
Penetrating captive-bolt	Alone or with an adjunct method (pithing) to ensure death if the brain is not immediately destroyed.
Nonpenetrating captive-bolt	Alone or with an adjunct method (pithing) to ensure death if the brain is not immediately destroyed.
Spinal cord severance immediately followed by pithing	Cord severance by itself is not an acceptable method. This can be accomplished within 3 seconds, but severance would be expected to be painful because the animal would be completely conscious.
Blunt force trauma to the head with a hard implement	In combination with an adjunct method (pithing) to ensure death.
Firearm	Shot placement is critical for this procedure to be humane.
Injection	Meat must be discarded.
Cervical dislocation	With proper technique and followed by another procedure to ensure death. Acceptable in animals under 200 g.
Decapitation immediately followed by adjunct method	Decapitation by itself is not an acceptable method.
Pithing	Adjunct method only. Should only be performed after prior stunning or decapitation and as method to ensure death.

agents, such as tricaine methane sulfonate (TMS, MS-222), may be used to euthanize amphibians (concentrations >500 mg/L). Before using, it is important to ensure that the MS-222 has been buffered with sodium bicarbonate at a 1 : 1 weight ratio or until the solution reaches a pH of 7 to 7.5. The buffered MS-222 can also be injected directly into the amphibian lymph sac or the coelomic cavity. Injection into the coelomic cavity may cause pain or discomfort so that should be a consideration. Benzocaine hydrochloride can also be used for euthanasia at a concentration exceeding 250 mg/L, used either in a bath or in a recirculating system.

In an emergency situation, aquatic amphibians can be euthanized by placing them in water that contains dissolved carbon dioxide (with the addition of sodium bicarbonate powder or Alka-Seltzer tablets to water).[5] Rapid freezing, such as dipping in liquid nitrogen, is approved and effective in reptiles and amphibians of less than 4 g.[1]

A recent study evaluated a two-step process of amphibian euthanasia by first cooling toads in a refrigerator for approximately 60 minutes followed by freezing for 30 minutes.[10] Brain activity as measured by EEG declined through the procedure. Based on this it was suggested that the animals did not feel pain and that this technique should be considered humane. The use of EEG's to assess pain in humans is a complex field with conflicting information. The use of EEGs to assess pain in amphibians has not been validated. In addition this study did not include a control group. Therefore the use of this method should be approached with caution until more data is available that validates the methodology and conclusions of the study.

REFERENCES

See www.expertconsult.com for a complete list of references.

Sedation

Rodney W. Schnellbacher and Molly Shepard

Sedation of reptiles has become an increasingly common strategy to provide immobilization, reduce trauma, and mitigate the stress response caused by physical restraint. Additionally, it facilitates clinical procedures such as physical examination, blood collection, and noninvasive or minimally invasive procedures. Sedatives act to induce the depression of the central nervous system while ideally preserving airway reflexes, hemodynamic stability, and a patient's ability to respond to repetitive or painful stimuli. Depending on patient selection and protocol design, a combination of sedation and local anesthesia can provide a safe alternative to general anesthesia for procedures such as wound care, placement of an intraosseous/intravenous catheter, some diagnostic endoscopy procedures, and minor surgery. Although the basis for sedation is to provide light to moderate narcosis, many sedation drugs also may serve as analgesics or premedications in the context of a general anesthetic event. The reader is directed to subsequent chapters on anesthesia (49) and analgesia (50) for elaboration on these topics.

Drugs used for sedation should ideally be short acting or reversible to avoid prolonged or unpredictable recoveries. Drug selection and administration technique should be determined based on the desired level of narcosis, the general condition of the patient (e.g., signalment, comorbidities, handling risks for personnel safety), environmental factors (facility limitations, weather), the monitoring modalities available, and the diagnostic and/or therapeutic procedures to be performed. Adverse events in the context of a sedation procedure may include compromise of upper airway patency, ventilation, or cardiovascular stability. Dosages should be adjusted according to the condition of the animal, with appropriate dose reduction and other special considerations for debilitated, gravid, pediatric, and geriatric patients, as well as patients in seasonal or metabolic states that may increase their sensitivity to tranquilizers.[1-3] Sedation requirements can vary widely between patients and species. In general, sedation dosages are lower than dosages required for anesthetic induction, and many tranquilizers, regardless of dose, cannot serve as single-agent anesthetics. Due to the paucity of published literature describing reptilian sedation, dosages are frequently extrapolated from other species, and many recommendations are based on anecdotal reports. The authors of this chapter recommend a multimodal approach to sedation, when possible, whereby a variety of injectable tranquilizers and analgesics are administered at subanesthetic doses to minimize the side effects of each agent.

MAINTAINING BODY TEMPERATURE

Due to their ectothermic nature, sedated reptiles should be maintained at temperatures and humidity levels appropriate for their species (their Preferred Optimal Temperature Zone, hereafter POTZ). Pharmacokinetic properties including clearance time and area under the curve (AUC) can be influenced significantly by a reptile's body temperature.[4] Maintenance of the POTZ is therefore crucial for the safety of the patient and reliability of the protocol (e.g. onset, duration and intensity of clinical effects) (see Chapters 49 and 50). Body temperature should be monitored throughout the procedure and can be actively maintained through the use of conductive (heating pads, circulating hot water blankets, heated examination tables, warm lavage fluids), convective (forced air warmers, incubators), and radiative (radiative infant warmers, sunshine) heating strategies. Body heat can also be preserved passively by reduction of evaporative heat loss (e.g., covering the patient after surgical preparation or minimizing surgical time while body cavities are exposed) (see Chapters 49 and 50).

INDUCTION AND RECOVERY

Indicators of sedation depth in reptiles are fairly consistent. Loss of withdrawal reflex and muscle tone is expected to start cranially and move caudally in the following sequence: pectoral limbs, pelvic limbs and neck, loss of the righting reflex, tail and cloaca, and often lastly jaw tone.[5] Reptiles maintain the ability to react to painful stimuli until lingual and palpebral reflexes are absent,[6] which signifies a deeper state of narcosis (anesthesia). In snakes and some lizards, palpebral and corneal reflexes cannot be elicited due to the presence of a spectacle. The reflexes described above allow practitioners to subjectively gauge sedative depth and predict features of recovery.

Recovery time from sedation is variable and depends on the drug protocol and patient condition. Debilitated animals may experience a more prolonged recovery presumably due to changes in hepatic blood flow or metabolic processes. Many drugs used for sedation (e.g., benzodiazepines opioids, and alpha-2 agonists) can be reversed, if necessary. Like induction of sedation, clinical signs of recovery in reptiles are uniform, with restoration of muscle control and withdrawal reflexes typically occurring in a caudal to cranial direction.

In order to improve the safety of sedation, it is necessary to evaluate sedation features, that is, via sedation scoring, which may allow the practitioner to target a sedation depth in a reproducible manner. The authors of this chapter suggest sedation scoring systems based on locomotion, muscle relaxation, and body position.

ROUTES OF ADMINISTRATION

Oral, intramuscular, intravenous, intraosseous, intranasal, subcutaneous, topical, cloacal, and intracoelomic routes are available. Routes of sedative administration should be selected based on ease of administration, size of animal, reliability of absorption, and rate of metabolism. Although oral, cloacal, intracoelomic, and subcutaneous routes of drug administration have been investigated, these routes are less reliable and characterized by poor absorption, delayed onset of action, protracted clinical effects, and occasionally, lack of clinical effect.[7]

Intravenous (IV) administration is considered the preferred method for sedation in reptiles, whenever possible, due to its predictability of drug action and recovery time. Unfortunately, IV administration can be technically difficult and can increase stress in small or fractious patients, or those difficult or dangerous to restrain. With experience, good technique, appropriate patient selection, and skilled physical restraint it is possible to approach the caudal (ventral coccygeal) vein in most snakes and lizards and the dorsal coccygeal vein, radial sinuses, and jugular vein in chelonians. The subcarapacial sinus is also a common target for IV administration in chelonians but should be approached with caution, due to the possibility of inadvertent intrathecal administration.[8] Lizards have a prominent ventral abdominal vein that can be used for the administration of sedatives. Intracardiac injections should only be given in emergency situations for administration of emergency drugs. However, one study in ball pythons (*Python regius*) showed that intracardiac injection of propofol is safe and only produced mild histopathological lesions to heart tissues.[9] Intraosseous routes of administration may provide a substitute for IV administration in some chelonian and saurian cases.[10,11]

In most reptiles, intramuscular administration of sedative agents is most practical and often effective. Although a renal portal system has been identified in reptiles, the clinical significance of this anatomic feature has little clinical impact on sedatives or analgesics injected into the caudal half of the body.[12] The epaxial muscles provide a suitable injection site in most snakes. In lizards, the muscle mass of the forelimb (triceps and biceps), hind limb (quadriceps, semimembranosus, and semitendinosus), and tail can be used. Caution should be used during handling of species known to autotomize their tails. In chelonians, intramuscular injections are recommended in the proximal pectoral limbs, targeting the triceps or pectoral muscles. However, some chelonian species lack significant muscle mass in this area, and intramuscular injection can inadvertently become subcutaneous.

Intranasal administration of sedatives has been utilized as a safe and effective route for short-term sedation and restraint in veterinary and human medicine.[13,14] Its appeal for reptile practitioners arises from its tendency to be less technically demanding than IV administration, less painful and stressful for patients than intramuscular injections, and its theoretical circumvention of hepatic first-pass metabolism. The nasal mucosa is a highly permeable port of entry for different drugs, presumably due to the relatively large mucosal surface area available for absorption and its proximity to the brain. Recent studies of intranasal sedation in chelonians have yielded variable results. One study of dexmedetomidine/ketamine in yellow-bellied sliders (*Trachemys scripta scripta*) showed positive sedation results[15] (Table 48.1), while another study of intranasal medetomidine/midazolam in the red-footed tortoise (*Chelonoidis carbonaria*) and Indian star tortoise (*Geochelone platynota*) showed little sedation benefit.[16] This administration route may offer a less invasive alternative to IM administration but requires more investigation with a greater range of drug species.

BENZODIAZEPINES

Benzodiazepines produce anticonvulsant and hypnotic effects through their enhancement of the neurotransmitter, gamma-aminobutyric acid (GABA) at the $GABA_A$ receptor, and anxiolytic and muscle relaxant effects through glycine-mediated inhibitory pathways in the brain and spinal cord. Their high margin of safety makes them appealing for use in compromised patients. Benzodiazepines such as midazolam and diazepam have been used alone and in combination with other sedatives to produce mild to deep narcosis in reptiles.

Midazolam has been investigated in many aquatic and terrestrial chelonian species. Intramuscular midazolam 1.5 mg/kg has been shown to produce sedation and muscle relaxation suitable for minor manipulations in red-eared slider turtles (*Trachemys scripta elegans*), with onset of 5 minutes and duration of approximately 80 minutes.[17] Other chelonian studies of IM midazolam sedation have described variable effects ranging from no sedation to profound sedation in the following species: common snapping turtle (*Chelydra serpentina*), red-footed tortoise, and Indian star tortoises.[16-21] Case reports have also described the use of midazolam combined with other agents (e.g., ketamine, medetomidine, dexmedetomidine) to produce standing sedation in the Galapagos tortoise (*Chelonoidis nigra*) and three African spurred tortoises (*Centrochelys sulcata*; see Table 48.1) (unpublished data).[22]

Midazolam appears to provide useful sedation for handling and minor nonsurgical procedures in several squamate species, as described in a recent retrospective study.[21] An average dose of 0.3 mg/kg (range 0.1–1.0 mg/kg) produced median onset time of 10 minutes and median time to maximal effect of 20 minutes (Fig. 48.1). Midazolam 2 mg/kg combined with medetomidine was also used to achieve standing sedation in the komodo dragon (*Varanus komodoensis*) (unpublished data).

Midazolam provides a proven benefit for restraint and handling of crocodilians. Routine capture of this species for transport or diagnostic events can cause significant stress, intense muscular exertion, lactic acidosis, and, in worst cases, capture myopathy and postcapture death.[23] Additionally, captive crocodilians frequently display abnormal interactions, basking, and feeding behavior for several days post-handling. One study of juvenile saltwater crocodiles (*Crocodylus porosus*) showed that those administered 5 mg/kg IM midazolam prior to physical examination, sample collection, and translocation had lower heart rates, respiratory rates, blood glucose, lactate, and acidosis during sedation, and faster recovery, compared to crocodiles under manual restraint alone.[20]

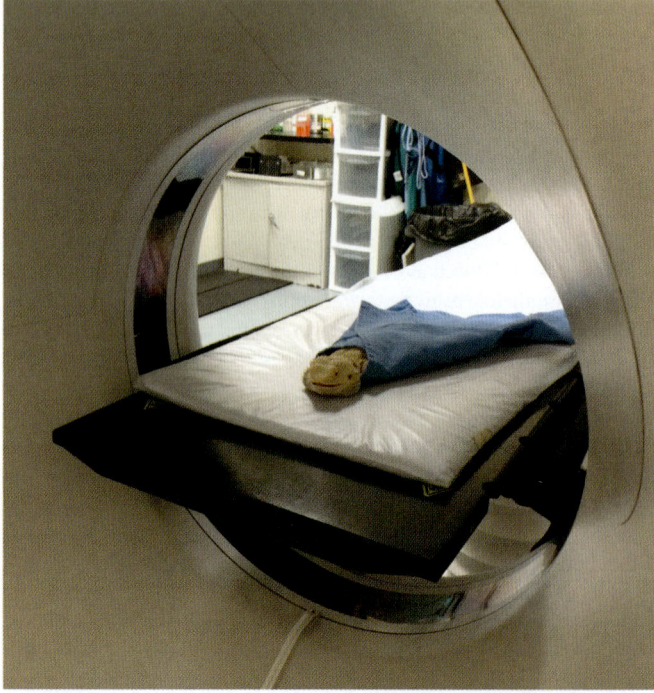

FIG 48.1 A bearded dragon (*Pogona vitticeps*) sedated with midazolam for advanced imaging. (Courtesy of Emi Knafo.)

TABLE 48.1 Sedation Protocols Commonly Used in Reptiles

	Dose (mg/kg)	Route	Species	Comments	Reference
Chelonians					
Midazolam	0.5–2	IM	Red-eared slider, snapping turtle, red-footed tortoise, Indian star tortoise	Mild to moderate sedation for minor procedures and handling; medium maximum effect 20 mins	17, 21
Dexmedetomidine	0.1	IM	Red-eared slider, North American box turtle	Mild to moderate sedation, completely reversible; rapid recovery after reversal	*
Midazolam	1				
Dexmedetomidine	0.1	IM, SC	Red-eared slider	Moderate sedation, partially reversible; rapid recovery after reversal, suitable for intrathecal injection and endotracheal intubation	7, 22
Midazolam	1				
Ketamine	2				
Medetomidine	0.1–0.2 5	IM, IN	Red-eared slider turtle, yellow-bellied slider	Deep sedation, suitable for intubation	15, 27, 29
Ketamine					
Medetomidine	0.15	IM, SC	African spurred tortoise	Deep sedation to light anesthesia, partially reversible; rapid recovery after reversal	22
Ketamine	2.5				
Morphine	1				
Medetomidine	0.2	IM, SC	African spurred tortoise	Deep sedation to light anesthesia, completely reversible; rapid recovery after reversal	22
Midazolam	2				
Morphine	1				
Alfaxalone	10	IM	Red-eared slider	Moderate sedation, suitable for intubation	2, 3
Alfaxalone	10 and 20	IM	Horsfield's tortoise	Moderate to deep sedation, intubation not possible in about half of the tortoises	52
Propofol	2 to 5	IV		Moderate sedation; light anesthesia	11, 29, 42, 43
Lizards					
Midazolam	0.1–2	IM	Bearded dragon, Merten's water monitor, spiny-tailed monitor, frilled lizard, Eastern water dragon, Hosmer's skink, Komodo dragon	Mild to moderate sedation for minor procedures and handling; medium maximum effect 20 mins	21
Dexmedetomidine	0.1–0.2	IM	Bearded dragon, green iguana	Moderate sedation, completely reversible; rapid recovery after reversal	*
Midazolam	1				
Dexmedetomidine	0.05–0.1	IM	Bearded dragon, spiny-tailed lizard, blue iguana	Moderate to deep sedation, partially reversible; rapid recovery after reversal	*
Midazolam	1				
Ketamine	3				
Alfaxalone	10	IM	Green iguana	Light to moderate sedation, maximum effect after approximately 5 min; duration of effect, approximately 10 min	45
Alfaxalone	9	IV	Australian lizards	Induction agent; maintain with gaseous anesthetic	54
Propofol	3–5	IV, IO		Deep sedation to light anesthesia	†
Snakes					
Midazolam	1–2	IM	Black-headed python, carpet python, water python, emerald tree boa, eyelash palm pitviper	Mild to moderate sedation for mild procedures and handling; median time to maximal effect was 20 minutes	21
Tiletamine/ zolazepam (Telazol)	2–5	IM	Large snakes	Mild to moderate sedation, endotracheal intubation	†
Ketamine	5–10	IM		Mild to moderate sedation, endotracheal intubation	†
Propofol	3–5	IV		Moderate sedation to light anesthesia	9†
Crocodilians					
Midazolam	1–2	IM	Juvenile saltwater crocodile	Moderate sedation handling; reduction of lactic acidosis post handing	23
Tiletamine/ zolazepam (Telazol)	1–2	IM	Crocodilians	Mild to moderate sedation	†
Xylazine	1–2	IM	Adult alligator	Partially sedated or no effects	†
Ketamine	50–60				
Medetomidine	0.15–0.3	IM	Adult alligator	Mild to moderate sedation	†
Propofol	3–10	IV	Alligator	Mild to Moderate sedation to light anesthesia	†

IM, Intramuscular; *IV,* intravenous; *SC,* subcutaneous; *IN,* intranasal.
Atipamezole is used to antagonize medetomidine/dexmedetomidine in 1:1 volume, SC or IM. Flumazenil is used to antagonize midazolam: 0.01 to 0.1 mg/kg SC, IM, or IV. Naloxone is used to antagonize morphine or hydromorphone: 0.04 to 0.2 mg/kg SC, IM, or IV.
*Anecdotal dosages used in practice.
†See Chapters 49 and 50.

Although midazolam at high dosages can provide variable sedation, combinations with other drugs (dissociative agents, opioids, alpha 2 agonists) are recommended to produce stronger and more reproducible results. Midazolam at 2 mg/kg in combination with 20 to 40 mg/kg ketamine, administered to common snapping turtles, provided better sedation than either agent alone or exposure to isoflurane. Combination of midazolam with the lower dose of ketamine produced levels of sedation for extensive manipulation for a minimum of 25 minutes.[18]

Diazepam appears to be an appropriate alternative to midazolam; however, this agent is less frequently used due to a longer anticipated duration of action and its hydrophobic properties, which cause a delay and reduction in IM absorption. Intramuscular diazepam (0.22–0.62 mg/kg) administered 20 minutes prior to IM succinylcholine chloride in American alligators (*Alligator mississippiensis*) resulted in reduced drug volume and decreased stress and lowered the dosage of succinylcholine chloride required for adequate immobilization for the purposes of safe handling.[24]

Flumazenil, an imidazobenzodiazepine derivative, antagonizes the actions of benzodiazepines by competitively inhibiting activity at the GABA receptor. Renarcotization can occur, especially if high concentrations of long-acting benzodiazepines such as diazepam were used, which may necessitate additional doses of this agent for sustained reversal.[21] While the recommended dosages in reptiles range from 0.01 to 0.3 mg/kg IM or IV, there are currently no pharmacokinetic studies of flumazenil in reptiles.

α2-ADRENERGIC AGONISTS

α2-Adrenergic agonists are a class of major tranquilizer drugs that selectively stimulate alpha adrenergic receptors, with sedative effects attributable to their activity in the central and peripheral nervous system and antinociceptive properties attributable to their activity within the spinal cord. α2-adrenergic agonists facilitate handling and synergistically combine with other sedative agents to facilitate short procedures such as abscess debridement, minor repair procedures, and collection of diagnostic samples. In most species, α2 adrenergic agonists initially produce a period of hypertension resulting from receptor activity on vascular smooth muscle and subsequent vasoconstriction. Hypertension is accompanied by bradycardia and decreased cardiac output as a result of reflex vagal activity and α2-mediated inhibition of norepinephrine release in the sympathetic nervous system. The α2 adrenergic agonists produce dose-dependent cardiovascular depression in reptiles. Significant decreases in mean heart and respiratory rates; systolic, diastolic, and mean ventricular pressures; and mean ventricular partial pressure of oxygen have been documented following administration of medetomidine 0.15 mg/kg in desert tortoises (*Gopherus agassizii*).[25] Due to the respiratory depressant effects attributed to these drugs, supplemental oxygen is recommended for extended procedures. While α2 adrenergic agonists may be used as single agents with variable efficacy (see Table 48.1), these agents are more commonly administered in combination with ketamine, benzodiazepines, and opioids to produce safe, reliable, and reversible sedation/anesthesia.

Xylazine, as a sole sedative agent or in combination with other agents, produces more variable clinical results than (dex)medetomidine. Xylazine sedative combinations, however, have been investigated for sedation in reptiles. Red-eared sliders given xylazine 2 mg/kg in combination with ketamine 60 mg/kg produced adequate sedation for minor procedures, however, xylazine appeared to provide no benefit over the group receiving ketamine alone.[19] Giant Amazonian turtles (*Podocnemis expansa*) administered xylazine 1.5 mg/kg IM followed by propofol 5 to 10 mg/kg IV produced deep sedation of approximately 150-minute duration, which provided adequate restraint for physical examinations, venipuncture, and minor surgery.[26]

The use of medetomidine and dexmedetomidine in reptiles has been well documented, primarily by the IM route. In the desert tortoise, medetomidine 0.15 mg/kg IM produced light to heavy sedation within 20 minutes post injection, with leg and neck reflexes significantly slowed. For tortoises given atipamezole at a dose of 0.75 mg/kg, reflexes were considered normal within 30 minutes of reversal.[25] Medetomidine 40 to 300 mcg/kg combined with ketamine 4 to 15 mg/kg IM have been used to produce light sedation followed by inhalation anesthesia in lizards, alligators, sliders, and other tortoises[27,28] (Fig. 48.2).

Yellow-bellied sliders administered dexmedetomidine 0.2 mg/kg and ketamine 10 mg/kg intranasally resulted in moderate to heavy sedation within 30 to 45 minutes post administration, without any adverse effects and with safe, reliable recovery within 19 minutes of atipamezole administration[15] (Fig. 48.3).

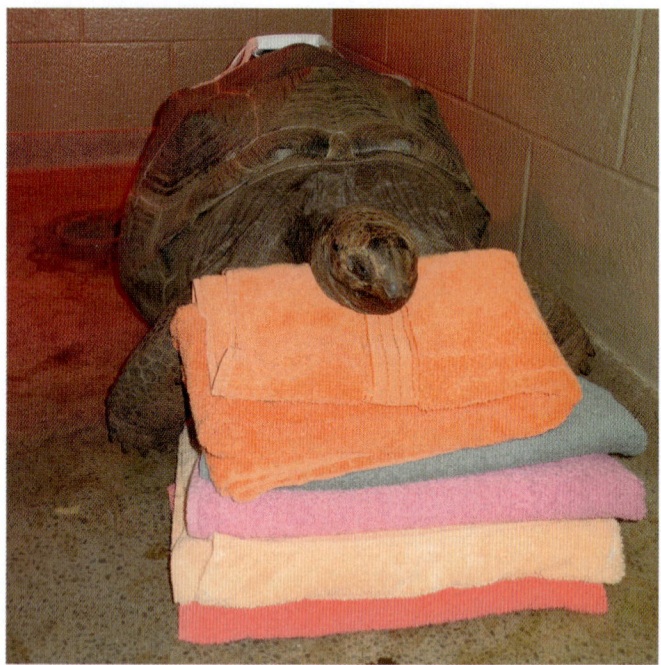

FIG 48.2 An Aldabra tortoise (*Aldabrachelys gigantea*) sedated with dexmedetomidine and ketamine for blood collection. (Courtesy of Stephen J. Divers.)

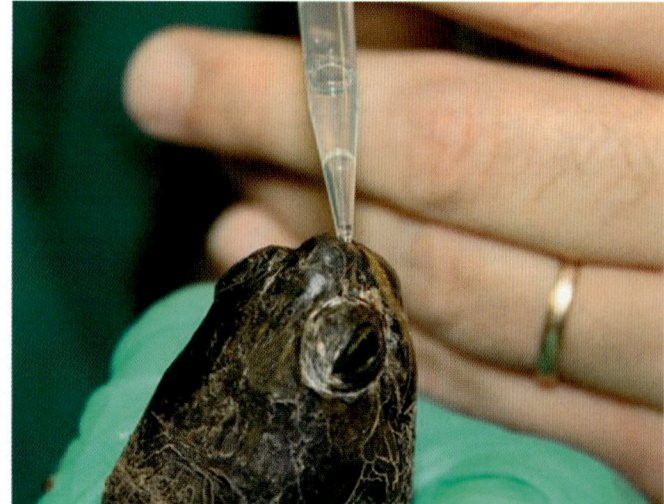

FIG 48.3 Intranasal administration of medetomidine and ketamine in a yellow-bellied turtle (*Trachemys scripta scripta*). (Courtesy of Rodney W. Schnellbacher.)

PHENOTHIAZINES (ACEPROMAZINE)

Acepromazine is a phenothiazine derivative, antipsychotic drug, which produces sedative effects mediated primarily by blockade of dopamine receptors in the basal ganglia and limbic system. Acepromazine also binds to adrenergic and muscarinic receptors. Systemic hypotension occurring as a result of this drug in mammals is typically attributed to antagonism of α1 adrenergic receptors in the peripheral vessels.

Although acepromazine can be used, little information has been published on its use in reptiles, either for sedation or as a premedicant prior to general anesthesia.[30,31] The irreversible character and prolonged effects of this drug make it less desirable as a tranquilizer in reptiles.

OPIOIDS

Opioid drugs, when administered alone, have variable sedation effects in reptiles. Butorphanol at 2 mg/kg IM in green iguanas did not reduce induction times, and when used as a premedication did not have isoflurane-sparing effects.[32,33] Additionally buprenorphine did not significantly increase iguana hind-limb withdrawal latencies at any time point when compared with saline. However, in chelonians the effects of opioids appear more profound. In a study of African spurred tortoises administered morphine at 2.0 mg/kg and midazolam at 1 mg/kg subcutaneously (SC), adequate sedation was achieved to allow physical examinations and blood collection to be performed.[22] Furthermore, red-eared slider turtles administered a high dose of tramadol at 25 mg/kg orally exhibited limb and neck flaccidity, as well as respiratory depression, within the first 12 hours after administration.[34] Moreover, red-eared sliders administered either butorphanol at 28 mg/kg or morphine at 1.5 mg/kg IM exhibited respiratory depression for 1 to 3 hours.[35] For this reason, oxygen supplementation should be considered for reptilian patients exhibiting reduced respiratory rates under morphine sedation.

SEDATION USING LOW-DOSE ANESTHETIC AGENTS

The following drug classes (dissociatives; sedative hypnotics, e.g., propofol; and steroid anesthetics, e.g., alfaxalone) are described in the literature and are clinically used as sedatives or anesthetics in reptiles. While the purpose of this chapter is to report evidence-based approaches to reptilian sedation, differentiation between sedation and anesthesia is difficult, given the challenges of determining depth of central nervous system depression in any vertebrate species and particularly reptiles. The authors of this chapter ask readers to recognize the inevitable overlap of information regarding protocols for sedation versus anesthesia and refer readers to Chapter 49, which addresses protocol design, monitoring, and other management issues surrounding general anesthesia in reptilians.

Dissociatives (Ketamine, Tiletamine)

Ketamine hydrochloride is a dissociative agent commonly used in sedative or anesthetic protocols for many species. The mechanism of action is by antagonism of the N-methyl-D-aspartate (NMDA) receptor, a glutamate receptor and ion channel protein residing in the central nervous system. It may be administered by IM or IV routes, and while its lower pH has been anecdotally noted to irritate tissue, especially when injected IM into smaller muscle bellies, it remains an important component of tranquilizer combinations for many species. Bienzle et al.[18] demonstrated that IM ketamine 20 to 40 mg/kg combined with midazolam 2 mg/kg provided sedation for physical examination of common snapping turtles, which was superior to

that achieved by 5% inhaled isoflurane. Medetomidine 0.1 mg/kg and ketamine 5 mg/kg provided short-term, adequate sedation, with moderate hypoventilation, for minor diagnostic procedures in gopher tortoises (*Gopherus polyphemus*).[36,37] Furthermore, IV administration of atipamazole precipitated severe hypotension in this study population, and IM administration is recommended. Additional studies describing ketamine use in reptiles were described above, in combination with other tranquilizer agents.

A combination of the dissociative anesthetic, tiletamine, and the benzodiazepine tranquilizer, zolazepam, produces sedation, mild analgesia, and muscle relaxation in many mammalian species. Tiletamine/zolazepam is commonly characterized by a prolonged, mildly to moderately dysphoric recovery in mammals compared to recovery from ketamine combinations.[38,39] The clinical efficacy of tiletamine/zolazepam in reptiles, however, can be unpredictable, and recovery from this drug may be prolonged, especially at higher doses.

Sedation in green iguanas is reportedly unreliable, with some animals remaining sedated for up to 16 hours.[40] Similar sedation levels were achieved at all doses investigated (4.4, 22, 33, 44, 66, 88 mg/kg), with the majority never reaching a "surgical" depth of anesthesia. Water snakes administered higher doses in this same study exhibited unreliable, prolonged sedation (>8 hours) or death.[40] Tiletamine/zolazepam can be useful for sedation of large or dangerous species (e.g., crocodilians, large monitor lizards), and although not recommended for routine use in most species, some have reported consistently good results. Doses of 1 to 2 mg/kg have been recommended for crocodilians and produce sedation but responsiveness.[41] Given the irreversible nature and unpredictable response to this drug, caution is required.

Propofol

Propofol (2,6-diisopropylphenol) is a short-acting, lipid-soluble sedative hypnotic used frequently as an injectable general anesthetic in mammals. General advantages of propofol include quick induction and recovery with minimal to no dysphoria. Disadvantages of this drug include a dose-dependent depression of respiratory function. In mammals, it has been shown to cause reductions in cardiac contractility and vascular tone, the latter two properties frequently leading to hypotension.[42] Propofol is not reversible and requires intravascular administration, which may represent a significant limitation in reptile species for whom IV or IO access is difficult. Some formulations are available in multidose bottles with storage for up to 28 days at room temperature.

Propofol has been paired with various tranquilizers for successful and safe reptile sedation.[29] Chelonian species safely sedated with IV propofol include red-eared sliders, giant Amazon turtles (*Podocnemis expansa*), and loggerhead sea turtles (*Caretta caretta*), who develop rapid narcosis and dose-dependent depth and duration of sedation under the influence of propofol.[29,43,44] Both species demonstrated respiratory depression, a common finding among other species. Ball pythons (*Python regius*) administered intracardiac propofol demonstrated rapid sedation but a prolonged recovery when compared to sedation or anesthetic induction with isoflurane gas.[44]

The significance of apnea is controversial in reptiles, particularly for aquatic species that exhibit profound dive reflexes. Intracardiac shunting, which is thought to cause blood to bypass the lungs during a dive, may also occur during times of iatrogenic physiological stress, for example, sedation. Arterial blood is difficult to sample in most reptiles, and in the event that arterial samples are available for blood gas analysis, demonstration of hypoxemia in these samples may not correlate with a systemic state of metabolic distress. Given the logistical difficulties inherent to monitoring oxygenation, manual ventilatory support in apneic reptiles is recommended.

Alfaxalone

Alfaxalone is an injectable anesthetic found in a novel cyclodextrin excipient, which conceals this lipid-soluble compound in a water-soluble exterior, thereby facilitating its absorption following IM injection. Alfaxalone has gained recent popularity as an injectable sedative or anesthetic agent in reptiles due to its smooth induction properties and utility as an IM or IV single agent or part of a combination protocol for minor or noninvasive procedures.[54] The lack of a preservative mandates disposal of a vial after it has been breached.

When administered IM to green iguanas, alfaxalone showed a dose-dependent narcosis, with 10 mg/kg providing light sedation appropriate for examination or venipuncture, 20 mg/kg sufficient for endotracheal intubation, and 30 mg/kg providing surgical anesthesia for durations up to 40 minutes.[46] Another study evaluated 5 mg/kg IV in green iguanas and found this protocol to provide a smooth anesthetic induction prior to intubation and gas anesthesia.[45] While cardiovascular parameters remained stable during sedation in both studies, respiratory rates under IM sedation uniformly decreased; meanwhile, respiratory rates increased during the IV alfaxalone anesthesia.

In red-eared sliders and Horsfield's tortoises (*Agrionemys horsfieldii*), IM alfaxalone provides a smooth induction of dose-dependent sedation, which clinically becomes deeper and longer in duration at lower ambient temperatures.[2,3,53] Alfaxalone 10 mg/kg caused light sedation for shorter periods of time (<20–30 minutes), providing a depth suitable for examinations, venipuncture, and other noninvasive procedures. This drug was reliable when administered IM and also provided a smooth recovery.

Disadvantages of this drug include its apparent lack of (or yet unproven) analgesic properties, high expense, locomotor activity that can occur during recovery (turtles), and the large volumes required (when used as a single agent) that often necessitate multiple IM injections at different locations to administer an adequate clinical dose. Additionally, the lack of a preservative mandates disposal of a vial after it has been breached. In some countries, refrigeration for up to 1 week is acceptable; however, in the United States the FDA has mandated that a vial must be discarded within 6 hours of opening. Unless used extensively alfaxalone is often an expensive agent to work with for a single, small reptile patient.

NON-PHARMACEUTICAL METHODS

Vasovagal Response

Besides pharmaceutical forms of restraint, the vasovagal reflex may also be used for mild sedation for short, nonpainful procedures. Pressure

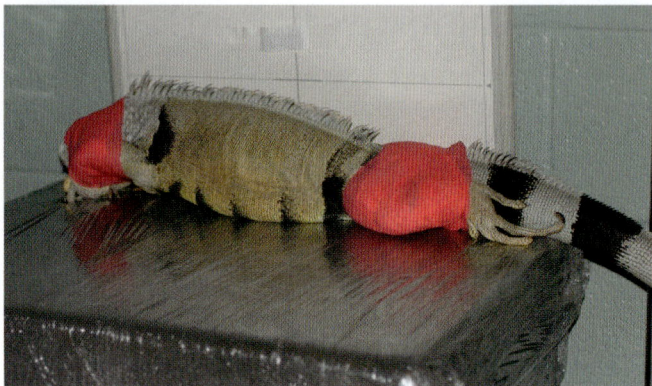

FIG 48.4 Vagal response for a green iguana (*Iguana iguana*) undergoing radiographs. (Courtesy of Stephen J. Divers.)

over the eyes of most lizards and crocodilians or placement of the animal in dorsal recumbency can stimulate a vagal response and decrease in heart rate, blood pressure, and activity. This physical sedation can last up to 40 minutes in some species of lizards and can be a useful supplement to chemical restraint (Fig. 48.4).

Cold Narcosis

Despite its historical use, cold narcosis is not considered an acceptable form of sedation for reptilians. Hypothermia may exacerbate underlying metabolic diseases and weaken the immune system,[47] reduce the ability to respond to nociceptive stimuli,[48–51] and cause tissue injury. Additionally, necrotic changes in the brain have been reported in snakes and turtles restrained with cold narcosis.[51,52]

MONITORING PATIENTS UNDER SEDATION

Recommendations for monitoring sedated reptiles include intermittent measurement and documentation of respiratory rate and effort, heart rate, reflexes, and body temperature until narcosis has decreased to a level allowing ambulation and the return of normal behaviors. At this point, patients are frequently transferred to a heated enclosure for visual monitoring until fully recovered.

REFERENCES

See www.expertconsult.com for a complete list of references.

49

General Anesthesia

Christoph Mans, Kurt K. Sladky, and Juergen Schumacher

Historically, managing anesthesia in reptiles has been problematic for three primary reasons. First, there is an enormous diversity of species across the class *Reptilia*, one of the most phylogenetically diverse animal classes with four extant orders (*Crocodylia, Testudines, Squamata,* and *Rhynchocephalia*) and more than 9600 species worldwide. Second, there is a lack of systematic research dedicated to advancing our understanding of effective anesthetic/analgesic induction and maintenance drugs, dose-dependent effects, duration of drug efficacy, interspecies differences, and potentially fatal drug-related adverse effects, such as cardiopulmonary depression. Lack of funding in support of such research has hampered the field and limited the application of anesthetic/analgesic agents in reptiles when compared with mammals. Third, the reptile literature is rife with anecdotal information, which has persisted and, in many cases, has grown to be widely accepted dogma for clinicians. The diversity of reptiles in terms of natural history, size, anatomy, and physiology presents a unique clinical challenge to the veterinarian.[1] Safe and effective anesthesia of the reptilian patient is a requirement for procedures, including physical examination of large or dangerous species, collection of diagnostic samples, and application of various imaging modalities, as well as for surgical procedures. The anesthetic management of the reptilian patient, including the design of the anesthetic protocol, represents unique challenges due to marked anatomic and physiologic differences between taxa. Responses to frequently used anesthetic agents and dosages are often variable between taxa, and individual differences are also commonly observed. Additionally, anesthetic and analgesic protocols, including monitoring techniques to evaluate cardiopulmonary performance, are often derived from domestic animals and then applied to the reptilian patient. These techniques are often of limited value and should be interpreted by clinicians with caution.

ANATOMY AND PHYSIOLOGY

Thermoregulation and Environmental Temperature

Reptiles differ from mammals physiologically and anatomically, and therefore it is difficult to directly extrapolate from methods used in mammalian anesthesia. Most importantly, reptiles are ectothermic, meaning that their body temperature is directly dependent on environmental temperature and associated behaviors to modify that body temperature. Changes in body temperature significantly affect metabolic rate and many other physiological processes. Therefore the temperature at which one maintains a patient is an important factor in reptilian anesthesia due to the fact that the absorption, distribution, metabolism, and excretion of drugs in reptiles is directly related to environmental temperature.[2–4] Consequently, it is important to maintain the reptile patient within its preferred optimal temperature zone (POTZ) to be able to better predict the physiological effects of anesthetic drugs. POTZ is generally considered to be 20° to 25°C (68°–77°F) in temperate and aquatic species and 25° to 35°C (77°–95°F) in tropical species.[5] In

red-eared sliders, the induction, duration, and recovery times after alfaxalone administration (10 and 20 mg/kg IM) were significantly shorter at 35°C (95°F) compared with 20°C (68°F).[6] At 20 mg/kg IM the induction times were 19 ± 6 (20°C, 68°F) and 7 ± 5 minutes (35°C, 95°F), and the plateau phase lasted 28 ± 13 (20°C, 68°F) and 8 ± 5 (35°C, 95°F) minutes.[6] Crocodiles administered medetomidine (0.5 mg/kg IM) for anesthesia were induced significantly faster at higher temperatures (32°C, 90°F) compared with lower temperatures (22 and 27°C, 72° and 81°F), while at 17°C (63°F) no anesthetic effects were observed.[7] In contrast, recovery times following atipamezole administration were not different between animals maintained at different temperatures.[7] In estuarine, but not in freshwater crocodiles, the duration of effect of intravenous alfaxalone was shorter at higher temperatures (32°C, 90°F) compared to lower temperatures (22°C, 72°F).[8] In neotropical rattlesnakes (*Crotalus durissus*) lower body temperature (22°C, 72°F) did not have an effect on induction times following administration of ketamine (80 mg/kg IM) when compared to animals maintained at 30°C (90°F). However, recovery times were significantly shorter at the higher temperatures (3.5 hours) compared to lower temperatures (5.5 hours).[3]

Cardiopulmonary Systems

The reptile cardiovascular system is characterized by several unique anatomic structures and physiological functions. In chelonians (turtles, tortoises), lizards, and snakes, the heart is 3-chambered, composed of a single ventricle and two atria. The two atria are completely separate, and the ventricle is divided longitudinally into two chambers by an incomplete intraventricular septum. The incomplete septum allows mixing of oxygenated and deoxygenated blood and shunting of blood from both left-to-right and right-to-left. All reptiles have two aortic arches, right and left. While cardiac shunting is considered detrimental in birds and mammals, it is an important physiological mechanism in reptiles during apneic periods (e.g., diving). The functional significance of cardiac shunts in reptiles has been the subject of debate for decades and is beyond the scope of this clinical review.[9,10] However, the clinician should be aware that cardiac shunting can play a role in inhaled anesthetic uptake and elimination, potentially causing delayed induction and delayed or an unexpectedly rapid recovery. In addition, cardiac shunts may affect systemic blood pressure and arterial/venous oxygen concentration, which, in turn will impact anesthetic monitoring (e.g., blood pressure, pulse oximetry, expired gases).

Hepatic First-Pass Effect. The hepatic first-pass effect following hind limb administration of anesthetic and other drugs has not received much attention in the literature. However, its pharmacodynamics and pharmacokinetic significance may be more clinically important than that of the renal portal system.[11] The venous blood flow from the hind limb in chelonians, lizards, and crocodilians drains into the ventral abdominal vein(s), which either passes directly to the liver or indirectly via the hepatic portal vein.[12–14] Hence, any liver-metabolized or excreted drug administered in the hind limb first enters the liver before reaching the systemic circulation, resulting in a hepatic first-pass effect. In turtles and crocodiles, the hepatic first-pass effect following hind limb administration leads to lower bioavailability of drugs, resulting in lower plasma concentrations and/or reduced or no clinical efficacy.[11,15,16] However, despite the published evidence of the clinical significance associated with the hepatic first-pass effect, pharmacokinetic and pharmacodynamic studies continue to be published without taking this anatomic factor into consideration with respect to study design.[15,17]

In leopard geckos (*Eublepharis macularius*), as well as red-eared sliders, hind limb administration of dexmedetomdicine-ketamine resulted in significantly less, or no, anesthetic effects compared to administration of the same dosages in the forelimbs (Lahner, Proc AAZV, 2011, p 136).[18] A suspected hepatic first-pass effect was also reported in estuarine crocodiles (*Crocodylus porosus*) following medetomidine administration.[16] In contrast, broad-snouted caimans (*Caiman latirostris*) administered ketamine (30 mg/kg IM) and xylazine (1 mg/kg IM) in both the forelimb and hind limb did not exhibit any differences in sedation scores, induction, recovery, or physiological and behavioral responses.[19] In ball pythons (*Python regius*) the subcutaneous administration of alfaxalone in the caudal body half, just cranial to the cloaca, had significant less cardiovascular and sedative effects than administration in the cranial body half, at the level of the heart (Yaw, Proc ARAV, 2017, p 145). Since many drugs commonly used in reptiles, particularly analgesics and anesthetics, undergo hepatic metabolism and/or excretion, one must consider the hepatic first-pass effect, since the majority of venous blood from the hind limbs and caudal body half drains directly into the liver before entering the systemic circulation.[11,14] Therefore it is advised to avoid administration of anesthetic drugs by intramuscular or subcutaneous injection in the caudal body of reptiles. Intravenous administration of anesthetics in the coccygeal (caudal ventral tail) vein of lizards does not result in an hepatic first effect, because it drains directly into the caudal vena cava.[13] In turtles the venous drainage from the tail is less consistent, with some blood entering the ventral abdominal vein and some entering the caudal vena cava.[14]

Respiratory Anatomy and Physiology. The structure and function of the reptilian respiratory system not only differs considerably from mammalian and avian species, but differences are also apparent between reptile orders and families.[7,8] All reptiles lack a functional diaphragm, and the force to move air during inspiration and expiration comes from movement of skeletal muscles, resulting in changes of intrapulmonary pressure. Chelonians use pelvic and pectoral muscles, which are functionally analogous to a mammalian diaphragm. Snakes use a combination of smooth muscle in the lung walls, as well as intercostal muscles, while lizards use lung smooth muscle, intercostal, pectoral, and abdominal muscles for respiration. The glottis of snakes is located rostrally, and air enters through the external nares, the nasal sinuses, and the internal nares.[9] The trachea consists of incomplete cartilagenous rings and bifurcates into short bronchi at the level of the heart. The lungs are elongated saclike structures lined with respiratory epithelium. Most snakes have a vestigial left lung and a functional right lung, which ends distally as an airsac that is lined with nonrespiratory epithelium. Boid snakes have functional right and left lungs (although the left tends to be smaller) and distally caudal air sacs.

The glottis of carnivorous lizards is located more rostrally when compared to herbivorous species, where it is commonly found at the base of the tongue. Lizards have incomplete tracheal rings, and the trachea bifurcates approximately at the base of the heart. The lungs of most lizard species are single-chambered organs that extend caudally into an air sac. Some iguanids, varanids, and chameleons have multichambered lungs that consist of an anterior and posterior chamber.

In chelonians, the glottis is located at the base of a fleshy tongue. The trachea has complete tracheal rings, is relatively short, and bifurcates into a left and right intrapulmonary bronchus at the level of the thoracic inlet. Turtles and tortoises have paired, multichambered, relatively rigid lungs. In crocodilians, the glottis is located behind the epiglottal (gular) flap. The lungs of crocodilians are complex and multichambered, and the bronchi branch into multiple internal lobes.

Physiologically, reptiles have lower metabolic, cardiac, and respiratory rates because of their lower oxygen demands. Reptilian respiration is controlled by hypoxia, hypercapnia, and environmental temperature. Specific receptors increase ventilation during periods of low O_2 and high CO_2. In most reptiles, hypercapnia causes an increase in tidal volume, and hypoxia increases respiratory rate. In reptiles, the stimulus to breathe comes from low oxygen concentrations. Respiratory rate has been shown in tortoises to increase during hypercapnia but decrease during hypoxia. The higher demand for oxygen during increased temperature, or after prolonged dives in aquatic species, is met by increasing the tidal volume and not the respiratory rate. In an oxygen-enriched environment, reptiles decrease ventilation, characterized by a decrease in respiratory rate and tidal volume. Intrapulmonary shunts, which represent the portion of pulmonary blood bypassing gas exchange, reduce the efficiency of gas exchange in the lungs and result in a reduction of arterial oxygen concentrations (PaO_2).

PREANESTHETIC EVALUATION

A thorough and complete evaluation of the patient should be conducted to design an effective anesthetic and analgesic protocol. A complete history and critical review of husbandry practices, including diet, temperature, and humidity, should be obtained since they will provide valuable information on the health status of the patient. The medical record of the patient, including past anesthetic episodes, should be reviewed, followed by a complete visual and physical examination. Specific attention should be paid to evidence of systemic disease, as well as signs of cardiovascular or respiratory compromise, which will affect the patient's performance under anesthesia.

Diseases of the respiratory tract are commonly observed in reptiles and may affect both the upper and lower respiratory tract.[20] Most commonly, a viral or bacterial etiology is identified, and the patient may require effective antimicrobial therapy prior to induction of general anesthesia. Determination of respiratory rate and effort will provide limited information on the presence of respiratory tract disease. Imaging modalities such as radiography or computed tomography, as well as collection of diagnostic samples, will assist in identifying the severity and etiology of respiratory tract disease.

Assessment of cardiovascular performance should be part of the physical examination. Unfortunately, few studies have determined normal cardiovascular performance (e.g., heart rate, arterial blood pressures) in reptiles. Although reference values for various cardiac parameters need to be established in common reptile species, determination of heart rate and rhythm, and radiographic evaluation of cardiac morphology, as well as echocardiography will give valuable information on cardiac performance and abnormalities.[21,22]

Diagnostic samples such as fecal screens, hematology, and plasma biochemistries should be collected, before anesthesia if possible, to determine the health status of the reptile. Reference values for common reptile species have been published and should provide important information on organ function and presence of infectious and noninfectious disease processes. Imaging modalities such as radiography, ultrasonography, and computed tomography are performed as indicated by medical history and physical examination findings.

Some attempt should be made to objectively classify and document patient anesthetic risks, and the following physical status classification system created by the American Society of Anesthesiologists (ASA) can be useful.

ASA 1: A normal healthy patient

ASA 2: A patient with mild, systemic disease

ASA 3: A patient with severe systemic disease

ASA 4: A patient with severe systemic disease that is a constant threat to life

ASA 5: A moribund patient who is not expected to survive without the operation

It is useful to calculate all possible intraoperative and emergency drug requirements prior to premedication and induction. A simple spreadsheet can, after inputting the reptile's weight, produce a printable list of all potential emergency drugs. This should be attached to the anesthesia record and be constantly available during the premedication, induction, maintenance, and recovery phases.

Supportive Measures

Many reptiles require supportive care prior to anesthesia due to underlying chronic disease processes and dehydration, often identified during preanesthetic evaluation. Elective procedures should be delayed until underweight, dehydrated, or debilitated animals have received treatment to improve their condition. For nonelective procedures, dehydration and electrolyte imbalances should be corrected prior to anesthesia (see Chapter 87). Even the most moribund dystocic reptile will usually benefit from stabilization for 24 to 48 hours before embarking on general anesthesia. In the authors' experience, reptiles that fail to stabilize prior to surgery tend to succumb intraoperatively or postoperatively. Effective fluid therapy is indicated to correct fluid and electrolyte imbalances and return the patient to a normovolemic state. Intravenous or intraosseous fluid therapy are most effective and should be administered as a constant rate infusion if vascular or intraosseous access has been established (Fig. 49.1). Intravenous catheters can, following surgical cut-down, be placed percutaneously in the jugular veins of chelonians; jugular, cephalic, ventral abdominal vein, or ventral tail veins of lizards; and cranial vena cava or jugular vein of snakes. In lizards, the tibia or femur are common sites for intraosseous catheterization when IV access is not possible (see Chapter 44).

In cases of suspected or confirmed bacterial and fungal infections, effective antimicrobial/antifungal therapy should be initiated following the collection of material for culture and prior to the anesthetic event if possible. Particular attention should be paid to signs of respiratory or cardiovascular compromise, since compromise of these systems will affect the anesthetic plan, including selection of drugs, dosages, monitoring equipment, and requirement of supportive care measures during anesthesia.

INJECTABLE ANESTHETIC AGENTS

Prior to administration of any anesthetic or sedative drugs, reptiles should be maintained within their preferred optimal temperature zone (POTZ), and the core body temperature should be monitored throughout the anesthetic period. A variety of agents representing different classes of drugs are frequently used, either alone or in combination, depending on the desired level of sedation or anesthesia. It is recommended to avoid administration of high dosages of a single anesthetic agent (e.g., ketamine, alfaxalone), and instead, consider protocols in which multiple drugs are combined with synergistic actions, thereby requiring lower dosages for each drug. Additionally, using readily reversible drug protocols

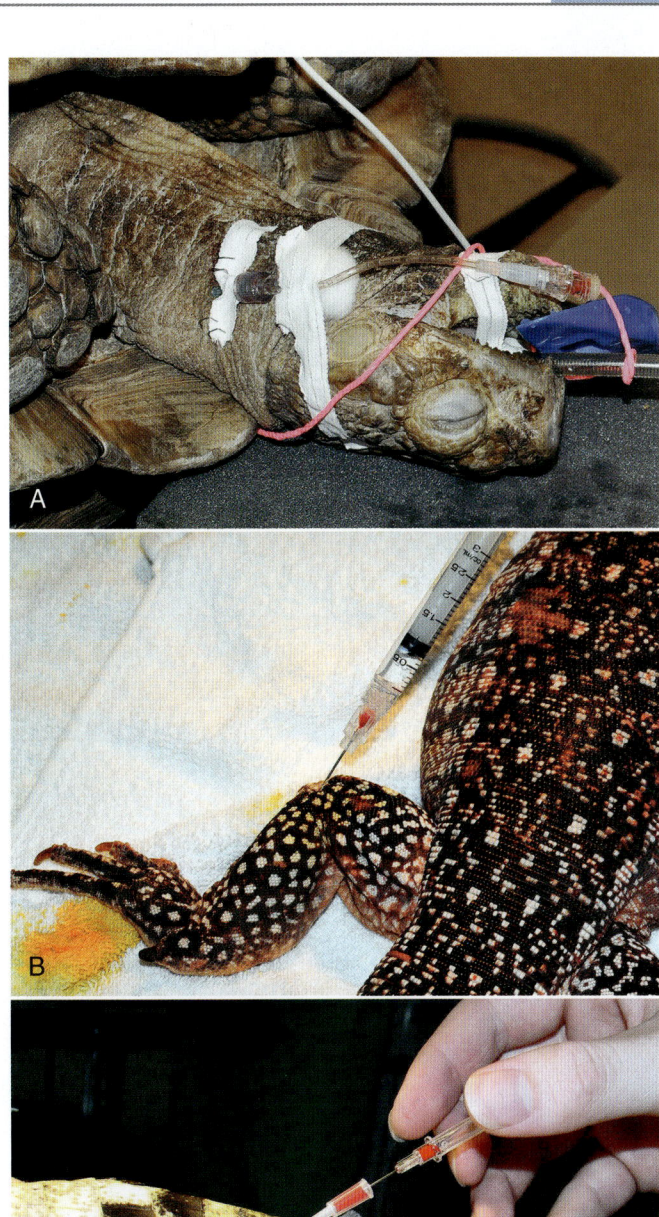

FIG 49.1 Intravascular access in reptiles. (A) Intravenous catheter in the jugular vein of an African spurred tortoise (*Centrochelys sulcata*). (B) Intraosseous catheter in the left tibia of a red tegu (*Tupinambis rufescens*). Correct intraosseous catheter placement is confirmed by aspiration of hemorrhagic aspirate (needle hub), consistent with bone marrow. (C) Intravenous catheter placement in the tail vein of a green anaconda (*Eunectes murinus*). (C, Courtesy of Stephen J. Divers.)

will provide for more rapid recoveries. Since most deleterious side effects (e.g., prolonged recovery, cardiopulmonary depression) associated with anesthetic and sedative drug administration are dose dependent, individual drug dosage reduction and reversibility will result in fewer complications and improved recoveries. Similar drugs and drug combinations can also be chosen for premedication/sedation prior to induction of general anesthesia. If the patient is scheduled for a painful procedure, it is recommended to include an analgesic agent such as an opioid in the preanesthetic protocol. Many injectable protocols in reptiles include the administration of an α-2 agonist (e.g., [dex]medetomidine) with ketamine and/or midazolam. A μ-opioid receptor agonist (e.g., morphine, hydromorphone) should be added to the protocol if additional analgesia is required in chelonians and lizards. One must keep in mind that many factors (e.g., site of injection, underlying disease, dehydration, body temperature, gravidity, etc.) may affect the onset, recovery, and efficacy of anesthetic drugs.[2–4] Therefore an individualized approach

in selecting appropriate drug combinations and dosages should be considered.

Injectable agents alone can be used to facilitate a variety of short diagnostic and surgical procedures, as well as for induction of general anesthesia. Maintenance of a surgical plane of anesthesia for prolonged, invasive procedures is frequently based on administration of an inhalational agent, such as isoflurane or sevoflurane. In aquatic freshwater turtles and terrestrial chelonians, injectable protocols containing (dex) medetomidine-ketamine, with or without opiates and local anesthetics, were successfully used to induce and maintain surgical anesthesia, without the need of gas anesthesia (Tables 49.1 to 49.4), and these protocols are preferred by the authors.[23–26]

Routes of Parenteral Drug Administration

While historically the intramuscular route of drug administration is recommended in reptiles, it is considered more painful, and less

TABLE 49.1 Anesthetic Protocols Reported in Tortoises and Freshwater Turtles

Protocol	Species	Dosage (mg/kg)	Route	Comments
Alfaxalone	Red-eared slider (*Trachemys s. elegans*)[56]	5	IV	Surgical anesthesia for 30 ± 15 minutes, following induction within 22 ± 8 seconds. Intubation possible in 100%. Recovery by 34 ± 5 minutes at 25°–30°C.
	Macquarie river turtle (*Emydura macquarii*)[15]	9	IV	Deep sedation to light anesthesia for 14 ± 5 minutes. Intubation possible in 100%.
	Red-eared slider[6]	10	IM	Moderate sedation within 16 ± 8 (20°C) and 5 ± 2 (35°C) minutes. Duration of maximum effect 13 ± 12 (20°C) and 8 ± 5 (35°C) minutes. Intubation possible in 80% (20°C) and 0% (35°C). Recovery by 105 ± 22 (20°C) and 41 ± 8 (35°C) minutes.
		20	IM	Anesthesia within 19 ± 6 (20°C) and 7 ± 5 (35°C) minutes. Duration of maximum effect 28 ± 13 (20°C) and 8 ± 5 (35°C) minutes. Intubation possible in 100% (20°C) and 30% (35°C). Recovery by 105 ± 22 (20°C) and 41 ± 8 (35°C) minutes.
	Russian tortoise (*Agrionemys horsfieldii*)[58]	10	IM	Moderate sedation within 15 ± 5 minutes. Duration of maximum effect 46 ± 23 minutes. Intubation not feasible. Recovery by 116 ± 39 minutes at 25°C.
		20	IM	Moderate to deep sedation within 14 ± 6 minutes. Duration of maximum effect 99 ± 74 minutes. Intubation possible in 56%. Recovery by 187 ± 30 minutes at 25°C.
Alfaxalone + medetomidine	Russian tortoise[58]	10 (A) + 0.1 (Me)	IM	Light anesthesia within 15 ± 5 minutes. Duration of maximum effect 99 ± 74 minutes. Intubation possible in 67%. Recovery by 223 ± 85 minutes at 25°C after administration of atipamezole at 60 minutes. Use cautiously—cardiovascular depression reported.
		20 (A) + 0.05 (Me)	IM	Light anesthesia within 13 ± 4 minutes. Duration of maximum effect 103 ± 49 minutes. Intubation possible in 89%. Recovery by 275 ± 108 minutes at 25°C after administration of atipamezole at 60 minutes. Use cautiously—cardiovascular depression reported.
Dexmedetomidine + ketamine	Red-eared slider[34]	0.1 (D) + 10 (K)	IM, SC	Light anesthesia. Suitable for intubation. Rapid recovery after reversal with atipamezole.
Dexmedetomidine + ketamine + midazolam	Red-eared slider[34,35]	0.1 (D) + 2 (K) + 1 (Mi)	SC	Light anesthesia, rapid recovery after reversal with atipamezole and flumazenil.
	Gopher tortoise (*Gopherus polyphemus*)[44]	0.075 (D) + 8 (K) + 1 (Mi)	IM	Light-moderate anesthesia within 22 ± 5 minutes. Recovery after low-dose atipamezole 93 ± 6 (10–266) minutes.
Dexmedetomidine + ketamine + morphine	Herman's tortoise (*Testudo hermanni*)[23]	0.1 (D) + 10 (K) + 1.5 (Mo)	IM	Surgical anesthesia induced within 30 minutes, cystoscopy in hatchlings, reversal with atipamezole (0.5 mg/kg IM) and naloxone (0.2 mg/kg IM). Recovery after reversal: 3–21 minutes.
Isoflurane	Most species	1%–4%		Maintenance agent. Not suitable for induction by mask in chelonians. Prolonged recovery possible, which can be shortened by administration of epinephrine 0.1 mg/kg IM.[74]

TABLE 49.1   Anesthetic Protocols Reported in Tortoises and Freshwater Turtles—cont'd

Protocol	Species	Dosage (mg/kg)	Route	Comments
Medetomidine + ketamine	Gopher tortoise[41]	0.1 (Me) + 5 (K)	IV	Light anesthesia.
	Red-eared slider[24]	0.1 (Me) + 5 (K)	IM	Light anesthesia, suitable for intubation, recovery by 60 minutes after reversal.
		0.2 (Me) + 10 (K)	IM	Surgical anesthesia, recovery by 60 minutes after reversal.
	Galapagos tortoise (*Chelonoidis nigra*)[43]	0.1 (Me) + 10 (K)	IV	Anesthetic induction within 11 ± 8 minutes. Required propofol (1.7 ± 1 mg/kg) in 50% for intubation. Maintained on isoflurane. Recovery by 120 ± 53 minutes after reversal.
Medetomidine + ketamine + morphine	Map turtles (*Graptemys* spp.)[a]	0.15 (Me) + 10-20 (K) + 1.5 (Mo)	IM	Surgical anesthesia by average induction time of 42 minutes. Reversal with atipamezole and naloxone. Naloxone at 0.02 mg/kg was insufficient and recovery was >3 hrs. Renarcotization noticed.
	Red-eared slider[26]	0.1 (Me) + 10 (K) + 1 (Mo)	IM	Surgical anesthesia by average induction time of 12 minutes. Reversal with atipamezole and naloxone (0.2 mg/kg). Mean recovery time 6 minutes.
		0.15 (Me) + 15 (K) + 1 (Mo)	IM	Surgical anesthesia by average induction time of 9 minutes. Reversal with atipamezole and naloxone (0.2 mg/kg). Mean recovery time 10 minutes.
	Chinese box turtles (*Cuora flavomarginata*)[25]	0.1 (Me) + 10 (K) + 1.5 (Mo)	IM	Surgical anesthesia, coelioscopy in hatchlings. Median reversal time 6 (0–21) minutes following administration of atipamezole and naloxone (0.2 mg/kg IM).
Medetomidine + hydromorphone + ketamine + midazolam	African spurred tortoise[76]*	0.15 (Me) + 0.5 (H) + 10 (K) + 0.5 (Mi)	SC	Light surgical anesthesia, maintain with gaseous anesthetic if necessary.
Midazolam + Ketamine	Common snapping turtle (*Chelydra serpentine*)[45]	2 (Mi) + 20-40 (K)	IM	Light anesthesia recovery up to 210 minutes without flumazenil administered.
Propofol	Most species[36,37]*	2–10	IV	Induction agent; use lower dose in large tortoises.
	Common snapping turtle[74]	5	IV	Induction agent.
	Red-eared slider[49]	10	IV	Light anesthesia within 1.7 ± 2.4 minutes. Duration of maximum effect 41 ± 20 minutes. Intubation possible in 70%. Recovery by 63 ± 24 minutes.
		20	IV	Surgical anesthesia within 0.9 ± 1.4 minutes. Duration of maximum effect 53 ± 32 minutes. Intubation possible in 100%. Recovery by 91 ± 32 minutes.

Atipamezole is usually dosed at 10 times the amount of dexmedetomidine or 5 times the amount of medetomidine in mg. Lower doses of atipamezole have been reported in reptiles. Recommended dose of flumazenil is 0.05 mg/kg in most cases. Lower dose (0.01 mg/kg) should be considered in large animals to reduce injection volume. Naloxone is used to antagonize morphine or hydromorphone: 0.04–0.2 mg/kg SC, IM, or IV.
*Information based on limited number of animals reported in case reports or based on anecdotal information.
[a]Hernandez-Divers SM, Proc ARAV, 2007, pp 34–35.
SC, Subcutaneous; *IM*, intramuscular; *IV*, intravenous.

space is provided in small muscle bellies for larger drug volumes when compared to the subcutaneous route. Recommended injection sites are summarized in Table 49.5. In snakes, the epaxial muscles are used, while in lizards and chelonians, muscles of the front limbs are a common intramuscular injection site but provide only limited space to administer anesthetic drugs (Fig. 49.2). The intramuscular injection of anesthetics may result in more rapid and less variable onset times compared to subcutaneous injection, depending on the drug administered. However, in red-eared sliders (*Trachemys scripta elegans*) administered dexmedetomidine-ketamine, the depth of anesthesia was not significantly different (~45 minutes) after either IM or SC injection.[1] In leopard geckos, the administration of alfaxalone-midazolam by subcutaneous injection resulted in first anesthetic effects within 5 to 10 minutes.[27] Furthermore, subcutaneous opioid absorption has been shown to be rapid in red-eared sliders.[1] Therefore the subcutaneous administration of anesthetic and analgesic drugs offers several advantages over intramuscular injection, including access to a variety of subcutaneous sites requiring minimal manual restraint or patient manipulation, suspected less discomfort on injection, and the capability of administering larger volumes in a single location (Fig. 49.3).

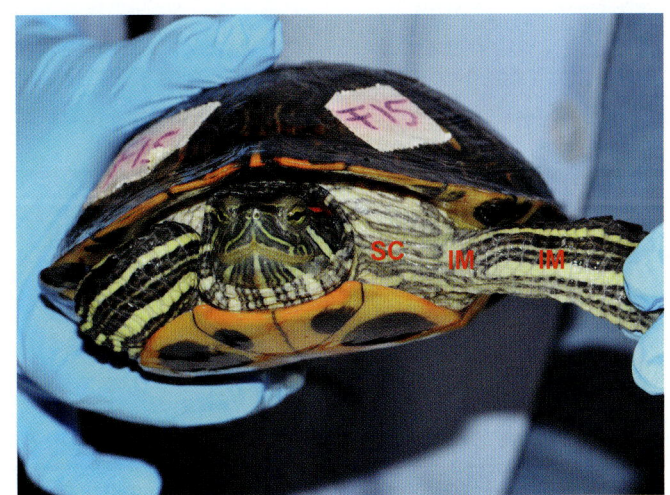

FIG 49.2 Red-eared slider turtle (*Trachemys scripta elegans*) demonstrating injection sites in the front half of the body. The SC (subcutaneous) site highlights the skin between the forelimb and neck. The IM (intramuscular) site highlights the muscle bellies of the forelimb.

TABLE 49.2   Anesthetic Protocols Reported in Lizards

Protocol	Species	Dose (mg/kg)	Route	Comments
Alfaxalone	Bearded dragon (*Pogona vitticeps*), Chinese water dragons (*Physignathus cocincinus*)[77]	5	IV	Induction agent, allows for endotracheal intubation in all animals. Loss of righting reflex within 12–45 seconds.
	Veiled chameleon (*Chamaeleo calyptratus*)[a]	5	IV	Surgical anesthesia within 2 minutes. Duration of maximum effect 5–10 minutes. Intubation possible in 100%. Recovery by 20 ± 5 minutes. Animals received butorphanol (2 mg/kg IM) prior to induction.
	Australian lizards[55]	9	IV	Moderate sedation—light anesthesia in most species; duration of effect <30 minutes, intubation possible, apnea reported, maintain with gaseous anesthetic if needed.
	Green iguana (*Iguana iguana*)[78]	5	IV	Surgical anesthesia within <1 minute. Duration of maximum effect 2–9 minutes. Intubation possible in 100%. Recovery by 14 ± 4 minutes.
	Green iguana[54]	10	IM	Light-moderate sedation within 8 ± 2 minutes. Duration of maximum effect 11 ± 4 minutes. Intubation possible in 40%. Recovery by 29 ± 36 minutes at 28°C–32°C.
		20	IM	Light anesthesia within 5 ± 2 minutes. Duration of maximum effect 22 ± 7 minutes. Intubation possible in 100%. Recovery by 45 ± 8 minutes at 28°C–32°C.
		30	IM	Surgical anesthesia within 4 ± 1 minutes. Duration of maximum effect 39 ± 12 minutes. Intubation possible in 100%. Recovery by 68 ± 9 minutes at 28°C–32°C.
	Leopard gecko (*Eublepharis macularius*)[27]	10–20	SC	Light-moderate sedation, inconsistent effects.
	Bearded dragon (*Pogona vitticeps*)[b]	20	SC	Light anesthesia within 5–10 minutes. Righting reflex lost and intubation possible. Maintained spontaneous respiration. Duration of maximum effect for ~30–45 minutes. Recovery by ~60 minutes at 25°C.
Alfaxalone + midazolam	Leopard gecko[27]	15 (A) + 1 (Mi)	SC	Moderate sedation, intubation possible in 33%, prolonged recovery (56 ± 29 minutes) after reversal with flumazenil at 26.0°C–28.0°C.
Dexmedetomidine + ketamine	Bearded dragon[b]	0.1 (D) + 20 (K)	SC	Light—surgical anesthesia within 5–20 minutes. Righting and limb withdrawal reflexes lost. Spontaneous breathing maintained. Reversed after 45 minutes. Recovered by 10–20 minutes after reversal at 25°C.
	Leopard gecko[18]	0.1 (D) + 10 (K)	IM/SC	Light anesthesia within 5–10 minutes. Righting reflex absent. Reversed after 45 minutes. Recovery by ~ 15 minutes at 26.0°–28.0°C.
Dexmedetomidine + midazolam	Bearded dragon[b]	0.1 (D) + 1 (Mi)	SC	Moderate sedation within 10–20 minutes. Righting reflex maintained, intubation not consistently possible.
	Leopard gecko[27]	0.1 (D) + 1 (Mi)	SC	Moderate sedation, intubation possible in 33%, completely reversible; rapid recovery by 6.1 ± 2.2 minutes after reversal with flumazenil + atipamezole at 26.0°–28.0°C.
Dexmedetomidine + ketamine + midazolam	Bearded dragon[b]	0.1 (D) + 10 (K) + 1 (Mi)	SC	Light—surgical anesthesia within 10–20 minutes. Righting and limb withdrawal reflexes lost. Spontaneous breathing maintained. Reversed with flumazenil and atipamezole after 45 minutes. Recovered by 10–20 minutes after reversal at 25°C.
	Bearded dragon, Uromastyx, blue iguana[76]*	0.05–0.1 (D) + 3 (K) + 1 (Mi)	SC	Deep sedation–light anesthesia, intubation possible, partially reversible; rapid recovery after reversal. Righting and limb withdrawal reflexes lost.
Isoflurane	Green iguana[59,60]			MAC: 2.0% ± 0.6 %, 1.8% ± 0.3%
	Dumeril's monitor (*Varanus dumerilii*)[79]			MAC: 1.54% ± 0.17%
Propofol	Green iguana[37,80,81]	5–10	IV, IO	Induction agent, apnea common, requires intubation and IPPV.
Sevoflurane	Green iguana[59]			MAC: 3.1% ± 1.0%
	Dumeril's monitor[82]			MAC: 2.51° ± 0.46%
Zolazepam-Tiletamine (Telazol)	Green iguana[83]	10.5 ± 4.2	IM	Light anesthesia, induction by 6.5 ± 0.7 minutes, intubation possible, initial excitement phase, long recovery times
	Large lizards[81]	5–10	IM	Premedication

Atipamezole is usually dosed at 10 times the amount of dexmedetomidine or 5 times the amount of medetomidine in mg. Lower doses of atipamezole have been reported in reptiles. Recommended dose of flumazenil is 0.05 mg/kg in most cases. Lower dose (0.01 mg/kg) should be considered in large animals to reduce injection volume. Nalaxone is used to antagonize morphine or hydromorphone: 0.04–0.2 mg/kg SC, IM, or IV.
*Information based on limited number of animals reported in case reports or based on anecdotal information.
[a]Knotek Z, Proc ARAV, 2011, p 179.
[b]Mans C, unpublished data

IM, Intramuscular; *IO,* intraosseous; *IPPV,* intermittent positive pressure ventilation; *IV,* intravenous; *MAC,* minimum anesthetic concentration; *SC,* subcutaneous.

TABLE 49.3 Anesthetic Protocols Reported in Snakes

Protocol	Species	Dose (mg/kg)	Route	Comments
Alfaxalone	Australian snakes[55]	9	IV	Light anesthesia, intubation possible
	Ball python (*Python regius*)[a]	5	SC	Light anesthesia, loss of righting reflex, intubation possible
Alfaxalone + midazolam	Ball python[b]	5 (A) + 0.5 (Mi)	SC	Light anesthesia, intubation possible
Dexmedetomidine + midazolam	Ball python[b]	0.1 (D) + 0.5 (Mi)	SC	Light anesthesia, intubation possible
Isoflurane	Radiated rat snake (*Elaphe radiata*)[c]			MAC: 1.68% ± 0.30%
Midazolam	Most species[36]*	1–2	SC, IM	Mild sedation, inconsistent effects
Ketamine	Most species[38]*	5–10	SC, IM	Mild-moderate sedation, endotracheal intubation
Propofol	Most species[36,37]*	3–5	IV	Moderate sedation—light anesthesia
	Most species[35,41,92,96]	5–10	IV, IC	Induction agent, short-term anesthesia, maintain with gaseous anesthetic is needed
Sevoflurane	Radiated rat snake[c]			MAC: 2.42% ± 0.57%
Telazol	Most species[36]*	2–6	IM	Induction agent; maintain with gaseous anesthetic
Zolazepam-Tiletamine (Telazol)	Large snakes[38,81]*	2–5	SC, IM	Mild-moderate sedation, endotracheal intubation
		5–10	IM	Moderate sedation

Atipamezole is usually dosed at 10 times the amount of dexmedetomidine or 5 times the amount of medetomidine in mg. Lower doses of atipamezole have been reported in reptiles. Recommended dose of flumazenil is 0.05 mg/kg in most cases. Lower dose (0.01 mg/kg) should be considered in large animals to reduce injection volume. Nalaxone is used to antagonize morphine or hydromorphone: 0.04–0.2 mg/kg SC, IM, or IV.
[a]Yaw T, Proc ARAV, 2017, p 145.
[b]Yaw T, Proc ARAV, 2017, p 144.
[c]Maas A, Proc ARAV, 2002, pp 306–307.
*Information based on limited number of animals reported in case reports or based on anecdotal information.
IM, Intramuscular; *IV,* intravenous; *SC,* subcutaneous.

TABLE 49.4 Anesthetic Protocols in Crocodilians

Protocol	Species	Dose (mg/kg)	Route	Comments
Alfaxalone	Australian freshwater crocodile (*C. johnstoni*)	3	IV	Light anesthesia for 25 (10–55) minutes at 22°C. Induction agent. Administered in dorsal occipital sinus.
	Estuarine crocodiles (*C. porosus*)[8]	3	IV	Light anesthesia for 30 (10–60) minutes at 22°C. Induction agent. Administered in dorsal occipital sinus.
	Johnson river crocodile (*C. johnstoni*)[84]	4	IV	Surgical anesthesia for 40–60 minutes. Administered in dorsal occipital sinus.
Isoflurane	Most species[85]*	1-5%		2%–3% for maintenance. Prolonged recovery possible, which can be shortened by administration of epinephrine 0.1 mg/kg IM.[86]
Ketamine + medetomidine	American alligator (*Alligator mississippiensis*)	10 (K) + 0.1 (Me)	IM	Juvenile animals required higher doses compared to adults.
Ketamine + xylazine	Most species[85]*	7.5–10 (K) + 1–2 (X)	IM	Reversal with yohimbine at 0.1 mg/kg IM.
	Broad-snouted caiman (*Caiman latirostris*)[19]	30 + 1	IM	
Medetomidine	Australian freshwater (*C. johnstoni*) and estuarine crocodiles (*C. porous*)[7]	0.5	IM	Moderate sedation. Rapid recovery after reversal with atipamezole.
Propofol	Most species[85]*	3–10	IV	Start at low dose, administer to effect until intubation is possible. Apnea possible.
Zolazepam-Tiletamine (Telazol)	Most species[85,87]*	5–15	IM	Prolonged recovery possible.

Atipamezole is usually dosed at 10 times the amount of dexmedetomidine or 5 times the amount of medetomidine in mg. Lower doses of atipamezole have been reported in reptiles. Recommended dose of flumazenil is 0.05 mg/kg in most cases. Lower dose (0.01 mg/kg) should be considered in large animals to reduce injection volume.
*Information based on limited number of animals reported in case reports or based on anecdotal information.
IM, Intramuscular; *IV,* intravenous.

TABLE 49.5   Preferred Anesthetic and Analgesic Injection Sites in Reptiles

Chelonia

SC drug administration sites include the skin between the neck and forelimbs.

IM drug administration sites include the forelimb and pectoral muscles.

IV access recommended includes the jugular vein, brachial vein, or ventral coccygeal vein.

Lizards

SC drug administration sites include the dorsum, overlying the epaxial muscles. Stay in the cranial half of the body.

IM drug administration sites include the forelimb and epaxial muscles in the cranial half of the body.

IV access includes the ventral coccygeal vein (i.e., ventral tail vein), jugular vein, ventral abdominal vein, and cephalic vein.

IO administration requires catheterization of the distal femur or proximal tibia.

Snakes

SC drug administration sites include the dorsum, overlying the epaxial muscles. Stay in the cranial half of the body.

IM drug administration sites include the epaxial muscles in the cranial half of the body.

IV access includes the ventral coccygeal vein (i.e., ventral tail vein) and the palatine veins in the oral cavity of larger species.

IM, Intramuscular; *IO*, intraosseous; *IV*, intravenous; *SC*, subcutaneous.

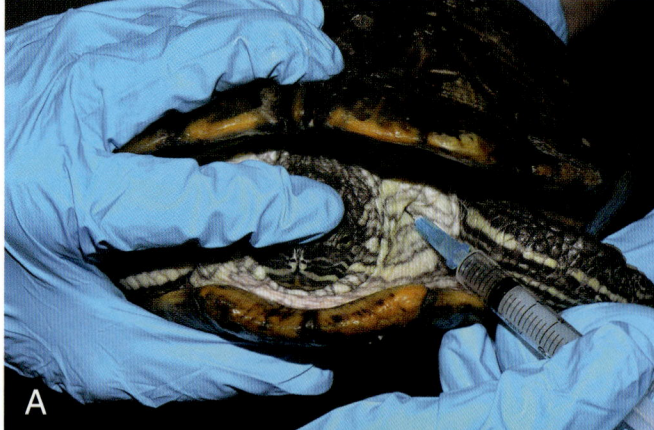

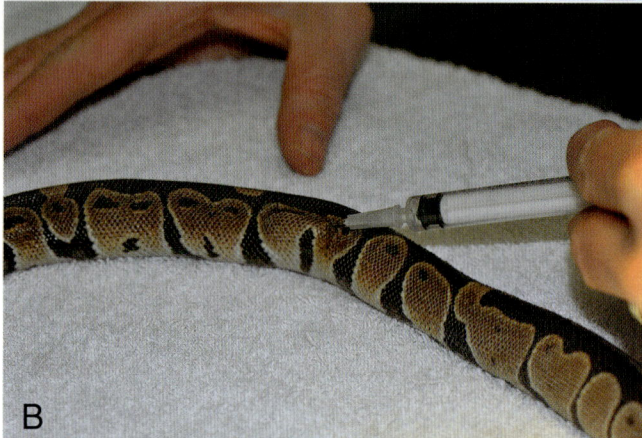

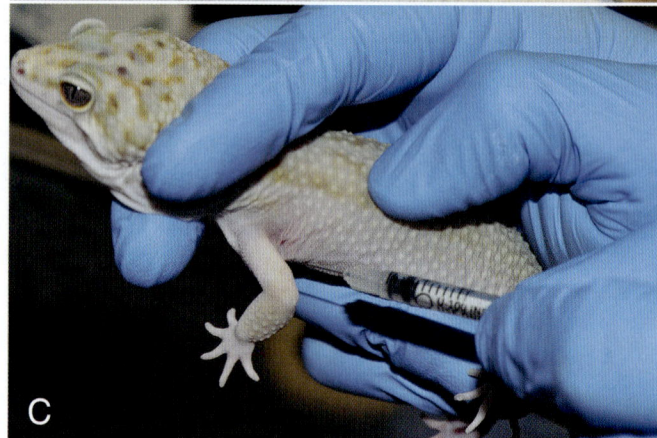

FIG 49.3 Subcutaneous drug administration in reptiles: (A) Red-eared slider (*Trachemys scripta elegans*), (B) ball python (*Python regius*), and (C) leopard gecko (*Eublepharis macularius*).

The intravenous route offers an excellent route of administration for anesthetic agents and results in rapid onset of anesthesia. However, depending on the species, patient size, and level of cooperation, intravenous access may be challenging or impossible to obtain, making the subcutaneous or intramuscular route more feasible. In lizards, intravenous injections are most commonly administered into the caudal (ventral tail) vein (Fig. 49.4). In most tortoises and nonmarine turtles, the jugular vein is preferred for intravenous drug administration, but the brachial plexus is also practical. The subcarapacial sinus and dorsal coccygeal vein cannot be recommended for intravenous drug administration in chelonians due to the risk of accidental administration of anesthetic agents into the intrathecal space, which may lead to severe neurologic complications including permanent paralysis and death.[28,29] In addition, the dorsal coccygeal vein is not consistently developed across chelonian species, and while present in red-eared sliders, it is absent or poorly developed in several tortoise species. Therefore it should be assumed that a well-developed dorsal coccygeal vein is the exception, rather than the rule, among chelonians. Hence, the authors advise against drug administration into the subcarapacial sinus or the dorsal tail vein in chelonians. Intravenous injection sites in snakes are limited to the caudal (ventral tail) vein and the jugular vein following a cut-down procedure. Intracardiac administration of propofol has also been reported in snakes and results in rapid onset with no significant complications reported in a controlled study.[30] However, cardiac tamponade after cardiocentesis in snakes has been reported, and the increased risk of intracardiac injections should be considered.[31]

Intranasal administration of anesthetic agents has been investigated in chelonians.[32,33] Intranasal administration of dexmedetomidine (0.2 mg/kg) and ketamine (10 mg/kg) only induced mild to moderate sedation in yellow-bellied sliders (*Trachemys scripta scripta*) at dosages that would

result in surgical anesthesia if administered IM or SC.[33] In red-eared sliders, the complete intranasal delivery of dexmedetomidine (0.1 mg/kg) and ketamine (10 mg/kg) was not possible due to the exhibited defense behavior of the turtles, and anesthesia was not induced (in contrast to IM or SC injection of the same doses of drugs). However, for administration of atipamezole in anesthetized red-eared sliders the intranasal route has been shown to be as effective as the IM or SC routes. In large chelonians in particular, large volumes of the anesthetic agent are a limiting factor.

As mentioned above, all IM or SC injectable anesthetic or analgesic agents should be administered in the cranial body half in order to avoid

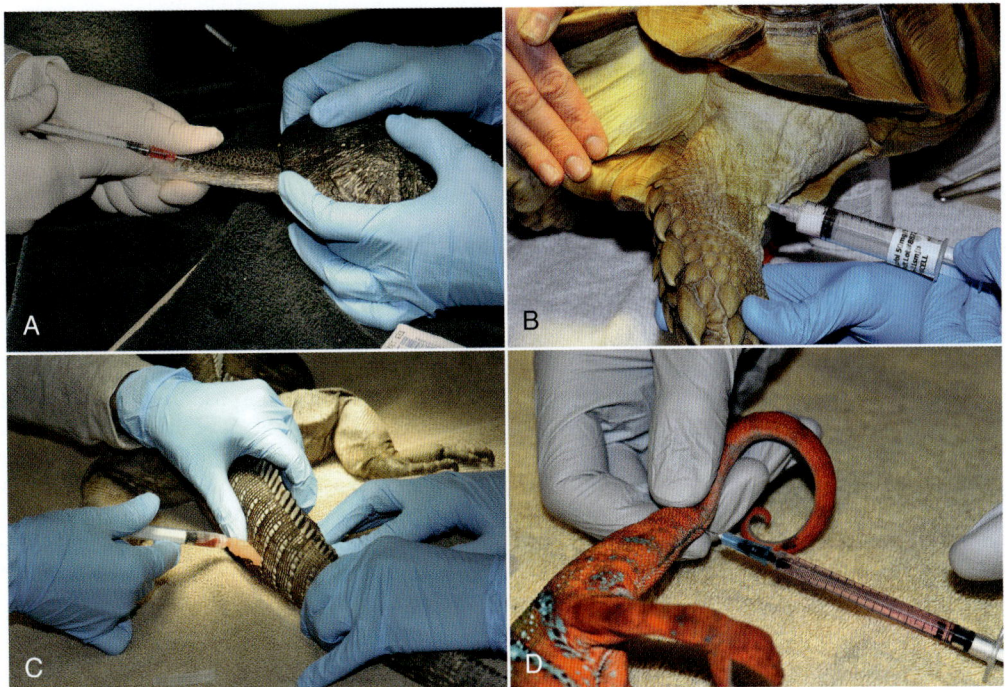

FIG 49.4 Intravenous drug administration in reptiles. (A) Intravenous injection in the left jugular vein of a side-necked turtle (Pleurodira). (B) Intravenous propofol administration in the left brachial plexus of a sedated African spurred tortoise (*Centrochelys sulcata*). (C) Lateral approach to the ventral coccygeal vein in a blue iguana (*Cyclura lewisi*). (D) Ventral approach to the ventral coccygeal vein in a panther chameleon (*Furcifer pardalis*).

a hepatic first pass effect and reduced or lack of anesthetic/analgesic effects.[16,18]

Drugs

Ketamine, a dissociative agent with dose-dependent anesthetic, sedative, and analgesic properties, is frequently used in reptile anesthesia. However, when administered alone, muscle relaxation is considered inadequate and recoveries excessively prolonged, especially when high dosages (>50 mg/kg) are used. Administration of an α-2-adrenergic agonist (e.g., dexmedetomidine) and/or a benzodiazepine (e.g., midazolam), in conjunction with ketamine, allows for reduction of ketamine dose. Additionally, these protocols have the benefit of partial reversibility, leading to more rapid recoveries and increased safety (see Tables 49.1 to 49.4). Even at lower, subanesthetic dosages (<5 mg/kg), ketamine can provide additional sedation and analgesia if combined with other anesthetic drugs.[34,35]

Tiletamine/zolazepam is a commercially available drug combination, which is composed of the dissociative anesthetic, tiletamine, and a benzodiazepine, zolazepam. Dosages of 2 to 10 mg/kg have been recommended for sedation, induction of general anesthesia, or facilitation of intubation.[36-38] The anesthetic efficacy of tiletamine/zolazepam can be unpredictable and recovery may be prolonged. In dehydrated patients, or those with underlying renal or metabolic disorders, the use of this drug combination is contraindicated.[37] Tiletamine/zolazepam is also useful in large or dangerous species (e.g., crocodilians, large monitor lizards, etc), especially when remote darting techniques are required (see Tables 49.1 to 49.4).

α-2-adrenergic agonists, such as medetomidine and dexmedetomidine, provide sedation, muscle relaxation, and analgesia in reptiles. Dose-dependent cardiovascular depression was documented in reptiles after α-2 agonist administration.[18,39-41] α-2-adrenergic agonists are commonly used in combination with ketamine, especially in chelonians, for safe, reliable, and reversible anesthesia, but can also be combined with benzodiazepines for procedural sedation.[24,25,27,42,43] Combining ketamine with medetomidine, or dexmedetomidine, allows reduction of both drug dosages, and reversibility of the α-2-adrenergic agonist with atipamezole will lead to faster and more predictable recoveries. Morphine or hydromorphone can be added to α-2 adrenergic agonist plus ketamine protocols in cases in which analgesia is needed.[23,25,26,44] If morphine is used, reversal with naloxone (0.04–0.2 mg/kg, SC) should be considered if respiratory depression persists after termination of the anesthetic procedure or recovery is delayed. In gopher tortoises anesthetized with dexmedetomidine-ketamine-morphine, administration of naloxone was not necessary, and animals recovered within ~90 minutes after administration of atipamezole.[44] Concentrated formulations of medetomidine (e.g., 20 mg/ml, Zoopharm Inc) are available and are more suitable for giant species, such as large chelonians, crocodilians, and komodo dragons (*Varanus komodoensis*).

Benzodiazepines, such as midazolam and diazepam, have sedative and muscle-relaxant properties. Midazolam is water soluble; can be administered SC, IM, and IV; and is considered a more appropriate choice than diazepam, which is not recommended for IM or SC injection.[9] Midazolam, used alone, is anxiolytic and provides mild, but highly variable, sedation, which may be sufficient for minor clinical procedures.[45-47] Midazolam, combined with ketamine and/or an α-2-adrenergic agonist, reduces all drug dosages and attenuates the dose-dependent cardiovascular depressant effects and prolonged recoveries commonly observed with high dosages of ketamine. Midazolam (1 mg/kg) has also been combined with alfaxalone (15 mg/kg) for subcutaneous administration in leopard geckos, and provides improved anesthesia, instead of using alfaxalone alone at higher doses (see Table 49.2). The effects of benzodiazepines can be antagonized using flumazenil (0.05 mg/kg, SC, IM), which shortens recovery from sedation or anesthesia.[27,48] Concentrated formulations of midazolam (e.g., 50 mg/ml, Zoopharm Inc) are available and are more suitable for administration of midazolam in giant reptile species.

Propofol, a short-acting, nonbarbiturate anesthetic agent can be administered intravenously or intraosseously to provide short-time anesthesia, facilitating procedures such as placement of an esophagostomy tube or abscess debridement, or to induce general anesthesia and allow for endotracheal intubation and maintenance of anesthesia with an inhalational agent. Respiratory depression is more profound when propofol is administered rapidly.[37,49] Since propofol does not accumulate in tissues and is rapidly metabolized, recovery can be expected with assisted ventilation in cases of overdose. Propofol requires intravascular administration, which can be challenging. Recently, published reports have described complications secondary to accidental extravascular injection of propofol intrathecally and into the subcarapacial sinus or the coccygeal vein of chelonian species.[28,29] Complications associated with intrathecal propofol injection included fore and hind limb paralysis, coma, and spinal necrosis.[28,29] In addition, complications with propofol in sea turtles were reported, which included respiratory arrest and death several hours post anesthesia (Mader: Pers. comm.). Two different formulations are available. The original preservative-free formulation should be discarded within 6 hrs of first use, while a newer formulation, containing 2% benzyl alcohol, can be used for up to 28 days after initial use.

Alfaxalone is a short-acting steroid anesthetic, which is labeled for induction of anesthesia in dogs by intravenous administration. However, alfaxalone can be administered by either the intramuscular or subcutaneous route at higher doses. Alfaxalone is rapidly cleared and its metabolism is independent of organ function; however, pronounced temperature-dependent difference in anesthetic induction, plateau, and recovery times have been reported.[6] Similar to propofol, alfaxalone administration is associated with dose-dependent cardiovascular and respiratory depression in mammals.[50–52] Recovery from alfaxalone induced anesthesia is dose-dependent, and at high dosages, prolonged recoveries are to be expected.[27,53] The major advantage of alfaxalone over propofol is that it can be administered intramuscularly as well as subcutaneously, in addition to the intravenous route.[6,27,50,54,55] Due to the high dosages needed for nonintravenous administration in chelonians and lizards, the resulting drug volumes are usually inappropriately large due to the low concentration of the available alfaxalone formulation (10 mg/mL). Therefore the authors recommend SC injection if large volumes of alfaxalone are to be administered. The subcutaneous administration of alfaxalone in reptiles has been associated with rapid induction times. In the United States, the USDA mandates that, following initial use, any unused drug must be discarded after 6 hours and cannot be stored.

The intravenous administration of alfaxalone in green iguanas (*Iguana iguana*) (10 mg/kg) and red-eared sliders (5 mg/kg) resulted in rapid induction of light to surgical anesthesia, which allowed endotracheal intubation.[55,56] Alfaxalone can be administered by subcutaneous administration, which results in comparable onset of effects as after intramuscular injection (see Table 49.2). Since large volumes usually need to be administered, the subcutaneous route should be used. The effects of intramuscular administration of alfaxalone was investigated in red-eared sliders, Russian (Horsfield's) tortoises (*Agrionemys horsfieldii*), and green iguanas (see Tables 49.1 and 49.2).[6,54,57] Induction times ranged between 5 to 15 minutes following intramuscular alfaxalone administration.[6,54] The induction times after intramuscular administration in green iguanas were short (approximately 5–10 minutes at 24°–27°C, 75°–81°F) and recovery was smooth. The induction and duration of effect following intramuscular administration were significantly shorter

at 35°C (95°F) compared with 20°C (68°F) in red-eared sliders.[6] At 20 mg/kg IM, the induction times were 19 ± 6 (20°C, 68°F) and 7 ± 5 minutes (35°C, 95°F), and the plateau phase lasted 28 ± 13 (20°C, 68°F) and 8 ± 5 (35°C, 95°F) minutes.[6] Recovery times following intramuscular administration were prolonged, in particular at room temperature, lasting approximately 60 to 90 minutes following 10 mg/kg IM and 2 hours or longer after 20 mg/kg IM at room temperature.[6,54] Increasing body temperature to 35°C (95°F) significantly shortened recovery times in red-eared sliders by >50%.[6] Green iguanas maintained at 28° to 32°C (82°–90°F) body temperature displayed a dose-dependent recovery between approximately 10 to 30 minutes after intramuscular administration of alfaxalone (10–30 mg/kg).[54]

Alfaxalone has been used in other species in combination with other drugs such as butorphanol, dexmedetomidine, and midazolam. In reptiles, the combined use of alfaxalone with medetomidine (0.1 mg/kg) was evaluated in Russian (Horsfield's) tortoises and resulted in deep anesthesia and cardiovascular depression (severe if combined with high doses of alfaxalone).[58] In leopard geckos, alfaxalone (15 mg/kg), in combination with midazolam (1 mg/kg), given by subcutaneous injection was evaluated.[27] This combination resulted in deep anesthesia with no clinically significant cardiovascular depression and allowed for use of lower alfaxalone doses, since 10 and 20 mg/kg of alfaxalone did not result in consistent chemical restraint in this species.[27] However, compared to dexmedetomidine-midazolam (0.1 + 1 mg/kg SC) the alfaxalone-midazolam protocol resulted in much longer recovery times.[27]

Inhalational agents, such as isoflurane and sevoflurane, can be used for both induction and maintenance of anesthesia. Both agents offer the advantages of relatively fast induction and recovery times, as well as limited organ toxicity, especially in patients with renal or hepatic impairment. Sevoflurane is commonly used in human and domestic animal anesthesia, has a low blood solubility, and a rapid increase in alveolar concentration can be observed during induction with this agent. The low blood solubility allows for rapid changes in anesthetic depth. Investigations of sevoflurane in various reptile species have shown variable results, with some species not achieving a surgical plane of anesthesia. Few studies have investigated comparative cardiopulmonary effects of sevoflurane versus isoflurane in reptiles. Administration of inhalational agents follows similar principles as those established for domestic animal anesthesia. Following induction of anesthesia, the trachea should be intubated with an appropriately sized endotracheal tube, which should be connected to a nonrebreathing (body weight <10 kg) or rebreathing system. Intermittent positive pressure ventilation should be performed in all reptiles. The concentration of the inhalational agent necessary to maintain a surgical plane of anesthesia depends on the health status of the patient. Minimum anesthetic concentrations (MAC) of isoflurane and sevoflurane were determined in green iguanas and are 1.8% to 2.1% and 2.1% to 4.1%, respectively.[59,60] Maintenance requirements for a surgical plane of anesthesia were reported to be 2% to 3% for isoflurane and 3.5% to 4.5% for sevoflurane.[36] Both isoflurane and sevoflurane have a dose-dependent, depressive effect on the cardiovascular system. Isoflurane was shown to significantly reduce blood pressure in green iguanas and ball pythons.[61,62] Therefore significant cardiovascular depression can occur with normal maintenance concentrations of isoflurane. No significant differences were detected between sevoflurane and isoflurane in cardiopulmonary function of green iguanas.[63] However, use of sevoflurane resulted in faster induction and recovery compared with isoflurane.[63]

Due to right-to-left cardiac shunting in some reptiles, reduced lung perfusion can occur, and therefore concentrations of inhalant anesthetic gases in the lungs do not necessarily reflect the concentrations in the blood or brain.[9] Sudden changes in shunting directions can lead to sudden changes in inhalant anesthetic blood concentration, which can lead to significant changes in anesthetic depth, evidenced by slow induction, sudden arousal from anesthesia, inability to deepen a lightly anesthetized reptile, or prolonged recovery from anesthesia.[1] In lizards and snakes, changes in gas concentration can be used to control anesthetic depth, but in chelonians, particularly aquatic turtles, a change in gas concentration will not lead to measurable changes in anesthetic depth as a function of cardiac shunting, breath-holding ability, and ventilation-perfusion mismatch.[1]

GENERAL ANESTHESIA

Induction

Induction of anesthesia can be accomplished with injectable or inhalational agents. In patients with established, reliable vascular access, slow administration of propofol (3–10 mg/kg IV, IO) or alfaxalone (5–10 mg/kg IV) will induce rapid induction of anesthesia (see Fig. 49.3 and 49.4). Alternately, intramuscular or subcutaneous administration of various combinations of ketamine, midazolam, α-2-agents, alfaxalone, and opioids will induce a dose-dependent plane of anesthesia adequate for endotracheal intubation and maintenance with an inhalational agent, if required. Mask or chamber induction with an inhalational agent can be used in snakes and lizards, and for handler safety reasons these are particularly useful in venomous species (Fig. 49.5). Mask or chamber inductions require high concentrations of gas anesthetic, which is associated with environmental contamination and can contribute to unpredictable and prolonged induction times. In monitor lizards, induction times of >10 minutes were noted following isoflurane and sevoflurane delivery by mask.[64] In reptile species that are able to breath-hold for extended periods, in particular semiaquatic and aquatic turtles and crocodilians, induction times will be prolonged and/or induction with inhalant agents may be ineffective.

Endotracheal intubation is relatively easy to perform in most snakes and lizards. In these species, the glottis is located rostrally in the oral cavity, and the trachea can be intubated with an appropriate-sized endotracheal tube (Fig. 49.6). Most chelonians have a fleshy tongue, and the glottis is located at the base of the tongue, thus making visualization difficult. Good muscle relaxation is necessary to open the mouth wide enough to visualize the glottis and intubate the trachea. Care should be taken not to intubate the left or right primary bronchus since the tracheal bifurcation is cranial in some chelonians. In crocodilians, the glottis is located behind the epiglottal (gular) flap, which has to be reflected ventrally to visualize the glottis and allow for intubation (Fig. 49.7). The reptile glottis is only opened during active respiration and is therefore likely to remain closed for prolonged periods following induction. A stylet may help in advancing the endotracheal tube through the closed glottis.

Securing the endotracheal tube is critical (Fig. 49.8) to avoid accidental extubation during anesthesia and excessive movement, which could lead to irritation of the tracheal mucosa. In some species, a mouth gag should be used to protect the endotracheal tube (see Fig. 49.1A) and

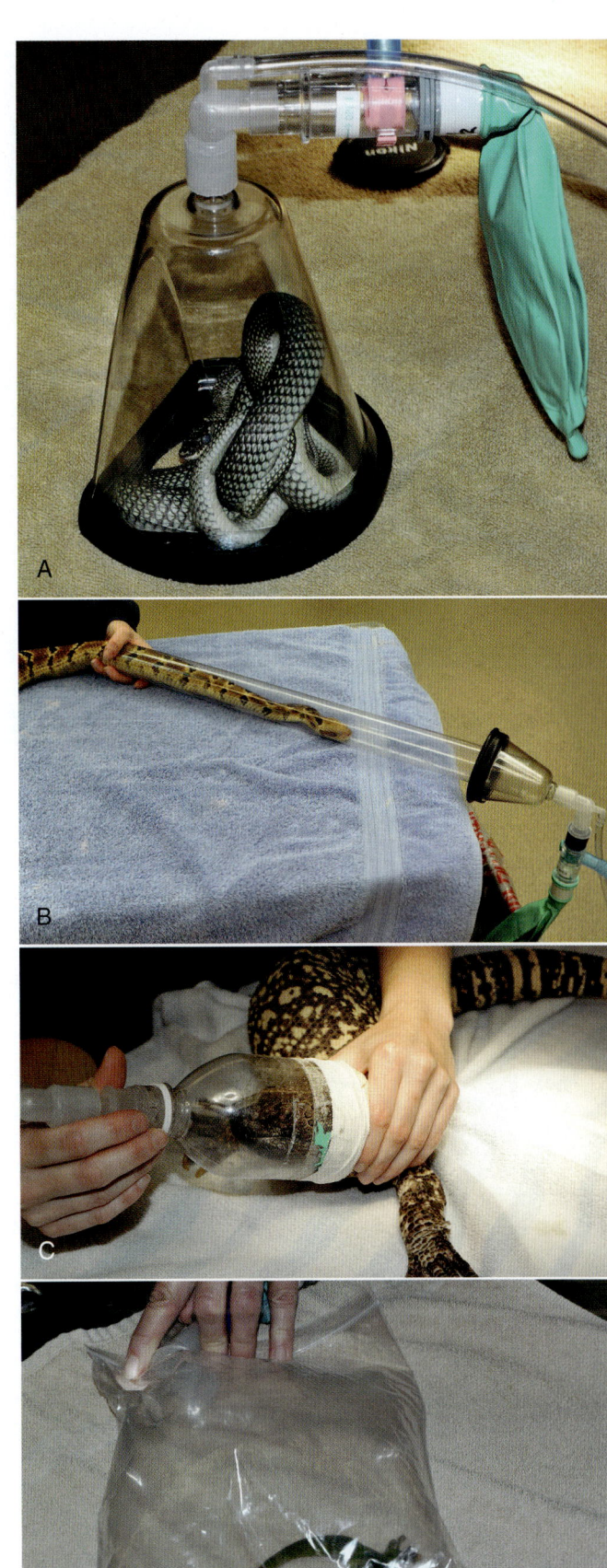

FIG 49.5 Anesthetic chamber and mask induction in reptiles. (A) Anesthetic induction of a snake using a canine face mask. (B) Induction of an Eastern massasauga rattlesnake (*Sistrurus catenatus catenatus*) in a snake tube attached to an anesthesia mask. (C) Mask induction a beaded lizard (*Heloderma horridum*). (D) Use of a resealable zipper storage bag for anesthetic induction of a Madagascan day gecko (*Phelsuma madagascariensis*). The bag is filled with anesthetic gas delivered in oxygen, and the bag is sealed.

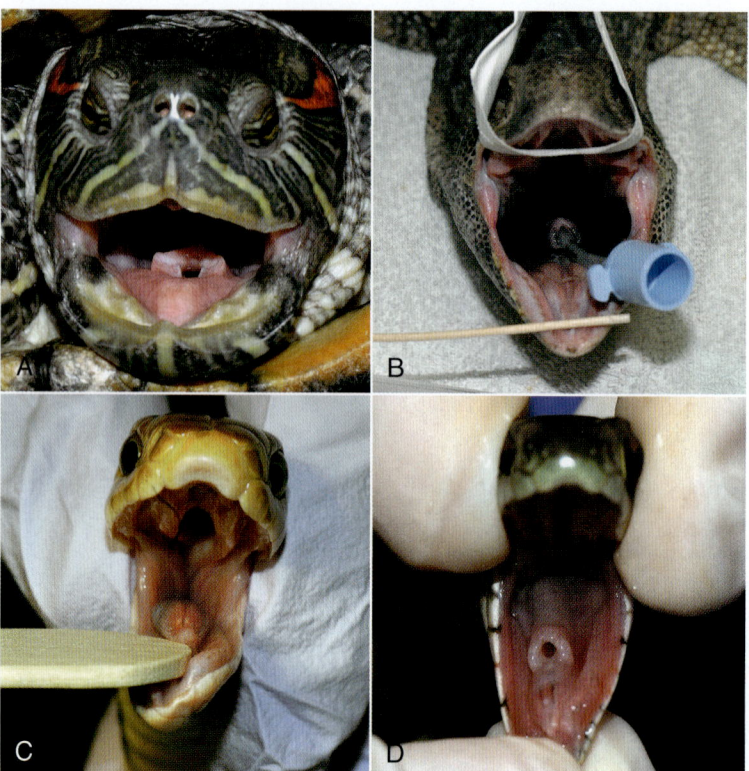

FIG 49.6 (A) Glottis of a red-eared slider (*Trachemys scripta elegans*). (B) Intubation of a savannah monitor (*Varanus exanthematicus*) with an uncuffed endotracheal tube. (C and D) Glottis of colubrid snakes in closed (C) and open (D) positions.

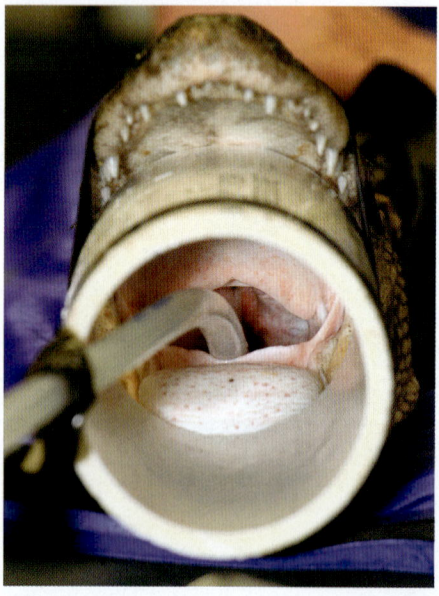

FIG 49.7 Intubation of a juvenile American alligator (*Alligator mississippiensis*). Note that the epiglottic flap has been dislodged ventrally to allow for endotracheal intubation. (Courtesy of Grayson Doss).

facilitate placement of monitoring devices (e.g., pulse oximeter probe). The trachea in chelonians has complete cartilaginous rings, while in lizards and snakes the cartilaginous rings are incomplete. Uncuffed endotracheal tubes are recommended in chelonians and in small lizards and snakes. In larger squamates, cuffed tubes can be used. It is important

to use the widest endotracheal tube possible, especially in smaller reptiles, to reduce airway resistance ($Resistance \propto 1/r^4$) and anesthetic gas leakage.

Maintenance

During maintenance of anesthesia the patient should be monitored regularly for depth of anesthesia, cardiopulmonary performance, and evidence of pain. If indicated, the anesthetic level should be adjusted and additional analgesic therapy may be warranted. Similar to domestic animals, cardiopulmonary depression is dose dependent in reptiles, and a decrease in heart rate and arterial blood pressure will be observed, although blood pressure monitoring is difficult and frequently impractical.

All reptiles require intermittent positive pressure ventilation (IPPV) at a surgical plane of anesthesia to maintain $EtCO_2$ between 10 and 25 mm Hg. Overventilation (decreased $EtCO_2$) causes respiratory alkalosis and delays return to spontaneous ventilation during recovery. Ventilation can be performed manually or more accurately with a mechanical ventilator (Fig. 49.9). Any anesthetized reptile that is breathing spontaneously is light. Pressure-driven ventilators are commercially available (e.g., SAV04 Vetronic Services, Ltd, UK, http://www.vetronic.co.uk/products/article/sav04; Small Animal Ventilator, Vetronics, BASi US, https://www.basinc.com/products/vetronics/products/smvent), which will accurately ventilate even small reptilian patients. To avoid overinflation of the lungs and air sacs, inspiratory pressure should not exceed 12 cm H_2O. While anecdotally, it has been recommended to ventilate anesthetized reptiles at 4 to 6 breaths per minute, the rate of IPPV needs to be adjusted to each individual patient based on the preanesthetic examination and $EtCO_2$ values. For example, in anesthetized neotropical rattlesnakes (*Crotalus durissus*) five breaths per minute lead to respiratory alkalosis and was considered excessive, while 0.67 breaths per minute led to mild hypercapnia and mild respiratory acidosis. Therefore a

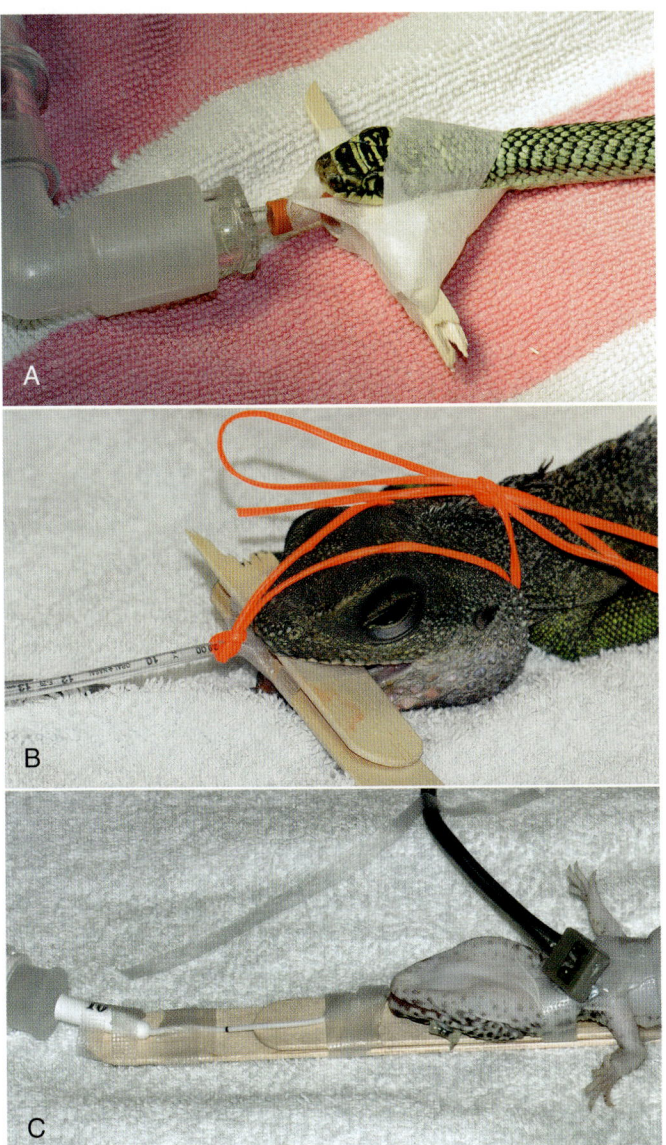

FIG 49.8 Securing endotracheal tubes in small reptile patients. (A) Tongue depressors are used (as with this colubrid snake) to protect the tube and to allow for application of tape, instead of placing it directly around the tube. (B) Tie-in technique for securing an endotracheal tube in a Chinese water dragon (*Physignathus cocincinus*). (C) In small lizards (such as this leopard gecko, *Eublepharis macularius*) and snakes a tongue depressor can be used to secure the patient and the endotracheal tube to avoid accidental extubation during anesthesia.

respiratory rate of one to two breaths per minute at a tidal volume of 30 ml/kg was recommended for this species.[65]

Intraoperative fluid therapy : Following standard practice in human and domestic animal anesthesia, intraoperative fluid therapy is recommended and anecdotally infusion rates of 3 mL/kg/hr are often suggested for reptiles, which are lower than those used for mammals (5–10 mL/kg/hr). Rates of balanced isotonic crystalloids are most frequently used (e.g., lactated ringer's solution), although specific solutions, colloids, and even blood products may be used with justifications similar to that of human and domesticated animal fluid therapy.

Depth of anesthesia: Depth of anesthesia should be evaluated regularly, and adjustments should be made if the patient is determined to be too deep or too light (Table 49.6). Response to a painful stimulus, such as

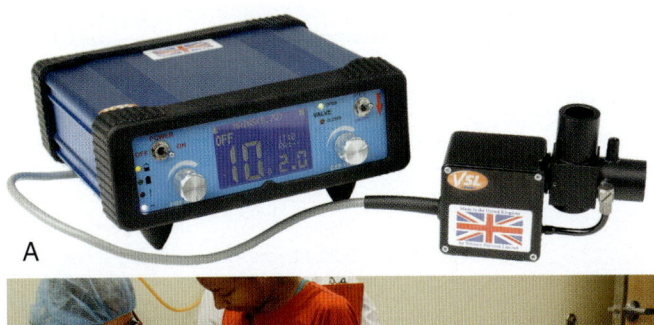

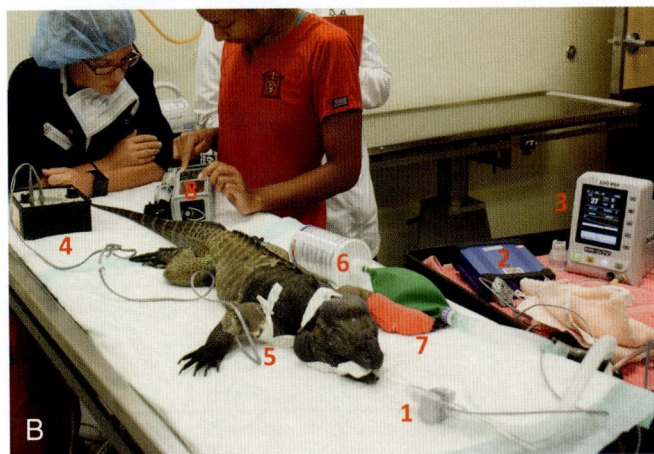

FIG 49.9 (A) The small animal ventilator (SAV4) offers accurate, consistent, uncomplicated pressure-cycled ventilation for reptiles from 35 g to 80 kg. The unit features main power and battery back-up for mobility; inspiratory time, respiratory rate, and pressure displays; overpressure and apnea alarms; and respiratory rate ranging from 1 to 120 breaths per minute with expiratory phase ranges of 0.1 to 60 seconds. (B) Large, anesthetized *Cyclura* lizard intubated (1) and connected to the SAV4 ventilator (2) with mainstream capnography and pulse oximetry unit (3); Doppler monitoring (4) with the probe placed close to the heart (5); mobile, passive scavenging of anesthetic gases using activated carbon (6); and intravenous cephalic catheterization (7) with connection to a syringe pump (8) for fluid support throughout the anesthetic event. (A, Courtesy of Keith Simpson, Vetronics Services Ltd; B, courtesy of Stephen J. Divers.)

movement and increase in heart rate, should be followed by an increase in the concentration of the inhalant anesthetic agent, or additional systemic or regional analgesic should be administered.

Body temperature: Response to anesthetic and analgesic agents is dictated by body temperature, and the reptile should be maintained within the preferred optimum temperature range prior, during, and after anesthesia.[6] A hypothermic reptile will have compromised metabolic function, and recovery from the anesthetic event will be delayed. It was demonstrated in several studies that body temperature has a profound effect on respiration, blood gases, and acid-base status in reptiles.[66,67] In freshwater turtles (*Chrysemys picta bellii*), oxygen uptake increased disproportionately when compared with pulmonary ventilation, with increasing temperatures.[66] Body temperature should be measured and recorded with an esophageal or cloacal temperature probe, not a mammalian rectal thermometer. Every effort should be made to maintain the patient in its optimal temperature range during anesthesia and the recovery period. Heat lamps, circulating water blankets, warm air blankets, and other equipment is available to accomplish this.

MONITORING TECHNIQUES

Accurate monitoring of anesthetic parameters is essential to safely and effectively anesthetize the reptilian patient. An accurate anesthesia record,

TABLE 49.6 Assessing Anesthetic Depth

Stage of Anesthesia	Behavior	Respiration	Cardiovascular Function	Response to Painful Stimuli	Depth	Muscle Tone	Reflex Response
Stage I	Disorientated	Breath hold, normal, or rarely hyperventilating	HR unchanged, may be hypertensive	Struggle	Not anesthetized	Good	All present
Stage II	Excitement, struggling	Irregular, breath hold, or hyperventilating	HR may increase, often hypertensive	Struggle	Not anesthetized	Good	All present, may be exaggerated
Stage III plane 1 (light)	Immobile	Normal, regular, or decreased	HR normal, normotensive	May respond with movement	Light	Good	Righting absent / Palpebral present may often be slowed / Limb and tongue withdrawal present / Cloacal reflex present / Corneal reflex present
Stage III plane 2 (surgical)	Immobile	Apnea	HR decreased, strong pulse, increasing hypotension	HR and blood pressure may increase	Moderate (surgical)	Relaxed	Righting absent / Palpebral absent / Limb and tongue withdrawal absent / Cloacal reflex may be present but greatly reduced / Corneal reflex present
Stage III plane 3 (deep)	Immobile	Apnea	HR decreased, pulse strength reduced, significant hypotension	None	Deep	Greatly reduced	Righting absent / Palpebral absent / Limb and tongue withdrawal absent / Cloacal reflex absent / Corneal reflex reduced or absent
Stage III plane 4	Immobile	Apnea	HR decreased to basal level, pulse weak, severe hypotension	None	Overdose	Flaccid	No reflex activity / Pupils often dilated
Stage IV	Immobile	Apnea	Cardiovascular collapse to slow intrinsic, basal HR, peripheral pulse often not appreciated	None	Dying	Flaccid	No reflex activity / Pupils widely dilated

HR, Heart rate.

including preanesthetic findings, anesthetic techniques and drugs, cardiopulmonary parameters, and recovery data, should be completed. Application and interpretation of many monitoring techniques in reptiles is in its infancy, and some devices and techniques may only be of limited value.[68] Monitoring of cardiopulmonary performance in the anesthetized reptilian patient presents challenges, and further work is needed to establish reference data for common reptile species. One should be familiar with the applications and limitations of various monitoring devices developed for human and veterinary anesthesia. Anesthesia-monitoring techniques such as pulse oximetry, arterial blood gas analysis, and capnography are commonly used in human and veterinary anesthesia, but not all have been validated for use in reptiles. In addition, reference values for common reptile species and common anesthetic protocols are scant. Therefore knowledge of the anatomy, physiology, and pathophysiology is essential. Also, the pharmacology of sedative and anesthetic agents being used, as well as their effects on cardiopulmonary performance and organ function, must be known. To accurately interpret cardiopulmonary performance, there is a need for normal values in conscious reptiles; however, few studies have investigated normal cardiopulmonary parameters in conscious, nonanesthetized reptiles. Most published reports have collected data on cardiopulmonary function from anesthetized animals. Comparison of data requires consideration of the different effects of the anesthetic agent used. A study in green iguanas determined selected cardiopulmonary values in conscious animals including respiratory rate, heart rate, and direct arterial blood pressures, as well as arterial and venous blood gas parameters.[69] In addition, the effects of 100% oxygen inspiration were measured. Comparison was also made between arterial blood gas analysis and pulse oximetry readings in conscious green iguanas. It was shown that oxygen saturation, as measured by pulse oximetry, underestimated saturation calculated by arterial blood gas analysis.[69]

Determination of the degree of sedation and depth of anesthesia is commonly performed by assessment of the presence or absence of reflexes such as head or limb withdrawal, righting reflex, palpebral and corneal reflexes, and toe/tail pinch reflex, as well as cloacal tone. However, significant anatomic differences exist between snakes, chelonians, and lizards. The corneal and palpebral reflex is present and useful in many reptiles but cannot be assessed in snakes and most geckos (one exception being leopard geckos), due to lack of eyelids and presence of spectacles. The righting reflex should be absent in snakes and lizards during a surgical plane of anesthesia but is not as useful in turtles and tortoises.[36] Assessment of head withdrawal and neck tone may provide useful information in turtles and tortoises. Snakes tend to lose muscle tone from head to tail during induction and regain muscle tone from tail to head during recovery.[37] In general, a surgical plane of anesthesia, including effective analgesia, is determined when there is no response to a painful stimulus, such as a skin incision and, consequently, no changes in cardiopulmonary parameters such as tachycardia, hypertension, or increase in respiratory rate. A classification system to determine anesthetic depth is provided in Table 49.6.

Cardiovascular Monitoring

Monitoring of cardiovascular performance is challenging in reptiles. Heart rate can be influenced by a variety of factors, including environmental temperature, metabolism, and presence of noxious stimulation.[70] Many parameters commonly recorded in mammalian species are either impractical to determine in reptiles, or reference values have not been established. Assessment of mucous membrane color and capillary perfusion time are inaccurate in reptiles, and measurement of cardiac output has limited clinical applications. The most accurate assessment of cardiac output in reptiles is determination of heart rate. An esophageal stethoscope or Doppler can be used in most reptiles for direct measurement of heart rate under anesthesia. Both tachycardia and bradycardia can decrease cardiac output and reduce flow of blood to peripheral tissues. A baroreceptor reflex has been demonstrated in conscious green iguanas.[69]

Ultrasonic Doppler flow devices are the most useful and reliable monitoring devices in reptile anesthesia and allow for noninvasive recording of heart rate and rhythm in both conscious and anesthetized animals. Values derived from the conscious patient prior to induction of anesthesia should be used as reference values during anesthesia. Flat and pencil probes are available (Figs. 49.8C and 49.10). The ultrasonic Doppler probe can be placed over the heart in snakes and lizards or over the carotid arteries in lizards and chelonians. In lizards, the heart is located cranially between the forelimbs (except in monitor lizards, Fig. 49.10B), and the probe can either be positioned ventrally on the cranial coelom or in the axillary region. In chelonians, the placement of a Doppler probe for heart rate measurement can be more challenging. Placing a flat or pencil probe on either side of the neck, at the coelomic inlet, can be effective in detecting the pulse rate via the carotid artery. If a Doppler device is not available, echocardiography, using an appropriate-sized probe/clip/needle, can serve as an effective way to monitor cardiac function and measure heart rate.

Electrocardiography (ECG) can be performed to monitor cardiac function (Fig. 49.11).[22] Unfortunately, limited data are published to establish reference parameters in commonly maintained species. The reptilian ECG is similar to a mammalian ECG with a P, QRS, and T wave, and, in some species, an SV wave is present before the P wave. Low electrical amplitudes may make interpretation of a reptilian ECG challenging. In snakes, electrodes should be attached two heart lengths cranial and caudal to the heart. In larger species, an esophageal ECG can be placed. Factors influencing heart rate, such as environmental temperature and painful stimuli, should be considered when interpreting a reptilian ECG. However, persistent baseline ECG and heart rate can also be detected in reptiles following CNS death, and therefore ECG

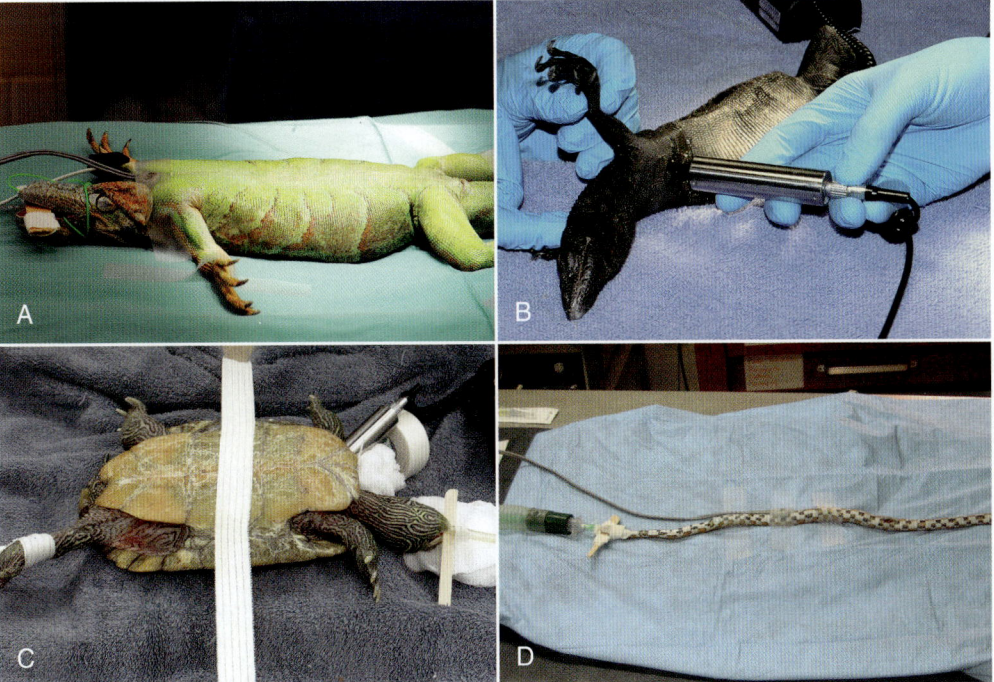

FIG 49.10 Placement of an ultrasonic Doppler flow device at the level of the heart in (A) an anesthetized green iguana (*Iguana iguana*) and (B) a black tree monitor (*Varanus beccarii*). Note that in monitor lizards the heart is located more caudad compared with other lizards, and therefore the Doppler probes are placed at different levels in these two animals. (C) Placement of an ultrasonic Doppler pencil probe in the coelomic inlet in a common map turtle (*Graptemys* spp.). (D) Placement of an ultrasonic Doppler flat probe ventrally over the heart in an anesthetized snake.

alone to monitor cardiac activity of anesthetized reptiles is of limited value, especially at a low basal rate.

Indirect blood pressure measurements are possible in many species of reptiles but have poor correlation with values obtained via direct blood pressure measurements.[61,71] Arterial blood pressure is a function of heart rate, blood volume, stroke volume, and arterial compliance. All anesthetic agents will compromise cardiovascular homeostasis to varying degrees. Direct arterial blood pressure measurements were reported in both conscious and anesthetized reptiles. Baseline arterial pressures were established in conscious green iguanas and gray rat snakes.[69,71,72] Green iguanas had lower baseline arterial blood pressures (MAP: 62 ± 12 mm Hg to 79 ± 13 mm Hg) than those reported for mammals. Direct arterial blood pressure measurements require surgical exposure of an artery, is time consuming, and therefore is largely impractical for clinical practice; however, these techniques are certainly of value for research purposes. Even though accurate pressure monitoring is not possible clinically, it is important to appreciate that reptiles maintained using inhalants are likely hypotensive. For example, compared to conscious mean arterial pressures of 79 ± 13 mmHg, iguanas anesthetized using 1.5% and 3% isoflurane were profoundly hypotensive at 47 ± 2 and 32 ± 10 mmHg, respectively.[71] Increasing blood pressure with dopamine and dopbutamine has been shown to be ineffective, but norepinephrine at 0.4 µg/mL/min resulted in normotension in anesthetized iguanas; however, clinically a more cautious rate of 0.1 µg/mL/min is used routinely (Divers, unpublished data).

Respiratory Performance

Determination of respiratory rate and effort prior to induction of anesthesia will provide valuable information with respect to the respiratory status of the patient, including evidence of underlying respiratory disease processes, and will provide baseline values for the rate of ventilation during anesthesia. Respiratory movements of the body wall in snakes and lizards can be easily visualized and measured in breaths/min if transparent drapes are used for surgery. In chelonians, movement of the skin overlying the prefemoral fossae, and at each side of the coelomic inlet, can be observed and measured during the respiratory cycle. The mean baseline respiratory rate of healthy green iguanas is 28 ± 6 breaths/min.[69] Supportive measures, such as administration of antimicrobial agents for confirmed infections, tracheal suctioning, and administration of oxygen should be initiated prior to anesthesia, if indicated. Once the reptile is anesthetized, monitoring of respiratory performance is limited to pulse oximetry, venous blood gas analysis, and capnography. Unfortunately, most devices have not been validated for reptiles but can provide valuable information on respiratory trends and metabolic status of the patient. Pulse oximetry was validated in green iguanas.[69] Inherent respiratory rate and effort cannot be determined because all reptiles require assisted ventilation during surgical anesthesia, either by means of manual ventilation or a mechanical ventilator. While the accuracy of these monitoring modalities have yet to be validated in reptiles, investigations were performed in some reptile species, mainly green iguanas, to determine usefulness and accuracy.[69]

Pulse oximetry is a noninvasive technique routinely used in mammalian patients to calculate relative arterial oxygen hemoglobin saturation (SpO_2). Accuracy of pulse oximetry is influenced by poor tissue perfusion, as well as pigmentation of the skin. In reptile anesthesia, use of pulse oximetry is associated with several concerns and potential erroneous readings (see Fig. 49.10A and 49.11A). Skin thickness and pigmentation often reduces signal strength, and the reported values should only be recorded if there is a good pulse wave. Pulse oximeters are calibrated based on the human oxygen hemoglobin dissociation curve, and SpO_2 values are calculated. High levels of methemoglobin have been reported for reptiles and will affect pulse oximeter readings. A further concern is the pronounced difference in respiratory physiology and function among reptile species. Therefore reference values derived from one taxa may be of limited value in other taxa. Reflectance pulse oximeter probes are most useful and can be placed into the oral cavity (Fig. 49.12), the

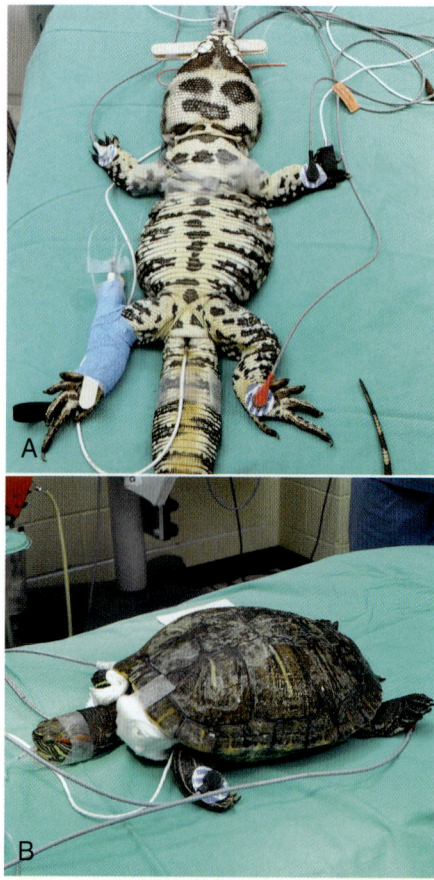

FIG 49.11 Electrocardiographic (ECG) monitoring in reptiles. (A) Argentine black and white tegu (*Salvator merianae*). Note the placement of the Doppler probe over the heart and pulse oximetry probe in the cloaca. (B) Red-eared slider (*Trachemys scripta elegans*).

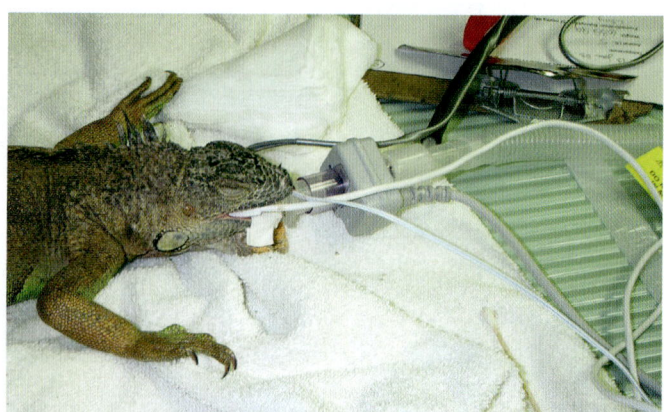

FIG 49.12 Anesthetized green iguana (*Iguana iguana*) with placement of an esophageal pulse oximeter probe connected to a pediatric mainstream capnography device.

esophagus at the level of the carotid artery, or in the evacuated cloaca (see Fig. 49.11A). In sevoflurane-or isoflurane-anesthetized green iguanas, a comparison of arterial blood oxygen saturation, as determined by pulse oximetry (SpO_2) versus arterial blood gas analysis (SaO_2), showed no significant differences between the two monitoring modalities over time. Although not significant, SpO_2 values were lower than SaO_2 values at all time points in isoflurane-anesthetized iguanas.[63] A study in conscious green iguanas showed that oxygen saturation, calculated by pulse oximetry (86% ± 6%), was lower than the SaO_2 (92% ± 5%) measured by arterial blood gas analysis.[69] Baseline SaO_2 values in conscious iguanas were reported to be >90%.[69]

Blood gas analysis: It has been well established in human and veterinary anesthesia that arterial blood gas analysis allows for accurate assessment of pulmonary function, including ventilation, oxygenation, and acid-base status. Venous blood gases will give an assessment of metabolic status. Venous blood gases are affected by local tissue metabolism and low blood flow, but in humans venous blood gas analysis can predict arterial blood gas values for pH, PCO_2, and bicarbonate concentrations. Baseline venous blood gas values in green iguanas are similar to those reported in humans and domestic animals.[69] In reptiles, collection and interpretation of arterial blood gas parameters is challenging due to poor accessibility and lack of normal reference values, as well as physiological features such as intracardiac shunting, the ability to tolerate varying degrees of hypoxia, and the capability to convert to anaerobic metabolism. Intrapulmonary shunts will bypass gas exchange in the lungs. In reptiles, many factors will influence arterial blood gas composition, including taxonomic differences (e.g., aquatic vs. terrestrial species), inspired concentration of oxygen, and temperature. At present, application of mammalian arterial blood gas values to reptiles is considered inappropriate because reptiles are more tolerant to changes in arterial partial pressures of oxygen and carbon dioxide. As mentioned above, intracardiac shunting and ventilation/perfusion mismatching in reptiles may also result in inaccurate interpretation of arterial blood gases. In green iguanas premedicated with butorphanol and maintained with sevoflurane or isoflurane, arterial blood oxygen saturation, as determined by arterial blood gas analysis, was >90% throughout the anesthetic event.[63] In the same study, significant decreases in pH values were observed over time. A study in conscious green iguanas demonstrated that $PaCO_2$ values (32 ± 7 mm Hg) were similar to those reported in mammalian species.[69] Arterial blood gas values were similar to mammalian species; however, baseline SaO_2 values were lower than in a similar study in gray rat snakes.[72] Circadian changes in arterial PO_2 and SaO_2 were reported in green iguanas, with values being significantly lower in the morning than in the afternoon. In most studies, blood gas values are determined at 37°C (98.6°F) and corrected for the body temperature of the reptile.[69]

Capnography is used in mammals as a noninvasive tool to determine concentrations of CO_2 in expired air and assess ventilation. In reptiles, capnography is associated with several limitations, which may provide erroneous results. End-tidal CO_2 concentrations will provide an estimate of arterial CO_2 tension; however, this technique needs to be validated for reptiles.[63] Right-to-left intracardiac shunts can make $EtCO_2$ difficult to interpret in reptiles. Another concern in small reptiles relates to the use of side-stream units with high sampling rates, which are likely to produce inaccurate, diluted results. Portable side-stream capnography units are available with low sampling rates adequate for even small patients, while pediatric mainstream units avoid the complication of side-stream dilution altogether (see Fig. 49.12). In green iguanas maintained with either sevoflurane or isoflurane, $EtCO_2$ decreased over time, but no differences were observed between groups.[63] $EtCO_2$ concentrations, in both isoflurane and sevoflurane anesthetized green iguanas, reflected $PaCO_2$ values at the beginning (10 minutes) of the

anesthetic event. However, over time $PaCO_2$ values were significantly higher than $EtCO_2$ concentrations. Therefore $EtCO_2$ appears to underestimate $PaCO_2$ but is a useful tool to monitor trends in arterial CO_2 tension.

Further studies are indicated to validate the aforementioned monitoring modalities in other species. In the meantime, it is recommended that values obtained with the use of pulse oximetry, arterial, or venous blood gas analysis and capnography should be interpreted with caution. However, all the above-mentioned techniques will provide information on trends in respiratory and metabolic performance so that corrective and supportive measures can be initiated.

ANESTHETIC EMERGENCIES

The principles and techniques of managing anesthetic emergencies, established in domestic mammalian veterinary medicine, also apply to reptiles. While topics such as effective fluid therapy, cardiopulmonary support techniques, and administration and selection of emergency drugs have been reported for reptiles, currently there is still a need for further investigation into effective drugs and dosages. The preoperative calculation and printing of an emergency drug sheet helps improve the speed and accuracy of emergency treatments. The need for effective cardiopulmonary resuscitation may arise in any anesthetized reptilian patient, especially in critically ill animals undergoing diagnostic or surgical procedures. The same concepts established for domestic animals apply, and the reptile should be assessed for respiratory status and cardiovascular status. The principles of airway (A), breathing (B), and circulation (C) apply. An airway should be (re)established immediately, and respiratory support should be provided, either by manual ventilation or a mechanical ventilator. Devices to monitor cardiac and circulatory function should be utilized, including ECG and Doppler flow device, and vascular access should be (re)established. If venous access is not possible, an intraosseous catheter can be placed to administer emergency drugs and fluids, while intratracheal administration can be used if no IV/IO access is possible. Unfortunately, little information is available on effective dosages of emergency drugs commonly used in mammalian species. Atropine is indicated during episodes of severe bradycardia and should be administered intravenously or intraosseously. Doxapram is a respiratory stimulant and should also be administered via the intravenous or intraosseous route to be most effective. Doxapram administration may result in reduced CNS oxygen delivery and long-term brain damage if the patient is hypoxic; therefore the use of doxapram is not recommended for cerebral-pulmonary resuscitation. In the rare case of true cardiac arrest, epinephrine is the drug of choice and can be administered either intravenously, intraosseously, or diluted with sterile saline via the endotracheal tube. Supportive measures such as effective fluid therapy and provision of heat and oxygen should accompany resuscitation efforts.

RECOVERY

Following cessation of the procedure, inhalant anesthesia should be discontinued and reversal drugs administered (taking care to provide alternative analgesia if using naloxone). Room air administered with an Ambubag (Fig. 49.13), instead of 100% oxygen, has, historically, been recommended for ventilation of reptiles during recovery. It was suggested that high oxygen concentrations in the lungs delay return to spontaneous respiration.[36] However, recent studies could not demonstrate any statistical or clinical significant difference in recovery times in monitor lizards or bearded dragons ventilated with 100% oxygen, compared with animals ventilated with room air during recovery from gas anesthesia.[64,73] As is standard protocol for domestic animals, fluid

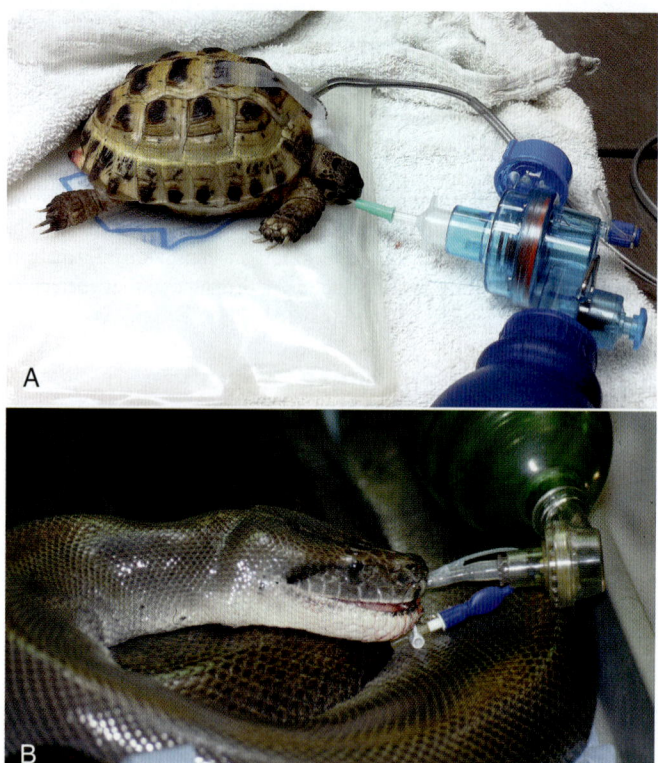

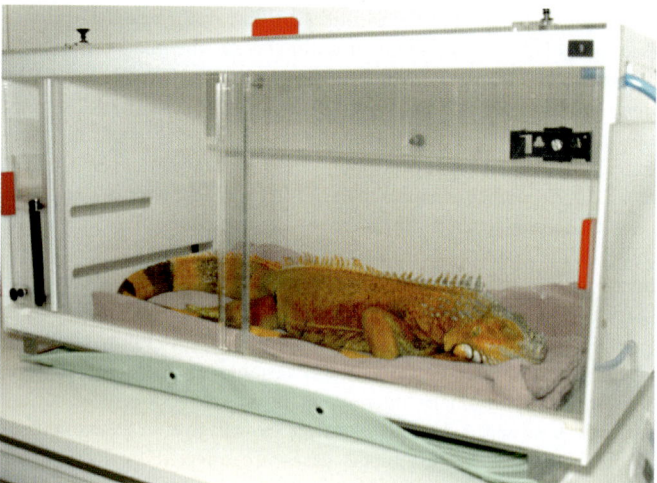

FIG 49.14 Postanesthetic recovery of a green iguana (*Iguana iguana*) in an incubator to ensure the patient is maintained within its preferred optimal temperature zone.

FIG 49.13 Use of an Ambubag during anesthetic recovery in reptiles. (A) Russian tortoise (*Agrionemys horsfieldii*) intubated with an intravenous catheter. (B) Burmese python *(Python bivittatus)* intubated with a cuffed endotracheal tube.

therapy and pain management should be continued during the recovery period, and additional analgesia should be provided as necessary.

Prolonged anesthetic recoveries are common in reptiles, especially if high dosages of nonreversible injectable drugs are administered (e.g., tiletamine/zolazepam). Isoflurane anesthesia in chelonians is also frequently associated with slow recoveries, which is suspected to be due to hypotension, right-to-left shunting, and reduced lung and tissue perfusion.[10,74] Administration of epinephrine (syn. adrenalin, 0.1 mg/kg IM) in common snapping turtles (*Chelydra serpentina*) significantly reduced time to return of spontaneous breathing and complete recovery following isoflurane anesthesia.[74] It was demonstrated that an increase in adrenergic tone of the pulmonary vasculature leads to shunting of blood away from the pulmonary circulation during episodes of apnea in turtles and that, by increasing the sympathomimetic tone of the systemic vasculature through administration of epinephrine, pulmonary

shunting is reduced, leading to accelerated recovery in turtles anesthetized with isoflurane.[74,75] Stimulation of the acupuncture point GV-26 also hastens snapping turtle recovery from isoflurane, comparable to the administration of epinephrine.[74]

During recovery the patient should be kept in a temperature-controlled environment (Fig. 49.14). For most reptilian patients, dedicated reptile or small animal incubators are ideal since they are designed for accurate temperature maintenance. It is not recommended to exceed the species-specific POTZ, since this will result in an increased metabolic rate and oxygen demand. Reptiles recovering from general anesthesia will be in a state of respiratory compromise, and it may be difficult to meet the increased demand of oxygen by spontaneous respiration. During the recovery period, it is essential to assess respiratory status of the patient and continue assisted ventilation until the patient is breathing spontaneously, has regained reflexes, and can be extubated.

Spontaneous breathing and ambulation are reliable indicators of anesthetic recovery. Reptiles should be extubated once spontaneous breathing is observed and oropharyngeal reflexes (e.g., jaw tone, tongue movement) have returned.[36] If spontaneous breathing has not returned, IPPV should be continued. Even following extubation, monitoring should continue, as it is not unheard of for a spontaneously breathing reptile to slip back into unconscious apnea.

REFERENCES

See www.expertconsult.com for a complete list of references.

50

Analgesia

Kurt K. Sladky and Christoph Mans

Veterinary clinical medicine typically lags behind human clinical medicine by several decades. Veterinary analgesia is one such discipline. While the focus in human analgesia is on chronic and neuropathic pain, as well as the molecular mechanisms associated with pain, the focus in veterinary medicine continues to be associated with whether reptiles experience pain, the measurement of pain, analgesic drug efficacy, duration of drug action, and appropriate routes of administration. Our current understanding of reptile pain and analgesia has advanced considerably in the last 5 to 10 years; however, there is much to be learned. Many veterinary clinicians still continue to debate whether reptiles experience pain and how best to treat pain in different reptile species.

To put the issue into historical perspective, less than 4 decades ago it was routine for human physicians to forego administering analgesic drugs to human infants, even after undergoing invasive surgical procedures. Before the late 1970s, clinical and empirical research on human pain and pain management focused entirely on adults. Pain management for infants and young children was nonexistent, and surgery was typically performed with only paralytics on board. For example, one of the most common surgical procedures performed on premature babies was thoracotomy for ligation of a patent ductus arteriosus, which most surgeons and anesthesiologists believed was best accomplished using oxygen and pancuronium as the sole anesthetic regimen.[1] At the time, it was hypothesized that human infants had an immature central and peripheral nervous system, which was neither structurally nor functionally capable of receiving and processing noxious stimuli. Because infants were nonverbal, measurement of pain was considered difficult, if not impossible. The thinking was that analgesic drugs would not only be ineffective, but that they contributed to deleterious physiological side effects, which further jeopardized the recovery and, ultimately, the health of the child. During the 1980s and 1990s, clinical analgesia research focusing on human full-term and premature babies blossomed, and we now understand the following: nociceptive neural pathways are fully developed and in place in humans by 22 to 24 weeks' gestation[2]; and nonverbal human infants can respond to pain using vocalizations, facial expressions, body movements, changes in respiratory and heart rate, changes in skin color, and metabolic changes. With this in mind, is it any wonder that we are just beginning to understand nonhuman mammalian pain and analgesia? The acceptance of nonverbal human infants being able to perceive and express pain was a breakthrough and a prelude to a new focus on veterinary analgesia.

Many veterinary clinicians continue to argue that the administration of analgesics is risky to the patient and may mask behavioral signs of pain, which are considered evolutionarily adaptive for survival. This remains particularly true when nonmammalian patients are considered. This issue was expressed in a survey of members of the Association of Reptile and Amphibian Veterinarians.[3] Most respondents (98%) believed that reptiles were capable of experiencing pain, but relatively few clinicians administered analgesics to reptiles under conditions in which they would administer analgesics to mammals. The implication from the survey data collected was that there were too many unknowns; recognition of pain was difficult, there was concern about detrimental side effects from analgesic administration, dosages and duration of effect were anecdotal, no pharmacokinetic data were available, and, at the time of the survey, published efficacy data were uncommon. Since that survey, we now recognize that, at some level, reptiles experience pain, and while there is interest in treating pain in reptile patients, we remain unsure if the chosen drugs, dosages, or duration of administration are effective or whether the chosen analgesic will have deleterious consequences. Added to this, the diversity of the class *Reptilia* makes it difficult to extrapolate analgesic efficacy from one species to the next. Regardless, veterinarians have an ethical obligation to treat painful conditions in all animals. Effective pain management reduces stress-induced disruption to homeostatic mechanisms and can decrease morbidity and mortality associated with trauma or surgery. Therefore the primary objective of this chapter is to describe and highlight the most current information with respect to pain and analgesia in reptiles.

REPTILE NOCICEPTION OR PAIN?

Do reptiles feel pain? Can we recognize pain in reptiles? Is the perception of pain by a reptile equivalent to that of a mammal? Does it make anatomic or physiological sense that the ability to perceive and respond to an aversive stimulus is evolutionarily limited to mammals? We will never be able to objectively answer these questions because reptiles simply cannot tell us. However, like nonverbal human infants or nonhuman mammals, should the inability to communicate dictate whether pain is being perceived or whether an analgesic drug should be administered? We would argue, emphatically, NO. By anthropocentric definition, the word "pain" implies higher level cortical processing of information, and therefore nociception and antinociception are used when referring to pain and analgesia in most nonmammalian species. This stems from the controversy concerning whether or not nonmammalian species have the appropriate central and peripheral nervous system structures and pathways, capable of "receiving and processing" noxious stimuli and responding appropriately. In other words, can nonmammals "experience" pain, or are they merely capable of demonstrating a "reflexive" response to a noxious stimulus, that is, nociception? Based on published neuroanatomic, neurophysiologic, and behavioral data, there is plausible evidence to suggest that, structurally and functionally, reptiles have the capacity to experience pain. Therefore as clinicians, it is our contention that, because of limited understanding of pain and analgesia in reptiles, we should err on the side of reptile patient well-being and assume that conditions considered painful in humans and other mammals are painful across all other vertebrate species, including reptiles.

Neuroanatomic and Neurophysiological Evidence

Nociceptive Pathways. It is adaptive for all animals to avoid aversive stimuli in the environment as an ultimate mechanism for survival, and therefore all vertebrates have specialized sensory receptors, nociceptors, which are capable of detecting noxious stimuli (e.g., thermal, mechanical, chemical receptors) and afferent pathways relaying this information to the central nervous system. Efferent pathways exist to initiate a response, typically a movement away from the noxious stimulus. Therefore for any vertebrate organism to "perceive" a painful stimulus, there must be the following: a peripheral sensory receptor (e.g., nociceptor), a sensory pathway to the spinal cord, initial processing of the painful stimulus within the spinal cord dorsal horn, ascending pathways to the brain, processing of the painful stimulus by the brain, and descending pathways, which exert control over the withdrawal, escape, or defensive or immobile responses. Like mammals, reptiles have all of the anatomic structures considered critical for the recognition of pain: peripheral nociceptors, appropriate central nervous system structures and pathways, opioid receptors and endogenous opioids, reduction of nociceptive response with analgesics (although data are sparse), pain avoidance learning, and suspension of normal behavior with pain.[4–6] Recent research in fish, amphibians, reptiles, and birds has demonstrated that the transmission of peripheral sensory signals, via the spinal cord, to midbrain and forebrain regions are homologous to mammalian cortical and limbic structures.[7–10] Thus the physiological and anatomic requirements for pain and analgesia appear to be remarkably similar among all vertebrate species.

Nociceptors. Although peripheral nociceptors have not been identified, specifically, in reptiles, nociceptors are highly conserved across phyla, from invertebrates to fish, amphibians, birds, and mammals.[9,11] Nociceptors have been identified in aquatic and terrestrial invertebrates, teleost fish, amphibians, and birds.[9,10] The only reason nociceptors have not been specifically identified in reptiles is, simply, because nobody has looked.

Functionally, all nociceptors do not respond to the same stimuli. Some may be specifically mechanoreceptors, chemical receptors, or thermoreceptors, and some nociceptors may be multimodal and respond to a variety of different noxious stimuli. Unfortunately, the Reptilia are among the least studied taxa with respect to presence of nociceptors, nociceptive pathways, and central nervous system involvement. In pit vipers, touch, thermosensitive, and thermo-mechanosensitive nociceptive neurons were identified in the trigeminal ganglia.[12] Mechanonociceptors were identified in the cutaneous plantar nerve of the alligator, *Alligator mississippiensis*, and some of these mechanoreceptors also responded to a noxious thermal stimulus (>40°C) as well.[13]

Ascending (Afferent), Cerebral Cortical, and Descending (Efferent) Pathways. We know from the mammalian literature that noxious sensory information is initially detected by cutaneous afferents, the cell bodies of which are in the dorsal root ganglia of the spinal cord, and can be separated into two main groups according to axon caliber and myelination: large-diameter, myelinated A-fibers and small-diameter, unmyelinated C-fibers.[9] As with mammals, fish, amphibians, and reptiles have myelinated and unmyelinated afferent fibers running together in sensory nerves: large, myelinated A fibers (Aβ); small, myelinated A fibers (Aδ); and small, unmyelinated C fibers (C).[10,14] In amphibians, small, slowly conducting fibers (Aβ and C) transmitted the majority of all impulses induced by noxious heat, pinching, pin pricks, and the application of dilute acetic acid to the skin.[14] There are limited published data for reptiles. In pit vipers, Aβ-fibers were shown to respond to nonnoxious mechanical stimuli and to have larger somata, whereas Aδ-fibers responding to noxious mechanical stimulation have smaller somata.[12]

Sensory information detected by nociceptors, and carried by the cutaneous afferents, is transmitted to the dorsal horn of the spinal cord and continues to the brain to activate systems responsible for producing the sensation of pain and the motivational-affective responses that accompany the experience of pain. In mammals, substance P, a peptide that is present in small primary afferent nerves and in the dorsal and ventral horns of the spinal cord, is expressed in direct association with painful stimuli. Substance P is highly conserved in mammalian and nonmammalian species, including invertebrates, fish, amphibians, reptiles, and birds. Specifically, in reptiles, substance P is present in the nervous system of several turtle species.[15,16]

Transmission of sensory information moves from spinal cord to brain. In mammals, pain-related activity detected by the thalamus spreads to the insular cortex (believed to process the feelings that distinguish pain from itch, for example) and by the anterior cingulate cortex (believed to control the motivational element of pain). The transmission of nociceptive information from peripheral to central nervous system is likely the function of several different ascending pathways originating from neurons located within the spinal cord gray matter. The axons of these neurons travel within the spinal cord white matter, and they terminate in higher centers, including several parts of the thalamus and the brain stem reticular formation.[17] In mammals, the ascending tracts in the anterolateral quadrant of the spinal cord that seem most likely to mediate pain are the spinothalamic, spinoreticular, and spinomesencephalic tracts.[18] Neurons belonging to these pathways project chiefly contralaterally, and recordings in mammalian experiments have demonstrated the presence of nociceptive neurons among the cells of origin of all of these pathways.[18] It was hypothesized that the sensory aspects of pain are mediated primarily by the spinothalamic tract and that the motivational-affective aspects result from activity in all three of these pathways. In reptiles, while the same basic ascending sensory pathways for the visual, auditory, and somatosensory systems are present, they involve fewer cell groups or subdivisions of cell groups in the thalamus and pallium compared with homologous pathways in birds and mammals.[19–23]

The telencephalon of reptiles, birds, and mammals consists of two major subdivisions: the pallium and the subpallium. The subpallium, also called the basal ganglia, is further divided into two main subdivisions: the striatum and pallidum. The striatum and pallidum are also thought to contribute to the septum and subpallial amygdala (central and medial nuclei). The subpallial components are relatively con-served in its organization among amniotes.[24,25] The neocortex of mammals, as a derivative of the dorsal pallium, is homologous as a field only to the hyperpallium of birds and the dorsal cortex of lizards/turtles. The dorsal pallium is present in all amniotes and shares a number of similar cell types and connections across phyla.[26] The organization of the reptile pallium is not yet as well-defined, but it consists of the dorsal cortex and the dorsal ventricular ridge (DVR), as well as olfactory, hippocampal, and pallial amygdala regions. The reptile anterior dorsal ventricular ridge (ADVR) is a large intraventricular protrusion in the reptilian forebrain, which receives information from many different sensory modalities, and, in turn, projects massively into the striatum. The ADVR possesses functional similarities to the mammalian isocortex and may perform complex sensory integrations. The ADVR in lizards is composed of three longitudinal zones, which receive visual, somatosensory, and acoustic info. These projections are relayed by the thalamic nuclei.[8] The posterior part of the dorsal ventricular ridge (PDVR) is considered an associative center that projects to the hypothalamus, thus being comparable to the amygdaloid formation. Evidence suggests that the PDVR and neighboring structures constitute the reptilian basolateral amygdala and indicate that an emotional brain was already present in the ancestral amniote.[27]

The descending motor pathways from the hypothalamus and brain stem to the spinal cord in the quadrupedal reptiles studied (turtles, *Pseudemys scripta elegans*, and *Testudo hermanni*, and the lizards, *Tupinambis nigropunctatus* and *Varanus exanthematicus*) appear to show remarkable similarities to pathways in mammals as regards their cells of origin as well as their spinal cord trajectory.[28] In the reptiles studied, the presence of interstitiospinal, vestibulospinal, and reticulospinal pathways could be demonstrated. The crossed reticulospinal tracts regulate the sensitivity of flexor responses to ensure that only noxious stimuli elicit the responses. A crossed rubrospinal tract has been shown in the turtles and in the lizard but could not be demonstrated in the python.[29] A small rubrospinal tract was demonstrated in a colubrid snake species (water snake).[30] The nonexistent or reduced rubrospinal tract in snake species is believed to be associated with limblessness. In the large *Psammodromus* lizard, efferent fibers from the dorsal cortex reach the rostral midbrain tegmentum, and it was suggested that this was the reptilian representation of the sensorimotor cortex.[31] A similar corticoefferent pathway was described in turtles after lesions in the general cortex.[31] In gecko species, anterograde-labeled fibers were observed in the same tegmental area after a tracer injection into different locations of the dorsal cortex.[31] Although axon terminals were not described in the gecko (*Gekko gekko*) midbrain tegmentum, thus far, reptile data strongly suggest the presence of a cortico-reticulo-spinal motor pathway. This pathway originates from the rostral dorsal cortex, and it may represent the anatomical substrate for a motor pallium in reptiles, which is comparable to the avian "motor pallium," both topologically and with respect to the organization of efferent pathways.[31] In addition, in pond turtles (*Pseudemys scripta elegans*), the determination of a descending pathway linking cortical regions with the red nucleus via the hypothalamus suggested indirect cortical control of the reptilian rubrospinal system.[32] Altogether, these findings suggest that the presence of functionally segregated thalamocortical projections is a conserved feature of brain organization among amniotes.

Opioid Receptors and Endogenous Opioids. The opioid receptor gene family is highly conserved across multiple vertebrate orders (e.g., bovids, chickens, bullfrogs, and teleost and elasmobranch fishes),[11] but there is limited information on opioid receptors in reptiles. The three main opioid receptors, μ, δ, and κ, were cloned and sequenced in three nonmammalian vertebrates: the zebrafish, the Northern grass frog, and the rough-skinned newt.[33–35] In aquatic turtles, μ- and δ-opioid receptors are located throughout the brain, and δ-opioid receptors are more abundant than μ-opioid receptors.[36] However, results of our study did not determine the location and distribution of μ- and δ-opioid receptors in the spinal cord (where nociceptive inputs enter the CNS) of turtles, nor were κ-opioid receptors examined anywhere in the CNS. With respect to endogenous opioid-related neurotransmitters, proenkephalin-derived peptides are present in turtles with a distribution similar to that in mammals and birds.[37] In addition, the reptilian brain (aquatic slider turtles, American alligators, and anole lizards) was found to contain large quantities of endogenous enkephalins, also known as endorphins (Met-enkephalin, Leu-enkephalin, and Met-enk-Arg-Phe or MERF).[38]

MEASUREMENT AND QUANTIFICATION OF PAIN AND ANALGESIA IN REPTILES

Measuring pain in any species, particularly reptiles, is the most difficult hurdle in the study of pain and analgesic efficacy. For example, as veterinarians, do we assume that this bearded dragon and sea turtle are experiencing some level of pain and should we attempt to provide an analgesic to make them more comfortable (Figs. 50.1 and 50.2)? In mammals, it is well established that perioperative pain management facilitates recovery and healing, reduces morbidity and mortality, and contributes to more rapid return to normal behavior.[39–41]

Why not consider this as salient in nonmammalian species? If measuring pain in mammals is challenging, how do we begin to decipher pain-related behavior in reptiles? An objective understanding of normal behavior of a particular species and the ability to differentiate the presence of abnormal behavior indicative of discomfort are critical to the study of pain and analgesia. Therefore one must first have an understanding of normal species-specific behavior within the environmental context in which that behavior is being displayed or observed, in order to be able to discriminate behavior associated with pain. For example, observing the postovariectomy behavior of an adult female green iguana in its own home cage may be different than behavior of the same animal under the same postovariectomy conditions observed in a hospital setting. This is certainly true in some mammalian species.[42] Methods for assessing and measuring pain in reptiles have been described previously.[41] Ideally, a combination of appropriate behavioral and physiological parameters might best be employed to measure pain and analgesia in reptiles. Along those same lines, the development of a species- and context-specific

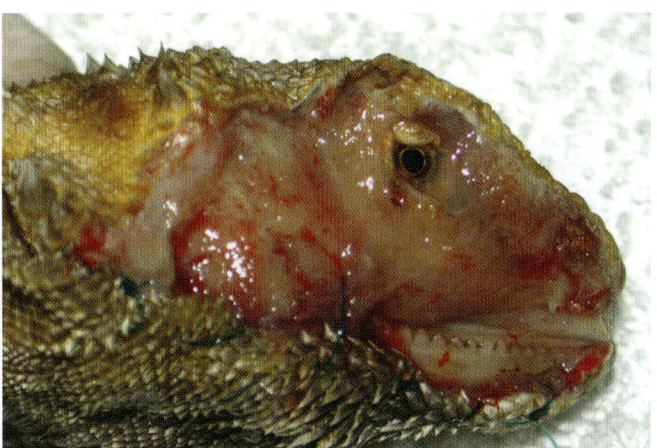

FIG 50.1 Bearded dragon (*Pogona vitticeps*) with complete skin sloughing of the right side of the face due to *Chrysosporium* anamorph of *Nannizziopsis vriesii* (CANV) infection. (Courtesy of Kurt K. Sladky.)

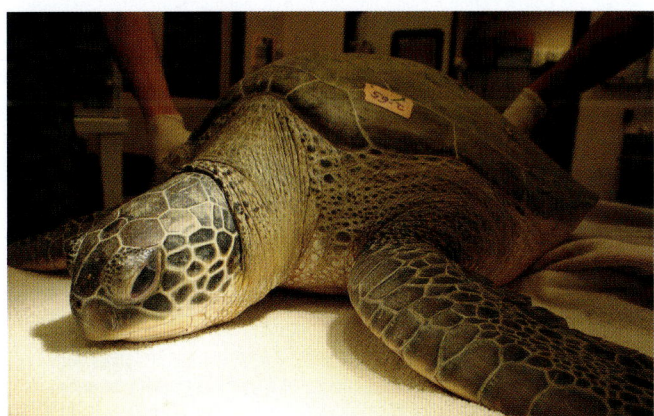

FIG 50.2 Green sea turtle (*Chelonia mydas*) shortly after being brought into the Georgia Sea Turtle Center, St. Catherines Island, Georgia, for treatment associated with being struck by a boat propeller. (Courtesy of T. Norton.)

ethogram for each species being evaluated would provide the best method for distinguishing normal versus abnormal (e.g., painful) behaviors. Most commonly, animal pain, or lack thereof, is assessed before and after some invasive procedure, such as a surgical procedure. This method requires the development of a behavioral ethogram, which, in turn, requires the observer to become well versed in subtle behavioral differences through many hours of observation and analysis (videotaped or live observation). Behaviors must be operationally defined, which will provide objectivity and reproducibility (Table 50.1). For example, in a recent study, our laboratory developed a behavioral ethogram to evaluate preoperative and postoperative behavioral responses to food intake, willingness to swim, and breathing in red-eared slider turtles following a unilateral orchidectomy.[43] We were able to compare postoperative behavior in turtles with and without analgesic administration using morphine, butorphanol, and saline. Our hypothesis was that preoperative behaviors would return to normal more rapidly in those turtles receiving a mu-opioid receptor agonist analgesic. We demonstrated that those turtles receiving morphine and undergoing unilateral gonadectomy returned to normal preoperative behavior more quickly than those receiving saline or butorphanol. An alternative to studying postsurgical pain is to measure pain under strictly controlled laboratory conditions using established behavioral models during which noxious stimuli (e.g., mechanical, thermal, chemical) are applied to an anatomic location on the reptile subject.[44–48]

Analgesic drugs can be administered and the response compared with baseline responses. The application of a noxious thermal stimulus provides a well-established behavioral model for assessing pain and analgesia in rodents.[49] In our own studies, we have successfully adapted this classic thermal nociception model developed for use in rodents and determined that reptiles show unambiguous, easily quantifiable withdrawal responses indistinguishable from rodents.[6,44–46] The thermal hind limb withdrawal latency model uses a noxious thermal stimulus applied to the plantar surface of the hind limb or the ventral surface of the body (e.g., snake species) of different reptile species (Figs. 50.3 and 50.4). A withdrawal latency is automatically determined when the animal withdraws its limb or tail from the noxious stimulus. This model has many advantages over other noxious stimulus paradigms, including rapid application and decay of the noxious stimulus (thereby not causing long-lasting inflammation), instant latency quantification, and unambiguous behavior after stimulus exposure (either the animal does or does not withdraw its limb). Most importantly, the animal can escape the noxious stimulus by simply withdrawing its limb. While some might argue that a withdrawal response to a noxious stimulus is not equivalent to pain, there is evidence in a variety of species that noxious thermal stimulation caused molecular and cellular changes in the central nervous system.[50–52] As a qualification to the noxious thermal, some have suggested that reptiles are prone to thermal burns, and therefore they are less likely to respond to a noxious thermal stimulus. While our understanding of thermal burns in reptiles is inadequate, there is no doubt that all reptile species studied in our laboratory perceive and respond to the focal heat source in an identical manner as a mammal. In fact, of the hundreds of healthy reptiles across multiple species subjected to a noxious thermal stimulus applied to either the plantar surface of the hind limb or various areas of the ventral body surface of limbless snakes in our laboratory, we have observed 100% response rate to this stimulus paradigm.

Physiological changes have been used to quantify stress and pain in mammals, and this approach has been adapted for reptiles as well.[53,54] For example, heart rate significantly increased in ball pythons after subcutaneous capsaicin administration.[54] In this study, opioid analgesic drugs did not alter this physiological response.

TABLE 50.1 Behavioral and Physiological Parameters Associated With Pain in Reptiles

1. Absence of normal behavior
2. Hunched posture
3. Increased aggression with manual manipulation
4. Rubbing/scratching affected area (e.g., incision site, wound, etc.)
5. Skin color changes, especially general darkening
6. Head extended away, and ventrally directed, from body, especially obvious in chelonians
7. Lameness: graded as 0 (no lameness), 1 (barely perceptible lameness), 2 (lameness always perceptible), and 3 (non-weight-bearing lameness)
8. Changes in consumptive behavior (food consumption):
   a. Scored as % of total food consumed in a 24-hour period
      i. Food intake can be quantified based on quantity or weight of food source within a given time limit (e.g., number of pellets consumed/number of pellets offered within 24 hours in aquatic turtles).
9. Lack of activity:
   a. Duration (in seconds/minutes) of spontaneous and voluntary movement within the tank during each observation period
      i.) Active versus complete reluctance to move
   b. Location within the enclosure during each observation period
10. Interactive behavior: immediate response to approaching observer/object
    a. Oblivious to environment, nonresponsive to interaction
    b. Partial retreat: attempted movement away from observer/object
    c. Full retreat: unambiguous movement away from the observer/object
11. Rate of respiration: scored as number of breaths per minute at each observation period
12. Heart rate: Not particularly useful in reptiles. Scored as beats per minute using a stethoscope or Doppler flow probe, although handling may confound the results.

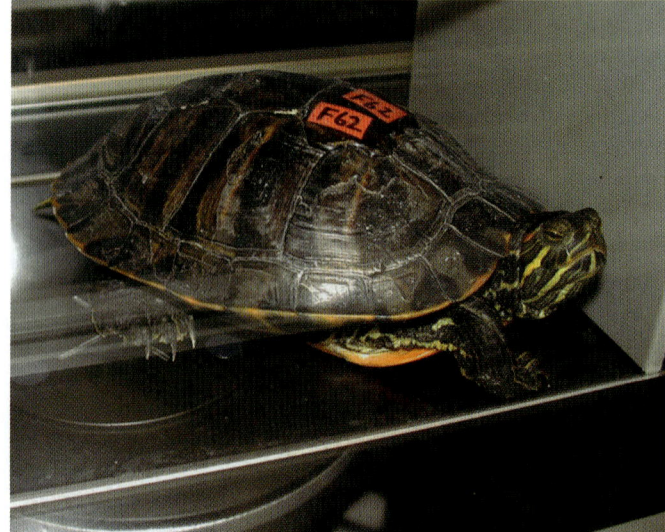

FIG 50.3 Red-eared slider turtle (*Trachemys scripta elegans*) at rest in the Hargreaves apparatus (noxious thermal hind limb withdrawal apparatus) during research testing of analgesic responses to opioid administration. The turtle has the plantar surface of its right hind limb placed directly over the infrared heat source. (Courtesy of Kurt K. Sladky.)

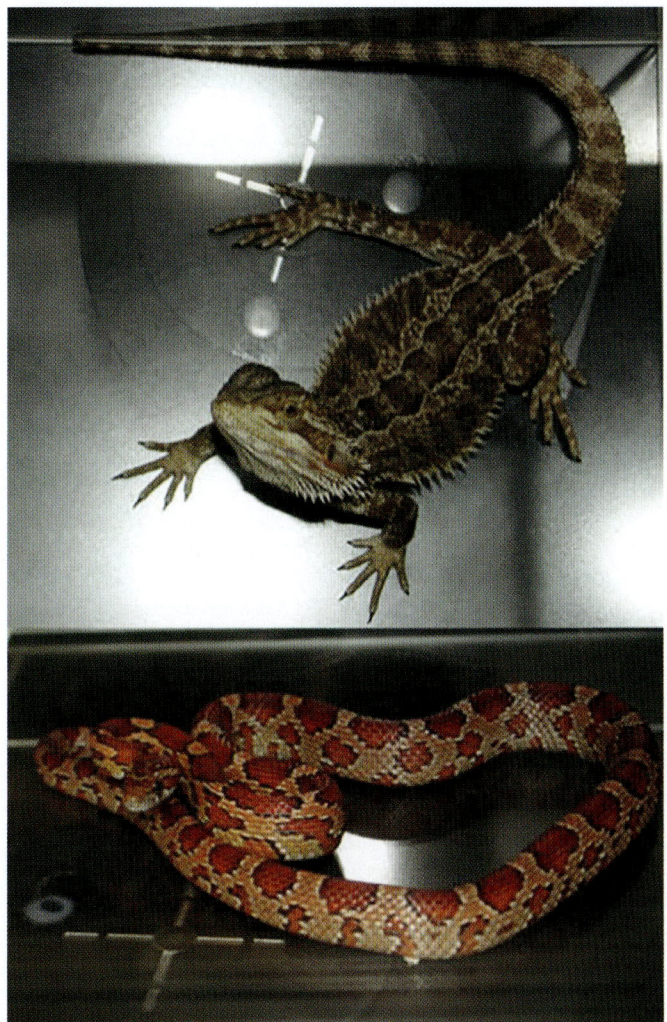

FIG 50.4 Bearded dragon (*Pogona vitticeps*; top image) and corn snake (*Pantherophis guttatus*; bottom) at rest in the Hargreaves apparatus (noxious thermal hind limb withdrawal apparatus) during research testing of analgesic responses to opioid administration. The bearded dragon has the plantar surface of its right hind limb placed directly over the infrared heat source. Note the circular region at the center of the "X" in the corn snake image, just in front of the snake's head, which is the focal infrared heat element. (Courtesy of Kurt K. Sladky.)

ANALGESIC DRUGS

Methods of Administration

It is difficult to describe the most appropriate methods for administering analgesic drugs in reptiles because analgesic pharmacokinetic and/or pharmacodynamic data in reptiles are scarce. Whether an analgesic drug is administered intravenously (IV), intramuscularly (IM), subcutaneously (SC), orally (PO), or transcutaneously (TC) is partially dependent on the size and temperament of the individual reptile. Anatomic location is another consideration, because there is pharmacologic evidence that drug administration to the hind limbs or tail of a reptile may cause rapid clearance by the renal portal system or, in the case of opioids, the hepatic first-pass effect.[41,55] However, whether this more rapid clearance has any implication for efficacy remains unknown.

Historically, and anecdotally, intramuscular administration was the preferred route for most analgesics and anesthetics in reptiles.[41,56,57] Many veterinarians believed that the subcutaneous space of reptiles was not well vascularized and therefore drug absorption would be prolonged. However, advantages associated with SC drug administration include access to a variety of subcutaneous sites requiring minimal manual restraint or patient manipulation and therefore increased safety and the capability of administering larger volumes in a single location. Currently there are no published data demonstrating that intramuscular administration results in superior analgesic efficacy compared with SC administration, and results from our laboratory indicate that drug effects can be measured rapidly after SC administration.[43–46] We determined that meperidine, an opioid analgesic with rapid absorption and excretion in humans, administered SC in red-eared slider turtles causes measurable behavior changes within 30 minutes of administration.[44] Therefore the authors routinely administer analgesic drugs and their antagonists SC in chelonians, lizards, and snakes, particularly if larger volumes of anesthetic drugs need to be injected.

Other routes of administration are also useful in reptiles. Transdermal fentanyl patches have been applied to two reptiles species for pharmacokinetic analysis, and plasma concentrations were detectable in both species.[58,59] Recently, our laboratory has evaluated the efficacy of transdermal fentanyl patch (12.5 mcg/hr) administration in ball pythons and corn snakes and determined that fentanyl patches may be the most promising analgesic approach for use in some snake species (Gutwillig, et al, Proc ARAV 2012, p 66). A new form of transdermal fentanyl, Recuvyra topical solution, is available for dogs and cats, has a 96-hour duration of effect, and may be a useful fentanyl application for reptiles in the future. Oral administration is an uncommonly used method for analgesic administration in reptiles, because there is concern that a potentially slow gastrointestinal transit time will delay onset, peak efficacy, and clearance. However, we have found just the opposite in our laboratory. Tramadol and metabolite plasma concentrations can be detected within hours of oral administration in loggerhead sea turtles,[61] and thermal hind limb withdrawal latencies increased in red-eared slider turtles within 4 hours of oral tramadol administration.[6] Table 50.2 summarizes commonly used analgesic protocols in reptile species.

Opioids and Opioidlike Analgesics

Opioids, the most effective drugs for controlling pain in mammals, are classified according to receptor subtypes—μ (mu), κ (kappa), and δ (delta) (Table 50.3). The μ, δ, and κ opioid receptors, abbreviated MOR, DOR, and KOR, mediate the analgesic effects of opioids, while the role of the fourth type of opioid receptor, the nociceptin or orphanin FQ receptor (ORL), is less clear.[62,63] For pain management in mammals, many clinicians prefer administering either a μ-opioid receptor agonist (e.g., morphine, fentanyl, hydromorphone, etc.); a partial μ-opioid receptor agonist (e.g., buprenorphine); or a mixed-opioid, κ-receptor agonist–μ-receptor antagonist (e.g., butorphanol). For exogenous opioids to be effective analgesics in reptiles, opioid receptors must be present. The gene family for opioid receptors (μ, κ, and δ) is highly conserved across multiple vertebrate orders.[11] Two snake species have endogenous brain opiates,[64] and red-eared slider turtles have both proencephalin-derived peptides and functional μ- and δ-opioid receptors in the brain.[36,37]

Although opioid receptors are expressed in reptiles, we are just beginning to understand the efficacy of commonly used opioid drugs. Butorphanol tartrate was considered to be the most commonly administered analgesic drug in reptiles.[3] In a published survey of veterinary medical clinicians, the applied reptile dosage range for butorphanol varied from 0.02 mg/kg to 25 mg/kg.[3] However, there were no clinical data to substantiate that butorphanol was an effective analgesic drug in reptiles. Butorphanol was, and still is, being used as a primary analgesic in reptiles because everyone was reporting that it worked. In 2005, our laboratory began to ask the first question: How do we know that butorphanol has analgesic properties in reptiles? Using our own noxious thermal stimulus paradigm, and through a series of controlled

TABLE 50.2 Analgesic Protocols for Use in Reptiles

	Dosage (mg/kg)	Route	Frequency	Comments
Opioids				
Buprenorphine[47,55,72]	0.075–0.1 0.02–0.1 0.1–1.0	SC, IM	q24h	No evidence of analgesic efficacy; plasma concentrations equivalent to those effective for analgesia in mammals; respiratory depression not studied
Butorphanol[43,45–48,65,66]	1.0–20.0 0.4–8.0	SC, IM	NDA	No evidence of analgesic efficacy; significant respiratory depression in RES (>10 mg/kg NOT RECOMMENDED)
Hydromorphone[72]	0.5	SC, IM	q24h	Good analgesic efficacy in RES; respiratory depression not studied, but thought to be significant
Fentanyl (Gutwillig, et al, Proc ARAV 2012, p 66)[58,59,71]	12.5 mcg/hr 2.5 mcg/hr	TC	One patch for 24–72 h	Transdermal patch; provided antinociception in ball pythons and corn snakes; plasma concentrations detected in ball pythons and prehensile-tailed skinks
Meperidine (pethidine) (Sladky K, unpublished data)[67,68]	1.0–5.0 10.0–50.0	SC, IM	q2-4h	Analgesic efficacy short-lived in RES; respiratory depression not studied
Methadone (Vaughan, personal communication)[102]	3.0–5.0	SC, IM	q24h	Good analgesic efficacy in RES; administered without evidence of efficacy in Australian Krefft's river turtle; anecdotal evidence in lizard species; respiratory depression not studied
Morphine[43–47,68–70,87]	1.0–5.0	SC, IM,	q24h	Good analgesic efficacy in RES & bearded dragons; unknown efficacy in snakes; significant respiratory depression (>5 mg/kg NOT RECOMMENDED)
	0.1–0.2	IT		Antinociceptive for >24 h in red-eared sliders
Naloxone[43–46]	0.04–2.0	IM, SC		All species; antagonizes μ-opioid agonists (e.g., morphine)
Oxymorphone (Sladky K, unpublished data)	NDA			As a μ-opioid agonist, analgesia presumably achieved, but no dosage information
Tapentadol[80,81]	5.0	IM		Analgesic efficacy in yellow-bellied sliders; pharmacokinetics indicated 10 h duration of effect
Tramadol[6,61,79]	5.0–10.0	PO	q48-72h	Good analgesic efficacy with relatively long duration when administered PO in chelonians; less respiratory depression than other opioids in RES, YBS; in loggerhead sea turtles, 10 mg/kg PO q 48–72 h
NSAIDs				
Carprofen[5,41]	0.1 1.0–4.0	SC, IM	NDA	No data regarding analgesic efficacy, safety, nor phamacokinetics/pharmacodynamics in any reptile species
Ketoprofen (Norton, Harms, personal communication)[99]	2.0	PO, SC, IM	NDA	Pharmacokinetic data in green iguanas; no evidence of analgesic efficacy in any reptile species, but an NSAID frequently used by sea turtle clinicians as an antiinflammatory due to apparent safety
Meloxicam[66,92–98,103,104]	0.1–0.5	IV, SC, IM, PO	NDA	Pharmacokinetic data in loggerhead sea turtles at 0.1 mg/kg; did not reach plasma concentrations indicative of analgesia in mammals; not recommended at these dosages; pharmacokinetic data in green iguanas at 0.2 mg/kg IV; no evidence of analgesic efficacy in any reptile species; no physiological changes in ball pythons administered postoperatively; aquatic turtles (0.2–0.4 mg/kg) IM, IV; ball pythons (0.3 mg/kg) IM; pharmacokinetic data in RES
Local Anesthetics				
Lidocaine (1% or 2%)[87,89]	1–2 (keep <5.0) 4.0	SC, IM IT	NDA	Appears to be a good local nerve block and effective IT in chelonians
Bupivicaine (0.5%)[87]	1.0 (keep <2.0) 1.0	SC, IM IT	NDA	Appears to be a good local nerve block and effective IT in chelonians
Mepivicaine (2%)[13]	1.0	SC	NDA	Used as a mandibular nerve block in alligators
Proparacaine Ophthalmic Solution (0.5%)[105–107]		Topicalcorneal	NDA	Blocked corneal sensitivity within 1 min of application with duration of effect at least 45 min. in Kemp's ridley turtles; green iguanas; bearded dragons; caiman

TABLE 50.2 Analgesic Protocols for Use in Reptiles—cont'd

	Dosage (mg/kg)	Route	Frequency	Comments
Other Anesthetics				
Medetomidine/ dexmedetomidine[41,108,109,111]	0.05–0.3 0.1–0.2	SC, IM	NDA	No evidence of analgesic efficacy; frequently combined with ketamine, midazolam, or an opioid in sedation/anesthesia protocols
Ketamine[108–110]	2	SC, IM, IV	NDA	No evidence of analgesic efficacy; low dose as an analgesic is extrapolated from the mammalian literature; frequently combined with an alpha-2, benzodiazepine, or an opioid in sedation/anesthesia protocols
Midazolam[110,112–114]	0.5–3.0	SC, IM, IV	NDA	No evidence of analgesic efficacy; frequently combined with an alpha-2, ketamine, or an opioid; enhances analgesic properties of dexmedetomidine in mammals

h, Hours; *IM,* Intramuscular; *IT,* intrathecal; *IV,* intravenous; *Lg,* large; *NDA,* no data available; *PO,* oral; *RES,* red-eared sliders; *SC,* subcutaneous; *TC,* transcutaneous; *YBS,* yellow-bellied sliders.

TABLE 50.3 Opioid Receptor Subtypes, Exogenous and Endogenous Opioids

Receptor Subtype	Exogenous Opioid Agonist	Endogenous Opioid Agonist	Exogenous Antagonist
Mu (μ)-opioid receptor (MOR) agonists	Morphine, hydromorphone, fentanyl methadone, oxymorphone, experimental drugs (DAMGO)	Endorphins (enkephalins), endomorphins	Naloxone, naltrexone
Kappa (κ)-opioid receptor (KOR) agonists	Butorphanol (kappa-agonist/μ-antagonist), nalbuphine (kappa agonist/ partial mu antagonist), experimental drugs (U50488, U69593)	Dynorphin A	Naloxone, naltrexone
Delta (δ)-opioid receptor (DOR) agonists	Only experimental drugs (DADLE, DPDPE, deltorphan II)	Endorphins (enkephalins)	Naltrindole, naloxone, naltrexone

DAMGO-[D-Ala 2, MePhe 4, Gly(ol) 5]enkephalin; DPDPE-[D-Pen 2, D-Pen 5]enkephalin; DPDPE-[D-Pen2,5]Enkephalin, [D-Pen2,D-Pen5] Enkephalin; U50488-trans-(-)-3,4-Dichloro-N-methyl-N-[2-(1-pyrrolidinyl)cyclohexyl]benzeneacetamide hydrochloride; U69593-N-methyl-2-phenyl-N-[(5R,7S,8S)-7-(pyrrolidin-1-yl)-1-oxaspiro[4.5]dec-8-yl]acetamide.

experiments, we determined that butorphanol had no analgesic efficacy in red-eared slider turtles when administered at dosages of 2.8 and 28 mg/kg SC or in bearded dragons when administered at dosages of 2 and 20 mg/kg SC.[44–46] Our butorphanol data in corn snakes was too variable to make any firm conclusions, but an unfortunate consequence of that publication[46] was that several clinicians decided to administer butorphanol (20 mg/kg) to debilitated snakes, which had fatal consequences in some cases. Consistent with our turtle and bearded dragon data, butorphanol administered IM at a dosage of 1 mg/kg had no analgesic efficacy (determined by use of a thermal noxious stimulus method)[48] and no isoflurane-sparing effect in green iguanas.[65] In ball pythons, butorphanol administered at 5 mg/kg IM had no effect on physiological parameters compared to saline.[66] Conversely, one study demonstrated that butorphanol may provide analgesia in green iguanas exposed to a noxious electrical stimulus.[47] On the other hand, morphine sulfate was an effective analgesic in bearded dragons (1 and 5 mg/kg) and turtles (1.5 and 6.5 mg/kg) using the thermal noxious stimulus method, but data were not as clear in corn snakes, even when administered morphine at a dosage of 40 mg/kg.[46] Similarly, morphine (5, 7.5, 10, and 20 mg/kg) and pethidine (10, 20, and 50 mg/kg) provided analgesia in Speke's hinged tortoises (*Kinixys spekii*) exposed to formalin administered into a limb, which was reversible after naloxone administration.[67] In further support of morphine analgesic efficacy in reptiles, morphine increased limb withdrawal latencies in crocodiles[68,69] and increased tail flick latencies in anole lizards.[70] Related to morphine, hydromorphone is a semisynthetic, μ-opioid receptor agonist, which was demonstrated to provide analgesia in red-eared sliders using the

thermal hind limb withdrawal nociception model at 0.5 mg/kg SC for up to 24 hours.[71]

Fentanyl is a μ-opioid receptor agonist, with 75 to 100 times the potency of morphine, which can be administered either transcutaneously as an impregnated patch or intravenously (Figure. 50.5). Two separate studies have evaluated the pharmacokinetics of fentanyl in two reptile species. In ball pythons, fentanyl plasma concentrations reached 1 ng/ml within 4 hrs of application of a transdermal fentanyl patch (12.5 mcg/hr)[59] and were detectable by 4 to 6 hours and for greater than 72 hours in the plasma of prehensile-tailed skinks (fentanyl dose was applied at 10% exposure of total surface area of a 25 mcg/hr patch for 72 hours).[58] It remains unclear whether there is any biologic significance to these plasma fentanyl concentrations. A recently completed study in our laboratory evaluated the efficacy of transdermal fentanyl patch (12.5 mcg/hour) administration in ball pythons.[72] The results demonstrated that the mean latency associated with withdrawal from a noxious thermal stimulus was not statistically different after fentanyl patch application compared to controls without a fentanyl patch. We also confirmed that fentanyl was readily absorbed through the skin of the snakes and remained at very high plasma levels during patch application. In the same study, we determined that fentanyl patch application decreased respiration in the same snakes, so we know that fentanyl is biologically active in the snakes, even though we cannot definitively determine analgesic efficacy.

Buprenorphine is an effective analgesic in many mammalian species and used extensively due to its longer duration of action compared with other opioids. Buprenorphine has partial agonist activity at the

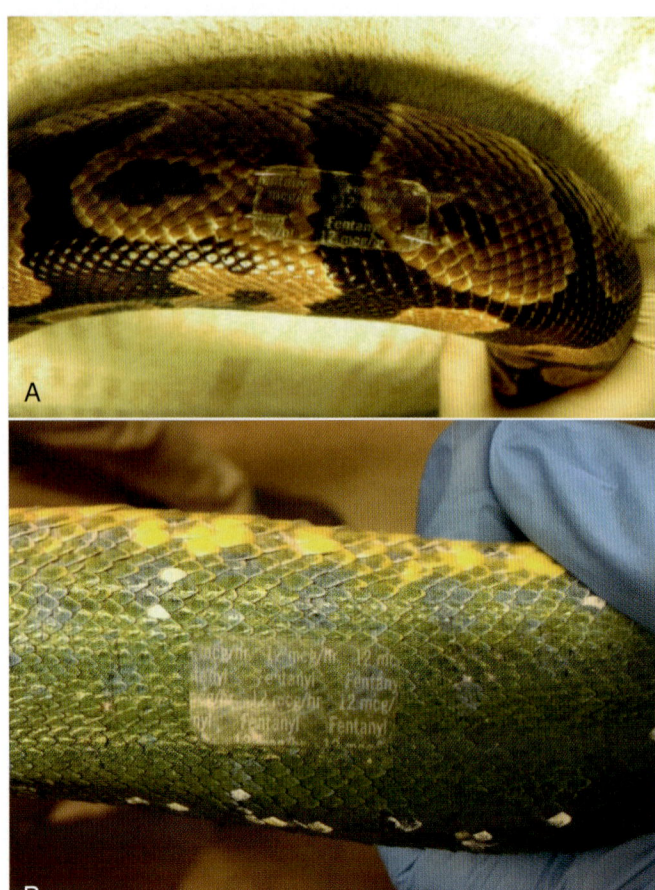

FIG 50.5 Fentanyl patch (12.5 mcg/hr) application on the skin of (A) a ball python (*Python regius*) and (B) a green tree python (*Morelia viridis*). (Courtesy of Kurt K. Sladky.)

μ-opioid receptor, partial or full agonist activity at the δ-opioid receptor, and antagonist activity at the κ-opioid receptor. Buprenorphine pharmacokinetics in reptiles were determined after SC administration in red-eared slider turtles, and effective dosages ranged from 0.075 to 0.1 mg/kg, which provided plasma concentrations at those associated with analgesic efficacy in humans for approximately 24 hours.[55] Interestingly, plasma concentrations of buprenorphine were reduced by approximately 70% when the drug was administered in the hind limb compared to the forelimb, indicating a significant hepatic first-pass effect. The analgesic efficacy of buprenorphine has not been demonstrated in reptiles. Buprenorphine did not alter responses to an electrical noxious stimulus in green iguanas.[47] Similarly, in our laboratory, buprenorphine (0.1, 0.2, and 1.0 mg/kg, SC) provided no analgesic efficacy in red-eared slider turtles exposed to a noxious thermal stimulus.[71]

Tramadol has become a widely used analgesic alternative to other opioids in veterinary medicine, because it can be administered orally and due to its relatively long duration of action. Tramadol and its major active metabolite, O-desmethyl-tramadol (M1), produce analgesia in mammals by activating μ-opioid receptors, but also by inhibiting central serotonin and norepinephrine reuptake.[73,74] Parent tramadol has μ-opioid activity, but O-desmethyl-tramadol, the active metabolite of tramadol, has up to 200 times greater affinity for μ-opioid receptors.[75] Overall, tramadol binds μ-opioid receptors with 6000 times less affinity than morphine,[75] thus having the potential for producing fewer μ-opioid–induced side effects. In fact, tramadol does not appear to alter breathing in humans[76]

and produces significantly less respiratory depression than morphine in cats and dogs.[77,78]

In mammals, the analgesic effects of tramadol typically begin within 30 minutes after oral administration and last for 6 hrs. In contrast, tramadol (5.0 mg/kg; PO) administered to turtles significantly increased withdrawal latencies for 12 to 24 hours postdrug administration and 6 to 96 hours after administration of the higher tramadol dosages (10 or 25 mg/kg; PO or SC).[6] In loggerhead turtles (*Caretta caretta*), plasma concentrations of tramadol and O-desmethyl-tramadol remained above the target concentration of ≥100 ng/mL for approximately 48 hours at a dose of 5 mg/kg PO and for 72 hours when tramadol was administered at 10 mg/kg PO.[61] Subjectively, appetite, swimming, and general activity level did not change after drug administration. Most human and nonhuman mammalian studies consider the tramadol target analgesic plasma concentration to be 100 ng/mL. Recently, tramadol pharmacokinetics and efficacy were evaluated in yellow-bellied slider turtles (*Trachemys scripta scripta*) after a single intramuscular dose (10 mg/kg) administered in either the hind limb or forelimb.[79] Using a thermal hind limb withdrawal latency test, antinociceptive efficacy appeared to last approximately 48 hours regardless of whether the tramadol was administered in the forelimb or hind limb, and tramadol and O-desmethyl-tramadol (M1) remained above an atypically high target plasma concentration (1 μg/mL or 1000 ng/mL) for approximately 48 hours.[79] Of interest was that the pharmacokinetic trends were similar for tramadol administration in forelimbs and hind limbs, but the concentration of M1 was approximately 20% higher in the plasma of the group receiving tramadol in the hind limbs compared with those receiving tramadol in the forelimbs.

With respect to deleterious side effects, respiratory depression associated with tramadol administration in red-eared slider turtles was approximately 50% less than that measured after morphine administration.[6] Therefore tramadol appears to be a promising analgesic alternative to traditional opioids in reptiles. As mentioned, one of the significant deleterious side effects associated with tramadol, and all opioid drug administration in mammals, is respiratory depression. This problem is paralleled in reptile studies. Our laboratory determined that both butorphanol and morphine caused profound respiratory depression in turtles,[45] whereas respiratory depression was significantly less when turtles were administered tramadol. The bottom line is that it is imperative that clinicians continue to monitor respiration during and after procedures in which any opioid drugs are administered to reptile species.

Tapendatol, similar mechanistically to tramadol, is a human drug that shares μ-opioid receptor activation and norepinephrine reuptake inhibition with tramadol, but tapendatol has only weak serotonergic reuptake and has more potent opioid properties without an active metabolite. Tapendatol was administered to red-eared and yellow-bellied slider turtles to determine analgesic efficacy using a thermal noxious stimulus model and pharmacokinetics.[80,81] After intramuscular administration (5 mg/kg), tapendatol plasma concentrations were detectable for approximately 24 hours, and the duration of antinociceptive effects was approximately 10 hours in both turtle species.[80,81] The shorter duration of antinociceptive efficacy, compared with tramadol, may be due to the lack of an active metabolite. Although respiratory depression has not been investigated after tapendatol administration in reptiles, in humans it is thought to cause less respiratory depression compared with commonly administered μ-opioid agonist drugs.

Parenteral Anesthetics

There are no published data demonstrating analgesic efficacy associated with administration of anesthetic drugs, such as ketamine, dexmedetomidine, medetomidine, midazolam, or propofol in reptiles. Combinations of these drugs are excellent for sedation and induction of anesthesia, but one can only extrapolate from the mammalian literature with respect to analgesic efficacy. In mammals, for example, there is interest in the fact that low-dosage ketamine provides analgesia.[82] Ketamine has an antagonistic effect on N-methyl-D-aspartate (NMDA) receptors, decreasing the wind-up effect and central sensitization, especially for chronic pain.[83] These receptors have been demonstrated in chelonians.[84] Unfortunately, nothing is currently known about ketamine as an analgesic in any reptile species. Combining ketamine with an alpha-2-adrenergic agonist (e.g., medetomidine, dexmedetomidine) increases the level of sedation in reptiles, as in mammals. Although such combinations provide analgesia in mammals, it can only be speculated that the same is true in reptiles, as no data are available.

Local Anesthetics as Analgesics

Local anesthetics can be used alone or as part of a multimodal anesthetic/analgesic approach. These include lidocaine, bupivacaine, and mepivacaine, which block peripheral nerve transmission to the dorsal horn by inhibiting sodium influx into the neurons and therefore blocking the nociceptive signal from traveling along the nerve fibers.[85] For all local anesthetics, the pain transmission is blocked as long as the local anesthetic nerve block lasts, but inflammation and pain will still develop at the site of injury and will be transmitted to the central nervous system after the effect of the block has ceased. Because of its significant analgesic effect, any local block that is correctly executed will significantly decrease the required amount of other anesthetic agents, but additional analgesia is warranted for postoperative pain management in certain cases. The limitations associated with local anesthetic administration include a focal nervous block and short duration of action.

With respect to local anesthetics, there is only one published reptile study, in which mepivacaine was used as a mandibular nerve block in an alligator.[13] In this study, a nerve locator was used to facilitate the procedure. Lidocaine (2%) (up to 5 mg/kg total dose) can be used for local ring blocks or line blocks. Lidocaine may be diluted with bicarbonate or sterile water at a 1:1 ratio or greater to decrease the pain of injection and allow increased volume to be infused without reaching a toxic dose. In addition, topical lidocaine (4%) is commonly administered directly to wounds before and after debridement for local analgesia, particularly in chelonian species. Proparacaine was demonstrated to be effective in blocking corneal sensitivity in Kemp's ridley turtles for up to 45 minutes, with a 1-minute onset to effect.[86] Similarly, intrathecal analgesia was reported in chelonians.[87] Intrathecal administration is useful for surgical procedures of the tail, phallus, cloaca, and hind limbs.[87] Lidocaine (2% at 4 mg/kg; <1 hour duration), bupivacaine (1 mg/kg; 1–2 hours duration) or preservative-free morphine sulfate (0.1–0.2 mg/kg; duration of up to 48 hours) can be administered intrathecally between the coccygeal vertebrae of turtles. For example, bupivicaine (0.1 mL for each 10 cm of carapace) was administered intrathecally in order to facilitate surgical excision of fibropapillomas from the posterior flippers of a green sea turtle.[88] In a different study, 2% lidocaine (1 mL/20–25 kg) was administered intrathecally in hybrid Galapagos tortoises prior to phallectomy surgery.[89] Coelioscopic orchiectomy was performed on adult male desert tortoises, and intrathecal lidocaine (2 mg/kg), in combination with morphine sulfate (0.1 mg/kg) were administered intrathecally prior to the surgical procedure.[90]

Nonsteroidal Antiinflammatory Drugs (NSAIDs)

While not as potent as the opioids, nonsteroidal antiinflammatory agents are used widely in reptile clinical practice as analgesics, as well as for their antiinflammatory properties. Nonsteroidal antiinflammatory drugs provide analgesia in mammals by blocking the binding of arachidonic acid to cyclooxygenase enzyme (COX), preventing the conversion of thromboxane A2 to thromboxane B2 (TBX), thus preventing production of prostaglandins (PG), potent mediators of inflammation.[91] Nonsteroidal antiinflammatory drugs are often classified based on their relative specificity. There are two COX enzymes, COX-1 and COX-2, that participate in renal and gastric protection and inflammation, respectively.[91] The NSAID ketoprofen is equipotent against both isoenzymes, although carprofen is slightly more COX-2 specific and meloxicam is COX-2 specific.[91] Therefore the degree of efficacy and side effects may vary with each of the three NSAIDS selected.

Although many NSAIDS appear to be relatively safe when used in reptiles, there is only one published study with respect to analgesic efficacy.[92] Ball pythons administered meloxicam (0.3 mg/kg, IM) prior to a surgical placement of an arterial catheter showed no physiological changes (e.g., heart rate, blood pressure, plasma epinephrine, and cortisol) indicative of analgesia. With respect to the pharmocokinetics of NSAIDS in reptile species, plasma concentrations of meloxicam (0.2 mg/kg, PO) administered as a single dose to green iguanas were at levels considered analgesic in mammals, and these levels were measurable out to 24 hours postadministration.[92] In loggerhead turtles, meloxicam (0.1 mg/kg) administered both IM and IV did not reach plasma concentrations consistent with analgesia in humans, horses, or dogs, and the half-life was short.[93,95] In a pharmacokinetic study in which meloxicam (0.2 mg/kg IM and IV) was administered to red-eared slider turtles, the IM dose provided a therapeutic concentration range necessary for meloxicam to provide analgesic and antiinflammatory effects equivalent in mammals for approximately 48 hours.[96] In a different study evaluating the pharmacokinetics of meloxicam (0.2 mg/kg PO, ICe, and IM) in red-eared slider turtles, only the ICe and IM routes, but not the PO route, provided mean blood concentrations of meloxicam that were above those considered effective to induce antiinflammatory effects in mammals for approximately 8 hours (IM) or 12 hours (ICe).[97] Ketoprofen (2 mg/kg, IV), administered to green iguanas, had a long half-life (31 hrs) compared to ketoprofen phamacokinetics in mammals, but the bioavailability after IM administration was 78% with a relatively short half-life (8.3 hours).[98]

Since no efficacy data and few pharmacokinetic data are available with respect to NSAID administration in reptiles, appropriate dosages and frequency of administration can only be extrapolated. Additionally, clinicians should be aware of the deleterious side effects documented in avian and mammalian species (e.g., renal impairment, gastrointestinal ulceration/inflammation, hematological abnormalities), and assessment of suitability for this class of drugs for the individual patient is prudent.

Acupuncture

Although acupuncture has been used as an analgesic across a variety of domestic species, including equine, canine, and rodent patients, systematically derived data collected under controlled conditions have not been described. The analgesic efficacy of acupuncture applied to nondomestic species has not been well documented. Electroacupuncture involves application of an electrical stimulus to peripheral nerves via acupuncture needles applied to specific acupuncture points.[99] Electroacupuncture-induced analgesia is attributable to stimulation of mu, sigma, and kappa receptors in rats.[100] However, little to nothing is known about the efficacy of electroacupuncture as an analgesic technique in reptiles. One study effectively transposed canine acupuncture points to a red-footed tortoise in order to successfully treat a locomotor disability associated with an injury.[100] In bearded dragons, morphine is considered to be the most effective antinociceptive agent, and μ-opioid agonists appear to be the most effective antinociceptive agents across many reptile species.[44,46] Since electroacupuncture also acts on μ-opioid receptors, electroacupuncture may be a promising method for providing analgesia (i.e., antinociception) to bearded dragons. The Chi institute of Traditional Chinese Veterinary Medicine in Florida has effectively treated bearded dragons for a variety of ailments such as malnutrition and anorexia with electroacupuncture (Sladky K, personal communication). In our

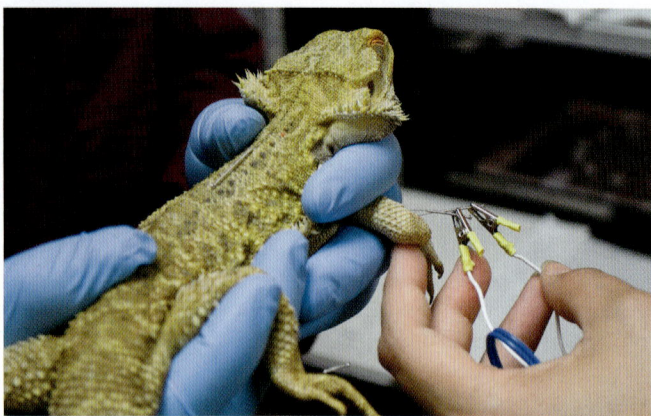

FIG 50.6 Bearded dragon (*Pogona vitticeps*) undergoing electroacupuncture. Needle placement sites were extrapolated from the veterinary mammalian literature. (Courtesy of Kurt K. Sladky.)

laboratory, we recently completed a study in which bearded dragons were subjected to electroacupuncture, followed by application of a thermal noxious stimulus to determine whether electroacupuncture provided thermal antinociception (Fig. 50.6). Preliminary data suggest that the bearded dragons relaxed under the influence of electroacupuncture and demonstrated a trend toward delayed limb withdrawal after exposure to a thermal noxious stimulus. However, the data are not statistically different from controls.

Multimodal Analgesic Approaches

In reptiles, multimodal drug paradigms may be the best approach for managing pain. Multimodal analgesia refers to the administration of multiple drugs, which have analgesic efficacy at different levels in the central and peripheral nervous system. For example, opioids will have greatest efficacy at opioid receptors in the central and peripheral nervous systems, whereas NSAIDs administered at the same time as the opioid will have greatest efficacy as antiinflammatory agents at the peripheral tissues.[101] Local anesthetics can enhance multimodal analgesic protocols by blocking the initial pain cascade at the peripheral level. In concert, all of these drugs have the potential to minimize transmission of pain signals to the brain, especially when administered preemptively, before a potentially painful procedure is established.

CONCLUSION

While our understanding of reptile pain and analgesia has advanced significantly during the past 10 years, there is a great deal of theoretical and clinical research to conduct, and our ability to extrapolate across orders and species remains a major limitation. In other words, an effective analgesic drug administered to a leopard tortoise may not have the same efficacy in a ball python. Our inability to have a "one size fits all" model for reptile analgesics stems from the fact that the class *Reptilia* is incredibly diverse. Continued research focusing on effective analgesic drugs, dose-dependent effects, duration of drug efficacy, interspecies differences, and potentially detrimental drug-related adverse effects will advance the field and begin to reinforce, or abolish, the perpetuation of anecdotal information, which remains pervasive in the reptile clinical medicine literature.

Butorphanol tartrate (a κ-opioid receptor agonist), administered at mammalian-derived dosages, was once believed to be the most effective analgesic drug for use in reptiles. More recently, however, our systematic investigation into pain and analgesia in a variety of reptile species has demonstrated that μ-opioid receptor agonists, such as morphine, hydropmorphone, fentanyl, or tramadol, provide effective analgesia, while butorphanol appears to be no more effective than saline. Extrapolation of analgesic efficacy across orders and species remains a major limitation, and there is a clear need for evaluating analgesic drugs across a variety of clinical situations, particularly as they apply to postsurgical pain. We believe that objectively derived methods for evaluation of pain in animals are critical, but these methods must be species and context specific. In addition, determining pharmacokinetic parameters, duration of drug efficacy, species-specific requirements, and deleterious side effects of opioid drugs in different reptile species remains critical to continue to advance the field of reptile analgesia.

ACKOWLEDGMENTS

Significant portions of this chapter were published previously in: Analgesia. In *Current therapy in reptile medicine and surgery* (3rd ed). Mader DR, Divers S (eds). St. Louis: Elsevier-Saunders; 2014:217–228.

REFERENCES

See www.expertconsult.com for a complete list of references.

51

Regional Anesthesia and Analgesia

Christoph Mans, Paulo Steagall, and Kurt K. Sladky

Regional anesthesia and analgesia are currently underutilized in reptile medicine but offer significant benefits, for example, in the ability to reduce injectable, inhalant anesthetic and sedative drug requirements and to produce preemptive analgesia in the perioperative period without deleterious side effects, such as respiratory depression. In addition, drugs used for regional anesthesia are widely available and often do not fall into controlled drug categories (e.g. Drug Enforcement Agency scheduling in the USA). Finally, in mammals, local anesthetics have the potential to blunt a surgery-induced neuroendocrine (stress) response. Knowledge of anatomic landmarks and basic pharmacology of local anesthetics is required for safe and effective nerve blocks. Regional anesthesia can be used as a sole anesthetic modality in manually restrained or sedated reptiles for minor surgical procedures (Fig. 51.1A and B). Common indications for the use of local anesthetics as part of an anesthetic protocol include distal limb surgery, cloacal procedures (e.g., prolapse), phallectomy, and celiotomy. Local anesthetics can be administered as part of topical or incisional (infiltration) anesthesia, peripheral or cranial nerve blocks, or neuraxial (intrathecal, spinal) anesthesia.

MECHANISM OF ACTION

Local anesthetics are expected to have a similar mechanism of action among reptiles as they have in other vertebrates. Local anesthetics block neuronal, voltage-gated Na^+ and voltage-dependent Ca^{2+} and K^+ channels. This results in a blockade of generation and propagation of electrical impulses in a reversible manner. These drugs will produce loss of sensory, motor, and autonomic function. Clinical experience shows that autonomic responses are inhibited before sensory (loss of sensation, pain, and light touch) and motor blockade. Resolution of blockade occurs in the reverse order. Local anesthetics have a pKa (dissociation constant) between 7.5 and 9 and are formulated as hydrochloride salts. When local anesthetics are injected into body tissues with a physiologic pH (7.4), the nonionized lipid-soluble form will prevail. This allows local anesthetics to cross biological membranes. In inflammation, the ionized form prevails due to acidic pH, and these drugs may not produce an appropriate anesthetic effect ("patchy" block).

Clinical experience demonstrates that local anesthetics have similar onset and duration of action in reptiles when compared with mammals. Dosages, volumes, and concentrations of local anesthetics are crucial in determining the magnitude and quality of the anesthetic block. High concentrations are preferred, but sufficient volume of tissue distribution should be considered. Site of injection will be an important factor in inducing the onset of block. For shorter onset of anesthesia, local anesthetics should be administered as close as possible but not directly into a nerve. Physical and chemical characteristics of the local anesthetic explain the slow onset, but some lipophilic drugs (e.g., bupivacaine) provide a long duration of action.

ADVERSE EFFECTS

Local anesthetics can produce irreversible or reversible nerve damage. Neurotrauma occurs during intraneural injections. A local anesthetic should never be injected if resistance to injection is observed. Systemic toxicity is produced by accidental intravascular injection of local anesthetics. Toxic dosages associated with adverse effects have not been determined in reptiles, but maximum dosages used in mammals, particularly in small reptiles, should be used as a guide. Adverse effects can include seizures, cardiorespiratory depression, and death. Only preservative-free drug formulations should be used for intrathecal injections.

LOCAL ANESTHETICS

Lidocaine

Lidocaine (2%) is an amino-amide local anesthetic that is commonly used in reptile medicine. Dosages associated with toxicity were reported to be between 5 to 20 mg/kg in mammals.[1] In reptiles, lidocaine was administered at up to 4 mg/kg intrathecally without side effects (Table 51.1).[2] Concentrations of 0.5% and 1% are also available. In addition, a commercial mixture of lidocaine (2.5%) and prilocaine (2.5%) in gel preparation (EMLA cream) is available and used for venipuncture in small animals. Its use was reported in turtles and tortoises undergoing phallectomy, with a dose of 1g/10 cm^2 applied to the phallic mucosa.[3] Onset of action was approximately 20 minutes and other anesthetic-analgesic techniques should be used in combination.[3] Infiltration of the prefemoral fossa in chelonians with lidocaine has been reported and is frequently used by biologists for coelioscopy. However, it has been documented that this technique using 1 mg/kg of lidocaine results in insufficient anesthesia and analgesia compared to general anesthesia and is therefore not recommended.[4]

Bupivacaine

Bupivacaine is a highly lipophilic, amino-amide local anesthetic that produces significant cardiotoxicity when injected intravenously. It is not clear what dosages will produce these deleterious effects in different reptile species, but negative aspiration of blood into the needle hub is always recommended prior to bupivacaine administration. Bupivacaine was used for tissue infiltration in garter snakes during cloacal procedures, for the study of mating behavior, and by the intrathecal route of administration in turtles (see Table 51.1).[2,5]

LOCAL ANESTHETIC TECHNIQUES

Tissue Infiltration (Incisional Anesthesia)

Local anesthetics are used for incisional anesthesia and can be infiltrated in the subcutaneous tissue in association with a surgical field, for example,

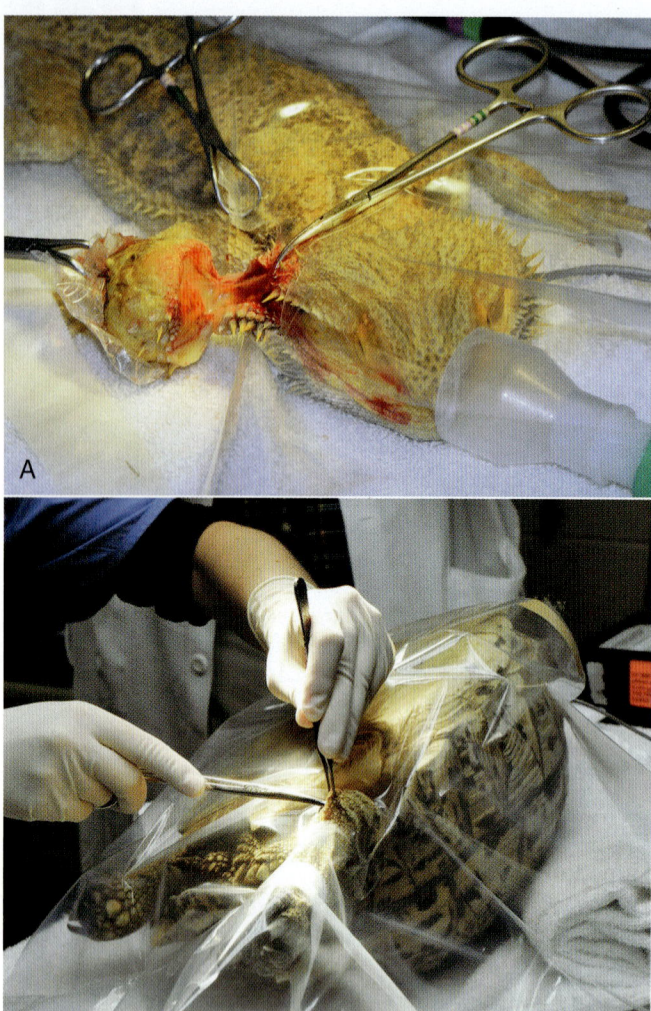

FIG 51.1 Regional anesthesia combined with procedural sedation in reptiles. (A) Bearded dragon (*Pogona vitticeps*) undergoing removal of a facial mass. Lidocaine was locally infiltrated after moderate sedation was induced with the administration of dexmedetomidine and midazolam. The skin mass was surgically excised. The animal continued breathing spontaneously and recovered without complications. (B) Sedated leopard tortoise (*Stigmochelys pardalis*) undergoing subcutaneous abscess removal, following the local infiltration of the surgical site with lidocaine.

prior to celiotomy ("line block"), skin biopsies, or laceration repair. However, local anesthetics should not be administered in proximity to neoplastic tumors, since the process can spread neoplastic cells. In small animals, this technique is used most frequently before laparotomy and as part of a multimodal analgesic approach, during which NSAIDs are also administered systemically. Aseptic techniques are always employed.

Nerve Blocks

Local anesthetic techniques of the head and limbs are not commonly reported in reptile literature. This is likely due to the large number of reptilian species and paucity of information on their specific neuroanatomy and the efficacy of locoregional techniques.

In crocodilians, dental blocks can be used as part of the clinical investigation, for tissue biopsies, draining abscesses and surgery, and to improve anesthetic recovery.[6] An electrical nerve locator was attached to an insulated needle and generated an electric field in the tissues surrounding a target nerve; in this particular case, the mandibular nerve.[6] This resulted in depolarization and muscle contractions that are used to confirm correct needle placement before drug administration. Theoretically, the use of a nerve locator reduces the dose of a local anesthetic required for an effective block and increases the rate of success. In large crocodilians, the positive electrode of the nerve locator is attached to an area of softer skin immediately behind the front leg. The external mandibular foramen is palpated, and after aseptic preparation, the needle attached to the negative electrode is inserted from a lateral approach into the cranial aspect of the external mandibular foramen. Alternatively, a different technique can be used when the needle is inserted (attached to the negative electrode) ventrocaudally along the lingual surface of the mandibular ramus toward the mandibular foramen. In crocodilians, the mandibular nerve branches travel past the cranial aspect of the external mandibular foramen. The nerve locator is set to deliver an initial current of 2 mA with frequency at two pulses per second. Higher currents may produce pain in the conscious patient. Movement of the intermandibularis muscle, during stimulation, is considered to be the end point. Mepivacaine 2% (1 mg/kg per side) was injected when responses were observed at 0.5 mA but not at 0.2 mA (risk of intraneural injection). Negative aspiration of blood should be confirmed before injection.[6] The use of nerve locators has great potential for reptile medicine, and further studies are warranted using this technique for locoregional anesthesia.

For surgical procedures involving the forelimbs, a nerve block should be considered. In an eastern box turtle (*Terrapene carolina*) a nerve block was used to perform an incisional biopsy of a forelimb digit swelling (Grioni et al, Proc ICARE, 2015, p 284).

Spinal Anesthesia

Spinal (also referred to as *intrathecal* or *subdural*) anesthesia offers substantial advantages, if used as part of a balanced anesthetic protocol, by reducing injectable and volatile anesthetic requirements needed to perform surgery. Consequently, the dose-dependent cardiorespiratory depressant effects of general anesthetics are reduced, and analgesia of longer duration can be provided. Local anesthetics are injected intrathecally (subdurally), which results in autonomic, sensory, and motor blockade. Opioids are commonly combined with local anesthetics for spinal analgesia. In this case, they bind to opioid receptors in the spinal cord and reduce release of excitatory neurotransmitters and hyperpolarize cell membranes, blunting nociceptive afferent input. Opioids do not produce motor blockade or impair proprioception and will increase duration of action providing sustained postoperative analgesia. In mammals, possible indications for spinal (or epidural) anesthesia include surgical procedures caudal to the diaphragm, including the tail, perineum, external genitalia, hind limbs, and caudal abdomen.[8,9]

Spinal anesthesia and analgesia of the spinal cord is currently in its infancy in reptiles and has only been reported in turtles and tortoises (see Table 51.1).[2,10–12] In chelonians, epidural anesthesia is not possible due to the lack of a sufficiently developed epidural space. However, a well-developed intrathecal (subdural) space, which directly surrounds the spinal cord and is filled with cerebrospinal fluid (CSF), has been reported (Fig. 51.2) and allows for intrathecal administration of various anesthetic and analgesic drugs.[2] The presence of the carapace, and the fusion of the vertebral column to the carapace, limits access only to the cervical and coccygeal intrathecal space in chelonians, but only intrathecal injections in the coccygeal region are of clinical interest.[2]

In turtles and tortoises, the cloaca, external genitalia, and hind limbs are innervated by caudal branches of the sacral plexus and coccygeal nerves.[13,14] The sacral plexus arises from spinal nerves XVII through XXI, located at the last dorsal and sacral vertebrae.[13,14] Within the sacral

TABLE 51.1   Spinal Anesthesia Studies Performed in Turtles and Tortoises

Species	Gender	Body Weight (kg)	N	Indication	Sedation	Drug(s) Used	Dose (mg/kg)	Duration of Effect	Comments
Galapagos tortoise (Chelonoidis nigra)[10]	Male	32–97	15	Phallectomy	No	Lidocaine 2%	0.8		No effects on hind limbs
Red-eared slider (Trachemys scripta elegans)[2]	Female	0.5–1	15	Experimental	Yes	Lidocaine 2%	4	76 ± 46 minutes	57% success after 1st injection, 83% success after 2nd injection of same dose
Red-eared slider (Trachemys scripta elegans)[2]	Male	0.5–0.8	13	Experimental	Yes	Lidocaine 2%	4	67 ± 24 minutes	60% success after 1st injection, 90% success after 2nd injection of same dose
Red-eared slider (Trachemys scripta elegans)[2]	Male	0.5–0.8	13	Experimental	Yes	Bupivacaine 0.5%	1	121 ± 57 minutes	
Red-eared slider (Trachemys scripta elegans)[2]	Male	0.5–0.8	20	Experimental	Yes	Morphine 0.1%	0.1–0.2	Up to 48 hours	Administered with lidocaine (4 mg/kg).
Black-bellied slider (Trachemys dorbigni)[11]	Female	1.1 ± 0.4 kg	10	Experimental	No	Lidocaine 2%	3	81 ± 10 minutes	

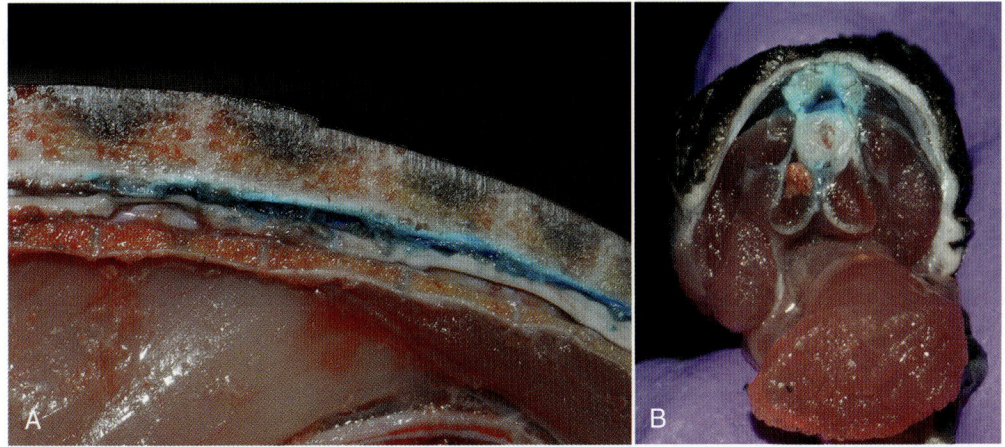

FIG 51.2 Methylene blue injection in the intrathecal (subdural) space of the spinal canal in red-eared slider (*Trachemys scripta elegans*) carcasses: (A) longitudinal view of the dorsal segment of the spinal canal, and (B) cross-section of the proximal tail base. Note the close proximity of the skin overlying the neural arch dorsally.

plexus, the nerves interconnect and subdivide several times before terminating in the inguinal, pelvic, and hind leg muscles.[13,14] Therefore the temporary desensitization of these nerves by intrathecal injection of local anesthetics and analgesics can provide regional anesthesia and analgesia sufficient for a variety of surgical procedures involving the cloaca, urinary bladder, genitals, and hind limbs in turtles and tortoises. More cranial spreading of intrathecally administered anesthetics will lead to desensitization of spinal nerves located more cranially, which supply the prefemoral fossae and caudal coelomic organs and may allow for surgical procedures via the prefemoral approach. A head-down body position should be avoided during and following intrathecal drug administration to avoid excessive cranial spread of the injected drugs.

Spinal anesthesia techniques are used, clinically, in a variety of turtles and tortoises. In conscious, male Galapagos tortoises (*Chelonoidis nigra,*

body weight 32–97 kg), 3-cm hypodermic needles were placed in the mid to distal dorsal coccygeal region after aseptic preparation (Fig. 51.3A).[10] Needle placement was performed through an intervertebral space, which had been identified by palpation. Correct intrathecal needle placement was confirmed by aspiration of CSF before intrathecal injection of 2% lidocaine at an average dose of 0.8 mg/kg (0.04 mL/kg body weight or 1 mL of 2% lidocaine per 20 to 25 kg body weight). In all 15 animals, the level of regional anesthesia was graded as excellent and allowed for successful completion of phallectomy in all tortoises. At the reported dosage, no hind limb paralysis was induced, and no side effects were reported.

In a green turtle (*Chelonia mydas*), spinal anesthesia was used to facilitate the surgical removal of a cutaneous fibropapilloma from the posterior flipper. In this case report, bupivacaine (0.5%), at a dose of

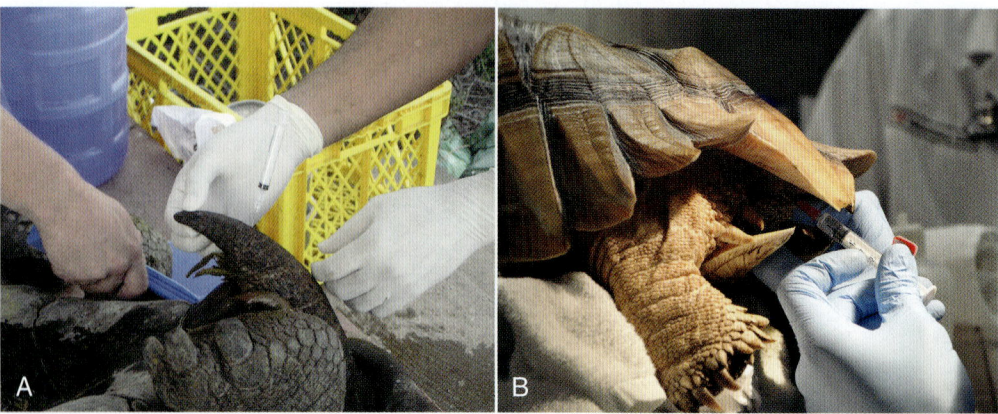

FIG 51.3 Spinal anesthesia in tortoises. (A) Intrathecal injection of lidocaine in a conscious male Galapagos tortoise (*Chelonoidis nigra*) positioned in dorsal recumbency for phallectomy. The needle is placed in the intervertebral space at the distal third of the tail. (B) Intrathecal injection of lidocaine at the proximal tail in a sedated female African spurred tortoise (*Centrochelys sulcata*) before prefemoral cystostomy. (A, Courtesy of Sam Rivera.)

0.1 mL per 10 cm of carapacial length, was administered following induction of anesthesia with midazolam and propofol.[12]

Black-bellied slider (*Trachemys dorbigni*) turtles were evaluated after the spinal administration of lidocaine in an observational study, without a control group using saline.[11] Ten healthy female animals, with an average body weight of 1.1 ± 0.4 kg, were used for this study, in which lidocaine, without epinephrine (3 mg/kg, 2%, or approximately 0.2 mL of lidocaine for each 10 cm of carapacial length), was administered while turtles were in dorsal recumbency. Motor and sensory block of the tail, cloaca, and hind limbs was successfully induced in all turtles. Onset times of spinal anesthesia were 0.4 ± 0.1 minutes for the cloaca and tail, and 2.6 ± 0.4 minutes for the hind limbs. The average duration of motor and sensory block was approximately 80 minutes for analgesia and muscle relaxation. Responses to toe pinch returned approximately 100 minutes after drug administration.[11]

In red-eared sliders (*Trachemys scripta elegans*), the feasibility of spinal anesthesia using lidocaine or bupivacaine was systematically evaluated.[2] Spinal anesthesia was successfully induced in turtles of both sexes, with body weights ranging from 0.5 to 1.0 kg. Injections were performed in sedated turtles, which allowed for proper restraint of the tail and correct intrathecal administration at the level of the mid-to-proximal coccygeal vertebrae. The turtles were positioned in ventral recumbency, and the tails were aseptically prepared before insertion of 28-g needles, attached to 0.5-mL insulin syringes (Fig. 51.4).[2] After penetration of the neural arch, the needle was advanced into the intrathecal space, and careful aspiration was performed. If significant amounts of blood were aspirated, the needle was inadvertently placed in the prominent intravertebral venous plexus surrounding the intrathecal space. The needle position was readjusted until no aspiration of blood occurred, followed by administration of anesthetic and analgesic drugs over approximately 3 to 5 seconds. Successful intrathecal injection and induction of spinal anesthesia was confirmed by complete motor block (relaxation) of the tail, cloacal sphincter, and hind limbs. The onset to motor block ranged from 1 to 5 minutes. Following the initial injection of either preservative-free lidocaine (4 mg/kg, 2%) or bupivacaine (1 mg/kg, 0.5%), spinal anesthesia was successfully induced in approximately half of the turtles. In turtles showing no evidence of spinal anesthesia after the initial injection, a second intrathecal injection, of the same drug and dosage, was administered approximately 15 minutes after the first. The repeated intrathecal injection increased the overall success rate to approximately 80% to 90%.[2] In male and female red-eared sliders,

the duration of motor block of the tail, cloacal sphincter, and hind limbs was approximately 1 hour following intrathecal lidocaine administration (4 mg/kg, 2%).[2] Intrathecal bupivacaine injection (1 mg/kg, 0.5%) in male red-eared sliders caused motor block of the tail, cloacal sphincter, and hind limbs, which lasted approximately 2 hours.[2] There was a large variation in duration of spinal anesthesia in turtles of both genders. A possible explanation for this variability was associated with the well-developed and prominent intravertebral venous plexus, which is located within the spinal canal directly overlying the intrathecal space, both dorsally and laterally. Therefore in some cases, a shorter duration of spinal anesthesia was attributed to a partial intrathecal dose delivery, secondary to an inadvertent IV administration into the intravertebral venous plexus. Consequently, care should be taken with needle placement within the intrathecal space by means of repeated aspiration before, and during, intrathecal injection.

In addition to the administration of anesthetic drugs, drugs with primary analgesic properties can also be administered intrathecally for provision of long-term spinal analgesia. Intrathecally administered morphine relieves somatic and visceral pain by selectively blocking nociceptive impulses without interfering with sensory and motor function or causing sympathetic nervous system blockade, which may lead to hypotension. Morphine is a highly hydrophilic drug that tends to induce long duration of action after intrathecal administration because of delayed systemic absorption and longer maintenance in the spinal cord.[15,16] In male red-eared sliders, intrathecal administration of preservative-free morphine (0.1–0.2 mg/kg, 4 mg/mL) and lidocaine (4 mg/kg, 2%) resulted in thermal antinociception of the hind limbs for up to 48 hours.[2] Sedation was not observed after intrathecal morphine administration. This drug combination has the advantage of providing intra- and postoperative analgesia since lidocaine has short anesthetic onset and duration of action, whereas morphine induces prolonged onset and duration of analgesia due to its physicochemical properties. Postoperative analgesic requirements are commonly reduced in this case. It is currently unknown if intrathecal morphine contributes to respiratory depression in turtles, as has been documented for systemically administered morphine.[17]

In summary, spinal anesthesia and analgesia are clinically feasible techniques in turtles and tortoises. However, significant anatomic differences exist, particularly the presence of a prominent intravertebral venous plexus in turtles. This makes general recommendations regarding technique and dosages across chelonian species challenging. Furthermore,

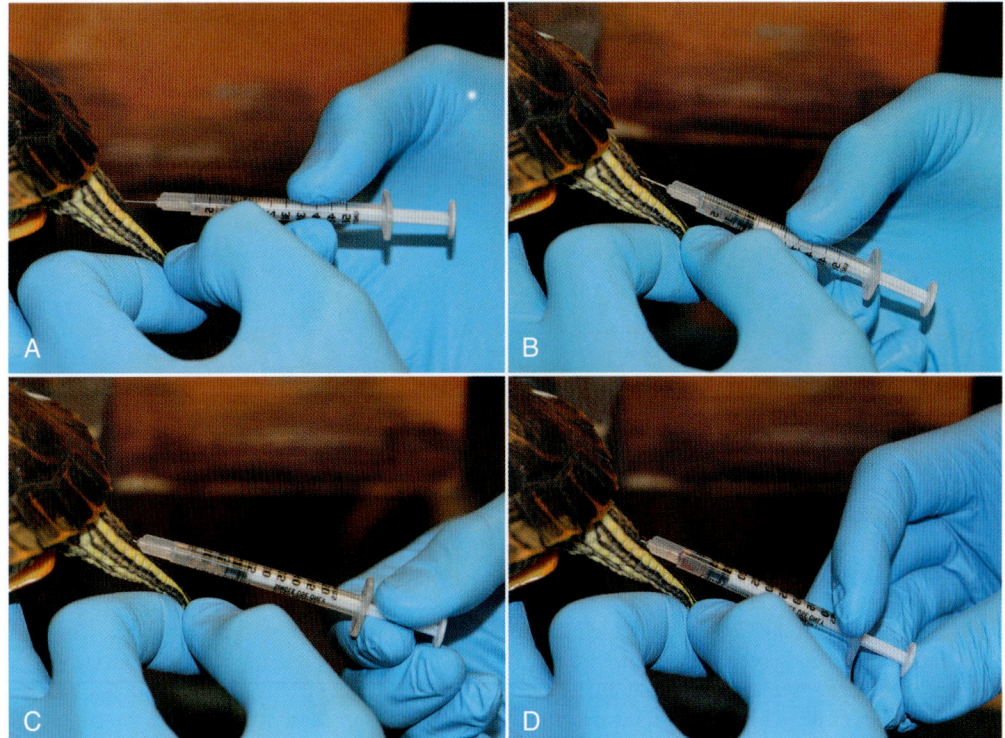

FIG 51.4 Intrathecal administration of anesthetic agents to induce spinal (intrathecal) anesthesia and analgesia in a red-eared slider (*Trachemys scripta elegans*). (A) Penetration of the skin and neural arch with the needle in approximately a 45-degree angle. (B) Advancement of the needle into the spinal canal at about a 20-degree angle. (C) Aspiration is performed to ensure correct placement in the intrathecal place. If an excessive amount of blood is aspirated the needle is repositioned until no further blood is aspirated. (D) Injection of the drug into the intrathecal space over 5 to 10 seconds.

the quantity of drug administered intrathecally will affect the extent of the sensory and motor block. Therefore different procedures will require different volumes of anesthetics and analgesics to be administered intrathecally. The technique may have to be repeated depending on the outcome of the first dose administered. Strict aseptic techniques should be used to avoid iatrogenic complications, and only preservative-free drugs should be administered into the intrathecal space, so that spinal toxicity and secondary neurologic complications are avoided. In contrast to mammals, in which the spinal cord terminates in the distal lumbar or lumbosacral region, the spinal cord in chelonians extends caudal to the last coccygeal vertebrae, and a cauda equina is not present.[18] Therefore

intrathecal needle placement in chelonians can potentially lead to iatrogenic mechanical trauma of the spinal cord in the coccygeal region, with accompanying neurological deficits. Sedation, prior to intrathecal drug administration, is recommended so that the tail is sufficiently restrained and immobilized and the caudal scratch/kick reflex is reduced. This reflex is commonly observed in chelonians and can make intrathecal injections in conscious turtles and tortoises challenging.

REFERENCES

See www.expertconsult.com for a complete list of references.

52

Amphibian Anesthesia

Izidora Sladakovic and Stephen J. Divers

Amphibians represent a vast and varied taxonomic class, with more than 6000 species occupying many ecological niches, including adaptations for both aquatic and terrestrial life. Amphibians are the "coal mine canaries" of the current times and are frequently evaluated as markers of ecosystem health. The changes that have occurred in the natural world, along with emergence of certain diseases, has seen amphibian populations decline dramatically. To provide a high level of care and to better understand and conserve these sentinel species, there is a need to deliver safe and effective anesthesia and analgesia. Anesthesia may be required for evaluating a patient not amenable to physical restraint or to perform various diagnostic and therapeutic procedures, including surgery.

ANATOMY AND PHYSIOLOGY

Amphibian anatomy and physiology is described in greater detail in Chapter 12. Aspects relevant to anesthesia will be briefly mentioned here. Amphibians are divided into three orders: anurans (frogs and toads), urodeles (salamanders, newts, and sirens), and caecilians. Amphibians are unique in their respiratory anatomy and physiology, between species and between life stages as they go through metamorphosis. Respiration can occur via four modes: lungs, skin, buccopharyngeal mucosa, and gills. The presence and extent of these modes contributing to respiration varies between species. In general, all amphibians utilize skin for respiration to varying degrees. The permeable and highly vascular skin of amphibians is unique in its ability to function as an organ for gas exchange and play a vital role in water and electrolyte homeostasis. Some amphibians have structural adaptations of the skin that increase its surface area, which maximize its ability to efficiently carry out multiple functions. All larval forms utilize gills for respiration. Adult anurans and most adult caecilians rely on lungs and buccopharyngeal mucosa. Pedomorphic urodeles retain gills in adulthood and rely on them for respiration, whereas in metamorphic urodeles, gills are resorbed and lungs develop to varying degrees. In some aquatic urodeles, both gills and lungs are present. Some species of urodeles lack lungs completely and rely on cutaneous respiration as a primary mode of gas exchange. Gas exchange also occurs across the highly vascularized buccopharyngeal mucosa via gular pumping, which has a higher rate of pumping than lung inflation. The mode of respiration should be researched and considered for a species when devising an anesthetic plan, particularly as there are many exceptions. For example, species that rely primarily on cutaneous respiration, such as hellbenders (*Cryptobranchus alleganiensis*), require a lower concentration of immersion agent. In lunged species, the trachea is composed of complete cartilaginous rings and is generally short in anurans, and the lungs are simple and delicate. Therefore care must be taken with intubation and ventilation to avoid bronchial

intubation, tracheal trauma, and overinflating the lungs because rupture can occur.[1,2]

ANESTHETIC AGENTS AND MODES OF ADMINISTRATION

Most studies on amphibian anesthesia have been performed using research species, predominantly African clawed frogs (*Xenopus laevis*) and leopard frogs (*Rana pipiens*), with less data available on other frog species and urodeles. At this time, the author could locate no peer-reviewed studies on anesthesia in caecilians. Therefore caution should be exercised when extrapolating the literature to the different species within the class Amphibia. Amphibians are a highly varied group of animals with great divergence time gaps between species, and marked differences have been observed between species using the same anesthetic agents and doses. When faced with an unfamiliar species for which peer-reviewed literature is lacking, the veterinarian is encouraged to reach out to colleagues with experience of the species in question.

Due to their multiple modes of respiration, delivery of anesthetic agents in amphibians has been investigated via various routes. Administration of anesthesia via immersion has traditionally been the method of choice for anesthetizing amphibians due to their permeable integument. There is ongoing research in this field, with agents designed for parenteral or inhalational administration being investigated as both immersion agents and via the route for which they are intended.

Tricaine Methanesulfonate

Tricaine methanesulfonate (MS-222) is one of the most commonly used anesthetic agents in amphibians. MS-222 is available in many countries through various suppliers but is banned in some countries due to toxicity reports. Depending on the country, it is licensed for use in amphibians. It is a water-soluble benzocaine derivative that blocks the sodium channels. Although it is a local anesthetic, when administered as an immersion it results in depression of the central nervous system compatible with anesthesia.[3] It comes as a white powder that is dissolved in water and administered as an immersion. It is buffered to a neutral pH with sodium bicarbonate to offset its acidity, which is irritating to the patient, and to aid absorption. Induction with MS-222 can range from a few minutes to approximately 30 minutes, during which time erythema of the ventral skin, agitation, and leaping may be observed (Fig. 52.1A). Respiration often slows, and by the time induction is achieved, respiration often ceases completely. Once the desired level of anesthesia is achieved, the patient is removed from the immersion, rinsed, and kept moist with anesthetic-free water. Induction with MS-222 often provides a surgical plane of anesthesia of approximately 30 minutes or longer depending on the dose and species. Time to induction and recovery is also dependent on the dose used. Higher concentrations

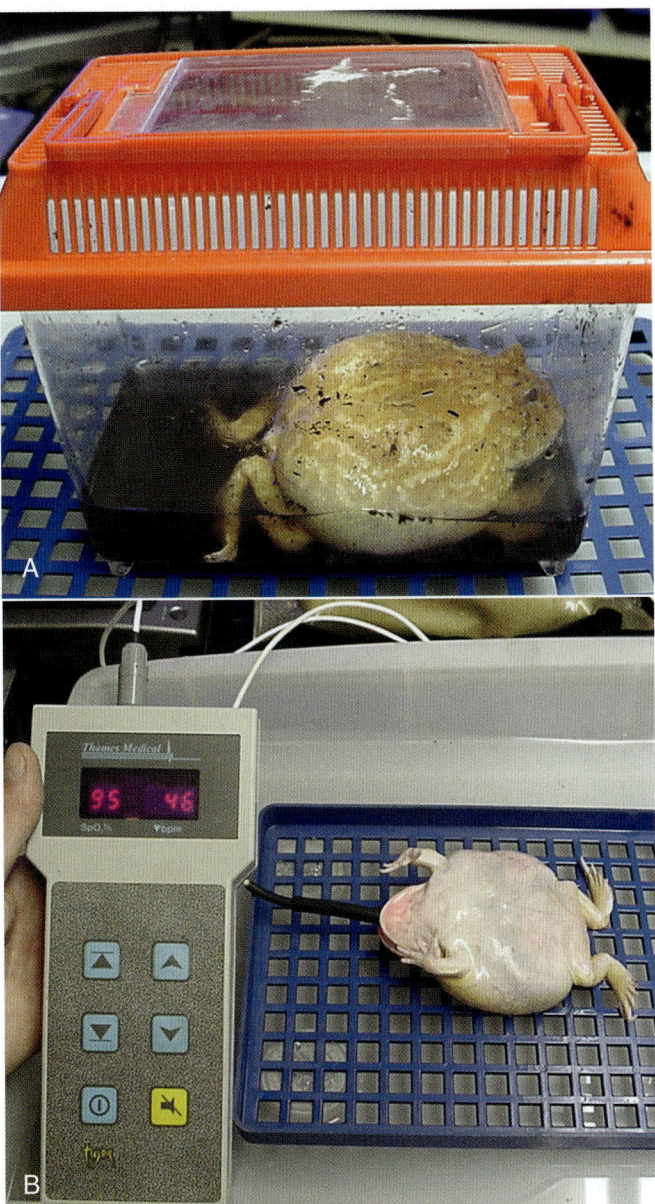

FIG 52.1 (A) Induction of an albino Argentine horned frog (*Ceratophrys ornata*) using an MS-222 immersion. The frog defecated during the excitatory phase of induction and contaminated the water. (B) Same frog after induction. The animal has lost righting and withdrawal reflexes. The intraoral reflectance probe and pulse oximeter indicates a pulse of 46 bpm and a spO₂ of 95%. Although the spO₂ values should be viewed sceptically, a robust waveform provides confidence in the pulse rate. (Courtesy of Stephen J. Divers.)

result in a shorter induction time but a longer recovery time. If ongoing anesthesia is required, the desired anesthetic depth can be achieved by partial immersion or trickling of MS-222 on the patient at half or less than the induction concentration.

In some studies a buffer is not used, which should be taken into consideration when interpreting the results. The dose of MS-222 per liter of water required varies with the life stage and species. Tadpoles, gilled species, and species that rely primarily on cutaneous respiration generally require lower doses than adult frogs. In leopard frogs, a 1 g/L immersion resulted in a surgical plane of anesthesia, with apnea and an average of 18% decrease in heart rate. No deaths occurred in the study.[4]

In African clawed frogs, 1 g/L and 2 g/L immersions resulted in a surgical plane of anesthesia for 30 and 60 minutes, respectively, with marked respiratory depression. The heart rate dropped significantly in the 1 g/L group but was unaffected in the 2 g/L group. Excess struggling in the 1 g/L group occurred prior to anesthesia, and it is suspected that stress tachycardia occurred as baseline mean heart rate was significantly higher than in the 2 g/L group. No histologic lesions were observed in euthanized frogs.[5] Heart rate reduced with MS-222 at concentrations of 400 mg/L in leopard frogs, but in this study the frogs were kept anesthetized for 4 hours at this dose, which is unlikely to occur in a clinical setting.[6] It is often stated that toads require higher doses of MS-222 due to their thicker and less permeable integument. In cane toads (*Rhinella marina*), a dose of 3 g/L was used, and mean time to induction was 40 minutes. No deaths were reported.[7] However, in Sonoran desert toads (*Bufo alvarius*), a dose of 1 g/L resulted in a mean time to induction of 20 minutes and surgical depth of anesthesia.[8] In Fowler's toads (*Bufo fowleri*), the use of unbuffered MS-222 at a dose of 0.5 g/L resulted in a 12% mortality rate. In this study, many of the toads urinated during handling prior to anesthesia, and it is speculated that in response to this water loss, the toads absorbed excess amount of the anesthetic agent through the pelvic patch.[9] Terrestrial anurans have a hypervascularized ventral pelvic region and increased skin surface area over this region;[1] therefore when using MS-222 immersion, higher doses may not be required for all species of toads and may result in excess depth of anesthesia, particularly if the patient is in negative water balance prior to immersion. In a study investigating surgical implantation of coelomic radio transmitters in Chinese giant salamanders (*Andrias davidianus*), 0.6 g/L immersion of MS-222 was sufficient to induce a surgical plane of anesthesia, and a 0.1-g/L shallow bath was sufficient for maintenance. Higher doses resulted in prolonged recoveries.[10] In hellbenders, 0.25 g/L of MS-222 is sufficient to induce anesthesia.[11] Within species, smaller individuals are often more rapidly induced, and a greater anesthetic effect is observed due to a larger surface area to body weight ratio.[4,10,12]

Eugenol

Eugenol, the active ingredient in clove oil, is also commonly used as an immersion agent. It acts by blocking sodium channels, vanilloid receptor TRPV1, and activating GABA A channels.[13] There are different formulations of clove oil with other ingredients often present, so the percentage of eugenol can differ between products. As far as the authors are aware, eugenol is not licensed for use in amphibians. No buffering is required for eugenol. An Aqui-S meter is available for accurately monitoring the concentration of anesthetic. This device is expensive but may be worthwhile for large institutions.

In leopard frogs, 255 mg/L immersion resulted predominantly in immobilization, with some frogs reaching light and deep levels of anesthesia. Apnea was observed in some of the frogs, and bradycardia was observed in all the frogs.[4] In African clawed frogs, 350 mg/L immersion resulted in a surgical plane of anesthesia lasting 30 minutes, with respiratory depression but no effect on the heart rate. There were no histologic lesions in euthanized frogs.[14] This is in contrast to a study where the same dose of the same formulation of eugenol resulted in renal tubule apoptosis and pulmonary hyaline membranes after a single anesthetic episode, and hepatic necrosis after three consecutive daily anesthetics.[15] Topical application of eugenol in African clawed frogs has also been reported to cause cutaneous necrosis.[16] Gastric prolapse and vomiting have been reported in leopard frogs and African clawed frogs, respectively, with the use of eugenol immersion.[14,17] In cane toads, 0.3 ml/L immersion resulted in 30% mortality rate, respiratory distress, and noncardiogenic pulmonary edema on necropsy.[7] In tiger salamanders (*Ambystoma tigrinum*), a 10-minute immersion at 450 mg/L resulted in a surgical plane of anesthesia in 67% of the animals. Bradycardia was observed, but there was no change in respiration and no other adverse effects were noted.[18] Isoeugenol was used to anesthetize tadpoles of the southern brown tree frog (*Litoria ewingii*). Three concentrations were used (10 μl/L, 20 μl/L, and 50 μl/L) and all were effective. No mortalities or adverse effects were noted, and 20 μl/L concentration was most suitable.[19]

Inhalant Agents

Anesthetic effects of inhalant agents have been investigated using the conventional route, immersion, bubbling vaporized inhalant through water, topical application, and parenteral administration. Inhalational induction in lunged amphibians can be used to induce anesthesia, however, the time to induction can be excessively long,[20] and during this time desiccation of skin can occur. In a study investigating effects of isoflurane in African clawed frogs, the frogs showed avoidance behavior when isoflurane was bubbled through water. None of the frogs became anesthetized when isoflurane was bubbled through water or delivered in air.[21] If using inhalational anesthesia for induction, the procedure should be stopped if the patient is showing signs of discomfort and an alternative anesthetic plan followed. In the same study, parenteral administration (intracoelomic, subcutaneous, and intramuscular) produced highly variable results, including mortalities with intracoelomic and subcutaneous administration. Topical application, using a pad with a vapor-barrier backing saturated with liquid isoflurane and placed on the frog's back, produced the most reliable results, with rapid induction, consistent recovery times, and no mortalities.[21] Isoflurane and sevoflurane mixed with water-based jelly and water creates a gel that reduces vaporization and increases skin contact time. In *Xenopus* and *Bufo* species, isoflurane gel provided consistent levels of surgical anesthesia (Stetter, unpublished data). However, in the American green tree frogs (*Hyla cinerea*), higher isoflurane doses caused unacceptable mortality levels when applied to the ventrum.[22] In addition to the higher dose, *Hyla* frogs have granular skin on the ventrum, increasing surface area available for absorption, which may have contributed to increased absorption of the isoflurane jelly.[1] In the same study, sevoflurane gel caused a rapid loss of the righting reflex and no mortalities.[22] In cane toads, sevoflurane gel applied to the dorsum of the toads resulted in a reliable and rapid loss of the righting reflex.[23]

Cotton balls soaked with isoflurane and placed in a porous pill vial, which is then placed in a plastic induction chamber, has been used to induce anesthesia in Australian green tree frogs (*Litoria caerulea*) (Fig. 52.2). Induction was achieved within 5 to 10 minutes, and signs of discomfort or excitation were not observed. Once induced using this method, the frogs retained gular respiration (Simpson S: Pers. comm.). It is possible that this method provides a higher percentage of isoflurane in the chamber due to lack of air flow, therefore ensuring a more rapid induction time while reducing the discomfort associated with fresh flow of dry anesthetic gas. Lack of direct topical application of jelly-based mixture may also avoid inhibition of cutaneous respiration. Isoflurane or sevoflurane can also be used for anesthetic maintenance in intubated patients (Fig. 52.3), which is discussed further in the Maintenance section of this chapter.

The risk to personnel needs to be considered when using inhalants, and all such procedures should use sealed chambers and have a scavenging system in place.

Injectable Agents

Various injectable agents, including propofol, ketamine, tiletamine/zolazepam, and medetomidine have been administered intracoelomically, intramuscularly, and/or as immersion agents. The results of these studies have produced variable results, however, extensive investigation of different dosages and in different species is lacking. In frogs, propofol

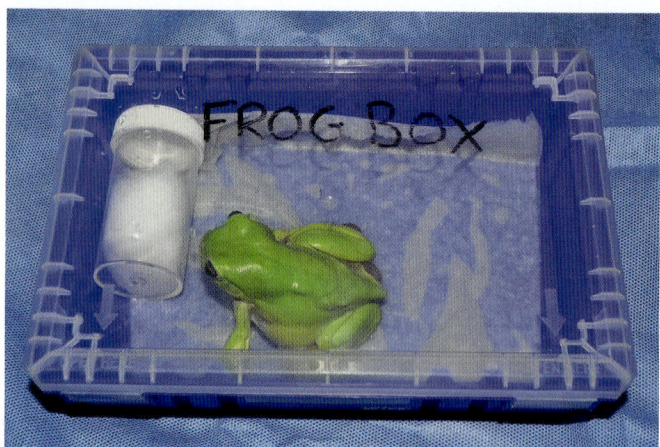

FIG 52.2 An Australian green tree frog (*Litoria caerulea*) in a plastic induction chamber. The chamber is lined with moistened paper towels. A pill vial lid is porous and contains isoflurane-soaked cotton balls. (Courtesy of Shane Simpson.)

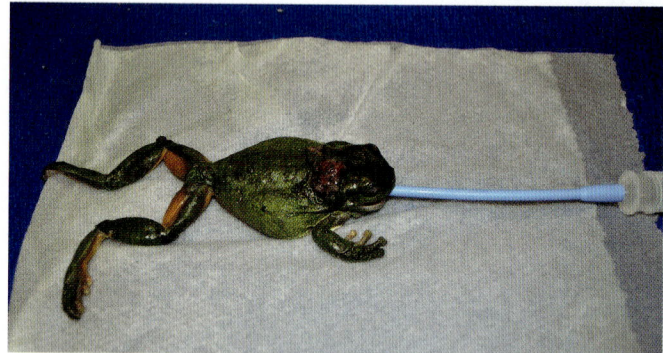

FIG 52.3 An Australian green tree frog (*Litoria caerulea*) anesthetized and intubated with a Cole endotracheal tube. Anesthesia is being maintained with isoflurane delivered via an intermittent positive pressure ventilator (not shown in picture). (Courtesy of Shane Simpson.)

as an immersion and as an intracoelomically administered agent has shown to have a narrow safety margin, with mortalities reported.[24,25] In tiger salamanders, intracoelomically administered propofol was found to produce a surgical plane of anesthesia; however, time to surgical anesthesia was prolonged.[18] Prolonged recoveries have also been reported with injectable agents.[7,8,18] There has been increased research on the use of alfaxalone in amphibians. While the agent has shown promise as an alternative to MS-222 and eugenol immersion and inhalant induction, the results appear to be species specific. Doses of 20 mg/kg and 30 mg/kg administered intramuscularly produced sedation and light anesthesia in three species of *Litoria* frogs.[26] Doses ranging from 10 mg/kg to 17.5 mg/kg administered intramuscularly immobilized bullfrogs (*Lithobates catesbeianus*), while immersion at 2 g/L was ineffective.[27] Conversely, immersion at 200 mg/L immobilized oriental fire-bellied toads (*Bombina orientalis*) but did not provide a surgical plane of anesthesia.[28] The addition of dexmedetomidine to the immersion did not increase the depth of anesthesia.[29] Topical application of a pad saturated with 1 ml of 10 mg/ml alfaxalone and placed on the dorsum of African clawed frogs, weighing on average 27 grams, resulted in loss of the withdrawal reflex (surgical plane of anesthesia) in 75% of the frogs (Fiddes, unpublished data). The use of alfaxalone was reported

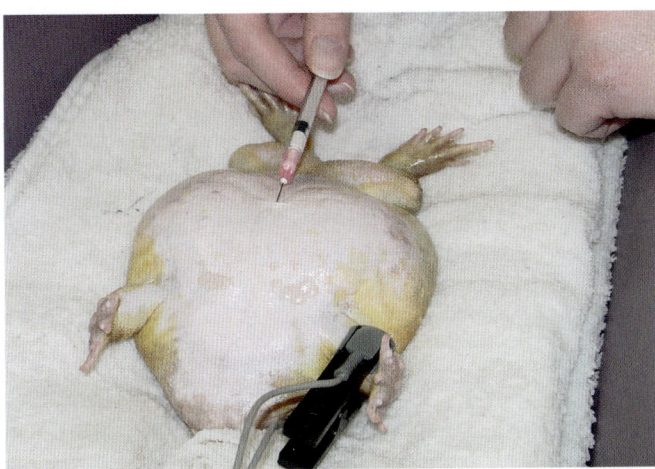

FIG 52.4 Intravenous administration of propofol into the ventral abdominal vein of an albino Argentine horned frog (*Ceratophrys ornata*). (Courtesy of Stephen J. Divers.)

in a case report as an intramuscularly administered induction agent, which resulted in sedation in a bullfrog. This was followed by a lidocaine block, allowing for surgical removal of a nuptial pad.[30] Alfaxalone immersion, followed by branchial and transcutaneous irrigation of additional alfaxalone, was used successfully in an axolotl (*Ambystoma mexicanum*) undergoing exploratory coeliotomy.[31] Although there are no studies evaluating intravenously administered agents, anecdotally alfaxalone and propofol administered intravenously have been effective in some species (Fig. 52.4).

Miscellaneous Drugs

Various other agents have been through trials with mixed results. Benzocaine cream (Orajel) used topically was effective in immobilizing leopard frogs,[4] and when used as an immersion was effective in anesthetizing Northern cricket frogs (*Acris crepitans*), mole salamanders (*Ambystoma talpoideum*), and northern dusky salamanders (*Desmognathus fuscus*).[9] However, it caused unacceptable mortality rates in Fowler's toads, presumably due to excessive anesthetic uptake after water loss from urination during handling.[9] Lidocaine:prilocaine cream (EMLA) resulted in a high mortality rate when used topically in leopard frogs.[4] Metomidate in leopard frogs failed to produce surgical anesthesia and prolonged recoveries were observed.[32]

MONITORING

Anesthetic depth classification system has not been clearly defined in amphibians as it has in domestic animals, and there is inconsistent use of terminology in the literature with regard to defining depth of anesthesia. This may be in part due to the different mechanisms of action of anesthetic agents and the variety of species in this taxa. In addition, much of the available monitoring equipment is either impractical or unable to be used in amphibians. Nevertheless, direct assessment of the patient can yield vital information and ensure that the patient remains under the appropriate level of anesthesia.

Cardiopulmonary Parameters

Monitoring respiration can be difficult in amphibians because many species become apneic under anesthesia. On induction, pulmonic (coelomic) respiration often disappears first, followed by buccal (gular) respiration. In some cases, gular respiration remains. During periods of apnea, the patient relies on skin for gas exchange. Although the skin

is capable of ventilating off carbon dioxide, it is a less effective means of oxygen uptake and the blood pH can drop, presumably due to metabolic acidosis from anaerobic metabolism.[33] Some species are physiologically adapted to cope with this as they undergo naturally occurring periods of apnea (such as during torpor). It should, however, be mentioned that anesthesia can suppress these cardiopulmonary adaptations. In cane toads, a significant drop in PaO_2 and an increase in $PaCO_2$ levels occurred during anesthesia.[34] Although these toads were presumed healthy and all recovered after the experiment, in a clinical setting unhealthy individuals may have reduced compensatory abilities, and oxygenation and ventilation support may be warranted.

The heart rate is often the most useful parameters that can be easily monitored during anesthesia in amphibians. It can be monitored by visually observing the cardiac impulse or using an ultrasonic Doppler flow detector placed over the heart. A resting heart rate should be obtained prior to anesthesia. Depending on the anesthetic protocol used, some agents will cause bradycardia once the patient is anesthetized, however, with most agents, the heart rate will remain unaffected. A slowing heart rate compared to baseline (more than 20% decrease) or loss of cardiac impulse is a sign of excessive anesthetic depth and should prompt lightening of anesthesia or resuscitation efforts.

Pulse oximetry has not been validated for use in amphibians and its usefulness is questionable (see Fig. 52.1B). A pulse oximeter was used in a study on MS-222 in African clawed frogs, and percentage saturation remained unchanged from baseline, despite marked respiratory depression, including apnea.[5] However, in an investigation of blood gases in anesthetized cane toads, apnea resulted in a decrease in PaO_2 to below 30 mmHg. Once breathing resumed, PaO_2 increased.[34] Arterial cannulation for blood gas monitoring has been performed in experimental studies and may be applied to a clinical setting, however, due to large physiological fluctuations of blood gases in amphibians, interpretation may be challenging.[34]

Reflexes

Assessing reflexes is useful in determining the depth of anesthesia in amphibians. The righting reflex is assessed by placing the animal on its back and observing its ability to correct its position. This is often the first reflex to disappear, and the patient is usually defined as being immobilized or sedated if the reflex is lost or delayed. Withdrawal reflex is assessed by pinching the toe of the patient. If the withdrawal reflex is lost, the patient is defined as being at a surgical plane of anesthesia. Reduced withdrawal reflex and lack of righting reflex is often classed as a light plane of anesthesia.

The presence and absence of the corneal reflex appears to vary between studies. The loss of corneal reflex is usually associated with excessive depth of anesthesia across species; however, in amphibians this is often cited as a feature of a light plane of anesthesia. It is possible that the use of MS-222 causes loss of corneal sensation due to its topical, local anesthetic effects, and that the lack of corneal response is merely a local effect unrelated to the anesthetic depth. However, loss of corneal reflex has also been observed with the use of intracoelomic propofol in Sonoran Desert toads under a surgical plane of anesthesia.[8]

Some studies have reported a transient darkening of skin color while the patient is sedated or anesthetized (Fig. 52.5).[14,26,27]

ANESTHETIC PROCEDURE

Preparation

A complete history should be collected and a physical examination performed, paying particular attention to the cardiopulmonary and integumentary systems. Obtaining an accurate weight and baseline parameters are essential. It is preferable to obtain a resting heart rate with

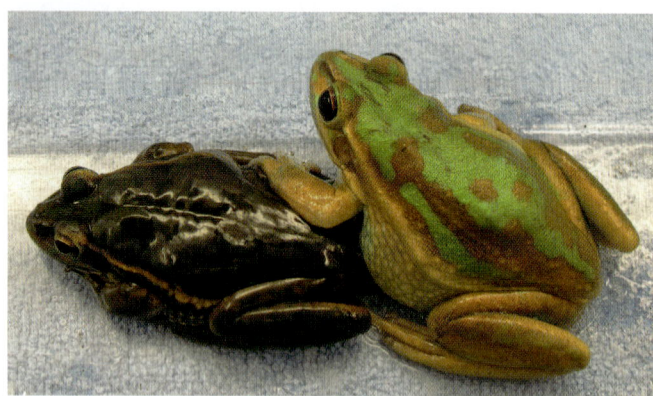

FIG 52.5 Two green and golden bell frogs (*Litoria aurea*). The sedated individual's skin is significantly darker. (Courtesy of Robert Johnson.)

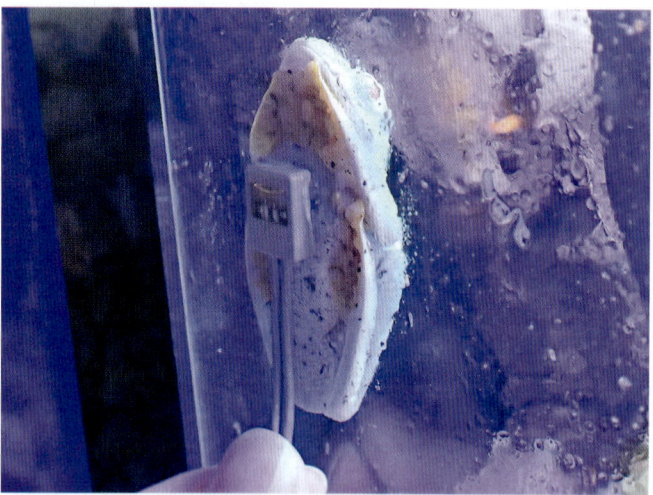

FIG 52.6 A red-eyed tree frog (*Agalychnis callidryas*) resting in its enclosure. A baseline heart rate being obtained through the wall of the enclosure to minimize stress-induced tachycardia. (Courtesy of Izidora Sladakovic.)

no or minimal handling (Fig. 52.6), because tachycardia can occur with holding, affecting interpretation of heart rate during anesthesia compared with the baseline.[5] Dermatologic diseases are common in amphibians and may affect the stability of the patient by interfering with osmoregulation, cutaneous respiration, and the uptake of immersion anesthetic agents.

Gloves should be worn when handling amphibians for the health and safety of both the patient and personnel. Rinsed and moistened nonpowdered gloves are recommended for adult amphibians. Tadpoles are particularly sensitive to gloves, with deaths observed after handling with latex, nitrile, and vinyl gloves. Although all gloves can potentially be toxic to tadpoles, well-rinsed vinyl gloves appear to be least harmful.[35]

Aspiration does not appear to be a risk factor for amphibians under anesthesia because their larynx remains tightly closed; however, they are able to vomit, and therefore fasting should be considered if the need for anesthesia is not urgent. The length of the fasting period depends on the species. The authors recommend skipping one meal as a general guide.

Plastic bags (such as disposable ziplock bags) and plastic containers are ideal induction chambers. These must be clean and free of chemicals and toxins that may be harmful if absorbed across the skin by the patient. They should be enclosed and padded to prevent injury if an excitation phase of anesthesia occurs. If working with inhalant agents, a scavenger or a fume hood should be used for personnel safety.

Chlorine-free, toxin-free water at the animal's preferred temperature is essential for use in the induction chamber, as are rinsing and keeping the animal moist during anesthesia. It is ideal to use water from the animal's environment if available, as long as the water quality parameters are acceptable. A water parameter testing kit is required to assess water quality and ensure appropriate buffering if using MS-222. Oxygenation can be provided by bubbling oxygen through water or via an anesthetic machine in an intubated patient. Uncuffed tubes, such as Cole tubes, and intravenous catheters can be used to intubate amphibians. Due to their tendency to remain apneic during the surgical plane of anesthesia, a ventilator is required.

Induction

For induction using an immersion agent, ziplock clear plastic bags provide an ideal induction chamber, because they are disposable and provide a cushion during the excitatory phase of anesthesia. The bag should be partially filled with an induction agent, enough to cover the ventrum of the animal is sufficient and not too deep as to cover the nostrils in lunged species. During induction, the animal should be monitored continuously because drowning is a risk in lunged species. Once the animal has reached the desired plane of anesthesia, it is removed from the immersion container and rinsed with anesthetic-free water. Lengthy immersion at MS-222 can result in excessive depth of anesthesia, even at low doses.[6]

For parenteral drug administration, intramuscular injections can be given in the thigh muscles of anurans or epaxial muscles in urodeles. To avoid damaging the integument, use gentle restraint with gloved hands and moistened cloth or net/plastic bag if required.

Maintenance

Mode of anesthetic maintenance is dependent on the type and length of the procedure and on the species. Animals induced with MS-222 can remain anesthetized for approximately 30 to 60 minutes. If additional length of anesthesia is required, the solution can be trickled over the animal, generally at 10% to 50% of the induction concentration. Lunged species can be intubated and maintained on an inhalant agent, delivered via an intermittent positive pressure or volume cycle ventilator. Lunged amphibians generally have a short trachea, so the endotracheal tube should not be placed too far as to intubate a bronchus. The lungs are saclike and delicate, so ventilator pressure should be set low, initially starting at 2 to 4 cmH₂O. There are no studies evaluating this mode of anesthetic delivery, although it is often utilized by practitioners. In an axolotl, anesthesia was successfully maintained by dripping alfaxalone over the gills and skin.[31] If the patient is partially immersed in water, it is ideal to bubble oxygen through the water to provide additional oxygenation.

During anesthesia, the skin needs to be kept moist. This ensures the skin does not desiccate and also maintains cutaneous respiration. Water-based lubricants should not be used to keep the skin moist, because this can impede cutaneous respiration.

Recovery

On completion of anesthesia, the patient should be rinsed with anesthetic-free water (Fig. 52.7), monitored until all reflexes and cardiopulmonary parameters have returned to normal, and kept in a moist environment at the preferred temperature for the species.

ANALGESIA

Literature on nociceptive pathways in amphibians is available and advocates that there are no major differences between amphibians and mammals.[36] The most widely used pain model in amphibians is the

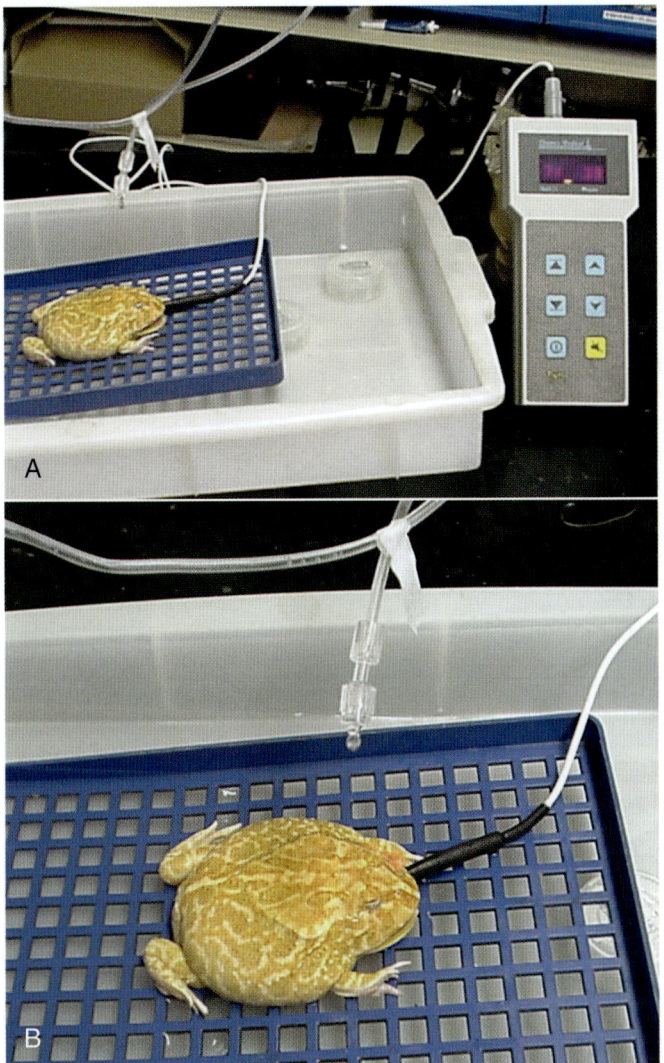

FIG 52.7 (A) Albino Argentine horned frog (*Ceratophrys ornata*) recovering from MS-222 anesthesia. (B) Close-up demonstrating an IV infusion set slowly but continuously dripping fresh water onto the frog's dorsum to speed anesthetic excretion and recovery, and keep the skin moist. (Courtesy of Stephen J. Divers.)

acetic acid test, in which acetic acid is applied cutaneously, on the thigh, and the area observed for a wiping response with the hind limb. Using this model, increased nociceptive threshold has been demonstrated for various opioid and nonopioid analgesics, with doses often being much higher than those used in mammals.[36]

There are few studies in amphibians evaluating analgesia using surgical pain. Buprenorphine and butorphanol were evaluated for analgesic effect by assessing food consumption and behavior following bilateral forelimb amputation in eastern red-spotted newts (*Notophthalmus viridescens*). Buprenorphine at 50 mg/kg administered intracoelomically at completion of surgery, and at 24 and 48 hours postsurgery, and butorphanol at 0.5 mg/L administered as an immersion both resulted in significant recommencement of normal behavior compared with the control group for 72 hours postoperatively.[37]

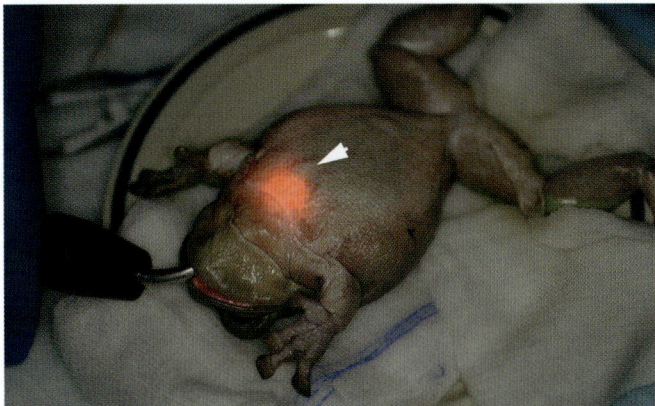

FIG 52.8 Use of a light source inserted through the mouth to transilluminate the heart (white arrow) of this green tree frog (*Litoria* sp.). This is a useful and rapid technique for visualizing the heart in emergent situations and where intracardiac injection is necessary. (Courtesy of Stephen J. Divers.)

A study in bullfrogs demonstrated a reduction in circulating serum PGE2 levels induced by surgical injury following intramuscular administration of meloxicam 0.1 mg/kg.[38] Flunixin meglumine injected into the dorsal lymph sac at 25 mg/kg significantly increased the nociceptive threshold in African clawed frogs using the acetic acid and Hargreaves (thermal stimulus) tests; however, the results after surgical oocyst harvest were equivocal. One frog died, and kidney congestion was observed on histopathology.[39]

EMERGENCIES

In the event of an anesthetic-related complication, principles of cardiovascular and respiratory support may be extrapolated from other species. Bradycardia may be responsive to atropine. Cardiac compressions should be performed in the event of asystole. Exogenous catecholamines may be administered for cardiovascular support, although there are no studies evaluating these agents in amphibian resuscitation. Although some references suggest doxapram for treatment of apnea, this has fallen out of favor in human and domestic animal medicine due to its side effects and worse long-term outcomes. In the event that respiratory support is required, the authors suggest endotracheal intubation and ventilation in lunged species. For gilled species, ventilation can be provided by flowing anesthetic-free water over the gills. Skin should be continuously rinsed of any anesthetic agent. Oxygenation can be provided by increasing ambient oxygen level, bubbling oxygen through water, or via an endotracheal tube in an intubated patient. Useful sites for gaining venous access are the ventral abdominal vein, femoral vein, axillary venous plexus, and lingual venous plexus in anurans. In tailed species, ventral tail vein can be used. Transillumination can be used to visualize the vein or the heart (Fig. 52.8). Cardiocentesis and intraosseous access are also options when peripheral venous access cannot be achieved. Intratracheal administration of emergency drugs at higher doses can also be considered in intubated patients.

REFERENCES

See www.expertconsult.com for a complete list of references.

53

Radiography—General Principles

Shannon P. Holmes and Stephen J. Divers

This chapter will focus on the production of radiographic images of reptiles, including equipment and interpretation principles. The individual radiography chapters on lizards, snakes, chelonians, and crocodilians provide species-specific information with respect to indications for radiography, radiographic positioning, standard views, radiographic anatomy, and interpretation.

In reptiles, as is true for all other species, radiographic diagnostic imaging is universally available and the most common first-line diagnostic imaging test performed. However, radiography is underused in reptile clinical practice compared with its use in dogs and cats.[1] Although this imaging modality can contribute greatly to the medical and surgical management of reptiles, there are numerous important factors that can affect its use and must be considered. Clinician comfort is undoubtedly one of the biggest factors, not just in interpreting radiographs but also in obtaining them. Specific training and experience with reptile radiography as a veterinary student is more limited compared with other species, and there are fewer accessible reference materials. The concern for sources for interpretation of reptile radiographs can be minimized in this age of digital radiology (DR) and teleradiology.[2] Numerous teleradiology groups offer specialists in this area for interpretation of these examinations. An additional benefit of DR is proven superior performance in avian reptiles and presumed extrapolation to non-avian reptiles.[2,3] Another challenge is the different interpretation principles that must be employed because reptiles possess a coelomic cavity rather than a distinct thorax and abdomen.[1,4] The most common radiographic feature of the coelom is its inherent poor tissue contrast, which can be displeasing to view and frustrating to interpret.[1] It also can lead to the erroneous assumption that poor coelomic detail will limit the diagnostic value of radiography to the extent that it will be of no diagnostic benefit. In spite of its limitations, the benefit of radiography as a first-line diagnostic should be appreciated over the subsequent chapters, as its applications are numerous.

RADIOGRAPHIC EQUIPMENT

Most radiographic units used routinely in clinical practice for mammalian species can be adapted to reptile radiographic procedures. The tube stand and design of the radiology area are important. Ideally, there is sufficient space around the X-ray unit to allow all personnel to work around the patient safely and move in and out of the room to minimize exposure (Fig. 53.1A).[5] A particularly important feature for X-ray units utilized in reptile radiography is the ability to rotate the X-ray tube 90

degrees to obtain horizontal beam radiographs (see Fig. 53.1B). These are a component of every standard reptile radiographic examination, whereas they are rarely performed in other small animal species.[1,6–9] The rotation of the X-ray tube to a horizontal projection results in the X-ray beam being directed parallel to the table top and toward a film-screen cassette or DR plate, which is stabilized in a cassette stand or other device.[1,4,10] Wall-mounted and table-mounted cassette holders are available. The cassette can also be supported in the vertical position with tape and radiolucent objects. When using technique chart values for mAs and kVp, it is important to maintain the distance between the radiograph tube and the cassette or DR plate at a focal film distance of 100 cm (40 inches). Some of the DR systems do not have the ability to do horizontal beam radiographs, because the DR plate has been permanently built into the table. Fluoroscopy units offer another form of diagnostic radiography studies (see Fig. 53.1C and D). These are primarily used in interventional procedures in small mammalian species but are more commonly used in reptile species to assess an anatomic area in a dynamic manner.

There are three options for making radiographs of reptiles. Previously, high-quality radiographs relied on film-screen systems. A few practices still use these systems and as a result their radiographic studies are viewed on a light box. Digital radiographic systems are currently more commonplace in most general and all specialty practices.[11] These systems include computer radiography and direct digital radiography; the end product of both is a digitized radiograph that is viewed on a computer monitor.[2,10,12] The ideal DR system for reptiles has a sufficiently large detector plate, spatial resolution (defined by pixel size) of 5 line pairs per millimeter, and high detector quantum efficiency (DQE).[2] A third option is limited to radiography of smaller patients or smaller anatomic areas, which can be imaged with dental radiography units. These can be either film or digital format.

The equipment used must be adjusted appropriately for the species and size of the patient. DR techniques will perform better than film-screen in adapting the technique charts developed for mammalian species to a reptile application.[2,13] With film-screen techniques, the exposure setting for a certain thickness of mammalian tissue will need to be adjusted to account for the thick shell of a tortoise, as an example, because the shell will more greatly attenuate the X-ray beam. In contrast, DR systems can produce diagnostic images over a wider range of exposure values than film-screen and therefore adjustment of the technique chart values may not be necessary.[2,3] This is not to say that exposure errors are not an issue in DR, but the number of retake images is significantly

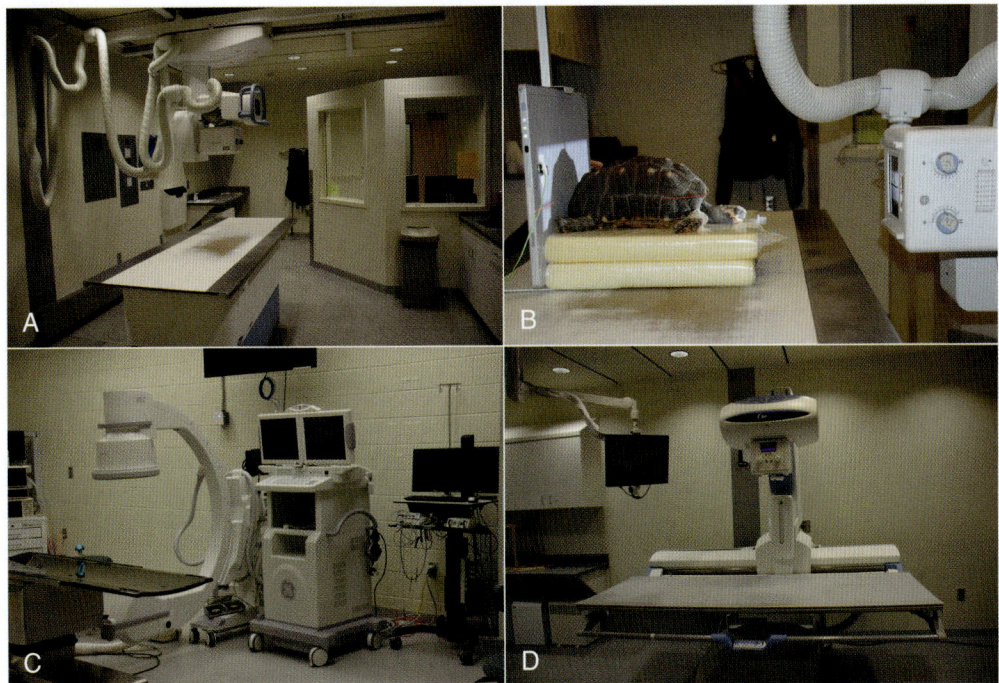

FIG 53.1 Small animal digital radiology (DR) suite with a moveable tube head capable of vertical (A) and horizontal (B) X-ray beams and protected technician control area. Such facilities are suitable for the vast majority of reptiles and amphibians, but giant chelonians and crocodilians may require equipment designed for large domesticated species. Fluoroscopy units come in different forms. C-arm units (C) are increasingly being used for interventional radiography and intraoperative assessments (e.g., orthopedic implants). Some units are capable of both fluoroscopy and digital radiography (D). Both have the ability to rotate to obtain horizontal beam or oblique images. Reptile fluoroscopic techniques are most useful for dynamic assessments of gastrointestinal, vascular, and urinary studies. (Courtesy of Stephen J. Divers.)

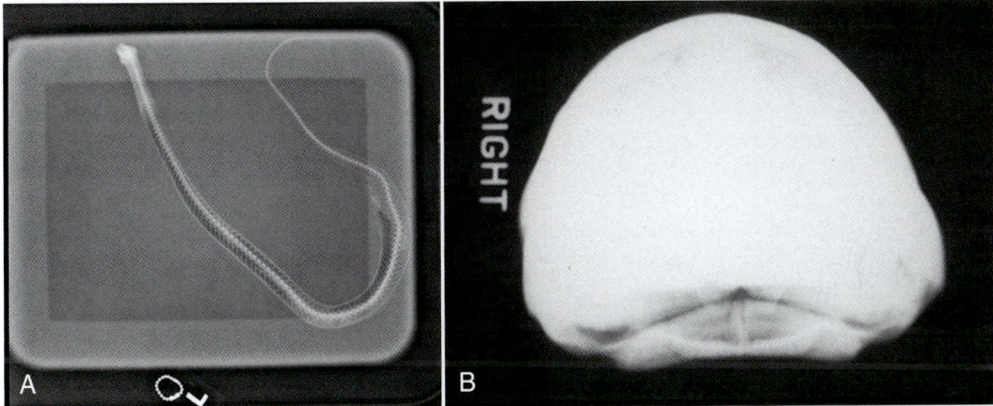

FIG 53.2 Examples of poor radiographic technique. (A) Dorsoventral vertical beam radiograph of a snake that has been constrained in a transparent plastic box, which partially attenuates the X-ray beam. Positioning is poor and evaluation for anything other than a large foreign body or egg is futile. (B) Craniocaudal horizontal beam radiograph of a tortoise. This radiograph is severely underexposed, such that the shell has essentially attenuated the X-ray beam and no internal anatomy is distinguishable.

reduced.[10,11] Underexposure of the aforementioned tortoise in film-screen system will result in less film blackening and potentially further reduced detail of the coelomic cavity (Fig. 53.2). Correcting over- and under-exposure in film-screen systems is important to optimizing image quality and follows specific rules for changing the milliampere/second (mAs) or kilovolt potential (kVp).[10] If your practice performs numerous reptile studies and uses film-screen systems, it may be beneficial to develop a species-specific technique chart. DR systems have more limited technique charts because of sensitivity to X-rays, conversion of information to digital format, and postpossessing techniques. Underexposure in digital films results in an image having a grainy, diffuse appearance superimposed on the anatomy and background. Overexposure will result in black areas that are described as saturated; there is no manipulation to the appearance of the image that can be made to retrieve the image anatomy in saturated areas.[2,14-16] It is beyond the scope of this chapter to thoroughly review all components of a DR systems that affect image quality. More comprehensive reviews of the application of DR systems with comparison to traditional screen-film systems, some focused on exotic pet radiography, are available and should be considered before purchase of a DR system.[2,3,10,11]

It is important to consider the internal or external anatomical areas of interest when planning a radiographic study. Reptile radiography generally follows the standard radiographic convention mandating that two orthogonal radiographs are necessary for anatomy depiction (see Fig. 53.2). The orthogonal radiographs remove summation of anatomy from different angles and give depth and spatial location information.[1,4,10] Single image studies are rarely indicated, as can be seen in Table 53.1. For example, the chelonian lungs are best evaluated in the craniocaudal projection, which allows comparison of the right and left lungs for degree of aeration versus abnormal accumulation of soft tissue representing pathological change. A lateral radiograph of the chelonian respiratory system can also be made to evaluate the spatial distribution of the lungs from cranial to caudal, given that this cannot be assessed on the craniocaudal view. In contrast, a single lateral projection of the respiratory system may be useful in snakes with only a right lung, because it allows complete system evaluation of the trachea through their saclike lungs

with minimal superimposed anatomy.[1] However, when dealing with boas and pythons that possess both left and right functional lungs, the dorsoventral view is also essential to differentiate between left, right, and bilateral disease. Species-specific considerations for radiographic positioning, including restraint techniques, will be discussed in subsequent chapters.

IMAGE INTERPRETATION

Some of the same principles of image interpretation that are used in mammalian species can be used in reptiles. For example, there are only five radiographic opacities that can be depicted; these include metal, bone, soft tissue, fat, and air.[10] However, reptiles generally have minimal diffuse fat located around their visceral organs; instead, most is localized within discrete fat bodies.[1,4,6,7] Diffuse peri-organ fat in mammalian species provides radiographic contrast; thus mammalian abdominal fat facilitates distinction, shape, and margination evaluation of organs. Radiographs of reptiles are often characterized by poor coelomic contrast (Fig. 53.3). The poor contrast in reptiles is exacerbated by close anatomic proximity of internal organs (increased silhouetting of structures), a coelom rather than separated body cavities (i.e., thorax and abdomen), and image degradation that is associated with their often heavily keratinized skin, scales, or osteoderms.[1] Similar to mammalian interpretation, increases in soft tissue within the coelom can produce a mass effect and further reduce regional serosal detail. This is an example of a mammalian radiographic interpretation principle that can be used

TABLE 53.1	Initial Radiographic Views Required for Reptiles		
	Vertical Beam Dorsoventral	**Horizontal Beam Lateral**	**Horizontal Beam Craniocaudal**
Chelonians			
Respiratory tract	X	X	X
Gastrointestinal tract	X	X	
Urogenital systems	X	X	
Carapace and plastron	X	X	X
Head and spine	X	X	
Pectoral and pelvic girdles	X	X	X
Limbs[b]	X		
Snakes			
Respiratory tract	X[a]	X	
Gastrointestinal tract	X	X	
Urogenital systems	X	X	
Head and spine	X	X	
Lizards			
Respiratory tract	X	X	
Gastrointestinal tract	X	X	
Urogenital systems	X	X	
Head and spine	X	X	
Limbs[b]	X		
Crocodilians			
Respiratory tract	X	X	
Gastrointestinal tract	X	X	
Urogenital systems	X	X	
Head and spine	X	X	
Limbs[b]	X		

[a]Boas and pythons have two functional lungs, and therefore a dorsoventral view is essential to differentiate between left and right pulmonary disease. The dorsoventral view is less valuable for most other snakes that only possess a functional right lung.
[b]Orthogonal views of the limbs are required, particularly if any lesions are identified on the dorsoventral view.

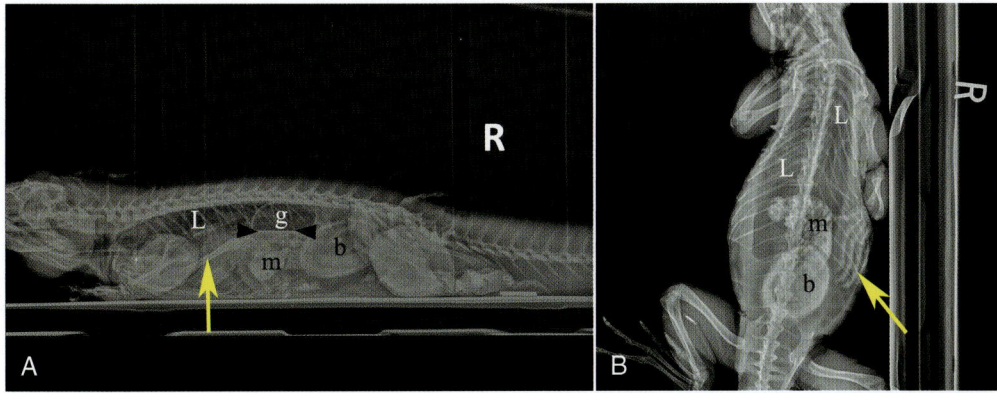

FIG 53.3 (A and B) Grand Cayman iguana (*Cyclura lewisi*). The poor inherent tissue contrast commonly seen in reptiles is demonstrated. Four radiographic opacities are shown: metal opaque label (R) in the dorsoventral image, skeleton and mineral opaque amorphous material (m) in the mid and caudal coelom, coelomic soft tissue caudoventral to the lungs and gas opacity within the aerated lungs (L), and nondependent area of the stomach (g). This degree of poor serosal detail in the caudoventral coelom is normal. In this case it makes it difficult to definitively localize the abnormal mineralized material. The caudal portion was suspected to be in the urinary bladder (b) based on the shape, but there was concern that the more cranial mineral material could be within the gastrointestinal tract because it extends cranial to the stomach that has a gas-fluid line (black arrowheads). Surgery confirmed all mineral material was within the urinary bladder. Note also the suboptimal positioning of the right pectoral limb (yellow arrow); it is superimposed on the coelom but more significantly over the area of interest on the lateral image. (Courtesy of Christine Fiorello, Albuquerque BioPark.)

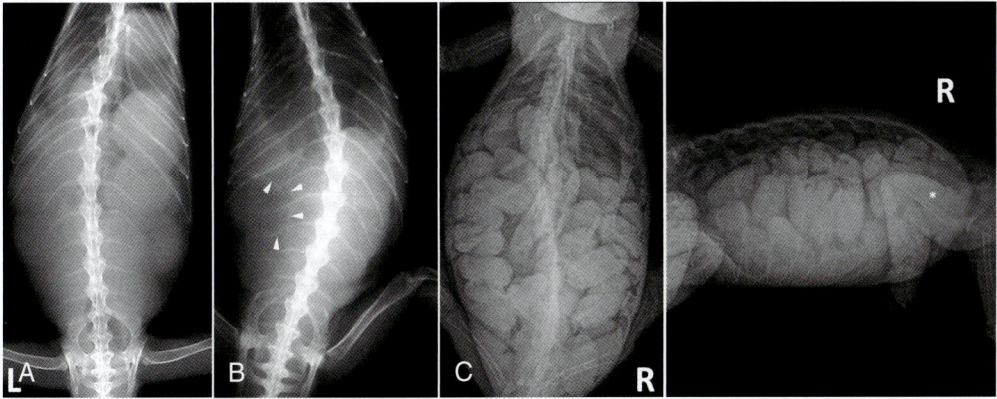

FIG 53.4 (A) Dorsoventral (screen-film) radiograph of a green iguana (*Iguana iguana*) demonstrating multiple, spherical, soft tissue densities consistent with preovulatory follicles. The ova produce a mass effect that further reduces serosal detail in the coelom. (B) Another green iguana dorsoventral (screen-film) radiograph demonstrating multiple soft tissue densities; however, note that the structures are more oval and surrounded by thin shells (arrows), indicating that they must be postovulatory eggs. (C) Dorsoventral and right lateral radiographs of a gravid old-world chameleon (Chamaeleonidae) made with a digital radiography system. The contrast resolution can be enhanced with postprocessing techniques, which explains why the shelled eggs are better seen with digital systems. (A and B, Courtesy of Stephen J. Divers; C, courtesy of Shannon P. Holmes.)

in reptiles but also requires knowledge of baseline poor coelomic detail (Fig. 53.4).

A systematic approach is critical for all radiographic interpretations. Because whole body radiographic examinations are more common in reptiles than focused system examinations routinely done in mammalian studies, the systematic approach used must be adapted. It is best to approach the coelom in anatomic components, such as cardiovascular, pulmonary, gastrointestinal, coelomic organs (liver, pancreas, and spleen), urogenital, and musculoskeletal systems, with each area more specifically evaluated similar to mammals. The evaluation of the respiratory system, for example, could include oral cavity, nasal cavities, trachea, and lungs.

Accurate radiographic interpretation requires a strong understanding of anatomical and physiological variations in different species, as these produce different radiographic appearances. For example, the chelonian lung contains muscular bands of tissue throughout, whereas the snake lung is divided into vascular (faveolar) and avascular (saccular) regions.[1,6,17] The alveolar, pleural, and bronchial patterns used in mammalian radiographic interpretation are not applicable to reptiles. Capturing anatomy in certain states is also critical for accurate interpretation, and evaluating inspiratory lungs is important. Artifactual increased opacity of deflated lungs can be misinterpreted as pathologic change (Fig. 53.5). It is important to assess the quality of the radiographic

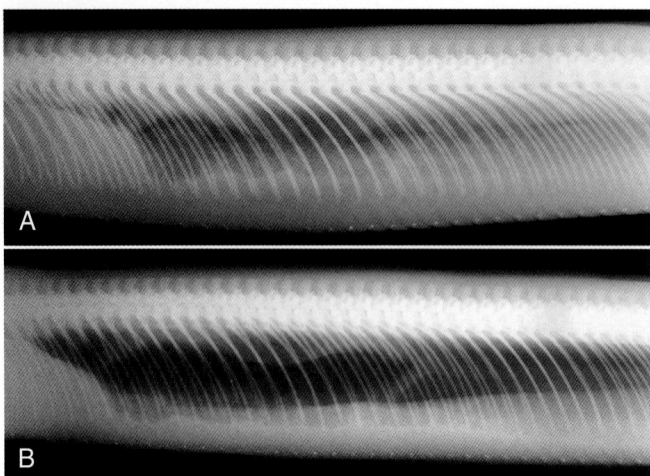

FIG 53.5 Boa constrictor (*Boa constrictor*). The radiograph (horizontal beam, lateral view) was made with the patient during expiration (top) and at peak inspiration (bottom). The lungs are more lucent and expanded on the inspiratory radiograph. This greatly improves the ability to evaluate the lungs for pathological change and is the reason general anesthesia and positive pressure ventilation is recommended for assessing the respiratory system. The cardiac silhouette on the left of the images serves as a point of reference.

study for the body system of interest, as this will impact the systematic approach. General considerations include extent of superimposed pectoral limbs that may interfere with assessment of the heart; degree of inspiration for evaluating the lungs; presence of ingesta in the gastrointestinal tract producing opacities that superimpose the coelomic anatomy to be evaluated; or detectable changes in mineralization of skeletal structures versus inappropriate technique.

REFERENCES

See www.expertconsult.com for a complete list of references.

54

Radiography—Lizards

Shannon P. Holmes and Stephen J. Divers

Radiography offers clinicians a minimally invasive tool to look inside their reptile patients using equipment that is readily available in virtually all veterinary practices. As with any diagnostic imaging test, there are benefits and limitations. A major benefit of radiography is that it is inexpensive relative to other diagnostic imaging tests. In lizards, one limitation that can significantly affect interpretation is the inherently low soft tissue contrast within the coelom. The resulting radiographs can be challenging to evaluate and successful diagnostic ability will be governed by the interpreter's knowledge of lizard anatomy, physiology, and pathological conditions. These factors differ significantly from mammalian species, and interpretation principles must be adapted to these unique lizard patients.

RESTRAINT AND POSITIONING

Restraint is a necessity in all aspects of diagnostic imaging. Motion is a major source of image quality degradation. Lizards can be radiographed while conscious with appropriate restraint of their limbs.[1–3] A self-adhesive bandage can be used to secure the pectoral and pelvic limbs away from the area of interest, often to create an uninhibited view of the coelom (Fig. 54.1).[2] It is important to consider the area of interest when securing the limbs to avoid superimposition.[1] This technique is feasible in patients with low activity. Incorporation of slight pressure over the closed eyes to induce a vasovagal response can also be effective in some lizards, especially iguanids.[6] Radiographic accessories can also aid in acquiring radiographs in conscious lizards.[1,4,5] These can include using radiolucent tubes or troughs for smaller lizards to positioning sponges and plexiglass positioners for larger animals. Chameleons will often remain motionless if permitted to perch on a rod or stick.[4] Care must be taken when using positioning aids so that any device extends the length of the area of interest to avoid additional variations in radiopacity that hinder interpretation. It is important that none of these accessories affect the patients' position relative to the cassette or detector. Specifically, none should be abnormally thick to cause the patient to be positioned further from the cassette or detector; this causes magnification and image degradation through blurring.[1,7] This can be a greater issue with the horizontal beam projections.

In those patients with higher activity level or requiring special radiographic views, chemical restraint is likely needed. Although greater preparation time and sedation/anesthesia risks are considerations, the increased efficiency in the radiographic room is beneficial through improved image quality, less retake radiographs, and ease for positioning the patient to obtain specific images.[1,8] The latter is most commonly encountered when the axial or appendicular skeleton of the lizard needs to be imaged and requires positioning in an abnormal posture and/or with limb extension.[8] Specifics on chemical restraint techniques that can be used are available in Chapters 48 and 49. Chemical restraint considerations for radiographic procedures should include the expected length of the procedure, if additional tests are to be performed or if dynamic studies are needed. When general anesthesia is required for other diagnostics, it is best to plan radiographic procedures to precede these and be performed under premedication/sedation if possible. If general anesthesia is required, radiographs should be acquired immediately following induction, because they can often be taken under light anesthesia, with anesthetic depth subsequently increased in preparation for surgery or more invasive procedures. Some drugs can interfere with gastrointestinal motility in mammalian species and therefore should be avoided in reptilian gastrointestinal contrast studies. To date, the effects of drugs on reptile GI motility and radiographic studies have not been investigated.

The ideal radiographic study of most systems consists of dorsoventral vertical x-ray beam and lateral horizontal x-ray beam images.[1,2] Optimal radiographic technique has the lizard positioned as close to the cassette or detector as is possible. The tabletop is as close as possible for systems that have the cassette or detector built into the unit. Otherwise, patients can be placed directly on the cassette or detector for the dorsoventral view (Fig. 54.2). For the lateral horizontal beam image, positioning the cassette or detector close to the patient is hampered if the laterally protruding extremities are not extended cranially or caudally (see Fig. 54.1). For machines that cannot perform horizontal beam imaging, the vertical beam lateral radiograph will be needed and requires greater restraint (Fig. 54.3). This will alter the confirmation of the coelomic structures from the typical published appearance (Fig. 54.4), and this

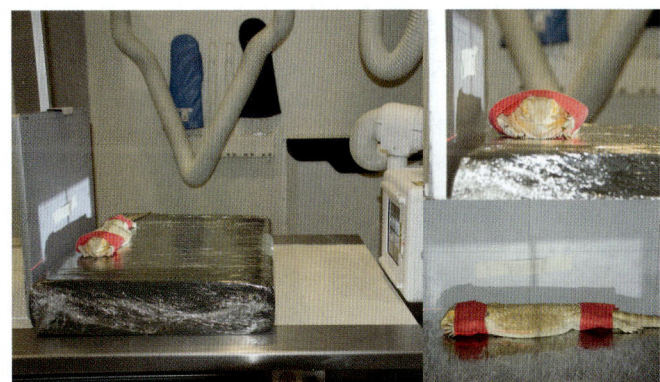

FIG 54.1 Positioning a sedated bearded dragon (*Pogona vitticeps*) for a standard right lateral, horizontal beam radiograph. This is the preferred positioning for lateral radiographs, because visceral displacement is avoided and fluid lines can be appreciated. The limbs have been taped to provide an unobstructed view of the coelom. Radiolucent positioning devices must often be used to elevate the patient from the table and center the x-ray beam. (Courtesy of Stephen J. Divers.)

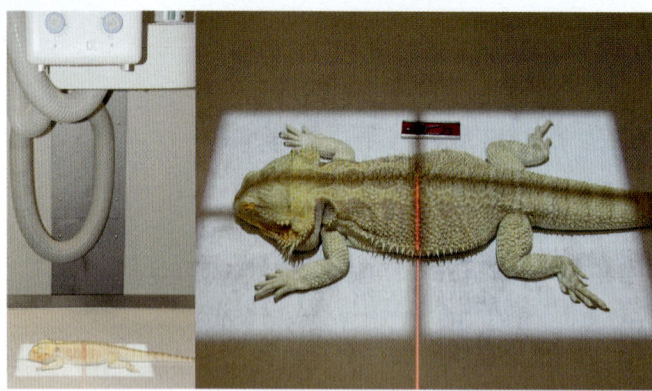

FIG 54.2 Positioning a sedated bearded dragon (*Pogona vitticeps*) for a standard dorsoventral radiograph. (Courtesy of Stephen J. Divers.)

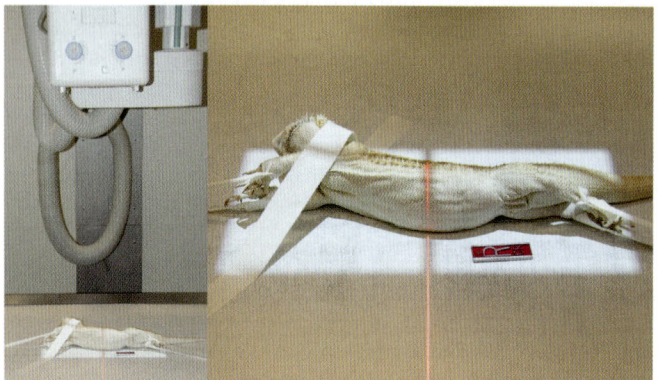

FIG 54.3 Positioning a sedated bearded dragon (*Pogona vitticeps*) for a right lateral vertical beam radiograph. Such positioning is not advised because of the displacement of visceral structures. (Courtesy of Stephen J. Divers.)

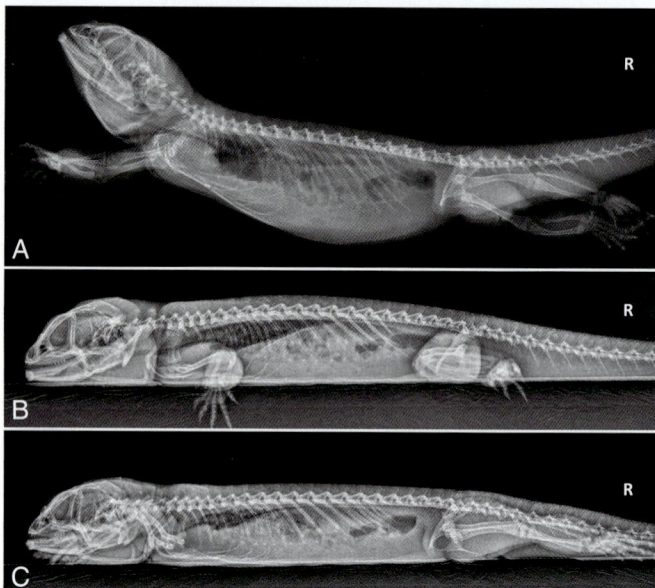

FIG 54.4 Right lateral radiographs of the same bearded dragon (*Pogona vitticeps*) comparing (A) vertical beam, (B) horizontal beam without limb retraction, and (C) horizontal beam with limb retraction to avoid super-imposition. Lung definition is poor in the vertical beam radiograph due to visceral displacement by gravity, whereas limb retraction provides a superior view of the cranial and caudal aspects of the coelom without superimposition of the limbs. With the lizard in sternal recumbency, there is some compression of the coelomic contents. (Courtesy of Stephen J. Divers.)

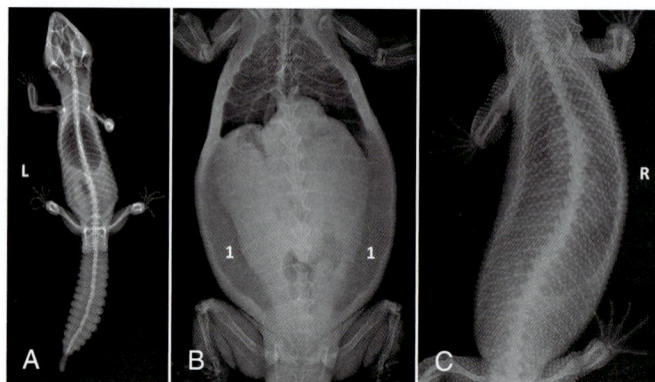

FIG 54.5 Common difficulties encountered in lizard radiology. (A) Small patient size, as demonstrated by this 55 g leopard gecko (*Eublepharis macularius*), may be overcome by using magnification, either by raising the lizard on a perspex platform above the radiographic plate or magnifying the image after acquisition. It should be remembered that detail may be sacrificed with any magnification process. (B) Most reptiles store fat in discrete coelomic fat bodies (1) rather than diffusely around visceral organs, which results in poor serosal detail. (C) Heavy scalation and osteoderms, as demonstrated in this helodermatid lizard, often obscure other radiographic details. (Courtesy of Stephen J. Divers.)

is a less ideal technique.[2,9] The positioning of the limbs must be considered with respect to the area of interest. Extension of the limbs cranially is important for evaluation of the heart and lungs, whereas the limbs may be preferably left in a neutral position or extended caudally to examine the head and neck region (see Fig. 54.4). In larger lizards, both right and left lateral views are recommended for respiratory tract evaluation; the lung and any pathology will be best resolved when it is closest to the cassette or detector.[1] Similarly, superimposition of the pelvic limbs over caudal coelom and pelvic girdle can hamper evaluation of these areas on the horizontal beam images. Extending the pelvic limbs caudally minimizes this effect.

There are some additional challenges in lizard radiography that cannot be overcome with technique. Some patients are extremely small (Fig. 54.5A). This is less of an issue with good-quality digital systems given that magnification of the resulting image is feasible.[10,11] Lesser-quality systems can limit the extent to which a radiograph can be magnified before pixilation is evident. With film-screen systems, it is ideal to use slower speed film to optimize resolution.[1,4] An air-gap technique has also been described to "enlarge" the patient, but this magnification technique can result in image blurring. For smaller body parts, such as the oral cavity or a distal extremity, dental film or digital systems can be used (Fig. 54.6). Another challenge is the inherent low serosal detail in the coelom of lizards (see Fig. 54.5B), which is attributed to the localization of fat in the coelom.[1,2,12] Minimal fat exists between

or around organ systems, and fat between serosal surfaces is necessary to provide radiographic contrast between different soft tissue opaque structures.[7] There are typically more discrete fat bodies within the caudolateral coelom. Their location does not aid in providing contrast; rather, it will tend to compress the organs together more, and this can worsen soft tissue contrast resolution regionally in the coelom. Fat body size is useful for evaluating body condition. Finally, it can be difficult to see the coelomic structures with radiopaque or dense scales or cutaneous osteoderms. Osteoderms have mineral deposits in the cutaneous or dermal layers that will obscure the internal anatomy on radiographs to varying degrees (see Fig. 54.5C).

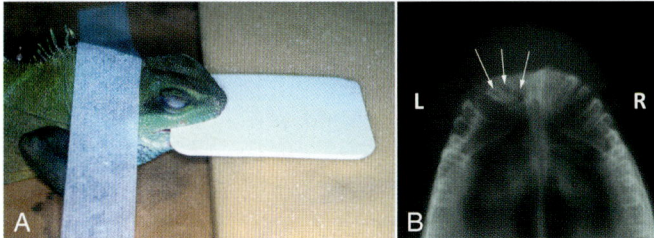

FIG 54.6 Dental radiography units and intraoral films often provide superior detail of oral structures, as they are designed for high-resolution output of smaller structures. In this Chinese water dragon (*Physignathus cocincinus*), small focal areas of osteolysis (*arrows*) are visible. In reptile practice, they can also be used to take survey radiographs of small reptiles or anatomical regions. However, care should be taken to ensure sufficient anatomy can be included for interpretation purposes. (Courtesy of Stephen J. Divers.)

CARDIOVASCULAR SYSTEM

The cardiac silhouette is positioned in the most cranioventral aspect of the coelom in most lizards, except for monitor lizards where it is more caudally positioned.[1,2] The heart can easily be obscured on the horizontal lateral view if the pectoral limbs are not taped forward. The heart and greater vessels are best visualized on this horizontal lateral image, but there are areas of the heart that may remain poorly visualized, including apex, base, and cranial margin.[13] Generally, the heart is poorly seen on the dorsoventral radiograph due to its close proximity to the coelomic inlet and the summation affect associated with the pectoral musculature and superimposition of the spine, ribs, and sternum. The cardiac silhouette of most lizards does not normally have discrete borders, especially on the dorsoventral image, because it is not surrounded by aerated lungs that typically provide margin contrast in mammalian species. The lungs efface the dorsal and, in some species, the caudal contour of the lizard cardiac silhouette (see Fig. 54.4C and 54.7A). Changes in the relationship of the trachea and lungs can be used to evaluate cardiac size (see Fig. 54.7D).[1] Typically, the width of the cardiac silhouette is increased with enlargement, or there is more soft tissue filling the cranioventral coelom. Because the normal cardiac silhouette has indistinct margins, increased marginal conspicuity due to greater

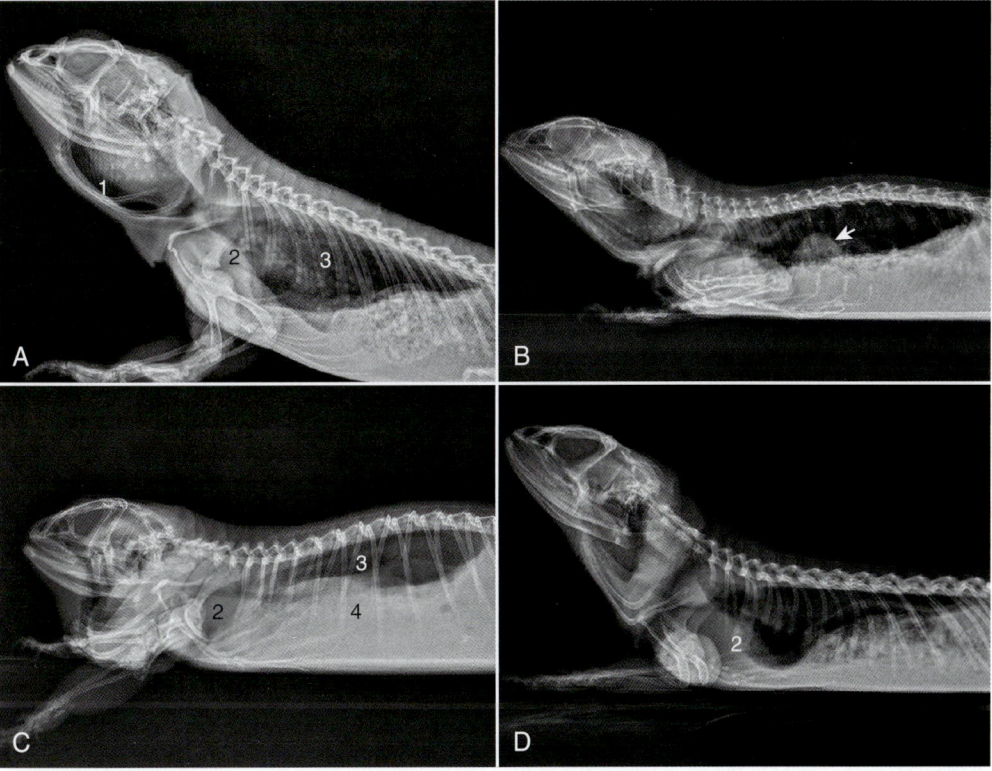

FIG 54.7 Horizontal beam, right lateral radiographs of four bearded dragons (*Pogona vitticeps*) that presented with respiratory signs. (A) Normal radiographic anatomy with unremarkable trachea (1), heart (2), and lungs (3). The apparent soft tissue densities within the cranial lungs are due to superimposition of large keratinized scales and dermal projections. The respiratory signs in this case were determined to be of environmental etiology. Note the effect of pectoral limb superimposition and how the cardiac silhouette is obscured in the cranioventral coelom. (B) Focal soft tissue density in the midventral pulmonary region (arrow). Possible differential diagnoses include abscess, granuloma, or extrapulmonary mass associated with the stomach or liver. (C) Possible enlargement of the cardiac silhouette (2) or increased soft tissue seen in the space between the heart and liver, causing compression of the lungs (3) and dorsal displacement of the trachea due to soft tissue mass effect within the cranioventral coelom (4). Ultrasonography indicated gross obesity and associated coelomic changes of hepatomegaly due to hepatic lipidosis, enlarged fat bodies, and increased pericardial fat. (D) Enlargement of the cardiac silhouette (2) was subsequently identified as ventricular enlargement due to bacterial endocarditis. (Courtesy of Stephen J. Divers.)

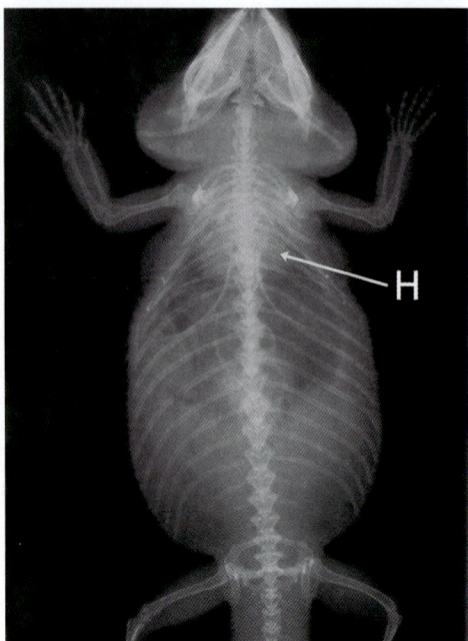

FIG 54.8 (A) Dorsal ventral view of a bearded dragon (*Pogona vitticeps*) with increased soft tissue in the area of cardiac silhouette, indicative of cardiomegaly or pericardial effusion. Fluid within the heart (H) (i.e., blood) cannot be distinguished from fluid around the heart because both silhouette or efface the same radiopacity (i.e., the soft tissue muscle of the heart). The ultrasound examination confirmed pericardial effusion was responsible for radiographic appearance. The fluid was aspirated (3 mL of cloudy yellow fluid) and was found to be inflammatory in nature, but no infectious organisms were identified. (Courtesy of Sam Silverman.)

effacement with the lungs can indicate enlargement of the silhouette (Fig. 54.8).[1,14] Enlargement in lizards is most commonly due to pericardial effusion or structural heart disease. Echocardiography provides the most specific structural and functional information about the heart (see Chapter 68).[13,15]

RESPIRATORY SYSTEM

The radiographic appearance of the lungs is highly influenced by the degree of inspiration or ventilation (see Fig. 53.4).[7] If the respiratory system is a primary concern, general anesthesia in stable patients may be elected, since positive pressure ventilation can be used to optimally inflate the lungs during exposure.[2] Because ventilation affects pulmonary radiopacity, it is important to use consistent pressure levels during inflation, especially when doing serial examinations. Overinflation of the lungs could be misinterpreted as a positive response to therapy.[1]

The lungs of lizards may be more radiolucent than mammalian species due to their larger air spaces (see Fig. 54.7A). Others, specifically more advanced lizards like many skink species, have more faveolar parenchyma in addition to the chambered lungs.[2,16] The radiolucency of the lungs should be uniform aside from pulmonary vasculature. The airways caudal to the trachea are not easily detected.[1] Lizard lungs are most easily evaluated on the lateral horizontal beam images. If the patient's coelom exceeds 6 cm in width, right and left lateral views are recommended.[1] The utility of dorsoventral vertical beam radiograph is hampered due to summation with the other coelomic structures, but it is the only view in which the right and left lungs can be individually evaluated. Hoey reported a unique presentation of unilateral lung hyperinflation in a New Caledonian giant gecko (*Rhacodactylus leachianus*) due to pulmonary-tracheobronchial prolapse that demonstrated the value of obtaining the dorsoventral image in addition to the lateral.[9]

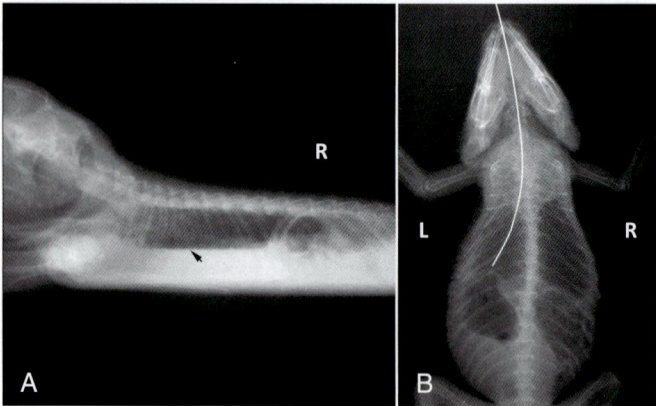

FIG 54.9 (A) Horizontal beam right lateral view of the cranial coelom of an adult bearded dragon (*Pogona vitticeps*) with an acute history of dyspnea. A distinct fluid line (arrow) can be seen. This is possible in lizards because of the more saclike conformation of the lungs. (B) Dorsoventral view of the same lizard following the introduction of a catheter with wire stylet and aspiration of lung exudate. (Courtesy of Stephen J. Divers.)

Radiographic examinations can be performed to investigate all portions of the respiratory tree. Infectious pneumopathies, including abscesses and granulomas, can produce areas of soft tissue consolidation(s) (see Fig. 54.7C).[16] These cannot be distinguished from neoplasia on radiographs. Pneumonia is uncommon in lizards but will also manifest as increased soft tissue opacity or in some cases as fluid accumulations.[2] Due to the saclike or chambered conformation of the saurian lung, fluid can accumulate and will be dependent on the horizontal beam radiograph (Fig. 54.9) producing a distinctly marginated gas-fluid line. This anatomical variation and the appearance of a lung cavity with gas and fluid differ greatly from the appearance of similar cavitations within mammalian lungs and may be misinterpreted if mammalian interpretation principles are applied. As in other species, computed tomography (CT) is a superior diagnostic modality for respiratory tract evaluation of reptiles (see Chapter 59).[7,16,17]

DIGESTIVE SYSTEM

The digestive system is more spread apart on the dorsoventral image, whereas the caudal coelomic anatomy is often dorsoventrally compressed (especially under sedation/anesthesia) on the lateral horizontal beam image. Therefore the spatial relation of the digestive tract is better visualized on the dorsoventral image.[1] Anatomically, the lizard digestive tract is reactively short (especially in carnivorous and insectivorous species) compared with mammals, but the transit time of ingesta is generally much longer. Some lizards are hindgut fermenters (i.e., green iguanas, chuckwallas [*Sauromalus* spp.]) and will therefore have large colons that may contain much fluid and/or gas.[2] Since there is no diaphragm, the relationship of the lungs and the stomach is dynamic. With lung hyperinflation, the stomach can be seen between the caudal aspect of the lungs (Fig. 54.10A and B). The duodenum extends from the pylorus in a caudal to cranial path between the stomach and the cecum. This is a unique variation of the lizard digestive tract that should be considered in interpretation.[6] The visibility of the gastrointestinal tract is highly influenced by the presence or absence of luminal content. An empty digestive tract, as well as the liver and pancreas, are poorly visualized on survey radiographs due to the low inherent soft tissue contrast within the coelom.[1,3,6] The introduction of coelomic gas (i.e., negative contrast coelomography) has been reported as a method to increase detail but is rarely utilized.[18] The presence of gas (often aerophagia) or ingesta aid in identifying the stomach. Therefore fasting

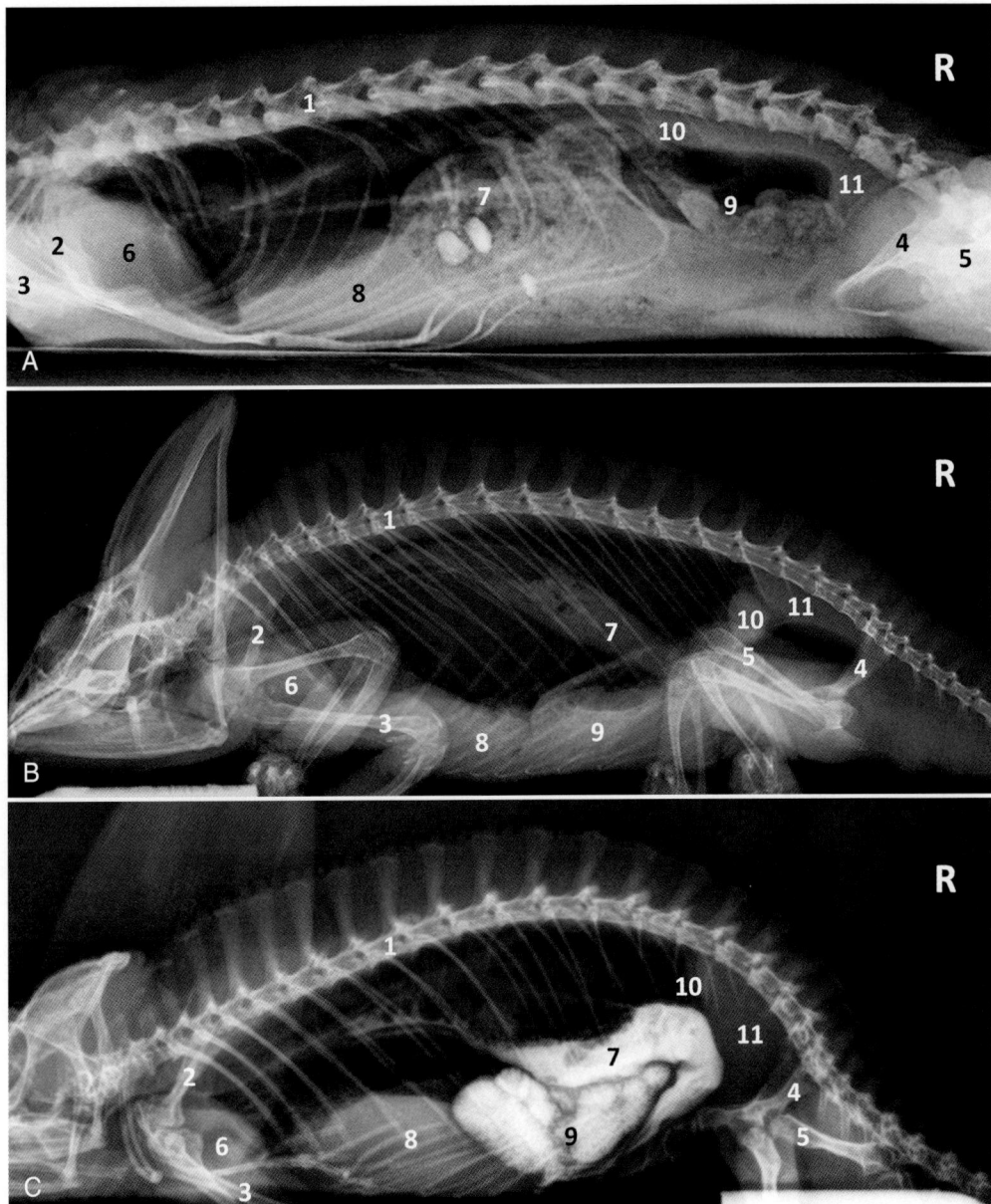

FIG 54.10 Right lateral horizontal beam radiographs of (A) green iguana (*Iguana iguana*), (B) veiled chameleon (*Chameleo calyptratus*), and (C) panther chameleon (*Furcifer pardalis*) following oral barium administration. Visible structures include the spine (1), scapulae (2), humeri (3), pelvis (4), femurs (5), heart (6), stomach (7), liver (8), intestinal tract (9), gonads (10), and kidneys (11). The contrast study demonstrates a variation from mammalian anatomy that is seen in lizards; the stomach extends caudally in the mid coelom, and the intestines largely occupy the ventral coelom rather than being positioned caudal to the stomach in the midcentral and midventral abdomen as is seen in mammals. (Courtesy of Stephen J. Divers.)

before radiography is not considered as important in lizards in that it improves visibility of the digestive tract. However, interpretation can be more challenging, since it requires decisions on the appropriateness of the food and its location in the gastrointestinal tract. The administration of barium or iodinated contrast can also be used to delineate the gastrointestinal tract (see Fig. 54.10C).

Radiographic examinations of the digestive system include the esophagus to cloaca. Disease processes commonly investigated with radiography include obstruction, foreign body ingestion, gastroenteritis, constipation, hepatomegaly or hepatic masses, and renomegaly, which can affect the gastrointestinal tract function.[2,3] Lizards often have mineral opaque bodies (such as rocks, gravel, or sand) in their digestive tract, which in moderation is noted as an incidental finding. Large volumes

of these materials can result in impaction. Gastrointestinal dilation should be evaluated in terms of generalized versus segmental ileus.[7] When generalized (e.g., enteritis), a functional problem is more common and disrupts motility, resulting in progressive distention (Fig. 54.11). Segmental dilation is suggestive of obstruction and is characterized by orad enlargement of the digestive tract. This is most common with foreign body ingestion.[2,19] A variety of objects have been reported (including substrate) and tend to be dependent on accessibility within their habitat. Coins or other metallic items and gravel/sand accumulations are readily identified with radiography (Fig. 54.12A and B), but soft tissue opaque foreign bodies such as textiles can be more challenging (see Fig. 54.12C). Radiolucent objects or those having the appearance similar to ingesta are masked, and combinations of diagnostic imaging

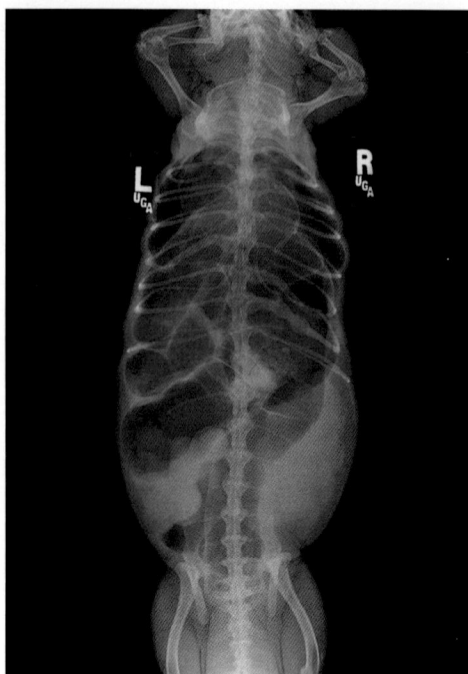

FIG 54.11 Dorsoventral radiograph of the coelom of a female green iguana (*Iguana iguana*) demonstrating extensive gastrointestinal gas from stomach to cloaca, as well as early ovarian activity. There is no evidence of a foreign body, and severe ileus secondary to bacterial gastroenteritis was later confirmed. (Courtesy of Stephen J. Divers.)

modalities have been advocated in these cases.[3,12,20] An obstructive gas pattern is not always seen and one must rely on knowledge of anatomy to determine whether a portion is inappropriately enlarged (see Fig. 54.12C). Sites to interrogate for foreign objects (i.e., where they become lodged) include the gastric lumen, intestines, or cloaca (see Fig. 54.12B). Masses in the saurian gastrointestinal tract follow similar interpretation rules as mammals. Identification of a mass effect is more difficult in lizards because of the poor serosal detail. Displacement of adjacent structures and abnormal gas foci are indicators of a soft tissue mass (Fig. 54.13). Depending on the origin of the mass, an obstructive pattern may also be present.

Numerous digestive tract radiographic contrast procedures have been discussed to improve contrast and anatomy identification, as well as to diagnose intestinal obstruction, foreign bodies, masses, and ileus. These procedures are time consuming because of the prolonged gastrointestinal transit times (which can take multiple days or even weeks) and the need to ensure that any delayed movement is indeed abnormal. Careful planning of these studies is important since it is not possible to remove the contrast once administered. These include positive (barium or iodinated) or negative (air) contrast. The most commonly performed contrast study is an upper gastrointestinal positive contrast study.[1,6,12,21,22] Typically, barium (25% weight/volume) is administered via an oroesophageal tube, and 25 mL/kg is administered. Alternatively, the volume of contrast medium administered should be similar to the volume used to tube feed a particular patient. It is important to sufficiently distend the stomach to initiate normal gastric reflexes for motility studies. These tests are preferred for evaluating motility or detecting obstruction; however, this volume of barium can mask gastric foreign material. Gastric masses or foreign bodies are better assessed with a double contrast study, using barium and air to distend the stomach. Since this improves contrast, it is reported that the study can be continued antegrade for intestinal evaluation as well.[1] If the issue involves the

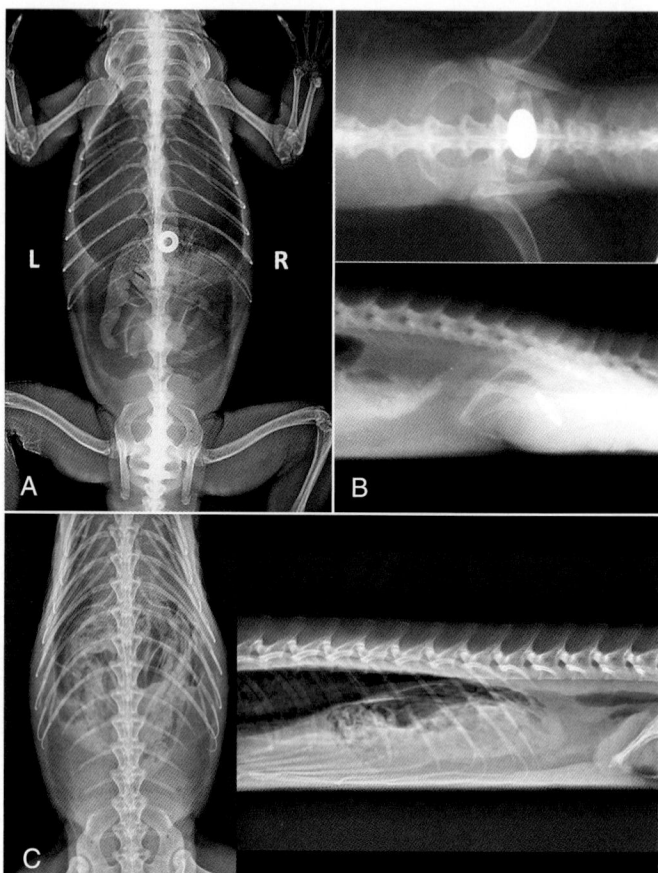

FIG 54.12 (A) Dorsoventral radiograph of a green iguana (*Iguana iguana*) after ingestion of a metal washer. Based on its position and the size of the foreign object, it is likely a gastric foreign body. (B) Green iguana (*Iguana iguana*) with intermittent signs of obstruction over several months. The foreign body (penny) is present in the cloaca of the lateral projection, but it is more obvious on the dorsoventral. (C) Dorsoventral and right horizontal beam lateral coelomic radiographs of a rock iguana (*Cyclura* sp.) that ingested a sock. The heterogeneous and fibrous nature of the textile can be appreciated, but it could be easily confused with fibrous food material. (A and C, Courtesy of Stephen J. Divers; B, courtesy of Sam Silverman.)

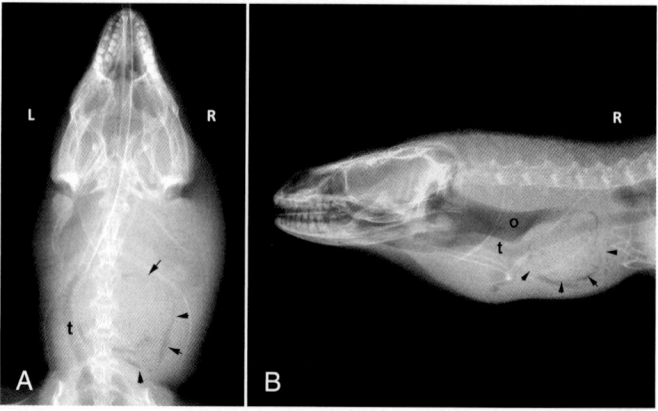

FIG 54.13 Dorsoventral (A) and right lateral (B) radiographs of a savannah monitor (*Varanus exanthematicus*) demonstrating a soft-tissue mass with intermixed and heterogeneous surrounding gas foci that is located within the right caudal cervical area (black arrows). Note that the trachea (t) is displaced to the left around this mass and the esophagus (o) is gas-filled, and the gas ends in a tapered manner around the craniodorsal aspect of the mass. Surgical exploration confirmed this mass to be an esophageal abscess. (Courtesy of Stephen J. Divers.)

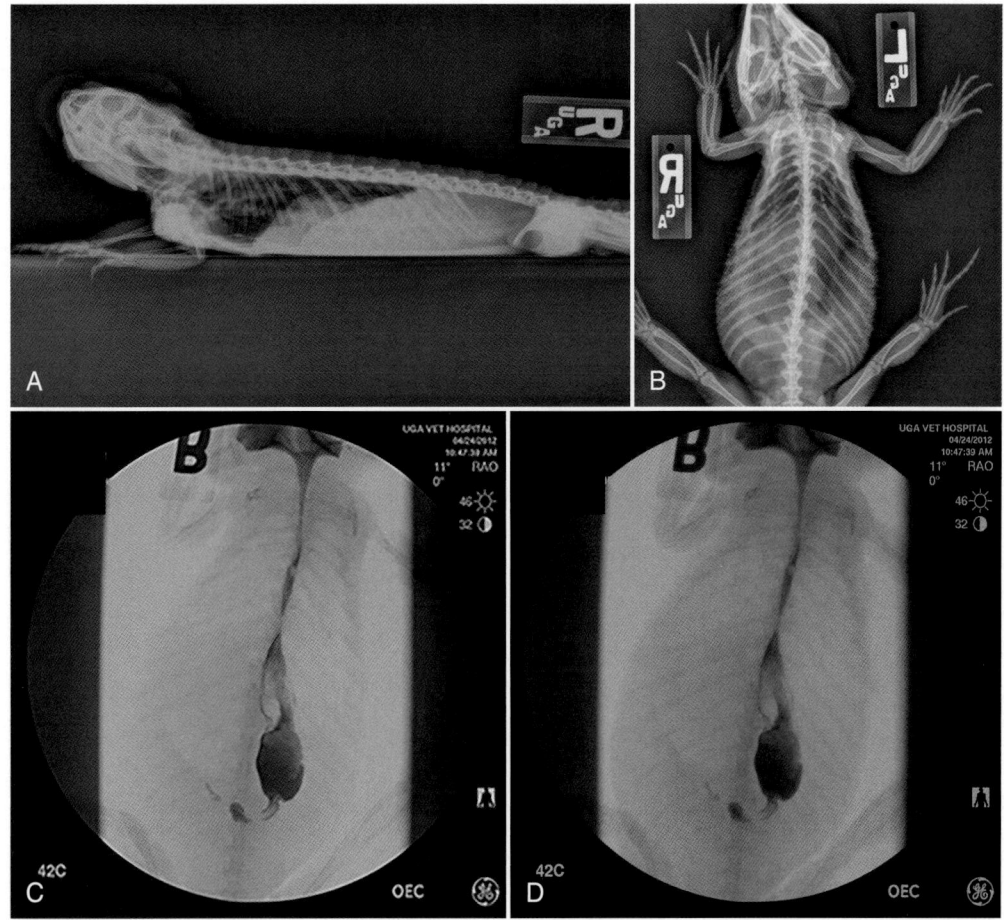

FIG 54.14 Orthogonal whole-body radiographs (A, right lateral horizontal beam; B, dorsoventral) of a bearded dragon (*Pogona vitticeps*) and two nonconsecutive fluoroscopic dorsoventral images (C and D) made after per os barium administration. There is a convex soft tissue opacity seen at the midcaudal aspect of the lungs, which is essentially midline on the dorsoventral image. It is seen in the area of the liver and stomach, and the lungs in this area are normal. In the positive contrast study, a persistent eccentric filling defect is present in the right lateral aspect of the stomach, which was confirmed to be a mural gastric mass. The remainder of the soft tissue in this area is enlarged liver with infiltrative nodules. Contrast is also seen in the first part of the duodenum. It should also be appreciated that respiration in lizards does not alter coelomic anatomy; the stomach is unchanged between end expiration (C) and end inspiration (D). (Courtesy of Shannon P. Holmes, Animal Cross-Sectional Imaging Specialists.)

cloaca, it is better to instill the contrast into the cloaca directly. Double contrast cloacograms, made following the instillation of nonionic iodinated contrast and air into the cloaca, have been used to define radiolucent cloacal foreign bodies or masses. These techniques can also be used with CT imaging to improve delineation of the digestive tract.

Contrast gastrointestinal studies have been described in a limited number of lizards. The normal appearance and transit times have been reported in the green iguana (*Iguana iguana*), bearded dragon (*Pogona vitticeps*), and partially in the common tegu (*Tupinambis teguixin*).[3,6,21] Radiographs are sufficient for upper gastrointestinal studies in lizards; however, fluoroscopy can also examine motility or persistence of a gastrointestinal abnormality, such as a mass or foreign body (Fig. 54.14). It is important that a large volume of barium contrast does not persist in the distal digestive tract given that it could, in rare instances, cause constipation.[1] Nonionic iodinated agents can be used; these have been shown to move through the gastrointestinal tract faster in other reptiles but have not been reported in lizards.[12,22,23]

In the age of ultrasonography and CT, the use of radiographs and contrast studies has diminished in the evaluation of the digestive system. However, there are important aspects to consider in continuing to use radiography and contrast. Radiographs offer a more global assessment of the coelom and can be easily sent in digital format for second opinions, compared with ultrasonograms. Contrast studies provide more longitudinal temporal information that is not possible with plain radiography, ultrasonography, or CT. The benefit of both ultrasonography and CT is not just in removing superimposition, but the parenchyma of the digestive organs (liver and pancreas) and the mural appearance of the gastrointestinal tract can be more thoroughly evaluated. As discussed previously, there is often great value in a multimodal imaging approach.

REPRODUCTIVE SYSTEM

Evaluation for gravidity (pregnancy) and dystocia are the most common reason for radiography of the reproductive system. This includes monitoring gravidity, detecting issues related to dystocia, or other conditions. Follicular stasis appears more common in lizards than other reptiles.[5] Normal developing ova are seen as spherical, soft tissue opacities in the caudal coelom bilaterally (Fig. 54.15).[5] They will summate or overlap and resemble a cluster of grapes.[1] Following ovulation, ova develop thin mineralized shells and become eggs. These eggs may develop a more ovoid appearance and fill the caudal coelom to displace the intestines cranially. It is important to accurately describe the appearance of the eggs; abnormally large, irregularly shaped, or inappropriate mineralization is indicative of an issue that merits further investigation and possibly surgery.

Radiography can also be used for sex identification in lizards. Specifically, positive contrast introduced through the vent can be used to delineate the presence or absence of hemipenes.[24] Monitor lizards may have mineralized hemipenes and can be seen without contrast.[2] Case reports of radiography used in the clinical diagnosis of reproductive disorders include an ovarian teratoma and follicular torsion.[25] In both cases, radiography was the first line diagnostic imaging modality, and soft tissue masses or a mass effect were identified. Ultrasonography provided more specific details of the anatomy contributing to the radiographic appearance. Like the digestive tract, assessment of the reproductive tract benefits from a multimodal approach, especially where poor radiographic detail hampers the imaging diagnosis.

URINARY SYSTEM

Normal green iguana kidneys may be difficult to visualize as they are located within the pelvis; however, most lizard kidneys are located within the dorsocaudal coelom. The bladder (if present) may be difficult to identify because of poor coelomic detail.[1-3] Both kidneys and bladder should exhibit soft tissue opacity. A caudodorsal coelomic mass effect can be seen with renomegaly.[1,18] The cranial aspect of enlarged iguanid kidneys become visible cranial to the pelvis (Fig. 54.16A). Mineralization of the renal parenchyma makes identification of the kidneys easy

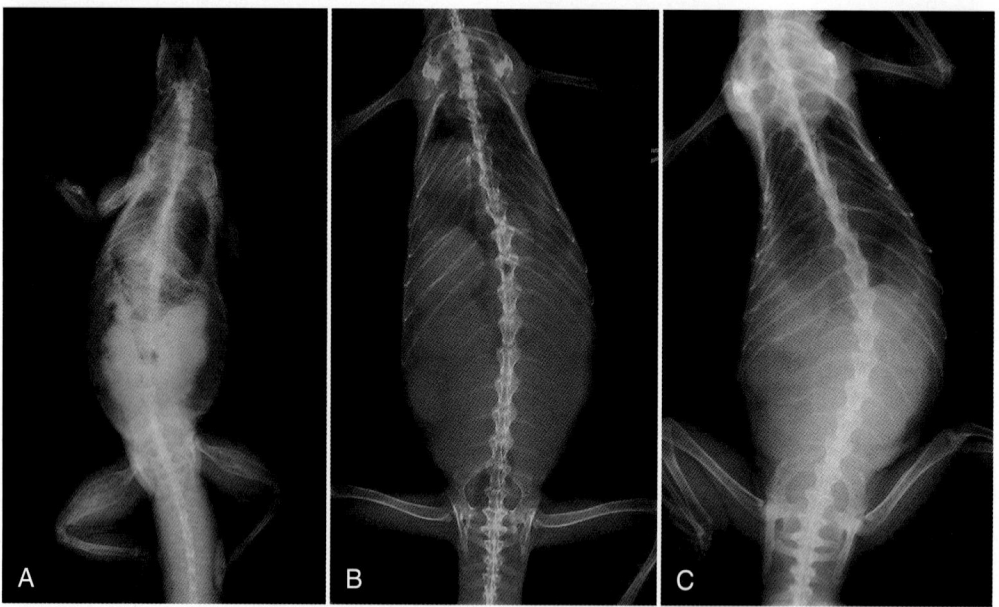

FIG 54.15 Dorsoventral radiographs of reproductive stages in iguanid lizards. (A) Early ovarian development and folliculogenesis with multiple small, rounded, soft tissue densities within the caudal coelom. Note the femoral changes consistent with nutritional secondary hyperparathyroidism, which is often unmasked when a female becomes reproductively active with increased calcium demands. (B) Preovulatory follicles are larger, spherical soft tissue densities that can occupy most of the coelomic cavity. (C) Postovulatory, thinly shelled eggs. (Courtesy of Stephen J. Divers.)

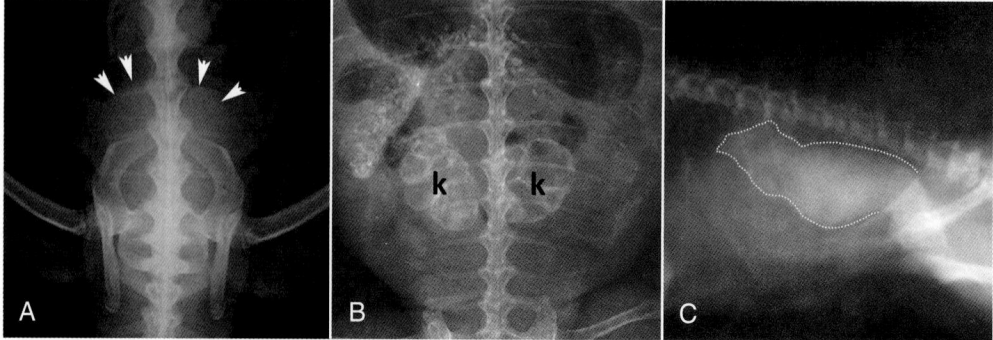

FIG 54.16 (A) Dorsoventral radiograph of the caudal coelom of a green iguana (*Iguana iguana*) demonstrating protrusion of the renal silhouettes (*arrows*) cranial to the pelvic rim, suggestive of renal enlargement. (B) Dorsoventral radiograph of the caudal coelom of a spiny-tailed lizard (*Uromastyx aegyptius*) demonstrating mineralization of both kidneys (*k*). (C) Lateral radiograph (excretory urogram) of a Chinese water dragon (*Physignathus cocincinus*) demonstrating an irregular cranial margin to the renal silhouette (dotted line) after intravenous iohexol administration. (Courtesy of Stephen J. Divers.)

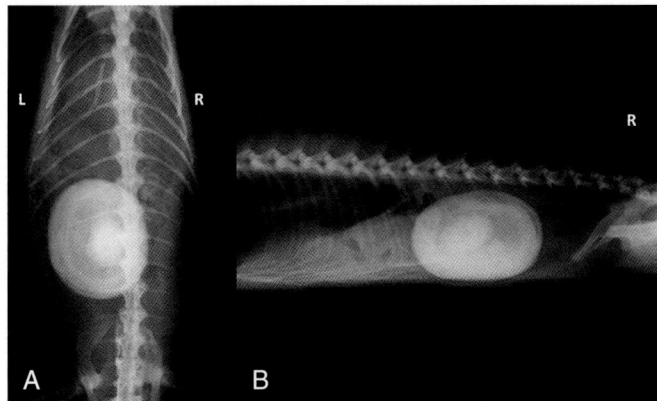

FIG 54.17 Dorsoventral (A) and right horizontal beam lateral (B) radiographs of an adult male green iguana (*Iguana iguana*) with a large urinary calculus. The calculus is composed of uric acid and mineral complexes, and the concentric rings of deposition can be appreciated. (Courtesy of Stephen J. Divers.)

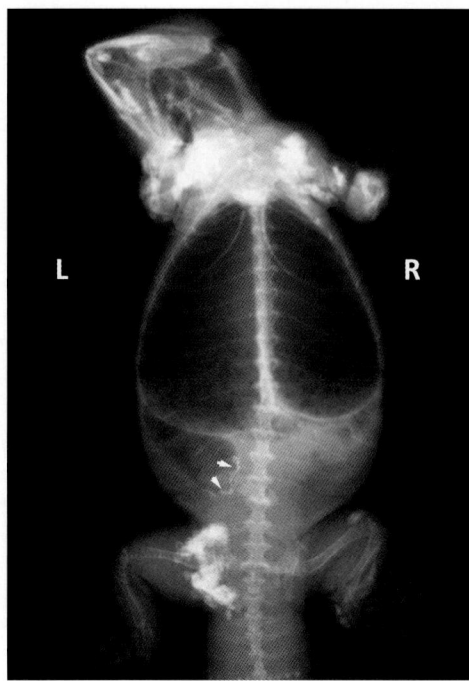

FIG 54.18 Dorsoventral radiograph of a spiny-tailed lizard (*Uromastyx* sp.) with hypervitaminosis D₃ due to excessive oral supplementation. Note the soft tissue calcification associated with the musculature of the pectoral girdle, forelimbs, left thigh, and gastric wall (*arrows*). There is also greater heterogeneity in the mineral opacity of the medullary bone, and the endosteal contours are irregular, which is most notable in the femurs. (Courtesy of Stephen J. Divers.)

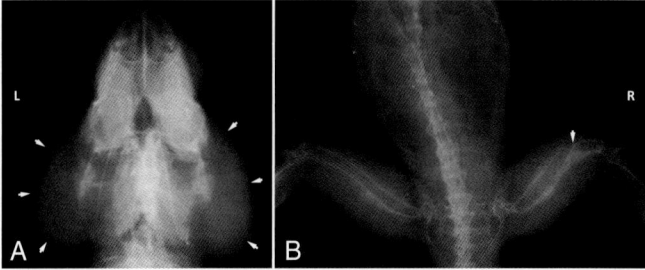

FIG 54.19 (A) Dorsoventral skull radiograph of a green iguana (*Iguana iguana*) with nutritional secondary hyperparathyroidism. Note the pronounced periosteal and fibrous proliferations associated with the mandibles (arrows), as well as generalized skeletal demineralization. (B) Dorsoventral radiograph of the pelvis and hind limbs of the same iguana. Note the poor skeletal mineralization, femoral periosteal reactions and fibrous changes seen as areas of soft tissue enlargement, and pathological folding fracture of the distal right femur (arrow). (Courtesy of Stephen J. Divers.)

(see Fig. 54.16B).[2] The visibility of the renal silhouettes can also be enhanced with negative contrast cloacography or excretory urography. The intravenously administered iodinated contrast will opacify the renal silhouettes to increase their conspicuity (see Fig. 54.16C).[18] An important consideration in the interpretation of renomegaly in iguanids is its effect on the lower intestine; these cohabitate in the pelvic canal, and enlargement of the kidneys can cause extramural compression of the colon.[26]

Urinary bladder calculi are not uncommon. Potassium or calcium salts are typically complexed with uric acid, making them radiographically detectable.[27] The presence of calculi can indicate dietary issues (e.g., excessive protein, dehydration), urine retention, or bacterial infection. When calculi are present, they can be more cranially positioned within the coelom than would be expected if extrapolating from mammals (see Fig. 53.3). They are typically irregularly marginated in shape or have an irregular, lamellated appearance and an irregular, rounded shape (Fig. 54.17).

Cloacal calculi are occasionally seen in lizards. After gentle irrigation and evacuation of the cloaca with warm saline solution, a radiographic double contrast cloacogram can be performed to identify masses, foreign bodies, strictures, and perforations.[1] The use of nonionic iodinated contrast media is preferred, because introduction of barium into the ureters or kidneys should be avoided. Contrast medium in a volume equal to 50% of the estimated cloacal volume is infused first, followed by infusion of room air in a volume equal to 100% to 200% of the estimated cloacal volume. Sometimes introduction of additional volumes of air between radiographic studies is necessary.

MUSCULOSKELETAL SYSTEM

The musculoskeletal system is one of the most common radiographic examinations in lizards. Radiographs are excellent for evaluating bones and, to a lesser extent, the associated soft tissues. They are most commonly used to evaluate for metabolic bone diseases (especially nutritional secondary hyperparathyroidism), trauma, infection, and neoplasia. The normal radiographic appearance of the musculoskeletal system in the green iguana, bearded dragon, common tegu, and leopard gecko (*Eublepharis macularius*) have been reported and are excellent references to have when embarking on interpretation.[28,29]

Metabolic bone diseases are common.[2] Oversupplementation with vitamin D₃ and calcium or renal disease can result in soft tissue

mineralization (Fig. 54.18). Decreased mineral opacity of the skeleton is more common and frequently encountered as a consequence of poor diet or inadequate lighting (Fig. 54.19), or less commonly due to renal secondary hyperparathyroidism (Fig. 54.20).[1,2,27] This will affect both the axial and appendicular skeleton, but will be most obvious in the long bones (that normally exhibit distinct corticomedullary regions), pelvis, and spine. In addition to decreased bone opacity, the radiographic features of metabolic bone disease can include soft tissue enlargement associated with fibrous proliferation, thinned cortices, long bone bowing, and pathological fractures.[1,4,30] In contrast to mammalian species, the

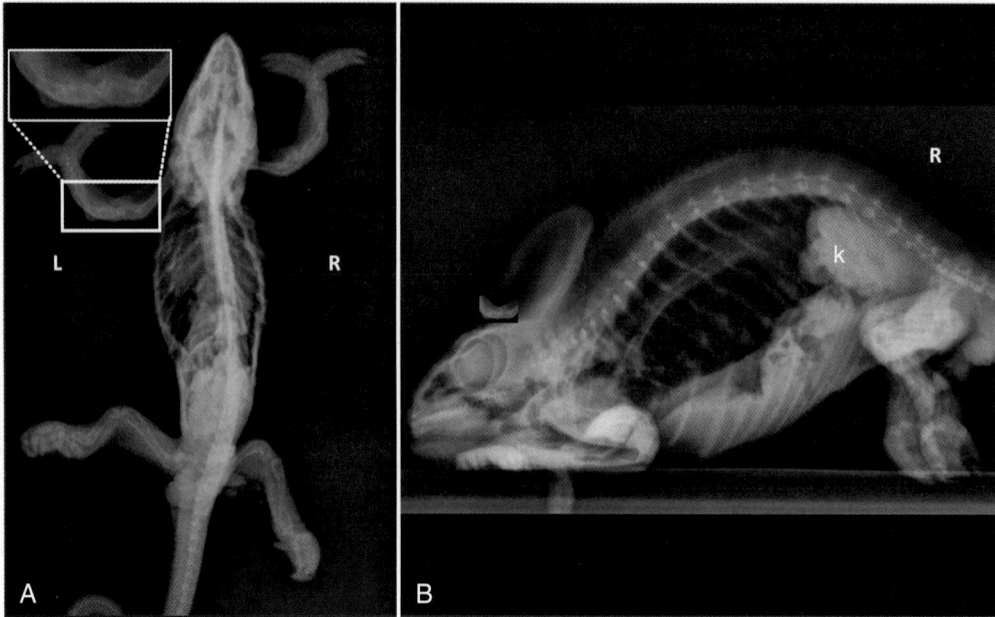

FIG 54.20 Dorsoventral (A) and right horizontal beam lateral (B) radiographs of a veiled chameleon (*Chameleo calyptratus*) with generalized skeletal demineralization, thin cortices, and pathological folding fractures of the long bones. There is increased soft tissue presence in the caudodorsal coelom in the region of the kidneys (k), suggestive of renal enlargement. Renal biopsy confirmed severe pathology and therefore the skeletal changes were associated with renal secondary hyperparathyroidism. (Courtesy of Stephen J. Divers.)

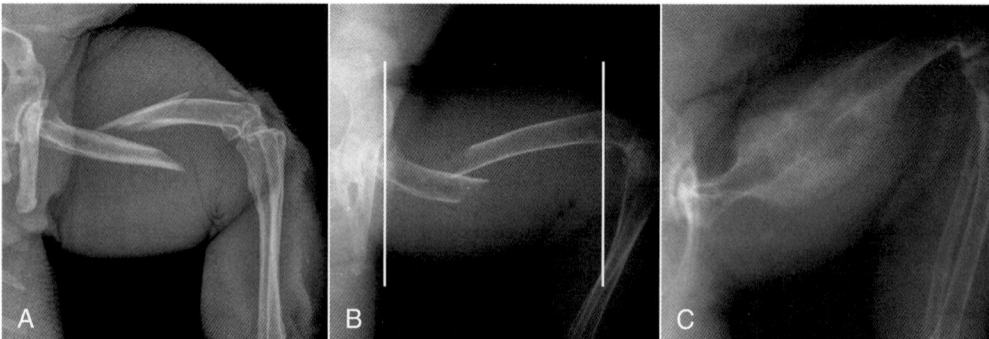

FIG 54.21 (A) Dorsoventral radiograph of an adult varanid lizard demonstrating a middiaphyseal fracture of the right femur. The fracture is comminuted and appears closed. The sharp fracture ends suggest an acute trauma and bone quality is suitable for internal fixation. (B) Lateral radiograph of a juvenile green iguana (*Iguana iguana*) demonstrating a middiaphyseal fracture of the right femur. There is no comminution, and the fracture appears closed. However, although the fracture ends are sharp, indicating an acute trauma, the thin cortices and reduced bone mineralization are consistent with nutritional secondary hyperparathyroidism, and external coaptation is more suitable. (C) Lateral radiograph of the same iguana's right femur 4 months later. The pronounced callus formation and remodeling is common after external coaptation. The appearance of the bone margins are smooth, indicating a healed fracture. Neither the periosteal proliferation nor the internal radiolucent areas are associated with infection in this case. (Courtesy of Stephen J. Divers.)

periosteal reaction seen in lizards with metabolic bone disease appears to be a unique reptilian manifestation.[1] With sufficient demineralization, angular limb deformities or pathological fractures develop due to bone softening. Clinical correlation in assessing metabolic bone diseases is important, since radiographic differentiation between different metabolic diseases and between active vs inactive disease can be challenging. With treatment, an increase in bone opacity and cortical thickness occurs, but the bones often have a decreased trabecular pattern and indistinct cortical borders compared with normal.[1]

Trauma can result in soft tissue injury, joint subluxation/luxation, or bone fracture. Digital luxations occur commonly and often require

radiographs for detection, since they can be missed on physical examination.[1] Fractures are the most common traumatic injury evaluated radiographically. They can involve the appendicular or axial skeleton, but the former is more common. Initially, the fracture fragment edges have distinct margination (Fig. 54.21). If internal or external stabilization is performed, immediate postoperative radiographs are essential and will establish the baseline.[7] The alignment, apposition, apparatus, and activity of the bone ("the four A's") should be compared over recheck examinations. The appearance of healing bone, however, differs in lizards compared with mammalian species.[1] Bone healing involves the formation of a mixed fibrous and mineralized callus.[1] Thus, clinical healing usually precedes radiographic healing. This healing process should also be considered when performing recheck radiographic examinations. Initial recheck radiographs are sometimes recommended to assess if a change in the fracture following surgical intervention has occurred in the patient after recovery from anesthesia. Osteomyelitis is a common complication and radiographic evaluation 2 to 6 weeks after surgery is recommended. To assess fracture healing, longer postoperative periods are recommended, such as 8 to 16 weeks after the injury/repair (as opposed to mammalian recheck examinations after 4–8 weeks). This is to allow sufficient time for detectable mineralized callous formation in addition to the fibrous callous. A third set of radiographs can be acquired at 30 weeks.[1] Radiographic confirmation of complete bony healing may not be evident for more than 6 months.[31] It is also noted that lucent areas at or around the fracture site may be visible in a completely healed fracture (see Fig. 54.21C). This is not seen in normally healed mammalian species and is attributed to the mixed fibrous and mineral callous formed in lizards.[1,7] Trauma can also produce fractures in the skull and spine (Fig. 54.22). The clinical significance and possible therapeutic options are difficult to estimate from radiographic examinations. Therefore CT or magnetic resonance imaging (MRI) examinations could be considered (see Chapters 59 and 60). In lizards, it has also been noted that an exuberant periosteal response occurs with any insult (trauma or infection) on the vertebrae or ribs, compared with mammals (Fig. 54.23).[1,29] As a result, focal or diffuse regions of spinal rigidity may be identified clinically, with dramatic radiographic changes. The radiographic changes are often more dramatic than the clinical signs. The vertebral hyperostosis in lizards may secondarily occlude blood vessels, and some cases of tail necrosis from vascular occlusion have resulted.[1]

Since the osteoproductive component can have a similar appearance between prior trauma and infection/inflammatory bone disease, identification of vertebral lysis or irregularly contoured widened disc space(s) is more indicative of infection or inflammation. Skull infections are most commonly localized to the cranial maxillary or mandible (unless there is another cutaneous defect) and are often associated with cage-associated trauma. With mandibular and maxillary infection, there is progressive cortical and medullary bone lysis, consistent with osteomyelitis (Fig. 54.24). Periosteal new bone production and soft tissue enlargement are other features. Expansile deformities appear more common in the mandible, and teeth are frequently lost.[1] Appendicular osteomyelitis and infectious arthritis also produce aggressive and progressive lytic changes (Fig. 54.25).[2] Similar to fracture healing, bone healing

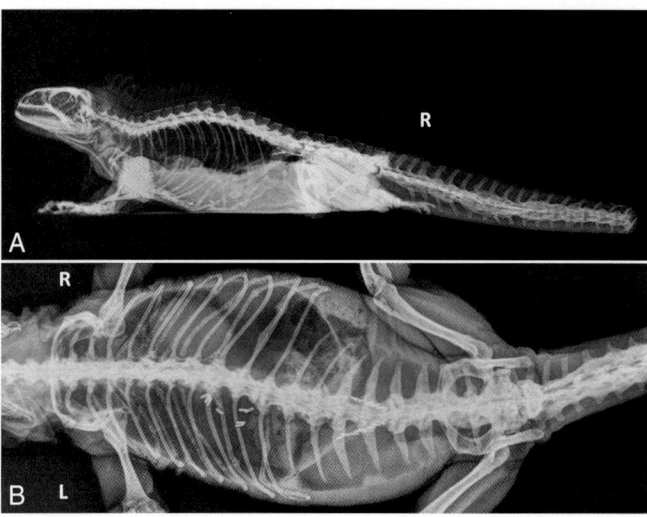

FIG 54.23 Horizontal beam right lateral (A) and dorsoventral (B) radiographs of an adult, spayed female green iguana (*Iguana iguana*) that presented with a rigid tail and reduced locomotion. The proliferative, expansile, and osteolytic changes associated with the caudal spine are characteristic of chronic osteomyelitis. In this case, the disease process has advanced into the caudal coelomic spine. (Courtesy of Stephen J. Divers.)

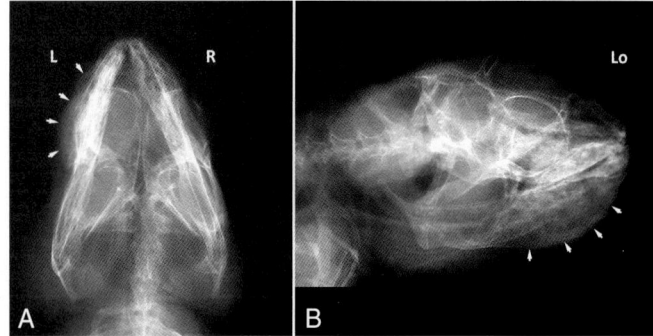

FIG 54.24 Dorsoventral and left lateral oblique radiographs of an iguanid with left mandibular osteomyelitis. Note the osteolysis, proliferative changes (*arrows*), and loss of definition associated with the left mandible. (Courtesy of Stephen J. Divers.)

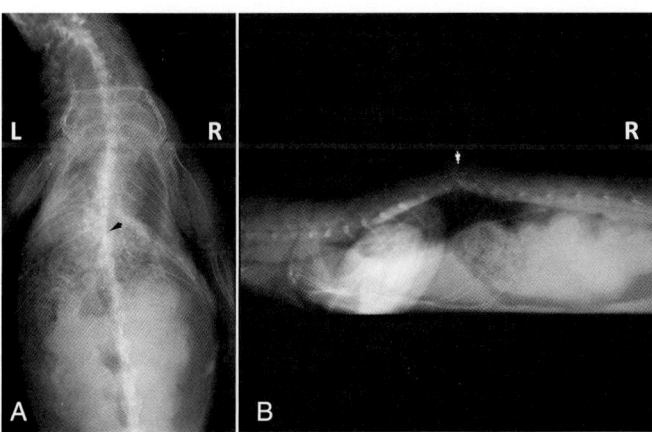

FIG 54.22 Dorsoventral (A) and right lateral horizontal beam (B) radiographs of an iguanid lizard with a vertebral fracture (arrows). There is evidence of generalized reduction in bone mineralization, which, given the obvious ovarian activity, is likely secondary to the increased calcium demands of reproduction. (Courtesy of Stephen J. Divers.)

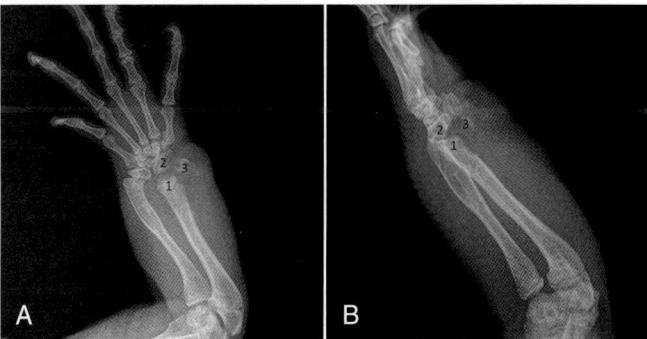

FIG 54.25 Dorsopalmar (A) and lateral (B) radiographs of the right forelimb of a green iguana (*Iguana iguana*) demonstrating osteolysis associated with the distal ulna (1), ulnar metacarpal bone (2), and accessory carpal (or pisiform) bone (3). There is also pronounced soft tissue swelling associated with the carpus. These radiographic findings are consistent with osteomyelitis and septic arthritis, but cytology or biopsy and culture are required for confirmation. (Courtesy of Stephen J. Divers.)

after osteomyelitis can have persistent lucent defects; this can make determination of resolution more challenging radiographically, and clinical correlation is essential. This lucency can be a focus of inflammation or nonossified fibrous tissue without infection or sequestration. Septic arthritis is also a largely lytic process in lizards (Fig. 54.26). Lysis

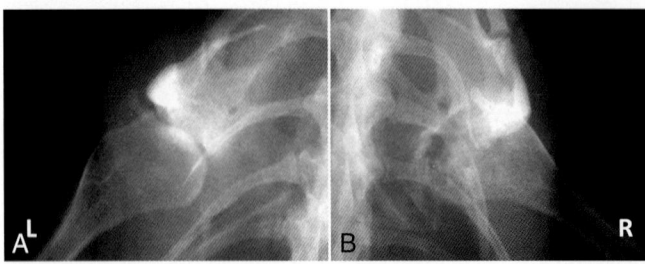

FIG 54.26 Dorsoventral radiographs of the left (A) and right (B) scapulohumeral joints of a green iguana (*Iguana iguana*) that presented with right forelimb lameness. Note the obvious irregularities and articular losses associated with the right humeral head and glenoid cavity. Joint aspiration confirmed septic arthritis. (Courtesy of Stephen J. Divers.)

is seen in the subchondral bone plate predominantly and extending into the epiphysis. Concurrent detection of synovial effusion, proliferation, intraarticular fibrous proliferation, or joint distention is dependent on accurate joint assessment. For example, it is difficult to detect intracapsular changes in the glenohumeral joint because of its position, whereas soft tissue enlargement of the distal joints is easier to detect due to the lack of adjacent anatomy.

MISCELLANEOUS

Abscess formation is common in lizards, and radiography is a critical step before surgical debridement in most cases.[2] Primarily, radiographs are used to evaluate involvement of regional tissues, such as detection of osteomyelitis. The extent of an early abscess might also be delineated with iodinated contrast injection into the abscess, although the inspissated nature of chronic forms renders this technique ineffective.

REFERENCES

See www.expertconsult.com for a complete list of references.

55

Radiography—Snakes

Jessica R. Comolli and Stephen J. Divers

Diagnosing internal disease in snakes can be challenging even for experienced veterinarians. Clinical signs are often subtle, and physical examination findings are seldom pathognomonic. Radiography is an essential tool; however, a thorough knowledge of snake anatomy, physiology, and pathology is required for proper acquisition and correct interpretation of images. The large number of snake species and the considerable morphologic and anatomic variability that exists contributes to the challenge.[1] Moreover, there is a relatively small amount of published information regarding imaging techniques and interpretation and a lack of clear guidelines for normal and abnormal radiographic parameters for these species. Additionally snakes have poor radiographic visceral contrast related to the close anatomic proximity of internal organs, the lack of periorgan fat (which is localized into discrete fat bodies), the absence of a clearly demarcated thorax and abdomen, and image degradation from heavily keratinized scales.

Fortunately, with a recent increase in published imaging information and studies, and now more affordable and improved digital radiology technology available, practitioners are capable of producing high detail images that can be electronically shared. The goals of this chapter are to describe proper techniques for radiographic positioning, illustrate normal radiographic anatomy, and discuss the principles of radiographic interpretation in snakes.

RESTRAINT AND POSITIONING

When conscious, snakes are relatively difficult to position and restrain for radiographic examinations. General anesthesia or heavy sedation is typically required (see Chapters 48 and 49). When relaxed, positioning is easier and eliminates spinal curvatures associated with normal muscular contractions. Furthermore, if detailed examination of the skeletal, respiratory, and digestive system is desired, the snake must be fully extended (Fig. 55.1). Radiographs of a coiled snake are not recommended because the internal organs are distorted and symmetry of the spine and ribs is compromised. However, if the purpose of the examination is to confirm a specific structure (e.g., radiodense foreign body or eggs/fetuses), then a coiled positioning study may be acceptable.

Unanesthetized snakes may be taped to a padded board or restrained with sand bags; however, care should be taken to avoid scale damage or bruising, and most snakes will still distort and create positional artifacts. Alternatively, the snake can be placed inside an acrylic tube, although this may also produce radiographic artifacts, and positioning will rarely, if ever, be ideal (see Fig. 55.1). A slight increase in the kilovolt peak to compensate for the acrylic's filtration of the radiograph beam may be necessary. The diameter and wall thickness of the tube should be as small and as thin as possible to minimize the object-film distance

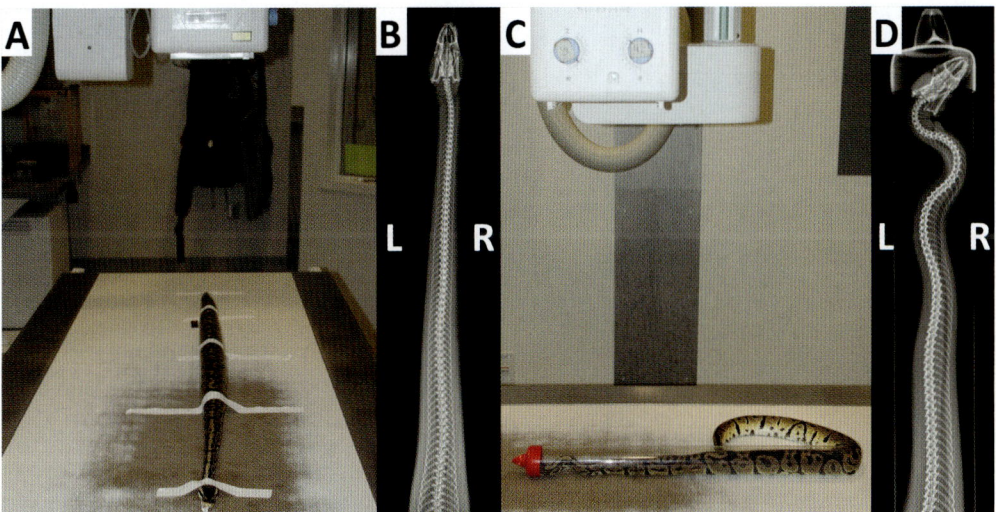

FIG 55.1 Positioning and corresponding dorsoventral radiographs of an anesthetized (A and B) and conscious, tubed (C and D) adult female ball python (*Python regius*). Although the use of plastic, radiolucent tubes does permit radiography of conscious snakes, positioning is still less than ideal. In this case the conscious snake radiograph exhibits significant spinal rotation to the left, and the cervical spine is not straight. (Courtesy of Stephen J. Divers.)

and to immobilize the patient effectively. The acrylic tube should not have perforations or other openings over the radiographed area, because these may produce image artifacts.

Radiography of most snakes requires the acquisition of serial films of the whole body or can be limited to a region of interest (e.g., the respiratory tract, stomach, kidneys). Familiarity with internal anatomy is essential for localization of the radiograph beam (Fig. 55.2).[2] Localization of the cardiac apex motion on the ventral abdominal wall can be used as a reference point for the beginning of the lung tissue in most snakes (Fig. 55.3). Accurate labeling of serial films is essential to relate a radiographic lesion with a specific body region or organ. Radiopaque markers can be taped to the skin, and metallic number markers are ideal for this purpose.[3] The numbers are attached to the skin in a sequential manner so that the contiguous segments can be identified on the multiple images.

Orthogonal views are recommended for evaluation of major organ systems, with dorsoventral projections obtained using vertical x-ray beams and lateral projections using horizontal beams. Lateral views are best taken using a horizontal beam to avoid displacement artifact of the viscera and to more accurately detect fluid lines (Fig. 55.4). Unlike most other reptiles, when positioning snakes for horizontal radiograph beam studies, their bodies can be placed very close or even in direct contact with the radiograph cassette, thus increasing radiographic detail and decreasing magnification. However, standard (vertical beam) lateral views can still be useful where horizontal beams are not possible or safe to undertake, but these technique details must be shared with the interpreter. The interpretations of dorsoventral views are hindered by the spine and ribs but are still useful when dealing with obvious structures, such as eggs, or pathology, such as mineralized masses or bony lysis.

CARDIOVASCULAR SYSTEM

Depending on species, the heart generally lies between 20% to 36% snout-to-vent length (SVL); however, it has been found to be more cranial in some arboreal snakes and caudal in aquatic snakes due to

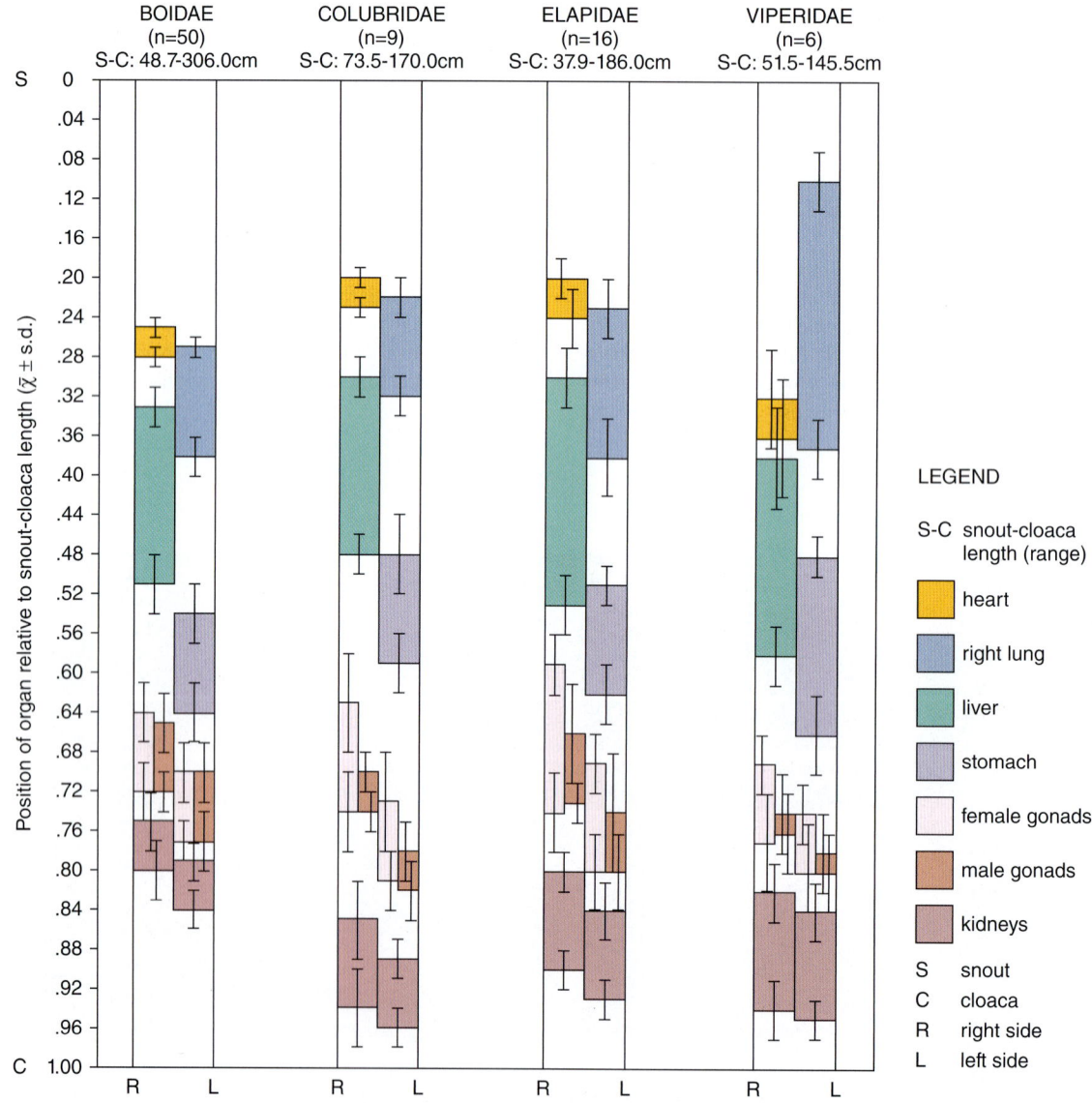

FIG 55.2 Position of internal organs relative to body length; family mean data. (Adapted with permission from McCracken HE. Organ location in snakes for diagnostic and surgical evaluation. In Fowler ME, Miller RE, eds. *Zoo and Wildlife Medicine: Current Therapy*, 4th ed. Philadelphia: WB Saunders; 1999;243–248.)

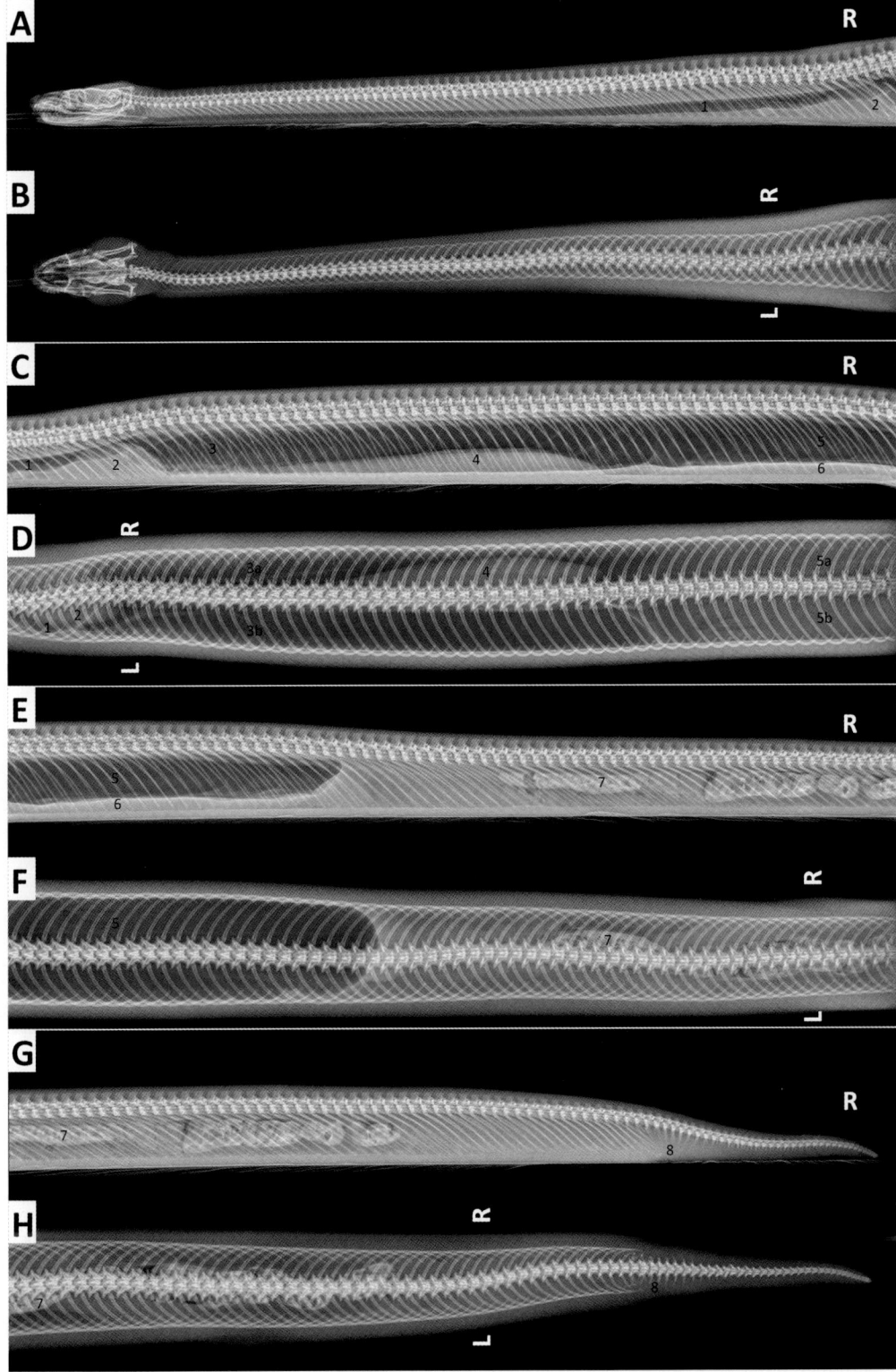

FIG 55.3 Horizontal beam right lateral (A, C, E, G) and corresponding dorsoventral radiographs (B, D, F, H) of a clinically healthy, fasted, adult female ball python (*Python regius*); (1) trachea, (2) heart, (3) vascular lungs (a right, b left), (4) liver, (5) saccular lungs (5a right, 5b left), (6) empty stomach, (7) feces within large intestine, and (8) cloaca. (Courtesy of Stephen J. Divers.)

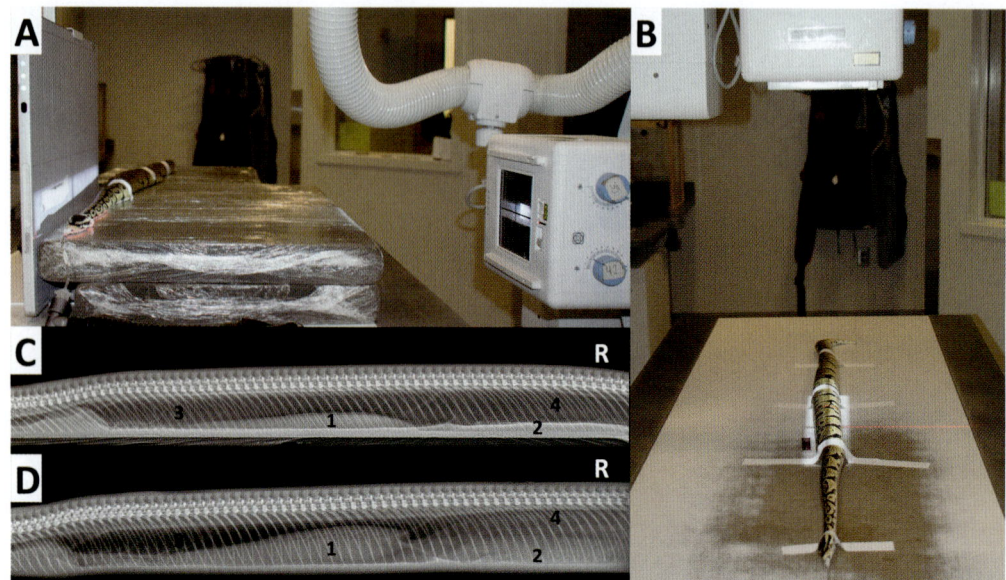

FIG 55.4 Positioning and corresponding horizontal beam (A and C) and vertical beam (B and D) right lateral radiographs of an anesthetized ball python (*Python regius*, 25%–65% snout-to-vent length). Note the displacement of the liver (1) and stomach (2), which has resulted in an apparent reduction in the size of the vascular (3) and saccular lungs (4). Visceral displacement and an inability to detect fluid lines are the primary reasons for recommending horizontal beam lateral views over the more usual vertical beam technique used in small animal practice. (Courtesy of Stephen J. Divers.)

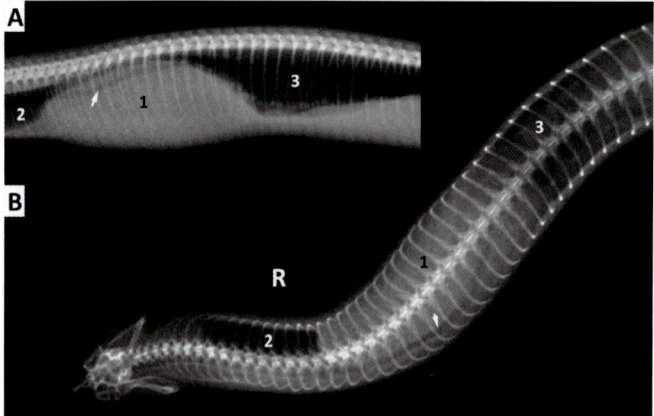

FIG 55.5 Right lateral (A) and dorsoventral (B) radiographs of a western hognose snake (*Heterodon nasicus*), centered over the heart (25% snout-to-vent length). The trachea (arrow) has been displaced dorsad and left laterad by a gross enlargement of the cardiac silhouette (1), which is bordered by an air-filled esophagus (2) and the primary faveolar lung (3). Enlargement of the cardiac silhouette can be associated with pericardial effusion, cardiomegaly, or other soft tissue masses adjacent to the heart. (Courtesy of Stephen J. Divers.)

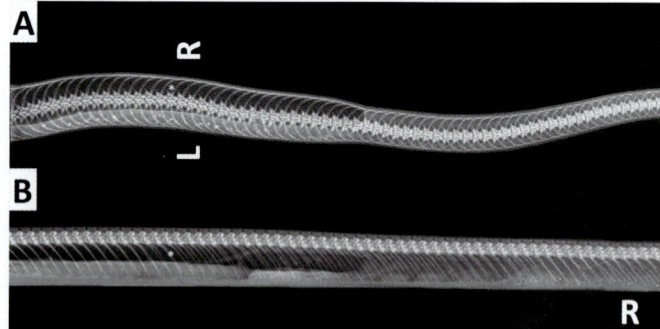

FIG 55.6 Dorsoventral (A) and horizontal right lateral (B) radiographs of a corn snake (*Pantherophis guttatus*, 50%–85% snout-to-vent) demonstrating the single, right lung (*) typical of most snakes. (Courtesy of Stephen J. Divers.)

gravitational effects and evolution in these species (see Fig. 55.2).[4–7] Radiographically, the heart is not usually well visualized on the dorsoventral view unless grossly enlarged but can be consistently evaluated on the lateral view (horizontal X-ray beam preferred) (see Fig. 55.3). Air within the trachea and cranial lung usually provide good contrast for the dorsal and caudal margins of the cardiac silhouette. Enlargement can indicate pericardial effusion or cardiomegaly. Cardiomyopathy, congenital etiologies, neoplasia, and congestive heart failure have been reported to cause cardiomegaly in snakes (Fig. 55.5).[8–15] Echocardiography is recommended after radiographic identification of enlargement of the cardiac silhouette. Postprandial concentric cardiac hypertrophy has been reported in boids and should be considered in species that consume large, infrequent meals.[16,17] Metastatic mineralization of large blood vessels around the heart can also be seen radiographically due to the negative contrast associated with the adjacent lungs.

RESPIRATORY SYSTEM

The lung(s) of snakes generally lie caudal to the heart at approximately 25% to 60% SVL in most species; however, in those species with tracheal lungs, the pulmonary tissue may start as cranial as 6% SVL (see Fig. 55.2). Most snakes, with the exception of boas and pythons, have only a single functioning right lung, with the left either absent or vestigial (Fig. 55.6).[3,18] Radiographically, snake lung(s) are visualized on the lateral view, and horizontal beams are again preferred to detect fluid lines and avoid organ displacement changing the appearance of the pulmonary

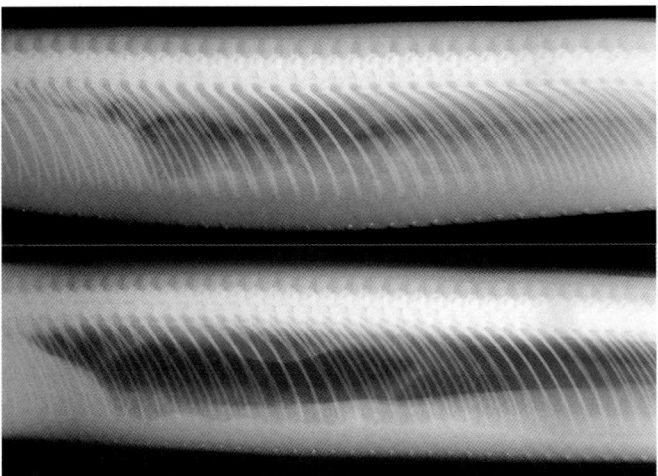

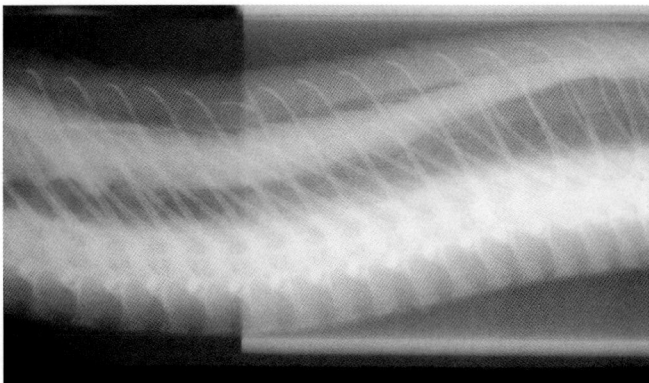

FIG 55.8 Acrylic positioning devices (right side) can increase radiopacity and decrease image detail.

FIG 55.7 Boa constrictor (*Boa constrictor*). The radiograph (horizontal radiograph beam, lateral view) was made with the patient during expiration (top) and at peak inspiration (bottom). The lungs are more lucent and larger on the inspiratory radiograph. The cardiac silhouette on the left of the images serves as a point of reference.

structures. If the patient's diameter exceeds 6 cm, both right and left lateral views are recommended.

The trachea can be visualized as a radiolucent line in the cranial third of the body extending from the head to the cardiac silhouette (see Fig. 55.3). Tracheal masses can often be appreciated if present. The lung becomes a thin-walled saccular structure caudally and may extend close to the level of the cloaca in some species. Overlap of other organs such as liver and stomach over the lung fields can make the radiographic interpretation of respiratory disease challenging, especially with vertical beam lateral views.

The phase of the respiratory cycle at which the radiographic exposure is made is critical and ideally should coincide with the peak of inspiration (Fig. 55.7). Endotracheal intubation and positive pressure inflation of the lungs (10–15 cm of water) for radiography are highly recommended; however, positive pressure ventilation does influence the radiographic appearance of the lungs. The volume of the lungs can be increased with positive pressure ventilation far in excess to what is present with spontaneous respiration. A subsequent diffuse decrease in pulmonary radiopacity has been seen with hyperinflation and in positive pressure studies (see Fig. 55.7). Thus care must be taken when evaluating these films, as they can be misinterpreted as an indicator of a positive response to therapy. The effect of positioning devices on lung opacity and detail must also be considered (Fig. 55.8). Additionally, radiographic studies should not be performed in close proximity to feeding, as distention of the digestive tract often compromises pulmonary inflation, and the radiopacity of the ingesta may obscure detail of superimposed structures.

Common indications for evaluating the respiratory system are rhinitis, stomatitis, and suspected neoplastic and infectious disorders of the trachea and lungs, as well as abscesses or granulomas (Fig. 55.9; also see Chapters 76 and 162).[19–21] As in other reptiles, because the structure of snake lungs (faveolar and saccular) differs greatly from mammals, the standard radiographic patterns (i.e., alveolar, interstitial, bronchial, pleural) used to describe the radiographic appearance of the mammalian lung are not applicable. Snake lungs have a relatively homogeneous radiopacity with more prominence to the pulmonary structure in the cranial vascular region. Airway markings are generally indistinct to indistinguishable throughout, but the intrapulmonary bronchus

can sometimes be appreciated. The radiographic manifestation of consolidative pulmonary disease (e.g., pneumonia) is increased pulmonary opacity, either diffuse (most common), focal, or multifocal.[22] Exudate or fluid accumulation may be appreciated as a fluid line on horizontal beam lateral views. Radiographic appreciation of respiratory disease may be limited, however, as changes may not become obvious until advanced.[1,18] Further examination by endoscopy, computed tomography (CT), or magnetic resonance imaging (MRI) may be indicated for snakes with less-advanced disease (see Chapters 59, 60, and 64).

GASTROINTESTINAL SYSTEM

The snake digestive tract is relatively short in length but has a longer transit time than mammals.[23] Snakes are ectothermic with low metabolic rates, and intervals between feedings are much longer than in mammals and many other reptiles. Many gastrointestinal diseases can affect snakes. Most etiologies are related to husbandry (e.g., improper temperature, inappropriate nutrition); gastrointestinal parasitism; gastroenteritis; or intestinal obstructions caused by foreign bodies, impaction, intussusceptions, or tumors.[24–26] Common clinical indications for evaluating the digestive system include chronic regurgitation and any coelomic swelling (e.g., hypertrophic gastritis, foreign body ingestion/impaction, constipation, hepatomegaly and hepatic masses, and other intracoelomic masses) (Fig. 55.10).

The digestive tract and the accessory organs (i.e., liver and pancreas) are poorly visualized on survey radiographs. Poor tissue contrast and serosal detail is seen because of the close apposition of internal organs and the paucity of periorgan fat. The stomach can be easily identified if gas-filled (usually from aerophagia) or radiopaque food was recently ingested, but there is often superimposition of the liver cranially and the gonads caudally. The appearance of the digestive tract is significantly affected by the time of previous feeding, the nature of the ingesta, and the species of the patient. In snakes, ingesta can often be identified as a bolus of material that produces a regional enlargement of the digestive tract. As the ingesta becomes more digested, the bolus becomes less distinct and is more diffusely distributed. Fecal material can often be identified by its heterogeneous presence due to the hair within.

The esophagus extends from the oral cavity to the stomach and is not normally visualized unless gas or contrast material is present. The stomach is located in the middle third of the body, approximately 45% to 65% SVL (see Fig. 55.2 and Fig. 55.3). Often, the radiodense skeletal remains of recently ingested prey can be visualized in the stomach. Ingesta of varying opacities can be observed in the small and large intestines in the caudal third of the body (positioned approximately 65%–100% SVL). Large

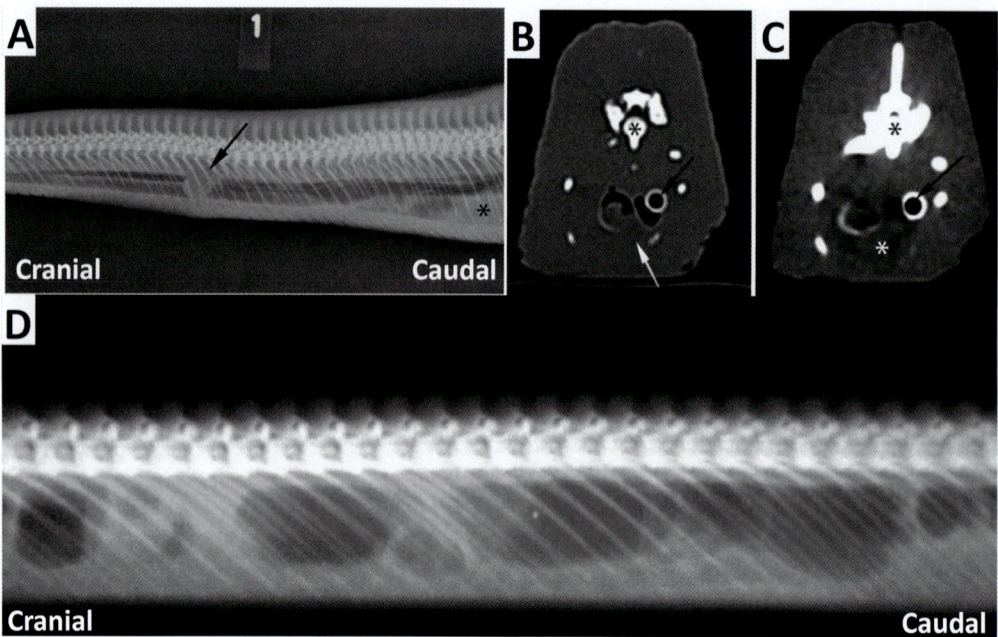

FIG 55.9 (A) Right lateral radiograph of the tracheal region of an 8-year-old boa constrictor (*Boa constrictor*). A round, soft-tissue mass (black arrow) is invading the tracheal lumen at the level of the midtrachea, cranial to the heart (asterisk). (B and C) Transverse computed tomography images of the cervical area of a boa constrictor in a lung algorithm (B) and soft-tissue algorithm (C) revealed a soft tissue mass partially obstructing the tracheal lumen (white asterisk). The mass extends ventrally and medially beyond the tracheal wall (white arrow), close to the esophagus (black arrow). A rubber tube has been inserted into the esophagus to delineate this structure during image acquisition (black arrow). The black asterisk indicates the cervical vertebrae. (D) Horizontal beam, right radiographic view of the cranial coelom (30%–50% snout-to-vent length) of a ball python (*Python regius*) demonstrating multifocal areas of increased soft tissue density throughout the vascular lung due to mycobacteriosis. (A–C, Reproduced with permission from Summa NM, Guzman DS-M, Hawkins MG, et al. Tracheal and colonic resection and anastomosis in a boa constrictor *[Boa constrictor]* with T-cell lymphoma. *J Herp Med Surg.* 2015;25:87-99; D, courtesy of Stephen J. Divers.)

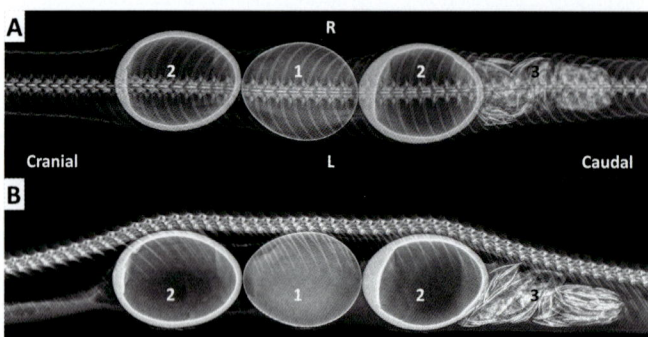

FIG 55.10 Dorsoventral and horizontal beam right lateral radiographs (40%–65% snout-to-vent length) of an eastern black rat snake (*Pantherophis alleghaniensis*) that was found poorly responsive with a pronounced midbody swelling. Note the normal chicken egg (1) along with two artificial ceramic eggs (2) and additional collapsed chicken eggs caudad (3). Gastric foreign bodies are not uncommon in snakes and often require endoscopic or surgical removal. (Courtesy of Stephen J. Divers.)

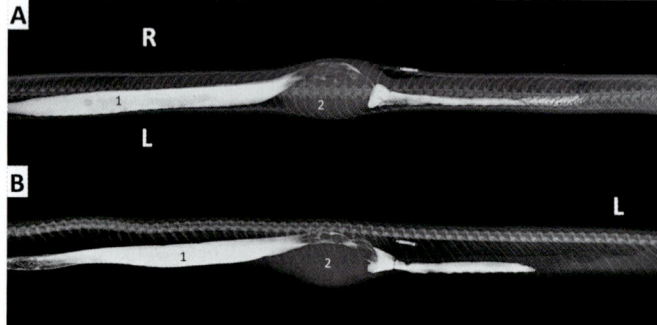

FIG 55.11 Dorsoventral (A) and vertical beam left lateral (B) radiographs of a speckled king snake (*Lampropeltis getula holbrooki*, 45%–65% snout-to-vent). The snake presented with a midbody swelling and films were taken after barium administration. Note the barium within the stomach (1) and the gastric compression by a soft tissue mass effect (2). A microchip is also visible. The mass was confirmed as a gastric leiomyosarcoma. (Courtesy of Rodney W. Schnellbacher, Dickerson Park Zoo.)

intestinal gas, if present, is often the only contrast visible in plain films of the caudal coelom. The cloaca lies at the level of the last pair of ribs.

Although orthogonal projections are recommended in all cases, the lateral view provides the best visualization of the digestive tract in snakes. Digestive tract radiographic contrast procedures can be helpful for documentation of gastroenteritis diagd gastric hyperplasia and are often necessary for intestinal obstruction and foreign bodies. In addition, contrast material in the gastrointestinal tract can often outline

and help determine the origin of nonspecific intraluminal or extraluminal intracoelomic masses (Fig. 55.11).

CONTRAST RADIOGRAPHY

Contrast media can be used in many instances to increase the yield of radiographic diagnostic information. Gastrointestinal studies with contrast agents enable detection of partial or complete obstructions, intraluminal masses originating from the digestive tract, enhancement and differentiation of extraluminal masses, and the evaluation of the digestive transit time.[24] For gastrointestinal contrast studies in snakes, standard orthogonal views should be routinely used, although oblique radiographs may be needed to assess a particular abnormality (Fig. 55.12).

Contrast agents include barium products (suspension and impregnated markers) and organic iodinated liquid (low and high osmolality). Barium sulfate is a noniodinated compound that is the standard agent for routine contrast studies of the upper and lower gastrointestinal tract. Barium is ideal in that it provides excellent detail of the gastrointestinal structures, is readily available, and inexpensive.[27] However, it can become desiccated in the digestive tract and result in intestinal obstruction, especially if a large volume of contrast medium is used and remains in the digestive tract for a long time. Although this is not a common complication, it should be considered in patients with preexisting ileus or dehydration. If a large volume of contrast medium is present in the distal colon or cloaca after completion of the study, it should be gently massaged out with external digital pressure. Alternatively, it can be evacuated by cloacocolonic catheterization and lavage using sterile saline. In mammalian radiography, barium sulfate is contraindicated if gastrointestinal perforation is suspected because of the risk of severe peritonitis.[28,29] Although not evaluated in snakes or other reptiles, alternative water-soluble iodinated agents should be used in cases of suspected perforation and intestinal adhesions, as they are known to be quickly absorbed from the peritoneal cavity with little to no adverse effects in mammals.[30,31]

Iodinated contrast water-soluble agents can be separated into two groups: ionic (high osmolarity) or nonionic (low osmolarity). Iodinated agents have a more rapid gastrointestinal transit time, which may be beneficial in patients where a faster diagnosis is required.[32,33] Ionic iodine-based contrast media consists of agents such as diatrizoate sodium and diatrizoate meglumine (Gastrografin). Due to its hyperosmolarity (1900 mOsm/L), it can draw interstitial fluid into the intestinal lumen, and therefore should not be used in young, dehydrated, hypovolemic, or renal-compromised patients.[3,33,34] Furthermore, these agents should not be used in patients with an increased risk of aspiration, as they cause chemical pneumonitis.[35] Nonionic, iodinated contrast mediums such as iohexol (Omnipaque™) have a lower osmolality (520 mOsm/L) and are preferentially used when other contrast media are contraindicated. Although often more expensive than barium sulfate, iohexol provides excellent mucosal detail in birds and mammals, even if partially diluted.[31,36,37]

Gastrointestinal transit times can vary greatly in snakes due to many factors, including their ectothermic nature, species, environmental factors

such as temperature and season, food composition, metabolic factors, and stage of digestion.[3,24,27] Comprehensive studies have been conducted on the digestive physiology of snakes; however, few studies have evaluated contrast gastrointestinal radiography. A study in ball pythons (*Python regius*) evaluating gastrointestinal anatomy, normal digestive transit time, and contrast radiographic quality of three different concentrations (25%, 35%, and 45% [w/v]) of barium sulfate concluded that the 35% concentration of contrast medium yielded the best imaging quality.[24] Similarly in bearded dragons (*Pogona vitticeps*), good-quality images were obtained with a concentration of 35% w/v.[27] Ball pythons had an average esophageal transit time of 6.89 ± 6.74 hours, onset of gastric filling time of 0.94 ± 0.54 hours, gastric emptying time of 40.67 ± 14.92 hours, onset of small intestine transit of 2.05 ± 1.70 hours, small intestine transit time of 50.82 ± 12.34 hours, and onset of large intestine transit of 28.94 ± 21.70 hours. However, interpretation of results may not translate well in other species due to anatomic and physiological differences.[24]

Snakes should be maintained at their species-specific preferred optimum temperature zone to ensure that contrast will pass through the gastrointestinal tract at an appropriate rate.[38,39] The contrast medium should be warmed to the approximate body temperature of the patient before administration (often 27°C–29°C, 80°F–85°F). Dose rates have not been determined for all species, but the volume of contrast medium administered should not exceed the volume that would be used to tube-feed the patient. In small animals, a dose of 6 to 16 mL/kg of barium is recommended.[31] Doses of 5 to 20 mL/kg have been suggested in reptiles.[40] In the study mentioned previously, a dose of 25 mL/kg of barium was administered to ball pythons based on the unique capacity for the distention of the gastrointestinal tract in snakes. Four of 18 ball pythons regurgitated immediately after administration, however, possibly indicating that this dose could be excessive and should be reduced, although no additional complications were observed.[24]

Double-contrast upper and lower gastrointestinal radiographic studies can be useful to document mucosal disease, foreign bodies, strictures, and partial or complete obstruction in the esophagus, stomach, and intestines (Fig. 55.13). The procedure uses a smaller volume of positive contrast agent and allows for a more rapid evaluation of the digestive tract, because the gas used propels the positive contrast medium rather than relying on peristalsis. In small animals, double-contrast studies produce superior radiographic mucosal detail over single contrast studies; although in humans, a study comparing diagnostic accuracy in both techniques indicated that the two methods were equal and complemented each other.[41,42] In upper double-contrast studies, a tube is passed into the stomach, and 100% barium sulfate or nonionic iodinated contrast is infused into the stomach at a volume estimated to be one third to

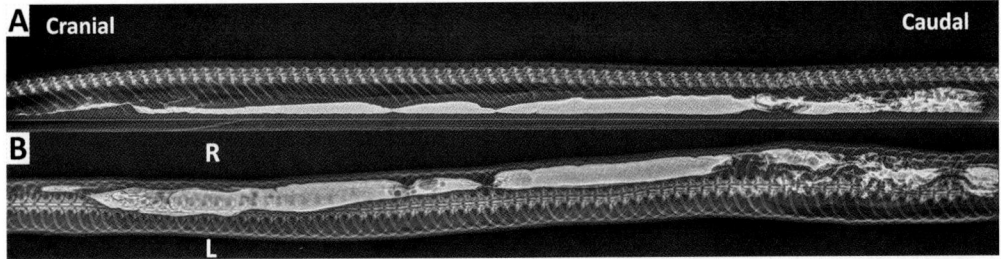

FIG 55.12 Right lateral (A) and dorsoventral (B) radiographs of a colubrid snake at 50% to 90% snout-to-vent length during a barium gastrointestinal study. Gastrointestinal contrast can be useful for evaluating motility, transit, partial obstructions, and coelomic soft tissue mass effects that may be impinging on intestinal function. Transit times are often prolonged requiring repeated radiography over several days or even weeks. (Courtesy of Stephen J. Divers.)

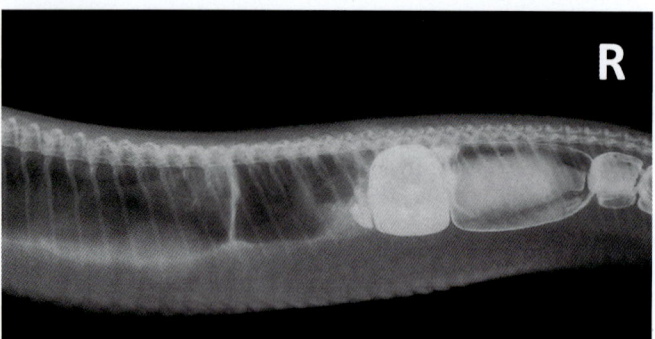

FIG 55.13 Emerald tree boa (*Corallus caninus*) with chronic abdominal distention. The retrograde double contrast study shows an angular constriction caused by an intestinal adenocarcinoma.

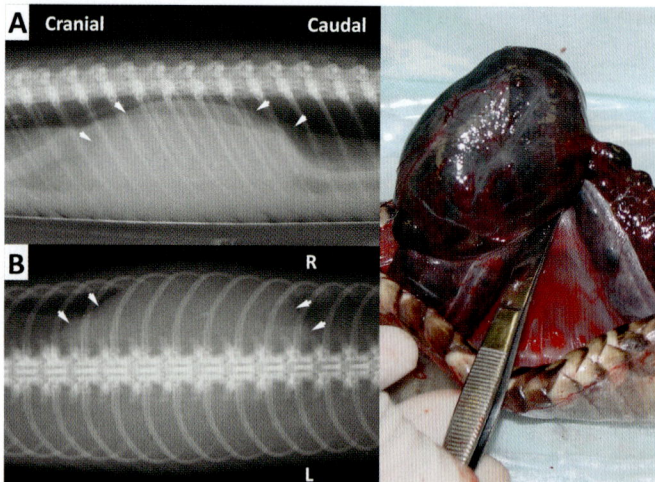

FIG 55.14 Right lateral (A) and dorsoventral (B) radiographs of a king snake (*Lampropeltis getula*) centered at 45% snout-to-vent length. (C) Surgical exploration confirmed a large hepatic mass, as well as numerous smaller nodules throughout the liver. (Courtesy of Stephen J. Divers.)

one half of the gastric volume. Room air is then infused into the stomach in an amount equal to the normal gastric volume. Contrast medium equal to one fourth of the gastric volume is infused into the esophagus as the tube is slowly retracted. When the distal tip of the catheter is in the cranial esophagus, an equal volume of air is infused into the esophagus (one-fourth the gastric volume). The catheter is then removed, and radiographs are taken.

If the intestines, especially the colon and cloaca, are the primary region to be evaluated, a retrograde study should be performed. These procedures usually require anesthesia because the intestinal distention stimulates peristalsis. A flexible catheter is introduced into the cloaca and advanced into the distal colon. Contrast medium is administered until resistance is encountered. A potential but infrequently encountered complication of retrograde studies is accidental introduction of the contrast medium into the ureters and subsequently the kidneys. This could represent a problem with barium sulfate if ureteral or renal concretions develop, especially in dehydrated patients.

Although contrast radiographic studies are helpful for documentation of mucosal disease, ultrasonography can also be useful in the diagnosis of gastrointestinal tract disease, especially if mural thickness is abnormal and the intestines are not filled with gas or fecal material. Endoscopic evaluation of the gastrointestinal tract may be superior in the diagnosis of mucosal disease, providing direct visualization and biopsy capability of the affected area (see Chapters 58 and 64).

LIVER

The liver in snakes is an elongated, poorly lobed organ that usually varies in color from pale tan to black depending on species and other external factors. It is the largest organ of most snakes, comprising of 3% to 4% of body weight, which can fluctuate by season, nutritional status, and reproductive activity.[43] It is located approximately 30% to 60% SVL and may be superimposed upon the heart cranially and stomach caudally (Figs. 55.2 and 55.3). Hepatomegaly, microhepatica, and discrete liver masses can have a variety of etiologies and are often difficult to differentiate from the gastrointestinal tract without contrast or ultrasonography (Fig. 55.14).[44–46] Nevertheless, the hepatic silhouette is often appreciable using horizontal beam techniques (see Chapter 67 for a more in-depth discussion of hepatic disease in snakes).

REPRODUCTIVE SYSTEM

Radiography is often helpful for diagnosing reproductive issues of snakes, especially if shelled eggs or developed embryos are present.[47] The gonads typically lie approximately 60% to 80% SVL (see Fig. 55.2).

In oviparous species (and some viviparous species) late gestation can be appreciated on radiographs with the identification of rounded, soft tissue opacity structures in the caudal coelom that are arranged in a linear overlapping pattern resembling a clumped string of pearls (Fig. 55.15A). They are bilateral in location. The ova can be well visualized and may have poorly mineralized calcified shells.[48] As the eggs develop, they enlarge and fill the caudal coelom, compressing the intestines. Radiographic evaluation for the presence, morphology, calcification, and abnormalities of eggs can be useful, especially in combination with ultrasonography.[47,48] Retained eggs can appear more radiopaque due to increased calcification. In viviparous species, fetal skeletons become visible as they mineralize late in gestation (see Fig. 55.15B). Common indications for evaluating the reproductive system include dystocia, apparent infertility, and reduced fecundity. It is important to note that it is usually not possible to diagnose dystocia with radiography alone. A detailed history, clinical signs, and other diagnostic techniques including ultrasonography are often necessary.[48–50]

The hemipenes of some species may appear mineralized and can be detected on radiographs. Contrast has also been used to radiographically highlight the hemipenes of snakes for gender identification.[51] A discrete soft tissue swelling at the level of the cloaca may also indicate cloacitis, abscessation, or fat deposition.

Neoplasia of the reproductive tract is common in snakes, with various tumors observed affecting the ovary, oviduct, and testes.[48] Clinical signs may include infertility, coelomic swelling, cloacal bleeding, and extramural intestinal obstruction. Caudal coelomic radiographs and contrast gastrointestinal studies (oral or per cloaca) are often useful in demonstrating soft tissue mass effects outside of the intestinal tract (Fig. 55.16). Ultrasonography is often preferred for reproductive evaluation and should be used along with radiography (see Chapter 58).[1]

URINARY SYSTEM

The kidneys of snakes are located dorsal to the intestinal tract in close association with the intracoelomic fat bodies, in the caudal coelom approximately 75% to 95% SVL (see Fig. 55.2). They are not always radiographically evident, unless enlarged or mineralized (Fig. 55.17). Disease processes that can cause renomegaly include renal gout infection, and neoplasia (also see Chapter 66). Secondary signs of renomegaly

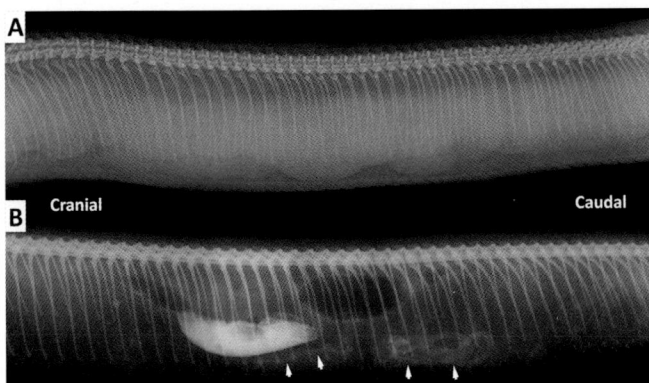

FIG 55.15 (A) Right lateral radiograph of the caudal coelom (65%–80% snout-to-vent length) of an adult female boa constrictor (*Boa constrictor*). The numerous, coalescing, soft tissue masses are consistent with ova, although it can be challenging to differentiate ovarian follicles from ovulated eggs as shells are poorly mineralized in oviparous snakes; in viviparous species, such as this boa constrictor (*Boa constrictor*), fetus development may not yet be evident. (B) Right lateral radiograph of the caudal coelom (70%–90% snout-to-vent length) of a Kenyan sand boa (*Eryx colubrinus*) demonstrating two retained fetuses (arrows). Barium can also be seen within the large intestine. (Courtesy of Stephen J. Divers.)

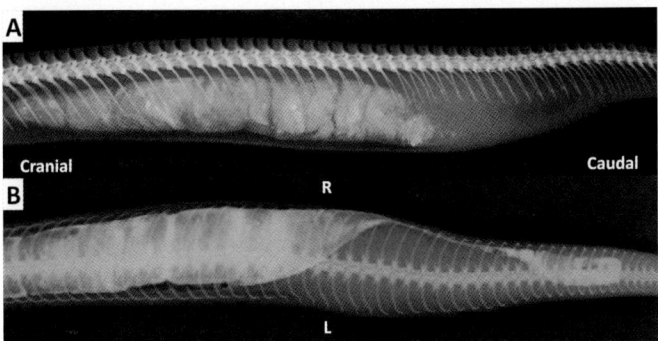

FIG 55.16 (A) Right lateral radiograph (65%–100% snout-to-vent length) of an adult female corn snake (*Pantherophis guttatus*) that presented with constipation. Note the indistinct increase in soft tissue density caudal to the fecal accumulation. (B) Dorsoventral radiograph of the same area after a barium enema. Note that the distal colon has been displaced and compressed by an extraluminal mass effect. Surgical removal was curative, and histopathology confirmed a granulosa cell tumor. (Courtesy of Stephen J. Divers.)

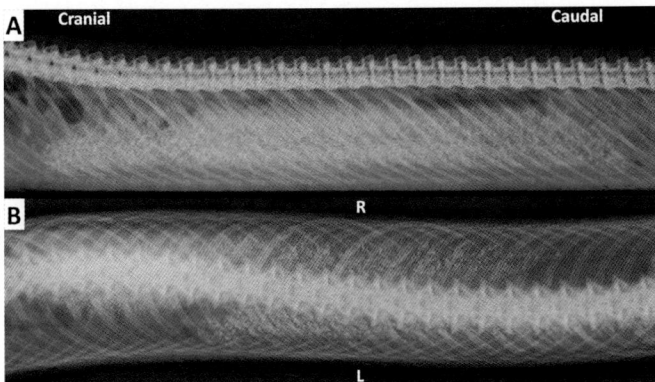

FIG 55.17 Dorsoventral (A) and right lateral (B) radiographs of a hyperuricemic boa constrictor (*Boa constrictor*) at 70% to 90% snout-to-vent. Note the radial, star-burst mineral pattern associated with the left and right kidneys. Although uric acid is radiolucent, chronic renal gout and mineral complexes resulted in increased radiopacity. (Courtesy of Stephen J. Divers.)

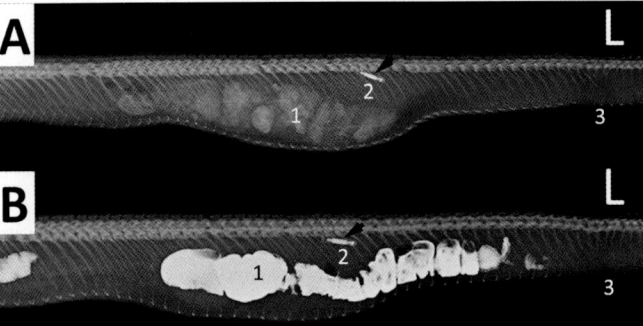

FIG 55.18 Vertical beam left lateral radiographs of a California king snake (*Lampropeltis getula californiae*, 70%–100% snout-to-vent). Noncontrast (A) and gastrointestinal barium contrast (B) radiographs demonstrating constipation (1) cranial to a dorsal coelomic soft tissue mass effect (2). The position of the vent (3) has been indicated and a microchip is also visible (arrow). The mass was identified as a renal mass on exploratory surgery and, after surgical removal, was confirmed as a tubuloepithelial tumor. (Courtesy of Rodney W. Schnellbacher, Dickerson Park Zoo.)

may be constipation or dystocia due to extramural compression. Contrast gastrointestinal studies might be useful in demonstrating renal involvement and location of mass effects (Fig. 55.18). Ultrasonography and advanced diagnostic imaging such as CT and MRI may be needed to further investigate and localize renal lesions.

MUSCULOSKELETAL SYSTEM

Musculoskeletal or, more specifically in snakes, spinal disease is a common indication for radiographic examination. Traumatic fractures, spondylitis/spondylosis, osteomyelitis, neoplasia, and congenital abnormalities are potential issues. Musculoskeletal deformities caused by nutritional secondary hyperparathyroidism have not been reported in snakes fed whole vertebrate prey. Exceptions may be found among insectivorous snakes (e.g., rough green snake, *Opheodrys aestivus*) fed unsupplemented invertebrates. In humans, an estimated 30% decrease in bone mass density is necessary before changes in radiographic bone opacity are recognized.[52] This has not been substantiated in reptiles, but it does emphasize the magnitude of disease necessary to produce radiographic changes. Evaluation of bone radiopacity in snakes is based on rib radiopacity as a reference point.

Traumatic skeletal fractures are common and are usually assessed by plain radiography. Fracture stability usually occurs before radiographic healing is evident due to a mixture of fibrous tissue and osseous callus during the bone healing process.[1,53] Displaced rib fractures with no sign of radiopaque calluses are common but are usually incidental findings. The edges of the fracture fragments may be rounded, and distortion of the fracture end is another sign of chronicity. Variable distortion, proliferation, and osteolysis can also be features of osteomyelitis.

Proliferative spinal osteopathy has been described in snakes and is characterized by proliferative segmented spondylosis, with adjacent vertebrae fused dorsally, ventrally, or laterally by foci of irregular proliferative bone. It is a radiographic description, not a definitive disease diagnosis. Bacterial osteomyelitis has been confirmed in a number of cases, but other possible etiologies include trauma, viral infections, dietary deficiencies, prolonged inactivity, and neoplasia (Fig. 55.19).[54] The radiographic appearance of osteomyelitis can be variable and include osteolysis, proliferative changes, and a loss of normal corticomedullary distinction.[54–56] These changes are not dissimilar to those seen in cases of bone neoplasia or osteitis deformans.[1,57-59] Therefore radiographic changes should not be considered pathognomonic for any of these particular bone diseases. Ultimately biopsy is required, but, in cases of suspected spinal osteomyelitis, blood culture may be more practical (see Chapter 81 for more information). Advanced imaging, such as CT and MRI, which can create three-dimensional reconstructions, can be especially helpful for further evaluation of complex fractures, as well as the extent of osteomyelitis and neoplasia, especially in the skull (see Chapters 59 and 60).

Soft or hard tissue swellings of the face and oral cavity are common indications for skull radiography. Radiographic examination is also performed in cases of suspected fractures, osteomyelitis, inflammation, or neoplasia. A variety of tumors have been identified in the oral cavity in snakes, including squamous cell carcinoma, fibroma, melanoma, and ameloblastoma (Fig. 55.20)[60-63] Radiographs can be useful in determining whether oral lesions in snakes have underlying bony involvement.

The serpentine skull is complex with the fixed regions comprised of the snout and neurocranium. The palatomaxillary apparatus (homologous to the maxilla), along with the supratemporal, quadrate, articular, suprangular, dentary, coronoid, and splenial bones, are mobile (Fig. 55.21). The two sides of the mandible are divided and lack a mandibular symphysis. Snakes have the most teeth of any reptile. The teeth are generally located on the mandibles and the maxillae, palatines, pterygoids, and premaxillae of the upper jaw. Venomous snakes also have fangs.[23] Obtaining symmetrical radiographs of the head of snakes can be difficult due to the flexible joints between the supratemporal, quadrate bones and the mandible. Therefore symmetry is best evaluated by centering the radiographic beam over the snout and neurocranim due to their fixed position.[64] Chemical restraint is typically required to obtain straight, orthogonal views. Lateral and dorsoventral should be standardized diagnostic views; however, oblique radiographs may be necessary to highlight areas of concern. For smaller snakes, digital dental radiographic systems may be necessary to obtain sufficient detail.

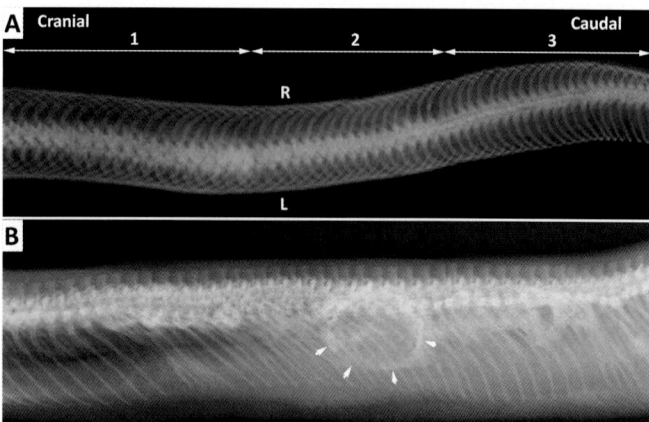

FIG 55.19 Dorsoventral radiograph of a boa constrictor (*Boa constrictor*) at 40% to 60% snout-to-vent length demonstrating moderate (1) and mild (2) spinal osteopathy, with normal spine (3) for comparison. (Courtesy of Stephen Divers, UGA.) (B) Right lateral radiograph of another boa constrictor (50%–70% snout-to-vent length) demonstrating more profound proliferative and osteolytic changes of the spine, with an aggressive expansile lesion also evident (*arrows*). These lesions are typically associated with chronic bacterial osteomyelitis. (Courtesy of Nancy Harrington, All Pets Animal Hospital.)

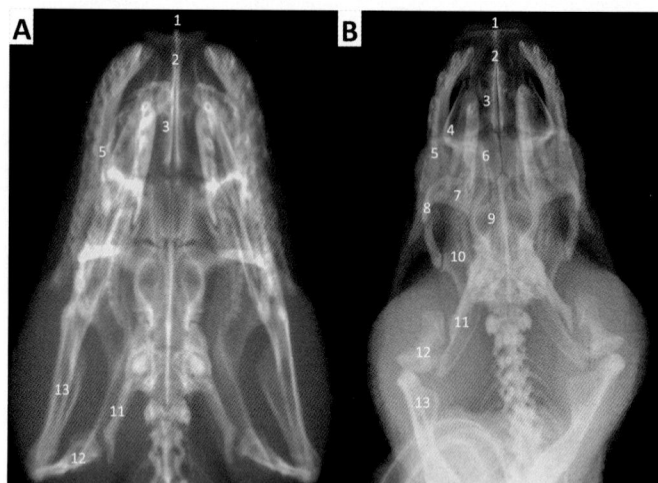

FIG 55.21 Whole skull dorsoventral radiograph (A) and open-mouth ventrodorsal view of just the maxilla (B) of a healthy boa constrictor (*Boa constrictor*) illustrating the major bones: (1) premaxillary, (2) vomer, (3) nasal, (4) prefrontal, (5) dentary, (6) frontal, (7) postfrontal, (8) transpalatine, (9) parietal, (10) pterygoid, (11) supratemporal, (12) quadrate, and (13) articular. (Courtesy of Stephen J. Divers.)

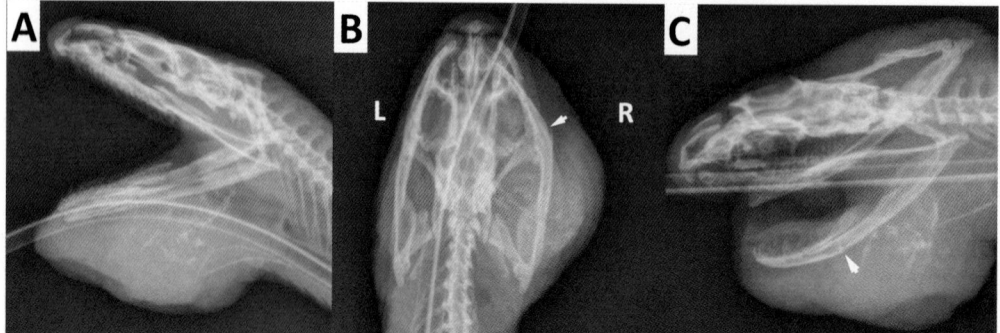

FIG 55.20 A free-ranging eastern black rat snake (*Pantherophis alleghaniensis*) presented with a 3-cm in diameter solid mandibular mass that was partially ulcerated. Lateral (A), dorsoventral (B), and oblique (C) radiographs demonstrated an ill-defined, lobular mass with amorphous intralesional mineral arising from the soft tissues and irregular margins with partial osteolysis and mild periosteal reaction of the adjacent mandible (arrow). Histopathology confirmed ameloblastoma. (Courtesy of Stephen J. Divers.)

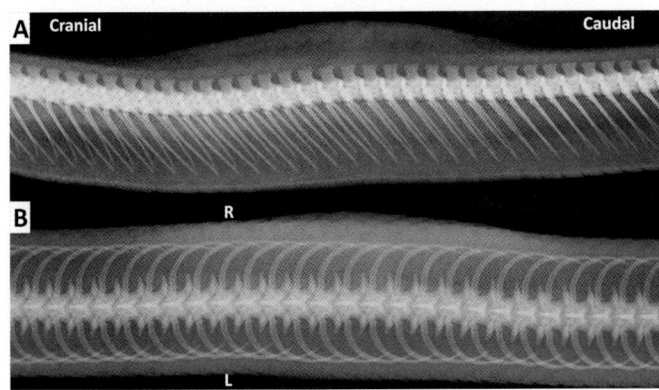

FIG 55.22 Right lateral (A) and dorsoventral (B) radiographs of a black rat snake *(Elaphe obsoleta)* at 50% to 70% snout-to-vent length. A diffuse, fat density can be appreciated dorsal to the spine and right of the midline. Surgical removal and histopathology revealed an infiltrative lipoma. (Courtesy of Stephen J. Divers.)

MISCELLANEOUS

The presence of any physical abnormality can be an indication for radiography. Abscesses, which can either be extracoelomic or intracoelomic and associated with a specific organ or the coelomic wall, are common findings in snakes. Steatitis (inflammation of fat) may be visualized radiographically as an increase in both size and density of the fat bodies. Cutaneous and subcutaneous tumors including lipomas and soft tissue sarcomas have also been reported and may be identified radiographically (Fig. 55.22).[65,66]

REFERENCES

See www.expertconsult.com for a complete list of references.

56

Radiography—Chelonians

Shannon P. Holmes and Stephen J. Divers

The hard shell typical for most chelonians will limit the clinician's ability to examine the coelom even more so than other reptilian species. Therefore radiography may be one of the only noninvasive mechanisms for clinicians to "look below the shell." Radiology units and the clinicians' comfort using them is more ubiquitous than other imaging modalities. Ultrasound equipment is also common in practice, but the shell limits these examinations to specific areas that can be visualized from the openings for the appendages. In practice, computed tomography is also becoming more popular, although the added expense may not be acceptable to some clients.

RESTRAINT AND POSITIONING

Acquisition of radiographs is generally easier to perform in chelonians, because the shell aids in patient restraint and positioning. The shell (and visceral structures within) can be positioned and remain motionless in conscious patients for the majority of radiographic exposures. The patient may retract the head and limbs into the carapace, which is suboptimal for image evaluation due to superimposition. We have found elevation of the chelonian by placement of the plastron on an appropriately narrow lucent structure, referred to as a central plastron stand, will encourage the head and limbs to extend and hang ventrally, even in conscious animals (Fig. 56.1). This does not hamper lateral image acquisition but can degrade acquisition if used for the dorsoventral radiograph. Securing the patient

to the table or using lucent positioning devices are also helpful.[1-3] If the area of interest is the head or limbs, general anesthesia will be needed to obtain diagnostic images. Manual restraint with adhesive tape around the limb for retraction during radiography has also be described in loggerhead sea turtles; this technique may be feasible given the patient size.[4] However, sedation or general anesthesia may also be elected if multiple procedures are to be performed, and at least one of those procedures requires anesthesia. Generally, similar to other reptiles, radiography of chelonians is easier and more efficient with anesthesia.[2] Therefore, developing a plan for the radiographic examination is an important first step before entering the radiography suite.

In order to obtain high-quality radiographs of chelonians, they must be positioned as close to the cassette or detector as possible. The carapace edge of chelonians is rounded so when the lateral edge is adjacent to the detector, there are internal structures that are more distant. This increased object-film distance detracts from radiographic detail in the lateral and craniocaudal images. Structures further away will be magnified or blurred, which is a greater issue for larger chelonians. Therefore obtaining right and left lateral images is helpful, especially for larger animals.[1]

Following radiographic standards, orthogonal radiographs should be obtained for all chelonian body systems (see Table 53.1). The shape of the shell and internal anatomy necessitates a horizontal radiographic beam for both lateral and/or cranial caudal images (Fig. 56.2), in addition to the dorsoventral vertical beam images (Fig. 56.3). For all radiographs,

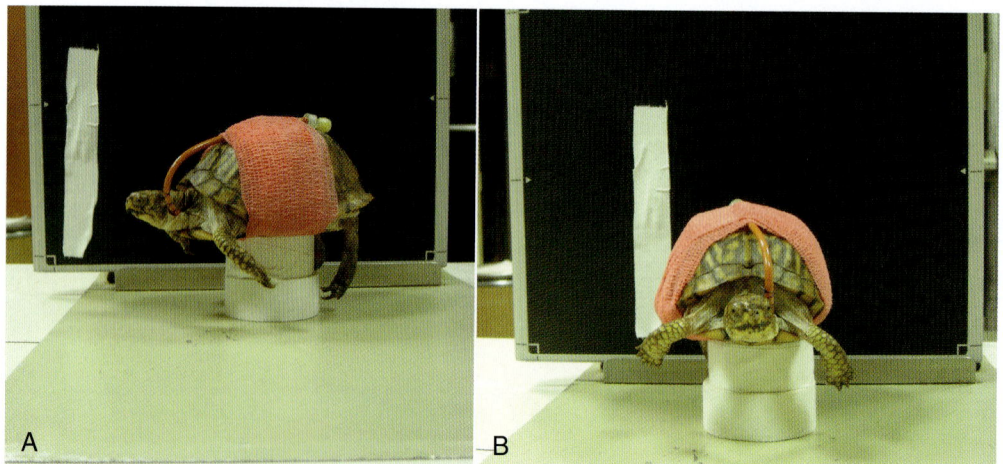

FIG 56.1 Suspended positioning of an eastern box turtle (*Terrapene c. carolina*) to facilitate extension of the limbs and head out of the shell. The additional advantage of this technique is the head and limbs can be better evaluated because they are not superimposed. Orthogonal horizontal beam lateral (A) and craniocaudal (B) radiographs of the carapace will effectively produce lateral and craniocaudal images of the limbs with this positioning technique and patient cooperation by extending limbs ventrally. (Courtesy of Shannon P. Holmes.)

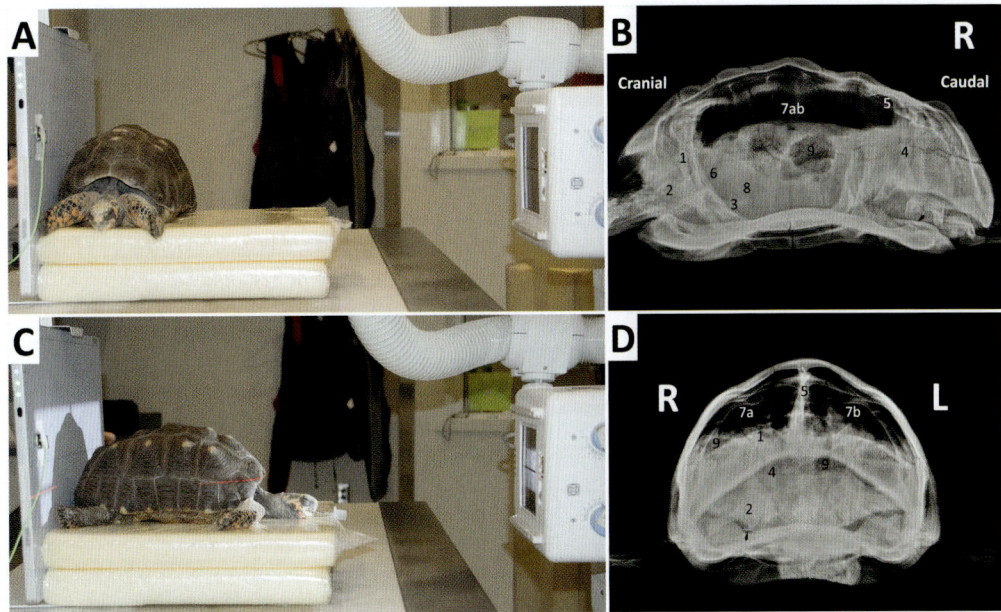

FIG 56.2 Positioning and corresponding horizontal beam right lateral (A and B) and craniocaudal radiographs (C and D) of an adult red-footed tortoise (*Chelonoidis carbonaria*), demonstrating the scapulae (1), humeri (2), coracoids (3), ilia (4), spine (5), trachea (6), right lung (7a), left lung (7b), cardiohepatic silhouette (8), gastrointestinal tract (9), and microchip (arrow). Note the poor serosal detail throughout the ventral coelom; however, these radiographs are most useful for evaluation of the lungs. (Courtesy of Stephen J. Divers.)

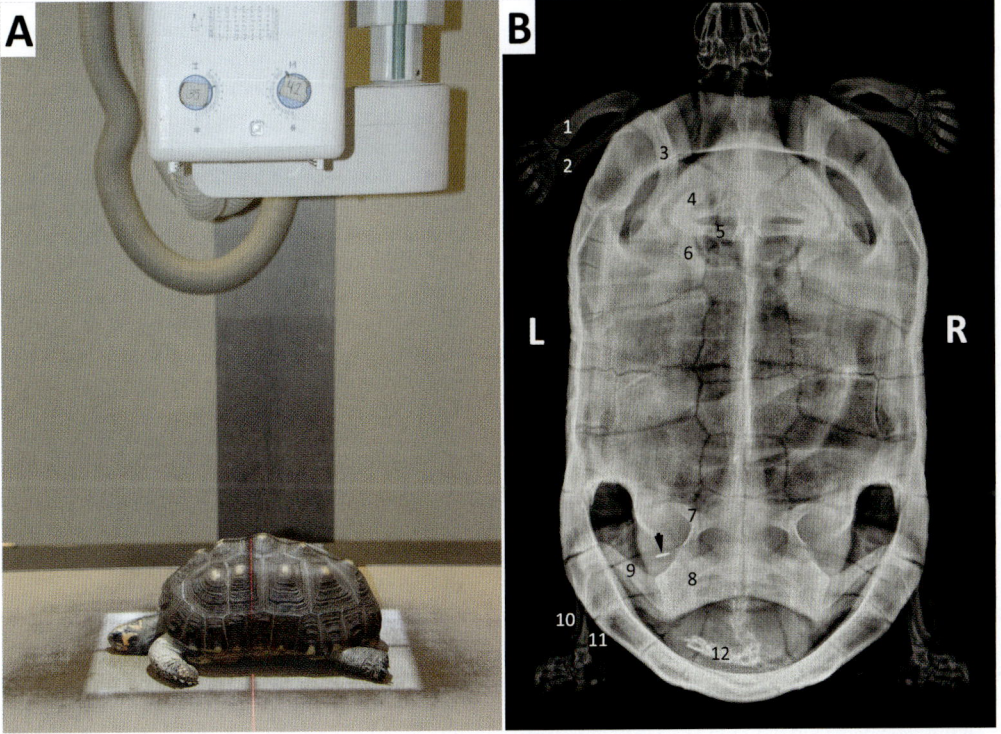

FIG 56.3 Positioning (A) and dorsoventral radiograph (B) of an adult red-footed tortoise (*Chelonoidis carbonaria*) demonstrating the major skeletal structures, including left radius (1), ulna (2), humerus (3), acromion process (4) of the scapula (5), coracoid (6), ilium (7), pubis (8), femur (9), tibia (10), fibula (11), and caudal vertebrae of the tail (12). Note the poor serosal detail throughout the coelom, gas within the gastrointestinal tract that is superimposed on the lungs, and the microchip (*arrow*). (Courtesy of Stephen J. Divers.)

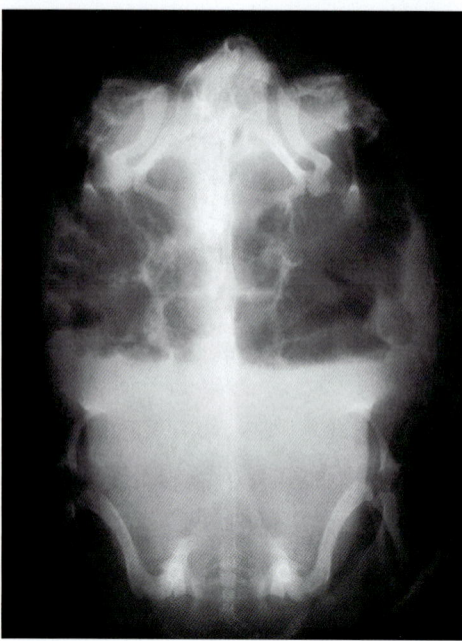

FIG 56.4 Cooter (*Pseudemys* sp.). Coelomic fluid is present from coelomitis and pneumonia. The ventrodorsal radiograph was made with the patient in the erect position with a horizontally directed radiograph beam. The straight gas–fluid interface level is helpful to evaluate the volume of coelomic fluid.

it is easiest, and least stressful to the patient, to position them in sternal recumbency or the prone position.[1,2] As outlined in Table 53.1, the anatomy of an organ system of primary interest, suspected pathological change, presence of coelomic fluid, degree of digestive tract distention, and the contents of the female reproductive tract determines the radiographic images needed. For example, evaluation of the chelonian lungs requires horizontal beam images of both craniocaudal and lateral radiographs. The dorsoventral radiograph does not provide the best evaluation of the lung due to the superimposed digestive tract anatomy. However, it does facilitate evaluation of the craniocaudal length of the right and left lungs individually. The craniocaudal horizontal beam also allows for comparison of the right and left lungs, but the cranial right lung is summated with the caudal right lung tissue. Finally, the right and left lungs are superimposed on the lateral horizontal beam image, such that a lateralized soft-tissue pulmonary focus cannot be localized without an orthogonal image. Determination of the needed radiographic images and radiograph beam orientation is dictated by the goal of minimizing superimposition of nonessential anatomy over the area of interest and to effectively recreate three-dimensional anatomy using two-dimensional radiographs. It is sometimes possible to move or redistribute obscuring structures through changing the patient's position from the standard. An example is the redistribution of coelomic fluid via erect positioning (i.e., as if the chelonian were vertical and resting on the tail and caudal shell) and horizontal beam orientation (Fig. 56.4). The fluid will become gravity dependent, and there will be less superimposition in the cranial coelom, resulting in improved aeration and visibility of the pulmonary parenchyma craniad. These can also be useful for estimation of the volume of coelomic fluid.[1]

One other technical consideration when planning chelonian radiographs is the effect of the shell. A prescribed radiographic technique developed for mammals assumes a soft-tissue body wall and adjusts the technique (i.e., kVp and mAs) according to patient thickness. The shell, and the density of the tissue of which it is composed, will cause greater attenuation of the x-ray beam relative to a mammalian patient of similar thickness. Therefore initially increasing mAs to account for the shell would be beneficial; this will increase the number of x-rays penetrating the shell.

CARDIOVASCULAR SYSTEM

Radiography is not commonly used as a diagnostic tool to evaluate chelonians for heart disease. The heart is poorly visualized due to indistinct borders. It rests on the plastron in the cranial third of the coelom.[2] The location of the heart can be identified as the soft-tissue opaque structure ventral to the tracheal termination.[1] In the loggerhead sea turtle (*Caretta caretta*), the triangle formed by the scapula and coracoid bones was determined to be an extracoelomic landmark.[5] Evaluation of cardiac size, chamber volume, and contractility are best performed with echocardiography.

RESPIRATORY SYSTEM

Evaluation of the respiratory system, especially the lungs, by radiography is a common application. The chelonian lung is an arborized structure characterized by small airways terminating in spongy (edicular) air spaces.[6] Another unique feature is the adherence of the dorsal lung to the carapace parietal serosa.[1,6] As a result, the lungs should never become ventrally displaced or collapsed ventrally. This also means that dorsal carapace trauma will often be complicated by pulmonary involvement. The shell, in addition to the digestive tract or other coelomic content such as coelomic fluid or eggs, will limit the expansibility of the lungs.[1] Muscular fibrous bands are interspersed throughout the parenchyma; these are typically not distinctly seen but contribute to the soft-tissue opacity of normal chelonian lung. The pulmonary vasculature should be visible in normal chelonian lungs, and loss of visibility can be used to confer pulmonary pathological change. Collateral pulmonary vasculature may also be identified.[5]

There are three standard radiographs needed to evaluate the lungs; the craniocaudal horizontal beam, lateral horizontal beam, and dorsoventral views. Some radiographic units are not capable of orienting the x-ray beam horizontally. In this instance it is important to be aware of the changes that result with laterally recumbent lateral radiographs. The lungs are most affected by coelomic organs moving dependently to cause pulmonary compression (Fig. 56.5). It is less intuitive that the head and limb position are important considerations in pulmonary interpretation, but retraction of the appendages will further reduce coelomic volume and increase lung compression. Therefore limb extension is important, and optimal lung inflation is crucial for accurate pulmonary interpretation.[2] Positive pressure ventilation can be used to inflate the lungs, and due to the unique chelonian anatomy, there is less risk of misinterpreting overinflation as absence of disease compared with snakes and lizards.

A wide variety of diseases can affect the respiratory system, including infection (viral, bacterial, fungal, or parasitical), trauma, or neoplasia.[6] Virtually all pulmonary pathological changes in chelonians will result in some degree of increased pulmonary soft-tissue opacity. With the exception of cold-stunned Kemp's ridley sea turtles (*Lepidochelys kempii*), distribution and pattern of pulmonary infiltrates have not been reported with disease/condition specificity as they have with mammals. The aforementioned Kemp's ridley turtles had pulmonary changes, but the most consistent (and normal) finding was a reticular or honeycomb pattern that conformed to the lung trabeculae and ediculae.[7] Changes consistent with disease processes like pneumonia tend to appear as focal, multifocal, or diffuse areas of increased soft-tissue opacification.[1,8] However, it is not possible to reach a definitive pulmonary disease

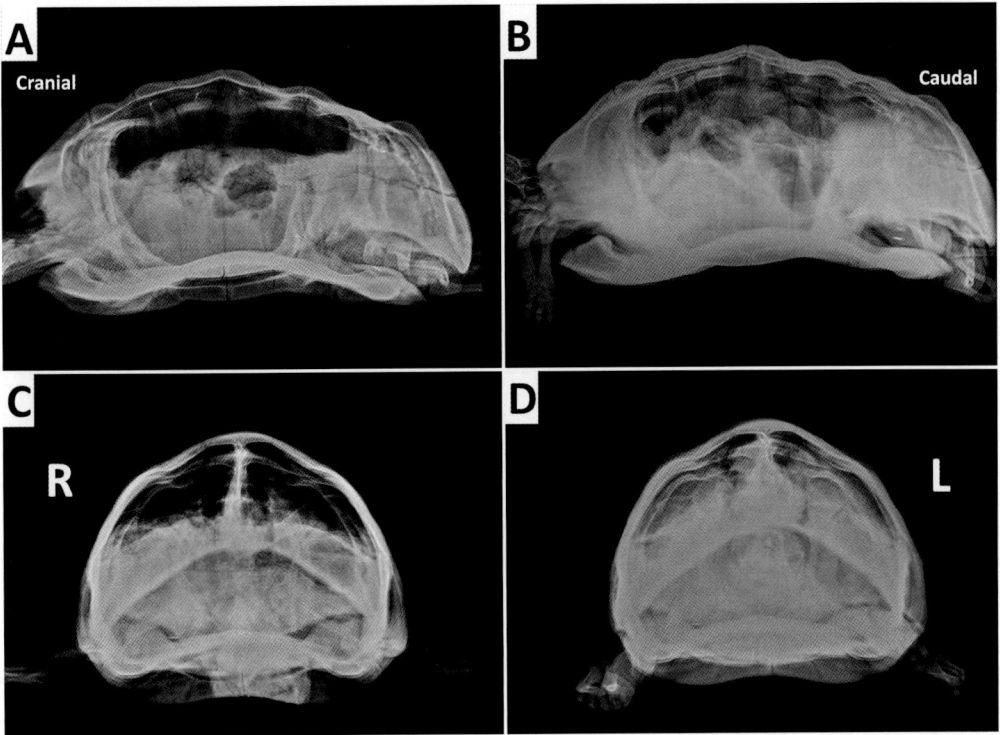

FIG 56.5 Comparison between right lateral (A and B) and craniocaudal (C and D) radiographs using horizontal (A and C) versus vertical (B and D) x-ray beams in an adult tortoise. Note the significant visceral displacement associated with rotating the animal to use a vertical beam, and the subsequent reduction in lung volume (B and D). Consequently, horizontal beam techniques (A and C) are recommended for lateral and craniocaudal radiographs. (Courtesy of Stephen J. Divers.)

diagnosis with radiography alone; clinical correlation and sampling for cytology/histopathology and microbiology are crucial for planning further diagnostics and devising appropriate treatment strategy.[2]

Infectious pneumonopathies are the most frequently encountered in clinical practice. A common feature with pulmonary infection is focal or multifocal ill-defined areas of pulmonary consolidation (Fig. 56.6). The localization of abnormal pulmonary soft tissue is best seen on the horizontal beam images. To accurately estimate the extent of lung involvement, all three radiographic projections are important. A differential diagnosis for a diffuse or multifocal soft-tissue pulmonary pattern could be fibrosis.[2] Solitary or more discrete soft-tissue lesions can also be seen. In this instance the differential diagnosis would include focal/consolidated pneumonia, granuloma, abscess formation, or neoplasia. The distinct margination of these lesions is an important identifier for a pulmonary location and is created by the gas–soft tissue interface. Apart from gas-distended segments of intestine, this would not be seen with other coelomic masses protruding dorsally. The ventral margin of these lesions may not be discrete. These are often better visualized on the dorsoventral image than on the horizontal beam; it is likely the soft tissue–gas interface is more tangential to the x-ray beam, which increases margin conspicuity (Fig. 56.7). Radiographs represent an important diagnostic assessment in monitoring response to therapy for pulmonary disease (Fig. 56.8). The initial radiographs form the baseline for comparison. Direct comparison and accurate interpretation are more reliable if all imaging parameters are kept constant through serial studies, such as the radiographic technique prescribed (mAs and kVp), patient positioning, and conscious free breathing versus anesthetized and ventilated. Computed tomographic (CT) studies are the optimal diagnostic technique for respiratory tract evaluation of reptiles (see Chapter 59). This is especially true for solitary lesions, because these can have distinguishing features in contrast-enhanced CT examinations.

GASTROINTESTINAL SYSTEM

Radiographic evaluation for digestive disease investigations are common in clinical practice. It can be a challenging system to evaluate due to the poor serosal detail in the coelom, which can limit the value of survey radiographs.[9] Radiographic evaluation is further complicated because factors such as temperature, nutritional status, time since last meal, and diet must also be considered.[2] In mammalian imaging, fasting is commonly recommended before imaging, but the presence of ingesta in the gastrointestinal tract aids in its identification in chelonian studies. However, the reviewer must decide if the ingesta is normal in appearance, which is why the previously mentioned factors must be considered. The inherent low contrast in chelonians is mostly due to minimal periorgan fat but is exacerbated by the limited space within the shell and greater effacement of coelomic structures.[1] Regardless, survey radiographs remain a first-line diagnostic step in clinical practice. These must be performed and serve as a baseline, even if contrast studies are needed to increase contrast within the digestive tract.

The standard radiographic images acquired for evaluation of the digestive system include dorsoventral vertical beam and lateral horizontal beam images. Radiograph units that are unable to make horizontal beam images will likely result in radiographs that will affect interpretation of the gastrointestinal system and can lead to misinterpretation when organ displacement obscures the mass effect of a

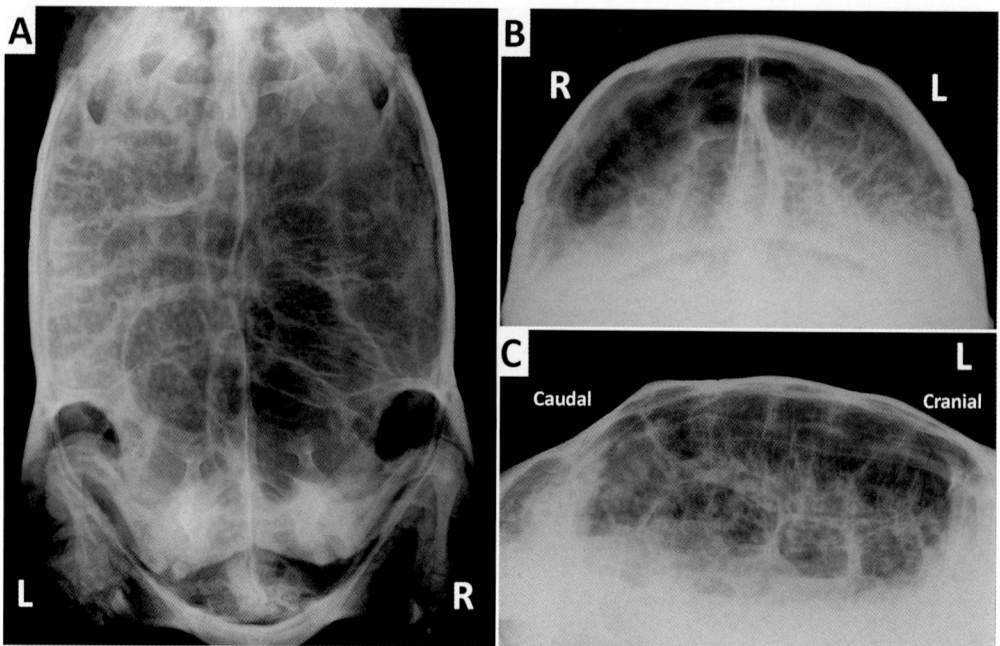

FIG 56.6 Dorsoventral (A), horizontal beam craniocaudal (B), and left lateral (C) radiographs of an adult male box turtle (*Terrepene*) with poorly defined areas of increased soft-tissue opacification of both lungs. The left is more affected, which can be seen on the craniocaudal image, but the extent throughout the left lung is better appreciated on the dorsoventral radiograph, even with the other coelomic structures superimposed. There are no obvious fluid lines. These changes are consistent with pneumonia. (Courtesy of Patrick Leadbeater, Douglas Chang, and Emma Kaiser, Kahala Pet Hospital.)

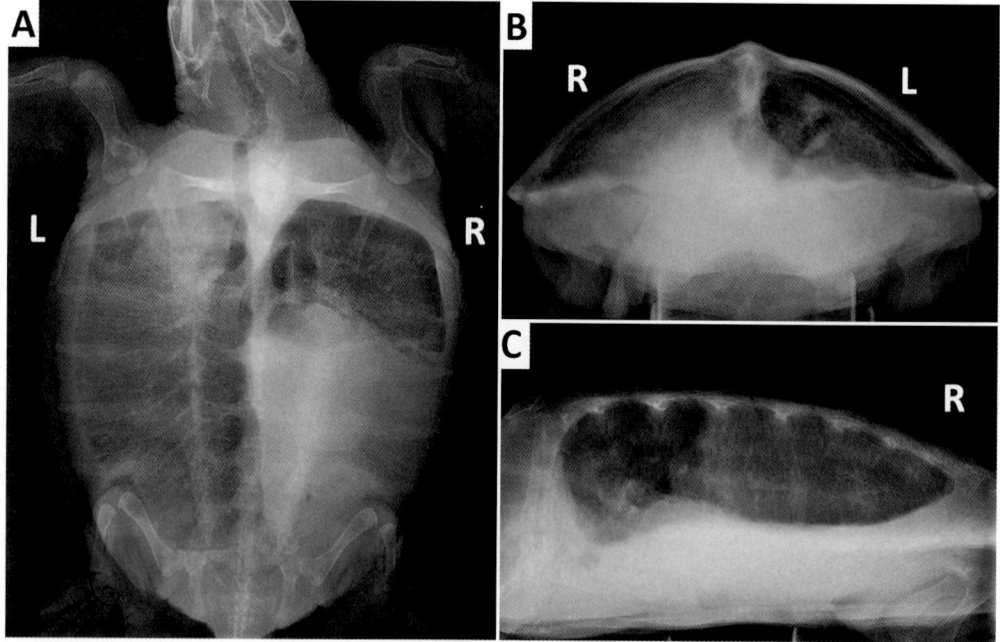

FIG 56.7 Dorsoventral (A), horizontal beam craniocaudal (B), and right lateral (C) radiographs of a juvenile loggerhead sea turtle (*Caretta caretta*). There is a well-defined increase in soft-tissue opacity occupying the mid to caudal right lung. Endoscopic biopsy confirmed a fungal granuloma. (Courtesy of Stephen J. Divers.)

lesion.[10] Generally, the gastrointestinal tract is better visualized on dorsoventral radiographs due to less superimposition. The stomach is located in the left midportion of the coelom on survey radiographs, and the large intestinal luminal contents often have a heterogeneous mixed soft tissue and gas appearance or a more granular look. In our experience the gastrointestinal tract is uncommonly empty in normal chelonians, which is associated with dietary behaviors and the slow transit time. Additionally, in the normal chelonian, minimal gas should be present in the stomach. Increased gastric gas is usually indicative of aerophagia, fermentation, or obstruction. Visualization of the

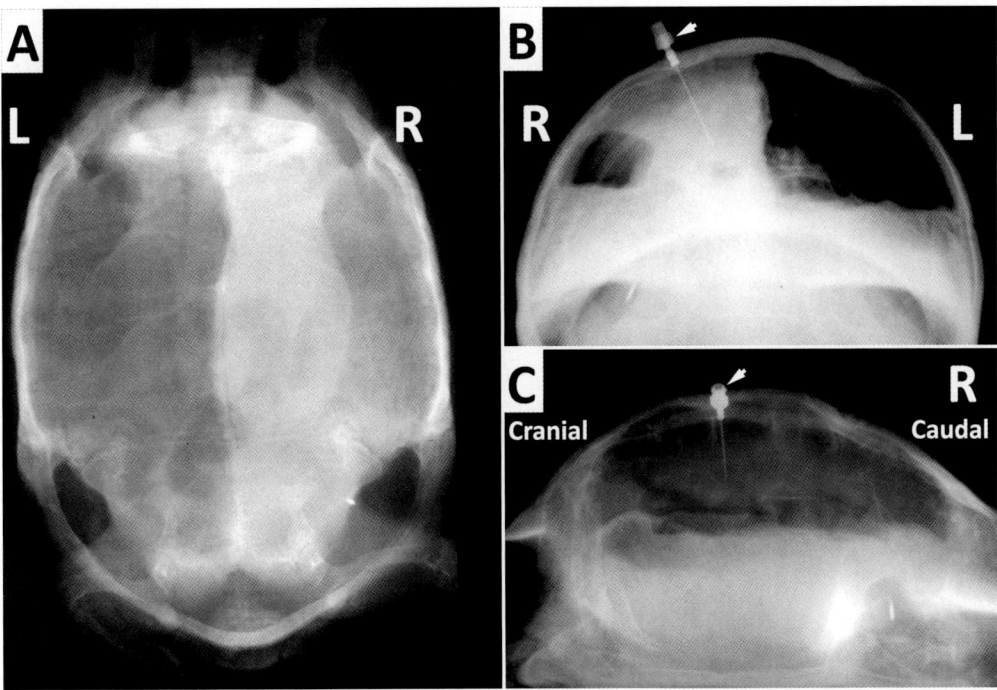

FIG 56.8 Dorsoventral (A), horizontal beam craniocaudal (B), and right lateral (C) radiographs of an adult Greek tortoise (*Testudo graeca*) with mycotic pneumonia. There is an obvious and distinctly marginated solitary soft tissue mass-like focus in the right lung (A and B). It is less opaque on the recheck examination made 4 weeks after the institution of intralesional therapy (C) via an intrapnuemonic catheter (arrows). This increased radiolucency of the right lungs indicates partial resolution. (Courtesy of Stephen J. Divers.)

intestines is more difficult to evaluate than the stomach or lower portions of the digestive tract.

The administration of radiographic contrast agents to delineate the gastrointestinal tract has been investigated and is used frequently in clinical practice. It is necessitated by the low contrast of the coelom. Complete evaluation with ultrasonography is also more difficult (than in squamates) because of the shell. For positive-contrast upper gastrointestinal studies (Fig. 56.9), barium sulfate and iodinated-based contrast are common. Barium sulfate studies have been reported in the red-eared slider (*Trachemys scripta elegans*), leopard tortoise (*Stigmochelys pardalis*), Geoffroy's side-necked turtle (*Phrynops geoffroanus*), yellow-spotted river turtle (*Podocnemis unifilis*), and Arrau river turtle (*Podocnemis expansa*), whereas iodinated contrast studies have been reported in the red-eared slider and Greek tortoise (*Testudo graeca*).[9,11–15] The barium sulfate dose used in the red-eared slider was 30% weight/volume (w/v) and 8 mL/kg at a temperature of 26° to 28°C and in the leopard tortoise was 5 mL/kg at 29°C. For other chelonian studies 70% w/v and a 10 mL/kg dosing rate was administered in mineral oil at a temperature of 26° to 28°C.[13] Di Bello used 60% barium sulfate and iodinated contrast mixed with saline to investigate foreign body obstructions.[14] The addition of food will influence transit time but can be useful for this purpose. For the iodinated contrast studies, Gastrografin (Diatrizoate Meglumine and Diatrizoate Sodium Solution—water-soluble iodinated radiopaque contrast medium for oral or rectal administration) has been used consistently. This contrast is rarely stocked in most veterinary practices in comparison to other iodinated contrast agents such as Iohexol (Nycomed Inc, Princeton, NJ). However, because these papers established transit times, it is important to strictly follow the technique outlined for each species.[16] The transit times were long for barium sulfate, ranging between 72 to 192 hours in the red-eared slider, 144 to 166 hrs in the leopard tortoise, 72 to 156 hours in Geoffroy's

side-necked turtle, 365 to 480 hours in the yellow-spotted river turtle, and 360 to 696 hours in the Arrau river turtle. For Gastrografin, the red-eared slider transit time was 48 to 192 hours versus 1.5 to 24 hrs for the Greek tortoise. The effect of temperature was nicely demonstrated in the Greek tortoise study, with faster times in patients maintained between 27° to 34°C. The contrast agent comparison study performed in the red-eared slider also demonstrated the differences in these contrast agents. In addition to faster transit with iodinated contrast agents, there is also poorer mucosal coating and dissipation of the contrast as it transits the gastrointestinal tract.

Contrast studies should be considered as an adjunct to survey radiographs that are inconclusive. It is also important to ensure proper administration of contrast into the alimentary system, because respiratory administration can be fatal. Ensuring successful passage beyond the upper esophageal sphincter and gastroesophageal sphincter is critical. Gastric gavage is used and fluoroscopic guidance is valuable in ensuring correct placement, along with placement of other therapeutic devices (Fig. 56.10).[14] In addition to upper gastrointestinal studies, the double contrast and cloacograms discussed in the taxa-specific chapters can also be performed.

With respect to clinical diagnosis of digestive disease, foreign body ingestion and/or obstruction is among the most common applications (fig. 56.11A–C). Examination of the esophageal area is important in free-ranging chelonians, because fish hooks are one of the more common foreign objects ingested.[17] Identification of an obstructive pattern consisting of orad distention of the gastrointestinal system is made more challenging because the gastrointestinal tract is shorter in length, especially in carnivorous species. Determination of distention due to obstruction versus generalized ileus is important, because surgical intervention is likely needed in the former and not in the latter. Generalized distention, referred to as ileus, can be due to progressive accumulation of ingesta in chelonians (see fig. 56.11D) or due to abnormal motility

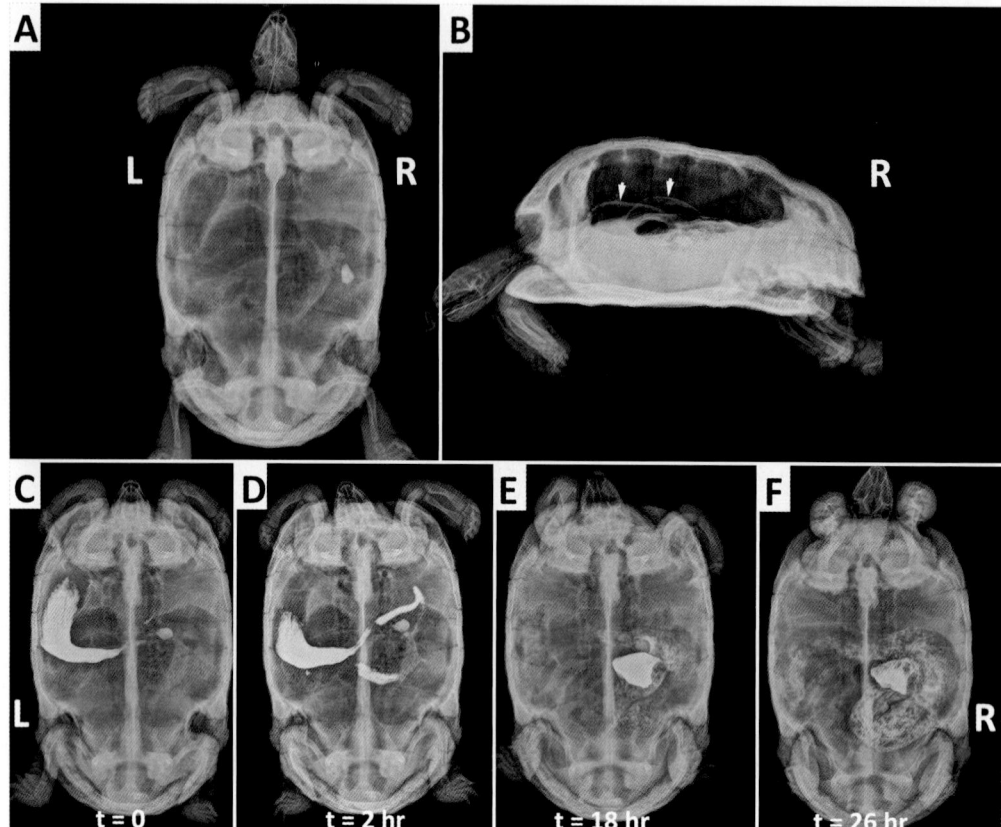

FIG 56.9 Dorsoventral (A) and horizontal beam right lateral (B) radiographs of a red-footed tortoise (*Chelonoidis carbonaria*) with gaseous distension of the gastrointestinal tract but without obvious obstruction. Note the gas-filled intestine impinging dorsally into the lung fields (arrows). Dorsoventral radiographs of the same tortoise immediately after the administration of oral barium (C), and 2 hours (D), 18 hours (E), and 26 hours (F) later. Barium progress is unimpeded, and there is no evidence of an obstruction. Gastrointestinal barium studies can take several days or even weeks to complete. (Courtesy of Stephen J. Divers.)

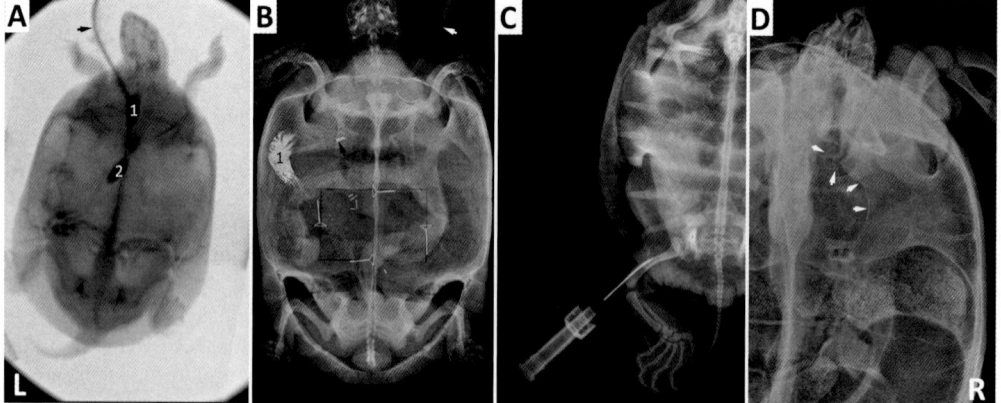

FIG 56.10 (A) Dorsoventral fluoroscopic image of an aquatic slider (*Trachemys*) after the placement of an esophagostomy tube (arrow). The initial test administration of barium (1) indicated that the tube was in the esophagus and was therefore advanced to enter the stomach (2). (B) Dorsoventral radiograph of a tortoise (*Gopherus*) after transplastron surgery and placement of an esophagostomy tube (arrows). Note the test administration of barium entering the stomach, metal vascular clips within the coelom, and the wire suture closure of the replaced section of plastron. (C) Dorsoventral radiograph of a diamondback terrapin (*Malaclemys terrapin*) to confirm placement of an intraosseous catheter into the left femur. (D) Dorsoventral radiograph of the cranial right coelomic quadrant of an aldabra tortoise (*Aldabrachelys gigantea*) to confirm correct placement of a central venous line in the right external jugular. (Courtesy of Stephen J. Divers.)

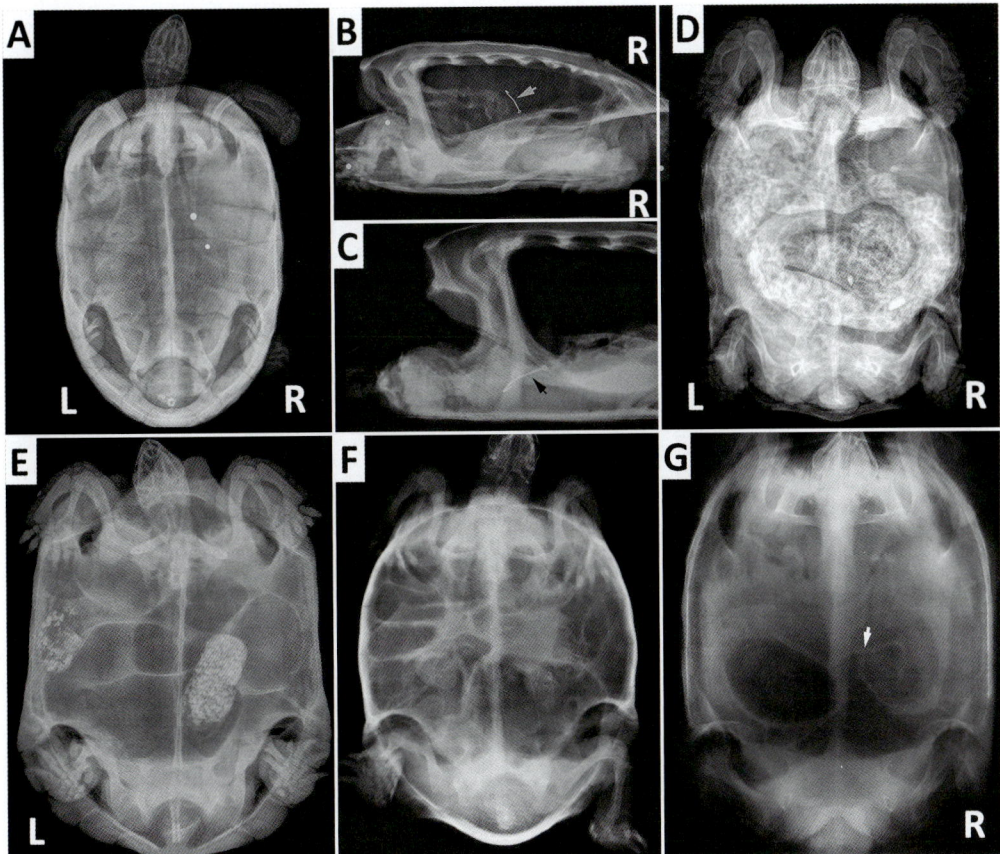

FIG 56.11 (A) Dorsoventral radiograph of a tortoise that ingested two spherical metallic objects. Given their location on the right of the coelom, they are unlikely to be in the stomach. (B and C) Horizontal right lateral radiographs of a free-ranging snapping turtle (*Chelydra serpentina*) that has ingested a fishing hook (*arrows*). The hook is closely associated with the cervical vertebrae, and when the head of the anesthetized turtle is extended (C) the hook moves position, confirming location within the esophagus. (D) Dorsoventral radiograph of an African spurred tortoise (*Centrochelys sulcata*) with severe constipation but without evidence of complete obstruction. (E) Dorsoventral radiograph of a desert tortoise (*Gopherus agassizii*) with a focal area of constipation. The gaseous distension is concerning and can indicate obstruction. (F) Dorsoventral radiograph of a Greek tortoise (*Testudo graeca*) demonstrating severe gas accumulation throughout the gastrointestinal tract. There is no evidence of an obvious obstruction and ileus due to gastroenteritis or generalized ileus is more likely. (G) Dorsoventral radiograph of an African spurred tortoise (*Centrochelys sulcata*) with gaseous distension of the large intestine and a visible stricture aboral (arrow). Surgical exploration revealed an intussusception. (A, Courtesy of S. Shaw, Broadview Animal Hospital; B–G, courtesy of Stephen J. Divers.)

that results in progressive gas distention (see fig. 56.10F). Severe gas distention with obstruction within the more distal portion of the small intestine is the most challenging to distinguish from a generalized pattern. A wide range of conditions are reported in which radiography and/or contrast studies were part of, or pivotal in, the diagnostic process and directed therapeutic intervention; these include foreign body obstructions, lead poisoning, coelomitis due to perforation, hematochezia with constipation, volvulus, and strictures.[18–22] Additionally contrast studies are valuable in detecting a persistent abnormality over serial studies in a manner that is not possible with other imaging modalities.[19]

REPRODUCTIVE SYSTEM

Radiographic examinations of the reproductive tract require dorsal and lateral horizontal beam images, with the dorsal image generally considered most useful. This is commonly performed for reproductive monitoring and conditions such as dystocia. Radiographic examination is limited regarding detection of follicles and ova due to the poor detail in the coelom.[23] Ultrasonography and CT provide a more thorough evaluation of the entire reproductive tract and can be employed as a second line diagnostic, especially if any pathologic change is suspected in the ovaries, salpinx, or testes.[23–25]

Since late-stage eggs have a variably mineralized shell, they are readily identifiable on radiographs in spite of poor coelomic detail (Fig. 56.12).[1,23] It is important to critically evaluate the shape, thickness, continuity, and uniformity of the mineralized egg shell, distribution of eggs within the coelom, uniformity in the size of eggs, and the presence of abnormal soft tissue associated with the egg or the reproductive tract. Before mineralization, follicular enlargement can produce a midcoelomic mass effect and compress the lungs craniodorsally.[23] The radiographic signs of dystocia include enlarged eggs, fractured egg shells, follicular stasis, or normal eggs outside of the reproductive season.[23] Eggs with increased but even shell mineralization and smooth shells are typically associated with prolonged retention within the lower reproductive tract. However, thickened and rough shells are often an indication of uric acid and mineral deposition on the shells of eggs that have been retained within the urinary bladder.

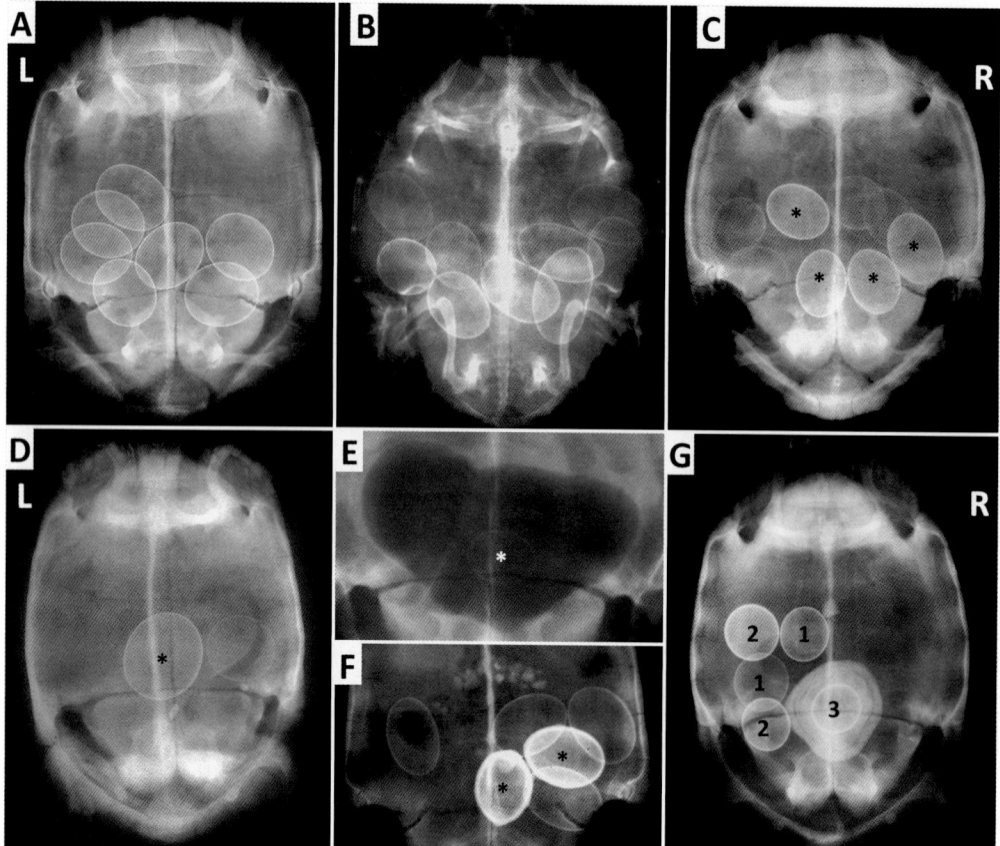

FIG 56.12 (A) Dorsoventral radiograph of a Greek tortoise (*Testudo graeca*) demonstrating normal eggs during the reproductive season. (B) Dorsoventral radiograph of a red-eared slider (*Trachemys scripta elegans*) demonstrating normal eggs during the reproductive season. Note the more elongated appearance of the eggs in this species. (C) Dorsoventral radiograph of a Greek tortoise (*Testudo graeca*) demonstrating normal (thin-shelled) eggs and abnormal eggs (*) with increased, even shell thickness consistent with prolonged retention within the oviduct. (D) Dorsoventral radiograph of a *Testudo* tortoise exhibiting a normal egg (in terms of size and shell thickness) and a significantly larger egg with increased shell thickness (*). Although some species of chelonian naturally produce a few large eggs, this is abnormal in *Testudo*. (E) Dorsoventral radiograph in a tortoise demonstrating a poorly mineralized egg (*) within the bladder by pneumocystography. (F) Dorsoventral radiograph of a Greek tortoise (*Testudo graeca*) demonstrating four normal (thinly shelled) eggs and two abnormal eggs (*). In this case the shells are irregularly thickened, which is commonly associated with eggs retained in the bladder and acting as a nidus for uric acid deposition. (G) Dorsoventral radiograph of a *Testudo* tortoise demonstrating two relatively normal eggs (1), two eggs with increased shell thickness (2), and a third egg (3) that has been retained in the bladder and acted as a nidus for a large calculus. (Courtesy of Stephen J. Divers.)

Abnormal soft tissue accumulation associated with the reproductive tract should produce areas of further reduced coelomic detail, which can be an interpretative challenge. It is important because these soft-tissue changes are sentinel indicators of disease processes such as follicular stasis or yolk coelomitis. For example, follicular stasis can be inferred from radiographic examinations when a soft-tissue-mass effect is persistently seen in the mid coelom.[2]

URINARY SYSTEM

When radiographically evaluating the chelonian urinary bladder, it is important to remember that it is extremely expansive in volume and bilobed in shape. It can extend into the midcranial coelom (Fig. 56.13) and can be in close proximity to the stomach. In a normal state, the urinary bladder is indistinct and difficult to identify, because the soft tissue is effaced by adjacent organs and there is poor coelomic detail.[2] Similar to the remainder of the coelom, the standard examination of

the urinary system consists of dorsoventral and lateral horizontal beam images. Contrast studies can also be used to improve visualization.

Radiographic examinations of the urinary tract are most commonly performed to evaluate for urinary calculi. Urate calculi are the most common in chelonians, and although urate is radiolucent, these calculi are typically visible on radiographs because of their size, density, and deposition of additional mineral complexes over time (Fig. 56.14).[2] The calculi tend to occur with greater frequency in the left lobe of the bladder.[1,26] They have an irregularly lamellated appearance and an irregularly rounded shape. Obstruction of the urinary bladder due to calculi is uncommon, but obstruction at the level of the cloaca can cause ureteral obstruction. Severe urinary bladder distention due to a spinal fracture has been reported; this demonstrates the importance a systematic review of whole body examinations because both of these conditions are clinically significant, but the urinary issues may require more emergent intervention.[10] Contrast cystography (Fig. 56.15) is an option to define the urinary bladder, as well as for detection of other

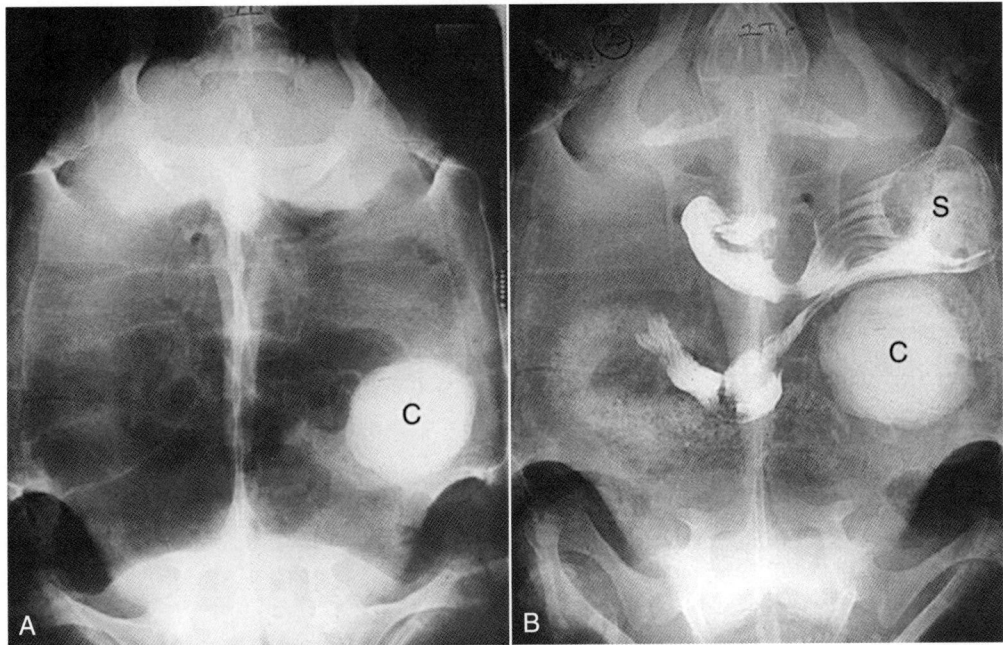

FIG 56.13 Desert tortoise (*Gopherus agassizii*). (A) A large mineral, opaque, rounded structure is seen in the mid right lateral coelom. It is located in a position that should be considered for a urinary calculus based on the degree of expansion that is possible in the chelonian urinary bladder. It is positioned near the caudal contour of the stomach based on the presence of fine amorphous soft tissue that is likely ingesta. The appearance is also suspicious, because calculi in chelonians are typically highly radiopaque, irregularly margin-ated, and can have a lamellar internal architecture. (B) In radiographs made 4 years later, the calculus is slightly larger. Its position adjacent to the stomach is better seen with the positive contrast in the gastric lumen, which was administered to rule out the possibility of a gastrointestinal foreign body. (Courtesy of Sam Silverman.)

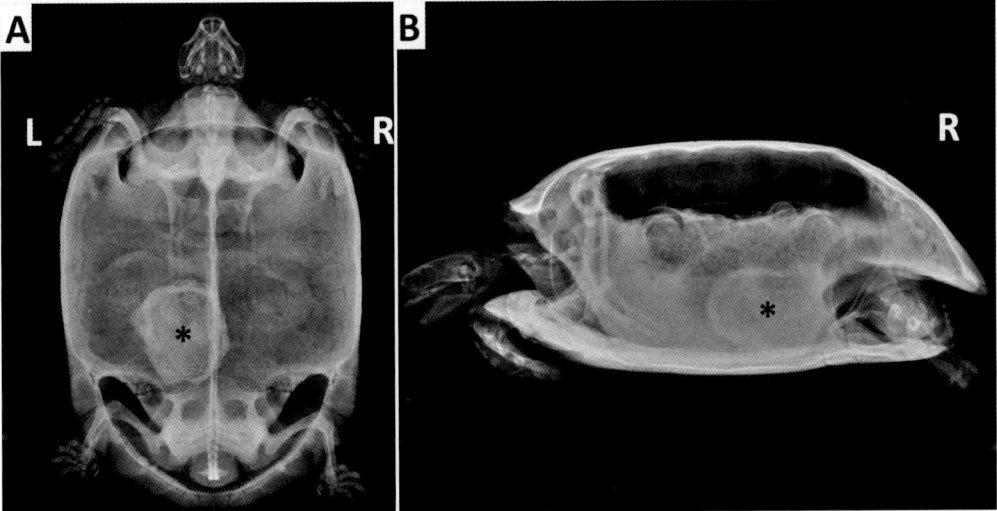

FIG 56.14 Dorsoventral (A) and horizontal beam right lateral (B) radiographs of a gopher tortoise (*Gopherus polyphemus*) demonstrating a large mineralized structure (*) in the caudoventral coelom that was confirmed as a urinary calculus by ultrasonography. (Courtesy of Stephen J. Divers.)

pathological conditions like small, radiolucent urate calculi, rupture, herniation/displacement, or masses (granuloma or neoplasia).

In survey radiographs, the location of the kidneys in the dorsocaudal aspect of the coelom severely limits their visibility.[2] Renal calcification is not commonly seen in chelonians, but increased opacity would increase their visibility. Similarly, intravenous iodinated contrast can be admin-istered to evaluate the kidneys and ureters.

MUSCULOSKELETAL SYSTEM

Evaluation of appendicular skeleton and shell in chelonians may be necessary to investigate disease processes like trauma, osteomyelitis or septic arthritis, metabolic bone diseases, or neoplasia (Fig. 56.16). Of the systems discussed, radiography is particularly useful in chelonians, because the shell and bones are the most opaque structures in the body.

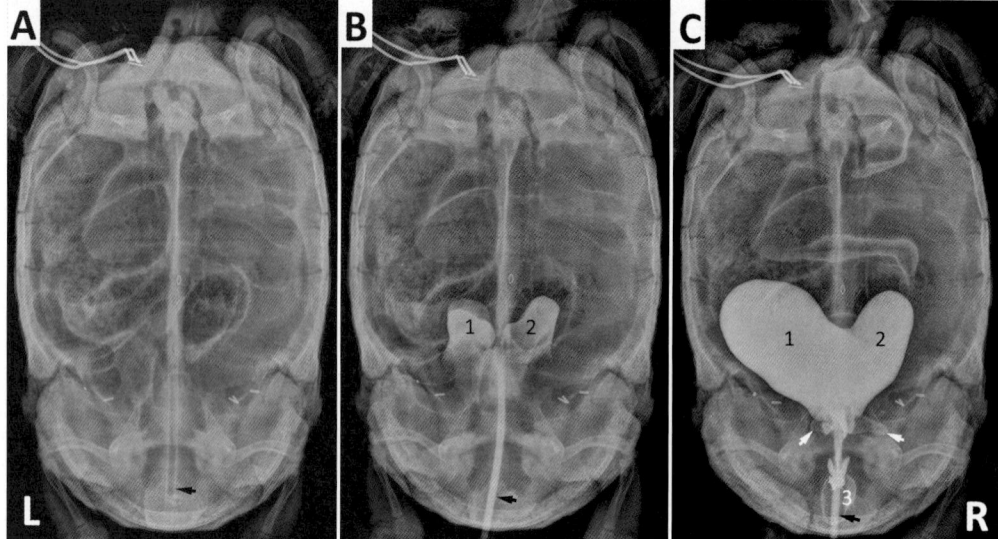

FIG 56.15 Serial dorsoventral radiographs demonstrating positive contrast cystography in a red-footed tortoise (*Chelonoidis carbonaria*) using a 12Fr red rubber catheter (black arrows) and iohexol. (A) Immediately after catheterization of the bladder. (B) Initial infusion of contrast demonstrates the left (1) and right (2) lobes of the bladder. (C) Submaximal infusion demonstrates greater distension of the bladder (1, 2), with contrast also backflowing into the accessory bladders (white arrows) and proctodeum (3). Cystography can be used to evaluate for possible bladder rupture, radiolucent calculi, bladder masses/neoplasia, and anatomical defects or displacements. (Courtesy of Stephen J. Divers.)

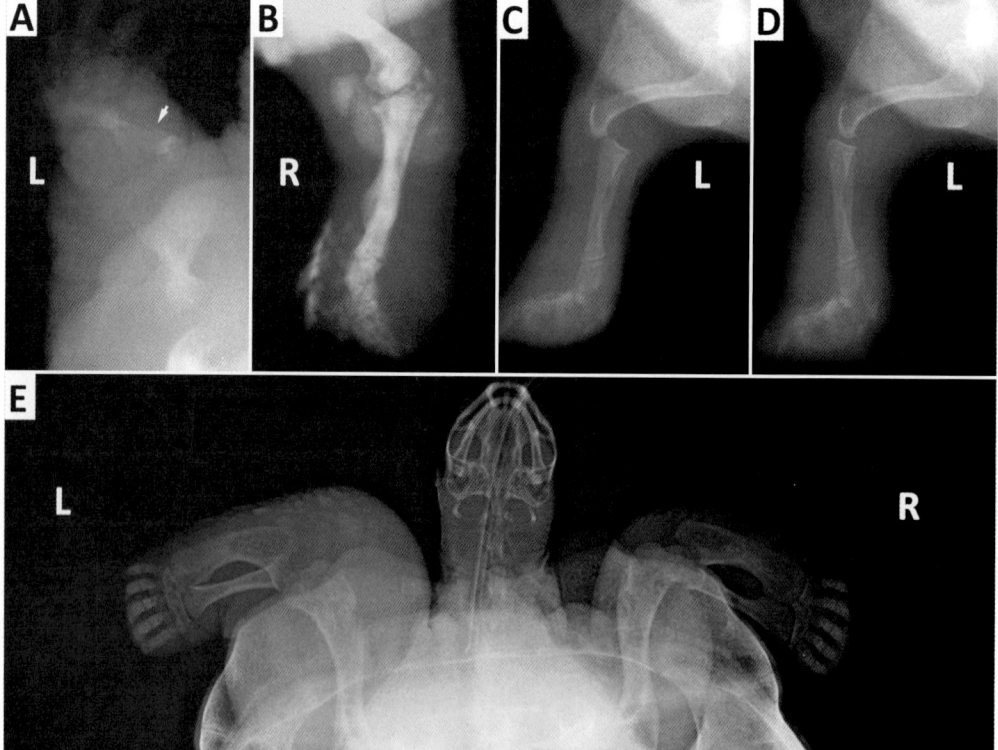

FIG 56.16 Dorsoventral radiographs (lateral view of limbs) of chelonians. (A) Reduced bone mineralization and pathological fracture of the left radius (arrow) associated with nutritional secondary hyperparathyroidism in a juvenile snapping turtle (*Chelydra serpentina*). (B) Effusion, swelling, and osteolysis associated with the right stifle of a *Testudo* tortoise due to septic arthritis and osteomyelitis. (C) Left stifle luxation in a *Testudo* tortoise that was associated with struggling against straw wrapped around the limb. (D) The same limb after cruciate ligament repair and joint imbrication. (E) Gross soft-tissue swelling and luxation of the left elbow in a radiated tortoise (*Astrochelys radiata*) due to an undifferentiated sarcoma. (Courtesy of Stephen J. Divers.)

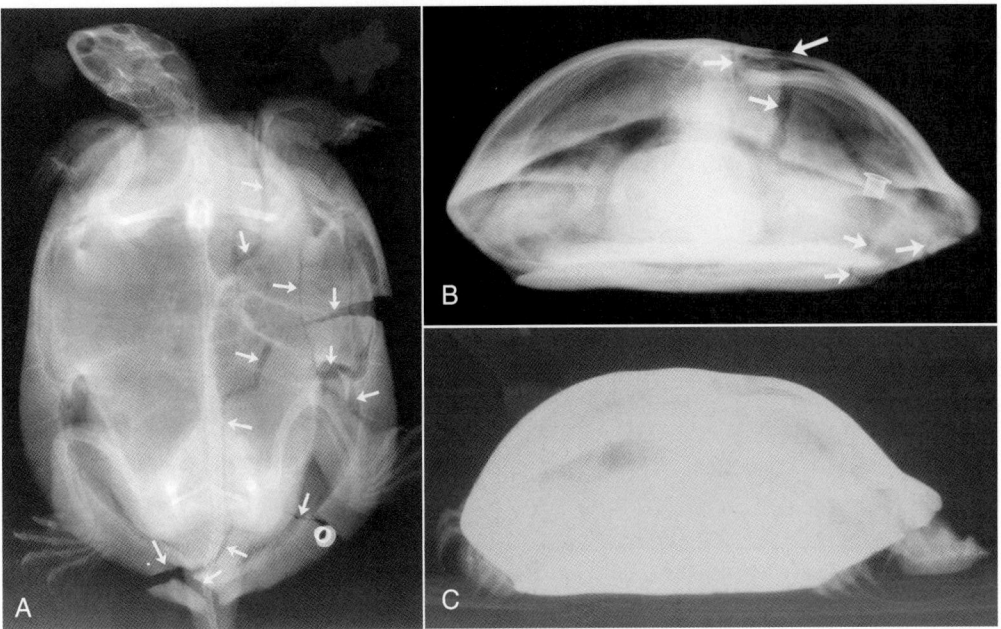

FIG 56.17 Multiple carapacial fractures with varying degrees of displacement (arrows) are present. The value of images with different image orientations noted as well. The slight depression of the carapace lateral to the near midline fracture is only seen on the craniocaudal. The effect of image quality is also demonstrated in this examination. The dorsoventral image (A) is the most appropriate exposed image. The craniocaudal image (B) is diagnostic as well, and fractures are more easily seen in the areas of the lungs and are superimposed over coelomic soft tissue; more critical evaluation is needed in this area since the human eye is best at detecting lesions on a black background. These are film-screen images, which would almost necessitate different exposures for the dorsal aspect of the patient compared with the ventral part. In contrast, digital radiography better corrects for these differences through postexposure processing. The lateral image (C) is severely underexposed to the extent that the fractures are barely visible. (Courtesy of Sam Silverman.)

Interpretation principles used in mammalian species are also more easily extrapolated, with a few notable additions. Obviously, systematic review of the shell is critical in chelonians. The long bones should have distinction between the cortical and medullary bone areas, but the transition between these is less distinct than is seen in normal mammal long bones.[1] In chelonians, the opacity of the pectoral girdle is used as a reference point in evaluating the quality of the radiograph and the bones; pectoral girdle bones should be clearly visualized with sharp margins, a small medullary canal, and a homogeneous cortical radiopacity.

Injuries to the chelonian shell are common. Because these are often visible on examination of the patient, the role of radiography is to document the degree of displacement and extensiveness of shell trauma, as well as to investigate for concurrent soft-tissue abnormalities associated with the injuries, especially pulmonary involvement.[3] Detection of minimally displaced fractures can be challenging if the x-ray beam is not tangential to the orientation of the fracture through the carapace or plastron. A complete examination of the carapace and plastron for fractures includes the dorsoventral, horizontal beam lateral, and horizontal beam craniocaudal images (Fig. 56.17). Additional oblique radiographs may be needed for detection of non- or minimally displaced fractures. This is more commonly needed in larger chelonians or those with greater carapacial curvature. CT can be extremely helpful in documentation of such injuries. Radiographs are also frequently utilized for serial postoperative evaluations (Fig. 56.18). However, monitoring healing of the shell is challenging, because healing occurs primarily through a fibrous callus, and the fracture lucent line can persist for years. It has been recommended that radiographs be repeated 10 to 20 weeks after stabilization, but complete healing and remodeling may

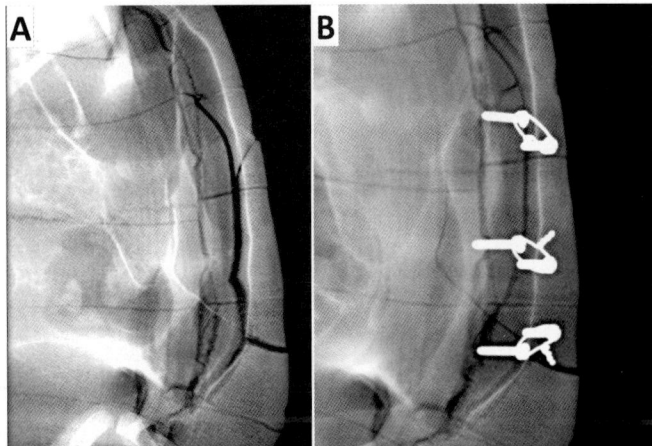

FIG 56.18 Dorsoventral radiographs of the fractured right plastrocarapacial bridge in an aquatic turtle before (A) and after repair (B). Note the radiolucency around the screws, which in this case is a software artifact and not indicative of osteolysis. (Courtesy of Stephen J. Divers.)

take 12 to 18 months.[2] If the carapace fracture crosses midline, concurrent spinal fracture should be expected, because the spine is intimately associated with the ventral surface of the carapace. CT, myelography or magnetic resonance imaging would be needed to evaluate the integrity of the spinal cord.[27]

Musculoskeletal trauma can result in fractures, luxations, subluxations, or soft-tissue injury (i.e., tendon/ligament tearing or muscle strain/

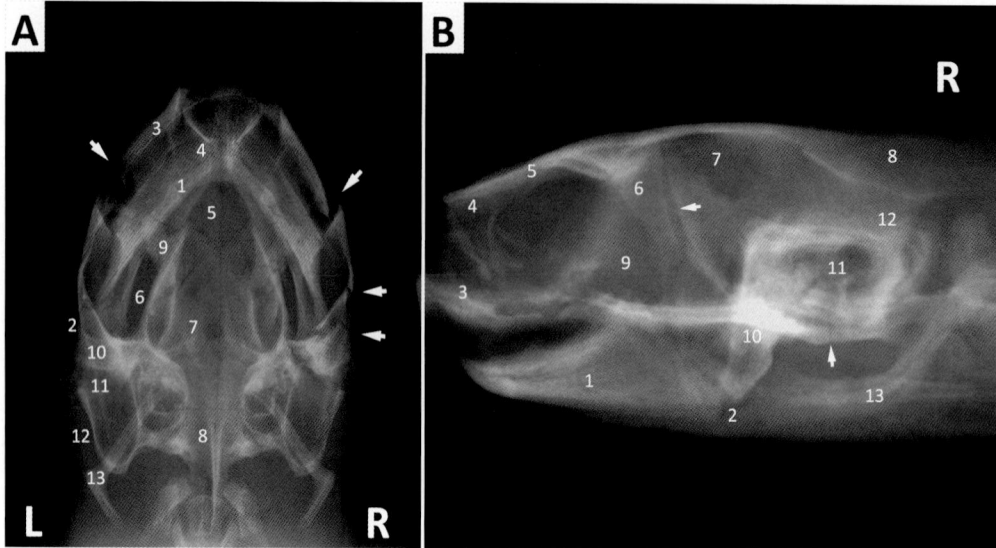

FIG 56.19 (A) Dorsoventral and right lateral radiographs of a *Testudo* tortoise skull demonstrating multiple fractures (*arrows*) and the major bones and structures including mandible (1), temporomandibular joint (2), maxilla (3), prefrontal (4), frontal (5), postorbital (6), parietal (7), supraoccipital (8), jugal (9), quadrate (10), auditory canal (11), squamosal (12), and ceratobrachial of hyoid apparatus (13). (Courtesy of Stephen J. Divers.)

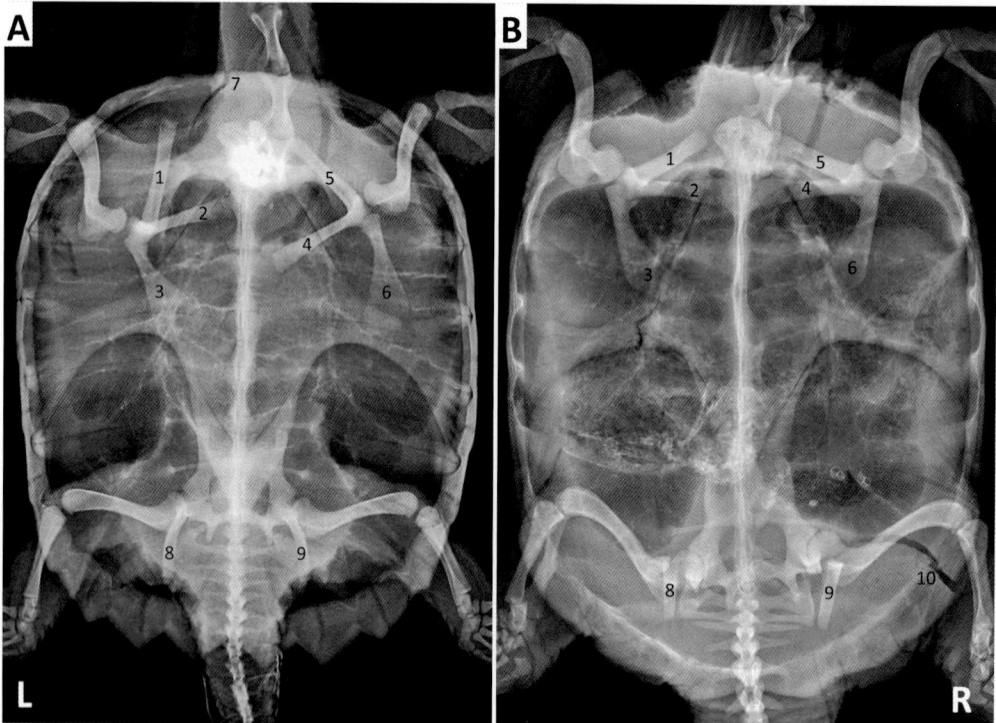

FIG 56.20 Dorsoventral radiographs of two traumatized snapping turtles (*Chelydra serpentina*). (A) The left acromion process (1) has fractured and is overriding the scapula (2) near the scapulohumeral joint. The left coracoid is unremarkable. The right scapula (4) has luxated from its normal attachment to the first fixed vertebra and has rotated caudad. Consequently, although the associated acromion process (5) and coracoid (6) retain their normal anatomical relationship with the scapula, they have also been rotated medially and laterally, respectively. A fracture of the cranial carapace is also visible (7). These injuries are commonly associated with a dorsoventral compressive force applied to the cranial carapace. The same pectoral structures in their usual positions have been labeled in (B) for comparison. (B) There are bilateral fractures of both left and right ilia (8 and 9), and an obvious fracture of the right caudal carapace (10) is present. These injuries are commonly associated with a dorsoventral compressive force applied to the caudal carapace. The same pelvic structures in their usual positions have been labeled in (A) for comparison. (Courtesy of Stephen J. Divers.)

sprain). Orthogonal radiographs of the limb(s) are needed for evaluation of the appendicular anatomy, consisting of lateral and craniocaudal/dorsopalmar/dorsoplantar images. The axial skeleton should be evaluated with dorsoventral and horizontal beam lateral images (Fig. 56.19). General anesthesia is needed for positioning the limb in extension and away from the carapace but should also be considered in traumatic cases for patient comfort. Fractures in the long bones are more easily seen than fractures involving the pectoral or pelvic girdles (Fig. 56.20). It is helpful to have a normal comparison series of radiographs of different species, especially for the interpretation of these more complex anatomical areas. CT can also be helpful in identifying fractures but can also aid in surgical planning. In chelonians, CT has also been shown to better define abnormalities that correlate with clinical presentation and were underestimated by radiography.[28] Dislocations or luxations can be encountered in chelonians in association with mishandling or predation. Similar to fracture detection, scapulohumeral or coxofemoral luxations may be more difficult; the addition of a horizontal beam craniocaudal radiograph may be beneficial in evaluating these areas.[2] Radiography is repeated for monitoring treatment of musculoskeletal disease in chelonians, similar to other species.

Osteomyelitis and septic arthritis are common. The radiographic features of osteomyelitis may include lytic and osteoproliferative changes in the affected bone(s). In contrast to mammalian species, the degree of lytic changes is greater, especially relative to periosteal reaction.[1,3] It is often accompanied by caseous abcessation.[2] Soft-tissue enlargement is prominent and causes regional distortion of anatomy. In the early stages, soft-tissue changes may be the only abnormality associated with osteomyelitis or septic aarthritis.[3] In the author's experience, critical evaluation of soft tissue is often skipped in musculoskeletal interpretation; it should be conceptualized as directing one's attention to an area that may not have osseous changes and therefore may be the most important to critically evaluate in the absence of bone changes.

Metabolic bone disease, specifically nutritional secondary hyperparathyroidism, is commonly seen in chelonians due to husbandry-related issues. Evaluation for nutritional secondary hyperparathyroidism requires good-quality radiographs to prevent erroneous diagnosis associated with bad technique (i.e., overexposure to reduced contrast). It also requires clinical experience with the expected degree of skeletal mineralization seen in different species at different ages (neonates and juveniles often exhibit reduced mineralization for up to the first year). Assessment of the pectoral or pelvic girdles provides the best assessment of skeletal mineralization. Diffusely decreased opacity of the bones is the primary abnormality (Fig. 56.21). Cortical bone thinning, shell, and less commonly, limb thickening due to fibrous proliferation and pathological fractures can further support the radiographic diagnosis.[2,3] Soft-tissue mineralization, mineralized gout tophi, or pseudogout

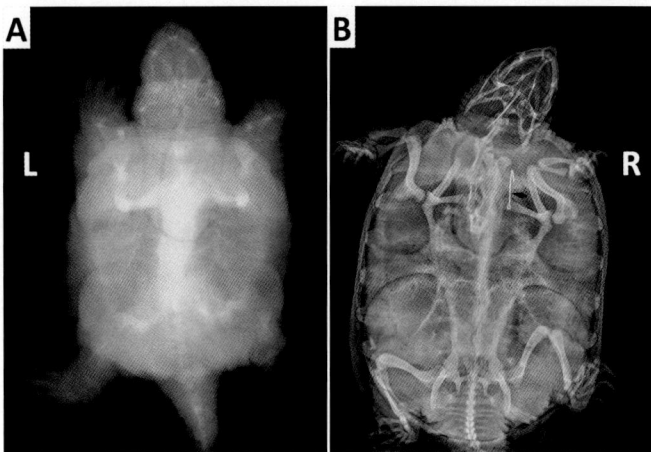

FIG 56.21 Dorsoventral radiographs of a juvenile common snapping turtle (*Chelydra serpentina*) with nutritional secondary hyperparathyroidism (A) and comparison to a normal animal of the same species (B). The generalized decrease in skeletal mineralization and reduced contrast between bone and soft tissues are characteristic of this condition. (Courtesy of Stephen J. Divers.)

represent other metabolic diseases that are often associated with nephropathy or excessive dietary protein.

Finally, degenerative joint disease is an increasingly encountered abnormality in radiographic examinations of older animals or those with previous musculoskeletal trauma.[2] This is partly associated with their lifespan, as they are some of the longest living animals encountered in veterinary practice. The radiographic features include periarticular mineral proliferation, forming osteophytes.[29] With advanced disease, there is more extensive soft-tissue mineralization around the joint, which is not a common feature in mammals. This can limit range of motion. Grossly, dense fibrous tissue accompanies this proliferation. Infrequently, in cases of severe coxofemoral degenerative joint disease femoral head and neck arthroplasty, can be performed as a salvage procedure.[30] Degenerative joint disease can be an age-related issue but can also be seen in association with prior disease processes like septic arthritis that have subsequently resolved. It should be noted that it can be difficult to distinguish active septic arthritis from degenerative changes in the early stages.

REFERENCES

See www.expertconsult.com for a complete list of references.

57

Radiography—Crocodilians

Nathalie Rademacher and Javier G. Nevarez

Standard equipment such as digital or computer radiography (DR or CR) can be used in crocodilians to acquire standard orthogonal views. In field situations, portable x-ray tubes are feasible, however, that will depend on the size of the animal. Depending on the history and clinical presentation, each body part can be radiographed with a similar technique and positioning used in small animals and will be described in more detail below. Radiation safety principles are the same as for small animals, and positioning devices such as foam pads or wedges, radiolucent tape, paper towels, sandbags, and PVC pipes should be used whenever possible with proper collimation for correct positioning to obtain high-quality diagnostic radiographs. Keep in mind that sandbags are of mineral opacity and need to be collimated out of view.

RESTRAINT, PREPARATION, AND POSITIONING

Crocodilians can be powerful animals, even at a small size. Proper restraint is essential for safety of the personnel and the animals, and sedation or anesthesia may be required to obtain the best views. Manual restraint should include keeping the mouth taped shut and the legs tied together. Even with the mouth taped, some teeth remain exposed and can inflict damage to personnel, so care must be taken when working with the head. Taping the eyes closed and inducing a vasovagal response is often effective.

In preparation for imaging, make sure the animal is clean, dry, and free of debris. In general, a minimum of two orthogonal views of each body part should be obtained. Additional views may be obtained as needed. Positioning for standard orthogonal views is similar to other animals. Based on the size of the animal and indication for performing the study, multiple views may be necessary for certain body areas or the whole body can be included in one image. The region of interest must be centered in the image, with proper collimation being used. Patient identification and directional markers must be clearly incorporated, not handwritten on the finished radiograph.

WHOLE BODY

Whole body imaging generally includes all structures except the tail, skull, and distal part of the limbs, although in small animals it may encompass most body structures. For the lateral projection, the crocodilian is placed in sternal recumbency with the legs in a neutral position or restrained away from the coelom and a horizontal beam directed through the patient (Fig. 57.1A). In crocodilians, a traditional lateral projection with the animal in lateral recumbency is also acceptable because the organs are compartmentalized and will not shift within the coelomic cavity as in other reptile species. For the dorsoventral

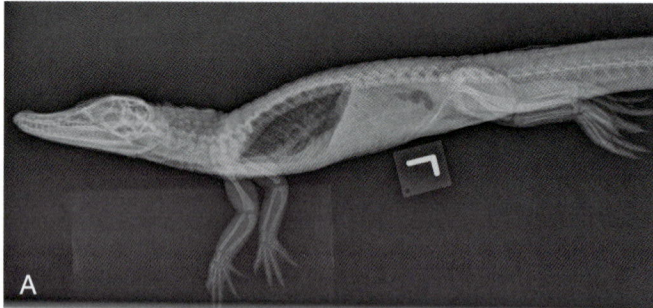

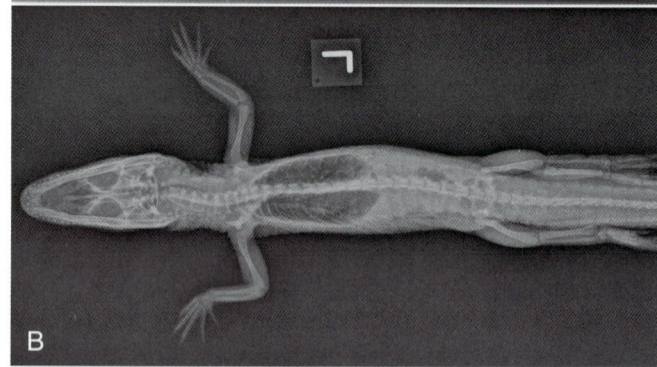

FIG 57.1 Whole body radiographs of an alligator (*Alligator mississippiensis*) brought in for head tilt and circling. (A) Left lateral (vertical beam) radiograph was acquired with the legs in neutral position. (B) VD projection with the patient in dorsal recumbency. Alternatively, a DV view with the patient in sternal recumbency can be acquired as well. No abnormalities were seen. (Courtesy of Natalie Rademacher.)

(DV) or ventrodorsal (VD) projection, place the animal in sternal or dorsal recumbency (see Fig. 57.1B). These views are generally used to assess injuries after trauma or to assess bone density in cases of metabolic bone disease (e.g., nutritional secondary hyperparathyroidism) (Fig. 57.2). These studies should not be used when evaluating specific areas, such as cranial coelom, caudal coelom, or the skeleton, due to technique differences as well as x-ray beam divergence that will result in improper centration.

CRANIAL COELOM

Orthogonal views, including right (and potentially left) lateral(s) (Fig. 57.3A) and DV (and potentially VD) views (see Fig. 57.3B), are recommended. The front limbs should be extended cranially to avoid superimposition with the lungs in the lateral view. In some cases, both

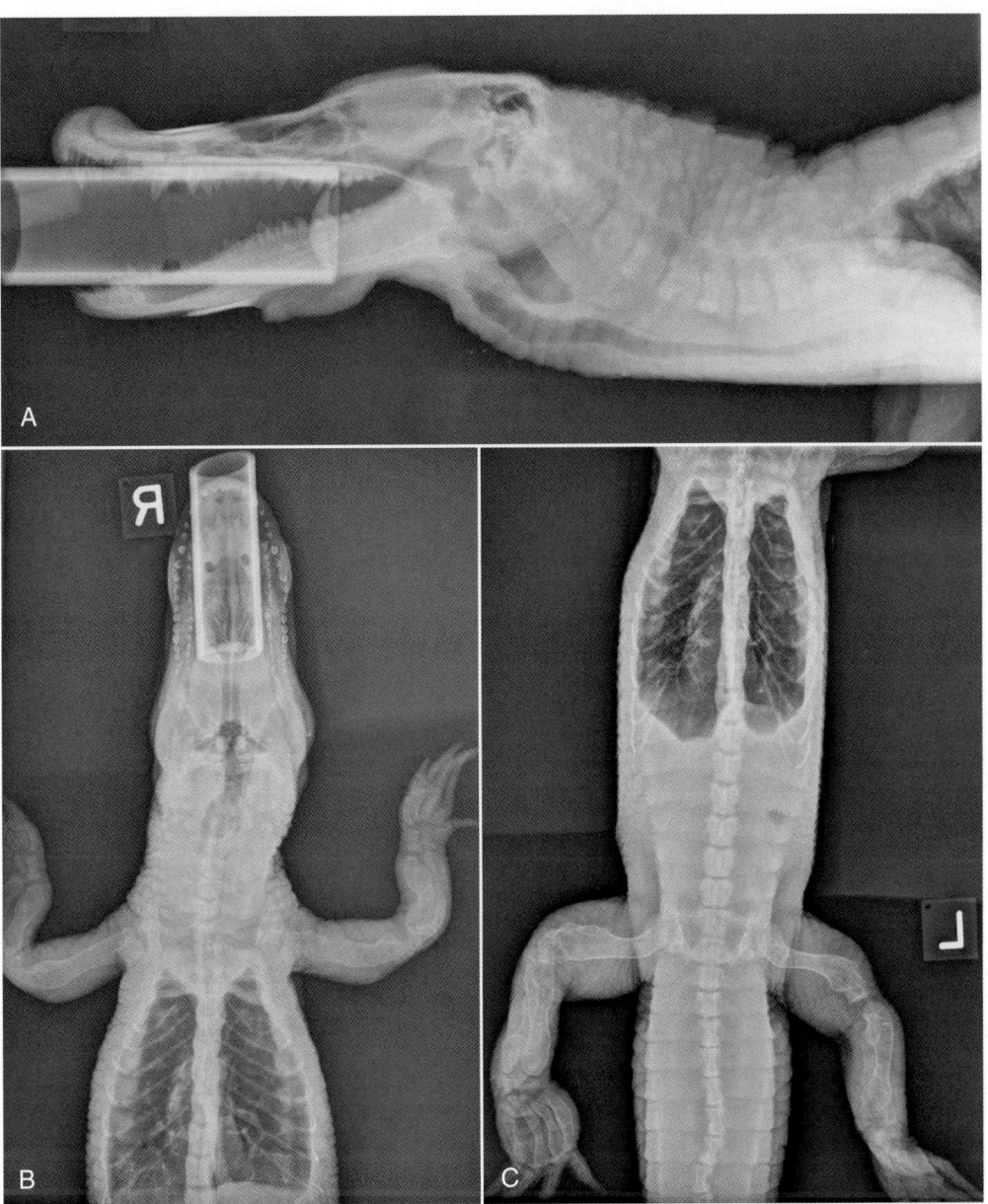

FIG 57.2 (A) Lateral and (B) dorsoventral views of the skull of an alligator (*Alligator mississippiensis*) that presented with a hunched posture and stiff legs at 1 week duration. (C) Dorsoventral whole body view. Overall, severe decreased bone opacity with thin irregular cortices is noted. Moderate folding of multiple long bones, most pronounced in the left radius as well as the tibias and fibulas bilaterally. Moderate leftward and rightward angulation of several caudal vertebral bodies throughout the length of the tail. Diagnosis of a nutritional secondary hyperparathyroidism was made with multiple chronic folding fractures. (Courtesy of Natalie Rademacher.)

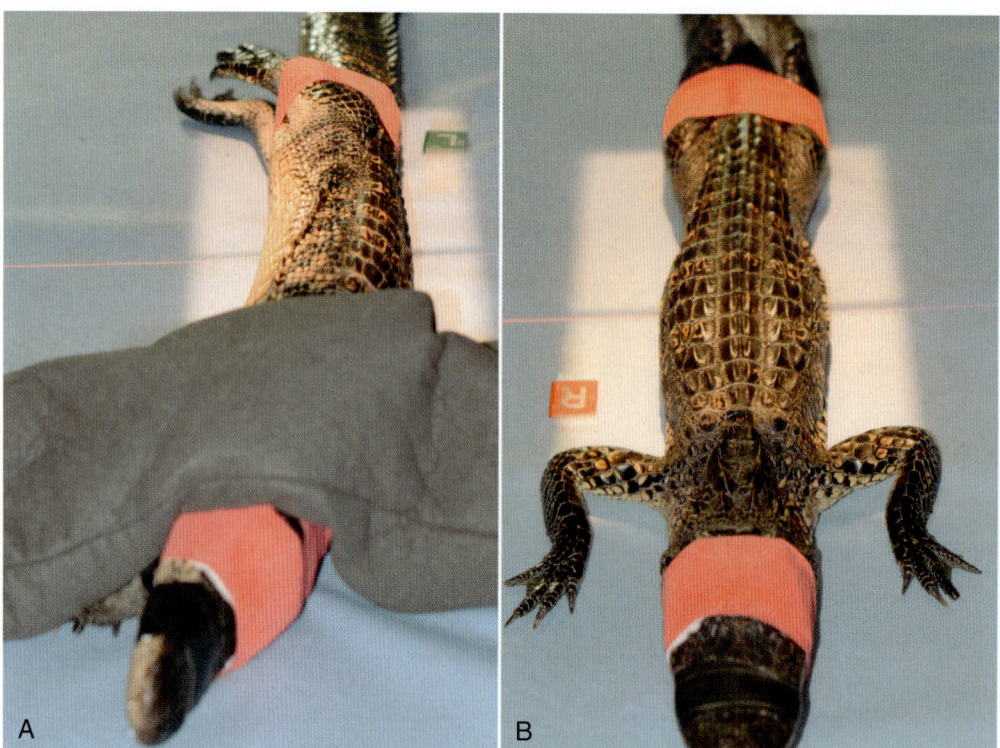

FIG 57.3 Photographs demonstrating positioning for coelomic and spinal projections in an alligator (*Alligator mississippiensis*). (A) Left lateral recumbency. A sandbag has been placed over the cranial half to stabilize the animal in lateral recumbency, and the legs have been secured with tape (not shown). Additionally, vet wrap has been placed over the eyes to calm the animal down. Care must be taken to align the alligator perpendicular to the tabletop in order to acquire straight radiographs. This positioning can be used to acquire total body, coelomic, and/or abdominal radiographs with a shift in the center of the field of view and collimation. (B) Sternal recumbency to demonstrate positioning for the DV view for total body, coelomic, abdominal, or spinal radiographs. Due to the shape of crocodilians, the DV view is usually easier to acquire. (Courtesy of Natalie Rademacher.)

lateral radiographs might be useful for evaluation. Respiratory motion artifacts are not usually a problem. If the patient is large, multiple views of the area of interest may be needed. Exposure at peak inspiration is ideal to maximize contrast by increased aeration. Care must be taken to include all pulmonary boundaries (Fig. 57.4).

CAUDAL COELOM

Right lateral and DV radiographic views are standard, with similar positioning for the cranial coelom (Fig. 57.5). Hind legs can be left in neutral positions or taped caudally along the tail base, out of the coelomic field as shown in Fig. 57.3. Exposure should be acquired at expiration (see Fig. 57.4). In large animals, multiple views will be needed for a complete evaluation.

SKULL

Lateral and VD or DV views are the minimum required projections to evaluate the skull. Given the lack of mobile soft tissues, vertical beam laterals are acceptable. Care must be taken for optimal and accurate positioning of the skull to obtain symmetric diagnostic radiographs. For the lateral projection, place the animal in left or right lateral recumbency with front legs against the body and away from the head. The head is

extended in a 90-degree angle perpendicular to the tabletop. A thin foam wedge or paper towels are placed to elevate the tip of the nose so its perpendicular to the tabletop (Fig. 57.6A). The mandibles should be superimposed with each other to check for symmetry (see Fig. 57.6C); however, this might be difficult in cases of mandibular or maxillary trauma. The orthogonal view can be acquired in either the DV or VD projection, depending on specific area of interest (see below) (see Fig. 57.6B and D). Foam wedges or paper towels should be used to elevate the tip of the nose so it is parallel with the table or cassette when in dorsal recumbency, whereas it is not necessary when placing the animal in sternal recumbency, making this view easier to acquire.

Open-mouth images are acquired with the use of a mouth gag (Fig. 57.7A and C) for separation and evaluation of the dental arcades. In cases of trauma and more specifically suspected fractures, the use of mouth gags must be done carefully to prevent injury. Oblique images are acquired in right and left lateral recumbency with rotation of the head by 20 to 45 degrees (see Fig. 57.7B), which highlights the left maxillary and the right mandibular arcades (see Fig. 57.7D). Fig. 57.7E depicts the contralateral maxillary and mandibular arcades and should be acquired for comparison. A case example of a traumatic injury to the right maxilla, also affecting the dental arcade, hard palate, and nasal bone that extends over to the right side, is shown in Fig. 57.8.

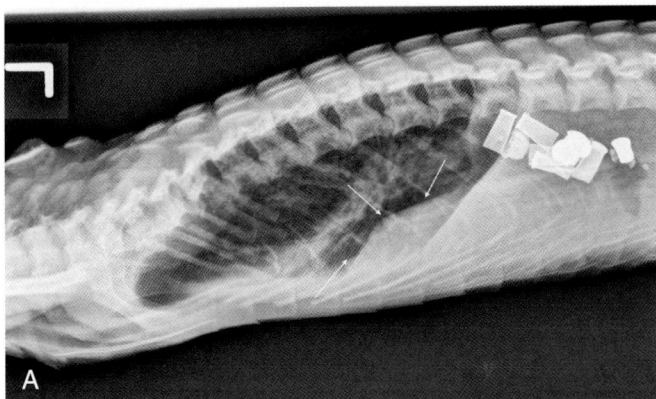

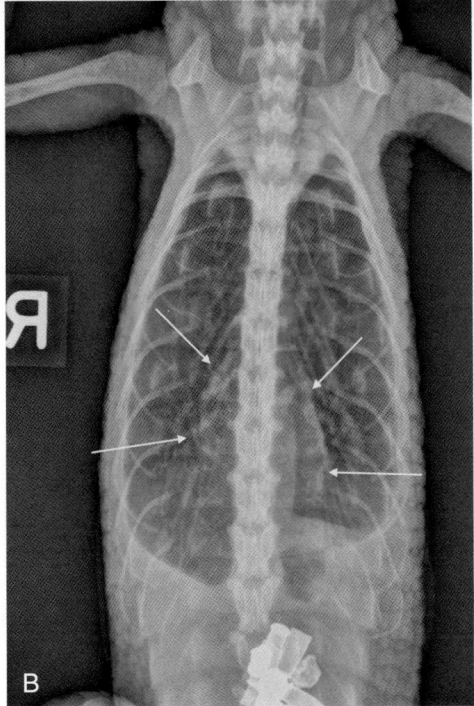

FIG 57.4 (A) Left (vertical beam) lateral and (B) DV cranial coelomic radiographs are shown from the same alligator (*Alligator mississippiensis*) as in Fig. 57.3. The front legs have been positioned out of the field of view cranially to avoid superimposition with the cranial coelom to allow identification of the most cranial part of the lungs. The cardiac silhouette (arrows) is indistinct and silhouettes with the diaphragmatic muscle at its caudal border. The alligator ingested multiple bullets and bullet casings. (Courtesy of Natalie Rademacher.)

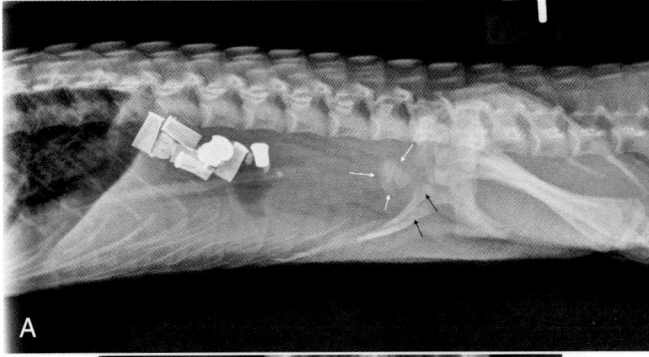

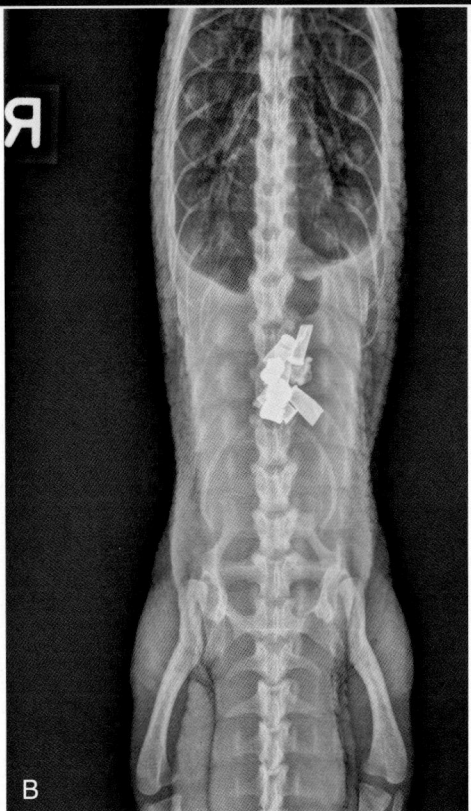

FIG 57.5 (A) Left lateral and (B) DV caudal coleomic radiographs of the same alligator (*Alligator mississippiensis*) shown in Figs. 57.3 and 57.4. The hind legs have been pulled and taped caudally to avoid superimposition with the caudal coelom. Note the multiple bullets and shell casings in the stomach. A well-defined, round mineral opacity is present in the caudal coelom (white arrows) with differentials of a urolith or bates body (calcified fat). The black arrows are pointing at the elongated pubic bone that is characteristic of crocodilians. (Courtesy of Natalie Rademacher.)

SPINE/TAIL

Lateral and VD/DV views are the minimum required projections to evaluate the spine. For the cervical spine, the front legs should be positioned caudally to prevent superimposition and allow evaluation of the entire cervical region (Fig. 57.9A, B, and D). The reminder of the spine must be acquired in separate segments to avoid beam divergence and are acquired in a similar position as shown in Fig. 57.3 (see Fig. 57.9C, E, and F). The total number of radiographs will depend on the size of the animal and available detector size. Fig. 57.10 shows positioning for tail radiographs. Additional views may be needed depending on lesion localization and suspected underlying disease process. As with the skull, care must be taken for optimal and accurate positioning to obtain symmetric diagnostic radiographs.

LIMBS

Lateral radiographs can be acquired either in sternal (Fig. 57.11A and B) or dorsal recumbency (see Fig. 57.11C and D). With the animal in lateral recumbency, the affected limb is placed down and the contralateral limb is pulled caudally away from the field of view to avoid superimposition (see Fig. 57.11A). Joint studies should include the proximal and distal third to the joint, whereas long bone studies should include the proximal and distal joints. Front or hind limb overview studies can be acquired for trauma evaluation or to rule out a lytic process. If lameness

Text continued on p. 540

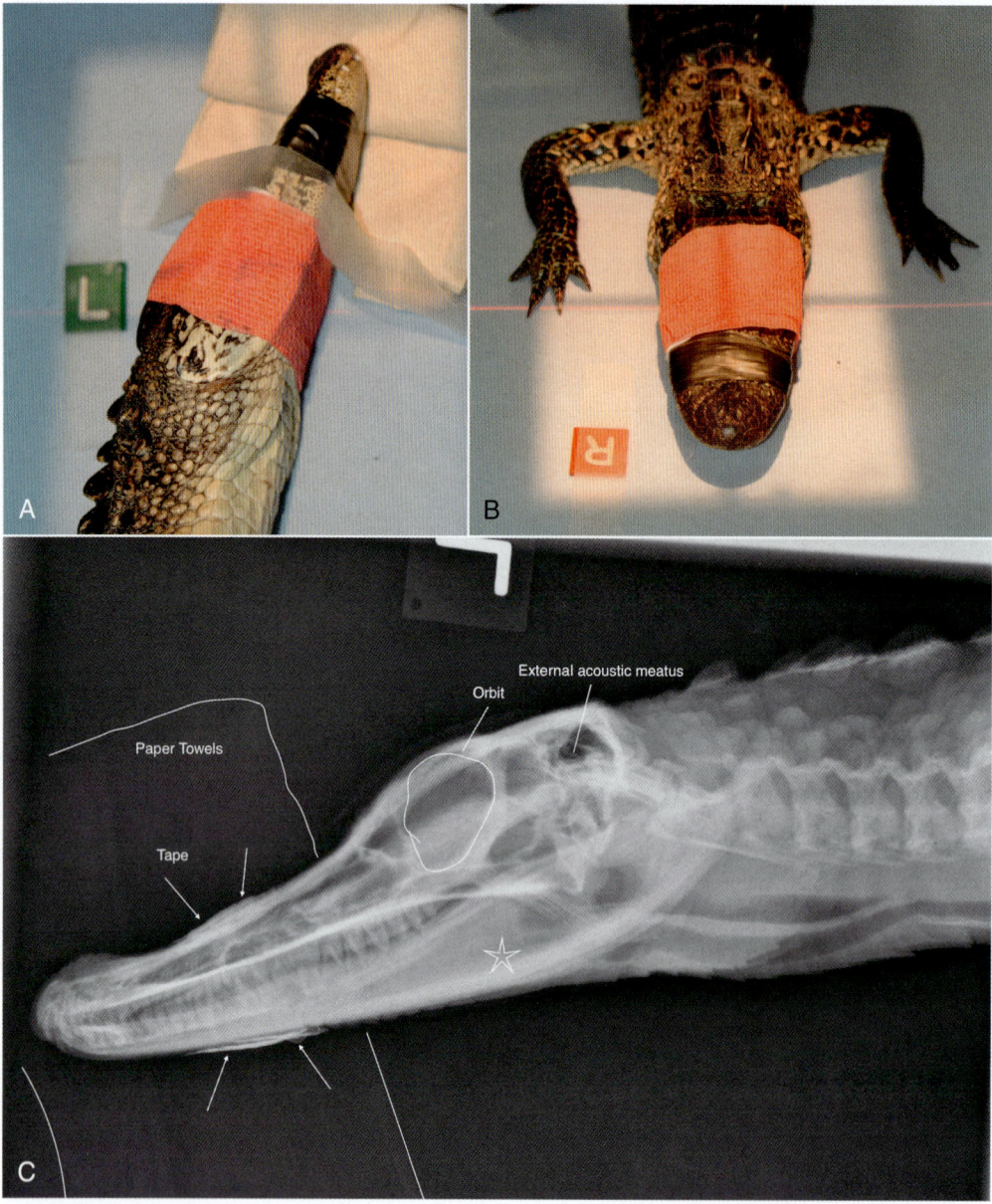

FIG 57.6 (A) The alligator (*Alligator mississippiensis*) is positioned in left lateral recumbency for a lateral skull radiograph, with paper towels placed under the tip of the nose to align the nose parallel with the tabletop. Radiolucent electrical tape has been used to secure the snout and tape the skull to the table. The front legs are pulled caudally away from the collimated field. (B) Alligator is in sternal recumbency with vet wrap covering its eyes and the center of the collimated view on the skull. Legs are in neutral position outside the collimated field. (B) Left lateral skull radiograph. Both mandibles are aligned and superimposed, indicating a straight view (white star). The paper towels (white outline) and duct tape (white arrows) are faintly visible. (Courtesy of Natalie Rademacher.)

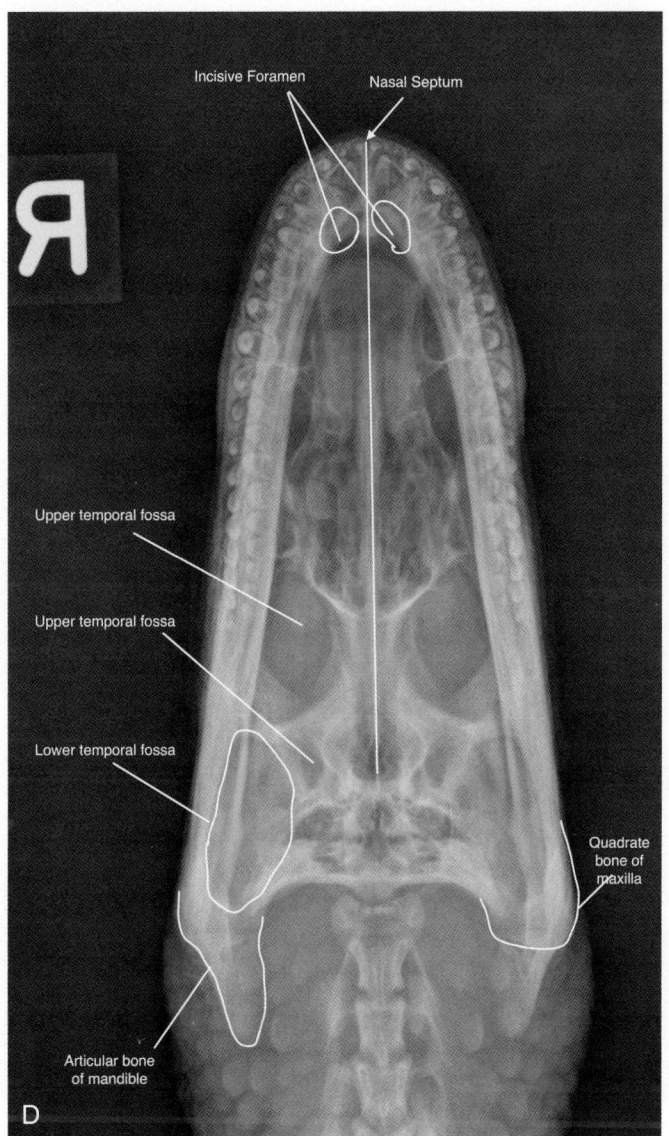

FIG 57.6, cont'd (D) DV radiograph of the skull. Care must be taken to align the entire animal in a straight line with the skull to acquire perfectly symmetrical radiographs. The nasal septum is straight and the mandibles are superimposed with the maxilla, and all other boney structures of the skull are symmetrical. (Courtesy of Natalie Rademacher.)

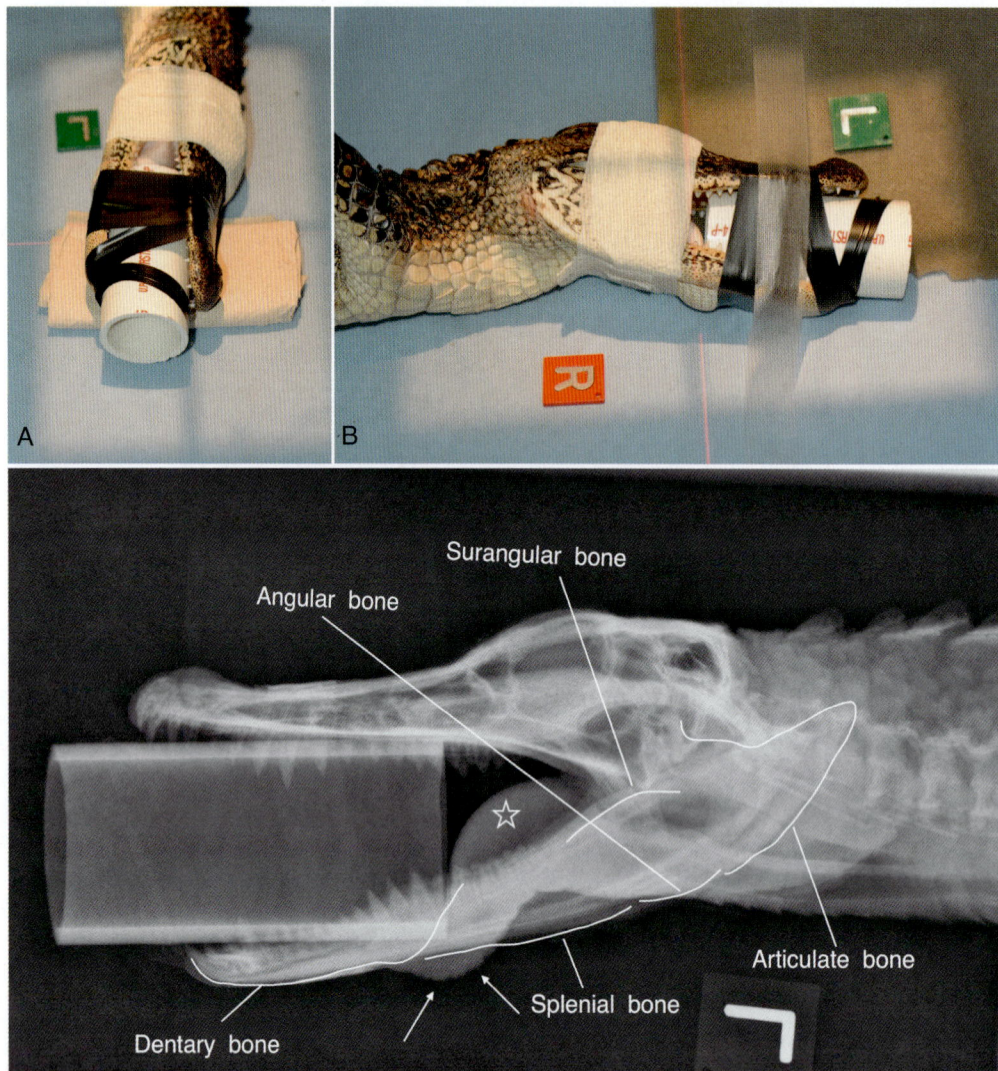

FIG 57.7 (A) Lateral recumbency with PVC pipe to acquire a lateral open-mouth view of the alligator skull (*Alligator mississippiensis*). (B) The alligator is placed in left lateral recumbency with a foam pad under the maxilla to create a 20- to 45-degree angle of the mandible with the table. Place the affected mandible closer to the table. (C) Left lateral open-mouth radiograph. The tongue has been pushed caudal by the PVC pipe and can be seen as a soft tissue opacity in the caudal oral cavity (star) and causes a fake soft tissue swelling ventral to the mandible (arrows). (Courtesy of Natalie Rademacher.)

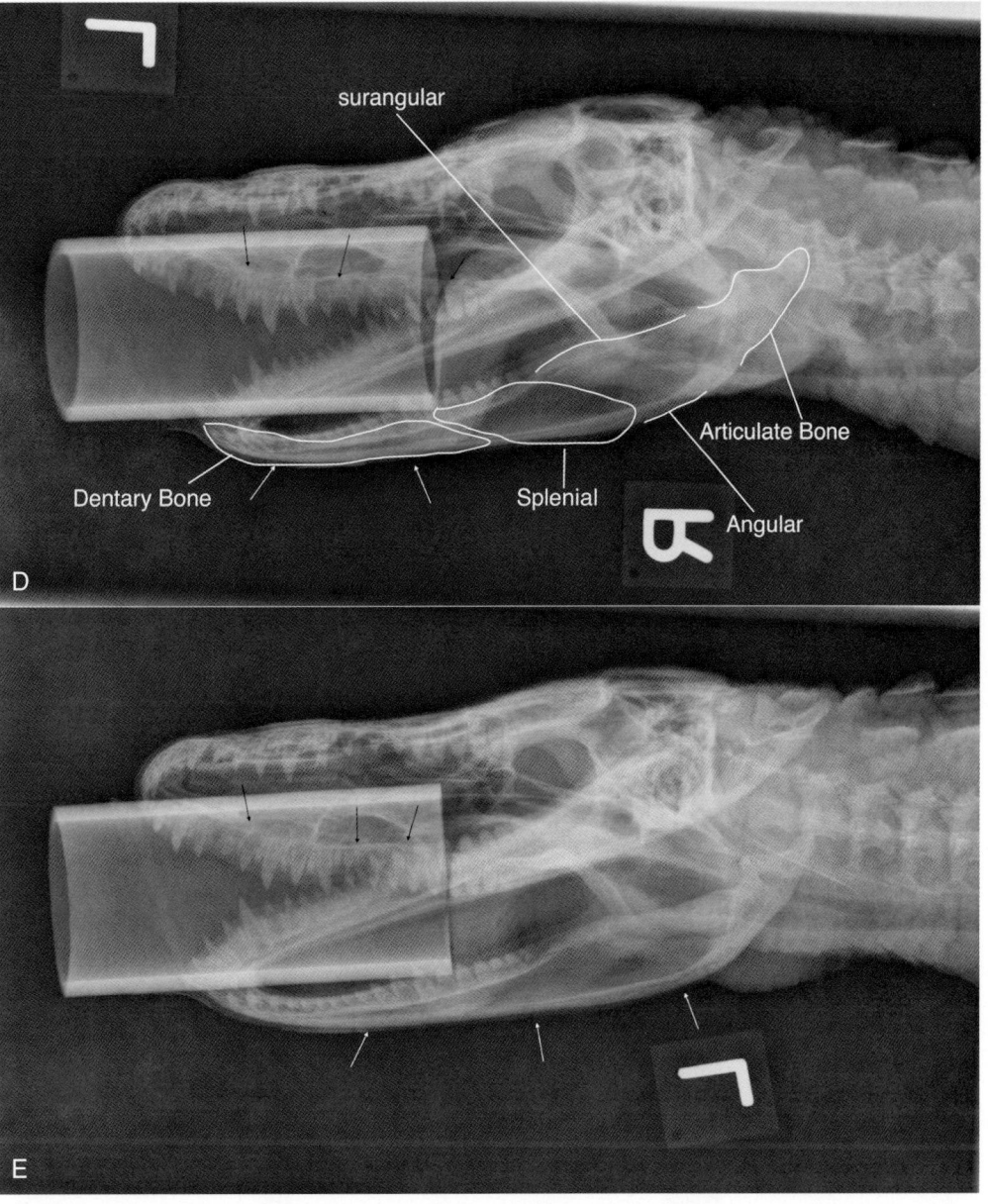

FIG 57.7, cont'd (D) Left lateral open-mouth oblique radiograph. With this view, the left maxillary (black arrows) and the right mandibular (white arrows) arcades are highlighted. (E) Right lateral open-mouth oblique to highlight the right maxillary (black arrows) and the left mandibular (white arrows) arcades. (Courtesy of Natalie Rademacher.)

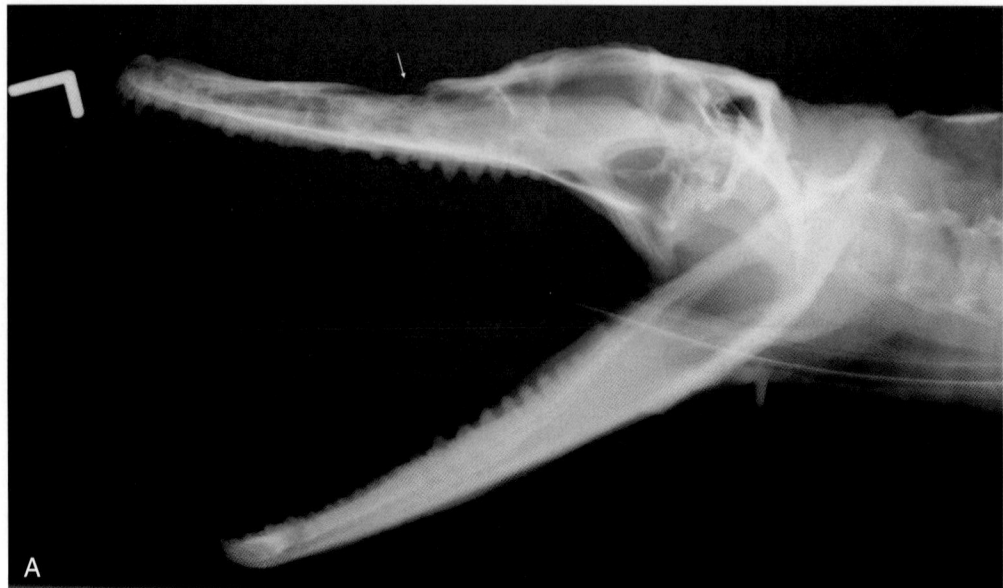

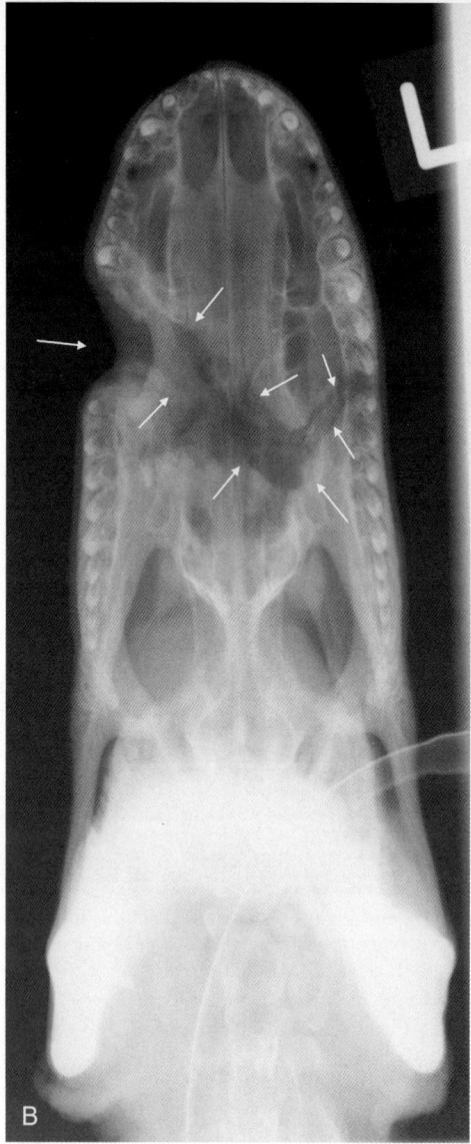

FIG 57.8 Left lateral open-mouth (A) and DV (B) radiographs of an alligator (*Alligator mississippiensis*) found with a wound to the rostral skull and suspected propeller damage. Radiographs were taken to characterize the extent of the damage. The anesthetized alligator is intubated. A defect of the right maxilla, also affecting the dental arcade, hard palate, and nasal bone that extends over to the right side, is noted with rounded margins (arrows). The damaged bone is better visualized in the DV view. (Courtesy of Natalie Rademacher.)

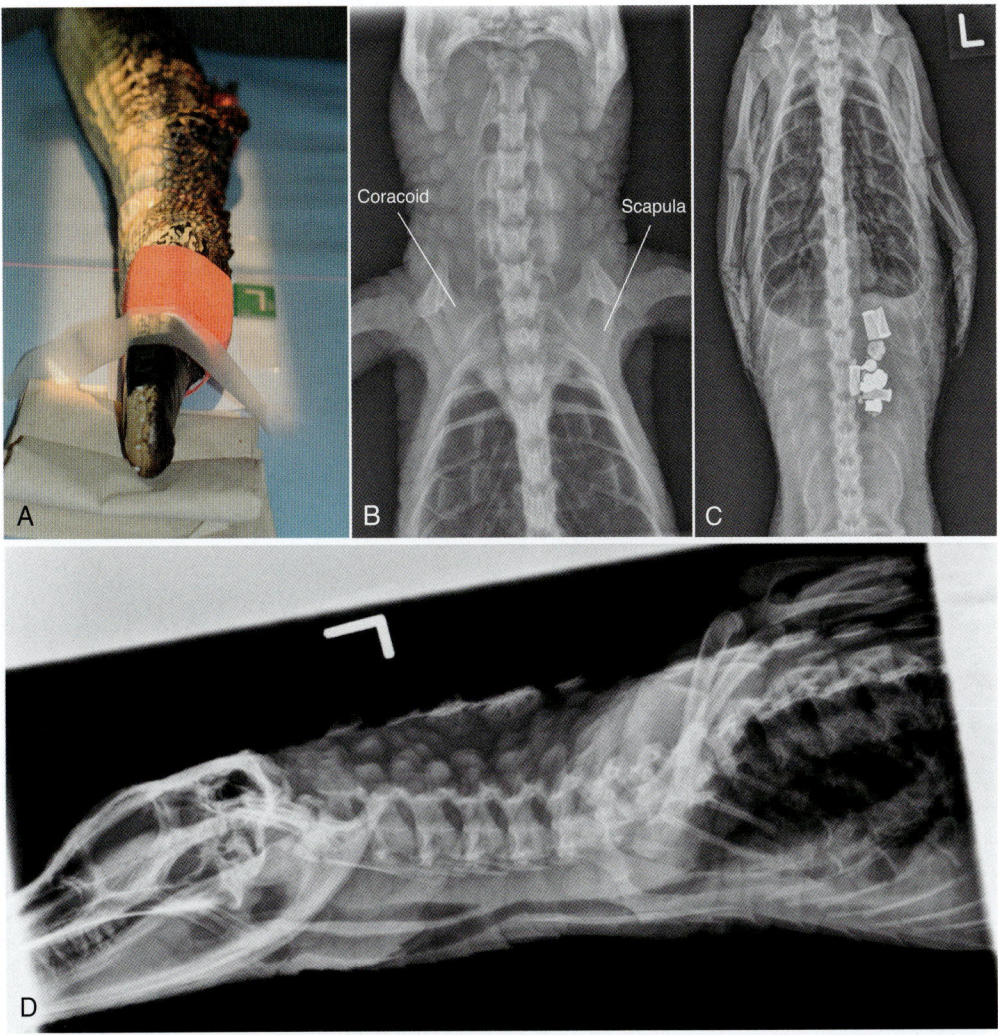

FIG 57.9 (A) Alligator (*Alligator mississippiensis*) positioned in left lateral recumbency for cervical spinal radiographs. The front legs should be positioned caudally to prevent superimposition and allow evaluation of the entire cervical spine. As with the skull, care must be taken to acquire straight and symmetric radiographs. (B) VD cervical spinal radiograph. (C) VD of the trunk spine. (D) Lateral cervical spinal radiograph. The scales of the neck are superimposed with the lateral cervical spine and can hinder evaluation, especially if the animal is wet or dirty. (Courtesy of Natalie Rademacher.)   *Continued*

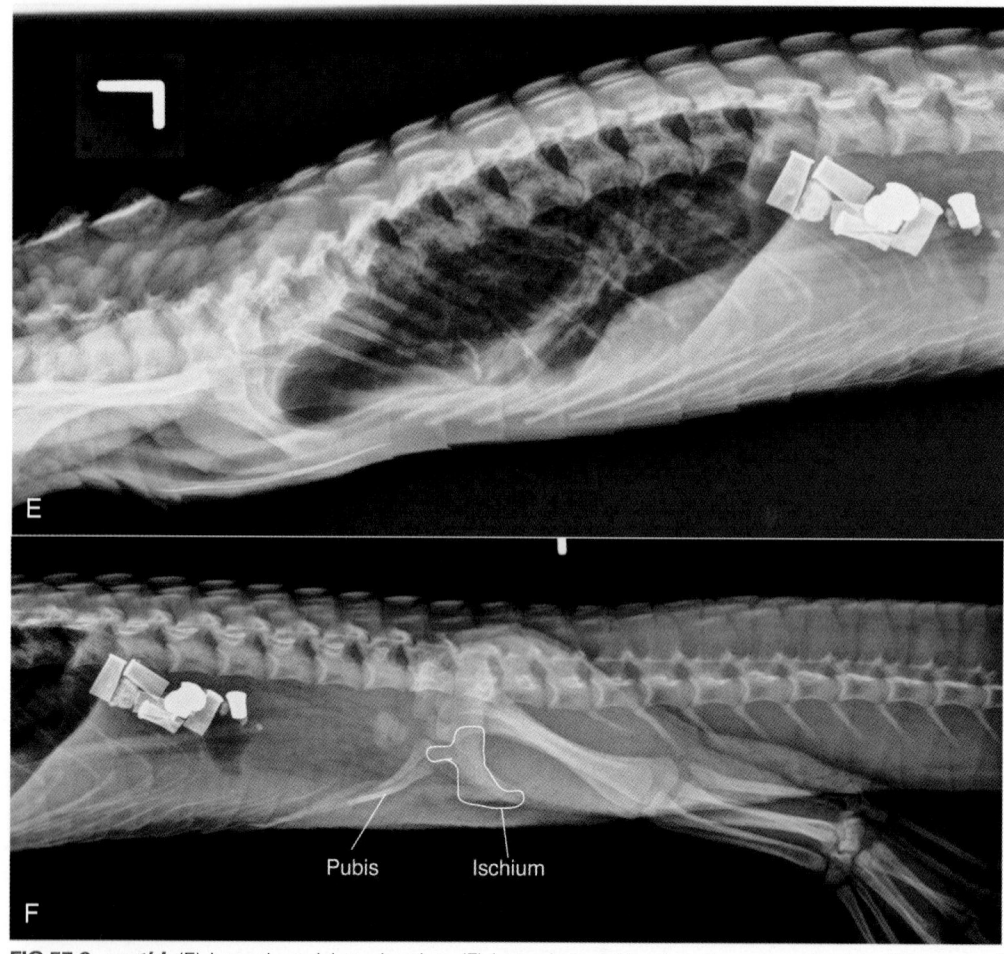

FIG 57.9, cont'd (E) Lateral cranial trunk spine. (F) Lateral caudal trunk and coccygeal spine. (Courtesy of Natalie Rademacher.)

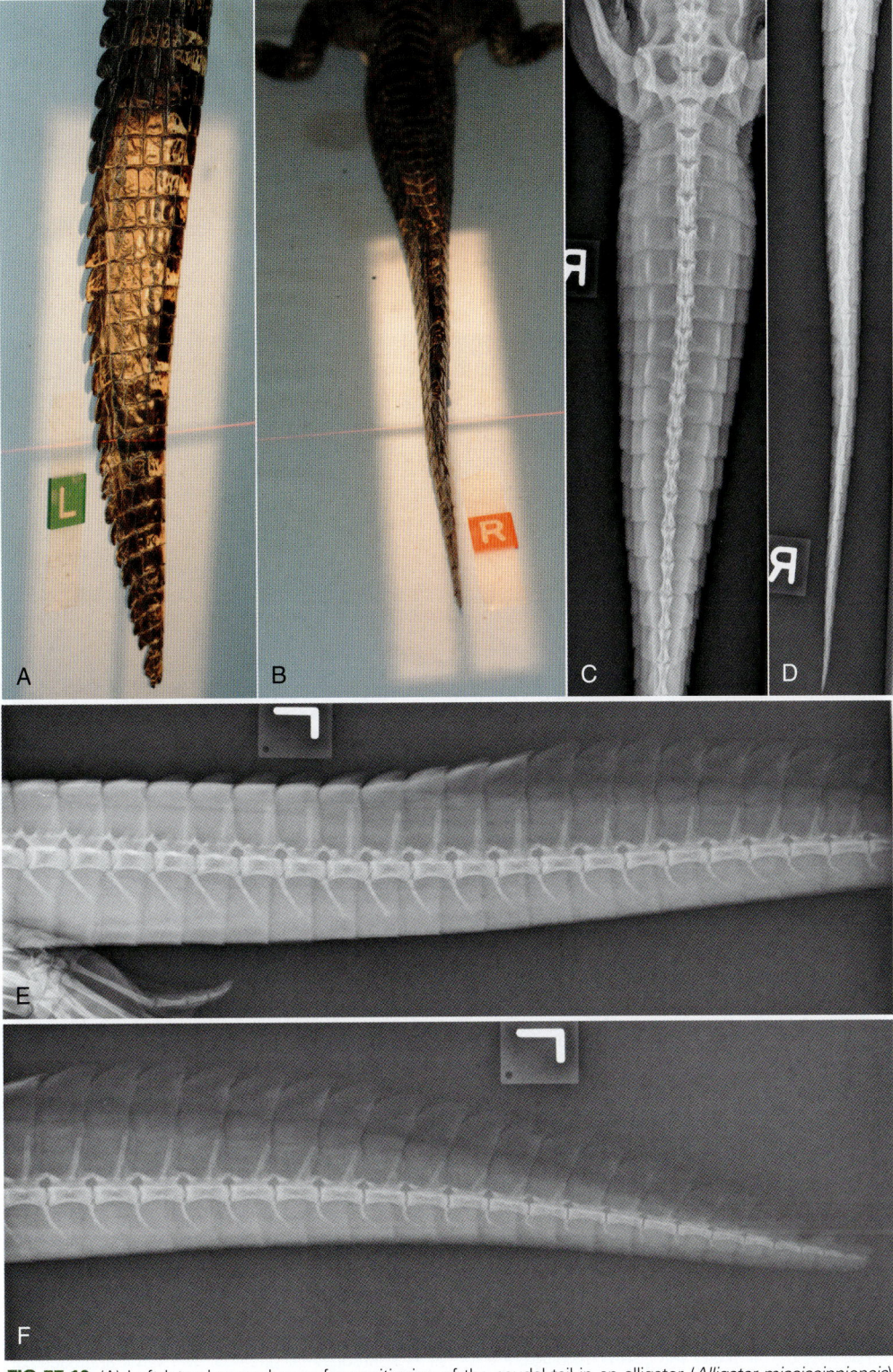

FIG 57.10 (A) Left lateral recumbency for positioning of the caudal tail in an alligator (*Alligator mississippiensis*). Depending on the length of the tail, multiple radiographs will be needed to cover the entire tail. (B) Sternal recumbency for the tail. (C and D) DV radiographs of the tail. The osteoderms and scales are clearly seen, as well as the coccygeal vertebral bodies. (E and F) Lateral radiographs covering the tail. (Courtesy of Natalie Rademacher.)

is present and can be localized to a specific joint or bone, or if a soft tissue swelling or skin defect/laceration is present, collimated views of affected areas should be acquired (Fig. 57.12). Contralateral radiographs of the unaffected side should be acquired for comparison. The orthogonal craniocaudal or caudocranial views are best acquired in dorsal recumbency (Fig. 57.13) with the leg angled away from the body to avoid superimposition with the body wall. This is important for the evaluation of soft tissues, as otherwise soft tissue swelling can be missed.

PELVIS

Proper evaluation of the pelvis requires good positioning and collimation of orthogonal views (Fig. 57.14). Evaluation of the pelvis and femur should be done with the limbs extended and in neutral positions (see Fig. 57.14).

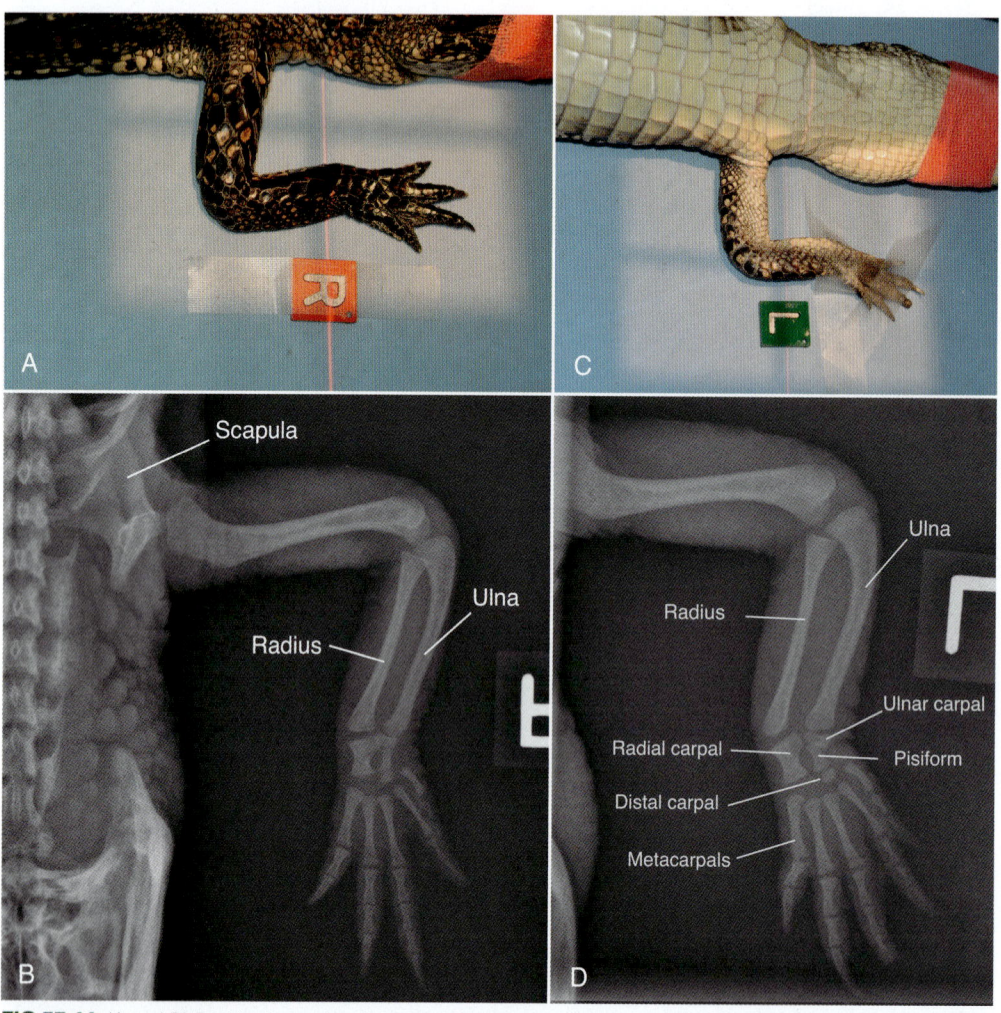

FIG 57.11 (A and B) Positioning and radiograph of the lateral projection of the right front leg with the alligator (*Alligator mississippiensis*) in sternal recumbency. Alternatively, the animal can be placed in lateral recumbency, as shown for the left front leg (C and D). The contralateral leg has been taped caudally along the body wall to avoid superimposition, and the foot has been secured with radiolucent tape to the table. The resulting views are the same and are good overviews of the skeletal structure of the front leg. Note that while a lateral view of the radius and ulna is acquired, the foot is in a dorsopalmar position. The same approach can be used for the hind limbs. (Courtesy of Natalie Rademacher.)

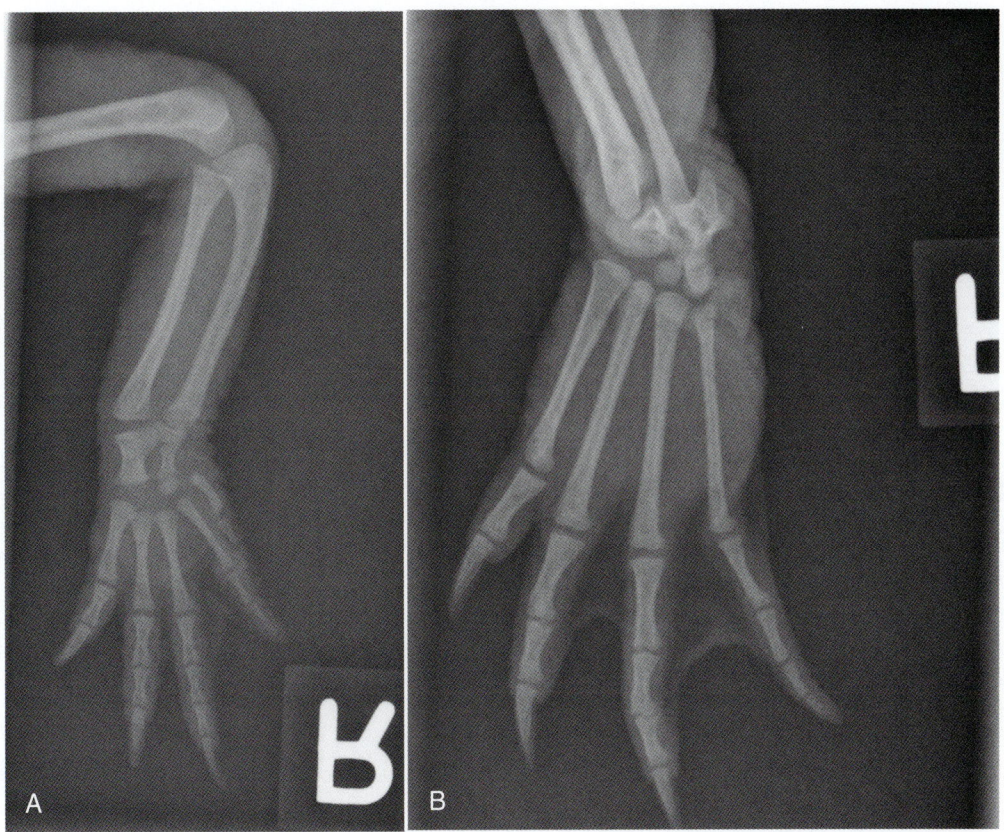

FIG 57.12 (A) Collimated lateral view of the right radius and ulna while the foot is in a dorsopalmar position (American alligator, *Alligator mississippiensis*). (B) Collimated dorsopalmar view of the right front foot. This allows higher resolution in cases where lameness can be localized or a soft tissue swelling is detected. (Courtesy of Natalie Rademacher.)

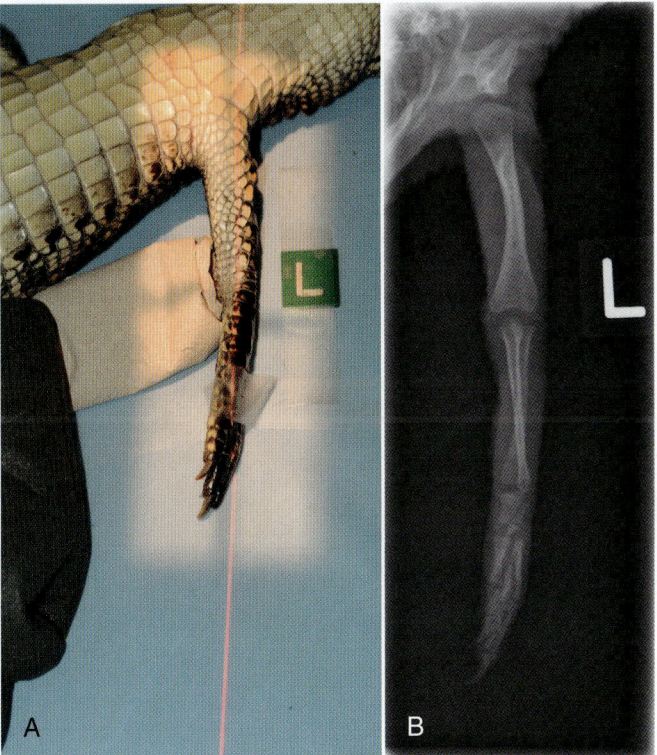

FIG 57.13 (A) The alligator (*Alligator mississippiensis*) has been placed in dorsal recumbency, and positioning is shown for the craniocaudal view of the left front leg. Paper towels have been used to angle the front leg away from the body wall, and it is secured with tape. (B) Craniocaudal view of the left front leg, acquired in the position shown in (A). (Courtesy of Natalie Rademacher.)

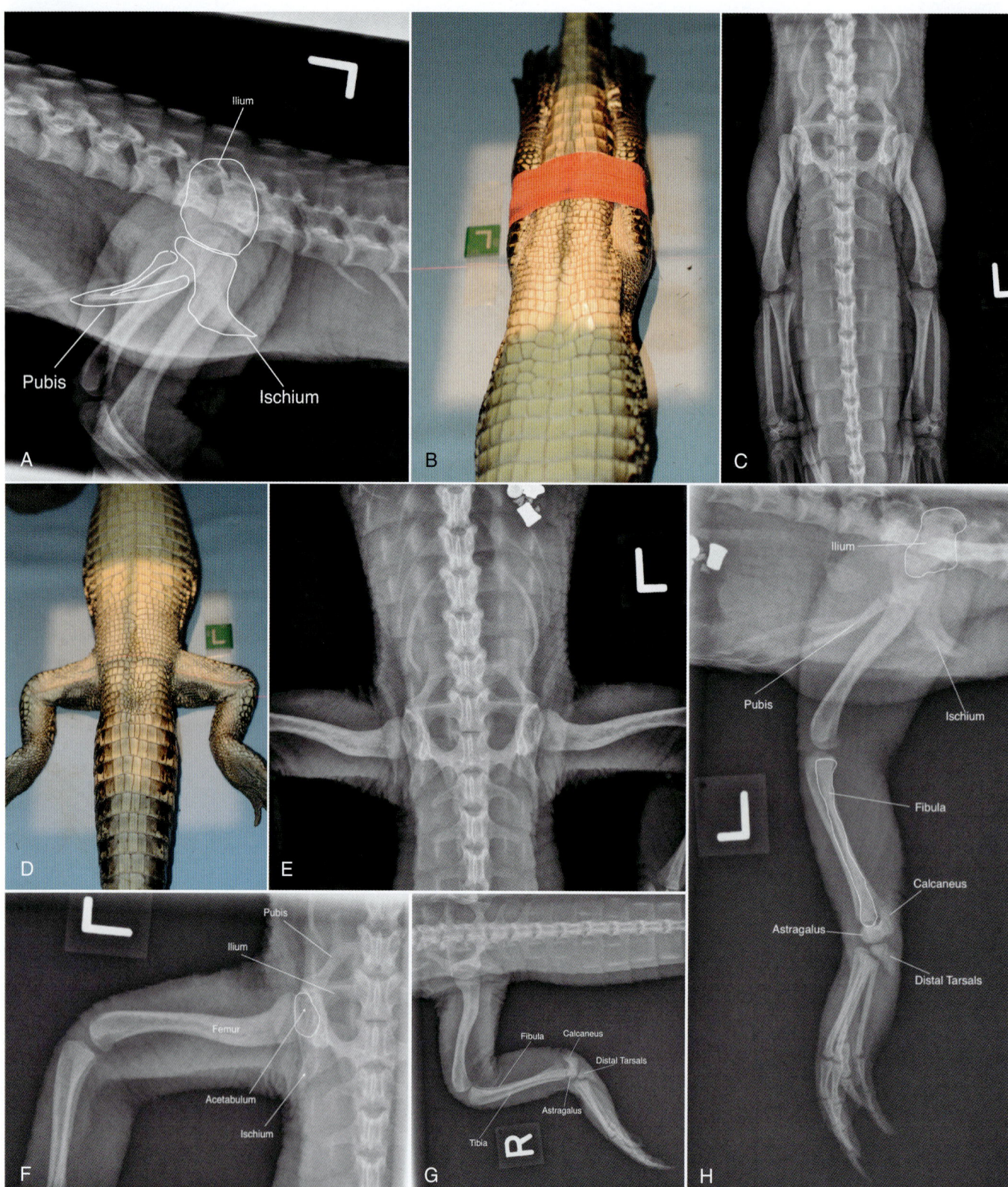

FIG 57.14 (A) Lateral radiograph of the pelvis with hind legs in a neutral position (American alligator, *Alligator mississippiensis*). (B) Positioning is shown for the VD pelvis extended radiograph. With the alligator in dorsal recumbency, the legs are taped parallel to the body wall without being distorted or rotated. (C) The VD extended pelvic radiograph, positioned with the alligator in dorsal recumbency. (D) Photograph of the alligator in dorsal recumbency with the hind legs in a neutral position. This positioning can also be used for lateral radiographs of the hind legs. (E) VD radiographs with hind legs in neutral position as in (D). This view highlights the femoral heads and acetabula. (F) Lateral radiograph of the femur and stifle. (G) Lateral view of the right hind leg. (H) Lateral radiograph of the left hind leg. The alligator was positioned in lateral recumbency versus (G), which was in dorsal with the right hind leg at 90-degree angles of the joints. (Courtesy of Natalie Rademacher.)

58

Ultrasonography

Claudia Hochleithner and Ajay Sharma

Ultrasonography has been used in small animal medicine routinely for more than 25 years. It has become a valuable imaging technique. Early sonographers of reptile patients adapted established small animal imaging techniques to the special anatomic features encountered within the wide range of animals in this class.[1–7] With continuing advances in ultrasound machines and transducers, the often small size of reptilian or amphibian patients is less of an obstacle. It is possible to perform ultrasonography even in small geckos or chameleons, with transducer frequencies of 10, 12, or even 18 and higher MHz. However, several unique considerations still must be kept in mind during ultrasonography of these species and will be discussed.

EQUIPMENT

Given the advances in ultrasound technology and equipment over the last several decades, good-quality scanners with high-frequency transducers are available for a reasonable price. A single, all-encompassing transducer does not exist because of the wide range of anatomic situations that may be encountered. Relatively inexpensive portable ultrasound units are now available, and selection should be based on image quality and intended use. Transducer selection is equally important and is based on patients' body shape and size. Three commonly used transducers are linear, microconvex, and convex probes (Fig. 58.1). The name refers to the shape and footprint of the transducer and is often associated with the frequency. Typically, linear transducers have flat surfaces and high frequencies (12–18 MHz); microconvex transducers have small curved surfaces and midrange frequencies (8–11 MHz) and convex transducers have large curved surfaces and low frequencies (1–5 MHz). Sector transducers have largely been replaced by modern electronic transducers. The range of frequencies varies with manufacturer. For snakes and lizards the linear transducers are generally recommended (Fig. 58.2). In lizards, alternating between linear and microconvex transducers may be required to evaluate the cranial coelomic cavity and liver due to the convexity of the rib cage. For chelonians, a microconvex transducer or convex transducer with a small footprint is advantageous because it fits in the curved contours of the small sonographic windows cervical and axillary to the thoracic limbs and cranial to the pelvic limbs. The frequency of the transducer depends on the size of the animal to be examined. High-frequency transducers have the advantage of superior spatial resolution, yielding excellent detail of superficial structures but have limited depth of penetration. Lower frequency transducers, although lacking in fine anatomic resolution, have the ability to penetrate deeper. Therefore, in smaller lizards high-frequency transducers (12–18 MHz) yield the best results. In larger lizards, such as iguanas, (8–11 MHz) linear or microconvex transducers are recommended. For larger patients such as giant tortoises, frequencies from 2.5 to 5 MHz are recommended.[1–3, 8–18]

SPECIAL CONSIDERATIONS

Not only must the equipment and sonography suite be adapted to the special requirements of reptiles, but the practitioner must also be aware of the wide variation in norms among the various species that may be encountered. There is a tendency to overinterpret normal structures in unfamiliar species. Whenever possible, known standards should be consulted, whether it be a different animal of the same or similar species or a published description of normal findings in that species.[1–20]

It is difficult to accumulate expertise and perform a thorough evaluation when sonographic evaluations are limited by the short periods of time typically available between appointments. Ultrasonography, especially in unfamiliar species, is not a quick procedure. Therefore the examination room and furniture should be ergonomically comfortable

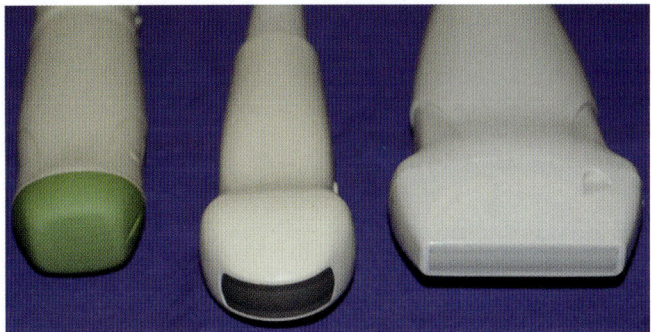

FIG 58.1 Ultrasound probes from left to right: phased array probe 5 to 7.5 MHz; microconvex probe 5 to 8 MHz; linear probe 10 to 18 MHz from Haslauer-Medizintechnik/Esaote Europe.

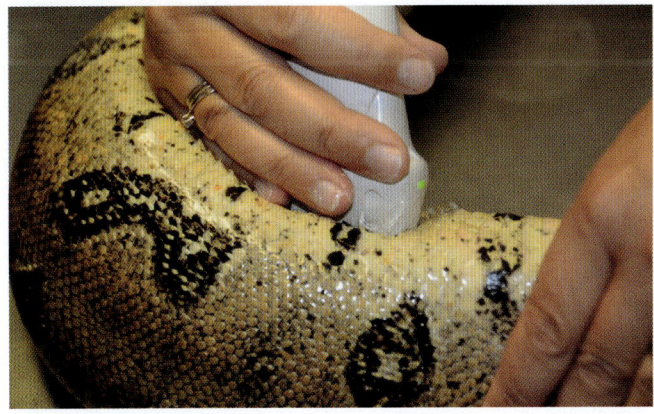

FIG 58.2 Performing ultrasound with a linear probe on a boa constrictor in a longitudinal plane; the green light indicates the cranial orientation of the indicator mark.

for the sonographer and the client, as well as for the persons handling the patient. A dim but not completely darkened room provides the best environment for viewing the monitor during the examination.

Proficiency in reptile ultrasonography is not easily acquired. Basic technical ultrasound skills needed to use the equipment and accurate interpretation of the findings are necessary. It is advantageous to have training/experience in small animal ultrasonography in order to gain familiarity with the scanning technique and operation of the machine. Small animal patients are, in general, easier to evaluate and have a more uniform, familiar anatomy.[1–7] When the sonographer has accumulated this basic knowledge, the more variable anatomy and unique sonographic appearances of reptile organs are more easily interpreted. Published literature in peer-reviewed journals and material acquired from books, seminars, conferences, and laboratories can be invaluable.[1–3] To improve image interpretation skills, one may also evaluate the organs of postmortem specimens in a water bath (Fig. 58.3). This reduces artifacts caused by skin, scales, and other surrounding tissues and allows a more thorough evaluation of the viscera. Any abnormalities detected should ultimately be correlated with surgical, necropsy, and histopathological findings (Fig. 58.4A and B) to clarify the etiology of the disease process.

INDICATIONS

Ultrasound is often used as a tool for further imaging of a suspected abnormality; although, in many circumstances, ultrasonography has a clear advantage over radiology or endoscopy and may be chosen as the primary imaging modality.

Coelomic enlargements of unclear origin (e.g., tumors and ascites), along with reproductive monitoring, are the most common indications for ultrasonography. Any kind of enlargement on the animal's body can be scanned and interpreted to better characterize the nature of the swelling. Ultrasound-guided aspirates and biopsies may also be performed, but the need for these procedures should be evaluated in

conjunction with possible risks such as organ perforation and hemorrhage.[15,16] Reptile echocardiography is a relatively young field, but with improving equipment and continuing publications, the practical clinical utility of this ultrasound application will continue to increase.

PATIENT PREPARATION

Positioning of the patient must be adapted to what the patient will tolerate while allowing access to the anatomic regions of interest. Typically, dorsal recumbency is the most useful position, but an upright position may also be helpful, especially in weak lizards and in iguanas (Fig. 58.5). Large snakes need more personnel to hold them comfortably for this procedure. In aggressive reptiles, sedation should be used to minimize the stress for the animal and the risk to the patient and veterinary staff. Sedation or anesthesia can facilitate positioning and reduce movement artifacts.

It is important to develop a routine scanning technique that allows evaluation of all typically detectable organs so that an important sonographic finding is not missed. Whenever possible, each organ should be scanned in two planes: usually transverse and sagittal/longitudinal. Oblique scanning planes are also frequently used to evaluate organs and pathology of variable shape and anatomic location. The probe

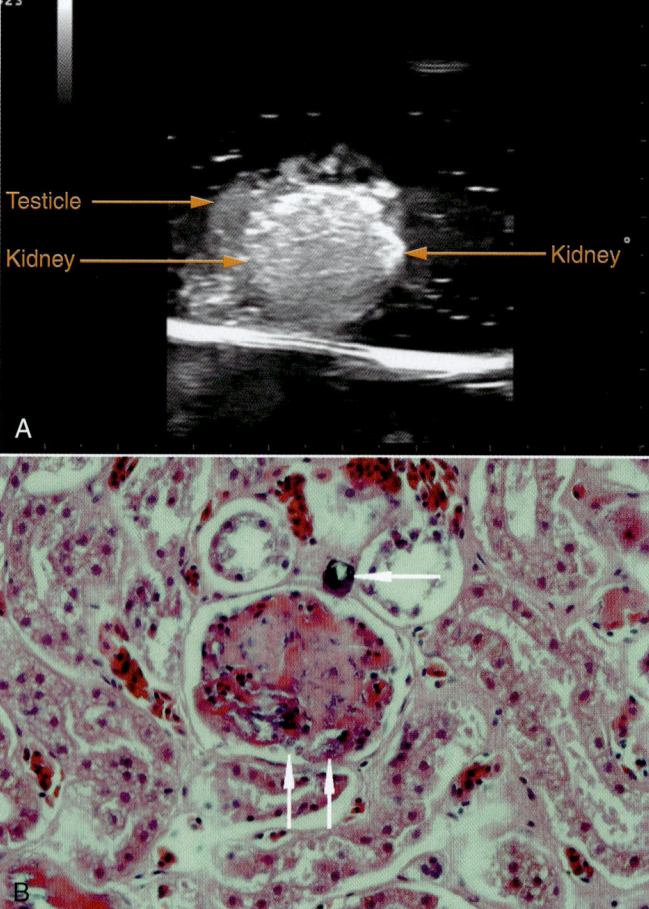

FIG 58.4 (A) Postmortem ultrasonographic images of kidney and testis of a Greek tortoise (*Testudo hermanni*) in a water bath. (B) Histopathology of the same kidney, demonstrating interstitial (a) and glomerular (b) calcium deposition. (H&E, ×400). (Courtesy of Dr. Anna Kübber-Heiss Research Institute of Wildlife Ecology, University of Veterinary Medicine Vienna).

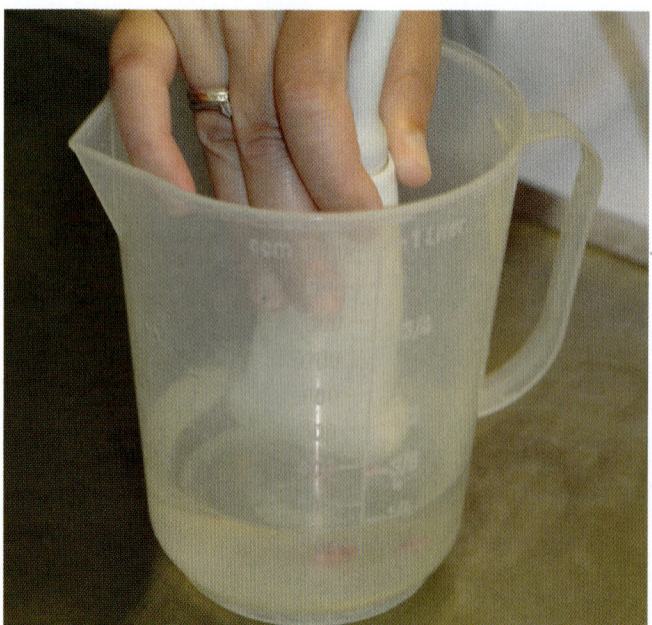

FIG 58.3 Water bath for investigating postmortem organs or tumors after surgery; results can be compared with histopathologic findings or can be used for self-training.

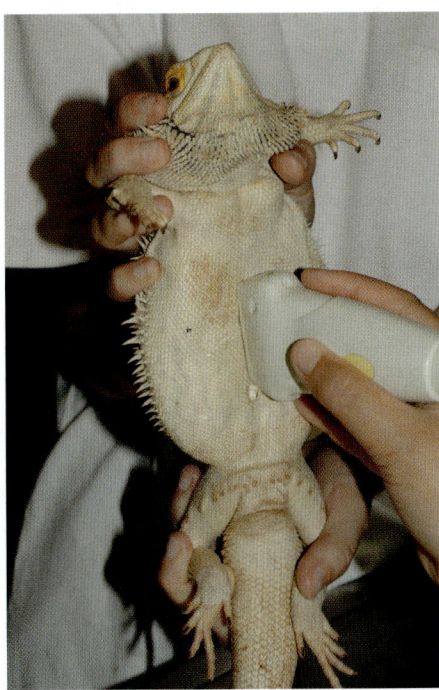

FIG 58.5 Upright positioning for weak patients. A bearded dragon (*Pogona vitticeps*) is held while ultrasonography is performed.

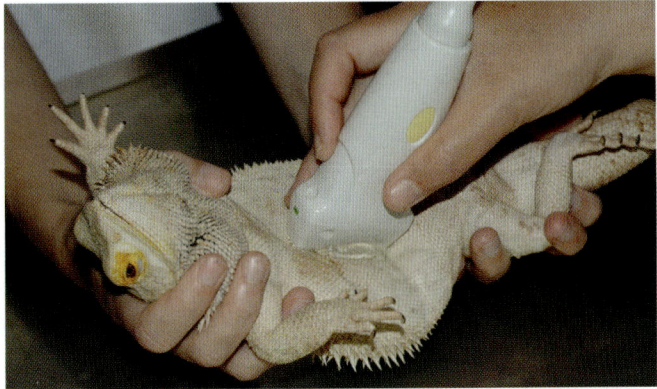

FIG 58.6 Positioning of the probe in a longitudinal view of a bearded dragon (*Pogona vitticeps*).

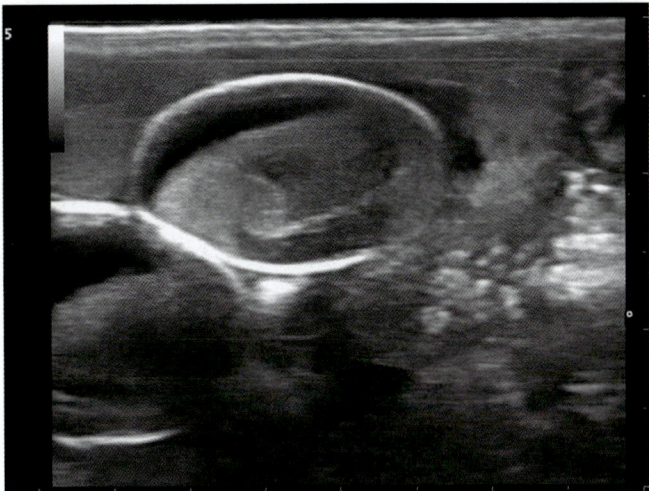

FIG 58.7 Sagittal plane image of an egg in the bearded dragon (*Pogona vitticeps*) from Fig. 58.6. The hyperechogenic oval structure is the shell, the hypoechoic part is the albumin, and the rest of the content is the developing vitellogenic mass shortly before laying.

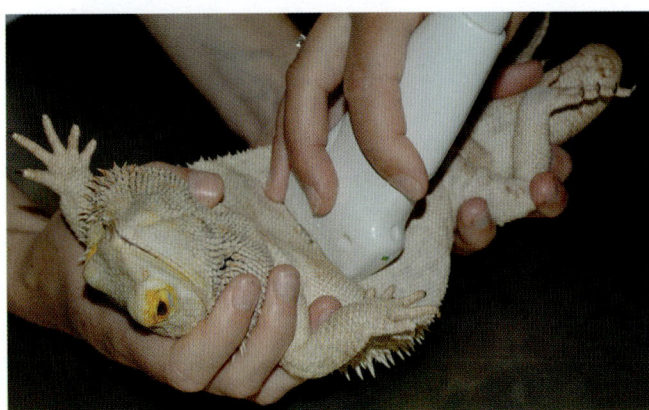

FIG 58.8 Positioning of the probe in a transverse imaging plane in a bearded dragon (*Pogona vitticeps*).

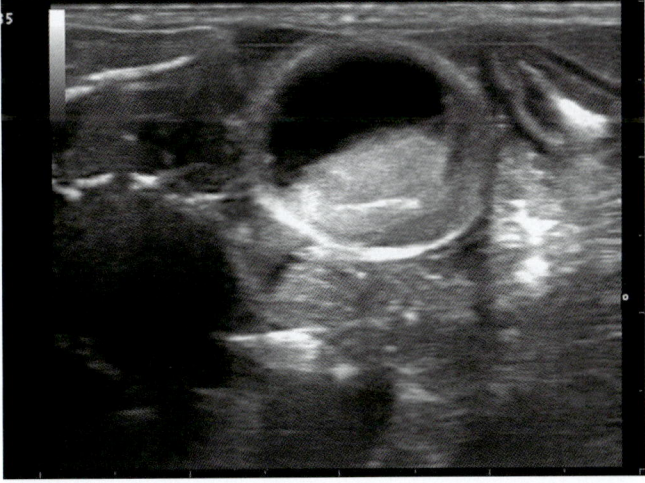

FIG 58.9 Transverse plane image of an egg in the bearded dragon (*Pogona vitticeps*) from Fig. 58.8.

should always be held in the same fashion such that the sonographer is oriented to the spatial relationship between the tissues being scanned and their appearance on the screen.[8–12,16,17,18] Standard convention dictates that when the patient is in dorsal recumbency, the head is on the left side or facing away from a right-handed sonographer, and the transducer is gripped so that the indicator of the probe shows either cranially or to the right side of the patient's body (Figs. 58.6–58.9). When this technique is used, the left side of the image on the monitor is cranial in a longitudinal/sagittal view and represents the patient's right in a transverse view (Fig. 58.10). Ample coupling gel must be applied to the skin surface. A gel bottle warmer should be used to prevent cooling of the patient. Better images can be obtained if the skin is moistened with warm water before the coupling gel is applied, because contact is improved and trapped air bubbles that can attenuate the sound beam are reduced. In smaller patients, a stand-off pad to fill the space between the skin and the transducer surface may be helpful. An examination glove filled with warm water is a useful substitution for an expensive stand-off that can easily conform to the desired shape (Fig. 58.11). Coating the standoff pad with coupling gel further enhances the image quality.

If the pressure of the probe on the patient's body is excessive, artifacts and inaccurate findings may result; excessive transducer pressure can result in compression and displacement of organs from their normal position, especially in snakes.

Although ultrasonography is an excellent tool to investigate the organs of the coelomic cavity, some circumstances can complicate this procedure. Patients undergoing or soon to be undergoing ecdysis are

poor candidates, because air between the layers of the skin attenuates the majority of the sound waves, resulting in poor penetration of deeper tissues. Some species with ossified scales (e.g., *Tiliqua* spp. and *Heloderma* spp.) are also poor candidates, because the ossified scales hinder penetration of the ultrasound beam. Additional limitations may be associated with increased intestinal gas or coelomic gas due to recent surgical or laparoscopic procedures.

SCANNING PATTERN

The geometrically simple shape of the snake lends itself to the most straightforward method of sonographic examination.[19] The heart is a useful starting point for establishing appropriate depth and settings on the machine. Blood in the vessels and chambers should be relatively hypoechoic to the cardiac muscle, and the valves should appear as hyperechoic lines. The body must to be scanned in sagittal, transverse, and dorsal (coronal) views caudally to the level of the cloaca (Fig. 58.12).

In lizards, the liver and the gallbladder should be evaluated first. Adjustments should be made to the machine at this time to optimize image quality before proceeding with the rest of the examination. Next, the examination should move cranially to investigate the heart and then back again caudally with transverse and longitudinal views to investigate the fat bodies, gastrointestinal tract, gonads, urinary bladder (if present), and, finally, the kidneys.[18,20]

Chelonians, except for soft-shelled species, are more challenging because they only have three useful acoustic windows to the coelomic cavity.[12] The three accessible sonographic windows are cervico-brachial (between the forelimb and caudal neck to investigate the heart and the liver); axillary (between the caudal aspect of the forelimb and the cranial margin of the plastrocarapacial bridge for the heart and the liver); and prefemoral (between the caudal margin of the plastrocarapacial bridge and the cranial aspect of the pelvic limb to assess the intestine, reproductive, and urinary systems (Fig. 58.13). In soft-shelled chelonians (e.g., *Apalone* spp.), it is possible to scan the coelomic viscera through the plastron. This is occasionally also possible in neonates or diseased chelonians with poorly mineralized plastrons (Fig. 58.14A and B).

Organs are evaluated by measuring size, shape, and margination. Changes in echogenicity, either focal or diffuse, should be visualized and recorded. The gastrointestinal tract is investigated as in small

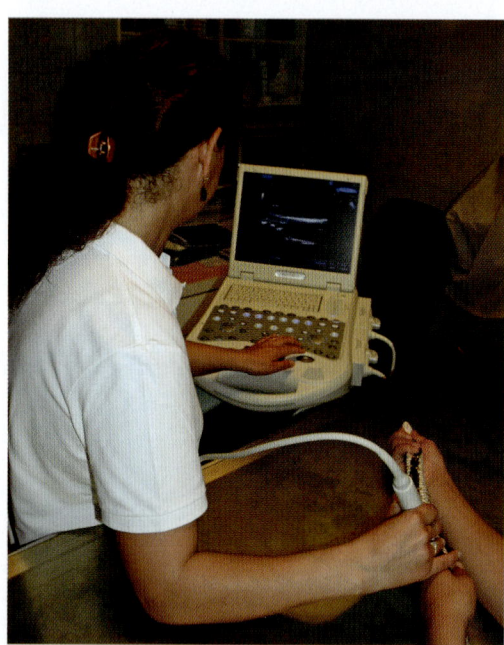

FIG 58.10 In dorsal recumbency, the head of the reptile is on the left side or facing away from a right-handed sonographer, so the indicator of the probe shows either cranially (in this picture) or to the right side of the patient's body.

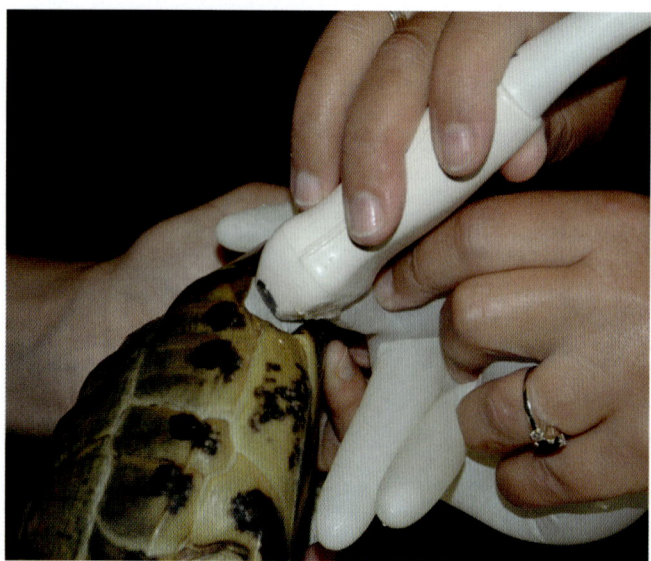

FIG 58.11 In tortoises, an examination glove filled with warm water can be used as a standoff pad in the prefemoral window.

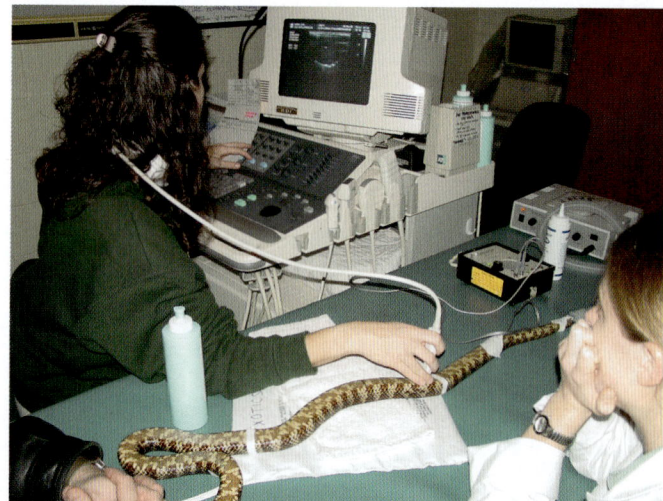

FIG 58.12 The simple shape of the snake lends itself to the most straightforward method of sonographic examination from cranial to caudal. All three planes should be scanned: sagittal, transverse, and dorsal.

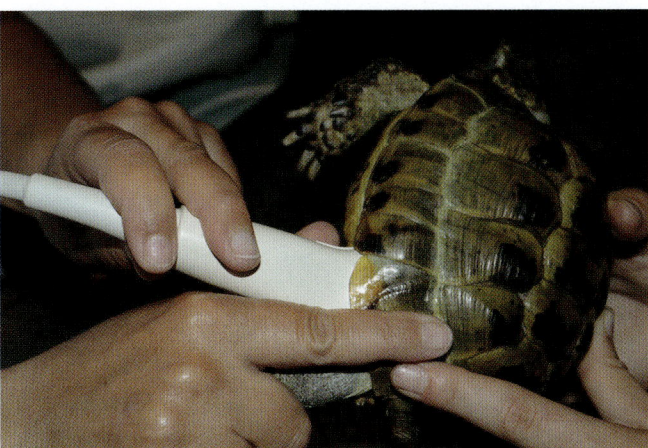

FIG 58.13 Prefemoral window to assess the intestine, urogenital tract, and the bladder in chelonians.

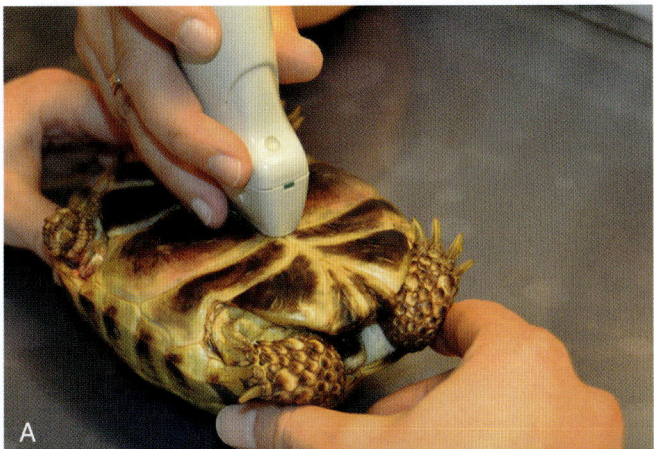

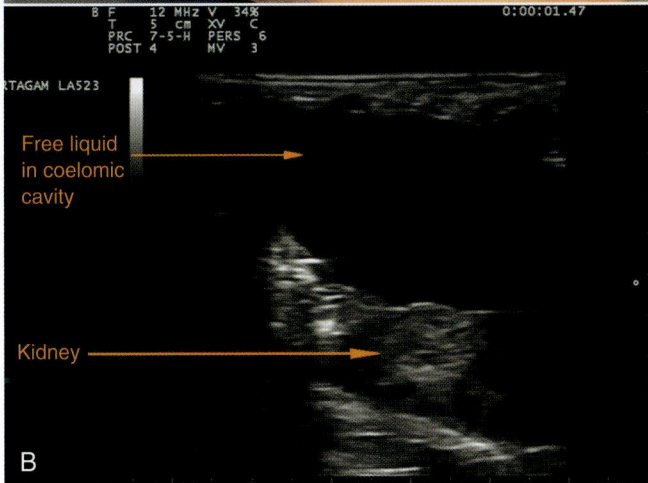

FIG 58.14 (A) In diseased tortoises, it may be possible to scan the coelomic viscera through the plastron. (B) Ultrasound image of the coelomic cavity of a diseased tortoise (histologic findings in Fig. 58.4B) with renal failure due to secondary nutritional hyperparathyroidism.

animals for motility, mural thickness, patency, and foreign content. With high-frequency transducers, intestinal wall layering can be appreciated (Fig. 58.15).

The gonads are evaluated for size and shape to interpret the reproductive stage in both sexes. The kidneys are assessed for size and changes

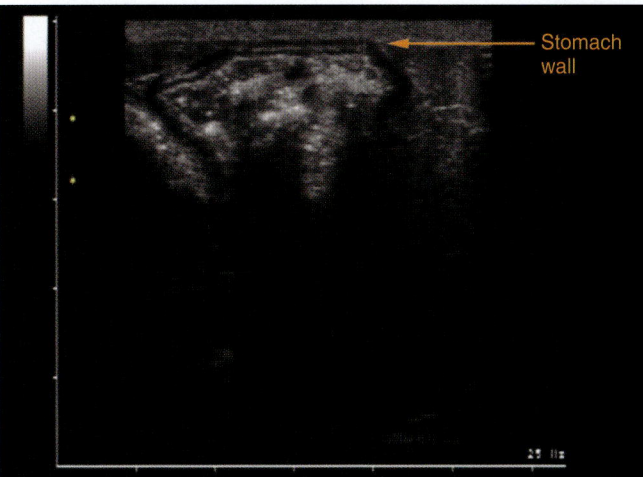

FIG 58.15 Ultrasound image of the different layers of the wall of the stomach of a Savannah monitor (*Varanus exanthematicus*). The first layer is the small hyperechoic line of the serosa, followed by the low echogenic muscularis layer; next is the higher echogenic submucosa, then the less echogenic mucosa, and the last layer is the highly echogenic mucosal surface, beneath which is seen the content of the stomach as a heterogeneous mass, with some parts showing distal attenuation of the ultrasound beam (gas).

in echogenicity. The urinary bladder, when present, should be investigated for foreign material (e.g., calculi or ectopic eggs). Free coelomic fluid can be detected and assessed for echogenicity, amount, and cellular or presence of flocculent material.

CARDIOVASCULAR SYSTEM

Ultrasonography can also be helpful for identifying blood vessels and guiding cannulation. Real-time ultrasound needle guidance with an in-plane/long-axis technique optimizes the probability of catheter placement. Ultrasound guidance can be used not only for central venous cannulation but also in peripheral and arterial cannulation.[17] For echocardiography, see Chapter 68.

THE LIVER

The liver is characterized by a homogenous relatively hypoechoic appearance compared to the fat body, and with anechoic vessels. Anechoic vessels. In lizards and chelonians, the liver is bilobed. The anechoic gallbladder is attached to the right lobe[1–3,11,18] (Fig. 58.16). With proper equipment, the portal vein, hepatic veins, and the caudal vena cava can be individually assessed (Fig. 58.17).

In snakes, the liver extends caudally from the level of the lungs, where it occupies approximately the middle third of the length of the body. Two large vessels (the hepatic portal vein located dorsally and the ventral hepatic vein ventrally) run from cranial to caudal through the length of the organ (Figs. 58.18 and 58.19). The anechoic gallbladder is not associated with the hepatic parenchyma as it is in lizards and chelonians. Rather, the gallbladder is separate, caudal to the liver, and is visible as an anechoic round or slightly oval structure[8,9] (Fig. 58.20). The liver can usually be easily differentiated from the fat body (Fig. 58.21 and 58.22).

Size and echotexture of the liver should be assessed; changes can be either focal, multifocal (see Fig. 58.21), or diffuse throughout the organ. These changes can be distinctly or indistinctly marginated, which can give a hint to the underlying process. Hyperechogenicity and enlargement of the liver are seen with fatty liver degeneration (Fig. 58.23). A heterogeneous pattern of the liver parenchyma with anechoic areas is common with focal necrosis or inflammation (Fig. 58.24). Anechoic round or oval structures can be visualized in connection with cystic change (Fig. 58.25). Hyperechoic particles in the gallbladder can be visualized as signs of thickening of the bile. Hyperechoic and heteroechoic lesions, usually focal and occasionally attached to the gallbladder, may represent abscessation[14] (Fig. 58.26).

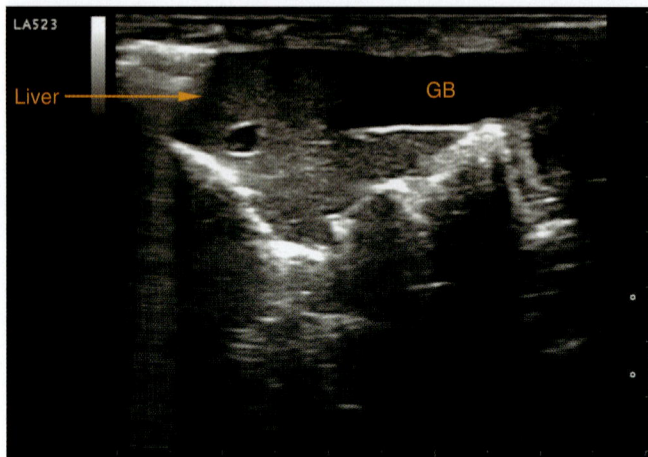

FIG 58.16 Ultrasound image of the homogenous hypoechogenic texture of the liver with the anechoic gallbladder (GB) attached to the right lobe in a green iguana (*Iguana iguana*).

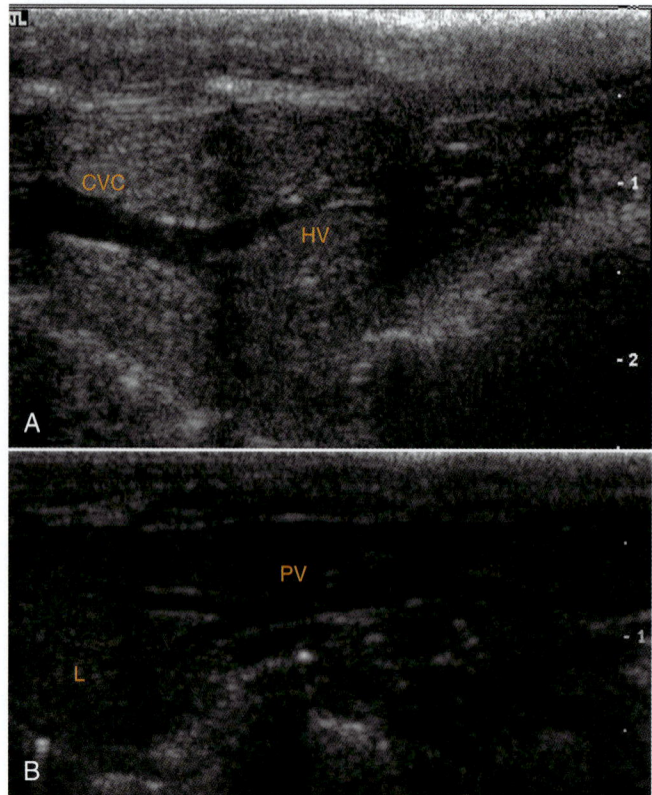

FIG 58.17 (A) Oblique plane ultrasound image showing a hepatic vein (*HV*) entering the caudal vena cava (CVC) within the liver of a healthy green iguana (Iguana iguana). (B) Sagittal plane ultrasound image showing the portal vein (PV) in a healthy green iguana originating in the caudal coelom and arborizing into the liver (L) on the left side of the image. (Courtesy of Mason Holland).

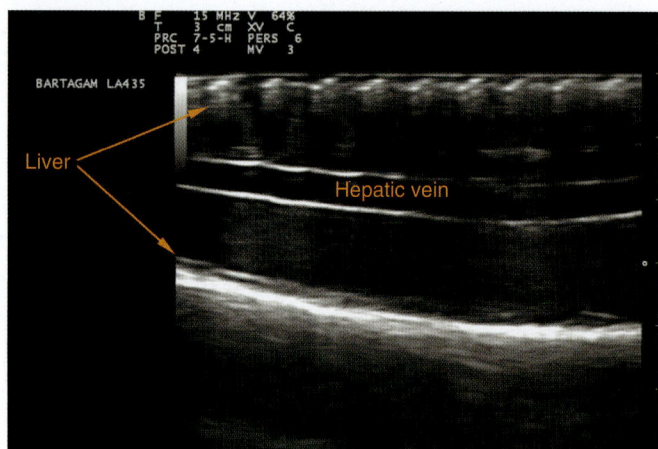

FIG 58.18 Sagittal plane image of the homogenous hypoechoic liver with the central hepatic vein in a ball python (*Python regius*). In this image, only the ventral vein is seen as the probe is held slightly paramedian.

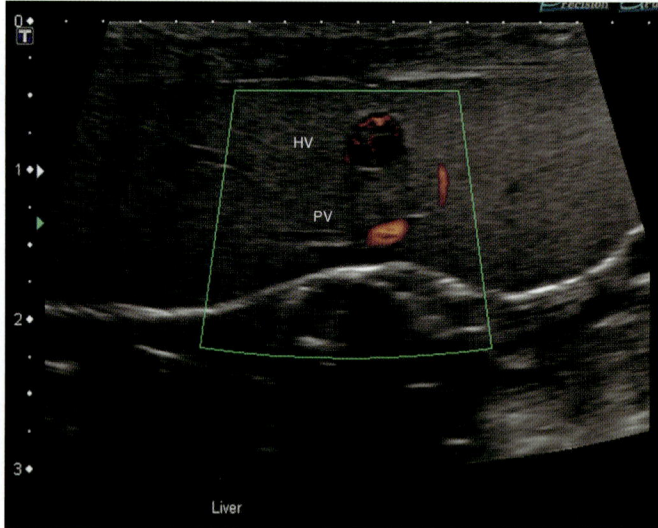

FIG 58.19 Transverse image of a liver showing two large vessels (the hepatic portal vein located dorsally and the vena hepatica ventrally) in a timber rattlesnake (*Crotalus horridus*).

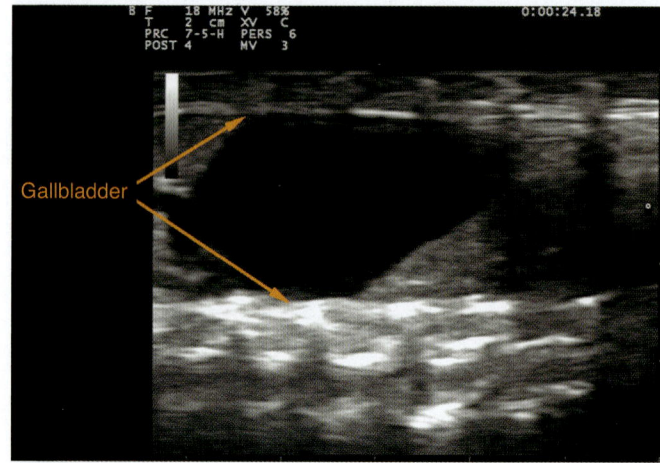

FIG 58.20 The gallbladder of snakes, here a western hognose (*Heterodon nasicus*), appears as a round to oval anechoic structure caudally separated from the liver.

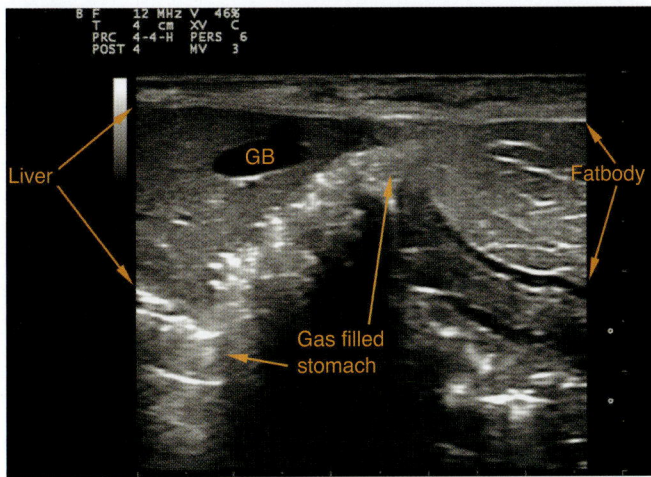

FIG 58.21 Ultrasound image of the echotexture of the liver in comparison with the higher echogenicity of the fat body and the characteristic hyperechoic lines in between the fat in a green iguana (*Iguana iguana*). Between the liver and the fat body is the gas-filled stomach, causing distal attenuation of the ultrasound beam. GB, Gall bladder.

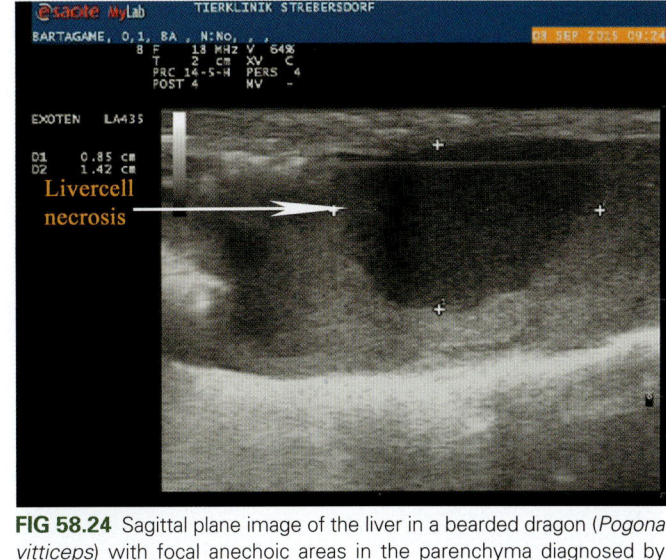

FIG 58.24 Sagittal plane image of the liver in a bearded dragon (*Pogona vitticeps*) with focal anechoic areas in the parenchyma diagnosed by cytology as focal necrosis.

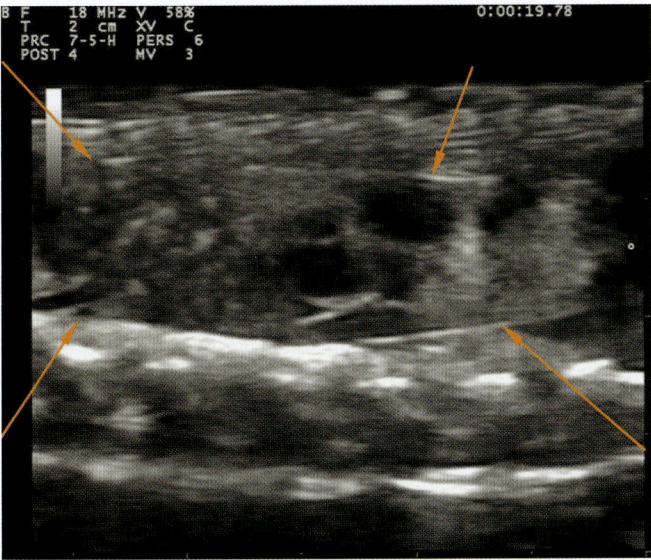

FIG 58.22 Ultrasound image of the liver (margins indicated with *arrows*) of a western hognose (*Heterodon nasicus*) showing a highly heterogeneous pattern throughout the whole liver with round to oval anechoic structures, characteristic of cystic change. Histopathology confirmed liver carcinoma with cystic abnormalities.

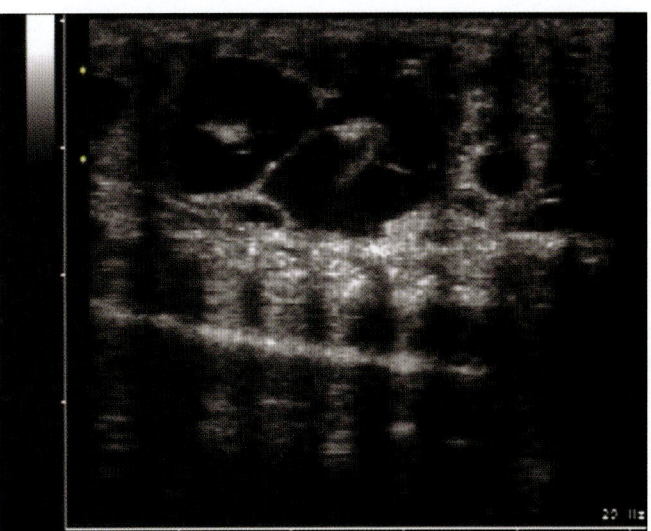

FIG 58.25 Ultrasound image of multiple anechoic structures in the liver of a kingsnake (*Lampropeltis* sp.) consistent with cysts (sagittal plane). Histopathology confirmed hepatic cystic adenocarcinoma.

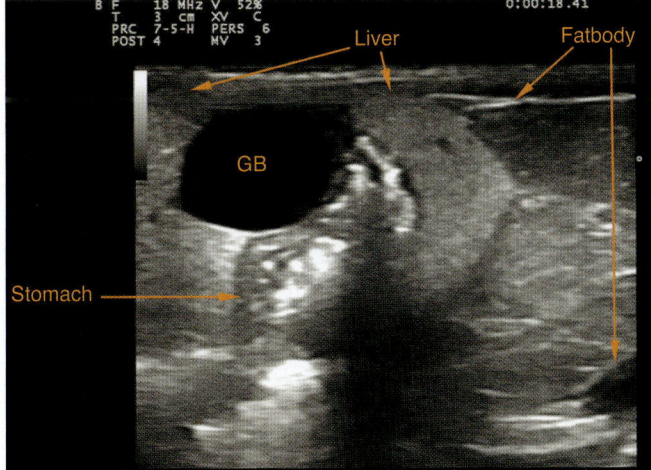

FIG 58.23 Sagittal plane image of fatty liver degeneration in a bearded dragon (*Pogona vitticeps*). The liver shows greater echogenicity than the fat body. In the middle of the figure, deep to the gallbladder (GB), the stomach filled with ingesta and gas is visible.

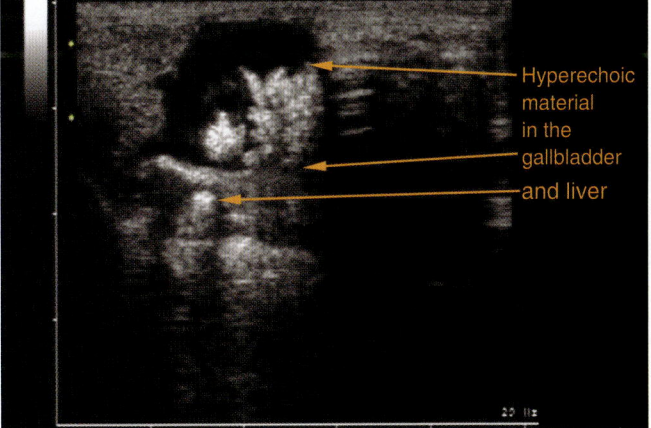

FIG 58.26 Ultrasound image of hyperechoic material in the lumen of the gallbladder and the surrounding liver tissue secondary to an abscess in a bearded dragon (*Pogona vitticeps*).

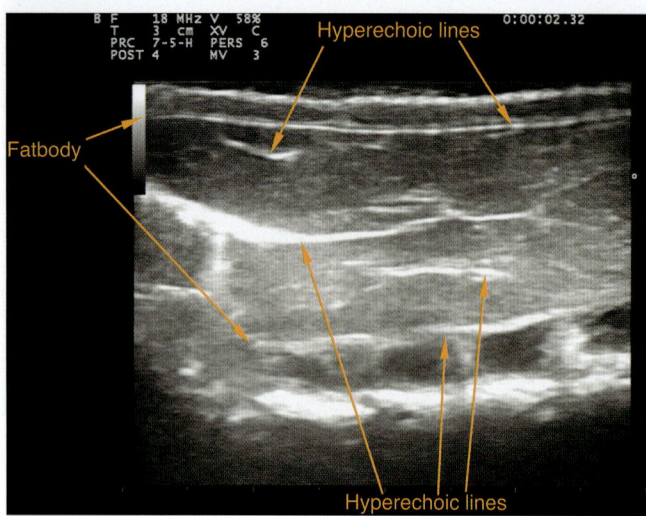

FIG 58.27 Ultrasound image of the fat body in a bearded dragon (*Pogona vitticeps*) with normal hyperechoic lines in between the fat.

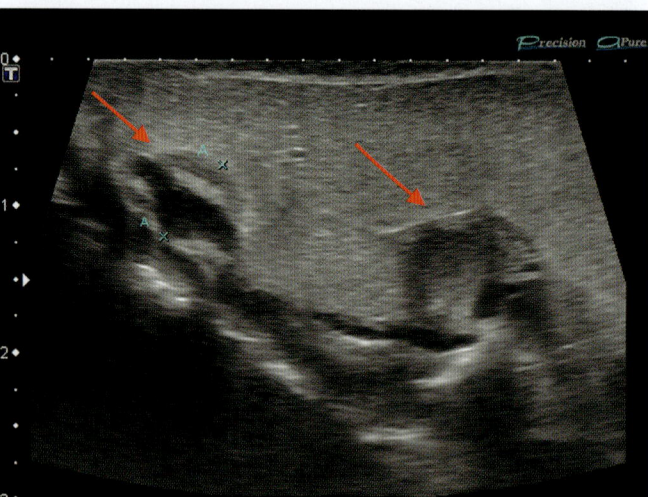

FIG 58.29 Sagittal image of heterogeneous cavitary nodules (*arrows*) in the fat body of an 8-year-old bearded dragon (*Pogona vitticeps*).

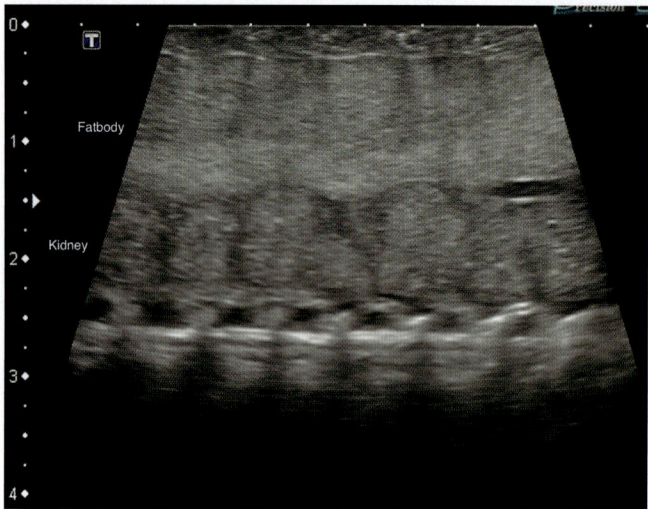

FIG 58.28 Sagittal image of the fat body (near field) and kidney (far field) in a timber rattlesnake (*Crotalus horridus*).

THE FAT BODY

The fat body varies in size, shape, and location depending on the species and body condition of the patient. Normally, they are paired structures that lie laterally within the coelom, extending cranially from the caudolateral coelom. They are hyperechoic to the liver and contain curvilinear hyperechoic septae between fat lobules (Figs. 58.27 and 58.28). Internal vasculature of the fat bodies will be less than that seen within the liver, which is useful to differentiate these two structures. The size of the fat bodies can provide a general assessment of the body condition of the animal (from emaciation through obesity). If a small amount of free fluid is present in the coelomic cavity (a common, normal finding), the fat bodies are easily distinguished. Abscesses, granulomas, or neoplasia (Fig. 58.29) can be visualized as round, sometimes hyperechoic, sharply delineated structures with central hypoechoic/anechoic regions. Dystrophic mineralization or crystal formation in the fat pads are discernible by evidence of hyperechoic foci.

GASTROINTESTINAL TRACT

The gastrointestinal tract and the relationship between the size of the different portions varies greatly depending on dietary classification (whether herbivore, omnivore, or carnivore). In carnivorous reptiles, the stomach is large, and longitudinal folds can be visualized; the intestine is smaller and shorter compared with herbivores. In herbivores, the stomach is smaller and has a thin wall, and the intestine (especially the large intestine) is elongated and often voluminous with mucosal folds. Depending on the size of the animal and the frequency of the transducer, intestinal wall layering can be visualized, similar to mammals and birds (Fig. 58.30A and B). Changes in motility, foreign bodies (Fig. 58.31), and large amounts of gas (Fig. 58.32) or impacted ingesta (such as sand impaction) can be visualized. Intestinal gas typically results in complete reflection of ultrasound waves, preventing assessment of deeper structures. This is especially true in herbivorous species.

Ultrasonography is often used after radiography, but it should be undertaken before gastrointestinal barium studies. Barium has the same effect as gas or stones in the gastrointestinal tract, absorbing and reflecting the sound waves and limiting evaluation. Iodinated contrast media is, however, typically sonolucent.

THE SPLEEN

The spleen is difficult to visualize because the organ is often located deep to the intestine, and evaluation is frequently limited by the presence of intestinal gas. Depending on the species, it is round to elongated and of variable, generally small size; the texture is homogenous with medium echogenicity and fine granular echotexture similar to the testes.[8–13,16,18,19,20] (Fig. 58.33) In male green iguanas (*Iguana iguana*) during breeding season, the spleen may be more easily seen because much of the adjacent intestine is displaced by hypertrophy of the adjacent testes (Fig. 58.34).[18]

THE GONADS

Ultrasonography is the noninvasive imaging modality of choice for evaluation of reproductive function, stage, and disease in (sub)adults

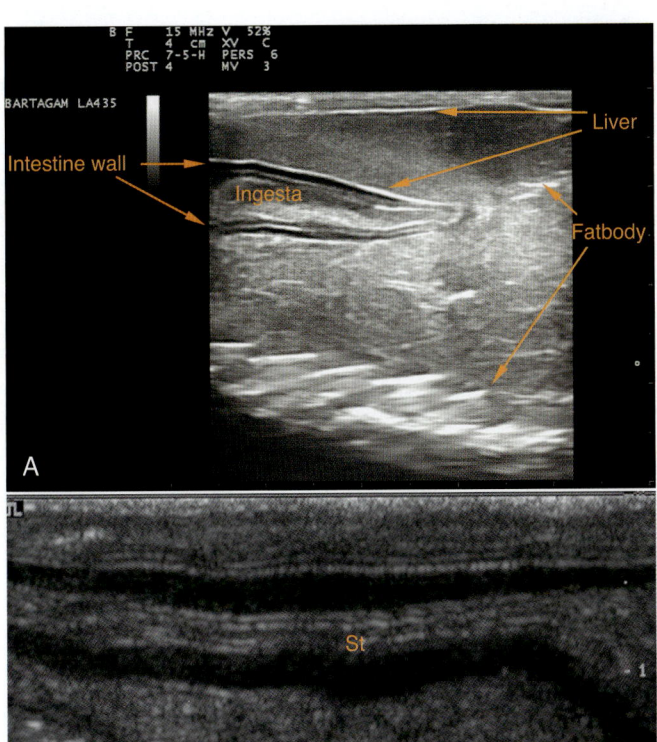

FIG 58.30 (A) Sagittal plane image of a portion of the intestine in a bearded dragon (*Pogona vitticeps*) filled with ingesta. Intestinal layering is visible. The first small hyperechoic layer next to the liver is the small line of the serosa, followed by the low echogenic muscularis layer; next is the higher echogenic submucosa, the low echogenic mucosa, and the highly echogenic mucosal surface, beneath which is seen the contents of the intestine (ingesta) as an heterogenous mass. Below the ingesta is the intestinal wall: small highly echogenic line of the mucosal surface, the low echogenic pattern of the mucosa, and the higher echogenic submucosa, followed by the low echogenic muscularis layer; next to the fat body, as the last outside layer, is the small hyperechoic line of the serosa. (B) Sagittal ultrasound image of the pyloric portion of a nondistended stomach (St) in a normal green iguana (*Iguana iguana*) showing prominent wall layering. A thick hypoechoic muscularis layer is present. Orad is to the right of the image.

and adults. Other applications include gender determination, evaluation of reproductive potential, and directing and assessing the efficacy of therapeutic interventions.[18–25]

Juvenile gonads are poorly visualized because they are obscured by the intestines and are frequently small in size (Fig. 58.35). The gonads lie in the caudal third of the coelom lateral to the aorta, with the right gonad slightly cranial to the left. Depending on the age of the patient and stage of reproductive cycle, the testes are ovoid and vary in size from barely visible to large and obvious; they are especially pronounced in bearded dragons (*Pogona vitticeps*) and green iguanas during breeding season (Fig. 58.36A–D). They show a fine, granular, homogenous echogenicity and are isoechoic to slightly hyperechoic to the liver.

The ovaries may be visualized, depending on their size. At the beginning of the reproductive cycle, the follicles are round and anechoic

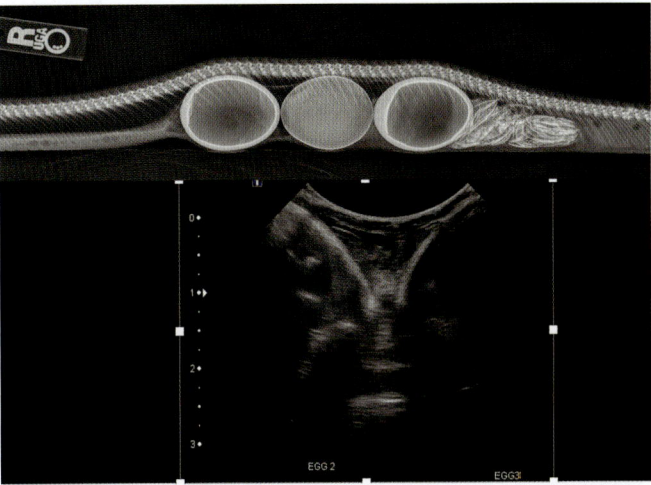

FIG 58.31 Sagittal image of the intestinal tract of a wild black rat snake (*Pantherophis obsoletus*) showing a natural egg (egg 2, echogenic contents) and a ceramic egg (egg 3, clean distal acoustic shadowing) and comparative radiography.

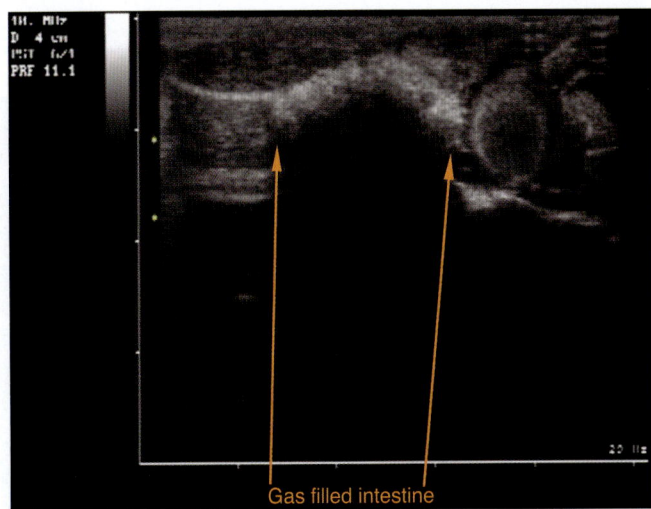

FIG 58.32 Ultrasound image of gas in the intestines with (distal) attenuation of the ultrasound beam in a bearded dragon (*Pogona vitticeps*).

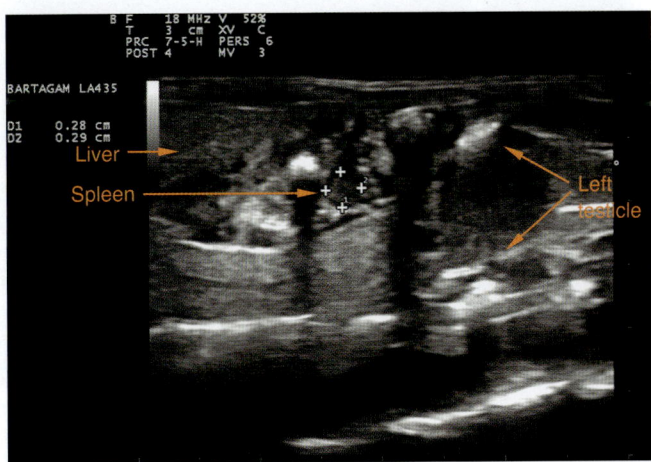

FIG 58.33 Ultrasound image of the spleen (+) in a bearded dragon (*Pogona vitticeps*) with adjacent intestine, liver, and left testis.

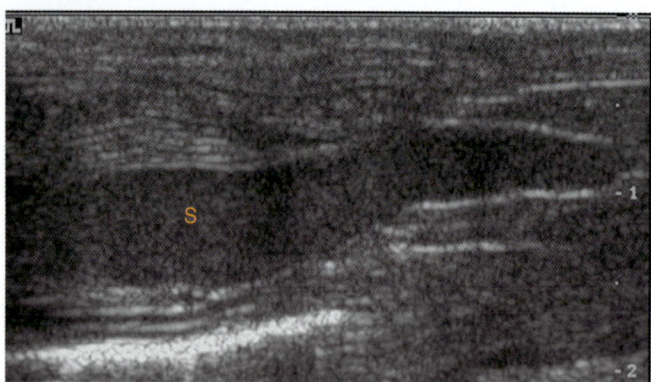

FIG 58.34 Sagittal image of the spleen (S) in a healthy male green iguana (*Iguana iguana*). Physiologically enlarged testes have displaced overlying intestine but are not visible in this image because they were displaced from the plane by transducer pressure.

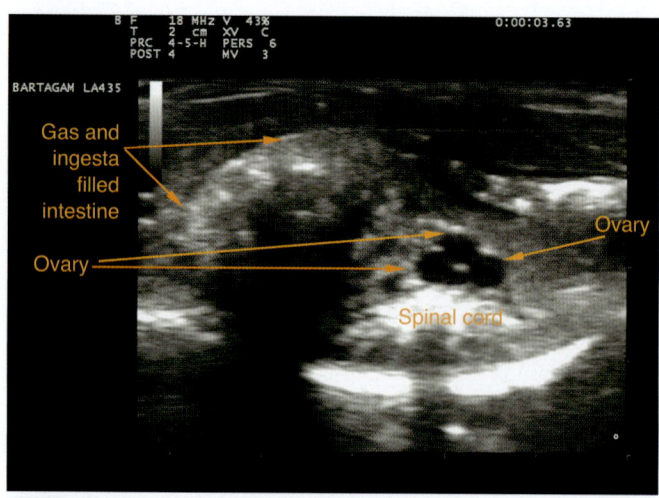

FIG 58.35 Ultrasound image in a transverse plane of the ovary as round anechoic structures ventral and lateral to the spinal cord in a 9-month-old Rankins dragon (*Pogona henrylawsoni*).

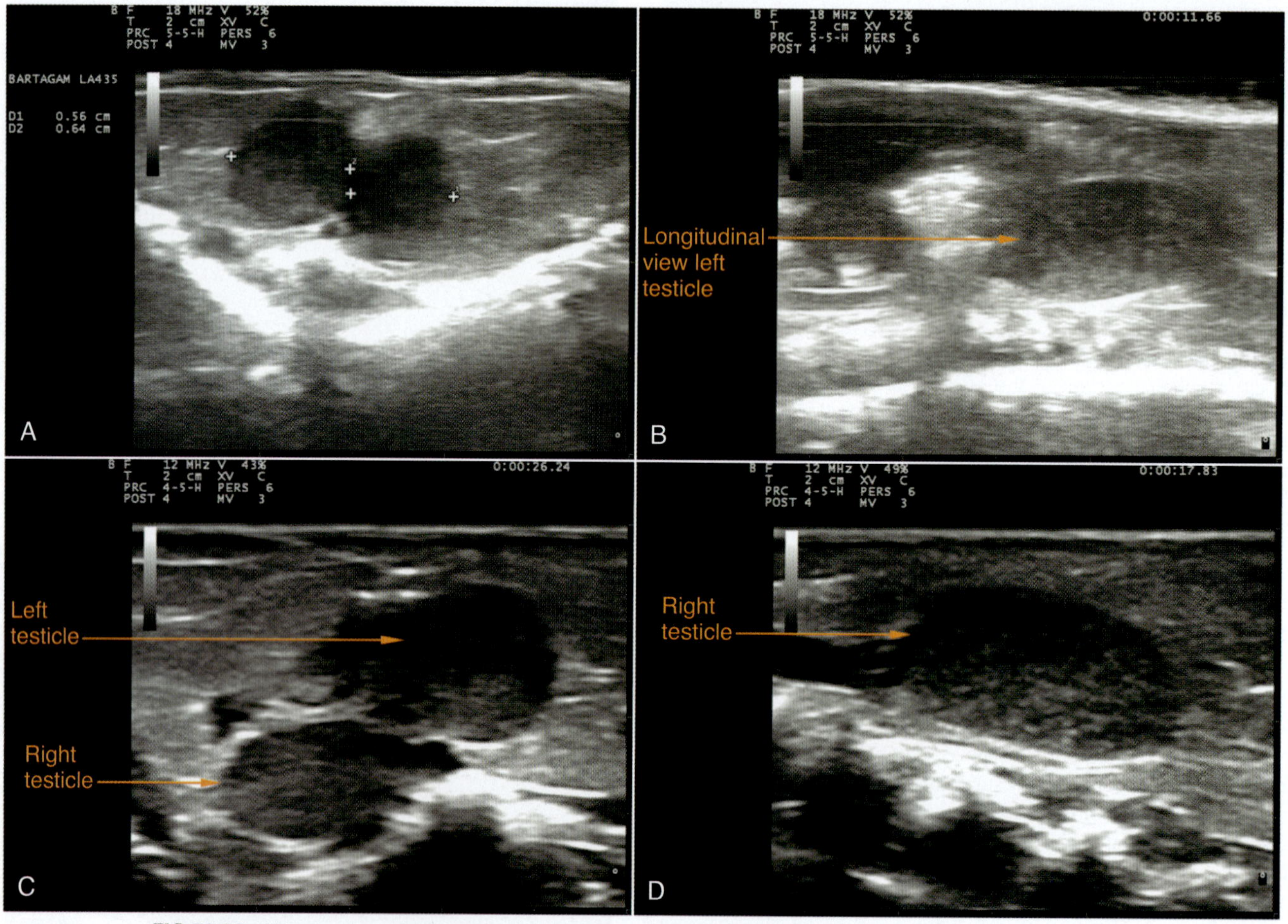

FIG 58.36 (A) Transverse plane image of the testes in a 9-month-old Rankins dragon (*Pogona henrylawsoni*). The right testis lies slightly cranial to the left, showing finely granular and homogenous echotexture. (B) Longitudinal ultrasound image of the left testis in the Rankins dragon from panel (A). (C) Transverse plane ultrasound image of the testes in an adult reproductively active bearded dragon (*Pogona vitticeps*). (D) Longitudinal view of the right testicle in the bearded dragon of panel (C).

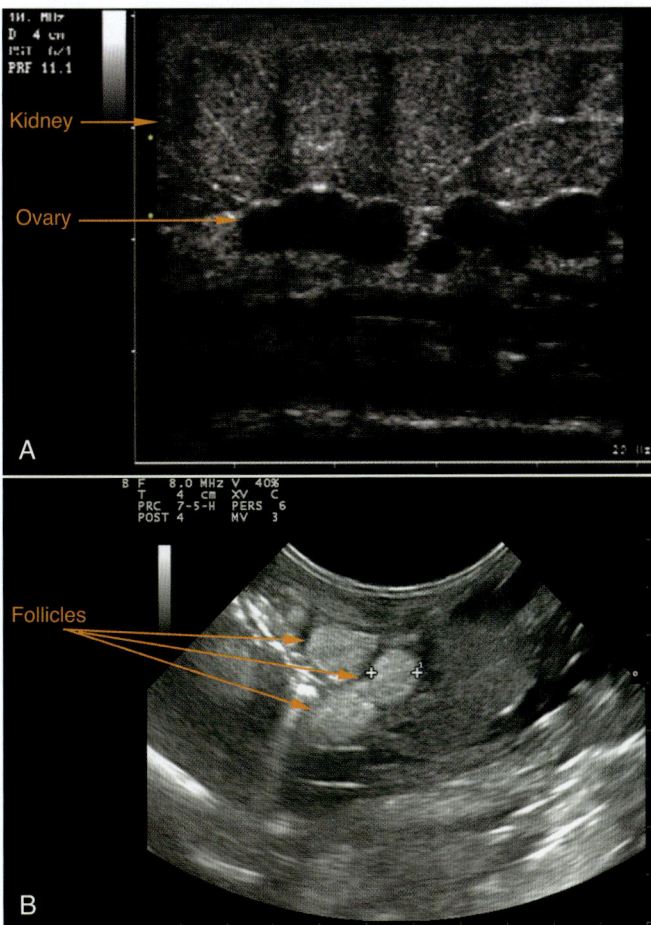

FIG 58.37 (A) Longitudinal slightly paramedian ultrasound image of the ovary in a green tree python (*Morelia viridis*). This is the beginning of the reproductive cycle, and different sizes of round, anechoic structures are aligned cranially to caudally. Laterally to the ovary, the right kidney is visualized. (B) Ultrasound image of the follicles in a red-eared slider (*Trachemys scripta elegans*). In tortoises, unlike snakes and lizards, the follicles already show a higher echogenicity at this early stage.

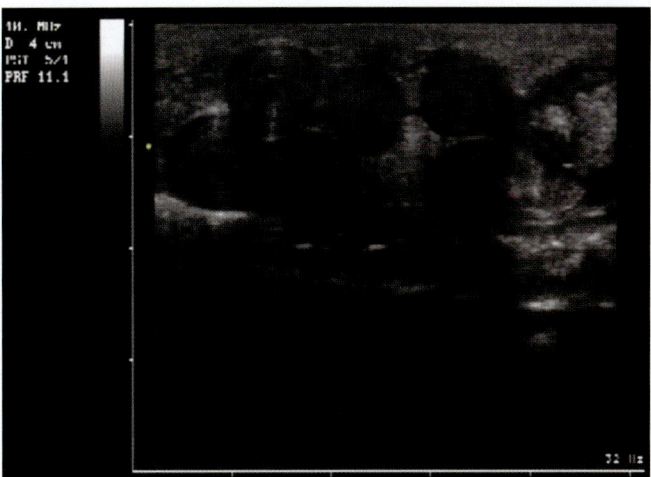

FIG 58.38 Ultrasound image of the ovary before ovulation in a bearded dragon (*Pogona vitticeps*). Round structures are starting to change from anechoic to more echogenic content. In this case, the bearded dragon developed preovulatory follicle stasis due to mismanagement.

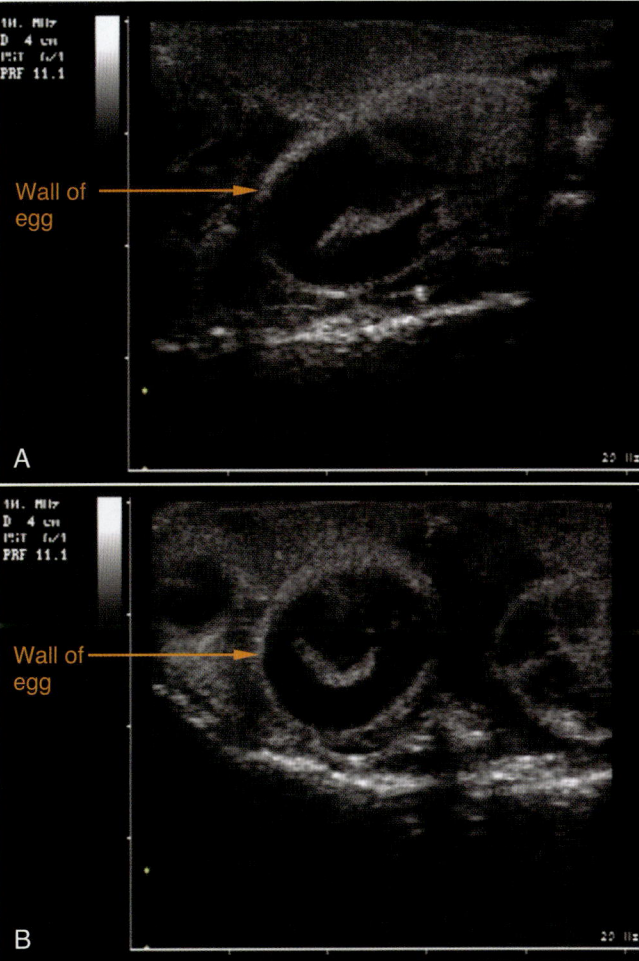

FIG 58.39 (A) Ultrasound image (sagittal plane) of a postovulatory egg with higher wall echogenicity in a bearded dragon (*Pogona vitticeps*). (B) Ultrasound image of the same egg in panel (A), in a transverse plane.

(Fig. 58.37A). In chelonians, they show higher echogenicity at this early stage (see Fig. 58.37B). The size varies from one to a few millimeters. Before ovulation they grow to large round structures, and their echogenicity increases. In snakes, many anechoic, round structures can be visualized before ovulation, depending on the size of the snake (up to 2 cm in diameter in large pythons). In the late preovulatory state, nearly the entire caudal coelom may be filled with round follicles (Fig. 58.38). After ovulation, the ova elongate, and a slightly hyperechoic wall is produced. Depending on the species, the egg wall will range from noncalcified to calcified (Fig. 58.39A and B). Depending on the degree of shell calcification, egg development can often be monitored. At the beginning of gravidity, the anechoic layer of albumin can be differentiated from the hyperechoic yolk (Fig. 58.40A and B). Occasionally, a small embryo can be visualized. In viviparous snakes and lizards, the development of the embryos can be monitored by the stage of development, activity, and heartbeat (Fig. 58.41A and B).

Pathologic changes can be monitored in all stages of the reproductive cycle. It is important to distinguish preovulatory follicles (e.g., follicular stasis) from postovulatory eggs (e.g., dystocia). Normally, preovulatory follicles are uniform, round, and either anechoic or hypoechoic. As the

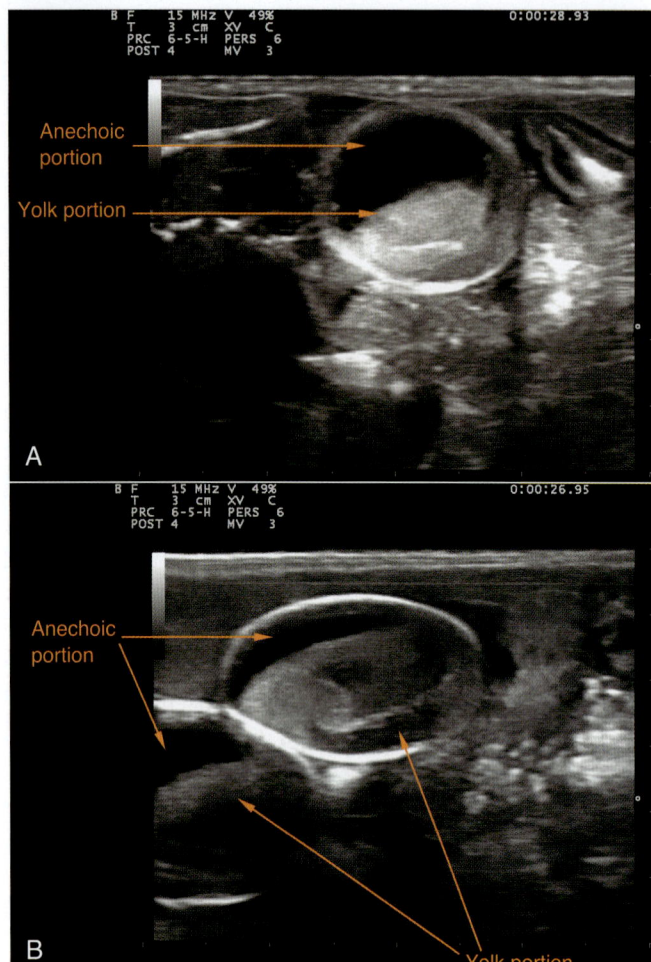

FIG 58.40 (A) Ultrasound image of eggs in a bearded dragon (*Pogona vitticeps*) in a transverse plane with differentiation of the yolk portion (more echogenic) from the albumin, visualized as the anechoic part of the egg. (B) Ultrasound image of one of the eggs from (A) in a bearded dragon in a sagittal plane with differentiation of the yolk portion and anechoic part of the egg.

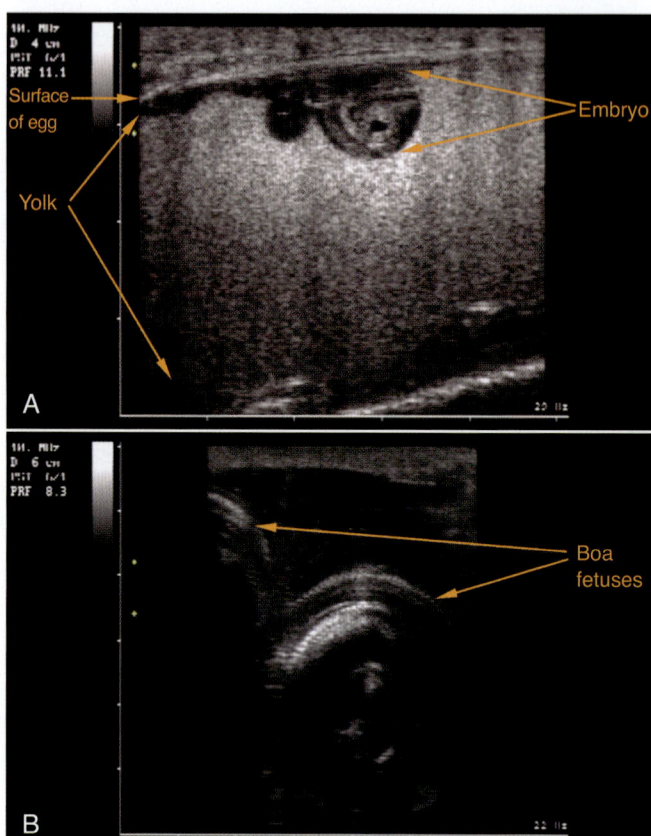

FIG 58.41 (A) Ultrasound image of an egg filled with highly echogenic yolk and a small embryo developing in a ball python (*Python regius*). (B) Ultrasound image just before birth in a viviparous boa constrictor; it is also possible to see the movements of the fetuses and the beating hearts at this stage.

follicles mature within the ovary, more echogenic layers appear. In addition, the echogenicity changes to a heterogeneous pattern, the surfaces of the follicles are no longer smooth and well demarcated, and anechoic fluid can be seen surrounding the follicles. Echogenic free-floating debris within this anechoic fluid often indicates inflammation (Fig. 58.42A and B).

After ovulation, the ova change to a more elliptical, echogenic structure. The wall of the egg is normally smooth, and irregularity of the surface can suggest delayed transit and likely dystocia. A heterogeneous pattern to egg contents combined with free fluid in either the distal oviduct (shell gland or uterus) or coelomic cavity generally indicates a poorer prognosis for successful laying. Pyometra may be associated with the complications of dystocia and may be evidenced with ultrasound (Fig. 58.43A and B).

Ultrasonography may also be useful in monitoring pathologic changes in the gonads.[22–24] Coelomic neoplasia of gonadal origin is often difficult to confirm because of the variable appearance of the gonads. Consequently, this may be a diagnosis of exclusion after successful identification of other normal coelomic structures (Fig. 58.44A and B).

URINARY BLADDER

The urinary bladder, when present, lies in the caudal portion of the coelomic cavity and has a thin, smooth, hyperechoic wall. The contents are generally anechoic with hyperechoic particles or larger aggregates of uric acid (Fig. 58.45).[25] Urate aggregates show a typical snowflakelike pattern, especially when the patient is moved. Calculi can be distinguished by their more solid structure and the distal shadowing of the ultrasound beam. Pathologic changes can be seen in tortoises with eggs within the bladder. They appear as large, round, multilayered structures within the urinary bladder. In these cases, the outer surface of the egg displays an irregular wall, with internal echogenic material. The urinary bladder wall may also be thickened because of mechanical irritation (Fig. 58.46A and B).

KIDNEYS

The kidneys show a higher echogenicity than the liver and fat bodies, with a clear granular echotexture and a distinctly marginated surface. In snakes, they are elongated and lobes can be visualized; however, no hyperechoic septae can be seen, unlike in the fat bodies, and this helps to differentiate between these structures (see Fig. 58.28). In some lizards, like the green iguana or bearded dragon, the kidneys lie largely within the pelvis and are not easily seen (Fig. 58.47). In other groups, such as the varanids, the kidneys are midcoelomic and readily scanned.

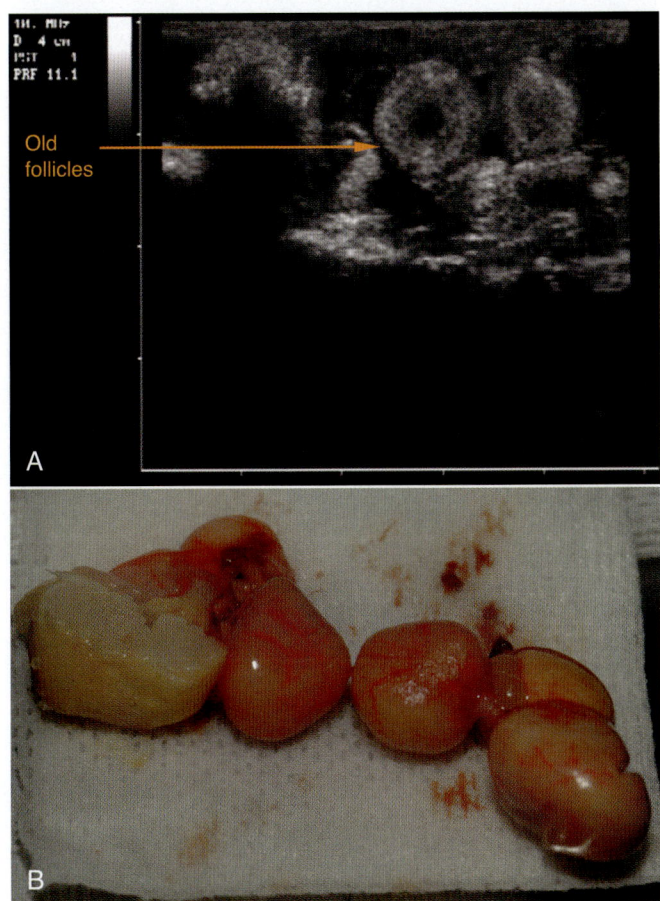

FIG 58.42 (A) Ultrasound image of older preovulatory follicles before surgery in a bearded dragon (*Pogona vitticeps*). The echogenicity increases and becomes slightly heterogeneous with aging of the follicles. (B) Preovulatory follicle stasis was identified surgically and removed in the bearded dragon from panel (A). The content of the follicles often solidify with progression of stasis.

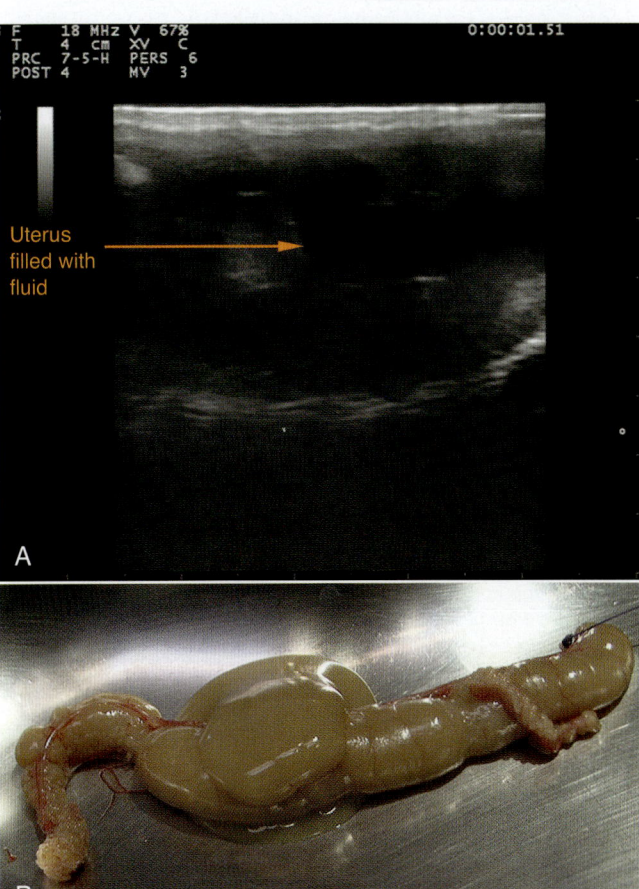

FIG 58.43 (A) Ultrasound image of the coelom of a veiled chameleon (*Chamaeleo calyptratus*). The curved tubular structure with anechoic content visualized on the left side of the caudal coelom represents an accumulation of purulent material in the fluid-filled salpinx. (B) Salpinx from the veiled chameleon in panel (A) filled with purulent exudate after surgery.

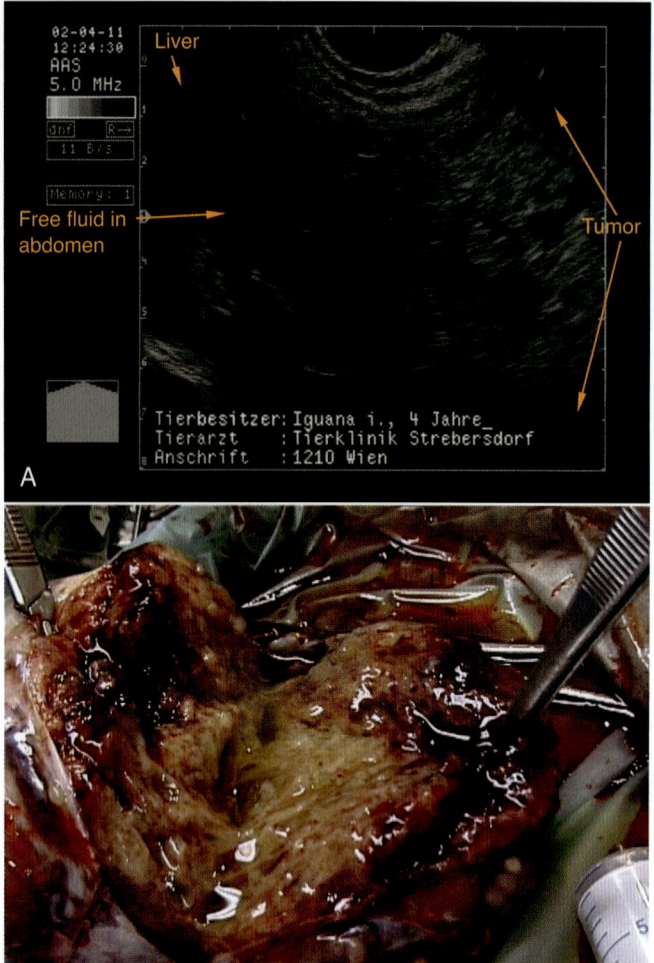

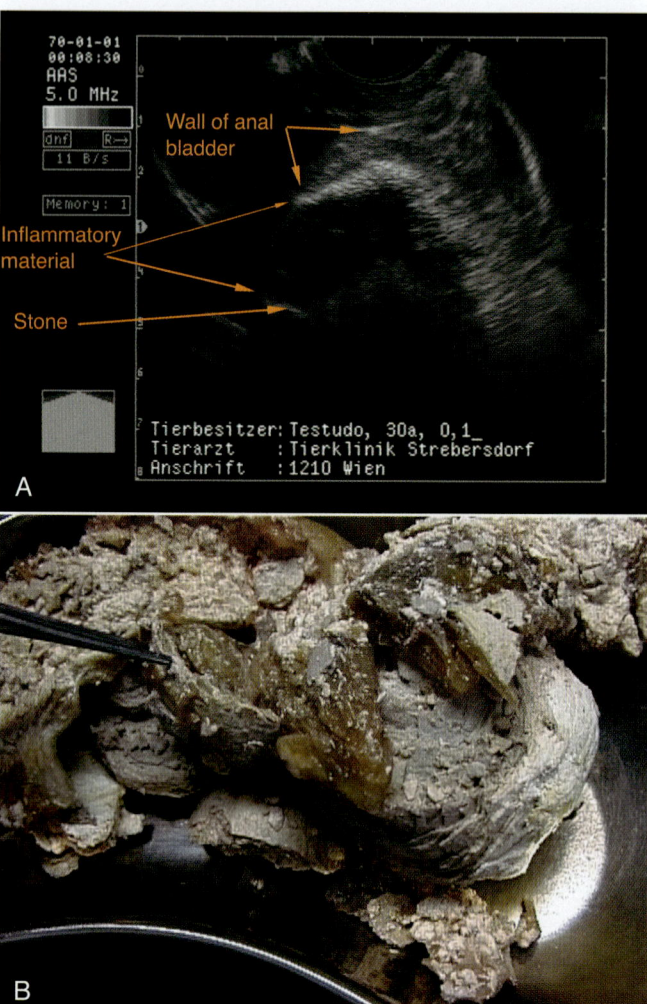

FIG 58.44 (A) Ultrasound image of a heterogeneous mass with anechoic patches distributed multifocally throughout the mass. A large amount of anechoic free fluid was found in the coelomic cavity of this green iguana (*Iguana iguana*). (B) After aspiration of 750 mL free fluid the surgical neoplasm was removed. Histopathology confirmed a cystic ovarian adenocarcinoma.

FIG 58.46 (A) Ultrasound image of the urinary bladder in a 30-year-old Greek tortoise (*Testudo hermanni*). The hyperechoic tissue of the urinary bladder is thickened, and a calculus is visible as a line with distal extinction of the ultrasound beam. Between the two structures is a thick layer of inflammatory reaction and fibrin. (B) The calculus with gel-like material on the surface. The cause of the calculus was determined to be the long-term presence of an egg in the lumen of the urinary bladder.

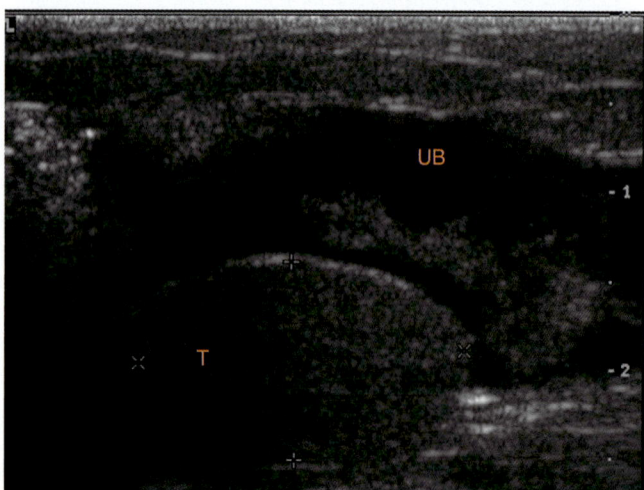

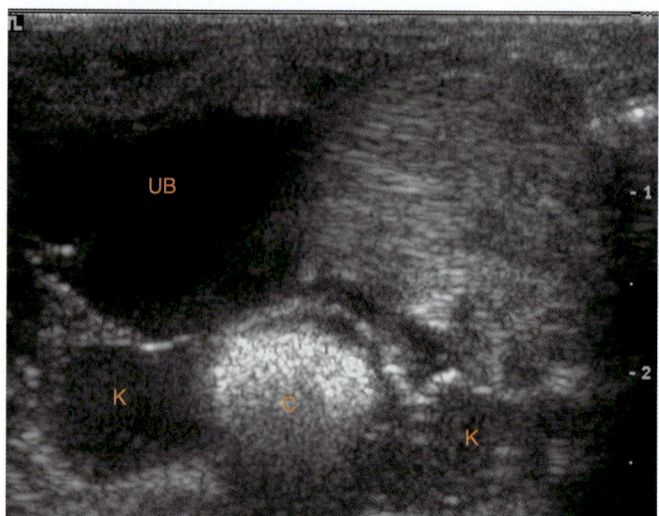

FIG 58.45 Sagittal plane ultrasound image in a healthy green iguana (*Iguana iguana*) showing an aggregate of echogenic urates suspended within the urinary bladder (UB). A testis can also be seen (T). The urinary bladder is thin walled and conforms to the surrounding organs.

FIG 58.47 Transverse plane ultrasound image in a healthy green iguana (*Iguana iguana*). The cranial poles of the kidneys (K), which lie within the pelvic cavity in this species, can occasionally be seen by angling the transducer caudally at the pelvic inlet, as in this image. C, Colon; UB, urinary bladder.

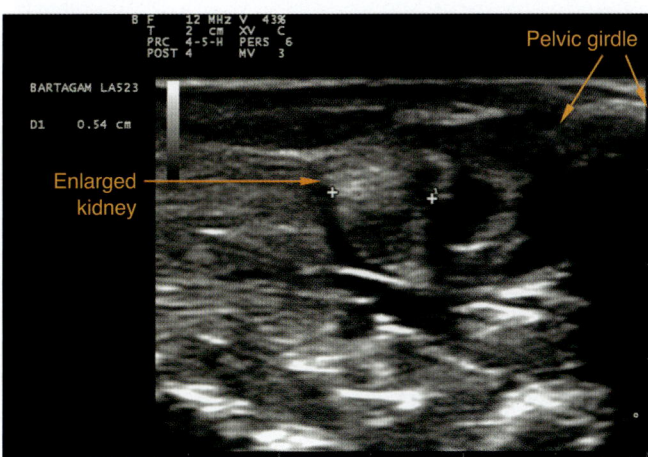

FIG 58.48 Ultrasound image of an enlarged kidney (+) in a bearded dragon (*Pogona vitticeps*) protruding cranially from the pelvic cavity.

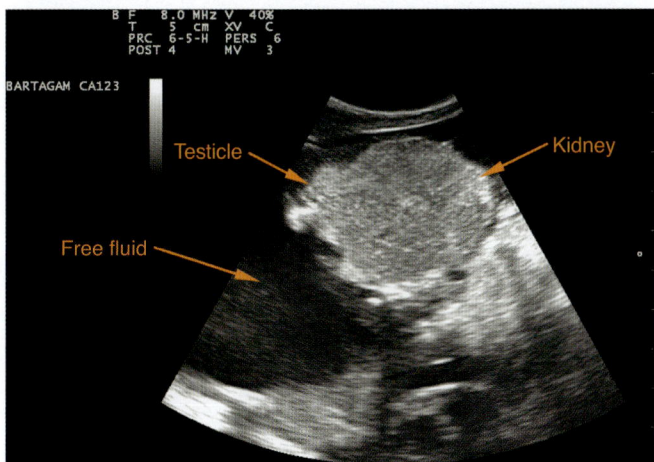

FIG 58.49 Ultrasound image of an enlarged kidney in a Greek tortoise (*Testudo hermanni*) with large hyperechoic granules in the tissue, as a result of renal failure. A large amount of free fluid was found in the coelomic cavity (same tortoise as Fig. 58.14).

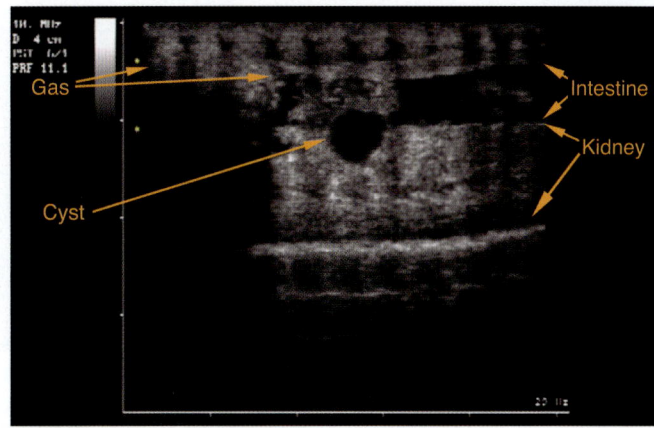

FIG 58.50 Ultrasound image of the kidney of a kingsnake (*Lampropeltis* sp.) with anechoic spherical structures in the tissue. A cystic abnormality of the renal tubules is seen on the surface of the kidney (same animal as Fig. 58.25). The intestine is filled cranially (on the left of the picture) with gas and caudally with fluid ingesta.

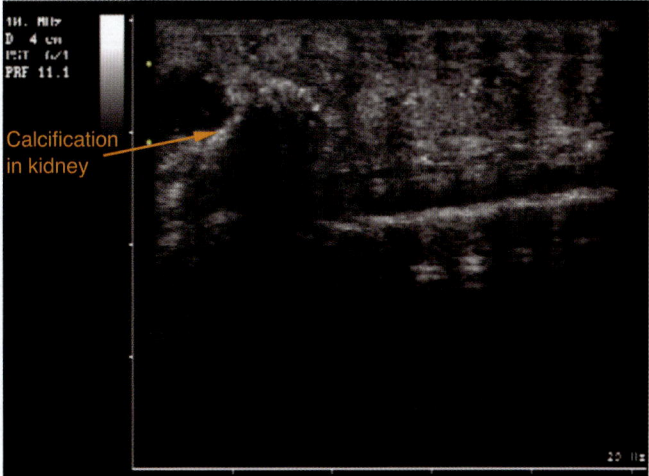

FIG 58.51 Ultrasound image of the kidney of the kingsnake (*Lampropeltis* sp.) from Fig. 58.25 and 58.50. The whole organ shows a slightly heterogeneous pattern. Focally there is a highly echogenic structure with distal attenuation of the ultrasound beam. On histopathologic examination, the changes in the kidneys were consistent with cystic adenocarcinoma with focal calcifications.

In patients with intrapelvic kidneys, when renomegaly is present, the cranial renal poles can be visualized cranial to the rim of the pelvis[25] (Fig. 58.48). In the iguana, an acoustic window just caudal to the pelvis may provide the best visualization of the kidneys.

Often small-to-large hyperechoic granules due to the presence of urate tophi can be detected and monitored in enlarged kidneys (Fig. 58.49). Anechoic spherical structures, occasionally multifocal throughout the organ, indicate cystic changes (Fig. 58.50). Mineralization, with the characteristic appearance of distal attenuation of the ultrasound beam, can be seen; tumors may also be detected (Fig. 58.51).

THE EYE

Because of the small size of the normal reptilian globe, high-frequency transducers with a small footprint should be used to obtain a good image of the structures of the eye and the surrounding tissues. Probes with frequencies from 40 to 60 MHz will give even more detailed images. In ophthalmology, this technique is referred to as *ultrasound biomicroscopy*.[26] The coupling gel and the probe can be placed either directly on the cornea, the spectacle, or the eyelids (as in chameleons). Both eyes should always be investigated in sagittal, dorsal, and transverse planes for a thorough evaluation and bilateral comparison.

The image of the normal cornea and the attached spectacle in snakes is a small, parallel, hyperechoic two-lined structure. Posterior to the cornea, the anechoic anterior chamber is visible. The lens is an oval, anechoic structure with thin hyperechoic margins. The iris is slightly heterogeneous of medium echogenicity, and, especially in small reptiles, not easily distinguished from the ciliary body. The vitreal body should be anechoic, and the fundus of the globe should be uniformly concave. The conus papillaris is visualized as a higher echogenic structure reaching from the posterior pole of the wall into the vitreal body. Its size ranges from small to large, almost reaching the posterior lens capsule wall (Fig. 58.52). Changes associated with dysecdysis in snakes, intraocular hemorrhage, abscesses, and tumors of the structures of the eye and the orbit can be visualized (Fig. 58.53A–E).

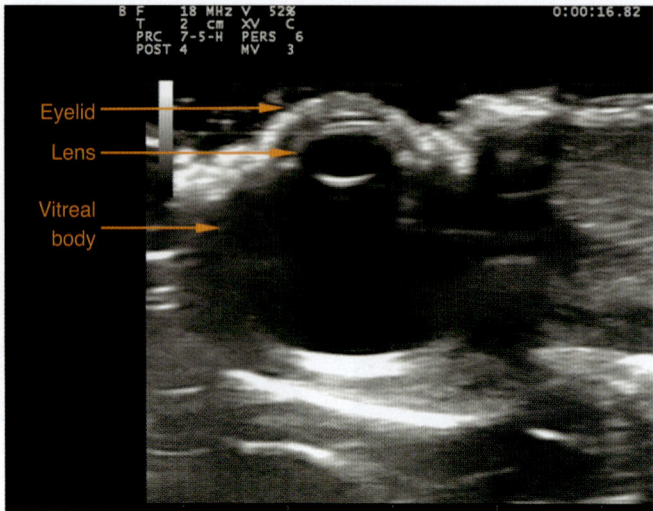

FIG 58.52 Ultrasound image with an 18 MHz transducer of a healthy eye in a veiled chameleon (*Chamaeleo calyptratus*). The most superficial echogenic structure is the eyelid; the lens appears as an oval, anechoic structure with thin hyperechoic margins; the vitreal body is anechoic; and there is a round border to the fundus.

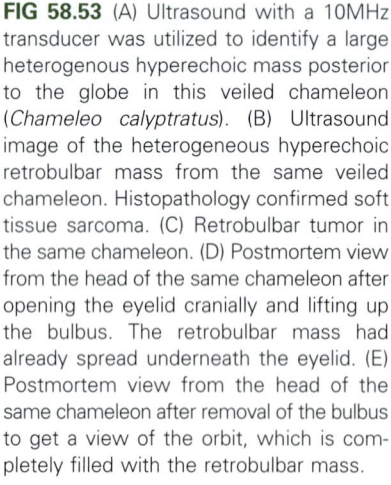

FIG 58.53 (A) Ultrasound with a 10MHz transducer was utilized to identify a large heterogenous hyperechoic mass posterior to the globe in this veiled chameleon (*Chameleo calyptratus*). (B) Ultrasound image of the heterogeneous hyperechoic retrobulbar mass from the same veiled chameleon. Histopathology confirmed soft tissue sarcoma. (C) Retrobulbar tumor in the same chameleon. (D) Postmortem view from the head of the same chameleon after opening the eyelid cranially and lifting up the bulbus. The retrobulbar mass had already spread underneath the eyelid. (E) Postmortem view from the head of the same chameleon after removal of the bulbus to get a view of the orbit, which is completely filled with the retrobulbar mass.

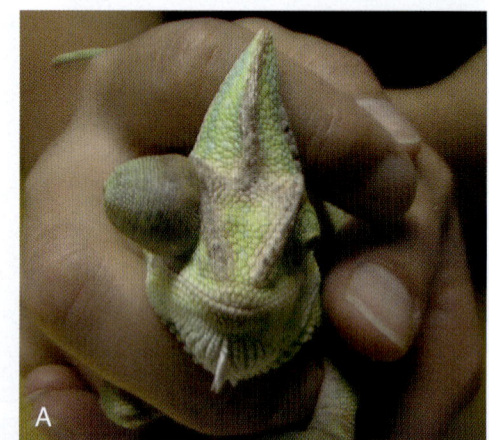

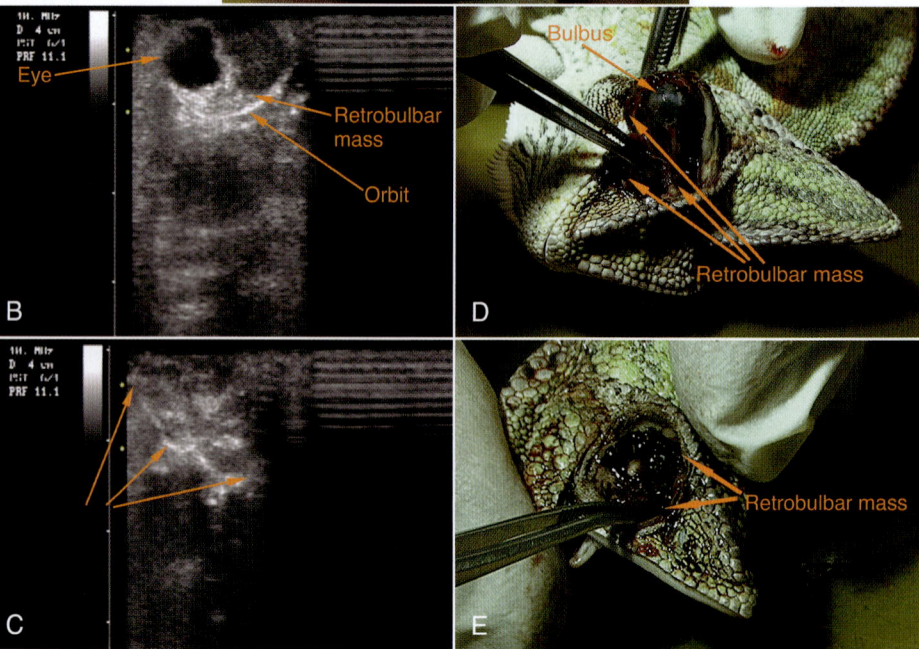

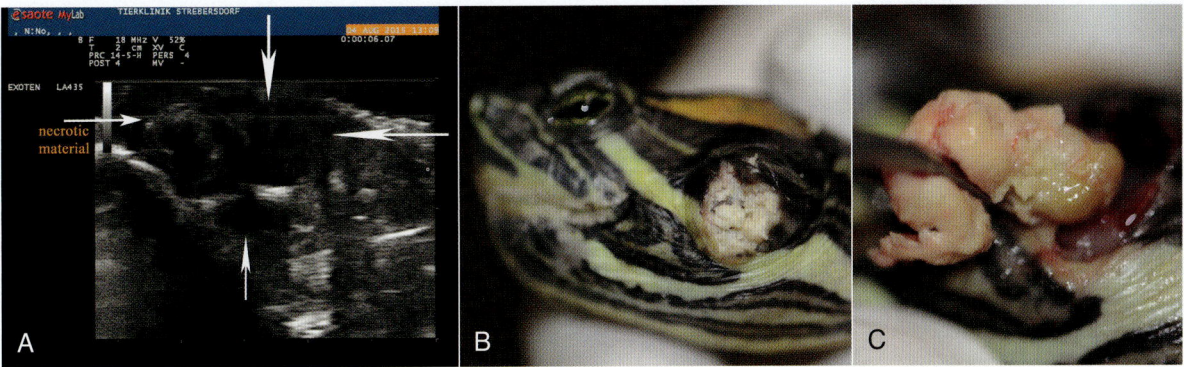

FIG 58.54 (A) Ultrasound image of the inner ear filled with purulent and necrotic material in a red-eared slider (*Trachemys scripta elegans*) associated with suspected hypovitaminosis A. (B) Gross view of necrotic material seen in the region of the ear of the same red-eared slider. (C) Necrotic material removed from below the tympanic scale in the same red-eared slider.

ABSCESSES

Internal abscesses can be challenging to image and diagnose.[27,28] Normally they have an inhomogenic pattern with a well-distinguished capsule. Size and shape of the necrotic area, as well as demarcations between healthy tissue, should be evaluated (Fig. 58.54A–C).

REFERENCES

See www.expertconsult.com for a complete list of references.

59

Computed Tomography

Ajay Sharma and Jeanette Wyneken

Reptile medicine and surgery is becoming multidisciplinary in keeping up with the expectations of pet owners, zoological collection managers, and conservationists. Diagnostic imaging is essential for providing clinically useful data in a noninvasive manner. Until recently, diagnostic imaging was limited to radiography and ultrasonography. Radiography, although providing excellent spatial resolution, is often limited by the two-dimensonality and superimposition of soft tissue and osseous structures. Additionally relatively poor soft-tissue contrast resolution limits assessment of coelomic organs. Ultrasonography, although a good noninvasive, real-time imaging modality, requires a high level of operator knowledge and proficiency and is limited for evaluation of gas-filled structures such as the gastrointestinal tract and lungs. In the past decade, there has been a tremendous increase in the use of advanced cross-sectional imaging in veterinary medicine. Computed tomography (CT) and magnetic resonance imaging (MRI) are now indispensible diagnostic imaging modalities in many academic and referral institutions.

The appropriate acquisition of CT images is equally, if not more, important than the clinician's interpretive ability. Standard CT imaging requires good restraint to avoid patient movement and selection of appropriate acquisition parameters, including slice thickness, pitch, anatomical region to be imaged, processing algorithm (soft tissue, bone, lung, etc.), contrast medium type, dose, rate of infusion, and timing of imaging relative to contrast administration. The precise acquisition parameters vary between CT machines and depend on manufacturer, age of the machine, and number of detector elements (e.g., 2-, 8-, 16-, or 64-slice CT). Computed tomography units that provide isotropic resolution are preferred for diagnostic quality 3D and multiplanar reconstructions. Multiplanar reconstructions (MPR) are the display of transverse images in sagittal and dorsal planes with the ability to triangulate a lesion on all three views (Figs. 59.1 and 59.2).

New multidetector CT (MDCT) machines provide good isotropic resolution and rapid multiplanar reconstructions and postprocessing in different windows/algorithms, such as soft tissue, bone, or lung. Other terms used to denote the window width/level include soft, sharp, and ultrasharp algorithms.

Assessment of a CT study includes quality control and diagnostic value. Quality control verifies that the entire anatomical region of interest is included, and appropriate slice thickness and processing algorithms have been selected. These are typically evaluated in real-time or immediately postacquistion using the transverse images. Evaluation of diagnostic quality includes presence or absence of motion and adequate contrast enhancement of normal tissues and cardiovascular structures. Intravascular access may be difficult in some patients, and the lack of contrast enhancement may be due to loss of vascular access and extravasation of contrast media, bradycardia, hypotension, and/or

dyssynchrony between time of injection and start of the CT scan. Some CT machines have an inherent delay when using automatic injectors for contrast administration, resulting in mistiming of the start of the CT scan relative to contrast injection.

Once the CT images are acquired and are deemed to be of diagnostic quality, the next step is interpretation. Due to the large volume of data and relative infancy of CT in reptiles, image interpretation requires a quiet viewing area with appropriate ambient lighting and a high-resolution computer monitor and a good knowledge of relevant normal anatomy. Diagnostic evaluation should be performed on the transverse images, with use of MPR to help triangulate difficult or small lesions. 3D reconstructions are useful for publications and gross assessment/ demonstration of organs or vasculature; however, during the reconstruction process, resolution is reduced due to the software process of smoothing various "edges" to create the pretty picture. This smoothing or interpolation process results in the loss of fine anatomical details. If 3D reconstructions are used for diagnostic purposes, it is imperative that these lesions be verified on the transverse images and further corroborated using MPR if available.

The use of proper nomenclature and anatomic terminology in interpretive reporting is essential to avoid ambiguity and confusion. Anatomical descriptors should follow Nomina Anatomica Veterinaire as closely as possible. Correct directional anatomical terminology includes cranial/rostral, caudal, dorsal, and ventral when referring to the head and body. Terms that are specific for limbs are proximal and distal and should not be used when describing lesions of the head/body/coelom. Because CT machines are designed for humans, correlative terms are: superior = cranial; inferior = caudal; anterior = ventral; and posterior = dorsal.

In humans (bipeds) it is appropriate to use terms proximal and distal when discussing the body; however, in quadripeds, the terms cranial and caudal are preferred.

In addition to knowledge of the physics, hardware, and software capabilities of CT, the application of CT in the diagnostic imaging of clinical patients requires a thorough understanding of normal imaging anatomy. Several excellent references are available that describe both CT acquisition and normal anatomy of several reptilian species.[1–10] With rare species, normal anatomic form may be undescribed. Although dissection of fresh dead animals for reference can provide a wealth of information, including important landmarks, species-specific organ structure, and the arrangement of organ systems, access to these specimens may be limited and may not be ethically appropriate.[6–13]

CT uses a rapidly rotating x-ray tube to acquire multiple projections in a 360-degree manner around the subject. The use of x-ray radiation results in images that represent the attenuation characteristics of structures. Dense tissues, such as bone, attenuate the incident x-rays

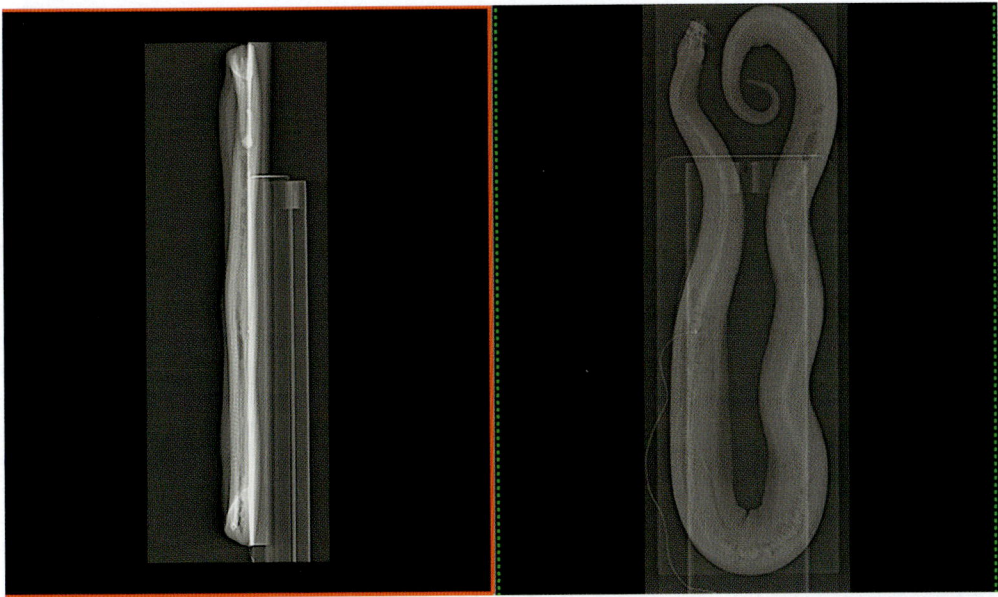

FIG 59.1 Computed tomography examinations are planned based on a short exposure or x-ray scout image using the CT machine. On the CT machine/computer monitor, the software provides reference lines that allow the imager to select regions of interest based on external topographical anatomy. These are often acquired in two planes. This image shows localizer/scout images of a snake in sagittal and dorsal planes. The localizer provides a guide for choosing the field of view using external anatomical landmarks when planning the CT scan. Because most commercially available CT machines have software specifically for human or large mammalian patients, one must carefully explain to the technician what planes of view are needed for reptilian patients. (Courtesy of Ajay Sharma.)

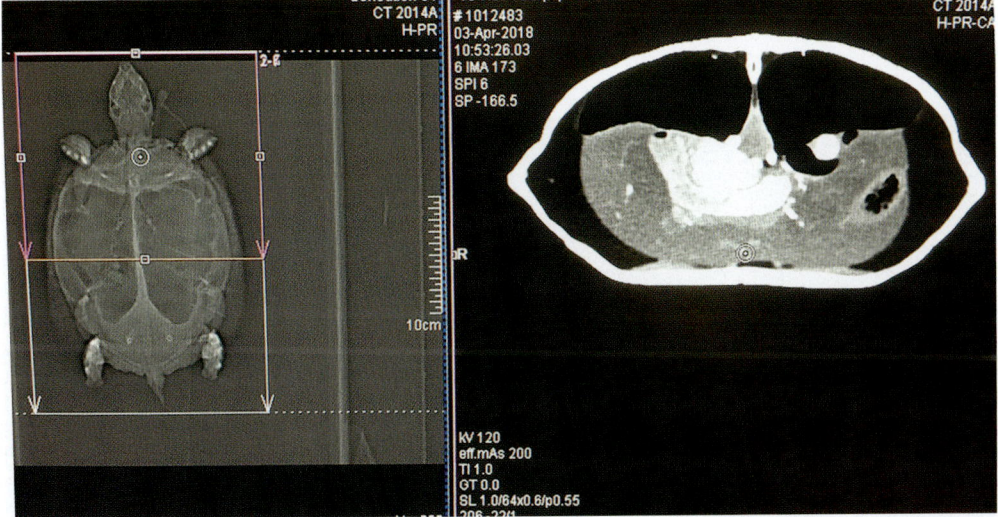

FIG 59.2 Screen capture showing the field of view (pink lines) and yellow grid line on a dorsal scout image and the corresponding transverse CT image at the level of the grid line in a chelonian patient. (Courtesy of Ajay Sharma.)

to a greater extent, resulting in a brighter image. Houndsfield units (HU) are the mathematical/numerical representation of structural densities on CT images. Structures/lesions are described in terms of their attenuation characteristics/HU values. For example, normal lungs are described as hypoattenuating or hypodense whereas bone is described as hyperattenuating/hyperdense. Typical HU values range from −500 for air to +1000 for bone, with a central value of 0 for water. Soft tissue structures range in density/HU values from 30 to 80. If there is contrast enhancement of a particular organ or structure, the HU value is often twice or three times the precontrast values (see Figs. 59.1 through 59.4). Modern multidetector CT (MDCT) machines provide complete imaging of large patients relatively quickly (seconds to minutes). Current MDCT uses helical or continuous image acquisition during movement (translation) of the patient/table through the gantry. This provides extremely rapid acquisition with minimal loss of spatial resolution using modern software and advanced reconstruction algorithms.[1] Older CT machines often used axial image acquisition. This is accomplished by acquiring one slice of data followed by automatic patient/table translation, before acquiring the next data slice. Axial imaging increases imaging time (and therefore also sedation and anesthesia) with no diagnostic advantage. Postprocessing reconstructions to obtain fine details of bone or soft tissue structures is available as needed (Fig. 59.5). The ability to acquire complete diagnostic imaging data quickly is useful in critical patients or in patients in whom general anesthesia is difficult or contraindicated.

Imaging data is reconstructed in two or three dimensions using standalone or proprietary software associated with the CT machine. Examples of standalone DICOM viewers include OsiriX (Pixmeo SARL, Geneva, Switzerland) or Horos (The Horos Project) and are available for Mac operating systems or Windows-based software such as RadiAnt (Medixant, Poznan, Poland). CT provides excellent anatomic detail and good spatial resolution; its resolution of osseous and pulmonary structures is exceptional, and soft tissue resolution is good. Because the images are collected serially along the axis specified by the clinician, CT scans can provide 2D section images, or the images are reconstructed as three-dimensional studies (see Figs. 59.5, 59.6, and 59.7). The same CT data can be reviewed in serial sections (Fig. 59.8) or reconstructed in a variety of ways to allow for the retention of three-dimensional landmarks (see Figs. 59.5 through 59.16).

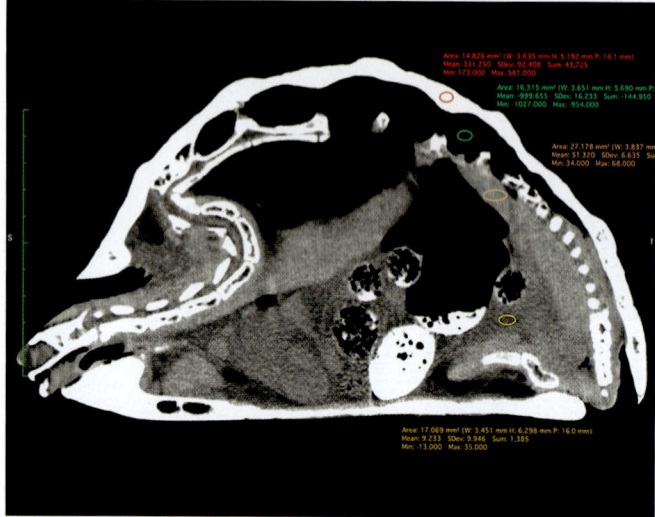

FIG 59.3 Sagittal image of a tortoise showing the different HU of various structures: Bone (*red oval*) mean HU = 331, Gas/air (*green oval*) mean HU = −999, soft tissue (*orange oval*) mean HU = 51, and coelomic fluid (*yellow oval*) mean HU = 3. (Courtesy of Ajay Sharma.)

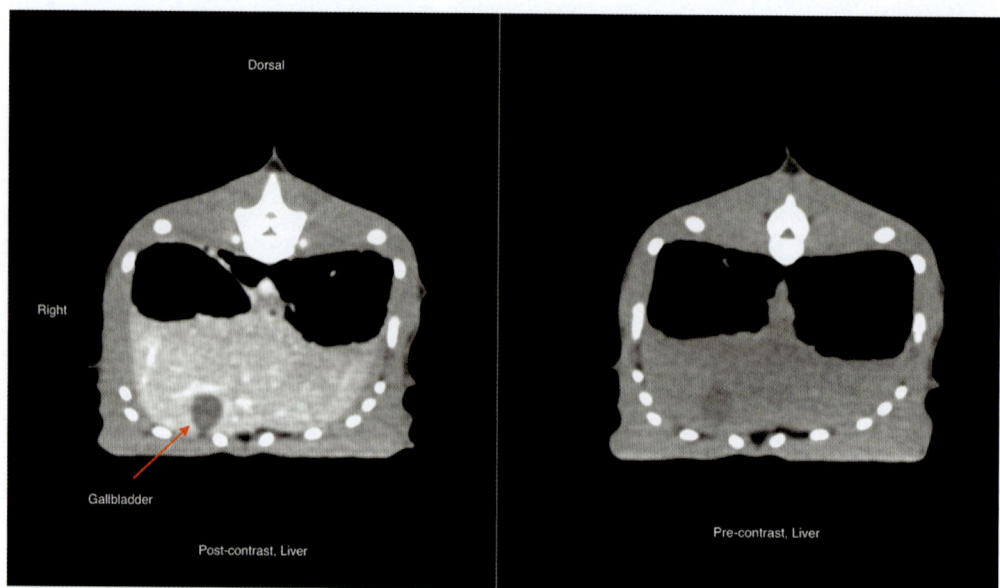

FIG 59.4 Transverse image of the cranial abdomen of an iguana (*Iguana iguana*) showing the strong contrast enhancement of the liver, the hepatic veins, and the fluid attenuating gallbladder. Noncontrast enhanced liver HU = 55; postcontrast enhanced liver HU = 150. (Courtesy of Ajay Sharma.)

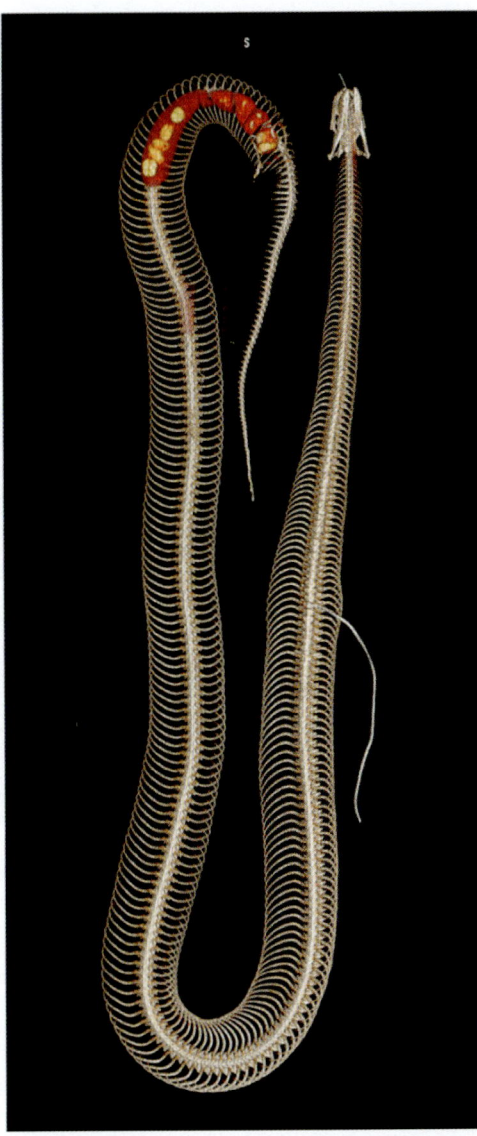

FIG 59.5 Precontrast 3D reconstruction of a Burmese python (*Python bivittatus*). The white-red material in the caudal aspect is feces. The white linear wire in the cranial third of the snake is a Doppler wire with the sensor placed on the heart. (Courtesy of Ajay Sharma.)

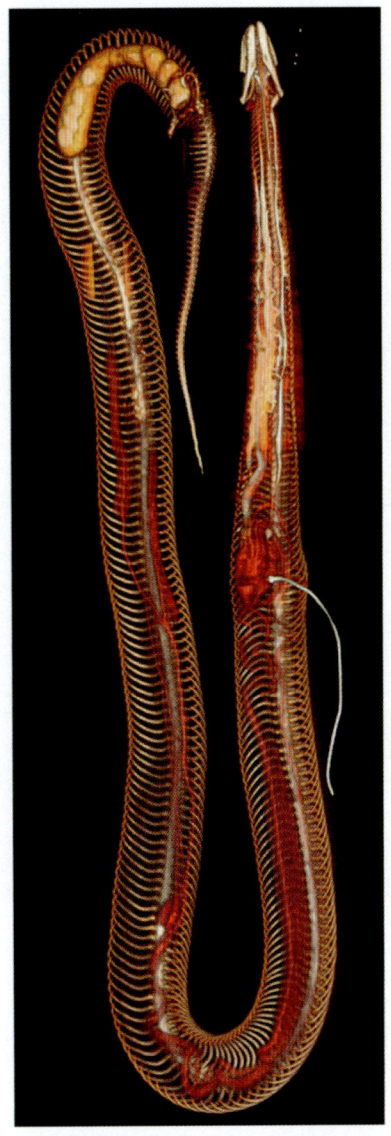

FIG 59.6 Postcontrast 3D reconstruction of the same patient as in Fig. 59.5 showing contrast enhancement of the heart, aorta, liver, renal arteries, and kidneys in a Burmese python (*Python bivittatus*). (Courtesy of Ajay Sharma.)

Computed tomography is essential for evaluating the lungs and airways and highly recommended for imaging the skeletal system, gastrointestinal tract, and reproductive organs in a variety of reptilian species (see Figs. 59.6 through 59.9 and 59.11 through 59.20). The technology is invaluable for assessment of the relative positions and sizes of organs and their functions, particularly for dynamic organ systems. Computed tomography is extremely beneficial in the management of patients with extensive osseous abnormalities such as osteomyelitis or trauma (see Figs. 59.18 and 59.20). CT is also used to assess the coelomic cavity, abnormalities of the urinary tract, and extracoelomic soft tissues (see Figs. 59.19, 59.21, 59.24, and 59.25). Virtual endoscopy is possible with appropriate software (Fig. 59.26).[13–20]

The use of positive contrast media and 3D reconstructions provides enhanced soft-tissue detail and good resolution of cardiovascular structures (see Figs. 59.3 through 59.6, 59.22, and 59.23). Positive contrast media include water-soluble iodinated compounds for intravascular injection and barium sulfate liquid for the gastrointestinal tract.

Over the past decade, the development of integrated videography, cineradiography, and CT imaging has enabled functional studies of a variety of vertebrate XROMM (x-ray reconstruction of moving morphology). Most address locomotion or feeding by manually and computationally merging motion data from in vivo x-ray video with skeletal data from CT scans into precise and accurate animations of bones moving in 3D space.[21–26] This contemporary rotoscoping provides contextual information to interpret skeletal function. Although generally used in functional anatomical studies of larger vertebrates, the approach has clinical utility in orthopedics and podiatry.[27,28]

Text continued on p. 570

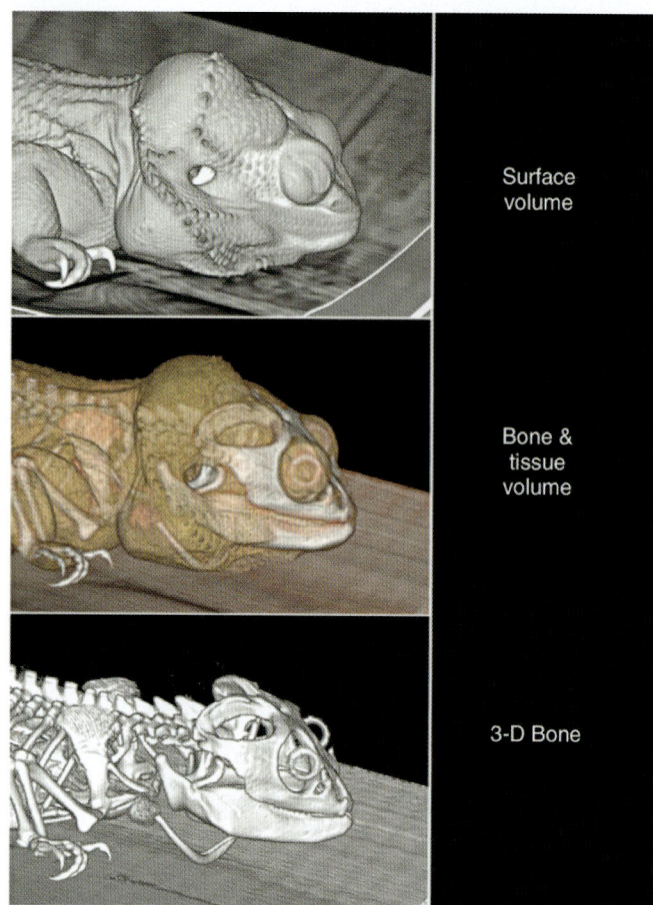

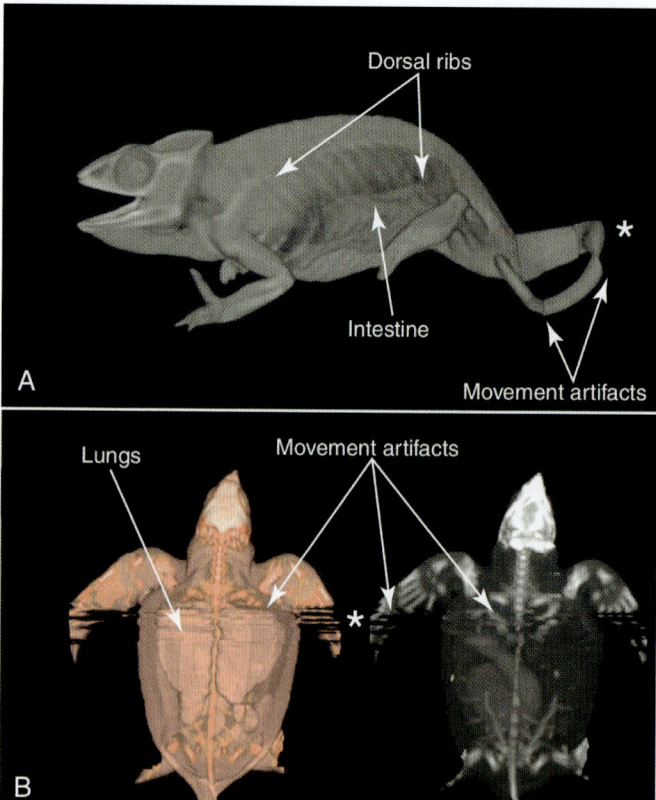

FIG 59.7 These lateral views of a bearded dragon's head and torso show the versatility of CT data. They may be reconstructed in three dimensions to emphasize different structure densities and to allow understanding of external landmarks and the internal structures (skeleton in this case). The same data set from a single CT scan shows the results of three reprocessing modes. Different threshold settings allow the same data set to be reconstructed as a surface image, showing the whole volume of the animal (surface volume), a translucent tissue image of the whole volume with the skeleton detected (bone + tissue volume), and a three-dimensional image of the skeleton alone. Bony sutures are not seen in this image because their small size was below the level of sampling resolution. Cartilage cannot be seen when reprocessing for bone but is included with other reconstruction settings that include the denser soft tissues. *Pogona vitticeps* snout-vent length was 22.5 cm. (Courtesy of Jeanette Wyneken.)

FIG 59.9 Chameleons have thin bones and large saclike lungs. The ribs are jointed at the articulations of the dorsal ribs, spine, and ventral ribs (Gastralia) from the belly. Chameleon ribs extend along the length of the trunk. These CT scans show the large areas of low-density lungs and the large numbers of ribs. *Furcifur pardalis* snout-vent length is 12.6 cm; in (A), the data were reconstructed from 0.6-mm serial images and reprocessed so that both skeletal and airway data could be seen. Postprocessing of the CT image data with false color (B) shows the lung field and skeleton of a posthatchling leatherback turtle. There is a movement artifact through the cranial lungs and distal flippers when the animal took a breath. *Dermochelys coriacea* straight carapace length is 5.7 cm. (Courtesy of Jeanette Wyneken.)

FIG 59.8 Two-dimensional transverse images along the body of an alligator. At the level of the eyes (A), the jaws form the boniest parts of the skull. Teeth can be seen extending from the lower jaw upward. The bony palate ventral to the choanae resides between spaces that are the palatal vacuities. The vitreous and the tongue are dark. The scleral ossicles appear light. (B) Posterior to the orbits, the palate is complete and the internal choanae can be seen joining the glottis. Dorsally is the oval braincase with posterior temporal bars extending ventrally and laterally. At the level of the shoulders (C), the vertebrae are mostly surrounded by the scapulae and procoracoids. The single element ventral to the trachea is the interclavical. (D) Posterior to the forelimbs, the body wall is supported by dorsal ribs and ventral ribs. The sternum is not detected. The dark heart can be seen ventral to the paired lungs. Two osteoderms are visible dorsal to the trunk vertebra. (E) The hind limbs are supported by robust ilia articulating with sacral vertebrae. The anterior aspect of the paired pubic bones can be seen ventrally. (F) The tail vertebra and ventral Y-shaped chevron bone are surrounded by muscle (gray) and tendon (black). *Alligator mississippiensis* snout-vent length is 22 cm. (Courtesy of Jeanette Wyneken.)

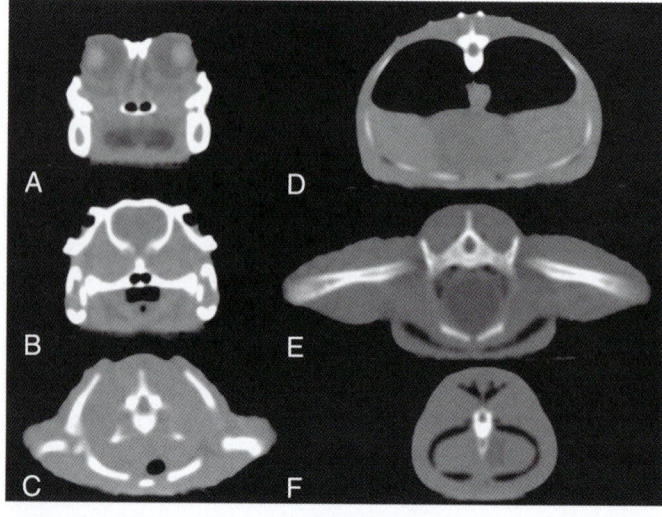

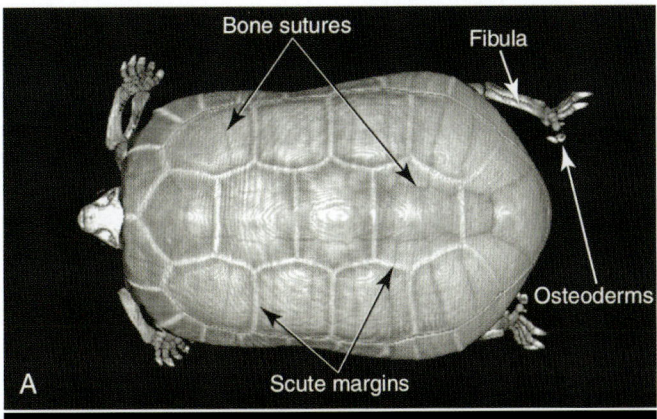

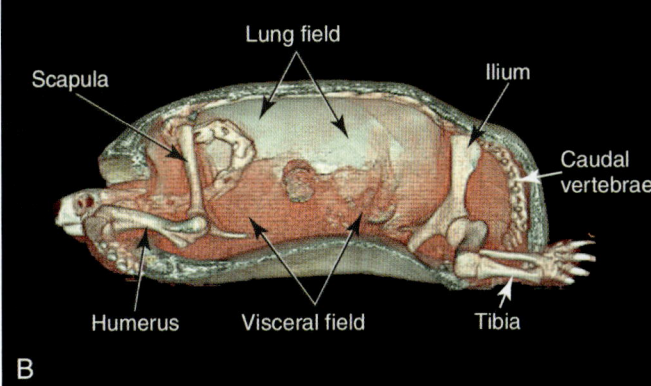

FIG 59.10 CT data can be reconstructed to show three-dimensional skeletal anatomy. Postprocessing software allows for the reconstructed images as whole skeletons that then can be cut virtually to show internal anatomy. Tortoise (Testudinidae genus and species unidentified) straight-line carapace length unknown, adult. (Courtesy of Jeanette Wyneken.)

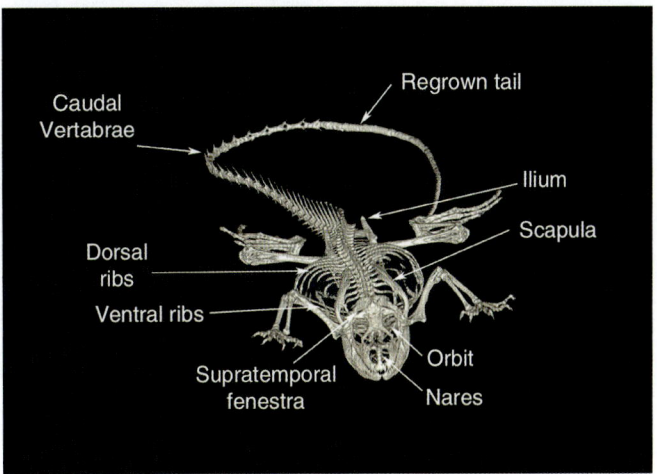

FIG 59.12 This three-dimensional reconstruction of an adult iguana skeleton shows normal anatomy, including the multiple fenestrae in the skull, arrangement of the vertebral spinous processes, and the dorsal limb girdle elements and a few common artifacts found in CT images. First, rib elements appear to be missing laterally. The thinnest rib ends and cartilaginous parts between the dorsal and ventral ribs are not detected in this kind of reconstruction. The thin nasal bones just behind the nares also appear to be missing. Their data fall outside of the threshold used by the software to make this kind of reconstruction. The striping, most apparent on the skeleton, is from reconstruction of sequential two-dimensional images. *Iguana iguana* snout-vent length = 41.8 cm. (Courtesy of Jeanette Wyneken.)

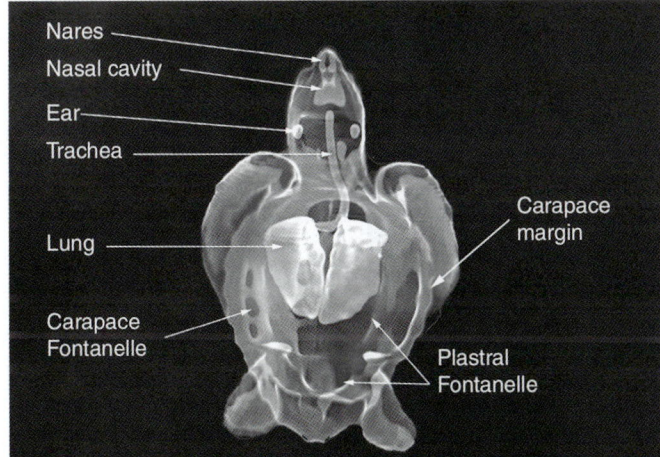

FIG 59.11 This CT scan of a small juvenile sea turtle was reconstructed applying threshold values to the data to make the bones and airways translucent and the surfaces and margins appear as outlines. The partial secondary palate of sea turtles allows the nares to be seen clearly and separately from the trachea, which opens at the base of the tongue. The lungs attach to the carapace and along the vertebral column. Unossified fontanelles are in the margin carapace and make up the center of the plastron. The otic chamber (labeled *ear*) is air filled. Other areas of trapped air appear in the neck and inguinal pockets. *Caretta caretta* straight-line carapace length is 6.3 cm. (Courtesy of Jeanette Wyneken.)

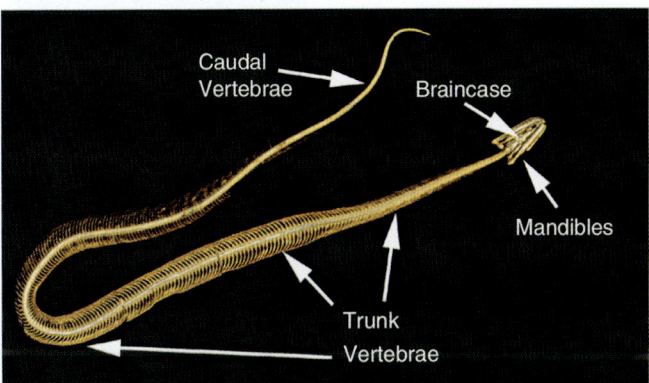

FIG 59.13 Ventral view of a ball python skeleton. This 3D reconstruction shows normal anatomy. The separate mandibles are easily seen. Snakes lack a secondary palate, so the roof of the mouth is also the floor of the braincase. Cervical vertebrae are limited to the anterior two and cannot be distinguished in this CT reconstruction. Trunk vertebrae have ribs and extend most of the length of the snake. Snakes lack ventral ribs. Caudal vertebrae lack ribs. The slight shift in registration of the reconstructed sections in the midbody are associated with one breath taken by the snake during scanning. *Python regius*, adult. Snout-vent length unknown. (Courtesy of Jeanette Wyneken.)

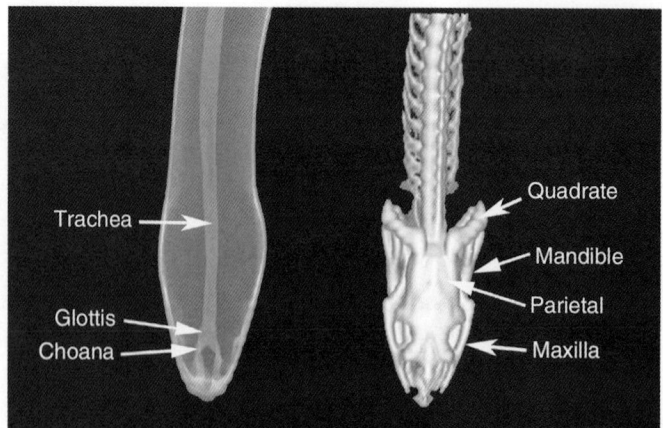

FIG 59.14 This close-up CT scan of the head structure shows the relationship of the airways in a corn snake to its skull and neck. Although snakes lack a secondary palate, the airways through the choanae and to the glottis are confluent. The reconstruction of the same CT scan as the snake's skull shows the bones that make the skull highly kinetic. Joints between the parietals, quadrate, and mandibles contribute to the snake's large gape. Highly mobile maxillae assist in prey capture and manipulation for swallowing. No rigid joint is found between the two mandibles or the maxillae. *Pantherophis guttata*, adult. Snout-vent length is unknown. (Courtesy of Jeanette Wyneken.)

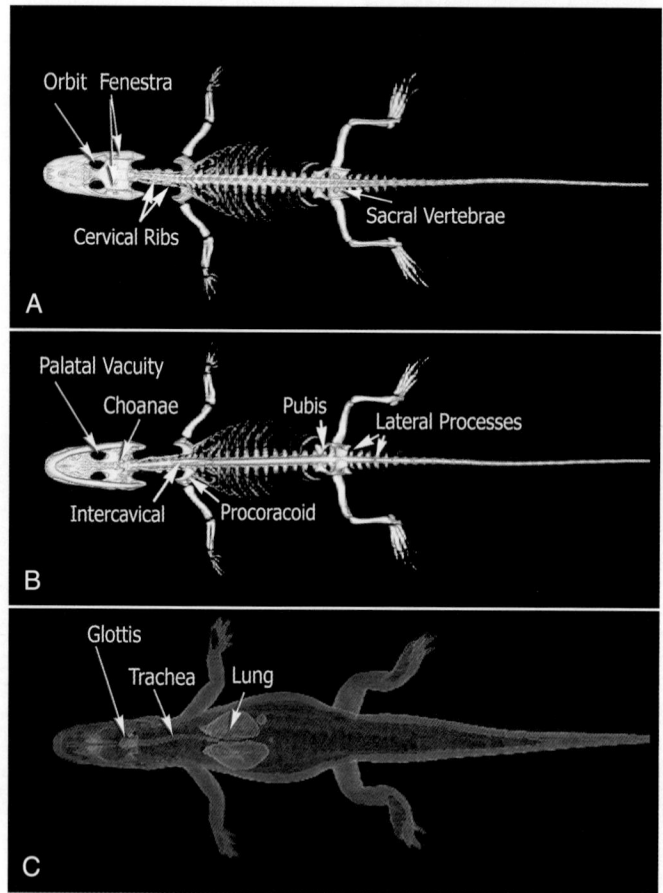

FIG 59.15 The skeleton of a small juvenile alligator from a CT scan. The scan shows normal anatomy of a small juvenile reconstructed for bones and airways. The diapsid skull architecture, in dorsal view (A), includes paired superior and lateral fenestrae located posterior to the large orbits. The ventral view (B) shows the large secondary palate separating nasal and oral passages. Paired palatal fenestrae (palatal vacuities) occur ventral to the orbits. The internal choanae, posterior to these openings, appear unpaired along the midline because of the resolution of this scan. The glottis in this lung volume reconstruction (C) aligns with the internal choanae. Crocodilians have cervical ribs (B), dorsal ribs that attach to a sternum, and extensive ventral ribs; the latter are not detected in this construction. The pectoral girdle of crocodilians is simple, with paired scapulae dorsally (A) and procoracoids ventrally (B); primitively it retains an unpaired interclavical. The pelvis is attached to the axial skeleton by robust sacral vertebrae (A). The more proximal caudal vertebrae have prominent lateral processes; these are absent near the end of the tail (A and B). The alligator's lungs occupy a relatively small volume in the body (C). *Alligator mississippiensis* snout-vent length is 22 cm. (Courtesy of Jeanette Wyneken.)

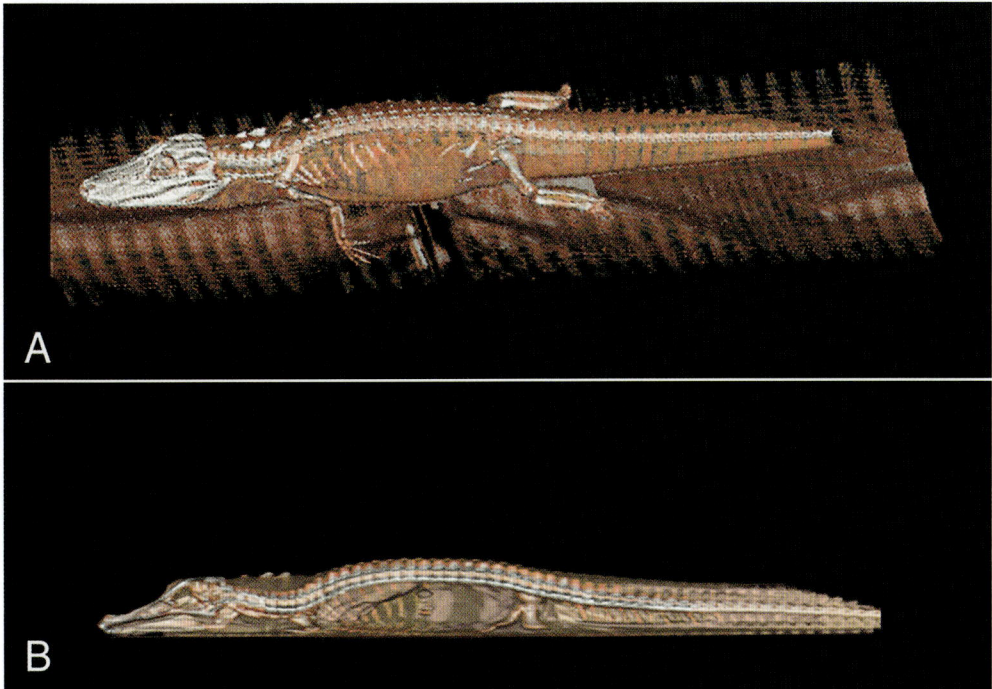

FIG 59.16 (A) The CT data of a small juvenile alligator are reconstructed in three dimensions. The bone and soft tissue together provide landmarks. (B) The reconstruction is cut virtually, showing the skull's internal architecture, spine, lungs, and pelvis. In both views, the terminal tail vertebrae were beyond the scanned field. *Alligator mississippiensis* snout-vent length is 22 cm. (Courtesy of Jeanette Wyneken.)

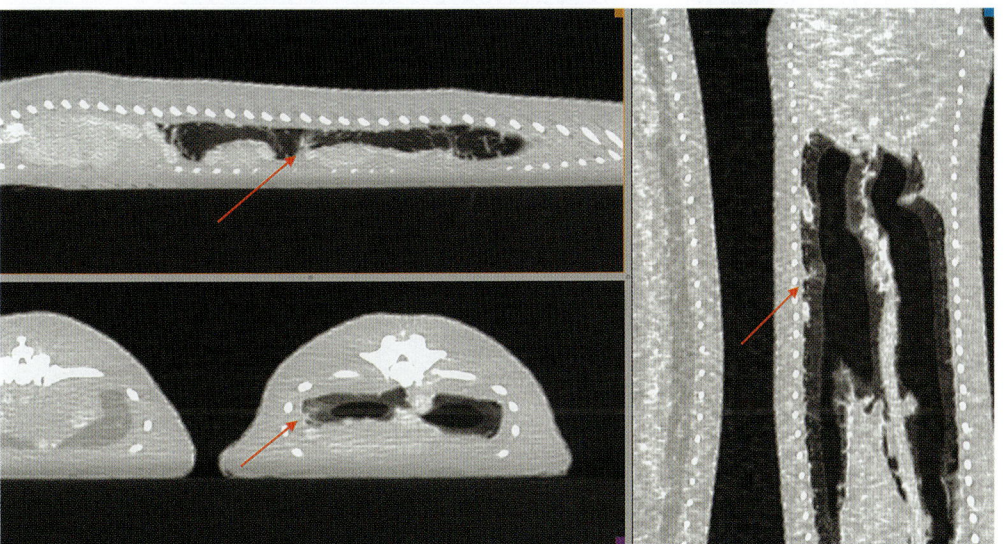

FIG 59.17 3D multiplanar reconstruction (3D MPR) of a Burmese python (*Python bivittatus*) showing localized pneumonia (*arrows*) in the right lung. (Courtesy of Ajay Sharma.)

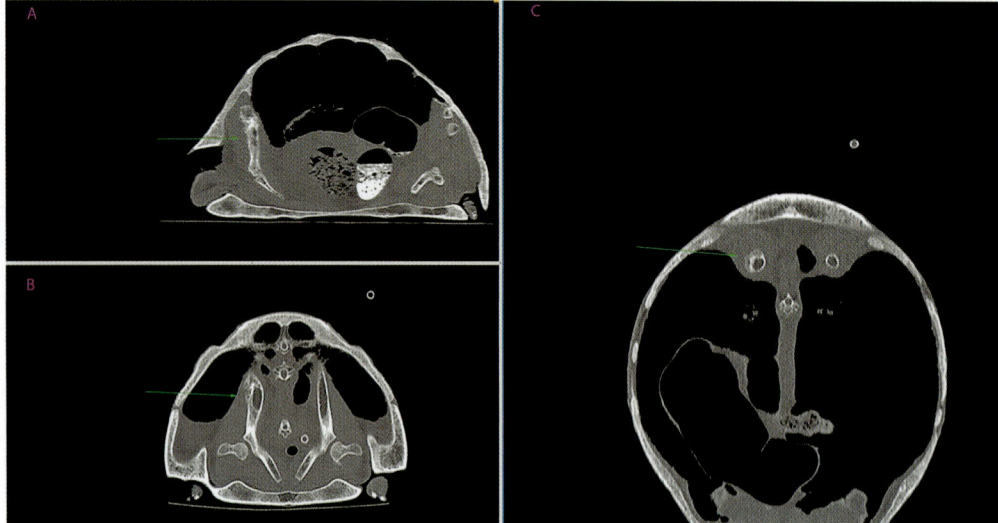

FIG 59.18 3D MPR of an aggressive bone lesion in the right scapula (arrows) of a radiated tortoise (*Astrochelys radiata*). Differential diagnoses include osteomyelitis and neoplasia. A, sagittal plane; B, transverse plane; C, dorsal plane. (Courtesy of Ajay Sharma.)

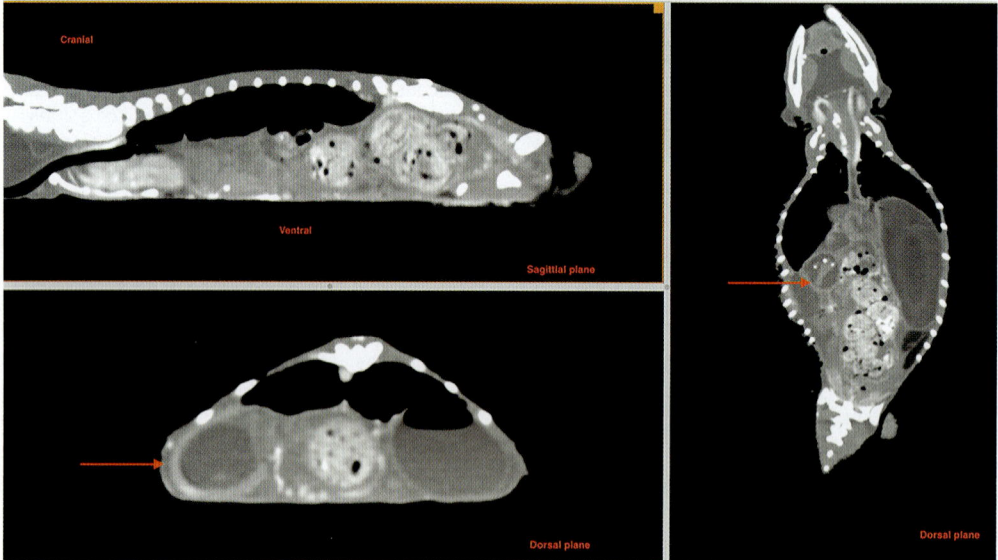

FIG 59.19 Gastrointestinal foreign material in a West Indian rhinoceros iguana (*Cyclura* spp.) Arrows indicate enlarged small intestine with foreign material. (Courtesy of Ajay Sharma.)

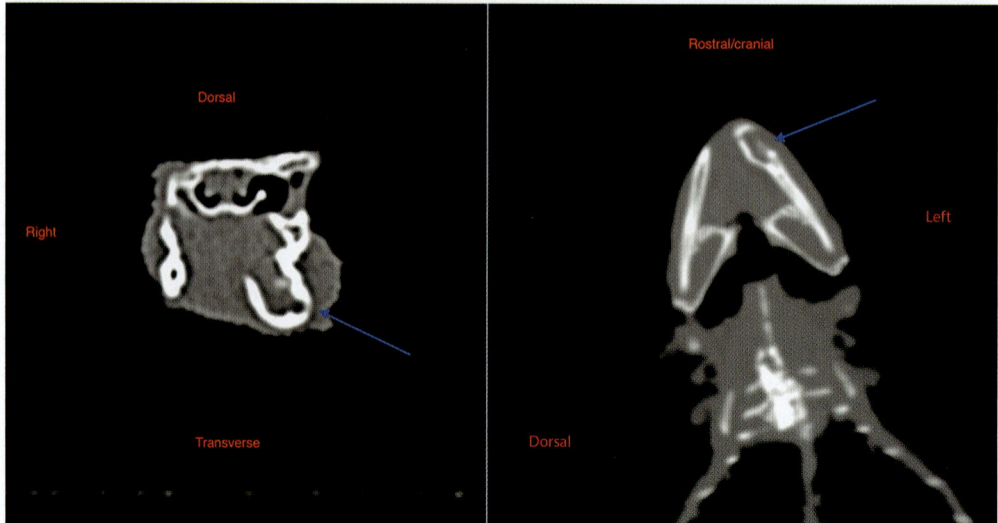

FIG 59.20 Aggressive bone lesion in the left rostral mandible of a bearded dragon (*Pogona vitticeps*). Primary differential diagnosis is osteomyelitis secondary to dental disease. The blue arrows indicate the expansile osteolytic lesion in the left mandible on transverse and dorsal plane images. (Courtesy of Ajay Sharma.)

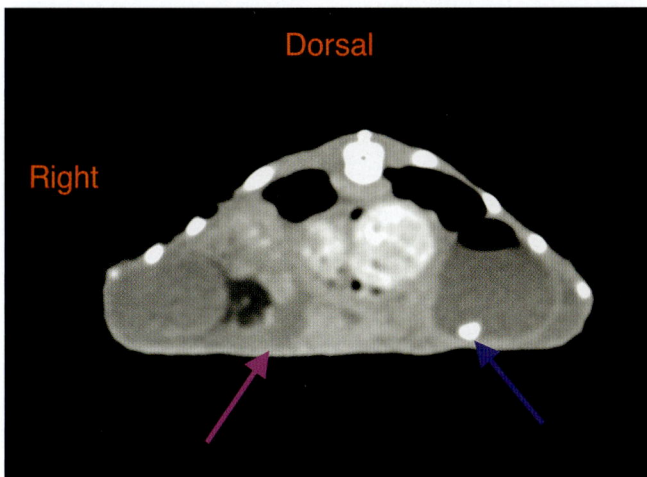

FIG 59.21 Egg yolk coelomitis, yolk granuloma/abscess, and urate calculi in a bearded dragon (*Pogona vitticeps*). The purple arrow indicates the hypoattenuating coelomic fluid, and the blue arrow indicates the urate calculi/density in the descending colon. (Courtesy of Ajay Sharma.)

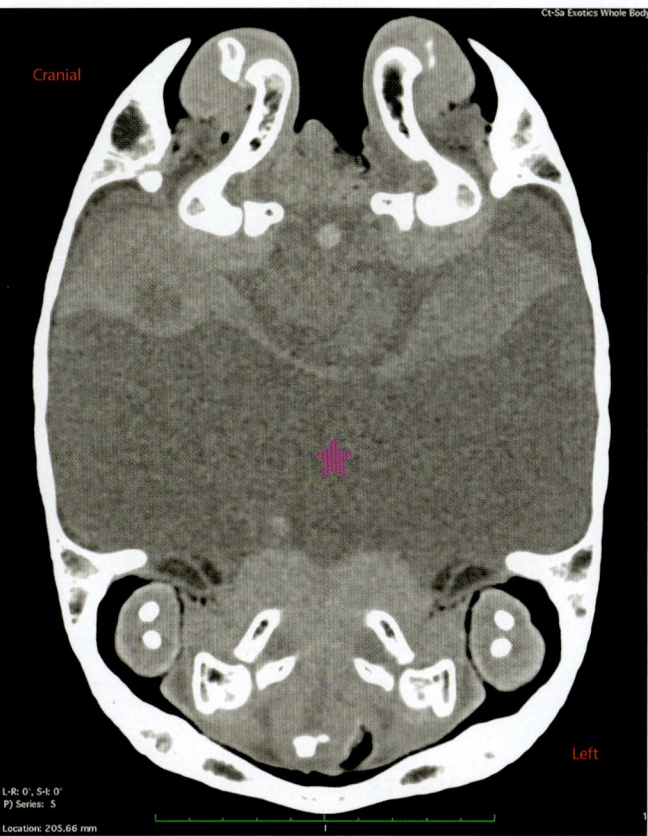

FIG 59.24 Dorsal plane CT image of a tortoise (Testudinidae) showing coelomic effusion. This is the same patient as in Fig. 59.3. The purple star identifies fluid accumulation in the midcaudal coelom (HU of 3). This region is noncontrast-enhancing compared with the muscles and other soft tissues. The low HU value and lack of contrast enhancement is consistent with fluid. (Courtesy of Ajay Sharma.)

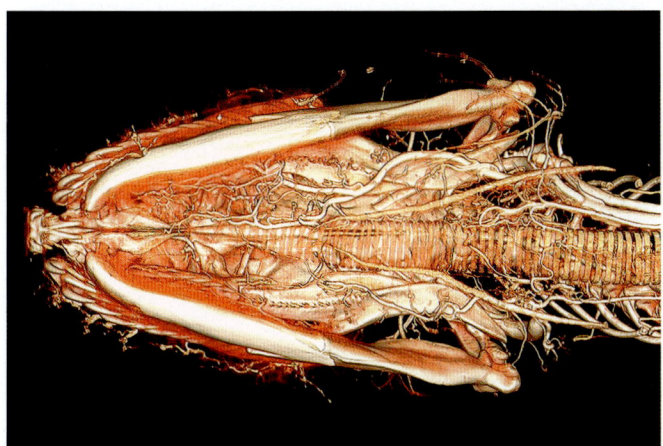

FIG 59.22 Postcontrast volumetric 3D reconstruction of the skull of a ball python (*Python regius*) perfused with BriteVu contrast agent (Scarlet Imaging, Murray, Utah) showing vascular structures of the gular region, jaw muscles, and palate. (Courtesy of Scott Echols.)

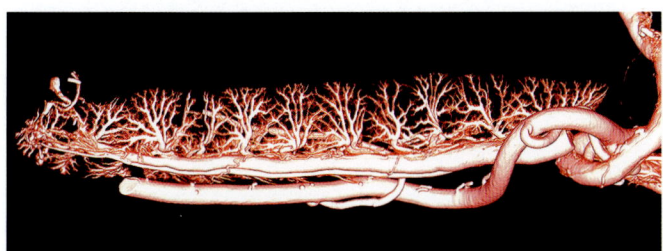

FIG 59.23 Postcontrast volumetric 3D reconstruction of the kidney of a ball python (*Python regius*) perfused with BriteVu contrast agent (Scarlet Imaging, Murray, Utah) showing the extensive afferent vasculature. (Courtesy of Scott Echols.)

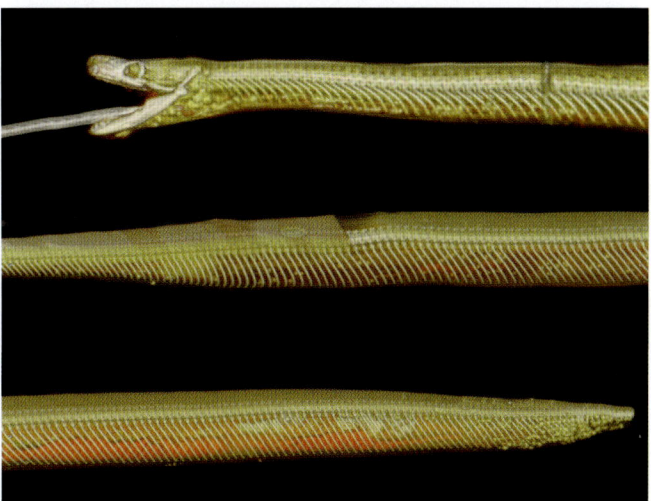

FIG 59.25 3D volumetric reconstruction of a ball python (*Python regius*) with severe generalized granulomata in the extracoelomic soft tissues. The lesions are worse around the neck and cloaca and are seen as yellow round structures in this reconstruction algorithm. (Courtesy of Stephen J. Divers.)

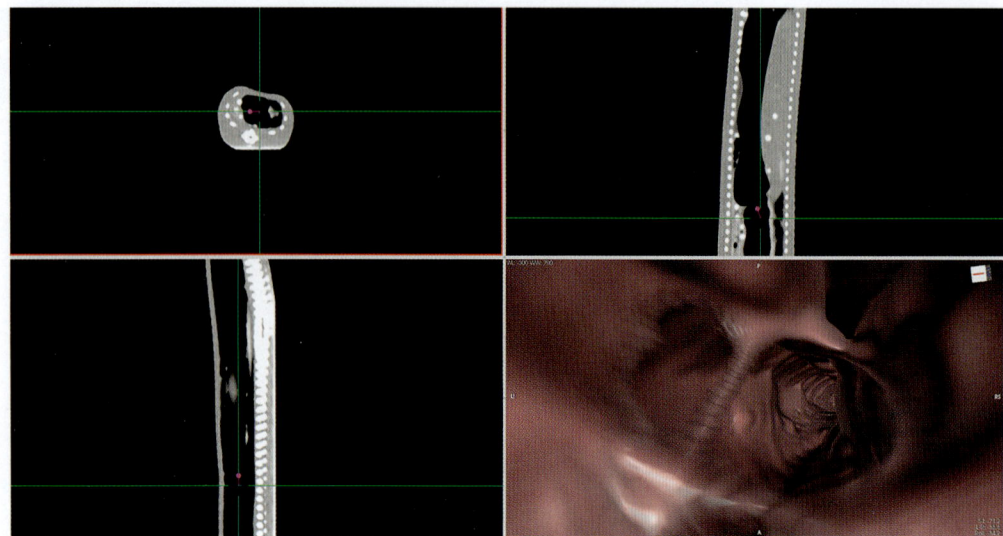

FIG 59.26 Virtual endoscopy and MPR images of the air sacs of a ball python (*Python regius*). The MPR images permit localization of the lesion(s). This is the same patient as in Fig. 59.25, and the deformation of the air sacs by the adjacent granulomas is evident on the virtual endoscopy as focal rounded bumps in the lumen of the air sac. (Courtesy of Ajay Sharma.)

ACKNOWLEDGMENTS

The authors thank Fred Steinberg, MD, Medical Director, University MRI, Boca Raton, for providing access to high-resolution CT equipment and software. Gina Boykin, Andrew Kaufman, and Steve Rubel collected the images at UMRI Boca Raton. The authors thank the faculty and clinicians in the departments of Zoological Medicine and Diagnostic Imaging, College of Veterinary Medicine, University of Georgia. Special thanks to Drs. Stephen Divers, Joerg Mayer, and Scott Secrest for their dedication and expertise in providing case material and interpretation of clinical images presented here. The authors are grateful to these talented individuals for fine mentorship, assistance, and willingness to work with reptiles.

REFERENCES

See www.expertconsult.com for a complete list of references.

60

Magnetic Resonance Imaging

Shannon P. Holmes and Jeanette Wyneken

The progressive development of cross-sectional imaging techniques, such as magnetic resonance imaging (MRI) and computed tomography (CT) in veterinary medicine continues as the value of these modalities are realized and increasingly used in zoological species, including reptiles.[1] Historically, radiographic examinations have been the main diagnostic imaging tool and will remain a generally available first-line diagnostic. Summation of similar tissue opacities, the inherent low coelomic contrast of reptiles, and superimposition of structures represent the major limitations of radiography. MRI overcomes both limitations in an unparalleled manner. There is no other clinical imaging modality that provides the soft tissue contrast resolution with high spatial resolution like MRI. The value of detailed anatomical and tissue chemistry information are beneficial in clinical practice, as well as in a diversity of research areas.

The main strength of MRI is the soft tissue contrast provided. Depiction of tissue in shades of gray is fundamental to diagnostic images, yet MRI also provides information on normal and altered tissue chemistry (function).[2-4] The manner in which a tissue interacts with magnetism confers a specific shade of gray in its normal state, and thus deviations in the shade of gray indicate a chemical change in the tissue that is associated with a pathologic process. These shifts in shades of gray across time or compared with known normal values can herald specific pathologic processes.[5] Therefore MRI will delineate disease processes that may not alter anatomy sufficiently to be detectable with other modalities. It can be thought of as a sensitive and specific noninvasive diagnostic modality.[3] In clinical patients and research animals, the normal relative positions and sizes of living organs in vivo and their functions, as well as pathologic changes, can be evaluated in a manner that previously relied on radiographs, ultrasound, or dissection. In addition to superior contrast resolution relative to the other main cross-sectional modality CT, the other advantages of MRI include multiplanar acquisition and numerous pulse sequences that can delineate different tissue characteristics and disease processes with nonionizing radiation.[6]

MRI units that can be used to evaluate reptiles are increasing in availability, and owners have increased interest in pursuing advanced imaging.[1] This includes greater numbers of clinical high-field units that are better for evaluating many reptiles of small body size or body weight. There is also continued development of MR techniques that can be advantageous to advancing our understanding of anatomy and disease detection in even the most unusual species. Further advances within MRI have been developed and applied to reptile species. These advanced imaging modalities include functional MRI (fMRI), which uses changes in blood oxygenation to detect areas of activation (tissue activity), and MR microscopy for investigation of signal alterations in very small anatomic regions or cellular alterations.[7,8]

The following section provides descriptions of MRI with basics for understanding this modality. The examples provided will function as an introduction into applications in reptile MRI, while providing baseline reptile anatomy in several taxa.

PRINCIPLES OF MAGNETIC RESONANCE IMAGING

A comprehensive review of MRI physics and principles is beyond the scope of this chapter. The focus is to provide sufficient understanding of image degeneration and specific challenges encountered in reptile MRI studies.

MRI is unique among imaging modalities in that it does not involve the interaction of ionizing radiation or ultrasound waves with tissue. The signal that is produced to form MR images is caused by responses of hydrogen protons within the body to magnetism and radiofrequency pulses; specifically, the relaxation of protons back to an equilibrium state following excitation. Hydrogen protons exhibit magnetism due to their nucleus being composed of an odd number of neutrons and protons.[2,3,9] These hydrogen protons vary in number and in the chemical environments of the tissue they reside within (i.e., fat with long chains of hydrogen protons versus more bound protons within muscle fibers); these factors bestow distinct biochemical and biophysical properties to tissues that are represented in the MR image. Following excitation by the MRI unit, energy is released from the excited protons and used to produce MR images. Specifically, the protons relax back to an equilibrium state and the relaxation rate releases an energy equivalent that is converted into a grayscale signal intensity and used to generate the image. The process of excitation and relaxation must be repeated numerous times to generate the image, which is one reason MRI scans take longer than CT.[1,10] The pulse sequence, which defines the timing of radiofrequency pulse delivery to cause proton excitation and reception of signal to compose images, determines the kind of images that will be obtained, and imaging protocols consist of numerous different pulse sequences.[1-3] Different types of pulse sequences are used to depict different biochemical properties of tissues, as well as some that are used for specific pathologic change detection (i.e., hemorrhage detection).

The subject must be placed within the strong magnetic field of the MRI unit, and pulses of radiofrequency (RF) energy are delivered to excite the protons in the body.[9,10] It should be noted that in contrast to the ionizing radiation of radiographs or CT, no harmful effects have been associated with the high magnetic fields used in the MRI, nor in association with the radiofrequency energy deposition.

MR images are serial, two-dimensional representations of the sectioned three-dimensional anatomy, which are more commonly referred to as slices. Slices refer to the orientation of image acquisition, and slices can be oriented in any direction within the X-Y-Z Cartesian planes. The image, or slice of tissue representation, is composed of pixels similar to a television or computer screen. The higher the number, the better the spatial resolution.[2,3] The pixels in an MR image are grayscale representations of small boxlike sampled volumes of tissue, called voxels.[3,4] The amount of signal available to create the image is determined by the number of protons in the cubic sample or voxel of tissue, which is computationally translated into a grayscale number, and the displayed image is a composite of pixels. If the sampling boxes through the anatomy are made too small, there may not be sufficient signal to produce diagnostic images.[3,11] This can be a significant issue in smaller patients, such as geckos, where high spatial resolution is also desired to evaluate the proportionally smaller anatomy. A major advantage of the MRI is that the amount of signal per voxel increases substantially with increasing field strength. MRI units are described by the magnet strengths, with clinical units having field strengths of 0.3 Tesla (T), 1.5 T, 3.0 T, or less commonly 7.0 T.[2,11] Imaging smaller animals at 3.0 or 7.0 T is easier than at 1.5 T, but the 1.5 T units are the most commonly available strength of veterinary clinical MRI units.[3] There can be successful imaging of smaller reptiles with 1.5 T units or less. Successful reports of MRI using low field strengths (i.e., <1.0 T) have been reported and diagnostic for the delineation of a mass in a tortoise.[12] However, these weaker magnets make diagnostic imaging of smaller patients a challenge. Thus, field strength needs to be a consideration in planning MR in reptiles of various sizes.

The MRI unit produces the strong magnetic field and can come in a bore (closed) or open conformation.[2] The bore units are characterized by a long tubular area within the MRI that completely encircles the patient (Fig. 60.1). These have more uniform magnetic fields at their isocenter, where the imaging of the patient occurs, than do open units. The clinical images presented here were all collected with a closed MRI system. The MRI unit is the source of the applied energy (RF energy) that is used to excite the protons. For some units and for very large patients, the MR unit itself can also collect the signal, but this generally produces poorer quality images than when using a receiver coil. The most standard methods of MRI employ the use of a receiver coil to collect the signal.[3,9,10] The coils can be rigid and encircle the patient or they can be flat or flexible to conform to a surface of the patient. The former is ideal, as the signal throughout the anatomy is uniform, whereas the surface or flexible coils are only able to collect signal over a certain depth. It is critical to use an appropriately sized coil for the patient or the part of the patient to be imaged.[1,3] Signal loss occurs if there is distance between the patient and the coil. Another factor to consider with coil selection is the number of available channels; the more channels the better the signal reception. In veterinary medicine, the most commonly used coil for smaller patients is the knee coil.[3] These encircle the patient and are rigid. The reference to human anatomy allows one to estimate the size of the patient that can be imaged in these coils. In the authors' experience, the bore or closed MRI units with a rigid coil are most commonly used in reptile imaging (see Fig. 60.1B–D).[1] Focal areas of anatomy or smaller patients can often be imaged with a surface or flex coil. We have used these more in our 7.0 T MR unit. The aim with all coils is to position the receiver as close to the patient as possible to optimize the received signal.

Generally, in veterinary medicine, general anesthesia is necessary for most MRI examinations. It is critical that there is no patient movement, because movement degrades image quality.[3] Another factor that undoubtedly influences the need for anesthesia is the length of MR studies. An examination in reptile patients typically includes at least six pulse sequences that are between 4 to 8 minutes long. MR imaging these species can differ from dogs and cats, because some species will move little when handled or in certain environments. With restraint of the limbs via wrapping the body and/or with light pressure applied with cotton balls over closed eyes and wrapping around the head (see Fig. 54.1), we have been able to image iguanas without anesthesia for a 45-minute examination. The cold environment of the MRI unit likely contributes to low movement. More active patients will require anesthesia. Anesthesia is often elected for ease, because movement during a pulse sequence will render the images nondiagnostic and necessitate repeating the entire pulse sequence.[2,3] Securing the patient within the coil through use of MR-compatible positioners and medical tape is helpful. A final patient consideration is metal. Ideally, no metal can be on or in the animal. Metals with magnetic susceptibility are of greatest concern (e.g., most forms of stainless steel), because they produce large artifacts that distort or obscure the anatomy of interest.[2,3,13] In veterinary medicine, the most commonly encountered artifact is associated with microchips, and removal of the chip may be necessary in smaller patients because it is positioned close to the anatomy of interest. To avoid radiofrequency burns, it is important that the patient not contact the magnet or be wrapped in microfiber materials, as some technical fabrics contain metal fibers. Focal tissue heating and/or patient discomfort have been reported in human patients but have not been reported in veterinary medicine.

An MRI protocol consists of multiple pulse sequences designed to detect various physiochemical features of tissue and detect pathologic change. Patient data, MRI information, and annotations are included, not only to enhance the reader's appreciation of MRI utility in clinical reptile scanning but also to provide an introduction to its versatility. The most important of these is likely a T2-weighted (T2w) fast spin echo (FSE) sequence, which is present in all MR protocols of various body parts.[3,6,14] The value of the T2w-FSE is attributed to its sensitivity to changes in intracellular and extracellular fluid, which are components of virtually all pathologic disease processes. The grayscale in MRI is described as signal intensity, and anatomy would be described as hyper- or hypointense for a given pulse sequence. T2w images provide high contrast between different tissue types (Fig. 60.2A–B); for example, fluids and fat are hyperintense (or less formally bright or white), muscle is hypointense (or dark gray), and intraabdominal parenchymal organs are various shades of intermediate signal intensity (or shades of gray that are less than muscle).[2,3,11] Some tissues will be hypointense (or black) on imaging series. This is true for dense bone, such as cortical bone, because the protons within this tissue are so tightly bound they cannot resonate and emit signal intensity. Bone marrow is different because of the fat and hematopoietic constituents within the trabeculae, and it appears bright or hyperintense. Lungs are also hypointense on all MR images, because they essentially lack detectable protons. However, MRI is uncommonly used for interrogation of the lungs because CT is superior for this body system.

Another pulse sequence used frequently is T1-weighted (T1w) SE or FSE sequences. These sequences produce lower contrast images; their strength is in the depiction of anatomy and following contrast administration.[2,3] In T1w images, fat remains hyperintense, fluids are hypointense, and soft tissues and muscle are similar intermediate signal intensity (see Fig. 60.2C). Gadolinium-based contrast agents shorten T1 proton relaxation, and organs that undergo enhancement (e.g., heart, liver, kidney) will have varying degrees of increased signal intensity compared with the precontrast T1w images (see Fig. 60.2D). In the authors' experience, the standard dose for gadolinium-based contrast agents of 0.1 mmol/kg (Magnevist, gadopentetate dimeglumine [Bayer HealthCare Pharmaceuticals Inc.] or Prohance, gadoteridol [Bracco Diagnostics Inc.]) produces detectable contrast enhancement to detail the circulation and enhance the parenchyma in several species of turtles, pythons, and agamid lizards with no detectable adverse effects. This dose is similar to that which produces good results in dogs and cats.[3] In small patients, gadolinium generally increases the emitted signal, and therefore it can

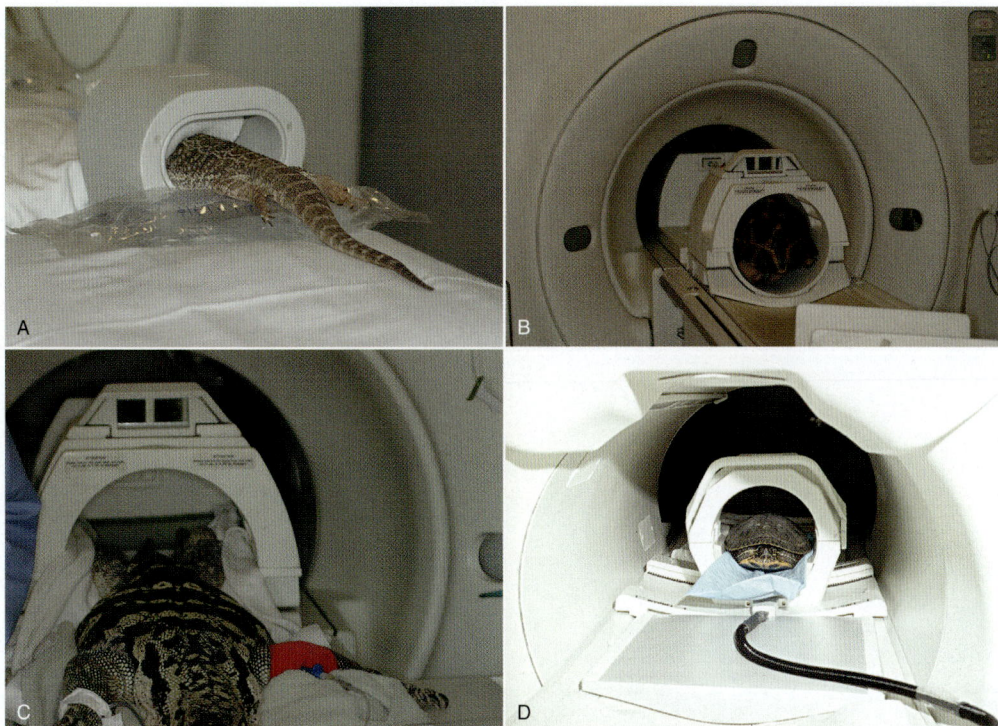

FIG 60.1 Closed MRI unit with two different receiver coils. The receiver coils are positioned at the bore opening of the MRI unit, and they will be advanced into the tube to the isocenter. The receiver coil optimizes the received signal when sized appropriately for the patient. If the receiver coil is too large for the patient, the released signal from the patient has to travel farther to be detected and will degrade. The phenomenon is similar to radio signal detection and improves with proximity to the radio station antenna. (A) A bearded dragon (*Pogona vitticeps*) is positioned in a wrist coil that wraps around the cranial coelom. As a result, only this portion of anatomy can be examined with this configuration. Positioning of the patient within the center of the coil is also important; a saline bag is elevating the caudal coelom and a towel is wrapped around the cranial coelom. The positioner within the coil aids in patient restraint. (B) A radiated tortoise (*Astrochelys radiata*) is positioned within a head and neck coil. In this instance the carapace is in contact with the coil. To avoid tissue heating, normally a layer is placed between the patient and the coil, but heating should not occur due to the tough keratinous and bone carapace composition; soft tissues are more vulnerable. The turtle will be moved into the bore head first so that it is positioned at isocenter for imaging. (C) The head and neck coil is used to examine the pelvis of this large water monitor (*Varanus salvator*). The width of the pelvis necessitates use of this coil, but the long distance between the dorsum of the patient is suboptimal. The caudal body is dorsoventrally compressed, and the pelvis is narrowed in this patient; a surface coil, such as a spine coil, could have been used. (D) A slider turtle (*Trachemys scripta*) is positioned in a receiver coil designed for human knees, and the receiver has been moved into the bore of the MRI. This shows how far in the magnet the isocenter is located (A, B, and C, Courtesy of Stephen J. Divers; D, courtesy of Jeanette Wyneken, Florida Atlantic University.)

be beneficial to repeat or acquire T2w sequences after contrast administration. This is not a standard practice in MR imaging because of concern for distortion by gadolinium contrast agent of representative tissue signal intensities in the T2w images. Gadolinium is mostly considered a T1 contrast agent with minimal effect on T2 relaxation. However, all possible techniques to increase signal intensity may be needed to image smaller reptiles, particularly when using the lower strength high-field (1.5 T) MR units.

There are almost endless numbers of pulse sequences that an MRI user can choose from, and the mixture of different pulse sequences acquired in different planes is responsible for the longer scan times associated with MRI. For example, inversion recovery (IR) sequences are extremely useful for depicting specific tissue chemistry features.[6,15] This kind of sequence uses MR physics and the application of an additional RF pulse to suppress the signal from a specific tissue or fluid.

In the neurocranium, fluid attenuation inversion recovery (FLAIR) sequences are useful in suppressing the signal intensity from CSF or other pure fluids. These IR pulse sequences can be acquired as a T2w or T1w FLAIR series. Periventricular parenchymal high signal intensity is more easily distinguished on T2w FLAIR images compared with T2w images.[3,16] T1w FLAIR images are necessary at higher MR field strengths (i.e., 3.0 T or more) to distinguish the areas of ventricular fluid, since T1 relaxation is affected by field strength.[17] Short tau inversion recovery (STIR) images are another form of inversion recovery sequence in which tissues composed of fat are suppressed (see Fig. 60.2E).[3,6,11]

Gradient-recalled echo (GRE) sequences are the second-most commonly used group of pulse sequences after FSE sequences. These have greater issues with artifacts, but like FSE, sequences can provide specific tissue information.[2] These can be run as T2w or T1w, but the most commonly used GRE sequence in veterinary medicine is T2*-weighted

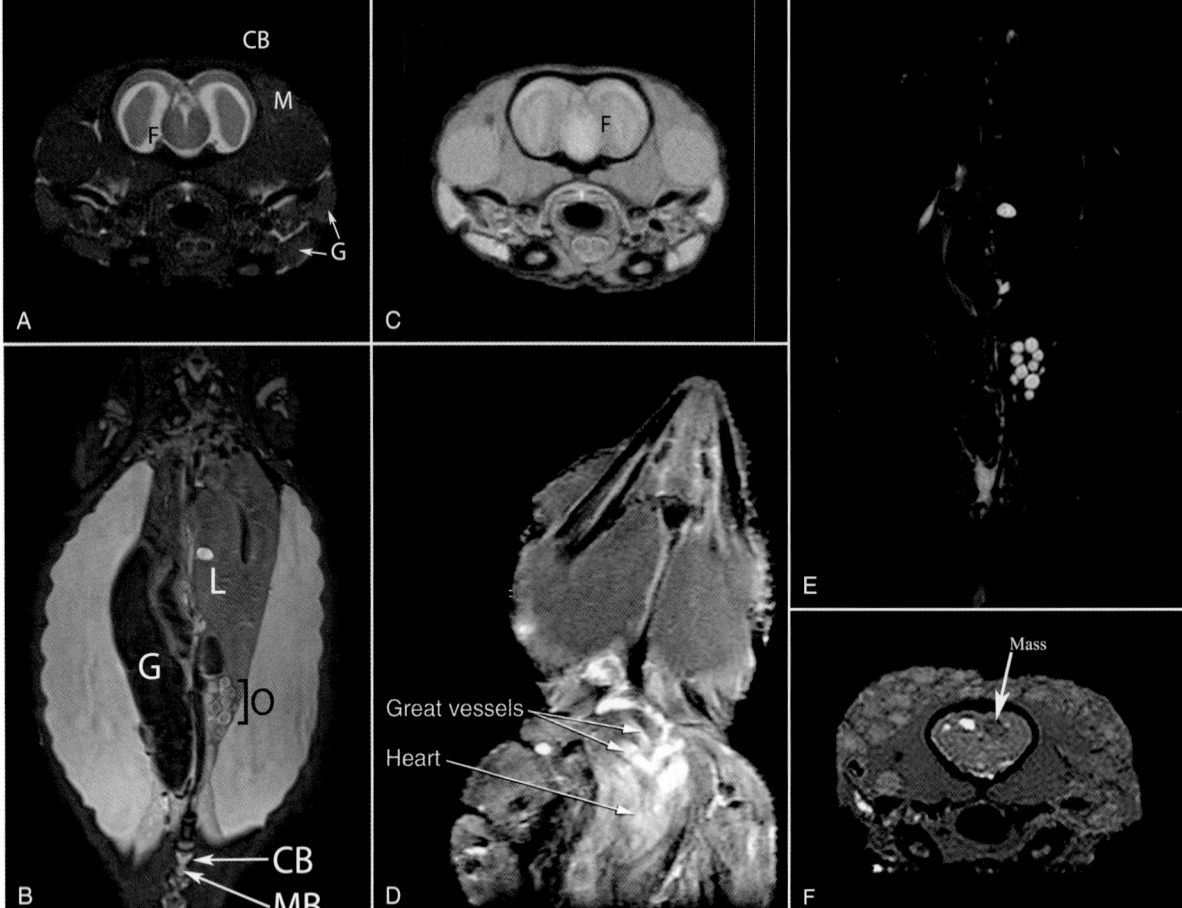

FIG 60.2 Examples of commonly used MR pulse sequences in reptile MRI. (A) T2w FSE transverse image centered on the brainstem of a ball python (*Python regius*). The CSF fluid (F) is markedly hyperintense, and fat would also be hyperintense if present. T2w are beneficial in the nervous system because of the enhanced distinction between the gray and white matter regions in the brain. Some hyperintense fluid is seen in the quadrate-articular joint. Cortical bone (CB) is most hypointense with muscle (M) being less hypointense. Glandular salivary tissue (G) is intermediate signal intensity. (B) T2w 3D FSE dorsal plane image of female lace monitor lizard (*Varanus varius*) centered in middorsal coelom. Bilateral large hyperintense fat pads (F) are identified and gas (G) in the colon is black because no protons are present. The liver (L) has uniform intermediate signal intensity with arborizing intraparenchymal foci that are both hyper- and hypointense, which is due to blood flow artifact. The gallbladder within the liver is hyperintense. The relative hyperintensity of medullary (MB) to cortical bone (CB) is seen in the included thoracic limbs (top of image) and vertebrae (bottom of image). The immature ova (O) have alternating signal intensity consistent with the parenchymal achitecture. (C) Precontrast administration T1w 2D GRE at the same level of the ball python brain in (A). The CSF fluid (F) is relatively hypointense to brain tissue. Note there is minimal to no distinction between the gray and white matter regions. (D) Dorsal plane postcontrast administration T1 images of a bearded dragon (*Pogona vitticeps*). The presence of gadolinium contrast in the circulatory system causes these structures to have increased signal intensity relative to precontrast. The hyperintensity in the heart is less than the greater vessels, which is most likely due to flow artifacts superimposed on the contrast-enhanced blood. (E) STIR dorsal plane image of the female lace monitor lizard matched to the coelomic image in (B). The fat pads are severely hypointense, which is due to complete suppression of all signal from fatty tissues. Interestingly, the liver is also markedly suppressed; this is not commonly seen in dogs or cats but would be expected in female reptiles with increased fat content within the liver in preparation for folliculogenesis, or secondary to hepatic lipidosis, which is common in many captive reptiles. The follicles and gallbladder are more conspicuous on the black background. This increased conspicuity of fluid areas is the primary benefit of this sequence. (F) T2*w transverse image of a ball python brain with an intraventricular mass that has a heterogeneous rim of hypointensity that was not present on any other imaging series performed. This rim of hypointensity was therefore most likely a rim of hemorrhage. Mineral can also be low signal intensity on this sequence but is similarly low signal intensity on other sequences. GRE sequences are more susceptible to artifact, and T2*w amplifies this susceptibility, making very small accumulations of hemorrhage visible. It is noted that this patient also has numerous intermediate signal intensity cysts encircling its head, which are abnormal and discussed in greater detail in Fig. 60.14. (D, Courtesy of Jeanette Wyneken, Florida Atlantic University.)

(T2*w). With T2* weighting, the sequence can be specifically used for hemorrhage detection and is capable of detecting microhemorrhagic foci (see Fig. 60.2F).[3,6,18] GRE sequences can be acquired as 2D or 3D acquisitions; the latter seems to be more frequently used in reptile imaging, especially on low field MRI units to optimize spatial resolution.[1,4] Although improvements in spatial resolution are one of the benefits of this sequence, the increased artifacts associated with this sequence compared with FSE sequences make it less useful and therefore is not commonly used in our reptile examinations. With MRI, angiography is possible both before and following contrast administration with the application of specific GRE sequences. 3D time-of-flight sequences are the easiest to use, because they do not require knowledge of the flow velocities, nor is the injection of contrast needed.[3]

Table 60.1 provides examples of pulse sequence protocols used to scan specific regions of the body. Each is designed to evaluate the tissue for both anatomical and biochemical appearance. The information gained from the different pulse sequences has been established in human, canine, and feline imaging and then extrapolated to reptils. The pulse sequence protocol for the neurocranium is a good example of how the appearance of a single tissue is depicted with different signal intensities or shades of gray on different pulse sequences (see Fig. 60.2).

Some newer pulse sequences have been developed and are particularly beneficial for imaging smaller patients, because they can acquire submillimeter slices. These are similar to 3D GRE sequences, but these possess contrast similar to FSE sequences.[19,20] Traditional MR slices for FSE sequences used in veterinary medicine usually need to be 2 to 3 mm thick.[15] One of the new sequences is essentially a 3D FSE sequence, with the name varying between MR companies (called CUBE in GE units, SPACE in Siemens units, VISTA in Philips units, and MVOX in Toshiba units).[20] These can be acquired as isotropic voxels, meaning the box sampling tissue in the anatomy is equal in all dimensions. The benefit of this form of acquisition is they can be reconstructed after the scan into different plans (Fig. 60.3), which is more similar to CT

TABLE 60.1 Examples of Pulse Sequence Protocols Used by the Authors to Evaluate Two Commonly Imaged Body Systems

Neurologic System	Coelom†
T2w sagittal and transverse	T2 sagittal and transverse
T2w FLAIR*	STIR dorsal
T2*w transverse	T1 dorsal and transverse
T1w transverse	Postcontrast T1w dorsal, transverse
Postcontrast T1w transverse, ± sagittal & dorsal	& sagittal
3D FSE or GRE, especially for small animals	

These are protocols used in reptile scanning but are similar to those outlined in human standard operating MRI protocols from the American College of Radiology (ACR). Some pulse sequences are more commonly used in different areas because of the biochemical information that is provided. For example, T2-weighted images are used in all MR imaging protocols, and this is attributed to their optimal soft tissue contrast and "fluid sensitivity" because abnormal fluid accumulations accompany most pathologic processes.

*T2w FLAIR images can be challenging in smaller patients since this sequence has low signal-to-noise inherently; it may need to be omitted in small patients scanned with a 1.5 T or less MRI unit.

†Negating effects of respiration (through respiratory gating) is rarely needed in reptiles.

acquisitions. 3D sequences historically have been GRE or angiographic sequences, which offer less desirable tissue contrast than FSE. Therefore these newer 3D FSE sequences maintain the superior soft tissue contrast of 2D FSE sequences and can obtain thinner slices (i.e., submillimeter) within a clinically feasible time.[21] Therefore, ideal contrast resolution is maintained and spatial resolution is optimized over 2D FSE sequences.

MRI APPLICATIONS IN REPTILES

Based on current literature, there are more numerous MRI examinations of reptiles for anatomic studies and research than for clinical diagnostic purposes. This pattern follows the development of MR in human, canine, feline, and equine medicine. The number of clinical cases examined with MRI has increased in recent years with the increased accessibility to MRI units and likely as clinicians have realized the clinical benefit of this modality. Glodek et al. went further and indicated that MRI was the preferred imaging modality in exotic animals.[1]

Cross-sectional imaging modalities have transformed our knowledge of in vivo anatomy. With the superior soft tissue contrast resolution offered by MRI, detailed anatomy can be delineated. Obviously, the superimposition of anatomy associated with radiography is removed with cross-sectional imaging. Both MRI and CT imaging provide excellent spatial positioning of organs. The benefit of the soft tissue contrast resolution of MRI is that the anatomy is defined by specific signal intensity characteristics, and the parenchymal architecture within organs is identifiable without the need to administer gadolinium contrast intravenously. CT can depict the positioning of anatomy but is more dependent on the intravenous administration of iodinated contrast to depict finer anatomical details, such as parenchymal architecture. Basic reptile MRI anatomy examples are provided (Figs. 60.4–60.13) to illustrate both the spatial and contrast resolution features encountered at different MR unit strengths.

The MR anatomic appearance has been reported for crocodile musculature, testudine middle ear, snake venom system, and head and body of loggerhead sea turtles.[22–26] However, the varied research applications demonstrate the sensitivity and specificity of this modality, which is most likely associated with its soft tissue contrast resolution. MRI is considered the gold standard for noninvasive examination of the neurological system. Using MRI, researchers were able to detect differences between male and female dragon lizard (*Ctenophorus* spp.) primary nuclei (medial peroptic nucleus, MPON) and the ventromedial hypothalamic nucleus, VMN), as well as evolving changes in brain volume.[27] Nonneurologic and neurologic reptile soft tissue structural details have been delineated using MRI, including the structural features that facilitate lizard tail autotomy, fiber-type distribution in the lizard tongue, and crocodile brain volume changes.[28–30] We have used MRI to test changes in the liver of the green iguana (*Iguana iguana*) following carbon tetrachloride administration (Schnellbacher et al, unpublished data). These studies demonstrate the ability to acquire both morphologic and quantitative data from reptiles using MRI, with the latter often being critical for research credibility. All MR images can provide quantitative data if the signal intensity is assessed relative to established normal values. Additional morphologic and quantitative sequences that can be used include diffusion-weighted imaging (DWI) for strokes, diffusion tensor imaging (DTI) for assessment of fractional anisotropy in white matter tracts, and T2 or T1 relaxation time mapping to provide visual representation of tissue alterations.

The use of MRI in clinical applications is similar to human and veterinary patients. For neurologic system evaluation, Brady et al. used MRI to determine whether structural brain disease was responsible for seizures in a crocodile.[31] With smaller brain sizes, higher field MR units are ideal. The spatial resolution, as well as the contrast resolution, can

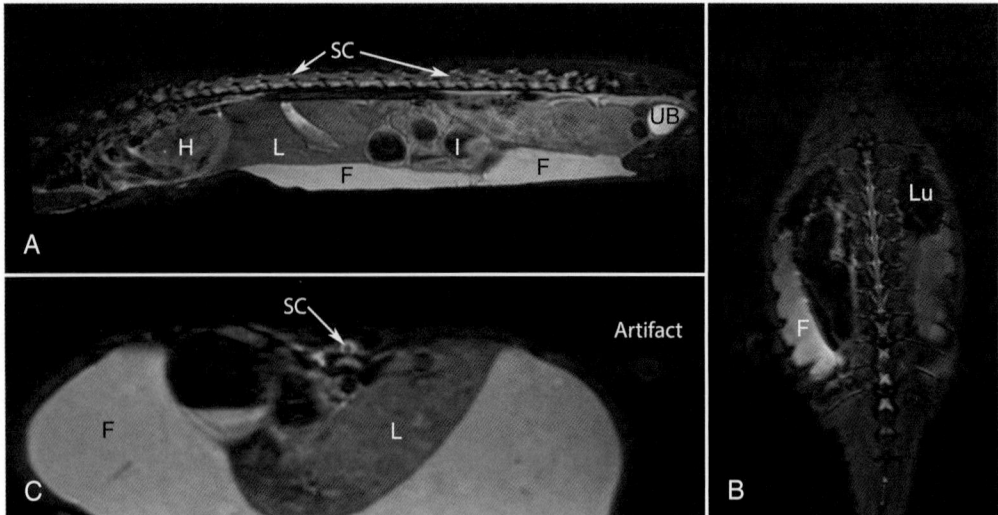

FIG 60.3 Standard MR imaging planes from a 3D FSE T2w sequence, consisting of sagittal (A), dorsal (B), and transverse (C) planes of a green iguana (*Iguana iguana,* snout to vent 30 cm). Unlike CT, which only acquires transverse plane images, MRI can acquire images in any plane. Historically, this meant that each plane had to be acquired separately. 3D FSE sequences acquire isotropic voxels in one plane, in this instance, in the dorsal plane (B), and then the voxels can be reconstructed into any plane. In this sequence, the voxel dimensions were 0.3 mm^3, which means the spatial resolution is 0.3 mm^2. This also means the slice thickness is 0.33 mm; contrast this to routine 2D FSE slice thicknesses of 1 mm at 7.0 T and 3.0 mm at 1.5 T. For reference, this lizard measured 43 cm in length by 7 cm in diameter. The spinal cord (SC) is distinguishable with this resolution. For reference, the coelomic anatomy (H, heart; Lu, lung; L, liver; F, fat; I, intestine; UB, urinary bladder) can also be well evaluated with this sequence.

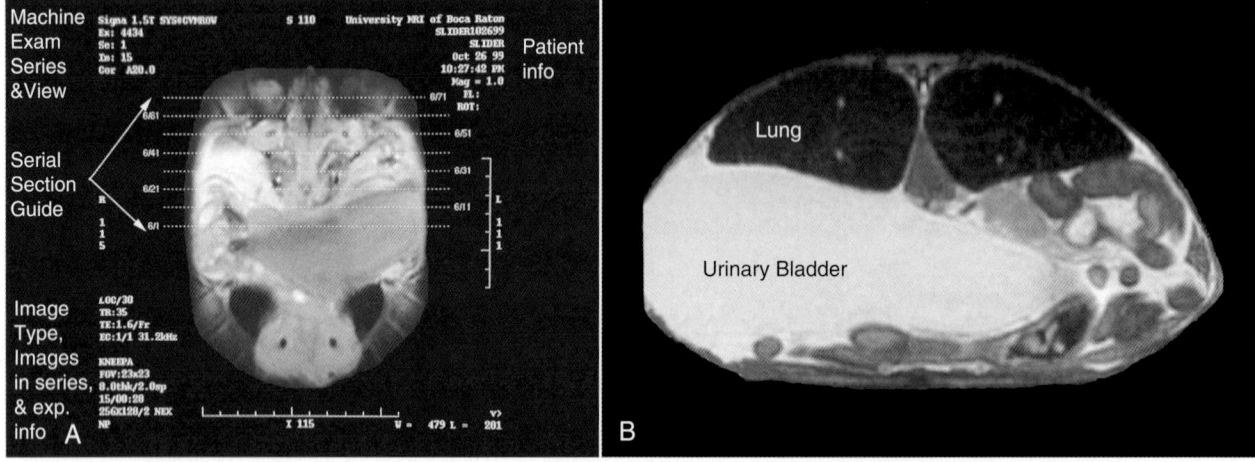

FIG 60.4 (A) Low-resolution "localizer" image is used to plan slices or the image planes. In this case, transverse T2w images are planned throughout the body of a slider turtle midbody. The turtle was oriented with the plastron down; left and right are not reversed in the image. (B) This image section represents localizer line labeled 6/1; the large fluid-filled urinary bladder (hyperintense) extends anteriorly and occupies most of the left half of the image. Bone is barely visible as a thin dark (hypointense) outline. Dorsally, the hypointense spaces are lung tissue with the paired pulmonary artery and vein seen as hyperintense dots. To the right are intestines with intermediate signal intensity; fat, intracoelomic fluid, and mesenteric blood are the most hyperintense areas. The darker gray caudal tip of the liver is ventral. The left side of the turtle was outside of the scanned area. This image was magnified slightly in processing the data. *Trachemys scripta,* adult.

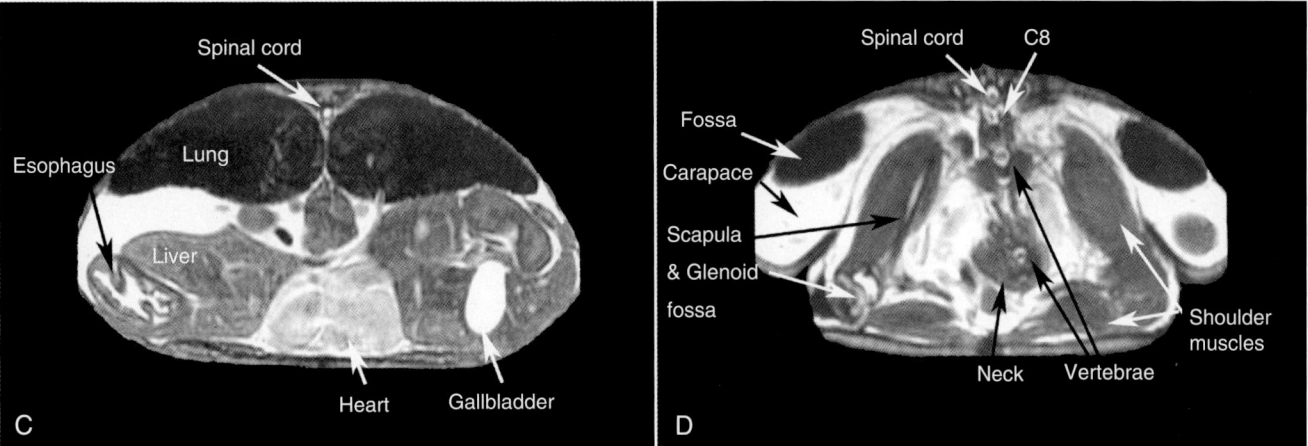

FIG 60.4, cont'd (C) This image is 20 slices more cranial (localizer line 6/21). At this level, the esophagus can be seen to the left. The liver has two large lobes that fill much of the ventral half of the body and one small lobe dorsal to the heart. The heart would be described as being hyperintense to the liver and is found midventrally. The hypointense lungs are dorsal and abut the vertebrae and carpacial bone. The spinal cord can be seen as a hyperintense (white) dot between the medial and dorsal parts of the lungs. (D) This image is another 30 slices more cranial (localizer line 6/51). Note the artifactual thickened appearance of the carapace; this is a partial volume artifact and is because the carapace passes through the slices oblique (i.e., along its curvature). The hypointense (black) spaces dorsolaterally are air-filled fossae where the forelimbs may retract. Medullary bone is hyperintense because of marrow fat. Muscle is among the most hypointense tissues but is less hypointense than cortical bone. Both sets of shoulder muscles and the left scapula are in this plane. In the middle of the body is the retracted neck at the level where the vertebrae form an s-curve. As a result, parts of vertebrae C8, C7 or C6, and C3 are seen from dorsal to ventral. (Courtesy of Jeanette Wyneken, Florida Atlantic University.)

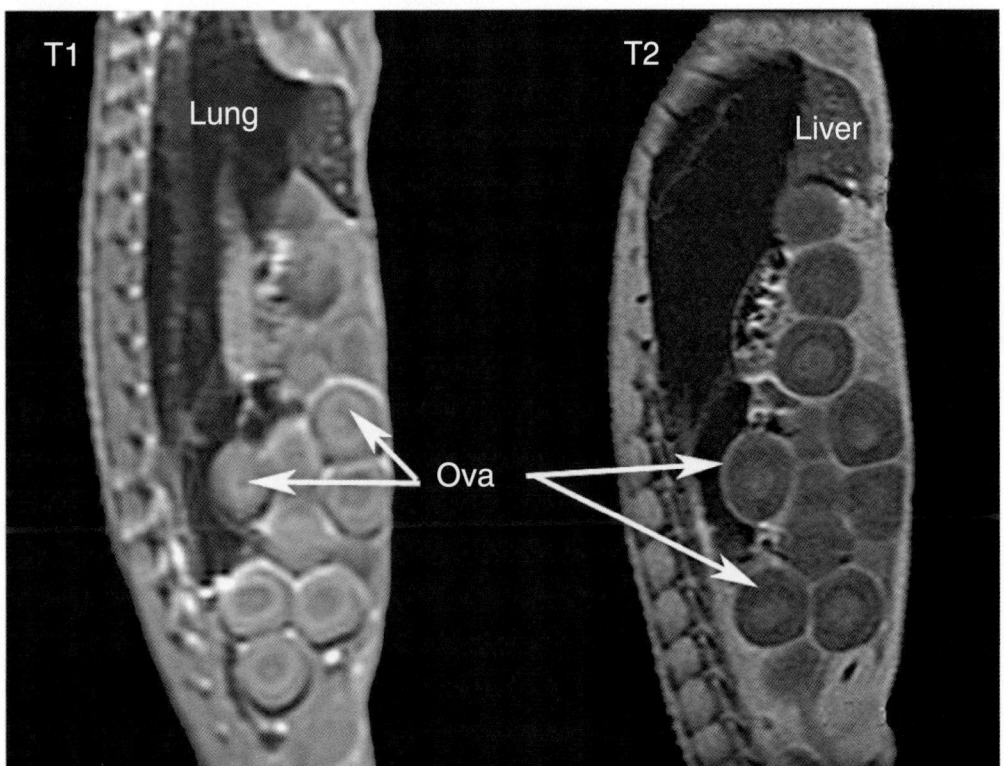

FIG 60.5 Two sagittal images of a female green iguana (*Iguana iguana*) torso taken at roughly the same position. Cranial is toward the top of the image. In the T1 image, fat is hyperintense, air is black, fluid (blood, edema, cerebrospinal fluid [CSF], or yolk) is hypointense, and cortical bone is the most hypointense tissue and will be on all images. Parts of the spinal nerves can be seen as the white dots running along the spine on the left side of the image. In T2 images, fluids are hyperintense; fats are also hyperintense not as hyperintense as fluid. The posterior trunk vertebrae and muscles are easy to identify. This T2 section caught little blood flow (seen immediately to the left of the more anterior ova). The more liquid centers of the yolked ova are clear in both images. (Courtesy of Jeanette Wyneken, Florida Atlantic University.)

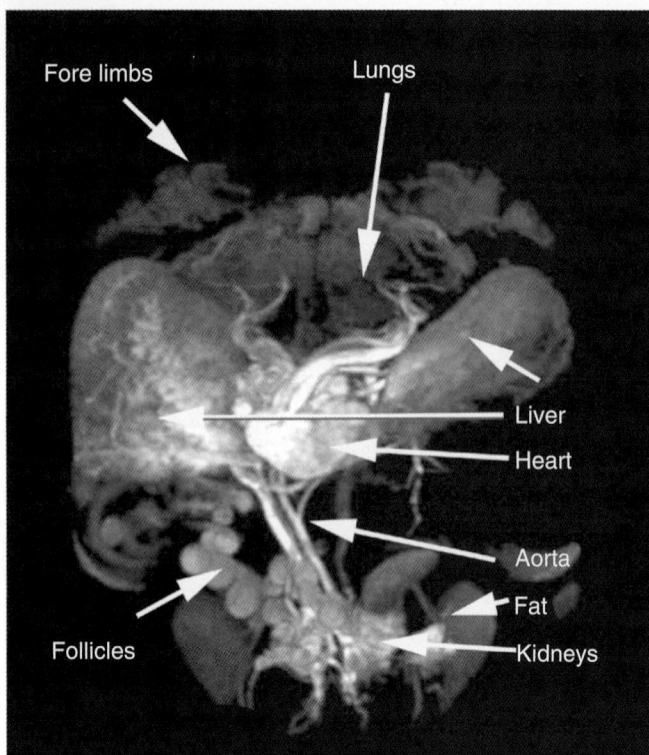

FIG 60.6 Soft tissue anatomy of a slider turtle (*Trachemys scripta*) in dorsal plane is outlined in this T2*-weighted MR image with the vasculature highlighted by the intravenous gadolinium contrast agent (acquired as part of a fMRI examination). The heart plus the highly vascular liver, pulmonary arteries and veins, and kidneys are clearly outlined. Forelimbs are outlined less densely. The two aortic arches join in the midbody as the single dorsal aorta. The larger vessel paralleling the dorsal aorta is the post caval vein. Follicles and fat pads are shown caudally. (Courtesy of Jeanette Wyneken, Florida Atlantic University.)

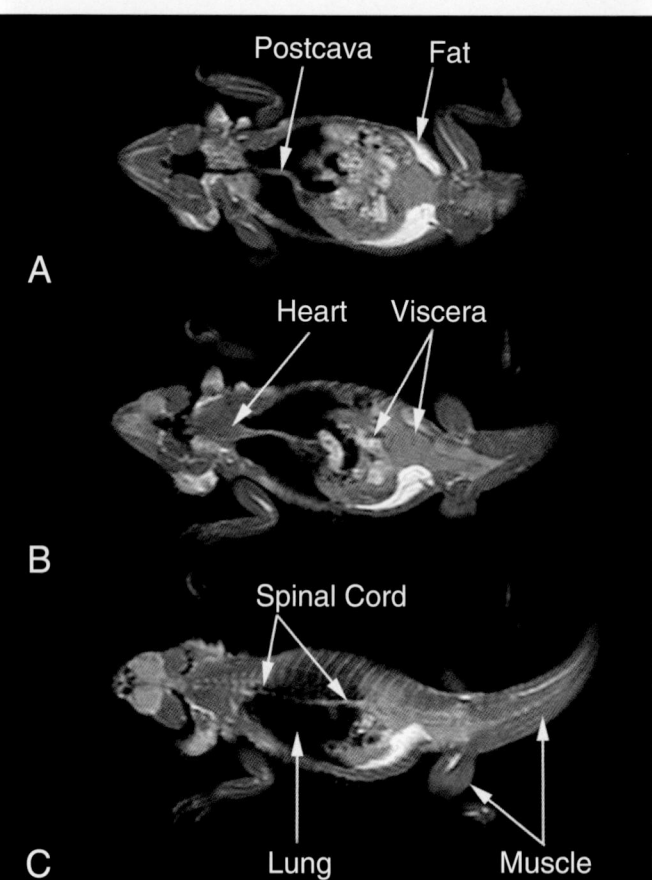

FIG 60.7 These three images are of an adult male bearded dragon (*Pogona vitticeps*, snout-to-vent length 17.6 cm) viewed serially from ventral to dorsal in dorsal plane T1w images, so fat and medullary bone are hyperintense. Fluid and nonfatty tissues appear gray. Air appears black. The most ventral section (A) passes dorsal to the tongue and through the trachea, lungs, postcava, liver, viscera, and through the proximal tail. Long bones and muscles of the limbs can be seen. More dorsally, (B) the lungs, heart, aorta, liver, viscera, and fat pads are clear. In the most dorsal view, (C) the air-filled nasal passages, the eyes, left lung, parts of the spinal cord (light), abdominal fat pads, and tail muscles and tendons can be discriminated. (Courtesy of Jeanette Wyneken, Florida Atlantic University.)

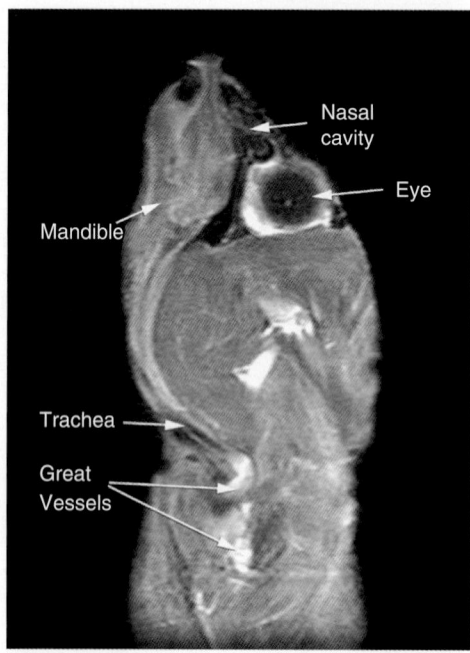

FIG 60.8 This two-dimensional parasagittal image of a bearded dragon (*Pogona vitticeps*, snout-vent length 22.5 cm) shows muscle, the medial edge of the mandible and the nasal cavity. The temporomandibular joint and part of the adjacent circulation (external jugular vein) appear hyperintense (white). This is a T1w image made after gadolinium contrast administration. Parts of the great vessels are caught in this plane of section, as is a small section of the trachea. (Courtesy of Jeanette Wyneken, Florida Atlantic University.)

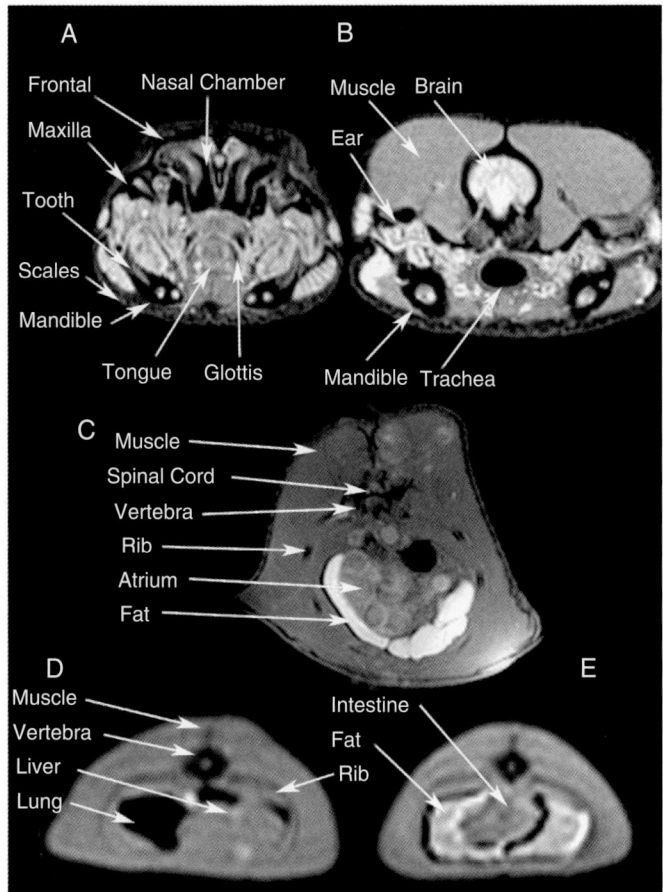

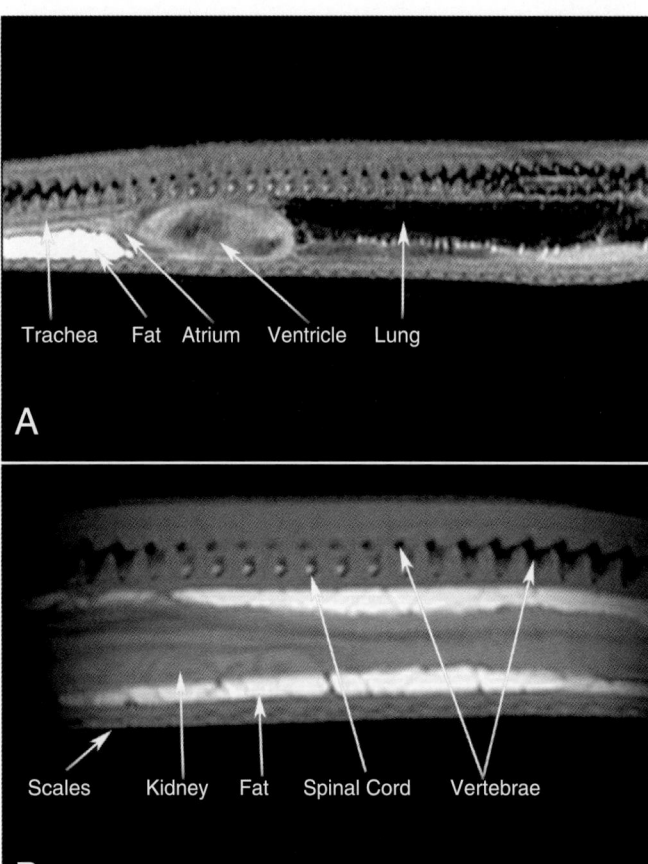

FIG 60.9 Transverse MRI of an adult male Burmese python (*Python bivittatus*, total length 2.9 m) made at multiple levels. MRI of whole snakes is difficult because of the tubular geometry of the animals. Often the snake must be examined in a series of sequential parts to avoid losing image quality (A–C). Snake images taken without the aid of a small imaging coil or in an open MRI may be of limited value, because they tend to have low signal to noise artifacts (D and E), resulting in a grainy appearance. For an MRI machine to have sufficient range to scan a whole snake, or even part of a large snake, the distance between the snake and receiver needs to be minimized. The entire length could only be examined if the snake fit the length of the longest coil in an MRI unit, which is the spine coil. These T1-weighted transverse images show nasal passages and mouth (A), more slices of the head show the brain is hypointense (white), and muscles are moderately hyperintense as various shades of gray (B). Sections through the trunk show the vertebrae and ribs as dark foci seen in part by the plane of view; the spinal cord is hyperintense. (Courtesy of Jeanette Wyneken, Florida Atlantic University.)

FIG 60.10 Sagittal or parasagittal T1w MR images of an adult male Burmese python (*Python bivittatus*, total length 2.9 m) demonstrating major structures of the cranial (A) and caudal trunk (B). The head is to the left in both images. A large hyperintense fat pad is located cranial to the heart. The heart (moderately hypointense) and lungs (hypointense) have less detail than the (moderately hypointense) lobular kidney tissues. Because the heart beats throughout image acquisition, some movement artifacts are seen in the cranial body. The thyroid and parathyroid glands could not be distinguished from the fat; this may be due to the pulse sequence or image resolution. (Courtesy of Jeanette Wyneken, Florida Atlantic University.)

be optimized for extremely small anatomy (Fig. 60.14), such as 1.5-kg ball python with a neurocranium diameter measuring less than 3 cm. The spine can also be examined. Spinal cord compressive lesions can be visualized well with MRI and used in determining feasibility of intervention.[32] We have used MRI to localize and diagnose spinal cord compression in a snake (Fig. 60.15), skink (Fig. 60.16) and monitor lizard (Fig. 60.17). The effect of field strength can be appreciated in this series of figures. The snake was 3 cm in diameter with the vertebral column width of 5 mm and a spinal cord width of 1.7 mm; therefore the 7.0 T MRI unit was needed to obtain high-resolution images in a clinically acceptable time. In contrast, the blue-tongued skink (6 cm in diameter with vertebral column width of 8 mm) was imaged with a 1.5 T MRI unit. If a patient this small is to be successfully imaged on a 1.5 T unit, it is necessary to scan for a longer period of time per pulse sequence to get sufficient signal, and the number of sequences may have to be reduced to those that are most diagnostically useful (i.e., T2w) to avoid prolonged anesthesia. The skink case demonstrates maintenance of the sensitivity of MRI because of superior soft tissue contrast resolution, but the specificity in characterizing the lesion is diminished with poorer image spatial resolution. The monitor lizard, with a neck thickness of 4 cm in diameter and spinal cord 3 mm in diameter, was also scanned on a 1.5 T MRI unit. This examination demonstrates the benefit of using 3D FSE and GRE sequences in patients with small anatomy. For reference, convention sagittal plane 2D FSE sequence obtained a single slice through the spinal cord, whereas the sagittal plane 3D FSE sequence produced 10 slices through the spinal cord at the level of the lesion, and these could be reconstructed into transverse and dorsal plane images after the examination was complete.

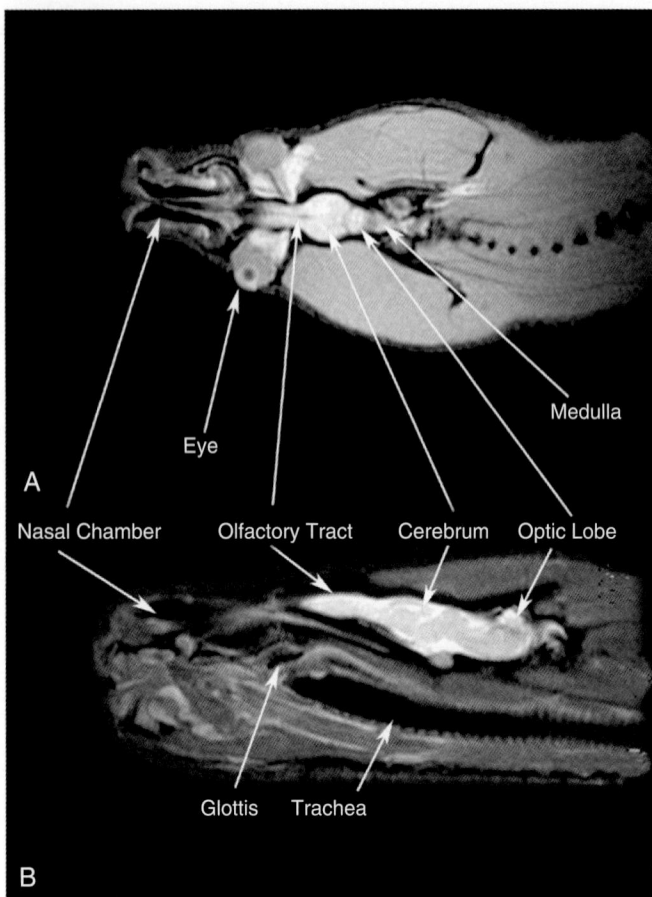

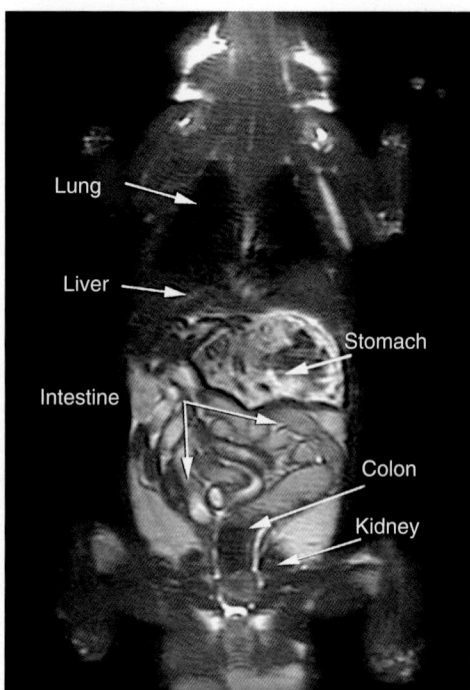

FIG 60.11 Dorsal and sagittal plane T2w MR images of the adult male Burmese python head (*Python bivittatus*, total length 2.9 m). This pair of images shows the major brain anatomy and some of the landmarks associated with the mouth and airway. The two images show the musculature surrounding the brain and calvarial vault (A) and the close proximity of the brain to the primary palate structure (B). (Courtesy of Jeanette Wyneken, Florida Atlantic University.)

FIG 60.12 This T2w GRE magnetic resonance image (MRI) of a juvenile alligator (*Alligator mississippiensis*, snout-vent length 29 cm) torso is a two-dimensional image. The plane of view is a dorsal section of the ventral one-third of the animal. The gastrointestinal tract and its contents are clearly visible as moderately hypotense shades of gray. Fluids in the coelomic cavity and throat are hypertense. Fat is dark gray, and air in the lungs is hypotense (black). Portions of the kidneys are visible adjacent to the colon. (Courtesy of Jeanette Wyneken, Florida Atlantic University.)

Therefore the lateralization of a lesion can be better defined, and additional planes can be made without extending anesthesia.

Reptiles can more greatly benefit from MRI and its superior soft tissue contrast resolution relative to many other species. Body MRI is more common in humans than in dogs and cats, yet, the number of case reports on body MRI of reptiles show its great value. For example, MRI has been used to diagnose coelomic masses (seminoma in a Greek tortoise, *Testudo graeca*), hepatocellular carcinoma in a green iguana, *Iguana iguana*) and cloacal stricture in a green sea turtle (*Chelonia mydas*).[12,33,34] In the Greek tortoise with a seminoma, the reported benefit of the MRI was localizing the mass within the coelom, discriminating and evaluating adjacent coelomic organs, and using the signal intensity characteristics of the mass to diagnose seminoma as the primary or more specific differential diagnosis. Knotek et al. were able to extrapolate the MR appearance of hepatocellular carcinomas in other species to reach a more specific noninvasive diagnosis in the iguana.[35] In our experience, neurological and coelomic MRI examinations are the most common clinical application in reptiles. This is due to its sensitivity in disease detection of the nervous system similar to that seen in other species and for the ability to provide a better distinction between

normal coelomic anatomy (based on signal intensity characteristics) and alterations in coelomic organ signal intensities, which can represent different disease processes. Some examples showing coelomic MRI applications in clinical practice are provided (Figs. 60.17 and 60.18). The benefit of higher field strength with smaller patients is also demonstrated (Fig. 60.19).

Radiographic imaging of the reptile coelom is often challenging due to poor serosal detail. MRI negates this concern in clinical practice. Therefore the major advantage realized to date with MRI in reptiles is the ability to depict anatomical and pathologic processes with great specificity. It does generally require anesthesia and is the most expensive of all diagnostic imaging modalities. These disadvantages can be outweighed by the effective digital antemortem-like examination provided by MRI. Increased usage of MRI in reptile diagnostics is expected, with an increasing accessibility to MR units that are capable of imaging a wide range of reptile sizes and as reptile owners and clinicians gain better knowledge about MRI.

An important final note is that most diagnostic MR imaging studies will benefit from the involvement of a radiologist as well as an MRI technologist. Diagnostic scans are often challenging to obtain, especially in smaller reptiles where acquiring sufficient signal is needed to create diagnostic images. The anatomic variation, in addition to signal intensity variations in tissue, is a further challenge in reptile MR image interpretation that can be partially mitigated by a radiologist with expertise in this area. Lack of MR experience can lead to misinterpretation or the possibility of missing lesions because reference material on the normal

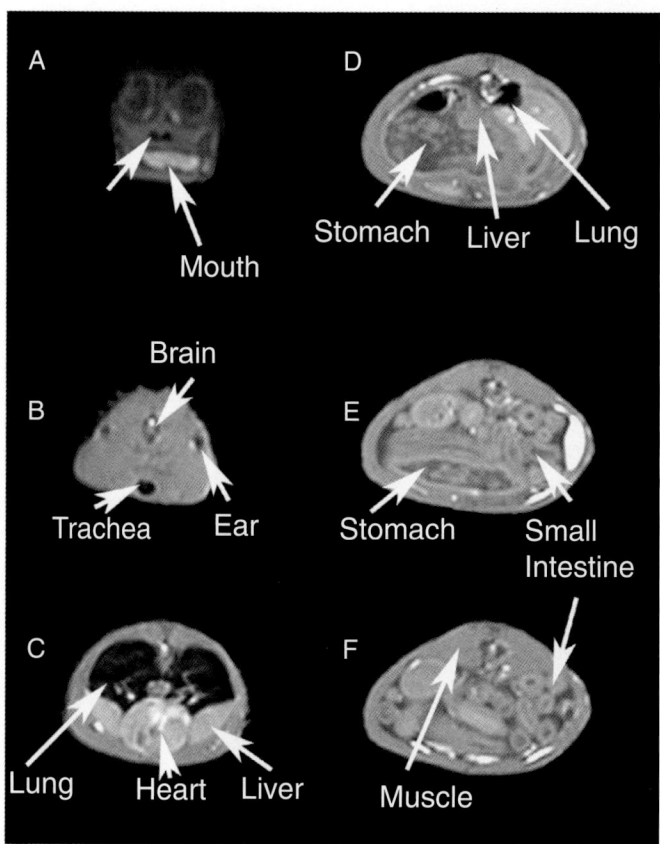

FIG 60.13 These MRI axial sections of a small alligator (*Alligator mississippiensis*, snout-vent length 22 cm) provide a survey of different parts of the animal from the head to the lower abdomen. They were collected using a 1.5 T unit to both deliver and receive signal. This approach provides information but limits the resolution. The eyes appear as light gray ovals with moderately hypointense (dark) gray centers (the vitreous); air in the nares, trachea, and ear cavities is hypointense (black); and the brain is hyperintense with gray surrounding bone (A and B). At the level of the heart (C), great vessels and the pulmonary circulation appear bright; the lungs are hypointense; muscles and liver appear moderately hypointense; and the spinal cord and cerebrospinal fluid (CSF) appear hyperintense. At the midbody, the lung sections are small. The stomach and liver are large, and major vessels including the abdominal veins and aortae can be seen (D). More posteriorly, the remainder of the gastrointestinal tract can be seen, and moderately hypointense (gray) epaxial muscles occupy much of the dorsal body (E and F). (Courtesy of Jeanette Wyneken, Florida Atlantic University.)

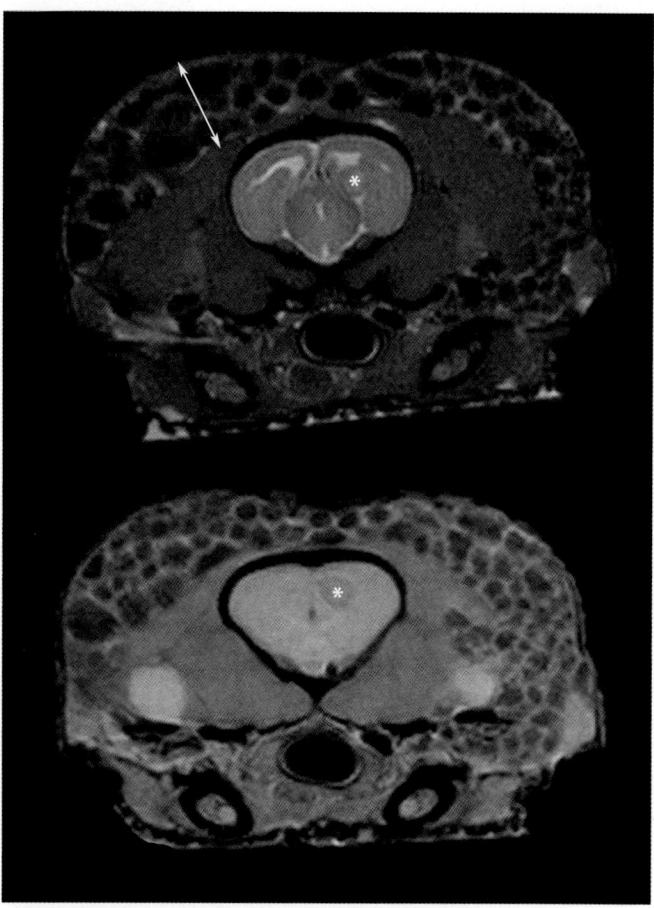

FIG 60.14 Transverse T2-weighted (*top*) and T1-weighted images acquired on a 7.0 T MRI unit of a 13-year-old ball python (*Python regius*, snout-to-vent length 95 cm) presenting with inappetence and facial swelling associated with the right cranium and left maxilla. Extensive distinctly marginated low signal intensity nodules (between arrowheads) are present just deep to the cutaneous layer and superficial to the temporal musculature. No evidence of infiltration into these structures was detected except extension into the deeper anatomical regions, such as into the area of the left maxilla. Because these nodules were hypointense in all imaging series, they were interpreted as consistent of dense tissue that exhibited minimal resonance. This included fibrous, keratinized, or less likely, mineralized foci. Biopsy confirmed extensive keratinized cysts. An intraventricular mass (*) was also identified in the left lateral ventricle. It was considered an incidental finding because there were no associated neurological abnormalities or deficits. For reference the images were acquired with field of view, 5.0 cm; slice thickness, 1 mm; pixel resolution, 0.2 mm^2. (Courtesy of Shannon P. Holmes.)

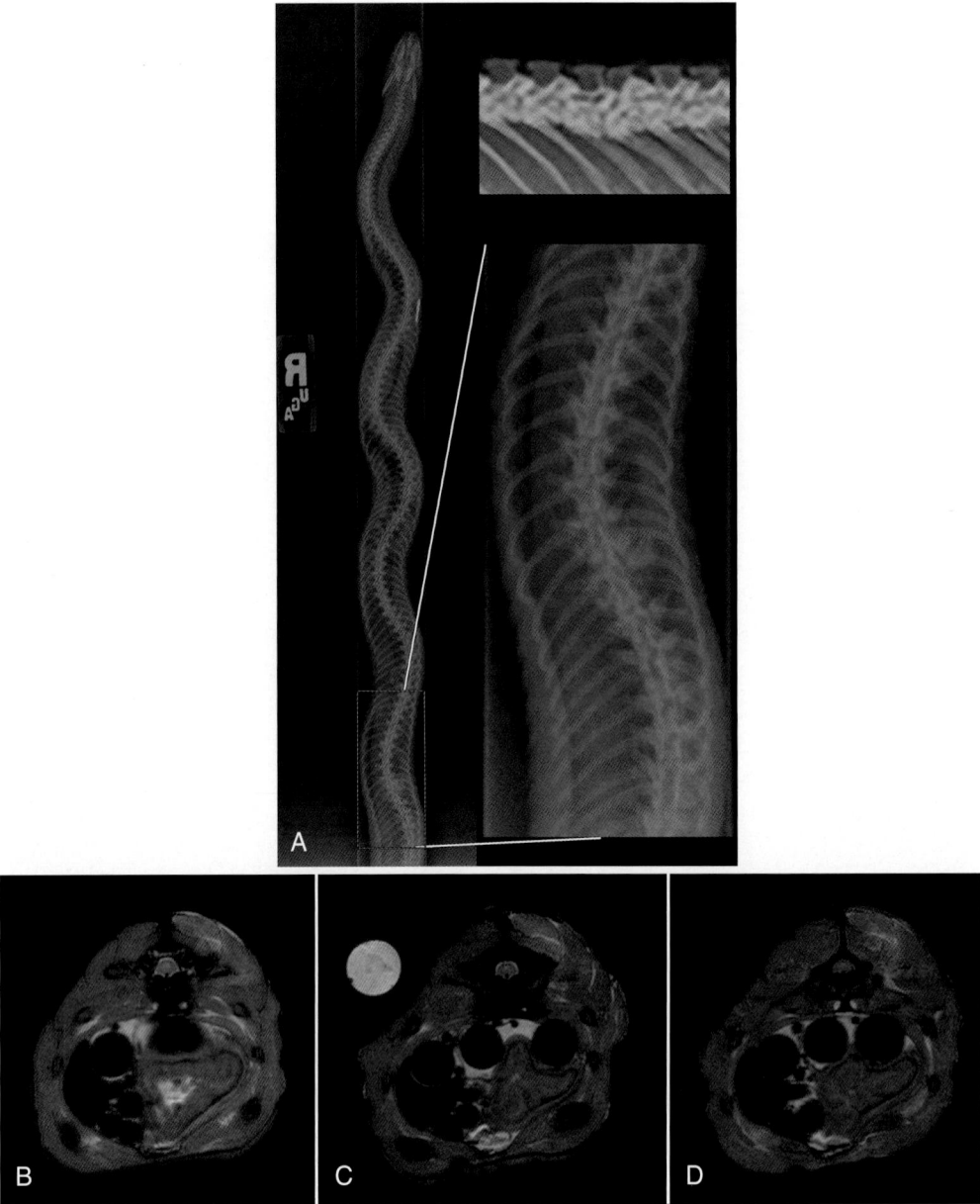

FIG 60.15 Dorsoventral and horizontal beam lateral radiographs (A) and 7.0 T T2-weighted MR images (B–D) of a 4-year-old female Florida king snake (*Lampropeltis getula floridana*, 96 cm total length) presented for evaluation of multiple areas of dull and wrinkled scales, and chronic dysedysis, inappetence, and severe weight loss. The spinous processes were abnormal on physical examination and multiple neurological deficits were exhibited, including flipping dorsally and delayed righting. Multifocal areas of exuberant osseous proliferation were present in association with the vertebral bodies, as well as areas of smooth periosteal proliferation on multiple ribs. Radiography was crucial for planning the areas to examine by MRI, because it is not possible to scan the entire length of the patient (maximum length dictated by the surface coil was 7 cm). The transverse images were acquired in the area seen in the lateral radiography where there was collapse of the interspinous space and mild focal lordosis. In the transverse images centered at this level, (D) there is moderate narrowing of the vertebral canal and mild to moderate dorsoventral spinal cord compression. Muscular asymmetry is also present with the left being swollen and having multifocal areas of hyperintense striations indicative of myositis. The normal appearance of the vertebral canal is seen distant to this lesion (A). There were also areas of canal narrowing that did not have associated spinal cord compression (B). For reference the images were acquired with field of view, 3.5 cm; slice thickness, 1 mm; pixel resolution, 0.1 mm². Notice the increase noise caused by decreasing field of view.

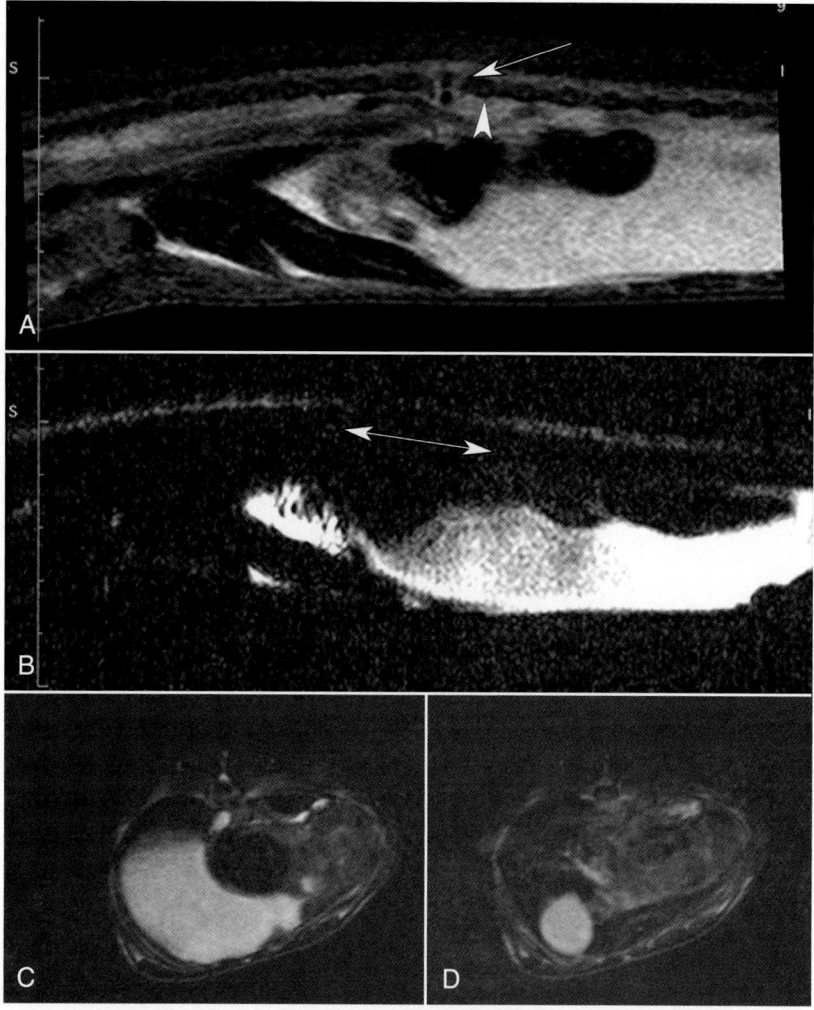

FIG 60.16 Multiplanar MR images of a blue-tongue skink (*Tiliqua scincoides intermedia*) acquired on 1.5 T MRI unit for evaluation of the spinal mass. (A) STIR sagittal, (B) sagittal MR myelogram, (C and D) 3D T2-weighted transverse of a normal vertebra (C), and at the level of the lesion (D). STIR sequences are often used to detect masses and are known for increasing lesion conspicuity. The vertebral mass is seen as an ovoid hyperintense lesion with central hypointensity. Extension in the canal is seen in the STIR images, but the myelogram shows the length of spinal cord change centered around the mass, causing attenuation of the signal from leptomeningial CSF (B). It is extremely difficult to see the spinal lesion in the transverse plane images due to poor resolution. For reference the images were acquired as follows: STIR sagittal series field of view: 14 cm; slice thickness, 1 mm; pixel resolution, 0.5 mm^2; and T2 3d transverse series field of view: 12 cm; slice thickness, 3 mm; pixel resolution, 0.65 mm^2. These images have increased image noise in spite of measures taken to increase the signal, such as increased field of view and slice thickness. The effect of field strength is most likely responsible. Good acquisitions on a 1.5 T are possible in these small patients but require longer scan times to get sufficient signal.

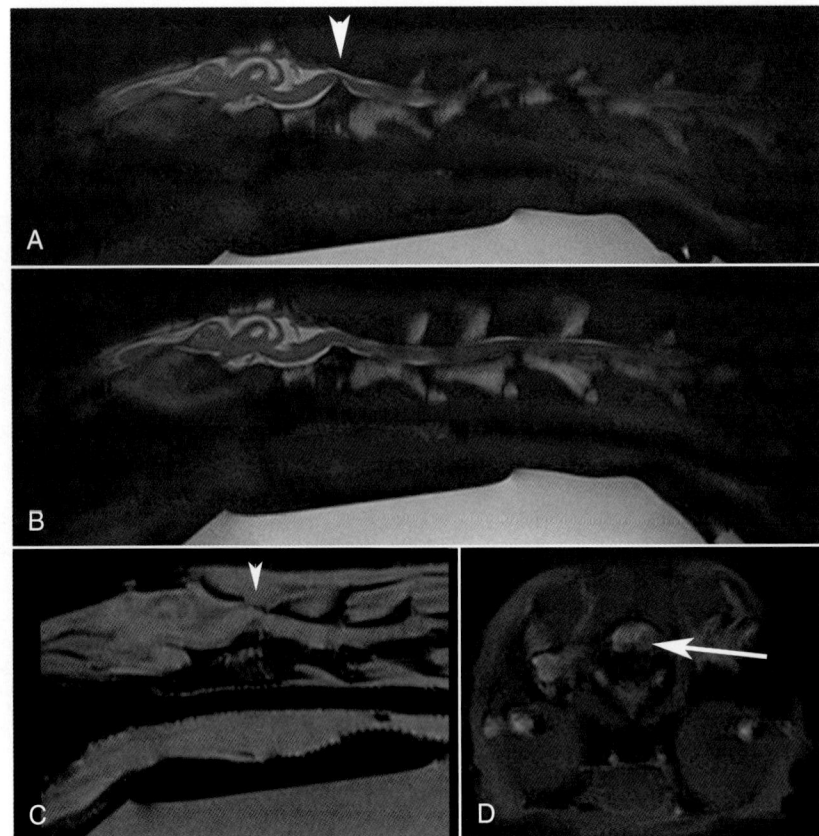

FIG 60.17 Multiplanar MR images of a lace lizard (*Varanus varius*) acquired on a 1.5 T MRI unit evaluated for prehension issue, stargazing, weight loss, and decreased appetite, as well as marked lethargy noted on physical examination. (A and B) 3D T2-weighted sagittal, (C) 3D T1-weighted sagittal, and (D) T2-weighted transverse images. Asymmetrical spinal cord compression is seen at the level of the C1-2 disc. The left half of the spinal cord (arrowhead in A and arrow in D) is compressed in association with disc herniation and/or degenerative proliferation associated with the endplate of the vertebrae. The right portion of the cord (B) is dorsally displaced by the disc and only mildly compressed. The value of 3D fast-spin echo series is demonstrated in small patients such as this; the slice thickness of 0.5 mm better resolves the tiny spinal cord in multiple slices (contrast to STIR sagittal in Fig. 60.16A). T1-weighted images (C) are excellent for evaluation of the osseous anatomy; the compressive material is less hypointense than the vertebrae, indicating greater fibrous content and/or heterogeneous mineralization. For reference and comparison to Fig. 60.17 (arrowheads in A and C), the 2D T2 transverse series field of view, 10 cm; slice thickness, 2.0 mm; pixel resolution, 0.4 mm², with an acquisition time of 6.5 minutes.

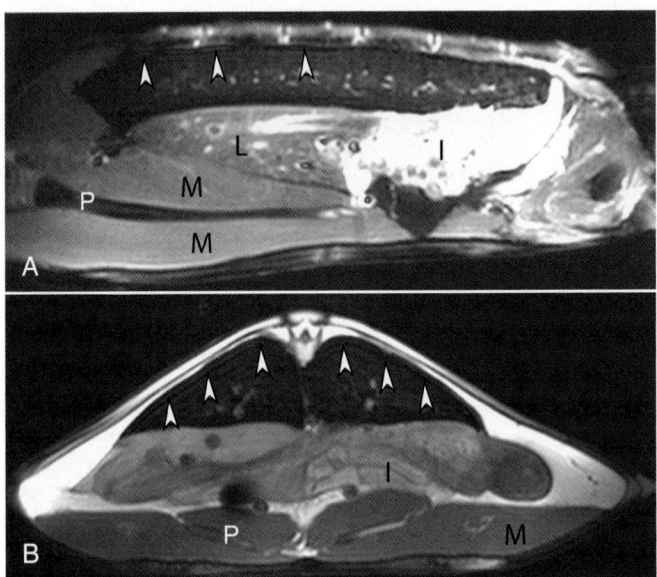

FIG 60.18 STIR sagittal (A) and T2-weighted transverse (B) images acquired on a 1.5 T MRI unit of a 6- to 8-year-old green sea turtle (*Chelonia mydas*) evaluated for persistent buoyancy issues. A thin rim of coelomic gas (*arrowheads*) is seen dorsal to the lungs and conforming to the carapace. The area is uniform and more hypointense than the lung parenchyma. The appearance of the lung parenchyma is a combination of the aerated regions with interstitium and vasculature. An artifact called chemical shift actually aids in visualization through the appearance of a surrounding hypointense rim. The liver (L), muscle (M) surrounding the procoracoid (P), and fluid-filled intestines (I) are distinguished based on appearance of parenchymal architecture and more unique on MRI because different types of soft tissues have different signal intensity. This differs from CT imaging where effacing soft tissues are less distinguishable. The compaction of these structures together is also seen in the transverse image (B), which visually demonstrates the cause of poor serosal detail noted in this area on radiographs.

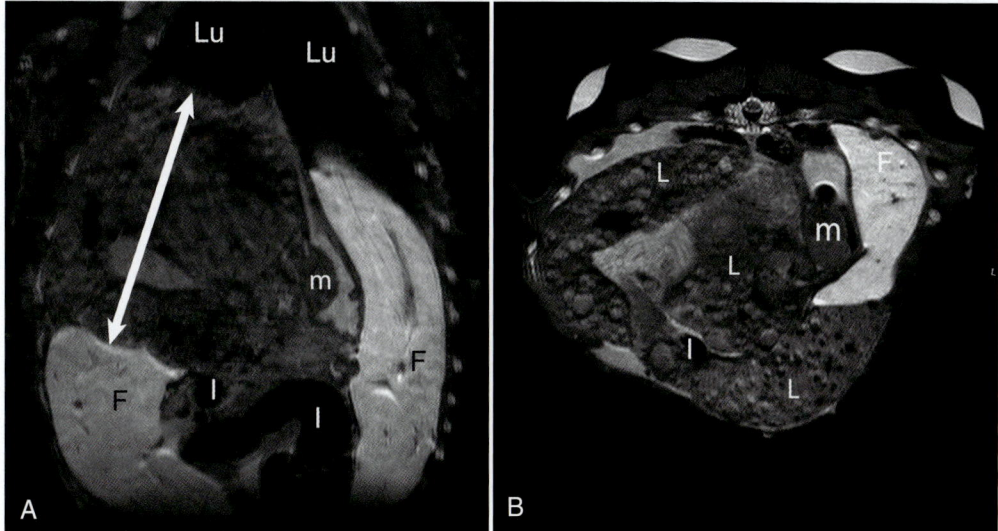

FIG 60.19 T2-weighted dorsal (A) and transverse (B) images of a bearded dragon (*Pogona vitticeps*) acquired on a 7.0 T MRI unit. The 3-year-old lizard presented with a 2-month history of anorexia, weight loss, and severe hyperglycemia. Radiographs were initially performed (see Fig. 54.14), and a soft tissue mass effect was present in the area of the liver. MRI was performed to better distinguish organ involvement and extent of disease in the coelom. Extensive nodular infiltrate was seen throughout the liver (L). The liver mass was extensive (double-headed arrow) and infiltrated into the area of the pancreas such that the pancreatic tissue was indistinguishable. A discrete mural mass (m) was also present in the medial wall of the stomach and is encircled by hyperintense fluid within the lumen (seen to right and dorsal of mass in A and B respectively). The fat pad (F) and intestine (I) are markedly caudally displaced in association with the mass effect. No soft tissue nodules were seen in the lungs (Lu), though small nodules were detected on gross evaluation of the lungs. Histopathologic diagnosis was a metastatic neuroendocrine carcinoma.

appearance is infrequently available in each species. With the availability of teleradiology services, the ability to involve a radiologist is easily accessible and recommended in both the planning of the MRI examination and in the interpretation.

ACKNOWLEDGMENTS

The authors thank Fred Steinberg, MD, Medical Director, University MRI, Boca Raton, for providing access to his high-resolution fMRI equipment and software. Gina Boykin, Andrew Kaufman, and Steve Rubel collected the images at UMRI Boca Raton. Dale Wilke (OMI of Jupiter) collected most of the turtle images presented here. Khan Hekmatyar, PhD, University of Georgia & 7.0 T MRI manager Bio-Imaging Research Center (BIRC), provided expertise and patiently operated the 7.0 T MR for our clinical reptile cases Animal Scan provided images of reptiles from their clinical MRI database. With special thinks to Stephen Divers, University of Georgia, who promotes the use of MRI for reptiles and provided cases to a veterinary radiologist with a special interest in MRI. The authors are grateful to these talented individuals for fine assistance and willingness to work with reptiles.

REFERENCES

See www.expertconsult.com for a complete list of references.

61

Scintigraphy

Mauricio Solano

Scintigraphy is a well-established imaging technique in which a pharmaceutical is tagged with a radioactive tracer, usually a gamma emitter, to obtain an image of an organ. To image the kidneys,[1] diethylenetriamine pentaacetic acid (DTPA) tagged with a gamma ray emitter known as technetium pertechnetate (^{99m}Tc) is used. Macro-aggregated albumin (MAA) is tagged with ^{99m}Tc to image the lungs,[2] and in skeletal scintigraphy, hydroxymethylene-diphosphonate (HDP) is tagged with ^{99m}Tc to obtain an image of the bones.[3] The gamma rays emitted by these radiopharmaceuticals are detected by a large scintillation crystal within the gamma camera. The crystal converts the gamma rays into light photons, which in turn are converted into a cascade of electrons. The stream of electrons is then used to form the image.[4]

SKELETAL SCINTIGRAPHY

A skeletal scintigram consists of three distinct phases designed to detect a radiopharmaceutical in the vasculature, soft tissues, and the bone matrix.[5] Skeletal scintigraphy is a commonly performed imaging technique for the diagnosis of bone diseases in veterinary medicine. While its primary use has been in equine orthopedics[6–8] and, to a lesser extent, in dogs[9–11] and cats,[12–14] little has been reported in reptiles. This chapter focuses on skeletal scintigraphy in Kemp's ridley sea turtles (*Lepidochelys kempii*). However, the information contained in this chapter can be applied to other reptile species. In turtles, skeletal scintigraphy has been used to stage osteomyelitis in an Aldalabra tortoise (*Aldabrachelys gigantea*),[15] Russian tortoise (*Agrionemys horsfieldii*; Hernandez-Divers et al, Proc ARAV, 2002, pp 103–104), and as an adjunct to radiography in cases of cold-stunned Kemp's ridley sea turtles.[16]

SCINTIGRAPHIC TECHNIQUES

Chemical restraint is usually required for all phases of the examination. However, it may not be necessary with cooperative animals. At the author's institution, propofol (Butler Healthcare Co., Irvine, CA) at 5 mg/kg IV, or a combination of medetomidine (Domitor, Pfizer, Exton, PA) 30 μg/kg IV and ketamine (Ketaset, Fort Dodge, Fort Dodge, IA) 3 mg/kg IV, are the standard protocols.

Images shown in this chapter were acquired using a 55 photomultiplier tube, rectangular large field-of-view planar gamma camera system (IS2 Medical Systems Inc. Ottawa, Canada) mounted on a mechanical gantry interfaced with a dedicated computer system (Segami Corporation, Columbia, MD) for image postprocessing. The patient is placed in ventral recumbency (Fig. 61.1) with the camera positioned underneath; 111 to 370 MBq of ^{99m}Tc-HDP is injected intravenously into the left or right dorsal cervical sinus (external jugular vein). The vascular phase is started at the time of injection in dynamic mode with 1-second-long frames, up to a total of 125 frames. The soft tissue phase can be performed in dynamic acquisition or static modes. For the dynamic mode, 60 seconds per frame for 8 frames are acquired, while in static acquisition mode images between 500,000 to 800,000 counts per image can be taken. For the bone phase of the scans, static images of 500,000 counts each are acquired 3 hours after radiopharmaceutical injection. After imaging, turtles are considered radioactive and remain in quarantine for a period of 24 hours until radioactive levels measure less than 2mR per hour at contact, typically after urination.

CASE 1

A 2.34 kg, juvenile, cold-stunned Kemp's ridley sea turtle (*Lepidochelys kempii*) was rescued off the coast of Massachusetts in late autumn. During the rehabilitation process, the turtle developed a fungal (*Penicillium* sp) infection with associated superficial perivascular lymphocytic-plasmacytic inflammation in the area of the left shoulder and neck with lameness and swelling of the elbows. Radiographs were taken at several intervals after the onset of clinical signs (Fig. 61.2). Due to the persistent lucencies noted between serial radiographs, skeletal scintigrams were performed at 7 and 9 months after the onset of clinical signs (see Fig. 61.2).

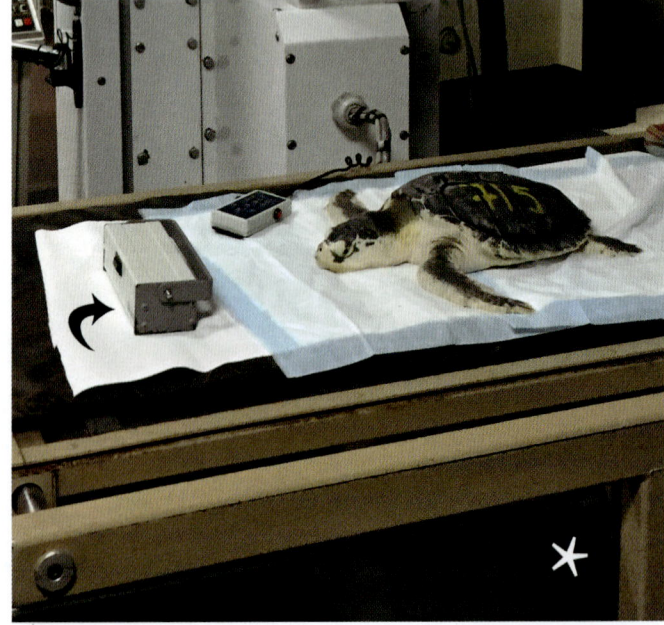

FIG 61.1 Image acquisition. The camera (*) is positioned below and as close as possible to the patient. Only a thin fiberglass tabletop and mat separates the camera from the patient. The radiopharmaceutical is placed in a syringe and is maintained inside a lead container (curved arrow) until delivered by intravenous injection. (Courtesy of Mauricio Solano.)

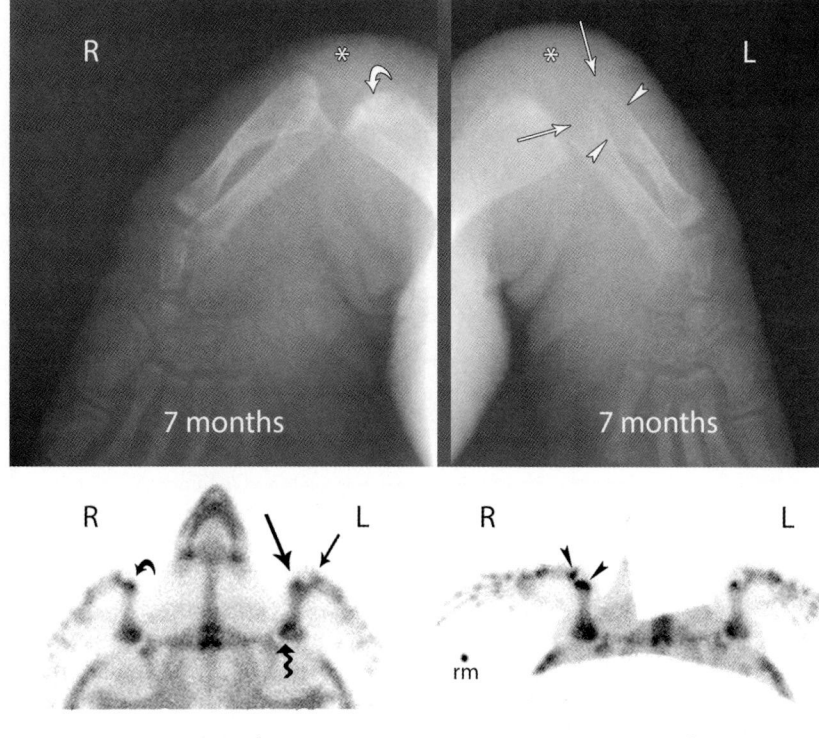

FIG 61.2 Dorsoventral radiographs and bone phase scintigrams performed 7 and 9 months into the rehabilitation process of a Kemp's ridley sea turtle (*Lepidochelys kempii*). The radioactive marker (rm) indicates the right flipper. There is bilateral soft-tissue swelling surrounding the elbow joints (*). Severe lysis of the proximal left radius and ulna (white arrows) is noted. The radial head and articular surface of the ulna are no longer present. Thinning of the proximal radial and ulnar cortices proximally (white arrowheads) and bilateral sclerosis of the distal end of the humeri is present. Sclerosis is more severe in the right humerus (curved white arrow). At 7 months, there is an ill-defined mild increase in radiopharmaceutical uptake associated with the proximal left radius and ulna (small black arrow) and moderate uptake in the distal left humerus (large black arrow). The right elbow uptake (curved black arrow) was initially deemed questionable as it did not appear to be as intense as the normal uptake of other long bones (wavy arrow). However, at 9 months, a more intense radiopharmaceutical uptake in the right humerus and radius was noted (black arrowheads), indicating that the right elbow lesion was already established at 7 months. Unchanged radiopharmaceutical uptake in the proximal left radius and ulna, and a persistent more localized uptake in the distal left humerus, were also noted at 9 months. (Courtesy of Mauricio Solano.)

Nuclear imaging studies taken at 7 months indicated the right-sided elbow lesion was at its early stages of development. At 9 months, the left elbow lesions were at the late stage of healing, somewhat quiescent, while the right-sided lesions were actively undergoing bone remodeling. The dynamic nature of the bone reaction was noticeable with the scintigrams but not with serial radiographs. While radiographically the left elbow lesion appeared more severe, it was the right elbow that showed a higher rate of bone changes and hence was more severe than the left elbow.

CASE 2

A captive 6-year-old Kemp's ridley sea turtle developed a slowly progressive soft tissue swelling along the right caudal aspect of the neck and bilateral decrease range of motion in the forelimbs. A CT exam confirmed the presence of large cranial coelomic masses in addition to loss of bone mass (Fig. 61.3). Ultrasonography through the left and right cervicobrachial areas revealed large fluid-filled space occupying lesions. *Mycobacterium chelonae* was confirmed following ultrasound-guided sampling. To further assess the affected bones a skeletal scintigram was also acquired (Fig. 61.4).

While initially not intended to be useful to assess the effects of these soft tissue masses on surrounding structures, the soft tissue phase of the scintigram revealed these large masses were extensive and were causing a left-sided displacement of the heart. The lesions were void of radiopharmaceutical uptake (photopenic), which indicated lack of blood supply consistent with the presence of necrotic tissue. There was no abnormal radiopharmaceutical uptake in the right humerus or the bones of the pectoral girdle, indicating the remaining bone was no longer actively responding to the large soft-tissue inflammatory reaction. This suggested the lesion was more chronic than originally expected. On the other hand, active bone remodeling was detected in the bones of the left shoulder joint.

The main advantage of skeletal scintigraphy over radiographs is the ability to detect bone lesions before they are apparent in radiographs.[10] The appearance of the scintigram is largely dependent on a patent vascular supply and the increased osteoclastic and osteoblastic activity of the bone.[3,17] In the management of cold stunned sea turtles, radiographic changes may lag behind the insult by several weeks, and once radiographic changes develop, they may persist for months in spite of resolution of the clinical signs.[16] Skeletal scintigraphy can be used in combination with radiographs to determine if animals can be released

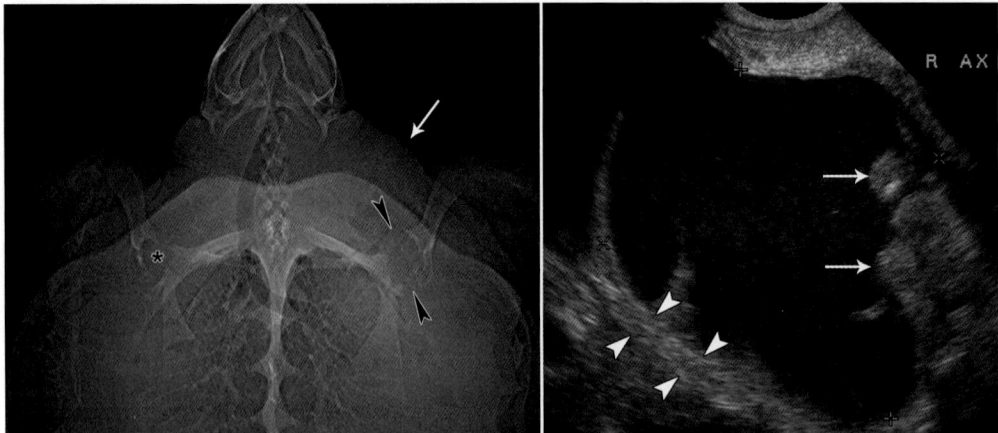

FIG 61.3 Dorsal CT scout projection and parasagittal ultrasound image of case 2 Kemp's ridley sea turtle (*Lepidochelys kempii*). Severe loss of bone mass is noted in the left and right shoulders. The right shoulder joint space (arrowheads) is obviously widened. The humeral head is no longer present, and the articular surfaces of the coracoid and scapula are irregular. A less-severe degree of loss of bone mass is also noted in the left shoulder (*). Soft-tissue swelling of the right cervicobrachial area is present (arrow). The ultrasound image depicts a large, fluid-filled mass in the right cervicobrachial area. The mass exhibits a thick wall (arrowheads), which in some areas is irregular and heterogeneous in echogenicity (*arrows*). The lesion is filled with homogenously echogenic contents. (Courtesy of Mauricio Solano.)

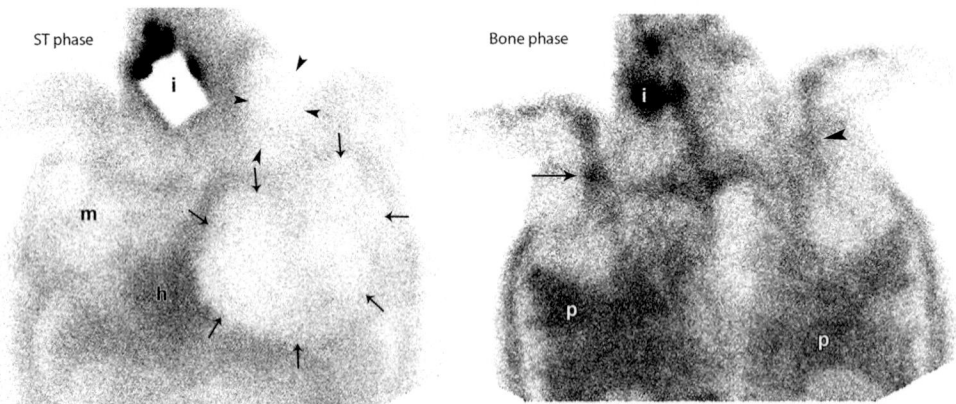

FIG 61.4 Soft tissue (left) and bone phase (right) scintigrams of case 2, Kemp's ridley sea turtle (*Lepidochelys kempii*). The rectangular photopenic area (i) represents a small lead shield that partially covers radiopharmaceutical activity at the injection site. In the left image, three large photopenic lesions are detected. The larger mass (arrows) displaces the heart (h) to the left of the midline. The smaller lesion (arrowheads) is the fluid-filled mass depicted in Fig. 61.3. The third mass (m) associated with the left shoulder is poorly defined but remains photopenic. In the bone phase of the scan (right image), the injection site (i) is no longer covered by the lead shield and indicates some perivascular leakage. A mild degree of poorly defined abnormal uptake is noted in the left shoulder (arrow). No abnormal uptake is present in the right shoulder area (arrowhead). The larger areas of diffuse bilateral moderate uptake caudally (p) represent the pattern of the plastron medial to the marginal scutes. (Courtesy of Mauricio Solano.)

in spite of the presence of radiographic lytic lesions. Other applications of skeletal scintigraphy in reptiles include cases of trauma to assess healing and viability of bone fragments. However, skeletal scintigraphy should not be used to assess fine anatomic detail, as the images are inherently of low resolution. Nuclear medicine offers an insight into the pathophysiology of bone that cannot be obtained by radiography or CT.

RENAL SCINTIGRAPHY

In an experimental study involving green iguanas (*Iguana iguana*),[18] the intravenous administration of ^{99m}TC-DTPA was followed by scan acquisition over a 20-hour period. However, scintigraphy was considered nondiagnostic for renal function because of serum protein binding and poor renal uptake of the isotope. Renal uptake and soft tissue clearance of ^{99m}TC-DTPA was $11.31 \pm 3.06\%$ at 20 hours. Nevertheless, renal uptake did produce distinct visualization of both kidneys. The percentage of radiopharmaceutical uptake in the kidneys has also been studied using different routes of administration in 16 iguanas. The route of administration did not change the dose accumulated in the kidneys.[19]

REFERENCES

See www.expertconsult.com for a complete list of references.

62

Diagnostic and Surgical Endoscopy Equipment

Stephen J. Divers

Despite the advances in flexible endoscopy equipment, rigid endoscopy still maintains a central role in reptile diagnostics largely because of its ability to gain access to areas of interest in most, including the smallest, reptiles. However, given variation in reptile size, species-specific anatomy, and a variety of procedures (including endosurgery and endoscope-assisted surgery) that may be performed, a selection of different endoscopes and instruments is recommended. This can be specifically tailored to suit individual practice needs (Table 62.1).[1,2] All rigid endoscopy equipment used by the author was supplied by Karl Storz Veterinary Endoscopy America, Inc. (Goleta, CA), and purchased by, not donated to, the Veterinary Teaching Hospital. Other manufacturers exist that can likely supply similar equipment.

TABLE 62.1 Diagnostic and Endosurgical Endoscopy Equipment	
Equipment Description	**Primary Indications**
Visualization and Documentation	
Endovideo camera and monitor	Required for all endoscopy procedures
Xenon light source and light guide cable	
Digital capture device (e.g., AIDA-DVD)	
Rigid Telescopes and Endoscopes	
1 mm x 20 cm semirigid miniscope, 0°	Stomatoscopy, otoscopy, rhinoscopy, tracheoscopy in animals up to 500 g
1.9 mm x 18.5 cm telescope, 30° oblique, with integrated 3.3 mm operating sheath	Stomatoscopy, otoscopy, rhinoscopy, tracheoscopy, gastroscopy, colonoscopy, cloacoscopy, and coelioscopy in animals up to 2–3 kg
2.7 mm x 18 cm telescope, 30° oblique, with 4.8 mm operating sheath	Stomatoscopy, otoscopy, rhinoscopy, tracheoscopy, gastroscopy, colonoscopy, cloacoscopy, and coelioscopy in animals between 100 g and 20 kg
3 mm x 14 cm telescope, 0°	
5 mm x 29 cm telescope, 0°, with 6 mm x 6.5 cm Ternamian EndoTip cannula	Coelioscopy of animals over 20 kg
5 mm x 29 cm telescope, 30° oblique, with 6 mm x 6.5 cm Ternamian EndoTip cannula	Coelioscopy of animals, especially chelonians, over 20 kg
5 mm x 8.5 cm otoendoscope, 0°, with integrated operating sheath	Stomatoscopy and otoscopy in animals between under 50 kg
Flexible Instruments for Use With Rigid Telescopes and Operating Sheaths	
1 mm biopsy forceps	For use with 1.9 mm telescope and integrated sheath
1 mm grasping forceps	
1.7 mm biopsy forceps	For use with 2.7 mm telescope and 4.8 mm operating sheath
1.7 mm single-action scissors	
1.7 mm remote injection needle	
1.7 mm grasping/retrieval forceps	
1.7 mm wire basket retrieval	
1.7 mm needle end radiosurgery electrode	
1.7 mm polypectomy snare	

Continued

TABLE 62.1 Diagnostic and Endosurgical Endoscopy Equipment—cont'd

Equipment Description	Primary Indications
Insufflation	
Dedicated CO_2 insufflator, capable of insufflation pressures as low as 3 mm Hg and flow rates as low as 0.1 L/min; CO_2 compressed gas with regulator; silicone supply tubing to endoscopy equipment	Used for insufflation during reptile coelioscopy
Sterile saline suspended above endoscopy table with intravenous drip line to a port on the operating sheath	Used for sterile saline infusion for cystoscopy, cloacoscopy, coelioscopy
Flexible Endoscopes	
Fiberscope, 2.5 mm x 100 cm working length, 1.2 mm instrument channel, 2-way tip deflection	Respiratory and gastrointestinal evaluations
Video bronchoscope, 5.9 mm x 61 cm working length, 2.2 mm instrument channel, 4-way tip deflection, suction, and irrigation	Respiratory and gastrointestinal evaluations
Video gastroscope, 9 mm x 140 cm working length, 2.2 mm working channel, 4-way tip deflection, suction, insufflation, and irrigation	Gastrointestinal evaluations in large reptiles
Instruments for Use With Flexible Endoscopes	
Grasping forceps, 1 mm x 120 cm	For 2.5 mm fiberscope
Biopsy forceps, 1 mm x 120 cm	
Biopsy forceps, round cupped jaws, diameter 1.7 mm, working length 120 cm	For 5.9 mm video bronchoscope
Grasping forceps, alligator jaws, 1.7 mm x 120 cm	
Biopsy forceps, round cupped jaws, diameter 1.8 mm, working length 180 cm	For 9.0 mm video gastroscope
Grasping forceps, alligator jaws, 1.8 mm x 180 cm	
Endosurgical Instrument Handles	
2 plastic handles without rachets	These ClickLine handles are interchangeable and can be used with most instruments from 2 mm to 5 mm
1 plastic handle with Mahnes-style rachet	
1 plastic handle with hemostat-style rachet	
Cannulae, Trocars, and Endosurgical Instruments	
3.9 mm graphite and plastic cannula and trocar, with silicone leaflet valve and luer-lock insufflation port	Accommodates 2.7 mm telescope and 3.5 mm protection sheath
2.5 mm x 4 cm, graphite and plastic threaded cannula and trocar, with silicone leaflet valve, and luer-lock insufflation port (for 2 mm instruments, typically two required)	For endosurgery in animals 0.1–5 kg Instruments are all 20 cm in length
2 mm Reddick-Olsen dissecting forceps	
2 mm Metzenbaum scissors	
2 mm Babcock forceps	
3.5 mm graphite and plastic threaded cannula and trocar, with silicone leaflet valve, and luer-lock insufflation port (for 3 mm instruments and 3 mm telescope, typically 2 required)	For endosurgery in animals 0.5–10 kg Instruments are all 20 cm in length
3 mm fenestrated grasping forceps	
3 mm Reddick-Olsen dissecting and grasping forceps	
3 mm short curved Kelly dissecting and grasping forceps	
3 mm atraumatic dissecting and grasping forceps	
3 mm Babcock forceps	
3 mm Blakesley dissecting and biopsy forceps	
3 mm scissors with serrated curved double action jaws	
3 mm micro-hook scissors, single-action jaws	
3 mm Mahnes bipolar coagulation forceps	
3 mm irrigation and suction cannula	
3 mm palpation probe with cm markings	
3 mm distendable palpation probe	
3 mm ultramicro needle holder	
3 mm knot tier for extracorporeal suturing	

TABLE 62.1 **Diagnostic and Endosurgical Endoscopy Equipment—cont'd**

Equipment Description	Primary Indications
6 mm x 5.5 mm Ternamian EndoTip cannula, with silicone leaflet valve and insufflation stopcock (for 5 mm instruments, typically two required) 5 mm biopsy forceps 5 mm Blakesley dissecting forceps 5 mm curved Kelly dissecting & grasping forceps 5 mm Babcock grasping forceps 5 mm curved Metzenbaum scissors 5 mm suction and irrigation cannula 5 mm needle holders 5 mm hook scissors 5 mm bipolar forceps	For endosurgery in animals 10–100 kg Instruments can be 36 cm or 43 cm in length
Hemostasis Equipment Ellman 3.8 or 4.0 MHz dual radiofrequency unit with foot pedal Monopolar lead to connect to plastic instrument handles Bipolar lead to connect to 3 mm Mahnes bipolar coagulation forceps LigaSure Force-Triad energy platform with foot pedal 5 mm x 37 cm LigaSure laparoscopic instrument	Enables many endoscopic instruments to be used as monopolar devices and facilitates bipolar coagulation using bipolar forceps. A wide variety of 2 mm, 3 mm, and 5 mm instruments available Only available in 5 mm or 10 mm instrument sizes, but a useful instrument that combines sealing and cutting. The instruments are disposable human items but most veterinarians clean and reuse

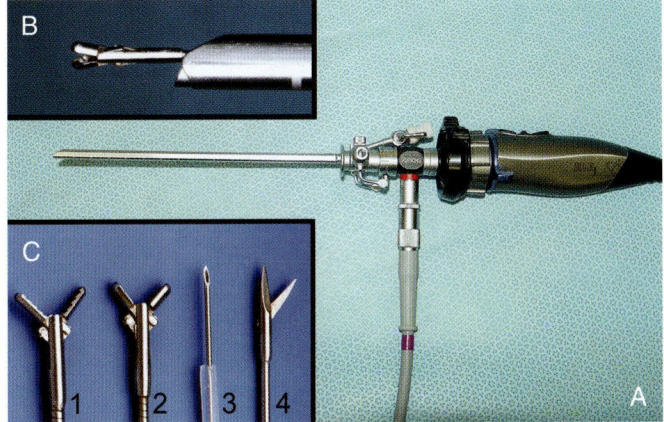

FIG 62.1 A 2.7-mm telescope system. (A) A 2.7-mm telescope housed within a 4.8 mm operating sheath, connected to a light cable and an endovideo camera. (B) 1.7-mm biopsy forceps inserted down the instrument channel and emerging directly in front of the telescope. (C) A variety of 1.7-mm instruments can be used through the operating channel, including retrieval forceps (1), biopsy forceps (2), remote injection/aspiration needle (3), and single-action scissors (4). (Courtesy of Stephen J. Divers.)

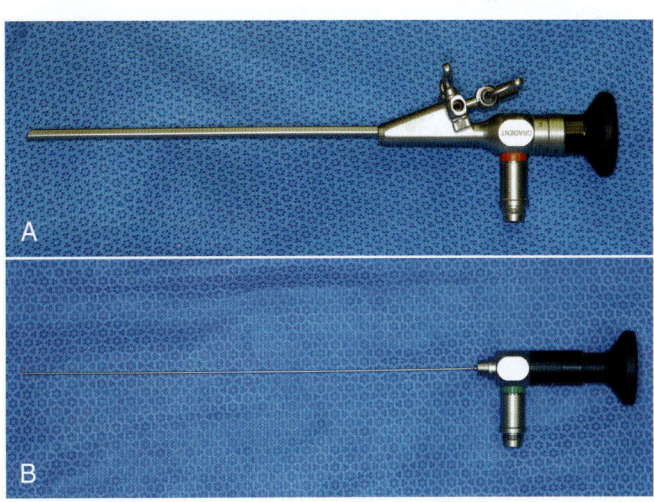

FIG 62.2 (A) A 1.9-mm telescope with integrated operating sheath. (B) A 1.0-mm semirigid miniature straight endoscope. (Courtesy of Stephen J. Divers.)

DIAGNOSTIC ENDOSCOPY EQUIPMENT

Telescopes and Sheaths

The 2.7-mm telescope system, first championed by Michael Taylor for avian species, still remains the workhorse in exotic animal practice because of its versatility and ability to be expanded as individual practice caseload dictates.[3–5] The 2.7-mm Hopkins telescope can be used with a 3.5-mm protection sheath or with a 4.8-mm operating sheath that possesses ports for gas or fluid infusion and an operating channel for the introduction of 1.7-mm (5Fr) instruments (Fig. 62.1). A smaller 1.9-mm telescope with an integrated sheath (3.2-mm) that can

accommodate introduction of 1 mm (3Fr) instruments and a 1.0-mm semi-rigid (fiberoptic) miniature straight endoscope are particularly useful for smaller species (Fig. 62.2), while 4-mm, 5-mm, and even 10-mm telescopes can be used with large-to-giant reptiles.

Flexible Endoscopes

There are two main classifications of flexible endoscope; the fiberscope (which transmits the image via a bundle of fiberoptic fibers) and the video-endoscope (which transmits the image electronically from a charge-coupled device [CCD] stationed at the distal tip). Fiberscopes are less expensive and are available in smaller diameters but suffer from pixelation and poorer image quality compared to video-endoscopes (Fig. 62.3). Video-endoscopes have tended to be larger in diameter

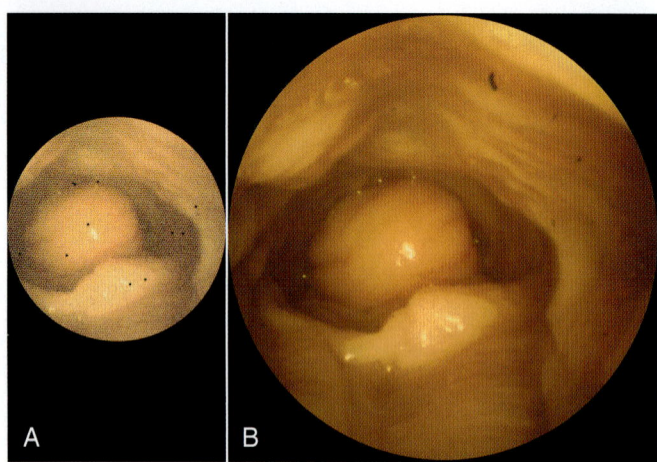

FIG 62.3 Relative comparison in endoscopic views of a snake's stomach using a 2.5-mm fiberscope (A) and 5.9-mm videobronchoscope (B). Note the smaller image, increased pixelation, and black dots (broken fibers) associated with the fiberscope. (Courtesy of Stephen J. Divers.)

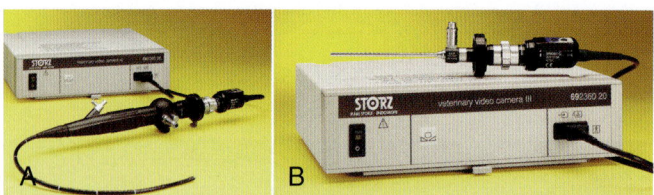

FIG 62.4 Both flexible (A) and rigid (B) endoscopes can now be connected to the same camera system and light source, thereby reducing and refining equipment requirements. (Courtesy of KARL STORZ GmbH & Co. KG.)

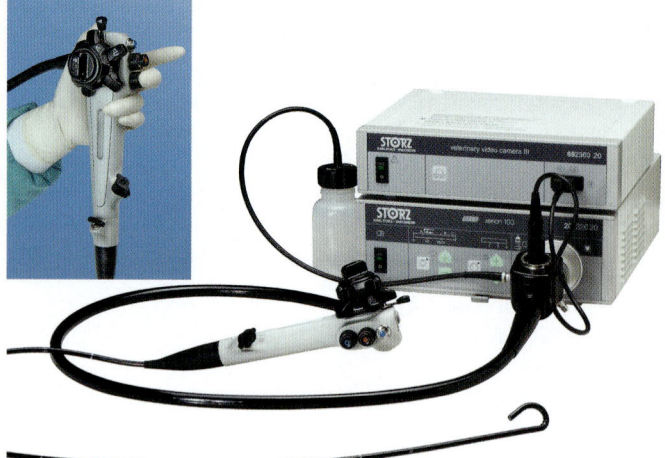

FIG 62.5 A 9 mm x 140 cm video-gastroscope with 2.2-mm working channel attached to a xenon light source and endovideo camera. (*Inset*) Handling technique that permits the endoscopists to control four-way tip deflection using their thumb, while their first finger operates the 2 buttons that control air insufflation, suction, and fluid irrigation. (Courtesy of KARL STORZ GmbH & Co. KG.)

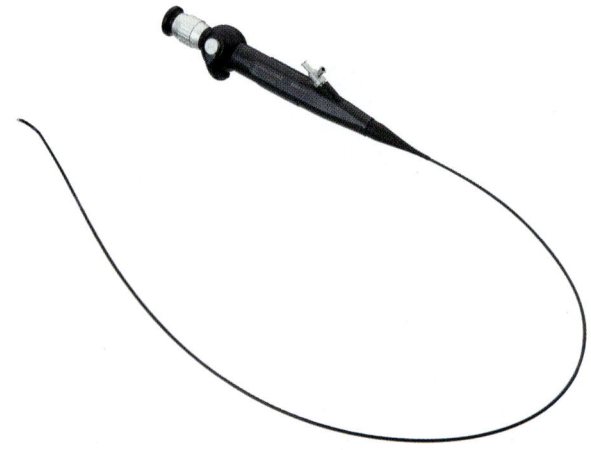

FIG 62.6 A 2.5-mm x 100-cm fiberscope with 1.2-mm instrument channel and two-way tip deflection. (Courtesy of KARL STORZ GmbH & Co. KG.)

because of the need to accommodate the terminal CCD chip, and their initial purchase costs have been considerably higher. Furthermore, until relatively recently, flexible and rigid endoscopy light sources and cameras were generally incompatible, which necessitated separate rigid and flexible tower systems. This undoubtedly forced practitioners to make a choice for one or the other. Fortunately, the advent of modern cameras and light sources now enables practitioners to invest in just one endoscopy tower that can be used with both rigid and flexible endoscopes (Fig. 62.4). Consequently, the ability to offer both flexible and rigid services has substantially increased in practice.

Flexible endoscopes vary from 14 mm to less than 1 mm in diameter, and those greater than 2 mm often offer tip deflection and possess a working channel (for instruments). Larger flexible scopes greater than about 6 to 8 mm often have four-way tip deflection, working channels as well as air insufflation and suction (Fig. 62.5). Current commercial video-endoscopes are limited to around 2.5 mm with a 1.2-mm instrument channel (although technology now exists to produce a <1-mm video camera). Therefore smaller fiberscopes (0.5 to 2.5 mm and considerably cheaper) still have a role in small reptile flexible endoscopy, although they often have just one- or two-way tip deflection and smaller working channels (Fig. 62.6).

Light Sources

The telescope is connected via a fiber-optic light guide cable to a light source (Fig. 62.7). While halogen light sources are far cheaper and effective for small animals <2 kg, xenon light sources provide better quality light and an intensity that can illuminate the body cavities of larger animals. The LED light source of the mobile Karl Storz Telepak Vet X has an

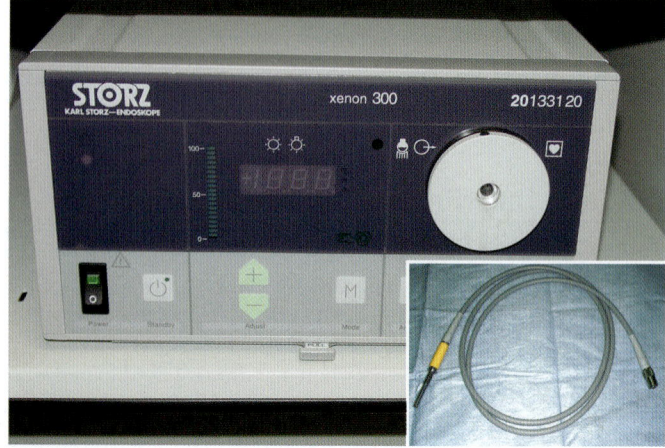

FIG 62.7 Xenon light source (300 watt) and fiber-optic light cable (*inset*). (Courtesy of Stephen J. Divers.)

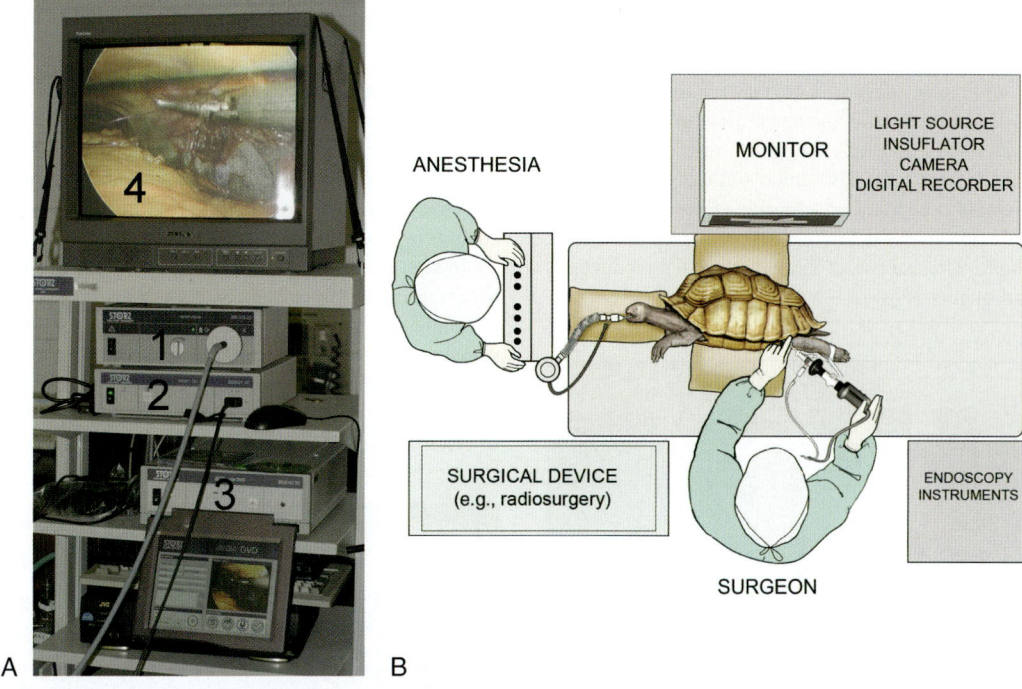

FIG 62.8 (A) Rigid endoscopy tower with xenon light source (1), endovideo camera base unit (2), DVD digital capture device (3), and monitor display (4). (B) Operating room layout demonstrating the preferred ergonomics and positioning for a right-handed surgeon performing chelonian coelioscopy. Note how the surgeon is facing the monitor with endoscopy instruments within easy reach on the right side. (A, Courtesy of Stephen J. Divers; B, courtesy of Educational Resources, University of Georgia.)

extended life expectancy of up to 30,000 hours, and these mobile units have been used to perform coelioscopy in giant tortoises up to 100 kg.

Cameras

An endovideo camera connected to the eyepiece of the telescope, although once considered a luxury addition, is an integral part of the endoscopy system and greatly facilitates the surgeon's performance (see Fig. 62.4; Fig. 62.8A). Cameras, available in both European PAL and American NTSC formats, can vary dramatically in cost from budget single-chip cameras to three-chip digital high-definition models. The traditional video system provided a resolution of 720×480, and therefore inevitably led to some cropping of the image for display on a traditional 4:3 aspect monitor. The advent of HD (high-definition) systems has increased the video size to 1920×1080 pixels. In addition, the new 16:9 aspect ratio provides a 33% wider field of view while progressive (as opposed to interlaced) scan produces improved resolution, color clarity, and refresh rates. Additional camera advances including 4k high-resolution, 3D, light filters, fluorescence imaging, and chromoendoscopy are already available, and, although typically outside of the veterinary hospital budget, secondhand equipment may make these items a practical option for some hospitals. The fact remains that any camera will greatly improve performance compared to using the eyepiece and will also facilitate photodocumentation. Operating room setup is important, and the monitor should be positioned directly in front of the endoscopist, with instruments within easy reach (see Fig. 62.8B).

Photodocumentation

The ability to record stills and videos of procedures is becoming increasingly important for maintaining accurate medical records, as well as

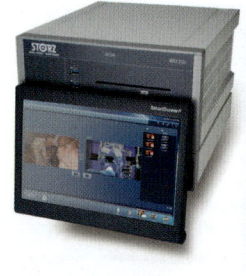
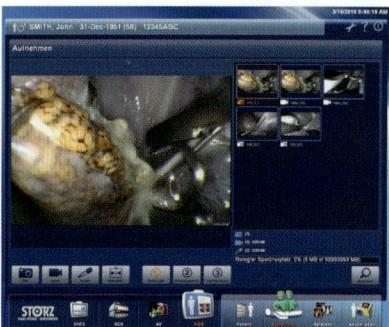

FIG 62.9 (A) Documentation devices such as this AIDA™ with SMART-SCREEN® can record still images and videos, including DICOM-compatible formats, and upload them to a previously defined network location or export them to a USB stick, CD, or DVD (B) Close-up of the interactive display. (Courtesy of KARL STORZ GmbH & Co. KG.)

for generating pictures for brochures, presentations, or scientific publications. Most camera systems generate s-video or digital outputs that can be connected to myriad nonprofessional, commercial recording devices (e.g., laptops, DVD recorders) that can ultimately save material in various formats to digital media. Professional-grade devices, although more expensive, provide dedicated functions that are important in medicine (Fig. 62.9). For example, most professional endoscopy recording devices will support still images (tiff, bmp, jpeg) and video (SD and HD) with audio voice-over (WAV). Modern systems can also provide network and web-based storage and file sharing, including industry-standard DICOM (digital imaging and communications in medicine) support.

Mobile Units

The Tele Pack Vet X system (Karl Storz Veterinary Endoscopy) combines an LED light source, endovideo camera, 38 cm (15″) color liquid crystal display (LCD) with digital image and video capture onto SD memory cards or USB drives into a portable unit that is well suited for veterinarians working in the field (Fig. 62.10). This unit has also become popular in practice as it supports both rigid and flexible endoscopy systems. An even more mobile option is the Endogo HD camera and battery-powered light, which provides real pocket-mobility albeit with reductions in light intensity and quality (Fig. 62.11).

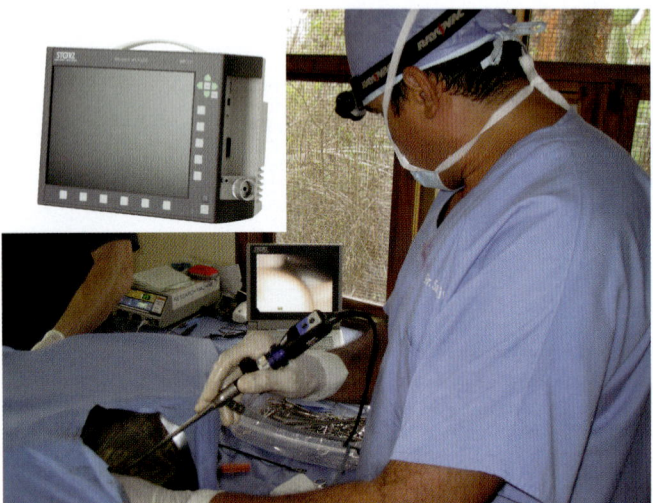

FIG 62.10 The Tele Pack Vet X LED is a mobile unit that can be readily transported and used in field situations. In this example, the endoscopist is performing coelioscopy in a Galapagos tortoise at the Charles Darwin Research Station, Santa Cruz Island, Galapagos Islands (Courtesy of Stephen J. Divers). (*Inset*) A close-up of the Tele Pack Vet X LED mobile endoscopic video system, which integrates every component necessary for endoscopic imaging: camera, LED light source, monitor, insufflation pump and image capture. This device is compatible with all types of endoscopes, including video endoscopes, rigid endoscopes, fiberscopes, and exoscopes. (Courtesy of KARL STORZ GmbH & Co. KG.)

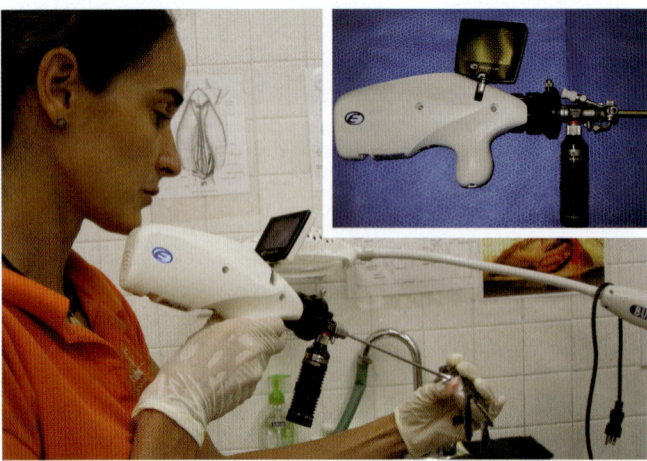

FIG 62.11 The EndoGo is a compact, battery-powered endoscopy camera and LED light system that offers true pocket-sized mobility. In this example, the endoscopist is performing an upper gastrointestinal examination in a neonate green sea turtle (*Chelonia mydas*) at the Grand Cayman Turtle Farm, British West Indies. (*Inset*) Close-up of the EndoGo camera and E-Zenon LED light source attached to a 2.7-mm telescope. (Courtesy of Stephen J. Divers.)

CO₂ Insufflation and Saline Infusion

Some form of insufflation is required for most coelioscopic procedures. CO_2 gas delivered by a dedicated endoflator is preferred (Fig. 62.12), but air delivered by syringe or a small aquarium air pump has been used with limited success. The risks associated with the use of air, specifically air emboli, cannot be ignored but appear rare. Dedicated endoflators precisely maintain the set insufflation pressure within the coelom by matching gas inflow with any leakage.

In some situations, the use of sterile saline can be especially helpful for creating mild distension. Saline infusion is particularly useful when dealing with a hollow viscus (e.g., upper gastrointestinal tract, bladder, cloaca, etc.), or when performing coelioscopy in small reptiles (e.g., juvenile chelonian gender identification). Saline infusion may also be preferred for coelioscopy of certain aquatic reptiles where there are potential ill-effects of residual insufflation gas on postoperative buoyancy (Fig. 62.13).

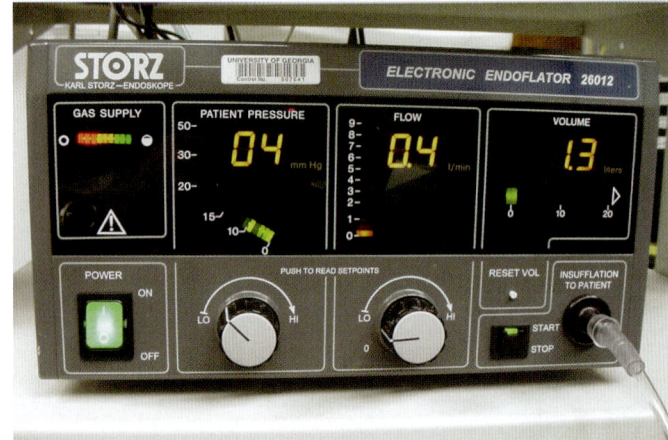

FIG 62.12 Electronic endoflator designed to precisely control the delivery of CO_2 for insufflation. In this example, the patient pressure has been set to 4 mmHg, with a CO_2 flow rate set to 0.4 L/min and a total gas consumption of 1.3 L. (Courtesy of Stephen J. Divers.)

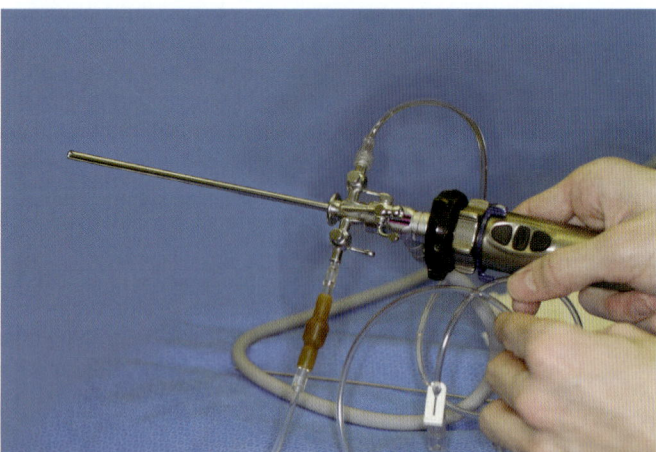

FIG 62.13 A simple saline infusion system requires a bag of sterile saline to be suspended above the animal (not shown) and an ingress fluid delivery line attached to one of the ports on the 4.8 mm operating sheath. A second intravenous line is used as an egress and empties into a bucket under the table. By adjusting the sheath ports, the endoscopist can control the rate of fluid entering and leaving an area. Such a system works well for neonate turtle coelioscopy, cloacoscopy, and gastrointestinal evaluations. It is important that the temperature of the saline is appropriate to the patient to avoid inducing hypothermia. (Courtesy of Stephen J. Divers.)

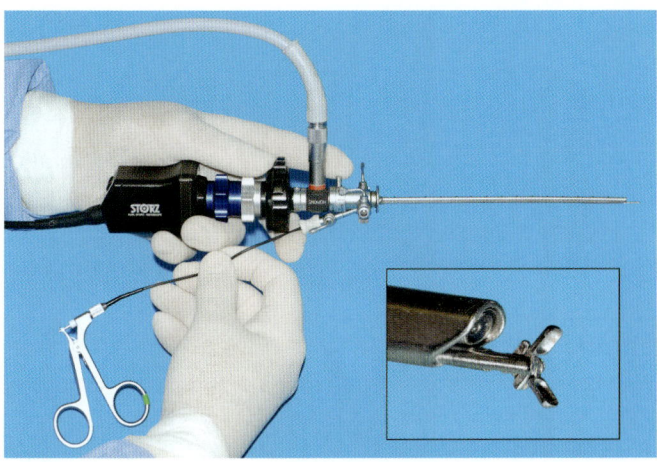

FIG 62.14 A 2.7-mm telescope within a 4.8-mm operating sheath, with TriCam 3-chip endovideo camera and light guide cable attached. Biopsy forceps (1.7 mm) passed through the working channel emerging in front of the terminal lens *(inset)*. (Copyright 2017 UGARF, photography Christopher B. Herron.)

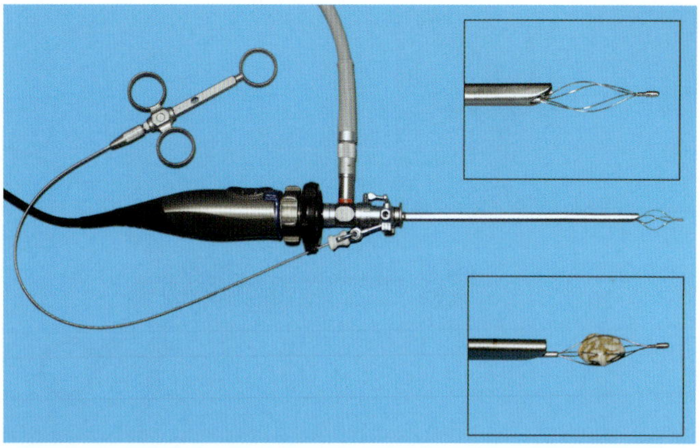

FIG 62.15 A 2.7-mm telescope within a 4.8-mm operating sheath, with Image-1 endovideo camera and light guide cable attached. Wire-basket retrieval device (1.7 mm) passed through the working channel with close-up views of the device opened and closed around a stone *(insets)*. (Copyright 2017 UGARF, photography Christopher B. Herron.)

Flexible Instrumentation

The basic and most frequently used instruments include biopsy forceps, retrieval forceps, scissors, and needle (see Fig. 62.1C). The 1.0 and 1.7 mm (3 and 5 Fr) grasping forceps are useful for manipulating tissues, debridement, and retrieving foreign objects or parasites. The fine aspiration/injection needle can be used for the aspiration of fluid from cystic structures where biopsy may be contraindicated due to postsampling leakage. The needle can also be used for irrigation and endoscopic drug administration. The 1.0- and 1.7-mm flexible biopsy forceps are used to harvest tissue samples for histopathology and microbiology in patients as small as 30 g. The small sample size usually permits the collection of several biopsies for multiple laboratory tests and serial biopsies to monitor disease progression over time to assess response to treatment. To take a tissue sample, the biopsy forceps are inserted down the operating channel and into the field of view (Fig. 62.14). It is much easier to advance and manipulate the sheath-telescope-instrument as a single device than to try and keep the sheath-telescope still and independently move the biopsy forceps back and forth. With the biopsy forceps held open, the sheath-telescope-instrument is advanced to the tissue of interest and when tissue enters the biopsy cup, the handle is released. These instruments are delicate and the biopsy handle is typically only required to open the biopsy jaws. The handle's spring mechanism is usually sufficient to take a soft-tissue biopsy without much additional manual pressure, if the instrument is sharp. Clamping down with force on the handle will damage the forceps and increase biopsy crush artifact. Some organs may be protected by a more fibrous membrane. The fixed blade of the scissors is inserted at a shallow angle through the membrane, and the sheath-telescope-scissors are advanced as a single unit, cutting the membrane as they proceed. The scissors can then be replaced by the biopsy forceps to take a sample through the capsular incision. Other instruments that can be invaluable in specific situations include a wire basket retrieval device (for removal of fibrous foreign bodies or stones; Fig. 62.15), polypectomy snare (for removal of small growths and polyps; Fig. 62.16) and radiosurgical needle electrode (for pinpoint ablation or coagulation).

ENDOSURGICAL EQUIPMENT

To operate inside the reptilian coelom, in addition to the telescope it is necessary to introduce additional, yet independent, instruments.[6]

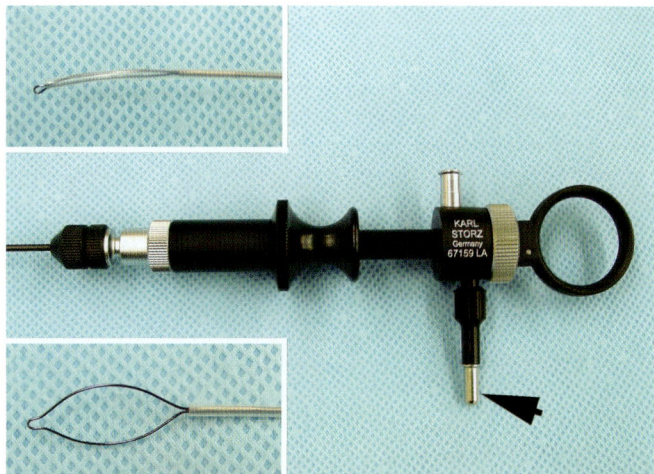

FIG 62.16 Polypectomy snare (1.7 mm) with radiosurgical connection *(arrow)*, and close-ups of the retracted and extended snare *(insets)*. (Courtesy of Stephen J. Divers.)

These instruments, and the cannulae through which they pass, are grouped into various size classes that are often color coded. For example, 2-mm instruments are used in conjunction with 2.5-mm cannulae, 3-mm instruments with 3.5-mm cannulae, and 5-mm instruments with 6-mm cannulae (Fig. 62.17). In addition, the 2.7-mm telescope housed within a 3.5-mm protection sheath will pass through a 3.9-mm cannula. Alternatively, a 3-mm telescope can be used through a 3.5-mm cannula. A listing of available equipment is provided in Table 62.1.[6]

Cannulae and Trocars

Cannulae are used to provide additional access ports (Fig. 62.18). They are of surgical steel or graphite/plastic construction and have internal leaflet valves and optional insufflation stopcocks for CO_2 delivery. These valves are designed to prevent loss of gas during insufflation. Insufflation stopcocks are optional, but at least one is required for the attachment of the insufflation line. The metal cannulae are more robust and heavier

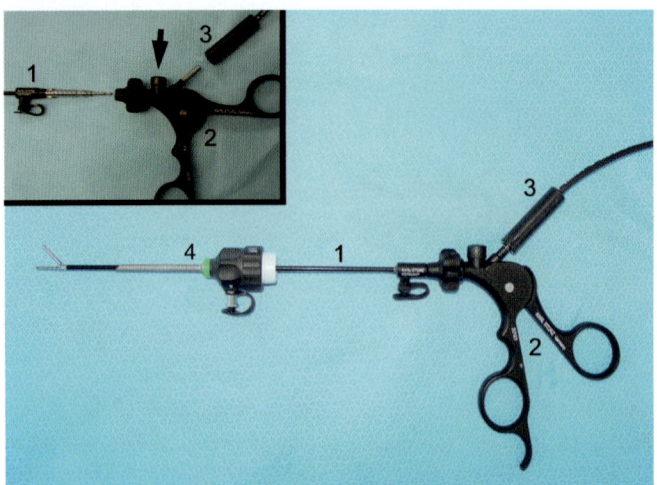

FIG 62.17 Miniature 3-mm laparoscopy equipment. A 3-mm instrument (1) attached to a standard ClickLine handle (2). The instrument, attached to a radiosurgery unit via a connector on the handle (3), has been inserted through a 3.5 mm graphite/plastic cannula (4). (*Inset*) Instrument (1) and handle (2) can be quickly exchanged by pressing on the release button (arrow). The radiosurgical connection is also shown (3). (Courtesy of Stephen J. Divers.)

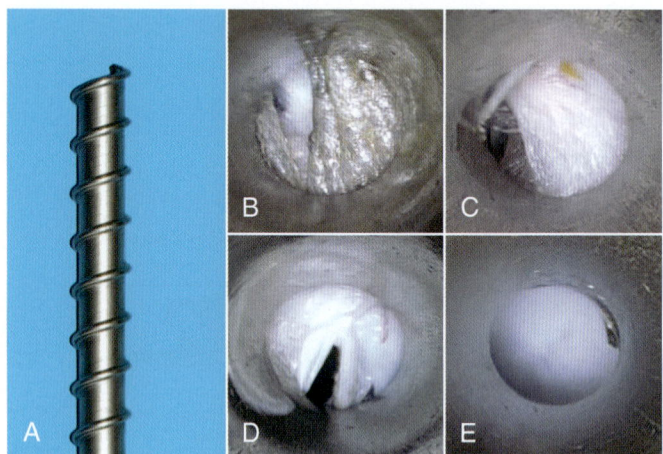

FIG 62.19 (A) Terminal end of a 6-mm threaded cannula. Screwed entry of the threaded cannula through an initial skin incision (B), subcutaneous tissue (C), and finally the coelomic membrane (D) before entering the coelomic cavity (E). (Courtesy of Stephen J. Divers.)

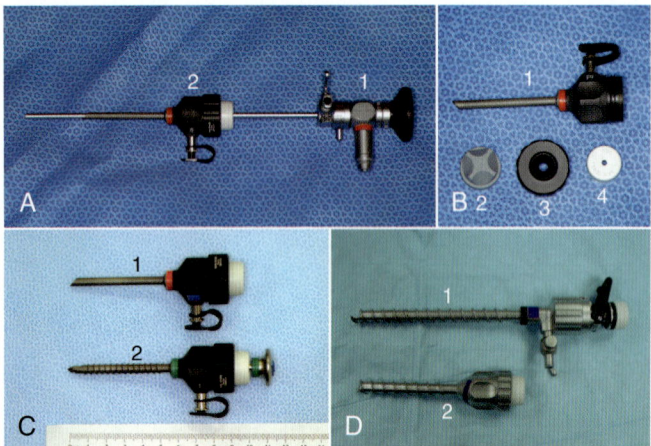

FIG 62.18 Cannulae and trocars. (A) A 2.7-mm telescope within a 3.5-mm protection sheath (1) inserted through a 3.9-mm x 10-cm graphite/plastic cannula with insufflation side-port (2). (B) A 3.9-mm x 10-cm graphite/plastic cannula disassembled to illustrate the graphite cannula (1), leaflet valve (2), screw cap (3), and instrument seal (4). (C) A 3.9-mm x 10-cm graphite/plastic cannula with insufflation side-port (1), and a 3.5-mm x 10-cm threaded cannula with insufflation side-port and trocar inserted (2). The 3.9 mm cannula can accommodate the 2.7-mm telescope housed in a 3.5-mm protection sheath while the 3.5-mm cannula can accommodate 3-mm instruments and telescopes, and, thanks to the threaded design, resists dislodgement in small exotic species. (D) Threaded (Ternamian endotip) cannulae: 6-mm x 15-cm with insufflation side-port and multifunctional valve (1), and a 6-mm x 10.5-cm cannula with silicone leaflet valve. These metal cannulae are heavier and best restricted to animals >10 kg. (Courtesy of Stephen J. Divers.)

and therefore are reserved for larger animals over 10 kg (i.e., 6-mm cannulae for 5-mm instruments). The plastic-graphite models are extremely light and ideally suited to most smaller reptiles (i.e., 2.5-mm and 3.5-mm cannulae for 2-mm and 3-mm instruments, respectively). Most cannulae are used in conjunction with trocars. A trocar is a solid,

often sharp and pointed metal rod that is inserted into the cannula to assist with placement. Most are sharp to facilitate perforation of the body wall when axial and penetrative force is applied.

The threaded cannula (e.g., EndoTip) is a recent improvement that has an external screw-thread to enable gradual advancement by rotation (Fig. 62.19).[7] These threaded cannulae are available in 3.5-mm, 3.9-mm, and 6-mm sizes and do not require a trocar or much in the way of axial penetrative force for insertion. A telescope positioned inside the cannula provides a magnified view during entry into the coelom. As the cannula is advanced, the fascia and then the muscle fibers spread radially and are transposed onto the cannula's outer thread. The thin coelomic membrane is transilluminated so that viscera, vessels, and/or adhesions are visualized before entry into the coelom. The risks of iatrogenic visceral damage are therefore greatly reduced. In addition, the threads also provide greater security, and such cannulae are less prone to being dislodged.

Instruments and Handles

At least one, generally two, and rarely three instruments are inserted through cannulae and into the endoscopic field of view. Instruments must be triangulated to bring the instrument tips together (convergence) and enable surgery within the reptilian coelom. There is a huge assortment of 5-mm instruments available, initially developed for humans but equally applicable for animals over 10 to 20 kg. However, it was not until the development of human pediatric laparoscopy that smaller 2- and 3-mm instruments became available and multiple-entry endosurgery became feasible in smaller reptiles.[8]

Currently, 2-mm instruments are limited to Babcock forceps, Reddick-Olsen forceps, and scissors. A greater selection of 3-mm instruments is available, including a variety of dissection forceps, grasping forceps, scissors, biopsy forceps, and palpation and irrigation probes (Fig. 62.20). All these instruments have a standard attachment that enables them to be used interchangeably with a selection of ClickLine handles (Fig. 62.21). Handles are of plastic or metal construction and can possess a radiosurgical connection that enables scissors or forceps to be used as monopolar devices. An optional hemostat, Mahnes, or disengageable-style rachet mechanism is available to maintain firm hold of tissue, even if endoscopists release their grip on the handle.

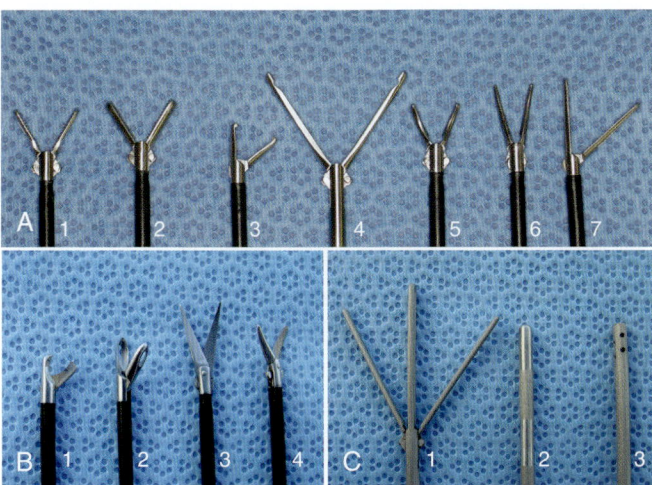

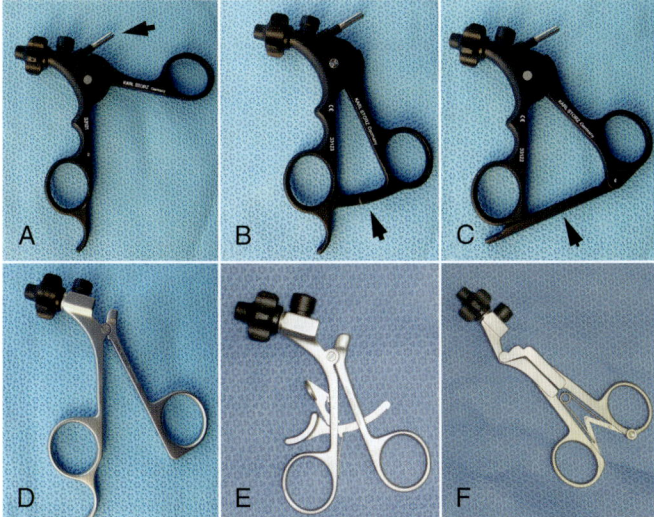

FIG 62.20 A selection of 3 mm instruments. (A) Forceps: fenestrated atraumatic grasping forceps (1), Reddick-Olsen dissecting forceps (2), small Babcock forceps (3), large Babcock forceps (4), short curved Kelly dissecting and grasping forceps (5), long curved Kelly dissecting and grasping forceps (6), and atraumatic dissecting and grasping forceps with single-action jaws (7). (B) Scissors and biopsy instruments: micro-hook scissors with single action jaws (1); Blakesley dissecting and biopsy forceps (2); long scissors with sharp, curved double-action jaws (3); and short scissors with serrated, curved double-action jaws (4). (C) Probes: distendable palpation probe (1), palpation probe with cm markings (2), and irrigation and suction cannula (3). (Courtesy of Stephen J. Divers.)

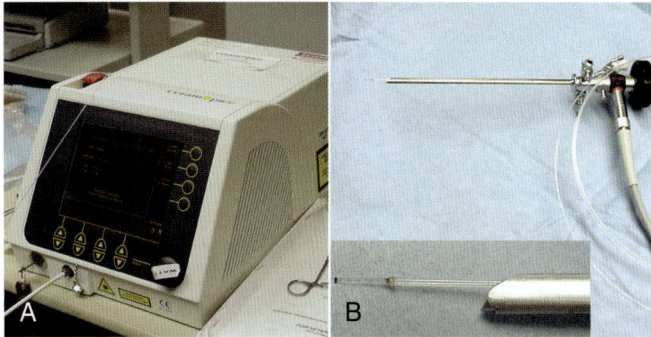

FIG 62.22 (A) A 980-μm diode laser unit. (B) A 600-μm diode laser fiber inserted down the instrument channel of the 4.8-mm operating sheath and emanating from the terminal end of the sheath in front of the terminal telescope lens *(inset)*. (Courtesy of Stephen J. Divers.)

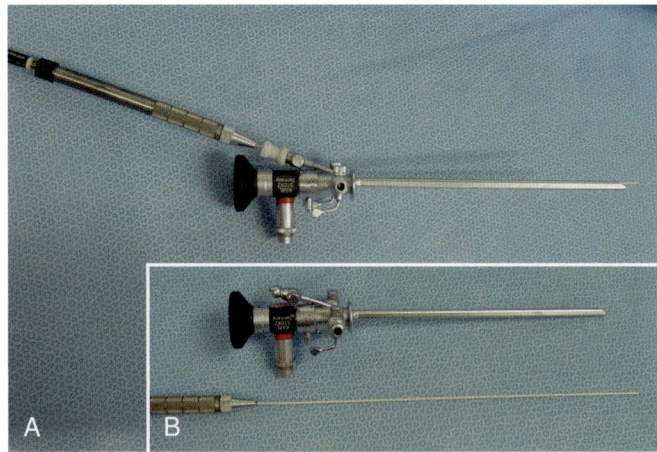

FIG 62.23 (A) Elongated ceramic CO_2 laser tip inserted down the instrument channel of the 4.8-mm operating sheath. (B) The same ceramic tip alongside the sheath. (Courtesy of Stephen J. Divers.)

FIG 62.21 Endoscopy instrument handles. (A) Plastic handle (without rachet) with radiosurgery connector (arrow). (B) Plastic handle with hemostat-style rachet (arrow). (C) Plastic handle with Mahnes-style rachet (arrow). (D) Metal handle without rachet or radiosurgery connection. (E) Metal handle with disengageable rachet but no radiosurgical connection. (F) Metal Y-handle with spring action. (Courtesy of Stephen J. Divers.)

Surgical Devices and Hemostasis

To effectively and safely perform endosurgery, accurate hemostasis becomes increasingly critical as the mere act of clamping a bleeding vessel or dabbing with gauze may be impossible. Surgical devices including radiosurgery and laser have become available and facilitated the ability to incise and debride internally while controlling hemorrhage. Diode lasers (e.g., AccuVet Lumenis Inc, Norwood, MA) are by design able to pass through flexible fiber-optic probes that can be inserted through instrument channels or cannulae (Fig. 62.22).[9,10] A variety of diode laser probes are available; however, 400- to 600-μm conical or flat tips at 2 to 10 watts are generally most useful (SurgiMedics Inc, The Woodlands, TX). Until recently CO_2 lasers (AccuVet Lumenis, Inc) could not be used via endoscopic instrument channels because of the inflexible nature of the ceramic delivery probes. The development of a long semirigid probe (AccuVet Lumenis, Inc), however, has enabled the use of the CO_2 laser via the 1.7-mm instrument channel of the 4.8-mm operating sheath, but, although functional, it is rather cumbersome (Fig. 62.23). Probably the most versatile, especially when using ≤3 mm instrumentation systems, is radiosurgery because a wide variety of tools is available for use with foot-pedal-activated units (e.g., 3.8 and 4.0 MHz Surgitron, Ellman International Inc, Oceanside, NY; Autocon III 400, Karl Storz Veterinary Endoscopy America, Inc.) (Fig. 62.24)[11]; the most useful of which include various needle electrodes, bipolar forceps, and retractable polypectomy snares. The degree of radiosurgical power required during endosurgery varies with operating conditions and the instrument being used, but due to the microsurgical nature of most endosurgical procedures, lower settings are generally required compared to open surgery. Considerable growth in endoscopic radiosurgery has

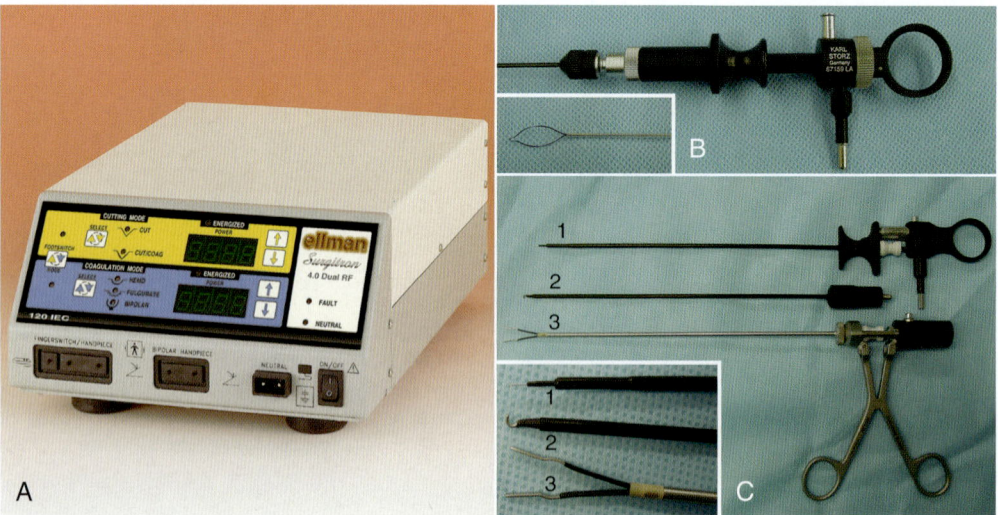

FIG 62.24 (A) A 4.0-MHz dual frequency radiosurgery unit. (B) Polypectomy snare hand-piece with extended end shown (*inset*). (C) Various radiosurgical endoscopic devices: retractable needle (1), dissecting hook (2), and bipolar forceps (3). Close-up of instrument ends also shown (*inset*). (Courtesy of Stephen J. Divers.)

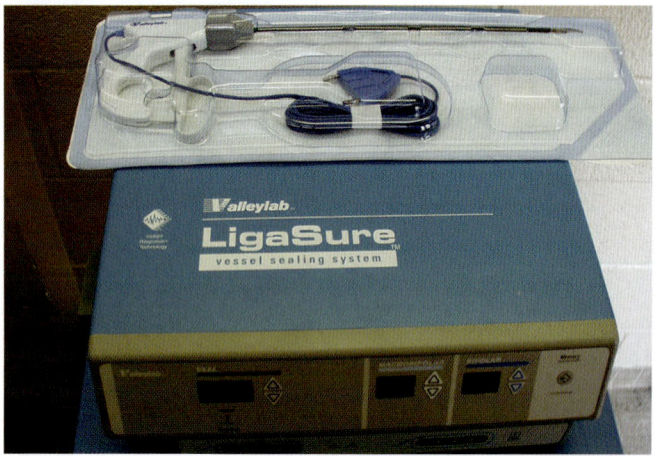

FIG 62.25 The LigaSure vessel-sealing system and a disposable 5-mm endoscopic sealing and cutting instrument. (Courtesy of Stephen J. Divers.)

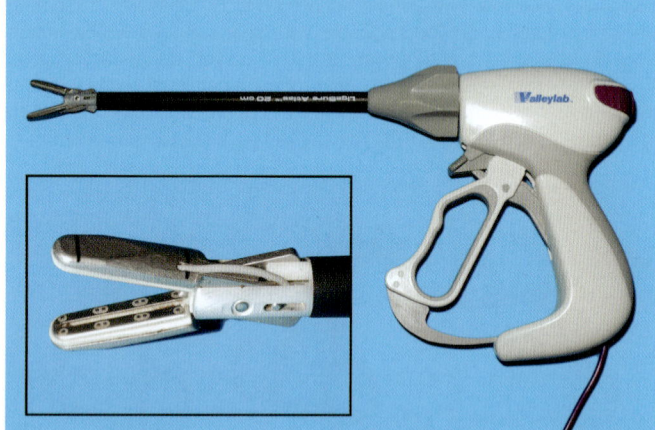

FIG 62.26 A LigaSure Atlas hand-piece. This 10-mm instrument has a working length of 20 cm and is capable of sealing and transecting vessels up to 7 mm in size. The smallest-diameter endoscopic instrument currently available is 5 mm, restricting this device to the largest of reptiles. (Copyright 2017 UGARF, photography Christopher B. Herron.)

led to the availability of many monopolar and bipolar devices. One particularly favored device amongst human and veterinary endosurgeons is the Ligasure Force-Triad (Covidien, 5920 Longbow Drive, Boulder, CO) (Fig. 62.25). This system detects the thickness (by measuring electrical impedance) of tissue to be coagulated and automatically defines the amount of energy required and the delivering time. An acoustic signal informs the surgeon when vessel obliteration is complete and transection is possible. Unfortunately, endoscopic handpieces below 5 mm are not available, limiting its usefulness to 5-mm systems and the largest of reptiles (Fig. 62.26).

Another useful item from human and domestic animal laparoscopy is the endoscopic vascular clip applicator (Fig. 62.27). These devices contain a cartridge of clips that can be rapidly used without having to remove from the patient and reload. Again, the smallest available size is 5 mm, which restricts their use to large reptiles.

Endoscopy Tables and Support Arms

Tilting tables are utilized to modify patient positioning and create advantageous organ displacement during surgery. Most of the table-mounted configurations used in veterinary medicine are designed for

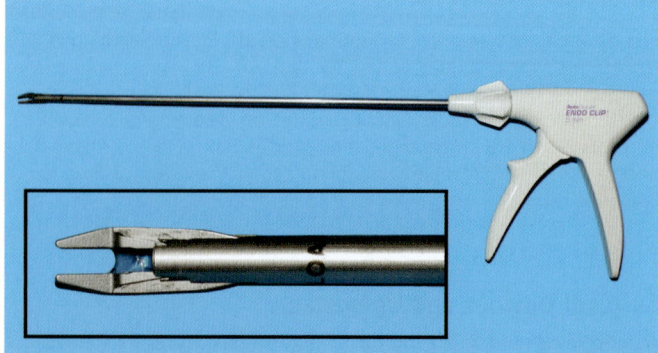

FIG 62.27 This 5-mm endoscopic vascular clip has a working length of 28-cm and contains 12 titanium clips. (Copyright 2017 UGARF, photography Christopher B. Herron.)

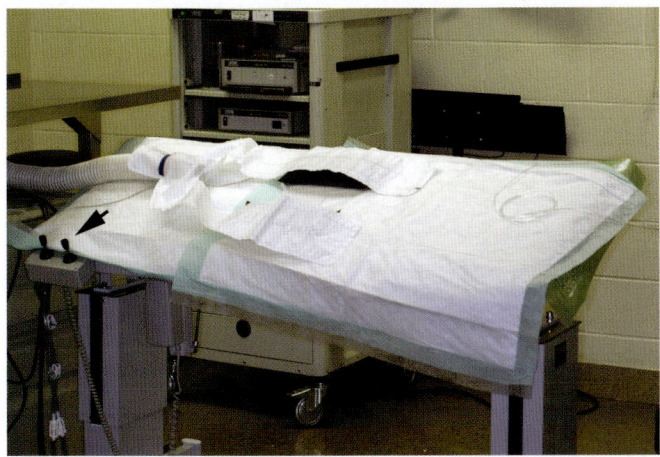

FIG 62.28 Electronic tilting table with joy-stick control (arrow). (Courtesy of Stephen J. Divers.)

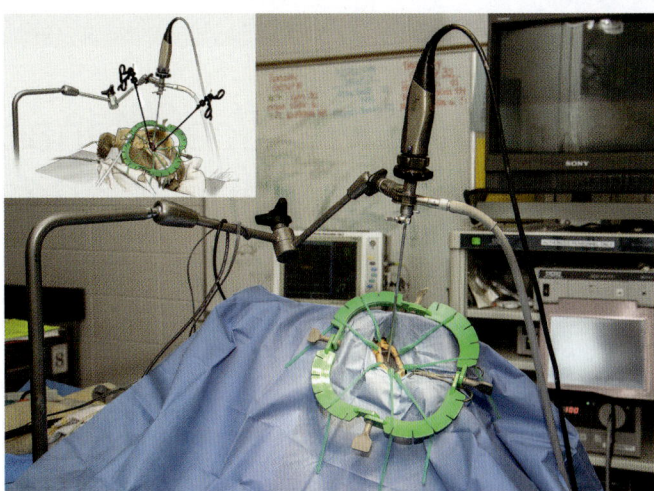

FIG 62.29 A mechanical arm being used to hold a 2.7-mm telescope through the left prefemoral fossa of a tortoise in preparation for orchidectomy. (Copyright 2017 UGARF, illustration Kip Carter, photography Christopher B. Herron.)

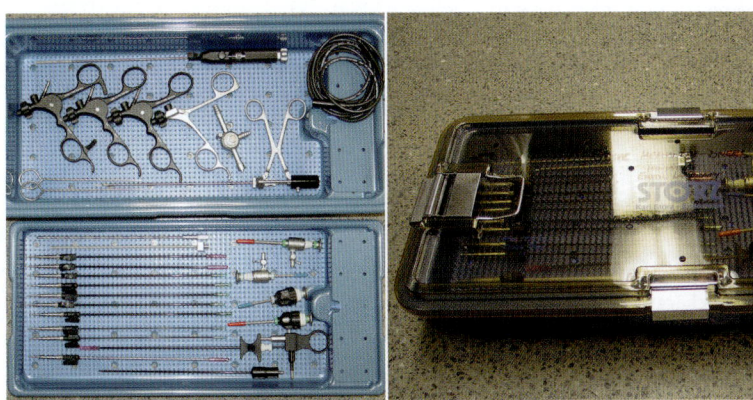

FIG 62.30 Plastic storage cases help protect equipment during storage and sterilization. (Courtesy of Stephen J. Divers.)

mammals and are less compatible with most reptiles. In addition, joystick-controlled tilting surgery tables (Fig. 62.28) are helpful but expensive and likely to be limited to teaching hospitals and other major referral institutions. Most practitioners can probably achieve similar positioning, albeit with less intraoperative versatility, by using towels, sand bags, vacuum pads, tape, and various other positioning aids.

It is often necessary to have an assistant hold the camera to permit the primary surgeon freedom to utilize two separate instruments during endosurgery. Alternatively, mechanical holding arms (e.g. VITOM, Karl Storz Veterinary Endoscopy America Inc) can be used to secure and hold the telescope when operating as a single surgeon (Fig. 62.29).

EQUIPMENT CLEANING, STERILIZATION, AND STORAGE

Specific and detailed cleaning instructions provided by manufacturers should always be followed. In general, endoscopes are first wiped and flushed to remove gross debris and tissue fluids before being soaked in a neutral pH enzymatic detergent. Ultrasonic cleaners are useful for many endoscopy items but should not be used with any optical equipment. High-level disinfection or sterilization can be achieved using ethylene oxide gas sterilization or cold sterilization using a 2%, 14-day,

low-surfactant glutaraldehyde solution (Cidex or MetriCide). Cold-sterilized equipment must obviously be thoroughly rinsed with sterile water before use. While most modern telescopes are autoclavable, some optical devices, including older endoscopes and camera heads, may be irreversibly damaged by high-pressure, high-temperature steam. Equipment should be stored in a safe and secure manner, and a variety of metal and plastic containers have been designed to purposefully house items and withstand sterilization (Fig. 62.30). It can be a disadvantage to store equipment sterilized, as this may dissuade the novice endoscopist from reaching for the endoscope to practice.

ACKNOWLEDGMENTS

Although the author uses Karl Storz Veterinary Endoscopy equipment, it should be noted that other companies can likely provide similar items. All hospital equipment used by the author was purchased, not donated, from Karl Storz, and the author receives no payment from any endoscopy company.

REFERENCES

See www.expertconsult.com for a complete list of references.

63

Endoscopy Practice Management (Fee Structures and Marketing)

Stephen J. Divers

While the clinical virtues of diagnostic and surgical endoscopy in herpetologic practice are obvious, appropriate management including a fiscally responsible fee structure appears to be more challenging. The costs of a basic rigid endoscopy system for a herpetologic practice can range between $10,000 and $30,000 (average around $25,000) and is not an insignificant capital investment; therefore a suitable fee structure is required to help recoup costs associated with purchase (or lease), use, repair, replacement, technician time, and practice facilities. A survey of veterinarians indicated reliance on the 2.7 mm telescope system (Table 63.1).[1] From discussions with various colleagues, it became obvious that there was widespread variation in endoscopy practice management. In addition, concerns regarding fee structures were frequently raised by attendees at endoscopy courses.

EQUIPMENT CHARGES, ANCILLARY FEES, AND PROCEDURAL FEES

There will obviously be considerable variation in charging mechanisms between practices and different countries. However, whatever charging system is employed it is important to identify the costs involved with providing the service:

1) Use of an endoscopy or operating room
2) Setup, cleaning, and storage of equipment
3) Operating supplies (e.g., surgical pack, drape, gloves, caps, mask)
4) Equipment wear and replacement
5) Anesthesia supplies and equipment use
6) Laboratory submissions (e.g., histopathology, microbiology)
7) Technician or nurse time

When it comes to actually charging for endoscopy procedures, there are a variety of options that veterinarians have used. Some use a tiered fee structure based on complexity and likely duration (e.g., level 1–6, see Table 63.2), while others may prefer an individual fee for every specific procedure (e.g., coelioscopy, tracheoscopy, gastroscopy, etc.). The advantage of a tiered fee structure is that it provides flexibility to increase or decrease fees depending upon difficulty and duration, is simple and easily utilized by staff and doctors, and avoids numerous fee codes and individual descriptors in computer systems. A major advantage of using detailed descriptors is that electronic medical record searches can be more targeted; however, this is at the expense of inputting considerably more data into a computerized accounting system.

Table 63.3 lists a number of exotic animal endoscopy procedures and the mean fees charged by veterinarians who responded an internet survey in 2014. It must be appreciated that, just like any fee structure, there was considerable variation between low and high levels (approximately 50%–150% of stated means) that was probably related to geographic location and the associated costs of living. An audit of the

TABLE 63.1 Endoscopy Equipment Ownership by Surveyed Exotic Animal Veterinarians	
Endoscopy Equipment Items	**Ownership %**
Separate xenon light source	60%
Separate halogen light source	34%
Separate standard-definition camera and monitor	66%
Separate high-definition camera and monitor	34%
All-in-one integrated light source, camera, and monitor system (e.g., TelePak)	23%
CO_2 insufflator	40%
Tilting endoscopy table	25%
Integrated operating theater with endoscopy equipment on drop-down ceiling booms	3%
Mobile endoscopy tower with endoscopy equipment on a mobile cart	60%
<1.9 mm rigid or semirigid endoscope	40%
1.9 mm telescope, sheath, and instruments (e.g., biopsy, retrieval forceps, scissors)	40%
2.7 mm telescope, sheath, and instruments (e.g., biopsy, retrieval forceps, scissors)	86%
3 mm endosurgery instruments (e.g., handles, instruments, trocars/cannulae)	17%
4 mm telescope, sheath, and instruments (e.g., biopsy, retrieval forceps, scissors)	20%
5 mm telescope	26%
5 mm endosurgery instruments (e.g., handles, instruments, trocars/cannulae)	20%
10 mm telescope	14%
10 mm endosurgery instruments (e.g., handles, instruments, trocars/cannulae)	17%
>10 mm telescopes and instrumentation	6%
Endoscopic radiosurgery or electrocautery	34%
Endoscopic laser (e.g., diode)	14%
Flexible endoscopes <3 mm in diameter (with biopsy/retrieval instruments)	14%
Flexible endoscopes 3–4.9 mm in diameter (with biopsy/retrieval instruments)	29%
Flexible endoscopes 5–9 mm in diameter (with biopsy/retrieval instruments)	29%
Flexible endoscopes >9 mm in diameter (with biopsy/retrieval instruments)	17%
Separate, dedicated, flexible endoscopy tower	11%

Data from Divers SJ: Endoscopy practice management, fee structures, and marketing, *Vet Clin North Am Exot Anim Pract.* 2015:18:579–585.

practice's exotic animal case load can be especially useful to identify likely endoscopy revenue streams (Table 63.4).

MARKETING

Whenever a practice develops a new service area, appropriate marketing is essential. The ability to capture images and video for documentation makes it relatively simple to showcase the procedure to the client or referring veterinarian. It is important that the name and telephone number of the practice accompanies any image or video, as clients will frequently show their friends and family. Past materials can also be used in the examination room to demonstrate a proposed diagnostic plan to a new client (Fig. 63.1). These images should also be incorporated into letters sent to other veterinarians regarding cases that they referred for endoscopy, or for referral brochures. Some practices have also discovered the benefits of holding an open house, where the public can take a behind-the-scenes tour and see demonstrations, including the use of endoscopy equipment (Fig. 63.2).

When marketing endoscopy to clients, verbal delivery is critical. Take the following as an example.

Mrs. Smith, your ball python appears to have respiratory disease, most likely bacterial. We could anesthetize for a radiograph and even perform endoscopy, or we could start treatment today with broad-spectrum antibiotics.

Compare the above delivery with the following and consider (a) which would be more convincing for the client and (b) more medically appropriate.

Mrs. Smith, your ball python appears to have respiratory disease, but there are several possible causes and different treatments. We need to stabilize before briefly anesthetizing for radiographs, and then consider endoscopy and biopsy to determine the best approach to treatment. Precise diagnosis will maximize treatment success.

The second delivery is more convincing and avoids the inappropriate use of antimicrobials. However, it does depend on the veterinarian having confidence in his or her endoscopic abilities. Therefore it is as important to invest in the appropriate training as it is in the appropriate equipment. Fortunately, there are a variety of training opportunities within the United States and Europe, and short 4- to 8-hour workshops are frequently available at veterinary conferences (e.g., ARAV, AAV,

TABLE 63.2 Tiered Endoscopy Fee Structure Used at the University of Georgia by All Services Including Zoologic Medicine

Endoscopy Fee Level	Cost (June 2018)	Examples of Exotic Animal Procedures
1	$96.87	Basic stomatoscopy, tracheoscopy, otoscopy
2	$215.96	Complicated stomatoscopy, tracheoscopy, otoscopy Basic rhinoscopy, gastroscopy, cloacoscopy
3	$314.96	Complicated gastroscopy, cloacoscopy Basic coelioscopy with biopsy
4	$414.45	More complicated coelioscopy, bilateral entries, basic endosurgery (e.g., granuloma removal)
5	$513.68	More complicated endosurgery, multiple ports, surgical assistant
6	$60.74	Reptile gender identification fee per animal belonging to the same owner (in addition to a $500 setup fee)

These fees only represent the procedure. Anesthesia, equipment, and laboratory tests are additional.

TABLE 63.3 Mean Fees Charged for Specific Herpetologic Endoscopy Procedures Performed by 35 Experienced Clinicians (2014 Values Adjusted for Inflation to 2018)

Reptile tracheoscopy	$159
Reptile tracheoscopy with biopsy or debridement	$287
Reptile esophagoscopy/gastroscopy	$205
Reptile esophagoscopy/gastroscopy with biopsy or debridement or foreign body removal	$326
Reptile coelioscopy	$262
Reptile coelioscopy with biopsy or debridement	$335
Reptile coelioscopy and gonadectomy	$456
Reptile juvenile gender identification by coelioscopy	$148
Reptile juvenile gender identification by cloacoscopy	$99
Reptile cloacoscopy for disease investigation	$181
Reptile cloacoscopy with biopsy or debridement	$240
Reptile pulmonoscopy (transcutaneous lung examination)	$265
Amphibian tracheoscopy	$142
Amphibian orograstroscopy	$58
Amphibian coelioscopy	$64
Amphibian cloacoscopy	$49

Data from Divers SJ: Endoscopy practice management, fee structures, and marketing, *Vet Clin North Am Exot Anim Pract* 2015: 18:579–585.

TABLE 63.4 Example of a Case Audit Used to Determine Approximate Monthly Revenue (Using the Mean Fees From Table 63.3)

Case	Procedure	Anesthesia	Procedural Charge	Lab Fees	Monthly Revenue
Cloacal prolapse	Cloacoscopy	$188	$181	$175	$544
Snake with respiratory disease	Transcutaneous pulmonoscopy	$188	$265	$295	$748
Anorectic lizard	Coelioscopy	$188	$262	$175	$625
Total monthly revenue					$1917

Note: This calculation is based upon only three reptile cases in a month and does not take into account any other exotic species, dog, or cat cases; most practices would probably do more. Just one of these streams would cover the $300 to $400 monthly equipment lease.

Reptile Endoscopy

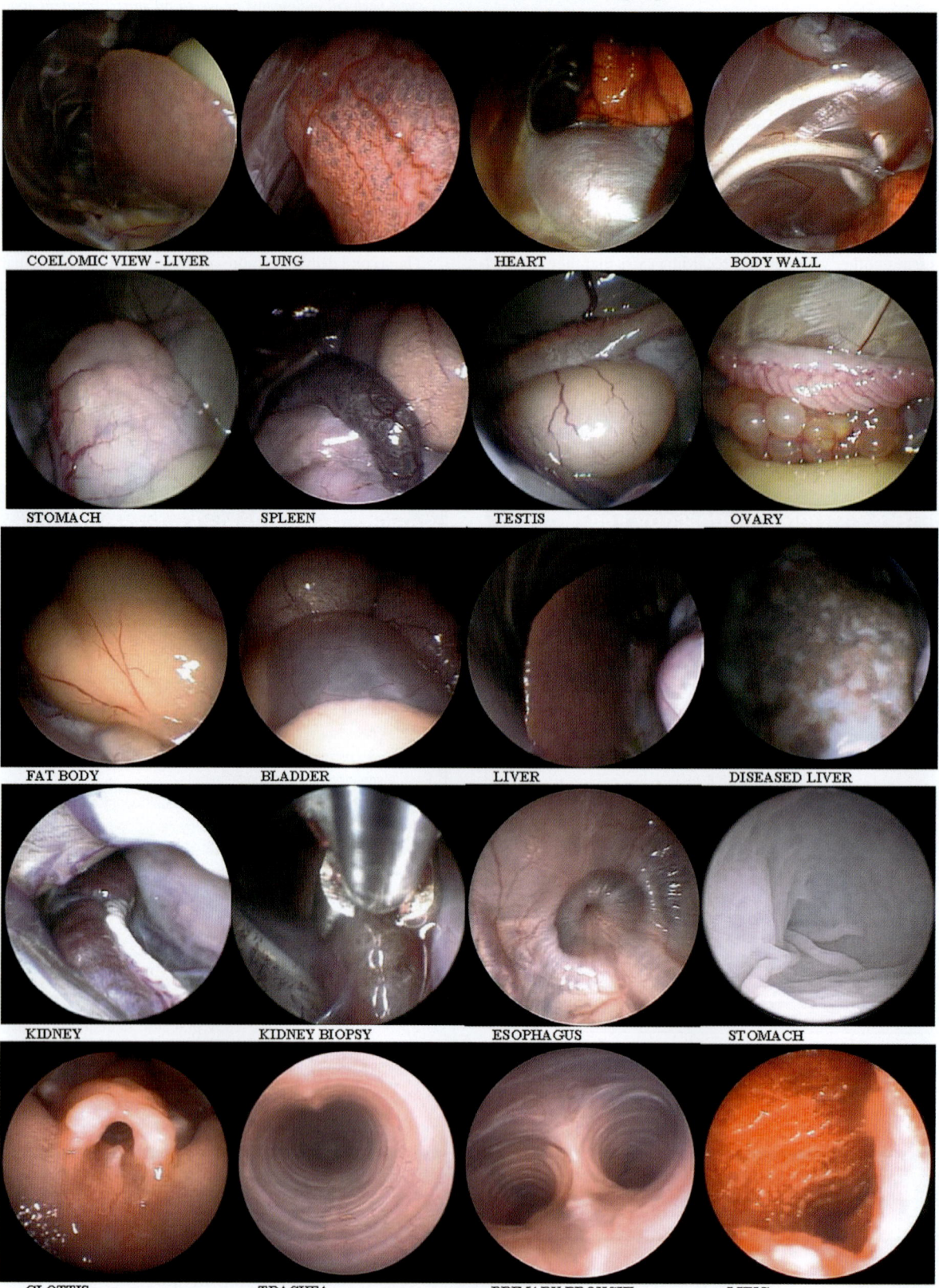

FIG 63.1 A laminated chart of reptile endoscopy images can be useful for client education and marketing purposes. (Courtesy of Stephen J. Divers.)

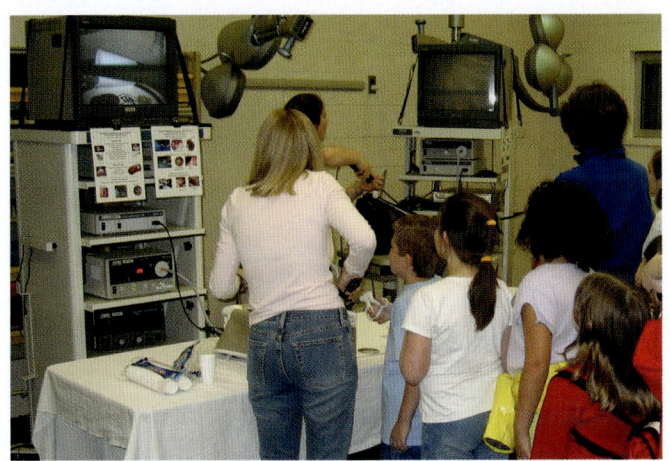

FIG 63.2 Endoscopy station at the annual open house day at the University of Georgia's Veterinary Teaching Hospital. Under veterinary staff supervision, children get to play various endoscopy games using old (autoclaved) disposable instruments. Such events can showcase practice facilities and staff, and improve client awareness and appreciation. (Courtesy of Stephen J. Divers.)

AEMV, AAZV, ICARE). More extensive 2- to 3-day courses on reptile/avian or small mammal endoscopy are regularly provided at the University of Georgia (http://www.vet.uga.edu/ce).

CONCLUSION

With a capital investment of around $15,000 to $25,000 (or $300 to $400 monthly lease) and basic training, a practice can offer endoscopy services to their herpetological clientele to create new and exciting revenue streams.

REFERENCES

See www.expertconsult.com for a complete list of references.

64

Diagnostic Endoscopy

Stephen J. Divers

A definitive diagnosis is important to maximize treatment success, but reptile cases are frequently mismanaged simply because of a failure to identify a specific problem and provide appropriate therapy. Definitive diagnosis relies on the demonstration of a host pathologic response (by histopathology, less reliably cytology, or with paired rising antibody titers) and the causative agent (by microbiology, parasitology, or toxicology). There are few reliable serologic tests available for reptiles, and those that are available require a minimum of 6 to 9 weeks to demonstrate the necessary twofold increase in titers. It is therefore clear that tissue samples offer the most expedient means to a diagnosis, and endoscopy offers a visually accurate, minimally invasive, antemortem method to collect such material. Previously plagued by vague medical histories, nonpathognomonic physical examinations, indistinct diagnostic images, and non-conclusive clinical pathology results, many clinicians have discovered that diagnostic endoscopy offers an unparalleled ability to facilitate antemortem diagnosis and maximize treatment success.

The class Reptilia consists of over 10,000 species, but preference has been given to those species and procedures that are most commonly performed in clinical and zoological practice. Prior to the 1990s there were only sporadic reports of reptile endoscopy. The majority of earlier reports described the use of endoscopy to examine or retrieve foreign objects from the gastrointestinal tract, along with case descriptions of coelioscopy, bronchoscopy, and urogenital endoscopy.[1–11] More recently, there has been further development and reviews of single- and multiple-entry techniques that have expanded endoscopic applications in the Reptilia.[12–16] In particular, validation of endoscopy procedures in lizards (e.g., liver and renal biopsy in iguanas), chelonians (e.g., renal biopsy in various species, neonate sex identification), and snakes (e.g., pulmonoscopy in ball pythons, *Python regius*) have helped confirm safety and diagnostic value.[7–11,17] Given the often small and delicate nature of small reptile species, the continued development of minimally invasive endoscopy appears assured in these taxa.

Since Taylor's original chapter on reptile endoscopy was published in the second edition of this book, the 2.7-mm telescope system has continued to gain popularity as an invaluable diagnostic tool in reptile practice.[18] Endoscopy has continued to grow and evolve with multiple journal publications, conference proceedings, and continuing education events dedicated to reptiles. Probably the greatest hindrance to undertaking endoscopic evaluations is lack of equipment and confidence, and here attendance at training courses can be beneficial. However, once confidence and skill are attained, endoscopy becomes a primary diagnostic modality that should be undertaken early in the course of disease investigation—not as a last resort.

PREOPERATIVE EVALUATIONS AND ANESTHESIA

Patient Selection, Evaluation, and Contraindications

Most reptiles are presented in a state of advanced, often chronic disease, and therefore medical stabilization is important prior to anesthesia and surgery. The most common endoscopic procedures performed by the author include coelioscopy, gastroscopy, cloacoscopy, tracheobronchoscopy, and pulmonoscopy. However, most of the procedures described (or necessary modifications thereof) can be undertaken in most reptiles assuming equipment can be matched to patient size. In addition to anesthetic complications, small patient size often presents the greatest challenge. Obesity is less of an issue in chelonians and lizards, because they store fat in discrete fat bodies rather than diffusely around organs like mammals do. Obesity in snakes can still be a significant hindrance during coelioscopy, however, due to their more widespread coelomic fat reserves.

The benefits of endoscopy are numerous but mostly center on the fact that traditional approaches are more invasive, require longer anesthetic periods, and can carry significantly greater procedural risks (e.g., coeliotomy vs coelioscopy). With the ability to internally examine the patient and collect tissue samples, the array of antemortem diagnoses has increased considerably, with accurate diagnosis resulting in more appropriate targeted therapy and improved clinical success.

Knowledge of species-specific anatomy, physiology, husbandry, and nutritional requirements are vital to properly evaluate the reptile patient. Inexperienced clinicians are directed to various chapters throughout this text and should prepare in advance.[19,20] Complete physical examination, including accurate body weight, is essential but may require sedation or anesthesia for aggressive, venomous or uncooperative reptiles. Serial clinicopathologic data can be helpful to quantify dehydration and indicate infection/inflammation and organ damage or dysfunction. However, most published reference ranges are too broad to be of value unless patient data is severely abnormal. Complete blood counts and biochemistry panels are recommended. Even in animals <100 g, hematocrit and total solids can still be obtained.

Patient Preparation and Anesthesia

In most cases, the sick reptile presents with anorexia of days to months duration, and fasting is usually not a concern. However, when dealing with animals that are still feeding, fasting should be in accordance with body size and feeding strategy. For example, a 20-kg python would typically be fasted for 2 to 3 weeks, whereas a 50-g gecko would require only 1 to 2 days. Likewise, fasting a carnivorous turtle for 1 to 3 days would reduce the volume of food in the stomach, whereas fasting an herbivorous tortoise for the same period would have little effect given the majority of digesta is located within the large intestine. As a general guide, a single feeding cycle should be avoided prior to anesthesia and surgery. In general, fluid therapy is the mainstay of stabilization, and rehydration using crystalloid fluids (with an osmolarity of 260–290 mOsm/L) at 25–45 mL/kg/day is recommended.[21] Fluids may be given intravenously or intraosseously for critical cases, or intra-coelomically, subcutaneously or orally. It is advisable to avoid oral fluids within 24 hours of gastroscopy, and intracoelomic fluids within 72 hours of coelioscopy.

Certain examinations (e.g., stomatoscopy, cloacoscopy) may be possible in the conscious or sedated patient using appropriate restraint (including a mouth gag for oral approaches), but complete immobilization is preferred to avoid risking damage to equipment, patient, or staff. General anesthesia is recommended for all endoscopy procedures (including oral and cloacal examinations) and is required for any invasive procedures (including coelioscopy).[9,22] Conscious coelioscopic examinations may be acceptable in research animals or wildlife under an appropriate experimental license, but in clinical practice, analgesia and anesthesia are mandatory. Although some authors have reported using only local anesthesia for chelonian coelioscopy, this provides inadequate analgesia for more involved coelioscopic procedures.[23] In a recent comparison of local versus general anesthesia for chelonian coelioscopy, struggling was significantly reduced for procedures conducted under general anesthesia compared to local lidocaine alone.[9] For a detailed description of sedation, anesthesia, and analgesia, see Chapters 48 to 52. Careful consideration should be given to intubation and adequate ventilation, especially when insufflating the coelom during coelioscopy. Opiate and nonsteroidal antiinflammatory drugs are used routinely to relieve or minimize any pain or discomfort associated with these endoscopic procedures.

OPERATING ROOM PREPARATION, ERGONOMICS AND EQUIPMENT HANDLING

Some consideration should be given to room setup and positioning, which will greatly facilitate procedural success. Procedural technique (incl whether the surgeon is left or right handed) and species anatomy are key factors in animal positioning and are dealt with under each individual procedure. The endoscopy tower and especially the video monitor should be positioned directly in front of the endoscopist (Fig. 64.1). Trying to observe a monitor to one side, or even worse over a shoulder, creates confusion, frustration, and discomfort. For right-handed surgeons, the instrument table should be placed on the right (and vice versa for those who are left handed).

The fact that most reptiles weigh <2 kg necessitates careful control of the telescope, with the eye-piece and camera supported using the superior hand and the distal shaft of the telescope held by thumb and forefinger of the inferior hand (Fig. 64.2A). Handling the telescope in this fashion provides fine control without tremor; however, for a single surgeon to be able to use instruments a modified hold is required. In order to insert and manipulate instruments through the operating sheath, it is necessary to change from a two-handed to a one-handed technique. The usual thumb and forefinger support of the telescope shaft is now adjusted so that the inferior hand takes the entire weight of the sheath-telescope-camera system. The thumb is slid up the shaft of the sheath, and the fingers are curled over the top to encircle the sheath. Now that the sheath is grasped in a fist-like grip with the sheath further supported by the thumb to prevent rotation, the superior hand can be removed to manipulate an instrument down the operating channel (see Fig. 64.2B). This can only be performed using a correctly sheathed telescope; damage will otherwise occur to the telescope.

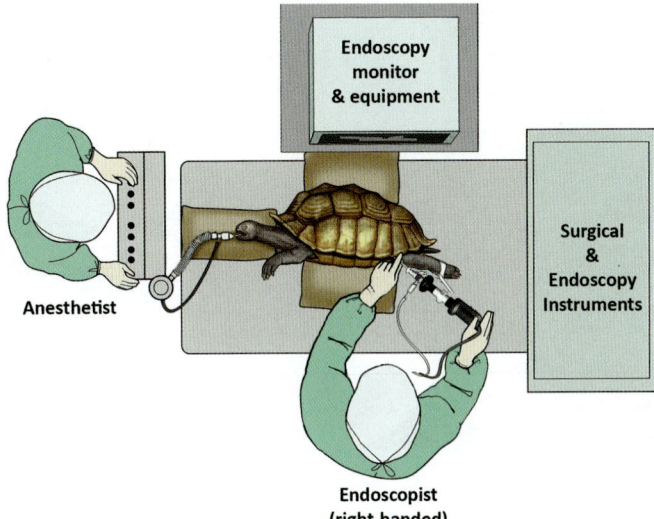

FIG 64.1 Operating room layout for a right-handed surgeon performing a left prefemoral approach for coelioscopy in a tortoise. (Courtesy of Educational Resources, University of Georgia.)

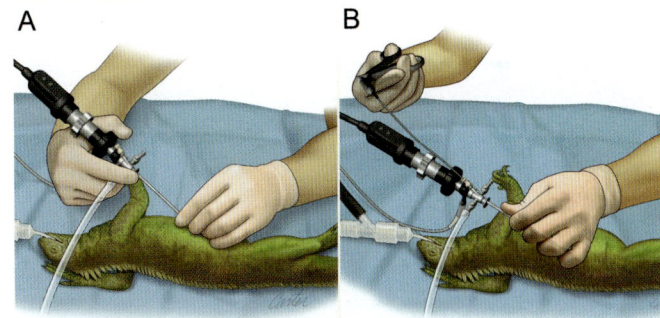

FIG 64.2 Correct handling of the 2.7-mm telescope housed within the 4.8 mm operating sheath. (A) The two-handed technique for general evaluation involves supporting the sheathed telescope and camera with the superior hand while the thumb and forefinger of the inferior hand provide fine motor control and prevents tremor. (B) The one-handed technique facilitates instrument use by a single surgeon and involves the inferior hand taking the weight of the sheathed telescope and camera by gripping the entire shaft, with the thumb slid up the sheath to prevent rotation. The inferior hand is now free to manipulate an instrument into the operating channel. (Courtesy of Educational Resources, University of Georgia.)

DIAGNOSTIC ENDOSCOPY PROCEDURES

Tracheoscopy and Pulmonoscopy

Depending upon the size of the reptile, a suitably sized rigid or flexible endoscope can be used to examine the glottis and at least part of the anterior trachea of most lizards, chelonians, and snakes (Fig. 64.3).[12] It is always preferable to use a protection sheath with the finer telescopes, but the increased diameter may be prohibitive. Rigid scopes of sufficient length can usually be directed into the lungs of lizards by careful manipulation of the lizard's head, neck, and body. It is often beneficial to provide a large breath immediately prior to inserting the endoscope. For large snakes and chelonians, fine diameter flexible endoscopes or videoscopes will permit a deeper examination into the lungs (Fig. 64.4).[18,24]

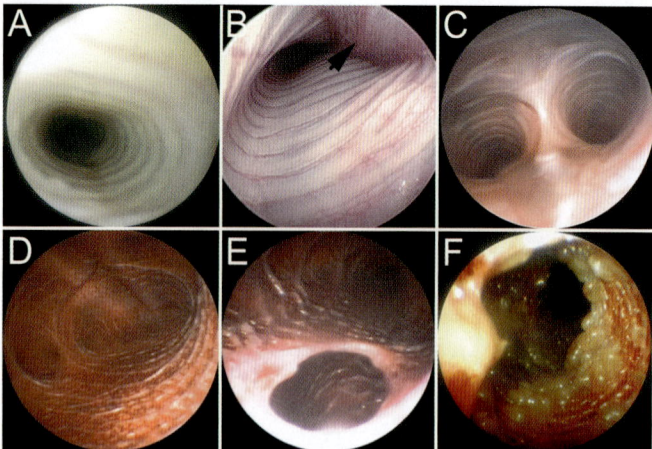

FIG 64.3 Tracheobronchoscopy. (A) Greek tortoise (*Testudo graeca*) trachea with complete tracheal rings. (B) Ball python (*Python regius*) trachea with obvious dorsal ligament (arrow). (C) Tracheal bifurcation and primary bronchi in a green iguana (*Iguana iguana*). (D) Simple saclike lung in a green iguana. (E) Compartmentalized lung in a panther chameleon (*Furcifer pardalis*). (F) Granulomatous pneumonia due to *Mycobacterium* spp in a ball python. (Courtesy of Stephen J. Divers.)

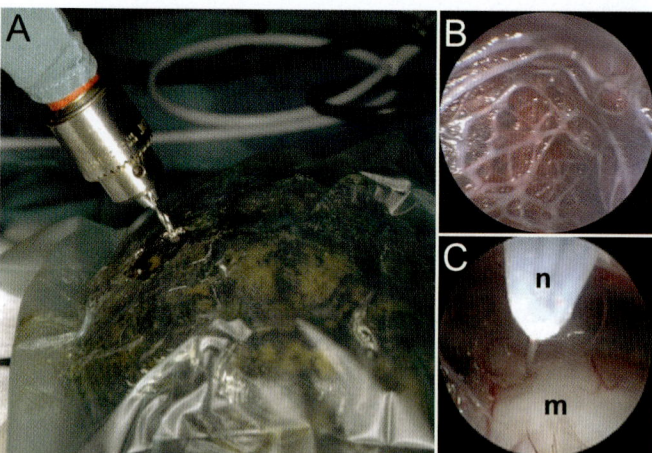

FIG 64.5 Chelonian transcarapacial pulmonoscopy. (A) Drilling a 4-mm temporary osteotomy through the carapace of a Greek tortoise (*Testudo graeca*) to access the lung. (B) Normal view of the chelonian lung through the temporary osteotomy. (C) Large mass (m) within the lung of a juvenile loggerhead sea turtle (*Caretta caretta*) via a temporary carapacial osteotomy. Aspiration is first attempted using an endoscopic needle (n) and, if not fluid-filled, biopsies are taken. In this case the lesion was an encapsulated fungal granuloma. (Courtesy of Stephen J. Divers.)

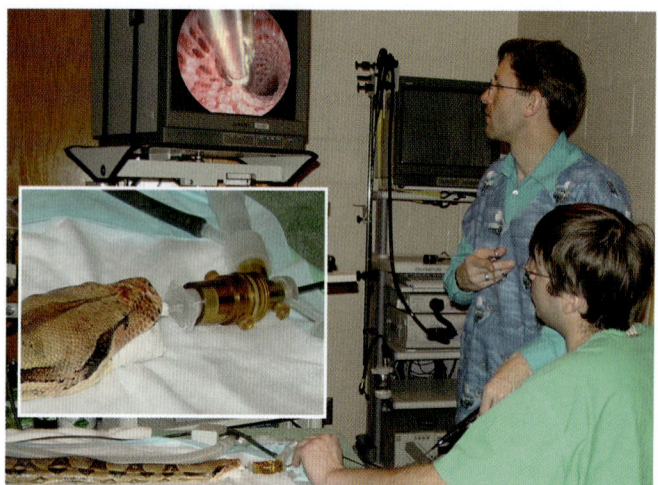

FIG 64.4 Tracheobronchoscopy in a boa constrictor (*Boa constrictor*) using a 2.5-mm fiberscope. Note the endotracheal adaptor (*inset*) that facilitates introduction of the fiberscope while maintaining anesthesia. (Courtesy of Stephen J. Divers.)

The anesthetized reptile is positioned in dorsal or sternal recumbency, with head and neck extended. A mouth gag is recommended to guard against a lightly anesthetized reptile from biting down on the endoscope. The endoscope should be inserted through the glottis and gently advanced under direct visual control to avoid damaging the mucosa. Complete tracheal occlusion for several minutes is well tolerated, and there is no need to provide an alternative airway. The incomplete (Squamata) and complete (Chelonia, Crocodilia) tracheal rings and mucosa can be clearly seen. Parasites, abscesses, granulomas, trauma, and mucosal defects, as well as chondromas and other neoplasms, can be readily appreciated.

A tracheal approach to the chelonian lung is particularly difficult because of the narrow trachea and meandering primary bronchi. It is possible in the largest species (e.g., giant tortoises, sea turtles) using

fine flexible endoscopes, but not in smaller specimens, and therefore two alternative approaches to the chelonian lung have been developed: carapacial and prefemoral.[12] The carapacial approach requires a 4- to 5-mm temporary osteotomy over the suspected pulmonary lesion, pinpointed by diagnostic imaging (Fig. 64.5A). The pleuropulmonary membrane is punctured using a trocar or straight hemostats while the animal is held at maximal inspiration. Leakage of anesthetic gases confirms entry into the lung, and additional anesthetic gas scavenging should be positioned close to the surgical site, or ventilation should be temporarily suspended during the procedure. The sheathed telescope can then be inserted into the lung for examination, remembering that, due to the rigid nature of the shell, telescope movements will be restricted (see Fig. 64.5B and C). Following endoscopy, the osteotomy can be closed using epoxy or acrylic, but it may be advantageous to secure a capped, intravenous catheter within the hole to permit intrapulmonary therapy. Following successful treatment, the catheter is removed and the hole sealed. The shell typically heals within 12 weeks.

The second, prefemoral approach to the chelonian lung is particularly suitable for those species that have a relatively large prefemoral fossa, which facilitates surgical entry into the coelom and identification of the caudolateral aspect of the postpulmonary membrane (septum horizontale) and caudolateral lung. A small (2–4 cm) craniocaudal incision is made in the craniodorsal aspect of the prefemoral fossa (Fig. 64.6A). The coelomic membrane is perforated and opened using hemostats. By frequently and maximally ventilating the lungs, the caudolateral lung can be readily identified. Two stay sutures are placed through the caudoventral border of the lung to facilitate elevation to the level of the skin incision. A stab incision through a thin, avascular portion of the exposed lung provides access for the telescope. Due to the soft tissue nature of this approach, greater endoscope maneuverability is possible and the pulmonary examination can proceed from caudal to cranial, and in some species it is possible to visualize the opening of the primary bronchus (see Fig. 64.6B and C). Upon withdrawal, the lung must be closed using fine suture material to avoid postoperative pneumocoelom, and this is most easily achieved by using the preplaced stay sutures. Coeliotomy closure is otherwise routine.

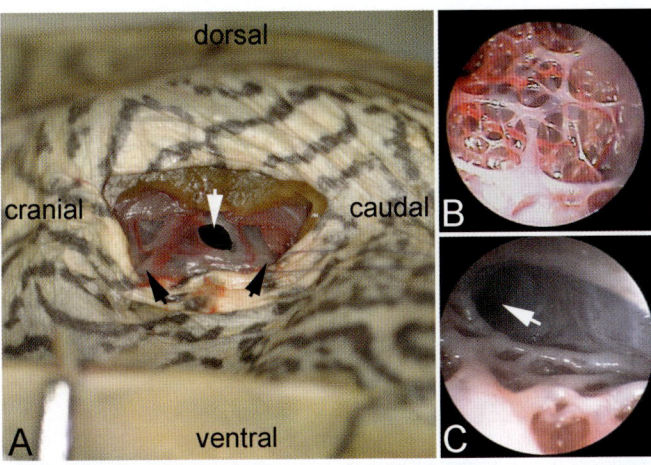

FIG 64.6 Chelonian transcutaneous pulmonoscopy. (A) Surgical view of the prefemoral fossa of a map turtle (*Graptemys* sp) following a mini-coeliotomy incision. Two fine stay sutures (black arrows) have been placed to elevate the lung to the skin incision, and a small stab incision has been made through an avascular window of the lung (white arrow). (B) Endoscopic view from within the lung of a map turtle demonstrating the characteristic edicular nature of the tissue. (C) Endoscopic view from within the lung of a Greek tortoise (*Testudo graeca*), demonstrating the opening to the left primary bronchus (arrow). (Courtesy of Stephen J. Divers.)

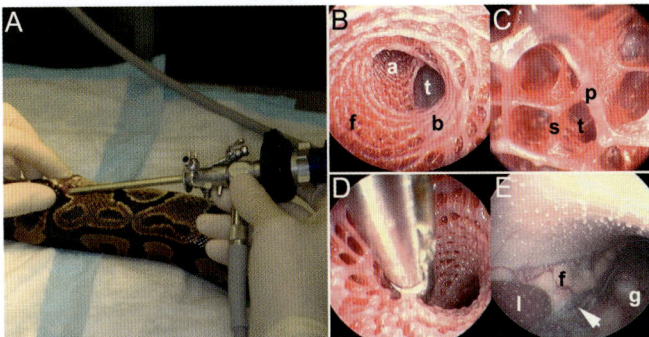

FIG 64.7 Ball python (*Python regius*) transcutaneous pulmonoscopy. (A) The sheathed 2.7-mm telescope inserted through the lateral body wall and introduced into the cranial lung of a research python that has not been draped to permit visualization of the snake's position and surgical entry site. (B) View of the cranial lung demonstrating the distal trachea (t), intrapulmonary bronchus (b), anterior lung lobe (a), and the faveolar lung tissue (f). (C) Close-up view of the faveolar region demonstrating the primary (p), secondary (s), and tertiary (t) septae of the anterior vascular lung. (D) Lung biopsy using the 1.7-mm biopsy forceps. (E) View of the thin, transparent, caudal air sac through which the caudal edge of the liver (l), fat body (f), gastrointestinal tract (g), and caudal vena cava (arrow) can be seen. (Courtesy of Stephen J. Divers.)

A transcutaneous approach to the lung of snakes has also been described.[11,25] This involves a minicoeliotomy approach approximately 35% to 45% from snout-to-vent, on the right side in boids and colubrids (or either left or right side for boas and pythons because they have two lungs). Following a 1-cm skin incision, and blunt dissection through an intercostal space, the lung is identified as it is ventilated, grasped, secured, and punctured using a scalpel blade before insertion of the telescope. Depending on the size of the snake, this approach can facilitate evaluation of the distal trachea, primary and intrapulmonary bronchus, cranial faveolar lung, transitional zone, and the caudal air sac (Fig. 64.7). In giant boids, a flexible endoscope can be inserted and advanced cranially and caudally to examine most of the unilateral pulmonary system. Lung and skin are closed routinely as separate layers. This technique has been thoroughly evaluated in ball pythons (*Python regius*), where the surgical approach and visualization of the distal portion of the trachea; primary bronchus; intrapulmonary bronchus; cranial lung lobe; and faveolar, semisaccular, and saccular lung regions were excellent.[11] This study also evaluated faveolar biopsy specimens collected using 1.7 mm biopsy forceps and concluded that the diagnostic quality of specimens that were shaken from biopsy forceps into physiological saline solution before fixation in 2% glutaraldehyde or neutral-buffered 10% formalin was good to excellent. Reevaluation of the same snakes a year later confirmed complete healing of the previous entry and biopsy sites with no apparent deleterious effects.

Stomatoscopy and Gastroscopy

Sternal or dorsal recumbency with head and neck extended is preferred for stomatoscopy and gastroscopy. It is often helpful to have the reptile close to the table edge or positioned on a raised surface. The rigid telescope-sheath system can be used to examine the buccal cavity, esophagus, and stomach of small lizards, crocodilians, and chelonians (Fig. 64.8). Flexible endoscopes are required to gain access to the stomach for most snakes and larger reptiles of other orders (Fig. 64.9). Air insufflation can be used to dilate the tract, which provides good exposure

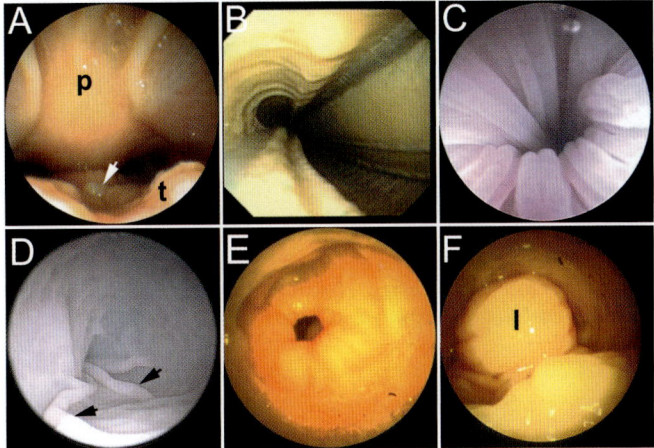

FIG 64.8 Stomatoscopy, esophagoscopy, and gastroscopy. (A) Oral cavity of a radiated tortoise (*Astrochelys radiata*) demonstrating the choana and hard palate (p), fleshy tongue (t), and larynx (arrow). (B) Air-distended esophagus of a Burmese python (*Python bivittatus*). (C) Saline-infusion view of the green iguana (*Iguana iguana*) distal esophagus. (D) Stomach of a savannah monitor (*Varanus exanthematicus*) with normal rugal folds (arrows). (E) Gastric hypertrophy in a corn snake (*Pantherophis guttata*) with cryptosporidiosis. (F) Leiomyoma (l) obstructing the pyloric outflow in another corn snake that presented with chronic regurgitation. (Courtesy of Stephen J. Divers.)

for detecting gross lesions and foreign bodies. Warm saline irrigation provides superior clarity, especially when examining for mucosal detail, although tracheal intubation is essential to avoid aspiration. Whether air or saline is used, it is important to gently dilate the tract as the endoscope is advanced to avoid damage and laceration to the wall. Foreign bodies can be readily retrieved, and biopsy collection should be undertaken with care to avoid perforation of the intestinal tract, which is more likely in the thin-walled esophagus than the stomach.

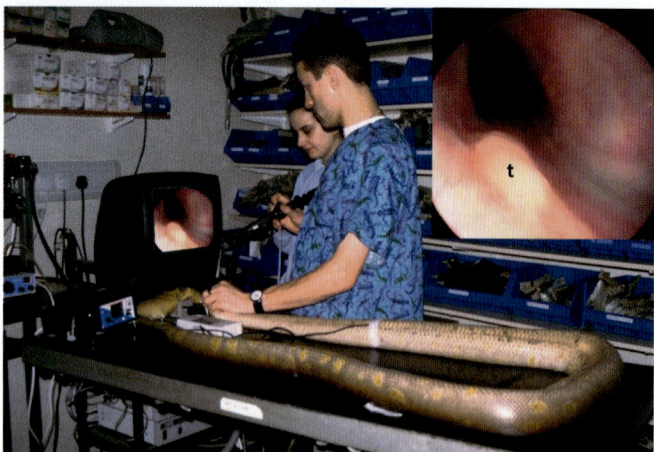

FIG 64.9 Flexible gastroscopy in a color-mutant burmese python (*Python bivittatus*). *(Inset)* Endoscopic view of an esophageal lymphoid aggregate ("esophageal tonsil"). (Courtesy of Stephen J. Divers.)

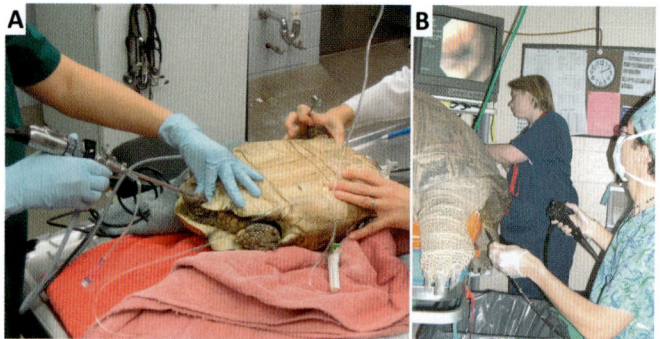

FIG 64.10 Chelonian cloacoscopy. (A) Cloacoscopy using a 2.7-mm telescope and saline infusion in an African spurred tortoise (*Centrochelys sulcata*). (B) Cloacoscopy using a 9.0-mm video gastroscope in an Aldabra tortoise (*Aldabrachelys gigantea*). (Courtesy of Stephen J. Divers.)

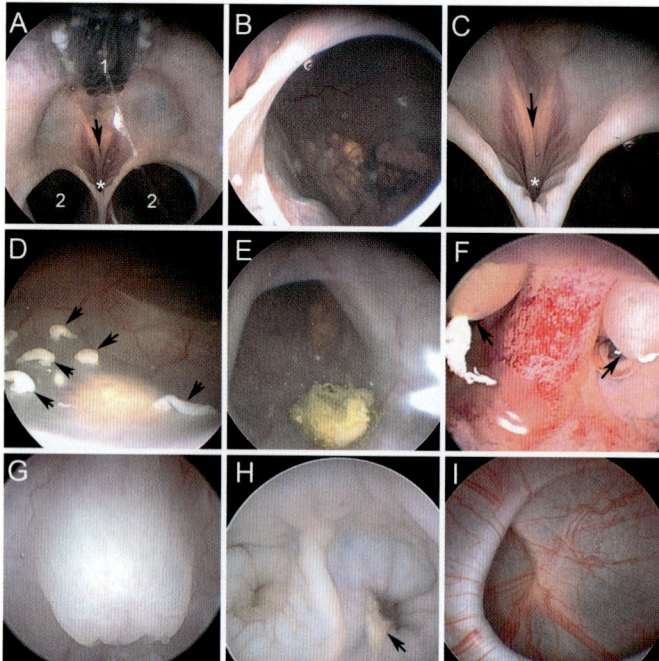

FIG 64.11 Cloacoscopy. (A) Endoscopic view of the cloaca of a female yellow-bellied slider (*Trachemys scripta*) demonstrating the clitoris lying on the ventral wall (1), bilateral accessory bladders (2), openings to the colon (*), and the urodeum (arrow), where the genital openings and urethra are located (dorsal recumbency using saline infusion). (B) Close-up of one of the accessory bladders. (C) Close-up of the openings to the urodeum and urethra (arrow), and the colon (*). (D) Cystoscopy in a female yellow-bellied slider demonstrating several trematode parasites (arrows) attached to the bladder wall. (E) Colonoscopy of a yellow-bellied slider with a small fecal mass visible. (F) View within the urodeum of a green iguana (*Iguana iguana*) with uric acid emerging from the urogenital papillae (arrows). (G) The single urogenital papilla within the urodeum of the ball python (*Python regius*). (H) View within the urodeum of a hognose snake (*Heterodon nasicus*) demonstrating the oviductal openings. Note the discharge emanating from one of the oviducts (arrow) that was associated with retained egg material. (I) Colonoscopy of a ball python (*Python regius*) demonstrating the normal spiral folds. (A-E, G, and I, Courtesy of Stephen J. Divers; F and H, courtesy of Scott J. Stahl, Stahl Exotic Animal Veterinary Services.)

Cloacoscopy

Although snakes can also be positioned in sternal or dorsal recumbency, chelonians and lizards are generally easier in dorsal (Fig. 64.10). Endoscopy using warm saline irrigation promotes unparalleled examination of the proctodeum, urodeum, and coprodeum. Detailed appraisal of the distal colon, cloacal mucosa, urogenital papillae, oviductal openings in females, and (when present) the urethral opening and bladder (Fig. 64.11) are possible. With practice, the endoscope can be directed through the urethra into the thin-walled bladder in chelonians and some lizards. It is also possible to enter the distal oviducts of reproductively active females. Cloacoscopy has been used to remove shell and egg material from the distal oviducts and bladder, guide exteriorization of partially prolapsed tissue and resection, and facilitate bladder catheterization. Mucosal biopsies should be taken with care, especially from the colon and bladder due to their thin nature and the risks of perforation. More recently, a technique for neonate gender identification that centered on observing the gonads through the bladder wall via a cloacoscopic approach has been described in Hermann's tortoises (*Testudo hermanni*).[26] This technique has the advantage of avoiding entry into the coelomic cavity but, because examination is through a membrane, may not be as sensitive as direct coelioscopic visualization. In addition, research at

UGA involving sliders (*Trachemys*) indicated that perforation of the urethra and bladder were common and the technique could not be recommended (Proenca, unpublished data). There may be species-specific safety limitations for this cystoscopic technique.

Coelioscopy

As reptiles lack a true abdomen, the term coelioscopy is preferred over laparoscopy. For a detailed discussion of generic laparoscopy methodologies the reader is referred to the dedicated literature, as only reptile specifics will be highlighted here.[27–30] Laparoscopy has been shown to offer significant advantages over traditional surgical options, both in human and veterinary medicine. In particular, laparoscopy is, with practice, faster, less traumatic, and causes less postoperative pain, with a more rapid return to normal function.[31–42] Until the advent of 2- and 3-mm human pediatric equipment, coelioscopy was limited to a single-entry system using the sheathed telescope; however, multiple-entry techniques are now possible and practical for animals over 500 g (see Chapter 65).[43]

Precise positioning for coelioscopy depends upon the reptile's body shape and confirmation, the structure(s) of interest, and the preferences of the endoscopist.[13] The entry site is aseptically prepared and draped, and adhesive clear plastic drapes permit better visualization of the patient. Insufflation is essential for lizards and snakes and, although the shell prevents coelomic collapse, can still be helpful in many chelonians. Typically CO_2 insufflation pressures of 3 to 5 mm Hg are used, which are lower than those recommended for mammals (8–12 mm Hg). In some situations, saline infusion may be preferred over gas. In the author's experience this is especially true when dealing with neonates, juveniles, and other very small reptiles, or aquatic species, where residual gas may have a negative effect on postoperative buoyancy.

Lizards. Dorsoventrad compressed lizards (e.g., bearded dragons) are more easily positioned in dorsal recumbency, while laterally compressed lizards (e.g., old world chameleons) in lateral. Round-bodied lizards (e.g., green iguanas) can be easily placed in either lateral or dorsal recumbency, but lateral is generally preferred and allows easier access to both ventral and dorsal structures. Given the relatively small size of most lizards, a single paramedian or paralumbar entry point will usually permit examination of most, if not all, organ systems.

While anatomic differences exist between families, the green iguana serves as a useful model for saurian coelioscopy.[7,44] In the iguana, there is no significant difference in visualization of lung, liver, pancreas, small intestine, large intestine, ovary, oviduct, testis, epididymis, vas deferens, bladder, fat body, or kidney from either left or right approaches. However, a left lateral approach to the heart, stomach, and spleen, and a right lateral approach to the gallbladder, are preferred.[7] Right-handed surgeons will find that a left paralumbar approach is easier, while left-handed surgeons will prefer a right paralumbar approach. Unless physical examination, diagnostic imaging, clinicopathology or anatomy suggests an asymmetric location the endoscopist's preference can prevail. For a left lateral approach, which is often favored by right-handed surgeons, the iguana is positioned in right lateral recumbency, with the left pelvic limb taped caudad against the tail base. The entry area is bordered craniad by the ribs, dorsad by the spine, and caudad by the pelvic limb (Fig. 64.12). However, in larger lizards an intercostal approach is also practical. Aseptically, a small skin incision is made in the center of the defined area. The skin and underlying muscle is grasped and elevated away from the coelomic viscera and the sheath (with obturator), aimed parallel to the table and toward the head, are gently forced through the coelomic musculature and into the coelomic cavity. It is wise to temporarily cease artificial ventilation until the telescope has been introduced into the coelom, thereby reducing the possibility of damage to an inflated lung or viscus. The obturator is replaced by the telescope and the insufflation line attached to one of the sheath ports. By making a small skin incision and breach in the muscle, the sheath will be tight fitting, and insufflation gas leakage will be minimized if there is any gas leakage, a mattress suture can be placed through the skin and around the sheath. Once a pneumocoelom has been created, it may be necessary to gently touch the tip of the telescope against a coelomic membrane to clean the terminal lens of condensation or tissue fluid. If there is fat or blood on the lens it is often necessary to remove the telescope from the sheath, clean with gauze moistened with sterile saline, and replace. It is unwise to continue with poor visualization.

Upon entry via a left paralumbar approach in the iguanid lizard, the first organ to note is the large brown liver lying in the midventral coelom (Fig. 64.13A). Advancing the telescope craniad will reveal the heart at the cranioventral extent of the coelom, close to the cranial coelomic inlet (see Fig. 64.13B). There are no diaphragmatic, postpulmonary, or longitudinal membranes in iguanas. However, these membranes do exist to a greater or lesser extent in tegus, monitors, and certain other saurians (see Fig. 64.13C). Minor perforation of these membranes by the telescope will not cause any harm, but care is required

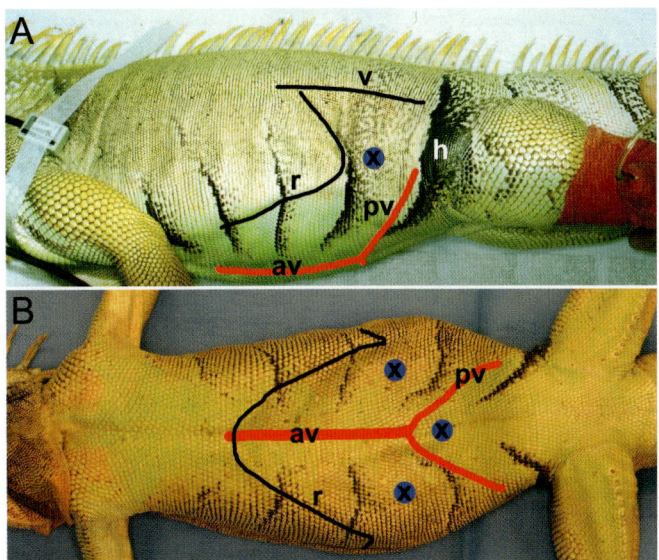

FIG 64.12 Common telescope entry sites for coelioscopy in lizards. (A) For a lateral entry into the coelom, the entry point (x) is bordered craniad by the last rib (r), dorsad by the lateral processes of the lumbar vertebrae (v), caudad by the musculature of the hind limb (h), and ventrad by the ventral abdominal (av) and pelvic veins (pv). (B) For a ventral approach to the coelom, insertion points (x) may be in the midline, behind the anastomoses of the lateral pelvic veins (pv), or lateral to the ventral abdominal vein (av), caudal to the last rib (r), and cranial to the pelvic veins (pv). (Courtesy of Stephen J. Divers.)

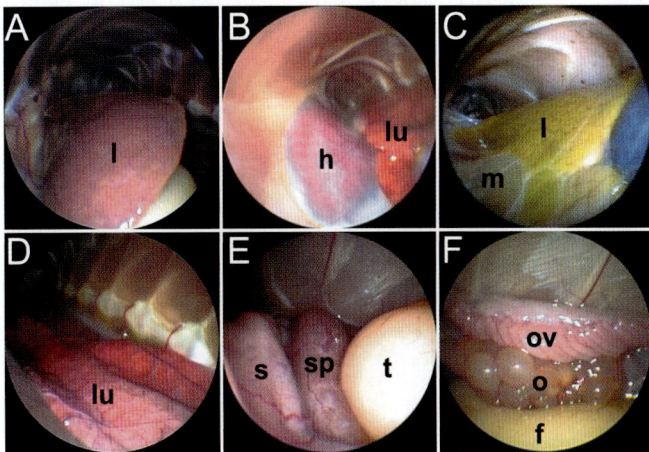

FIG 64.13 Lizard coelioscopy. (A) Left liver lobe (l) in a green iguana (*Iguana iguana*) (left lateral approach). (B) Heart (h) and lung (lu) in a green iguana—note the absence of a postpulmonary membrane (left lateral approach). (C) Left liver lobe (l) behind the post-hepatic membrane (m) in a monitor lizard (*Varanus* sp.) (left lateral approach). (D) Lung (lu) in a green iguana; note the absence of a postpulmonary membrane in this species (left lateral approach). (E) Stomach (s), spleen (sp), and testis (t) in a green iguana (left lateral approach). (F) Oviduct (ov), ovary (o), and fat body (f) in a green iguana (left lateral approach). (Courtesy of Stephen J. Divers.)

to avoid perforating the underlying viscera. Dorsal to the heart and extending to midcoelom are the paired lungs (see Fig. 64.13D). Lung ventilation will be substantially reduced during CO_2 insufflation, and careful communication with the anesthetist is required to balance ventilation and coelomic pressures. Caudal to the lungs, in the midcoelom, is the stomach with the spleen, an elongated dark red organ in iguanas, situated close behind (see Fig. 64.13E). Careful examination medial to the stomach and spleen will reveal the splenic limb of the pancreas. The gonads are located just caudal to the spleen, on either side of dorsal midline. Rigid endoscopy can be utilized to determine the gender of reptiles, even at a very early age. This is extremely useful in monomorphic species or when involved in an endangered species breeding program that requires gender identification of neonates or juveniles.[9] Endoscopy also provides feedback on reproductive activity and disease. The testis is usually ovoid and smooth, and size may vary dramatically with season (see Fig. 64.13E). The immature or inactive ovary appears as a cluster of small, fluid-filled follicles (see Fig. 64.13F). As the ovary matures some of the follicles will enlarge and appear yellow to orange in color as they fill with yolk. Some species of lizards have thin post-hepatic or postpulmonary membranes that may be pigmented and obscure the gonads. The membrane can be breached to allow better visualization by grasping and tearing with retrieval forceps or incising using scissors. Care must be taken not to damage the follicles because leakage results in coelomitis.

Dorsal to the gonads are the adrenal glands, which lie adjacent to the renal veins (see Fig. 64.14A). The vas deferens of males and oviducts of females are also visible and can be followed caudad to the pelvic inlet. The kidneys of most lizards are situated in the caudodorsal coelom; however, those of the iguana are intrapelvic but can still be visualized (see Fig. 64.14B). Moving ventrad from the pelvic inlet the bladder (if present) and fat body can be seen (see Fig. 64.14C). A left paralumbar approach will reveal the small intestine and terminal colon; however, a right paralumbar approach will provide access to the gallbladder and caecum (see Fig. 64.14D). The majority of the pancreas is easier to locate via a right approach, residing caudal to the liver and gallbladder and closely associated with the duodenum (see Fig. 64.14E). On the right side, the heart is partially obscured by the ascending vena cava (see Fig. 64.14F).

This approach to saurian coelioscopy has been validated, at least in the green iguana, and found to be both safe and effective.[7] In addition, endoscopic biopsies of liver and kidney have also been demonstrated to be safe and capable of producing samples of diagnostic quality.[8,10]

Snakes. Snakes are less commonly subjected to coelomic endoscopy because (1) they have more extensive coelomic fat, (2) it is impossible to examine all the major organs via a single entry point, and (3) insufflation is generally more difficult; however, targeted coeliotomy can be readily performed along the entire length of the coelom. If a targeted endoscopic approach to a single coelomic region is required, lateral entry between the ribs in larger snakes, and ventrolateral entry just medial to the ribs in smaller snakes, are practical options (Fig. 64.15A).[13] A recently developed technique for liver biopsy entails access via the pulmonoscopy approach to the serpentine air sac. From within the air sac it is possible to visualize and biopsy the liver (see Fig. 64.15B–D).

Chelonians. With the chelonian supported in lateral recumbency, the most useful coelioscopic approach is via the left or right prefemoral fossa (Fig. 64.16).[13] Right-handed surgeons will generally find it easier to enter the left prefemoral fossa, and left-handed surgeons the right. Again, unless unilateral pathology or organ asymmetry exists, the surgeon's preference can prevail. A large bladder can hinder coelioscopy, and chelonians should be encouraged to urinate prior to surgery. This can be achieved by bathing the animal or by gentle digital stimulation of the cloaca prior to anesthetic induction.

The pelvic limb is retracted and taped caudad to expose the prefemoral fossa. In chelonians with a well-developed plastron hinge (e.g., box turtles), it is wise to place a wedge between the caudal plastron and carapace to maintain exposure. Following aseptic preparation, a small (2–4 mm) craniocaudal skin incision is made in the center of the prefemoral fossa. The subcutaneous fat and connective tissues are bluntly

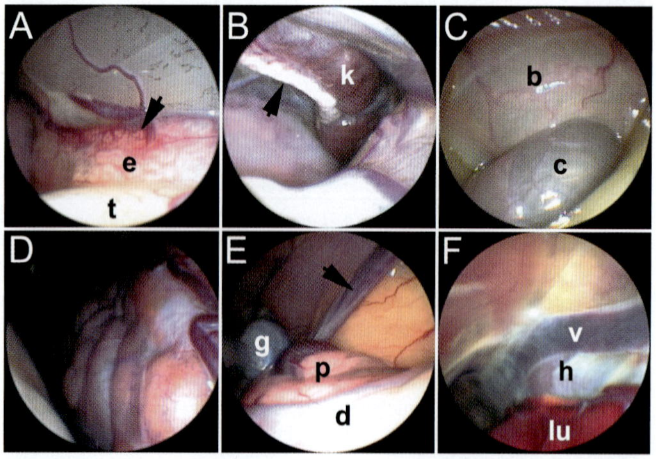

FIG 64.14 Green iguana (*Iguana iguana*) coelioscopy. (A) Epididymis (*e*) and adrenal (*arrow*) lying dorsal to the testis (t) in a male (left lateral approach). (B) Normal vas deferens (arrow) and kidney (k) emerging from the pelvic inlet (left lateral approach). (C) Bladder (b) and distal colon (c) (left lateral approach). (D) Loops of small bowel (left lateral approach). (E) Gall bladder (g), pancreas (p), duodenum (d), and ventral abdominal vein (arrow) (right lateral approach). (F) Cranial lung (lu) and caudal vena cava (v), partially obscuring the heart (h) (right lateral approach). (Courtesy of Stephen J. Divers.)

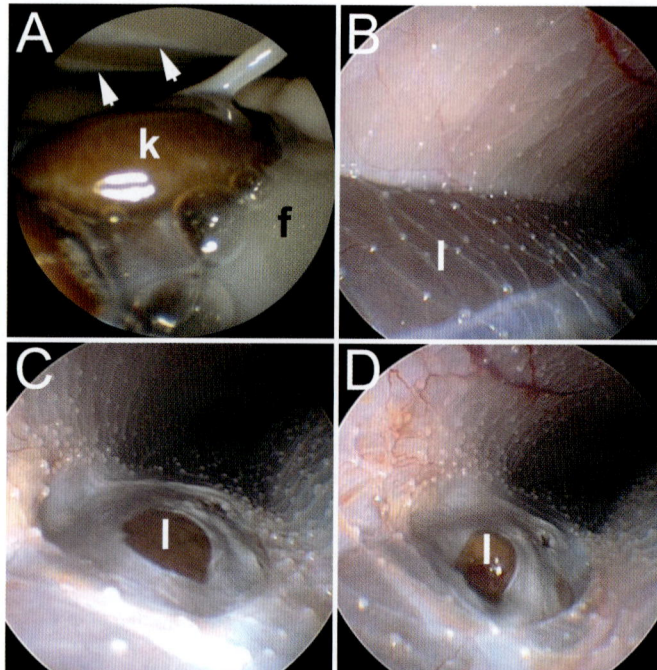

FIG 64.15 Snake coelioscopy. (A) Left lateral approach 82% snout-to-vent revealing the caudal pole of the left kidney (k), fat body (f), and ribs (arrows) in a boa constrictor (*Boa constrictor*). (B) Ball python (*Python regius*) liver (l) viewed from within the air sac of the right lung. (C) The air sac and serosal membranes have been incised to expose the liver parenchyma (l). (D) View of the liver (l) following biopsy using 1.7-mm forceps. (Courtesy of Stephen J. Divers.)

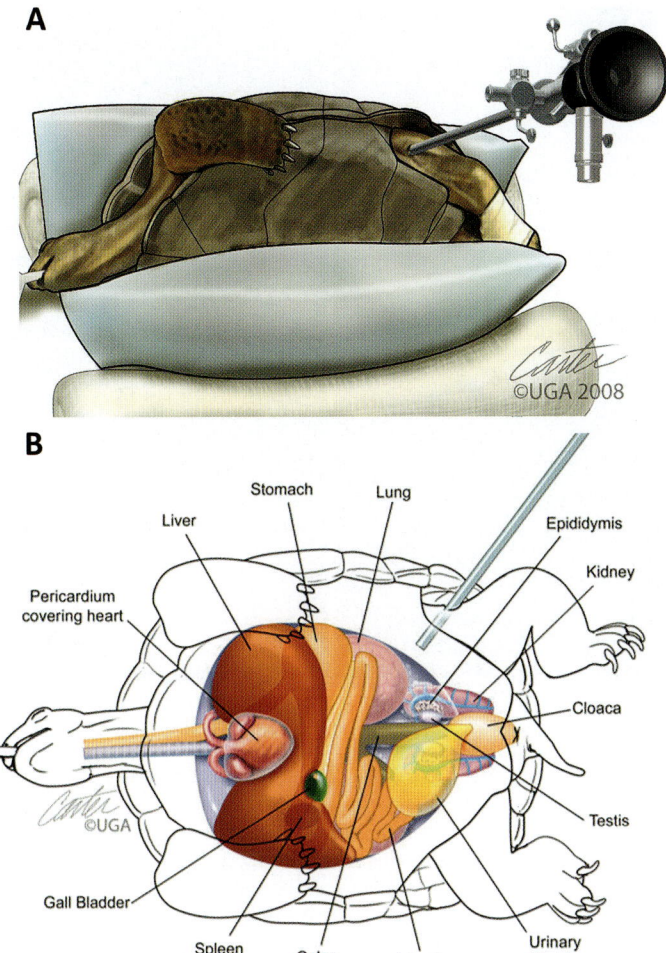

A

B

FIG 64.16 Chelonian coelioscopy. (A) Positioning for a left prefemoral approach (in front of the left pelvic limb) in order to access the chelonian coelomic cavity. (B) Diagram to illustrate position and orientation of coelomic viscera inside a male chelonian. Note the entry position of the telescope through the prefemoral fossa and the asymmetry of certain organs. (Courtesy of Educational Resources, University of Georgia.)

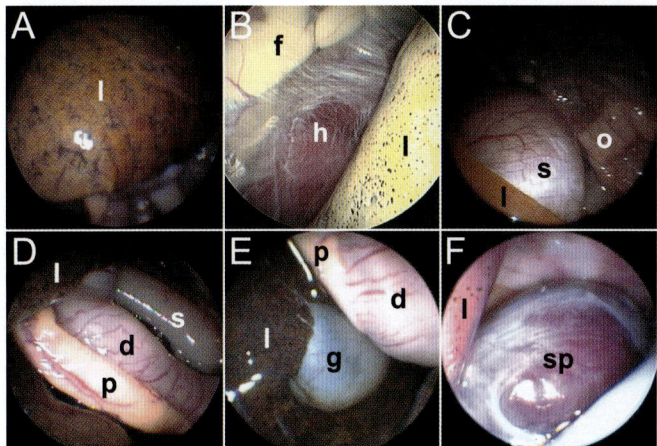

FIG 64.17 Chelonian coelioscopy. (A) Normal liver (l) in a radiated tortoise (*Astrochelys radiata*) (left prefemoral approach). (B) Heart (h) and pericardial fat (f) behind the coelomic membrane of a yellow-bellied slider (*Trachemys scripta scripta*). Note the pale liver (l) within the coelomic cavity (left prefemoral approach). (C) Stomach (s), liver (l), and oviduct (o) in a red-foot tortoise (*Chelonoidis carbonaria*) (left prefemoral approach). (D) Liver (l), pancreas (p) with closely associated duodenum (d), and stomach (s) of a red-eared slider (*Trachemys scripta elegans*) (left prefemoral approach). (E) Pancreas (p), duodenum (d), and gallbladder (g) embedded within the caudal aspect of the right liver lobe (l) in a red-eared slider (right prefemoral approach). (F) Spleen (sp) lying under the right liver lobe (l) in a yellow-bellied slider (right prefemoral approach). (Courtesy of Stephen J. Divers.)

dissected using hemostats down to the coelomic aponeurosis (formed by the broad tendinous portions of the transverse and oblique abdominal muscles), being careful to remain cranial to the sartorius muscle and ventral to the iliacus muscle that lies between the femur and ventral surface of the ilium. The coelomic aponeurosis is penetrated by advancing hemostats (or the sheath with obturator) toward the head (i.e., parallel, not perpendicular, to the table). Some force is required to breach the coleomic membrane and gain access to the coelomic cavity. An objective evaluation of coelioscopy in freshwater turtles (*Trachemys scripta* spp) has been published.[45] This study evaluated the ability of the 2.7 mm telescope to visualize the coelomic viscera of red-eared and yellow-bellied sliders and collected diagnostic biopsies from liver and kidney. Ease of entry and organ visualization were satisfactory to excellent for all observed structures, except the spleen, which could only be located from the right side.[17]

The dark red-brown to tan liver is the most obvious organ to use for orientation (Fig. 64.17A). The heart is cranioventral to the liver and partially obscured by a prominent pericardium (see Fig. 64.17B). The stomach is most prominent on the left (see Fig. 64.17C) and, while potentially seen from either lateral, the pancreas and closely associated duodenum are easier to see from a right approach (see Fig. 64.17D). The gallbladder is obvious and associated with the caudal edge of the right liver lobe (see Fig. 64.17E), but the spleen is often hard to locate

under the right liver lobe, close to the duodenum and pancreas (see Fig. 64.17F). The ventral aspects of the lungs are located dorsad and are most obvious in those species that lack a prominent postpulmonary membrane (Fig. 64.18A). The colon, gonads, oviducts (in females), bladder, and kidneys can be viewed from either side. The bladder is situated in the most dependent area, while the ovaries and oviducts of reproductively active females can occupy much of the coelom (see Fig. 64.18B and C). The male testes (cream, yellow, or brown in color) are situated in the caudodorsal coelom and are closely associated with the vasa deferentia, epididymides, adrenal glands, and retrocoelomic kidneys (see Fig. 64.18D). Recently, coelioscopy using saline-infusion has been shown to be accurate for identifying gender in hatchling and neonate chelonians. A study in Chinese box turtles (*Cuora flavomarginata*) concluded that gonads could be visualized and sex easily identified in animals as small as 10 g (see Fig. 64.18E and F).[9] More than 300 individual juveniles of various chelonian species have been subjected to early gender identification by coelioscopy (Fig. 64.19) (Divers S, unpublished data). Thus far, this technique has been found to be accurate and safe and has become established as a significant clinical service to breeders as well as curators of head-start conservation programs.

The kidneys are retrocoelomic, residing behind an often transparent coelomic membrane (Fig. 64.20A). When presented with a pigmented coelomic membrane, the close association with the testis (or immature ovary) can help indicate their location (see Fig. 64.20B). However, in adult females where the ovary and suspensory ligament have enlarged and fallen away from the pigmented coelomic membrane, it can be challenging to locate the kidneys unless they are grossly abnormal (see Fig. 64.20C).[17] An extracoelomic approach to the chelonian kidney is also possible in those species with a more flattened carapace and negates the need to enter the coelomic cavity. The sheathed endoscope is gently advanced from the same prefemoral skin incision in a caudodorsal

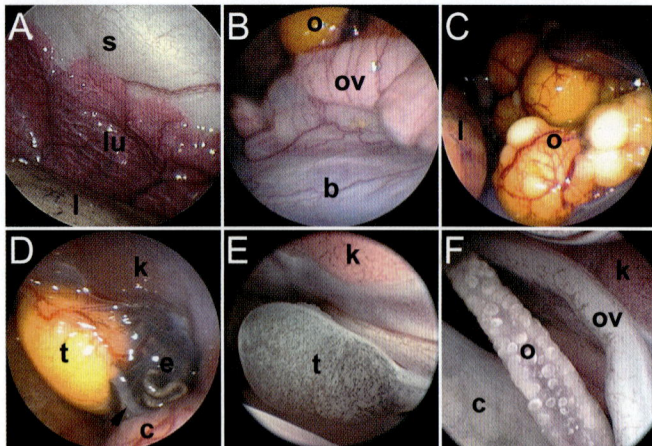

FIG 64.18 Chelonian coelioscopy. (A) View of the serosal surface of the dorsal shell (s), left lung (lu), and liver (l) in a red-eared slider (*Trachemys scripta elegans*) (left prefemoral approach). (B) Urinary bladder (b), oviduct (ov), and ovary (o) in an African spurred tortoise (*Centrochelys sulcata*) (left prefemoral approach). (C) Mature ovary (o) extending to the caudal edge of the left liver lobe (l) in a Hermann's tortoise (*Testudo hermanni*) (left prefemoral approach). (D) Testis (t), epididymis (e), and vas deferens (arrow) in the caudodorsal coelom of a red-eared slider. Note the closely associated retrocoelomic kidney (k) and the distal colon (c) (left prefemoral approach). (E) Immature testis (t) closely associated with the kidney (k) in a hatchling Chinese box turtle (*Cuora flavomarginata*) (left prefemoral approach with saline infusion). (F) Immature ovary (o) and oviduct (ov) closely associated with the kidney (k) and distal colon (c) in a hatchling Chinese box turtle (left prefemoral approach with saline infusion). (Courtesy of Stephen J. Divers.)

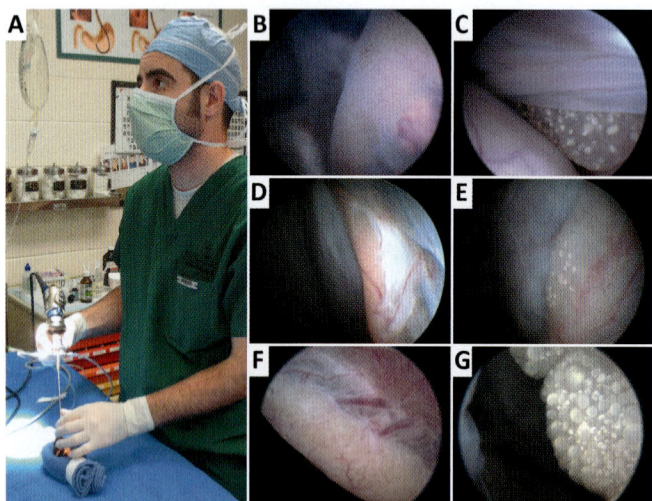

FIG 64.19 Juvenile chelonian gender identification. (A) Endoscopist using saline infusion and a 1.9-mm telescope with integrated sheath to perform sex identification in a juvenile tortoise. Juvenile male (B) and female (C) radiated tortoises (*Astrochelys radiata*). Juvenile male (D) and female (E) Galapagos tortoises (*Chelonoidis nigra*). Juvenile male (F) and female (G) Hermann's tortoises (*Testudo hermanni*). (Courtesy of Stephen J. Divers.)

direction between the coelomic aponeurosis and the broad iliacus muscle. A combination of gentle lateral movements of the telescope tip and intermittent insufflation are used to further separate the coelomic aponeurosis from the adjacent musculature to reveal the kidneys (see Fig. 64.20D).

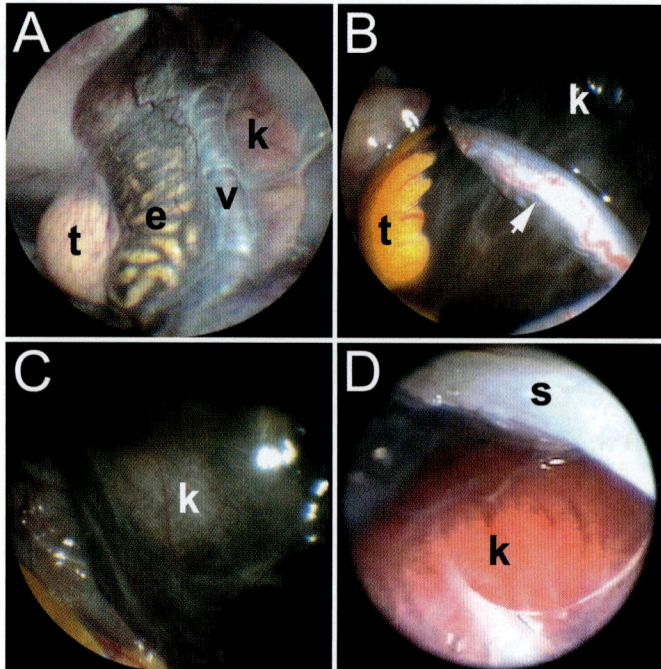

FIG 64.20 Chelonian renal examination. (A) View of the retrocoelomic kidney (k), renal vasculature (v), and closely associated testis (t) and epididymis (e) in a male red-eared slider (*Trachemys scripta elegans*). Note that renal visualization is possible thanks to the transparent nature of the coelomic membrane (left prefemoral approach). (B) View of the same caudodorsal region in an adult male Greek tortoise (*Testudo graeca*). The retrocoelomic kidney (k) is obscured by the pigmented coelomic membrane; however, its position can be determined by the obvious testis (t) and vas deferens (arrow) (left prefemoral approach). (C) View of the same caudodorsal region in an adult female Greek tortoise with the retrocoelomic kidney (k) obscured by a pigmented membrane. With no closely associated gonad to indicate the kidney's location, the endoscopist must rely on accurate anatomical knowledge alone (left prefemoral approach). (D) Direct, extracoelomic view of the kidney (k) and internal surface of the caudodorsal carapace (s) in a loggerhead sea turtle (left prefemoral approach). (Courtesy of Stephen J. Divers.)

Natural Orifice Transluminal Endoscopic Surgery (NOTES)

Natural orifice transluminal endoscopic surgery (NOTES) is an experimental surgical technique whereby "scarless" abdominal operations can be performed with an endoscope passed through a natural orifice (e.g., mouth, urethra, anus) then through an internal incision in the stomach, vagina, bladder, or colon, thus avoiding any external incisions or scars.[46] An increasing number of clinical procedures have been published in the human literature, and NOTES is considered the next frontier of human endoscopic surgery.[47] To date, the only reptile NOTES that the author is aware of involves the evaluation of gonads through the transparent bladder wall of juvenile tortoises (*Testudo marginata*).[26] This technique has the advantage of being less invasive (as the coelom is not entered), but it does not provide the same degree of visual acuity as direct examination and has been found to be unsafe in juvenile sliders (Proenca, unpublished data). Therefore in species where the immature gonads appear very similar or the bladder wall is less transparent, accuracy may be decreased (Fig. 64.21).

Pathology and Endoscopic Biopsy

A variety of pathologies may be appreciated endoscopically, often with surprisingly few clinicopathologic or discernible radiographic or

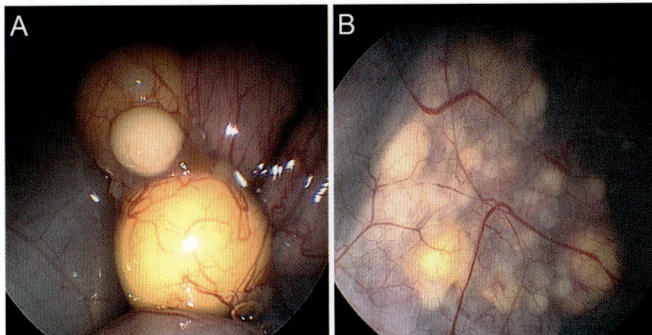

FIG 64.21 Endoscopic gender identification in the same adult female yellow-bellied slider (*Trachemys scripta scripta*). A comparison between direct examination by coelioscopy using CO_2 insufflation (A) and indirect examination using sterile saline and a translumenal technique across the accessory bladder wall (B, natural orifice translumenal endoscopic surgery). Note the reduced clarity of the ovary using the transluminal technique, which may be clinically significant when dealing with immature and less developed gonads. (Courtesy of Stephen J. Divers.)

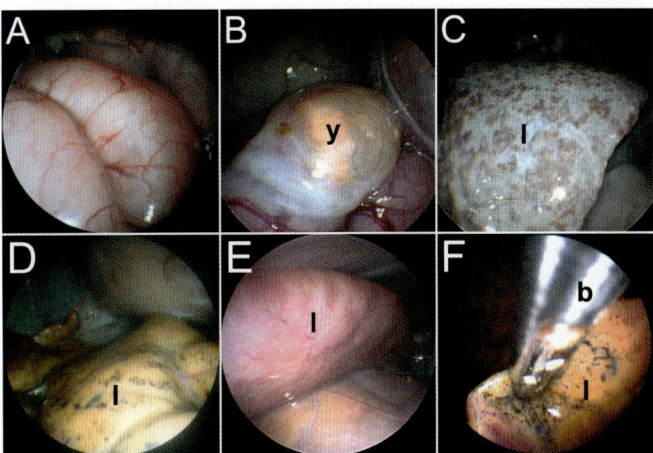

FIG 64.22 Endoscopic pathology and liver biopsy. (A) Grossly distended small intestine in a Russian tortoise (*Agrionemys horsfieldii*). This herbivorous tortoise was fed dairy products, which resulted in fermentative enteritis (left prefemoral approach). (B) Retained, inspissated yolk sac (y) in a juvenile radiated tortoise (*Astrochelys radiata*) that presented for intermittent anorexia and poor growth. Clinicopathology and diagnostic imaging were unremarkable but endoscope-assisted removal proved curative (left prefemoral approach). (C) Chronic hepatic fibrosis in a green iguana (*Iguana iguana*) that presented for anorexia and occasional regurgitation. Diagnostic imaging and clinicopathology were unremarkable. Endoscopic biopsy confirmed the diagnosis of severe hepatic fibrosis with cholestasis (left lateral coelioscopy). (D) Pale liver (l) in an Aldabra tortoise (*Aldabrachelys gigantea*) that presented with intermittent anorexia. All liver parameters were unremarkable, but severe hepatic lipidosis was diagnosed following liver biopsy (left prefemoral approach). (E) Diffuse hepatomegaly (l) in a green iguana that presented with lethargy and anorexia. Diagnostic imaging and liver biochemistry were unremarkable; however, moderate leukocytosis, predominantly heterophilia and azurophilia, was evident. Endoscopic liver biopsy confirmed the diagnosis as bacterial hepatitis due to *Klebsiella*, and appropriate treatment proved curative (left lateral coelioscopy). (F) Biopsy from the edge of the chelonian liver (l) using 1.7-mm biopsy forceps (b) (left prefemoral approach). (Courtesy of Stephen J. Divers.)

ultrasonographic changes (Fig. 64.22A–E). Tissue samples can be easily harvested from most organs and, in general, any abnormal soft tissue structure. Liver disease may be focal or diffuse, and although the caudal edge is easiest to sample, biopsies can also be taken from the surface by first incising the serosal covering (see Fig. 64.22F). A variety of renal diseases have also been described (Fig. 64.23A and B).[17,48] In lizards and snakes the lobulated kidney is easy to approach and biopsy directly (see Fig. 64.23C). However, in chelonians its flattened retrocoelomic position first requires incision of the coelomic membrane via a coelioscopic approach (see Fig. 64.23D–F). Endoscopic liver and kidney biopsies have been objectively assessed in freshwater turtles and green iguanas.[10,45,49] These studies have confirmed the ability of the 2.7-mm telescope to visualize and harvest samples from liver and kidney using the 1.7-mm biopsy forceps. No significant iatrogenic trauma was reported, and biopsy specimens were consistent with tissues collected at necropsy and were considered acceptable for histologic interpretation. Furthermore, the ability to diagnose renal diseases using endoscopic biopsy has also been demonstrated for a variety of chelonian species.[17]

Various studies have concluded that endoscopic biopsies are more diagnostic than ultrasound-guided aspirates or biopsies.[31,38,50] Endoscopic biopsies are delicate and measure approximately 1 mm^3 when collected using 1.7-mm forceps. Handling and other histologic artifacts are reduced by gently dislodging the tissue from the biopsy cups into a small volume of sterile saline, before then decanting into a biopsy cassette or bag, and submitting in 10% neutral buffered formalin (Fig. 64.24A).[11] Picking the biopsy out of the instrument using a needle will cause severe damage, and even moistened cotton-tipped applicators have been shown to cause tissue alteration (see Fig. 64.24B and C). Biopsies for microbiology are best submitted in sterile saline for immediate processing. Alternatively, if mailing to a laboratory, they should be submitted in appropriate transport media. For the submission of samples for toxicology or parasitology, it is wise to consult with the laboratory prior to sample collection.

POSTOPERATIVE CARE, COMPLICATIONS, AND OUTCOMES

Reptiles should be continuously maintained within their species-specific preferred optimum temperature zone and closely supervised until fully recovered from anesthesia. Opiates and meloxicam are often relied on for postoperative analgesia. Continued fluid therapy is more important than an immediate return to feeding. Typically, reptiles return to normal function and behaviors more quickly after endoscopic procedures compared with traditional surgeries. Sutures are removed at 6 to 8 weeks.

The major complications encountered are typically associated with anesthesia and advanced states of disease. The importance of a thorough preoperative evaluation and stabilization cannot be ignored but early endoscopic evaluation to reach a definitive diagnosis cannot be overemphasized. Minor hemorrhage following tissue biopsy is common but clinically insignificant. Return to normal behaviors and weight gain are often the most useful indicators of overall improvement. Serial clinicopathology can also be useful if abnormalities were detected preoperatively. Serial endoscopic evaluations can be used to monitor patients, especially because some diseases (e.g., hepatic lipidosis, glomerulonephrosis) may have a protracted course. Most endoscopy issues are related to poor or inappropriate equipment and/or operator error until competency has been achieved. To facilitate endoscopy caseload without compromising patient welfare, it is recommended that the surgeon obtains training and retains the option to convert to a traditional surgical approach if required.

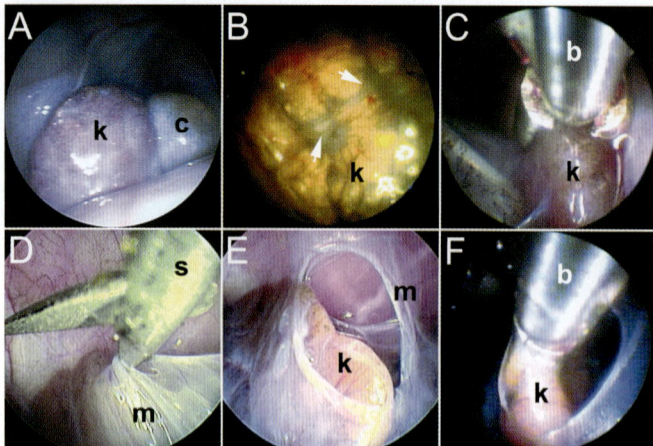

FIG 64.23 Endoscopic pathology and kidney biopsy. (A) Enlarged kidney (k) with associated renal cyst (c) in a green iguana (*Iguana iguana*) that presented with anorexia and cachexia. Radiography and ultrasonography confirmed renomegaly, while plasma biochemistry revealed reversed calcium:phosphorus ratio and elevated uric acid. Endoscopic biopsy confirmed the diagnosis of glomerulonephrosis with renal gout and mineralization (left lateral coelioscopy). (B) Abnormal kidney (k) with fibrous bands (arrows) in a female Greek tortoise (*Testudo graeca*) that presented with anorexia, lethargy, and polyuria. Diagnostic imaging and clinicopathology were unremarkable; however, renal biopsy confirmed the diagnosis as severe tubulonephrosis (left prefemoral approach). (C) Biopsy of an iguanid kidney (k) using 1.7-mm biopsy forceps (b) (right lateral coelioscopy). (D) Incising the caudodorsal coelomic membrane (m) of a yellow-bellied slider (*Trachemys scripta scripta*) using 1.7-mm endoscopy scissors (s) to gain access to the retrocoelomic kidney (left prefemoral approach). (E) View of the incised coelomic membrane (m) revealing the kidney (k) (left prefemoral approach). (F) Biopsy forceps (b) being passed through the incision to collect a biopsy from the kidney (k) (left prefemoral approach). (Courtesy of Stephen J. Divers.)

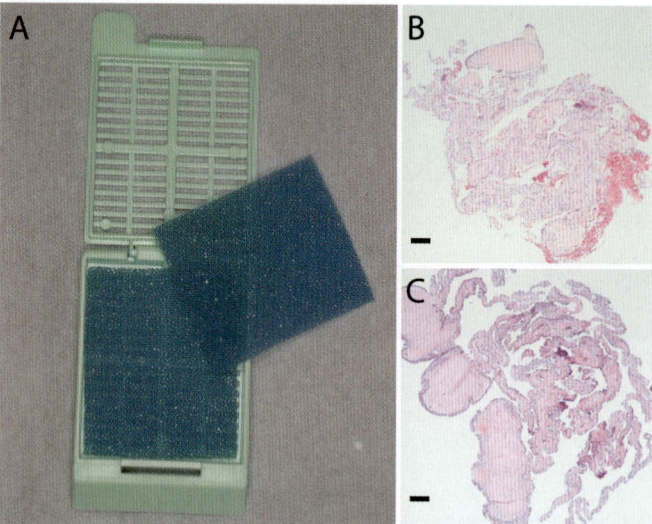

FIG 64.24 (A) Endoscopic biopsies are best sandwiched between foam and secured within a histology cassette. (B) Crush artifact in a snake lung biopsy caused by a cotton-tipped applicator used to transfer the tissue from forceps to histology cassette (H&E, bar = 300 μm). (C) Another snake lung biopsy exhibiting reduced artifact because it was shaken from the forceps into sterile saline before being decanted into the histology cassette (H&E, bar = 300 μm). (Courtesy of Stephen J. Divers.)

ACKNOWLEDGMENTS

The author would like to thank Karl Storz Veterinary Endoscopy and, in particular, Dr. Chris Chamness, Mike Bateman, and Dan McMahon for supporting endoscopy research, development, and training at the University of Georgia. In addition, I am indebted to Drs. Scott Stahl, Charles Innis, Sam Rivera, and Jörg Mayer, as well as the large number of residents, for their collegiality and support in various endoscopic ventures. I am also fortunate to work with highly motivated and dedicated technicians, including Ashley Schuller, Nia Chau, Danielle Stewart, and Robert Miller, who collectively ensure that equipment is clean, functional, and protected from overzealous veterinarians.

REFERENCES

See www.expertconsult.com for a complete list of references.

65

Endoscope-Assisted and Endoscopic Surgery

Stephen J. Divers

In human medicine, endosurgery has been credited with numerous advantages over traditional open procedures, including reductions in pain, operating time, hospital stay, and convalescence periods.[1,2] Although such advantages may be less easily quantified or documented in zoological medicine, over the past decade there have been considerable advances in minimally invasive endosurgery of exotic species, including reptiles.[3–8] Considering that most reptiles weigh less than a few kilograms, the development of minimally invasive endosurgery would seem a logical evolution in their surgical care, particularly given the hindrances of the chelonian shell.[7–9]

The transition from a technique that is purely diagnostic (see Chapter 64) to one that is more complex and allows surgical manipulation requires additional equipment (see Chapter 62), and even more taxing, a more refined surgical skill set. It is no exaggeration that the technical difficulty associated with multiple-port endosurgery is a magnitude greater than that required for single-entry diagnostic endoscopy. This chapter is an extension of the previous chapter and should not be read in isolation. Only supplemental techniques are covered here, and a firm grounding in diagnostic endoscopy is assumed.

Endosurgical Principles and Techniques

As already indicated, endosurgery requires placement of the telescope and triangulation of additional instruments (Fig. 65.1). Advanced endosurgical skills can only be built upon a firm foundation in single-entry diagnostic endoscopy. Minor errors or inadequacies that can be tolerated in single-entry procedures are likely to become magnified, resulting in serious problems during endosurgery. Well-executed and atraumatic placement of the telescope is essential and can only come from practice. Poor technique will result in tissue damage, increased tissue fluid including blood on the terminal lens, and decreased visibility. The need to practice instrument triangulation and develop fine motor skills with limited tactile feedback in a three-dimensional environment may exceed the endoscopy caseload, at least initially. Therefore the reptile endoscopic surgeon must find additional means to practice and maintain skills. One method is to maintain equipment in a clean, yet nonsterile, state. This will not dissuade the veterinarian from using equipment to practice on a cadaver, as opening a sterile pack would. In addition, inexpensive artificial trainers can be readily made from supplies found at local hobby and home-improvement stores. A clear plastic Tupperware container can serve as the basis for such a trainer. First, a large square hole is cut from the lid and replaced with rubber matting. Several 4 mm holes can be made in the rubber top and in the front of the container to provide a selection of instrument access ports (Fig. 65.2). A variety of "endoscopy games" can be devised to be completed inside the box. These can include dissection of a drawn shape on tissue paper, picking up felt discs off one pin and transferring to a second pin, or even endoscopic suturing (Fig. 65.3).

Surgeon ergonomics also become increasingly important when fine motor control now becomes more complicated by the need to triangulate and establish a perception of depth using a two-dimensional monitor. The monitor should, whenever possible, be directly in front of the surgeon, who should be comfortably standing on a padded mat or sitting (Fig. 65.4). Finally, the usual degree of tactile feedback experienced when handling tissues with standard instruments is greatly reduced when working with endoscopic instruments at distances of 20 cm or more from the tissues (Fig. 65.5).

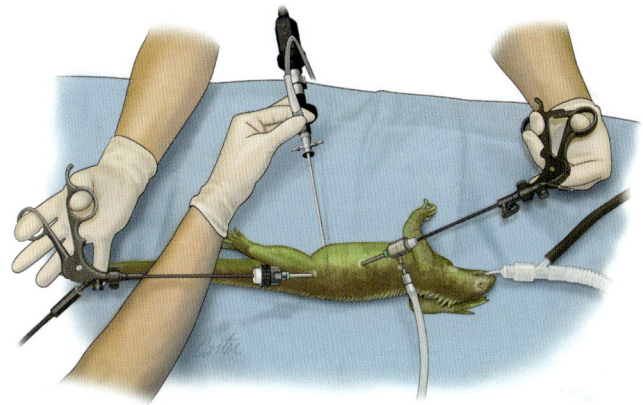

FIG 65.1 Illustration demonstrating instrument triangulation during left orchiectomy in an iguanid lizard. (Courtesy of Educational Resources, University of Georgia.)

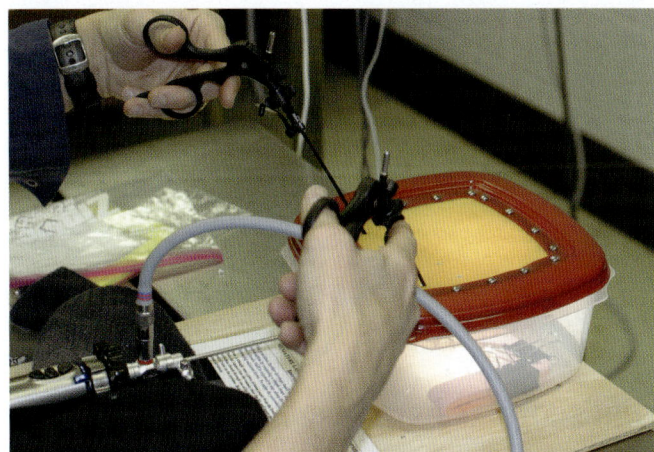

FIG 65.2 An endoscopy trainer fashioned from a modified plastic Tupperware container. Holes at the front permit the introduction of the telescope, which is supported using sand bags. The top has been largely replaced by a sheet of rubber containing several holes for the introduction of instruments. (Courtesy of Stephen J. Divers.)

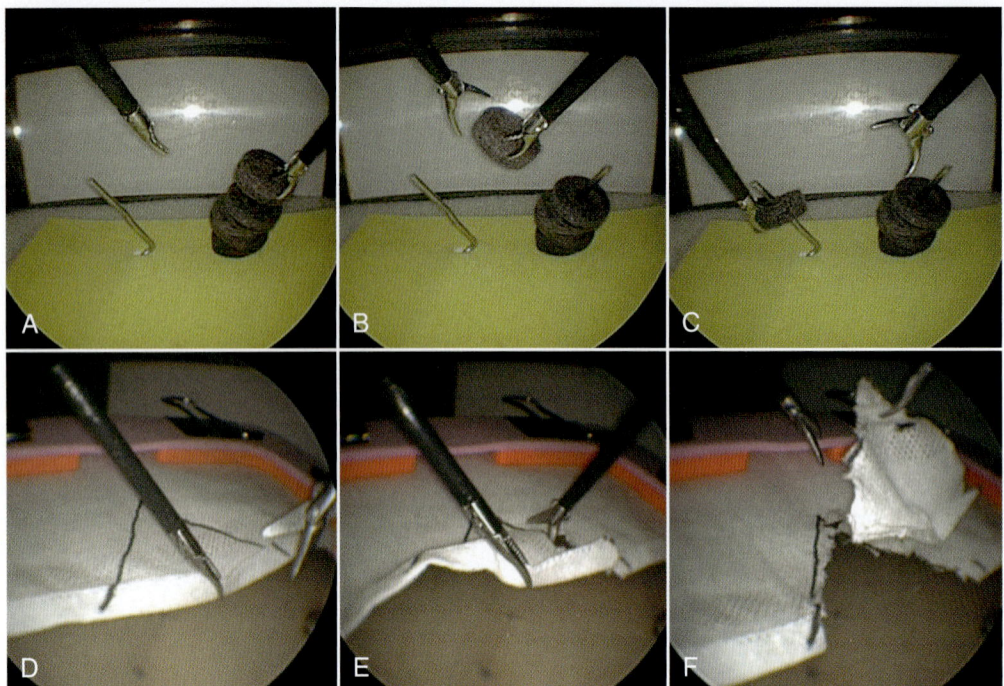

FIG 65.3 Endoscopy training exercises. (A–C) This basic exercise involves picking up a felt ring from one pin using forceps, exchanging the ring to a second pair of forceps, and then placing the ring on a second pin. This game helps with depth perception, instrument triangulation, and instrument to instrument transfer. It can be made more difficult by changing the orientation and direction of the pins. (D–F) This more difficult exercise involves using forceps and scissors to dissect a shape from a piece of tissue paper. This game helps with depth perception, instrument triangulation, and instrument dexterity. It can be made more difficult by increasing the complexity of the shape and by swapping the scissors and forceps. (Courtesy of Stephen J. Divers.)

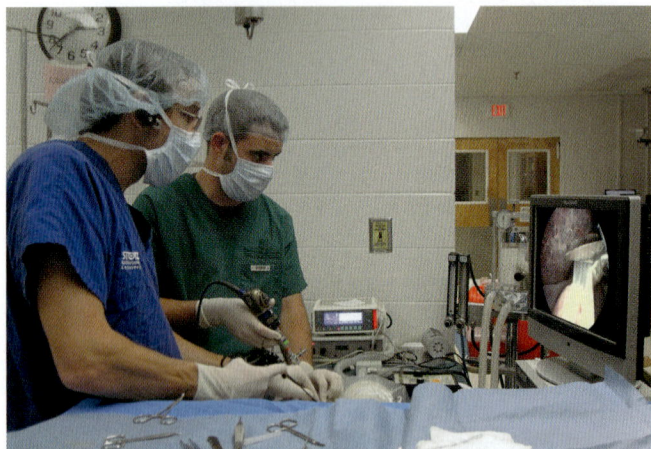

FIG 65.4 Proper positioning and orientation of the surgeon(s) to the patient and monitor becomes increasingly critical with endosurgery. In this example, the two surgeons are perpendicular to the monitor while they perform endosurgery in a small chelonian. (Courtesy of Stephen J. Divers.)

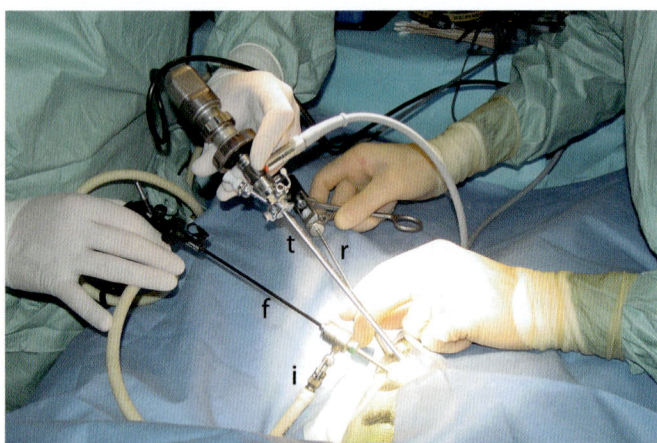

FIG 65.5 Tactile feedback and sensation is reduced during endosurgery because tissues are manipulated at a greater distance than with traditional surgery. This photograph also demonstrates the concept of triangulation with the two instruments on either side of the camera but converging toward the common endoscopic field of view. (Courtesy of Stephen J. Divers.)

ENDOSCOPE-ASSISTED PROCEDURES

An endoscope-assisted procedure is a hybrid that combines elements of endoscopy with traditional surgery. In its simplest form, an endoscope-assisted procedure uses endoscopy to identify and grasp an internal structure, which is then exteriorized through a miniature coeliotomy incision for completion of the procedure outside the body cavity. The advantages of endoscope-assisted procedures are that they decrease the size of the coeliotomy incision and exposure of internal viscera to the environment. An assortment of endoscope-assisted coelomic procedures, including enterotomy, enterectomy, cystotomy, salpingotomy, and salpingohysterectomy, are now possible. These techniques rely on the ability to exteriorize the tissue of interest out through a small, targeted coeliotomy incision. If the tissue cannot be exteriorized then the procedure cannot be completed externally, and a true endosurgical technique is required.

Endoscope-assisted procedures have been most commonly used in chelonians, where a soft tissue prefemoral approach has now superseded the need for transplastron coeliotomy in many situations. Of particular practical relevance is endoscope-assisted, prefemoral oophorectomy (or ovariectomy) of mature female chelonians that negates the need for a transplastron coeliotomy.[10] By virtue of the extensive mesovarian found in mature females, an endoscope-assisted procedure is practical in animals weighing a few hundred grams to 100 kg or more (Fig. 65.6).[10,11] With the chelonian in dorsal recumbency, a unilateral surgical approach to the coelom is made via one prefemoral fossa. The telescope is inserted into the coelom and used to locate the ipsilateral ovary. Then, using the telescope to guide atraumatic forceps (or even long hemostats in small chelonians), the interfollicular tissue is grasped and gently elevated to the skin incision. Once the first follicle is exteriorized, the telescope is no longer required, as the ovary is carefully manipulated out of the coelom. Once the entire ovary is exteriorized, oophorectomy proceeds using traditional techniques. The same procedure is repeated for the contralateral ovary, but it is usually not necessary nor recommended to remove the oviducts unless diseased. In most species, both ovaries can be removed from the same incision; however, in some terrestrial tortoises with particularly restrictive prefemoral fossae or voluminous large intestinal tracts or bladders, it may be necessary to perform a bilateral procedure. The prefemoral approach is closed routinely. This technique has several advantages over traditional transplastron approaches, namely, less invasive with faster healing.

Similar endoscope-assisted procedures have also been accomplished for the removal of retained eggs, bladder calculi, and gastrointestinal foreign bodies. The general technique and endoscopy skills are very

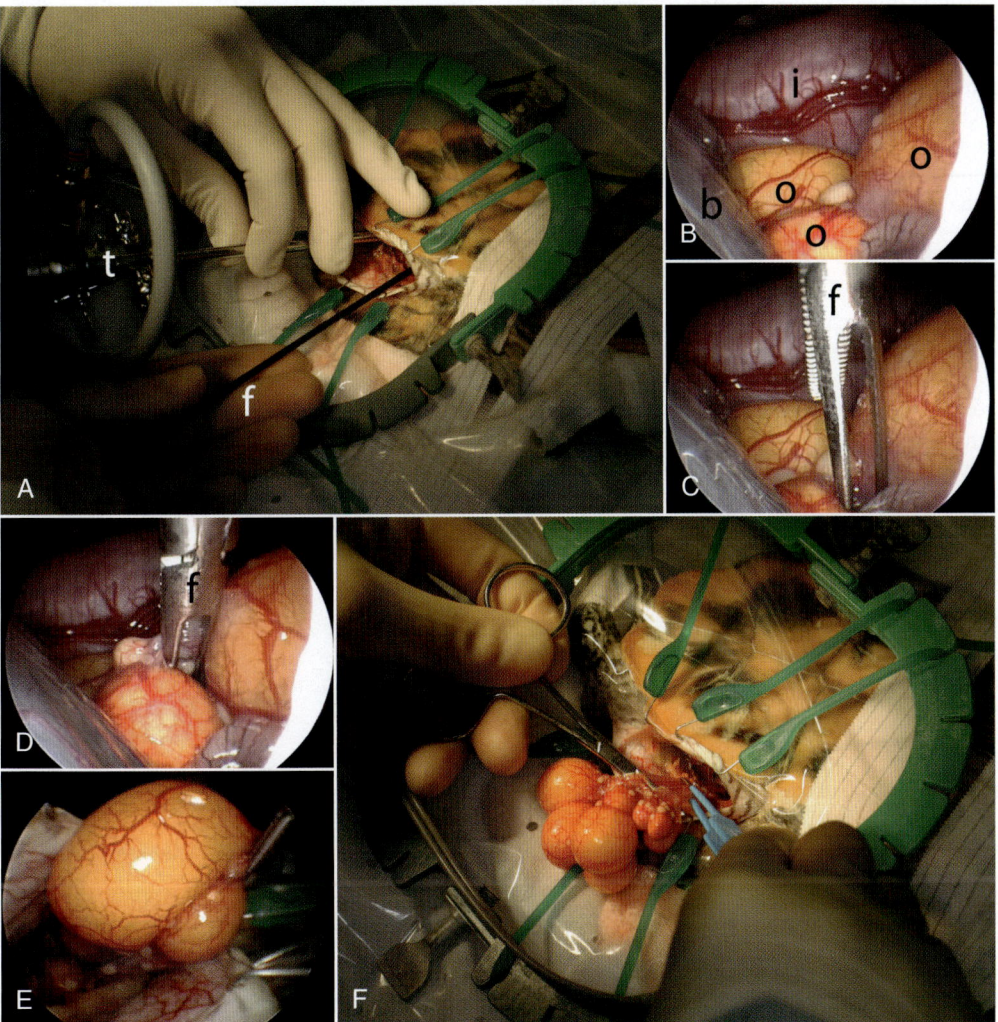

FIG 65.6 (A) Endoscope-assisted oophorectomy in an adult red-eared slider (*Trachemys scripta elegans*). (A) Following a prefemoral approach to the coelom, the ipsilateral ovary is located and retracted to the incision using the telescope (t) and 3 mm atraumatic forceps (f). (B) Endoscopic view of the caudal coelom demonstrating the ovary and three large ova (o), closely associated with the bladder (b) and gastrointestinal tract (i). (C) Endoscopic view of 3 mm atraumatic forceps (f) being used to grasp the interfollicular tissue. (D) Endoscopic view of the ovary being gently retracted toward the prefemoral incision. (E) External view (taken using the telescope) demonstrating the first two follicles of the ovary exteriorized through the prefemoral incision. (F) Continued manipulation to exteriorize the whole ovary precedes surgical oophorectomy using radiosurgery. In many species, the contralateral ovary can also be removed through the same prefemoral incision. (Courtesy of Stephen J. Divers.)

similar. First, diagnostic imaging is used to determine which side is favored for the approach. Then following a prefemoral coeliotomy, the telescope is used to identify the structure of interest and guide atraumatic tissue forceps. While any tissue that is due to be resected and removed can be grasped using Kelly or Babcock forceps (or similar), any tissue that is to ultimately be replaced should ideally be handled using atraumatic or fenestrated forceps. This is especially important when handling the bladder, gastrointestinal, or reproductive tracts.

ENDOSURGERY

To date, endosurgery has been more commonly performed in chelonians, although endosurgical orchiectomy of iguanids has also been described.[7] Although established endosurgical dogma dictates that telescopes are often placed through the umbilicus or linea alba and instrument ports are placed far enough apart to facilitate triangulation, reptile anatomy often necessitates a modified approach.

Endosurgical procedures usually commence with the placement of the telescope cannula, and two main techniques are commonly used. Either the telescope cannula is surgically placed via a mini-coeliotomy incision, after which the CO_2 line is attached and the coelom insufflated, or a Veress needle can be used. Placing the telescope cannula surgically, as preferred by the author, ensures intracoelomic placement, reduces the risks of iatrogenic trauma, but does require a mattress suture around the cannula to close the incision and prevent gas leakage.

Chelonians

Due to the constraints of the chelonian shell, it is seldom possible to place the telescope and ports where established protocols would suggest. There are two major approaches, depending upon the size of the animal. For larger chelonians, the telescope and instruments may all be inserted through one prefemoral fossa (Fig. 65.7), while in smaller animals the telescope and instruments may be placed through one or both fossae (Fig. 65.8). There are advantages and disadvantages to both approaches. Placing all instrumentation through a single fossa enables the surgeon to control both instruments even in large animals, but instrument triangulation and coordinated use can be more difficult due to the acute angles involved (often ≤20 degrees) because instruments run more parallel. Nevertheless, compared to a bilateral fossa technique, a unilateral approach is less invasive, with only a single surgical approach required, and in addition enables the animal to be positioned in lateral recumbency, which may aid organ visualization. A single surgeon can utilize both prefemoral fossa in smaller animals, but here the angle of triangulation is often obtuse (90–180 degrees), again making coordinated instrument manipulation more challenging. If the target structure is cranial to the bladder and the chelonian is less than 20 kg, it is often preferable for one instrument and telescope to be inserted through one prefemoral fossa, while the second instrument is inserted through the contralateral fossa. For such procedures, the animal is in dorsal recumbency and enjoys the advantage that instruments can be more easily triangulated within the cranial to mid coelom. However, in larger chelonians it can be difficult to impossible for a single surgeon to operate through both prefemoral fossa simultaneously, and in such cases a second surgeon is required to operate through one fossa. The endosurgical approach to caudal structures (e.g., bladder, kidney, adrenal, gonad) is more problematic as it is often difficult to access the same structure simultaneously from both fossae. Therefore where a caudal structure is the focus of the procedure, insertion of telescope and instruments through a single prefemoral fossa is often preferable. In such cases, the chelonian is generally positioned in dorsal or lateral recumbency, which provides greater accessibility as the intestines and bladder fall away into the more dependent areas of the coelom. This approach is easier in those animals

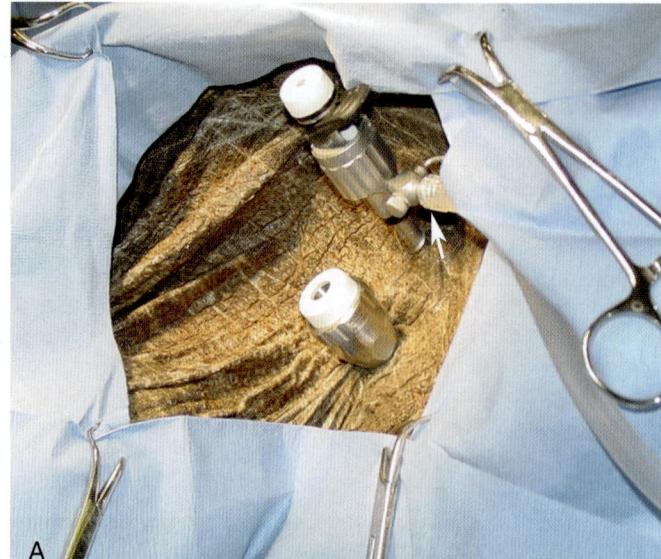

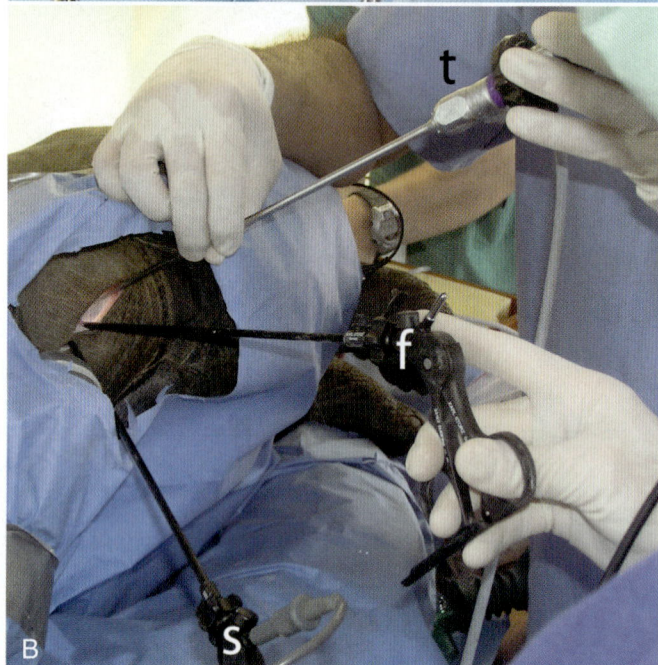

FIG 65.7 (A) Placement of two 6-mm Ternamian endotip cannulae, one with an insufflation port and CO_2 line attached (arrow) through the prefemoral fossa of an Aldabra tortoise (*Aldabrachelys gigantea*). (B) Surgical view of a juvenile Galapagos tortoise (*Chelonoidis nigra*) undergoing endoscopic oophorectomy. The telescope (t), held by an assistant, with grasping forceps (f) and radiosurgical scissors (s) operated by the primary surgeon, have all been introduced via a single prefemoral incision, rather than using separate cannulae. (Courtesy of Stephen J. Divers.)

with a large prefemoral fossa, but even so the close placement and parallel nature of instrumentation can make triangulation more difficult. In addition, it is often easier (especially in smaller animals) to make a single large prefemoral incision for the insertion of all instruments, rather than place three cannulae adjacent to one another (see Fig. 65.7). Insufflation is seldom essential due to the noncollapsible nature of the chelonian shell, and therefore endoscopic devices can still be used through an incision without the need for cannulae.

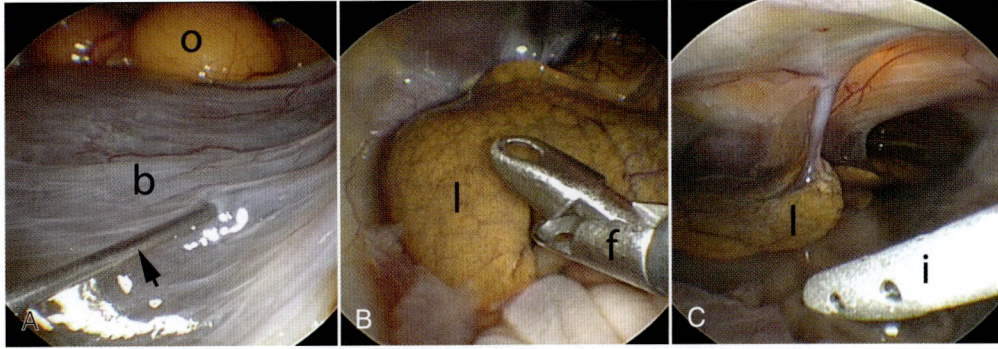

FIG 65.8 (A) Endoscopic view of the caudal coelom demonstrating the bladder (b) and right ovary (o) as seen through a left prefemoral approach in a box turtle (*Terrapene carolina*). In this example, an aspiration needle has been placed through the same left fossa and is being used to perform cystocentesis and collapse a full bladder. (B and C) Endoscopic views of the cranial coelom and liver (l) of another box turtle with ascites, as seen through the left prefemoral fossa. Biopsy forceps (f) and irrigation/suction cannula (i) have been introduced through the right fossa, which provides greater instrument triangulation. (Courtesy of Stephen J. Divers.)

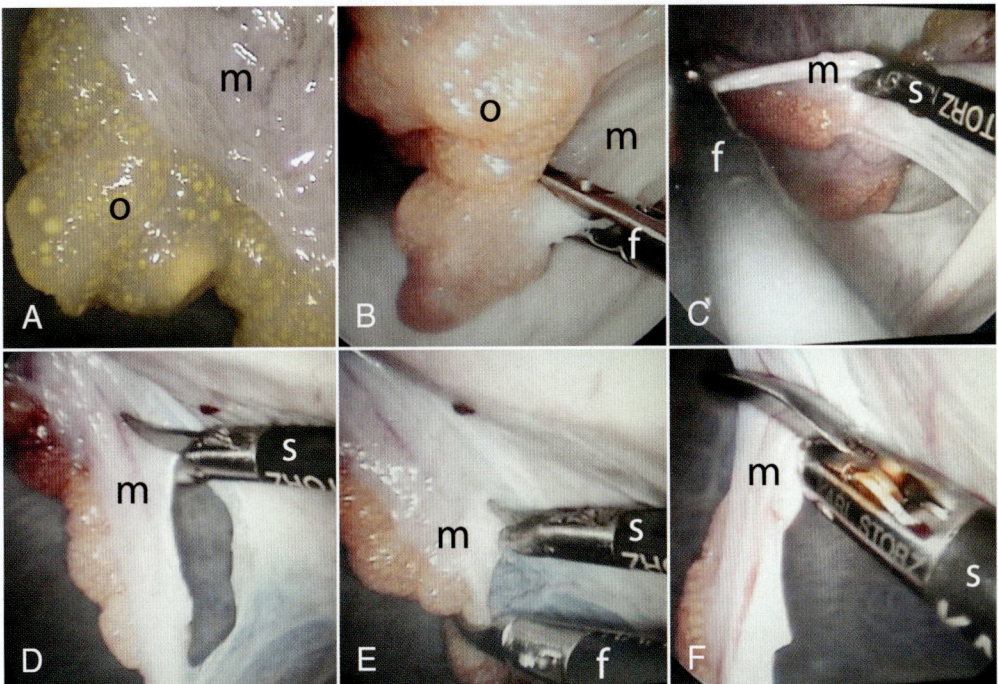

FIG 65.9 Endoscopic left oophorectomy in a juvenile Galapagos tortoise (*Chelonoidis nigra*) with all instrumentation inserted through the left prefemoral fossa as shown in Fig. 65.7B. (A) Normal, immature, left ovary (o) suspended from the caudodorsal body wall by a short mesovarium ligament (m). (B) Grasping forceps (f) are introduced and used to grasp the mesovarium (m) but not the friable ovary (o). (C) The mesovarium (m) is stretched by moving the forceps (f) cranially, while radiosurgical scissors (s) are used to incise through the suspensory ligament. (D–F) Dissection through the mesovarium (m) continues using forceps (f) and scissors (s) until the ovary is dissected free and can be removed through the prefemoral incision. The incision is closed before the procedure is repeated via the right prefemoral fossa to remove the contralateral ovary. (Courtesy of Stephen J. Divers.)

Oophorectomy of Immature Females

Intracorporeal oophorectomy has been described in immature, Galapagos tortoises (*Chelonoidis nigra*) using 5 mm instrumentation.[11] However, there is no reason why this same technique could not be applied to smaller chelonians with suitably sized (3 mm) instrumentation. In addition, this technique provides a model for other possible endosurgical procedures. The paired, immature ovaries reside within the caudodorsal coelom, and in close association with the retrocoelomic kidney. The bladder often obscures the contralateral ovary, and so a bilateral endosurgical approach is often necessary. With the animal in lateral recumbency, a prefemoral approach to the coelom is made in order to accommodate the telescope and two instruments via a single incision (see Fig. 65.7B). Cannulae generally are not helpful because the instruments are so closely aligned and insufflation is not required. The telescope is positioned and held by a surgical assistant or mechanical arm in order to maintain the view of the ovary. The immature ovary is elevated away from the serosal surface of the kidney and caudodorsal shell using Babcock or Kelly forceps, and monopolar scissors are used to dissect the ovary free from its mesovarian attachments (Fig. 65.9). The prefemoral incision is closed routinely, and the procedure is repeated on the opposite side.

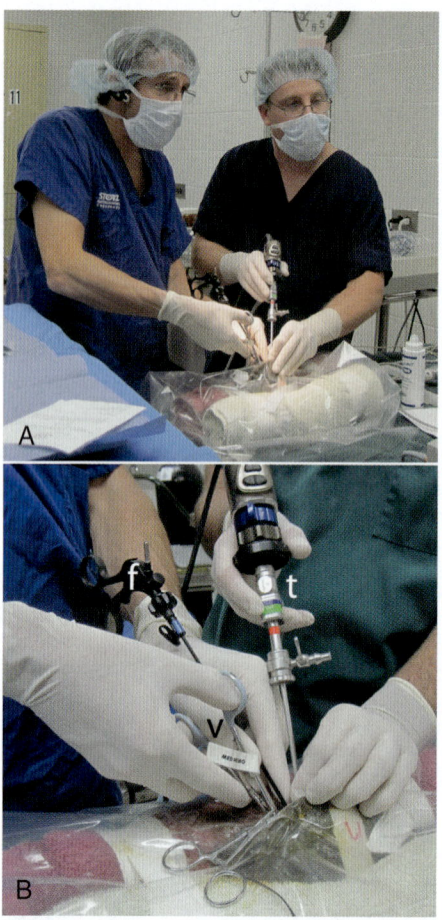

FIG 65.10 (A) Endoscopic orchiectomy in a red-eared slider (*Trachemys scripta elegans*). (B) Close-up of the surgical site. Note that the assistant controls the camera and telescope (t) while the primary surgeon uses 3 mm grasping forceps (f) and a vascular clip applicator (v) to perform the orchiectomy. (Courtesy of Stephen J. Divers.)

Orchiectomy

Researchers originally developed a similar approach for safe and effective orchiectomy, using the red-eared slider (*Trachemys scripta elegans*) as a model.[12] The animal is again positioned in lateral recumbency and, following prefemoral coeliotomy, a surgical assistant identifies and maintains a clear view of the testis (Fig. 65.10). The endosurgeon then uses Babcock or Kelly forceps to grasp and elevate the testis away from the kidney and epididymis to expose the mesorchium and associated vessels. Both monopolar radiosurgery and vascular clips have been used to ensure hemostasis before scissors are used to dissect the testis free (Fig. 65.11). At least in *Trachemys* it is possible to remove both testes via a unilateral prefemoral approach.

Further procedural development was required to permit orchiectomy in larger tortoises where the mesorchial attachments are typically more substantive and require extensive dissection to free the testis. Using the desert tortoise (*Gopherus agassizii*) as a model, a single-surgeon technique was developed that employed a mechanical support arm for the telescope, freeing the surgeon to utilize a combination of endoscopic vascular clips and radiosurgical dissection to dissect each testis free (Figs. 65.12 and 65.13).[13]

Lizards

It is particularly important to remember that the standardized placement of cannulae through the linea alba cannot be applied to most lizards due to the presence of the midline abdominal vein; however, placement of a midline cannula, caudal to the umbilicus, is certainly practical and often preferred, particularly in iguanids (Figs. 65.14 and 65.15).

Orchiectomy

With the iguana in right lateral recumbency, the telescope and protection sheath are inserted, just lateral to the ventral midline, close to the anastomosis of the left and right pelvic veins as they form the ventral abdominal vein. The first cannula is placed cranial to the telescope, just caudal to the last rib, while the second cannula is placed caudal to the anastomosis of the pelvic veins in the ventral midline (see Figs. 65.14C and 65.15). Grasping forceps are inserted through one cannula and used to elevate the testis, while scissors (attached to monopolar radiosurgery) are inserted through the other cannula and used to coagulate and cut through the mesorchium and associated vessels (Fig. 65.16). In larger iguanas, bipolar forceps are used to coagulate blood vessels prior to scissor dissection. The testis is extracted through the forceps cannula hole, which can be enlarged using hemostats if necessary. The cannula holes are closed with a single suture or tissue adhesive. The iguana is rotated into left lateral recumbency, and using the same telescope entry site, the procedure is repeated for the second testis.

ENDOSCOPY TRAINING

The ability to perform diagnostic endoscopy and endosurgery is not innate, and training is certainly required. Fortunately, various continuing

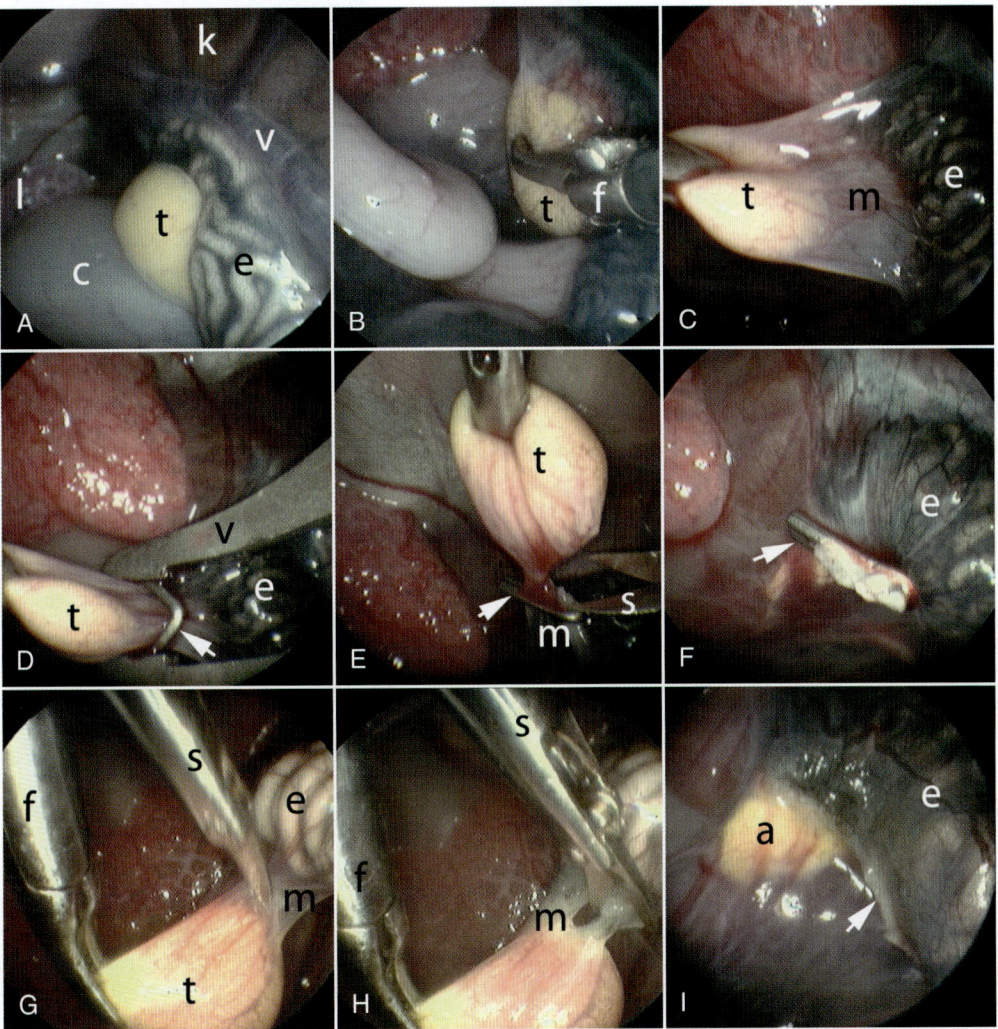

FIG 65.11 Endoscopic orchiectomy of a red-eared slider (*Trachemys scripta elegans*) via a unilateral prefemoral incision. (A) View of the left testis (t) and epididymis (e) closely associated with the kidney (k) and renal vein (v). The descending colon (c) and caudal lung (l) are also visible. (B) Three-mm Kelly forceps (f) are introduced and used to grasp the testis (t). (C) The forceps (f) are angled to retract the testis (t) cranially away from the epididymis (e) to expose the mesorchium (m) and associated vascular supply. (D–F) Orchiectomy using vascular clips. A vascular clip applicator (v) is introduced and a single clip (arrow) is placed across the mesorchium, between the testis (t) and the epididymis (e), before the testis is dissected free using 3 mm scissors (s). (G–I) Orchiectomy using radiosurgery. While retracting the testis (t) away from the epididymis (e), monopolar scissors (s) are used to coagulate the mesorchial vessels, prior to dissecting the testis free and removing with forceps (f). Following orchiectomy, the adrenal gland (a) can be seen. (Courtesy of Stephen J. Divers.)

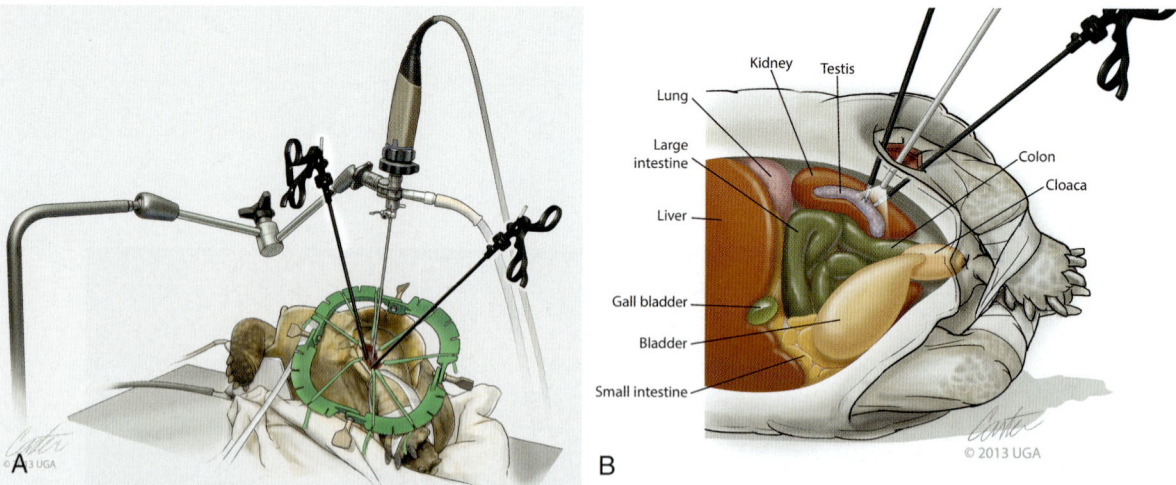

FIG 65.12 Illustrations depicting left orchiectomy in a tortoise. (A) The tortoise is positioned in right lateral recumbency, and a left prefemoral coeliotomy has been performed. The telescope is supported by a mechanical arm, freeing the surgeon to use two independent instruments. (B) Internal view demonstrating the position of the testis, telescope, and instruments. (Courtesy of Educational Resources, University of Georgia.)

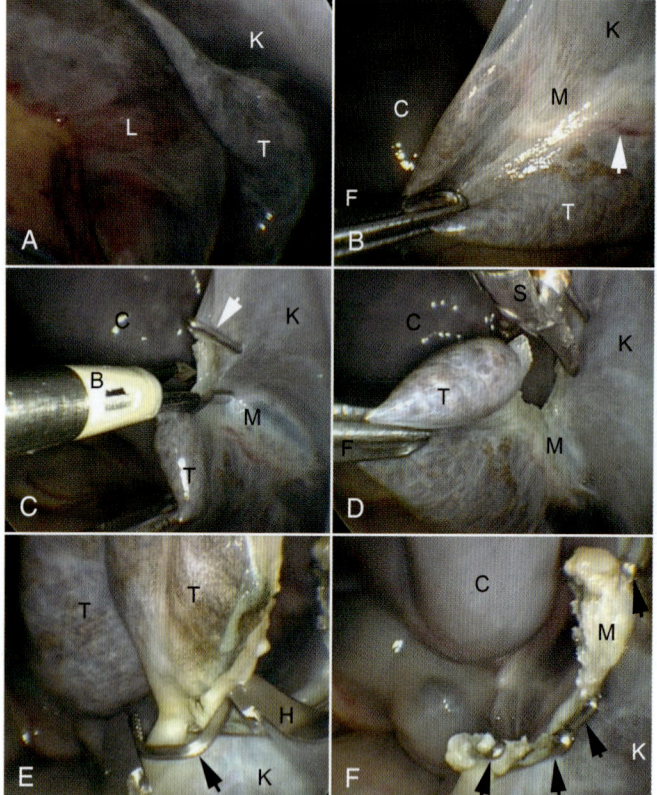

FIG 65.13 Endoscopic orchiectomy of a desert tortoise (*Gopherus agassizii*) via sequential vascular clip ligation and radiosurgical dissection. (A) Telescope view of the caudal coelom via a left prefemoral approach. (B) Atraumatic endoscopic forceps (F) used to expose the mesorchium and associated vasculature (arrow). (C) Stainless steel vascular clip (arrow) has been placed on the caudal aspect of the mesorchium, close to the kidney, prior to mesorchial coagulation using bipolar forceps (B). (D) Mesorchial dissection using short curved Metzenbaum scissors (S). (E) Placement of vascular clip (arrow) across the cranial aspect of the mesorchium. (F) View of the ligation clips (arrows) across the mesorchium remnant following excision of the testis. Lung (L), kidney (K), testis (T), colon (C), and mesorchium (M). (From Proença LM, Fowler S, Kleine S, et al. Single surgeon coelioscopic orchiectomy of desert tortoises [*Gopherus agassizii*] for population management. *Vet Rec.* 2014;175:404.)

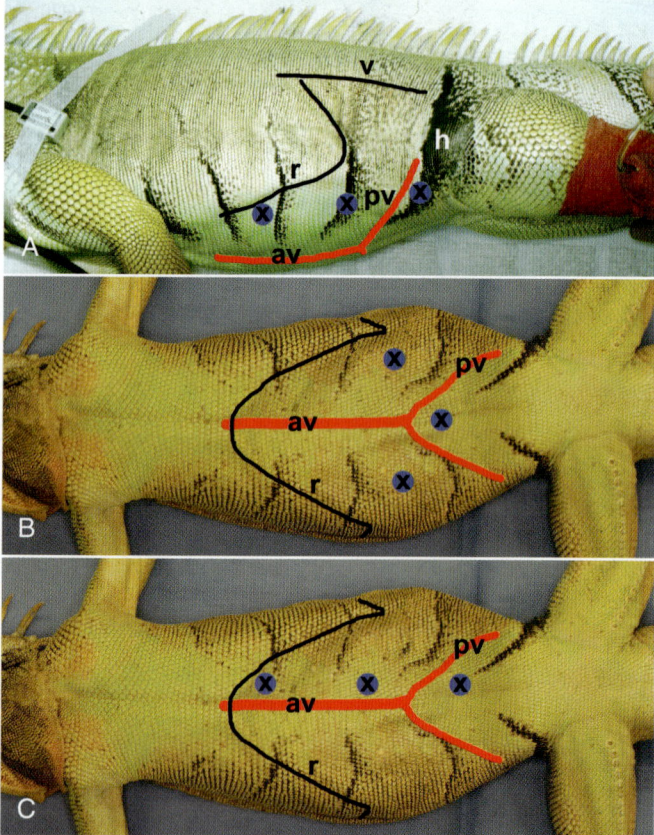

FIG 65.14 Lateral (A) and ventral (B,C) views of an iguanid lizard illustrating the possible cannula insertion points (*x*) for performing multiple-entry endosurgery in lizards. The positions of the vertebral spine (v), last rib (r), ventral abdominal vein (*av*), and pelvic veins (pv) have been shown to indicate anatomic landmarks that should be appreciated. (Courtesy of Stephen J. Divers.)

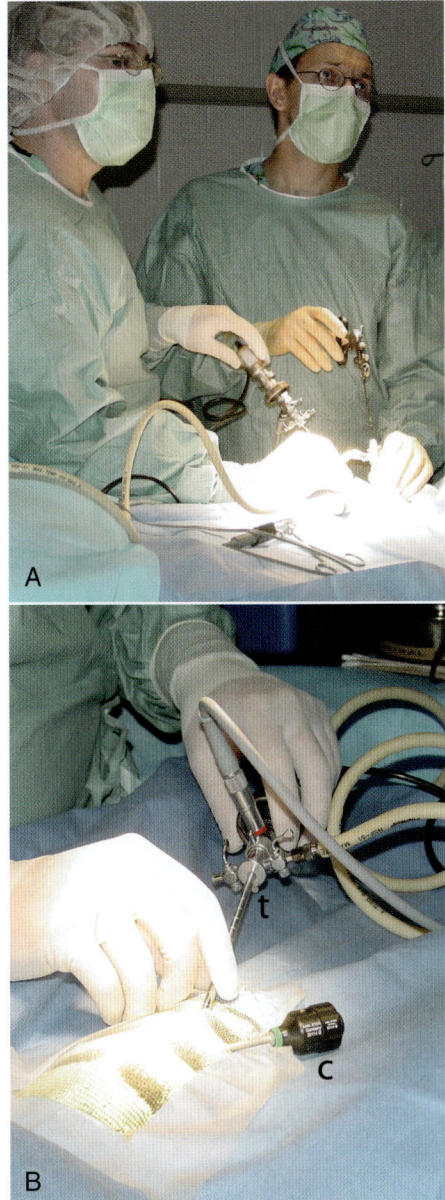

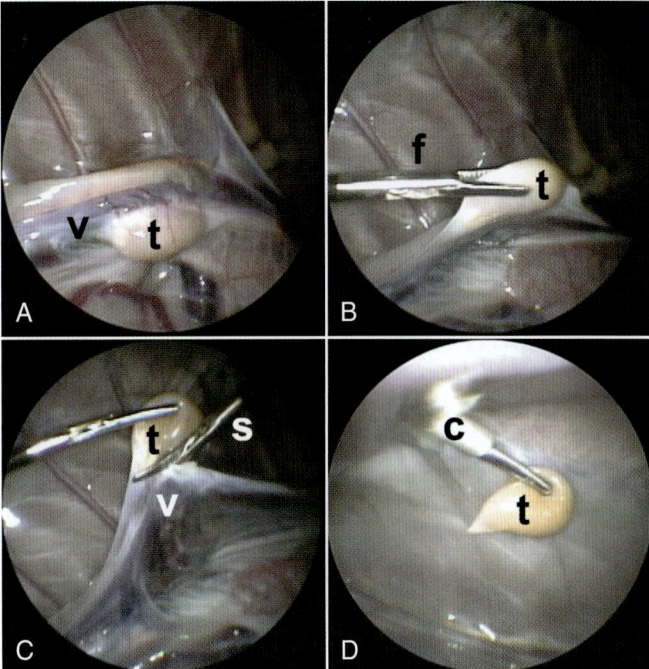

FIG 65.16 Endoscopic orchiectomy in a green iguana (*Iguana iguana*). (A) View of the dorsal coelom showing the right testis (t) and closely associated renal vein (v). (B) Forceps (f), introduced through a caudal cannula, are used to grasp and elevate the testis (t) away from the body wall. (C) With the testis (t) elevated away from the renal vein (v), monopolar scissors (s) are used to coagulate and cut across the mesorchium. (D) The freed testis (t) is then retracted to the cannula (c), which is slid up the shaft of the forceps before the testis is removed through the cannula hole. If the testis is large, hemostats can be used to temporarily stretch the cannula hole to facilitate removal. (Courtesy of Stephen J. Divers.)

FIG 65.15 (A) A primary surgeon and assistant performing endosurgery in a green iguana (*Iguana iguana*). (B) Close-up of the surgical site demonstrating the placement of the sheathed telescope with insufflation line attached (t) and a 3.5 mm cannula (c). (Courtesy of Stephen J. Divers.)

education courses offer training in the United States, Europe, and less commonly elsewhere. The Association of Reptilian and Amphibian Veterinarians (https://www.arav.org) regularly offers a 4-hour introduction to reptile endoscopy at the annual conference. In addition, the University of Georgia offers a 2- to 3-day course in reptile, avian, and small mammal diagnostic endoscopy and endosurgery every December (http://www.vet.uga.edu/CE/).

ACKNOWLEDGMENTS

The author would like to thank Karl Storz Veterinary Endoscopy, especially Mike Bateman and Chris Chamness, for supporting endoscopy research, development, and training at the University of Georgia. In addition, I am indebted to Drs. Scott Stahl, Charles Innis, Sam Rivera, Randon Feinsod, Joe Flanagan, and Joerg Mayer, as well as numerous students, interns, and residents for their collegiality and enthusiasm in pursuing various endoscopic ventures at the University of Georgia.

REFERENCES

See www.expertconsult.com for a complete list of references.

66

Urology

Stephen J. Divers and Charles J. Innis

Continued strides in captive husbandry and nutrition have resulted in many reptiles surviving to adult and geriatric ages. Nevertheless, renal disease remains a major cause of morbidity and mortality, particularly among older reptiles, and continues to be of significant concern to veterinarians and owners alike.[1-3] Protein excess, dehydration, overheating, and secondary nutritional hyperparathyroidism are considered common predisposing factors for the development to chronic renal disease, while acute renal failure, infectious or toxic in nature, tends be less common and sporadic.[1-4]

GROSS ANATOMY

The reptilian urinary tract consists of paired kidneys, ureters, urodeum, and the bladder or cloacocolon (Fig. 66.1). In those species with a bladder, urine enters the bladder via the urodeum of the cloaca and urethra, not directly from the ureters. In those species without a bladder, urine storage may occur within distal, dilated ureters, or within the cloacocolonic region (Table 66.1). Unlike mammals, reptiles do not have separate external orifices for the discharge of urinary and digestive wastes. The cloaca is divided into three regions: (1) the coprodeum is most anterior and receives waste products from the large intestine; (2) the middle section, or urodeum, receives the ureters, urethra, and genital ducts and in some species the genital ducts and ureters enter the urodeum separately, however in other species they fuse before entering the urodeum (Fig. 66.2); and (3) the last, posterior section, proctodeum, receives waste and urogenital products, which are discharged through the vent.

Order Squamata: Suborder Sauria

The saurian kidneys may be located within, or cranial to, the pelvis (Fig. 66.3). The kidneys are paired, symmetrical, elongated, slightly lobulated, and often flattened, dorsoventrally in most species and laterally in chameleons.[5] In some species, the caudal aspects of the kidneys are fused (e.g., iguanas), while in others (e.g., water monitors) they remain separate. The kidneys of mature males can undergo hypertrophy of the distal convoluted tubules (sexual segment) to produce secretions for seminal fluid.

A fully developed bladder, connected to the urodeum by a urethra, is present in many saurians; however, in others the bladder may be small, rudimentary, or absent (Table 66.1, Fig. 66.4). A rudimentary bladder exists in some agamas, Australian dragons, banded geckos, zebra-tailed lizards, collared lizards, spiny lizards, tree lizards, and night lizards. Apart from a single report of a bladder in western whiptail lizard (*Cnemidophorus tigris*), members of the Teiidae do not possess a bladder, nor do snake lizards or horned lizards. Most monitors appear to lack a bladder, although there is some controversy with ultrasonography demonstrating a bladder in water monitors (*Varanus marmoratus*) but not in savannah monitors (*Varanus exanthematicus*).[6-8]

Like all reptiles, the saurian kidney is supplied by both arterial and portal venous supplies (Fig. 66.5).[9,10] Arterial blood is supplied by a variable number of renal arteries that branch off the aorta. These arteries form an interlobular arterial supply that deliveries blood to the afferent arterioles of the glomeruli. The efferent arterioles from the glomeruli then supply the peritubular capillary network. The portal venous supply is formed by the returning blood from the tail (via the caudal vein)

TABLE 66.1 Presence of Urinary Bladders in Different Reptiles

Taxa With Well-Developed Urinary Bladders	Taxa With Rudimentary Urinary Bladders	Taxa Without Urinary Bladders
Chelonia	**Lizards**	**Snakes**
Rhynchocephalia	Agamidae	**Crocodilians**
Lizards	Gekkonidae	**Lizards**
Anguidae	Coleonyx	Teiidae (except
Chamaeleonidae	Iguanidae	*Cnemidophorus*
Gekkonidae	Callisaurus	*tigris*)
Gekko	Cophosaurus	Varanidae* (except
Phelsuma	Crotaphytus	*V. marmoratus*)
Hemidactylus	Sceloporus	Pygopodidae
Helodermatidae	Urosaurus	Iguanidae
Iguanidae	Uta	Phrynosoma
Anolis	Xantusiidae	
Iguana		
Lacertidae		
Scincidae		
Xantusiidae		

*Most monitors and tegus appear to lack a bladder, although there is some controversy because ultrasonography and dissections have demonstrated a bladder in whiptails (*Cnemidophorus tigris*) and water monitors (*Varanus marmoratus*) but not in savannah monitors (*Varanus exanthematicus*).[6-8]

From Beuchat CA. Phylogenetic distribution of the urinary bladder in lizards, *Copeia* 1986(2):512–517, 1986.

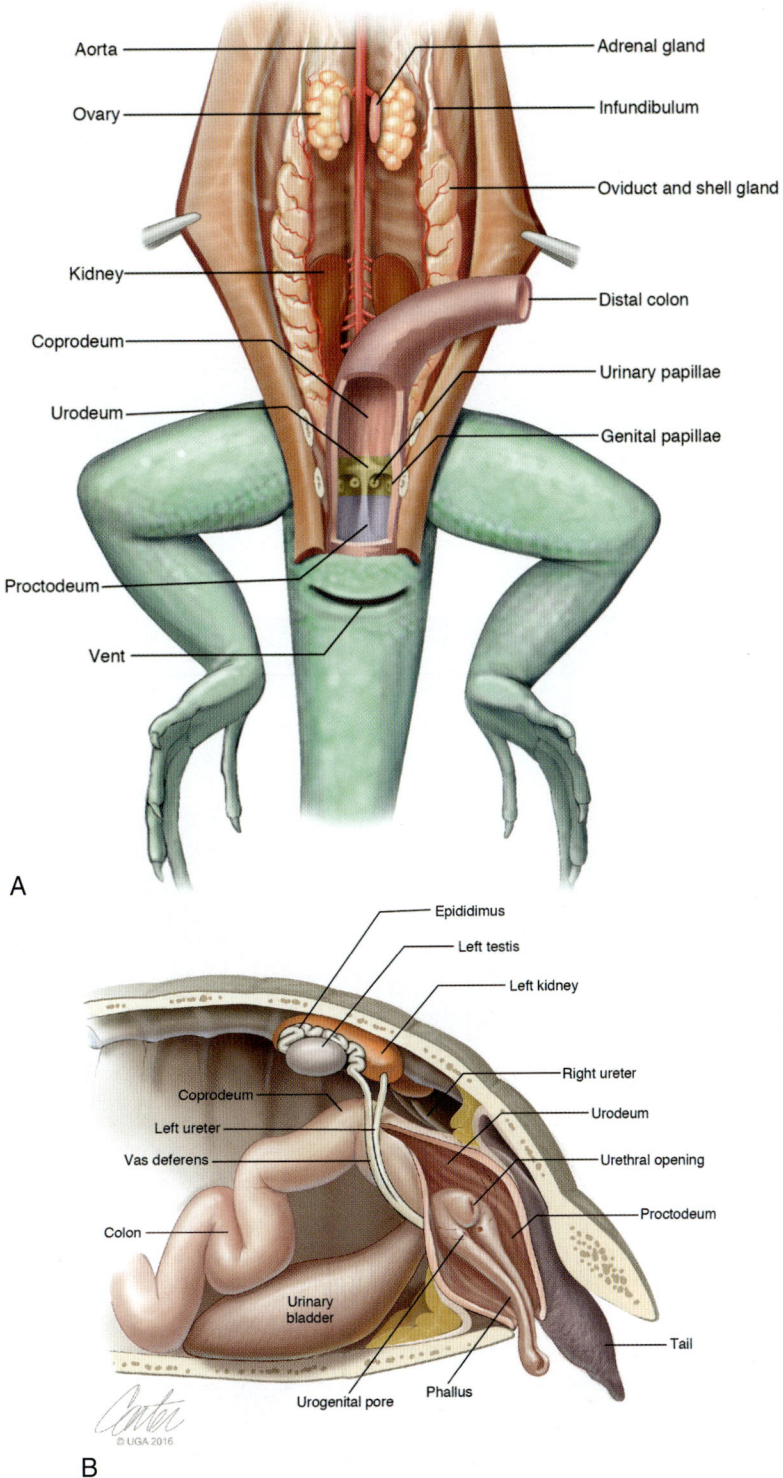

FIG 66.1 Gross urogenital anatomy of a lizard (A) and chelonian (B). (Courtesy of Educational Resources, University of Georgia.)

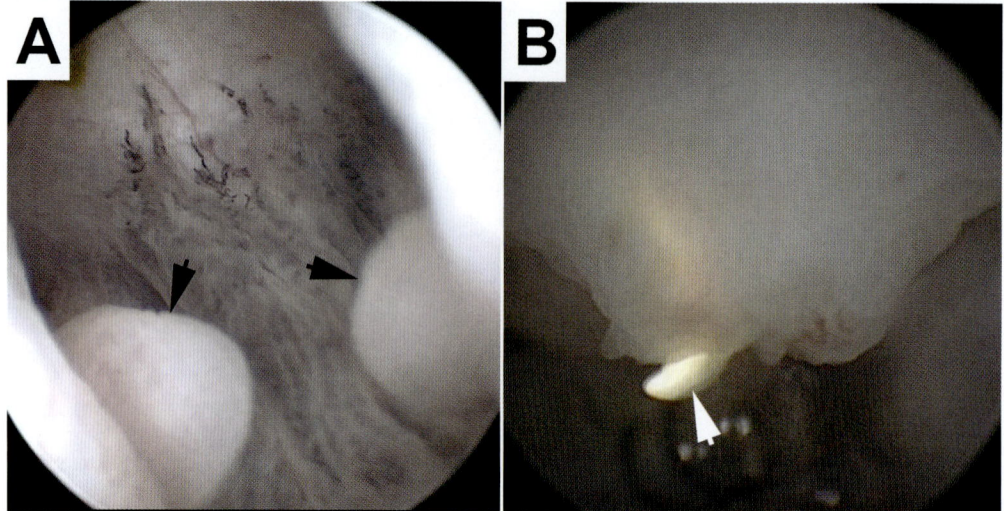

FIG 66.2 (A) Endoscopic view of an iguanid (*Iguana* sp.) urodeum (dorsal recumbency) shows two separate, dorsolateral urogenital papillae (black arrows). (B) Endoscopic view of a ball python (*Python regius*) urodeum (ventral recumbency) shows a single dorsal urogenital papilla containing both ureteral openings. Uric acid can be seen emerging from the left ureter. (Courtesy of Stephen J. Divers.)

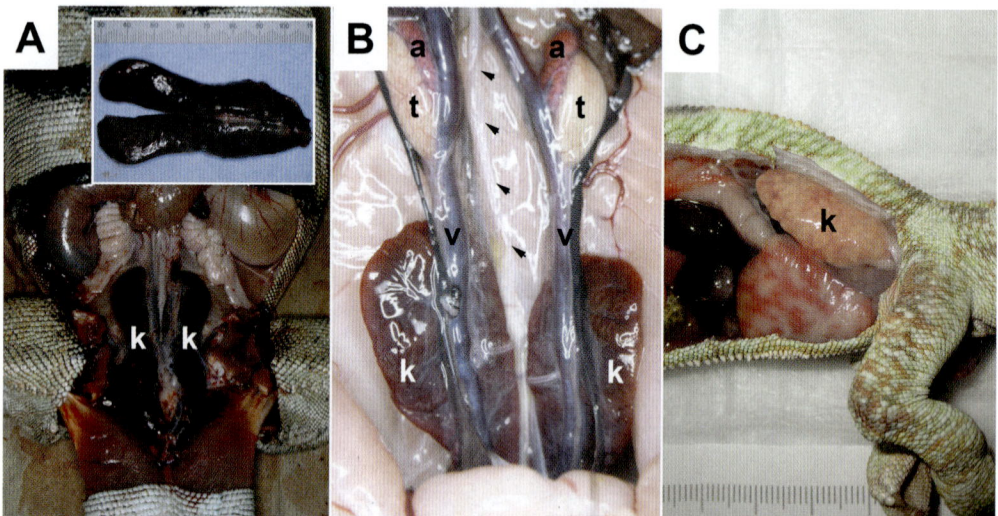

FIG 66.3 Saurian kidneys. (A) The pelvis has been removed to reveal the ventral view of the normal intrapelvic kidneys (*k*) in a female iguana (*Iguana iguana*). (*Inset*) Note how the caudal poles of the kidneys are fused. (B) Ventral view of normal (healthy) kidneys (k) in the caudal coelom of a in a monitor lizard (*Varanus* sp.). Note the close association with the renal veins (v), dorsal aorta (arrows), testes (t), and adrenal glands (a). (C) Left lateral view of the caudal coelomic left kidney (k) in a chameleon (*Chamaeleo* sp.). This kidney is not normal and demonstrates renomegaly and pallor due to glomerulonephrosis, renal calcification, and gout. (Courtesy of Stephen J. Divers.)

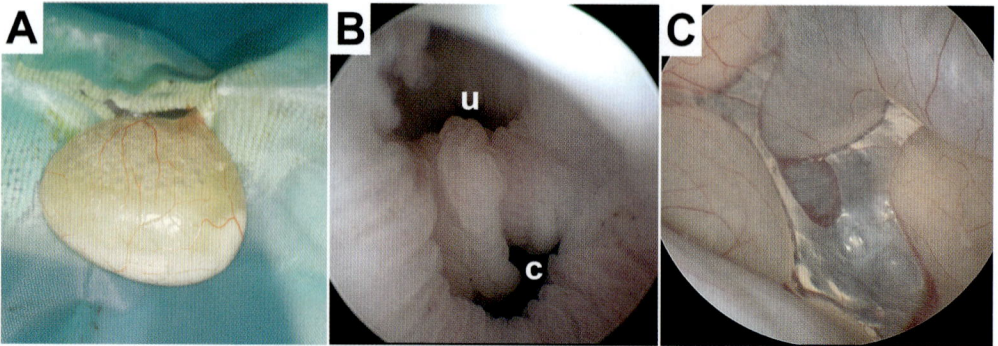

FIG 66.4 Lower urinary tract of a green iguana (*Iguana iguana*). (A) Intraoperative view of the bladder exteriorized through a coeliotomy incision. (B) Endoscopic view from within the urodeum of the cloaca (dorsal recumbency) shows the dorsal opening to the coprodeum (c) and ventral opening to the urethra (u). (C) Endoscopic view from within the saline-distended bladder. (Courtesy of Stephen J. Divers.)

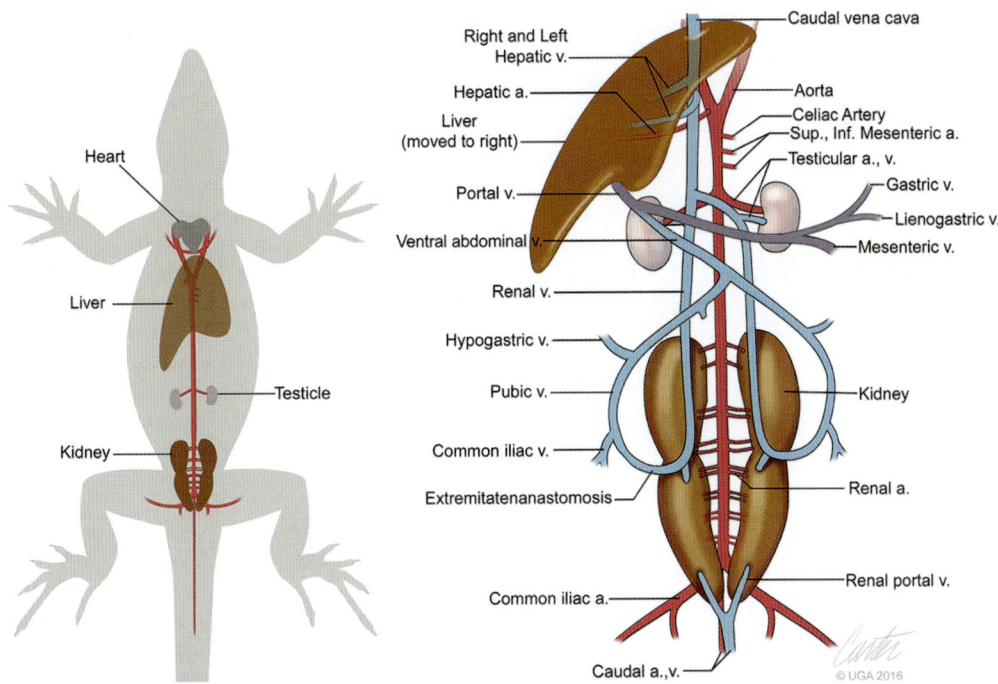

FIG 66.5 Gross vasculature of the hepatic and urogenital systems of a generic lizard. (Courtesy of Educational Resources, University of Georgia.)

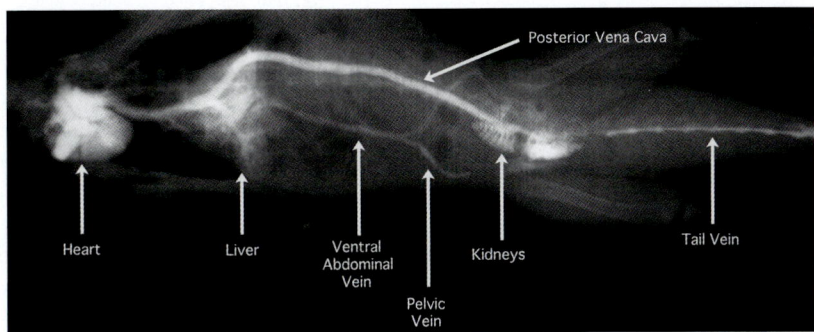

FIG 66.6 Contrast angiography showing the major vascular anatomy of the green iguana (*Iguana iguana*). Renografin-60 (Diatrizoate Megulime and Sodium, Squibb, NY), a high osmolar contrast medium (292 mg I/ mL), was injected at a dose of 2 mL/kg body weight into the caudal tail vein. The radiograph was exposed immediately after the injection was administered. (Courtesy of L. Pace.)

and hind legs (via the iliac veins). This venous blood enters the left or right afferent renal portal veins that supply their respective kidneys. In the kidneys, this portal blood enters a series of capillaries that perfuse the renal tubule cells but not the glomeruli. Venous blood from the renal tubules drains into the interlobular efferent veins and then into the renal veins before fusing to form the postcaval vein, which conveys blood back to the heart (Fig. 66.6). Pelvic veins connect to the iliac veins before their attachment with the afferent renal portal veins and can divert blood around the kidneys into the single ventral abdominal vein. From here, the blood flows to the liver.

Suborder Serpentes

Boid kidneys are paired, flattened, and elongated organs that contain 25 to 30 lobules (Fig. 66.7A), except for dwarf and rough boas (Tropidophiidae), whose kidneys are not lobulated.[5,11] The right kidney lies cranial to the left, and studies have reported renal position as a proportion or percentage of the distance between the snout and the cloaca (76%–84% in boids, 84%–96% in colubrids, 80%–92% in elapids, and 84%–96%

in viperids).[11,12] The kidneys occupy approximately 10% to 15% of the snake's body length and can hypertrophy and become paler due to sexual segment development in mature males (see Fig. 66.7B). A ureter connects each kidney to the urodeum (see Fig. 66.2B). There is no urinary bladder, but urine may be stored in the distal colon or in dilated distal ureters.[5]

Arterial blood supply is similar to that of the Sauria (Fig. 66.8). The venous blood flow is also similar except for the absence of iliac veins. Blood can bypass the kidneys through the mesenteric vein, which receives connections directly from the afferent renal portal veins. The mesenteric venous blood is carried to the liver. The abdominal vein is present and is connected to the afferent renal portal veins in some species (e.g., African rock python, *Python sebae*), while in others it originates in the fat bodies.[9]

Order Rhynchocephalia

The kidneys of the Tuatara (*Sphenodon punctatus*) are similar to those of lizards. They are paired, single-lobed, and crescentic in outline, located

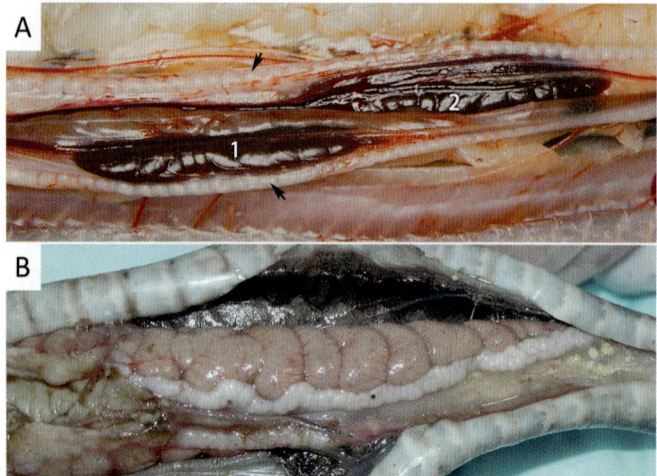

A

B

FIG 66.7 (A) Right (1) and left (2) snake kidneys with closely associated vasa deferentia (*arrows*). (B) Pronounced swelling and pallor of the left kidney due to sexual segment proliferation in a reproductively active male snake. (Courtesy of Stephen J. Divers.)

dorsally within the pelvic canal. The 2 kidneys meet posteriorly, but they do not fuse.[5] The blood supply is also similar to lizards; however, no direct connection exists between the iliac veins and the abdominal vein. A connection to the abdominal vein has been postulated to exist within the body of the kidneys.[13] A bladder is present.

Order Testudines

Chelonian kidneys are paired, retrocoelomic, and lie in the caudodorsal coelom just ventral to the caudal carapace (Fig. 66.9A). In marine turtles, the kidneys are cranial to the pelvic girdle. The kidneys are flattened, lobulated, and symmetrical (see Fig. 66.9B). Ureters leave the kidneys and enter the urodeum, close to the opening of the urethra, which connects the bladder to the urodeum (see Fig. 66.9C).[5] The bladder is a single large or bilobed structure, and smaller bilateral accessory bladders usually exist on either side of the urodeum. Arterial and venous blood supply is similar to that of the lizards; however, two abdominal veins are found that are linked by a transverse anastomosis (Fig. 66.10).[9]

Order Crocodilia

Crocodilians have paired lobulated kidneys that lie against the dorsal body wall adjacent to the spinal column. The left kidney may be larger than the right kidney. Ureters enter the cloaca at the urodeum. No urinary bladder exists.[5] Arterial and venous supply is similar to the

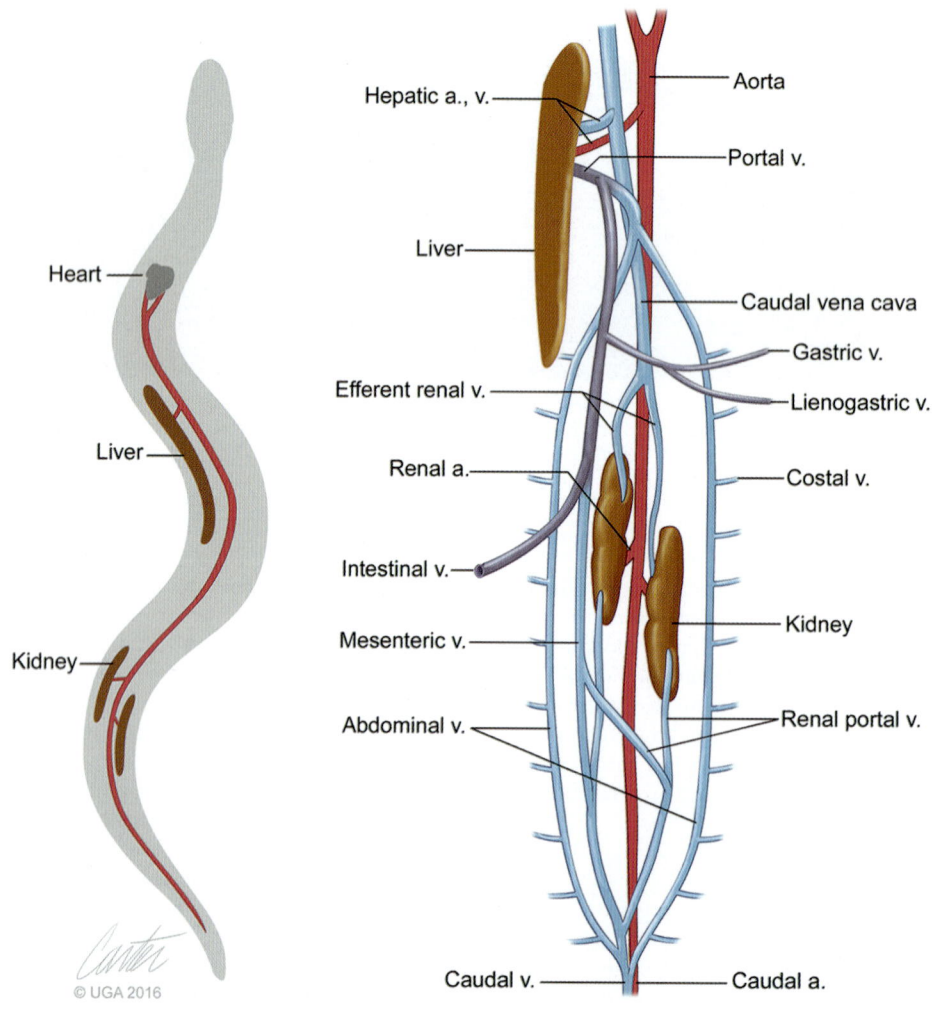

© UGA 2016

FIG 66.8 Gross vasculature of the hepatic and urinary systems of a generic snake. (Courtesy of Educational Resources, University of Georgia.)

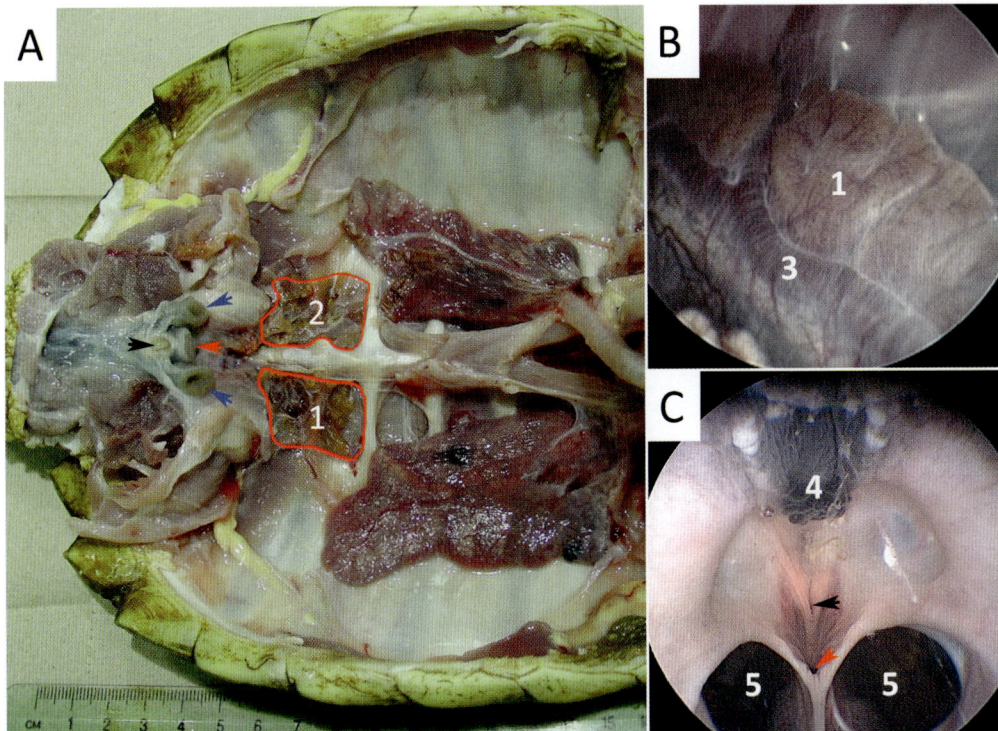

FIG 66.9 (A) Ventral view of a common snapping turtle (*Chelydra serpentina*) with the gastrointestinal, bladder, and reproductive organs removed. The transected ends of the oviducts (blue arrows), colon (red arrow), and urethra (black arrow) are visible. The outlines of the left (1) and right kidneys (2) are indicated in red. (B) Coelioscopic view of the left kidney (1) and renal vein (3) from a left prefemoral approach. (C) Cloacoscopic view with the turtle in dorsal recumbency illustrating the ventral clitoris (4) and accessory bladders (5). The opening to the urethra (black arrow) and colon (red arrow) are also shown. (Courtesy of Stephen Divers.)

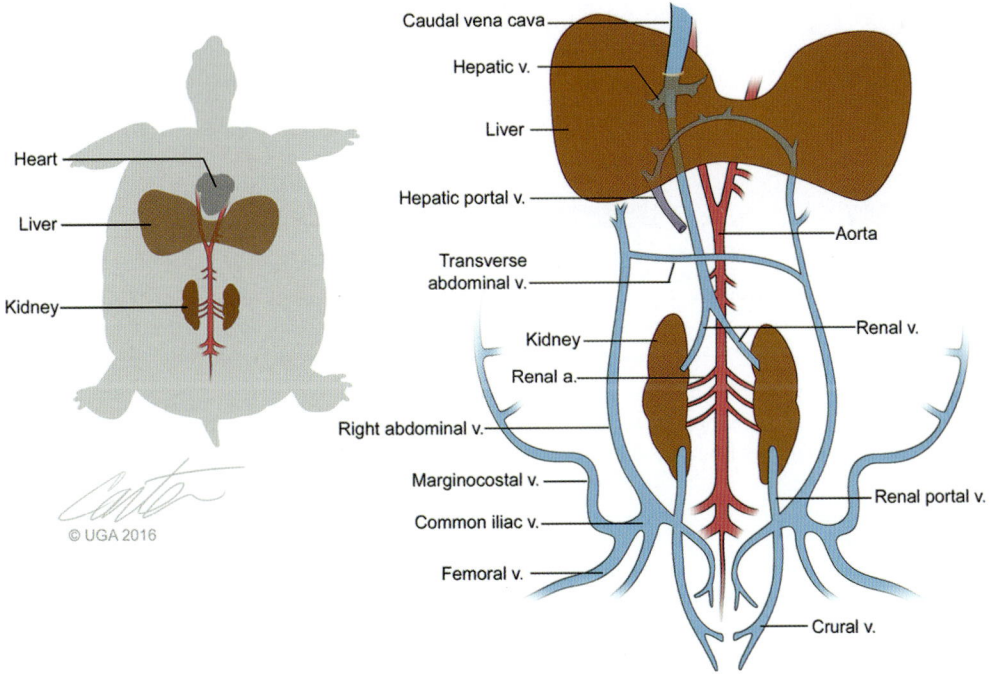

FIG 66.10 Gross vasculature of the hepatic and urinary systems of a generic freshwater turtle. (Courtesy of Educational Resources, University of Georgia.)

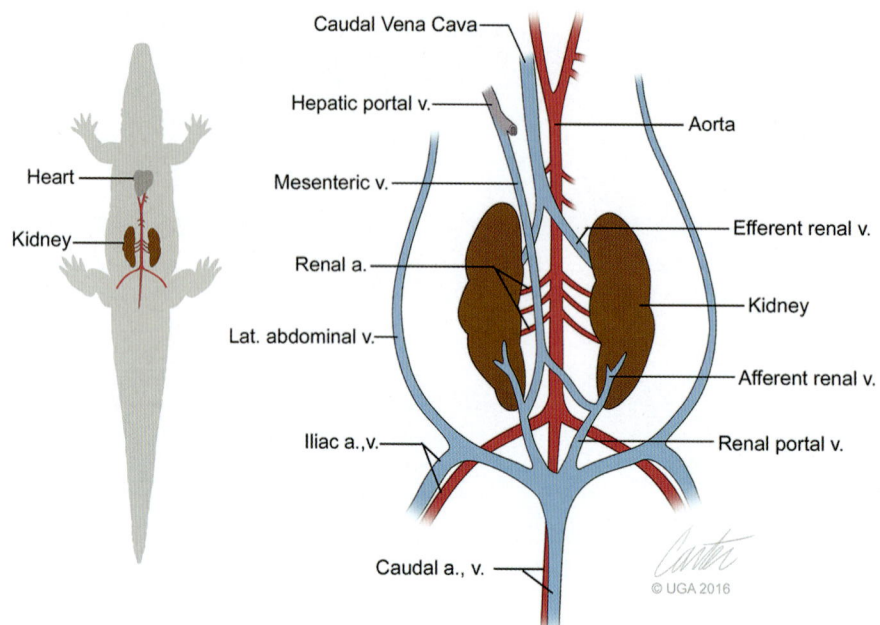

FIG 66.11 Gross vasculature of the hepatic and urinary systems of a generic crocodilian. (Courtesy of Educational Resources, University of Georgia.)

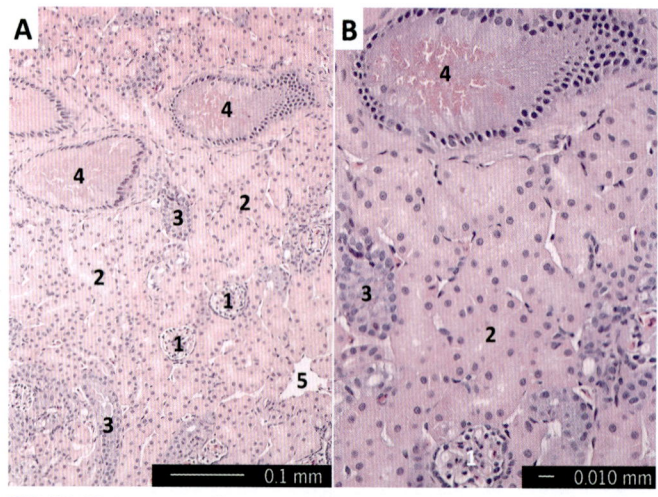

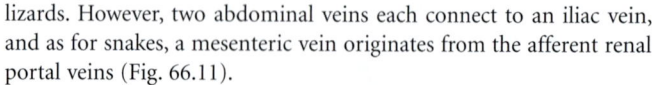

FIG 66.12 Low-magnification (A) and high-magnification (B) histomicrographs of an adult male iguana (*Iguana iguana*) kidney illustrating the glomeruli (1), proximal tubules (2), distal tubules (3), sexual segment (4) and collecting duct (5) (H&E). (Courtesy of Stephen J. Divers.)

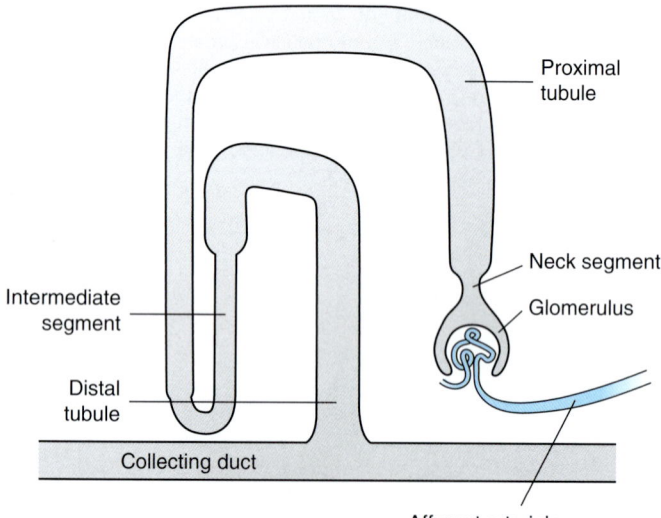

FIG 66.13 The reptilian nephron. The glomerulus is followed by the neck segment, the proximal tubule, the intermediate segment, and the distal tubule.

lizards. However, two abdominal veins each connect to an iliac vein, and as for snakes, a mesenteric vein originates from the afferent renal portal veins (Fig. 66.11).

MICROSCOPIC ANATOMY

Reptilian kidneys have no pelvis or pyramids and are not divided into medulla and cortex (Fig. 66.12). They contain a few thousand nephrons, compared with the typical million or so of mammalian kidneys.[5] Where measured, reptilian nephrons are 2 to 8 mm long, compared with bird nephrons that are approximately 18 mm and human nephrons that are 30 to 38 mm.[14] Each nephron is oriented at right angles to the long axis of the kidney and enters the collecting duct at right angles. The renal corpuscles lie in a circular pattern near the midportion of each lobule.[15]

Structurally, reptilian glomeruli are less developed, with a lower number of capillaries per gram body weight compared with birds.[14] The glomerulus is followed by the neck segment, proximal tubule, intermediate segment, and distal tubule (Fig. 66.13). There is no loop of Henle (ansa nephroni). All of the segments, except the distal tubule, consist of ciliated cuboidal cells. The cells of the distal tubule lack cilia. The distal tubule is followed by the sex segment in male squamates. The cells are flat and filled with mucus during the nonbreeding season; however, during reproductive activity, these cells increase in height two to four times and are filled with large refractile granules that stain brightly eosinophilic with hematoxylin and eosin.[16] They contain acid phosphatase, phospholipids, glycoprotein, mucoprotein, and amino acids. The function of the sex segment secretions has not been definitively determined; however, a number of theories have been proposed, including

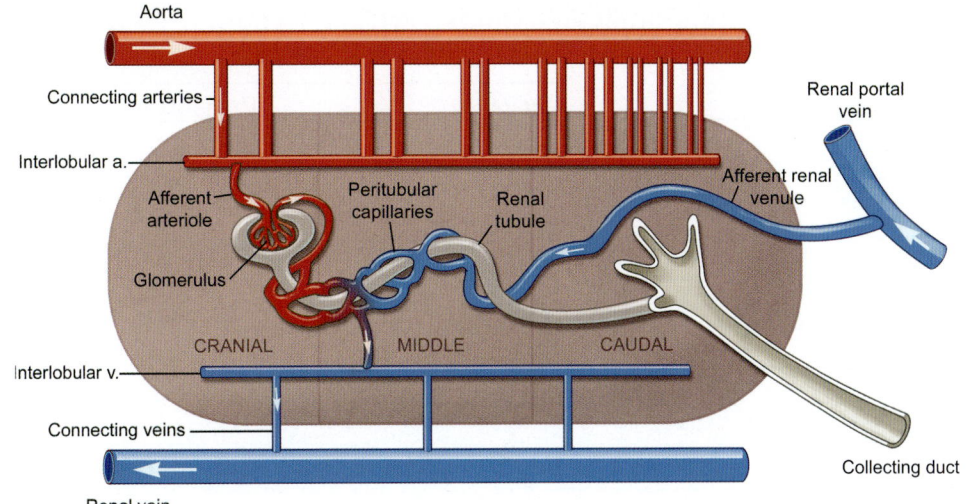

FIG 66.14 Schematic illustration of the nephron and associated vasculature in a green iguana (*Iguana iguana*) kidney. (Courtesy of Educational Resources, University of Georgia.)

(1) creation of a copulatory plug to prevent rivals from mating successfully, (2) blockage of the tubules during copulation to functionally separate semen and urine, or (3) as an activator or source of sustenance for sperm survival.[16]

After the sex segment, the nephron terminates with the collecting duct. These cells are similar to those contained within the sex segment, except mucus is only present at the tip of the cell. The collecting ducts are oriented at right angles to the long axis of the kidney. They originate on the dorsolateral surface of each lobule, wrap around the lateral margin of the lobule, and pass ventrally into the ureter, which lies on the ventromedial surface of the kidney.

Blood supply to the nephron consists of an afferent arteriole that forms the glomerular capillary tuft, which is surrounded by Bowman's capsule. Blood exits in the efferent arteriole, which supplies blood to the tubule cells. Venous blood, via the renal portal system, mixes with the arteriolar blood at the start of the proximal tubule (Fig. 66.14).

PHYSIOLOGY

The metabolism of protein and amino acids results in the production of nitrogen, which must be excreted as ammonia, urea, or uric acid (Table 66.2). The production and excretion of ammonia is the simplest method for this task. However, ammonia is toxic to the central nervous system and requires large amounts of water for its excretion. Hence, its production in reptiles is limited to aquatic species of turtles and crocodilians.[14,17] Urea is less soluble than ammonia but 40,000 times more soluble than uric acid. It must also be excreted with water and is most common in aquatic species; however, significant amounts can be found in some terrestrial chelonians. Reptile kidneys lack a loop of Henle (ansa nephroni) and so cannot produce urine hypertonic to that of plasma. Consequently, other means of water conservation are employed, including a greater reliance on uric acid production and decreases in glomerular filtration rate (GFR).

Reptiles have reduced GFRs to the order of 5 to 25 mL/kg/hr compared with those of birds and mammals (100–200 mL/kg/hr).[3,14] GFR has been reported for several species using clearance methods (Table 66.3). The differing physiological challenges of marine, freshwater, and terrestrial environments, combined with methodologic differences, may explain the differences reported from different species.

During dehydration (experimentally studied with the intravenous infusion of hyperosmotic saline solution), GFR tends to decrease, and water-loading (experimentally studied with the intravenous injection of sterile water) increases GFR; however, considerable variation exists between different species from different habitats. As an example, GFR of the Puerto Rican gecko is 3.33 ± 0.37 mL/kg/h with dehydration and 24.3 ± 1.67 mL/kg/h with water loading.[14] In some species that possess an alternate method for salt excretion (e.g., nasal salt glands of the sand monitor, *Varanus gouldii*), dramatic elevations of plasma osmolarity may not cause the expected decrease in GFR because mechanisms for postrenal reabsorption of water from the cloaca, colon, or bladder are usually well developed.[14]

Few studies have evaluated the effects of temperature on GFR in reptiles, but in two saurian species (*Tiliqua rugosus* and *Sauromalus obesus*), significant increases in GFR have been associated with increasing temperature from 5°C to 25°C, mediated by increases in mean arterial pressure.[14] However, these same studies also indicate that within the preferred optimal temperature zone, mean systemic arterial pressure and urine flow appear to be virtually independent of temperature.

The concept that overall GFR is mediated by changes in the number of filtering glomeruli rather than subtle variations in individual nephron filtration rates appears justified, because the maximum rate for renal tubular transport of para-amino-hippurate (PAH) has been shown to vary directly with GFR.[14] If changes in GFR resulted from changes in the amount filtered by each glomerulus with all glomeruli continuing to function, the renal tubular transport for PAH would not be expected to change because the mass of tissue transporting PAH would not have changed. In addition, microscopic studies in various reptile species, including the eastern blue-tongue skink (*Tiliqua scincoides*), have indicated that the ratio of open-to-closed proximal tubular lumina correlates with GFR. A tubule collapses when the glomerulus ceases filtering, supporting the concept that changes in GFR result from changes in the number of functioning nephrons.[14] The cessation of blood flow through the glomerulus would place a nephron at risk from ischemic necrosis. To prevent this from happening, reptiles evolved a renal portal blood supply that continues to perfuse the tubules despite low GFR. As discussed previously, blood from the caudal regions of the body can be diverted through the kidneys or bypass the kidneys. Presumably more blood is shunted through the renal portal system during times

TABLE 66.2 Nitrogenous End-Products Excreted by Selected Reptiles

Species	% TOTAL NITROGEN[a]		
	Ammonia	Urea (BUN)	Uric Acid
Chelonia			
Common slider (*Trachemys scripta*)	4–44	45–95	1–24
West African mud turtle (*Pelusios castaneus*)	19	24	5
Common snapping turtle (*Chelydra serpentina*)	11	80	10
European pond turtle (*Emys orbicularis*)	14	47	3
Forest hinge-back tortoise (*Kinixys erosa*)	6	61	4
African spurred tortoise (*Centrochelys sulcata*)	3	20	55
Kleinmann's tortoise (*Testudo kleinmanni*)	4	49	34
Yellow-footed tortoise (*Chelonoidis denticulata*)	6	29	7
Greek spur-thighed tortoise (*Testudo graeca*)	4	22	52
Indian star tortoise (*Geochelone elegans*)	6	9	56
Western or ornate box turtle (*Terrapene ornata*)	23	47	30
Desert tortoise (*Gopherus agassizii*)	3–18	15–50	20–50
Squamata (Serpentes)			
Eastern racer (*Coluber constrictor*)	0	0	58
Diadem snake (*Spalerosophis diadema*)	4	2	69
Kenyan sand boa (*Gongylophis colubrinus*)	6	0	63
Squamata (Sauria)			
Cuban rock iguana (*Cyclura nubila*)	<1	1	98–99
Carolina anole (*Anolis carolinensis*)	13	13	73
Sandfish skink (*Scincus scincus*)	3	0	93
Crocodilia			
Nile crocodile (*Crocodylus niloticus*)	66	5	21
Spectacled caiman (*Caiman crocodilus*)	53	6	27
Saltwater crocodile (*Crocodylus porosus*)	77	21	2

[a]Calculated as % sum of the ammonia, urea, and uric acid when total nitrogen data was not available. Molecular weights of 18, 60.1, and 168.1 and percentages N of 83%, 46.7%, and 33.3% were used respectively, in calculations.[17]
From Campbell JW: Excretary nitrogen metabolism in reptiles and birds. In: Walsh PJ, Wright P, editor: *Nitrogen Metabolism and Excretion*, London: CRC Press; 1995:147–178.

TABLE 66.3 Glomerular Filtration Rates (GFRs) of Selected Reptiles

Species		GFR (mL/kg/hr)
Green iguana[3]	*Iguana iguana*	16.6 ± 3.9
Puerto Rican gecko[14]	*Hemidactylus mabouia*	10.4 ± 0.8
Blue-tongued skink[14]	*Tiliqua scincoides*	15.9 ± 1.0
American crocodile[14]	*Crocodylus acutus*	9.6 ± 1.0
Kemp's ridley turtle[52]	*Lepidochelys kempii*	12.9 ± 2.9
Green sea turtle[14]	*Chelonia mydas*	14.3
Red-eared slider[14]	*Trachemys scripta elegans*	4.7 ± 0.7

of water deprivation. A valve responsible for regulating the direction of blood flow has been tentatively described in red-eared sliders (*Trachemys scripta elegans*).[18]

Arginine vasotocin (AVT), released from the posterior pituitary, causes a significant reduction in GFR by vasoconstriction of the afferent glomerular arteriole, which appears to be independent of systemic arterial pressure. More recent studies have suggested that AVT may also stimulate dilution of urinary fluid in the thin-intermediate segment and facilitate water reabsorption along an osmotic gradient as the urine passes through the final segments of the nephron.[19] Antidiuretic effects

and reductions in GFR have been attributed to high doses of oxytocin, while prolactin increases GFR. However, at least in some species, these effects appear to be mediated by reductions in systemic arterial blood pressure.[14]

Tubular function includes the regulation of water, sodium, potassium, hydrogen ions, calcium, phosphorus, and nitrogenous compounds. Uric acid is freely filtered by the glomeruli and actively secreted into the proximal tubule against a concentration gradient. Instead of dissolving in solution, like urea, uric acid complexes with protein and either sodium, potassium, or ammonium cations to form a colloidal suspension.[14,17] This suspension contains spheres that are composed of about 65% uric acid and range in diameter from 0.5 to 15 µm. The kidney secretes mucoid substances that contain glycoprotein or mucopolysaccharides that aid in sphere formation and prevent clogging of collecting ducts with urates.[14,17]

Only 30% to 50% of the filtered water is absorbed in the proximal tubules, compared with 60% to 80% in mammals. The rest is absorbed in the distal tubules, colon, cloaca, and where present, bladder. The acidification of urine through hydrogen ion secretion or bicarbonate absorption, combined with water reabsorption in the cloaca or bladder, enhances the formation of urate precipitates from the colloidal material present in the aqueous phase of urine.[17] Failure to adequately excrete urate leads to hyperuricemia, gout, and death. Electrolytes, including sodium and potassium, are freely filtered by the glomerulus. Most of the ultrafiltrate sodium (and water) is reabsorbed from the nephron, collecting duct, colon, cloaca, or bladder. Studies in hydrated geckos (*Hemidactylus* sp.) and iguanids (*Phrynosoma* sp. and *Tropidurus* sp.) have indicated that only 15% to 46% of sodium filtered by the glomeruli is actually excreted in urine.[14] Isosmotic sodium reabsorption occurs in the proximal tubule. However, because the osmolarity of ureteral urine is generally lower than plasma, fluid reabsorbed from the distal tubule varies from isosmotic to hyperosmotic. In many species, the colon, cloaca, and bladder are more important sites for the regulation of sodium excretion and water reabsorption than the kidneys. Control of sodium and potassium regulation has been poorly studied in reptiles, but AVT, aldosterone, and temperature have been shown to exert significant effects.[14] The theoretic ineffectiveness of furosemide (as a loop diuretic) in the reptile kidney, lacking a loop of Henle, has not been confirmed experimentally. Indeed, studies in chelonians and lizards have shown that furosemide exerts significant diuretic effects by increasing sodium, chloride, potassium, and water losses from the kidney (probably at the site of the intermediate segment), colon, cloaca, and bladder.[20–22]

While the injection of renal-tubularly excreted drugs (e.g., carbenicillin) into the caudal body of a reptile may result in a statistically significant effect on some pharmacokinetic parameters, the effect on plasma drug concentrations and hence clinical efficacy are likely inconsequential.[23] However, the possibility of high-dose first-pass effects of renally toxic drugs (e.g., aminoglycosides) may still suggest avoidance of the caudal body, despite a lack of obvious pharmacokinetic effects.

As well as functioning as an excretory organ, the reptilian kidney is also responsible for vitamin C synthesis and the conversion of 25-hydroxycholecalciferol to the active forms, 1,25-dihydroxycholecalciferol or 24,25-dihydroxycholecalciferol.[24,25]

In summary, because reptiles represent the first group of vertebrates to adapt to a wholly terrestrial lifestyle, their kidneys have evolved to maximize water conservation. This is accomplished with comparatively few nephrons, reliance on uric acid production (in squamates), and a low GFR with tubular blood flow maintained by a renal portal supply.

CLINICAL INVESTIGATION

Diagnosis of urinary tract disease in reptiles is made on the basis of history, physical examination, hematology, biochemistry, urinalysis, diagnostic imaging, and ultimately histopathology, microbiology, and evaluation of renal function.

History and Physical Examination

Reptiles affected by urinary tract disease may present with acute onset of depression, anorexia, and sometimes cessation of urine and urate output. Such cases often involve individuals that are poorly managed and often in unhygienic conditions. Recent exposure to nephrotoxins, including aminoglycoside antibiotics and high doses of vitamin D₃, may be inferred from a detailed case history and previous medical or owner records. Total water deprivation, severe dehydration, or hemorrhage could also lead to poor renal perfusion and acute renal failure.

Reptiles with chronic urinary tract disease have often suffered from long-term mismanagement. High-protein diets rich in purines and in particular the use of canned dog or cat foods can lead to azotemia and hyperuricemia, with increased demands for effective nitrogenous waste excretion. Likewise, persistently inadequate humidity or inappropriate water provision (e.g., for some species, water bowl instead of misting) can result in chronic dehydration. The regular use of oral vitamin D₃ as a substitute for broad-spectrum (including UVB) lighting can cause soft tissue mineralization, including nephrocalcinosis. Reptiles that recover from secondary nutritional hyperparathyroidism as juveniles

may have sustained chronic renal damage from the cytotoxic effects of excess parathyroid hormone.[26] Affected animals tend to have a more protracted history, including deteriorating body condition, capricious appetite, and reduced activity that may extend over weeks or months, and as a result, most cases present dehydrated and emaciated. Only rarely do owners report polydipsia or polyuria.

A thorough physical examination is always indicated and should include an accurate measurement of weight and body condition assessment. Reptiles with severe renal compromise present in a depressed and weakened state (Fig. 66.15). Those with acute renal failure often exhibit better body condition than those with chronic renal compromise. Dehydration may be inferred from reductions in skin elasticity, salivary, and ocular secretions. Pharyngeal edema is not uncommon and lizards may present with bilateral exophthalmia and/or increased scleral vascularity. Digital palpation of the kidneys percutaneously, or in larger animals, per cloaca, is possible in some species, and the size, shape, and contours of the kidneys may be appreciable. Pronounced renomegaly may cause constipation and cloacal prolapse.

Clinical Biochemistry

Azotemia, hyperuricemia, or uremia seldom ensue before the majority of renal function has been lost and renal failure is evident. In clinical practice, creatinine is considered a poor indicator of renal disease in reptiles because of low production and variable excretion.[17] Creatinine

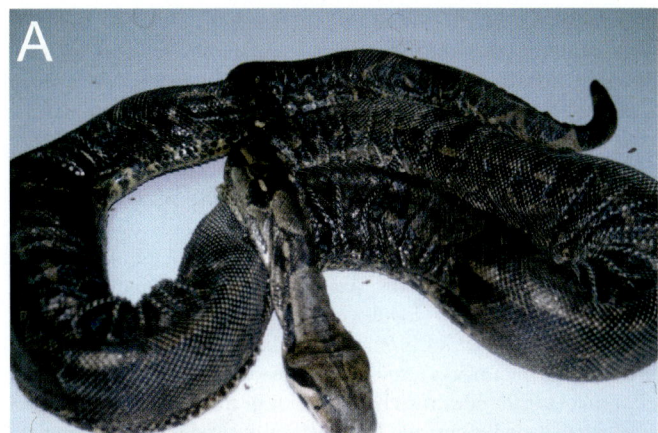

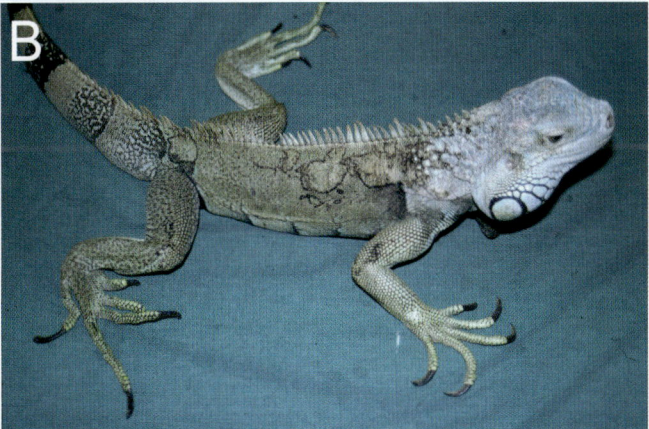

FIG 66.15 Physical presentation of reptiles with chronic renal disease. (A) Boa constrictor (*Boa constrictor*) with severe nephrosis and renal gout. (B) Green iguana (*Iguana iguana*) with tubulonephrosis and glomerulonephrosis attributed to high-protein diet, low humidity, and inappropriate water provision. (Courtesy of Stephen J. Divers.)

and creatine values have been described in a limited number of healthy iguanas and individuals with renal disease (Boyer, 1996, Proc ARAV, pp113). Creatinine production and excretion appear to be too variable for useful clinical value, and creatine, like uric acid, only rises during renal failure in iguanids. For most squamates, uric acid is the principle nitrogenous metabolite to measure. However, urea and ammonia quantification may be important in many chelonians and crocodilians (see Table 66.2). To complicate matters further, the relative proportions of ammonia, urea, and uric acid may vary with hydration status, postprandial effects, and hepatobiliary disease.[17] Serial measurements of relevant nitrogenous metabolites probably offer the greatest clinical value. Reliance on uric acid alone to assess nitrogenous excretion in many reptiles is flawed, with urea and ammonia often deserving consideration in some species. While urea and uric acid assays are typically available from commercial laboratories and using in-practice equipment, ammonia presents more of a challenge because it must be collected into cold heparinized syringes, kept on ice, and analyzed within an hour.[27]

In some species, notably the green iguana, calcium/phosphorus ratios may become inverted in many, but not all, cases of renal failure. Other electrolytes, including sodium, potassium, and magnesium, may also be informative; however, significant regulation of sodium and potassium is possible at extrarenal sites in some species (e.g., nasal salt glands). Hyponatremia and hyperkalemia may be expected from dysfunction of the distal tubules, cloaca, colon, bladder, or extrarenal salt glands. Other plasma biochemical parameters, including aspartate aminotransferase (AST), creatinine phosphokinase (CPK), and lactate dehydrogenase (LDH), may be elevated during renal disease, but their wide tissue distribution makes them non-specific markers of renal damage.[28] Tubular disease may be expected to result in increased urinary loss of the brush border enzyme, gamma glutamyl transferase (GGT); however, further studies are necessary to confirm this theory. Severe glomerular disease may increase urinary loss of albumin and lead to hypoalbuminemia (protein-losing nephropathy); however, albumin determinations by anything other than electrophoresis are likely inaccurate.[29] Fibrinogen may also be useful for identifying inflammation, and, although an observed range has been documented for the red-eared slider (*Trachemys scripta elegans*), elevation due to inflammation could not be demonstrated.[30] Chronic disease may lead to renal secondary hyperparathyroidism as a result of either inadequate renal hydroxylation of calcidiol to 1,25-dihydroxycholecalciferol, or from phosphate retention resulting in hypocalcemia and increased parathyroid hormone secretion. While accurate measurement of reptile-specific parathyroid hormone is difficult, a measurement of 1,25-dihydroxycholecalciferol is available commercially (Heartland Assays, Iowa State University Research Park, Ames, IA). Normal reference ranges for 1,25-dihydroxycholecalciferol are unavailable, and therefore comparison with conspecifics kept under the same management would be necessary.

Gender, season, nutrition, and management can significantly affect many biochemical values, even within the same species, and therefore published ranges must be interpreted with caution. Furthermore, most published ranges do not meet the criteria of the American Society of Veterinary Clinical Pathologists for true reference interval designation.[31] Given these variations, biochemical values derived from a healthy reptile during regular health examinations may prove to be the most useful comparison for that individual patient during times of illness. In addition, serial sampling offers the best approach for ongoing evaluation.

Hematology

Pathologic elevations of packed cell volume are usually related to dehydration. The clinician must also be aware that chronic renal disease may lead to a nonregenerative anemia that may mask hemoconcentration.

Unless immunosuppression is present, acute infection or inflammation usually results in heterophilia and/or azurophilia. In cases of chronic renal disease, a decreased, normal, or mildly increased total white blood cell count, often with monocytosis, is more common. Reptiles constantly exposed to temperatures below the preferred optimum temperature zone may become immunocompromised and fail to show an appropriate leukocyte response, even in the face of overwhelming infection. Although hematologic ranges have been published for many species, few comply with the criteria for reference range generation and should be used with caution.[31]

Urinalysis

The reptilian kidney cannot concentrate urine, and so urine-specific gravity is of limited use in the assessment of renal function. Furthermore, renal urine passes through the urodeum of the cloaca before entering the bladder, and therefore bladder urine is often not sterile. The clinical picture is further complicated by electrolyte and water changes that can occur across the bladder (or cloacocolonic) membrane.[18] Nevertheless, despite these biochemical drawbacks, urine samples are useful for cytologic assessments of inflammation and infection, and for the identification of renal casts.

Urine Collection. The urinary, genital, and intestinal tracts empty into a common cloaca, and therefore any samples voided from the vent may represent material derived from, or contaminated by, any of these systems. Voided urine and urates, although useful for cytology, must be critically evaluated whenever a culture is obtained. Urine microbiology results must be particularly scrutinized if the sample was collected from the floor of the enclosure or the examination table. Fresh urine and urate samples can be collected as a free catch. Many reptiles spontaneously void urine and urates (often with fecal material) when handled. More stoic individuals may be encouraged to urinate with gentle digital stimulation of the cloaca.

Cystocentesis prevents the gross contamination associated with free catch or collection from the floor or table. However, given the thin, fragile nature of the bladder, the potential for postsampling leakage and coelomitis must be appreciated. Given the passage of urine through the cloaca and the electrolyte and water changes that can occur in the bladder, urine collected by cystocentesis may not be representative of renal urine with respect to electrolyte composition and osmolarity. Such samples are often unsterile, although a heavy pure growth should alert the clinician to a potentially significant infection. The saurian bladder can be approached laterally or ventrally just anterior to the pelvis, aiming the needle anteromedially (Fig. 66.16A). The caudal extent of the liver on the right side of the chelonian coelom makes a left prefemoral approach preferable (see Fig. 66.16B). Rotation of chelonians may allow the bladder to fall dependently toward the prefemoral fossa and increase the chance of success. A 22-g to 25-g needle is appropriate, but the smaller needle sizes may become clogged. Ultrasound-guided cystocentesis may reduce the chances of iatrogenic trauma to other structures, including the intestines.

In general, catheterization of the bladder is challenging, although dilation of the cloaca with a nasal or vaginal speculum may be helpful, while cloacoscopy (often requiring saline infusion) will allow visualization of the urethral opening ventral to the opening of the large intestine (see Figs. 66.4B and 66.9C). Following endoscope-guided placement, the urethral catheter can be secured in place to permit estimation of urine output and repeated acquisition of samples (Fig. 66.17).

Urine Evaluation. Standard urinalysis technique can be used to evaluate reptilian urine. Ideally, urinalysis should be performed immediately after obtaining a sample because changes in pH and bacterial populations,

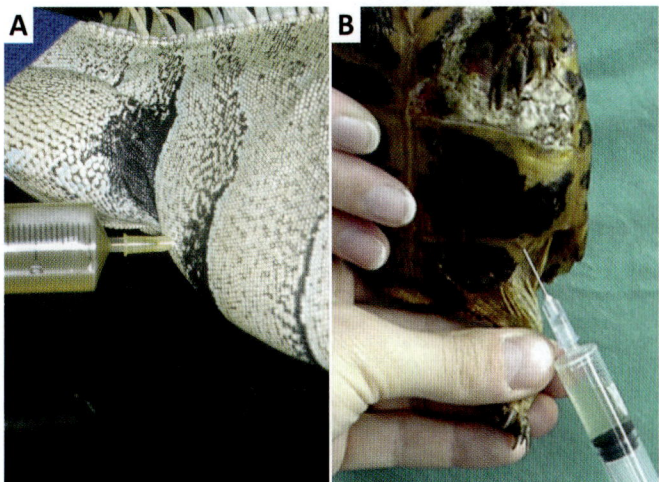

FIG 66.16 (A) Cystocentesis in a green iguana (*Iguana iguana*). (B) Cystocentesis in a Greek tortoise (*Testudo graeca*). Following aseptic preparation, the smallest gauge needle should be used and ultrasound guidance is recommended. (Courtesy of Stephen J. Divers.)

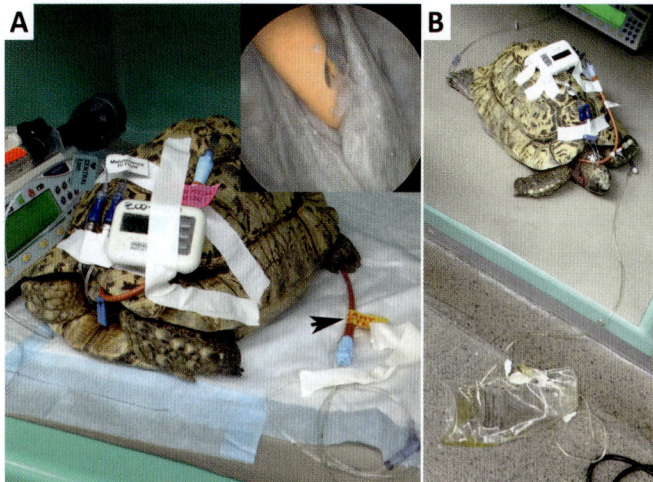

FIG 66.17 (A) Critical leopard tortoise (*Stigmochelys pardalis*) with central line, esophagostomy tube, and indwelling bladder catheter (arrow). (*Inset*) Endoscopic view of the red rubber catheter being directed through the urodeal fold and into the urethra. (B) Same patient with collection bag containing urine. (Courtesy of Stephen J. Divers.)

lysis of cells, and precipitation of crystals could occur as the urine ages. As in mammalian medicine, a complete urinalysis should include gross observation, biochemical testing, specific gravity measurement, and microscopic sediment evaluation. A gross evaluation of the urine is the appropriate first step. Much can be learned regarding the patient's well-being with evaluation of the appearance of the urine sample. Starvation and hepatic disease promote the production of biliverdin, which may turn urine a lime green color (Fig. 66.18).

Standard urine chemistry dipsticks appear to be useful, albeit not validated. Although not all dipstick assays are of value, several appear to provide important information. Unless otherwise specified, detection of abnormalities with urinalysis should prompt the clinician to consider any and all causes of the abnormal values as seen in other species. For example, severe proteinuria may be seen with protein-losing nephropathy, and hematuria may be seen with cystic calculi.

Urine pH. Initial studies in chelonians indicate that urine pH may have significant diagnostic value. Unpublished data suggest that the urine pH of several herbivorous tortoise species is normally alkaline (Innis, Proc ARAV, 1997, pp 109–112; Kolle, Proc ARAV, 2000, pp 111–113), while that of omnivorous box turtles (*Terrapene*) is slightly acidic (Gibbons et al, Proc ARAV, 2000, pp 161–168). However, published data indicate mean urine pH of 5.6 to 7.3 in desert tortoises (*Gopherus agassizii*), 6.7 in red-eared sliders, and 5.9 to 6.2 in hawksbill turtles (*Eretmochelys imbricata*).[32-34] Published reports of the urine pH of lizards and snakes are lacking. Acidic urine has been observed in herbivorous tortoises under conditions of drought, with high-protein diets, near the end of hibernation, or during prolonged periods of anorexia from illness.[32] Although the pathogenesis of acidic urine production in these tortoises is unclear, protein catabolism and ketogenesis may contribute. In most cases, tortoise urine pH has been shown to return to the alkaline range within several weeks of active foraging after hibernation or recovery from illness. As such, monitoring the urine pH of herbivorous reptiles may be a simple means of monitoring recovery from illness and return to positive energy balance. Acidic urine and dehydration may be predisposing factors for precipitation of urate crystals and uroliths. If so, attempts to alkalinize the urine through dietary change and medical therapy may be of use in preventing recurrence of such stones after surgical removal. Although not yet proven, alkaline urine in a carnivorous

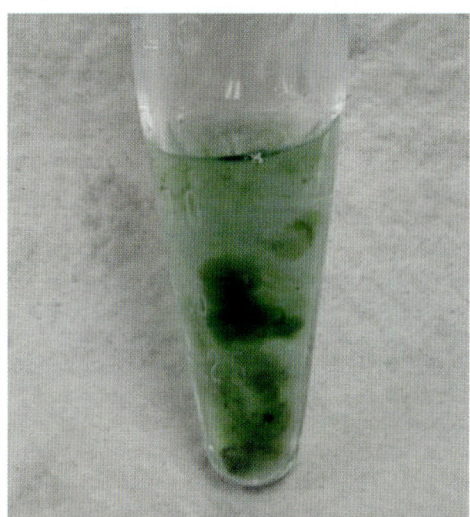

FIG 66.18 Urine from a cachectic reptile demonstrating green biliverdin pigment. (Courtesy of Charles J. Innis, New England Aquarium.)

reptile could indicate the presence of urinary tract infection from a urease-positive bacteria. This situation has been well-documented in human and domestic animal urology.[35]

Protein. Urine dipstick protein assays primarily respond to the presence of albumin. False-positive protein readings may occur with hematuria and pyuria or in the presence of reproductive secretions.[35] Unpublished observations of tortoise and box turtle urine indicate that zero to trace protein levels are detected in active healthy specimens. Protein levels of 30 mg/dL or higher have been noted during hibernation or during illness.

Glucose. Glucosuria is not normally present in significant amounts in those reptiles that have been studied. Glucosuria was noted by Koelle (Proc ARAV, 2000, pp 111–113) in 12 of 25 tortoises with renal disease and by Gibbons (Proc ARAV, 2000, pp 161–168) in several box turtles, including one that was hyperglycemic (plasma glucose 372 mg/dL). Better documentation of glucosuria and correlation with plasma glucose and organ pathology are needed to ascertain the significance of glucosuria.

Potential causes of glucosuria include diabetes mellitus, liver disease, stress/excitement, and renal tubular diseases.[35]

Occult blood. Free hemoglobin, myoglobin, or intact erythrocytes may produce a positive reaction for "blood." A positive dipstick reaction should be verified with urine sediment microscopy. Hematuria may also be associated with cystocentesis and excessive force during bladder expression. Free hemoglobin may be caused by transfusion reactions, hemolytic anemia, disseminated intravascular coagulation, and heat stroke. Myoglobinuria may occur secondary to severe rhabdomyolysis associated with crushing injuries.

Ketones. The role of ketones in reptile physiology is largely unstudied, but there is evidence of increased plasma and urine β-hydroxybutyrate in desert tortoises in response to drought but not hibernation, indicating that this may be a clinically important ketone in reptiles.[32] Unfortunately, most urine dipsticks utilize a nitroprusside reagent and respond to acetoacetic acid and, to a lesser extent, acetone, but not to β-hydroxybutyrate.[35] Further studies on the pathophysiology of reptile ketogenesis and the relative amounts of various ketones produced are needed. Trace ketonuria has been detected with dipstick in the urine of tortoises emerging from brumation (hibernation) but resolved within several weeks of resumed activity and feeding. Abnormal urine color may result in false-positive ketone reaction on dipsticks.[35]

Leukocyte esterase reaction. The leukocyte test on urine dipsticks reacts to the presence of esterases produced by granulocytes, and although accurate in humans has poor sensitivity in dogs and poor specificity in cats.[35] Its utility in reptile urinalysis has not been evaluated.

Nitrite. The nitrite assay reacts to the presence of nitrite produced by nitrate-reducing bacteria. Although useful in humans it has not been validated in other species, including reptiles. The significance of positive reactions in reptiles is unclear as urine is not typically sterile.

Urobilinogen and bilirubin. The role of urobilinogen in reptiles is unclear, and it has not been reported to be present in their urine. Only snakes appear capable of producing bilirubin in significant quantities, but the renal threshold for urinary bilirubin is unknown.[36] Most reptiles produce very little bilirubin, and so the bilirubin assay is largely useless. A biliverdin assay has been developed but is currently not commercially offered.[37]

Urine-specific gravity. Although validated for human urine, dipstick-specific gravity correlates poorly with refractometric results in various domestic animals.[35] Therefore for an accurate determination of specific gravity in reptile urine, a refractometer should be used; however, the value of specific gravity for evaluation of renal function is questionable as reptiles cannot concentrate urine above that of plasma. Urine-specific gravity may provide an indirect method of evaluating plasma specific gravity.

Urine sediment evaluation. Microscopic evaluation of the urine sediment is an important part of reptile urinalysis and should be performed on fresh samples as casts and cellular elements degenerate rapidly. Urine should be spun in a centrifuge at 1000 to 1500 rpm for 5 minutes and examined both unstained and stained using Sternheimer-Malbin stain, although Romanowsky and Gram stains may also prove useful.[35]

Erythrocytes, leukocytes, epithelial cells, microorganisms, spermatozoa, crystals, and casts may be identified (Fig. 66.19). In clinically healthy tortoises, urine may reveal small numbers of leukocytes and epithelial cells but is generally acellular. Erythrocytes are not routinely seen unless catheterization or cystocentesis has been performed. Some reptile bladder epithelial cells are ciliated, and finding such cells in the urine sediment in small numbers is not surprising.[38] The numbers of leukocytes, erythrocytes, or epithelial cells are reported per high power field, and large numbers should prompt further investigation.

Because urine passes through the urodeum of the cloaca to enter the bladder, some degree of bacterial contamination is often present in bladder urine. With experience, however, the microscopist may become comfortable with subjectively assessing the relative numbers and morphology of the urine flora. A mixed population of moderate numbers of rods and cocci may be normal, but a huge number of monomorphic bacteria or yeasts should be concerning, especially if combined with a prominent inflammatory response (see Fig. 66.19A). In such cases, urine culture may be useful; however, qualitative and quantitative data on reptile urine flora are currently lacking, and clinical judgment should be used when interpreting microbiological results. Pure, heavy cultures are generally more clinically significant than mixed, scant growth. As renal biopsy becomes more common, data correlating renal tissue culture and histopathology with urine culture results should better define the value of urine culture in diagnosing bacterial nephropathies.

Occasionally, protozoan or metazoan parasites may be detected (see Fig. 66.19B). The flagellated protozoan and renal parasite *Hexamita* has been reported from chelonian urine samples.[39] Myxozoan parasites (*Myxidium, Myxobolus*) have been reported to cause dilated renal tubules and interstitial nephritis in a variety of aquatic turtles.[39] In snakes and crocodilians where urine is stored in dilated, distal ureters and/or in the colon, urine evaluation may serve as a useful substitute for fecal testing in an anorectic animal that is not producing feces.

The presence of casts and crystals in reptile urine may be significant, but more data are needed before definite recommendations can be made. Urinalysis in mammals is useful for the demonstration of

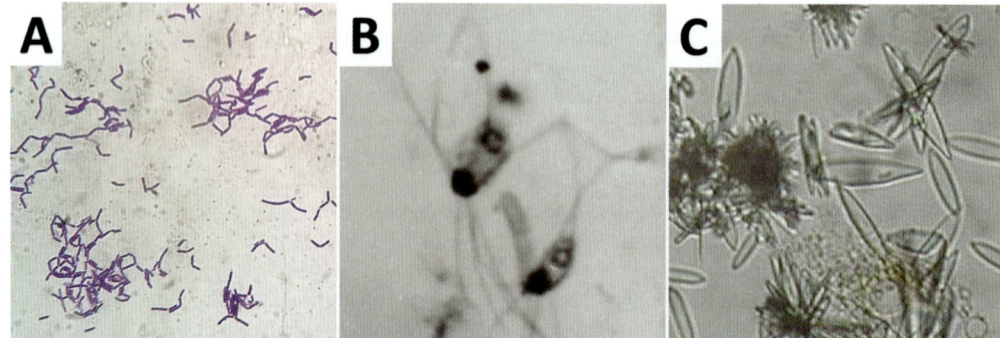

FIG 66.19 Urine sediment evaluation. (A) Gram-positive rods in urine from a radiated tortoise (*Astrochelys radiata*) collected by cystocentesis (Gram stain, ×1000 original magnification). (B) *Hexamita parva* in urine from a leopard tortoise (*Stigmochelys pardalis*) (direct wet-preparation, ×1000 original magnification). (C) Urate crystals in the urine from a green iguana (*Iguana iguana*) (direct wet-preparation).

ammonium biurate crystalluria and uric acid; however, given the variable expectation for such nitrogenous products in many reptiles, their diagnostic usefulness is probably limited as an adjunct to hepatic disease diagnosis. Although crystals and casts may be seen, one should be cautious in assuming that these have the same significance as their mammalian counterparts on the basis of appearance alone. For example, biochemical assays to determine the chemical composition of various crystals and histochemical staining to determine the nature of cast components have not been performed on reptile urine. In many reptilian urine sediment samples, small spherical urate crystals may be seen (see Fig. 66.19C).[14,17] Other crystals that have been identified on the basis of morphology include calcium oxalate, cholesterol, cystine, hippuric acid, leucine, sodium urate, tyrosine, bilirubin, and triple phosphate.[14]

Radiography

Normal reptile kidneys are not always readily appreciable on plain radiographs, especially in chelonians; however, dorsoventral and lateral (horizontal beam) views are generally the most useful (see Chapters 54 through 57). Radiographs can reveal renomegaly, radiopaque uroliths, macroscopic soft tissue mineralization, and chronic (mineralized) gout (Fig. 66.20). Renomegaly can cause extramural obstruction of the colon with resultant constipation and/or prolapse. This constipation or prolapse is often radiographically more obvious than the renomegaly. Intravenous urography can be used to highlight the kidneys, identify masses (abscesses, neoplasia, calculi), and show renal or ureteral damage or obstruction. Bolus intravenous injection of 800 to 1000 mg/kg of aqueous iodine contrast media (e.g., iohexol) is followed by serial dorsoventral and lateral radiographs at 0, 2, 5, 15, 30, and 60 minutes, with the reptile maintained within the species-specific-preferred optimum temperature zone.[2,40]

Ultrasonography

Ultrasonography permits an appreciation of normal tissue and mineralization, cysts, and other gross pathologic changes (see Chapter 58). Ultrasonography also aids kidney visualization for transcutaneous biopsy, although the risks of iatrogenic damage to renal vasculature and ureters must be considered. In the iguana, the bony pelvis is a barrier to ultrasound waves, and therefore the transducer must be angled caudad from a prepelvic location in the ventral midline just cranial to the hind limbs or craniad from a cloacal position at the ventral tail base. Sonographic evaluation of the kidney is often more rewarding than radiography alone, especially in snakes and chelonians (Fig. 66.21). Transcloacal imaging should be considered in giant reptiles.

Scintigraphy

Technetium has been shown to be useful to evaluate renal function in healthy green iguanas. Experimental scintigraphy studies involving 10 normal iguanas documented normal renal uptake of technetium-99m dimercaptosuccinic acid (99mTc-DMSA), and iguanas with reduced functional renal mass were postulated to exhibit a decrease in technetium uptake.[41] However, the expense of such equipment combined with radiation regulations makes this an impractical method for most private practices.

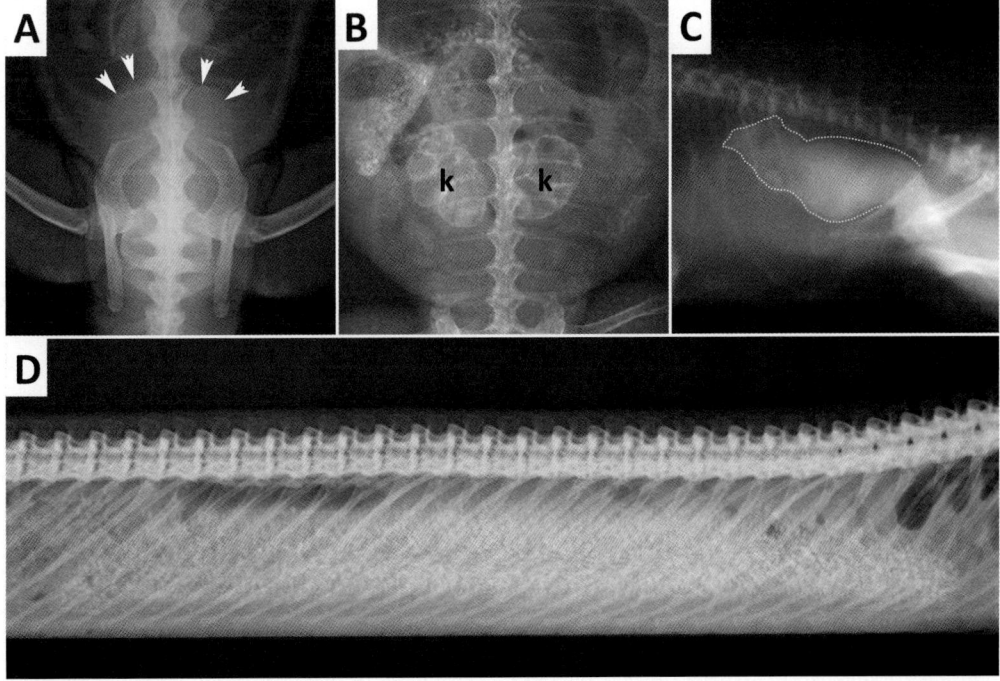

FIG 66.20 (A) Dorsoventral radiograph of the caudal coelom of a green iguana (*Iguana iguana*) demonstrating protrusion of the renal silhouettes (arrows) cranial to the pelvic rim, suggestive of renal enlargement. (B) Dorsoventral radiograph of the caudal coelom of a spiny-tailed lizard (*Uromastyx aegyptius*) demonstrating mineralization of both kidneys (k). (C) Lateral radiograph (excretory urogram) of a Chinese water dragon (*Physignathus cocincinus*) demonstrating an irregular and enlarged kidney (dotted line) following intravenous iohexol administration. (D) Lateral radiograph of a boa constrictor (*Boa constrictor*) with chronic renal gout demonstrating a characteristic starburst pattern along the length of the kidney due to dilation and impaction of the renal tubules. (Courtesy of Stephen J. Divers.)

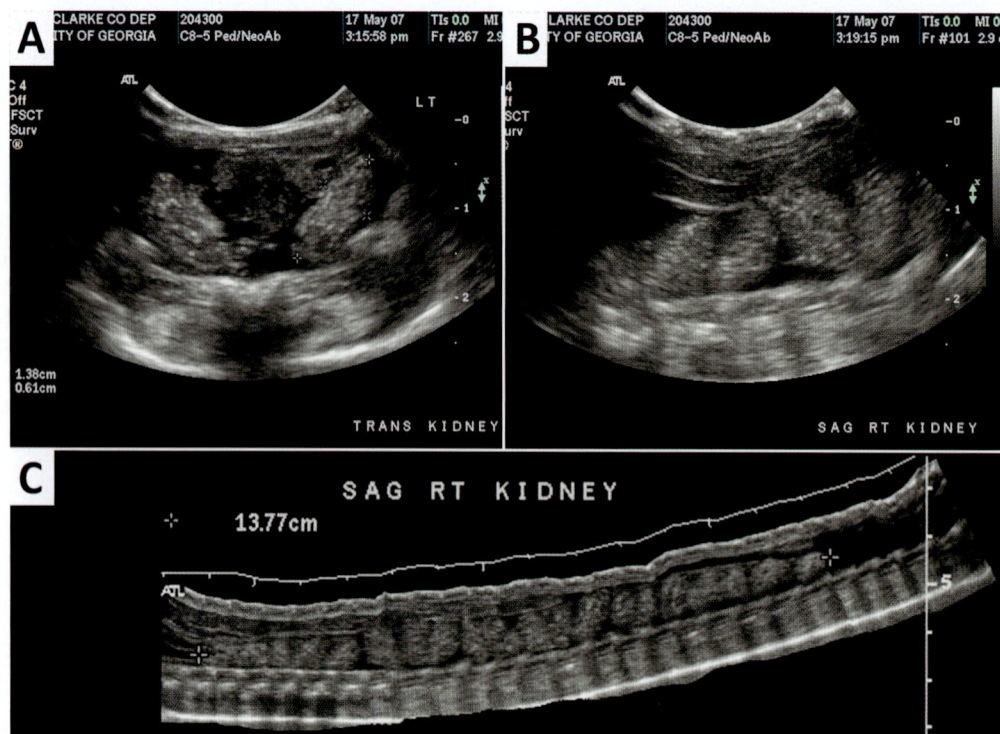

FIG 66.21 Renal ultrasonography of a yellow rat snake (*Pantherophis obsoleta quadrivittata*) with hyperuricemia. (A) Transverse view of the kidneys with the left kidney measuring 1.38 cm × 0.61 cm. (B) Sagittal view of the right kidney. (C) Sagittal sonographic reconstruction of the entire right kidney measuring 13.77 cm in total length. Note the multiple, hyperechoic pinpoint areas throughout the renal parenchyma in all views. Renal biopsy subsequently confirmed heterophilic nephritis with tubular and glomerular degeneration, tubular mineralization, and interstitial fibrosis. (Courtesy of Stephen J. Divers.)

Computed Tomography (CT) and Magnetic Resonance Imaging (MRI)

Advanced cross-sectional imaging can be useful for the evaluation of renal size, shape, and space occupying lesions. CT is typically faster, less expensive and often offers greater resolution; however, MRI can also provide information on parenchymal changes and renal blood flow. The acquisition of pre- and postcontrast images can be particularly useful when evaluating a renal mass and planning surgical removal or radiation therapy. CT can also be used to triangulate biopsy needles. See Chapters 59 and 60 for more details.

Endoscopy

Endoscopic techniques for the evaluation of the chelonian and saurian coelom have been well described (see Chapters 63 and 64).[3,42,43] The use of fine-diameter rigid endoscopes has permitted the direct visualization of a color-magnified image of visceral organs, including the kidneys, through a small surgical entrance into the coelomic cavity (Fig. 66.22).[1,3,43] Equipment should be matched to patient size; the 2.7-mm telescope with 4.8-mm operating sheath is appropriate for most reptiles <10 kg. Insufflation, preferably with carbon dioxide, is essential for lizards and snakes and preferred for chelonians. General anesthesia, lateral positioning, aseptic preparation, and paralumbar (in lizards) or prefemoral (in chelonians) entry permits examination of the coelomic cavity. In most lizards the kidneys are viewed cranial to the pelvis but are intrapelvic in iguanids. In chelonians they are intimately associated with the caudodorsal carapace, behind the coelomic membrane, which if opaque can make visualization difficult. In those turtles with a more flattened carapace, it is possible to approach the kidneys retrocoelomically without entering the coelom.[1] Adequate examination of both kidneys from a single entry point is possible, although visualization of the contralateral organ is more difficult. The endoscope entry site requires a single suture for closure. Endoscopy offers an unrivaled appreciation of renal size, surface contours, color, and lesions, which should be documented as focal, multifocal, or diffuse. Endoscope-guided fine needle aspiration for cytology or endoscopic biopsy are practical options for obtaining diagnostic samples.[1,3,43]

Needle Aspiration and Cytology

Palpably enlarged squamate kidneys may be aspirated transcutaneously with or without ultrasound guidance. Aspiration of normal-sized or smaller squamate kidneys may be more challenging, and aspiration cannot be recommended in chelonians without imaging guidance. Needle aspirates produce relatively small amounts of diagnostic material in comparison to biopsy samples. In addition, the lack of tissue architecture often complicates pathologic evaluation and interpretation. Nonetheless, needle aspirates often provide enough material for culture and may produce sufficient material for cytology.

Renal Biopsy

The relatively poor diagnostic value of urinalysis, the late detection of renal disease by blood biochemistry, and the poor regenerative capabilities of the diseased kidney exemplify the importance of renal biopsy early in the diagnostic process. Furthermore, renal biopsy is preferred over cytologic evaluations because cellular architecture is maintained and pathologic interpretations are often more reliable.

Ultrasound-Guided Biopsy. Ultrasound-guided needle biopsies may be possible in many squamates, but anesthesia is mandatory,

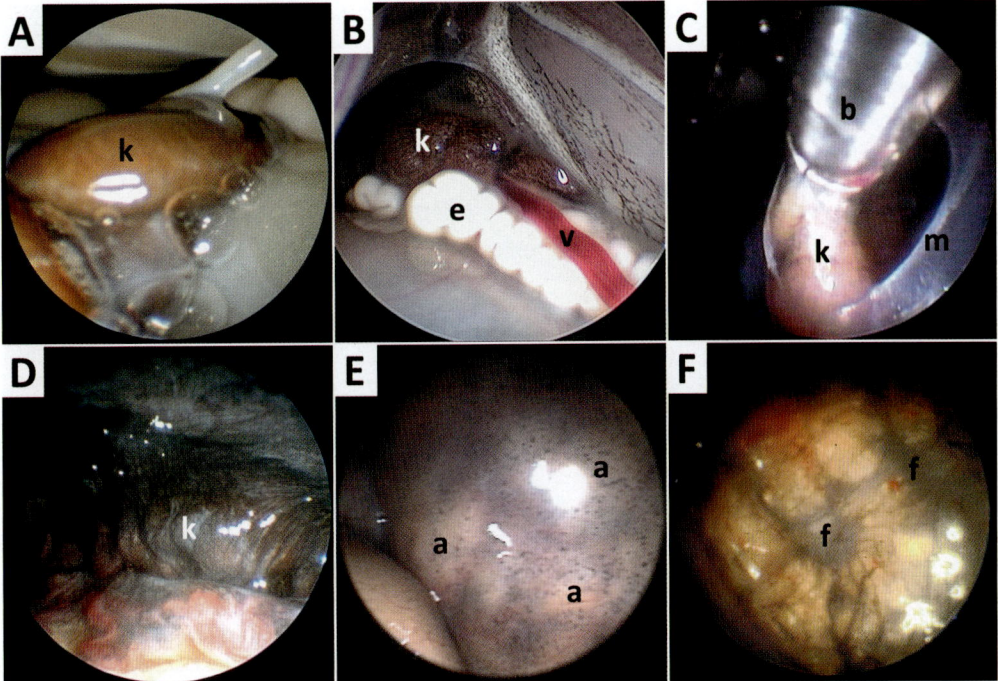

FIG 66.22 Endoscopic views of reptile kidneys using a 2.7-mm telescope. (A) Cranial pole of the left kidney (k) of a boa constrictor (*Boa constrictor*). (B) Cranial pole of the right kidney (k), epididymis (e), and renal vein (v) of a green iguana (*Iguana iguana*). (C) Biopsy of the left kidney (k) of a freshwater turtle (*Trachemys scripta*) using 1.7-mm biopsy forceps (b) introduced through an incision in the coelomic membrane (m). (D) Enlarged kidney (k) protruding into the coelom of a leopard tortoise (*Stigmochelys pardalis*). (E) Kidney of a male red-eared slider (*Trachemys scripta elegans*) exhibiting areas of pallor (a) that were confirmed as microabscesses following biopsy. (F) Kidney of a female Greek tortoise (*Testudo graeca*) exhibiting fibrous bands (f) across the surface. Biopsy confirmed tubulonephrosis with fibrosis. (Courtesy of Stephen J. Divers.)

and imaging is required for appropriate targeting in chelonians, and lizards with intrapelvic kidneys. Even so, there are still significant risks associated with iatrogenic trauma to the ureters, bladder, large intestine, reproductive tract, and major blood vessels. Depending on the quality of the equipment and skill of the ultrasonographer, multifocal or focal lesions may be appreciated or missed. Needle biopsy techniques have not been evaluated for reptile kidneys, but hepatic needle biopsy in anesthetized snakes and iguanids have resulted in gastrointestinal perforation (6%) or hemorrhagic death (12%).[45,46] The risks associated with renal biopsy would appear even greater, and therefore extreme caution is required.

Endoscopic Biopsy. The endoscope permits evaluation of renal size, color, and shape via a single, small surgical entry in anesthetized snakes, lizards, and chelonians. Studies have evaluated endoscopic renal biopsy techniques in freshwater turtles and iguanid lizards and concluded that they are rapid, safe, and effective for acquiring diagnostic samples without any reported mortality or morbidity.[1,3,43] Endoscopic scissors and biopsy forceps, under direct visual control, permit the incision of the coelomic membrane or thickened renal capsule and the collection of quality samples with less risk to surrounding structures (Fig. 66.23). The excellent optics of the telescope also permit an assessment of focal and multifocal disease and the selection of appropriate biopsies that may otherwise be difficult to ascertain without a color, magnified image. Endoscopic samples can be submitted for histology, microbiology, parasitology, or toxicology.

Surgical Biopsy. Coeliotomy provides access to the kidneys for harvesting surgical biopsies. The advantage of open surgical access is

the ability to collect larger samples, as well as an improved opportunity to more completely evaluate and sample other visceral structures. Surgical access to the chelonian and intrapelvic iguanid kidneys can be particularly challenging using traditional surgical approaches, and in all cases increased surgical exposure and duration of anesthesia must be considered. Surgical biopsies can be collected using a standard wedge technique in snakes, while small biopsy forceps or needle biopsy devices can also be used (Fig. 66.24A and B). Hemorrhage must be controlled, and radiosurgery, hemostatic materials (e.g., GelFoam), and digital pressure are effective.

A relatively simple technique to biopsy the intrapelvic kidneys of iguanids requires a cranial tail cut-down procedure under local or, more commonly, short-term general anesthesia. A small longitudinal incision is made in the lateral midline just below the lateral processes of the coccygeal vertebrae at the tail base. The incision extends for 1 to 3 cm caudad, starting just behind the hind limb. Blunt dissection between the dorsal and ventral coccygeal muscles permits exposure of the caudolateral aspect of the kidney that can then be sampled (see Fig. 66.24C). This technique is particularly valuable when the kidneys are not enlarged, surgical approach to the intrapelvic kidneys is difficult, and endoscopy is not available. It is limited to unilateral biopsy unless bilateral cut-down procedures are undertaken. Furthermore, because only a small area of the caudal kidney can be visualized and sampled, this technique is best reserved for diffuse or focal diseases of the caudal kidney.

Functional Renal Evaluation

Elevations of nitrogenous metabolites in plasma are poor indicators of renal function, because they can be affected by hydration status,

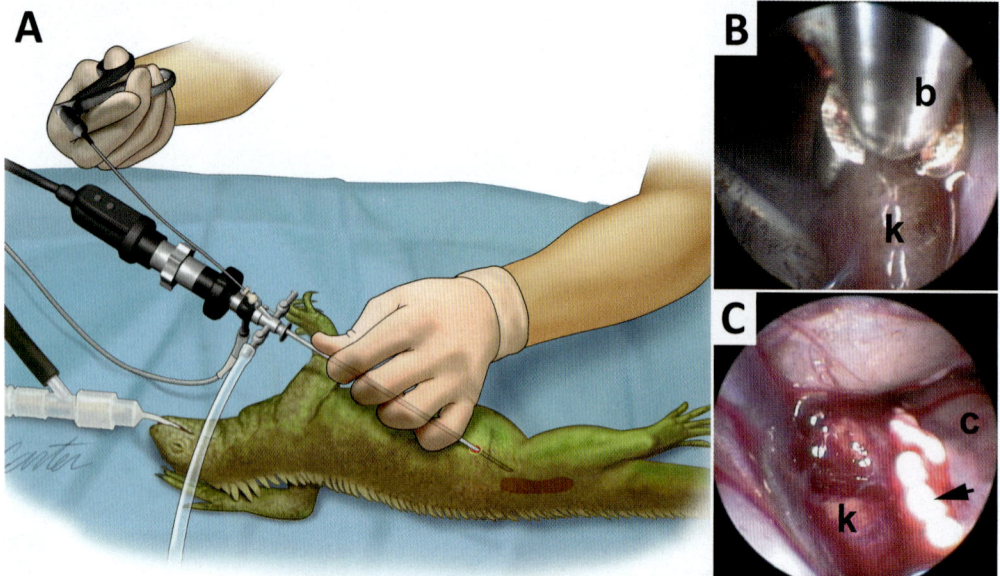

FIG 66.23 (A) Endoscopic biopsy in an iguanid lizard using a 2.7-mm telescope, 4.8-mm operating sheath, and 1.7-mm biopsy forceps. (B) Endoscopic view of the biopsy forceps (b) being advanced onto the kidney (k). (C) Postbiopsy view of the kidney (k) demonstrating minor hemorrhage. Note the lack of trauma to the closely associated epididymis (arrow) and colon (c). (Courtesy of Stephen J. Divers.)

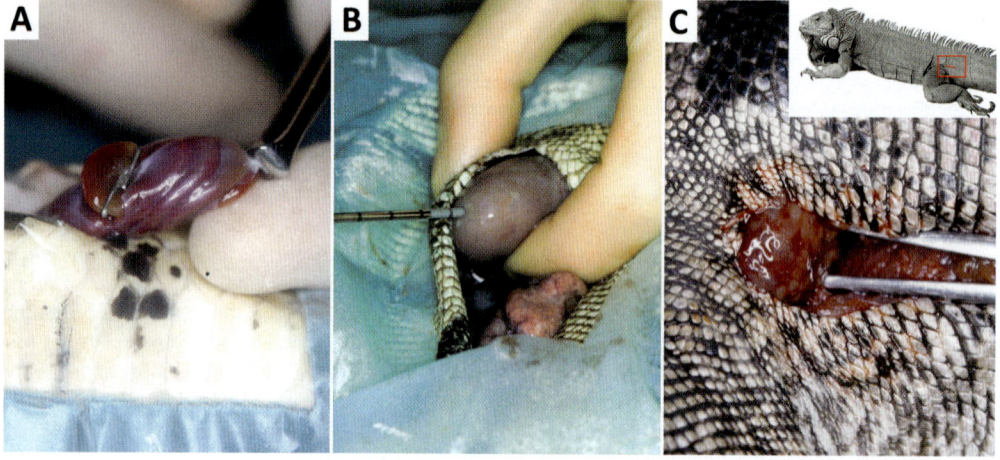

FIG 66.24 (A) Kidney biopsy in a boa constrictor (*Boa constrictor*) using two vascular clips to isolate a small wedge of tissue for sharp resection. (B) Needle biopsy from an enlarged kidney in a large saurian. (C) Cranial tail cut-down access to the left kidney in a green iguana (*Iguana iguana*). (Courtesy of Stephen J. Divers.)

and pathologic changes tend to only occur once the majority of renal function has been lost. In human and domestic animal medicine, measurement of renal function has been established as an important tool in the diagnosis and surveillance of kidney disease. Advanced imaging modalities, including scintigraphy, and magnetic resonance imaging to measure renal blood flow or renal clearance of radioactive nuclides or contrast agents have been used in human and veterinary medicine. Other techniques relying on the plasma clearance of an exogenous compound (e.g., phenolsulfonphthalein, inulin, creatinine) have also been used in veterinary medicine but require bladder catheterization for urine collection. Postrenal modification of urine occurs in the bladder, while many reptiles lack a bladder, and therefore catheterization of the ureters would likely be required.

Glomerular function assessment is essential in the diagnostic approach to animals with suspected renal disease because GFR is directly related to functional renal mass.[35] Iohexol clearance has proven to be useful for determining GFR in mammals and is the only renal function test that has been evaluated in reptiles.[3,47–52] Iohexol is a nonionic radiographic iodine contrast medium of low osmolarity that is excreted solely by glomerular filtration with negligible extrarenal elimination in mammals. The plasma clearance of iohexol can be determined with analysis of plasma iohexol concentration over time after a single intravenous injection (Fig. 66.25). The rate of clearance of iohexol from plasma can be used to estimate GFR by dividing the iohexol dose by the area under the curve (AUC). In addition, this methodology has the advantages of (i) requiring just three small blood collections over 24 hours, (ii) not requiring urine collection, and (iii) being practical for reptiles as small as 300 g.

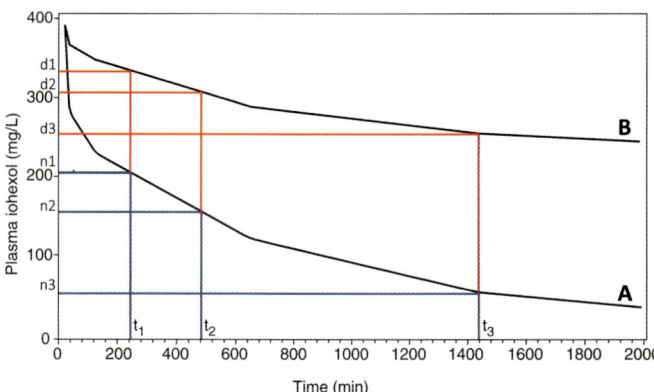

FIG 66.25 Iohexol excretion curves for a healthy iguana (A) and one with significant reductions in glomerular filtration rate (GFR) but no other changes on blood biochemistry (B). Timed blood samples are collected at 4 (t1), 8 (t2), and 24 (t3) hours post iohexol administration. Plasma levels of iohexol for the normal (n1–n3) and unhealthy lizards (d1–3) were then used to calculate GFR values of 16.5 mL/kg/hr and 8.2 mL/kg/hr, respectively. (Courtesy of Stephen J. Divers.)

TABLE 66.4 Protocol of Glomerular Filtration Rate (GFR) Determination in Reptiles

1. In the United States, contact the Diagnostic Center for Population and Animal Health (DCPAH, Michigan State University, East Lansing, MI 48824, 517-353-1683, https://www.animalhealth.msu.edu/) to check for any changes to the blood collection and/or submission requirements for iohexol assay and GFR calculation. Additional laboratories that offer iohexol assays are often available and include the following; however, they should be contacted to ensure appropriate sample volumes are collected:
   The Royal Veterinary College, University of London (http://www.rvc.ac.uk/pathology-and-diagnostic-laboratories/therapeutic-drug-monitoring)
   IDEXX Reference Laboratories (test code 3384), available in the United States, Europe, Australia, Africa, and Asia (https://www.idexx.com/small-animal-health/products-and-services/reference-laboratories.html)
2. Ensure the reptile is hydrated and fasted for 24 hours.
3. Obtain an accurate body weight to the nearest gram and inject 75.0 mg/kg iohexol intravenously at time 0.
   IV administration is critical and catheterization should be considered to reduce the risks of perivascular injection that will invalidate the results.
4. Collect 0.5 mL blood sample into heparin at 4 hours and record the exact time of blood collection. Spin down the blood, separate, and freeze the plasma. At least 0.2 mL of plasma is required.
5. Repeat blood collection, plasma separation, and freezing at 8 hours and 24 hours postiohexol administration. Again, record the exact times of blood collection. Given that a total of 1.5 mL of blood is required (at least for DCPAH), this protocol is limited to reptiles weighing approximately 300 g or more.
6. Send frozen plasma samples on ice overnight to the laboratory.

Calculation of GFR by iohexol clearance has been validated in green iguanas and sea turtles.[3,47] In healthy green iguanas, GFR was reportedly 16.56 ± 3.90 mL/kg/h, with a 95% confidence interval of 14.78 to 18.34 mL/kg/h. Iguanas with renal disease exhibited significant reductions in GFR even in the absence of other clinical or biochemical signs.

Similarly, Kemp's ridley sea turtles with histologically confirmed renal disease showed GFR reductions that correlated to the severity of renal disease.[47] Notably, for turtles, renal function testing allowed for prognostic determination such that treatment could be continued or the patient could be euthanized, as appropriate. Iohexol clearance testing confirmed that naturally cold-stunned Kemp's ridley turtles were affected by 75% decreased renal function even after several days of hospitalization, while convalescent GFR were normal.[52] A suggested protocol for GFR determination has been published and summarized in Table 66.4, while published reptile GFR values are included in Table 66.3.[3] Unlike most other clearance techniques, iohexol excretion does not require bladder or ureteral catheterization, and unlike scintigraphy, it does not require expensive equipment or radioisotopes to perform. Given that iohexol assays are commercially available, functional renal evaluation in reptiles can be easily undertaken in private practice.

GENERAL APPROACH TO TREATMENT

Medical management of urinary tract diseases of reptiles largely relies on extrapolation of principles used in mammalian species. The reader is referred to various chapters throughout this book that are likely to be ancillary to the therapeutic management of renal disease cases. Success is more likely if a definitive diagnosis has been obtained and targeted, specific therapy can be provided.

Fluid therapy is used routinely and should be tailored to correct any electrolyte imbalances, with serial biochemistry and weight used to evaluate hydration and progress. Other treatments that may be considered include antimicrobials, diuretics, intestinal phosphate binders, allopurinol, colchicine, enalapril, calcitriol, or other agents used for management of renal conditions in other species. Aside from some antimicrobials and allopurinol, there are no pharmacokinetic/pharmacodynamic data for use of these drugs in reptiles.[53] Although the use of certain diuretics (e.g., furosemide) could be questioned in species that lack a loop of Henle, there is evidence in freshwater turtles that furosemide and ethacrynic acid are effective in increasing urine volume and urine electrolyte excretion by tubular effects.[22] Furosemide (2 and 5 mg/kg) produced no changes in blood pressure, hematocrit, plasma electrolytes, GFR, or plasma renin activity; however, sodium excretion increased 20-fold, whereas chloride and potassium excretion increased 12-fold. Dehydration by administration of furosemide and withholding fluid therapy has been reported as a successful treatment for brevetoxicosis in sea turtles.[54]

Oral allopurinol (xanthine oxidase inhibitor) at 25 mg/kg once daily has been shown to decrease uric acid levels by 45% in green iguanas.[53] Probenecid and sulfinpyrazone act by inhibiting uric acid reabsorption from the proximal tubule; however, given that very little, if any, reabsorption occurs in reptiles, the efficacy of these medications is questionable. Hypocalcemia should be treated with oral calcium supplementation with food (which also competes with phosphate absorption). Injectable calcium therapy should be avoided because most cases exhibit concurrent hyperphosphatemia, and the sudden elevation of calcium with high phosphorus can elevate the solubility index and precipitate soft-tissue mineralization. If calcium therapy for tetany is required, then it should be given slowly, preferably IV or IO, to effect with concomitant diuresis and phosphate binders. Oral phosphate binders (e.g., oral aluminum hydroxide) should be given between meals or they may interfere with dietary calcium absorption.[55] Human chronic renal failure can be treated with low, carefully titrated doses of cholecalciferol (vitamin D_3) to reduce the nephrotoxic effects of increased intracellular calcium within renal cells.[56] In reptiles, such accurate and titrated dosing is unlikely to be practical, and therefore it is safer to provide access to broad-spectrum lighting, preferably unfiltered sunlight. Antimicrobials should be used

TABLE 66.5   Selected Nutritional Compositions of Various Food Items That Deserve Consideration in Reptiles With Renal Disease

Invertebrates	Cricket *Acheta domesticus* Adult	Juvenile	Mealworm *Tenebrio molitor*	Superworm *Zophobas morio*	Silkworm *Bombyx mori*	Waxworm *Galleria mellonella*	Earthworm *Lumbricus terrestris*
Protein (% DM)	40–68	40–50	35–55	40–50	65	27–41	73

Vertebrates	Mouse *Mus musculus* Adults	Pups	Rat *Rattus norvegicus*	Meadow Vole *Microtus pennsylvanicus*	Smelt *Sprinchus lanceolatus*	Herring *Clupea harengus*	Chicken *Gallus gallus domesticus* Adult	Day-Old
Protein (% kcal)	48	29	55	63	63	39	47	52

Plants	Romaine Lettuce	Iceberg Lettuce	Alfalfa Sprouts	Mushrooms	Sweet Potato	Squash	Forage & Hays	Prickly Pear	Clover	Apple	Cantaloupe
Protein (% DM)	36	25	37	30	5	17	15–17	5	19	1	8

Plants	Lettuce	Cabbage	Cauliflower	Endive	Sweet Potato	Kale	Raisins	Apple	Cantaloupe
Total purine load (mg uric acid/100g)	13	37	51	17	16	48	107	14	33

Plants	Romaine Lettuce	Iceberg Lettuce	Mustard Greens	Collards	Broccoli	Kale	Spinach
Na (mg/100g)	8	9	25	18	18	27	79
K (mg/100g)	290	158	358	169	325	447	558

only when infection has been demonstrated, with drug selection based on culture and sensitivity or, better still, MIC testing. The indiscriminate and widespread misuse of antimicrobials is unfortunately all too common.

In humans and domesticated animals, emphasis is placed on nutritional management. Protein restriction and the selective provision of pyrimidines (thymine and cytosine) over purines (guanine and adenosine) may help to reduce uric acid production. In addition, potassium supplementation may also be beneficial. Until concrete dietary recommendations for chronic renally impaired reptiles are forthcoming, the data in Table 66.5 may help clinicians make informed decisions regarding dietary choices. Further detailed information on human food compositions can be easily obtained from the USDA National Nutrient Database (https://ndb.nal.usda.gov/).

SPECIFIC UROLOGIC DISEASES

Gout

Gout is a metabolic disease characterized by overproduction or underexcretion of uric acid, resulting in hyperuricemia and deposition of positively birefringent monosodium urate (MSU) crystals in tissues.[57]

Clinical Significance. Although gout is frequently seen in humans and primates, it is not a common problem in general veterinary medicine. As a result, veterinarians who specialize in avian and reptilian patients must rely on the human medical literature for information regarding diagnosis and treatment.[58–60] Gout, in any of its forms (visceral, articular, and periarticular), is a common affliction in reptilian patients. Few studies cite the incidence of gout in reptiles, but unpublished data of 280 European tortoise necropsies indicated 64.3% had evidence of renal disease and 16% showed gout Kolle and Hoffman, 2002, Proc ARAV, pp 33–35).

Known Etiological Cause(s). In vertebrates, uric acid is derived from both exogenous and endogenous nucleic acids that are degraded in the liver to yield free purine and pyrimidine bases.[17] If these free bases are not reused by the body, they are further degraded and ultimately excreted. The pyrimidines are catabolized to the end products CO_2 and NH_3 that enter the ornithine cycle (Fig. 66.26). In some vertebrates, including primates, the dalmatian dog, birds, squamates, and some chelonians, purine degradation can produce significant quantities of uric acid.[17] Degradation of the major purines, adenine and guanine, starts initially with a conversion to hypoxanthine and then to xanthine for adenine and directly to xanthine for guanine. Both of these pathways require the flavoprotein, xanthine oxidase, to form uric acid (see Fig. 66.26). While carnivores are well adapted to high-protein diets and may even experience normal postprandial hyperuricemia, herbivorous reptiles may be overwhelmed by excessive animal protein, which results in pathologic hyperuricemia.[53]

In reptiles, uric acid is cleared from the blood by glomerular filtration but mainly by secretion from the proximal renal tubules. Urates are poorly water soluble and precipitate at low concentrations. While uric acid secretion is independent of glomerular filtration, in cases of dehydration where glomerular filtration and tubular flow are decreased, secretion of uric acid eventually ceases, and the renal tubule becomes blocked with uric acid. The reptilian nephron actively secretes three times more urates when normally hydrated.[14]

In blood, uric acid is present predominantly as MSU. Both free uric acid and urate salts are relatively insoluble in water. When the concentration of either or both of these forms becomes elevated in the blood (hyperuricemia) or in other body fluids (e.g., synovial fluid), MSU crystallizes, forming insoluble precipitates that are deposited in various tissues. Crystallization in synovial fluid results in acute, painful inflammation of the joint, a condition called gouty arthritis. Crystals can also

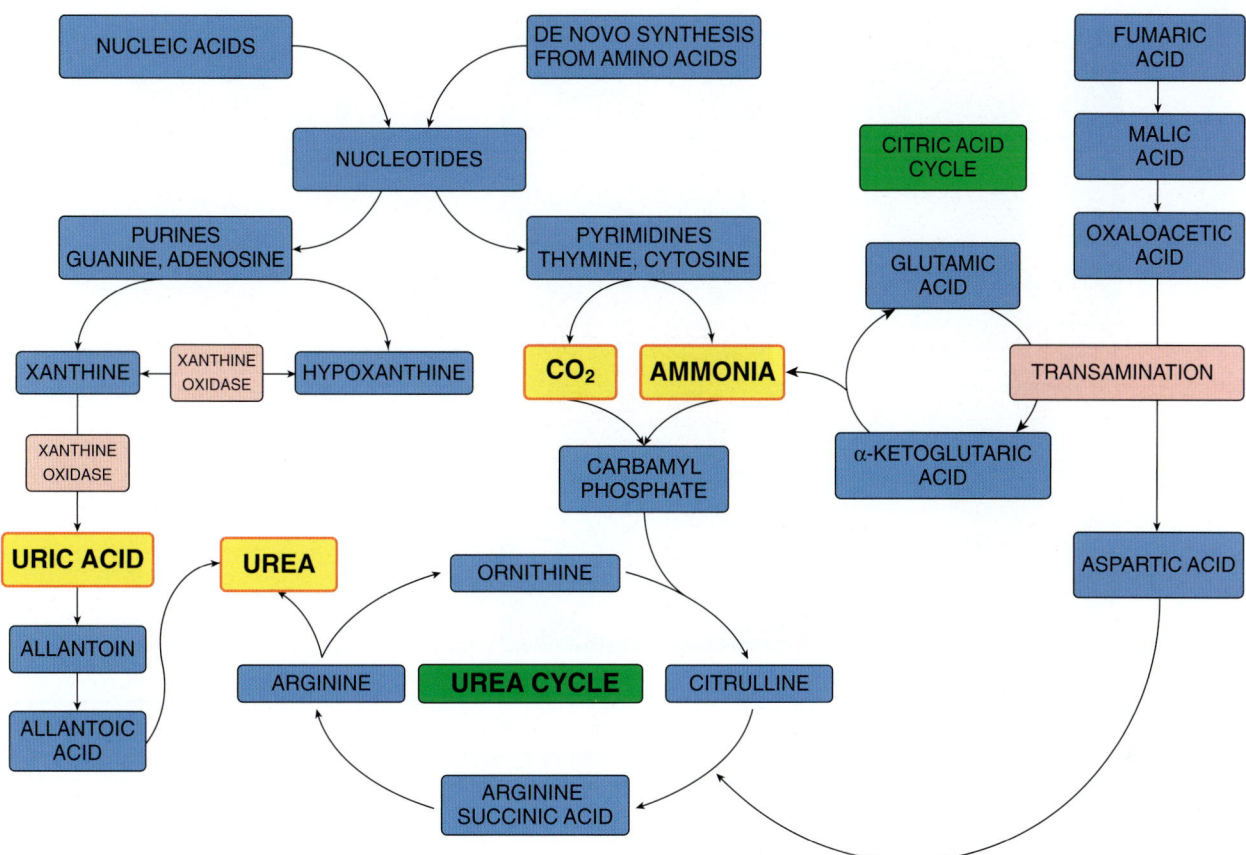

FIG 66.26 Hepatic nucleotide, amino acid, and nitrogenous metabolism in reptiles.

deposit around the joints (periarticular gout) and in other subcutaneous and internal tissues (visceral gout). The MSU crystals form small, macroscopic white nodules called tophi.

Most cases of gout involve the final stage of chronic renal failure and/or dehydration; however, hypovitaminosis A has also been suggested as a predisposing factor in crocodile hatchlings by reduced uric acid secretion due to squamous metaplasia of tubular cells.[61] True gout is caused by the presence of MSU, while pseudogout occurs as a result of any other precipitate (e.g., calcium hydroxyapatite, calcium pyrophosphate dihydrate), which can also cause an acute articular or periarticular inflammatory response.[62]

In primary gout, hyperuricemia results from overproduction of uric acid. Secondary gout occurs when hyperuricemia results from an acquired chronic disease or a drug that interferes with the normal balance between the production and excretion of uric acid. Diuretics are the drugs most commonly implicated in causing gout in humans. Furosemide decreases the renal tubular excretion of uric acid and is contraindicated in dehydration, hyperuricemia, or cases of suspected gout. Misuse of potentially nephrotoxic antibiotics (e.g., aminoglycosides and sulfonamides) can cause tubular nephrosis and predispose the patient to hyperuricemia, especially if dehydrated.

Clinical Presentation. In reptilian patients, common sites for MSU tophi deposition include the pericardial sac, kidneys, liver, spleen, lungs, subcutaneous, and other soft tissues (Fig. 66.27A–C). Clinical signs are typically related to the structures affected and may include anorexia, lameness, joint swelling, and organ dysfunction.

Diagnostic Confirmation. Presumptive diagnosis of gout is made based on history and clinical examination. Laboratory sampling may or may not demonstrate plasma hyperuricemia, depending on the state of health at the time of sampling. Radiographs may reveal lytic lesions in, around, or near the joints. Soft tissue tophi are generally radiolucent and may go unnoticed; but more chronic lesions often become complexed with calcium and may be radiographically visible (see Fig. 66.20D). Ultrasonography may demonstrate MSU deposits as hyperechoic lesions without posterior acoustic shadowing, which enables their differentiation from calcifications (see Fig. 66.21). While standard CT may show crystal aggregates, it does not enable specific identification of MSU crystals; however, dual-energy CT can distinguish MSU crystals from deposits containing calcium.[63] Endoscopic evaluation of the coelomic viscera enables a minimally invasive means of identifying lesions (see Fig. 66.27B and C).

A definitive diagnosis of gout is made by demonstrating MSU crystals in affected joints or tissues. Cytologic examination by phase contrast microscopy of joint aspirates is useful to identify MSU crystals. Visceral gout can be diagnosed by histopathologic examination of soft-tissue biopsies collected by traditional or endoscopic techniques (see Fig. 66.27D). When using polarized light, the tissues must be fixed in absolute ethanol, because MSU crystals tend to degrade and wash out during formalin (aqueous solution) fixation.[64] However, even though MSU may be lost from formalin-fixed tissues, histologic diagnosis is usually still straightforward. If there are no obvious lesions to biopsy then renal function assessments using iohexol clearance should be considered, as GFR measurements are still directly related to functional renal mass.

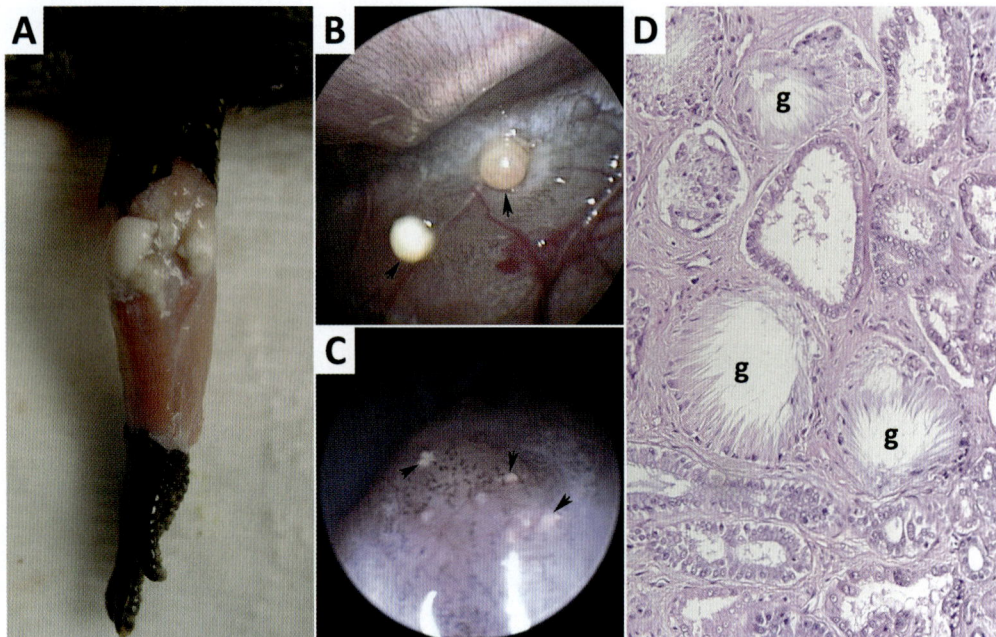

FIG 66.27 (A) Gouty arthritis of the left stifle of a blue-tongued skink (*Tiliqua gigas*). (B) Gout tophi (arrows) associated with the coelomic wall in a green iguana (*Iguana iguana*). (C) Small gout tophi (arrows) visible on the surface of a veiled chameleon's (*Chamaeleo calyptratus*) kidney. (D) Renal biopsy histology from the same chameleon, demonstrating the characteristic appearance of tophi (g). Note that the urate material has been largely washed away from this formalin-fixed sample, but the appearance is still considered pathognomonic (H&E, original magnification ×400). (Courtesy of Stephen J. Divers.)

Prognosis and Prevention. The overall prognosis for patients with severe gout is grave. Advanced cases can be maintained for a short period with suppportive care. In humans, acute gouty attacks are painful, and one should assume that antiinflammatories and analgesics are required for reptiles. Localized disease may be managed surgically.

Appropriate nutrition, particularly the provision of appropriate protein, both in terms of amount and type (animal vs plant) is important. In addition, appropriate provision of water (both dietary and free) to prevent dehydration, and species-specific thermal environments to maintain renal metabolism, are essential.

Specific Treatment. Treatment of gout is threefold: (1) lower blood uric acid levels with antihyperuricemic drugs such as allopurinol, (2) promote urate excretion by diuresis, and (3) manage localized inflammatory tophi through surgical removal (or amputation), and/or antiinflammatory drugs such as colchicine and, if necessary, corticosteroids. Allopurinol at 25 mg/kg PO daily has been shown to decrease plasma uric acid levels in hyperuricemic iguanas by 45%, and there are case reports to confirm its clinical value.[53,65,66] While human drugs such as probenecid act by blocking urate reabsorption from the proximal tubule, there is no evidence of net urate reabsorption along any part of the reptile nephron, and therefore efficacy is more doubtful.[17] The need for analgesics should not be overlooked, and opiates are preferred over nonsteroidal antiinflammatory drugs (NSAIDs) if renal function is questionable.

Newer drugs may have potential for use in herpetologic medicine, but minimal clinical use has been reported to date. Newer xanthine oxidase inhibitors such as oxipurinol and febuxostat are first-line treatments for human patients with renal calculi, renal insufficiency, and hyperuricemia. In humans, they appear safe and well-tolerated with few side effects.[67] Recombinant urate oxidase is used for the treatment of tumor lysis hyperuricemia in human cancer patients, while pegylated urate oxidase shows promise in patients with hyperuricemia and gout.[68] If the patient has severe gouty arthritis, surgically entering the affected joint and physically removing the MSU crystals is possible. However, by the time the crystals have formed, severe joint damage is usually present, and permanent arthopathy ensues. In these cases, treatment may be attempted with long-term allopurinol therapy or amputation.

Glomerulosclerosis, Nephrosclerosis, Glomerulonephrosis, and Tubulonephrosis

Clinical Significance. Degenerative nephroses represent the most common renal diseases encountered and are usually characterized by variable degeneration or necrosis of the glomeruli (glomerulonephrosis) or tubules (tubulonephrosis) (Fig. 66.28). When the majority of renal function has been lost, gout and aberrant calcium metabolism may result in MSU crystals within soft tissues, including the kidney. Calcification of the great vessels and myocardium can lead to congestion of peripheral blood vessels (especially obvious on the sclera of the eye), poor circulation, and ischemic necrosis of the tail or digits. Fracture of mineralized vessels can lead to severe internal hemorrhage. Gastrointestinal effects may include vomiting and passing poorly digested food.

Known Etiological Cause(s). High-protein diets are considered a predisposing cause of hyperuricemia, gout, and nephrosis in herbivorous reptiles. Blockage of the renal tubules with secreted urate in the proximal tubule is another process that impairs renal function and has been associated with chronic dehydration in snakes. The maintenance of high-humidity rainforest species in dry, overheated, captive conditions may result in chronic dehydration and nephropathy.

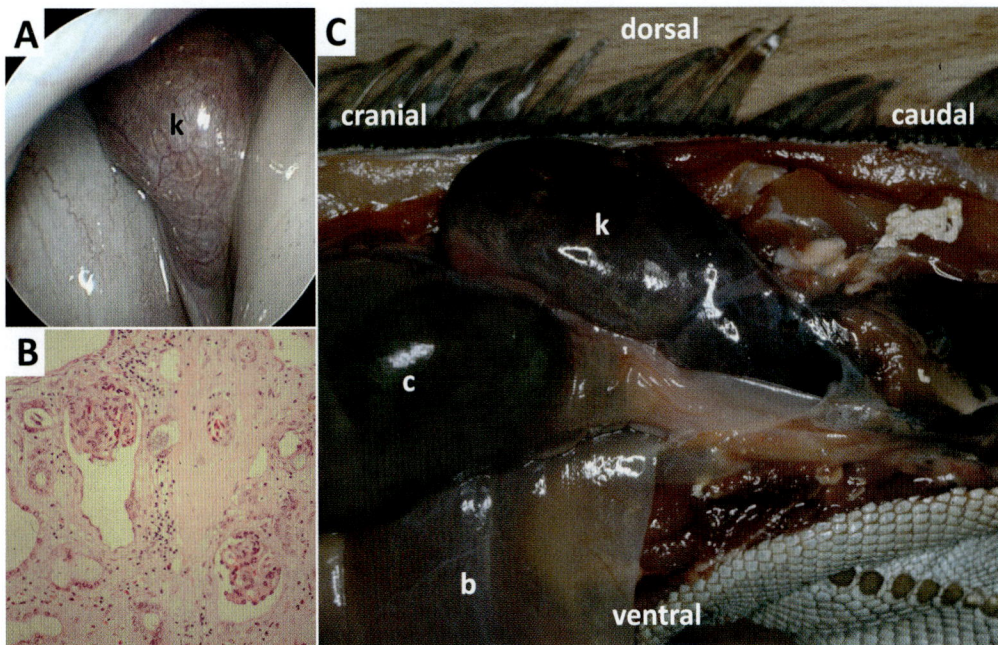

FIG 66.28 Glomerulonephrosis and tubulonephrosis in iguanid lizards. (A) Endoscopic view of an enlarged kidney. (B) Histology section of an endoscopic kidney biopsy revealing glomerulonephrosis, tubulonephrosis, and fibrosis (H&E, original magnification x400). (C) Saggital necropsy view of the pelvic region with the left pelvic limb and pelvis removed revealing a grossly enlarged kidney (k), bladder (b), and constipation of the colon (c) due to extramural pressure. (Courtesy of Stephen J. Divers.)

Clinical Presentation and Diagnostic Confirmation. Typically, reptiles present late in the course of disease when the majority of renal function has been lost, and clinical signs typically include anorexia, weight loss, and poor body condition (see Fig. 66.15). Unlike chronic renal disease in mammals, affected reptiles often present with enlarged, not small, fibrotic kidneys (see Fig. 66.20). Renal biopsy is required for a definitive diagnosis (see Figs. 66.23 and 66.24), but functional evaluation by iohexol clearance is also useful for prognosis.

Prognosis, Prevention, and Treatment. Prognosis depends on the degree of renal function remaining and the extent of the pathologic changes, but is generally guarded to poor. Prevention usually centers on good husbandry, including suitable thermal environment, appropriate humidity/temperature, and removal of animal protein from herbivorous diets. Treatment is supportive and often includes efforts to increase water intake (i.e., soaking plant foods and feeding wet, injecting vertebrate prey with water), decrease purine loads, decrease nitrogenous waste levels, and increase potassium intake.

Interstitial Nephritis, Glomerulonephritis, Tubulonephritis, and Pyelonephritis

Clinical Significance. Inflammatory conditions of the kidneys appear to be less commonly encountered but have been associated with bacterial, viral, fungal, and parasitic infections in reptiles.[4] In addition, drug-induced nephritis has been reported in humans and may be possible in reptiles. Severe, acute infections can cause acute renal failure; thus it is important to diagnose these conditions accurately because prompt and appropriate therapy may result in reclamation of temporarily lost renal function and complete recovery.

Known Etiological Cause(s). Various bacteria, including *Citrobacter, Escherichia, Moraxella, Salmonella, Serratia, Aeromonas, Listeria, Leptospira, Streptococcus, Mycobacteria,* and *Chlamydia* have been isolated from reptile kidneys, either as primary agents of nephritis or secondary to generalized sepsis (Fig. 66.29A). Renal geotrichosis, phaeohyphomycosis, cryptococcosis, coccidioidomycosis, and candidiasis have also been identified in select individuals with renal pathology. *Entamoeba invadens, Hexamita parva, Myxidium, Klossiella,* and *Caryospora* are documented protozoan causes of nephritis and renal necrosis, while *Spirorchis* nematodes have been reported from aquatic chelonians, and filarial nematodes from lizards (see Fig. 66.29B). Herpesviruses, adenoviruses, arenaviruses, and iridoviruses have been associated with inflammatory or necrotic renal lesions.[4]

Clinical Presentation and Diagnostic Confirmation. Many of these conditions may result in chronic debilitation, chronic renal disease, and renal insufficiency, whereas acute conditions can result in acute renal compromise and even renal failure. Such acute cases usually present in good body condition, and aggressive case investigation is warranted because appropriate treatment can regain lost renal function and recovery. Pronounced inflammation and/or infection may induce leukocytosis. Ultimately, renal biopsy is required for definitive diagnosis, although urinalysis, especially sediment evaluation, can provide valuable clinical insight in cases of parasitic, bacterial, or fungal nephritis. In cases of bacterial or fungal nephritis, culture and sensitivity or, better still, MIC testing, is always indicated.

Prognosis and Prevention. Prognosis is dependent on the degree of renal damage and the success of treatment. Following treatment, iohexol clearance can be repeated to monitor renal function for long-term prognosis. Some conditions are associated with obligate pathogens, and strict attention to quarantine and preventative health programs should be effective for prevention. Many bacterial infections, however, are opportunistic and involve commensal flora. In these cases, some degree of immunosuppression is often considered a predisposing factor and may include inappropriate environment, poor nutrition, inappropriate multianimal grouping, and unsanitary conditions.

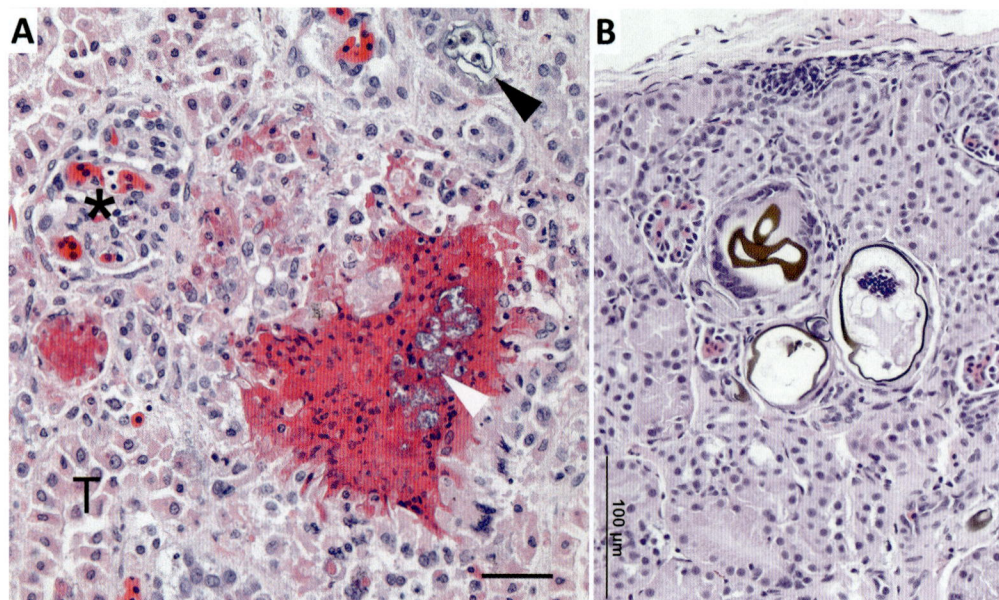

FIG 66.29 (A) Kemp's ridley turtle (*Lepidochelys kempii*), bacterial nephritis. Heterophils and macrophages infiltrate tubules (T) and the renal interstitium, forming heterophilic granulomas containing bacteria (white arrowhead). Also shown are a tubule containing mineralized material (black arrowhead) and a glomerus (asterisk) bordering the inflammation (H&E, bar = 50 µm). (B) Histologic section demonstrating a *Spirorchis* nematode within the kidney of a *Trachemys* slider (H&E, bar = 100 µm). (A, Courtesy of Brian Stacy, National Oceanic and Atmospheric Administration Fisheries; B, courtesy of Stephen J. Divers.)

Treatment. In addition to general supportive measures, a definitive diagnosis will dictate specific antibacterial, antifungal, antiparasitic, or antiviral therapies. The appropriate use of culture and sensitivity or MIC data to direct treatment cannot be overemphasized. In humans with severe renal insufficiency, there are specific drug dose reductions/ modifications that have been formulated when using drugs that are renally excreted. Although no such determinations have been made for reptiles, it would be wise to monitor for potential drug accumulation and toxicity if using renally excreted drugs. Serial monitoring of drug levels probably provides the most accurate means of therapeutic management.

Toxic Nephropathy

Toxic nephropathies have been associated with aminoglycosides and exogenous vitamin D_3 supplementation. While any aminoglycoside can cause nephrotoxicity, gentamicin has been well-documented in snakes.[69,70] Heavy metals, including lead, tend to bioaccumulate in liver and kidney tissues and might be expected to compromise function.[71] Exogenous vitamin D_3 supplementation may be used by some to avoid the expense of providing broad-spectrum lighting; however, this can result in soft tissue mineralization, including the kidneys (see Fig. 66.20B). Radiographic demonstration of metallic gastric foreign bodies with elevated blood levels are diagnostic for heavy metals. Vitamin D_3 (25-hydroxcholecalciferol) assays are available commercially. Other toxicities are difficult to confirm because assays and testing are toxin-specific. Preserving frozen tissues following necropsy can be helpful if, following histological evaluation, further toxicological investigations are warranted. Diuresis, physical removal, and chelation therapy for heavy metals, and preventing further exposure, are the mainstays of treatment.

Renal oxalosis has been documented in both health and unhealthy green turtles (*Chelonia mydas*) and desert tortoises (*Gopherus agassizii*).[72,73] While it is often stated that captive herbivorous reptiles should not be fed plants that contain substantial amounts of oxalate (e.g., spinach), it is highly likely that herbivores have evolved tolerance for modest oxalate ingestion. It is notable that no cases of oxalate urolithiasis have yet been documented in reptiles. However, the diagnosis of subclinical oxalosis in two herbivorous chelonian species suggests that additional investigation of oxalate tolerance is indicated.

Urolithiasis

Urolithiasis (cystic calculi, ureteroliths, cloacal uroliths) has been reported in chelonians and lizards.[74–77] Urolith location may be anywhere along the urinary tract, including the kidneys, ureters and cloaca; however, cystic calculi are most common.[78] Most uroliths are composed of urate salts, however, calcium-phosphate, -carbonate, -oxalate, and mixed compositions have been reported.[74–77] Postrenal obstruction, either by ureteroliths or uroliths lodged within the urodeum, can result in renal failure.[76]

Clinical Significance and Known Etiological Cause(s). It has been proposed that chronic dehydration, high-protein diets, and overheating may factor in the etiology of urolithiasis.[74] Urine modification occurs across the bladder epithelium with water reabsorption along a concentration gradient resulting in further urine concentration (but not exceeding that of plasma).[33,79] Therefore chelonians will often not urinate until they have the ability to drink and replenish their bladders. Consequently, chronic dehydration, overheating, and lack of drinking water are likely to increase water absorption from the bladder, leading to supersaturation of urates, which, along with prolonged urine retention, may predispose to urolith formation. Small cystic calculi probably do not cause significant problems other than minor irritation. Larger stones, because of their size and weight, can act as space-occupying lesions and result in severe cystitis, pressure necrosis of the bladder wall and internal viscera, and coelomitis.

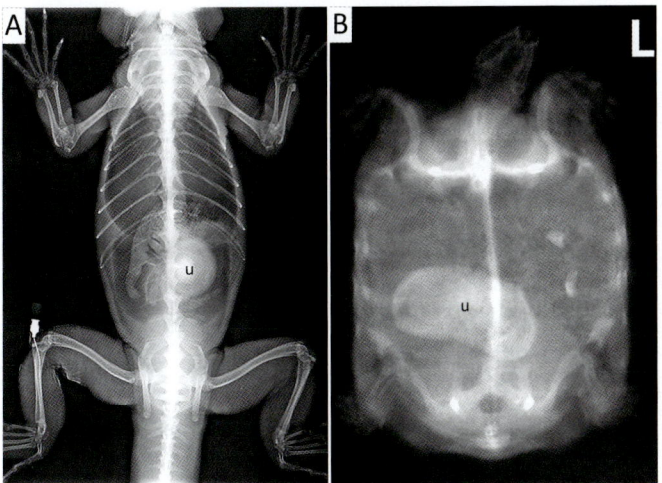

FIG 66.30 Cystic uroliths (*u*) within the bladders of (A) *Iguana* lizard and (B) *Testudo* tortoise. (Courtesy of Stephen J. Divers.)

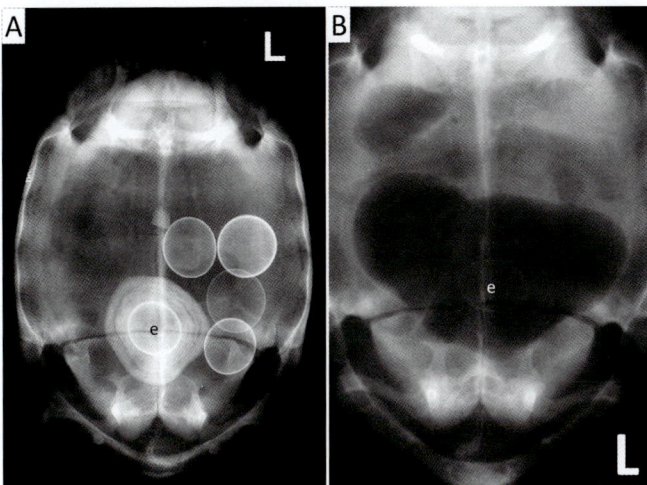

FIG 66.31 (A) *Testudo* tortoise with several retained eggs; however, one egg (*e*) is within the bladder and, as a nidus, has led to the development of a cystic calculus. (B) Pneumocystography to demonstrate the presence of a poorly mineralized egg (*e*) within the bladder of a *Testudo* tortoise. (Courtesy of Stephen J. Divers.)

Clinical Presentation and Diagnostic Confirmation. Many cystic calculi probably have protracted subclinical courses; however, anorexia, constipation, tenesmus, dystocia, dysuria, poor growth, cloacal prolapse, lethargy, hind limb paresis, and lack of fecal/urine production may become apparent. Palpation of the prefemoral fossae of chelonians, caudal coelom of lizards, or per cloaca may reveal a hard structure. Gentle rocking of the patient from side to side often allows for digital ballottement of large calculi. There may be a predisposition, in chelonians, for cystic calculi to be located in the left lobe of the urinary bladder.[74] Hematology, plasma biochemistry, and urinalysis do not appear to be routinely beneficial in the diagnosis of urolithiasis in reptiles; however, obstructive uroliths may cause biochemical changes indicative of postrenal obstruction, and severe cystitis may result in leukocytosis and hematuria.

Urinary calculi are most easily confirmed by radiographic demonstration of radio-opaque, rounded laminar structures in the caudal coelom, intrapelvic, or cloacal regions (Fig. 66.30). While urate calculi are sometimes radiolucent in mammals, reptilian stones are often composed of potassium or calcium urate salts and are radiodense. Variable mineral complexes result in variable radiographic appearances and, rarely, calcium apatite or calcium phosphate stones have been reported.[74,76,80] Ultrasonography, CT, MRI, or cystoscopy can also be useful in select cases. Urolith evaluation can include chemical analysis, infrared spectroscopy, optical crystallography, radiographic microanalysis, and scanning electron microscopy, with radiographic microanalysis and scanning electron microscopy providing nondestructive, rapid analysis, for both the exterior and interior of stones.[81]

Preferred Medical or Surgical Treatment(s). There are no medical dissolution recommendations for reptile uroliths, and surgical removal is recommended. Cystic calculi can be removed during coeliotomy and cystotomy, with recurrent cases managed with cystectomy (see Chapters 97 through 101 and 104).[82] Care must be taken to avoid contamination of the coelom as bladder contents are seldom sterile, and in addition to perioperative antibiotics, thorough irrigation of the coelom should be performed after bladder surgery. Cystic and cloacal calculi can be endoscopically removed through the vent.[78] There are few reports of endoscopic laser lithotripsy in reptiles, which describe variable success; however, extracorporeal shockwave lithotripsy does not appear to have been tried but may be worthy of consideration given reported success in humans.[83,84]

Prognosis and Prevention. The prolonged subclinical stage of cystic calculi has prompted many clinicians not to treat this condition. However, a retrospective study has indicated urolithiasis as a cause of death in 50% of chelonians necropsied with urolithiasis.[74] The prognosis following surgical removal is good, although recurrence is possible. Reducing dietary protein of herbivores, ensuring appropriate thermal and humidity gradients, and adequate provision of water are probably important for prevention.

Ectopic Eggs in the Urinary Bladder

Retrograde displacement of shelled eggs into the urinary bladder has been documented in chelonians (Fig. 66.31).[85,86] In some cases there is a previous history of oxytocin therapy to induce laying. Like cystic calculi, ectopic eggs can traumatize the bladder mucosa and act as a nidus for infection and urolith formation. Egg removal from the chelonian bladder can be pursued via traditional plastronotomy or prefemoral coeliotomy but has also been successfully performed cystoscopically.[85,86] Saline-infusion cystoscopy is used to identify and isolate the egg, and a variety of techniques have been used to fragment and remove egg material. Thorough lavage of the bladder ensures complete removal of egg fragments and contents. Endoscopic snares and baskets may be useful for retrieving eggs during cystoscopic visualization.

Neoplasia

A variety of urinary neoplasias have been reported from snakes, lizards, and chelonians, but not, as yet, crocodilians. Renal adenomas, adenocarcinomas, neofibroblastoma, fibroma, myxofibroma; cloacal carcinoma, transitional cell carcinoma, sarcoma, and ureteral transitional cell carcinoma have been reported (Fig. 66.32).[87] Few clinical signs have been reported and have typically been nonspecific; however, firm swellings associated with the caudal coelom (75%–95% snout-to-vent) of snakes, or the caudodorsal coelom or tail base dorsal to the cloaca of lizards, should be treated with suspicion.

Miscellaneous Diseases

Renal cysts, fibrosis, renal edema, renal amyloidosis, and cholesterol deposition have been reported.[4,88,89] Patent urachus and yolk coelomitis was diagnosed in a neonate prehensile-tailed skink (*Corucia zebrata*). Clinical signs included coelomic swelling, weakness, and dehydration. Diagnosis was confirmed by contrast radiography per cloaca, and surgical ligation was successful.[90]

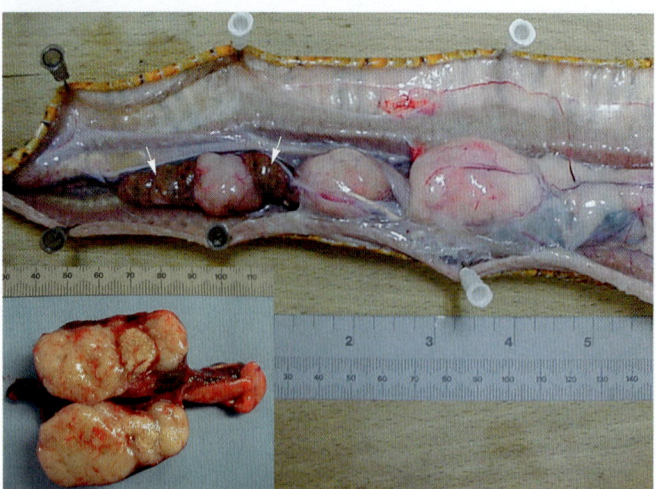

FIG 66.32 Renal carcinoma in a corn snake (*Pantherophis guttatus*) with little normal renal tissue visible (arrows). (*Inset*) Cut surface of the neoplasm again demonstrating replacement of normal renal tissue with neoplasm. (Courtesy of Stephen J. Divers.)

CONCLUSION

Urinary tract disease remains an important veterinary consideration; however, much remains to be learned about reptile urologic pathophysiology. In many cases, initiating causes are often inferred from poor management or extrapolated from histopathologic interpretations made late in the course of the disease or too often, at necropsy. The link between parathyroid hormone and renal disease in humans has been well documented, and given the high prevalence of clinical (and subclinical) nutritional secondary hyperparathyroidism in many captive-reared reptiles, this certainly warrants further investigation. Along with hyperparathyroidism, chronic dehydration, overheating, and protein excess appear to be common predisposing factors, especially in herbivores.

In cases of chronic renal disease, clinical signs and biochemical changes are unlikely to become apparent until late in the disease. Iohexol clearance appears to be a safe and practical method for estimation of GFR in practice. Endoscopic evaluation provides a safe and effective means for visualization and biopsy of kidneys. Appropriate therapeutic and surgical decisions (including euthanasia) can only be made after an accurate diagnosis.

ACKNOWLEDGMENTS

The authors would like to acknowledge the profound influence of those that have contributed to our clinical knowledge of reptile urology, notably Doug Mader and Peter Holz, whose efforts in producing the previous chapter and edition have remained foundational for the current chapter.

REFERENCES

See www.expertconsult.com for a complete list of references.

67

Hepatology

Stephen J. Divers

The reptilian liver is similar in structure and function to that of other vertebrates. It is the largest single visceral organ and may be elongated in snakes and some lizards, or transverse in testudines and other lizards. Liver disease is not uncommon in reptiles, and yet a review of spontaneous hepatopathies indicates that the vast majority of cases have been diagnosed postmortem.[1–11] This implies deficiency in the current clinical approach to hepatobiliary disease diagnosis. Therefore the aim of this chapter is to familiarize the clinician with hepatic anatomy and physiology and provide clear guidance on antemortem diagnosis of hepatobiliary diseases in reptiles.

ANATOMY

The embryonic liver originates from the endodermal gut with the hepatic diverticulum branching as it advances, giving rise to the bile ducts and gallbladder.[12] The formed organ is typically (except in snakes) bilobed, dark brown to almost black in some species, and comprises about 4% to 5% of body weight in most squamates. In temperate species, the liver tends to weigh more in the fall before hibernation when glycogen and intrahepatic fat stores are maximal; however, great interspecies variation exists. The liver of snakes typically lies alongside the right lung or is retroperitoneal along the dorsal body wall, 30% to 58% snout-to-vent depending on taxa, with the heart cranial and the stomach caudal (Fig. 67.1A).[13] The saurian liver is often divided into left and right lobes, although some species may possess a large middle or even accessory lobes. The liver of lizards is usually triangular in shape and traverses the cranial to mid coelom (see Fig. 67.1B).

The chelonian liver is large and traverses the cranial coelom. The smaller, left lobe is connected to the concave side of the stomach by the gastrohepatic ligament, and the right lobe is attached to the duodenum by the hepatoduodenal ligament (Fig. 67.2). The coronary ligament connects the chelonians liver to the transverse septum, while the pericardial sac rests in the depression between the left and right lobes. A very short mesentery, equivalent to the falciform ligament of other vertebrates, attaches the liver to the parietal peritoneum. This mesentery contains the ventral abdominal veins that carry blood from the caudal coelom and viscera to the portal vein. In crocodilians, the liver occupies a large portion of the cranial to mid coelomic cavity, more so on the right. During inspiration, the liver is pulled caudad, allowing the lungs to expand, and although not homologous to the mammalian diaphragm, there are certainly some functional similarities.

The blood supply to the liver includes the portal vein and hepatic artery (Fig. 67.3). The portal vein is variably formed by the anastomosis of the anterior abdominal, gastric, lienogastric, and intestinal veins.[12] Additional venous supplies may come from the dorsal gastroesophageal and parietohepatic veins.

Although the parenchyma is one continuous mass of cells, it is not functionally homogenous. However, the reptilian liver is less clearly divided into lobules compared to its mammalian counterpart, and metabolic zonation, common in mammals, is difficult to appreciate in reptiles. Portal tracts may consist of a bile duct and a portal vein branch surrounded by a small amount of connective tissue; however, the distribution of portal tracts is not uniform (Fig. 67.4). Histologic cross-sections suggest that the hepatocytes are arranged in a tubular or trabecular fashion, but most of these cords are arranged in sheets or plates. The reptilian hepatocyte shares many similarities with its mammalian counterpart, and there are three additional main cell types that form the hepatic sinusoids, namely the endothelial cells, macrophages (including Kupffer cells), and stellate or Ito cells. The sinusoids are lined by a thin layer of endothelial cells, and filamentous material between these cells and the hepatocytes may play an insufflating role in ectotherms, maintaining metabolism despite variations in body temperature. The Kupffer cell is an intraluminal macrophage attached to the endothelium, charged with clearing the portal blood of intestinally derived endotoxins. A second macrophage is perisinusoidal and is variably pigmented. Clusters of these macrophages or melanomacrophages are numerous in a parasinusoidal position in amphibians and reptiles and are believed to be responsible for the removal of free radicles. The stellate cell, Ito cell, or lipocyte has been well-studied in various reptiles. They lie between the endothelium and sinusoidal surface of the hepatocyte and are numerous in crocodilians but less so in testudines. The cytoplasm of the resting form contains round, fat droplets, which, being rich in vitamin A ester, are the main site of vitamin A storage.

The bile canaliculi form a meshwork throughout the parenchyma. Most reptiles have a gallbladder embedded within the caudal margin of the right lobe; however, in snakes it is distinct and caudal to the liver. The gallbladder of colubrid snakes splits into many branches, forming a biliary plexus that joins the cystic duct. The common bile duct passes to the right of a small spherical gallbladder and through the pancreas to the ampulla of Vater, where it is joined by the pancreatic duct before entering the small intestine. In some lizards, the common bile duct does not go through the pancreas but enters the ampulla directly. In chelonians, peristaltic contractions have been noted in the gallbladder and common duct, beginning at the fundus and proceeding down to the duodenum. These contractions are stimulated by the presence of fat in the duodenum.

PHYSIOLOGY

Hepatic metabolism changes as the reptile develops from egg to hatchling to adult. In addition there are annual cycles in those animals that hibernate. The rate of hepatic metabolism in adult reptiles is similar to that of the kidney and only slightly less than that of the heart. Liver function is sensitive to changes in temperature and decreases sharply in a linear fashion when core body temperature falls. One of the most important functions of the liver is to supply glucose. The normal precursor of glucose in the hepatocyte under aerobic conditions is glycogen. Glycogenolysis is a multistep enzymatic process similar to that documented in mammals. The liver can produce glucose from pyruvate, lactate, fats, and some amino acids by gluconeogenesis. Blood glucose levels typically vary between 25 and 150 mg/dL (1.38–8.26 mmol/L). Reptiles do not incur cerebral cortical damage at the very low blood glucose levels measured during hibernation and after prolonged dives. Some reptiles maintain blood glucose during prolonged fasting as well

as glycogen stores (mainly derived by gluconeogenesis) from protein sources. Consequently, metabolic reserves are depleted and insulin levels fall. Hepatic glycogen storage is maximal in the fall in those animals that hibernate and becomes quickly depleted during hibernation. When glycolysis switches from aerobic to anaerobic, hepatic and muscle tissues produce lactate, which under aerobic conditions is converted to pyruvate in the liver. The resulting lactic acidosis causes a drop in blood pH and heart rate, even if the animal is active (e.g., during a dive).

Unlike mammals, fat is not stored in subcutaneous sites, but instead reptiles tend to possess discrete intracoelomic fat bodies. The main purpose of this fat is to supply material for vitellogenesis during the reproductive cycle and as an energy supply during most of hibernation,

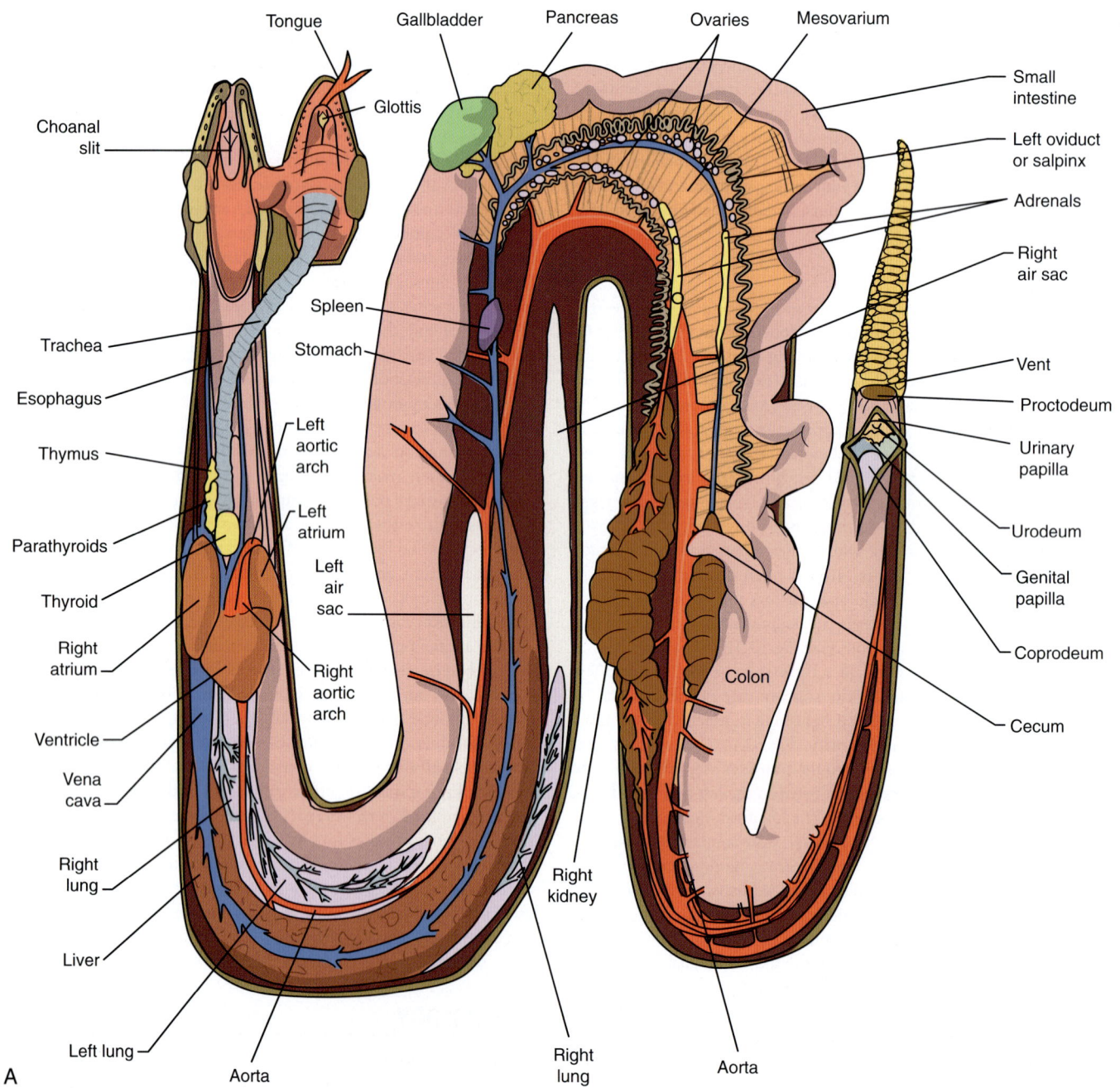

FIG 67.1 (A) Snake coelomic anatomy.

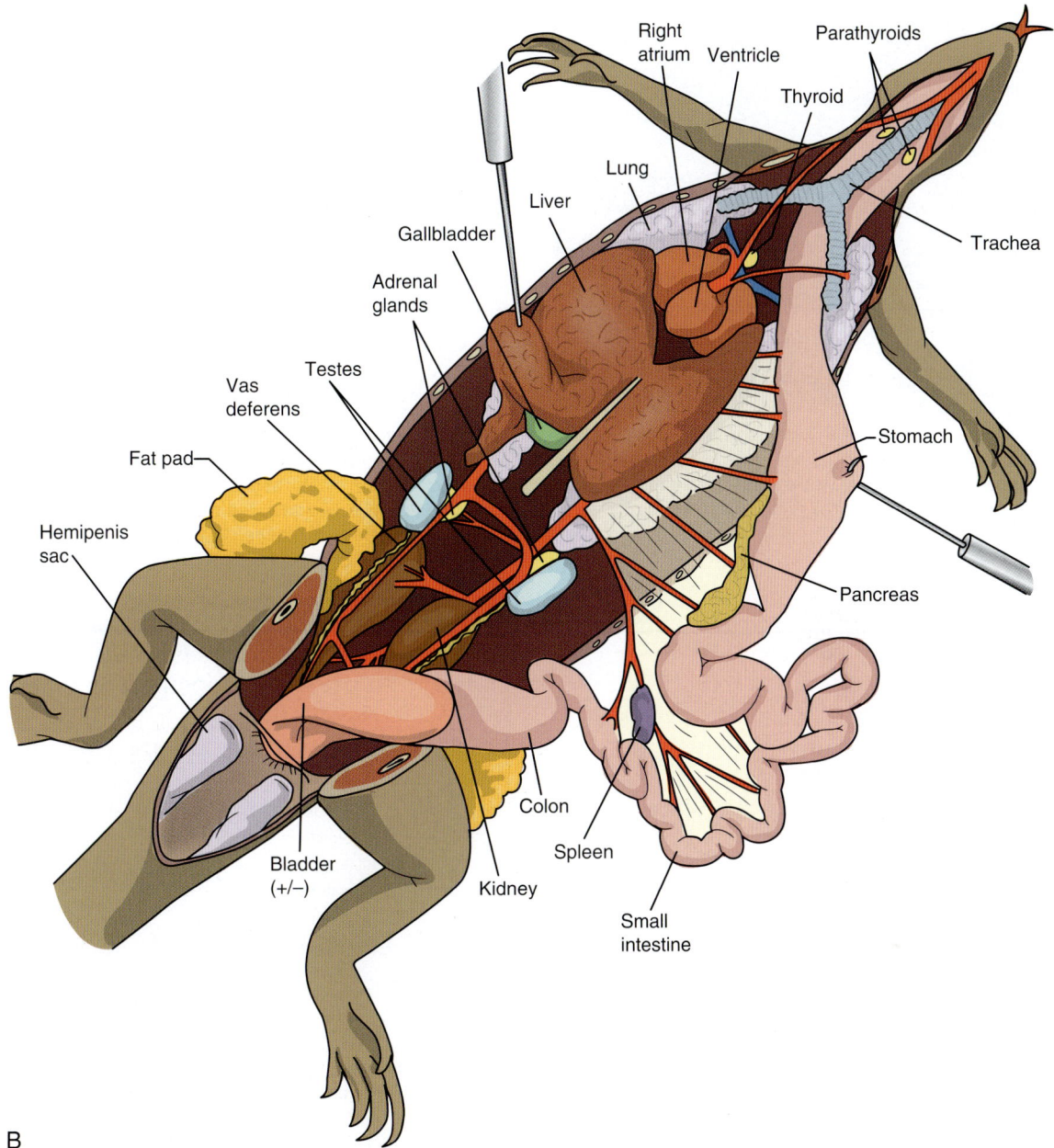

FIG 67.1, cont'd (B) Lizard coelomic anatomy.

periods of prolonged fasting, and in hatchlings following the absorption and translocation of yolk lipids. The fat content of the liver is highest just before hibernation and lowest at emergence. Typically, the livers of females tend to contain more fat than those of males; however, this additional fat should naturally become depleted after reproduction. Captive, temperate reptiles that are not permitted to hibernate, and females that are not permitted to reproduce, may go through annual cycles of increased fat deposition, resulting in obesity and hepatic lipidosis. Fat is transported to the liver as unesterified fatty acids and becomes esterified and lipoprotein-bound before entering the circulation. The liver also exports phospholipids and cholesterol.

Bile acids, derived from cholesterol, are only formed in hepatocytes and are important in lipid digestion and absorption. Bile acids of reptiles have been extensively studied from an evolutionary perspective with the most primitive bile acid, 3α-hydroxyl bile acids, found in all reptiles studied (Table 67.1). This is convenient as bile acid assays used in veterinary medicine measure this 3α-hydroxyl metabolite.

Reptiles can develop hyperbilirubinemia with jaundice/icterus due to impairment of bile flow, either intrahepatic or posthepatic. Most reptiles lack the biliverdin reductase and are reportedly unable to reduce biliverdin to bilirubin. However, snake plasma contains bilirubin and not biliverdin, although biliverdin may still be the predominant pigment in serpentine bile. The enzyme responsible for conjugation of bilirubin with glucuronic acid is less prominent, and the hepatic uptake of unconjugated bilirubin is much slower in snakes than in mammals. The plasma of indigo snakes (*Drymarchon* sp) contains 10 times more unconjugated bilirubin in the absence of hemolysis than that of other species of snakes. In addition, the bile of these snakes contains more than 95% biliverdin.

The liver is central to protein metabolism as it processes alimentary amino acids and peptides for the reptile's own distinctive proteins. The majority of the synthesis occurs in the endoplasmic reticulum of hepatocytes. During hibernation of temperate species, protein metabolism may actually increase with formation of more amino acids and amides.

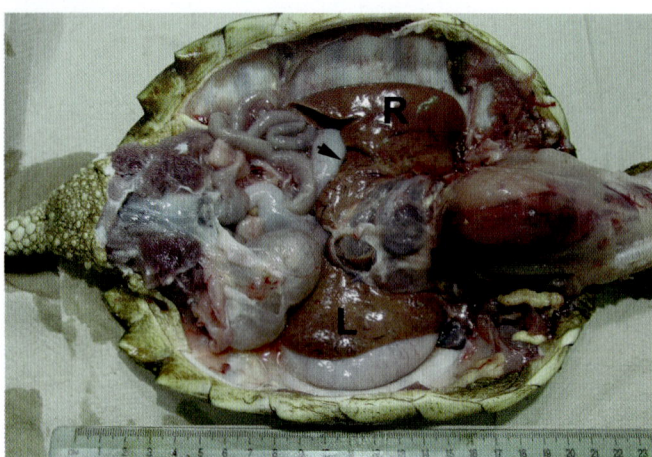

FIG 67.2 Gross coelomic anatomy of a juvenile snapping turtle (*Chelydra serpentina*) illustrating the smaller left (L) and larger right (R) liver lobes. The edge of the gallbladder is barely visible, embedded into the caudal aspect of the right lobe (arrow). Scale = cm. (Courtesy of Stephen J. Divers.)

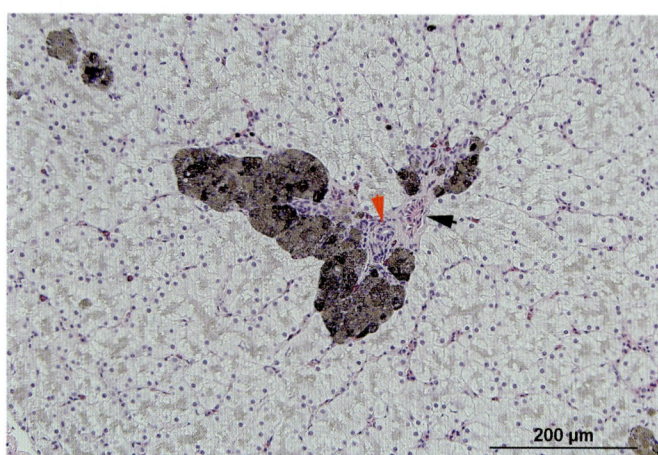

FIG 67.4 Histologic section of a healthy liver from an aquatic turtle (*Trachemys scripta*). In the center there is a portal tract containing a portal vein (black arrow) and bile duct (red arrow), surrounded by aggregates of heavily pigmented melanomacrophages. H&E, ×10, bar = 200 μm. (Courtesy of Stephen J. Divers.)

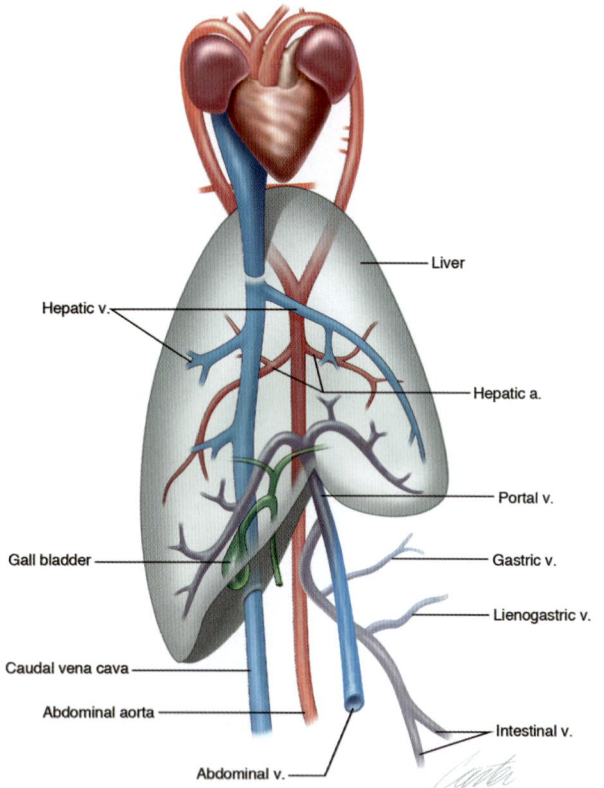

FIG 67.3 Diagram of the blood supply to the iguanid liver. (Courtesy of Kip Carter, Educational Resources, University of Georgia.)

TABLE 67.1	**Common/Known Bile Acids Found in Reptiles**						
		POSITION OF HYDROXYL GROUPS					
Order	**Family**	**3α**	**7α**	**12α**	**16α**	**22**	**23**	**24**
Turtles	Cheloniidae	X	X	X		X		
	Emydidae	X	X	X		X		
Lizards	Varanidae	X	X	X				X
	Iguanidae	X						
Snakes	Pythonidae	X		X	X			
	Viperidae	X	X	X			X	
	Crotalidae	X	X	X				
Crocodylians		X	X	X				

The liver is the only source of albumin, which is required for the carriage of many endogenous (e.g., calcium) and exogenous substances, and for maintaining the colloid osmotic pressure of plasma. The liver produces clotting proteins (including fibrinogen; prothrombin; and factors V, VII, VIII, IX, and XI) and is also responsible for the synthesis and degradation of carrier proteins. These include transferrin; ferritin; various hormone-transporting proteins for secretions of the thyroid, adrenal cortex, and pituitary, and more. During acute liver injury, carrier proteins may rise in plasma and behave like acute phase reactants. Fibrinogen and enzymes of hepatocellular origin may also participate in the response to acute hepatic injury. This is the basis for the widely used measurements of alanine transaminase (ALT), aspartate transaminase (AST), and sorbitol dehydrogenase (SDH) activities for assessing hepatocellular damage. Enzymes related to bile secretion include alkaline phosphatase (ALP), gamma glutamyl transferase (GGT), 5′ nucleotidase, and leucine aminopeptidases. The range of normal or observed activities of these and other hepatocellular enzymes has been documented in only a few reptilian species (see Chapters 34 and 35), although very few, if any, conform to the requirements for the establishment of reference ranges published by the American Society of Veterinary Clinical Pathologists.[14]

The liver also processes proteins prior to recycling or removal from the body. The amino groups may be used in transamination or converted to urea by the ornithine–citrulline-arginine cycle (Fig. 67.5). Urea is formed in hepatocellular mitochondria, and although the kidneys excrete most, some enters the intestinal tract, either in bile or by diffusion. Urea production in reptiles tends to be low and variable, having a more significant function in chelonians and crocodilians, especially aquatic species. Nucleic acids, especially those of purine origin, are degraded to uric acid by the liver and then secreted by the proximal renal tubules. This uricotelic process is present in some terrestrial chelonians but is most pronounced in the lizards and snakes. The most toxic nitrogenous waste product, ammonia, is produced by pyrimidine degradation and

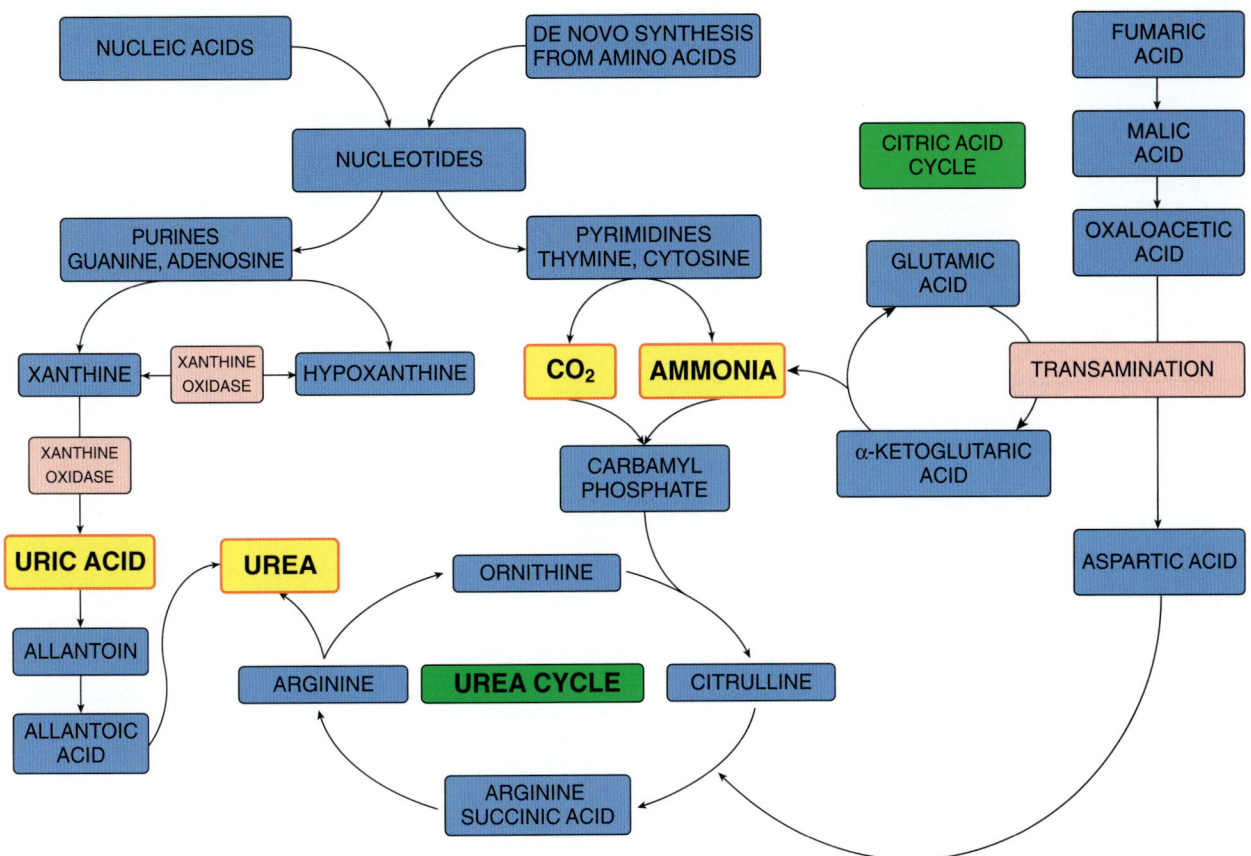

FIG 67.5 Hepatic nucleotide, amino acid, and nitrogenous metabolism in reptiles.

deamination of glutamate within hepatocytes. However, ammonia is combined with carbon dioxide to form carbamyl phosphate, which drives the urea cycle. The variability of ammonia, urea, and uric acid excretion is variable between species and affected by ecology (desert vs rainforest vs aquatic) and even the season (Table 67.2).[15] It would be a mistake for clinicians to rely solely on uric acid (often the only nitrogen parameter in commercial biochemistry reptile profiles) and to ignore the significant contributions of ammonia and urea in non-squamates.

The liver removes and degrades many hormones from the circulation, a process that may involve oxidation, reduction, and conjugation. The hepatic metabolism of progesterone has been examined in Shingle-back lizards (*Tiliqua rugosa*) and was found to be similar to that of mammals. Estrogen receptors have been identified within the liver of painted turtles (*Chrysemys picta*), with levels varying during the year but highest in the spring (preovulatory), with a smaller peak in the fall (vitellogenesis). Seasonal variations in the hepatic metabolism of adrenal hormones have been studied in some agamids (*Calotes* sp), with levels greatest in the spring and lowest in the fall. Epinephrine increases, and thyroidectomy decreases, hormonal metabolism by the liver. Vitellogenins, stimulated by estrogen, are the yolk protein precursors that are formed exclusively in the liver and transported to the ovaries by the general circulation.

CLINICAL INVESTIGATION

History and Physical Examination

The approach to hepatic disease investigation in reptiles is similar to that in mammals. Recently, the World Small Animal Veterinary

Association (WSAVA) published guidelines for the diagnosis of known hepatic diseases in dogs and cats.[16] Although these guidelines relate specifically to dogs and cats, they serve as a useful guide for the appropriate investigation of hepatobiliary disease in reptiles. They also serve as a useful reminder that just because a specific disease process has not been identified in reptiles, it does not mean that it cannot occur. As clinicians involved in the evolution of herpetologic medicine, we must continually strive to watch for the first case of a portal systemic shunt or hepatocutaneous syndrome.

Detailed information on performing a physical examination is covered elsewhere (see Chapter 42). Clinical signs, physical examination findings, and clinicopathologic abnormalities associated with hepatobiliary disease often reflect disruptions in normal structure and function. The liver possesses a large functional reserve, and therefore the appearance of potentially hepatic-associated signs such as icterus and ascites typically represents exhaustion of these reserves that occur late in the course of disease. Therefore any reptile exhibiting such signs should be investigated as a matter of urgency. Nonspecific signs including intermittent anorexia, vomiting, and lethargy can occur with diseases associated with the liver or a variety of other organ systems. Therefore diagnostic investigation is also required to differentiate from hepatic and nonhepatic diseases.

Historical events such as the ingestion of known hepatotoxic substances (e.g., aflatoxins, pyrrolizidine alkaloids) or treatment with potentially hepatotoxic drugs (e.g., NSAIDs, glucocorticoids) may suggest the presence of hepatobiliary disease. An obese reptile that becomes anorectic may be predisposed to hepatic lipidosis, while chronic hepatic disease often predisposes to gastrointestinal ulceration, hematemesis, coelomic pain, and melena.

TABLE 67.2   Nitrogenous End-Products Produced by Reptiles[15]

Species	% TOTAL NITROGEN[a]		
	Ammonia	Urea (BUN)	Uric Acid
Chelonia (freshwater aquatic to semi-aquatic)			
Common slider *(Trachemys scripta)*	4–44	45–95	1–24
West African mud turtle *(Pelusios castaneus)*	19	24	5
Common snapping turtle *(Chelydra serpentina)*	11	80	10
European pond turtle *(Emys orbicularis)*	14	47	3
Forest hinge-back tortoise *(Kinixys erosa)*	6	61	4
Chelonia (terrestrial)			
African spurred tortoise *(Centrochelys sulcata)*	3	20	55
Kleinmann's tortoise *(Testudo kleinmanni)*	4	49	34
Yellow-footed tortoise *(Chelonoidis denticulata)*	6	29	7
Greek spur-thighed tortoise *(Testudo graeca)*	4	22	52
Indian star tortoise *(Geochelone elegans)*	6	9	56
Western or ornate box turtle *(Terrepene ornate)*	23	47	30
Desert tortoise *(Gopherus agassizii)*	3–18	15–50	20–50
Squamata (Serpentes)			
Eastern racer *(Coluber constrictor)*	0	0	58
Diadem snake *(Spalerosophis diadema)*	4	2	69
Kenyan sand boa *(Gongylophis colubrinus)*	6	0	63
Squamata (Sauria)			
Cuban rock iguana *(Cyclura nubila)*	<1	1	98–99
Carolina anole *(Anolis carolinensis)*	13	13	73
Sandfish skink *(Scincus scincus)*	3	0	93
Crocodilia (freshwater)			
Nile crocodile *(Crocodylus niloticus)*	66	5	21
Spectacled caiman *(Caiman crocodilus)*	53	6	27
Crocodilia (marine)			
Saltwater crocodile *(Crocodylus porosus)*	77	21	2

[a]Calculated as % sum of the ammonia, urea, and uric acid when total nitrogen data were not available. Molecular weights of 18, 60.1, and 168.1 and percentages N of 83%, 46.7%, and 33.3% were used, respectively, in calculations.
From Campbell JW: Excretary nitrogen metabolism in reptiles and birds. In Walsh PJ, Wright P, eds. *Nitrogen Metabolism and Excretion.* London: CRC Press; 1995;147–178.

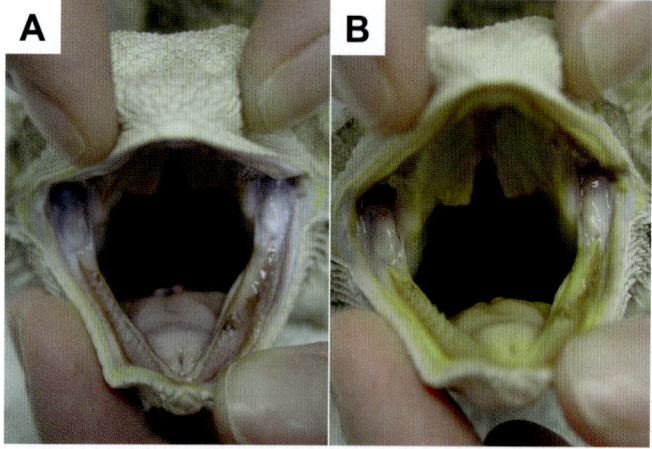

FIG 67.6 (A) Normal and (B) icteric appearance of the oral cavity in two bearded dragons *(Pogona vitticeps)*. (Courtesy of Stephen J. Divers.)

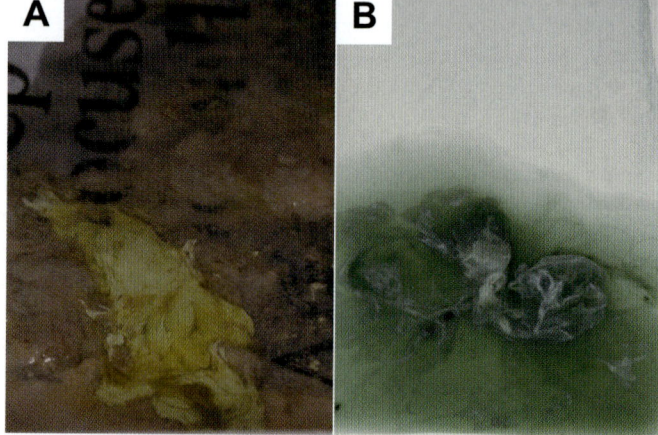

FIG 67.7 Voided urine from (A) a boa constrictor *(Boa constrictor)* and (B) a Greek tortoise *(Testudo graeca)*. Note the yellow to green pigmentation of the urine/urates. (Courtesy of Stephen J. Divers.)

The presence of icterus is the most significant and specific sign associated with hepatobiliary disease. In those squamates that produce bilirubin, a yellow discoloration to the mucus membranes may be obvious, while in other species, a more green pigment, especially in urine/urates, is often appreciated (Figs. 67.6 and 67.7). However, in many cases, mucous membrane pigmentation often complicates evaluation. Commonly reported in mammals, polyuria/polydipsia is seldom appreciated in reptiles; however, coelomic enlargement due to ascites or hepatomegaly, anorexia, poor body condition, neurologic depression, and lethargy might also be indicators of an underlying hepatic disorder.

TABLE 67.3 Plasma Enzyme Changes Following Hepatotoxin (Carbon Tetrachloride) Administration in Green Iguanas (*Iguana iguana*)

Enzyme	MEAN VALUES IN U/L					SUBJECTIVE DIAGNOSTIC VALUE	
	0 hrs (Pretoxin)	24 hrs	48 hrs	96 hrs	144 hrs	Sensitivity	Specificity
AST (aspartate transaminase)	28	1337	1022	1157	124	+++	++
ALT (alanine transaminase)	35	116	136	135	21	+	++
ALP (alkaline phosphatase)	16	17	17	21	16	-	+
SDH (sorbitol dehydrogenase)	12.0	178.0	156.4	106.0	5.6	++	+++
GGT (γ-glutamyltransferase)	<3	<3	<3	<3	<3	-	++
LDH (lactate dehydrogenase)	230	25,445	11,914	8107	688	+++	-

Data from Schnellbacher R et al, unpublished data.

Clinical Enzymology

Although evaluations of hepatobiliary enzymes (e.g., ALT, AST, ALP, GGT, and SDH) are routine in human and domesticated animal medicine, it would be wrong to assume that they are as reliable in reptiles (Table 67.3). All of the commercial enzyme measurements are designed for mammals and are run at 37°C. Very few studies have attempted to objectively measure hepatocellular enzyme activities in healthy reptiles, and even fewer have attempted to demonstrate changes following an hepatic insult. Very few, if any, of the published studies have managed to satisfy the requirements of the American Society for Veterinary Clinical Pathologists (ASVCP) for reference range determination. Therefore clinicians should be cautious of including or excluding hepatobiliary disease on the basis of plasma biochemistry results. Taking the green iguana (*Iguana iguana*) as an example, moderate activities of LDH and AST were found in many tissues, making differentiation between hepatic and nonhepatic (especially muscle) sources impossible.[17] Whereas, ALT and ALP activities were also generally low but again found in a variety of tissues. Recent research at the University of Georgia demonstrated significant elevations in a number of parameters, compared to controls, following an acute hepatotoxic insult (Schnellbacher et al, Proc ARAV, 2014, pp 127–128). AST, SDH, and LDH activities increased more than 15-fold and ALT increased 4-fold, whereas ALP and GGT did not change significantly (see Table 67.3). Nonhepatic tissue trauma (especially involving muscle) can also cause increases in AST and LDH, and these parameters are considered less specific. Enzyme activities remained high for at least 48 hours after insult, but decreased by day 6 in most cases. Therefore elevation of AST, ALT, LDH, and SDH are consistent with the initial phase of acute liver injury, but there is little information on the plasma half-lives of reptile hepatic enzymes. Furthermore, although the degree of enzyme activity is considered proportional to the degree of hepatobiliary damage, they are not predictive of hepatic function and therefore do not indicate prognosis.[19]

Plasma Proteins

Albumin is exclusively produced by the liver, but because of functional capacity and protein half-life, hypoalbuminemia is typically only seen during chronic hepatic disease. Liver cirrhosis may result in hypoalbuminemia, sodium, and water retention, and lead to ascites. Hypoalbuminemia is not specific and can occur secondary to protein-losing nephropathies/enteropathies, exudative cutaneous lesions (e.g., severe burns), vasculitis, acute blood loss, or excessive blood collection. Inadequate nutrition and systemic inflammatory conditions can curtail albumin synthesis. Unfortunately, the measurement of albumin by the bromocresol green dye-binding method has been shown to be inaccurate in turtles when compared to the gold standard of protein electrophoresis.[20] Recent work at the University of Georgia has also demonstrated inaccuracies between albumin measurements by bromocresol green when compared to electrophoresis in the bearded dragon (*Pogona vitticeps*) (Comolli et al, Proc ICARE, 2017, pp 575–576). Based upon current knowledge, the measurement of albumin in chelonians and bearded dragons by bromocresol green is inaccurate. Until proven otherwise, the accuracy of albumin measurements in all reptiles by anything other than protein electrophoresis should be considered questionable.

The plasma globulin fraction is composed of immunoglobulins and nonimmunoglobulins, and hepatic impairment can result in decreases in α- and β-globulins. However, because many immunoglobulins are acute phase proteins and hepatic production is increased during systemic response to inflammatory disease, hepatitis may actually lead to hypergammaglobulinemia.[22] Some commercial laboratories are able to offer acute phase protein assays, including C-reactive protein, haptoglobin, and amyloid A, although their accuracy and relevance to reptile diseases have not been proven.

Coagulation abnormalities are common in mammals with severe hepatopathy, but appear to be rare in reptiles where the extrinsic and common pathways are thought to play major roles in coagulation. The extrinsic pathway can be assessed using prothrombin times (PT); however, the use of commercially available tests using mammalian thromboplastin results in prolonged coagulation times or lack of coagulation. Recent investigations into PT in green iguanas (*Iguana iguana*) and red-eared sliders (*Trachemys scripta elegans*) using reptile-derived thromboplastin have demonstrated clotting times in the range of 22 to 37 seconds, which are not dissimilar to those reported in endotherms (Sladakovic et al, Proc ICARE, 2017, p 570). The value of activated partial thromboplastin time (APTT) in reptiles is likely negligible due to the relative lack of intrinsic pathway clotting factors. Although not completely understood, the impacts of temperature and calcium need to be considered when assessing coagulation in reptiles.

Ammonia

The liver is responsible for detoxifying ammonia of intestinal bacterial origin through the urea cycle (see Fig. 67.5). Ammonia is an important, but not exclusive, cause of hepatic encephalopathy; however, it is currently the only measureable toxin. Hepatic failure or shunting of portal blood away from the liver can result in hyperammonemia, although in mammals test sensitivity is greater for shunting disorders. The greatest issue facing testing is sample handling as blood must be collected into cold heparinized tubes and transported on ice for immediate laboratory evaluation. Currently, there is very little information on the use of ammonia in reptiles.

Uric Acid and Blood Urea Nitrogen

Decreased urea levels have been documented in mammals with severe hepatic fibrosis due to decreased hepatic production. It would also seem likely therefore that urea and uric acid levels, in ureotelic and uricotelic reptiles, would also be decreased due to decreased hepatic production. A recent study investigating hepatotoxin-induced hepatopathy in iguanas reported resting levels of urea and uric acid of 3.5 mg/dL and 4.1 mg/dL, respectively (Schnellbacher et al, Proc ARAV, 2014, pp 127–128). Peak levels of 11.5 mg/dL and 4.4 mg/dL were recorded at 96 hours postinsult. These elevations (rather than decreases) emphasize the many confounding variables that can influence urea and uric acid levels, which include hydration status, dietary protein content, recent feeding, gastrointestinal hemorrhage, glomerular filtration rate, drug therapy (e.g. allopurinol), and diuresis.

Bilirubin and Biliverdin

In those snakes that can reduce biliverdin to bilirubin, hepatobiliary disease would be expected to cause an elevation in unconjugated bilirubin. Although elevated bile pigments are more specific for hepatobiliary disease, they are generally less sensitive than hepatocellular enzymes. Hyperbilirubinemia and hyperbiliverdinemia can be prehepatic, hepatic, or posthepatic. Prehepatic causes include severe hemolysis and can be confirmed by demonstrating a decrease in packed cell volume. Hepatic causes can be due to impaired uptake, conjugation, or excretion, which cause severe intrahepatic cholestasis. Differentiation between hepatic and posthepatic causes is difficult but important as posthepatic conditions typically require surgical decompression of the gallbladder, and intrahepatic cases are treated medically. A recent experimental study in iguanas documented resting bilirubin levels of 0.2 ± 0.1 mg/dL, rising to 0.6 ± 0.1 mg/dL 96 hours following the administration of hepatotoxin (Schnellbacher et al, Proc ARAV, 2014, pp 127–128). However, for most nonserpentine reptiles measurement of biliverdin is required and, despite the existence of validated assays, few are commercially offered.[24]

Bile Acids

In normal animals during fasting, when the enterohepatic recirculation of bile acids is low, total serum or plasma bile acids are also low. In dogs and cats, bile acids are highly specific for hepatobiliary disease and are an ideal hepatic function test. However, with the exception of portosystemic shunts, the sensitivity of bile acids is insufficient to warrant use as a screening test, and the same may be true for reptiles.[19] In clinically healthy green iguanas and bearded dragons, mean fasting levels of 7.5 (range 2.6–30.3) µmol/L and 4.6 (range 0.8–33.7) µmol/L, respectively, have been documented (Cusack LM, Divers SJ, unpublished data).[25] Significant postprandial effects have also been demonstrated, and in iguanas, mean elevations to 33.3 ± 22.0 µmol/L have been recorded 3 hours postfeeding. In bearded dragons, mean elevations to 6.9 (range 1.4–37.6) µmol/L and 11.9 (4.3–31.0) µmol/L have been documented at 4 and 24 hours postfeeding. The duration of this postprandial effect has not been determined but suggests that reptiles should be fasted for several days prior to sampling, probably longer in large carnivorous species. A number of factors can affect total plasma bile acids, including degree of gallbladder emptying, rate of gastric emptying, intestinal transit rate, efficiency of ileal bile acid reabsorption, frequency of enterohepatic cycling, fat and amino acid content of the test meal, and amount of test meal consumed. Therefore a consistent approach to performing a bile acid stimulation test is important (Box 67.1).

BOX 67.1 **Recommend Bile Acid Stimulation Procedure for Reptiles**

Fast insectivorous and herbivorous lizards and chelonians for 3 days.

Fast carnivorous lizards, snakes, and small crocodilians for 7 days.

Fast large boids and crocodilians for 14 days.

Calculate daily maintenance calorific requirements and prepare full daily calorific provision using a commercial carnivore, omnivore, or herbivore critical care feeding diet.

At time 0, collect blood into heparin and then immediately assist feed by gavage tube.

(If ammonia testing is available, heparinized blood should also be submitted immediately for blood ammonia levels.)

Centrifuge and harvest plasma for resting 3α hydroxyl-bile acids.

At 4 hours, collect a postprandial sample.

(If ammonia testing is available, heparinized blood should also be submitted immediately for blood ammonia levels.)

Centrifuge and harvest plasma for resting 3α hydroxyl-bile acids.

Glucose

Hypoglycemia occurs in mammals with hepatic failure but is rare in cases of chronic disease. Given the already low resting glucose levels of most reptiles, and the effects of nutrition and handling stress, the detection of hypoglycemia may be difficult unless accurate baseline values for a specific patient have been repeatedly documented over time. Following hepatotoxin insult to iguanid livers, no significant changes in glucose levels were appreciated over a 6-day period (Schnellbacher et al, Proc ARAV, 2014, pp 127–128).

Cholesterol, Triglycerides, and Lipids

The liver converts fatty acids into triglycerides, which are either stored or released from the liver as very low-density lipoproteins (VLDL). Cholesterol may be synthesized within the liver or acquired through chylomicron remnants and low-density lipoproteins (LDL). Hepatic cholesterol can be esterified and secreted in lipoproteins or stored in the liver. Hypercholesterolemia can be associated with excessive production or decreased excretion (e.g., extrahepatic biliary obstruction). Normal female reptiles undergoing vitellogenesis often exhibit increases in cholesterol and triglycerides; however, sustained elevations or elevations in males are often seen in cases of hepatic lipidosis. There is a variable postprandial effect on triglyceride levels (less so for cholesterol) in bearded dragons, and fasting prior to sampling is recommended (Cusack LM, Divers SJ, unpublished data). In addition to cholesterol and triglycerides, some commercial laboratories offer lipoprotein profiles.

Urinalysis

Urinalysis in mammals is useful for the demonstration of ammonia biurate crystalluria and uric acid; however, given the variable expectation for such nitrogenous products in many reptiles, their diagnostic usefulness is probably limited as an adjunct to hepatic disease diagnosis. Bilirubinuria is considered abnormal in cats but not dogs. Only snakes appear capable of producing bilirubin in significant quantities, but the renal threshold for urinary bilirubin is unknown.

Hematology

Coagulopathies are rare, but bleeding could result in regenerative anemia. Nonregenerative anemia may be present in cases of chronic hepatobiliary disease, and normocytic, normochromic anemia would be expected

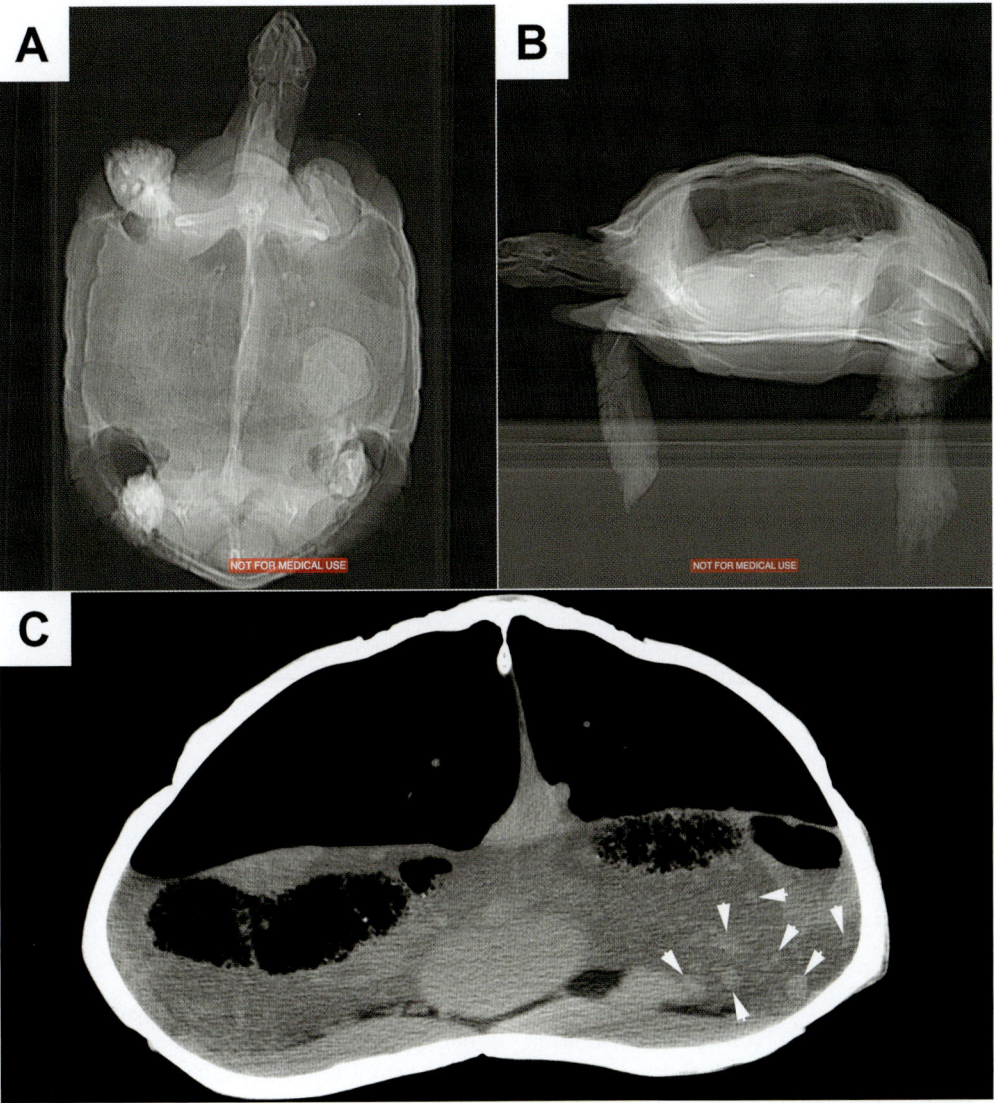

FIG 67.8 Radiographic and CT images from a male Texas tortoise (*Gopherus berlandieri*) that presented with an AST of 178 U/L. (A and B) Survey radiographs demonstrating a cystic urolith, but the hepatic region looks unremarkable. (C) CT image showing multiple nodules (arrows) throughout the left liver lobe. (Courtesy of Stephen J. Divers.)

because of inefficient utilization of systemic iron stores (anemia of chronic disease).

Radiography

The size, shape, and position of the liver can sometimes be determined from plain radiographs of the cranial coelom (see Chapters 54 through 57). Unfortunately, due to lack of diffuse, peri-organ, fat, serosal detail is typically poor in reptiles, and evaluation of liver margins is often not possible (Fig. 67.8A and B). In addition, although hepatomegaly can cause displacement of the stomach, there is little appreciation of changes in gastric axis in reptiles. Hepatomegaly commonly occurs due to infiltrative disease (e.g., neoplasia, lipidosis, amyloidosis) and inflammatory disease (e.g., bacterial hepatitis). Focal enlargement due to a neoplasm, cyst, granuloma, or abscess may be appreciated by displacement of adjacent tissues. Microhepatica, often associated with fibrosis and atrophy (including chronic cachexia), is seen as a decrease in the size of the liver silhouette. Normally the liver is homogenous in appearance. Mineralization can be diffuse (choledocholithiasis), or a focal discrete

opacity associated with the right liver lobe in lizards and chelonians, or just caudal to the liver in snakes. Gas opacities may be associated with abscesses or as a grave sign associated with severe necrotizing gastroenteritis.

Computed Tomography (CT)

The size and structure of the liver can be assessed using CT, in much the same way as in mammals (see Chapter 59) (see Fig. 67.8C).[27,28] Pre- and postcontrast images in both soft tissue and bone algorithms should be collected. Computed tomography can be used to detect alterations in the X-ray attenuation of hepatic parenchyma. In healthy juvenile sea turtles (*Chelonia mydas*) a mean attenuation value of 60.09 ± 5.3 Hounsfield units (HU) has been reported, and in general values between 50 to 70 HU are considered normal for chelonians.[29,30] However, in male captive red-footed tortoises (*Chelonoidis carbonaria*) hepatic values were much lower at 11.2 ± 3.0 HU and were attributed to multiple cases of hepatic lipidosis in the group, although this was not confirmed histologically.[31]

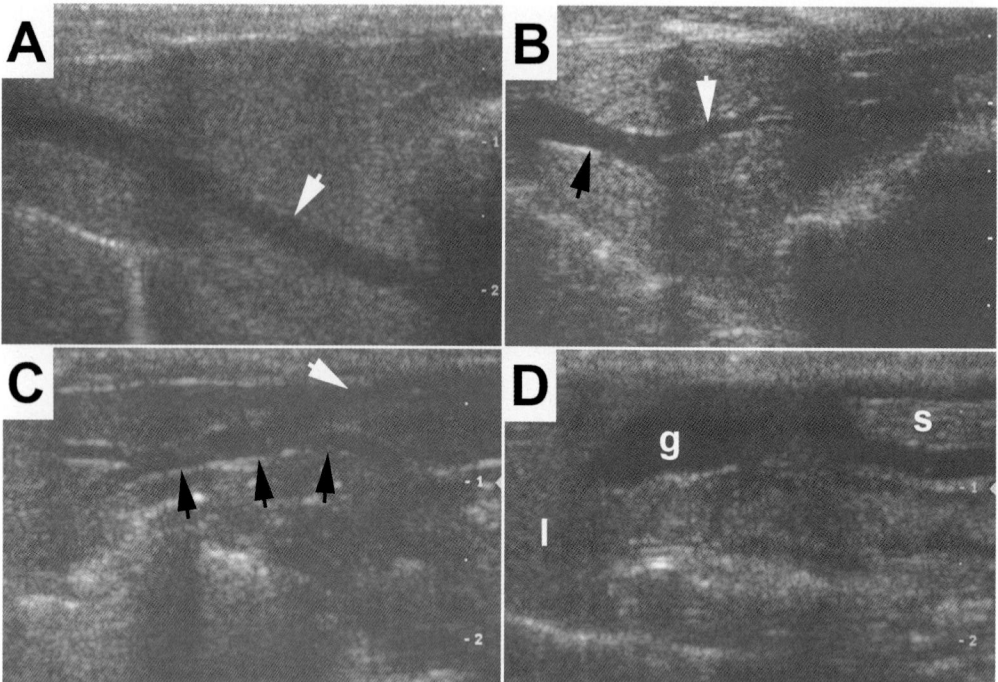

FIG 67.9 Ultrasonographic anatomy of the iguanid liver. (A) Saggital view of the right liver lobe with the intrahepatic portion of the vena cava visible (arrow). Note the homogenous hepatic echotexture. Cranial is to the left. (B) Oblique plane showing entry of a hepatic vein (white arrow) into the caudal vena cava (black arrow). Note the echogenic walls of the hepatic vein. Acoustic shadows from ribs are also present. Right cranial is to the left. (C) Saggital view of the portal vein at the porta hepatis. The portal vein (black arrows) can be seen accepting the ventral abdominal vein (white arrow) and then entering the liver. Cranial is to the left. (D) Saggital plane image of the gallbladder (g), which lies adjacent to the caudoventral surface of the liver (l), slightly to the right of midline. The aboral aspect of the pyloric portion of the stomach (s) is seen caudal to the gallbladder. Cranial is to the left. (Courtesy of Stephen J. Divers.)

Ultrasonography

Ultrasonography is useful for the evaluation of coelomic viscera, including the liver (see Chapter 58). However, despite the relatively few descriptions of ultrasonographic anatomy, it is generally considered useful for the differentiation between focal and diffuse disease, as well as assessment of displacement/compression, parenchymal changes, gallbladder disease, and vascular abnormalities.[32]

In the green iguana, hepatic parenchyma is of uniform echotexture with medium echogenicity, similar to that of the spleen, testes, and fat bodies (Fig. 67.9).[33] Hepatic lobation is generally indistinct. The gallbladder is easily identified adjacent to and partially embedded in the caudoventral border of the liver, right of midline. Gallbladder contents are normally anechoic, but small amounts of dependent material of mineral echogenicity can sometimes be identified. The subadult iguanid gallbladder is an elongated oval in the sagittal plane with mean ± SD long-axis dimensions of 1.67 ± 0.40 cm (1.00 to 2.72 cm), and mean short-axis dimensions in the sagittal plane of 0.67 ± 0.16 cm (range, 0.34 to 1.00 cm). However, significant linear correlations between body weight and gallbladder dimensions appear to be lacking. Preliminary investigations into contrast-enhanced hepatic ultrasonography have indicated that peak enhancement of 19.9% ± 7.5% (11.7%–34.6%) is achieved after 134.0 ± 125.1 seconds (59.6–364.5). However, as the distribution of contrast medium in iguanas differs from that of mammals, specific reference ranges of hepatic perfusion for diagnostic evaluation of the reptilian liver are still needed.[34]

Ultrasonographic liver anatomy has also been briefly described for the desert tortoise (*Gopherus agassizii*) via left and right mediastinal or cervicobrachial acoustic windows.[35] No descriptions of hepatic

parenchymal structure or measurements were given, although visualization of the gallbladder was limited by the amount of gastrointestinal gas present. The liver of the boa constrictor (*Boa constrictor*) has been described as uniformly heterechoic, fusiform, and primarily located on the right side of the coelom, with the vena cava ventral and hepatic vein dorsal.[36] The gallbladder, anechoic with hyperechoic wall, is located just caudal to the caudal margin of the liver, in close association with the pancreas, spleen, and fat body.

Magnetic Resonance Imaging (MRI)

The hepatobiliary system can be evaluated using MRI, with most current descriptions involving chelonians (see Chapter 60).[37,38] Image quality is largely dependent upon the size of the animal, strength of the magnet, and scanner software. In general, units capable of generating magnetic fields of 3+ tesla provide better quality images for most reptiles. The liver is more signal intensive in T_1-weighted images compared to those that are T_2-weighted (Fig. 67.10). In addition to hepatic size, parenchymal homogeneity can be assessed, and its fat content compared to that of fat bodies. The internal parenchymal structure is interrupted by vessels, which, along with the biliary system, are better evaluated using T_2-weighted images.

Endoscopy

Endoscopic techniques for the evaluation of the chelonian and saurian coelom have been well described (see Chapter 64).[39-41] Endoscopic evaluation of the liver provides magnified, color visualization of the

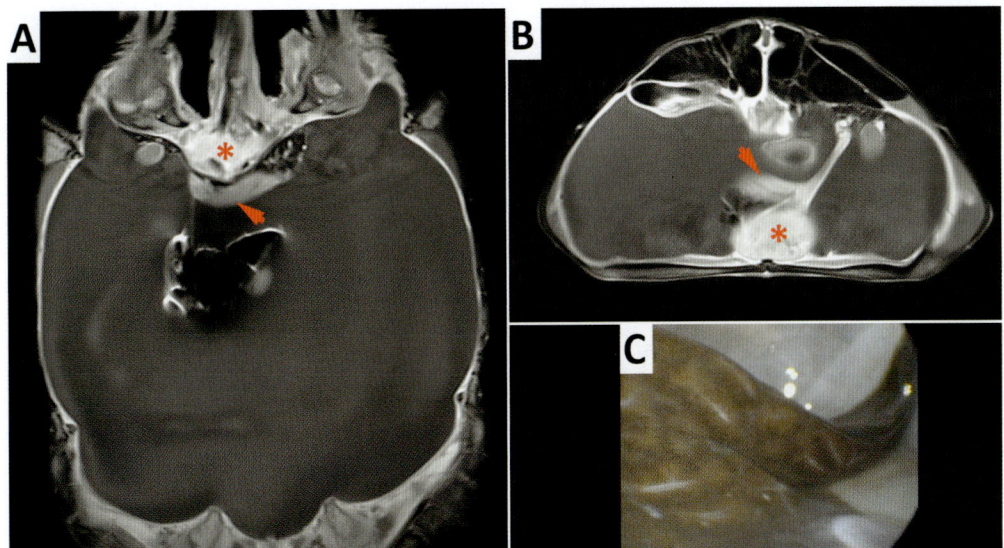

FIG 67.10 MRI of a desert tortoise (*Gopherus agassizii*) with microhepatica. (A and B) T1 postcontrast coronal (dorsal) and transverse images at the level of the heart (*) demonstrating microhepatica (arrow) and a coelom largely filled with fluid. (C) Endoscopic image of microhepatica. Histopathology demonstrated marked atrophy, hemosiderosis, and an absence of glycogen and lipid stores. (Courtesy of Stephen J. Divers.)

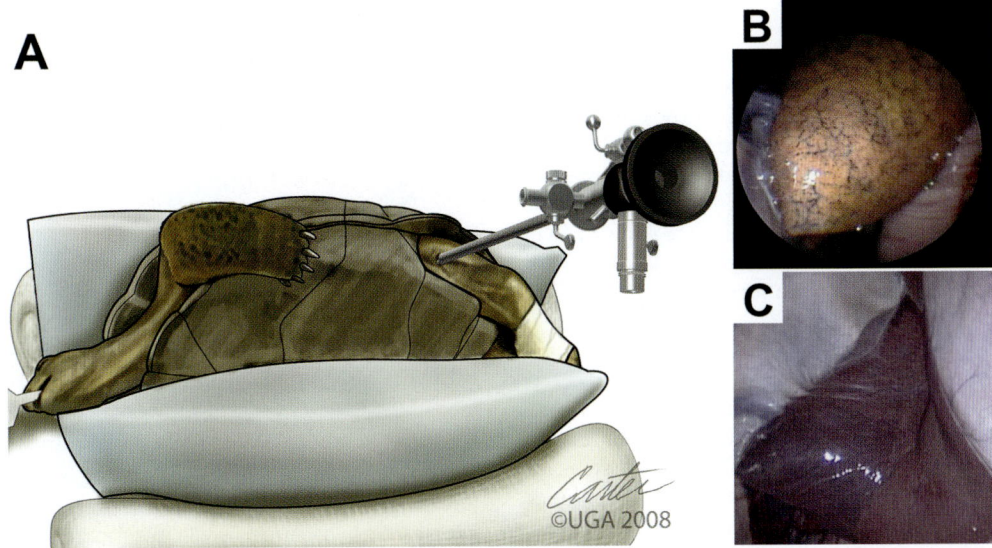

FIG 67.11 (A) Endoscopic examination of a chelonian from a left prefemoral approach. (B) Endoscopic view of the liver of an adult female slider (*Trachemys scripta*). Note the pale parenchyma and prominent sinusoidal pattern outlined by the melanomacrophages. This increased intrahepatic fat is physiologically normal in females preparing for folliculogenesis. (C) Endoscopic view of the liver in juvenile male Aldabra tortoise (*Aldabrachelys gigantea*). The parenchyma is not as pale due to reduced intrahepatic fat content, which is characteristic of healthy males. Intrahepatic fat would be expected to increase in males of temperate species during fall, in preparation for hibernation. Cranial is to the left. (Courtesy of Stephen J. Divers.)

hepatic surface and gallbladder, although deeper lesions can often be appreciated, especially if large. In addition, significant lesions can often be identified endoscopically, despite the lack of obvious clinicopathologic, radiographic, ultrasonographic, or cross-sectional imaging abnormalities. In laterally recumbent chelonians and lizards, a lateral prefemoral or paralumbar approach provides visualization of the ventral and dorsal surfaces of the ipsilateral liver lobe (Figs. 67.11 and 67.12). In dorsal recumbency, a prefemoral/paramedian approach provides access to the ventral surface of the entire liver. In green iguanas and red-eared sliders, entry of a 2.7-mm telescope within a 4.8 mm operating sheath and visualization of the liver from both left and right paralumbar approaches was easily performed without complications; however, the gallbladder could only be reliably seen from a right approach (see Fig. 67.12).[40,41] In snakes, a targeted coelioscopic approach is often required because, in most cases, no single entry can permit examination along the length of the entire liver. However, examination from within the air sac does permit evaluation over a much greater hepatic length.

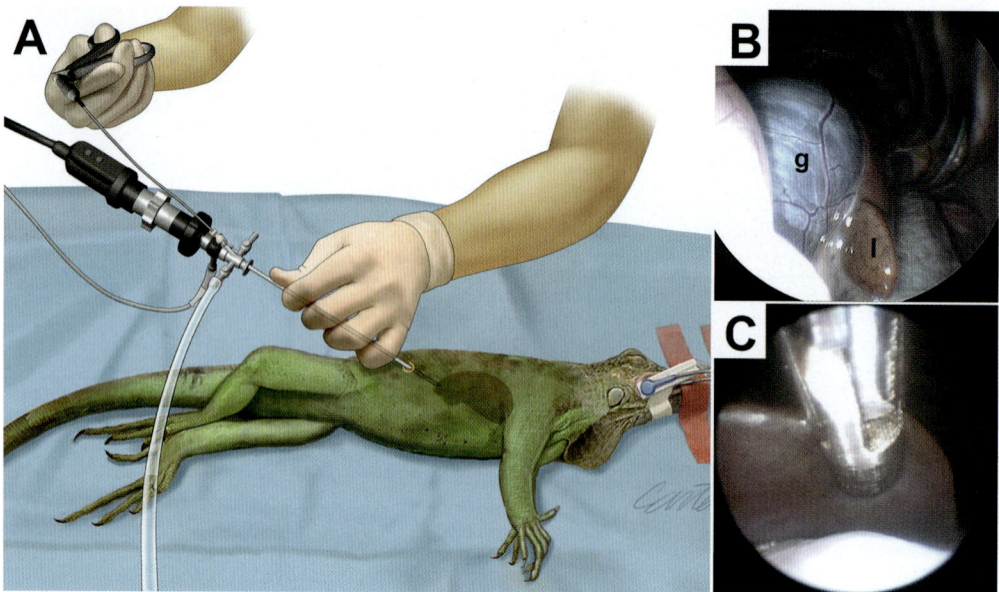

FIG 67.12 (A) Endoscopic examination of an iguanid liver via a right paralumbar approach. (B) Endoscopic view of the caudal edge of the right liver lobe (l) and the gallbladder (g). (C) Endoscopic biopsy of the liver using 1.7 mm (5 Fr) biopsy forceps. (Courtesy of Stephen J. Divers.)

Fine Needle Aspirate Cytology

Fine needle aspiration from the liver is possible under ultrasound or CT guidance. However, due to the loss of tissue architecture, such cytologic aspirates are generally inferior to endoscopic or surgical biopsy.[42,43] A recent study investigated hepatotoxin-induced disease in green iguanas, and invariably, ultrasound-guided fine needle aspirates were of poor diagnostic value (Fig. 67.13) (Schnellbacher et al, Proc ARAV, 2014, pp 127–128). Fine needle aspirates may be more useful in disease processes that are highly cellular (e.g., neoplasia) and for microbiologic evaluation, as well as when longer periods of general anesthesia carry unacceptable risks.

Biopsy

Clinicopathological changes may be attributable to hepatobiliary disease; however, they do not reliably differentiate between different disease processes and do not provide an accurate prognosis. In order to reach a definitive diagnosis it is essential to demonstrate both (1) an accurate host pathological response and (2) the etiologic or causative agent. While paired rising titers are definitive, there are few commercial assays available for reptiles, and those that are available typically require samples 6 to 9 weeks apart. Given the poorer diagnostic value of cytology compared to histopathology, tissue biopsy is generally preferred. Tissue biopsies can be used for histopathologic, microbiologic, parasitologic, and toxicologic evaluations and can typically provide a definitive diagnosis within days of collection. Indications for hepatic biopsy include elevations of hepatic enzymes (especially AST and SDH), bile acids, biliverdin/bilirubin, unexplained coelomic effusion/ascites, and hepatomegaly.[44] The most common complication concerning hepatic biopsy (especially following needle biopsy) is hemorrhage, and therefore consideration should be given to platelet count, PT, PTT, and buccal mucosal bleeding time. Biopsy samples may be collected using cutting biopsy needles (e.g., Tru-Cut), endoscopically, or by standard wedge or excisional surgical techniques.

Handling of biopsies must be undertaken with atraumatic instruments to minimize damage. Small endoscopic and needle biopsies should be gently shaken free into sterile saline, and not removed using cotton-tipped

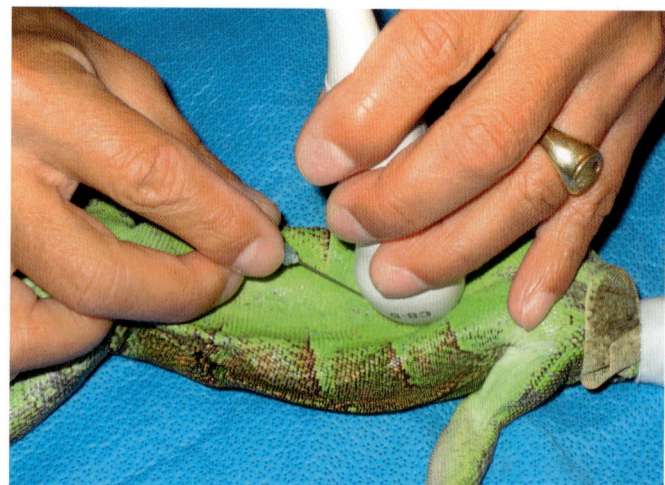

FIG 67.13 Ultrasound-guided fine needle aspiration of an iguanid liver using a 22-g hypodermic needle. Cytologic quality of hepatic aspirates were consistently poor and nondiagnostic. (Courtesy of Stephen J. Divers.)

applicators, or worse still, a hypodermic needle. Small samples are placed into labeled histology filters before being submitted in 10% neutral buffered formalin for histopathology. For transmission electron microscopy (TEM), glutaraldehyde is often preferred, while ethanol or methanol may be preferred for urate tophi or parasite evaluations. Tissue samples for microbiology often need to be sent in appropriate transport media depending upon whether fungal, bacterial, or viral investigations are most important. Additional biopsies can be frozen at −20°C while histopathology results are pending. Then, if histopathologically indicated, such frozen tissue can be submitted for specific microbiological (often virologic) investigations.

Ultrasound-guided, percutaneous hepatic biopsies have been reported from 1 to 25 kg boid snakes using an 18-g × 20-cm biopsy needle.[45] All collected biopsies were considered diagnostic, and all snakes survived; however, multiple biopsy attempts were required for some snakes and iatrogenic gastric perforation was documented in at least one animal.[45] Although general anesthesia is seldom employed for such biopsies in humans and dogs, it is still recommended for reptiles to ensure adequate restraint. Automated needles are preferred and operated by the ultrasonographer to ensure that vessels and other organs are not in the path of the needle. Holding an anesthetized reptile at maximum inspiration tends to improve localization and visualization of the liver. The biopsy site should be evaluated for postsample hemorrhage. Comparison between needle biopsies and wedge biopsy (gold standard) in dogs and cats has indicated an overall agreement on only 48%, and similar results would might be expected for reptiles.[46]

Endoscopic liver biopsies have been experimentally evaluated in green iguanas and freshwater chelonians (Fig. 67.14).[39,41] Biopsies were collected using 1.7-mm biopsy forceps, and each contained a mean of 1.9 and 3.1 portal tracts in iguanas and sliders, respectively. Although peripheral crush artifact was common, it was minimal, and all samples were considered diagnostic. No adverse effects of endoscopic hepatic biopsy were reported. Multiple samples can be readily collected and should be routinely submitted for histopathology, bacterial (aerobic/anerobic), and fungal cultures. Additional parasitic or toxicologic analyses can also be considered on an individual case basis. This technique enables gross evaluation of most, if not all, of the liver, extrahepatic biliary system, and surrounding structures. The ability to collect multiple samples from various hepatic locations decreases the risks of sampling artifact in cases of regional diversity within the liver. The standard oval/round cup biopsy forceps also produce less hemorrhage than biopsy needles, but if hemorrhage is encountered direct pressure can be applied by the closed biopsy forceps or a blunt probe, or radiosurgical coagulation can be used. Direct visualization of the hepatic parenchyma enables the clinician to correlate clinical data with liver appearance and histopathology to adjudicate the most accurate diagnosis.

Coeliotomy provides access to the liver for harvesting surgical biopsies. The advantages of open surgical access include the ability to collect larger liver samples, as well as an improved opportunity to completely evaluate and sample other visceral structures (e.g. intestines). Nevertheless, increased invasion and duration of anesthesia must be considered. Surgical biopsies can be collected using a standard wedge technique.[44] Hemorrhage can be controlled using hemostatic material (e.g., GelFoam) and digital pressure. Advantages and disadvantages are similar to those of endoscopy.

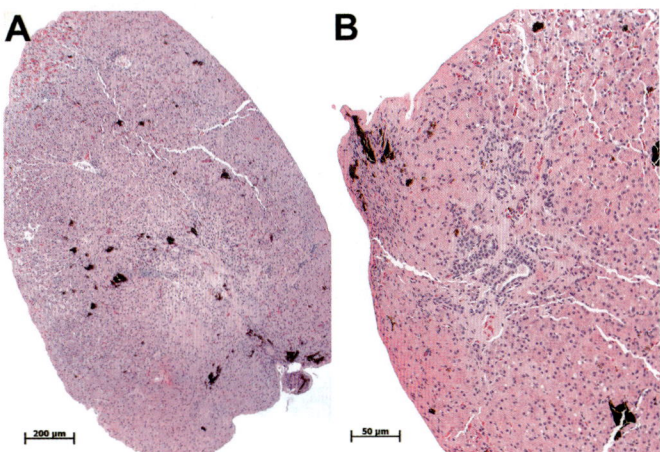

FIG 67.14 Iguanid liver biopsy collected using 1.7-mm (5Fr) biopsy forceps. (A) The specimen has minimal crush artifact confined to the periphery of the section. H&E, bar = 200 μm. (B) Mild hyperplasia of the biliary ductules is apparent. H&E, bar = 50 μm. (Courtesy of Stephen J. Divers.)

GENERAL APPROACH TO TREATMENT

Provision of species-specific thermal requirements must be provided initially. The route of drug therapy will be directed by the animal's condition at the time of presentation. Mild to moderate cases of hepatic lipidosis are usually anorectic on presentation but in good condition, and in these cases oral fluids are often adequate. Reptiles with more severe/acute hepatobiliary disease will often require intracoelomic, intravenous, or intraosseous fluid and drug administration. In cases of severe liver pathology it may be wise to avoid solutions containing lactate. Other medications may be employed at the clinician's discretion, but care should be taken not to invalidate future diagnostic investigations. For example, blood samples should be collected prior to fluid therapy, while antibiotic medication should be delayed until after liver biopsy and culture.

There are many different therapeutic approaches to treating liver disease. In general, for a treatment to be recommended there must be a well-established connection between pathophysiology and medicinal effects. For example, to appropriately treat a green iguana with clostridial hepatitis, the clinician would first and foremost need to make the definitive diagnosis by hepatic biopsy for histopathology and bacterial cultures (or PCR). Only then could the case be treated with an antimicrobial drug with demonstrated efficacy (either through disc sensitivity, minimum inhibitory concentration, or inherent biologic efficacy) against the organism and for which pharmacokinetic drug data for that species was known. In this case, such data is available to advocate the use of metronidazole for the treatment of clostrial hepatitis in the iguana.[47,48] The second, and indeed preferable, way a therapy can be scientifically proven to be effective is through randomized, double-blinded, and placebo-controlled clinical trials. Currently, as far as this author is aware, no such studies have been published for the treatment of any reptile disease. Table 67.4 provides an overview of medications that have been subjectively advocated for the treatment of liver disease in reptiles.

Ascites is typically a late decompensatory sign in the course of chronic liver disease due to portal hypertension and/or hypoalbuminemia. Diuretics should be used with caution in cases of concurrent hepatic encephalopathy, because alkalosis and hypokalemia both exacerbate the production of more toxic forms of ammonia. Indeed, ammonia levels may be low because the toxic form enters cells, becomes ionized, and subsequently sequestered. This cellular ammonia trap is best avoided by using potassium-sparing diuretics such as spironolactone.[49] Free coelomic fluid can account for more than the entire circulating volume, and the renin-angiotensin-aldosterone system is likely activated during this time, resulting in sodium and water retention and potassium loss. Cautious coelomocentesis is the best approach to avoid complications of hepatic encephalopathy. While in animals that are anorectic, fluid therapy and potassium supplementation are required. Sodium restriction should be considered if portal hypertension (e.g., secondary to hepatic fibrosis) is likely.

Intestinal protein digestion produces ammonia and aromatic amino acids that must enter the general circulation to cause encephalopathy. In dogs, the functional reserve of the liver is sufficient, such that concurrent portosystemic collateral circulation is required for clinical signs. However, cats with hepatic lipidosis can also develop encephalopathy due to metabolic derangements. It is unknown whether portosystemic collateral circulation or hepatic lipidosis can result in encephalopathy in reptiles; however, it may be a key factor in the signs of depression that are frequently observed in cases of severe hepatobiliary disease, including hepatic lipidosis. While reduction in dietary protein may be helpful, catabolism is even more problematic and must be avoided. Lactulose and soluble fiber may help reduce ammonia uptake from the large intestine and should be administered at a dose sufficient to cause

TABLE 67.4	**Drugs of Potential Value for the Treatment of Liver Disease**	
Drug Class/Name	**Indications**	**Precautions/Comments**
Prednisolone Prednisone	Autoimmune hepatitis	Immunosuppressive, contraindicated in cases of infectious disease
Azathioprine	Autoimmune hepatitis, where steroid-induced side effects are unacceptable	Can cause bone marrow suppression More expensive Potentially toxic in humans
Ursodeoxycholic acid	Natural, nontoxic, bile acid that, in humans, prevents mitochondrial damage and cellular apoptosis, increases bile flow, reduction in immune response, increases production of glutathione (GSH) and metallothionein to reduce oxidative damage	Only really proven in chronic severe cholestatic diseases and cholangitis Contraindicated in cases of extrahepatic bile duct obstruction
Antioxidants		
Vitamins C and E	Natural antioxidants	No proven efficacy, but little risk
L-Carnitine	Normally synthesized endogenously from methionine, lysine, and SAMe, but can be derived from diet. Essential cofactor for fatty acid oxidation, may prevent hepatocellular accumulation of free fatty acids and help remove toxic acetyl groups from mitochondria	Surmised that in hepatic lipidosis a relative deficiency of hepatocellular carnitine exists Use medical grade as solubility may limit oral availability
S-adenosyl-L-methionine (SAMe)	Natural hepatic metabolite and precursor to cysteine and GSH. Important in defense against free oxygen radicals. Basically replaces methionine (precursor to SAMe) to restore GSH in deficient hepatocytes	Some evidence of positive effects in domesticated animals with liver toxicity
Silymarin/silibinin (milk thistle extract)	Strong free-radical scavenger, with proven effects against oxidative liver intoxication, for a variable time	Most useful against oxidative stress and intoxication
Colchicine	Antifibrotic via stimulation of collagenase activity	Rarely vomiting, diarrhea, and neurological side effects reported. Clinical trials in humans failed to demonstrate any effect
Anticopper Medications		
D-penicillamine Trientine	Copper toxicity maybe more of a clinical concern in aquatic reptiles and amphibians. Chelators that bind copper and increase renal excretion	Give with food to reduce inappetance, nausea, vomiting. Treat for 3–6 months then reassess
Zinc	Induces metallothionein in enterocytes, which sequests copper and is eliminated by senescent cells in feces	Give 1–4 hours before food. Avoid concurrent use with chelators

stool softening but not diarrhea. Neomycin has also been advocated in humans and appears to be synergistic with lactulose to alter intestinal flora. Gastrointestinal bleeding can acutely elevate ammonia levels and encephalopathy, necessitating the use of protectants and antiulcer medications. Glucocorticoids are contraindicated because they stimulate lipolysis and fatty acid accumulation in the liver and induce catabolism and the risk of hyperglycemia. Anabolic steroids have been advocated in an attempt to increase hepatic metabolism.

SPECIFIC HEPATIC DISEASES

Hepatic disease can be classified as acute or chronic, inflammatory (hepatitis) or degenerative (hepatosis), and a variety of hepatobiliary diseases have been reported in the literature. Most reports involving free-ranging or large collections focus on infectious etiologies, especially viral diseases, while individual companion reptiles are more likely to suffer from degenerative hepatopathies, especially hepatic lipidosis, or abscesses/granulomas. A full investigation is essential to differentiate accurately between acute and chronic liver disease, and it is important that pretreatment blood samples are collected prior to initiating fluid therapy and other treatment measures. Antimicrobial therapy should not be started until material has been obtained for microbiology.

Hepatic Lipidosis
Clinical Significance. Hepatic lipidosis is a well-recognized condition that is frequently diagnosed post mortem in numerous species.

Unfortunately, there is a paucity of information concerning the pathogenesis of hepatic lipidosis in reptiles, and until relatively recently, the collection of biopsies for definitive antemortem diagnosis presented a challenge to clinicians. Although many of the difficulties of sample acquisition have now been overcome, the practitioner is still faced with the problems of microscopic (histopathologic and electron microscopic) interpretation. A logical case investigation is described with particular emphasis on histologic interpretation through the grading of microscopic lesions.

Hepatic lipidosis is probably one of the most frequently stated and misunderstood diagnoses made, both ante- and postmortem. For example, increased hepatic fat in an adult male Greek spur-thighed tortoise (*Testudo graeca*) in October might not be pathologic, as many temperate reptiles will normally increase intrahepatic fat levels prior to hibernation. In addition, many female reptiles will naturally increase intrahepatic fat in preparation for vitellogenesis. Therefore the problem is more complex and extensive than perhaps has been previously appreciated from our knowledge of domesticated mammals. In addition to diet and body condition, consideration must also be given to age, gender, reproductive status, and ecology.

Known Etiological Cause(s). Hepatic lipidosis is a metabolic derangement and not a single clinical disease. There are a host of factors that can predispose to increased hepatic fat. Classically, the high-fat diet (e.g., obese laboratory rats, waxworms, etc) have been implicated in obesity, an increase in the size of coelomic fat bodies, and an increase in hepatic fat. Equally, reduced activity and energy expenditures are common in captive reptiles that are maintained in small enclosures with little opportunity to roam, exercise, or forage. Another predisposing factor is the apparent prevalence in nonbreeding adult to aged females. Many female reptiles undergo seasonal cycles of lipogenesis in preparation for vitellogenesis. Those females that do not have the opportunity to reproduce and lose this fat through egg production appear more prone to obesity in captivity. Males and females of temperate regions are also known to increase hepatic and fat body stores in preparation for periods of reduced environmental temperatures, reduced food intake, and hibernation. When not given the opportunity to go through these natural fasting periods, temperate and subtropical species, with these annual cycles of increased fat deposition, are likely to become obese. Finally, acute hepatosis is rare but can occur secondary to toxic insult, and ivermectin-induced hepatic lipidosis is a documented example.[50]

Clinical Presentation. Hepatic lipidosis is usually chronic, and therefore observant owners and keepers who maintain accurate records may report a gradual reduction in appetite, activity, fecundity and fertility, weight gain (or later weight loss), hibernation problems including posthibernation anorexia, and changes in fecal character and color (Fig. 67.15). However, it may only be during episodes of increased physiological demand (e.g., hibernation, breeding, concurrent disease) that the underlying hepatic dysfunction becomes clinically apparent. Unfortunately, many caretakers miss these early signs of disease. As a result, veterinary attention is usually only sought once the animal has deteriorated to a life-threatening condition. When lipidosis is advanced, most affected reptiles are in poor condition, lethargic and weak. The body weight (mass) is usually below normal but can be elevated due to large fat bodies or ascites. Diarrhea is uncommon, as most affected animals will have been anorectic for a prolonged period of time.

Diagnostic Confirmation. Presumptive concerns regarding hepatic lipidosis can arise when plasma biochemical changes, including elevations in triglyerides, cholesterol, and lipoproteins, are appreciated.[51] There is usually minimal to no elevation in hepatocellular enzymes because cellular damage is usually minimal; however, reduced hepatic function can result in elevations of bile acids and hypoalbuminemia. Cholestasis is not usually a feature, and elevations of biliverdin would not be expected. Hemoconcentration can result in elevations of packed cell volume, but there is generally little to no inflammatory response in the leukogram. Radiographic evidence of hepatomegaly may be discernible in lizards and snakes but is challenging in chelonians. Ultrasonography and CT are more useful, especially when the hepatic parenchyma is compared to fat bodies. Reptiles with hepatic lipidosis typically exhibit hyperechoic livers and reduced radiographic attenuation (<20 HU).[31]

It is important to identify the primary cause of liver disease, which may remain undiscovered when the diagnosis of lipidosis is based on fine needle aspirates of the liver rather than biopsy. At present, there appears to be nothing to surpass the diagnostic value of hepatic biopsy for both microscopic and, where infectious agents may be present, microbiologic culture. Endoscopic hepatic biopsy is straightforward and well proven (Fig. 67.16).[39,41] In addition to facilitating a definitive diagnosis, serial biopsies offer the best means of monitoring disease progression and response to treatment and are invaluable for providing an accurate prognosis.

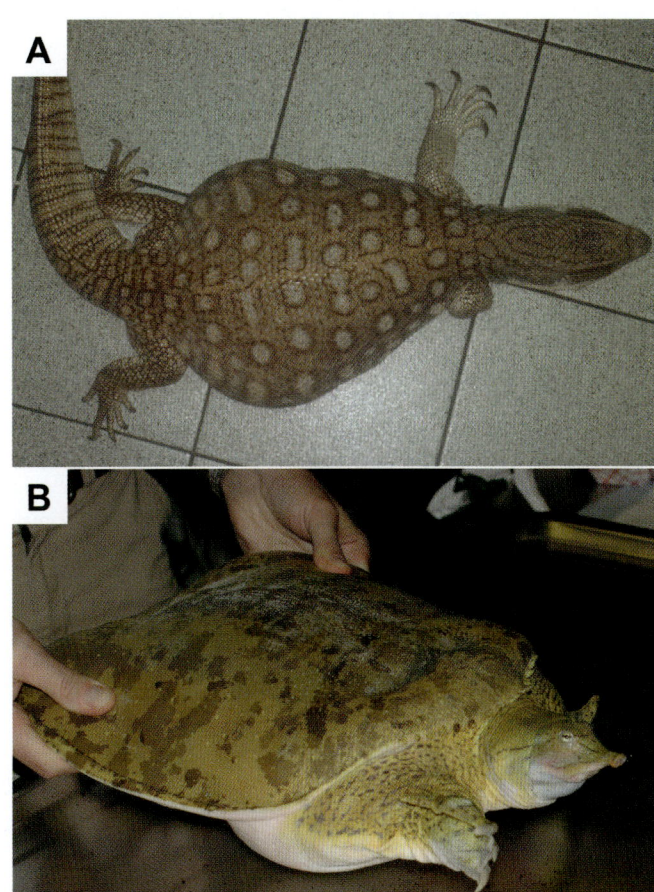

FIG 67.15 Grossly obese monitor lizard (*Varanus exanthematicus*) (A) and spiny softshell turtle (*Apalone spinifera*) (B). (Courtesy of Stephen J. Divers.)

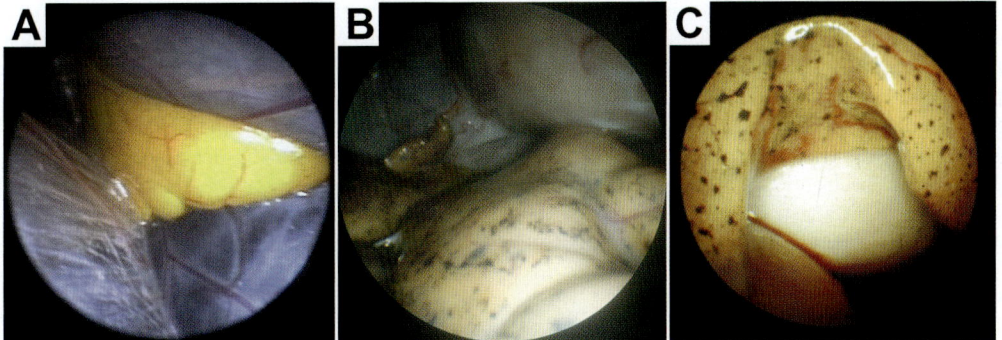

FIG 67.16 Endoscopic views of hepatic lipidosis in (A) a bearded dragon (*Pogona vitticeps*), (B) a Greek tortoise (*Testudo graeca*), and (C) a leopard tortoise (*Stigmochelys pardalis*). (Courtesy of Stephen J. Divers.)

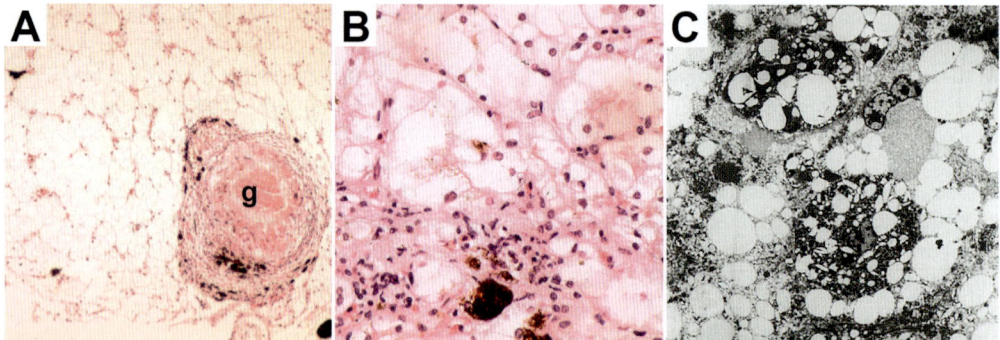

FIG 67.17 (A) Histologic section of the liver of a Greek tortoise (*Testudo graeca*) shows marked vacuolation of hepatocytes. A bacterial granuloma (*g*) is also evident. H&E, x20. (B) Higher magnification of the same liver demonstrating nuclear margination and pyknosis. H&E, x200. (C) Transmission electron micrograph (TEM) of the liver of a Round Island gecko (*Phelsuma guentheri*) shows a mixture of microvesicles and macrovesicles. Some lipid has been phagocytosed by granulocytes. x3000. (A and B, Courtesy of Stephen J. Divers; C, courtesy of John E. Cooper.)

When performing a necropsy on a hepatic lipidosis suspect, care must be taken to ensure that all other body organs are meticulously examined. In particular, note should be taken of (1) other fat deposits, including the size and weight of fat bodies and presence or absence of adipose tissue under the skin and around the heart, and (2) changes in other organs, such as the pancreas, that may have been predisposed to fatty change.

In hepatic lipidosis, the liver color may be pale tan to almost white (see Fig. 67.16). The color may also be affected by the natural color of fat in the species, and that, in turn, can be influenced by diet. A "fatty liver" is usually swollen, with rounded, nonangular edges, and may weigh more than normal—organ weights can be helpful in this respect. Markedly fatty livers will have a soft fatty "feel" when held for cutting and are friable—easily torn. Both the surfaces of the scalpel and the touch preparation, even before staining with specific stain (ORO, Sudan), may show greasy fat droplets.

There can be both normal and pathologic deposition of fat within the liver. Schaffner,[12] writing specifically about the reptilian liver, states categorically that "small fat droplets normally may be found in cytoplasm." He goes on to emphasize that the amount of fat can vary depending on such factors as gender and season. Thus the presence of fat in the liver of reptiles is not, per se, indicative of lipidosis. A more accurate description would be "fatty change" but not necessarily "lipidosis."

The detection of fat in a reptile's liver is not usually difficult. In a standard paraffin-embedded section, the lipid will appear as "holes"— vacuoles or vesicles—and usually these can be assumed to be fat (Fig. 67.17A and B). However, some caution is needed since vacuoles can, on occasion, contain water, glycogen, or other nonlipid material. Sometimes light microscopy will per se permit a distinction to be made, but often other tests are needed, such as special stains or even TEM. Once it has been ascertained by histology that fat is present, a number of subsidiary questions need to be asked before a diagnosis (tentative or definite) of hepatic lipidosis can be made. These include an appreciation of the precise location, position, and size of the fat vacuoles. Evidence of hepatocellular dysfunction or degeneration, and inflammatory changes, must also be noted. It should be mentioned in passing that other techniques could also be used to investigate fatty change in the liver of reptiles. TEM is hardly suitable for routine diagnosis but has an important role to play when working with valuable or endangered species—for instance, where lipidosis is a feature of a disease "outbreak," perhaps linked with other metabolic changes, such as xanthomatosis. In such cases TEM can provide essential information on pathogenesis, including the presence or absence of changes in intracellular organelles or the

presence of pathogens (see Fig. 67.17C).[52] TEM is also one of the keys to more research on fat metabolism in reptiles.[53]

Even when the presence of what appears to be "excess" fat has been established, a diagnosis of hepatic lipidosis cannot usually be confirmed without taking into account the following.

1. The clinical history and the clinician's assessment of the case (including other laboratory results).
2. The patient's details and circumstances (e.g., species, age, sex, reproductive status, hibernation status, estivation, diet).

Specific Treatment(s). In advanced, severe cases correction of dehydration with nonlactate, nonglucose-containing fluids is advisable. Vitamin K administration can be considered, especially if coagulopathy has been confirmed. In many instances, hepatic lipidosis is a chronic disease that may take months, if not years, to reverse. Therefore a means of providing long-term fluid and nutritional support (e.g., esophagostomy tube) is typically required.

The importance of nutritional support cannot be overemphasized and, given the available literature in human and veterinary medicine, appears to offer the best therapeutic approach to hepatic lipidosis. When providing nutritional support it is important to consider (1) the patient's energy and nutritional requirements and (2) the patient's natural dietary preference (e.g., herbivorous, omnivorous, carnivorous), as well as (3) attempt to use natural foods for long-term support and only rely on artificial, critical care substitutes during initial stabilization. Total calorific requirements and total daily food requirements (see Chapter 122) should be calculated. However, these calculations are mere estimates, and actual requirements could vary by ±50%. Care is also required to avoid refeeding syndrome and gastric overload in reptiles that have been anorectic for prolonged periods. In general, it is safer to start feeding at 10% of calculated daily requirements using a dilute formula and increase slowly with the aim of achieving 100% of daily requirements by 10 to 30 days. Efforts should be made to correct hypokalemia and hypophosphatemia during initial stabilization. Subsequent adjustments should be based upon monitoring weight, defecation, and plasma biochemistry. The esophagostomy tube is also useful for oral drug delivery.

Supplementation with L-carnitine (a derivative of lysine and required for the transportation of acyl-CoA across the inner mitochondrial membrane of hepatocytes) may improve hepatic metabolism of fat. A daily dose of 100 mg/kg L-carnitine mixed with the tube-feeding formula appears to be safe in reptiles. Supplementation with water-soluble vitamins may also be beneficial and appears to be safe. Antioxidantas, such as SAMe (which replaces the previous recommendation of methionine) and vitamin E, may also be beneficial, and because no reptile-specific doses have been produced, allometric calculation from mammalian doses is probably appropriate.

Prognosis. If the condition is diagnosed early prior to the onset of obvious clinical signs (e.g., during annual health evaluations or routine sterilization surgery), then the prognosis is good, and resolution, although taking months or even years, is often possible with appropriate improvements in husbandry and nutrition. However, once clinical signs develop and hepatic dysfunction is advanced, then the prognosis becomes more guarded and often requires prolonged nutritional support, medication, and nursing for months until the animal regains appetite. Such cases can often take years to resolve excessive hepatic fat, fat body size, and body condition.

Prevention. Although there are no clear guidelines established for the treatment of hepatic lipidosis in reptiles, addressing the following factors can often help reduce or prevent occurrence.

1. Provide a suitably large enclosure to facilitate exercise and foraging. This is often the most difficult change to make given the culture of maintaining reptiles in small enclosures.
2. Avoid excessive feeding, both in terms of frequency and calorific quality of food items. For example, snakes are often fed on a predetermined weekly schedule whether they show hunger (foraging/hunting) behaviors or not. It may be preferable to feed well-adjusted reptiles when they actually show hunger and increased foraging behaviors. Another example would be feeding arid land tortoises (e.g., *Testudo graeca*, *Centrochelys sulcata*) high-quality grocery fruits and vegetables, when lower energy items, including hay, are preferable.
3. Facilitate the natural loss of fat, both hepatic and fat body, by permitting temperate species to fast and hibernate and intact females the ability to reproduce.
4. Caretakers should be encouraged to keep health logs (including monthly weight and body lengths [straight carapace or snout-to-vent]) for their reptiles and seek annual or biennial health evaluations (including physical examinations and routine blood testing).

Hepatitis

Clinical Significance. Hepatitis (an inflammatory change) is not uncommon in reptiles and often associated with infectious agents. The condition can be acute (often viral) or chronic (often parasitic, bacterial, or fungal). If several animals are affected simultaneously, a common etiology is most likely.

Known Etiological Cause(s). Herpesvirus (*Boa*, *Testudo*), adenovirus (*Boa*, *Pogona*), orthoreovirus (*Boa*), hepatitis B virus (*Mauremys*), and West Nile Virus (*Alligator*) are viral infections that have either, naturally or experimentally, been shown to cause liver disease in reptiles.[2,5,6,8,10,54–56] Most of these viral diseases have been reported to cause acute hepatitis or hepatocellular necrosis. Bacterial and mycotic hepatopathies tend to be more chronic and cause granulomatous hepatitis. *Providencia rettgeri* (*Varanus*), *Salmonella typhimurium* (*Testudo*), *Mycobacterium* spp (*Caiman*, *Phrynops*, *Trionyx*, *Gonyosoma*, *Pituophis*), *Chlamydia* (*Bitis*), *Coccidioides* (*Pituophis*), *Penicillium* (*Geochelone*, *Chamaeleo*), and unidentified anerobic *Bacillus* (*Natrix*) have been reported; however, the actual list of potential bacterial and fungal pathogens is probably far longer.[1,4,9,57–62] In some cases, the involvement of the liver is likely secondary and a reflection of systemic infection and generalized sepsis. Acute bacterial hepatitis is less common, but chlamydial hepatitis has been reported in hatchling crocodiles (*Crocodylus*), and the author has seen diffuse hepatic swelling due to acute bacterial infections (Fig. 67.18A).[8] Parasitic hepatitis has also been reported; histiocytic hepatitis due to microsporidia in bearded dragons, necrotizing hepatitis due to *Entamoeba* in snakes and tortoises, and granulomatous hepatitis due to *Hepatozoon* meronts in water snakes.[7,63,64] Metazoan larval migrations have also been reported through the reptilian liver.[65] Hepatitis can be aseptic and associated with surface/serosal inflammation in response to yolk proteins and coelomitis (see Fig. 67.18B).

Clinical Presentation. Reptiles with acute liver disease usually present in good body condition, and may exhibit depression, anorexia, regurgitation, or acute mortality. Severely affected animals will usually be

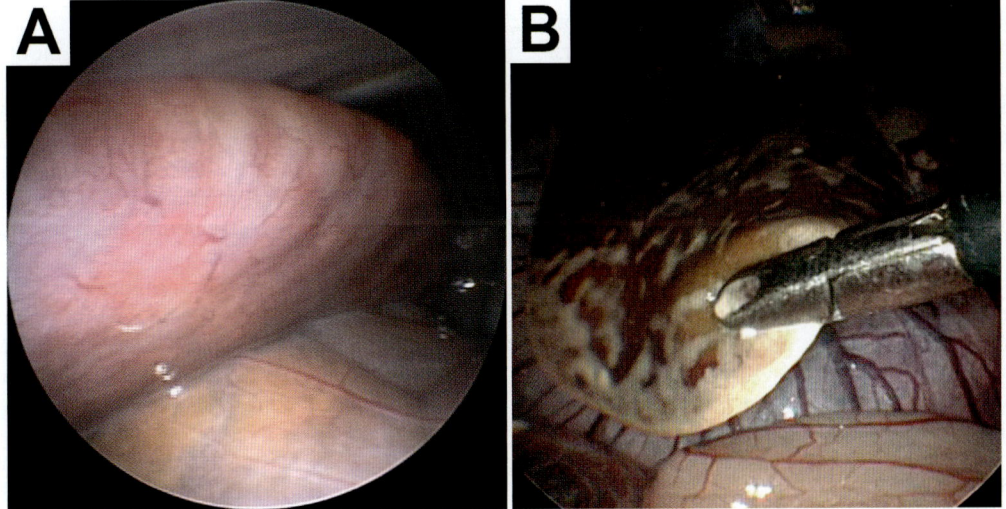

FIG 67.18 (A) Diffuse hepatic swelling with loss of the sharp caudal border associated with acute bacterial hepatitis in a green iguana (*Iguana iguana*). (B) Multifocal areas of pale, proteinaceous material and hepatitis that were inflammatory reactions to yolk coelomitis in a female box turtle (*Terrapene carolina*). This pathology was not appreciable on radiographs, CT, or ultrasonography. Note the use of 3-mm biopsy forceps to obtain a biopsy. (Courtesy of Stephen J. Divers.)

depressed, lethargic, and weak, while mucous membranes may be pale, hyperemic, or icteric. As already stated, the early signs of chronic disease may be missed; this, in conjunction with the rapid onset of severe clinical signs, may confuse and convince the clinician that this is an acute hepatitis rather than the end-stage presentation of a chronic condition.

Diagnostic Confirmation. This author could not find any documented cases of naturally occurring hepatitis that included appropriate antemortem diagnostic testing with histopathologic confirmation. This is obviously an area of clinical medicine that can be improved with the adoption of endoscopic or surgical biopsy (see Fig. 67.18). Nevertheless, plasma increases in AST, ALT, LDH, and SDH may be seen in cases of hepatitis; however, AST and LDH are also found in muscle, and potential nonhepatic sources must be appreciated. Elevation in bile acids or ammonia would not be expected unless there was major functional impairment. Hematology may reveal a leukocytosis characterized by heterophilia, azurophilia, or monocytosis, depending upon the acute or chronic nature of the condition. Eosinophilia might be seen in cases of parasitic hepatitis. Ultimately, liver biopsy is required for a definitive diagnosis, accurate prognosis, and to direct specific therapy.

Specific Treatment(s). Early definitive diagnosis is a prerequisite for, and typically dictates, selecting appropriate drug therapies. Consequently, any drug that can affect histopathology, microbiology, parasitology, and toxicology should not be started until after samples have been collected. Initial antimicrobial drug selection can be based on Gram-stained impression smears, clinical knowledge and experience, likely causative organisms, and host-drug preferences. The routine use of advanced broad-spectrum drugs, including fluoroquinolones, implies a low level of clinical expertise. First-line drugs include tetracyclines, macrolides trimethoprim-sulfa and amoxycillin-clauvulanate with subsequent modification-based culture and sensitivity or MIC testing. Successful treatment relies on the selection of an effective drug and effective delivery of an appropriate dose to maintain tissue levels well above MIC for a period of time. Consequently, MIC testing is preferred because it not only provides more reliable sensitivity data but can also be used to determine the actual dose required (assuming volume of distribution, Vd) (Box 67.2). Even so, actual drug levels can often deviate from pharmacokinetic research, and it is still wise to measure antimicrobial blood levels and adjust dose and frequency, as and where necessary.

Prognosis. The paucity of reported cases makes establishment of an accurate prognosis impossible. However, early diagnosis of acute bacterial or mycotic hepatitis probably has a better chance of successful treatment compared to chronic cases with innumerous, encapsulated granulomas that are more resistant to antimicrobial penetration.

Prevention. Appropriate husbandry, nutrition, preventive health programs (including quarantine), and regular veterinary evaluations can help reduce the incidence of disease or ensure that it is detected early. Appropriate diagnosis and treatment of dermatological, gastrointestinal, and pulmonary infections can help to reduce systemic spread to other visceral structures including the liver.

Toxic Hepatopathy
Clinical Significance. The only clinical reports of toxic hepatopathies relate to ivermectin usage in chelonians, where there was an association with (but not proven to cause) hepatic lipidosis.[50] Meloxicam at 5 mg/kg daily for 12 days failed to induce hepatic changes in green iguanas.[66] Experimental studies using carbon tetrachloride induced hepatocellular

---

BOX 67.2   Determination of Required Antimicrobial Drug Dose Using Minimum Inhibitory Concentration (MIC) and Volume of Distribution (Vd)

Hepatic biopsy reveals Salmonella hepatitis in a slider (*Trachemys scripta*)

	Disc Sensitivity	MIC (µg/mL)	Vd (L/kg)	Calculated Dose* (mg/kg)
Carbenicillin	Intermediate	16	0.24	31 mg/kg required[a]
Enrofloxacin	Sensitive	1	2.48	20 mg/kg required[b]
Metronidazole	Resistant	128	0.74	758 mg/kg required[c]

*Calculated drug doses from MIC calculated as follows: MIC (µg/mL = mg/L) × Vd (L/kg) × treatment factor (often 4–10, using 8 in this example). If drug is given orally, then the bioavailability needs to be considered (e.g., if oral availability is 82%, calculated drug dose should be increased by 100/82).
[a]The calculated dose (31 mg/kg) is well below the pharmacokinetically evaluated, published dose (200 mg/kg).[82] Therefore use of the published dose would easily achieve high tissue levels and greater likelihood of treatment success, despite the *intermediate* disc sensitivity.
[b]The calculated dose (20 mg/kg) is greater than the pharmacokinetically evaluated, published dose (10 mg/kg).[83] Therefore use of the published dose would fail to achieve adequate tissue levels and result in treatment failure, despite the *sensitive* disc sensitivity. The high calculated dose may achieve adequate tissue levels at the expense of causing drug toxicity.
[c]The calculated dose (758 mg/kg) is far greater than the pharmacokinetically evaluated, published dose (20 mg/kg).[84] Therefore use of the published dose would fail to achieve adequate tissue levels and result in treatment failure, and is consistent with the *resistant* disc sensitivity. It would likely be impossible to achieve such high tissue levels, and attempts to do so would cause drug toxicity.

---

necrosis in green iguanas (Fig. 67.19) (Schnellbacher et al, Proc ARAV, 2014. pp 127–128). Many bacterial toxins, compounds, and environmental pollutants might be expected to affect reptiles in similar ways to other vertebrates.

Known Etiological Cause(s). Chronic exposure of arsenic-, cadmium-, selenium-, strontium-, and vanadium-contaminated fish (coal-ash contaminated site) results in hepatic accumulation and hepatic fibrosis in watersnakes (*Nerodia*).[67] Organic pesticide residues (including methoxychlor, aldrin, dichlorodiphenyltrichloroethane [DDT], endosulfan I, endosulfan II, and lindane) have been reported within the hepatic tissues of viperids, colubrids, and heloderms.[68]

Clinical Presentation. In the experimental carbon tetrachloride study, lethargy, reduced food intake, and weight loss were noted in some iguanas. Chelonians with ivermectin toxicity typically display profound neurologic depression, which is thought to be associated with the GABA agonist effects within the CNS, rather than hepatic encephalopathy.

Diagnostic Confirmation. Most toxins cause hepatocellular leakage and necrosis, and therefore elevation in hepatocellular enzymes, and possible functional impairment and elevation of bile acids may be expected. Hepatic biopsy is required to demonstrate histologic changes, although the precise etiologic agent cannot be demonstrated without employing toxicologic analyses for likely agents (see Fig. 67.19C). Such toxicologic sampling typically requires the harvesting of larger biopsies

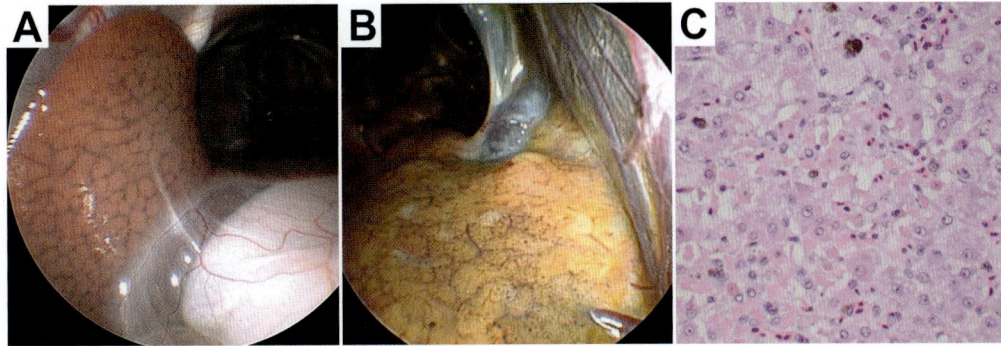

FIG 67.19 Carbon tetrachloride hepatic toxicity in green iguanas (*Iguana iguana*). (A) Endoscopic view of the normal liver. (B) Endoscopic view of the liver 6 days after toxic insult. (C) Liver biopsy histopathology demonstrating hepatocellular necrosis. (Courtesy of Stephen J. Divers.)

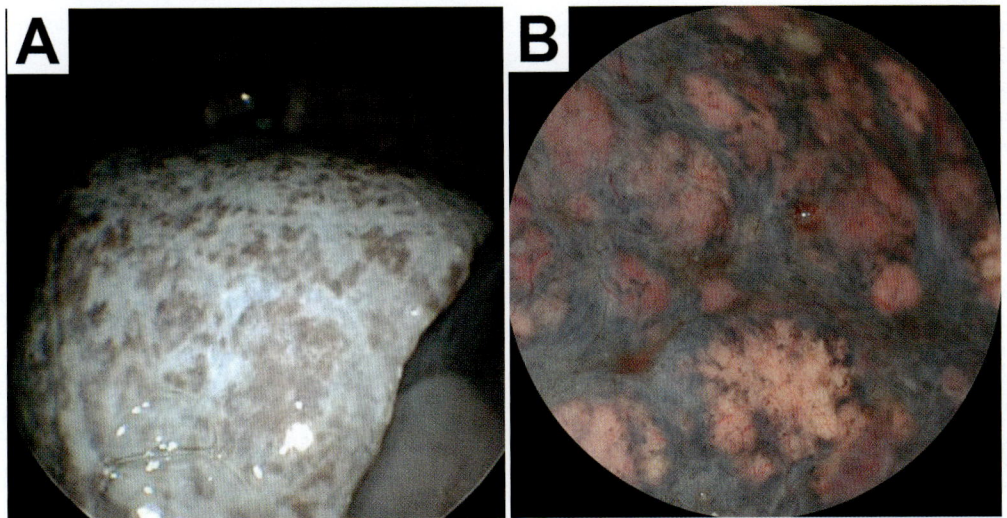

FIG 67.20 (A) Endoscopic view of the liver of a green iguana (*Iguana iguana*) demonstrating bands of pale fibrosis. The liver was enlarged but functionally deficient due to extensive fibrosis. (B) Close-up endoscopic view of the hepatic parenchyma of a Texas tortoise (*Gopherus berlandieri*) demonstrating fibrous bands and nodular hyperplasia. (Courtesy of Stephen J. Divers.)

and some idea of which class(es) of toxins may be involved. Survival from acute insults or chronic, intermittent exposure may result in fibrosis and nodular hyperplasia (Fig. 67.20).

Specific Treatment(s). Treatment is generally supportive; however, if there is a known antidote to a specific toxin then its administration may be beneficial.

Prognosis. Prognosis is unknown but probably guarded to poor once clinical signs are established. Serial sampling and improvement in clinicopathological results would give cause for continuing therapy.

Prevention. Preventing access to environmental pollutants/chemicals and avoiding inappropriate or unnecessary drug use will be beneficial.

Cholangitis, Cholecystitis, and Cholecystolithiasis

Clinical Significance. Inflammatory conditions involving the biliary system have been reported from terrestrial chelonians, large iguanid lizards, and snakes.[69] In most cases, the lesions are coincidental findings at necropsy, but chronic disease can lead to gross distension of the gallbladder, wall thickening, and fibrosis. Choleliths and cholecystoliths

are uncommon but have been reported in association with trematode infestation of the liver and gallbladder.

Known Etiological Cause(s). Several metazoan (trematodes) and protozoan parasites (e.g., *Hexamita, Eimeria, Trichomonas*) have been associated with the bile ducts and gallbladder, probably due to migration from the gastrointestinal tract.[69]

Clinical Presentation. Intra- and posthepatic biliary obstruction can cause icterus.

Diagnostic Confirmation. Elevation of bilirubin (snakes) or biliverdin is likely following intrahepatic or posthepatic biliary obstruction. Leukocytosis, characterized by heterophilia, azurophilia, and/or monocytosis might be expected given the granulomatous inflammation that often accompanies cholecystitis. Ultrasonographic evaluation of the biliary system may help identify thickened biliary walls and cholecystoliths. Routine fecal evaluations for protozoan and metazoan parasites should be performed.

Specific Treatment(s). Cholecystectomy remains the treatment of choice in humans. A variety of treatments have been advocated in humans and laboratory animal studies, including ursodiol, ursodeoxycholic acid, hyodeoxycholic acid, ezetimibe, aspirin, and dietary cholesterol restriction.[70–72] Most of these therapies were geared toward preventing gallstone development rather than dissolution of existing stones. Extracorporeal shock wave lithotripsy has been used successfully in some human patients; however, reptile cholecystoliths tend to be soft and friable rather than lithic and therefore may be less affected by such therapy.[73] Parasitic infections should be treated accordingly.

Prognosis. The prognosis is unknown as most cases appear to be identified postmortem.

Prevention. Unknown in reptiles, but in humans and domesticated animals lean body condition, exercise, and regular meals have been advocated for prevention.

Hepatic Neoplasia

Clinical Significance. Neoplasia is not uncommon, and indeed recent surveys have indicated that hepatic neoplasia (hepatic adenoma and adenocarcinoma) is particularly prominent in squamates.[11,74–80] However, there have been very few antemortem diagnoses and no documented cases describing successful management.

Known Etiological Cause(s). There are no known carcinogens, although genetic/taxa predispositions have been suggested.[81]

Clinical Presentation. In snakes with a solitary hepatic mass, a firm midbody swelling may be appreciated 28% to 60% snout-to-vent, depending on species. A large liver or associated soft tissue mass effect may be palpable in lizards but is difficult to impossible to appreciate in chelonians due to their shell. More discrete nodular disease is more difficult to evaluate without advanced imaging, endoscopy, or surgical exposure (Fig. 67.21).

Diagnostic Confirmation. Elevation of hepatocellular enzymes and bile acids may be appreciated.[11] Ultimately, biopsy is required for a precise diagnosis, and even then staging is recommended but has not been previously reported for hepatic neoplasia in reptiles (see Chapter 78).

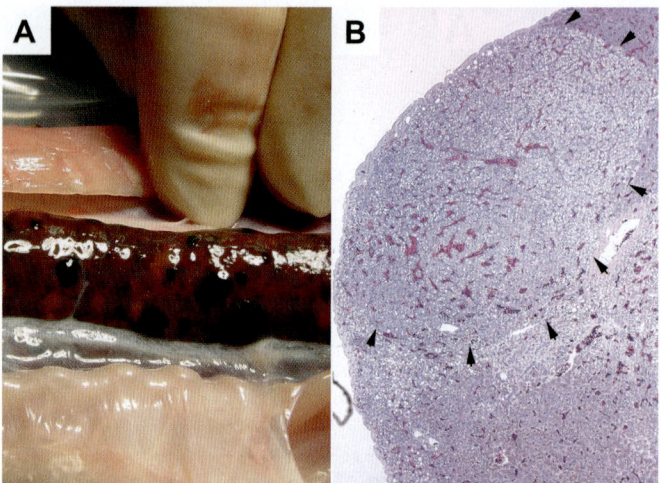

FIG 67.21 California king snake (*Lampropeltis getula californiae*) with hepatic melanomas. (A) Gross appearance of the liver intraoperatively. (B) Histologic photomicrograph of a melanoma nodule. H&E, ×20. (Courtesy of Stephen J. Divers.)

Specific Treatment(s). Oncologic treatments can include surgery, chemotherapy, and radiation, with the specific recommendation dependent upon a histological diagnosis and staging. In general, oncological therapy is often aimed at prolonging quality of life rather than cure.

Prognosis. Prognosis is dependent upon histopathology and determination of malignancy. A solitary, benign hepatoma may be resectable and carry a good prognosis. The prognosis for carcinomas and other malignancies is probably poor.

Prevention. No specific preventative measures have been identified.

REFERENCES

See www.expertconsult.com for a complete list of references.

68

Cardiology

Lionel Schilliger and Simon Girling

Until recently, primary cardiovascular conditions were rarely considered to affect ectotherms. This assumption is now challenged by the increased availability of diagnostic tools that have improved our knowledge of reptile cardiovascular anatomy, physiology, and pathology. Diagnostic techniques such as auscultation, electrocardiography, radiography, and, in particular, ultrasonography are now readily available in general practice. Despite a good basic understanding of reptilian cardiac anatomy and physiology, cardiology remains a poorly developed subspecialty in herpetological medicine compared to some other disciplines. The etiology, diagnosis, and treatment of cardiac conditions in reptiles are often poorly understood. However, translating our present knowledge of physiology and pathology into clinical practice will allow us to advance the discipline.

Cardiac physiology and anatomy differs markedly between mammals and reptiles and also between reptile taxa.[1–4] As in mammals, the reptilian heart is part of the circulatory system. The circulatory system consists of both a cardiovascular system that distributes blood pumped by the heart and a lymphatic system that distributes lymph throughout the body via a well-developed set of coelomic, muscular, cutaneous, and vertebral lymphatic vessels.[2,5–7]

The circulatory system is connected to all organ systems and plays a crucial role in homeostasis. In association with the respiratory system, it provides transport of gases between sites of external and internal respiration. Additionally, the circulatory system distributes products of digestion for metabolic use or energy storage, waste products to the kidneys, and electrolytes and hormones to target tissues. The circulatory system also plays a key role in the distribution of heat and immune system components throughout the body and adapts to variations of blood pressure.[8,9]

Reptiles in general have a smaller ratio of heart size to body mass than birds or mammals.[1,10] The presence of a single undivided ventricle in the heart of noncrocodilian reptiles originally thought to represent a simplistic or primitive precursor to the mammalian heart is now understood to be a complex, compartmented, and specialized chamber that confers physiological benefits to these animals, which have a low basal metabolic rate and a high tolerance for anaerobic respiration.[8,11]

CARDIAC ANATOMY AND PHYSIOLOGY

The reptilian heart is very similar to the early embryological heart of mammals and birds before ventricular septation.[2,12] It is grossly composed of two atria and one ventricle in noncrocodilians.

The basic embryonic pattern common to reptiles, birds, and mammals includes six aortic arches, of which arches III, IV, and VI persist in reptiles.[2,4,9] During embryonic development, the right aortic arch, left aortic arch, and the pulmonary trunk (the latter incorporating the base of the paired sixth arch) are formed from the ventral aorta. The right and left systemic arches (the right one being the most prominent of the two) merge caudally to form the common dorsal aorta.[2,4] Thus, these three efferent arterial trunks produce one pulmonary circuit and two systemic circuits, each of which arises independently from the heart.

Most publications of reptilian cardiac anatomy describe a small range of species that show variable designs in anatomy and physiology.[13–19] Little is known about the cardiac anatomy and physiology of the other 10,000 species of reptiles, and generalizations should be avoided whenever possible.

Cardiac Size, Shape, and Position

Heart mass compared to total body mass ranges between 0.2% and 0.3% in reptiles, similar to that found in amphibians (0.16%–0.32%).[1,12] This ratio is variable according to the degree of physical activity. For example, in "athletic" tree snakes, which also experience higher pressures due to gravitational and behavioral effects, the heart mass can reach 0.45% of the body weight, compared to 0.16% in slow-moving species such as the Brisbane short-necked turtle (*Emydura macquari*) or the European slow-worm (*Anguis fragilis*).[1]

Despite minor variations, the external anatomy of the reptilian heart tends not to vary significantly between species, but the position of blood vessels (efferent arteries and afferent veins) (Fig. 68.1) and inner structures can vary among groups and be more species specific.[4] The shape of the heart is broad and globoid in chelonians, elongated in ophidians, and ovoid in lizards and crocodilians.[1,10]

The location of the heart varies between taxa reflecting their phylogenetic position and ecological niche (Fig. 68.2).[20] In most species, the heart is roughly positioned along the axial midline and relatively cranially within the coelom. In snakes, the heart is found along the midline axis, but its longitudinal position varies with species. In marine and freshwater snakes, it is positioned nearer to the middle of the body. In non-tree-dwelling snakes it is found at about 25% snout-to-vent length (svl) and even more cranially in arboreal species (up to 15% svl).[1,4,9,21] These differences can be understood by considering the different physical forces to which the heart is subjected in different environmental conditions. A cranially positioned heart reduces the hydrostatic pressure above the heart and stabilizes variations in cephalic blood pressure.[1,4,9] Some studies have shown that those species of snakes that spend time raising their heads (arboreal and other climbing snakes) possess relatively shorter vasculature between the heart and head than do terrestrial species. The reverse is true in aquatic species, where the effect of gravity in water is minimal.[22]

Because of the absence of a diaphragm, the ophidian heart is mobile within the coelomic cavity. This probably facilitates the movement of large whole prey inside the esophagus.[1] In the coelom, the heart is found adjacent to the caudal tracheal rings, caudal to the thyroid, cranial to the bronchial bifurcation, close to the cranial pole of the lung(s), and just cranial to the liver.[1,4,23,24] Externally, the position of the heart

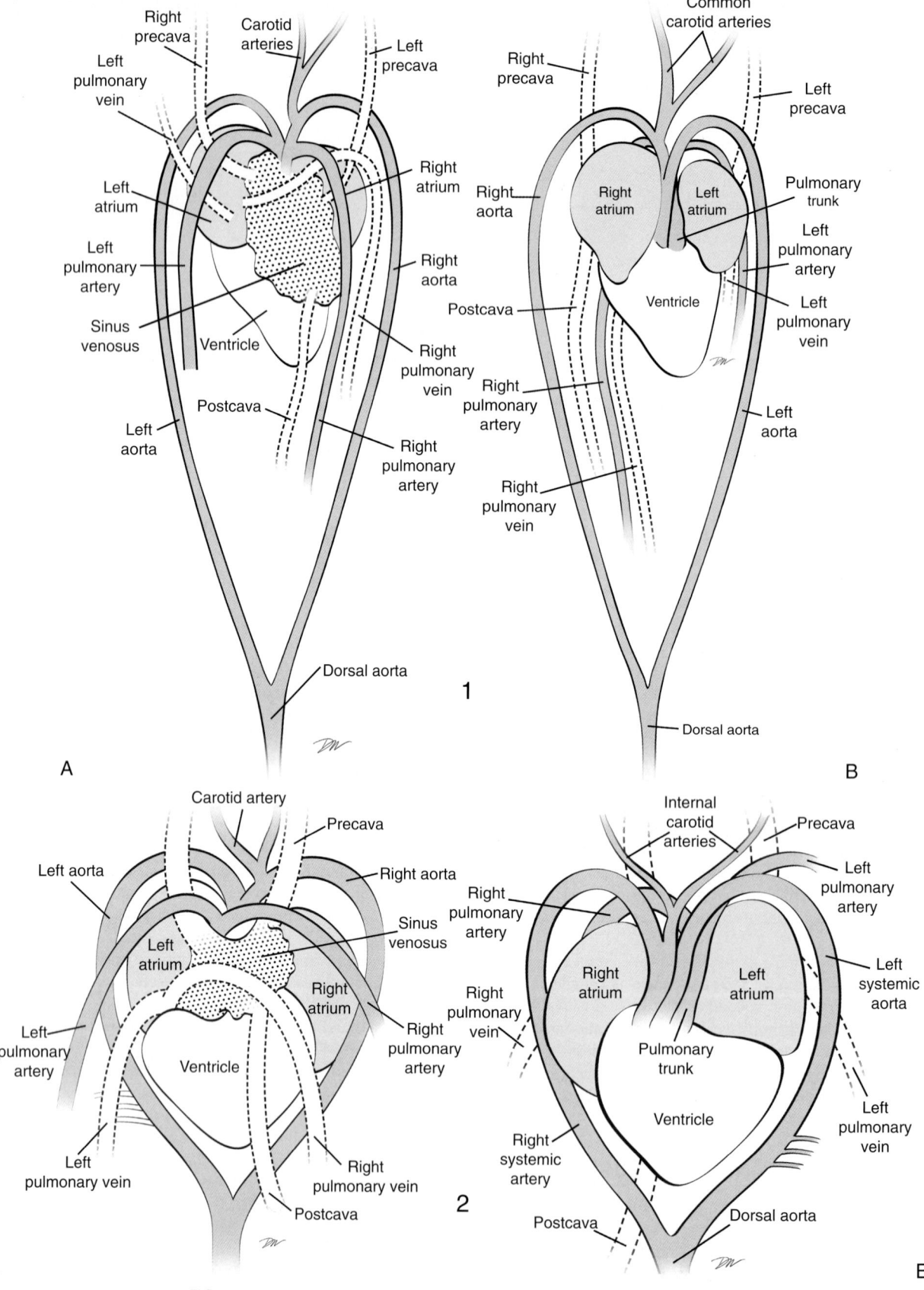

FIG 68.1 (1) Snake heart. (2) Lizard heart. (A) Dorsal view. (B) Ventral view.

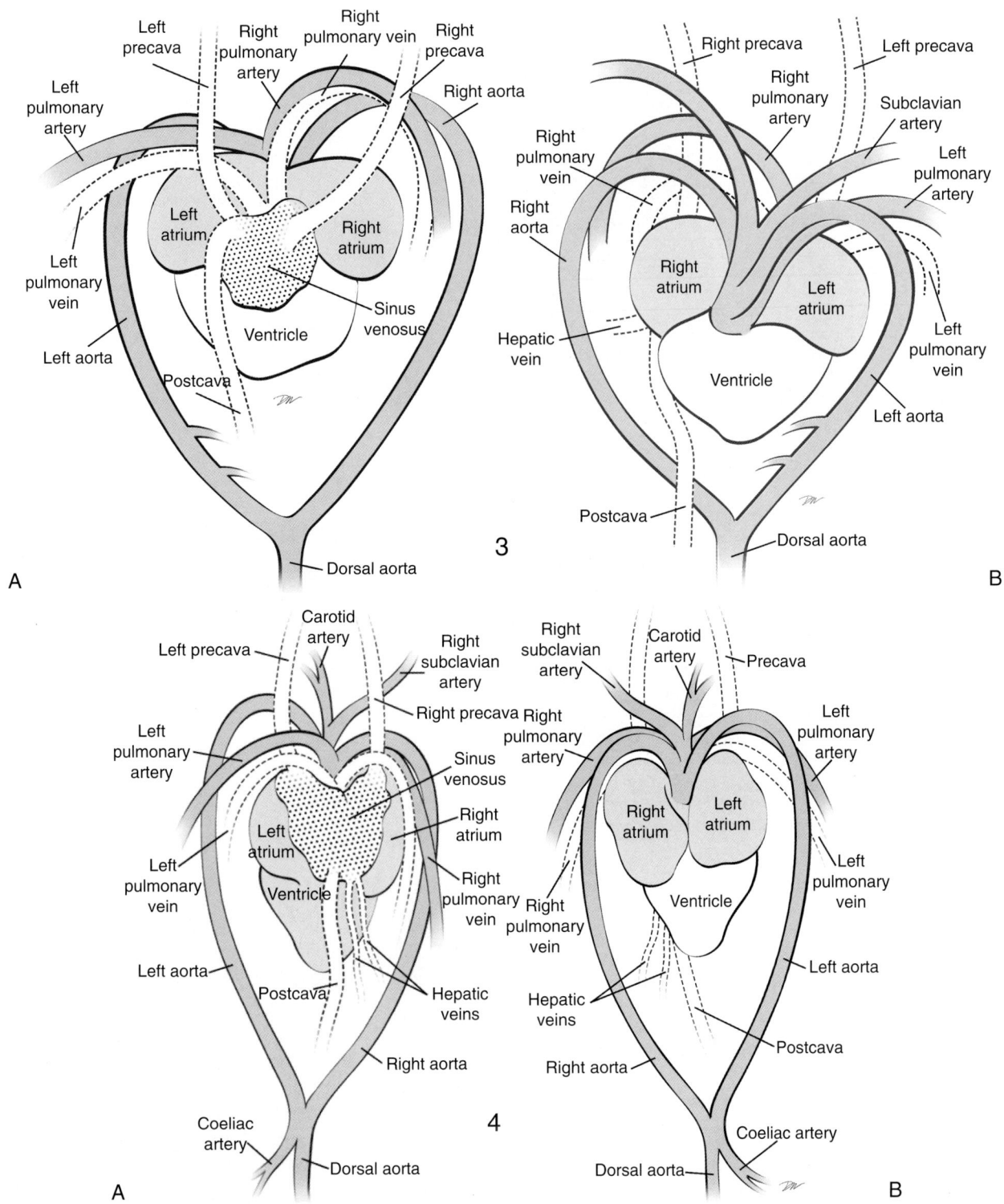

FIG 68.1, cont'd (3) Turtle heart. (4) Crocodilian heart. (A) Dorsal view. (B) Ventral view. (Reprinted from Murray MJ, Wyneken J. Cardiopulmonary anatomy and physiology. In Mader D, ed. *Reptile Medicine and Surgery.* 2nd ed. St. Louis: Elsevier; 2006:124–134, with permission from Elsevier.)

is indicated by percutaneous visualization of the ventral precordial tap when stretching the animal and placing it in dorsal recumbency. This is particularly obvious in the anesthetized and relaxed reptile.[23]

In chelonians, the heart is located in the ventral midline at the level of the intersection of the humeral, pectoral, and abdominal scutes of the plastron.[4,25] In some species it is positioned more caudally, above

the junction of the humeral-pectoral and pectoral-abdominal scute lines.[25] This may, however, be an unreliable landmark, as the positions of the pectoral and humeral scutes differ widely among species.[4] In the coelom, the heart is bordered dorsally by the septum horizontale and the cranial lungs, laterally by the liver lobes, and ventrally by the coelomic membrane and plastron.[23] In soft-shelled turtles (*Trionychidae*), which

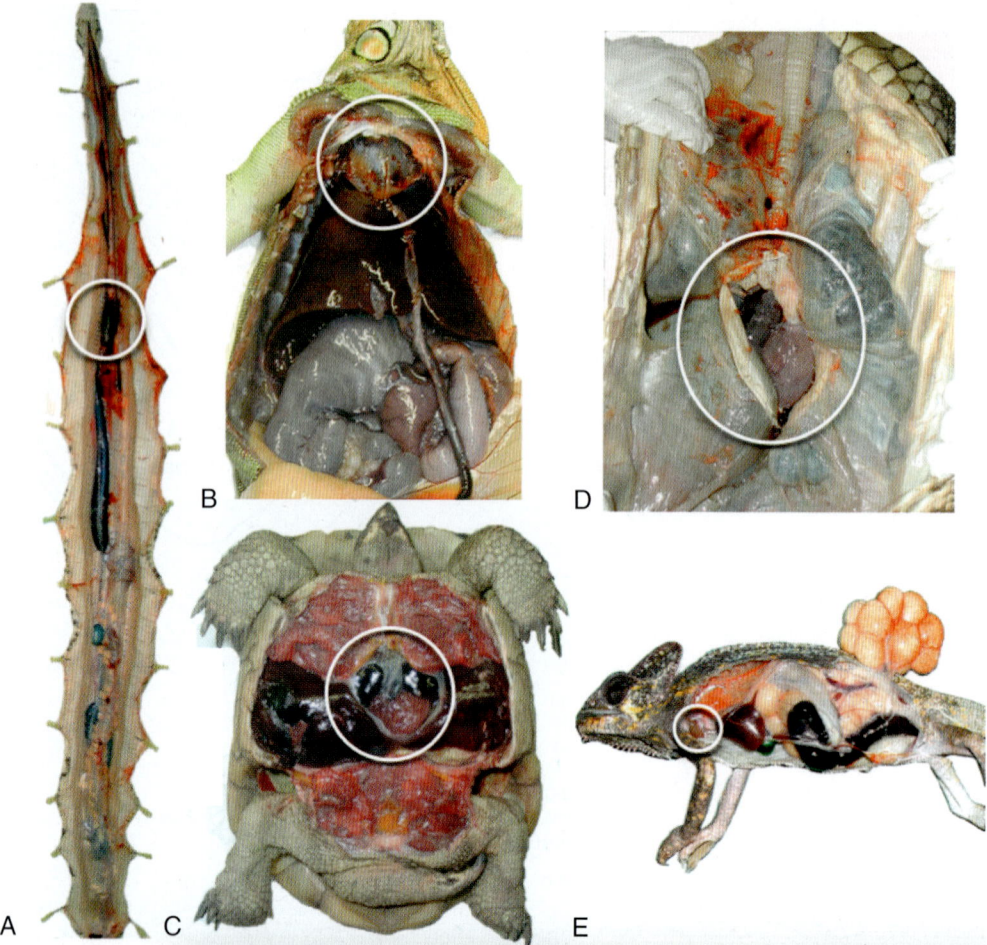

FIG 68.2 Topographic anatomy of the heart (white circles). (A) Ball python (*Python regius*); (B) green iguana (*Iguana iguana*); (C) eastern Hermann's tortoise (*Testudo hermanni boettgeri*); (D) saltwater crocodile (*Crocodylus porosus*); and (E) veiled cameleon (*Chamaeleo calyptratus*).

possess a very streamlined carapace and hence vertically compressed coelomic cavity, the heart is displaced to the right.[4,26] This is due to a long protractile neck, which when retracted into the carapace causes a displacement of the heart and liver to the right and of the stomach to the left.[1]

In most lizards, the heart is encased within the pectoral girdle of the gular region. In tegus (*Teiidae*), Gila monsters (*Helodermatidae*), and monitor lizards (*Varanidae*), the heart is located more caudally in the coelomic cavity.[1,4,9,23]

In crocodilians, the heart lies midline approximately midway between the pelvic and pectoral girdles.[1,4,15,27] The apex lies deep between the right and left medial aspect of the hepatic lobes, adjacent to the liver isthmus. The base of the heart extends slightly cranial to the cranial border of the liver and lies within the mediastinum, ventral to the primary bronchi and esophagus.[28]

Pericardium

As in mammals, the heart lies in a visceral space known as the pericardial cavity and is covered by the pericardium (Fig. 68.3). The innermost layer of the pericardium is the epicardium, and immediately adjacent to this is the myocardium. The heart apex is attached to the pericardium by a ligament termed the *gubernaculum cordis*, except in snakes and varanids where the ventricle remains free within the pericardial space.[1,2] The pericardial sac lies within the caudoventral part of the thoracic cavity in crocodilians.[1,4,15,28]

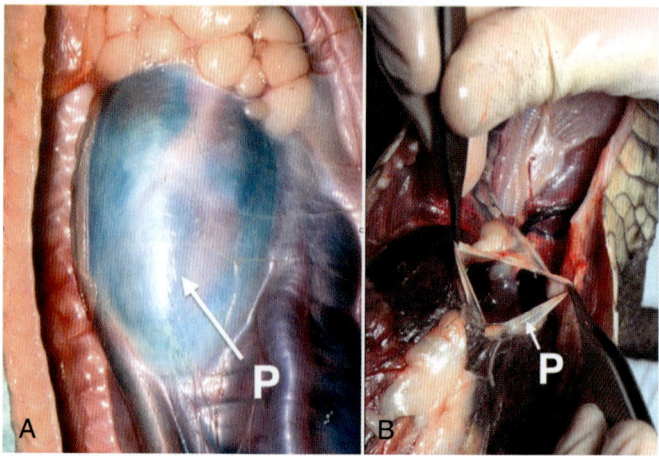

FIG 68.3 External aspect of the pericardial sac (A) in a Burmese python (*Python bivittatus*) and (B) (after incision) in a spectacle caiman (*Caiman crocodilus*). P, Pericardial sac. (Courtesy of Lionel Schilliger.)

Heart Anatomy

Reptilian hearts can be loosely classified into two basic patterns: the noncrocodilian heart (in squamates and chelonians) and the crocodilian heart (in crocodiles, alligators, gavials, and caimans) (Figs. 68.4 and 68.5).[1,4,9,29]

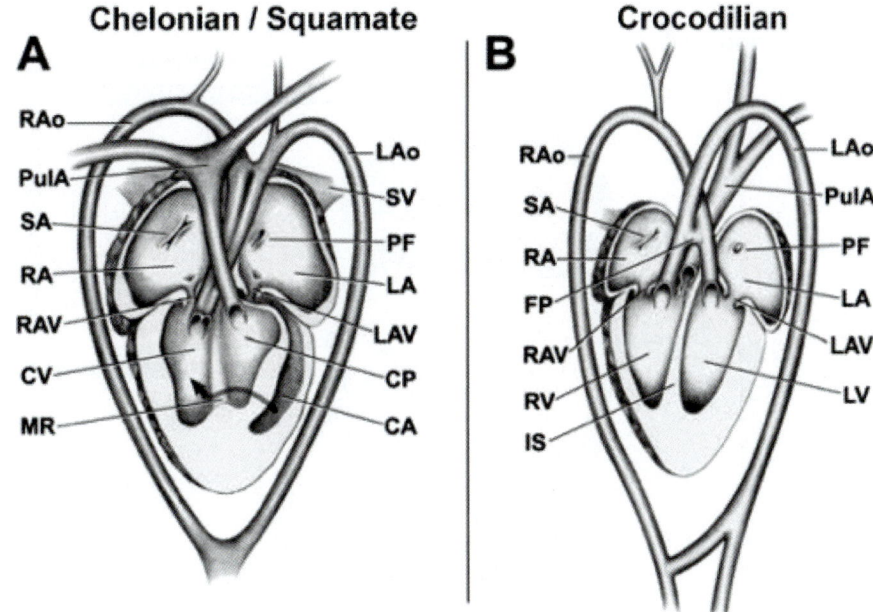

FIG 68.4 Anatomical drawing of the two reptilian cardiac configurations. (A) Chelonian and squamate pattern and (B) crocodilian pattern. CA, Cavum arteriosum; CP, cavum pulmonale; CV, cavum venosum; FP, foramen of Panizza; IS, interventricular septum; LA, left atrium; LAo, left aorta; LAV, left atrioventricular valve; LV, left ventricle; MR, muscular ridge; PF, pulmonary vein foramen; PulA, pulmonary artery; RA, right atrium; RAo, right aorta; RAV, right atrioventricular valve; RV, right ventricle; SA, sinoatrial valve; SV, sinus venosus. (Modified from Wyneken J. Normal reptile heart morphology and function. *Vet Clin North Am. Exot Anim Pract.* 2009;12:51–63, with permission from Elsevier.)

Noncrocodilians. The noncrocodilian heart has historically been described as a three-chambered organ composed of two atria and one single ventricle (Fig. 68.6). The ventricle is morphologically considered as a single chamber due to the lack of a complete interventricular septum. It is only partially partitioned by muscular ridges (see later) that incompletely subdivide it with various degrees of structural and functional compartmentalization depending on adaptations to specific ecological and physiological parameters. This contrasts with the four-chambered crocodilian heart, where the presence of a complete interventricular septum anatomically and functionally separates the ventricle into two chambers.

The ophidian heart is substantially asymmetric with a larger right atrium extending caudally and covering a larger area of the right side of the ventricle than the left atria covers the left side of the ventricle. Three arterial trunks—the left aortic arch, the right aortic arch, and the pulmonary trunk—are visible on external examination (Fig. 68.7A). They run from the ventricle and emerge between the two atria, rotate toward the right, and form a 180-degree angle. The right (but not the left) aorta branches off several major arteries (including the right and left carotid arteries) and fuses caudally with the left aorta to form the common abdominal aorta (dorsal aorta) (see Fig. 68.7B).[1,2,4,9,23,25,27,30] The pulmonary artery later divides into left and right pulmonary arteries to supply the left and (where present) right lungs respectively. In species that only have one predominant right lung (e.g., most ophidians) the left pulmonary artery is absent or vestigial.[1,2]

The sinus venosus is situated on the dorsal aspect of the heart and is attached to the dorsal wall of the ventricle by the dorsal ligament (see Fig. 68.7C). It is composed of spontaneous contractile tissue and contains the pacemaker. It receives deoxygenated blood from the two cranial vena cavae and the caudal vena cava and drains into the right atrium through a sinoatrial orifice guarded by a pair of small flap valves, termed the sinoatrial valves. In some species, the hepatic vein or jugular vein also drain directly into the sinus venosus. In most squamate species, the sinus venosus possesses a partial septum.[1,2,4] As the sinus venosus can be considered as an additional chamber, the noncrocodilian heart may also be regarded as an atypical four-chambered heart.[1,2,8,9,26]

The left atrium is generally smaller than the right atrium and receives blood from the two pulmonary veins. In some species, paired valves are found in the pulmonary veins as they enter the atria.[23] The atria communicate with the ventricle via the atrioventricular funnels separated from the ventricle by monocuspid atrioventricular valves. This AV valve-complex is made of connective tissue and is bell-shaped with the concave side facing the ventricle.[23] Fibrous strands similar to chordae tendinae join the atrioventricular valves to the ventricular musculature in some species.[1,2,4]

In noncrocodilian reptiles, the ventricle is subdivided into three subchambers: the cavum pulmonale, the cavum venosum, and the cavum arteriosum (see Fig. 68.6).[1,2,4,23] The internal structure of the ventricle is complex. Two-dimensional anatomical illustrations may give an incomplete understanding of its structure, especially considering the anatomical and topographical diversity among species. Essentially, the cavum venosum and arteriosum are mostly dorsal (often collectively referred to as the *cavum dorsale*) and to the cavum pulmonale is ventral (sometimes named *cavum ventrale*).[1] The left and right aortic arches arise from the cavum venosum at two orifices with bicuspid valves (rather than tricuspid valves as in mammals). The pulmonary trunk is a continuation of the cavum pulmonale, and its base also contains small semilunar valves.[1] In some species of turtles and squamates, a foramen connects the left and right aortas. The functional significance of this is unknown, as both aortas originate from the cavum venosum.[16]

Noncrocodilian reptiles have two ventricular septa. One is the muscular ridge (also called the *horizontal septum*), which runs from the apex to the base of the heart and is incomplete toward the base. It separates the cavum pulmonale from the cavum venosum/cavum

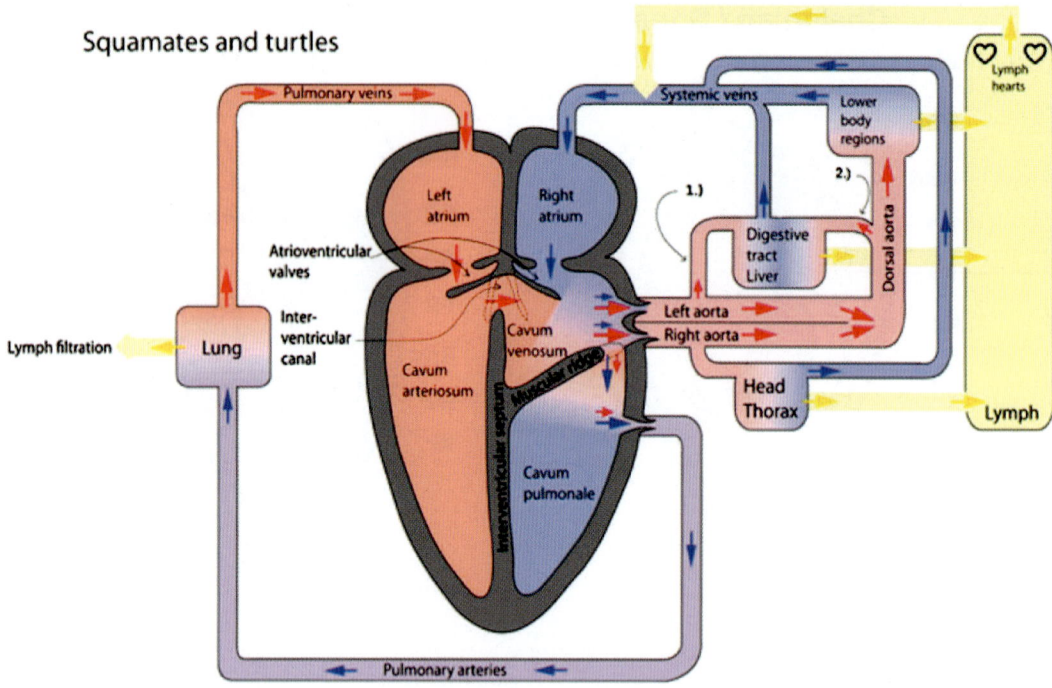

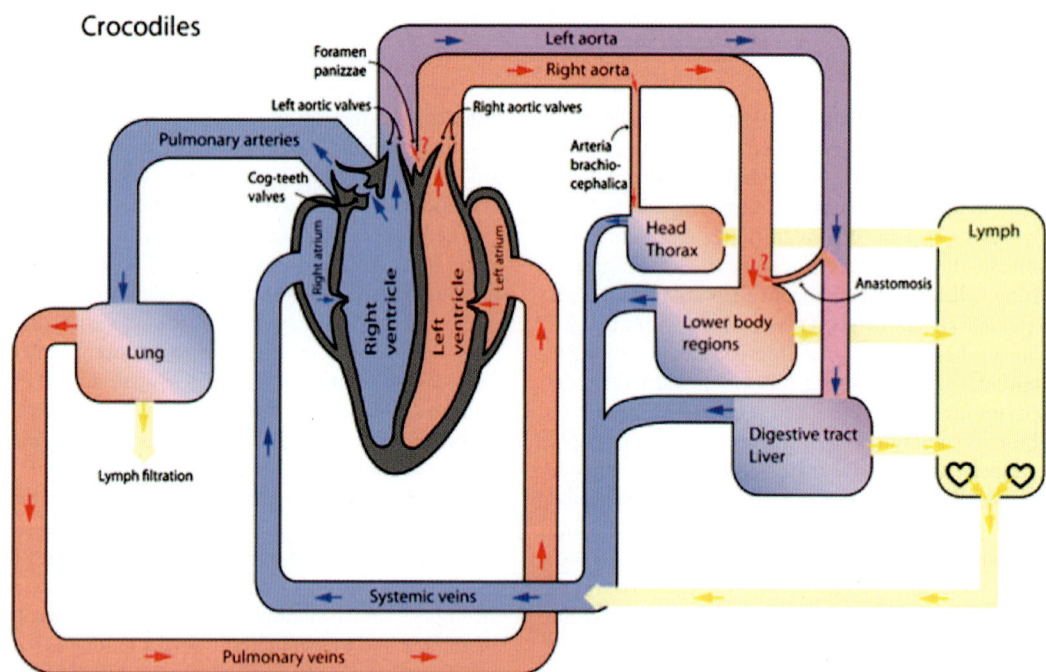

FIG 68.5 Schematic illustration of the circulatory and lymphatic systems in squamates/turtles and crocodiles. Red color indicates O_2-rich, CO_2-poor blood; blue color indicates O_2-poor, CO_2-rich blood. Different shades of violet stand for different degrees of mixing. Lymph is drawn in yellow. Arrows indicate the direction of blood/lymph flow. (Modified from Campen R, Starck M. Cardiovascular circuits and digestive function of intermittent-feeding sauropsids. In McCue M, ed. *Comparative Physiology of Fasting, Starvation, and Food Limitation.* Berlin: Springer-Verlag; 2012;133–155, with permission from Springer-Verlag.)

arteriosum predominantly during the ventricular systole. This muscular ridge is relatively inconsistent in structure and position across species. It is poorly developed in chelonians, except marine turtles and giant tortoises.[1] It is more developed in varanids and pythons compared to other squamates and many species of chelonians.[1,14,16] In evolutionary terms, the interventricular septum present in archosaurs (crocodilians and birds) seems to have evolved from this muscular ridge.[1,10,27]

An incomplete muscular septum (also called the *vertical septum* or *interventricular septum*) divides the cavum dorsale into the cavum arteriosum to the left and the cavum venosum to the right and often

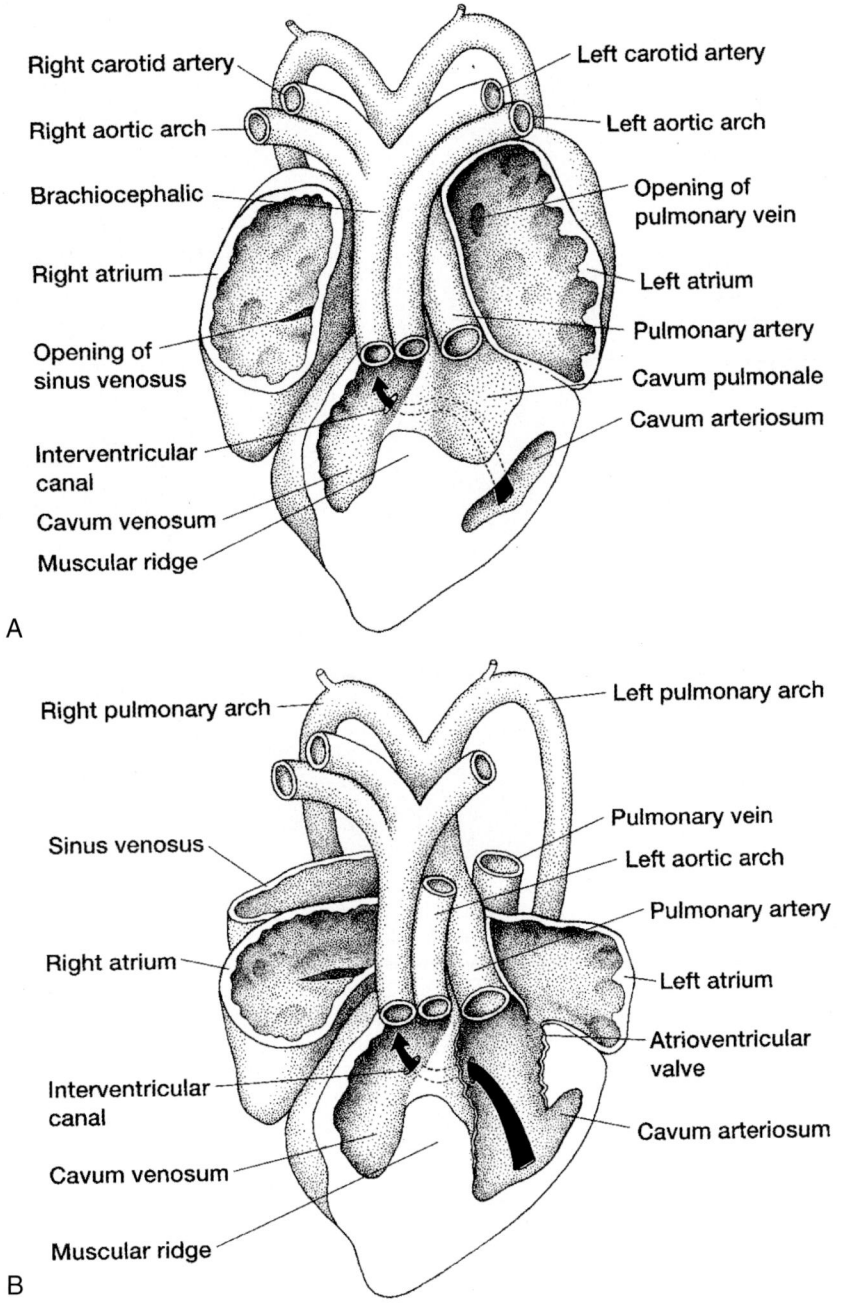

Right carotid artery

Right aortic arch

Brachiocephalic

Right atrium

Opening of
sinus venosus

Interventricular
canal

Cavum venosum

Muscular ridge

Left carotid artery

Left aortic arch

Opening of
pulmonary vein

Left atrium

Pulmonary artery

Cavum pulmonale

Cavum arteriosum

A

Right pulmonary arch

Sinus venosus

Right atrium

Interventricular
canal

Cavum venosum

Muscular ridge

Left pulmonary arch

Pulmonary vein

Left aortic arch

Pulmonary artery

Left atrium

Atrioventricular
valve

Cavum arteriosum

B

FIG 68.6 Lizard heart, ventral view. (A) Part of the ventral wall of the heart has been removed to show its three interconnected compartments (cavum venosum separated by a muscular ridge from the cavum pulmonale and deeper cavum arteriosum. The solid arrow indicates the blood flow from the cavum arteriosum via the interventricular canal into the cavum venosum entering at the base of the aortic arches. (B) The wall of the cavum pulmonale has been cut away to better reveal the association of the deeper cavum arteriosum. Trimming of the atria and left aortic arch permits better viewing of the sinus venosus and pulmonary artery. (Reprinted from Kardong KV. The circulatory system. In Kardon KV, editor. *Vertebrates. Comparative Anatomy, Function, Evolution*, ed 6. New York: McGraw-Hill; 2012:451–498, with permission from McGraw-Hill).

joins the muscular ridge at its base. It contributes to the separation of pulmonary venous blood from systemic flow during ventricular diastole.[1]

Another septum, the bulbus lamelle, lies opposite the muscular ridge, curving over and around it. It is situated immediately to the right of the vertical septum.[18]

A large interventricular canal, located below the atrioventricular valves, is the only connection between the cavum arteriosum and the cavum venosum (see Fig. 68.6). The atrioventricular valves are positioned in such a way that, when pressed toward the midline (i.e., opened),

they partially or completely obstruct the interventricular canal. This system allows a certain functional separation of the systemic and pulmonary circulation, with the cavum pulmonale (cavum ventrale) being the functional homologue to the mammalian, crocodilian, and avian right ventricle, and the combined cavum venosum and arteriosum (cavum dorsale) being the functional homologue to the mammalian, crocodilian, and avian left ventricle.[1,2,4]

The cavum venosum is a relatively small cavity that receives both oxygenated and deoxygenated blood at various times during the cardiac

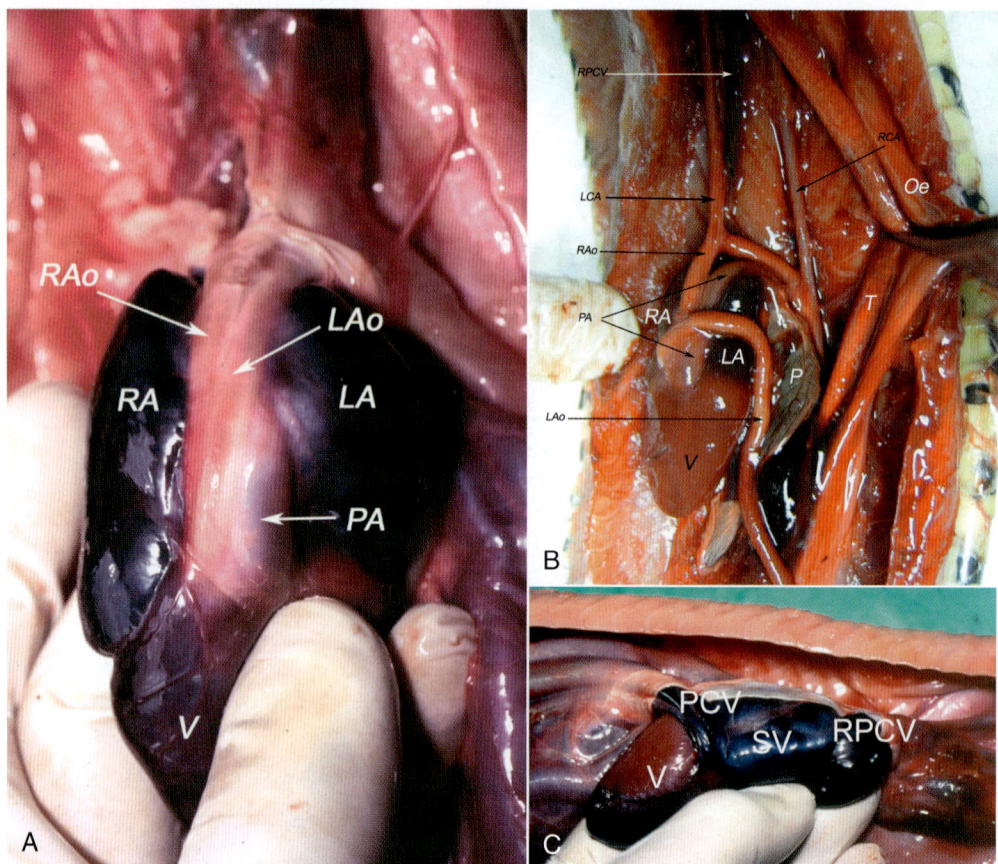

FIG 68.7 (A) Ventral aspect of the heart in a Burmese python (*Python bivittatus*) after resection of the pericardial sac: note the two atria (the right one [RA] being more developed than the left one [LA], separated from each other by the three arterial trunks, the pulmonary artery [PA], the right aortic arch [RAo], and the left aortic arch [LAo], rotating toward the right) and the single ventricle (V). (B) Efferent arterial trunks arising from the ventricle and adjacent anatomical structures in a carpet python (*Morelia spilota variegata*). LA, Left atrium; LCA, left carotid artery; Oe, esophagus; P, pericardium; PA, pulmonary artery; RA, right atrium; RAo, right aortic arch; RCA, right carotid artery; RPCV, right precaval vein; T, trachea; V, ventricle. (C) Photograph showing the aspect of the tubular-shaped sinus venosus (SV) in a Burmese python, located on the dorsal face of the right atrium, at the confluence of the three venae cavae. PCV, Postcaval vein; RPCV, right precaval vein; V, ventricle. (A, Courtesy of Lionel Schilliger, from Hochleitner C, Holland M. *Ultrasonography.* In Mader D, Divers S, eds. *Current Therapy in Reptile Medicine and Surgery.* St. Louis: Elsevier; 2014:107–127, with permission from Elsevier; B, courtesy of Lionel Schilliger; C, courtesy of Lionel Schilliger, from Schilliger L, Tessier D, Pouchelon JL, et al. Proposed standardization of the two-dimensional echocardiographic examination in snakes. *J Herp Med Surg.* 2006;16[3]:76–87, with permission from the *Journal of Herpetological Medicine and Surgery*).

cycle. This is particularly marked in varanids and pythons.[1,16,19,31] Thus, two kinds of cardiac morphologies can be roughly defined in noncrocodilian reptiles:

1. The typical noncrocodilian heart has a ventricle that is a continuous single chamber, operating as a single pump during the entire cardiac cycle. This is seen in most chelonians, such as freshwater turtles and tortoises, and in squamates, including aquatic snakes, grass snakes, rattlesnakes, and most lizard species. In this type of heart, the muscular ridge is relatively small and not well developed.[1,2,4,9,10,32] The right aortic and the intraventricular pressures are equal (Fig. 68.8).[1,19]

2. The varanid and python heart possess a large, well-developed muscular ridge, which almost forms a complete ventricular septum that can be visualized as an asymmetric thick wall. This is also found in at least one species of marine turtle, the leatherback turtle.[1] Moreover, in these reptiles, the cavum arteriosum is enlarged and the cavum venosum is reduced. In this heart model, the cavum pulmonale becomes functionally separated from the cavum venosum and from the cavum arteriosum during systole. Thus, this kind of ventricle functions as a double pump, with higher pressures in the cavum venosum and the systemic arches than in the cavum pulmonale and pulmonary arteries (Fig. 68.9).[19] This complete separation of the pulmonary and systemic circulations has been clearly shown in varanids (*Varanus exanthematicus* and *Varanus niloticus*), in the Burmese python (*Python bivittatus*), and in the ball python (*Python regius*).[10,16,19,31,33,34]

Crocodilians. The four-chambered crocodilian heart has a complete interventricular septum that anatomically and functionally separates the ventricle into two chambers. It resembles that of mammals and divides pulmonary and systemic flow (Fig. 68.10).[1,4,9,27] The gubernaculums cordis is a ligament that extends from the right ventricle (not from the apex as in Testudines and Sauria) and anchors the heart to the pericardium. The sinus venosus is much reduced and possesses a partial septum internally. It resembles an elongated pyramid, with the base lying cranially and the apex caudally. The right and left atria are of similar size. Both aortic arches remain. The left ventricle ejects blood

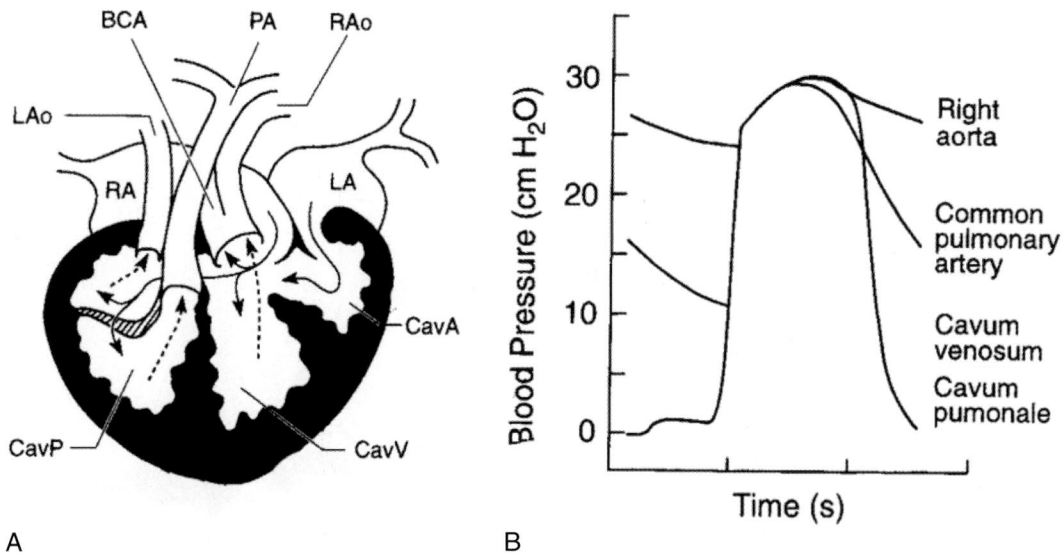

FIG 68.8 (A) Generalized anatomy and blood flow patterns in the chelonian heart (solid arrows indicate flow during ventricular diastole; broken arrows indicate flow during ventricular systole). (B) Intraventricular and aortic pressures during a cardiac cycle indicating that the ventricular cava function as a single pump. BCA, Base of carotid arch; CavA, cavum arteriosum; CavP, cavum pulmonale; CavV, cavum venosum; LA, left atrium; LAo, left aortic arch; PA, pulmonary artery; RA, right atrium; RAo, right aortic arch. (Reprinted from Farrel AP, Gambrel AK, Francis ETB. Comparative aspects of heart morphology. In Gans C, ed. *Biology of the Reptilia*. Vol. 19. Morphology G. Visceral Organs. Ithaca, NY: Society for the Study of Amphibians and Reptiles; 1998:375–424, with permission from the Society for the Study of Amphibians and Reptiles).

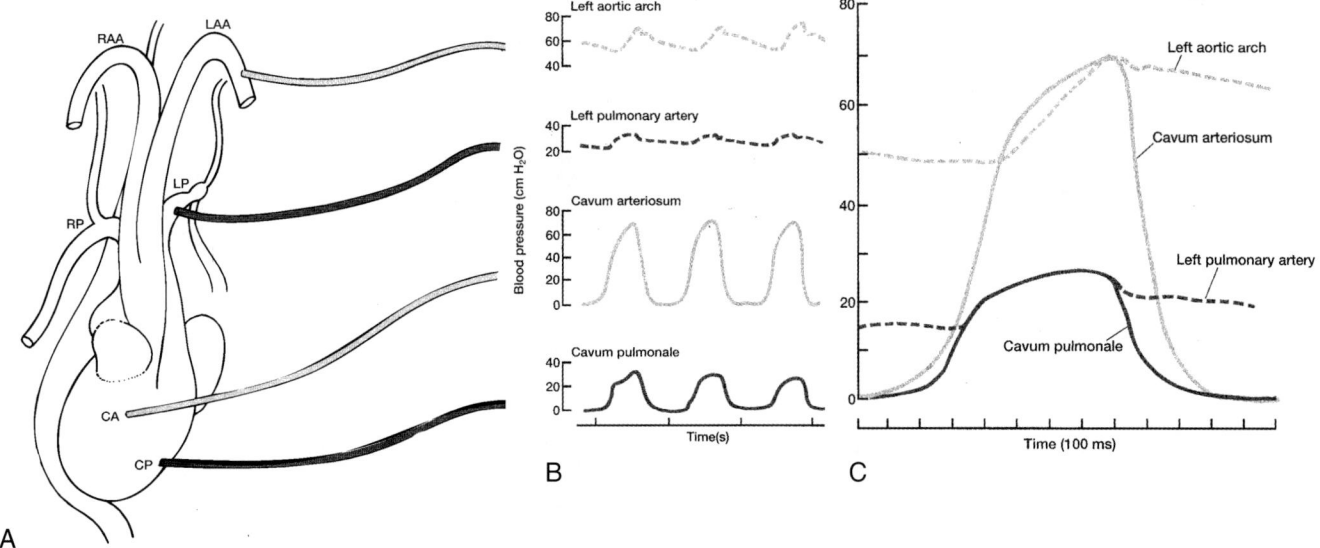

FIG 68.9 Hemodynamics of blood flow through the heart of the varanid lizard (*Varanus exanthematicus*). (A) Cannulae placed in the lizard heart (monitoring of blood pressures). (B) Tracings of pressures recorded at these locations (CP, CA, LP). (C) Tracings of pressures from different vessels are superimposed. During ventricular contraction, the peak pressure in the aortic arch is over twice that in the pulmonary arch. This provides evidence that the ventricle operates as a dual pressure pump, simultaneously producing high pressures in the systemic circuit and low pressures in the pulmonary circuit. CA, Cavum arteriosum; CP, cavum pulmonale; LAA, left aortic arch; LP, left pulmonary artery; RP, Right pulmonary artery; RAA, right aortic arch. (Reprinted from Kardong KV. The circulatory system. In Kardong KV, ed. *Vertebrates: Comparative Anatomy, Function, Evolution,* ed 6. New York: McGraw-Hill; 2012:451–498, with permission from McGraw-Hill.)

into the right aorta while the right ventricle ejects blood into the left aorta and the pulmonary artery. As they exit the ventricle, all three vessels are of similar diameter. As they run cranially, the aortae and the pulmonary artery are bound together by a connective tissue sheath. The base of each efferent artery has a bicuspid valve, the medial cusp being longer than the lateral one. A narrow channel, called the foramen of Panizza, creates a connection between the left and the right aortic arches, shortly after their exit from the ventricules.[1,2,4] The bicuspid atrioventricular valves, which guard the connection between the atria and ventricles, are composed of a left septal and a right marginal cusp. The left atrioventricular valves are membranous and the marginal cusp of the right atrioventricular valve is a thick, liplike structure. As in

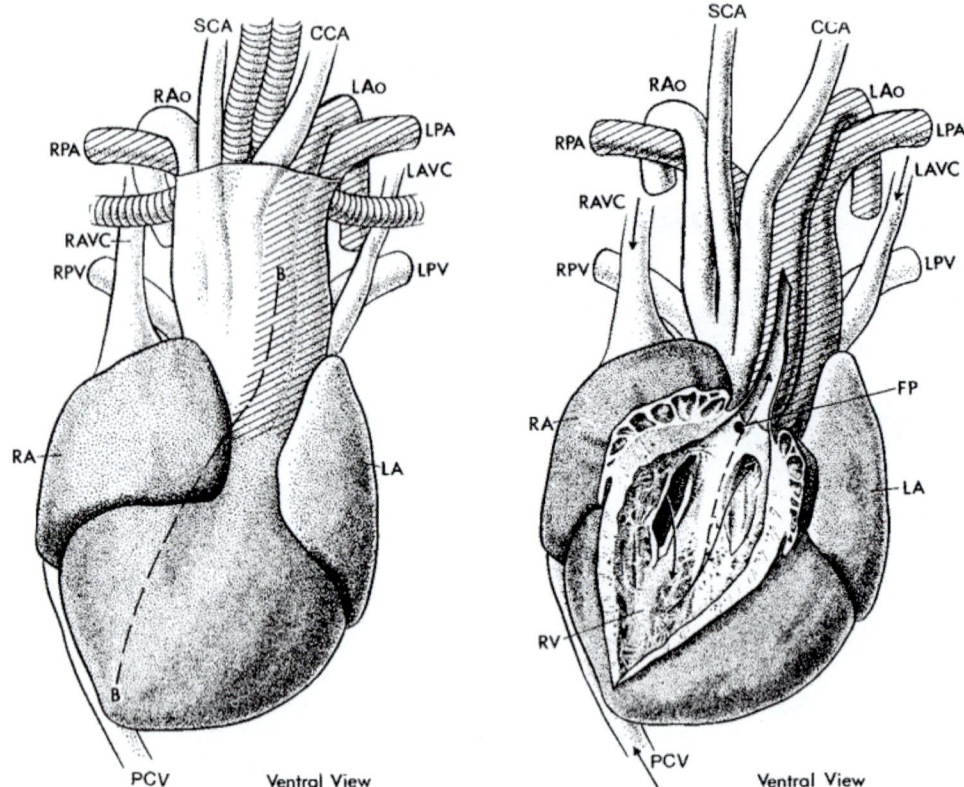

FIG 68.10 Schematic diagram of the crocodilian heart (*Crocodylus porosus*). The right side of the figure shows the heart opened ventrally along the line B. The solid arrows show the direction of flow during normal air breathing from right atrium to right ventricle to pulmonary arch. The dashed arrow, from right ventricle to left systemic arch, indicates the direction of blood flow when the pulmonary bypass shunt operates (e.g., during diving). CCA, Common carotid artery; FP, foramen of Panizza; LA, left atrium; LAo, left aortic arch; LAVC, left anterior vena cava; LPA, left pulmonary artery; LPV, left pulmonary vein; LV, left ventricle; PCV, postcaval vein; RA, right atrium; RAo, right aortic arch; RAVC, right anterior vena cava; RPA, right pulmonary artery; RPV, right pulmonary vein; RV, right ventricle; SCA, subclavian artery; SV, sinus venosus. (Reprinted from Farrel AP, Gambrel AK, Francis ETB: Comparative aspects of heart morphology. In Gans C, ed. *Biology of the Reptilia*. Vol. 19. Morphology G. Visceral Organs. Ithaca, NY: Society for the Study of Amphibians and Reptiles; 1998:375–424, with permission from the Society for the Study of Amphibians and Reptiles).

mammals, the pulmonary veins are devoid of valves. The right and left aortic arches anastomose at two locations, first at the foramen of Panizza and second at the level of the midcoelomic cavity by the dorsal connecting artery.[1,2,4] Opening of the foramen of Panizza is actively controlled and is discussed below.

Cardiac Physiology

Pacemaker and Heart Rate. Unlike mammals, reptiles do not have a specialized cardiac conduction system such as pacemaker nodes and Purkinje fibers.[1,35] Instead, the contractions are initiated by cardiac muscle. The contractions originate in fibers within the sinus venosus of the right atrium, which spread in sequential coordination, first to the left and then toward the apex caudally.[36] The ventricle is depolarized starting at its base and then proceeding to the left. Repolarization starts from the base and spreads symmetrically to the right and left toward the apex. It is believed that specific areas of cardiomyocytes slow conduction between different heart compartments, creating marked delays in electrical conduction. Such delays are clearly visible on the ECG of all researched reptile species with a characteristic rapid systolic phase and far slower diastolic one. Thus, the spongy myocardium of the ventricle functions as a medium for both conduction and contraction.[35]

The heart receives innervations from both parasympathetic and sympathetic fibers. The parasympathetic fibers run in the vagus nerve and provide cholinergic (inhibitory) control. The less-developed sympathetic fibers cause positive chronotropism and inotropism via adrenergic innervation.[1,4]

The heart rate (HR) is generally slower in reptiles than in mammals or birds. HR is dependent on numerous factors.[4] Myocardial efficiency is optimum when the reptile is within its preferred optimal temperature zone and at its preferred body temperature. Tachycardia occurs when the animal is exposed to higher temperatures, and, together with peripheral vasodilatation, increases heat loss from cutaneous vascularization. Conversely, lower temperatures stimulate bradycardia, and, together with peripheral vasoconstriction, reduce heat loss. This mechanism, which often anticipates internal temperature variations, is regulated by cutaneous thermoreceptors. HR is proportional to metabolic level and inversely proportional to body size. Reptiles that experience hypovolemia (e.g., as a result of surgery or trauma) may become tachycardic to maintain cardiac output and tissue oxygenation. Bradycardia is observed during apnea as pulmonary resistance increases and blood flow to the lungs decreases, effectively creating a right-to-left cardiac shunt.[37] Other effects on HR include digestion, gravidity, sensory stimulations (such as handling, postural, and gravitational stress), méthylatropine, and certain anesthetics and sedatives (e.g., α-2 agonists).[1,4,38]

Blood Flow During Normal Breathing

Noncrocodilians. In noncrocodilian reptiles (Fig. 68.11A.a and B), the ventricle is not physically divided, but pulmonary and systemic blood flow are separated and regulated by functional plasticity.

Oxygenated and deoxygenated blood flowing from the aortic arches are partially mixed, the amount of mixing being determined by the degree of development of the muscular ridge and interventricular septum.

During early ventricular diastole, both atrioventricular valves open simultaneously and block the interventricular canal between the cavum arteriosum and the cavum venosum. The cavum venosum and pulmonale receive deoxygenated blood from the right atrium, and the

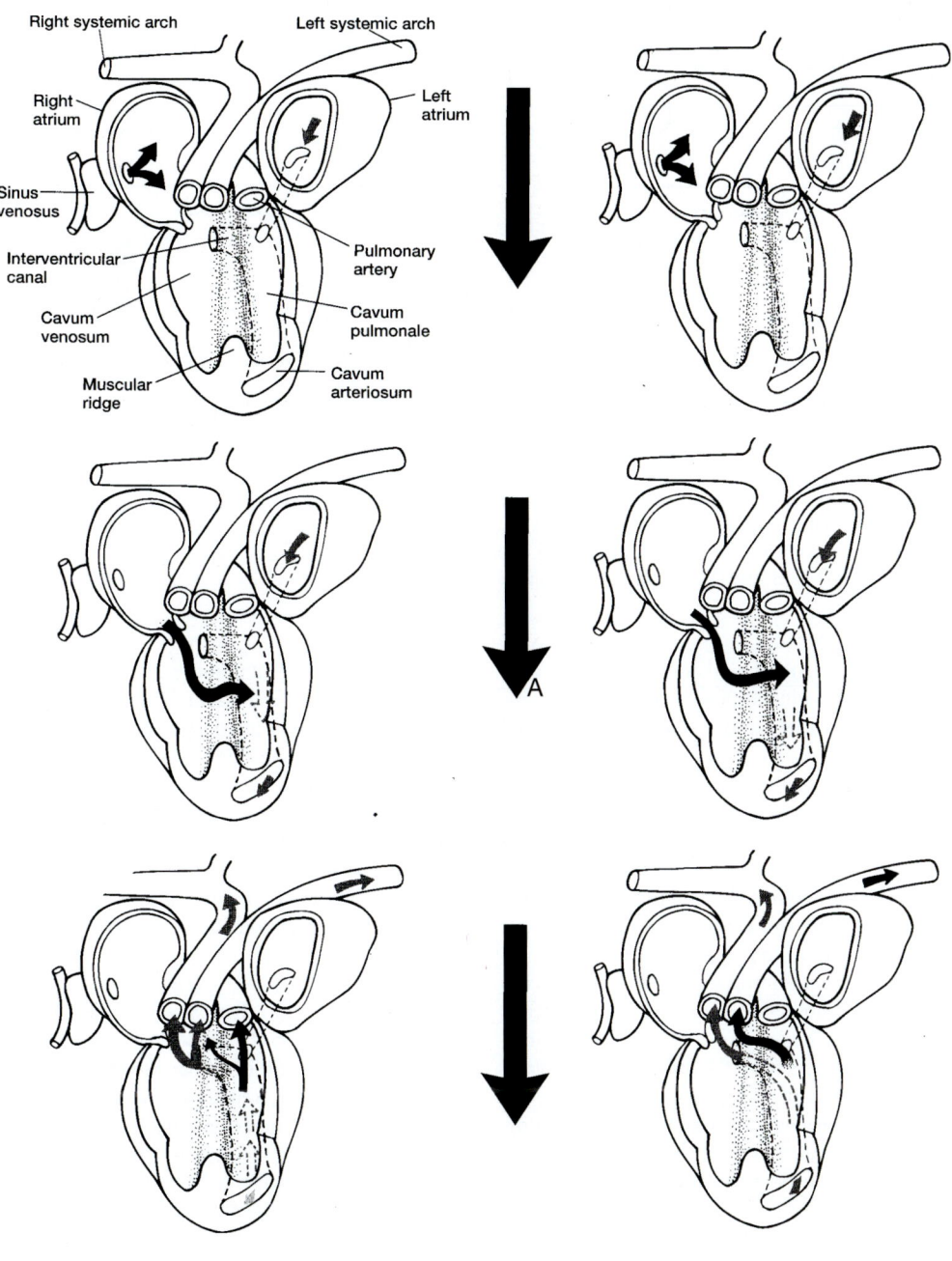

A   (a) Air breathing   (b) Diving

FIG 68.11 Blood flow through the noncrocodilian (squamate and chelonian) heart. (A) (a) When squamates breathe air on land, venous blood from the right atrium enters the cavum venosum of the ventricle and crosses a muscular ridge to fill the cavum pulmonale momentarily. Upon ventricular contraction, most of this blood exits via the pulmonary artery. Simultaneously, blood from the left atrium enters the cavum arteriosum. Contraction of the ventricle moves this blood through the interventricular canal, and then the blood departs via the left and right systemic arches. (b) When squamates and turtles dive, resistance to pulmonary blood flow encourages blood that would normally exit to the lungs to move instead across the muscular ridge and depart primarily via the left aortic arch. *Continued*

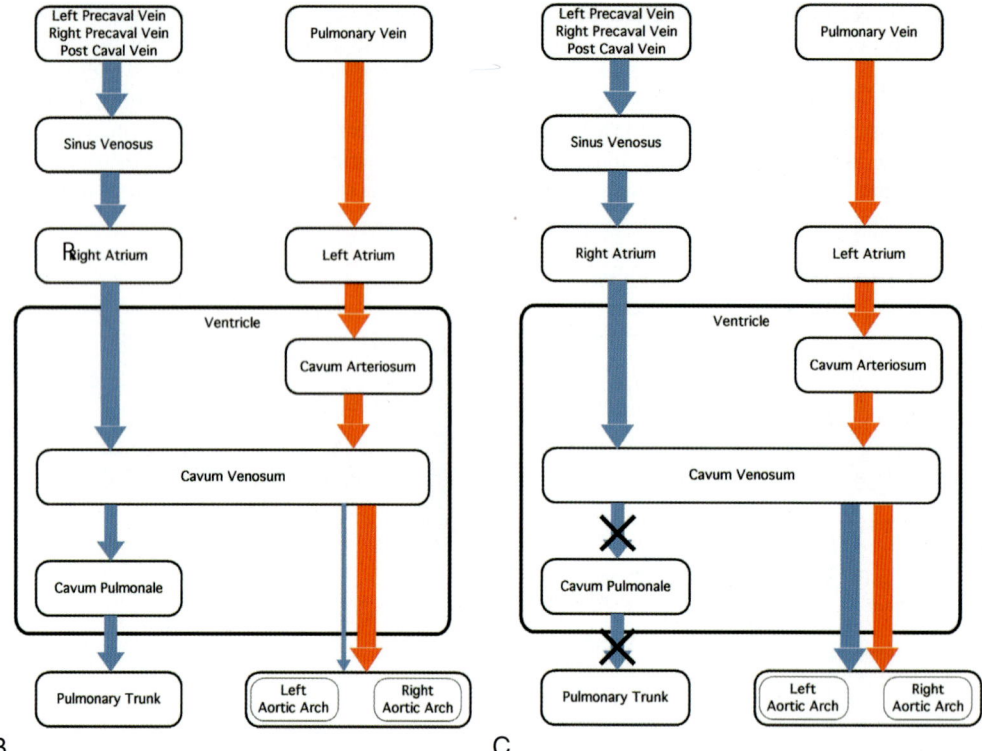

FIG 68.11, cont'd (B) Schematic drawing of blood flows during normal breathing. (C) Schematic drawing of blood flows during apnea. (Reprinted from Kardong KV. The circulatory system. In Kardong KV, ed. *Vertebrates. Comparative Anatomy, Function, Evolution*, ed 6. New York: McGraw-Hill; 2012:451–498, with permission from McGraw-Hill; B and C, courtesy of Lionel Schilliger.)

cavum arteriosum receives oxygenated blood from the left atrium. During the late ventricular diastole, blood flow from the atria ceases, and deoxygenated blood from the cavum venosum flows into the cavum pulmonale. During ventricular systole, the atrioventricular valves close the atrioventricular funnels. This opens the interventricular canal and allows blood flow from the cavum arteriosum into the cavum venosum. During late systole, the muscular ridge moves cranially and separates the cavum venosum and the cavum pulmonale. Oxygenated blood is then pumped out of the cavum venosum into the left and right aortic arches, and deoxygenated blood is pumped out from the cavum pulmonale toward the pulmonary arterial trunk (see Fig. 68.11A.a and B).[1,2,4,16,29] Because the diastolic blood pressure is lower in the pulmonary arches than in the systemic ones, blood flows first in the pulmonary arteries and then in the systemic arteries. Ventricular systole tends to be long and diastole is short. As already mentioned, the muscular ridge nearly completely separates the two sides of the ventricle in varanids and pythons. This produces a more pronounced separation of blood flow and allows for higher systemic pressures. In many chelonians, the cavum venosum is much larger, and so more blood mixing occurs between the left and right sides of the ventricle.[1,25,27] Unlike mammals, the reptilian atria make an active contribution to ventricular filling. On a cellular level, the atrial and ventricular walls are composed of an inner, thick, spongy and outer, compact myocardium. The spongy cardiomyocytes receive nutrition by diffusion from luminal blood via intramural flow, and a coronary circulation supplies the compact myocardium of the ventricles.[17]

Crocodilians. When crocodilians have free access to air, the heart functions in a similar way to mammals with separate systemic and pulmonary circulations (Fig. 68.12a). Because the blood pressure in the pulmonary vasculature is much lower than in the systemic vasculature,

the pressure generated in the right ventricle is much lower than in the left ventricle. The blood pressures in the left and right aorta are equalized via the foramen of Panizza (which opens during ventricular diastole) and the dorsal connecting artery. Consequently, the bicuspid valve at the orifice of the left aorta (which exits the right ventricle) remains closed, as the right ventricular pressure does not exceed left aortic pressure. Hence, all the blood in the right ventricle is pumped into the pulmonary circulation. In addition, the blood in the left ventricle goes primarily into the right aorta, as one of the valves guarding the right aorta folds back to completely cover the foramen of Panizza during systole.[1,4,5,24,27,30]

Cardiac Shunting. Given their unique anatomy, reptiles have the ability to regulate blood shunting in the ventricle based on their metabolic needs.[39,40] While cardiovascular shunting is detrimental in birds and mammals and is only seen in congenital abnormalities, it serves important physiological functions in reptiles.[8]

The extent of shunting is determined by differences in pulmonary and systemic vascular resistance, which is partially regulated by parasympathetic and sympathetic tones. During periods of high parasympathetic tone (e.g., during rest, fasting, diving, apnea, hibernation), vasoconstriction causes an increase in pressure in the pulmonary artery and a decreased blood pressure in the pulmonary veins. These results in high pulmonary outflow resistance, and a right-to-left (R-L) shunt may occur, decreasing pulmonary perfusion. The R-L shunt ensures blood perfusion to vital organs during anoxia (see Fig. 68.11A.b and C).[1,2,39,40]

Inversely, increased sympathetic tone as a result of physiological or environmental events causing an increase in metabolism (such as increases in temperature, exercise, or digestion) causes a left-to-right shunt. This facilitates pulmonary perfusion and increases blood oxygenation and

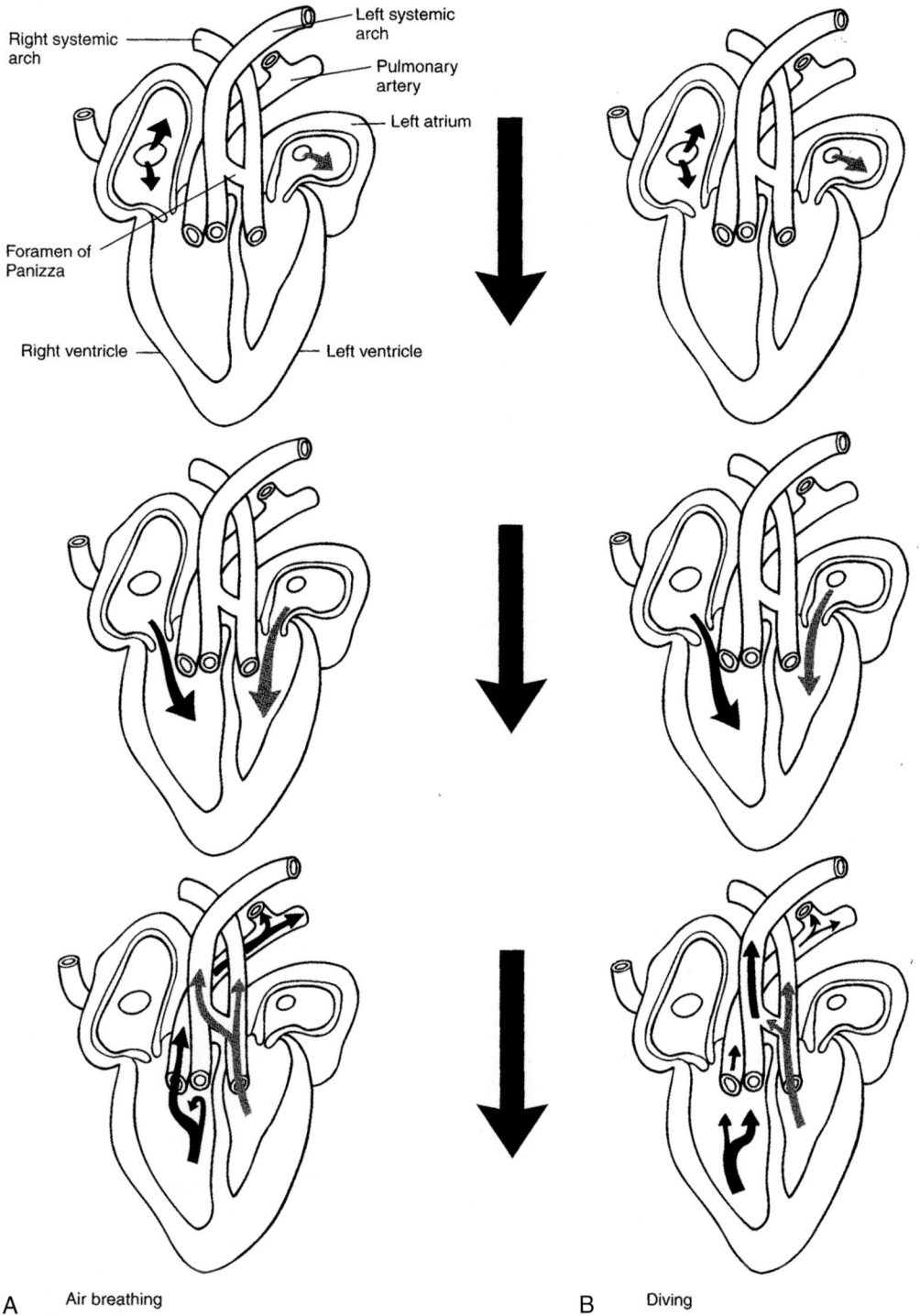

FIG 68.12 Blood flow through the crocodile heart. (A) Systemic and pulmonary blood flow when the crocodilian breathes air. (B) Internal changes that result in decreased pulmonary flow when the crocodilian dives. (Reprinted from Kardong KV. The circulatory system. In Kardong KV, ed. *Vertebrates. Comparative Anatomy, Function, Evolution,* ed 6. New York: McGraw-Hill; 2012:451–498, with permission from McGraw-Hill.)

gaseous exchange. In most reptiles breathing is intermittent with long, nonventilatory phases of apnea. The ability to shunt blood in both directions may therefore be optimal to limit ventilation/perfusion mismatch.[1,2,39,40]

This kind of cardiac shunting mechanism is observed in chelonians and also in most squamates, where the heart acts as a single-chamber pressure pump. This is termed "pressure difference shunting," whereby

the balance between R-L or L-R shunts depends essentially on the ventilatory state of the animal (i.e., the pulmonary and systemic vascular resistances). "Washout shunting" may also be responsible for cardiac shunting in reptiles. The main difference between these two shunting mechanisms depends on the ability of the muscular ridge to separate the cavum pulmonale from the cavum venosum and cavum arteriosum during systole. "Pressure difference shunting" only occurs in crocodiles, whereas in turtles, both "pressure difference shunting" and "washout shunting" occurs.[1,40]

The "washout" mechanism is probably the primary physiological determinant of intracardiac shunting in species with a partially developed "double pressure" pump (varanids and pythons). In varanids and pythons, the separation between the cavum pulmonale and the two other cava prevents any resistance in outflow pressure to influence intracardiac shunting during ventricular systole (as is the case in other squamates). "Washout shunting" occurs when the residual volume of blood remaining in the cavum venosum is mixed within the pulmonary or systemic circuit during the cardiac cycle. During right atrial systole, even though most of the systemic venous blood passes into the cavum pulmonale, a residual amount of deoxygenated blood remains in the cavum venosum. During ventricular systole, the cavum arteriosum injects blood into the cavum venosum and into the systemic arches. This results in the mixing of the two atrial supplies and thus creates an R-L shunt. At the end of ventricular systole, oxygenated pulmonary venous blood may remain in the cavum venosum (i.e., end-systolic volume of the cavum venosum is not zero). During the next diastole, deoxygenated systemic venous blood pumped out from the right atrium through the cavum venosum and the cavum pulmonale will mix with this oxygenated pulmonary venous blood, resulting in a L-R intracardiac shunt. This end-systolic oxygenated blood is washed from the cavum venosum into the cavum pulmonale during the following diastole. Thus, the degree of R-L shunt depends on the volume of deoxygenated blood in the cavum venosum at end diastole in addition to the volume of blood ejected from the cavum arteriosum during systole. The degree of L-R shunt depends on the volume of oxygenated blood in the cavum venosum at the end of systole in addition to the volume of systemic venous blood.[1,40] Thus, "washout shunting" is dependent on preload, contractility of the heart, and afterload. This has been demonstrated in the ball python, in which shunting occurs in the cavum venosum, when the atrioventricular valves open but the muscular ridge is not yet closed. During fasting and resting, up to twice as much blood flows into the systemic circulation than into the pulmonary one (R-L shunt), whereas during digestion, more blood is pumped through the pulmonary circulation (L-R shunt) because of increased oxygen demand.[16]

The direction and degree of cardiac shunting in squamates and chelonians may also be influenced by internal and/or external factors, including temperature, disease/healing, digestion, vascular sphincters, hibernation, and, in aquatic species, the dive reflex. Various investigative approaches have been followed in order to better understand the potential physiological benefits.[4,25,29,39,40] It is also reasonable to assume that anesthetic drugs, pulmonary ventilation, and the composition of inhaled air may have an effect on cardiac shunting during anesthesia. This is likely to vary between species and may impact the duration of anesthetic recovery and anesthetic gas excretion.

In crocodilians, despite a complete ventricular separation, cardiovascular shunting can still occur via the foramen of Panizza, which joins the two aortae originating from separate ventricles.[1,4,40] During apnea (see Fig. 68.12b), increased pressure in lung tissue together with coglike valves at the base of the pulmonary artery causes an increase in pulmonary resistance. This results in the pressure of the right ventricle overcoming that of the pressure in the left systemic aorta, and blood from the right ventricle enters the left aorta and pulmonary artery. During apnea, most of the blood follows the course of the left aorta. However, some blood passes into the right aorta via the foramen of Panizza and, at the confluence of the left and right aortic arches, results in some mixing of oxygenated and deoxygenated blood in the systemic circulation.[1,4,40]

Other cardiac physiological parameters, such as heart rate, stroke volume, and blood pressure, greatly depend on environmental and behavioral parameters (e.g., temperature, oxygen demand, and activity).

Different cardiovascular variables are important in reptilian thermoregulation, such as heart rate and cutaneous vasodilation.[4,9] For instance, green iguanas (*Iguana iguana*) exposed to heat experience tachycardia, and about 20% of blood flow is shunted from right-to-left to increase thermal diffusion across the body. The presence of two aortae is beneficial in reptiles: shunting toward the left aorta contributes to thermal diffusion while the right aorta (having more branches, including the carotid arteries) still supplies the brain and major organs with well-oxygenated blood.[5]

Aside from cardiac shunting, another important physiological benefit is postprandial cardiac hypertrophy of intermittent feeders. In large, postprandial boids, blood flow to the intestines and portal system can increase by up to 30% and 300%, respectively.[29,41,42] This is supported by an increase in ventricular mass to support the postprandial increase in metabolism and blood flow. Heart mass can increase by 40% within 48 to 72 hours of a fasted Burmese python (*Python bivittatus*) ingesting a large meal. Such an increase in cardiac mass seems to be promoted by the presence of certain plasma fatty acids.[42]

DIAGNOSTIC TOOLS IN REPTILE CARDIOLOGY

Physical Examination

Ambient temperature can influence cardiopulmonary parameters in reptiles, so it must be considered during examination.[4] When cardiac pathology is suspected, the clinician should initially evaluate for concurrent disease to determine if any cardiac issue is primary or secondary.

In general, clinical signs of cardiovascular diseases in reptiles are similar to those in mammals, but certain differences exist due to differing cardiovascular physiology and anatomy. They include swelling around the cardiac region (cardiomegaly) (Fig. 68.13), cyanosis, peripheral edema (e.g., gular) (Fig. 68.14A), pulmonary edema, ascites (see Fig.

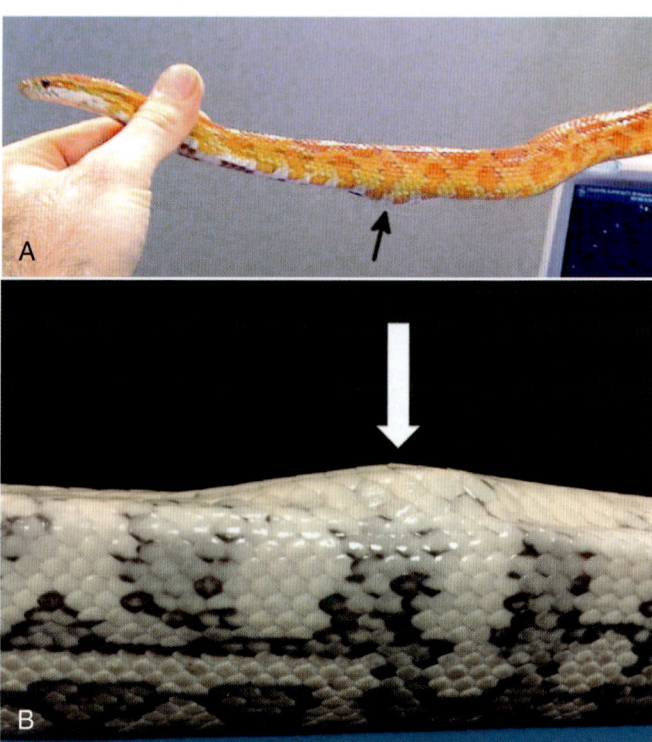

FIG 68.13 Cardiomegaly. (A) Corn snake (*Pantherophis guttatus*), black arrow, and (B) McDowell's carpet python (*Morelia spilota mcdowelli*), white arrow. (Courtesy of Valérie Chetboul.)

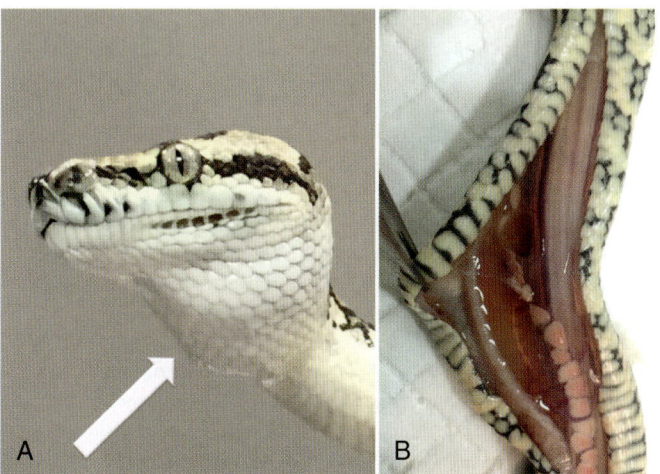

FIG 68.14 Congestive heart failure in a McDowell's carpet python (*Morelia spilota mcdowelli*). (A) Gular edema and (B) coelomic effusion. (Courtesy of Valérie Chetboul and Lionel Schilliger.)

68.14B), and exercise intolerance.[4,11] Decreased cardiac output can cause exercise intolerance, syncope, tachycardia, cyanosis, decreased peripheral perfusion, and arrhythmias. Brain anoxia, secondary to heart failure and atherosclerosis, may cause neurological signs, such as ataxia and head tilt.[43]

Because reptiles lack a true diaphragm, coughing is not a feature of congestive heart failure (CHF) as observed in mammals.[11,23] The pathophysiology of CHF is likely to be similar across vertebrate taxa because of shared neuroendocrine regulation of cardiovascular circulation and hemodynamic constraints. However, some differences exist between mammals and reptiles, mainly regarding physiological regulation of the cardiovascular system and the relative importance of neural versus humoral influences. For instance, in mammals, blood volume is regulated principally by the renal and gastrointestinal systems, whereas some reptiles (especially lizards) possess additional osmoregulatory organs such as salt glands. Additionally reptile respiratory physiology and their ability for cardiac shunting differs greatly from mammals and influences the pathophysiology of heart failure, notably edema formation.[8]

Clinical signs of CHF result from chronic, excessive compensatory mechanisms to maintain cardiac output and blood pressure. Increased preload leads to pulmonary edema and coelomic effusion, and increased afterload further impairs cardiac output and cardiac remodeling. The ability to shunt blood (of major physiological importance) and having a single cardiac ventricle (and consequently a different mechanism of blood ejection) are two major differences between mammals and reptiles that will be greatly affected by cardiac pathology and will have implications for blood oxygenation and ventilation/perfusion mismatch.[8]

Auscultation

Heart sounds in reptiles are muffled and may be difficult to auscultate with a standard stethoscope. A pressure-sensitive acoustic stethoscope (e.g., Ultrascope-Parker Medical Associates LLC, aka Ultrascope Inc., Charlotte, NC) allows for the diagnosis of heart murmurs but is only suitable in large snakes and lizards where the heart lies in the midcoelomic region and not within a bony pectoral girdle (e.g., monitor lizards). A continuous Doppler ultrasonic probe (8 MHz) can be used for cardiac "auscultation" in all reptiles. The probe is placed with an acoustic coupling gel coating on the epidermal surface at the level of the heart or large efferent arteries (Fig. 68.15). Doppler only indicates blood flow and not valve closure but allows determination of heart rate and rhythm.[4,11]

Heart rate (HR) varies but can be roughly estimated using an allometric formula; $HR(bpm) = 33.4 \times W_{(kg)}^{-0.25}$ in general, and HR(bpm)

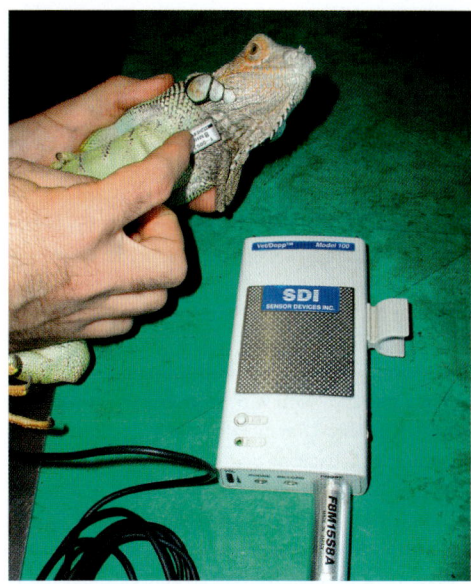

FIG 68.15 Continuous Doppler ultrasonic probe (8 MHz) used as an auscultation technique in a juvenile green iguana (*Iguana iguana*). (Courtesy of Lionel Schilliger.)

$= 20.6 \times W_{(kg)}^{-0.229}$ more specifically for snakes.[44] This formula should be used in conjunction with known HR parameters (if available), as it tends to overestimate heart rates in some species such as bearded dragons (*Pogona vitticeps*).[45] The reptile should be within its preferred optimum temperature zone for assessment of HR.

Blood Pressure Measurement and Pulse Oximetry

Measuring arterial pressure with a typical cuff and Doppler probe is not reliable. The thick and highly keratinized skin in the limb and tail regions constitutes a major obstacle to the penetration of acoustic waves from the Doppler probe. Oscillometric techniques using a cuff and Doppler probe in boid snakes and green iguanas were determined to be unreliable.[46,47] Direct blood pressure measurements are accurate and consistent but require surgical exposure of a large artery and are impractical for clinical practice.[38] Pulse oximetry machines use mammalian hemoglobin algorithms and are less helpful in reptiles, owing to the different structure of the hemoglobin molecule. It may be possible to assess changing trends in SpO_2 using a pulse oximeter that may provide limited information on response to treatment.[38]

Clinical Pathology

Creatine kinase (CK) and lactate dehydrogenase (LDH) may increase with conditions affecting cardiac muscle, such as myocarditis or infarct. However, increased plasma CK can also result from skeletal muscle damage from traumatic injuries, loss of body condition, and intramuscular injections (in particular, caustic drugs such as enrofloxacin).[4,11] Several LDH isoenzymes have been described but, unlike mammals, none have thus far been utilized for reptile clinical cardiology. Dyslipidemias such as hypercholesterolemia have been associated with atherosclerosis in a bearded dragon.[43] Hypocalcemia, commonly seen with nutritional disorders, can affect striated cardiac muscle and be visualized as electrocardiographic abnormalities.[11] Cardiac troponins have been used to detect myocardial damage in humans and domestic animals. There are two main troponins measured—troponin I and troponin T—and both are cardiac regulatory proteins that control the calcium-mediated interaction between actin and myosin. Elevation in cardiac troponin levels are the standard mammalian test to diagnose myocardial infarction. Point-of-care analyzers currently available in the veterinary field predominantly test for cardiac troponin I.[48] Currently, cardiac troponins have not been assessed in reptiles, but one of the authors (Girling) has found their measurement useful to assess progressive trends/worsening of clinical cases of cardiac dysfunction/failure. Leukocytosis, lymphocytosis, and heterophilia may be present and indicate underlying infections (such as vegetative or septic endocarditis) or hematopoietic neoplasia with secondary cardiac effects.[49]

Electrocardiography

Electrocardiography (ECG) is valuable, particularly in reptile species where the heart is difficult to observe using conventional radiography and echocardiography.[4,11] Widened QRS complexes and lengthened Q-T intervals were found in a green iguana (*Iguana iguana*) with aortic stenosis and atrioventricular dilatation. Tall and wide QRS complexes were reported in a carpet python with atrioventricular valve insufficiency, and increased P-R intervals associated with decreased Q-T intervals were seen in a boa constrictor (*Boa constrictor*) with atrioventricular valve insufficiency.[50]

The main challenges associated with the use of ECG in reptiles are the low electric amplitudes (usually <1.0 mV) that do not always provide readings of diagnostic quality. Moreover, standard parameters are not established for many species, thus interval and segment values may not always be of much use (Tables 68.1 and 68.2). Where reference ranges do exist they may not be reproducible because lead placement and temperature have not been clearly described. Even slight alterations in lead placement may alter an ECG. Performing routine ECGs on healthy reptile patients (with electrode positions and ambient temperature precisely identified) can help build up baseline values for future comparison.[4,11,36,51,52]

Reptile ECG interpretation is very similar to that of mammals, with similar P, QRS, and T complexes. An SV wave is represented by the depolarization of the sinus venosus (and the caudal vena cava) and is measured just before the P wave (Fig. 68.16). The SV wave is followed by sinusal contraction, the P wave is followed by atrial contraction, and the R wave is followed by ventricular contraction. The T wave indicates ventricular repolarization (Fig. 68.16).[4,11,36,51–53] Common findings in the normal reptilian ECG include P wave pleomorphism, very reduced Q and S deflections, and prolonged Q-T intervals as compared to similar-sized mammals.[4,11,36,51–53] Being of low amplitude (typically 0.1 mV or less), the SV wave may be obscured by background interference associated with skeletal muscle activity. When the SV wave is detected, it occurs after the T wave and before the P wave. In some cases the SV wave is difficult to separate from the preceding T wave.[55]

Correct electrode placement is essential to avoid erroneous ECG readings. The electrodes can be attached to the reptile by using self-adhering skin electrodes, stainless steel hypodermic needles, stainless steel suture material, or alligator clips (although care should be taken with the latter, as skin damage can occur). Placement of the electrodes varies according to species, but usually the traditional four-limb lead placement prevails. In snakes, the cranial limb leads should be placed two heart lengths cranial and the caudal limb leads two heart lengths caudal to the heart (Fig. 68.17). The negative lead can also be placed on the right side, one heart length cranial to the heart, and the positive lead can be placed on the left side, roughly 60% to 75% the distance from the head. The neutral or ground lead should be placed on the right side, across from the positive lead. In lizard species where the heart is within the pectoral girdle (e.g., Iguanidae, Agamidae, Chamaeleonidae, Scincidae), the two cranial limb electrodes should be placed on the cervical region instead of the forelimbs (yellow lead on the left, red lead on the right), and the caudal electrodes should be placed on the lateral body wall, cranial to the pelvis (green lead on the left, black lead on the right) (Fig. 68.18). In those species in which the heart is caudal to the pectoral girdle (Crocodilia, Teiidae, Varanidae), cranial

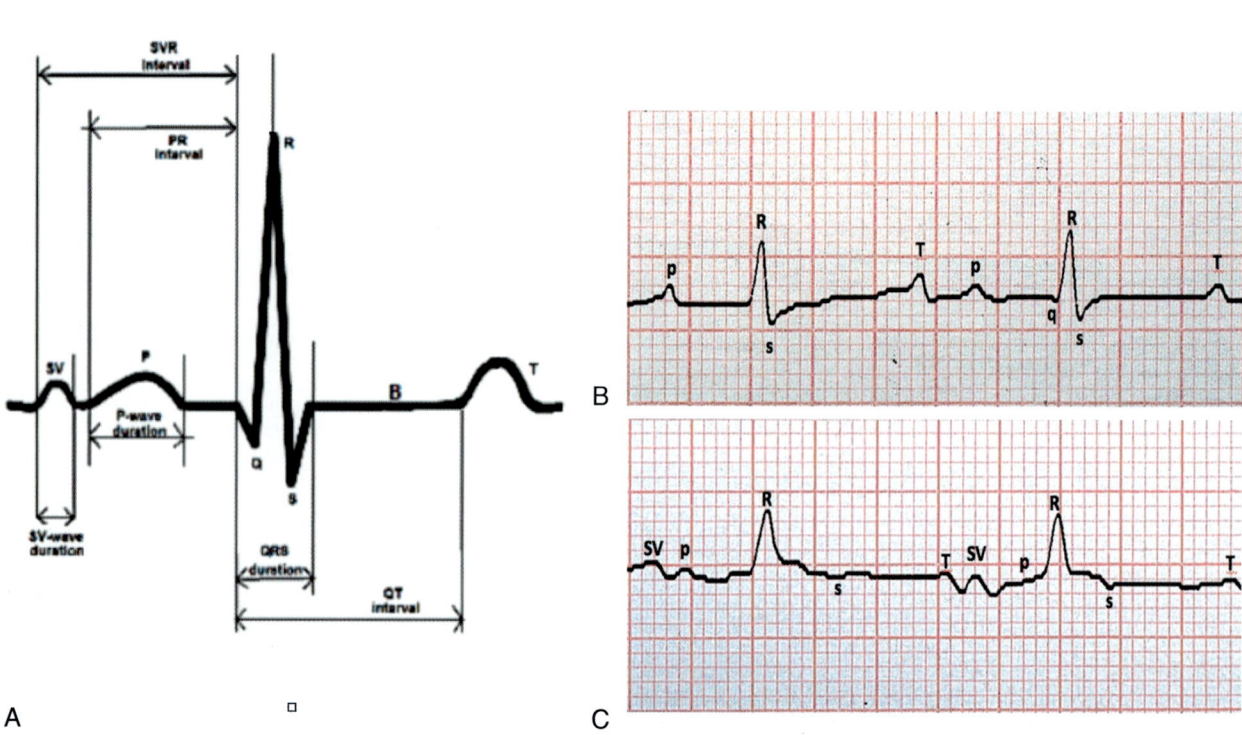

FIG 68.16 (A) Typical ECG complex in reptiles. B, Baseline. P, P wave; QRS, QRS wave; SV, SV wave; T, T wave. (B) ECG tracings in a green iguana *(Iguana iguana)*. (C) ECG tracings in a Dumeril's Madagascar boa *(Acrantophis dumerili)*. (A, Courtesy of Craig Hunt; B and C, courtesy of Lionel Schilliger.)

TABLE 68.1 ECG Measurements (Lead II) From Select Reptiles*

| Species | BOA CONSTRICTOR[52] | | | Snakes[53] | Lizards[53] | American Alligator[54] |
	Unanesthetized	Metofane	Pentobarbital			
n	6	6	12	101	321	10
Heart rate	11–42	11–37	5–34	22–136	45–230	
SV-P interval		0.24–1.3	0.40–0.60	0.29	0.19	
SV duration		0.04–0.35	0.04–0.18			
P amplitude				Inconsistent	Inconsistent	Inconsistent
P duration	0.06–0.1	0.05–0.2	0.04–0.11	0.02–0.07	0.02–0.06	Inconsistent
PR interval	0.38–0.90	0.40–1.04	0.35–0.56	0.26	0.16	Inconsistent
R amplitude				Inconsistent	Inconsistent	0.03–0.43
QRS duration	0.1–0.24	0.1–0.2	0.11–0.16	0.02–0.12	0.02–0.14	0.064–0.148
T amplitude				Inconsistent	Inconsistent	0.06–0.18
QT interval	0.8–2.0	0.84–1.74	1.16–2.40	0.30–1.36	0.18–1.30	0.93–1.45
MEA				96	95	60–108

Amplitude in mV, duration in s, MEA in degrees.
*Room temperature was 22°–26°C during ECG recording.
n, Sample size.
From Beaufrère H, Schilliger L, Pariaut R. Cardiovascular system. In: Mitchell MA, Tully TN, eds. *Current Therapy in Exotic Pet Practice.* St. Louis: Elsevier; 2016:151–220, with permission from Elsevier.

TABLE 68.2 Electrocardiographic Measurements of the Bearded Dragon (*Pogona vitticeps*) Recorded at 25 mm/sec and 0.5 mV/cm

	Mean or [Median]	Range	Standard Deviation or [IQR]
Weight (g)	335	66–517	140
Age (month)		4–30	
Snout-vent length (cm)	18.9	11.5–23.0	3.0
Cloacal temperature (°C)	32.7	27.7–37.9	2.0
Ambient temperature (°C)		26 & 35	
Heart rate (beats/minute)	90	24–170	39
R-R interval (mS)	[723]	353–2520	[533–1020]
P wave duration (mS)	56	30–100	13
P wave amplitude (mV)	0.03	0.01–0.06	0.01
P-R interval (mS)	145	75–253	38
SV wave duration (mS)	[57.5]	30–125	[50–67]
SV wave amplitude (mV)	0.03	0.01–0.07	0.01
SV-R interval (mS)	243	130–440	62
QRS duration (ms)	85	60–120	15
R wave amplitude (mv)	0.23	0.08–0.57	0.11
S wave amplitude (mV)	0.04	0.01–0.13	0.02
Q-T interval (mS)	355	120–980	139
T wave amplitude (mV)	0.04	0.01–0.14	0.02
MEA		+60–+110	

Postrecording digital enhancement was used to improve accuracy.
IQR, Interquartile range.
From Hunt C, unpublished data.

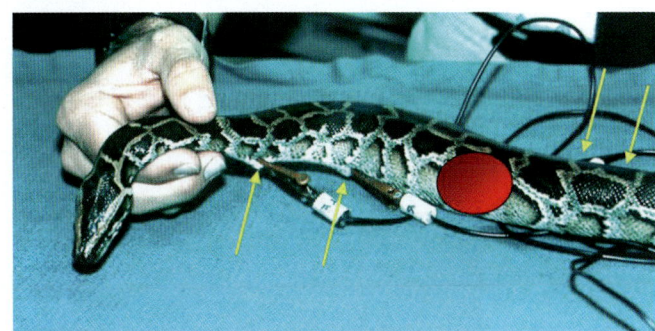

FIG 68.17 Lead placement in a snake can be a challenge because of the lack of limbs. Placing the two forelimb leads cranial to the heart (shown as a red circle) and the rear limb leads caudal to the heart yields a tracing similar to a standard lead II in dogs and cats. (Courtesy of Douglas R. Mader.)

electrodes should be placed on the forelimbs or cranial coelom and caudal electrodes on the hindlimbs or torso. The four-limb placement is not appropriate in chelonians because of the low surface voltage, and the two cranial electrodes should be placed in the cervical region, lateral to the neck and medial to the forelimbs. The caudal leads can be placed on the cranial skin fold of the stifles or caudally to the pelvic limbs.[4,11]

The mean electrical axis (MEA) is difficult if not impossible to determine in reptiles due to low potentials and is of limited value due to inconsistent placement of electrodes.[11]

Diagnostic Imaging

Radiography. Although radiography is central to reptile disease diagnosis, it remains challenging to produce images of high diagnostic value, especially when assessing the cardiac silhouette. Radiographs can rarely be used alone to evaluate the reptilian heart, mainly due to reduced tissue contrast and anatomical location. In chelonians and crocodilians, for example, the heart cannot be visualized, as it is superimposed with other visceral soft tissues and masked by osteoderms.[11,56] In lizards, particularly agamids and iguanids, the heart is obscured by the bony pectoral girdle (Fig. 68.19). Some of these difficulties may be overcome by using different settings; however, the use of computed tomography (CT) and digital radiography allow post-acquisition enhancement (level and window parameters) that can greatly improve image quality. Despite these limitations, radiographs can be used to evaluate the size of the cardiac silhouette in monitor lizards (Fig. 68.20) and snakes (Fig. 68.21).

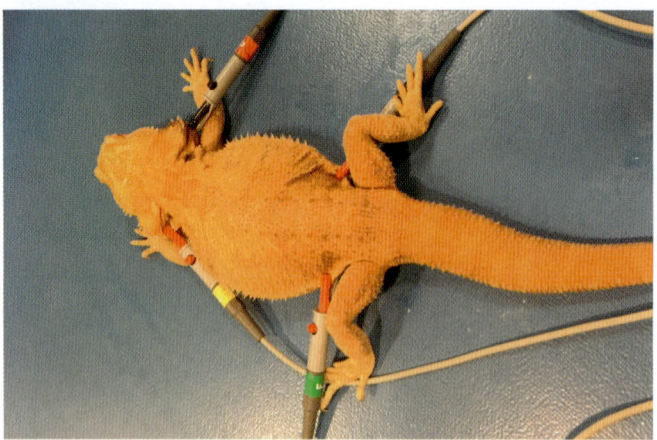

FIG 68.18 ECG in a bearded dragon *(Pogona vitticeps)*. The two cranial electrodes should be placed in the cervical region instead of on the forelimbs and the two caudal ones on the lateral body wall, cranial to the pelvis. (Courtesy of Lionel Schilliger.)

The paucity of normal reference parameters is another limitation to cardiac radiography. This can be overcome by archiving radiographs performed for other indications or during routine health evaluations in order to acquire a database of standard parameters.[57] Normal physiological variations in heart size should be taken into account when assessing cardiac enlargement (see anatomy and physiology section). As with any routine radiographic examination, two orthogonal projections should be taken: a dorsoventral view and a horizontal beam lateral view. In chelonians, a craniocaudal view can be useful but is most valuable for visualizing lung fields.[11,52,53,55] Mineralization of the great vessels may be observed as a result of hypervitaminosis D_3 or other metabolic disturbances.[9]

Computed Tomography and Magnetic Resonance Imaging. CT typically offers greater resolution than MRI and is particularly valuable for visualizing lung tissue (e.g., for pneumopathy, lung traumas induced by road accidents) and bone tissue (trauma, osteomyelitis, metabolic bone disease). Due to its ability to differentiate, MRI is generally preferred

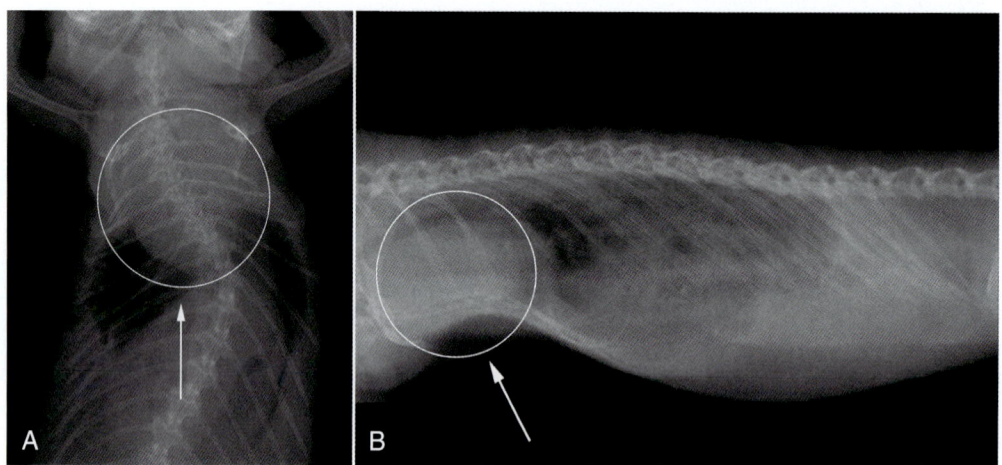

FIG 68.19 In lizards that have their heart located close to the pectoral girdle, the cardiac silhouette (white circles) is lost behind the surrounding bones and soft tissue on the dosroventral (A) and lateral (B) views. (Courtesy of Lionel Schilliger, with permission from the *Journal of Veterinary Diagnostic Investigation*.)

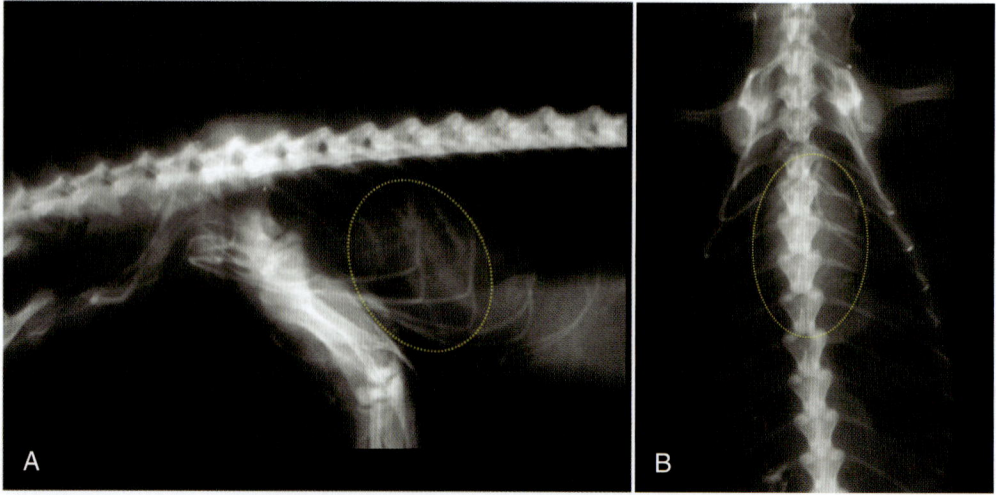

FIG 68.20 In lizards with a more caudally placed heart (e.g., varanids), both the lateral (A) and dorsoventral (B) views are useful, with the former giving the best cardiac image. (Courtesy of Douglas R. Mader.)

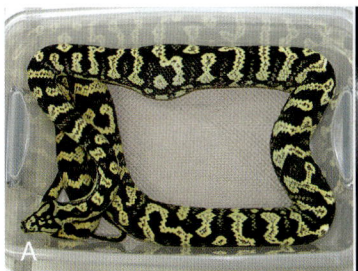 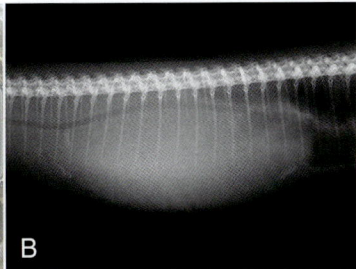 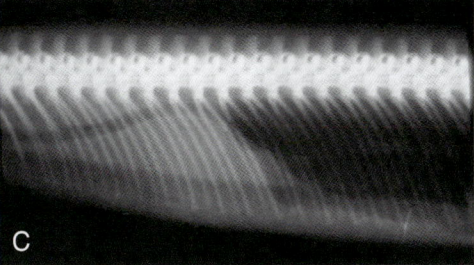

FIG 68.21 (A) This carpet python (*Morelia spilota variegata*) was seen for cranial coelomic swelling. (B) Radiograph of the patient shows an enlarged cardiac silhouette. (C) Radiograph of a normal python for comparison (A and B, Courtesy of Stephen Barten; C, courtesy of Douglas R. Mader.)

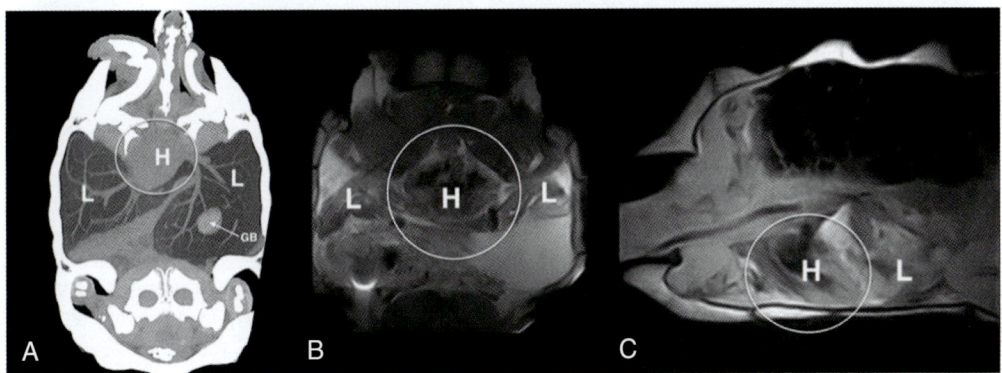

FIG 68.22 (A) CT scan in a radiated tortoise *(Astrochelys radiata)* showing the cardiac silhouette (H) between the two liver lobes (L). (B and C) MRI (T2 = spin-spin or transverse relaxation time) in a spur-thighed tortoise *(Testudo graeca)* with better contrasts. H, Heart; L, liver; GB, gallbladder. (A, Courtesy of M. Huynh; B and C, courtesy of L. Cauzinille.)

for soft tissue evaluations (Fig. 68.22). MRI is indicated for the examination of soft tissues, especially the central nervous system, liver, the reproductive system, and the kidneys. Apart from obvious cardiomyopathy, neither CT nor MRI (unless using very high magnetic field strengths) is of use for visualizing moving cardiac structures. Depending upon the equipment available and the speed of image acquisition, sedation or general anesthesia are typically required to ensure patient immobility and may be contraindicated in cases of heart failure.[56]

Echocardiography

Ultrasonography with Doppler is often the most practical diagnostic tool for antemortem evaluation of reptilian heart diseases and allows visualization of blood flow within the heart.[56,58–65] Patterns of normal blood flow in ball pythons (*Python regius*) and cardiac anatomy in Hermann's tortoises (*Testudo hermanni*) and Russian tortoises (*Agrionemys horsfieldi*) have been documented through the use of a combination of B-mode, color-Doppler, and contrast-echocardiography.[16,66,67]

A great range of ultrasound equipment is currently available, and many of these units are suitable for reptiles. The size and depth of the structures of interest dictate the transducer probes needed to perform echocardiography. Reptiles less than 250 g will require a 15 to 20 MHz or greater transducer; reptiles between 250 g to 2 kg can be scanned using a 10 to 15 MHz transducer; a 5 to 8 MHz transducer is used for reptiles between 2 to 20 kg; and a 3 to 5 MHz probe may be warranted for large crocodilians, lizards, or chelonians over 20 kg. A linear array is often used in snakes and lizards, while a biconvex sector scanner is recommended for chelonians because of their small acoustic windows. A thick layer of acoustic coupling gel should be applied at least 10 minutes prior to the examination to allow it to penetrate between the scales and obliterate any air pockets.[56,59,61,65,68,69]

Ultrasonography is challenging in most lizards and chelonians where boney obstructions (e.g., pectoral girdle, plastron) restrict the penetration of ultrasound waves. In lizards where the heart is located in the cranial coelom within the pectoral girdle (e.g., iguanids, chamaeleonids, lacertids, agamids), the acoustic window is craniocaudal and the probe must be positioned in front of (or behind) and above the bony pectoral girdle (Fig. 68.23A and B). This window is relatively narrow and restricts visualization of the entire heart. To counter this issue, the probe can be placed in the left or right axillary region in sternal or lateral recumbency (see Fig. 68.23C and D).[70] In the *Varanidae* and *Teiidae*, the heart can be easily accessed via a ventral midline approach caudal to the sternum (see Fig. 68.23E and F).[56,65]

In chelonians, the transducer is placed in the cervicobrachial area (Fig. 68.24A and B).[71] The heart lies immediately dorsal to the plastron and is caudal to the thyroid. The left and right atria are of similar size with thin walls. The ventricle is thick walled, and the two atrioventricular valves echogenic with their movement clearly discernible. In soft-shelled turtles (e.g., *Trionyx, Apalone, Cyclanorbis*) and pancake tortoises (*Malachochersus*), the heart is located more to the right side so the probe can either be placed in the right axillocervical fossa or pressed directly on the plastron, which is cartilaginous and so will permit, albeit it reduced, ultrasound wave penetration (see Fig. 68.24C and D). Echocardiography can also be performed on neonate or juvenile chelonians and crocodilians when ventral scutes have yet to become mineralized.

A standardized, two-dimensional echocardiography approach, based on established procedures used in mammals, has been advocated from work in boid snakes and bearded dragons (*Pogona vitticeps*).[58,60,70] Chelonian echocardiography techniques, including intravenous contrast, have been described in freshwater and terrestrial species (*Trachemys scripta elegans, Testudo hermanni,* and *Agrionemys horsfieldi*).[67,72]

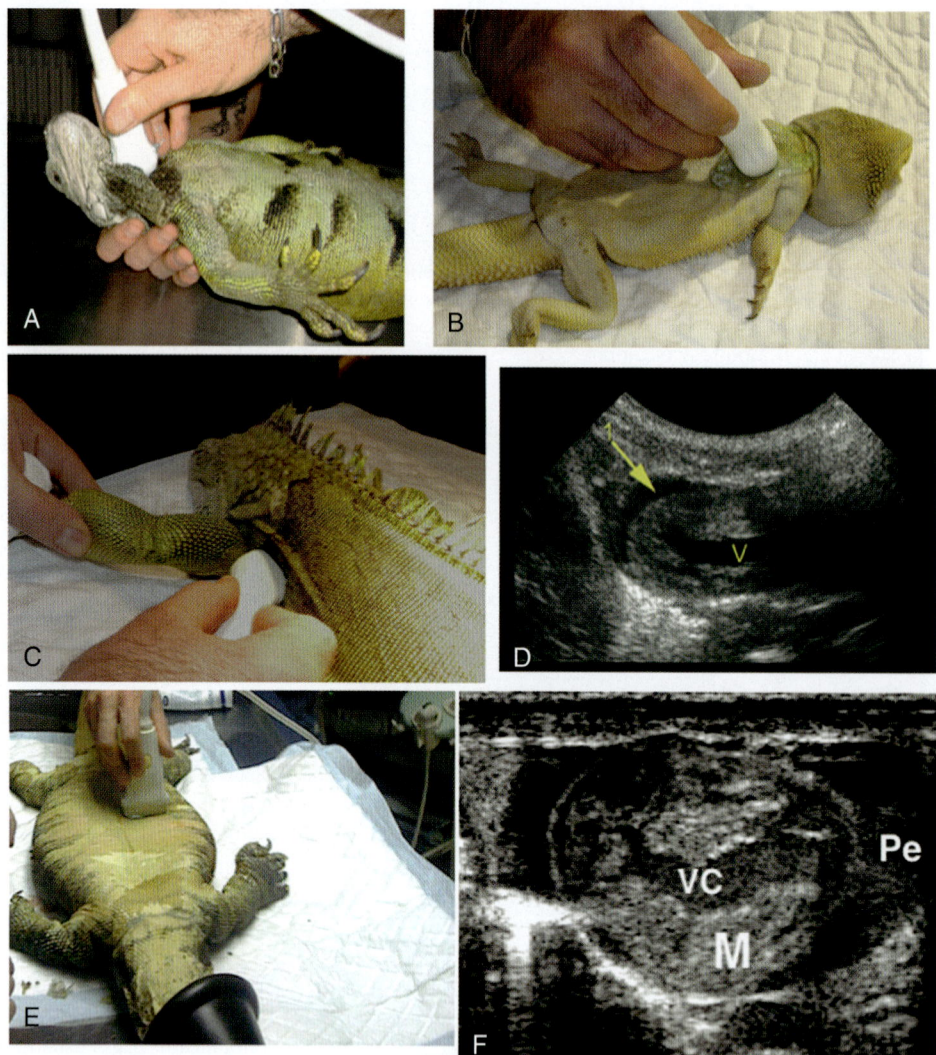

FIG 68.23 Acoustic windows that enable visualization of the heart in saurians. (A) Gular window in a green iguana (*Iguana iguana*); (B) caudocranial window in a bearded dragon (*Pogona vitticeps*); (C) left axillary window in a green iguana; (D) long-axis view of the heart by ventral approach in a bearded dragon demonstrating pericardial fluid (arrow) and the normal ventricle (V); (E) ventral approach, caudally to the heart, in a monitor lizard (*Varanus salvadori*); (F) short-axis section of the ventricle in a monitor. M, Myocardium; Pe, pericardial fluid; VC, ventricular cavity. (Courtesy of Lionel Schilliger, D with permission from the *Journal of Veterinary Diagnostic Investigation.*)

In snakes, three approaches are used in succession to define the ultrasound windows (Fig. 68.25).[60]

1. Ventral examination with the probe ventral to the heart to view (i) the organ from the caudal ventricular apex to the cranial atria, (ii) the sinus venosus, (iii) the atrioventricular junctions, and (iv) the three arterial trunks.

2. and 3. Right and left intercostal approaches obtained by lateral positioning of the probe to obtain lateral visualization of (i) the three arterial trunks, (ii) both atria, and (iii) the single ventricle.

By placing the probe ventral to the heart, the operator can scan or "sweep" the organ from the apex to the arterial trunks along its short axis (short-axis views). Thus, two transventricular views can be obtained by ventral approach:[58,60]

1. The apical or transapical short-axis view shows a transverse view of the apical myocardium and the pericardium from behind, in the form of an echogenic line (Fig. 68.26.1a).

2. The transventricular, subarterial, short-axis view shows a transverse view of the three cava surrounded by the peripheral myocardium (the ventral cavum pulmonale, the right dorsal cavum venosum, and the left dorsal cavum arteriosum) (see Fig. 68.26.1b). The interventricular (vertical) septum, located in the ventricular cavity between the cavum arteriosum and the cavum venosum, can be partially visualized, as can the muscular ridge (horizontal septum) marking the separation between the cavum venosum and the cavum pulmonale.

By moving the probe cranially, a transarterial short-axis view is obtained, giving a transverse view of the three large arterial trunks: the two aortic arches of equal diameter and the pulmonary trunk of larger diameter (producing a "Mickey-Mouse-head" figure) (see Fig. 68.26.2).

The probe is then kept in a ventral position but moved slightly to the right. The resultant right transatrial short-axis view shows the opening of the sinus venosus into the right atrium and enables assessment of both sinoatrial valves (see Fig. 68.26.3).[58,60]

Long-axis views are obtained by turning the probe 90 degrees in relation to the previous projections. Starting from the transventricular or subarterial view, the rotation of the probe provides two long-axis views of the heart. These are the atrioventricular sections, and they show both atrial cavities

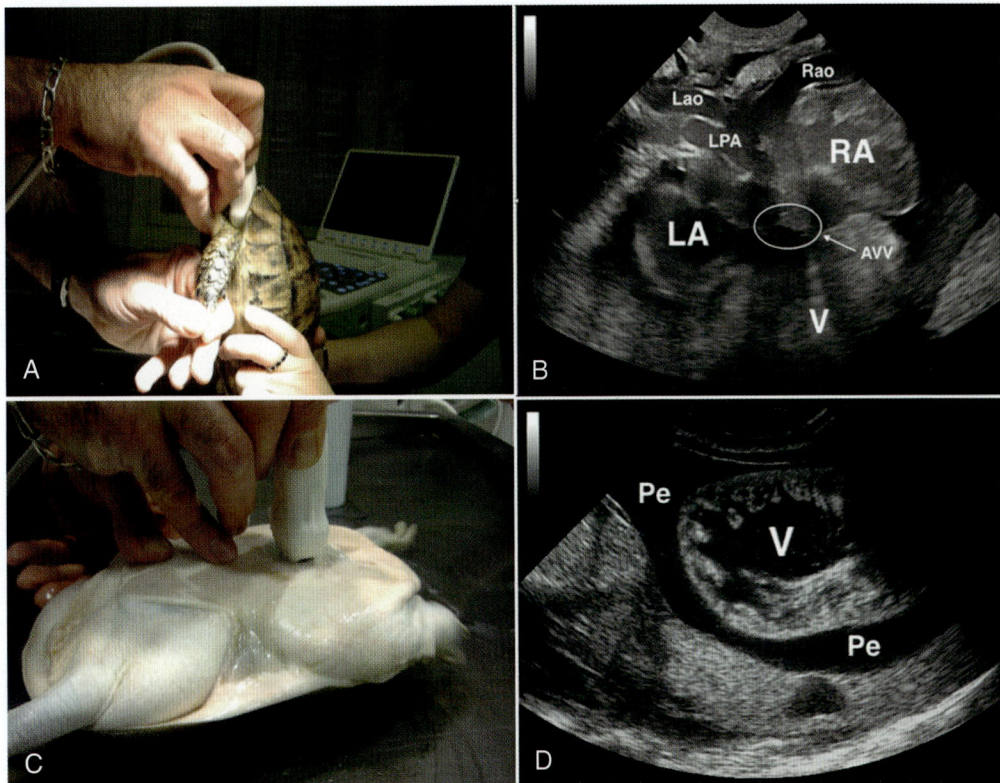

FIG 68.24 Acoustic windows that enable visualization of the heart in chelonians. (A) Cervicobrachial window in a spur-thighed tortoise (*Testudo graeca*). (B) Echocardiographic image from an African spurred tortoise (*Centrochelys sulcata*). (C) Ventral approach through the plastron in a Chinese soft-shell turtle (*Pelodiscus sinensis*). (D) Echocardiographic image of the same chinese soft-shell turtle, demonstrating pericardial fluid around the ventricle. LA, Left atrium; Lao, left aortic arch; LPA, left pulmonary artery; Pe, pericardial fluid; RA, right atrium; Rao, right aortic arch; V, ventricle. (Courtesy of Lionel Schilliger.)

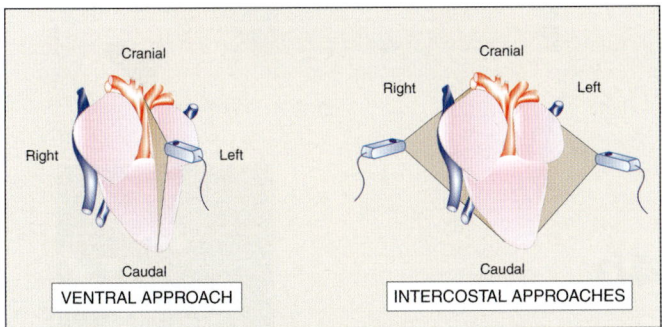

FIG 68.25 The three acoustic windows for echocardiography of ophidians: ventral, right, and left intercostal approaches. (From Schilliger L, Tessier D, Pouchelon JL, et al. Proposed standardization of the two-dimensional echocardiographic examination in snakes, *J Herp Med Surg.* 2006;6[3]:76–87, with permission from the *Journal of Herpetological Medicine and Surgery.*)

opening into the single ventricle. The left atrioventricular junction can be observed by orientating the ultrasound plane ventrodorsally from the right to the left (see Fig. 68.26.4a). The right atrioventricular junction can be observed by orientating the ultrasound plane ventrodorsally from the left to the right (see Fig. 68.26.4b). The atrioventricular valves, also known as septal monocuspid valves, can be visualized.[58,60]

Similarly, starting from the short-axis transarterial view, the probe is rotated by 90 degrees to obtain a long-axis transarterial section. This reveals the right aortic arch and the pulmonary trunk with parallel paths (see Fig. 68.26.5). The path of the pulmonary artery can be located by moving the probe caudally. The path of this artery comes closer to the probe ventrally and then opens out on the right with the cavum pulmonale. Finally, starting from the right transatrial short-axis view, the probe is rotated again by 90 degrees and moved caudally to give the long-axis transcaval section. This shows the caudal vena cava from the level of the sinus venosus running parallel to the pulmonary vein (see Fig. 68.26.6).[58,60]

In the case of small snakes, the examination is completed with two intercostal approaches. The transarterial long-axis section is obtained by the right intercostal approach, and the probe is placed laterally on the right so that the cross-section is parallel to the animal's body and the left atrium is removed from the proximal field occupied by the large arterial trunks. This provides clear visualization of the left atrium. Conversely, the left symmetrical intercostal section provides a good approach for observing the right atrium.[58,60]

In bearded dragons, echocardiography can be performed through windows in the left and right axillae (Fig. 68.27), with the animal in lateral recumbency.[70] The window in the left axilla allows for a subjective and objective assessment of cardiac structure and function. The right axillary window allows for evaluation of pulmonary artery flow. Both views provide data for the presence of pericardial effusion or valvular insufficiency. With optimized imaging planes, cardiac chambers and fractional area change, along with fractional shortening in the longitudinal and transverse planes, can be calculated (Table 68.3). Body weight and cardiac chamber dimensions of males were significantly larger than for females. Ventricular fractional area change was the most consistent functional assessment (Table 68.4). The majority of animals were found to have no evidence of valvular insufficiency, while approximately half had evidence of pericardial fluid. Pulmonary artery flow was assessed in all patients.

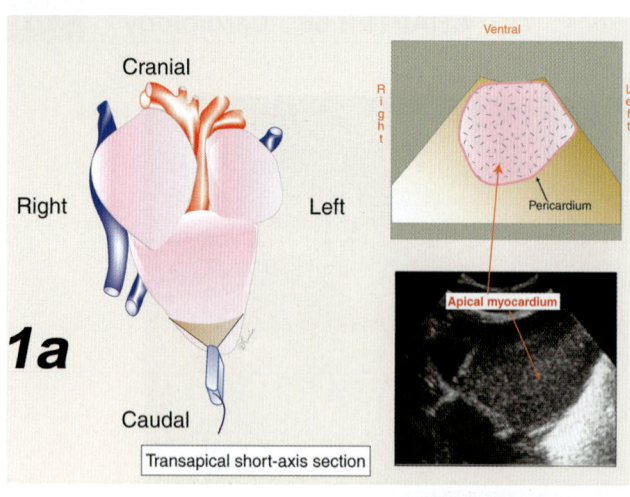

1a

Apical myocardium

Pericardium

Transapical short-axis section

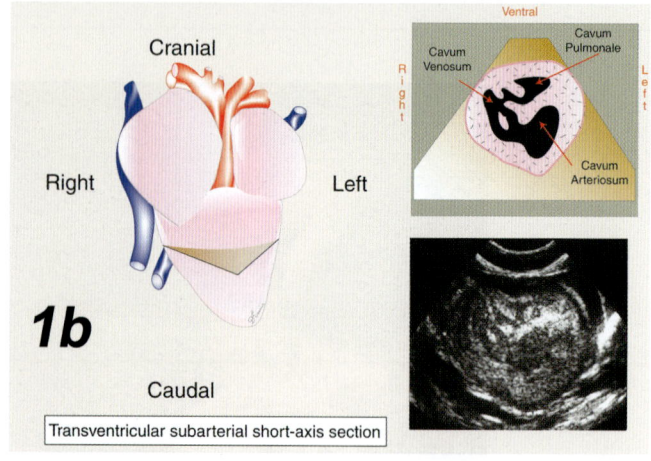

1b

Cavum Venosum
Cavum Pulmonale
Cavum Arteriosum

Transventricular subarterial short-axis section

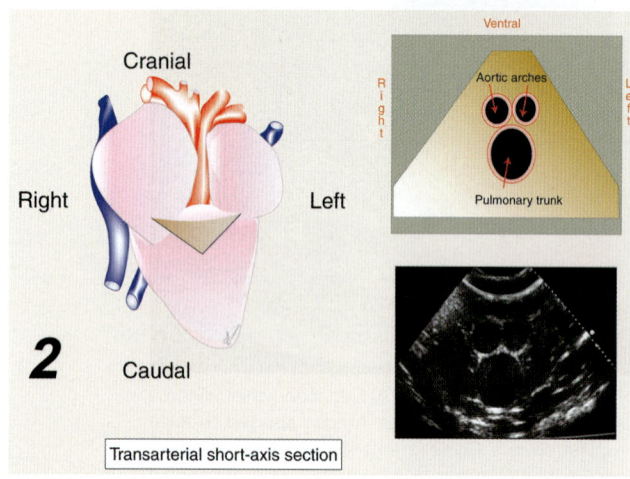

2

Aortic arches

Pulmonary trunk

Transarterial short-axis section

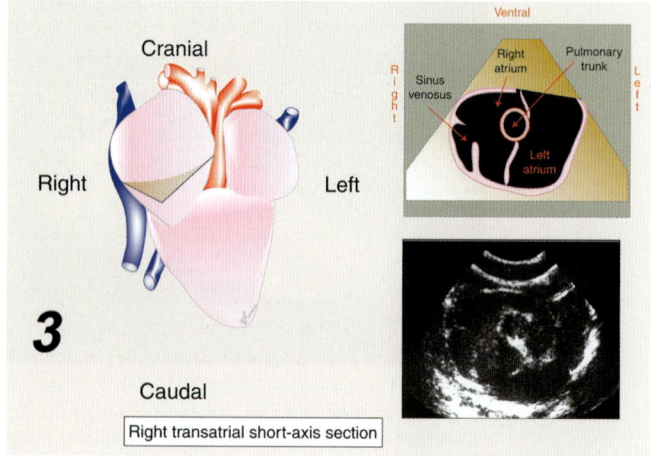

3

Sinus venosus
Right atrium
Pulmonary trunk
Left atrium

Right transatrial short-axis section

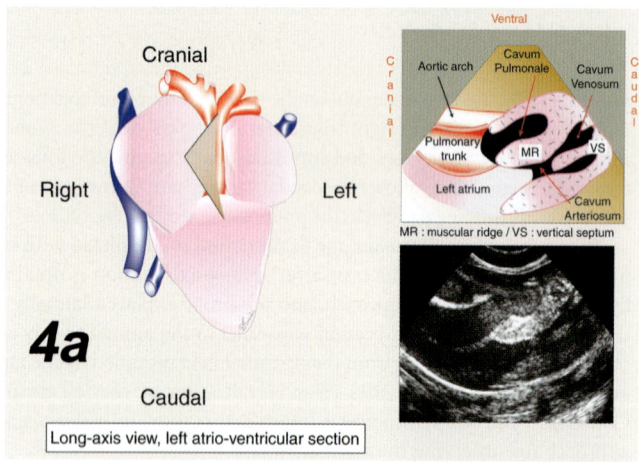

4a

Aortic arch
Cavum Pulmonale
Cavum Venosum
Pulmonary trunk
MR
VS
Left atrium
Cavum Arteriosum

MR : muscular ridge / VS : vertical septum

Long-axis view, left atrio-ventricular section

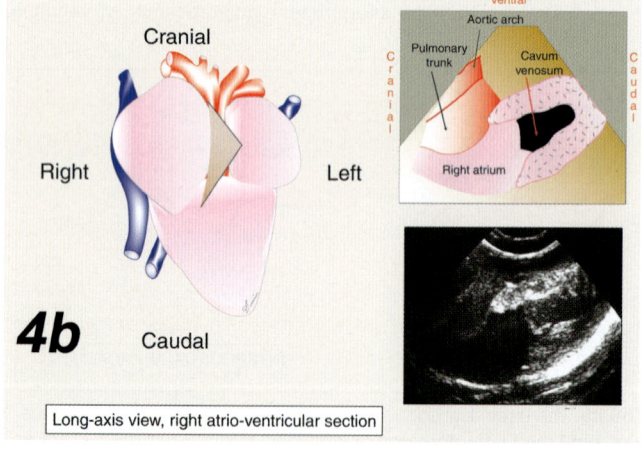

4b

Aortic arch
Pulmonary trunk
Cavum venosum
Right atrium

Long-axis view, right atrio-ventricular section

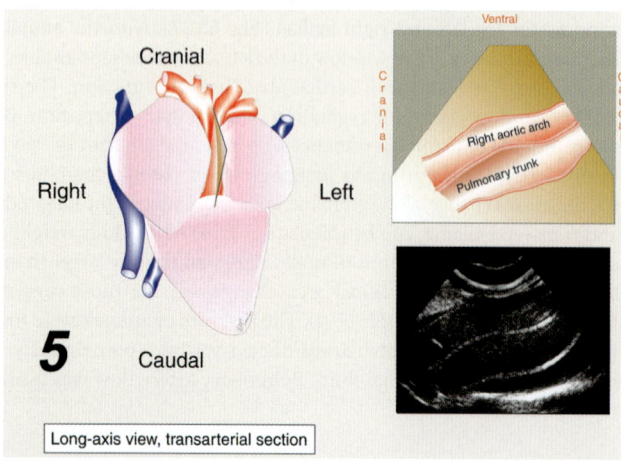

5

Right aortic arch
Pulmonary trunk

Long-axis view, transarterial section

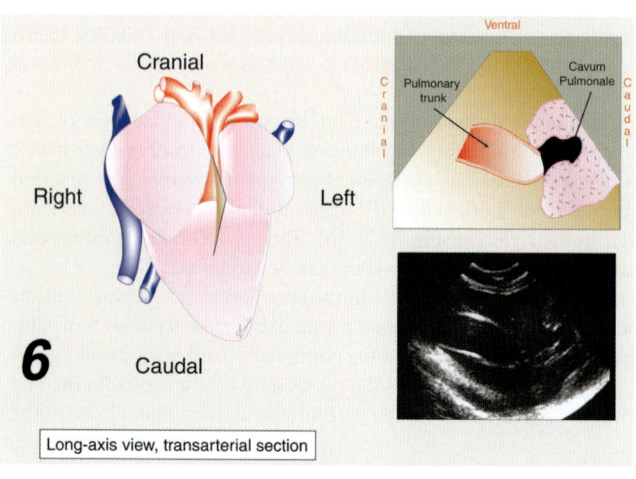

6

Pulmonary trunk
Cavum Pulmonale

Long-axis view, transarterial section

FIG 68.26 (1a) Transventricular apical (or transapical) short-axis section. This apical short-axis view shows a transversal section of the apical myocardium. (1b) Transventricular subarterial short-axis section showing the three cava (cavum pulmonale, cavum venosum, cavum arteriosum). (2) Transarterial short-axis section. This short-axis view shows the two aortic arches and the pulmonary trunk. (3) Transatrial short-axis section. This short-axis view shows the right atrium, the sinoatrial valves, and the sinus venous on the right and the left atrium on the left. (4a) Long-axis section of the left atrioventricular junction. One of the two aortic arches and the pulmonary trunk are observed. (4b) Long-axis section of the right atrioventricular junction. (5) Transarterial long-axis section. The distal view shows the path of the dorsal pulmonary trunk parallel to the ventral right aortic arch. (6) Transcaval long-axis section. This long-axis lateral view shows the ventral caudal vena cava parallel to the more dorsal pulmonary vein. (From Schilliger L, Tessier D, Pouchelon JL, et al. Proposed standardization of the two-dimensional echocardiographic examination in snakes. *J Herp Med Surg.* 2006;6[3]:76–87, with permission from the *Journal of Herpetological Medicine and Surgery*).

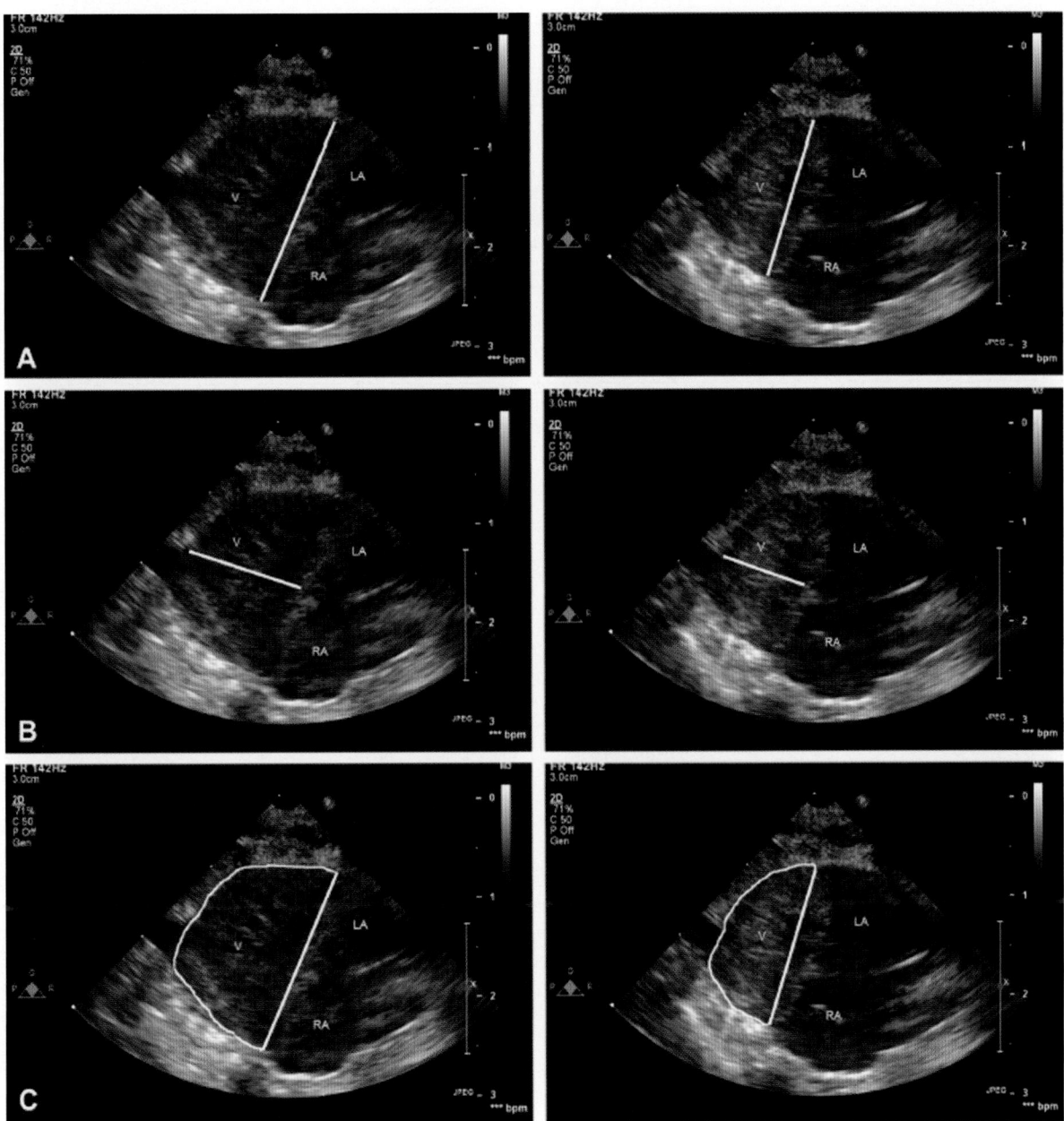

FIG 68.27 Left axillary views showing ventricular diastole (left of image) and systole (right of image) in the heart of a central bearded dragon (*Pogona vitticeps*) with (A) a representative line where the transverse dimension was measured, (B) a representative line where the longitudinal dimension was measured, and (C) tracing of the ventricle for area. LA, Left atrium; RA, right atrium; V, ventricle. (From Silverman S, Sanchez-Migallon Guzman D, Stern J, et al: Standardization of the two-dimensional transcoelomic echocardiographic examination in the central bearded dragon (*Pogona vitticeps*). (From *J Vet Cardiol.* 2016;18: 168–178, with permission from Elsevier).

TABLE 68.3 **Measured Variables From Two-Dimensional Echocardiographic Evaluation in Central Bearded Dragons (*Pogona vitticeps*)**

Variable	Males (*n* = 9)	SD	CV (%)	Females (*n* = 7)	SD	CV (%)	*p* Value
LA (cm)	0.860 (0.805–0.956)	0.09	10.35	0.812 (0.749–0.858)	0.06	7.35	0.09
RA (cm)	1.16 (1.03–1.25)	0.15	13.29	0.859 (0.839–0.981)	0.08	8.96	0.0012
Total Atrial Diameter (cm)	2.04 (1.89–2.17)	0.19	9.45	1.67 (1.58–1.84)	0.14	8.08	0.0052
Ventricular Transverse Diastole (cm)	2.02 (1.86–2.17)	0.16	8.21	1.66 (1.49–1.70)	0.10	6.05	0.0002
Ventricular Transverse Systole (cm)	1.677 (1.54–1.88)	0.17	10.02	1.39 (1.29–1.49)	0.11	7.83	0.0002
Ventricular Longitudinal Diastole (cm)	1.48 (1.36–1.58)	0.11	7.26	1.23 (1.14–1.31)	0.08	6.13	0.0003
Ventricular Longitudinal Systole (cm)	1.18 (1.03–1.23)	0.09	8.19	1.04 (0.94–1.08)	0.09	8.44	0.054
Ventricular Internal Chamber Transverse (cm)	1.56 (1.35–1.61)	0.14	8.97	1.11 (1.06–1.15)	0.04	3.95	0.0045
Ventricular Area Diastole (cm²)	2.30 (2.19–2.77)	0.33	13.24	1.63 (1.43–1.71)	0.15	9.41	0.0002
Ventricular Area Systole (cm²)	1.48 (1.39–1.90)	0.28	17.54	1.15 (0.968–1.27)	0.18	16.26	0.0007
PA Flow Velocity (m/sec)	0.649 (0.621–0.731)	0.11	15.66	0.572 (0.503–0.652)	0.09	15.31	0.0311

CV, Coefficient of variation; *LA*, left atrium; *PA*, pulmonary artery; *RA*, right atrium; *SD*, standard deviation.
The values reported are the median and interquartile ranges.
The *p*-values are reported to assess for significant differences between males and females. A *p*-value of <0.05 is considered statistically significant.

TABLE 68.4 **Calculated Measurements for Ventricular Fractional Shortening and Fractional Area Change in Central Bearded Dragons (*Pogona vitticeps*)**

Variable	All (*N* = 16)	Males (*n* = 9)	SD	CV (%)	Females (*n* = 7)	SD	CV (%)	*p* Value
Transverse FS (%)	14.08 (11.04–18.30)	14.25 (11.07–18.73)	5.20	34.34	13.13 (10.25–18.44)	4.40	30.69	0.805
Longitudinal FS (%)	20.37 (14.22–23.56)	22.31 (20.37–24.48)	6.10	28.4	16.00 (12.69–20.04)	4.60	27.5	0.0545
Fractional Area of Change (%)	33.00 (27.46–38.37)	36.89 (28.52–40.49)	6.40	18.0	31.67 (26.19–33.29)	6.00	19.82	0.171

CV, Coefficient of variation; *FS*, fractional shortening; *SD*, standard deviation.
The values reported are the median and interquartile ranges.
The *p*-values are reported to assess for significant differences between males and females. A *p*-value of 0.05 is considered statistically significant.

In red-eared sliders (*Trachemys scripta elegans*), the best imaging was obtained through the right cervical window (Fig. 68.28), which facilitated base-apex inflow and outflow views, as well as measurements of ventricular size, ventricular wall thickness, and ventricular outflow tracts. Fractional shortening was calculated. Pulsed-wave Doppler interrogation enabled the diastolic biphasic atrioventricular flow and the systolic ventricular outflow patterns to be recorded. The following Doppler-derived functional parameters were calculated: early diastolic (E) and late diastolic (A) wave peak velocities, E/A ratio, ventricular outflow systolic peak and mean velocities and gradients, velocity-time integral, acceleration and deceleration times, and ejection time (Table 68.5).[72]

Endoscopy. Endoscopy is limited in its ability to aid in the evaluation of cardiac disease. It can be used to evaluate the surface of the heart (and the myocardium if the pericardium is transparent). In general, only changes of the pericardium can be appreciated: for example, gout deposition, neoplasia, or pericardial effusion.

CARDIAC DISEASES

A variety of pathological lesions have been reported involving the reptilian cardiovascular system, including cardiomyopathy,[73,74] septic endocarditis,[64,74,75] valvular insufficiency,[50,63] myocarditis,[62,76–80] pericardial effusion,[43,81] infarcts,[82] atherosclerosis,[43] aneurysms,[82] gout,[83,84] arterial calcification,[11,85] thrombus,[74] parasitic infestation,[86–90] congenital heart defects,[57,82,91] and even tumors.[43,92–95] In many cases, the definitive diagnosis was made postmortem. Inadequate husbandry, resulting in chronic stress, immune suppression, and malnutrition, is the most likely common predisposing factor for the development of cardiovascular conditions in captive reptiles.[96] Cardiac diseases can be classified as noninfectious, infectious, or parasitic.

Noninfectious Cardiac Disease

Congenital Defects. Congenital cardiac diseases are considered rare in reptiles. A secundum atrial septal defect located on the craniodorsal portion of the interatrial septum was reported in a Komodo dragon (*Varanus komodoensis*).[57] Various congenital conditions have been reported in several species of snakes: ventricular mural hypoplasia with plasmacytic pericarditis (Burmese python); aortic valvular stenosis with secondary cardiomyopathy (Children's python, *Liasis childreni*); and enlarged/abnormally shaped cardiac chambers, bifid ventricles, and reduced muscular ridge causing inadequate ventricular pressure separation with pronounced hemodynamic consequences (ball pythons, *Python regius*).[91]

Aortic and subaortic stenosis have been reported in other species: histopathological examination of the heart of a green iguana (*Iguana iguana*) with aortic stenosis associated with dilatation of the right atrium and the ventricle revealed atrophy of myocardial fibers and a thickening of the intima of both aortic arches with consequent narrowing of the lumen. No diagnosis was established, but chronic congenital lesion was suggested as a differential diagnosis. Bilateral subaortic stenosis was also described in an alligator (*Alligator mississippiensis*).[97]

Cardiomyopathies. Cardiomyopathies have been described in various species of snakes. A black king snake (*Lampropeltis niger*) that presented with marked cardiomegaly, dilatation of the ventricle, and congestive heart failure (CHF) was diagnosed with dilated cardiomyopathy upon necropsy.[96] CHF was also reported in a Deckert's rat snake (*Pantherophis obsoleta deckertii*) with degeneration and necrosis of myocardial fibers and mineralization of blood vessels with focal aggregates of lymphocytes within the lamina.[77] CHF was diagnosed in a mole king snake (*Lampropeltis calligaster rhombomaculata*) with myocardial collagen proliferation and osteoidlike material. The etiology of this disorder was unclear;

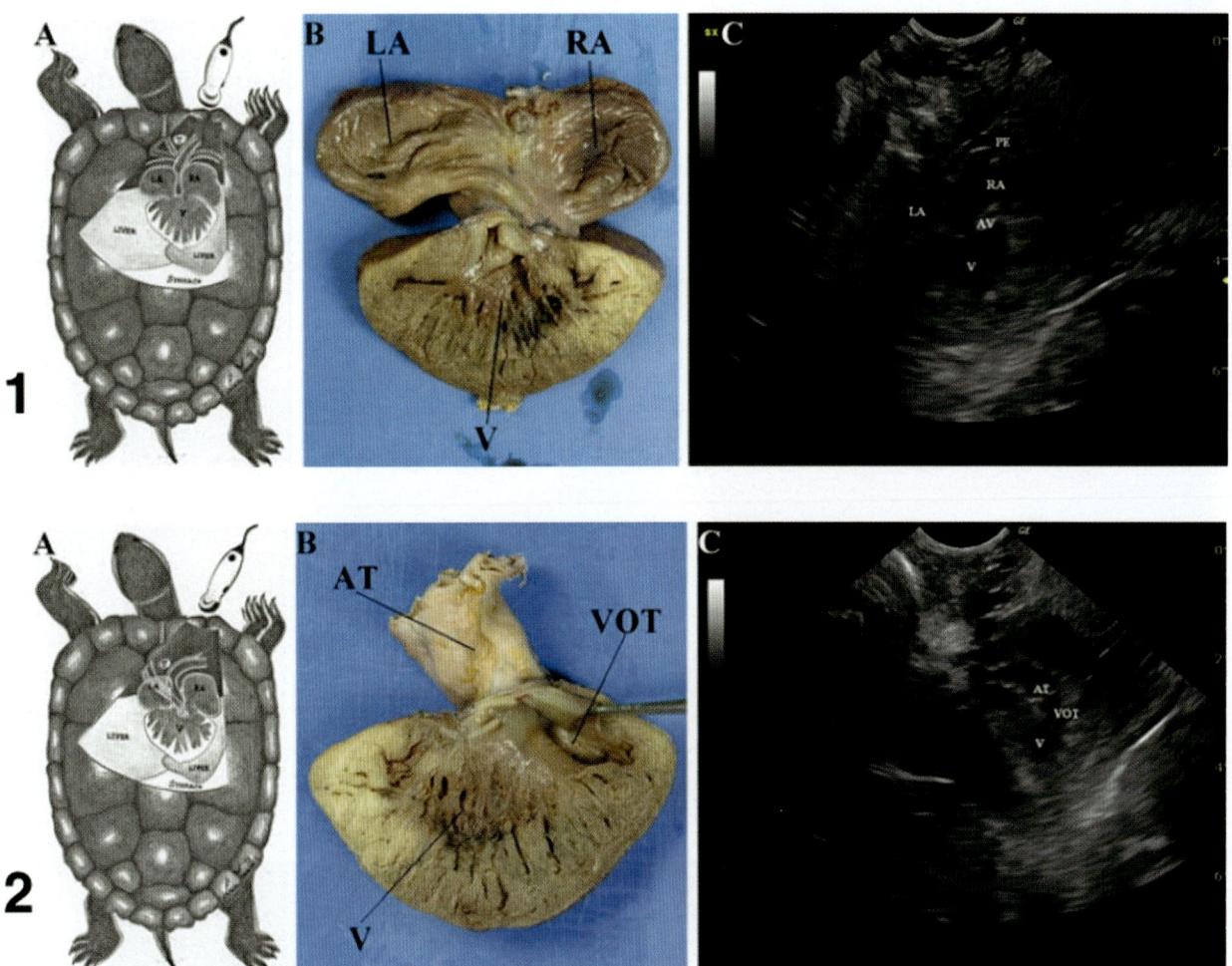

FIG 68.28 (1): (A) Probe positioning at the cervical-brachial acoustic window to visualize the base-apex inflow (*Trachemys scripta elegans*). (B) Preserved specimen of the *Trachemys scripta elegans* heart. (C) Echocardiographic image of the *Trachemys scripta elegans* heart obtained through the right cervical-brachial acoustic window (long-axis inflow view). (2): (A) Probe positioning at the cervical-brachial acoustic window to visualize the base-apex outflow. (B) Preserved specimen of the *Trachemys scripta elegans* heart. (C) Echocardiographic image of the *Trachemys scripta elegans* heart obtained through the right cervical-brachial acoustic window (long-axis outflow view). AT, Arterial trunk; AV, atrioventricular valves; LA, left atrium; PE, pericardial effusion; RA, right atrium; T, thyroid; V, ventricle; VOT, ventricle outflow tract. (From Poser H, Russello H, Zanella A. Two-dimensional and doppler echocardiographic findings in healthy non-sedated red-eared slider terrapins. *Vet Res Commun.* 2011;35:511–520, with permission from Springer).

TABLE 68.5 **Doppler-Derived Echocardiographic Parameters of Adult Female Red-Eared Sliders (*Trachemys scripta elegans*)**

Parameter	Mean ± SD	Range (min-max)	95% CI
V_{max} E-wave (m/s)	0.33 ± 0.05	0.27–0.42	0.27–0.38
V_{max} A-wave (m/s)	0.50 ± 0.07	0.42–0.64	0.43–0.57
E/A	0.66 ± 0.08	0.54–0.76	0.58–0.74
E-wave deceleration time (ms)	542.46 ± 278.71	258.79–997.00	249.97–834.94
V_{max} outflow (m/s)	0.52 ± 0.07	0.43–0.62	0.44–0.59
V_{med} outflow (m/s)	0.33 ± 0.05	0.24–0.37	0.27–0.37
G_{max} outflow (mmHg)	1.09 ± 0.31	0.72–1.54	0.76–1.41
G_{med} outflow (mmHg)	0.53 ± 0.14	0.29–0.68	0.38–0.67
VTI (cm)	24.30 ± 4.87	15.22–28.63	19.19–29.42
Outflow acceleration time (ms)	149.22 ± 51.65	93.80–223.34	95.02–203.43
Outflow deceleration time (ms)	557.52 ± 41.17	479.06–598.55	514.32–600.73

CI, Confidence interval; *SD,* standard deviation.

however, microscopic examination of this snake's kidneys and liver revealed severe heterophilic inflammation.[73,98] Cardiomyopathy of undetermined origin was also reported in two pythons: a Children's python (*Liasis childreni*) and a juvenile Burmese python (*Python bivittatus*) (Frye FL, personal communication).

Restrictive cardiomyopathy with alteration of the myocardial compliance and CHF was diagnosed for the first time in a 2-year-old captive lethargic Carpet python (*Morelia spilota variegata*), based on echocardiography, Doppler, and histopathology. The disease was characterized by left atrial dilation, displacement of the interatrial septum, subsequent right atrial collapsus, and sinus venosus dilation with thrombosis in the sinus venosus (Fig. 68.29).[99]

Myocardial degeneration can occur as a result of metabolic disorders and can be observed grossly. For example, gout (of metabolic,

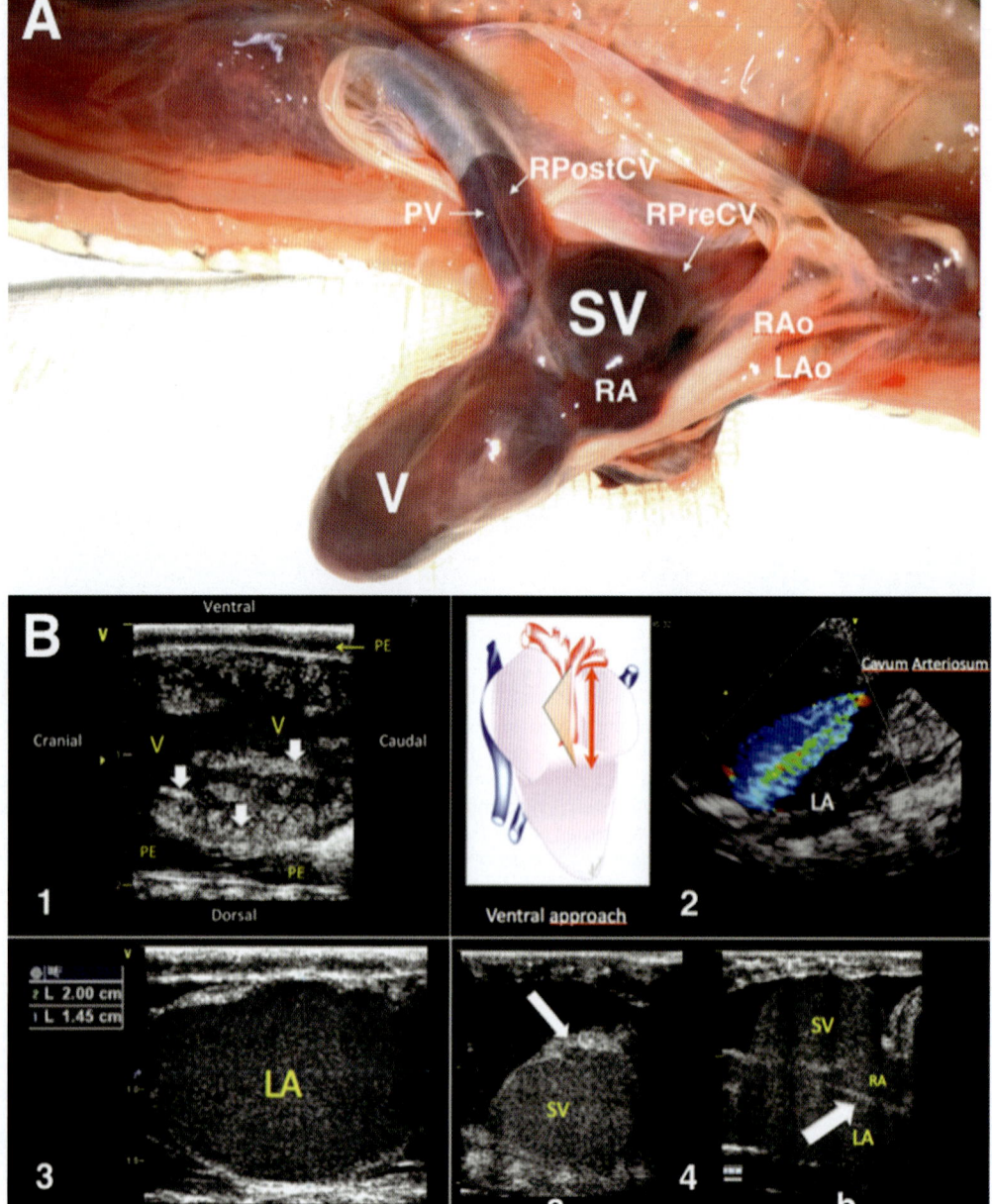

FIG 68.29 (A) Necropsy: restrictive cardiomyopathy associated with SV dilation and thrombosis within the SV in a McDowell's carpet python (*Morelia spilota macdowelli*). (B): (1) Long-axis transventricular section obtained by ventral approach. Note the abnormal heterogeneous myocardium characterized by the presence of diffuse hyperechoic lesions mainly within the left myocardium (arrows). (2) Color Doppler flow examination. Long-axis left transatrioventricular section obtained by ventral approach showing a severe left atrioventricular insufficiency characterized by an aliased signal encoded in blue. (3) Left intercostal approach. Marked dilatation of the LA responsible for localized swelling of the coelomic cavity. (4) (Right intercostal approach) (a) thrombus within the dilated SV (white arrow). (b) Severely dilated SV and displaced interatrial septum toward the RA (white arrow) during the systolic time with secondary right atrial compression. LA, Left atrium; LAo, left aortic arch; PE, pericardial effusion; PV, pulmonary vein; RA, right atrium; RAo, right aortic arch; RPostCV, right postvacal vein; RPreCV, right precaval vein; SV, sinus venosus; V, ventricle or ventricular cavity. (Courtesy of Lionel Schilliger and Valérie Chetboul.)

nutritional, or iatrogenic origin) can cause deposition of urate crystals in multiple tissues, including the myocardium.[81,82,97] With vitamin E and selenium deficiencies, the myocardium undergoes degeneration with loss of myocytes replaced by fibrous stroma and gross whitish/grey discoloration.[3,4,11,98]

The myocardium and the major arteries may also be subject to mineralization (calcification) when a diet contains excessive levels of calcium and vitamin D$_3$.[11,98] Aortic rupture associated with mineralization of the aorta attributed to nutritional secondary hyperparathyroidism is reported in lizards.[3]

Noninfectious Valvulopathies (Valvular Endocardiosis).
There is no current evidence for primary degenerative endocardiosis occurring in reptiles. However, occasionally reported cardiac conditions of undetermined etiology suggest that this might be a possibility. For example, right atrioventricular insufficiency resulting in bilateral heart failure was observed in a young carpet python.[50] The lack of septation in squamates may cause sufficient elevation in diastolic pressure to cause bilateral heart failure. Valvular regurgitation can be confirmed with echocardiography (see Fig. 68.29B.2).[63,99]

Pericardial Diseases.
Visceral gout can lead to thickening of the pericardium with urate deposition, which is easily recognizable by endoscopy or during postmortem examination.[84] Traumatic hemopericardium with the formation of hematomas can occur as a result of cardiac blood sampling in snakes.[100,101] It has also been reported in a green iguana (*Iguana iguana*) in conjunction with a myocardial abscess.

Pericardial effusion can be inferred from radiography but can only be confirmed by ultrasonography. It can also be an unexpected finding during necropsy (Fig. 68.30).

Pericardial effusion has also been reported in tortoises. A Californian desert tortoise (*Xerobates agassizi*) with cervical fractures and osteomyelitis also had pericardial effusion, but no attempt was made to investigate the implication and underlying cause.[102] Echocardiography, radiography, and necropsy of an 80-year-old male spur-thighed tortoise (*Testudo graeca*) with posthibernation anorexia and lethargy revealed pericardial effusion, atrial dilatation, six liver lesions containing choleliths, pneumonia, and/or pulmonary edema.[81] These findings were confirmed by postmortem after nonresponse to treatment. Pericardial effusion has also been reported in a 2-year-old male bearded dragon suffering from atherosclerosis in the major arteries of the base of the heart.[43] Pericardial effusion can also be secondary to neoplasia,

as was the case in a female reticulated python (*Malayopython reticulatus*) diagnosed with endocardial fibrosarcoma at the base of the aorta.[103] A small amount of fluid within the pericardial sac may be normal, and therefore volume measurement is advised during postmortem examinations.[70]

Neoplasia.
Primary neoplasia of the cardiovascular system is uncommon in reptiles. Cardiac tumors in snakes are frequently visible as a distinct mass located approximately 15% to 25% svl, depending on species. Reported cases include a cardiac rhabdomyosarcoma in a boa constrictor and a black king snake (*Lampropeltis getula nigrita*), a cardiac hemangioma of the left atrium in a corn snake (*Pantherophis guttatus*), a cardiac hemangiosarcoma in a copperhead (*Agkistrodon contortrix*) and a Madagascar giant hognose snake (*Leioheterodon madagascariensis*), a fibrosarcoma in a Gaboon viper (*Bitis gabonica*), and an endocardial fibrosarcoma in a reticulated python.[81,92,96,103–106]

Metastasis to the heart has also been reported; metastatic chondrosarcoma (Schmidt, RE, and Reavill, DR, personal communication) and oviductal adenocarcinoma have been reported in a corn snake with metastasis to the heart.[107] Similarly, a disseminated mast cell tumor in an eastern king snake (*Lampropeltis getulus getulus*), multicentric lymphoblastic lymphoma in a loggerhead sea turtle (*Caretta caretta*), and lymphoblastic malignant lymphoma in a boa constrictor affected the heart as well as other organs.[47,94] Disseminated coelomic papillomas affecting various organs, including the heart, were found in 39% of 255 stranded green turtles (*Chelonia mydas*) with fibropapillomatosis.[108]

Infectious Cardiac Disease
Bacterial (Endocarditis, Myocarditis, and Pericarditis).
In captive reptiles, infections of the cardiovascular system are often secondary to systemic infections. Where it cannot be attributed to a specific bacteria, endocarditis is most commonly associated with aerobic gram negative infections.[62,63,64,74] *Salmonella* spp., for example, has been isolated in various species of snakes: ultrasonography and angiography revealed a blood flow obstruction in the right atrium of a Burmese python; postmortem isolation confirmed *Salmonella arizonae* in addition to *Corynebacterium* spp.[74] *S. arizonae* was also isolated in a coelomic culture in a Dumeril's boa (*Acrantophis dumerili*).[62] This was concomitant with a granulomatous myocarditis associated with a fibrinous and necrotic pericarditis, as well as hepatitis, pneumonia, and thyroiditis with bacterial infiltration (Fig. 68.31). *Salmonella enterica* was also diagnosed in a

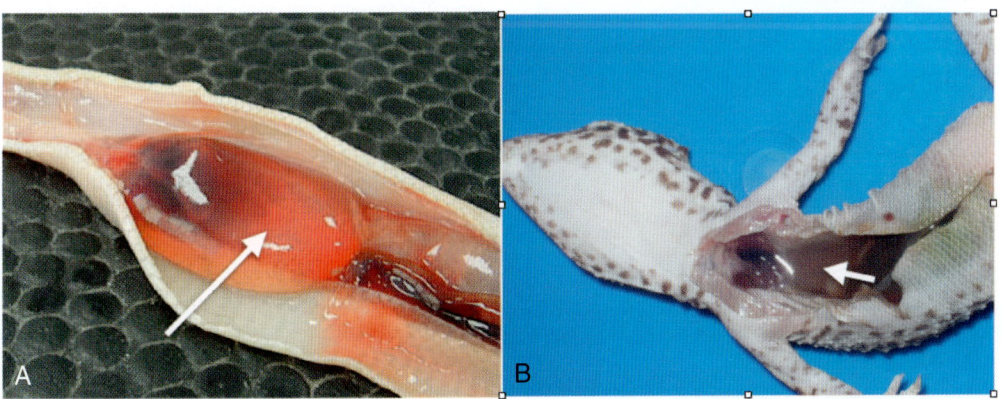

FIG 68.30 Pericardial effusions (white arrows) in (A) an albino boa (*Boa constrictor*) and (B) a leopard gecko (*Eublepharis macularius*). (Courtesy of S. Girling.)

Burmese python with valvular endocarditis and dilated pulmonary trunk and sepsis.[64] Pericarditis can also be associated with fibrinonecrotic lesions (Fig. 68.32).

Concomitant bacterial pneumonia and valvular insufficiencies suggesting bacterial endocarditis can be observed (but without a

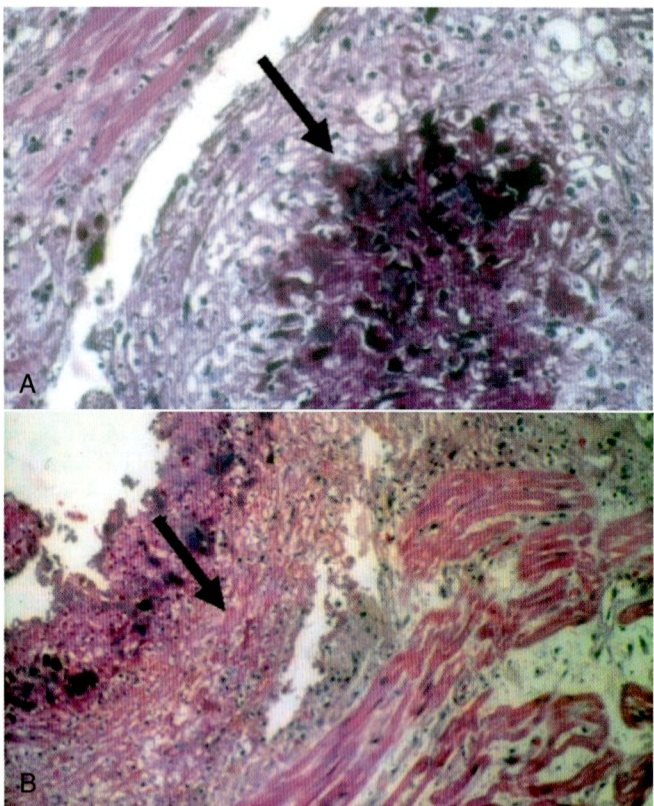

FIG 68.31 (A) Myocardial granuloma (H&E, x40) and (B) pericarditis (H&E, x 20) due to *Salmonella enterica arizonae* in a Madagascarian Dumeril's boa (*Acrantophis dumerili*). (From Schilliger L, Vanderstylen D, Pietrain J. Granulomatous myocarditis and coelomic effusion due to *Salmonella enterica arizonae* in a Madagascarian Dumeril's boa [*Acrantophis dumerili*, Jan. 1860]. *J Vet Cardiol.* 2003; 5:43–45, with permission from Elsevier.)

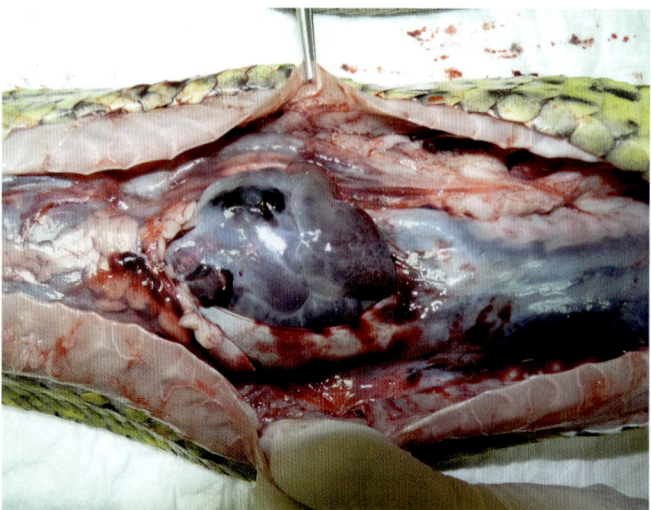

FIG 68.32 Diffuse fibrinonecrotic bacterial pericarditis in a green anaconda (*Eunectes murinus*). (Courtesy of Lionel Schilliger.)

demonstrated cause-effect relationship); sinoatrial (Fig. 68.33.1) and atrioventricular (see Fig. 68.33.2) insufficiencies were diagnosed on echocardiographic examination in a Burmese python suffering from concurrent pneumonia caused by *Pseudomonas aeruginosa*. Histopathological examination of the valve was not performed as the snake survived.[63] An Argentine boa (*Boa constrictor occidentalis*) presenting with cardiomegaly, pneumonia, and inclusion body disease showed a large vegetative lesion on the right atrioventricular valve with valvular insufficiency, a mildly dilated right atrium, and pulmonary hypertension on echocardiographic examination. Cultures of a tracheal wash sample resulted in growth of *Ochrobactrum intermedium* and *Pseudomonas putida*. Postmortem examination confirmed the presence of pneumonia and bacterial endocarditis with dystrophic mineralization of the right atrioventricular valve, with different bacteria (gram-positive) than those cultured from the tracheal wash.[75]

Flavobacterium meningosepticum and *Vibrio damsel* have been isolated from the myocardium of a Barber's map turtle (*Graptemys barbouri*) and a vegetative thrombus attached to the left atrioventricular valve and interventricular wall of a stranded leatherback turtle (*Dermochelys coriacea*).[80] *Mycobacterium* spp. was reported in granulomatous myocarditis in a frilled lizard (*Chlamydosaurus kingii*).[11] *Chlamydophila* (*Chlamydia*) spp. has also been associated with cardiovascular disease. Reported cases include granulomatous pericarditis and myocarditis in a puff adder (*Bitis arietans*),[108] necrotizing myocarditis in green sea turtles,[74] and histiocytic granulomas (determined by transmission electron microscopy) in the heart and organs of an emerald tree boa (*Corallus caninus*).[74,78,108] *Mycoplasma alligatoris* is responsible for pericarditis (and for pneumonia and arthritis) in American alligators (*Alligator mississipiensis*).[109]

A diagnosis can be obtained with ultrasound, hemoculture, postmortem tissue culture, and/or histopathological examination (valves, myocardium, pericardium). In cases where bacterial infection is confirmed, antimicrobial treatment can be attempted.

Viral (Myocarditis, Degeneration, Necrosis). Inclusion body disease (IBD), thought to be caused by an arenavirus, affects snakes and causes large eosinophilic intracytoplasmic inclusion bodies in many different organs, including the heart.[110] Acute deaths of a Savannah monitor with myocarditis and Rosy boas (*Lichanura trivirgata*) with hepatitis and endocarditis were attributed to an adenovirus.[111,112] Flaviruses have been reported to cause myocardial degeneration and necrosis in farmed American alligators.[79,113]

Parasitic. Encapsulated cestodes have been reported within the heart of lizards, with one study finding a prevalence of 5% in 220 wild whiptail lizards (*Cnemidophorus* spp.).[90] Filarial nematodes within the cardiovascular system can cause edema, thrombosis, and necrosis.[3,114] *Macdonaldius oschei* has been observed in fresh blood smears and myocardial histology in various species of reptiles.[98] Trematodes have been reported in the heart chambers and major vessels of chelonians (attached to, or found freely floating within, the lumen) in wild and wild-caught chelonians.[87] Green sea turtles can be infested with spirorchid flukes that cause arteritis, endocarditis, thrombosis, and aneurysms.[88] Similarly, spirorchid eggs and adult *Learedius learei* were observed inside the heart of black sea turtles (*Chelonia mydas agassizii*).[86] Spirorchid eggs were observed in multiple organs and associated with granulomatous lesions in the myocardium of *Trachemys scripta elegans* and *Chrysemys picta*.[89] Besnoitiosis and sarcosporidiosis have also been observed in histological sections of ophidian hearts.[98] All these parasitic diseases were diagnosed postmortem. The use of targeted anthelminthic drugs may be a treatment option when antemortem parasite identification is performed (fecal examination, blood smear cytology).

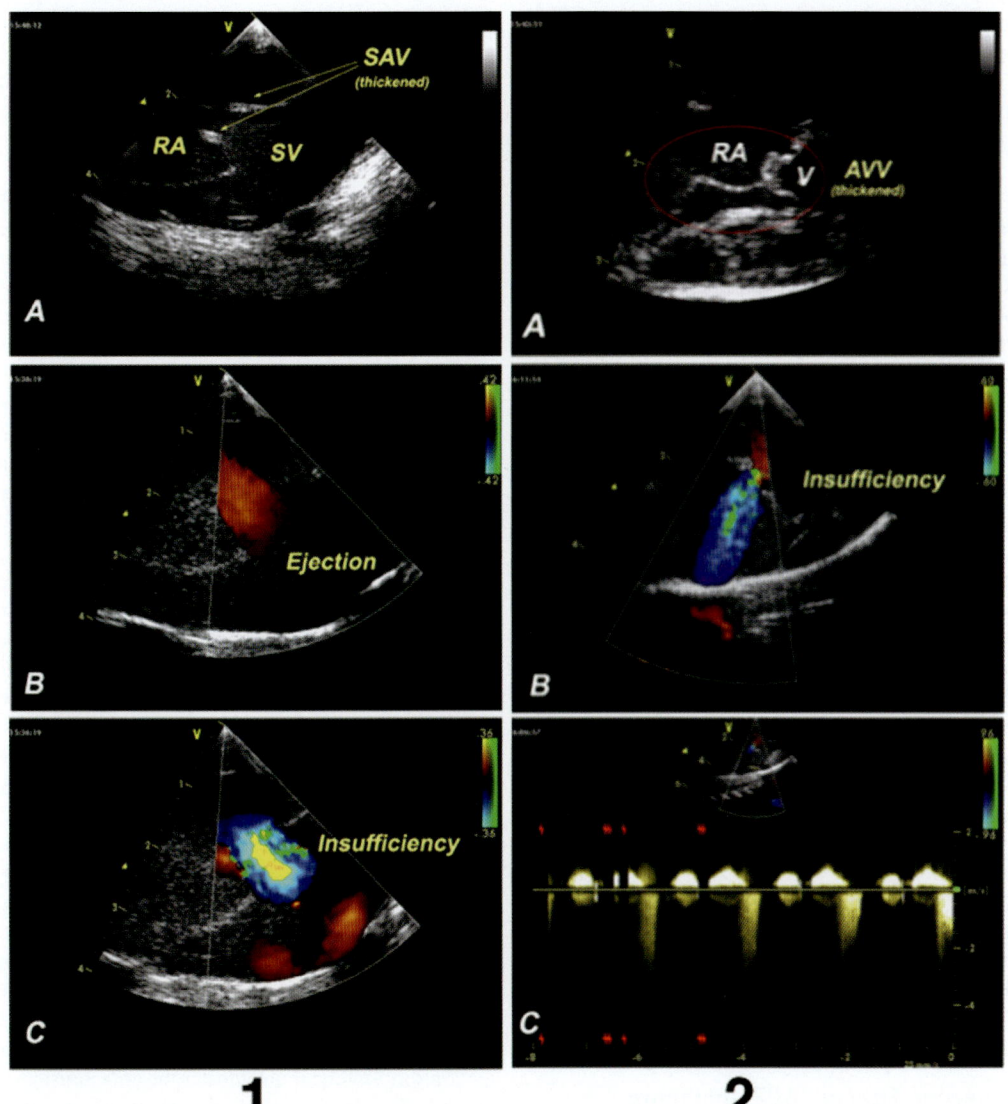

FIG 68.33 (1): (A) Two-dimensional echocardiography (right transatrial short-axis view) showing the abnormal sinoatrial valves (*SAV*) during atrial diastole in a Burmese python *(Python bivittatus)* with bacterial pneumonia. (B and C) Color Doppler examination of the sinoatrial valve showing a normal ejection flow colored in red (B) and an abnormal regurgitation with aliasing (C) during atrial systole. (2): (A) Two-dimensional echocardiography (right atrioventricular long-axis view) showing the abnormal right atrioventricular valvular leaflet (AVV). (B) Color Doppler examination of the atrioventricular valve showing a marked aliased regurgitation in the right atrium during ventricular systole. (C) Continuous-wave Doppler mode examination confirming a high-velocity regurgitant jet (peak velocity of 4 m/s, arrows). RA, Right atrium; SV, sinus venosus; V, ventricle. (From Schilliger L, Tréhiou-Sechi E, Petit AMP, et al. Double valvular insufficiency in a Burmese python suffering from concomitant bacterial pneumonia. *J Zoo Wildl Med.* 2010;41:742–744, with permission from the *Journal of Zoo and Wildlife Medicine.*)

TREATMENT/MANAGEMENT OF CARDIAC DISEASE

Little information exists regarding cardiovascular treatment, and the pharmacological actions of cardiac drugs in reptiles. Future advances in herpetological medicine will likely improve knowledge in the diagnosis and treatment of cardiovascular diseases.

As a rule, pharmacological agents exert their effect on the heart (effect on contractility and rate), blood vessels (causing constriction or dilatation), and/or blood volume (increase or decrease in volume). Different drugs are often used in combination in mammals, but extrapolation from canine and feline cardiac management may be inappropriate due to reptile differences in size, metabolism, anatomy, and physiology. However, basic principles remain applicable. Non-drug-related management of cardiac disease in reptiles may also include reducing metabolic rates by maintaining the reptile at the lower end of its preferred optimum temperature zone, reducing stress by minimizing handling and separating from cage mates, and using caution not to overfeed, as this has resulted in the death of snakes with cardiomyopathy.[77,82]

The cornerstone of managing congestive heart failure rests on reducing the volume of extracellular fluid and reducing preload. This is achieved through the use of diuretics and vasodilators in mammals, but reptiles suffering from cardiac disease are often diagnosed postmortem and thus are rarely subject to therapeutic trials. Oxygen supplementation should be instituted for dyspneic animals, especially if pulmonary edema is present, but in reptiles this may alter blood shunting, and the response to therapy is often difficult to assess.

Inotropes

Inotropes are pharmacological agents that alter the force of muscular contractions. Positive inotropes enhance cardiac contractility. Pimobendan is commonly used in small animal cardiology and has been shown to increase both survival time and quality of life in canine dilated cardiomyopathy.[115] Digoxin is a positive inotrope, negative chronotrope, and positive lusitrope. It increases the cytosolic calcium concentration by inhibiting Na/K ATPase pumps, resulting in increased contractility.[116] It is mainly indicated for atrial fibrillation. Beta-blockers (e.g., atenolol, propranolol) and calcium channel blockers (e.g., diltiazem) are negative inotropes. They are mainly indicated in the treatment of hypertrophic cardiomyopathy in cats and supraventricular arrhythmias. Side effects include bradycardia and hypotension.[117] Beta-blockers can be used for treatment of supraventricular tachycardia and atrial fibrillation, but these are uncommon in reptile patients, and their effectiveness is unknown in reptile patients.

Atenolol administration significantly reduced resting HR and the range of the baroreceptor reflex in 15 conscious healthy juvenile green iguanas (*Iguana iguna*) but did not alter their upper or lower mean arterial blood pressure thresholds, indicating that atenolol did not affect baroreceptor reflex function per se.[38] As expected, the upper HR plateau (i.e., tachycardia) was substantially lower after administration of atenolol, whereas the lower plateau (i.e., bradycardia) was unaffected by the β-adrenoceptor antagonist.

In the same study, methylatropine administration resulted in an increase in the iguanas' resting HR but did not significantly affect the mean arterial blood pressure recorded at the midpoint of the heart rate range. After injection of methylatropine, the mean sensitivity of the baroreceptor reflex was substantially diminished, and consequently, the range of the baroreceptor reflex was substantially reduced.[38]

Angiotensin-Converting Enzyme (ACE) Inhibitors

In mammals, ACE inhibitors block the formation of angiotensin II, which promotes venous and arterial vasodilation, and block aldosterone production and reduce preload and afterload through venous and arterial vasodilation. Enalapril and benazepril are the most commonly used ACE inhibitors in dogs and cats because of their longer half-life, but it is unknown if this is also the case in reptiles. Enalapril inhibited angiotensin I conversion in alligators, and at 0.5 to 0.7 mg/kg once every 24 hours (combined with spironolactone and furosemide) briefly managed CHF in a spiny-tailed monitor (*Varanus acanthurus*) (Clayton, LA, Hadfield, CA, Gore SR, et al., personal communication).[118]

Diuretics

Diuretics increase water excretion and so reduce fluid overload and decrease edema and effusions. In mammals the principle diuretic is furosemide, a loop diuretic that acts by inhibiting sodium, potassium, and chloride cotransporters in the ascending limb of the loop of Henle of the kidney. Reptiles have a metanephric kidney that lacks a loop of Henle; however, furosemide has shown a diuretic effect in chelonians and ophidians.[119–122] Two main mechanisms of action have been suggested in reptiles: the first is that in those species that possess a urinary bladder, sodium:potassium pumps in the wall of the bladder can be influenced by furosemide.[123] A second hypothesis is that furosemide may act upon the sodium:potassium pumps present in the terminal colon and cloaca, as many reptiles reflux urine from the cloaca into the distal colon to absorb water in conjunction with NaCl.[124]

A spur-thighed tortoise with atrial dilatation and pericardial effusion was administered furosemide at a dose of 5.2 mg/kg on two occasions, 3 weeks apart, which resolved peripheral edema.[81] A carpet python diagnosed with atrioventricular insufficiency and secondary pulmonary edema and pericardial effusion failed to respond to furosemide at 5 mg/kg.[50] Furosemide should be used with caution in reptile patients with renal disease, and biochemical parameters including potassium, phosphorus, and the major nitrogenous waste product (ammonia, urea, or uric acid) should be monitored.

Information on other diuretics in reptiles is lacking. Hydrochlorothiazide has been used as a diuretic in lizards with renal disease (Divers SJ, personal communication). Methylated xanthines (aminophylline and theophylline) have successfully induced diuresis. Their diuretic effect may be partly due to their stimulatory effect on cardiac function, increased renal blood flow, and increased glomerular filtration rate. The major diuretic effect of these compounds is apparently due to increased rates of excretion of sodium and chloride ions by renal tubules.[23]

Spironolactone is an aldosterone antagonist and a weak diuretic in mammals.[125] It is a potassium-sparing diuretic that can either be used alone or in conjunction with furosemide to offset the loss of potassium. Nothing is known about its potential use in reptiles.

REFERENCES

See www.expertconsult.com for a complete list of references.

69

Dermatology—Skin

T. Franciscus Scheelings and Tom Hellebuyck

The immense variation observed in modern vertebrates can be attributed to two pivotal moments in the history of Earth's biodiversity. Firstly, and probably most profoundly, the advent of the amniotic egg severed the reliance that animals had on water for reproduction and paved the way for unprecedented terrestrial evolutionary radiation. However, this momentous biological accomplishment was insufficient on its own to support terrestrial vertebrate life, and the early terrene conquerors had to devise an array of strategies in order to resist the challenges that their potential new environment presented. The second crucial stratagem for terrestrial exploitation came in the form of the reptilian integument. Reptile skin had to evolve as a protective barrier to conserve body fluids from deeper tissues and prevent their exposure to the dehydrating external environment; it had to combat ultraviolet (UV) irradiation, protect against an invading army of novel pathogens, and withstand the daily mechanical trauma that accompanies a terrestrial existence. The dawn of the reptilian integument occurred during the late Devonian period and was necessitated by the warming and drying of Earth's climate. By the late Triassic period, reptiles were the most dominant vertebrates on Earth, and they have managed to survive in myriad forms today, on every continent except for Antarctica.

There are over 9000 species of extant reptiles, and as such, there has been enormous diversity in scalation as the class has undergone rapid change to fill various ecological niches. Not only does the integument of reptiles act as a protective barrier to environmental and biological threats, it has further been adapted to trap and conserve thermal energy and collect water, and has evolved important appendages for communication and defense. In addition, the skin of reptiles has played an integral part in the psyche of human history. In various cultural myths and legends, the periodic shedding and renewal of reptilian skin has been portrayed as both sinister and rejuvenating, and as such, reptiles have been depicted as either heroic or evil, with important ramifications for their conservation. Furthermore, the value of many captive-bred animals is inherently linked to their skin color and patterns.

Pathological conditions of the reptilian integument are common, particularly in captive animals. They may be primary in nature, secondary to systemic illness, or as a consequence of inadequate husbandry conditions. Therefore a sound understanding of the pathophysiology of reptile dermatological disease, as well as the husbandry requirements of captive animals, is critically important for veterinarians who treat reptiles.

ANATOMY

Fundamentally, the skin of reptiles is similar to that of other amniotes in that it consists of two layers: the outer epidermis and the underlying dermis. The epidermis is covered by either α- or β-keratin.[1] β-keratin is a durable, lightweight material that is critical for increasing the mechanical resistance of the reptilian epidermis.[2] The epidermis of

reptiles is a stratified squamous epithelium comprised of multiple distinct layers. From superficial to deep these are (Fig. 69.1)[3] as follows:
- Outer epidermal generation
  - Oberhautchen: the outermost portion of the β-layer and characterized by serrations, surface ornaments, and pits
  - ß-keratin: inelastic, tough, stratified epithelial layer, composed primarily of β-keratin (the hinge area between scales is lacking this layer)
  - Meso stratum: transitional cells between the α- and β-layers
  - α-keratin: soft, flexible epithelial layer composed primarily of α-keratin
  - Lacunar stratum: innermost layer of outer portion of skin, tightly adhered to newly forming oberhautchen
- Inner epidermal generation
  - Presumptive β-keratin layer
  - Presumptive meso layer
  - Presumptive α-keratin layer
  - Stratum germinativum: deepest basal layer of progenitor columnar epithelium

The scales of reptiles represent a folding of the epidermis and, for the most part, cover the entirety of the reptile integument. The β-keratin

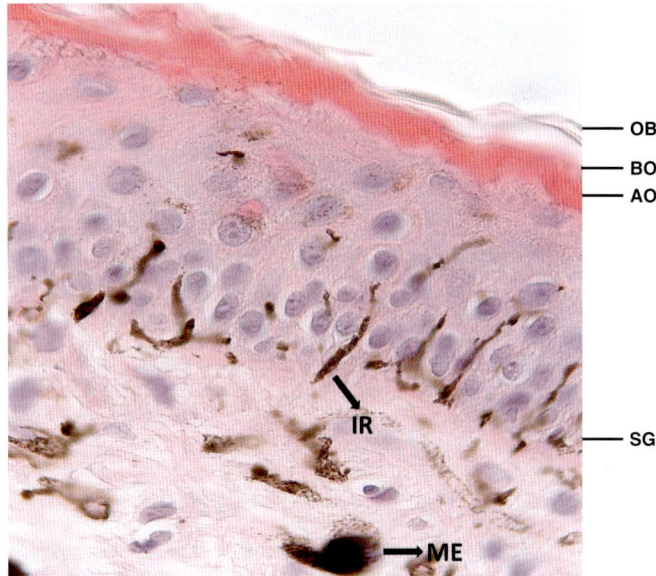

FIG 69.1 Higher magnification photomicrograph of the skin of a boa constrictor (*Boa constrictor*). The epidermis consists of oberhautchen, α-layer (AO), β-layer (BO), and stratum germinativum (SG). Two types of pigment cells are seen in the dermis: melanophores (ME) and iridophores (IR). (Courtesy of Tom Hellebuyck.)

forms the outer exoskeleton layer, which protects the underlying soft inner stratum of connective tissue containing α-keratin. This layer is usually thinner, and less rigid, and forms the "joint" or hinge at the base of the scale.[2] Such an arrangement provides greater flexibility than the completely rigid exoskeleton seen in insects.[2]

There are four extant orders of modern reptiles, Crocodilia (crocodiles and alligators), Chelonia (turtles and tortoises), Squamata (snakes and lizards), and Rhynchocephalia (tuataras),[1,4,5] with each group employing one of three scalation types (Fig. 69.2).[2,5,6] Morphologically, the scales

of crocodilians show little variation and only minor overlapping.[5] Chelonians have a soft, folded skin in the limbs, tail, neck (most aquatic turtles), and a scaled/scute form of the shell.[7,8] In the limbs and tail of terrestrial turtles, hard scales containing β-keratin are also present, but β-keratin is decreased or absent in the hinge regions.[5] In most chelonians the shell is covered by β-keratin, except for soft-shelled chelonians in which α-keratin covers the carapace and plastron.[9] In squamates, the most frequently occurring scale type is the overlapping scale, which is found on the body. These scales are asymmetric and have distinct outer

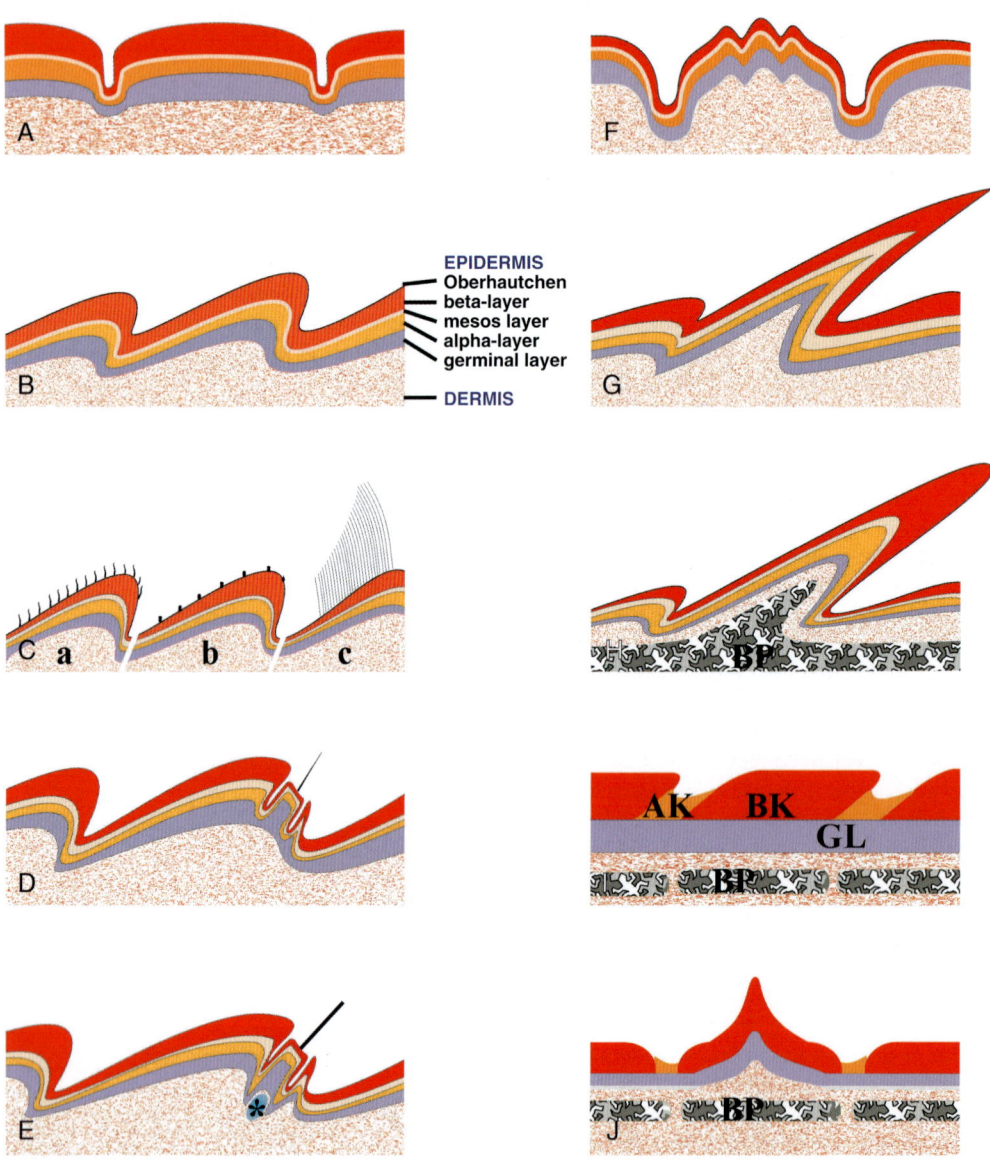

FIG 69.2 Schematic drawings showing different types of reptile scales. (A) Nonoverlapping tuberculate type scales. (B) Overlapping scales commonly seen in squamates. (C) Variations of microstructures from the oberhautchen layer, illustrating short spines in a and b and long setaes in c (such as those in the adhesive pad lamellae in geckos). (D) Pits on the scales of anole, gecko, and iguana (mainly epidermal sensory organs). (E) Tactile sensory organ on the hinge side of a scale in agama. Some follicle-like structures have clustered dermal cells associated to their base. (F) Scales with ridges are seen on the back of skink or the neck of anole. (G) Frills, or very elongated scales, are seen on the back of iguana. (H) The horn on the head of the chameleon contains a bony element core (osteoderm). (I) Scales on the limb of crocodilians show only minor overlapping. (J) Keeled scales with a central, elevated corneous ridge are seen on the dorsal body of crocodilians and some armored agamid lizards (e.g., Australian spiny desert lizard or moloch). Legends: a, fine "hair" on scales of anoles; b, microornamentation on scales of snakes; c, toe pad of anole or gecko; AK, α-keratin; BK, β-keratin; BP, bone element; *, dermal cells clustered at the base of sensory organs in Agama. (Reproduced with permission of UPV/EHU Press [Bilbao, Spain] from Chang et al. [2009]. Reptile scale paradigm: Evo-Devo, pattern formation and regeneration. *Int J Dev Biol* 53:813-826.)

and inner surfaces and a hinge at the caudal end.[5] In contrast, the head scales of squamates are nonoverlapping and do not exhibit cranial-caudal polarity. These cranial scales are typically arranged in precise, exquisite patterns and usually form the basis for species identification in this order. In chelonians and crocodilians, α- and β-keratins in epidermal scales alternate horizontally while the keratins in the outer portion of squamate scales alternate vertically.[9]

The skin of reptiles contains relatively few glands, and is generally dry. Some species have musk glands adjacent to the cloaca, while in crocodilians they are medial to the dentary bone. Mental or chin glands are present in some chelonians, and specialized glands are associated with the angle of the jaw in chameleons.[9] The exact function of these glands is unknown, but they may play a role in scent marking or predator deterrence. In many lizards the males develop prominent femoral or precloacal pores associated with sexual maturity (Fig. 69.3). These glands are located along the ventral surface of the hind limbs or cranial to the vent, and their function is to secrete pheromones and a thick waxy substance that aids in adhering the male to the female. Another secretory gland that is used for defense against predation is the paired Rathke's gland of chelonians, located between the dorsal corners of the bridge/carapace junction, caudal to the foreleg and cranial to the hind leg. In some species this gland emits a foul-smelling liquid when the animal has been disturbed. Integumentary sense organs located in the postcranial and ventral scales have been described in a range of crocodilian species, and it has been hypothesized that they may serve as either mechanoreceptors or chemosensory organs.[10]

Boas, pythons, and vipers possess specialized pits that are utilized to sense infrared radiation to aid in the location of prey. In pythons and boas, they are located along the edges of the labial scales and cover almost the entire upper or lower lip (Fig. 69.4). In vipers they are found bilaterally, midway between the nostril and the eye, and are focused in a forward direction (Fig. 69.5).

The parietal eye is a structure unique to lizards and is most well developed in the tuatara. It is located on the dorsal head and consists of a rudimentary lens and retina. Its function is to relay environmental cues to the pineal gland, thus controlling hormone production and influencing thermoregulation. In some species it is also important for spatial relation, helping animals return to their homerange.[11,12]

Deep to the epidermis, and separated by a basement membrane, lies the dermis, which is a highly vascular structure that contains sensory tissue, chromatophores and osteoderms in some species. It is the complex arrangement (both vertically and horizontally) of pigment cells within the dermis that gives each reptile its unique coloration. Four basic chromatophores have been identified in reptiles and include melanophores containing melanin, erythrophores and xanthophores containing pteridines and carotenoids, and iridophores containing reflecting platelets of guanine, adenine, hypoxanthine, and uric acid.[13,14]

Entrenched within the dermis of many reptiles are bony plates known as osteoderms (Fig. 69.6). Osteoderms are pleisomorphic for reptiles

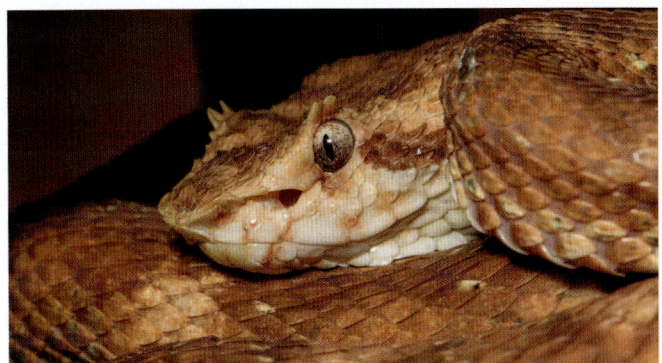

FIG 69.5 In vipers, the heat-sensing pits are focused in a forward direction and are located between the eye and the nostril. (Courtesy of T.F. Scheelings.)

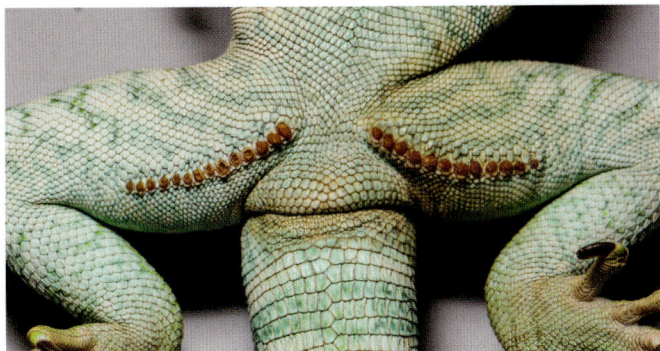

FIG 69.3 Femoral pores are associated with sexual maturity in males of many lizard species. (Courtesy of T.F. Scheelings.)

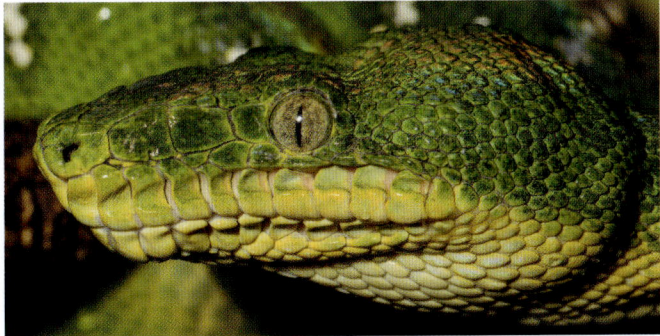

FIG 69.4 In pythons and boas, heat-sensing pits are located along the edges of the labial scales. (Courtesy of T.F. Scheelings.)

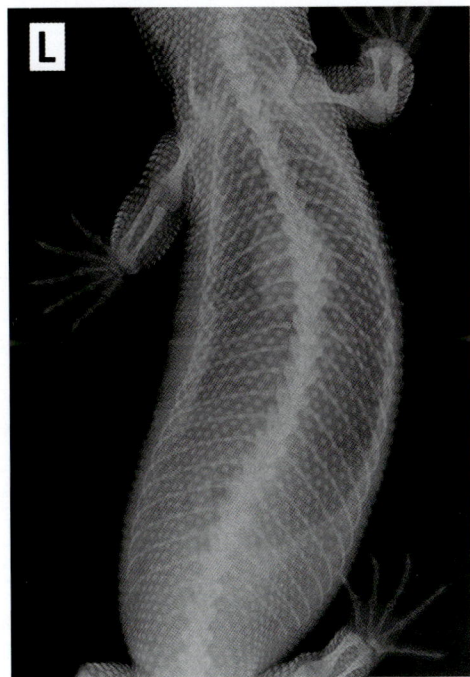

FIG 69.6 Osteoderms are mineralized dermal tissue and are commonly seen in many reptiles, like this heloderm lizard. They may be evident when radiographing animals. (Courtesy of Stephen J. Divers.)

but demonstrate considerable lineage-specific variability in size, shape, and composition.[15] The most extreme example of osteoderm development is the carapace and plastron of chelonians. All osteoderms share embryonic origins with other dermal tissues and are predominately comprised of osseous material. Histologically, osteoderms are not uniform and contain variable amounts of mineralized and nonmineralized connective tissue and bone marrow.[15] Osteoderms are an evolutionary relic of the fully mineralized skins of ancient, now extinct, fish species.

PHYSIOLOGY

Undoubtedly the most identifiable physiological trait of reptilian skin is the periodic process of sloughing and renewal known as ecdysis (Fig. 69.7). In most chelonians and archosaurs (crocodiles and birds), desquamation is continuous, while in other species such as lepidosaurs (lizards, amphisbaenids, sphenodontids, and snakes) and some chelonians, the process is discontinuous, where shedding of epidermal areas of variable dimensions occurs.[16] In lepidosaurs, skin sloughing is cyclical, and, depending on the species, an animal may shed its entire skin at once (snakes and some lizards) or in small portions over a 1- to 2-week period. A cycle consists of a resting stage (consisting of three subdivisions) followed by five stages of renewal.[9,16,17] The resting phase follows a slough and is the normal state. During this time there is little cellular activity. The renewal phase is characterized by cellular divisions in the epidermis that results in the generation of a new skin. Once the old skin is ready to be replaced, the two layers are separated by enzyme-induced digestion of the bonds holding the old skin to the new, and at this time animals may appear dull or have a bluish hue.[9,16,17] In contrast to lepidosaurs, the large, flat, keratinous scutes of chelonians and crocodilians are shed fragmentally. Continued epidermal growth adds keratinous material over the inner surface of individual scutes, compensating for wear. When the outer layer of scutes becomes excessively worn, there is a switch from β to α–keratin production, resulting in the formation of a shedding layer. There is then a slow intracorneous detachment of the more external layers, with the surface of the scute being sloughed, followed by the formation of a new β-keratin layer.[2,18]

No matter the species, skin sloughing appears to be under hormonal control from the pituitary-thyroid axis and may be influenced by factors such as age, temperature, UV-B exposure, skin trauma, and frequency and amount of food consumption.[9,16,17,19]

Although most reptiles exhibit a changeless or slowly changeable color pattern (morphological color change), some species of reptiles possess the ability to rapidly change color in response to environmental stimuli such as background color, light intensity, or changing social context.[20] This color alteration is known as physiological color change and is achieved by repositioning of the pigment granules within the cytoplasm of chromatophores by microscopic intracellular microorganelles. This process is affected by the nervous and endocrine systems, and depending on the species they may use one or a combination of both systems.[20] For example, in the green anole (*Anolis carolinensis*), chromatic transformation is solely controlled by hormonal activity. In response to a dark background, visual cues sent to the brain result in a release of melanocyte-stimulating hormone (MSH) from the pituitary gland, leading to stimulation and dispersal of melanin granules within melanocytes and a resultant darkening of the skin. Conversely, when placed onto a light background, MSH is no longer released and the animal pales.[21] Additionally, stress hormones such as adrenalin and noradrenalin may also affect the color of green anoles.[21] In contrast, color change in the old world chameleon is under sympathetic nervous regulation and contrary to popular belief evolved primarily as a social signaling system with camouflage being a secondary concern.[22,23] In the horned lizard (*Phrynosoma* spp.), both nervous and hormonal agents appear to play a role in the regulation of chromatophores.[21]

Morphological color change, such as the ontogenetic color adjustment that occurs in the green tree python (*Morelia viridis*) and the emerald tree boa (*Corallus caninus*), usually reflects a shift in life-stage requirements and an adaptation to a new ecological niche. It results from altered pigment cell number and/or amount of pigment within cells.[24]

Another extraordinary skin adaptation of some species of desert-dwelling reptiles is the ability to harvest free-standing water or rain. For example, the thorny devil (*Moloch horridus*) inhabits much of arid Australia, where rainfall is sporadic and surface water is in low supply.

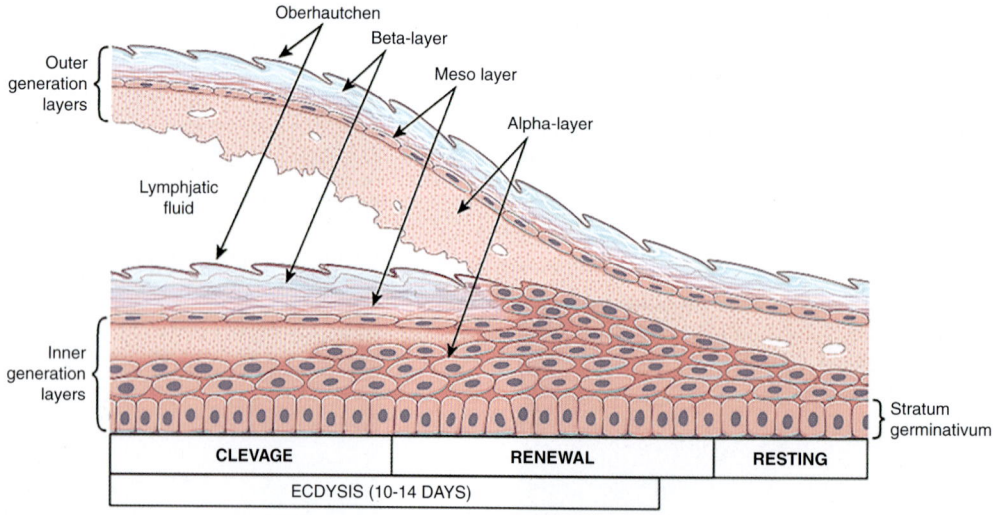

FIG 69.7 The normal shedding cycle of reptilian skin is characterized by two major phases: the resting phase and the renewal phase. The process of ecdysis (from midresting to the conclusion of the renewal phase) takes approximately 10 to 14 days in most species. The length of the resting phase is variable and is dependent on extrinsic factors such as environment and diet. The old skin is cleaved from the newly formed layer by the enzymatic activity of lymphatic fluid that floods the space between the two layers. It is this process that gives the skin of shedding reptiles a blue hue.

Subsequently, the skin of thorny devils has developed hygroscopic properties that allows direct uptake of water from dew, wet foliage, standing water, and damp sand.[25–27] This process is achieved by the presence of minute interscalar capillary channels about 5 to 50 μm wide that support a pressure head of about 10 cm of water.[26,27] As water is drawn into these conduits, it is directed toward the labial scales where it is mixed with saliva and imbibed.[24–27] The existence of these interscalar capillary channels is not unique to the thorny devil, as they have also evolved independently in other species such as the sunwatcher toadhead agamid (*Phrynocephalus helioscopus*) and the Texas horned lizard (*Phrynosoma cornutum*). However, in these species the scalation does not have the same drawing power as in the thorny devil and cannot facilitate movement of ground water into the capillary channels. Instead, these animals rely on rainfall to capture water and exhibit distinctive behavioral postures during storms to maximize their dorsal body surface area and thus increase the volume of water that they are able to collect. This phenomenon is known as "rain harvesting" and is not seen in thorny devils.[26–28]

CLINICAL DISEASES

Infectious Dermatoses

Viral Diseases. Reptile virology is a dynamic and rapidly evolving discipline in herpetological medicine, with new viruses identified regularly. A number of viral diseases have been described in which a component of the disease process affects the integument (Fig. 69.8). A summary of these has been provided in Table 69.1. A diagnosis of viral infection usually requires the examination of biopsies with light and/or electron microscopy as well as molecular techniques. Clinicians should remember to include these on their list of differential diagnoses especially in cases unresponsive to conventional treatment. See Chapter 30 for more information.

Bacterial Diseases

Clinical significance. Various bacterial agents have been associated with dermatological diseases in reptiles. Demonstrating a causative relationship between the isolation of bacteria and the observed dermatological disorder, however, should be based on a multidirectional diagnostic approach to demonstrate a host pathological response (e.g., cytology or histopathology) in combination with the pathogen. Consideration should be given to possible underlying disease and environmental stressors, leading to immunosuppression and secondary bacterial dermatitis.[29–31] In addition to secondary invaders, a relatively small number of bacterial agents have been implicated as primary pathogens of reptiles.[31] Appropriate precautions may need to be instigated in view of the zoonotic potential of some of the organisms associated with dermatological disorders in reptiles. Nevertheless, the risk must be seen in the context of other dangers, including the fact that other apparently less pathogenic bacteria may cause disease in immunocompromised humans.

Known etiological cause(s) and clinical presentation. *Aeromonas, Pseudomonas, Flavobacterium, Staphylococcus, Salmonella, Morganella, Edwardsiella, Klebsiella, Micrococcus, Neisseria, Proteus, Serratia,* and *Enterobacter* spp. are commonly isolated from dermal lesions in reptiles.[29–32] Anaerobic bacteria, including *Bacteroides, Fusobacterium, Peptostreptococcus* and *Clostridium* spp., have been demonstrated to be part of the normal microbiota in reptiles and are frequently reported to cause dermal disease following bite lesions, scratches, or septicemia.[33]

Several bacterial agents belonging to the Actinobacteria have been reported to cause primary dermatological disease in a wide array of taxa.[31] Infection with *Dermatophilus congolensis* has resulted in cutaneous ulceration, hyperkeratosis, necrosis, and subcutaneous abscesses in lizards, snakes, and saltwater crocodiles.[34–37] *Austwickia chelonae,* formerly referred to as *D. chelonae,* has been cultured from skin lesions in chelonians.[38,39]

Devriesea agamarum has been designated as the causative agent of devrieseasis, a dermatological disease entity that is mainly characterized by chronic proliferative dermatitis and septicemia, especially in desert-dwelling (Fig. 69.9) and dry land lizard species.[40] While certain saurian taxa such as dab lizards (*Uromastyx* spp.) show high morbidity, mortality remains low. In other lizard species such as collared lizards (*Crotaphytus* spp.) and Agamid (*Agama* spp.) lizards, entire collections may be eradicated in a few weeks or months.[40,41] Persistence of devrieseasis in lizard collections has been attributed to the presence of asymptomatic carriers, especially bearded dragons, and long-term environmental survival of the bacterium under relatively moist environmental conditions and relatively low ambient temperatures.[41,42] In dab lizards as well as tropical lizard species, such as basilisks (*Basiliscus* spp.) and water dragons (*Physignathus* spp.), *D. agamarum* has been associated with the development of chronic subcutaneous abscesses and septicemia.[43,44]

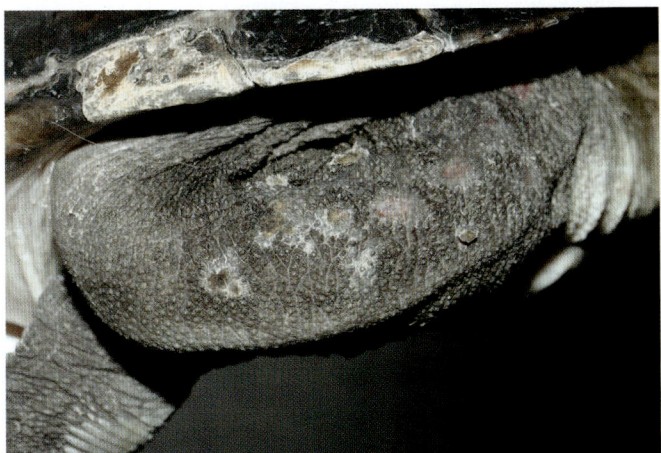

FIG 69.8 Papilloma virus–associated skin lesions in an Eastern long-necked turtle (*Chelodina longicollis*). (Courtesy of Tom Hellebuyck.)

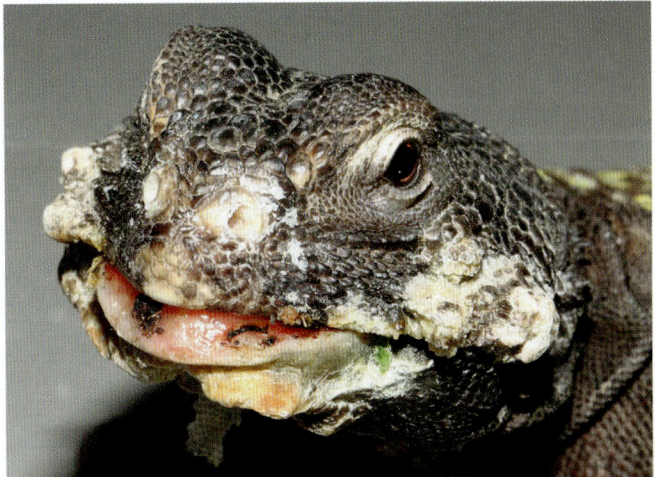

FIG 69.9 Hyperkeratotic skin lesions presenting as cheilitis associated with *Devriesea agamarum* infection in a dab lizard (*Uromastyx acanthinura*). (Courtesy of Tom Hellebuyck.)

TABLE 69.1 Reptile Viral Diseases That Often Have a Dermatological Manifestation

Virus	Species Affected	Clinical Signs
Poxviridae		
Chelonian poxvirus	Hermann's tortoise (*Testudo hermanni*)	Small, white-yellow papular lesions of the lower eyelids and the rostrum.
Crocodilian poxvirus (CRV)	Caimens, Nile crocodile (*Crocodylus niloticus*), saltwater crocodile (*Crocodylus porosus*), freshwater crocodile (*Crocodylus johnstoni*)	Typically present as brown wartlike lesions that may affect any part of the body. Some crocodilians may develop grey-white patches of skin. An atypical form has been identified in Nile crocodiles, with genetic analysis revealing it may be related to but not identical to CRV.
Tegu poxvirus	Tegu lizard (*Tupinambus teguixin*)	Multiple brown-colored papules distributed over the integument.
Iridoviridae		
Ranavirus	Predominately chelonians, but other species include green pythons (*Morelia viridis*) and occasionally lizards	Lethargy, nasal and ocular discharge, subcutaneous cervical oedema, gastrointestinal disease, granulomatous inflammation of the tail. High morbidity and mortality.
Invertebrate iridoviruses	Frilled lizard (*Chlamydosaurus kingii*), various other lizard species	Poxlike lesions of the skin, sudden death.
Herpesviridae		
"Grey Patch Disease" (ChHV-1)	Green sea turtles (*Chelonia mydas*)	Areas of patchy, gray discoloration of the skin in aquaculture-reared young turtles. Associated with chronic illness and death.
Fibropapillomatosis	Green, loggerhead (*Caretta caretta*), hawksbill (*Eretmochelys imbricata*), and olive ridley (*Lepidochelys olivacea*) sea turtles.	Papillary, arborizing neoplasms on the external surface of the body.
Herpesvirus of crocodiles (CrHV-1, 2 and 3)	Saltwater crocodile, freshwater crocodile	Lymphonodular skin proliferations.
Lacertid lizard papilloma	European green lizard (*Lacerta viridis*)	Papilloma lesions covering the skin with varied distribution associated with sex. No abdominal lesions observed.
Papillomaviridae		
Chelonian papilloma virus (Cc-PV-1, Cm-PV-1)	Bolivian side-neck turtle (*Platemys platycephala*), Russian tortoise (*Testudo horsfieldii*), loggerhead turtle, and green turtle	Circular papular skin lesions with occasional skin necrosis.
Lizard papilloma virus	European green lizard	Benign wartlike neoplasms on the surface of the skin.
Reoviridae		
Lizard reovirus	European green lizard	Papillomatous skin lesions and death.
Flaviviridae		
West Nile Virus	Crocodilians	Neuropathies and death. Lymphohistiocytic proliferative cutaneous lesions in American alligators (*Alligator mississippiensis*).

Adapted from Marschang RE: Viruses infecting reptiles. *Viruses*. 2011;3:2087–2126; Jacobson ER: Viruses and viral diseases of reptiles. In Jacobson ER, editor: *Infectious Diseases and Pathology of Reptiles*, Boca Raton, FL: CRC Press, 2007; and Hernandez-Divers SJ: Reptile viral diseases—summary table. In Mader DR, editor: *Reptile medicine and surgery*, 2nd edition. St. Louis: Saunders Elsevier, 2006.

Mycobacterium spp. are considered ubiquitous in the environment and may infect animals following a breach of integrity of the skin or through ingestion.[45,46] The pathogenicity of these acid-fast bacteria seems to vary significantly and may be associated with granulomatous inflammation of the skin but systemic disease may also develop.[45,46]

Skin lesions characterized by the presence of subcutaneous erythema, fluid-filled vesicles, and bullae typically (but not always) on the ventrum are often referred to as blister disease, necrotizing dermatitis, and "scale rot." The condition is most frequently seen in captive snakes, and occasionally in lizards, and is considered to be induced by inadequate environmental factors such as poor ventilation, excessively high humidity levels, and inadequate hygiene. If confined to the ventrum and there is associated ventral heat source (or dorsum with a radiant heat source), thermal damage may need to be excluded. Efficient treatment necessitates elimination of predisposing factors, topical antiseptics, and antimicrobial treatment.[17,29,32]

Diagnostic confirmation. Diagnosis is usually based on the detection of bacteria in scale samples, touch preparations, squash preparations, swabs, or biopsies.[29–32] Cutaneous granulomas comprised of multinucleated giant cells coupled with the presence of acid-alcohol fast bacteria typify mycobacterial infections. PCR can be used to confirm the diagnosis.[45] See the section on diagnostic testing at the end of this chapter for more information on diagnostic testing and the selection of relevant microbial isolates from skin samples.

Medical therapy. Besides systemic antimicrobial treatment, based upon culture and sensitivity testing, and debridement of hyperkeratotic skin lesions and abscesses, factors promoting persistency of the disease should also be eliminated.[29,31,43] Accordingly, identification and correction of husbandry issues and treatment of concurrent diseases, the use of effective disinfection procedures for the captive environment and identification of asymptomatically infected animals are essential for establishing a holistic therapeutic approach for the treatment of microbiological causes of skin disease in reptiles.[31,32,42] Debridement of proliferative and necrotic lesions is invaluable because of the limited penetration of these poorly vascularized tissues, resulting in the establishment of inadequate drug concentrations at the target sites.[31,43,47]

Prognosis. Taking into account the overall multifactorial nature of bacterial skin disease in reptiles, the prognosis largely depends on correct identification and elimination of the etiological agent involved combined with the correction of factors that promote the onset of the disease.

Prevention. As most bacterial skin infections are secondary to substandard husbandry and underlying disease, providing an optimal captive environment is essential in the prevention of bacterial skin disease in reptiles.[31] The introduction of bacterial agents acting as primary agents causing high morbidity in captive collections may be prevented through clinical examination of newly acquired reptiles and correct sampling of skin lesions for microbial examination. The importance of adequate quarantine measures and the identification of asymptomatically infected carriers cannot be overemphasized.[45]

Mycotic Diseases

Clinical significance. As for bacterial infections, dermatomycosis in reptiles is often secondary to inadequate environmental conditions or underlying disease. Clinical signs may be similar in appearance to dermatitis, abscesses, and granulomas caused by bacteria.[30–32,48] Several dermatomycoses in reptiles on the other hand are caused by obligate pathogenic fungi of different orders and have been associated with high mortality and morbidity in captive and free-living reptiles.[49,50]

Known etiological cause(s) and clinical presentation. Various fungal species have been reported to cause dermatomycoses in reptiles, including *Aspergillus, Basidobolus, Chamaeleomyces, Geotrichum, Lecanicillium, Mucor, Saprolegnia, Penicillium, Fusarium, Purpureocillium (Paecilomyces;* Fig. 69.10), *Trichophyton, Trichosporon, Oospora,* and *Alternia.*[31,32,51] Infections with yeasts and yeastlike fungi such as candidiasis, cryptococcosis, and trichosporonosis are less commonly observed.[31] Many of these fungal agents use a breach of skin integrity as a portal of entry and initially attack superficial areas of skin but can quickly develop into a subcutaneous mycelial growth, eventually leading to deep and disseminated mycosis.[31,48]

Primary pathogenic fungi, formerly referred to as *Chrysosporium* anamorph of *Nannizziospsis vriessii* (CANV), have been reassigned to the family Onygenaceae based on phylogenetic studies. Currently, the CANV-complex comprises nine different species, clustered in three phylogenetic lineages. One lineage represents the genus *Nannizziopsis* including isolates from saurians and crocodiles; two other lineages represent the genus *Ophidiomyces* with *Ophidiomyces ophiodiicola,* the etiological agent of a cutaneous fungal disease syndrome known as snake fungal disease (SFD), occurring in free-ranging and captive snakes, and *Paranannizziopsis* spp. infecting squamates and tuataras.[48–50] In general, clinical infections are characterized by the development of localized, crusty, yellow to brown skin lesions, vesicles, and hyperkeratotic lesions evolving to necrosis of extensive areas of skin.[48,52–59] Although considered as obligate fungal pathogens, substandard environmental conditions seem to determine disease initiation and progression. *Nannizziopsis guarroi* infection is frequently associated with severe and sometimes fatal dermatomycosis in inland bearded dragons (Fig. 69.11) and green iguanas (Fig. 69.12).[52] The pericloacal and mandibular region seem to be predilection sites for the development of associated skin lesions.[52,57–59] SFD is an emerging disease characterized by superficial

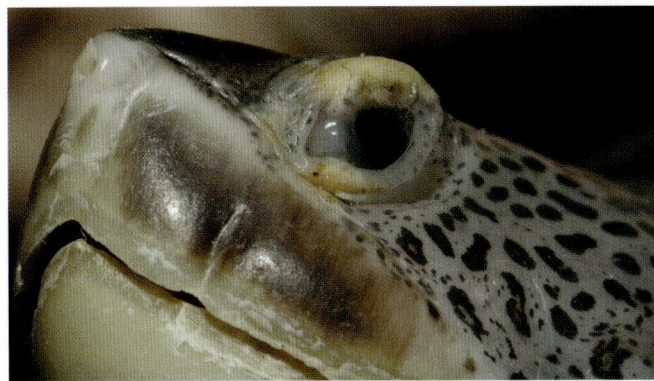

FIG 69.10 *Purpureocillium (Paecilomyces) lilacinus*–associated dermatitis of the eyelids in a diamondback terrapin (*Malaclemys terrapin*). (Courtesy of Tom Hellebuyck.)

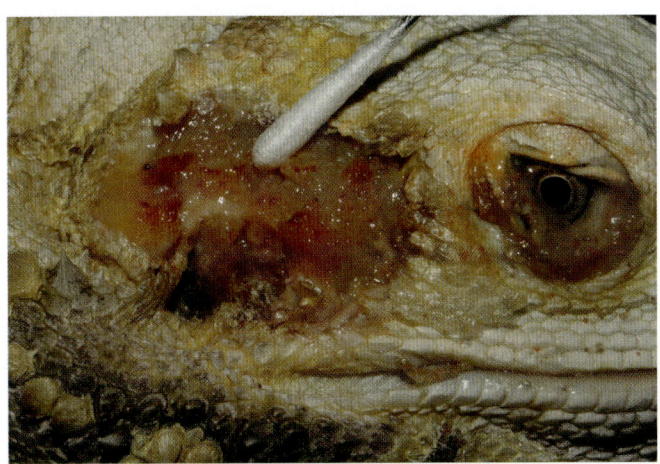

FIG 69.11 Microbiological sampling of *Nannizziopsis guarroi*–induced skin lesions in an inland bearded dragon (*Pogona vitticeps*). (Courtesy of Tom Hellebuyck.)

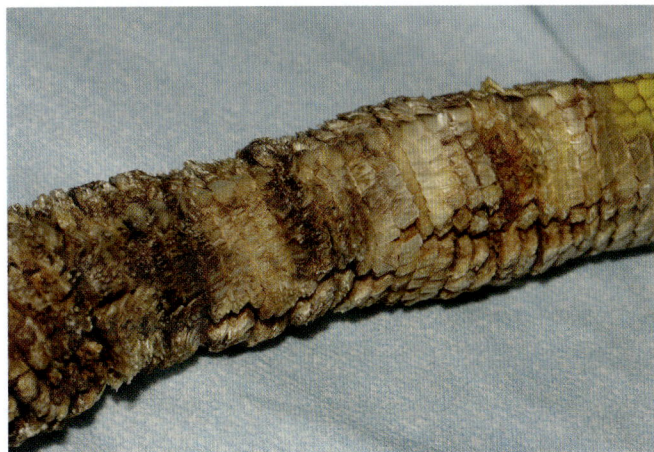

FIG 69.12 Fungal granuloma at the tail of a green iguana (*Iguana iguana*). (Courtesy of Tom Hellebuyck.)

dermatitis and subcutaneous nodules with subsequent morbidity and mortality.[53–55]

Diagnostic confirmation. Many of the considerations made toward the diagnosis and treatment of bacterial skin disorders equally apply for dermatomycosis. Diagnosis is usually based on the detection of fungi with a host inflammatory response in skin samples. Incubation of fungal cultures derived from reptile patients often require specific temperature conditions, and fungal growth may be relatively slow in comparison to mycotic agents that are isolated from dermatological lesions in domesticated mammals.[48] Obtained isolates may be a part of the skin microbiota in healthy reptiles.[31,32,56]

Except for fungal isolates with a known primary pathogenicity, repetitive and correct sampling of skin lesions, adequate culture, histopathological examination of skin and underlying tissue, the use of molecular methods to identify fungal isolates to the species level, and demonstration of a host pathological response are mandatory to assign a fungal isolate as the causative agent of an observed dermatological disorder.[31,32,48]

Medical therapy. Besides the systemic use of triazole antimycotic agents, such as ketoconazole, itraconazole, terbinafine, fluconazole, and voriconazole for the treatment of filamentous fungi infections, debridement of skin lesions and treatment with topical terbinafine or 0.125% chlorhexidine solution may facilitate the treatment of dermatomycosis.[31,57,60] If possible, susceptibility testing of fungal isolates should be performed as resistant clones have been demonstrated.[60] As dermal and deep mycosis often require long-term treatment, the effectiveness of antimycotic treatment and signs of toxicity should be carefully monitored, especially for itra- and ketoconazole.[31,58,60] Voriconazole is recommended as a safe and effective alternative, but the use of the latter agent should be investigated in species such as chameleons that seem to be poorly tolerant to the recommended dosages.[48] When confirmed fungal lesions are isolated to appendages, amputation may also be considered as a viable treatment option, as potential toxicity and antifungal treatment failure are not uncommon.

Efficacy of antimycotic treatment should be confirmed by regular sampling of skin lesions to confirm elimination of the causative agent.[31,60]

Abscesses

Known etiological cause(s) and clinical presentation. The lesions in reptiles that are usually termed abscesses generally appear as raised, hard, and demarcated cutaneous or subcutaneous nodular swellings (Fig. 69.13).[17,31,47] Although mostly gram-negative bacteria are involved, infection with gram-positive bacteria, anaerobic bacteria, or mixed infections may be encountered. Dermal abscesses may also originate from hematogenous spread of bacterial infection, especially when a multifocal distribution is observed.[17,31] Most reptilian abscesses are well encapsulated and show a lamellar appearance on cross-sectional cut. Histological examination of such lesions usually reveals a central core containing bacteria surrounded by inflammatory cells and fibrosis, presumptively to entrap bacteria and prevent systemic spread and resulting in the typical solid appearance. These lesions might be better termed fibriscesses.[61] Similar processes with a more cellular component are essentially granulomas. If *Salmonella* or *Mycobacterium* spp. are isolated from dermal abscesses or granulomas, the presence of concurrent infectious osteoarthritis, osteomyelitis, or soft tissue abscesses should be considered.[30,47,62] Neoplastic disorders, parasitic cysts, fungal granulomas, epidermal cysts, hematomas, and aneurysms might show a similar appearance and should be differentiated from bacterial abscesses.[30]

Cellulitis is a deep suppurative infection characterized by dissemination through the skin and can result in a whole network of infected sinuses and tracts within the dermis (Fig. 69.14). The presentation is similar to that of a large abscess, but as the caseous core is often missing the swelling is soft and fluid can often be aspirated.[17]

Pododermatitis and abscessation of the feet are regularly observed in large saurians such as monitors (*Varanus* sp.), iguanas (*Cyclura* spp., *Iguana iguana*) (Fig. 69.15), and chelonians following bacterial infection of skin lesions caused by inappropriate husbandry such as excessive

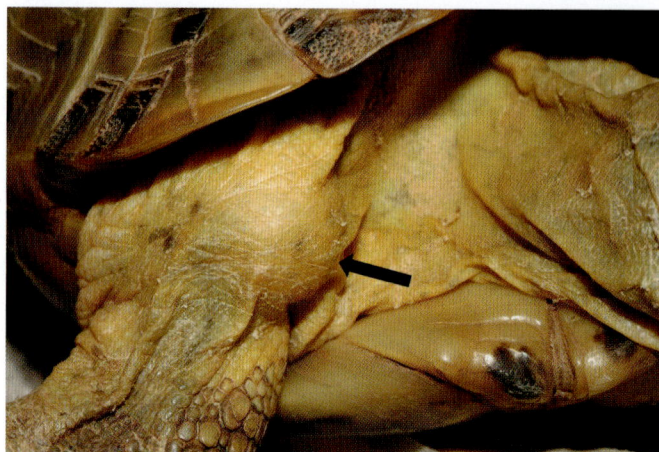

FIG 69.13 Subcutaneous abscess (*arrow*) in a Russian tortoise (*Agrionemys horsfieldii*) following anaerobic infection of a foreign object penetration. (Courtesy of Tom Hellebuyck.)

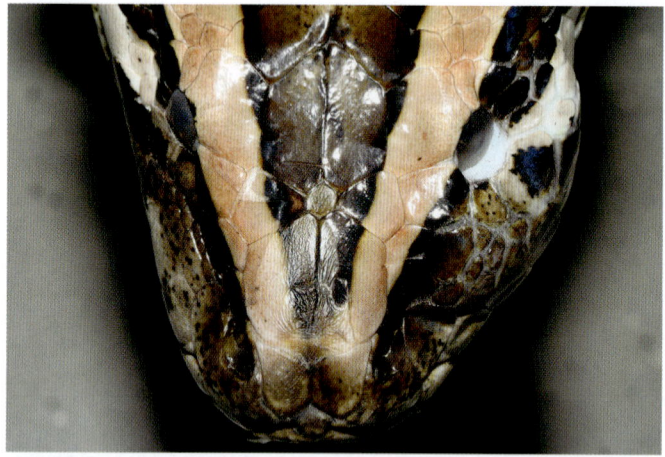

FIG 69.14 Periocular cellulitis in a Burmese python (*Python bivitattus*) associated with *Proteus* sp. infection. (Courtesy of Tom Hellebuyck.)

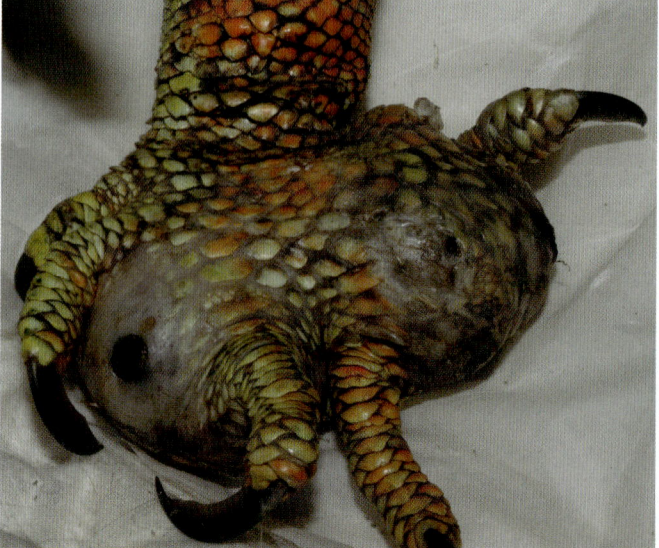

FIG 69.15 Pododermatitis and abscessation in a green iguana (*Iguana iguana*). (Courtesy of Tom Hellebuyck.)

humidity and exposure to an abrasive substrate.[63] In chronic stages, deeper tissues may be affected and osteomyelitis can develop.

Diagnostic confirmation. Definitive diagnosis of an abscess usually requires aspiration or collecting swabs from the inside wall of the fibrous capsule for cytology and culture/sensitivity testing. Anaerobic and fungal cultures should be performed as well as gram, Wright-Giemsa, periodic acid shift, and acid-fast staining of cytological preparations or histopathological sections.[17,32] If the involvement of bony structures with the development of osteomyelitis is suspected, the use of radiography is essential toward installing an appropriate treatment.

Medical and surgical therapy. Due to the presence of caseous pus and thick capsules in most abscesses, these lesions are poorly penetrated by antimicrobial agents.[43] Accordingly, abscesses and granulomas are best excised in toto. If complete excision is not possible, surgical exposure, followed by marsupialization and/or the removal of a large area of epidermis, is important. These techniques will allow continued debridement, aggressive flushing, topical antiseptic treatments, and prolonged topical antimicrobial therapy (when possible based on culture and sensitivity testing).[31,43] Systemic antimicrobials are seldom warranted for the treatment of a discrete abscess.

Parasitic Diseases

Clinical significance. External parasites frequently infest both captive and wild reptiles. Pathology associated with these infections can range from subclinical to severe debilitation depending on the species of parasite and the overall health of the affected reptile. Importantly, external parasites have been implicated as vectors for transmission of serious infectious diseases such as arenavirus.[64,65]

Known etiological cause(s). The most important external parasites in reptiles include ticks and mites. Aquatic reptiles may additionally have to contend with leech infections but these are rare. Ticks and mites are acari parasites, of which over 400 species have been described in reptiles.[65] Parasites within this taxon are characterized as having three pairs of legs as larva and four pairs of legs as nymphs and adults. The head, thorax, and abdomen are fused. Ticks and mites show variable host specificity with some being generalists, while others are highly species specific. Mites from the families Macronyssidae, Paramegistidae, Heterozerconidae, Trombiculidae, and Leeuwenhoekiidae have all been described in reptiles.[65] Of the Macronyssidae, only the genus *Ophionyssus* are ectoparasites of reptiles, and the snake mite, *Ophionyssus natricis*, is the most common species seen.[65] More than 100 soft- and hard-bodied ticks belonging to eight genera of the families Argasidae and Ixodidae have been collected from reptiles worldwide.[65]

The life cycle of acarid parasites of reptiles are varied, with some species spending their entire life on the host, whereas others may have intermittent periods as free-living stages.[65] For example, in the snake mite, *Ophionyssus natricis*, five life periods are recognized: the egg, larva, protonymph, deutonymph, and adult. Only the protonymph and adult are parasitic, feeding on the blood of the host, while the other stages are free-living in the environment.[66]

Clinical presentation. Clinical signs associated with external parasites are typically nonspecific. Mite or tick infestations may result in behavioral changes such as continued rubbing on cage furnishings or prolonged soaking in water bowls. Mite-infected animals often appear dull, or dirty, and may be covered in small, white, powderylike dots, which are mite feces. Dysecdysis or increased frequency of shedding may be observed in affected animals. In severe infestations animals may become lethargic, anorectic, septicemic, or anemic.

Diagnostic confirmation. Diagnosis is confirmed by observation of parasites on the animal. Mites have areas of predilection, including the periocular region, in the folds of skin under the chin, around the cloaca, in the thermosensory pits of snakes, and in the axillae and tympanic recesses of lizards.[67] Ticks often bury themselves under scales, with their presence being disclosed only by slight raising of the scale that they are embedded beneath. Once parasites have been located, they should be removed for microscopic examination. Although most clinicians will readily be able to distinguish between mites and ticks, further identification beyond this level can be difficult in-house and may require specialized training. For submission to a parasitologist, mites and ticks should be stored in an eppendorf container in 70% to 90% ethanol. Where possible, it is best to get as many different life stages and sexes to aid in identification.

Medical therapy. Successful therapy relies on a combination of treating the host, as well as environmental management to break the life cycle. A number of chemicals have been proposed for the treatment of acarid infections in reptiles;[68] however, some carry inherent toxicity risks and are not recommended. The most effective treatments are fipronil spray (Frontline Spray Treatment, Merial, Duluth, GA; active ingredient 0.29% fipronil) or a pyrethroid spray (Provent-a-Mite, Coulston Products Inc, Safety Harbor, FL; active ingredient 0.5% permethrin and the only ectoparasiticide licensed for reptiles in the United States). Although these compounds are relatively safe, care should be taken when using them, as inappropriate application may still result in toxicity to the reptile host. Some clinicians advocate the use of macrocyclic lactones (e.g., ivermectin, moxidectin) as either a spray or an injection, but it should never be used in chelonians and great care taken in crocodilians. In addition, the first author (FS) of this chapter has seen instances of toxicity with their use in some lizard species, in particular those belonging to the genus *Tiliqua*. If a topical treatment is used, it is recommended to wipe the drug off the animal prior to returning it to its enclosure. Reptilian ticks can easily be removed manually, and in most circumstances this is the best method for eliminating them. All topical treatments should also be accompanied by aggressive treatment of the environment to eradicate any free-living stages. Methods suitable for sanitation include applying an acaricide such as a pyrethrin, pyrethroid, carbaryl, or organophosphate to enclosure surfaces and cage furnishings. Other acceptable methods include immersion in boiling water or washing with a 3% bleach solution. No matter which compound is used, it is important that the enclosure is rinsed thoroughly afterward in order to remove any chemical residues and prevent inadvertent toxicity when reptiles are placed into it.

Prognosis. For the majority of cases, acarid infections in reptiles carry an excellent prognosis provided that the animal is not severely debilitated.

Prevention. Preventing infections from entering collections is best achieved with sound quarantine protocols. New animals should be isolated from the existing animals, preferably in a separate room or facility, for a minimum of 3 months. Where possible, it is also a good idea to have enclosures within the quarantine area further isolated by surrounding them with a moat to prevent acarids from dispersing.[45] All animals should be thoroughly examined prior to entering quarantine for the presence of external parasites. At this time, prophylactic treatment may also be administered. Unauthorized personnel should be excluded from entering the quarantine facility, and ideally anyone servicing isolated animals should change clothes before having any contact with the main collection. All enclosures and cage furnishings (water bowls, hides, etc.) used for quarantined animals should be sanitized between occupants, and most importantly before these are used in acarid-free enclosures.[45]

Noninfectious Dermatoses
Dysecdysis

Definition. Dysecdysis is the term given to abnormal or impaired shedding of the outer layer of skin.

Clinical significance. Although one of the most commonly observed dermal problems in reptiles, this disorder should be considered as a nonspecific clinical finding.[31]

Known etiological cause(s). Dysecdysis may be associated with numerous infectious diseases that directly or indirectly affect the skin as well as inappropriate environmental conditions, nutritional deficiencies, dehydration, and traumatic injuries that interfere with the normal shedding process. Dehydration may starve the cleavage zone of the fluids necessary for normal segregation and new epidermal layers. Hypoproteinemia may interfere with the normal enzyme production necessary for the breakdown of the fission layer.[31,69]

Clinical presentation. Retention of sloughed skin may affect the entire integument or may be restricted to retained spectacles in snakes and constricting bands of old skin on the digits or the tail.[69] The latter may eventually result in avascular necrosis or dry gangrene and inevitable loss of distal extremities if left untreated. Dysecdysis should be differentiated from normal fragmented ecdysis as observed in many lizard species.[31]

Diagnostic confirmation. Besides taking into account the history and shedding habits of the affected patient, a thorough assessment of captive husbandry and identification of any underlying or concurrent diseases is often necessary to discern the origin of the observed shedding problems and to instigate appropriate therapeutic measures.

Medical therapy. The therapeutic approach for dysecdysis is often directed by the chronicity of the problem, the number of layers of retained skin, and the size and location of the affected skin site. Aggressively peeling back retained or shed skin as well as premature removal of older epidermal layers should be avoided, as this may result interfere with normal skin integrity and cause considerable loss of fluids and proteins.[69] See Chapter 71 on reptilian ophthalmology for a more detailed discussion on the diagnosis and treatment of the retained spectacle.

Increasing the environmental humidity by spraying the animal and its environment may be sufficient to accomplish the removal of relatively small pieces of retained skin. For snakes, retained skin sloughs are often readily removed with gentle 20-minute soaks in warm, shallow tap water.

Prevention. Applying optimal husbandry protocols based on a sound knowledge of the captive requirements of commonly kept species and eliminating any condition that may interfere with a normal shedding cycle are essential for prevention of this secondary skin disorder.

Prognosis. If the actual source of dysecdysis is left unidentified, captive reptiles are doomed to repeat the problem with each subsequent shed. Once the primary problem is diagnosed and treated, normal ecdysis should return within two or three cycles. If the problem is detected and dealt with early, most animals have an excellent chance of recovery.[69]

Burns

Clinical significance. Reptiles are frequently presented to veterinarians for treatment of thermal burns. These can range from mild to life threatening. It is not completely understood why reptiles are prone to burns but their behavior (not moving away or off of heat devices causing thermal damage) predisposes them to this type of injury.[70] Less common burn injuries include electrical and chemical burns. All serious burns should be considered medical emergencies, and treatment is essentially the same regardless of the initiating cause.

Known etiological cause(s). Burn injuries are typically caused by provision of inappropriate heat sources. Most burn injuries occur when animals are given direct access to heating elements, such as "hot rocks" or heat mats. These devices are unreliable and frequently overheat or have electrical faults. A second important source of potential injury comes from heat lamps placed too close to animals or inside enclosures without any screen guards. An uncommon source of burns are fan heaters and hot water, but nonetheless, they still pose a significant risk if used improperly.

Clinical presentation. Burns are classified based on the degree of tissue damage.[70] Superficial (first-degree) burns only involve the epidermis and are painful but heal quickly if treated appropriately. In some cases, small blisters may be seen. Superficial partial-thickness or deep partial-thickness (second-degree) burns are very painful, resulting in the patient adopting an abnormal posture to relieve pressure on the affected areas. There is complete destruction of the epidermis with marked swelling and blister formation. Full-thickness (third-degree) burns involve both the epidermis and dermis. These are usually painless due to loss of sensory nerve endings and are very slow to heal. The final category, fourth-degree burns, involve the skin and underlying tissue such as muscle and bone and may extend into the coelomic cavity in severe cases.

Diagnostic confirmation. Diagnosis and confirmation is based on a combination of clinical signs (Fig. 69.16) and investigation into husbandry practices.

Medical or surgical therapy. The diagnostic plan and management of reptile wounds should follow standard protocols described for domestic animals. It is important to realize that in many instances the full extent of the burn injury may not be apparent until a few days to a week after the initial trauma. Particularly in circumstances of acute presentation, the client must be made aware that the wound may first look worse before it improves. A complete blood count and plasma biochemistry are useful tools in assessing the physiological state of burnt reptiles. Burns that affect large surface areas are likely to result in significant fluid loss as well as electrolyte imbalances, and so provision of fluids is essential in these cases. Under most circumstances lactated ringer's solution is appropriate for fluid replacement in reptiles as osmolarities are similar to mammals. Intravenous or intraosseous fluid administration is by far the most effective way to correct fluid deficits, and it can be administered as boluses in small patients or via indwelling catheters in larger animals. It is also important to remember that burn injuries typically lose a significant amount of protein, so nutritional support is of paramount importance to prevent animals from becoming hypoproteinemic. In inappetent animals, this may require assisted feeding. For superficial burns, first aid should comprise of rinsing it under a cold tap or applying a cold compress to the affected area. In these cases, topical application of an antimicrobial ointment such as silver sulfadiazine is usually all that is required to prevent contamination of the wound.

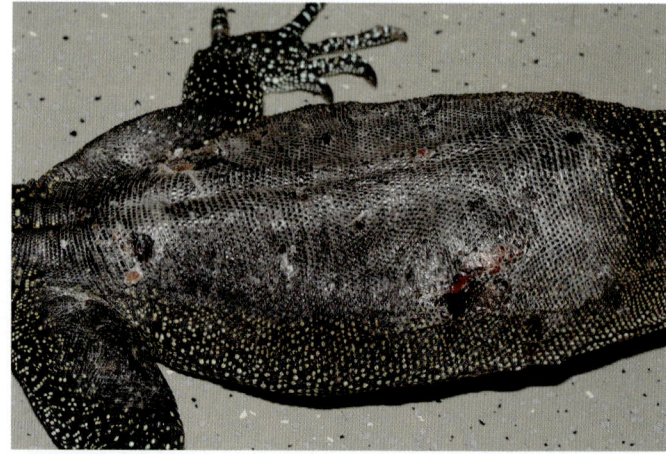

FIG 69.16 Second-degree burn in a peach-throated monitor (*Varanus jobiensis*) resulting from the inappropriate installation of heat sources. (Courtesy of Tom Hellebuyck.)

For any burn that is more severe than superficial, more involved treatment is required and will be dependent on the extent of tissue damage. Such wounds may require surgical debridement or daily bandage changes. These wounds are prone to infection with possible septicemia, so systemic antibiotics may be warranted if extensive. Wounds should be covered with a protective layer that promotes healing and inhibits microbial growth. Suitable products include silver-impregnated gels or ointments or honey/sugar bandages. This initial layer then needs to be further protected using an absorbent bandage material, and finally, covered with a more robust layer to prevent rubbing. Initially, bandage changes should be performed daily, as wounds will leak significant amounts of fluid, but this can be extended out to every 3 or 4 days once the wound has stopped oozing. No matter the type of burn, analgesia should be provided to all animals. A combination of NSAIDs and opioids are recommended. For bandage changes, the clinician should routinely consider general or local anesthesia prior to cleaning wounds.

Prognosis. Superficial to deep partial-thickness burns have a good prognosis, full-thickness burns carry a guarded prognosis, while fourth-degree burns have a grave prognosis. When embarking on management of burn injuries, the client should be well-informed that treatment and healing times are often prolonged and require a significant commitment on their behalf.

Prevention. Reptiles should not be given direct access to heat sources. It is not recommended to use hot rocks or heat mats inside enclosures. Where possible, heat lamps should be placed outside enclosures or covered with a protective cage. Aquarium heaters can be placed inside a PVC pipe to prevent aquatic reptiles touching the heating elements.

Bites From Prey

Clinical significance. Live prey items offered to reptiles may inflict serious injuries if left unattended in enclosures (Fig. 69.17). Bites may occur from rodents or invertebrate prey. In extreme cases wounds may result in the death of the reptile.

Known etiological cause(s). Live prey items left in enclosures for extended periods of time may attack predators in self-defense, or they may inflict damage on the reptile as they are being captured. Invertebrates may start biting or feeding on reptiles if they are not consumed. Reptiles may become inappetent for a variety of reasons and a thorough investigation into general health and husbandry is recommended for any animal that consistently refuses food items.

Clinical presentation. Wounds may range from superficial abrasions to deep and contaminated bites with extensive soft-tissue damage. They may be singular, or as is often the case in invertebrate bites, they may be disseminated over the entire body. Infections may lead to septicemia and/or severe debilitation.[29]

Diagnostic confirmation. Confirmation occurs by discussing husbandry practices with the client.

Medical therapy. The general principles of decontamination, antibiosis, and analgesia apply to any wounds arising from bites by prey.

Prognosis. Prognosis is dependent on the extent of the injuries.

Prevention. Offering live rodents should be discouraged (and is illegal in many areas). Ultimately, feeding freshly killed or frozen/thawed rodents is more humane for the prey item and is also more cost-effective for the hobbyist. Invertebrates not eaten within 15 minutes of being placed into an enclosure should be removed and reoffered at another time.

Rostral Abrasions

Clinical significance. Captive reptiles are particularly liable to the development of rostral abrasions. In chronic cases and if left untreated, affected animals may be unable to feed or succumb to osteomyelitis and systemic infection.

Known etiological cause(s) and clinical presentation. Rostral abrasions are commonly caused by rubbing on glass or wire surfaces, especially in lizard species that show explosive bursts of flight behavior (e.g., *Physignathus* and *Basiliscus* spp.; Fig. 69.18) and nervous snake species. If left untreated, these lesions may develop into deep abscesses, and in severe cases necrosis or osteomyelitis of underlying bone may occur.

Diagnostic confirmation. Besides taking into account the species predisposition, the location and appearance of these lesions, confirmation is by assessment of the captive environment.

Medical therapy. Topical antiseptic or antimicrobial therapy and wound care should prevent the entry of pathogens. In those cases where deep infection occurs, surgical intervention and prolonged systemic antimicrobial therapy (based upon culture and sensitivity testing) is often required.[17,29,31]

Prognosis. Prognosis is dependent on the extent of the injuries, especially the involvement of bony structures and the establishment of environmental adjustments.

Prevention. These injuries can be prevented by providing animals with adequate housing and an environment in which they feel secure and unthreatened.

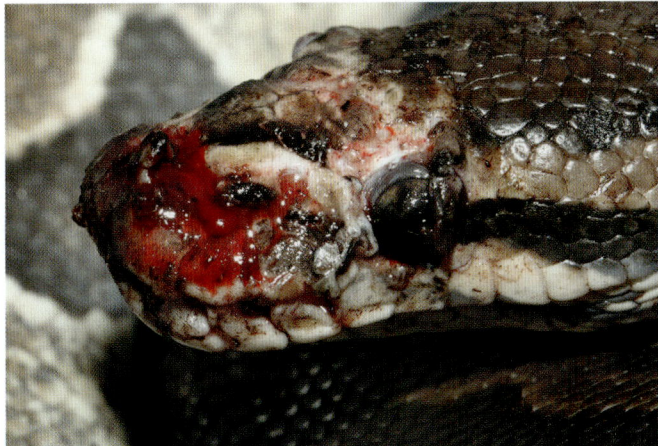

FIG 69.17 Prey item trauma at the head of a royal (ball) python (*Python regius*). (Courtesy of Tom Hellebuyck.)

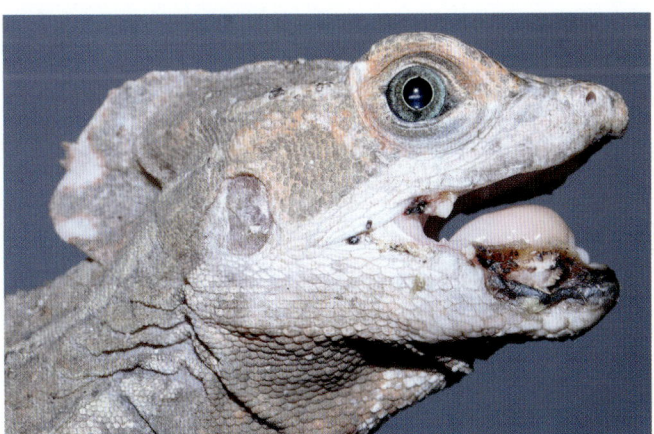

FIG 69.18 Rostral trauma in a *Basiliscus* sp. is typically caused by explosive bursts of flight behavior. (Courtesy of Tom Hellebuyck.)

Nutritional Dermatoses

Clinical significance. Nutritional dermatoses are frequently observed, especially in captive lizards and chelonians, due to the considerable interspecies differences in nutrient requirements. These may present as abnormal color changes, dysecdysis, abrasions, or keratinization disorders resulting in an abnormal appearance to skin texture. Delayed wound repair of the skin may indicate general malnutrition.[31,71–73]

Known etiological cause(s) and clinical presentation. Hypovitaminosis A in reptiles is primarily recognized as a disease of chelonians, although the prevalence of hypovitaminosis A may be underdiagnosed in saurians (Fig. 69.19). Palpebral edema, conjunctivitis, cheilitis, and aural abscesses in chelonians, especially in aquatic species, are common indicators of this nutritional disorder. Impaction of precloacal and femoral pores as well as the development of hemipenile plugs with secondary infection may be associated with hypovitaminosis A in lizards.[31,72–74] Tissues that have been pathologically altered as a consequence of hypovitaminosis A are prone to secondary bacterial and mycotic infection.[62]

Abnormal fragility of the skin with separation and skin tearing has been anecdotally reported in snakes and is associated with poorly organized collagen and vitamin C deficiency. However, there is little scientific evidence to support these diagnoses. Steatitis of the skin with necrosis and sloughing is observed in piscivorous reptiles fed diets high in polyunsaturated fats, especially when rancid.[17]

Diagnostic confirmation. Diagnosis of nutritional causes of dermatological problems are often presumptive and based on clinical history, assessment of the management, and response to therapy.[72,73,75]

Medical therapy. As for other fat-soluble vitamins, parenteral administration of vitamin A should be carefully dosed to avoid iatrogenic hypervitaminosis A, and dosing intervals based on clinical response to treatment should be respected. Doses of 2000 to 5000 IU/kg vitamin A are considered safe in those patients showing signs related to hypovitaminosis A.[62,63,75] Alternatively, nutritional improvement and oral supplementation are safer. Metaplastic abscesses should be surgically removed and local or systemic antimicrobials may be required.[31,72–75]

Prognosis. Nutritional dermatoses have a good prognosis if adequate treatment is initiated and dietary imbalances are corrected.

Prevention. β-carotene-rich food sources should be included in the diets of susceptible species as a part of the prevention and long-term treatment of vitamin A deficiency. In primarily insectivorous lizard species (geckos, chameleons), supplementation with preformed vitamin A may be necessary, as clinically they appear to have a decreased ability to utilize beta carotenoids as vitamin A precursors.

Cutaneous Neoplastic Disorders

Known etiological cause(s). Cutaneous neoplasms are regularly diagnosed in reptiles and include fibrosarcomas, liposarcomas, chromatophoromas, epitheliomas, mast cell tumors, and squamous cell carcinomas (SCC; Fig. 69.20).[31,76–30] In chelonians, the shell may be directly or indirectly involved. Papillomatosis and fibropapillomatosis associated with viral infection have been discussed previously.

Chromatophoromas are classified as melanophoromas or melanomas, iridophoromas, xanthophoromas, erythrophoromas or mixed depending on the type of pigment-producing cells involved.[79] Although once considered uncommon, melanophoromas (Fig. 69.21) and iridophoromas seem to show a relatively high incidence, especially in diurnal species. As for SCC, continuous exposure to high doses of artificial UV radiation has been proposed as a predisposing factor in the development of chromatophoromas.[78,79]

Clinical presentation. While most skin neoplasms present as cutaneous or subcutaneous demarcated proliferative or nodular processes, diffuse skin masses may be observed. Secondary microbial infections

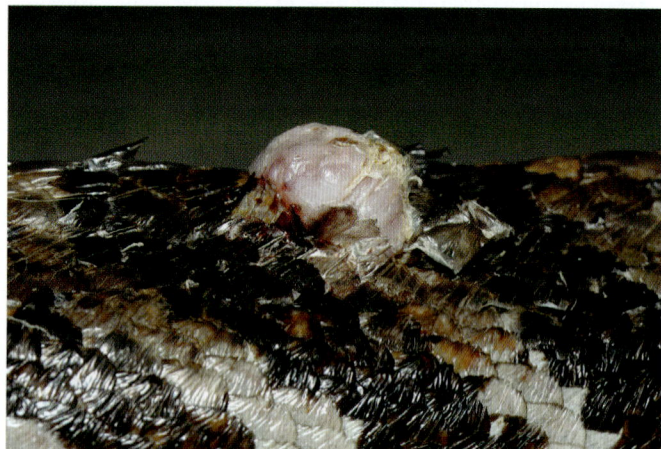

FIG 69.20 Squamous cell carcinoma located at the dorsal skin in a blue-tongued skink (*Tiliqua gigas*). (Courtesy of Tom Hellebuyck.)

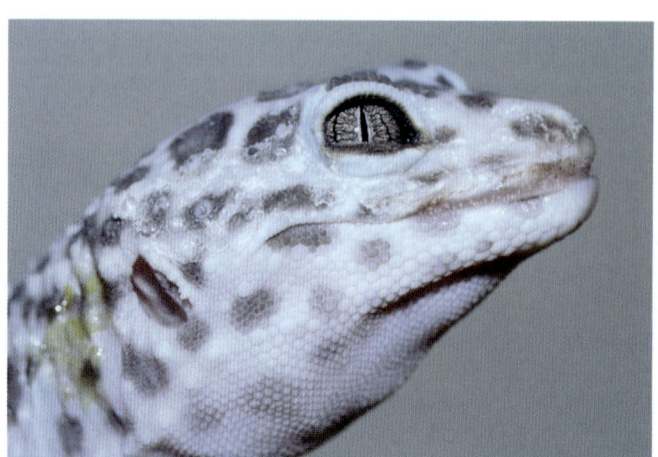

FIG 69.19 Vitamin A responsive cheilitis in a leopard gecko (*Eublepharis macularius*). (Courtesy of Tom Hellebuyck.)

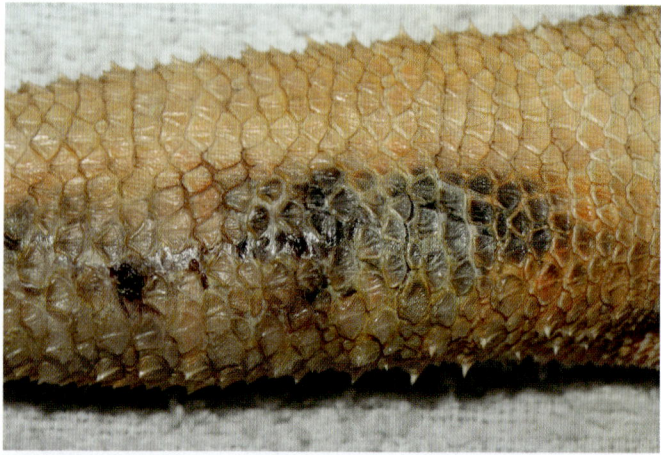

FIG 69.21 Cutaneous melanophoroma located at the dorsal side of the tail in a bearded dragon (*Pogona vitticeps*). (Courtesy of Tom Hellebuyck.)

may complicate the clinical picture, especially when the integrity of the epidermis has been breached. Although most of these types of skin neoplasms exhibit locally aggressive behavior, they show a relatively low tendency to metastasize.[31] Mast cell tumors, squamous cell carcinomas, and melanophormas may show a multicentric appearance.

Diagnostic confirmation. Cytological or histopathological examination is usually essential to distinguish a neoplasm from other lesions such as abscesses and granulomas. Immunohistochemistry is a valuable tool toward the differentiation of dermal neoplasms in human and traditional small animal medicine but is left largely unexplored in reptiles. Evaluation for metastases should be investigated in each patient with a confirmed diagnosis of cutaneous neoplasia.

Medical or surgical therapy. In addition to, or as an alternative to, surgical excision, cryotherapy, laser ablation, or radiation may be of value in some patients. Intralesional and systemic chemotherapy protocols have been described for the treatment of some neoplastic disorders in reptiles with variable effectiveness.

Prognosis. In general, the selection of appropriate therapies on the basis of the stage and biological behavior of the tumor in question determines the prognosis. Those cases where complete surgical excision is possible carry a fair prognosis. Nevertheless, long-term monitoring is often required, as many reptile skin neoplasms show a moderate to high recurrence rate. If complete resection is deemed impossible because vital structures are involved or the presence of metastases exist, the prognosis is worse.

DIAGNOSTIC TESTING

Evaluation of the reptilian integument necessitates a holistic approach with particular attention paid to both the animal and its environment. A general physical examination should be accompanied by detailed analysis of husbandry. Where possible, pieces of shed skin may provide valuable information so clients should be encouraged to bring these to the appointment if available. As many reptiles are small, magnification may aid in diagnosis. For detailed information on clinical examination of reptile patients, refer to earlier chapters.

The collection of skin samples plays an important role in diagnosis. Many of these tests can be performed in-house by clinicians. Tests that should be performed at the initial examination include swabs or impression smears of wounds, skin scrapes, and sticky-tape preparations. Samples can be stained with Romanowski stain (Diff-Quick or similar) and examined immediately. Laboratory diagnostics may then be necessary depending on these results, and consideration should be given to collect samples for microbiological culture, PCR, and skin biopsies for histological examination.

Skin biopsies can be collected under a combination of sedation/manual restraint and local anesthesia, or while the animal is under general anesthesia. The decision of which method to utilize depends on the competency of the handler and the behavior of the animal, as well as the scenario in which the procedure is being performed (i.e., in the hospital or in field conditions). Once the area to be biopsied has been identified, care must be taken not to surgically prepare the site as this may potentially eliminate etiological agents such as bacteria or fungi. However, sterile saline flushing and a sterile drape should be used to isolate the area, and the surgeon should prepare themselves as for other surgical procedures. In most instances, biopsy punches (Fig. 69.22) are an effective method for obtaining diagnostic samples in reptiles, but in rare cases (e.g., tough skin, larger biopsy required) a section of skin may need to be removed using a scalpel blade. Once the biopsy has been obtained, it should be placed gently into 10% neutral buffered formalin for histopathological examination. Larger areas of skin should be placed on card to prevent rolling before being

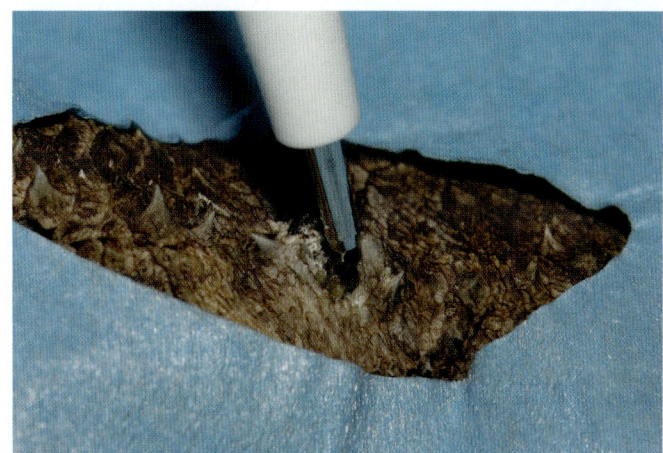

FIG 69.22 Collection of a full-thickness skin biopsy using a biopsy punch. (Courtesy of Tom Hellebuyck.)

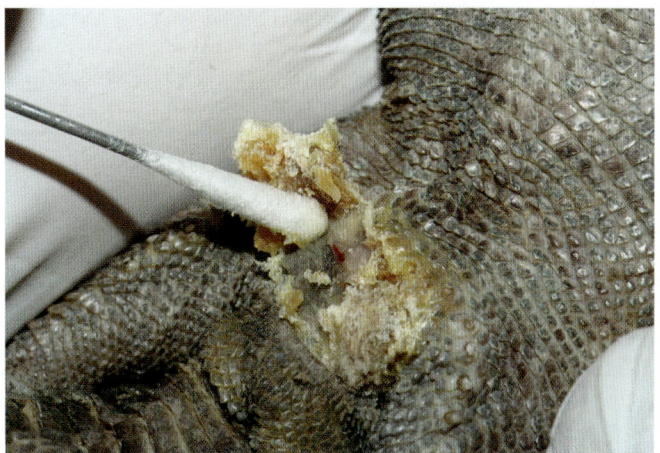

FIG 69.23 Debridement of dried scabs associated with skin lesions allows sampling of the deeper infected tissue, which results in more accurate microbiological isolates from culture. (Courtesy of Tom Hellebuyck.)

placed in formalin. Where appropriate, an additional biopsy sample should also be collected into a sterile pot for microbiological culture. Care must be taken not to crush biopsy samples after they have been collected. If the clinician is having difficulty retrieving the sample from the biopsy tool, then flushing it with sterile saline from a 25 g needle into the formalin pot is usually the easiest way to extricate the tissue. The resultant wound can be closed with sutures or alternatively by covering it with a small dressing and allowing it to heal by secondary intention.

Cultured bacteria and fungi from skin lesions, especially superficially, do not always represent the primary causative agents as contamination from the environment, together with secondary infection, can complicate the picture. Moreover, relatively little is known concerning the normal microbiota of reptile skin and adnexa.[31,32] The correct selection of dermal sampling sites and methods may facilitate the selection of clinically important bacterial and fungal isolates (Fig. 69.23).[29] In addition, the identification of microbiological agents should always be correlated with the results of other tests (e.g., hematology, cytology, and histopathology).

REFERENCES

See www.expertconsult.com for a complete list of references.

70

Dermatology—Shell

Jean Meyer and Paolo Selleri

Chelonian anatomy is unique as it contrasts with the anatomy of other tetrapods by encasing the shoulder girdle into the rib cage, providing an unprecedented way of protection. The exact evolutionary steps that lead to the formation of the shell are mostly speculative, as transitional forms of fossils are missing from the fossil record.

Four major index fossils are the basis for the tentative decryption of the evolution of the chelonian body plan: *Eunotosaurus* (260 million years [myr]), *Pappochelys* (240 myr), *Odontochelys* (220 myr), and *Proganochelys* (214 myr). The first three taxa share the common feature of craniocaudally broadened ribs and elongated trunk vertebrae, shortening the trunk to nine dorsal vertebrae.[1,2] The axial arrest of the dorsal ribs (see also Embryonic Development of the Shell) can be demonstrated in *Odontochelys*, going hand-in-hand with the incorporation of the clavicle and interclavicle into the plastron. The final encapsulation of the scapula within the shell, as well as the metaplastic ossification of the carapace and the presence of peripherals suggesting the formation of a carapacial ridge (see Rib Growth Mechanisms), are the most striking features of *Proganochelys*.[3] Broadened gastralia in *Pappochelys* might be at the origin of a fully developed plastron that is already present in *Odontochelys*. Fossils of *Odontochelys* and *Proganochelys* demonstrate that their shells were already covered by scutes.[2]

ANATOMY

The chelonian shell consists of the dorsal convex carapace and the ventral flatter plastron. The carapace and the plastron are usually rigidly joined laterally by the bridge formed by the conjunction of lateral extensions of the carapacial and the plastral bones (plastrocarapacial bridge).

Embryonic Development of the Shell

The mechanisms involved in the embryonic development of the chelonian shell are a source of numerous debates and are still not completely resolved. Chelonian anatomy is unique as it contrasts the anatomy of other tetrapods by encasing the shoulder girdle into the rib cage. Two main different hypothetical approaches to the development of this topographic peculiarity are proposed. The first emphasizes the role of the growth pattern of the ribs, which leads to roofing of the shoulder girdle and thus enclosing it into the rib cage,[4–7] whereas another approach is based on evolutionary morphologic changes in the shoulder girdle itself, being independent of specific alterations in rib growth.[8]

Rib Growth Mechanisms

To elucidate the former theory, new investigational strategies are warranted by a multimodel approach using immunohistochemistry and genetic analysis. These sophisticated methods permitted to demonstrate that the rib growth patterns differ between studied hard-shell (red-eared slider turtle, *Trachemys scripta elegans;* Reeve's pond turtle, *Chinemys reevesii;* loggerhead sea turtle, *Caretta caretta;* snapping turtle, *Chelydra serpentina*) and softshell (Chinese softshell turtle, *Pelodiscus sinensis*) chelonians. Both groups share two common features in embryonic development: First the formation of a carapacial ridge (CR) bilaterally along the flanks extending craniocaudally between the limb buds (Fig. 70.1) and second the flabellate primaxial growth of the ribs, which in contrast to other vertebrates do not grow ventrally to encompass the viscera but enter into the dermis and extend over the pectoral and pelvic girdle. The CR is a unique structure in vertebrates and seems to influence rib growth by two different strategies. In hard-shell turtles, rib precursor cells seem to be attracted by means of paracrin signaling pathways to the CR. This model shows some evidence that fibroblast growth factors (FGF) secreted by CR cells lead to migration of the rib precursor cells laterally through the muscle plates. The developing ribs extend centrifugally in a peripheral direction. Reaching the CR mesenchyme, their tips fold beneath the ridge and ultimately unite with the peripherals, taking shape in the CR at the periphery of the shell. In softshell turtles, by contrast, no FGF could be demonstrated immunohistochemically in the CR area. Furthermore, rib growth is characterized by "axial arrest" hypothetically promoted among other factors by the CR.[5] The ribs are subjected to ossification early in the development, impeding further longitudinal growth. In these turtles, the carapacial disc is likely to grow independently of the ribs, leading to an inward

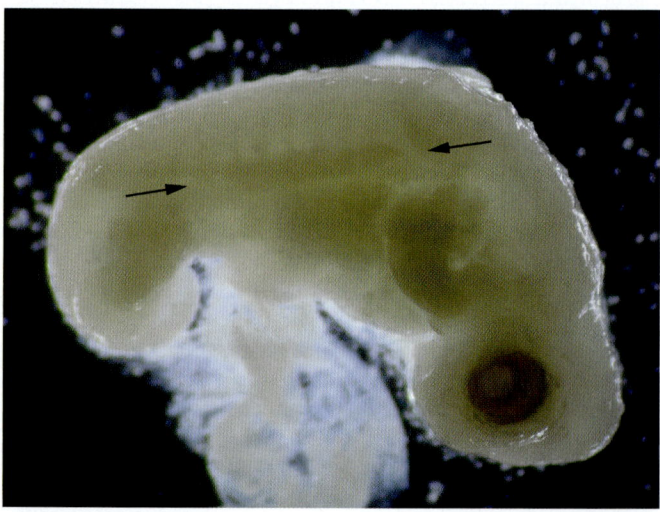

FIG 70.1 Carapacial ridge in a *T. hermanni* embryo, extending between the limb buds in craniocaudal direction (between the arrows). (Courtesy of Jean Meyer.)

folding of the lateral body wall thus enclosing the shoulder girdle in the carapace. A number of studies aimed at deciphering the genetic basis for the axial arrest of rib growth but demonstrated missing similarities in the expression of these genes between different turtle species.[9–12] However, again, differences between softshell turtles (*P. sinensis*) and hard-shell turtles (*T. scripta, E. orbicularis*) could be highlighted.

Formation of the Solid Carapace

Rib growth alone is insufficient to elaborate a solid carapace. Further ossification is necessary to fill in the gaps between the ribs and form the interdigiting plates. Putatively, two different mechanisms find their expression depending on whether the turtle develops a hard or a soft shell.[4] Hard-shell chelonians rely on exo- and endoskeletal ossification. Formation of the shell starts with small bony protrusions budding in cranial and caudal directions from the periosteum surrounding the ribs (Fig. 70.2). It is suspected that bone morphogenic proteins (BMPs) are secreted by the ribs and induce metaplastic ossification of the surrounding intramembranous dermal cells, thus leading to formation of the dermal plates embedding the ribs. The overwhelming part of this process takes place after hatching. In softshell chelonians the growth of costal bony plates is rudimentarily concentrated to the area close to the vertebrae and seems to be solely derived from extensions of the periosteum of the ribs.[5] The unique plywood-like arrangement of bony crystals in the cortex of the shell of *Trionychids*[13] might have its origin in a new bone formation modality in soft shells, which still needs to be elucidated.

Formation of the Plastron

In hard-shell chelonians the plastron is composed of nine bony plates, which develop by dermal ossification.[14] The ossification starts in nine separate ossification centers, which grow in the direction of the midline and form long spicules. As the hatchling grows, these spicules cross the midline and interdigit without immediately fusing. Recent investigations on the origin of the plastral bones in red-eared sliders (*Trachemys scripta*) using immunohistochemistry suggests that they are derived from late emigrating populations of trunk neural crest cells.[15]

Development of the Scutes

The scutes overlying the dermal bone originate from local epithelial thickenings called placodes. Placode arrangement follows a pattern of somatic segmentations and is highly conserved throughout the taxa.

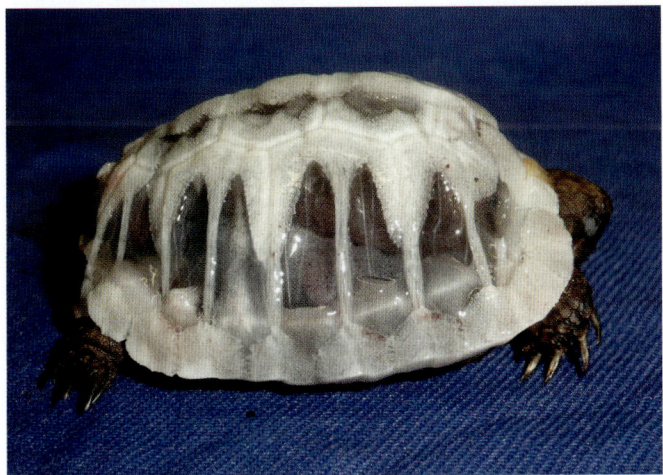

FIG 70.2 Carapacial bony structure of an 8-week-old *T. hermanni*, showing the ongoing ossification of the carapace in caudal and cranial direction starting from the ribs. (Courtesy of Jean Meyer.)

They appear early during embryonic development, first at the carapacial ridge, followed by the costals and vertebrals on the carapace, and the peripheral plastral placodes.[16] The scutes grow radially and contiguously in the epidermis until they contact the adjacently forming scutes.[17–19] Scute growth is potentially governed by the expression of a number of genes for growth factors, and morphogenic proteins. Inhibition of these proteins lead to loss of scute placodes. The loss of epidermal scutes in softshell turtles may be owed to the evolutionary loss of these placodes.[19] Where scutes meet, a small furrow is formed, impressing a sulcus into the underlying bones thus reinforcing the cohesion of the shell structures. Of clinical importance, the location of the scute seams does not show a one-to-one conformance to seams of their bony counterparts (Fig. 70.3A and B).

Dermal Bones

The shell is in general formed by 58 bony plates (49 carapacial and 9 plastral) of dermal origin and covered by epidermal keratin scutes (see Fig. 70.3A and B). A large number of species- or family-specific variations exist.[20] The shapes and the size of the bone plates determine the overall cross-section and size of the shell, whereas the numbers stay relatively constant. The bony dorsal midline of the carapace covering the spine is formed by an unpaired row of up to 12 smaller neural bones. The most cranial bone of this row is called the nuchal, and the most posterior is the pygal. Interposed between the pygal and the last neural lies the suprapygal. On either side of the neurals the costals form the dome of the carapace and verge laterally on the peripherals, composing the outer ventral rim of the carapace. An odd number of bony plates form the ventral plastron with the unpaired entoplastron lying ventral to the pectoral girdle. The entoplastron may be absent in mud turtles (*Kinosternidae*). Cranial to the entoplastron the paired epiplastron shapes the cranial edge of the plastron. Posteriorly to the foresaid plates follow the paired hyoplastron, hypoplastron, and xiphiplastron, divided by a central seam. All bony plates of the shell are deeply interlocked by bony sutures. The leatherback turtle *Dermochelys coriacea*, as well as *Trionychidae*, shows a large variety of reductions of the ossified shell (see Plastral Pecularities in this chapter).

Scutes

The dermal bony shell is in general covered by keratin scutes or shields of epidermal origin. In softshell turtles (*Trionychidae*), the Fly River turtle (*Carettochelys insculpta*), and the leatherback turtle (*Dermochelys coriacea*), the scutes are completely reduced. The epidermal layer of hard-shell turtles generally consists of 38 carapacial and 16 plastral scutes (see Fig. 70.3A and B). The size and shape of these scutes do not show a one-to-one conformance to their bony counterparts and bear a divergent designation. The dorsal unpaired midline scutes are called vertebrals, lined on either side by the pleurals that are bound in turn by the marginals. Cranially, a cervical scute may be present. The absence or presence of the cervical may be one of the few distinguishing marks between the Indian star tortoise (*Geochelone elegans*) (absent) and the South African geometric tortoise (*Psammobates geometricus*) (present). On the plastron all scutes are paired with the gular or the intergular, being the most cranial, followed by the humerals, pectorals, abdominals, femorals, and anals in caudal direction. An axillary and inguinal scute lines the cranial and caudal rim of the bony bridge. Inframarginals are present between the marginals and pectorals and abdominals in all families other than *Trionychidae* and *Testudinidae*. Alligator snapping turtles (*Macrochelys temminckii*) may feature a row of supramarginals between pleurals and marginals. The seams, also called epidermal hinge regions, where the keratin scutes are joining do not line the bony sutures but in contrary indent into the dermal structures, reinforcing the shell structure (see Fig. 70.3A and B). Individual variations in scalation

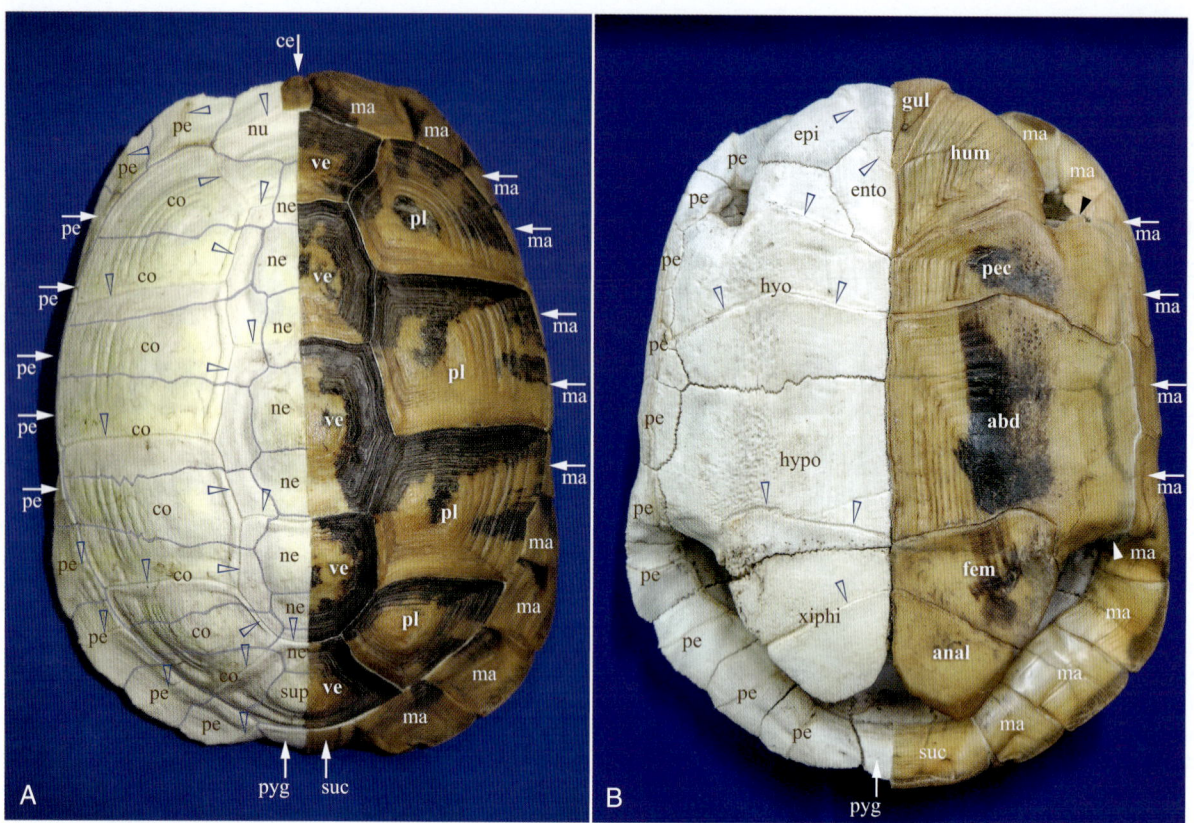

FIG 70.3 (A) Carapace of a *Testudo hermanni*, bones (left) and scutes (right). The bony sutures are highlighted with thin blue lines. Indentations of the scutal seams in the bone, reinforcing the shell structure (blue arrows). Scutes: ce, cervical; ma, marginals; pl, pleurals; suc, supracaudal; ve, vertebrals. Bones: co, costals; ne, neurals; nu, nuchal; pe, peripherals; pyg, pygal; sup, suprapygal. (B) Plastron of a *Testudo hermanni*, bones (left) and scutes (right). Indentations of the scutal seams in the bone, reinforcing the shell structure (blue arrows). Scutes: abd, abdominal; anal; fem, femoral; gul, gular; hum, humeral; ma, marginals; pec, pectoral; axillary (black arrowhead); inguinal (white arrow head). Bones: ento, entoplastron; epi, epiplastron; hyo, hyoplastron; hypo, hypoplastron; pe, peripherals; xiphi, xiphiplastron. (Courtesy of Jean Meyer.)

are common and may on one hand be the result of impairments during ontogenetic development (see previous section, Embryonic Development of the Shell) and on the other hand represent morphologic variation. A number of publications deal with these variations in terms of localization and frequency in different genera.[21] Pigmentation and color patterns of the scutes may be characteristic for a certain species and even allow the gender differentiation in certain *Pseudemydid* species, where males gradually become melanistic with age.

Kinesis—Flexible Skeletal Hinges

Kinesis of the shell describes the development of a certain flexibility of the shell by means of skeletal hinges. These skeletal hinges allow either partial or total closure of the shell, thus enhancing its protective function, or facilitate oviposition if posterior plastral elements are involved. Plastral, carapacial, or pankinesis may be distinguished.

Plastral kinesis can be localized just cranially (e.g., *Pyxis arachnoides*), just caudally (e.g., *Homopus, Rhinoclemmys, Testudo* spp.), or at both ends by a transverse central hinge (e.g., *Terrapene, Cuora* spp.). The unique carapacial hinge in *Kinixys sp.* requires special anatomic adaptations like the replacement of peripheral bones by pliable soft tissue, a floating neural plate, and the transversal alignment of the lumbar bony sutures.[20] These specific anatomic features should not be mistaken for fractures.

A unique feature is the carapacial pankinesis of the Malayan softshell turtle *Dogania subplana*, which develops with maturity by breakdown

of sutures[22] and should not be misinterpreted as progressive metabolic bone disease.

Fontanels

Fontanels are generally defined as membranous gaps between growing bony segments of the shell, thus allowing certain flexibility (Fig. 70.4). Fontanels may be extremely large in hatchlings of *Leucocephalon yuwonoi* and *Heosemys spinosa* or completely absent in the side-necked turtles of the family *Pelomedusidae*. During growth, the gaps decrease in size and become completely ossified. Pritchard describes the enormous variability of these fontanels.[20] In the south East Asian genus *Batagur*, males will retain lifelong large porthole-like structures in the ventrolateral aspect of the costal bone plates. These can be used for ultrasonographic, endoscopic, or surgical approaches.

Plastral Peculiarities

The plastron may be reduced to a cross-shaped entity (e.g., *Macrochelys, Chelydra, Sternotherus, Staurotypus, Claudius* spp.), enhancing the range of motion of extremities as well as of their large head and neck. Another form of plastral reduction is the arrangement of the plastral bones in the form of a ring, leaving a central soft-tissue window as in the pancake tortoise (*Malacochersus tornieri*). A flexible nonossified midline opening in the plastron is also present in hard-shelled marine turtles and *Trionychidae*. The latter present additional features in the form of intermembranous sesamoid bones in addition to the regular plastral bones.

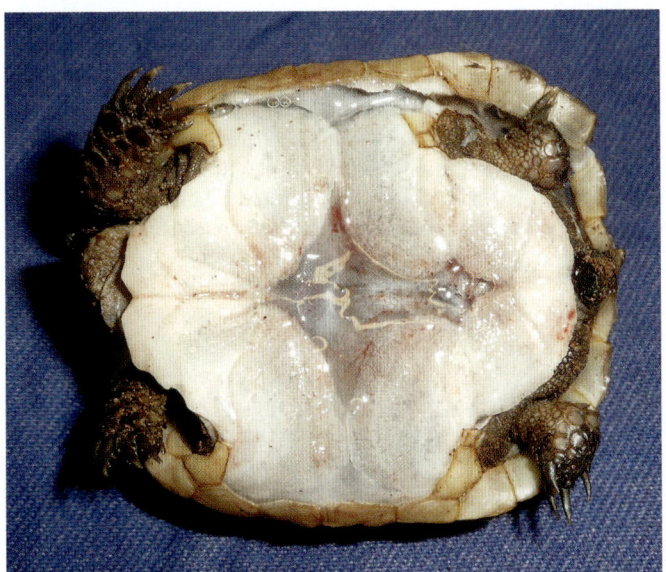

FIG 70.4 Bony plastron of an 8-week-old *T. hermanni*. Growth of the bony plastron is starting at the periphery during late embryonic development. A fontanelle in the center of the plastron is still present at hatching. (Courtesy of Jean Meyer.)

In the leatherback turtle (*Dermochelys coriacea*) the plastron is vestigially reduced to a very narrow ossified ring structure. Ventral soft tissue windows are often present in the form of fontanels in juvenile specimens of most chelonians. Plastral reductions facilitate endoscopic or surgical approaches to the coelomic cavity.

PHYSIOLOGY

Scute Growth

The scutes are produced by the corneous epidermis covering the dermal bone. In the Hermann's tortoise (*Testudo hermanni*), scute growth mainly occurs in the hinge region where neighboring scutes adjoin each other forming a visible seam. During the growing season, beta-keratin–producing cells proliferate at the epidermal hinge region and form a thick new corneous layer, which becomes visible as a growth ring.[17,18] In *Chrysemys picta* the scute is growing along the whole surface, producing beta-keratin during the growing season and a thin layer of alpha-keratin in late fall, shortly before hibernation. When resuming growth in the following spring, new beta-keratin layers are produced underneath the alpha-keratin layer. The latter will serve as a scission layer, allowing shedding of the outer, older scute. It takes corneocytes 5 to 9 days to migrate from the base to the outer surface.[18] In *Graptemys* spp. the transition between epithelium and keratin is abrupt and lacks a discernable cornification zone.[23] In softshell turtles (*Trionychidae*) where dermal scutes are absent the body armor is guaranteed by a leathery dermis. The dermis consists of highly ordered plywood-like arrangements of collagen fiber bundles, which even find their reflection in the inner zone of the outer cortex of the underlying lamellar bone.[13] This plywood-like pattern of skin and bone reduces the weight of the shell and provides an outstanding biomedical stability and flexibility.

Scutes and Age Determination

The growth cycle of the keratinous scutes reflects metabolic conditions of the turtle. The resulting ring pattern, which is most obvious in species from temperate regions, may temptingly be used for age estimation. A literature survey[24] based on 145 publications dealing with this subject concludes that aging turtles by counting their rings is generally inaccurate but might be useful in some species, at some locations, up to a certain age. Scute surfaces are worn off superficially depending on environmental conditions, leading to erroneous results. In many aquatic species, an alpha-keratin layer is produced regularly between the normal beta-keratin layers. The superficial scute is shed along this scission layer, leaving a smooth outer surface.

Sexual Dimorphism

In general, females tend to grow larger than males and have a more vaulted carapace in order to host the produced clutch. In many chelonians, the concavity of the plastron is gender related, with males showing a greater concave curvature to accommodate the caudal aspect of the female's carapace during mating. Increased kinesis of the posterior end of the plastron aiding in oviposition is present in a number of species (e.g., *Rhinoclemmys*, *Testudo*, *Homopus*, *Leucocephalon* spp.). In male bowsprit tortoises (*Chersina angulata*) and African spurred tortoises (*Geochelone sulcata*) the epiplastron is impressively elongated cranially and aids in courtship fights. Fontanels may be retained for longer periods in female *Graptemys* spp. when compared with males.[20]

Role of the Shell in Anoxia Tolerance in Freshwater Turtles

During long-term submergence (hibernation), freshwater turtles are accumulating high concentrations of lactic acid. The shell acts as a buffer reserve by uptaking lactic acid in exchange with carbonates and bicarbonates. Interspecific anoxia tolerance differences exist with *Chrysemis picta* and *Chelydra serpentina* being more tolerant than *Stenotherus odoratus*, *Graptemys geographica*, and *Trachemys scripta*.[25] During submergence at 5°C, an alpha-adrenergic vasoactivity regulating the blood flow to shell and liver is evident.[26]

CLINICAL DISEASES

Scute Anomalies

Clinical Significance and Known Etiological Cause(s). These anomalies typically represent morphological variations without pathologic significance. The anomalies result from a developmental disruption of the embryonic arrangement of the placodes (see Embryonic Development of the Shell). The tessellation pattern of the keratinous scutes is well-conserved phylogenetically but is subject to significant individual variability.[27,28] The highly variable scutation in olive loggerhead sea turtles (*Lepidochelys olivacea*) opposes the determination of an exact number of scutes. A genetic determination of developmental anomalies could not be ascertained. The disruption of signaling pathways in early morphogenesis leads to a loss of the normal segmented distribution of scute primordia.[19] Environmental factors like high temperatures, desiccation,[29] and pollution[28] are hypothesized triggers to scute anomalies. The most frequent anomaly is the presence of supernumerary scutes. Their formation may be triggered by altered distances between placodes, resulting in vacant areas where supernumerary scutes form.[16]

Clinical Presentation, Treatment, and Prevention. Clinical presentations may include supernumerary scutes, missing scutes, or abnormal scute shapes due to the fusion of adjacent scutes. No therapy is indicated, but prevention includes the correction of unfavorable environmental conditions.

Ankylosis—Distorted Growth

Clinical Significance and Known Etiological Cause(s). Ankylosis is defined by the closure of bony sutures, thus impeding further growth. This may be generalized and physiological during the aging process in a number of species (e.g., *Terrapene*, *Cuora*, *Batagur*, *Callagur*, *Kachuga*,

Dermatemys, and *Kinyxis*).[20] Irregular growth of bony plates is a common feature in chelonians. They mostly pose a cosmetic problem and may only lead to health concerns if the shape of the shell is substantially deformed, impairing organ function (especially breathing) and interfering with limb and neck movement or oviposition due to narrowing of the cranial or caudal shell.

Scoliosis, kyphosis, and lordosis or combinations thereof are rare conditions in chelonians and might reflect unfavorable conditions during incubation (humidity, dessication, temperature), or dietary and ambient inadequacies after hatching. Abnormalities in growth may be partly genetically based or a result of trauma in the pre- or post-hatching stage (see also Embryonic Development of the Shell). Severe scoliosis, kyphosis, and lordosis (impinging on spinal cord) can result in rear-limb paresis and chronic or acute prolapse of colon, cloaca, oviduct, and phallus. When ankylosis is confined to single suture areas of the growing shell, distortions of the carapace may result, as adjacent areas pursue their normal development. Trauma or developmental abnormalities may lead to premature ankylosis (see Chapter 113, Fig. 113.7b).

Clinical Presentation and Treatment. Irregular disproportionate growth, or distortions of carapace and plastron, are usually obvious. Surgical therapy is warranted if dystocia might result. In the early stages of deformation, dental expansion screws can be glued between the caudal carapace and plastron on either side of the cloaca to allow gradual widening of the caudal shell opening. Ovariectomy would also be an option to prevent dystocia.

Pyramiding
Clinical Significance and Known Etiological Cause(s). Pyramidal growth of the shell describes a condition characterized by the humped appearance of the carapace. This is physiological in the tent tortoise (*Psammobates tentorius*) but is pathological in most other tortoise species. The humps are the result of trabecular bone thickening between the inner and outer bone cortices of the shell. Scutes remain thin and just outline the dorsal shape of the bones. Pyramiding is usually a cosmetic problem if not accompanied by distorted growth (see Ankylosis—Distorted Growth) but does indicate captive mismanagement.

Many factors have been implicated in the cause of these changes: high dietary protein, inappropriate dietary calcium:phosphorus ratios, improper UV lighting, elevated temperature, low dietary fiber. or simple overfeeding. Research in African spurred tortoises (*Centrochelys [Geochelone] sulcata*) has indicated that low humidity appears to play a crucial role in the development of pyramidal growth. At higher humidity levels, the tortoises produced significantly smoother carapaces.[30] Dietary protein had only questionable influence when combined with dry ambient conditions. The underlying pathologic mechanisms remain hypothetical and abide their histologic elucidation. It is theorized that during dry seasons the intra- and intercellular pressure in growth zones is reduced by dehydration and that the tissues are ossified in this collapsed condition. In captive-raised leopard (*Stigmochelys pardalis*) and African spurred tortoises, the application of supplemental nocturnal heat can lead to increased growth rates and pyramiding.[31]

Clinical Presentation, Treatment, Prognosis, and Prevention. Clinically the carapace displays multiple humps or dorsal projections. Once formed, the deformed pyramid shaping is irreversible. Deficiencies in husbandry, especially low humidity, high nocturnal temperature, and diet should be corrected.

Softening of the Shell in Juvenile Herbivorous Tortoises
Clinical Significance and Known Etiological Cause(s). Described in juvenile *Testudo hermanni, T. graeca, T. marginata, Geochelone elegans,*

Geochelone pardalis, pathology has been demonstrated in association with picornavirus infections, although adults may test PCR positive but appear healthy.[32] Cryptosporidiosis, *Balantidium*, and *Hexamita* spp infestations have also been reported in association with softening of the shell.[33,34] Picornavirus infections and *Hexamita* infection are often seen in conjunction with nephropathy leading to renal secondary hyperparathyroidism and osteodystrophy. Metabolic bone diseases of other origins must also be considered as differentials.

Clinical Presentation and Diagnostic Confirmation. Hatchlings thrive well up to the age of 6 to 8 weeks, when they start to present with signs of rhinitis, conjunctivitis, and anorexia, paired with translucency of the grayish plastron. The gallbladder may become visible as a dark spot on the right side, and there is progressive softening of the entire shell (Fig. 70.5). Pharyngeal swabs (for picornavirus PCR), fecal evaluations (for *Cryptosporidium* and *Balantidium*), and urinalysis (for *Hexamita*) are recommended. Postmortem examinations may permit picornavirus isolation from liver, lung, kidney, spleen, heart, brain, tongue, and intestine.

Treatment, Prognosis, and Prevention. Supportive care (fluid therapy, nutritional support) is the mainstay of therapy. In animals that present with distended bladders (that can cause ventilator compromise), catheterization and voiding the bladder can be beneficial. Prognosis is guarded. Quarantine and strict barrier nursing of affected animals are recommended.

Secondary Hyperparathyroidism (Metabolic Bone Disease)
Clinical Significance and Known Etiological Cause(s). Commonly seen in animals maintained indoors or in conjunction with improper dietary management (e.g., calcium deficient diets, unsuitable dietary Ca:P ratios, lack of UVB light exposure), or less commonly as a sequela to chronic liver and/or kidney failure.

Clinical Presentation and Diagnostic Confirmation. Softening of the shell and humped or distorted growth are common clinical presentations. (Fig. 70.6). Often there is collapse of the caudal carapace due to

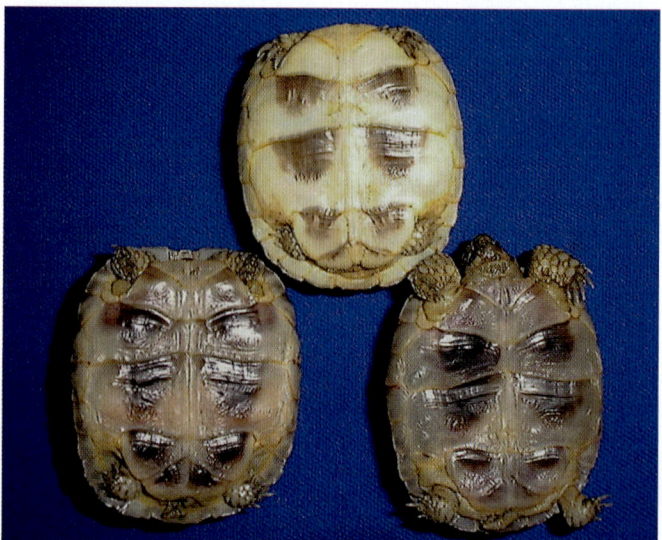

FIG 70.5 Softening of the shell of juvenile *Testudo graeca*, resulting from a picornavirus-induced nephropathy. Healthy clutch mate (*above*); affected animals with translucent shell (*below*) due to osteodystrophy. (Courtesy of Jean Meyer.)

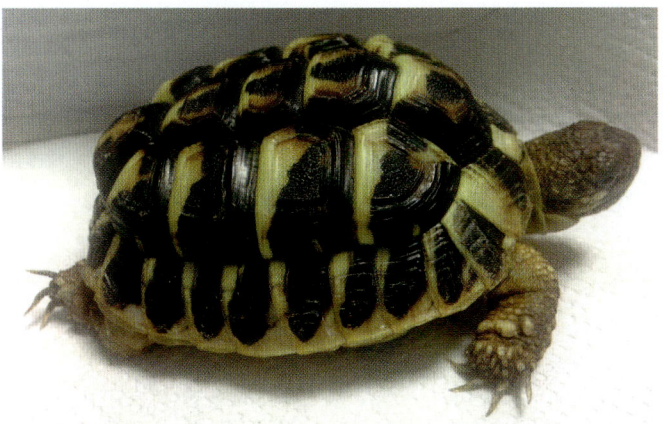

FIG 70.6 Nutritional secondary hyperparathyroidism in a young *Testudo hermanni*. Note the pyramiding and the collapse of the caudal carapace. The nails are overgrown due to the abnormal gait. (Courtesy of Paolo Selleri.)

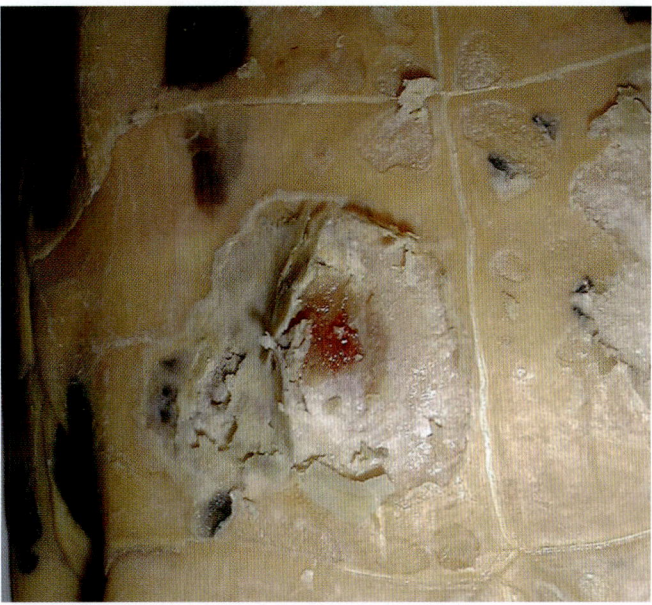

FIG 70.7 Deep ulcerative shell lesion on the plastron of a *Trachemys scripta*. *Aeromonas hydrophila* was cultured from freshly exposed tissue of the debrided lesions. (Courtesy of Jean Meyer.)

hind limb muscles pulling on their insertion points at the caudodorsal aspect of the carapace. These severe shell distortions may result in scoliosis, kyphosis, and lordosis (impinging on the spinal cord), causing rear limb paresis and chronic or acute prolapse of colon, cloaca, oviduct, and phallus. Additionally, dystocia may result. Survey radiographs typically reveal generalized reductions in skeletal opacification, consistent with demineralization. Total plasma calcium tends to only decrease late in disease progression, while ionized calcium tends to remain stable until the terminal stages. Elevations in phosphorus may also occur. Hypovitaminosis D_3 (25-hydroxy-cholecalciferol) assays are commercially available (Heartland Assays, Ames, IA) and decreases confirm UVB light deficiency.

Treatment, Prognosis, and Prevention. Therapy usually includes oral or parenteral calcium therapy, diuresis, and phosphate binders, but the mainstays are environmental and dietary improvements. (See Chapter 84 for more details.) Prognosis is good to poor depending on the stage of disease at which animals are presented and whether hepatic/renal failure is involved in the pathogenesis. Carapacial deformations are irreversible. Appropriate environment (especially UVB light and thermal provision) and diet are usually the best preventive measures.

Bacterial Shell Dermatitis/Osteomyelitis (Including Septicemic Cutaneous Ulcerative Disease)

Clinical Significance and Known Etiological Cause(s). Lesions of the carapace and the plastron have been historically termed "septicemic cutaneous ulcerative disease" (SCUD) or "shell rot" and are quite common in chelonians.[35] Although this condition is suspected of being of bacterial etiology,[36] few bacteria have been reported to be primary causative agents. In early reports of SCUD, the original causative agent was identified as *Escherichia freundii* (currently *Citrobacter freundii*); however, despite extensive clinical investigations, the primary cause of dermatitis and osteitis in chelonians often remains undetermined,[37–39] and currently SCUD is considered more as a syndrome associated with various bacteria, rather than a single obligate pathogen. In a study in which 19 bone biopsies were obtained from map turtles with shell lesions, six samples yielded aerobic isolates (*Chryseobacterium indologenes*, *Aeromonas hydrophila*, *Ralstonia pickettii*, and *Morganella morganii*), whereas 11 samples yielded various clostridial anerobes[23]; however, it was unclear if the bacteria were the cause of lesions.[23] In a zoologic collection, the gram-negative bacterium *Beneckea chitinivora* resulted in an outbreak of ulcerative shell disease in sliders, musk turtles, softshell turtles,

side-neck turtles, and painted turtles.[40] *Serratia* may allow other bacteria (e.g., *Citrobacter freundii*) to invade tissues due to its lipolytic and proteolytic activity.[41] Generalized *Mycobacterium kansasii* infection may result in white carapacial lesions.[42]

Clinical Presentation and Diagnostic Confirmation. Cutaneous lesions of the shell often penetrate through the keratin layer into the underlying bone, resulting in dermatitis and osteomyelitis (Fig. 70.7; Fig. 70.8a and b). Presumptive diagnosis is based on clinical appearance, but definitive diagnosis requires shell biopsy for microbiology (bacterial and fungal cultures) and histopathology.[23] Shell biopsies should be collected under general anesthesia using a bone trephine, preferably with fine teeth to reduce crushing artefacts of the biopsy samples. Dilute chlorhexidine may be used for mild antiseptic preparation of the biopsy site.[23] Obtained samples are to be submitted for microbiology and histology to evaluate the involvement of the cultured microorganisms in the shell pathology. The biopsy sites are closed with methylmethacrylate containing bone cement. As a more objective means to quantify shell lesions, a shell scoring system has been developed that divides the 54 scutes into six regions, with each region scored for lesion extent and severity and summated to produce a total shell disease score (TSDS).[23] The plastron is divided into three scutal regions, with the first including the gulars, humerals, and pectorals; the second being composed of the abdominals; and finally the third caudal region encompassing the femorals and anals. The carapacial regions are formed by a peripheral region containing all marginal scutes, the second region comprising the eight pleurals, and the third consisting of the vertebral scutes. A regional shell disease score is calculated by multiplying the regional score for the extent of the visible lesions (0 = absent, 1= minor [occupying <10% of the region], 2 = moderate [10%–50%], 3 = severe [>50%]), with a regional shell disease score for the severity of the lesions (0 = no lesion; 1 = superficial, only involving the keratin layer; 2 = intermediate, involving keratin and partial bone; 3 = deep, involving keratin and full thickness bone). The TSDS is calculated by adding all six regional scores.[23] The TSDS allows an objective evaluation of the extent and severity of shell lesions in relation to general body condition or other biometric data as hematology and biochemistry results.

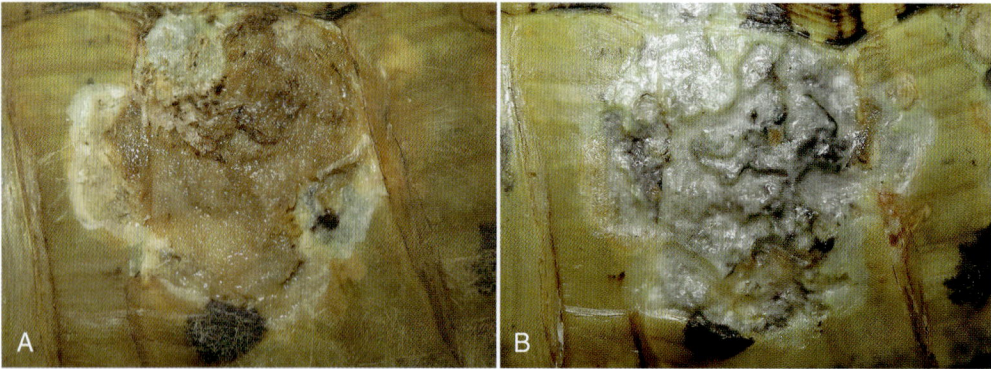

FIG 70.8 (A) Subscutal dermatitis and osteomyelitis (overlying scutes have been removed in the course of debridement). *Sphingobacterium mizutani, Brevundimonas diminuta, Corynebacterium* sp., and the fungus *Metarhizium anisopliae* were isolated from the necrotic bony material. (B) Progression was stopped by debridement followed by local antibiotic and antifungal treatment based on sensitivity testing. Beginning keratinization of the ingrowing epidermal surface is visible. The physiological color pattern of the scutes will not be restored. (Courtesy of Jean Meyer.)

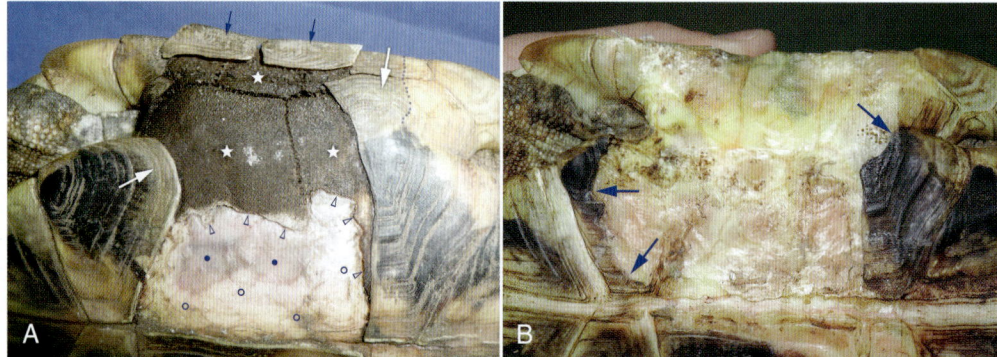

FIG 70.9 (A) Healing stages of a necrosis of the plastron in a tortoise. Detachment of the scutes (blue arrows). Subscutal bony necrosis visible through discoloration (white arrows). Scutes should be left in place and may be cut back to the dotted line. Bony necrosis (stars) and demarcation (blue arrowheads). Thickening of the semitranslucent soft coelomic membrane (blue dots). Fibrosis with subsequent calcification of the coelomic membrane (blue circles). (B) Same tortoise as in (A), but 1 year later. Well-calcified and keratinized solid scar tissue. Scutal definiton and colorization is lost. Old scutes were cut back to the level of intact contact with the epidermis (blue arrows). They should never be entirely removed if only margins detach from the epidermis. (Courtesy of Jean Meyer.)

Treatment. Treatment usually includes surgical debridement, dry docking aquatic species, bandages, and topical and systemic antimicrobials based on culture and sensitivity testing. Treatment of shell ulcerations using photopolymerizable nanohybrid composite appears to prevent relapses and allows faster return of aquatic turtles to their environment.[43] Low-level laser (photobiomodulation) therapy may also be used. We suggest two different approaches based on the severity of the disorder.

Fresh-contaminated wounds should be copiously flushed with antiseptic solutions (e.g., Nolvasan, Zoetis, Octenisept, Schülke & Mayr, Prontosan, Braun). Care must be taken that these solutions do not enter the body cavity through perforating bony lesions. Minor debridement can be achieved by the use of tooth brushes and wet-to-dry dressings. Fresh superficial wounds should be bandaged and changed daily. Silverdiazine cream or povidone-iodine containing ointments can be used on wounds. Exudative lesions benefit from absorptive dressings (e.g., Melolin, Smith & Nephew, UK). The wounds typically heal by second intention, and systemic antimicrobial therapy is seldom required.

Contaminated-infected wounds require more radical debridement, under general anesthesia with appropriate analgesia, using scalpel, dental units and descalers, bone burrs, or Dremel-type rotational hobby tools.

The use of water-cooled systems prevent thermal damage and aid in flushing contaminated material. Swabs or tissue biopsies taken from freshly exposed, infected areas will give the most reliable culture results. Wet-to-dry dressings will help with further debridement. Filling the thoroughly debrided and disinfected areas with dental composite may promote healing in aquatic species.[43] Antibiotic treatment should be based on gram stains initially and subsequently culture and sensitivity testing. Metronidazole or ceftazidime should be considered where anaerobes are suspected or confirmed. The use of vacuum-assisted wound closure with silver impregnated bandaging materials promotes faster healing.[44] Deep-shell necrosis with substantial loss of bony shell will heal by metaplastic calcification of the coelomic membrane and subsequent keratinization of the ingrowing epidermal surface (Fig. 70.9A and B).

Prognosis and Prevention. Prognosis is dependent upon severity, nature of the pathogen(s) involved, and response to treatment. Prevention relies on proper management. Anecdotally, high humidity, low temperatures, poor nutrition, under-floor heaters, and traumatized skin or shell tend to be predisposing factors for the development of shell infections.[36]

Mycotic Shell Dermatitis/Osteomyelitis (Including White Spot Disease in Softshelled Turtles)

Clinical Significance and Known Etiological Cause(s). Fungal infections of the shell resulting in white or pale discoloration (e.g., "white-spot disease" in softshelled turtles) are not uncommon and are often secondarily infected with various bacteria.[45] Softshelled turtles artificially infected with the zoospores of *Aphanomyces sinensis* showed the typical whitish maculae on the carapace and high mortality.[45]

A ubiquitous saprophytic mold, *Purpureocillium lilacinum (Paecilomyces lilacinus)*, was the etiological agent of hyalohyphomycosis, characterized by white to gray spots on the carapace, plastron, and skin, diagnosed in Chinese softshelled turtles (*Pelodiscus sinensis*)[46] and Fly River turtles (*Carettochelys insculpta*).[47] In 1996 an *Aphanomyces* sp. infection was diagnosed as being responsible for white, cottonlike lesions in two juvenile softshelled turtles (*Pelodiscus sinensis*).[48] Mucormycosis has been described in softshelled turtles in Japan and in the United States.[49,50] White papular carapacial lesions could also be seen in conjunction with a generalized *Mycobacterium kansasii* infection and should be considered as differential.[42]

Clinical Presentation and Diagnostic Confirmation. Lesions are typically characterized as white to gray cottonlike spots or discolorations on the carapace, plastron, and skin. Diagnosis is confirmed by biopsy for fungal culture and histopathology, although secondary bacterial infections are common, and concurrent bacterial culture is also recommended (see Fig. 70.8A and B).

Treatment, Prognosis, and Prevention. Several antifungal treatments are reportedly effective. Hyalohyphomycosis has been successfully treated in Fly River turtles with 0.038% malachite green and 4.26% formaldehyde dips (Rid Ich+, Kordon, Hayward, CA), 0.15 mg/L for 15 minutes, twice a day, in combination with systemic itraconazole therapy at 10 mg/kg PO every 48 hrs for 20 days.[47]

Prognosis is generally guarded. In a mucormycosis outbreak affecting approximately 400 Florida softshell turtles showing circular gray integumentary lesions, death rate exceeded 50%.[50] However, timely treatment with topical and systemic therapy (i.e., described in the medical therapy previously), clinical resolution has been obtained.[47] Fungal overgrowth may develop as a consequence of indiscriminate, broad spectrum antibiotic use and may be favored by certain anatomic characteristics (e.g., the peculiar carapace of softshelled turtles (see previous discussion on scute growth) and by compromised immune functions due to inappropriate thermal provision, poor hygiene, or high population density.[45,46] Different species of fungus have different growth characteristics. The fungus *Aphanomyces* sp. found in two juvenile softshelled turtles had optimal growth at a temperature of 30°C, while the fungus *Aphanomyces sinensis* had maximal growth at 25° to 30°C and between pH 6–9, and mycelial growth declined and ceased at incubation temperatures of 35° and 40°C, respectively.[45,48]

Dyskeratosis in Tortoises

Clinical Significance and Known Etiological Cause(s). Shell dyskeratosis has been described worldwide in a number of species, including Texas tortoises (*Gopherus berlandieri*) and Mediterranean tortoises (*Testudo* sp.).[51,52] In Texas tortoises, *Fusarium semitectum* is responsible for characteristic lesions of the carapace and plastron.[52] The pathogenicity of *F. semitectum* was confirmed by isolation from affected individuals and cultivation in keratin-enhanced agar.[51] Hyalohyphomycosis by *Acremonium strictum* and *F. semitectum* caused whitish areas and fissures in the plastron and to a lesser extent on the plastrocarapacial bridges of nine privately owned Hermann's tortoises.[52] Cultures of soil samples from the garden where the animals lived also yielded *F. semitectum*.[52] In an adult male Aldabra

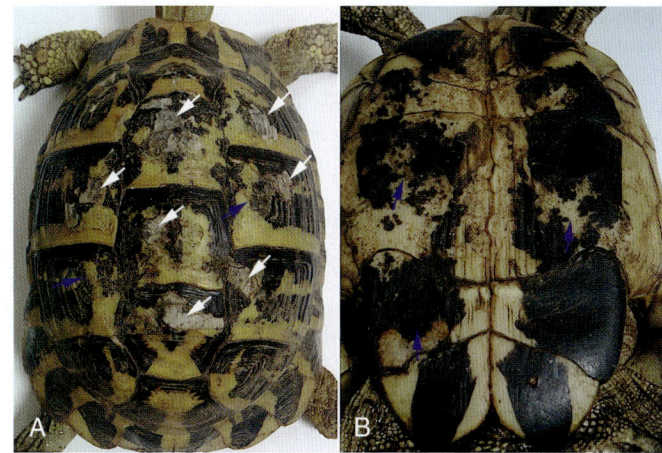

FIG 70.10 Dyskeratosis in an adult Hermann's tortoise (*Testudo hermanni*). Notice the different stages of alterations of several scutes on the carapace (A) and on the plastron (B) (loss of scute cover, white arrows; recornification, blue arrows). (Courtesy of Paolo Selleri.)

tortoise (*Aldabrachelys gigantea*), phaeohyphomycosis due to *Exophiala oligosperma* was responsible for a deep flaking area of the carapace.[53]

Clinical Presentation and Diagnostic Confirmation. Shell dyskeratosis lesions may be small, affecting a single scute, or extensive white blemishes affecting most scutes, in various stages of necrosis.[51] Fungal infections of the carapace typically result in corrosion of the epidermal lamellae of the scutes and scute sloughing (Fig. 70.10). Whitish blemishes may develop on the keratinaceous epidermal scutes (epidermal lamellae) that overlay the bones, such that the affected areas of the carapace appear whitish.[51]

Fungi may be diagnosed by culture or PCR. The degree of deep-bone involvement may be assessed through histological examination and nuclear scintigraphy bone scanning.[53]

Treatment, Prognosis, and Prevention. Treatment includes weekly debridement of the lesions and oral and topical antifungal agents with appropriate bandaging. In captive individuals, changes in management (e.g., improving substrate, sun exposure, and hygiene in the environment) and soil disinfection have been suggested.[52] Lesions typically resolve over several months.[53]

Dyskeratosis caused by *F. semitectum* is usually self-limiting although may result in corrosion of most of the carapacial scutes. Other fungal diseases (e.g., phaeohyphomycosis by *E. oligosperma*) may progress and spread to numerous sites on the carapace with severe deep-bone involvement. Systemic mycoses involving visceral structures have the worst prognosis. Because this disorder is caused by ubiquitous fungus, proper management of chelonians (e.g., avoiding excessive humidity, poor hygiene) may prevent the infection.[52]

Burns

Clinical Significance and Known Etiological Cause(s). Defective under-floor heaters and heating lamps might expose captive chelonians to hyperthermia, leading to various degrees of tissue damage of the plastron or carapace. Knocked over heating devices are prone to causing fire in shelters and entrapping the animals therein. In the case of blazes, free-ranging tortoises tend to seek shelter by digging into the ground and often incur carapacial burns.

Clinical Presentation and Diagnostic Confirmation. The keratinous scutes of the shell resist overheating or open fire to some extent, and affected tortoises might, at first glance, appear unharmed. As the heat destroys the underlying epidermis, scutes will start do detach at the thinner scutal seams days or weeks after the insult. Mild exudation may be initially seen at the scutal margins, which will dry up in the course of the disease process. Affected scutes should not be removed immediately as they often remain well attached in the center where the keratinous layer is thickest and heat damage to the underlying epidermis less pronounced. In chelonians exposed to open fires, smoke intoxication may result in respiratory distress with excessive salivation.

Treatment, Prognosis, and Prevention. Intensive supportive care with IV fluids, analgesics (e.g., Hydromorphone 0.5 mg/kg q 24 h) and nutritional support is vital. Radical debridement of loosening scutes is contraindicated, painful, and might result in substantial bleeding. In the course of the healing process, curved-up scute margins can be cut or debrided to prevent accumulation of devitalized tissue (Fig. 70.11). Infestation with fly larvae below the detached scutes must be prevented by bandaging the affected shell areas and/or by keeping the affected animals in pest-free environments. A combination of systemic and local antibiotic treatment is preferred, as systemic antibiotics alone might not reach peripheral sites with poor blood supply. Fungal overgrowth on necrotic tissues is a common sequel and must be treated with topical antifungals (e.g., Terbinafin ointment). Systemic antifungal drugs tend not to reach minimal therapeutic concentrations in the damaged tissues. Where scutes detach, granulation occurs and will subsequently keratinize. This tissue will not resemble a regular scute in contour or color. In deep burns, new bone will form below, and the necrotic tissue may take years to completely slough (see Fig. 70.9A and B).

Prognosis is good to poor depending on the degree and extension of burns and smoke intoxication. Financial implications of prolonged recovery and ongoing veterinary care should be considered. Fire detection devices should be installed in reptile areas with electrical heaters. Heating lamps and their installation must meet electrical and fire control regulations.

Frostbite
Clinical Significance and Known Etiological Cause(s). The exposure of parts of the body to freezing temperatures causes frost damage

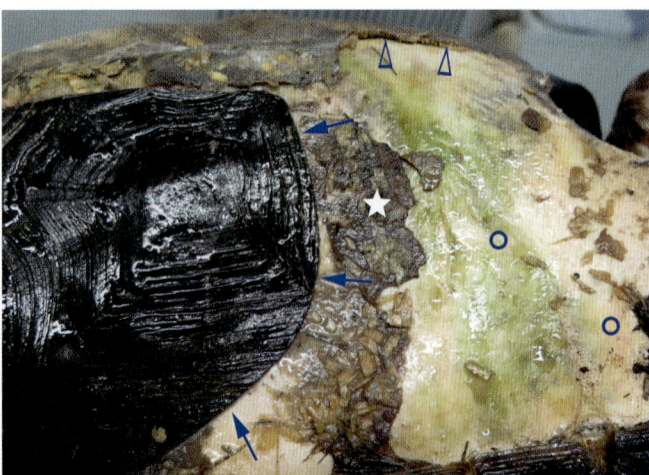

FIG 70.11 Deep burns on the plastron of an *Aldabrachelys gigantea*. The margins of the scutes detach as the underlying epidermis suffered a thermal necrosis (star). Scute margins are cut back (blue arrows). As necrotic bone is demarcated (arrowheads), scar tissue (circles) is formed underneath. The greenish tinge resulted from fecal material trapped below detached scute margins. (Courtesy of Jean Meyer.)

to the skin and peripheral tissues. This happens periodically when animals are hibernated under natural/outdoor conditions. Irregular stratification of the soil with interposed layers of stones and gravel might impede the digging efforts, causing hibernation too near the surface. At very low temperatures the dorsal carapace will undergo vascular and cellular injury.

Clinical Presentation and Diagnostic Confirmation. Clinical signs of anorexia and ecchymosis of the shell, often paired with other nondermatologic presentations (e.g., pneumonia, rhinitis, cataracts, corneal opacities) are the main reasons for the owner to seek veterinary assistance. Because no specific diagnostic test for frostbite exists, the history of inadequate outdoor hibernation under long-lasting freezing weather conditions prompts the diagnosis of frostbite. Viral and bacterial infections with subsequent organ failure must be considered as differentials.

Treatment, Prognosis, and Prevention. Patients should be warmed up slowly to the species-specific preferred optimal temperature zone (POTZ) and provided with fluid therapy, analgesics, and nutritional support. In cases with concurrent lower respiratory tract disease, an antibiotic treatment is warranted. Subscutal ecchymosis will resolve. Scutes should be left in place even if exudation is present at the scutal seams. Local antimicrobial treatment may prevent secondary infection in these cases. If the damage to the capillary supply is irreversible, scutes will loosen, exposing necrotic epidermis and bone. In affected areas granulation tissue will grow and undergo subsequent keratinization.

The prognosis for the dermatologic conditions is good, but a concurrent pneumonia downgrades the prognosis for the patient. Frostbite can easily be prevented by providing monitored hibernation conditions at temperatures between 5° to 8°C. See Chapter 23 for detailed information.

Neoplasia of the Shell
Clinical Significance and Known Etiological Cause(s). Two cases of invasive, osteolytic, nonmetastatic squamous cell carcinomas (SCC) of the shell of *Testudo hermanni* have been described.[54]

Clinical Presentation and Diagnostic Confirmation. A 28-year-old and 55-year-old male *Testudo hermanni* presented with soft tissue swelling dorsal to the base of the tail and an ulceration of the caudal plastron, respectively. The extensive osteolysis of the caudal carapace of the first animal could only be detected by CT scan because the overlying scutes were still intact. The plastral SCC most likely originated from the shell, whereas the carapacial SCC originated from the skin at the dorsal base of the tail.

Full thickness biopsies or fine needle aspiration cytology are the diagnostic tests of choice for proliferative masses. Radiography and CT should be used for further evaluation of the extent of the bone and soft-tissue involvement.

Treatment, Prognosis, and Prevention. A surgical excision is the treatment of choice and may be combined with other modalities, such as cryosurgery, radiotherapy, and chemotherapy.[55–57] Squamous cell carcinomas have metastatic potential in chelonians,[58] which should be accounted for when the further therapeutical approach is to be elaborated. Furthermore, the prognosis is guarded to poor due to the highly invasive nature of SCCs.

REFERENCES
See www.expertconsult.com for a complete list of references.

71

Ophthalmology

Martin P.C. Lawton

Reptilian ophthalmology is still in its infancy, especially compared with the same subject in other taxa. However, it is slowly growing and becoming an established and appreciated discipline. Ensley et al.[1] stated that "The veterinary clinician does not routinely find himself examining the eyes of snakes"; a mere 5 years later, disease of the eye and the adnexal structures was considered commonly encountered in reptiles.[2] The difference in these statements probably has more to do with the lack of a routine and thorough ophthalmic examination as part of the standard clinical examination of all reptile cases than with a sudden advance in knowledge within such a short period of time.

The eye is a barometer that reflects the health of the animal, and therefore many systemic diseases can produce ocular signs even though they are not primary ocular diseases. The reptilian eye can also be an environmental barometer, as toxicity can affect many aspects of the eye. Organochlorine pesticides have been associated with ocular discharge, conjunctivitis, and blepharitis in eastern box turtles (*Terrapene carolina carolina*)[3] Always remember that the ocular responses to injury vary between different species and have a profound influence on the type of inflammatory responses and healing capabilities that may be expected.[4]

The eye is considered to clearly show how various species have modified their basic structures to current conditions and evolutionary opportunities.[5] The anatomy of the reptilian eye (with the exception of snakes) has many general anatomic similarities, with only minor variations between the groups.[2,6] In snakes, many structural differences (other than just spectacles, which some lizards also have) are seen in comparison with the rest of the reptiles and are covered separately.

ANATOMY AND PHYSIOLOGY

In considering the evolution, development, diversity, and function of the reptilian eye, there are two texts[6,7] that must be considered as the foundations of reptile ophthalmology and should be consulted before any other sources when studying this subject.

Parietal Eye

The parietal eye is also known as the third eye, median eye, or pineal accessory apparatus. It is found in two distinct groups of reptiles (order Squamata, suborder Sauria [Lacertillia], and order Rhynchocephalia) but is absent in crocodilians.[8] This is the remnant of the median eye of provertebrates, which was originally a paired visual organ on the roof of the head.[6] In reptiles, it still appears as an eyelike structure, on the top of the head, situated in a hole beneath the parietal bone (Fig. 71.1).[9] Some lizards have a superficial parietal eye, which is just below the skin in the parietal foramen at the junction between the parietal and frontal bones.[8] Supporting evidence has shown that dinosaurs had a pineal foramen that was thought to have contained a parietal eye.[10] The overlying scales show varying degrees of transparency (almost clear in the tuatara, *Sphenodon punctatus*) and are described as a cornea-like apparatus.[10] Lacertillia, which have a prominent parietal eye, include slow worms, monitors, lacertids, some iguanids, and skinks.[11]

Histologically, the parietal eye is variable in complexity and design but has been shown to always have a neurological input and to contain a primitive retina. In the tuatara (*Sphenodon punctatus*), *Anguis* spp., *Varanus* spp., and *Sceloporus* spp., the retina is cup-shaped and surrounded by a fibrous capsule with a lens-like structure above and attached to the retina on both sides.[6,11] The posterior space between the lens and the retina is filled with a material that resembles the vitreous of the lateral eyes. No irises, lids, or muscles are found.[11] The retina of the parietal eye, unlike that of the lateral eye, has fewer but larger ganglion cells, and the photoreceptoral processes protrude forward into the lumen.[10] The retinal innervation leads to the parietal nerve, which is a small nonmyelinated structure that may have two branches and a not entirely known distribution of the fibers.[10]

Although the true function of this organ remains a mystery,[12] a relationship and connection exists between the parietal eye, the pineal body,[10] the diencephalons of the forebrain, and especially the habenular nucleus.[6,11] In families with no parietal eye (gekkonids), the pineal body has been noted to be reduced in size.[10] The parietal eye is thought to play a role in both hormone production and thermoregulation[6,8] by acting as a dosimeter[9,11] with an ability to sense changes in intensity and wavelength of light then convert photic stimuli into neuroendocrine messages,[8] allowing optimal timing for reproduction and other activities.[10]

The parietal eye has also been shown to act as a "compass" for orientation and navigation within their home environment, a function that

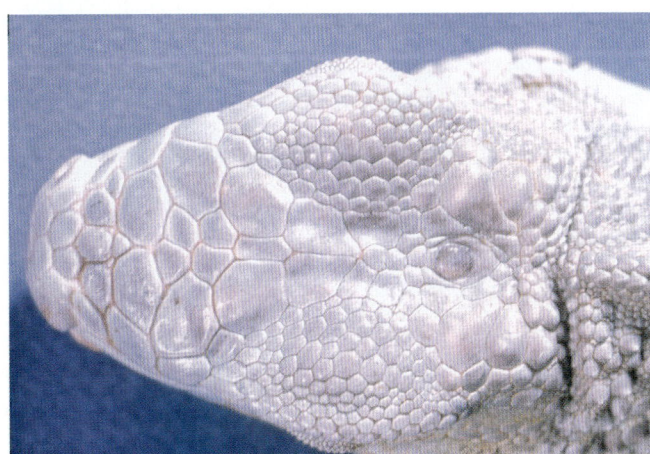

FIG 71.1 Parietal eye of an iguana. (Courtesy of Martin P.C. Lawton.)

was lost on the organ being covered, temporarily, with nail varnish.[13] Electroretinographic (ERG) studies suggest that the parietal eye has a slower response (latency) to light than do lateral eyes and that this is irrespective of light wavelength.[10] The experimental effects of removal of the parietal eye in various lizards have shown changes in basking behavior and activity cycles[11] and a lower thermal tolerance.[10] This is probably because of the close physiological relationship between the parietal eye and the pineal body. The pineal body is responsible for producing melatonin and serotonin, both of which have marked effects on the sleep and awake cycles, and the parietal eye has been reported as having high levels of melatonin-forming enzymes (hydroxyindole O-methyltransferase).[10] This connection between the parietal eye acting as a dosimeter is further supported by the natural absence of the parietal eye in nocturnal lizards, although exceptions exist, such as in teiids and some geckos.[10]

Eyelids

Eyelids within the class Reptilia could well fill a chapter in themselves. Reptiles are divided into those with functional eyelids with a normal palpebral fissure; those with immobile and fused eyelids (spectacle) with no palpebral fissure; and all the possible variations in between.[14] Even within the group of reptiles with functional eyelids and normal palpebral fissures continued variation exists, and this group is further divided on the basis of various adaptations and changes that occur within the lower eyelid. Chelonia and Crocodilia all have functional eyelids with normal palpebral fissures, and the main variation to functionality of the eyelids and size of the palpebral fissure is mainly found in the squamates. Reptiles with spectacles are not dealt with in this section but have a separate heading of their own (Spectacles).

In most reptiles, the upper eyelid is the smaller and less mobile of the two,[1,9] with the lower eyelid moving up to cover the majority of the globe,[8] which is the reverse of the mammalian situation. The lizards are no exception, with the lower eyelid being the more moveable.[2] Most species have a third eyelid (Fig. 71.2). In Lacertidae, Teiidae, Scincidae, *Cordylosaurus, Lanthanotus,* and *Anolis,* some of the lower eyelid has become transparent,[2,7] with reduced or absent scales.[7] Some iguanids just have a few scales that are semitransparent when the eyelid is closed but are hidden within folds when the eyelid is open.[7] These are a protective mechanism to allow varying degrees of vision when the eyelids are closed, especially in adverse conditions, providing protection from sand or grit.[2,7]

Some lizards have a tarsal plate in the lower eyelid that offers support and is made of fibrous tissue.[7] *Ablepharus* and ground geckos often

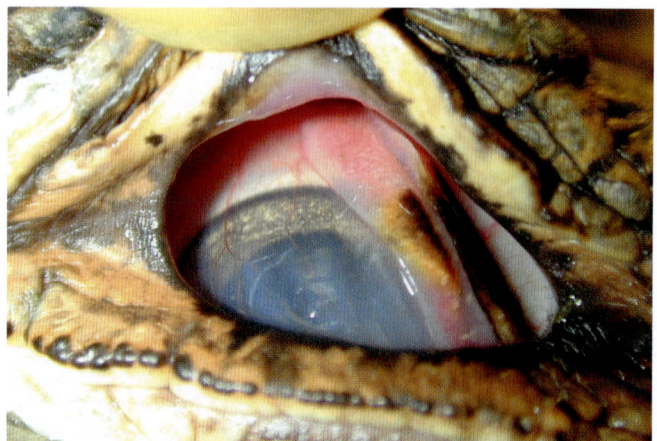

FIG 71.2 Semitransparent third eyelid in a caiman. (Courtesy of Martin P.C. Lawton.)

have fused eyelids that form a spectacle (discussed under the heading Spectacle). If any doubt exists as to the presence of true mobile eyelids or not, one should look for a nictitating membrane within the medial canthus, because whenever the eyelids are mobile, it is present.[7]

Similar to most lizards, the lower eyelid of chelonians is larger and more mobile than the upper eyelid.[7] The presence of a transparent window in the eyelid is rare in Chelonia and is only found in Chelodina or Emydidae.

The crocodilian eye is more of an exception in the reptile form as the upper eyelid is more mobile and, like humans, has a well-developed tarsal plate (tarsus),[7,15] which often becomes ossified with age.[16] The nictitating membrane (third eyelid) of crocodilians is well developed but semitransparent with a cartilaginous plate[7] (see Fig. 71.2). The presence of this third eyelid and the ability to close it across the globe even when the eyelids are open can make examination difficult but is a highly desirable protective feature. In aged alligators, calcium or other salt deposits can lead to an opacification of the normally clear third eyelid.[2]

Spectacles

When the eyelids are fused, they form a transparent membrane over the globe, which is known by many terms, including spectacle, brille, eyecap, eye scale, watchglass, and goggle.[6,9,14] Spectacle is the term that will be used here. Three types of spectacles have been described[6]; the type found in squamates is the tertiary spectacle. Embryologically, a circular lid fold forms for all vertebrates, but in squamates that have spectacles this gradually closes over the globe, with the aperture moving dorsally and shrinking until it vanishes.[6,7] This dorsal movement of the aperture means that most of the squamate spectacle is composed of the lower eyelid. In the uropeltid snake (*Rhinophis* spp.) a small horizontal slitlike palpebral fissure is present in the newborn.[6,7]

All snakes, Amphisbaenidae, some geckos, some Lacertilia (*Ablepharus* sp., *Ophisops* sp., *Aniella* sp., Dibamidae, Anelytropidae, Euchirotidae), some Teiidae, *Uroplatus,* Pygopodidae, and Xantusiidae have fused eyelids with no palpebral fissure.[6] Although sometimes incorrectly reported as having spectacles, *Eublepharis* and *Coleonyx* geckos have normal eyelids, confirmed by the existence of their nictitating membranes.

The spectacle is composed of skin and therefore is a dry horny scale that is transparent. The spectacle has been referred to as a fixed window covered by the *stratum corneum* of the epidermis.[5] The surface of the spectacle is insensitive (compared to a cornea), as expected for hornified (cornified) skin. Lizards with spectacles are often seen cleaning this surface with their tongues.[9]

Microsilicone injection of the spectacle has shown it to be highly vascular,[2] and although in normal circumstances these vessels are not readily seen, they become apparent with inflammation.[14] The vascularity increases during ecdysis (Fig. 71.3B), and fluorescein studies[17] have showed that there is an increase permeability and leakage from these vessels. This transepidermal water loss causes the change in color of the spectacle prior to and aiding in the separation of the new and old layers of the epidermis. The permeability of the blood vessels is not found during the resting stage between cycles of ecdysis.[17] The spectacle becomes transparent again just before shedding.[2]

The most important point to remember is that the spectacle is not part of, nor is it attached to, the cornea.[14] There is always a space that separates the spectacle and the cornea—the subspectacular space (Fig. 71.4). This space has also been referred to as the intraconjuctival space.[6] The spectacle functions like a contact lens[7] under which the eye is fully mobile and independent. The subspectacular space is the equivalent of the conjunctival sac or space in mammals, except it is enclosed by the spectacle.[14] The space is filled with the secretions of the Harderian gland (see Lacrimal System), which provides lubrication

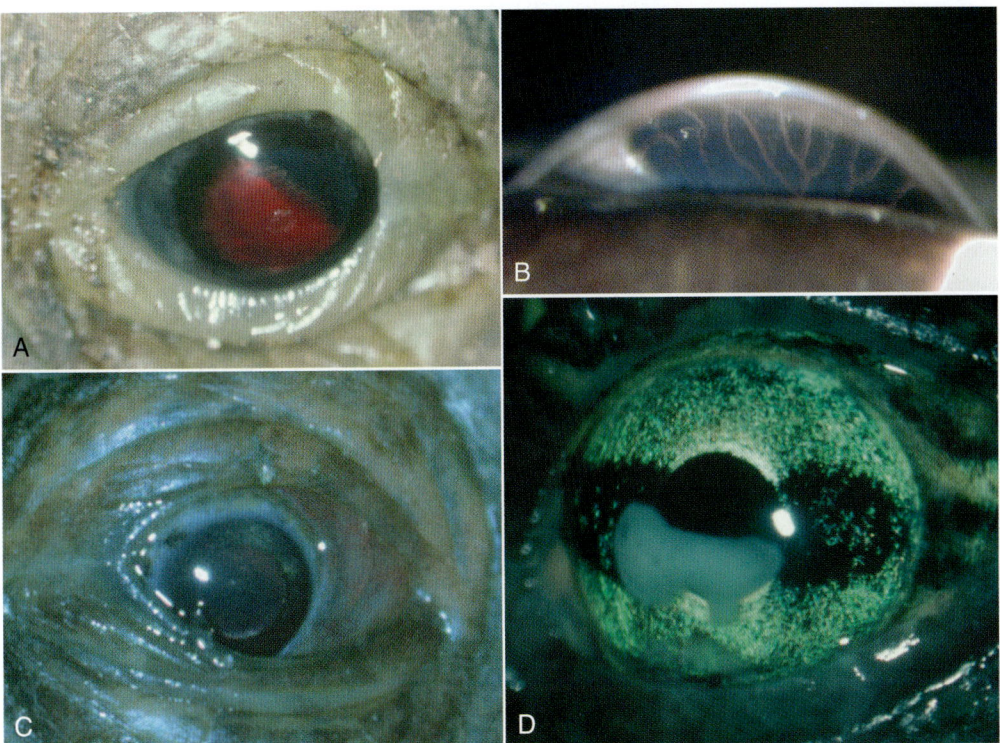

FIG 71.3 (A) Post-hibernation hyphema in a Mediterranean tortoise *(Testudo)*. (B) Vascular structure of the spectacle. (C) *Arcus lipoides cornea* in a Mediterranean tortoise. (D) Corneal stromal dystrophy with cholesterol deposits in a red-eared slider *(Trachemys scripta elegans)*. (Courtesy of Martin P.C. Lawton.)

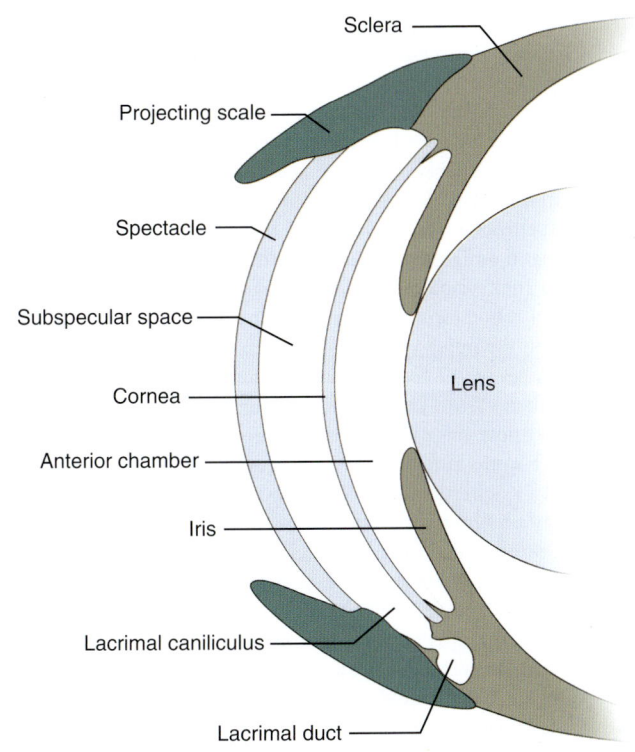

FIG 71.4 Diagram of the anterior structures of the spectacled reptile eye. (Courtesy of Educational Resources, University of Georgia.)

and easy movement of the globe (although this is limited) beneath the spectacle. Despite this anatomic arrangement to allow movement, spontaneous movements of the globe are not frequently noted because the *bursalis* and *retractor bulbi* muscles are absent.[7] The thick, oily Harderian secretions do have a high reflective index and are thought to have some optical importance.[6]

Lacrimal System

The lacrimal (also cited as lachrymal or ophthalmic) glands are variable within the class Reptilia.[18] Most Sauria and Chelonia have a Harderian (Harder's) gland in the orbitonasal (medial) region[18,19] and a lacrimal gland in the orbitotemporal (lateral) region.[18] Conjunctival glands are also found and are mainly associated with the upper lid.[7]

The Harderian gland is firmly fixed in the medial part of the orbit, with the duct normally opening on the surface of the nictitating membrane (where present).[19] This is common to all groups of terrestrial vertebrates and was first described by Johan Harder in 1694, after whom the gland was named. Histologically, an enormous similarity is seen in reptiles between the lacrimal and Harderian glands that makes it difficult for them to be identified, even on histologic examination.[18] In Chelonia, confusion exists over which is the Harderian gland and which is the posterior lacrimal gland; the literature names both.[19] This has caused much doubt on claims such that the Harderian gland is absent in many geckos and chameleons.[2,7] In various Chelonia (*Testudo graeca*, *Trachemys scripta*, and *Chelonia mydas*), salt-secreting cells have been shown within the Harderian glands; these play a part in osmoregulation.[2] A large number of immunocompetent cells are also in the Harderian gland.[19]

Snakes are generally accepted as having no lacrimal gland[2,5,6,9]; however, Williams[20] appears to be alone in considering that snakes have both lacrimal and Harderian glands, although this appears to be based on assumption rather than histologic studies. This lack of a lacrimal gland in snakes is an odd arrangement, because the lacrimal glands are usually associated with the upper and lower lids, and the Harderian gland is usually associated with the nictitating membrane,[19] which is absent in snakes. The Harderian gland is mainly posterior to the orbit and is large except in sea snakes, where it is reduced but still present.[2] The Harderian gland produces an oily secretion, and the lacrimal gland produces a watery secretion. The tear production in snakes is from the Harderian gland, which enters and fills the subspectacular space. The oily Harderian secretion is superior in lubrication properties to the watery lacrimal tears. Thus the retention of the Harderian gland and loss of the lacrimal gland is of advantage to the squamates with spectacles, where the globe may otherwise rub on the dorsal aspect of the spectacle. The duct of the Harderian gland opens directly into the lacrimal duct in *Natrix natrix*, but in more primitive snakes, it opens into the subspectacular space by several small ducts with a main duct opening into the lacrimal duct.[2] This oily secretion flows from the subspectacular space through the nasolacrimal duct first to the nose and then to the mouth.[6] In the family Dasypeltis (egg-eating snakes), the large Harderian gland's oily secretion contributes to the lubrication that is essential for swallowing eggs whole.[19] In chameleons there is a reverse movement of drinking water from the oral cavity through the nasolacrimal duct to flush the conjunctival sac.[21]

The nasolacrimal duct is absent in all Chelonia.[9] In crocodilians, the lacrimal ducts open in the front section of the nose, similar to mammals.[9]

Globe

The globe of most reptiles, unlike that of birds, is almost spherical. The scleral bones (scleral ossicles), when present, number between 6 to 17, with Mediterranean tortoises having 6 to 9, chameleons 11, and tuatara 16 or 17.[6] The bones are compactly placed and overlap their neighbors such that they form an almost immobile cup. In Chelonia, in addition to the scleral ossicles that may extend to the corneal rim,[6] a scleral cartilage is seen, up to 1 cm thick. In chameleons, the scleral cartilage is reduced to the foveal region, but in most other lizards it extends from the posterior pole of the globe to beyond the equator.[7] The scleral ossicles serve to maintain the convexity of the globe, allowing the ciliary body to be close to the lens and play a more important part in accommodation by changing the shape of the eye, therefore altering the distance between the cornea and fundus. Scleral ossicles are absent in crocodilians, but scleral cartilage extensions are found well into the *ora serrate*,[2,7] forming a cartilaginous cup.[6] The snake eye is totally different from all other reptiles in that it is slightly elongated along the visual axis.[7] The eye also has no scleral ossicles or cartilage but retains the spherical shape with the presence of tendinous connective tissue.[6] Pigmentary cells are found throughout the sclera.

Movement of the eye (except in chameleons) is limited because of the poor development of the rectus muscles, although, unlike birds, the *retractor bulbi* muscle is well developed. Chameleons have well-developed ocular muscles that allow a wide range of vision both monocular and binocular with 180 degrees in the horizontal plane and 90 degrees in the vertical plane.[9,21] Crocodilia have eyes situated dorsally so that even when they are in the water they can see above water level.[7] Land tortoises, crocodiles, and many diurnal lizards have narrow binocular vision of 25 degrees or less and thus rely on monocular vision.[9] Binocular vision is better in freshwater Chelonia (up to 30 degrees) and is most marked in the snapping turtle (*Chelydra serpentina*).[9]

The position of the eye in relation to the body has been shown[22] to affect intraocular pressure in juvenile loggerhead sea turtles (*Caretta caretta*). In dorsoventral and ventrodorsal positions the turtle has lower intraocular pressures compared with a head-down position; this is a response that is also seen in humans and is the result of venous pressure gradients within the eyes and the head. The normal intraocular pressure of reptiles is far lower than in mammals, with an average of about 6 mm Hg, whereas some land tortoises may have an average of 14 mm Hg.[22,23] A nonlinear negative relationship between body length and intraocular pressure was found in American alligators (*Alligator mississippiensis*).[24] The intraocular pressure was found to decrease as the body length increased, with a relationship to length and age; therefore a direct correlation may exist between the age and the intraocular pressure as has been found in some mammals.

The snake eye does not follow the normal reptilian format. Paleontologists and researchers generally agree that the snake evolved from the Varanidae. Because of evolutionary changing lifestyles to involve a nocturnal, burrowing, or subterrestrial existence, modification to the serpentine eye occurred. The changes involved were many, but of particular importance were the formation of the spectacle and development of a yellow lens and loss of the scleral ossicles. These changes in the eye occurred at the same time as the loss of limbs, parietal eye, and ears. The eye is considered to have degenerated to a vestigial organ, only to later evolve into its present structure as the snakes came back to the surface.[6] This certainly explains the major differences (not just in the spectacle) of the snake eye when compared with other reptilian species.

Cornea

The reptilian cornea is usually thin with no Bowman's membrane (layer). The crocodilian cornea is typically reptilian and thin.[7] In squamates with spectacles, the cornea is even thinner with only a single layer of corneal epithelium being found,[6,7] which is all that is necessary due to the protection provided by the presence of the spectacle. In lizards, the Descemet's membrane is present in all but a few geckos.[7] In land Chelonia, the cornea is thick with a prominent Descemet's membrane.[6]

The corneas of Chelonia have small radii of curvature and are therefore optically powerful in air, contributing dioptric power to the eye. In aquatic species, the cornea is optically ineffective when in water, but they are able to overcome this loss and still focus.[25] Freshwater turtles have exceptionally well-developed ciliary and iris musculature and a highly flexible lens that provides a wide dioptric range, giving high visual acuity in both air and water despite the loss of corneal refraction.[26] They are able to squeeze the lens (which is soft) through the pupil aperture,[6,7,25] which is similar to the accommodative changes seen in some diving birds. Two investigations have been undertaken of the visual acuity of the various Chelonia. The first was a retinoscope assessment of green sea turtles (*Chelonia mydas*), which were compared with a freshwater turtle (*Clemmys insulpta*) and a gopher tortoise (*Gopherus polyphemus*)[26]; the second study involved anatomic dissection, the use of a streak retinoscope, and schematic eye calculations in the red-eared slider (*Trachemys scripta elegans*) and marine turtles (*Chelonia mydas*, *Dermochelys cariacea*, and *Eretmochelys imbricata*).[25] Both studies came to the conclusion that the eyes of the marine turtles varied significantly compared with those of the freshwater turtles and land tortoises. The severe hyperopia of underwater is compensated by the accommodative changes of the lens.[25] The green sea turtle was found by Ehrenfeld and Kock to be emmetropic in water but extremely myopic when out of water.[26] Conversely, Northmore and Granda[25] considered marine turtles as emmetropic out of water as they were able to see coastlines, which they could not if they were myopic out of water. The difference in opinion was considered by Northmore and Granda[25] to be due to the actively accommodating eye. The land tortoises were found to be similar to humans in that they are not able to overcome the loss of the corneal refraction in water.

As part of the normal aging process of *Testudo, arcus lipoides cornea*, seen as a white infiltration of cholesterol crystals into the peripheral cornea (see Fig. 71.3C),[27] is not unusual. Corneal cholesterol dystrophy can also occur in reptiles (such as terrapins) on a high polysaturated fat diet and is usually noted in the center of the cornea (see Fig. 71.3D).

Anterior Chamber and Uveal Tract

The reptilian iris has a well-developed sphincter of striated muscles that allows rapid control over papillary movement[2] and is resilient to the effects of mydriatics.

Naturally occurring miosis is sluggish.[8] Voluntary control of the iris is important where the sphincter iris is responsible for accommodation by deforming the lens, such as in Chelonia.[6] The voluntary control also means that there is no consensual pupillary light reflex.[8] A peculiar sexual dimorphism is shown in the color of the iris of most (but not all) *Terrepene* spp., where the male has a red iris and the female a brown iris.[7]

In lizards, differences in pupil shape are common, depending on whether a reptile is nocturnal (slit pupil) or diurnal (round pupils). *Heloderma spp.* are the exception as they have a round pupil.[7] In the Gekkonidae, often several tiny notches are paired off along the opposite margin of the iris.[6] In bright light, the pupil (normally a single slit) closes completely, leaving a series of pinholes (stenopeic openings)[7] that are very small oval pupils formed by these apposed notches. These stenopeic openings allow a sharp image to form on the retina, irrespective of distance, and it is a far sharper image than that of a single aperture.[6] Stenopeic openings are most obvious in the tokay gecko (*Gekko gecko*), in which its presence is considered to allow the formation of a clear image without any other accommodative adjustments.[7] The crocodilian iris, although more mobile and responsive than in lizards or chelonians, is also able to form a stenopeic slit in bright sunlight.[7]

The snake iris is generally a thick, heavily pigmented structure. It is highly mobile as, with the absence of eyelids, it plays a more important role in light protective function.[7] The East Indian long-nosed tree snake (*Dryophis mycterizans*) and the African bird snake (*Thelotornis kirtlandi*) have a horizontal keyhole-shaped pupil with the slot of the keyhole pointing forward beyond the rim of the lens. This is to position the slot of the keyhole (nasally) in line with the fovea (two of only three genera that have a fovea).[6] These two species are thought to have the sharpest sight and most accurate distance judgment of all snakes.[6]

Lens and Accommodation

Most reptiles have some sort of annular pad (ringwulst or annular ring), which is a thickened area of epithelial cells, usually at or near the equator, that allows the lens to connect directly to the ciliary body, usually by zonular fibers. The lizards have a thick equatorial annular pad formed by radial growth of the subcapsular epithelium that is largest in chameleons.[7] The ciliary body has a broad zone of firm contact with the lens in lizards.[6] Unlike lizards, chelonians have well-formed ciliary processes that attach to the lens,[7] although a small but weakly developed annular pad is found.[6,7] The crocodilians have ciliary processes that connect with the equator of the lens, where a small annular pad is found.[7] The snake has no equatorial annular pad,[6,7] but an anterior pad is formed from the subcapsular epithelial cells on the anterior surface.[7]

The reptile lens is flatter than that found in fish and amphibians.[28] The lenses of lizards are soft.[2] A larger lens is seen in nocturnal species.[7] In lizards, accommodation depends on the deformation of the lens.[7] Nocturnal and diurnal gekkonids differ in the biochemical composition of their lenses.[29] Nocturnal animals have colorless lenses, and yellow crystalline (water soluble protein) is found exclusively in lenses of diurnal geckos and gives their lenses a yellow coloration.[29]

The lens capsule is thin in chelonians, and the lenses are extremely soft and almost fluidlike in consistency.[6,7] The land tortoises have a flat lens that is less flat in the terrapins and more spherical in sea turtles.[6] Turtles are able to accommodate when submerged by squeezing the soft lens through the pupil aperture.[6,7,25]

The snake lens is pigmented yellow, spherical, and firmer than that of other reptilian lenses.[7] In snakes, the oil droplets in the rod cells of the retina do not have any color, so the yellow lenses take over this function of ultraviolet protection.[6] Accommodation in the snake is unique compared with other reptiles,[7] because it relies on the lens moving backward and forward in response to pressure changes within the vitreous and aqueous.[12] This is aided by the ciliary muscles that have migrated into the root of the iris, where they can apply pressure to the lens without altering its shape.[9]

Retina and Visual Tracts

Reptiles, like birds, have an anangiotic (avascular) retina (Fig. 71.5A). Nutrients are supplied and metabolic wastes removed by choroidal blood vessels or modified vessels protruding into the vitreous. All reptiles have a choriocapillaris and, during development, had a hyaloid vascular system.[30] The major differences found in the various reptile orders occurred as the hyaloid system regressed.

In chelonians there is total regression of both the hyaloid system and the choriocapillaris, with sole reliance on remaining choroidal blood vessels. An early avascular conus did develop above the optic disc in some turtles, but this regressed and is absent in all adults.[7]

In lizards, a structure similar to the avian pecten develops but is known as the *conus papillaris*. The *conus papillaris* usually protrudes into the vitreous from the optic disc[2] (Fig. 71.6), consisting of a vascularized glial tissue,[30] and is ectodermal in origin.[6] As in the avian pecten, the inner limiting membrane (vitreoretinal border) covers the *conus papillaris*.[31] It consists mainly of tiny blood vessels that are heavily pigmented.[6] The *conus papillaris* entirely obscures the fundoscopic view of the optic disc.[7] The conus is absent in Amphisbaenidae.[7]

In snakes, the conus has regressed in all but a few species and is replaced by a preretinal vascular meshwork derived from the hyaloid vessels known as the *membrana vasculosa retinae*,[30] which is mesodermal in origin.[6] This is a branching array of vessels derived from the choroid running into the posterior vitreous near and originating from the optic disc but just above the retina. In colubrids, the capillaries of the *membrana vasculosa retinae* penetrate the retina and become an intraretinal vessel.[7,30]

In adult crocodilians, the *conus papillaris* is functionless and is reduced to a glial pad consisting of one or two capillary loops that scarcely protrude into the vitreous and are on the optic nerve head.[2,6,7] In alligators, the conus has regressed even more into a layer of melanocytes found on the optic nerve head.[30]

The retina of reptiles, like other vertebrates, is composed of five primary cell types:
i.   Photoreceptors,
ii. Outer segment,
iii. Inner segment,
iv. Nuclear and connecting fibers
v.   Synaptic pedicles.

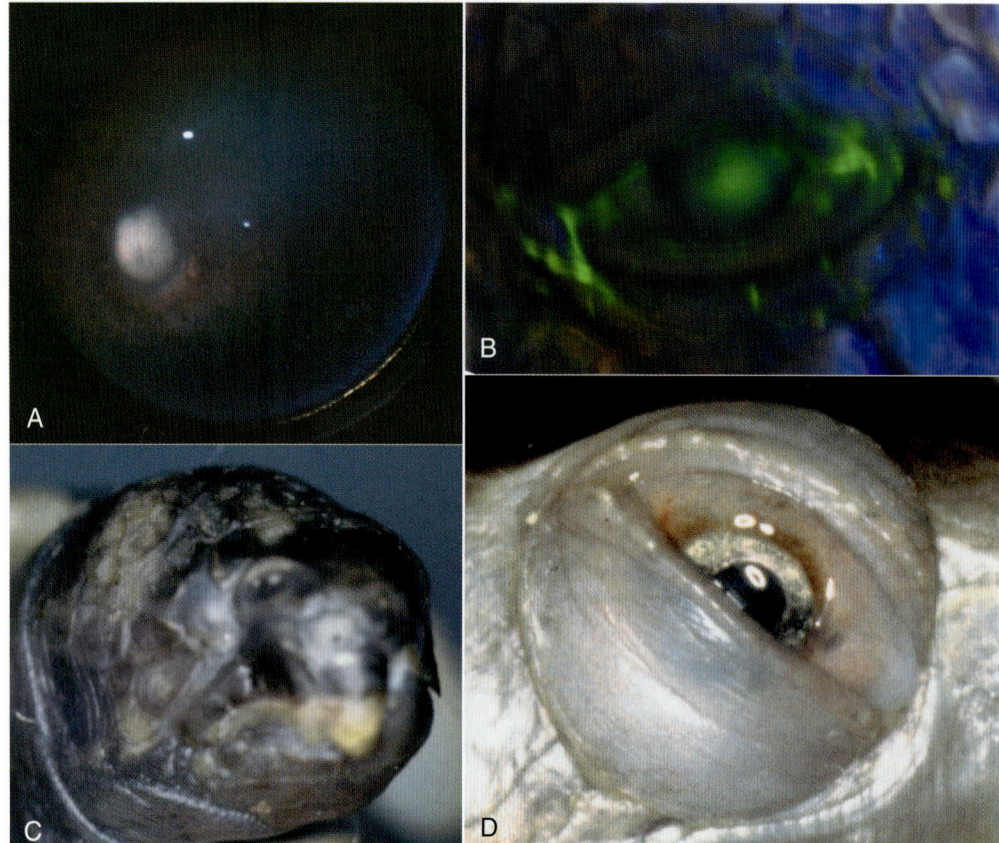

FIG 71.5 (A) Anangiotic retina of a Mediterranean tortoise (*Testudo*). (B) Fluorescein dye to show a corneal ulcer in a Mediterranean tortoise. (C) Microphthalmous in a Mediterranean tortoise. (D) Blepharoedema in a red-eared slider (*Trachemys scripta elegans*) with hypovitaminosis A. (Courtesy of Martin P.C. Lawton.)

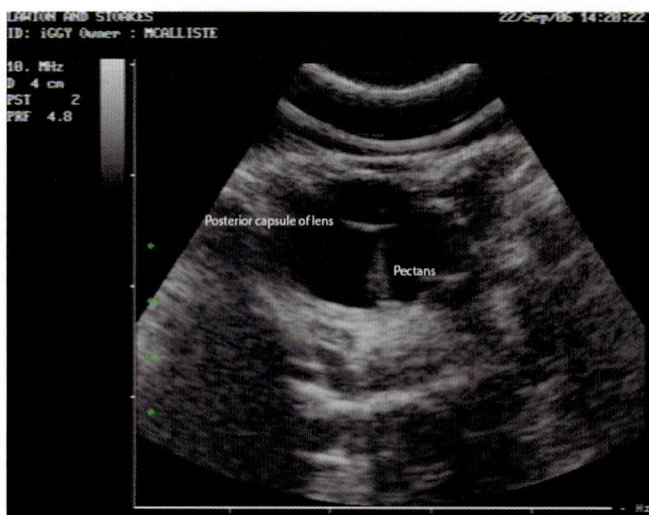

FIG 71.6 Ultrasound (annotated) of an iguana (*Iguana iguana*) eye showing the *conus papillaris* (pectans) in the vitreous reaching almost to the posterior aspect of the lens. (Courtesy of Martin P.C. Lawton.)

In the inner segment there are oil droplets with a high refractive indices that contribute to light collection in the visual cells and enhance retinal sensitivity as well as contrast and motion detection.[32] The reptile retina has rods and cones.[2,9] Many diurnal species have lost their rods,[8] for example, new world chameleons (*Chamaeleo* sp.) have a cone-rich retina.[33] In chelonians, cones predominate the retina.[7] In diurnal reptiles, yellow oil droplets are associated with the rod or certain cone cells (except for snakes), which act as ocular filters and are able to absorb ultraviolet and shortwave blue radiation to protect underlying cells[34] and reduce glare.[9] Where colored oil droplets are not found in the rod cells of the retina (such as in snakes) this function can be undertaken by yellow lenses.[6] Extra retinal photoreceptors allow circadian rhythms to be initiated and controlled, and the eyes have an inhibitory role.[5]

An *area centralis* is found in most species where the cones are smaller and more densely packed. Vision in all animals is improved by the presence of *areae centrales* or *foveae*. The *area centralis*, despite its name, is not always in the center of the fundus other than in humans (*macula lutea*). The *area centralis* is an area that has a marked increase in resolving power compared with the rest of the retina. A foveal depression in the retina is associated with a thinning of the retina and allows for a magnifying action and thus increased visual acuity; however, it is only present in a small number of reptiles.[6]

Fovea are present in *Amyda* spp. (the only turtles to have a fovea), *Sphenodon punctatus* (a medium, pure rod fovea), some diurnal skinks and varanids, and three genera of snakes (*Dryophis*, *Dryophiops*, and

Thelotornis). The fovea is absent in all crocodilians.[6] In nocturnal species of lizard, the fovea is absent (heloderms and most geckos) or reduced to the remnant of a foveal pit (*Xantusia*).[7] In diurnal species of lizards with a fovea, it has elongated cones that are closely packed, and some species (mainly arboreally diurnal) may have a second fovea temporally, as is also seen in some bifoveate birds.[7]

The crocodilian retinal epithelium has a tapetum formed by guanine crystals[6,7] that are hyperreflective at night when lights are shone into their eyes and is often used against them while being hunted. Rods greatly outnumber the cones in the periphery, with the cones resuming in the tapetal area. Near the ventral border of the tapetum, a horizontal oval *area centralis*, mainly of rods, exists.[7]

The optics and ocular physiology of *Trachemys scripta elegans* have been extensively studied.[25,35–37] They were found to have good vision; with the photoreceptors being 90% cones, they are able to see colors[36,38] and are particularly sensitive in the red region of the spectrum.[36] Although they have a high number of cones, they are thought to have a similar optic range to the duplex system of humans.[25]

The fibers within the optic chiasm do not completely cross in reptiles; however, most squamates and some turtles have ipsilateral projections providing good binocular vision.[39] There is nearly complete crossover of the optic nerves at the optic chiasm in *Trachemys scripta*.[35] This allows accurate panoramic vision and improved detection of movement, although only limited binocular vision is present and restricted to directly in front (25–30 degrees). The more lateral the eye, the more independent each eye, and greater panoramic field of vision. Optokinetic studies in *Trachemys scripta*[35] showed that transection of the tectal commissure caused no significant change in vision, suggesting that visual movement detection is a relatively independent function of the two eyes.

Many differences are seen in the neural pathways of reptiles. Blind snakes (which, despite their names, are sensitive to light and therefore not blind) of the families Typhlopidae and Leptotyphlopidae have a different retinal efferent system from that of higher snakes.[40] The blind snakes lack retinotectal connections, and the *nucleus rotundus* (the major thalamic nucleus receiving tectal efferens in reptiles and birds) is barely distinguishable.[40]

Boidae and Crotalinae (not Viperinae) have two electromagnetic radiation imaging systems, which although very similar, evolved independently.[41] The first is the lateral eyes, responsible for visible light, and the second are the pit organs, responsible for seeing infrared radiation.[42] These are the only animals known to image two distinct parts of the electromagnetic spectrum at the same time. Both the visual and infrared information obtained are probably involved in prey targeting. Experiments have shown that although vision is not necessary for accurate targeting (shown in experimentally blinded snakes), it is necessary for precise targeting in association with the infrared perception.[41] The infrared and visual information merge in the optic tectum where the individual neurons are found to be sensitive to both stimulation of the eyes (by visible light) and stimulation of the pit organs (by infrared radiation) from the same points in space.[41] A lateral descending nucleus of the medulla oblongata also is unique to infrared-imaging snakes. The combination of the electromagnetic radiation imaging system is important in triggering the guiding of the strike toward the prey by supplying accurate information on the position of the prey.[42] Accurate location of the prey requires the snake to move from a lateral to a rostral position and thus not only sensing the heat form of the prey but also the position and direction of any movement before striking.[42]

The pit organ in boidae is simple, consisting of a shallow depression in the labial scales (Fig. 71.7) in comparison to Viperidae, which have a concave membrane suspended within a cavity within a depression of the maxillary bone.[42] Both types of pit organs are innervated by a

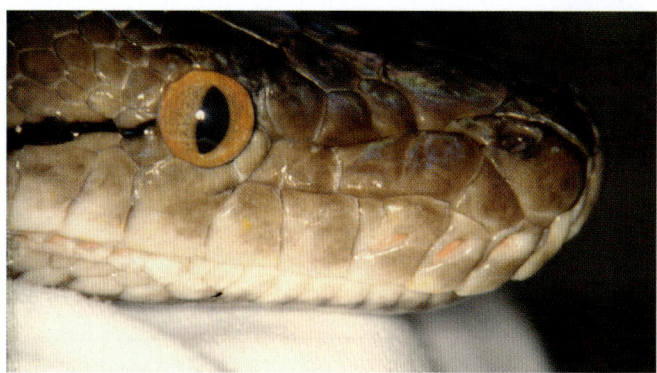

FIG 71.7 Pit organs associated with labial scales of a reticulated python (*Malayopython reticulatus*). (Courtesy of Martin P.C. Lawton.)

branch of the trigeminal nerve (ophthalmic, mandibular, and maxillary branches).[8,42] Electrophysiological studies demonstrate these organs are sensitive to temperature changes of 0.003°C, and the distance assessment is a basic trigonometrical surveying of the intensity profiles perceived by the various pits.[42] The pit organs may also be sensitive to microwave energy.[42]

OPHTHALMIC EXAMINATION

Reptilian ophthalmology requires an understanding of the normal state to recognize the abnormal. The veterinarian who desires to be proficient in reptilian medicine should perform a full ophthalmic examination in all cases, not only to gain the experience of the normal but also because systemic disease is often represented in lesions noted in the eyes and related structures.

The ophthalmic examination should be systematic, as for any other animal or any other part of the body. The examination should start with an assessment of the eyelids (fused or mobile), the tear film (where a spectacle is not present), the size and position of the globe, the cornea, anterior chamber, iris, lens, and finally the fundus. Both eyes, when present, should always be examined so that they can be compared and contrasted. If an obvious or suspected problem is seen with one eye, it is important to examine the other eye first as subtle changes or early lesions associated with a disease process may be more noticeable in the apparently normal eye than in the abnormal eye.

A brief examination with some form of focal illumination should be used (pen light, auroscope, etc). This allows a simple assessment of the clarity of the cornea and anterior chamber and highlights any adnexa or globe abnormalities. Any pupillary light response should be noted. Although the presence of striated muscles within the reptilian iris could prevent a pupillary light reflex, it is seldom absent unless substantial ocular disease exists[43]; indeed, a rapid direct light response is generally noted. Reptiles do not have a consensual light response, although they show a normal direct pupillary light response.[44]

A more detailed examination of the eye is not possible without some form of magnification (magnifying loupe, slit-lamp biomicroscope, or +10 to +15 diopter lens of the direct ophthalmoscope). The small size of the reptile eye leads to a high likelihood of subtle changes being missed if magnification is not employed. Magnification and slit-lamp use are essential to also aid the clinician in examination of snakes and lizards with spectacles, to distinguish between the anterior chamber and the subspectacular space, which is essential in reaching an accurate diagnosis of the site of any pathology (Fig. 71.8).[45,46] The use of a slit-lamp biomicroscope will allow an accurate placement of a lesion within the

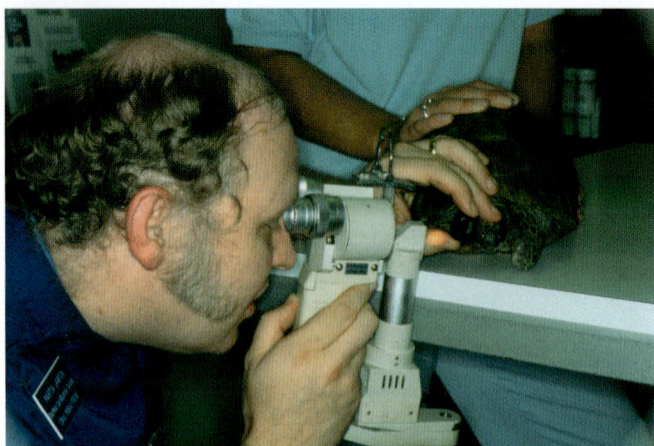

FIG 71.8 Slit-lamp biomicroscopic examination of a Mediterranean tortoise (*Testudo*). (Courtesy of Martin P.C. Lawton.)

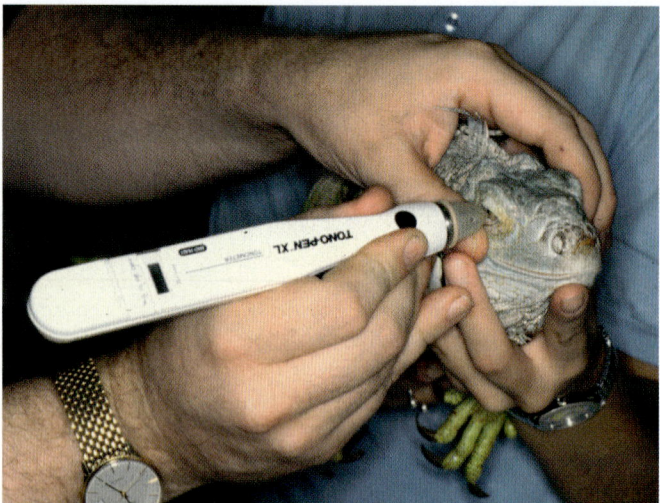

FIG 71.9 Tonometry in an (*Iguana iguana*). (Courtesy of Martin P.C. Lawton.)

anterior segment when an angled slit illumination is used to cut a "segment" of the area being examined.

Fundoscopy is often best achieved with indirect ophthalmoscopy and a 90-diopter lens or a panophthalmoscope (Welch Allen) that allows vision even through a small, often undilated pupil, as found in reptiles. The striated muscle in the iris allows voluntary control of the pupil size, which is unaffected by topical mydriatics routinely used in mammals.[2] Two ways of inducing mydriasis are with general anesthesia or with intracameral injection of neuromuscular blocking agents. Topical application of neuromuscular blocking agents has been shown to be ineffective in achieving mydriasis that may be related to a lack of corneal penetration of the drugs. The intracameral injection is performed under local anesthesia (proxymetacaine, applied topically to species without a spectacle) or with sedation (for those with spectacles). The technique requires a 27-gauge to 30-gauge needle to be advanced through the limbal conjunctivia and the cornea, into the anterior chamber where the neuromuscular blocking agent is administered in small volume. Reports of 0.05 to 0.1 mL of d-tubocurarine[15] or 0.1 mL of 20 mg/mL curare are effective.[2] The resulting mydriasis may last from 30 minutes to several hours for d-tubocurarine[15] to even days for curare.[2] In snakes and lizards that have a spectacle (as discussed later), an injection into the subspectacular space is ineffective and should not be confused with an intracameral injection (requiring the needle to first penetrate through the spectacle and then the cornea into the anterior chamber).[2]

Diagnostic Tests Specific to Ophthalmology

Ancillary ophthalmic aids, such as tonometry (Fig. 71.9), stains (see Fig. 71.5B), bacteriology, cytology, histopathology, electronmicroscopy, or ERG (electroretinography), all have application in evaluating the reptilian eye. Additionally as ophthalmic pathology often reflects systemic disease, ancillary diagnostics should be routinely utilized, including hematology, biochemistry, radiography, CT/MRI, and ultrasonography. Special mention should be made of the usefulness of ultrasonography (a minimum of 10 MHz is necessary) for the assessment of the globe or retro-orbital evaluation (see Fig. 71.6), which is easily performed, in most species, with manual restraint alone.[43,47]

Testing Patency of the Nasolacrimal System

The lacrimal system can be tested with fluorescein. In reptiles with a palpebral fissure, the stain is placed into the conjunctival fornix, and where it drains into the mouth is noted. In squamates with a spectacle, the patency of the lacrimal ducts can still be shown with injection of

0.05 mL of fluorescein through a 30-gauge needle into the subspectacular space.[15] The technique requires the needle to pass through the spectacle near the lateral canthus with visualization of the eye, with some form of magnification to prevent damage to the underlying (and very thin) cornea. The dorsal/maxillary mouth area just rostral to the Jacobson's organ should be evaluated for evidence of patency.[14] One must remember that tear-staining syndrome seen in tortoises is the result of the lack of a functional nasolacrimal system and is not indicative of an abnormality.[27] The tears of chelonians naturally spill over the eyelids and down the side of the face to eventually evaporate away, and any fluorescein placed into the eye does the same. Biopsy and cytology may be valuable[28] in determining disease etiology and assist in the treatment requirements.

CLINICAL DISEASES

Congenital and developmental ocular diseases are uncommon,[28] although microphthalmous (see Fig. 71.5C), anophthalmous, various colobomata, and failure of fusions can occur.

Eyelid Trauma

Trauma frequently affects the eyelids and may occur in any species. Trauma is particularly noted in red-eared sliders as a result of a feeding frenzy.[48] In most cases, traumatized lids need only topical antiseptic treatment (povidone-iodine) and cleaning to allow healing. More substantial lesions need surgical intervention (see Chapter 91).

Blepharoedema and Blepharitis

Swollen eyelids can be the result of a fluid edema (blepharoedema) or more solid swelling (blepharitis) (see Figs. 71.5D and 71.10A). Often one can lead to the other. A blepharospasm is often the presenting clinical sign of any irritation or abnormality of the eyelids (Fig. 71.11). Blepharospasm may be present in association with other ocular pathology or disease (as discussed later). Only primary blepharoedema and blepharitis are dealt with here. As always, samples should be taken for further investigation and to reach a definitive diagnosis and facilitate correct treatment.

Blepharoedema is a common finding in reptiles, especially freshwater chelonians,[18] and is often associated with hypovitaminosis A (see Fig. 71.5D). Hypovitaminosis A is the most common problem that affects the ocular adnexa.[2,18] The lack of vitamin A leads to squamous metaplasia

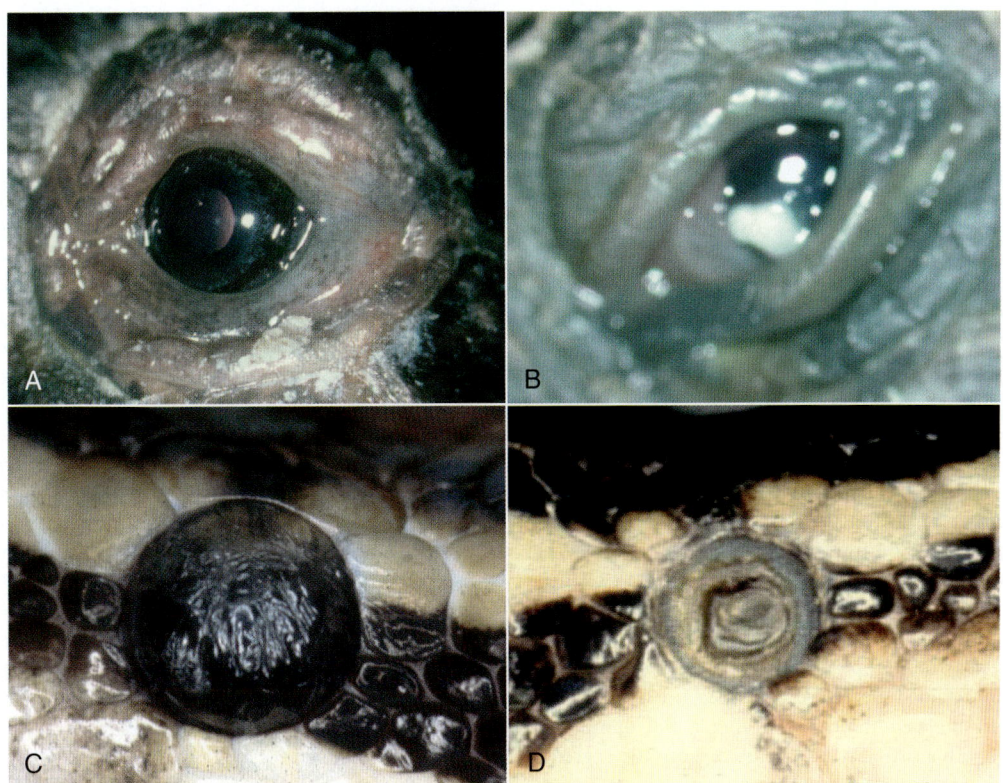

FIG 71.10 (A) Blepharitis in a Mediterranean tortoise (*Testudo*). (B) Bacterial keratitis in a Mediterranean tortoise. (C) Abrasion of a spectacle in a ball python (*Python regius*). (D) Desiccation and ulceration of cornea due to loss of a spectacle in a ball python. (Courtesy of Martin P.C. Lawton.)

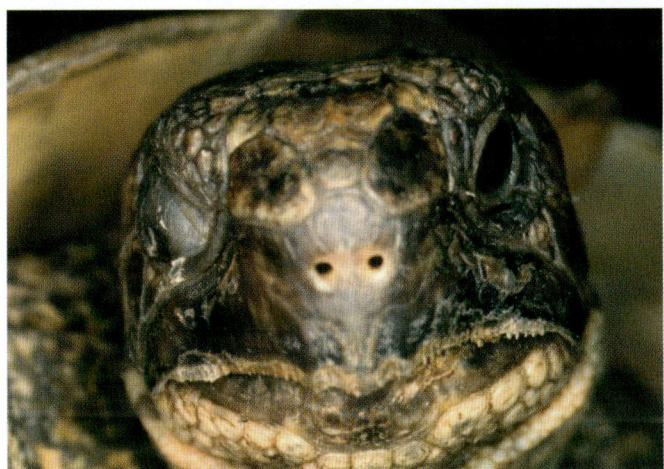

FIG 71.11 Right blepharospasm in a Mediterranean tortoise (*Testudo*). (Courtesy of Martin P.C. Lawton.)

of the orbital glands and their ducts. This leads to replacement of mucus-secreting cells by flattened keratinized squamous epithelium, and the gland lamina become dilated and filled with keratinaceous and cellular debris.[49] Once the cells have undergone squamous metaplasia, they no longer perform their protective functions, and opportunistic bacterial infection is common. Lack of tears and metaplasia cause blepharoedema and a secondary blepharitis and conjunctivitis.[2,18] A good clinical history often allows the diagnosis to be suspected and

response to treatment used for confirmation. Where treatment does not improve the condition, biopsies for histopathology prove useful. Treatment with vitamin A is dose related, and care must always be taken to prevent iatrogenic hypervitaminosis A. Swollen eyelids have also been documented in a colony of green anoles (*Anolis carolinensis*)[49] and are implicated in gecko retained eyecap syndrome. Blepharitis and closure of the eyelids associated with hypovitaminosis A is partly the result of the increase in bulk of the eyelids caused by enlargement of the ophthalmic glands.[18] Blepharitis (see Fig. 71.10A) can also be associated with a wide range of bacteria and can result in granulomata or abscess formation. Blepharitis may be caused by parasitic infestations, and five parasites (*Foleyella*) removed surgically from a newly imported Oustalet's chameleon (*Furcifer oustaleti*) have been described.[50] Eyelid scrapes for stained cytology should always be the first approach. Where bacteria are shown, samples for culture and sensitivity are advised. Where granuloma or abscess formation has occurred, surgical removal is necessary but with care to preserve the anatomic position of the eyelids. Sliding graft for eyelid reconstruction in reptiles is possible but is more involved than in mammals and is reason for referral.

Eyelid Neoplasia

Viral neoplasia of the eyelids has frequently been reported in a number of species. Although there are no published reports of non-viral-related neoplasia of the eyelids, these can occur. Viral neoplasias include fibropapilloma in green sea turtles, papillomata in green wall lizards (*Lacerta viridis*), and papillomata associated with poxvirus in the spectacled caiman (*Caiman crocodilus*).[2,15] Poxvirus in the caiman can be seen as focal raised papules anywhere on the skin, including the eyelids.[2]

Herpesvirus infection of green sea turtles may cause severe ocular, cutaneous, and visceral disease.[51] Proliferative ulcerative lesions have been reported to affect the cornea, eyelids, periocular skin, and conjunctiva, and are typically pedunculated or polypoid with verrucous surface composed of hyperplastic epithelium overlying a collagenous stroma containing reactive fibroblasts.[2,51] This condition is often complicated by secondary bacterial infections, usually gram-negative organisms. Surgery may be attempted, although recurrence is common, and even recovered individuals are a potential source of infection for others in a colony. Diagnosis can often be made on the basis of gross appearance, but histopathologic examination is definitive.

Abrasions and Ulcers of the Spectacle

The spectacle is a physical barrier derived from the skin, and as such it is impervious to most topical medicaments,[2] making treatment of the underlying cornea or globe difficult, if not impossible, without a subspectacle injection or application.

Spectacles are protective in function, and therefore some trauma naturally occurs and is noted on routine examination of the spectacle but are often lost with subsequent ecdysis (see Fig. 71.10C). Damage to the spectacles of snakes may occur from a variety of causes. Factors that can lead to damage include the hazards of feeding live prey (especially to captive breed species), inappropriate environment, dysecdysis, and incorrect treatment of retained spectacles.[14] The spectacle is also subject to infectious or parasitic conditions. Only after a full ophthalmic examination, ideally with a slit-lamp biomicroscope can the degree of damage be assessed. Further investigations may also be necessary, including the use of scrapings for cytology or bacterial culture and sensitivity. In severe or chronic conditions, biopsy may be necessary for histopathologic examination.

In most circumstances, minor damage to the spectacle is normal and of little consequence, as the spectacle renews at every shed. Abrasions can normally be seen on the surface of the older spectacle (see Fig. 71.10C). Scratches and minor abrasions regularly occur without any discomfort and should never be misdiagnosed as a "corneal ulcer." If loss of transparency of the spectacle occurs, then the underlying cause should be assessed; causes include ecdysis, inflammatory deposits on the inner surface,[52] exposure to chemicals, or retention of spectacles and bacterial or fungal infection. The use of organophosphate insecticide or volatile polyurethane organic solvents for chemical fogging of the vivaria has been implicated in a thickening of the deeper cellular layers of the spectacle and a resulting loss of transparency in *Lampropeltis* sp.[53]

Deeper abrasions can, in some circumstances, be more correctly referred to as ulcers once the epidermis has been breached,[14] but they should more correctly be referred to as dermatologic ulcers to distinguish them from corneal ulcers. These more noticeable abrasions are always secondary to an underlying husbandry or disease problem, such as low humidity, parasites, or dysecdysis. Increased and often constant rubbing of the face against rocks, branches, or other objects in the vivaria results in abrasions to the spectacle. This appears as loss of clarity of the spectacle, with abrasions varying from superficial scratches to deep ulcers. The accumulation of substrate (particularly wood chips, fine sand, and walnut shell pieces) also may be forced under the superficial layers of the spectacle. Once the spectacle is damaged, associated vascularization or secondary infection may also be seen.

Providing the abrasions are not full thickness (see section, Loss of Spectacle), treatment is with topical antibiotics (ophthalmic or dermal), and correction of the underlying problem usually leads to no permanent damage. Steroidal combinations should be avoided because these could lead to delayed healing or predisposition to secondary infection, particularly fungal. Surgical debridement may be necessary with excessive

roughness or pocketing or looseness of the edges of the skin or with accumulation of substrate under the surface layer of the spectacle (see Chapter 91). Rarely does damage or treatment of abrasions result in permanent opacity to the spectacle.

Loss of Spectacle

More substantial trauma to the spectacle usually involves avulsion, which is serious because it may result in corneal desiccation from a lack of continuity of the tear film and may ultimately result in loss of the eye, despite topical antibiotic therapy.[1,14] The spectacle is important for maintaining the tear film within the subspectacular space. The loss of a small part of the spectacle may have only minimal effects by increasing overflow (through the deficit) or evaporation of tears until regrowth occurs. If there is a total loss of the spectacle then this leads to the loss of the tear film and eventual desiccation of the cornea or panophthalmitis. The loss of the protective spectacle and the underlying fluid leads to damage of the single delicate layer of corneal epithelium (see Cornea section). The resulting damage to the cornea by drying leads to infection, ulceration, scarring, rupture, and permanent opacity with loss of vision (see Fig. 71.10D). In severe cases, shrinking of the globe (*phthisis bulbi*) occurs.

Loss of the spectacle can occur from a number of causes. The most common cause of the loss of the whole spectacle is associated with an inexperienced herpetologist (or veterinarian) attempting to remove a normal spectacle (wrongly diagnosed as a retained spectacle) with cellophane tape or forceps.[14] Other causes of loss include trauma (particularly as a sequel to long-term abrasion of the spectacle) or infection (as discussed later). Feeding of live prey (rodents) could also result in injury or penetration of the spectacle and should be avoided.

Treatment may be attempted with topical antibiotics and artificial tears, a cut-down soft contact lens, or transposition of an oral mucosa flap over the eye.[27,48] The use of a mucosal flap may save the eye but seldom allows normal vision, even though (like conjunctival grafts to the cornea in mammals) some long-term clearing may be seen (Fig. 71.12A). Some success has been achieved with a collagen graft material.

Infection of the Spectacle: Bacterial and Fungal

Although it is transparent, the spectacle is dermal, and this fact should not be forgotten at any stage of the assessment. Swabs, scrapes, and even biopsies can be performed to allow cytologic, histopathologic, bacterial, or fungal examinations, as indicated for any other dermal abnormality on the body.[14] Topical dyes routinely used for the examination of the cornea (such as Rose Bengal or fluorescein) have little advantage for assessment of the spectacle. For infection beneath the spectacle, see Subspectacular Abscess section.

Infections of the external surface of the skin are a common problem. Bacterial infections usually involve opportunistic gram-negative bacteria. In some cases, the epidermal layer may become infected with bacteria and result in an intraspectacular dermatitis.[20] In severe cases, such infections may be noted to spread beyond the margins of the spectacle.[14] This is often caused by retained spectacles or poor hygiene. Such an infection, in itself, could lead to spectacle retention or even loss of a spectacle or the eye. Treatment may require surgical incision to allow debridement and application of a suitable antibiotic agent. Where systemic spread is suspected, parenteral antibiotics may also be necessary.

Fungal infections are often encountered and are considered to be a reflection of poor management.[2] They are usually slower to develop, with the resulting infection causing more deformity of the spectacle, particularly thickening and pigmentary changes (see Fig. 71.12B).[14] The changes are seldom restricted to just the spectacle and often involve surrounding scales or even the whole head. Fungal infections need to

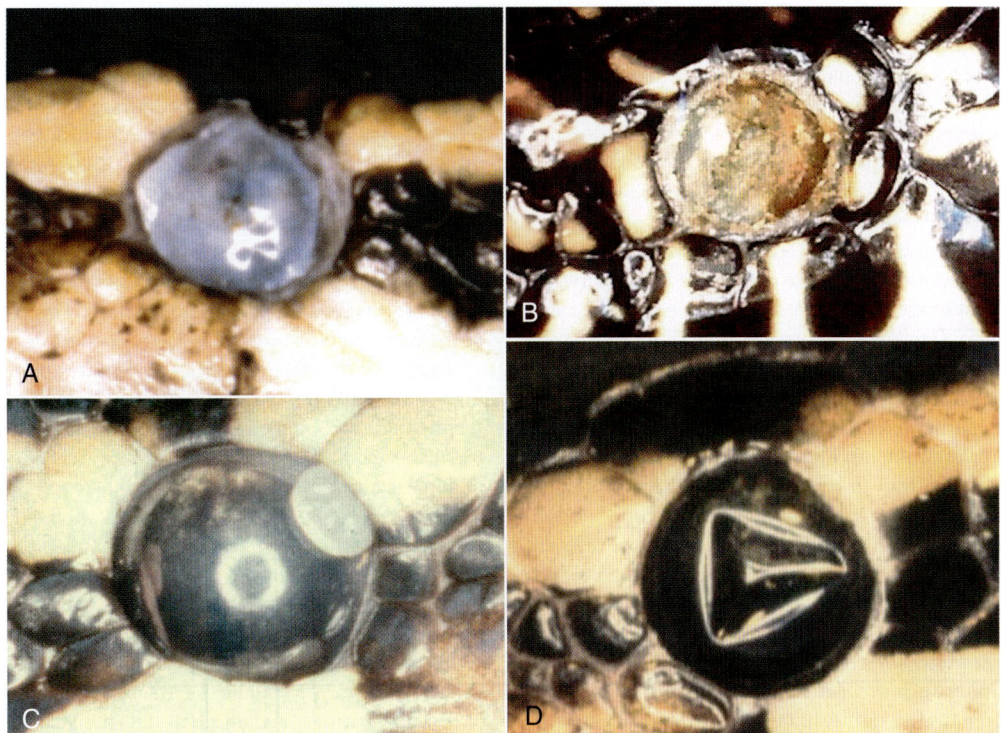

FIG 71.12 (A) Loss of spectacle after surgical and medical treatment in a ball python (*Python regius*). (B) Fungal infection of the spectacle in a king snake (*Lampropeltis* sp.). (C) Tick in the perispectacle sulcus of a ball python. (D) Indented spectacle associated with a retained spectacle in a ball python. (Courtesy of Martin P.C. Lawton.)

be identified and treated at an early stage or they may spread further. Diagnosis is based on cytology, culture, and sensitivity. These infections, if diagnosed early enough, can be treated with topical dermal antifungal creams, lotions, or ointments. A fungal infection from *Fusarium oxysporum* was reported[54] as penetrating the spectacle, and treatment required enucleation.

Subspectacular Abscess

Infection under the spectacle, involving the subspectacular space, is a common problem and can be due to one of four causes: (i) ascending infection from the oral cavity (via the nasolacrimal ducts), (ii) septicemia with hematogenous spread, (iii) penetrating trauma through the spectacle, or (iv) as a sequela to conjunctivitis.[2,15,28,52,55] In cases of primary infection or trauma, only one eye is affected, but with septicemic spread the infection is more often bilateral (Fig. 71.13).

The spectacle appears cloudy or white (leukoria) and may sometimes be distorted.[14] In cases of unilateral involvement, determining whether the infection is local or secondary to septicemia is important. White blood cell counts and blood cultures are necessary for differentiation. If the infection is secondary to septicemia, then locating and treating the primary infection at the same time as dealing with the subspectacular abscess is important.

Obtaining diagnostic material and effecting treatment requires making a surgical incision through the spectacle (see Chapter 91). Following the collection of diagnostic material, the subspectacular space should be flushed with balanced salt solution (or another suitable solution) often repeated until clear and an ophthalmic antibiotic solution such as gentamicin applied once or twice daily until infection is cleared. Depending on the culture and sensitivity results, systemic antibiotic

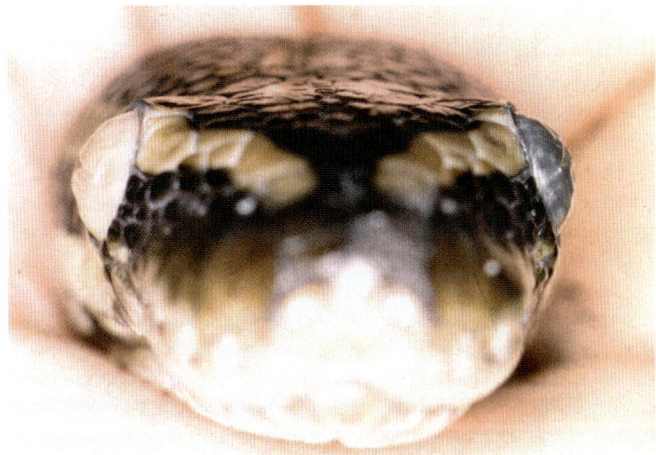

FIG 71.13 Established subspectacular abscess in right and developing subspectacular abscess in left eye of a ball python (*Python regius*). (Courtesy of Martin P.C. Lawton.)

treatment may also be necessary. In cases where severe disease of the oral cavity is involved, such as bacterial stomatitis, aggressive therapy to treat the underlying stomatitis must also be initiated. Gentle debridement and removal of caseous material in the oral cavity may be required. Additionally husbandry-related issues that have resulted in damage to the oral cavity and secondary bacterial stomatitis and subsequent subspectacular abcessation must be addressed. A common example is mature boids housed in inappropriate caging with screen mesh tops or wide spacing in a rack system resulting in tauma to the rostrum as they attempt to "push out." This often occurs in the breeding season when male and female snakes are housed near each other and males are desperate to get out to breed females.

Parasites Affecting the Spectacle

Parasites, especially mites or ticks, are not uncommonly found around the adnexa.[56] Mites (*Ophionyssus* spp.) are commonly found between the thin skin in the area of the sulcus formed by the periorbital scales and the spectacle. Ticks (*Ixodidae*) are usually only found on newly imported species. Although ticks may be found anywhere on the body, they are more often found around the cloaca or head. They usually attach to the softer skin between scales or at the junction where the spectacle meets the scales of the head (see Fig. 71.12C).

Parasitic infestation can lead to retained spectacles and potential spread of bacterial or viral disease. Slit-lamp biomicroscopy is often necessary to detect mites, but even then visualization may prove difficult because they are often deep within the sulcus. Parasites may be physically removed (to thus confirm the diagnosis) by flushing with a suitable solution (such as balanced salt solution) via a fine 24-gauge cannula.[14] They may also be noted after the removal of a retained spectacle.

Direct-life cycle mites such as *Ophionyssus* are always an environmental problem and removal alone is insufficient. Any residual parasites or eggs must also be removed from the environment. Flushing with ivermectin (Ivomec, MSD Agvet) is a good method of physical removal of mites from the sulcus of the spectacle.[14] This technique requires the instillation of a small amount (0.2 mL) of undiluted ivermectin flushed around the sulcus, which, 2 minutes later, is followed by a thorough flushing with saline solution to remove the parasites. Although transdermal absorption is possible, the small volume of ivermectin and the thorough flushing appears sufficient to prevent any toxic effects.

Retained Spectacle

Retained spectacle is the most common ocular problem of snakes.[14,57,58] There is a syndrome in geckos referred to as retained eye caps.[28] However, this is a misnomer as it is often described in species without a spectacle. In these cases there is often underlying hypovitaminosis A with secondary bacterial infection and a resulting failure to shed the conjunctival lining underneath the eyelids, with the accumulation of cell debris within the palpebral fissure.[28]

The rest of this section concentrates only on the condition in snakes. Among multiple etiologies, environmental conditions are contributory if not the primary cause.[48] The condition arises because of a failure of the old spectacle to be shed during ecdysis.[14,48] The most common cause is a dry environment or dehydration (such as associated with systemic illness).[2] Other factors, such as inadequate nutrition or systemic disease, may also be contributory.[15] Scarring and the presence of mites may also lead to dysecdysis and retained spectacles. It is not unusual upon removal of a retained spectacle to find the mite (*Ophionyssus natricis*) still clinging to the spectacle or embedded within the sulcus formed from the spectacle and the protruding scales of the orbit ridge. Any cause of skin disease could also lead to the retention of spectacles,[14] including a suggestion of thyroid dysfunction.[46]

Temporary visual impairment may result from the retention of several spectacles. The retained spectacles may become secondarily infected, resulting in blindness. If not removed, subsequent shedding is also inhibited, and the spectacles build up to form a thickened mass of dead skin that affects the snake's vision and may affect its willingness or ability to feed.[14] The more retained layers, the easier the diagnosis of retained spectacle. A single retained spectacle may have only limited effects on the vision of the snake and is often missed by the owner, being picked up only during routine clinical examination at the time of presentation for other reasons. Often an associated creasing of the spectacle is seen as a dent in the surface when a spectacle has been retained. Ball (royal) pythons (*Python regius*) seem to be particularly prone to this phenomenon (see Fig. 71.12D). Although the absence of denting cannot be used to eliminate the possibility of a retained spectacle, the denting of a healthy spectacle (without a retained spectacle) is in itself pathognomonic of a previously retained spectacle. The denting decreases with time and usually disappears after the next slough, providing the spectacle is shed easily at that stage. This creasing or indenting of the new spectacle appears to have no effect on vision.

Diagnosis of a retained spectacle requires more than examining a slough and failing to find spectacles. Where dysecdysis is seen with retained skin still on the head and around, or leading to, the spectacle, the diagnosis is straightforward. Diagnosis is also easily made when multiple retained layers are found. The difficulty arises with the possibility of only one retained layer, when no indentation or opacification is seen. Examination with magnification (ideally with a slit-lamp illumination or biomicroscope) allows visualization of the increased thickness of the spectacle associated with extra layers.[14] Examination of the edges of the spectacle is useful because often tags of skin may be seen, especially if the head skin has been sloughed but only the spectacle is retained. Failure to confirm a retained spectacle before attempting treatment may lead to iatrogenic damage to the spectacle and corneal exposure (see previously). If any doubt exists as to whether or not a spectacle is retained, no treatment should be attempted but to wait until after the next shed and reexamine at that time.

Treatment involves soaking the retained spectacle to aid removal. This is best done with a wet cotton swab and rubbing from the medial and lateral canthi toward the center of the spectacle (Fig. 71.14). If the spectacle does not detach after gentle manipulation with a cotton swab, then artificial tears (hypromellose, Tears Naturale; Alcon or Ilube, Morfields) are applied several times daily for a few days to soften the spectacle before the technique is repeated. Although Frye[59] advised the use of forceps or other instruments to remove a retained spectacle, this author considers instrument use rarely indicated and should only be undertaken by an experienced veterinarian using magnification to reduce the risks of damage to, or even avulsion of, the underlying spectacle. The inadvertent removal of a new spectacle, as opposed to a retained spectacle, if unmanaged, leads to exposure keratitis[1,2] and eventual loss of the eye. If the retained spectacle cannot be removed easily, then waiting until the next shed to try again is best.

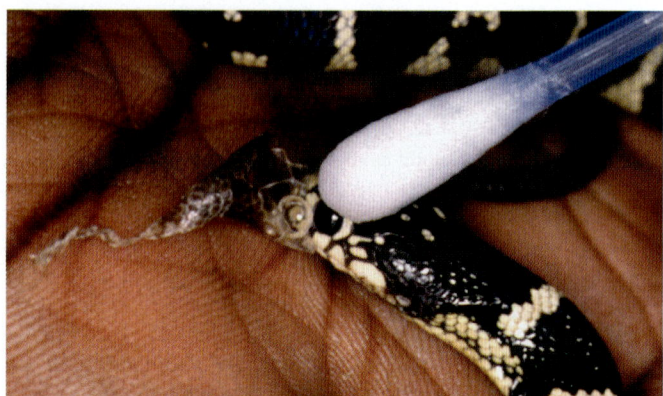

FIG 71.14 Removal of a retained spectacle with gentle rubbing, utilizing a moist cotton bud (swab). (Courtesy of Martin P.C. Lawton.)

Pseudobuphthalmos

Blockage of the nasolacrimal system is more commonly encountered as a clinical problem in snakes and geckos.[2,44] Any fluid not draining down the nasolacrimal ducts is incapable of overflowing the sealed eyelid margins and accumulates in the subspectacular space. If fluid accumulation in the subspectacular space is due to a failure of nasolacrimal drainage, then the spectacle will bulge (see Chapter 91). This is correctly referred to as pseudobuphthalmos.[60] The resultant stretching of the spectacle has also been incorrectly referred to in the literature as a bullous spectaculopathy,[20,61] as it was considered similar to bullous keratopathy of mammals, where bullae or vesicles form within the epithelial cells of the cornea and can become large and even pendulous with the possibility of rupture.[62,63] The definition of a bulla is a cavitation, larger than a vesicle, within the epidermis.[64] The buildup of fluid within the subspectacular spaces cannot therefore be referred to as "bullous," nor indeed does it involve the spectacle per se. It should not therefore be referred to as bullous spectaculopathy but pseudobuphthalmos.

This condition was first incorrectly described[1] in an indigo snake (*Drycmarchon corais*) as "acute proptosis," but slit-lamp biomicroscopy confirms the accumulation of a clear, colorless fluid between the spectacle and the cornea, causing the spectacle to protrude with a noticeable enlargement in the subspectacular space biomicroscopy.[48] Pseudobuphthalmos is differentiated from subspectacular abscesses in that the fluid is clear and uninfected; if in doubt, stained cytology of aspirated fluid can be performed to document bacterial/inflammatory elements.

Investigation of nasolacrimal duct patency is possible with an injection of a small amount of fluorescein dye through the lateral canthus of the spectacle into the subspectacular space, as mentioned previously. However, when blockage is present, the increased pressure is likely to push fluid out through even the smallest hole in the spectacle. Chronic increase in pressure can eventually lead to damage of the cornea or even the globe itself.[14]

This condition may be only a temporary problem, and in one case, the eye returned to normal within 3 days without any therapy.[1] However, if it persists, then other causes, including masses in the maxillary region, may need to be ruled out by radiography or CT. Surgery may be required for persistent problems (see Chapter 91).

Keratoconjunctivitis Sicca (Dry Eye)

Keratoconjunctivitis sicca (dry eye) is seen in reptiles that do not have a spectacle (Fig. 71.15A). It is related to a reduction or failure of production of the aqueous phase of the tear film and is usually associated with changes in the lacrimal and Harderian glands associated with vitamin A deficiency.[18] The deficiency also causes conjunctival and corneal epithelial metaplasia and hyperkeratosis. Changes are reversible, but this is dependent on the length of time that the deficiency has existed. Often by the time the condition is presented to the veterinarian, permanent changes may have developed. Definitive diagnosis of the dry eye is made with cut down Schirmer tear test strips, phenol red thread, or the standardized endodontic absorbent paper point tear test placed into the conjunctival fossa to measure the aqueous phase of the tear film over a minute. Treatment of keratoconjunctivitis is similar to that

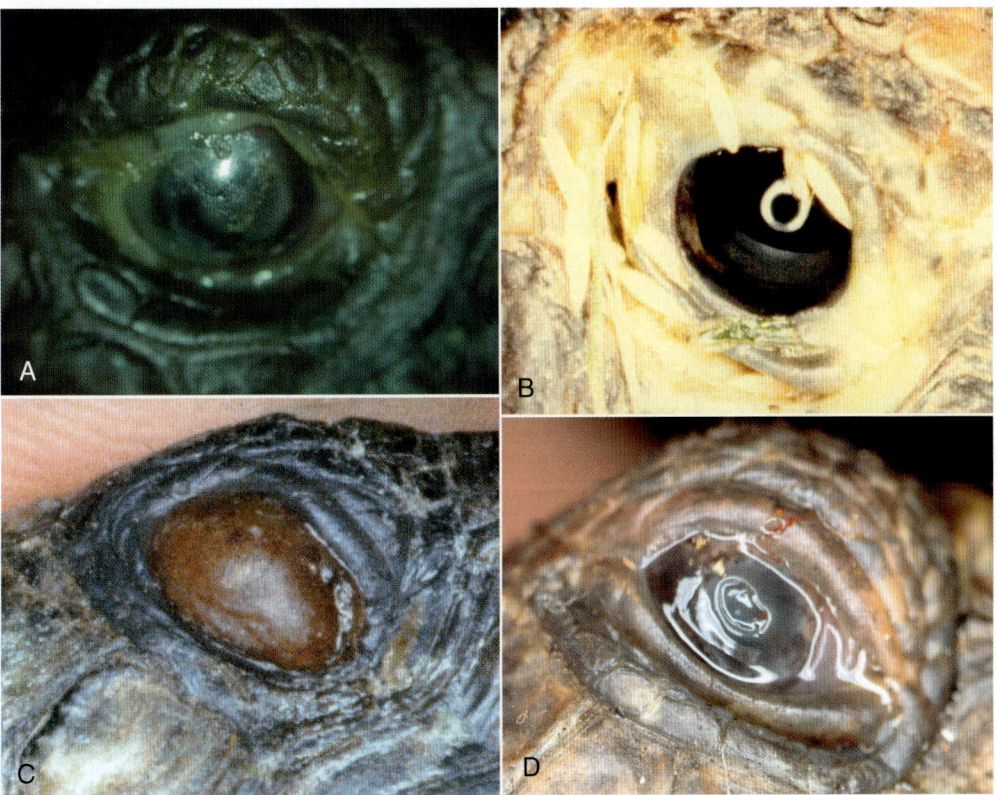

FIG 71.15 (A) Keratoconjuntivitis sicca (xerophthalmia) in a Mediterranean tortoise (*Testudo*). (B) Foreign body (seed) in eye of a Mediterranean tortoise. (C) Conjunctival swelling extending beyond the eyelid margins in a Mediterranean tortoise. (D) Corneal ulceration in a Mediterranean tortoise. (Courtesy of Martin P.C. Lawton.)

used in mammals, with artificial tear preparations, and when xerophthalmia (no tear production) is from vitamin A deficiency, administration of vitamin A and dietary correction is advised.[27,65]

Congenital Abnormalities of the Globe

Of the few congenital abnormalities described for the reptilian globe, microphthalmia is the most common disorder particularly in snakes,[2,16] although cyclopia and anophthalmia have been noted.[2] Five cases of bilateral and two of unilateral microphthalmia in a clutch of 16 eggs from 2 red-headed rat snakes (*Elaphe moellendorffi*) have been reported.[1] On histopathologic examination, normal structures were found within the small globes, with the only abnormalities being the absence of lenses.[1] Factors implicated in microphthalmia include genetics, nutrition, incubation temperatures and oxygen concentrations. Anophthalmia is rare but has been reported in several northern pine snakes (*Pituophis melanoleucus melanoleucus*).[2] The occurrence of true anophthalmia is rare, and a reptile that appears not to have eyes should always be considered as a case of microphthalmia unless histopathology confirms the absence of an eye (see Fig. 71.5C).[48]

Exophthalmos

Any retro-orbital mass or swelling can result in exophthalmia. Ultrasonographic examination with 10 to 20 MHz or greater probe is a useful tool to investigate, diagnose, and even allow guided biopsy for the collection of samples for cytology, histopathology, and culture. Abscessation is the most common cause of exophthalmos or periorbital swelling, and surgery is always indicated.[47] In chameleons, exophthalmos is often caused by periorbital swelling, which may be related to husbandry issues (reduced ventilation and humidity), irritants, vitamin A deficiency, and foreign bodies, as well as infection.[21]

An orbital varix (pathologic enlargement of one or more venous channels) has been described as a cause of an acute progressive swelling of one eye associated with an aneurysm of the retrobulbar vein in a green iguana (*Iguana iguana*), probably as a result of trauma.[43] Hypertension secondary to renal disease in iguanas, bearded dragons (*Pogona vitticeps*), and chameleons may also result in exophthalmia. This condition is often misdiagnosed in snakes and is really pseudobuphthalmos, with the subspectacular space being enlarged and causing enlargement of the globe.[1] A true unilateral congenital exophthalmia has been described, with histopathology demonstrating a cystlike structure with abundant eosinophils.[57]

Infection of the Globe

Bacterial infection can lead to a widespread degeneration within the globe and granulomatous response, often with the infection spreading beyond the globe itself.[66] Orbital infections can occur from hematogenous spread, penetrating injury, or foreign body.[67] The granulomatous response usually causes an enlargement of the globe, but as in other animals, severe trauma, inflammation, or infection can also lead to a shrinking of the eye (*phthisis bulbi*). A fungal infection in a rainbow boa (*Epicrates chenchria maurus*) has been reported as a cause of *phthisis bulbi*.[54]

Conjunctivitis

The examination of the conjunctiva should be routine in all reptiles with nonfused eyelids. Visual examination can still be performed (especially with magnification) in reptiles with a spectacle but is often limited because most of the conjunctiva is hidden from view. The frequent occurrence of foreign bodies within the conjunctival fornix is often linked to environmental conditions. In tortoises, ocular foreign bodies are a common finding in those that hibernate in hay (see Fig. 71.15B) or sand.[48] Lizards kept on peat or sand may occasionally get these materials into their eyes, resulting in blepharospasm.[48] Treatment is the

removal of the foreign body by grasping it, often under topical local anesthesia with the aid of magnification and fine forceps or by physically flushing it out with a suitable solution (such as balanced salt or Hartmann's [lactated Ringer's] solution) via a soft fine-gauge intravenous cannula. Any ulceration or abrasion of the cornea should be treated with topical antibiotic.

A nonspecific inflammatory response due to a variety of ocular insults or disease can result in hyperemia, edema, and, it has been claimed, chemosis, but this is more subtle than in mammals and more associated with conjunctival swelling, extending beyond the eyelid margins (see Fig. 71.15C).[28]

Conjunctivitis is a common problem, although primary bacterial conjunctival infections are rare[2] and secondary opportunistic bacteria are more frequently encountered. In a survey of bacteria isolated from nondomesticated species with eye infections at a zoological collection, 5 of the 19 reported cases involved reptiles and included infections associated with *Aeromonas* spp., *Pasteurella* spp., and *Pseudomonas* spp.[68] In a laboratory colony of mixed lizards, an outbreak of conjunctivitis (with some developing respiratory disease) was associated with *Aeromona liquefaciens*.[69] A catarrhal conjunctivitis in a large group of Russian (Horsfield's) tortoises (*Agrionemys horsfieldii*) was secondary to debilitation and characterized by infection with *Proteus vulgaris*, *Citrobacter intermedium*, and a heavy infestation with oxyurids.[70]

Bacterial conjunctivitis in mammals is frequently suggested by mucopurulent discharge, but reptiles, like birds, lack granulocytic lysosomes, and therefore discharge is rarely seen. Infectious conjunctivitis usually results as caseous plaques, often retained within the conjunctival fornix but more commonly on the corneal surface (as discussed later).[48] Cases of keratoconjunctivitis (where both the cornea and conjunctiva are involved) are more likely to be associated with poor hygiene.[46] Ocular discharge and blepharospasm have been noted with bacterial infections of the conjunctiva in lizards.[69] Local extension of any infection could result in panophthalmitis and loss of the eye or even eventual septicemia and death.

The presence of plaques within the conjunctival fornix can cause a foreign body reaction. Any caseous material within the conjunctival fornix should be examined carefully with a microscope and, where indicated, submitted for culture and sensitivity. Occasions also exist where conjunctival biopsies should be taken for histopathologic or electron microscopic examination to differentiate between infection and metaplasia (vitamin A deficiency). Hypovitaminosis A causes displacement of the conjunctiva by desquamated cells that leads to the production of an amorphous mass or pseudoabscess and multiple retention cysts.[18] The material that accumulates in the conjunctival sac is a mixture of keratinous lamellae and eosinophil granulocytes.[18] One should always remember that this condition is a systemic disease.

Caseous conjunctivitis is part of the herpesvirus-related lung, eye, and trachea disease reported in green sea turtles.[71] An underlying secondary infection often involves gram-negative bacteria and a resultant keratoconjunctivitis. Affected turtles also have respiratory signs and may be unable to dive.[71]

Where conjunctivitis was noted in a survey of reptiles in a zoological collection, blepharitis (blepharoconjunctivitis), corneal disease, or other problems were found.[68] Any reptile (except those with spectacles) with blepharospasm warrants a careful examination of the conjunctival fornix with magnification and wetted endodontic paper points to remove any caseous plaques. Routine flushing with an appropriate solution, via a fine soft cannula (24-gauge), and antibiotics usually controls bacterial infections.[48] Conjunctivitis in snakes presents as a subspectacular abscess[14] and has been covered previously.

Certain plants (*Ficus, Pothos*) have been found to cause conjunctivitis in chameleons due to the oxalates in their leaves.[21] Viral infections, such as fibropapilloma or herpesvirus infection of green sea turtles, may cause proliferative or ulcerative lesions of the conjunctiva.[2,51] Leeches (*Ozobrancus* sp.) have been found to parasitize the conjunctiva of green sea turtles.[2] Six species of *Neopolystoma* spp. were isolated from the conjunctival sac of freshwater chelonians, with a high prevalence rate (80% in one study) but low intensity (one to three worms per animal).[72]

Corneal Disease

Ulceration of the cornea may be associated with foreign bodies, prolonged infection, and trauma, as encountered in other taxa (see Fig. 71.15D). Corneal ulceration in snakes is rare because of the protective effects of the spectacle; generally only infection or severe trauma may cause this problem. Diagnosis of a corneal ulceration is made with the uptake of fluorescein dye into the stroma (see Fig. 71.5B). In reptiles with spectacles, topical fluorescein is not useful unless it is injected into the subspectacular space. Corneal lacerations are usually traumatic[73] and can be surgically repaired (see Chapter 91) but should always be treated prophylactically with topical ophthalmic antibiotics.

Keratitis

Excessive exposure to UV light may contribute to an induced photo-keratoconjunctivitis and eventually lead to corneal ulceration.[74] In addition, care is required when using surgical or low-level therapeutic lasers.

Corneal inflammation/infection (keratitis) in tortoises may present as a white corneal mass (see Fig. 71.10B), is often associated with the immunosuppressive scenario of hibernation, and may be the result of infection with *Moraxella* spp., *Pseudomonas* spp., or *Aeromonas* spp.[27] Such keratitis is infectious and contagious and should be considered a herd problem. Treatment consists of removal of the plaque from the cornea (see Chapter 91) and topical therapy based on culture and sensitivity of the removed material. Severe keratitis can lead to scarring and pigmentation of the cornea, similar to that seen in mammals.

The presence of the spectacle in snakes does not preclude the development of corneal disease. A mycotic keratitis in a reticulated python has been described[75] where a firm mass was palpated under the spectacle and required enucleation together with the removal of some surrounding tissue. Histopathologic examination showed the corneal stroma to be infiltrated with spores and mycelia with branching filaments and septation. If fungal hyphae are seen on corneal scrapings, then treatment with topical miconazole is a possibility. Fungal keratitis, however, can cause a panophthalmitis,[44,54] which is only treatable with enucleation.[54] Topical corticosteroid therapy[44,54] and trauma[44] are possible underlying causes of fungal keratitis.

There are a number of viral infections that can cause keratitis, including herpesviral-induced proliferative or ulcerative lesions of the cornea of green sea turtles that can involve the entire cornea.[2,51,76] The lung-eye-trachea disease also causes changes to the cornea, usually involving a white plaque or opacification.[77]

Uveitis

Uveitis is infrequently reported and may be due to systemic disease, trauma, infection (bacteria, fungi, or virus), or neoplasia.[28] The clinical signs and treatment are similar to those noted in mammals. Hyphema and hypopyon are often present after exposure to freezing temperatures in chelonians (see Fig. 71.3A).[27,48] Hypopyon is a secondary feature of reptiles with an underlying systemic infection[2] such as a bacterial septicemia; *Klebsiella pneumoniae* has been associated as one possible cause.[45] All reptiles with hypopyon should have a thorough investigation for potential infectious causes. Where septicemia is confirmed, the prognosis is guarded.

Cataracts

As in all taxa, cataracts may occur for a variety of reasons, including senility. Cataracts in tortoises have been associated with freezing episodes.[27,48,78] They are hypothesized to be particularly prone to damage from low temperatures because of the soft and fluidlike nature of their lenses.[7] In some cases, these changes are reversible, although up to 18 months may be necessary for the lens to clear.[27,48] Cataract surgery in reptiles can be performed (see Chapter 91).

Retinal Disease

Our knowledge of retinal disease in reptiles is still very much in its infancy and sadly lacking when compared with that of mammalian and avian species. Often the effects are not noticed until the patient is totally blind, when medical intervention to restore vision is futile.[79] Retinal damage associated with vitamin A deficiency and freezing have been reported in tortoises.[78] In certain circumstances, early treatment with vitamin A may result in clinical improvement. Retinal degeneration has been reported in tokay geckos,[45,80] although it is thought to be a sporadic finding in most reptile families.[52]

Ocular Therapeutics

There are no specific medications licensed for ophthalmic use in reptiles, and therefore off-label treatments of human and other veterinary preparations are required. The range of antimicrobial ophthalmic preparations are often appropriate for the potential bacterial pathogens encountered and include several fluoroquinolones as well as gentamycin. The frequency used should mirror that for other species (usually three to four times per day). The size of the drop is appropriate for mammalian species (including humans), and owners should be warned that despite spillover from the small reptilian fornix, effectiveness is not reduced. Where the ocular presentation is part of a systemic infection, oral or injectable antibiotics are also indicated.

Vitamin supplements, especially vitamin A, can be used as an adjunctant therapy for a wide range of ocular conditions for which the case history is suggestive of nutritional deficiency. Overuse should be avoided to prevent possible toxic effects (e.g., hypervitaminosis A), and dietary correction is the mainstay of long-term treatment and prevention.

Inflammatory conditions, such as trauma and uveitis, should be treated with nonsteroidal anti-inflammatories (NSAIDs), either topically or systemically, or both. Topical drugs such as flubiprofen and bromfenac appear to be well tolerated. Corticosteroids should be avoided unless there is a real justification (e.g., unresponsive NSAID uveitis or corneal vascularization, immune-mediated disease).

For reptiles with spectacles, the potential penetration of topical medications may require a systemic treatment protocol or subspectacular injections in order to provide effective administration to the target area to be treated.

Lubricating drops (artificial tears) and N-acetylcystine may help to soften and dislodge retained spectacles.[28]

REFERENCES

See www.expertconsult.com for a complete list of references.

72

Otorhinolaryngology

Michelle Kischinovsky, Stephen J. Divers, Lori D. Wendland, and Mary B. Brown

The anatomy and physiology of reptiles differ greatly from avian and mammalian species but also between its orders, genera, and species. Knowledge of normal anatomical structures, their functions, physiological capabilities, and pathophysiology is essential in differentiating between the healthy and diseased.

Diseases affecting the ear, nose, and throat often follow similar disease patterns or have similar clinical signs, although different etiologies. Many are multifactorial, have nutritional, infectious or noninfectious causes or a combination thereof, as well as involving multiple areas of the body; therefore disease complexes or syndromes are often described in relation to these body systems. Although pathologies of the ear and nose involve key sensory organs, some reptiles appear to have great plasticity in thriving with sensory alteration, although welfare aspects should not be ignored. Disease differentiation can be difficult, time-consuming, and expensive. A systematic approach to the clinical examination combined with knowledge of the available and appropriate diagnostic tools will aid the investigatory process. With the threat of antibiotic resistance, emerging novel viruses and other infectious agents, as well as an increase in the incidence of zoonotic diseases, we should aim to treat a definitive diagnosis rather than a clinical manifestation.

ANATOMY AND PHYSIOLOGY

The structures of and within the laryngo-pharynx, aural, and nasal cavities vary greatly in size, shape, and function, between and even within orders. Taxonomic differences significant for disease identification will be highlighted, but unfortunately some generalizations will be made as detailed anatomical and physiological adaptations are beyond the scope of this chapter.

Ear

The reptilian ear is located caudoventral to the eye and is covered either by an enlarged cutaneous scale or a semitransparent tympanum of varying thickness. There are species-specific adaptations; however, the ear generally consists of three divisions (Fig. 72.1 and Fig. 72.2).

The external ear comprises the depression (external auditory meatus) extending from the lateral surface of the head to the tympanic membrane and collects sound waves from the environment. It is usually no more than a few millimeters deep, if present at all. The external ear is absent in chelonians, snakes, amphisbaenians, and tuataras, as well as some lizards.[1] In most species of gecko a meatal closure muscle is present, offering further protection to the tympanum.[2] In crocodilians a similar muscle is present in the dorsal of two skin folds (earflaps) overlaying and hiding the external meatus and tympanum.[3]

The middle ear transmits and amplifies sound waves from the tympanic membrane, creating vibrations transmitted through a chain of bony ossicles—the columella (an elongated version of the stapes)—and

in some species also the cartilaginous extracolumella. The incus and malleus are absent in reptiles. The ossicles are suspended in the air-filled tympanic cavity and extend medially from the tympanic membrane to the oval window of the cochlea (Fig. 72.2 and Fig. 72.3). The tympanic cavity and structures vary widely in shape and size between orders, merely a narrow fissure in snakes and absent in amphisbaenians and tuatara. Snakes, lacking Eustachian tubes, have a quadrate bone connecting the mandible to the stapes and can receive low-frequency vibrations. In turtles, the large cavity extends caudally into a blind pouch within the squamosal bone. Crocodilians have an extensive channel system linking the right and left middle ears.[4]

In most lizards the differentiation between the tympanic cavity and pharyngeal space is indistinguishable, though in some chameleons this division is marked by a thin membrane with a small fenestration believed to correspond to the Eustachian tube.[1,5] The pharyngeal orifice of the Eustachian tube can be identified on the buccal oral mucosa just caudal to the angle of the jaw of the chelonian (Fig. 72.4).

The inner ear comprises the organs related to equilibrium/balance (the semicircular canals, utricle, and saccule) and auditory perception (cochlear duct). The vibrations received are transmitted via fluid oscillations to the cochlear hair cells. These movements are subsequently transmitted to the brain via the vestibulocochlear nerve (cranial nerve VIII) for interpretation. Species adaptations are extensive, and their individual anatomical and physiological descriptions are beyond the scope of this chapter.[1,6] In general, species with a well-developed

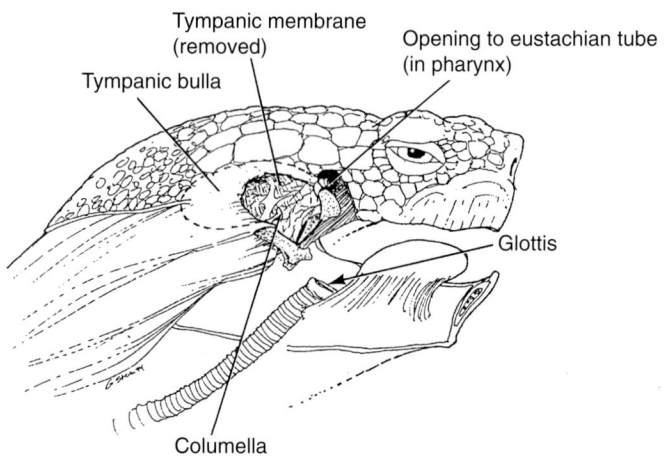

FIG 72.1 Head of a box turtle (*Terrapene* sp.) with the right lower jaw removed. Note the extent of the middle ear cavity demarcated by the *dashed line*. (Adapted from Boyer TH: Common problems of box turtles [*Terrapene* sp.] in captivity, *Bull ARAV*. 1992;2[1]:11.)

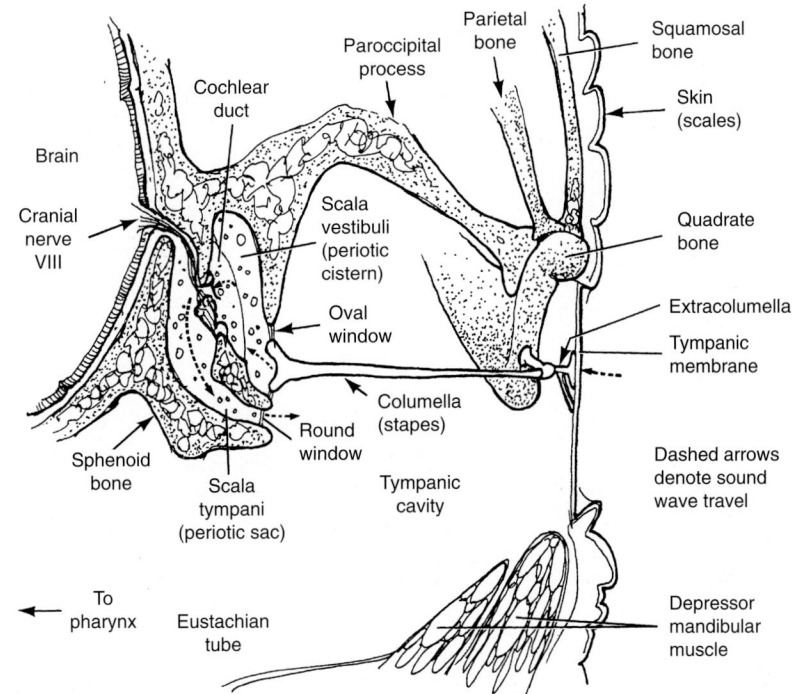

FIG 72.2 General relations of the middle and inner ear structures in the lizard *Scleroporus magister*. Coronal view of the right ear as viewed from behind. (Adapted from Wever EG: *The reptile ear,* Princeton, NJ: Princeton University Press; 1978.)

tympanum have a good sense of hearing, and atympanic species have hearing limited to low-frequency ranges of 150 to 600 Hz—generally the groundborne (somatic) or waterborne vibrations as opposed to airborne sound.[1,7] Furthermore, hearing does not seem dependent on the tympanic cavity size but more so on the conductive mechanism of the columella. It is supposed that reptilian ears are more important for balance than for hearing.[1]

Nasal Cavity

The upper respiratory tract consists of the rhinarium and the nasal cavity (Fig. 72.5). Within the nasal cavity are the external nares (Fig. 72.6), vestibulum nasi, cavum nasi proprium, conchae (turbinates), ductus nasopharyngeus, and the choanae (internal nares).[8–10] Furthermore, some species have a vomeronasal (Jacobson's organ) and nasal salt glands (Fig. 72.7). Reptiles typically breathe in air through the external nares with their mouth closed. Air enters the relatively short vestibulum and passes across the conchae in the nasal chamber then enters the pharynx via the choana(e), which is in close anatomical association with the larynx.

The tubular vestibulum nasi extends from the external nares to the cavum nasi proprium with the border often distinguishable by the difference in diameter and, in most, demarcated by a ridge in the lateral nasal wall. Turtles and many species of squamates, both aquatic and terrestrial, have erectile tissue in the vestibulum to close the opening during water or sand submersion.[11,12] In most reptiles and amphibians the cavum nasi proprium is the largest nasal structure and is usually subdivided into smaller cavities or parts by ridges, membranes, or cartilaginous septae. It is the portion that lies between the vestibulum and the nasopharyngeal duct and is partially covered by sensory epithelium. In chelonians the dorsal area is lined with multilayered olfactory epithelium and ventrally with nonsensory or respiratory epithelium.[11] The chonchae, projections from the lateral wall of the cavum nasi proprium, are present in varying degrees in crocodilians, tuataras, lizards, and most snakes, however, are

lacking in chelonians.[11] The nasopharyngeal duct is a simple tubular connection between the cavum nasi proprium and the choana(e). The tuatara lack this structure; it is short in lizards and increasingly longer and more developed in snakes, turtles, and crocodilians, and even more so in aquatic species. It is lined by nonsensory epithelium.[11]

The vomeronasal organ, also referred to as Jacobson's organ, is generally located in the ventral nasal cavity (as opposed to the olfactory epithelium which generally lies dorsally). It is innervated by a branch of the olfactory nerve (cranial nerve I) and is rich in chemoreceptors. It is absent in crocodilians. In tuatara it remains in the nasal septum as a duct in the choanae connected with both the oral and nasal cavities, whereas it is associated with the mouth in squamates.[11,13] Turtles appear to have similar sensory cells scattered across the dorsal nasal epithelium and believed to be the homolog of the organ found in other reptiles. Semiaquatic turtles, crocodilians, and some lizards perform buccal oscillation (sometimes referred to as gular pumping), when air is passed over nasal epithelium by pharyngeal contractions. It is believed to serve an olfactory, rather than a respiratory, function, analogous to mammalian "sniffing."[14–16] In snakes and some lizards it is present just rostral to the choana(e) as a pair of pits in the roof of the mouth into which the tongue transfers chemical scents. The nasolacrimal ducts open either within (some snakes) or adjacent (some lizards) to the organ and drains from the medial canthus of the eye.[11]

Several nasal glands are present and vary greatly in shape, size, and function between species. The nasal salt glands are present in some desert-living, herbivorous, and marine lizards, such as the green iguana (*Iguana iguana*) and chuckwallas (*Sauromalus* sp.).[17,18] Excessive sodium, potassium, and chloride is excreted by these glands when plasma osmotic concentration is high and allows water conservation. The lizards can expel a clear fluid that dries into a fine white sodium-potassium salt powder, which can sometimes be seen deposited around the nares or on glass enclosures.

The choana(e) (palatine-like structure) divide the nasal, oral, and/ or pharyngeal cavity. It is visible in the dorsal oropharynx and varies in shape and length from a narrow oval slit to a larger triangular opening.

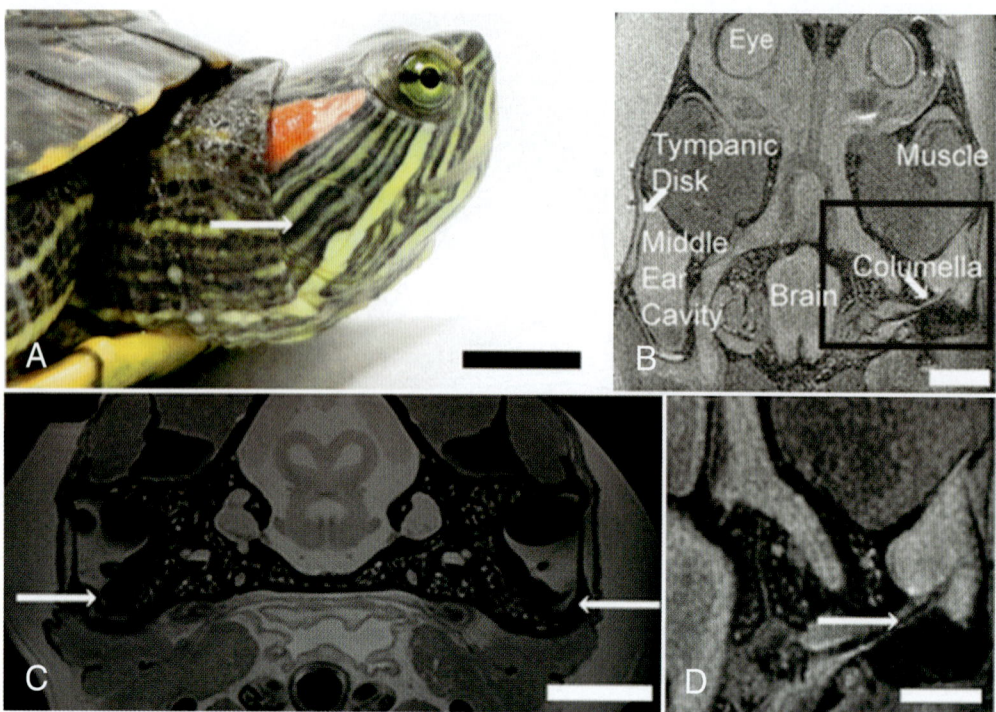

FIG 72.3 Anatomical structures of the testudine auditory system in *Trachemys scripta elegans*. (A) Lateral view of head (1 cm scale bar). *Arrow* indicates the tympanic membrane. (B) Horizontal MR image (5 mm scale bar). "Muscle" is the splenius capitus. (C) Transverse MRI at the level of the tectum. *Arrows* indicate Eustachian tubes (5 mm scale bar). (D) Horizontal MR image, enlarged from box in (B). The columella runs through the middle ear cavity to the inner ear. *Arrow* indicates the columella (3 mm scale bar). (Courtesy of Katie L. Willis, University of Oklahoma. From Willis KL, Christensen-Dalsgard J, Ketten DR, et al. Middle ear cavity morphology is consistent with an aquatic origin for Testudines. *PLoS ONE*. 2013; 8[1]:e54086.)

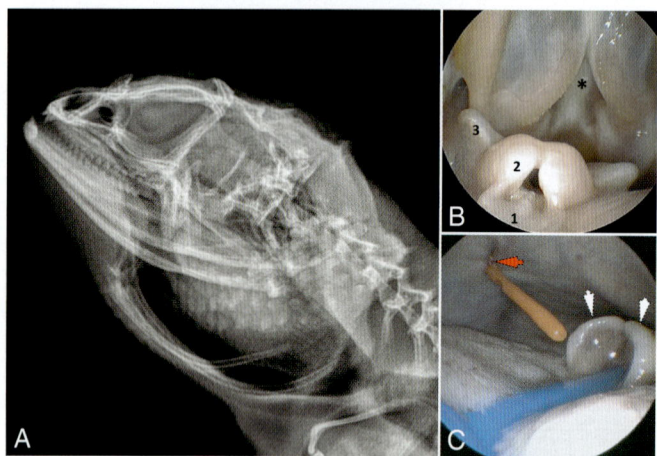

FIG 72.4 (A) Lateral radiograph of a conscious bearded dragon (*Pogona vitticeps*) illustrating the continuous airway from external nares to trachea thanks to the close approximation of the larynx and choana when the mouth is closed. (B) Endoscopic view of the iguanid larynx illustrating the epiglottis (1), paired arytenoid (2), and cricothyroid (3) cartilages. The dorsal choanal opening (*) is also visible. (C) Endoscopic view of the larynx and pharynx of a leopard tortoise (*Stigmochelys pardalis*). The blue Cole endotracheal tube has been retracted to provide a better view of the arytenoid cartilages (white arrows) and the right Eustachian opening (red arrow), which has been catheterized with a red catheter (as part of a surgical resolution for bacterial otitis). (Courtesy of Stephen J. Divers.)

It can be either a single opening or a paired structure. Most chelonians have ridges, flaps, or papillae along the lateral choanal margins.[11] Crocodilians have a unique structure visible in its place, the basihyal valve and velum palate, which isolate the oral cavity from the nasal cavity, pharynx, and larynx when partly submerged.

Pharynx/Larynx

The larynx is the section of the respiratory tract connecting the pharynx to the trachea. Its primary function is to protect the lower airways by closing upon mechanical stimulation. It allows reptiles to breathe while consuming food. There is a complex skeletal, muscular, ligamental, and neurological relation between the larynx, tongue, glottis, and palate that allow swallowing, inhalation, and vocalization, which is beyond the scope of this section.[19,20]

The larynx is situated on top of the hyoid bone, which is technically not part of the laryngeal structure, yet without it laryngeal motion would not be possible. Typically, the larynx is made up of several cartilaginous structures—often including the thyroid cartilage, cricoid cartilage, and paired arytenoid cartilages. In most reptiles, including chelonians and crocodilians, the thyroid and cricoid are fused to create the cartilago thyreocricoidea or cricothyroid cartilage (see Fig. 72.4B and C). As the larynx lies on the corpus of the hyoid apparatus, this part of the hyoid of turtles and crocodilians assumes the functions of the mammalian thyroid cartilage. Some reptiles have a membrane at the tongue-base equivalent to the epiglottis; others have a cartilaginous structure, which aids in vocalization sounds. Crocodilians lack an epiglottis. Snakes have one of the most specialized laryngeal structures, with a muscular hyoid-type attachment allowing forward movement of the upper trachea (glottal tube) pulling the larynx forward. This allows breathing during a lengthy prey-swallowing process.[21]

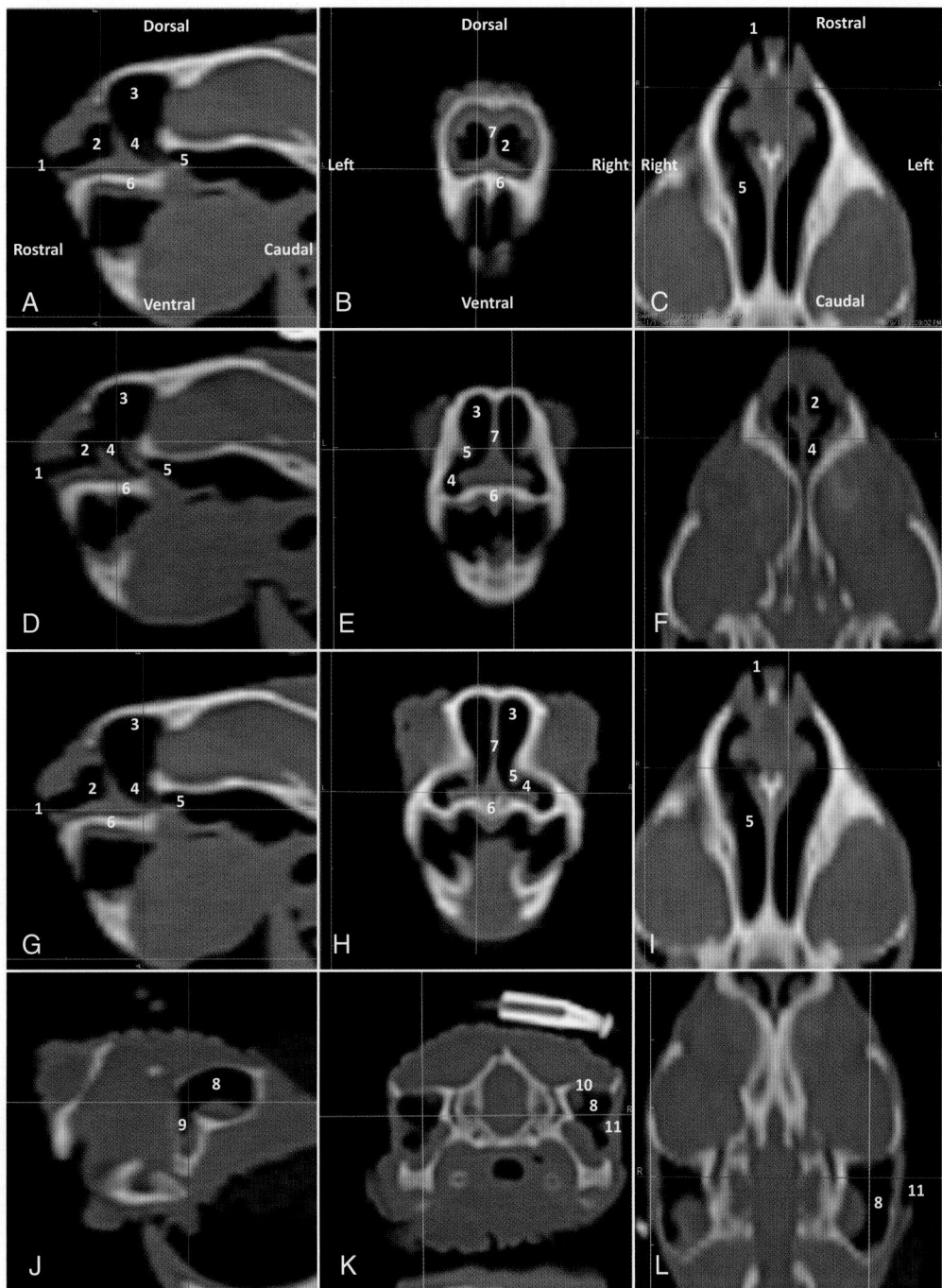

FIG 72.5 Skull CT of a desert tortoise (*Gopherus agassizii*, 0.6 mm slices, post-contrast bone algorithm, WW: +4000; WL: +400). Images A–C, D–F, and G–I represent corresponding sagittal (A, D, G), transverse (B, E, H) and coronal (C, F, I) planes through the skull. Yellow, purple, and blue lines indicate sagittal, transverse, and coronal planes, respectively; external nares (1), nasal vestibule (2), regio olfactoria (3), and regio intermedialis (4) make up the nasal cavity, choanal tube (5), palatine bone (6), and nasal septum (7). Images (J–L) represent corresponding sagittal (J), transverse (K), and coronal (L) at the level of the ear. Yellow, purple, and blue lines indicate sagittal, transverse, and coronal planes, respectively; also represented are the tympanic cavity (8), auditory or Eustachian tube (9), paraoccipital process (10), tympanic membrane (11). (Courtesy of Stephen J. Divers.)

GENERAL APPROACH TO CASE MANAGEMENT AND TREATMENT

The foundation for any successful case management is a thorough understanding of the clinical signs displayed. A detailed anamnesis will often identify anatomical areas that require further investigation, as well as understanding of the urgency and "aggressiveness" necessary in diagnostic and treatment planning. As many reptilian disease processes occur as a direct result of suboptimal husbandry, knowledge of individual species requirements is paramount, and detailed questioning into these conditions is necessary (e.g., temperature, humidity, ultraviolet lighting, daylight hours, air quality/draft, as well as feeding/dietary circumstances). See section 3 for further details.

During evaluation, care should be taken not to cause injury to the animal or the handler. Furthermore, many infectious agents are spread through the serous discharges produced in these body systems, hence appropriate protection and sanitation is necessary, especially when handling multiple specimens (see Chapter 42).

Clinical examination of the aural, nasal, and pharyngeal/laryngeal cavities should include inspection for symmetry and any pain response. All cavities should be free from lesions, discharges and swellings, parasites, and foreign objects. An oral inspection is necessary to evaluate the internal nares (choanae/choanal slit) as well as the pharyngeal space.

A complete blood count (biochemistry and hematology) may allow differentiation between an infectious and an inflammatory process as well as the overall function of vital organ systems. Such clinicopathologic data can be useful if general anesthesia or prolonged medical treatment is anticipated. Advanced diagnostic equipment has become available for aiding the investigation into these cavities, which are otherwise often difficult to impossible to evaluate antemortem.[22] Endoscopy, radiology, CT, and MRI facilitate visualization and sample collection for cytology, microbiology, or histopathology (see Fig. 72.6).

SPECIFIC DISEASES

Otitis

Generally, diseases of the reptilian ears are not extensive. Conditions that in other species would most certainly cause sequelae or noticeable behavioral changes caused by impaired hearing or balance do not appear to affect reptiles in a notable way. Congenital abnormalities have not been described.

Tympanic Protrusions. Aural polyps in the middle ear and aural-pharyngeal region of the green iguana (*Iguana iguana*) have been associated with cryptosporidial infections (Fig. 72.8B). The protozoan, commonly seen as a reptilian gastric pathogen, is not known to be part of the normal aural microflora in iguanas. Progressive protrusion of the tympanic membrane is typical, but anorexia and head swelling can occur. Histologically the masses consist of dense fibrous connective tissue with hyperplastic epithelium and mixed cells (heterophils,

lymphocytes, and plasma cells), with scattered ducts, cysts, and glands.[23,24] The lesions resemble the inflammatory, nasopharyngeal polyps located in the tympanic cavity or auditory tube of cats.[25] Transmission electronmicroscopy has been used to identify cryptosporidial trophozoites. It is unknown whether *Cryptosporidium* was involved in inducing the polyp formation or a secondary invader.[24] Data surrounding best-practice treatment are deficient. Surgical removal has been attempted, but recurrence has been reported.

Aural Abscess

Clinical significance. Aural abscessation is a condition characterized by an accumulation of caseous material within the middle ear or tympanic cavity, resulting in a protrusion of the tympanum (Fig. 72.9). The condition exists in both free-ranging and captive reptilian populations and is most commonly seen in chelonians (tortoises and semiaquatic turtles) as well as occasionally in lizards.[26–32] It is commonly encountered in private practice and, although usually not an emergency, should be addressed with promptness. During an active infection/episode or postoperatively there appears to be no notable vestibular or hearing-related sequelae.

Known etiological cause(s). No known cause has been identified. Aural abscess formation appears to be multifactorial and a result of several predisposing factors. It is generally accepted that there exists a correlation between abscess formation and improper husbandry (e.g., suboptimal habitat temperatures, poor hygiene) leading to

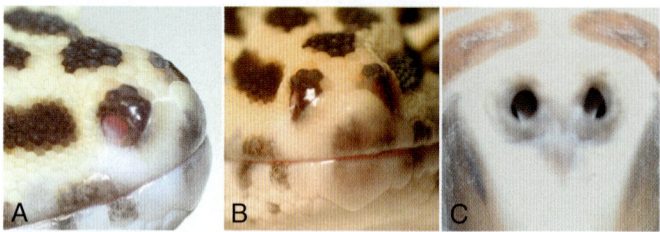

FIG 72.6 Normal external nares in a (A and B) leopard gecko (*Eublepharis macularius*) and (C) loggerhead sea turtle (*Caretta caretta*). (Courtesy of Stephen J. Divers.)

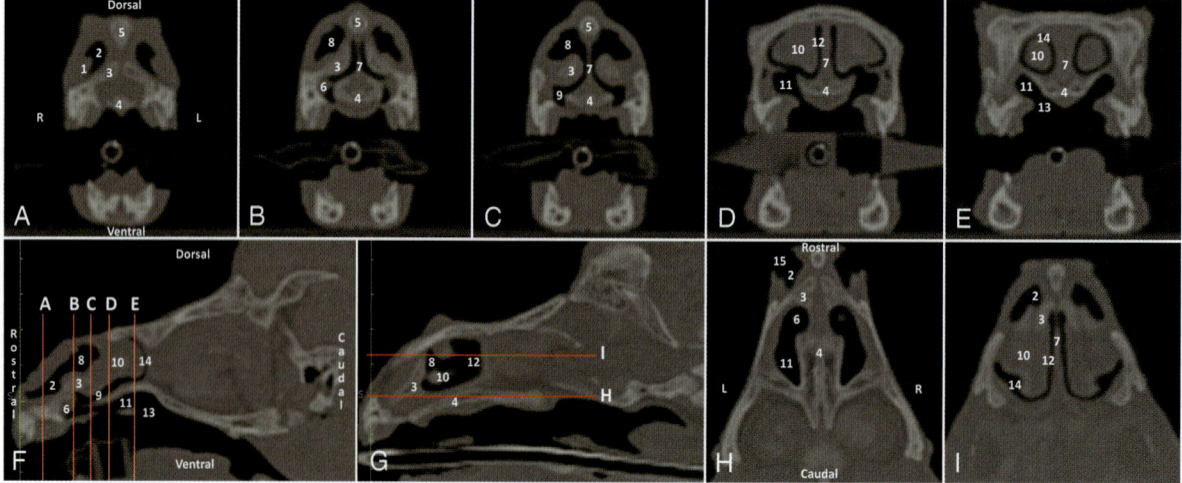

FIG 72.7 Computed tomography of the skull of a rock iguana (*Cyclura* sp.) demonstrating nasal anatomy (0.6 mm slices, post-contrast, bone algorithm, WW: +4000; WL: +400). (A–E) Cranial to caudal transverse sections demonstrating the alar fold (1), nasal vestibule (2), vomer bone (3), palatine bone (4), nasal bone (5), vomeronasal organ (6), nasal septum (7), supraconchal recess (8), subchonchal recess (9), concha (10), choanal tube (11), stammteil (12), orochoanal opening (13), caudal chonchal recess (14), and anterior or external nares (15). (F and G) Sagittal sections through the maxilla with red lines to indicate the level of transverse planes for images A–E, and coronal planes for images H and I, respectively. (H and I) Coronal sections through the maxilla. (Courtesy of Stephen J. Divers.)

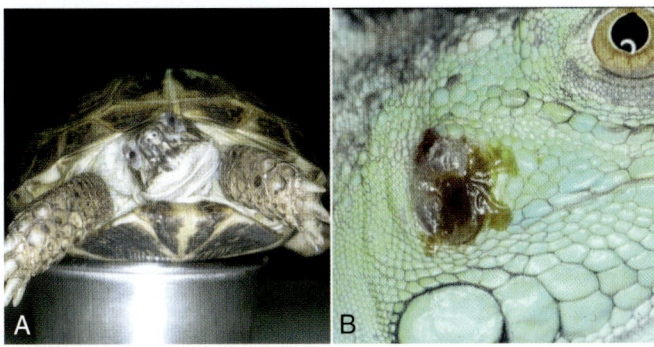

FIG 72.8 (A) Right-sided head tilt associated with otitis in a *Testudo* tortoise. (B) Otitis in a green iguana (*Iguana iguana*) due to cryptosporidiosis. (Courtesy of Stephen J. Divers.)

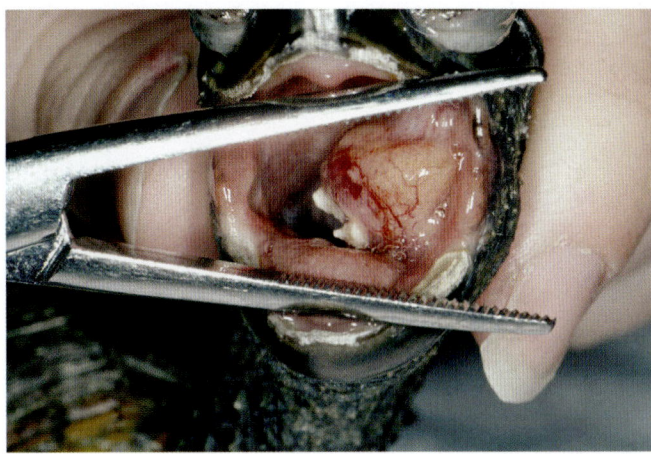

FIG 72.10 The Eustachian tube connects the middle ear to the oropharynx. Digital pressure on the tympanic membrane may force inflammatory debris through the passage into the pharynx. (Courtesy of Stephen Barten.)

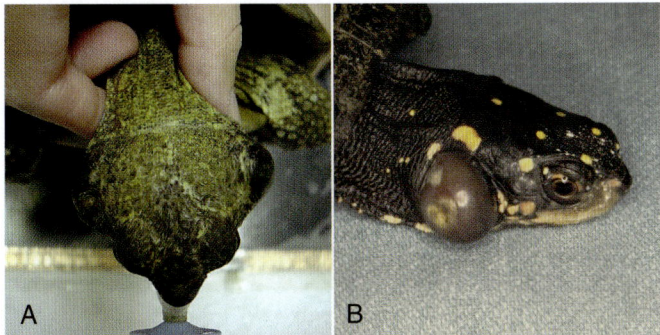

FIG 72.9 (A) Bilateral aural abscessation and otitis in a *Testudo* tortoise. (B) Unilateral aural abscess in a Chinese spotted turtle (*Clemmys guttata*). (Courtesy of Stephen J. Divers.)

immunosuppression as well as inadequate nutrition resulting in vitamin A deficiency.[32] Hypovitaminosis A causes hyperplasia and squamous metaplasia of epithelial tissues, including those of the pharynx, trachea, middle ear, and Eustachian tube, leading to an accumulation of exfoliated squamous cells and keratin-like debris within the tympanic cavity, which eventually results in abscess formation.[27,32–34]

This assumed relationship is supported by free-ranging Eastern box turtles (*Terrapene carolina carolina*) with pathological aural changes in association with organochloride-containing pesticides known to cause vitamin A metabolism disruption in other species.[33–36] However, other studies have been unable to induce tympanic squamous metaplasia and therefore experimentally could not replicate the correlation between abscess formation and organochlorine compounds in vitamin A–deficient red-eared sliders (*Trachemys scripta elegans*).[37,38]

The Eustachian tubes, connecting the oropharynx to the middle ear, may provide a pathway for ascending pathogens into the tympanic cavity, which in an immunocompromised animal may contribute to abscess development (Fig. 72.10). However, no consistent bacterial pathogen has been isolated, and most (mainly aerobic gram-negatives) are believed to be opportunistic commensals from the oral cavity.[27,31,39] Though less likely, hematogenous spread and traumatic etiology are possible.

The anatomical differences between the chelonian ear and other reptilian taxa may also be a factor in the increased incidence of aural abscesses in chelonians, as this condition is rarely seen in lizards that lack Eustachian tubes and snakes where the tympanic cavity is reduced to a narrow fissure.[1] Aural abscesses have never been reported in species lacking a tympanic cavity.

The absence of lysosomes (within their granulocytic leukocytes) in reptiles results in a caseous, inspissated pus. Histologically, cases range from mild squamous metaplasia and hyperplasia to more severe cases involving pronounced inflammation and osteolysis.[27,33,39,40]

Clinical presentation and diagnostic confirmation. The tympanic swelling(s) may present as unilateral or bilateral, semifirm to firm, and cause protrusion of the tympanic membrane rather than rupture. Caseous debris may be seen entering the pharynx through the Eustachian openings. Obvious vestibular signs are generally lacking, though head tilt can occur (see Fig. 72.8A).

Diagnosis can often be made solely by visual assessment. Additional tests may add therapeutic or prognostic value and can include fine-needle aspiration cytology (to aid differentiation from neoplasia and cryptosporidiosis) as well as hematology and blood chemistry to evaluate systemic disease involvement. Radiography and computed tomography may aid in determination of severity and appropriate management.[40]

Specific therapy. Surgical intervention is required (see Chapter 92 for details on surgery of the ear). Due to the avascular and inspissated structure of the abscess, it is easily manipulated out of the tympanic cavity in its entirety. Vigorous cleaning with a curette is not advised, as it may damage the structures of the middle ear (columella) responsible for sound conduction.[41] The deficit is lavaged daily to twice daily and the tympanum is often left to heal by second intention, though reports of successful outcomes from sutured tympanums do exist. Placing an irrigation cannula can assist frequent flushing, especially in uncooperative tortoises (Fig. 72.11). Antibiotics, particularly systemic, are seldom necessary. Vitamin A supplementation as adjunct therapy has been suggested; however, no scientific evidence exists confirming that supplementation alone will add relief to the condition. Furthermore, a risk exists in development of iatrogenic hypervitaminosis A if given parenterally (see Chapter 84). It is difficult to reliably diagnose a deficiency of vitamin A as blood levels generally remain stable unless liver stores are severely depleted.[42]

Prognosis and prevention. Complete excavation of aural debris, appropriate wound management, and correction of any concurrent suboptimal husbandry conditions results in a good prognosis. Recurrence does occur and is typically due to inadequate surgical debridement or failure to address the underlying predisposing factors.[32] Education with regard to appropriate husbandry, sanitation, and nutrition is beneficial for prevention.

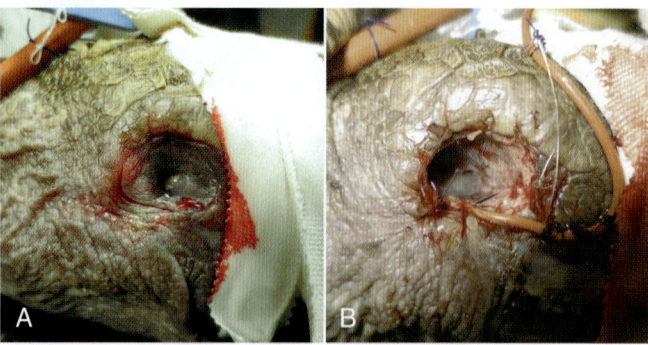

FIG 72.11 Aural ulceration and chronic otitis in a leopard tortoise (*Stigmochelys pardalis*), right lateral view. (A) The central ulcer is visible and an incision has been made around the tympanic membrane in preparation for surgical debridement. (B) Postoperative view demonstrating an irrigation cannula sutured in place to permit frequent flushing and topical therapy in this recalcitrant tortoise. (Courtesy of Stephen J. Divers.)

Rhinitis
Mycoplasmosis

Clinical significance. In general, respiratory mycoplasmosis in animal hosts is associated with chronic lower respiratory tract disease (pneumonia or pleuropneumonia) and can be accompanied by extrapulmonary manifestations, including synovitis/arthritis, otitis, and central nervous system sequelae.[43,44] In contrast, mycoplasmosis in turtles (also known as upper respiratory tract disease [URTD]) presents with clinical signs including nasal discharge, conjunctivitis, ocular discharge, and palpebral edema but not pneumonia.[45] Mycoplasmal infection can cause fulminant lethal sepsis and synovitis/arthritis in alligators and in experimentally infected caimans and synovitis/arthritis in crocodiles, and has been implicated in pneumonia in snakes.[7,46–51] *Mycoplasma* has been isolated from vertebral abscesses in green iguanas, but experimental infection studies were inconclusive as to the pathogenic potential.[52,53]

Mycoplasmosis is one of the most extensively characterized infectious diseases of free-ranging chelonians. Although a great deal of progress has been made to establish the etiology and distribution of the disease and the development of diagnostic assays, information is currently lacking with regards to the long-term effects of this disease within tortoise populations. Nearly catastrophic declines in desert tortoise (*Gopherus agassizii*) populations located in and around Kern County, California, that occurred in the late 1980s may have been associated with mycoplasmosis and contributed to the listing of desert tortoises north and west of the Colorado River as "threatened" by the federal government.[45,54] Similar morbidity and mortality events have been reported in gopher tortoise (*Gopherus polyphemus*) populations.[55–61] The extent to which mycoplasmosis is a contributing factor in these die-offs is presently unknown; however, many of these populations are the focus of extensive investigations attempting to determine the cause of increased tortoise mortality. Mycoplasmosis in virtually all animal species studied is typically characterized by chronic and life-long morbidity, with mortality observed during initial outbreaks or when stressors exacerbate the disease.[43,62,63] Therefore mortality events in wild populations are likely the result of synergism between the pathogen and external stressors such as drought and habitat degradation. Additional long-term studies evaluating mycoplasmal disease dynamics, influences on population demographics and individual tortoise survival, and anthropogenic influences on disease are critical for the development of sound, scientifically based management recommendations for free-ranging tortoises.

Known etiological cause(s). *Mycoplasma agassizii* and *M. testudineum* are recognized as distinct species and are the only confirmed, independent etiological agents of URTD in chelonians.[64–68] An unidentified but proposed third *Mycoplasma* sp. has been reported, in some cases in concert with clinical signs of URTD, in several members of the Emydidae family, most notably in *Terrapene* spp.[69–74] Mycoplasmas from the Emydidae family were not cultured and were identified only by partial 16S rRNA sequences that have 97% to 98% similarity to *M. agassizii*; however, based on the available GenBank sequences, Emydidae-specific signature mutations are present in the 16S rRNA gene.[70,72,73] Partial 16S rRNA sequences from members of the Geoemydidae also had 97% to 98% similarity to *M. agassizii*.[75,76] The PCR 16S rRNA sequence determined for members of the Emydidae and Geoemydidae ranged from only 15% to 66% of the gene with no clinical isolates obtained. Therefore it is unclear if these are new, but closely related, species or in fact *M. agassizii*. Clinical isolates will be required to fully address this issue.

Coinfections with herpesvirus and ranavirus have been reported.[70,77–79] Environmental stressors and concurrent infections with other bacterial and viral organisms may also be involved in the pathogenesis of this disease, as has been observed in mycoplasmal diseases affecting other host species.[62,80–83]

Although other microorganisms, including *Pasteurella testudinis*, iridovirus, herpesvirus and several fungal organisms have been isolated from tortoises with overlapping clinical signs; none have been demonstrated as independently resulting in URTD.[84–89]

Both *M. alligatoris* and *M. crocodylii* are confirmed as etiological agents of arthritis and pneumonia in Crocodylians; additionally, *M. alligatoris* is associated with multiorgan sepsis and mortality in alligators and caimans.[47,48,50,90–92] Although *Mycoplasma iguana* is generally considered pathogenic, the etiology has not been as rigorously confirmed.[52,53]

Experimental studies suggest that the primary route of transmission for mycoplasmas in both wild and captive tortoises is through direct contact, particularly when an animal is exhibiting a nasal discharge.[45,67,68,93,94] Vertical transmission occurs at a very low rate in mycoplasmal infections of poultry and is likely similar in chelonia.[94,95] It will be influenced by the time of infection in the female tortoise, the stage of oogenesis when the animal is clinically ill, and the virulence of the organism. In the wild, animals do not become seropositive until the age of sexual maturity.[61] Additional studies involving a large number of tortoises infected at different times during the reproductive cycle would be required to completely rule out vertical transmission in tortoises. Environmental transmission is unlikely in wild populations, since mycoplasmas lack a cell wall and are highly susceptible to desiccation in natural environments. In captive conditions, however, increased tortoise densities and higher loads of organic material could facilitate the persistence of the organism outside the host.

A *Mycoplasma* was isolated from a Burmese python.[49] Additionally, *Mycoplasma* sp. have been detected by 16S rRNA PCR and isolation from Boidae and Pythonidae snakes.[51] The clinical isolates appear to be new species, with only 90% reported similarity to *M. agassizii*; available GenBank sequences for Boidae and Pythonidae snakes were only 95% similar to both *M. agassizii* and *M. tesudineum* as well as to *Mycoplasma caviae*, a commensal of guinea pigs.[49,51] All cases presented as tracheitis and pneumonia; however, although these anecdotal reports are suggestive, the pathogenic potential and clinical significance remain unclear.[49,51]

Clinical presentation. URTD in tortoises is characterized by a rhinitis and conjunctivitis. Clinical signs, including nasal discharge, ocular discharge, palpebral and periocular edema, and conjunctival hyperemia and edema, may develop as early as 2 weeks postinfection (Fig. 72.12).[45,67,68,94] It is important to note that clinical signs may appear alone or in concert with other signs. The clinical presentation of URTD in tortoises is somewhat unusual in that tissue damage and disease

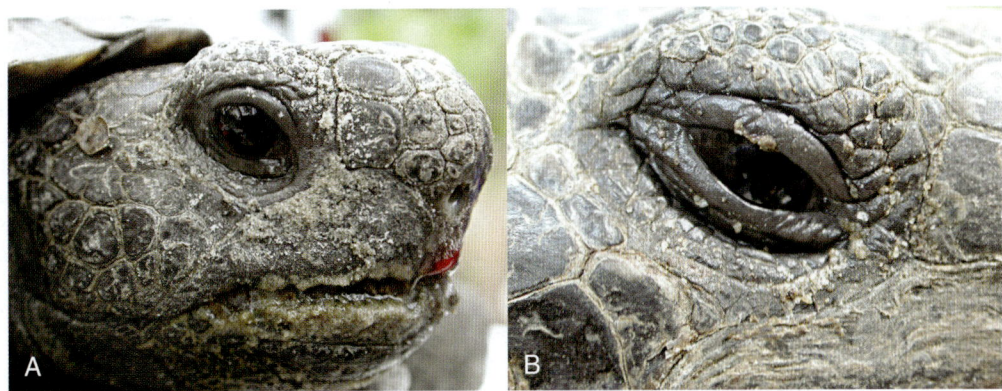

FIG 72.12 (A) A wild gopher tortoise (*Gopherus polyphemus*) with acute mycoplasmosis exhibiting a severe, hemorrhagic nasal discharge. (B) Gopher tortoise with conjunctivitis, ocular discharge, and palpebral edema due to mycoplasmosis.

appear localized to the upper respiratory tract. Mycoplasmal infections in other reptiles present primarily as pneumonia or arthritis.[47,48,52,91,92]

Experimental infection studies in gopher and desert tortoises suggest the following course of disease: (1) primary colonization of the upper respiratory tract with *Mycoplasma*; (2) host immune response to infection resulting in a reduction of *Mycoplasma* numbers and the development of clinical disease; and (3) progression to a chronic disease state where clinical signs and shedding of *Mycoplasma* occur intermittently. In chronically infected tortoises, it is typical for clinical signs to intensify and then abate cyclically.[45,75,94,96] Grooves extending ventrally from the nares, eroded nares, and depigmentation around the nares can be observed in tortoises that have repeatedly exhibited clinical signs (Fig. 72.13). Subclinical infections have also been documented; where the animal has a detectable serological response, histopathological lesions are present and *Mycoplasma* can sometimes be recovered on culture, but the tortoise does not exhibit overt disease.[45,85,94,96,97] Such tortoises could serve as a source of infection for naïve animals within the population or collection.

Decreased activity, irregular basking and burrowing behaviors, and reduced foraging have been documented in experimentally infected gopher and desert tortoises as well as a limited number of wild gopher tortoises.[58,98]

It is not certain which factors trigger the recrudescence of clinical signs in asymptomatic tortoises; however, environmental stressors have been shown to play a major role in mycoplasmal infections of other hosts.[44,63] Modeling of the impact of duration and time between recrudescent epizootic events suggested that the length of time between recrudescence events was a key component to minimizing adverse population impacts.[99] Anthropogenic factors such as habitat degradation, habitat destruction, and tortoise relocation, as well as climatic factors including drought or excessive rainfall, have all been suggested as potential influences that may result in increased morbidity and mortality in wild tortoises.[45,54,100] Increased tortoise densities, inappropriate temperature, and poor nutrition may all exacerbate mycoplasmosis in captive tortoises.

A specific antimycoplasmal antibody response develops and can be detected by 6 to 8 weeks after experimental infection.[67,68] The immune response generated may not be protective, however, and may in fact exacerbate the disease. In experimental studies, infected gopher tortoises that were challenged a second time with *M. agassizii* developed more severe clinical signs and had a more intense antibody response than from the initial infection.[45,94] This is consistent with the immunopathology associated with most mycoplasmal infections, where the host immune

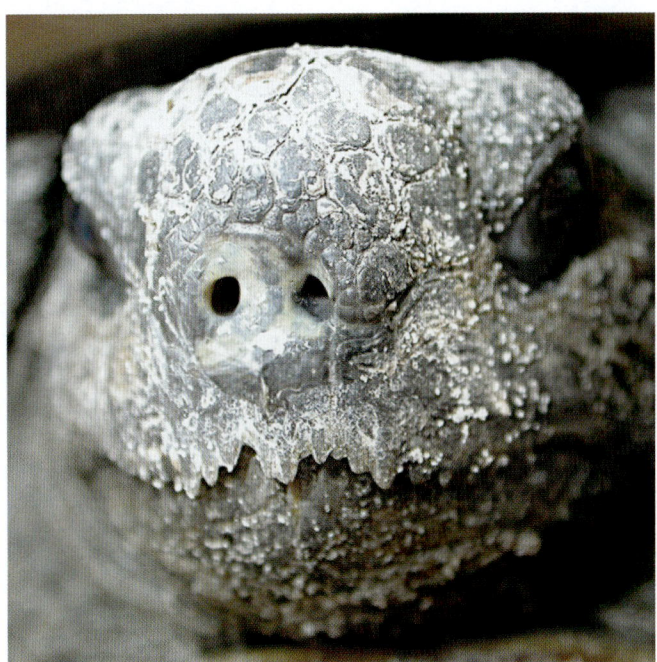

FIG 72.13 A wild gopher tortoise (*Gopherus polyphemus*) with severely eroded and depigmented nares. *Mycoplasma agassizii* was cultured from this individual.

response is a key contributor to disease severity.[63] Studies evaluating the role of the immune response in the pathogenesis of this disease are difficult because very little is known about reptilian immunology and the reagents needed for such investigations are limited.

Pathology. *Mycoplasma agassizii* adheres to the ciliated mucosal epithelium of the tortoise upper respiratory tract and causes severe disruption of the normal tissue architecture and function.[54,67,68,85,96] Gross, postmortem examination of infected animals may reveal no apparent clinical signs or a serous to mucopurulent nasal and ocular discharge, edematous and erythemic conjunctiva, and periocular and palpebral edema. Severely affected tortoises may have one or both nasal cavities completely obstructed with a thick, caseous discharge and varying degrees of nasal cavity erosion. Such animals may also have reduced coelomic fat or cachexia, thymus atrophy, hepatic hemosiderosis, and lymphocytic inflammation in the splenic sinusoids.[54,67,68,85,96] Histopathological lesions in the nasal cavity can also vary dramatically in severity and may include multifocal to focally extensive subepithelial lymphoid aggregates, a mixed inflammatory cell infiltrate consisting of heterophils, lymphocytes, plasma cells and macrophages, basal cell hyperplasia, mucous and olfactory epithelial metaplasia, and erosion of the ciliated epithelium.[54,67,68,85,96] Although *M. testudenium* can cause clinical signs of URTD, it does not appear to be as virulent as *M. agassizii* and the associated pathology and damage to the respiratory tract appears to be more focal and less severe.[45,101] In a study of 24 gopher tortoises, animals with URTD were more likely to have gram-negative bacteria isolated from their nasal cavity than tortoises without URTD, strongly suggesting that mycoplasmosis increases susceptibility to secondary infections.[96] This is consistent with other well-established mycoplasmal infections in mammalian and avian hosts.[63] Moribund tortoises with mycoplasmosis are often cachectic, have multisystemic disease, and death may be associated with secondary infectious, metabolic, or nutritional factors.[45,54,85,96]

For nonchelonian mycoplasmal infections of reptiles, pathology is primarily associated with the lower respiratory tract, joints, or sepsis-related multiorgan lesions. In naturally infected alligators, prominent findings included multifocal abscesses of the coccygeal and thoracic vertebrae, with degeneration of the spinal cord white matter, fibrosis, vertebral osteomalacia, and epaxial myofiber degeneration.[50,91] In lungs, airways, and small venules, a mixed inflammatory infiltrate of lymphocytes, plasma cells, and heterophils was present, typically extending into the adjacent connective tissue, which was often edematous with a similar inflammatory infiltrate. The bronchial epithelial lining was hyperplastic. Significant pericardial fluid and, in some cases, fibrinous adhesions of parietal and visceral pericardia were common, and the fibrin strands contained a mixed population of heterophils and lymphocytes.[91]

Although the etiological and clinical significance of mycoplasmosis has not been confirmed, tracheitis with concomitant pneumonia of suspected mycoplasma origin has been observed in snakes. Primary pathology attributed to *Mycoplasma* in snakes was proliferative lymphocytic tracheitis and pneumonia. Submucosal infiltrates consisted primarily of lymphocytes in the lungs and trachea, with heterophils seen in the trachea. Epithelial hyperplasia of airway mucosa with blunting or loss of cilia was observed in the respiratory tract, which is consistent with other respiratory mycoplasmal infections.[49,51]

Diagnostic testing and confirmation. Three diagnostic tests exist for the identification of *Mycoplasma* in reptiles: (1) direct mycoplasmal culture; (2) detection of mycoplasmal chromosomal DNA by polymerase chain reaction (PCR and qPCR); and (3) detection of antimycoplasma antibodies by enzyme-linked immunosorbent assay (ELISA). Each assay has strengths as well as limitations. The ELISA for tortoises has been extensively validated.[102] An ELISA is also available for *M. testudineum*.[101] ELISA tests for antibodies to other reptilian pathogens (*M. alligatoris, M. crocodylii, M. iguana*) have been developed, but these infections have not been widely studied so validation is limited.[46,103,104] Serological assays for other potential mycoplasmal pathogens of reptiles are not available. Therefore detailed information is provided here only for URTD diagnostics.

For URTD diagnosis, ELISA may not detect tortoises in the earliest stages of infection but is the most likely to detect clinically silent, intermittently shedding, and chronically infected animals. PCR/qPCR may detect animals in early stages of infection or those currently shedding *Mycoplasma*; however, false negative results can occur in chronically affected, intermittently shedding, or clinically asymptomatic animals or with inadequate sampling of nasal passages. Therefore optimal diagnostics include use of ELISA serology, culture, and PCR coupled with health assessment and observations for clinical signs, which may be intermittent or absent depending on the stage of infection.[45,102,105–107]

These assays have been widely utilized for epidemiological surveys and for captive tortoise management; however, certain features of mycoplasmal infections in tortoises and other species create a diagnostic dilemma. For example, more than one *Mycoplasma* species can cause similar clinical disease, but exposure to these mycoplasmas is not necessarily detectable with the existing serological test. Further, individual strains of a given species may vary in virulence but have overlapping serology. Therefore diagnostic results must be interpreted cautiously and in the context of the clinical picture for each patient.

Either tortoise serum or plasma can be used for ELISA. Numerous sampling techniques can be used to collect specimens for PCR/culture, including swabs of choana(e) or nares, direct aspirates of a nasal discharge, or flushes of the nasal cavity. *Mycoplasma* preferentially colonizes the ventrolateral depression of the tortoise nasal cavity, and this area is difficult to access in a live animal. Nasal flushes can be performed with 0.5 to 5.0 mL sterile saline or sterile PBS (phosphate buffered saline) or using 0.5 to 1 mL sterile SP4 broth. If saline or PBS is used for the nasal flush, enrichment of the flush sample with 10% sterile bovine serum albumin, horse or fetal calf serum, SP4 medium, or glycerol before shipping is recommended. Unless the animal is exhibiting a significant nasal discharge, swabbing or even flushing the nasal cavity may be uninformative and result in false negative results. However, some recent studies have used oral swabs for PCR with similar to higher effectiveness than nasal lavages.[93,105,107] This method of collection may be less stressful and easier to perform, but the swab should be taken as close to the choanal opening as possible. It is important that swabs are protected in sterile transport medium, *Mycoplasma* SP4 medium, 10% sterile bovine serum albumin, or sterile glycerol before shipping, especially if cultural isolation is desired.

Elisa. Specific antibodies to *M. agassizii* in tortoise plasma are detected using an enzyme-linked immunosorbent assay, or ELISA with a sensitivity of 0.985 to 0.983, and a specificity of 0.999 to 1.0. A positive ELISA result has been positively correlated with the presence of histological lesions as well as the presence of clinical signs, especially a nasal discharge.[45,55,57,61,96,102,105,108] The ELISA was originally developed and validated for gopher and desert tortoises; however, there is evidence that the monoclonal antibodies utilized in the assay do recognize immunoglobulins from numerous other tortoise species. As with other serological assays, the ELISA can be performed on plasma or serum, and results are reported as a titer. A single positive result indicates that the animal has been exposed to *M. agassizii*, but it does not confirm that the animal was actively shedding at the time of sampling. Because it takes a minimum of 6 to 8 weeks postinfection for antibodies to reach a level that can be accurately detected by the assay, false negatives are more likely in the early stages of infection. The ELISA positive predictive value drops below 90% only at a seroprevalence of <9%, and the negative predictive value drops below 90% at a >85% seroprevalence, making the ELISA particularly useful for population studies.[109]

The current ELISA uses *M. agassizii* whole-cell lysate antigens in the analysis. The specificity of the assay is based on the affinity and avidity of antibodies produced by the tortoise in response to infection by *M. agassizii*. Because other *Mycoplasma* species have been documented to share immunogenic antigens, there is a potential for limited cross reactions to occur in any serological test. However, sera from >1000 wild gopher and desert tortoises with documented isolation of the two pathogens had relatively few serum samples that reacted to both *M. agassizii* and *M. testudineum*.[101,102,109] Importantly, those samples that did react with both *Mycoplasma* spp. were from tortoises in populations with documented presence of both pathogens supporting that cross reactions are unlikely. As new species of *Mycoplasma* are isolated from tortoises, validation and standardization of serological assays will be required. Therefore the current ELISA assays may miss infections by other *Mycoplasma* species. This demonstrates the importance of interpreting diagnostic results in the context of the individual patient. If a tortoise with clinical signs consistent with mycoplasmosis has a negative ELISA result but positive PCR, and the complete 16S rRNA gene is <97% identical to that of *M. agassizii,* then infection with other mycoplasmal species that do not cross-react with the current ELISA must be considered. The culture and PCR tests discussed below may help clarify the clinical picture in such an animal.

Western blots. Western blot banding patterns obtained using a single strain (*M. agassizii* PS6) have been interpreted as being able to distinguish between uninfected tortoises with natural antibodies and exposed tortoises with acquired antibodies.[100,110] However, studies in swine, poultry, and ruminants document extensive strain variability and the necessity to use multiple *Mycoplasma* strains as antigens in Western blots in order to avoid false negatives.[111–119] The importance for using multiple strains of *M. agassizii* in a Western blot was confirmed using sera from culture-positive gopher tortoises with histopathological evidence of URTD.[109] When using heterologous strains of *M. agassizii* as antigens in Western blot, approximately 25% of proven URTD-positive gopher tortoises had binding patterns similar to those reported by Hunter et al. as natural antibodies; [110] however, all sera had strong banding patterns when the homologous strain was used as antigen.[109,110] Thus, Western blot analysis using a single antigen (PS6) failed to detect gopher tortoises known to have URTD, whereas an ELISA using the PS6 strain as antigen was strain independent and reliably detected all infected tortoises. The need for multiple strains in Western blot analysis, but not in ELISA, is consistent with findings for other *Mycoplasma* species.[113,119] The concept of natural antibody must also be considered in light of new findings that identified immunobinding proteins in *Mycoplasma* species.[120,121] Similar to other well-known immunoglobulin-binding proteins such as Protein A, a new immunoglobulin-binding protein (Protein M) that binds with high affinity to all types of human and nonhuman immunoglobulins, has been identified in mycoplasmosis.[121] At least one other system has been described in which a *Mycoplasma* immunoglobulin-binding protein binds to IgG from a wide range of hosts and a second Ig protease then is able to cleave off the VH domain of the bound IgG.[120] Interestingly, an immunobinding/blocking protein homolog is present in *M. agassizii* (SMC19080.1, GI: 1174984488) and could confound interpretation of Western blots. Therefore Western blots are recommended only as a confirmatory test and only if either multiple strains or the homologous strain is used as antigen. Further, appropriate diluents should be added to the reagents to minimize nonspecific binding to the newly recognized immunoglobulin-binding proteins. A Western blot assay has been used to identify immunoreactive proteins of *M. crocodylii* but not for other mycoplasmas of reptile origin.[122]

Culture. *Mycoplasma* is extremely fastidious and require very specific medium and growth conditions. Therefore use of a laboratory with experience culturing this organism and established quality control procedures is essential. Tortoise mycoplasmas (*M. agassizii* and *M. testudineum)* must be cultivated at 30°C and grow slowly, requiring up to 6 weeks for primary isolation in many cases.[64–66] SP4 medium is used for culture and can be obtained from the laboratories that provide this service or large-scale manufacturers (Remel Laboratories, Lenexa, KS). Colonies on agar are small and can only be reliably seen by 50× magnification. There is a color change to broth medium, but caution should be taken if turbidity is observed, as this indicates bacterial or fungal contamination. In direct contrast, both *M. alligatoris* and *M. crocodylii* grow rapidly, producing visible colonies and color change to broth medium within 24 hours.[47,90] *Mycoplasma alligatoris* does not grow above 32°C, whereas *M. crocodlyii* has an optimal growth temperature of 37°C.[47,90] *Mycoplasma iguana* was first isolated on blood agar after 4 days but grows best on SP4 agar with an optimal growth at 37°C.[52]

PCR. Testing using PCR has many advantages for the diagnosis of mycoplasmosis, including high specificity and rapid detection. All current PCR assays target the 16S rRNA gene. A positive PCR provides direct proof of the presence of mycoplasmal genomic material at the time of sampling. Important considerations for diagnostic tests targeting the presence of the pathogen are that the microbial load may be decreased when clinical signs are absent and that inadequate sampling of the upper respiratory passages may lead to false-negative results. Although contamination of samples by other organisms will not generally interfere with the PCR test, swabs containing calcium alginate may inhibit the reaction and thus should not be used. The conventional PCR uses primers that amplify virtually the full ~1440 bp 16S rRNA gene.[61,64,102] Many reports suggest finding novel species based on sequence coverage of 15% to 60% of the gene; caution should be used unless the majority of the 16S rRNA gene sequence is obtained or a clinical isolate is available for confirmation of species differences. For *M. agassizii* and *M. testudineum,* restriction fragment length polymorphism (RFLP) analysis of the 1400 bp PCR product using AgeI and NciI yields a unique pattern for each species.[64] In the event that an aberrant pattern is observed, complete sequencing of both strands of the 16S rRNA gene using a minimum coverage of reads obtained from two primers is recommended. The nature of the qPCR assay targets shorter regions of genes. The qPCR protocols for tortoise *Mycoplasma* target specific regions of the 16S rRNA gene and have the advantage of providing a quantitative assessment of gene copies.[105,123] However, the amplicons cover only a small region of the gene and may not detect strains of the pathogen or closely related species that differ in genomic content in that target region; therefore specificity should be assessed stringently. For example, full sequence of the *M. agassizii* clinical isolate from an Indian star tortoise (*Geochelonia elegans;* GenBank KY212533) showed that virtually all of its sequence differences occurred in one variable region, which was included in the target for qPCR assays. Finally, molecular techniques do not provide clinical isolates for further testing, including determination of antimicrobial sensitivity. Combining either conventional or qPCR with culture would provide optimal pathogen detection.

Specific therapy. Although being one of the most extensively researched infectious chelonian diseases, antimicrobial treatment recommendations are largely empirically derived or based on information extrapolated from what is known about mycoplasmal infections in other species.[124–126] Limited studies are available to inform dosage and drug delivery in reptiles.[30,127–146] Further, all of the listed treatment protocols are considered extralabel use because none of these chemotherapeutic agents have been specifically licensed for reptiles.

Anecdotal reports of *Mycoplasma* clearance after treatment with various protocols exist; however, differentiation between clearance and subclinical infections can be exceedingly difficult and limitations of the diagnostic assays and sampling techniques add additional difficulty. In a recent study, even long-term oral therapy over 3 months failed to clear *Mycoplasma* from subclinical tortoises.[76] Chronically infected animals may remain asymptomatic for years before clinical signs recur. Further, antibody titers may decrease, and cultures may be negative because *Mycoplasma* numbers may be below the detectable limits of the assay or in such low numbers that they are difficult to recover by nasal flushing techniques. Captive tortoises as well as snakes with suspected mycoplasmosis should be isolated and treated with appropriate supportive care and antimicrobials to alleviate clinical signs and decrease the risk of disease transmission.

Mycoplasma lack a cell wall, and therefore antibiotics targeting cell wall development will be ineffective. Antibacterial classes typically used to treat mycoplasmal infections in numerous hosts include tetracyclines, fluoroquinolones, lincosamides, macrolides, and certain aminoglycosides.[125,147,148] Most pharmacokinetic studies have only been performed with a single-dose administration using intravenous, intramuscular, subcutaneous, rectal, or oral routes of administration. In chelonians, pharmacokinetics are available for enrofloxacin in gopher, Indian star, Hermann's (*Testudo hermanii*) tortoises, and loggerhead (*Caretta caretta*) sea turtles; for marbofloxacin and danafloxacin in loggerhead sea turtles; for clarithromycin and tulathromycin in desert tortoises; and for oxytetracycline in loggerhead sea turtles.[129,134–137,139,140,144,149,150] For nonchelonian reptiles, pharmacokinetic studies have been performed for azithromycin in ball pythons; for enroflaxacin in alligators, crocodiles, Burmese pythons, bearded dragons, and green iguanas; for marbofloxacin in ball pythons and crocodiles; and for tetracycline and oxytetracycline in alligators.[131,138,141,145,151–156] Although limited minimum inhibitory concentration data are available for mycoplasmas of reptile origin, minimum inhibitory concentrations are available for *Mycoplasma* originating from other species using macrolide, tetracycline, and quinolone classes of antibiotics.[125,126,143,157] Tetracyclines should be considered the first-line drug while pending sensitivity results. Advanced drugs like enrofloxacin and clarithromycin have frequently and inappropriately been advocated, and resistance is likely to become an increasing issue. In one study, oral clarithromycin treatment for 3 months failed to clear *Mycoplasma* from all but one subclinical animal.[76] The long-lasting macrolide tulathromycin may provide an additional treatment option.[134] New delivery methods such as the osmotic pump may provide an alternative route of antibiotic administration for long-term treatment.[158,159] Given the immunopathology associated with URTD, topical antibiotic-corticosteroid combinations are often used in conjunction with oral or parenteral antibiotics to minimize the local inflammatory response.[45,133,142,158,160,161] Providing necessary supportive care in terms of hydration and nutritional support, as well as maintaining the tortoise in the upper ranges of the preferred optimal temperature zone (POTZ) for that species, will all improve the animal's response to treatment.

Table 72.1 lists the various treatment regimens for antimicrobials with efficacy against mycoplasmas that have been reported in reptiles (see Chapter 127 for more details).[45,127,128,132,133,146,158,161] With minor clinical disease, oral medications are generally initially used and topical therapies are added as necessary. Animals with severe disease may have reduced enteric absorption of drugs and should be administered parenteral medications. Topical ophthalmic drops or ointments containing antibiotics such as tetracycline, oxytetracycline, gentamicin, or ciprofloxacin applied to the eyes may minimize ocular signs and provide more rapid relief. Therapeutic nasal flushes using gentamicin/betamethasone, gentamicin/DMSO/saline, and enrofloxacin/saline combinations or nebulization using an enrofloxacin/saline solution have all been described.[45,128,132,142,146,158] A retrograde flush technique has been reported in tortoises that involves placing the animal in dorsal recumbency, stabilizing the head, opening the beak by applying continuous pressure to the chin, and flooding the choanae with the gentamicin/betamethasone solution.[45,142] The tongue is then used to expel the fluid by applying digital pressure to the intermandibular area, forcing the tongue against the choanae. Chemical restraint may or may not be needed to perform this technique. Alternatively, the solution can be applied directly into the external nares. Some clinicians anecdotally report that the corticosteroid-antibiotic nasal flushes performed every 48 to 72 hours may reduce recurrence of clinical disease; however, long-term oral treatment with clarithromycin did not eliminate shedding of *Mycoplasma* from subclinical tortoises.[45,76]

Prognosis. Inadequate data on reptiles other than tortoises precludes rigorous prognoses, but observed clinical pneumonia in snakes suggests that if left untreated, adverse outcomes might be expected.[49,51] Acute mortality has been reported but is exceedingly rare except for alligators, where the septic disease was lethal.[91] Acute arthritis has been observed in farmed crocodiles, with 10% morbidity but low mortality.[48] Mortality was more commonly observed in chelonian hatchlings during the initial

transmission studies.[94] Some tortoises may actually clear the infection, although this is not believed to occur very often.[68] Mycoplasmal infections involving other hosts usually are not cleared; however, numbers of *Mycoplasma* may be significantly reduced during chronic phases of infection when clinical signs are not exhibited.[44,63] Most tortoises develop chronic disease with intermittent expression of clinical signs. The bacteria persist in the nasal cavity and damage the mucosal tissue of the upper respiratory tract, resulting in increased susceptibility to secondary infections.[45,85,94,96] In cases of chronic mycoplasmosis, mortality is presumed to be due to severe debilitation and multisystemic disease.[45,85,94,96] Although not definitive, current data strongly suggest that the long-term effects of this disease may play a role in tortoise die-offs in selected populations, may shorten the longevity of individual tortoises, and may lower the reproductive potential of female tortoises, particularly if animals are sick during the reproductive season (Rostal et al Proc Desert Tortoise Council Symposium, 2001, pp 81–82, available at: https://deserttortoise.org/ocr_DTCdocs/2000-2001DTCProceedings-OCR.pdf).[94] This could result in profound impacts on the long-term survival of rare species.

The species or strain of *Mycoplasma* present in an individual or population is an important consideration when attempting to assess prognosis and develop appropriate management strategies. *Mycoplasma* in other hosts are known to vary in virulence, and preliminary evidence suggests that this occurs in reptiles as well.[67,94,162,163] Early transmission studies showed that different strains of *M. agassizii* differed in terms of the number of organisms required to colonize and cause disease.[67,94] Unfortunately, knowledge of the virulence potential is available for only a limited number of isolates. Therefore developing strategies to minimize risk from *Mycoplasma* in general is probably the safest approach. Actions taken will depend on the ultimate disposition of the animals and the risk to cohorts.

Prevention. Once a reptile has been diagnosed with mycoplasmosis, it is safest to consider that animal as persistently infected and a potential source of infection for other animals in the collection or population. In captivity, individual animals with confirmed mycoplasmosis should be housed independently from others, with efforts made to minimize the chance of cross-contamination using appropriate disinfection and sanitation protocols. Intermittent clinical disease can be treated periodically as discussed previously. Although the impact of this disease on overall longevity is unknown, many infected reptiles have continued to live and thrive for over a decade since their original exposure. However, the full impact of chronic disease in a long-lived species may take decades to become apparent.

Fomite transmission has been documented for other mycoplasmal infections.[164,165] Fomite transmission, particularly if equipment is contaminated with nasal exudates, should be considered possible in reptiles as well. Routine disinfection of all equipment using a 3% to 5% bleach solution or other appropriate commercial disinfectants will minimize the chance of cross-contamination.

Efforts should be made to separate eggs and hatchlings, as the hatchlings may be more likely to develop acute, fulminant disease. Further, keeping hatchlings separate may result in a noninfected group of animals. Managing a large group of infected reptiles will be significantly more challenging, as the presence of clinically ill animals within the same enclosure may exacerbate disease in the nonclinical animals, because those exhibiting a nasal discharge are more likely to transmit the organism. Empirical experience in the management of URTD outbreaks in group-housed tortoises, as well as standard infection control practices for other infectious diseases, suggest that the most effective management strategy is to separate the clinically ill animals for treatment. Isolation of ill reptiles for more intensive monitoring and treatment may help contain flare-ups. Ensuring adequate husbandry practices to minimize

TABLE 72.1 Drugs Commonly Used to Treat Mycoplasmosis in Reptiles

Drug Class	Dosage[127,132,142,146,158,189]	Notes
Aminoglycosides (bacteriostatic)		Aminoglycosides are potentially nephrotoxic, maintain hydration
Gentamicin	10–20 mg/15 mL saline solution: nebulize for 30 min q12h[133,142]	Chelonians
	40 mg/1 mL DMSO/8 mL saline solution: use for nebulization[132,142]	
Gentamicin/betamethasone ophthalmic drops	1–2 drops to eyes, q12–24h[133]	Chelonians
	Drops applied to external nares q12–24h[133]	
	Reverse nasal flush q48–72h: Drops applied to choanae and flushed-out nares as described in text[45,133,142]	
Gentamicin	1.75 mg/kg IM q4d[189]	American alligator
	10 mg/kg IM q2d[189]	Painted turtle
	6 mg/kg IM q25d[189,190]	Red-eared terrapin
	2.5 mg/kg IM followed by 1.5 mg/kg q96h[191]	Python
Tobramycin	10 mg/kg IM q24–24h[189]	Chelonians
	2.5 mg/kg IM q24–72h[189]	Most species
Tylosin	5 mg/kg/day IM[189]	Most species
Fluoroquinolones (bacteriocidal)		
Danofloxacin	6 mg/kg IM/SC q48h	Loggerhead sea turtles[136]
Enrofloxacin: IM injection likely causes necrosis, so using a single IM followed by oral dosing should be considered[189]	5–10 mg/kg IM q12–48h[132,138,140,141,145,150,152,156,157,189,192]	Most species, including chelonians,[140,150,192] crocodylia,[138,152] bearded dragons,[141] iguanas,[193] and snakes
Enrofloxacin	Nasal flush: 50 mg per 250 mL sterile water, use 1–3 mL for nasal flush per nostril q24–48h	Use with oral or parenteral antibiotics until no nasal discharge[146,158,161]
Marbofloxacin	2–10 mg/kg PO/IM/IV q24–48h[135,137,151,154,194,195]	Loggerhead sea turtles[135,137] Chinese soft-shelled turtle[195] Ball pythons[151,194] Freshwater crocodiles[154]
Macrolides/Azalide (bacteriostatic)		
Azithromycin	10 mg/kg PO q5d[131,158,189,196]	Ball python[131,196]
Clarithromycin	15 mg/kg PO q48–72h[144,158,189]	Desert tortoises[133,144,189,197]
	20 mg/kg PO q48–72h for 90 days[76]	Forsten's tortoise, Sulawesi forest turtles[76]
Tylosin	5 mg/kg IM q24h for 10–60d[132,133,189]	
Tetracyclines (bacteriostatic)		
Oxytetracycline	5–10 mg/kg IM q24h[132,133]	Tortoises
Doxycycline	5–10 mg/kg q24h PO[189]	Most species
	25–50 mg/kg IM[142]	Most species
	50 mg/kg IM, then 25 mg/kg q72h[149,189]	Hermann's tortoises[149]

Please note that the routine use of broad-spectrum antimicrobials like fluoroquinolones should be avoided in favor of first-line drugs like tetracyclines.

d, Day; *DMSO*, dimethyl sulfoxide; *h*, hour; *IM*, intramuscularly; *IV*, intravenously; *PO*, orally; *q*, every; *SC*, subcutaneously.

stress within the colony may also help decrease the frequency of clinical disease expression.

Determining the disposition of seropositive or culture/PCR-positive wild tortoises, particularly those that end up in rehabilitation centers, is problematic. There is presently inadequate scientific data to provide definitive guidelines for such animals. In some cases, state and federal guidelines exist that specify protocols for rehabilitation and repatriation of these animals. Often tortoises in rehabilitation facilities are exposed to other chelonians either directly by combined housing or indirectly in common grazing areas. Such practices could potentially expose tortoises to a myriad of pathogens and parasites that these animals would not normally encounter in the wild. Although *Mycoplasma* does not survive long outside the host unless protected in organic material, there are numerous other pathogens, viruses in particular, that persist for extended periods in the environment. Rehabilitated animals that are exposed to such circumstances pose a serious threat to wild populations when they are released.

Potential options that have been considered for the repatriation of tortoises with mycoplasmosis include the release of tortoises back to the exact site of origin; relocation to recipient populations with high prevalence of infection; and with resident tortoises that already express clinical signs of URTD, admission into captive breeding programs, adoption as pets, or euthanasia for animals showing severe morbidity.[45,106] Unauthorized relocation of URTD-positive gopher tortoises into a naïve population with subsequent mortality events has been documented.[55,61] Each of these options has inherent problems and no single solution is applicable for every situation. The unique circumstances of each population should be considered. The ultimate disposition of the animal will depend on the rarity of the species, the value of that animal to the population, the potential risk that animal poses to the population, and any existing regulations pertaining to that species. Certainly, decision making for such tortoises should be flexible and change as new scientific information becomes available.

Infectious Rhinitis (Excluding Mycoplasmosis). Discharges can range from clear serous discharge with bubbles to thick and mucoid (see Fig. 72.7A). Due to their position anterior to the oropharynx, stomatitis and pneumonia might also result in nasal discharge. It is important to distinguish nasal discharge from gastric reflux, as these have different causes and treatments. The long-nosed snakes (*Rhinocheilus* spp.) and dwarf boids (*Tropidophis* spp.) have been known to squirt blood from their nostrils as part of a defense mechanism (autohemorrhage); however, epistaxis is uncommon and should always be considered an abnormality that requires further investigation (Fig. 72.14A).[166] Metastatic mineralization of the nasal vasculature has been the cause of bleeds in green iguanas. Iatrogenic hypervitaminosis D$_3$ and hypercalcemia can result in mineralization of blood vessels, making them rigid and prone to rupture.

In addition to mycoplasmosis (mentioned previously), other agents identified in association with rhinitis include herpesviruses, ranaviruses, adenoviruses, reoviruses, intranuclear coccidiosis, *Pasteurella testudinis*, iridovirus, and chlamydiosis.[84–89]

Fungal infection and/or chronic upper respiratory tract disease may cause erosion or depigmentation of the nares (see Figs. 72.13 and 72.15C). Obstructive rhinitis usually occurs in conjunction with ulcerative stomatitis and/or bronchopneumonia and can be either uni- or bilateral, partial, or complete. The obstruction is most often caused by exudates, caseous material, and/or mucosal inflammation. This disease complex caused high mortality rates in hatchling and juvenile green turtles (*Chelonia mydas*) and loggerheads due to the inability to breathe and feed. The bacteria *Vibrio alginolyticus*, *Aeromonas hydrophila*, and *Flavobacterium* sp. were repeatedly isolated from cases of ulcerative stomatitis and obstructive rhinitis.[167]

Radiography and particularly CT can be useful for evaluating the nasal cavity, and sample collection for histopathology (or cytology) and microbiology cannot be overemphasized. Treatment should be based upon demonstration of a host pathological response and the causative agent. The routine use of advanced, broad-spectrum antimicrobials (e.g., fluoroquinolones, third- or fourth-generation cephalosporins) is not recommended.

Noninfectious Rhinitis. Noninfectious causes of nasal discharge include foreign bodies (e.g., grass awns or foxtails), congenital orofacial abnormalities (e.g., oronasal fistulae), or inhalant irritants. Some herbivorous, marine, varanid, and iguanid lizards can at times be seen with white, sometimes dried discharge surrounding their nostrils. This can be normal physiological excretion of sodium and potassium chloride crystals, produced by their nasal salt glands, but should, however, be differentiated from an upper respiratory or fungal infection.[17,18]

Complete or partial obstruction of the nare(s) can be attributed to various processes (Fig. 72.15B and D and Fig. 72.16C). Rhinoliths are seen infrequently, even in burrowing species where dirt could be an obvious nidus. However, on occasion, dysecdysis (retained shed) can occur within the nares, uni- or bilaterally (see Fig. 72.16B). This does not usually create a problem, unless allowed to accumulate over several sheds, causing obstructions. It is important to recognize that this may be an indication of an underlying condition and possibly caused by inappropriate husbandry. The retained shed usually dislodges on its own accord; however, it can be gently manipulated out, sometimes aided by moist cotton buds. If solidified within the cavity, a small hook

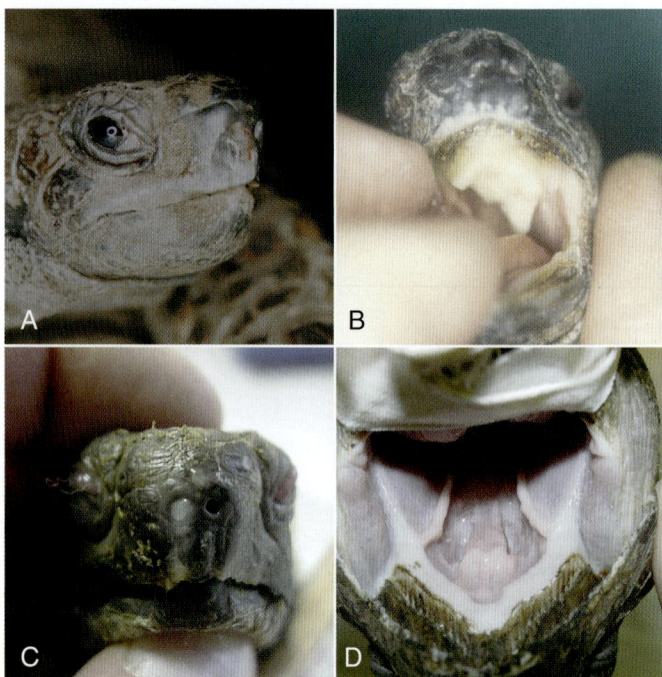

FIG 72.14 Rhinitis and related issues in chelonians. (A) Unilateral hemorrhagic, serous discharge from a Greek tortoise (*Testudo graeca*) associated with a nasal foreign body. (B) Inspissated infection associated with the choanae and choanal tubes in a Hermann's tortoise (*Testudo hermanni*). (C) Purulent nasal discharge associated with mycoplasmosis in a *Testudo* tortoise. (D) Choanal hyperplasia in a gopher tortoise (*Gopherus polyphemus*) is often associated with chronic rhinitis, including mycoplasmosis. (Courtesy of Stephen J. Divers.)

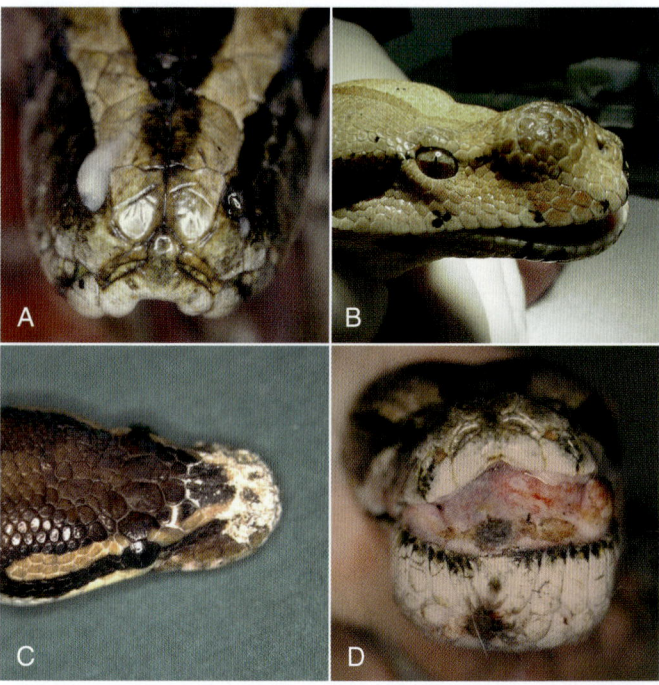

FIG 72.15 (A) Unilateral nasal discharge in a Burmese python (*Python bivittatus*). (B) Nasal abscess in a boa constrictor (*Boa constrictor*). (C) *Fusarium* sp. infection around the external nares of a ball python (*Python regius*) with extension of infection into the nasal vestibule. (D) Rostral lymphosarcoma in a Burmese python, causing local destruction and compression of nasal structures. (Courtesy of Stephen J. Divers.)

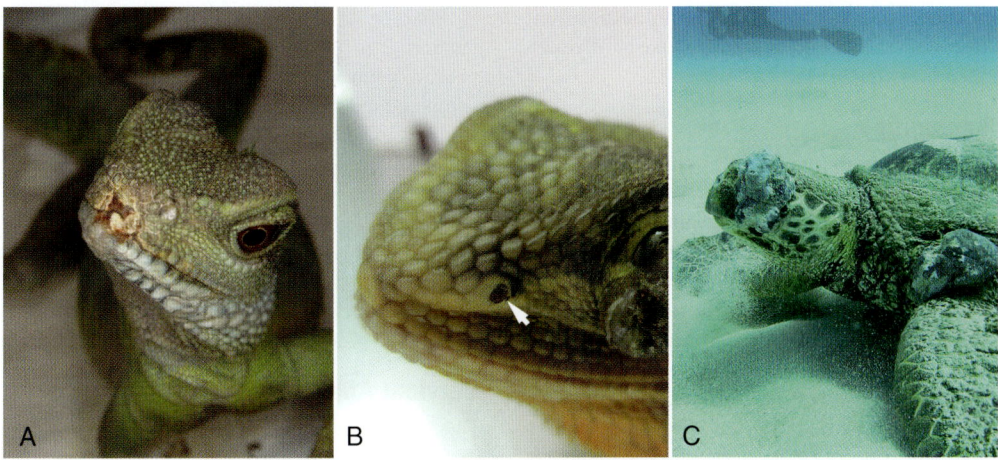

FIG 72.16 (A) Rostral trauma, as seen in this Chinese water dragon (*Physignathus cocincinus*), can result in damage to the external nares. (B) Dysecdysis resulting in nasal obstruction (arrow) in this bearded dragon (*Pogona vitticeps*) was probably associated with debilitation secondary to the lower palpebral squamous cell carcinoma. (C) A large fibropapilloma obstructing the left external nares in a loggerhead sea turtle (*Caretta caretta*). (Courtesy of Stephen J. Divers.)

instrument or forceps can be used, but care should be taken not to traumatize the surrounding tissues. No further local treatment should be necessary.

Foreign bodies or discharge can easily lodge in the choanal slit (see Fig. 72.14B). Not infrequently will lizards present with abnormal mouth movements or mucoid discharge from mouth and/or nare(s). Bearded dragons appear overrepresented, and most often ingesta is the culprit and detected on clinical examination of the oral cavity. Among others, inflammation, petechiae, and icteric changes may also be noted on clinical examination of the choanal region (Fig. 72.17).

Sea turtles have been described with both a plastic straw and a fork occupying this space.[168,169] Removal was done in situ with pliers using forceful retraction and cleaned with a betadine solution before immediate release. It is believed that a fork was ingested, and thereafter regurgitation resulted in the fork entering the choana and lodging within the nasal turbinates. This highlights the importance of a thorough clinical examination and the use of appropriate imaging modalities (radiography, MRI, CT). It is also a site for fish-hook trauma in aquatic and semiaquatic species. Endoscopic evaluation and retrieval may be useful in larger reptiles. Rhinoscopy is invaluable in the investigation of the narrow nasal passage and cavity.

Rostral trauma, as a result of excessive rubbing or striking against enclosure sides, is not uncommon in captive amphibians and reptiles (see Fig. 72.16A). Fast-moving and fractious animals are at greater risk of injury, hence water dragons (*Physignathus* sp.), bearded dragons (*Pogona* sp.), and terrestrial snakes appear overrepresented. Mature male snakes housed near mature female snakes during the breeding season will commonly damage the rostral area by excessive attempts to "push out" of their enclosure, presumably in response to pheromones. Enclosure overcrowding, conspecific mismatch causing flight behavior, inappropriate caging, and inadequate furniture/enclosure design are primary causes.

The injuries span from superficial, self-limiting abrasions to damage so extensive that the external nares suffer long-term disfigurement and/or physiological consequences. Damage to the rostral area often leads to disruption of air movement through the nares, which results in open-mouth breathing. This results in drying of the oral mucosa, making it more susceptible to secondary infections, which may lead to nasal obstruction, stomatitis, and osteomyelitis, with loss of or even fractures of the maxillary bone.[170] Although challenging, due to the anatomical

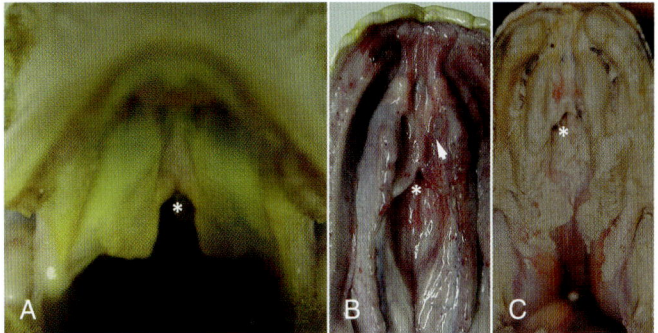

FIG 72.17 (A) Icteric appearance of the choanal mucosa in a bearded dragon (*Pogona vitticeps*) with severe hepatopathy. (B) Petechial hemorrhage and inflammation of the choana and surrounding mucosa in a Burmese python (*Python bivittatus*), with blockage of the left lacrimal duct (*arrow*). (C) Severe caseous, bacterial infection of the choana in a boa constrictor. The choanal opening in all three images is denoted by an asterisk (*). (Courtesy of Stephen J. Divers.)

restrictions surrounding the rhinarium, repairing the tissues to allow patency of the nares is critical to success (see Chapter 93). Inability to create nasal patency may result in the animal becoming an obligate mouth breather. Some affected animals may become anorectic, presumably due to interference with olfaction and may need nutritional support. Once lesions are established they should be treated immediately and aggressively. Daily to twice-daily flushing using topical antiseptics is essential (e.g., dilute chlorhexidine or betadine or saline-containing antimicrobials). Topical ointments may be considered (e.g., Manuka honey, silver sulfadiazine, antibiotic ointments) and if necessary adjunct systemic antibiotic therapy; however, these are no substitutes for accurate surgical debridement and reconstruction. Stress to the animal must be considered when determining the frequency of these treatments.

Prevention, or limitation, of rostral trauma can often be accomplished by husbandry changes, either directly, relating to the choice of specimens housed together (i.e., quantity, gender, age, size), or in enclosure design (i.e., adequate and species-appropriate furniture, removal of materials such as metal screens or "invisible" glass barriers). Although prohibited in most countries, feeding live prey can also result in significant rostral trauma, as reptiles, snakes especially, will repeatedly strike hard/rough surfaces before apprehending prey.

Laryngitis and Pharyngitis

Laryngeal swelling and laryngitis are not uncommon; however, they usually occur in conjunction with other clinical signs (Fig. 72.18). A pharyngitis/laryngitis/conjunctivitis syndrome has recently been described in Australian farmed saltwater crocodiles (*Crocodylus porosus*), primarily hatchlings and juveniles.[171,172] In severe lesions there were frequently mixed gram-negative and -positive bacteria, as well as occasional hyphae in the necrotic exudates. PCR detected (a 55% prevalence of) *Chlamydia* spp. and (of these, 81% also harbored) a concurrent herpesvirus infection. There was a poor response to trialed treatments, with further research needed to identify the specific causative agent(s) and etiology. Crocodiles were prone to starvation and susceptible to laryngeal obstruction by fibrinous exudate due to their anatomical features (including the gular seal and their inability to cough). High mortality rates were common.[171]

Multifocal necrotizing ulcerative pharyngitis, with concurrent extensive tracheitis, pneumonia, and esophagitis, was seen in a gopher tortoise (*Gopherus polyphemus*). On transmission electron microscopy, intracytoplasmic viral particles were morphologically resembling an *Iridovirus*.[89] A similar respiratory syndrome involving pharyngitis, sinusitis, stomatitis, tracheitis, and a proliferative interstitial pneumonia with caseous material in the choana in ball pythons (*Python regius*) has been attributed to a novel *Nidovirus*.[173]

Rhabdias spp., nematode lungworms with a direct life cycle, are a common cause of respiratory infections in captive anurans. Eggs or first-stage larvae may sometimes be detected in oropharyngeal mucus. Several trematode species have been found in the oropharynx of frogs and toads, although clinical infections rarely arise from these infections.[174]

Myiasis is well known in wild amphibians (toads, frogs, salamanders) where the larva of two fly species, *Bufolucilia*, parasitize the nasal passages and cause extensive destruction of the mucosa, often leading to fatality.[175] Pharyngeal myiasis with the sarcophagid flesh fly larvae (Diptera) has been reported in two common ameivas (*Ameiva chrysolaema*).[176] And larval ascarids (presumed *Hexametra* sp.) has caused severe purulent, abscess-forming pharyngitis in the green-striped tree dragon (*Japalura splendida*) concurrently infected with multiple viruses.[177]

Pharyngeal and Submandibular Edema and Cellulitis

Swelling of the mandible can become so extensive, it interferes with normal breathing and swallowing mechanisms (Fig. 72.19A and B).

Pharyngeal edema has been associated with renal disease in green iguanas. It is not uncommon due to hypoproteinemia, secondary to protein-losing nephropathy.[178] It is relevant to note that a presenting complaint may be dysphagia due to laryngeal/pharyngeal extra-luminal compression. Edema of the pharyngeal submucosa in combination with nasal mucosa ulceration, hepatic necrosis, and severe necrotizing inflammation was documented in green pythons (*Morelia [Chondropython] viridis*) as a result of ranavirus infection.[179]

Some Old World chameleons have an accessory lung lobe projecting from the anterior trachea. It can appear as a swelling of the ventral cervical region if it becomes filled with fluids, parasites, or inflammatory exudates. Its function is not fully understood.

Cervical Aneurysm

Dissecting aneurysms, or pseudoaneurysms, arising from the internal carotid artery or the aorta are not uncommon in adult bearded dragons but have also been reported in a green iguana and Burmese python (see Fig. 72.19C).[180] The clinical presentation in these cases was a large unilateral fluctuant to firm swelling on the dorsolateral neck or dorsal to the temporal muscles. Affected animals behave and forage normally unless the structure becomes a physical encumbrance. Aspiration yields whole blood and immediately refills after draining. In chronic cases, the blood may coagulate and cannot be aspirated. Doppler ultrasonography, radiography, CT, and MRI have been performed in preparation for surgical treatment.[181] Surgical removal is extremely challenging, but one successful surgical case has been anecdotally reported (Barten et al, Proc ARAV, 2006, pp 43–44). The etiology of the syndrome is unknown; trauma, hypertension, or genetic predisposition are possible.

Laryngeal Paralysis

A laryngeal paralysis-like condition was observed in a loggerhead sea turtle.[182] Stertorous upper airway sounds were caused by a partial airway obstruction due to unilateral laryngeal paralysis—similar to that seen in dogs. MRI, CT, and electromyography revealed abnormalities of the

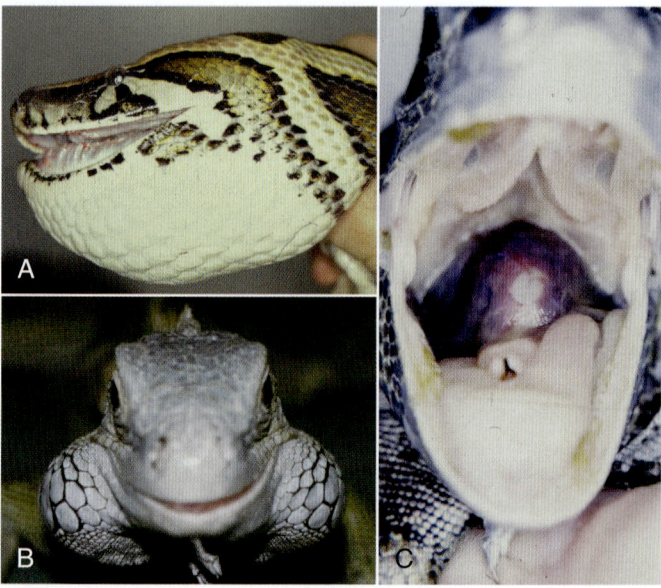

FIG 72.19 (A) Submandibular and cervical bacterial cellulitis in a Burmese python (*Python bivittatus*). (B) Bilateral fibrous swellings of the mandible secondary to nutritional secondary hyperparathyroidism, which interfered with swallowing. (C) Cervical aneurysm and edema in a green iguana (*Iguana iguana*) protruding into the esophagus and oropharynx. (Courtesy of Stephen J. Divers.)

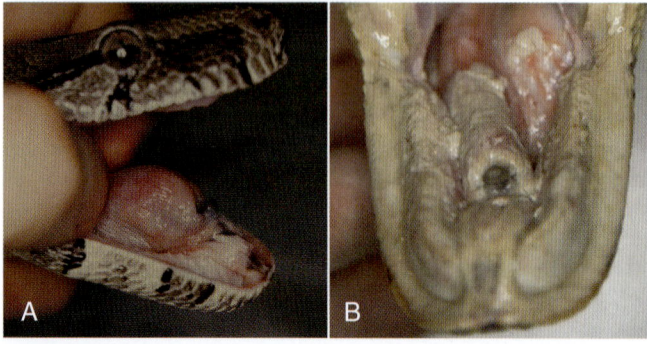

FIG 72.18 Laryngeal disease in two boa constrictors (*Boa constrictor*). (A) Laryngeal swelling and (B) bacterial laryngitis with generalized stomatitis. (Courtesy of Stephen J. Divers.)

abductor arytenoideae or dilator laryngis muscle.[19,182,183] Hepatic and muscle biopsies were collected for histological and toxicological assessment, which showed unilateral myofiber atrophy as the predominant histological finding. The etiology was unknown, however, but suspected to be related to denervation atrophy. Iatrogenic cause from topical lidocaine to the glottis could not be excluded, though no other reports of this adverse effect exists (to the authors' knowledge).

Neoplasia

Primary neoplasms do not commonly originate from the ear, nose, or throat region of reptiles or amphibians. As with other swellings or growths, they should be systematically approached with aspiration cytology or, better still, biopsy histopathology before considering the most appropriate medical and/or surgical plan. Neoplasms are more frequently encountered in snakes, followed by lizards, chelonians, and crocodilians.[184,185] Lymphoma (with secondary infection) was diagnosed in the cranial cervical area of a green iguana and was diagnosed through histology and microbiology. Successful remission was achieved with a multimodal radiation and chemotherapy.[186] An incisional biopsy of a mass in the caudoventral pharyngeal region of a Madagascar ground boa (*Boa madagascariensis*) was confirmed as a squamous cell carcinoma. CT and MRI was performed to evaluate tumor invasion and planning for radiation therapy; however, therapy resistance was evident and the snake euthanized.[187] Thyroid adenoma in a green iguana presented as a ventral cervical mass and was successfully removed.[188]

Neoplasms originating from the nasal epithelium/mucosa are rare. One report of a well-differentiated esthesioneuroepithelioma of the olfactory epithelium (olfactory neuroblastoma) with involvement of the vomeronasal organ (Jacobson's organ) was diagnosed on histology in a blue-tongued skink (*Tiliqua scincoides*) (Zwart et al, Proc EAZWV and EWDA, 2002, pp 81–84). However, growths originating in adjacent organ systems can impede on the structures of the ear, nose (see Fig. 72.15D), and throat as seen with fibropapillomas in sea turtles (see Fig. 72.16C).

REFERENCES

See www.expertconsult.com for a complete list of references.

73

Gastroenterology—Oral Cavity, Esophagus, and Stomach

Ryan De Voe

Just about every imaginable feeding strategy is employed by members of the class Reptilia, with carnivores, herbivores, omnivores, and a variety of specialized feeders represented (Fig. 73.1). As expected, there is tremendous variation in gastrointestinal anatomy and physiology. Lack of knowledge of these differences and how they affect husbandry, captive nutrition, and medical management can significantly limit a clinician's ability to provide effective care. It is impossible for even the most knowledgeable reptile veterinarian to be familiar with all possible variations of anatomy and physiology. Therefore the interested clinician should become intimately familiar with the anatomy and feeding strategies of commonly seen species. When unfamiliar species are presented, the clinician should recognize the need to research specific information regarding gastrointestinal anatomy and function or at the very least extrapolate from what is known about a similar species.

ANATOMY AND PHYSIOLOGY

One of the most important features of reptilian gastrointestinal physiology is the effect of ectothermy. Many of the unique adaptations revolve around the ectotherm's ability to efficiently process calories. Similarly sized reptiles, birds, or mammals have extremely different caloric and nutrient requirements to function and grow. Though variation occurs between taxa, in general, reptiles use approximately 10% the energy of mammals and birds with comparable feeding strategies and niches.[1,2] Some species of reptiles eat infrequently in nature; others will forage/graze and eat frequently but can often survive extended periods of anorexia without suffering the acute consequences that would be encountered in most mammals or birds. Understanding the feeding ecology of a species in the wild is paramount for maintaining them in captivity.

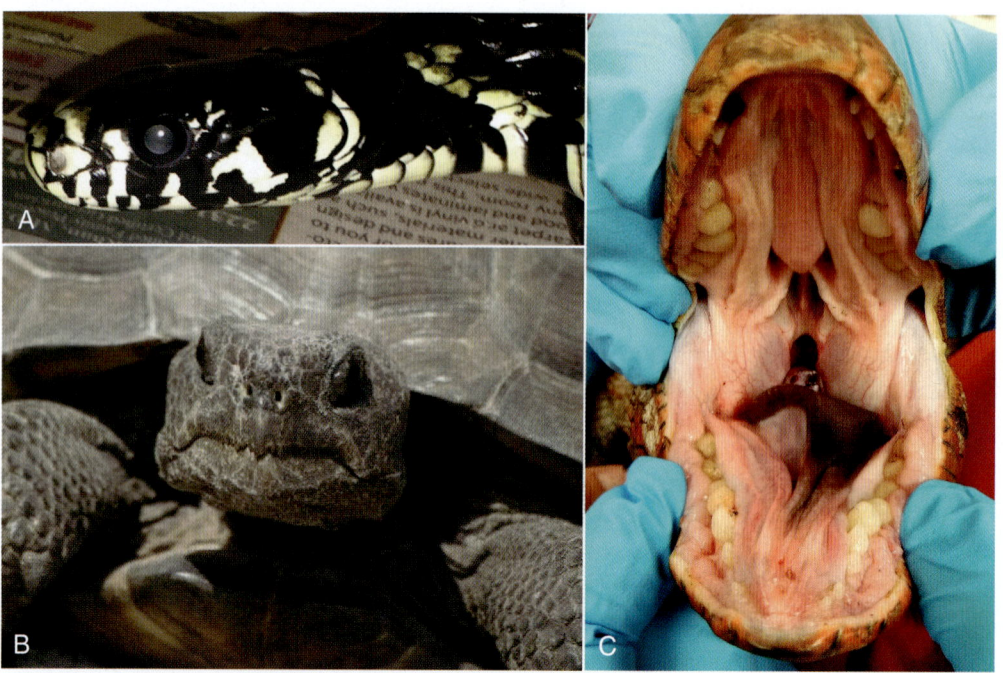

FIG 73.1 Many different feeding strategies are represented in the class Reptilia. As examples, snakes are exclusively carnivorous, some tortoises are grazing herbivores, and caimen lizards are specialized mollusk feeders: (A) tiger rat snake (*Spilotes pullatus*), (B) gopher tortoise (*Gopherus polyphemus*), and (C) caimen lizard (*Dracaena guinanensis*). (Courtesy of K. Ranos.)

Diseases of the gastrointestinal tract are relatively common in reptiles. Both primary gastrointestinal disease and dysfunction secondary to other disease processes and husbandry deficiencies are encountered.

Oral Cavity

The anatomy of the reptilian oral cavity varies dramatically according to taxa. Squamates have lips that protect the gingiva and teeth. Lizards typically possess two maxillary and two mandibular dental arcades, whereas snakes have two additional palatal arcades for a total of six arcades (Fig. 73.2). The vomeronasal organ is located in the rostral maxilla. In the roof of the mouth, snakes and lizards have a choana in which the tubular larynx sits when the mouth is closed. The lingual structure varies drastically in different species of lizards. Some lizards, such as chameleons, have specialized tongues and hyoid apparatus for capture of prey from a distance, whereas others have fleshy tongues in a form similar to that of mammals. Varanid lizards and snakes have specialized telescoping, forked tongues with keratinized epithelium that are used for collection and delivery of scent particles to the vomeronasal organ. The forked tongue facilitates tracking of prey scent trails.[3]

The dentition of squamate reptiles also shows great anatomical diversity. Lizards possess either acrodont or pleurodont dentition. With acrodont dentition, the teeth are fused to the maxillary and mandibular ridges. With advanced age, the teeth of some lizards with acrodont dentition may become worn down to the point where only the bony ridges of the mandibles and maxillae remain. Agamid lizards, such as bearded dragons (*Pogona vitticeps*), and chameleons possess acrodont dentition. With pleurodont dentition, the replaceable teeth are seated in grooves on the medial aspect of the maxilla and mandibles. Iguanid lizards have pleurodont dentition (Fig. 73.3). Snakes are considered to have modified pleurodont dentition, and teeth are constantly shed and replaced throughout life. Snake dentition is further defined according to the presence of fangs and, when present, venom delivery systems. Aglyphous snakes do not have specialized fangs for venom delivery and represent many of the nonvenomous species frequently kept in captivity. Solenoglyphous snakes are the viperids, which have hollow fangs. These fangs are mobile and lie folded against the roof of the mouth when not in use. Proteroglyphous snakes are the elapids; the fangs are fixed in

an erect position. Opisthoglyphous snakes are rear-fanged venomous snakes, where the fixed erect fangs are typically found at, or caudal to, the level of the eye.[3]

Lizards have numerous mucous glands as well as labial, lingual, sublingual, palatine, and dental salivary glands. Snakes are similar but do not possess dental salivary glands.[4] Lizards and snakes are capable of producing copious amounts of saliva and mucous in the oral cavity, which lubricates food items for swallowing.[5] There are specialized oral glands in the various venomous species, including the labial venom glands of helodermatid and varanid lizards[6] and the venom glands of some snakes, which are associated with the maxillae.[4,7]

Chelonians possess keratinized beaks instead of lips and teeth. Most chelonians have broad, fleshy, relatively mobile tongues. Some aquatic turtles, such as alligator snapping turtles (*Macrochelys temminckii*), have lingual appendages that mimic worms that they use to bait prey. Other chelonians that specialize in eating crustaceans and mollusks have keratinized palatal plates that are used for crushing the shells of the prey. Chelonians also have a tubular glottis and palatal structure similar to that of avian species.[3]

Crocodilians have no lips and the teeth are exposed when the mouth is closed (Fig. 73.4). The tongue in crocodilians fills the entire intermandibular space and is immobile, being firmly attached ventrally. A palatal fold arises from the base of the tongue and can effectively seal the pharyngeal region so the crocodilian can open its mouth and prehend food without introducing water to the pharynx. The laryngeal opening is found just caudal to the palatal fold and is similar in appearance to that of mammals, albeit with a much reduced epiglottis. Crocodilians possess thecodont dentition, in which the teeth are seated in sockets in the maxilla and mandibles similar to what is seen in mammals. Thecodont teeth are replaced throughout the life of the animal.[8]

Esophagus

The structure of the reptilian esophagus varies across taxa but is generally similar to that of mammals. The esophagus is variably distensible and typically has longitudinal folds extending the entire length. The esophagus of snakes is quite distensible and relatively longer than that of other taxa. In snakes, the stomach may be too small to completely accommodate a large prey item or items, therefore the esophagus may assist in food storage. Reflux of digestive enzymes may allow digestion

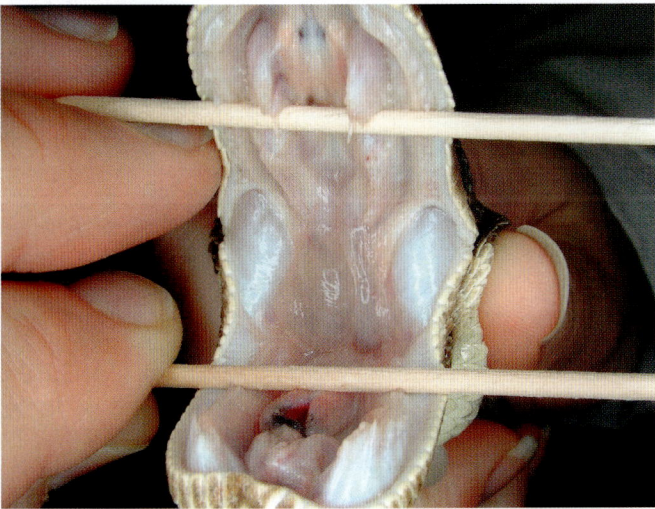

FIG 73.2 Snakes have palatine dental arcades in addition to mandibular arcades. Several teeth in this palatine arcade are hooked on a wooden tip applicator during the oral examination of this boa (*Boa constrictor* sp.). (Courtesy of Scott J. Stahl, Stahl Exotic Animal Veterinary Services.)

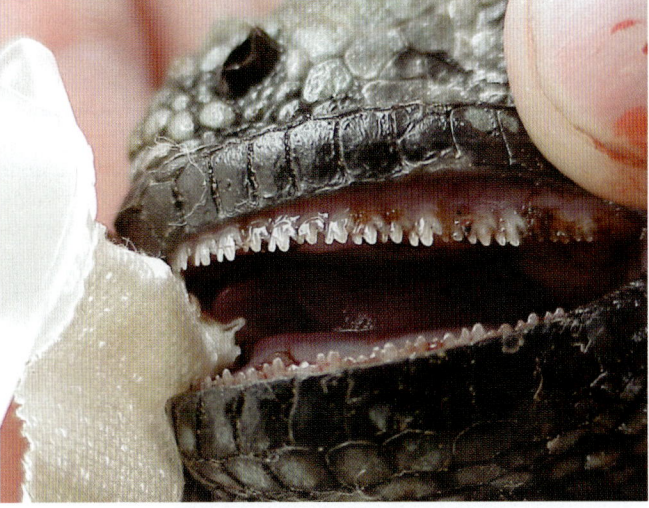

FIG 73.3 Pleurodont dentition of an iguanid lizard. These teeth are shed and replaced throughout the animal's life.

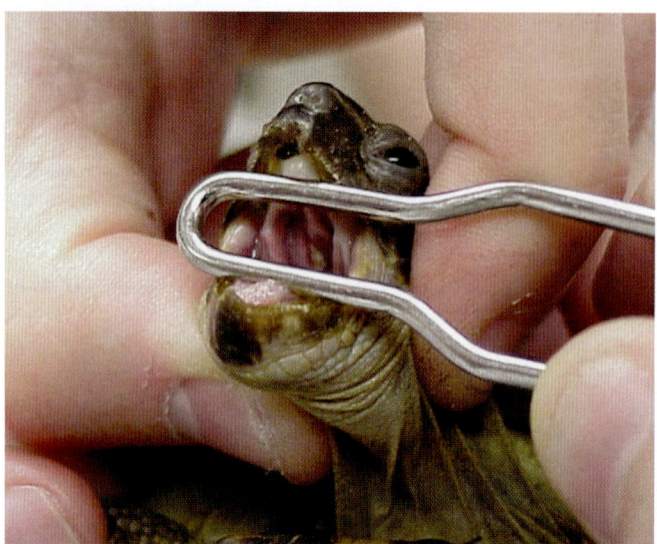

FIG 73.4 Competent handling technique and proper equipment are necessary for a safe and thorough oral examination in reptiles. Gentle use of an appropriate oral speculum, as is used here with this tortoise, is important to avoid iatrogenic damage to the oral structures.

to begin in the esophagus.[9] The esophagus of sea turtles is uniquely lined by conical, keratinized, caudally directed papillae. These papillae are thought to facilitate the movement of slippery food items aborad and facilitate mechanical digestion in the esophagus.[9] There are submucosal lymphoid aggregates throughout the esophagus of reptiles, which may be organized into esophageal tonsils in some species. Endoscopic biopsies of the esophageal tonsils of boid snakes[10] are often collected for histopathology and/or molecular diagnostics in screening for arenavirus infections.[11] The tunica muscularis is variably developed in different taxa. In some it is quite robust, allowing for some degree of mechanical digestion in the esophagus of some chelonians, whereas in others it is relatively thin and fragile and can easily be damaged if care is not utilized when administering medications, gavage, or assist-feeding.[9]

Stomach

The reptilian stomach is divided into cardiac, fundic, and pyloric regions, which are variably developed according to taxa. The snake stomach represents one end of the spectrum, as it can be difficult to differentiate from the esophagus and duodenum. The stomachs of "sit and wait" predators are extremely distensible in order to accommodate large, intermittent meals. The gastric mucosa has mucosal folds or rugae to varying degrees. The fundic portion of the crocodilian stomach is quite muscular with keratinized mucosa similar to the avian ventriculus. Gastroliths are commonly encountered in crocodilians.[8,9] The stomach functions to store and begin digestion of ingesta via both mechanical and chemical means. The mucosal glands produce hydrochloric acid and pepsinogen, which is cleaved to the active product pepsin. The pH of the stomach can drop dramatically in response to ingestion of a meal, especially in animals that have not eaten recently (from 7–2 in Burmese pythons, *Python bivittatus*). The typical pH of the reptilian stomach during digestion appears to be between 2 and 2.5. The presence of secretory glands in the gastric mucosa tends to be regionally variable; in some snakes the largest number of glands are present in the middle portion of the stomach with relatively nonglandular regions in the cranial gastric mucosa.[9,12]

Reptilian gastric conformation can also depend on recent feeding history. The stomach of reptiles has adapted to consume occasional large meals and will vary in mass and structure depending on the stage of digestion. Sit-and-wait predators such as Burmese pythons best represent this digestive strategy. The digestive function of Burmese pythons has been extensively studied, revealing that in between meals the stomach is maintained in an atrophied, quiescent state. No acid or enzymes are secreted and the actual mass of the stomach is significantly reduced.[13] Species that forage or graze and feed daily represent the other end of the reptile extreme. In these species, gastric anatomy and function is maintained and relatively static in health.

Digestive function in the stomach and other organs is dependent on access to temperatures capable of supporting these processes. If the reptile is not allowed to thermoregulate effectively, gastric activity can be inhibited, resulting in maldigestion.

CLINICAL INVESTIGATION

History and Physical Examination

History is paramount in the evaluation of reptile patients. Even seemingly minor deficiencies in husbandry and nutrition can dramatically impact a reptile's health. Thus specific information should be collected regarding environmental parameters and stressors, dietary composition, and consumption. Evaluation of appetite and fecal output can be especially difficult based on the intermittent feeding and defecation behaviors of some species. Differentiation between a physiological fast (seasonal, reproduction-related) and anorexia due to illness is often challenging.

Lizards with acrodont dentition appear uniquely predisposed to the development of periodontal disease due to the relatively thin and fragile gingival tissue found along the lateral surfaces of the maxillary and mandibular bones. When the gingival tissue is disrupted due to trauma or dessication, secondary infection may occur, leading to periodontitis/stomatitis and occasionally osteomyelitis.[14]

Many cases of stomatitis can ultimately be attributed to husbandry issues. Identification and correction of the inciting cause is critical for successful management of the condition. Trauma to the tissues of the rostrum and oral cavity due to interactions with the environment can lead to trauma and stomatitis. Abrasive or sharp surfaces within the animal's environment, especially those associated with potential escape routes (screen tops on aquaria), are important risk factors. Factors that result in efforts by the animal to escape from its enclosure can lead to incessant nose-pressing and pacing along and crashing into barriers, resulting in trauma even in the absence of inappropriate surfaces. Causes of continued escape efforts can include, but are not limited to, enclosure size and configuration, inappropriate thermal and light gradients, the presence of cagemates or conspecifics housed in close proximity (especially during breeding seasons), and lack of hide areas. Some species, such as basilisks (*Basiliscus basiliscus*) and water dragons (*Physignathus cocincinus*), can be nervous in captivity and have long flight distances, predisposing them to crashing into enclosure walls in response to environmental disturbances. Nervous snakes will sometimes strike repeatedly against glass barriers when disturbed. Environmental humidity and water availability can also be important factors in the development of stomatitis. Dehydration and dessication of the oral mucous membranes as well as dysecdysis with retention of exuviae along the lip margins can predispose to stomatitis.

Short of dysphagia, regurgitation (from the esophagus), and vomiting (from the stomach), the clinical signs associated with disease of the upper gastrointestinal tract are often vague. Lethargy, anorexia, and weight loss are frequently encountered and are nonspecific signs. A thorough oral examination is always indicated. Oral examination is often daunting due to dangers working around the mouth in large or venomous species, or simply the inability to access and open the mouth of many chelonians. The diminutive size and fragile nature of the oral structures of some species can also create challenges. At the very least, competent and firm handling should be utilized; however, sedation or anesthesia may be necessary. Struggling with a reptile to open the mouth can potentially result in injury to both animal and handler, not to mention that a thorough examination is often impossible with an uncooperative patient. Many reptiles will gape when handled, which may allow at least a visual examination. Decisions regarding measures to facilitate oral examination should be made on a case-by-case basis.

Thorough palpation of the neck and coelom can occasionally yield useful information about abnormalities of the esophagus and stomach. Snakes and some lizards have anatomy that allows for meaningful palpation with adequate knowledge of anatomy. Palpation of the coelom is possible in chelonians through the prefemoral or inguinal space, though it is typically difficult to access the stomach and structures cranial to the level of the liver. Crocodilians and lizards with osteoderms, gastralia, or heavy scalation are challenging to palpate, with only dramatic abnormalities of the stomach detected.

Clinical Pathology

A minimum database consisting of hematology and plasma biochemistry configured for reptilian species is often indicated. Hematology may show evidence of inflammation via leukocytosis, toxic changes to the leukocytes, and changes in the differential cell count. The differential cell count may show changes to suggest chronicity of the disease process (monocytosis, nonregenerative anemia). Changes in the plasma biochemistry panel that may be associated with disease of the upper gastrointestinal tract should theoretically mirror what would be expected in a mammal with similar pathology. Alkalosis, hypokalemia, and hypochloremia are possible, with vomiting or obstruction of the small gastrointestinal tract. Elevations in creatine kinase and aspartate aminotransferase are also possible due to damage/necrosis of the smooth muscle of the gastrointestinal tract and potentially catabolism of muscular tissues associated with severe catabolic conditions. Elevated nitrogen waste products (ammonia, urea, uric acid) may also be encountered as a nonspecific change associated with dehydration and reduced renal excretion or gastrointestinal hemorrhage. Severely wasted, chronically anorexic reptiles may have low blood uric acid, urea, or ammonia levels despite decreased renal excretion due to decreases in protein catabolism and nitrogen waste production.

Diagnostic Imaging

Various diagnostic imaging modalities are commonly utilized in the evaluation of the gastrointestinal tract and coelomic viscera. Radiography, computed tomography, magnetic resonance imaging, and ultrasonography all have utility in clinical evaluation of the gastrointestinal tract and should be applied based on the specific details of the case. Knowledge of normal anatomy for a particular species is important for thorough and subtle evaluation of the patient regardless of modality. When dealing with unfamiliar species, extrapolation from knowledge of related taxa is often the only course of action.

Administration of contrast material via gavage can highlight the gastrointestinal tract, identify filling defects within, help identify adjacent visceral organs, and determine gastrointestinal transit time. A number of studies are published that describe the radiographic anatomy of the gastrointestinal tract and transit time in various species.[15–19] Gastric emptying and transit times can vary considerably in relation to body temperature, with slower transit times corresponding with lower body temperatures. Parenteral administration of iodinated contrast material may also prove useful in increasing soft tissue contrast when imaging

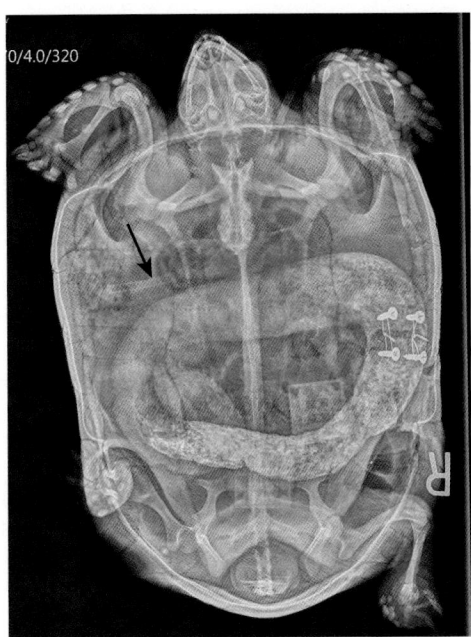

FIG 73.5 Constipated gopher tortoise (*Gopherus polyphemus*) with fecal mass highlighted following administration of barium sulfate via esophagostomy tube at approximately 30 mL/kg. The arrow shows the tip of a tube in the stomach lumen on the left side. Also note the metal screws and wire on the right side (associated with a shell repair). (Courtesy of Ryan De Voe.)

via computed tomography. If administering oral medications or gavage feeding, the author will often add contrast material (barium sulfate or iohexol) to facilitate radiographic documentation of gastrointestinal motility, patency, and transit time if desired (Fig. 73.5). Iohexol provides the benefit of faster emptying and transit time than barium but often becomes diluted in the lower gastrointestinal tract, limiting its usefulness for evaluation of the large intestine.[17]

Ultrasonographic examination of the gastrointestinal structures can be useful in certain instances. Infusion of saline into the gastrointestinal tract via gavage to provide contrast is often helpful, especially for novice ultrasonographers. Ultrasonography can also facilitate collection of samples via aspiration for cytology, microbiology, or DNA-based diagnostics. Some reptiles are difficult to image due to characteristics of their skin (heavy scalation, osteoderms, etc.); however, in most cases these challenges can be overcome or at least minimized (see Section 7 for more information on diagnostic imaging).

Endoscopy

Endoscopy is commonly employed in evaluation of the upper gastrointestinal tract. Endoscopic evaluation of the oral cavity allows the clinician to visualize areas and structures that might not otherwise be accessible. Also, the magnification provided by most of the available imaging systems may allow for identification of lesions that would otherwise be overlooked. Endoscopy has the additional benefit of facilitating the collection of diagnostic samples and implementation of therapy.

Endoscopic examination of the esophagus and stomach is routinely performed in many patients with signs of upper gastrointestinal disease.[20] If the correct equipment is available, endoscopic retrieval of gastric foreign bodies can be relatively straightforward.[21] Smaller, rigid telescopes may be adequate for endoscopic evaluation of the oral cavity, esophagus, and stomach in small species/individuals; however, flexible endoscopes will likely be necessary in larger specimens (including most snakes over approximately 75 cm). The anatomy of certain taxa, such as crocodilians and some lizards, allows relatively easy removal of gastric foreign bodies per os due to the relatively short and broad nature of their esophagus.

Endoscopic biopsy of the oral, esophageal, and gastric mucosa is possible, but caution should be utilized to avoid perforation, as the esophageal tissue is especially thin in certain taxa. A common procedure for screening boid snakes for inclusion body disease is collection of biopsies from esophageal lymphoid aggregates.[11]

CLINICAL DISEASES

Stomatitis, Esophagitis, and Gastritis

Stomatitis, esophagitis, and gastritis are all encountered with relative frequency in reptile practice. In these cases, a thorough diagnostic investigation is paramount, especially when populations of animals are at risk. Collection of swabs and tissue samples for culture, polymerase chain reaction, and cytology/histology (and possibly immunohistochemistry) is typically indicated. Cytology and histology are critical pieces of the diagnostic investigation, as the clinical significance of potential pathogens may be otherwise difficult to assess. Specific diagnostic testing should of course be directed by clinical presentation, though many times no clear direction is recognized early in the investigation. Occasionally a primary infectious etiology can be revealed; however, in most cases the etiology is likely multifactorial with various pathogens involved. Eastern box turtles with stomatitis have been documented with coinfections of herpesvirus, ranavirus, and *Mycoplasma* sp.[22]

Lizard species with acrodont dentition appear uniquely predisposed to the development of periodontal disease due to the relatively thin and fragile gingival tissue found along the lateral surfaces of the maxillary and mandibular bones. When the gingival tissue is disrupted due to trauma or dessication, secondary infection may occur, leading to periodontitis/stomatitis and occasionally osteomyelitis.[23]

Viral Diseases

Herpesviral infections are a common cause of stomatitis and esophagitis in various species. Herpesviruses that cause pathology in chelonians are fairly well described, with novel isolates being commonly encountered.[24] Several chelonian herpesviruses have a predilection for mucoepithelial cells and are commonly associated with stomatitis/glossitis.[24] Herpesvirus-associated stomatitis/glossitis is reported in lizards[25] and may cause predisposition to development of oral squamous cell carcinoma in some species, such as green tree monitors (*Varanus prasinus*).[26] Many viral pathogens can cause oral, esophageal, and/or gastric lesions in addition to other pathology. Adenoviral infection is reported to cause mucosal ulcerations/erosions in Sulawesi tortoises (*Indotestudo forsteni*).[27] Necrotizing stomatitis and glossitis are reported in American alligators (*Alligator mississippiensis*) suffering from West Nile virus infection as part of the disease presentation.[28]

Viral esophagitis is occasionally encountered. Ball pythons (*Python regius*) with nidovirus infections are reported to suffer from esophagitis, as well as tracheitis and pneumonia.[29,30] Ranaviral infections in chelonians frequently cause necrotizing stomatitis and esophagitis[31] (Fig. 73.6). Though esophagitis is not typically part of the disease process, boid arenavirus infections are often detected by biopsies of lymphoid aggregates found in the esophagus of boas and pythons.[11] Atadenoviral infections in colubrid snakes (*Lampropeltis* and *Pituophis* species) are reported to cause gastritis as well as pathology in other organs.[32]

Bacterial Diseases

Bacteria often play a role in reptilian stomatitis, esophagitis, and gastritis, but infections are thought to typically be secondary. Regardless, it may be necessary to provide appropriate antibiotic therapy (based upon

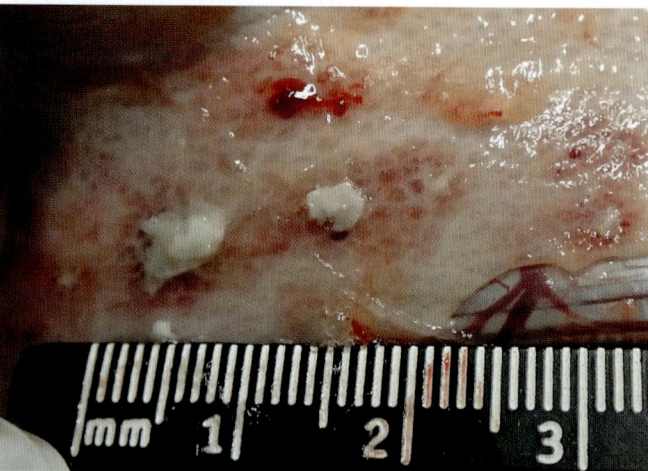

FIG 73.6 Pharyngeal plaques in an eastern box turtle (*Terepene carolina carolina*), associated with ranaviral infection. (Courtesy of Ryan De Voe.)

culture and sensitivity) to effectively treat a reptile suffering from disease of the upper alimentary tract. A wide variety of bacterial isolates may comprise normal oral/gastrointestinal flora, though the same bacteria can create clinically important infections under certain circumstances. The majority of isolates include gram-negative species such as *Pseudomonas* spp., *Aeromonas* spp., *Alcaligenes* spp, *Acinetobacter* spp, *Stenotrophomonas* spp., and *Salmonella* spp. Gram-positive isolates are also encountered with *Staphylococcus* spp. and *Clostridium* spp., as reported in some investigations.[33–36]

Cheilitis associated with *Devriesea agamarum* is reported in lizards from the genus *Uromastyx*. *Devriesea agamarum* is considered a facultative pathogenic bacterium and is found in the oral cavity of some healthy bearded dragons (*Pogona vitticeps*) but is also capable of causing infection in abraded skin experimentally in the same species.[37]

Mycobacterial infections of the upper gastrointestinal tract are occasionally reported and are likely more common than the literature suggests. Atypical species such as *Mycobacteria marinum*, *M. chelonae*, and *M. fortuitum* are usually isolated from mycobacterial lesions. *Mycobacterium* species typically involved in infections are ubiquitous environmental organisms; some manner of predisposition to infection is likely required to effect clinical disease. Histopathology or cytology with acid-fast staining and collection of samples for mycobacterial culture should always be considered, especially in cases that become chronic and/or do not respond as expected to conservative therapy.[38]

Chlamydophila-associated disease is reported in emerald tree boas (*Corallus caninus*) with "regurgitation syndrome," which is a relatively common syndrome in this species. Based on clinical experience and anecdotal data, it does not appear that chlamydiosis is the sole cause of regurgitation syndrome. Gastric atrophy and fibrosis is the end state of emerald tree boas with regurgitation syndrome and can likely occur as a sequela to any condition causing chronic gastritis.[39]

Mycotic Diseases

There are occasionally mycotic components to stomatitis, esophagitis, and gastritis. It is likely that most of these mycotic infections in captive reptiles are secondary to compromised defense mechanisms due to poor husbandry. Mycotic coinfections with other pathogens are also possible, as well as secondary infection of traumatic injuries or neoplastic lesions. Prolonged, broad-spectrum antibiotic use may predispose to dysbiosis and mycosis.

Some fungal organisms capable of causing infections of the upper gastrointestinal tract are thought to be primary pathogens. *Metarhizium viride* and *Metarhizium granulomatis* are reported to cause disseminated mycosis in veiled (*Chamaeleo calyptratus*) and carpet chameleons (*Furcifer lateralis*), panther chameleons (*Furcifer pardalis*), and bearded dragons, including granulomatous glossitis and stomatitis. These fungi are grouped in the family Clavicipitaceae and are thought to be primary pathogens.[40–43] *Purpureocillium lilacinum* (*Paecilomyces lilacinus*) is another potential pathogen of reptiles capable of causing infections of the upper gastrointestinal tract, which is in the family Ophiocordycipitaceae. *Purpureocillium lilacinum* is a ubiquitous, saprophytic fungi frequently encountered in moist, humid environments.[44] *Candida* spp. infections of the upper gastrointestinal tract are reported. Cytology, histology, culture, and PCR are used to detect *Candida* spp. and other yeast species in diagnostic samples.[45]

Parasitic Diseases

Helminthiasis. Parasitism of the oral cavity and esophagus with digenetic trematodes from the families Ochetosomatidae and Plagiorchiidae is relatively common in wild reptiles that consume intermediate amphibian hosts (Fig. 73.7). The adults of these species are also often found in the lungs. There is usually very little if any pathology associated with the presence of oral flukes in healthy animals, although they can cause localized inflammation where they attach to the epithelium. The lesions at the attachment sites may become secondarily infected and lead to morbidity, especially in compromised animals.[46] There are numerous helminths that inhabit the upper gastrointestinal tract of various species and can cause pathology. Parasite-associated gastritis has been reported in a number of species of crocodilians, chelonians, and squamates, free-ranging and captive.[46–48] Ascarids and strongyles, including parasites from the genera *Ophidascaris* and *Kalicephalus*, will infect the esophagus and stomach of snakes, occasionally causing gastritis, ulceration, and secondary bacterial infections.[46] Gastric impactions with helminths have also been reported (Fig. 73.8).[49] Helminths that normally reside in the nasal cavity, esophagus, and stomach may sometimes be encountered in the oral cavity and can be associated with stomatitis (see Chapter 32).

Cryptosporidiosis. Cryptosporidiosis is a potentially devastating disease of captive reptiles. In susceptible species, infection leads to a chronic wasting syndrome caused by the parasite's impact on the stomach or intestinal tract and subsequent maldigestion. *Cryptosporidium* species

are ciliated protozoa assigned to the phylum Apicomplexa. A number of *Cryptosporidium* species are identified as reptile pathogens, including *C. serpentis*, *C. varanii/saurophilum*, and *C. ducismarci*.[50] There appears to be significant variability in the genetic identity of *Cryptosporidium* isolates obtained from reptile species, with novel species/variants routinely identified. It is reasonable to assume that not all *Cryptosporidium* organisms harbored by reptile species are uniformly pathogenic and cause consistent clinical signs. *Cryptosporidium* species than infect reptiles have not been documented as capable of causing infection or disease in mammals and birds and are therefore not known to cause zoonotic infections. Conversely, *Cryptosporidium* species that cause infections and disease in mammals (including *C. muris* and *C. parvum* of rodents) and birds are not known to infect reptiles. *Cryptosporidium* organisms can pass through the gastrointestinal tract of nonsusceptible species with no ill effect to the animal and remain viable.[51] This discussion will focus on cryptosporidiosis in snakes and lizards.

Many species of snakes are fed domestic rodents in captivity, which often harbor *Cryptosporidium* species such as *C. muris* or *C. parvum*. These organisms may traverse the gastrointestinal tract and pass in the feces, being microscopically indistinguishable from *Cryptosporidium* species that are pathogenic to reptiles. Molecular characterization is typically required to identify the species of *Cryptosporidium* and subsequently assign significance to its presence. Coinfections may occur that predispose animals to clinical *Cryptosporidium* sp. infections when they might otherwise not be susceptible.[52–54] A conundrum can occur when novel *Cryptosporidium* species are identified in asymptomatic individuals. Pathogenicity can be difficult to predict both in the species harboring the organism and others that may be exposed.

Clinical signs observed in reptiles suffering from cryptosporidiosis may vary according to host species and likely the particular *Cryptosporidium* species. Vomiting, anorexia, and chronic wasting leading to emaciation (Fig. 73.9) are fairly consistent clinical signs. Diarrhea is also seen; however, decreased fecal output due to anorexia can make observation of this clinical sign difficult. On physical examination snakes with advanced disease will often be emaciated with a palpably firm stomach, which may cause a grossly visible soft tissue mass effect (Fig. 73.10).[46] Snakes with cryptosporidiosis typically suffer from hypertrophic gastritis (Fig. 73.11), which leads to fibrosis and ultimately maldigestion. Occasionally cryptosporidial enteritis with or without gastritis may be encountered in snake species.[55] Infection of the gall bladder and intrahepatic bile ducts has also been reported in corn snakes (*Pantherophis guttata guttata*).[56] Although it is suggested that some animals may be

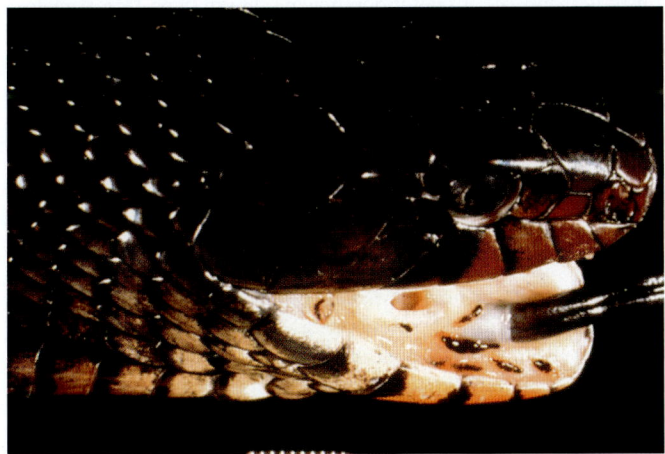

FIG 73.7 Trematodes in the oral cavity of an indigo snake (*Drymarchon couperi*). (Courtesy of M. Loomis.)

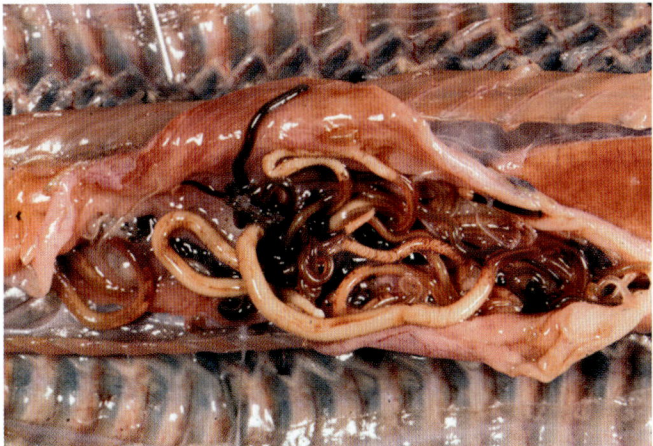

FIG 73.8 Gastric impaction with various helminth species in a colubrid snake. (Courtesy of M. Loomis.)

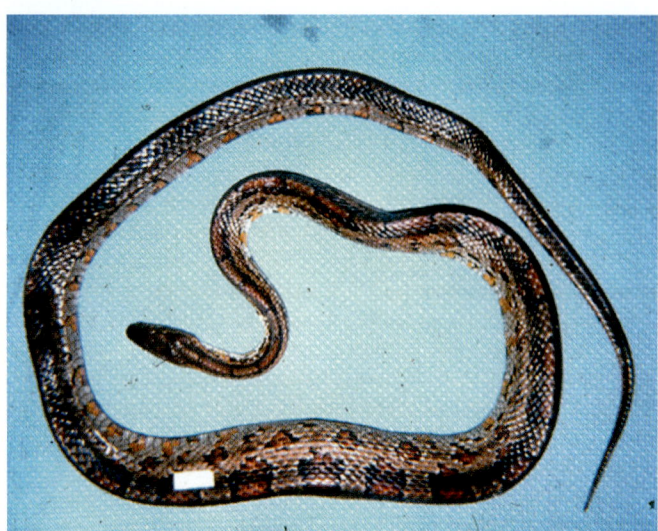

FIG 73.9 Emaciated corn snake (*Pantherophis guttata guttata*) with cryptosporidiosis. (Courtesy of Ryan De Voe.)

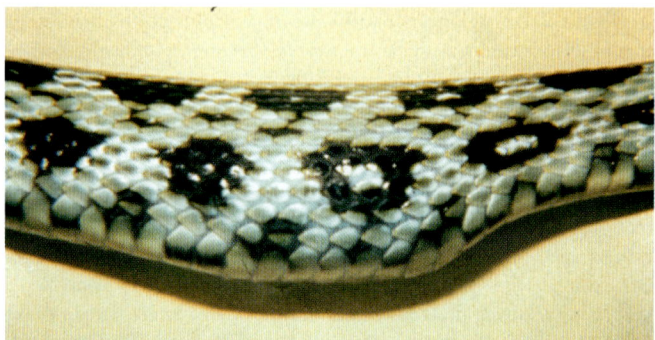

FIG 73.10 Externally visible gastric hypertrophy due to cryptosporidiosis in a fox snake (*Pantherophis vulpinus*). (Courtesy of Ryan De Voe.)

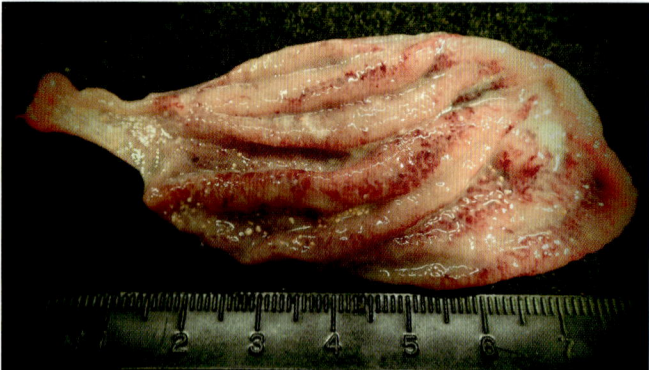

FIG 73.11 Hypertrophic gastritis with thickened, edematous gastric rugae due to cryptosporidiosis in a rosy boa (*Lichanura trivirgata*). Note the multiple petechial hemorrhages in the mucosa. (Courtesy of C. Rodriguez.)

able to recover from cryptosporidiosis, with or without supportive care and treatment, in most animals the disease process is progressive and eventually leads to death.

Diagnosis of cryptosporidiosis in snakes can be challenging. Examination of feces via direct smear cytology, fecal floatation, and acid-fast staining is useful in screening suspect animals. Polymerase chain reaction

of samples for DNA detection is sensitive and specific.[57] In addition to feces, gastric lavage or gastroscopy may provide useful samples for screening snake species. Typically, gastric lavage is performed 2 to 3 days after feeding, as this practice enhances recovery of organisms.[46] The mucus from vomited prey items may also be used for detection of *Cryptosporidium* spp. organisms. Fecal antigen assays for *C. parvum* are occasionally used as a screening tool because cross-reaction may occur with other *Cryptosporidium* species. Confirmation of the *Cryptosporidium* species should be pursued in an effort to assign clinical significance, especially in asymptomatic patients. Species identification is typically accomplished via molecular characterization of the organism. Gastric biopsy with histopathology, performed either surgically or endoscopically, can help confirm a definitive diagnosis of clinical cryptosporidiosis in snake patients.[58] Assays to detect antibodies to *Cryptosporidium* sp. organisms are described in the literature, but antibody titers can fluctuate, showing alternating positive and negative results in infected animals.[59] If antibody titers are measured, diagnosis should not be based only on a single antibody titer to *Cryptosporidium* sp.

Management of asymptomatic animals that are diagnosed as carriers of *Cryptosporidium* sp. (*C. serpentis, C. varanii/saurophilum, C. ducismarci,* or other species/genotypes) should be based on risk assessment of the specific situation. In cases where the animal is a pet in a single-reptile household, the animal may live an acceptable life, so no actions may be warranted as long as the animal remains clinically normal. If the animal is a part of a larger population, either of the same species or a cosmopolitan collection, the health of the population as a whole must be considered. Culling of carrier animals may make sense if the existing population is devoid of carrier animals or the carriage rate is low. In cases where animals are considered valuable from a genetic/conservation standpoint, a permanent quarantine situation may be indicated.

A number of treatment approaches are described to address cryptosporidiosis in reptiles; however, none are uniformly effective, and usually amelioration of clinical signs for a period of time is the best that can be expected. Treatment with paromomycin can result in improvement of clinical signs and a decrease or cessation of shedding in some animals, but progression of the disease and shedding typically resumes when treatment is discontinued. At least one study reports clearance of *Cryptosporidium* infection in asymptomatic bearded dragons treated with paromomycin, though similar information is not available for snakes.[60] Other therapies such as halofuginone, spiramycin,[61] and trimethoprim/sulfamethoxazole can also induce decreases or cessation of cryptosporidial shedding but do not appear effective in clearing infections. Treatment with hyperimmune bovine colostrum created utilizing *C. parvum* isolates appears effective in clearing infections in subclinical animals but not those showing clinical signs. Unfortunately, this treatment option is not readily available and beyond the capabilities of most clinicians.[62] Supportive care in the form of fluid and nutritional supplementation may improve clinical signs and/or slow progression of the disease.

Disinfection of *Cryptosporidium* sp. can be difficult. Mechanical cleaning and removal of organic material before application of chemical agents is necessary for effective disinfection. Standard bleach solutions, quaternary ammonium compounds, phenols, alcohol, iodine, and glutaraldehyde are typically ineffective against *Cryptosporidium* oocysts. High kill rates can be reached with application of 3% hydrogen peroxide or ammonium hydroxide solutions for 20 to 30 minutes. Information regarding disinfection is typically based on studies with *C. parvum* isolates, so some variation may exist between different *Cryptosporidium* species.

Due to the lack of consistently effective therapeutics for treatment of cryptosporidiosis in snakes, control hinges on effective screening of animals and implementation of appropriate biosecurity measures.

MALNUTRITION

Hypovitaminosis A can result in squamous metaplasia of tissues of the oral cavity and upper gastrointestinal tract. Structural abnormalities and dysfunction of these tissues can predispose reptiles to secondary infections, cheilitis, and stomatitis. Captive chameleons, geckos, and other lizard species fed diets without supplementation of preformed vitamin A often present with clinical signs suggestive of hypovitaminosis A.[63,64] Nutritional secondary hyperparathyroidism can lead to skeletal deformities of the skull, resulting in chronic exposure of oral mucous membranes. Dessication of mucous membranes and/or increased incidence of trauma may increase risk of developing stomatitis.

MALDIGESTION DUE TO ENVIRONMENTAL AND DIETARY ISSUES

Ingestion of meals that are too large and/or consumed when the animal is too cool, dehydrated, etc. can cause vomiting or even morbidity and mortality due to putrefaction of ingesta in the gastrointestinal tract. Vomiting is typically a protective response when the environment cannot support the physiological conditions necessary for effective digestion. Animals that are not able to expunge a putrefying food item often suffer from associated gastritis/enteritis and potentially endotoxemia and/or septicemia (Fig. 73.12). Gas-producing bacteria often proliferate in these conditions, causing bloating, which can be severe. Passage of fetid gas from the oral cavity or vent may also be appreciated. Effective therapy is based on removal of any decomposing food items in the gastrointestinal tract via lavage or catharsis, correction of dehydration, and improvements in captive management. Local gastrointestinal protectants such as bismuth subsalicylate, and sucralfate may also be indicated.

Handling or significant stress can also induce vomiting, especially in snakes and carnivorous lizards. It is usually advisable to avoid handling of carnivorous reptiles during at least the gastric phase of digestion. Typically, there is no lasting consequence following an isolated incident of handling or stress-induced vomition. However, the event can be quite unpleasant for the personnel in attendance.

FOREIGN BODIES

Foreign bodies are occasionally encountered in the oral cavity, esophagus, and stomach (Fig. 73.13). Sometimes it can be difficult to tell if a foreign body in the stomach is clinically significant and requires intervention. Reptiles, especially those that are not fed frequently, may not show recognizable clinical signs associated with foreign bodies of the upper gastrointestinal tract until the condition is quite advanced. Oral and esophageal foreign bodies may induce ptyalism, retching, clawing at the mouth, and reluctance or inability to feed. Regurgitation or vomiting may occur with esophageal or gastric foreign bodies, but many animals will simply become anorectic and lose body condition.

Many animals will incidentally pick up and swallow small stones or other pieces of substrate when they eat. Pica can also occur due to calcium-deficient diets and nutritional secondary hyperparathyroidism. Calcium carbonate sands that are touted as "digestible" can cause problems as readily as any other particulate substrates. If particle size is small and the material is not consumed in large amounts, incidental consumption of substrate is typically not a problem. Sharp pieces of mulch from the substrate can cause traumatic injury to the mucosa and rarely perforation. Dehydrated polyacrylamide hydrogels can also act as foreign bodies if ingested.

Pet reptiles that are allowed to free-roam in the household often consume inappropriate items they come in contact with. Not only can these items cause trauma or obstruction in the gastrointestinal tract, but toxicosis is also possible. Other animals that are indiscriminate or aggressive feeders will sometimes ingest inappropriate items that require recovery. Snakes will often consume items that smell like a prey item. The classic history is a snake that was fed a rodent on a towel and went on to swallow the towel after the rodent. Egg-eating snakes will occasionally consume indigestible "dummy eggs" that are used in aviculture or other foreign bodies that resemble eggs. Depending on the size of the snake and the foreign body, it may be possible for the animal to naturally pass the item through the gastrointestinal tract. Especially large foreign bodies that are present in the esophagus or stomach for long periods of time can cause pressure necrosis of the esophagus or gastric wall.[65] Recovery of foreign bodies from the stomach of snakes can be relatively easy, and nonsurgical techniques should always be considered before surgical intervention. In many cases, the snake is anesthetized, intubated, and following instillation of a water-soluble lubricant into the stomach via gavage, the item is "milked" orad and removed via the mouth. This

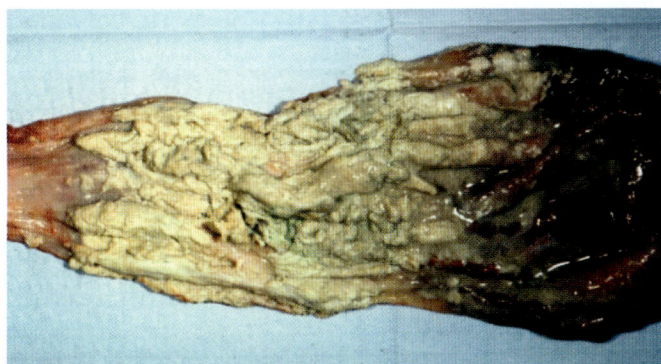

FIG 73.12 Necrotic gastritis in a python secondary to putrefaction of a prey item in the stomach. Putrefaction of prey items in the stomach may occur when the reptile does not have access to appropriate environmental temperatures. (Courtesy of Ryan De Voe.)

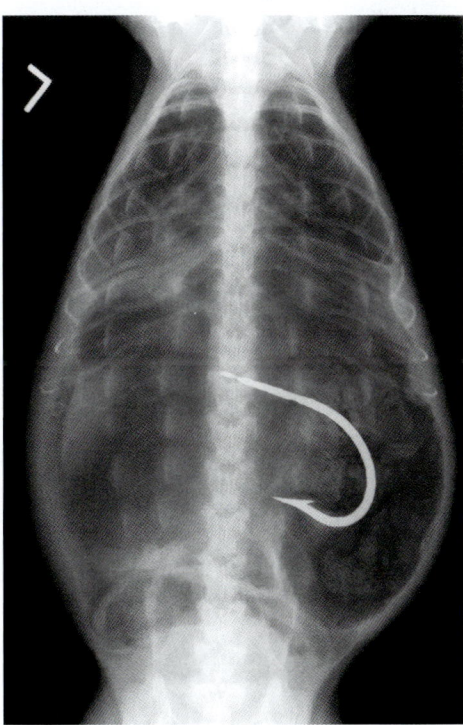

FIG 73.13 Radiograph of an alligator with a fishing hook in the gastrointestinal tract.

method is not appropriate for items that could potentially cause trauma or those that have traveled aborad to the stomach.

With other taxa, endoscopic retrieval of esophageal or gastric foreign bodies is usually possible. The limiting factor is typically the size of the animal, as with diminutive species the available equipment is simply not suitable. With very large lizards and crocodilians, manual retrieval of foreign bodies may be possible. For both animal and human safety concerns, this technique should only be utilized with a properly anesthetized and/or restrained animal. Surgical removal of foreign bodies via esophagotomy or gastrotomy are both relatively straightforward procedures for competent veterinary surgeons.[65]

NEOPLASIA

A variety of neoplastic conditions are described involving the upper gastrointestinal tract of various reptile taxa.[66–68] Neoplasia should be a differential for any mass associated with the upper gastrointestinal tract, especially in older animals. Nonhealing ulcers/erosions, recurrent abscessation, or nonspecific inflammatory conditions should also raise suspicion of a neoplastic process. Typically, assumptions of how reptilian neoplasms will behave and what treatment is most appropriate are based on information available for domestic animals.

Gastric neuroendocrine sarcomas have been described specifically in bearded dragons (*Pogona vitticeps*). Metastasis to the liver is frequently identified. A number of these neoplasms have been identified as somatostatinomas, though some tumors have exhibited multihormonal expression. Hyperglycemia, weight loss, and anemia are typical symptoms associated with these neoplasms.[69,70]

REFERENCES

See www.expertconsult.com for a complete list of references.

74

Gastroenterology—Small Intestine, Exocrine Pancreas, and Large Intestine

Kevin Eatwell and Jenna Richardson

The identification of primary enteric or pancreatic disease in reptiles can be difficult. Clinical signs such as emaciation, anorexia, or altered fecal consistency may suggest disease but are often nonspecific. Confirmation of specific disease processes can be challenging, and overinterpretation of fecal microbiology and parasitology can occur.

ANATOMY AND PHYSIOLOGY

Small Intestinal Tract

Reptiles are adept at surviving and thriving in a variety of environmental niches. To do this, they have evolved selective anatomical and physiological differences compared with mammals and birds. Even within different reptile orders, there can be variation in anatomy and function of the digestive tract. These differences can pose challenges to the practitioner when interpreting physical examination findings, diagnostic imaging, and determining appropriate therapeutic regimes.

The reptilian gastrointestinal (GI) tract has many similarities to higher vertebrates with an oral cavity, oropharynx, esophagus, stomach, small intestine, and large intestine. The terminal GI tract, the cloaca, is similar to that found in avian species. The length of the reptilian GI tract varies between species and generally is dependent on the composition of the natural diet. Carnivorous reptiles have a shorter GI tract length, followed by omnivorous species, and the longest GI tracts are found in herbivores.

Within the intestines, longitudinal muscular folds are present. This allows for distention of the lumen to cope with the consumption of large volumes of ingesta. As the intestines are the primary site for absorption of nutrients, the folds also increase the surface area to facilitate this. The pH of the intestines varies, from being slightly acidic to slightly alkaline (pH 6.5–8).[1]

Chelonian small intestines are located in the caudal coelomic cavity. In many species there is no clear divide between the duodenum, jejunum, and ileum. The small intestines function similar to that of mammals; however, proportionally the tract is shorter. A connection between the blood supply of the intestines and the parenchyma of the liver is seen in most species, creating a hepatoportal system. As would be expected, there is an aboral decline in digestive enzyme activity.[2]

In snakes, the small intestine empties directly into the colon, with the exception of boid snakes, which generally have a small cecum located at the proximal colon. In most reptiles, the large intestines are composed of the cecum and colon, before terminating in the coprodeum of the cloaca. With lizards and chelonians, the cecum is usually found in the right caudal coelomic cavity. The cecum may be difficult to differentiate visually from the colon. It appears as a widening of the colon wall, rather than a distinct separate organ, as seen in mammalian species. In chelonians, the cecum is not well developed.

In herbivorous species, the colon can appear sacculated, with multiple subchambers in which fermentation occurs. Differentiation is seen between juvenile and adult animals of some species. With iguanas, there is a marked difference dependent on age, with more defined saccules in the adult. This accounts for the dietary changes that occur as the lizard matures. Complex carbohydrates—for example, cellulose—are broken down via fermentation to simple sugars and fatty acids. In iguanids, the principle protozoon, *Nyctotherus* sp., are believed to serve as beneficial commensals required for the processing of dietary cellulose and other complex carbohydrates in the sacculated colon.[3] This ciliated organism is an important commensal in hind-gut fermenters. Herbivorous reptiles generally have a higher optimal body temperature range compared with carnivorous reptiles, which helps promote microbial fermentation. Examples of hind-gut fermenters include the iguanas (*Iguana*, *Cyclura*), prehensile-tailed skink (*Corucia zebrata*), spiny-tailed lizard (*Uromastyx* spp.), and chuckwalla (*Sauromalus* spp.) In those species that lack a bladder, urates can travel into the distal colon where they are retained along with fecal material before they are voided.

Pancreas

In lizards, the pancreas is trilobed, with each lobe extending toward the gallbladder, duodenum, and spleen, respectively.[4] In chelonians, the pancreatic and bile ducts enter the pylorus instead of the duodenum. A study characterizing pancreatic lipase in turtles showed no significant differences between it and known mammalian pancreatic lipases.[5] In snakes, the pancreas is located caudal to the stomach in the area of the gallbladder and spleen. It is often pyramidal in shape and is more consolidated than in other reptiles.[4] In some species, it is intermixed with the splenic tissues to form a splenopancreas.[6] Even when closely related species are considered, there are variations of the macroscopic structure.[7]

The function of the reptilian pancreas is comparable to that of mammals, and it produces a similar range of enzymes. The pancreas is composed of both endocrine and exocrine tissue. The endocrine component lacks a sharp demarcation from the exocrine pancreas, as seen in mammals. The pancreatic islets of lizards and snakes are larger than those of crocodilians and chelonians.[7] Alpha cells are more abundant in lizards, with alpha and beta cells equally present in snakes, chelonian, and crocodilians. The exocrine pancreas secretes digestive enzymes, including lipolytic, proteolytic, and amylolytic enzymes. Insectivorous reptiles also produce pancreatic chitinase.[8] The exocrine parenchyma consists of branching tubules, unlike mammalian species that display typical acini.

Reptile pancreatic "juice" contains alkaline secretions, as well as these digestive enzymes. The alkaline secretions neutralize the acidic stomach contents as they enter into the duodenum. This buffer provides an ideal environment for the digestive enzymes to act, further breaking down ingesta. In one study in the Burmese python (*Python bivittatus*), the effects of feeding on pre- and postprandial pancreatic trypsin and amylase saw respective 5.7- and 20-fold increases in the peak activities following feeding. The pancreas also doubled in mass during this time.[9] The production of the different ratios of digestive enzymes appears linked to the diet and feeding strategy of the reptile.

CLINICAL INTESTINAL DISEASES

Nematodiasis

Clinical Significance and Etiology. Common parasites vary depending on the species of reptile and its origins. Wildlife casualties, recently imported specimens, or those housed outside in their native region have access to intermediate hosts and parasites with indirect life cycles. Long-term captive animals or captive-bred individuals usually lack access to intermediate hosts, and so only parasites with direct life cycles are typically problematic. Parasite identification can prove helpful in determining the origins of a purchased animal. A wide variety of nematodes can be seen, and the important species are summarized in Table 74.1. (See Chapter 32 for more details.)

Clinical Presentation. The clinical presentation of enteric parasites can vary. Parasitism may be identified when performing routine fecal evaluations (fecal flotation, direct smears) in apparently healthy individuals or in patients where enteric disease is a differential diagnosis. For owners, often the first indication of parasitism in their pet is the visible presence of worms in feces. Adult oxyurids are commonly seen, presenting as small white threads, and measure 1.5 to 7 mm in length. Ascarids are large (up to 10 cm in length) and can be yellow in coloration (Fig. 74.1).

Common clinical signs associated with enteric disease include anorexia, emaciation, diarrhea, regurgitation, vomiting, coelomic discomfort, colonic prolapses through the cloaca, stunted growth, and death.[10,11] Heavy burdens of ascarids or strongylids can lead to intussusception, ulceration, avascular necrosis and fatal intestinal impactions.[12–14] Visceral migration can lead to damage in other tissues.[15]

Oxyurids are commonly seen in juvenile lizards and chelonians (Fig. 74.2). Snakes are less commonly affected. Factors such as small enclosures, poor environmental hygiene, or exposure to natural substrate where the nematode eggs can overwinter can be significant.[16] The need for treatment is usually based on parasite load (rather than mere presence) and the physical condition of the reptile. Low levels of oxyurids are often inconsequential.[17] Generally all individuals housed in a group are

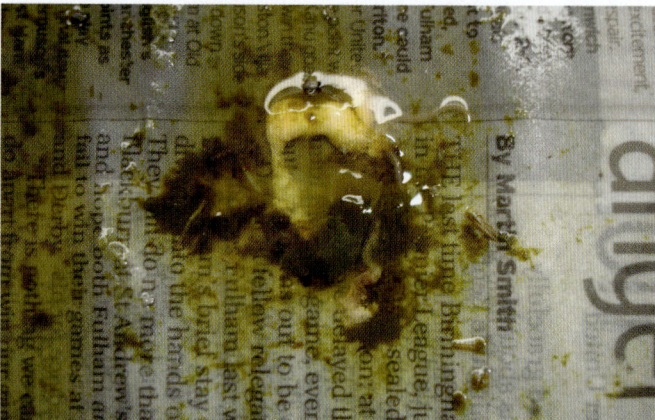

FIG 74.1 Ascarids in the feces of a spur-thighed tortoise (*Testudo graeca*). (Courtesy of Kevin Eatwell.)

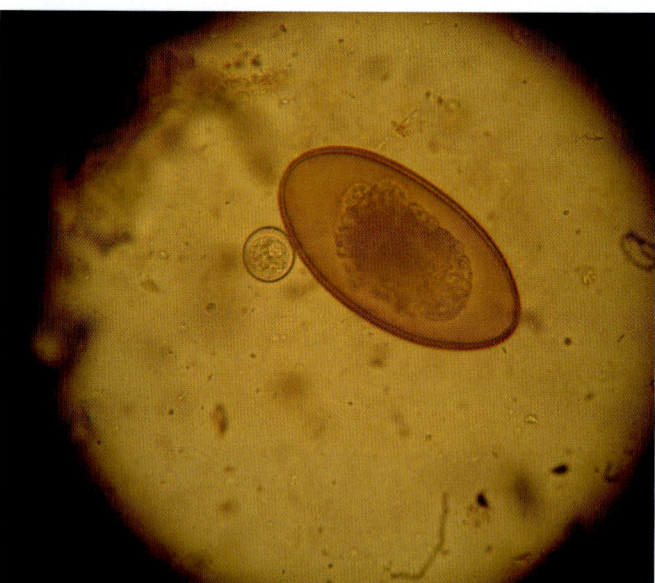

FIG 74.2 An oxyurid egg (large, ovoid) and a coccidial oocyst (small, round) identified on a wet preparation fecal analysis (400× magnification) from a bearded dragon (*Pogona vitticeps*). (Courtesy of Kevin Eatwell.)

TABLE 74.1	**Common Enteric Nematodes Seen in Captive Reptiles**				
Helminth	**Examples**	**Species**	**Life Cycle**	**Common Hosts**	**Clinical Signs**
Oxurids	*Oxyuris, Tachygonetria, Ozolaimus*	All	Direct	Juvenile lizards and chelonians	Only if heavy burdens
Ascarids	*Angusticaecum, Sulcascaris* (chelonians), *Ophidiascaris, Polydelphis* (snakes)	All	Direct, chelonians; indirect, others	Adult chelonians	Only if heavy burdens
Rhabditids	*Strongyloides, Rhabdias*	All	Direct	Snakes and lizards	Migrate via (or adults live in) the lungs so respiratory signs can also be seen
Strongylids	*Kalicephalus, Diaphanocephalus*	All	Direct	Snakes	Only if heavy burdens
Trichuroidids	*Capillaria*	All	Indirect	Snakes and lizards	Only if heavy burdens
Acanthocephalans	Spiny-headed worms		Indirect	Freshwater turtles	Only if heavy burdens

treated, and a pooled fecal sample can be used when testing a group. If treatment is not warranted, ongoing routine monitoring of parasite levels is still advised.

Ascarids typically utilize an intermediate host, although some chelonian ascarids have a direct life cycle. These species undergo extensive tissue migration resulting in significant pathology. *Ophidiascaris* and *Polydelphis* are present in snakes feeding on amphibians and rodents, which are intermediate hosts. Ascarids are also a common finding in crocodilians.[18]

Rhabditid nematodes have a direct life cycle and typically inhabit areas outside the intestinal tract, but *Strongyloides* can be found in the small intestine of snakes. Diarrhea and weight loss can be seen. *Kalicephalus* and *Diaphanocehalus* are strongyloid nematodes with direct life cycles. Hemorrhagic ulceration, malabsorption, diarrhea, and obstruction can be seen with heavy burdens. Capillaria can be found in lizards, snakes, and crocodilians. Spiny-headed worms (Acanthocephalans) have an indirect life cycle and can be seen in the small intestine of freshwater turtles.

Diagnostic Confirmation. Fecal analysis remains one of the most commonly performed tests in veterinary practice. Samples should be fresh, free from contamination, and not desiccated. Samples need to be kept moist and can be stored in a plastic container. If not processing the sample immediately, it should be refrigerated to slow bacterial overgrowth and parasite development.

An anorectic presentation, combined with the typically slow GI transit time, can result in difficulty obtaining a fecal sample. This is particularly true for larger, carnivorous reptiles. Assisted orogastric tube feeding can provide nutritional support while also encouraging gastrointestinal motility and the passing of fecal material. Warm water baths may stimulate bowel movement (Fig. 74.3), whereas some patients (i.e., chelonians) may void a fecal sample during handling.

For those patients that are still challenging, cloacocolonic flushes can be performed (Fig. 74.4). The lubricated, smooth-ended tube (an avian metal crop tube, red rubber catheter, or, for small reptiles, a plastic feline urinary catheter is appropriate) should be directed dorsally through the cloaca. Warmed water or physiological saline is infused slowly at a volume determined by the size of the animal (1–2 mL per 100 g body weight).[7] The reptile is gently massaged in the caudal coelom before the sample is aspirated. In this situation, the sample should be centrifuged to allow analysis of the sediment of fecal material.

Gross visual assessment is required to first confirm adequate fecal material for analysis but also to evaluate the nature of the feces compared with that expected for the species and the diet fed. Fresh or digested blood, mucus, adult parasites, or segments may be visually apparent.

For fecal parasitology testing, qualitative analyses (wet preparation and flotation) are routine and provide a general overview of the burden of parasites present, including identification of eggs and motile organisms. Flotation methods help concentrate parasite numbers so that low burdens are not missed. A modified McMaster technique can be used to quantify egg counts following qualitative evaluation and can also aid identification by reducing contaminants (Fig. 74.5).[16] Different flotation solutions can be used and are detailed in Table 74.2. Other, less commonly used protocols include fecal sedimentation and centrifugation techniques for small samples (e.g., cloacocolonic wash) or specific parasites (e.g., spiny-headed worm ova). These tests require minimal equipment to perform, with standard protocols readily available (see Table 74.3).[19,20]

Oxyurid ova have a variable appearance but are generally thin-walled, measuring ~130 × 40 µm, and may appear either oval or asymmetrical (D-shaped). Ascarid eggs are round with a thick shell and typically measure 80 to 100 × 60 to 80 µm. Strongylid eggs appear thin-walled with blunt ends, with the developing embryo filling most of the shell. They measure ~70 to 100 × 40 to 50 µm. Rhabditid ova are thin-walled embryonated eggs and measure ~60 × 35 µm. Capillaria ova have a typical lemon shape with end caps at each pole.

Specific Therapy. Owners are often aware of the need for prophylactic parasite control in dogs and cats and therefore may apply similar

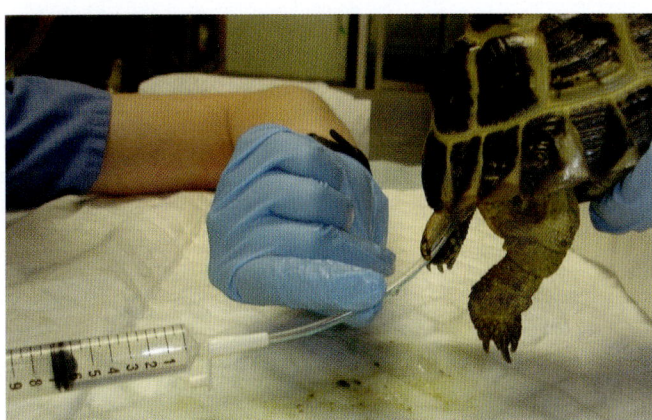

FIG 74.4 Cloacal flush being performed in a Russian tortoise (*Agrionemys horfieldii*). (Courtesy of Kevin Eatwell.)

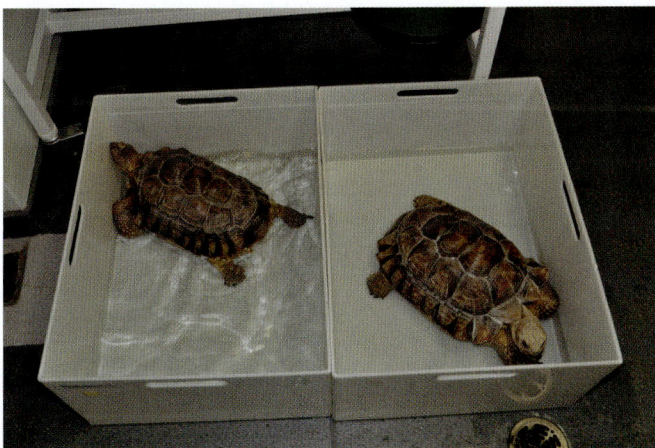

FIG 74.3 Two sulcata tortoises (*Centrochelys sulcata*) having a warm water bath to encourage defecation for fecal sample analysis. (Courtesy of Jenna Richardson.)

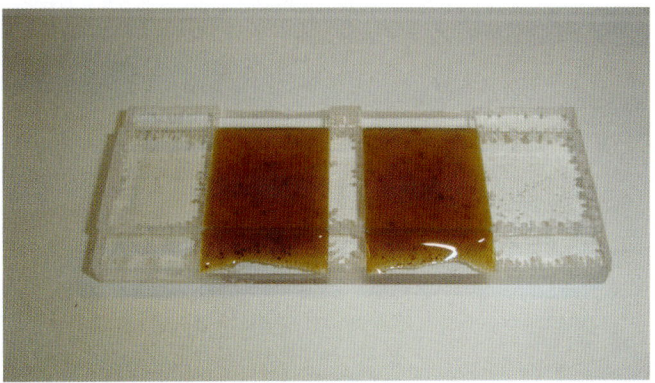

FIG 74.5 Modified McMasters technique for flotations using a small amount of fecal material. (Courtesy of Kevin Eatwell.)

principles to their reptile pets. There are many "(de)worming" products available, both online and in pet stores. These can often be purchased and administered without veterinary consultation. Owners should be encouraged to seek veterinary advice and present their reptiles for routine health checks. Routine fecal parasitology testing can be performed at this time, which prevents unnecessary treatments of reptiles without parasite burdens.

Routine prophylactic treatment for enteric parasites is not advised. Unnecessary treatment courses may not be benign, with side effects reported with commonly used antiparasitic drugs. Instead, treatments should be tailored to the health status of the patient and the results of fecal parasitology screening tests.

Benzimidazoles are commonly used to treat helminthiasis in reptiles, with fenbendazole, oxfendazole, and albendazole being commonly available. Fenbendazole is metabolized by the liver to the more active oxfendazole, and therefore lower doses given daily for 3 to 5 treatments are generally more effective than a single high dose. Fenbendazole toxicity leads to radiomimetic signs and has been reported in a number of reptiles.[21] Oxfendazole is generally considered less toxic in a number of species[22,23] and, as the more active compound, would be expected to be more efficacious following a single dose. Research at the University of Georgia demonstrated the ability of oxfendazole (25 mg/kg PO once) to reduce oxyurid egg counts to zero in green iguanas (Kehoe, Divers, Verocai, unpublished data).

Levamisole has a narrow margin of safety, and so oral treatment is recommended over parenteral use. Neurological signs can be seen with toxic doses.[24] Pyrantel is very similar in action to levamisole and is a substituted imidazothiazole derivative. It has been used orally to treat nematode infections.

Ivermectin toxicity in chelonians is well known.[25] Caution has also been advised in indigo snakes and skinks.[26] Ivermectin is generally not advised for treatment of enteric helminths.

Monitoring fecal samples routinely is important to evaluate the effectiveness of any treatment regimen, and repeat samples are usually recommended 3 to 4 weeks after treatment. Ongoing monitoring to identify any increases in burden from the environment is also advised every 6 months.

After treatment, the worm egg count in the feces must diminish before moving the animal to a new enclosure or placing/replacing the

TABLE 74.2 Flotation Solutions

Salt flotation	Sodium chloride salt flotations are used most commonly but can severely distort parasite eggs. Heavier eggs (such as fluke eggs) will not float in this solution, and alternative methods would be preferred for imported specimens or wildlife casualties. It is easy and economical to make up the saturated solution from salt, which is added to water until no more dissolves (usually 40 g/100 ml).
Zinc sulfate flotation	Add 371 g of zinc sulfate to 1 liter of water while stirring continuously (mild heating can be used to hasten the dissolution process).
Sodium nitrate flotation	Add approximately 400 g of sodium nitrate to 1 liter of water while stirring continuously (mild heating can be used to hasten the dissolution process).
Sugar flotation	Pour 355 mL of **warm** water into a beaker and place onto a hot plate. Heat water on high but **do not boil**. Slowly add 454 g granulated sugar, stirring constantly until dissolved completely. Remove from heat and cool.

TABLE 74.3 Common Fecal Analytical Methods

Technique	Details
Wet preparation	A small amount of fecal material is thoroughly mixed in warmed saline on a glass slide. Large pieces of fecal material are removed. This is examined under the ×10 objective for eggs and larvae and then under ×40 for motile protozoa and cysts. If the sample has been chilled, it can be rested on a heated coin to encourage motility on the slide.
Fecal flotation	Feces are added to the flotation solution and gently mixed thoroughly. This is poured through a tea strainer (or alternative), and large particulate matter is discarded. The filtered liquid is titrated into a small container and topped up with flotation solution to form a meniscus. A cover slip is gently placed on top of the tube. The tube is allowed to rest for 20 minutes. The cover slip is then removed by pulling it vertically off the top and is placed onto a glass slide. This is then examined under ×10 and ×40 objectives.
Modified McMaster technique	Weigh out 1 g feces and mix with 15 mL of flotation solution. Strain through a tea strainer and fill up both sides of the McMaster slide. Leave to stand for 20 minutes. Examine both grids. Count all eggs that lie within the lined 1 cm² of the counting chamber and repeat for the second side. Each side is filled with 1% of the original volume. So multiplying the total by 50 gives the eggs per gram.
McMaster technique	Weigh out 3 g of feces and mix with 42 mL of flotation solution (approximately 45 mL total volume) and strained through a tea strainer. Leave the solution to stand for 20 minutes. Remove the meniscus with a pipette and load the McMaster chamber on both sides. Count all eggs that lie within the lined 1 cm² of the counting chamber and repeat for the second side. The calculation is based on the fact that the depth of the chamber is 1.5 mm, and the volume of fluid examined is 0.15 mL, which is 1/300 of the original volume of 45 mL. Therefore each egg counted represents 300 per 3 g of feces, which is equivalent to 100 eggs/g. When done in duplicate, the total count of the two chambers is multiplied by 100 and divided by 2.
Sedimentation technique	This is ideal if a cloacal flush has been performed and the sample is dilute. Strain the mixture (adding saline if needed) through a tea strainer and pour into a centrifuge tube. Centrifuge the tube for 3 minutes at 1500 rpm. Decant the supernatant off, and transfer a small amount of the sediment to the microscope slide and dilute with saline if needed.
Formalin and ethyl acetate concentration	Place 6 mL of 10% buffered formalin into a centrifuge tube. Add feces and emulsify thoroughly. Leave overnight. Cysts and ova will be preserved by the formaldehyde, although motile forms will not survive. Then mix gently and strain the sample through a tea strainer. Add 5 mL ethyl acetate and mix gently, leave for 10 minutes for the fat globules to dissolve, and centrifuge at 1500 rpm for 30 seconds. Decant the supernatant off, resuspend the deposit by agitation, and place a drop on the slide and dilute with saline if needed.

cage furniture or substrate. This can take a protracted time, up to 31 days in chelonians.[27] Timing of treatment is important, as the reptile must be metabolically active for treatment to be effective. As a result, do not treat close to hibernation or brumation. Those reptiles with high parasite burdens should not be hibernated until treatment has proven effective.

Prognosis and Prevention. Nematode infections can have varying outcomes depending on the health status of the reptile and the level of parasite burden. In severely affected cases, supportive care including fluid therapy and nutritional support may be required, together with antiparasitic treatment.

Environmental management is of utmost importance for prevention of parasites with direct life cycles. Prompt removal of feces from cages is recommended, whereas those maintained in larger outdoor enclosures would benefit from strategic treatment and movement (similar to pasture management of domesticated horses and ruminants). Generally, several days are required for life stages to become infective, and therefore daily cleaning is usually adequate. Fecal material left in the tank can easily be spread around the enclosure and contaminate food sources. Housing reptiles on newspaper with minimal cage furniture is advised for those undergoing antiparasitic treatment until repeat fecal samples have confirmed effective control of the parasite. Live prey can become contaminated with fecal material from the enclosures. To reduce the risk of environmental contamination, the reptile can be fed in a separate area from their regular housing.

Trematodiasis

Trematodes (flukes) can occur in a wide variety of tissues. Only a few species inhabit the GI tract. Of these, *Aspidogastreas* can be identified in chelonians. These require an intermediate host in their life cycle (aquatic snails) and are limited to recently caught, wild reptile specimens. No clinical signs have been reported. Digenetic trematodes are more commonly seen and also rely on an intermediate host (typically snails). Again clinical signs are not reported. Transmission is via eggs passed in the feces or urine of the host animal. Diagnosis is based on the observation of adult fluke in the feces, cloaca, or mouth. Fluke eggs can be found in the feces and are large and yellow/brown with a single operculum.[28]

Flukes can be treated with parenteral praziquantel, with a repeated dose required 14 days later. Prognosis is usually favorable.[12] Prevention involves prevention of access to intermediate hosts. Amphibians (e.g., frogs) fed to reptiles should be frozen for at least 3 days before feeding to prevent potential transmission.[28]

Cestodiasis

Tapeworms are not an uncommon finding in the GI tract of reptiles. All reptilian tapeworms require an intermediate host. Three orders of cestodes are of significance in the GI tract. The proteocephald tapeworm, *Ophiotaenia*, is the most common tapeworm found in wild-caught North American snakes.[29] Frogs serve as the intermediate host. In reptiles the eggs or adult tapeworms can be identified in the feces. Diphyllobothrid tapeworms (*Bothridium* sp.) are found as adults in pythons, whereas other species use reptiles as intermediate hosts. Mesocestoidid tapeworms can be found as adults in the GI tract of snakes and lizards, but most tapeworms of this family use them as intermediate hosts.

Often reptiles with tapeworm infections are asymptomatic; however, if numbers are large enough, enteritis, malnutrition, and intestinal obstructions can occur. The diagnosis rests on the identification of segments or whole parasites in fecal samples. Adult cestodes are

treated using parenteral praziquantel, with a repeated dose required 14 days later.

Cryptosporidiosis

Clinical Significance, Etiology, and Presentation.
Cryptosporidium is a small coccidian parasite frequently encountered in a wide variety of wild and captive reptiles worldwide. Unlike other coccidia, pathogenicity does not appear to depend on number of parasites, but instead is due to the reduced immunocompetence of the host or presence of concurrent disease. *Cryptosporidium serpentis* causes gastric disease in snakes; however, *C. varanii* and *C. saurophilum* in lizards causes enteric disease.[30] The parasite has a direct life cycle but is also able to replicate within the host. Ingested sporulated oocysts each produce four sporozoites in the intestine that develop into trophozoites in parasitophorous vacuoles within intestinal epithelial cells. Merozoites are formed and further cycles continue alongside the formation of oocysts that arise from sexual reproduction. These can be autoinfective or can be shed in the feces. Shedding in the feces is often intermittent, which can result in false negative fecal results. Cysts shed in the feces are immediately infective and are extremely resistant within the environment. All of these factors make *Cryptosporidium* difficult to eradicate from a collection.

Unlike snakes, in which gastritis is the norm, in lizards enteritis is the more common form, with associated anorexia, diarrhea, weight loss, and death (Fig. 74.6).[31] Passing undigested food and regurgitation are also possible.[32] An asymptomatic carrier state is also common, which can make the diagnosis of clinical disease problematic.[32,33] Enteric disease is unusual in snakes and chelonians.[16]

Diagnostic Confirmation.
Cryptosporidia can be identified as part of a routine fecal examination. A simple screening method is to analyze repeat fecal samples, as the agent can be intermittently shed. A thin wet preparation is made and then air dried. *Cryptosporidium* staining kits are available commercially (Pro-Laboratory Cryptosporidium staining kit, Pro-Laboratory Diagnostics, Toronto, Canada) and are essentially a modified cold Ziehl-Neelson stain (see Table 74.4). Oocysts appear as bright red ovals approximately 4 to 8 μm in length, whereas bacteria and yeasts stain pale green (Fig. 74.7). Cryptosporidia can also be detected

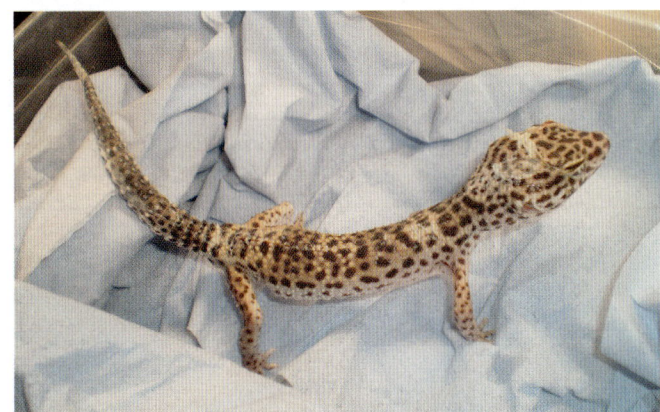

FIG 74.6 This emaciated leopard gecko (*Eublepharis macularius*) tested positive for *Cryptosporidium* oocysts on fecal acid-fast staining. (Courtesy of Jenna Richardson.)

TABLE 74.4 Modified Cold Ziehl-Neelson Stain Technique

1. Make a thin smear of fecal material on the slide and allow to dry.
2. The slide should be placed on the staining rack and covered with methanol (to fix the smear) before being allowed to air dry for 10–15 minutes.
3. Flood the dried slide with strong carbol fuchsin and leave for 10 minutes.
4. Gently wash the carbol fuchsin from the slide with deionized water and before flooding with hydrochloric acid.
5. Wait 1 minute then gently wash the hydrochloric acid from the slide with deionized water.
6. Repeat step 5 until the slide appears light pink in color.
7. Cover the smear with malachite green and leave for 30–60 seconds.
8. Rinse the slide for a final time with deionized water and allow to dry.
9. Examine under the ×100 oil-immersion objective.

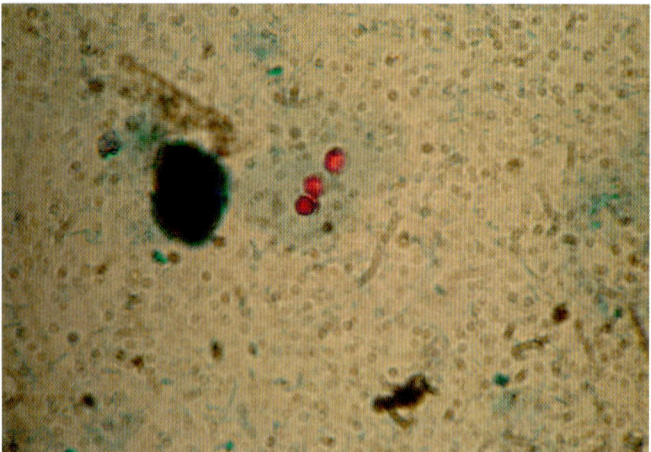

FIG 74.7 *Cryptosporidium* oocysts staining red on a ZN-stained fecal sample from a leopard gecko (*Eublepharis macularius*). The oocysts measure 4 to 8 microns in length. (Courtesy of Kevin Eatwell.)

by immunofluorescent staining using a commercially available test kit, which is 16 times more sensitive than acid-fast staining.[34]

These techniques do not differentiate *Cryptosporidium* species. This is a concern in species-fed mammalian prey, as *C. parvum* and *C. muris* can be passed incidentally in reptile fecal samples.[35] Correctly identifying the species is important, and this can be confirmed by polymerase chain reaction (PCR).[36] Pathogenicity can also be confirmed using histopathology of gastric or intestinal biopsies or samples collected postmortem, with immunofluorescent antibody testing to confirm the species of *Cryptosporidium*.[32,34]

Postmortem examination findings in lizards with enteric disease often show poor body condition. Cytology of the intestinal lumen can confirm large numbers of oocysts. Ultimately histopathology of the intestine is required to confirm a host pathogenic response. The organisms reside in the brush border of epithelial cells, and typically there is a marked infiltrative enteritis.[32]

Specific Therapy. Effective treatment is challenging, and no completely successful treatment regime has been reported. Paromomycin treatment in a small study of infected bearded dragons (*Pogona vitticeps*) was found to prevent oocyst shedding.[37] Bovine hyperimmune colostrum has shown

more promise, with small studies in monitors showing a significant reduction in oocyst shedding, in addition to histopathological resolution of disease after a course of treatment. In geckos, however, in which intestinal cryptosporidiosis is common, colostrum treatment appeared less efficacious, possibly owing to changes to the structure of colostrum immunoglobulins after passing through the stomach.[38] Hyperimmune colostrum is not commercially available.[38] Other treatment options include ionophores, but severe side effects can be seen.[34] Treatments to stimulate the immune system (increasing temperature, immunomodulators) and provide nutritional and fluid support may help support the patient.[26] In severe cases or in collection management, euthanasia may be recommended.

Environmental control is therefore of critical importance to control cryptosporidiosis in a collection. The prompt removal of fecal material with disinfection of the environment is important, but even then oocysts can be difficult to eliminate. Routine disinfectants (iodophors, cresylic acid, sodium hypochlorite, benzalkonium chloride, sodium hydrochlorite) are all ineffective. Ammonia (5%) and formalin (10%) appear effective, but with a contact time of 18 hours at 4°C these may not be the most practical solutions.[39] Currently, moist heat (45°–60°C for 5–9 minutes), freezing, or desiccation appear to be the most effective ways to clear the environment.[40]

Prognosis and Prevention. In reptiles with clinical signs, prognosis is poor, with species-dependent chronic enteritis, and wasting disease seen. Asymptomatic reptiles may never show clinical disease but can act as source of infection with intermittent shedding of oocysts.

Quarantine and multiple testing of new arrivals (three examinations are recommended over a 60-day period) to reduce the risk of introduction to an existing collection is advised. Routine monitoring of animals in the collection by fecal screening and postmortem examination (including histopathology) is also recommended. Animals shedding oocysts should be isolated from the rest of the collection and undergo strict barrier nursing. Intermittent excretion may limit the effectiveness of this method. Removal of positive animals from the collection may be required. Vertical transmission does not appear to occur.

Amoebiasis

Clinical Significance, Etiology, and Presentation. *Entamoeba invadens* is a well-recognized pathogen of reptiles and has a worldwide distribution, although other *Entamoeba* species may also be pathogenic. A number of reports have described fatal amoebiasis in a variety of species, including carnivorous and herbivorous species, although the infection appears less common now than historically.[41] A variety of clinical signs may occur, but mucoid dysentery appears characteristic in most cases. Other signs include anorexia, wasting, dehydration, and eventual death. Tissue invasion by trophozoites is possible, with ulceration of the gastrointestinal tract and abscesses forming in the liver.[41] Entamoeba is spread via the ingestion of feces contaminated with cysts. It has a direct life cycle and can rapidly spread through a collection.

Diagnostic Confirmation. Diagnosis is based on detection of cysts or trophozoites in feces. A fresh wet preparation is made and should be examined immediately. The diagnosis of amoebiasis is possible by identification of amoebae, trophozoites (9–39 μm), or quadrinucleate cysts (9–24 μm) in a fresh fecal smear stained with Lugol's iodine. Carrier animals can be difficult to detect due to the low numbers of parasites shed.

Culture techniques are available but are not practical for clinical settings.[42] PCR is also available.[41] A variety of human diagnostic techniques exist but are yet to be applied to reptile amoebiasis.[32] On histopathology (or postmortem examination), signs of severe pathology can be seen. *Entamoebiasis* causes thickening and edema of the intestine wall, erosions, ulcers, and infection, which can extend to the liver, creating abscesses. Histopathologically, the organisms can be seen invading the bowel submucosa, causing a marked enteritis and, where infection of the liver is present, hepatitis.

Specific Therapy. Treatment for amoeba should target both trophozoites and cysts (so combination therapy is often recommended). Metronidazole is effective against trophozoites but has no effect against cysts. High doses have traditionally been recommended, but caution is advised in indigo snakes (*Drymarchon corais*), rattlesnakes (*Crotalus* sp.), and king snakes (*Lampropeltis getulus* sp.), as toxicity has been reported.[43,44] Paromomycin, diloxanide furoate, or iodoquinol are used to target cysts.

Adjunctive therapy with antibiotics may be considered due to the opportunistic invasion of lesions by bacteria; however, antibiotics have not been shown to improve survival in cases of gut-associated sepsis in humans.[45] Analgesia should also be considered given the severity of pathology induced by the organism.

Prognosis and Prevention. Morbidity and mortality can be high, with infection most commonly found in lizards and snakes and with chelonians usually acting as reservoir hosts. *Entamoeba* has been identified in herbivorous chelonians with no clinical signs.[43] Quarantine, cleaning, and effective disinfection of the environment is critical alongside routine screening for amoebiasis. Amoebic trophozoites and cysts are resistant and can survive in the environment for more than 14 days.[46]

Coccidiosis

Clinical Significance, Etiology, Presentation, and Diagnostic Confirmation.
Coccidia are commonly identified in fecal samples, particularly those from lizards. Various coccidian species may be seen, and types of oocysts are generally differentiated by the number of sporocysts contained within an oocyst.[47] *Eimeria* oocysts normally contain four sporocysts, *Isospora* and *Sarcocystis* contain two, and *Caryospora* contains one. When ingested, the oocyst releases sporozoites that invade the cells and mature into schizonts. The cell then ruptures and releases merozoites that invade more cells. Merozoites also undergo sexual reproduction to form zygotes, which release the oocysts.

Low numbers of coccidia are rarely of concern, but numbers can escalate in juveniles in association with poor hygiene, overcrowding, or concurrent disease. *Isospora amphiboluri* is a common problem in young bearded dragons and may result in enteritis in high numbers (Fig. 74.8). Heavy numbers can also be seen associated with concurrent adenovirus infections.[48] This can lead to a wide range of clinical signs, including anorexia, lethargy, weight loss, diarrhea, tenesmus, prolapses, and death may occur if untreated. Stunting of juveniles is also a feature of heavy burdens. The diagnosis is made by fecal examination using the same techniques as described for helminths.

Specific Therapy, Prognosis, and Prevention.
Treatment of coccidia is recommended for young animals or those with a moderate to high parasite burden. There is a variety of treatment options, with toltrazuril commonly used. It is alkaline and best diluted before oral administration. Trimethoprim/sulphonamides are also commonly used and are widely available as oral suspensions. Other options include the use of clazuril (see Chapter 120). Prognosis is dependent on the health status of the individual reptile and the coccidia burden. Prevention involves fecal screening of new reptiles to avoid introduction of disease, and environmental control with prompt removal of fecal material and good

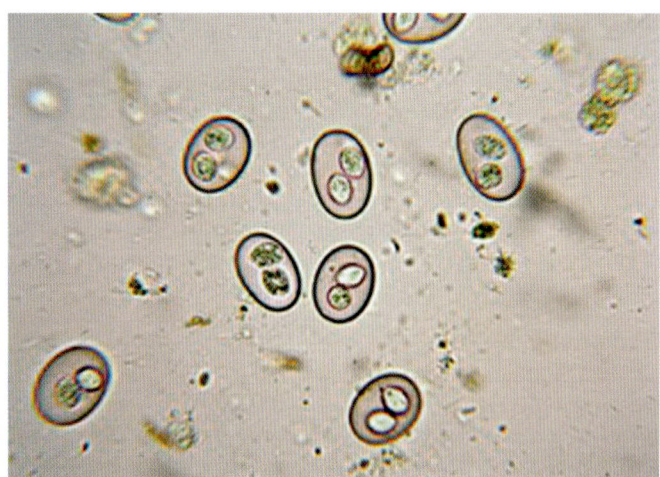

FIG 74.8 *Isospora* oocyst on a fecal flotation from a bearded dragon (*Pogona vitticeps*). Viewed under a 400× magnification. Oocysts measure 10 to 40 microns in length. (Courtesy of Kevin Eatwell.)

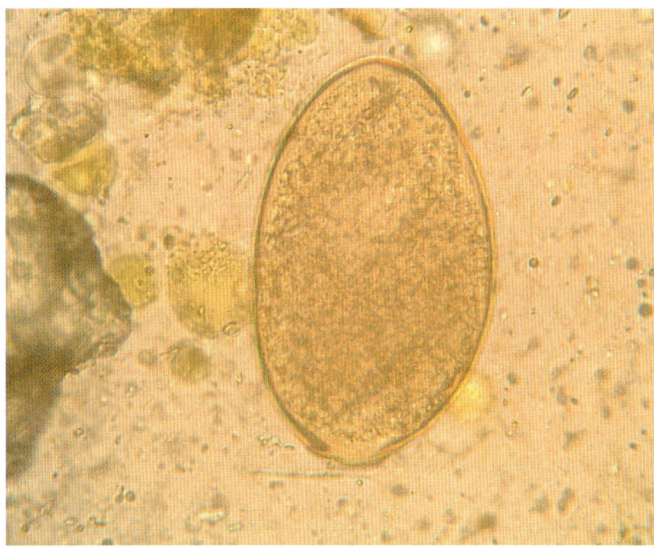

FIG 74.9 Ciliates, such as *Nyctotherius* (400× magnification), are a common finding in fresh fecal samples from chelonians and require no treatment. (Courtesy of Kevin Eatwell.)

hygiene. Oocysts can be inactivated by freezing or exposure to high temperatures.

Nonpathogenic Protozoa (Amoeba, Flagellates, and Ciliates)

Various amoebae, flagellates (typically *Trichomonas*, *Hexamita*, or *Giardia*), and ciliates (such as *Balantidium* and *Nyctotherus*) are often found in fecal samples and are generally considered nonpathogenic commensal organisms (Fig. 74.9). Larger burdens, however, can be associated with (but are often not the cause of) anorexia, weight loss, and diarrhea.[26,49] Higher levels may be found in animals housed on soil substrates.[16] Treatment of animals with clinical signs of enteritis is recommended.

A fresh wet preparation is used to detect motility in fecal samples. This ideally should be examined immediately. Once prepared, the slide can be gently warmed to stimulate motility. This is particularly important if the fecal sample had been refrigerated before assessment.

Specific Therapy, Prognosis and Prevention. Although rarely indicated, oral metronidazole or ronidazole can be used to treat flagellates and ciliates. Care is advised in indigo snakes, rattlesnakes, and king snakes, as toxicity has been seen.[42,44] Repeat fecal assessment can be used to confirm effectiveness.

The presence of large numbers of protozoa can be indicative of an underlying disease process; however, mortality from primary protozoal overgrowths is not well supported in the veterinary literature. Good environmental hygiene, along with prompt treatment of episodes of diarrhea and anorexia, may prevent protozoal overgrowths.

Bacterial Enteritis

Clinical Significance and Presentation. Bacterial diseases are often blamed for illness in reptiles; however, clinical reports where specific bacterial pathogens have been implicated as a cause for intestinal disease are rare, with only one report of *Pseudomonas* recorded.[50] *Salmonella* can be isolated from reptile feces. Some reports state prevalences as high as 90%, whereas others have failed to identify any *Salmonella*.[51,52] Routine screening of reptiles for *Salmonella* is not recommended, as they are generally not pathogenic and are considered part of the normal intestinal flora.[53] Eradication is problematic due to vertical transmission and prompt horizontal transmission to juveniles after hatching.[53–56] *Salmonella* is a zoonotic concern, and there are a large number of reports of reptile-associated salmonellosis in humans (see chapter 174).[57–59] *Salmonella* has been associated with clinical disease in reptiles, most notably in an outbreak of Nile crocodiles where *Salmonella* was isolated from the gastrointestinal tract on postmortem examinations.[60] *Salmonella* has also be reported to cause enteritis in red-tailed boas (*Boa constrictor* spp.).[61]

Anaerobic infections are probably more common than currently reported, and consideration should be given to comparing fecal gram stains with culture results. *Clostridium perfringens* has been implicated in a case of diarrhea in a red-footed tortoise (*Chelonoidis carbonaria*).[62] Other agents such as *Mycobacterium* or *Chlamydia* may be identified in cultures or samples from the intestinal tract. *Chlamydia*-like organisms have been implicated in clinical enteritis in snakes and iguanas.[63–65]

Diagnostic Confirmation. Routine culture of feces will invariably yield positive culture results with a combination of aerobic (typically gram-negative, such as *Pseudomonas* and *Escherichia coli*) and anaerobic bacteria likely.[66,67] These often exhibit multidrug resistance. Infections caused by gram-negative aerobes are generally considered more common.[68] It is often assumed that these are primary or opportunistic pathogens that require treatment (Fig. 74.10). Confirming that a specific bacteria isolated from a fecal sample is pathogenic can be difficult. Hematology may yield altered white cell counts or toxic activity on blood films, indicating systemic inflammation. Confirmation of pathology relies on the identification of a host pathological response. This essentially means that serology, cytology, or histopathology (ideally) is required to confirm pathogenicity.

Specific Therapy, Prognosis, and Prevention. Antibiotic therapy, if indicated, should be based on culture and sensitivity results. The local/topical administration of antibacterials that are not absorbed from the GI tract (e.g., aminoglycosides) is often more efficacious. Repeat testing of the reptile is required to determine when treatment can be discontinued. Prognosis is dependent on the severity of dehydration and duration of the disease. Prevention is aimed at appropriate husbandry with suitable temperature ranges, environmental hygiene, and appropriate dietary items. Long-term oral antibiosis should also be avoided.

Fungal Enteritis

Fungal pathogens are typically opportunistic and have been reported in the GI tract; however, none are primary pathogens.[7] Knowledge of

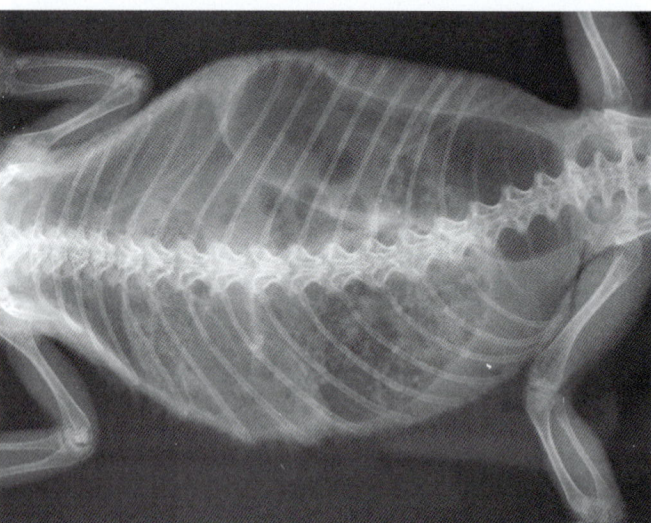

FIG 74.10 This radiograph shows a bearded dragon (*Pogona vitticeps*) with a marked bacterial enterocolitis with gas formation. The animal was in significant coelomic discomfort. (Courtesy of Kevin Eatwell.)

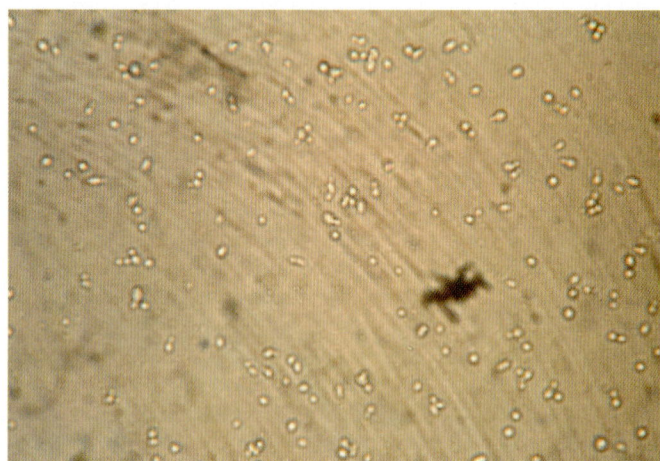

FIG 74.11 This overgrowth of *Candida* was found on fecal analysis from a Chinese water dragon (*Physignathus cocincinus*) that had been treated with oral enrofloxacin for 2 weeks. (Courtesy of Kevin Eatwell.)

the normal intestinal microbiome of reptiles is scant, although likely to be highly varied.[69] In crocodilians and agamid lizards a wide variety of fungal species have been identified.[70,71] Yeasts are considered part of the normal flora, particularly in herbivorous species.[72,73] Overgrowths are often directly associated with the use of prolonged antibiotic therapy in reptiles, and isolates identified include *Aspergillus, Fusarium, Mucor, Candida, Penicillium, Basidiobolus*, and *Paecilomyces/Purpureocillium* (Fig. 74.11).

The diagnosis rests on the growth of organisms on fecal culture or identification of fungal elements on fecal cytology. The decision to treat should be based on the presence of a host pathological response on cytology or histopathology. This is not always possible, and generally clinical judgment is required based on the numbers identified. Nystatin is often used as a locally acting antifungal agent; however, systemically acting agents such as itraconazole or voriconazole may be required in advanced or disseminated cases.

Prognosis is good with low-grade infections but poor with major organ involvement or disseminated disease.[8] Prevention is aimed at

TABLE 74.5 Common Enteric Viral Infections Seen in Captive Reptiles

Virus	Species	Gross Findings/ Clinical Signs	Histopathological Findings	Virus Isolation/ Electron Microscopy
Adenovirus[75]	Nile crocodiles	Enteritis/sudden death	Necrotizing enteritis, basophilic intranuclear inclusion bodies in epithelial cells	
Adenovirus[76]	Rosy boas	Hemorrhage on serosa of the intestinal tract/sudden death	No enteric inclusion bodies	
Adenovirus[77]	Chameleons	None	Basophilic intranuclear inclusions in epithelial cells	
Adenovirus[78]	Bearded dragons		Inclusions seen in enterocytes	
Adenovirus[79]	Geckos		Lymphoplasmacytic enteritis	
Adenovirus[79]	Skinks		Enteric inclusion bodies	
Reovirus[80]	Chinese vipers	None/sudden death/enteritis	No enteric inclusion bodies	
Reovirus[81]	Rattlesnake	Neurological disease		Yes
Herpesvirus[82]	Chelonians	Enteritis		Yes
Iridiovirus[83]	Chelonians		Basophilic intracytoplasmic inclusion bodies in enterocytes	
Iridioviruses[84]	Chameleons			Yes
Iridioviruses[85]	Bearded dragons			Yes
Parvovirus[78,86]	Bearded dragons			Dependoviruses identified alongside adenoviruses
Parvovirus[87]	King snakes		Basophilic inclusions in the enterocytes	
Parvovirus[88,89]	Snakes			Yes
Inclusion body disease (IBD) arenavirus[90]	Snakes		Enteric eosinophillic intracytoplasmic inclusion bodies	
Mixed viral infection, adenovirus, parvovirus, picornavirus & herpesvirus[83]	Gastroenteritis	Sudden death	Inclusion bodies	

appropriate husbandry with suitable temperature and humidity levels, as well as stringent environmental hygiene.

Viral Enteritis

Viruses may be provisionally or definitively identified within the intestinal tract by the presence of enterocyte inclusion bodies or by viral particles in digesta or feces. In many cases the involvement of viral disease is identified on histopathology of intestinal biopsies or on postmortem examination. The difficulty arises when identifying the significance of the viral infection and relating this to the clinical presentation. Many viral infections are found associated with other pathogens such as bacteria or enteric parasites.[74] A summary of the enteric viral infections of reptiles is listed in Table 74.5 (also see Chapter 30, Virology).

Nutritional Disorders

Clinical Significance, Etiology, and Presentation. Metabolic bone disease, specifically nutritional secondary hyperparathyroidism, is common in captive reptiles. Gastrointestinal transit and motility are dependent on calcium concentrations, and reduced ionized calcium levels can lead to reduced GI motility and ileus. This can lead to increased fermentation of digesta, especially in herbivorous species, with marked gas production. The increased transit time can lead to progressive dehydration of bowel contents, obstipation, and the production of firm fecoliths. Husbandry-related problems can also play an important role in intestinal transit time. When environmental temperatures are too low, they can lead to a reduction in both appetite and fecal output, as the animal's metabolic rate and GI motility are reduced. Sudden dietary change can also lead to diarrhea, primarily due to the increased water

or simple carbohydrate content of the food being offered, or associated with dysbiosis in herbivores. Greater levels of dietary fiber also increase transit time.

Diagnostic Confirmation. Investigation of obstipation or diarrhea can include imaging to evaluate the intestinal tract. Plain radiography can be helpful in identifying the quantity of fecal material or the build-up of intestinal gas. Contrast agents such as liquid barium, or barium-impregnated polyspheres (BIPS, Medical I.D Systems, Inc., MI), can be used (Fig. 74.12). Computed tomography can provide detailed images (Fig. 74.13). Ultrasonography of the intestinal tract can yield useful results; however, increased intestinal gas can severely hamper examination.

Flexible endoscopes of appropriate size are typically required to enter the duodenum and small intestine. Cloacal endoscopy is of use in the investigation of patients with obstipation. A rigid endoscope can be passed into the colon under general anesthesia, allowing direct visualization of the colonic mucosa and fecal contents. Coelomic endoscopy can also be used to evaluate the serosal surface of the intestinal tract (see Chapter 64).

Specific Therapy. Resolution relies on improvement in husbandry and nutrition. Providing a suitable diet for the species long term is important. Fluid therapy (initially parenteral, but progressing to oral) to rehydrate and soften GI contents is often a critical first step. Agents such as lactulose have been used as a bulk laxative alongside prokinetic agents such as metoclopramide and cisapride. The use of prokinetics in reptiles may have limited clinical benefit, and the true efficacy is unknown.

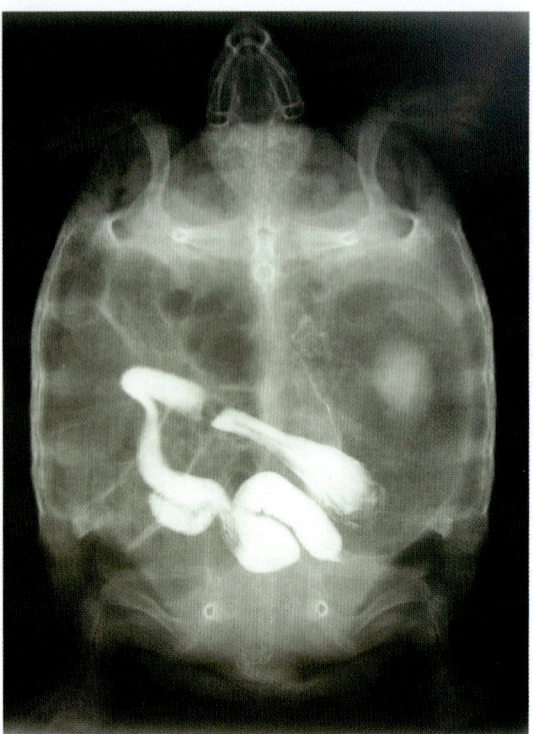

FIG 74.12 Barium contrast study of a horsfield tortoise (*Agrionemys horsfieldii*) showing normal filling of the small intestine. (Courtesy of Kevin Eatwell.)

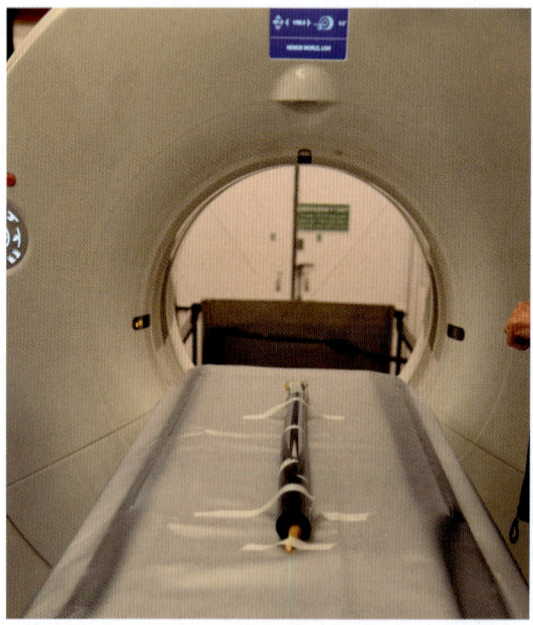

FIG 74.13 Computerized tomography being used to evaluate a conscious corn snake (*Pantherophis guttatus*). (Courtesy of Jenna Richardson.)

If obstipation is severe, then more invasive techniques may be indicated to alleviate the blockage. This can be achieved under general anesthesia, using colonic irrigation with saline and gentle manipulation of the large bowel either externally or per cloaca to remove content. Endoscopic guidance may be useful for direct visualization of the

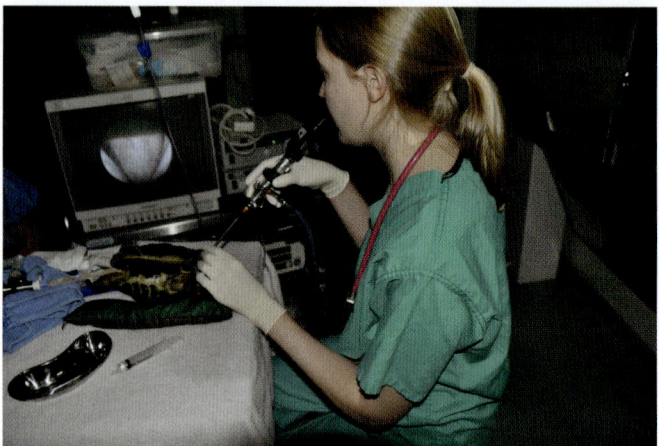

FIG 74.14 Cloacal endoscopy performed on a Hermann's tortoise (*Testudo hermanni*). Endoscopy is a useful tool to examine the distal intestinal tract. (Courtesy of Jenna Richardson.)

intestinal mucosa and blockage (Fig. 74.14). It is important to evaluate for any signs of iatrogenic damage to the intestinal tract. Long-term oral fluid therapy may be necessary, and in nonresponsive cases, surgical intervention is indicated.

Foreign Bodies

Clinical Significance and Presentation. Ingestion of foreign material is relatively common. Pica, lithophagy (ingestion of stones), and geophagy (ingestion of earth or soil-like substrate, e.g., sand, chalk, or clay) are reported in both captive and wild reptiles (Fig. 74.15A).[91] Feeding practices can increase the risk of foreign body ingestion. Housing on sand can result in contamination of food items. Over time, the volume of sand ingested accumulates, which can lead to sand impactions within the intestines (see Fig. 74.15B). Chelonians appear prone to ingesting rocks and wood materials (Fig. 74.16 and Fig. 74.17).[6] They are also attracted to brightly colored objects, which can result in plastic or metal ingestion, particularly in grazing animals or those with outdoor access (Fig. 74.18). Chelonians will also readily accept being hand-fed foreign objects or consume newspaper substrate. Sharper material (e.g., aspen, bark, etc.) can puncture the GI tract and lead to coelomitis or abscess formation. Consumption of skin shed (dermatophagy) (Fig. 74.19) could act as a potential obstructive material, and reptiles may also ingest ectoparasites from the exuvium[92] (Fig. 74.20).[92] In reproductively active females, ingestion of stones, etc. may be associated with an increased demand for calcium. There are many cases reported in the literature of novel and enclosure-related foreign body ingestion in captive reptiles.[93–95]

Snakes do not appear to deliberately ingest foreign material; however, when consuming prey, they can swallow substrate (e.g., aspen or bark) that has become attached to their food. In general, feeding directly on particulate substrates should be avoided. Feeding can occur in a separate container or on particulate-free surfaces (e.g., slate tiles).

Depending on the size and composition of the ingested foreign material, it can either pass through and be voided in feces or lodge within the intestinal tract, leading to a partial or complete obstruction. In many cases this can be life threatening. Rarely impactions can lead to physical distention of the coelomic cavity (Fig. 74.21). Foreign bodies within the large intestine typically continue and pass uneventfully.

Clinical signs are similar to other species with foreign body ingestion; however, the duration can be extended and appear more chronic. The

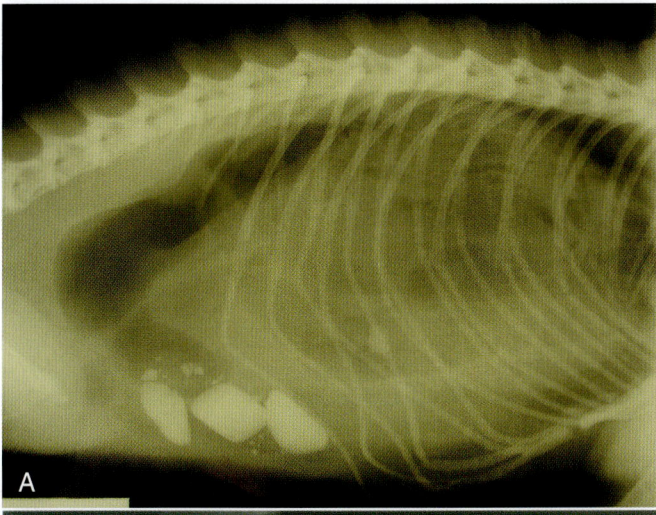

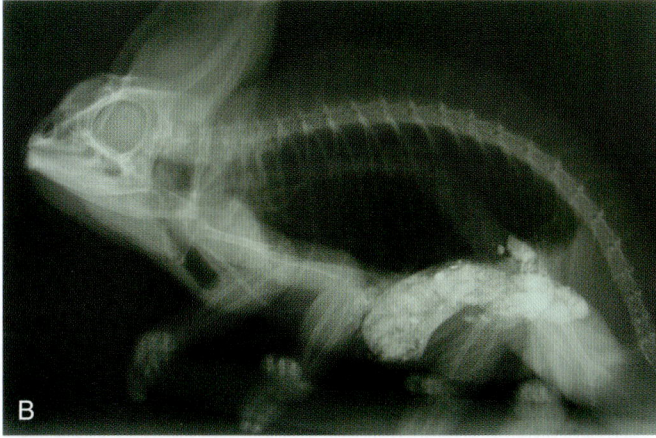

FIG 74.15 Substrate ingestion is commonly seen in reptiles. (A) This green iguana (*Iguana iguana*) had ingested stones that passed uneventfully. (B) This veiled chameleon (*Chamaeleo calyptratus*) had ingested small stones that required surgical intervention. (Courtesy of Kevin Eatwell.)

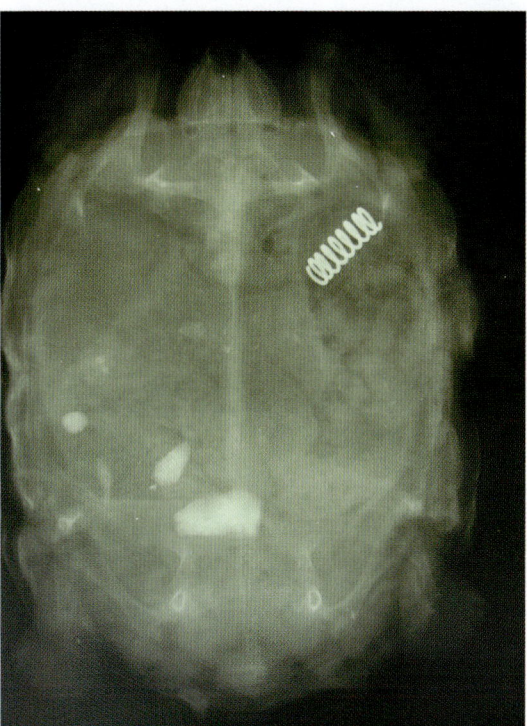

FIG 74.16 This radiograph of a horsefield tortoise (*Agrionemys horsfieldii*) shows stones and a metal spring the animal had ingested while loose in the owner's garden. (Courtesy of Kevin Eatwell.)

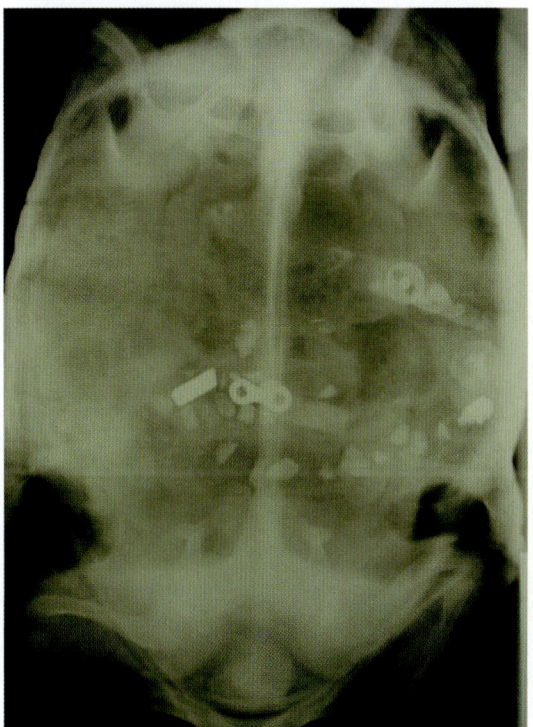

FIG 74.17 This is a radiograph of a leopard tortoise (*Stigmochelys pardalis*), which was hand-fed household items by small children. It readily accepted whatever was offered to it. Surgical intervention was not required. (Courtesy of Kevin Eatwell.)

reptile can appear subdued and lethargic, and there may be a recent history of anorexia. Vomiting can be seen with small intestine involvement. The clinical history may be vague and include anorexia, weight loss, and lethargy, which can extend over weeks to months. Constipation, reduced or absent fecal production, bloating, cloacal prolapse, and diarrhea are possible. Reptiles with chronic disease are often dehydrated and cachectic. Intestinal atony has been reported in green iguanas (*Iguana iguana*), caused by ingestion of foreign bodies.[96]

Diagnostic Confirmation. Survey radiography is useful for the detection of an intestinal foreign body. Horizontal beam radiography can be useful, as foreign bodies are often located ventrally, whereas gaseous distention can lead to dorsal displacement of bowel loops and provides further evidence of possible obstruction (Fig. 74.22). Sand obstipation can be readily identified by radiography; wooden, rubber, or plastic materials can be difficult to detect without contrast or ultrasonography.[95] Coelomic ultrasonography can be used for further clarification; however, a build-up of intestinal gas may affect image quality. Gastrointestinal contrast studies can be performed, but they are not without their own limitations (Fig. 74.23). The GI motility time in reptiles is generally longer than that of mammalian and avian species. In some cases (e.g., large constrictors), transit times can extend over several weeks to more than a month (Fig. 74.24). For smaller species, contrast studies may extend over 2 to 5 days.

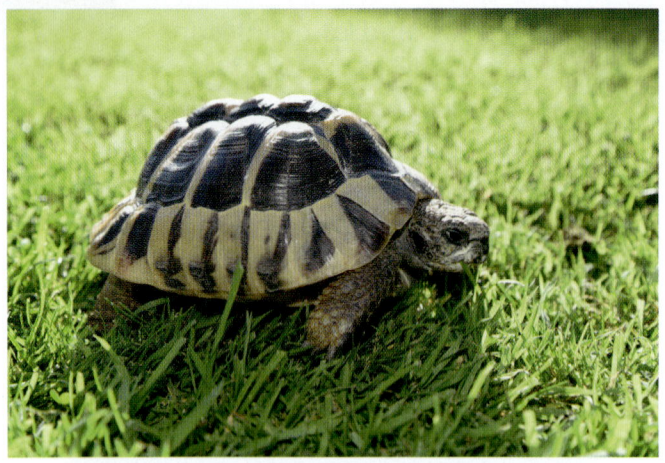

FIG 74.18 Tortoises, like this Hermann's tortoise (*Testudo hermanni*) with access to outdoors, are likely candidates for foreign body ingestion. (Courtesy of Jenna Richardson.)

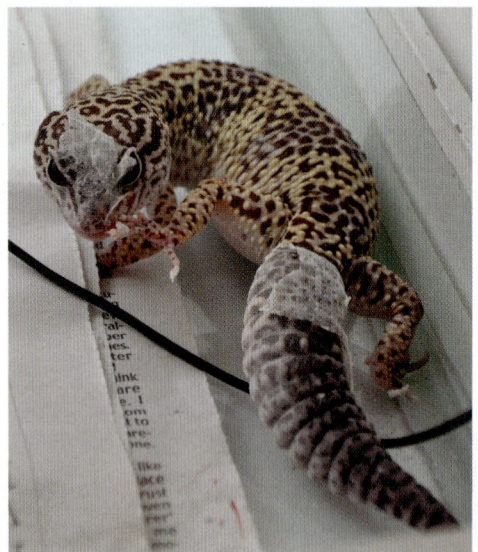

FIG 74.19 Dermatophagy, as seen with this leopard gecko (*Eublepharis macularius*), could act as a potential obstructive material during time of shed. (Courtesy of Jenna Richardson.)

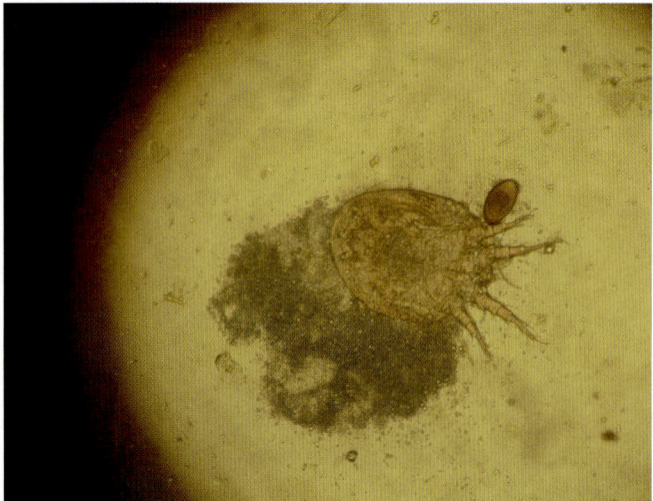

FIG 74.20 Snake mites can be ingested by the host reptile from their shed skin and the environment (400× magnification). This sample is from a Chinese water dragon (*Physignathus cocincinus*). (Courtesy of Kevin Eatwell.)

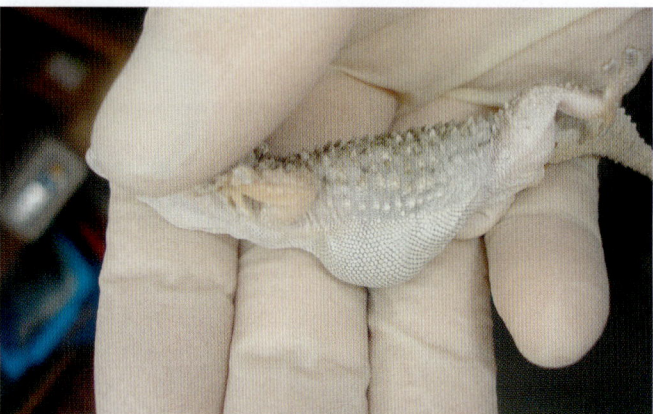

FIG 74.21 Intestinal impaction can cause coelomic distention, as seen here in this Moorish gecko (*Tarentola mauritanica*). (Courtesy of Kevin Eatwell.)

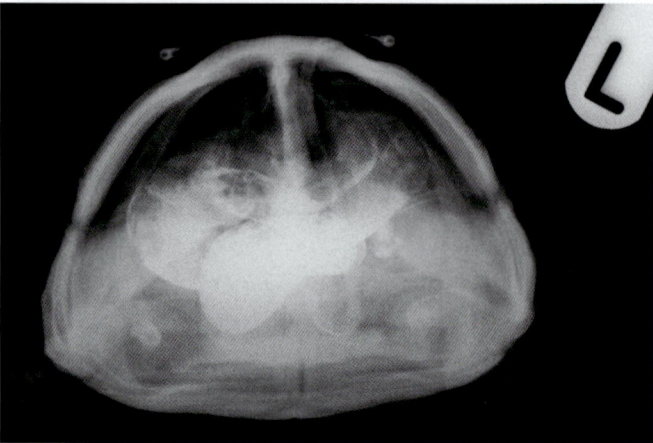

FIG 74.22 Horizontal beam radiography can demonstrate gas-filled intestinal loops encroaching on the lung fields in chelonians. This craniocaudal view of a barium study on a spur-thighed tortoise (*Testudo graeca*) shows markedly dilated bowel loops, compressing the lung. (Courtesy of Jenna Richardson.)

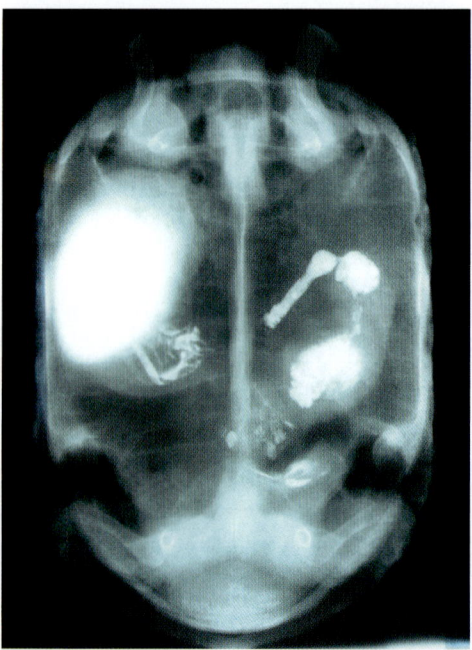

FIG 74.23 This dorsoventral radiograph of a red-footed tortoise (*Chelonoidis carbonaria*) shows a failure of barium sulfate to pass through the small intestine due to a total obstruction. A complete section of small intestine had become necrotic and was identified on postmortem examination. (Courtesy of Kevin Eatwell.)

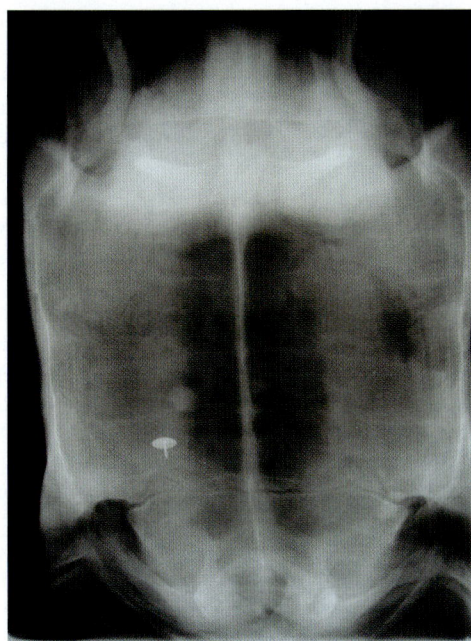

FIG 74.24 This thumbtack took 28 days from ingestion to pass in the feces of this marginated tortoise (*Testudo marginata*). (Courtesy of Kevin Eatwell.)

TABLE 74.6 Neoplasia of the Intestinal Tract and Pancreas

Species	Tumor Type	Tumor Location	Treatment (if any)
Northern water snake[100]	Adenocarcinoma	Splenopancreas	Euthanasia
Western hognose[101]	Adenocarcinoma	Splenopancreas	Surgical excision—
Leopard gecko[102]	Adenocarcinoma	Colon	Euthanasia
Savannah monitor[103]	Lymphosarcoma	Intestinal and hepatic	Euthanasia
Komodo dragon[104]	Carcinoma	Colon	—
Komodo dragon[104]	Colon carcinoma (with concurrent islet cell tumor and thyroid adenoma)	Colon	

Specific Therapy. Foreign body removal requires endoscopic or surgical intervention. Patients should be stabilized initially with fluid therapy, analgesia, and a suitable temperature range. Surgical approach varies with species; for example, a paramedian incision is performed in many lizards, whereas in a chelonian, a large intestinal foreign body may require a plastronotomy. Removal of the foreign material is by standard enterotomy; however, in cases of intestinal devitalization, enterectomy and anastomosis are required.

Prognosis and Prevention. The prognosis is dependent upon foreign body composition and potential toxicity (e.g., heavy metals), location, duration of obstruction, and degree of damage (e.g., perforation, devitalization). In cases with coelomitis, the prognosis is guarded, even with emergency surgery. Prevention is better than cure, and during routine health check consultations, enclosure substrate and furniture should be discussed, with removal of potentially hazardous, high-risk materials recommended.

Intestinal Neoplasia

Clinical Significance and Presentation.
With continued advancements in captive management and herpetological medicine, increased reptile longevity is to be expected. This increase in life expectancy leads to an aged population at increased risk of developing neoplastic disease. Based on a necropsy review, captive reptiles have an incidence of neoplasia comparable with that of birds and mammals.[97] Neoplastic disease should always be considered as a differential diagnosis in any unresolving or multifactorial presentation, regardless of the age of the patient.[6] Intestinal neoplasia has been reported in all orders of the Reptilia.[98–100] More commonly, case reports or small case series are published in the literature. Christman et al. published a review of all reported reptile oncology cases between 2004 and 2017.[98] Of the 59 case reports reviewed, only three involved the intestinal tract or pancreas (Table 74.6). Hernandez-Divers reviewed 1287 lizard pathology cases, of which 81 displayed neoplastic conditions.[103] Of these, only four were pertaining to the intestinal tract, of which one animal, a komodo dragon (*Varanus komodoensis*), had multiple tumor types.[104]

The clinical signs attributed to GI neoplasia in reptiles can vary and may include palpable intestinal masses or thickenings, anorexia, weight loss, wasting, caudal coelomic distention, melena, asymmetrical cloacal enlargement, and constipation. If tumor size is large, partial or complete intestinal obstruction can result.

Diagnostic Confirmation.
Case investigation and management can prove challenging and expensive. Routine hematology and plasma biochemistries can provide some insight into the physiological status of the patient; however, in many instances results are nonspecific and vague. Where neoplasia results in ulceration or hemorrhage, hematochezia, melena, and anemia may be appreciated. Hematological findings associated with gastrointestinal neoplasia include lymphopenia or lymphocytosis, heterophilia, and monocytosis.[6]

Survey radiography is useful and widely available in practice.[103] Soft tissue structures can be difficult to differentiate from one another due to superimposition and lack of diffuse fat; however, gross enlargements should be readily visible. Ultrasonography can be very useful for both assessing structures within the coelomic cavity and for guiding fine-needle aspirates or core biopsies. Pre- and postcontrast computed tomography (CT) is a superior modality that provides cross-sectional images and three-dimensional reconstructions in conscious or sedated patients. Unfortunately, CT is often restricted to referral institutions.

In stable patients, surgical exploration is advised, either by coelioscopy or coeliotomy. Endoscopy is minimally invasive and can facilitate the collection of biopsy samples while allowing direct visualization of the coelomic cavity. A definitive histological diagnosis and staging is preferred before considering treatment options (surgical resection, chemotherapy, radiation). Where mass removal is warranted, a coeliotomy allows for improved access and visualization. Recovery times and discomfort from incision size are greater with a coeliotomy technique.

Therapy and Prognosis.
Sadly, a large number of neoplastic conditions in reptiles are diagnosed postmortem. Our current understanding for treatments of neoplasia in reptiles is limited. Surgical removal of intestinal tumors without prior histological diagnosis and staging is unfortunately the most common clinical approach. Further work is required to assess the use of chemotherapy or radiation therapy in the treatment of

neoplasia in reptiles. In many cases with advanced or metastatic disease, euthanasia is often indicated on welfare grounds.

CLINICAL PANCREATIC DISEASES

Diseases of the reptile pancreas appear to be generally uncommon (or underdiagnosed), with few clinical reports in the literature. Further research may be required to better understand the diagnosis of these conditions.

Pancreatitis

Clinical Significance, Etiology, and Presentation. Pancreatitis is not commonly seen in reptiles, although cases have been reported.[4] Acute necrotizing pancreatitis is similar to that seen in mammals. Digestive enzymes escape from a damaged pancreas, resulting in severe, necrotizing inflammation of the pancreatic tissues. Pancreatic damage can be caused by infection, trauma, or migrating parasites. In severe cases, with extensive inflammation, both the endocrine and exocrine pancreas can be involved. This painful condition can lead to altered posture, reluctance to be handled, lethargy, anorexia, and weight loss.

Intranuclear coccidiosis has been described in a number of chelonian species, with variable clinical signs including anorexia, lethargy, wasting, and oculonasal discharges.[105] Numerous organs may be affected, including the liver, kidneys, and pancreas. Histopathology is required for diagnosis.[106] Treatment with standard anticoccidials so far appears ineffective for nonintestinal coccidiosis. *Cryptosporidium* has been reported in the pancreas of corn snakes.[2]

In a group of red-eared slider turtles (*Trachemys scripta elegans*) pancreatitis was found to be associated with nematode infection.[107] Migratory nematodes and trematodes found in pancreatic tissue are typically walled off and phagocytized.[12] They appear to cause minimal damage to the pancreas but can result in secondary infection with the introduction of bacteria.[4] Diagnosis is often incidental at postmortem examination.

Inclusion body disease (IBD, arenavirus) is a common condition affecting boas and pythons and has also been identified in colubrid snakes and vipers. Clinical signs are varied and can include neurological disease, regurgitation, and weight loss. The disease, believed to be an arenavirus, produces eosinophillic intracytoplasmic inclusion bodies. The diagnosis is largely dependent on histological demonstration of inclusion bodies, which can be found in the pancreas as well as the kidneys, the liver, and, more commonly, the central nervous system. Herpes viral inclusion bodies in the pancreas have been identified in boa constrictors.[108] Two of five wild-caught rough green snakes (*Opheodrys aestivus*) had subacute to chronic pancreatitis associated with orthoreovirus infection.[109]

Diagnostic Confirmation and Therapy. Diagnosis can be complicated, as clinical signs are often nonspecific, with lethargy and inappetance. Coelioscopy to visualize the pancreas, along with biopsy collection, is advised. Treatment is largely dependent on the inciting cause; however, supportive care with nutritional support, fluid therapy, and analgesia should always be considered. Often cases of pancreatitis are diagnosed postmortem.

Radiography, ultrasonography, coelioscopy, or exploratory coeliotomy can be used to assist with the diagnosis; however, biopsy of the affected pancreatic tissue is recommended.[4] Treatment includes aggressive supportive care, alongside addressing the inciting cause.

Pancreatic Neoplasia

Pancreatic neoplasia is not commonly reported.[4] Disease is often advanced by the time of presentation, and treatment options are limited. Euthanasia on welfare grounds is commonplace. Multihormonal pancreatic islet cell carcinomas were found in one female and two male captive geriatric Komodo dragons (*Varanus komodoensis*). The animals presented with lethargy, weakness, and anorexia. Gross changes in the pancreas were visible in two of the three cases.[110]

REFERENCES

See www.expertconsult.com for a complete list of references.

75

Gastroenterology—Cloaca

Stuart McArthur and Ross A. Machin

Cloacal organ prolapse is a common veterinary emergency and is seen in both first opinion and referral practice. It occurs in all classes of reptiles. A cloacal prolapse is a clinical sign, not a condition; as in most cases, a pathological prolapse is associated with deeper clinical issues and significant debility. The gastrointestinal, reproductive, and urinary systems end in the cloaca, and therefore a wide variety of disorders may manifest as abnormalities around these anatomic structures, especially if they become obstructed at the cloaca. Prolapses have been described in wild, as well as captive, reptiles (McArthur and Machin, Personal Observation, 2017).[1–12]

Treatment of all cloacal prolapses involves a simultaneous balance of medical and surgical interventions. The presentation draws upon many of the techniques described across all clinical disciplines.[11,12] Information that will assist a clinician facing this presentation is located within several sections of this book; surgical management is covered in Chapter 106 and throughout Section 10. Medical management is included here and throughout Sections 5 and 9, and a case summary of the approach to the cloacal prolapse is described in Chapter 143.

ANATOMY

Three different body systems terminate at the reptilian cloaca. These are the reproductive, urinary, and gastrointestinal tracts. Cloaca anatomy is mildly variable between the orders, but the cloaca is divided into three compartments, which lie between the body of the caudal colon and the vent.[14–22] The cloaca acts as a vestibule to collect, modify, and prepare the output from each of these three organ systems. It therefore helps the reptile to manage both the quantity and the quality of fecal and urinary output, and it is involved in the output of the male or female reproductive systems (i.e., sperm release, live birth, oviposition)[14,22–24] (Figs. 75.1 and 75.2)

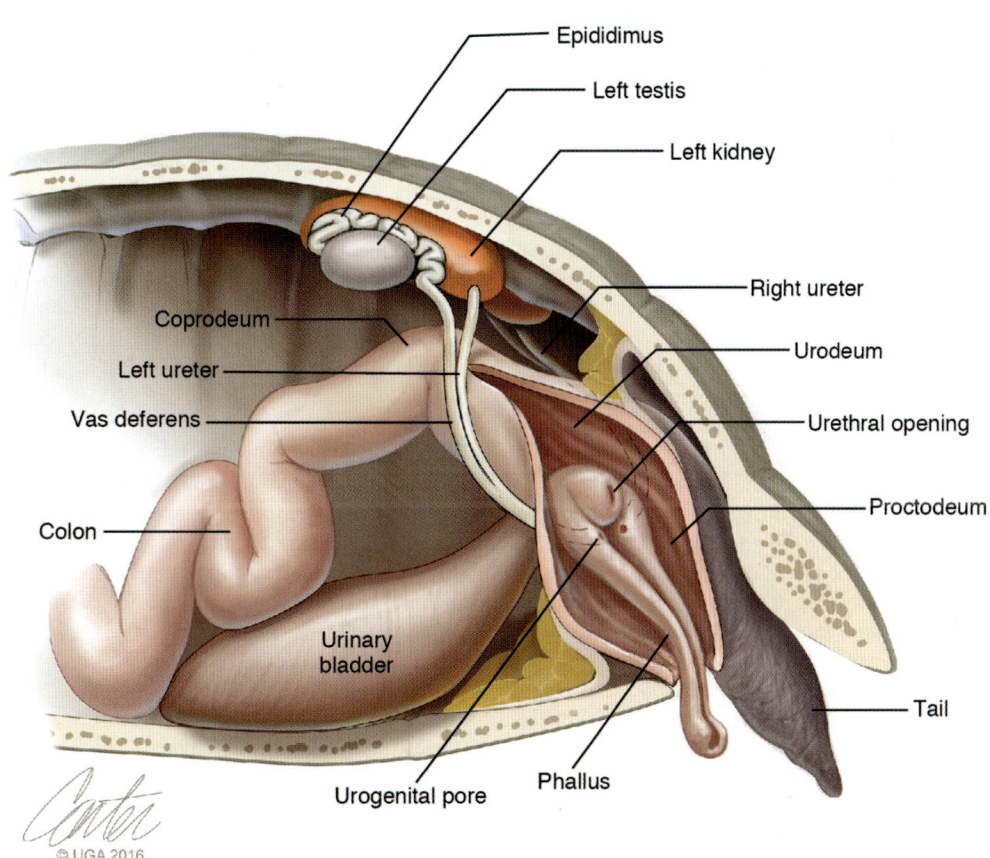

FIG 75.1 Caudal coelomic and cloacal anatomy of a male *Testudo* sp. (Courtesy of Educational Resources, University of Georgia.)

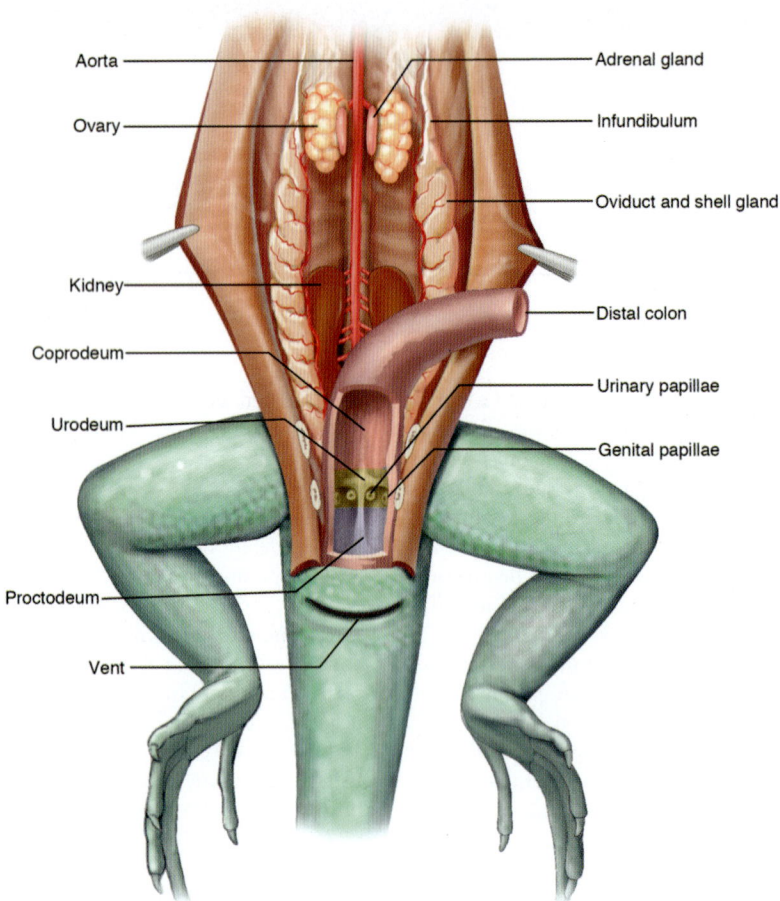

FIG 75.2 Caudal coelomic and cloacal anatomy of the female *Iguana iguana*. (Courtesy of Educational Resources, University of Georgia.)

The cranial compartment of the cloaca is called the coprodeum. The coprodeum receives the outflow of the large intestine. In chelonians, the ventral surface of both the coprodeum and urodeum also houses the nonengorged male copulatory organ or a similar smaller clitoral organ in the female. During sexual activity, the male organ(s) can enlarge considerably through vascular engorgement.[6,22,23]

The midsection of the cloaca is called the urodeum. The urodeum lies between the coprodeum and proctodeum, which is the most caudal part of the cloaca. The urodeum contains the openings to the ureters (urinary pores), the genital openings of the oviducts/vas deferens (genital pores), and the bladder, when present. Sometimes the urodeum is separated by an incomplete partition where the ureters end. The genital ducts arise from the mesonephric Wolffian duct and the paramesonephric Mullerian ducts. In males, the Wolffian duct develops but remnants of the Mullerian duct may remain. The paired male copulatory organs in snakes and lizards are sacs, extending from and just distal to the proctodeum to be housed within the base of the tail, and in females these regress or are less developed.[14–16,19,20,26]

The proctodeum is the most caudal part of the cloaca and opens to the outside at the vent. This structure receives the outflow of the bladder, urodeum, coprodeum, genital organs, and ureters and serves as the reservoir for fecal and urinary waste before excretion.[15,20–24] The openings of any musk glands are also located within this compartment.[21,24]

Snakes

Cloacal anatomy in snakes is relatively simple as divisions are less defined as other reptile groups. No urinary bladder is present; ureters empty into the urodeum via urinary pores. Paired hemipenes are located as invaginations just inside the mucocutaneous junction medial to the lateral edges of the vent. The functional surface of the hemipenis is the lumen of this invagination. When erect, the hemipenes evert through the vent. Scent glands or anal sacs are found in both sexes in snakes and empty into the caudal proctodeum. Secretions are used in "active" and "passive" marking. Specialized exocrine glands elaborate behaviorally active chemicals, similar to the chin glands of some tortoises (see Chapters 80 and 171).[15,20,21,24–26]

Lizards

Lizards have variable anatomy depending on genre or species. Where a bladder is present, it empties via a short urethra into the ventral urodeum. Hemipenes like those of snakes evert from their usual position within hemipenile sacs, through the vent. Remnants of the Mullerian duct may remain in some males. Some gecko species may have cloacal bones present.[15,20,27]

Chelonians

Chelonians have relatively consistent cloacal anatomy across the species. Cloacal divisions are well defined. The bladder empties via a short urethra into the ventral urodeum, and accessory bladders or bursae, if present, empty into the lateral wall of the urodeum. A single copulatory organ (or a female equivalent) originates from the ventral urodeum, and when engorged, this protrudes through the vent. The chelonian cloaca has extensive physiological interactions with both the bladder and large intestine, enabling fluid recycling, especially in uricotelic and hibernating species. Such animals may remain relatively healthy, yet not take on fresh fluids for up to 6 months. This feature is virtually unparalleled in any other vertebrate.[6,20,28–31]

PHYSIOLOGY

Reptiles utilize the cloaca as a common outflow for the gastrointestinal, urinary, and reproductive systems. Reptile kidneys cannot form urine that is hyperosmotic to the plasma, and therefore a greater renal water loss is experienced with the excretion of solutes in solution.[30,32] In many species, renal losses are balanced by fluid resorption in the lower urinary tract.[28–32]

Uricotelic reptiles mainly excrete uric acid and urates, whereas ureo-uricotelic reptiles produce uric acid and urea. Typically, uricotelic species live in arid environments or hibernate. Uric acid is barely soluble and therefore can be excreted with minimal volumes of water. Ureotelic animals mainly excrete urea, whereas amino-ureotelic excrete ammonia and urea. Typically, amino-ureotelic species reside in aquatic or fresh water. Reptiles that live in areas of limited water supply will excrete urates, as these are relatively insoluble and therefore require much less water than urea and ammonia to excrete. Excess sodium and potassium may also be precipitated in the cloaca as urate salts.[28–39]

Depending on species and hydration status, reptile urine may be directed toward either the urodeum or proctodeum after exiting the ureters. Water resorption may occur in the colon or proctodeum, and urine may be directed into the bladder where electrolyte and fluid exchange occurs. In species without a bladder, urine ultimately mixes with fecal material, which is then voided simultaneously.[20,28–33]

In chelonians, a bladder connects with the cloaca. This may hold large volumes of water. In many species, postrenal modification of urine occurs as fluid is resorbed across the bladder wall and ions such as potassium are excreted in the opposite direction.[28–33] In these species, the cloaca is often a route of water intake, and dehydration and some electrolyte imbalances can be addressed, at least in part, through regular baths where soak water can be drawn into the bladder, stored for long periods, and then absorbed via the physiological recovery system there.[23,28,29] Some semiaquatic turtles also absorb oxygen through cloacal bursae, a mechanism used during underwater hibernation.[22]

In crocodilians and snakes, the bladder is absent. Therefore postrenal modification of urine occurs in the urodeum or proctodeum. The functions of the accessory bladders in these species may include water and electrolyte regulation, respiration, and absorption of solutes.[35] In lizards, anatomy and therefore physiology is variable with a bladder present in only some species.[20]

For more detail on the role of the lower urinary tract in the management of appropriate hydration, see Chapter 66.

CLOACAL ORGAN PROLAPSE

This common condition is regarded as a true reptilian emergency, because the prolapsed structure will quickly devitalize from ischemic necrosis if not protected and reperfused rapidly following prolapse. With the exclusion of prolapses of the male copulatory organ(s), untreated prolapses involving the colon, bladder and oviduct are likely to be fatal because of the combined effects of ischemic tissue necrosis and compromised body system functions.[1–12] The cloacal organ prolapses encountered in the various reptile classes are summarized in Table 75.1.

Conditions that predispose to a cloacal organ prolapse are also summarized in Table 75.2. It is important to assess both the identity and viability of any prolapse, as well as the underlying health issues that have led to it and that may persist beyond its resolution.

Occasionally a cloacal prolapse case is presented because of the appearance of a normal cloacal structure that is externalized through

TABLE 75.1 Types of Reported Prolapse

Snakes[1,4,5,7,11,12]	Lizards/ Crocodilians[1,7,8,10–12]	Chelonians[1–3,6,7,9,11,12,40]
Hemipenes (males)	Hemipenes (males)	Phallus (males)
Oviduct with or without eggs/ fetuses (females)	Oviduct with or without eggs/fetuses (lizards), (females)	Oviduct with or without eggs (females)
Colon/rectum	Colon/rectum	Ovarian prolapse (female marine sp)
Cloacal mass/ neoplasia	Cloacal mass/neoplasia	Colon/rectum
Cloacal tissue	Cloacal tissue	Bladder
		Cloacal mass/neoplasia
		Cloacal tissue

TABLE 75.2 Cloacal Prolapse Causes and Associations[1–12]

Intestinal conditions	Infection
	Parasites
	Constipation
	Fecoliths
	Foreign bodies
Urinary tract conditions	Infection
	Uroliths/calculi
Reproductive conditions	Dystocia
	Abnormal eggs
	High reproductive output
	Prolapse of the phallus or hemipenis is often the result of trauma (e.g., sexing/probing, cohort bites, inappropriate mating separation, substrate contamination)
	Chronic sexual activity
	Constipation
	Paraphimosis
	Neurologic dysfunction
	Prolapse due to coelomic tumor and chronic debility
Metabolic conditions	Debility/metabolic disease/collapse
	Hypocalcemia
	Dehydration/water deprivation
	Electrolyte derangements
Coelomic conditions	Ascites
	Coelomitis
	Coelomic masses (e.g., neoplasia, granuloma, cloacolith, eggs, urolith/calculus)
Cloacal conditions	Infection
	Cloacal masses (e.g., neoplasia, granuloma, cloacolith, eggs, urolith)
Neurological conditions	CNS or spinal trauma
	CNS neoplasia
	Infection
Anesthesia	Incidental—nonpathogenic and often associated with stimulation and flaccidity/reduced tone

CNS, Central nervous system.

normal behavior. For example, in chelonians it is not uncommon for a normal engorged clitoris or phallus to protrude through the vent during handling, bathing, urination, or during chemical restraint. Normal structures usually return to the cloaca quickly, without assistance, prior to clinical presentation, whereas a pathologic prolapse does not.

Clinical Presentation

All reptiles with a cloacal prolapse require urgent veterinary examination and attention. Immediate emergency presentation to the nearest suitable clinician is recommended.[1–4,7–12] Structures that can potentially prolapse include the cloaca itself, colon, bladder, oviduct, intestine, rectum, and copulatory organs (phallus or hemipenes) (McArthur and Machin, Personal Observation, 2017).[1–12]

The goal of intervention is threefold:

1) Provide analgesia and emergency stabilization; simultaneous provision of patient support and analgesia, such as the options described in Table 75.3 and Table 75.4, should be the clinician's primary clinical goal.
2) Identify, clean, and protect the anatomic structure and then replace or remove the prolapse. Reduction is described in Table 75.5.
3) Identify, plan, and treat the underlying cause(s) of the prolapse.

Triage

At the first point of veterinary contact, both the prolapse and any systemic health issues should be assessed simultaneously. Information gathered during a primary survey, which may involve telephone triage, questioning a client or the referring veterinarian, and direct clinical examination, allows planning for patient stabilization.[11,12]

TABLE 75.3 Patient Stabilization Measures for a Cloacal Prolapse

- **Fluid support:** Correct perfusion and hydration issues. Where significant intervention and long-term support is anticipated, early placement of an esophagostomy tube or intraosseous, intracoelomic, or epicoelomic fluid administration may be necessary.
- **Nutritional support:** Identify and support any chronic malnutrition and energy deficits.
- **Thermal support:** Provide suitable warmth throughout stabilization transportation and interventions. Few reptiles with prolapses will benefit from desiccating basking heat, so alternative methods of maintaining core body temperature should be employed—maintaining temperatures at the upper end of the preferred optimal temperature zone (POTZ) is generally recommended. This may involve critical vivarium units, heat pads, and similar veterinary thermal heat sources. Continuous measuring thermometer probes are ideal to measure and monitor core body temperatures.
- **Environment support:** Appropriate humidity should also be provided alongside the thermal support plan. Avoid conditions that may lead to dehydration or desiccation of the prolapse.
- **Metabolic support:** Electrolyte imbalances, calcium, or glucose deficiencies may be identified following initial blood work due to dehydration, poor husbandry, sepsis, or other underlying pathologies. Some hypocalcemic reptiles may require vitamin D_3/calcium treatment prior to further intervention.
- **Infection/sepsis:** Topical diluted antiseptics or antibiotics may be considered in combination with systemic antibiotics. When possibl,e antibiotic choice should be choice based on culture and sensitivity. As culture is time consuming, broad-spectrum antibiotics may be prescribed following local and national antimicrobial-use guidelines.
- **Pain management:** Ensure the reptile is being assessed for pain using a local pain score protocol, and ensure analgesia options such as those given in Fig. 75.4 have been considered.
- **Monitoring of in-patients:** Ensure that for all hospitalized in-patients, the hospital records show vital signs, appetite, demeanor, urination, defecation, activity, baths, medications and pain score, fluid administration rates, fluid balance calculations, and weight.

Clinical options available at first presentation following emergency stabilization, may include temporary prolapse protection, prolapse reduction, prolapsed retention, removal of a prolapsed organ, pexy of a reduced structure or euthanasia (McArthur and Machin, Personal Observation, 2017).[1–12] Inexperienced clients and staff should not attempt complex prolapse reduction or removal techniques but should be encouraged to preserve and protect a prolapse, while stabilizing the patient in preparation for referral (McArthur S, Machin R, personal observation, 2017).[11–12]

Prolapse Protection

While developing a treatment plan, prolapses can be cleaned using a saline or warm-water lavage and then protected temporarily by wrapping the caudal body and prolapse in cling film, moist toweling, or dampened swabs. These, in turn, can be taped in place or retained using traditional veterinary dressings. Temporary protective dressings may include an osmotic reduction solution, lubricant, and local anesthetic agents to facilitate future treatment options.[40]

Diagnosis

An initial workup should incorporate a complete history, including husbandry, physical examination, hematology, biochemistry, fecal parasite analysis, radiography and ultrasonography, initially, and if indicated cytology, histopathology, CT scan, MRI, and endoscopy.

History

Attempt to ascertain the patient's general condition and ASA status (American Society of Anaesthesiologists physical status classification)[52] through analysis of a comprehensive history, as covered in Chapter 42. Often owners will report straining associated with an abnormal organ prolapse, and imaging of the caudal body as well as enteric parasite screening is recommended. Survey radiography is recommended in all cases of cloacal organ prolapse. Where possible, use the anamnesis to explore and identify potential disease associations, such as those listed in Table 75.2. The cloacal mucosa is usually moist, and examination

TABLE 75.4 Analgesia Measures Suited to a Cloacal Prolapse

Local Analgesia

Typically, lidocaine and bupivacaine. Local application may aid organ reduction and reduce straining. These can be applied locally, via infiltration or as an intrathecal block.

Consider local anesthesia, topically or by infiltration, especially when there has been persistent tenesmus/straining (McArthur S, Machin R, personal observation, 2017).[49–51]

Systemic Analgesia

Once hydration and perfusion concerns have been addressed, systemic drugs, including tramadol and meloxicam, can be used for pain and are ideal for perioperative use.

- **Tramadol:** 10 mg/kg, PO, q48h (range 2–10 mg/kg, SC, PO, q6–96h or PRN)[42–44,49,50]
- **Meloxicam:** 0.1–0.3 mg/kg PO, SC, IM, IV, q24 h–48 h[45,46,49,50]

Sedation and Anesthesia

Deep multimodal sedation or anesthesia may be required to facilitate handling and reduce stress and may also reduce straining during primary prolapse reduction; IV alfaxalone, or midazolam and ketamine, are preferred by the author. (See Chapters 48 through 51 for more details.)

may help determine the patient's hydration status if considered with other hydration markers.[11–12,23,40]

Because husbandry and nutritional related issues may have led to the prolapse, intervention is usually required, and important husbandry deficiencies or problems should be identified during the anamnesis and reported to the client. The client must also be informed of the costs of diagnostic options, such as serum biochemistry and hematology screening and traditional and advanced imaging, as well as possible surgical costs. While establishing estimated costs, an honest prognosis must be conveyed to the owner.

Physical Examination

Follow a logical examination protocol, such as that covered in Chapter 42. Where possible, ascertain patient species, sex and life stage, core body temperature at presentation, weight, body condition, hydration and perfusion status, and, where realistic, a pain score. Identify the organ that has prolapsed, as this may suggest conditions that have predisposed to prolapse. A guide to prolapse identification is provided in Figs. 75.3 through 75.24.

Combine the physical examination with the data from the anamnesis to help identify signs suggestive of dehydration, emaciation, sepsis, parasitism, hypocalcemia, or toxemia. Immediate management of core temperature, pain, hydration status, sepsis or toxemia, and electrolyte derangements are equally as important as protecting and dealing with the prolapse. Suitable stabilization measures are summarized in Table 75.3 and covered in depth in Chapter 87.

Perform any further diagnostic tests (clinical pathology and imaging) as indicated following the primary survey (anamnesis combined with initial physical examination).

Clinical Pathology

At the commencement of treatment, knowledge of organ function, possible azotemia, the patient's hematocrit, and the systemic inflammatory state will help the clinician to monitor the patient over time.

As fecal and urinary output may both be impaired by the presence of a cloacal prolapse, and severe metabolic derangements, dehydration, and hypocalcemia associated with nutritional or renal secondary hyperparathyroidism may have predisposed the patient to the presentation, a serum biochemistry profile to assess hydration and metabolic stability is recommended. Ideally a complete blood count should also be obtained.

If a parasitic, protozoan, or bacterial infection is suspected as an underlying cause of a prolapse, direct microscopy, cytology, and microbiologic examination of cloacal washes may be helpful. See Section 4 for more details.

Imaging

All reptiles experiencing a prolapse should be examined using some form of imaging. Survey radiography is mandatory in all reptiles with prolapses, and where facilities and experience are available, additional imaging such as sonography, CT, or MRI can be also be performed.

Imaging will help the clinician assess whether cystic calculi, eggs, or space-occupying masses are present, and the presence of unexpected

TABLE 75.5 Summary of Temporary Prolapse Reduction

- Assess the patient and ensure it has been adequately stabilized using the techniques summarized in Table 75.3.
- Ensure that a pain management plan has been made (e.g., through analgesia techniques such as those summarized in Table 75.4).
- Consider the use of additional future local anesthetic agents.
- Examine survey radiographs and pay special attention to evidence of metabolic bone diseases or coelomic states that may have predisposed to the prolapse, for example, cystic calculi, pelvic or ectopic eggs. (In many cases radiographic findings may indicate a need for coeliotomy in addition to any reductive techniques used.)
- Provided the reptile is adequately hydrated and metabolically and thermally stable, consider general anesthesia or deep sedation to mitigate patient distress during handling. Suitable options include multimodal protocols (e.g., combinations of midazolam 1–2 mg/kg, medetomidine 40–200 µg/kg, and ketamine 5–10 mg/kg—either IV or IM),[48,50,51] or alfaxalone (2–7 mg/kg, IV),[47,51] and as detailed in Chapters 48 and 49.
- Ensure the patient remains thermally stable and monitor core body temperature throughout.
- Glove up before handling the prolapse and manage potentially infected or necrotic material carefully to limit cross-contamination.
- Remove all substrate contamination and clean the prolapse using copious warm water or saline lavage.
- Assess prolapse viability. Only employ reductive prolapse-sparing techniques where prolapse tissue is considered viable. Reduce prolapses with caution if the tissue is only regarded as potentially viable.
- Resect and remove any unviable, necrotic, or avascular material (e.g., a traumatized penile organ).
- Apply osmotic reductants as necessary, for example, 50% dextrose or sugar solution, and, at this point, consider the application of temporary pressure dressing across the prolapse if the volume of tissue swelling present needs considerable osmotic reduction. In these cases, it may be necessary to let the patient recover from sedation or anesthesia and then continue reduction at a later point.
- Where conditions for reduction are favorable, apply further sterile lubricant. Mix in a local anesthetic agent(s) and ensure dosages are subtoxic.
- Reduce the prolapse, for example, use through pressure from multiple moist tongue depressors, cotton buds, or swabs. Apply even force over the base and body of the prolapse, as this will often result in significant hydrostatic reduction. The process will be similar to kneading bread.
- Pressure applied evenly across damp swabs can be useful in addition to digital compression, and swabs can be taped in place under pressure, if time is available.
- Once the prolapse has been reduced, consider cloacal flushing with warmed fluids to remove further debris and involute any inverted organ.
- Involution of bladder oviduct and colon will almost certainly require further celiotomy.
- Where reduction is not possible, consider amputation and celiotomy. Ensure the client is comfortable with any surgical escalation to this level.
- Retention sutures or staples can now be used to temporarily support the vent and prevent a recurrence of the prolapse.
- Ensure the patient can still urinate and pass feces.
- Insertion of a damp compression swab/tampon soaked with saline and diluting local anesthetic agent may aid both retention (e.g., reduction for transit to a referral site or during initial stabilizing hospitalization).
- Continue the patient stabilization techniques summarized in Table 75.3.

free fluid within the coelomic cavity may encourage fine-needle aspirate/coelomocentesis and additional cytology and fluid examination.[41] See Section 7 for more detail.

Prognosis

For many reptiles suffering a cloacal organ prolapse, the prognosis for stabilization and future quality of life are reasonable, provided secondary trauma is moderate and response time is short (e.g., within 24–48 hours). The prognosis for a cloacal organ prolapse is dependent on multiple factors; most importantly underlying causes, the patient's condition, and the prolapse viability and duration of the prolapse. Prognosis varies from excellent to grave and euthanasia should be considered in serious cases.

An informed decision should be made by the client and clinical team together, to choose between further patient stabilization or euthanasia, and the clinician must recommend the treatment most likely to address patient welfare.

Occasionally, euthanasia may be advised or performed at the initial presentation because no viable welfare-orientated treatment is possible, affordable, or available. Advice regarding reptile euthanasia is provided in Chapter 47.

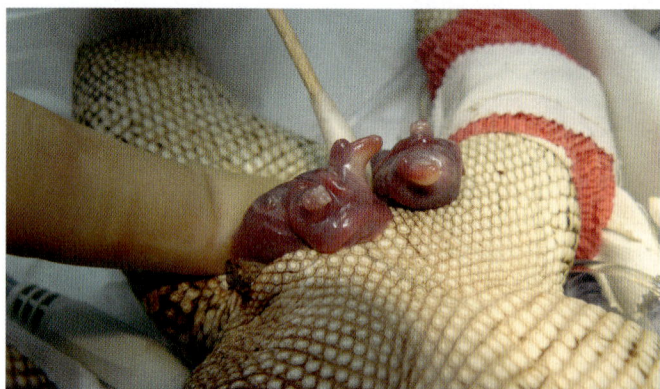

FIG 75.5 Monitor lizard (*Varanus* spp.) with bilateral prolapse of the hemipenes. (Courtesy of Stephen J. Divers.)

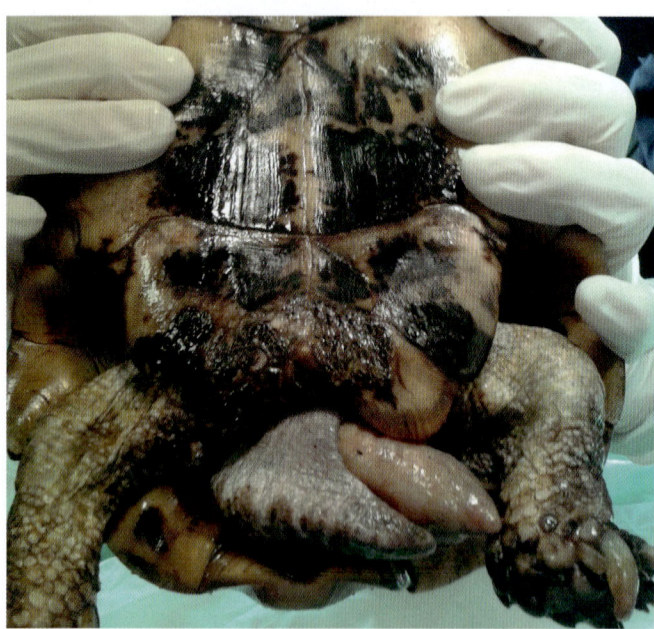

FIG 75.3 *Testudo* sp. tortoise with a phallus prolapse. A mild phallus prolapse like this is typical of a debilitated male *Testudo* species with hypocalcemia. Correction can be achieved by restoring electrolytes, blood calcium levels, and core body temperature. (Courtesy of S. Brown.)

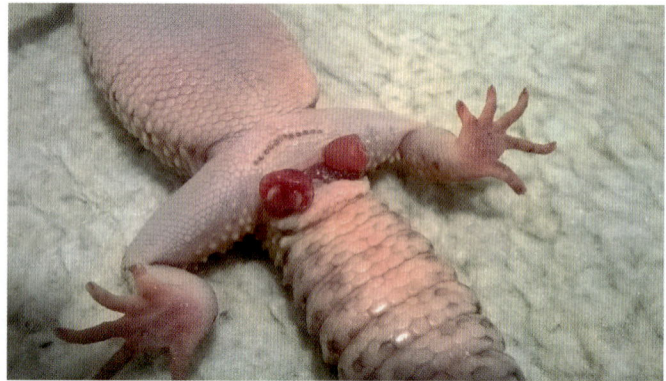

FIG 75.6 Leopard gecko, *Eublepharis macularius*, with bilateral hemipenile prolapses. (Courtesy of Sarah Pellett.)

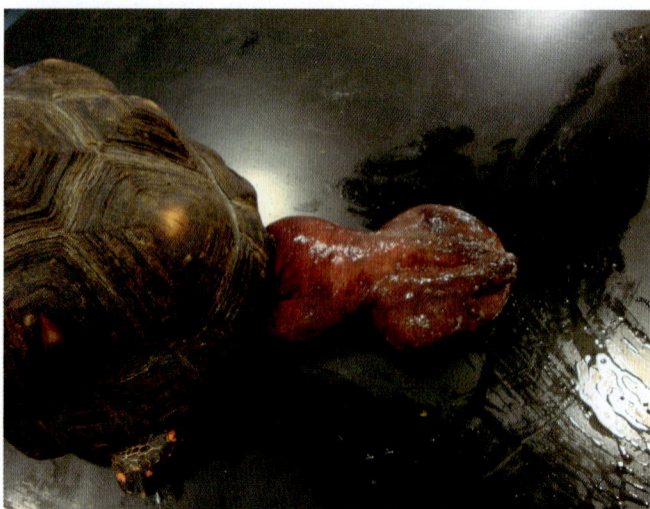

FIG 75.4 Red-footed tortoise, *Chelonoidis carbonaria*, with a large phallus prolapse. This can be amputated with a good prognosis if predispositions are also addressed. (Courtesy of S. Brown.)

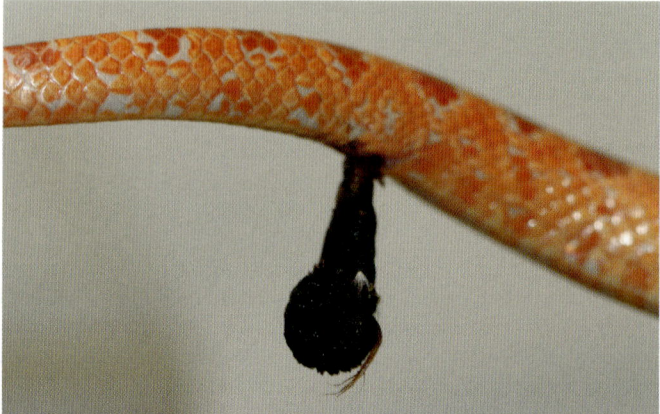

FIG 75.7 Corn snake, *Pantherophis guttatus*, with a necrotic hemipenile prolapse. This can be surgically removed; however, the underlying cause for the prolapse must be addressed. (Courtesy of A. Raftery.)

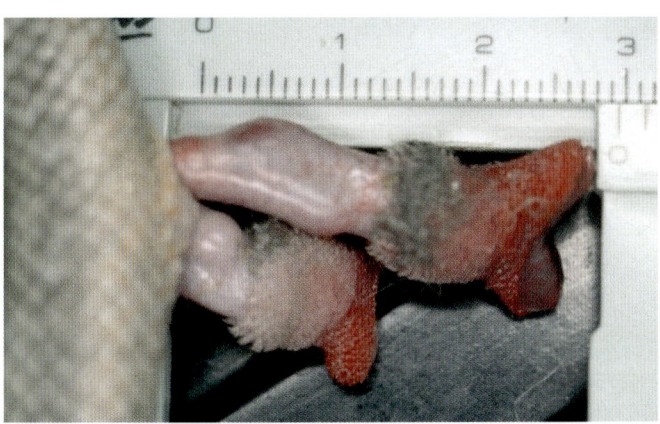

FIG 75.8 Bilateral recent hemipenile prolapse in a snake. (Courtesy of A. Raftery.)

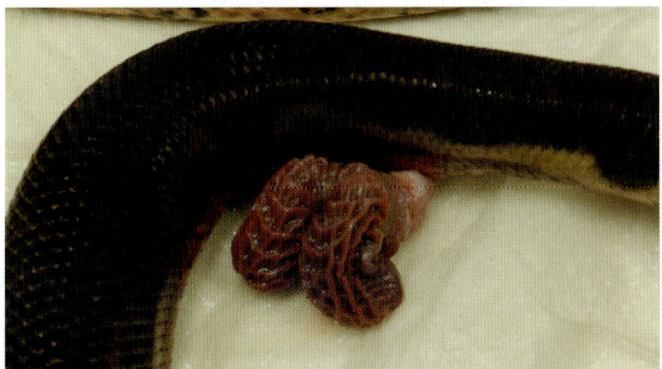

FIG 75.9 *Boa constrictor* with recent hemipenile prolapse. (Courtesy of J. Chitty.)

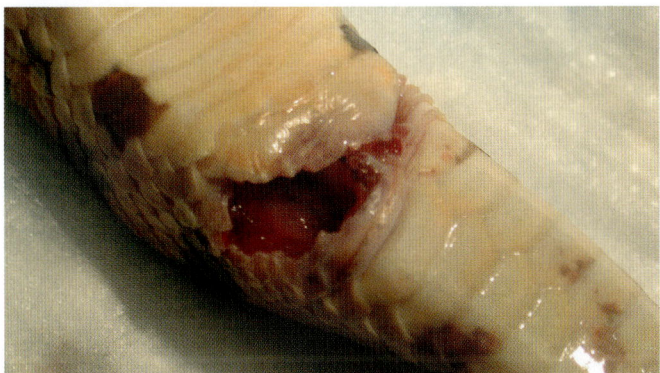

FIG 75.10 Corn snake, *Pantherophis guttatus*, with a necrotizing cloacitis. (Courtesy of Stephen J. Divers.)

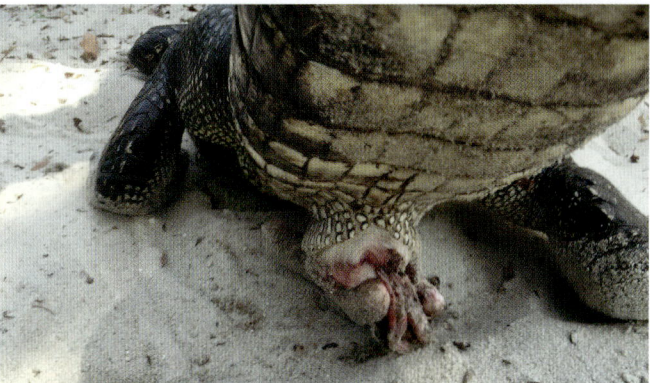

FIG 75.11 *Alligator mississippiensis* with traumatized cloacal tissue. Sometimes a swollen cloacal protrusion cannot be easily identified without removal or coeliotomy. Cloacal granulomas, renal granulomas and masses, and even ingested foreign material have all been presented as cloacal organ prolapse at the authors' hospital(s). (Courtesy of Douglas R. Mader.)

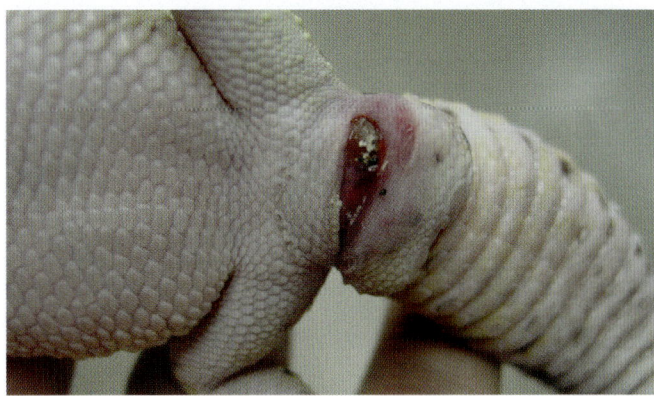

FIG 75.12 Leopard gecko, *Eublepharis macularius*, with a hemipenal plug associated with cloacitis. (Courtesy of Stephen J. Divers.)

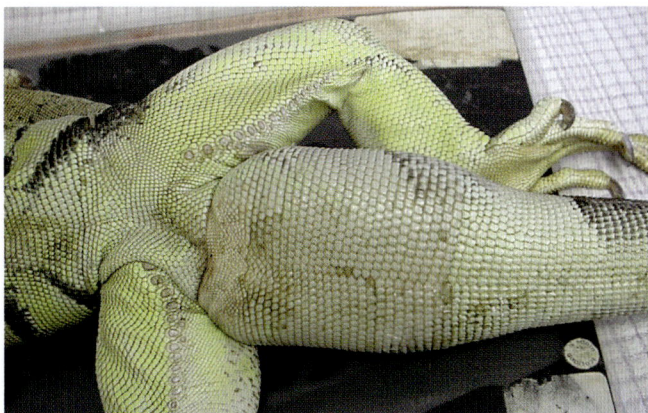

FIG 75.13 *Iguana iguana* with large hemipenal plugs and associated hemipenal abscessation. (Courtesy of Stephen J. Divers.)

Treatment

While a reptile experiencing a prolapse may not show obvious indications of pain as mammals do, all will benefit from a carefully considered pain management program.[7–12] Analgesia is always advised (see Chapter 50). Suitable analgesia protocols for managing a cloacal prolapse are provided in Table 75.4.[42–46]

After addressing patient stabilization using techniques summarized in Table 75.3, the prolapse should be protected from desiccation, substrate contamination, or further trauma. This usually involves lavage, application

of lubricant gels, application of osmotic gels, and protective wraps such as cling film or toweling. The longer a prolapse is contaminated with substrate, strangulated, engorged, and traumatized, the less likely it is to be viable and the more likely it will require surgical removal or necessitate euthanasia. Early lavage using warm sterile saline, reduction, and stabilization is advised in combination with general patient

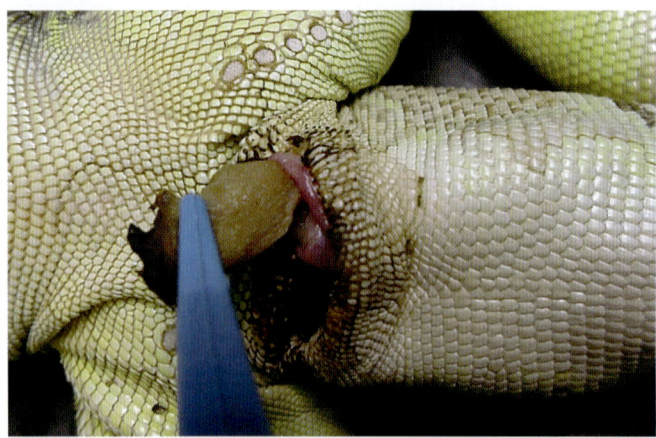

FIG 75.14 Removal of a large hemipenal plug associated with a hemipenal abscessation in the same iguana shown in Fig. 75.13. (Courtesy of Stephen J. Divers.)

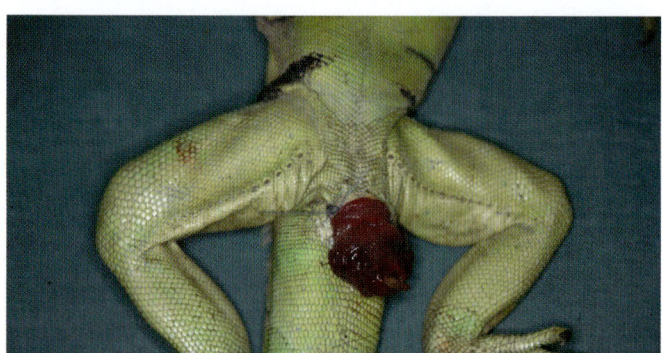

FIG 75.17 *Iguana iguana* with a prolapsed oviduct. Longitudinal striations are present on the surface of the oviducts but absent on the colon. (Courtesy of Stephen J. Divers.)

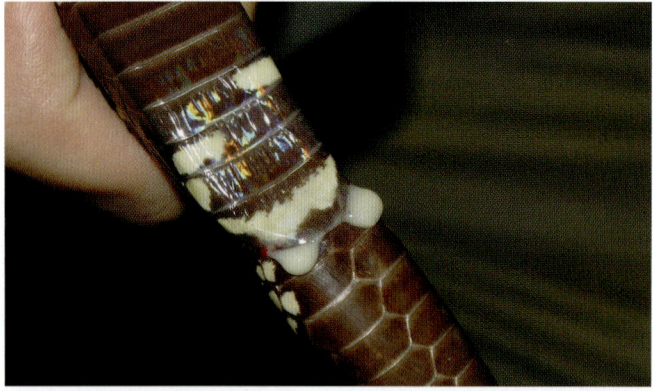

FIG 75.15 California king snake, *Lampropeltis getula californiae*, showing secretions expressed from the scent glands. This normal discharge can easily be confused with discharge associated with cloacitis or hemipenile plugs or infection. (Courtesy of Stephen J. Divers.)

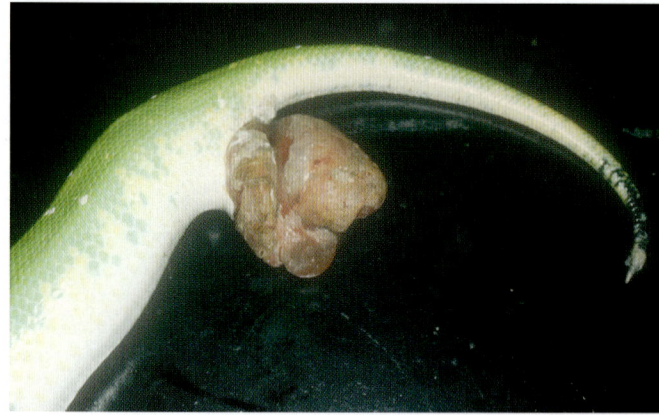

FIG 75.18 Green tree python, *Morelia viridis*, with a prolapsed oviduct with secondary changes due to dessication and strangulation. Longitudinal striations are present on the surface of the oviducts but absent on the colon. Both oviduct and colon will have a lumen. (Courtesy of Stephen J. Divers.)

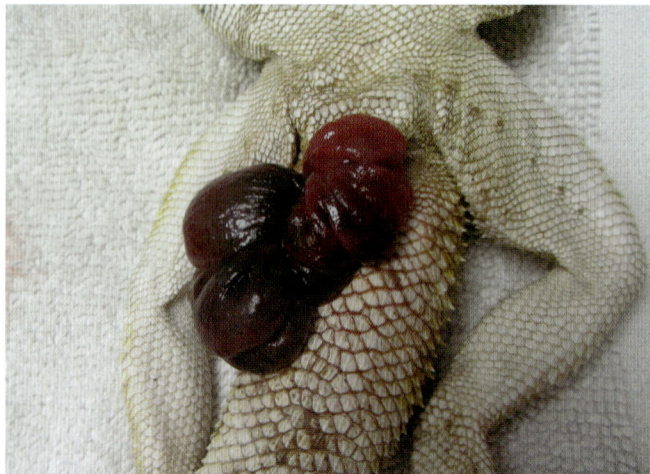

FIG 75.16 Bearded dragon, *Pogona vitticeps*, with a prolapsed oviduct. Longitudinal striations are present on the surface of the oviducts but absent on the colon. Prolapse of the salpinx can occur because of egg binding, dystocia, retained eggs or fetuses, hypocalcemia, salpingitis, neoplasia, or intracoelomic disease or mass effects. (Courtesy of J. Hedley.)

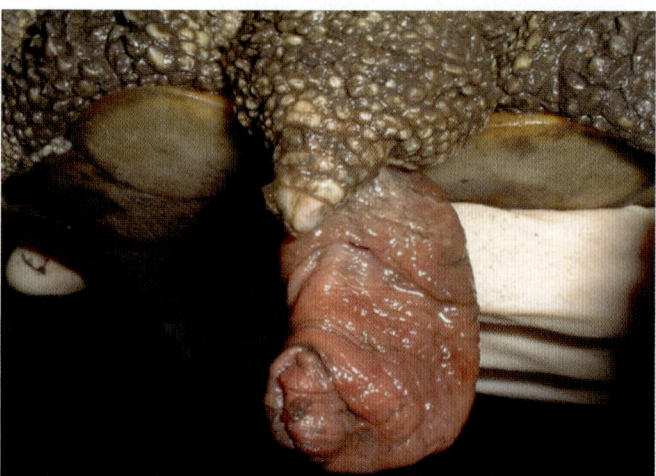

FIG 75.19 *Testudo hermanni* with a prolapsed oviduct. The oviduct is soft, flaccid, and tubular and has a lumen. There is some fecal contamination evident. This prolapse requires a celiotomy and an investigation into the underlying cause, such as dystocia. (Courtesy of Stuart McArthur.)

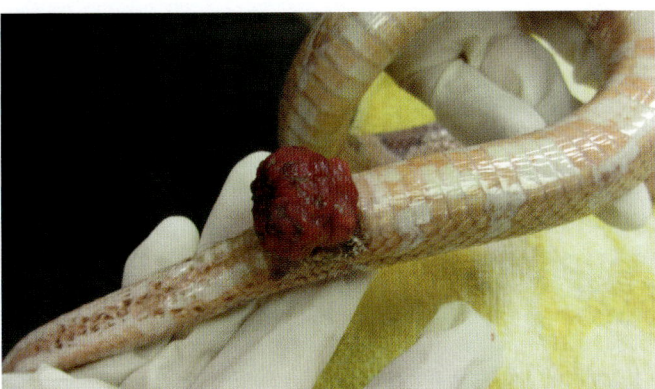

FIG 75.20 Corn snake, *Pantherophis guttatus*, with a prolapse of the colon. This is usually the result of tenesmus, caused by conditions such as colitis, endoparasites, foreign body/fecaliths, renomegaly, hypothermia, hypocalemia, or physical deformity. (Courtesy of J. Hedley.)

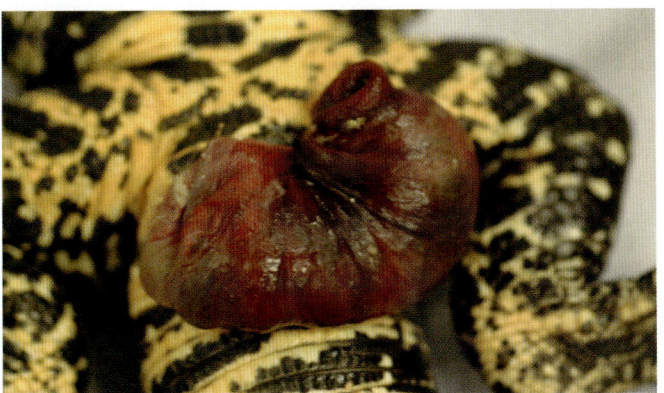

FIG 75.21 Black and white tegu, *Salvator merianae*, with a colonic intussusception. (Courtesy of J. Chitty.)

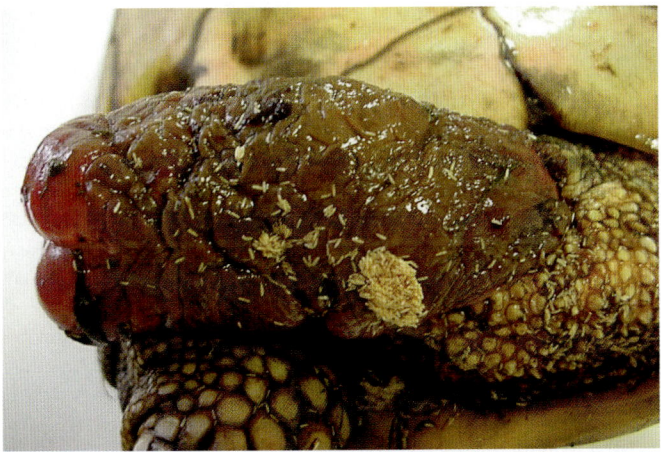

FIG 75.22 *Testudo* tortoise with a colonic prolapse and associated fly eggs laid on the surface. Ideally this requires thorough lavage and removal of all alien and necrotic tissue and then correction of the prolapsed intussusception via a coeliotomy. Where there is a lack of suitable finance, experience, or motivation, euthanasia should be considered or resection of the prolapsed intussusception and reduction of the anastomosis attempted; however, the owner must be given a guarded to grave prognosis. (Courtesy of Stephen J. Divers.)

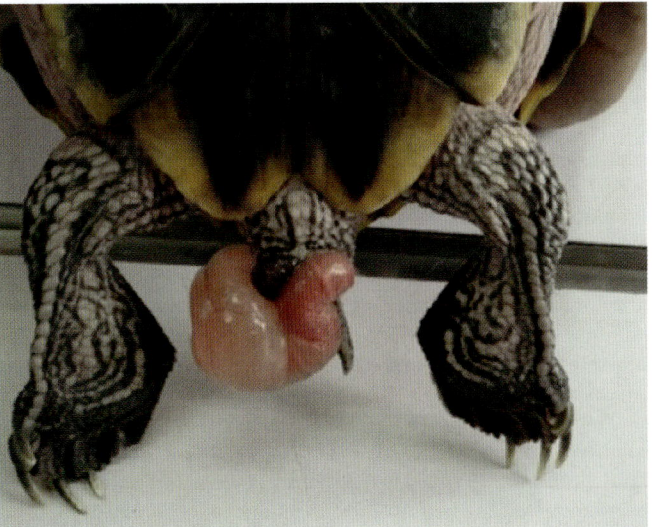

FIG 75.23 Bladder prolapse in a female red-eared slider, *Trachemys scripta elegans*. In all chelonians and most lizards, prolapse of the bladder may occur. This organ is thin, and it has an obvious vascular pattern. It is easily ruptured. The bladder, if still intact, is a fluid-filled, saclike structure. If exposed for a long time, the bladder may become devitalized and rupture, thus appearing as thin, shredded tissue. (Courtesy of Dinesh Vinherkar.)

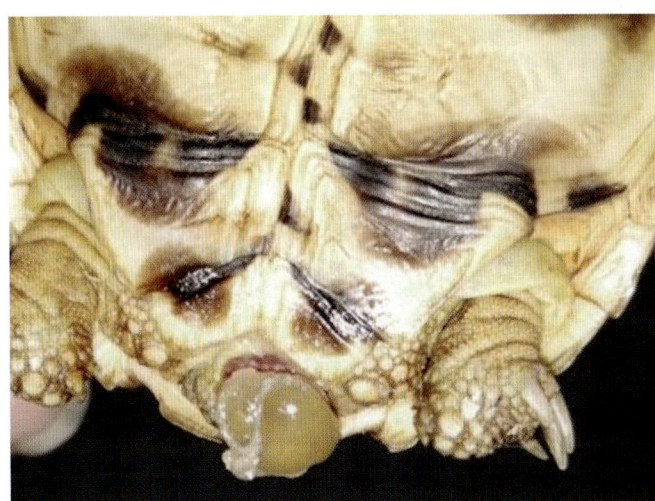

FIG 75.24 Juvenile leopard tortoise, *Stigmochelys pardalis*, with severe nutritional secondary hyperparathyroidism and associated hypocalcemia that has prolapsed a small portion of its bladder. (Courtesy of Dinesh Vinherkar.)

stabilization. If prolapse handling is likely to distress the patient, a risk-benefit analysis may favor sedation or general anesthesia (McArthur S, Machin R, personal observation, 2017).[12,40]

Where dystocia or coelomic masses such as cystic calculi have predisposed to a cloacal prolapse, a coeliotomy is always indicated. Prolapses of the large intestine and oviducts are invariably surgical conditions.[8,40] Medical management will help in all cases where there is sepsis or significant local infection, parasitism, nutritional secondary hyperparathyroidism/hypocalcemia, other electrolyte derangements, and dehydration, and often supports future surgical management (McArthur S, Machin R, personal observation, 2017).[12,40]

Prolapse Reduction

It is important that clients understand that simply reducing the prolapse is not comparable with the resolution of the prolapse. Few oviduct or colonic prolapses will resolve by simply forcing them back into the cloaca, and most animals left with a partially reduced prolapse will experience life-threatening future complications.

Initially a prolapse can be irrigated with sterile fluid or even gently washed with warm running water to clean and remove any contamination. Physical manipulation and osmotic reduction benefit from medical lubrication to which a clinician may add local anesthetic agents (e.g., lidocaine or 2.5% bupivacaine).[50,51] Lubricating gels may allow a fresh prolapse to simply be returned to the cloaca for transportation or until an experienced reptile clinician is available. Osmotic reduction of organ swelling is aided by application of sugar, honey, or concentrated dextrose solutions. These shrink edematous tissues, allowing organ reduction through sustained gentle manual compression or surgery. Tissues can be protected during transport using osmotic reduction agents applied beneath dressings.[2,7,8,40]

The male reproductive organs of all reptiles can be reduced and retained, or removed, without the need for coeliotomy. In some cases, where calculi are not involved in the etiology, a bladder prolapse can also be reduced without coeliotomy. However, all tubular or intussuscepted prolapses (those with a lumen) will require coeliotomy to be correctly reduced and retained via sutures or removed along with additional associated structures such as retained eggs, ectopic eggs, cystic calculi, ovaries, follicles, etc.[2,8,40] (see Chapter 106).

Specific Prolapse Management Plans

Phallus (Chelonian)

Known etiological cause(s). Etiological causes of phallus prolapse in chelonians (Figs. 75.3 and 75.4) include male courtship trauma, balanoposthitis, mating injuries, dystocia, chronic sexual activity, constipation, paraphimosis, neurologic dysfunction, substrate contamination, hypothermia, hypocalcemia, dehydration, cloacoliths, and neoplasia. Only males are affected.

Clinical presentation. This prolapse is not life-threatening, but it often indicates deeper issues influencing debility.

Diagnostic confirmation. The prolapsed chelonian phallus presents as a single, large, engorged, nontubular structure protruding through the vent. There is no lumen. The prolapse may be a considerable size in comparison to the animal. The presentation is pathognomonic; however, additional investigations should be made into the underlying etiology. Survey radiography is recommended.

Prognosis. The prognosis with or without conservation of the phallus is good, provided any other underlying issues are correctable.

Suggested treatment. Recent viable prolapses can be reduced and replaced as described earlier in this chapter and in Table 75.5. Plenty of lubrication should be used during reduction, which is accomplished by applying even pressure across the structure. Temporary retaining sutures may be required across the vent opening to hold the prolapse in place for the first 24 to 48 hours (or longer in severe cases or relapses). Surgical removal, as described in Chapter 106, is preferred for avascular traumatized, necrotic, or infected prolapses, where reduction is not regarded as feasible or with relapse. Postoperative care will be minimal.

Prevention. The reptile's environment and nutrition should be optimized. Parasitic infestations require elimination from the patient, cohorts, and the environment.

Hemepenis(es) (Squamate)

Known etiological cause(s). Etiological causes for hemepenal prolapse (Figs. 75.5 through 75.9) include male courtship trauma, balanoposthitis, mating injuries, dystocia, chronic sexual activity, constipation, paraphimosis, neurologic dysfunction, substrate contamination, hypothermia, hypocalcemia, dehydration, cloacoliths, and neoplasia. Only males are affected.

Clinical presentation. This prolapse is not life-threatening but often indicates deeper issues influencing debility.

Diagnostic confirmation. The prolapsed hemipene(s) presents as a single or paired small, nontubular structure protruding through the vent at its lateral edges. It is a small size in comparison to the animal, even when strangulated or desiccated. There is no lumen. The presentation is pathognomonic; however, additional investigations should be made into the underlying etiology. Survey radiography is recommended. Do not confuse cloacitis (Fig. 75.10), cloacal trauma (Fig. 75.11), hemipenile plugs (Figs. 75.12 through 75.14), or scent gland secretion (Fig. 75.15) with hemipenal prolapse.

Prognosis. The prognosis with or without conservation of one or both hemepenes is good, provided other underlying issues are correctable.

Suggested treatment. Recent viable prolapses can be reduced and replaced as described earlier in this chapter. Any plugs or contaminating material should be gently removed. Plenty of lubrication should be used during reduction, which is accomplished by applying even pressure across the structure. Temporary retaining sutures may be required about the vent opening to hold the prolapse in place for the first 24 to 48 hours (or longer in severe cases). Surgical removal, as described in Chapter 106, is preferred for avascular traumatized, necrotic, or infected prolapses, where reduction is not regarded as feasible or with relapse. Postoperative care will be minimal.

Prevention. The reptile's environment and nutrition should be optimized. Parasitic infestations require elimination from the patient, cohorts, and the environment.

Oviduct (Oviparous Species)

Known etiologic cause(s). Etiological causes of oviductal prolapse in reptiles (Figs. 75.16 through 75.19) include hypocalcemia, dehydration, dystocia (e.g., uterine rupture, ectopic eggs, abnormally sized or shaped eggs), infections (parasitic, mycotic, bacterial, or viral), uroliths, and neoplasia. Most animals will have follicular stasis, urinary calculi, or be in dystocia. Only females are affected.

Clinical presentation. A oviductal prolapse is considered life-threatening and usually indicates deeper medical issues.

Diagnostic confirmation. A prolapsed oviduct often presents as a modest flaccid, intussuscepted structure. It is usually solid and linear. It has a lumen. Where tissues are exposed they may have become traumatized and necrotic. It may be large in size in comparison to the animal. Survey radiography is recommended, and additional investigations as indicated should be made into the underlying etiology.

Prognosis. The prognosis with or without conservation of the prolapsed oviduct tissue is poor. Few oviduct prolapse cases will return to a normal quality of life. However, where a prolapse is recent it may be possible to reduce and remove it via a celiotomy.

Suggested treatment. A celiotomy and entire ovariosalpingectomy are advised. Alternatively, the prolapse can be amputated and then the residual tissue addressed via a coeliotomy. These surgical procedures are described in Chapters 80 and 106. Where future breeding of an endangered species is an issue, a minimum of unilateral salpingectomy is advised, and this must include an ipsilateral ovariectomy. Fresh viable prolapses, without coelomic masses (e.g., cloacoliths, dystocia, or ectopic eggs), can occasionally be reduced and replaced without coeliotomy. A coeliotomy is always advised by the authors to correctly unravel any intussusception, correctly return it to the coelomic cavity, and immobilize it to prevent immediate recurrence. Additional conditions, such as uroliths and obstipation, will also require appropriate management. Postoperative care will be significant.

Prevention. The reptile's environment and nutrition should be optimized. Dystocia, follicular stasis, and any concurrent urinary calculi issues will all warrant appropriate investigation and treatment.

Colon (All Species)

Known etiological cause(s). Etiological causes of colonic prolapse in reptiles (Figs. 75.20 through 75.22) include hypocalcemia, dehydration, constipation, infections (parasitic, mycotic, bacterial, or viral), and neoplasia. Some animals may have bladder stones, fecoliths, or uroliths within the urodeum or be in dystocia. Cachectic and emaciated animals with low body fat may be overrepresented.

Clinical presentation. A colonic prolapse is considered life-threatening and usually indicates deeper medical issues.

Diagnostic confirmation. The prolapsed colon often presents as a large, rigid, engorged, and, intussuscepted structure. It is usually solid and linear, has a lumen, and, where tissues are exposed, may have become traumatized and necrotic. It may be a considerable size in comparison to the animal. Survey radiography is recommended, and additional investigations as indicated should be made into the underlying etiology.

Prognosis. The prognosis with or without conservation of the intestinal prolapse is generally grave. Few colonic prolapse cases will return to a normal quality of life. However, where a prolapse such as an ileocolic intussusception is relatively fresh and recent, it may be possible to reduce it via a coelomic celiotomy approach.

Suggested treatment. Recent viable prolapses without coelomic masses (e.g., cloacoliths, ectopic eggs) can be reduced and replaced. However, a celiotomy is always advised to correctly unravel any intussusception, properly return it to the coelomic cavity, and to immobilize it to prevent immediate recurrence. Surgical management is described in Chapter 106. Additional conditions such as uroliths and dystocia will also require appropriate management. Once reduced the colon can be fixed using colopexy sutures to the coelomic wall (see Chapter 106). Postoperative care will be significant.

Prevention. The reptile environment and nutrition should be optimized. If thought to be a contributing factor, parasitic infestations need elimination from the patient, cohorts, and the environment. Predispositions such as constipation, dystocia, or urolith formation should be addressed and managed.

Bladder (All Chelonians and Some Lizards)

Known etiological cause(s). Etiological causes of prolapse of the reptilian bladder (Figs. 75.23 and 75.24) include hypothermia, hypocalcemia, dehydration, uroliths, ectopic eggs, bladder and cloacal infections (parasitic, mycotic, bacterial, or viral), and neoplasia. Cachectic and emaciated animals with low body fat may be overrepresented. Reptiles of any sex or age may be affected.

Clinical presentation. A bladder prolapse is considered life-threatening and usually indicates deeper medical issues.

Diagnostic confirmation. The prolapsed bladder often presents as a large, engorged, fluid-filled structure. It may be thin-walled, and liquid may be apparent within it. There is no lumen and the structure is not tubular. Urate deposits may be apparent within any cystic structures or distributed across any visible prolapsed mucosa. If the bladder wall has ruptured, a bladder prolapse may present as a long, stringy, non-specific, nontubular structure protruding through the vent. It may be a considerable size in comparison to the animal. Survey radiography is recommended, and additional investigations as indicated should be made into the underlying etiology.

Prognosis. The prognosis with or without conservation of the bladder prolapse is grave. Few bladder prolapse cases will return to a normal quality of life.

Suggested treatment. Recent viable prolapses, without coelomic masses (e.g., cloacoliths and ectopic eggs) can be reduced and replaced, as described in Table 75.5. Fluid can be gently and consistently infused into the cloaca to reverse the organ involution. The sheath of a rigid endoscope is ideal for this, and the scope can be used to visualize appropriate coelomic reduction and cloacal patency. Temporary retaining sutures may be required across the vent opening to hold the prolapse in place for the first 24 to 48 hours (or longer in severe cases). Surgical replacement is preferred for avascular traumatized, necrotic, or infected prolapses and where reduction is not regarded as feasible. (See Chapter 106 for the surgical approach to bladder prolapse repair.) Where the bladder wall is severely damaged, the bladder wall can be resected and viable edges of the bladder wall closed together. Braided suture materials are best avoided in uricotelic species. Postoperative care will be significant.

Prevention. The reptile's environment and nutrition should be optimized. If thought to be a contributing factor, parasitic infestations will need elimination from the patient, cohorts, and the environment. Predispositions such as constipation, dystocia, or urolith formation should be addressed and managed.

REFERENCES

See www.expertconsult.com for a complete list of references.

76

Pulmonology

Zdenek Knotek and Stephen J. Divers

The respiratory tract includes the nares, rhinarium, choana, larynx, tracheobronchial tree, and lungs; however, for the purposes of this chapter the focus will be the larynx, trachea, and lungs, with the nasal cavity included in Chapter 72.

Recent movement through the wholesale/retail trade, importation, severe parasitism, malnutrition, and suboptimal temperature are all stressors that can predispose to primary or secondary respiratory disease.

ANATOMY

A basic understanding of the normal anatomy and physiology of the respiratory tract of reptiles is important for clinicians to successfully diagnose and manage respiratory disease in these patients. The reptilian respiratory tract is anatomically and physiologically different among the various taxa.[1–3]

Snakes

The larynx is situated rostrally in the oral cavity. It opens in the floor of the mouth caudal to the lingual sheath opening and is generally easily visualized (Fig. 76.1A). The larynx consists of two small vertical arytenoid cartilages laterally, connected by a large azygous and rounded ventral cricoid cartilage.[1] The glottis is the opening to the trachea and controls airflow and permits hissing. A preglottal keel is obvious in some species (e.g., *Pituophis*) (see Fig. 76.1B). The cranial part of the trachea, or glottal tube, is composed of 3 to 16 fused cartilaginous rings and can, during large prey ingestion, be pushed craniolaterad to maintain ventilation. The glottis is actively opened and closed by the dilator and sphincter laryngis muscles, respectively. Excluding the glottal tube, the trachea is composed of 70 (*Thamnophis*) to 1120 (*Hydrophis*) incomplete cartilageous rings; however, there are exceptions, with *Python bivittatus* and *Crotalus viridis* having up to 30 and 25 complete cartilaginous rings, respectively, following the glottal tube. All the remaining rings are incomplete and possess a significant dorsal ligament, which is thin, composed of collagenous and elastic connective tissue, but lacking muscle fibers (Fig. 76.2). This dorsal tracheal membrane proliferates to form a tracheal lung and is particularly common in the Elapidae, Viperidae, Hydrophiidae, and Colubridae. Tracheal lungs facilitate additional gas exchange and can be used to inflate the neck (but not spread the hood of cobras). The trachea normally courses ventrad or dextrolaterad to the esophagus, and either dorsal or left of the heart. The trachea enters the right lung in two distinct ways (although intermediate variations exist): (1) *subterminal*, in which the trachea enters the medial side of the lung, caudal to the anterior tip or lobe (e.g., boids); and (2) *terminal*, in which the trachea enters the most cranial portion of the lung and an anterior lobe is absent.[1] In most snakes with a single lung, the trachea becomes an intrapulmonary bronchus upon entry into the right lung; however, in boids, the differentiation is at the level of the bifurcation.

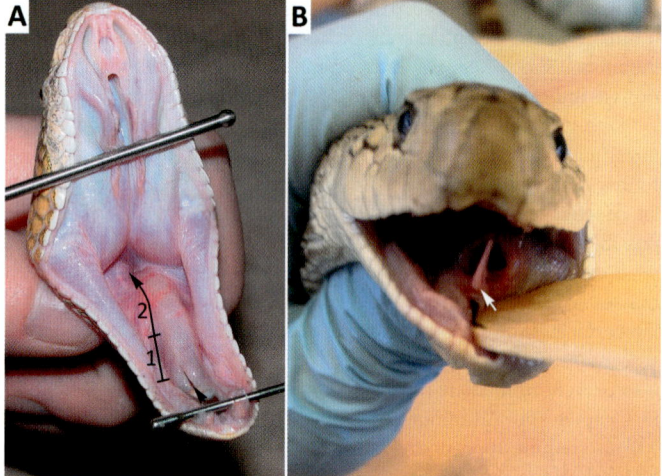

FIG 76.1 Snake larynx, glottis, and glottal tube. (A) The laryngeal region of a timber rattlesnake *(Crotalus horridus)* depicting the closed glottis (arrow), glottal tube (1), and incomplete cartilaginous rings of the cranial trachea (2). (B) Preglottal keel *(arrow)* in a *Pituophis* snake. (Courtesy of Stephen J. Divers.)

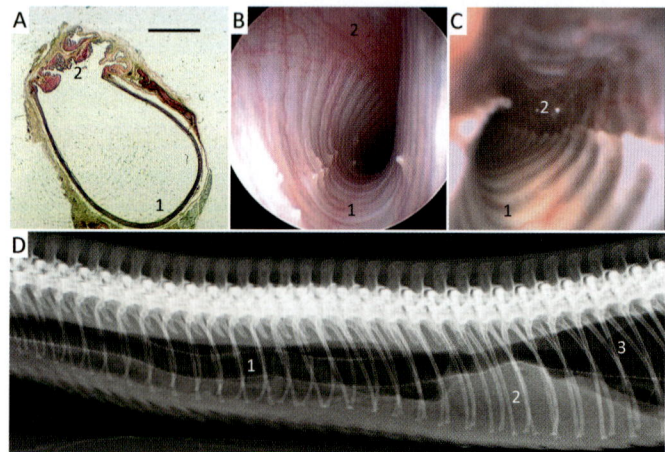

FIG 76.2 Snake trachea. (A) Histologic cross-section of a trachea demonstrating the incomplete cartilaginous ring (1) and dorsal ligament expansion into the tracheal lung (2) of a colubrid (bar = 1 mm). (B) Endoscopic view within a boid trachea demonstrating the incomplete tracheal rings (1) and dorsal ligament (2). (C) Endoscopic view within a colubrid trachea demonstrating the incomplete tracheal rings (1) and expanded dorsal ligament expansion into the dorsal tracheal lung (2). (D) Lateral radiograph (horizontal beam) of a boid snake illustrating the trachea (1) coursing dorsad over the heart (2) and terminating in the vascular lung (3). (Courtesy of Stephen J. Divers.)

The bronchus terminates proximally within the faveolar region but can extend far caudally in some species.[1] The epithelium has relatively fewer cilia, which diminishes the ability to remove foreign material from the respiratory tract. A poorly developed mucocilliary escalator in the airways reduces the ability of the reptile to clear discharges.

All snakes have a right lung, located dorsal to the liver and lateral to the stomach, which typically measures 25% to 60% of the total snout-to-vent length (SVL). The left lung (present in boids) is generally smaller but can be comparable. In all snakes (except some typhlopids) the lung is unicameral (single chamber). The right lung (and left lung of boids) is divided into a thick-walled, highly vascular respiratory portion (vascular lung) and a thin-walled, transparent, avascular, nonrespiratory portion (air sac or saccular lung), which is variably demarcated by a transitional zone (semisaccular lung) (Fig. 76.3D and

E). This air sac may act as an oxygen reservoir during periods of apnea and as a buoyancy organ in aquatic snakes.[1]

Three different types of reptilian lung parenchyma have been described: (1) *trabecular*, consisting of a single layer of low-relief branching muscular structures (trabeculae); (2) *edicular*, composed of a single layer of trabeculae with raised walls or septa that form cubicles (ediculae) that are wider than they are deep; and (3) *faveolar*, single- or multiple-layered faviform parenchyma, the compartments (faveoli) of which are deeper than wide and have a honeycomb appearance[1] (see Fig. 76.3D and E).

The vascular lung is typically located starting at 20% to 30% SVL and ending approximately 40% to 60% SVL.[4] This respiratory region is rich in faveolar parenchyma, heavily perfused, and red in color and can easily be distinguished from the reduced vascularization of the

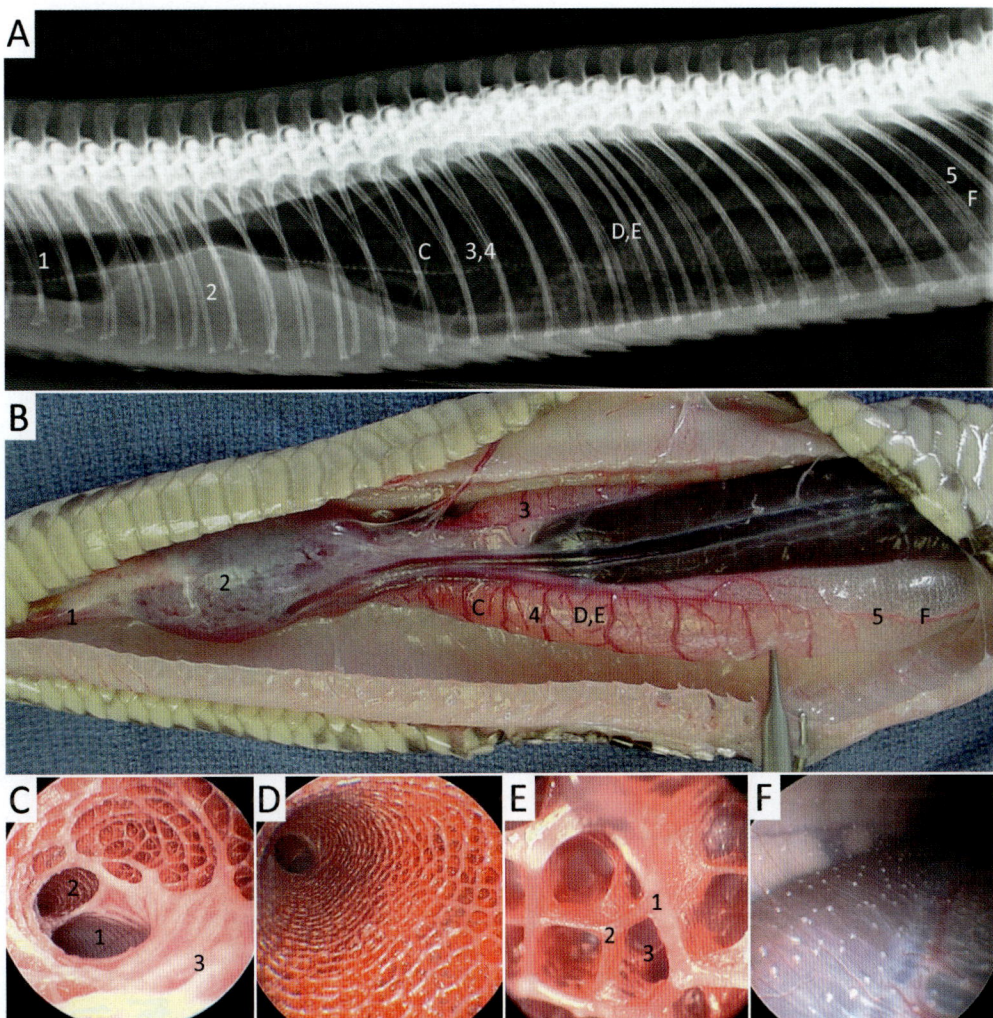

FIG 76.3 Python (*P. regius*) lungs. Radiographic (A) and anatomic (B) views of the distal trachea (1), heart (2), vascular left (3) and right (4) lungs, and semisaccular right lung (5). The location of endoscopic images (C–F) are also indicated. (C) Endoscopic view of the anterior right lung illustrating the distal trachea (1), anterior lobe (2), and intrapulmonary bronchus (3). (D) Endoscopic view of the entire right vascular lung. (E) Close-up endoscopic view of the faveolar parenchyma illustrating the primary (1), secondary (2), and tertiary (3) divisions. (F) Endoscopic view of the right saccular lung. (A and C–D, Courtesy of Stephen J. Divers; B, courtesy of Scott J. Stahl, Stahl Exotic Animal Veterinary Services.)

gray-white air sac. This saccular portion extends caudally for a variable length, depending on species.[1] These two clearly defined regions are separated by a transitional zone of varying magnitude in which the parenchyma gradually becomes less concentrated, and the faveoli exhibit larger diameters, lower and thinner walls, and fewer horizontal tiers.[1] In some snake species (*Gonyosoma* sp., *Naja* sp., *Boiga* sp., and other arboreal colubrids) the transition from the vascular lung to the avascular air sac is abrupt. The air sac may constrict to 10% to 20% of its cranial diameter and continue to its tip as a very slender tail. The position of the air sac tip is sexually dimorphic in most species of snakes, with the tip more caudally placed in males than in females.[1]

The respiratory cycle of the snake involves both active and passive components. Elevation of the ribs, caused by contraction of levator costarum and retractor costarum muscles, increases coelomic volume, decreases intrapulmonary pressure, and results in the active component of inspiration. Expiration is controlled by dorsolateral (transverse dorsal and superior internal intercostal) and ventrolateral (transverse abdominal and internal abdominal oblique) muscles. Relaxation of the expiratory muscles results in initial, passive inspiration, whereas limited passive expiration occurs as a result of relaxation of the inspiratory muscles.[1–3]

Lizards

The larynx of the lizard is variable in its location within the oral cavity. It is found in the rostral aspect of the mouth in carnivorous species, or it is located more posterior at the base of the fleshy tongue (Fig. 76.4). The glottis is normally closed except during inspiration or expiration. Gular pumping does not mirror ventilation rate but is associated with forcing air into the lungs (positive pressure ventilation) and may also have a role in olfaction and cooling.[5] The trachea, composed of incomplete rings in most species, remains a single structure until it enters the coelomic cavity near the base of the heart (Fig. 76.5). Some chameleons have an accessory lung lobe that projects from the trachea cranial to their forelimbs. This may fill with secretions when infected, resulting in swelling of the ventral neck.

Most lizards possess single-chambered lungs (Eublepharoidea, Amphisbaenia, Gymnophthalmidae, Teidae, Lacertidae, Xanthusiidae, Scincidae, and Anguidae), whereas others (Chamaelonidae, Agamidae, Iguanidae, Gekkonoidea, Xenosauridae, and Lanthanotus) exhibit transitional lung morphology in which a short, troughlike intrapulmonary bronchus extends from the hilus to the base of a septum, which divides the lung into smaller anterior and larger posterior chambers.[2] The intrapulmonary bronchus present in the *Iguana* is absent in the *Pogona, Uromastyx,* and *Physignathus,* but these species all exhibit a posterior lung that is variably divided by two or three large septae into lobes. Chameleons exhibit specific septal arrangements and caudal diverticulae resembling air sac appendages (see Fig. 76.5). Varanids and helodermatids are unique among lizards in that they possess the most complex, multichambered lungs, which are large, heterogeneously partitioned, and possess cartilage-reinforced secondary bronchi.

Faveolar lung parenchyma is typical in the scinomorph, iguanid, and agamid lizards.[2] Edicular patterns are common in varanid, chamaeleonid, and some gekkonid species but are also present in distal pulmonary regions in iguanid and agamid lizards.[2] The terminal saclike regions of many lizards are lined by trabecular parenchyma (Fig. 76.6).

Lizards lack a diaphragm and move tidal volume with expansion and contraction of the ribs, facilitated by the intercostal muscles. In some lizards, an incomplete (Helodermatidae) or complete (Varanidae) postpulmonary fascialike septum divides the coelom into cardiopulmonary and visceral compartments but does not aid respiratory movements.[3] Most lizards complete the expiratory-inspiratory cycle with a nonventilatory period of varying length.

Chelonians

The larynx is located caudally in the oropharynx at the base of the fleshy tongue, making it difficult to visualize on occasion (Fig. 76.7A). The trachea is composed of complete cartilaginous rings with mucous, ciliated,

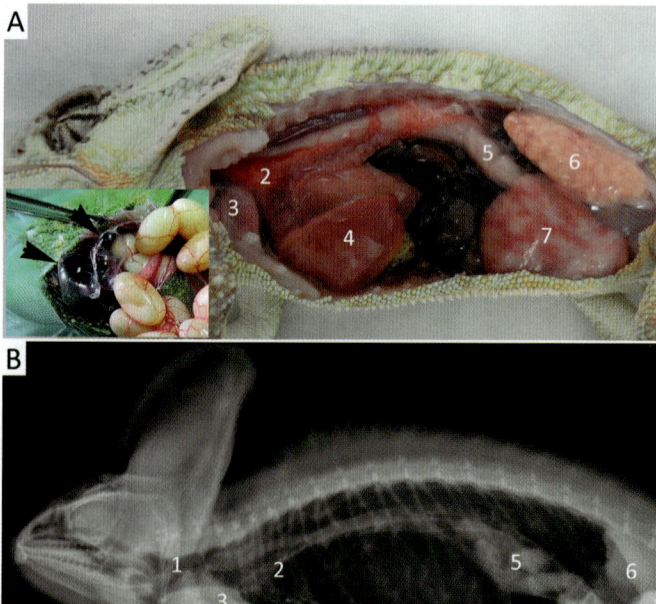

FIG 76.5 Gross lateral anatomical (A) and radiographic (B) views of a veiled chameleon (*Chamaeleo calyptratus*) illustrating the trachea (1), lung (2), heart (3), liver (4), stomach (5), kidney (grossly enlarged and pale in A) (6), and fat body (7). Note that the lungs are collapsed at necropsy but fully inflated in the radiograph of a live lizard. (Insert) this intraoperative view illustrates the caudal saccular projections characteristic of this genus. (Courtesy of Stephen J. Divers.)

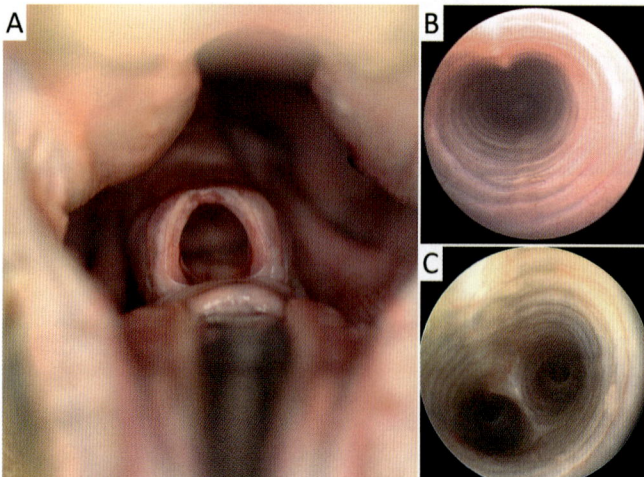

FIG 76.4 Lizard larynx, glottis, trachea, and primary bronchi. (A) View of the larynx of a large varanid during active inspiration. (B) Endoscopic view of the iguanid trachea demonstrating the incomplete cartilaginous rings. (C) Endoscopic view of the iguanid tracheal bifurcation and primary bronchi. (Courtesy of Stephen J. Divers.)

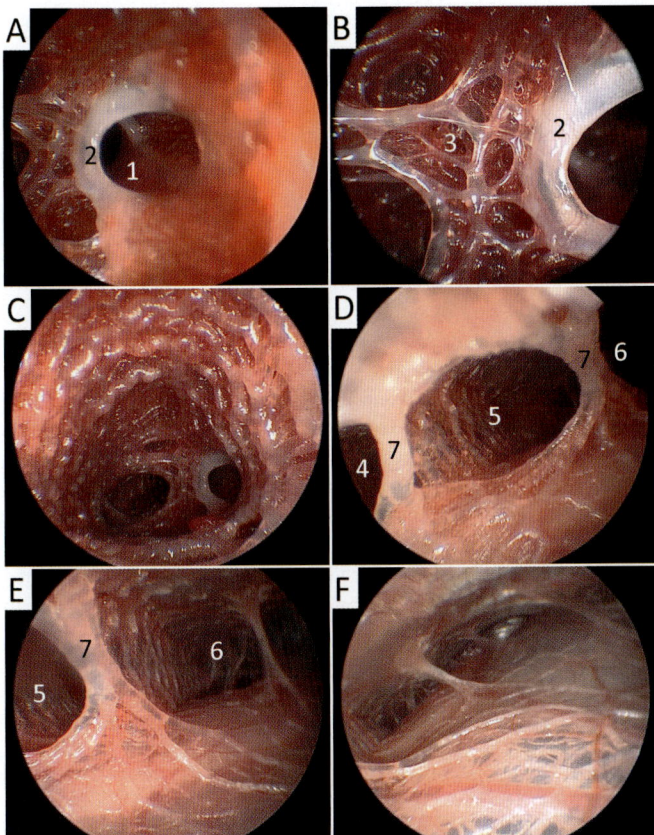

FIG 76.6 Green iguana (*Iguana iguana*) endoscopic lung morphology. (A) Anterior view of the intrapulmonary bronchus (1) and hyaline cartilaginous support leading into the ventral chamber where the endoscope is located. (B) Close-up view of the hyaline cartilaginous support (2) and faveolar parenchyma (3). (C) View of the cranial lobe of the ventral lung chamber. (D and E) Views of the cranial (4), middle (5), and caudal (6) lung lobes that are separated by large septa (7). Notice how the lung parenchyma becomes progressively edicular. (F) View of the most caudal aspect demonstrating the trabecular pattern characteristic of caudal saccular lung. (Courtesy of Stephen J. Divers.)

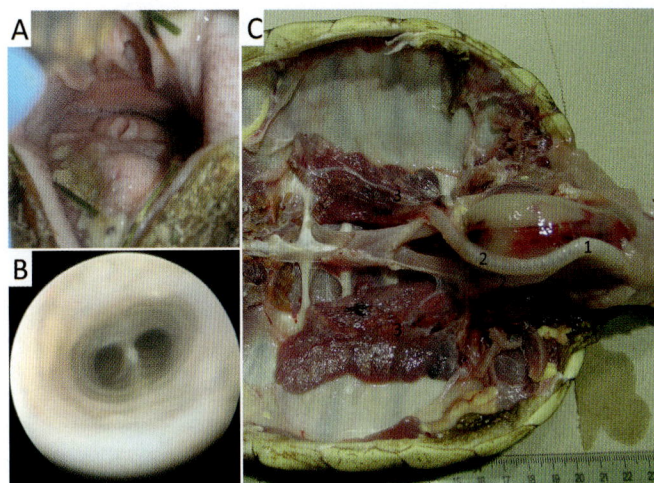

FIG 76.7 (A) View of the larynx and glottis of a large terrestrial tortoise. (B) Endoscopic view of the distal trachea and bifurcation in a *Testudo* tortoise. Gross dissection of a common snapping turtle (*Chelydra serpentina*) demonstrating the trachea (1) and the long primary bronchi (2) that enter the lungs (3) craniomedially. Note that there is no obvious postpulmonary membrane in this species. (Courtesy of Stephen J. Divers.)

and basal cells lining the epithelial wall (see Fig. 76.7B).[6] The chelonian suborder Cryptodira which includes most turtles and tortoises, retract their head and neck straight back into the shell, and the trachea is relatively short and quickly bifurcates into two main-stem bronchi that open directly into the lungs. The cranial bifurcation of the trachea enables chelonians to breathe unimpeded when the neck is withdrawn.[7] The suborder Pleurodira which includes side-neck turtles, fold their necks sideways along the body, and the trachea is generally longer with more caudal bifurcation. The paired bronchi are also significantly longer than those of squamates and enter the lungs cranio medially (see Fig. 76.7C).

The rigid chelonian shell necessitates a unique process of ventilation. Ventilation involves the activity of antagonistic pairs of muscles, which decrease or increase coelomic volume and thus lung volume.[7] This action is supplemented with limb and head movements. Chelonians accomplish the movement of air through a variety of methods. Both inspiration and expiration are active processes. Groups of muscles are involved—contraction of the diaphragmatic and transverse abdominal muscles compress the coelomic cavity, thus causing expiration. The testocoracoidus and abdominal oblique muscles expand the cavity and cause inspiration.[7] In some terrestrial species, movements of the pectoral girdle are the primary muscles of respiration; inspiration occurs with

contraction of the serratus and abdominal oblique muscles, whereas expiration occurs with contraction of the transverse abdominal and pectoralis muscles.[7]

The lungs attach dorsally to the ventral surface of the carapace and ventrally to a postpulmonary membrane (*septum horizontale*) that is weighted by attachments to the liver, stomach, and intestinal tract (Fig. 76.8A). Chelonians have no true diaphragm.[7] The membraneous separation is most obvious in terrestrial species and is often indiscernible or lacking in aquatic turtles like the common snapping turtle (*Chelydra serpentina*), where the lungs are attached dorsomedially by means of a broad ligament to the vertebral column (see Fig. 76.7C).

All testudines have multichambered lungs with an unbranched, intrapulmonary bronchus that is reinforced by cartilage (see Fig. 76.8B).[2] Each primary bronchus gives rise to 3 to 11 groups of chambers, most consisting of a medial (to ventral) and lateral (to dorsal) chamber. The *Testudo* tortoises have the simplest lungs, with just four groups of dorsal and ventral chambers, with intermediate forms like *Trionyx* (soft-shelled turtles) having seven groups of medial and lateral chambers (see Fig. 76.8B–D). The most complex lungs are found in sea turtles, with parenchyma-rich, 10 or 11 groups of dichotomously bifurcating medial and lateral chambers.[2] The lung surface is reticular and interspersed with bands of smooth muscle and connective tissue. Edicular parenchyma extends throughout the lung, and unlike most reptiles, testudines possess goblet cells rather than serous secretary cells on the trabeculae and intrapulmonary bronchus.

Crocodilians. The full development of a bony hard palate is seen only in the crocodilians where the nasopharynx opens at the back of the mouth in close proximity to the larynx. The larynx is located caudal to the prominent epiglottal flap (*velum palati*) (Fig. 76.9A). Air can be held in the respiratory tract for an extended period by closure of the glottic valve, allowing submersion for extended periods. The trachea is lined with a pseudostratified, ciliated, columnar epithelium with varying numbers of goblet cells.

Crocodilians have complex, multichambered lungs located in the cranial coelom. Though not a true thorax, the term thorax could legimately be used because of the functional separation between the lungs and other viscera by a substantial membraneous postpulmonary membrane (see Fig. 76.9B).[2] Ventilation is accomplished with the intercostal muscles and muscles attached to the nonmuscular diaphragm. Active expiration occurs due to a reduction in volume caused by transverse muscles. The cranial aspect of the liver is attached to the postpulmonary membrane. Caudally, the liver is connected to the pelvic girdle by a pair of diaphragmatic muscles. Contraction of these muscles causes caudal movement of the liver, which, combined with the action of the intercostal muscles, causes active inspiration. Parabronchi further divide the lungs into a series of chambers. The *individual* chambers tend to be tubular, and the most cranial chambers extend well craniad of the hilus. The edicular paranechyma appears to be more densely partitioned in alligators than crocodiles.[2]

PHYSIOLOGY

The following is a summary; a more detailed explanation of respiratory function has been published.[3] Although most gas exchange is pulmonary,

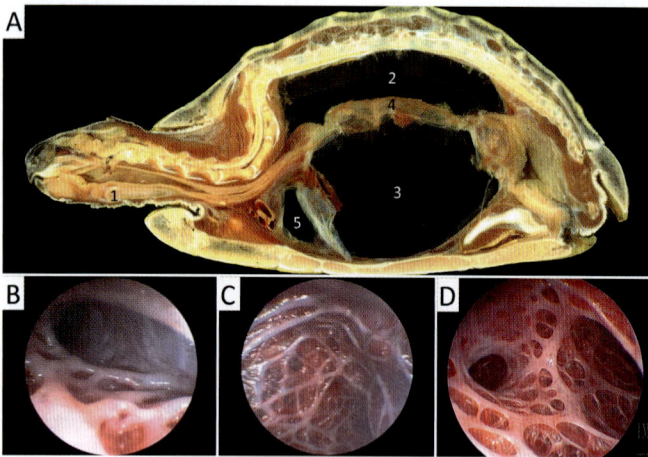

FIG 76.8 (A) Midline saggital section of a *Testudo* tortoise illustrating larynx and anterior trachea (1), pulmonary (2). and visceral (3) cavities, separated by the postpulmonary membrane (4). This membrane is much more substantial and often opaque in terrestrial species. The cardiac cavity (5) is also shown. (B and C) Endosocpic views of the left lung of a *Testudo* tortoise (via a left prefemoral approach to the coelom and caudolateral lung). Note the cartilage supported intrapulmonary bronchus (B) and simplified lung structure (C). (D) Endoscopic view of the left lung in an emydid turtle demonstrating the more complex, compartmentalized lung of aquatic species. Note the characteristic edicular parenchyma. (A, Courtesy of Udo Hetzel; B, courtesy of Stephen J. Divers.)

it is important to appreciate that cutaneous (skin, gular, cloacal) gas exchange may be significant in many terrestrial species (5%–15% of total gas exchange) but is most utilized in aquatic species where it can account for up to 35% of total gas exchange. During periods of inactivity, especially hibernation at low temperatures, it is possible for all gas exchange requirements to be met through nonpulmonary routes.

The arrhythmic breathing pattern of reptiles may appear abnormal compared with mammals. Reptile metabolism and, hence, needs for oxygen and carbon dioxide exchange are reduced, and therefore two options are available for reducing respiration rate: (1) maintain a continuous, but slow, inspiratory/expiratory breathing pattern, or (2) maintain a normal inspiratory/expiratory breathing pattern (largely based on the intrinsic elasticity of lungs and associated tissues) but have periods of nonventilation and therefore breathe intermittently. Option 2 prevails in most resting reptiles because it is more energy efficient, and therefore the respiratory pattern of reptiles can be divided into ventilatory and nonventilatory periods. Nevertheless, reptiles experience and are tolerant of greater variations in blood pH and are capable of prolonged periods of anoxia.

Increasing inspired CO_2 or decreased O_2 results in less or shortened nonventilatory periods. In general, hypercapnia causes an increase in tidal volume (due to suppression of pulmonary stretch receptors), whereas hypoxia acts to increase breathing frequency (due to arterial and pulmonary chemoreceptors) (Table 76.1). However, exceptions exist, and acute hypercapnia can result in sudden breath holding. These

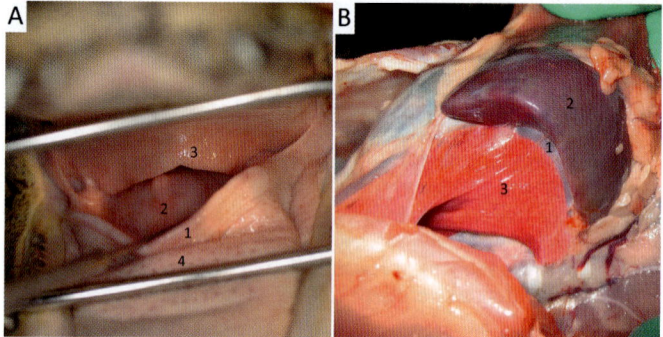

FIG 76.9 American alligator (*Alligator mississippiensis*). (A) Oral view with the epiglottal flap (1) ventrally displaced to reveal the larynx and closed glottis (2). The caudal soft palate (3) and caudal tongue (4) are also visible. (B) Necropsy view of the anterior coelom demonstrating the prominent postpulmonary membrane or septum (1) and its attachments to the liver (2) and lungs (3). (Courtesy of Stephen J. Divers.)

TABLE 76.1	**Clinical Effects of Changes in Physiologic Parameters**			
	Increase Causes	**Decrease Causes**	**Effected by**	**Clinical Significance**
Carbon dioxide	Elevation in tidal volume and minute volume	Decrease in tidal volume and minute volume	Intrapulmonary stretch receptors and chemoreceptors; central chemoreceptors; upper respiratory chemoreceptors	Carbon dioxide generally has a lesser effect on respiration than oxygen
Oxygen	Decrease in respiratory rate	Increase in respiratory rate	Arterial chemoreceptors	Reptiles on 100% oxygen will have dramatically reduced respiratory rates, which complicates spontaneous breathing during anesthetic recovery and nebulization therapy
Temperature	Increased responses to hypoxia and hypercapnia	Decreased responses to hypoxia and hypercapnia	General thermodynamics	Reptiles must be maintained within their POTZ, and this is especially true during anesthesia
pH	Decrease in tidal volume and minute volume	Elevation in tidal volume and minute volume	Intrapulmonary chemoreceptors; central chemoreceptors	pH and CO_2 are intrinsically linked

effects are also significantly impacted by temperature, with more robust responses to hypercapnia and hypoxia at higher temperatures.[7]

Chelonians seem particularly adept at tolerating hypoxia, which is the primary stimulus for ventilation in this group and is most pronounced in the aquatic species, such that increasing inhaled CO_2 has less effect on respiration. Conversely, most (nonaquatic) lizards and snakes appear to be more sensitive to elevations of CO_2 than hypoxia. For most reptiles, $PaCO_2$ values range between 15 to 35 mm Hg and should be maintained during anesthesia.[7]

In aquatic species, there are often significant differences between blood gas measurements from alveolar and arterial sources, which is an indication of the significant intracardiac shunting that can occur. Ventilation-perfusion mismatch can also result in similar differences and can often be induced by placing large reptiles (especially chelonians) into dorsal recumbency.

Numerous studies have demonstrated that dives involving reptiles are performed aerobically, not anerobically, and that most reptiles inhale as the last ventilatory act before submerging. Therefore lung oxygen reserves appear as important (if not more so) as hemoglobin and myoglobin oxygen storage. Arterial PCO_2 is predominantly determined by pulmonary ventilation, and plasma pH shows only minor deviations among reptiles and other vertebrates, provided comparisons are made at identical temperatures. In general, arterial pH decreases consistently with increasing temperature predominantly from an increase in arterial PCO_2 production (due to relative decrease in pulmonary ventilation relative to CO_2 production).[7]

CLINICAL INVESTIGATION

A presumptive diagnosis of respiratory tract disease may be made on the basis of historical analysis, physical examination, and a variety of ancillary diagnostic techniques.[8–11] However, a definitive diagnosis typically requires demonstration of both a host pathologic response (cytology, histopathology, paired rising titers) and the causative agent (microbiology, parasitology, toxicology).

History and Physical Examination

The historical data collected from owners usually confirms significant deficiencies in husbandry or nutrition. Optimal temperature and humidity regimens are often overlooked. Excessively high humidity (often at the expense of ventilation) may result in bacterial and fungal proliferations with heavy environmental exposure predisposing to pneumonia. Nutritional imbalances, particularly hypovitaminosis A, are often anecdotally associated with respiratory disease. Significant ectoparasite loads are often associated with poor environmental hygiene. Snake mites (*Ophionyssus natricis*) have been implicated as vector of several infectious causes of pneumonia, including aeromoniasis. Lack of appropriate quarantine is a common cause of infectious disease outbreaks.

Clinical signs of respiratory disease can include open-mouth breathing, dyspnea, and tachypnea. In addition to upper respiratory obstructions and lower respiratory tract disease, and (because of a poor functional separation between the lungs and the other viscera) space-occupying lesions within the coelom (e.g., ascites, neoplasia, granuloma, gastrointestinal distension, gravidity) can prevent normal lung expansion and cause dyspnea. Agonal respiration in terminal patients may also resemble dyspnea, while pulmonary edema secondary to cardiac or hepatic disease and hypoproteinemia can also occur.

Snakes. Increased respiration or respiratory noise associated with acute disturbance, shedding, or defensive hissing should be differentiated from a disease presentation. Blocked nares from shed, debris, discharge,

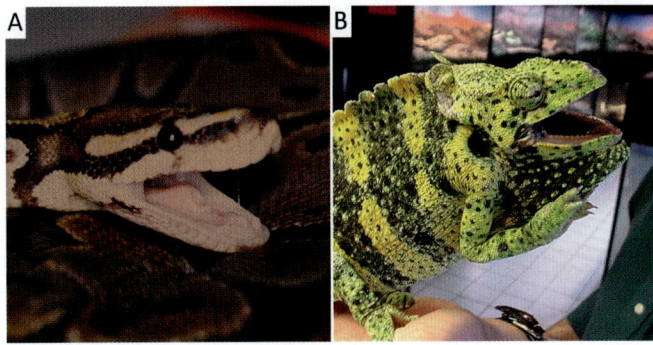

FIG 76.10 (A) Dyspnea and open-mouth breathing in a ball python (*Python regius*) with mycobacterial pneumonia. (B) Open-mouth threat displays and hissing, like this Meller's chameleon (*Trioceros melleri*), should not be confused with respiratory disease. (Courtesy of Stephen J. Divers.)

or trauma can result in open-mouth breathing. Choana must be evaluated to differentiate upper from lower respiratory disease. Abnormal respiratory signs may include abnormal posturing with head and neck elevated, forced nasal exhalations, dyspnea including open-mouth breathing, swollen or distended cervical region nasal/oral/choanal/glottal discharge, and increased respiratory sounds (Fig. 76.10A). Inflammatory debris may accumulate within respiratory (vascular) or nonrespiratory (saccular) portions of the lung. Infectious material can persist within the lower respiratory tract because the saccular lung is minimally vascularized, poor mucociliary transport and ability to cough. Many snakes with respiratory illness are anorectic and lethargic.

Lizards. Open-mouth panting associated with threat/defensive displays, hyperthermia, and nasal salt gland excretion are not considered primary respiratory issues (see Fig. 76.10B). Both the external and internal nares must be examined for discharge, which may be serous, mucoid, or purulent. Blocked nares result in open-mouth breathing. Respiratory sounds may result from any fluids within the respiratory tract as a result of pneumonia, aspiration, or near drowning. These must be differentiated from hissing and snorting as a defensive gesture in response to a perceived threat. Conversely, complete lack of lower respiratory sounds might be noted in a fully consolidated lung.

Chelonians. Clinical signs of upper respiratory tract disease include clear to colored discharge or bubbling from the nares, ocular discharge, and palpebral edema. Concurrent clinical signs of rhinitis, stomatitis, and conjunctivitis are not uncommon. Dietary history is important to exclude hypovitaminosis A in carnivorous and omnivorous chelonians, which can cause squamous metaplasia and predispose to secondary infections. This is not an issue, because hypovitaminosis A is very rarely present. Excess salivation and inhaled irritants such as pollen or foreign bodies, such as foxtails or grass awns, can also lead to foreign body reactions and discharge. Chronic upper respiratory tract disease may erode or depigment the nares. Any lesion that compromises the larynx and glottal opening, such as abscesses or neoplasia of the oral cavity, can cause dyspnea.

Dyspneic chelonians may stretch their necks and open their mouths with obvious labored effort. Abnormal breath sounds, such as slight whistle, may be appreciated. Wheezing, tachypnea, or dyspnea may or may not occur with fungal pneumonia or tracheitis. Clinical signs of pneumonia are often not apparent until they are advanced (Fig. 76.11A). Most patients are depressed and lethargic, but the most dramatic clinical presentation involves inspiratory and expiratory dyspnea. The respiratory rate is generally elevated with a reduction in the nonventilatory period

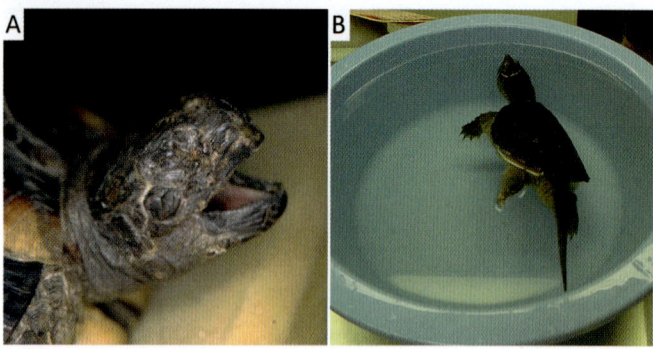

FIG 76.11 (A) Dyspnea in a *Testudo* tortoise due to mycotic pneumonia. (B) Assymetrical floatation in this snapping turtle (*Chelydra serpentina*) could be associated with right lung consolidation, right extrapulmonary coelomic mass, or increased gas in the left coelom. (Courtesy of Stephen J. Divers.)

and exaggerated respiratory movements of the limbs. Affected tortoises tend to breathe with the head and neck extended, and aquatic species may spend less time in the water. Nasal discharge may or may not be associated with lower respiratory tract disease. Ausculation is often difficult and results vary; however, use of moistened gauze between the stethoscope diaphragm and the shell may be helpful. The clinician should pay particular attention to the presence of abnormal sounds and asymmetry during auscultation. In aquatic species, asymmetrical lung consolidation often results in abnormal position in the water column or an inability to submerge (see Fig. 76.11A). Any unilateral mass (e.g., abscess, neoplasm, bladder stone) or asymmetrical gas presence (e.g. gastrointestinal bloat, obstruction) can cause similar signs. Any serious carapacial fracture that enters the dorsal coelom has the capacity to involve the lungs.

Crocodilians. Clinical signs are often nonspecific and range from subclinical infection to apparent peracute mortality. More often, however, a chronic course of intermittent anorexia with progressive weight loss, lethargy, and weakness precedes death. Clinical signs associated with respiratory disease in crocodilians include abnormal swimming (either in circles or on one side of the body), dyspnea, tachypnea, excessive basking, nasal discharge, and anorexia.

Hematology, Biochemistry, and Serology

Collection of blood, before starting therapy, for routine hermatology and plasma chemistry profiles can be informative, although seldom specific. Infectious disease may result in leucocytosis, often charcaterized by hereophilia and monocytosis (including azurophilia). Eosinophilia may be expected but is not invariably associated with verminous pneumonia. Most reptiles with pneumonia are critically ill, and evaluation of hydration, as well as renal and hepatic function, is necessary before initiating specific treatment. Serologic assays (ELISA) and PCR for ophidian paramyxovirus and tortoise mycoplasma infection methods are available in the United States and some European countries.

Radiography

Radiographic evaluation of the respiratory tract requires orthogonal views (see radiology Chapters 53 through 57 for more details). Digital imaging techniques allow the clinician to alter brightness or contrast and reverse the image, which can help highlight otherwise indistinct changes. In addition to dorsoventral views, lateral views should be obtained using a horizontal beam, and, in chelonians, a third craniocaudal view, also taken with a horizontal beam, is required (Fig. 76.12).

Quality radiographs permit the clinician to evaluate the trachea and bronchi in the cervical region and as they enter the lungs in the cranial coelom, often near the heart (Fig. 76.13A). Increased soft tissue densities, focal, multifocal, or diffuse within one or both pulmonary areas suggest exudate or increased tissue presence that can be consistent with infection or tissue proliferation (Figs. 76.13B and 76.14). Horizontal beam projections may reveal fluid lines.

Computed Tomography and Magnetic Resonance Imaging

Computed tomography (CT) scans and magnetic resonance imaging (MRI) are useful techniques for evaluating the lungs and localizing pulmonary lesions (Figs. 76.15 and 76.16) (see Chapters 59 and 60).[8,9] Reptiles typically require sedation or short-term anesthesia to ensure the necessary immobility during image acquisition, with both pre- and postcontrast images obtained. CT is most useful for evaluating soft tissue and air interfaces, often at higher resolution, whereas MRI provides detailed images of various respiratory soft tissues, albeit at usually lower resolution (see Chapters 59 and 60). CT and MRI scan data are collected in series and can be reconstructed in a variety of ways. Postprocessing software allows for the reconstruction of the cross-sectional image series into a complete 3D respiratory tract; however, consultation with a diagnostic imaging specialist is strongly recommended to avoid misinterpretation.

Cytology and Microbiology

The ability to diagnose pathologic changes within the respiratory system of reptiles is relatively straightforward if initial reliance is placed on the collection of material for cytology/histopathology and microbiology. Reptiles should not be treated with broad spectrum antimicrobials unless attempts to demonstrate and characterize a bacterial disease have been undertaken.

The upper respiratory tract, including the nares, choana, larynx and cranial trachea, can be visualized and often sampled directly without anesthesia. Small-diameter culturettes permit the collection of samples, direct from the anterior trachea although care is required to avoid contamination by oral commensals. Swabs can be submitted for cytologic evaluation, microbiologic staining, and culture.

The transtracheal lavage is often preferred as the initial diagnostic tool for investigating lower respiratory tract disease and can be safely performed in most reptiles. Patients should be appropriately stabilized before short-term sedation or anesthesia, and the lavage should be undertaken after radiography or CT. The glottis is identified and intubated with a sterile endotracheal tube, then a sterile catheter of appropriate diameter and length is passed through the sterile endotracheal tube and down the trachea, past the bifurcation, and into a lung. If the disease is unilateral then a curved metal stylet can be used to guide entry into the left or right lung (Fig. 76.17A). Sterile saline (5 mL/kg) of 0.9% sterile saline (without any preservative) is instilled into the lung while the animal is restrained in the horizontal position. It is helpful to draw up the saline into a larger syringe to provide greater aspiration ability (i.e., for a 1 kg reptile, draw up 5 mL into a 60 mL syringe). The patient is then gently inverted, rolled, or rocked for 10 to 15 seconds before attempting aspiration. If no fluid is aspirated, then a second dose of saline is infused. It is often helpful to tilt the reptile head down and continue aspiration as the catheter is withdrawn up the trachea. Any residual saline is readily absorbed from the lungs. In cases of severe pneumonia, it may be possible to aspirate without the need for instilling saline, or quantities greater than the amount infused may be retrieved. In snakes the catheter should ideally be inserted to

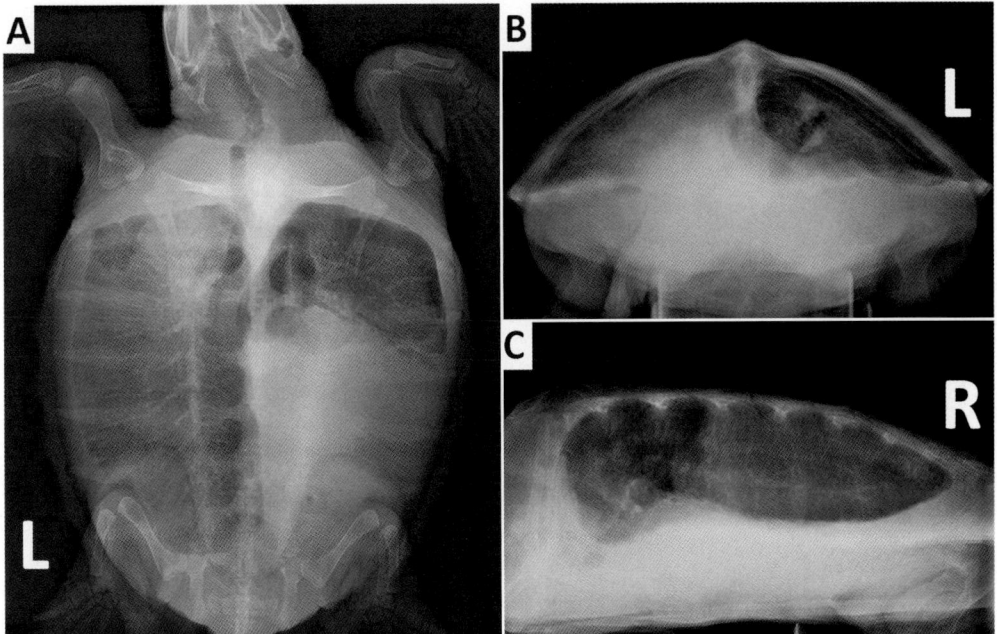

FIG 76.12 Dorsoventral (A), horizontal beam craniocaudal (B), and right lateral (C) radiographic views of a loggerhead sea turtle (*Caretta caretta*) with pronounced consolidation of the mid-to-caudal right lung. (Courtesy of Stephen J. Divers.)

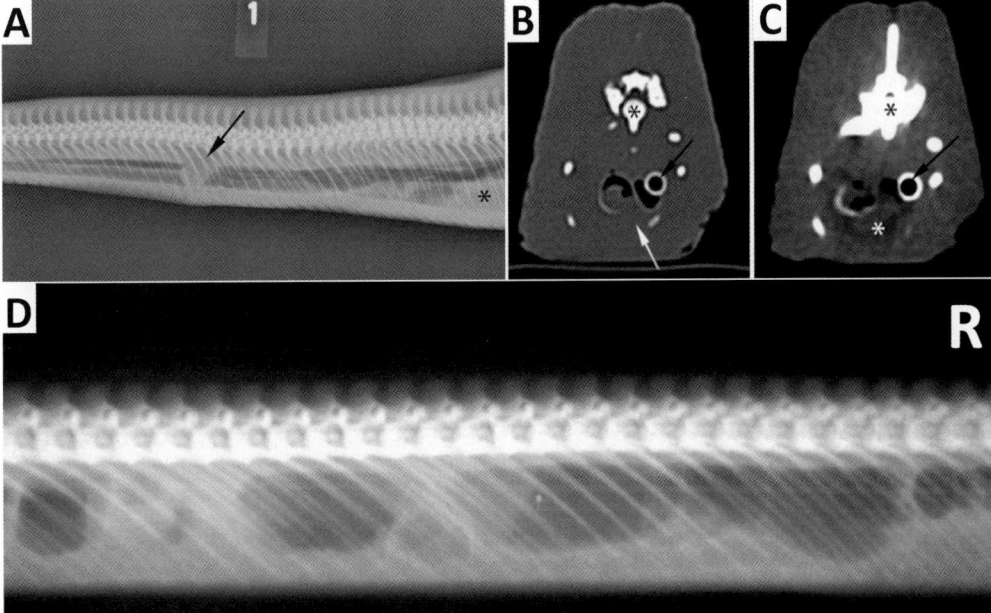

FIG 76.13 (A) Right lateral radiograph of the tracheal region of an 8-year-old boa constrictor (*Boa constrictor*). A round, soft-tissue mass (*black arrow*) is invading the tracheal lumen at the level of the midtrachea, cranial to the heart (asterisk). (B and C) Transverse computed tomography images of the cervical area of the same boa constrictor in a lung algorithm (B) and soft-tissue algorithm (C) confirms the soft tissue mass to be partially obstructing the tracheal lumen (white asterisk). The mass extends ventrally and medially beyond the tracheal wall (white arrow), close to the esophagus (black arrow). A rubber tube has been inserted into the esophagus to delineate this structure during image acquisition (black arrow). The black asterisk indicates the cervical vertebrae.[17] (D) Horizontal beam, right radiographic view of the cranial coelom of a ball python (*Python regius*) demonstrating multifocal areas of increased soft tissue density throughout the vascular lung due to mycobacteriosis. (A–C, Reproduced with permission from *Journal of Herpetological Medicine and Surgery;* D, courtesy of Stephen J. Divers.)

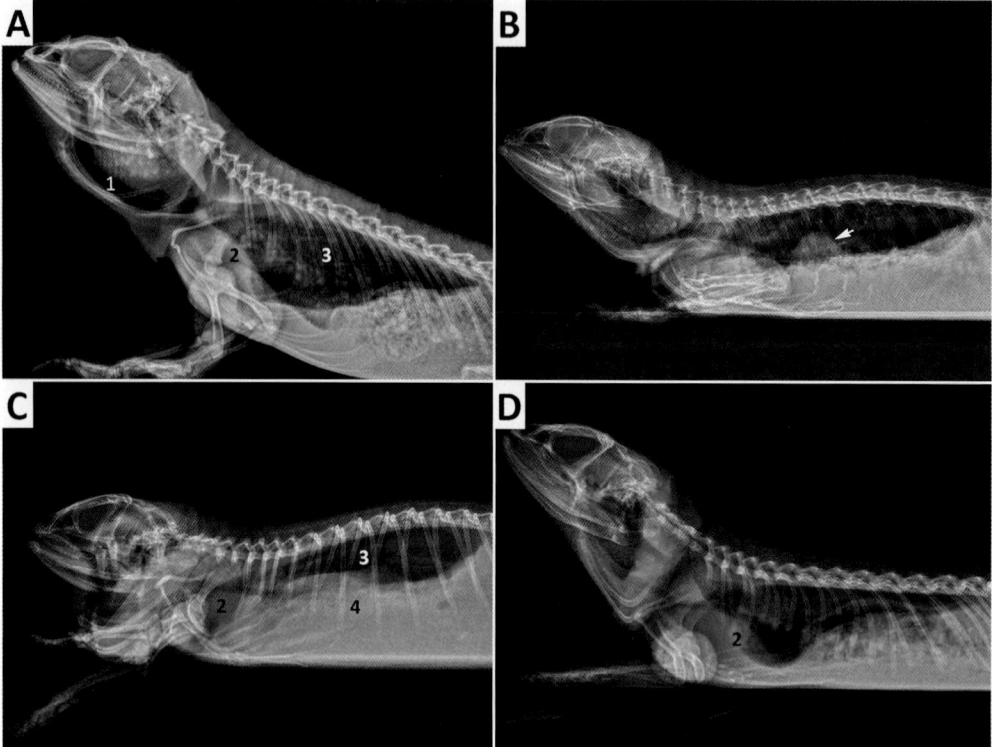

FIG 76.14 Horizontal beam, right lateral radiographs of four bearded dragons (*Pogona vitticeps*) that presented with respiratory signs. (A) Normal radiographic anatomy with unremarkable trachea (1), heart (2), and lung (3). The apparent soft tissue densities within the cranial lungs are due to superimposition of large keratinized scales and dermal projections. The respiratory signs in this case were determined to be of environmental etiology. (B) Focal soft tissue density in the midventral pulmonary region (arrow). Possible differential diagnoses include abscess, granuloma, or extrapulmonary mass associated with the stomach or liver. (C) Apparent enlargement of the cardiac silhouette (2) with compression of the lungs (3) due to increased soft tissue mass effect within the ventral coelom (4). Ultrasonography indicated gross obesity with hepatic lipidosis, enlarged fat bodies, and increased pericardiac fat. (D) Mild enlargement of the cardiac silhouette (2) subsequently identified as ventricular enlargement due to bacterial endocarditis. (Courtesy of Stephen J. Divers.)

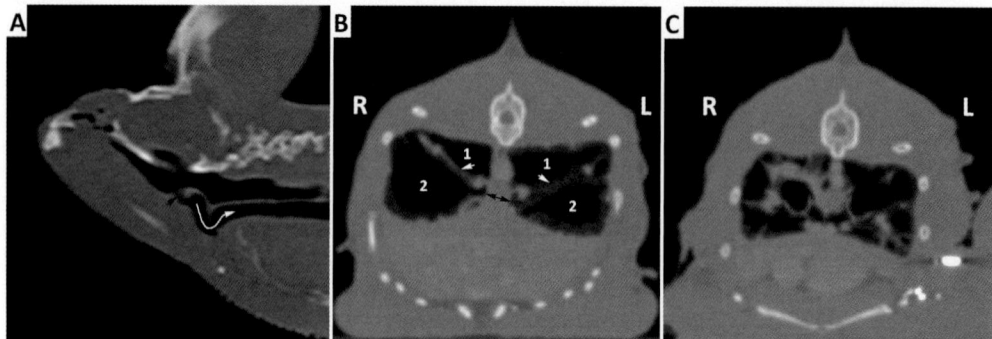

FIG 76.15 (A) Saggital CT reconstruction of a veiled chameleon (*Chamaeleo calyptratus*) demonstrating the larynx (black arrow) and the normal, deviated path of the anterior trachea (white arrow), which often makes intubation difficult. (B) Transverse CT image of a healthy iguanid lizard at the level of the eighth trunk vertebrae demonstrating the intrapulmonary bronchi (black arrows), pulmonary septa (white arrows), and dorsal (1) and ventral (2) lung lobes. (C) Transverse CT image of another iguanid with respiratory signs demonstrating bilateral disruption of the normal lung anatomy with increased soft tissue presence particularly evident in the right lung. (Courtesy of Stephen J. Divers.)

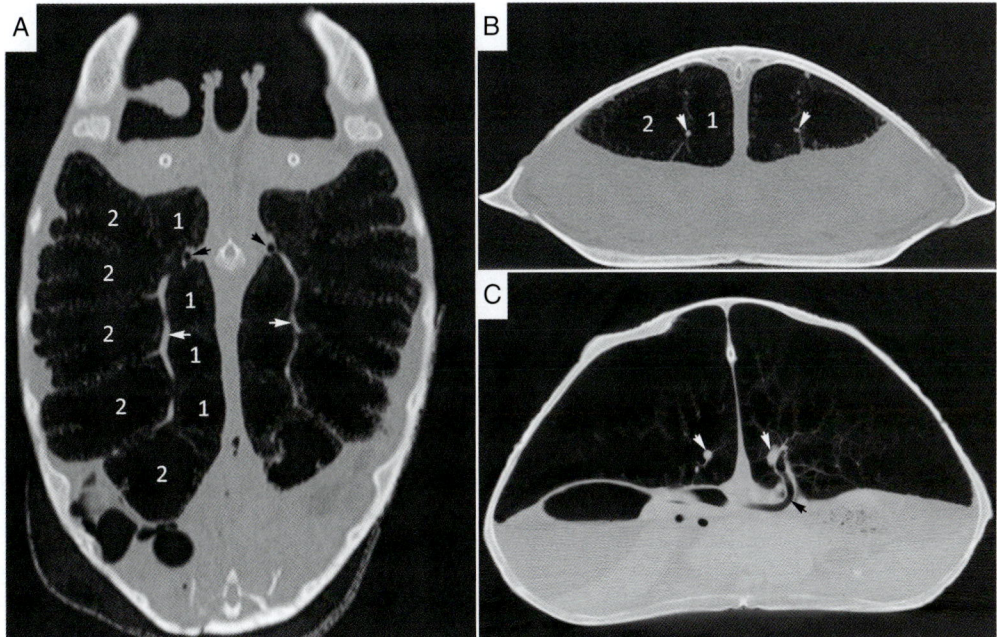

FIG 76.16 Coronal CT reconstruction (A) and transverse CT images (B) of a healthy emydid turtle demonstrating normal lung anatomy including the primary bronchi (black arrows), intrapulmonary supporting cartilage (white arrows), and medial (1) and lateral (2) lung chambers. (C) Transverse CT of a Galapagos tortoise (*Chelonoidis nigra*) illustrating a primary bronchus (black arrow), intrapulmonary supporting cartilage (white arrows), and a less ordered lung structure, more typical of land tortoises. (Courtesy of Stephen J. Divers.)

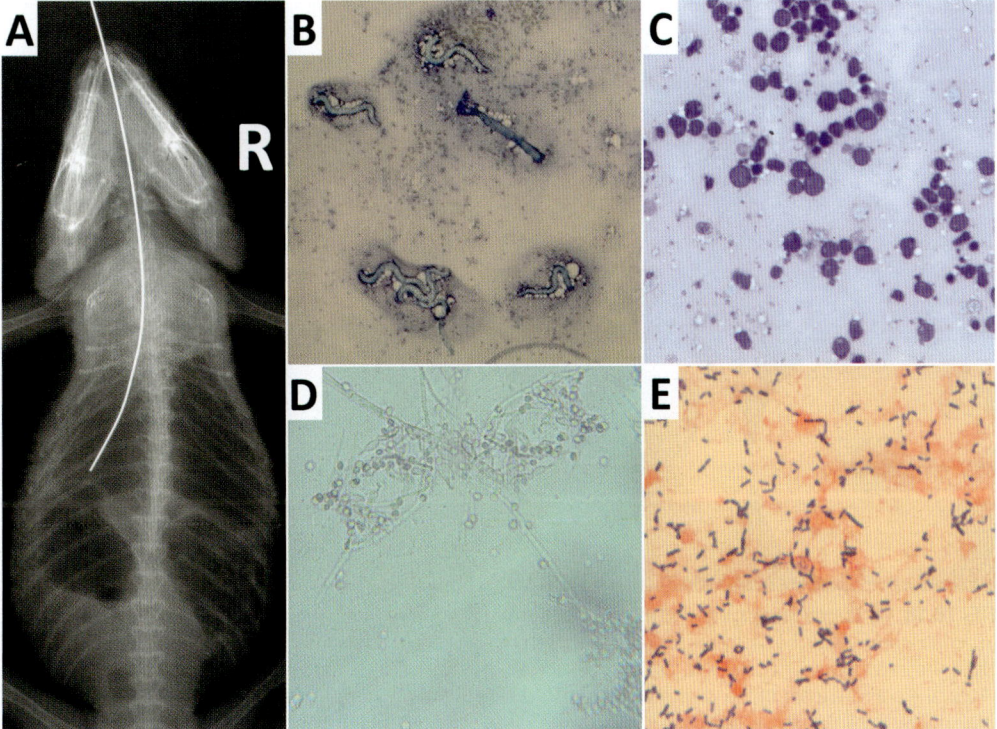

FIG 76.17 (A) Use of a curved stylet to ensure catheterization and lavage of the left lung in a bearded dragon (*Pogona vitticeps*). (B) Lung lavage cytology from a snake with verminous pneumonia demonstrating multiple nematode larvae (DiffQuik, x200). (C) Lung lavage cytology from a tortoise with mycotic pneumonia demonstrating large gram-positive structures consistent with yeast (DiffQuik, x1000). (D) Lung lavage cytology from a sea turtle with mycotic pneumonia demonstrating fungal hyphae and conidia (wet prep, x1000). (E) Lung lavage from an agamid lizard with bacterial pneumonia demonstrating gram-positive bacilli (gram stain, x1000). (Courtesy of Stephen J. Divers.)

30% to 40% SVL; however, in larger snakes a tracheal lavage may be all that is possible. In lizards, the catheter is advanced to a point just caudal to the forelimbs, and no further than 1/3 of the length of the coelom. In chelonia, the catheter can be advanced to a midcoelom position. The collected fluid can be used for cytology and microbiology (including bacterial and fungal cultures, or PCR) (see Fig. 76.17B–E). Depending on the volume and quality of the sample obtained, material should be divided and submitted as requested by the laboratory.

In chelonians, a percutaneous lung lavage can also be performed with a long intravenous catheter. Following aseptic preparation and while holding the animal at maximum inspiration, the catheter is positioned in the dorsocranial area of the prefemoral fossa and advanced in a dorsomedial direction. Aspiration of air confirms entry into the lung. The needle is removed before performing lavage through the catheter. Similar techniques are possible in lizards and snakes.

Endoscopy

Depending on the size of the animal and the equipment available, endoscopic examination of the larynx, trachea, bronchi, and lungs are often practical and provide a minimally invasive means of direct examination and biopsy for microbiology and histolopathology (see Chapters 62 through 64 for more details). Routine considerations before general anesthesia and endoscopy should be undertaken. Transglottal endoscopy of the larynx, trachea, bronchi, and lungs is a noninvasive procedure that can be undertaken during short-term anesthesia. Transcutaneous pulmonoscopy requires a more involved, albeit minimally invasive, surgical approach and longer anesthesia times.[10,11]

Transglottal Endoscopy. The use of fine-diameter rigid telescopes and flexible fiberscopes or videoscopes permits endoscopic access to, and biopsy of the lower respiratory tract tissues in many reptiles.[10,11] Semirigid

or rigid endoscopes 1 to 4.0 mm can be used to evaluate the larynx and trachea as far as their diameter and length permits (Fig. 76.18A). In small lizards and snakes this may include access to the cranial aspect of the lung(s). However, in chelonians the long, meandering bronchi make rigid endoscopy access to the lungs difficult to impossible in animals <5 kg. In larger reptiles, the 1.9- and 2.7-mm rigid endoscope can be used with an operating sheath to permit the use of 1- to 1.7-mm (3–5 Fr) instruments including biopsy forceps. In smaller animals these instruments can still be used, with difficulty, using the trachea as the sheath to guide the advancing instrument. For deeper access, flexible endoscopes (often uretheroscopes or bronchoscopes) 2 to 6 mm can be used with the instrument channel for biopsy forceps or cytology brushes (see Fig. 76.18B). To avoid handling artefacts, endoscopic biopsies should be gently shaken from the biopsy forceps into sterile saline and then decanted into histology filters before placing into formalin.[10] Individual laboratory requirements should always be followed, but in general biopsies for microbiology are often submitted in enrichment or transport broth, whereas ethanol is generally preferred for parasitology.

Transcutaneous Endoscopy. These endoscopic approaches were developed to permit practitioners that have access to established avian and exotic rigid endoscopy systems the chance to examine the lower respiratory tract of reptiles. For snakes, depending on available equipment and the size of the snake, endoscopic evaluation of the distal trachea, intrapulmonary bronchus, vascular, semisaccular, and saccular lung may be possible (see Fig. 76.18C–H). In most snakes a right lateral approach with the snake in left lateral recumbency is preferred, whereas in boids (with two lungs), left, right, or bilateral examinations can be performed. With the anesthetized snake in lateral recumbency and following aseptic preparation, a small (1–2 cm) skin incision is made at the level of the semisaccular lung (or transitional zone) to avoid

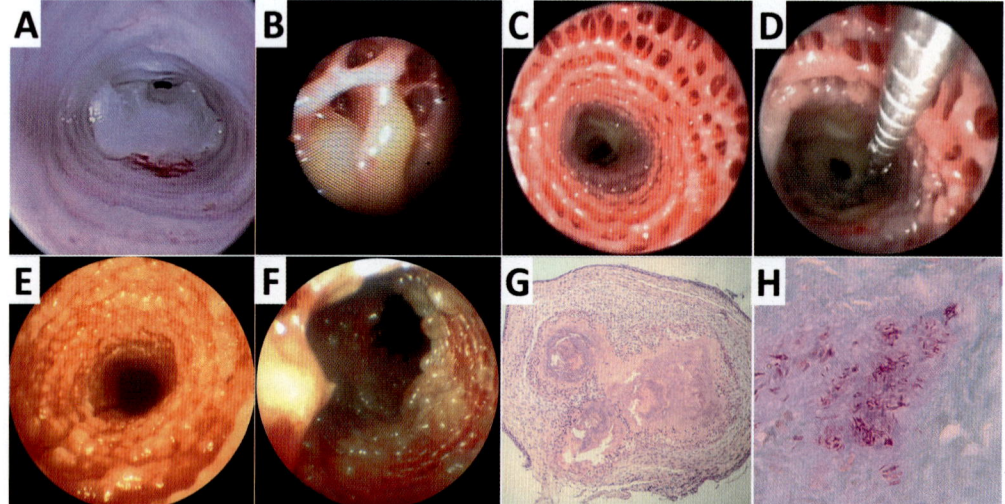

FIG 76.18 (A) Tracheoscopic view of a chondroma in a ball python (*Python regius*) using a 2.7-mm telescope. (B) Endoscopic view of exudate associated with the cranial vascular lung in a boa constrictor *(Boa constrictor)*. Note the reduced image size and pixilation associated with this 2.5-mm fiberscope. (C) Purulent exudate within the cranial aspect of the vascular lung of a Burmese python (*Python bivittatus*). (D) Endoscopic collection of exudate from the same Burmese python. (E) Transcutaneous pulmonoscopy of the right lung of a boa constrictor using a 2.7-mm telescope. Note the severe inflammation of the faveolar parenchyma associated with acute bacterial pneumonia. (F) Endoscopic view of the left vascular lung of a ball python with chronic pneumonia characterized by granulomatous change. (G) Endoscopic biopsy of the same snake demonstrating the typical histological form of a granuloma (H&E, ×20). (H) Acid-fast stain of the same biopsy illustrating acid-fast bacteria consistent with *Mycobacterium* sp. (Ziehl-Neelson, ×1000 oil immersion). (A, Courtesy of Scott J. Stahl, Stahl Exotic Animal Veterinary Service; C and D, courtesy of Zdenek Knotek; B and E–H, courtesy of Stephen J. Divers.)

major hemorrhage (approximately 35%–45% SVL) (Fig. 76.19).[10,11] A ventrolateral approach can made after a craniocaudal incision between the second and third rows of lateral scales, or dorsoventrally over an intercostal space. The subcutaneous coelomic muscle and coelomic membrane are bluntly dissected. When the wall of the lung (transparent avascular membrane) is reached, two fine stay sutures can be placed to elevate it to the level of the skin incision (this is often not necessary with the more lateral approach). Following perforation of the lung, the endoscope (rigid with or without the operating sheath, or, in large boids, a flexible scope) is introduced through the incision and directed cranially toward the vascular lung, anterior lung lobe, intrapulmonary bronchus, and distal trachea (see Fig. 76.3C–F). By directing the endoscope caudally, various visceral organs can be viewed through the transparent saccular lung wall. If there are pathologic changes, the affected part of the lungs can be sampled for further testing (cytology, histopathology and microbiology).[10,11]

Subsequent to examination via the ventrolateral approach, the lung is closed with a single simple interrupted suture using absorbable material, with the muscle and skin closed routinely. The lateral, intercostal approach does not typically require closure of the lung or the muscle, just the skin.[10] Biopsies should be gently shaken from biopsy forceps into sterile saline before fixation in 10% formalin (or 2% glutaraldehyde) to ensure the best diagnostic quality.[10] The aforementioned techniques have been performed in colubrids, pythons, and boas with good to excellent results.[10,11] Reevaluation of snakes a year later confirmed complete healing of the previous entry and the biopsy sites.[10] The authors have not experienced any negative consequences associated with pulmonoscopy in snakes; however, greater hemorrhage would be expected if a more cranial approach through the vascular lung was performed.

With the exception of fine diameter flexible endoscopy in large chelonians, the short trachea and long, narrow bronchi make entry into the chelonian lung extremely difficult via an oral approach. Two nonglottal approaches to the chelonian lung can be used, prefemoral (soft tissue) and carapacial (osteotomy). Both approaches require orthogonal radiographs or CT to determine which side is primarily affected, and in the case of carapacial approaches, precise targeting is needed because of the bony restriction to endoscope movements. The prefemoral approach is a soft tissue surgical approach to the caudal lung. The chelonian is anesthetized and placed in lateral recumbency with the pelvic limb retracted caudad and the prefemoral area aseptically prepared. A 2- to 5-cm craniocaudal incision is made close to the craniodorsal margin of the prefemoral fossa. Upon entry into the coelom, the caudal aspect of the lung is identified (aided by increased ventilation rate and maximal tidal volume), gently grasped, and two retaining

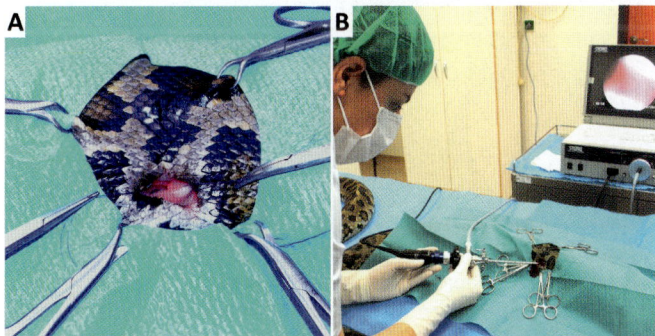

FIG 76.19 (A) Identification and isolation of the semisaccular lung using stay sutures in a Burmese python (*Python bivittatus*). (Courtesy of Zdenek Knotek). (B) Endoscopic evaluation of the right lung of a Burmese python. (Courtesy of Zdenek Knotek.)

sutures are placed to hold the lung close to the skin incision. A small stab incision through an avascular window permits entry of the endoscope (Fig. 76.20). Careful advancement of the endoscope can often permit examination of most of the lung, sometimes to the level of the primary bronchial opening. Closure of the lung after biopsy is important to prevent pneumocoelom.

The carapacial approach requires a temporary osteotomy. With the chelonian anesthetized and placed in ventral recumbency, the area of carapace over the site of lung pathology is aseptically prepared. A 3.5-mm (for the 1.9-mm integrated telescope) or 5-mm (for the 2.7-mm telescope and 4.8-mm operating sheath) osteotomy is then created with a sterile orthopedic drill with the patient at maximal expiration (Fig. 76.21). Entry into the lung is accomplished using small straight hermostats with the animal held at maximal inspiration. Escape of gas confirms entry into the lung. Examination proceeds with the endoscope, although there is far less manoeuvrability. After examination and sample collection, the osteotomy site may be closed with an epoxy resin, or a catheter can be secured in place to facilitate intrapulmonic drug administration. Appropriate samples must be submitted for cytology/histopathology and bacterial/fungal cultures before starting antimicrobials. Untreated or inappropriately treated chronic respiratory tract disease often spreads to other areas, resulting in septicemia and systemic abscess/granuloma formation in remote tissues, notably the liver.

Surgical Biopsy

If minimally invasive endoscopic techniques are not possible, then surgical access to the lung can be achieved by coeliotomy. There is no functional diaphragm or negative pleural pressure to preserve. In snakes the vascular lung is typically located between 12% and 45% SVL; however, great species variation exists.[1,2] Preoperative radiography can easily determine the margins of the respiratory tract and should be performed before surgical biopsy to ensure a correct, targeted approach. Biopsy of the vascular cranial lung commonly results in hemorrhage unless appropriate measures are taken. Biopsy of the thinner posterior lung (or air sac) is not complicated by hemorrhage but is seldom a site for primary pathology. In lizards, the cranial lung is also more highly vascularized than the caudal areas. A cranial coeliotomy may permit sufficient exposure; otherwise, a lateral, intercostal approach between ribs may offer better exposure for biopsy of the cranial lung. The tuatara (*Sphenodon punctatus*), some varanids, and crocodilians possess significant postpulmonary membranes that should be respected with large surgical breaches sutured closed. In chelonia, the lungs are protected by the carapace, which makes surgical access more difficult. Creation of a 4-mm to 5-mm temporary osteotomy in the carapace, directly over the area of interest, does permit the use of biopsy needles, either blind or using radiographic/CT guidance (Fig. 76.22). A ventral approach to the chelonian lungs is not recommended due to obstruction by the coelomic viscera and the need to close the lung and septum horizontale if surgically incised or penetrated in any way.

GENERAL APPROACH TO TREATMENT

Early diagnosis and aggressive therapeutic measures, including intensive nursing, are often necessary. Patients should be maintained at the upper end of their preferred optimum temperature zone or range, and with appropriate humidity to facilitate immunologic and mucociliary functions. The use of hospital oxygen cages should be reserved for those cases in which hypoxemia is present or suspected. Fluid therapy is often required due to increased insensible losses from exacerbated respiratory rate and effort. Route of fluid administration should be consummate with urgency and degree of deficit. Anorexia is not uncommon, but

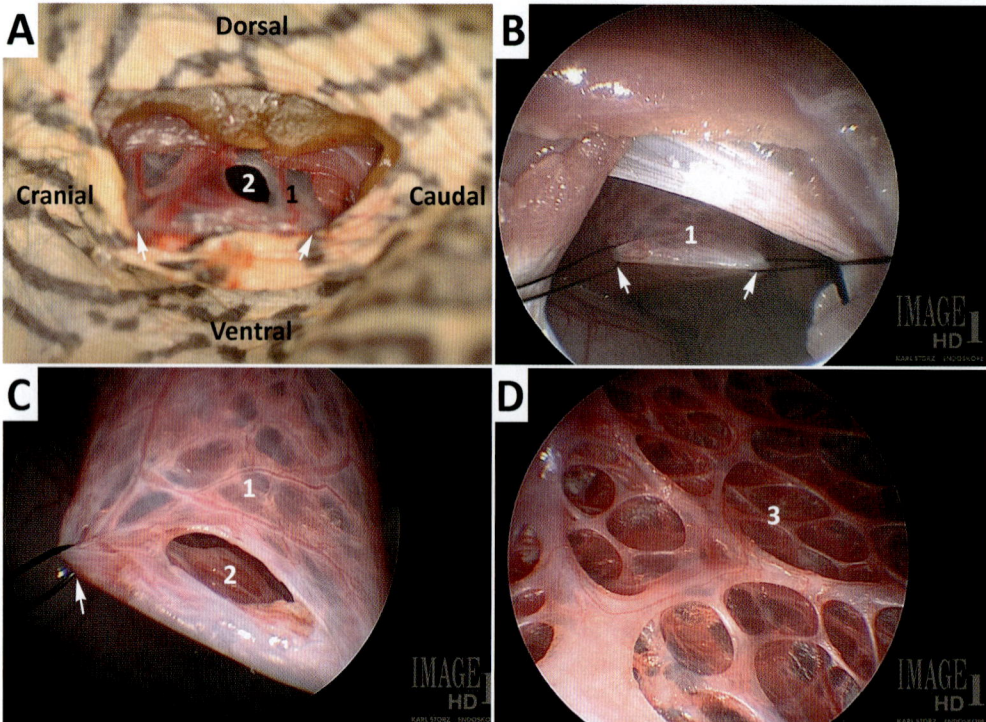

FIG 76.20 Left prefemoral transcutaneous pulmonoscopy in chelonians. (A) Surgical approach via a prefemoral coeliotomy in an emydid turtle. Stay sutures (arrows) have been placed through the left lung (1), which has been elevated to the skin incision. A small stab incision has been made through an avascular edicular window (2) to permit endoscope access. (B–D) Prefemoral coelioscopic view of the left lung (1) of a *Trachemys* turtle. Again, note the use of stay sutures (arrows) to elevate the lung, and the small stab incision (2) to facilitate entry of the endoscope to examine the edicular parenchyma (3). (Courtesy of Stephen J. Divers.)

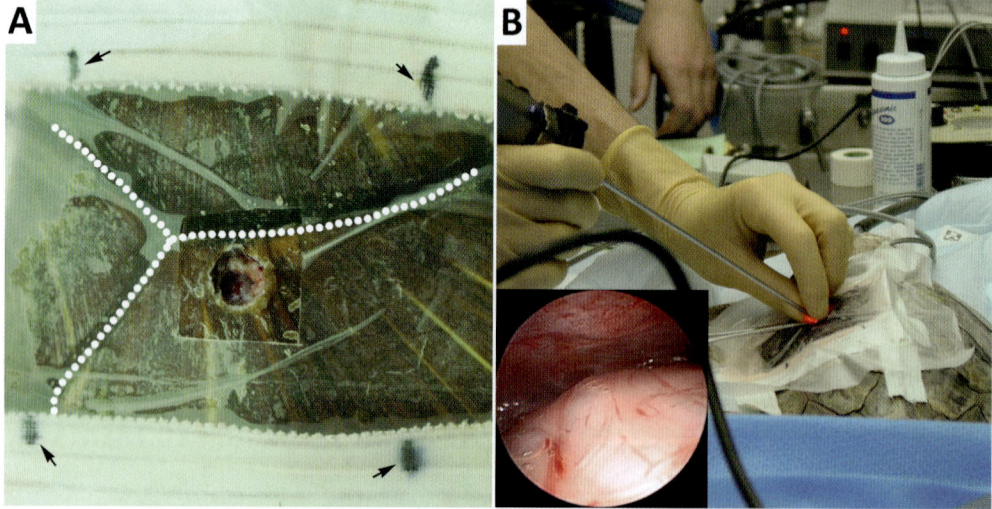

FIG 76.21 Transcarapacial pulmonoscopy in a juvenile loggerhead sea turtle (*Caretta caretta*). (A) View of the surgical site illustrating the position of the osteotomy through the carapace over the radiographically targeted lesion. The margins of the lesion were marked on tape (arrows). The hole was created close to the intersection of the keratin scutes (white dotted lines) as this would avoid disrupting a bony growth plate. (B) Surgical view of the telescope being placed through the osteotomy site. (*Inset*) endoscopic view of a large granuloma. Biopsy and intraoperative cytology indicated fungal granuloma, and consequently the surgical plan was modified to create a larger carapacial flap and remove the granuloma. (Courtesy of Stephen J. Divers.)

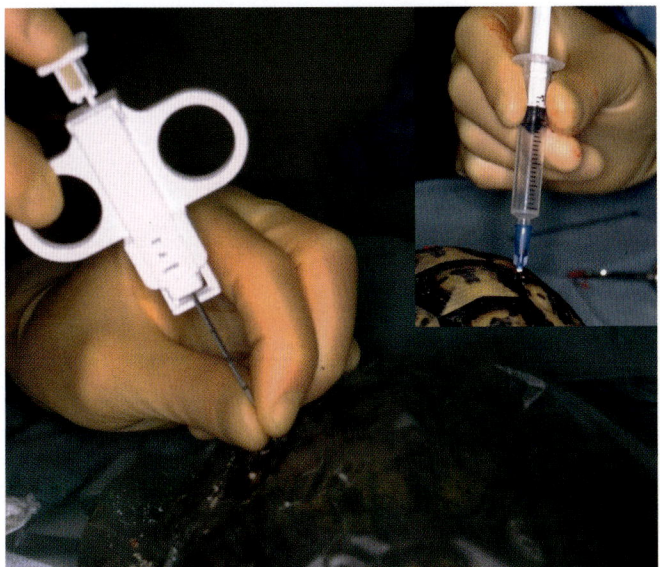

FIG 76.22 Needle biopsy of the lung of a Greek tortoise (*Testudo graeca*) via a 4-mm carapacial osteotomy, targeted using radiography. (Insert) Fine-needle aspiration can be useful for microbiology and cytology. (Courtesy of Stephen J. Divers.)

TABLE 76.2 **Suggested Drugs for Nebulization of Reptiles**	
Drug	**Dose**
Amikacin	50 mg in 10 mL saline
Tobramycin	50 mg in 10 mL saline
Ceftazidime	100 mg in 10 mL saline
Amphoteracin B	10 mg in 10 mL saline
Benzalkonium/polyhexanide (F10)	54 mg/4 mg (1 mL) in 250 mL saline
Acetylcysteine	20% solution

In humans the mg quantity of drug is entirely inhaled and therefore most useful. However, reptiles are placed in a nebulization chamber such that drug concentration and duration of exposure (typically 2–4 hours) are more important than the mg of drug used.

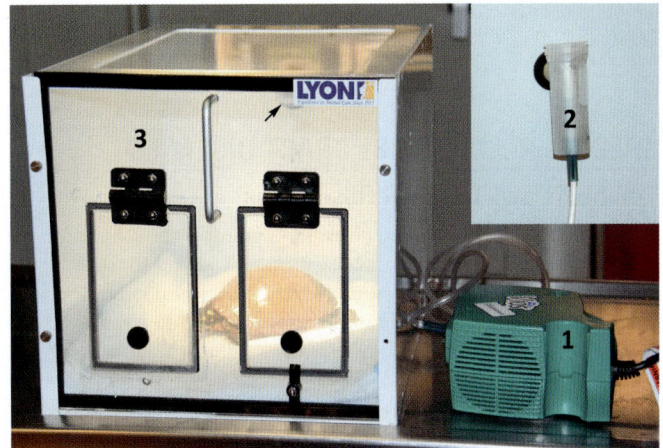

FIG 76.23 Nebulization set-up suitable for reptiles. The compressor (1) forces air through the drug reservoir (2), located on the external rear wall, to form a fine mist that is delivered through a port (arrow) into the nebulization chamber (3), which has rubber seals around the front access door to reduce drug vapor escape. (Courtesy of Stephen J. Divers.)

there is rarely an urgent need to provide nutritional support during initial case management. Assisted feedings should be delayed until dehydration has been corrected and diagnostics (that often require sedation or anesthesia) have been performed.

Antimicrobial Therapy

A variety of bacterial and fungal organisms can cause disease and therefore culture (or PCR), and sensitivity (disc diffusion or MIC) testing is important. While awaiting microbiology results, gram-stained smears should be used to direct initial antimicrobial choice. Antimicrobials should only be prescribed when a bacterial or fungal disease has been identified. Inappropriate use of broad-spectrum antimicrobials implies a low level of clinical expertise and predisposes to drug resistance (see Chapters 29, 115 and 116).

Nebulization. Nebulization can be useful to deliver antimicrobials, especially those that may be systemically toxic, topically to the respiratory tract. Small particle size to ensure penetration deep into the respiratory tract, appropriate solution (in sterile water or saline), and air as the carrier are important to maintain ventilation. Using oxygen as a carrier gas tends to suppress respiration and reduce drug delivery. Although there have been no direct studies to date, the results involving avian reptiles suggest that successful nebulization requires particle sizes of ≤3 μm delivered for 30 minutes (if anesthetized and ventilated) or 2 to 4 hours (if conscious).[12,13] Once- or twice-daily treatments are recommended. In addition to antimicrobials (often aminoglycosides, amphoteracin B), mucolytics (acetylcysteine), and benzalkonium-polyhexanide solutions (F10 Antiseptic Solution Concentrate, Health and Hygiene Ltd, South Africa) are often nebulized but should not be mixed (Table 76.2). However, there is no evidence to suggest that antimicrobial nebulization is more effective than intravenous administration or that bronchodilators or mucolytics have any beneficial effects. If nebulization is pursued, a dedicated chamber should be used to facilitate creation of a thick fog for the reptile while preventing human exposure (Fig. 76.23).

Intrapulmonic Treatment. Transcutaneous catheterization of the lung can provide an alternative airway in cases of tracheal obstruction or to provide a route for direct drug delivery to the lungs.[14,15] In one case of tracheal obstruction in a ball python (*Python regius*), local anesthesia was used, and after a 1.5-cm surgical cut-down, the saccular lung was identified, stab incised, and a 4-mm endotracheal tube was inserted and sutured in place.[14] Although this endotracheal tube functioned as an alternative airway for 13 days before being removed and the site surgically closed, a smaller catheter could be employed for drug delivery. Following transcarapacial pulmonoscopy in an anesthetized Greek tortoise (*Testudo graeca*), the osteotomy site was not closed, but a 20-g teflon IV catheter was inserted into the diseased lung, capped, and secured in place using epoxy or acrylic (Fig. 76.24).[15] *Candida albicans* pneumonia was confirmed, and intrapulmonary therapy using amphoteracin B via the catheter for 3 weeks proved effective. Irritating drugs should be avoided; however, this technique can provide a route for delivering drugs that may be systemically toxic but that are poorly absorbed across the respiratory epithelium (e.g., aminoglycosides, amphoteracin B). After removal of the catheter, the site should be covered with acrylic or epoxy and allowed to heal by second intention.

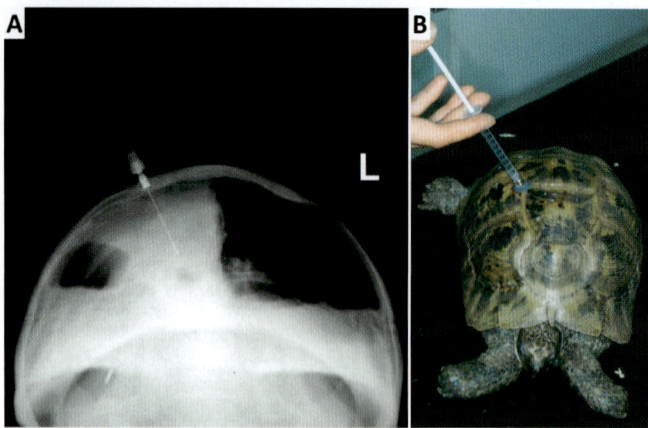

FIG 76.24 Intrapulmonic therapy in a Greek tortoise (*Testudo graeca*). (A) Craniocaudal (horizontal beam) radiograph demonstrating the position of the catheter and stylet into the diseased right lung. (B) Giving amphoteracin B by intrapulmonic injection. (Courtesy of Stephen J. Divers.)

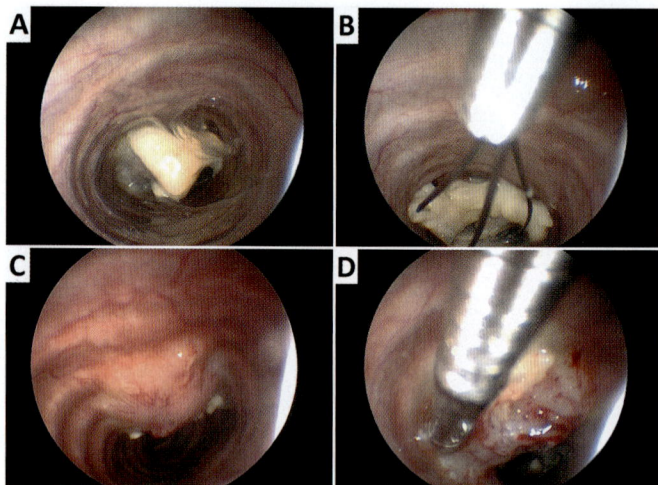

FIG 76.25 Tortoise tracheoscopy. (A) Caseous exudate within the tracheal lumen causing severe dyspnea. (B) Removal of the caseous plug using a wire basket retrieval device. (C) Submucosal fungal granuloma. (D) Biopsy of a tracheal granuloma. (Courtesy of Stephen J. Divers.)

SPECIFIC RESPIRATORY TRACT DISEASES

Tracheitis and Tracheal Obstruction

Clinical Significance. Inflammation, granulomas, chondromas, lymphomas, and exudates can be associated with the trachea.[16–18] If obstructive, these can lead to dyspnea, which tends to be poorly responsive to oxygen; however, dramatic improvement would be expected after creation of an alternative airway (e.g., lung catheter).

Known Etiological Cause(s). *Mycoplasma* have been reported to cause tracheitis in a number of chelonians (*M. agassizii*, *M. testudineum*) and proliferative tracheitis in a Burmese python (*Python bivittatus*).[18] *Salmonella arizonae* was considered the etiologic cause of tracheitis in a double-headed king snake (*Lampropeltis hondurensis*).[19] Nidovirus was seen in association with tracheitis in a group of ball pythons that also had bacterial pneumonia.[20,21] Iridoviral tracheitis was identified in a gopher tortoise (*Gopherus polyphemus*).[16] Tracheal chondromas and lymphoma have been reported in several boid snakes.[17,22,23]

Clinical Presentation and Diagnostic Confirmation. Most publications have involved postmortem evaluations, but lethargy and respiratory compromise, including dyspnea and open-mouth breathing, are common.

Most published reports have described patients as presenting dead or being euthanized shortly after presentation for postmortem investigations. Ideally, endoscopic evaluation of the trachea permits evaluation and selective biopsy of specific lesions for histopathology and microbiology (culture, PCR) (Fig. 76.25). If unavailable, radiography, CT, and tracheal lavage may be useful, but diagnoses may be missed (Fig. 76.26).

Specific Treatment. Exudates should be suctioned from the trachea, whereas firm, space-occupying masses (chondromas, granulomas) typically require endoscopic debridement or tracheal resection and anastomosis. Antimicrobial therapy is based upon culture and sensitivity or MIC results, and treatment for 3 to 6 weeks is often required. Reevaluation is important to determine the effectiveness of treatment.

Prognosis. Endoscopic and tracheal resection have been curative for single chondromas.[23] Multiple masses/granulomas carry a less favorable prognosis. Bacterial tracheitis can often be treated. Fungal infections tend to be more granulomatous and more resistant to medical therapy.

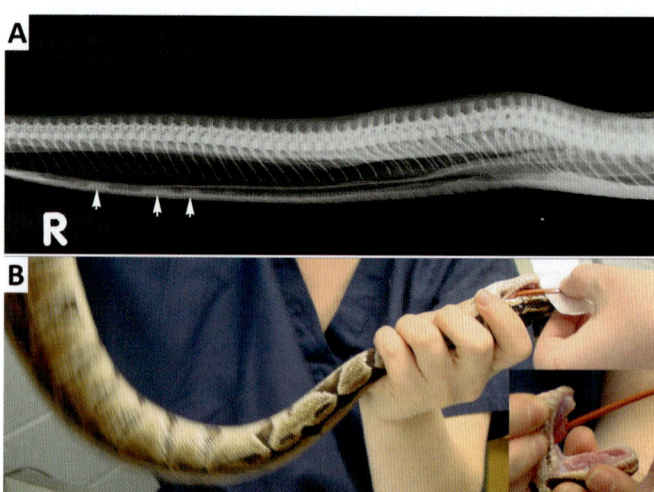

FIG 76.26 (A) Lateral radiograph (horizontal beam) of a ball python (*Python regius*) demonstrating multiple solitary masses within the tracheal lumen, consistent with chondroma. (B) Tracheal lavage in a ball python. In larger reptiles a sterile endotracheal tube should be placed into the trachea before inserting the lavage catheter. (A, Courtesy of Scott J. Stahl, Stahl Exotic Animal Veterinary Services; B, courtesy of Stephen J. Divers.)

There are no reports of successful treatment of viral tracheitis, and supportive care is often all that can be provided.

Bacterial Pneumonia

Clinical Significance. Bacterial pneumonia may occur as a primary entity, secondary to stomatitis and aspiration, by hematogenous spread (e.g., endocarditis), or by direct/close anatomic association (e.g., hepatitis, coelomitis). Bacterial pneumonia can be focal, multifocal, or diffuse, and unilateral or, in boids, bilateral. Many infections involve commensal or environmental organisms that become pathogenic in an immunocompromised host.

Known Etiological Cause(s). Bacterial pneumonia is common in snakes, less so in lizards and chelonians. Microbiologic results have included *Mycoplasma, Aeromonas, Alicaligenes, Chlamydia, Citrobacter, Corynebacterium, Enterobacter, Escherichia coli, Klebsiella, Morganella, Moraxella, Pasteurella, Proteus, Pseudomonas, Acinetobacter, Brevibacterium, Achromobacter, Bacillus, Stenotrophomonas, Empedobacter, Salmonella,* and *Mycobacterium.*[24–29] Compared with healthy snakes with a predominance of *Providencia rettgeri* and coagulase-negative *Staphylococcus* spp., those with pneumonia exhibit moderate to heavy growth of aerobic gram-negative bacilli.[25] Anaerobic organisms (including *Bacteroides, Clostridium, Fusobacterium,* and *Peptostreptococcus*) have been rarely reported.[30]

Mycoplasma (*M. agassizi* and *M. testudineum*) are important respiratory pathogens of tortoises, and pneumonia appears to be intimately involved in the upper respiratory disease complex of these species. Other *Mycoplasma* spp. have been associated with pneumonia in crocodilians (*M. alligatoris, M. crocodyli*) and pythons.[28]

Clinical Presentation and Diagnostic Confirmation.
Cases of acute or peracute pneumonia may present as sudden death, although lethargy, anorexia, and respiratory signs, including dyspnea and open-mouth breathing, are common.

Although diagnostic imaging may provide convincing evidence of lung disease, a definitive diagnosis relies on the collection of material for histopathology (or cytology) and microbiology. Therefore endoscopic evaluation or lung lavage is typically required.

Specific Treatment.
High-volume lung lavage and aspiration, or coupage, have been used to remove considerable quantities of exudate from the lower respiratory tract of anesthetized or sedated squamates (Fig. 76.27). Systemic and local application of antimicrobials are typically required, and selection should be based upon disc sensitivity or MIC results. Prolonged treatment is often required, along with correction of any predisposing husbandry or nutritional components. Pharmacokinetic studies have been performed for clarithromycin and oxytetracycline, which should be used in preference to fluoroquinolones for mycoplasmosis.[31–35]

Prognosis.
If left untreated most cases progress to generalized sepsis and death, although chronic granulomata or abscesses can develop. Severe cases, especially involving *Mycobacterium* and *Chlamydia* sp. have a more guarded to poor prognosis.

Fungal Pneumonia
Clinical Significance.
Mycotic pneumonia is occasionally diagnosed in captive reptiles (see Chapter 31). Typically, fungal infections occur due to high mycotic exposure (poor environment), immunosuppression (hypothermia, hatchlings, concurrent disease), or long-term, broadspectrum antibiotic abuse. Environmental temperature appears to be critically important; for example, cold-stunned sea turtles appear particularly prone to fungal pneumonia.[36]

Known Etiological Cause(s).
A number of fungi have been associated with pneumonia in reptiles, including *Aspergillus, Candida, Fusarium, Mucor, Geotrichum, Penicillium, Cladosporium, Rhizopus, Chrysosporium, Paecilomyces,* and *Beauveria.*[37–40] The systemic deep mycoses occasionally diagnosed in mammals, such as blastomycosis and histoplasmosis, have not been diagnosed in reptiles to date.

Clinical Presentation and Diagnostic Confirmation.
Most cases are presented dead or terminal, but severe respiratory compromise would be expected. A diagnosis of fungal pneumonia is often difficult to make antemortem without biopsy. Recovery of fungal elements, hyphae, or spores or culture of fungal agent (in combination with cytologic evidence

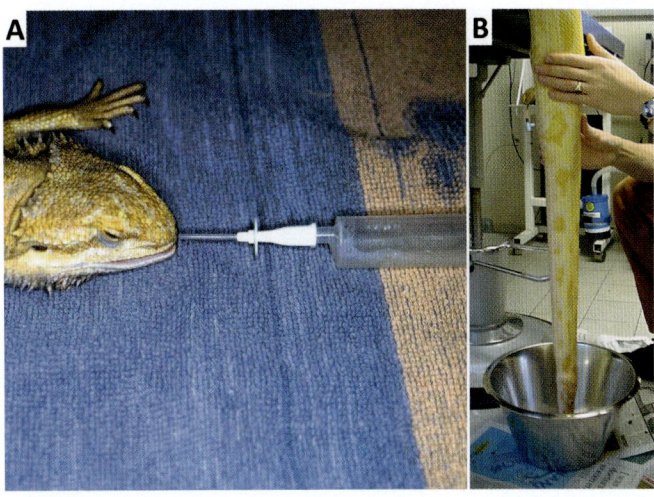

FIG 76.27 (A) Aspiration of large volume of exudate from an anesthetized bearded dragon (*Pogona vitticeps*). (B) Coupage (percussion therapy) in a sedated albino Burmese python (*Python bivittatus*) to facilitate drainage of pulmonary exudates. (Courtesy of Stephen J. Divers.)

of inflammation/infection) from a transtracheal wash is supportive of a diagnosis. However, lesions may be encapsulated and not productive. Endoscopic evaluation and biopsy is more effective and less invasive than traditional surgical approaches. Gross pathologic changes of mycotic pneumonia include pulmonary granulomata, lung consolidation, and occasionally extension of the disease to adjacent organs.

Lesions in chelonians typically consist of nodular, caseous to firm masses within the tracheal wall, pulmonary parenchyma, or over the mucosa or serosal surfaces. Sometimes, pale plaques or fungal mats are present over tracheal and bronchial mucosae, and caseous exudate within air passages is less common unless secondary bacterial infection is present. In severe cases, a whole lung or part of the lung may be consolidated and emphysematous bullae may be observed. In crocodilians, pneumonia also presents as multifocal necrotic to granulomatous foci in the substance of the lung.

Specific Treatment.
Large encapsulated lesions require surgical removal, and even small encapsulated granulomas are often resistant to drug therapy (Fig. 76.28). In acute cases and those where encapsulation is absent, antifungal medication may be effective, and both local and systemic administration should be combined. It is often wise to obtain antifungal MIC results and to check antifungal drug blood levels to ensure they are exceeded.

Prognosis.
Typically the prognosis is poor when dealing with extensive disease. Single granulomas that can be surgically removed carry a fair to good prognosis, especially when combined with postoperative antifungal therapy.

Viral Pneumonia
Clinical Significance.
Several viruses have been identified in association with peracute to chronic pathology of the respiratory system; however, the majority of viruses identified have only been circumstantially incriminated as causes of disease, with few studies fulfilling Koch's postulates (see Chapter 30). Therefore the clinician must be cautious and attempt to differentiate between infection and disease. In addition, the clinical picture is frequently complicated by secondary bacterial or fungal infection.

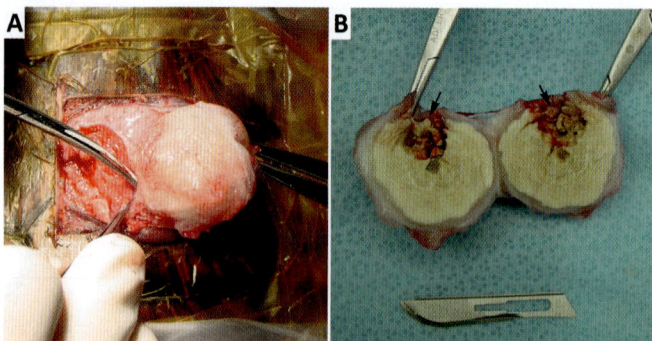

FIG 76.28 (A) Removal of a pulmonary fungal granuloma from the same loggerhead sea turtle (*Caretta caretta*) depicted in Fig. 76.21. (B) Gross dissection of the fungal granuloma reveals thick encapsulation that is resistant to drug penetration. Notice the sites of endoscopic biopsy (*arrows*). (Courtesy of Stephen J. Divers.)

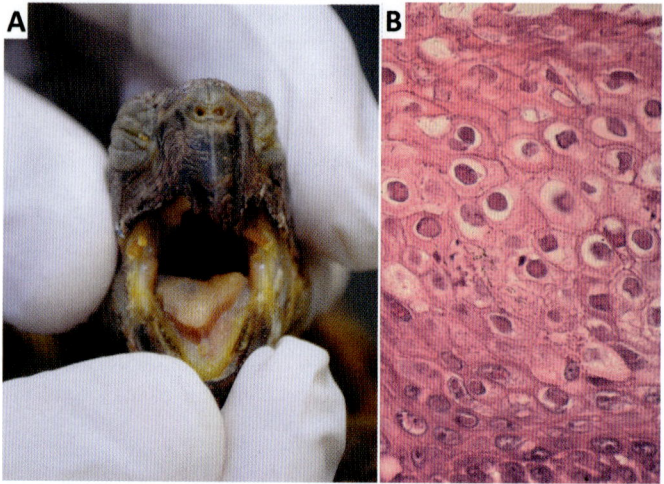

FIG 76.29 (A) Clinical presentation of herpesvirus infection and disease in a *Testudo* tortoise. (Courtesy of Zdenek Knotek.) (B) Laryngeal histology demonstrating multiple intranuclear inclusion bodies consistent with herpesvirus. (Courtesy of Stephen J. Divers.)

Known Etiological Cause(s). A variety of viruses have been detected in association with respiratory pathology.[41-45] Herpesviruses have been associated with rhinitis, tracheitis, and bronchopneumonia in green sea turtles (lung, eye, and tracheal virus of green turtles); fibropapillomas in green and loggerhead sea turtles (chelonid fibropapilloma–associated herpesvirus); and rhinitis, stomatitis, pharyngitis, glossitis, tracheitis, bronchitis, and pneumonia of various terrestrial tortoise species (herpesviruses of terrestrial tortoises, e.g., chelonid herpesvirus 4) (Fig. 76.29). Adenovirus infections of chameleons have been reported in association with proliferative tracheitis, whereas bronchopneumonia has been seen in association with poxvirus and secondary bacterial infection. Iridoviruses from tortoises and turtles have been associated with pharyngitis, tracheitis, and pneumonia. Paramyxoviruses (ferla-viruses) have been rarely implicated in saurian pneumonia (e.g., caiman lizards, *Dracaena guianensis*) but are more common pathogens in snakes (*Bothrops, Bitis, Crotalus, Trimeresurus, Vipera, Atheris*), where they have been associated with caseous necrotic debris, lung thickening, and edema (see Fig. 76.29).[43] Other species of colubrids and boids have also been affected.[44] Multiple isolates of "virus x" have been recovered from a variety of European tortoises with gastrointestinal and respiratory lesions. More recently, a nidovirus has been identified as a likely etiologic agent of severe respiratory disease in pythons.[45] It is important to stress, in the majority of cases, the association of virus with respiratory lesions is just that, an association, and a direct causal relationship has not been demonstrated.

Clinical Presentation and Diagnostic Confirmation. Typical signs of upper and/or lower respiratory tract disease are often reported. The extent that clinical signs can be attributed to the virus rather than secondary infections is open to debate in most cases. Many cases of viral pneumonia are determined by histopathology and electronmicroscopy, without virus isolation or genetic sequencing. However, where serologic tests exist (e.g., ophidian paramyxovirus) they should be utilized, and paired rising titers can be useful to differentiate between active infection versus past exposure. PCR testing has revolutionized the ability to identify viruses from oral/tracheal swabs, lung lavage, or biopsy samples. However, positive results only indicate the presence of the virus and not necessarily disease. Therefore it is important to demonstrate host pathologic response by serology, cytology, or histopathology. It may be wise to save additional biopsy or necropsy tissues at −20°C in case virologic investigations are subsequently required.

Specific Treatment. With the exception of acyclovir (and related drugs) against herpesviruses, there are few medical options available

(see Chapter 118). There are a number of human drugs that have been developed, but high costs and limited commercial interests have resulted in a lack of efficacy, pharmacokinetic, safety, and clinical trials in reptiles. When dealing with an outbreak, separation of diseased animals, barrier nursing, and disinfection are critical. In many cases, immunosuppression associated with poor husbandry and nutrition may be important and should be corrected. General medical support should include fluid therapy and nutritional supplementation. Appropriate quarantine with PCR and serologic testing (when available), remain the mainstays of prevention. In collections, euthanasia of affected animals should be considered.

Prognosis. Viral infections are able to persist for protracted periods, and treatment of clinical viral disease may not resolve persistent infection. Improvements in husbandry and nutrition may be important factors in the outcome.

Verminous Pneumonia

Clinical Significance. A number of parasites encountered in captive reptiles have a portion of their life cycle associated with the respiratory system. Except in cases with overwhelming parasite loads, most respiratory involvement is subclinical and minor, causing primarily localized inflammation.[46] However, heavy burdens or novel host-parasite interactions can lead to significant disease, often complicated by secondary infections.

Known Etiological Cause(s). Several genera of digenetic trematodes within the Ochetosomatidae and Plagiorchiidae (renifers) commonly inhabit the oral cavity, but adults often migrate via the glottis to the lungs and air sacs (Fig. 76.31A). Adults attach to the epithelial lining in the lower respiratory tract causing focal lesions that can become secondarily infected. Infection of aquatic turtles with digenetic spirorchid trematodes of the genera *Spirorchus, Henotosoma, Ullicaecum, Vasotrema*, or *Hapalorhynchus* may result in clinical signs suggestive of pneumonia. Substantial granulomatous reaction within the lungs may result in an asymmetrical position in the water, with the affected side floating lower than the contralateral side. Large trematodes (Hydrophidae) can infect the lungs of sea snakes, causing mucoid exudate with hyperplasia, hemorrhage, and necrosis.[46]

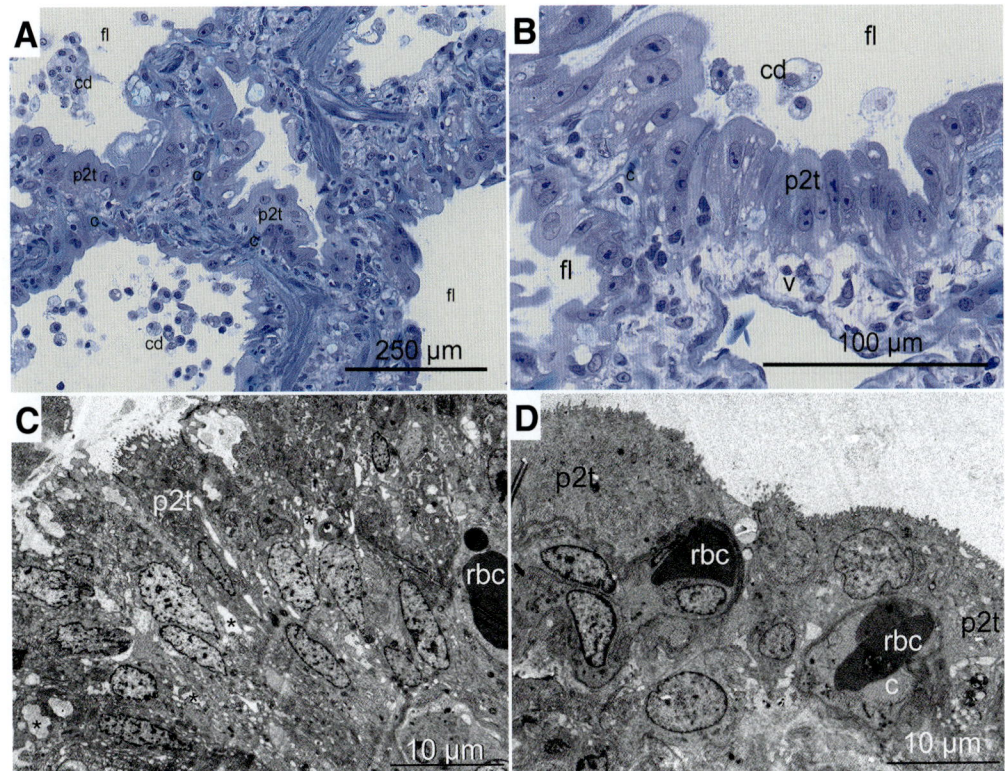

FIG 76.30 Histology and electron microscopy of pulmonary ferlavirus infection and disease in corn snakes (*Pantherophis guttatus*). (A) Thirty-five days postinfection: the respiratory epithelium is completely overgrown by transformed type-2 pneumocytes. Capillaries are hidden under several layers of transformed type-III pneumocytes. (B) Thirty-five days postinfection: the respiratory epithelium is overgrown by very large transformed type-II pneumocytes. Cells contain large vesicles, capillaries are deformed. Semithin sections. Methylene blue–thionine stain. bv, Blood vessel; c, capillaries; cd, cellular debris; fl, faveolar lumen; mf, myofibrillar bundle; p2t, transformed type-II pneumocytes; v, intracellular vesicle. (C) Thirty-five days postinfection: the respiratory epithelium is completely overgrown by transformed type-2 pneumocytes containing numerous vacuoles and forming large intercellular spaces (asterisks). (D) Thirty-five days postinfection showing a different part of the respiratory epithelium with capillaries overgrown by transformed type-II pneumocytes. TEM. Arrows, Diffusion barrier; bl, basal membrane; c, capillary; e, endothelium cell; hp, heterophil leukocyte; n, nucleus; p1, type-I pneumocyte; p2, type-II pneumocyte; p2t, transformed type-II pneumocyte; rbc, erythrocyte. (Original images Figs. 5G, 5H, 6G, and 6H from Starck JM, Neul A, Schmidt V, et al. Morphology and morphometry of the lung in corn snakes [*Pantherophis guttatus*] infected with three different strains of ferlavirus, *J Comp Pathol.* 2017;156[4]:419–435. ISSN 0021-9975. https://doi.org/10.1016/j.jcpa.2017.02.001.)

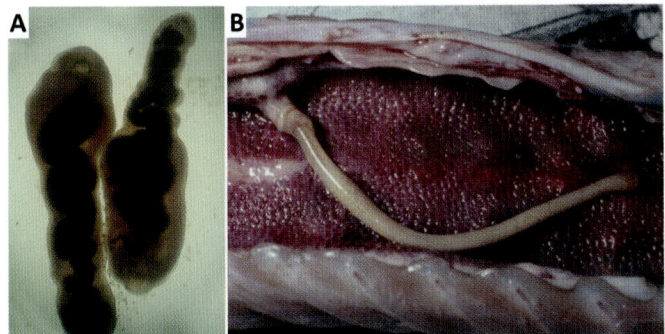

FIG 76.31 (A) Renifers (digenetic trematodes) recovered from the larynx of a free-ranging eastern black rat snake (*Pantherophis alleghaniensis*). (Courtesy of Stephen J. Divers.) (B) Pentastomid attached to the vascular (faveolar) lung of a large boid snake. (Courtesy of Zdenek Knotek.)

Migrating nematode larvae have caused respiratory signs or pulmonary lesions in tortoises (*Angusticaecum*), chameleons (*Hexametra*), and pythons (*Ophidascaris*). Adults of the Filarioidea and Dioctophymatoidea inhabit extraintestinal sites, including the lungs.

Adult lungworms (*Rhabdias*) reside within the lungs of snakes and lizards. The parthenogenic females lay their eggs within the lung. The eggs are then transported up the trachea, swallowed, and passed in feces. Migrating larvae (*Strongyloides*) may also be associated with pulmonary lesions.[46]

Pantastomids (parasitic crustaceans commonly known as tongue worms) undergo extensive visceral migrations before locating within the lungs (and less commonly the trachea and nasal passages) (see Fig. 76.31B). The most important genera are *Sebekia* (crocodilians), *Raillietiella* (lizards and snakes), *Kiricephalus, Porocephalus,* and *Armillifer* (snakes). Mammals, including humans, can act as intermediate hosts. Pentastomids can cause localized lesions, whereas moulting can induce antigenic responses. The adults feed on tissue fluids within the lung and pass embryonated eggs, which enter the oral cavity, before being swallowed and passed in feces.

Rarely, coccidians have been identified in crocodilian lungs, whereas *Hepatozoon* schizonts may be found in the lungs of squamates. Intranuclear coccidia have been reported in captive tortoises (*Geochelone*). The obligate intracellular Microsporidia have been identified within pulmonary cells of inland bearded dragons (*Pogona vitticeps*) dying of the systemic effects of the disease. Although the primary target organs appear to be the liver and kidney, the significance of pulmonary infection is yet to be determined.[46]

Clinical Presentation and Diagnostic Confirmation.

Although most trematode infestations are asymptomatic, heavy parasite loads may cause enough damage to predispose the animal to a secondary pneumonia. The diagnosis is made on the basis of the identification of the typical fluke eggs on transtracheal wash. Currently, no effective and safe treatment has been advocated, although praziquantel could be considered.

The diagnosis of spirorchid fluke infection is difficult. Typical fluke eggs may be identified in direct saline solution mounts from lung washes or by sedimentation concentration of fecal samples. Often, however, the diagnosis is made postmortem with the identification of adults within the cardiovascular system or in squash preparations of pulmonary tissue.

Although most parasitic infections are subclinical, heavy infestations of *Rhabdias* can be associated with open-mouth breathing, extended glottal tube, and severe pneumonia (including secondary bacterial pneumonia) in snakes. A mucus-laden exudate may accumulate around the nares. A proliferative pneumonia may be identified by histopathology. Antemortem diagnosis relies on the demonstration of embryonated eggs (60×35 µm) in a lung lavage or biopsy.

Clinical disease associated with pentastomids is rare, and they are often incidental findings. However, they may cause focal irritation and with a host antigenic response, more diffuse inflammation. Antemortem diagnosis depends on microscopic identification of the ova, which appear distended with a thinly walled capsule and may measure up to 130 µm in diameter. Larva and their hooklets may be seen within these eggs.

Specific Treatment.

Nematode infections may be treated with ivermectin (not chelonians), benzimidazoles, levamisole, or pyrantal. Pentastomids should ideally be treated by removing (often endoscopic) as anthelmintics such as ivermectin result in parasite death and massive antigenic release. Praziquantel can be considered for trematode infections (see Chapter 120). Prevention relies upon acquisition of captive-bred (instead of wild-caught) specimens, appropriate quarantine including fecal screening; use of captive-bred, clean food items; and sound hygiene.

Prognosis.

Cases of uncomplicated verminous pneumonia often respond to medical (anthelmintic and NSAID therapy) or, in the case of pentostomids, surgical removal. Secondary infections, especially if severe, can significantly reduce prognosis.

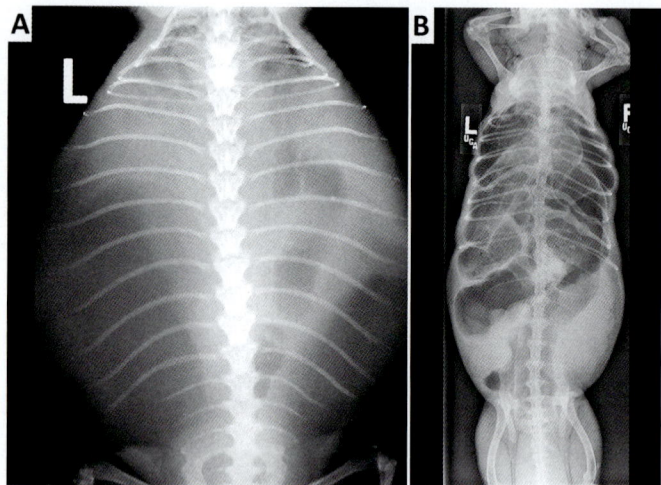

FIG 76.32 Dorsoventral radiographs of two lizards that presented with respiratory signs unrelated to respiratory disease. (A) Grossly obese savannah monitor (*Varanus exanthematicus*) with huge fat bodies and ascites causing lung compression. (B) Generalized gaseous distension throughout the gastrointestinal tract compromising respiratory function in a green iguana (*Iguana iguana*). (Courtesy of Stephen J. Divers.)

Noninfectious Pneumonia

Not all inflammatory diseases are infectious by nature. Aspiration of foreign material, either iatrogenically or by chance, is certain to cause significant inflammation within the lungs. Aspiration pneumonia begins as a foreign body reaction; however, if neglected, progresses rapidly to secondary bacterial pneumonia.

Diseases that compromise tidal volume may mimic primary respiratory disease, even though the respiratory tract itself is healthy. Obesity, ascites, and cranial coelomic space-occupying lesions (e.g., cardiomegaly, hepatomegaly) have the potential to cause respiratory compromise (Fig. 76.32). Significant respiratory disease may result in an increase in pulmonary vascular resistance. The shunting that may occur from pulmonary pathology could decrease oxygen delivery to peripheral tissues. Serious, life-threatening hypoxia and acidosis may result from overwhelming the blood's buffering systems as anaerobiosis becomes prolonged. Conditions as innocuous as the loosening of skin around the nares immediately before ecdysis, which can increase respiratory noise, may be misinterpreted as disease. The "problem" is self-resolving after completion of ecdysis.

REFERENCES

See www.expertconsult.com for a complete list of references.

77

Neurology

Simon R. Platt

A variety of clinical syndromes in reptiles have neurological manifestations. Traumatic injury, nutritional deficiencies, neoplasia, and toxicities can all affect the nervous system. In addition, many infectious diseases (e.g., bacterial and viral) may cause neurological dysfunction. Unfortunately, there is a paucity of information on clinical neurology syndromes affecting reptiles. Additionally, available information is often based on individual case reports or extrapolated from mammalian species.[1]

The manner in which a specific disease of the nervous system causes clinical signs depends very much on the functional neuroanatomy of the vertebrate affected. The reptilian nervous system is moderately simple in structure yet allows functional diversity in species-specific behavior. Although there is a certain amount of specialization of the nervous system of various reptilian species, it is more similar among reptile taxa than different. The most important clinical aspects of functional reptile neuroanatomy are detailed here.

The behavior and anatomy of the various reptile species may render the performance of the neurological examination difficult or impossible; in the case of the more dangerous reptiles, examination may be impossible without restraint or anesthesia. However, many of the principles and techniques employed for the examination of mammalian patients with neurological dysfunction can be adapted for use in reptiles, providing useful information on managing these cases. The specifics of how to practically perform and interpret a neurological examination in reptiles is presented.

Diagnostic aids used in mammalian neurology, such as cerebrospinal fluid (CSF) analysis, advanced imaging, and electrodiagnostic evaluations, may also be difficult to acquire and/or of limited value in reptile neurology on the basis of patient size and anatomic and physiological differences.[1] The premise and latest understanding of the diagnostic testing procedures that are possible and helpful are outlined.

FUNCTIONAL NEUROANATOMY

A basic understanding of reptile neuroanatomy helps the clinician understand the clinical manifestations of neurological diseases and provides an opportunity for the clinician to determine the location of a focal lesion.[1-4] The reptilian central nervous system (CNS) is tubular, organized linearly, and has some degree of dorsoventral flexure along its length.[4] (Fig. 77.1) The brain is located midsagitally and is housed within a tubular brain case bounded rostrally by the ethmoid cartilages, laterally by the otic bone series, ventrally by the basisphenoid and laterosphenoid, and caudally by the occipital bones.[4] There is a large amount of space between the brain and the roof and walls of the braincase in many lizards, aquatic turtles, and tuataras and a smaller but still substantial space in tortoises and crocodilians; minimal space exists is snakes. The anatomy of the skull and cervical vertebrae and their relationship to the CNS has been described using computed tomography in sea turtles, snakes, and several lizards.[5-7] The normal anatomy of the head of loggerhead sea turtles has been described using MRI.[8]

Reptiles are lissencephalic (having no cerebral gyri and sulci) but are the first group to have a developed cerebral cortex with two hemispheres that are separated by a deep median fissure.[3] Reptiles are also the first group of animals with a cephalic flexure such that the brain lies off-line with the spinal cord and grows back to partially cover the diencephalon.[3] In most reptiles, the neocortex is absent; however, in chelonians, there is some evidence that the internal dorsal ventricular ridge is homologous to the neocortex of mammals.[4] The brain is roughly divided into a forebrain, midbrain, and hindbrain (see Fig. 77.1). The forebrain is associated with olfaction, taste, and sensorimotor integration and mediation. The midbrain is associated with visual processing and neuroendocrine function. The hindbrain is associated with auditory function, balance, and physiological homeostasis. The cerebellum is part of the hindbrain, which integrates sensory and motor input as well as having a role in maintaining postural equilibrium.

There is a poorly studied blood-brain barrier formed by the meninges—endothelial lining of the brains blood supply—and the choroid plexus.[4,9]

The spinal cord of reptiles extends to the limit of the osseous spine (the tip of the tail), and no cauda equina exists. The cord is housed within the vertebral column but generally only fills a portion of the canal; less than 50% of the canal is occupied by the spinal cord in alligators and 66% to 71% in several lizard species.[4] The spinal cord is organized segmentally as in other vertebrates but lacks some of the functional regionalization seen in higher vertebrates. The cord is structured much like described in other vertebrates, with white matter tracts of myelinated axons surrounding inner gray matter formed of cell bodies and organized into bilaterally symmetrical dorsal and ventral horns. The dorsal horns include the dorsal roots and the ventral horns have motor neurons.[4]

Locomotor centers are found within the spinal cord, giving it a degree of functional autonomy from the brain. Because of this, reptiles with spinal cord injury have been said to have a better prognosis for recovery than higher vertebrates.

Spinal nerves are laterally paired and composed of dorsal nerve roots that are primarily sensory and ventral roots that contain visceral motor and somatic motor roots, comprising the reflex arc.[4] The nerves exit the vertebrae from the spinal cord via intervertebral foraminae. The number of spinal nerves is associated with the number of vertebral bodies, with snakes often having a greater number than other reptiles.[10]

Two networks of interconnected spinal nerves control limb functions; the cervical or brachial plexus and the sacral or lumbosacral plexus formed by ventral nerve roots and their branches.[4] For obvious reasons, snakes either lack or have reduced brachial and sacral plexi.[4] More than one branch of the plexus is usually responsible for individual muscle innervation. The cervical plexus typically includes the median nerve

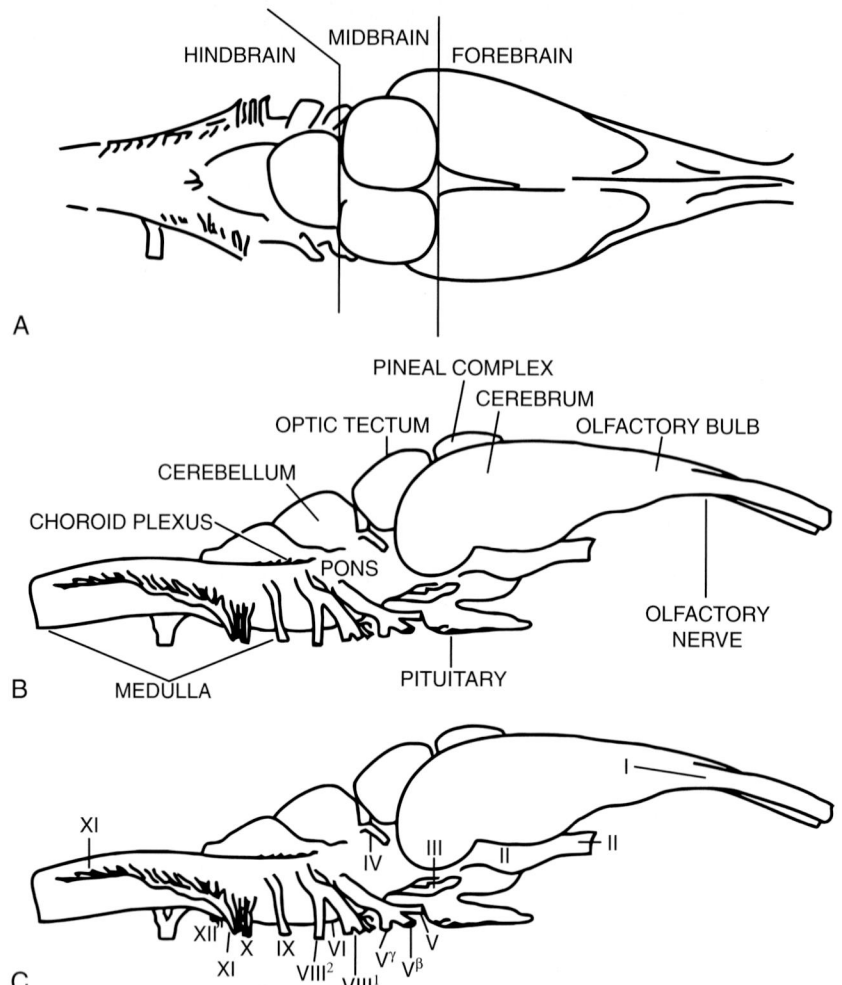

FIG 77.1 Illustration representing the gross structure of the reptilian brain, generalized from turtle and lizard anatomy. (A) Dorsal view depicting the major regions. (B) Lateral view with major external components identified. (C) The cranial nerves. Rostral is toward the right. (Reproduced with permission of Wyneken J. Reptilian neurology: anatomy and function. *Vet Clin North Am Exot Anim Pract.* 2007;10:837–853, vi.)

and the inferior brachial nerve, which divides to form the superficial and deep radial nerves to the shoulder and dorsal thoracic limb. The supracoracoideus, subscapular, and ulnar nerves innervate the pectoral muscles, subscapularis, and ventral thoracic limb muscles, while the deltoideus nerve innervates the shoulder.[4] The sacral plexus consists of up to six branches from spinal nerves associated with the caudal-most lumbar vertebra and the sacral vertebrae.[4] These nerves ultimately pass to the inguinal, pelvic, and pelvic limb muscles. The caudal nerve roots give rise to the obturator nerve innervating the ventral pelvic muscles and the ischiadicus nerve innervating muscles of the ilium before dividing into the peroneal and sciatic nerves. The more cranial nerve roots interconnect to provide major innervations (via crural, femoral, and tibial nerves) to the inguinal muscles, thigh adductors, and limb extensors.[4] There are also sacral branches going to the bladder (when present).

The visceral nerves function as the autonomic nervous system (ANS) with both sympathetic and parasympathetic components. The reptilian ANS differs from that of mammals in that the autonomic visceral nerves are not anatomically segregated into thoracolumbar sympathetic and craniosacral parasympathetic regions.[4] These nerves arise along the length of the spinal cord and may have both sympathetic and parasympathetic components.

Nerve endings in the skin of reptiles are similar to those identified in mammals and serve the same function, being responsible for cutaneous sensation. Some lizards have hairlike structures in the skin with sensory function as well.[1]

Most reptiles have 12 to 13 cranial nerves (CNs), although snakes only have 11 to 12.[4] The terminal nerves (nervus terminalis, cranial nerve 0), discovered after the classical human-based numbering and naming system was in place, travel with the olfactory nerves; these two are the most rostral CNs. The terminal nerve innervates the vasculature of the nasal epithelium and is not tested clinically. The functions of CN 0 are not characterized but are believed to be associated with the gonadotropin-releasing hormones.[4,11] The remaining cranial nerves have well-documented functions, which are summarized in Table 77.1.

The vestibulocochlear system detects sound or vibrations through the auditory apparatus and movement and orientation in space.[4] Auditory nerves from each lagena, which is equivalent to the cochlea of mammals, project to the auditory tectum. The vestibular apparatus (semicircular canals, sacculus, and utriculus) is innervated by branches of the stato-acoustic (CN VIII) nerve.[4]

Two meninges are found in reptiles, covering the brain and spinal cord. The outer dura mater is tough and largely avascular. The

TABLE 77.1 Reptilian Cranial Nerve Function and Evaluation[2,4,21,108]

Cranial Nerve		Function	Clinical Test
0	Nervus terminalis	Innervates vasculature of nasal epithelium; chemosensory for gonadotropin-releasing hormone (GnRH)	None
I	Olfactory	Olfaction; carrying sensory information from the nasal sacs and vomeronasal organ	Move head toward food when eyes are covered
II	Optic	Vision, carries sensory information from the retina to the thalamus and optic tectum	Menace response if patient has eyelids and/or behavioral response to threatening gesture
III	Oculomotor	Controls movement of eyes via dorsal, ventral and medial rectus muscles; moves eye medially; controls iris and ciliary body	Check for normal, coordinated eye movement, strabismus, and pupil shape; pupillary light reflex
IV	Trochlear	Controls movement of the eyes via dorsal oblique muscle of eyeball	Check for normal, coordinated eye movement (rotation of globe) and strabismus
V	Trigeminal	Sensory innervation of skin around eyes and mouth; sensory pits of pit vipers and boids; controls jaw adductor muscles, muscles of skin around teeth bearing bones in snakes, and intermandibularis (in floor of mouth). Innervates depressor palpebrae muscle, moving the lower eyelid.	Mandibular branch: check normal jaw closure and buccal pumping. Ophthalmic and maxillary branches: test ability to feel stimulus to face, lower lid, and nasal area with palpebral reflex and stimulus to the cornea with the corneal reflex.
VI	Abducens	Controls movement of eye via lateral rectus and retractor bulbi muscles	Check for normal, coordinated eye movement and strabismus; corneal reflex
VII	Facial	Motor to eyelid muscles and some jaw muscles. Sensory from skin and muscle around the ear, upper jaw, and pharynx, as well as taste receptors on rostral tongue. Controls superficial neck muscles and mandibular depressor.	Normal movement of eyelids if present, which can be elicited with the palpebral reflex. Monitor ability to open mouth voluntarily.
VIII	Vestibulocochlear (statoacoustic)	Balance and hearing: sensory from the inner ear.	Turn head left and right to check for spontaneous nystagmus; check for head tilts and/or poor righting reflex.
IX	Glossopharyngeal	Taste and sensation in the pharynx; controls tongue muscles	Examine tongue for active protrusion and retraction. Observe ability to swallow.
X	Vagus	Sensory and motor to glottis, heart, and viscera	Apply pressure to both eyes for several minutes and check for decreased heart rate. Observe ability to swallow, opening, and closure of glottis.
XI	Spinal accessory	Controls neck and shoulder musculature	Dorsal neck and shoulder muscles should have strong tone in lizards and crocodilians; difficult to assess in snakes and turtles
XII	Hypoglossal	Controls hyoid muscles and tongue	Look for deviation and/or weakness of the tongue to indicate defects

pia-arachnoid layer is vascular and lies in close contact with the surface of the central nervous system (CNS).[4] The space between the pia-arachnoid layer and the dura mater is the subdural space. Reptiles do not have a true subarachnoid space, an important fact in attempts to collect cerebrospinal fluid (CSF); in mammals CSF is collected from the subarachnoid space. CSF is produced by the tela choroidea, a specialized vascular structure located in the dorsal midbrain.[4] The epidural space contains veins located ventral or lateral to the spinal cord.

NEUROLOGICAL EXAMINATION AND LESION LOCALIZATION

Before the reptile patient is restrained, the clinician should observe the patient in its environment to evaluate its mental status, degree of alertness, and presence of abnormal posture. Stimulating the patient to move is helpful to evaluate for postural or ambulatory abnormalities, such as paresis or hemiparesis, likely indicating the presence of a neurological condition. As reptiles are ectothermic, it is important that the examination takes place at appropriate environmental temperatures. Low temperatures can result in reduced nerve conduction, weakness, sluggishness, behavioral changes, or frank neurological deficits.[2,12]

Many neurological diseases in reptiles can be related to inadequate husbandry. Therefore clinicians must be aware of proper dietary and environmental requirements needed for the species evaluated and owners questioned about care.[13,14] As an example, exposure to excessively low temperatures during hibernation or sudden drops in water temperature can result in neurological dysfunction in turtles and tortoises.[2] Additionally, low-calcium diets may lead to hyperparathyroidism, feeding fish-based diets may result in thiamine deficiency, egg-based diets may result in biotin deficiency, and leaf-based diets can lead to vitamin E or selenium deficiency, all of which can result in neurological dysfunction.[2,14] The owner must also be asked about the possibility of toxin exposure, as there are a considerable number of toxicities that can result in neurological dysfunction. Improper bedding, rhubarb or firefly ingestion, lead, ethylene glycol, antibiotics (such as metronidazole, aminoglycosides, and enrofloxacin), ivermentin, or other antiparasitic drugs can all lead to significant neurological disease.[2,15–17]

Assessment of mentation and responsiveness can provide an indication of an animal's level of consciousness, which can be graded as alert, obtunded, stupor, or comatose, which is suggestive of an intracranial lesion (Table 77.2). Such an assessment can be accomplished by opening an enclosure, attempts to handle, prodding with a pole or stick, and offering food.[18,19] However, the ease of assessment is certainly species related and requires knowledge of what behaviors would be expected in a normal animal (Fig. 77.2), some of which may actually mimic neurological disease.[2,12,19] An inappropriate and/or confused mentation would suggest forebrain dysfunction.

The position of the head and neck should be noted. Most reptiles are able to lift and move their head freely (Fig. 77.3). Abnormalities of head position may include head tilts, turns, or dorsal flexion

TABLE 77.2   Lesion Localization Within the Nervous System[2]

Lesion Localization	Localizing Clinical Signs
Forebrain	Seizures, altered mentation, behavioral changes, visual or olfactory deficits, contralateral limb postural reaction deficits
Midbrain	Altered mentation, contralateral or ipsilateral weakness, and/or postural reaction deficits, CN III or CN IV dysfunction
Hindbrain	Altered mentation, ipsilateral weakness, and/or postural reaction deficits, CN V-XII dysfunction
Cerebellum	Ataxia, intention tremors, dysmetria, possible head tilt, and nystagmus
Cervical spinal cord	Paresis and ataxia in all four limbs or trunk caudal to lesion; normal spinal reflexes
Spinal cord at level of the cervical intumescence	Paresis and ataxia in all four limbs or trunk caudal to lesion; reduced to absent thoracic limb spinal reflexes; normal pelvic limb spinal reflexes; possible severe muscle atrophy in thoracic limbs
Spinal cord between cervical and lumbar intumescences	Paresis and ataxia in pelvic limbs or trunk caudal to lesion; normal thoracic limb spinal reflexes; normal pelvic limb spinal reflexes; panniculus and/or righting reflex may be abnormal
Spinal cord at level of lumbar intumescence	Paresis in pelvic limbs or trunk caudal to lesion; normal thoracic limb spinal reflexes; reduced to absent pelvic limb spinal reflexes, cloacal reflex, and/or clasp reflex; possible severe muscle atropy in pelvic limbs
Spinal cord caudal to lumbar intumescence	Weak, paralyzed, and/or flaccid tail
Diffuse neuromuscular	Weakness in all four limbs; possible cranial nerve dysfunction; reduced to absent spinal reflexes in all four limbs; possible severe muscle atrophy in all four limbs

CN, Cranial nerve.

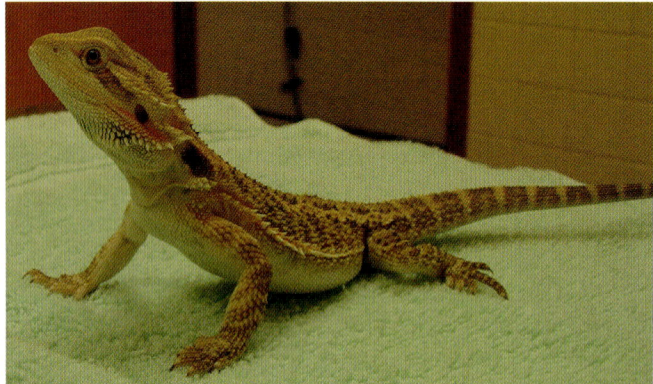

FIG 77.2 The posture and alert behavior demonstrated here in this bearded dragon (*Pogona vitticeps*) is normal. The evaluator should be aware of similar assessment parameters in each species. (Courtesy of Joerg Mayer.)

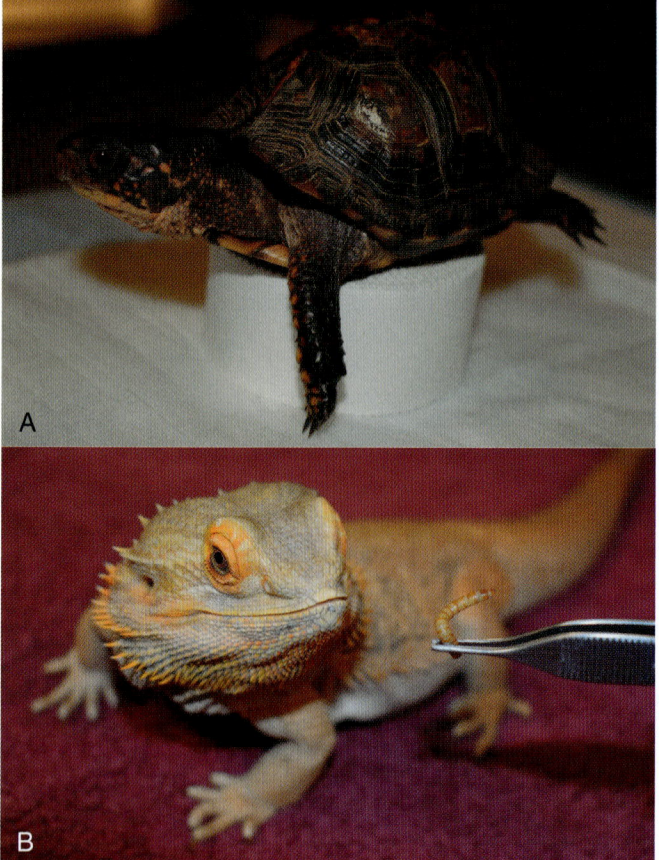

FIG 77.3 (A) The voluntary movement of the head and neck as well as the limbs can be seen in this eastern box turtle (*Terrapene carolina carolina*) by placing it on an object such as a tape roll, raising it off the ground. (B) Using food in species like this bearded dragon (*Pogona vitticeps*) can encourage them to move their head and neck, and it also helps assess vision. (Courtesy of Simon R. Platt.)

(opisthotonus, stargazing) and ventral flexion.[2] The latter may be related to generalized weakness rather than neurological dysfunction. Abnormal head movements can be due to tremors and seizure activity, although head bobbing while breathing has been associated with respiratory infections in box turtles and tortoises, which could be confused with neurological dysfunction.[2] Abnormal spinal curvature, such as kyphosis, lordosis, and scoliosis, can be due to neurological disease causing alterations in paravertebral muscle tone or caused by vertebral abnormalities, such as congenital malformations.[20]

Ataxia, paresis, or weakness and lameness may all be identified during a gait evaluation. Ataxia always indicates neurological disease but is often very difficult to identify in many reptiles due to their anatomical conformation. Weakness, however, may be due to muscle disease, or a systemic illness and lameness can indicate an orthopedic condition or a localized nerve dysfunction (Fig. 77.4).

An appropriate surface for the animal to move on must be provided, depending on the species, and in some species, evaluation of movement in water will be very helpful.[2,21,22] In most cases, tortoises are able to walk with their plastron suspended off the ground (see Fig. 77.3A). With paresis or motor weakness, this ability may be lost.

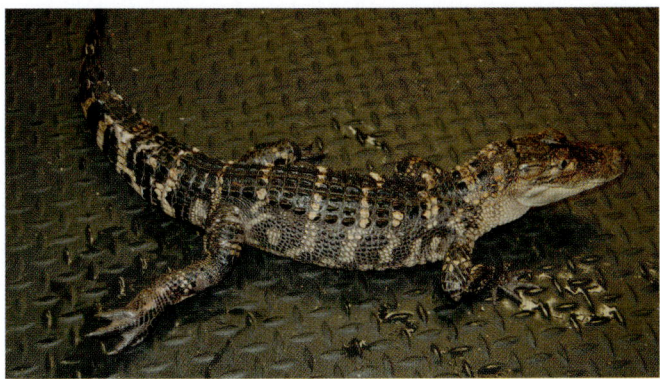

FIG 77.4 Injury to peripheral nerves can result in monoparesis, as is seen affecting the right pelvic limb of this crocodilian. (Courtesy of Simon R. Platt.)

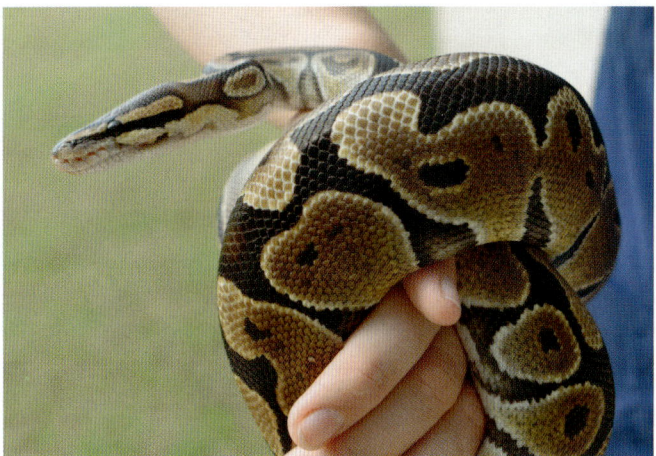

FIG 77.6 If the snake is held by the midbody, the ability to raise its head should be noted as seen in this picture of a ball python (*Python regius*). (Courtesy of Simon R. Platt.)

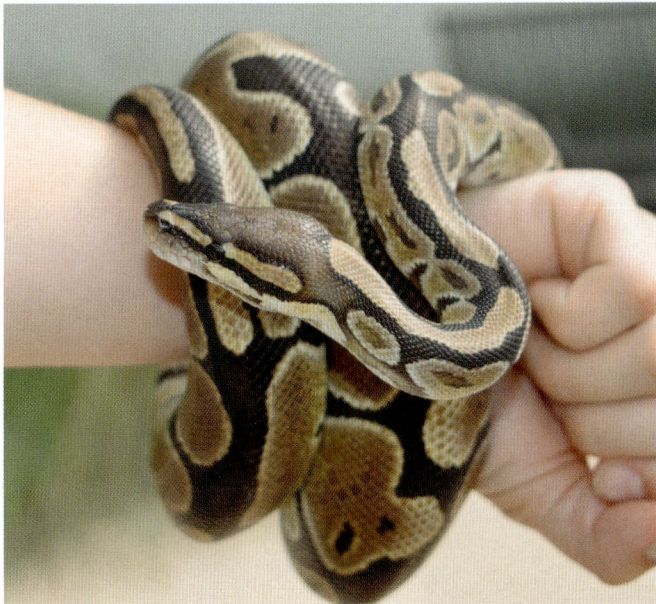

FIG 77.5 As this ball python (*Python regius*) wraps around an arm, the movement and gripping ability of its trunk can be assessed. (Courtesy of Simon R. Platt.)

Chelonians with neurological disease frequently circle and are unable to hold up their head or hold their head in cervical hyperextension. They may be unable to prehend food properly and may show dysphagia. With chelonians, the head and legs should be pulled from within the shell to evaluate the muscle tone of the extremities. Sea turtles or other aquatic species presented for swimming in circles, or in one direction, often have asymmetric buoyancy issues as a result of a mass or uneven gas distribution in the lungs or coelomic cavity and not a related vestibular disease.[21]

Snakes with central nervous system disease often have fine motor tremors and are unable to strike at prey with accuracy. Some snakes are unable to constrict prey because of the loss of muscle tone or may be unable to move the prey accurately toward their mouth after a kill. As a snake ambulates across the hand and arm, the gastropedges gripping the skin provide an indication of muscle tone (Fig. 77.5). Palpation is also useful for evaluation of general body muscle tone. When a healthy snake is suspended by its midbody, it should be able to lift its head straight and steady to search for a substrate (Fig. 77.6). With neurological disease, jerky, irregular movements are often present as the snake seeks a substrate.

In reptiles with limbs the assessment of postural reactions for the evaluation of proprioception can be relatively adapted from what is described in dogs and cats. Hopping, hemiwalking or hemistanding, wheel-barrowing, and tactile placing assessments can be attempted and interpreted based on what would be expected in a normal reptile of the species being evaluated (Fig. 77.7). Limb-placing responses as performed in dogs by turning over the digits and watching for an immediate correction are unlikely to be possible in many reptiles, apart from some of the larger lizards.

Cranial Nerve Examination

Olfaction (CN I) is a chemosensory system in reptiles mediated by sensory cells in the nasal cavity and by the Jacobson's organs, which have ducts that open into the mouth. The tongue brings odoriferous particles to the Jacobson's organ, where the vomeronasal branch of the olfactory nerve is stimulated, providing input to the brain. The Jacobson's organ is absent in crocodilians and modified or absent in chelonians. This system is rarely evaluated in clinical patients. Testing the patient's response to noxious odors such as alcohol may assess the functional status of the olfactory nerve, but care must be taken with interpretation as such substances may stimulate the trigeminal nerve. A healthy patient recoils or moves away from an alcohol-soaked pledget or cotton-tipped applicator. A history of a normal ability to locate food may also indicate a functional CN I, although other sensory functions may also play a role in food recognition.

The optic nerve (CN II) is responsible for vision. Reptiles with eyelids can be tested for vision, with a menace response confirming optic nerve (CN II) and facial nerve (CN VII) function, and this can be performed with a hand, finger, or an object such as a cotton-tipped applicator (Fig. 77.8). Most reptiles have eyelids and nictitating membranes; however, in snakes and some lizards (especially geckos), the eyelids are fused and transparent, forming the spectacle, and the nictitans is absent. Movement of the upper eyelid closes the eyes of crocodilians, and the eyes are closed by movement of the lower lid in other reptiles. One must not create air movement or vibrations; many reptiles are able to sense vibrations that are imperceptible to humans. Vision may also be assessed by observing the patient's ability to navigate around, and react to movement within, the environment. Some reptiles use vibrations or thermal sensors to locate prey and may not rely on their visual senses.

The oculomotor nerve (CN III) controls the iris, which is composed entirely of skeletal muscle in reptiles, allowing voluntary control of

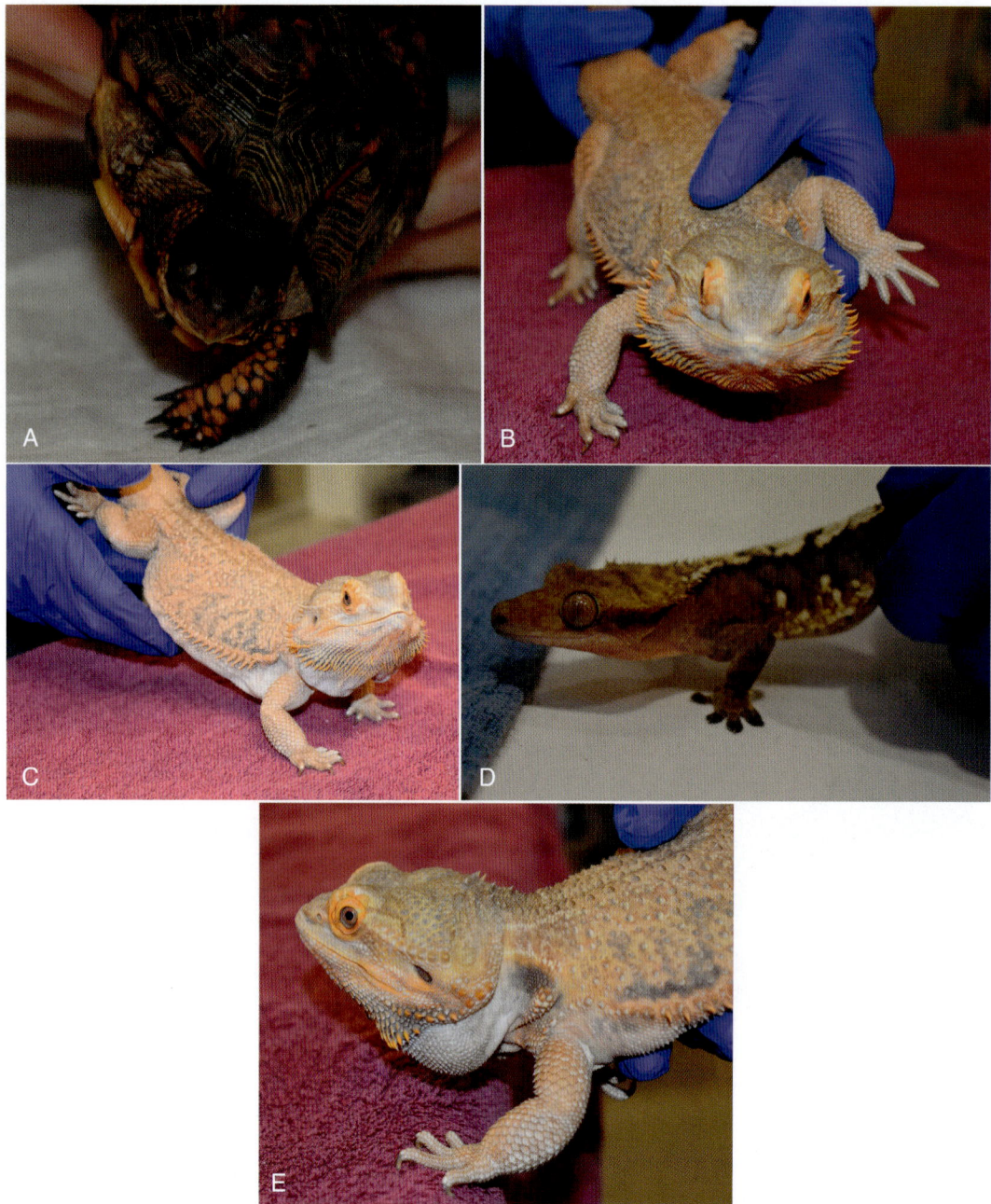

FIG 77.7 Supporting the animal and testing one limb at a time for hopping ability is a good way to test proprioception, demonstrated here in (A) an eastern box turtle (*Terrapene carolina carolina*) and (B) a bearded dragon (*Pogona vitticeps*). Holding the caudal body of the animal higher than the thoracic limbs and slowly pushing them forward encourages a wheel-barrowing test to evaluate the motor function and proprioception, shown here in (C) a bearded dragon and (D) a crested gecko (*Correlophus ciliatus*). Bringing the reptile to a table edge can test visual and tactile placing (E), which assesses vision, motor function, and proprioception, although, it is not uniformly reliable as in mammals. (Courtesy of Simon R. Platt.)

pupil size.[2] Dysfunction of the nerve may result in mydriasis and anisocoria (Fig. 77.9). The pupillary light response, which evaluates CNs II and III in mammals, is not very reliable in reptiles due to this voluntary override capability and the iris not being responsive to traditional mydriatics (Fig. 77.10); however, topical neuromuscular blocking agents can produce mydriasis. Intracameral injection of neuromuscular blocking agents, such as d-tubocurare, produces mydriasis but is somewhat invasive. Topical application of nondepolarizing neuromuscular blocking agents, such as vercuronium, on the cornea of species without a spectacle may produce mydriasis. The oculomotor nerve also innervates the extraocular muscles (dorsal, ventral, and medial rectus and the ventral oblique muscle), so dysfunction of this nerve may result in ventrolateral strabismus.

The trochlear nerve (CN IV) and the abducens nerve (CN VI) innervate the dorsal oblique, and the lateral rectus extraocular muscles respectively and are involved in coordination of ocular movements

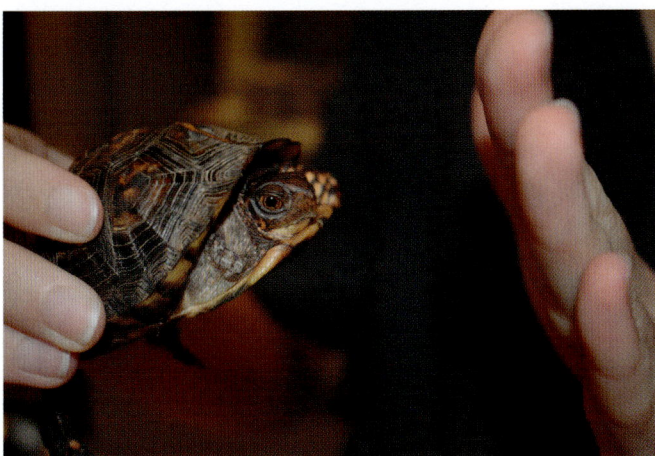

FIG 77.8 A threatening gesture is necessary to perform the menace response; in addition to observing for a blink in those species that have eyelids, a behavioral avoidance of the threat may also be observed, manifested in chelonians by withdrawal of the head into the shell. (Courtesy of Simon R. Platt.)

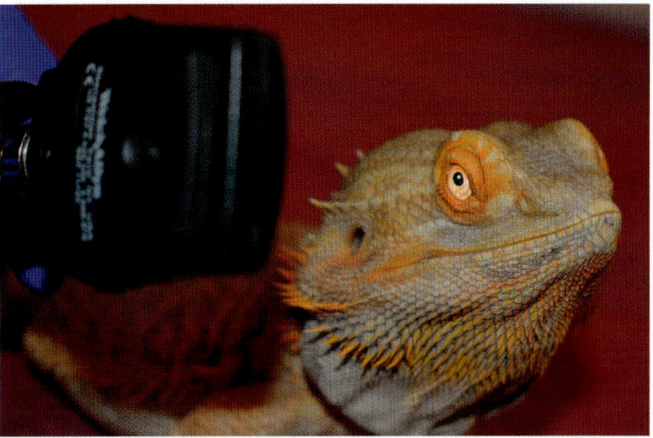

FIG 77.10 A bright light shone into each eye may elicit the pupillary light reflex in some, such as this bearded dragon (*Pogona vitticeps*); however, the skeletal muscle of the iris means that there is voluntary control of the pupil size, which makes this reflex difficult to interpret. (Courtesy of Simon R. Platt.)

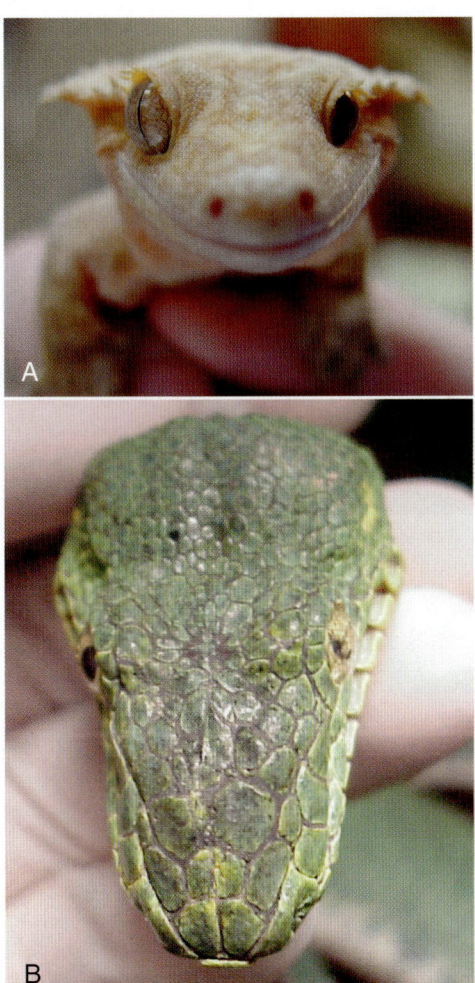

FIG 77.9 Anisocoria can be seen in reptiles due to ocular lesions, optic nerve, oculomotor nerve, or sympathetic supply dysfunction, which may result in either mydriasis or miosis. Anisocoria is seen in (A) a crested gecko (*Correlophus ciliatus*) due to left-sided mydriasis and (B) an Amazon green tree boa (*Corallus caninus*) due to left-sided miosis. (Courtesy of Joerg Mayer.)

along with CN III. Some reptiles (chameleons) are capable of moving their eyes independently, which makes assessment for the presence of strabismus difficult. Normal and coordinated eye movements indicate healthy function of these nerves. Medial strabismus may indicate dysfunction of CN VI. A branch of the abducens (CN IV) supplies the nictitans.

The trigeminal nerve (CN V) is composed of both sensory and motor fibers with mandibular, maxillary, and ophthalmic branches. The mandibular branch supplies motor fibers to the muscles responsible for jaw function. The anatomy of the trigeminal nerve has been mapped out in crocodylians using computed tomography.[23]

The presence of normal jaw function indicates healthy nerve function, and dysfunction may result in a dropped jaw if bilaterally affected, and masticatory muscle atrophy may be seen chronically in some species. The ophthalmic branch provides sensory innervation to the skin surrounding the eye and the mucosa of portions of the nasal and oral cavities. The maxillary branch is sensory to the upper jaw, nose, and lower eyelid. Its function may be tested by determining the patient's ability to feel a cotton-tipped applicator around the face; if the species has eyelids, a palpebral reflex may be used to evaluate this nerve in conjunction with CN VII, which causes the eyelids to close in species with eyelids (Fig. 77.11). If necessary, a painful stimulus such as a 27-gauge needle may be used. Additionally, a corneal reflex may be performed to evaluate corneal sensory innervation, resulting in globe retraction due to retractor bulbi muscle contraction, which is innervated by CN VI (Fig. 77.12). In some reptiles (pit vipers), CN V is also responsible for innervating the heat-sensing infrared receptors[2] (Fig. 77.13). In these snakes, the sensory fields overlap, creating three-dimensional heat perception used to locate prey. In boas and pythons, smaller simpler pits are present along the upper and lower labial scales and are innervated by the ophthalmic, maxillary, and mandibular branches of the trigeminal nerve (CN V).

The facial nerve (CN VII) supplies motor function to the muscles of the eyelids and can be assessed with the palpebral reflex. Snakes and many species of lizards have developed cranial kinesis, which is the ability to move the upper and lower jaw, facilitating capture and swallowing of prey. Cranial nerve VII innervates the muscles responsible for opening the jaw. The facial nerve also supplies sensory fibers to the taste buds of the cranial two-thirds of the tongue. These fibers form part of the chorda tympani, which is a branch of the facial nerve that passes through the middle ear.

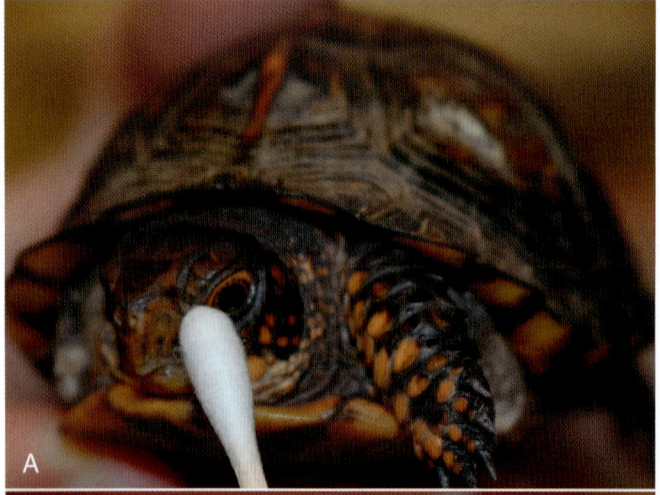

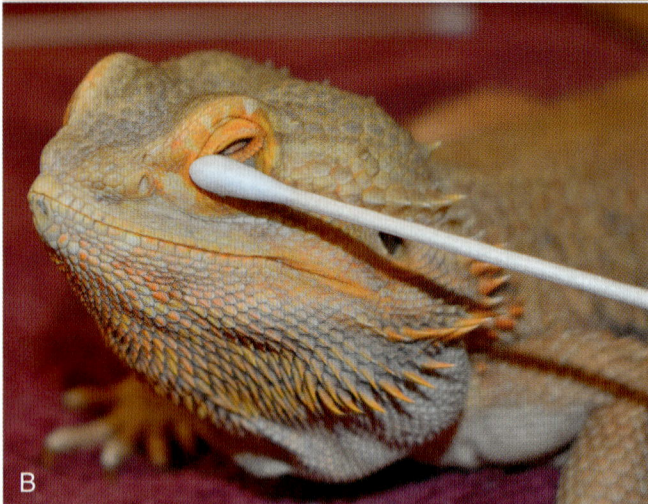

FIG 77.12 The corneal reflex can be elicited by gently touching the cornea with a sterile cotton-tipped applicator and watching for retraction of the globe, shown here in an eastern box turtle (*Terrapene carolina carolina*). (Courtesy of Simon R. Platt.)

FIG 77.11 A cotton-tipped applicator can be used to perform the palpebral reflex by touching each canthus of the eye and monitoring for eyelid closure, if possible, in the species being tested, demonstrated here in (A) an eastern box turtle (*Terrapene carolina carolina*) and (B) a bearded dragon (*Pogona vitticeps*). (Courtesy of Simon R. Platt.)

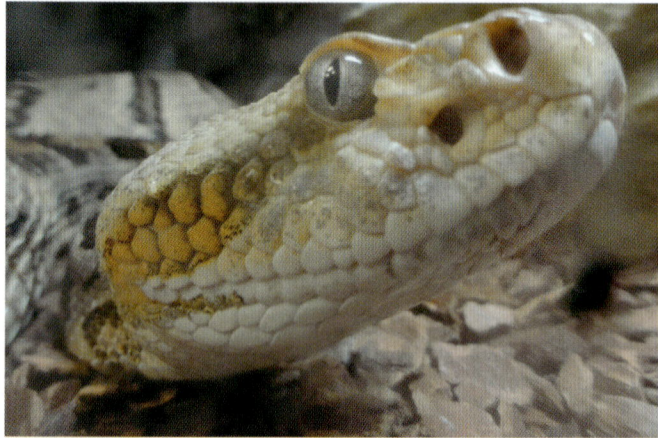

FIG 77.13 A close-up image of the pit organ in a rattlesnake (*Viperidae*). These pits can sense radiant heat so accurately that vision is not needed to strike the prey. (Courtesy of Joerg Mayer.)

The statoacoustic or vestibulocochlear nerve (CN III) is responsible for both hearing and the sense of balance or equilibrium. Hearing is well developed in most reptiles, especially those with an externally visible tympanum, although they are best able to perceive lower frequencies. Many reptiles may not have a pronounced response to auditory stimuli. This, coupled with their ability to sense vibration, makes assessment of the cochlear portion of CN VIII difficult. A defect in the vestibular system may manifest itself as spontaneous nystagmus, head tilt, rolling, ataxia, and an abnormal righting reflex[21,24] (Fig. 77.14). As in birds with nystagmus, the whole head may move with the fast and slow phases in conjunction with the eyes. The eyes should also be evaluated for the presence of normal physiological nystagmus and for evidence of positional nystagmus or strabismus, often characterized as a ventral strabismus with head elevation on the side of the lesion.[2]

The glossopharyngeal nerve (CN IX) innervates a chemosensory system analogous to taste with taste buds and sensory papillae throughout the oral mucosa, particularly on the caudal tongue and pharynx. Assessment of the ability of reptiles to taste is difficult. Many patients have a negative reaction to bitter substances placed into their mouth by holding

their mouth open, writhing, and pawing at their mouth. This nerve also innervates pharyngeal musculature and so in part is responsible for swallowing function.

The vagus nerve (CN X) in reptiles is responsible for pharyngeal, esophageal, and laryngeal musculature innervation and so is responsible for swallowing in conjunction with CN IX. Dysfunction is manifested as dysphagia and laryngeal paresis or paralysis.

The spinal accessory nerve (CN XI) supplies motor fibers to the larynx, pharynx, and the superficial cervical musculature (sternocleidohyoideus and trapezius) but is apparently absent in some snakes and some lizards.[2]

The hypoglossal nerve (CN XII) innervates the tongue musculature and can be assessed by watching for normal tongue movement, position, tone, and symmetry. Regular tongue "flicking" should be noted in snakes and some lizard species during examination. Opening the mouth to assess the tongue can be achieved using a plastic card, rubber spatula, or an avian beak speculum (Fig. 77.15). Some lizards will open their

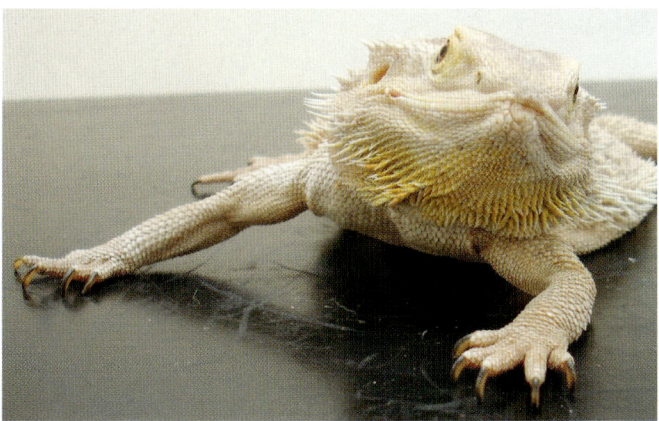

FIG 77.14 A head tilt is seen in this female bearded dragon (*Pogona vitticeps*). (Reproduced with permission by Hunt C. Neurological examination and diagnostic testing in birds and reptiles. *J Exot Pet Med.* 2015;24:34–51.)

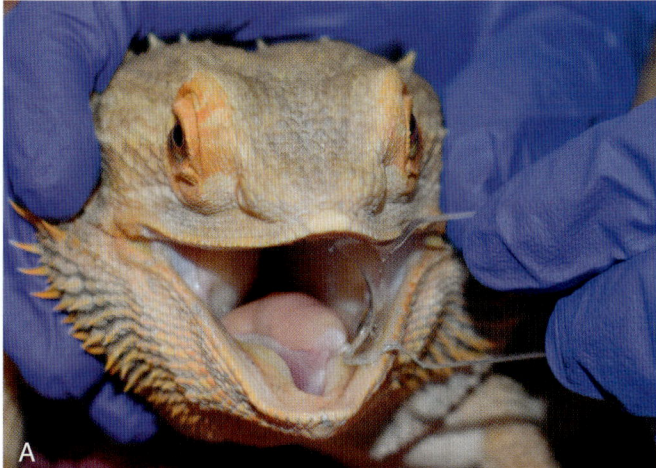

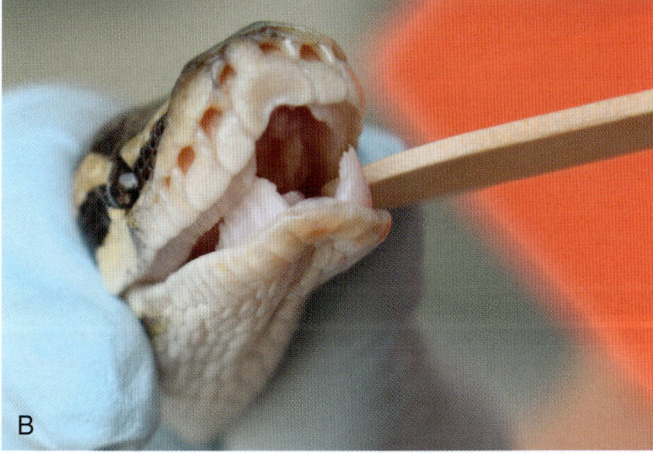

FIG 77.15 Opening the mouth of (A) a bearded dragon (*Pogona vitticeps*) and (B) a ball python (*Python regius*) can serve to test jaw tone and evaluate tongue size and function. (Courtesy of Simon R. Platt.)

mouths in response to tapping on the nose or with gentle traction on the dewlap.[2]

Reflex evaluations. Anatomical studies suggest that reflexes in reptiles should function segmentally in a similar fashion to that seen in mammals.[2] This means that they require afferent (sensory) and efferent (usually motor) peripheral nerves and a connection within the spinal cord at a certain level, without the need for ascending or descending control. Many myotatic reflexes in dogs and cats (and thus reptiles too?) are too subjective to be reliable and so should definitely be interpreted with caution if attempted.[21]

The withdrawal reflex can be elicited reliably from most reptiles with limbs (Fig. 77.16). The stimulus is performed usually by pinching on a digit manually or with hemostats or by pricking the plantar surface of the limb with something sharp. A healthy animal has a brisk withdrawal reflex. These reflexes are known to be temperature dependent. With a decrease in environmental temperature, a corresponding decrease is seen in conduction velocity within the peripheral nerves. During brumation (hibernation), conduction along peripheral nerves almost ceases.[25] Assessment of the patient's body or environmental temperature in conjunction with an evaluation of reflexes is therefore important. Reflexes are best evaluated with the animal in its optimum temperature range.

The cloacal reflex, similar to the anal reflex in mammals, can often be elicited by stimulation of the cloaca with a cotton-tipped applicator or hemostats (Fig. 77.17), resulting in contraction of the cloacal musculature in normal animals. In some reptiles, there may also be ventral movement of the tail as part of the reflex response, and in turtles the pelvic limbs normally will come together in a clasplike response.[21] The segmental nature of the cloacal reflex remains undocumented; a loss of cloacal tone has been reported for spinal cord injuries above the segmental level expected for innervation, which is dissimilar to what is documented in mammals.[2,21]

The panniculus reflex is present in reptiles and is particularly useful in snakes (Fig. 77.18). A hypodermic needle may be used to stimulate the patient's skin along the lateral margins of the body. A healthy patient responds with a twitch of the skin and so is obviously not possible in chelonian species. With spinal cord injury, the panniculus response is present cranial to the lesion and absent caudal to the lesion.

The righting reflex is frequently used to evaluate the neurological status of reptile patients. Squamate reptiles and crocodilians placed on their back should turn their head over first and then roll the body over to the normal position.[1] Chelonians placed on their back generally try to right themselves by pushing their head against the substrate and attempting to get their legs onto the surface (Fig. 77.19).

This provides a good opportunity to evaluate movements of the head, neck, and limbs as the patient attempts to right itself.[21] In snakes, the righting reflex is useful in identifying the location of a spinal cord injury. The snake rights itself to the level of the injury and is unable to right caudal to the lesion. Some animals, especially crocodilians and lizards, when placed on their back with their ventral coelom gently stroked, become sedate or flaccid, inhibiting the righting reflex.[2]

NEURODIAGNOSTIC TECHNIQUES

Imaging

Plain radiography is relatively easy to perform and useful for confirming osseous pathology that may be causing neurological dysfunction.[26–28] Traumatic lesions, congenital malformations, secondary hyperparathyroidism, osteomyelitis, osteoarthritis, and neoplastic disease may all cause visible lesions on radiographs.[14,16,20,29] The normal radiographic anatomy of the skull has been documented in several reptile species[5–7] (Fig. 77.20). Radiographs may be helpful to identify retention of eggs in female chelonians or other space-occupying caudal coelomic lesions, which may be responsible for pelvic limb neurological dysfunction.[2,29]

Intrathecal Contrast-Enhanced Imaging. This contrast-enhanced radiographic technique requires injection of an iodinated medium into the space normally occupied by CSF to identify compressive lesions affecting the spinal cord.[28] Currently, a lack of scientific evidence exists

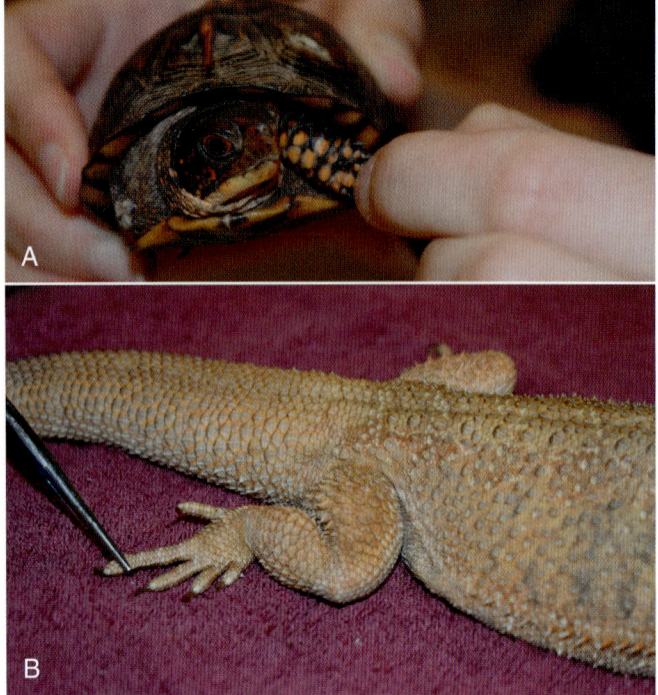

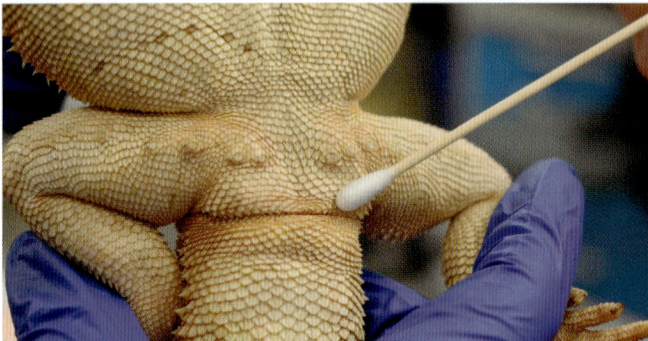

FIG 77.16 Pinching the limbs with (A) fingers in an eastern box turtle (*(Terrapene carolina carolina)* and (B) with hemostats in a bearded dragon (*Pogona vitticeps)* elicits the withdrawal reflex. (Courtesy of Simon R. Platt.)

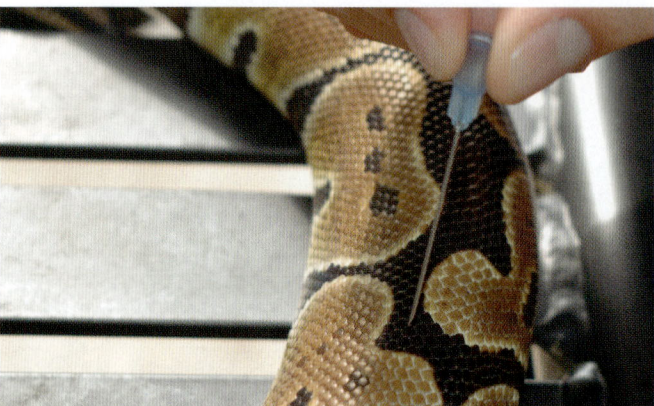

FIG 77.18 Lightly touching the skin on each side of the dorsum in the snake with a needle can elicit the panniculus reflex. (Courtesy of Simon R. Platt).

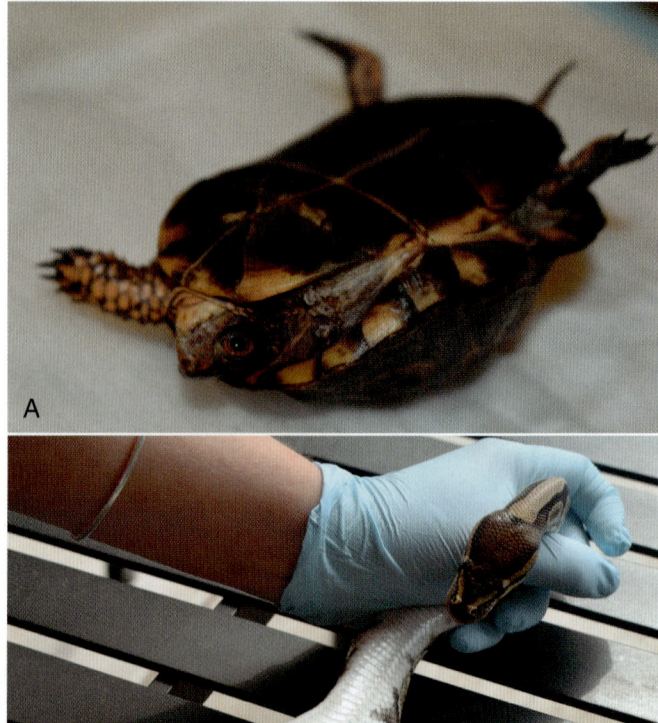

FIG 77.17 Stimulating around the vent with a cotton-tipped applicator, as seen in this bearded dragon (*Pogona vitticeps)*, can evaluate the reptile for vent tone and function. (Courtesy of Simon R. Platt.)

FIG 77.19 (A) Turning a box turtle (*Terrapene* sp.) on its back can stimulate the righting reflex, which is initiated by using the head, neck muscles, and one of the thoracic limbs; this is not possible in turtles with generalized weakness as well as nervous system disease. (B) Turning a snake on its back will also stimulate the righting reflex, initially seen as a reorientation and position of its head and neck, as seen in this ball python (*Python regius*). (Courtesy of Simon R. Platt.)

to confirm the presence of a subarachnoid space in reptiles. With no subarachnoid space, myelography is technically not possible. However, clinical reports indicate that CSF collection and intrathecal contrast-enhanced imaging are useful in examining the central nervous system of reptiles, albeit difficult to perform![2]

Computed Tomography (CT). CT scanning uses radiographs and computer technology to create cross-sectional images of the patient[30,31] (Fig. 77.21). CT scan provides superior soft tissue imaging with no superimposition of structures when compared with conventional radiography and provides good contrast images of calcified structures.[28,30] Contrast enhancement allows for better visualization of soft tissue structures with increased blood flow. CT scan also helps reveal changes in bony tissues and provides greater detail of imaged structures than

conventional radiography, even allowing guided biopsy of the lesions once identified.[28,32] Imaging of the caudal abdomen in animals for space-occupying lesions may be better accomplished using CT than radiography in many species.[28,33] The skull, head, and neck anatomy of sea turtles, crocodilians, snakes, and several lizard species has been described using CT, which can be useful to compare to when looking for structural disease.[5–7,23]

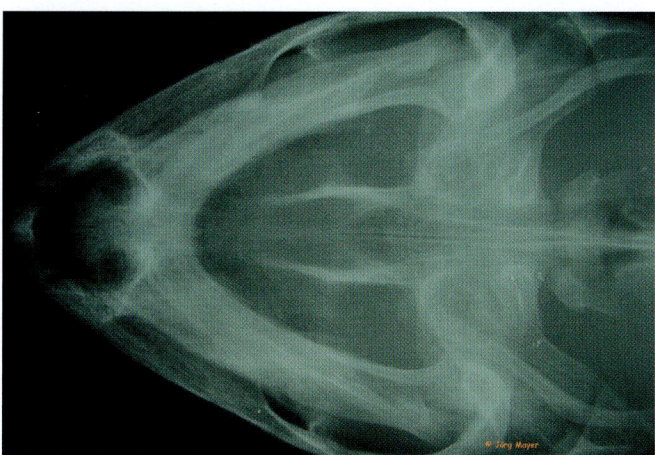

FIG 77.20 A ventrodorsal radiographic view of a bearded dragon (*Pogona vitticeps*) skull. (Courtesy of Joerg Mayer.)

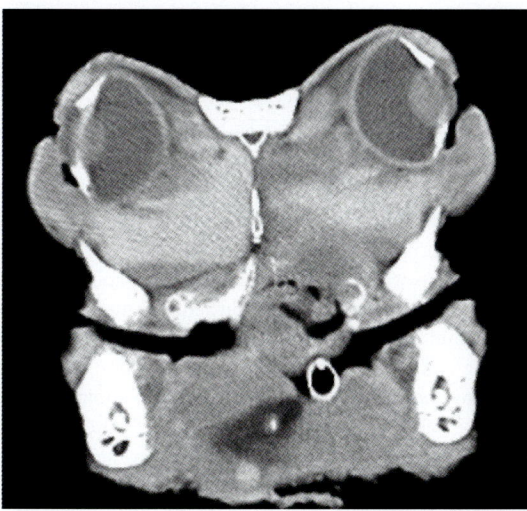

FIG 77.21 A transverse CT image of a bearded dragon (*Pogona vitticeps*) head at the level of the eyes, demonstrating the skull and soft tissue detail possible with this imaging modality. (Courtesy of Joerg Mayer.)

Magnetic Resonance Imaging (MRI). MRI uses a pulsating external magnetic field that produces radiofrequency signals to generate images.[34,35] The natural frequency of the hydrogen ion is used as the frequency for the magnetic pulse because of the high content of hydrogen ions in biological tissues.[28,35] Tissues with high hydrogen ion content are imaged, and regions of bone and air appear void. Contrast may also be used with this imaging method. The main advantages of MRI over CT include the ability to image the entire brain, an increase in soft tissue resolution, and the creation of true images in various planes.[28,34] MRI involves long scanning times, and the animal typically is immobilized by using general anesthesia.[34] Alternatively, heavy sedation may minimize respiratory movements and reduce related artifacts sufficiently in some species. General anesthesia poses a risk in all animal species, but the risk is greater in small animals, such as reptiles. Species-specific and interindividual differences may require the adaptation of standard anesthesia protocols. Protocols for the anesthesia and immobilization of reptiles for MRI are available in the literature, and they can be modified to suit individual needs. Turtles typically do not require pharmacological sedation, and only the head and limbs have to be mechanically immobilized during an examination. However, anxious turtles require

pharmacological sedation to prevent head and limb movements, and all turtles undergoing direct MRI examinations of the head or limbs must be sedated.[34] All snakes have to be sedated to prevent movement inside the coil.[36]

MRI has potential as an effective tool for reptile medicine and has been used for turtles and snakes in clinical practice.[34] Radiology has limited diagnostic potential in turtles due to the low contrast between soft tissues and shell scales. Similarly, ultrasound scanning is not highly effective in turtles because it does not visualize deep organs or those shielded by bones or gas. MRI appears to be an advantageous method in turtles because it is by far more effective in cross-sectional examinations of internal organs than is CT. The intravascular injection of an MRI contrast agent (gadolinium) further supports the visualization of organ vasculature.[37] Turtles can be placed in the dorsoventral position inside a human knee coil.[38] In low-field MRI, tissues should be scanned in T1-, T2-, and proton-density-weighted sequences in the sagittal, dorsal, and transverse planes.[34] Slice thickness should ideally not exceed 5 mm to enhance the visualization of the tissues; however, in very small patients and where the type of machine used allows, 1-mm slices or less would be necessary. In high-field MRI, a 3D gradient-echo sequence with 0.5-mm slice thickness is recommended.[37] Attention should be paid to the size of coil used to pick up the signal from the patient; specialized "extremity" coils obtain high-resolution images and include wrist and finger coils.

A recent study of a Burmese python (*Python bivittatus*) over time that ranged in weight from 227 to 635 g compared the antemortem MRI results with postmortem findings to describe normal anatomy.[39] The snake was placed inside the coil of a 1.5-T MRI scanner in a ventral position, with distal parts of the body folded parallel to the central part of the body. The entire body was scanned simultaneously, and images were compiled with the use of computer software. Imaging involved 2D, proton-density, multislice spin-echo (slice thickness, 1 mm; repetition time, 4220 ms; echo time, 73 ms, including a prepulse for fat suppression) and 3D, T1-weighted, gradient-echo (repetition time, 9.3 ms; echo time, TE 3.3 ms) sequences.[39] The normal anatomy of loggerhead sea turtles and the normal tail morphology of rattlesnakes have been described; the knowledge of the appearance of normal anatomy is essential when assessing clinical patients for structural abnormalities.[8,40] Clinical use of MRI to confirm cervical spinal cord compression has been described using MRI in Komodo dragons (*Varanus komodoensis*), but the lack of normal anatomical knowledge hindered interpretation of the imaging.[41]

Nuclear scintigraphy may help identify active bone lesions and can be feasible, safe, and relatively inexpensive. This technique uses radioactive tracers, which concentrate in areas of active bone modeling and are subsequently visualized with a detection device. The images obtained are of low-resolution, nonspecific, and come with the issues associated with handling of radioactive materials and waste. Infectious, traumatic, or neoplastic lesions affecting the skull and spine potentially may be identified with this modality.[2] Individual institution protocols regarding isolation of patients post-scintigraphy should be investigated prior to recommendation of this modality in case it is not feasible.

Cerebrospinal Fluid Analysis

Analysis of CSF is an important diagnostic tool in the evaluation of patients with neurological disorders. Reptiles do not have a true subarachnoid space, an important fact in attempts to collect cerebrospinal fluid (CSF); in mammals CSF is collected from the subarachnoid space. However, CSF flows caudally, from the ventricles, in a subdural space in reptiles, which is where the fluid should be collected for analysis.[2] A spinal needle or a hypodermic needle can be used (Fig. 77.22); however, in some species, such as crocodilians, a blood sinus may be present, overlying the dura and subdural space, and a stiletted needle is required

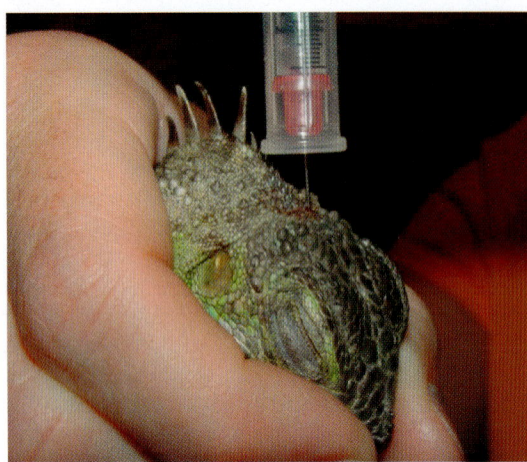

FIG 77.22 An anesthetized iguana (*Iguana iguana*) undergoing a cerebrospinal fluid tap with the head ventroflexed to the neck. A hypodermic needle is used, which is inserted between the occipital bones of the skull and the first cervical vertebra. (Courtesy of Joerg Mayer.)

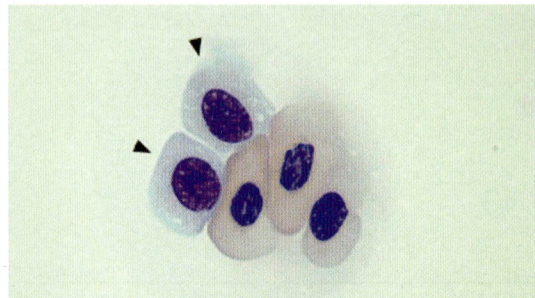

FIG 77.23 Cytological evaluation of a normal CSF sample obtained from the atlanto-occipital space in a bearded dragon (*Pogona vitticeps*). The erythrocytes seen here on the right are representative of blood contamination. Small mononuclear cells (arrowheads) are visible on the left. Scale bar = 20 um. (Reproduced with permission by Mariani CL. The neurological examination and neurodiagnostic techniques for reptiles. *Vet Clin North Am Exot Anim Pract.* 2007;10:855–891, vii.)

to traverse the sinus to obtain CSF.[2] As challenging as this technique can be, it may be more difficult to obtain an adequate volume of fluid for analysis, even when the needle is in the correct position. It is inadvisable to apply negative pressure to the needle used in an attempt to aspirate CSF; this may cause damage to the CNS.

Currently, no normal values are reported for reptilian CSF. In a study with American alligators (*Alligator mississippiensis*), CSF was collected percutaneously from the dorsal midline near the base of the skull with a spinal needle. The animals consistently showed gross body movement or a muscle twitch when the tip of the needle was in the proper position for fluid collection. The fluid was confirmed to be CSF on the basis of its constitution. Healthy alligator CSF was found to have a higher protein content compared with mammalian CSF.[2] Published reports of CSF analysis in reptiles with neurological disease are lacking, but it is suggested that mammalian values for cell counts should be used as a guideline; however, if a limited quantity is available, analysis should be restricted to cytology (Fig. 77.23). Special staining and PCR analysis may be possible when investigating patients for possible infectious agents.

Electrodiagnostics

Electrodiagnsotic techniques used for the evaluation of neurological disease in veterinary patients include electromyography, motor and sensory nerve conduction velocity, F-wave evaluation, repetitive nerve stimulation, spinal cord–evoked potentials, and electroencephalography. Because of their relative unavailability, these methods have not been used extensively in clinical reptile neurology. Reptiles are poikilothermic, and their nerve conduction velocity varies with the ambient temperature. Information regarding normal velocity for a given temperature and reptile species is lacking. If a specific control is available for comparison, a difference might support a tentative diagnosis of a conduction disturbance. Still, the size of many patients and difficulty finding a nerve to evaluate make this diagnostic tool of limited value.

Electromyography is used to determine whether muscle dysfunction is the result of nerve injury or a myopathy.[1] It is performed by inserting a needle into individual muscle bellies, which produces waveforms that can be visually and acoustically evaluated. The EMG of a normal muscle should be electrically silent, as the procedure is performed under general anesthesia. Denervation of muscle or intrinsic disease of the muscle itself produces abnormal electrical potentials that have characteristic

waveforms and sounds. It is easily performed and interpreted in reptiles as in other species. The needle often needs to be directed between dermal scutes or scales, but the muscle underneath typically is accessed without difficulty.[2]

Motor nerve conduction velocity involves the stimulation of a selected nerve at two or more points, with recording of a resulting compound muscle action potential within a muscle innervated by the nerve.[2] A velocity of conduction can be calculated for specific nerves; it is important to perform the test at appropriate body temperatures as low temperatures will reduce nerve conduction velocity.[42] Demyelinating peripheral nerve disease can result in reduced motor nerve conduction velocity, and in patients with trauma this test also can be useful to document anatomical or functional transection of a nerve. To perform this test on reptiles, the operator needs to know the anatomical course of the nerve, and the anatomy of the patient needs to be considered with respect to stimulating and recording site possibilities; it is most useful on appendicular nerves. Normal values for reptiles have not been established.

Spinal cord–evoked response, or somatosensory-evoked potential, is a waveform elicited after stimulation of a nerve of a pelvic or thoracic limb and recorded from the spinal cord itself at a point rostral to the stimulation site.[43] The recording electrode is placed ideally on the dorsal surface of the dura mater, or alternatively in contact with the dorsal lamina of a vertebra. This test may provide information regarding the speed of conduction of impulses in the spinal cord, and it has been used to detect areas of spinal cord injury.[2] The author and others have used this technique in an attempt to identify chelonian patients with functionally transected spinal cords (i.e., complete spinal lesions). Trauma to the shell of the tortoises and turtles can result in spinal cord trauma, because the carapace is closely associated with the vertebrae; this technique may provide an assessment of the integrity of the spinal cord and therefore possibility for recovery in these patients.

Brainstem auditory-evoked response (BAER) is a waveform produced after stimulation of the auditory nerve, and it corresponds to the transmission of impulses from this nerve, through associated nuclei, ascending to higher brain centers from the brainstem.[2] In mammals this response usually is recorded as a six-to-seven-peak waveform, typically elicited by playing a series of auditory clicks through headphones or tubal inserts into the ear canal. Recording, reference, and ground electrodes are placed on the skin of the head. This test may be of limited value in reptiles because of the anatomical variations present (reptiles have very short to nonexistent external ear canals), and the unique range of frequencies, it is believed, are detectable by the reptile auditory system (1.5–6 kHz).[44] As with other electrophysiological testing in reptiles, auditory responses seemed to be altered by temperature changes. Reports exist of responses in reptiles, including caiman and loggerhead sea turtles, to airborne sound, underwater sound, and vibrational stimulus.[2,45–47] In another study, hearing sensitivity was measured in five geckos and seven anoles.[48] The lizards were sedated with isoflurane, and BAERs were measured at levels of 1% and 3% isoflurane. The typical BAER waveform in response to click stimulation showed one prominent and several smaller peaks occurring within 10 months of the stimulus onset. BAERs to brief tone bursts revealed that geckos and anoles were most sensitive between 1.6 to 2 kHz and had similar hearing sensitivity up to about 5 kHz thresholds, typically 20 to 50 dB SPL. Above 5 kHz, however, anoles were more than 20 dB more sensitive than geckos and showed a wider range of sensitivity, 1 to 7 kHz. Generally, thresholds from BAERs were comparable to those of small birds. Best hearing sensitivity, however, extended over a larger frequency range in lizards than in most bird species.[48]

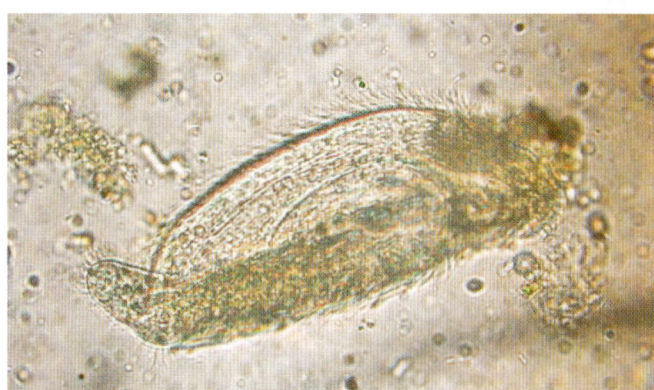

FIG 77.24 Microscopic view of an *Acanthamoeba* organism. (Courtesy of Joerg Mayer.)

DISEASES AFFECTING THE REPTILIAN NERVOUS SYSTEM

Neurological diseases in reptiles can result from a variety of causes, some of which have been well characterized, especially those of infectious, nutritional, and toxic origin. These diseases have been categorized below by the mechanism of disease responsible, as much as is possible.

Infectious Diseases

Bacterial, viral, fungal, and protozoan infections are known to cause neurological signs in reptiles.[1,14] In some cases, although an infectious agent is suspected, definitive determination may not be possible. As an example, infectious or toxic etiology was suspected to be responsible for the acute onset of neurological dysfunction seen in 12 Australian water dragons over a 2-month period.[49] The water dragons presented with obtundation, head tilts, loss of proprioception, loss of righting reflexes, ataxia, and hyperesthesia. No treatment protocols were effective, and all dragons died or were euthanized. Histopathology identified multifocal encephalomalacia, which is a nonspecific finding.[49] Diagnosis in such cases may necessitate an exclusion of causes rather than definitive identification of an etiology, and broad treatment regimens may need to be employed.

Protozoa

Acanthamoeba* *meningoencephalitis. Species of *Acanthamoeba* are generally pathogenic to humans[50] but can infect any soft tissue of reptiles.[1] Human infections are most commonly the result of contamination of recreational water sources. Organisms enter via the nasal mucosa and migrate through the cribriform plate or are transported to tissues by the vascular system.[1] Free-living Acanthamoeba have been encountered in the intestinal contents and during necropsies of amphibians and reptiles[1,51] (Fig. 77.24). Clinically, *Acanthamoeba* encephalitis was diagnosed in a boa constrictor (*Boa constrictor*) and a Pacific Coast rattlesnake (*Crotalus viridis oreganus*) with spasmodic opisthotonos.[1] Organisms were contained within the CSF in both snakes. Environmental stimulus exacerbated opisthotonos. The drinking water was proposed as the source of contamination. A diagnosis of *Acanthamoeba* meningoencephalitis is difficult antemortem, and no successful treatment has been reported.

Toxoplasmosis. Toxoplasma spp. have been reported to be associated with abscessation within the brain and meningoencephalitis in reptiles.[1,14] Toxoplasma is generally a parasite of homeotherms that can develop in reptiles when their body temperature is maintained near 37°C (99°F). Insects may serve as vectors or fomites for the transmission of toxoplasmosis, emphasizing the need for pest control. Diagnosis is based

on histopathology and polymerase chain reaction (PCR); molecular testing of 68 postmortem captive snake brains for *Toxoplasma gondii* revealed 81% to be positive.[52] Clindamycin has appeared to be beneficial in treating mammals with toxoplasmosis.[1] The recommended dose is 5 mg/kg by mouth daily; however, no studies are found regarding its efficacy against toxoplasmosis in reptiles.

Bacteria.
Bacterial infections may be a primary cause of nervous system disorders (encephalitis, meningitis, myelitis) or may secondarily affect the nervous system by infection of surrounding structures causing nervous tissue damage.[14] An example of secondary or indirect infection is vertebral osteomyelitis, often seen in snakes;[53–55] spinal cord compression can result from vertebral remodeling associated with the infection (as discussed later).[14] Gram-negative bacteria (e.g., *Salmonella* spp., *Staphylococcus* spp., *Listeria* spp., *Mycoplasma* spp., and *Mycobacterium* spp.,) are the most common isolates from nervous system isolates in reptiles.[14] Based on this, if culture and sensitivity of appropriate samples such as vertebral biopsy,[32] CSF, or blood culture, is not possible, selection of an antibiotic that has treatment activity against gram-negative bacteria and crosses the blood-brain barrier, such as enroflaxacin, should be utilized.

After septicemia, especially from respiratory infections, microabscesses or macroabscesses can develop within the brain. Histologically, these abscesses consist of areas of necrosis usually associated with a large number of mononuclear leukocytes.[1]

Mycobacterium generally produces a multisystemic disease that can involve the nervous system and/or muscles.[56–58] It induces a granulomatous inflammation with granulomas containing caseous cellular debris and acid-fast organisms.[1,57] Cytological preparations of granulomatous debris may be acid-fast stained to determine the presence of the organisms.[59] There is a significant prevalence of *Mycobacterium* species in clinical healthy pet reptiles;[60] treatment of mycobacteriosis in reptiles is controversial because of the zoonotic potential of the infection.

Spinal osteopathy/discospondylitis/osteomyelitis.
A lytic proliferative spinal osteopathy has been reported in members of the *Boidae* and *Viperidae*;[1] however, clinically it appears to be more widespread. Some believe it may be caused by a virus of snakes that is transmitted by mice, but other considerations include neoplasia, hypovitaminosis D, and prolonged inactivity associated with cage confinement.[1,20] Septicemia has also been implicated as a cause because often these lesions culture positive for bacterial organisms, leading to the concern that a significant proportion of these cases may have discospondylitis or osteomyelitis.[1,20,53–55,61]

The blood flow in the area of the intervertebral discs may favor seeding of infection in this location during episodes of septicemia. Another theory is that it is an immune-mediated disease caused by a septicemia that stimulates a polyclonal B cell proliferation.[1] *Pseudomonas fluorescens*, *Salmonella arizonae*, and *Staphylococcus* sp. have been implicated in inducing this type of gammopathy.

The potential role of bacteria in proliferative osteoarthritis and osteoarthropathy of the spine has been reported.[20] In all, 10 of the 15 snakes with histological evidence of bacterial osteoarthritis had positive bone cultures, and 8 of 10 snakes with positive bone cultures had corresponding positive blood cultures. *Salmonella* sp. and *Streptococcus* sp. were cultured from these patients. Three distinct groups were identified. Group 1 had strong evidence of active bacterial osteoarthritis, both histologically and on bone cultures. Group 2 was identified as having a noninflammatory osteoarthrosis without histological evidence of bacteria but with positive culture results of the bone. Group 3 had degenerative osteoarthrosis and ankylosis with minimal to no inflammation and lack of positive bone or blood culture results.[20]

Early in the course of the disease, focal or multifocal swellings may be identified along the dorsum associated with the spine (Fig. 77.25). Palpation of the spine may reveal segmental areas of ankylosis and kyphosis.[20] Digital pressure usually induces a pain response. Motor deficits, trembling, torticollis, and spinal deformity may be manifested.[1,20] Radiographically, in the early stages of the disease, sclerosis of the vertebral end plates is seen with evidence of bone proliferation that does not involve the adjacent ribs. The condition progresses with remodeling of vertebrae. The bony proliferation is usually periarticular at the costovertebral joints and the dorsolateral articular facets. As the disease progresses, the ribs may become affected and the costovertebral articulations often show evidence of ankylosis, making this condition different from spondylosis deformans or ankylosing spondylosis.[1,20]

With time, ankylosis of the spine occurs, often affecting large segments of the spinal column. Eventually, the animal becomes unable to move, constrict, or swallow prey. Histologically, the bone trabeculae in the vertebrae are thickened with irregular cement lines, and the intertrabecular spaces are usually filled with blood vessels and fibrous connective tissue.

Blood cultures are recommended for evaluation for septicemia; however, evidence shows that the lesions can develop as late as 22 to 36 months after an episode of septicemia.[1] Local cultures may be obtained with fine-needle aspirate or surgical exploration for debridement and sample collection.[14] Cultures should be submitted for aerobic and anaerobic evaluation and acid-fast staining.

In a California king snake (*Lampropeltis getula*) with vertebral osteopathy at the San Francisco Zoo, *Salmonella* sp., *Proteus mirabilis*, and *Bacteroides* sp. were isolated from samples collected during surgical debridement of the lesion.[1] A section of the spinal column was removed, and the snake remained neurologically healthy after surgery. This snake was followed radiographically for 6 months, during which time no evidence of reossification was found in the area where the vertebrae were removed.[1]

In summary, snakes with radiographic evidence of spinal osteopathy should be evaluated with blood cultures and local aspirates to identify bacteria present within the lesion or systemically. Treatment involves appropriate long-term antibiotic therapy and surgical debridement if lysis predominates. The prognosis of bacterial-induced osteomyelitis is guarded as the condition is often advanced by the time a patient is presented.[14]

Viruses

Paramyxovirus. Ferlaviruses, sometimes referred to as ophidian paramyxoviruses, are a significant viral infection in many snakes and

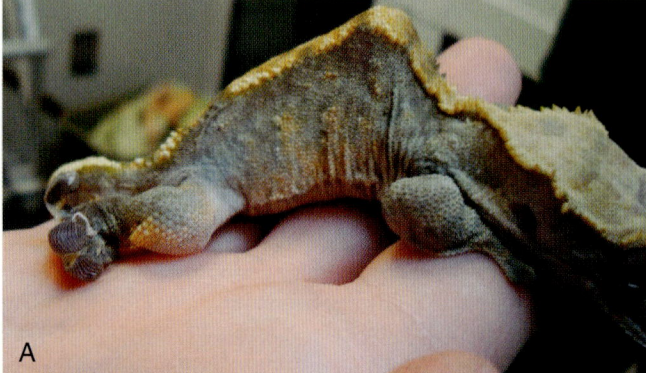
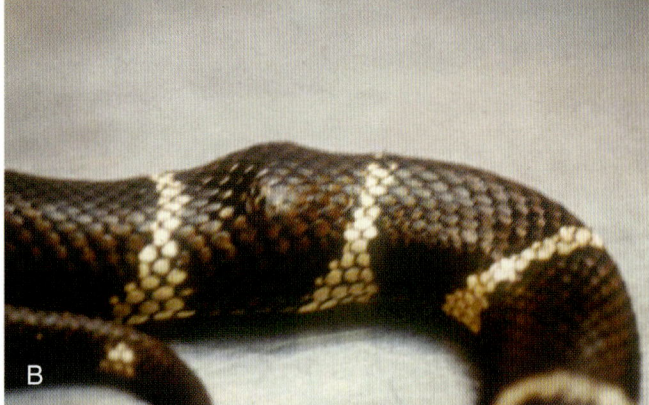
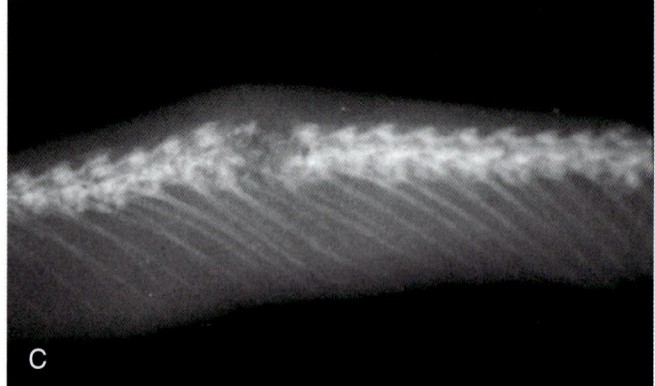

FIG 77.25 (A) Kyphosis secondary to spinal trauma in a crested gecko (*Correlophus ciliatus*) (Courtesy of Joerg Mayer) and (B) a visible swelling is present in this California king snake (*Lampropeltis getula californiae*) due to vertebral osteomyelitis, which can be seen as pronounced bone lysis radiographically (C). (Reproduced with permission by Bennett RA, Mehler SJ. Neurology. In DR Mader, ed. *Reptile Medicine and Surgery*, ed 2. St. Louis: Saunders Elsevier; 2006:239–250.)

is especially common in viperids, although this virus also affects elapids, boids, and colubrids.[14,62–65] The virus is mainly transmitted by direct contact with respiratory secretions, but there is also potential exposure via snake mites.[14] A variety of respiratory, gastrointestinal, and neurological signs may be observed when snakes are infected, including opisthotonus (Fig. 77.26), torticollis, a reduced righting reflex, and death.[14,66] A progressive central nervous system disorder manifesting clinically as head tremors and loss of equilibrium with opisthotonos has been described in rock rattlesnakes (*Crotalus lepidus*).[67] These snakes also lost the righting reflex and had irregular and slow tongue flick responses. The disease was linked to a paramyxolike virus that was identified with electron microscopy. The disease was believed to have been introduced

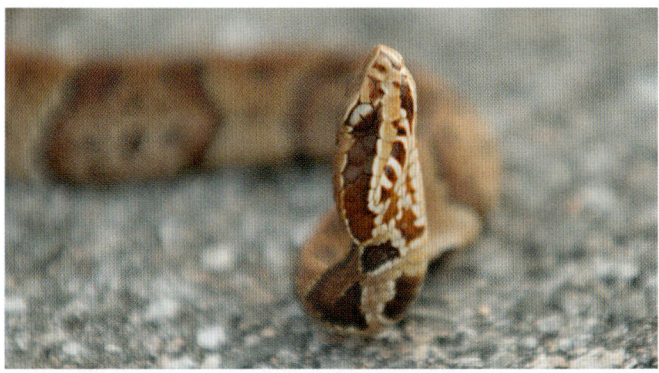

FIG 77.26 A water moccasin (*Agkistrodon piscivorus*) displaying an opisthotonus-like pose. Note that in some species this is not a pathological behavior. Sometimes this behavior is part of a courtship ritual. (Courtesy of Joerg Mayer.)

to the private collection with the addition of two wild-caught snakes that had signs develop within 14 days of their capture.

Histologically, gliosis and perivascular cuffing were identified in a variety of locations within the hindbrain. Demyelination, axon degeneration, and ballooning of axon sheaths were seen in the brain stem and spinal cord. In addition to the central nervous system lesions, the lungs also showed pathology consisting of cellular debris and exudate filling the primary bronchi and air spaces.[1] Antemortem diagnosis is possible with paired serology or PCR using either an oral or cloacal swab.[14] Supportive treatment may be provided to snakes exhibiting clinical signs, but euthanasia is generally advised.[14]

Sunshine virus is a recently discovered novel paramyxovirus that is associated with neurorespiratory illnesses in snakes.[64,68,69] It does not phylogenetically cluster within either of the two currently accepted paramyxoviral subfamilies. It is therefore only distantly related to the only other known genus of reptilian paramyxoviruses, ferlavirus, which clusters within the Paramyxovirinae subfamily.[68] During a natural outbreak of sunshine virus in a collection of 32 snakes, the virus could be detected in 5 out of 39 combined oral-cloacal swabs that were collected from 23 of these snakes over a 105-day period. All snakes that were infected with sunshine virus were negative for reovirus and ferlavirus by PCR. Snakes infected with sunshine virus reliably exhibited hindbrain white matter spongiosis and gliosis with extension to the surrounding gray matter and neuronal necrosis evident in severe cases.[68]

Inclusion body disease of boids. This condition is believed to be caused by an arenavirus and affects boas and pythons; however, the clinical syndrome is distinct between these two groups.[1,14,70,71] The neurological severity is significantly worse in pythons than in boas, underscoring the recommendation to not mix boas and pythons in the same collection. Boas may be inapparent carriers. The snake mite, *Ophionyssus natricis*, is suspected as one of the vectors incriminated in the spread of the disease. Other modes of transmission include direct contact and venereal spread.[1]

Clinical signs are generally multisystemic, including gastrointestinal, respiratory, and neurological signs. In juvenile boas, the condition is often quickly fatal with an acute onset of flaccid paralysis. Adult boas have a more chronic manifestation of the disease, with central nervous system signs occurring only in the terminal stages. Early in the course of the disease, chronic regurgitation, cachexia, and chronic pneumonia are common.[14] Neurological signs are generally manifest as an inability to strike, constrict, and prehend food items. Dysecdysis may occur as a result of an inability to control body movements to rub off the shed skin.[1]

In pythons, the clinical course is much more rapid, progressing to a fatal CNS disturbance.[14] Pythons also have multisystemic disease, with pneumonia and infectious stomatitis common. Neurologically, they have a loss of righting reflex, hyperreflexia, disorientation, and loss of motor coordination. Some animals develop central blindness.[1]

Currently, a PCR test is available to screen for arenavirus infection from a blood sample and/or an esophageal swab.[14,72] Biopsy results of the liver, kidney, esophageal lymphoid tissue, and skin may show the typical eosinophilic intracytoplasmic inclusions.[14] Histologically, eosinophilic intracytoplasmic inclusion bodies have been identified within epithelial cells of the pancreas, kidney, esophagus, stomach, and liver. Occasionally, inclusion bodies are identified in white blood cells.[14] A nonsuppurative encephalitis with neuron degeneration and mononuclear cell infiltrates characterizes the lesions within the brain and spinal cord. In the white tracts of the spinal cord, areas of gliosis with extensive myelin degeneration and axon loss are seen. Intracytoplasmic eosinophilic inclusion bodies have been found within the neurons of the brain and the gray tracts of the spinal cord. The degree of inflammation is much greater in pythons compared with that found in boas. Perivascular cuffing with degenerative myelopathy is evidence of a viral etiology; however, some bacterial infections also stimulate perivascular cuffing.[1]

No treatment has been shown to be successful for this viral disease. It may be mild in boas and may go undiagnosed. Therefore prevention of exposure of pythons to boas is best as they may be in apparent carriers. Identification and elimination of animals with known positive disease are recommended.

Agamid adenovirus. Agamid adenovirus-1 is considered endemic in the pet bearded dragon (*Pogona vitticeps*) and appears to be associated with both neurological and gastrointestinal signs, reduced growth, and death.[73] Alternatively, in some dragons the infections remain subclinical.[14] Transmission of the virus is via the fecal-oral route, with infection resulting in severe gastrointestinal and hepatic pathology.[14]

Young (6–10 weeks) juvenile inland bearded dragons from a breeding collection in southeast Queensland were recently described with neurological signs, poor growth, and occasional deaths.[74] Histopathological examination revealed that six of eight lizards had multifocal nonsuppurative hepatitis associated with 5 to 10 μm diameter, smudgy, basophilic, hyaline intranuclear inclusion bodies that marginated the nuclear chromatin. These histological lesions were considered consistent with adenoviral hepatitis. A definitive diagnosis is based on PCR testing of an oral or cloacal swab, and treatment is only supportive.[14]

West Nile virus (WNV). Reptiles may serve as reservoir hosts for western equine encephalitis and Venezuelan equine encephalitis.[75–77] WNV has been reported in reptiles as early as the 1960s in Israel.[1] More recently, WNV has been found to occur in alligator and crocodile species in the United States.[14,78,79] The mode of transmission to reptiles is thought to be from the ingestion of, or a bite from, the insect carrier (e.g., mosquito),[80] or from ingestion of infected horse meat.[79] Crocodiles are thought to be an amplifying host owing to high levels of viremia and viral shedding.[14] Affected animals have an acute onset of paresis, circling, head tremors, neck spasms, and a star-gazing appearance before death.[1,19] In reptiles with neurological disease, the presence of perivascular cuffing within the brain and spinal cord is indicative of viral infection, yet in many instances no agent has been identified.[1] Definitive diagnosis is based on viral isolation and PCR testing of postmortem samples. A WNV vaccine has been recently approved for use in alligators.[14]

Nutritional Diseases

When dealing with a patient with neurological disease, evaluation of the patient's nutritional status is important. Animals being fed intact whole prey diets rarely have nutritional deficiencies.[1]

Thiamine Deficiency. Thiamine deficiency (or thiaminase excess) may be observed in animals fed thawed frozen fish, clams, and some types of vegetation.[1,14] Freezing fish and subsequent thawing decreases the amount of available thiamine and potentially increases the activity of thiaminases.[14] Snakes of the genus *Thamnophis* and *Natrix* are piscivorous, as are some crocodilians and chelonians, which makes them more prone to leukoencephalopathy if fed frozen-thawed fish.[1] The consumption of thiaminase-positive gizzard shad (*Dorosoma cepedianum*), a commonly eaten wild fish, is thought to have been the cause of the low tissue thiamine and resulting mortalities in alligators in central Florida.[81,82] Herbivorous reptiles fed a diet high in vegetation containing phytothiaminases may develop thiamine deficiency.

Clinical signs are generally nonspecific and include muscle twitching, incoordination, blindness, seizure activity, torticollis, abnormal posture, spiral locomotion, jaw gaping, dysphagia, and potentially death.[1,14] Snakes frequently are unable to accurately strike prey. In chelonians, the most striking clinical sign is a sinking of the eye within the bony orbit (enophthalmos).[1] At necropsy, usually no gross lesions are seen. Histologically, cerebral cortical necrosis with peripheral neuritis and cardiomyopathy is frequently encountered.[1] Histological lesions also include a diffuse eosinophilia with severe demyelination and axon sheath fragmentation. Generally inflammatory cells are absent.

Treatment involves oral or subcutaneous supplementation of vitamin B_1 (thiamine) at 25 mg/kg/day. A dramatic response to therapy is usually seen. The longer the duration of clinical signs, the more severe the neurological compromise and the less likely it is to completely resolve. In addition to supplementation, the diet should be evaluated and, if possible, the patient should be placed on a fresh fish diet, although some fish will contain high levels of thiaminase (see Chapters 27 and 84 for more information). If frozen fish must be used, they should be supplemented with thiamine. Fish may also be heated to denature the thiaminase.

Herbivores fed plant material containing phytothiaminase should be placed on an appropriate diet containing alternative plant sources. From a theoretical standpoint, long-term antibiotic therapy has been suggested to induce clinical signs of thiamine deficiency by decreasing the intestinal microflora responsible for producing vitamin B_1 (see Chapter 122). Although this theory has not been confirmed scientifically, some believe placing patients receiving long-term antibiotic therapy on a thiamine supplement may be prudent.[1]

Biotin Deficiency. Biotin is a B vitamin readily supplied in most food sources. Raw egg whites contain avidin, which has antibiotin activity.[1] Deficiency may be induced in reptiles (usually in egg-eating snakes and lizards, for example, varanids) by feeding a diet of whole raw eggs. Because of the ubiquitous nature of biotin, the entire diet must consist of raw eggs to induce deficiency. Free-ranging, egg-eating reptiles do not generally have biotin deficiency because they eat fertile eggs, often with some degree of embryonic development. Embryonic tissue contains biotin, and the avidin in the egg is used up during embryonic development. In addition, most egg-eating reptiles also consume small animals that contain biotin.[1]

Clinical signs of biotin deficiency consist of muscle tremors and generalized muscle weakness. Treatment involves supplementing vitamin B complex orally or via injection and correcting the dietary deficiency by supplementing with biotin or diversifying the diet to include other items that contain adequate biotin.[1]

Hypocalcemia. Hypocalcemia is generally observed as the result of end-stage nutritional or renal secondary hyperparathyroidism.[1]

Inadequate dietary calcium or vitamin D_3, inadequate ultraviolet (UV)-B lighting, or low temperatures may lead to neurological signs

in affected reptile patients once the calcium reserves in the bone are depleted.[14,41] In chelonians and crocodilians, the deficiency is usually from a diet of exclusively red meat, which is deficient in calcium. The neurological manifestations of hypocalcemia include weakness, inability to withdraw the tongue, muscle twitching or tetany, and seizures, which may be seen in any class of reptiles.[14] Treatment of hypocalcemic tetany entails the parenteral administration of a calcium gluconate solution after confirmation with a blood ionized calcium level.[29]

Hypovitaminosis E. Vitamin E/selenium deficiency has been described in iguanas exhibiting clinical signs of weakness, paresis, and ataxia, as well as in a veiled chameleon (*Chamaeleo calyptratus*) that was unable to open its mouth and move its tongue.[14] A similar nutritional deficiency has been seen in bearded dragons, which responded to vitamin E supplementation, which is necessary to support the diagnosis of this condition.[14]

Trauma

Reptiles are susceptible to trauma from a variety of causes, which can be direct (e.g., head trauma) or indirect (e.g., chelonians with paraparesis secondary to dystocia).[1,29] Regardless of the etiology, trauma to the nervous system is often categorized for assessment and therapeutic purposes into brain injury, spinal cord injury, and peripheral nerve injury. The clinical signs and prognosis are referable to both the location of the injury and its severity. Grading systems for clinical severity are documented for canine and feline trauma but not for trauma to the reptile nervous system. However, it is proposed that a similar grading system can be applied and a similar prediction of prognosis may be possible. The assessment and management described in the following subsections is predominantly what is documented in canine and feline medicine unless otherwise stated.

Brain Injury. Head trauma pathophysiology can be divided into primary and secondary injury.[83] Primary injury to the brain cannot be reversed, occurs immediately, and describes the physical disruption of brain tissue; this includes contusions, hematomas, lacerations, and diffuse axonal injury leading to vasogenic edema.[84] The underlying vascular and cellular pathophysiology of head trauma is similar to that described for spinal cord trauma but is complicated by elevations in intracranial pressure (ICP). This secondary injury is delayed and progressive, potentially providing targets for treatment. In addition to excitatory neurotransmitter release, ATP depletion results in cytotoxic edema, intracellular calcium accumulation causing activation of intracellular enzyme systems, and oxygen radical production resulting in lipid peroxidation. Traumatic brain injury is associated with a marked inflammatory response. The secondary injury "cascade" is exacerbated by systemic abnormalities present in the patient, which includes hypotension, hypoxia, hypo- or hyperglycemia, hypo- or hypercapnia, and hyperthermia.

After head trauma, the volume of the brain tissue compartment increases, usually due to edema or hemorrhage. As the brain tissue compartment increases, the CSF and the blood compartments must decrease or ICP will increase.[85] Compensation for increased brain tissue volume initially involves the translocation of CSF out of the skull; this is followed by decreased production of CSF and, eventually, decreased cerebral blood flow. These compensatory mechanisms prevent increases in ICP for an undetermined period. Once the ability for compensation is exhausted, a further small increase in intracranial volume will result in dramatic elevations of ICP, with the immediate onset of clinical signs.[85] Increases in ICP are often responsible for clinical decline after head trauma. Marked increases in ICP lead to an elevation of mean arterial blood pressure (MABP) and reflex bradycardia (Cushing reflex). In addition to a drop in heart rate coupled with an elevated MABP, other clinical manifestations of ICP elevation include anisocoria, miosis, mydriasis, altered mentation, and loss of motor function with the development of vertical nystagmus and extensor rigidity toward the end stages.[85]

Imaging of the patient's head is often indicated, especially in animals that fail to respond to aggressive medical therapy or deteriorate after initially responding. Skull radiographs are unlikely to reveal clinically useful information about brain injury but may occasionally reveal evidence of calvarial fractures. CT is the preferred modality for imaging the head in cases of severe head injury associated with fractures. Even patients with "mild" head trauma can exhibit abnormalities on the CT scan, and so the initial decision to image the patient's head should not be based on the neurological examination alone. CT image acquisition time is faster and often less expensive than MRI, and CT also demonstrates bone detail better than MRI. However, MRI has been shown to provide key information relevant to the prognosis based on its ability to detect subtle parenchymal damage not evident on CT imaging. The detection of midline parenchymal shift and ventricular obliteration on MR images are associated with a poor prognosis for survival, based on a recent canine study.[86] Furthermore, lesions of the intracranial structures that may benefit from surgical therapy, such as hematomas and pneumocephalus, can be accurately identified using advanced imaging. Cervical spinal radiographs or CT are also advised at the time of any skull imaging to rule out concurrent spinal lesions.

Accurate assessment is important for determining the way in which treatment is tailored to the individual patient. Systemic and neurological assessment must be undertaken rapidly and continually reassessed. In humans, traumatic brain injury is graded as mild, moderate, or severe on the basis of an objective scoring system (e.g., Glasgow coma score, GCS). A modification of the GCS has been proposed for use in veterinary medicine.[87] The modified scoring system incorporates three categories of the examination (level of consciousness; motor activity; brainstem reflexes), which are assigned a score from 1 to 6, providing a total score of 3 to 18, with the best prognosis being the higher score.

The most important consideration in head injury is maintenance of cerebral perfusion by treatment of hypotension and elevated ICP. The basic goal of fluid management of head trauma cases is to maintain a normovolemic to slightly hypervolemic state to ensure an adequate cerebral perfusion pressure. Initial resuscitation usually involves IV administration of hypertonic saline and/or synthetic colloids. Use of these solutions allows rapid restoration of blood volume and pressure while limiting the volume of fluid administered. In contrast, crystalloids will extravasate into the interstitium within an hour of administration and thus larger volumes are required for restoration of blood volume. If isotonic crystalloids are chosen for administration (appropriate in mild head trauma), an aliquot of the shock dose can be given rapidly and repeated until improved tissue perfusion is achieved. Hypertonic saline administration draws fluid from the interstitial and intracellular spaces into the intravascular space, which improves blood pressure and cerebral blood pressure and flow, with a subsequent decrease in ICP. Colloid solutions can be administered after hypertonic saline is used to maintain the intravascular volume, possibly due to retention of fluids in the intravascular compartments, maintaining an intravascular oncotic gradient.

Osmotic diuretics are very useful in the treatment of intracranial hypertension. Use of mannitol is recommended once vascular volume has been stabilized. Mannitol has an immediate plasma-expanding effect, which reduces blood viscosity, increasing cerebral blood flow and oxygen delivery. This results in vasoconstriction within a few minutes, causing an almost immediate decrease in ICP. The better known osmotic effect of mannitol reverses the blood-brain osmotic gradient, thereby reducing extracellular fluid volume in both normal and damaged brains. Mannitol

should be administered as a bolus over a 15-minute period, rather than as an infusion, in order to obtain the plasma-expanding effect; its effect on decreasing brain edema takes approximately 15 to 30 minutes to establish and lasts between 2 and 8 hrs. These times may be extended in reptiles but are unknown.

Oxygen supplementation is recommended for most acutely brain-injured animals. Supplemental oxygen should be administered via flow-by or oxygen cages, which (although often inadequate for mammals) may be suitable for reptiles with their slower metabolism. The target 40%-inspired oxygen recommended for mammals may cause reptiles to significantly decrease their respiratory rate, and lower levels may be clinically acceptable.

The use of steroids in brain-injured patients is controversial. The original rationale for use of glucocorticoids in central nervous system trauma came from the thought that they would reduce edema and intracranial pressure and counteract oxidative damage.[85] Methylprednisone sodium succinate may exert further actions, such as preventing progressive ischemia and reversing intracellular calcium accumulation.[85] Current human and veterinary literature indicates that the use of steroids in central nervous system trauma shows no specific benefit, and their use may actually increase morbidity.[88] Some of the side effects observed in patients with head trauma or spinal cord trauma treated with steroids include increased blood pressure, lowered seizure threshold, decrease in platelet aggregation, muscle weakness, and gastric ulceration. Glucocorticoids stimulate gluconeogenesis, and hyperglycemia has been associated with increased mortality rates in humans with severe head injury.

Surgical therapy of head-injured patients is suggested when (1) medical therapy has not been successful, (2) there is a penetrating injury, or (3) there is an open fracture with risk of infection necessitating immediate decontamination. A recent report documented an adult male Fly River turtle (*Carretochelys insculpta*) that presented with dull mentation and a proptosed right eye due to severe head trauma.[89] Injuries included rostral mandibular, left mandibular, left maxillary, and bilateral orbital fractures. The right orbital fracture was repaired immediately. Radiography and computed tomography (CT) were performed to evaluate the extent of the fractures. The use of CT provided complete evaluation of the skull fractures, was a guide for surgical planning, and allowed for monitoring of fracture healing. The turtle returned to normal behavior 2 months after surgery. The fractures were either healed or almost healed 6.5 months after surgery.[89] Another recent study evaluated the use of a plant-derived dressing (1 Primary Wound Dressing) in three sea turtles with severe lesions of the skull, exposing the brain.[90] Following surgical curettage, the treatment protocol involved exclusive use of the plant-derived dressing applied on the wound surface as the primary dressing, daily for the first month and then every other day until the end of treatment. The wound and surrounding skin were covered with a simple secondary dressing without any active compound (nonwoven gauze with petroleum jelly). The report described an excellent healing process in all three cases and no side effects due to contact of the medication with the cerebral tissue.[90]

Overall there is not enough data to know what level and speed of recovery is possible following brain injury in reptiles. However, evidence accumulated over the last few decades demonstrates that all healthy reptiles continuously add neurons at a high rate and in many regions of the adult brain throughout their life.[91] This so-called adult neurogenesis has been described in the olfactory bulbs, rostral forebrain, all cortical areas, anterior dorsal ventricular ridge, septum, striatum, nucleus sphericus, and cerebellum. The rate of neuronal production varies greatly among these brain areas. In addition to producing new neurons in the adult brain, lizards, and possibly other reptiles as well, are capable of regenerating large portions of their telencephalon damaged as a result of experimentally induced injuries, thus exhibiting an enormous potential for neuronal regeneration.[91]

Spinal Cord Injury. Chelonians are susceptible to spinal cord injury secondary to carapace trauma[1,29] (Fig. 77.27). Pathological spinal fractures can occur in association with metabolic bone disease[1] (Fig. 77.28).

Results of the neurological examination are used to determine neuroanatomic localization and severity of the spinal cord injury (Fig. 77.29). Reptiles with spinal cord injury generally have a loss of panniculus response caudal to the site of injury and a loss of tail or vent stimulation reflex.[1] In some cases, they have hypertonia cranial to the site of the injury.[2] It is important to perform the neurological examination with care to prevent further injury and displacement of the spine. The neurological examination findings are most important in establishing the prognosis irrespective of radiographic findings. Plain radiography of the entire spine should be performed. Results of survey radiography are used to determine the precise lesion location(s) and extent, demonstrate multiple lesions, and guide appropriate management[29] (Fig. 77.30). Intrathecal contrast-enhanced imaging or cross-sectional imaging is used when the radiographic findings do not correlate with the neurological examination, to evaluate spinal cord swelling in concussive injuries, and to further assess severity of spinal cord compression. CT or MRI is useful for further evaluating bone and spinal cord tissues, respectively, and provide a three-dimensional configuration of the fracture/luxation extent for assessment of spinal stability.

The critical factor in determining whether conservative or surgical management of spinal fracture and luxation is appropriate depends on the presence of instability. Priority is placed on treatment of extraneural injuries, beginning with management of shock and hemorrhage. Management of an animal with spinal trauma focuses on the prevention of secondary injury to the spinal cord parenchyma. Indications for nonsurgical management include minimal neurological deficits, minimal vertebral displacement, and lack of advanced imaging evidence of spinal cord compression. Principles of conservative management are appropriate confinement for 6 to 18 weeks and use of external coaptation. The aim of external support is to provide immobilization of the vertebral segments cranial and caudal to the damaged area. It is important to follow principles of bandage care when using methods of external support. The patient will need to be carefully managed and kept clean from urates and feces.

Surgical management often provides a better chance for more rapid and complete neurological recovery. However, the role of surgery for reptile spinal trauma remains unclear. Indications include severe neurological deficits and deteriorating neurological status, imaging evidence of compression, and damage of two or more vertebral

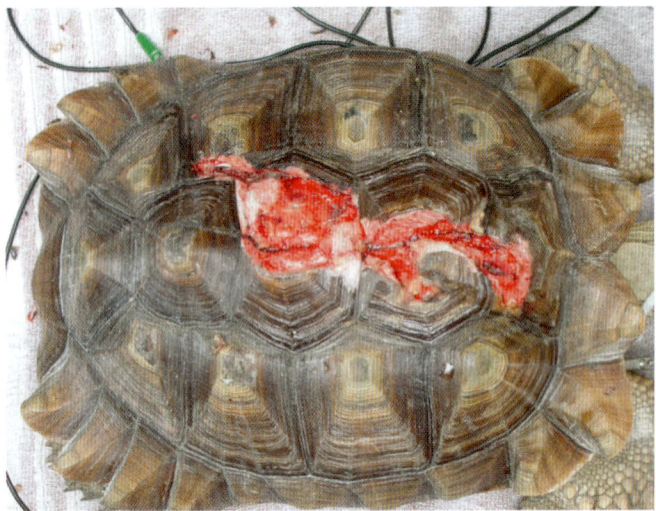

FIG 77.27 A severe carapace injury resulting in damage to the underlying spinal cord can be seen in this African spurred tortoise (*Centrochelys sulcata*). (Courtesy of Joerg Mayer.)

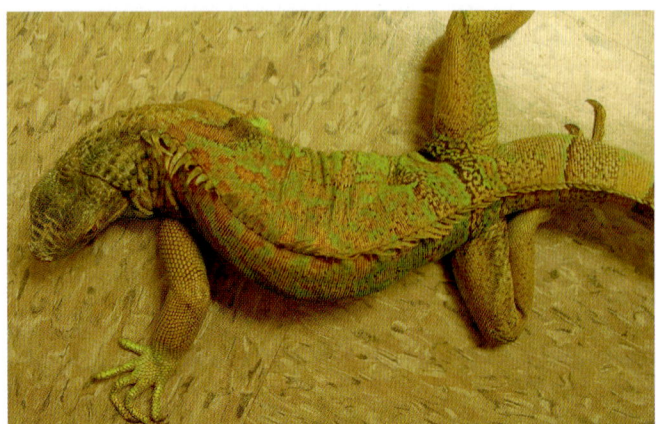

FIG 77.28 An iguana with secondary nutritional hyperparathyroidism exhibits scoliosis secondary to a pathological vertebral fracture. (Courtesy of Joerg Mayer.)

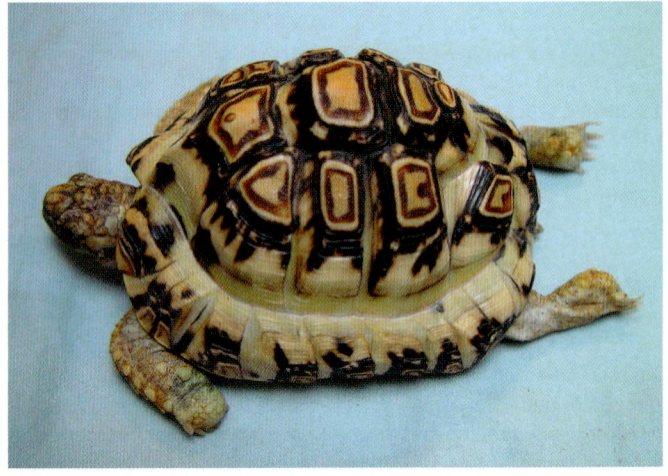

FIG 77.29 Severe tetraparesis can be noted in this juvenile leopard tortoise (*Stigmochelys pardalis*) with cervical spinal injury. (Courtesy of Joerg Mayer.)

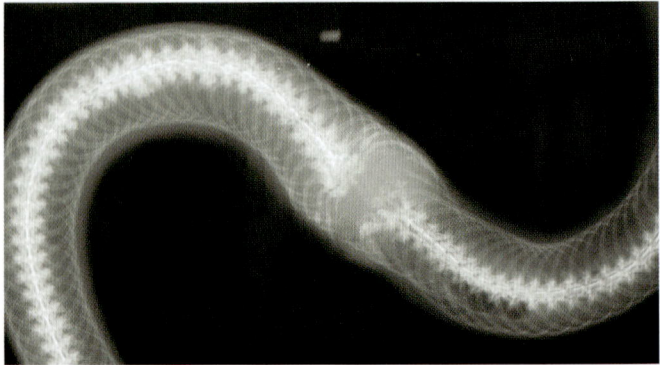

FIG 77.30 A chronic spinal fracture associated with osteolysis is seen on radiographs of this ball python (*Python regius*). (Courtesy of Joerg Mayer.)

compartments. Timely surgical intervention is important to allow for maximal recovery. The objectives for surgical management of spinal trauma are decompression, realignment, and stabilization. The decompressive procedure should be conservative so as not to disrupt further the integrity of the vertebrae but large enough to allow for removal of compressive material. Successful outcome after surgical fixation depends on the type and strength of fixation, the surgeon's skill and knowledge of the spinal anatomy, and the accuracy of vertebral column alignment (which becomes increasingly difficult as patient size decreases). Surgical fixation of a vertebral fracture has been reported in a coastal taipan (*Oxyuranus scutellatus*), and attempts to surgically decompress vertebral disc material to treat cervical subluxation and compressive myelopathy have been performed in Komodo dragons.[41,92]

Careful attention to postoperative care is imperative for the well-being of the patient.[93] Potential complications include cloacitis, urine/fecal retention, urinary tract infections, decubital ulcers, and implant failure. Physical rehabilitation is important in the recovery process (see Chapter 131).

The prognosis for animals with acute spinal injury is dependent on the results of the neurological examination. The prognosis for recovery from a spinal fracture or luxation that results in paraplegia with loss of nociception is considered poor. Patients that maintain pain perception may still require months to recover and have residual neurological deficits, including urinary and/or fecal incontinence.

The prognosis may be better in some reptiles than in mammals due to the documented neurogenesis that occurs within the cord following injury.[94] However, it has been reported that following spinal cord injury in a snake, the cord is repaired by ingrowth of connective tissue, and nerve fibers do not regenerate.[1] The clinical impact of spinal neuronal regeneration in some injured reptiles is currently unknown. Even with complete spinal transection, some reptiles may still exhibit coordinated hind limb movements, and as long as they are able to ambulate, urinate, and defecate, quality of life is often acceptable.

Peripheral Nerve Injury. Trauma to the soft tissues of the limbs or fractures of the extremities can injure peripheral nerves, which may just affect the function of one limb (monoparesis/monoplegia). This can also occur with any trauma that causes traction or stretching of the peripheral nerves. Paraparesis due to bilateral peripheral nerve injury occurs in reptiles, especially chelonians, with dystocia, presumably as a result of nerve compression.[1] A history of forelimb monoparesis after a traumatic incident should raise a high suspicion of brachial plexus avulsion (Fig. 77.31). Every animal unable to use one forelimb after

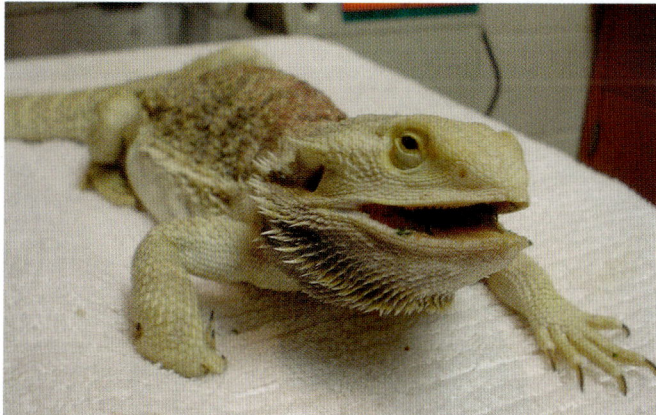

FIG 77.31 Right-sided thoracic limb monoparesis suggestive of brachial plexus nerve injury in a bearded dragon (*Pogona vitticeps*). (Courtesy of Joerg Mayer.)

trauma should be examined carefully to detect orthopedic as well as neurological abnormalities. MRI of the affected plexus may provide information on the degree of nerve and associated soft tissue trauma. Electromyography allows detection of spontaneous electrical activity in the denervated muscles 7 to 10 days after the injury. Nerve conduction velocity studies of the radial and ulnar nerves allow determination of the degree of injury. Since the radial nerve is commonly injured in brachial plexus avulsions, serial electrodiagnostic evaluations of this nerve may provide useful diagnostic and prognostic information.

Treatment of acute peripheral nerve trauma is primarily supportive. Unfortunately, there is no routinely effective treatment for this type of injury. The degree of recovery depends only on the severity of the nerve lesion at the time of injury. In mammals, if nociception is present in the medial and lateral digits, prognosis for recovery is good and aggressive physiotherapy should be recommended. If nociception is absent, prognosis will depend on the severity of the axonal injury, being good for neurapraxic lesions but guarded to poor for axonotmetic (nerve injury to axon while sparing the myelin) and neurotmetic (disruption of axon, myelin sheaths, and connective tissue) lesions. Pure axonotmesis occurs rarely, so the potential for recovery, although present, is low and prognosis poor.

When the proximal branches of the radial and musculocutaneous nerves are spared—so that the elbow flexor and extensor muscles are not denervated—corrective surgery can be used to provide carpal extension and prevent the distal part of the limb from collapsing. Tendon transplantation or carpal arthrodesis procedures could be considered in larger lizards.

Animals with caudal and complete brachial plexus avulsions have a poor to guarded prognosis if neurotmesis has occurred. Only those with neurapraxic (temporary loss of sensory and motor function due to nerve injury) injuries show improvement and recover completely. However, most animals do not improve but go on to show severe limb atrophy, eventually developing serious complications such as trophic ulcers, joint contractures, limb trauma due to loss of control and secondary environmental injury, or abnormal sensation in the affected areas produced by regeneration of sensory nerves. In these cases, amputation of the limb is necessary. The best predictor of complete recovery seems to be nociception. Preservation of nociception is an indicator of a milder type of injury and should prompt the clinician to recommend supportive therapy while waiting for motor function to recover. However, if no improvement is seen during the first 3 to 6 months, recovery is unlikely to occur.

Vascular Diseases and Circulatory Disturbances

Gout may cause neurological dysfunction due to circulatory abnormalities and directly by the formation of tophi within nervous tissue. A decrease in blood flow to the central nervous system as a result of gout may result in neurological signs.[1]

Granulocytic leukemia in a gopher snake (*Pituophis melanoleucus*) at the San Francisco Zoo caused thrombus formation and infarction of the spinal cord. The patient showed paralysis caudal to the site of the infarction, which was identified histologically.[1]

Metabolic Diseases

Xanthomatosis. Xanthomatosis has been reported in captive female leaf-tailed Geckos (*Uroplatus henkeli*) with hydrocephalus secondary to obstruction caused by a brain xanthoma.[1,95] Clinical signs of brain xanthomas, also reported in snakes and water dragons, include opisthotonus, torticollis, dorsal recumbency, and seizures.[1,95–98] Xanthomas are cholesterol-laden granules that develop in various organs and are thought to be caused by hypercholesterolemia and hyperlipidemia.[14] Xanthomatosis is suspected to be frequently accompanied and exacerbated by renal disease. Metabolic derangements associated with hyperuricemia, hypercholesterolemia, and hyperlipidemia are suspected in cases of xanthomatosis. A dietary correlation is suspected but currently unable to be identified.[14] Most cases occur in females, and the condition is thought to be exacerbated by folliculogenesis, follicular degeneration, and yolk coelomitis. By the time animals are seen with neurological signs, they appear to be unresponsive to supportive care.

Freeze Damage.   This condition is most commonly observed in tortoises coming out of brumation (hibernation).[1] The cause is unknown but may be related to water crystals forming in neurological tissue. Additional predisposing factors may include hepatic lipidosis or sepsis and micro-abscessation within the brain. Clinical signs include circling, head tilt, and blindness with hyphema. Ocular lesions include lenticular change and retinal damage. These lesions may improve with vitamin A supplementation.[1] Many cases improve clinically with time; however, a head tilt usually does not resolve.

Hypoglycemia.   A syndrome caused by hypoglycemia that appears to be stress induced has been reported in crocodilians.[1] Clinical signs include muscle tremors, loss of righting reflex, and mydriasis. The pathophysiology of this syndrome is unknown. Animals respond to oral glucose administered at 3 g/kg and elimination of the stress-inducing factor.[29]

Hepatic Encephalopathy.   Reptiles with hepatic disease may show a wide variety of clinical signs. Lethargy, chronic anorexia, weight loss, and gastrointestinal and neurological signs are common. The last stage of liver disease often results in hepatic encephalopathy (HE).[99] Clinical signs of HE are extremely variable (e.g., circling, weakness, ataxia, ptyalism, seizures, and coma). The pathophysiology of HE is not completely understood, but there is a proposed synergistic effect involving liver failure and ammonia detoxification, increased cerebral inflammatory proteins, impaired brain perfusion with development of astrocytic swelling, and neuronal edema.[99]

Hematology of the HE-affected patient often shows anemia, heterophilia, and monocytosis. Biochemistries frequently reveal high values of aspartate aminotransferase, gamma glutamyltransferase, alkaline phosphatase, alanine aminotransferase, and lactate dehydrogenase, but none of these analytes are truly liver-specific enzymes in reptiles. Bile acids may eventually prove to be a promising hepatic marker.[99]

Diagnostic imaging techniques are also clinically useful to detect changes in size or appearance of the liver. An endoscopically obtained tissue biopsy sample is considered as a useful diagnostic tool.[99] Prognosis of the patient exhibiting clinical signs of HE is guarded at best. Recommended treatment for snakes that are diagnosed with HE involves fluid administration (avoidance of solutions that contain lactate), along with more specific hepatic therapeutic agents. Carnitine (250 mL/kg orally) is a derivate of the amino acid lysine, which is involved in the transport of the acetyl coenzyme A through the cellular membrane of the hepatocyte. Lactulose is commonly used in treating hyperammonemia, which is believed to be one of the underlying causes of HE. Lactulose (0.5 mL/kg orally) is fermented by the gut flora into metabolites that acidify the colon. An acidic environment turns freely diffusible ammonia (NH_3) into ammonium (NH_4^+), which can no longer be absorbed.[99] Silymarin (milk thistle) has a long history of use in the treatment of liver disease, predominantly in controlling inflammation and limiting uptake of toxins. In the human patient, silymarin exerts membrane stabilizing and antioxidant activity and promotes hepatocyte regeneration; furthermore, it reduces the inflammatory reaction and inhibits fibrogenesis in the liver.[100] The use of silymarin to treat HE in reptiles appears to be promising. Antioxidants, such as SAMe and vitamin E, may also be

beneficial, and as no reptile-specific doses have been produced, allometric calculation from mammalian doses may be appropriate (see Chapter 67 for more details).

Congenital Diseases

Congenital neuropathies in reptiles are frequently associated with poor maternal and sometimes paternal husbandry or improper gestational incubation conditions. Most embryonic neuropathies lead to an early fetal or neonatal death.

Caudal Coiling Syndrome.   Congenital neuropathic anomalies reported in snakes include axial bifurcation, kyphosis, and fusion of adjacent coils.[1] (Fig. 77.32). A congenital neurological condition exists in newborn boa constrictors that grossly appears like a vertebral malformation. Though the vertebrae are normal, these snakes appear to have kyphosis, scoliosis, or lordosis. Affected snakes are seen with single to multiple coils of their spine, compromised locomotion, abnormal posturing, and anorexia. The condition frequently affects only the caudal half of the snake and has been termed "caudal coiling syndrome."[14] Radiographically, the vertebral bodies themselves appear to be normal and not the cause of the condition. When anesthetized, the snake's body is able to be manually stretched and uncoiled. The condition can be a cause of acute mortality in neonates or a chronic debilitating syndrome in juveniles. Affected animals have shown no response to assist-feeding and supportive care, ultimately progressing and succumbing to the disease. The unaffected portions of the snake's body appear to function normally, and normal voluntary muscle contractions are observed as the snake attempts to drag its disfigured body. The disorder does not appear to involve the brain or CNS, and structures caudal to the lesion maintain sensory and motor function.

Necropsy examination confirms the radiographic findings; no gross abnormalities of the vertebrae are identified. Histologically, the dorsal epaxial musculature contains multiple leukocytic infiltrates surrounding the nerves and vessels within the perimysium.[1] Potential causes of this condition include infectious agents, an inflammatory process, neoplasia, and improper incubation conditions. All attempts to culture or isolate an infectious organism have been unsuccessful, and the husbandry associated with the gestation of the neonates is reportedly appropriate.[1] Further investigations into the cause of this condition are indicated.

Toxicities

Information on toxins that adversely affect reptile species usually originates from case reports, and so the true risks of the various toxins to different reptile species can be difficult to determine.[14] However, with the development of animal poison hotlines and the efforts of the

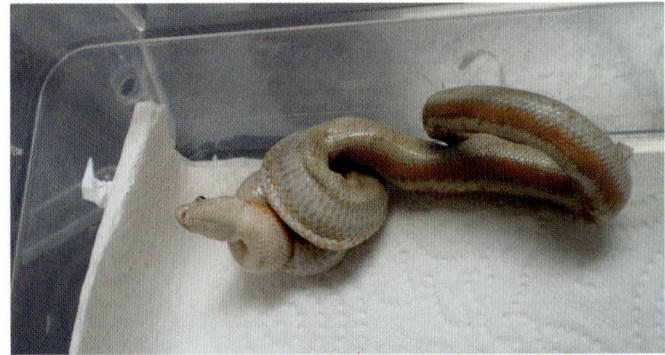

FIG 77.32 Congenital coiling deformity in a rosy boa (*Lichanura trivirgata*). (Reproduced with permission by Hedley J. Neurologic diseases of birds and reptiles. *J Exot Pet Med.* 2015;24;6–20.)

American Board of Veterinary Toxicology, the knowledge of poisonings in reptiles has blossomed significantly (see Chapter 88 for more details).[101]

Chlorhexidine.

There are reports of 0.024% chlorhexidine solution as a topical medication or soaking solution in reptiles with cutaneous disease.[1] At this concentration, the agent appears to be safe. However, the use of the 2% stock solution as a therapeutic bath has caused acute neurological disease and death in reptiles. Chelonians appear to be extremely sensitive to the toxic effects of the solution.[101]

Clinical signs include acute flaccid paralysis and progress to loss of the righting reflexes and diminished withdrawal reflexes. Signs do not resolve, and death from neurological and respiratory collapse readily ensues.

Insecticides.

Reptiles appear to be especially sensitive to insecticide toxicosis.[101] Birds are reportedly 10 to 20 times more sensitive to insecticides than mammals, and reptiles appear to be more sensitive than birds.[1] Many forms of insecticides, including sprays, powders, and pesticide strips, have been used to control external parasite problems in reptiles. Their use may result in neurological signs.[1]

Organophosphates are the most commonly used insecticides worldwide. This group of insecticides includes chlorpyrifos (Dursban), dichlorvos (Vapona, No-Pest), diazinon, cythioate (Proban), fenthion (ProSpot), malathion, ronnel, parathion, and metrifonate.[101] The closely related carbamates include aldicarb, carbaryl (Sevin), bendiocarb, methiocarb, propoxur, and carbofuran. As newer, safer insecticides are marketed, these two groups are involved in fewer accidental poisonings, but they still account for a large number of intoxications.[101]

Organophosphates and carbamates interfere with metabolism and breakdown of acetylcholine at synaptic junctions. Acetylcholinesterase is the enzyme responsible for breaking down the neurotransmitter at these sites. Acetylcholinesterase is inhibited by organophosphates and carbamates at these cholinergic sites. As a result, acetylcholine accumulates at the synapses, first exciting and then paralyzing transmission in these synapses.[101] This inhibition of the synapse is irreversible with organophosphates but is reversible with carbamates. Organophosphates are readily absorbed by all routes: dermal, respiratory, gastrointestinal, and conjunctival. Overdose with organophosphates may happen more readily if they are given together with imidothiazoles, such as levamisole.[101] Neurological signs can be autonomic (bronchospasm, bronchosecretion, lacrimation, diarrhea), neuromuscular (weakness, tremors, muscle fasciculations), or CNS related (seizures, depression).

Pyrethrin is the oldest used botanical insecticide originating from *Chrysanthemum cinerariifolium*. Pyrethroids are synthetic derivatives of pyrethrin and are widely available.[101] Pyrethroid insecticides have enhanced stability, potency, and half-life compared with the parent molecule. A variety of dilute pyrethrin- and pyrethroid-containing sprays have been recommended for reptiles, and one is even licensed for reptiles in the United States (Provent-A-Mite).[102] Pyrethrins and pyrethroids have the same mechanism of action. These molecules affect parasites by altering the activity of the sodium ion channels of nerves. These poisons prolong the period of sodium conductance and increase the length of the depolarizing action potential, resulting in repetitive nerve firing and death. With the right conditions or at higher doses, these compounds can intoxicate exposed animals. Because of the potential for transcutaneous absorption, pyrethrin and pyrethroid sprays must be thoroughly rinsed from the animal immediately after their application.[101] Rinsing with lukewarm water usually is sufficient. Clinical signs have been reported for pyrethrins and pyrethroids, particularly with the use of sprays that also contain insect growth regulators (e.g., methoprene).[101] Signs can develop in animals within 15 minutes of application and include salivation, ataxia, inability to right themselves, and muscle fasciculation;[103] the reptile's body temperature can influence the sensitivity to toxicity.[104] Idiosyncratic reactions to pyrethrins can happen at much lower doses than expected. If caught early enough, treatment for pyrethrin and pyrethroid toxicity involves dermal decontamination (bathing in copious amounts of water), isotonic fluids, and diazepam for tremors and seizures.[101] Care must be taken to keep pyrethrin and pyrethroid sprays away from the reptile's eyes and mouth to prevent intoxication. The prognosis depends on the strength of the agent used, the duration of the exposure, and the size of the animal involved.

Ivermectin.

Ivermectin is a macrocyclic lactone derived from *Streptomyces avermitilis*, which acts at gamma-aminobutyric acid (GABA) synapses to stimulate excess release of GABA.[17] In nematodes, GABA is an inhibitory neurotransmitter. It binds irreversibly to the receptors, thus requiring that it be metabolized before its effects diminish. In most mammals, unless there is ap-glycoprotein abnormality, ivermectin is not able to cross the blood-brain barrier and therefore shows no effect. Ivermectin has been used successfully in a variety of reptilian species; however, it appears to be toxic primarily in chelonians, with crocodilians, lizards, and snakes also occasionally affected.[14,16,17] Ball pythons (*Python regius*), in particular, may show mild neurological signs when treated.[101] Ivermectin has been postulated as able to cross the blood-brain barrier in chelonians, or GABA may be a more important peripheral neurotransmitter in chelonians.[17]

Clinical signs associated with ivermectin intoxication are primarily related to general neuromuscular weakness.[14] Death is a function of paralysis of the respiratory muscles. Some variation appears in species susceptibility, and leopard tortoises (*Stigmochelys pardalis*) are especially sensitive, with paresis occurring at a dose as low as 0.025 mg/kg.[17] Because ivermectin binds irreversibly, it takes at least 7 days for reversal of clinical signs. Further, a cumulative effect may be observed if the drug is administered at frequent intervals. Treatment is primarily supportive, with particular attention paid to the respiratory, hydration, and nutritional status. Most animals need ventilatory support for several days. In general, the use of ivermectin in chelonians is contraindicated.[1,101]

Milbemycin is safe and effective for use in some chelonians.[1] This agent is related to and acts similar to ivermectin on the GABA receptors and was effective in red-eared sliders (*Trachemys scripta elegans*), Gulf Coast box turtles (*Terrepene carolina major*), and ornate box turtles (*Terrepene ornata*).[1] No toxic side effects have been observed, but the drug has not been evaluated in all chelonians. Milbemycin was effective at 0.5 to 1 mg/kg subcutaneously.

Antimicrobials.

Metronidazole is an antibiotic and antiprotozoal agent commonly used in reptile medicine. The half-life of metronidazole in iguanas is longer (12.7 +/- 3.7 hours) than that reported for mammalian species (dogs, 4–5 hrs; humans, 6–10 hrs).[1] At high doses, metronidazole may induce clinical signs of vestibular disease with head tilt, circling, and dysequilibrium[101] (Fig. 77.33). In snakes, severe neurological signs and death have been associated with administration of metronidazole above 100 mg/kg.[1,14] Treatment is supportive and clinical signs are reversible.

Polymyxin and the aminoglycocides (streptomycin, kanamycin, gentamicin, and neomycin) at high doses cause neuromuscular blockade and may induce neurological signs such as paralysis.[1]

Heavy Metal Intoxication.

Plumbism was diagnosed in a tortoise after ingestion of lead-based paint chips.[1] Diagnosis was made on the basis of clinical signs of generalized central nervous system disease and

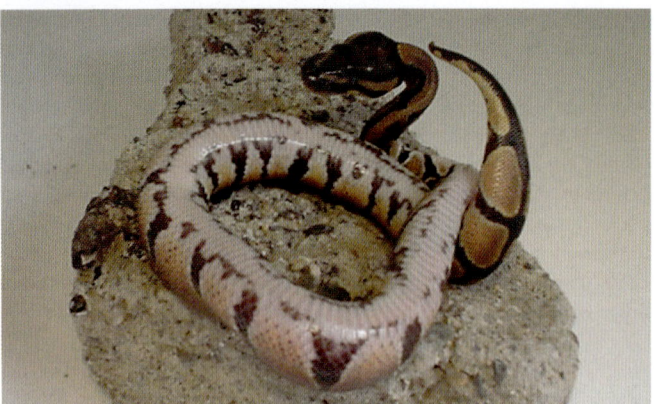

FIG 77.33 Metronidazole toxicity resulting in a loss of righting in this ball python (*Python regius*).

supported by high blood lead levels. Blood samples from a control animal must be submitted for comparison purposes. Treatment should involve eliminating the lead from the gastrointestinal system with gastric lavage and catharsis in conjunction with calcium ethylenediamine tetraacetic acid therapy at 10 to 40 mg/kg intramuscularly twice a day.

Apparent zinc toxicity was observed in a green iguana (*Iguana iguana*) that had ingested pennies.[1] The patient was seen with anorexia, weakness, and anemia. Blood zinc levels were elevated compared with normal ranges published for other species. The iguana recovered uneventfully after chelation therapy and surgical removal of the pennies from the cecum.

Bromethalin. Bromethalin is one of the newer rodenticides. It is formulated in baits of pelleted grain and may be dyed green or turquoise. Bromethalin is a neurotoxin, but because of its name it can be confused with the long-acting anticoagulants bromadiolone and brodifacoum. Clients should be encouraged to bring in original containers to obtain valuable label information concerning ingredients.[101] The mechanism of action of bromethalin is the uncoupling of oxidative phosphorylation. The brain is the primary target for bromethalin because of its unique dependence on oxidative phosphorylation. The drug causes brain electrolyte disturbances and results in the development of cerebral edema.[101] Clinical signs include hind-limb paralysis, abnormal postures, fine muscle tremors, and seizures. Severely poisoned animals are comatose. Clinical signs are usually seen within 24 hrs of ingestion. Bromethalin is a nonselective vertebrate poison. No antidote exists, and treatment is directed initially at reducing gastrointestinal absorption and providing supportive care. Treatment also must aim at controlling cerebral edema seen in severe poisonings. Administration of dexamethasone and mannitol has been recommended to control bromethalin-induced cerebral edema. Unfortunately these agents are not very effective in controlling bromethalin-poisoned animals. Animals showing severe signs, such as seizures, paralysis, or coma, generally have a grave prognosis.[101]

Other Toxins. A variety of other environmental agents are potentially toxic to reptiles and amphibians, including iodoforms, nicotine, naphthalene, paraffin, and paint solvents.[1] Sometimes toxicity can only be suspected even after extensive investigations. An example of this situation is described in a report on loggerhead sea turtles presenting with neurological dysfunction in south Florida.[105] Despite a heavy spirorchiid

parasitism existing in these turtles, a chronic exposure to a novel toxin in the diet was suspected. Similarly, severe neurological signs in a group of Australian water dragons (*Physignathus lesueurii*) with encephalomalacia was suspected to be due to a toxic etiology, although a viral infection could not be excluded.[49]

Wood shavings with high resin content such as cedar shavings may cause a reversible ataxia. Ingestion of fireflies of the genus *Photinus* is lethal to inland bearded dragons.[1] These fireflies contain lucibufagins, a steroidal pyrone, and ingestion of one insect is enough to be fatal to an adult bearded dragon. The toxin is actually thought to be cardiotoxic, but affected animals show signs of focal facial seizures, violent head shaking, mouth gaping, and protrusion and biting of the tongue. Although fireflies have been shown to be nontoxic in certain lizards, it is recommended not to use fireflies as food items.

Neoplasia

Neoplasia affecting the nervous system is uncommon in reptiles, but brain and spinal cord cancers have been described.[14,106,107] Pituitary adenomas have been reported in multiple snake species with clinical signs of brain dysfunction becoming evident in the late stages of the disease.[14] Advanced imaging techniques such as MRI are necessary to detect CNS neoplasia antemortem.

A 22-year-old red-tailed boa constrictor was evaluated for neurological abnormalities, including cervical weakness and right-sided optical and thermal blindness.[107] Magnetic resonance imaging (MRI) with the use of both a 7-T research unit and a 1.5-T clinical unit was performed and confirmed the diagnosis of a large mass within the diencephalon and mesencephalon causing hydrocephalus and asymmetry of the lateral ventricles. Necropsy and histopathology confirmed the presence of an intracranial mass likely to have an ependymal or astrocytic origin based on immunoreactivity of neoplastic cells to glial fibrillary acidic protein.[107]

CONCLUSION

Much remains to be learned about neurological diseases of captive reptiles. In many instances, neurological manifestations are caused by improper husbandry, trauma, or infectious disease. Clinical signs associated with neurological disease in reptiles are often nonspecific, and localization of the site of the lesion and the etiology may be difficult. Evaluating the patient for known causes of neurological dysfunction helps the clinician develop a diagnostic and therapeutic plan appropriate for the species. A complete diagnostic evaluation both antemortem and postmortem is vital especially in treatment of animals within a collection.

ACKNOWLEDGMENTS

The author would like to thank Drs. R.A. Bennett and S.J. Mehler for permission to use some of the material previously published in the last edition of this textbook. The author would also like to thank Dr. Izidora Sladakovic, Kelsey Weeks, Thomas Campbell, Clark Broughton, Shelbe Harry, and Ashley Mcgaha for assistance in photographing the normal neurological examination and loaning their pets for this purpose.

REFERENCES

See www.expertconsult.com for a complete list of references.

78

Oncology

Joerg Mayer and Antony S. Moore

While some of the earliest evidence of cancer in humans dates back to the time 2000 BC,[1] some of the earliest recorded cases date back 70 million years.[2] It is not surprising then to realize that cancer can affect even the most primitive animals such as corals.[3] Contrary to older beliefs, which suggested that cancers are rare in reptiles, more systematic analysis and longitudinal studies have noted that cancers in reptiles have an overall prevalence of 9.8%.[4]

In veterinary oncology, quality of life for the patient is always the top priority. Some cancers can be cured by treatments compatible with good quality of life. In other cases, anticancer treatment may significantly extend good quality survival time even if the patient is not permanently cured. However, for other patients, palliation may be a more appropriate goal, and because it delays the need for euthanasia, effective palliation can significantly enhance survival time as well as quality of life in veterinary medicine. Even in those cases where hospice care or euthanasia is the best option, performing this with compassion and skill can be one of the most valuable services a veterinarian can provide to help both patient and client.

As a subspecialty, oncology is increasingly important in veterinary practice, as client demand for advanced cancer care increases. To meet that need, the treatment of cancer in pets has evolved to parallel treatment in humans, with certain differences. One of the most important differences is in the goal of therapy. In humans, many cancers are cured, and cancer survivors may enjoy many decades of comfortable life. For this reason, treatment of cancer in humans is aggressive and often associated with severe side effects. On the other hand, most pet owners prefer to avoid severe side effects and prolonged hospitalization for quality of life reasons. In addition, the intense, specialized supportive care units and strategies for human cancer patients are not available for pets even in private practice specialty centers and university veterinary hospitals. Therapies are therefore primarily directed at maximizing quality of life, and the aim is often tumor control, or remission, rather than cure at any cost. "Remission" means partial or complete reduction of any outward evidence of cancer on examination or routine laboratory analyses and imaging (i.e., radiography, ultrasonography, CT, MRI), and relief of any clinical signs, making the pet appear as normal as possible. It is important for the veterinarian to inform the owner of the differing goals for cancer therapy in pets with cancer; that is, that the treatment (including surgery) should not cause the patient what is considered undue toxicity, as defined by the veterinarian and the owner. For some owners this definition may be *any* loss of quality of life, for others it may be hospitalization. In either situation the veterinarian should establish the goals of therapy in advance of starting treatment. If owners understand that quality of life will take precedence in their pets' treatment, they are more likely to trust the veterinarian and to treat their pets. It is important to recognize that although a pet's cancer may not be curable, he or she can enjoy a high quality of life. In this sense cancer is similar to other chronic illnesses such as nephrosis or cardiomyopathy, which can often be controlled providing a high quality of life, although they may not be curable.

DIAGNOSIS

The finding of a mass on any species does not immediately mean the lesion is neoplastic (Fig. 78.1), and without a histologic or cytologic confirmation of the neoplasia appropriate management is not possible. This is particularly true of reptiles. Due to the slow metabolic rate, a slow-growing mass can actually be an abscess or a granuloma. If such a process is suspected, biopsy material should be processed for bacterial and/or fungal culture and sensitivity, as well as histology. Some parasites, such as plerocercoids, larval dracunculids, acanthocephalans, cryptosporidiosis, and spiruroids, can mimic tumors. Other conditions associated with poor husbandry, such as steatitis, or infectious stomatitis, may also mimic neoplastic diseases (Fig. 78.2). Being able to obtain diagnostic samples and establish definitive diagnoses are crucial to developing an effective treatment plan. Therefore identifying veterinary pathologists that excel in zoologic/oncologic pathology is a major priority. The two main areas of pathology important in cancer diagnostics are

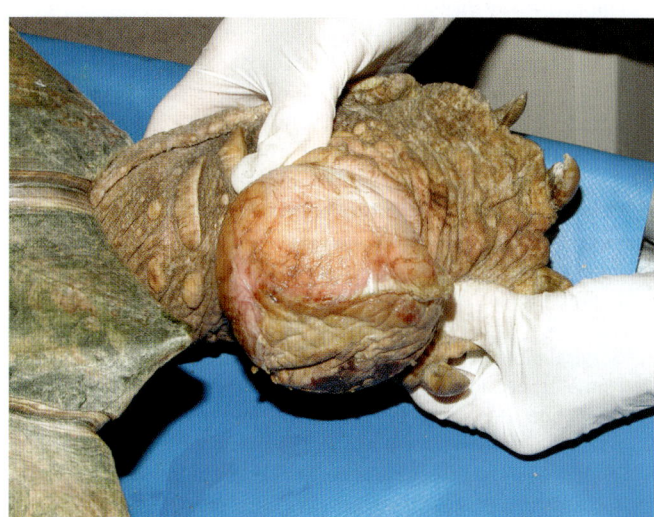

FIG 78.1 An alligator snapping turtle *(Macrochelys temminckii)*, 56.8 kg (125 lb), with a fibroid mass on the plantar surface of the hind foot is caused by a rough concrete surface and an enclosure too small for the size of the turtle. Reptiles commonly have large tissue reactions that mimic neoplasia development. (Courtesy of Stephen Barten.)

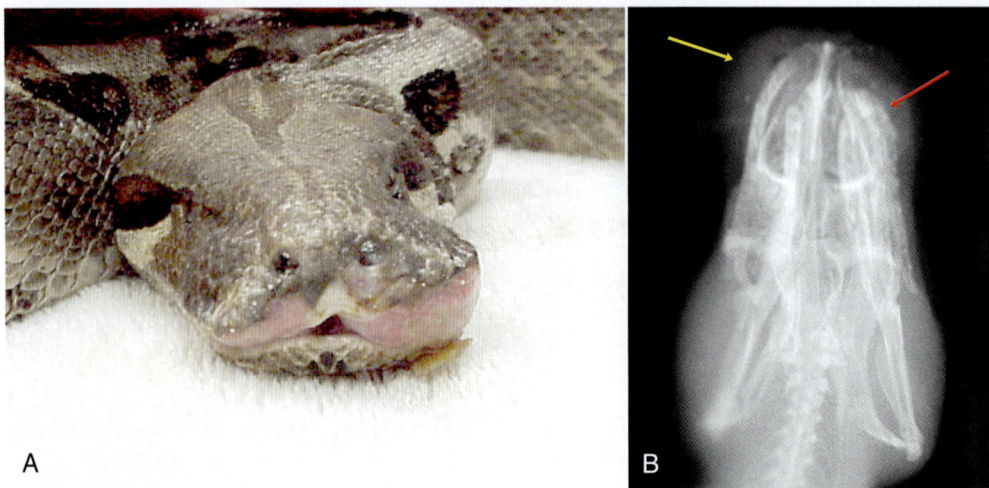

FIG 78.2 (A) A red tailed boa *(Boa constrictor)* with chronic infectious stomatitis. (B) The granulomatous tissue, which is secondary to infection and inflammation, has grossly disfigured the maxillary region (yellow arrow). The inflamed tissue on the lower jaw has displaced the mandible medially. Diagnosis in presentations like these can be difficult but ultimately depends on biopsy with microbiologic testing. (Courtesy of L. Pace.)

cytopathology and histopathology. Cytopathologists are specialists at examining individual cells obtained by fine-needle aspirate or impression smear to determine the identity of a disease process. Histopathologists examine intact tissue samples and associated architecture to determine the underlying pathologic process.

Choosing either diagnostic modality, or both, to apply in a given reptile with cancer depends on the individual case variables. Some of the advantages and disadvantages of cytopathology compared to histopathology include:

- Cytopathology samples of peripheral tissues can be easily obtained preoperatively, often without general anesthesia and sometimes even without sedation, and can be used to screen patients for more comprehensive diagnostics.
- Fine-needle aspiration cytology is less costly than surgical biopsy in both sample collection and laboratory analysis.
- The procedure of fine-needle aspiration is less likely to result in adverse effects when compared to tissue biopsy.
- Cytopathology requires less sample processing than histopathology and thus provides earlier results than histopathology.
- Cytopathology is more difficult to interpret and more prone to sample damage and "non-diagnostic" results.
- Surgical biopsy is generally more accurate and more representative of the entire tissue of concern than fine-needle aspiration cytology.
- Surgical biopsy provides information on tissue architecture, which cannot be obtained from cytological specimens. In some neoplasms evaluation of tissue architecture/tissue invasion is essential to differentiate between benign and malignant neoplasms.
- The relatively large tissue sample provided by biopsy enables further specialized testing such as histochemistry (special stains), immunohistochemistry, electron microscopy, and polymerase chain reaction to be performed, if required, to achieve a definitive diagnosis.
- For these reasons histopathology is generally more likely to provide a definitive diagnosis and is preferred; although the "investment" in time, client cost, and invasiveness of sample collection is greater.

A definitive diagnosis will help guide the treatment plan and, with staging, allow an estimate of the prognosis for any given patient. For example, knowing whether a tumor is a benign sebaceous adenoma or a malignant soft tissue sarcoma is extremely important. This is because, even though they may have the same outward appearance, the latter requires an extensive surgical resection and additional staging procedures to determine the extent of disease. In contrast, a benign adenoma may need a simple resection. The methods that the surgeon can use to diagnose the malignant condition or the extent of this disease are needle-core biopsy, punch, incisional biopsy, and excisional biopsy (Figs. 78.3 and 78.4).

A needle-core biopsy can be obtained with a simple needle or with a spring-loaded device (e.g., TruCut) and is primarily useful for externally palpable masses. In many reptiles with a thicker epidermis, it might be wise to cut down to the mass prior to the biopsy procedure. A spring-loaded 14-gauge needle will collect a piece of tissue, about 1 mm wide and 1.0 to 1.5 cm long. If these devices are used on internal masses the procedure should be performed with ultrasound guidance and with the reptile anesthetized; however, iatrogenic trauma and severe hemorrhage are significant risks. An alternative approach is to use endoscopy guidance to collect biopsies from internal lesions; such techniques are well described in the herpetologic literature.[5] Endoscopic biopsies of internal structures are often faster than traditional coeliotomy approaches. Although surgical mass resections can be performed endoscopically in humans and some domesticated animals, they are not routine in reptiles. Endoscopic biopsies should be large, or multiple smaller biopsies should be collected to ensure an accurate histologic diagnosis.

When performing a biopsy, it is important to plan the procedure with future definitive treatment in mind.

1. Needle tracts or biopsy incisions should be placed with careful thought so that the entire biopsy tract can be removed when the definitive surgical procedure is performed.
2. Care should be taken to not distribute cancer cells into surrounding tissues or through tissue planes during the biopsy procedure. For example, care must be taken to avoid the formation of a hematoma or a seroma, because the hematoma or seroma might spread cancer

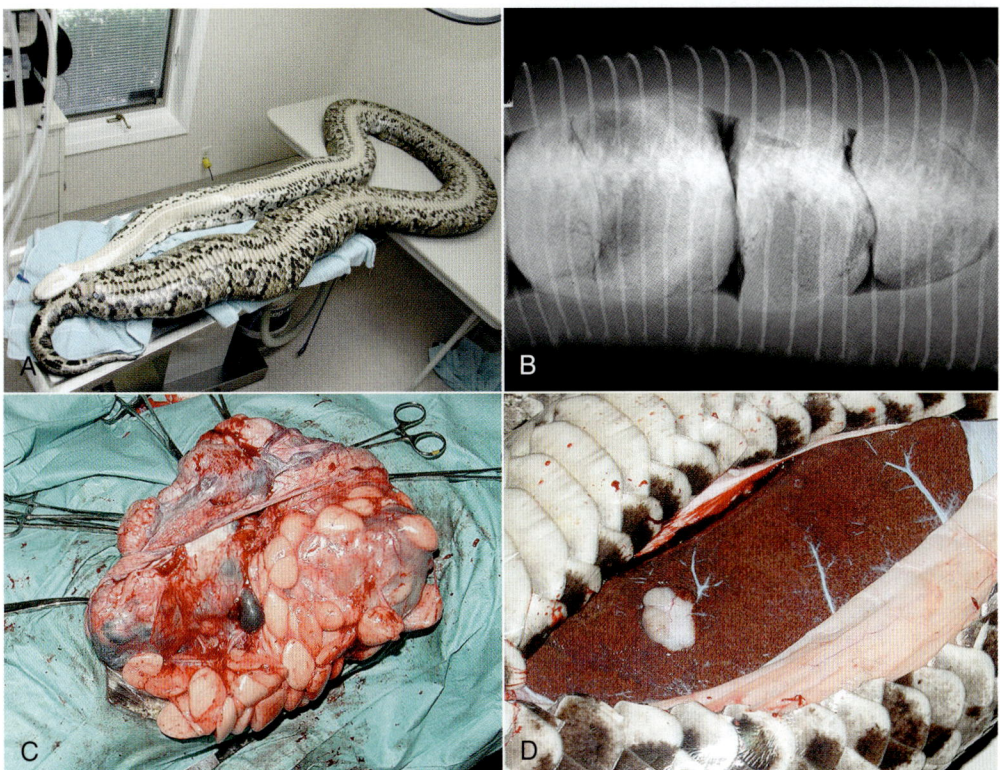

FIG 78.3 (A) A Burmese python *(Python bivittatus)* with renal adenocarcinoma. The snake was 26 years old, 5.56 m (18 ft, 3 inches), and 90 kg (198 lb). It presented for anorexia, weight loss, and a visible caudal coelomic mass. (B) Lateral radiograph of massive chronic constipation caused by gastrointestinal obstruction by a metastatic lesion in the cloaca. (C) This is the primary tumor seen during celiotomy. It obliterates the left kidney and measures 28 × 20 × 20 cm (11 × 8 × 8 inches). Coelomic fat bodies are adhered to the ventral half of the tumor in this view, and the ovduct is adhered as it crosses the middle of the tumor. Virtually no normal kidney tissue remains. (D) A large, pale metastatic lesion is seen in the liver at necropsy. (Photographs courtesy of Stephen Barten.)

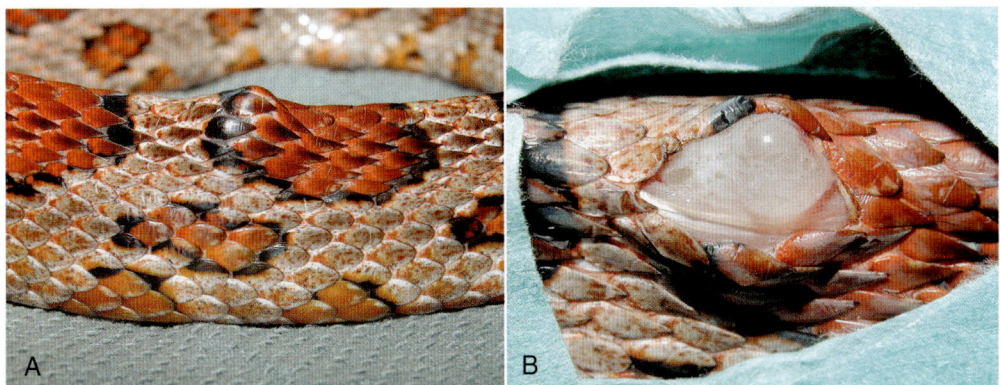

FIG 78.4 (A) A cornsnake *(Pantherophis guttata)*, 12 years old, with a subcutaneous mass. (B) The mass consisted of multilobular cysts filled with clear gelatinous fluid that were nestled between, but not attached to, bands of muscle. Simple surgical incision was used to remove the mass, which was diagnosed as a myxosarcoma. (Photographs courtesy of Stephen Barten.)

cells as it dissects between fascial planes, which would require a more extensive definitive resection. When multiple biopsy specimens are taken from different sites, care should be taken to change instruments so that tumor cells are not transplanted from one site to another by the surgeon (Figs. 78.5 and 78.6).

3. Biopsy techniques should be carefully selected to allow the acquisition of sufficient tissue to make a histopathologic diagnosis. Obtaining multiple biopsy specimens increases the likelihood of an accurate diagnosis if an excisional biopsy is not being planned. Surgical lasers (including CO_2), electrocautery, and 4.0-MHz radiosurgery can

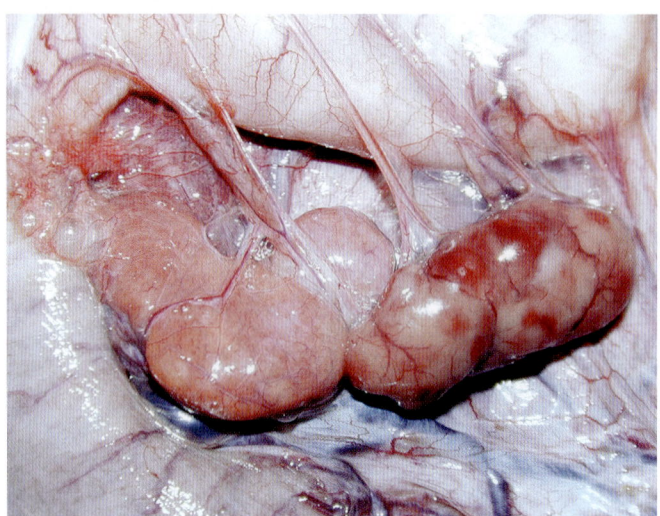

FIG 78.5 A savannah monitor *(Varanus exanthematicus)*, 5 years old, with lymphoma. The lizard presented for anorexia and lethargy. It had a white blood cell count of $100,000 \times 10^3$/uL or $\times 10^9$/L with 97% lymphocytes including young and blast forms. Pronounced hepatomegaly was visible on dorsoventral radiographs and was also confirmed at necropsy. All the parenchymatous organs, such as the pancreas (left) and spleen (right), were grossly enlarged and heavily infiltrated with neoplastic lymphocytes. (Courtesy of Stephen Barten.)

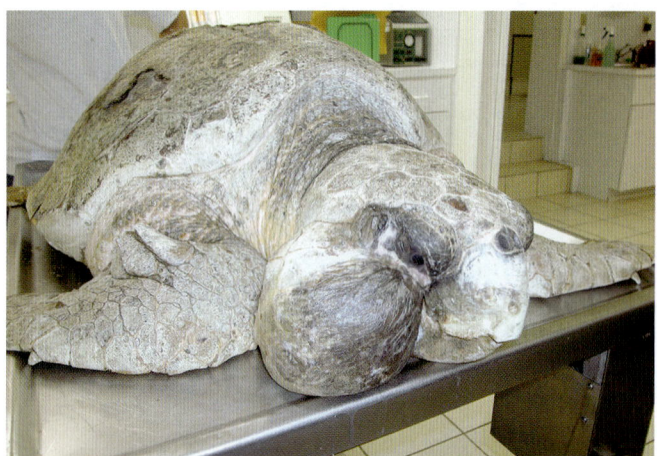

FIG 78.6 An adult loggerhead seaturtle *(Caretta caretta)* with a histiosarcoma effacing the maxillary region below the eye. Similar lesions were noted in the heart, liver, and kidneys on necropsy. (Courtesy of Douglas R. Mader.)

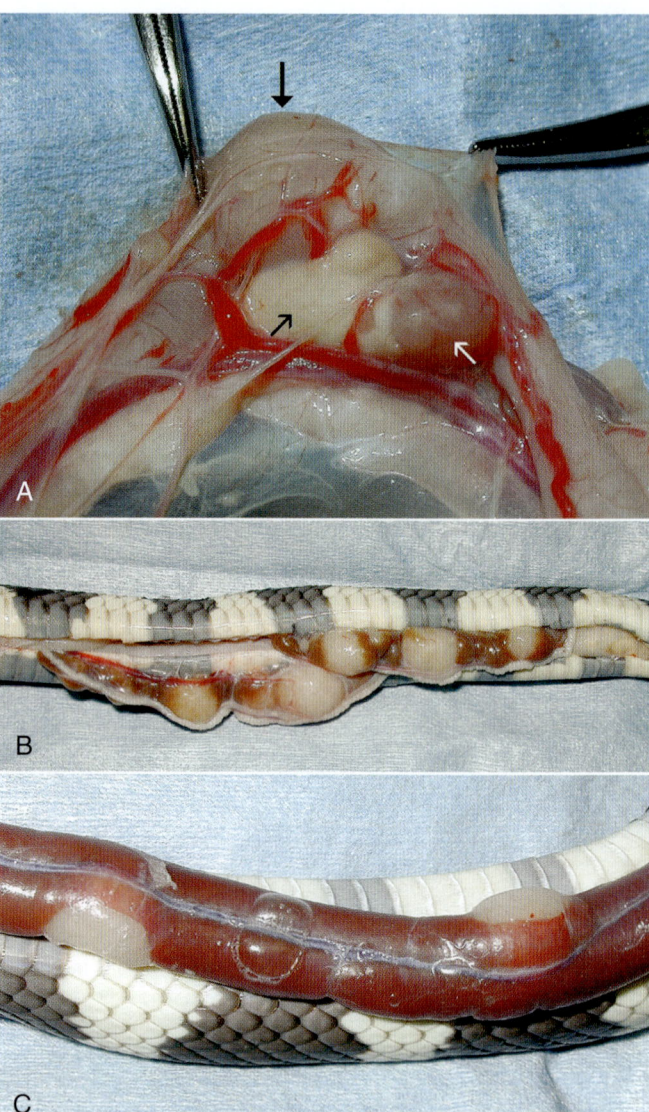

FIG 78.7 (A) The primary neoplastic lesion in this California kingsnake *(Lampropeltis getula californiae)* was an intestinal adenocarcinoma (large black arrow). The light-colored pancreas (small dark arrow) is just ventral to the tumor, and the spleen (white arrow) is to the right. (B) Metastatic lesions are visible throughout both kidneys. (C) Two metastatic lesions are visible in the liver. (Courtesy of Stephen Barten.)

significantly alter tissue, preventing an adequate evaluation of the margins, and may even hinder a diagnosis.[6] In general, such surgical devices should be reserved for controlling hemorrhage following the biopsy procedure but not used for harvesting the biopsy.

4. The biopsy specimen should be handled carefully to prevent crushing, artifact, or alteration of the orientation of the tissue specimen. Submitted tissues should be prepared in such a manner as to allow adequate evaluation of the tissue by the histopathologist using different procedures, such as immunohistochemistry. Specimens should be placed in enough preservative to allow complete fixation (a good rule is 1 part tissue to 10 parts formalin); however, prolonged fixation or storage in formalin may reduce the chances for future successful immunohistochemical staining. Using inked margins or

sutures may give the pathologist information regarding orientation of biopsy tissue within the body, which can be helpful when planning a further procedure for an incompletely excised tumor. Check with your pathologist to determine their preferred method of marking tissue.

5. The surgeon should have an understanding of reptile anatomy and the biologic behavior of malignant conditions to ensure that all possible sites of metastases are evaluated prior to a definitive procedure being performed (Figs. 78.7 and 78.8).

SUITABILITY OF THE PATIENT FOR TREATMENT

When evaluating an animal for treatment of cancer, it is important not only to obtain a definitive diagnosis but also to assess the general health

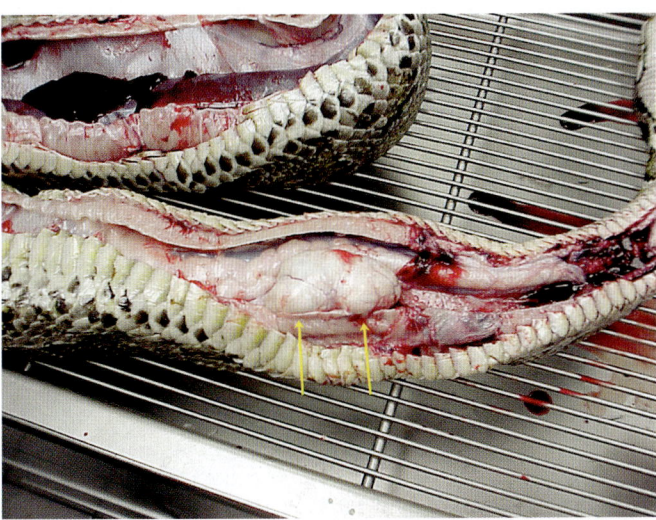

FIG 78.8 This red tailed boa *(Boa constrictor)* presented with a large firm mass firmly attached to the ribs. Necropsy and tissue analysis revealed a chondrosarcoma (between the yellow arrows). (Courtesy of Douglas R. Mader.)

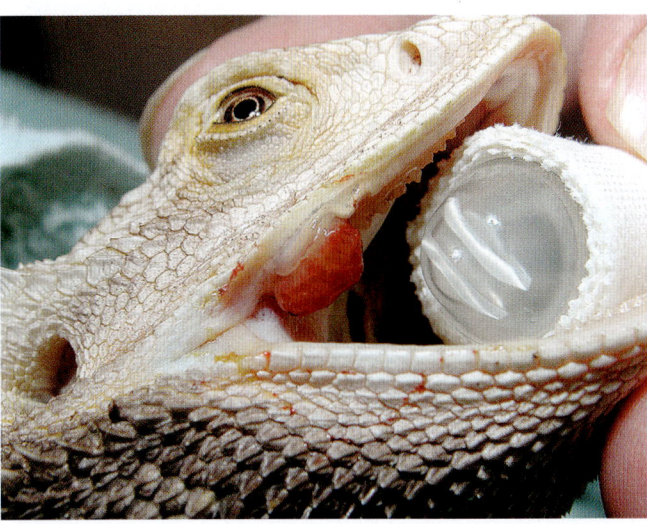

FIG 78.9 A bearded dragon *(Pogona vitticeps)* with a mass arising from the mucocutaneous junction of the right upper lip. Biopsy of the lesion confirmed a nerve-sheath tumor. (Courtesy of Stephen Barten.)

of the patient by clinical examination and ancillary diagnostics. The prognostic information gained by determining the extent of organ involvement with the tumor, as well as identifying unrelated or secondary conditions that need to be treated or controlled before instituting appropriate therapy is mandatory to determine the suitability of a patient for chemotherapy. This information is also vital for individualizing the type and intensity of a treatment regimen. A full diagnostic investigation of the patient is essential due to the stoic and cryptic nature of reptiles and to assess the animal's condition prior to any therapy.

STAGING

Staging is a clinical process that enables the veterinarian to quantitate the extent of cancer involvement in the patient. Staging is sometimes confused with *grading*, which characterizes histopathologic features of the tumor. Staging often carries prognostic significance and enables the veterinarian and client to make informed and rational decisions as to the type of therapy best suited for the patient. In mammalian species, most staging systems are based on an assessment of three major components of the malignant process (TNM): the size of the primary tumor (T), lymph node metastasis (N), and distant metastasis (M). However, because most reptiles lack a well-defined lymphatic system, a modified TM process is more appropriate here.

Most of the information can be obtained from physical examination, but ancillary diagnostics (radiography, ultrasonography) are very important and can often incorporate sophisticated imaging techniques (CT, MRI) (Figs. 78.9, 78.10, and 78.11). Particularly for patients where superimposition of structures hinders interpretation of regular radiographs and access to internal viscera by ultrasonography is limited (e.g., carapace in chelonians), CT may be very helpful and is rapidly becoming established as a primary imaging modality. The value of cross-sectional imaging can be in identifying unsuspected metastatic disease (that can influence the types of treatment being offered and their likelihood of success), or it may allow assessment of resectability of a tumor, which can help in planning surgery. This information may help with a decision not to proceed with surgery based on a poor likelihood of success, allowing the veterinarian and owner to focus on other approaches or

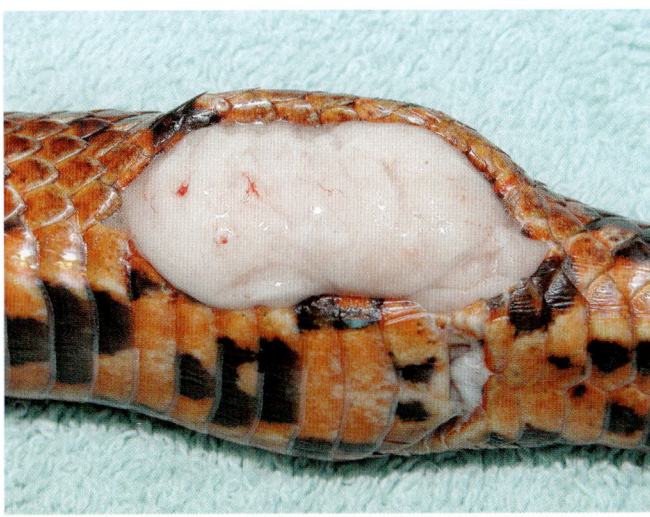

FIG 78.10 Older captive cornsnakes *(Pantherophis guttata)* sometimes have lipomas and liposarcomas can develop. These tumors are usually located subcutaneously on the lateral aspect of the trunk adjacent to and anterior to the cloaca. They may be locally invasive but rarely metastasize. (Courtesy of Stephen Barten.)

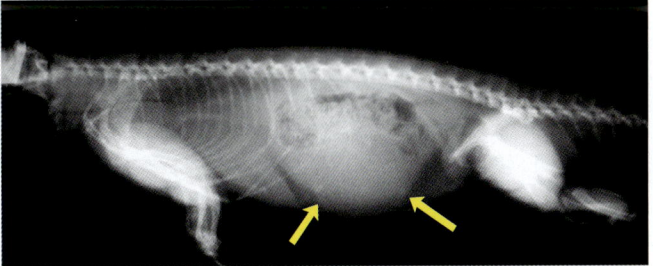

FIG 78.11 This green iguana *(Iguana iguana)* presented with a swollen coelom. The lateral radiograph shows a large circular mass in the caudal coelom. A 7-cm diameter (yellow arrows) mass was removed. The diagnosis was ovarian carcinoma. The contralateral ovary was not removed, and the patient had a complete recovery. (Courtesy of Douglas R. Mader.)

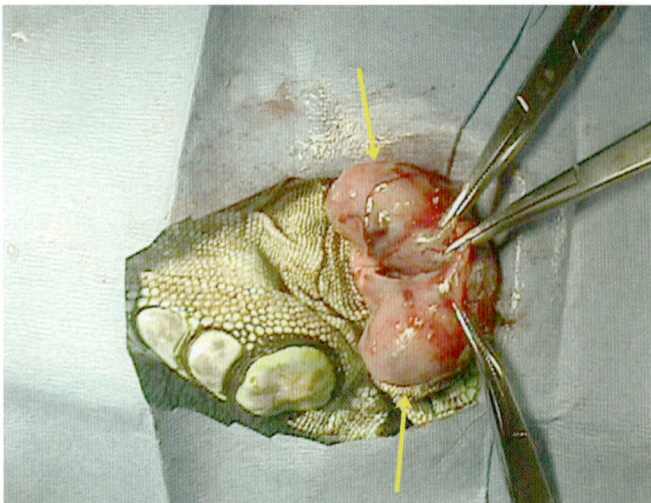

FIG 78.12 Bilateral thyroid adenomas (yellow arrows) in a green iguana *(Iguana iguana)*. (Courtesy of Douglas R. Mader.)

TABLE 78.1	Definitions of Objective Tumor Remissions and Responses Following Anticancer Therapy
Tumor Response	**Criteria**
Complete (CR)*	Disappearance of all evidence of cancer in all sites for a defined period of time (e.g., one intertreatment interval of 3 weeks).
Partial (PR)*	Decrease in size of all tumors by 30% or greater as measured by the sum of the products of two diameters for target lesions. There should be sustained decrease in tumor size, as defined for CR, and no new tumors should arise.
Stable disease (SD)	Decrease of <30% or an increase of <20% in the sum of the products of the target diameters as measured for PR.
Progressive disease (PD)	Increase of 20% or more in the sum of the target diameters *or* the appearance of a new tumor.

*CR + PR = Objective or overall response rate.

palliative strategies. If radiation therapy is available, CT or MRI will allow the treatment field to be defined and the risk for side effects to be reduced or avoided, improving outcomes for the patients.

The majority of patients for whom chemotherapy may have therapeutic benefit will have systemic or metastatic disease that is either physically evident or presumed through historical knowledge of tumor behavior (e.g., osteosarcoma,[7] hemangiosarcoma[8]) (Fig. 78.12).

The likelihood of a successful outcome for a patient treated with chemotherapy is as dependent on drug metabolism and elimination (and drug absorption for orally administered chemotherapy) as it is on the sensitivity of the tumor. This information is severely lacking for reptiles. In addition, information gained during staging (hematology, serum chemistry profile, and urinalysis) may identify problems that will impact the type and dosage of chemotherapy to optimize efficacy while limiting toxicity. For example, hepatic dysfunction may lead to delayed drug elimination (e.g., vinca alkaloids, doxorubicin) and therefore lead to greater toxicity such as myelosuppression. In contrast, cyclophosphamide is activated in the liver, so hepatic dysfunction may result in poor efficacy.

Similarly, renal dysfunction may worsen toxicity for some drugs that are themselves renally toxic. For example, cisplatin should not be used in patients with renal azotemia. Reduced renal excretion of carboplatin will exacerbate myelosuppression. For more details regarding chemotherapy side effects, see Chapter 123.

DESCRIBING THE PROGNOSIS WITH STATISTICS

Some terms that are often used when describing the prognosis for a patient with cancer follow. These are statistical terms and provide a guide as how the population of animals with the same cancer type will respond to treatment; such numbers can never tell you how an individual patient will respond to therapy, and how long they will survive.

The currently used criteria for response assessment by anatomic imaging modalities (World Health Organization [WHO] and response evaluation criteria in solid tumors [RECIST]) are defined in Table 78.1. In RECIST, only 1 to 5 "target lesions" that are greater than 10 mm in the longest dimension (for clinical examination or CT/MRI), or >20 mm (for radiographs or ultrasonography) are measured for response.

TREATMENT

Some private practice specialty centers and university veterinary hospitals are equipped to provide high levels of care to animals with a wide variety of malignancies. For the primary care veterinarian it is important to have resources to provide information that will allow the caregivers to decide between rational, evidence-based treatments that will maximize their pet's quality of life. It is important to remember that every patient can be helped regardless of finances, time, and the specific diagnosis with supportive care, curative treatment, palliative therapy, and hospice care or euthanasia. Furthermore, the veterinarian should provide realistic, honest information in both written form and thorough face-to-face discussions with the owner/caretaker.

In the setting of zoologic practice, that information may need to be extrapolated from similar tumor types in other species and often is based on single case reports or small series of cases. In addition, many reptiles are valuable for their breeding potential, and that may limit the type of treatment and the intensity of treatment for some patients. On the other hand, reptiles can live a long time, and for pets where breeding is less important, there is potential for meaningful outcomes from more aggressive treatment.

Palliative Intent Treatment

For many older veterinary patients, the diagnosis of cancer is obtained at a time when other diseases may limit their long-term survival already. For these patients, palliative care may be most appropriate, and the choice of chemotherapy must be weighed against the risk of toxicity. Such patients may benefit from supportive care and pain relief.

Curative Intent Treatment

For younger patients that are in good health, have no concurrent illnesses, and for which treatment holds the possibility of a long tumor control with little risk of toxicity, curative intent therapy may be undertaken.

Surgery

Surgery is still the modality most likely to cure an animal of cancer if the tumor is localized (not metastasized and not invading into sensitive structures). However, it is not only with curative intent that surgery is

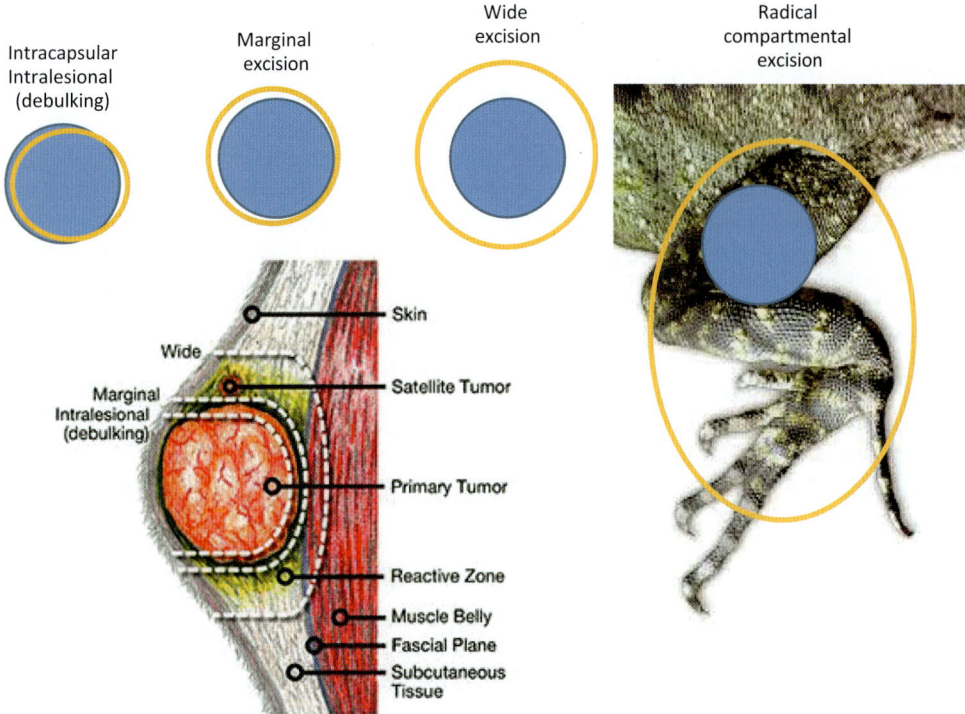

FIG 78.13 Intracapsular/intralesional and marginal surgery are very likely to fail to control a malignancy but can provide palliation for pain or bleeding. Curative intent surgery is preferred whenever anatomically possible, with radical excisional surgery preferred if a more localized curative surgery is not possible. Surgical margins should be confirmed by histopathology, whichever method is chosen.

applied to pets with cancer. Biopsy, debulking, and palliation are achieved through surgery, and each needs to be carefully performed to minimize the impact on the patient's quality of life while still achieving the appropriate goal.

Careful preparation of the patient, as well as anticipation of complications (especially dehiscence), can be as important as the surgery itself in leading to a good outcome for the patient. Fig. 78.13 illustrates the different excisional techniques that could be used to treat cancer in reptilian patients.

Intracapsular Surgery. Also known as debulking or cytoreduction, this technique will never lead to a cure for a cancer but can have a role in preserving surrounding normal tissues and structures that, if damaged, could negatively affect the patient's quality of life. Debulking will often leave behind visible tissue at the site but can provide palliation when a tumor is causing obstruction (say to the upper respiratory tract or the gastrointestinal tract) or pain (retrobulbar tumors or spinal tumors). Most debulking surgeries require adjunctive therapy if the patient is to be cured or have a long-term remission. For some cancer types, debulking of the tumor, followed by radiation therapy (see Chapter 124), could be considered to have a high probability of long-term control.

Marginal Surgery. By this surgical technique the tumor is removed along the pseudocapsule. The pseudocapsule is formed when the tumor expands, compressing the peripheral tumor cells against the surrounding normal tissue. Grossly, the tumor appears to "shell out," but microscopic compressed (but viable) tumor cells remain and will regrow if no further treatment is performed. Again radiation therapy

is indicated for marginally removed tumors where metastasis has not occurred, and cure is still a possibility with that additional therapy.

Curative Intent Surgery. When preparing a patient for curative intent surgery, it is important to plan the surgery to include any biopsy needle tracts and incisions, as well as drain holes and tracts, which will need to be removed as these could be a source of future recurrence.

Wide Excisional Surgery. Excisional surgery removes a "cuff" of normal tissue along with the tumor contained within. Ideally, the tumor is removed en bloc, and the lateral or deep margins of the tumor are never exposed. If the margin is wide enough, a cure is possible. However, often what appears to be a wide surgery to the cancer care team may still not be adequate. Placing ink or sutures at the areas the surgeon feels least confident about will assist the pathologist to specifically section and examine those sites.

Most investigators feel a clear histologic margin of 5 mm to 10 mm (depending on the tumor type) is adequate. To achieve this, wider surgical margins of macroscopically normal-appearing tissue need to be removed. Clearly in very small reptiles this will not be feasible, especially for larger tumors or those located around sensitive or vital structures. For these smaller patients, surgery should have the aim of achieving the maximum margins that will allow quality of life to be preserved. In mammalian species a technique of proportional margins has been successful for smaller patients, where the peripheral and deep margins are equal to the measured diameter of the tumor.[9] This may be a reasonable approach, if feasible, in smaller reptiles. For larger patients, similar criteria to those used for other pet animals apply. The margins reported in the pathology report should always be interpreted in light of the clinical impression of the surgery. If the surgeon was not confident that clear margins were achieved, the best option is a second, "scar revision" surgery to remove margins around the remaining scar. If the surgeon feels confident, but the pathologist finds tumor cells at the margin, the pathology report should take precedence; whereas if the surgeon feels it is unlikely the excision was complete, but the pathology report does not find tumor cells at the margins, the surgeon's impression should take precedence. On the other hand, if the deep margin includes underlying fascia or muscle that has not been penetrated, these may act as a barrier to tumor invasion, particularly early on in tumor growth. Aggressive surgery such as partial pneumonectomy and/or partial hepatectomy are feasible and may be curative in some reptiles.[10]

Radical Excisional Surgery. Radical surgery removes a complete compartment organ or structure to achieve complete margins. The most commonly seen example is a limb amputation that could cure a soft tissue sarcoma and be palliative for pain from, or curative for, a bone cancer such as chondrosarcoma or osteosarcoma.[11,12]

Such aggressive surgical procedures may be viewed as "mutilating" by some owners, as they anthropomorphically project their interpretation of their own well-being onto their pets. It is important to remember that animals often have a great quality of life with little regard for the cosmetic changes such surgeries cause.

Chapter 123 of this book focuses on the chemotherapy of various tumor types in the reptilian patient, and Chapter 124 focuses on the option of radiation therapy. Much more scientific data must be collected in an attempt to fully understand how reptilian physiology is affected by cancer cells and how it responds to chemotherapy and radiation treatment. The authors encourage clinicians to collect and publish data on reptilian oncology patients, especially in cases involving chemotherapy or radiation therapy.

REFERENCES

See www.expertconsult.com for a complete list of references.

79

Endocrinology

Paul Raiti

Similar to other vertebrates, the reptilian endocrine system consists of ductless glands that synthesize, store, and release polypeptide hormones directly into the circulatory system. Specific target cells form surface complexes with these hormones prior to intracellular metabolism. This chapter includes the hypothalamus, pituitary, thyroid, ultimobranchial, parathyroid, splenopancreas, and adrenal glands. Gonadal physiology and reproduction are discussed elsewhere in Chapter 80.

HYPOTHALAMUS AND PITUITARY GLAND (HYPOPHYSIS)

The hypothalamus is the ventral part of the anterior brainstem or diencephalon. On the ventral surface of the hypothalamus is the optic chiasma and just caudal to this the pituitary stalk emerges. The pituitary gland is located in a boney cavity of the floor of the cranium (sella tursica).[1] In reptiles, as in other vertebrates, the hypothalamus controls the pituitary gland, through nerve impulses and secretion of neurohormones. The hypothalamic/pituitary axis regulates the endocrine system via positive and negative feedback systems. Several hypothalamic-pituitary axes have been described, including the hypothalamic-pituitary-thyroid (HPT) axis, the hypothalamic-pituitary-adrenal (HPA) axis, and the hypothalamic-pituitary-gonadal (HPG) axis.[2] Release or release-inhibiting hormones produced by the hypothalamus controlling the pituitary gland are thyrotropin-releasing hormone (TRH); corticotropin-releasing hormone (CRH); dopamine (DA); prolactin (PRL)-inhibiting hormone; growth hormone–releasing hormone (GHRH); GH-release-inhibiting hormone (GHIH), also called somatostatin (SS); gonadotropin-releasing hormone (GnRH); melanocyte-releasing hormone (MRH); and melanocyte release-inhibiting hormone (MRIH).[2]

The anterior lobe (adenohyphysis) of the pituitary gland is composed of three structures (pars intermedia, pars tuberalis, and pars distalis) and produces growth hormone, prolactin, ACTH (adrenocorticotropic hormone), TSH (thyroid stimulating hormone), MSH (melanophore-stimulating hormone), beta endorphans, and gonadotropins.[2] Beta endorphins influence temperature regulation, respiration, and cardiovascular function.[3] Beta endorphins are also thought to act synergistically on chromatophores to potentiate the action of MSH in promoting physiological color change.[3] Prolactin is involved in a wide variety of physiological functions, which are mainly associated with reproduction, behavior, osmoregulation, and immunoregulation.[4] In squamates (lizards and snakes), injections of ovine prolactin-releasing hormone increased appetite, growth, tail regeneration rate, and frequency of sloughing.[5] The posterior lobe (neurohypophysis) of the pituitary gland produces vasotocin (arginine-oxytocin),[6] a hormone similar to mammalian antidiuretic hormone.

Several cases of pituitary neoplasia have been reported in snakes.[7,8] Pituitary adenomas and cystadenoma were described in adult snakes

with variable clinical signs, including decreased mentation, postural abnormalities, ataxia, decreased muscle tone, enterolipidosis, polydipsia, cutaneous mycotic infection, and partial-to-complete loss of righting reflexes consistent with central nervous system disease. Diagnoses were made on postmortem with tumors located in the anterior lobe of the pituitary, causing compression of adjacent pituitary and brain. To date, no cases of diabetes insipidus have been reported in reptiles. Improved brain evaluation at necropsy and further investigation into the diagnostic value of ACTH are required.

THYROID GLAND

Chelonians and snakes possess single thyroid glands. The thyroid glands of lizards may be single, bilobed, or paired among different members of the same family.[9] In the green iguana and crocodilians, the paired thyroid glands are joined by a narrow bridge of tissue (Fig. 79.1). In snakes, the thyroid gland is located ventral to the trachea, cranial to the heart base, and caudal to the thymus (Fig. 79.2).[9] In chelonians and lizards, the thyroid gland is generally located ventral to the trachea and near the base of the heart (Fig. 79.3). The Nile crocodile (*Crocodylus*

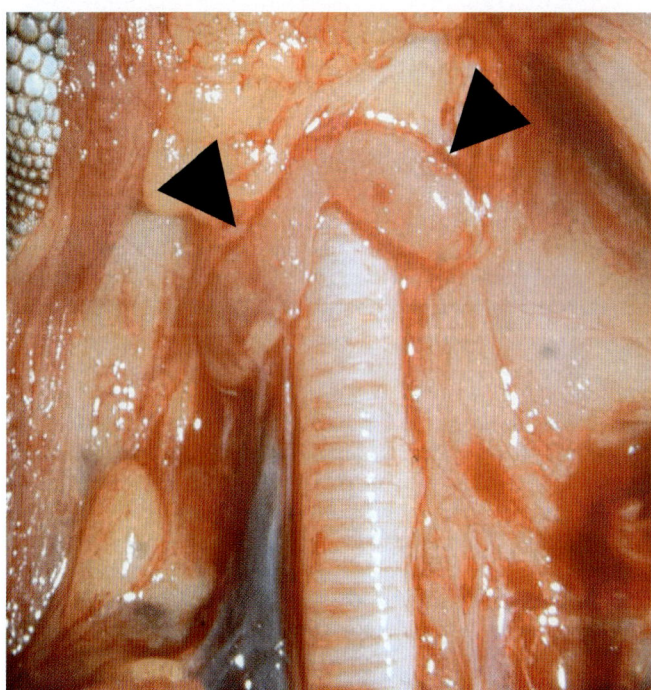

FIG 79.1 The bilobed thyroid gland (*arrows*) of the green iguana (*Iguana iguana*) is located in the cervical area immediately ventral to the trachea.

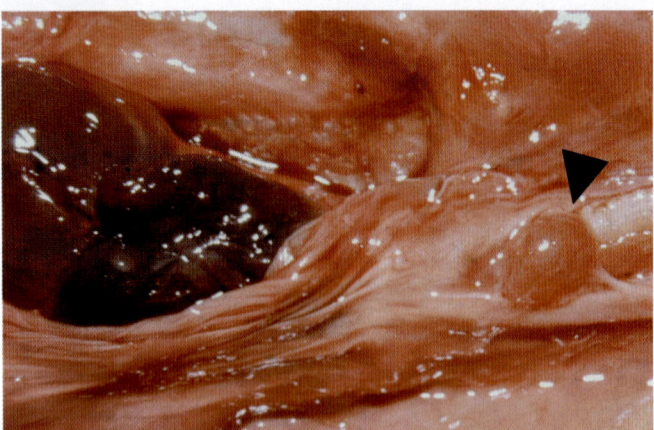

FIG 79.2 The single-lobed thyroid gland (*arrow*) of the boa constrictor (*Boa constrictor*) is located anterior to the cardiac base.

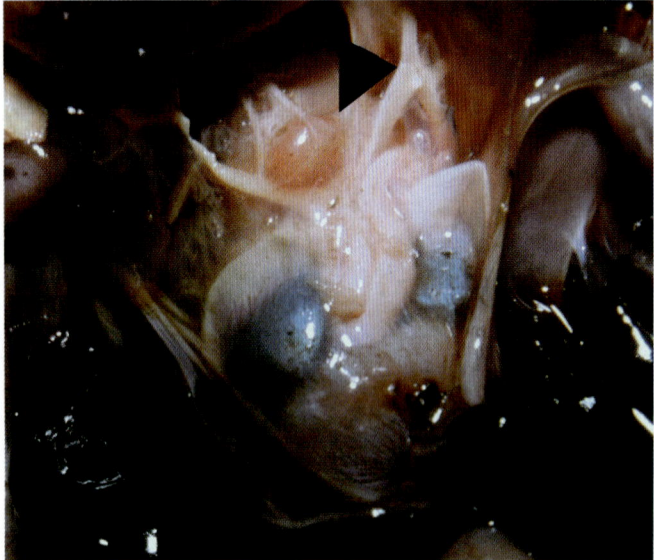

FIG 79.3 The single-lobed thyroid gland (*arrow*) of the Russian tortoise (*Agrionemys horsfieldi*) is located just anterior to the cardiac base.

niloticus) possesses two separate asymmetric lobes found not on the trachea but attached to the lateral side of each bronchi, the right closer to the right bronchus where it enters the lung and the left closer to the bifurcation of the trachea.[10] The tuatara has a single transversely elongate thyroid gland.[9] Unlike mammals, the reptilian thyroid glands are anatomically distinct from the parathyroid glands.[9] Thyroid glands are capable of regeneration if damaged or incompletely removed.[11]

Though small, the thyroid gland receives one of the largest relative blood supplies of any organ.[9] The thyroid gland has dual arterial supplies on both sides. In *Lacerta* and *Xantusia* the superior thyroid arteries (or right and left thyroid arteries) branch off the external or internal carotid's (respectively) and attach to the lateral thyroids.[9] The inferior thyroid arteries (or right and left laryngotracheal arteries) are short, large vessels that attach to the dorsal thyroid body. The thyroid glands are drained by one or two medial thyroid veins into the right tracheal or right internal jugular veins. The thyroid gland itself is contained in a large lymphatic sac and surrounded by lymph tissue.[9] Innervation of the thyroid gland is from the laryngeal branches of the vagus nerve and fine branches of the cervical sympathetics.[9] The thyroid gland has a dense irregular connective tissue capsule enveloping it. It consists of follicular acini of varying size lined by simple cuboidal or columnar

epithelium that may show seasonal/cyclic variation association with reproduction.[12] In mammals, the thyroid gland also secretes calcitonin; however, in reptiles calcitonin is secreted by a separate gland called the ultimobranchial gland.[13]

Reptile thyroid physiology is similar to other vertebrates; however, mammalian thyroid shows greater secretory activity than the reptilian thyroid.[14] Thyroid function is mediated centrally via TRH from the hypothalamus and TSH released from the pituitary gland. TSH controls the synthesis and release of T_4 and T_3 from the thyroid gland. Dietary iodine, an essential trace element, is absorbed in the small intestine and plays an essential role in metabolism as a component of thyroid hormones.[15] The follicular cells concentrate iodides from the thyroid's vascular supply and convert iodide to iodine. One or two molecules of iodine then attaches to the amino acid tyrosine to form either monoiodotyrosine (MIT) or diiodotyrosine (DIT). MIT and DIT can be coupled to form triiodothyronine (T_3), or two DITs can couple to form tetraiodothyronine (thyroxine or T_4).[16] These reactions depend on a glycoprotein that the follicles produce called thyroglobulin. As the thyroglobulin is secreted into the follicular lumen, iodination and coupling occurs and thyroglobulin stores all these molecules as eosinophillic colloid. In reptiles, T_4 accounts for approximately 80% of thyroid hormones in the thyroid gland and plasma. Hence, T_4 is considered a storage and transport form of thyroid hormones, while T_3 is the more metabolically active form.[16] T_4 is converted to T_3 in skeletal muscle, liver, brain, and other target tissues by removal of an outer layer ring 5′iodine (deiodination).[16] Among reptiles, thyroid levels in snakes are generally the lowest and chelonians the highest; crocodilians are similar to birds.[14] In sea turtles and other reptiles, most T_4 in plasma is bound to carrier proteins; only the unbound or "free" T_4 (fT_4) is available to tissues for conversion to T_3 via deiodinases.[17] Free T_4 has been recommended as the most informative measure of thyroid function in reptiles, yet most publications have measured total T_4 due to a lack of validated fT_4 assays for reptiles.[17]

In reptiles, the hypothalamic/pituitary/thyroid axis influences many processes, such as shedding, growth, development, reproduction, metabolic rate, nutrient assimilation, and activity. The studies on cyclic changes in the thyroid in connection with the reproductive cycle indicate that thyroid activity may play a part in sexual behavior as well as gonad maturation depending on day length and temperature.[18] Thyroid hormones are critical for normal bone growth and development, as T_3 stimulates both osteoblast and osteoclast activities.[19,20] The thyroid gland exhibits both direct and indirect effects on the heart and cardiovascular system (i.e., influences myocardial contractility and hemodynamics).[21] The effects caused by thyroid hormones on the heart result from interactions with specific nuclear receptors in cardiac myocytes.[21] Low thyroid hormones are known to inhibit activity and feeding in many ectotherms, with thyroidectomized individuals generally showing sharp reductions in activity, feeding, and metabolic rate. In lizards (*Lacerta, Hemidactylus, Gekko*), thyroidectomy caused either a decrease or cessation of shedding with a build-up of the horny layer, while administration of thyroxine caused increased shedding frequency.[9] In snakes (*Thamnophis, Python, Natrix, Ptyas, Chionactus*) excess thyroxine caused shedding to cease, while hypophysectomy or thyroidectomy increased shedding frequency.[9]

Many factors influence thyroid values including age, sex, diurnal changes, seasonal changes, day length, shedding, illness, stress, and breeding.[18] Chelonians (*Agionemys, Lissemys, Trachemys*) exposed to prolonged or continuous illumination exhibit a gradual decline in T_4, while shorter or variable conditions stimulate T_4 production.[9,22] Interestingly, the genera *Chrysemys, Pseudemys*, and *Trachemys* appear to have significantly higher thyroid values than other reptiles (see Table 79.1), and females in these genera have higher levels than males, perhaps

TABLE 79.1   Normal Thyroid Values in Reptiles

Species	T₄ nmol/L (μg/dl)	T₃ nmol/L	fT₄ pmol/L	fT₃ pmol/L	Sex #	Temp °C	Month	S
American Alligators (*Alligator mississippiensis*)[45]	4.18 ± 0.31 (0.32 ± .02)	ND	ND	ND	U	ND	May	ND
Freshwater crocodiles (*Crocodylus johnstoni*)[14]	3.24 ± 0.6 (0.25 ± 0.04)	0.51 ± 0.02	ND	ND	U, 5	30–32	ND	C
Common cobra (*Naja naja*)[46]	12.87–25.74 (1.0–2.0)	ND	ND	ND	M, 6	ND	June–April	D
Corn snakes (*Pantherophis guttata*)[17]	0.45–6.06 m = 2.75 (0.03–0.47) m = 0.21	ND	ND	ND	U, 10	ND	ND	TV
Milk snakes (*Lampropeltis triangulum*)[17]	0.27–2.94 m = 1.88 (0.02–0.23) m = 0.14	ND	ND	ND	U, 10	ND	ND	TV
Ball pythons (*Python regius*)[17]	0.93–4.79 m = 2.58 (0.07–0.37) m = 0.20	ND	ND	ND	U, 11	ND	ND	TV, C
Boas (*Boa constrictor*)[17]	≤0.24–3.98 m = 2.50 (≤ 0.02–0.31) m = 0.19	ND	ND	ND	U, 11	ND	ND	TV, C
Eastern fence lizards (*Sceloporus undulatus*)[47]	4.81–6.78 (0.37–0.52)	3.8 ± 0.80	ND	ND	M, 17	23–41	July	IO
Western fence lizards (*Sceloporus occidentalis*)[48]	6.2 ± 0.60 (0.48 ± 0.04)	ND	ND	ND	U, 59	21–26	Jan	IO
Six-lined racerunners (*Cnemidophorus sexlineatus*)[29]	1.3–5.4 (0.1–0.4)	ND	ND	ND	M, 102 F, 140	5–31	YR	TV
Desert iguanas (*Dipsosaurus dorsalis*)[49]	12.2 ± 2.8 (0.94 ± 0.2)	ND	ND	ND	M, 8	2–30	May	IO
Indian garden lizards (*Calotes versicolor*)[50]	0.21–5.96 (0.02–0.46)	0–2.70	ND	ND	M, 128–160	ND	YR	C
Green iguanas (*Iguana iguana*)[42]	3.81 ± 0.84 (0.29 ± 0.06)	ND	ND	ND	M, 3 F, 4	ND	ND	TV
Leopard geckos (*Eublepharis macularius*)[a]	6.05–19.3 m =12.48 (0.47–1.49) m = 0.96	ND	ND	ND	M, 2 F, 4	ND	ND	TV
Green sea turtles (*Chelonia mydas*)[51]	11.4–13.5 (0.88–1.04)	ND	ND	ND	M, 73	ND	Jan Mar Sept	DCS
Shingleback skinks (*Tiliqua rugosus*)[14]	1.48 ± 0.42 (0.11 ± 0.03)	0.14 ± 0.03	ND	ND	U, 9	20–22	ND	C
Shingleback skinks (*Tiliqua rugosus*)[14]	2.62 ± 0.30 (0.20 ± 0.02)	0.28 ± 0.05	ND	ND	U, 9	30–32	ND	C
Snake-necked turtles (*Chelodina longicollis*)[14]	0.69 ± 0.11 (0.05 ± 0.01)	0.31 ± 0.03	ND	ND	U, 10	20–22	ND	JV
Snake-necked, turtles (*Chelodina longicollis*)[14]	0.55 ± 0.11 (0.04 ± 0.01	0.28 ± 0.05	ND	ND	U, 10	30–32	ND	JV
Painted turtles (*Chrysemys picta*)[52]	13.0 ± 2.3 (1.01 ± 0.12)	<0.192	ND	ND	M, 24	17–29	June	TC
Painted turtles (*Chrysemys picta*)[52]	24.0 ± 6.0 (1.86 ± 0.04)	ND	ND	ND	F, 20	17–29	June	TC
Painted turtles (*Chrysemys picta*)[18]	6.0–97.0 (0.4–7.53)	ND	ND	ND	M, 128	ND	May–Oct	TC
Green sea turtles (*Chelonia mydas*)[51]	11.4–13.5 (0.88–1.04)	ND	ND	ND	M, 73	ND	Jan Mar Sept	DCS
Desert tortoises (*Gopherus agassizii*)[28]	0.46–3.15 (0.03–0.24)	<0.15	ND	ND	M, U	ND	YR	JV
Desert tortoises (*Gopherus agassizii*)[28]	0.55–3.69 (.04–0.28)	< 0.15	ND	ND	F, U	ND	YR	JV

Continued

TABLE 79.1	Normal Thyroid Values in Reptiles—cont'd							
Species	T$_4$ nmol/L (μg/dl)	T$_3$ nmol/L	fT$_4$ pmol/L	fT$_3$ pmol/L	Sex #	Temp °C	Month	S
African spurred tortoises (*Centrochelys sulcata*)[53]	2.0–9.0 (0.15–0.69)	0–0.8 (10%–90%)	3.0–6.0 (10%–90%)	1.5–4.8 (10%–90%)	M, 4 F, 8	ND	ND	JVSCP
Galapagos tortoises (*Chelonoidis nigra*)[b]	10.39 ± 18.72 (0.08 ± 1.45)	ND	ND	ND	M, 2 F, 3	ND	ND	BV
Hermanns tortoises (*Testudo hermanni*)[32]	12.8 ± 7.0 (0.99 ± 0.54)	0.2 ± 0.1	<0.45	8.1 ± 2.9	69	ND	YR	TV
Greek tortoises (*Testudo graeca*)[32]	12.3 ± 3.9 (0.95 ± 0.30)	0.2 ± 0.04	<0.45	7.2 ± 1.7	11	ND	YR	TV
Russian tortoises (*Agrionemys horsfieldii*)[32]	9.9 ± 4.1 (0.76 ± 0.32)	0.1 ± 0.03	<0.45	5.6 ± 1.4	11	ND	YR	TV

Values listed as mean ± standard deviation, range, or 10 to 90 percentiles.
Adapted from Boyer TH, Steffes ZJ, unpublished data.
Unpublished data by: [a]Boyer TH; and [b]DiGesualdo CL.
BV, Brachial vein; *C*, cardiocentesis; *D*, decapitation; *DCS*, dorsal cervical sinus; *F*, female; *JV*, jugular vein; *m*, mean; *M*, male; *ND*, no data; *OS*, orbital, infra, or suborbital sinus; *S*, blood collection site; *SCP*, subcarapacial plexus; *TC*, tail cut; *TV*, tail vein; *U*, unknown sex; *YR*, year round.

because of a thyroxine-binding protein (TBP), which may cause marked seasonal variation.[23,24] This high-affinity T$_4$-binding protein (TBP) appears to be the major component of T$_4$ transport in these turtles.[23,24] Thyroxine-binding protein was minimal upon emergence from hibernation and maximal in late summer (July–August), about a month after the peak in plasma T$_4$.[23,24]

Seasonal thyroid patterns are typical in reptiles and are believed to be necessary for the normal functioning of the thyroid gland and immune system. In a wide variety of temperate reptiles (*Lacerta, Dipsosaurus, Natrix, Vipera, Gopherus, Chrysemys, Trachemys, Pseudemys*), thyroid activity is high during summer's higher temperatures and low during winter's lower temperatures.[25–29] Tropical species (*Anolis*) have higher thyroid values in the cooler months and decreased values in the warmer months when they are often less active.[9] Both T$_4$ and T$_3$ tend to decline during stress, particularly if the stressor involves decreased body temperature, starvation, or both.[30]

Thyroid Testing

Mammalian thyroid function is assessed using basal total and free thyroxine (T$_4$, fT$_4$), basal total and free triiodothyronine (T$_3$, fT$_3$), T$_3$ suppression, TSH response, and TRH stimulation tests. High TSH levels with low T$_4$ concentration and accompanying symptoms are considered diagnostic for hypothyroidism; however, this test has not been validated in reptilian species.[17,31] Conversely, low values of TSH and high T$_4$ concentration are indicative of hyperthyroidism. Total T$_4$ and T$_3$ values in reptiles are roughly 20% and 25%, respectively, of the average values in mammals; however, determining/detecting thyroid hormone values for reptiles is complicated because assays are designed for the higher levels found in mammals.[17] T$_3$ is often undetectable even by radioimmunoassay (RIA). For these reasons, total T$_4$ is most typically assayed in reptiles, and ranges have been published for several species.[31] (See Table 79.1.) Significant "normal" variations in T$_4$ are seen in reptiles, which complicates interpretation; hence, subnormal T$_4$ levels alone may be suggestive of but not diagnostic for hypothyroidism. In the past, reptilian fT$_4$ values (i.e., *Testudo* spp.) were frequently below the limits of detection (<0.45 pmol/L) of mammalian thyroid assays.[32] Total T$_4$ and T$_3$ concentrations circulate at nanomolar (nmol) concentrations and are considerably easier to measure than fT$_4$ and fT$_3$, which circulate in minute concentrations that are measured at picomolar (pmol/L) or

picogram (pg/ml) concentrations.[33] (Note: pg/ml × 1.287 = pmol/L.) "Free" hormone immunoassays are based on the principle of using a specific antibody to sequester a small amount of the total hormone such that the fractional occupancy of antibody binding sites is determined by the free hormone concentration.[33] Currently, the Society for Comparative Endocrinology encourages the use of Standard International (SI) units (e.g., molar units such as nmol/L, pmol/L). Some veterinary laboratories still report T$_3$ and T$_4$ values as μg/dl. This unit of measurement can be converted to nmol/L by multiplying μg/dl by a factor of 12.87. Thyroid autoimmunity testing against thyroid-specific antigens (thyroid peroxidase [TPO], thyroglobulin [TG], and TSH receptors) is useful for the diagnosis of autoimmune thyroid disorders (hypothyroidism) in dogs and humans.[31] Currently, this diagnostic test is not available for other animal species.

In 2001, a high-sensitivity RIA procedure was validated to measure and establish initial reference ranges for T$_4$ concentration in select species of snakes.[17] Nuclear medicine has been used for the diagnosis of human thyroid dysfunction, specifically cases of hyperthyroidism. Taking advantage of the physiological iodine/iodide cycle, an isotope with high affinity to the thyroid gland is administered, and uptake by the thyroid gland is either quantified or compared with another organ.[31] Other imaging modalities used for thyroid diagnostic testing include ultrasonography (US), scintigraphy, computed tomography (CT), and magnetic resonance imaging (MRI), mainly for the diagnosis of neoplasia.[31] Although these tests have been used to assess the thyroid gland, they may not provide information regarding glandular function.

Overview of Thyroid Disease

Vertebrates with goiter or, more correctly, thyromegaly may be clinically hyperthyroid, euthyroid, or hypothyroid. In reptiles, thyroid malfunction has been associated with hypertrophy/hyperplasia (adenomas, colloid goiters), malignancies, euthyroid sick syndrome, and hypothyroidism. Proposed etiologies for proliferative thyroid disease (adenomatous disease) include iodine deficiency or toxicity, goitrogenic substances (e.g., *Brassica* spp. plants), endocrine-disrupting compounds, trace vitamin and mineral deficiencies (e.g., vitamin A, selenium, iron, and zinc in humans), autoimmune disease, genetic predisposition, age, temperature, and photoperiod.[34] Histological features of adenomatous hyperplasia consist primarily of hypertrophy of the follicular epithelium.

A zoo colony of Kirtland's snakes (*Clonophis kirtlandii*) were evaluated due to a historic high prevalence of thyromegaly (goiter) and mortality unrelated to gender.[36] Subjective thyromegaly was noted in most, while microscopic thyroid lesions (ademomatous changes) were observed in all snakes. Unfortunately, antemortem thyroid hormone testing was not performed due to small patient size. But suspected etiologies included suboptimal dietary iodine, other nutritional deficiencies, exposure to goitrogenic substances, exposure to and bioaccumulation of endocrine-disrupting contaminants from the environment, genetic predisposition, or a combination thereof. Supplementation with iodine was attempted in some snakes in various ways but was generally unsuccessful. In reptiles, most reported cases of hyperthyroidism are associated with thyroid neoplasia.

Thyroid adenomas and carcinomas have been reported in lizards, snakes, and several chelonian species.[35] Histological features of carcinomas include nuclear pleomorphism, mitotic figures, necrosis, local invasion, and metastases to the liver and lungs. Affected reptiles have evidence of concurrent diseases, including stomatitis, rhinitis, uveitis, conjunctivitis, cellulitis, epicarditis, pancreatic atrophy, pancreas islet cell tumor, colonic carcinoma, renal disease, and articular gout; however, no cause or effect relationships have been established. A group of three diplodactylid geckos with signs of intraoral mass, ventral throat swelling, oral bleeding, and weight loss were diagnosed with proliferative thyroid lesions.[37] Thyroid hormone assays were deemed impractical in these geckos due to their limited size. Thyroid carcinomas were confirmed in two geckos, with metastases to the liver and lungs in one animal. Thyroidectomy with replacement levothyroxine therapy was curative in the third gecko (marbled velvet gecko, *Oedura marmorata*) with adenomatous hyperplasia. Given the size of the animal, clinical response was used to assess therapy. Five other diplodactylid geckos in the collection remained unaffected, giving a 38% prevalence of proliferative thyroid lesions (3/8). The etiology remained undetermined. Many cases of thyroid disease have been serendipitously identified during necropsies of reptiles that presented with nonspecific symptoms of illness, hence the relative lack of abnormal T$_4$ values reported in the literature (Fig. 79.4).

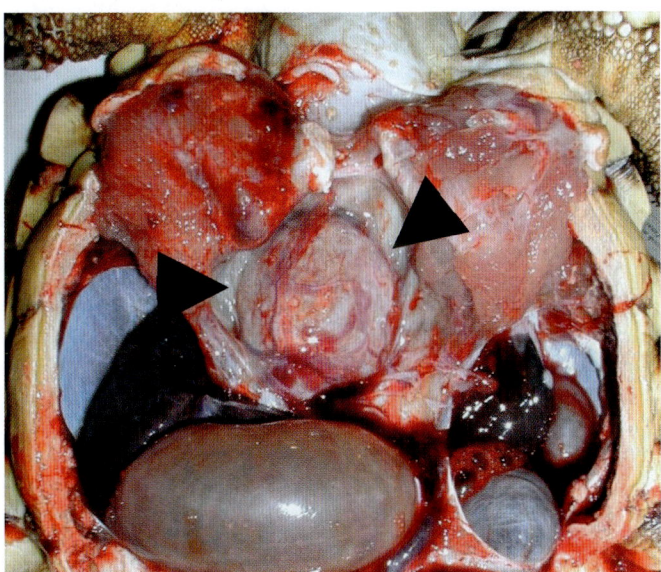

FIG 79.4 Massive thyromegaly due to an adenoma (arrows) in a Chaco tortoise (*Chelonoidis chilensis*). The heart lies beneath the adenoma and is not visible.

Euthyroid Sick Syndrome

"Euthyroid sick syndrome" or "nonthyroidal illness syndrome" refers to changes in serum TSH, serum thyroid hormones, and tissue thyroid hormone levels that occur in patients with various nonthyroidal conditions.[31,34] In humans, this syndrome occurs in cases of starvation, sepsis, surgery, myocardial infarction, bypass, bone marrow transplantation, and probably any severe disease.[31,38] In endotherms and probably in ectotherms, this shut-down of thyroid function at low ambient temperatures is thought to be an adaptive strategy to reduce energy costs.[31] Food restriction reduces thyroid hormones in green sea turtles (*Chelonia mydas*), desert tortoises (*Gopherus agassizii*), and several other reptiles.[31] It is thought that the relative hypothyroid state produced is a physiological means of conserving energy during times of food deprivation (starvation) and hibernation. In red-eared sliders (*Trachemys scripta elegans*), for example, low temperatures caused in vitro pituitary tissue to become almost completely unresponsive to hypothalamic TRH, and in vitro thyroid tissue also became less responsive to pituitary TSH.[30] In cold-stunned Kemp's ridley sea turtles it was found that upon admission, affected turtles' fT$_4$s were usually undectable.[39]

Hypothyroidism

Primary hypothyroidism, the result of idiopathic thyroid atrophy or lymphocytic thyroiditis, and secondary hypothyroidism, the result of iodine deficiency in the diet, are most commonly implicated in mammalian disease. The most commonly reported causes of hypothyroidism in reptiles have been associated with conditions that were thought to interfere with normal thyroid function, such as iodine deficiency or toxicity and feeding excessive amounts of goitrogenic food items. Proposed etiologies include feeding plants grown in iodine-deficient soil and/or dietary goitrogens found in bok choy, broccoli, cabbage, cauliflower, kale, mustard seed, rapeseed, soybean sprouts, and turnips. Iodine deficiency leads to decreased thyroxine levels, which subsequently activates the hypothalamo-pituatary axis leading to increased TSH production and resulting thyromegaly (goiter).[15] Clinical signs may be suggestive of hypothyroidism, but proper diagnosis should be based on measurements of total T$_4$ and TSH levels. In one study, thyroid values from normal Galapagos tortoises housed at the Oklahoma City Zoo were compared with suspected hypothyroid conspecifics that had been on loan to another zoo for 2 years. Results indicated reduced T$_3$ values (0.07 nmol/L compared with euthyroid controls of 0.51–2.53 nmol/L). Additionally, T$_4$ values (2.43–6.02 nmol/L were reduced compared with euthyroid controls of 13.9–19.82 nmol/L) (DiGesualdo CL, unpublished data). For the tortoises with cervical myxedema, treatment was instituted with levothyroxine at 0.02 mg/kg PO every 48 hrs. Previously, hypothyroidism has been suggested primarily in Galapagos (*Chelonoidis nigra*) and Aldabra (*Aldabrachelys gigantea*) tortoises that were thought to possess a higher metabolic requirement for iodine, which was deficient in diets formulated for captive animals.[40] Clinical symptoms have included anorexia, lethargy, and myxedema of subcutaneous tissues generally involving the head, neck, and proximal forelimbs. However, it should be noted that the chelonian thyroid gland is located just anterior to the cardiac base within the shell; hence, an enlarged thyroid is not visible or palpable in the ventral cervical area. In addition, thymic hyperplasia has been reported to cause cervical swelling in giant tortoises.[41]

Interestingly, a clinical syndrome has recently emerged based upon observations of captive F1 offspring from founder Galapagos tortoises over the past 30 years characterized by incorrect feeding combined with insufficient exercise, abnormal hind limb ambulation, inability of the tortoise to raise itself squarely on its limbs, and an edematous neck lesion (Hairston-Adams C, unpublished data). Thyroid testing of affected animals is currently being done to distinguish if these tortoises represent true hypothyroid cases or perhaps euthyroid sick syndrome secondary to poor husbandry practices.

Hyperthyroidism

Hyperthyroidism is a multisystemic disorder characterized by a state of abnormally high metabolism due to elevated concentrations of T_3 and T_4. Hyperthyroidism is most commonly caused by hyperfunctional thyroid nodules (adenomas), malignant thyroid neoplasms, oversupplementation of exogenous thyroid hormone, and/or increased TSH secretion due to pituitary dysfunction.[34] The diagnosis of hyperthyroidism is characterized by an elevated T_4 level and accompanying clinical symptoms. Current laboratory assays are able to measure reptilian T_4 by RIA; however, validated assays to test samples from many reptilian species have not been reported. Treatment options for proliferative thyroid disease in mammals include thyroid hormone inhibitors (e.g., methimazole, propylthiouracil), radiotherapy with injectable iodine (I-131), or surgical resection.[34]

Hyperthyroidism was reported in a 7-yr-old female green iguana with weight loss, polyphagia, hyperactivity, increased aggression, loss of dorsal spines, tachycardia, and a palpable bilobed mass in the ventral cervical region near the coelomic inlet.[42] The diagnosis was based on an elevated T_4 level (30.0 nmol/L; 2.33 µg/dl); controls 3.81 ± 0.84 nmol/L (0.29 ± 0.06 µg/dl). Excision was curative, and histopathology confirmed thyroid adenoma. Interestingly, T_4 values of the affected iguana returned to normal after surgery despite the absence of thyroid replacement therapy, suggesting incomplete removal or extraneous thyroid tissue.

A case of hyperthyroidism in a 14-yr-old female leopard gecko (*Eublepharis macularius*), with clinical symptoms consisting of anorexia, diarrhea, increased shedding frequency, and a unilateral midline cervical mass, was reported (Boyer T, unpublished data). Serial T_4 levels were elevated (20.59, 64.35 nmol/L; 1.59 µg/dl, 5.0 µg/dl) compared to normal conspecific levels (6.05–19.31 nmol/L; 0.47–1.5 µg/dl). Computed tomographic findings revealed a unilateral thyroid gland enlargement. Iodine-131 (0.1 mCi), injected subcutaneously in the ventral neck, decreased T_4 levels at 1 month (14.16 nmol/L; 1.1 µg/dl), 3 months (6.44 nmol/L; 0.5 µg/dl), and 5 months (12.61 nmol/L; 0.9 µg/dl). Diarrhea resolved posttreatment; the gecko resumed feeding and gained weight. The radioactive I-131 treatment resulted in a euthyroid state for 5 months posttreatment, resolution of diarrhea, return to normal appetite, and weight gain, but then T_4 increased again. This gecko later died of complications of systemic disease. Boyer and Bourdon subsequently recommended a dose of radioactive Iodine-131 of 0.2 mCi in affected geckos.

Miscellaneous Thyroid Conditions

Intranuclear coccidiosis with thyromegaly was diagnosed in a radiated tortoise, *Astrochelys radiata* (unpublished data), and a Bowsprit tortoise, *Chersina angulata*.[43] In the radiated tortoise the T_4 was 11.5 nmol/L and 0.89 µg/dl 11 days prior to necropsy, and the ventral neck, head, and front legs were edematous. Coccidial infections were systemic and involved alimentary, urogenital, respiratory, lymphoid, endocrine, and integumentary systems. Moderate numbers of birefringent calcium oxalate crystals, based on infrared and electron microscopy, were considered incidental findings identified in the thyroid glands and kidneys of necropsied wild desert tortoises (*Gopherus agassizii*).[44] The source of calcium oxalates was suspected to be of plant origin.

ULTIMOBRANCHIAL GLAND

The ultimobranchial gland (UBG) in vertebrates is derived from the pharyngeal pouch epithelium during embryonic development and secretes calcitonin (CT) from C-cells.[54,55] The gland is either separately located (nonmammalian vertebrates) from the thyroid gland or embedded in the thyroid (mammals). Adult reptiles possess one (usually on the left side) or two UBGs UBG's just anterior to the heart. The functional aspects of these glands in reptiles are similar to those of birds and mammals.[54,55] Calcitonin is involved in calcium and phosphorus homeostasis and skeletal remodeling, along with parathyroid hormone (PTH) and vitamin D_3.[54] Administration of mammalian CT had no effect on plasma calcium in turtles, snakes, or lizards.[57] In contrast, administration of salmon CT resulted in hypocalcemia and hypophosphatemia in young iguanas and snakes.[57] However, when salmon CT (200 IU/ml) was administered as a single dose at 50 IU/kg in the front leg of eight healthy adult green iguanas, and blood was collected at 0, 24, 48, 72, and 96 hours, plasma Ca concentrations were within reference intervals at all times and calcitonin did not appear to have influenced Ca concentrations on a long-term basis.[57]

Light and electron microscopy have shown the gland contains follicles and cell cords (cell aggregates). The follicular epithelium is lined by simple cuboidal or pseudostratified columnar cells. Ciliated and goblet cells may be present in the follicular epithelia in some groups. The lumen contains a colloid-like substance with desquamated cells or debris. Functions of calcitonin include neurotransmission, blood volume regulation, phosphate balance, and promotion of bone calcification.[55,58] Its secretion is regulated by serum calcium levels; elevated serum calcium levels stimulate the secretion of CT.[59] Calcitonin inhibits calcium resorption from the bone and acts in opposition to parathyroid hormone to reduce serum calcium levels.[58,59]

PARATHYROID GLANDS, VITAMIN D₃, AND CALCIUM HOMEOSTASIS

Unlike in mammals, the parathyroid glands (PTGs) of reptiles are not closely associated with the thyroid gland.[13,34,56] The location of the parathyroid gland varies among different reptilian species; generally, the anterior pair is associated with the carotid artery and the posterior pair is associated with the aortic arch.[13,34] In snakes, the anterior pair is associated with the carotid artery near the mandibular ramus. Lizards may have one or two pairs of PTGs (Fig. 79.5A and B). In green iguanas, the anterior PTGs are located along the medial surface of the mandibular rami, and the posterior pair is located at the origins of the internal and external carotid arteries.[13] Chelonians have two pairs of PTGs. The anterior pair is located within the thymus, and the posterior pair is caudal to the aortic arch and cranial to the heart. Crocodilians may have one or two pairs of PTGs located near the common carotid artery.[13] The parenchyma of the parathyroid gland in reptiles consists largely of chief cells, which are arranged in cords separated by connective tissue that contains a capillary network.[13] The chief cells are involved in the production and release of parathyroid hormone (PTH). The PTGs have a similar role to those of mammals and are responsible for the minute-to-minute regulation of calcium.

Within the body, calcium exists intracellularly in all tissues and extracellularly as brushite and hydroxyapatite (in bone).[60] Skeletal bone comprises >99% of total body calcium, while nonbone calcium is <1%.[60] Nonbone calcium is generally maintained within a narrow range.[60] The total calcium in the general circulation is composed of two fractions: protein bound and ionized. The biologically active ionized calcium (iCa) plays a major role in many biological processes, including muscle contractions, blood coagulation, enzyme activity, neural excitability, hormone release, and membrane permeability.[60,61] It is preferable to evaluate iCa levels for an accurate evaluation of

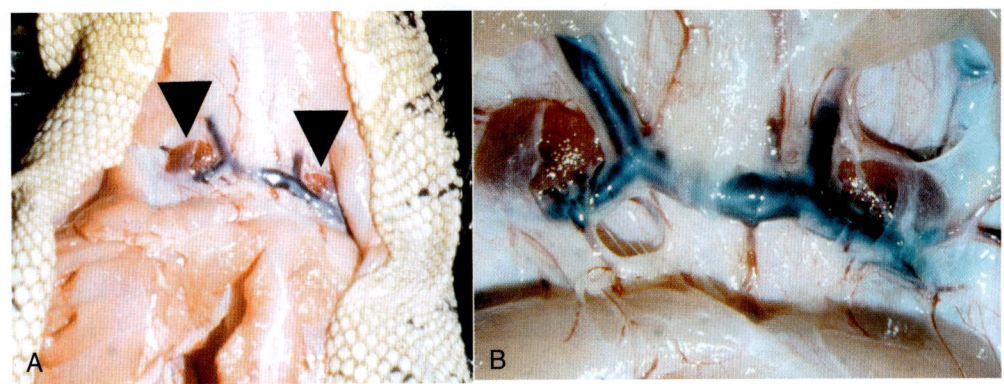

FIG 79.5 (A) Paired parathyroid glands in the cervical area of a water monitor (*Varanus salvator*); (B) magnified view of the same structures.

TABLE 79.2 Ionized Calcium Values From Select Reptiles

Species	Ionized Calcium (mmol/L) Mean ± SD, Range
Wild green sea turtles (*Chelonia mydas*)[76]	1.05, 0.87–1.23
Green iguanas (*Iguana iguana*)[77]	1.47 ± 0.105
Green iguanas[78]	1.38 ± 0.1
Ball pythons-females (UVB) (*Python regius*)[71]	1.84 ± 0.05 (day 0); 1.78 ± 0.07 (day 70)
Ball pythons–males/females (no UVB)[71]	1.79 ± 0.07 (day 0); 1.81±0.05 (day 70)

SD, Standard deviation; *UVB*, ultraviolet B.

calcium status (Table 79.2). Serum calcium, magnesium, and phosphate levels are closely regulated by the combined effects of several hormones (e.g., PTH, vitamin D_3, calcitonin, and cortisol), the gastrointestinal tract, bone, and kidneys.[59] Magnesium, also essential for proper function of muscles and nerves, is a cofactor in over 300 enzymatic reactions, particularly those involving the metabolism of food components, and it is required by all enzymatic reactions involving the energy storage molecule ATP.[61] Phosphorus is a structural component of nucleotide coenzymes: ATP and creatine phosphate.[61] Hypomagnesemia can cause a secondary hypocalcemia, which remains resistant to calcium supplementation until magnesium levels are corrected.[61] Magnesium deficiency in humans induces reversible failure of PTH secretion and increases peripheral PTH degradation and resistance to PTH.[59,61]

Decreased levels of ionized calcium in the blood stimulate the release of PTH, which results in calcium resorption from the bones and kidneys and increased intestinal absorption.[59] Increased iCa in the general circulation has a negative effect on the release of PTH. Parathyroidectomy will result in hypocalcemia and tetanic convulsions.[62]

The two naturally occurring vitamin D forms are cholecalcifrol (vitamin D_3) from animal sources and ergocalciferol (vitamin D2) from plants. Vitamin D can also be synthetized in exposed skin. Provitamin D_3 (7-dehydrocholesterol, 7-DHC), a cholesterol-like precursor, is converted into previtamin D_3 (cholecalciferol) by sunlight (ultraviolet B [UVB] radiation, 290–315 nm) and temperature-dependent isomerization (Fig. 79.6).[63] PTH stimulates hydroxylation of cholocalciferol to 25-hydroxycholecalciferol (25-OH-D_3) or calcidiol in the liver. Calcidiol is the major metabolite of vitamin D and represents the storage form, which is then converted to 1,25-hydroxycholecalciferol (1,25 OH-D_3 or calcitriol) in the kidney by renal 1α-hydroxylase.[59,64] Calcitriol has a very short half-life and is the active form of vitamin D_3, which is responsible for maintaining calcium balance in the body. Major physiological effects of 1,25-OH-D_3 are increasing calcium, magnesium, and phosphate intestinal absorption; increasing renal calcium and phosphate reabsorption; and increasing bone resorption.[59,60] In general terms, 1,25-OH-D_3 assists PTH in performing its functions.

Calcidiol is generally measured for determining vitamin D status because its longer half-life makes it more stable and reliable (Table 79.3).[64–66] Liquid chromatography–mass spectrometry (LC/MS/MS) represents the gold standard, is preferred over radioimmunoassay, and is available commercially (Heartland Assays, Ames, IA). In juvenile black-throated monitor lizards (*Varanus albigularis*), deprivation of dietary vitamin D_3 resulted in significant decreases of circulating levels of calcidiol (25-OH-D_3) (25%–35%), calcitriol (1, 25-OH-D_3) (73%–76%), calcium (60%), and phosphorus (16%).[67] The half-life of circulating calcidiol during deprivation was estimated to be from 128 to 139 days. Single weekly doses of 10 to 20 minutes of UVB exposure to a Spectroline EB-28 UVB lamp (Spectronics Corp., Westbury, NY) failed to prevent 25-OH-D_3 decline; however, the rate of decline was reduced. Conversely, weekly oral vitamin D_3 (10,000 lU/kg) caused an excessive increase (600%) in circulating calcidiol levels that could result in intoxication.[67] Levels of vitamin D were restored and maintained in monitors by (a) daily exposure to UVB gradients generated with a Westron 100-watt mercury-vapor lamp (Westron Corp., Oceanside, NY) and (b) feeding crickets gut-loaded with a commercial vitamin D–supplemented diet along with whole mice. Experimental evaluation of UVB sources in Hermann's tortoises (*Testudo hermanni*) concluded that exposure to sunlight was superior to UVB-emitting mercury vapor and fluorescent lamps.[68] Mean calcidiol concentrations for tortoises exposed to the mercury vapor and fluorescent lamps were significantly lower (155.69 ± 80.71 nmol/L and 134.42 ± 51.42 nmol/L, respectively) when compared to sunlight (411.51 ± 189.75 nmol/L).

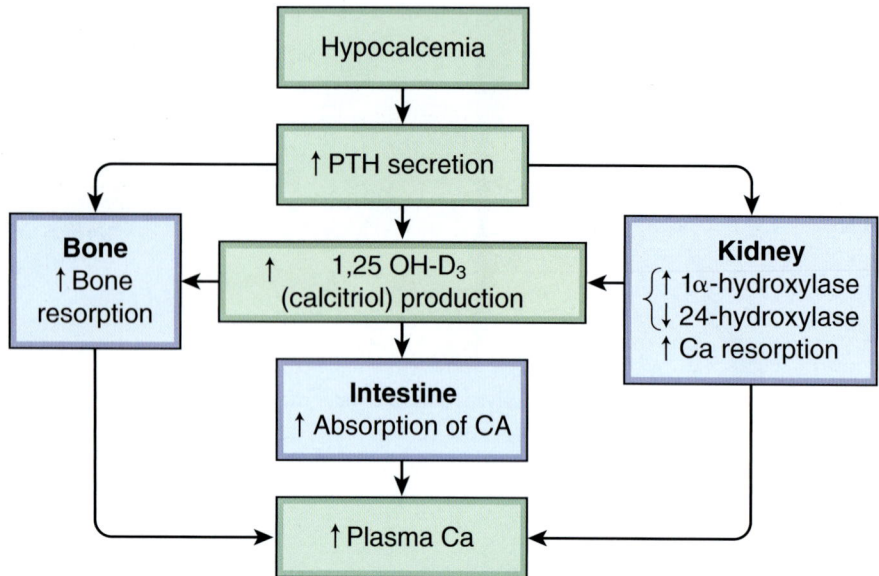

FIG 79.6 The control of hypocalcemia. Calcium blood concentrations are restored mainly by the actions of PTH and 1,25 OH-D$_3$ (calcitriol) in the bone, kidneys, and intestinal tract. ↑, Upregulation; *Ca*, calcium; *PTH*, parathyroid hormone. (From de Matos R: Calcium metabolism in birds, *Vet Clin North Am Exot Anim Pract.* 2008;11:59–82.)

TABLE 79.3 Calcidiol (25-OH-D$_3$) Values From Select Reptiles

Species	Calcidiol (25-OH-D) (nmol/L) Mean ± SD, Range
Wild Ricord's iguanas (*Cyclura ricordii*)[79]	554, 250–1118
Wild rhinoceros iguanas (*Cyclura cornuta cornuta*)[79]	332, 260–369
Captive rhinoceros iguanas[79]	317, 220–519
Captive rhinoceros iguanas (housed outdoors in summer)[80]	239, 157–314.2
Captive rhinoceros iguanas (no UVB in winter)[80]	32.2, 16.2–49.5
Komodo dragons (*Varanus komodoensis*)[81]	150–325
Wild green sea turtles (*Chelonia mydas*)[76]	36, 16.1–72.1
Testudo spp tortoises[82]	28.41 ± 2.0
Captive corn snakes (no UVB) (*Pantherophis guttata*)[70]	57.17 ± 15.28
Captive corn snakes (with UVB)[70]	196 ± 16.73
Ball pythons–females (UVB)[71] (*Python regius*)	197±35 (Day 0); 203.5±13.8 (Day 70)
Ball pythons–males/females (no UVB)[71]	77.7±41.5 (Day 0); 83.0±41.9 (Day 70)
Hermann's tortoises (outdoors) (*Testudo hermanni*)[68]	387.74 ± 114.56

SD, Standard deviation; *UVB*, ultraviolet B.

Studies of UVB and dietary calcium/vitamin D in several reptile species have shown that there is considerable variation in the requirement for dietary vitamin D and for UVB.[31] Some species are able to modulate their endogenous D$_3$ production to complement dietary intake by adjusting their UVB exposure, while crepuscular species may exhibit increased skin sensitivity to UVB.[69] High concentrations of vitamin D within iguanid embryos and egg yolks suggest a role for this compound in embryogenesis in these species and perhaps indicate that there is a mechanism for vitamin D delivery to eggs comparable to that found in the domestic chicken.[65,69] Vitamin D status may be important in animals that are being affected by infectious diseases such as ranavirus and mycoplasma, since vitamin D can play a significant role in immune function. It has been thought that snakes were capable of obtaining their vitamin D exclusively through dietary means rather than photobiosynthesis. However, corn snakes (*Pantherophis guttata*) can increase plasma calcidiol concentrations significantly when provided with supplemental UVB.[70] No association was demonstrated between exposure of ball pythons to UVB radiation, plasma calcidiol, and iCa concentrations.[71]

Hyperparathyroidism

The most common conditions that lead to PTG disorders in reptiles are inadequate calcium or vitamin D$_3$ (nutritional or UVB) leading to nutritional secondary hyperparathyroidism (NSHP) or, less commonly, severe chronic renal disease causing a disturbance in the production of calcitriol and calcium/phosphorus homeostasis, leading to renal secondary hyperparathyroidism (RSHP).[72] Common predisposing factors for the development of NSHP include decreased dietary calcium, vitamin D$_3$ deficiency, improper dietary calcium/phosphorous ratio, inadequate thermal provision, and/or inadequate exposure to ultraviolet radiation in diurnal/nocturnal species.[31,72] Common clinical signs associated with NSHP include thickening and swelling of the long bones and mandibles, pathological fractures of long bones and spine, tetany, muscle fasciculations, hyperreflexia, constipation, cloacal or rectal prolapse, anorexia, and stunted growth.[31] Initial therapy should address presenting complaints, such as fractures and life-threatening hypocalcemia. Many cases require husbandry (adequate UVB light and thermal provision) and nutritional improvements (oral calcium supplementations) for months before recovery is complete. Initial supplementation of parenteral vitamin D$_3$ (100 IU/kg IM once and repeat in 2 weeks) may be useful, followed by UVB exposure.[72]

Renal secondary hyperparathyroidism (RSHP) is a condition that is a consequence of chronic renal failure. Two mechanisms have been proposed. The first is that impaired renal function leads to hyperphosphatemia.[64] As the concentration of phosphorus increases, blood calcium levels decrease, leading to increased PTH secretion and subsequent decreased calcium absorption from the intestines. The second mechanism is that kidney disease results in a relative or absolute deficiency of calcitriol.[64] Since calcitriol is necessary to enable intestinal absorption of dietary calcium and phosphorus, less calcitriol leads to progressive hypocalcemia, which then stimulates PTH secretion. Both ionized calcium and calcitriol must be present in the blood at appropriate levels to inhibit gene transcription of PTH; reduction in either or both leads to PTH synthesis and secretion.[64] Uncontrolled release of PTH leads to skeletal demineralization (rickets, osteomalacia), nephrotoxicity, and subsequent metastatic mineralization. The prognosis for RSHP is guarded. In reptiles, RSHP has been managed with fluid therapy, phosphorus binders, xanthine oxidase inhibitors, and carefully titrated calcitriol supplementation.

While administration of excess vitamin D₃ can result in hypercalcemia and metastatic mineralization, soft tissue mineralization associated with hypovitaminosis D₃ has also been reported in *Iguana* and *Uromastyx* (Richman LK, unpublished data; Raphael BL, unpublished data). In cases of hypovitaminosis D₃, reduced negative feedback by calcitriol commonly associated with RSHP leads to excessive production of PTH with subsequent metastatic mineralization. The provision of vitamin D₃ through UVB (especially sunlight) is certainly safer than routine D₃ supplementation; however, most, if not all, artificial lights are a poor substitute for natural sunlight.

Primary hyperparathyroidism is a disease in which excessive and inappropriate secretion of PTH occurs, and it is most often associated with a solitary functional adenoma or, less commonly, a PTG carcinoma. Parathyroid adenomas or adenocarcinomas have been identified in green iguanas, red-foot tortoises (*Chelonoidis carbonaria*), spur-thighed tortoises (*Testudo graeca*), and desert tortoises (*Gopherus agassizi*).[73–75] Parathyroidmegaly was present in all cases, and affected animals had significant osteomalacia presumably due to elevated levels of PTH. The blood calcium and phosphorus ratios were often reversed and renal calcinosis was present.

PANCREAS

The exact location and anatomical relationships of the pancreas show much variation among reptile species. The pancreas of lizards is more complex than snakes in that it is extended and often trilobed (Fig. 79.7).[83] One portion runs along the bile duct toward the gallbladder, one portion runs to the small intestine, and typically a thin limb with a distinct distal lobe runs to the spleen.[83] In some lizards, such as the house gecko (*Hemidactylus*), a thin diverticulum of pancreas tissue extends anteriorly from the ventral portion of the pancreas and encircles the common bile duct. This is known as the hepatic portion and may actually enter the hepatic parenchyma.[83]

The pancreas of snakes is consolidated and simpler, often pyramid shaped, and attached to the first portion of the duodenum.[83] It generally lies posterior to the spleen and may be in contact with the spleen. The pancreas is usually posterior or adjacent to the gallbladder and lies just posterior to the caudal tip of the liver. In snakes, the association of the pancreas, spleen, and gallbladder is often referred to as the "triad" (Fig. 79.8). There are differences in the amount of pancreatic association with the spleen among species of snakes. In some snakes, such as some members of the Boidae, there is a limb of pancreas that runs forward to the spleen. In others, such as the emerald tree boa (*Corallus caninus*), this limb is interrupted or there is no splenic limb at all. In some snakes the spleen and pancreas are adjoined to form a splenopancreas.[83]

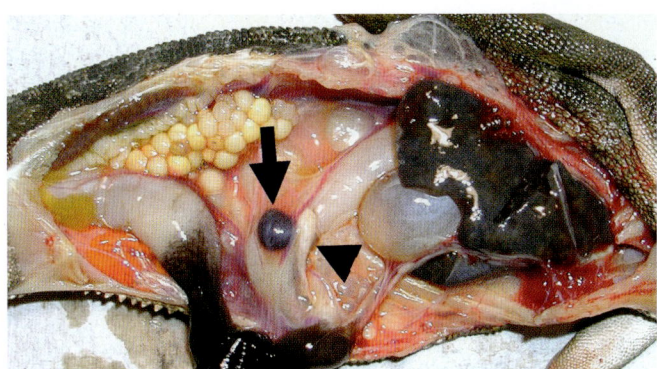

FIG 79.7 The pancreas of this Senegal chameleon (*Chamaeleo senegalensis*) is located between the stomach and duodenum. Note the proximity of the spleen (arrow) to the pancreas (arrowhead).

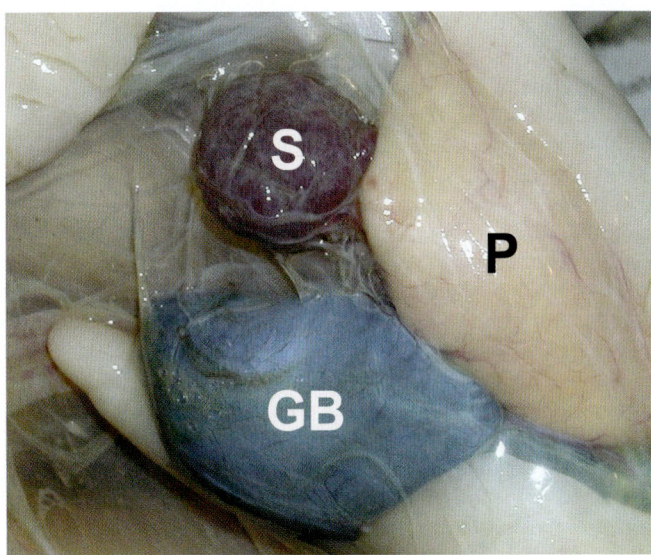

FIG 79.8 Gallbladder (GB), pancreas (P), and spleen (S) ("triad") of an indigo snake (*Drymarchon couperi*).

In the painted turtle (*Pseudemys scripta*) the pancreas is attached to the mesenteric border of the duodenum starting at the pylorus and ends by splaying out over the spleen (which is dorsal and more posterior).[83] In the snake-headed turtle (*Chelodina longicollis*) the proximal pancreas is associated with the proximal portion of the spleen.[83] Some turtles, such as the South American side-necked river turtle (*Podocnemius unifilus*), lack an association between the pancreas and the spleen.[83] In the alligator, *Alligator mississippiensis*, the ventral portion of the pancreas is between the limbs of the ventral duodenal loop. The body of the pancreas follows the dorsal portion of the duodenum and ends on the spleen, which is attached to the descending limb of the dorsal duodenal loop.

There is great variation in the pancreatic islet morphology among different reptile orders.[84] Lizards have large islets usually confined to the dorsal lobe and localized primarily in the splenic portion of the pancreas. In lizards and snakes there is no segregation of alpha and beta cells as in mammals, birds, or fish.[84–86] These cells lie adjacent to each other in an alternating pattern along vascular spaces. In snakes large islets are composed of both alpha and beta cells distributed in a mixed pattern.[85] Taxa-specific distributions of endocrine tissue have been reported and may be focal, regional, or evenly dispersed throughout the pancreas of most squamates or the spleen of colubrid snakes.[85] In some species insulin-immunoreactive (IR) cells have been located in the intestinal mucosa.[86]

The pancreatic islets of turtles are not as large as lizards and snakes, and they tend to be diffusely distributed throughout the pancreas.[83–84] In chelonians there is a marked segregation of the alpha and beta cells—similar to fish, some birds, and mammals. The endocrine cells of *Testudo graeca* are present throughout the pancreas; however, alpha and beta cell islets are larger and more numerous in the splenic region than in the duodenal one.[87] The alpha cells are peripheral in their distribution as opposed to a mixed distribution in most lizards and snakes. Seasonal and reproductive cycles can also influence cell-type prominence and distribution.[87] The relative number of alpha cells in reptiles is noticeably higher than in mammals, and the same is true for glucagon content.[84] In the alligator islet tissue is associated with first-order ducts at the periphery of the pancreas. Beta cells are often aggregated at the central portion of the islet, and alpha cells are clustered around the periphery.[83]

The endocrine pancreas secretes hormones for the regulation of blood glucose. Alpha cells are responsible for glucagon production, beta cells produce insulin and amylin, delta cells produce somatostatin, and F cells produce pancreatic polypeptide.[31,88] Insulin promotes the absorption of glucose from blood to muscle and adipocytes.[89] In the liver insulin promotes glycogen biosynthesis by stimulating glycogen synthetase and inhibiting glycogen phosphorylase.[89] Concurrently, insulin suppresses fuel mobilization by inhibition of glycogen breakdown by the liver, amino acid release from muscle, and free fatty acid (FFA) release from adipose tissue.[89] In adipose tissue glucose is converted to fatty acids, which provide hydrocarbons for triglyceride formation.[89] Mammalian adipose tissue is considered a metabolically dynamic organ that not only is the primary site of storage for excess energy but additionally serves as an endocrine organ capable of synthesizing a number of biologically active compounds that regulate metabolic homeostasis.[90] It is currently unknown if the same is true for reptiles. Glucagon, also a peptide hormone, has the opposite effect of insulin, leading to an increase in blood glucose when the animal is deprived of food.[31] This effect is mainly executed by the liver, because few glucagon receptors are found on other tissues.

Somatostatin, also known as growth hormone inhibiting hormone, regulates insulin and glucagon release in a paracrine fashion.[31] In other areas of the body somatostatin can affect neurotransmission and cell proliferation.

Due to the variability of pancreatic islet cell location in various taxa, submission of the entire pancreas, spleen, stomach, and small/large intestines is required at postmortem evaluation to ensure distant, nonpancreatic sites of islet concentration are not missed.[91] Furthermore, untargeted pancreatic biopsy may not be as useful to evaluate islet presence or activity, because the limited tissue available for antemortem analysis may or may not be representative of tissue pathology.[91]

Pancreatitis

Pancreatitis is defined as inflammation of the pancreas and in reptiles is typically the result of the presence of bacteria or metazoan parasites.[91,92] Acute necrotizing pancreatitis has been associated with trauma to the pancreas, abscesses or pyogranulomatous conditions, migrating helminthes, and obstruction of the pancreatic outflow ducts by masses or calculi.[92] Depending on the location and severity of the inflammation, both the exocrine and the endocrine portions of the pancreas may be involved. Pancreatic fibrosis or chronic fibrosing pancreatitis is a common histopathological finding (Fig. 79.9A and B).[92] On histopathology, the disease is characterized by fibroblasts and fibrocytes invading the interlobular septa. Clinical management of acute and chronic forms of pancreatitis includes supportive care such as fluid therapy, assisted alimentation, antimicrobials, and pain management. Unfortunately, due to the difficulty in diagnosing these cases, the disease is often not identified until necropsy.[91] Complete obstruction of the ductal outflow of a portion of the pancreas may result in either atrophy or autodigestion and resulting necrosis.[92] Frye describes two specific cases, one in a northern diamondback terrapin (*Malaclemys t. terrapin*), where complete obstruction of the interlobular ducts by amorphous crystalline material resulted in a loss of pancreatic tissue including islet tissue.[92] In another case involving a Pacific rattlesnake (*Crotalus viridis oreganos*), the majority of the pancreatic duct system was occluded, which resulted in chronic pancreatitis followed by pancreatic fibrosis.[92]

Trematodes and nematodes have occasionally been found to migrate into pancreatic tissue and are typically seen at histopathology.[91,92] The

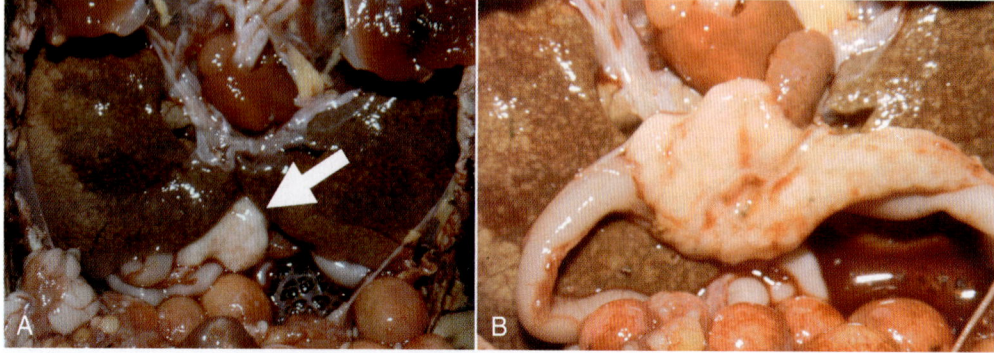

FIG 79.9 (A) Pancreatic fibrosis (arrow) associated with an unidentified protozoan infection in a wild-caught moribund Blanding's turtle (*Emydoidea blandingii*); (B) magnified view of the pancreas.

diagnosis is usually made at necropsy and histopathology by finding the helminthes or their characteristic ova on cross-section. Cryptosporidiosis involving the pancreas and biliary ducts has been reported in corn snakes (*Pantherophis guttata*).[93] Another report describes intranuclear coccidiosis in two radiated tortoises (*Geochelone radiata*) with histopathlogical evidence of pancreatitis.[94] Nephritis, hepatitis, and enteritis with similar intranuclear coccidiosis were also found in these tortoises. Intracytoplasmic inclusions are often present within the pancreas of snakes with boid inclusion body disease.[95] Pancreatic neoplastic diseases have been reported in snakes and are typically carcinomas or adenocarcinomas of the acinar or ductular epithelium.[96] A Komodo dragon (*Varanus komodoensis*) was reported to have a pancreatic islet cell tumor along with several other neoplasms, including a colonic carcinoma, a metastatic adenocarcinoma involving the spleen, and a thyroid adenoma.[96] Additional cases of pancreatic neoplasia are discussed in the following section.

HYPERGLYCEMIA

Reptile blood glucose appears to be regulated by insulin and glucagon as it is in mammals.[31,97] Reptiles with hyperglycemia are often presented for a variety of nonspecific clinical signs, including anorexia, weight loss, lethargy, and severe depression. Polyuria and polydipsia may be present but are not consistent.[97] Physical examination findings may also be nonspecific but may include loss of muscle mass, weakness, loss of righting reflex, stupor, and severe depression.[97] Some reptiles may present over-conditioned or obese. It is important to obtain a complete history, because blood glucose values in reptiles can be affected by physiological and environmental factors.[98] Husbandry information obtained should include housing, lighting, heating, diet, vitamin and mineral supplementation, and feeding history. Any recent changes in the environment, previous medical history, and treatment with any drugs should also be reviewed. Seasonal cycles including hibernation and reproduction, both past and present, are important variables that may reflect on blood glucose and thus should be noted.[99] Multiple sampling and/or serial sampling can be valuable in confirming true hyperglycemia, establishing general trends, and helping determine the clinical progression of the reptile patient.[97] Also, if other reptiles of the same species, in the same collection and kept under similar environmental conditions, are sampled, it can help establish a baseline for reptiles in the group.[97] Glucosuria may be noted in reptiles with persistent hyperglycemia.

Variations in blood glucose may be more common in reptiles due to variable metabolic rates, environmental influences and adaptations, and relative insulin resistance.[97] Stress-associated hyperglycemia has been reported in a number of species.[98] A normal seasonal variation in blood glucose levels may occur in many taxa.[99] Temperate reptiles generally have higher blood glucose levels during the breeding season.[99,100] In the fall when most temperate species are increasing fat storage, peripheral blood glucose is low. Tropical reptiles, however, may not show seasonal blood glucose variations.[100] In a study involving captive Mediterranean tortoises (*Testudo graeca* and *T. hermanni*) blood glucose values were found to have a statistically significant peak in April and May upon emergence from hibernation.[99] This elevated blood glucose provides a readily available energy source for tortoises until they begin to feed again. Fresh water turtles were found to show a marked hyperglycemia when diving, which is probably related to increased anaerobic metabolism.[100] Other studies indicate reptiles may exhibit hyperglycemia of several days' duration after a meal.[101] In a laboratory setting, 2 months of starvation (at approximately 21°C [70°F]) was necessary before blood sugar levels became hypoglycemic.[102] By contrast, in a study on savannah monitors (*Varanus exanthematicus*), starvation altered beta cell constituents, resulting in a reduction in the biosynthesis of insulinlike

material and subsequent hyperglycemia.[103] This may be clinically relevant in cases of sick reptiles that have been anorexic for extended periods. The inanition may result in damage to beta cells, with a subsequent reduction in insulin and possible clinical hyperglycemia.

It appears that reptile insulin has a high affinity for human and mammalian insulin receptors and may favorably react with mammalian radioimmunoassays.[104] The affinity of python insulin for human insulin receptors appears similar to that of human insulin.[105] Furthermore, a mammalian insulin radioimmunoassay was used with apparent success in a hyperglycemic bearded dragon (Griswold WG, unpublished data). In general, blood glucose values for normal reptiles are between 3.3 to 5.5 mmol/L (60–100 mg/dL).[106] In one study, a range of blood glucose values in various species was found to be between 1.6 to 11.3 mmol/L (30–205 mg/dL), with average values usually in the range of 5 to 5.5 mmol/L (90–100 mg/dL).[107] Blood glucose values above 300 mg/dL should prompt further investigation. In reptiles, hyperglycemia has not been established as a consistent or specific indicator of pancreatic disease or diabetes mellitus.[97] Reported cases of hyperglycemia have been associated with hepatic lipidosis, hepatic carcinoma, renal adenocarcinoma, chronic glomerulonephritis, interstitial nephritis, granulomatous pancreatitis, gastrointestinal adenocarcinoma, pancreatic glucagonoma, gastric somatostatinoma, and diabetes mellitus (Table 79.4). Gastric somatostatinoma (neuroendocrine gastric carcinoma) is a recently identified neoplasia of bearded dragons and usually arises from the gastric or pyloric mucosa with aggressive metastasis to the liver, kidney, heart, pancreas, ovary, and oviduct.[108,109] A genetic etiology for this disease is suspected. Although delta cells that produce somatostatin are found in the pancreas and stomach, the stomach appears to be the primary site of tumor origin. Reported cases have been young animals (less than 3.5 years old), and severe hyperglycemia is the most significant clinicopathological abnormality. The most clinically significant aspect of these tumors is the immunohistochemical demonstration of large reservoirs of somatostatin in the tissues.[108,109] Somatostatin suppresses the pancreatic secretion of insulin and lowers insulin receptor sensitivity, resulting in the hyperglycemia.[109]

Management of Hyperglycemia

Initially, management of a reptile with hyperglycemia should focus on making a diagnosis of what may be causing an elevation of blood glucose. The goal of the veterinary investigation should be to rule out physiological factors affecting blood glucose and identify underlying pathologies such as specific organ disease, particularly neoplasia.[97] Most reported cases of hyperglycemia in reptiles have been associated with malignancy.[97] Physiological effects that induce hyperglycemia do not appear to cause the severity of glucose elevations seen with neoplasia. Physical examination, biochemical analysis, radiology, ultrasonography, endoscopy, and surgery are all modalities that are utilized to identify diseases resulting in hyperglycemia. Research indicates that compared with mammals and birds, reptiles respond very slowly to the administration of mammalian insulin.[97] Currently it is unknown if the potential exists for inducing immune-mediated (islet-targeted) pancreatitis following the injection of heterologous insulin products in reptiles. Lizards and alligators have been shown to be much less sensitive to insulin than snakes or turtles.[97] If all factors indicate that the patient is truly a strong candidate for diabetes mellitus (a rare diagnosis in reptiles), and the clinician feels some glucose-regulating agent must be initiated, Stahl recommends the following as a starting point using regular mammalian insulin: Lizards and crocodilians 5 to 10 IU/kg body weight IM every 24 to 72 hours; snakes and chelonians 1 to 5 IU/kg body weight IM every 24 to 72 hours.[97] These doses are empirical and should be adjusted based on response to therapy and serial glucose sampling.

TABLE 79.4   Hyperglycemia Values From Select Reptiles

Species (Age)	Blood Glucose mmol/L (mg/dL)	Etiology
Warty chameleon (2 yr) (*Furcifer verrucosus*)[a]	52.68–57.18 (948–1029)	Hepatic lipidosis, nephritis
Bearded dragon (6 yr) (*Pogona vitticeps*)[b]	33.5 (604)	Hepatocellular carcinoma, pancreatic hyperplasia
Chinese water dragon (adult) (*Physignathus cocincinus*)[c]	38.1 (686)	Renal tubular adenocarcinoma, hepatic metastasis
Rhinoceros iguana (adult) (*Cyclura c. figgensi*)[d]	54.8 (987)	Pancreatic alpha cell glucagonoma
Bearded dragon (2.5 yr) (*Pogona vitticeps*)[e]	90.1 (1623)	Gastric somatostatinoma with hepatic metastasis
Red-eared slider (12 yr) (*Trachemys scripta elegans*)[92]	33.8 (610.7)	Diabetes mellitus (pancreatic beta cell islet atrophy)
North American western pond turtle (adult) (*Clemmys m. marmorata*)[d]	46.7 (842)	Diabetes mellitus (pancreatic beta cell islets infiltrated with lymphocytes/plasmacytes)
Desert tortoise (adult) (*Gopherus agassizii*)[92]	46.1 (830)	Gastrointestinal adenocarcinoma, granulomatous pancreatitis
Chinese water dragon (4 yr) (*Physignathus cocincinus*)[f]	44.1 (794)	Osteomyelitis, diabetes mellitus (pyknosis of pancreatic beta cell islets)

Unpublished data by: [a]Knotek Z; [b]Griswold WG; [c]Hanon D; [d]Frye FL; [e]Levine B; and [f]Heatley JJ.

HYPOGLYCEMIA

In reptiles, hypoglycemia has been associated with starvation, hepatobiliary disease, and septicemia.[106] Reported symptoms include weakness, depression, loss of righting reflex, mydriasis, and tremors.[106] A pancreatic islet cell tumor (beta cell insulinoma) with hepatic metastases and multifocal hepatic cholangiocarcinomas was reported in a 7.5-year-old captive born savannah monitor (*Varanus exanthematicus*) presented with lethargy, anorexia, constipation, and narcolepsy-like behavior.[110] Interestingly, multiple glucose levels obtained during a 2-month period (5.2, 2.9, 4.7, 3.7 mmol/L; 95, 53, 85, 67 mg/dL) (ISIS range: 2.2–8.8 mmol/L; 40–159 mg/dL) were considered unremarkable. Insulin immunoassay values from the affected monitor were compared to normal conspecifics. Serum insulin concentrations from the normal monitors were <2 μU/mL. Serum collected during clinical manifestation revealed an insulin level of 8.78 μU/mL. Normalized means and standard deviations for serum insulin analytes were based on information from Cornell University (Ithaca, NY). It should be noted that serum insulin reference ranges have not been established for *Varanus exanthematicus*.

ADRENAL GLANDS

In reptiles the adrenals are paired and vary in color from yellow to pink to red. In chelonians the flattened adrenals are adjacent to the craniomedial poles of the kidneys.[111] In crocodilians the adrenals are retroperitoneal and dorsolateral to the gonads.[111] In squamates the adrenals are located within the gonadal mesentery (mesorchium or mesovarium) (Fig. 79.10A and B). Blood supply includes a venous portal system.[111] The "medullary" tissue occupies a peripheral position, and the "cortical" tissue is centrally placed.[111] Currently, reptilian adrenal tissue is still called "interrenal," a term created by Balfour (1876) for the cytological

and functional equivalent in other vertebrates of the adrenal cortex of mammals.[111] In reptiles hematoxylin and eosin staining reveals the presence of predominantly two cell types: interrenal and chromaffin cells.[13] The pale-staining interrenal cells may either be located toward the periphery of the gland or scattered throughout the adrenal parenchyma. These cells are interspersed with clusters of basophilic-staining chromaffin cells. The interrenal cells secrete glucocorticoids (cortisol and corticosterone).[111] The chromaffin cells secrete catecholamines (epinephrine and norepinephrine).[111] It is suspected that reptiles possess a renin-angiotensin system that causes vasoconstriction, aldosterone release, and a subsequent increase in blood pressure.[112] Corticosterone is the primary glucocorticoid secreted in amphibians, birds, and reptiles.[113,114] In mammals corticosterone is the precursor molecule to the mineralocorticoid aldosterone, which with the renin-angiotensin system regulates blood pressure and sodium and potassium levels.[114] Sufficient serum levels of glucocorticoid hormones provide negative feedback to the hypothalamus and pituitary, causing a decrease in CRH and ACTH.

Glucocortocoids are subject to a circadian rhythm with maximum secretion occurring during the most active period. For example, free-living diurnal Galápagos marine iguanas (*Amblyrhynchus cristatus*) have lower corticosterone concentrations during the night than during the day while the opposite pattern occurs in nocturnal reptiles.[115] Corticosterone levels in reptiles may also vary between adult males and females and have been documented in crocodilians,[125,126] desert tortoise,[127] and Galápagos tortoise.[128] However, these differences were not found when comparing juvenile male and female loggerhead sea turtles (*Caretta caretta*) in Florida (Table 79.5).[129]

Stress can be defined as a normal biologically adaptive response of an individual to internal or external stimuli representing a threat to homeostasis.[113,116] The physiological response to stress includes activation of the sympathetic nervous system (SNS) as well as the HPA axis.[117,121]

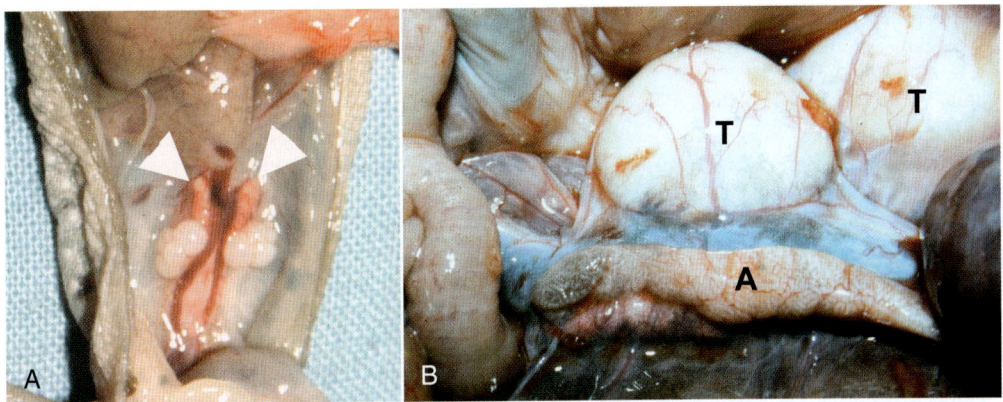

FIG 79.10 (A) The paired adrenal glands (arrowheads) of a female leopard gecko (*Eublepharis macularius*) are suspended in the mesovarium and located anteromedial to the gonads. (B) The paired adrenal glands (A) of a male green iguana (*Iguana iguana*) are suspended in the mesorchium and located medial to the testes (T).

TABLE 79.5	**Glucocorticoid Values From Select Reptiles**		
Species	**Plasma Corticosterone** **ng/ml, Mean ± SD, Range**	**Blood Cortisol** **nmol/L (ng/ml)**	**Fecal Corticosterone** **(ng/day)**
Captive gopher tortoises (*Gopherus polyphemus*)[37]	0.032–0.14		
Captive Hermann's tortoises (*Testudo hermanni*)[138]		Resting: 9.79–16.52 (3.54–5.98) Posttransport stress: 31.12–59.84 (11.27–21.6)	
Galápagos tortoises (*Chelonoidis nigra*)[128]	Adult males: 0.3–2.9 Adult females: 0.0–2.0		
Desert tortoises (*Gopherus agassizii*)[127]	Adult males: 0.58–6.45 Adult females: 0.20–4.08		
Captured wild Kemp's ridleys (*Lepidochelys kempii*)[39]	Juveniles: 20.0–25.0 Hypothermic adults: 39.3 ± 2.5, 12.7–75.6 Convalescent adults: 0.10		
Captive green iguanas (*Iguana iguana*)[135]			Rest: 2–30; handling: 8–150; deprived of climbing: 6–300

SD, standard deviation.

Accurate measurement of catecholamines (i.e., epinephrine and norepinephrine) released as a result of SNS activation is difficult because these substances are only available for transient periods of time.[120] Thus, evaluation of the HPA axis, most commonly by measurement of its end-product glucocorticoids, has traditionally been the primary means to evaluate the stress response in animals.[121] Glucocorticoids (GCs) are metabolized by the liver prior to excretion both through urine and feces via bile.[118] Glucocorticoids are normally bound to a carrier protein, corticosteroid-binding globulin (CBG), and only the free form (5%–10% of the total) is biologically active.[119] In mammals, free unbound cortisol has been measured in conjunction with total cortisol levels. However, to obtain free levels, it is necessary to measure both the CBG levels and to know the binding coefficients.[119] This author is unaware of any published "free" glucocorticoid levels of reptiles.

In reptiles, studies have shown that corticosterone and cortisol increase dramatically during stressful events coordinated by the hypothalamus and anterior pituitary.[113] In most vertebrates, this response is triggered by a wide variety of stressors such as cold stress, nutritional stress, social aggression, crowding, predator presence, transport, drought, infection, and injury.[113,121] Evaluating hormone responses to stress in reptiles relies on acquiring baseline corticosterone levels; however, restraint stress associated with blood collection can obviously affect results.[122] It is important to obtain a blood sample in a relatively short time after capture. In some avian and reptilian species, a "3-minute rule" has been determined, suggesting that blood samples collected within 3 minutes of capture are more likely to represent baseline corticosterone levels.[122] In reptiles, increased glucocorticoids levels are associated with heterophilia and lymphopenia (stress leukogram), and in some species glucocorticoids can affect degranulation of the granulocytes (e.g., heterophils and eosinophils).[124,131,132] Creatine phosphokinase also increases during stress due to capture.[130] Hyperglycemia has been reported in stressed crocodilians and ophidians, while increased hematocrit, red blood cell count, sodium, chloride, and potassium levels have been reported in aquatic chelonians subjected to hyperosmotic stress.[131]

Although corticosterone levels are usually determined through blood sample measurements, fecal, urine, and saliva samples have also been used to measure stress in nonreptiles.[123,133,134]

Various sea turtle species have shown a significant corticosterone stress response on exposure to stressors such as capture and handling, coeliotomy, infection, overcrowding, overheating, and being inverted.[131–132] A study of cold-stunned Kemp's ridley sea turtles demonstrated that affected turtles had significant elevations of corticosterone and excessively decreased levels of thyroxine.[39] Plasma corticosterone concentrations were determined by quantitative radioimmunoassay (Corticosterone Double Antibody 125-I RIA Kit #07–120103, MP Biomedicals). During recovery from cold-stunning, all Kemp's ridleys showed a significant decrease in corticosterone.

An alternative method to assess stress levels is the use of fecal glucocorticoid metabolite concentrations.[134] Fecal samples offer the advantage that they can be easily collected and the procedure is feedback free. Studies have shown that fecal glucocorticoid metabolites reflect free, biologically active glucocorticoid concentrations in the blood, and that fecal glucocorticoid metabolites are an excellent predictor of the responsiveness of an animal to a stressor.[133–134] In a longitudinal study (analyses on repeated individual measurements), fecal corticosterone metabolite levels (FCM) in captive green iguanas were quantified during periods of rest and exposure to hypothesized stressors.[135] FCM levels were measured using the Corticosterone ELISA Kit (DRG Instruments, Marburg, Germany). FCM quantification was combined with behavioral analysis to further interpret the measured increases. It was shown that both daily 5-minute handling/restraint as well as housing devoid of climbing opportunities resulted in increased FCM excretion. Behavioral analysis suggested that the iguanas were chronically stressed by the lack of climbing opportunities, whereas handling induced only a transient stress response. The study provided insight into the functioning of the hormonal stress response in green iguanas for refining housing and handling practices.

Adrenal neoplasia has been reported in green iguanas (Fitzgerald SD, unpublished data), Komodo dragons,[35] and woma pythons (*Aspidites ramsayi*).[136] Tumors were identified as carcinoma, pheochromocytoma, and interrenal cell adenocarcinoma, respectively. Neoplasms were highly malignant with metastases. The Komodo dragon also had a colon carcinoma, thyroid gland adenoma, and pancreatic islet cell tumor. Ultrasonography of the woma python revealed significant tumor regrowth eighteen months postsurgery.

REFERENCES

See www.expertconsult.com for a complete list of references.

80

Theriogenology

Scott J. Stahl and Dale F. DeNardo

The reptilian reproductive tract has similarities in structure and function to other vertebrates but also differs in many ways. The most obvious are two diverging reproductive strategies, oviparity, similar to avian species, and a more evolved mammalian-like strategy with varying degrees of viviparity.

With continued advances in husbandry and nutrition, captive reptiles are living longer, are healthier, and are better adapted and thus exhibit natural reproductive drive and activity. The successful breeding of many species of reptiles has become common both commercially (pet market and herpetoculture) and for conservation efforts in zoos and private institutions to establish captive colonies of threatened and endangered species. Reproductive disease is common in captive reptiles, and clinicians must familiarize themselves with their normal reproductive anatomy and physiology. A review of important unique parameters of reptile reproductive biology will be discussed in this chapter. Additionally, reproductive diseases will be reviewed, including diagnostic and management considerations for these conditions. Surgery of the reproductive tract is covered in Chapter 105.

Many advances in reptile theriogenology have occurred in the last 20 years, especially with the successful captive reproduction of many species for the first time. This is the result of a better understanding of breeding strategies, including environmental manipulation, cycling, hormonal influence, and an improved knowledge in perinatology, including egg incubation and neonatal management (see Chapter 85). Additionally, with concerns on preserving and protecting the growing number of endangered species, developments in semen collection, semen storage, and artificial insemination have advanced and are summarized. Identifying the sex of many reptiles has always been challenging, and many novel and less invasive techniques have been developed and are discussed.

Popularity of reptiles as pets has grown tremendously, resulting in a dramatic increase in animals presented to veterinarians. Single female pets with follicular activity or true dystocia involving infertile eggs, and sexually mature males exhibiting aggressive hormonal behaviors, are common clinical problems. Clients and institutions that are attempting to breed reptiles may rely on their veterinarian as a resource to understand a reptile's general reproductive physiology, captive breeding strategies, and husbandry requirements. Reptile clinicians must familiarize themselves with this information and be prepared to provide both consultation and important theriogenology services such as sexing, routine sterilization, health assessment of breeding animals, gravidity determination/management, and assistance with artificial insemination, as well as diagnosis and correction of reproductive disease.

ANATOMY AND PHYSIOLOGY

Male Reproductive Tract

Testes. The reptilian testes are paired organs that are embryonically derived from the medullary region of the germinal ridge.[1,2] The testes are located dorsally in the mid to caudal coelom adjacent to the adrenal glands and near the cranial portion of the kidneys in chelonians (Fig. 80.1), crocodilians, tuatara, and most lizard species. In lizards with intrapelvic oriented kidneys the testes are considerably more cranial to the kidneys. In chelonians, crocodilians, and the tuatara the testes are generally symmetrical.[1,2] In snakes and many lizard species the right testis is cranial to the left. In snakes the right testis is located just caudal to the gall bladder in the cranial portion of the lower one-third of the body. In a study on anatomical organ positioning in multiple snake species the right and left testes were found between 65% to 82% of the total snout-to-vent length (SVL) depending on taxa, with the right testis cranial to the left but with a high degree of overlap.[3] The testes vary in color from white and yellow to tan-brown and black (e.g., old world chameleons) and are generally smooth and ovoid or flat in shape except in snakes and legless lizards where they are elongated. In mature reptiles the size of the testes varies seasonally and correlates with reproductive activity. Active spermatogenesis results in testicular enlargement whereas a reduction in size is associated with spermatogenic quiescence.[1,2,4] The mesorchium supports and attaches the testis, surrounded by a protective tunica albuginea, to the dorsal wall of the coelom. In squamates the adrenal glands are contained within the mesorchium.[1] The dorsal aorta gives rise to the testicular arteries, which then extend to the ductus deferens. The testicular vein empties into the renal vein, which then drains into the post cava.[1,5]

The testis proper consists primarily of seminiferous tubules and the interstitium, which is made up of interstitial cells, fibroblasts, blood vessels, and lymphatics. The seminiferous tubules have a lining of epithelium containing Sertoli cells and germ cells in different stages of development. Generally, there are three organized layers of germinal cells from immature, along the basement layer (spermatogonia); to developing, the middle layer (spermatocytes); to mature, in the center (spermatids and free spermatozoa).[1,2]

Epididymis/Vas Deferens. The genital ducts of reptiles arise initially from the mesonephric Wolffian ducts and the paramesonephric Mullerian ducts. In males, the Wolffian duct develops and persists with the Mullerian ducts regressing under the influence of testosterone; however, in some species remnants of the Mullerian duct may remain.[1] The epididymis is a flat tubular structure lateral to each testis and makes up the anterior

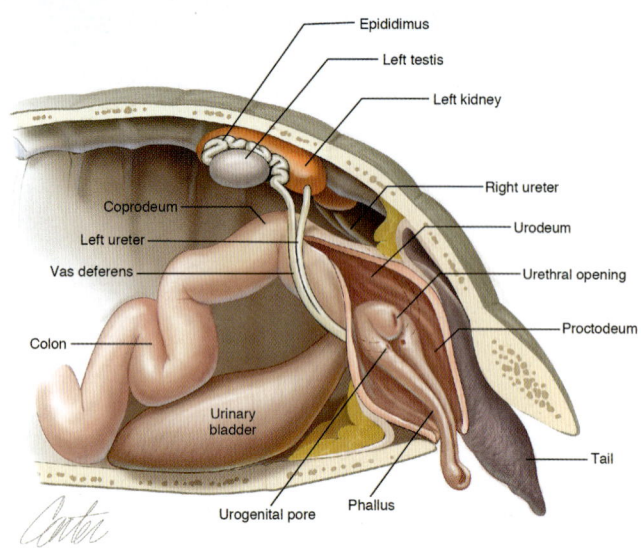

FIG 80.1 Male tortoise reproductive anatomy: testis, epididymus, ductus deferens, and phallus. (Courtesy of Educational Resources, University of Georgia.)

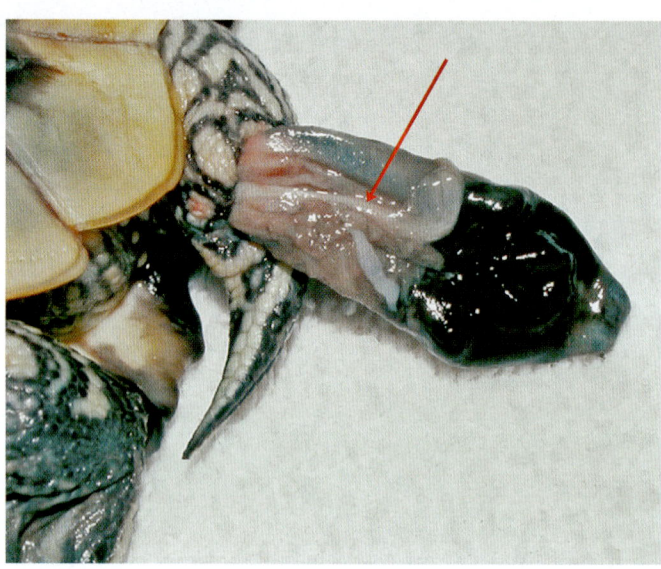

FIG 80.2 The muscular phallus in chelonians extends from the ventral urodeum of the cloaca. The seminal groove in this slider turtle (*red arrow*) transports sperm during copulation. (Courtesy of Stephen Barten).

portion of the ductus deferens (see Fig. 80.1). The epididymis is not typically present in snakes.[1] The ductuli efferentia from the testis passes through the mesorchium into the epididymis. The seminiferous tubules release sperm into ductuli efferentia, which are lined with a single layer of flattened cells and then into the ductus epididymis, and finally sperm empties into the ductus deferens. To assist in movement of sperm, the walls of these ducts contain ciliated cells and a muscular layer.[1,2] The vas deferens courses caudally, generally running along the ventral portion of the kidney, then empties into the urodeum at the genital papillae (see Fig. 80.1). In some species the vas deferens and the ureters will join to form a common urinogenital papillae in the urodeum.[1,4,5]

Renal Sexual Segment. The kidney of male squamates possesses an enlarged (when active) sexual segment, which is composed of hypertrophied distal and collecting tubules. It is absent in crocodilians and chelonians.[1] Seasonal activity in this portion of the kidney can dramatically change gross renal appearance (to a white-yellow color change) and should not be mistaken for pathology. During sexual quiescence the sexual segment of the squamata kidney is involuted and cannot be distinguished from other tubular regions of the kidney. However, in response to seasonal change and hormonal (androgen) influence this sexual segment hypertrophies, and secretory cells fill with numerous granular inclusions.[1] Lizards appear to have more of a seasonal change in the activity of this renal sexual segment than snakes.[1] The large secretory granules of these cells produce a secretion that varies from holocrine to merocrine and contains proteins, amino acids, and phospholipids.[1] The true role of these sexual segment secretions in squamates is not understood. However, some functions have been confirmed, including a role in the production of copulatory plugs in some snake species (*Thamnophis* spp. and *Nerodia* spp.). In these species, after breeding a copulatory plug remains in the female's cloaca and prevents rival males from copulating with the same female.[6] Renal sexual segment secretions have also been shown to activate sperm,[7] serve as a source of energy for sperm, and help with survival of sperm in the female oviduct.[8] This renal sexual segment is thought to correlate well with

the mammalian seminal vesicle due to similarities in embryologic origin, relationship with the vas deferens, and response to androgens.

Copulatory Organ(s). Copulatory systems are different among reptile taxa, with chelonians and crocodilians having a single median phallus that originates from the floor of the urodeum and resides in the ventral aspect of the proctodeum of the cloaca (see Fig. 80.1).[1,4] However, squamates have elaborate paired copulatory organs known as hemipenes located laterally in the ventral tail base and held there by retractor muscles. The morphology of the hemipenes is variably ornate, with structural differences utilized for taxonomy purposes in squamates.[4] The tuatara has no specialized copulatory organ.[1,4] The copulatory organs do not contain a urethra and have no direct connection with the ductus deferens. However, the hemipenes of squamata have a seminal groove, the sulcus spermaticus, located on the everted surface (eversion occurs for copulation and no actual erectile tissue is present), which functions to direct sperm into the female cloaca.[4,5] In chelonians and crocodilians, the copulatory organ does not invert, but the tissue becomes engorged and a pair of spongy longitudinal ridges on the dorsal surface form a seminal groove that directs semen toward the vent. In chelonians these longitudinal ridges are formed from coelomic canals and the corpus cavernosa. With erection the corpus cavernosa become engorged with blood (from the internal iliac vessels) resulting in dorsal and medial curling of the seminal ridges forming a tubelike seminal groove to direct sperm down the phallus (Fig. 80.2).[1] Additionally, the chelonian phallus has a spade-shaped glans at the distal end with three folds, the plica externa, plica media, and plica interna, which direct sperm and help maintain the phallus in the female's cloaca.[1] The erectile ability combined with muscle action extends the phallus out of the vent and into the female cloaca.[4]

Female Reproductive Tract

Ovaries. The ovaries are paired and embryonically derived from the cortex region of the germinal ridge.[1,2] They are located dorsally in the mid to caudal coelom adjacent to the adrenal glands and near the cranial portion of the kidneys in chelonians, crocodilians, tuatara

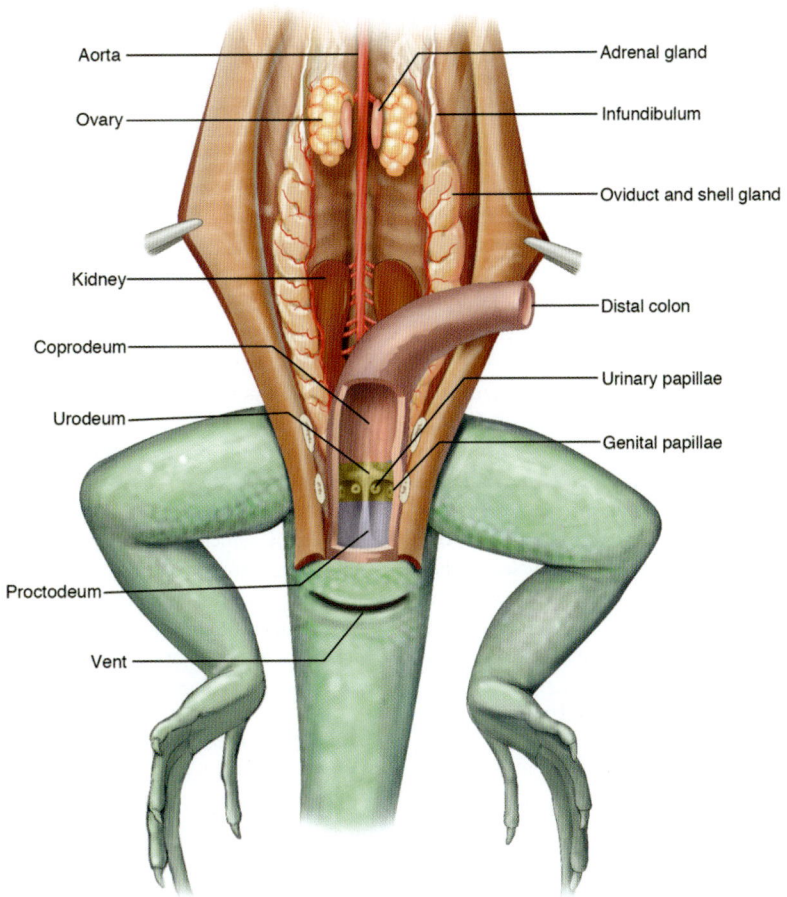

FIG 80.3 Female lizard reproductive anatomy: ovaries, oviducts, genital papillae. (Courtesy of Educational Resources, University of Georgia.)

and most lizard species.[1] In lizards with intrapelvic-oriented kidneys the ovaries are more cranial to the kidneys (Fig. 80.3), as in the green iguana (*Iguana iguana*) with the right ovary just caudal to the tip of the right liver lobe.[5] In chelonians, crocodilians, and the tuatara the ovaries are generally symmetrical; however, in squamates the right ovary is cranial to the left.[1] In snakes the cranial pole of the right ovary is located just caudal to the gall bladder in the cranial portion of the lower one-third of the body (Fig. 80.4). In a study on anatomic organ positioning in multiple snake species the right and left ovaries were found between 58% to 80% of the total SVL length depending on taxa, with the right ovary cranial to the left but with a high degree of overlap.[3] The ovaries vary in color depending on maturity and seasonal activity. Immature ovaries are flat and granular in appearance but with adulthood the presence of different stages of maturing follicles results in a variable appearance (see Fig. 80.4). The ovary is made up of intrafollicular stroma with an associated hierarchy of follicles at different stages of development and atresia.[1,2] Previtellogenic follicles are small and clear to white in color, whereas vitellogenic follicles are larger and yellow to orange in color as they develop yolk. Depending on the species and the reproductive cycle, generally the ovary will be inactive for large portions of the year with only previtellogenic follicles present during these periods.[1,2]

The ovaries are supported by the mesovarium, which is attached to the dorsal wall of the coelom. In squamates the adrenal glands are contained within the mesovarium (see Fig. 80.3). In crocodilians and chelonians, the adrenals are retroperitoneal, dorsal to the gonads, and closely related to the kidney.[2,9] The dorsal aorta gives rise to the ovarian

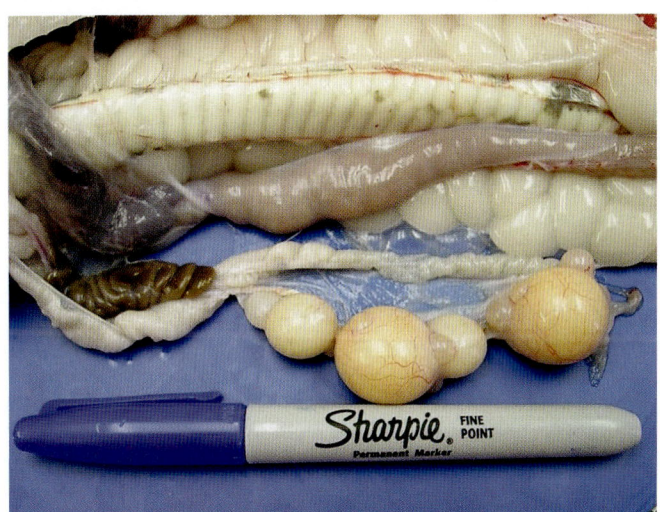

FIG 80.4 Adult female ball python (*Python regius*) at necropsy. The left side of the reproductive tract has been removed from the body cavity and is adjacent to and displayed in the normal anatomical position it would appear within the snake. Note the ovary (just above marker) and ovarian follicles at different stages of development (yellow follicles are vitellogenic) and oviduct just above ovary, with kidney (brown) laying across the more distal oviduct. The lower gastrointestinal tract and fat bodies are between the oviduct thend the body. (Courtesy of Scott J. Stahl, Stahl Exotic Animal Veterinary Services.)

arteries. The ovarian vein empties into the renal vein, which then drains into the post cava.[1,2]

The ovary proper consists of epithelial cells, connective tissue, nerves, blood vessels, and germinal cell beds encased in an elastic tunic.[1,2] The primordial follicles of the ovary are made up of a nucleus, ooplasm, and a simple squamous follicular epithelial layer.[2] Inactive (previtellogenic follicles) do not contain yolk as do vitellogenic follicles. Within the follicle the ooplasm and the granulosa are separated by the acellular zona pellucida.[1,2] Ovarian follicular development (influenced by season) has two distinct phases known as previtellogenic and vitellogenic. Vitellogenesis is the movement of yolk into a maturing ovarian follicle, and the liver is hormonally influenced to produce yolk precursors to support vitellogenesis.

Much variability occurs in this follicular cycle in reptiles but eventually vitellogenic follicles will either ovulate, regress, or rarely become static and potentially inspissated (follicular stasis). Once ovulation occurs, actively proliferating granulosa cells establish the corpora lutea, producing progesterone and remaining active through the gravid cycle.[2,10] After oviposition or birth the corpora lutea regresses, becoming a corpora albicans, which can remain for years.[2] If vitellogenic follicles do not ovulate they will typically begin a cycle of regression (atresia). During this atresia phase the granulosa becomes variable with associated hypertrophy and hyperplasia as granulosa cells, infiltrative histiocytes, and leukocytes phagocytize yolk material.[2,10] The occurrence and frequency of follicular atresia is variable by species and influenced by exogenous factors such as season.[2,10]

Oviducts. The genital ducts (oviducts, salpinges) of female reptiles arise from the mesonephric Wolffian duct and the paramesonephric Mullerian ducts.[1] Reptiles generally have a right and left oviduct; however, there are two genera of snakes (*Typhlops* and *Leptotyphlops*) that are missing the left oviduct.[1] The oviducts are flattened tubular structures positioned adjacent to each ovary (see Figs. 80.3 and 80.4). In immature reptiles the structures appear as thin bands of tissue; in adults with previous reproductive activity the oviduct is more distinct, with notable "concertina" or "accordion" appearance demonstrating contraction from previous enlargement/stretching of gravidity. The mesosalpinx is the supportive mesentery of the oviduct and may contain a prominent oviductal ligament. The presence of this ligament can be useful in determining the sex of some immature reptiles endoscopically as no grossly recognizable ligament is present in males, and the gonads may be difficult to differentiate at this age.[11] The infundibulum is the opening of the oviduct located on the dorsal body wall just craniad to each ovary. The oviducts then course caudally, passing ventromedial to the kidneys and terminating individually in the dorsal wall of urodeum at the genital papillae (see Fig. 80.3).

Histologically the oviduct is made up of two layers of smooth muscle enclosed by an outer serosa. Five regions of the oviduct (from cranial to caudal) are recognized histologically: the infundibulum, the uterine tube, the isthmus (a-glandular portion), the uterus (glandular), and terminally the vagina (thick muscular portion).[2,12] Not all species have each oviduct division, and there is variability. Fertilization takes place near the cranial end of the oviduct (infundibulum) and occurs before deposition of the egg envelopes by the oviduct glands. Copulation occurs before ovulation, and sperm must be stored by the female; seminal receptacles for this purpose have been identified in the posterior uterine tube, isthmus, and anterior vagina of many reptiles.[1,13]

The oviduct has ciliated and nonciliated mucous cells, along with glands below the epithelial lining. These glands generally have both an albumen-secreting and calcareous-secreting (shell and shell membranes) function, and no true uterus exists. However, differences among reptile orders exist.[2,12,13] Generally, the albumen layer provides both physical support to the embryo and assists with water storage. Additionally, a recent study reported that antimicrobial peptides, secreted by the oviduct and found in the albumen of some avian and reptile species, may protect the developing embryo from infection.[14]

In oviparous reptiles the oviduct contains mucosal glands that produce calcium and fibrous portions of the shell membrane and the egg shell.[1,2,12] In viviparous species these glands are few or not present. A relationship exists between the types and abundance of glands and glandular activity in the oviduct and the reproductive strategy of the female. One difference in the evolution of viviparity in reptiles relates to the origin of calcium for the developing embryo. In oviparous species mineral for bone is primarily derived from the shell and shell membranes; however, with viviparity calcium minerals are derived from the yolk material.[1]

The last portion of the oviduct is represented by the vagina, which contains ciliated cuboidal cells with no glandular structures.[1] The vagina empties into the urodeum through the genital papilla (see Fig. 80.3).

Copulatory Homologue. Female reptiles have a phallic/hemipenal homologue, which is located anatomically in the same position as the male. The clitoris and hemiclitoris (squamates) are smaller and less elaborate structures than the copulatory organs of males. However, in some female squamates the hemiclitores are more developed, such as in monitor lizards (*Varanus* spp.),[15] larger skink species (*Tiliqua, Corucia*), and some boids (e.g., short-tail pythons, *Python curtus*).

Cloacal Scent Glands (Snakes)

Cloacal scent glands in snakes are specialized exocrine glands that produce a thick semiliquid material containing pheromones (intraspecific) and/or semiochemicals (interspecific) used to actively mark an object/substrate/organism.[16] These paired cloacal scent glands are uniquely ophidian and generally larger in females, but present in both sexes and in all species of snakes.[16]

Some snakes such as the copperhead (*Agkistrodon contortrix*) have a unique liquid gland material with an ability to void the material as a defensive spray.[17] These paired glands are located within the tail base just dorsal to and attached to the hemipenes in males and in a corresponding position in females (see Chapter 171, Fig. 171.1A). A duct positioned at the anterior portion of the gland curves laterally and opens adjacent to the opening of the hemipenis/hemiclitoris.[16] The glands are ovoid to spherical in shape and vary in color from white/yellow to tan/brown. A muscular sphincter is associated with the duct itself, and the entire gland is surrounded by a muscular sheath, which assists in discharge of contents. Cloacal scent glands are holocrine and the tan brown to black material consists of mostly (90%) free fatty acids (the source of the musk odor), primarily palmitic, oleic, and linoleic acids with mucopolysaccharides and mucoproteins also present.[18]

The function of these glands is complex and more research is necessary, but secretions are likely associated with behavior, including sex attractant, defensive/repellant, aggregation cues, alarm/alert, and territorial marking.[16] The fatty acid composition of these secretions are different among species and within the same species depending on sexual maturity; however, only some species have differences in composition *between* sexes.[18] Therefore these secretions may not represent an intraspecific sexual attractant effect in all species, but may be valuable to assess sexual maturity within the same species or useful to identify the presence of a different species. An example of the complexity and multifunctional properties of these cloacal secretions is evident in the burrowing blind snake (*Leptotyphlops dulcis*). When attacked by ants these snakes will cover their bodies in a thin film of cloacal scent-gland secretion, which repels and thus protects them from ant predation. In this same species, these secretions were found to function as an *intraspecific* sex attractant and an *interspecific* snake repellant.[18] The uniqueness of these scent gland lipids in snakes may prove useful as taxonomic indicators.[19]

REPRODUCTIVE CYCLES

The timing of reproductive events in reptiles is influenced by endogenous and exogenous factors. Examples of exogenous factors include the effects of environmental temperatures on spermatogenesis and embryogenesis, availability of nutritional requirements for vitellogenesis, and timing of oviposition or birth with favorable conditions for newborn survival.[20] These seasonal changes in temperature, photoperiod, and rainfall (food availability) affect endogenous control of reproductive cycles by influencing the hypothalamic-pituitary-gonadotropin endocrine system, similar to mammals.[1,4,21,22] In temperate species the breeding season is short and occurs during the annual cycle. In the tropics, however, reptiles may breed more frequently and may remain reproductively active throughout the year; however, seasonal cycles of rainfall and food availability can influence reproduction.[4,21,22]

Spermatogenic Cycle

The spermatogenic cycle is quite variable in reptiles and has been studied in many species.[1,4,21,23] A full discussion of all spermatogenic cycle strategies utilized by reptiles is not within the scope of this chapter but basic concepts are summarized. In temperate reptiles the breeding cycle typically begins with individuals emerging from hibernation in the spring. Active spermatogenesis is usually associated with increased testicular size; however, the timing of gonadal recrudescence and regression in the annual cycle varies greatly among species.[2,21] These differences often relate to the ability of males to store sperm in the epididymis or vas deferens for extended periods of time, even overwinter. This ability allows insemination and fertilization to occur even when testes are in regression. The three most important environmental factors that influence endogenous control of spermatogenesis and thus breeding cycles are temperature, rainfall, and photoperiod.[21,23] The hypothalamic-pituitary-gonadotropin endocrine system is influenced by these environmental cues, and the spermatogenic cycle and thus sexual steroid production is controlled by the release of pituitary gonadotropins (see Vitellogenic Cycle discussion). Many variations in the reptile spermatogenic cycle exist, but two basic strategies commonly utilized are termed "prenuptial" and "postnuptial" spermiogenesis.[1] With prenuptial spermiogenesis testicular recrudescence occurs in the spring after emerging from hibernation and ends in late spring or summer *before* mating. With postnuptial spermiogenesis testicular recrudescence begins in the spring but continues through the summer, with spermiogenesis occurring at the end of summer. In this case spermatozoa are often *stored* overwinter in the vasa deferentia for use the following spring. This allows reptiles to breed immediately on emergence from hibernation, often when females are present in abundance (communal hibernation), and is an effective strategy utilized by many species and is well studied in garter snakes (*Thamnophis* spp.).[1] An example of the environmental influences on the spermatogenic cycle (even within a species) is the common snapping turtle (*Chelydra serpentina*). Snapping turtles in Tennessee store spermatozoa overwinter in the vasa deferentia for breeding in the spring (postnuptial), but snapping turtles living in the warmer climate of Louisiana have sperm in the vasa deferentia year round (prenuptial and postnuptial).[1] Tropical and subtropical reptiles may have more frequent reproductive cycles, often have a second breeding season, or may breed throughout the year.[20]

Vitellogenic Cycle

As with the spermatogenic cycle the vitellogenic cycle in female reptiles varies greatly among species. One major difference is the dependence on adequate amounts of energy required for folliculogenesis compared with spermiogenesis.[1,20] A major step in the maturation of the ovarian follicle is the accumulation of yolk, or vitellogenesis. The energy for vitellogenesis comes primarily from fat stores in the body of the female but in some species can also be derived from calories taken in during vitellogenesis.[20] However, many reptiles, especially snakes, are capital breeders where energy necessary for reproduction is derived exclusively from fat stores rather than food intake. This regulation ensures that a female can complete a reproductive effort without consuming a meal, which is critical when food availability is unpredictable.[24] If females have insufficient energy stores, they may forego reproduction that season.

As with mammalian species the vitellogenic cycle including follicular development, ovulation, and the production of sexual steroids is controlled by pituitary gonadotropins. This hypothalamic-pituitary-gonadotropin endocrine system is influenced by the environmental cues mentioned for males but also with a greater dependence on energy reserves in females. In squamates a follicle-stimulating hormone (FSH)–like pituitary gonadotropin has been identified, and in crocodilians and chelonians gonadotropins similar to FSH and luteinizing hormone (LH) have been identified.[10] These gonadotropins appear to play similar roles in reptiles as with other vertebrates and an increase in LH, progesterone, and testosterone levels have been documented with ovulation in many chelonian species.[2,21]

Additionally, like mammals, the steroid hormones estrogen, progesterone, and testosterone (androgens) are important in the reproductive cycle of female reptiles. The secretion of intrafollicular estrogen in anolis lizards (*Anolis carolinensis*) with active vitellogenesis results in increased follicular hyperemia and encourages the progression of folliculogenesis.[25] Additionally, this increased vascularity leads to greater yolk deposition in the most hyperemic follicles.[2,25] The mature ovum becomes 10 to 100 times larger than its previtellogenic size.[26]

In a group of captive female veiled chameleons (*Chameleo calyptratus*) fecal hormone values were utilized to evaluate sex steroid hormonal patterns associated with both nonovulatory and ovulatory phases of the reproductive cycle.[27,28] Estrogen levels were found to rise during vitellogenesis and peaked in late vitellogenesis. Progesterone concentrations rose during the late vitellogenic cycle, peaked at midgravidity, and fell to baseline values at oviposition. Testosterone levels varied during the previtellogenic and vitellogenic phases, but similar to progesterone reached peak concentrations during ovulation and gravidity. Ovulation was found to occur in these chameleons with a decreasing estrogen/progesterone ratio.[27,28]

Estrogen (and progesterone) plays a role in vitellogenesis but also in stimulating the liver to convert lipid from the body's fat stores to vitellogenin. Estrogen receptors have been identified in the liver of painted turtles (*Chrysemys picta*), with levels varying during the year but highest in the spring (preovulatory activity) with a smaller peak in the fall (vitellogenesis).[29] During this time the liver enlarges dramatically and takes on a yellow color (physiological increase in intrahepatic fat, not pathological hepatic lipidosis). This vitellogenin (yolk protein) is then selectively absorbed from the bloodstream by ovarian follicles. Calcium is predominantly supplied to the embryo via the yolk in reptiles, and plasma calcium levels are elevated during vitellogenesis.

Progesterone is important in supporting egg and embryo development in reptiles.[29] After egg deposition, concentrations of estrogen, progesterone, and testosterone have been found to decrease in many chelonian species.[2,21] Other hormonal factors affecting reproduction in reptiles include thyroid activity with the hypothalamic/pituitary/thyroid axis influenced by temperature and photoperiod, resulting in effects on gonadal maturation and sexual behaviors.[30] (See Chapter 79.)

There is much variation in the ovarian cycles of reptiles and a detailed discussion is not within the scope of this chapter, but some basic concepts are summarized. As described for the testicular cycle many external and internal factors affect the ovarian cycles. The estrus period usually corresponds with active vitellogenesis, occurring early in the vitellogenic cycle in snakes and in the later stages in lizards.[20] However, vitellogenic cycles do not necessarily coincide with active spermatogenesis, as stored sperm from previous months is often used for breeding.[1,2,4,21] Temperate species tend to have a single seasonal estrus cycle, with an interseasonal period of hibernation. Although temperate males are often consistent with annual spermatogenic cycles, females may have a biennial estrus cycle, dependent on energy sources. These energy sources are often affected by climate, and one example includes the variable cycling of the female European viper (*Viperia berus*) from southern Britain.[1,20] Tropical and subtropical species have more frequent reproductive cycles, are often polyestrous, may have a second breeding season, or breed throughout the year.[20] Exceptions in reproductive cycling do exist, and one noteworthy variation includes tropical boids. The common boa (*Boa constrictor*) and Burmese python (*Python bivittatus*) tend to breed during the cooler periods of the year; however, temperature variations in their natural habitat is mild compared with temperate species. In habitats where rainfall is seasonal, many species key their reproduction cycle to rainfall rather than temperature.[20] Even when environmental cues are appropriate, reproduction may still be inhibited due to other limiting factors. The role of the male in influencing the reproductive cycle of females is not well understood but varies between species. In some species (parthenogenic), females can proceed through the entire oogenic cycle in the abscence of a male (although in some species psuedo-copulation between females is required to stimulate follicular growth), but in other species female snakes may require the male's presence, and possibly the act of copulation, to proceed beyond previtellogenic follicular growth.[31,32] Although the requirement for male presence before vitellogenesis is premature for fertilization, it assures the female of a mate before mobilizing substantial energy stores into reproduction.[32]

FECUNDITY AND CLUTCH DYNAMICS

Differences in reproductive strategies exist for females of different species and are dependent on exogenous and endogenous factors; however, three basic ovulation strategies have been described.[10,33] Polyautochronic ovulation refers to simultaneous ovulation of many ova from both ovaries and includes many squamata and chelonian species seen in clinical practice, including iguanids, bearded dragons (*Pogona vitticeps*), boids, colubrid snakes, red-eared sliders (*Trachemys scripta elegans*), and many box turtle

and tortoise species. Monoautochronic ovulation involves a single ovum simultaneously from each ovary and is common in Gekkonidae. Lastly, monoallochronic ovulation results when one ovum from either the right or left ovary ovulates, and the ovaries alternate between each single egg clutch. This is the reproductive strategy for *Anolis* spp.[2,25]

Clutch size or fecundity is related to and controlled by anatomical and physiological limitations of the species.[1,2] A limited amount of energy is available for reproduction, and consequently, a trade-off is seen between offspring size and clutch size. As described previously, some species have predetermined clutch sizes that may be limited to one, two, or many with polyautochronic ovulators. Thus, a small amount of energy can be allocated to each of many offspring, or large amounts of energy to only a few. The total amount of energy utilized for reproduction can be extraordinary in reptiles, especially in snakes where more than 40% of a female's body mass can be allocated to reproduction. Clutch size is extremely variable, ranging from one (Anoles [*Anolis* spp.], pancake tortoises [*Malococchersus tornieri*]) to 200 (green sea turtles [*Chelonia mydas*]) in oviparous species, and one (shingleback skinks [*Tiliqua rugosus*]) to up to 92 (garter snakes [*Thamnophis radix*]) for viviparous species.[34] Experimental techniques have been developed to alter the clutch size of reptiles. Ablating some developing follicles during early vitellogenesis reduces clutch size and allows for a greater allocation of energy to the remaining ova.[35] The result is the production of larger and presumably hardier offspring. Alternatively other studies have shown that the use of FSH at the onset of the reproductive cycle will increase clutch size while decreasing offspring size.[35] These manipulative strategies could be useful in the preservation and conservation of endangered species.

COURTSHIP

Copulation is usually preceded by specific and often elaborate courtship behavior in reptiles. A great deal of variability exists in the courtship interactions and behaviors. Intermale rivalry with visual displays (of colors and/or head and leg movements), vocalizations, physical fighting, and chemical cues (pheromones) are utilized to establish territory or influence females to breed.[4,34] Male snakes use their bodies and especially their tail and spurs for tactile stimulation of the female, and male lizards use species-specific postures and movements to impress females. Chelonians use both visual and tactile stimulation in the form of head bobs (tortoises), forepaw fluttering (turtles), and biting. Minor injuries are relatively common during courtship and copulation and can become quite serious in the confines of captivity (Fig. 80.5A). Chelonians often bite at the limbs and shell of females to discourage them from walking

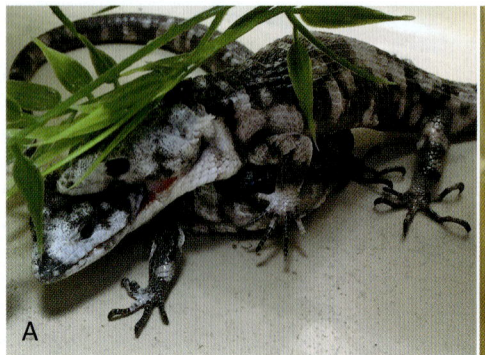
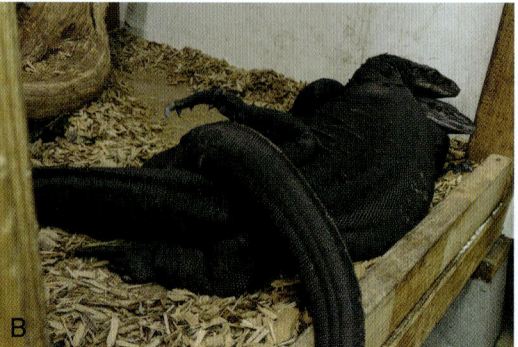

FIG 80.5 (A) Courtship can be aggressive in reptiles. A male alligator lizard (*Ambronia lythrochila*) bites a female's nape to hold her in position while attempting copulation. (Courtesy of Scott J. Stahl, Stahl Exotic Animal Veterinary Services.) (B) Black water monitors (*Varanus salvator*) copulating. Notice the orientation of the male's pelvis (on top) to allow insertion of the hemipenis into the females cloaca. (Courtesy of Cory Aymar, Toothless Reptiles.)

or swimming. Some species of squamata have evolved to engage in mate-guarding behavior as a technique to improve sexual selection. See Chapter 13 for a more detailed discussion.

COPULATION

All fertilization in reptiles occurs internally. Copulatory behavior in males does not necessarily coincide with peak spermatogenesis and testicular development, as sperm for reproduction is often stored in the epididymides or vasa deferentia for extended periods of time.[1,28] Copulation frequently occurs during mid vitellogenesis in females but may occur before vitellogenesis in some species. Male chelonians and crocodilians use their single phallus, whereas male squamates use one of their paired hemipenes to facilitate movement of sperm from the vasa deferentia into the females' cloaca during intromission (see Fig. 80.5B). The tuatara has no copulatory organ and like many avian species copulates by pressing the vent lips together for sperm transfer.[1] Copulation behavior is quite variable. It can be quite short as with many lizards (seconds) or longer (hours to days) in chelonians and snakes (Fig. 80.6A). Aquatic turtles breed in the water, box turtles and tortoises on land. The chelonian phallus is quite elaborate and increases in size dramatically to lock into the female cloaca whereas the more concave plastron allows the male chelonian to "fit" on top of the female's carapace. Male box turtles will utilize their rear feet by placing them between the plastron and carapace to keep the female from closing the plastron on the phallus (see Fig. 80.6B). Male lizards routinely bite and hold the nape of the neck to secure a position on the back of the female during copulation. Additionally, male lizards and chelonians will bite at a female's limbs and tail if she is avoiding advances. Generally, females are more likely to receive the brunt of the trauma during courtship; however, female blue-tongued skinks (*Tiliqua* spp.) are known for aggression toward advancing males. Snakes are less aggressive with courtship and copulation; however, they may intertwine their bodies, often with the male biting (colubrids) the neck area in an attempt to secure the female while inserting a hemipenis into the female's cloaca. Some male snakes (primarily boas and pythons) will use cloacal spurs as a tactile tool to stimulate females during courtship and copulation. Injury during courtship and copulation may be exacerbated by the confinement of captive reptiles to a cage that limits their ability to escape.

FERTILIZATION

Fertilization is internal in all reptiles and takes place near the cranial end of the oviduct (infundibulum) before any deposition of egg envelopes. The timing of fertilization, in terms of the female's reproductive cycle, is not well understood. Because copulation occurs before ovulation, sperm must be stored by the female, and seminal receptacles have been identified in many species in the posterior uterine tube, isthmus, or anterior vagina.[1,13]

Some reptiles can store sperm for up to 6 years; however, fertility is highest when copulation occurs in concert with the female's reproductive cycle.[34] Similarly, second clutches can be produced without a second mating, but fertility is greater if copulation occurs during the development of the second clutch.[34] Using copulation as the onset of gestation often results in exaggerated times for fetal and egg carriage. To further complicate the issue of gestation time, multiple breedings are commonplace. This is especially true for boid snakes, where a pair may repeatedly copulate over a period of 1 to 2 months. In these instances, copulation is obviously occurring at varied stages of the female's reproductive cycle. Additionally, female chelonians are known to store sperm from several males, simultaneously resulting in clutches of eggs with multiple paternity.[36,37] To accurately determine the gestation of a reptile, more advanced techniques such as ultrasonography must be used. The postfertilization developmental pattern a female follows will involve one of two basic reproductive strategies, reptiles that lay eggs (oviparous) and those that are live bearers (viviparous).[38]

REPRODUCTIVE STRATEGIES

Oviparity

Oviparity represents the ancestral mode of reproduction in reptiles and characterizes all living chelonians, crocodilians, the tuatara, and most squamates (Fig. 80.7). Once ovulation takes place, usually little transfer of nutrients is thought to occur between the female and the ova. However in squamates embryos have often completed 25% to 30% of their development at oviposition. This is clinically relevant because the health of the offspring is dependent not only on environmental conditions during (external) egg incubation but also (as with viviparous species) on the conditions a female experiences post-ovulation and prior to

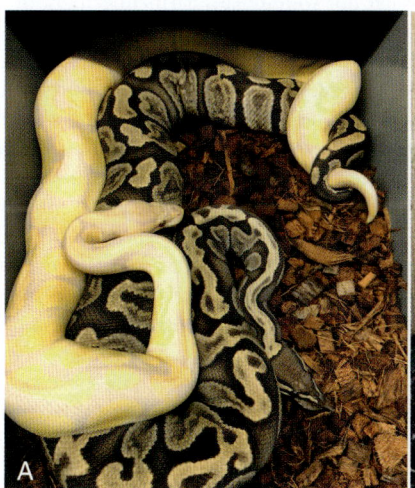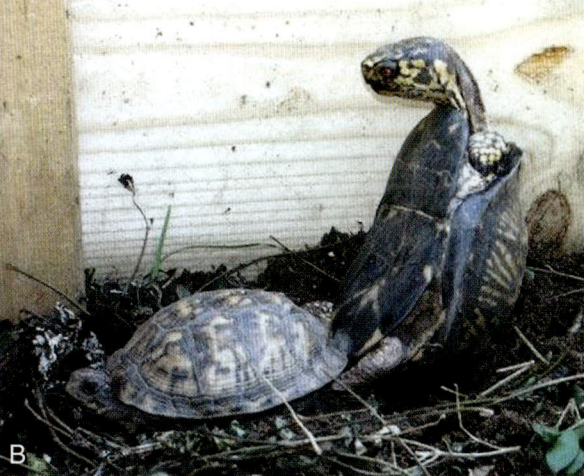

FIG 80.6 (A) Ball pythons (*Python regius*) copulating. This pair is "locked up" as breeders refer to it, with the amelanistic (lavender GHI) male on top and tails intertwined, with the male having one hemipenis inserted into the female's cloaca. (B) Male box turtles (*Terrapene* spp.) often incline the body beyond the vertical to achieve intromission during breeding. The male will wedge his rear feet between the plastron and carapace to keep the female from closing the plastron on his phallus. (A, Courtesy of J. Kobylka Reptiles.)

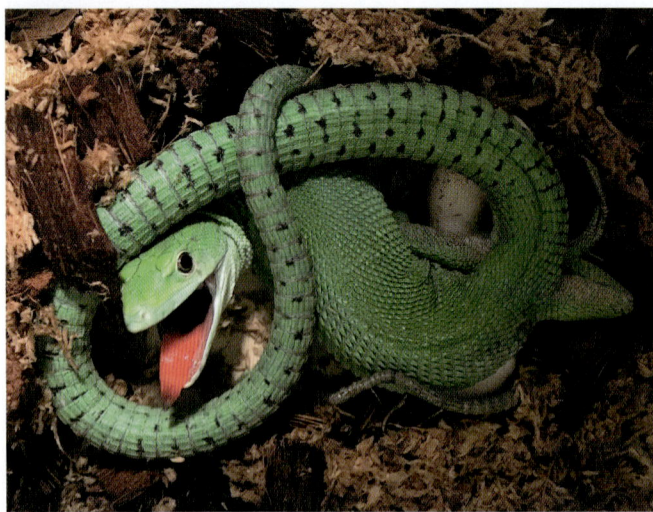

FIG 80.7 A green keel-bellied lizard (*Gastropholis prasina*) with her recently laid clutch of eggs. (Courtesy of Scott J. Stahl, Stahl Exotic Animal Veterinary Services.)

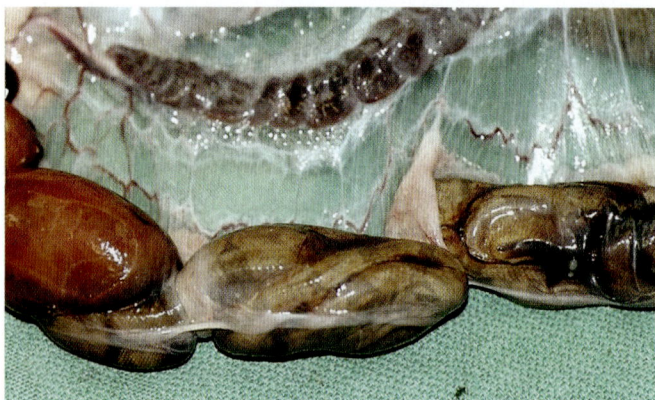

FIG 80.8 One of the most commonly kept captive snakes is the boa constrictor (*Boa constrictor* spp.), which is a live-bearing (viviparous) species. This female died, and dead, full-term fetuses were found at necropsy. The fetuses show normal orientation in the oviduct. The kidney can be seen just above the mesosalpinx and oviduct/fetuses. To the left of the fetuses are several infertile eggs (yellow/orange solid masses) often referred to as "slugs." (Courtesy of Scott J. Stahl, Stahl Exotic Animal Veterinary Services.)

oviposition. The ovum becomes an egg when albumin and a shell are added in the oviduct. The degree of shell calcification varies among species, ranging from minimal, resulting in pliable eggs (snakes, most lizards, and some turtles) to pronounced, resulting in rigid eggs (crocodilians, tortoises, and many geckos). An example of the variation in shell rigidity is evident in geckos, in which egg type is phylogenetically based. Geckos in the family Gekkonidae have rigid eggs, however, Diplodactlidae (i.e., Australian and New Zealand geckos) and Eublepharidae (eye-lid geckos) have pliable eggs. Clinically, ultrasonography can be used to distinguish the general stages of gonadal inactivity, early previtellogenic follicle growth, vitellogenesis, ovulation, and either shelling or fetal development. See ultrasonography later in this chapter and in Chapter 58.

Viviparity

Many species of lizards and snakes have developed the ability to produce live young (Fig. 80.8). These live-bearing reptiles are often subdivided into ovoviviparous and viviparous, depending on the degree to which the female contributes nutrients to the developing embryos.[39,40] In this chapter the term viviparous will be synonymously used with live-bearing. In addition, although the term pregnant is oftentimes reserved for viviparous species and gravid for oviparous species, in this chapter the term gravid will include all females, whether incubating eggs or fetuses. Nutrients are provided to the developing embryos either by lecithotrophy (via yolk during follicular development) or matrotrophy (during embryonic development such as across a placenta). The degree of matrotrophy in squamates can be variable, with the most extreme example being skinks (*Mabuya* spp.) that contribute more than 99% of the neonatal mass through a chorioallantoic placenta.[41] Besides providing gas and possibly nutrient exchange to the developing offspring, viviparity provides some protection to the developing embryos and permits a female to adjust developmental temperature by simply moving between warm and cold locations.[42] Viviparity also has energy costs, and by retaining the developing fetuses within the body for an extended period of time, the female is limited to a single clutch per year.[39] The space occupied by fetuses (and eggs in oviparous species) also limits the function of the gastrointestinal tract, and females usually reduce intake or cease feeding during the latter stages of gestation. Postpartum females are often in poor condition, having mobilized virtually all energy stores for production of offspring. Because sufficient lipid stores are

necessary for reproduction, reptiles that are unable to rapidly restore lipid often reproduce biennially or even triennially (see Vitellogenic Cycle and Fecundity and Clutch Dynamics).[43] In captivity, however, extensive postpartum feeding may allow for naturally biennially breeding species to produce annually. Oviparous species may also suspend feeding during the latter stages of egg development; however, the length of time is shorter (weeks versus months) and less significant. Although all viviparous species cannot possibly be listed, Table 80.1 provides a list of common viviparous and oviparous species seen in practice. Clearly, the reproductive mode of a reptile has a phylogenetic component (e.g., all pythons are oviparous, all rattlesnakes are viviparous). However, reproductive mode is a plastic trait that has evolved independently at least 100 times in squamates,[41,42] and both viviparity and oviparity can be present within a genus (e.g., *Rhacodactylus*, *Eryx*, *Charina*) and even a single species (e.g., *Sceloporous aeneus*).

Parthenogenesis

Although not widespread, parthenogenesis, or asexual reproduction, has been reported in about 30 plus species of lizards and has been extensively studied in whiptails (*Aspidoscelis* [*Cnemidophorus*] spp.), where parthenogenic species have evolved from the hybridization of two species. These lizards reproduce asexually, but females still show courting and pseudocopulation, and these behaviors have a positive effect on reproductive output.[44]

More recently the Komodo dragon (*Varanus komodoensis*) has also been found to have the ability to reproduce by parthenogenesis.[45] Genetic finger printing was utilized to determine this in captive hatchling Komodo dragons, and the use of this technology will likely result in identifying more species with this ability. Parthenogenesis has also been discovered in snakes, and all blind snakes (*Indotyphlops* [*Rhamphotyphlops*] *braminus*) are triploid females.[46] Other snake species can switch between asexual and sexual reproduction, and a recent report indicates there may be an emerging phylogenetic pattern for parthenogenesis in snakes, especially with more species being continually identified.[47] Some species with this ability include certain garter snakes (*Thamnophis elegans* and *T. marcianus*), rattlesnakes (*Crotalus horridus* and *C. unicolor*),[47] copperheads (*Agkistrodon contortrix*) and cottonmouths (*Agkistrodon piscivorus*),[47] file snakes (*Achrochordus arafurae*),[48] and Burmese pythons (*Python bivittatus*).[49]

TABLE 80.1 Reproductive Modes of Commonly Kept Reptiles

Oviparous (Egg-Laying)

All crocodilians
All chelonians
Lizards
    All monitors (*Varanus* spp.)
    Iguanids (majority)
    -Iguanas (*Iguana, Cyclura, Ctenasaur* spp.)
    -Water dragons (*Physignathus* spp.)
    Geckos (majority)
    Chameleons (majority)
    -Veiled chameleon (*Chamaeleo calyptratus*)
    -Panther chameleon (*Furcifer pardalis*)
Snakes
    All pythons
    Colubrids (majority)
    -King snakes and milk snakes (*Lampropeltis* spp.)
    -Rat snakes and corn snakes (*Pantherophis* spp.)

Viviparous (Live-Bearing)

Lizards
    Geckos
    -New Caledonian rough-snouted gecko (*Rhacodactylus trachyrhynchus* spp.)
    Skinks
    -Blue-tongued skink (*Tiliqua* spp.)
    -Shingle-backed skink (*Tiliqua rugosus*)
    -Prehensile-tailed skink (*Corucia zebrata*)
    Chameleons
    -Jackson's chameleon (*Trioceros jacksonii*)
Snakes
    Boas (except *Charina reinhardti, Eryx jayakari*)
    Vipers (majority)
    Colubrids
    -Garter snakes (*Thamnophis* spp.)

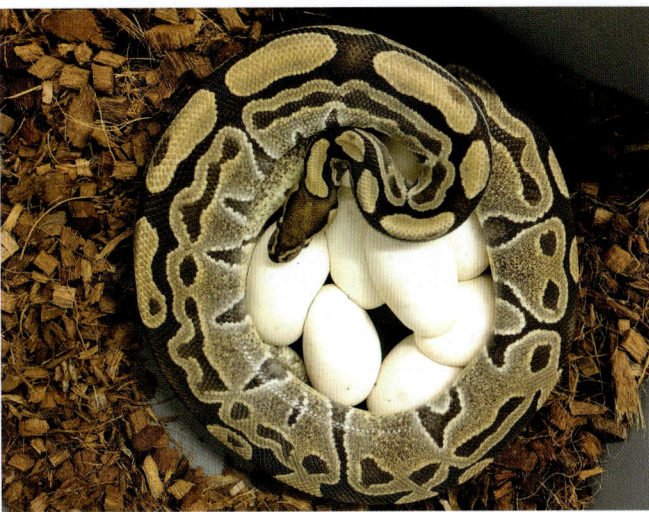

FIG 80.9 A female ball python (*Python regius*) coiled around her eggs after oviposition. (Courtesy of J.Kobylka Reptiles.)

Parental Care

Most reptiles show no parental care of their eggs or offspring beyond choosing an appropriate nesting site and concealing the eggs; however, some degree of care has been documented in more than 100 species.[50] In the few cases of parental care, the investment is usually limited and nonessential for survival of the offspring.

Many female pythons coil around their eggs until hatching, protecting eggs from predators and providing temperature and humidity regulation (Fig. 80.9). Some python species have the ability to twitch muscles to generate heat.[51] Recent research with children's pythons (*Antaresia childrenii*) showed this maternal brooding instinct to be strong, as female pythons were willing to brood the eggs of other females or even rocks similar in size to their eggs.[52]

Nest building and guarding has been documented in several species, including turtles (e.g., Burmese mountain tortoise [*Manouria emys*]), lizards (e.g., skinks [*Eumeces* spp., *Mabuya* spp.] and glass lizards [*Ophiosaurus* spp.]), snakes (e.g., king cobra [*Ophiophagus hannah*] and cobras [*Naja* spp.]), and especially crocodilians (virtually all species). Female king cobras use their coils to build an elaborate nest out of branches and bamboo leaves and will guard their eggs for up to 3 months.[53]

Crocodilians guard their nest but also assist neonates in emerging from the nest and guard them for some time after hatching. Some viviparous species also show some maternal care. Rattlesnakes remain with their offspring until the neonates first shed, which is approximately 1 week after birth.[54] In addition, some females assist neonates in escaping from their amniotic sacs (skinks [*Mabuya* spp.] and night lizards [*Xantusia* spp.]) or consume infertile yolk sacs (common boas [*Boa constrictor*] and sand boas [*Eryx* spp.]). More extensive postnatal, parental care has also evolved in many species. A study on wild populations of long-tailed skinks (*Eutropis longicaudata*) found that populations with a higher predation pressure on the offspring provided maternal care, whereas populations under less predation pressure did not.[55] See Chapters 13 and 85 for more discussion on maternal and paternal behaviors.

SEXUAL MATURITY

Sexual maturity in reptiles is determined primarily by size, with age playing a less significant role.[34] Although standard ages for sexual maturity can be found in the literature, these numbers are usually based on free-ranging reptiles, where all individuals in a population have similar environmental influences. However, in captivity, care and diet can vary dramatically, often resulting in captive reptiles reaching sexual maturity at considerably different ages. For example, many boid species are "power fed" by ambitious breeders to encourage them to grow quickly to reach early maturity with the hope to breed them as young as 18 months to 2 years. In contrast, reptiles provided with poor husbandry and diet can have slow and stunted growth, delaying sexual maturity.

The interspecific variation in maturation size is greater than the intraspecific variation in growth rate, making discussion on specific maturation sizes difficult. To provide some reference, the following generality is provided; snakes raised under optimal conditions usually mature in 2 to 3 years, small lizards take 1 to 2 years, and large lizards 3 to 4 years. Chelonians take longer to mature, usually 5 to 7 years.

SEX IDENTIFICATION

Reptiles do not possess external genitalia, so sex identification is not always obvious. The proper method to identify the sex of a reptile varies greatly among species and the age of the individual. Sex can often be identified with various methods that differ in simplicity or accuracy. When choosing a sexing method, understanding the accuracy of that method is important. If identifying the sex of an individual is not critical, such as a pet reptile not utilized for breeding, safety and simplicity

---

TABLE 80.2   Practical Techniques for Sex Identification by Major Taxa

Snakes
Sexual dimorphism

Thickened and longer tail in males (paired hemipenes located in the base of the tail)

Larger spurs in males (boas and pythons)

Size (females of some species may be larger as adults, e.g., ball python, [*Python regius*])

Everting hemipenes ("popping") (primarily neonates/juveniles)
Probing (most reliable technique)

Lizards
Sexual dimorphism

Larger head, jowls, crests, spines, body size in males

Thicker tail, paired hemipenes located at base of tail in males

Femoral/preanal pores larger in males

Color

Unique anatomy (male), rostral horns (Jackson's chameleon, *Trioceros jacksonii*), heel spur (veiled chameleon, *Chamaeleo calyptratus*)

Probing (not reliable in most species)
Everting hemipenes "popping" (more reliable/safest with anesthesia)
Transillumination (light-colored species, several to compare differences between male/female)
Radiography

Some monitor species calcified hemipenal hemibaculae with maturity

Contrast solution introduced into hemipenal/clitoral sulcus (male spiral, female flat/straight)

Ultrasonography

Mature females may note clusters of anechoic ovarian follicles

Male more difficult to identify testes

If ovary not seen, identification of sex not definitive, not useful for immature lizards

Not useful in large monomorphic skinks (*Tiliqua, Corucia*) due to keratinized scales

Endoscopy (coelioscopy)

Most definitive with visualization of the gonad, and biopsy possible

Requires anesthesia and is more invasive

Chelonians
Sexual dimorphism

Longer nails on front feet in male aquatic turtles (e.g., red-eared sliders and painted turtles)

Concavity to plastron in males

Tail larger and longer, vent opening more distal on tail

In some tortoises the plastron anal scutes curve inward in female, outward in male

Female larger body size in some species (e.g., leopard tortoises, *Stigmochelys pardalis*)

Male larger body size in some species (e.g., eastern box turtle, *Terrapene carolina*)

Red/orange iris color in male eastern box turtle

Ultrasonography (mature females but not immature/juvenile)
Endoscopy

Coelioscopic, gonad is directly visualized, most definitive for immature/juveniles

Cystoscopic, gonad visualized through bladder, can be definitive but not direct visualization

Procedures require anesthesia and are more invasive

All
Molecular/DNA sexing
Sex hormone analysis (plasma and fecal)

---

are important considerations. However, when captive breeding is intended, one must choose an identification method that provides virtually 100% accuracy. Obviously, accuracy of a given procedure is dependent on the ability of the individual performing the procedure, and proper training and experience enhances success.

The various methods used to identify sex in reptiles are discussed. Important variables to consider when choosing a particular technique include: species, age, safety versus invasiveness, and need for high accuracy. Table 80.2 provides a quick reference to the preferred method(s) of sex identification in common species maintained in captivity.

Secondary Sexual Characteristics

In some species, sex can be easily identified based on obvious secondary sexual characteristics that anatomically distinguish adult males from females. This is most prevalent in lizards and to a lesser extent chelonians. Other than differences in maximal body size, secondary sexual characteristics are rare in snakes and crocodilians. The accuracy of secondary sexual characteristics in sex identification varies dramatically, depending on species, age, characteristic being examined, and the experience of the observer.

Some species have obvious coloration or ornamentation that distinguishes the sexes. This is best exemplified in chameleons, such as Jackson's chameleon (*Trioceros jacksonii*), where the male possesses 3

large rostral horns that are absent in females. Unfortunately, most secondary sexual characteristics are more subtle, involving minor differences between sexes.

Generally, male reptiles have a larger more robust appearance, especially of the head area. This may include ornamentation of the head such as crests, spikes, protruberances, jowls, dewlaps, (Fig. 80.10A) and increased coloration in these areas; examples include the colorful dewlap of the male anolis and the black beard of an alarmed bearded dragon (*Pogona vitticeps*). However, these differences are often minor and large females can easily be confused with small males. Common species where general appearance and head size are frequently used in sex identification, with mixed accuracy, include iguanas, Gila monsters (*Heloderma suspectum*), and beaded lizards (*Heloderma horridum*), and many of the larger skinks (*Tiliqua* spp., *Egernia* spp.).

A recent study in eastern blue-tongued skinks (*Tiliqua scincoides*) utilized morphometrics of head size compared with body size to establish an accurate technique for identifying sex.[56] This large popular lizard has unique, heavy keratinization of body scales, which makes ultrasonography and other sexing techniques challenging. Sexual dimorphism in this species is subjective but typified by mature males having a larger head than females, and females generally having a longer snout-to-vent length (SVL) than males. The study evaluated 69 free-living eastern blue-tongued skinks and utilized noninvasive body measurements to develop a formula

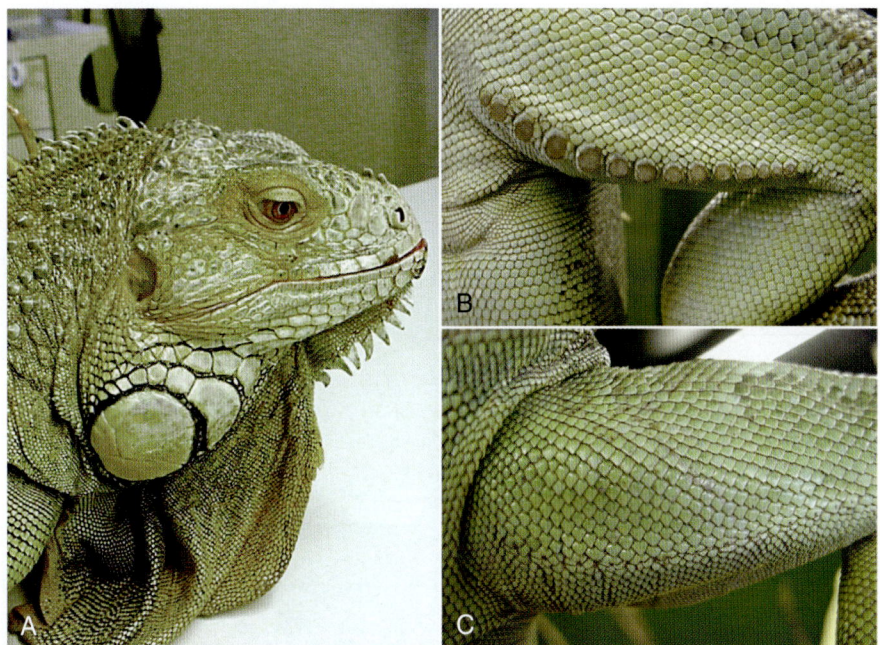

FIG 80.10 Secondary sexual characteristics in the green iguana (*Iguana iguana*). (A) Mature males often have larger, broader heads with more developed crests, dewlaps, and jowls. (B) Mature males have more developed femoral pores, with a definitive wax secretion containing pheromones for marking territory. (C) Females tend to have reduced or absent femoral pores. (Courtesy of Stephen J. Divers.)

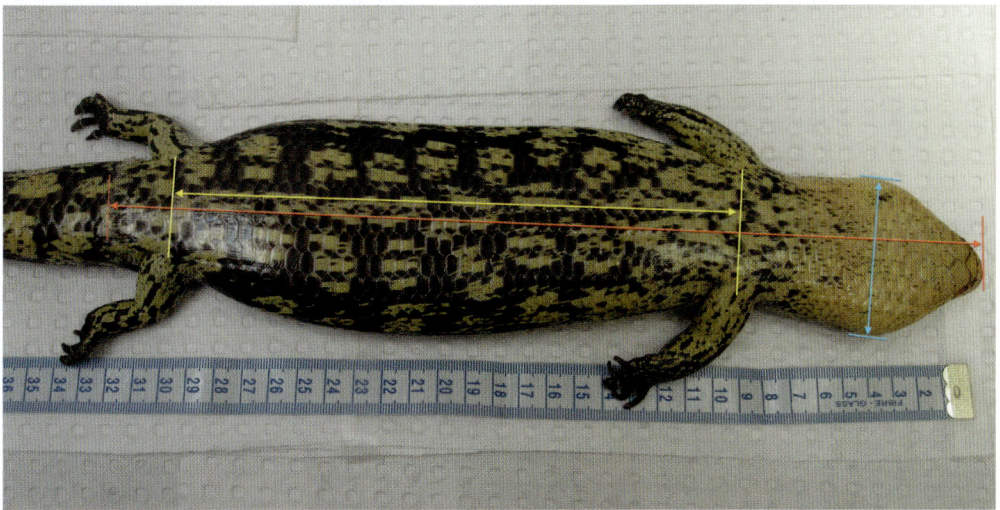

FIG 80.11 Measurement points for morphometrics calculations in blue-tongue skinks are demonstrated on this blotched blue tongue skink (*Tiliqua nigrolutea*) in dorsal recumbency. The blue line is head (H), red line is snout-to-vent (SVL), and the yellow line is trunk (T). (Courtesy of Robert Johnson.)

for sexing them. Ratios of morphometric measurements—head width measurement/SVL (H/SVL)% and head/trunk (H/T)%—showed significant predictability with respect to sex identification in both adult and subadult skinks.[56] Smaller numbers of other blue-tongued skink species were also evaluated and similar results found, suggesting these ratios may be useful in other *Tiliqua* species. To apply the technique, measurements of the H, SVL, and T are taken (Fig. 80.11). Ratios are then calculated for H/SVL% and H/T%, and these measurements are then compared with the confidence intervals (CI) found in the study to identify the sex of the skink.[56] The CI ranges found were for H/SVL% (males: 15.35–15.99; females 13.20–13.94) and for H/T% (males: 23.79–25.31; females 20.03–21.35).[56] Further work may validate the use of this noninvasive technique in other lizard species.

In chelonians, the plastron of males is often concave (Fig. 80.12A and B). This plastron concavity allows the male to closely appose his cloaca to the female's during mounting. The degree of plastron concavity and gender differences show considerable intraspecific and interspecific variation.

Many inconspicuous but notable secondary sexual characteristics are located near the cloaca. Many iguanid and gekkonid lizards possess either femoral or preanal pores that excrete a waxy substance used for marking territory. Although present in both sexes, these pores are more pronounced in mature males and even moreso with seasonal hormonal influence (see Fig. 80.10 B and C).

Many boas and pythons possess spurs located just lateral to the vent. The spurs are vestigial hind limbs, and in males, they are used for tactile

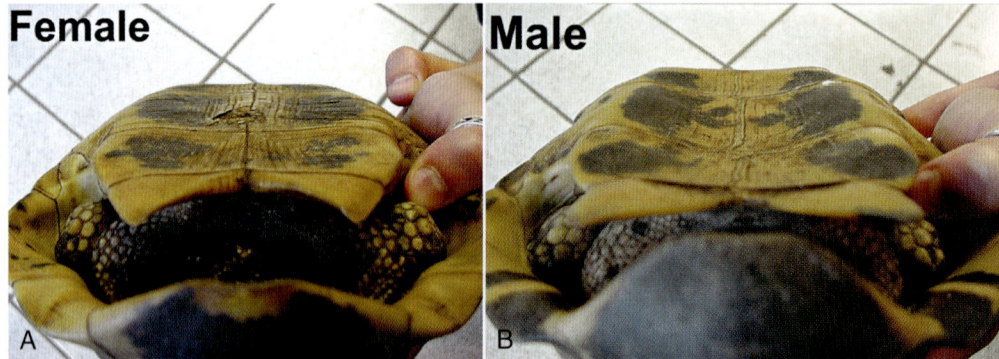

FIG 80.12 (A and B) Gender identification in red-footed tortoises (*Chelonoidis carbonaria*) is based on plastron concavity and shape of the plastron anal scutes. Notice the female's anal scutes curve inward while the male's point outward. Also note the concavity in the male's plastron. This concavity helps the male to "fit" on top of the female's carapace during copulation. (Courtesy of Stephen J. Divers.)

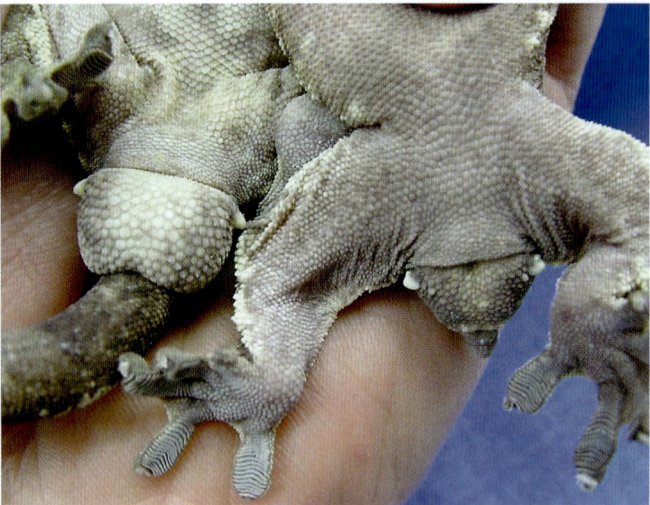

FIG 80.13 Adult male (left) and female crested geckos (*Corellophus ciliatus*) showing sexual dimorphism. The male has normal bilateral hemipenal enlargement at the tail base compared with the female. Note the female has lost her tail, and this species does not have tail regenerative abilites. (Courtesy of Scott J. Stahl, Stahl Exotic Animal Veterinary Services.)

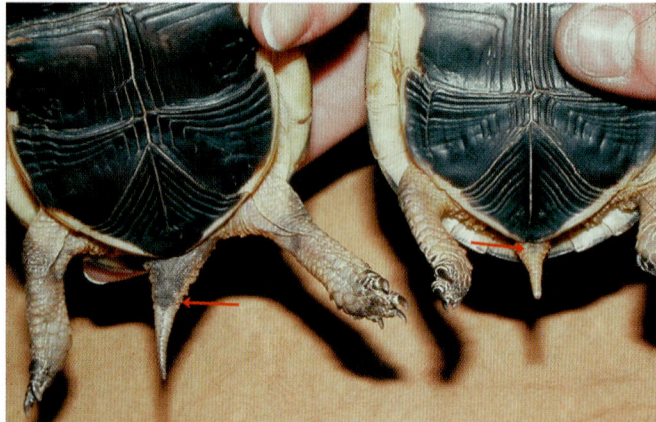

FIG 80.14 One consistent distinguishing characteristic between male and female turtles and tortoises is the length of the tail. In these box turtles (*Terrapene* spp.) the male's tail is longer and broader and the vent opening is further out on the tail, usually past the edge of the cara-pace. In the female the vent opening is between the edges of the plastron and carapace. See red arrows identifying the vent. (Courtesy of Douglas R. Mader.)

stimulation of the female during courtship. Spurs are usually larger in males, but the difference in size is variable by species. In some species, such as the rosy boa (*Charina trivirgata*) and sand boas (*Eryx* spp.), spur size is a highly reliable predictor of sex. However, in other species, the reliability is reduced. In the ball python (*Python regius*), spur size is extremely variable in both sexes and therefore has little value as a sex identifyer.

The tail is a critical reproductive structure for many male reptiles, because it provides both a storage location for hemipenes (squamates) and a muscular appendage to help position the male's cloaca adjacent to the female's. Because of these traits, the size and shape of the tail is often sexually dimorphic. In squamates the prescence of hemipenes may result in symmetrical bulging at the base of the tail, which can often be quite dramatic, sometimes visible without picking up the individual. The extent of this dimorphism is usually greater in lizards than snakes, especially smaller species like geckos (Fig. 80.13).

Male chelonian tails, although not enlarged due to housing the phallus, are usually much larger and longer than the females'. In addition, the vent is usually located more distally along the tail of males (Fig. 80.14). The larger tail provides better access to the female's cloaca, which, with the presence of the shell, is important. Some tortoises also use the tip of the tail for tactile stimulation of the female's cloacal region.

Other secondary sexual characteristics located near the tail but specific to individual species include enlarged postanal scales of many iguanid lizards (e.g., spiny lizards [*Sceloporus* spp.]) and the pelvic protuberances of the banded geckos (*Coleonyx* spp.). In some chelonians, especially many tortoises the anal scutes on the plastron, tend to curve inward toward the cloaca in females and point outward in males (see Fig. 80.12A and B).

In many mature male aquatic turtles, notably the red-eared slider and painted turtle (*Chrysemys picta*), the nails on the front feet grow significantly longer than females and are used in courtship by waving them in front of females as they swim backward in front of them. Male box turtles (*Terrapene* spp.) often have a much brighter red/orange iris color compared with females (Fig. 80.15). Veiled chameleons (*Chameleo calyptratus*) can be sexed at hatching, as the male has a definitive spur pointing caudally at the heel of the rear foot.

In addition to the challenge of being familiar with species-specific dimorphism these (hormonally influenced) secondary sexual charac-teristics are usually not developed in juveniles. Thus juveniles of many species that may have obvious sexual differences as adults will not develop these features until maturity and must have their sex identified by other methods. Some of the sexing techniques described later, such as endoscopic sex determination, were developed as a result of the need

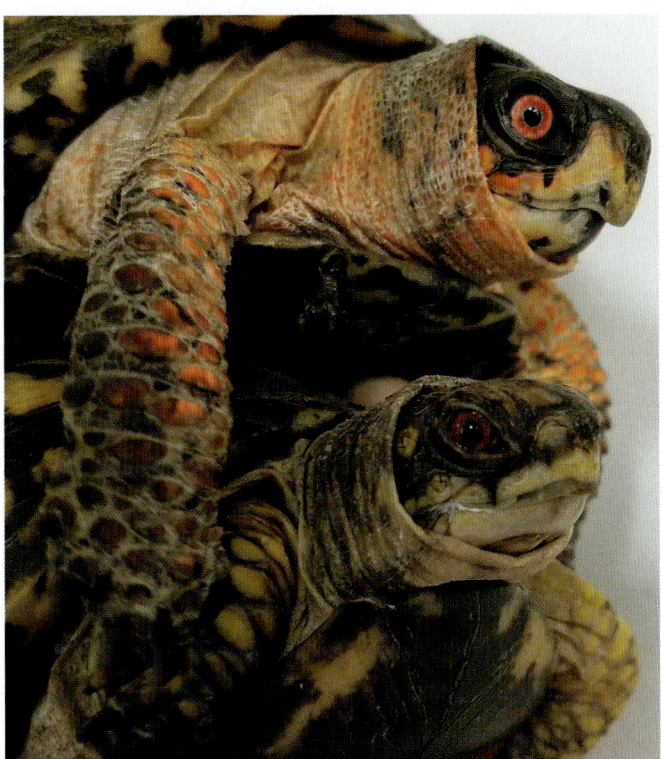

FIG 80.15 A male (*top*) and female eastern box turtle (*Terrapene c. carolina*) showing the darker red/orange iris color of mature males. (Courtesy of Scott J. Stahl, Stahl Exotic Animal Veterinary Services.)

to definitively sex these neonatal and juvenile animals for economic or conservation reasons.[11]

Tail-Base Transillumination

A novel, noninvasive technique popular among reptile breeders for sexing small lizards, especially those with light-colored skin, involves tail-base transillumination to visualize the hemipenes. This technique is especially useful if several reptiles of the same species are evaluated at the same time to compare differences between sexes. With transillumination the males' hemipenal structures have an increased tissue and vascular prescence compared with the females' hemiclitores. Smart phones with a "flashlight" mode can be used to transilluminate smaller species such as geckos. The cool light source is placed dorsally at the tail base with the light passing through the base of the tail and peri-cloacal area to highlight tissues. Stronger flashlights or an endoscopy light source in the veterinary practice may be useful in larger lizard species such as bearded dragons. Caution must be used to avoid thermal damage to the lizard when utilizing this technique, as some light sources can produce significant heat (http://www.beardeddragon.org).

Cloacal Probing

Probing the cloaca with a slender blunt instrument is the most common method of sex identification in adult snakes and some large lizards (e.g., monitors [*Varanus* spp.]) and was first described by Lazlo.[57] This procedure identifies the presence of the hemipenes. The particular instrument used is not critical as long as it is long, smooth, and blunt on the probing end. Commercially manufactured probes are available in various sizes from several sources (Fig. 80.16A). Cloacal probing is a straightforward technique that can be easily mastered with practice.

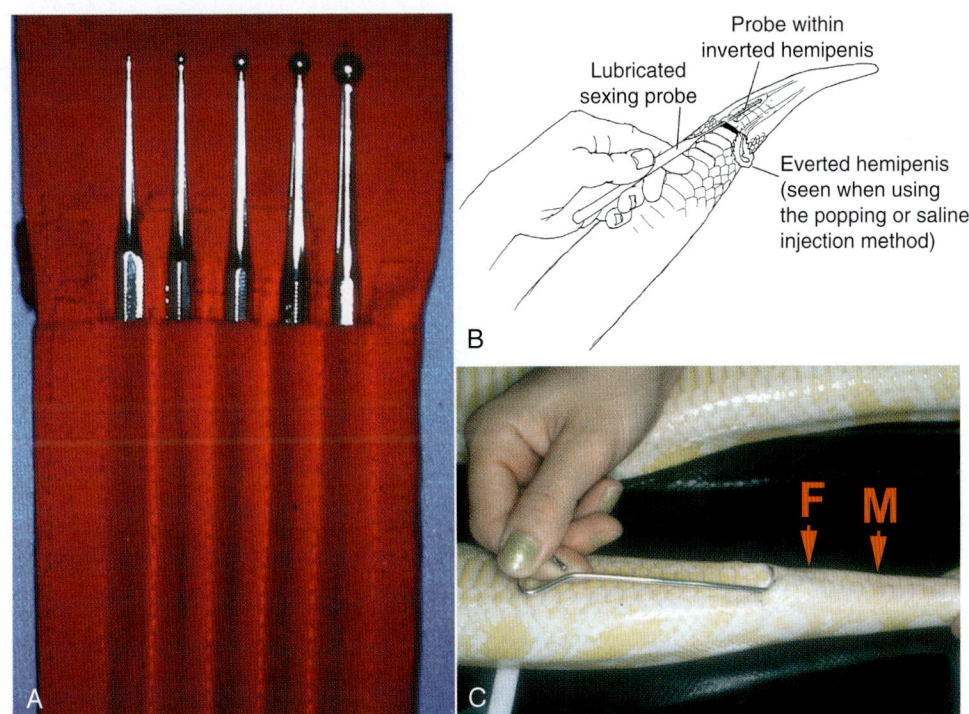

FIG 80.16 (A) Sexing probes can be purchased commercially as a probing kit with different sizes and appropriate rounded balls at the probing end. (B) Probing method for sex determination; the illustration depicts probing of a male snake. (C) Probing of a male albino Burmese python (*Python bivittatus*), showing depth of probe in reference to subcaudal scale probe depth of male (M) and female (F). (A and B , Courtesy of Douglas R. Mader; C, courtesy of Stephen J. Divers.)

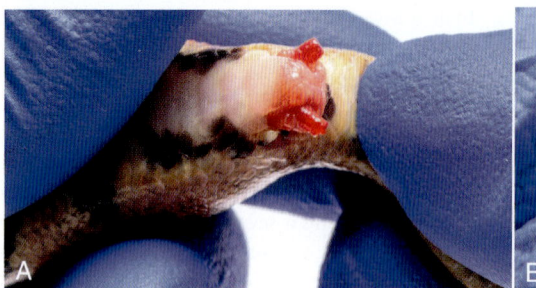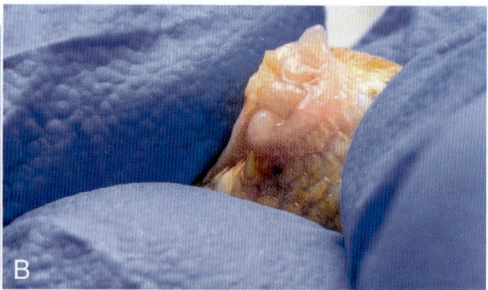

FIG 80.17 Hemipenal eversion (known by breeders as "popping") in juvenile ball pythons (*Python regius*). (A) Note the distinct "tubular" structures that identify this as a male. (B) A female showing the scent gland "papillae" but no distinct tubular structure as with the male. This technique takes practice but can be quite accurate in experianced hands with juvenile snakes. (Courtesy of Mike Schultz.)

With the reptile properly restrained, the probe is inserted into the cloaca and directed caudally. Many lubricants have been found to be spermicidal, so caution must be used when probing reptiles that are actively breeding or are expected to breed in the near future.[58] Saline is the safest lubricant to use in these cases.

With gentle maneuvering of the probe just lateral to midline, the probe enters the inverted hemipenis in a male and freely advances within the hemipenal sulcus (see Fig. 80.16 B and C). The depth to which the probe enters the tail is dependent on the species. Probing females results in shorter depth of penetration because the female has a hemipenal homologue or hemiclitoris, which is shorter in depth and smaller in diameter than the hemipenis. A properly sized probe allows the probe to enter the inverted male hemipenis and the female hemiclitoris without puncturing or damaging the tissue. If a probe is too small or sharp or excessive force applied a female could inadvertently be probed as a male as the probe perforates through the hemiclitoris. Common species in which female hemiclitores are well developed and misidentification of sex is likely include short-tailed (blood) pythons and monitor lizards (*Varanus* spp.).[15] This technique does not work as well in lizards as in snakes because many lizards have increased musculature in this area and contraction hinders probe advancement.

Manual Eversion of Hemipenes

The most common method used for identifying the sex of neonatal colubrid snakes is to manually evert the hemipenes. This procedure, frequently referred to as "popping" by snake breeders, entails firmly rolling one's thumb proximally up the tail base toward the cloaca. The pressure forces the hemipenes to evert laterally at the caudal edge of the cloaca (Fig. 80.17A). To avoid injury, care must be taken to roll the thumb rather than simply apply pressure.

In females, the scent gland openings/papillae can sometimes be identified during popping with the openings located laterally in the cloaca (see Fig. 80.17B). These scent gland papillae are especially visible in female king snakes (*Lampropeltis* spp.); however, females of most species are identified merely by the lack of hemipenes. This negative result in identifying females can lead to the misidentification of males as females. However, with experience, the sex of most neonatal colubrids can be determined with nearly 100% accuracy using this technique. Sometimes this technique can be utilized in juvenile or small- to medium-sized lizards, but care must be taken not to injure the lizard, and it should not be used in species that perform tail autotomy. For heavy-bodied juvenile snakes, including many of the boas and pythons and some colubrids (e.g., hognosed snakes [*Heterodon* spp.]), everting the hemipenes is more difficult or not possible and may risk injury.

This same technique can be performed under anesthesia (see Chapter 49) to relax the reptile enough to overcome the retractor muscles (usually sedation alone is not enough) and allow eversion of the hemipenes or hemiclitores. This approach is more definitive, may eleviate stress and

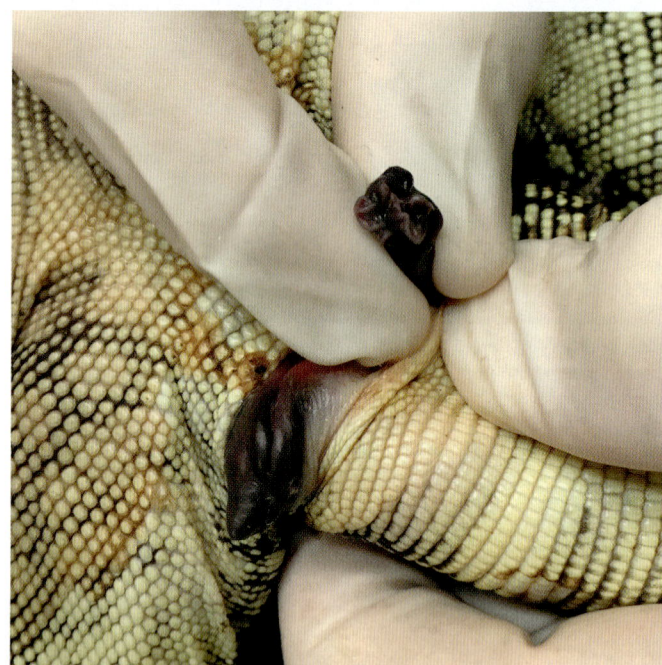

FIG 80.18 A yellow-headed water monitor (*Varanus cumingi*) under general anesthesia allowing the left hemipenis to be manually everted. Note the elaborate spiral/flowering distal end. The partially everted right hemipenis in this figure looks similar to the hemiclitoris in female monitors, showing the importance of completely everting the structure to see the male spiral portion to acurately identify the sex with this method. (Courtesy of Juliet Mejia, Stahl Exotic Animal Veterinary Services.)

discomfort, and reduces the likelihood of injury from an awake reptile struggling during eversion attempts. On evaluation the hemiclitoris of the female can look similar to the hemipenis of a male in some species, and close examination may be necessary to differentiate the two, especially in neonatal specimens. Hemipenes are more ornate and larger in length and diameter compared with the hemiclitores of females (Fig. 80.18).[15]

Hydrostatic Eversion of the Hemipenes

Hydrostatic eversion by saline injection is more invasive and uncomfortable and has increased risk for injury; therefore other techniques discussed should be considered first. However, if done properly this technique can be accurate and safe.

Like manual eversion, this procedure relies on the eversion of the hemipenes from the base of the tail to identify males. However, unlike manual eversion, the technique provides a definitive anatomic indicator of females rather than the mere absence of the male trait. Procedurally, sterile isotonic saline solution is injected into the tail just distal to where the hemipenes would be located if the individual was a male. The fluid is injected into the tail until either sufficient eversion has occurred or resistance can be felt at the plunger. Placement of the needle too proximally on the tail may direct the fluid into a hemipenis rather than behind it, therefore making the procedure not only ineffective but also potentially injurious. The hydrostatic pressure created within the tail not only forces the hemipenes to evert but also causes swelling of the tissue surrounding the cloaca. This swelling partially everts the cloaca through the vent, allowing visualization of the oviductal papillae in females. This technique is useful for neonatal snakes in which manual eversion is ineffective and for many lizard species. For large specimens, including monitors, iguanas, and heloderms, the strength of the retractor penis muscle can counteract the hydrostatic pressure and prevent eversion of the hemipenes. In these species, the muscle must be relaxed using a surgical level of anesthesia. With eversion the hemipenis is more ornate and larger in length and diameter compared with the hemiclitoris of females (see Fig. 80.18).

Digital Palpation of Cloaca

The preferred method for sex identification of crocodilians involves digitally palpating the ventral aspect of the cloaca for the presence of a phallus. With the animal appropriately restrained in dorsal recumbency, the cloaca can be easily explored with a gloved finger. The presence of a phallus is obvious, because it is the only structure that can be felt in the otherwise smooth-walled cloaca. If desired, the phallus can be everted through the vent for visualization.

Plasma Sex Hormone Evaluation

Sex hormone evaluation to identify sex may be valuable in chelonians and lizards. In a study in hatchling and immature desert tortoises (*Gopherus aggassizii*), tortoises that were confirmed to be males by visualizing testes endoscopically had significantly higher plasma testosterone levels than female tortoises, with a 98% correletion between the two different techniques.[59] A hormone stimulation study was described for sexing hatchling giant river turtles (*Podocnemis expansa*) where one unit of FSH was injected intracoelomically and blood was drawn 4 hours later to measure plasma testosterone. Male chelonians had testosterone levels >0.5 ng/mL, whereas females had plasma testosterone values <0.2 ng/mL.[60]

A study in monitor lizards evaluated the use of plasma sex hormone levels in conjunction with hemipenal eversion as a possible technique to increase the accuracy of sexing Merten's water monitors (*Varanus mertensi*) in the field.[61] This monitor species is semiaquatic with significant tail musculature for swimming, and thus traditional hand-pressure-induced hemipenile eversion is difficult and may result in inaccurate sexing. Sixty-two different, field-captured adult monitors were examined between January 2001 and February 2003 in the tropical north of Western Australia. On examination manual hemipenal eversion was attempted and recorded as eversion (yes or no) and plasma was collected and later measured for androgen (An) and estradiol-17β (E2) levels. The final sex of individuals was determined using a combination of plasma (An: E2) ratio and field eversion result. With the additional plasma hormone information, it was possible to determine the sex of 37.0% of males and 31.2% of females that could not be determined through hemipenal eversion and thus increased the accuracy of sex identification in the field.[61] More work needs to be done in evaluating plasma sex hormone levels as a reliable technique for sexing monomorphic reptile species (knowing that many extrinsic and endogenous factors affect these hormones), but this report shows there may be clinical value, especially when combined with other sexing techniques. Several studies evaluating fecal sex hormone levels to monitor the ovarian follicular cycle in a group of captive female veiled chameleons was successful and this same technology (less invasive and expensive then

blood analysis) could possibly prove useful in sex identification in sexually monomorphic reptiles.[27,28]

Radiography

Many but not all species of monitors (*Varanus* spp.) possess mineralized hemibacula within their hemipenes, which are easily recognizable on radiographs.[62] Monitor species in which these structures occur are listed in Chapter 9, Table 9.2, and depicted in Fig. 9.13 in that chapter. Unfortunately this calcification occurs with age and maturity and is not often evident in young monitors when sex identification is most valuable. Another study found pelvic measurements taken from radiographs in Gila monsters (*Heloderma suspectum*) was useful to differentiate the sexes.[63]

A recent study involving 20 eastern blue-tongue skinks (*Tiliqua scincoides scincoides*) utilized a noninvasive radiographic technique for sex identification by introducing radio-opaque solutions into the hemipenal/hemiclitoral sac (Mallett, Proc UPAV, 2015a, pp 40–46). Contrast medium (1 mL of iohexal; Omnipaque, GE Healthcare) was introduced into the postcloacal sulcus with a syringe and attached tom-cat catheter or 22 g intravenous catheter with stylet removed (similar to the sexing probe technique with insertion of the catheter to the full depth of the sulcus), and the contrast material was injected continously as the catheter was slowly withdrawn. Excess contrast was wiped away, and the skinks were radiographed utilizing horizontal beam lateral and dorsoventral views. The positive contrast images showed repeatable differences in the definition of the hemipenes and hemiclitores in the skinks. On the dorsoventral view the hemipenes were wider and showed a spiralling outline compared with the hemiclitores, which had a thinner and sharply angled outline. On the horizontal view the hemipenes were larger and showed a spiral shape (related to the ornate nature of the hemipenis), whereas the hemiclitores were thin and straight/horizontal (Fig. 80.19A–D). The technique had 100% correlation with the definitive sex identification of skinks using breeding records or coeliscopic sexing. This procedure was felt to be effective for skinks of 15 cm SVL and larger.

Another imaging study looked at the sensitivity of hemipenes identification with several imaging modalities, including ultrasonography,

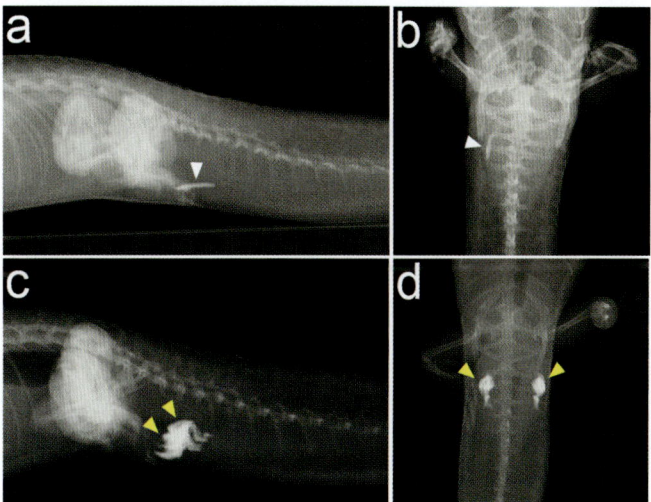

FIG 80.19 Contrast radiographs of a female and male eastern blue-tongue skink (*Tiliqua scincoides scincoides*). (A) Horizontal beam view of female, (B) dorso-ventral view of female, (C) horizontal beam view of male, and (D) dorso-ventral view of male. Note in female images (A and B) the hemiclitores (white arrowheads) are identified as thin, sometimes sharply angled structures, compared with images of the male (C and D), where hemipenes show a spiraling effect indicative of the more elaborate hemipenes (yellow arrowheads). (Courtesy of Steven Mallett.)

radiography (with contrast introduced into the cloacal sulcus), and CT (with and without introduced contrast) in four different lizard species (*Pogona vitticeps, Uromastyx aegyptia, Tiliqua scincoides, Gerrhosaurus major*).[64] In this study 19 lizards were evaluated and the accuracy of cloacal sulcus contrast radiography was 94.7%. In male lizards radiographs showed distinct spindle-shaped opacities associated with the contrast medium within the inverted hemipenis lumen. This study concluded that contrast radiography and contrast CT (see later) were effective, noninvasive, but more costly, techniques for gender identification in lizards.[64]

Ultrasonography

The value of ultrasonography is limited to identifying females, as ovarian follicles (spherical anechoic to hypoechoic structures based on cycle) are the only easily recognized reproductive structures (Fig. 80.20). Therefore only reproductively active females can be identified with confidence, leaving immature females, acyclic females, and all males often undistinguishable.[36,65]

One study in mature heloderms found ultrasonography to be useful for identifying the presence or absence of hemipenes in the proximal tail base.[66] However, a more recent study evaluated hemipenal identification using several imaging modalities in 19 lizards of 4 different species and concluded that the accuracy of ultrasonography to identify gender was poor at 64.3%.[64]

CT/MRI

Advanced imaging techniques such as CT and MRI are becoming more affordable technologies in clincal practice and can be offered to clients as a possible tool for sexing reptiles. Resources and guidance on the normal imaging anatomy of many reptile species with these advanced imaging modalities is increasingly available. In the hemipenal imaging study mentioned earlier noncontrast CT had poor accuracy (63.1%), and hemipenes were identified in only two lizards, both of which had spindle-shaped kinked structures consistent with smegma within the hemipenal sulcus.[64] However, with the use of contrast, CT accuracy improved to 100% with hemipenes being correctly identified in all 9 males. With more research CT and MRI may continue to prove to be

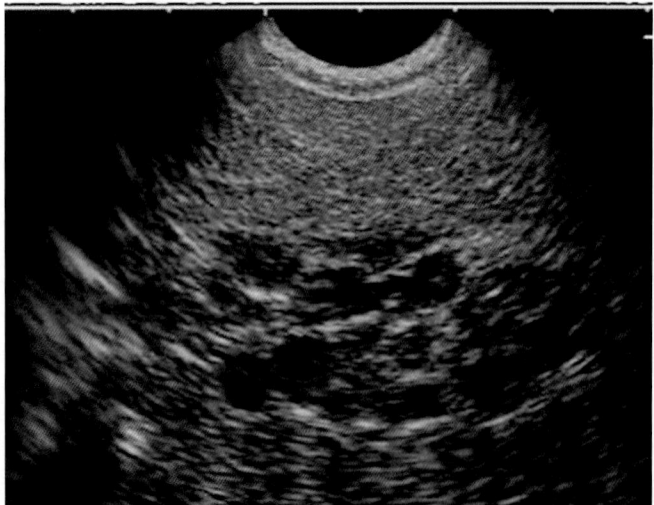

FIG 80.20 Ultrasonography for sex identification in monomorphic species can be useful if distinct ovary follicles are noted but if *not seen* the sex can still be in question. This sonographic image shows immature ovarian follicles (clustered ovoid anechoic structures) in a green iguana (*Iguana iguana*). (Courtesy of Scott J. Stahl, Stahl Exotic Animal Veterinary Services.)

valuable, noninvasive, but more costly, tools to accurately sex monomorphic reptile species.

Surgical or Endoscopic Sex Determination

Visualization of the gonads via surgery or coelomic endoscopy (coelioscopy) is a definitive method for determining the sex of reptiles.[67,68] Endoscopy is less invasive than traditional surgery, and the basic rigid endoscopic equipment (2.7-mm telescope and 4.8-mm sheath system) in most veterinary facilities can be utilized for gender identification in many reptiles, even at an early age. Coelioscopic sexing is indicated in monomorphic reptile species (lizards and chelonians) where less invasive techniques lack accuracy. It is especially useful to breeders and for endangered species breeding programs, where early gender determination in juveniles is critical.[11,59] Coelioscopy using saline infusion was shown to be accurate in identifying sex in hatchling and neonate chelonians. A study in Chinese box turtles (*Cuora flavomarginata*) concluded that gonads could be visualized and sex identified in animals as small as 10 g (Fig. 80.21A–C).[11] More than 300 individual juveniles of various chelonian species have been safely and successfully subjected to early gender identification by coelioscopy (Divers SJ, unpublished data). Coelioscopic sexing is not useful in snakes because of their unique anatomy and the intimacy of coelomic organs. Along with accurately identifying sex through direct visualization of the gonad, in mature reptiles coelioscopy can provide feedback on the status and health of the reproductive tract.

Another endoscopic approach to sexing reptiles was recently published and involved evaluation of the gonads through the transparent bladder wall of juvenile tortoises (*Testudo marginata*).[69] This technique has the advantage of being less invasive (coelom is not entered) but does not provide the same degree of visual acuity as direct coelomic examination and has been found to be unsafe in juvenile sliders (Proenca L, unpublished data).With more research this technique may prove useful in many chelonians but in species where the immature gonads appear similar, or the bladder wall is less transparent, accuracy may be decreased. For details on coelioscopic and cystoscopic sexing techniques in reptiles, see Chapter 64.

Temperature-Dependent Sex Determination

Many reptile species have temperature-dependent sex determination (TDSD), where the sex of the developing embryo is determined by the temperature at which the eggs are incubated. TDSD occurs in all crocodilians, most chelonians, and a few species of lizards, most notably for clinical practice the bearded dragon (*Pogona vitticeps*), leopard gecko (*Eublepharis macularius*), and crested gecko (*Correlophus ciliatus*).

The exact temperatures at which each sex is produced is species-dependent. In some, warmer temperatures produce males, and in others, warmer temperatures produce females. In still other species, bimodal variation is seen, with one sex produced at moderate temperatures and the other sex produced at high and low temperatures. In all cases, the shift from one sex to the other is not absolute, but instead a range of temperatures exists at which both sexes are produced in varying proportions. Because these intermediate temperature ranges exist and incubator thermometers may not be accurate, predicting sex solely based on incubator temperature can be flawed. Sex should be confirmed in these species using one of the previously mentioned techniques. See Chapter 85 for more information on TDSD.

Genotyping (DNA/Molecular Sexing)

For reptile species where sex is determined genetically, identifiying the sex of an individual using a genetic code unique to their heterogametic chromosome is possible.[70] Unlike mammals where the male is the heterogametic sex in all species, the heterogametic sex varies among

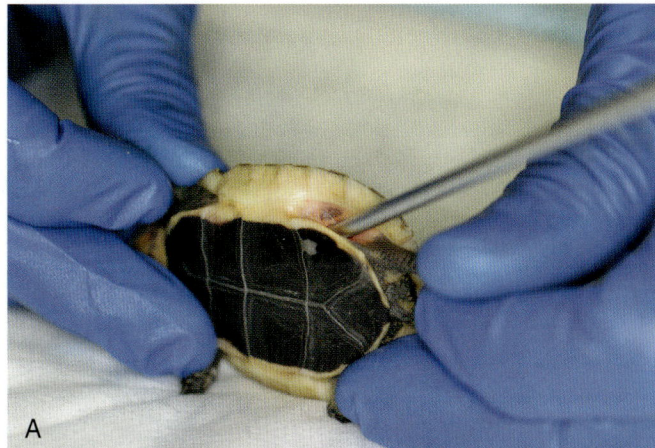

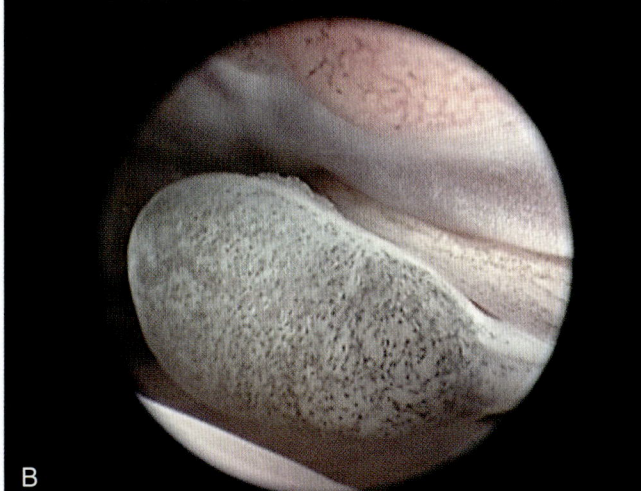

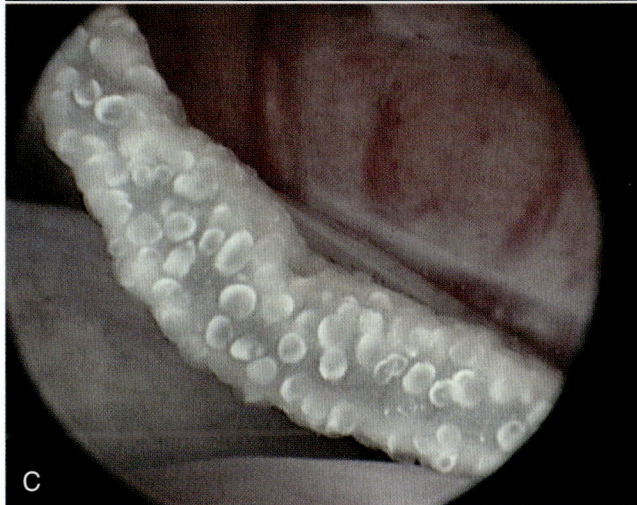

FIG 80.21 (A) A juvenile Chinese box turtle (*Cuora flavomarginata*) undergoing coelioscopy for sex identification. (B) Coeloscopic image of immature testis in a juvenile male Chinese box turtle. (C) Coelioscopic image of immature ovary in juvenile female Chinese box turtle. (Courtesy of Stephen J. Divers.)

species of reptile. Reptiles have different modes of sex determination, including both temperature-dependent determination and chromosomal sex determination. With chromosomal determination in reptiles some genera have XY sex chromosome, some genera have ZW sex chromosome, some genera have no recognizable sex chromosome, and some may show all three variations.[70] Therefore it is unlikely that a DNA marker

found in one species or genus will be sufficiently conserved to be broadly applicable to other reptiles.[70] Thus this technology, at least currently, may be limited to threatened or endangered species and has been reported as a potentially useful conservation tool.[70] In the Komodo dragon specifically, these molecular techniques have been further evaluated, and PCR analysis consistently resulted in the amplification of a male-specific longer fragment found to be useful for molecular sex identification.[71]

CAPTIVE BREEDING

Understanding the anatomy and reproductive physiology of reptiles, along with the ability to accurately identify their sex, are clinically important. Knowledge of reproductive anatomy and physiology of reptiles is considerd a science; however, the captive reproduction of these animals in many ways is an art. Veterinarians must have the ability to combine the science and art to effectively help clients with captive breeding and management of their reptiles. References on captive breeding are readily available, and an exhaustive discussion of all captive-breeding parameters is beyond the scope of this chapter but some important principles are summarized. Much of the information shared here is derived from the snake-breeding industry, which has historically been successful and can be used as a template for other taxa.

Breeding Stock

The three components of good breeding stock are: (1) at least 1 individual of each sex is needed, (2) the individuals in question must be sexually mature, and (3) they must be healthy. Although these points seem obvious, it is not uncommon for owners to present breeding "pairs" of the same sex or breeding individuals in poor health. These three requirements are essential for captive breeding but are not sufficient to ensure positive results. Successfully breeding reptiles involves a series of events occuring in succession, and failure of any one may lead to poor results.

Seasonal Cooling

As discussed previously, a period of cooler temperature is necessary for most species to initiate reproductive behavior. This seasonal cooling is commonly referred to as brumation, hibernation, or cycling. A reptile's physiology is greatly affected by the imposed cooler ambient temperature. Most body systems, including the immune system, operate best at an optimal temperature. When body temperature differs substantially from the optimal temperature, such as during seasonal cooling, these systems are less effective. The goal is to safely provide the seasonal cooling stimuli necessary (based on natural history) while putting the reptile at the lowest risk. To stimulate an appropriate reproductive response in the spring, temperate species must be subjected to lower temperatures reaching a constant low winter temperature of 10° to 13°C (50° to 55°F) for 8 to 12 weeks. High latitude and high elevation species may need lower temperatures. Subtropical and tropical species need less drastic temperature drops, usually to 20° to 24°C (68° to 75°F) and primarily at nighttime with an available (yet optional) focal heat source during the daytime hours. Significant nighttime cooling appears to be the critical component to stimulating reproduction in many subtropical and tropical species. A similar cool night, with an available (yet optional) focal heat source during the day, approach to seasonal cooling can also be effective and safer for small temperate lizards.

All reptiles should undergo a physical examination and fecal evaluation before seasonal cooling. Unhealthy animals should not be cooled. Both the immune system and digestive system are dramatically affected by body temperature. For temperate reptile species that will experience a dramatic/constant temperature reduction, first ensuring that the digestive tract is empty is essential. Lower body temperature reduces the ability to digest food; therefore any material in the gut can lead to severe and sometimes fatal enteritis. Snakes should have food withheld for at least 2 weeks before extended cooling, and lizards and chelonians usually require several days to a week to clear the intestinal tract. Seasonal cooling is usually coordinated with the natural weather pattern, but animals can be phase-shifted to respond at other times. The required duration of the cooling period to assure reproductive conditioning is unknown. Common lengths range from 4 to 12 weeks. Energy demands of a cooled reptile are variable; however, losses in body weight during seasonal cooling are usually less than 10%.[72]

All reptiles seasonally cooled at a constant low temperature should be checked weekly or biweekly. Although reptiles may be sluggish, they should not show any physical or behavioral signs of illness. In addition, water, if not offered ad libitum, should be offered during these evaluations. If water is offered continuously, precautions must be taken to assure that it does not spill. High humidity during seasonal cooling is a frequent cause of respiratory infections. Reptiles showing any signs of potential illness must be returned to an optimal temperature immediately. Most importantly, caution must be utilized during these temperature transition times, because maintaining reptiles at intermediate temperatures, between the optimal temperature and a target cooling temperature, may be deleterious as such temperatures are nonconducive to feeding or immune function. Reptiles held at these intermediate temperatures may lose significant weight and be prone to illness. Like the precooling period, the postcooling period is a time of careful observation. Many problems occurring before or during seasonal cooling often fulminate with the return to active temperatures. Quick detection and correction of such problems is essential for maximizing reproductive potential and even survival.

Other Stimuli of Reproduction

Other environmental parameters that may also affect reproductive activity can also be utilized in conjunction with or as a possible alternative to seasonal cooling. Such stimuli include increased cage humidity, artificial raining, increased feeding, repeated introduction to multiple potential mates, adding shed skins from conspecifics, and male-male combat. Although these methods seem to provide benefits in certain species, the details and the universality of their use are not well known.

Frequency of Reproduction in Captive Reptiles

The frequency with which a captive reptile reproduces is dependent on species, environmental conditions, and nutritional status (see Reproductive Cycles and Fecundity). These factors can be manipulated in the captive situation to influence breeding, reproductive cycling, and fecundity. Most importantly the female must be in good health with adequate energy stores to reproduce. Reproduction is costly and nonessential for individual survival, so it is usually bypassed when body condition is poor.

Many oviparous species have the ability to produce more than one clutch per year. This is true for many turtles and lizards but is less common in snakes. Some tropical geckos produce a clutch of two eggs once a month throughout the year. More commonly, however, only two to three clutches are laid during a more defined breeding season, lasting only a few months. Whether a second clutch is laid is dependent on the time of year and the condition of the female. Although females may not attain the weight they were before producing the first clutch, females must regain sufficient energy stores after oviposition to commit to another clutch. Reinsemination is not necessary between clutches, but it can lead to increased fertility. Viviparous species commit a greater amount of time to a single reproductive event. Gestation lasts from 1.5 to 6 months, and the female feeds sparingly or not at all during this time. As a result of this lengthy investment, viviparous reptiles are generally limited to the production of a single clutch per year.

Determination of Gravidity (Pregnancy)

See earlier in this chapter for details on courtship, copulation, and fertilization, which all lead to gravidity. Gravidity can often be determined by observing the appearance and behavior of a captive female. Midbody swelling is apparent in gravid snakes and lizards; however, obese animals can cause both false-negative and false-positive assessments. The change in appearance is more obvious in smaller and less robust species. In some geckos, the eggs can be seen through the semitransparent skin covering the ventral aspect of the coelom. Realizing that the right ovary/oviduct is located more cranial to the left aids in differentiating developing follicles/eggs from similarly colored but symmetrically located fat bodies (Fig. 80.22).

Behavioral signs can be used in conjunction with appearance to aid in gravidity determination. Classic behaviors of gravid reptiles include an increase in basking time that correlates with an increase in selected body temperature, partial or complete anorexia, and a change in body positioning. In snakes, body-positioning changes often include looser coiling and lying in semilateral or even dorsal recumbency. Later in gravidity, restlessness and nesting behavior can be observed.

Coelomic palpation can provide a more reliable determination of gravidity and is straightforward in most snakes (except heavy-bodied ones) and with practice sometimes possible in lizards. In chelonians, the shell makes palpation difficult but not impossible. Holding the chelonian vertically (head up), fingers are directed craniomedially in the prefemoral fossa and the chelonian is gently tilted side to side, often allowing detection of shelled eggs (Fig. 80.23).

In snakes, a firm but careful thumb is run down the ventrum from approximately midbody to the cloaca and may reveal the presence and often an estimate of the number of follicles, eggs, or fetuses. Follicles

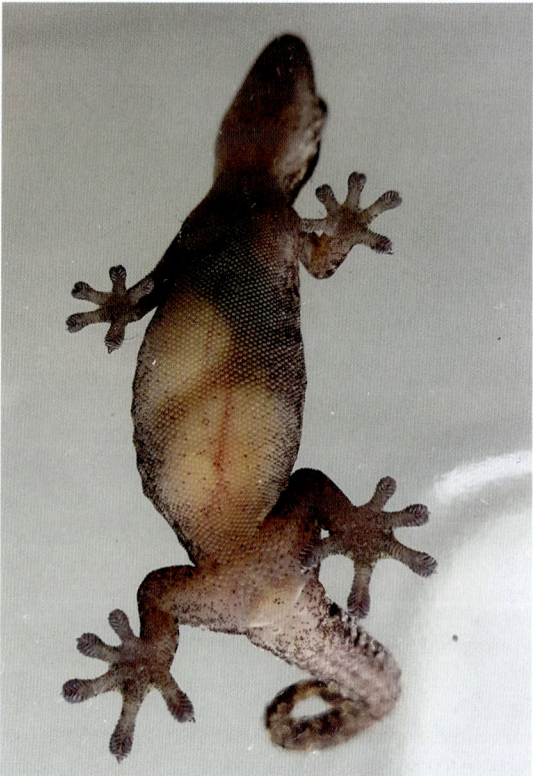

FIG 80.22 A female mourning gecko (*Lepidodactylus lugubris*) showing eggs through the ventral skin over the coelom. In the normal situation the right oviductal egg is cranial to the left and helps to differentiate the presence of eggs from the paired coelomic fat bodies. (Courtesy of Jennifer Hutchins, Stahl Exotic Animal Veterinary Services.)

are firm and often easily differentiated from softer eggs or fetuses. Lizards are palpated with a thumb and forefinger placed ventrolaterally on the relaxed coelom. As with snakes, follicles are differentiated from eggs by their firmness. Lizards are more difficult to palpate than snakes, leading to an increase in false negatives, and if one is not gentle, possible iatrogenic injury with follicle or egg rupture.

Currently radiography and ultrasonography are the most accessible and exacting methods of gravidity determination in reptiles. Radiography is useful in determining gravidity in chelonians, because the hard calcium-rich eggshells are clearly visible on radiographs and alternative methods are more limited. There are no reports to date that (limited) radiographic exposure has any detrimental effects on the developing embryos.

For lizards and snakes, the lower amount/lack of calcium in the softer eggshell makes radiographic identification more difficult. Therefore ultrasonography is often preferred and can reveal all stages of ova

development. In snakes the gallbladder can be used as a marker, because it is readily identified as a large echolucent sphere about 60% SVL. The right ovary is located just distal to the gallbladder and the left ovary just distal to the right. Vitellogenesis in squamates is signified by the follicles becoming larger and progressively more echogenic but remaining clustered (lizards). In chelonians similar changes occur except the follicles are not as clustered due to a larger fan-shaped mesovaria. Ovulated follicles and eggs are linearly arranged, occupying nearly the entire caudal half of the reptile. With practice, the pliable egg shells of squamates can be detected, and the densely mineralized shelled eggs of chelonians are readily identified on ultrasound scanning (Fig. 80.24). The ultrasonographic appearance of viviparous species is similar in appearance to oviparous species until after ovulation. Immediately after ovulation, developing fetuses are dominated mostly by yolk and therefore appear similar to ovulated eggs. However, as the embryo grows, an amniotic sac is seen as a small echolucent sphere on the periphery of the larger echogenic yolk mass. Eventually, in larger specimens, fetuses can be seen (Fig. 80.25A and B). See imaging under Reproductive Diseases, Clinical Investigation later in this chapter and Section 7 for more information on imaging of the reproductive tract.

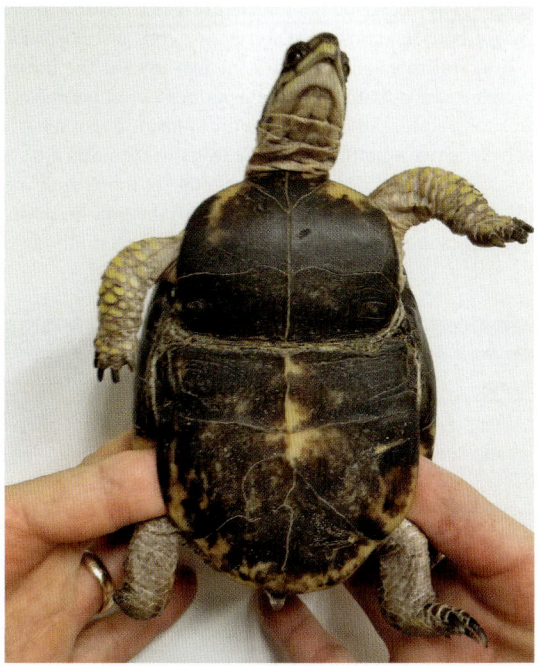

FIG 80.23 A female eastern box turtle (*Terrapene c. carolina*) is palpated digitally in the prefemoral fossa for possible eggs. (Courtesy of Katie Willis, Stahl Exotic Animal Veterinary Services.)

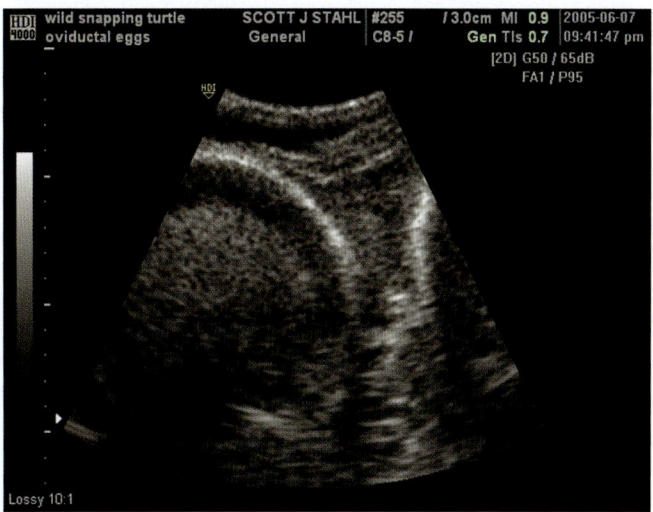

FIG 80.24 Normal oviductal eggs in a snapping turtle (*Chelydra serpentina*). Note distinctly round eggs and heavily calcified (hyperechoic) shell. (Courtesy of Scott J. Stahl, Stahl Exotic Animal Veterinary Services.)

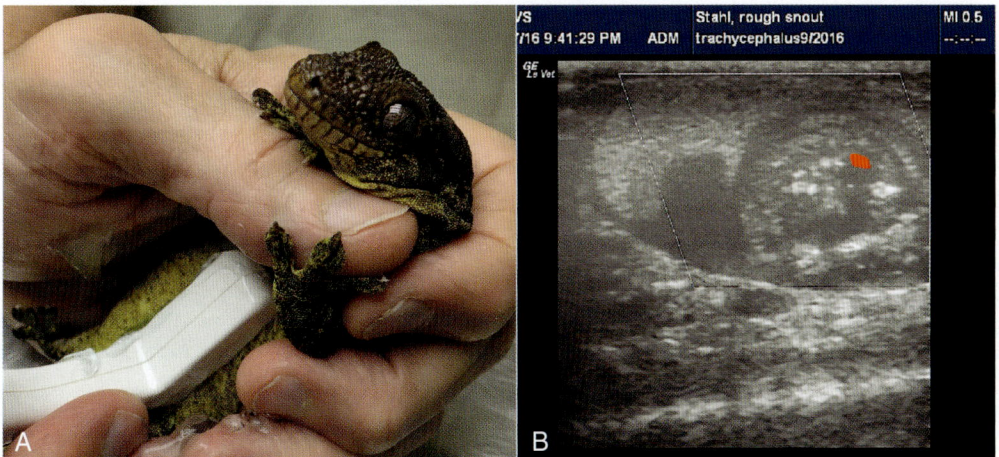

FIG 80.25 (A) Performing a coelomic ultrasonographic evaluation on a gravid lesser rough-snouted gecko (*Rhacodactylus trachyrhyncus trachycephalus*). This is one of the few gecko species that are live-bearing. (B) Sonographic image showing hyperechoic fetal spine dorsal to the heart with a heartbeat (red). (Courtesy of Scott J. Stahl, Stahl Exotic Animal Veterinary Services.)

Gestation and Oviposition

Gestation is a critical time for both the female and the developing offspring. A great demand is placed on a gravid female because gravidity requires energy (although much of the energy reserve was already invested with folliculogenesis prior to ovulation) but oftentimes limits food intake. The drastic imbalance between energy intake and energy demand is satisfied by energy reserves, including the breakdown of muscle mass. In addition, gravidity can affect immune function.[73] The combined effect of the energy deficit and altered immune function can lead to clinical disease during gravidity. Persistent, low-grade infections often fulminate during gravidity, jeopardizing both the female and the offspring. No reports have been found nor have the authors observed any negative effects of any drugs on gravidity, neither as an abortifacient nor a teratogen.

True gestation time can be difficult to determine in reptiles for a multitude of reasons. Among these are (1) the temporal separation between copulation and ovulation, (2) the prevalence of multiple copulations, and (3) the temperature-dependent effect in which warmer temperatures may decrease gestation time. Reported gestation lengths for viviparous reptiles range from 1.5 to 6 months. Most snakes undergo ecdysis before oviposition, which is likely associated with concurrent thyroid hormonal activity and influence.[30] This "prelay shed," as it is termed, provides a relatively reliable predictor of oviposition date for snakes. Snake breeders utilize this prelay shed (also called postovulatory shed) along with other markers to estimate oviposition. Much data appear in the popular literature describing these markers, and veterinarians should be familiar with these reproductive parameters for the most common snakes seen in practice. These and other useful reproductive parameters for commonly bred snakes are listed in Table 80.3.

However, colubrid snakes usually oviposit 8 to 14 days after this prelay shed, and pythons oviposit 24 to 49 days after, with some variation. The prelay shed date is used by many reptile breeders as the time to offer the female a nesting site.

Van Mierop and Bessette first reported another gestation marker in ball pythons, which they described as a notable "midbody swelling" and concluded was associated with ovulation.[74] Many snake breeders utilize this marker and, like the "prelay shed," use it to estimate oviposition. The Barkers' in their book on breeding the ball python call this gestational marker "the lump" and describe its appearance as a dramatic midbody swelling that lasts 8 to 24 hours and is the result of ovulation (Fig. 80.26).[75] They describe the female using her posture to compress her posterior body, creating tight serpentine coils just posterior to the mass of ova, and this action pushes the ova toward the infundibula. The movements are pulsatile, with long periods of rest between contractions (an action similar to that seen in the anterior portion of the body when a snake is regurgitating). During this time females are stoic and unresponsive to stimuli. Subsequently, female pythons appear smaller afterward, which is supposedly associated with the eggs becoming more linearly arranged and spread out in the oviduct. This midbody swelling

TABLE 80.3	Important Breeding and Gestation Parameters for Common Captive Snakes		
Species	**Introduction for Breeding**	**Gestation Markers***	**Ovipositon/Gestation/Fecundity**
Ball python[75–76,79] *Python regius*	Pairs placed together in late December, 1 male with up to 4/5 females continuously or introduce males/females weekly for 3-day intervals until late March (breeders may manipulate cycle to breed year-round) Ultrasound: introduce males when female follicles (15–25 mm)	Ovulation from mid-March to April or typically 6–30 days after the last observed copulation Ovulation lasts about 24 hours Approx. 20 days after ovulation start of postovulatory shed cycle Ultrasound: once follicles at 30 mm ovulation likely occurred, move male to another female	Oviposition 24–34 days after postovulatory shed (avg. 28 days) Eggs usually laid at night Females will coil around eggs Average clutch size is 6.5 eggs Range of 1–11 eggs Clutch 17%–65% female body wt. Avg. clutch 50% female body wt.
Boa constrictor[163–164] *Boa constrictor*	Males are introduced to females 1–2 weeks after females' last meal One strategy is to introduce for 3–5 days if no courting activity then separate, offer female a small meal, and reintroduce in 3 weeks Keep repeating this cycle until courtship behavior begins Several different males can be introduced at different times during these cycles	Typically 3–8 weeks after courtship behavior a preovulation swelling in posterior midbody will be observed, and this takes place about 2–3 weeks before ovulation Female boas will appear uncomfortable during ovulation, laying in unusual positions Female boas may ovulate from each ovary at different times, thus extending the opportunity to observe ovulation Boas shed 16–20 days after ovulation	Boas give birth approx.105 days after postovulatory shed Approx. 123 days after final ovulation Most babies born June/July Usually give birth at night, associated with barometric pressure change/rain Birthing takes 10 min to 6 hours A 6 foot boa will give birth to 25 neonates (avg.) Litter size represents between 10%–40% female body wt.
Corn snake[165] *Pantherophis guttata* **Rat snake**[165] *Pantherophis obsoleta* spp. **King snake**[166] *Lampropeltis getulus* spp.	Introduce males and females after female's first posthibernation shed Females are at maximum receptivity after this first shed	Ovulation may or may not be observed in colubrids, but females usually lay their eggs 7–14 days after prelay shed	Oviposition 31–45 days after mating (avg. 39), 7–14 days after prelay shed Typically all eggs are laid within 24 hours Average clutch size is 20–25 eggs Range 1–50 Can produce 2nd clutch in same season (smaller clutch size)

*Gestation markers: Ovulation in this table is used synonymously for "midbody swelling" or "the lump," which has anecdotally been thought to be an indicator for ovulation. Postovulatory shed is used synonymously for "prelay" shed. See discussion under Captive Breeding for more information about these markers.

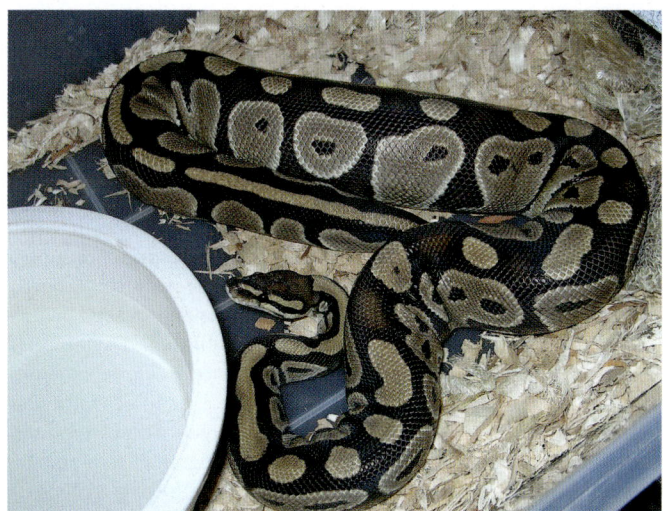

FIG 80.26 A gravid female ball python (*Python regius*) exhibiting the midbody swelling (considered to represent ovulation), which is used as a gestation marker in snakes to predict oviposition. (Courtesy of J. Kobylka Reptiles.)

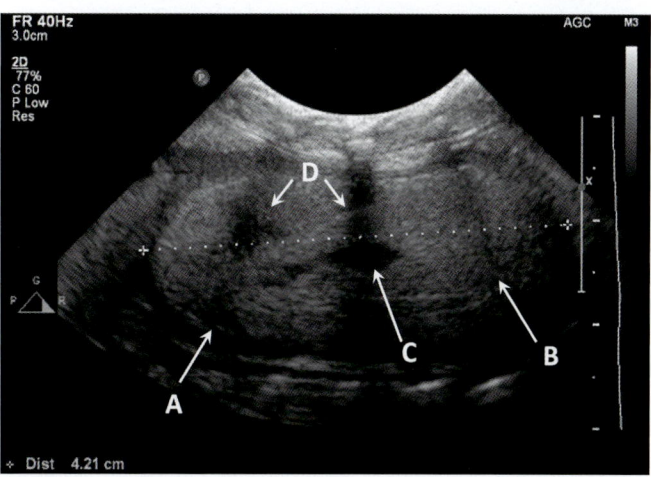

FIG 80.28 Long axis, ventral approach of the mid coelom of a ball python (*Python regius*), utilizing 8 MHz microconvex probe. (A) A postovulatory 42-mm oviductal egg. Note the increasing elongated elliptical shape with no apparent shell deposition. (B) The contents of the follicle are similar to a soft tissue echogenecity. (C) An anechoic center develops within the follicle before egg shell deposition. (D) Note the rib shadowing, a common artifact. (Courtesy of Emily Nielsen.)

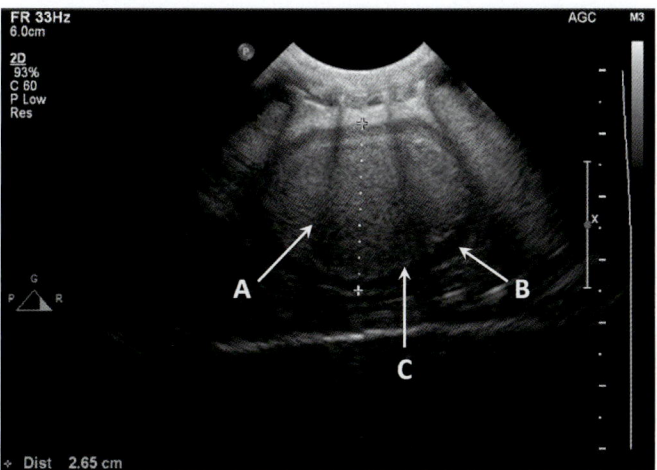

FIG 80.27 Long axis, ventrolateral approach of the mid coelom of a ball python (*Python regius*), utilizing 8 MHz microconvex probe. (A) A 26-mm follicle consistent with a postovulatory follicle (egg). Note the elliptical rather than circular shape. (B) The hypoechoic outer rim and (C) the thin hyperechoic inner rim. (Courtesy of Emily Nielsen.)

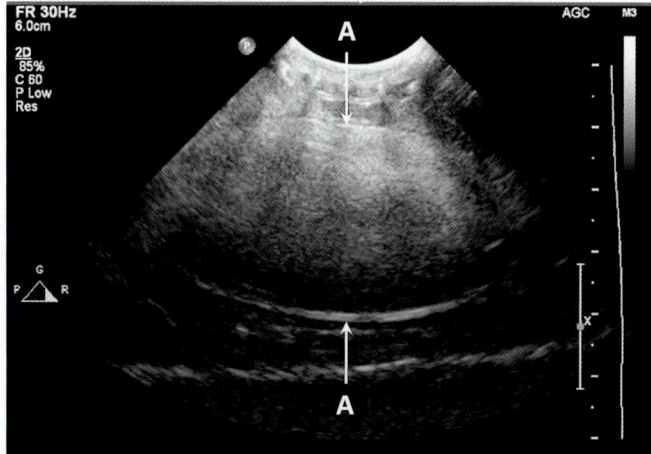

FIG 80.29 Long axis, ventrolateral approach of the mid coelom in a ball python (*Python regius*), utilizing 8 MHz microconvex probe. A hyperechoic ring (A) representing egg shell deposition is seen surrounding the egg. Egg shell mineralization is occuring, resulting in the associated distal acoustic shadowing and overall darker appearance. (Courtesy of Emily Nielsen.)

has been witnessed in more than 20 python species and several boa and colubrid species.[75] More recently, a ball python ultrasonography study has challenged this theory and suggests that this midbody swelling occurs *after* true ovulation and may be associated with egg shell deposition/mineralization.[76] In this study ovulation was thought to occur once follicular size was 20 to 25 mm, with consistent changes seen on ultrasound scanning at this size, including the appearance of an anechoic outer ring (presumed free fluid around follicles), a more elliptical shape versus round shape, evidence of a hypoechoic outer rim, and a hyperechoic inner ring with soft tissue echogenecity centrally (Fig. 80.27). The sonographic changes for these presumed postovulatory follicles were consistent with sonographic descriptions for postovulatory ova in studies in Borneo short-tailed pythons (*Python curtus*)[32,77] and red-tailed boas (*Boa constrictor occidentalis*).[78] Furthermore, in the ball python study, the "midbody swelling" was associated with oviductal eggs reaching their maximum size of 40 to 45 mm with a notable anechoic

center (Fig. 80.28).[76] Within 1 to 2 weeks after the midbody swelling, mineralization and egg shell formation was identified sonographically as a thin hyperechoic rim surrounding each ova (Fig. 80.29).[76]

Many snake breeders are utilizing ultrasonography, not only to detect gravity but also to evaluate a female's follicular cycle to determine the best time for pairing.[75,79] If a female has ovulated or has follicles undergoing atresia, pairing will be less beneficial. Snake breeders often use one male to breed multiple females, and ultrasonography provides an effective tool to improve the efficiency of a limited number of males.

Sonographic studies on multiple snake species describing ovarian anatomy, follicular activity, and gravity have been reported,[32,75,77,78] but a description of the *entire* follicular cycle and gestation period in a single species, the ball python, has only recently been published.[76] This sonographic study identified three distinct stages of the follicular cycle, which could routinely be found in ball pythons, and they described them as follicular quiescence, atresia, and development to oviposition (maturation).[76] Follicular quiescence involved nonvitellogenic (anechoic) follicles that were generally less than 10 mm in size. Follicles that reached 10 mm had two possible end points; they could increase in size to become dominant follicles and proceed to ovulation, or they will undergo follicular atresia. Follicular atresia was characterized by nonvitellogenic follicles that developed into vitellogenic follicles between 10 to 20 mm but then remained static for 50 days or more and eventually regressed.[76] Oviposition (maturation) was predictable for follicles that reached 20 mm in diameter, and follicles that reached 22 to 27 mm allowed an acurate determination for timing of oviposition. In this study, once follicles reached 30 mm in size it was possible to predict with 100% accuracy the number of eggs at oviposition. Based on this study the best timing to ensure fertilization of the female ball python would be to introduce the male when follicles are between 15 to 25 mm in size.

A sonographic study describing follicular development and ovulation in the viviparous lizard *Barisia imbricata* has been published,[80] and studies in some chelonian species[81] are described as well. More studies similar to these will prove beneficial to the future of captive reproduction, especially involving threatened and endangered reptile species. See Imaging in Reproductive Diseases, Clinical Investigation later in this chapter and Section 7 for more information.

Nesting Sites/Ovipositoria

Provision of an appropriate oviposition site is critical for many species. Not providing a female with the proper laying conditions can lead to dystocia in an otherwise healthy reptile. Many reptiles use an ovipositorium or "nest box." A nest box can simply consist of an opaque container with a small entrance hole in the side (for lizards) or top (for snakes). The container should be half filled with lightly moistened substrates; the most commonly used are sphagnum moss, vermiculite, or a sand/soil combination (for a proper consistency) to allow nest site excavation, which is important for some species (lizards, chelonians). For most species the nest box should be situated so that

the temperature inside is 28° to 30°C (82° to 86°F). Although snakes usually use the provided nest box, lizards oftentimes ignore it, laying their eggs in another area of the cage where they can rapidly desiccate. To avoid this, gravid lizards can be moved to a separate cage that is set up entirely as an ovipositorium. In such setups, the substrate, moistened vermiculite, or soil/sand combination should be reasonably deep, and a basking platform should be provided. The platform, a tray that covers approximately one-quarter to one-third of the substrate allows the lizard to avoid the moist substrate if desired and provides an object under which to dig. A basking light is provided over the platform. Properly designed large-scale ovipositoria can house lizards for extended periods and greatly increase the success in obtaining viable eggs. Dystocias are common in green iguanas and other lizard species, including monitors and old-world chameleons, and frequently are a result of inadequate nesting sites. For example, in nature, gravid iguanas and monitors exhibit extensive nesting behavior, including migration to a suitable nest site and digging a relatively deep nest for the eggs (Fig. 80.30A–C). In captivity, homologous conditions to allow such behavior are difficult to replicate. Minimally, gravid iguanas and other large lizards should be provided a large ovipositorium with substantial amounts, 30 to 60 cm (1–2 ft), of substrate. Chelonians lay eggs in excavated holes, which they carefully cover. A general rule for chelonians is to provide a nest box depth that is 1 to 2 times the length of the female's carapace. A week or two before oviposition, chelonians usually show increased activity, commonly digging several incomplete nest holes before selecting the ultimate nest site. This preovipository behavior can be used to signify that a female is gravid. See Chapter 85 for a discussion of egg evaluation, incubation, and neonatal management.

ARTIFICIAL INSEMINATION

With greater than 1000 species of reptiles considered threatened and more than 250 species critically endangered, there is a need for the development of artificial insemination (AI) techniques. Reptile

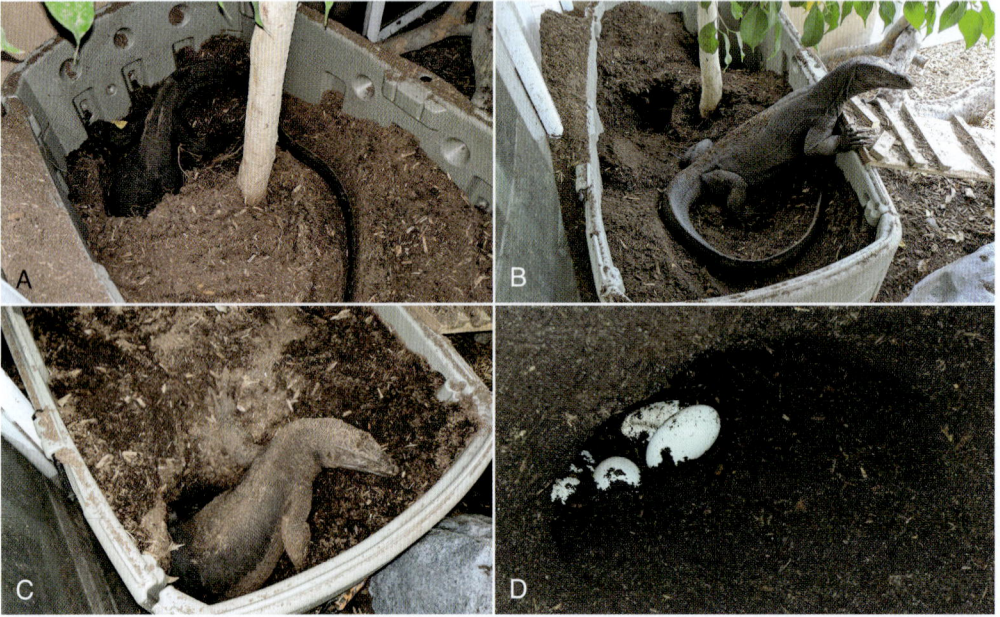

FIG 80.30 Adequate nesting sites must be provided for gravid reptiles, especially lizards and chelonians. The lack of an appropriate nest site can result in egg retention and dystocia. (A and B) A female black water dragon (*Varanus salvator*) is provided a large, deep nesting site and spends hours/days digging multiple nests before (C and D) finally laying her eggs. (Courtesy of Cory Aymar, Toothless Reptiles.)

conservation and breeding programs continue to increase, and the success of these programs is dependent on maintaining genetic variation. Important techniques to ensure and protect such genetic diversity include identifying genetically significant males through sperm sampling, utilizing techniques such as cryopreservation for long-term sperm banking, and successfully using that sperm to fertilize females.[82–84] Unfortunately, sample collection, cryopreservation, and successful fertilization are all challenging and limiting factors with AI. A full discussion of all parameters of artificial insemination in reptiles is not possible in this chapter, but some basic concepts and recent advances will be summarized. Some of the earliest work with artificial insemination included the American alligator (*Alligator mississipiensis*), the Angolan python (*Python anchietae*), Gaboon viper (*Bitis gabonica*), and the checkered garter snake (*Thamnophis marcianus*), and was met with limited success.[58,85,86] Since that initial work, AI in many species has been evaluated to help advance these capabilities. Successful techniques developed for avian, fish, and amphibians have not worked well in reptiles. One complicating issue relates to the unique effects of seasonal, environmental factors (and thus hormonal influences) on the reproductive cycle of reptiles, including temperature, photoperiod, rainfall, and barometric pressure changes. Another critical obstacle with AI has been the fragile nature of reptile spermatozoa and poor results from cryopreservation techniques and storage.[58,85,87,88] Finally, insemination timing and techniques have not been fully elucidated for maximal fertilization ability. Ideally, to maximize success, artificial insemination should be coordinated with the female's follicular cycle, and more work is necessary in this area.

Semen Collection

One of the most important factors for successful AI is the safe collection of sperm. A variety of techniques have been utilized in reptiles to accomplish semen collection with varying results. In crocodilians success has been achieved with manual collection.[85] The manual technique involves placing the crocodilian in ventral recumbency and manipulating the phallus digitally. Sedation can be utilized in crocodilians if necessary but often alligators can be trained to allow the procedure.[85] Electroejaculation (EEJ) can also be utilized in crocodilians, but the less-invasive manual technique is often successful and EEJ unnecessary.[89] In chelonians EEJ has been utilized to successfully collect semen from many different species including the green turtle (*Chelonia mydas*),[90] hawksbill turtles (*Eretmochelys imbricata*),[91] the black marsh turtle (*Siebenrockiella crassicollis*),[92] and the leopard tortoise (*Stigmochelys pardalis*).[93] A vibrational device (vibrator) was successfully utilized to collect semen in three different species of turtle, the painted turtle (*Chrysemys picta*), the wood turtle (*Glptemys insculpta*), and Blanding's turtle (*Emydoidea blandingii*).[94] Generally, an erection was elicited by setting the vibrator at the highest frequency and moving it along the carapace in a linear or circular motion.[94] In snakes, manual sperm collection has been successful in many boids, colubrids, and vipers.[58,88,95] This manual collection technique can be performed in conscious snakes and involves a repeated stripping/stroking motion with firm pressure starting in the lower third of the coelom and continued distally toward the cloaca in a smooth repeated fashion. The hemipenes are often everted, and semen samples can be collected at the cloaca.[58,88,95] EEJ was also successfully used to collect sperm from the checkered garter snake (*Thamnophis marcianus*) and may be a useful technique for larger snakes, where size and strength may not allow manual stripping.[86] In lizards a manual extraction technique has been described for the collection of spermatozoa in the McCann's skink (*Oligosoma maccanni*).[96] A similar manual technique has been described for many Australian skinks.[97] EEJ has been successfully performed in the green iguana and other lizards under anesthesia to reduce stress and minimize any discomfort (Perry S, Mitchell M, personal communication).[98] In one study, weekly EEJ events were evaluated in veiled chameleons (*Chamaeleo calyptratus*) over a 1-month period (Fig. 80.31A and B). The EEJ procedure showed only transient cloacal mucosa inflammation after each EEJ event, and no chronic changes were observed. All animals included in this study survived, and these repeated EEJ events were determined to be safe (Perry S, personal communication).

Sperm Analysis

Sperm analysis is important to evaluate male fertility and sample quality for insemination. Techniques developed to evaluate sperm in mammals

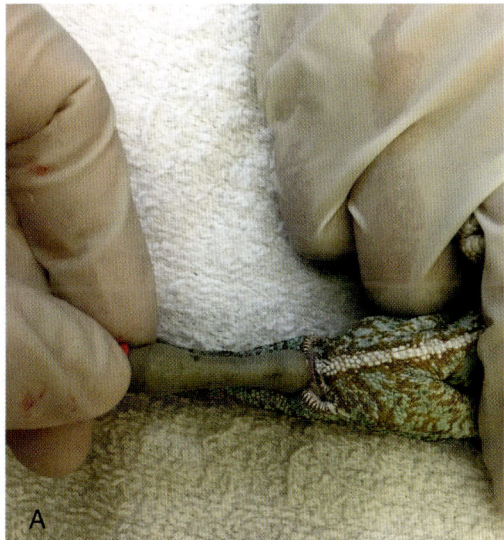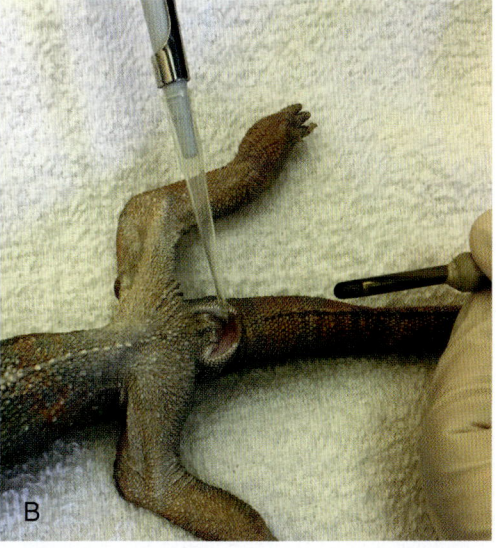

FIG 80.31 (A) An ejaculation probe is placed within the cloaca of a veiled chameleon (*Chameleo calyptratus*). Mild pressure is placed dorsally to engage nerve roots innervating the reproductive tract, stimulating ejaculation into the cloaca. Appropriate placement is estimated by establishing concurrent hind-limb movement when the electrode is discharged. (B) Semen collection from the cloaca of a panther chameleon (*Furcifer pardalis*) utilizing a micropipettor following electroejaculation. Semen can be successfully collected following electroejaculation without everting the hemipenes. (Courtesy of Sean Perry, Louisiana State University.)

can be utilized in reptiles. Ejaculates must be evaluated for three major parameters: concentration, motility, and morphology. Evaluating a neat (fresh/direct) sample is difficult because of the high spermatozoa concentration. As an example, snake semen has approximately 1.5 billion sperm cells/mL compared with dog semen at 500 million/mL.[58] The average volume of ejaculate from adult Angolan pythons and Timor pythons (*Malayopython timorensis*) was found to be only 0.1 to 0.4 mL.[58] In leopard tortoises spermatozoa samples collected with EEJ techniques under sedation averaged 0.26 ± 0.16 mL.[93] Reptile ejaculates collected either manually or by EEJ are comparatively much lower in volume than those produced by mammals, and for proper evaluation, reptile ejaculate should be extended to a 1:10 dilution or 1:100 dilution to facilitate accurate counts (although clumping may still be exhibited). Due to the spermatozoa's fragility extender type (yolk based, milk based, etc) should be taken into consideration. Each chamber of a hemocytometer is loaded with 10 μL of diluted sample. A Maklersperm counting chamber can be used to evaluate concentrated samples. Formal buffered saline can be used to extend a sample to inhibit motility for counting. Spermatozoa/mL is the standard for most animals when quantifying sperm concentration; however, it is more correct to quantify it per ejaculate (spermatozoa/ejaculate) because of the small volumes reptiles produce.[88,93,95,98] Motility of spermatozoa in semen samples can be estimated by placing a drop of semen or diluted semen on a slide with a coverslip (2 μL is the recommended minimum) and estimating the percentage of progressively motile spermatozoa to the nearest 5% in 5 hpfs (magnification, 400×).[58,88,98] Motility is dramatically affected by time and cooling and should be evaluated as quickly as possible. In leopard tortoises where spermatozoa were collected with EEJ, average motility at time of collection was found to be 57.3%, similar to other reptiles.[93] In a study evaluating sperm motility as a determination of sperm quality in the Argentine boa (*Boa constrictor occidentalis*) samples manually collected had 63% motility at the time of collection.[99] Generally a lower spermatozoa motility percentage (compared with higher vertebrates) may be normal/acceptable for reptiles. In the checkered garter snake a 0.05 mL sample of spermatozoa with 50% motility was successful in producing offspring via artificial insemination.[86] Morphology should be evaluated 1000× magnification under phase contrast or normal microscopy. Generally, a 100-cell count can be performed with morphological abnormalities noted, including bent tails, coiled tails, detached heads, and presence of droplets.[58,88,93,98] More research is needed to understand and validate spermatozoa abnormalities in reptiles and whether they truly compare with those described for other vertebrates. Advanced systems (computer-assisted analysis and epifluorescences microscopy) do exist and may prove applicable for evaluating reptile semen in the future.[93]

Sperm Storage and Cryopreservation

Much research is still needed in this area, as reptile semen has generally been difficult to preserve. Extenders or media for short-term storage that have been utilized include Hamm's F-10, egg yolk buffer, lactated ringers solution, phosphate-buffered saline, and TCG-Tris-citrate-glucose. Extenders have only been scientifically evaluated in crocodilian species. Storage temperature has been evaluated in snakes, lizards, and chelonians.[88,93,98] Cooled short-term semen storage has been successful in crocodilians for up to 2 days[85] and for a shorter duration in snakes.[88,100] Chelonian semen appears to be quite fragile and does not store well.[93] Cryopreservation techniques utilized for other vertebrates have not worked well for reptiles. The most common cryopreservatives utilize glycerol and dimethyl sulfoxide (DMSO), and results with these and other extenders have been poor with reptiles.[58,85,87,88,98] More research is needed into the use of extenders, cryopreservatives, and associated techniques, which may be species specific. For example, semen from

Argentine black and white tegus (*Salvator merianae*) extended in 12% DMSO and frozen at a slow rate (0.3°C min) exhibited the best post-thaw viability.[101] Vitrification, a technique where spermatozoa are frozen quickly in liquid nitrogen, may be a promising technology but is not yet tested in reptiles. This procedure prevents ice crystal formation, thus eliminating damage to the spermatozoa plasma membrane.

AI Procedures and Techniques

Reports of successful artificial insemination in reptiles are rare. Difficulty with sperm extension and preservation are important reasons for these limitations. Hopefully, as semen-handling techniques are further refined, improved capabilities with AI will follow. Artificial insemination does show promise, fresh semen and short-term cooled semen has been successfully used in the American alligator.[85] In the saltwater crocodile (*Crocodylus porosus*), AI was successful with oviductal catheterization. Visualization of the oviduct was achieved with a tilt table and vaginal speculum. Semen was deposited using either a sheep AI pipette or a 3.5-Fr gauge "tom-cat" catheter. Success was low, with only one out of five inseminated females producing fertile eggs and only one egg hatching.[89] AI has also been successful in corn snakes using fresh semen.[100,102] In the checkered garter snake, artificial insemination utilizing sperm collected by electroejaculation was also successful.[86] Artificial insemination of the giant Yangtze softshell turtle (*Rafetuss winhoei*) has been attempted several times both via cloacoscopy into the urodeum and then via coelioscopy into the oviduct. To date, the female has laid clutches of eggs; however, none have been fertile (Kuchling, Turtle Survival Alliance Symposium, 2016). Successful AI has recently been reported in two corn snakes and an Amazon tree boa (*Corallus hortulanus*).[103] Semen was collected from males using the massage method and diluted 1:5 with normal saline and stored short term at room temperature. Females were monitored with ultrasonography, and insemination was timed with the presence of preovulatory follicles. Fresh diluted semen was introduced with a catheter into the females' oviduct using cloacoscopy. Two out of three corn snakes inseminated with this method laid 14 and 16 eggs, respectively, and all went on to successfully hatch. One Amazon tree boa inseminated with this technique gave birth to two healthy babies and five infertile ova 4 months after AI.[103] Much work is still needed in the field of artificial insemination in reptiles. However, as this most recent successful study indicates, endoscopically guided semen deposition, delivered to specific regions of the oviduct, with timing based on sonographic monitoring of the female's follicular cycle, may improve AI success.

REPRODUCTIVE DISEASES

Clinical Investigation

Historical Information and Presentation. Historical information and presentation can vary dramatically; however, regardless of the issue, clinicians must obtain a detailed history, complete a thorough husbandry review, and have a good understanding of species-specific reproduction. All chelonians and crocodilians are oviparous, as are most squamates; however, some lizard and snake species are viviparous (see Table 80.1). It is often challenging to differentiate normal reproductive activity (expected seasonal behavior for healthy intact reptiles) from reproductive diseases such as a follicular stasis or dystocia. For example, chelonians are known to be able to retain eggs in the oviduct for extended periods of time in their natural environment waiting for the right nesting site or conditions to lay.[104] Therefore differentiation between pending oviposition and true dystocia is often difficult. Historically owners often report reproductively active reptiles as becoming restless in their cages, pacing and climbing, presumably looking for possible mates or nesting sites. Oviparous lizards and chelonians may dig in planters or substrate.

Aquatic turtles may spend extended time out of the water. Appetite and water intake are often reduced or absent. Coelomic distention in females may be noted in conjunction with reduced body condition, and owners may or may not be aware of their animal's gender, let alone reproductive activity. For dystocia cases, tenesmus without successful oviposition or parturition may occur or females may have produced a smaller clutch or litter than expected and still appear gravid due to retained eggs/fetuses. Alternatively, the breeder's records may indicate that the female is past her due date. With more serious or chronic conditions such as yolk coelomitis, ectopic ova, oviductal or hemipenal/phallic prolapses, reptiles may present lethargic, depressed, and even obtunded. Seasonally, owners may present mature male reptiles for increased aggression, especially large lizard species such as the green iguana. Many of these lizards are free roaming in the home and can become territorial, attacking humans or other household pets.[105]

Physical Examination.

Detailed information on performing a physical examination is covered elsewhere (see Chapter 42); however, reproductive specific parameters are discussed here. First and foremost, the sex of the animal in question should be identified. In reproductive female squamates, palpation of preovulatory ova may be possible, but it may be difficult to differentiate large preovulatory follicles from postovulatory ova. Ovarian follicles tend to be more dorsal and spherical and not as mobile as oviductal eggs. Preovulatory follicles are generally not palpable in chelonians and crocodilians. Postovulatory ova (oviductal eggs) in squamates can often be differentiated from follicles because eggs are less firm, larger, more oblong, and more caudally located in the coelom. However, in some oviparous lizards and viviparous squamates it can be difficult to differentiate between the two. Chelonians are more difficult to palpate but in smaller species digital palpation in the prefemoral area with the patient held vertically (head up) and gently tilting the chelonian side to side may allow shelled eggs to be detected (see Fig. 80.23). This technique is not accurate for determining numbers of retained eggs, and clinicians must be cautious to avoid personal injury from the powerful retraction of a rear limb or shell hinge closure. It is usually not possible to palpate developing fetuses in viviparous squamates and imaging will be necessary. The cloaca should be evaluated for any abnormalities as the reproductive tract terminates at the urodeum. Blood, discharge, and abnormal odors could all be indications of possible cloacitis or salpingitis. A digital cloacal examination may reveal an ova or mass in the pelvic area.

In males, evaluation of the phallus in chelonians or crocodilians is important to exclude trauma or infection as a source of abnormal cloacal signs (asymmetry, swelling, odor, or prolapsed tissue). Asymmetry or bilateral swelling distal to the vent is often associated with scent gland adenitis in both male and female snakes and hemipenal abscessation, impaction, or prolapse in male squamates. Seasonally active males may show increased evidence of secondary sexual characteristics (eg, green iguanas with increased orange coloration, bearded dragons with a black beard, larger femoral and preanal pores in many lizards, and increased mental gland size and activity in chelonians) and show an increase in seasonal sexually driven territorial behaviors such as head bobbing, dewlap displays, increased aggression, and mounting behaviors. With more serious and/or chronic conditions such as yolk coelomitis, ectopic ova, and oviductal or hemipenal/phallic prolapses, animals may be depressed, weak, cachexic, dehydrated, and obtunded.

Hematology and Biochemistry.

Abnormalities in the hemogram with reproductive disorders are usually associated with inflammatory changes and infection. Yolk coelomitis, ectopic ova, chronic dystocia with associated salpingitis, oviduct prolapse, or hemipenal/phallic prolapse/infection are conditions that can be associated with a leukocytosis and toxic morphological changes to granulocytes. Azurophils may also be elevated. In more chronic or severe cases, a leukopenia, heteropenia with left shift, and anemia may be present.[106,107] Serial hematology may be useful in monitoring response to procedures and therapy.

Plasma biochemical changes often include elevations of albumin, total protein, and alkaline phosphatase. Total calcium is usually elevated consistent with active folliculogenesis in females, but ionized calcium typically remains normal. However, in females with severe nutritional secondary hyperparathyroidism or hypovitaminosis D, ionized calcium may be low (<1.3 mmol/L). Normal females undergoing vitellogenesis will exhibit increases in cholesterol, triglycerides, and lipids. With laboratories making these tests more readily available, cholesterol, triglycerides, and lipoproteins could become a useful tool to monitor reproductive activity in females (see Chapter 34).

Radiography.

Radiography is an important tool in diagnosing reproductive activity, diseases, and disorders in reptiles.[108] Radiology can also be utilized in sexing some monomorphic species (see Sex Identification earlier in this chapter). Basic principles of radiography should be utilized including orthogonal studies and, for lateral views, horizontal x-ray beams for squamates and chelonians (see Section 7 for a review of proper techniques). Radiography is useful for determining the presence of, and differentiating between, preovulatory follicles and postovulatory eggs (Fig. 80.32). Radiographically preovulatory follicles (rarely seen in chelonians) are more spherical with no mineralized shell, clustered, and more dorsally positioned. With oviparous species, radiographs are useful to determine normal gravidity and, in cases of suspected dystocia, to identify obstructive or pathological conditions. Radiographs will identify mineralized eggs (squamate egg shells are generally much less calcified than chelonian eggs) and confirm egg numbers, abnormalities (e.g., shell thickening, breaks), ectopic eggs, comparative egg size, and pelvic diameter versus egg size. Additionally, radiography can identify underlying metabolic issues that may be contributing to the dystocia, including nutritional secondary hyperparathyroidism or concurrent coelomic pathology, such as cystic calculi, obstipation, or organomegaly. Oxytocin should not be used without radiographic confirmation that an obvious obstruction does not exist. With viviparous squamates radiography can still be useful, but not until late in gestation when skeletal structures become mineralized (see Section 7 for more information).

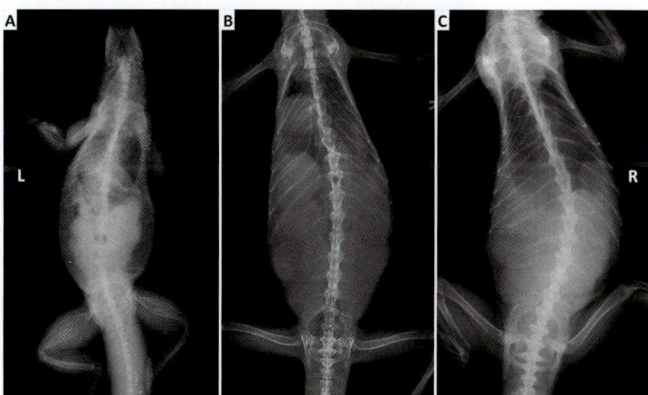

FIG 80.32 Dorsoventral radiographs of three different female green iguanas (*Iguana iguana*), all with varying stages of ovarian activity. (A) This female has early vitellogenesis evident with ovaries beginning to enlarge with yolking follicles. (B) This female has large ovulatory-sized ovarian follicles, round and clustered. (C) This female has ovulated, and oviductal eggs with a thin shell are evident. (Courtesy of Stephen J. Divers.)

Ultrasonography. Ultrasonography is well documented as the imaging modality of choice to evaluate the reproductive tract in squamates (see Chapter 58).[108,109] In chelonians, it is also useful for preovulatory conditions; however, radiography is preferred for postovulatory diagnostic evaluation.[108] Ultrasonography is noninvasive, can often be performed without sedation or anesthesia, allows evaluation of ovarian follicular activity (previtellogenic and vitellogenesis) and oviductal egg/fetus development, and can help identify reproductive disease and disorders such as follicular stasis and dystocia. Numerous reports on the use of ultrasound to evaluate the reproductive anatomy of reptiles have been published (see Chapter 58). A summary of some of this information is shared here. The immature gonads are difficult to visualize with normal clinical ultrasound machines and are generally not useful for sexing immature reptiles. Sonographically, the paired mature testes may be identified dorsally in the mid to caudal coelom as round to ovoid structures (elongated in snakes) that often vary in size and echogenicity depending on season and activity. Generally, the testes have a granular homogenous hyperechoic echogenicity similar to the liver and hypoechoic compared with the echogenicity of the kidneys. Hemipenes were also identified and described sonographically in Gila monsters.[66] With sexual maturity, ovaries are sonographically identified dorsally in the mid to caudal coelom and become obvious during follicular activity. Generally, early in the reproductive cycle previtellogenic follicles are small, distinctly round, and anechoic. In snakes they appear as a long chain of variably sized round anechoic structures, and in lizards as a cluster of round anechoic structures (like a bunch of grapes) (see Fig. 80.20). Ultrasonography has been utilized to determine the sex in mature female monomorphic lizards.[65] Chelonian ovaries are similar in appearance to lizards but are not as closely clustered, and follicles have an increased echogenicity even during the early stages of development.[108] As follicles mature and become vitellogenic they enlarge with yolk deposition and their echogenicity increases from anechoic to more hypoechoic. Depending on species, much of the coelom can be filled with large ovaries containing preovulatory follicles. Follicle size as an indicator for ovulation has been reported in the ball python, short-tailed python, boa constrictor, the viviparous lizard *Barisia,* American alligator, and many chelonian species.[76–78,80,81,110] See the Captive Breeding section of this chapter for more details. Postovulatory eggs become more elongated (squamata), and a hyperechoic wall is noted depending on the degree of species-dependent egg calcification (if oviparous) (see Fig. 80.27). Additionally, postovulatory eggs tend to be more uniformly linear, and anechoic material may be noted between and around the ova, indicating a small amount of normal fluid within the oviduct (see Fig. 80.28). Egg maturation within the oviduct can be monitored in oviparous reptiles depending on the degree of eggshell development, more so in squamates than chelonians (Figs. 80.24 and 80.29).[108,109] The anechoic albumin portion can be differentiated from the more uniform hyperechoic yolk, which decreases with maturation. Late in development a small embryo may sometimes be identified. For viviparous squamates, ultrasonography can be valuable late in gestation to determine whether fetuses are alive as fetal movement and heartbeats may be observed. Additionally, the loss of these indicators late in gestation may help to differentiate dead fetuses and dystocia (with the need for intervention) versus a normal pregnancy. Birth can be reasonably predicted with ultrasonographic monitoring of the loss of yolk. Birth usually occurs about a week after yolk is no longer detectable.

Ultrasonography is an invaluable tool for evaluating obstetric disease and/or complications.[108,111,112] Ultrasonography can be utilized to monitor the status of follicular stasis, as with active resorption or degenerate change the ova progress from a homogenous hypoechoic appearance to a more mixed heterogenic (hypoechoic and anechoic) echogenicity (Fig. 80.33). This progresses to a loss of shape, and follicles are no longer smooth and well demarcated. With resorption they continue to reduce in size; however, with stasis and degenerative change the follicles appear to coalesce, and anechoic fluid often surrounds the follicles. If echogenic free-floating debris is noted within this anechoic fluid, the follicles are likely degenerate and inflamed, and surgical intervention is indicated.[108]

With postovulatory disease such as dystocia or salpingitis, the normally smooth wall of the egg may become irregular with a notable heterogenous echogenicity change, and an increase in free fluid within the oviduct(s) and/or the coelom itself may be noted.[108] In these situations normal oviposition/birth is unlikely, and medical or surgical management is needed.

Ultrasonography can also be valuable for the identification of testicular abnormalities, including cystic or neoplastic changes (see Chapter 58).

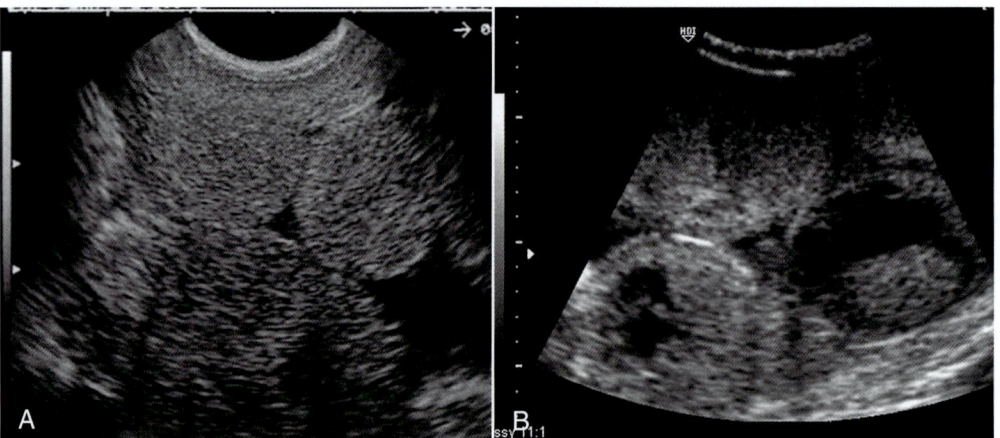

FIG 80.33 (A) Sonographic appearance of normal, homogenous, and hypoechoic, preovulatory ovarian follicles in a bearded dragon (*Pogona vitticeps*). (B) Sonographic appearance of ovarian follicles in a bearded dragon that are degenerative from chronic follicular stasis. Note the irregular hypoechoic/anechoic echogenicity of the follicles that several weeks earlier were uniformly hypoechoic. These changes are similar to those seen with normal follicular resorption so multiple sonographic examinations over time, along with monitoring the lizards condition, may be necessary to determine which condition is occuring. (Courtesy of Scott J. Stahl, Stahl Exotic Animal Veterinary Services.)

Computed Tomography (CT) and Magnetic Resonance Imaging (MRI). Advanced imaging techniques such as CT and MRI are becoming more affordable technologies in clincal practice and thus can be useful for evaluating reproductive disease. In a recent report on imaging of the reproductive tract of reptiles, CT (compared with other imaging modalities such as radiology and ultrasonography) was most informative with regard to the chelonian reproductive tract.[108] Another advantage with CT over radiography is its ability to evaluate each ovarian follicle and oviductal egg individually. Specifically CT was useful to identify advanced changes in follicular stasis, as a distinct horizontal leveling of the contents of static ovarian follicles was noted once degeneration started. Horizontal leveling was also evident in retained oviductal eggs with CT, and with more chronic retention a gas cap often formed within, and gas pockets around, the egg (Fig. 80.34A and B).[108] Unfortunately these advanced imaging modalities are not avaialable in most private clinical practices but are routinely available in referral hospitals. Resources for imaging techniques, normal anatomy, and diseases are becoming increasingly available.[108,113] See Section 7 for more information on advanced imaging.

Endoscopy. Endoscopic techniques for the evaluation and surgical manipulation of the chelonian and saurian reproductive tracts have been well described (see Chapters 64 and 65). Endoscopy is minimally invasive compared with traditional surgery, and the basic rigid endoscopic equipment (2.7-mm telescope with 4.8-mm operating sheath system) utilized in most veterinary facilities works well to allow coelomic evaluation of the reproductive tract. Unfortunately, due to unique anatomy, the intimacy of coelomic organs, and multiple membranes/compartments restricting movement, coelomic evaluation of the reproductive tract is more challenging in snakes and crocodilians except via cloacoscopy for evaluation of the urodeum and oviducts.

As described earlier, endoscopy is useful for sexing monomorphic species but coelomic evaluation of the gonads can also provide feedback on reproductive activity and disease or disorders. This is especially valuable when working with threatened or endangered species programs or private breeders relying on production.[114,115]

Generally, the gonads of chelonians and lizards are located dorsally in the mid to caudal coelom; the testis appears as ovoid and smooth and may dramatically vary in size with season and reproductive activity.

Some lizard species (e.g., monitors) have thin, pigmented, posthepatic, or postpulmonary membranes that may obscure the gonads and must be incised to allow direct gonad visualization. In cases of male infertility or abnormal appearance of the testes, endoscopic biopsies can be taken for histopathology and microbiological sampling. Depending on follicular activity, ovarian biopsy may be more challenging unless neoplastic or granulomatous changes have replaced the large yolk-filled follicles. Cloacoscopy may also be utilized to evaluate the urodeum, and in some situations the oviduct may be entered for evaluation and possible manipulation of retained eggs/fetuses.

Cytology/Biopsy. A definitive diagnosis of reproductive disease often requires demonstration of a host pathologic response and an etiologic agent. The diagnostic value of cytology is often more limited compared with histopathology, and tissue biopsy is preferred whenever possible. Where it is critical to maintain breeding ability and the abnormal reproductive tract cannot be removed, tissue biopsies can be used for cytology, histopathology, microbiology, parasitology, and even toxicologic evaluation. Biopsy samples may be collected at surgery using biopsy needles (eg, Tru-Cut), endoscopically with biopsy forceps, or with standard wedge or excisional surgical techniques. With reproductive disease, especially in nonbreeding pet or display animals, surgical removal and submission of the entire reproductive tract for laboratory evaluation is recommended.

Coeliotomy. In cases of reproductive disease/disorders surgical evaluation and the removal of all, or part, of the reproductive tract can provide valuable diagnostic information and therapeutic guidance and aid resolution. For pet or display reptiles this is likely the appropriate action either endoscopically or with traditional coeliotomy. With reproductive disorders such as follicular stasis, dystocia, oviductal disease/prolapse, ectopic eggs or yolk coelomitis, coeliotomy is the best surgical option because (1) the use of minimally invasive keyhole techniques are not practical if large amounts of biologic material must be removed, and (2) it allows a more thorough evaluation of the coelom. If one side of the reproductive tract is diseased or damaged (unilateral ovarian or testicular pathology and/or oviductal disease, damage, or prolapse), a unilateral procedure can be performed to preserve reproductive ability in valuable animals. The removed tissue is submitted for

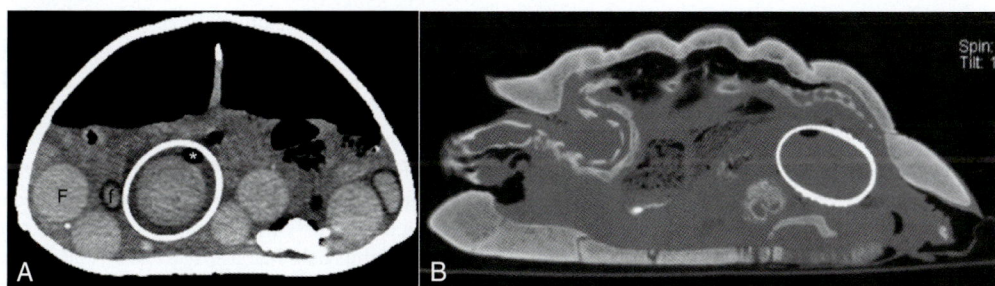

FIG 80.34 (A) Transverse CT image (soft tissue window) of a Hermann's tortoise (*Testudo hermanni*). A normally calcified shell with an unremarkable yolk is seen. A tiny dorsal gas cap suggests dystocia (asterisk). Adjacent to the egg some follicles (F) are visible. One small follicle (f) shows a hypodense peripheral rim indicating atrophy. (B) Sagital CT image (bony window) of another Hermann's tortoise. A thickened egg-shell (being denser then the skeleton) with a rough spiculated surface is positioned within the pelvis. The egg is wider than the maximal diameter of the shell opening near the cloaca. Chronic dystocia is not only indicated because of the egg-shell formation but also by the loss of proper egg contents, a gas cap within the egg shell, and multiple gas pockets around the egg shell. Surgery proved severe inflammation and adhesion of the egg shell to the oviduct. Note the thickened heterogenous shell and the pyramid-shaped neural bony plates indicating long-standing mineral imbalances and improper diet and husbandry. (Courtesy of Michaela Gumpenberger.)

histopathology and microbiological analysis. For the surgical approach to the coelom, see Section 10, Surgery, and for details on surgery of the reproductive tract, see Chapter 105.

General Approach to Treatment

Prevention. During health examinations of juvenile and subadult reptiles, clinicians should discuss maturation and hormonal influences on behavior, familiarize owners with signs of reproductive activity, and offer preventative options for management. Initial studies evaluating hormonal therapy to suppress reproductive activity in reptiles have had mixed results. Captive studies in female veiled chameleons and leopard geckos were performed to evaluate the clinical value of GnRH implants (deslorelin 4.7 mg) and were found to be ineffective in suppressing reproductive activity in these lizards.[116] Tamoxifen (antiestrogen) has been experimentally used to inhibit reproductive activity in leopard geckos, but its clinical value remains untested.[117] Mixed results have also been reported in the use of gonadotropin releasing hormone (GnRH) therapy in males to decrease aggression.[118,119] More research is necessary to determine whether medical hormonal therapy can be clinically useful in the management of reproductive activity and diseases in reptiles. Therefore at this time, offering owners preventative ovariectomy for lizards and chelonians may be the best option to avoid future reproductive problems. Surgical orchiectomy of those species that are particularly aggressive as adults may also be warranted[120] (see Chapter 105).

Initial Therapy. It is important initially to stabilize the patient by providing species-specific thermal support and correcting hydration (see Chapters 46 and 87). Initial therapeutic choices must also be considered carefully to not invalidate future diagnostic testing. For example, blood samples should be collected before fluid therapy and antibiotics delayed until after biopsy and culture whenever possible.

The reproductive tract is not essential for survival and in cases of severe disease, especially in reptiles where reproduction is not important, partial or complete surgical removal of the reproductive tract is often the most effective therapy. If not possible, treating the diseased and/or damaged reproductive tract with the most specific therapy is recommended. Therapy should be based on results of appropriate diagnostic procedures (described earlier) and when possible a well-established connection between pathophysiology and medicinal effects.

COMMON REPRODUCTIVE DISEASES/DISORDERS

Male

Seasonal Behavioral Aggression

Clinical significance. Seasonal *interspecies* aggression toward owners and keepers is a problem with larger species, such as green iguanas, rock iguanas (*Cyclura* spp.), and monitors (*Varanus* spp.).[105] This is a normal seasonal (hormonal) *intraspecies* behavior for these lizards in the wild and allows males to establish territorial hierarchies (see Chapter 13). However, in captivity humans or other family pets are perceived as an "intraspecific threat," and territorial aggression often ensues with physical attacks, including biting and tail whipping. These behaviors are generally not acceptable to pet owners. Seasonal intraspecies male aggression can also occur with cagemates and is usually associated with breeding groups of reptiles or when multiple mature males are housed together.

Known etiological cause(s). Androgen (testosterone and dihydrotestosterone) elevations associated with sexual maturity can result in seasonal behavioral aggression in male lizards.[120,121] Often, these male lizards are allowed to roam free in the owner's home. In these situations, the entire home becomes the lizard's territory, compared with confinement to a cage. During the breeding season these lizards may become

extremely territorial, and humans in the home domain are attacked. Male iguanas have been reported to be aggressive specifically toward women during their menstrual cycle.[122] Presumably male iguanas are detecting pheromones produced by their female owners. Human females are often bitten by iguanas in attempts at breeding, with attacks oriented toward the face or neck, as female iguanas' necks are often bitten and held to secure them during copulation. Often any human males in the household are considered competition, and aggression is oriented toward moving them out of the lizard's (the dominant male's) territory, and when this fails aggressive behavior escalates.[123] Conspecific aggression is usually associated with mature males being housed together during the breeding season. Male combat rituals are common in lizards, snakes, and chelonians. In the wild these interactions end in the submissive male fleeing; however, in captivity the subordinate male may not be able to escape the attack of the dominant male and serious injury or death can result. Owners may unknowingly be housing multiple males together and, with sexual maturity, combat and injury often occurs.

Clinical presentation and diagnostic confirmation. Seasonal aggression must be differentiated from defensive aggression, which occurs in response to being provoked or threatened, or from an animal that is generally aggressive with no seasonal influence. In the northeast United States, breeding typically occurs from the fall to the spring. However, this aggressive behavior can occur any time of the year, often associated with changes in temperature, light cycle, and barometric pressure changes. With conspecific aggression the owner usually presents an injured reptile, from a group (often of an unknown sex ratio) or after introducing an incorrectly sexed pair of reptiles for breeding.

History, presenting complaint, signalment, and proper sexing of the reptile are often diagnostic for this behavioral problem. Some species of lizards can be difficult to sex and may require advanced techniques for identification. Often the aggressive behavior change can be related to reaching sexual maturity, and there is a defined seasonal pattern to the aggression.

Preferred treatment(s). It is important to educate clients, so they can understand that this seasonal behavior is quite normal for a healthy mature (intact) male lizard. Behavioral management options can be considered to reduce seasonal hormonal aggression in lizards; however, often they are unsuccessful. Most importantly, reducing and/or controlling "territory" by not allowing the lizard to free roam in the house may help reduce aggression or allow more control of the behavior, and the owner can take protective measures when working with the lizard in the confined space or cage. Providing a surrogate object for the lizard to mate with such as a stuffed animal or colorful towel may help. Reducing the light cycle to 10 hours or less, avoiding red clothing/objects (or other colors that result in aggressive responses), and not having female family members work with the iguana during their menstruation cycle are all important to implement.[123]

Medical management. There are several reports in the literature evaluating the effectiveness of antiandrogens such as gonadotropin-releasing hormone (GnRH) agonist compounds to chemically castrate lizards and thus help manage aggression, and results have been mixed. In one study involving 18 captive, mature, male green iguanas, three groups were established, a control group, a group that received 0.2 mg/kg of mammalian leuprolide acetate IM, and a group that received 0.4 mg/kg IM. Blood was collected and testosterone levels were determined using radioimmunoassay at day 0, 1, 4, 7, 14, 21, 28, and 35 posttreatment.[118] No significant differences in testosterone levels were found between the groups, and although there were some statistical differences between days of sampling (all involving comparisons with day 0 vs. other days), in all cases testosterone levels were lower on day 0. This study concluded that mammalian leuprolide acetate at these doses did not significantly reduce testosterone levels in captive male green iguanas.[118] A male bearded dragon was implanted with a 4.7 mg deslorelin (GnRH agonist) implant, and subjectively appeared to be less aggressive toward the owner for 2 months after implantation, but no further follow-up was available.[119] Anecdotal reports have also indicated that GnRH agonist may be helpful in managing seasonal (testosterone driven) aggression in reptiles, but more research is necessary to determine efficacy of these hormones.

Surgery. Currently orchiectomy is the treatment of choice. Before considering orchiectomy, it is important to characterize the aggressive behavior. If before or after sexual maturity the lizard is consistently aggressive (year-round), then orchiectomy may not be effective, as the behavior is not likely solely androgen driven. However, in males where aggressive behavior began after sexual maturity and appears to be seasonal, orchiectomy may be beneficial. In iguanas the best results are achieved when orchiectomy is performed in prepubescent males.[124] Once iguanas are sexually mature and aggressive behavior has become established, orchiectomy may be less effective. One study involving 16 adult mature male iguanas, 3 experimental groups were studied; one group was castrated before the onset of breeding season aggression, another group was castrated during the breeding season while exhibiting aggressive behavior, and the last group was sham operated but no orchiectomy was performed.[120] The study found a statistically significant reduction in the aggressive behavior in the group orchiectomized before the onset of the breeding season. No significant reduction in aggression was found between the group orchiectomized during the breeding season and the control group. Thus orchiectomy was less succesful in managing aggression once hormonal behavior was initiated. However, the same authors reported that more than 60 male green iguanas were subsequently castrated and monitored for up to 3 years afterward, and orchiectomy reduced or eliminated aggression in 70% of the iguanas.[123] See Chapter 105 for details on performing orchiectomy.

Prognosis and prevention. Prevention provides the best prognosis, with orchiectomy being performed before sexual maturity.[124] Once sexually mature and aggressive hormonal behavior has already been established, orchiectomy may be less effective. For conspecific aggression, the prognosis is good if injuries can be successfully treated, reptiles are then properly sexed, and males separated to minimize future problems. In breeding colonies, providing enough space and visual barriers within the enclosure may reduce male combat interaction and aggression.

Veterinarians should educate owners about these potential behavioral changes at sexual maturity and discuss elective orchiectomy during young (male) lizard consultations (value of identifying the sex). However, with early orchiectomy, and the subsequent loss of testosterone influence, male secondary sexual characteristics will not develop. For example, prepubescent orchiectomized male iguanas will not develop the same large body and head size, larger dewlap, jowls, or crests and spikes that owners may desire with owning a "majestic" mature male iguana. This information should be understood by the owner before orchiectomy.

Having the owner initiate environmental changes before the start of the "season" may help to manage hormonal aggression. If the lizard is free-roaming in the house, restricting the lizard's territory to a single room or caging them, during this time of the year, may help with management. In some instances rehoming or euthanasia may have to be considered, often as a result of a severe injury to a (human) family member.

Testicular Disorders

Orchitis

Clinical significance and known etiological cause(s). Orchitis in male reptiles is uncommon. Presentation for low fertility or reproductive-related issues may result in evaluation of testes and a possible diagnosis of orchitis. However, damage and pathology of the copulatory organs

in male reptiles *is* common and infectious agents associated with these problems can result in cloacitis and scent gland adenitis with possible ascending infection. In breeding males venereal transmission of bacterial (and other infectious agents) organisms is possible. Adjacent coelomic pathology may involve the testes, and a variety of neoplasms have been described (see Neoplasia section later).

Clinical presentation and diagnostic confirmation. Physical examination may reveal coelomic distention/guarding, weight loss, lethargy and depression, pale mucous membranes, and dehydration. Orchitis may mimic changes associated with normal reproductive activity, such as seasonal testicular recrudescence, and must be differentiated from normal physiological changes.

Ultrasonography may be useful to detect morphological changes, especially in unilateral cases of orchitis. Ultrasound-guided aspiration may be possible but is potentially high risk. Radiography or advanced imaging modalities such as CT and MRI may be useful in some cases (see imaging in Clinical Investigation earlier).

Coelioscopy is minimally invasive and is useful to diagnose orchitis (less so in snakes) by allowing direct visualization. Most importantly, diagnostic confirmation can be achieved by collecting aspirates or biopsies for cytology, microbiology, and histopathology. Additionally, coelioscopy may allow therapeutic procedures as well. See Chapters 64 and 65, for more details on these endoscopic procedures. Exploratory coeliotomy is more invasive but can confirm a diagnosis, provides the most thorough coelomic evaluation, and allows therapeutic procedures.

Preferred treatment(s), prognosis, and prevention. In a reptile that is not part of a breeding program, surgical sterilization (orchiectomy) offers the best chance of resolution. In breeding males with unilateral disease, a unilateral orchiectomy can be performed. In these cases, microbiology and histopathology should be performed on removed tissues to direct therapeutics for any remaining reproductive tract (see Chapter 105). In mild cases or cases where future reproduction is critical and diagnostic evaluation has indicated that treatment may be effective, antiinflammatories and appropriate antimicrobial therapy may be initiated based on microbiology and histopathology.

The prognosis depends on the condition of the reptile at presentation, the duration of the condition, and the extent of pathology. Prognosis for survival may be good if orchiectomy is performed but eliminates future reproduction if bilateral. For breeding reptiles, providing appropriate husbandry, nutrition, preventive health programs (including quarantine), implementing safe breeding practices (breeding environment hygiene, not overextending males, etc), and regular veterinary evaluations (including necropsy and histopathology of losses and culls) can help reduce the incidence of reproductive disease.

Copulatory Organ Pathology (Prolapse and Abscessation)

Clinical significance and known etiological cause(s). Trauma, prolapse, and infection of the phallus or hemipenes is a common clinical presentation. In one study involving a review of 3000 reptiles presented for cloacal prolapses, 35% of the prolapses involved the male reproductive organ.[125] A good understanding of the anatomy and function of this organ is important for management. The organ does not house the urethra and plays no role in the urinary system, thus management is not as complicated as with mammalian species.

Typically prolapse occurs as a result of trauma. Traumatized tissue becomes engorged, making retraction difficult, and the exposed tissue is subjected to further damage, infection, and necrosis.

Prolapse, trauma, and infection/abscessation is seen most commonly in sexually mature, often actively breeding males. Thus the incidence of prolapse and trauma increases during the breeding season or with perceived seasonal changes. If breeding animals are housed on rough or contaminated particulate substrates such as mulch or wood shavings, the likelihood of trauma and infection is increased. Male snakes breeding too many females in a season (breeders typically move males from female to female) may develop hemipenal trauma, infection, and possible prolapse (Fig. 80.35). Single housed male chelonians may repeatedly attempt to mount and breed females or even inanimate objects in their environment, resulting in phallus trauma.

Trauma or pathology associated with the vertebral spine and spinal cord can result in neurological damage/dysfunction and organ prolapse. Prolapse of the hemipenes is common in young growing herbivorous and insectivorous lizards due to nutritional secondary hyperparathyroidism (NSHP) resulting in spinal deformities and fractures. NSHP in chelonians often results in carapacial deformities involving the vertebrae and spinal cord, resulting in neurologic damage/dysfunction and prolapse. Hypovitaminosis A in lizards may also contribute to hemipenal abscess and prolapse as squamous metaplasia may increase the incidence of

hemipenal plugs (accumulation of seminal material and sloughing skin).[116,126] This retained material results in swelling, inflammation, and secondary bacterial involvement with possible abscessation (Fig. 80.36).

Other known causes include metabolic disease, colonic/cloacal obstruction associated with urinary calculi, and renomegaly in lizards with intrapelvic kidneys (e.g., green iguana) resulting in obstipation and tenesmus.

Clinical presentation.   Owners are frequently alarmed by the appearance of a prolapse, and reptiles are often presented as an emergency. The prolapse is usually engorged and hemorrhagic with associated discharge from exposure trauma and, in severe cases, necrotic. The prolapsed phallus/hemipenis must be differentiated from other possible prolapsed tissue, including cloaca, colon, or bladder (in chelonians and some lizards). See Chapter 75 for details on determining the origin of prolapsed cloacal tissue. In squamates the hemipenal tissue is located within the base of the tail, so prolapsed tissue will originate from the caudal margin of the vent (Fig. 80.37A). In chelonians the phallus may be more difficult to differentiate as it originates from the floor of the urodeum but is generally a large, tubular, often elaborate structure (see Fig. 80.37B).

Squamates with hemipenal abscesses and impacted seminal plugs may be presented for asymmetry (although can be bilateral) and swelling

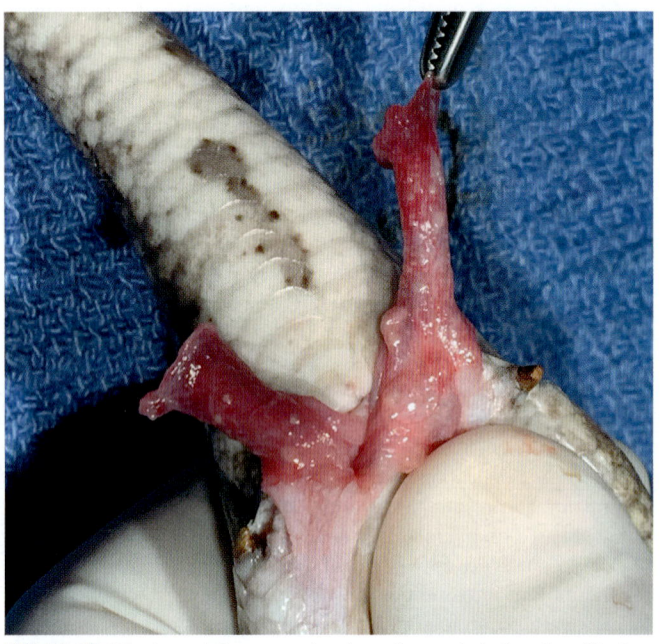

FIG 80.35 Hemipenal abscesses in a breeding male ball python (*Python regius*). Note the small multifocal white/tan lesions on both hemipenes; anesthesia is utilized to allow full inspection and delicate surgical removal of infected tissue. Amputation and/or multiple procedures may be necessary to remove all infected tissue. (Courtesy of Scott J. Stahl, Stahl Exotic Animal Veterinary Services.)

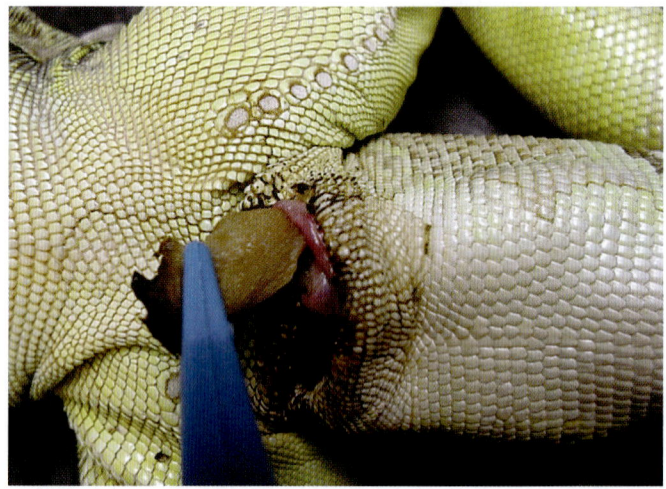

FIG 80.36 Removal of a hemipenal plug in a green iguana (*Iguana iguana*). Hypovitaminosis A in lizards may contribute to hemipenal abscess and prolapse, as squamous metaplasia may increase the incidence of hemipenal plugs (accumulation of seminal material and sloughing skin). (Courtesy of Stephen J. Divers.)

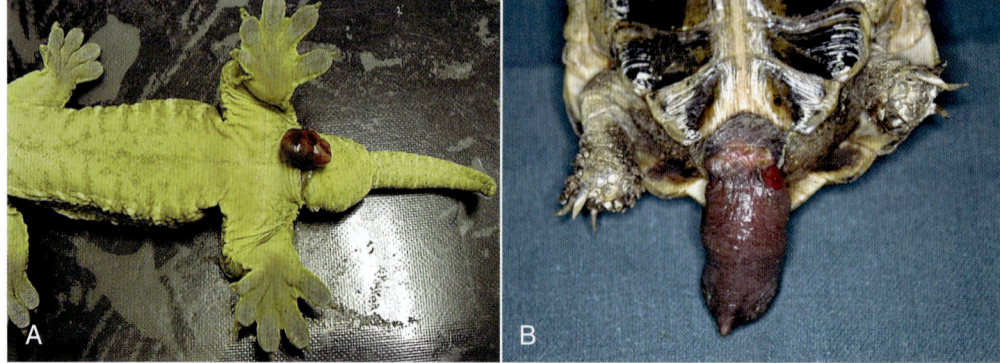

FIG 80.37 (A) Hemipenis prolapse in a giant New Caledonian gecko (*Rhacodactylus leachianus*). The hemipenis is inflamed, swollen, and hyperemic. (B) A phallus prolapse in a Hermann's tortoise (*Testudo hermanni*). The phallus is inflamed, congested, and hyperemic. (Courtesy of Stephen J. Divers.)

at the base of the tail, often with discharge and in severe cases ulceration of the skin. In snakes, scent gland adenitis may be concurrent.

Diagnostic confirmation. For copulatory organ prolapses, examination of the structure is usually diagnostic. For partial prolapses, hemipenal abscesses or hemipenal plugs, sedation, or anesthesia may be required for thorough evaluation. In cases with infection and abscessation, culture and sensitivity is useful to determine specific pathogens and direct therapy. In breeding squamates with hemipenal abscessation (especially if housed on mulch or soil) biopsy of debrided tissue or an amputated hemipenis (if not salvageable) can be collected for histopathology and microbiology. Radiography or advanced imaging such as CT or MRI may be useful to look for spinal involvement in cases where prolapse may be the result of neurological dysfunction. Also, imaging may be helpful to rule out other causes of prolapse such as coelomic obstructive disease (e.g., bladder stone, obstipation).

Preferred treatment(s). Evaluating the prolapsed copulatory organ to assess the extent of the damage, determining the underlying reasons for the prolapse, and understanding the goals of the owner are all important considerations when developing a therapeutic plan.

Often at presentation the prolapsed organ has extensive damage with desiccation and necrosis, and for most nonbreeding animals, amputation is often preferred. Amputation of the phallus/hemipenis does not affect the urinary system, and in squamates (with paired copulatory organs) reproductive potential is maintained with a second hemipenis. Anesthesia or sedation is required; see Chapters 105 and 106 for surgical techniques.

For breeding reptiles, attempting to repair and replace the copulatory organ(s) may be necessary. If the organ appears viable it can be gently cleaned with saline and the swelling reduced using hypertonic solutions such as 50% dextrose. Topical lidocaine or bupivacaine may help minimize discomfort during replacement. When replacing a prolapsed hemipenis it is critical for the tissue to be inverted back into the base of the tail rather than simply replaced into the cloaca. General anesthesia is often required for proper replacement, and stay sutures can be placed across the vent opening, either unilateral or bilateral, to help hold the copulatory organ in place. This allows organ protection and healing while underlying causes are addressed. With recurrent or chronic prolapse, amputation is recommended.

In lizards with hemipenal plugs, gentle removal of the adhered material and flushing of the hemipenis is necessary. Topical anesthesia or general anesthesia may be necessary to facilitate cleaning and evaluation. Topical wound gels or creams (e.g., 1% silver sulfadiazine cream) can be applied to the damaged tissues. With severe inflammation and secondary bacterial involvement, systemic NSAIDs and antimicrobials may be indicated. Dietary improvement and vitamin A supplementation in lizards is often important (see Chapter 122).

In breeding snakes with hemipenal trauma, cellulitis, and abscessation, general anesthesia is required to thoroughly evaluate the hemipenes. Magnification is helpful because delicate debridement of infected tissue is necessary to attempt to maintain normal architecture. Often hemipenal infections in these snakes present as invasive multifocal nodular abscesses (see Fig. 80.35); the organ is quite vascular, and hemorrhage makes it difficult to see all lesions as surgery progresses. Several surgeries may be necessary to ensure removal of all affected tissue and maintain as much healthy hemipenal tissue as possible.[127,128] One or both hemipenes may be involved, and sometimes one hemipenis may need to be amputated, based on severity, but the other hemipenis can be salvaged as described. Systemic broad-spectrum antimicrobials should be initiated based on initial cytology and modified based on microbiology and histopathology results.

Prognosis and prevention. Prognosis is good for survival as the phallus and hemipenes are not part of the urinary system and can be removed if they cannot be repaired. Additionally, because squamates have two hemipenes, amputation of one will still allow copulation and future breeding. Chelonians only have one copulatory organ thus amputation results in a loss of reproductive ability. If prolapse and damage of the copulatory organ is the result of neurological dysfunction due to spinal pathology, the prognosis is guarded to poor because obstipation and prolapse of the cloaca and colon often follow.

Breeding male reptiles should not service too many females as overuse of the phallus or hemipenis may increase the incidence of trauma, abscessation, and prolapse. Keepers should maintain a clean breeding environment and avoid using rough particulate substrates to minimize trauma to the copulatory organ. Maintaining adequate levels of vitamin A is important to reduce the incidence of squamous metaplasia and associated hemipenal plug problems in lizards.

Providing a diet with adequate calcium and vitamin D$_3$ in growing lizards and chelonians is important to prevent spinal abnormalities resulting from NSHP and subsequent prolapse from neurologic dysfunction.

Female

Behavioral Aggression.
In the authors' experience ovariectomy in female iguanas (and other lizard species), usually performed for preventative or medical reasons, may result in the development of androgen-driven characteristics, including the development of male secondary sexual characteristics and aggression.[126]

In a study involving free-living female mountain spiny lizards (*Sceloporus jarrovi*), females were ovariectomized and returned to their natural environment for behavior observation.[129] Females of this species aggressively defend territories from other females, and the effects of ovariectomy itself and the administration of a testosterone implant to ovariectomized females was evaluated. The study determined that estrogen and testosterone were both necessary to elicit the normal territorial aggression displayed by females of this species.[129] Interestingly, however, postovariectomized lizards' plasma estrogen levels in the study were reduced, but testosterone plasma levels remained the same as the sham ovariectomized lizards. This may explain what is seen clinically, as ovariectomized female lizards appear to develop androgen-driven changes associated with persistent testosterone but reduced estrogen. More research is necessary to understand what is occurring hormonally in these cases. Clinically, however, ovariectomy in lizards has been found to sometimes result in these issues, and owners must be warned about the potential for these behavior and morphological changes before surgery. Ovarian neoplasia/or disease could also result in pathological changes in sex hormone production which may also result in hormonal-based aggression.

Clinical presentation, preferred treatment(s), prognosis, and prevention. Generally, females presenting with this condition have a history of ovariectomy. Often these females will show evidence of male secondary sexual characteristics such as an increase in head size, larger jowls, dewlap, dorsal spines, and more obvious femoral/preanal pores. History, signalment, and presenting complaint will typically confirm a diagnosis. With ovarian neoplasia or pathology, signalment and presentation may be similar but without history of ovariectomy.

See discussion on male hormonal aggression for environmental changes that can be used to help reduce and mediate these behaviors. Many of these suggestions are based on utilizing safer practices to protect the owner when working with these aggressive lizards. Mixed study results and anecdotal reports have indicated that GnRH agonist may be helpful in managing seasonal (testosterone-driven) aggression in reptiles and thus may help these females, but more research is necessary. In cases where ovarian pathology is suspected to be causing hormonal changes, a thorough evaluation of the ovary and likely surgical ovariectomy is indicated.

Prognosis is good for survival; however, depending on the lizard's response to environmental manipulation or possible hormonal therapy, the prognosis for compatability as a pet or display animal may be poor. Prevention is a challenge, as in most cases these females have been ovariectomized due to reproductive diseases or disorders as a life-preserving procedure. It does add caution to the general recommendation of preventative ovariectomy in some lizard species. Eliminating one condition (reproductive disease) could create new issues with aggressive behavior. Owners should be forewarned about this possibility before ovariectomy.

Ovarian Disorders

Follicular stasis

Clinical significance and known etiological (causes). Ovarian (preovulatory) follicular stasis in reptiles occurs when mature follicles develop but do not ovulate or resorb, becoming static and eventually degenerative. This condition occurs commonly in lizards, chelonians, and less often in snakes kept as single pets or display animals. Follicular stasis is usually a seasonal problem because hormonal cycles, and thus reproductive activity and breeding of most captive reptiles (temperate species), occurs at specific times of the year. However, in captivity environmental factors may result in reproductive activity in reptiles at any time of the year.

Follicular stasis has an increased incidence and risk with single or pet reptile where, if the female is healthy and has adequate energy reserves, she will often proceed with active folliculogenesis. Under normal conditions the female would likely be courted and bred by a male and proceed to ovulation and oviposition. However in the captive environment this may not occur (although some of these females will ovulate and produce infertile eggs). In these captive single females, does the lack of a male play a role in contributing to this condition? A study using ultrasonography to monitor the development of ovarian follicles in captive short-tail (blood) pythons found that at the onset of the reproductive season all females initiated early follicular development; however, only females that were already housed with males actually initiated vitellogenesis, ovulated, and oviposited viable eggs.[32] Perhaps in other reptiles the male's presence is not always necessary for progression to vitellogenesis but plays an important role in influencing ovulation or resorption. Metabolic disease such as NSHP may contribute to follicular stasis because calcium plays an important role in the vitellogenic cycle. More research is needed to better understand this condition, as the etiologies for follicular stasis are multifactorial and complex, and the definitive cause in many of these cases is not determined.

Clinical presentation. Distinguishing follicular stasis (at least initially) from normal folliculogenesis can be challenging, and a diagnosis is sometimes made prematurely, and unnecessary treatment instigated. A clear understanding of the reproductive biology of the species, a thorough history, physical examination, and, in some cases, supplemental diagnostic tests may be necessary to determine the need for intervention.

Historically, reptiles with follicular stasis may be restless, pacing and climbing, looking for possible mates or nesting sites. Oviparous lizards and chelonians may dig in planters or substrate. Female aquatic turtles may spend extended time out of the water. Appetite and water intake may be reduced or absent. Coelomic distention with reduced body condition, anorexia, and behavior changes may be noted. Differential diagnoses for a coelomic mass include fecal masses, cystic calculi, abscesses, and tumors and should all be considered or ruled out.

On physical examination palpation may confirm preovulatory follicles in squamates, but sometimes it may be difficult to differentiate preovulatory follicles from postovulatory eggs. Ovarian follicles tend to be more dorsal and spherical and not as mobile as oviductal eggs, which are usually more oblong and ventral/caudal in the coelom.

Diagnostic confirmation

Hematology and biochemistry. Plasma biochemical changes often include elevations of total calcium; however, ionized calcium is often normal. Hematology may show a stress leukogram or, in cases of inflammation or infection, a leukocytosis, or leukopenia with left shift due to sequestration may be present. In more chronic cases anemia may be observed. In captive tortoises, clinical pathological findings consistently included elevations of calcium, albumin, total protein, alkaline phosphatase, and hematological changes including anemia, leukopenia, and heteropenia.[107]

Imaging. Radiography is an important tool to differentiate between follicular stasis and dystocia in squamates. (See Section 7 and associated radiography chapters.) Radiographically squamate follicular stasis often appears as a cluster of spherical, dorsal, homogenous, soft tissue structures that lack a shell. Radiography can also identify contributing, and/or concurrent, coelomic pathology, such as cystic calculi, obstipation, or organomegaly. Radiography may also help to identify abnormalities of bone associated with metabolic diseases such as NSHP or renal secondary hyperparathyroidism (RSHP) and the resulting calcium metabolism issues that may contribute to follicular stasis.

Ultrasonography is preferred for identification of follicular stasis and to differentiate between follicular stasis and poorly shelled postovulatory eggs. Sonographically, vitellogenic follicles show no hyperechoic shell and are uniformly hypoechoic and clustered. Ultrasonography can be utilized to monitor follicular progress. With active resorption or degenerate changes the ova progress from homogenous and hypoechoic to a more mixed (hypoechoic and anechoic) echogenicity (see Fig. 80.33A and B). This progresses to a loss of shape, and follicles become less spherical and poorly demarcated. With resorption they continue to reduce in size, but with stasis and degeneration the follicles coalesce with surrounding anechoic fluid often evident. If echogenic free-floating debris is noted within this anechoic fluid the ova are likely degenerate and inflamed, and surgical intervention is indicated.[108,111]

CT and MRI may also be indicated in some cases, and this technology is becoming more accessible. Specifically in managing follicular stasis, CT (versus radiography) allows each ovarian follicle to be individually evaluated. CT is more useful for identifying advanced changes, including distinct horizontal leveling of the contents of degenerating follicles indicating the need for intervention.[108]

Preferred treatment(s). Treatment for follicular stasis may differ depending on the species and objectives of the owner. If the reptile is a pet or display animal then ovariectomy as soon as (safely) possible is preferred. If maintaining the reptile's breeding ability is important, using the least invasive technique(s) to resolve issues and still allow future reproduction is the goal.

For pet or nonbred squamates, and chelonians with follicular stasis where the patient is considered healthy, a nest box can be provided and the reptile (except snakes) sent home on calcium glubionate (23 mg/mL) at 1 mL/kg PO SID-BID for 2 to 3 weeks depending on dietary history. Appetite and behavior should be monitored, and reevaluation is recommended in 2 to 3 weeks to determine whether resorption or ovulation has occurred. Ovariectomy may also be offered at initial presentation, as this may be the safest way to ensure health (owners often choose this option). If a breeding female (and healthy on examination), she can be paired with a male and a nesting/laying environment provided.

Once stable, or if returning with no change or follicular degenerative changes evident (utilizing ultrasonography or CT), ovariectomy is recommended. For follicular stasis cases if the patient is not considered

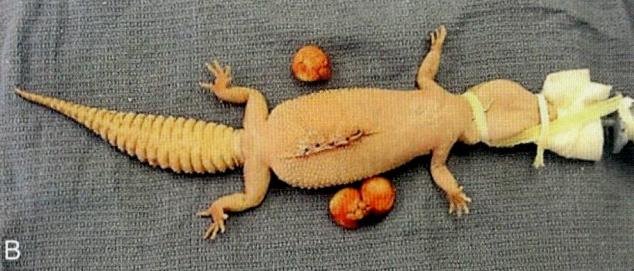

FIG 80.38 (A) Sonograph of a female leopard gecko (*Eublepharis macularius*) with follicular stasis. Note two preovulatory follicles (hypoechoic, spherical structures) on one ovary. (B) The same leopard gecko recovering from surgey after ovariectomy. (Courtesy of Scott J. Stahl, Stahl Exotic Animal Veterinary Services.)

healthy they must be stabilized by providing appropriate thermal support (for the species) and addressing hydration issues. After warming and hydrating the patient as necessary, additional medical therapy may be initiated, including calcium (lizards and chelonians), nonsteroidal antiinflammatories (NSAIDS), opiates (analgesia and mild sedation if necessary), and antimicrobials if infection is present. Once considered stable, ovariectomy is recommended (Fig. 80.38A and B). It is not useful to use oxytocin in cases of follicular stasis as ova are not in the oviduct. See Chapter 105, for details on performing ovariectomy.

Prognosis and prevention. Prognosis and outcome are favorable for follicular stasis cases with early diagnosis and intervention. Chronic cases are more likely to have associated pathology, including degenerative changes, and may require surgical intervention. The prognosis is good for survival but ovariectomy obviously renders the animal sterile, which may be unacceptable for breeders.

During health examinations of female reptiles, clinicians should discuss the likelihood of eventual hormonal influences, familiarize owners with signs of reproductive activity, and offer preventative ovariectomy to clients as an option to avoid future reproductive issues (see Chapter 105).

Since calcium plays an important role in successful reproduction, the diet of reproductively active reptiles should be reviewed to ensure adequate levels of calcium and vitamin D_3 (see Chapter 27). Breeding females that mature quickly (lizards) should be monitored closely for reproductive activity, and if noted, providing access to a male may help reduce the incidence of follicular stasis.

Oophoritis

Clinical significance and known etiologic cause(s). Oophoritis is usually associated with folliculogenesis or dystocia in captive reptiles. Follicular stasis often results in oophoritis when static follicles become degenerate and secondarily infected. Ovarian follicular stasis, yolk coelomitis, dystocia, and ectopic ova can be inflammatory disorders that predispose to opportunistic bacterial or fungal oophoritis.

Clinical presentation and diagnostic confirmation. See Clinical Presentation for Follicular Stasis and Ectopic Follicles and Yolk Coelomitis. Physical examination findings may include coelomic distention and sensitivity, weight loss, lethargy and depression, pale mucous membranes, and clinical dehydration.

As with follicular stasis, ultrasonography can be useful for diagnosis. Sonographically degenerate and inflammatory changes in ovarian follicles may include a loss of their typical round, well-demarcated shape, and follicles may appear to coalesce, often resulting in rupture and leakage (see Ectopic Follicles and Yolk Coelomitis). Ultrasound-guided aspirates of the ovary are possible but higher risk. Radiography or other advanced imaging modalities such as CT and MRI may be useful in some cases.

Coelioscopy is minimally invasive and is useful for allowing direct visualization of the ovary. Most importantly, diagnostic confirmation can be achieved with endoscopy by collecting aspirates or biopsies for cytology, microbiology, and histopathology. Additionally, coelioscopy may allow therapeutic procedures (see Chapters 64 and 65 for more details).

However, in cases of active coelomitis, yolk coelomitis, and ectopic eggs, exploratory coeliotomy is preferred over coelioscopy, because, in addition to diagnostic confirmation (direct sample collection), it facilitates complete coelomic evaluation and more extensive surgical intervention (e.g., removal of inflammatory material and ovariectomy). In the authors' experience microbiologic sampling using these techniques often results in the identification of gram-negative bacteria.

Preferred treatment(s), prognosis, and prevention. For a reptile that is not part of a breeding program, surgical sterilization (ovariectomy) is the best resolution. In breeding reptiles with unilateral disease, a unilateral ovariectomy can be performed. In these cases, microbiology and histopathology should be performed on removed tissues to direct therapy for the remaining reproductive tract. See Chapter 105 for details on performing these procedures.

In mild cases and/or cases in which future reproduction is critical and diagnostic evaluation has indicated that treatment may be effective, antiinflammatories and appropriate antimicrobial therapy may be initiated based on culture and sensitivity testing and histopathology.

The prognosis depends on the condition of the reptile at presentation, the duration of the disease, and the extent of the pathology (see Prognosis for Follicular Stasis and Ectopic Follicles and Yolk Coelomitis).

Additionally, for breeding reptiles, providing appropriate husbandry, nutrition, and preventive health programs (including quarantine) and implementing safe breeding practices (e.g., breeding environment hygiene, not overextending males) and regular veterinary evaluations (including necropsy and histopathology on losses and culls) can help reduce the incidence of reproductive disease.

Ectopic follicles and yolk coelomitis

Clinical significance and known etiological cause(s). Chronicity or complications associated with preovulatory follicular stasis can lead to ovarian follicles becoming degenerate or damaged, resulting in leakage or rupture, with the release of free yolk into the coelom resulting in coelomitis. Follicular stasis, and thus yolk coelomitis, is most commonly seen in lizards, followed by chelonians and less frequently in snakes.[37,116,126,130–132] Free yolk material results in an inflammatory response in the coelom, often with secondary bacterial infection and sepsis (Fig. 80.39).

See previous discussion for a description of follicular stasis and etiologies, however once the condition occurs the static ovarian follicles become degenerate, often coalescing and becoming friable. Trauma, continued degeneration, and secondary bacterial involvement can increase the risk of rupture and yolk leakage into the coelom.[37,116,130–132]

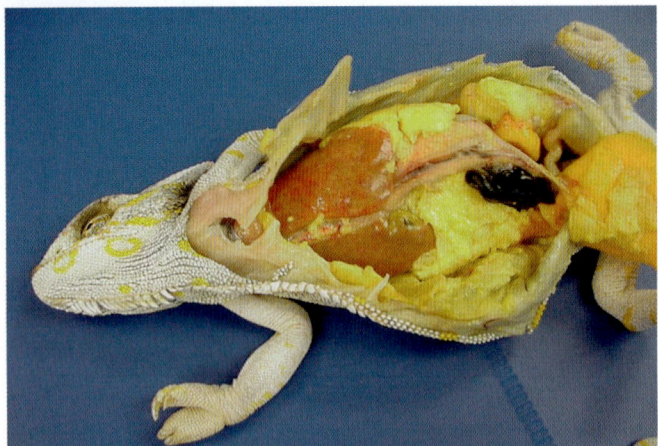

FIG 80.39 A female veiled chameleon (*Chamalaleo calyptratus*) with severe yolk coelomitis identified at necropsy. (Courtesy of Scott J. Stahl, Stahl Exotic Animal Veterinary Services.)

Clinical presentation and diagnostic confirmation. This condition is often a sequela to follicular stasis as previously discussed. Owners may have appreciated behavioral changes such as restle ssness, nesting, and aggressive behaviors. Tenesmus, anorexia, weight loss, and weakness may occur, and more advanced cases may present obtunded. Additional physical examination findings may include coelomic distention and sensitivity, pale mucous membranes, and dehydration.

Abnormalities in the hemogram and biochemistry are the same as described for follicular stasis and reflect severe inflammatory changes associated with coelomitis and sepsis. Dramatic leukocytosis (or leukopenia and a left shift) with toxic changes and azurophilia are common in squamates, whereas in more chronic cases anemi a and leukopenia may be noted.[106,107]

Imaging, especially ultrasonography, can be useful in diagnosing this condition. Sonographically degenerate follicles will have a loss of their round, well-demarcated shape and appear to coalesce (see Fig. 80.33A and B). Free anechoic fluid in the coelom with echogenic free-floating debris may indicate degenerative changes associated with the inflammatory response to yolk.[108,111,112] Ultrasound-guided aspiration of free coelomic fluid often yields yellow flocculent material, which is cytologically consistent with inflammation and proteinaceous debris. Other advanced imaging modalities can be utilized when necessary and available.

Coelioscopy may be used to confirm these conditions, but complications associated with free fluid, yolk, and possible adhesions make endoscopy more challenging, and coeliotomy is often preferred. Exploratory coeliotomy will confirm the diagnosis, facilitate thorough coelomic evaluation, and allow therapeutic procedures. Samples can be collected for micriobiological and histopathological evaluation during these confirmatory procedures.

Preferred treatment(s). Surgical intervention is usually required for treatment and resolution of yolk coelomitis. Once the patient is stable and under general anesthesia a coeliotomy is performed. The entire coelom is evaluated, paying particular attention to the reproductive tract, and any ectopic or diseased material debrided and removed. For pet or display reptiles a bilateral ovariectomy is performed to eliminate reoccurrence. In breeding reptiles a unilateral ovariectomy and salpingectomy can be performed if one side of the reproductive tract is diseased or damaged and cannot be repaired. Any damaged/abnormal reproductive tissue can be removed and submitted for microbiological analysis and histopathology to guide therapy. The coelom is thoroughly and copiously lavaged before closure. Aggressive postoperative support and systemic antimicrobials, antiinflammatories and analgesics are initiated as necessary.

Prognosis and prevention. Prognosis depends on the reptile's condition at presentation and duration, and the extent of the coelomic pathology. With surgical evaluation of the coelom; removal of the reproductive material; copius lavage of the coelom; aggressive postoperative support; and systemic antimicrobials, antiinflammatories, and analgesics, the prognosis is guarded to good. Lizards generally have a better prognosis than chelonians, likely due to easier access to the coelom and earlier detection.[37,126] In severe cases and/or chronic cases where the patient is presented in a debilitated state the prognosis is poor.

For pet or display reptiles, bilateral ovariectomy can prevent these conditions. For breeding reptiles, providing optimal management is important to reduce reproductive complications. Prebreeding health evaluation of females may be valuable to ensure they are sound before the stress of reproduction. In some species with high fecundity, alternating years of breeding may reduce reproductive complications.

Oviductal Disorders

Salpingitis and pyosalpinx

Clinical significance and known etiological cause(s). Dystocia, especially chronic egg retention, often results in inflammatory changes in the oviduct, with secondary bacterial involvement and subsequent salpingitis (Fig. 80.40A).[133] Yolk coelomitis, dystocia, and ectopic ova can all be inflammatory disorders that predispose to opportunistic bacterial salpingitis. Actively breeding females may develop cloacitis associated with copulation and develop an ascending bacterial salpingitis. This often occurs in snakes bred on unsanitary particulate substrates.[127] Venereal transmission of bacteria (and other infectious agents) to females by male snakes with hemipenal abscesses and/or scent gland adenitis is possible.

Clinical presentation and diagnostic confirmation. See clinical presentation for Dystocia, Oviduct Prolapse, and Oviductal Rupture and Ectopic Eggs. Ultrasonography can be useful, and the oviduct(s) may be thickened with increased echogenicity, with evidence of accumulated fluid or flocculent debris. Ultrasound-guided aspiration of fluid within the oviduct is often consistent with inflammation and proteinaceous debris. Sampling often results in the identification of gram-negative bacteria by culture and cytology of gram-stained slides. Radiography is often unrewarding unless there is mineralization or bacterial gas production within the oviducts. With CT/MRI especially, postcontrast studies may demonstrate increased size and volume of the oviducts and increased blood flow due to inflammation.

Coelioscopy can help directly visualize the serosal surfaces of the oviduct and detect gross enlargement, fluid accumulation, and abnormal soft tissue masses; however, salpingoscopy can provide access to the luminal surfaces via cloacoscopy using saline infusion. Careful evaluation of the oviductal mucosa and collection of biopsies for diagnostic evaluation are possible (see Chapters 64 and 65 for more details). Exploratory coeliotomy is more invasive but can confirm a diagnosis, provide the most thorough coelomic evaluation, and allow therapeutic procedures.

Preferred treatment(s), prognosis, and prevention. In nonbreeding reptiles, surgical sterilization (ovariosalpingectomy) is the best resolution (see Fig. 80.40B). In breeding reptiles, if conditions are unilateral, a unilateral ovariosalpingectomy can be performed. In these cases, microbiology and histopathology should direct additional therapeutics. In mild cases or cases where future reproduction is critical and diagnostic evaluation has indicated that treatment may be effective, antiinflammatories and appropriate antimicrobial therapy may be initiated based

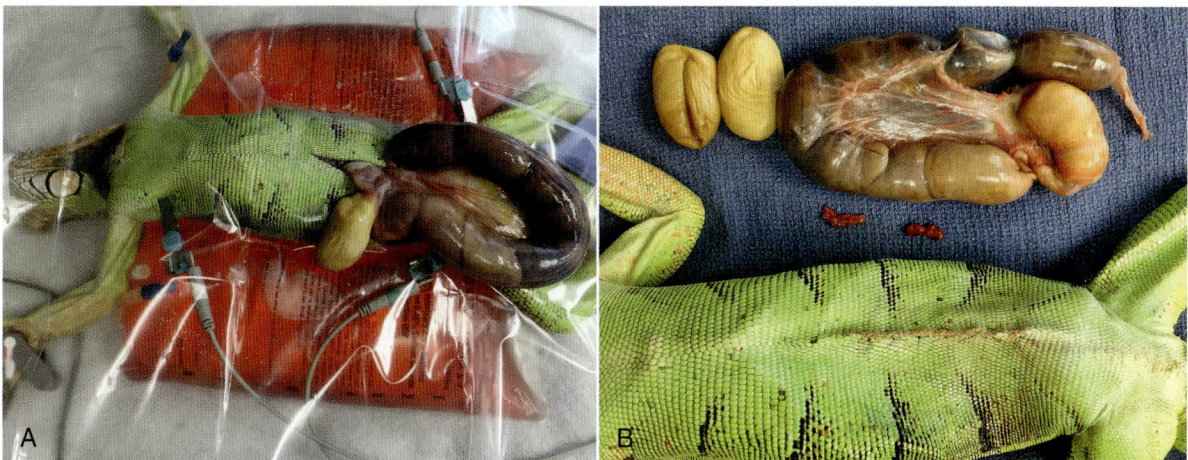

FIG 80.40 Exploratory coeliotomy performed on a green iguana (*Iguana iguana*) with a history of chronic dystocia (after laying a partial clutch of eggs weeks earlier). (A) At surgery one oviduct was filled with necrotic ova with an associated salpingitis. (B) The same iguana recovering after surgery with the affected oviduct, two ectopic eggs, and both ovaries removed. Note the small size of the postovulatory ovaries (between the iguana and the oviduct in the figure). (Courtesy of Scott J. Stahl, Stahl Exotic Animal Veterinary Services.)

on culture and sensitivity and histopathology.[133] Contrary to dogs and cats, there appears to be little to no information on the medical treatment of salpingitis/pyosalpinx in reptiles; however, if surgery is not possible, endoscopic oviductal lavage and progestogen therapy could be considered.[134]

The prognosis after ovariosalpingectomy is generally guarded to good, but dependent on the extent and severity of the condition. Preventative ovariosalpingectomy will help avoid future disease. Furthermore, salpingitis has not been reported in ovariectomized reptiles, where healthy oviducts were left in situ.

Oviductal rupture and ectopic eggs

Clinical significance and known etiological cause(s). Ectopic eggs usually occur with complications of dystocia involving rupture of the oviduct, releasing eggs into the coelom, and possible associated oviduct prolapse. The condition can be iatrogenic with owners attempting to manipulate retained oviductal eggs and/or damaging the oviduct with inappropriate use of oxytocin for obstructive dystocia.[127,131,135]

Chelonians may present with an ectopic egg(s) in the bladder; initially the egg is passed normally into the cloaca before being retropulsed into the bladder and retained.[37,132] Ectopic eggs often result in an inflammatory response in the coelom (or bladder), often with secondary infection and sepsis. Ectopic eggs in the coelom and bladder can contribute to retention of other eggs still present in the reproductive tract. See discussions on Dystocia and Oviductal Prolapse for more information on these conditions.

Clinical presentation and diagnostic confirmation. The clinical presentation, diagnostic testing, and confirmation are similar to those for the Dystocia discussion and should be reviewed for more detail.

Imaging is useful in diagnosing these conditions. Radiography can identify retained shelled or mineralized eggs or fetuses, but it may be difficult to determine whether they are within the oviduct or free in the coelom. Ectopic eggs in the bladder are not uncommon in chelonians and may have an abnormal shape, with irregularly thickened shells and a lamellar appearance due to uric acid and mineral deposition (Fig. 80.41).[108,132] Ultrasonography can also detect ectopic eggs/fetuses and the prescence of free anechoic fluid in the coelom. Echogenic free-floating debris indicates degenerative changes associated with the inflammatory response to ectopic eggs.[108,111,112] Ultrasound-guided aspiration of free

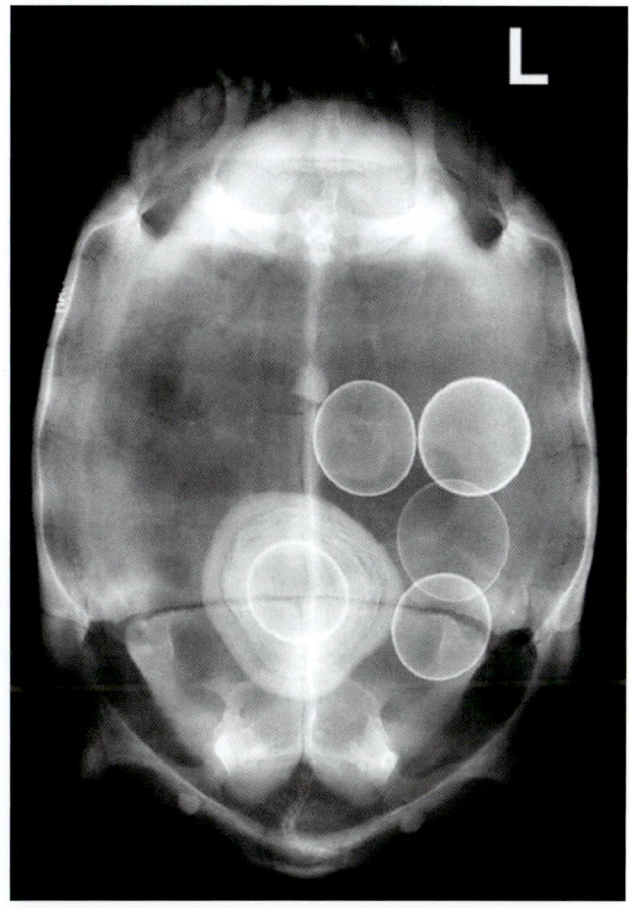

FIG 80.41 A radiograph of a tortoise that was presented for chronic dystocia. Numerous eggs are retained and one egg is ectopic in the bladder (center) and is easily identified with its irregular shape and lamellar appearance from uric acid and mineral deposition. The other retained eggs have abnormally thickened shells from chronic retention. (Courtesy of Stephen J. Divers.)

coelomic fluid often yields flocculent material, which on cytology is consistent with inflammation. Other advanced imaging modalities can be utilized when necessary and available (see CT and MRI in Dystocia section). However, with most imaging modalities it can still be challenging, due to the thin bladder wall, to differentiate between eggs in the bladder and any free in the coelom.

Coelioscopy may be used to confirm these conditions, but complications associated with free fluid, and possible adhesions, make endoscopy more challenging and coeliotomy is often preferred. Exploratory coeliotomy facilitates confirmation of diagnosis, thorough coelomic evaluation, and therapeutic/surgical resolution.

Preferred treatment(s). Coeliotomy and surgical removal of ectopic eggs is required. The coelom and especially the reproductive tract are thoroughly evaluated but it it not always possible to find the oviductal injury (which may have healed before diagnosis). Any ectopic eggs must be removed, and the coelom copiously lavaged before closure. If the oviducts are healthy, a bilateral ovariectomy is performed to eliminate reoccurrence. If there is any doubt regarding the status of the oviducts, then complete ovariosalpingectomy should be performed. In valuable breeding reptiles, surgical repair of the damaged salpinx can be undertaken using fine absorbable suture or, if the damage/disease is extensive, a unilateral ovariectomy and salpingectomy can be performed (see Chapter 105). Any damaged/abnormal reproductive tissue removed should be submitted for microbiologic analysis and histopathology to guide additional therapy. Aggressive postoperative support, antiinflammatories, and analgesics are initiated. Antimicrobials may be required and should be directed by sensitivity testing.

Prognosis and prevention. For simple ectopic eggs without evidence of coelomitis, surgical removal is typically curative. Lizards generally have a better prognosis than chelonians, likely due to easier access to the coelom and earlier detection.[37,126] In severe cases or chronic cases where the patient is presented in a debilitated state, the prognosis is guarded to poor. Ovariectomy or ovariosalpingectomy performed at the same time as egg removal prevents recurrence in pet or display animals. For breeding reptiles, providing optimal nutrition and husbandry practices is important to reduce reproductive complications. Prebreeding health evaluation of females may be valuable to ensure they are sound before the stress of reproduction. In some reptile species with high fecundity, alternating years of breeding may reduce reproductive complications. Veterinarians should educate snake clients not to attempt to manipulate eggs in cases of dystocia. Oxytocin should not be used for obstructive or chronic dystocias, and chelonians that appear to have nonobstructive dystocias but do not respond to oxytocin should be evaluated for possible ectopic eggs.[37,132]

Oviductal prolapse

Clinical significance and known etiological cause(s). Oviductal prolapse usually occurs as a result of dystocia and is primarily seen in oviparous reptiles.[125,127,131] Snakes are overrepresented with this condition, as oviduct damage and prolapse is a common sequela to breeders attempting to "manipulate" retained eggs out through the cloaca. Additionally, the inappropriate use of oxytocin in cases of obstructive dystocias or in squamates with chronic dystocia (see Medical Management in Dystocia) may result in oviduct torsion, rupture, and prolapse.[127,131,135] Other specific reproductive-related issues, including salpingitis, oviduct rupture/tear, abnormal shaped or sized ova, ectopic ova, and follicular stasis can lead to prolapse. Concurrent underlying metabolic disorders and diseases at the time of reproductive activity that may also predispose to oviductal prolapse include hypocalcemia (lizards and chelonians), dehydration, systemic or obstetrical infections (parasitic, mycotic, bacterial, or viral), uroliths/obstipation, and neoplasia.

Clinical presentation and diagnostic confirmation. Owners are frequently alarmed by an oviductal prolapse, and reptiles are often presented on emergency. An oviductal prolapse is a life-threatening concern and requires aggressive support and therapy. Snake owners may have attempted to manipulate retained eggs, resulting in iatrogenic damage and prolapse. Owners or referring clinicians may have attempted inappropriate oxytocin use in obstructive or chronic cases. Any history of reproductive activity, in conjunction with the physical appearance of the exposed organ, is confirmatory. If presented acutely the organ may be engorged, hemorrhagic, or discolored (Fig. 80.42A), but in more chronic cases it is often dark, necrotic, or even desiccated. Often the eggs are still retained within the prolapsed tissue (see Fig. 80.42B). A prolapsed oviduct appears as a linear soft tissue structure, often with a concertina appearance, and must be differentiated from other possible tissues including cloaca, colon, or bladder (see Chapter 75 for details on determining the origin of prolapsed cloacal tissue). Survey radiography is useful to determine whether more eggs are retained or whether other contributory issues may exist (e.g., cystic calculi). Hematology and biochemistry are useful to evaluate the patient before surgical intervention and assess for underlying conditions such as sepsis.

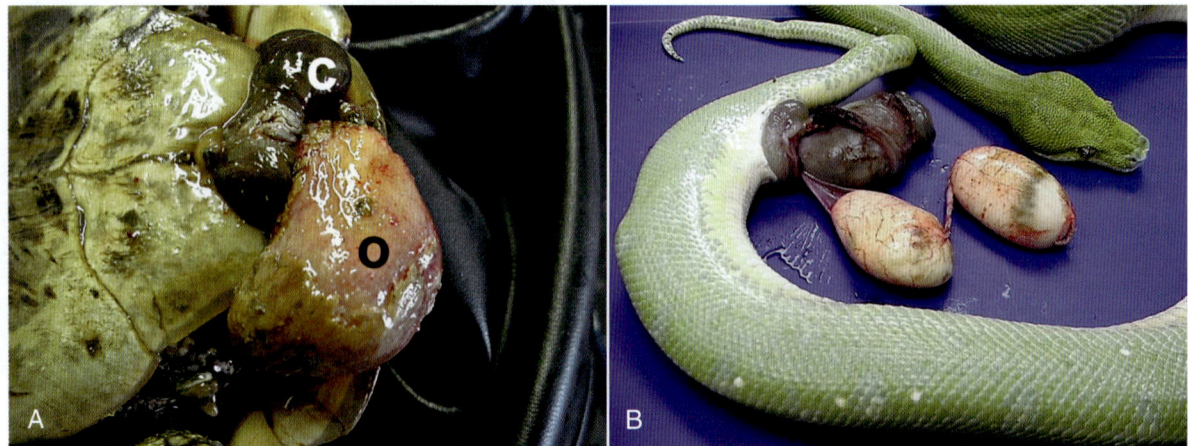

FIG 80.42 (A) A prolapsed oviduct (O) and cloaca (C) in a Greek tortoise (*Testudo graeca*). (Courtesy of Stephen J. Divers). (B) A green tree python (*Morelia viridis*) that presented with oviductal prolapse. Two eggs are still evident in the oviduct, and the cloaca and a portion of the colon are also prolapsed. The prolapse occurred after overzealous attempts by the owner to "manipulate" eggs out of the female. Humane euthanasia was performed in this case. (Courtesy of Scott J. Stahl, Stahl Exotic Animal Veterinary Services.)

Preferred treatment(s), prognosis, and prevention. Initially evaluating the prolapsed oviduct to assess the extent of the damage, determining the underlying reasons for the prolapse, and understanding the goals of the owner must all be considered when developing a therapeutic plan. Often at presentation the prolapsed oviduct has extensive damage, with desiccation and necrosis evident, and the ability to repair or replace the organ is not possible and amputation/removal is necessary (Fig. 80.43A and B). Where breeding is not important, amputation of the prolapsed oviduct followed by coeliotomy and ovariosalpingectomy is the best resolution. For breeding reptiles, attempting to repair and replace the oviduct may be considered if the tissue appears viable. Only acute, mild, partial oviductal prolapses can potentially be replaced per cloaca. The fragile externalized tissue must be kept moist, clean, and protected before being gently inverted and replaced; it cannot simply be pushed back into the cloaca. Inversion of tissue is best accomplished by placing a relatively large diameter blunt instrument through the exteriorized opening and carefully working the tissue back through the cloaca. Endoscopic assistance may be of value to assess replacement, but coeliotomy may be required for full evaluation and ensure proper replacement. However, even with fresh viable oviductal prolapses, rarely can the oviduct be reduced and replaced without concerns for adhesions, fibrosis, and reoccurrence. Often the prolapsed tissue is amputated at the cloaca and exploratory coeliotomy utilized to identify the remaining damaged oviduct internally. In most cases involving pet or display reptiles, in the likely event that the damaged oviduct cannot be repaired, a ovariosalpingectomy is performed. In important breeders, unilateral ovariosalpingectomy, leaving the undamaged ovary and oviduct intact, will maintain some breeding potential. See Chapters 105 and 106 for details on surgical techniques.

The prognosis after oviductal prolapse is poor to guarded but can be improved with early presentation and immediate surgical manipulation. Long-term survival improves after complete ovariosalpingectomy. Future reproductive potential of the affected oviduct is poor. If the oviductal prolapse is bilateral, future reproductive ability is lost and sterilization for survival is necessary. Veterinarians should educate clients not to attempt to manipulate eggs from dystocic females and ensure that oxytocin is used appropriately.

Dystocia

Clinical significance and known etiological cause(s). Dystocia is the inability to successfully expel term eggs or fetuses from the lower reproductive tract. The reasons for dystocia are poorly understood in reptiles but may include abnormal (especially large or fused) eggs/fetuses, failure of the distal reproductive tract to contract (especially metabolic causes), lack of suitable nesting/birthing sites, and lack of viable embryos. Dystocia has been rarely reported in wild reptiles.[136–138] This may be related to the inability to routinely detect dystocia before death in a wild reptile, however the lack of reports of dystocia in reproductive studies of wild reptiles suggests it is uncommon. Unlike conditions in the natural setting, dystocia is relatively common in captive reptiles and complications with laying or birthing are common. Additionally, like avian species, follicular activity and ovulation can occur without male presence/copulation in some species, often resulting in the production of infertile ova in solitary females. Dystocia in squamates and chelonians involving these infertile ova is common.

Dystocia is seen more commonly in oviparous reptiles than in viviparous species, but this could be related to captive population demographics. Dystocia is usually a seasonal problem because hormonal cycles, and thus breeding of temperate species (especially those exposed to seasonal changes), occur at specific times of the year. However, in captivity, environmental control may result in reproductive activity at any time of the year. The causes for dystocia in captive reptiles are often multifactorial and complex, and a definitive cause in many of these cases is not determined. Dystocias are divided into two broad groups: obstructive and nonobstructive.

Obstructive dystocia. An obstructive dystocia is the result of an anatomical barrier that prevents passage of one or more eggs/fetuses through the oviduct and cloaca. The cause may be a fetal or maternal abnormality. Fetal abnormalities include oversize, malformations, and adhesions. Maternal abnormalities include misshapen pelvis, oviductal stricture, or coelomic pathology, including cystic or cloacal calculi, obstipation, organomegaly, abscesses, or neoplasia. In addition, obstructive dystocias may result from complications during oviposition, such as malpositioning of eggs or broken/damaged eggs. Chronicity and salpingitis can result in fibrinous adherence of eggs to the oviduct mucosa.[127]

Nonobstructive dystocias. A large number of dystocias occur with no evidence of obstruction. In these cases, the eggs or fetuses appear to be of normal size and shape and the female appears anatomically normal. These nonobstructive dystocias have been attributed to many etiologies, unfortunately based primarily on association rather than proven causation. Improper nesting sites (common with lizards and chelonians), improper temperature, malnutrition, and dehydration may

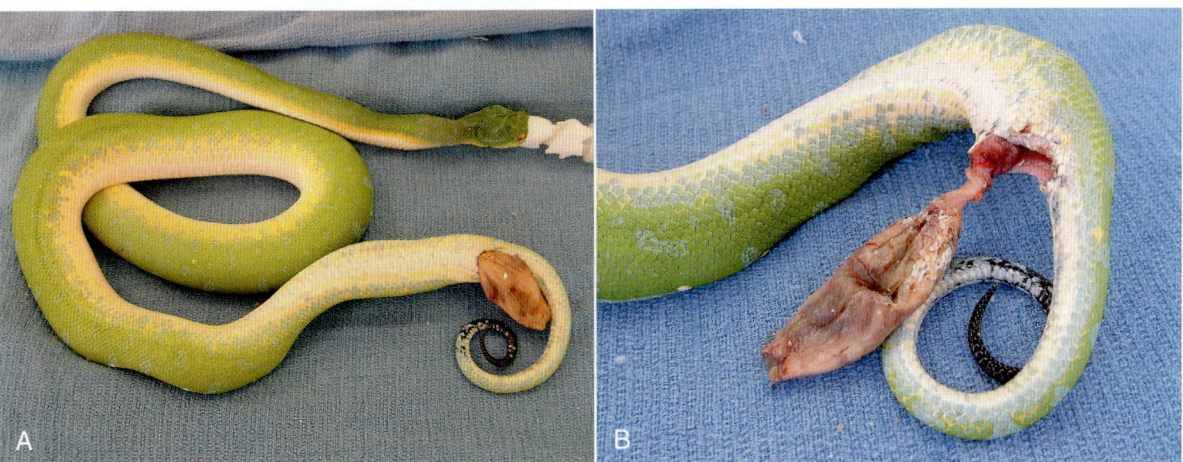

FIG 80.43 (A) A green tree python (*Morelia viridis*) was presented for a prolapse, with a history of recently laying a clutch of eggs, some of the eggs had appeared abnormal. (B) The prolapse tissue was identified as oviduct, coeliotomy was performed to remove the remaining (internal) damaged oviduct, and an ovariectomy performed on the ipsilateral ovary. (Courtesy of Scott J. Stahl, Stahl Exotic Animal Veterinary Services.)

lead to dystocia. Females must be provided with the proper environment during gestation and at oviposition/parturition, and often environmental requirements for gravid females are different than those of nonreproductive conspecifics.[139,140] One of the most common causes of nonobstructive dystocia in lizards and chelonians relates to calcium deficiency. High-energy diets fed in large volume to pet or breeder reptiles result in accelerated growth and early pubescence. However, these diets, usually low in calcium and with inadequate environmental lighting (or vitamin D_3), result in marginal or deficient levels. Hormonal activity ensues and mobilization of calcium for vitellogenesis causes a subclinical condition to become apparent. Depletion of bone calcium leads to orthopedic changes and associated weakness, lameness, anorexia, and dystocia due to poorly mineralized ova or weak contractions at oviposition/birth. Such conditions are most prevalent in herbivorous and insectivorous species where dietary balance is most challenging (see Chapter 84).

Another cause of dystocia may relate to poor physical condition of the female.[127,141] Captive reptiles are extremely sedentary compared with their wild counterparts and often possess poor muscle tone. In addition, some species may reproduce excessively and become exhausted throughout the season. Oviposition requires a substantial muscular effort, and if a female is in poor condition she may fail to complete the task. The predominant presentation in many dystocia cases involving oviparous snakes supports this theory where obese, poorly conditioned females will lay the majority of the clutch without complication but retain the last egg or two without any evidence of an obstruction. Infectious diseases may cause infection with resulting salpingitis, causing egg/fetus retention. The authors have seen several cases of dystocia and fetal death in several species of boa with a confirmed diagnosis of boid reptarenavirus.[127]

Although challenging and not always possible, it is important to attempt to determine the cause(s) of dystocia. The information can help define the prognosis for the case and guide prevention or recurrence in this patient and other females in the breeding collection. Regardless of the etiology the authors have found an increased prevalence of dystocia in snakes and lizards that are first-time breeders, have had a previous dystocia, or are carrying a predominantly infertile clutch.

Clinical presentation. Distinguishing a dystocia from a normal reproductive cycle/gravidity can be challenging. Mischaracterization of normal gravidity and inappropriate treatment is common and unnecessary. An example of the complexity of determining a true dystocia versus normal gravidity is evident with chelonians, where individuals may voluntarily retain oviductal eggs for up to 6 months until conditions are ideal for oviposition.[104,106] A clear understanding of the reproductive biology of the species, a thorough history, physical examination, and diagnostic tests may be necessary to ensure appropriate management. Historically, dystocic reptiles may be restless, pacing and climbing, looking for possible nesting sites. Oviparous lizards and chelonians may dig in planters or substrate. Female aquatic turtles may spend extended time out of the water. Appetite and water intake may be reduced or absent. Coelomic distention with reduced body condition and anorexia may be noted. Differential diagnoses for a coelomic mass include fecal masses, cystic calculi, abscesses, and tumors. Tenesmus without successful oviposition or parturition is a clear sign of dystocia. Females that have produced a small clutch or litter may still appear gravid due to retained eggs/fetuses. Alternatively, the breeder's records may indicate that the female is past her due date. Diagnosis of a true dystocia in females that contain the entire clutch can be challenging (Fig. 80.44).

Postovulatory retained eggs are usually palpable in most snakes and many lizards. However, in some oviparous lizards and in viviparous squamates it can be difficult to differentiate between ovarian follicles and oviductal eggs/fetuses. Postovulatory ova (oviductal eggs) in squamates can often be differentiated from follicles because they are less firm, larger, more oblong in shape, and more caudally located in the coelom. Chelonians are more difficult to palpate, but in smaller species digital palpation in the prefemoral area with the patient held vertically and gently tilted side to side may allow shelled eggs to be

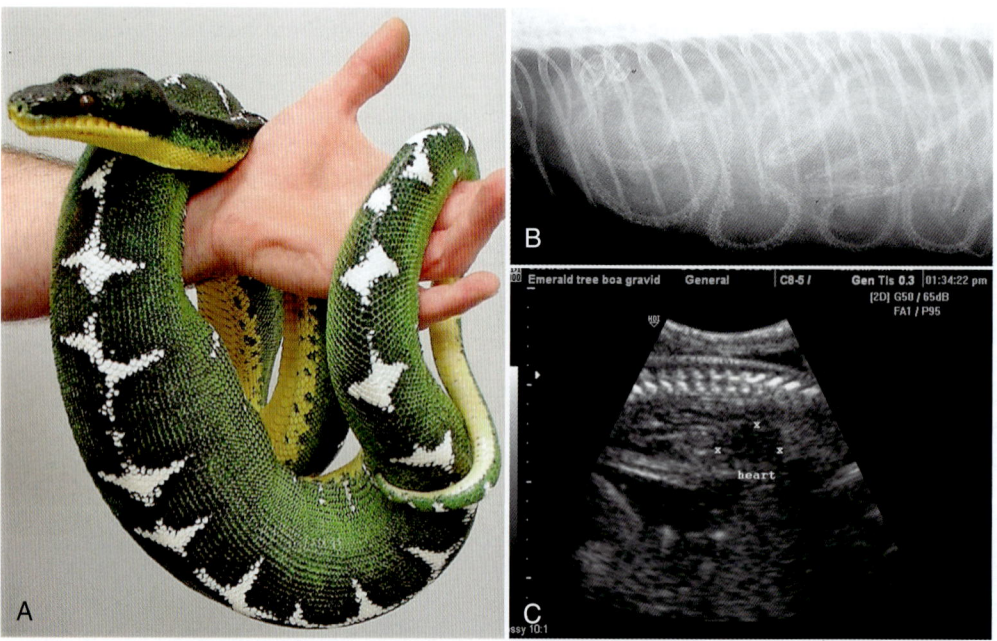

FIG 80.44 (A) A full-term gravid Amazon basin emerald tree boa (*Corallus batesii*) presented for possible dystocia based on the breeder's records. (B) Radiograph showing fetuses in a normal orientation with no indications of an obstructive process or abnormalities. (C) Ultraound showed heartbeats and fetal movement. The owner was concerned about being well past her due date so oxytocin was given and within 1 hour of administration a healthy litter was produced. (Courtesy of Scott J. Stahl, Stahl Exotic Animal Veterinary Services.)

detected (see Fig. 80.24). This technique is not good for determining numbers of retained eggs, and clinicians must be cautious to avoid injury as their fingers can be crushed by a retracting chelonian limb or hinged shell. It is usually not possible to palpate developing fetuses in viviparous squamates and imaging is necessary.

Diagnostic confirmation. Plasma biochemical changes often include elevations of total calcium; however, ionized calcium is often normal. Complete blood count may show a stress leukocytosis or, in cases of inflammatory/infectious change, a leukocytosis with left shift. In more chronic cases anemia and leukopenia may be observed.[106]

Radiography is essential and can help differentiate between follicular stasis (spherical, soft tissue structures) and dystocia (thinly shelled, oblong eggs) in squamates (see Fig. 180.33A–C). Radiographs are important to exclude obstruction (before the use of oxytocin); identify mineralized eggs (considerably less calcified in squamates, compared with chelonians); and confirm egg numbers, shell abnormalities (e.g., thickening, broken), ectopic eggs, and comparative egg-to-pelvic dimensions. Radiography can also identify contributing, and/or concurrent, coelomic pathology, such as cystic calculi, obstipation, or organomegaly (see Fig. 80.41). With viviparous squamates radiography can be useful late in gestation when skeletal structures become visible (see Fig. 80.44B). Typically, viable fetuses are coiled, whereas an uncoiled or linear appearance likely indicates fetal death and the need for surgical intervention (Fig. 80.45A and B).[127] Radiography may also help to identify abnormalities associated with nutritional or renal secondary hyperparathyroidism, with derangements in calcium homeostasis likely contributing to the dystocia.

Ultrasonography can be useful to differentiate between follicular stasis and postovulatory eggs. Sonographically, postovulatory eggs exhibit hyperechoic mineralized outer shells, and, in squamates, a more oblong appearance. A small amount of anechoic fluid may be visualized around and between eggs. With dystocia and salpingitis the normally smooth wall of the egg may become irregular, with a notable change in heterogenous echogenicity and an increase in both oviductal and coelomic free fluid.[108,112] In these situations normal laying/birth is unlikely, and medical or surgical management is needed. Late in gestation, ultrasonography is valuable in viviparous squamates to determine whether fetuses are alive, as they may be seen moving with an obvious heartbeat (see Fig. 80.25A and B). The loss of these indicators can also be helpful to differentiate a true dystocia from normal gravidity.

Compared with radiography, CT allows individual egg evaluation and can demonstrate indicators of dystocia such as distinct horizontal leveling of egg contents and oviductal gas accumulation (see Fig. 80.34A and B).[108] Thus, CT can be clinically useful to determine when

intervention is necessary, especially in chelonians that can electively retain eggs for extended periods.

Preferred treatment(s). Dystocia is rarely, the acute emergency that it is in mammals and birds. If the reptile is a pet or display animal then surgical removal of the reproductive tract (as soon as safely possible) is best. If maintaining breeding ability is important then the least invasive intervention required to resolve the issue while maintaining future reproduction is the goal. Often the procedures can be performed in a step-by-step fashion starting with the least invasive and safest procedures and proceeding to more invasive and/or surgery. In chronic or complicated cases, surgery may be preferable.

If a possible dystocia situation is suspected (versus normal gravidity) but the female appears healthy, a nest box and (depending on species, dietary history, radiographic, and clinicopathologic results) oral calcium therapy can be provided. These cases must be monitored closely and may need reappraisal within a few days to 1 to 2 weeks if no action occurs or sooner if tenesmus or deterioration becomes evident.

For dystocia cases where the patient is not considered healthy, medical stabilization should be prioritized, followed by additional medical therapy as indicated (e.g. calcium, nonsteroidal antiinflammatories, opiate analgesics, antimicrobials).

Medical management. Although studies have indicated that laying/birthing appear to be controlled by arginine vasotocin, it is rarely available, and oxytocin is used in cases of nonobstructive dystocia.[142] Inappropriate use of oxytocin may result in egg fracture, oviduct rupture, eggs forced into the bladder, or severe hemorrhage. This drug should only be used in individuals with a confirmed nonobstructive dystocia. Oxytocin is most effective if some portion of the eggs have been recently laid, attempts at oviposition are occurring, or obvious nesting behavior is ongoing. Because temperature influences the effect of oxytocin on oviductal muscles,[143] patients should be maintained at or near their optimal body temperature during treatment.

In squamates there is a small window of efficacy, usually within 48 to 72 hours of normal laying. Chronically retained eggs often develop a fibrinous adherence to the oviduct and oxytocin may be ineffective or result in oviduct torsion and damage (Fig. 80.46A, B).[127,130,135] Viviparous snakes may have a longer window of effectiveness, up to a week after a partial birthing.[144]

Chelonians are more responsive to oxytocin, even in more chronic cases of dystocia (Fig. 80.47). This may be related to their ability to electively retain eggs for extended periods of time from 9 days to 4 to 6 months depending on the species.[37,104] Oxytocin dosing differs considerably with chelonians responding well to lower doses (1–4 IU/kg)

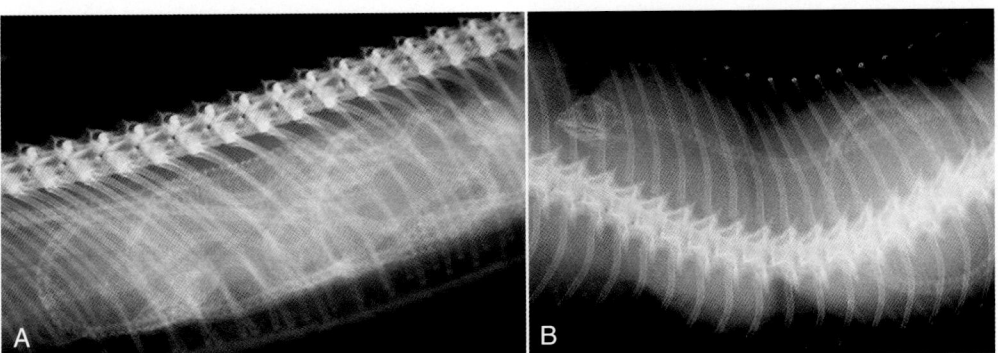

FIG 80.45 (A and B) With viviparous squamates radiography can be useful late in gestation when skeletal structures become visible. Typically, viable fetuses are coiled (see Fig. 80.44B), when fetuses are uncoiled or have an obvious linear appearance, as in these radiographs of a Boa constrictor (*Boa constrictor* spp.), it is usually an indication of fetal death and the need for surgical intervention. (Courtesy of Scott J. Stahl, Stahl Exotic Animal Veterinary Services.)

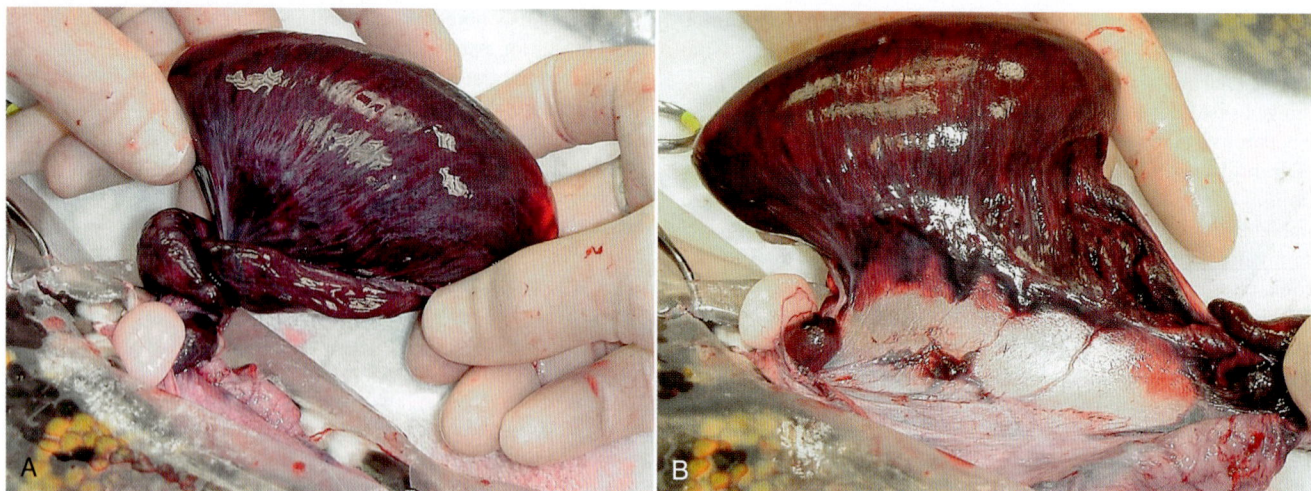

FIG 80.46 (A) A reticulated python (*Malayopython reticulatus*) presented for dystocia of several weeks. Oxytocin had been given (inappropriately based on chronicity) and upon referral, surgery identified an oviductal torsion. (B) Resolution of the oviduct torsion at surgery, note the severe inflammatory changes and poor color. Due to the extent of the damage a unilateral ovariosalpingectomy was performed. (Courtesy of Scott J. Stahl, Stahl Exotic Animal Veterinary Services.)

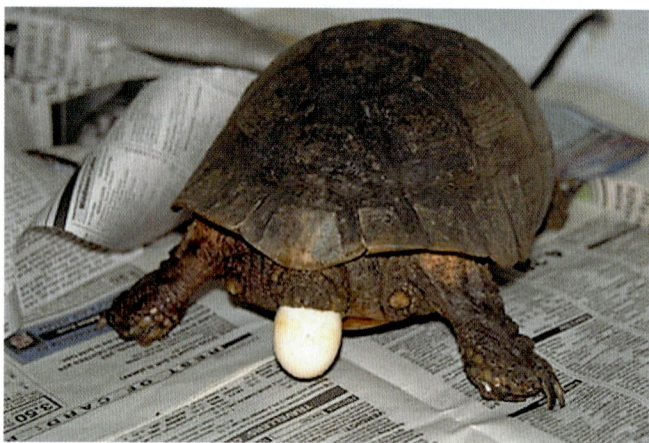

FIG 80.47 A spur-thighed tortoise (*Testudo graeca*) laying an egg in response to treatment with oxytocin. Radiographs had ruled out an obstructive dystocia and supportive medical treatment (fluid and thermal therapy) initiated followed by oxytocin resulting in oviposition. Chelonians often do not attempt to dig/nest when given oxytocin, so eggs (if fertile) should be protected from damage by the female after being laid. (Courtesy of Scott J. Stahl, Stahl Exotic Animal Veterinary Services.)

compared with higher doses necessary for squamates (10–20 IU/kg). Oxytocin administration should be slow and can be given intravenously or diluted in saline and given subcutaneously (SQ).[130] A nest box or nesting material should be offered after oxytocin treatment, however often eggs are expelled without nesting behavior. Dosing can be repeated and the dose increased (start at lower dose initially) every 6 to 12 hours; however, after 2 to 3 doses with no response oxytocin will likely not be effective.

Oxytocin causes elevations in prostaglandins and likely plays a role in lysis of the corpora lutea and is important in the physiology of laying/birthing.[145,146] Therefore, administration of prostaglandins F2a (injection) and E (gel administered per cloaca) may be helpful in augmenting the oxytocin response. Prostaglandin F2 alpha (1.5 mg/kg) administered SQ was used in combination with oxytocin (7.5 IU/kg) and found to be effective in inducing oviposition in red-eared sliders.[147] Additionally, topical use of prostaglandin E gel via cloaca in conjunction with oxytocin has been successfully used in many chelonian species.[132]

Beta-blockers may potentiate the effects of oxytocin, and atenolol has been used in conjunction with oxytocin successfully in many chelonian species for dystocia. McArthur recommends giving atenolol (7 mg/kg PO, in the evening) approximately 12 hours before giving oxytocin at 1 to 3 IU/kg SQ the following morning, repeating the dosing of the same drugs in the same pattern until all eggs pass.[148]

In cases of absolute or relative hypocalcemia, calcium can be given before oxytocin dosing, and NSAIDS may be indicated for inflammation and analgesia. In chelonians where eggs have been chronically retained and/or there is a suspicion of salpingitis, NSAIDS and antimicrobials may be indicated, especially when surgery is not an option.[130]

External egg manipulation. Due to the linear anatomy of snakes, egg manipulation may be possible and is noninvasive.[127] General anesthesia is required to determine whether retained eggs are adhered to the oviduct or can be gently manipulated toward the cloaca. If the first egg moves freely toward the vent, a vaginal speculum can be used to dilate the cloaca and allow visualization of the egg at the oviduct opening. Sometimes it can be gently grasped and removed with forceps, or ovocentesis, using a large-gauge needle (14–18 G), may be necessary to reduce size. The collapsed egg can then be removed with forceps or hemostats, and the procedure repeated for the remaining eggs (Fig. 80.48A–D). This procedure is only recommended in lizards and chelonians if the egg is visible within the cloaca. In these cases, however, the egg often breaks, requiring piece-meal removal of shell fragments.

Cloacoscopy. Cloacoscopy may be utilized to manipulate retained eggs/fetuses out of the cloaca if medical and/or less-invasive techniques have failed or are not appropriate.[127,130] This procedure can be useful in snakes and chelonians, less so in lizards, and is best utilized when only one or a few ova or fetuses are retained. General anesthesia is required, and standard rigid endoscopy equipment (2.7-mm rigid endoscope with 4.8-mm working sheath system) and warm saline infusion is utilized. The openings into the oviducts are located dorsolateral in the urodeum. In some cases, the oviduct(s) may be entered and eggs/fetuses identified. Gentle manipulation of the egg/fetus with the endoscope and/or grasping forceps, along with the infusion of warm saline, may allow all or portions of the egg/fetus to be removed. However, in some cases endoscopic entry into the oviduct is not possible, as the

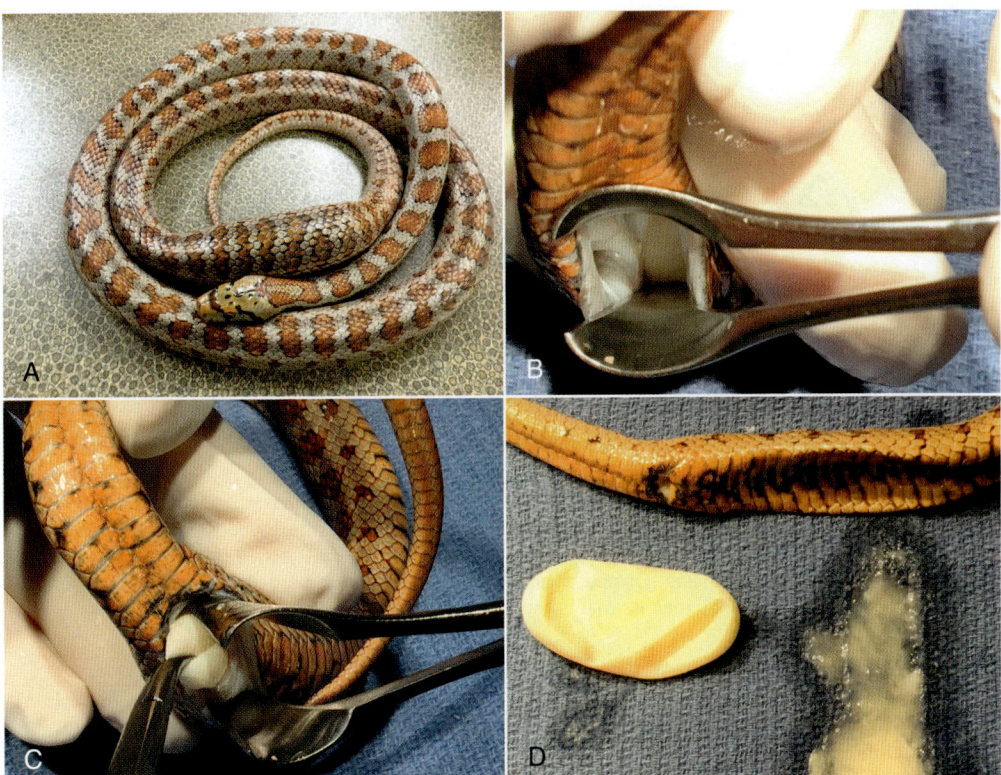

FIG 80.48 (A) A female leopard rat snake (*Zamenis situla*) was presented for a retained egg after laying the majority of her clutch several days earlier. (B) Under general anesthesia the egg was manipulated toward her cloaca, and a vaginal speculum was used to dilate the cloaca allowing visualization of the egg at the opening of the right oviduct. Note the empty left oviduct opening is dilated and open. (C and D) The egg was gently grasped with hemostats and removed; some egg contents were released on removal, deflating the egg. (Courtesy of Scott J. Stahl, Stahl Exotic Animal Veterinary Services.)

oviduct opening is tightly closed. Sometimes entry into the oviduct is possible but adhesions are present and cannot be safely broken down. If there is severe inflammation or infection of the oviduct and/or degenerative eggs/fetuses are present, then treatment with antimicrobials and NSAIDS for 14 to 21 days may be required to manage the active salpingitis before repeating endoscopy.[127,130] See Section 8 for more details on cloacoscopy.

Percutaneous ovocentesis. Percutaneous ovocentesis is a technique that can be considered in snakes. This technique has risks (possible leakage of egg contents into the coelom or iatrogenic needle trauma) and should be utilized only if other options are not feasible. Deep sedation to general anesthesia is recommended. The egg is isolated against the lateral body wall and the area aseptically prepared. The use of sonographic guidance is recommended. A 16- to 20-gauge needle (depending on the size of the patient) is inserted between the first and second row of lateral scales and into the egg (Fig. 80.49). The contents of the egg are aspirated using caution to avoid leakage of egg material into the coelom. After collapse, the snake will usually pass the egg within 12 to 24 hours of aspiration. Eggs cranial to the collapsed egg may pass on their own after the first egg passes or may also need aspiration. Postoperative analgesics such as NSAIDs are recommended. Antimicrobials are unlikely to prevent coelomitis if leakage occurs, but coverage using a first-line drug can be considered. Eggs retained more than several weeks are not likely to aspirate as the contents solidify, and surgical removal is required.[127]

Surgery. Surgical management by ovariosalpingectomy offers a permanent solution for resolving dystocia in chelonians and lizards (Fig. 80.50A and B). Where future reproduction is important, salpingotomy can be attempted if less-invasive methods have failed. Coeliotomy and salpingotomy often provides the best evaluation of the reproductive

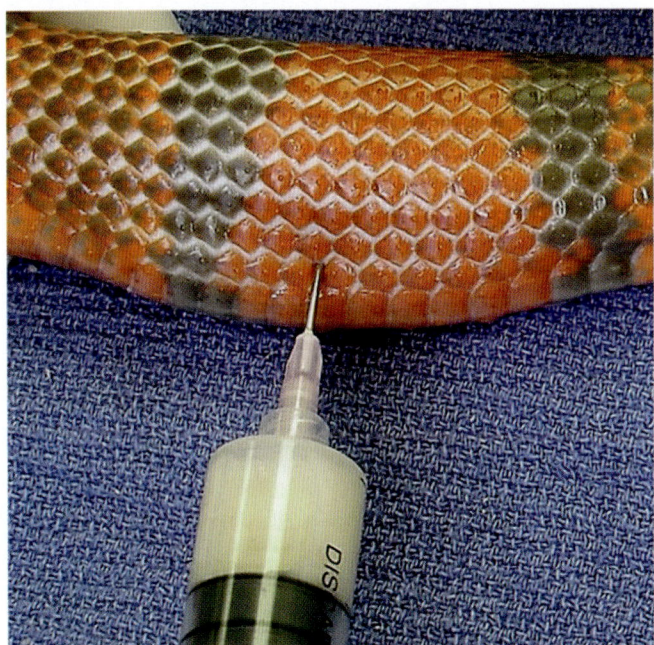

FIG 80.49 A Honduran milk snake (*Lampropeltis triangulum hondurensis*) with a retained egg. Under anesthesia the retained egg would not move caudally to the cloaca. Due to economic constraints not allowing coeliotomy, a percutaneous aspiration of the egg was performed. The aspiration site was surgically prepped, and a 20-g needle introduced between the lateral scale rows and directly into the egg. The contents were aspirated to collapse the egg and assist passage. (Courtesy of Scott J. Stahl, Stahl Exotic Animal Veterinary Services.)

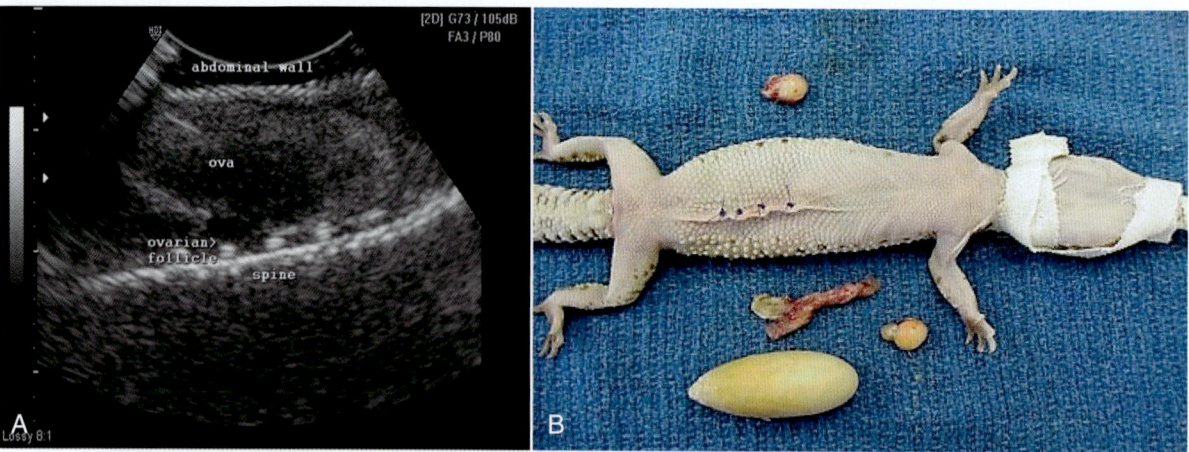

FIG 80.50 (A) Sonograph of a female leopard gecko (*Eublepharis macularius*) with dystocia. Note calcified elongated oviductal egg with hyperechoic shell (labeled: ova), also a small round ovarian follicle can be noted dorsal to the egg. (B) The same leopard gecko recovering from surgery after ovariosalpingectomy. Note abnormal changes to the chronically retained egg and inflamed oviduct. The inactive ovaries were removed to prevent future reproductive issues. Compare with Fig. 80.38 of a leopard gecko with follicular stasis. (Courtesy of Scott J. Stahl, Stahl Exotic Animal Veterinary Services.)

tract to allow a more informed therapeutic decision and improve the chances of future reproduction. If significant oviductal pathology is identified, a unilateral ovariosalpingectomy can be performed. See Chapter 105, for details on performing these procedures.

Prognosis and prevention. Prognosis and outcome are favorable for dystocia cases with early diagnosis and intervention. Chronic cases are more likely to have associated pathology and may require more invasive surgical intervention. Successful reproduction 1 year after a surgical correction of a dystocia has been reported,[149–150] but minimally a 1-year nonbreeding rest period is recommended. Dystocia involving prolapse of the oviduct(s) and/or cloaca is a more serious condition (see Oviductal Prolapse). The prognosis may be good for survival but poor for continued reproductive performance.

Although countless numbers of retained (and often fertile) eggs have been removed from reptiles, successful incubation of these removed eggs is rare. However, eggs passed after oxytocin induction are often successfully incubated.[151] The removal of viable fetuses during salpingotomy in snakes has been reported.[152]

Preventative ovariectomy should be considered for lizards and chelonians (see Chapter 105). Providing an appropriate environment and nesting site (ovipositoria) based on a good understanding of the natural history of the species is important to reduce the incidence of dystocia (see Nesting Sites/Ovipositoria/ in the Captive Breeding section). Since calcium plays an important role in successful reproduction and may contribute to issues with dystocia the diet of reproductively active reptiles should be reviewed to ensure adequate levels of calcium and vitamin D₃ (see Chapter 27).

For breeding reptiles, dystocias are often thought to be related to overconditioning and small cage size (reduced activity). Breeders and veterinarians should address these issues when evaluating dietary strategy and housing in the reptile breeding facility. Veterinarians working with squamate breeders should explain the limited time window for the use of oxytocin and encourage females be presented urgently if complications are suspected.

Reptiles that have presented for dystocia (notably snakes) may be more likely to present with dystocia in the future. Correcting associated husbandry issues or not actively breeding an affected female may be important to prevent recurrence. It is recommended that reptiles that have had eggs/fetuses removed from the oviduct should not be bred

the next season but given a rest period of at least 1 year before breeding again.

Scent Gland Adenitis (Snakes)

Clinical Significance and Known Etiological Cause(s). Cloacal scent gland adenitis has been reported in snakes and is not an uncommon presentation.[128] Clinically, scent gland adenitis appears to be more common in older female colubrids, and actively breeding snakes.[128] Causes include impaction of the gland, infection of the gland, and neoplastic changes. A recent review of six cases of cloacal scent gland impaction in snakes at several zoological collections included four colubrids, one viper, and one boid (Couture et al, Proc ARAV, 2017 p 352). The colubrids were all greater than 20 years old, all had bilateral involvement, and three of four were females. Three of four colubrids also had bacterial adenitis, one had mineralization of the affected gland, and one, a Taiwan beauty snake (*Orthriophis taeniura freese*) had a fibrosarcoma associated with one of its bilaterally affected glands. Increased frequency of scent gland adenitis in older snakes may be related to reduced general activity, and/or reduced muscular ability in the lower body. Without release the impacted scent material becomes thick and inspissated and the gland becomes secondarily infected, swollen, hard, and may rupture. If impaction is bilateral it may indicate functional issues associated with an inability or difficulty in the release of material. Captive-related environmental factors affecting glandular release include humidity, substrate (paper or carpeting versus a natural substrate), and presence or absence of conspecifics. Bacterial infection of the scent gland is a common cause of adenitis.[128] The opening of the scent gland is located at the caudal margin of the cloaca, near passing fecal and urate material that may predispose to infection. This is exacerbated if snakes are housed under poor sanitary conditions. The authors have found an increased incidence of scent gland adenitis associated with captive breeding in snakes.[128] Cloacitis in females and cloacitis and/or hemipenis infections in males are common during courtship and breeding, especially if housed on soiled particulate substrates, and can predispose to scent gland adenitis. Neoplasia should be considered with scent gland adenitis, especially in older snakes that present with unilateral involvement. One author (SJS) has seen several cases of neoplasia associated with scent glands, and a fibrosarcoma was associated with a scent gland adenitis in a colubrid (Couture et al, Proc ARAV, 2017, p 352).

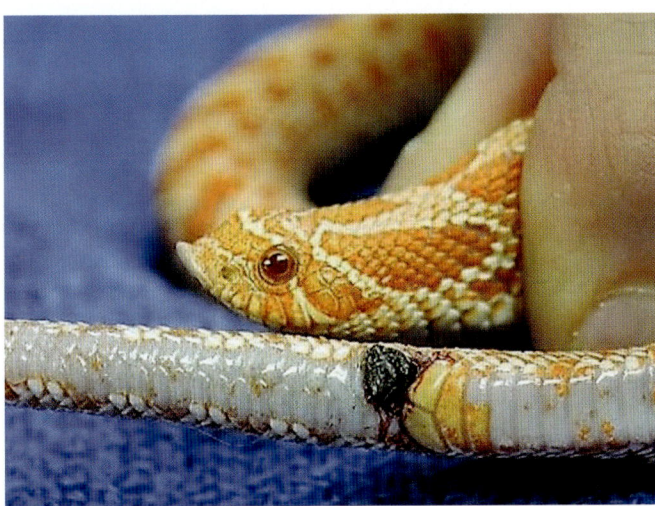

FIG 80.51 An albino male western hognose snake (*Heterodon nasicus*) with an abcessed and ulcerated scent gland. (Courtesy of Scott J. Stahl, Stahl Exotic Animal Veterinary Services.)

Clinical Presentation and Diagnostic Confirmation. Typically, older and/or actively breeding females are overrepresented. Physical examination is often diagnostic, with snakes presenting with unilateral or bilateral swellings caudal and lateral, and in chronic situations craniolateral to the cloaca. In severe cases rupture of the gland may occur (Fig. 80.51). On palpation the gland may be soft to hard depending on duration. Fine needle aspiration and cytology can confirm gland involvement and may indicate neoplasia. Radiography is less useful except to confirm mineralization. Ultrasonography can differentiate between neoplastic tissue and impaction. Biopsy for histopathology and microbiological testing at surgery is often necessary for a definitive diagnosis.

Preferred Treatment(s). In cases of mild impaction gently massaging the gland (after warm water soak) to move material toward the gland opening may allow release. In larger snakes, with sedation and/or local anesthesia, cannulation of the duct opening can be attempted with a urinary catheter or metal lacrimal duct cannula.[128] Unfortunately, with retention, gland material becomes thick, grainy, often inspissated, and cannot pass out of the narrow duct opening, necessitating surgery.

Under general anesthesia, surgery is performed by making an incision between the lateral scale rows over the enlarged gland. The gland is opened, impacted material removed, and biopsies of the gland collected for histopathology and microbiological culture. The gland can then be gently lavaged with saline and a catheter passed normograde through the opening of the duct to ensure patency. If the gland was successfully cannulated it can be closed or marsupialized to allow continued flushing and treatment.[128] Systemic antimicrobials and/or topical antimicrobials may be initiated based on histopathology and microbiological results along with local flushing with antiseptics. Surgical removal of the entire affected gland(s) is often the curative choice in cases that are severe, reoccurring, bilateral, or if neoplasia is suspected/confirmed (Couture et al, Proc ARAV, 2017, p 352).[128]

Surgical removal of the gland, if required, is performed by making an incision between the lateral scale rows over the enlarged gland. Sharp and blunt dissection is used to separate the gland from the associated muscle and connective tissue. When possible, the gland is left intact to minimize contamination of the surgery site and ensure removal of all glandular material. The gland is elevated out of the incision and hemostasis managed with hemoclips or radiosurgery. The duct is then ligated as far cranially as possible where it curves toward the vent opening. The other gland can be removed through the same incision by transecting the midline muscle that separates the left and right glands. Muscle and skin closure are routine. Postoperative analgesics are indicated. A recent review of six cases of cloacal scent gland impactions of snakes in several zoos found that surgical removal of the affected glands was successful (Couture et al, Proc ARAV, 2017, p 352).

Prognosis and Prevention. Prognosis is good with complete surgical removal of the gland(s) and if underlying conditions leading to blockage and/or adenitis are corrected after successful medical treatment. If neoplasia is confirmed, the type of neoplasm determines prognosis. Prevention involves correcting husbandry issues that may be contributing factors. Snakes should be observed closely during breeding to ensure they are kept in sanitary conditions and are not overbred.[128] Owners and keepers should be aware of this possible condition in older snakes and watch for indications of increased material in the cloacal scent glands.

Neoplasia

Clinical Significance. In one report involving 3500 reptile necropsies performed at a zoo over a 100-year span (1901–2002) showed neoplastic incidence to be only 2.3%; however, the study found there was a trending increase in neoplasia in the last 30 years especially in snakes and lizards.[153] In another study 5000 biopsy samples submitted to a specialty pathology service between 1994 to 2002 found a cancer incidence of 9.8% in reptiles, with snakes having the highest incidence of neoplasia (15.0%) followed by lizards (8.5%), chelonians (2.7%), and crocodilians (2.2%).[154] However, in this same study reproductive neoplasms were most commonly found in lizards, except for granulosa cell tumors, which were more common in snakes. No reproductive tumors were found in chelonians or crocodilians.[154] Ovarian adenocarcinomas were the most common reproductive tumors found, with an incidence of 3.7% in lizards and 2.7% in snakes. Ovarian adenocarcinomas had a higher incidence of metastasis in snakes compared with lizards. Granulosa cell tumors were more prevalent in snakes (1.5%) than lizards (0.6%), and the overall incidence of oviduct neoplasia (adenocarcinoma) was low in the study, with lizards having a higher incidence at 1.2% compared with snakes (0.6%).[154] Many individual case reports and reviews have reported ovarian carcinomas, fibromas, hemangiomas, dysgerminomas (red-eared sliders), and teratomas.[153–157] Oviductal neoplasms reported include leiomyosarcomas and leiomyomas.[153–156]

Testicular neoplasms are rare, with seminomas being the most prevalent (1.2% in lizards and 0.6% in snakes).[154] Interstitial cell adenomas, Sertoli and Leydig cell tumors, have also been reported[153–155,158] (see Chapter 78).

Known Etiological Cause(s). No known carcinogens have been determined for reptiles; however, genetic/taxa predispositions were suggested for a group of Egyptian spiny-tailed lizards (*Uromastyx aegyptius*) with a high incidence of lymphoid neoplasia.[159] The authors have seen multiorgan lymphoid neoplasia in snakes involving the reproductive tract. A malignant granulosa cell carcinoma was reported in a green iguana after an incomplete ovariosalpingectomy, suggesting a possible relationship with neoplastic change and an ovarian remnant.[160]

Clinical Presentation and Diagnostic Confirmation. Reproductive neoplasia may mimic changes associated with reproductive activity such as folliculogenesis or testicular recrudescence and must be differentiated from these normal physiological changes. Additionally, presentation may resemble other more common reproductive disorders, including follicular stasis, dystocia, yolk coelomitis, or ectopic eggs. Infertility and low fecundity could also result from reproductive tract neoplasia. Behavioral changes may also be noted if gonadal neoplasia affects sex hormone production.

Physical examination findings may indicate activity or enlargement in the mid to caudal coelom, where reproductive tract activity would occur. Radiography, ultrasonography, and/or advanced imaging including CT and MRI may be useful to identify reproductive tract neoplasia. Ultrasonography was valuable in diagnosing an ovarian teratoma in a green iguana.[157] A 13-year-old spur-thighed tortoise was diagnosed with a testicular seminoma antemortem using ultrasonography and MRI. Comparable MRI imaging changes in the affected tortoise's testis were similar to those seen in testicular seminomas in humans. The diagnosis was confirmed at postmortem and after histopathology.[161] In most cases endoscopy or coeliotomy with biopsy will be necessary to confirm an antemortem diagnosis. If histopathology confirms neoplasia, staging is recommended whenever possible.

Preferred Treatment(s), Prognosis, and Prevention. Oncologic treatments can include surgery, chemotherapy, and radiation, with specific recommendations dependent on a histologic diagnosis and staging. Surgical removal of the reproductive tract may be curative if diagnosed early, especially for benign disease. In cases where surgical removal of the affected reproductive tract is not possible, or metastasis has occurred, oncologic therapy will be aimed at prolonging the patient's quality of life rather than curing the patient (see Chapter 87).

The prognosis is dependent on histopathology and determination of malignancy. Since the reproductive tract can be removed, if a diagnosis is made before metastasis, the prognosis may be favorable. For advanced carcinomas with likely metastasis, the prognosis is poor even with aggressive surgery. Ovariectomy and orchiectomy at a young age may be preventative.

Infertility/Low Fecundity

Clinical Significance. The successful breeding of many species has become common both commercially (pet market and herpetoculture) and in conservation efforts to establish captive colonies of threatened and endangered species. Reptile veterinarians can play an important role in assisting these efforts by providing guidance on production management issues such as infertility and fecundity.[162] Interestingly, this has been an important veterinary service for the livestock and poultry industry for decades. Infertility can be divided into two basic categories: disorders of fertility (absence of egg/fetus production or production of infertile eggs/ova) and disorders of fecundity.[132,163] Infertility is generally defined as the inability to conceive, whereas fecundity measures reproductive performance and is determined by the number of live young produced. Infertility typically is the result of events that occur in either the male or female before conception.

Known Etiological Cause(s). Factors that influence fertility in reptiles include improper reproductive cycling (particularly temperature), an incompatible pair (incorrectly sexed, size mismatch, different species), an under- or overconditioned male or female, stress with excessive or aggressive copulation or copulatory attempts, abnormal (nonfunctional) reproductive anatomy of the male or female, and reproductive disease. External factors that may affect fertility include exposure to extreme temperatures (high or low), use of spermicidal lubricants during hemipenal probing, exposure to environmental toxins such as insecticides or disinfectants, and potentially excessive exposure to radiation (with diagnostic imaging) similar to mammals.[132,163]

Specifically, male infertility may be related to a lack of interest in copulation, inability to succesfully copulate, and a true lack of spermatogenesis.[132] A desert tortoise (*Gopherus agassizii*) diagnosed with a testicular intersticial cell adenoma did not produce viable sperm and was considerd sterile.[158]

Infertility in females is more commonly associated with a lack of appropriate environmental stimuli and/or underlying nutritional deficiencies. Females that commonly produce infertile eggs or (in viviparous species) infertile ova may have underlying nutritional issues or reproductive disease, assuming male issues have been excluded.[37,132]

In disorders of fecundity, conception occurs, but the clutch or litter size is smaller than normal. There may be high numbers of infertile eggs or stillborn young. The same environmental factors that affect fertility can be responsible for damage or death to developing embryos. Embryonic death is common and warrants a review of incubation conditions (oviparous species) and maternal nutrition/husbandry. A review of protocols for egg care/incubation and embryonic death investigation is disscussed in Chapter 85. Health issues that affect the female during gestation and result in embryonic death/decreased fecundity include low fat reserves, underlying disease (oophoritis, salpingitis, cloacitis, neoplasia), abnormal reproductive anatomy, and any other issues resulting in dystocia.

Clinical Presentation and Diagnostic Confirmation. If the reptile breeder has kept detailed records on breeding stock, problems associated with fertility and fecundity will become evident. A review of all aspects of the reproductive strategy for any given pair or breeding group must be performed and individual animals must have a thorough physical examination. Accurately identifying the sex of an individual is important, especially in monomorphic species where misidentification of sex is common (see (Sex Identification, earlier in this chapter). Additional tests to specifically evaluate the reproductive tract of the breeding individual may be required and include hematology and biochemistry, ultrasonography (allows evaluation of testicular, ovarian, and oviductal architecture) and other imaging modalities (CT and MRI), cloacoscopy and coelioscopy/celiotomy for biopsy/histopathology, and microbiological evaluation. See clinical investigation for reproductive diseases earlier in this chapter for more information on these procedures. Specifically for males the copulatory structure(s) should be evaluated for pathology. If males appear to copulate effectively, evaluation of semen may be necessary. A variety of manual techniques and/or electroejaculation can be utilized to collect semen samples from males (or the female's cloaca postcopulation), and the semen can be evaluated (see Artificial Insemination earlier in this chapter to review these techniques).[37] If no abnormalities are detected during semen evaluation then coeliscopy/coeliotomy may be necessary to evaluate the testes and perform a testicular biopsy for histopathology/microbiology. It is important to understand that spermatogenesis in most males occurs seasonally, and serial biopsies and plasma testosterone levels may need to be evaluated over time (several years) before a definitive diagnosis of sterility can be determined.[132]

For females, monitoring the vitellogenic cycle (over several seasons) with the use of ultrasonography will provide noninvasive information on seasonal folliculogenesis and cycling; however, coeliscopy/coeliotomy to evaluate the ovary and biopsy may be necessary to confirm disesase.

Preferred Treatment(s). Specific treatment for infertility and fecundity issues will be based on the confirmed diagnosis. If, on evaluation, breeding reptiles are appropriately sexed and determined healthy and "fit" for breeding then a discussion on managing external variables (based on natural history of the species involved), such as proper cycling techniques, minimizing social stress, providing a conducive breeding environment, etc., may result in improved success. However, in cases of reproductive disease and pathology specific treatment based on the diagnosis will be necessary. See previous sections on reproductive diseases for a review of the management of these conditions as they may contribute to infertility and reduced fecundity, especially in the early stages. In a breeding situation reptiles with poor reproductive performance or advanced reproductive pathology may need culling or rehoming (to a nonbreeding situation) to improve results in facility production.[162]

Ultimately the reptile veterinarian should approach the breeder with a comprehensive plan involving a review of proper husbandry, nutrition, record keeping, reproductive strategies utilized, and a thorough prebreeding evaluation of breeding reptiles. In addition, providing ultrasonography services (or instruction) to assist with timing of male introduction during the female follicular cycle, confirming and monitoring gestation, and reviewing any potential reproductive complications can improve reproductive success for the breeder or facility. See earlier section, Captive Breeding, for more details.

Prognosis and Prevention. If, on evaluation, the breeding reptiles are appropriatley sexed and determined healthy and "fit" for breeding, the prognosis is good, as management of external variables may resolve issues. However, in cases of reproductive disease and pathology the prognosis may be more guarded depending on possible resolution of these conditions.

For breeding reptiles, providing appropriate husbandry, nutrition, preventive health programs (including quarantine), implementing appropriate breeding practices (understanding natural history of species, breeding environment hygiene, not overextending males, etc), and regular veterinary evaluations (including necropsy and histopathology on losses and culls) can help reduce the incidence of reproductive disease and thus infertility and fecundity issues.

REFERENCES

See www.expertconsult.com for a complete list of references.

81

Musculoskeletal System

S. Emi Knafo

Musculoskeletal pathology and common disease states will be presented in this chapter, as well as the normal musculoskeletal anatomy and physiology of amphibians and reptiles. Musculoskeletal system reviews of amphibians and reptiles have mostly focused on disease processes, particularly metabolic bone diseases, traumatic injuries, and fractures. However, there is a paucity of information in the veterinary literature on the normal musculoskeletal anatomy and physiology. Therefore this chapter will also describe the form and function of reptiles by integrating basic biology, zoology, and physiology literature as it applies to clinical medicine. The author has attempted to present the anatomical features most likely to be of clinical significance in relation to medical and surgical procedures.

ANATOMY AND PHYSIOLOGY

Muscle

Across different orders of reptiles, there exists a general anatomical organizational plan, likely established with the first tetrapodal terrestrial vertebrates.[1] This musculoskeletal body plan served as the origin, from which modifications arose, connected to the shape and natural history of the species (i.e., carapacial or limbless body forms). Characteristics of the musculature of each reptile group reflect these modifications. Ophidia have highly specialized axial muscles, including subvertebral musculature, visceral cephalic muscles that insert more caudally, and hypaxial musculature of the body wall that extends cranially with the abdominal oblique and rectus abdominis muscles reaching the skull.[2] Amphisbaenia have subvertebral muscles restricted to the cervical region and lack musculature of the limbs as would be expected.[1] Sauria presents the greatest diversity, particularly in the hypaxial muscles, owing to the different respiratory mechanisms. Subvertebral musculature is restricted to the neck as described in legless lizards. Rhynchocephalia possess epaxial muscles with transverse linkages dorsoventrally via a network of tendons and aponeuroses.[1] The chelonians generally have reduced or absent axial muscles yet have well-developed hypaxial and subvertebral muscles in the neck. Lastly, the crocodilians have similar muscular anatomy as other saurian reptiles, with subvertebral musculature restricted to the cervical region, yet have well-developed, multilayered epaxial and hypaxial muscles.

Amphibians, reptiles, and birds possess three types of muscle fibers: broad white, narrow red, and intermediate. These fiber types may correspond to mammalian muscle fiber types, but this has not been clearly demonstrated.[3] Reptile muscle fibers are also classified as twitch and tonic fibers. The tonic fibers are slow, and their ultrastructure includes a sarcotubular system that is much less extensive than even the slow-twitch fibers of mammals.[3] The myofilaments are poorly bundled into fibrils. The membranes of these tonic fibers only support junction potentials, not action potentials, and show graded, rather than all-or-nothing, contractions.[3] It is likely that mammalian slow-twitch fibers may be tonic fibers that acquired characteristics of fast-twitch fibers but maintain lower ATPase levels.[3] More generally, the skeletal muscles of vertebrates follow a similar pattern in myofibrillar structure but differ in sarcomere length.[3] Longer sarcomeres may be characteristic of slower muscles. Within sarcomeres, the thick filaments (A bands) are conserved and similar in size across reptile groups, whereas thin filaments (I bands) demonstrate more variability and do not seem to correlate with speed of contraction.[3] Chelonians have longer thin filaments, which are believed to allow for greater ranges of length over which the muscle may contract.[3] The orientation of T tubules is such that two cisterna of the sarcoplasmic reticulum come together with the T tubules to form triads. Fast-twitch fibers of leg muscles typically have two triads regularly spaced between A and I bands to increase sensitivity to electrical stimulation and improve excitation-contraction coupling.[3] In contrast, the tonic fibers have few triads and often have diads (T tubules associated with a single sarcoplasmic cisterna). Twitch fibers also show distinct myofibrils in cross-section, whereas tonic fibers are more loosely organized. Lizard muscles typically have fewer tonic fibers compared with muscles of snakes, and tonic fibers are more common in postural muscles.[3]

Bone

Haversian bone is considered the basic structural unit of bone in mammals. However, the classic Haversian system is absent in many reptiles, including lizards and snakes, yet can be found in certain localized areas of cortical bone in chelonians and crocodilians.[4] Reptile bone can be primary vascular or nonvascular bone. The primary vascular bone has primary canals, which are oriented longitudinally when they are of periosteal origin. This is characteristic of bone that has been quickly laid down during periods of growth. Nonvascular bone is found in virtually all adult reptiles to some degree. Nonlamellar, woven, or fibrous bone is composed of a fibrous matrix with randomly oriented collagen fibers within. This is characteristic of parts of the skeleton undergoing rapid growth or fracture repair (deposition of bone in a short period of time). When nonlamellar bone is present on the cortex, it is considered fine-cancellous bone. This is in contrast to the coarse-cancellous bone of the medullary cavity. Fine-cancellous bone has small cancellous spaces that are filled with bone deposits and form standard diameter canals. Ultimately, this bone becomes compact. The process of compaction within the medulla also occurs by bone deposition within cancellous spaces. However, in the case of the medullary coarse-cancellous bone, it becomes engulfed by the growing, inward-moving cortex as it becomes compact. This compacted coarse-cancellous bone is identified in all reptiles.[4] As bones grow, new bone is deposited on periosteal or endosteal surfaces, depending on the direction of growth in a particular bone or part of a bone. Therefore the entire cortex, in different parts of any reptilian bone, may be made of periosteal tissue or endosteal bone. The alternating inward and outward direction of cortical growth produces a distinctive layering pattern.[4]

Chelonians and crocodilians have more comparable bone structure and conform to a basic body plan of organization. They undergo skeletal remodeling, which is similar to all tetrapods. The bones are composed of an outer cortex enclosing a central medullary cavity with cancellous trabeculae. The compact cortical bone lacks outer and inner lamellae and does not contain a Haversian system.[4] The more common cortical bone pattern in chelonians and crocodilians is a laminar structure containing laminae and primary vascular canals. This laminar structure is more pronounced as the animal matures, and circumferentially arranged laminae are accumulated during periods of growth.[4] Skeletal growth, and therefore cortical lamination itself in chelonians and crocodilians, takes place in seasonal waves, often corresponding to alternating periods of hibernation and activity, or seasonal differences in feeding habits or nutrition.[4] Metaphyseal and epiphyseal cortical bone can be thin and composed of mostly endosteal bone. Cancellous bone is found throughout the medullary cavities of long bones, including the metaphysis and diaphysis.[4] In mammals, cancellous trabeculae of the medullary cavity of long bones undergo remodeling and reorganization by way of resorption and secondary deposition of new bone. This secondary rebuilding of primary cancellous bone is limited or completely absent in the bones of chelonians and crocodilians.[4] Instead, reptilian bones grow as the endosteal cortex is expanded upon and moves inward. The process is followed by growth of the periosteal layer of the cortex, which creates diaphyseal widening.[4] By this mechanism, the cancellous trabeculae of the medulla can be composed of bone originating from the periosteal cortex rather than endosteal origin and has been relocated to the medulla by the increasing diameter of the bone.[4] Additionally, it is possible that the bands produced earlier in bone growth can be progressively removed by endosteal resorption as the bone continues to grow in size. Therefore there is no reliable way to correlate the number of bands of bone with the age of the individual.[4] This conversion from compact to cancellous bone, without secondary remodeling and reorganization, is exceedingly rare or entirely absent in mammals.[4] Haversian systems can be found in specific areas involving the insertion of muscle or tendon to the cortex. This is advantageous to a growing animal, as the secondary Haversian remodeling within this section of cortical bone provides continuous attachment by the formation and reformation of new Haversian systems, which are continuous with the inserting muscle or tendon.[4]

The bones of squamates differ from those of chelonians and crocodilians in two notable ways. First, the cancellous trabeculae in the mid diaphysis of long bones is limited (compared with chelonians and crocodilians); however, the ends of long bones have extensive cancellous trabeculae. This is because as bones grow longitudinally, there is a transition from metaphysis to diaphysis by decreasing bone diameter. Therefore the composition of bone at the metaphyseal-diaphyseal transition is compact cancellous bone of endosteal origin.[3,4] The cortices of snake and lizard bones contain a mix of both endosteal and periosteal origin, as in chelonian and crocodilian bone.[4]

The second main difference is that the compact bone of periosteal origin in lacertilians and ophidians is virtually nonvascular. Vascular canals do exist but are located in the endosteal deposits of the metaphysis.[4] Within compact bone, the sparse distribution of vascular canals results in a process called osteocytic necrosis. This cellular necrosis is usually isolated to the more remote locations between vascular canals where blood supply is distant. As a direct consequence of osteocytic necrosis, the network of canaliculi become filled with mineral deposits. The middiaphyses of long bones typically have a broad cortex, therefore this location is most likely to demonstrate cell necrosis in lacertians given the increased distance between the inner and outer surface blood supply.[4] This condition has been described in the *Iguana*, as well as in the nonvascular areas of chelonian and crocodilian bone. Avascular

bony tissue likely represents the result of a slower growth rate. The reduced cancellous trabeculae means that the previously described conversion from compact cortical to cancellous medullary bone seen in chelonians and crocodilians is not as prevalent in squamates. Additionally, since primary vascular canals are not present, the resorptive enlargement of primary cortical canals to form medullary spaces cannot occur, and formation of Haversian systems does not take place.[4]

Musculoskeletal Anatomy

Amphibia. The discussion of musculoskeletal anatomy of amphibians will focus on adult, postmetamorphosis amphibians. Caecelians resemble an earthworm in their body form and lack pelvic and pectoral girdles. No sacrum is present, and the ribs are uniquely double-headed.[5] The skull is solid compared with salamanders, which have a more intermediate skull. Siren salamanders lack a pelvic girdle, and some species of salamander lack digits.[5] Anurans are the most highly modified of the amphibians. Their skull is reduced, and there is no bony separation between the globe and oropharynx.[5] The sacrum is reduced, and there is a modified pelvic girdle. As an adaptation for jumping, many of the long bones are fused to create stronger bones to absorb landing impact or to add length to the legs to facilitate liftoff. These adaptations give rise to unique anuran anatomical terminology. The urostyle is composed of fused tail vertebrae retained within the pelvis; the radius and ulna are fused to form the radioulna; the tibia, fibula, and tarsal bones are fused to form the tibiofibula; and metatarsal bones are elongated and fused to form the calcaneum and astralagus.[5] The ileum is elongated and forms an additional joint with the sacrum, which is believed to aid in jumping.

Ophidia (Snakes). The most defining characteristic of the snake musculoskeletal system is the lack of legs for use in locomotion. Most snakes have pelvic remnants; however, only snakes in the infraorder Alethinophidia (e.g., Boidae) have vestigial limbs or spurs. The kinetic skull of snakes is a unique feature in which the ligamentous mandibular symphysis along with the quadrate bone allow the snake to open its mouth almost 180 degrees. The quadrate bone is an extra bone that articulates between the mandible and the skull, thus providing an extra joint.[6] Interestingly, snakes do not have cervical vertebrae yet have retained cervical musculature (Fig. 81.1).

Lacertilia, Amphisbaenia, and Sphenodontia (Lizards, Legless Lizards, and Tuatara). The Amphisbaenia are specialized in their morphology, as they are generally limbless. The total number of their vertebrae varies from 82 to almost 160, and the vertebrae themselves are typically flattened with no neural spines in the trunk region.[2] Differentiating the regions of the vertebral column is difficult. Although the vestigial pectoral and pelvic girdles are present, they have no connection to the vertebral column and serve as poor markers of anatomical region.[2] As the body form becomes more serpentine and the vertebral column elongates, lateral undulation as the main mode of locomotion increases. In contrast, bipedal lizards show shortening of the presacral vertebral column along with increased tail length. This serves as a counterbalance to the body, as locomotion becomes less reliant on lateral undulation. The shorter trunk increases lateral stability and moves the center of gravity over the hind limbs and pelvic girdle.[7] In lacertilia, the shoulder and pectoral girdle is complex, owing to its role in locomotion, ventilation, and feeding (Fig. 81.2). The pectoral girdle forms a system of braces to transfer forces and brace against forces. There is an indirect connection to the vertebral column, which includes the scapulocoracoid complex, interclavicle, clavicles, and sternum. The sternum meets the coracoid in a horizontal plane to brace the girdle from axial or inward-driving forces, whereas the clavicle braces against

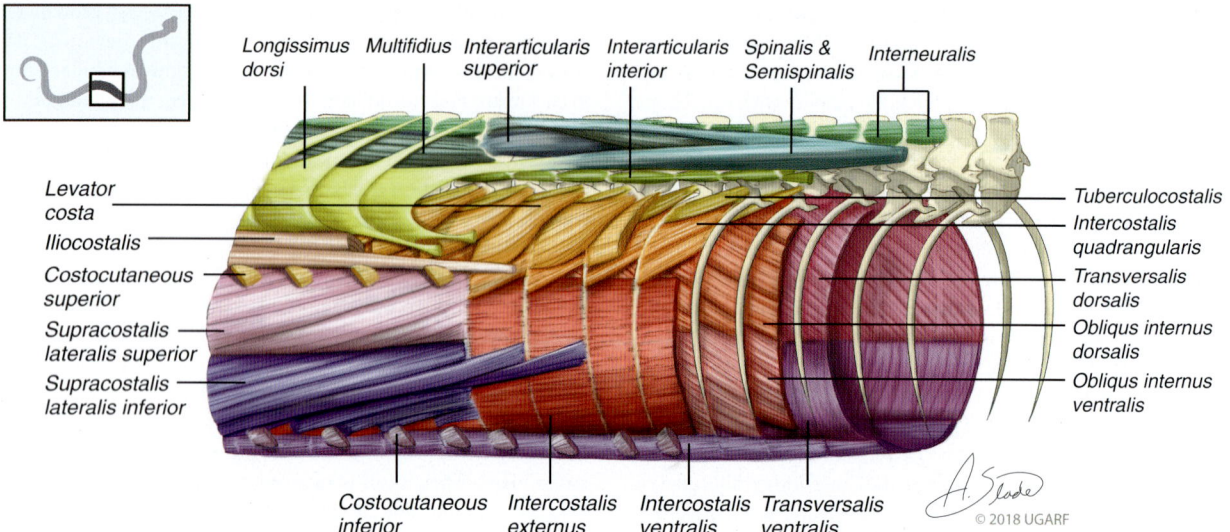

FIG 81.1 The axial musculature of a viperid snake, demonstrating the complex arrangement of muscles in relation to the numerous vertebrae and associated ribs, which facilitates coordinated locomotive patterns. (Redrawn with permission by Educational Resources, University of Georgia.)

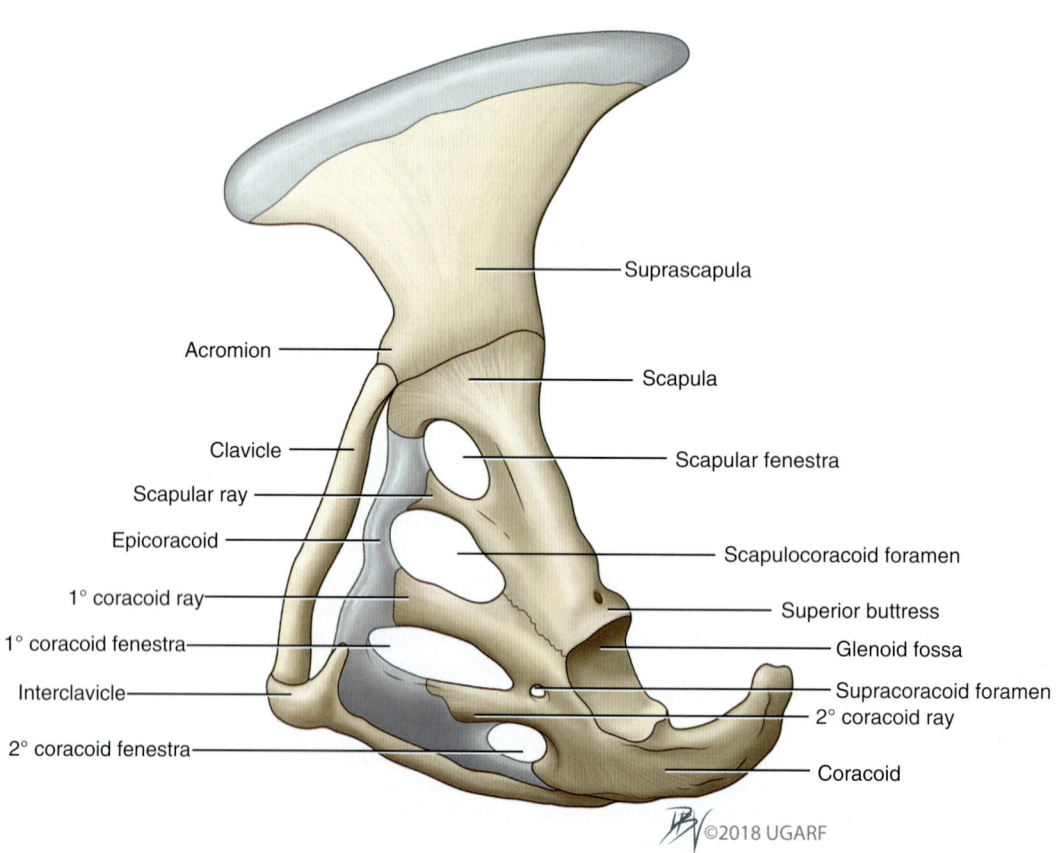

FIG 81.2 Pectoral girdle of the green iguana (*Iguana iguana*). (Redrawn with permission by Educational Resources, University of Georgia.)

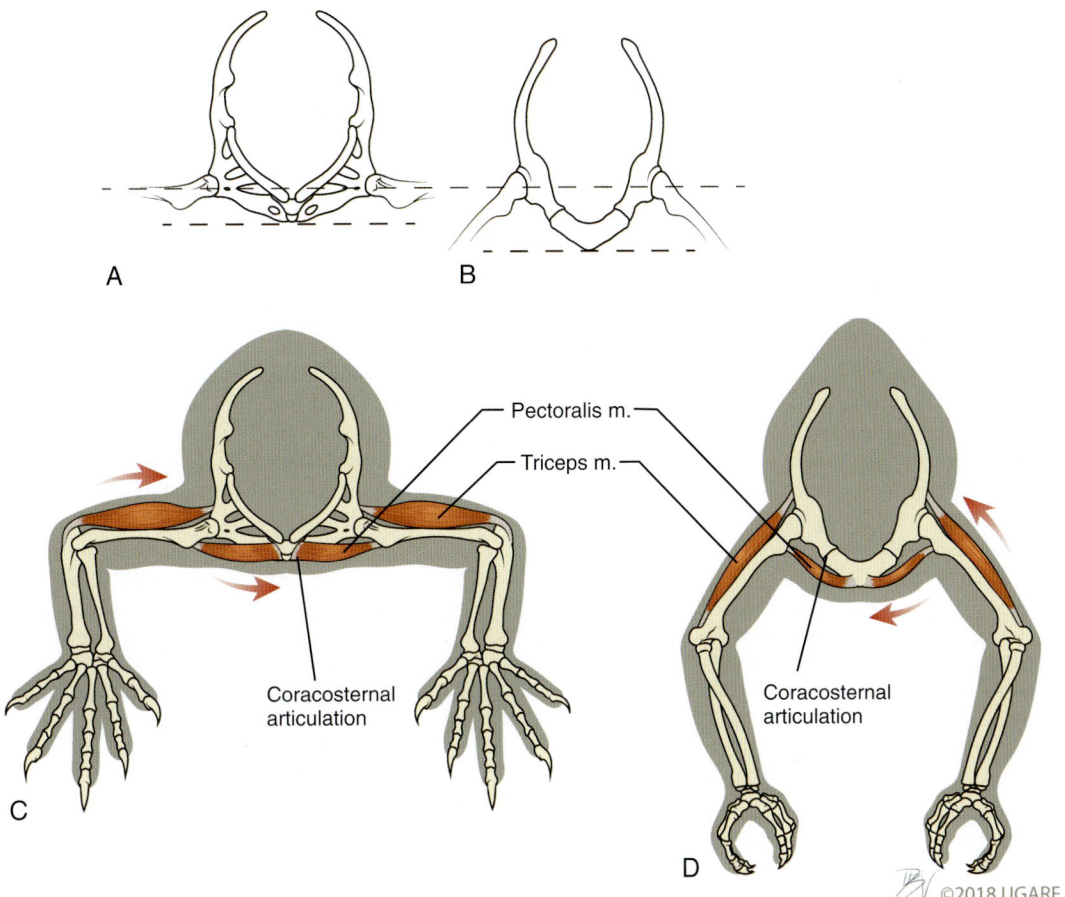

FIG 81.3 Comparative shoulder girdle of lizards of differing body conformation. (A) *Iguana*. (B) *Chameleo* showing the relative level of the glenohumeral joints (upper dashed line) and coracosternal articulation (lower dashed line). These different orientations affect weight transfer as depicted in (C) *Iguana* and (D) *Chameleo*. (C) Limbs in *Iguana* act as transverse struts and push coracosternal articulations together. *M. triceps* and *M. pectoralis* assist in this motion and actively force closed the coracosternal articulations. Weight bearing is only possible due to this active force applied. (D) Limbs in *Chameleo* are oriented more vertically, with the glenoid dorsal to coracosternal articulation. This orientation, along with body weight and the action of associated muscles, causes a passive closure of the coracosternal articulation. (Redrawn with permission by Educational Resources, University of Georgia.)

craniomedial forces. The exception to this arrangement is the chameleon, where the orientation of the articulation is turned dorsally (Fig. 81.3).[7] Finally, the scapulosternal ligament resists lateral forces. These three braces form a triangle around the scapulocoracoid to increase stability of the girdle in the absence of direct articulation with the vertebral column.[7] In the *Iguana* the clavicle articulates dorsally with the suprascapula, and the scapula does not bear a distinct acromion process. The suprascapula may or may not possess an acromion process depending on the body form of the species. In *Elgaria* it far exceeds the length of the scapula, whereas in *Xantusia* it is very short. In the *Uromastyx* and *Gallotia,* the suprascapula exhibits a number of holes along its dorsal border.[7] The clavicle attaches dorsally at the acromion zone, which is a calcified cartilaginous prominence on the suprascapula or an ossified process of the scapula. In dorsally compressed species, the scapula is fenestrated and the suprascapula bears the acromion process. Most fenestrae are occluded by a membranous tissue and are believed to be associated with the origin of muscles.[7] In laterally compressed species the scapula is thin, elongated, and bears the acromion process.[7] A great variety of fenestration anatomy has been described, including the presence or absence of fenestrae and foramina; the extent of osseous or cartilaginous borders surrounding the fenestrae; the shape and angle on

the scapula; the fenestration of the suprascapular itself; and the form of the coracoid.[7] However, the clinical significance of these anatomical details is unclear. Therefore the reader is encouraged to consult cited resources for more thorough discussions of this anatomy.[7] In lacertilians the interclavicle is associated with muscles of the neck and shoulder that attach in patterns responsible for the shape of the bone.[8] The interclavicle acts to link the sternum to the clavicles, the two elements that brace the pectoral girdle. The median strut of bone resists compression between the ventral ends of the clavicles and transfers this force to the sternum.[7] Laterally, there are paired ligamentous processes that support and prevent lateral bending between the girdle elements. Both the ligamentous and the bony portions of the interclavicle serve as attachment sites for muscle fibers. Stresses exerted on the clavicle at the acromion are directed caudally onto the median process of the interclavicle, and thus the major role of the median process is to resist this compression.[7] A relatively short interclavicle increases stability of the clavicle relative to the sternum because rotation forces are minimized. This, however, has a cost in terms of lateral undulation locomotion. A longer interclavicle process may be related to greater lateral undulation locomotion.[7] Clavicles are never straight, but the degree of curvature varies between species. Expanded clavicles generally are recognized in species that are strong climbers with robust forelimb musculature. In general, the pectoral girdle is capable of displacement relative to the body wall in arboreal species but to a lesser extent in terrestrial ones.[7] The relative immobility of the girdle in some terrestrial forms is an adaptation to enhance lateral undulation locomotion. In *Varanus*, however, there is considerable movement of the primary girdle during locomotion. The degree of mobility of the primary girdle varies with the magnitude of the coracosternal angle, and it is greatest when the angle is low.[7] In arboreal species, increased mobility of the pectoral girdle provides greater range of limb postures.[7] The humerus is a complexly sculpted bone that is able to swing back and forth in the glenoid fossa while also undergoing long axis rotation.[7] One of the most noticeable features of the lacertian humerus is its apparent torsion, in which the proximal and distal expansions do not lie in the same plane. The flat surface of the proximal end is at an almost right angle to the distal end, and this torsion is thought to ensure transition of muscle forces from the distal part of the brachium to the antebrachium, owing to the characteristics of a sprawling forelimb locomotion.[7]

The glenoid is defined dorsally by a supraglenoid buttress and ventrally by an infraglenoid buttress. The glenoid surface itself is saddle-shaped, and the humeral condyle matches the glenoid fossa. The articular capsule of the glenohumeral joint is thin, composed of four ligamentous bands that form cruciate pairs.[7] In arboreal species, the glenohumeral joint is modified to permit greater range of motion. The cranioventral ligament is oriented so that it is placed more laterally beneath the glenoid and does not tighten when sliding occurs (as occurs in terrestrial species). This, in addition to expansion of the articular surfaces, permits the humerus to slide laterally during extreme abduction. Excursion into the cranial quadrants of the glenoid is also increased by the more lateral orientation of the articular surface. In terrestrial species, the glenoid fossa faces caudolaterally, whereas in arboreal species it is turned laterally on the girdle and affects lateral orientation of the limb. In chameleons the glenoid faces ventrally, giving a more vertical limb orientation. The major articulatory condyle of the distal humerus is the radial condyle, whereas the rim of the ulnar condyle forms by a pulleylike structure to guide the action of the elbow joint. The depression separating the condyles is the condylotrochlear gutter. The proximal radius and ulna bear two facets, each separated by a ridge, thus creating two articular cavities.[7]

The long axis of the radius is slightly curved, such that it is gently turned around the long axis of the ulna. Thus, with the forelimb in the standardized position, the curvature carries the long axis of the radius from proximolateral to distomedial.[7] Pronation of the antebrachium is manifested by the curvature of the radius in conjunction with the relationship of the proximal versus the distal ends of the radius and ulna.[7] The elbow joint axis moves from medial to lateral, whereas the wrist joint operates dorsoventrally. The net result is the maintenance of a constant position of the manus as the humerus undergoes backswing because the glenoid, elbow, and wrist joints permit compensatory movements of the limb.[7] In standardized posture the ulna is functionally the lateral-most element of the antebrachium. At its proximal extremity, there is a prominent olecranon process on which inserts the common tendon of the triceps complex.[7] The ulna of chameleons differs from most other lizards in that the olecranon is not well developed, with a flat proximal aspect and a lateral buttress at the distal extremity, which is unique.[7] This allows the elbow joint to more fully extend and permit an erect posture. In the *Iguana*, there are nine carpals: three in the proximal row, one in the middle row, and five in the distal row. The proximal row, from medial to lateral, consists of the radial, ulnar, and pisiform. The middle row consists of the central only. The distal row consists of a series of carpal elements, each associated with a single metacarpal bone.[7] The carpus of chameleons is the only major departure

from the typical lacertian morphology. There are only two rows of carpals present; a proximal row of three elements consisting of a radial, ulnar, and pisiform, and distal row including a large central cartilage (postulated to be distal carpal 4) and a distal carpal 5.[7] No fusion of any distal carpals with metacarpals is observed. The functioning of the carpus in chameleons is very different from that in other lizards. Articulation takes place largely between the ulnar carpal bone and the large element of the distal carpal row. The wrist joint is thus mesocarpal and may be interpreted as mechanically equivalent to a ball and socket.[7] Only in chameleons is there any marked divergence from the basic plan of metacarpal structure. The metacarpals are depressed and expanded extremities and are divided into two bundles that articulate with the largest element of the distal carpal row. The first three digits comprise the medial aspect, whereas the fourth and fifth form the lateral parts of a "pincer" system.[7] The phalangeal formula varies somewhat both within and between families, but in general, phalanges are shorter than the metacarpal of their respective digit and also generally exhibit a progressive shortening distally.[7] The proportions of phalanges along the length of the digit vary between taxa, and the shortness of the intermediate phalanges in the longer digits (three and four) of certain taxa has been proposed as a modification associated with climbing.[7] Most geckos show digits of a more primitive type, with the acquisition of subdigital adhesive pads. The short metacarpals (and metatarsals) are important in the equalization of digit length and the spreading of the digits over a wide arc.[7]

The pelvic girdle has a direct connection to the vertebral column and includes the ilium, ischium, and pubis. Each of these elements, in part, compose the acetabulum. The pubis and ischium are separated ventral to the acetabulum by the thyroid foramen or fenestra.[7] The architecture of the lacertian pelvic girdle facilitates horizontal limb action, along with the adductor muscles, which aid in limb recovery (return to normal position).[7] Variations in pelvic girdle width have been correlated with locomotor patterns in lizards. Specifically, species that exhibit bipedalism generally have a narrower pelvis to allow the limbs to be adducted closer under the midline of the body.[7] The ilium of *Sphenodon* projects dorsocaudal, whereas in lizards it projects caudally. This arrangement results in the sacral vertebrae being located just above the acetabulum in *Sphenodon* and caudal to the acetabulum in lizards. Varanids have a steep, horizontally oriented iliac blade, whereas chameleons have an almost completely vertical iliac blade. The subsequent orientation of the hind limb is largely determined by pelvic girdle conformation and morphology of the femur.[7] In general, the femoral head is turned upward compared with the axis of the shaft, and the femur itself has a sigmoid curvature, which becomes clinically significant during fracture repair. The shaped femoral head is oval and confines the movement of the thigh to the horizontal plane. The acetabulum is larger than the femoral head, and therefore there is never complete contact over the entire acetabular surface at any one time.[7] In relation to bipedal locomotion, the internal trochanter acts as a lever on the ventral acetabular edge, which tends to pull the femoral head from the acetabular socket. This positioning precludes, to some degree, pulling the legs completely underneath the body, which would result in a more vertical posture during bipedal locomotion.[7]

The lacertian stifle is bicondylar as in mammals, yet it differs significantly. Mammalian femoral condyles are typically symmetrical and arranged in line with the long axis of the femur. Among lizards, this orientation is only seen in chameleons. In all other lizards, the femoral condyles are asymmetrical, with separate contact surfaces for the tibia and fibula.[7] The lateral femoral condyle has a cone or wedge shape in *Varanus*, *Tupinambis*, and *Lacerta* but takes a more cylindrical shape in *Basiliscus* and *Iguana*. Similarly, the patellar surface is well defined in *Varanus* and *Tupinambis* but is a shallow groove in

Lacerta and *Iguana*. In *Basiliscus* and *Chamaeleo* the patellar groove is essentially absent.[7] These differences in distal femur anatomy affect the structure and function of the stifle in different species. Within the stifle, the articular surfaces are defined proximally by the lateral and medial femoral condyles and distally by the meniscus and proximal tibial epiphysis. The meniscus increases the stability and congruence of the joint while aiding in lubrication. Laterally, the proximal fibula forms the margin of the stifle by articulating with the lateral femoral condyle via the cyamella sesamoid. The exact location and presence of a cyamella sesamoid is variable between species. The stifle joint is stabilized by the joint capsule, collateral ligaments, and cruciate ligaments, and part of the joint capsule is formed by the quadriceps femoris muscle. Continuous with the synovial cavity is a bursa created between the quadriceps tendon and the intercondylar groove.[7] The collateral ligaments are formed by the two lateral femorofibular collaterals and the medial femorotibial collateral ligaments.[7] The femorofibular collateral ligaments cross, and all collaterals are in tension throughout normal range of motion to maintain position and contact of the stifle joint.[7] The two cruciate ligaments originate in the ventral intercondylar groove of the femur and insert on the proximal tibial epiphysis, just medial to their point of origin.[7] The cruciate ligaments cross each other and are oriented lateral to medial.[7] This is in contrast to cruciate ligament anatomy in most small mammals (dogs and cats), which have two cruciate ligaments named for their insertion on the proximal tibia—the cranial and caudal cruciate ligaments. In reptiles, the fibula and tibia are well attached by the proximal and distal tibiofibular ligaments. Additionally, these bones are constrained from rotation due to their articulation with the astragalocalcaneum. As a result of this cumulative anatomy, and most importantly the asymmetry of the femoral condyles, the stifle joint is not perpendicular to the long axis of the femur. Rather, the line of motion

of the joint runs parallel to the contact surface between the meniscus and the femoral condyle, passing in a distolateral to proximomedial orientation.[7] The tarsus is reduced with only two tarsal bones in lizards (the third and fourth tarsals), and three in *Sphenodon* (the second, third, and fourth tarsals), which gives asymmetry of the tarsus and foot. The distal tarsals are functionally firmly bound by ligaments to the first four metatarsal bones and can be viewed as a tarsometatarsus. These metatarsals are enclosed in a cutaneous sheath and form the sole of the foot. The fifth metatarsal is specialized, shorter, and has an offset articulation with the fourth distal tarsal bone, which lends a "hooked" appearance to this toe.[7] This consolidation of the tarsus may improve transfer of forces into forward propulsion. There is an increase in metatarsal length, such that the distal tips of the first three metatarsals lie on a straight line, the metatarsophalangeal line (Fig. 81.4).[7] This striking asymmetry of the lacertian foot is an adaptation for sprawling locomotion and stands in contrast to the near symmetrical feet of crocodilians.[7] Phalangeal morphology is fairly uniform and the phalangeal formula is 2-3-4-5-4. Geckos, especially those species that exhibit subdigital adhesive pads, are unique in that they are the only group of normal-limbed lizards to exhibit claw loss, which may occur on one or all digits.[7]

Some species of lizards are capable of tail autotomy (iguanids, geckos). This is considered a predator avoidance strategy, in which the tail is self-detached along a preexisting fracture plane and is cast off with minimal hemorrhage.[9] The tail will regenerate in time, and the autotomized tail will wiggle on the ground, presumably to distract the predator. In species that undergo tail autotomy, each caudal vertebra has a cartilaginous fracture plane through the vertebral body and neural arch. Fracture planes are absent in the cranial part of the tail to protect the hemipenes and fat deposits.[9] The lost tail is regenerated with a

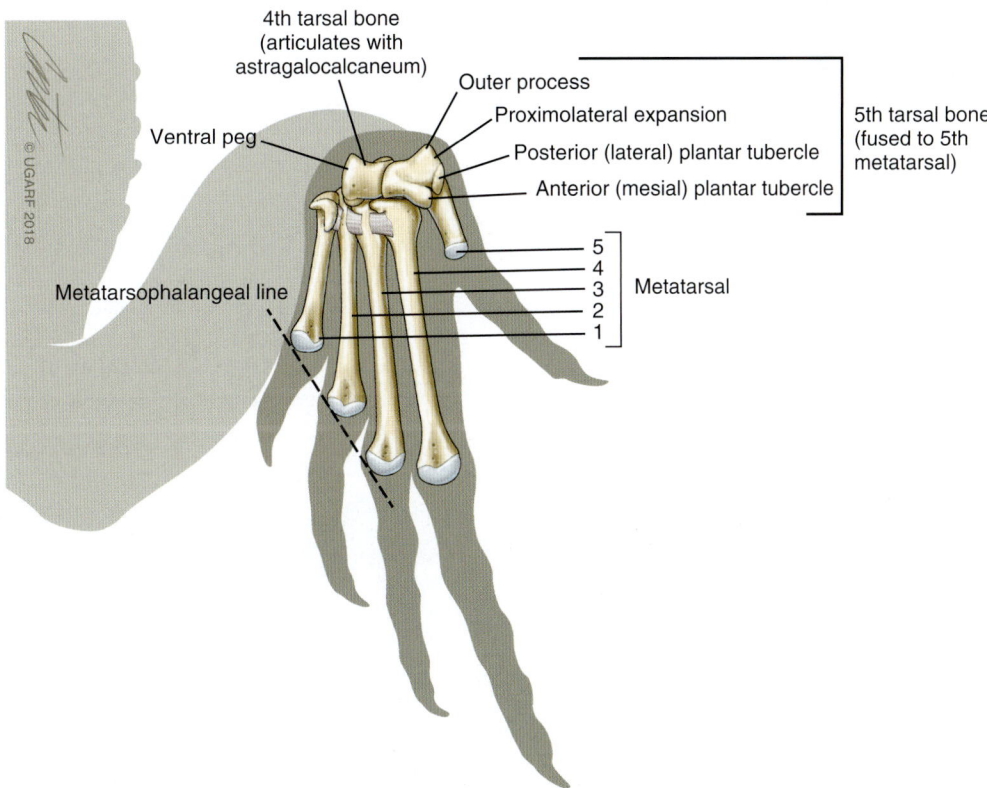

FIG 81.4 *Iguana* tarsometatarsus, demonstrating asymmetry of the metatarsals and the metatarsophalangeal line. (Redrawn with permission by Educational Resources, University of Georgia.)

cartilaginous rod for support and is covered with smaller darker scales in an irregular pattern compared with the original tail.[9] Tail autotomy is clinically relevant, as stress and handling can cause tail fracture. Additionally, tail autotomy should be considered in cases of surgical tail amputation. A study in leopard geckos, *Eublepharis macularius*, demonstrated that tail autotomization along a preexisting fracture plane or surgical amputation outside of a fracture plane resulted in scar-free wound healing and regeneration of the tail regardless of location or mode of detachment.[10] In leopard geckos, wound healing is characterized by transient myofibroblasts and highly proliferative wound epithelium, which is immunoreactive for wound keratin marker WE6.[10] New tails form from a blastema, which is a mass of mesenchymal cells. Unlike mammals, transforming growth factor B3 is not involved in wound healing in these lizards.[10] Tail autotomy generally does not occur in agamid lizards, monitors, or true chameleons, and these species do not regenerate tails that are lost from trauma or amputation. Other species of lizards may have prehensile tails, which aid arboreal movement.

Chelonians. The most unique anatomical feature of chelonians is the presence of a shell, including a dorsal arched disc, the carapace, and a ventral plate, the plastron. (See Chapter 70 for more detailed information.) Most turtles can retract their heads and necks into their shell, though *Pleurodira* species retract their head and neck horizontally, and *Cryptodira* species retract their head and neck vertically. Sea turtles cannot fully retract their head and neck under their shell.[11]

The vertebral column in chelonians is quite specialized, with 18 presacral vertebrae (8 cervical, 10 trunk; the lowest number among reptiles).[2] In the neck, the vertebrae are mobile, whereas within the carapace they are ankylosed to each other, and the ribs are connected to the carapace. Unique cervical anatomy is present in *Cryptodira*, in which the vertebrae articulate in such a way as to permit sagittal flexure of the neck.[2]

Within the carapace, the rigid ribs originate from the spine and extend laterally. They are engulfed in dermal bone. Each rib has a dorsal and ventral cortex, which enclose cancellous bone.[12] This arrangement aids in weight reduction of the shell. The ribs are also attached to each other via soft, unmineralized collagenous suture lines, which make up a zig-zag pattern.[12] This enables displacement caused by minor loads.[12] The sutures are located in such a way that the tissues take on a rib-suture-rib pattern in order to protect the compliant sutures from failure upon cranial-caudal bending forces. This further prevents any possible cracking from being propagated in a cranial-caudal direction. Cracks (from a focal force) typically originate in the brittle ribs and advance laterally, not from one rib to another. This pattern of rigid and compliant features helps to protect the carapace from catastrophic failure.[12]

The pectoral girdle of chelonians is unusual (Fig. 81.5). Dermal bone elements are incorporated into the plastron, with the clavicle contributing to the epiplastron, the first pair of lateral bony plates in the plastron.[13] The interclavicle is incorporated into the entoplastron, a median bony plate of the cranial part of the plastron.[13] The pectoral girdle is a triradiate complex within the cranial portion of the shell.[13] The scapula has long projections, which make it unique anatomically. The scapular prong is columnar and extends dorsomedially toward the carapace. A suprascapular cartilage connects the scapular prong by way of a ligament, to the cranial border of the first rib and carapace. The acromion is on the cranioventral aspect of the scapula, which extends craniomedially and ventrally almost perpendicular to the scapular prong. The acromion has a cartilaginous cap, which attaches to the entoplastron via a ligament.[13] The two almost vertical scapular prongs form a truss for the transfer of body weight from the vertebral axis and shell to the limbs. The scapula articulates with two small joints on the shell, between which the pectoral girdle rotates. This pectoral girdle rotation normally occurs with respiratory movements as well as locomotor patterns. A coracoid, which is considered the equivalent of a procoracoid of other

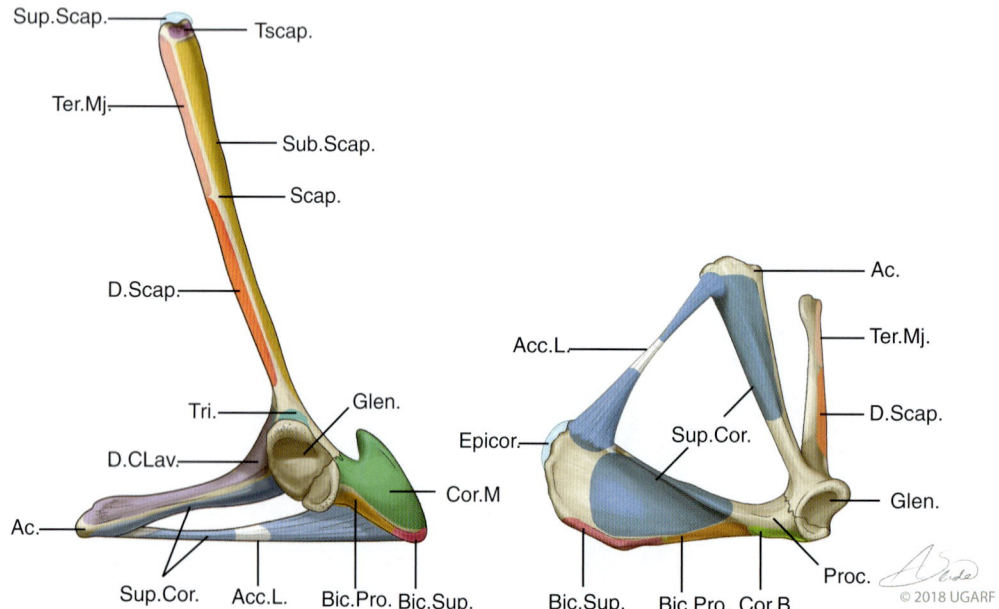

FIG 81.5 The pectoral girdle of *Trachemys scripta elegans* (lateral view left and ventral view right). The areas of attachment of major muscles are indicated. Ac, Acromion; AccL, acromiocoracoid ligament; BicPro, biceps profundus; BicSup, biceps superficialis; CorB, coracobrachialis brevis; CorM, coracobrachialis magnus; DClav, deltoideus clavicularis; DScap, deltoideus scapularis; Epicor, epicoracoid cartilage; Glen, glenoid cavity; Proc, procoracoid; SubScap, subscapularis; Scap, scapular prong; SupCor, supracoracoideus; Supscap, suprascapular cartilage; TerMj, teres major; Tri, triceps brachii; Tscap, testoscapularis. (Redrawn with permission by Educational Resources, University of Georgia.)

reptiles, extends from the scapula caudomedially in approximately the same plane as the acromion.[13] The coracoid is broader than the acromion and has a sickle-shaped epicoracoid cartilage on the medial edge. There is no ligament between the coracoid and the plastron, yet a connection exists between the acromion and the coracoid, the acromiocoracoid ligament.[13] In sea turtles, the coracoid is longer than the scapula, and this is correlated with swimming ability.[13] In some other families (mainly terrestrial), the coracoid is as wide as it is long, and there is also variability in the size of the epicoracoid cartilage. Limb morphology of chelonians also varies between species. Marine species have more flattened appendages with reduced or absent claws adapted for swimming, whereas terrestrial species may have flattened forelimbs with claws adapted for burrowing. Freshwater species have interdigital webbing to aid swimming, whereas this webbing is absent in terrestrial species.[11]

The chelonian humerus is unique in that the diaphysis arches and rotates around the long axis relative to the humeral head so that the morphological dorsal surface is directed cranially.[8,13] This unique feature allows the humerus to be protracted very far forward during locomotion and as the animal retracts into the shell. This degree of arching can vary slightly between species, and sea turtles have a notably stouter and flatter humerus compared with freshwater and terrestrial species.[8] These anatomical differences in humeral arching and rotation become clinically significant during fracture repair and other procedures. The ulna is broad and dorsoventrally flattened. The radius is more columnar and slender, and these forearm bones tend to vary less between species. The carpus is typically short. The metacarpals are unspecialized, with a row of five metacarpals proximally, and a phalangeal formula of 2-3-3-3-2. All toes are clawed and the foot is webbed in freshwater aquatic species. Terrestrial groups have further reduction of the phalangeal formula of 2-2-2-2-2 or 1, and no webbing is present. In highly aquatic species, the manus is elongated to form a flipper. The claws are retained (though reduced) except in the most aquatic species (*Dermochelys*).[8]

The pelvic apparatus includes the pelvis and bones of the hind limbs. The pubis and ischium act as struts to support a vertical ilium, which extends dorsally to the sacrum. The ilium of *Pseudemys* inclines posteriorly and expands distally to create an iliac blade. This articulates with the three sacral vertebrae and ribs. These caudal ribs expand to form a buttress with the carapace, which also articulates with the ilium. In species with reduced tail musculature, the iliac blade has smaller posterior expansion.[8] A thyroid fenestra (also called obturator fenestra or puboischiadic foramen) separates the pubis and ischium. This thyroid fenestra is associated with passage of the obturator nerve and the origin of the puboischiofemoralis externus muscle.[8] The degree of convergence of the pubis and ischium medial to the thyroid fenestra varies with species, thus affecting the distance between the fenestrae. The degrees of convergence are described as complete, nearly complete, partial, and no convergence. Emydinae and Testudininae have nearly complete convergence separated only by a small piece of cartilage. *Dermochelys* also has near-complete convergence, though the fenestrae are much smaller than other groups. In Cryptodira, the convergence is complete and the ischium and pubis are continuous. The most common conformation is partial convergence with separation achieved with a rod of cartilage as seen in Dermatemydidae, Chelydridae, Staurotypinae, and Plastysterninae. There is essentially no convergence in Cheloniidae, Carettochelyidae, and Trionychidae, where the fenestrae reach midline separated only by a ligament or a very thin rod of cartilage.[8] The pubic symphysis is separated from the ischiadic symphysis by a rhomboid cartilage. The caudal border of the ischium curves ventrally to rest on the plastron, and the pubis is extended cranially by epipubic cartilage. This epipubic cartilage can be ossified in Chelydridae, Kinosternidae, and some emydines. All pelvic girdle elements contribute to the formation of the acetabulum, though the ilium has the largest facet. The pelvic

girdle in Pleurodira is uniquely fused. The ilium ankyloses with the last one to two pleural plates, and the pubis and ischium are fused with the xiphiplastron.[8]

The femur is similarly shaped as the humerus but is longer, with a typically oval-shaped femoral head (except in testudinines, which have a round femoral head). The femoral head is offset from the long axis of the bone at an angle of approximately 120°.[8] Proximally, the minor trochanter corresponds to the internal trochanter seen in other reptiles. The major trochanter is unique to chelonians but is likely originated from the ventral ridge, as seen in other reptiles. The intertrochanteric fossa is deep, and the femoral shaft arches dorsally to a lesser extent as the humerus. The distal femur fans out and forms the large tibial condyle. A small fibular condyle is located caudoventral, with a fibular epicondyle located dorsal and proximal.[8] The typically arched femur is nearly flat in sea turtles. In aquatic species, in which the hind legs presumably have greater propulsive thrust than the forelimbs, the femur is subequal or longer than the humerus. In terrestrial species, in which the forelimbs are more important for burrowing, the femur is significantly shorter than the humerus.[8] The tibia and fibula are of similar length, though the tibia is somewhat thicker. The tibial head expands to articulate with the tibial condyle of the femur. The longitudinal cnemial crest, to which the patella tendon attaches, extends along the tibia's dorsal surface.[8] The fibular head articulates with the tibia and femur proximally and the tarsus and tibia distally. The stifle has less range of motion than in other reptiles and is limited to extension, flexion, and minimal rotation.[8] The crurotarsal joint has essentially no movement, whereas the tarsometatarsal joints do move.[8] The foot is bent at the mesotarsal joint, which keeps the sole of the foot flat on the ground. The astragulus and calcaneum of sea turtles is unique and provides extra flexibility to the ankle.[8] The additional rotation achieved allows the distal appendage to be used as a rudder. In other species, the astragulus and calcaneum are fused to form a single unit. The metatarsals are unspecialized, except for the fifth metatarsal, which is flattened, L-shaped, and broadens the foot.[8] This aids webbing, particularly between digits four and five. The fifth toe is clawless as it is completely included in the webbing.[8] During locomotion, the medial aspect of the foot makes firmest contact with the ground. The most common phalangeal formula is that of freshwater turtles, 2-3-3-3-3, though the fifth digit does not bear a claw and therefore the terminal phalanx is often very small or not present. Terrestrial species have short toes with stubby claws and no webbing. The reduced phalangeal formula is 2-2-2-2-1(0). In marine species, there is a tendency toward toe elongation and hyperphalangy. The phalangeal formula is 2-3-3-3-4 in *Chrysemys* and *Malaclemys* and 2-3-3-4(5)-3(4) in Trionychidae. *Pelomedusa* demonstrates fusion of the proximal two phalanges on the second digit, giving a stiffer foot and a phalangeal formula of 2-2-3-3-3. Most aquatic species have four claws, but Trionychidae has three, *Carettochelys* has two, Cheloniidae has one or two, and *Dermochelys* has none.[8]

The rectus abdominus muscle arises from the plastron and inserts on the lateral pubic process. This muscle is important because it, along with the testoiliacus muscle, which originates from the carapace and inserts on the ilium, helps anchor the pelvis to the shell.[8] The rectus abdominus muscle also plays a minor role in respiration. Both of these muscles are absent in *Pelomedusa*, in which the pelvic girdle is fused to the shell.[8] Typically, dorsal muscles are innervated by dorsal nerves (from the brachial and lumbosacral plexuses), and ventral muscles are innervated from ventral nerves from the plexus.[8] There are some muscle groups, typically large muscles like those in the thigh, which receive double innervation.[8]

Crocodilians. Likely, the most striking feature of crocodilians is their uniquely adapted skull. The general skull characteristics include an elongated snout and expanded premaxilla, which isolates the external nares from the maxilla.[14] The elongation of the jaw and narrow snout reflects adaptations to prey, with the longest-snouted species being specialized for ichthyophagy and the species with more moderate length snouts feeding on a greater variety of animals (reptiles, birds, fish, mammals).[14] As the elongation of the snout increases, so does the mandibular symphysis.[14] Width of the external nares is inversely related to length of the snout, as is orbit size. The skull is flattened, particularly the dorsal postorbital segment of the cranium (often called the cranial table), and has caudolateral protrusions.[14] The temporal fossa and middle ear are highly modified, with the quadrate and pterygoid bones expanded medially to contact the lateral aspect of the cranium.[14] The squamosal bones are laterally expanded to overhang the external ear, creating deep "pockets" across which the tympanic membranes are stretched.[14] These overhangs are thought to protect the tympanic membrane from injury. Further, the quadrate bones are inclined, which causes the jaw articulation to be displaced caudally, yet crocodilians do not possess a kinetic skull.[14] Thecodont teeth are found on the premaxilla, maxilla, and dentary bones. The most rostral teeth prehend prey, whereas the middle of the tooth row crushes the prey item.[15] Strong, quick muscles are necessary for feeding, and the placement of these muscles must not restrict the gape.[15] Therefore the adductor muscles are spread over the ventral surfaces and outside surfaces of the jaw.[15] There is a secondary palate formed by the palatal process of the premaxillae, maxillae, palatines, and pterygoids.[15] The long, narrow snout has undulations along the lateral margins.[14] These lateral margin undulations form three convex and two concave arches on each side. The convex arches of the mandible are opposed by concave arches of the maxilla and vice versa.[14] These undulating arches let the crocodilian hold captured prey more firmly and are more developed in shorter-snouted crocodilians than those species with longer snouts.[14]

The nasal passages are extended caudally and run the full length of the snout.[14] The palatine and pterygoid bone extensions permit this nasal passage extension, where they terminate in the secondary choanae ventral to the cranium.[14] The orbits themselves are displaced dorsally along with the external nares, which leads to confluence of the external nares into a common opening. This, along with the previously described flattening of the dorsal surface of the skull, permits the animal to remain inconspicuous in the water, as only the nostrils, eyes, and flat cranial roof are exposed.[14] The bones of the crocodilian skull are pneumatized, though the function is not completely understood. It has been hypothesized that this feature may increase the isolation of the internal ear from sounds transmitted by water.[14]

The appendicular skeleton has many distinguishing features. The femoral head is prominent and deviates medially from the shaft.[16] Distal condyles are also prominent and project caudally, though the fibular condyle is less prominent. The proximal tibia is flat, whereas the distal end is sloped.[16] This all serves to reduce the complexity of the stifle and hock to permit increased range of motion of these joints seen in crocodilian locomotive patterns.[16] The tarsal joints are characteristically oblique, and when the ankle is flat on the ground, the crus is angled medially.[16] The metatarsals overlap at the proximal end, creating a functional metatarsal wedge, which increases strength of the foot.[16] The foot is also mediolaterally compressed with reduced external digits to further increase lever capability. Interestingly, in the belly walk (described later), crocodilians may evert the fourth digit to use as a pivot point for pedal rotation, similar to the use of the fifth digit in lizard locomotion.[16]

Locomotion

Snakes. Snakes use five (at least) described modes of locomotion. The specific locomotion method depends on the surface on which the snake is moving and its speed. Remarkably, an individual snake can utilize different modes in different body segments. The five described modes of locomotion are lateral undulation, sidewinding, concertina, rectilinear, and slide-pushing.[17,18] Lateral undulation is the propagation of waves of lateral bending along the body. Sliding friction is a critical component of lateral undulation. The defining feature of lateral undulation is that as objects are contacted, a force is exerted against the object and deforms locally around it.[18] When a snake pushes against multiple objects simultaneously, the lateral force vectors are canceled out, which results in forward propulsion. Snakes possess fine sensorimotor control over the direction of force exertion by utilizing postural adjustments.[18] The large dorsal epaxial muscles are activated sequentially. These muscles are unilaterally activated with each bend of the body, from the convex side toward the straight and concave regions. This continues and each part of the body follows the path of the head and neck.[18] Sidewinding resembles lateral undulation in the pattern of bending but is otherwise quite different. The snake body segments are sequentially placed in static friction with the surface (vs. sliding), and the body segments are physically lifted off the ground between regions in static contact with the ground surface.[17,18] This moves the body forward by rolling from the neck to tail. The body moves diagonally relative to the track formed, and the tracks left by sidewinding snakes correspond to snake length. Epaxial muscles are active as in lateral undulation, though many times the muscles are active bilaterally during trunk lifting.[18] Concertina locomotion is when the front and back halves of the body alternate between bending and straightening. Forward movement is achieved as the body straightens away from the bends in a forward direction. This mode is used for moving through a narrow space or climbing.[19] The muscles are activated in bending segments unilaterally. Rectilinear locomotion is when the snake moves in a straight line. This is more typical of large snakes (boas, pythons, large vipers). The ventral scales are lifted up and forward, then pressed back down and backward, thus propelling the body forward over the scales. This occurs simultaneously in multiple body segments, and when the body has moved forward enough to result in stretching of the scales, the pattern repeats. This mode is reliant on the static friction between the ground surface and the ventral scales.[20] Bilateral muscular activity, specifically of the muscles connecting the skin to the skeleton, permit this locomotive pattern. It is dependent on active ribs and ventral scales and is not seen in *Tropidonotus*.[18] Slide-pushing is the result of vigorous lateral undulations as the body slides over a smooth surface. Irregular body bends and tail-pressing result in enough downward force onto the surface to move the body in a stepwise pattern. The movement is not regular, and slipping is encountered throughout the movement. There are moments of static contact, but slide friction is most important in slide-pushing. This is typically seen when a snake is startled on a smooth surface and tries to flee.[17]

Lizards. Lacertian locomotion is fundamentally different from mammalian locomotion, as lateral bending of the trunk is a defining feature. Limbless lizards rely entirely on lateral undulation for forward propulsion.[17,21] This may suggest that the limbs of lizards play a less important role in locomotion than in mammals. The typical posture of lacertians can be described as "sprawling," with the body slung between laterally oriented limbs, or "erect," with the limbs pulled more vertically under the body (Fig. 81.6).[7] The morphology of the femoral head and its relation to the acetabulum (as described previously) permit this change from horizontal to vertical femur orientation.[7] Hypaxial trunk muscles of *Iguana iguana* stabilize the trunk during slow speed walking, and lateral trunk bending is the result of activity of the rectus abdominus and external oblique muscles in *Varanus salvator*.[7] Lateral bending at low speeds serves to increase stride length, whereas at higher speeds it

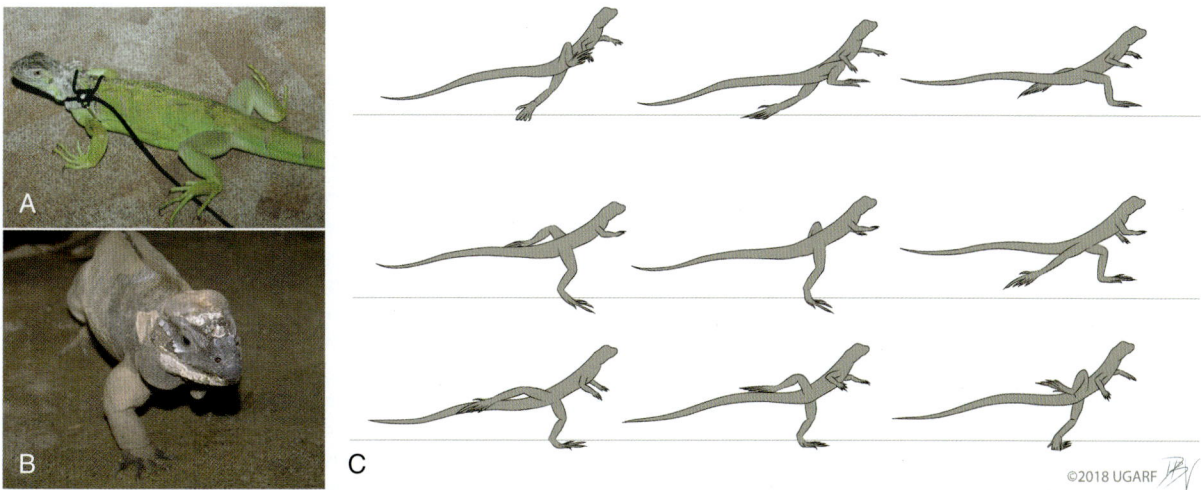

FIG 81.6 Lacertian locomotion. Sprawling, erect, and bipedalism. (A) Sprawling posture. (B) Erect posture. (C) Bipedal locomotion. Bipedal locomotion is accomplished by thrusting one or both hind limbs, rapidly followed by one hind limb swinging around in a lateral arc to catch and support the weight of the body, thus creating the first bipedal step. The forelimbs do not play a significant role, and the tail is used as a critical counterbalance to achieve coordination and propulsion. (A and B, Courtesy of Stephen J Divers; C, redrawn with permission by Educational Resources, University of Georgia.)

serves to produce propulsive force and provide limb support and coordination.[7] Simply, lizards typically use an "inverted pendulum" gait at slow speeds, and a bouncing gait (trot) at high speeds, similar to the main two gait types observed in mammals.[21] The inverted pendulum corresponds to walking and refers to the pendulumlike movement of the legs, as well as the exchange between the kinetic energy and the gravitational potential energy of the lizard's center of mass, with the legs acting as stiff struts.[21] As a result of this arrangement, the pendulum-like energy exchange reduces mechanical energy requirements in this gait by as much as 70%, thus making walking an energy-efficient mode of locomotion.[21] At higher speeds, bouncing gaits are used in which the legs behave as more compliant springs. There is no significant energy savings (between kinetic and gravitational potential energy) in bouncing gaits; however, the elastic energy storage present in muscles, tendons, and ligaments provides some energy savings in these higher-speed gaits.[21]

Sprawling posture has also been defined as a posture or gait in which the humerus and femur cannot attain an orientation with their long axes directed vertically. It has been considered "primitive" based on its evidence in the earliest tetrapods; however, it may offer an advantage in climbing; inclined movement; sprinting; and frequent, rapid acceleration of small-bodied lizards.[7] The propulsive limb stroke has five phases: humeral/femur backswing, long axis rotation, forearm/crus rotation, forearm/crus flexion, and forearm/crus extension.[7] The limb movements are coordinated in a diagonal manner, which allows the body to remain in equilibrium during all phases of the movement cycle. This diagonal coordination during walking means the diagonal forelimb leaves the ground before and touches back down before the diagonally opposite hind foot.[7] As previously described, the anatomy of the lacertian stifle is asymmetrical and prevents significant rotation of the crus. Therefore rotation of the crus occurs at the cruropedal articulation.[7] The asymmetrical tarsometatarsus permits enough flexion for the crus to orient almost perpendicular to the pedal long axis, and thus the foot can act as an additional limb lever.[7] In larger-bodied lizards, and as the limbs increase in length, this sprawling posture/gait is less effective, because the horizontal action of the limbs fails to vertically lift the center of body mass, and the hind limbs can physically interfere with the action of the forelimbs.[7] This means the span of time in which the body is "suspended" is very short or absent.[7] The inherent problems of sprawling

posture and gait in large-bodied lizards can be overcome by bipedal locomotion, as this provides vertical lift of the cranial body mass and increased stride length yet does not increase speed.[7]

Bipedalism, which is classically associated with *Basiliscus basiliscus*, is a locomotive behavior exhibited by more than 50 species of lizards.[22,23] During bipedal locomotion, the trunk is elevated and the hind limbs power forward movement. The epaxial muscles allow for the cranial torso to be elevated, and there is no significant contribution from the forelimbs.[24] *Basiliscus* can begin bipedal motion from a resting position by thrusting both hind limbs, rapidly followed by one hind limb swinging around in a lateral arc to catch and support the weight of the body, thus creating the first bipedal step. The hind limbs arc laterally with each step, the pelvis rotates to increase body length, and the spine undulates laterally.[22] The proximal portion of the tail is elevated during bipedal locomotion, though the tip of the tail may drag. Though the hind legs actively participate in propulsion, the tail is critical for bipedal-ism and acts as a counterbalance to the trunk and head of the body. With decreasing tail length, bipedal locomotion is negatively affected.[24] When the caudal one-third of the tail was removed, bipedalism was only possible for a short distance, and when the caudal two-thirds was removed, bipedalism was not possible.[7] This is because the most powerful muscles causing hind-limb retraction (including the caudofemoralis muscle) are in the base of the tail, and tail removal may also disrupt neural feedback mechanisms to coordinate bipedal locomotion.[7] There is no difference in bipedalism based on substrate; however, there are differences in terrestrial and aquatic bipedalism. Lateral undulation of the spine is exaggerated in the water, likely to counter drag.[24] Locomotion analyses have not shown any energy or speed advantage of bipedalism over quadrupedal locomotion, though bipedalism may be utilized as a defensive posture or when escaping predators.[21–25] *Varanus* species specifically have been noted to take a tripodal stance balancing on the hind limbs and tail during times of intraspecific aggression.[7]

In species that display a more erect posture, like chameleons (and crocodilians during rapid locomotion), the humerus and femur are further depressed during the stance phase compared with sprawling lizards.[7] The humerus and femur undergo backswing in a vertical orientation, which requires less muscle bracing because upward thrust is braced by skeletal components. This transition to a more erect posture in chameleons was likely associated with the need to navigate narrow branches and is further associated with the grasping modifications of the feet.[7]

Other modes of lacertian locomotion include aquatic and sand swimming. No physical adaptations or modifications have been observed to accommodate aquatic locomotion, even in the marine iguana, *Amblyrhynchus*.[7] Many species are able to swim and do so by using body and tail lateral undulations. Species that burrow and move over shifting sand display a variety of toe fringes. These fringes can exist in various shapes and be present on one or all toes. Fringe morphology has been strongly correlated with substrate and enhances locomotor performance over loose sand, which is likely to be advantageous in escaping a predator or apprehending prey.[7]

Crocodilians. Crocodilians utilize a belly walk in a sprawling posture and a high walk in an erect posture (Fig. 81.7).[26] The crocodilian sprawling posture is functionally different than the sprawling posture of more primitive lizards and amphibians (where limbs are held laterally to the body). Kinematic analysis of the crocodilian sprawl has suggested it is actually just a lower version of the high walk and could more correctly be termed a "low walk."[26] The transition from the belly or low walk to the high walk in crocodilians occurs as speed increases and as they transition from wet and muddy substrates (belly walk) to drier substrates (high walk).[26] The belly walk is only used for short distances, usually as a transitional behavior to a high walk. They can also transition into a gallop at higher speeds or on heterogeneous substrates.[26] Crocodilians increase speed by recruiting the distal limb elements rather than of the proximal limb.[26] This strategy is completely different from that of other terrestrial vertebrates.[26] The percentage of the stride that the foot maintains contact with the ground (duty factor) does not change as speeds increase but rather stride length increases. This is quite unique, as most tetrapods increase speed by altering the swing and stance proportions of the stride and decreasing duty factor.[26] In addition to a constant duty factor, axial bending does not alter as speed increases.[26] In order to accomplish this, the ankle must attain a more plantar-flexed position at high speeds to allow quick ankle extension to generate propulsive force and stride elongation.[26] As speeds increase, the knee is flexed less in the swing phase, which results in a longer limb at the foot-down stance phase. The stride length and speed are increased as the longer limb (resulting from a more extended knee) is retracted, and the more flexed ankle is more quickly and forcefully extended against the ground.[26] Given these unique features of posture and locomotion, it is postulated that crocodilians evolved from erect ancestors and independently evolved a variable semierect posture.[26]

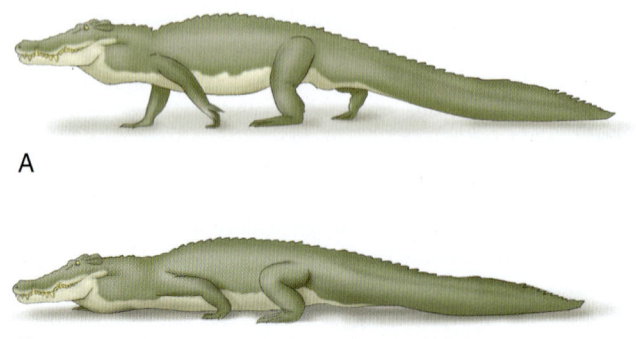

FIG 81.7 Representations of the "high walk" and "belly walk" or "low walk" postures of crocodilians. The "high walk" (A) is the primary posture for travel, whereas the "belly walk" or "low walk" (B) is a transitional posture typically used on wet or muddy surfaces. (Redrawn with permission by Educational Resources, University of Georgia.)

Bone Healing

A slower rate of fracture repair is expected, owing to the ectothermic nature of reptiles. The typical sequence of events in reptilian bone healing includes rapid epithelialization, sequestration of dead bony fragments, proliferation of the dural periosteum, organization and fibrosis of the callus, osteoblast differentiation, osteogenesis, and bony union.[27] Early fracture repair is defined by formation of proliferative periosteal, medullary, and intermuscular (parosteal) connective tissue (blastema) around the hematoma at the fracture site (Fig. 81.8A).[28] Cartilage and new bone are first deposited in the periosteal blastema, and later new bone is placed in the medullary blastema (Fig. 81.8B). The parosteal blastema develops similarly to granulation tissue. Cartilage is the primary tissue type in the periosteal blastema of amphibians and reptiles, whereas new bone replacement occurs slower than in mammals. New bone formation is also less regular, with invasion of new bone from all sides of the fracture. The vascular spaces are wider, with coarser endochondral bone trabeculae compared with mammals. The vascular spaces are eroded slowly, and the new bone matrix is deposited along the walls of these spaces. Calcification lags behind this process and depends on new ingrowth of blood vessels.[28] There is no evidence of secondary cartilage development in the fracture callus in reptiles and amphibians.[27] It is theorized that secondary cartilage arose late in vertebrate evolution and is limited to endothermic animals.[27]

GENERAL APPROACH TO CASE MANAGEMENT

Examination

A thorough clinical history and physical examination are critical to successful case investigation and management. Important husbandry data to discuss includes diet offered and diet eaten; vitamin and mineral supplementation including amounts, feeding method, and frequency; humidity range; temperature range; substrate; enclosure furniture; presence and type of water available (bowl, moving/filtered water feature, mister, fogger, dripper, etc); type of supplemental heat (heat mat, ceramic basking bulb, etc.) including location in/out of cage; use of thermostat, light timers, and associated settings; and light type (UVA, UVB, fluorescent, etc.), light cycle provided, and frequency of bulb replacement. It is also essential to establish a relationship of trust with the client or caretakers to permit effective client education in cases of inappropriate husbandry conditions. Management of caretaker expectations regarding case prognosis, time frame, required nursing care, need for referral, and financial investment is also critical.

Diagnostic Imaging

Clinical suspicion of musculoskeletal disease should warrant pursuit of diagnostic imaging for further injury or disease assessment. Radiographs are useful in evaluating bone cortical thickness and integrity, as well as presence and conformation of traumatic and pathological fractures and luxations. Osteomyelitis can also be evaluated radiographically, but it cannot be diagnosed solely based on radiographs. To diagnose osteomyelitis, demonstration of infection with histopathology and culture is required. In reptiles, osteomyelitis presents radiographically as lytic lesions. The periosteal reaction typically appreciated in mammals is not always a key feature in reptiles. Characteristic osteomyelitis in reptiles is defined as osteolysis with or without new bone formation or proliferation. This can resemble the appearance of neoplastic change in mammalian bone and can be misinterpreted as such in reptiles.

Computed tomography is often necessary to evaluate complex anatomical regions, fractures, osteomyelitis, and neoplasia. Chelonians may present a challenge to interpret bony structures radiographically due to the degree of bony superimposition with the carapace and plastron.

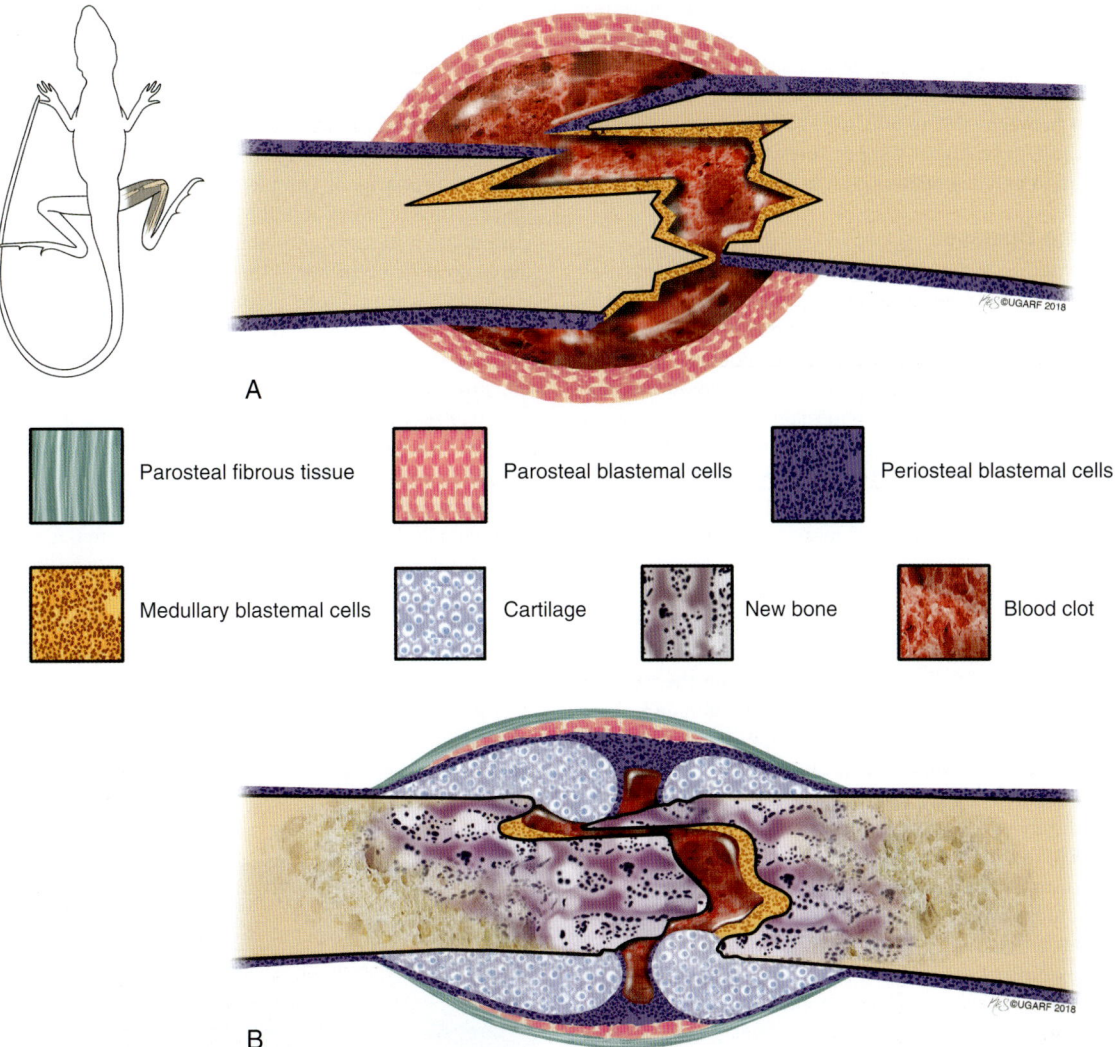

| Parosteal fibrous tissue | Parosteal blastemal cells | Periosteal blastemal cells |
| Medullary blastemal cells | Cartilage | New bone | Blood clot |

FIG 81.8 (A) The periosteal, medullary, and parosteal blastemal response of a fracture at early stage. (B) New bone, cartilage, and fibrous tissue at later stages of bone healing. (Redrawn with permission by Educational Resources, University of Georgia.)

Osteoderms in crocodilians can pose a similar challenge. Therefore CT may offer superior imaging in these species. For a more detailed discussion, see Chapters 53 through 57, 59 and 61.

Therapeutics

Therapeutics will depend on the underlying diagnosis. General assessment of patient condition by way of physical examination, clinical history, baseline clinicopathologic data (hematology and biochemistry profile), and imaging is important in guiding appropriate therapeutic choices. The most common therapeutics used in various musculoskeletal injuries or diseases include rest (strict confinement), splints, bandages, surgical fracture repair, amputation, low level laser therapy, physical therapy, nonsteroidal antiinflammatories, and correction of underlying mismanagement. Nutritional, thermal, and fluid support are critical in cases of metabolic bone diseases. In most cases, the use of analgesics and, when infectious agents are involved, antimicrobials is important. Appropriate tissue samples should be collected for cytology, histopathology, and culture to best guide antimicrobial choice, but initial selections with good bone penetration include tetracyclines and lincosamides.

MUSCULOSKELETAL DISEASES

Vitamin E and Selenium Deficiency

In reptiles, steatitis, fat necrosis, and muscular degeneration can be clinical and pathological signs of vitamin E deficiency. This typically occurs in animals fed diets high in polyunsaturated fatty acids (PUFAs) and/or rancid fats/oils. In crocodilians, deficiencies have been attributed to diets comprised of fish with high levels of PUFA and/or oxidative rancidity.[29] Vitamin E and selenium are antioxidants and protect from inflammatory damage. When diets high in PUFAs, rancid fish oils, or rancid fish are fed, these can cause fat necrosis, saponification, and resulting inflammation. Mortality from pansteatitis has been reported in crocodiles.[30] Clinical presentation is often vague, including lethargy, decreased intestinal motility, and presence of firm swellings (hardened fat deposits in coelom or tail).[10]

Diagnosis is made by biopsy or necropsy. Lesions may include yellow to brown discolored granulomatous steatitis and fat necrosis. Histological findings may include circumscribed zones of macrophages, multinucleated giant cells, ceroid, and hemorrhage.[31]

There is no effective treatment, though if caught early, vitamin E and selenium supplementation may be beneficial. However, steatitis generally carries a poor prognosis. Prevention is best accomplished by appropriate freezing and storage of fish fed to captive reptiles. Fish should be frozen between −18° to 30°C (0°–22°F) and used within 4 to 6 months, as storage at higher temperatures for longer durations can lead to oxidation and degradation of fish lipids.[32]

Metabolic Bone Diseases

Clinical Significance.

Metabolic bone disease is a general term used to describe a collection of medical disorders that affect the integrity and function of bones. The term metabolic bone disease (MBD) should always be accompanied by a qualifier such as "nutritional" or "renal." Metabolic bone diseases (MBDs) of various origins are the most common causes of lameness, skeletal, and spinal abnormalities in reptile patients. MBDs can manifest with a range of pathology, including nutritional secondary hyperparathyroidism (NSHP), renal secondary hyperparathyroidism (RSHP), fibrous osteodystrophy, osteomalacia, osteoporosis, osteopetrosis, pathological fractures, and more (see Chapter 84).

Known Etiological Cause(s) and Clinical Presentation

Nutritional secondary hyperparathyroidism. The most common of the MBDs is nutritional secondary hyperparathyroidism (NSHP). The layterm often used for NSHP, "rubber jaw," comes from the fact that animals with NSHP often have facial deformities that affect and soften the lower jaw. NSHP occurs as a result of an inappropriate diet and/or husbandry, with the most common factors being deficiency of dietary calcium or vitamin D_3, imbalance of the calcium-to-phosphorus ratio in the diet (usually an excess of phosphorus), or inadequate exposure to ultraviolet (UVB) radiation in diurnal animals. Nutritional secondary hyperparathyroidism can potentially affect all reptilian and amphibian species, but it is most commonly described in diurnal (herbivorous and insectivorous) lizards and chelonians. Affected animals may show thickening and swelling of the long bones and mandibles (Fig. 81.9), lameness, pathological fractures of the long bones and spine, horizontal (rather than the normal vertical) rotation of the scapulae, hypocalcemic tetany, tremors, muscle fasciculations, paralysis, paresis, hyperreflexia, cloacal or rectal prolapse, anorexia, inability or unwillingness to ambulate, and stunted growth. Swelling of the toes without evidence of external trauma may be noted. Fibrous osteodystrophy, trauma, gout, infection, and neoplasia should be considered as differential diagnoses. Affected joints are often firm, swollen, and have a limited range of motion. Long bone and/or joint swelling can result from healed or healing fractures, luxations, gout, pseudogout, neoplasia, osteomyelitis, septic arthritis, or NSHP. Degenerative joint disease related to trauma or aging may also be an underlying cause of digital swelling. Chelonians often present

with a misshapen and/or soft shell. Radiographs can reveal a variety of findings, including reduced cortical thickness and opacity of long bones, fibrous or periosteal proliferation, soft tissue swelling, and pathological or folding fractures (Fig. 81.10).

In most snakes, crocodilians, some chelonians, and some amphibians, a nocturnal lifestyle or ingestion of whole prey have allowed vitamin D_3 to be primarily or completely obtained from the diet.[33] However, diurnal, insectivorous, or herbivorous reptiles (particularly lizards, some chelonians, and some amphibians) require UVB exposure to activate the cholecalciferol pathway.[33] Under natural conditions, reptiles synthesize vitamin D_3 when exposed to sunlight. Ultraviolet light in the spectrum (290–320 nm) reacts to convert cholesterol to the inactive form of vitamin D_3 in the skin. This vitamin D_3 is then converted to 1,25 dihydroxycholecalciferol (calcitriol) through the liver and kidneys. Calcitriol is then used to facilitate absorption of calcium from the intestinal tract. In captivity, an alternative to natural sunlight that mimics the spectrum of natural light is required. A number of artificial lighting systems are available that provide an ultraviolet light spectrum (see Chapter 17). However, these UV lights are often a poor replacement for natural sunlight, and natural sunlight should be provided whenever possible. When an animal cannot be provided with proper exposure to ultraviolet light, vitamin D_3 supplementation can be considered; however, there are serious risks associated with hypervitaminosis D.

In clinical cases of NSHP, excessive production of parathyroid hormone from the parathyroid gland occurs in response to the diet or husbandry-related hypocalcemia. Calcium is then resorbed from the bones to compensate for this deficiency. Osteopenia results and weakens

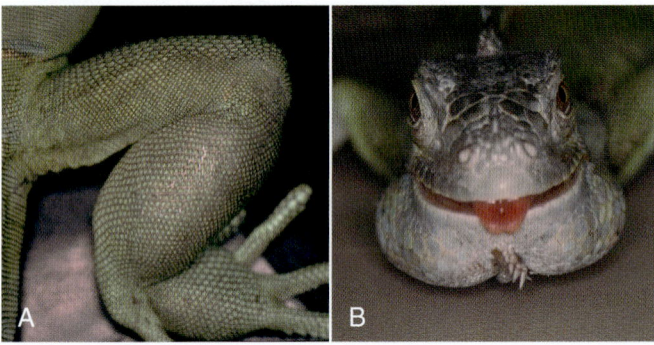

FIG 81.9 Subadult green iguanas (*Iguana iguana*) with nutritional secondary hyperparathyroidism. (A) Fibrous proliferation of the long bones often causes palpably firm limb swellings. (B) Mandibular swelling and shortening as a result of muscle tension and weakened bones. (Courtesy of Stephen J. Divers.)

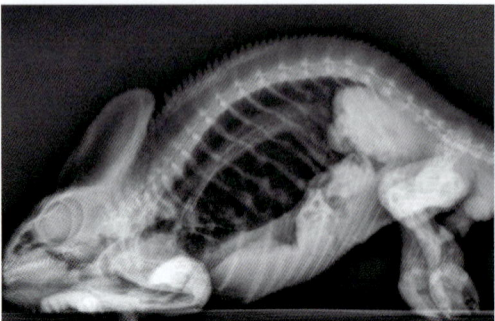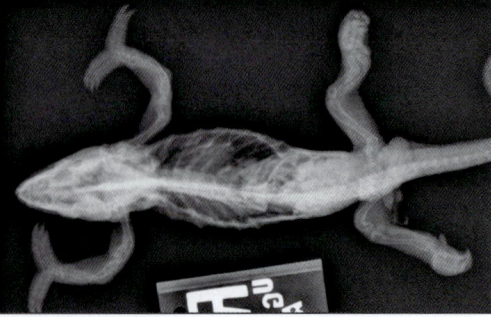

FIG 81.10 Orthogonal radiographs of a veiled chameleon (*Chamaeleo calyptratus*) with secondary renal hyperparathyroidism. Note the thin cortices, poor overall bone quality, and folding bone deformities consistent with osteomalacia and pathologic folding fractures. Enlarged kidneys in the caudodorsal coelom are also visible. (Courtesy of Stephen J. Divers.)

the bones. Clinical pathology findings often reveal low normal blood calcium levels late in the course of disease. As blood calcium decreases, parathyroid hormone (PTH) increases, which increases blood calcium by stimulating bone resorption and renal tubular reabsorption of calcium. Phosphate excretion in the urine is also increased. PTH stimulates formation of 1,25 dihydroxycholecalciferol, which increases absorption of intestinal calcium. Calcium deficiency can increase the threshold potential of nerves and muscles, thus causing partial depolarization. This can present as spastic tremors and twitching of the digits.

Various metabolic bone diseases are seen in young crocodilians and may manifest in different ways depending on the cause (e.g., nutritional, renal). Weakness, lethargy, kyphosis, scoliosis, paresis, tooth decalcification, and other skeletal abnormalities can be observed in crocodilians as well. This is seen less often as improved diets are offered to captive crocodilians. Nonetheless, some crocodilian operations may still fail to offer a source of calcium in the diet. The innate requirement of ultraviolet-B light as a source of vitamin D_3 in crocodilians is not known. They appear to be able to obtain appropriate levels from their diet, but research in this area is still needed. There are reports of adult alligators raised in enclosed buildings and offered a pelleted diet with some meat supplement that show no evidence of metabolic disease. However, anecdotal comments from various ranchers indicate that the animals appear to thrive better if exposed to sunlight. This is also true of captive amphibians, as historically it has been suggested they do not require UVB exposure. However, MBD is commonly diagnosed in amphibian species, and it is believed that exposure to UVB lamps or natural sunlight is important to overall health.

Renal secondary hyperparathyroidism. Renal secondary hyperparathyroidism (RSHP), a consequence of chronic renal disease, is characterized by hyperphosphatemia. The hyperphosphatemia is associated with low calcitriol levels, soft tissue calcification, renal osteodystrophy, and hypocalcemia. Because excretion of phosphorus is a sum of glomerular filtration and tubular resorption, in renal failure the decreasing filtration rate leads to phosphorus retention and resulting hyperphosphatemia. Phosphate retention along with decreased production of calcitriol result in low normal or low serum calcium levels.

Diagnostic Confirmation. Diagnosis is typically based on signalment and historical information regarding species, age, husbandry (temperature, humidity, UVB lighting), diet, clinical signs, and radiography. Radiographs typically show poor mineralization of the cortices and deposition of fibrous tissue and may show evidence of pathological fractures, either recent or healed. Exaggerated or abnormal long bone shape and curvature can be suggestive, as well as irregularity, lysis, or fractures of the ribs, jaw, spine, and other bones. Clinical pathology is also useful in advanced cases as changes in calcium, phosphorus, electrolytes, and other metabolites may further support the diagnosis. It is important to remember that total calcium may not accurately reflect the metabolically available calcium, and an ionized calcium level is much more informative but seldom decreases until the final stages. In cases of swollen joints, radiography, arthrocentesis, or fine-needle aspiration with cytology, culture, and fluid analysis are all warranted diagnostics to help guide appropriate treatment.

Most discussions of MBDs in reptiles focus on UVB light exposure, diet, and calcium supplementation. Although these are critical for overall health of captive reptiles, it has also been demonstrated that there is a critical interaction with vitamin A in the development of MBDs in captive chameleons.[34] UVB exposure is one of the most important aspects of proper captive reptile husbandry. Oral vitamin D_3 supplementation given to bearded dragons, even at high doses, was ineffective in producing plasma vitamin D_3 levels similar to bearded dragons who were exposed to UVB radiation.[35] Further, if previously adequate UVB exposure is provided, plasma vitamin D_3 levels can be maintained up to 83 days in bearded dragons.[36]

Specific Therapy. Initial treatment for NSHP should focus on stopping bone loss and promoting new bone production. Low blood calcium stimulates PTH secretion, and when the blood calcium concentration is above normal, PTH secretion is halted. Calcitonin, which is produced from the ultimobranchial bodies, then increases. Therefore the mainstay of treatment for MBDs includes oral or parenteral calcium supplementation. Some practitioners warn of increase risk of adverse effects with IV, IM, or SQ administration and recommend oral calcium supplementation.[33] The authors have not had any known adverse events from administering diluted subcutaneous calcium gluconate at 100 mg/kg every 24 hrs during the initial critical period. However, care should be taken to monitor calcium and phosphorus levels during treatment, with special attention paid to the solubility index, as renal function may be compromised. The ratio of calcium and phosphorus is a reliable indicator of (early) renal disease. The solubility index is calculated as the product of Ca (mmol/L or mg/dL) x PO_4 (mmol/L or mg/dL) and is normally less than 9 mmol/L (55 mg/dL). If the solubility index rises above 12 mmol/L (70 mg/dL), then healthy tissue will start to mineralize, whereas between 9 mmol/L (55 mg/dL) and 12 mmol/L (70 mg/dL), mineralization of diseased tissue (kidneys) occurs.[37]

Affected animals should be housed in enclosures with padded substrate or soft towels, and climbing branches and other enclosure furniture should be removed or lowered to a height that will reduce risk of fractures or other trauma should the animal fall. Hydration and oral supplementation of vitamin A are also important to support renal health. Parenteral supplementation of vitamin D_3 is not generally recommended, because overdose and vitamin D_3 toxicity may occur. Thorough evaluation of current husbandry and clear recommendations for corrections must be made to caretakers. In cases of long bone fractures, these may heal quickly once calcium homeostasis returns, but surgical repair should be avoided or considered carefully as the bones may be too soft to hold hardware, and any reptile suffering from MBD is at a higher risk for an anesthetic complication. Splints and bandages are typically best in these cases.

Prognosis and Prevention. Prognosis generally depends on the stage of disease at the time of diagnosis, as early intervention in some cases can result in resolution of clinical signs and provide a near-normal life expectancy when underlying causes are addressed. When there is significant organ function impairment (e.g., renal secondary hyperparathyroidism) and/or systemic infection, prognosis is guarded to poor. Tremors, ataxia, and cloacal prolapses are all early signs, whereas fibrous osteodystrophy, pathological fractures, and paralysis suggest significant disease and carry a worse prognosis. Female lizards and turtles that have severe deformities resulting from NSHP may have difficulty laying eggs due to the deformity of the pelvis and may benefit from elective ovariosalpingectomy. Fractures of the spine carry a more guarded to poor prognosis, especially if limb, intestinal, or bladder function is compromised.[33] In these cases, euthanasia may be appropriate. It is important to note that even animals with severe resulting scoliosis may survive, and although they will be deformed, they tend to do well as pets. Owners should be well advised of the nursing care required, risks of further complications, and realistic prognosis for recovery given the disease state of the individual. Pain medication and nutritional support should also be included in any treatment plan for MBD.

Trauma and Fractures

Fractures can be traumatic, infectious, or metabolic in origin. Traumatic causes can include bite wounds, closure in a cage door or lid, fall from a perch or branch, or interaction with a prey animal. Fractures should be accurately described as traumatic or pathological, complete (transverse, oblique, spiral, comminuted), incomplete (bowing, buckle, greenstick), or Salter-Harris (types I to V). In addition, the location of the fracture (diaphysis, metaphysis, epiphysis), whether it is displaced (angulation, translation, rotation, distraction, or impaction), open or closed, and whether there is any joint involvement should be documented.

Clinical Significance, Known Etiological Cause(s), and Clinical Presentation. Trauma and fractures are common presentations in captive reptiles and can be the result of a myriad of causes. Demineralization, osteomyelitis, abscessation, or neoplasia can weaken a bony area and result in an associated fracture. Large breeding male chelonians may traumatize a limb by falling off the female's carapace during courtship and copulation. Trauma is also common in captive crocodilians, usually the result of fighting, transport, or restraint. Limb fractures and partial amputations can be seen after altercations. On some crocodilian farms, animals have reportedly lost limbs after fights and demonstrated complete healing. Similar lesions can also be observed in wild alligators. These may also lead to nerve or muscle damage and consequent paresis or paralysis.

Fractures or trauma can also result in paresis or paralysis. However, paresis and paralysis can also result from neurological abnormalities. Spinal cord or vertebral lesions including those secondary to MBD, spinal abscesses, ossifying spondylosis, and spinal tumors have been reported.[38–42] Fecal and or urolith impactions can present as a caudal paresis and usually resolve with treatment. Neurologically related postural abnormalities may be mistaken for musculoskeletal signs. See Chapter 77 for a more detailed discussion.

Diagnostic Confirmation and Specific Therapy. Diagnosis is most often made using a combination of data obtained through a thorough clinical history, physical examination, and imaging. Radiography is the most common imaging modality, though ultrasound, computed tomography, and nuclear scintigraphy may all have utility (Fig. 81.11).

Principles of fracture fixation are similar to those utilized in mammals and are described in more detail in other chapters (including Chapters 108 through 110). Rib fractures generally do not need to be treated unless they are protruding or penetrate an organ. Head fractures in snakes may be difficult to detect on skull radiographs, and CT is preferred. However, the presence of pain, swelling, or palpable abnormalities may suggest trauma or fracture. Lower jaw fractures may heal if they are closed, reduced well, and the snake is not fed for a period of time to allow callus formation. Esophagostomy tube feeding may be required. External fixators can be constructed, but the cage must be kept bare so the fixators do not get caught on cage furniture or bedding.

Prognosis and Prevention. Prevention of trauma and fractures depends on maintenance of safe, secure, and appropriate enclosures, adequate husbandry, social groupings, and safe handling/restraint. Prognosis depends largely on the nature of the traumatic injury or fracture. When the animal is to be released back to the wild, there will be a different set of criteria used compared with a captive animal. Therefore careful consideration of the species, animal "occupation," healing potential, quality of life, and owner commitment should all be included when determining an individual animal's prognosis.

Osteomyelitis and Arthritis

Clinical Significance. Osteomyelitis is the localized or generalized inflammation and destruction of bone from pyogenic infectious agents (Antinoff, Proc ARAV, 1997, pp 149–152). Osteomyelitis can cause local inflammation, periosteal proliferation, stiffening of joints, bone destruction, reduced range of motion, septicemia, and death (Fig. 81.12). Septic arthritis and tenosynovitis refer to inflammation of the synovial structures, particularly joints. Most cases are infectious but articular gout can also cause joint inflammation. Clinical presentation of osteomyelitis and septic arthritis is unfortunately quite common, as inadequate husbandry and associated immunosupression are predisposing factors in many captive reptiles.

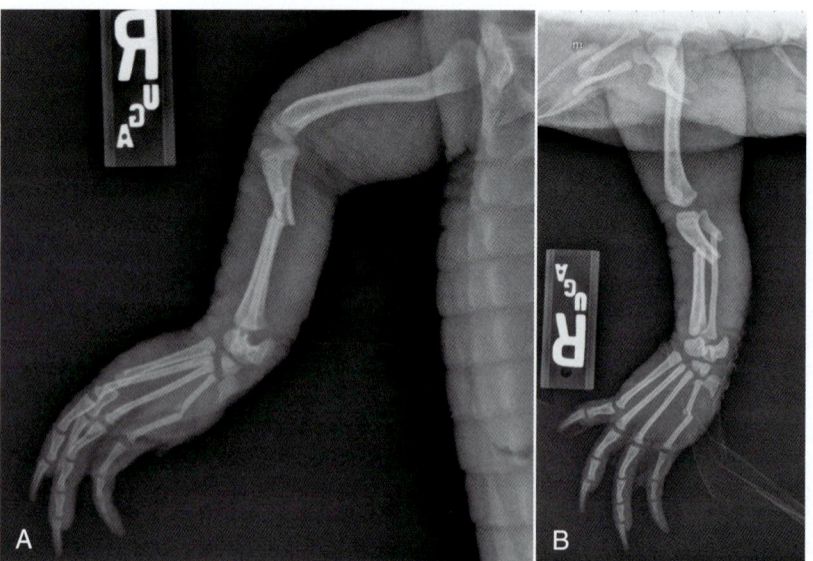

FIG 81.11 Orthogonal radiographs (A, dorsoventral; B, lateral) of the right pelvic limb of a juvenile American alligator (*Alligator mississippiensis*) demonstrating closed, complete, transverse fractures through the proximal diaphysis of both the right tibia and fibula. There is moderate to severe angulation and impaction but no evidence of osteolysis, metabolic bone disease, or joint involvement. Additionally, there is a closed, complete, transverse fracture through the middiaphysis of metatarsal IV, which demonstrates no evidence of osteolysis and only minor displacement. (Courtesy of Stephen J. Divers.)

Known Etiological Cause(s) and Clinical Presentation. In most cases, trauma and/or immunocompromise are predisposing factors. Inappropriate husbandry including low temperature, poor/unhygienic substrate, overcrowding, excessive humidity, poor diet, and stress all contribute to immunosuppression and bacterial colonization by opportunistic organisms (e.g., *Salmonella* spp., *Proteus*, *Pseudomonas*, *Citrobacter*, *E. coli*, and *Staphylococcus* spp.). Most microbial organisms involved in infectious processes in reptiles are normal flora, which become opportunistic pathogens during times of stress and immunosuppression. Introduction of pathogens to tissues and secondary vascular dissemination can occur as a result of traumatic injury.[43] Infection of the toes from external trauma and vascular compromise is common in reptiles that get caught in the wire mesh of the enclosure, or in carpeting/fabric in their environment, or in relation to dysecdysis with retained skin constricting the toes. Trauma and secondary infection of the mandible is also seen frequently in lizards (Fig. 81.13). When combined with poor husbandry, these local infections may progress and often become systemic. Generalized signs of illness, such as inappetence and lethargy, may result. Microorganisms such as *E. coli*,

Salmonella, and other coliform bacteria are often found in blood or joint cultures in such cases. Cuts and open wounds caused by improper housing often result in swelling, even once the external wounds have healed. In crocodilians, *Mycoplasma alligatoris* and *M. crocodyli* can cause polyarthritis, which may be evident antemortem. *Mycobacterium* spp. are common in the environment. Potentially pathogenic species in reptiles include *M. marinum*, *M. chelonei*, and *M. thamnopheos*. These bacteria are commonly isolated or identified from interdigital lesions. In addition to causing localized dermal infections, mycobacteria can also cause systemic disease that is usually fatal.

Diagnostic Confirmation. Diagnosis is typically made using a combination of clinical history, physical examination, radiography, culture and sensitivity, histopathology, and clinical pathology data. Radiographic changes associated with osteomyelitis in reptiles are quite different than mammalian lesions. Osteomyelitis in reptiles appears radiographically as lytic lesions, and this lysis may persist long after the infection has been cleared (Fig. 81.14).[43] Although mammals typically display a periosteal reaction on radiographs, this is often less recognizable in reptiles.[43] Lysis without new bone formation is often characteristic of osteomyelitis in reptiles. This can resemble neoplasia in mammalian bone, and it is important not to misinterpret this finding in reptiles. Arthritis if often associated with enlarged joint spaces and can progress to destruction of the articular surfaces and subchondral bone.

Bone biopsy and histology can be useful in demonstrating the presence of organisms, though special stains may be needed in cases of fungal or mycobacterial involvement. Affected bone may be osteolytic or osteoporotic.[43] Joint aspiration for cytology and microbiologic cultures are often useful. Microbial cultures or MIC levels are useful to direct antimicrobial therapy. Hematology may show a systemic heterophilia, indicative of an active inflammatory response. Toxic heterophils may also be present in cases of advanced bacterial infections. Monocytosis or azurophilia may be present in cases of infectious disease.[43]

Specific Therapy. Treatment should focus on surgical debridement of affected bone and soft tissues followed by aggressive antimicrobial therapy based upon culture and disc sensitivity, or better still, MIC testing. Given the granulomatous nature of the reptile inflammatory response, antimicrobial penetration of affected tissue and bone may be limited. Antimicrobial selection should be based on cytology (gram

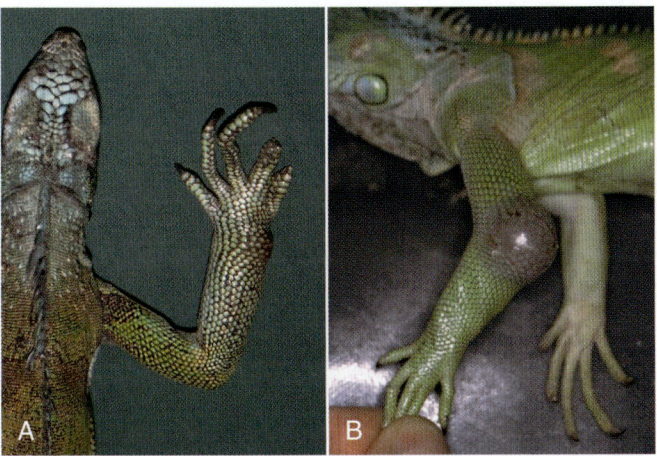

FIG 81.12 (A) Pronounced soft tissue swelling associated with distal ulnar and carpal osteomyelitis in a green iguana (*Iguana iguana*). (B) Pronounced elbow swelling due to septic arthritis in a green iguana. (Courtesy of Stephen J. Divers.)

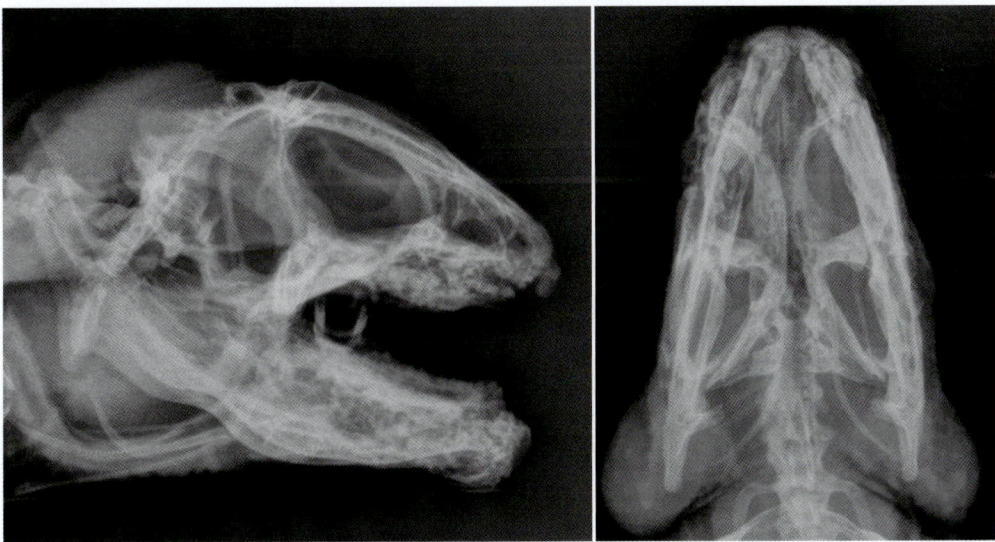

FIG 81.13 Lateral and dorsoventral radiographs of an iguanid skull demonstrating lytic and proliferative changes consistent with osteomyelitis. (Courtesy of Stephen J. Divers.)

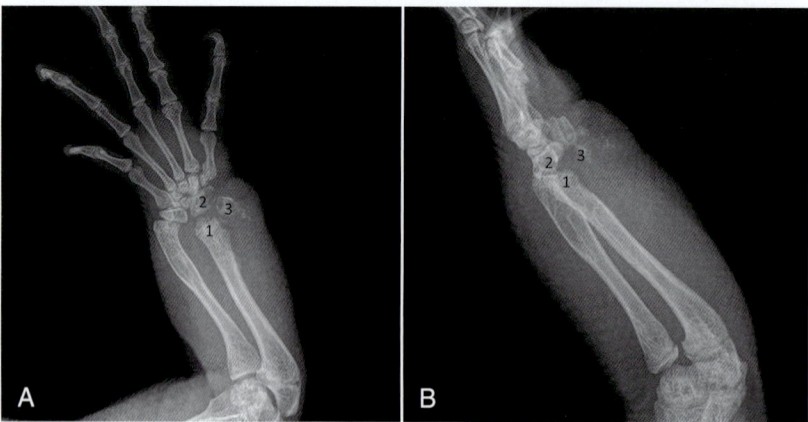

FIG 81.14 Dorsopalmar (A) and lateral (B) radiographs of the right forelimb of a green iguana (*Iguana iguana*) demonstrating osteolysis associated with the distal ulna (1), ulnar metacarpal bone (2), and accessory carpal (or pisiform) bone (3). There is also pronounced soft tissue swelling associated with the carpus. These radiographic findings are consistent with osteomyelitis but biopsy is required for confirmation. (Courtesy of Stephen J. Divers.)

stain), culture and sensitivity (or MIC), and histopathologic analysis. Oral versus injectable medications need to be selected with the species and owner abilities in mind. Antimicrobials should be selected for their ability to penetrate bone and initial gram-stain results. Acceptable initial choices include tetracyclines, first- and second-generation cephalosporins, basic and potentiated penicillins, potentiated sulfonamides or aminoglycosides. Modification of therapy should be based on culture and sensitivity data and may require fluoroquinolones, third-generation cephalosporins, or advanced penicillins. Intravenous or intraosseous administration of the first doses should be administered whenever possible, as this may establish therapeutic concentrations more rapidly than other administration routes. Thereafter, intramuscular, subcutaneous, or oral administration should be continued for a minimum of 4 weeks.[43] Cultures should ideally be repeated every 2 to 4 weeks to monitor response to treatment. Repeat radiographs may also aid case management decisions, though it is important to remember that radiographic changes can lag behind clinical changes. Septic joints should be thoroughly lavaged and antimicrobials can be instilled into the joint space. When the articular cartilage and subchondral bone have been destroyed, joint function cannot be regained. Therefore even if infection can be resolved, arthrodesis or amputation is typically required because of a persistently nonfunctional, painful joint.

Appropriate analgesia and supportive care should be included in the treatment plan as needed. Amputation, when necessary, may be a viable alternative to euthanasia in some patients. Treatment of mycobacterial infection is not recommended because of the risk of creating antibiotic resistance to a potentially zoonotic organism. If only the distal portions of an extremity are associated with the infection, amputation may be a realistic alternative to euthanasia.

Prognosis and Prevention. If diagnosis is made early and infection remains mild or localized, then aggressive treatment can be successful. However, clinical disease can also be severe and debilitating. If the diagnosis is made late in the disease process, where significant bone is affected or septicemia is present, then therapeutic efforts may not be successful. Mycobacterial infections carry a poor prognosis and euthanasia is typically recommended.

Noninfectious Arthropathy and Gout
Clinical Significance. Gout is a metabolic disease characterized by overproduction or underexcretion of uric acid resulting in hyperuricemia

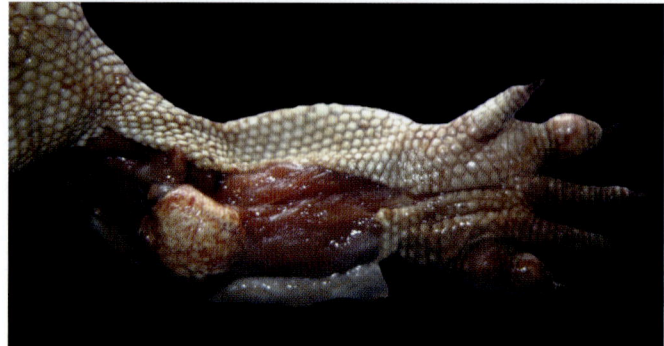

FIG 81.15 Periarticular gout in a savannah monitor (*Varanus exanthematicus*). Note the periarticular accumulation of tophi around the elbow and the swelling of several digits. (Courtesy of Jorge Orós.)

and deposition of positively birefringent monosodium urate (MSU) crystals in tissues.[44]

The most common noninfectious arthropathies seen in reptiles are articular/periarticular gout (MSU) and pseudogout (hydroxyapatite deposition disease, calcium pyrophosphate dihydrate deposition). These disease entities are significant in pet reptiles, as they often reflect deficiencies in captive husbandry and nutrition (e.g., dehydration, high-protein diets, inbalances of vitamins and minerals) or severe renal dysfunction.

Known Etiological Cause(s) and Clinical Presentation. Articular/periarticular gout and pseudogout have been reported in many lizard species. Gout consists of radiolucent MSU deposits in or around the joints, whereas pseudogout consists of radiopaque calcium deposits (Fig. 81.15). Deposits of urate crystals are called tophi and consist of a complex of MSU crystals surrounded by granulomatous inflammation. Differentiating between these diseases can be difficult with lysis and deposition of crystals/material often seen in the metatarsal/carpal-phalangeal joints. Gout also occurs in crocodilians as either the articular or visceral form. High-protein diets, dehydration, and stress are contributing factors. Deficiencies of vitamins A, B, C, or E can also lead to a variety of musculoskeletal disorders. These are not commonly seen when commercial diets are fed in addition to meat products. Clinical signs can be nonspecific in nature, but limb paresis/paralysis and joint enlargement may be observed. Tophi may also be noted in mucous membranes during the oral examination.

Diagnostic Confirmation. Plasma biochemistry, diagnostic imaging, fine-needle aspirate cytology, and often surgical biopsy and histopathology may be necessary to confirm a diagnosis. Whole-body survey radiographs or CT may demonstrate mineralization in other organs. CT shows crystal aggregates but does not enable specific identification of urate acid crystals. Dual-energy CT distinguishes urate crystals from deposits containing calcium.[45] Ultrasonography shows urate crystal deposits as hyperechoic images without posterior acoustic shadowing, which enables their differentiation from calcifications.

Cytological examination by phase contrast microscopy of joint aspirates is also useful to identify urate crystals. When using polarized light, the tissues must be fixed in absolute ethanol, because urate crystals tend to degrade and wash out during formalin (aqueous solution) fixation.[46] Determination of the glomerular filtration rate using iohexol excretion can also be useful to evaluate the renal function.[47] Differential diagnoses include hydroxyapatite deposition disease and pseudogout or calcium pyrophosphate dihydrate deposition and can be differentiated based on histological appearance, histochemical staining for calcium, and birefringence under polarized light.[46,48,49] See Chapters 66 and 84 for a more detailed discussion.

Specific Therapy, Prognosis, and Prevention. Treatment is aimed at slowing or stopping further progression rather than reversing existing damage or curing the disease. Fluid therapy and rehydration, as well as analgesic and antiinflammatory drugs, are typically indicated. Uricostatic drugs reduce uric acid production through competitive inhibition of xanthine oxidase, and allopurinol is most commonly used and has been shown to effectively reduce uric acid levels in iguanas.[50] Other uricostatic drugs (e.g., oxypurinol and febuxostat) are used in humans, but their efficacy in reptiles is unknown. Uricosuric drugs (e.g., sulphinpyrazone, probenecid, benzbromarone) are also used in human medicine to increase urinary uric acid excretion by blocking urate anion reabsorption by proximal renal tubule epithelial cells. However, such reabsorption is likely very low in reptiles, and so the efficacy of this therapeutic approach may be poor. Pegylated uricase therapy (pegloticase and pegadricase reserved for selected human patients) reduces urate levels by increasing its metabolism.[45]

In cases of localized gout, surgical removal by arthrotomy or amputation may be curative. Correction of vitamin deficiencies and any husbandry inadequacies is important.

Localized articular or periarticular gout carries a fair to poor prognosis depending on the state of progression and extent. When visceral gout or renal compromise is present, the prognosis tends to be poor to grave. In all cases of gout, the comfort of the animal and quality of life should be considered, as it is known to be a painful process in humans.

Spinal Osteopathy

Definition and Clinical Significance. Spinal osteopathy has been described in turtles, lizards, and snakes. Although it has been compared with osteitis deformans (Paget's disease) in humans, the condition in reptiles is believed to be a chronic bacterial osteomyelitis of the spine in most cases.[51] In reptiles, the lesions are progressive and proliferative, resulting in variable ankyloses. Eventually, reptiles are unable to move or feed.

Known Etiological Cause(s) and Clinical Presentation. In humans, a similar condition is known as osteitis deformans (Paget's disease), which is a localized disorder initially marked by excessive bone resorption followed by deformity and then excessive bone formation. These cycles cause the bone to become dense and fragile. Pathological fractures are common, and the condition is believed to be painful. Cases of osteitis deformans are most often associated with a septic or autoimmune condition of the spine.[51,52] Many snakes with this disorder have active inflammatory changes from which bacteria have been isolated, such as *Salmonella*, *Klebsiella*, *Morganella*, and *Providencia*.[51] Therefore this condition in reptiles is believed to be a chronic bacterial osteomyelitis of the spine (Fig. 81.16).[51]

Affected animals may present initially with focal swellings visible along the dorsum or sides of the body. Palpation of the spine may reveal segments of ankylosis, kyphosis, scoliosis, or lordosis. Digital pressure may also prove painful, with the animal resenting palpation. Kyphosis and scoliosis of the spine are often observed in green iguanas and other lizard species (Fig. 81.17), resulting from genetic defects, malnutrition, or pathology of the epaxial muscles. Spinal osteopathy, osteomyelitis, or metabolic abnormalities can all cause a lizard's spine and tail to become stiff, resulting in an altered gait. However, older iguanas may present with similar changes to the tail, which do not appear to be

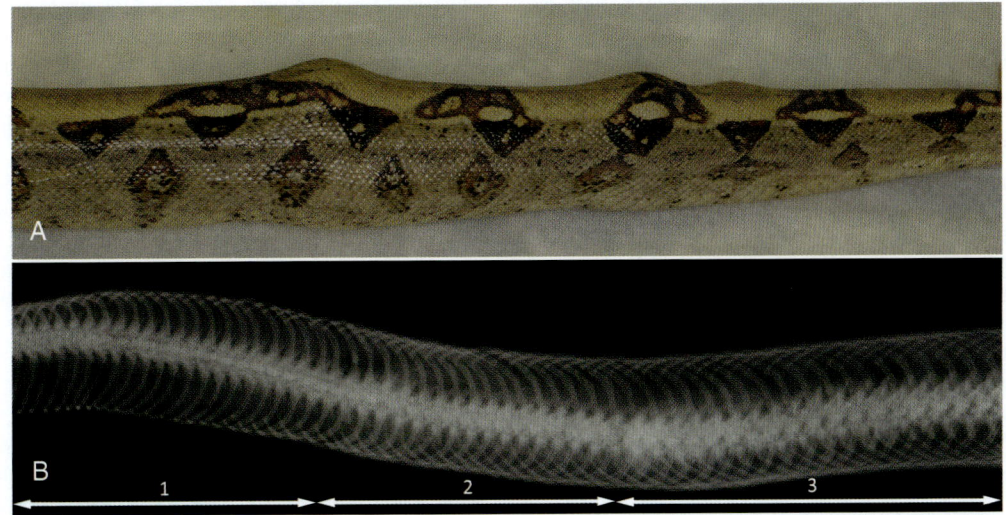

FIG 81.16 Spinal osteopathy in a *Boa constrictor*. (A) Clinical presentation demonstrating deformity and swellings associated with the spine. (B) Dorsoventral radiograph of the spine demonstrating normal spine (1), as well as mildly (2) and severely (3) affected regions of the spine. (Courtesy of Stephen J. Divers.)

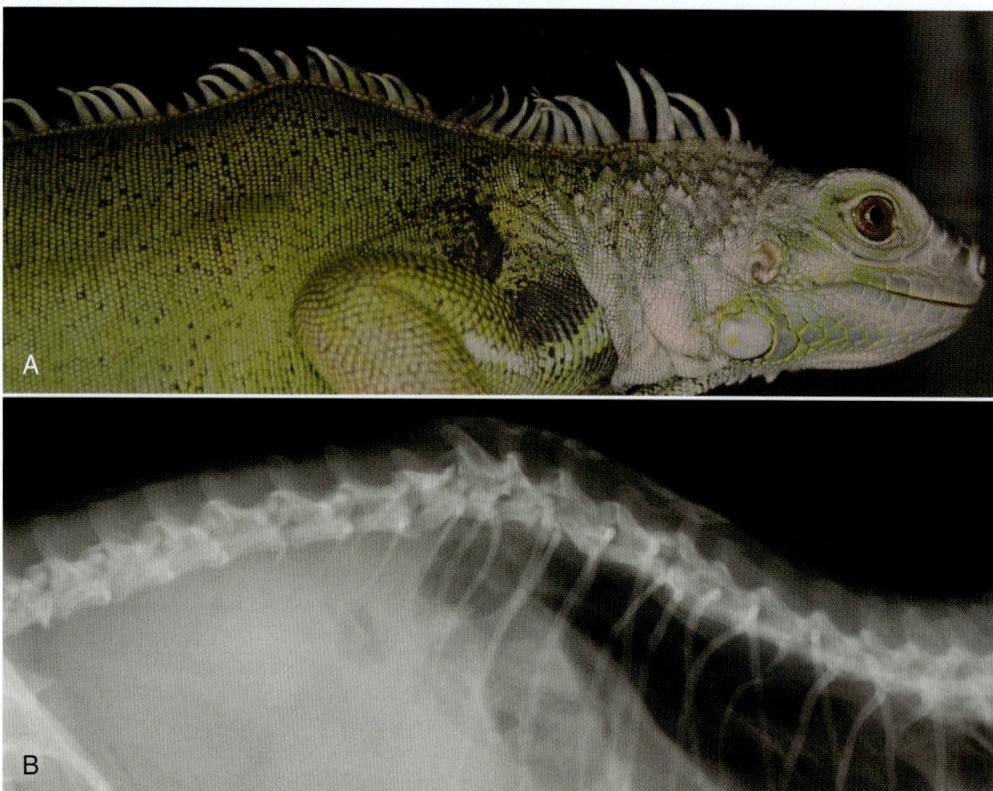

FIG 81.17 Pathological spinal fractures due to nutritional secondary hyperparathyroidism in green iguanas (*Iguana iguana*) presenting with kyphotic spines. (Courtesy of Stephen J. Divers.)

related to bacterial involvement. Therefore a thorough history and clinical investigation should help differentiate these disease processes.

Diagnostic Confirmation. Definitive diagnosis is accomplished by radiography or CT, biopsy, and bone or blood culture. Radiography is useful to confirm the presence of spinal disease but cannot identify active infection or inflammation. Comparison between pre- and postcontrast CT can assist in identifying inflammatory lesions. Bacterial culture (and sensitivity testing) of blood, bone biopsies, or joint fluid may help isolate bacteria and guide treatment. Histopathologic lesions include chondro-osseous metaplasia, active osteomyelitis, epidermal ulceration and necrosis, subperiosteal reactive bone, fibrocartilaginous metaplasia with bone resorption and osteoclasis, vascular thrombosis, infarction, spondylosis, granulomatous inflammation, and thrombosis.[53]

Specific Therapy, Prognosis, and Prevention. Most described therapies have been unsuccessful. However, effective treatment depends on early identification of causative agents, aggressive treatment with appropriate antibiotics, and delivery of antimicrobials to the affected bony site. In lizards, particularly green iguanas, amputation of a large portion of the tail can be a useful therapeutic option to help with pain.[53] Long-term antibiotic therapy may be helpful at slowing progression of disease, but the long-term prognosis is guarded to poor. Reptiles with spinal osteopathy carry a poor to grave prognosis, as most animals have advanced lesions by the time of diagnosis.[53]

Neoplasia
Clinical Significance. Neoplasia is defined as an abnormal growth of tissue.[54] The growth of neoplastic tumors may form a space-occupying lesion, invade organs, or inhibit or alter the function of the immune system.[54] Neoplasia is relatively uncommon in the literature, likely because it is underreported, with the incidence of neoplasia in reptiles reported as 12% to 26%.[55,56] Snakes are most commonly reported as affected by neoplasia. Reviews of reported tumor types in reptile species provide more thorough details on disease presentations and management.[54,56,57]

Known Etiological Cause(s) and Clinical Presentation. Most tumors in reptiles are spontaneous in origin, but some tumor types have a known cause. Several viruses have been identified for their carcinogenic potential in association with tumors, including herpesvirus, papovavirus, and poxvirus.[56] Reported tumors of musculoskeletal origin include chondrosarcoma in two related monitor lizards and a corn snake (*Pantherophis guttatus*), osteosarcoma in Woma python (*Aspidites ramsayi*), undifferentiated sarcoma in a radiated tortoise (*Astrochelys radiata*), periosteal chondroma in a spiny-tailed lizard (*Uromastyx*), chondroblastic osteosarcoma in a spiny-tailed monitor (*Varanus acanthurus*), rhabdomyosarcoma in a Galapagos tortoise (*Chelonoidis nigra*), adenocarcinoma in an Asian leaf turtle (*Cyclemys dentata*), and mucinous melanophoroma in a red-bellied cooter (*Pseudemys rubriventris*).[55,56] Musculoskeletal neoplasia often presents as a swelling or growth, lameness, or both (Fig. 81.18). Other clinical signs can include tremors, ataxia, lethargy, and anorexia.

Diagnostic Confirmation. Diagnosis is made based on histopathology; however, a thorough history, physical examination, clinical pathology, imaging, and cytology may be important diagnostic aids. Complete blood count and plasma biochemistry results should be performed to assess overall health of the patient, to determine the presence and degree of systemic involvement of disease, and for preanesthetic evaluation. Some hematopoietic tumors (lymphoma and leukemia) may also be associated with marked lymphocytosis.[56]

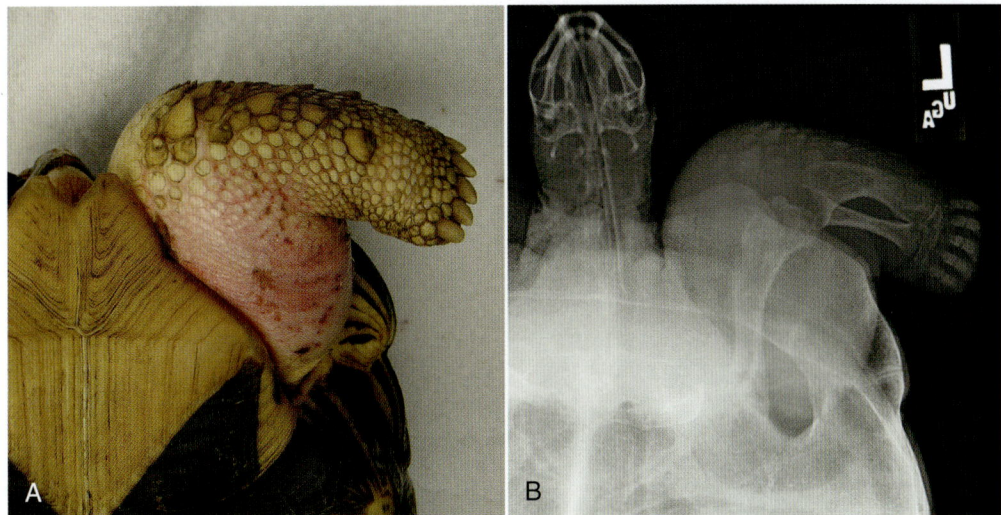

FIG 81.18 (A) Radiated tortoise (*Astrochelys radiata*) with gross swelling associated with the left pectoral limb. (B) Dorsoventral radiograph of the same limb demonstrating a pronounced increase in soft tissue associated with the limb musculature, which is causing subluxation of the left elbow. There is no evidence of calcification, mineralization, or gas. Histopathology revealed an undifferentiated sarcoma. The tortoise did well following amputation. (Courtesy of Stephen J. Divers.)

Orthogonal radiographs are always required for appropriate interpretation. Dorsoventral and horizontal beam lateral views of the whole body should be obtained, along with a cranial-caudal view in chelonian species. More advanced imaging technologies, especially pre- and postcontrast CT, often aid in diagnosis, assessment of the extent of disease, and surgical planning.

Specific Therapy, Prognosis, and Prevention. Cancer treatment plans for reptiles are similar to those of other species. Local disease is best treated with local therapy, whereas systemic disease should be treated with systemic therapies.[56] Chemotherapy and radiation may be curative or palliative, where the differences in protocol intent dictates different dosing strategies in terms of intensity and frequency of the chemotherapeutic agent or radiation. Thorough, well-documented client communication is important before pursuing chemotherapy or radiation so that the intent and goals are clear. There is a paucity of information available on effective chemotherapy and radiation in reptiles. Therefore it is important that owners understand that extension of life span or improved quality of life cannot be guaranteed.[56]

Surgical excision may be curative in cases of local tumors, and all excised tumors should be submitted for histopathology and margin evaluation. In some cases, amputation may be recommended, or follow-up treatment with chemotherapy or radiation may be indicated if there is evidence of tumor extension beyond the surgical margins. Prognosis depends on the tumor type, grade, and stage. Given the lack of information in published literature regarding case management, general prognostic guidelines may be borrowed from the small animal literature until more data are available regarding the outcomes of various neoplastic types in reptiles.

Disorders of the Tail
Clinical Significance, Known Etiological Cause(s), and Clinical Presentation. Disorders of the tail may result from a variety of causes, including mechanical or infectious agents. Tails generally hold an important function, either for social signaling or as a locomotive aid. Damage to, or disorders of, the tail are usually the result of congenital defect, nutritional secondary hyperparathyroidism, trauma,

or infection. Avascular necrosis of the tail is relatively common in lizards. The distal tail becomes hard, dry, stiff, and discolored. A zone of devitalized tissue characterized by swelling, erythema, and occasional serous discharge often exists between necrotic and healthy tissue. More than one etiology can cause these clinical signs. When the clinical signs occur after venipuncture of the ventral caudal vein, iatrogenic vascular damage may be a factor. Likewise, trauma and hematogenous spread of infection can be involved (Fig. 81.19). Swelling of the ventral tail base, adjacent and caudal to the cloacal opening, in male lizards usually involves the hemipenes. Some male lizards, such as green iguanas and various species of chameleons, undergo dramatic enlargement of the hemipenes with sexual maturity.

Diagnostic Confirmation, Therapy, Prognosis, and Prevention. Diagnostics should focus on determining an underlying cause and include a detailed history, physical examination, and husbandry information. Radiography, CT, hematology, biochemistry panel, tissue culture, blood culture, cytology, and/or histopathology should all be considered. Specific therapy depends on a definitive diagnosis but would likely include wound cleaning and debridement, treatment of any fractures or other trauma, appropriate selection of antimicrobials based on culture and sensitivity testing, analgesics, and modification of the environment if indicated. Additionally, in cases of poor peripheral circulation, low-level laser therapy has been used successfully by the author and is believed to increase perfusion and help support healing.

Supernumerary Limbs
Clinical Significance. Supernumerary limbs are caused by digenic trematodes, specifically *Ribeiroia ondatra,* and the condition most commonly affects the hind limbs of amphibians. It is a particularly prevalent cause of limb deformities in the western United States, including California, Oregon, Washington, and Montana, although the parasite has been detected across much of the United States.[58] In multiple species of frogs and toads, laboratory and field studies show that even low levels of *Ribeiroia* infection can induce 30% to 95% mortality, and frogs often do not survive to sexual maturity.[58–60] This high mortality has grave consequences for affected frog populations.

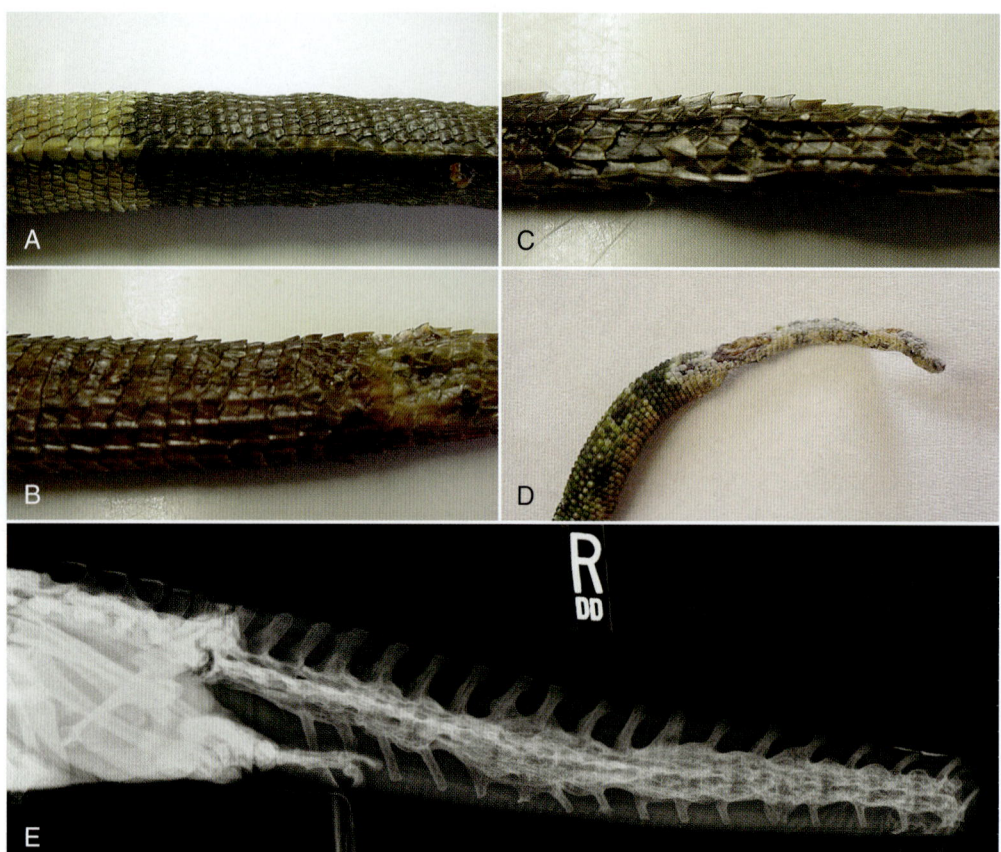

FIG 81.19 (A) Undulations and swellings along the tail of a green iguana (*Iguana iguana*) with bacterial osteomyelitis. (B) Sepsis and necrosis associated with the tail of a green iguana. (C) Ischemic, dry necrosis of the distal tail of a green iguana. (D) Tail necrosis in a chameleon several weeks following repeated venipuncture. (E) Lateral radiograph of a green iguana tail demonstrating proliferative and lytic changes characteristic of (but not pathognomonic for) osteomyelitis. (Courtesy of Stephen J. Divers.)

Known Etiological Cause(s) and Clinical Presentation. *Ribeiroia* has a predilection for limb buds and has been shown to cause polydactyly, polymelia, and jaw malformations in many anuran species.[58–60] The cercarial larval stage of the trematode penetrates the skin to form cysts (metacercariae), which are preferentially localized in the cloacal region, including the developing hind limb regions in larval amphibians. Frogs with parasite-induced deformities are less able to jump, swim, obtain food, or survive to maturity. Deformities have been reported in threatened or endangered amphibian species, including the California red-legged frog (*Rana draytonii*).[58] Given the high mortality associated with this deformity, the impact of infection on a given population can be significant. A single case report exists of encysted digenetic trematodes of the genus *Clinstomum* causing scoliosis in a tiger salamander (*Ambystoma tigrinum*).[61] The herbicide atrazine is the best predictor of larval trematode exposure in northern leopard frogs (*Rana pipiens*).[62] Field study data also supported a causal mechanism where agrochemicals atrazine and phosphate, which are used commonly in corn and sorghum production, increased exposure and susceptibility to larval trematodes by increasing snail intermediate hosts and suppressing amphibian immunity.[62]

Diagnostic Confirmation, Therapy, Prognosis, and Prevention. Little is known about the best strategies for early diagnosis and intervention. Currently, there is no effective treatment once supernumerary limbs have formed. Efforts should be focused on minimizing exposure of larval amphibians to trematodes and pesticides.

Spindly Leg
Clinical Significance, Known Etiological Cause(s), and Clinical Presentation. Spindly leg is a developmental abnormality of the forelimbs and occasionally hind limbs of amphibians, defined as skeletal and muscular underdevelopment. This disease process is only appreciated in captive anurans, which initially appear healthy as tadpoles and often initially develop normal hind limbs. As metamorphosis progresses, the forelimb buds may appear, and the hind limbs may develop valgus or varus deformity. Often one or both forelimbs will fail to erupt normally, and the limbs produced will be thin and delicate. Several factors are known to affect or interrupt metamorphosis, including antibiotics, goitrogenic substances, and other toxins. Additionally, limb malformation in froglets can result from trauma, environmental crowding, genetics, and nutrition. The exact nutrients that may be involved in normal metamorphosis are yet to be determined, but it is believed that deficiency in one or more B vitamins may be a contributing factor in spindly leg.[63] Criteria for staging the disease has been proposed from stage 0 (normal limbs) to 5 (rear limbs extremely stunted and forelimbs do not emerge) (Fig. 81.20).

Diagnostic Confirmation, Therapy, Prognosis, and Prevention. Froglets that survive complete metamorphosis typically die within a few days. The degree of severity can vary from mildly affected forelimbs with normal hind limbs to complete absence of forelimbs with deformity of hind limbs (see Fig. 81.20). It has been recommended to supplement

Stage	Affected Limb	Description
5	R	Rear limbs are extremely stunted or absent, remaining in Gosner stages 25–30 despite tadpole body development to metamorphosis (Stage 42–44). *
	F	Forelimbs do not emerge (Pre stage 40).*
4	R	Rear limbs are small, stunted, and stiff (Stages 31–35). Toes have not developed fully and are not sepaated.*
	F	Forelimbs emerge underdeveloped (stage 41–42), and are very thin. Toes on forelimbs may be underdeveloped or virtually absent.**
3	R	Rear limbs are stunted and stiff, and toes have developed (Stages 36–39). Legs do not bend and may splay outwards.*
	F	Forelimbs appear fully developed, but thin (Stage 42). In some cases, one forelimb may fail to emerge (Stage 40–41), or may emerge abnormally- i.e. both limbs emerge from the same side of the body.**
2	R	Rear limbs are fully developed, but thin (Stage 40). Legs splay outwards, and may be crossed.*
	F	Forelimbs emerge with developed toes (Stage 42), but are held abnormally- i.e. parallel ageinst the body. Forelimbs may be very thin and weak.**
1	R	Rear limbs are fully developed (Stage 40), but thin. At rest tadpole or metamorph does not fully bend legs, but legs do not splay outwords.*
	F	Forelimbs emerge fully developed (Stage 42) and normally positioned, but thin and weak. Metamorph is able to prop itself up, but mobility is compromised.**
0	R	Rear limbs are toes fully developed and appear normal (Stage 40). Tadpole may progress through remaining stages as normal, or metamorph may exhibit forelimb abnormalities.
	F	Forelimbs emerge compheteley and appear normal (Stage 42). Metamorph is able to hold itself up and move normally, and progresses through remaining stages as normal.

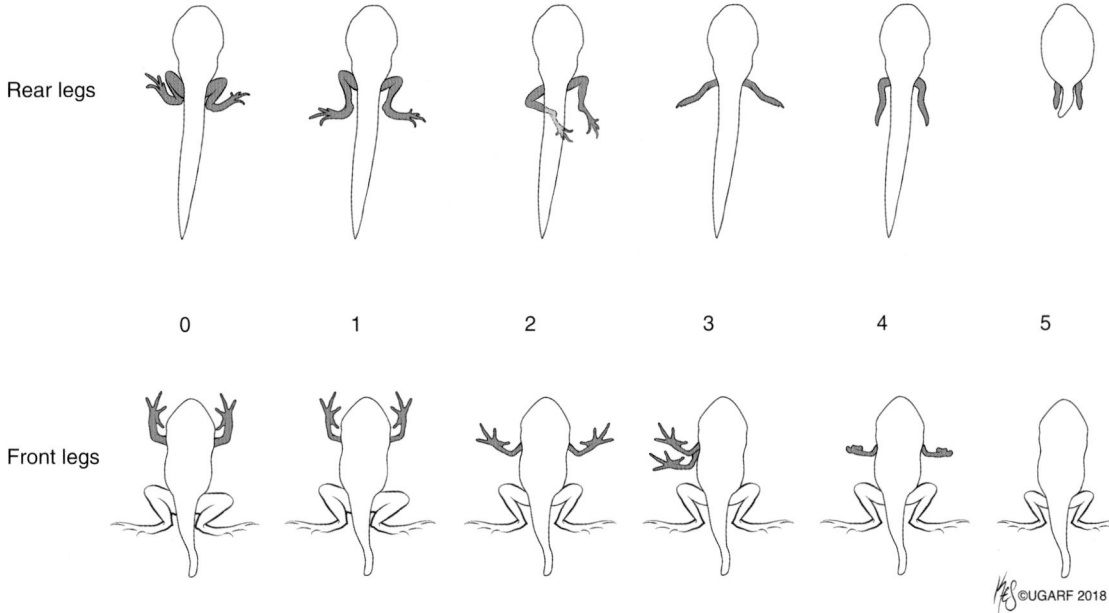

FIG 81.20 Spindly leg syndrome (SLS) classification scale for tadpoles and metamorphs.[63] A value of 5 represents the earliest detectable developmental stage at which SLS occurs, whereas 0 represents no clinical signs of SLS. In stages 1 to 5 affecting forelimbs: continued development up to tail resorption may occur while limbs remain stunted, although most will perish before reaching this point. Stages 1 to 4 affecting rear legs: most metamorphs are unable or struggle to hold their head above water or climb out of water, and they may not be able to pursue prey. High instances of drowning occur. R, Rear limb; F, forelimb. (Redrawn with permission by Educational Resources, University of Georgia, from Claunch N, Augustine L. Morphological description of spindly leg syndrome in golden mantella *(Mantella aurantiaca)* at the Smithsonian National Zoological Park. *J Herp Med Surg.* 2015;25:72–77.)

water with B complex for eggs and developing larvae. Most information to date has focused on tadpoles and froglets, but the nutrition of the parents must also be considered.[5]

Rhamphotheca and Digits

Overgrowth of the rhamphotheca and toenails may indicate an underlying nutritional deficiency such as nutritional secondary hyperparathyroidism or protein excess. Lack of wear in captivity has been suggested as a cause, yet overgrowth is generally not a problem in captive turtles on balanced diets.[4] Elongated nails (but not rhamphotheca) on the front or rear feet (not both) is a normal secondary sex characteristic in some aquatic chelonians. Overgrown nails and rhamphotheca may reflect lack of wear or protein excess.

Problems in the feet can be related to deficient husbandry, whether it be incorrect temperature, humidity, or diet. In cases of missing toes or nails, husbandry and shedding history of the patient should be obtained. Retained shed (dysecdysis) around the digits can form strictures that compromise circulation to the appendage, resulting in necrosis and sloughing of the toe. This condition can be exacerbated with inadequate humidity in the enclosure, which impedes proper shedding. Additionally, carpet fibers or hair can wrap around the digits with a similar effect. Chameleons frequently catch their nails in the mesh of the cage as they climb up the sides, which may lead to infections of the digits and joints.

Congenital Deformities

Congenital malformations of the head may include foreshortening of the upper jaw, cleft palate, and microphthalmia. Short, absent, or kinked tails may also be seen. Many of these deformities are seen in captive-bred snakes, including shortened jaws, restricted orbits, domed cranial vaults, arched necks or spines, and various types of spinal kinks and bends. Congenital defects may be a result of genetic defects or improper environmental conditions during incubation, primarily temperature levels that are too high or too low for some or all of incubation (see Chapter 85). Gravid ovoviviparous or viviparous females subjected to improper temperatures might also produce dead or deformed young. A possible role of inbreeding is often postulated but rarely well-documented. Defects that appear later in life may be genetic or the result of external factors, including infection, trauma, neoplasia, and malnutrition. Tail tips may be damaged by parasites, such as *Alaria* flukes or ticks, or by trauma (prey or predator bites).

ACKNOWLEDGMENTS

The author would like to thank Stephen Divers and Scott Stahl for their friendship and guidance over the years and Mike Karlin for his thoughtful review of this manuscript.

REFERENCES

See www.expertconsult.com for a complete list of references.

82

Vascular, Hematopoietic, and Immune Systems

Simon Girling

This chapter deals with the medical aspects of disease associated with the vascular, hematopoietic, and immune system. Discussion of the normal anatomy and physiology of these systems may be found in Chapters 7 through 12.

VASCULAR ANATOMY AND PHYSIOLOGY

Chemoreceptors

Chemoreceptors have been identified in the aortae, common carotid artery, and pulmonary artery of turtles, with oxygen-sensing cells innervated by the tenth cranial nerve.[1] The morphology and size of the cells resemble glomus cells in mammals and are thought to have a similar function in sensing changes in blood oxygenation and regulating respiration and blood cardiovascular shunting.

Vascular Shunting

It has been shown that reptiles can shunt blood through the heart and between the great vessels emanating from the heart depending on lung function and blood gas levels (see Chapter 68 cardiology). Blood flow from the caudal half of a reptile's body may pass through the parenchyma of the kidneys via the caudal, hypogastric, or iliac veins (renal portal system, RPS). Any drugs injected into the caudal half of the body may therefore potentially be excreted by the renal tubules (but not the glomeruli) before entering the general venous circulation. Nephrotoxic drugs (such as the aminoglycoside family) administered in the caudal half of the body may have greater nephrotoxicity, because it is theoretically possible for the drug to be directed into the kidney parenchyma very rapidly and at high concentrations, leading to enhanced toxic effects. The RPS shunting mechanism is not as straightforward as this, and many facets have not been fully elucidated. Common practice has been to avoid giving potentially nephrotoxic medications, or medications primarily removed from the body via the kidneys (e.g., ketamine), in the caudal half of the reptile patient.

In snakes, blood flow volume to the intestines and hepatic portal system can increase by up to 30% and portal venous flow up to 300% following feeding.[2–4] Blood flow may also be shunted preferentially to peripheral limbs and extremities when the reptile is warm or to the core of the reptile when its body temperature is cool, suggested to be due to decreased or increased vasomotor tone, respectively.[5]

VASCULAR DISEASES

Metabolic Vascular Disease

Hypervitaminosis D$_3$ or abnormalities associated with the calcium/phosphorus ratio (which may be caused by secondary or primary hyperparathyroidism) can lead to metastatic mineralization. In green iguanas (*Iguana iguana*) and a plumed basilisk (*Basiliscus plumifrons*), pulmonary vessel metastatic calcification in association with an erythroid response has been described.[6] The plumed basilisk also showed evidence of aortic mineralization. In the majority of these cases the following pathologic abnormalities were also noted: hyperphosphatemia with an inverted calcium/phosphorus ratio; chronic renal failure; and renal gout. Dystrophic vascular mineralization has also been suggested as associated with stress, high lipid diets, hypercholesterolemia, hepatic lipidosis, and low daily activity levels.[7,8]

Bacterial Thromboembolic Disease

Embolic septicemia caused by *Salmonella* spp. has been reported as a cause of atrial thromboembolism in a green iguana.[6] This may lead to showers of microthrombi in the bloodstream, likely affecting other vessels and vital organs. Other sources of bacterial thromboemboli include severe periodontal disease, which is commonly seen in lizards with acrodont dentition. One such example resulted in hepatic artery thromboembolism in inland bearded dragons (*Pogona vitticeps*) associated with *Pseudomonas* spp. bacteria seeding from the periodontal infection[9] (Fig. 82.1).

Congenital and Developmental Vascular Diseases

Congenital aortic stenosis has been reported in a green iguana with secondary ventricular dilation.[10] The iguana presented clinically with a history of inappetence, lethargy, increased respiratory rate, and a change in skin coloration.

Aneurysms have been reported in bearded dragons and Burmese pythons (*Python bivittatus*).[10,11] This author has seen aneurysms arising from the internal carotid artery or the aorta. A firm but fluctuant swelling is often seen on the dorsolateral neck or cranial coelomic cavity respectively. The etiology of aneurysms in reptiles is currently unknown.

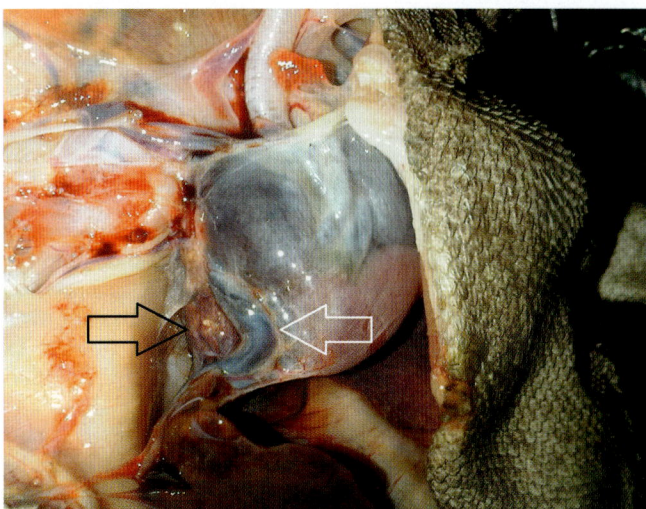

FIG 82.1 Lung bacterial granuloma due to *Pseudomonas aeruginosa* (black arrow) in a bearded drago, which had migrated into the wall of the caudal vena cava (white arrow). (Courtesy of Simon Girling.)

It has been suggested they may be the result of trauma to the affected vessels due to the superficial position of the carotid arteries in the dorsolateral pharyngeal area. However, this does not fully describe all cases of aortic aneurysms, and some may be associated with congenital wall defects in a high blood pressure vessel, as is seen in mammals and birds. These aneurysms have been successfully surgically removed, with patients surviving months to years afterward.

HEMATOPOIETIC SYSTEM AND IMMUNOLOGY

Cellular Immunology

Cellular immunity can be specific or nonspecific. Specific cellular immunity in vertebrates is associated with lymphocyte function. In reptiles, evidence of B and T lymphocyte equivalents has been known for some time.[12] There is also evidence of subsets of T and B lymphocytes, for example, T-helper lymphocytes.[13] Additionally, it has been found that variations exist in the population of subsets of lymphocytes and in the lymphocyte numbers themselves over the course of the year, particularly in species that undergo hibernation or aestivation. Non-specific cellular immunity is seen with mononuclear leucocytes, such as monocytes and azurophils, and granulocytes, such as heterophils, basophils, and eosinophils. Blood and bone marrow cell types are described in more detail in Chapters 33 and 37.

Humeral Immunology and Acute Phase Proteins

Humeral immunity may be specific or nonspecific. Specific humeral immunity is clearly associated with immunoglobulins and in lower vertebrates is assumed to be comprised of IgY (the equivalent of mammalian IgG but has facets of IgE activity) and IgM (which functions in reptiles as a combination of the IgM and IgA antibodies in mammals). So far IgE and IgD have not been proven to exist in reptiles, but subsets of IgY may cover some of their spectrum of functions.[14] Nonspecific humeral immunity is associated with interferons, transferrins, lysozymes, complement, and other acute phase proteins. As with birds, the accurate determination of albumin and globulin levels in reptiles should be performed using plasma protein electrophoresis. Standard dry chemistry systems are frequently inaccurate in this assessment because many reptiles, particularly but not exclusively chelonians (as with birds), have prealbumin and other proteins that appear to the left of albumin on the electrophoretogram. Many act as a carrier protein often for thyroxine.[15] Plasma is preferred for protein electrophoresis in reptiles, as one of the major acute phase inflammatory proteins is fibrinogen. As there are few serodiagnostic tests available for reptiles through commercial laboratories, plasma protein electrophoresis can be a useful aid to detecting infectious/inflammatory disease[16] (Figs. 82.2 and 82.3).[16]

HEMATOPOIETIC DISEASE

Hemoparasites

Hemoparasites are commonly seen in pet reptiles, particularly in wild-caught species. The majority of these parasites are nonpathogenic. Table 82.1 lists some of the more commonly seen protozoal hemoparasites of reptiles (see also Fig. 82.4). For further and more detailed information, readers are urged to consult Chapter 32.

Helminths—Family Ascarididae

Nematodes (e.g., Ophidascaris). A Papuan python (*Apodora [Liasis] papuana*) that was in captivity for a number of years died after a brief period of anorexia and at postmortem had adhesions between the aorta and esophagus.[22] The aortic wall contained numerous aneurysms and fibrous nodules along its length from which large nematodes were removed and identified as *Ophidascaris papuanus.* Similar nodules were seen in the peritoneum of the coelomic cavity.

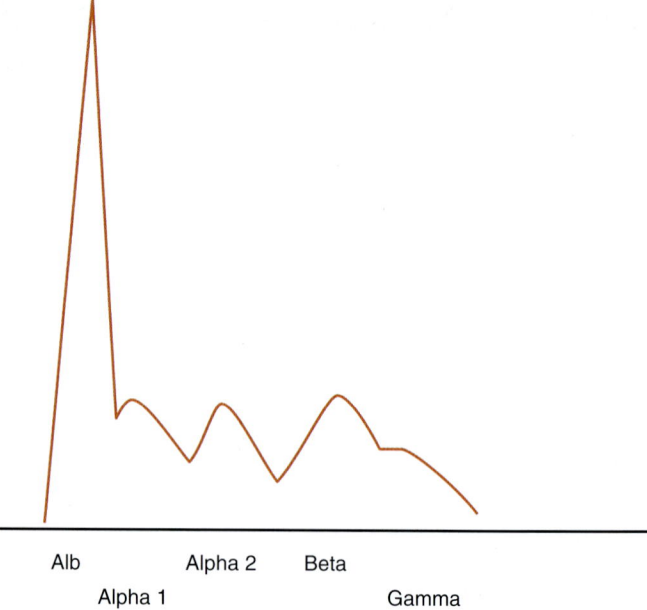

FIG 82.2 A plasma protein electrophoretogram from a clinically healthy bearded dragon (*Pogona vitticeps*). Alb, Albumin; Alpha 1, alpha 1 globulins; Alpha 2, alpha 2 globulins; Beta, beta globulins; Gamma, gamma globulins.

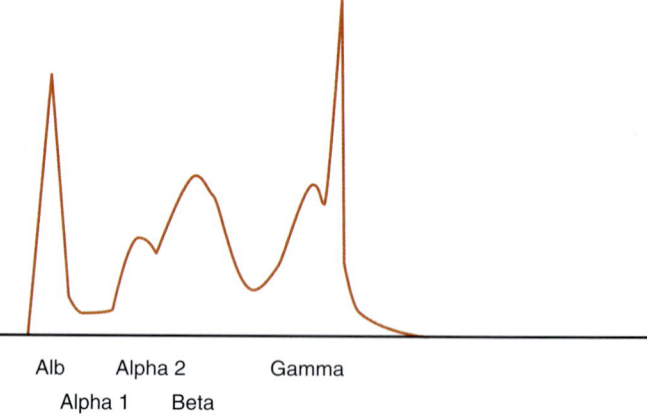

FIG 82.3 A plasma protein electrophoretogram from a bearded dragon (*Pogona vitticeps*) with lymphoma. Note the monoclonal antibody spike in the gamma globulin peak associated with the condition. Alb, Albumin; Alpha 1, alpha 1 globulins; Alpha 2, alpha 2 globulins; Beta, beta globulins; Gamma, gamma globulins.

Helminths—Family Onchocercidae, Subfamily Dirofilariinae

Microfilaria (e.g., Foleyella, Oswaldofilaria). Microfilaria are commonly seen in lizards but may affect any reptile. The intermediate host range includes ticks, mites, and mosquitoes. Filarid wormlike organisms may be seen free in the plasma. The parasite may cause blockage of terminal vessels. Treatment is by maintaining the affected reptile at environmental temperatures of 35° to 37°C (95°–99°F) for 24 to 48 hours to kill the adult worms, although with large worm burdens anaphylaxis may occur, and care should be taken to monitor the reptile for signs of heat stress.[23]

Trematodes—Family Spirorchidae

Digenetic Spirorchid Flukes (e.g., Spirorchis, Henotosoma, Vasotrema). These are seen most commonly in chelonians, particularly marine turtles. Aquatic snails (e.g., *Lernea* spp.) are believed to be the intermediate hosts. Trematode eggs are rarely seen in peripheral blood smears. Pulmonary tissue biopsy and squash preparation are often required to diagnose infection.[24] Adult flukes rarely cause clinical disease,

TABLE 82.1 Common Protozoal Hemoparasites of Reptiles

Hemoparasite Genus	Vector	Reptile Species Reported	Pathogenicity and Appearance in Blood	Treatment Reported
Order Haemosporida				
Plasmodium	Aedes or Culex spp. mosquitoes or Culicoides spp. midges. Other blood-sucking ectoparasites may also act as vectors, but scant information available.	Mainly chelonians but also reported in snakes, and Plasmodium relictum has resulted in fatalities in juvenile lizards.	In the blood, schizonts, micro-, and macrogametocytes in the cytoplasm of erythrocytes may be observed, as well as in mononuclear cells and endothelium of blood vessels.[17] These are often refractile. They can cause severe hemolytic anemia. It is possible to see extramedullary hematopoiesis, as well as vascular occlusive disease in the brain, heart, and so on due to swelling of the endothelium of vessels.	Treatment of chelonians with chloroquine at 125 mg/kg, orally every 48 hours for 3 treatments/occasions has been suggested as effective[18]
Haemoproteus	Dipteran biting flies and mosquitoes, possibly mites.	Mainly lizards, some turtles, and occasionally snakes.	Gametocytes seen in erythrocytes and are refractile. It is rarely pathogenic.	Rarely pathogenic, therefore treatments not reported.
Saurocytozoon	Believed to be mosquitoes.	Mainly lizards.	Resembles Leucocytozoon spp. in birds with gametocytes in leucocytes and immature erythrocytes. The organism lacks pigmentation. It is rarely pathogenic.	Rarely pathogenic, therefore treatments not reported.
Order Eucoccidiorida				
Haemogregarina	Leeches and possibly dipteran flies. On American alligators (Alligator mississippiensis) the leeches are Placobdella multilineata and P. papillifera.	It has been reported in aquatic species—mainly freshwater turtles (e.g., Haemogregarina stepanovi in Emys orbicularis), tortoises of the genera Geomyda and Testudo, the tuatara (Sphenodon punctatus), many snakes, and some crocodilians. Pathogenicity is seen occasionally with Haemogregarina crocodilinorum in wild American alligators.	Sporogeny occurs in an invertebrate ectoparasitic intermediate host (often leeches). The hemoparasite may also accumulate in the liver, spleen, and lung of the reptile as well as the bloodstream. Blood smears demonstrate erythrocytic inclusions, micro-, and macrogametocytes, which are rarely refractile.	Rarely required as considered nonpathogenic, with the exception of American alligators, which have occasionally resulted in disease, therefore treatments not recorded.
Haemolivia	Chelonian tick Hyalomma aegyptium is the definitive host (the reptile is the intermediate host).	Tortoises act as the intermediate host (e.g., Haemolivia mauritanica in Testudo graeca and T. marginata).[19]	Blood smears demonstrate erythrocytic inclusions, micro-, and macrogametocytes, which are rarely refractile.	Rarely pathogenic, therefore treatments not reported.
Hepatozoon	Arthropods such as the snake mite, Ophionyssus natricis, act as the vector.	Mainly seen in terrestrial snakes.	Sporogeny occurs in an invertebrate intermediate host. The organism may also accumulate in the reptile's liver, spleen, and lung, as well as the bloodstream. Blood smears demonstrate erythrocytic inclusions, microgametocytes, and macrogametocytes. (See Fig. 82.4).	Rarely pathogenic, therefore treatments not reported.
Karyolysus	Arthropods (e.g., the lizard mite, Hirstiella trombidiiformis) can act as vectors. It is transmitted through the feces of the intermediate host.	Mainly seen in old world lizards and tree snakes.[20]	Sporogeny occurs in an invertebrate intermediate host. The organism may also accumulate in the reptile's liver, spleen, and lung, as well as the bloodstream.	Treatment in snakes with quinacrine at 20–100 mg/kg orally every 48 hours for 2 weeks has been shown to be effective.[21]

Continued

TABLE 82.1   Common Protozoal Hemoparasites of Reptiles—cont'd

Hemoparasite Genus	Vector	Reptile Species Reported	Pathogenicity and Appearance in Blood	Treatment Reported
Lainsonia	Mites of dipteran biting insects thought to be intermediate hosts.	Primarily seen in lizards.	Clinical pathology shows unpigmented inclusions in leucocytes and thrombocytes. The parasite enters the reticuloendothelial system and sporozoites may be refractile. No pathology has been reported.	Rarely pathogenic, therefore treatments not reported.
Schellackia	Mites of dipteran biting insects thought to be intermediate hosts.	Generally seen in new world reptiles.	Clinical pathology demonstrates the parasite in leucocytes, but it is most commonly seen in erythrocytes. Ovoid unpigmented inclusions tend to deform the host nucleus. There may also be parasitism in the gut of lizards as a schizont. Sporozoites are released into the bloodstream and may be refractile. It has been reported to occasionally cause anemia.	Rarely pathogenic, therefore treatments not reported; quinacrine could be tried in cases of associated anemia.
Order Achromatorida				
Sauroplasma	Ticks and biting flies thought to be intermediate hosts.	Primarily seen in lizards.	Vacuoles with inclusions may be seen in circulating thrombocytes and erythroid cells.	Rarely pathogenic, therefore treatments not reported.
Serpentoplasma	Ticks and biting flies thought to be intermediate hosts.	Primarily seen in snakes.	Vacuoles with inclusions may be seen in circulating thrombocytes and erythroid cells.	Rarely pathogenic, therefore treatments not reported.
Order Kinetoplastida				
Trypanosoma	All forms of reptiles may be affected.	Intermediate hosts are thought to be dipteran and phlebotamine flies, and leeches for aquatic species.	The parasite may be seen free in plasma as a trypanomastigote with a classical undulating cellular membrane. It is rarely pathogenic.	Rarely pathogenic, therefore treatments not reported.
Leishmania	Common in wild-caught lizards.	Phlebotamine sandflies thought to be intermediate hosts.	Amastigote form is seen in erythrocytes; promastigote form found free in plasma. It is rarely pathogenic.	Rarely pathogenic, therefore treatments not reported.

although occasionally endothelial hyperplasia in major arteries have been reported. The main pathology is associated with blockage of end arterioles with fluke eggs and resultant ischemic necrosis.[25] Treatment with praziquantel at 8 mg/kg, orally, once has been suggested, but due to the embolic nature of the condition may not be effective in preventing clinical disease.[26] Controlling the aquatic snails, which act as the intermediate host, can reduce exposure and infection rates.

Other Parasites. A debilitated or sick reptile, as with any vertebrate, may as a consequence of its disease develop a chronic, generally non-regenerative anemia. Some parasites may cause anemia more directly, however, and may include:

- The ectoparasite *Ophionyssus natricis* (the snake mite) may cause anemia due to its blood-sucking nature.
- The endoparasite hookworm *Kalicephalus* spp. may also be associated with anemia and malnutrition, particularly in snakes.
- Leeches (Hirudinae) may cause anemia in aquatic species if the burden is sufficiently high. They may also act as vectors for hemogregarines and trypanosomes, which in turn may lead to hemolytic anemia.

Viruses Causing Anemia

Pirhaemocyton spp. was originally classified as a protozoal hemoparasite. However, it is now known that the erythrocytic metachromatically staining inclusions are associated with viral assembly factories, consistent with viruses of the family Iridoviridae. High levels of infection are known to cause hemolytic anemia, although morbidity is only occasionally reported and usually associated with another underlying medical condition. There has been a report of spontaneous resolution of the viremia in a chameleon.[27] A report of an erythrocytic virus causing an anemia with a PCV of 7% in a diamond python (*Morelia spilota spilota*) had nearly 100% of the erythrocytes demonstrating acidophilic intracytoplasmic inclusion bodies.[6]

Neoplasia of the Hemopoietic System

Lymphoid or other hemopoietic origin neoplasia has been reported with an incidence rate between 0% and 30.8% of cancers in reptile species.[28,29] Indeed, one report suggests that the hemopoietic system is the body system most commonly affected by neoplasia.[30] Another publication states that snakes (e.g., cobras and urutus, *Bothrops alternatus*)

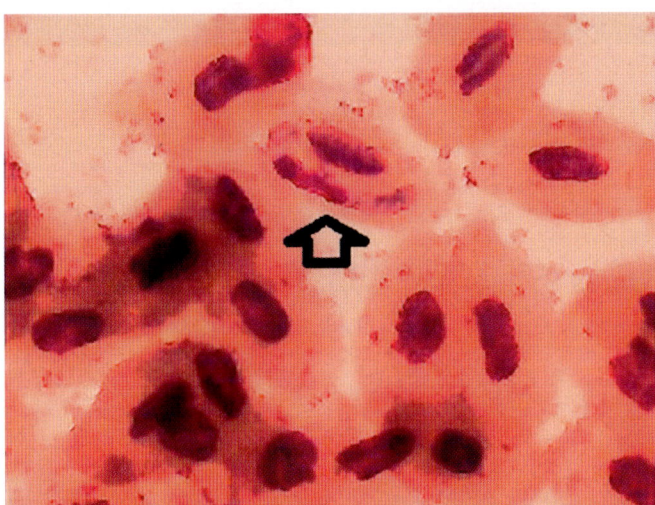

FIG 82.4 *Hepatozoon* spp. hemoparasite in the cytoplasm of an erythrocyte from a sand boa (*Eryx* spp.) (black arrow) (×1000 oil immersion, Romanowsky stain). (Courtesy of Simon Girling.)

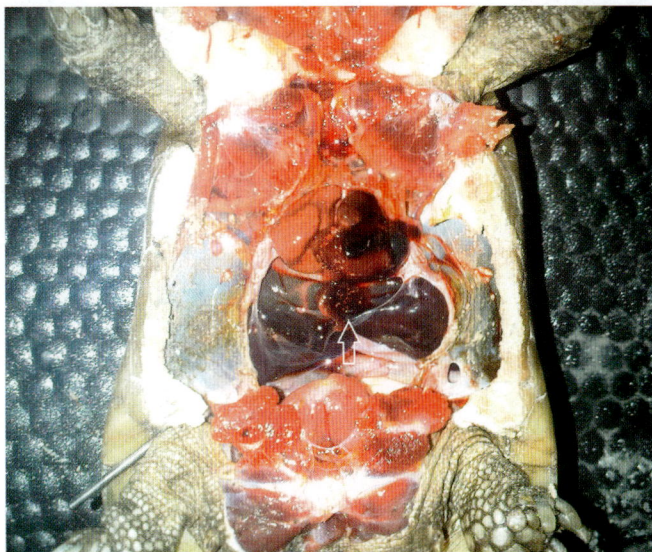

FIG 82.5 A hemangioma (white arrow) associated with the liver of a Greek tortoise (*Testudo graeca*) remained subclinical until rupture when cardiovascular collapse and the death of the reptile ensued. (Courtesy of Simon Girling.)

and lizards (e.g., savannah monitors, *Varanus exanthematicus*, and bearded dragons) are the most commonly reported species with hemopoietic system neoplasia.[31] It should be noted that lymphoid neoplasia may involve infiltration of body organs and often may not involve the bloodstream directly. Lymphoblasts are rarely found in the bloodstream of healthy reptiles and so, if seen in moderate to large numbers, are indicative of leukemia.

Leukemia has been reported in red eared sliders/terrapins (*Trachemys scripta elegans*) (in a myeloblastic form); a helmeted turtle (*Pelomedusa subrufa*) (in a myelogenous form); bearded dragons (chronic monocytic form; myelogenous form); a green iguana (immunoblastic form); a savannah monitor (associated with lymphosarcoma); a desert spiny lizard (*Sceloporus magister*) (in an undifferentiated form); an Indian python (*Python molurus*) (lymphocytic form); a common boa (*Boa constrictor*) (lymphocytic form); a broad banded copperhead (*Agkistrodon contortrix laticinctus*) (lymphocytic form); a diamond python (lymphocytic form with multicentric T-cell lymphoma); an Aruba Island rattlesnake (*Crotalus unicolor*) (lymphoid form in association with lymphosarcomas); a Russell's viper (*Daboia russelii*) (myelogenous form); and a Honduran milksnake (*Lampropeltis triangulum hondurensis*) (myelogenous form).[6,21,32–40]

Tissue-associated lymphomas/lymphosarcomas have been reported in a loggerhead turtle (*Caretta caretta*) (multicentric form, including the heart and aortae); green iguanas (disseminated form; pharyngeal lymphoma); East Indian water lizard (*Hydrosaurus amboinensis*) and an Asian water monitor (*Varanus salvator*); a savannah monitor (with leukemic profile); Egyptian spiny-tailed lizards (*Uromastyx aegyptius*) (multicentric form); a diamond python (multicentric T-cell lymphoma with leukemic overspill); an Aruba Island rattlesnake (lymphosarcomas associated with leukemia); and a red-tailed boa (*Boa constrictor constrictor*) (lymphoblastic lymphoma).[21,30,36,40–45] Plasma cell tumors have been reported in a Nile monitor lizard (*Varanus niloticus*) and an East Indian water lizard.[46,47]

Treatment of leukemia and lymphoma in reptiles is very much in its infancy. A number of reports have been published with differing regimes. In a case of lymphoma in a green iguana, radiation therapy at 10 Gy focused on the cervical lesion was used in combination with chemotherapy using vincristine, cyclophosphamide, and prednisolone.[42] The regimen was altered to doxorubicin (0.75 mg/kg IV once every 3 weeks) and prednisolone (2 mg/kg every 24 hours) after a relapse, and the case appeared in remission by day 1008. Another case of lymphoma in a king cobra (*Ophiophagus hannah*) used a regimen of prednisolone 40 mg/m² orally every 48 hours with L-Asparagine aminohydrolase at 10,000 IU/m²

given subcutaneously once during week one.[6] This was altered to prednisolone (40 mg/m²) orally every 48 hours with vincristine (0.5 mg/m²) intravenously once for week two. For week three the same regimen as week one was repeated. This regimen appeared successful, but regrowth occurred. A new regimen of 40 mg/m² prednisolone orally once every 48 hours plus chlorambucil at 2 mg/m² subcutaneously every 24 hours for 30 days was instituted. This seemed successful, but poor sloughing, anorexia, hypoalbuminemia, and hyperglycemia were noted side effects.

Neoplasia of the Vascular System

Hemangiomas have been reported in the corn snake (*Pantherophis guttatus*) and red-eared slider.[48,49] Most are subclinical until they rupture, usually after some form of blunt trauma, and with profound internal hemorrhage may result in the death of the reptile (Fig. 82.5).

Immune-Mediated Hemopoietic Disease

Immune-mediated hemolytic anemia has been reported in a Parson's chameleon (*Calumma parsonii*).[6] Clinically the chameleon showed signs of profound anemia (PCV 7%–8%), slide autoagglutination of erythrocytes, hemolytic serum with marked anisocytosis and polychromasia, and signs of lethargy and weakness. Therapy was initiated with prednisolone at 4 mg/kg, orally twice daily, and a blood transfusion was performed from sibling chameleons via the intraosseous route. Clinical resolution of signs was rapid but iatrogenic effects included osteomyelitis, which did respond to antibiotic therapy.

Toxic Anemia

Nonregenerative anemia has been seen in reptiles such as chelonians in association with the consumption of lead or other heavy metals. Chelation therapy is required and sodium calcium edetate has been advocated; however, there have been side effects with its usage (hemolysis). Care should be taken to ensure the reptile is well-hydrated, as renal damage is another sequela to both heavy metal and chelation agent toxicity.[50]

REFERENCES

See www.expertconsult.com for a complete list of references.

83

Clinical Behavioral Medicine

Teresa Bradley Bays and Leticia Mattos de Souza Dantas

Like many exotic species, reptiles have evolved to hide signs of illness as a survival mechanism. With their slower metabolic rates and physiological processes, reptiles exhibit a more gradual progression of clinical disease. This is especially true for prey species with which practitioners and caretakers are often presented. Behavioral changes that indicate illness are often not detected until late in the course of the disease. Frequently kept as single pets, with the lack of healthy conspecifics with which to compare, changes in behavior may not be detected until advanced.

Practitioners need to have a good understanding of the natural behavior of reptiles and amphibians but also how that behavior is affected by captivity. Understanding the medical implications of abnormal behavior can then help practitioners to diagnose medical conditions, assess captive welfare, and make recommendations to foster psychological well-being.[1,2] This chapter will focus on captive-related behaviors and relevant points of abnormal behavior in the most commonly kept species.

ANATOMY AND PHYSIOLOGY OF THE BRAIN AND BEHAVIORAL RESPONSES

As in other higher vertebrates the reptile brain can be divided into three sections: the forebrain (telencephalon and diencephalon), midbrain, and hindbrain.[3,4] The forebrain aids in smell, taste, rhythms, and sensory-motor integration and mediation. The diencephalon houses, among other things, the hypothalamus, thalamus, infundibulum, pituitary gland, and the pineal complex.[3] The midbrain or mesencephalon contains the areas for neuroendocrine roles and visual processing.[3,4] Hearing, balance, and physiological homeostasis are associated with the hindbrain.[4] Stress in all species induces activation of the sympathetic nervous system and also directs a neuroendocrine response, derived from activation of the hypothalamus/pituitary/adrenal (HPA) axis.[5] This neuroendocrine axis regulates physiological functions such as immune competence, reproduction, metabolism, and behavior.[5] The HPA axis is activated when the corticotrophin-releasing hormone produced by the hypothalamus is released following a threat, stimulating the pituitary to secrete adrenocorticotropic hormone (ACTH), which acts on the adrenal cortex to stimulate the production of glucocorticoids that effect the alteration of circulating levels of sex steroids and other hormones.[5] This stress response then maximizes energy available to body systems to face physiological challenges and simultaneously inhibits nonessential systems that, although critical for long-term survival, are not essential for the day-to-day survival of the animal, including growth and reproduction.[6]

Behavioral changes noted in reptiles in captivity are often a result of a response to stress. Most species are adapted to cope with specific, evolved challenges in their natural environment.[7] A single, sustained stress occurrence, whether physical (thermal), psychic (perceived predator), or physiological (adrenal response), may have long-term adverse consequences on the health and welfare of reptiles and amphibians.[7] Acute or intense stressors may predispose reptiles to emaciation, immune depression, and reproductive difficulty.[5] If the stressor continues, abnormal nonfunctional behaviors may occur, including stereotypical behavior, that can help the animal face the psychological aspect of the event and also reduce some of the associated physiological responses.[5] Chronic stress in reptiles may also predispose to obesity and hepatic lipidosis, aggression, anorexia, displacement behaviors,[8] and, in some lizards, a change in their skin color created by variations in the deposition of carotenes.[9]

Capture and restraint, and even the inability to escape from captivity, has been found to increase stress-related corticosterone levels in reptiles.[9] Captive conditions also typically replace many features of the natural world with artificial and frequently poorly matched alternatives that deprive animals of known normal behavior and associated biological needs.[7] Reptiles in captivity are also often kept in conditions that create understimulation, and the associated stress has been shown to be difficult to assess through more common physiological measurement such as corticosterone levels.[8]

APPROACH TO BEHAVIORAL APPOINTMENTS

A basic assessment of behavioral issues should be included with every reptile and amphibian examination. However, for dedicated behavioral consultations a behavioral history form (Table 83.1) should be filled out by the owner or caretaker prior to the visit, so pertinent information on which to make a diagnosis is not missed.[10] Photos of the enclosure and videos of the altered behaviors and postures should also be requested for the appointment. A visit to the animal holding facility may be necessary to assess conditions that may be causing behavioral issues and medical problems.

Anamnesis, Physical Examination, and Behavior

Most health problems in reptiles are the result of deficiencies in captive management, especially in relation to the environment and diet. Therefore a thorough, detailed history is vital for the evaluation of these patients. Information on any behavioral changes the owner or caretaker has noted is essential. While collecting the history, it is prudent to observe the behavior and posture of the patient before any handling (by the

TABLE 83.1 Reptile and Amphibian Behavioral History Form

Name of pet: _____ Date: _____

Common name or scientific name of species: _____

Reason for presentation? Please describe the signs that you have noticed that made you come in today. _____
_____

What changes in behavior have been noted in recent months and days? _____
_____

Have changes been noted in any of the following categories?

Appetite? _____

Foods eaten? _____

How food is eaten? _____

Placement in the enclosure? Where does the patient spend most of its time? Has this changed? _____
_____

Basking time? _____

Aggression to people or other reptiles? _____
_____

Level of mobility and activity? Changes in activity level? _____
_____

Nesting behavior? _____

Breeding behavior? _____

Swimming or diving changes (in aquatic species)? _____

Changes in respiratory rate or effort? _____

Excessive hiding? _____

Pacing or repetitive behaviors? _____

Any new or unusual behaviors noted? _____

Rubbing on objects in enclosure? _____

Gaping or open-mouthed breathing? _____

Biting at a body part? _____

More passive or easier to handle? _____

Repeated swallowing? _____

Scratching? _____

Excessive drinking? _____

Difficulty going to the bathroom? _____

Other changes in behavior? _____

Where does the patient spend most of its time in relation to heat and light sources and hiding places? How has this changed in recent days/weeks/months? _____
_____

Have there been any changes in social structure or occupants in the enclosure? _____
_____

Any new pets or people in the household? _____

Any changes in food or how it is provided? _____

Any changes in substrate or cage furniture? _____

Any changes in the environment? _____

Any other issues noted? _____
_____

client or doctor) (Figs. 83.1 and 83.2A). Watching how the patient responds during the physical examination and how it recovers postexamination is important (see Fig. 83.2B and C). The clinician's observations of the patient's behavior during the consultation are critical, as otherwise the patient's behavioral issues are solely dependent upon what is disclosed by the owner or caretaker, which may be inaccurate or biased.

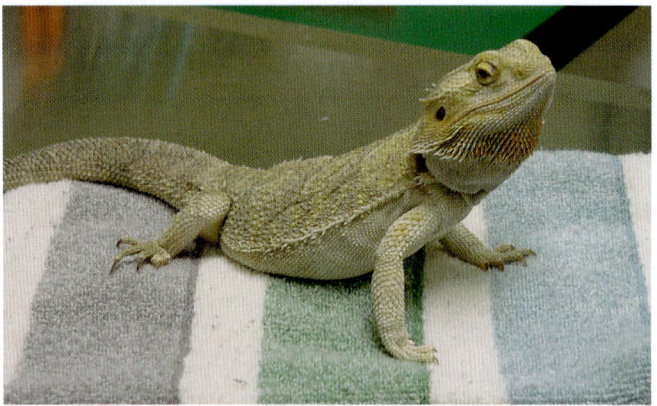

FIG 83.1 Normal posturing in a bearded dragon (*Pogona vitticeps*)—bright, alert, interested in the environment, and holding itself up well.

CLINICAL DISEASES

Husbandry-Related Behavioral Disorders

Understanding the importance of how husbandry affects reptile behavior is paramount to successful practice. Environmental decisions are often guided by the clients desire to make enclosures aesthetically pleasing without knowledge of species-specific needs or behaviors. Important husbandry factors that must be considered include substrate, heat sources, light, humidity, spatial needs, and dietary choices.

Assessing husbandry practices and having knowledge of enclosure size and design is necessary for understanding if behavior is affected by environmental conditions (see Section 3). Because reptile enclosures are often too large to bring into the veterinary clinic, it is helpful to encourage clients to bring in pictures of enclosures for evaluation. Several examples of how husbandry can affect behavior and therefore affect the practitioner's ability to best make a diagnosis are listed below.

Observation: Not moving away from direct heat sources despite thermal burns or hyperthermia.

Clinical significance: Reptiles not provided with radiant heat for basking may seek out a heat source, especially if ill, and could burn themselves on a hot rock or other in-the-cage heating element if this is the only heat source provided. This thermal nociception latency is not completely understood, but it is believed that heat receptors are not the same as pain receptors in reptiles, so they may not perceive pain until thermal damage has occurred, or they do not associate the pain with the object causing the thermal burn. Under-tank heaters may be especially

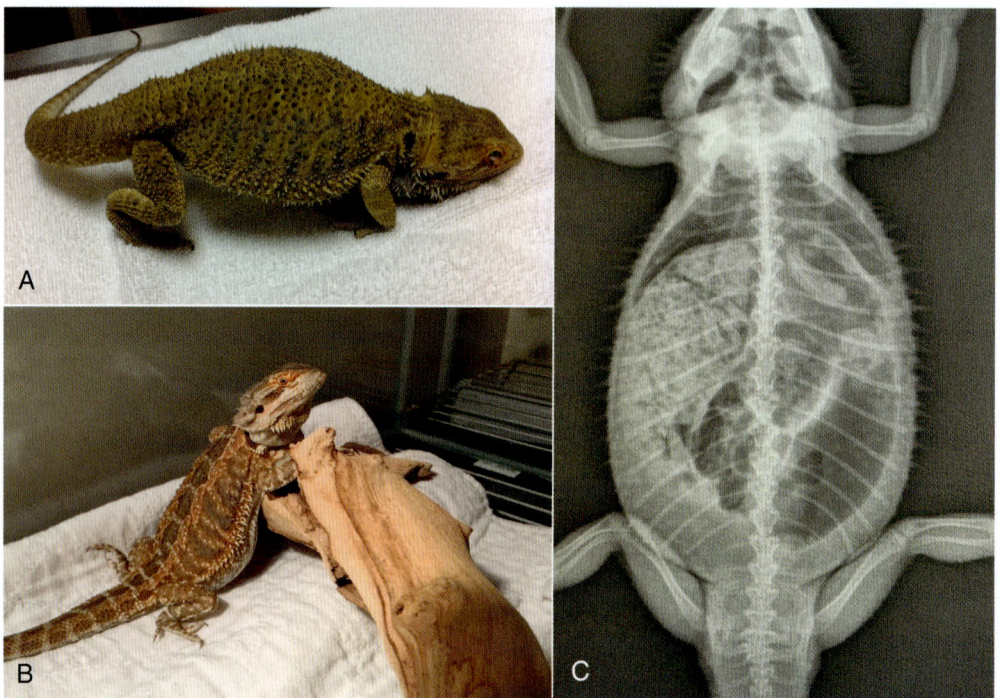

FIG 83.2 (A) Bearded dragon (*Pogona vitticeps*) with abnormal posture in response to palpation of the coelomic cavity, indicating severe pain. (B) Bearded dragon continuously holding itself up on enclosure furniture due to respiratory compromise from gastrointestinal obstruction and severe ileus compressing lungs. The distended coelomic cavity is evident in this profile. Intermittent behavioral changes should not be attributed to primary respiratory system pathology. (C) Ventral dorsal radiograph of the bearded dragon in B, indicating a severe ileus secondary to gastrointestinal obstruction creating a severe compression of the lungs.

inappropriate for burrowing reptile species that may expose themselves directly to the heat and be more likely to develop ventral burns.

The constant illumination associated with an incandescent light as the sole heat source, especially in nocturnal species, may result in creating conditions that result in stress and immune supression. Understanding the environmental needs of reptiles and amphibians, including whether they are nocturnal or diurnal and how they thermoregulate in their natural environment, is important. This information is helpful when evaluating the current captive enclosure to identify how thermal burns may have occurred and how to prevent them in the future.

Understanding how behavior can be affected by the environment can be useful in diagnosing medical issues. For example, gaping in a reptile patient can be associated with aggression or a response to a threat, overheating or thermoregulation, respiratory disease, pain, or a sign of nausea or other gastric or esophageal discomfort (especially if associated with repeated swallowing). However, if that patient is suffering from nutritional secondary hyperparathyroidism (NSHP) it may have difficulty ambulating and may be unable to move away from the heat source. A client or caretaker may interpret gaping in this patient as a respiratory or other issue when in fact the gaping is a direct result of hyperthermia. Resolution of the signs with cooling when removed from the enclosure, examination, clinical history, and diagnostics, including radiographs, can aid in a correct diagnosis.

Prevention: Providing a temperature gradient (horizontally or vertically depending on species) in an appropriately sized enclosure allows reptiles to thermoregulate as they move about the enclosure, as they would if free-ranging. In general, diurnal species fare better if given radiant heat sources from above with an appropriate day/night cycle. Nocturnal species may thrive better when under-tank heaters are provided, but care must be taken that they are not able to be burned by these heaters.

Observation: Shy or stressed species such as chameleons remain hidden rather than exposing themselves in order to bask or eat.

Clinical significance: If the shy reptile is spending most of its time in a hide box that is placed on the cooler side of the tank, then it may not thermoregulate, as the need for security may outweigh its desire to spend time basking. Also, the presence of other domestic pets such as cats, dogs, and birds can be perceived as threatening to captive reptiles and amphibians and create psychological stress that will lead to immune suppression and failure to thrive.

Thorough historical review about where the patient spends most of its time in relation to heat sources and hide boxes, and a description of exactly how the enclosure is set up, is needed to evaluate the problem.

Prevention: Appropriate space and hiding places for reptiles may alleviate some of the stress associated with captivity and provide for behavioral enrichment. Hide boxes, carved-out logs, or plants should be placed throughout the enclosure, allowing a shyer reptile to have the ability to thermoregulate and eat without feeling exposed. The clinician must have detailed knowledge of enclosure setup to know if the environment is adequate to avoid medical issues.

Observation: Rostral abrasions and other injuries from escape behaviors.

Clinical significance: Stereotypical behaviors related to escape attempts can cause rostral abrasions and other traumatic lesions in captive reptiles.[8] It has been found that the inherent psychological organization and adaptational constraints present in reptiles result in failure to recognize the abstract invisible barriers.[8] Chinese water dragons (*Physignathus concincinus*) are particularly prone to escape attempts that create rostral wounds. Mirrors, glass, and other reflective surfaces should be avoided in enclosures containing less social species, because a reptile's reflection may be perceived as a conspecific and create undue stress because it is perceived as competition (Fig. 83.3). The reptile may attack the reflection, causing injury as it strikes the surface of the

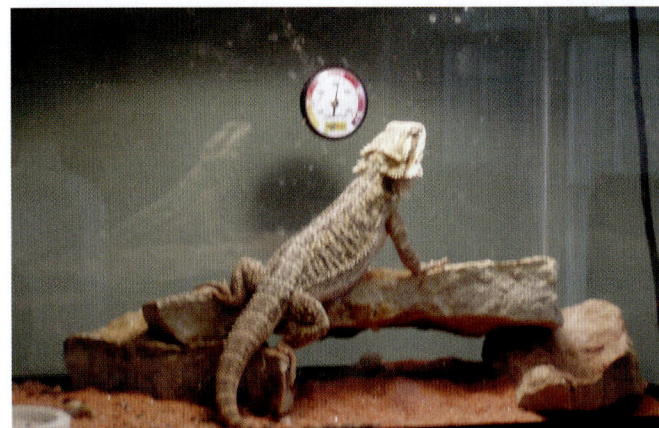

FIG 83.3 Glass and mirrored surfaces in enclosures can create reflections that can be stressful to reptiles such as this male bearded dragon (*Pogona vitticeps*) that perceives the reflection as a male conspecific and induces undue social stress.

enclosure. Mandibular lesions can also be seen and may be associated with arboreal species diving or dropping onto hard surfaces.[8]

Prevention: Placing a visual barrier such as black tape on a transparent enclosure and minimizing glare and reflection in an enclosure, as well as providing adequate space and hiding places, may decrease this behavior. Covering the glass with a less reflective paper, or using one-way glass can help to eliminate this problem.

Observation: Obstruction due to substrate ingestion and pica.

Clinical significance: Substrate ingestion can lead to intestinal impactions and may be associated with understimulating environments that are commonly found in captivity.[8]

Medical problems noted with substrate ingestion include obstruction, perforation, coelomitis, and cloacal prolapse from tenesmus. Particularly common in young bearded dragons (*Pogona vittiveps*), the authors have also seen it in chameleons, geckos, and uromastyx lizards.

Historical details are needed regarding substrates used currently and previously, as well as exposure to areas outside of the enclosure. Radiography and ultrasonography are useful to identify obstruction, impaction, and ileus. Pica can be noted secondary to mineral deficiency as seen with NSHP, so blood work should be performed to evaluate total calcium, ionized calcium, phosphorous, and vitamin D_3 levels. Radiography also allows for visualization of bone density to aid in diagnosis.

Prevention: A substrate that is not easily ingested, or is safe if ingested, is important in species that flick their tongues to investigate their environment or get substrate mixed in with food items as they are ingested. Even substrates that are designated as safe for reptiles, including bark, corncob, and calcium-containing sands, can cause gastrointestinal problems if ingested in large amounts. If a more naturalistic substrate is used to enhance environmental enrichment, then food should be offered on a plate or tray to minimize substrate ingestion.

Observation: Stress related to the environment.

Clinical significance: Many situations can create stress for reptiles and amphibians that can lead to immune suppression and disease over time. Captivity-related chronic stress behavior may be evidenced by increased abnormal behaviors, including behavioral inhibition, vigilance behavior, hiding, and fearfulness.[11] Additionally, an increased frequency of startle, aggression, and freezing behavior can be seen, as well as decreased exploratory behavior and reproductive behavior.[11] Green iguanas (*Iguana iguana*) are arboreal in nature and should be provided with a vertical enclosure to facilitate climbing. They also tend to be less stressed when their enclosure is at a reasonable height. Rock iguanas (*Cyclura* spp.) are ground dwellers and look for places to dig and burrow. Knowledge of whether a species is arboreal, terrestrial, or aquatic is necessary to provide the most natural environment for a reptile.

Captive conditions often deprive animals of known normal behavior and associated biologic needs, including hunting for food, spatial range, and macro-habitat exploration.[8] Home-range studies of reptiles in their natural setting have shown that reptiles are highly active and that they have been known to travel from several hundreds of square meters to hundreds or thousands of kilometers looking for food.[8] In addition, insectivorous species often need to feed more frequently and require a great deal of activity to catch their prey.[8] It is normal and healthy for an animal to spend hours of exploratory locomotor activity hunting for food[8] and interacting with the environment, and stress is created when small enclosures in captivity with plentiful food and minimalistic unnatural furnishings are substituted for a more natural environment.

All reptiles appear to seek out and occupy "angles" and orientation that allows them to find comfort in their environment and appear to play roles in delivering comfort and focused thermal needs, as well as in the amelioration of discomfort.[8] A snake that needs to adopt a straight-line posture to relieve intestinal discomfort cannot do so in a cage or enclosure that is shorter than the snake itself (Fig. 83.4).[8]

Mimicry, or blending in with the environment, is a strategy used by reptiles, and the chameleon is one of the more popular species using this method of crypsis (Fig. 83.5). When housing a species that relies on visual mimicry, it might be best to use cage furniture that has natural colors to afford the animal the opportunity to blend in with its environment.

Dramatic or rapid changes in ambient temperature may induce a stress response in an animal, whereas a slow change/increase over a period of time allows for physiological adjustments that allow the individual to better tolerate the change.

When advising on changes in the temperature of an enclosure, it is imperative that cage dimensions, existing temperatures, temperature gradients, and humidty levels are all considered. Without specific recommendations, clients may misconstrue directions, and inappropriate thermal changes in the enclosure could be detrimental to the patient.

It has been shown that snakes use pheromones in their environment to mark their territory. Thus constant rearrangement of cage furniture or cleaning the cage might add additional stress to captive snakes. Used in moderation, however, rearranging enclosures has been found to increase foraging and exploration behavior in snakes.

Prevention: The natural behaviors of the species kept in captivity must be taken into consideration when creating and furnishing enclosures appropriate for reptiles and amphibians. Also, the practitioner should have a working knowledge of enclosure set-up before making recommendations on changes in temperature and humidity. Experience has shown that some reptile species are easier to maintain in captivity, including leopard geckos (*Eublepharius macularius*), crested geckos (*Rhacodactylus ciliatus*), fat tail geckos (*Hemitheconyx caudicinctus*), bearded dragons (*Pogona vitticeps*), corn snakes (*Pantherophis guttatus*), king snakes (*Lampropeltis getulus*), and milk snakes (*Lampropeltis triangulum*). Reptiles have been found to possess the cognitive ability to be trained using desensitization and operant conditioning.[12] This training not only helps to facilitate veterinary care, it can also aid in eliminating some of the psychological stress associated with captivity.[12]

Providing environmental enrichment and creating foraging opportunities can decrease stress-related behavioral issues. A Nile soft-shelled turtle, *Trionyx triunguis*, at the National Zoo (Washington, DC) was given objects such as balls, sticks, and hoses in an attempt to reduce self-mutilation behavior often noted in response to stress.[13] The turtle

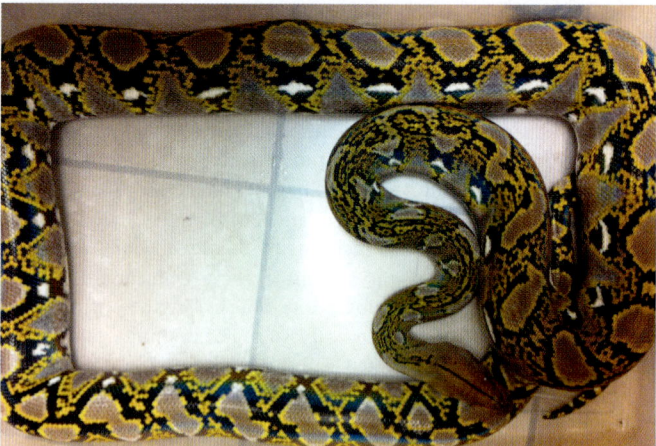

FIG 83.4 A reticulated python (*Malayopython reticulatus*) assuming a position that may indicate coelomic discomfort because it is unable to stretch out in this small container. Subtle changes in position of the body and placement in an enclosure can indicate medical issues or deficiencies in the environment.

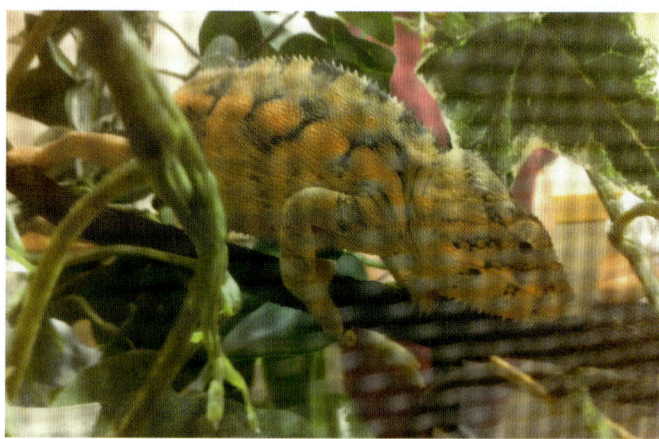

FIG 83.5 A panther chameleon (*Furcifer pardalis*) using visual mimicry of its environment as a form of crypsis. Using neutral and natural colors in the enclosure helps to make them feel more secure.

spent considerable time interacting with the objects, and the level of self-mutilation behavior decreased greatly over many months. Based on video recordings, an ethogram of the turtle's behavior was developed and showed that the turtle interacted with the objects for 20.7% of the time and was active for 67.7% of the time, much more time than was expected.[13]

Behavioral Issues Related to Feeding

Knowledge of how and what reptiles and amphibians naturally eat and drink, and how these are provided to captive reptiles, is imperative for helping them thrive. Understanding specifics about the diet, as well as how the food is prepared and presented, is helpful in aiding the practitioner to best serve the needs of the patient. Awareness of ontogenic shifts in feeding behaviors also allows practitioners to better advise clients. This is seen in bearded dragons (*Pogona vitticeps*), which are significantly more insectivorous as juveniles and more herbivorous as adults. Below are examples of how the knowledge of normal behavior can affect the decisions that should be made for feeding captive reptiles.

Observation: Anorexia, inappetance.

Clinical significance: Many situations lead to anorexia in reptiles and amphibians, including infection and other disease processes, competition from conspecifics, as well as overly restrictive and inappropriate environments[11] and maladaption to captivity. Social stress or intraspecific aggression from the presence of individuals that are aggressive or become aggressive or protective around resources may keep cage mates from eating as well or as often and cause failure to thrive. This is commonly seen in groups of captive lizards and in colonies of aquatic turtles. Overhandling shy species (e.g., chameleons, ball pythons) can cause anorexia due to stress. It is also not advisable to examine or perform diagnostic procedures on a snake shortly after feeding due to increased risk of regurgitation.

Undetected disease processes, often evidenced by behavioral changes that may go unrecognized by the owner or caregiver, may lead to anorexia. Pathologic conditions of the upper gastrointestinal tract that negatively impact the feeding response and oral, dental, and beak disorders of reptiles are common presentations.[14] Many reptile species become anorectic in cooler months, so it is important to distinguish seasonal anorexia/hypophagia from a pathologic etiology. Hormonal activity during the breeding season in both male and female reptiles and in gravid females may result in decreased appetite or anorexia. Feeding nocturnal species during the day may lead to anorexia. Knowledge of normal feeding behaviors will also help the owner to pick appropriate prey items and, with some imagination, help with behavioral enrichment.

Both infectious and noninfectious disease processes will often result in associated anorexia.[15–17] Incubation of these infectious diseases can be long (up to 6 months), making it difficult to associate anorexia with an infectious exposure or injury that leads to the infection. Medical problems can ensue if live prey items are left in the enclosure with uninterested or ill reptiles for lengthy periods of time. Crickets have been known to create conjunctival or corneal lesions in geckos, chameleons, bearded dragons, and anoles[18] as they look for a source of moisture. Rats and mice can chew on a snake, causing extensive damage to skin, underlying muscle, and even vertebrae. An anorexic blood python (*Python curtus*) that hasn't defecated for several weeks and has a distended caudal ceolomic cavity could have a gastrointestinal impaction, a foreign body, parasites, or a neoplastic mass. Because this species needs a particularly high humidity of 60% to 70%, constipation and impaction is a common problem when kept at temperatures too high and humidity too low.

Snakes, especially those that are wild caught, may refuse to eat albino laboratory rats or mice but be more likely to strike at brown rodents. Gerbils are often substituted for white mice in smaller snakes, especially ball pythons (*Python regius*), for which gerboas and other brown-colored rodents are natural prey. Anorectic reptiles that are hospitalized should be supported with species-appropriate food items. Syringe-feeding supplements are available for herbivores (i.e., Critical Care, Oxbow Pet Products), carnivores (i.e., Carnivore Care, Oxbow Pet Products), and insectivores (i.e., Insectivore Diet, Walkabout Farms). Esophagostomy tubes can be placed for long-term supplemental feeding or in those species that are difficult or dangerous to feed orally (see Chapter 45).

Prevention: Knowledge of the captive feeding habits is essential. Home-range defensive behavior appears to be most prevalent in the iguanian and gekkotan lizard,[19] so it is important to provide adequate resources (space, basking areas, hiding spaces, and food) for all communally housed individuals. Providing multiple feeding stations can reduce competition in enclosures that contain several reptiles, otherwise cage or tank-mate aggression can lead to severe injuries. Placing food in open, as well as visually protected, areas will encourage feeding even for shy species. It would be inappropriate and inhumane to place predators and prey in the same enclosure. Crickets and other insects should not be left in the enclosures of lizards in large quantities over long periods.

The feeding of live vertebrate prey is illegal in most countries; however, if live prey is provided to snakes, it is preferred that they be fed in a separate enclosure and removed if the snake has not eaten them within a few minutes. Captive reptiles and amphibians that are not eating prey quickly should be evaluated for clinical signs of disease and have the diet and environment scrutinized for problems that may be causing anorexia. Preferably frozen, thawed prey items should be provided.

Healthy lizards kept in proper environments may experience seasonal or hormonal anorexia that will not usually result in weight loss of more than 5% to 10% of body weight.[20] Monitoring weight during this normal physiological process is therefore important in assessing health status. Many captive lizards, however, are already somewhat compromised by poor diet, dehydration, less-than-optimal environment, and parasitism such that this period of anorexia may not be tolerable. Because of the risks associated with reproduction in females, consideration should be given to ovariectomize pet reptiles to avoid compromise created by reproduction.

Knowing the details of the environment and understanding the specific environmental needs of the species, as well as performing diagnostics including radiographs, ultrasound, intestinal parasite examination, and blood work, can lead to a quicker diagnosis, resolution of the problems involved, and prevention of reoccurrence. Providing adequate humidity and opportunities to soak help with constipation. Routine wellness checks and intestinal parasite exams may help with early diagnosis of other etiologies of anorexia.

Observation: Inability or unwillingness to drink water.

Clinical significance: How water is provided to different species must be taken into consideration when determining the cause of dehydration. Box turtles and many species of tortoises normally drink from water pooled on the ground during and after rain. The water is consumed by filtering it through overlying vegetation, so they may not recognize or be stimulated to drink from a bowl. In many lizards and most snake species, hydration is maintained more from moisture in the diet than from drinking. This is especially true for those reptiles on moist and vegetative diets, so appreciable amounts of free water may not be consumed. To provide water in a bowl to a species that naturally gets water from lapping morning dew, such as chameleons, may act as a stressor and lead to chronic dehydration over time. Such species often fare better if a misting or drip system is provided.

Dehydrated reptiles and amphibians will have dry (if skin is normally moist), loose skin, sunken eyes, and tacky mucous membranes. Diagnostic testing includes hematology and plasma biochemistry, including hematocrit. Treatment includes correcting fluid imbalances, evaluating how water is provided, and ensuring that competition for procuring water is minimized.

Prevention: For many species, a sprinkler system outdoors can be utilized to simulate rain if lack of water consumption or dehydration is of concern. Lizards that do not drink from a water bowl may lap water that has been spray misted on the inside of the enclosures or from a continuous drip system. Water can also be spray misted on food items to help maintain hydration.

Observation: Inactivity and overeating leading to obesity.

Clinical significance: Obesity is a common consequence of captivity due to lack of exercise, inappropriately small cage size and inappropriate or excessive calories. It is especially prevalent in sit-and-wait predators such as captive monitors and boids (Fig. 83.6A and B), which are offered frequent high-caloric food items without exercise to obtain the food. A lack of variety of diet items, especially those containing lower caloric value, may also contribute to obesity. Obese reptiles are more likely to

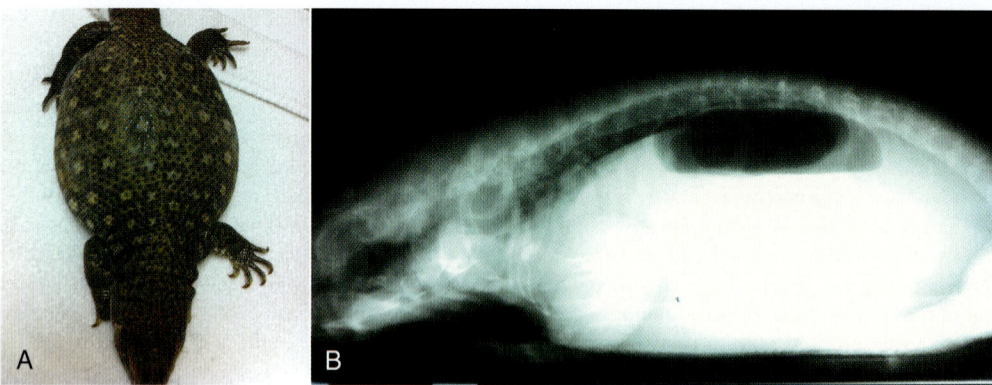

FIG 83.6 (A) This savannah monitor (*Varanus exanthematicus*) is so obese that its legs barely touch the ground. Coelomic fat is causing pressure on lungs and coelomic organs. (B) A lateral radiograph of the savannah monitor (*Varanus exanthematicus*) seen in A. Adipose tissue and fluid in the coelomic cavity is compressing the lungs and creating a mechanical ileus in the gastrointestinal tract. Hepatic lipidosis and ascites is common in this species when they become anorectic.

suffer from hepatic lipidosis if they become anorectic due to stress or disease.

Prevention: Obese reptiles do not live as long as healthy conspecifics and tend to be more immune suppressed. Providing variety in the diet, feeding less, and allowing the captive reptile to forage for food to increase exercise are all helpful in preventing obesity. Other forms of environmental enrichment also aid in prevention, including placing food in multiple areas around the enclosure and creating other foraging opportunities.

Social Behavior

It has been found that amphibians and reptiles exhibit traits commonly seen in birds and mammals, including sophisticated communication, problem-solving abilities, signs of parental care, as well as play and complex sociality.[21,22] Understanding the normal behavior of reptiles and amphibians that are kept in captivity is necessary in providing them with enclosures and a social structure that will allow them to thrive.

Sudden changes in the social structure of a group of animals, with the addition of conspecifics, can lead to stress and immune suppression. The animals within the group may readjust their social dynamics as the group changes and as new individuals are added, potentially leading to conflict around acquisition of mates and resources. It is also essential that caretakers are aware that if one or more of the reptiles in an enclosure is not developing as fast as the others, it may need to be separated in order to thrive. Wellness exams at least every 6 months, along with obtaining periodic weights, are helpful in determining if such discrepencies exist and if changes in social structure need to be made.

Observation: Intraspecific aggression and agnostic behaviors.

Clinical significance: Most reptiles are not considered to be social animals, and relatively few reptiles live constantly in social groups. The social tendencies of reptilian behavior vary both with species and with ontogenicity. While many reptiles show a significant increase in social behavior at breeding time, for most of the year even these species prefer a solitary lifestyle.

Social behavior of a given species must be taken into consideration when deciding on whether to cage conspecifics or members of different species together. Turtles appear to be solitary for most of the year and live only socially during the breeding season. Sick or injured chelonians should be housed individually, as the presence of another animal might

be an additional stressor to these animals. Severe injuries and fatalities from fighting occur more commonly in captivity with less opportunity to flee. Reptile species that are naturally gregarious such as leopard geckos (*Eublepharus macularis*) and bearded dragons (*Pogona vitticeps*) thrive better when kept in groups, especially when a single male is kept with multiple females. Lizards housed together for months to years may become aggressive toward each other and should be separated if such behavior is noted. Keeping male reptiles in cages that allow for visualization of other males is often socially stressful, so a setup where direct visual contact can be established should be avoided, especially for chameleons and iguanas. Sexual aggression toward humans by reptiles has been reported most commonly with the green iguana (*Iguana iguana*)[23,24] during the breeding season, when hormone levels are fluctuating, and is often initiated by the presence of a menstruating human female. After the breeding season is complete, some will revert back to their normal docile behavior, while others remain aggressive.

Individuals of any given species that control resources will often thrive more and grow faster than subordinates in the same enclosure. Since onset of adult behavior patterns is related to body size, the larger males also display adult behaviors much sooner, so separation of the other individuals is not only necessary for them to thrive but may become necessary for them to survive. The presence of aggressive conspecifics, predators, and perceived predators will significantly alter daily behavior in reptiles and amphibians. For instance, it was noted that eye contact between human observers and free-living iguanas resulted in significant disruption of normal hierarchical perching in the iguanas being observed.[25]

Prevention: Having a working knowledge of species-specific behaviors allows caretakers to provide an environment and social structure that better mimics what is seen in nature and more likely to be successful. Providing multiple basking areas for groups of reptiles may minimize social stress, as some individual males tend to take and defend the preferred spots,[26] grow more rapidly, and use the supplemental heat sources more often than subordinate males. Social stress can also be minimized when housing nongregarious reptile species together in environments by providing sufficient space, appropriate hiding spaces, visual barriers, and multiple feeding stations.

It has been suggested that sexually mature male iguanas that are showing signs of aggression may have some of these behaviors reduced by decreasing daylight hours, eliminating exposure to other male animals and female conspecifics, and decreasing environmental temperatures slightly. The practitioner should stress to the client, however, that aggression is a normal expected behavior for iguanas and that efforts to control behavior should not be extreme enough to cause harm to the iguana. Depo-Lupron and Depo-Provera have both been used with mixed results to decrease human-directed aggression in male iguanas. Castration of male iguanas prior to sexual maturity may help to decrease the chance of reproductive-related aggression toward people and other pets.[27] Clients should be counseled that castration prior to puberty would also decrease the development of secondary sexual characteristics including large jowls and crests. Castration after sexual maturity has occurred has variable but limited effect on decreasing aggression (see Chapter 80).

In green iguanas femoral gland pore size was positively correlated with the frequency of head-bob displays and the plasma levels of testosterone during the breeding season in males older than 12 months of age.[28] This behavior is part of the normal agonistic repertoire for this species.

These head bobs, not present when the iguana is first acquired as a juvenile, may be mistaken by a novice caretaker as an indication of illness such as hypocalcemic tetany or central nervous system disease. Because they are intermittent and stimulated by the presence of other male iguanas or in response to a threat makes them easier to distinguish as a normal behavior and not a clinical sign.

Handling and Behavior

As wild creatures, reptiles are not domesticated and may act and react instinctively and defensively. Any reptile that is approached too quickly or handled inappropriately may show signs of aggression or flight. Defensive aggression in reptiles can represent a safety hazard for your staff if employees are not instructed in proper restraint and handling. Early recognition of a stressed individual can help to deescalate the situation or to anticipate the next step and to avoid injury to the animal, the handler, or the examiner. Despite attempts to decrease stress, behavioral issues may be "masked" by acute arousal states in the clinical environment, which may make an accurate diagnosis more difficult.[8]

Observation: Behavioral issues related to handling.

Clinical significance: A green iguana (*Iguana iguana*), as well as other lizards, may sit with its head extended and its eyes closed as it is being petted. This behavior is often considered to be a sign of contentment; it may, however, be a sign of fear, illness, learned helplessness, or even the dissociative behavior of a patient that is highly stressed. The lizard may be "zoning out" in a strange environment riddled with strange sounds, smells, and potential predators, or it may be too ill to respond with curiosity to a new environment. This could also be a lizard that will readily strike if provoked—using teeth, claws, and whipping tail to defend itself against predators. This lizard may also be much sicker than it would appear, and any stressor such as handling, diagnostic procedures, or treatment may prove to be detrimental.

Defensive aggressive behaviors in reptiles include posturing that makes the aggressor appear to be more threatening, such as inflation of the body, standing more erect on all four legs, broadside posturing, dewlap extension, open-mouthed threat, and head bobbing. Biting, striking, and tail whipping may also be seen. Male frill-necked lizards (*Chlamydosaurus kingii*) will also kick and bite at each other while displaying extension of the frill around their necks.

Handling by owners, as well as by practice staff for medical diagnostics, causes psychological stress similar to that created by predators. Lizards that become frightened may roll like a crocodile in attempts to escape restraint or predators. Some lizards such as the basilisk lizard (*Basiliscus vittatus*) that normally ambulate with all four legs are able to run bipedally on their rear legs to escape predators, even across water.

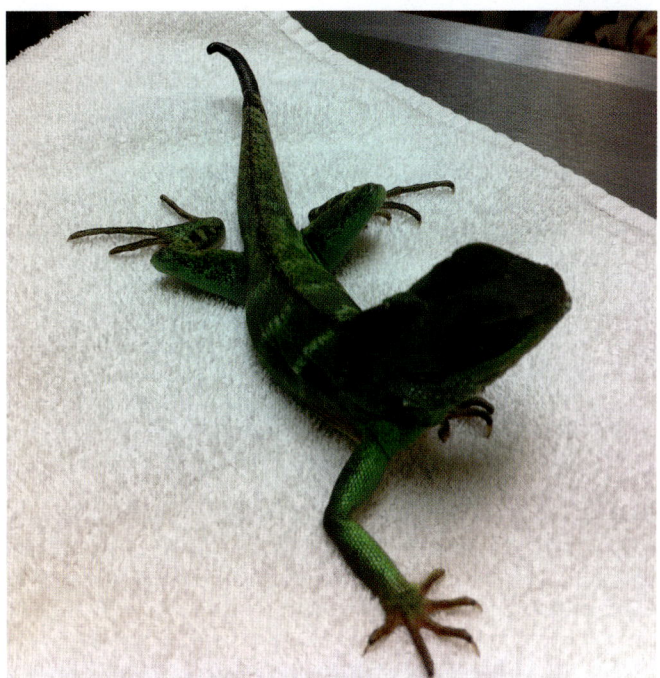

FIG 83.7 This Chinese water dragon (*Physignatus cocincinusis*) forming a u-shaped posture toward the perceived predator as a defense mechanism, ready to strike if necessary.

Chuckwallas (*Sauromalus obesus*) will crawl into crevices in rocks to escape predators and then inflate their bodies so that they cannot be pulled out from their hiding place. During manual restraint, snakes will usually exhibit negative taxis to the restrainer and try to work the body out of the grasping hold with constant forward movements and/or rotation on its own axis. Iguanas and other lizards that are placed on an exam table may assume a u-shaped position with their tail pointed toward the practitioner (Fig. 83.7), ready to defend themselves if needed.

All reptiles will struggle if not well supported during handling and may cause injury to the handler or to themselves (i.e., loss of tail, damage to vertebrae). Most lizards will exhibit a serpentine-type motion when struggling that can be minimized if both the thoracic and pelvic girdles are well supported and firmly but gently restrained. Turtles will often urinate during handling. This may be associated with fear, pain, a defensive behavior to repel a predator, or as a part of a flight reaction in an attempt to quickly decrease body weight. It has been proposed that the bladder in tortoises can function as a water reservoir,[29] so, when a chelonian patient has forcefully emptied the bladder, it is important to make sure the animal has proper facilities to replenish fluid. Snakes can empty their musk glands in the cloacal area when frightened during handling, especially milk snakes, which might detract predators due to the foul smell and taste.

Overhandling of shy species can lead to stress, anorexia, and ill health. Species such as chameleons and ball pythons may not be the best pet choice for owners that wish to handle their pets frequently. Snakes, especially ball pythons, that are handled soon after feeding often regurgitate. Regurgitation may also be seen in certain diseases such as cryptosporidia, cardiomyopathy, or various metabolic diseases. Chelonians or lizards will not normally regurgitate in response to handling.

It is advisable not to handle snakes and lizards just before a shed. The old keratin layer that is shed comes off after the new keratin layer beneath has completely formed, so shed should never be pulled off prematurely. In snakes that are preparing to shed, the eye caps will often become opaque, and the snake may be more apt to strike, probably due to decreased vision during this time. After a few days the eye caps will clear, and the skin over the entire body may appear dull. A novice snake owner may think that eye caps are retained when these changes are first noted.

Many lizards, including monitors and iguanas, will become more active and even aggressive when exposed to natural sunlight,[30] and owners must be warned that they may become dangerously aggressive or escape if they are not handled carefully. Usually once the lizard is out of the sunlight, normal behavior resumes. Much individuality in personality can be seen in different reptiles of a given species, depending on how much social contact they have been exposed to, how much environmental enrichment is provided, and how they are treated and handled. Frequently owners and caretakers, however, may mistake some atypical behaviors as a sign of domestication while not understanding that the aberrant behavior or new behavior may be a sign of illness, fear, or stress.

Prevention: Successful treatment of reptiles and amphibians must include not only treatment of disease but also the reduction or elimination of stressors while in the care of the practioner and, most importantly, in the animal's home environment. Teaching the staff and owners how to handle each species appropriately, as well as when it is best not to handle them, is important in ensuring their well-being. It has been found that reptiles possess the cognitive ability to be trained using desensitization and operant conditioning to facilitate veterinary care[12] and handling (see Chapters 14 and 121). Providing mental stimulation with this type of training may also help to eliminate some of the psychological stress for reptiles maintained in captivity.[12]

Reproduction and Behavior

Knowledge of normal reproductive behaviors in any given reptile or amphibian species that is kept in captivity is important for both providing optimal care, as well as for successful breeding and reproduction. Without the proper environment and nutrition, for instance, many reptiles cannot successfully reproduce, and pathologic conditions such as dystocia or preovulatory follicular stasis may result.

Observation: Behavioral issues related to seasonal/hormonal influence.

Clinical significance: Gravid females not provided with a proper place to lay eggs or kept under conditions of inappropriate temperature, humidity, and diet will often suffer from preovulatory stasis, egg binding, or dystocia. Gravid female reptiles will often initially be hyperactive, and, as they become visibly gravid, females of many lizard species tend to become lethargic and anorectic, spending more time basking. They may also become more aggressive and active as they attempt to find an appropriate nesting site. Gravid green iguanas will protect a nest site by acting aggressively toward cage mates, including biting and hissing.

As discussed previously (see Feeding and Behavior section), there are many etiologies that lead to anorexia. If anorexia is a presenting complaint, it is important for the clinician to be able to distinguish whether it is pathologic or associated with breeding condition in males or gravidity in females. The throat of male bearded dragons becomes dark black (Fig. 83.8), much darker than the females, during the breeding season.[31] Female chameleons will often become darker in color during gravidity. Female bearded dragons will perform an arm waving behavior where they stand on three legs and wave one front leg in a slow circular motion from front to back. It is thought that this is an appeasement display toward aggressive males during the breeding season and during copulation.[31]

Prevention: It is imperative to assess whether a reptile is in adequate physical condition to undergo what would be a normal period of anorexia

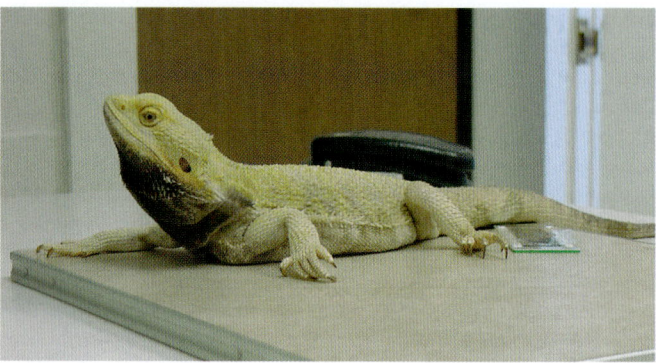

FIG 83.8 Black beards in bearded dragons (*Pogona vitticeps*) can signify many things. It can be present in males in breeding condition and can also be seen when bearded dragons are stressed, fearful, or in pain. This female is suffering from an intestinal obstruction and is presumably in significant pain.

associated with reproductive activity in that species. Environmental clues such as a proper moist or sandy substrate are needed for some females to induce egg-laying behavior. Knowledge of species-specific behaviors related to reproduction is important in ensuring the welfare of reptiles and amphibians in captivity, as well as in recognizing reproductive problems and responding to them sooner.

Behavioral Changes Associated With Medical Issues

Depressed demeanor in reptiles and amphibians is exhibited by half-closed, unfocused eyes, inability or unwillingness to move, extended head and limbs, lack of interest in the surroundings, and the lack of righting and proprioceptive reflexes. Many lizards will sit quietly with head extended, eyes closed, and feet planted firmly when being handled or placed on an examination table. The practitioner must be able to discern between what is normal and abnormal, as even subtle changes in behavior can be significant. Knowledge of abnormal behaviors in light of other clinical signs will aid the practitioner in determining if diagnostics such as blood work, radiographs, and/or ultrasound are needed to rule out the presence of medical issues.

Observation: A normally skittish or aggressive lizard that has suddenly become docile.

Clinical significance: A lizard that does not try to escape as it lays on its owner's chest may in fact be attracted to the warmth of the body in a situation where there is no other heat source. Lizards that suddenly allow handling may also have developed difficulty in ambulation. This is often a chronic gradual process that has been undetected by the caretaker. This could also be a lizard that is stressed or ill and may be perceived as becoming more "tame" to a novice owner or handler. If the lizard is typically more difficult to handle and suddenly becomes "tame," this behavior change may actually indicate lethargy or illness, and a complete physical exam and a full medical workup is needed, including blood work, radiographs (especially if ambulation is a problem), and intestinal parasite exam.

Observation: Snake soaking excessively in a water bowl.

Clinical significance: Rule-outs include a snake enjoying this behavioral enrichment, a stressed or insecure snake that has nowhere else to hide, or a snake that is infested with snake mites (*Ophionyssus natricis*) or trombiculid mites (*Hirstiella spp.*) that is trying to soothe irritated skin. Environmental temperatures may also be too high or humidity may be too low.

Along with a complete physical examination, a husbandry evaluation, including information on how the enclosure is set up and where in the temperature gradient of the enclosure the snake spends most of its time is helpful in determining a diagnosis. This may give the practitioner clues to environmental conditions that are causing immune suppression and disease.

CONCLUSION

Having a working knowledge of normal and abnormal behaviors of reptiles and amphibians is essential for successful practitioners. This information is useful to assess the general well-being of the patient, the appropriateness of the environmental enrichment and husbandry provided to the patient, and as an indicator of clinical disease when abnormal behavior is recognized.

It is important for us as clinicians to establish a "whole patient" approach to the presenting reptile or amphibian, providing guidance on their captive environment, handling, care, and behavior, and not just focusing on the specific presenting sign or symptom.

ACKNOWLEDGMENTS

Much of this chapter is an adaptation from Bradley (2002, Proc ARAV, pp 165–170) and Bays (2006).[32]

REFERENCES

See www.expertconsult.com for a complete list of references.

84

Nutritional Diseases

Thomas H. Boyer and Peter W. Scott

The most common reasons people seek veterinary care for reptiles and amphibians are for nutritional-related diseases. Thus nutritional disorders continue to be important in captive herpetologic medicine, from the all-too-common nutritional secondary hyperparathyroidism (NSHP), hypovitaminosis A, and obesity to the less common thiamine, biotin, vitamin E/selenium deficiencies, steatitis, gout, and corneal lipidosis. This chapter covers significance, etiology, presentation, diagnostic confirmation, and specific therapy of nutritional diseases. To better understand guidelines and recommendations for nutrition, see Chapter 27. For general nutritional therapy guidance, see Chapter 122.

NUTRITIONAL SECONDARY HYPERPARATHYROIDISM

NSHP, particularly rickets and osteomalacia, are the most common of the metabolic bone diseases seen in reptiles and amphibians. Renal secondary hyperparathyroidism (RSHP) was commonly seen in practice in older green iguanas (*Iguana iguana*) presenting in renal failure but is less common currently, as green iguanas are less frequently kept as pets. Hypertrophic osteopathy and osteopetrosis-like lesions have been described in lizards.[1,2] These unusual presentations need to be considered alongside others, such as gout and tumoral calcinosis (pseudogout), as potential differential diagnoses when investigating metabolic bone disease.

Clinical Significance and Known Etiological Cause(s)

NSHP, unfortunately, is still common, especially in amphibians and growing reptiles, except snakes. The most commonly affected reptiles include young growing tortoises (Testudinidae), leopard geckos (*Eublepharis macularius*), and bearded dragons (*Pogona vitticeps*), which is probably a reflection of demographic bias. In the 1990s green iguanas were popular and most commonly affected. Calcium (Ca) deficiency arises from inadequate dietary Ca, an unbalanced calcium:phosphorus (Ca:P) ratio, and/or a lack of vitamin D_3. Diagnosing a calcium deficiency would appear to be straightforward, but it can be a complex and multifactorial issue.

Reptiles require vitamin D_3, cholecalciferol, either in the diet or from dermal ultraviolet B (UVB) photochemical production. Vitamin D_3 is biologically inactive; activation requires hydroxylation in the liver and kidney. Synthesis of vitamin D_3 from UVB is regulated by a negative feedback loop that prevents toxicity. In the liver, D_3 is converted to calcidiol, or 25-hydroxyvitamin D_3, which is typically measured in serum/plasma to determine an animal's vitamin D_3 status. Calcidiol is converted by the proximal renal tubules of the kidneys to calcitriol, or 1,25-dihydroxycholecalciferol, the biologically active form of vitamin D_3. The conversion of calcidiol to calcitriol is catalyzed by the enzyme 1α-hydro, levels of which are increased by parathyroid hormone (PTH) due to low levels of Ca or increased P. Calcitriol circulates in blood as a hormone, regulating the concentration of Ca and P in the bloodstream,

promoting growth and remodeling of bones and also affecting neuromuscular and immune function. Secondary hyperparathyroidism is due to excessive secretion of PTH in response to hypocalcemia, usually from Ca or vitamin D_3 deficiency, or excessive P intake (such as with a low Ca:P ratio diets) and occasionally from chronic kidney failure and inadequate calcitriol production.

Dietary supplementation of D_3 is problematic because recommended daily allowances are unknown for reptiles and amphibians, and given the likely taxonomic variabilities, toxic hypervitaminosis D_3 would be a concern. For example, in growing bearded dragons plasma concentrations of UVB-exposed dragons, for just 2 hours/day, were 18 times higher for calcidiol and 5 times higher for calcitriol than in vitamin D_3-supplemented dragons at 6 months of age. This work is interesting in that whatever period of UVB exposure was used, the blood levels remained within a relatively close range, approximately 10x that of the highest level of supplementation.[3] Natural sunlight or artificial UVB exposure of Komodo dragons (*Varanus komodoensis*) significantly increased calcidiol levels compared with dietary supplementation of 450 IU vitamin D_3/kg feed, which resulted in no increase in any of the measured vitamin D metabolites.[4] Green iguanas also do not seem able to efficiently utilize dietary vitamin D without high doses, likely to cause toxicity in other species, and are dependent on UVB radiation for vitamin D synthesis.[5–7] Most of the iguanas housed indoors at the National Zoo in Washington, DC, fed a diet with 2000–3000 IU vitamin D_3/kg, dry matter basis (DMB), developed NSHP after 2 years (about 25% died) and had extremely low levels of calcidiol (0 to 20 nmol/L [0–8 ng/mL]), which increased rapidly after exposure to artificial UVB (mean = 746 nmol/L [299 ng/mL]) to levels of iguanas housed outdoors (374 to 998 nmol/L [150–400 ng/mL]).[7] Dietary vitamin D levels for other species range from 140 to 2500 IU/Kg, although some primates require higher levels.[7] In humans, serum calcidiol levels less than 50 nmol/L (20 ng/mL) are considered vitamin D deficient, and toxic effects of vitamin D are seen when vitamin D levels are greater than 374 nmol/L (150 ng/mL).[8] As arboreal folivores, iguanas appear far more dependent on UVB for vitamin D_3 production than on dietary vitamin D_3.[6,7] In contrast, researchers found that UVB was not required for western fence lizards (*Sceloporus occidentalis*) for normal bone growth.[9] The differences in metabolic routes of sourcing and use of D_3 shown by such diverse species undoubtedly implies differences will exist in other species, which, as yet, have not been identified. Vitamin D_3 is a fat-soluble vitamin, which means D_3 is stored in hepatic and adipose tissue for long periods of time and generally poses a greater risk for toxicity, when consumed in excess, compared with water-soluble vitamins. This, however, may not be a straightforward assumption because D_3 is inactive without kidney and liver activation.

For captive-raised veiled chameleons (*Chamaeleo calyptratus*) ideal calcidiol levels, based on bone mineral density, were thought to be >250 nmol/L (>100 ng/mL), but levels of 102 nmol/L (41 ng/mL) were sufficient to prevent NSHP.[10] Mean ± SD calcidiol levels of red-eared sliders (*Trachemys scripta elegans*) exposed to UVB for 1 month (71.7 ± 46.9 nmol/L, 29 ± 19 ng/mL) were significantly higher than those without UVB for a month (31.4 ± 13.2 nmol/L, 31 ± 13 ng/mL).[11] Mean ± SD plasma concentration of calcidiol in corn snakes (*Pantherophis guttatus*) that were provided with UVB (196 ± 16.73 nmol/L, 79 ± 7 ng/mL) differed significantly from values in corn snakes without UVB (57.17 ± 15.28 nmol/L, 23 ± 6 ng/mL).[12]

For years UVB light in the 280 and 320 nm wavelength has been recognized as essential for most reptiles, with peak vitamin D synthesis occurring between 295 and 297 nm in mammals. The only reptiles that do not seem to require UVB light, if they have dietary sources of vitamin D_3, are snakes and nocturnal geckos (such as leopard geckos and New Caledonian geckos [*Correlophus* spp. and *Rhacydactylus* spp.]). However, plasma calcidiol levels were increased with UVB radiation in corn snakes[12] but not in ball pythons (*Python regius*).[13] Some snakes (diamond pythons, *Morelia spilota spilota*; indigo snakes, *Drymarchon couperi*; water snakes, *Nerodia* spp.; and green snakes, *Opheodrys* spp.) seem to anecdotally do better with UVB exposure. In one study measuring the effects of UVB radiation on leopard geckos, erythema and increased ecydysis, consistent with sunburn, was noted.[8] Breeding colonies of leopard geckos have been maintained with no UVB exposure and only dietary sources of D_3; others have maintained leopard geckos in excellent health under UVB light without dietary supplements (Boyer T, personal observation., 1982–1994; Baines F, personal communication, 2016). One study suggested that some nocturnal geckos may rely on photobiosynthesis of vitamin D_3 and that they might have a more sensitive mechanism than diurnal lizards to compensate for their limited exposure to natural UVB radiation.[14] In general, broad-spectrum (including UVB) light is recommended for all reptiles and amphibians.

Six sources of ultraviolet light are currently available for reptiles: unfiltered sunlight, fluorescent tubes, compact fluorescent bulbs, mercury vapor spot lights, mercury vapor flood lamps, and light emitting diodes. Recent investigations have demonstrated the ability for LED lights to produce UVB and maintain calcidiol plasma levels in bearded dragons.[15] Sunlight is always recommended as the best source of UVB light, and although short periods may be sufficient, this is not always practical due to temperature. Hermann's tortoises (*Testudo hermanni*) exposed to mercury vapor or fluorescent UVB lights had significantly lower calcidiol plasma levels after 35 days (155.69 ± 80.71 nmol/L, 62.38 ± 32.34 ng/mL, and 134.42 ± 51.42 nmol/L, 53.85 ± 20.60 ng/mL, respectively) compared with tortoises with natural sunlight exposure (411.51 ± 189.75 nmol/L, 164.87 ± 76.02 ng/mL).[16] UVB light is almost completely filtered by glass or plastic, unless these materials are specifically UVB transmissible. UVB transmissible glass or plastics are available but costly, and rarely used outside zoos. Fluorescent tubes and compact fluorescent bulbs produce UVB light but little heat, thus the demand for and use of mercury vapor lights that can produce both heat and UVB light. This may be advantageous because vitamin D_3 activation requires both UVB light and heat. All spot lights seem prone to burning because they produce a focused beam. Mercury vapor flood lamps produce more diffuse heat. Manufacturers' recommended minimum distances should always be followed. UVB light intensity decreases with the inverse square law ($1/distance^2$), so a light that is twice as far away has one-fourth the UVB intensity. Consequently lights, especially those of lower power like fluorescents, should be kept close to the animal, no more than 30–60 cm (12–24 inches) away. UVB lights should be replaced every 6 to 12 months or when UVB output drops below 70% of the original output. UV meters are now available and are an important tool for testing bulb output and assessing efficacy of basking areas. Not all reptile lights produce UVB; practitioners must check products individually. Many reptile lights state "daylight," "broad spectrum," or "UVA" (320–400 nm) but lack critical UVB. See Chapter 17 for more information.

Bones are the main storage site of Ca in the body (99%). Total plasma Ca concentration consists of three fractions: 40% total Ca (which is albumin bound), 15% anion bound (Ca sulfate, phosphate, lactate, or citrate), and 45% as ionized (or free) Ca. The wide range in normal total plasma Ca concentration is probably due to variations in plasma albumin concentrations. When ionized Ca levels drop in blood, the parathyroid gland releases PTH, which increases Ca resorption from bone, reabsorption from kidneys, and absorption from intestines. If bone levels are not replenished from Ca intake, chronic hyperparathyroidism weakens bones, sometimes causing pathological fractures and/or fibrous osteodystrophy (lizards) or shell softening (chelonians). Life-threatening reductions in blood-ionized Ca can lead to seizures, tetany, and flaccid paresis (Fig. 84.1A and B). Mean ionized calcium concentrations in blood for iguanas were 1.47 ± 0.105 mmol/L (5.89 ± 0.44 mg/dL) and for Mediterranean tortoises (*Testudo* spp.) were 1.32 ± 0.14 mmol/L (5.29 ± 0.56 mg/dL). Significant differences were not detected among juveniles, males, and females.[17,18] When ionized Ca levels are high, calcitonin, from the ultimobranchial bodies, inhibits osteoclast activity and reduces renal tubular reabsorption of calcium and presumably provides negative feedback to the parathyroid glands to reduce PTH secretion. Ca is often deficient in the diets of insectivores (insects have little Ca), omnivores, and herbivores (vegetables and fruits are typically low in Ca) but usually not carnivores, because the bones within the whole animals they are feeding on generally provide a balanced source of Ca. Exceptions include feeding organs, meat without bone, or neonatal rodents (pinkies). Neonatal rodents have a borderline low Ca:P ratio depending on age and how long they have been nursing. Most carnivores grow quickly enough that they outgrow pinkies and begin to take larger prey with more calcified bone and avoid Ca deficiency. For more information on this, see Chapter 27.

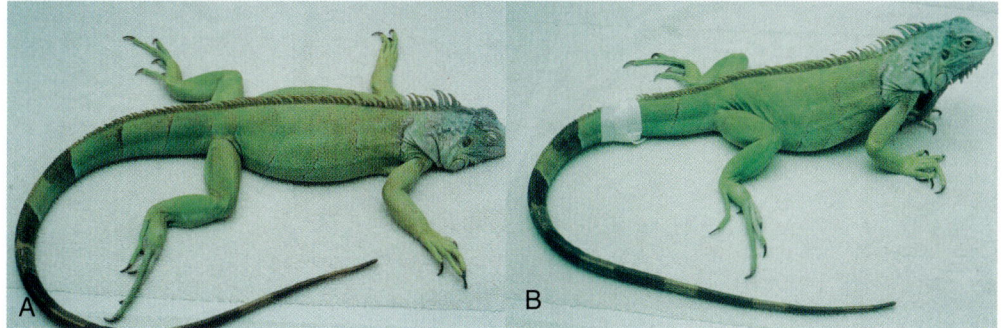

FIG 84.1 Hypocalcemic flaccid paresis in a green iguana (*Iguana iguana*), before (A) and minutes after (B), 100 mg/kg 10% Ca gluconate intracoelomically. Ca injections should only be given if neurological signs are present, usually as a result of a drop below normal of ionized Ca. (Courtesy of Thomas H. Boyer.)

Clinical Presentation and Diagnostic Confirmation

Symptoms of NSHP vary widely by individual and species. Common signs include lethargy, weakness, anorexia or decreased appetite, lack of growth, sprawl (Fig. 84.2A–D), and reduced ability to raise the body during ambulation. Lizards are prone to spinal injury from pathological vertebral fractures, which may result in paraparesis, paraplegia, or quadriplegia, depending on the location of the spinal lesion.

NSHP can cause the ribs and scapuli of lizards to flatten horizontally, away from the more normal vertical orientation. Iguanas and leopard geckos have similar clinical signs, including bowed long bones (especially the radius and ulna), walking on the antebrachiums (not plantigrade), long bone fractures, pliable mandibles and maxillae (Fig. 84.3A–D), kyphosis, scoliosis, lordosis, or rhoecosis (all three of the former). Iguanas sometimes bloat, can prolapse their colon/cloaca, and are particularly prone to fibrous osteodystrophy (Fig. 84.4), especially of the mandible.[19]

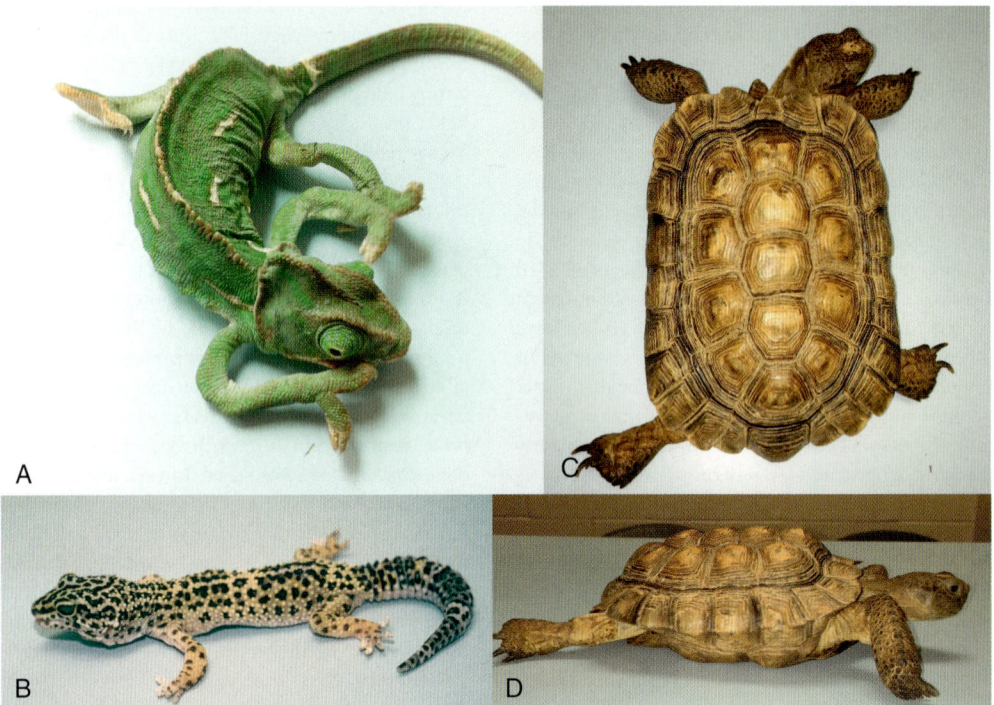

FIG 84.2 Sprawl (A–C) and lack of truncal (A and B) or shell lifting (D) are common signs of nutritional secondary hyperparathyroidism in lizards and chelonians. (Courtesy of Thomas H. Boyer.)

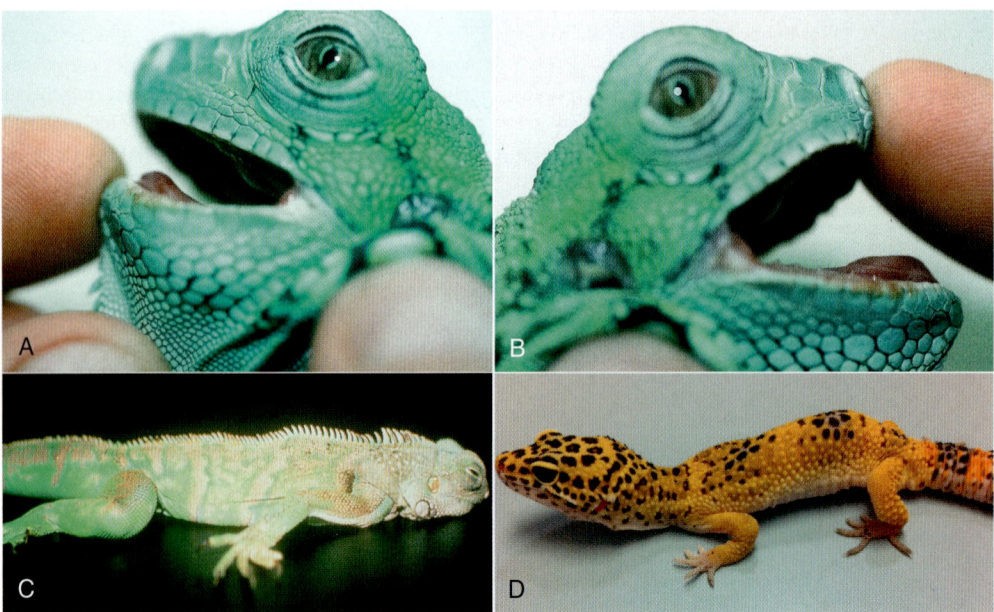

FIG 84.3 Iguanas (*Iguana iguana*) and leopard geckos (*Eublepharis macularius*) have similar clinical signs of nutritional secondary hyperparathyroidism, including pliable mandibles and maxillae (A and B); kyphoscoliosis, lordosis, or rhoecosis (C and D); bowed long bones (especially the radius and ulna, D); and walking on the antebrachium (not plantigrade, D). (Courtesy of Thomas H. Boyer.)

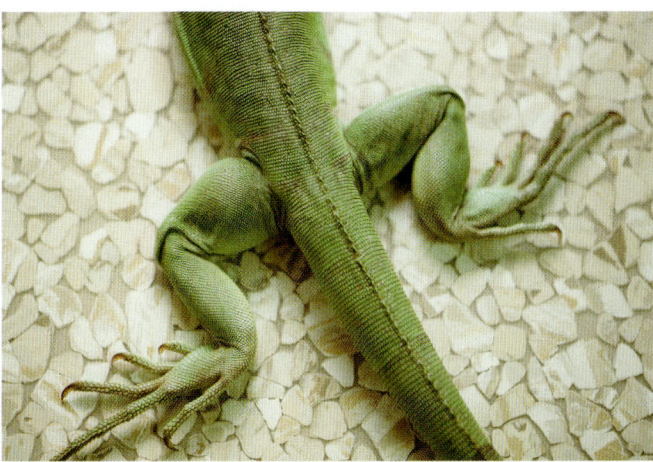

FIG 84.4 Fibrous osteodystrophy (in the left femur and right tibia/fibula of this iguana [*Iguana iguana*]) is common in lizards with nutritional secondary hyperparathyroidism but is not seen in chelonians. (Courtesy of Thomas H. Boyer.)

Chameleons have a noticeably weakened grip, fall repeatedly, and have bowed, distorted or fractured long bones, scoliosis of the parietal crest or vertebrae, cloacal distention, and tail weakness (Fig. 84.5A–D). In iguanas, bearded dragons, and monitors (Varanidae), when ionized Ca can no longer be maintained, tremors (especially in the digits, limbs, or large muscle masses), spasms, seizures, flaccid paresis, or death can occur (see Fig. 84.1A and B).[20]

NSHP is obvious in tortoises with soft or deformed shells, inability to lift the shell while walking, splayed legs, and decreased appetite. Tortoise shell should feel very much like skull, with no soft areas (except pancake tortoises and chelonians with shell kinesis [Fig. 84.6]. Shell pliability of neonates typically disappears within 6 to 18 months. Calcium-deficient females probably produce calcium-deficient eggs/hatchlings. Chelonians rarely develop fibrous osteodystrophy; they simply calcify their shell poorly. This is typically followed by anorexia and a reduced ability or inability to move, likely in relation to muscle weakness, from associated hypocalcemia, or bone pain. Clinical signs vary depending on age of exposure to a calcium-deficient diet. Small tortoises fail to grow or gain weight, have normal shell morphology except it is soft, splay out their legs, and have overgrown nails. Black areas beneath the scutes may represent normal coloration, but if the shell is soft, decreased shell ossification can result in transparency of scutes to an underlying darker tissue ("black spot disease") (Fig. 84.7A and B). In general, tortoises that are not eating carry a poor prognosis and typically die. In adult tortoises there is curving of the normally straight ventral or dorsal midline scutes, and the epiplastron projection may curve dorsally instead of anteriorly (Fig. 84.8A and B). The convex carapace may develop lordosis (Fig. 84.9). The central plastron may be flexible, or the anterior and posterior plastron flexes more than it should during palpation. The medial nails of the pelvic limbs wear excessively whereas the lateral nails overgrow because the tortoise walks on its heels, not plantigrade (Fig. 84.10). Pyramidal shell growth may accompany calcium deficiency; however, it appears to be multifactorial in origin, with humidity and growth rate also involved (see Fig. 84.9).[21,22] In box turtles (*Terrapene*), the marginal scutes curl dorsally; the seams between scutes collapse inwardly; the plastrocarapacial bridge widens vertically; the anterior rhamphotheca may curve more like a parrot's beak; the body may appear too large for the shell; and phallic, clitoral, or cloacal prolapse may occur (Fig. 84.11A–D). Curling of the posterior plastron also occurred experimentally in red-eared sliders fed a protein-deficient diet

(10% crude protein).[23] Protein deficiency may accompany Ca deficiency in chelonians and contribute to shell softening or curling.

Crocodilians with NSHP may move freely in water but are weak, sluggish, or ataxic on land and eventually are unable to come out of the water.[24] The upper jaw softens so much it can be bent upward. Long bones soften and deform, and posterior paralysis, kyphosis, scoliosis, lordosis, or rhoecosis may be present. The teeth may be translucent or diaphanous (glassy teeth), deviate horizontally, or fall out.[24] Disturbance may result in tremors or seizures; seizures in water may lead to drowning.[24]

Clinical signs in amphibians include abnormal posture (lack of truncal lifting, dorsal curling of the toes) and locomotion, anasarca/dropsy/subcutaneous edema, vertebral deformity, mandibular deformity, pathological fractures of long bones, and absence of radio-opaque calcium carbonate in the endolymphatic sacs.[25] Early signs may be limited to fractured bones, tetany, or subcutaneous (lymph sac) fluid accumulation; advanced cases have decreased bone demineralization and skeletal deformities.

Clinical signs and nutritional histories are typically informative in reaching a presumptive diagnosis of NSHP. Radiographs are useful to confirm suspicion of NSHP and whole body assessment of fractures. Only severe reductions in bone density are radiographically obvious, because 40% to 50% of bone mineralization must generally be depleted before it is visible radiographically.[26] In lizards with NSHP there is a general decrease in bone opacity and cortical thinning of long bones and flat bones, especially appreciated with poor contrast of pelvic bones.[20] Decreased opacity in thin bones, such as the caudal vertebral transverse processes and dorsal spinous processes, can result in poor contrast from the associated soft tissue. There may be bowing of long bones, absent metaphyseal trabecular markings or more radiolucent metaphyses, and extensive soft tissue swelling involving the limbs (fibrous osteodystrophy).[20] Transverse folding fractures of long bones and compression fractures of vertebrae may be present. In chelonians decreased opacity is difficult to appreciate in the shell and limb bones but may be present in the pectoral and pelvic girdles, which typically are in good contrast to the overlying shell.

Usually, total Ca is within normal limits until skeletal reserves have been depleted, whereas ionized Ca levels are maintained until terminal. One study found total serum Ca levels of veiled chameleons with NSHP to be 2.0 to 2.2 mmol/L (8.0–8.8 mg/dL), slightly below the reference range of 2.3 to 3.5 mmol/L (9.2–14.00 mg/dL).[10] Elevated nitrogenous byproducts (ammonia, urea, or uric acid) may indicate renal secondary hyperthyroidism or dehydration. Calcium-deficient females may have elevated Ca levels because of egg production. Conversely, a gravid oviparous female with normal Ca levels may be calcium deficient. With obvious clinical signs, further diagnostics, apart from radiography, are seldom required. The definitive diagnosis of hyperparathyroidism requires demonstration of elevated PTH, but commercially available mammalian assays do not appear to be accurate for reptiles and cannot be recommended. Plasma calcidiol values can be more easily measured to assess the potential deficiency of UVB or dietary D_3 deficiency.

The best ways to measure bone density are via quantitative computed tomography[27] or dual-energy X-ray absorptiometry (DEXA).[20] The latter has been described experimentally in green iguanas,[20] leopard tortoises (*Stigmochelys pardalis*),[28] and Hermann's tortoises.[27] Regression equations of bone density as a function of body weight are available for normal iguanas and iguanas with NSHP, with the skull, lumbar spine, and femurs being most useful.[20] In Hermann's tortoises, decreased bone mineral density of the shell was apparent with DEXA but not in the axial and appendicular skeleton,[27] which may explain why spinal and appendicular fractures or fibrous osteodystrophy are not seen in chelonians.

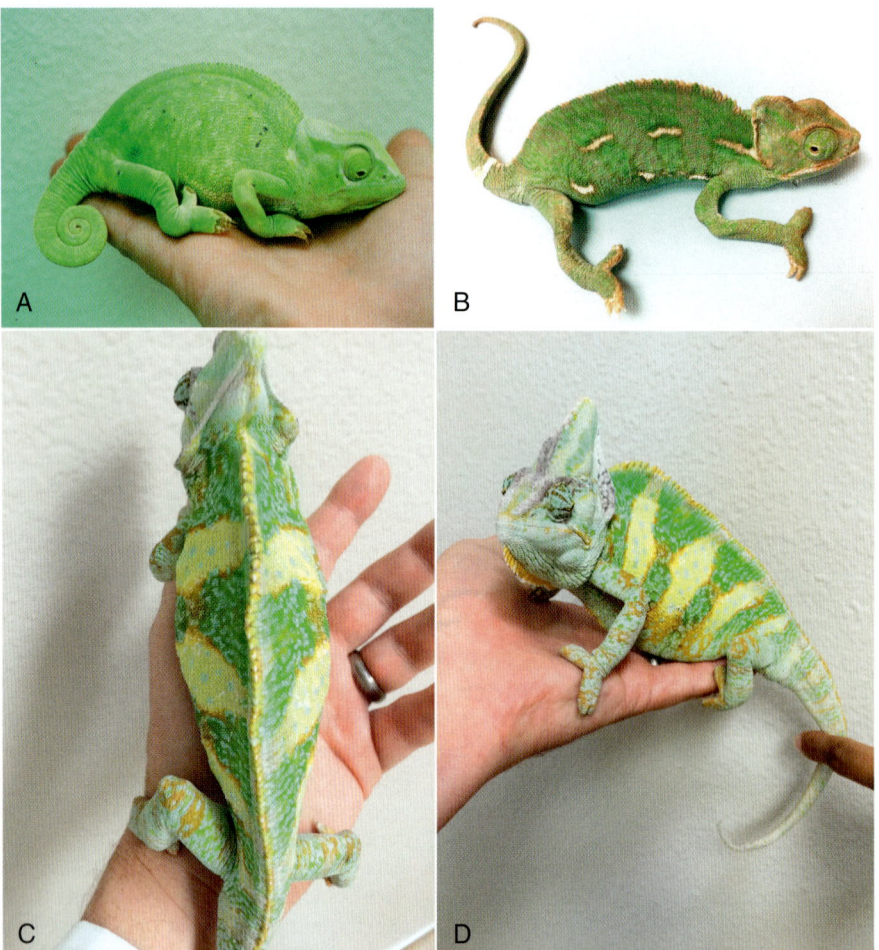

FIG 84.5 Chameleons with nutritional secondary hyperparathyroidism have a weakened grip; fall repeatedly; have bowed, fractured, or grossly distorted long bones (A and B); spinal kyphoscoliosis (C), lordosis (B), or rhoecosis; and tail weakness (D). A healthy chameleon would normally wrap its tail around the finger. (Courtesy of Thomas H. Boyer.)

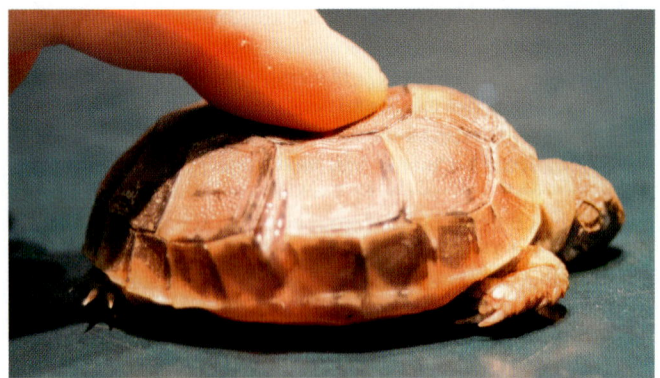

FIG 84.6 A soft shell is abnormal in almost all chelonian species (except for pancake tortoises [*Malacochersus tornieri*] and other exceptions noted in Chapter 7); the shell should feel like solid bone, much like a skull. (Courtesy of Thomas H. Boyer.)

Preferred Treatment(s)

Patients with NSHP should be strictly cage rested and handled carefully to prevent fractures or spinal trauma. All patients should have exposure to unfiltered sunlight (preferred, but be wary of overheating) or artificial UVB light (290–300 nm). Treatment includes calcium (Ca) supplementation, nutritional support, improved husbandry, analgesia, and calcitonin (although cost and availability may be an issue with the latter). Oral Ca supplementation is easiest via Ca-rich syrups, either Ca glubionate (1.8 gm/5 mL) or Ca gluconate (23% w/v); both are dosed at 1 mL/kg PO BID. Calcium doses are given in mL/kg, rather than mg/kg, because different Ca products vary in the amount of elemental Ca available and how Ca is measured (Ca salts vs elemental Ca, mg vs mEq, or mmol), which can lead to confusion, potential sources of medication errors, and delayed treatment. As mentioned, Ca gluconate is labeled as 23% w/v, which is 24 mg/mL elemental Ca, and Ca glubionate as 1.8 gm/5 ml, which is 21 mg/mL elemental Ca; neither is labeled as mg/mL (see Tables 27.10 and 27.11 in Chapter 27). Calcium supplementation is typically continued for 1 to 3 months or until the patient is consistently eating calcium-enriched foods, moving normally, and, if growing or in poor body condition, gaining weight. Powdered calcium supplements on foods are not recommended as a sole treatment unless the patient has minimal clinical signs and continues to eat voluntarily; however, if a viable option, it does reduce the risks associated with handling to medicate the patient. Calcium sprays available through pet stores have so little Ca present (1700 ppm Ca or 0.17% Ca) that they are of poor therapeutic value. Ideally, patients with hypocalcemic tetany should be treated by slow intravenous (or intraosseous) infusion (100 mg/kg 10% Ca gluconate), but this is often impractical. If IV or IO therapy is not possible, then intramuscular or intracoelomic administration at

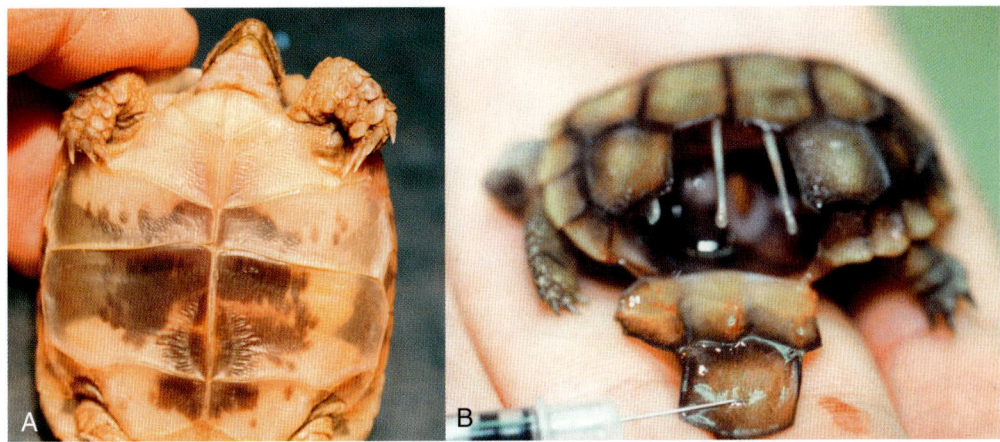

FIG 84.7 Black areas beneath the scutes in young tortoises (A) may represent decreased shell ossification (from nutritional secondary hyperparathyroidism) and transparency of scutes to underlying darker tissue ("black spot disease"), or may be normal coloration. Note the lack of rib ossification to form the shell in this juvenile tortoise (B). (Courtesy of Thomas H. Boyer.)

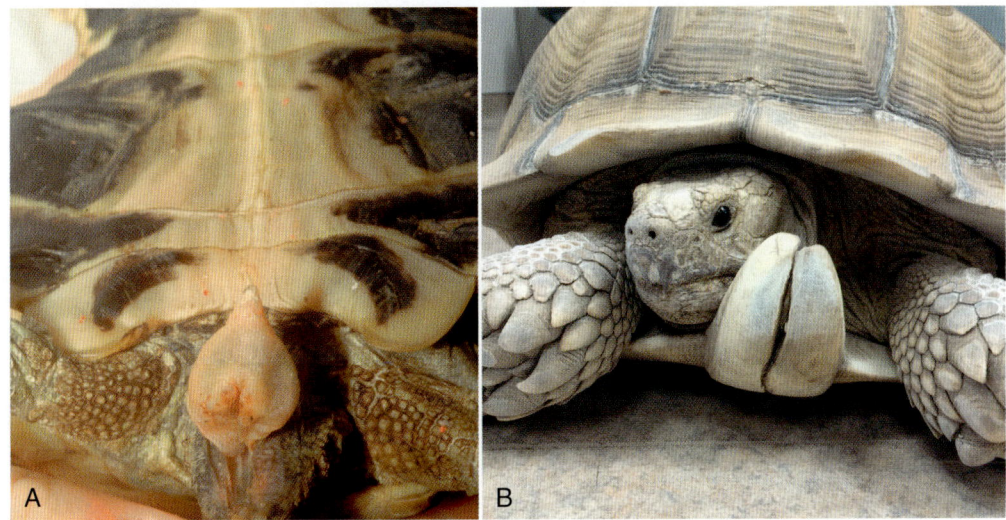

FIG 84.8 Curving of the normally straight ventral or dorsal midline scutes and associated prolapses (A) or the epiplastron projection (B) are telltale signs of Ca deficiency, currently or in the past. (Courtesy of Thomas H. Boyer.)

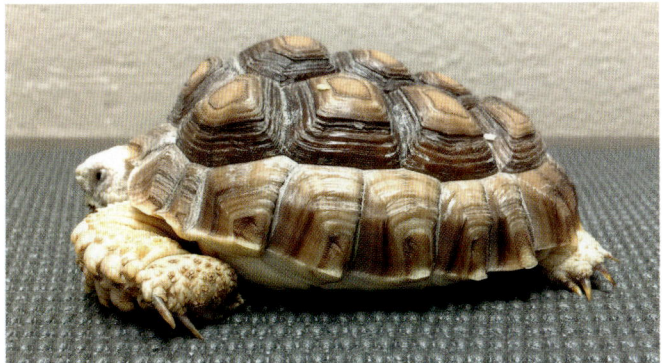

FIG 84.9 In chelonians with nutritional secondary hyperparathyroidism the normally convex carapace may have lordosis and/or pyramidal shell growth. Pyramidal shell growth appears to be multifactorial in origin, with humidity and growth rate being important factors. (Courtesy of Thomas H. Boyer.)

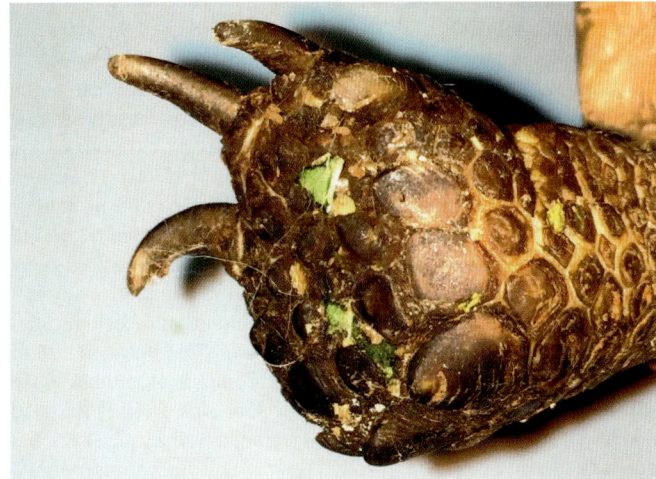

FIG 84.10 Sprawl causes tortoises to walk on their heels, which wears down the inner nails. Note the inner nails of this tortoise are worn smooth whereas the outer nails are overgrown. (Courtesy of Thomas H. Boyer.)

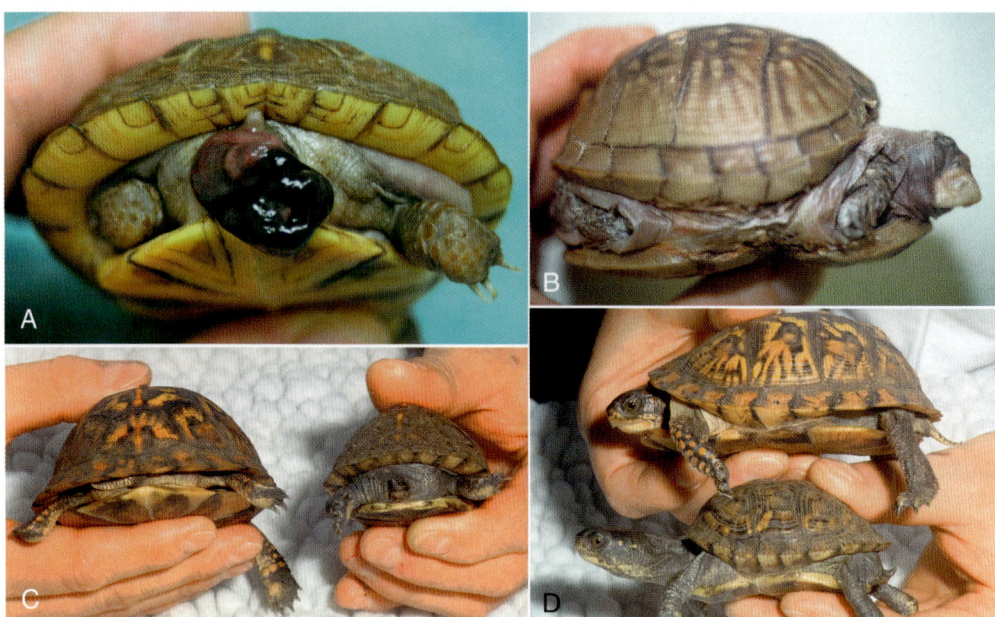

FIG 84.11 Nutritional secondary hyperparathyroidism in chelonians affects the shell and often spares the axial and appendicular skeleton. As a result, the turtle's body outgrows its shell, and chronic prolapse of the cloaca, phallus, or clitoris may result (A). Note the upturned marginal scutes (B), increased space between carapace and plastron bridge (C), and the anterior rhamphotheca, which may curve more like a parrot's beak. Normal wild-caught eastern box turtle (*Terrapene carolina carolina*) on the left, compared with a long-term captive on the right (C); note how much smaller the shell of the lower affected turtle is compared with the upper wild-caught turtle (D). (Courtesy of Thomas H. Boyer.)

100 mg/kg 10% Ca gluconate q 6 hours can be continued until tetany ceases and the patient can be given oral Ca.

Nutritional support is critical, allowing the patient to gain weight and begin to grow as a normal process. Although pathological fractures will usually heal, angular deformities typically persist. Weight loss in an already cachexic patient continues a downward spiral. Nutritional support is critical for successful treatment, and the use of nutritional enterals via stomach tube (or gentle hand feeding in some cases) once daily for most reptiles and up to twice daily for small lizards until the patient is eating unaided and maintaining or gaining body weight is important. These foods may contain vitamin D_3, so a vitamin D injection is not required.

Analgesics are recommended. Salmon calcitonin (SCT) injections have been recommended at 50 IU/kg IM; repeated in 1 week if normocalcemic, or 1 week after starting calcium supplementation.[19,29,30] Calcitonin is thought to act by stimulating negative feedback on the parathyroid gland, reducing parathyroid hormone, decreasing osteoclastic activity, stimulating osteoblasts, and decreasing blood Ca concentration, and may have an analgesic effect on skeletal pain.[31,32] However, there is little research to evaluate efficacy of SCT in reptiles. One study in aquatic turtles (*Pseudemys scripta, Graptemys kohni, Chelydra serpentina*) found that 4 micrograms/kg SCT 3x/wk for 11 to 19 weeks enhanced bone growth in turtles under Ca-deficient conditions by inhibiting osteolysis.[33] In green iguanas, a single dose of SCT (20 milliunits intracoelomically) stimulated a significant decrease in total plasma Ca levels from 20 to 120 minutes; blood Ca levels were back to normal at 240 minutes.[34] In another study with green iguanas, a single dose of SCT (50 IU/kg) had no effect on total Ca concentration long term; however, ionized Ca was not measured (which SCT affects) (Wagner and Bodri, unpublished manuscript, 1996). Do not give calcitonin if the patient is hypocalcemic or Ca status is unknown. Research evidence would suggest salmon calcitonin should be given more frequently.

Fractures can be treated with external coaptation (see Chapter 108). Lizards with dramatic spinal cord deformities can maintain an acceptable quality of life as long as paralysis, or urinary or fecal retention does not occur. Treatment generally takes months, so a long-term commitment by the owner is required. Reevaluations should be considered at 1, 2, 4, and 8 weeks, until weight is improving and it is clear the patient is recovering. Progress evaluations are important to discuss husbandry and ensure that clients are adopting permanent improvements to prevent recurrence. Radiography can help track response to therapy, especially with fractures, but are insensitive to subtle changes in bone radiopacity.

Prognosis and Prevention

Prognosis is dependent on severity of clinical, radiographic, and clinicopathologic changes. Multiple deficiencies, such as calcium and vitamin A deficiency, common with chameleons, are difficult to recover from. Lizards and crocodilians often respond better than chelonians. Early diagnosis and aggressive treatment is essential; chronic NSHP has a worse prognosis. Owners must be committed to several months of daily treatment. If no decreased radiopacity of bone is visible, the prognosis is good. Decreasing radiopacity of bone and hypocalcemia worsen prognosis. Paralysis, urinary retention, and obstipation are poor prognostic indicators. For small chelonians with soft shells, if they are not eating at presentation or soon after, the prognosis is typically poor. Even with intensive care, they typically die. NSHP can be prevented by good nutrition with adequate Ca and UV supplementation (for more information, see Chapter 27).

HYPOVITAMINOSIS A

Clinical Significance and Known Etiological Cause(s)

Vitamin A was the first fat-soluble vitamin to be discovered and is an essential nutrient required for normal vision, embryonic development, reproduction, immune function, bone metabolism, hematopoiesis, and epithelial tissues in all vertebrates.[35] In humans, vitamin A deficiency (VAD) causes nyctalopia (night blindness initially), xerophthalmia, keratomalacia, and eventually complete blindness.

There are several forms of vitamin A. Retinol is the alcohol form; replacement of the alcohol with aldehyde gives retinal, and replacement by an acid group produces retinoic acid.[36] Retinal combines with the protein, opsin, to form rhodopsin, the light-absorbing molecule of the retina, vital for vision. The retinoic acid form is an important hormone-like growth factor for normal epithelial cell differentiation. In humans, retinoic acid switches on genes that differentiate keratinocytes (immature skin cells) into mature epidermal cells.[37] Without retinoic acid, hyperkeratosis (an abnormal thickening of the outermost layer of the epidermis, the stratum corneum, associated with excess keratin) and squamous metaplasia (transformation of cuboidal, columnar, or ciliated glandular, or mucosal, epithelium into keratinizing stratified squamous epithelium) affect new epithelia, especially in the respiratory, ocular, endocrine, gastrointestinal, and genitourinary systems.[38]

Carotenoids (carotenes and xanthophylls) are fat-soluble pigments found in plants, many of which have provitamin A activity, especially the β-carotenes. Herbivores and omnivores, such as tortoises, iguanas, and bearded dragons, are apparently good at converting carotenoids to retinol because they do not suffer from hypovitaminosis A; plants are excellent sources of carotenoids. Enterohepatic circulation is an important means of vitamin A conservation before fecal excretion. Secondary hypovitaminosis A is rare but possible, with chronic malabsorption of lipids (such as with pancreatitis) or impaired bile production and release. In foods of animal origin, the major form of vitamin A is primarily retinyl palmitate, which is converted to retinol in the small intestine. Retinol is transported mainly with lymph chylomicrons to the liver, where it is converted back to retinyl palmitate for storage. In most species, more than 80% to 90% of the vitamin A in the body is stored in the liver.[35]

Clinical Presentation

In general, insectivorous and carnivorous reptiles and amphibians cannot convert carotenoids to vitamin A and rely on animal sources of vitamin A. Fish and mammalian liver are rich sources of retinyl palmitate, thus snakes, carnivorous reptiles, and amphibians that consume whole vertebrate prey regularly do not get VAD. Unfortunately, insects are deficient in vitamin A unless gut-loaded or dusted with multivitamins containing vitamin A and not β-carotene. VAD is well recognized in emydid turtles (aquatic turtles and box turtles) and is also seen in insectivorous lizards such as chameleons, leopard geckos, fat-tailed geckos (*Hemitheconyx caudicinctus*), and *Anolis* lizards not supplemented with preformed vitamin A.

Amphibians, being insectivores, are also prone to VAD. It is thought that amphibians do not synthesize vitamin A from β-carotene, but scientific evidence to support this is sparse.[25,38–40] Cane toads (*Bufo marinus*) and Cuban tree frogs (*Osteopilus septentrionalis*) were not able to convert β-carotene to retinol in liver and small intestines samples, suggesting a lack of β-carotene 15,15'-dioxygenase activity (Comb-Renjifo et al, unpublished data, 2011). However, tadpoles of the Asian common toad (*Duttaphrynus melanostictus*) and Indian bullfrog (*Haplobactrachus tigerinus*) were capable of converting β-carotene and lutein (another carotenoid) to retinol and dehydroretinol, respectively.[41] Mixed carotenoid (β-carotene, lutenin, canthaxantin, and xanthophylls) dietary supplementation for 9 weeks did significantly raise plasma retinol levels in tomato frogs (*Dyscophus guineti*), however, β-carotene alone did not.[39] Chiricahuan leopard frogs (*Rana chiricahuaensis*) developed conjunctivitis in the lower eyelid that was responsive to vitamin A supplementation because of a diet that lacked vitamin A (the multivitamin supplement

contained β-carotene but not vitamin A).[42,43] Carotenoids are not without benefit; they have been shown to improve development, fecundity, and reddish coloration in amphibians.[39,44–46]

In amphibians, VAD causes short tongue syndrome (STS).[43] STS results from replacement of the normal mucus-producing epithelium of the tongue tip with a keratinizing stratified squamous epithelium (squamous metaplasia), which makes their tongues less sticky. Anurans with STS repeatedly strike prey items with their tongue but are unable to prehend food, giving the appearance of a shortened tongue.[42,43,47] STS has been recognized in Bufonidae (toads), Dendrobatidae (poison dart frogs), Hylidae (tree frogs), Ranidae (true frogs), and Rhacophoridae (foam nesting frogs).[38] Amphibian lingual squamous metaplasia develops rostrally, then progresses caudally, therefore the entire amphibian tongue, bisected longitudinally, should be submitted for histopathology. Transverse sectioning could overlook early cases.[38,42,43] In addition to lingual and oronasal mucosal squamous hyperplasia, VAD also variably affects epithelium of the skin, conjunctiva, gastrointestinal, urinary, and reproductive tracts, contributing to poor reproductive success, reduced survival of tadpoles, and immune dysfunction.[38,47] For instance, lingual squamous metaplasia was not present in lemur leaf frogs (*Hyomantis lemur*) that had extensive squamous metaplasia in the cloaca and urinary bladder.[38] Periocular and conjunctival swelling, responsive to vitamin A supplementation, has been observed in ranid and dendrobatid frogs, as well as a tiger salamander (*Ambystoma tigrinum*).[38,43]

Many reptile multivitamins contain β-carotene instead of preformed vitamin A, a lasting influence of several inaccurate hobbyist articles (Chameleon Information Network Newsletter 1993, #9, pp 18-25, and #10, pp 15-18 that concluded consumption of small amounts of preformed vitamin A caused edema in the neck and throat areas of chameleons, bone decalcification, and birth defects. Currently about a third of the reptile and amphibian multivitamins on the market lack vitamin A or retinol esters (retinyl acetate or retinyl palmitate) and instead carry only β-carotene in the misguided notion that vitamin A is unnecessary, or dangerous. Several years after these hobbyist articles, researchers objectively demonstrated hypovitaminosis A induced gular edema in 15/16 panther chameleons given low dietary levels of vitamin A.[48] Although it is true that a high intake of carotenoids does not produce vitamin A toxicity,[35] many insectivores and carnivores cannot convert β-carotenes to vitamin A and thus require dietary vitamin A. Excess vitamin A has been shown to be toxic in most species studied, typically from chronic intakes of 100 to 1000 times the nutritional requirements, but also has been observed with intakes as low as 10 times the specific dietary requirement.[35] Presumed upper safe levels are 4 to 10 times the nutritional requirements but remain unknown for reptiles and amphibians. However, estimates for other species are useful, with estimated dietary levels of 8000 IU/kg feed or 56 IU/kg body weight daily for green iguanas (*Iguana iguana*).[6] Estimated dietary levels for cricket gut-loading diets were 5000 to 8000 micrograms retinol equivalents/kg as fed (8% moisture).[49]

In reptiles, hypovitaminosis A causes a series of changes, most noticeably to the eyes. The normal lacrimal and mucus-secreting cuboidal to columnar epithelium of the eye is replaced by a flattened keratinized epithelium (squamous metaplasia), which continually desquamate followed by the buildup of keratin debris (hyperkeratosis), which blocks lacrimal, salivary, and mucous glands. Plump amphophilic mucus-secreting cells are replaced by flattened, scalelike, keratinized squamous epithelium. Gland lumina dilate and fill with keratinaceous and cellular debris.[50] In *Anolis*, VAD caused decreased numbers of conjunctival goblet cells.[50] Decreased lacrimal production induces xerophthalmia (dry eye). In emydid turtles and leopard geckos, the lacrimal glands block and slowly swell, expanding under the palpebra, gradually swelling the palpebral fissure shut (Figs. 84.12 and 84.13). In chameleons, early signs are

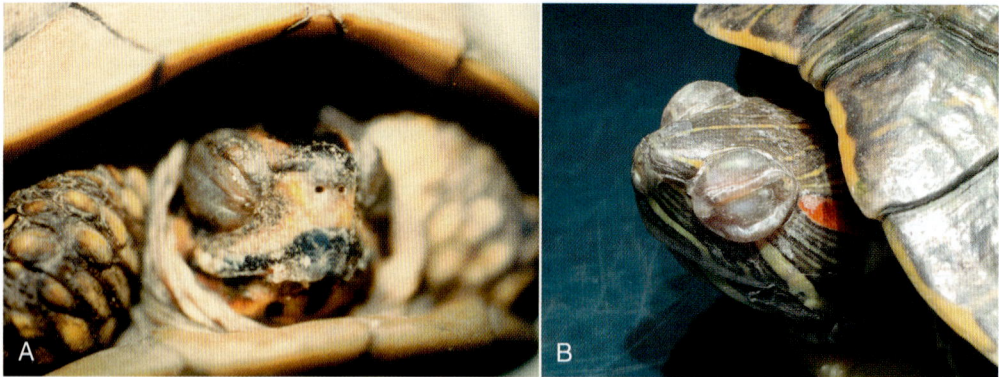

FIG 84.12 (A) Hypovitaminosis A in a three-toed box turtle (*Terrapene carolina triunguis*) and (B) a red-eared slider (*Trachemys scripta elegans*); note the blepharedema. (Courtesy of Thomas H. Boyer.)

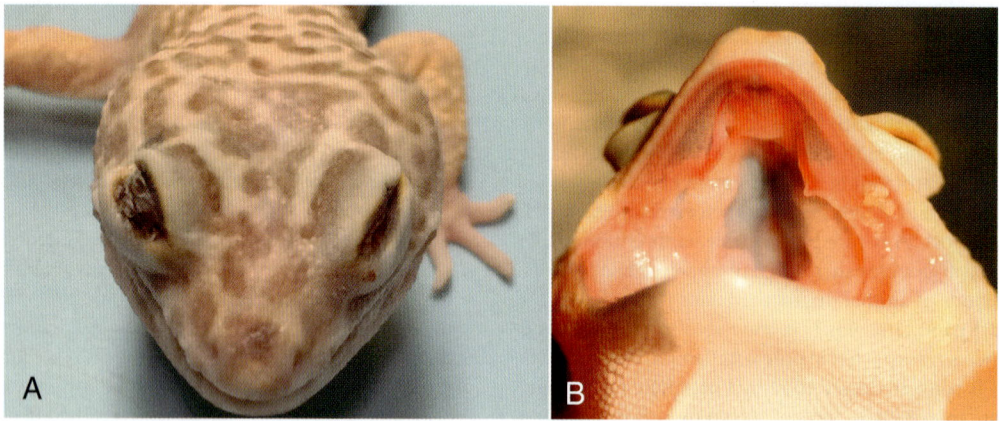

FIG 84.13 Hypovitaminosis A in a leopard gecko (*Eublepharus macularius*) with blepharedema (A), buildup of oral solid cellular debris, which is one of the few causes of stomatitis (B). (Courtesy of Thomas H. Boyer.)

decreased tear production with blepharospasm, thick ocular mucus, and thickened palpebral margins (Fig. 84.14A–C). Chameleons frequently have a history of worsening eye disease unresponsive to antibiotic therapy and eventually keep their eyes shut unless disturbed. Owners report poor aim and prehension, perhaps from squamous metaplasia of mucous glands in the tongue tip and/or retinal damage. With chronicity, multifocal minute distended glands swell and irregularly thicken the lips (see Fig. 84.14C) and sometimes the jaw commissures, and tail tip necrosis may develop.[48] Leopard geckos can have periocular glands distended with solid cellular debris and diffuse massive cellulitis (Fig. 84.15A and B). Decreased tear production causes keratitis, corneal erosion and ulceration, keratomalacia, and eventually permanent corneal scarring and perhaps blindness (Fig. 84.16). With chronic VAD, the eyelids swell shut and, in leopards geckos and emydid turtles, white to yellow, semisolid to solid, keratinaceous, inflammatory cellular debris and bacteria accumulate under the palpebrae (Fig. 84.17A–C). VAD in insectivorous lizards also results in decreased appetite, difficulty catching prey, retained and recurrent hemipenal plugs, dysecdysis, dull coloration (particularly in chameleons), and stomatitis (leopard geckos). Emydid turtles may have concurrent tympanic ear abscesses, pneumonia, or dystocia. Hatchling aquatic turtles typically have enough vitamin A yolk reserves for 6 months.[51]

Farm-raised freshwater and saltwater crocodiles (*Crocodylus johnsoni* and *C. porosus*) fed a vitamin A–deficient diet (125 IU vitamin A/kg dietary dry matter) had multifocal brown dorsal lingual nodules, up to 5 mm in diameter, as well as renal and visceral gout. Gout was thought to be induced by renal tubular squamous metaplasia and hyperkeratosis, classic symptoms of hypovitaminosis A.[52]

Vitamin A is also involved in osteoclast and osteoblast activity in epithelial cartilage. In mammals, joint involvement is associated with VAD. Constriction of nerve foramina during embryonic and early growth may result in blindness, deafness, and cerebellar herniation; other congenital malformations have also been seen in soft tissues.

Diagnostic Confirmation

Most cases in clinical practice are treated based on dietary history, clinical signs, biopsy histopathology, and response to therapy. Determining normal levels of Vitamin A is fraught with error based on what is measured (i.e., total Vitamin A [retinol + retinyl ester] vs. vitamin A [retinol]) and the method of measurement (high-performance liquid chromatography is currently the standard; techniques before the early 1980s were prone to experimental error and should be interpreted with caution), and assay differences among laboratories may give disparate values for similar levels.[53] Vitamin A also degrades with light exposure, high temperatures, and patient autolysis.[43] A study in amphibians found that determining a normal level of vitamin A is also problematic, as asymptomatic captive amphibians often have lower values than wild amphibians.[53] Patient size may prevent collection of sufficient blood for vitamin A analysis. With VAD, blood concentrations of vitamin A drop below 20 µg/100 mL but only after depletion of hepatic reserves.[35] Thus plasma vitamin A concentrations do not provide a linear indication of liver/whole body vitamin A status or intake.[35,54] As most vitamin A

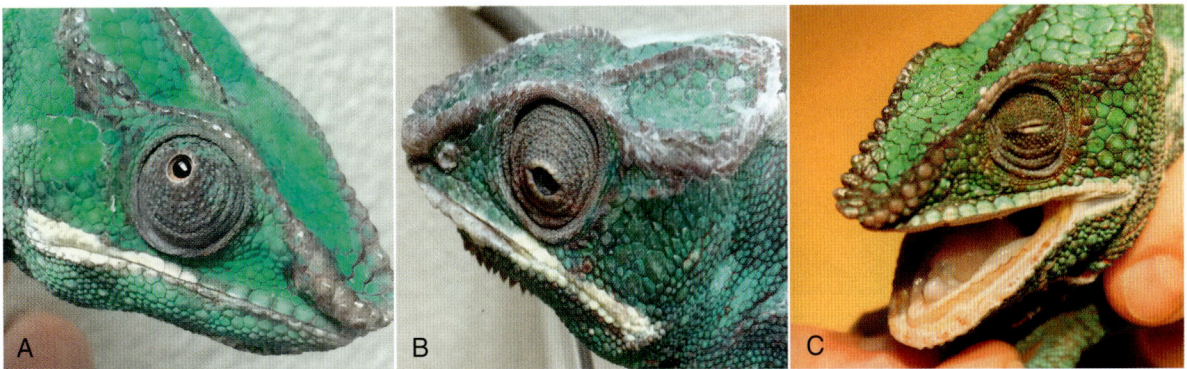

FIG 84.14 (A) Normal panther chameleon (*Furcifer pardalis*) compared with several panther chameleons with hypovitaminosis A (B and C); note the dull coloration, ocular mucus buildup, squinting, cheilitis, patchy dysecdysis, especially on eyelids (B), blepharospasm, and multifocal minute distended labial glands as a result of squamous metaplasia and hyperkeratosis (C). (Courtesy of Thomas H. Boyer.)

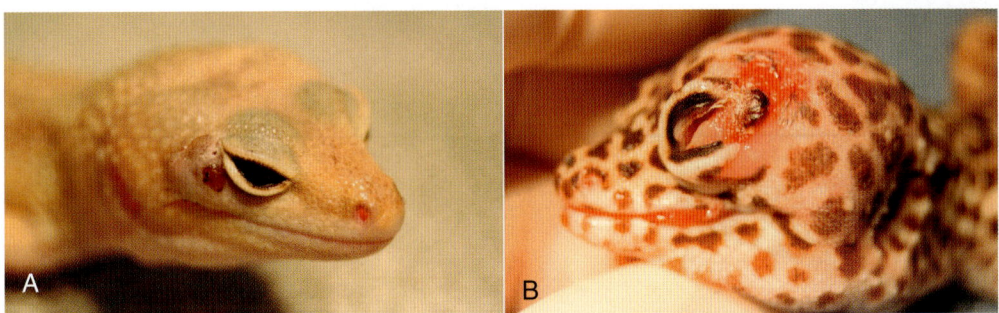

FIG 84.15 In leopard geckos (*Eublepharus macularius*) with vitamin A deficiency, periocular glands can also be affected (A and B) and may need to be lanced, flushed, and sutured. (Courtesy of Thomas H. Boyer.)

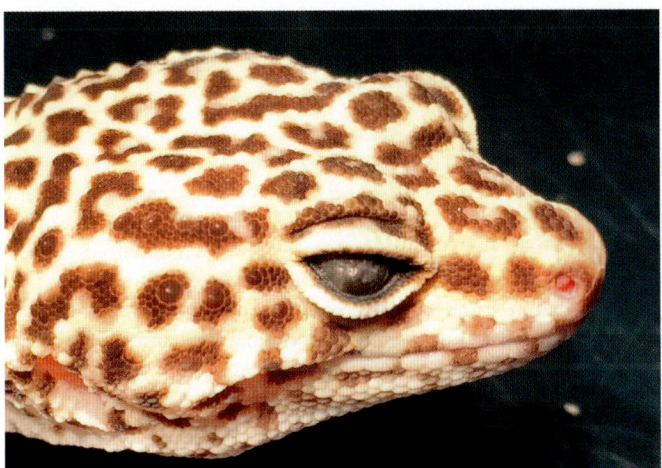

FIG 84.16 Chronic corneal scarring in a leopard gecko (*Eublepharus macularius*) from chronic hypovitaminosis A; chronic hypovitaminosis A may cause blindness. (Courtesy of Thomas H. Boyer.)

is stored in liver (≈80%–90%), liver levels are the best indication of whole body vitamin A status. Therefore liver biopsy, or postmortem liver analysis, are effective methods for diagnosis. Captive Wyoming toads (*Anaxyrus baxteri*) with STS had mean liver retinol levels of 1.5 μg/g, compared with free-ranging Wyoming toads without STS, which had mean liver retinol levels of 104.6 μg/g.[38,43] vitamin A levels

<5–10 μg are suspicious for hypovitaminosis A.[43] However, captive-born marine toads (*Bufo marinus*) without STS had significantly lower mean liver retinol levels of 0.58 μg/gram compared with wild-caught marine toads without STS of 61.89 μg/gram, so species variability likely exists with regard to critical levels and propensity to develop clinical signs.[54]

Preferred Treatment

Response to treatment is slow because mature epithelium cannot be repaired and must be replaced by differentiation of resident stem cells.[38] In effect, epithelium must be turned over to be repaired in an animal that has been chronically nutritionally compromised.

Vitamin A Therapy in Reptiles. One author (TB) has been using 0.01 mL of fat-soluble vitamin A and D SC (500,000 IU vitamin A palmitate/mL, 100,000 IU vitamin D/mL), repeated in 2 weeks, then discontinued (two doses total), for reversal of hypovitaminosis A in reptiles for several decades without visible signs of toxicity. Patients take 2 to 4 weeks to recover (Fig. 84.18A and B). This dose arose from the desire to give the smallest effective dose that can be measured and given with a 0.3 mL U-100 insulin syringe. For a 1 kg reptile this provides 5000 IU vitamin A/kg, but for a 50 gram reptile, this provides 100,000 vitamin A IU/kg, which is still at the lower end of dosages (100,000 or 400,000 IU vitamin A/kg) that did not elicit any clinical or histopathologic signs of hypervitaminosis A at 10 and 14 days with parenteral fat-soluble vitamin A in Hermann's tortoises (see Hypervitaminosis A section).[55]

Alternatively, a parenteral fat-soluble vitamin A and D solution (100,000 IU vitamin A palmitate/mL, 10,000 IU vitamin D₃/mL, and

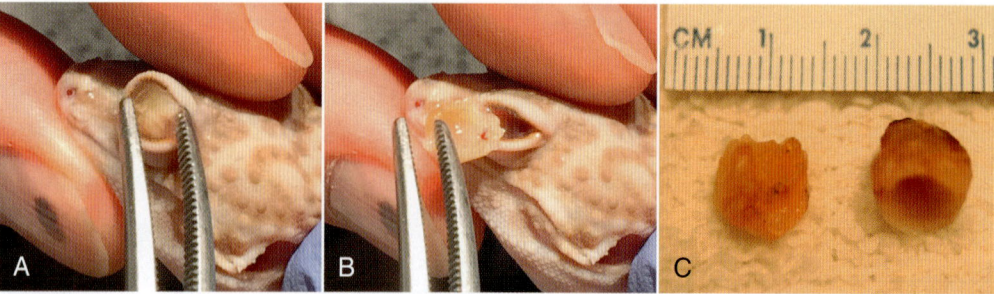

FIG 84.17 (A) Leopard gecko (Eublepharis macularius) with solid cellular debris under the palpebrae from chronic vitamin A deficiency. (B) The debris is gently removed after moisturizing with saline and grasping with hemostats or blunt probe, while applying digital ocular pressure. (C) The solid cellular debris can be larger than the patient's eye. (Courtesy of Thomas H. Boyer.)

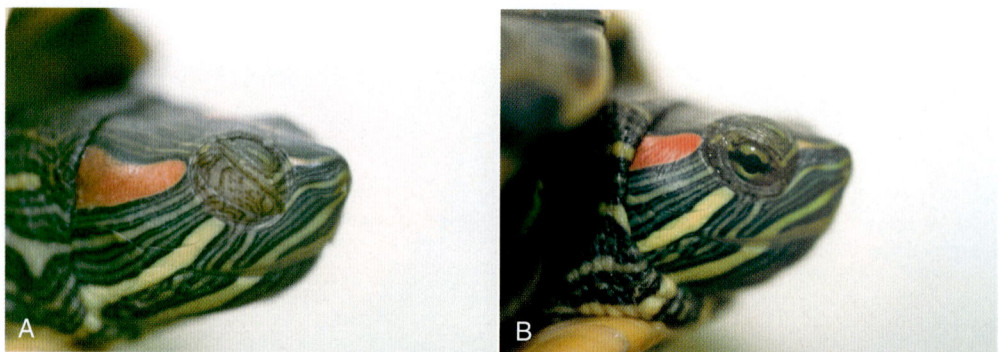

FIG 84.18 (A) Vitamin A deficiency in a red-eared slider *(Trachemys scripta elegans)* at presentation after months of treatment with topical and systemic antibiotics. Note the blepharedema and dull orange ear stripe. (B) The same turtle 2 weeks after a single SC dose of 0.01-mL fat-soluble vitamin A palmitate and discontinuation of antibiotics. Note the ocular resolution and improved color of the red ear stripe. (Courtesy of Thomas H. Boyer.)

20 IU vitamin E/mL) has been shown to work clinically in lizards and box turtles given orally at a dosing rate of 2000 IU/30 gm body weight once and repeated in 7 days. Clinically, the parenteral drug appears to be absorbed by the oral route and may be less toxic when given in this manner.[56]

Cellular debris under the eyelids can be carefully removed with a blunt probe or hemostats and digital pressure (see Fig. 84.17A–C).[57] The eyes should be flushed regularly with saline or ophthalmic rinses and kept moist with ophthalmic antibiotic ointment or drops, without steroids, as ulcerative keratitis is common. Patients do not resume feeding until their eyes are open, so fluid therapy followed by nutritional support should be provided.

Vitamin A Therapy in Amphibians. For amphibians topical or oral vitamin A can be given, or fresh mouse, rat, or fish liver can be fed whole or pureed. Many larger amphibians will eat whole pinkies. Prey insects should be fed a good-quality, gut-loading diet, with preformed vitamin A, before being fed to insectivores.

Parenteral treatment of amphibians is different compared with reptiles, most likely because smaller body size necessitates use of a less concentrated vitamin A formulation (such as 1:10 diluted Aquasol A) to improve dosing accuracy. Topical treatment with water soluble vitamin A (Aquasol A, Mayne Pharms, Paramus, NJ) at 50 international units every other day raised whole body levels of vitamin A in foam-nest tree frogs better than dusting insects with vitamin A.[58]

Prognosis and Prevention

Patients recover in several weeks, unless secondary disease is present, and resume feeding. Death is not uncommon. Severe corneal scarring and blindness worsens the prognosis. Insectivores and carnivores require preformed vitamin A in their diet. The liver in whole vertebrates is adequate to prevent VAD in carnivores. Insectivores must be fed a variety of insects that have been dusted with multivitamins that contain preformed vitamin A and mixed carotenoids (not just β-carotene), and/or insects fed a good-quality, gut-loading diet with vitamin A and mixed carotenoids. Additionally some insectivores can be fed pinkies. Most herbivores and omnivores seem resistant to VAD, perhaps because they can convert carotenoids into vitamin A.

HYPERVITAMINOSIS A

Clinical Significance and Known Etiological Cause(s)

Vitamin A injections continue to be given to tortoises in the mistaken notion that it may help with upper respiratory tract disease or improve appetite. Tortoises, being herbivores, are good at converting carotenoids to vitamin A and rarely, if ever, develop primary VAD. Emydid turtles, such as box turtles and red-eared sliders, being more carnivorous to omnivorous, are prone to VAD, either because they may be less capable of carotenoid conversion to vitamin A or from dietary deficiency. Chelonian differences are important, and veterinarians should be aware that giving vitamin A injections to tortoises is unnecessary and can cause iatrogenic toxicity.[51]

Clinical Presentation and Diagnostic Confirmation

Experimentally, hypervitaminosis A has been produced in Hermann's tortoises at doses of 100,000 to 400,000 IU/kg IM water-soluble vitamin A palmitate, but not with fat-soluble vitamin A palmitate at identical doses.[55] Blisters, or bullae, started forming around the neck and extremities, usually by 14 days, as the outer epithelium sloughed in large pieces.[51,55] Light and electron microscopy detected the stratum corneum separating from the stratum germinativum, subcorneal acantholysis (loss of intercellular connections, such as desmosomes, resulting in loss of cohesion between keratinocytes), intercellular edema, parakeratosis (retention of nuclei in the stratum corneum), and well-differentiated acanthosis (thickening of the skin).[55] Essentially, hypervitaminosis A causes chelonians to slough their outer epidermis (Fig. 84.19A and B).

Water-soluble vitamin A is resorbed more quickly than fat-soluble vitamin A from injection sites and accumulates faster in the liver, which may lead to greater potential for toxicity; until more is known, it may be prudent to avoid water-soluble vitamin A in reptiles.[55,57] With highly concentrated vitamin A products, empirical dosages, and unknown requirements, iatrogenic hypervitaminosis A is possible. Vitamin A injections will not boost immune status in reptiles, improve appetite, or treat upper respiratory tract disease, unless signs of hypovitaminosis A are present.[51] High intake of carotenoids from vegetables and fruits does not cause hypervitaminosis A, as conversion from carotenoids to the active form of vitamin A is regulated by the body.[35] The safest approach is to treat a nutritional disease with improved nutrition and oral supplementation. Injectable therapy should only be given to reptiles with clinical signs and dietary histories that support treatment.[51]

In amphibians, hypervitaminosis A is rare, but has been noted in African clawed frogs (*Xenopus* spp.) that were fed vitamin A–rich mammalian livers or whole immature rodents. In these circumstances, hypervitaminosis A may play a role in the development of metabolic bone disease and may cause anemia, liver damage, and chronic weight loss.[59]

Preferred Treatment

Treatment is similar to that of partial-thickness burns. The epidermal barrier is compromised, causing extracellular fluid loss and bacterial invasion. Hypovolemia and infection are primary concerns. Fluid support, nutritional therapy, and analgesics are indicated until the patient resumes drinking and eating. The patient, and areas where skin has sloughed, should be gently and thoroughly cleaned and flushed, initially with dilute chlorhexidine in sterile saline (1:30) and then 0.9% saline. Adherent necrotic skin should be debrided. Sloughed areas may or may not be treated with topical salves, such as aloe vera, 1% silver sulfadiazine cream, or antibiotic ointment. A number of dressings are thought to have some benefits over alternatives for the management of superficial and partial-thickness burns. There is some research evidence in humans to suggest that superficial and partial-thickness burns heal more quickly with silicon-coated nylon, silver containing dressings, and biosynthetic dressings (such as hydrogel) than with silver sulfadiazine cream.[60] Burns treated with hydrogel dressings healed more quickly than those treated with usual care.[60] The same recommendations apply to hypervitaminosis A patients; however, tortoises are difficult to bandage. Wounds should be flushed with sterile saline, and all residual topicals removed and redressed daily. Treatment should continue until skin has healed, which may take weeks to months.

Vitamin E appears to be an effective treatment for hypervitaminosis A, and in chicks and rabbits may prevent side effects of high doses of vitamin A.[61,62] Taurine significantly reduced vitamin A toxicity in rats, perhaps because retinoids can be conjugated by taurine, then excreted in the bile; conjugated retinol has little biological activity.[63–65] These supplements may be beneficial for treatment of hypervitaminosis A in reptiles as well.

Prognosis and Prevention

Avoid the use of injectable vitamin A in tortoises and other herbivorous species. The prognosis is dependent on the extent of clinical care, dosage, and type of vitamin A supplement used. Widespread epidermal sloughing carries a guarded prognosis. For amphibians, reduce feeding whole rodents and discontinue feeding whole liver.

OBESITY

Clinical Significance and Known Etiological Cause(s)

Obesity in captive reptiles is a common problem. As with humans, and many companion animals, it is usually the result of excessive caloric intake over expenditures. Captive animals forage less, are usually overfed, and are rarely exposed to reproductive demands, estivation, or hibernation. Limited cage space discourages activity and exercise. Some producers push-feed reptiles for rapid growth and early breeding. Excess caloric

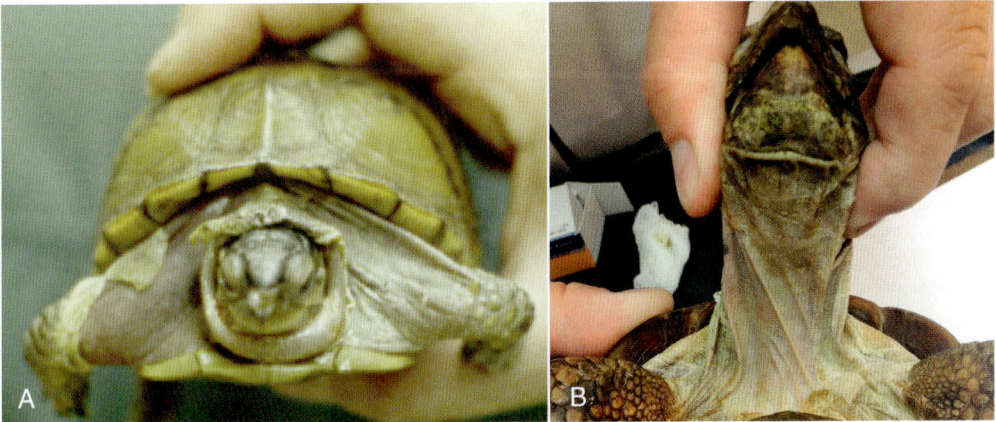

FIG 84.19 Epidermal sloughing in a three-toed box turtle (*Terrapene carolina triunguis*), caused by overdosage with water-soluble vitamin A (A), and in a tortoise (B), caused by fat-soluble vitamin A. Tortoises rarely, if ever, develop hypovitaminosis A and do not require vitamin A injections. (Courtesy of Thomas H. Boyer.)

intake also influences folliculogenesis, which is a substantial nutritional demand; however, many captive females are then not bred, leading to resorption of follicles, which may result in adding to fat reserves.[66]

Clinical Presentation and Diagnostic Confirmation

Obesity is especially common in monitors, bearded dragons, red-eared sliders, and larger boid snakes. Body condition scoring and graphing has been described for leopard geckos and chelonians.[67–73] As with all creatures, obesity is not a healthy state and often decreases longevity. Obesity is thought to predispose to hepatic lipidosis, yolk coelomitis, and dystocia. In obese monitors and other lizards, the coelomic fat pads can enlarge to such an extent that they constrict and compromise coelomic organs. For bearded dragons, fruits and berries rich in sugars are avidly, and eventually preferentially, consumed, as are high-fat mealworms, superworms, and waxworms (with a mean fat content of 31%–51% DM compared with 10%–23% DM for juvenile to adult crickets).[74] The consumption of these rich foods gradually results in a loss of interest in mobile insects and greens, less activity, and only consuming foods placed directly in front of them or hand-fed. For carnivores, domestic mice and rats produced for the market may well have larger fat stores than wild mice and rats. Similarly, older, larger, ex-breeder rats and mice have relatively greater fat stores than juvenile wild animals. Young, leaner rodents with lower fat levels (17% crude fat DM) are a better food source for obese reptiles than older animals (24% crude fat DM); however, pinkies may have a lower Ca content, which may not be ideal for rapidly growing animals.[75]

Preferred Treatment

Weight loss treatment consists of decreased caloric intake and increased caloric expenditure. Owners are skeptical that their pet is obese, so accurate monthly to quarterly weights and encouragement will help keep the owner on track. Gradual weight loss is the goal. It is difficult to increase exercise in reptiles, but providing a larger cage, more climbing surfaces, localized hotspots, and live insects, or insects hidden throughout the exhibit will help. Supervised time out of the cage helps, and large tractable monitors can be walked on a leash attached to a body harness, indoors, in an enclosed yard (be wary of predators), or be trained to chase retrieved objects. Treatment for bearded dragons consists of eliminating all fruits in the diet, restricting diet to gut-loaded crickets and Dubia cockroaches (avoid insect larvae that are high in fat), dark leafy greens, and flowers. Encourage activity and foraging behaviors by discouraging hand feeding. Feeding should be reduced to every other day and then twice weekly. If healthy, when winter approaches, dragons and red-eared sliders should be hibernated/brumated to consume excess lipid reserves. For adult sliders, feed less and offer more greens. For monitors, reduce rodents and meat (even low-fat turkey) and provide at least 50% mobile insects.[76] For further details, see Chapter 67.

Prognosis and Prevention

If the patient is still eating well, the prognosis is good and more dependent on owner compliance. If the patient is not eating, the prognosis is more guarded, and hepatic lipidosis is a frequent sequela. Reptiles that normally hibernate should be hibernated if healthy. Most reptiles are overfed in captivity, feeding less, less frequently; periodic fasting and increased exercise can help avoid obesity.

HEPATIC LIPIDOSIS

Clinical Significance and Known Etiological Cause(s)

Hepatic lipidosis is a pathological accumulation of lipid within hepatocytes. Storage of fat in reptiles is primarily divided between the fat bodies in the coelom and the liver. Squamates do not store subcutaneous fat.

Chelonia tend to use hepatic storage, although the prefemoral fossa is also used. Fat stores are used for vitellogenesis and as an energy source during hibernation, aestivation, or fasting. In hepatic lipidosis, the normal storage and use of lipids becomes disrupted; the metabolic changes are not well understood. Inciting factors include diets high in fat and carbohydrates, obesity, chronic hyporexia, lack of exercise, hibernation, or reproductive activity (see Chapter 67 for more information).[77] Certain vitamin or amino acid deficiencies may impact liver function. Reptiles that are chronically stressed (leading to higher corticosteroid production) may be more likely to become obese and develop hepatic lipidosis.

Starvation is a common cause of hepatic lipidosis in mammals. In cats, guinea pigs, and rabbits, even short periods of anorexia may cause hepatic lipidosis. This may be true for certain species of captive reptiles as well. Shortage of dietary glucose causes hormonal changes and sympathetic activity, resulting in decreased insulin release. This promotes increased peripheral lipolysis and release of free fatty acids into the circulation. The free fatty acids are taken up by the liver and metabolized into triglycerides. Because protein shortage causes a parallel decrease in lipoprotein synthesis, triglycerides are not efficiently converted to very-low-density lipoproteins (VLDL), thus triglycerides accumulate in the liver. Deficiencies of active amino acids such as methionine, arginine, and carnitine, which all play important roles in lipid metabolism, can result in the development of hepatic lipidosis. Insufficient or poor-quality dietary protein, exposure to hepatotoxins, anoxia, impaired carbohydrate, or volatile fatty acid metabolism can all lead to hepatic lipidosis (see Chapter 67 for more details).

Clinical Presentation and Diagnostic Confirmation

In general, early signs include developing lassitude; females may develop preovulatory stasis, as repeated lipogenesis and resorption occur. Liver function becomes deranged. Sudden-onset lethargy and anorexia are seen. Pathologically there is excessive accumulation of lipid within hepatocytes. The problem is determining when this is excessive because hepatic fat storage is normal and varies by gender and season. Pathologists inexperienced with reptiles may erroneously identify the normal increase in prehibernation or prereproductive hepatic fat as lipidosis. In hepatic lipidosis some degree of inflammatory reaction may be seen.

Dietary history of affected bearded dragons usually includes large amounts of fruit and non-gut-loaded insects, especially insect larvae. Dietary history for tortoises includes heavy reliance on grocery store fruits and vegetables (which are high in carbohydrates and protein) and insufficient hay. Clinical signs, other than anorexia and high body condition scores, are vague. Tortoises typically have a gradual reduction in appetite and activity; the tortoise may have a more selective appetite, eating only fruits. Posthibernation anorexia often involves hepatic lipidosis. Weakness, often present, manifests as dragging the plastron while walking. In advanced cases the patient may be flaccid, edematous (Fig. 84.20A and B), lethargic, weak (head and legs easily extended), anemic, hypoalbuminemic, or hypocalcemic, and rarely may have neurological symptoms from hepatic encephalopathy (altered mentation, stupor, incoordination). Hypoalbuminemia (<1 g/dL, 10 g/L), hypercholesterolemia, and hypertriglyceridemia are common. If the patient is dehydrated, packed cell volume (PCV) may be elevated. Leopard geckos may have a ventral, grossly visible, white liver surrounding the dark green gall bladder (Fig. 84.21A and B). In lizards, radiography and ultrasonography may reveal liver enlargement or hyperechogenicity; the liver can be readily compared with coelomic fat bodies. From clinical experience, the lateral liver silhouette of lizards should be less than half the dorsoventral coelomic space. Reptiles rarely vomit with hepatic lipidosis unless there is gastrointestinal obstruction or other causes. Elevated bile pigments (green urine or urates) and diarrhea are variably present. Anemia is not uncommon. Liver enzymes are often normal,

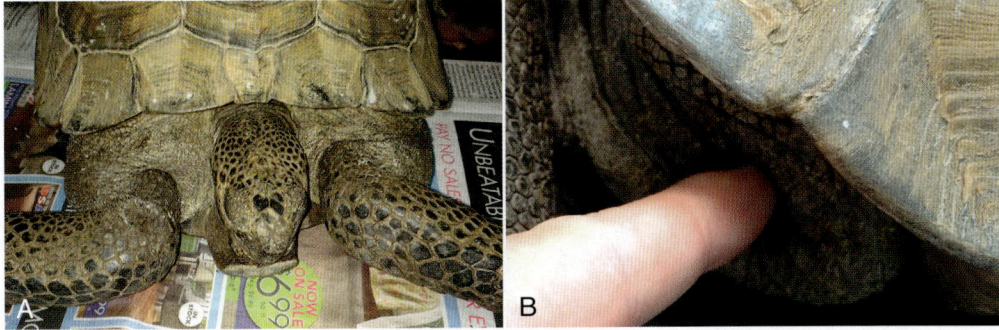

FIG 84.20 (A and B) Desert tortoise (*Gopherus agassizii*) with edema, lethargy, weakness (head and legs easily pulled out from shell, not lifting shell while ambulating), anemia, hypoalbuminemia, and hypocalcemia, all suggestive of hepatic lipidosis. (Courtesy of Thomas H. Boyer.)

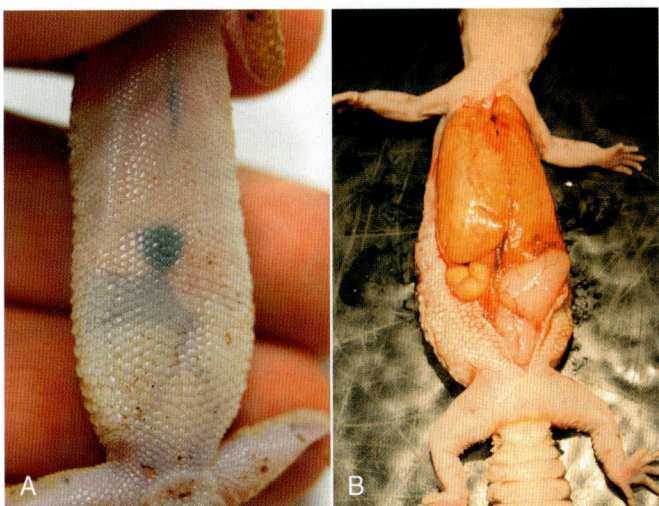

FIG 84.21 Hepatic lipidosis in leopard geckos (*Eublepharus macularius*) visible through ventrum (A) and at necropsy (B); note the dark green gall bladder in (A). (Courtesy of Thomas H. Boyer.)

as there is no breakdown of liver cells, whereas triglycerides and cholesterol may be elevated (but must be differentiated from vitellogenesis and prehibernation). One study found statistically higher levels of triglycerides in red-footed tortoises (*Chelonoidis carbonaria*), with endoscopic and histopathologically confirmed hepatic lipidosis, but no differences in AST, ALT, or GGT.[78] There are few studies on the diagnostic use of bile acids in reptiles; one study did not detect 24- and 48-hr postprandial increases in normal red-eared sliders,[77] another study detected significant increases in preprandial fasting bile acids at 3 and 7 hours postprandial in normal green iguanas.[79] The 3α-hydroxy-bile acid levels should be less than 60 μmol/L; unfortunately lipemia can interfere with analysis. Most reptiles (excluding some snakes) do not convert biliverdin to bilirubin. A definitive diagnosis can be obtained by liver biopsy and histopathology. Fatty livers are pale white, tan, or yellow (see Fig. 84.21); friable with swollen rounded edges; ooze greasy yellow brown fluid on cut surfaces; and float in formalin. Affected reptiles represent higher anesthetic risks, and drugs that rely on hepatic metabolism should be avoided.

Preferred Treatment

Treatment consists of long-term nutritional support via stomach tube for lizards or via esophagostomy tube for chelonians until the patient is eating well on its own, which may take weeks to months. Multiple small feedings are better than less frequent larger feedings. Several commercially available products have worked well, including Emeraid Omnivore or Herbivore (LaFeber Co., Cornell, IL), Critical Care and Critical Care Fine Grind (Oxbow Animal Health, Murdock, NE), and Critical Care Formula (Vetark Professional, Winchester, UK). Carnivore diets tend to be too high in fat. Other supplements, such as L-carnitine, methionine, taurine, S-adenosylmethionine, lactulose, and milk thistle extract, can also be used if not present in aforementioned foods (see Chapter 127 and 128 for dosages); however, no prospective clinical trials have been conducted to evaluate efficacy of any of these drugs in reptiles. The goal of dietary therapy is to maintain body weight until the patient starts eating on its own.

Prognosis and Prevention

The prognosis for patients that are still eating is guarded and guarded to poor for anorexic patients, depending on the extent of pathology. Prevention involves better nutrition. For tortoises this means less greens, vegetables, or fruits and more hays, grasses, and commercial tortoise diets. For bearded dragons, less fruit and more variety of gut-loaded insects, and the latter is also recommended for leopard geckos. Increasing opportunities for caloric expenditures (e.g., exercise, hibernation, reproduction) can also be beneficial. See Chapter 67 for additional information.

PYRAMIDAL SHELL GROWTH (PSG)

Clinical Significance and Known Etiological Cause(s)

PSG is a growth deformity of many tortoise species, resulting in pyramidal scute growth of the carapace (Fig. 84.22A and B). Many etiologies have been suggested, including improper humidity, various nutritional and mineral imbalances (particularly Ca and protein), endoparasites, overeating, lack of sunlight, increased growth rate, improper environmental temperature, lack of mechanical abrasion on the shell, and lack of exercise.[22] One of the few scientific studies on PSG was in African spurred tortoises (*Centrochelys sulcata*), reared under different humidity conditions ("dry" 24–58%, "mid" 31–75%, and "humid" 45–99) and different protein levels (14%, 19%, and 31% DM), and Ca:P ratios of greater than 3.7 : 1.[21] The study showed a trend for greater pyramiding under drier conditions, with higher protein having only a minor impact. Higher protein levels did lead to more rapid growth, and larger size, however, which led to the erroneous impression of more pyramiding to the researchers, which, when measured, were not relatively larger.[21] The least pyramiding was found in the experimental group with environmental humidity between 45% to 99%, and the most pyramiding was found in the group with 24% to 58% environmental humidity; both groups had identical dietary

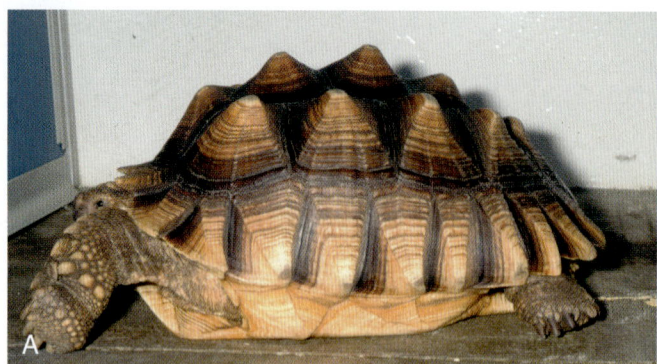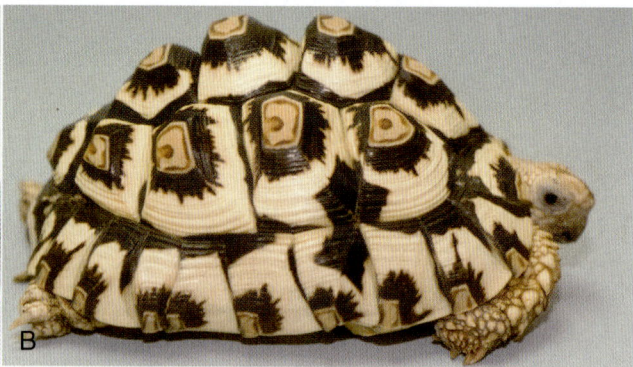

FIG 84.22 Pyramidal shell growth in an African spurred tortoise (*Centrochelys sulcata*) (A) and leopard tortoise (*Stigmochelys pardalis*) (B). (Courtesy of Thomas H. Boyer.)

protein levels (19% DM). The authors concluded that to keep PSG minimal, hiding areas with relatively high humidity should be provided at all times.[21] The nutritionists speculated that during humid seasons there is a concurrent increase in growth of plants with better nutritional value that can support rapid growth. Conversely, during dry seasons, nutritional quality decreases and growth slows. Many tortoises naturally seek humid refuge in burrows or under foliage at soil level. Thus, providing a dry environment with constant rich nutrition, in captivity, is unnatural and may contribute to PSG.[21] Another study with African spurred tortoises and leopard tortoises found increased nocturnal heat exposure leads to increased growth rate and a subsequent significant increase ($P < 0.05$) in PSG. Humidity and diet were the same between treatment and control groups (no nocturnal heat).[22] The authors suggested that an unnatural growth rate may lead to deposition of material between keratin scutes faster than the bone shell can spread, leading to a conical upgrowth of carapacial scutes.[22] Both studies point out that increased growth rates lead to more PSG. Most likely PSG has multifactorial etiologies but is largely independent of dietary calcium and phosphorus. Another study looked at animals using DEXA scans and demonstrated higher bone mineral density in affected tortoises.[27]

Clinical Presentation and Diagnostic Confirmation

PSG is a common affliction in captive tortoises but can be a normal morphological feature of some species, such as Indian star tortoises (*Geochelone elegans*) and some tent tortoise species (*Psammobates* spp.). PSG affects primarily the carapace, especially the central vertebral scutes (see Fig. 84.22), which have a knobby pyramidal shape rather than an evenly rounded smooth carapace. There is thicker bone underlying the scute annuli, and with pronounced PSG the vertebral column may separate from the dorsally domed dermal bone.[22] Diagnosis is via presenting clinical signs and husbandry review.

Preferred Treatment

There is no treatment for PSG. Shell deformities are permanent, and only new shell growth can be corrected.

Prognosis and Prevention

The prognosis is favorable, although shell deformities cannot be corrected. Future PSG can be reduced with better nutrition, such as more hay, grasses, and commercial tortoise diets (see Chapter 27), humid retreats for growing tortoises, and slowing growth rate, such as with a night time temperature drop. Concurrent anorexia or nutritional secondary hyperparathyroidism can also complicate treatment and prognosis.

THIAMINE DEFICIENCY

Clinical Significance and Known Etiological Cause(s)

Thiamine (Vitamin B$_1$) deficiency is probably the first documented deficiency disease (beriberi), described in China as early as 2600 BC. It has been reported across the animal kingdom as associated with feeding shellfish and fish-containing thiaminases, which destroy thiamine. Thiaminase is heat labile and boiling or cooking will destroy it. Freezing does not destroy thiaminase, and over time it will continue to break down thiamine. Phytothiaminases found in plants, such as bracken ferns (*Pteridum aquilinum*), horsetails (*Equisetum arvense*), nardoo (*Marsilea drummondii*), rock ferns (*Cheilanthes sieberi*), and kochia (*Kochia scoparia*), could also contribute to thiamine deficiency but are not typically fed to reptiles. Thiamine, being water soluble, is not generally stored in the body, thus deficiency can develop and resolve rapidly. No gross lesions are seen at necropsy; however, histopathology may reveal necrotizing encephalopathy.[80]

Clinical Presentation and Diagnostic Confirmation

Diagnosis is based on dietary history, clinical signs, and rapid response to thiamine therapy. Listlessness and acute loss of righting reflex was attributed to suspected thiamine deficiency in 20 out of 100 2- to 3-month-old juvenile farmed saltwater crocodiles (*Crocodylus porosus*) that were fed thawed frozen donkey meat and chicken heads, supplemented with calcium and multivitamins containing a low concentration of thiamine (3 mg/kg).[81] These juvenile crocodiles were found floating, or lying on their sides or backs, with their jaws open and responded quickly to thiamine injections within 1 to 2 days. Addition of dried Brewer's yeast, with 95 mg/kg thiamine, resulted in no further cases. Torpor, depression, and uncoordinated behaviors in alligators (*Alligator mississippiensis*) have also been related to thiamine deficiency.[80] Neural lesions characteristic of thiamine deficiency were noted in the telencephalon, particularly the dorsal ventricular ridge. Liver and muscle tissue concentrations of thiamine (vitamin B$_1$) were low, and the consumption of thiaminase-positive gizzard shad (*Dorosoma cepedianum*) was thought to have been the cause. Suspected thiamine deficiency has also been reported in garter snakes (*Thamnophis* spp.) and brown water snakes (*Nerodia taxisplilota*) fed frozen fish (Fig. 84.23). Clinical signs include anorexia, lack of accurate striking reflex, opisthotonus/torticollis, frantic curling, tremors, seizures, mydriasis, blindness, dysphagia, enophthalmia, and eventually death.[82–84]

Preferred Treatment

Initial thiamine injections followed by dietary thiamine supplementation results in rapid reversal of clinical signs. Saltwater crocodile juveniles

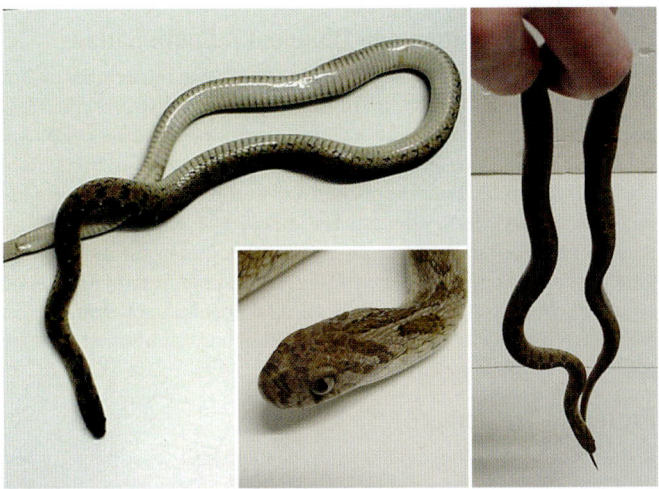

FIG 84.23 Neurological deficits and mydriasis in a mole kingsnake (*Lampropeltis calligaster*) fed goldfish (*Carassius auratus*). The clinical signs resolved within 24 hours of an injection of 100 mg/kg thiamin B1 and were prevented by converting to a rodent diet. (Courtesy of Stephen J. Divers.)

responded rapidly to 30 mg thiamine HCL (100 mg/mL) IM SID for two treatments. Recovery of righting reflex occurred within 24 hours, with full recovery by 48 hours.[81] Frye recommended 25 mg/kg thiamine tablets in the body cavity of fish for 3 to 7 days.[82]

Prognosis and Prevention

The prognosis is excellent if diagnosed and treated early. Long-term prevention includes feeding a better balanced, more diverse diet, and supplementation of 25 to 30 mg thiamine per kg of wet fish.[85] Thiaminases are not restricted to marine or freshwater fish; they can be found in either (see Chapter 27, Table 27.13, for more information). Trout do not contain thiaminases and do not require thiamine supplementation.

GOUT AND HYPERURICEMIA

Gout refers to the deposition of uric acid in tissues. Hyperuricemia refers to elevated blood levels of uric acid and may precede gout. Hyperuricemia and gout can be associated with excessive uric acid production (e.g., excessive dietary protein) and/or reduced uric acid excretion (e.g., renal failure).

Clinical Significance and Known Etiological Cause(s)

Most snakes and lizards are primarily uricotelic (>90% uric acid excretion), so anything that reduces renal excretion of uric acid can lead to gout. Many chelonians, including terrestrial species, produce significant urea, whereas marine and aquatic reptiles may produce significant ammonia levels. Contributing factors that can lead to elevations of uric acid are high intakes of purine-rich proteins, severe dehydration, and suboptimal temperature. Most carnivores eat a relatively high-purine diet; however, wild reptiles obtain food less frequently than captive reptiles. Overfeeding is typically a captive issue. Push feeding for rapid growth is a common risk factor, thus gout is a common problem seen in commercial alligator production. Nephrotoxic drugs, severe dehydration, and VAD can lead to uric acid deposition in renal tubules.

Clinical Presentation and Diagnostic Confirmation

Many reptiles with gout are hypophagic or anorexic, as well as dehydrated. Uric acid is relatively insoluble and can easily form white tophi deposits

in any tissue but predominantly in joints, spleen, kidneys, pericardial sac, liver, and even the CNS. Tophi, especially once mineralized, are often visible radiographically as areas of increased opacity around distal joints and surrounding tendons and tissues. Tophi may lead to chronic arthritis, due to bone erosion, and predispose to secondary infection. Hyperuricemia is suggestive, but not all patients with gout are hyperuricemic; severe dehydration can also cause hyperuricemia. Diagnosis of gout may be confirmed by seeing monosodium urate crystals in joint fluid or tissues. Under polarized light microscopy, urate crystals are needlelike and have strong negative birefringence. Synovial fluid must be examined relatively soon after aspiration, as temperature and pH affect solubility. Uric acid is routinely removed by formalin and histological processing, leaving characteristic "holes" with associated inflammation in tissue sections. Articular gout can be distinguished from pseudogout, abscesses, or septic arthritis by synovial fluid analysis or biopsy.

Preferred Treatments

Medical treatment of gout is indicated if uric acid levels are elevated. Allopurinol at 25 mg/kg PO SID in green iguanas (*Iguana iguana*) reduced uric acid levels by 45%[86] while 50 mg/kg PO SID x 30 days, then q 72 hours thereafter has been recommended in Mediterranean tortoises (*Testudo* spp.) (Kolle Proc ARAV, 2001, pp 185–186). Allopurinol blocks the enzyme xanthine oxidase, reducing breakdown of xanthine to uric acid, leading to the excretion of xanthine and hypoxanthine. These require more water for successful excretion, so fluid therapy and frequent soaking are recommended during treatment. These may be combined with judicious use of analgesics (e.g., colchicine, meloxicam, tramadol), although care should be exercised with NSAIDs if renal compromise is present. Visceral gout is difficult to treat and typically carries a poor to hopeless prognosis; however, there are scattered case reports of success.[87–89] Surgical removal of urate tophi from critical areas (e.g., joints, pericardial sac) may be beneficial. Unilateral renal gout was successfully treated in a monocellate cobra (*Naja kaouthia*) with unilateral nephrectomy.[89] See Chapters 66, 151, 163, and 164 for more information.

Prognosis and Prevention

Prognosis is poor as advanced gout is often an end stage state and generally considered incurable, with significant pain and suffering. Early cases with few indicators other than hyperuricemia, that are not dehydrated, often respond well to long-term allopurinol and dietary modulation. Prevention is through good husbandry, including access to water, appropriate humidity, diet, temperature, and avoiding overfeeding.

VITAMIN E/SELENIUM DEFICIENCY

Steatitis, fat inflammation, and necrosis, also known as yellow fat disease, occurs in carnivores fed diets high in polyunsaturated, or rancid, fat, or low in tocopherols or selenium.

Clinical Significance and Known Etiological Cause(s)

Crocodilians are most commonly affected, but steatitis, fat necrosis, and muscular degeneration have been reported in lizards and snakes.[24,90–95] Vitamin E and selenium are both antioxidants that protect against toxic effects of rancid fats.[96] Fish high in polyunsaturated fats, rancid fish, or rancid fish oils (either from putrification, overlong, or inadequate freezer storage) are toxic and cause fatty tissue in crocodilians to undergo necrosis and saponification (hardening).[24] Saponified fat elicits an inflammatory response (steatitis). Inadequate amounts of vitamin E or selenium can also cause muscles to degenerate (white muscle disease).

Widespread mortality from idiopathic pansteatis was noted in Nile crocodiles (*Crocodylus niloticus*), fish, and other apex predators in the Olifants River system in South Africa, including Kruger National Park.[97] Other studies suggest that an alien-invasive silver carp (*Hypophthalmychthys molitrix*) with high levels of n-3 polyunsaturated fatty acids, which other fish and crocodiles feed upon, could be the culprit.[98] Steatitis was also reported in three captive olive Ridley turtles (*Lepidochelys olivacea*), where it was ascribed to a long-term diet of frozen fish (Manawatthana and Kasorndorkbua, unpublished data, 2005).

Clinical Presentation and Diagnostic Confirmation

Hardened fat reduces tissue elasticity and can cause restriction of physical activity, which may be confused as lethargy. In crocodilians, large saponified intermuscular fat deposits in the tail may render the tail immobile, palpably firm, and the animal unable to swim. Saponification of intracoelomic fat may reduce intestinal motility.[24] In a *Ctenosaurus* lizard, bilateral hind-limb ataxia with muscle degeneration, interstitial fibrosis, and focal lymphocyte infiltration were consistent with white muscle disease.[90] A green iguana, with similar clinical signs, responded to vitamin E-selenium supplementation.[91] Feeding obese laboratory rodents raised on sunflower seeds also led to clinical signs of deficiency in a *Boa constrictor*.[82]

Diagnosis is typically postmortem with obvious round, red to yellow to brown, indurated, encapsulated nodules of granulomatous steatitis and fat necrosis; however, antemortem biopsy would be expected to be definitive in the live patient. Indurated fat has a greasy soaplike feel. Histologically, circumscribed zones of macrophages, multinucleated giant cells, ceroid, and hemorrhage are present.[93–95]

Preferred Treatment

There is no effective treatment to reverse fat saponification.

Prognosis and Prevention

Prognosis is poor for steatitis; most cases are diagnosed postmortem. Vitamin E is abundant in fresh fish, but fish lipids have a lower freezing point than mammalian fats and much of the vitamin E may be destroyed by oxidation after only a few weeks of freezing.[85,99] Degradation and oxidation of fish lipids, resulting in rancidity, can be accelerated by inappropriately high freezer temperatures, and therefore fish should be frozen between −18° to −30°C (0° to −22°F). Frozen fish should be used within 4 to 6 months.[85] Suggested levels of supplementation are 100 IU of vitamin E per kg of wet fish or 1 IU/kg/day for reptiles.[85,100]

Requirements and dosages of selenium for reptiles are largely unknown; mammals do best with diets containing 0.3 ppm selenium and should not exceed 0.5 ppm.[100] Several studies found exposing banded water snakes (*Nerodia fasciata*) and brown house snakes (*Lamprophis fuliginosus*) to diets containing about 1, 10, or 20 ppm Se, for 10 to 24 months, resulted in accumulation of Se in target organs and maternal transfer of Se to eggs at levels that exceeded established toxicity thresholds for other vertebrates.[101] A vitamin E–selenium responsive muscle condition in a green iguana was treated with 28 to 56 mg/kg vitamin E with 0.14 to 0.28 mg/kg selenium for 3 treatments.[91]

PROTEIN DEFICIENCY

Clinical Significance and Known Etiological Cause(s)

Protein deficiency usually results in hypoalbuminemia. Albumin is synthesized in the liver, and low albumin may be indicative of liver failure, such as with hepatic lipidosis, cirrhosis, or chronic hepatitis. Hypoalbuminemia can also result from malnutrition, protein-losing nephropathy, and enteropathy.

Clinical Presentation and Diagnostic Confirmation

Protein deficiency, from hepatic lipidosis, chronic malnutrition parasitism or renal insufficiency is common in tortoises. Tortoises are often less active, weak, eating more selectively, or anorexic, and may have peripheral edema or rarely signs of hepatic encephalopathy, such as stupor (see Fig. 84.20A and B). Long-term captive desert tortoises on inadequate diets often have blood albumin levels less than 1 mg/dL, as well as anemia and hypocalcemia. Measurement of albumin by the bromocresol green dye–binding method may lead to inaccurate results for plasma albumin concentration, especially in sick emydids and testudinids. Therefore for health assessment, in chelonians, albumin should be measured by protein electrophoresis.[102,103]

Preferred Treatment

If the tortoise is eating, dietary improvement, such as adding grasses, hays, and good-quality commercial pellets, will correct the problem. For patients that are not eating, further diagnostic investigation is indicated, as hepatic lipidosis, parasitism, or renal insufficiency may be present. Long-term nutritional support may be indicated (see Chapters 45 and 122).

Prognosis and Prevention

The prognosis is excellent if the tortoise is eating and the caregiver commits to improving the diet (see Chapters 23 and 27 for more information). If the patient is not eating the prognosis may be guarded to poor, depending on the extent of concurrent disease(s).

GEOPHAGY

Clinical Significance and Etiological Causes

Both free-ranging and captive tortoises, lizards, and crocodilians may consume stones (lithophagy), soil, and sand (geophagy). Desert tortoises, especially females, in the Mojave Desert, were found to selectively seek out and consume white calcite stones (not brown, gray, or other dull-colored stones), which were mostly calcium carbonate.[104] Eating bones, stones, and soil may be important for calcium acquisition, detoxification of toxic plants, or to expel parasites. Many reptiles incidentally ingest sand or gravel while eating.[104] Crocodilians ingest stones that may stay in their stomachs for months to years, and their significance is much debated. Some believe gastroliths are incidentally ingested and are nondetrimental, others believe they assist with ballast and/or mechanical breakdown of food.[105]

Clinical Presentation and Diagnostic Confirmation

Many tortoises have large numbers of stones in their GI tract normally; 60% of a large sample of free-ranging desert tortoises (n = 185) had stones in the gastrointestinal tract.[104] Intestinal obstruction is common in reptiles housed on sand, gravel, decomposed granite, aspen wood chips, or crushed walnut shells. Radiography and ultrasonography should be considered if complete obstruction is a concern.

Preferred Treatment

If the reptile is eating and defecating (therefore no obstruction is present), then no treatment is needed. If the reptile is not eating or defecating, but no complete obstruction can be identified, then aggressive rehydration (soaking, parenteral, and oral), enemas or stomach tubing with water, or mineral oil, may help. Many lizards will defecate with gentle colonic palpation. Severe cases often need an esophagostomy tube for long-term fluid and nutritional support. Regurgitation, or cases exhibiting radiographic or ultrasonographic evidence of complete obstruction, should be considered surgical. Gastroliths are not treated in crocodilians.

Prognosis and Prevention

Do not house reptiles on sand or gravel. As long as the reptile continues defecating, most stones can be defecated over time, and the prognosis is good. With surgery, the prognosis is good if secondary complications, such as hepatic lipidosis or colonic perforation, are not present.

GOITER

Goiter is the enlargement of the thyroid gland in an attempt to compensate for a deficiency in iodine. Toxic goiter refers to thyroid enlargement associated with alteration in thyroid function, whereas nontoxic goiter represents thyroid enlargement that does not result from an inflammatory or neoplastic process and is not associated with abnormal thyroid function.[106]

Clinical Significance and Known Etiological Cause(s)

Goiter is commonly misdiagnosed in Galapagos (*Chelonoidis nigra* complex) and Aldabra (*Aldabrachelys gigantea*) tortoises. More commonly these cases of ventral neck swelling represent thymic hyperplasia.[107] In other animals nontoxic goiters are the result of a dietary deficiency in iodine, or feeding foods high in iodine-binding goitrogens, which are found in cabbage, kale, broccoli, rapeseed, turnips, mustard seed, cauliflower, Brussels sprouts, and bok choy.[100,108] Excess dietary nitrates, the result of ingestion of fertilized grasses and hays, vegetables grown hydroponically, and iodine intoxication—the result of oversupplementation—have also been noted to predispose animals to goiter.[100,106] However, dietary goiter appears to be exceedingly rare in reptiles (see Chapter 79 for more information). Case reports of nontoxic goiter have been documented in giant tortoises, an eastern diamondback rattlesnake (*Crotalus adamanteus*), and Kirtland's snakes (*Clonophis kirtlandii*).[106,108,109] Two cases of intranuclear coccidiosis had nontoxic goiter, a radiated tortoise (*Geochelone radiate*) (Boyer, T, personal observation), and a Bowsprit tortoise (*Chersina angulata*).[110] Toxic goiter can be secondary to neoplasia.[111]

Clinical Presentation and Diagnostic Confirmation

A single (unpublished) case of nontoxic goiter in a Greek tortoise (*Testudo hermanni*) that was making whistling respiratory sounds had a sonographically enlarged thyroid gland compressing both atria (Buehler, 2006, unpublished data). Blood parameters and thyroid hormone concentrations were within established normal ranges. Biopsy of ventral cervical neck masses in giant tortoises can confirm thymic hyperplasia.[107]

Preferred Treatments

In the Greek tortoise, after 1 month of 1 mg/kg of potassium iodide PO daily, the whistling sound ceased and the sonographic thyroid diameter had decreased from 34 mm to 23 mm, and the atria were no longer compressed. After 4 months of therapy the ultrasonic thyroid diameter was 16.8 mm and remained 17.0 mm ± 0.2 mm for several more months, at which point the potassium iodide was reduced to twice weekly doses. The thyroid size remained unchanged sonographically for 6 additional years (Buehler I, unpublished data, 2006). See Chapter 79 for more information.

CORNEAL LIPIDOSIS/XANTHOMATOSIS

Corneal lipidosis, more properly termed corneal arcus, is a lipid storage disease in anurans associated with corneal lipid (especially cholesterol) deposition and, less commonly, deposition of cholesterol granulomas (xanthomas) elsewhere in the body (the later also in female lizards).[112–115]

Clinical Significance and Known Etiological Cause(s)

Corneal arcus is the most commonly reported corneal disease of captive amphibians, especially hylid frogs such as Cuban tree frogs (*Osteopilus septentrionalis*), and White's tree frogs (*Litoria caerulea*). Females are overrepresented in case reports. Experimentally, Cuban tree frogs fed diets high in cholesterol had significantly elevated serum cholesterol and LDL levels, which lead to significantly more corneal cholesterol deposition than in frogs on a lower cholesterol diet, or wild Cuban tree frogs.[113] Folliculogenesis, with associated hypercholesterolemia, nutrition, genetic predisposition, or trauma (cholesterol may be released from damaged cell membranes and induce a granulomatous response) may be involved in the pathogenesis of xanthomas.[110,115,116] Xanthomas are not neoplasms, but they can be locally invasive.[116]

Clinical Presentation and Diagnostic Confirmation

In anurans, corneal arcus starts as perilimbal, small, white, crystalline foci, which become denser, more raised, and slowly progress centrally, resulting in corneal haziness that progresses to opacity and blindness. Diagnosis is apparent with ocular examination. Xanthomas have been identified postmortem in the brain, viscera (especially liver), peripheral nerves, periarticular soft tissues, and digital pads. In lizards, xanthomas have been reported in coelomic surfaces and viscera, as well as the brains of female lizards (a northern green gecko, *Naultinus grayi*; leaf-tailed geckos, *Uroplatus* spp.; leopard geckos, a great plated lizard, *Gerrhosaurus major*; and green water dragons, *Physignathus cocincinus*), and associated with progressive neurological signs, such as seizures, vertigo, stargazing, circling, and/or torticollis (Boyer T, personal observation, 2013).[110,115,116]

Preferred Treatment, Prognosis, and Prevention

There is no treatment, and although low-cholesterol diets, such as limiting or avoiding larval insects, and improved husbandry may slow progression, existing lesions do not regress. Prognosis is poor for amphibians, as most patients eventually become blind, cannot feed independently, and die within 18 to 24 months of diagnosis. Lack of normal biology (e.g., thermoregulation, vitellogenesis, egg laying, mating behavior, hibernation, estivation), decreased activity, overfeeding, and poor diet (reduced dietary diversity, high cholesterol) may all predispose anurans to excess fat disposition.[113,117] The prognosis is poor for lizards with neurological signs, as xanthomas continue to expand within the confines of the skull; coelomic xanthomas may be amendable to surgical resection.

BIOTIN DEFICIENCY

Biotin (Vitamin B_7) deficiency can result from feeding raw unfertilized eggs exclusively. Raw eggs contain avidin, a tetrameric biotin-binding protein; cooking denatures avidin, and fertile eggs have embryos that are rich in biotin. Occasionally diagnosed in egg-eating species such as helodermids, varanids, teids, and egg-eating snakes (*Dasypeltis* spp.),[82] principle signs are muscle tremors and generalized weakness. Diagnosis is via clinical signs and dietary history. Multi-B injections should reverse clinical signs rapidly, and prognosis is typically excellent. Biotin deficiency can be prevented by feeding fertilized eggs and varying the diet to include whole prey, and by vitamin supplementation.

FIBER-RELATED DISORDERS

Most commercial greens, vegetables, and fruits are lower in fiber and higher in carbohydrates compared with their wild counterparts, which results in soft, semiformed, or liquid stools in captive herbivores. Clinical significance is unknown, but tortoises are commonly affected. Dietary history can be reviewed using Tables 27.1 to 27.3 in Chapter 27 for fiber content of foodstuffs, and routine fecal examination is indicated to exclude parasitic etiology.

Feeding less greens, vegetables, and fruits and more grasses, hays, and commercial diets with good fiber levels are indicated. Prognosis is excellent with dietary changes.

REFERENCES

See www.expertconsult.com for a complete list of references.

85

Perinatology

Krista A. Keller

In human medicine, perinatology is a branch of obstetric medicine encompassing the period of time surrounding childbirth. In reptile medicine, perinatology is the time period surrounding hatching for oviparous species, or immediately after birth for viviparous species. For the purposes of this chapter, the term perinatology will include relevant information regarding the egg, incubation period, and hatching (relevant for oviparous species), as well as hatchling and neonatal care and medicine. An understanding of reptile perinatology is important in the management of captive rearing programs within the pet trade, industry, research, or to bolster free-ranging populations. For instance, conservation efforts for Blanding's turtles (*Emydoidea blandingii*) in the United States include "head start" programs, allowing artificial incubation of eggs collected from the wild. Veterinarians aiding in these projects may be involved in diagnostic procedures involving eggs, investigation into causes of hatching failure, and evaluation and treatment of the sick hatchling.

THE REPTILIAN EGG

Oviparous species lay eggs in the environment that hatchlings emerge from. Viviparous species do not lay eggs but instead birth neonates. Ovoviparous species develop eggs, but the juvenile hatches from the egg while within the oviduct or very shortly after oviposition. The discussion of the reptile egg anatomy and physiology is relevant to oviparous and ovoviparous species. A full discussion of reproductive strategies can be found in Chapter 80.

The reptilian egg at oviposition is composed of the eggshell, extraembryonic membranes, albumen (or whites), and the yolk (Fig. 85.1). Each structure is involved in some support mechanism for the developing embryo. The shell of the reptilian egg can be categorized as being inflexible and hard or flexible and soft (leathery).[1] The structure of the eggshell is correlated with the environment where the eggs will incubate naturally; in general, hard-shelled eggs are laid by species that nest in

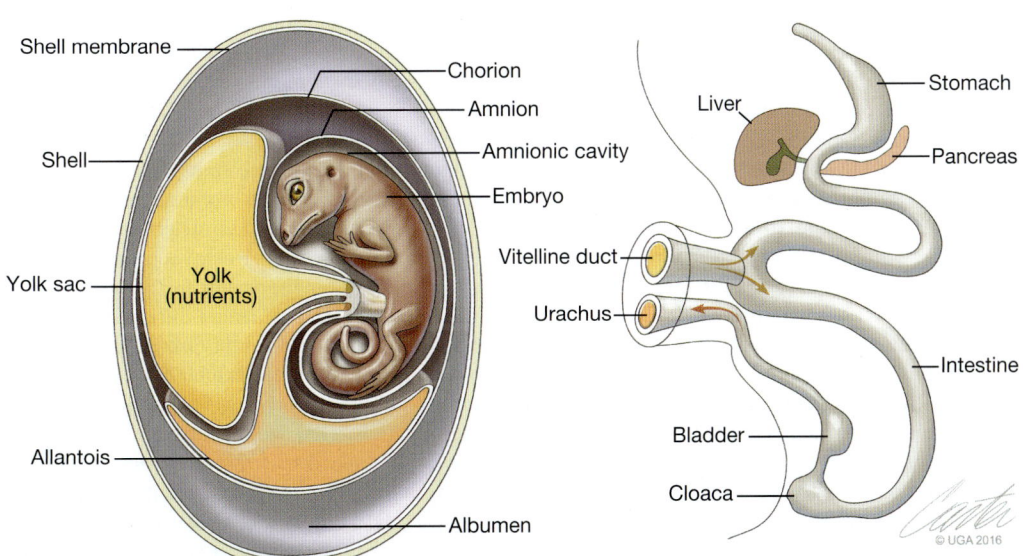

FIG 85.1 The image on the left depicts the diagrammatic appearance of a reptilian egg several weeks after embryonic and extraembryonic membrane development. Note the relationships of the amnion, allantois, chorion, yolk, and associated yolk sac with the embryo. The diagram on the right shows a magnified view of the body stalk, including the flow of yolk through the vitelline duct to the embryonic intestines for nutrient transfer and the flow of urine and urates through the urachus to the allantoic cavity for excretion. (Courtesy of Educational Resources, University of Georgia.)

arid and semiarid environments while soft-shelled eggs are laid by species that nest in moist environments.[1]

Physiologically, the eggshell functions as the boundary between the embryonic and external environments and provides calcium for embryonic development. Regardless of shell structure (hard or soft-shelled), the porous nature of the shell allows for gas and water exchange.[1,2] Softer-shelled eggs have a higher rate of oxygen exchange when compared to more solid-shelled eggs; however, this has no effect on the metabolism of the developing embryo, and mechanisms of how this is possible are unknown at this time.[2] Reptile embryos derive 20% to 25% of their calcium from the eggshell.[3]

The albumen is a viscous clear to slightly opaque proteinaceous material. Albumen, derived from specialized oviductal glands, has a high water content, although a variety of proteins are present.[4] In the leatherback turtle (*Dermochelys coriacea*), albumen makes up the largest mass component of the egg, whereas in the American alligator (*Alligator mississippiensis*), the mass is divided equally between the yolk and albumen.[4,5] Physiologically, the albumen layer provides the embryo with physical support and assists in water storage.[1] A class of antimicrobial peptides limited to bird and reptile species is secreted by the oviduct into the albumen layer and likely protects the developing embryo from infection.[6]

The extra embryonic membranes are composed of the amnion, allantois, and chorion (see Fig. 85.1). The amnion is the membrane that directly surrounds the embryo. Contraction of specialized amniotic smooth muscles at initiation of hatching causes retraction of the amnion and is ultimately responsible for the internalization of the yolk.[7,8] The allantois originates at the body stalk (paired with the vitelline duct and associated vessels) and is a continuation of the urachus external to the embryo. The allantoic cavity is the major storage site for protein catabolism excretion products, including urea and uric acid.[9] The chorion is the outermost membrane that encloses the embryo, amnion, allantois, yolk, and yolk sacs.

The yolk and its surrounding membrane, the yolk sac, are attached to the developing embryo at the body stalk via the vitelline duct (also referred to as the omphalomesenteric duct) (see Fig. 85.1). The vitelline duct is continuous with the embryonic intestines, allowing direct transfer of nutrients from the yolk. During incubation and embryonic development, as the yolk contents traverse the vitelline duct, the yolk size decreases while the embryo size increases.[9] Whereas avian yolks are liquid in composition, in corn snakes (*Pantherophis guttatus*), the yolk is solid for the last third of incubation due to the proliferation and invasion of endodermal cells and blood vessels from the yolk sac.[10]

Physiologically, the yolk is the primary energy source for the developing embryo and the hatchling.[1] The embryo obtains retinal (storage form of retinoids in reptiles), hormones, fatty acids, proteins, and minerals such as calcium, phosphorus, and magnesium from the yolk.[11–13] Maternal diet influences yolk fatty acid content and yolk size, thus affecting offspring nutrition. This should be considered when evaluating the hatchlings from a female with poor nutrition and captive care.[14–15] In addition, yolk can serve as maternal transfer of toxins (heavy metals, selenium, persistent organic pollutants) and antibodies as reported with *Mycoplasma agassizii* in desert tortoises (*Gopherus agasizzi*).[16–19] There is evidence for vertical transmission of sunshine virus, a neurorespiratory paramyxovirus of pythons, and *Hepatozoon* spp. in garter snakes (*Thamnophis elegans*).[20–21] Countless other pathogens likely have vertical transmission but have not been evaluated.

INCUBATION CONDITIONS

Natural incubation strategies among reptile species are extremely varied. For instance, the northern snake-necked turtle (*Chelodina rugose*) exhibits

a post-ovipositional developmental arrest; eggs are laid at the bottom of flooded wetlands and the embryos will not develop until after floodwaters subside. Consequently, these eggs require aquatic submergence prior to incubation for successful development.[1] In addition, many species of python and skinks exhibit egg-brooding behavior.[22,23] Understanding species-specific incubation conditions will improve hatching success in artificial conditions.

Outside of species-specific requirements, it is important to understand the basic conditions of incubation and how they can affect the egg and developing embryo to ultimately achieve successful hatching. The basic conditions of incubation include moisture and temperature.

Humidity

Hard- and soft-shelled eggs will respond differently to moisture in their environment. Soft-shelled eggs are more porous and are expected to enlarge and gain mass during incubation due to diffusion of water into the egg, as seen in the green iguana (*Iguana iguana*) egg that doubles in weight due to water absorption.[9] Hard-shelled eggs do not allow such impressive water diffusion; however, lack of moisture during incubation has been shown to influence hatchling size and performance.[24,25]

If conditions are too dry, soft-shelled eggs will lose water mass to the environment and begin to crinkle or collapse. Intervention with additional moisture at this stage may correct the dehydration; however, further dehydration may cause nonviability of the egg. This has been postulated to be secondary to buildup of toxic levels of nitrogenous wastes in the allantoic cavity.[1,9] At the other extreme, if the egg is surrounded by too much water, oxygen diffusion may cease, leading to hypoxia and death.[1]

Temperature

Species-specific incubation temperatures should be followed whenever available (Table 85.1). Studies show that abnormal incubation temperatures lead to hatchling performance deficits and reduced growth and immunity, and even latent effects on growth after hatching.[24,26–28] Specific syndromes, such as "failure to thrive syndrome," occurs in hatchling crocodilians and is 2.5 times more likely to occur in clutches that are incubated at lower air temperatures.[29] When kept within the species-specific temperature ranges, an inverse relationship exists between temperature and incubation length. For example, in the common wall lizard (*Podarcis muralis*) eggs incubated at a higher temperature (32°C) hatched more than 5 weeks earlier than eggs incubated at a lower temperature (24°C).[30]

Outside of appropriate embryonic development, temperature can be used to manipulate the sex of the developing embryo(s). Many reptiles exhibit temperature-based sex determination (TSD). Unlike genotypic sex determination (GSD), where sex phenotype is determined secondary to genes passed from the parents, in TSD gender phenotype is determined by specific temperature ranges during incubation.[31] Specific patterns of TSD exhibited by different taxon are presented in Table 85.2. Most chelonian species studied exhibit TSD, notable exceptions include the family Chelidae (Pleurodira).[32] Lizards exhibit mixed patterns of sex determination, even within taxonomic families. The leopard gecko (*Eublepharis macularius*) is a classically described TSD species, while other Eublepharid lizards are GSD. Another popular species in the pet trade, the bearded dragon (*Pogona vitticeps*), exhibits GSD.[33] Of the crocodilian and sphenodontia species studied to date, all follow a TSD pattern.[34,35]

While GSD and TSD are the classically discussed mechanisms for sex determination in reptiles, some species have been shown to exhibit multifactorial sex determination that include factors unrelated to temperature, such as yolk size, presence of exogenous hormones, and water availability.[36–38] Interestingly, a single species, the montane lizard

TABLE 85.1	Clutch Characteristics and Recommended Incubator Settings for Select Reptiles				
	Species	Typical Clutch Size	Humidity (%)	Temperature (°F/°C)	Expected Hatch Time (Days)*
Chelonian	Red-eared slider (*Trachemys scripta elegans*)	4–25	75–85	81–86/27.2–30.0	60–80
	Eastern box turtle (*Terrapene carolina carolina*)	3–8	80–90	72–90/22.2–32.2	70–120
	Greek tortoise (*Testudo graeca*)	2–7	50–80	82–90/27.8–32.2	60–80
	Russian tortoise (*Agrionemys horsfieldii*)	1–5	50–80	84–90/28.9–32.2	80–120
Squamate	Bearded dragon (*Pogona vitticeps*)	16–24	70–80	82–86/27.8–30.0	50–80
	Leopard gecko (*Eublepharis macularius*)	1–2	80–90	80–90/26.7–32.2	35–89
	Crested gecko (*Correlophus ciliatus*)	1–2	70–80	72–80/22.2–26.7	60–120
	Corn snake (*Pantherophis guttatus*)	10–30	75–90	78–88/25.6–31.1	60–80
	Ball python (*Python regius*)	4–9	90–100	86–92/30.0–33.3	52–65
Crocodilian	American alligator (*Alligator mississippiensis*)	35–90	90–100	82–95/27.8–35.0	65
	Nile crocodile (*Crocodylus niloticus*)	55–60	90–100	82–95/27.8–35.0	84–90
Rhynchocephalan	Tuatara (*Sphenodon spp.*)	1–18	75	64–72/17.8–22.2	180–720

*Lower temperatures will require longer incubation times, while higher temperatures will produce shorter hatch times.

(*Bassiana duperreyi*), exhibits both TSD and GSD.[39] These examples highlight that the traditional categorization of a species as exhibiting either TSD or GSD is likely oversimplified.

Keeping in mind that many reptile species exhibit TSD, the effect of the warming climate on sex ratios, and ultimately population health, is of concern. Effects of global warming could lead to skewing of the sex ratio, causing catastrophic population declines. For instance, in chelonian species that have more females created at higher temperatures, global warming conditions would create a lower percentage of males.[31] In contrast, with warmer ambient temperatures, the tuatara (*Sphenodon* spp.) would be expected to create more male offspring.[40] Outside of changing sex ratios, climate temperatures above the highest recommended incubation temperatures for a species may lead to reduced hatchling survivability.[26,28]

ARTIFICIAL INCUBATION

Incubators can either be constructed or purchased. Commercially available reptile incubators and chick incubators have been used successfully. Most incubators are designed with a double-chamber principle (Fig. 85.2). The inner chamber houses the eggs and substrate and is then suspended within a larger chamber. Either air or water can be present between the two chambers; when water is used, evaporation helps maintain the necessary high humidity. Separation of the inner chamber from the heat source and buffering the heat through the air or water medium has the advantage of creating a more homogenous temperature zone without associated "hot spots." When constructing an incubator, a waterproof container such as a plastic storage bin will work well for the inner chamber, while a larger plastic or Styrofoam ice chest would be appropriate for the outer chamber, with modifications for air flow.

Within the inner chamber, various substrates have been used with success. These include vermiculite, perlite, sterilized potting soil, sand, sphagnum moss, shredded paper, or a combination of the above. Substrates are recommended to be moist but not soaking wet. Concern with chlorine, chloramine, and other potential toxins have prompted many individuals to use bottled water in lieu of tap water. Other toxins that may be present in particulate substrates, particularly pesticides, may cause reduced hatchability or hatchling abnormalities.[41,42] Use of purchased and packaged substrate will remove the likelihood of pesticide exposure. Prior to incubation, discussion with an experienced individual

(breeder, zookeeper) will enable more precise information regarding successful substrate types used for the species in question. Typically, the eggs are half buried in the substrate (Fig. 85.3).

Various heat sources have been utilized to maintain incubator temperatures. Heating coils, strips, pads, and submersible aquarium heaters are available. Ideally, heaters with adjustable capacities should be used to maintain accurate temperatures within the inner chamber. Reliable thermometers, ideally digital, should be used that allow external evaluation of the temperature in the inner chamber, as repeated opening of the incubator will allow loss of heat and moisture. Fluctuating temperatures, as would be expected with frequent opening of an incubator, have been shown to delay hatching and affect hatchling body size in the smooth soft-shelled turtle (*Apalone mutica*), signifying the importance of consistent temperatures.[43] Daily monitoring and temperature recording is recommended. Successful species-specific incubation temperature ranges are reported in Table 85.1.

Moisture sources for the humidity required during incubation should come from the substrate and from the water bath used between the inner and outer chamber, depending on incubation design. Daily misting of the substrate may help increase humidity levels but requires opening the incubator, which leads to loss of heat and moisture; thus self-regulation of humidity with a closed incubator design is preferable. If misting is to be done, the misting bottle should be kept at the same ambient temperature as the internal incubation temperatures. Reliable hygrometers should be utilized that allow external evaluation of humidity of the inner chamber and daily monitoring of humidity concentrations. Although a closed system, it is crucial that incubators have appropriate air flow and ventilation. Hypoxia from a completely closed system would be a cause of embryonic death, either in the shell or soon after emergence from the shell. Successful species-specific incubator humidity concentrations are reported in Table 85.2.

The incubator, whether purchased or constructed, should be set up and operational several days before the expected arrival of the eggs to allow for equilibration of the temperature and humidity within the system. A window in the top of the incubator, which is standard in most commercial incubators, allows for observation during incubation and hatching.

During egg collection, care should be taken not to change the spatial orientation of the egg during transport or when placed into the substrate of the incubator. Although a previously controversial topic, it is now supported by a study in the water snake (*Natrix maura*) that showed

TABLE 85.2   Temperature-Based Sex Determination (TSD) Patterns that Are Exhibited by Different Reptile Taxa

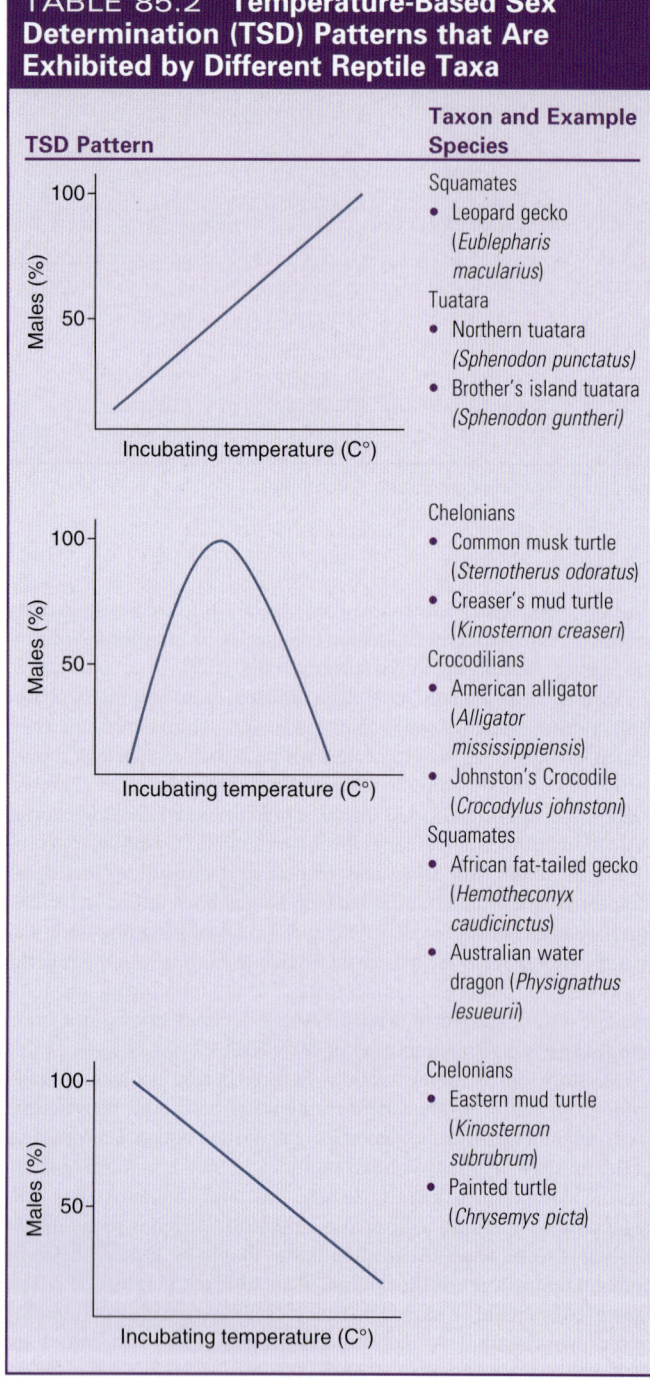

TSD Pattern	Taxon and Example Species
	Squamates
	• Leopard gecko (*Eublepharis macularius*)
	Tuatara
	• Northern tuatara (*Sphenodon punctatus*)
	• Brother's island tuatara (*Sphenodon guntheri*)
	Chelonians
	• Common musk turtle (*Sternotherus odoratus*)
	• Creaser's mud turtle (*Kinosternon creaseri*)
	Crocodilians
	• American alligator (*Alligator mississippiensis*)
	• Johnston's Crocodile (*Crocodylus johnstoni*)
	Squamates
	• African fat-tailed gecko (*Hemotheconyx caudicinctus*)
	• Australian water dragon (*Physignathus lesueurii*)
	Chelonians
	• Eastern mud turtle (*Kinosternon subrubrum*)
	• Painted turtle (*Chrysemys picta*)

that turning the eggs early in embryo development significantly increased post-hatching mortality.[44] In crocodilians, it has been shown that turning the eggs prior to embryo attachment (occurs within 24 hours of oviposition) has no effect on hatchability; however, rotation after this point will cause embryo death.[45] Because the effects of turning and the exact times of embryo attachment post-oviposition have not been elucidated for all species, the author recommends not changing the spatial orientation of any egg during transport.

NATURAL INCUBATION

In many situations, it is preferable and appropriate to allow natural incubation to occur. Knowledge of species-specific incubation strategies is important. Several species of python and *Eumeces* skinks are known for egg brooding, for instance.[22,23] Other species may create elaborate nests or excavate nests into substrate. Either in free-ranging or captive settings, if conditions support incubation change, eggs may be collected and moved to an artificial incubator setting. Egg collection should be done with caution in species that are known to guard nest sites such as crocodilians.

EGG DIAGNOSTIC PROCEDURES

There are several ways to evaluate egg viability: evaluation of the external appearance, candling, and noninvasive heart rate monitoring. Daily monitoring of the appearance of the eggs should be performed and recorded. A healthy, viable egg should stay a consistent color, although slight mottling to the surface is often not significant. Marked changes in color or texture, or growth of fuzzy mold usually indicates that the embryo has either died or that the egg was nonfertile (Fig. 85.4). Wrinkling and shrinking of the eggs does not always indicate embryo death, but that moisture levels are too low and the egg is dehydrating. Moistening of the surrounding substrate and checking humidity levels may be effective at rehydrating the egg, although severe dehydration often leads to embryo death. Viable crocodilian eggs will have a distinct band around the pole of the egg that increases in size with the growth of the embryo. This facilitates visual assessment of fertility and determination of the relative age of the embryo and is an important visual tool for viability in these species.[45]

Candling can be performed with a high-intensity light source, such as an ophthalmic transilluminator or a commercially available egg candler. The light should be placed in direct contact with the far side of the egg in a darkened room. Candled viable eggs will have a diffuse developing vascular pattern or the presence of an embryo (Fig. 85.5A). Nonviable eggs lack a vascular pattern and have a homogenous diffuse yellow-white appearance (see Fig. 85.5B). Care should be taken that the candling process is not prolonged, as heat from some light sources can damage the developing embryo and its membranes.

For soft-shelled eggs, a standard high-frequency (7.5–10 MHz) ultrasound transducer can be used to evaluate the heart rate of the developing embryo (Fig. 85.6). Standard water-soluble ultrasound gel can be used as an interface; however, because it may clog pores of the shell and prevent oxygen exchange, minimal gel should be utilized and removed afterward. In addition, a noninvasive commercially available infrared digital heart rate monitor can be used on both hard-shelled and soft-shelled eggs. Because an infrared light is used it can be a source of heat that may cause harm to the developing embryo if used for a prolonged amount of time.[46]

Additional diagnostics of the egg may be beneficial for research applications and investigation of reduced hatchability. A modified yolk biopsy technique has been described that allows for embryo survival.[47] Necropsy of the egg and collection of samples for histopathologic, bacteriologic, and/or toxicologic examinations can be a vital component of developing a successful incubation and hatching program. Assessment of records of daily temperatures and humidity can also be helpful in evaluation of causes of embryo death. Standard avian egg necropsy practices should be followed.

HATCHING AND MANUAL PIPPING

In the natural hatching process, immediately prior to hatching, the yolk sac is internalized into the coelomic cavity of the hatchling by retraction of the amnion. After successful yolk internalization, the body wall closes around the navel. From this point, gas exchange can no longer take place through the membranes, and the embryo must initiate gas exchange

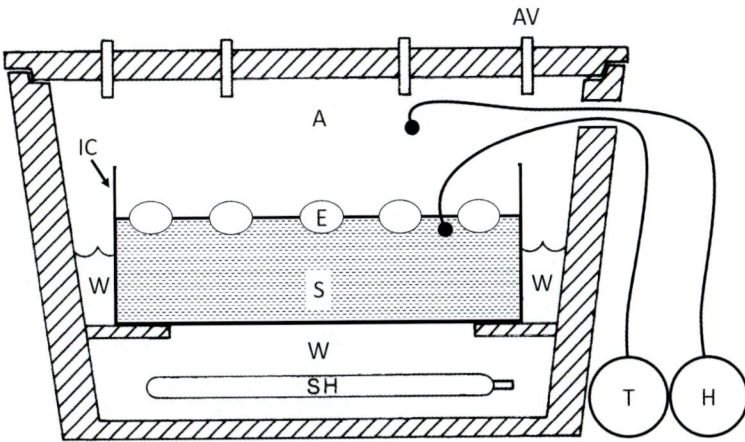

FIG 85.2 Diagram of appropriate reptile incubator utilizing an inner and outer chamber design. A, Air; AV, air vent; E, egg; IC, inner chamber; S, substrate; SH, submersible heater; W, water; T, thermometer; H, hygrometer.

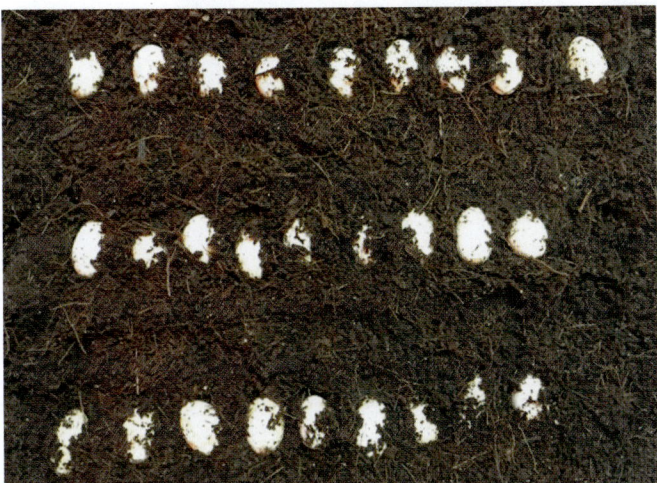

FIG 85.3 Incubating panther chameleon (*Furcifer pardalis*) eggs. The substrate used is a moistened coconut coir product. Note that the eggs are half buried in the substrate.

through its lungs. It is hypothesized that hypoxic conditions in the embryo during yolk internalization cause contraction of muscles in the neck of the hatchling, leading to pipping.[7] Pipping occurs when the egg tooth, or caruncle, (Fig. 85.7) is forced through the eggshell. Once the eggshell is broken, the process of emergence of the hatchling from the shell can take 24 to 48 hours.[7]

Hatching is expected to occur based upon calculated species-specific hatch times that are additionally influenced by incubation temperatures (see Table 85.1). In many instances, the specific hatch time will not be known and constant observation should be performed to investigate when the process should be expected. In some species of crocodilians, embryos will begin vocalizing from within the egg prior to pipping.[48] Environmentally cued synchronous hatching occurs in at least 43 species of reptiles and may include physical disturbances such as vibrations or hypoxia. Synchronous hatching may serve to dilute predation risk in natural environments.[49] Regardless of whether environmentally cued synchronic hatching has been documented in a species, most eggs from the same clutch will be expected to hatch within a few days of each other.

Manual pipping and intervention in the natural events of hatching should be reserved for situations where the viability of the embryo is

at risk. An example would be if vocalization was previously heard within an egg, as is the case with crocodilian species,[48] and other eggs in the clutch have been pipping, but this particular egg has not yet pipped. Another indication would be if the hatchling has pipped but not progressed to full emergence in the same amount of time as hatch mates or the expected time for that species. It is important to remember that the process of full emergence from the shell takes 24 to 48 hours,[7] and prematurely initiated emergence can lead to rupture of chorioallantoic membranes, bleeding, or incompletely internalized yolk sac, thus placing that hatchling at risk for infection and death.

In cases where manual pipping is indicated, sterile technique should be used with magnification. A small wedge incision is made in the top of the egg with sharp scissors (Fig. 85.8A). Care should be taken to avoid incising any internal vessels of the extraembryonic membranes (see Fig. 85.8B) When performed properly, the extraembryonic membranes are left intact. A blunt probe when placed in contact with the hatchling should cause movement if viable. If the extraembryonic membranes appear dry and tacky, rehydration can be performed with judicious use of a few drops of isotonic saline. After manual pipping is performed, the neonate should be allowed 24 to 48 hours to emerge from the egg on its own.

NEONATAL/HATCHLING CARE AND MEDICINE

The terms neonate and hatchling refer to the same time period but relate to the different reproductive strategies used by reptiles. Viviparous juvenile reptiles would be referred to as neonates, while oviparous juvenile reptiles would be referred to as hatchlings. The veterinary considerations during this time would be the same, whether caring for a hatchling or a neonate, and therefore the terms are often used interchangeably.

Maternal Care

Few reptile species are noted to provide protection and care to the hatchling. Among these species are the crocodilians and some skinks, to name a few.[50,51] The evolutionary advantages of providing maternal care includes protection of the young from predators and providing young with food, thus improving offspring survival. The parental costs of providing this care may include reduction of reproductive capacity due to loss of mating opportunities, lower energy intake, and in some cases reduced survival. A recent study evaluating long-tailed skinks (*Eutropis longicaudata*) found that populations experiencing higher predation pressure on offspring provided maternal care, while other

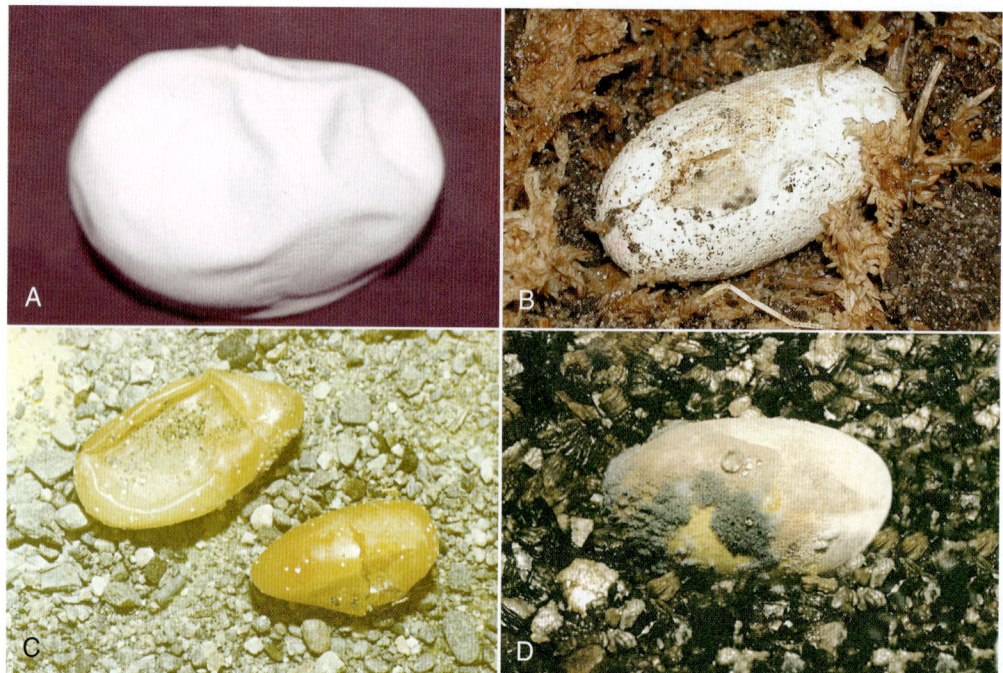

FIG 85.4 Egg viability should be visually assessed on a daily basis. (A) Collapsed or wrinkled appearance is a sign of dehydration and not necessarily egg death. These eggs can often be salvaged with rehydration of the substrate and increased humidity in the incubator. (B) Mottling or partial discoloration, although appearing lethal, can be normal in many cases. (C) Waxy yellow "slugs" may be passed from either viviparous or oviparous animals and represent unfertilized ova. (D) Mold on the surface of the egg is usually a sign of egg death. Nonviable eggs should be removed from the incubator immediately.

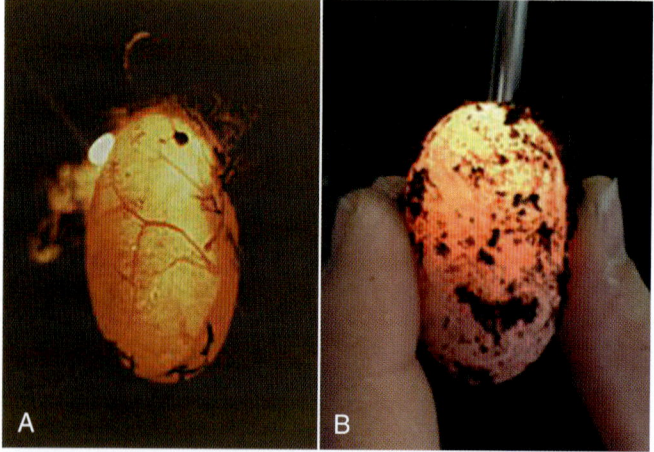

FIG 85.5 Egg viability can be evaluated by candling with a high-intensity light source. (A) Viable eggs readily show developing vasculature. As the embryo develops in later stages, movement can be seen within the egg (not shown). (B) Nonviable eggs lack developing vasculature and appear as homogenous yellow-white egg contents.

FIG 85.6 Egg viability can be evaluated by ausculting the heart rate of the developing embryo. Here, a commercially available 8-MHz ultrasound transducer is used to evaluate the heart rate of a snake embryo.

populations did not.[52] In the captive setting, the advantages of housing neonates with the parent of a species known to exhibit maternal care should be balanced with the disadvantages of group housing (conspecific predation, trampling, access to appropriate food sources, etc).

Husbandry

Reptile neonates are born precocious and find food, feed themselves, and perform normal functions as an adult. The housing and husbandry requirements of neonates will mirror those of adults, although temperature and humidity requirements tend to be higher. Neonatal growth rates are strongly affected by environmental temperatures.[53] Most breeders keep neonates in the incubator for the first few days of life at the incubation temperatures with a humidity of 90% to 100%, as neonates have a higher total body water loss rate than adults.[54] Neonates will do well on a simple substrate of moistened paper towels that are easy to monitor and clean fecal and urinary outputs. Group housing should only be pursued if appropriate for the species, and care should be taken to ensure that all individuals are eating. Cannibalism can be prevented by reducing stocking density and ensuring that neonates housed together are of similar size.

It is common for a neonatal reptile to not eat for the first few days to weeks of life. During this time period, the internalized yolk is providing nutrition. The time period that the yolk can sustain the neonate is species specific; in the Mitchell's water monitor (*Varanus mitchelli*), neonates eat after first ecdysis at 4 to 10 days post-hatching, while in the Lake Erie water snake (*Nerodia sipedon insularum*), the first meal may be delayed until after hibernation.[55,56] Inappropriately intervening with nutritional support during this physiological period of fasting is unnecessary and stressful.

In general, the neonate should be fed items that mirror what the adult would eat although in smaller sizes. Smaller versions of the adult diet should be offered, which may require insect breeding to obtain the smallest size for insectivores or finely chopped vegetation in the case of herbivorous species. There are some exceptions to this rule with species that exhibit ontogenetic diet shifts or changing dietary preferences with maturity. In the bearded dragon, adults ingest a diet of 90% plant matter and 10% animal matter, while juveniles consume 50% plant matter and 50% animal matter.[57] Other examples of species that exhibit ontogenetic dietary shifts include the yellow-bellied slider (*Trachemys scripta*), Australian eastern bearded dragon (*Pogona barbata*), green lizard (*Lacerta bilineata*), and the green turtle (*Chelonia mydas*) among others.[58-61]

Because neonates are fast growing and have high nutrient demands, supplementation of foods with additional calcium and a reptile-specific multivitamin, whether dusted, gut loaded, or both, is recommended. In addition, as hind gut–fermenting herbivores, green iguanas (*Iguana iguana*) require a complex population of large intestinal microbes. These microbes are shown to be transferred from the adult to the neonate in the wild, and this should be replicated in captivity by allowing access to fresh feces from a healthy adult.[62]

Techniques for stimulating "slow to eat" neonates are species or diet specific. For carnivorous and insectivorous neonates, visual cues, including prey motion, have significant effects on feeding in hatchling Komodo dragons (*Varanus komodensis*), and live prey should be offered whenever legally possible to resistant feeders.[63] Live prey left with small reptiles can easily harm the neonate, so care should be taken in these situations. The same study in komodo dragons also found that chemical cues were important to the feeding behavior of hatchlings.[63] For species that have feeding preferences that are difficult to recreate in captivity, such as certain frog-eating snakes, scenting easier to obtain food items (e.g., rodents) with the scent from the preferred food item may aid in prey acceptance. Other appetite-inducing techniques may include "slap feeding" in snakes, warming of food items, or placing food in the neonates' mouth. In cases where true assist- or force-feeding must be performed, care should be taken to carefully calculate stomach volume (typically 1%–3% of body weight) and to gently use a soft pliable tube with lubrication so as not to harm delicate tissues.

NEONATE DIAGNOSTIC PROCEDURES

In many cases, diagnostic techniques utilized for adults can be similarly used in the neonatal patient. Complete blood count and plasma biochemical reference intervals for neonates have not been evaluated for any species known to the author, although studies are available that have evaluated limited analytes.[64,65] Additionally, most neonates are of a size that precludes venipuncture or severely limits the amount of blood that can be collected. Radiography may be utilized, and dentistry radiographic units may be most appropriate given the small size of hatchlings. Sex identification of hatchlings is an important topic, and there are many techniques utilized including endoscopic methods in a variety of chelonian species.[66,67] See Chapter 80 for a detailed discussion on sex identification. Necropsy of deceased neonates is advisable, and standard techniques similar to those used for adults are recommended.

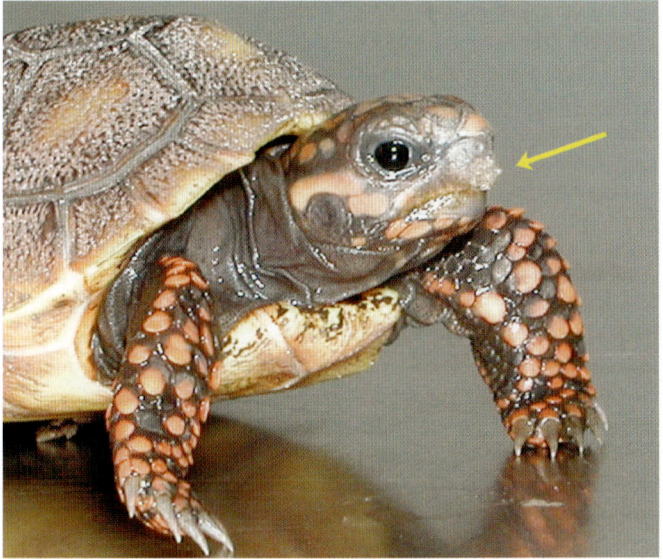

FIG 85.7 Most oviparous species, including this hatchling red-footed tortoise (*Chelonoidis carbonaria*), have a caruncle (arrow), or egg tooth, that is used to pip through the egg during hatching. This structure is not present in adult specimens and is lost after the first shed or within a couple weeks of hatching.

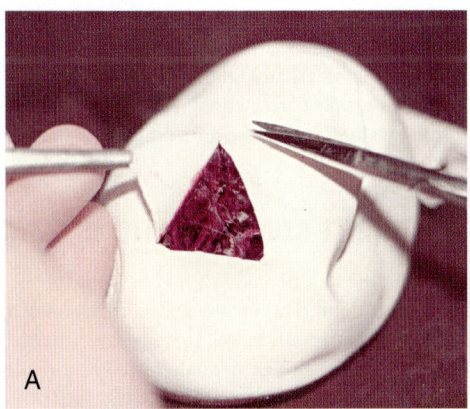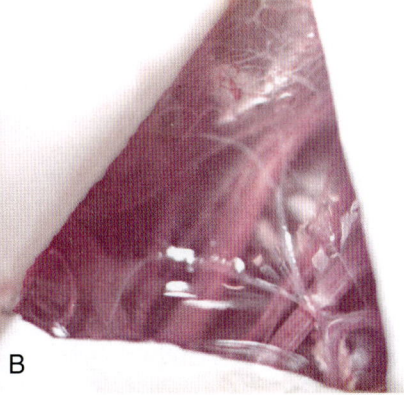

FIG 85.8 Occasionally, artificial pipping of the egg becomes necessary. (A) Using sterile technique and magnification, a triangular wedge is cut into the egg. (B) Extreme care is taken to avoid cutting or damaging the vessels of the extraembryonic membranes.

TABLE 85.3 Common Infectious Diseases and Associated Clinical Signs in Neonatal and Hatchling Reptiles

Etiological Agent	Species	Clinical Signs
Cryptosporidium saurophilum	Any lizard species, especially prevalent in the leopard gecko (*Eublepharis macularius*)	Poor body condition score, diarrhea, anorexia, failure to thrive
Agamid adenovirus 1	Bearded dragon (*Pogona vitticeps*)	Diarrhea, weight loss, anorexia, central nervous system dysfunction
Nannizziopsis sp.	Most lizard species	Crusting/ulcerative dermatological lesions; lesions often yellow in color in bearded dragons
Mycoplasma sp.	Chelonians	Conjunctivitis and ocular discharge, nasal discharge/bubbling, choanal inflammation
Ophionyssus spp.	Snakes and lizards	Increased shedding frequency, visible ectoparasites, increased soaking, anorexia, anemia
Testudid herpesvirus	Chelonians, especially Russian tortoises (*Agrionemys horsfieldii*)	Oronasal discharge, ocular discharge, fibrinous/necrotizing stomatitis

DISEASES

Yolk Sac Diseases

In most cases, the yolk sac has been absorbed into the coelomic cavity before hatching.[7] If this sac is not internalized at emergence, the neonate is at risk for yolk sac rupture and/or infection. If the internalization process has progressed to an advanced state, the natural progression of internalization may progress on its own if the neonate is closely monitored and maintained on a clean damp surface, such as a moistened paper towel. In cases where the umbilicus is pendulously attached to the neonate through the umbilicus, it is advisable to ligate and transect the yolk sac as proximal to the neonate as possible to reduce incidence of infection and allow the neonate to ambulate unencumbered. After transection, if the body wall is open, surgical closure should be performed. A strangulating umbilical cord that has not internalized the yolk must be addressed immediately.

Yolk sac infection may occur even if the yolk was internalized prior to emergence. The yolk may be infected prior to envelopment into the coelom, through an incompletely closed umbilicus and ascension from omphalitis, or it may become infected through ascension of intestinal bacteria from the vitelline duct. Infection of the yolk sac causes closure of the vitelline duct cutting off nutritional sources to the neonate, and the infected yolk and yolk sac may lead to generalized coelomitis. Affected neonates may have a palpable structure in the coelom and will show clinical signs of lethargy, anorexia, and general malaise. Exploratory coeliotomy with collection of bacteriologic samples after surgical removal of the yolk sac is indicated. Post-operatively, antibiotics, modified on culture and sensitivity results, should be administered.

Infectious Diseases

In general, any infectious disease that can affect the adult can also affect the neonate, although with their small size and incomplete immune function, neonates have a higher morbidity and mortality when exposed to these same pathogens. For example, the common snake mite (*Ophionyssus natricis*) may cause subclinical infections in adults, but this hematophagous mite can overwhelm and exsanguinate neonates in a short amount of time. Some classic species-specific pathogens in neonatal and juvenile reptiles are listed in Table 85.3.

The topic of salmonellosis should be discussed in more detail, because it is a common zoonosis (see Chapter 174). Despite a long-standing federal ban in the United States on the sale of turtles with a carapace length of less than 4 inches, continued multistate outbreaks of turtle-associated salmonellosis occur.[68] Although most reptile-associated salmonellosis in humans is linked with turtle contact, a variety of species have been implicated in infections, including bearded dragons, corn snakes (*Patherophis guttatus*), veiled chameleons (*Chamaeleo calyptratus*), and a variety of *Python* spp., among others.[68–70] Infection of the reptile neonate has been shown to occur transovarially and from salmonella-contaminated environments.[71] As it is considered a commensal in most reptiles, *Salmonella* spp. may or may not cause clinical illness in reptile neonates, the former being highlighted in a reported outbreak of salmonellosis in hatchling Nile crocodiles (*Crocodylus niloticus*) that was successfully controlled through supportive care, environmental decontamination, and systemic antibiotics.[72] Basic hygiene and awareness when dealing with neonatal reptiles is appropriate to reduce chances of outbreaks in reptile and human patients.

Husbandry-Associated Diseases

In general, any husbandry-related disease that can affect the adult can also affect the neonate; although, with rapid metabolism and growth, neonates have a higher morbidity and mortality when husbandry deficiencies are present. The most readily noted is nutritional secondary hyperparathyroidism (see Chapters 27 and 84) and is typically related to inadequate dietary intake of calcium and vitamin D3 (or lack of appropriate UVB lighting). Other common husbandry-associated diseases include sand/substrate impaction and predation by prey items and predation from cage mates due to inappropriate pairings or high stocking densities. See Section 3 for more details.

Congenital Diseases

Many congenital diseases have been reported in neonatal reptiles and may have a genetic or inappropriate incubation root cause. In the recent literature, two ball pythons were reported to have bifid ventricles secondary to an abnormally small-sized muscular ridge, and a patent urachus was diagnosed in a hatchling prehensile-tailed skink (*Corucia zebrata*) that was surgically corrected.[73,74] Diagnosis of a congenital lesion should prompt evaluation of the breeding stock and artificial incubation parameters.

TREATMENT CONSIDERATIONS

In general, the sick neonate should be afforded the same treatments as a similarly ill adult. This includes administration of appropriate analgesic and other medications, as well as nutritional, thermal, and fluid support. Due to the small size of neonates, medication administration can be challenging. Dosages for neonates that take into consideration differences that may exist in pharmacokinetics are lacking, and judicial use of dosages used in adults are often utilized. Concentrations of medications

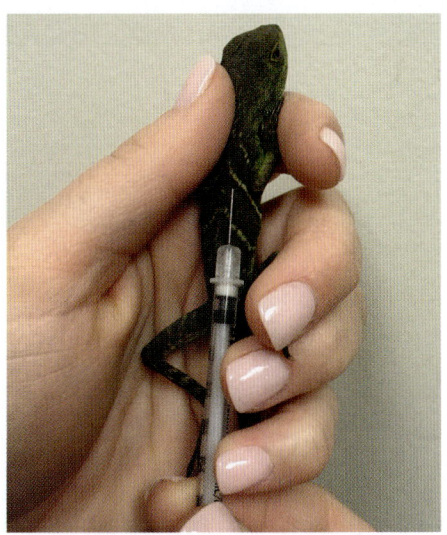

FIG 85.9 Subcutaneous injection of a hatchling Chinese water dragon (*Physignathus cocincinus*). A commercially available insulin syringe and needle are being utilized to prevent excessive tissue trauma.

may not be amenable to dosing and may require dilution. Consultation with a veterinary pharmacist may aid in developing medication-specific dilutions that are safe and efficacious. For instance, at least one injectable form of ivermectin (Ivomec 1% sterile solution, Merck & Co., Inc.) is suspended in a lipid carrier. Consequently, dilution with saline or sterile water may lead to nonhomogeneous distribution of the precipitated drug and potential patient overdose or underdose.

Injectable or oral administration of medications can be safely performed using the same guidelines as would be used in adults but with smaller instrumentation and greater care to prevent trauma. Injections can be given using insulin syringes that are available to measure to the nearest 0.005 mL (half unit on a U-100 syringe) (Fig. 85.9). These syringes have the added benefit of having small needle sizes to reduce tissue trauma. Oral medications can be given using insulin syringes after the needle is removed. A guitar pick can be an excellent tool to open small mouths.

REFERENCES

See www.expertconsult.com for a complete list of references.

86

Geriatric Medicine

Paul Raiti

The aging process (senescence) is defined as "a persistent decline in age-specific fitness components of an organism due to internal physiological deterioration."[1] Three patterns of senescence have been described for reptiles: rapid, gradual, and negligible.[2] An example of rapid senescence is observed in the African skink (*Trachylepsis buettneri*), which has an average longevity of 1 to 2 years. The majority of lizards and snakes undergo gradual senescence similar to most vertebrates. Chelonians and crocodilians are characterized by negligible senescence.[2] Reptiles have the record of the highest longevity among vertebrates (Table 86.1).[2] Growth rate of most reptiles declines with age. Age-related loss of organ weight and thymus atrophy have been considered secondary indications of senescence.[2] Most reptiles replace their teeth (polyphyodonty) throughout life, presumably to reflect the need for new sets of slightly larger teeth during the continuous growth of their jaws throughout their lifespan.[2] In most lizards and snakes, there is no evidence that tooth replacement ceases or slows down at advanced age, but in crocodiles the replacement rhythm becomes irregular and slower with increasing age. Decreased reproductive capability and the decline in capacity for regeneration are examples of morphogenetic senescence. Long-lived species live longer than short-lived counterparts, whether in natural surroundings or in captivity. Senescence occurs earlier in females with a high reproductive effort early in life compared to those with reproductive effort later in life; hence, there is a trade-off between early reproductive performance and longevity in reptiles.[3] Many reptile species exhibit increasing fecundity with advancing age through a direct physiological effect with increasing body size.[4] In addition to indeterminate growth, reptiles have the ability to shut down their metabolism for long periods of time.

Two theories have been used to characterize senescence. The first is the "oxidative stress" theory, whereby there is an age-related accumulation of cellular damage, and the second is the chromosomal "telomere attrition" theory, which accounts for the loss of DNA replication.[5] The oxidative stress theory of aging hypothesizes that senescence and death result from the accumulation of damaged biomolecules (free radicals) due to a declining ability to repair cellular damage with age.[5] Free radicals oxidatively damage the cellular components: DNA, protein, and lipid.[6] The damaging forces can be such stressors as UV radiation, heat, starvation, xenobiotics, pollution, pesticides, ozone, hyperoxia, etc.[6] Ascorbic acid and catalase have protective effects against lipid peroxidation and oxidative damage.[7] Telomeres are chromosome fragments that possess polarity, which prevents their reunion with any fragment after a chromosome has been broken; hence, they stabilize mitosis and meiosis.[8] Behavior is also an important aspect to consider in aging variation, as it relates to mating strategy,[9] mate choice,[10] and offspring dispersal.[11]

There are several hypotheses regarding the evolution of longevity. The relative reproductive rate hypothesis predicts traits that increase the reproductive output or survival rates of older compared to younger individuals, whereas the senescence hypothesis predicts a reduction in reproductive output or survival in older versus younger individuals.[12] Three traits—increased clutch size, reproductive frequency, and survivorship of individuals in the older age groups—support the relative reproductive rate hypothesis for evolution of longevity. Increases in survival and reproductive output are associated with larger body sizes of older individuals.[13] In many turtle species, increased reproductive output is associated with increased body size of females, because larger females produce larger eggs or larger clutches of eggs.[4] For example,

TABLE 86.1 Longevities of Assorted Reptiles and Amphibians

Species	Life Expectancy (yrs)
African skink (*Trachylepsis buettneri*)	<2
American alligator (*Alligator mississippiensis*)	30–50
Blue-tongued skink (*Tiliqua scincoides*)	15–20
Caiman (*Caiman crocodiles*)	25
Chinese water dragon (*Physignathus cocincinus*)	12–20
Crested gecko (*Correlophus ciliatus*)	15–20
Green iguana (*Iguana iguana*)	10–20
Inland bearded dragon (*Pogona vitticeps*)	8–14
Jackson's chameleon (*Trioceros jacksonii*)	5–10
Komodo dragon (*Varanus komodoensis*)	10–20
Leaf-tailed gecko (*Uroplatus* spp.)	10–15
Leopard gecko (*Eublepharis macularius*)	20–30
Savannah monitor (*Varanus exanthematicus*)	10–15
Uromastyx (*Uromastyx acanthinura*)	10–35
Veiled chameleon (*Chamaeleo calyptratus*)	2–5
Ball python (*Python regius*)	20–50
Corn snake (*Pantherophis guttatus*)	15–25
Red-tailed boa (*Boa constrictor*)	20–30
African spurred tortoise (*Centrochelys sulcata*)	50–100
Blanding's turtle (*Emydoidia blandigii*)	75
Box turtle (*Terrapene carolina*)	60–100
Red-eared slider (*Trachemys scripta elegans*)	45–65
Red-footed tortoise (*Chelonoidis carbonaria*)	22–50
Snapping turtle (*Chelydra serpentina*)	40–50
Green tree frog (*Hyla cinerea*)	3–6
Tomato tree frog (*Dyscophus* spp.)	3–5
Axolotl (*Ambystoma mexicanum*)	10–20

female Blanding's turtles postpone maturity to 14 to 21 years of age and produce a maximum of one clutch of 3 to 19 eggs annually.[4] Annual survivorship of adult females exceeds 93%, and some individuals can live in excess of 75 years.[4] Faster metabolic rates have been implicated with faster biochemical activity and a faster aging process.[14] The maximum amount of time a mammal can expect to live after maturity, even in captivity, is typically proportional to the amount of time it took that animal to reach maturity.[14] Species with low rates of mortality from extrinsic sources, such as predation, senesce more slowly and have longer maximum life spans than related species with higher rates of predation.[14] Studies of anurans and urodeles (salamanders, newts) have revealed that maximum body size is positively correlated with maximum life span in captivity.[15] Amphibians of northern regions (hibernation) have a longer life span than those of southern regions.[15] Chemically protected species (venomous or poisonous) generally live longer than their nonchemically protected counterparts of similar body sizes, and larger species are less likely to be chemically protected than smaller species.[16]

Morphometric criteria or growth curves/charts established for wild individuals may be skewed in captivity, as growth can be significantly affected by feeding regimen and husbandry.[17] Deficiencies lead to stunting whereas overfeeding, or power-feeding, accelerates growth.[17] Age determination is estimated by sclerochronology and skeletochronology using natural growth rings in epidermal scutes and bone, respectively. Counting growth rings through skeletochronological techniques involves harvesting bone from a live animal (distal phalange or tail) and using histology to estimate age. In a field study involving desert monitor lizards (*Varanus griseus*), it was determined that age could be estimated in adult specimens with an accuracy of ±2 years.[18] It should be noted that sclerochronology and skeletochronology reflect seasonal periodicity of growth and not necessarily yearly time sequences (Fig. 86.1). Under natural conditions, sclerochronological evaluation of geriatric tortoises can be problematic due to seasonal changes in growth, injuries, and abrasive forces associated with foraging, burrowing, etc., which tend to wear away growth rings. Additionally, some species of turtles lose the previous year's scute (*Chrysemys picta*), which affects reliability of growth ring counting. Under captive conditions, irregular growth rates

associated with inappropriate diets, lack of ultraviolet B, inadequate hydration, lack of basking areas for semiaquatic turtles, etc., can distort and obscure growth rings. Rattlesnakes (*Crotalus* and *Sistrurus*) add a segment to their rattle with each ecdysis so that a crude age may be estimated by counting segments, but shedding in snakes is irregular, may occur 2 to 3 times each year, and the rattle often breaks as it gains in length.[17] Captive-born reptiles are generally longer-lived than their wild counterparts, because captivity shields reptiles from adverse climatic pressures, starvation, and predation. Captivity can affect longevity negatively if husbandry parameters are inappropriate. As a rule, captive-born animals are better acclimated to captivity and handling, are better feeders, and do not come with the heavy parasitic burden that wild-caught reptiles often bear.[17]

Unlike many mammals, which clearly show the aging process, senescent reptiles and amphibians often show few signs—and even these are subtle—until their death from natural causes.[17] There may be pigmentary changes, decreased mobility, and slowing of actions and reactions (Fig. 86.2). Ecdysis is usually less frequent in older squamates due to decreased growth rate but may also be more frequent with disease. Dysecdysis, hyperkeratosis, cutaneous growths and excrescences, broken tails and regrowths, missing toes and/or nails, and overgrown beaks are more common in senescent animals (Fig. 86.3A–C).[17] Constipation is common and may be caused by dehydration, diminished mobility, and renomegaly/urinary calculi. Degenerative bone and articular changes may also be encountered in geriatric reptiles (Fig. 86.4). Spondylopathies are prevalent in green iguanas, Komodo dragons, and snakes.[19] Symptoms can include reduced mobility, scoliosis, kyphosis, and paraparesis. Articular gout causes painful swelling of the limbs (Fig. 86.5). Diagnosis is by radiography and arthrocentesis (Figs. 86.6 and 86.7). Visceral gout, insidious and difficult to diagnose, may cause death with no premonitory signs or may cause various degrees of lethargy, anorexia, and other nonspecific signs.[17] Tachypnea, bradypnea, and dyspnea may indicate pulmonary disease or may reflect pain or metabolic disturbances. Atherosclerosis and vascular mineralization are common in older squamates and chelonians (Figs. 86.8).[17] What constitutes "geriatric" for a reptile or amphibian varies dramatically by species. (See Table 86.1 for longevities of assorted reptiles and amphibians[20]). Diminished appetite, weight loss, and cachexia commonly accompany significantly advanced age. Geriatric reptiles may bask more, possess sunken eyes, be less active, ambulate in a plantigrade stance, and appear

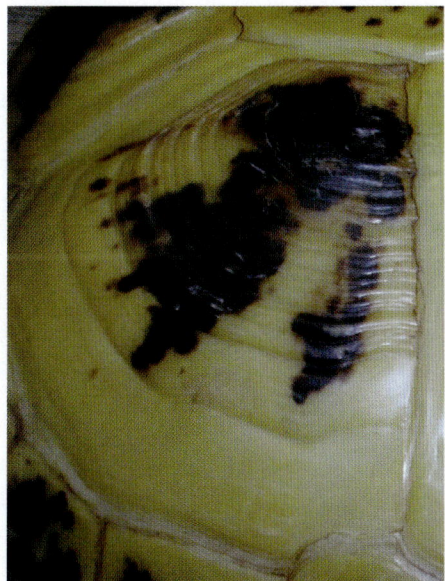

FIG 86.1 Note the wider growth rings of this captive adult Russian tortoise (*Agrionemys horsfieldii*) scute associated with accelerated growth compared to the narrower rings formed while living under natural conditions.

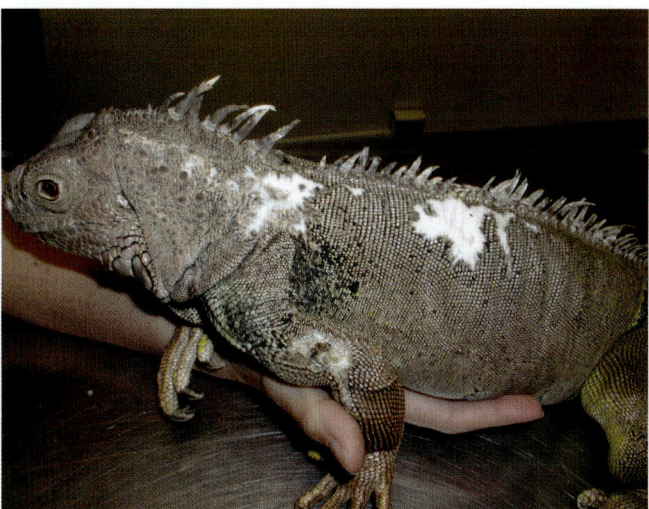

FIG 86.2 Idiopathic leukoderma in a green iguana (*Iguana iguana*) of 21 years. Eschars from excessive radiant heat can cause similar-appearing lesions.

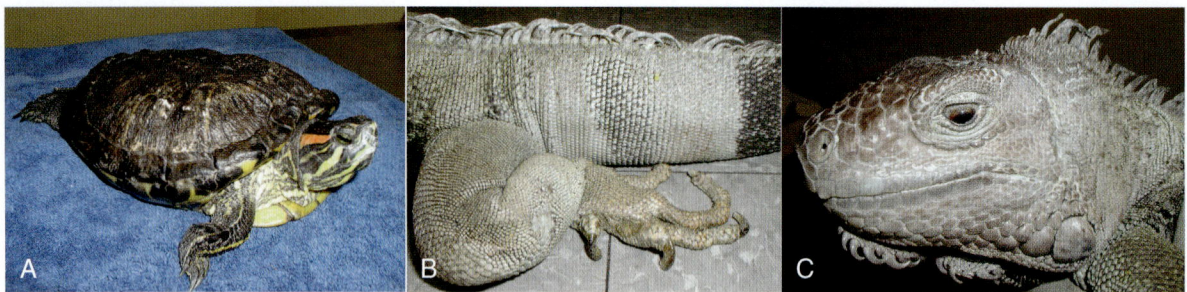

FIG 86.3 (A) Shell distortion and hyperkeratosis in a geriatric red-eared slider (*Trachemys scripta elegans*) of 50 years; (B) deformed appendages and drooping dermal spines in a geriatric green iguana (*Iguana iguana*) of 20 years; and (C) idiopathic strabismus in the same iguana.

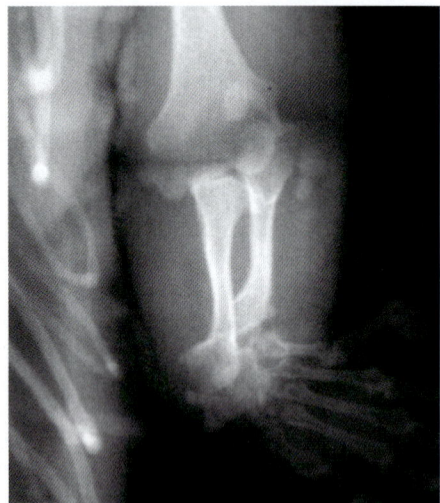

FIG 86.4 Caudocranial radiograph of the right elbow joint in a green iguana (*Iguana iguana*) of 22 years, revealing chronic degenerative joint disease.

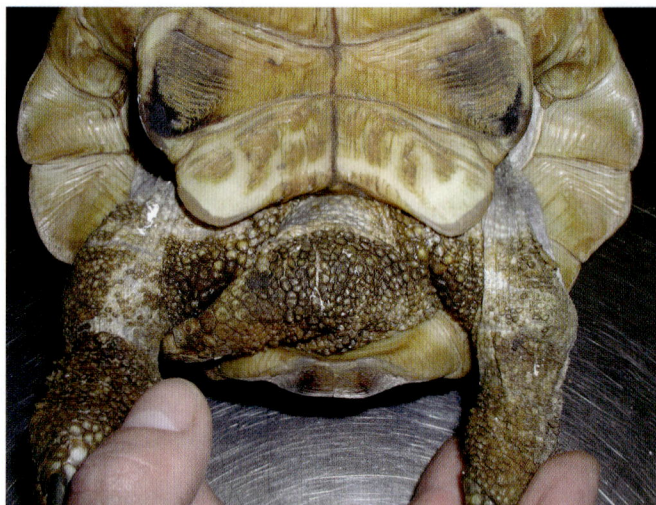

FIG 86.5 Bilateral swollen stifle joints secondary to articular gout in a Hermann's tortoise (*Testudo hermanni*) of 28 years.

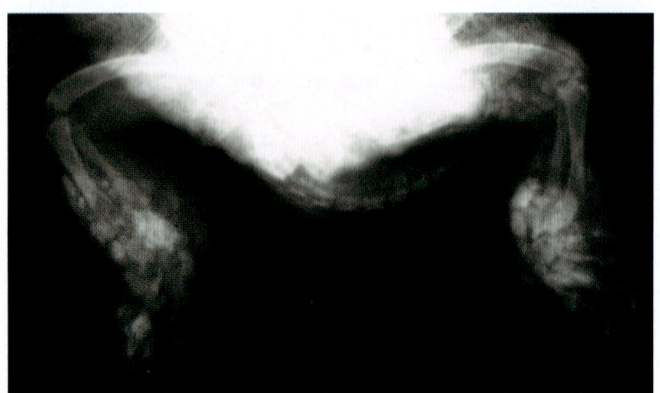

FIG 86.6 Radiograph of articular gout in a red-eared slider (*Trachemys scripta elegans*) of 40 years with renal secondary hyperparathyroidism (RSHP). Note the intraarticular and periarticular deposits (uric acid tophi) affecting multiple joints.

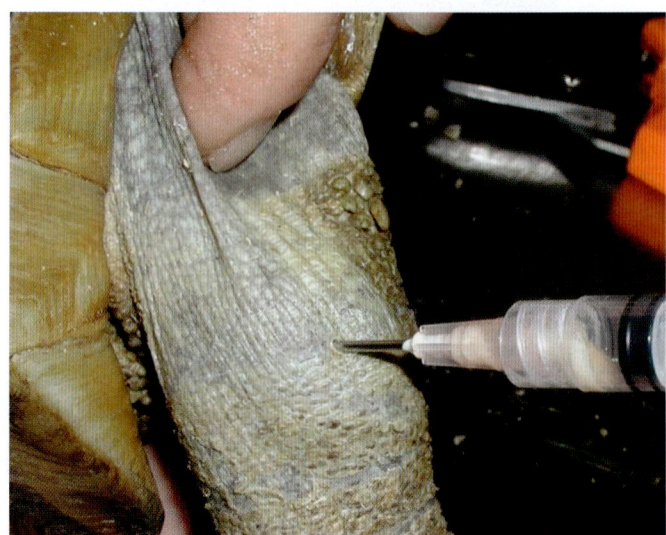

FIG 86.7 Arthrocentesis of the same tortoise in Fig. 86.5. Cytology of the joint effusion revealed urate crystals.

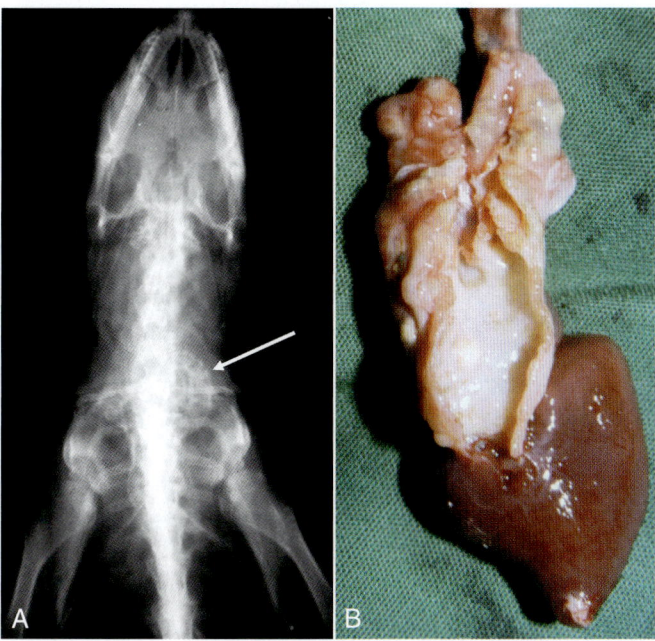

FIG 86.8 (A) Radiograph of soft tissue mineralization of an aortic arch (arrow) in a green iguana (*Iguana iguana*) of 10 years diagnosed with renal secondary hyperparathyroidism (RSHP). (B) Severe arthrosclerosis and soft tissue mineralization of a prosected aorta in a green iguana of 15 years with RSHP.

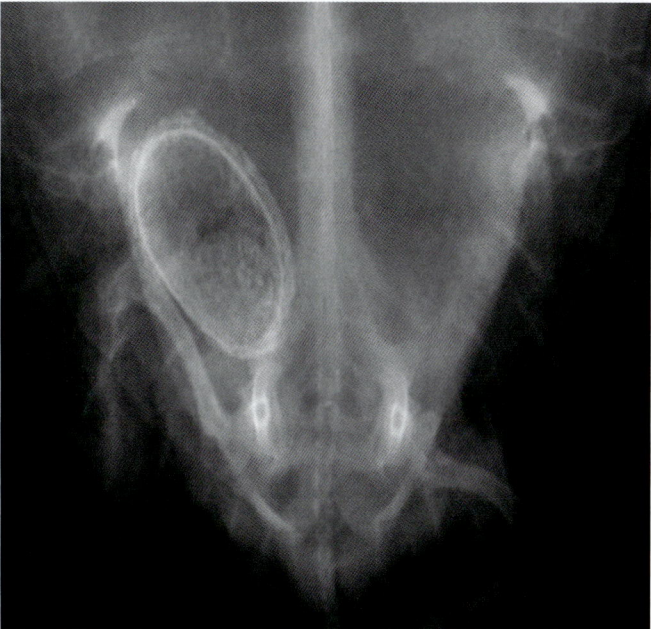

FIG 86.9 Dystocia due to a retained egg in a red-eared slider (*Trachemys scripta elegans*) of 48 years. Note the thickened shell due to chronic calcium deposition.

malnourished.[17] Breeding and reproduction usually decrease with advancing age. There may be fewer eggs or young and a diminished viability of those that are produced. Follicular stasis and egg retention can be problematic in geriatric reptiles (Fig. 86.9). Larger geriatric lizards such as green iguanas are more apt to sustain injuries associated with dyskinesia and/or fractures when they drop from their perches or accidentally fall while held (Fig. 86.10).

VETERINARY CARE OF THE GERIATRIC PATIENT

Geriatrics is defined as the branch of medicine that treats problems peculiar to old age and the aging, including the clinical symptoms of senescence and senility. Signs of senescence can mimic disease and should be distinguished with appropriate diagnostics such as hematology/plasma biochemical analysis and diagnostic imaging. Differentiating senescent-induced morbidity from active disease is not always a straightforward endeavor. Senescence itself is not a disease; however, there are diseases commonly associated with the aging process. Diagnosing age-related pathologies allows the clinician to suggest treatments and alternative husbandry methods that may improve the quality of life for aged reptiles. (See Table 86.2 for a list of common diseases of geriatric reptiles and amphibians).

External features or lesions suggestive of senescence in reptiles may be more a function of prior disease or trauma or may reflect inadequate or substandard husbandry.[17] Serial clinicopathology and radiographs establish baselines for each individual reptile and can be repeated every second year, yearly, or even more often, as the patient ages. Hematocrit, white blood cell count, hepatic and renal function, cholesterol, calcium/phosphorus, uric acid, T_4, and glucose are blood parameters that may change with age. Annual radiographs can optimize the odds of detecting bone and soft tissue changes in an individual reptile. In older females, egg-yolk coelomitis and ovarian neoplasia sometimes occur.

Fluid therapy and diuresis, xanthine oxidase inhibitors, dietary adjustments, and pain management are used to aid reptiles afflicted with articular gout. Infection or impaction of the femoral and perianal pores and hemipenal sulci in lizards, and scent glands and hemipenal sulci and hemipenes in snakes, tend to be seen more often in older individuals[17] (see Chapter 171). Tremors and fasciculations in geriatric reptiles are usually related to hypocalcemia secondary to renal secondary hyperparathyroidism (RSHP). Xanthomas (cholesterol granulomas) have been reported in the central nervous systems and coelomic cavities of geriatric reptiles, including geckos, green water dragons (*Physignathus cocincinus*), and snakes (Fig. 86.11).[21–23] Affected animals are usually sexually mature females. Xanthomas in the brains have been associated with various degrees of hydrocephalus; neurologic symptoms consist of opisthotonos, horizontal head bobbing, and incoordination.[21–23] A case of cerebral xanthomatosis was reported in a 13-year-old female long-nosed snake (*Rhinocheilus lecontei*) that presented for pronounced lethargy, anorexia, and diminished righting reflex.[21] Neoplasia, particularly lymphoproliferative disorders, is seen with increased frequency in older reptiles, especially chelonians and snakes. Neoplasia causes clinical symptoms that may be very slow to progress and vary according to the affected organ systems.[17] Lipid keratopathy (corneal lipidosis) occurs in some agamids and iguanids and has been seen in older green water dragons, plumed basilisks (*Basiliscus plumifrons*), and anurans.[17] This condition is usually associated with a high-fat diet. Ophthalmic age-related changes such as cataracts are similarly seen in reptiles as in other vertebrates (Figure 86.12). Additional diagnostic modalities, such as magnetic resonance imaging, bone scintigraphy, and endoscopy require immobilization to further define lesions or assess progression of disease in the older patient.[17] Short-acting or reversible drug combinations offer the widest safety margins for these geriatric reptiles. Tracheal intubation, placement of an intravenous or intraosseous access line, and the use of monitoring devices will help detect a complication and allow for early intervention.[17]

A literature search reveals a paucity of peer-reviewed sources addressing reptile geriatrics. One report describes cervical subluxation and compressive myelopathy resulting in nerve root and/or spinal cord

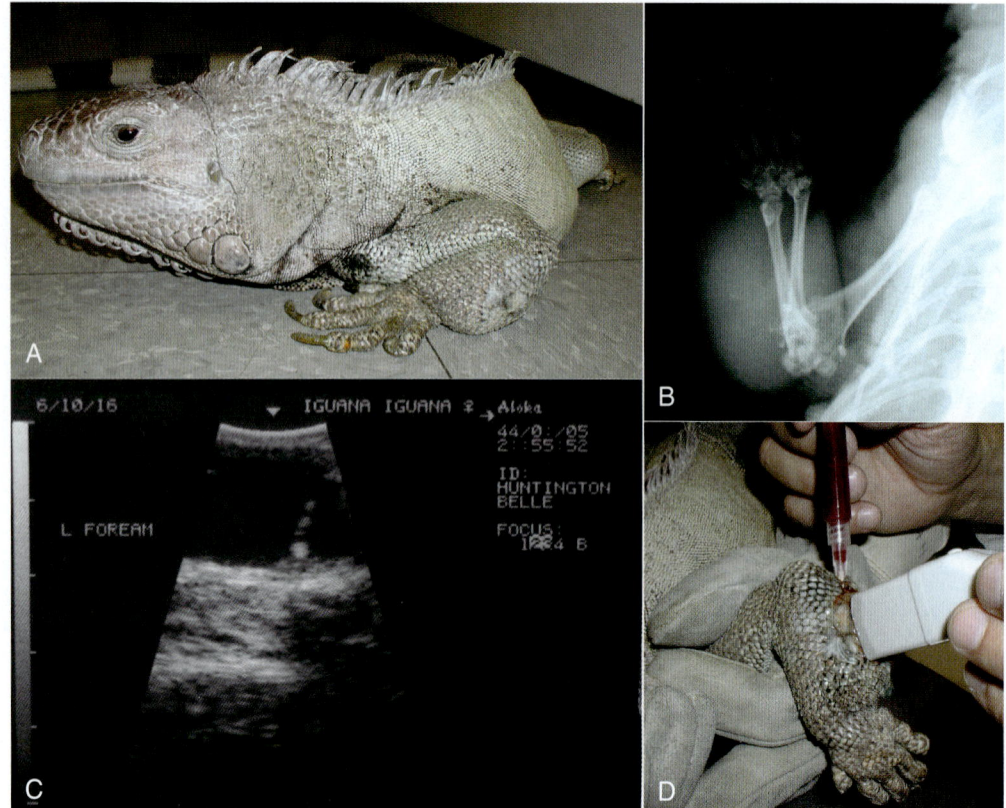

FIG 86.10 (A) Swollen antebrachium of acute onset in a green iguana (*Iguana iguana*) of 20 years; (B) radiograph of the affected limb revealed soft tissue swelling and chronic degenerative joint disease of the left elbow; (C and D) ultrasound-guided aspirate cytology was consistent with a hematoma secondary to suspected trauma.

TABLE 86.2 Common Conditions of Geriatric Reptiles and Amphibians	
Diseases	**Diagnostics**
Dysecdysis	Physical examination
Osteoarthritis	Radiography/CT
Renal secondary hyperparathyroidism (RSHP)	Hematology, plasma biochemistry, radiography/CT, ultrasonography, GFR evaluation, renal biopsy
Metastatic mineralization	Radiography/CT
Urinary calculi	Radiography, ultrasonography
Retained eggs	Radiography
Follicular stasis	Radiography/CT, ultrasonography
Cataracts	Physical examination
Overgrown rhamphothecae, toe nails	Physical examination
Neoplasia	Cytology, biopsy
Articular gout	Plasma biochemistry, radiography/CT, arthrocentesis
Lower respiratory tract disease (LRTD)	Radiography/CT/endoscopy
Impaction of hemipenal pockets	Physical examination
Lipid keratopathy	Physical examination
Xanthoma	Cytology, biopsy
Constipation	Physical examination, radiography

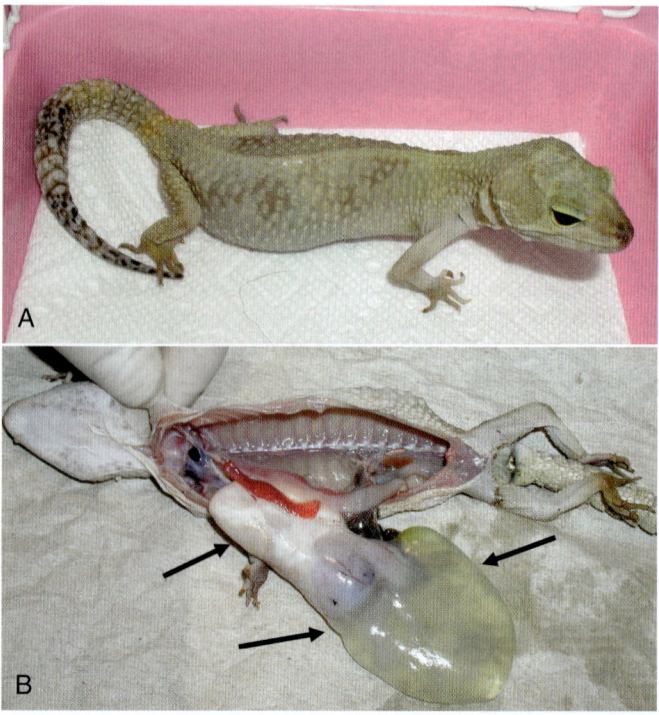

FIG 86.11 (A) Coelomic distention and cachexia in a male leopard gecko of 9 years due to a xanthogranuloma; (B) prosected cadaver revealing the massive size of the lesion (arrows).

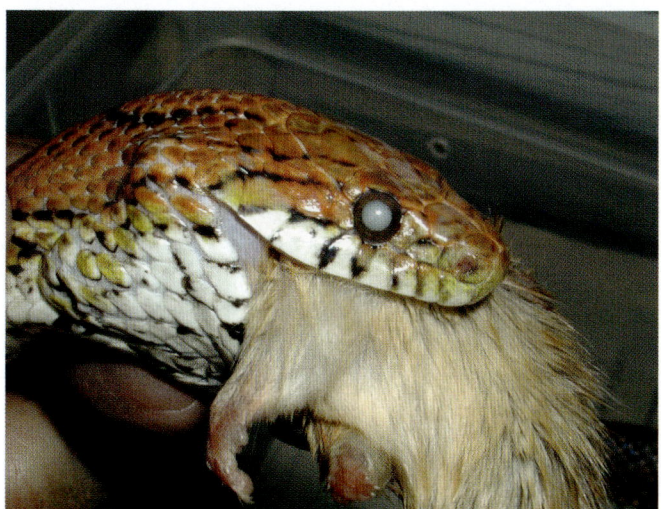

FIG 86.12 Cataracts (bilateral) in a corn snake (*Pantherophis guttatus*) of 17 years that was assist-fed by presentation of a thawed mouse held with tongs.

compression in four captive geriatric Komodo dragons.[24] Three were presumptively induced by trauma, and one had an unknown inciting cause. Two Komodo dragons had exhibited signs of chronic cervical instability. Clinical symptoms included ataxia; ambulatory paraparesis or tetraparesis to tetraplegia; depression to stupor, cervical scoliosis, and anorexia. Treatment ranged from supportive care to attempted surgical decompression. All dragons died or were euthanatized, at 4 days to 12 months postpresentation. The authors proposed that geriatric Komodo dragons may be anatomically predisposed, pathogenically predisposed, or both to cervical subluxation.[24] Arthritic animals may benefit from rearrangement of the enclosure/cage furniture, weight management, and judicious use of nonsteroidal antiinflammatory drugs.[17] Adjunctive techniques such as acupuncture, low-level therapeutic laser (photobiomodulation), massage, and physical therapy have been used in reptiles where improving blood flow aids healing.[25] Another report describes physical therapy, specifically the Wolf-Kinetic technique (WKT), as adjunctive therapy in the treatment of severe osteoarthritis in a 20-year-old Komodo dragon (*Varanus komodoensis*).[19]

The WKT is a gentle manual technique that is performed with the intent of changing movement patterns in a way that spreads out the work load of the body when the patient performs functional activities. The technique operates under the premise that the performance of the spine and core dictates the movement patterns of the extremities and that the spine and core must move normally for the extremities to move normally. This particular Komodo dragon had been managed with oral analgesics (meloxicam, tramadol, gabapentin, and chondroitin-glucosamine) for 3 years with fair to minimal response over time. Due to worsening of lameness and mobility, physical therapy was initiated. Ten treatment sessions were administered at 1-week intervals. Within 1 month the Komodo dragon exhibited marked improvement in gait and function, increased responsiveness to his environment, and increased mobility that continued to improve over the subsequent sessions. Physical therapy frequency was then reduced to every other week with no appreciable worsening of the animal's condition. By manually performing micromovements that harmonize with the patient's habitual movement patterns, the practitioner attempts to spread the workload throughout the body so that there is an appropriate, proportional amount of work being done as the body moves in functional patterns. Neural plasticity is the mechanism by which the damaged CNS relearns lost behavior

in response to rehabilitation and includes the capacity of neurons to change their structure and function in support of normal development and learning, as well as in response to injury or disease.[19,26] After spinal cord injury, plastic changes occur at all levels of the CNS, including the cortex, other areas of the brain, and the spinal cord.[26] At the spinal cord level, there may be normalization of reflexes and strengthening of motor-evoked potentials. Neuroanatomically, axonal and dendritic sprouting and even neurogenesis have been observed. Other causes of morbidity and mortality in captive geriatric Komodo dragons over the past 20 years have included vascular mineralization and follicle rupture in females; renal disease, gout, or both; generalized infection; gastroenteritis; paralytic ileus; and neurologic disorders.[19]

Pain scales are commonly used for human pain assessment, but their use in animals relies on interpretation by the observer and is subject to variability.[26] Because not all animals outwardly respond the same to painful stimuli, recognition and assessment of the level of pain in each individual animal requires skilled observation by the veterinarian and the keeper or caregiver.[26] Some of the pharmaceutical advances in human and companion animal medicine have been adapted for zoological patients.[17] These include major and minor tranquilizers; some in longer-acting formulations; nonsteroidal antiinflammatories; serotonin reuptake inhibitors; better formulations of narcotics, including fentanyl patches; and other drugs.[17] Gabapentin and tramadol are labeled for use in humans but have shown positive results when used for pain control in animals. Zoo and companion animal veterinarians may use multimodal drug strategies and creative dosing regimens for end-of-life comfort and pain control. Most medications used in pain modulation for animals are considered "off label."[27] Routine measures to prevent illness, minimize stress or boredom-associated health problems, and enhance the quality of life for captive individual wild animals and small zoo populations are widely utilized.[27]

The Farm Animal Welfare Council has proposed that an animal's welfare be evaluated in terms of "five freedoms": freedom from hunger and thirst; freedom from discomfort; freedom from pain, injury, or disease; freedom to express normal behavior; and freedom from fear and distress.[27] The following issues should be addressed on a case-by-case basis. To what extent is a disease process affecting normal behavior such as food consumption, mobility, excretion habits, sleeping habits, and presence of pain? Geriatric reptiles may require daily assistance to ensure adequate hydration, thermoregulation, and nutrition as they face the challenges of old age. Daily prolonged observance of the pet, maintenance of a weekly log, and provision of humane captive conditions can significantly reduce morbidity and mortality.[28] To accommodate an aging arboreal lizard (iguana, basilisk, chameleon, etc.), an elevated basking area of easier access can be provided. Branches provided for climbing and basking can be replaced with flat, ridged boards several inches wider than the lizard's body. Geriatric semiaquatic turtles can be provided with readily accessed flat-ridged boards on which they can easily leave the water. Reduction of stressful circumstances is also important. Agonistic displays are intended to intimidate conspecific males. Even when kept in separate terraria across a room, a geriatric male will be unnecessarily stressed if he can view ongoing territorial displays by younger males. Altering dietary needs for aging reptiles and amphibians may also have to be considered. For example, digesting large prey items may become difficult for geriatric snakes, especially if cage temperatures are not ideal and stable.[28] Be certain that cage temperatures are appropriate and give the snake smaller-sized prey. The vitamin and mineral requirements of reptiles, particularly lizards and chelonians, may have to be increased with advancing age. Geriatric heliothermic (sun-basking) species often bask for longer periods and may preferentially choose temperatures a little warmer than normal.[28] By learning to read and interpret "normal" behavior, the caretaker will be able to provide the reptile or amphibian with the best conditions possible throughout its life.[28]

PALLIATIVE AND HOSPICE VETERINARY CARE

Veterinary assessment combined with observations by the caregiver or owner should guide decisions about when declining quality of life may dictate euthanasia.[26,27] Increasingly, hospice services, palliative care, and grief and bereavement support are becoming incorporated into veterinary medical care.[27] The World Health Organization defines palliative care as "an approach that improves quality of life of patients and their families facing problems associated with life-threatening illness through the prevention and relief of suffering by early identification, impeccable assessment and treatment of pain and other problems, and physical, psycho-social and spiritual care."[29] For companion animals (including reptiles and amphibians), end-of-life issues, as interpreted from their owners' perspective, include addressing pain and symptom control, relationships with family and other animals, providing support and information for caregivers, and assisting with preparation for death and/or euthanasia.[27] These same issues also are applicable for captive wildlife in a zoological park setting. Those reptiles with hierarchical social structure and hospice patients may need to be removed from the group to reduce potential for injury because of aggression, or aggressive individuals may need to be removed from the group with a hospice patient.[27] The transition from curative medical intervention to palliative care should occur on a natural gradient; however, controversy exists regarding prolongation of life and "suffering."[27] In the zoo setting, a recognized hospice program can formalize who will be the animal's advocate and could even set up "advanced directives," such as no resuscitation. If worked out ahead of time, this can reduce the burden of decision making of others who may not be as able or as responsible from attempting to take on that role.[27] Primary concerns at the end of life include the following: adequate pain and symptom control, avoidance of inappropriate prolongation of dying, and ultimately achieving a good death.[29] Most of these goals are applicable and attainable for veterinary patients, including reptiles and amphibians.

The hospice movement is rooted in the centuries-old tradition of offering a place of shelter and rest or hospitality to the weary or sick traveler on a long journey.[30] Veterinary hospice is based on the same basic tenets as human hospice, which was developed during the late 1960s in the United Kingdom and during the early 1970s in the United States as an alternative to aggressive treatment or nontreatment of terminally ill people.[30] Central principles of hospice and palliative care emphasize comfort, relief of pain and anxiety, maintenance of the quality of life, and respect for the patient's needs and wishes.[27] In human medicine, hospice care most often is initiated when the physician believes that the patient is unlikely to live for more than 6 months; further curative medical treatment is unlikely to prolong the patient's life or would be so burdensome as to greatly reduce quality of life; or when the patient refuses such treatment and requests hospice care.[27,28]

For humans and animals, the most common condition necessitating hospice care is cancer. One key difference between humans and animals with regard to hospice care options is the availability of euthanasia for animals.[30] Veterinary hospice care includes 24-hour availability of the primary veterinarian, extended appointments involving supported decision-making and counseling, in-home care, and a wide variety of palliative and euthanasia options tailored to the needs of the client.[29] At-home hospice care gives family members more time to spend with the animal and may increase the animal's comfort and reduce any anxiety associated with being in the hospital. The AVMA Guidelines for Veterinary Hospice Care state, "Euthanasia service should be available if the client and veterinarian at any time believe this service is appropriate."[30] Most veterinarians consider timely euthanasia a part of hospice care. Euthanasia, derived from the Greek, "euthantos," literally means good or pleasant end of life. For reptiles and amphibians, the animal's caregivers, keepers, members of the public, and veterinarians and their staff must deal with the fact that euthanasia is an act intended to end life.[30]

Because the term hospice encompasses an increasing variety of end-of-life care philosophies and protocols, some veterinarians may find certain aspects of it controversial or problematic.[29] Some individuals and groups in the hospice movement believe that animals should not be euthanized or should be euthanized very rarely and will actively support a choice to not euthanize an animal if the client wishes. Thus veterinarians and clients must reach a shared understanding beforehand about the use of euthanasia.[30] When establishing a hospice program, legal advice should be sought regarding risk factors and insurance coverage for staff members, particularly staff members who travel to clients' homes.[30,31] Currently, many veterinarians are perceived as unfamiliar with hospice as a concept or practice, and the variety of uses of this word may compound this misapprehension.[30,31] Veterinarians and their support staff should be able to discuss hospice in such a way that they come to understand their clients' wishes.[28]

In recent years, two international symposia on veterinary hospice care organized by the Nikki Hospice Foundation for Pets and the Assisi International Animal Institute have begun to galvanize the veterinary profession on this issue.[30,31] By embracing hospice concepts and end-of-life care, veterinary practitioners can benefit from personal growth. It can help make one a better and more complete veterinarian, as well as improve relationships with animal care staff and strengthen our institutions.[31] Beyond providing pain relief and compassion, the formal recognition of hospice allows time for grieving, for celebration, and for saying goodbye.[30] With early recognition, the chances of treatment and/or attenuation of geriatric medical conditions increase dramatically. Factors such as genetic background, environment, nutritional history, and veterinary history influence the emergence of age-related conditions.[27,30,31] It has been stated that the quality of life in people and pets is a careful balance between pleasant and unpleasant feelings.[31] A number of progressive small animal veterinary practices, particularly those centered on oncology, have embraced hospice and make it a featured part of their practice.[27] It is only logical that in time reptiles and amphibians, particularly those maintained as companion animals, will become included in the practice of palliative and hospice veterinary care.

REFERENCES

See www.expertconsult.com for a complete list of references.

87

Emergency and Critical Care

Olivia A. Petritz and Tolina Tina Son

Do reptile emergencies actually exist? Yes, they most definitely do. However, reptiles are also presented on emergency for acute exacerbation of chronic diseases, seemingly more often than mammals. This, in combination with their slow metabolism, may present challenges for veterinarians and veterinary staff. Adequate staff training on the basics of triage (both on the phone and in person) is imperative. For example, prolonged anorexia in certain reptile species—for example, snakes—may not be a cause for an emergency presentation, which is the opposite for most mammalian species. Owners should also be instructed over the phone to secure their reptile in an escape-proof, ventilated container prior to transport. Ideally, the exact species should be determined prior to the animal's arrival. If the exact species is not known, at least an approximate weight, age, and taxa should be obtained, as some species' (chelonians especially) weights can vary greatly. Any reptile displaying one of the following clinical signs should be seen on an emergency basis: hemorrhage, seizures/tremors, moribund or unresponsive, organ prolapse, and dyspnea or open-mouth breathing. Emergencies should also include animals thought to be in pain or if a reptile experienced trauma, which would be considered painful in a mammal. And finally, regardless of the patient's condition, if an owner or caretaker is concerned about the animal's well-being and wishes it to be seen on an emergency basis, they should not be turned away.

PHYSIOLOGY AND OSMOLARITY OF BODY FLUIDS

In mammals, approximately 60% of an animal's body weight is water while 40% of the body weight is within the intracellular fluid compartment and 20% is within the extracellular fluid compartment.[1] In reptiles, excluding chelonians, approximately 71% to 75% of the body weight is fluid, with an equal distribution between the intracellular and extracellular fluid compartments.[2] The carapace and plastron of chelonians reduces their distribution of total body water closer to that of mammals, approximately 66%. The osmolal gradient maintains the fluid balance between the intracellular and extracellular spaces. An increase in extracellular fluid plasma osmolality will result in fluid shifting out of cells causing cellular dehydration. A decrease in extracellular plasma osmolality will cause fluid to shift into cells, resulting in cellular swelling. Rapid fluid shifts in either direction can have detrimental consequences.[1,2]

Osmolality refers to the number of osmoles per kilogram of solvent (expressed as milliosmoles per kilogram, mOm/kg), and osmolarity refers to the number of osmoles per liter of solution (expressed as milliosmoles per liter, mOm/L).[3] In biological fluids, the difference in osmolality and osmolarity is negligible, and the terms are often used interchangeably.[3,4] In clinical medicine, the term osmolarity is more commonly used and essentially refers to the concentration of osmotically active particles in a solution and is not related to the molecular weight,

size, shape, or charge. Knowledge of the patient's normal osmolarity, as well as their osmolarity on emergency presentation, would be helpful for determining appropriate fluid therapy and minimizing detrimental fluid shifts. Most of the intravenous fluid products readily available on the market are formulated based on the plasma osmolarity of humans. Selection of the appropriate crystalloid solution for reptiles is confounded by a paucity of information about species-specific plasma osmolarity. Documented plasma osmolality and osmolarity in reptile species is reported to have a wide range.[5,6] Commercially available electrolyte solutions isotonic with mammalian blood have been recommended for terrestrial and marine chelonian species, as they may tolerate a wide range of osmolarity without adverse effects.[5,7]

Most of the documented normal osmolality ranges in reptiles have been similar to mammalian osmolality. For example, the mean measured plasma osmolality in 11 healthy adult male bearded dragons (*Pogona vitticeps*) was 295.4 ± 9.35 mOsm/kg, which is similar to normal osmolality ranges reported in dogs, cats, and other desert lizards.[8] Documented normal canine osmolality is 290 to 310 mOsm/kg, and reported normal feline osmolality is 290 to 330 mOsm/kg.[4] Plasma osmolarities of green iguanas (*Iguana iguana*) are reported to be 327 ± 3.3 mOsm/L and 300 mOsm/L.[6,9] Reported plasma osmolality of the desert-dwelling squamates, the Gila monster (*Heloderma suspectum*), is 292 mOsm/kg (range 284–298 mOsm/kg),[10] and osmolarity of the desert iguana (*Dipsosaurus dorsalis*) is 300 mOsm/L.[11] The mean measured plasma osmolality in a study of American alligators (*Alligator mississippiensis*) was 269.3 mOsm/kg.[7] This value was within the range reported in two previous studies, one in American alligators[12] and another in Nile crocodiles (*Crocodylus niloticus*).[13] The study in the American alligators evaluated the effects of chronic salt exposure and found the mean plasma osmolality ranged between 253.5 to 291.1 mOsm/kg.[12] In the study on Nile crocodiles, the mean plasma osmolality of animals in freshwater ranged from 258 to 319 mOsm/kg.[14] Plasma osmolality in adult corn snakes (*Pantherophis guttata*) ranged from 304.5 to 373.0 mOsm/kg, with a mean value of 344.5 mOsm/kg.[13] These values are higher than those of commercially available fluids (see Fluid Therapy later in this chapter). This difference should be considered when administration of large volumes of fluids are needed to avoid rapid and large shifts in the patient's plasma osmolarity. Ideally the use of crystalloid solutions that are significantly hypo-osmolar or hyper-osmolar to normal osmolarity should be avoided.

Determination of plasma osmolality can be performed either by direct measurement with an osmometer or by calculation based on formulas utilizing biochemistry values. Studies have shown that directly measured plasma osmolality in reptiles such as the American alligator had poor agreement with calculated values.[7] The authors of that study do not recommend calculating plasma osmolality using previously reported formulas. There was also poor agreement between measured and initially calculated osmolalities in bearded dragons until a new formula was proposed to account for the differences in primary cations and anions in reptile plasma.[8] The authors of that study concluded that calculated values were not an accurate measure of the reptile patient's osmolality and recommend using those values with caution when administering fluids to a dehydrated or debilitated bearded dragon.

TRIAGE AND INITIAL ASSESSMENT

Emergency Anamnesis

A complete recount of the animal's history, including diet and husbandry, may seem impractical on an emergency basis. However, this information is vital to help determine the health status of the patient and can occur while general emergency support (e.g., oxygen, warm incubator) is being given. As previously stated, many emergency presentations are actually the result of chronic disease, with inappropriate husbandry still a large contributing factor. Therefore it is extremely important to ask detailed questions and critically evaluate the animal's diet, environmental temperature, humidity, cage setup, lighting, etc. Owners may even try to resolve any husbandry or dietary deficits just before the initial presentation, and as such, their answers to these questions may seem appropriate for the species, even though the animal still suffers from chronic disease resulting from poor husbandry. Additional standard historical information is also important to obtain, including duration and progression of any current abnormal clinical signs, recent additions or new exposure to another species, toxin exposure, previous medical/surgical problems, and a list of all current medications (including all supplements).

Temperature, Pulse, and Respiration (TPR)

Reptiles are ectothermic, and their body temperature varies with changes in the ambient environment. Each species has its own preferred optimal temperature zone (POTZ)—a temperature range in which all aspects of their metabolism and immune function are ideal. POTZ values for commonly seen reptile species have been published previously.[15] Medications should not be administered until a reptile has reached its POTZ, as their efficacy will be greatly diminished. Drugs administered during CPCR (cardiopulmonary-cerebral resuscitation) are an exception. Warming most reptiles to their POTZ should be achieved slowly over 4 to 6 hours and can be completed with various exogenous heating devices, including heated air blankets, warming blankets, incubators, and heat lamps. Larger reptiles, such as sea turtles, are typically warmed more slowly at approximately 1°C (1.8°F) per hour. The use of recirculating hot water blankets and warm water bottles should be used with caution due to risk of iatrogenic thermal burns. Reptiles should be housed in an appropriate thermal gradient, whether at home or in a hospital environment. Ill reptiles reportedly seek temperatures at the high end of their POTZ, and digital thermometers should be placed in multiple locations throughout the hospital enclosure.[16,17] Moribund animals unable to move and thermoregulate should be maintained at the upper end of their POTZ. A temperature range of 75°F to 85°F (24°C–29°C) is a good starting point for most reptile species if the POTZ is unknown (see Chapter 46).[17]

Respiratory rates can be obtained through visualization before handling, bearing in mind that they are usually much slower and may be intermittent. If no respirations are noted, a heart rate should be verified immediately and CPCR may be indicated. Opening of the mouth with each respiration is abnormal, and as in mammals, the clinician should determine whether the upper or lower (or both) respiratory tracts are affected. Dyspnea in chelonians may also manifest with extension of the head, neck, and forelimbs with each respiration. This should be differentiated from straining (to urinate, defecate, or pass an egg).

Auscultation with a stethoscope is challenging if not impossible in most reptiles, but their heart rate can be easily obtained with an ultrasonic

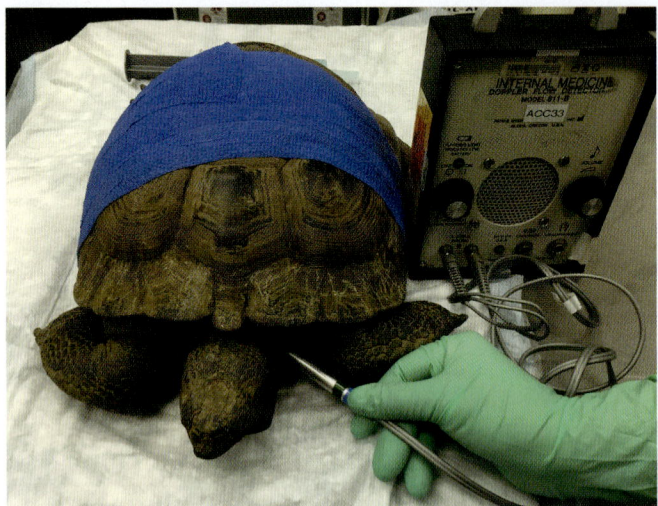

FIG 87.1 An ultrasonographic Doppler probe has been placed in the axillocervical (cervicobrachial) area of an adult male California desert tortoise (*Gopherus agassizii*) to monitor heart rate and rhythm. (Courtesy of Olivia A. Petritz, NCSU.)

Doppler probe directly over their heart or major artery. Distal arteries in extremities can also be used to assess pulse quality and rate, but flow may not always be detected, even in healthy, well-perfused reptiles.[17] In lizards, the probe is placed ventrally between their shoulder blades, or in larger species, in their axillary region. The hearts of varanids are more caudal than other lizards, and this affects Doppler probe placement. Thickened skin or osteoderms of larger lizards and crocodilians may inhibit standard ultrasonic Doppler use altogether, and then an ultrasound probe is required. In chelonians, a pencil ultrasonographic Doppler probe is recommended and can be placed in either axillocervical (cervicobrachial) area, directed ventrocaudally toward the heart (Fig. 87.1).

Confirmation of Death

Some reptiles presented for emergency evaluation may have already experienced respiratory or cardiac arrest, unbeknownst to the owners. According to the AVMA Guidelines for the Euthanasia of Animals, it is "difficult to confirm" death in reptiles and amphibians.[18] Certain reptiles, especially freshwater turtles, can tolerate prolonged periods of anoxia and corresponding severe bradycardia.[19] Corneal reflexes are difficult to assess in reptiles that lack eyelids, such as snakes and some geckos. Every reptile, even if unresponsive and in respiratory arrest, should be checked for a heartbeat using the methods described above. However, the presence of a heartbeat is not synonymous with "life," as reptile and amphibian hearts can and will continue to beat for hours after brain death.[18] An electroencephalogram (EEG) can determine brain activity in unconscious reptile patients that still maintain a heartbeat[20]; however, this test is not practical in most clinical settings. The reader is referred to Chapter 47 in this text for additional information on euthanasia.

DIAGNOSTICS AND MONITORING

Mucus Membrane Color, Capillary Refill Time, Blood Pressure

Routine physical exam assessments commonly used in mammals, such as mucous membrane color and capillary refill time, are not accurate reflections of perfusion in reptiles.[21] The most accurate and consistent assessment of a reptile's cardiovascular status is determination of the heart rate.[21] Because the heart rate is closely related to body temperature in reptiles, baseline heart rates should be recorded with temperature and while the patient is warmed to the POTZ. Noninvasive, indirect blood pressure measurement can be taken in reptiles using a sphygmomanometer and Doppler probe or oscillometric monitor, but readings are often inconsistent and inaccurate.[22,23] The most accurate assessment for arterial blood pressure measurement is the direct method, which is invasive and not practical for clinical use.

Blood Collection

Chapter 43 in this text reviews venipuncture techniques in all of the common reptile groups. Ethylenediaminetetraacetic acid (EDTA) is the anticoagulant of choice for hematologic studies, but it may cause lysis in certain species, especially chelonians. Blood volumes in reptiles vary from 4% to 8% of total body weight. Of this amount, up to 10% of this volume in a healthy patient can be safely collected for analysis.[16] As a rough approximation, the sample size should never be larger than 0.8% of the animal's total body weight. Estimation of blood loss through hemorrhage should be considered before taking blood from small animals. Pre-heparinizing needles and syringes before blood collection has been shown to cause significant and unpredictable hemodilution in packed cell volume and total solids and cannot be recommended.[24]

Assessment of Dehydration, Acid-Base, Electrolytes, and Perfusion

The severity of dehydration should be assessed to guide the fluid therapy plan. Subjective assessment of hydration should include evaluation of the eyelid turgor, skin turgor and elasticity, appearance of the eyes (sunken vs bright), mucous membrane tackiness, and saliva thickness. Mildly dehydrated reptiles may have dull skin with decreased skin turgor from loss of elasticity. Severely dehydrated reptiles (≥10%) may have sunken eyes, thick durable strands of saliva, durable skin wrinkles, dry mucous membranes, and a doughy abdomen (Fig. 87.2).[17] Sunken eyes can also be seen in severely emaciated animals. If the patient's healthy weight was known prior to becoming ill, the degree and rapidity of weight loss may also primarily reflect fluid loss.

Blood, if available, is preferred for an objective evaluation of dehydration. Evaluation of packed cell volume (a direct measurement and therefore preferred over a calculated hematocrit), total protein/solids, blood urea nitrogen (especially chelonians and crocodilians), uric acid

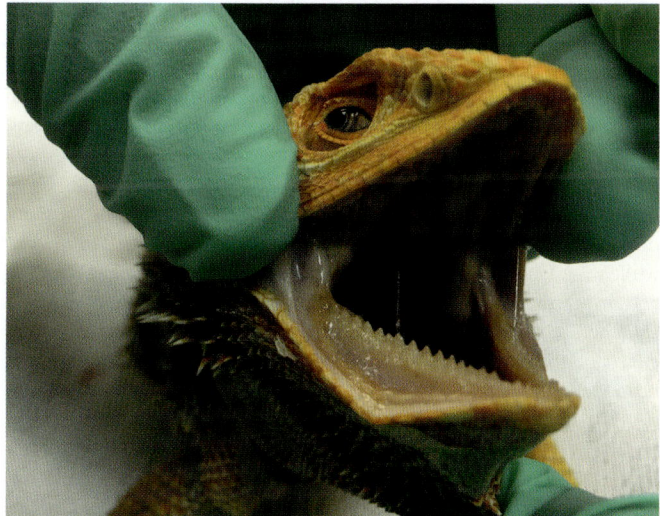

FIG 87.2 A severely dehydrated juvenile inland bearded dragon (*Pogona vitticeps*); note the sunken eyes and thick strands of saliva. (Courtesy of Olivia A. Petritz, NCSU.)

(especially lizards and snakes), plasma sodium, and plasma chloride are helpful, and values should be correlated to the normal range for the given species, or indeed the same individual when healthy.[2] Urine-specific gravity is not as useful for assessment of prerenal dehydration as it is in mammals. Reptiles normally have hypo- to isosthenuric urine, and the urine-specific gravity does not increase above plasma osmolality during dehydration.[25] Also, significant post-renal modification of urine can occur across the bladder or cloacocolonic membranes. Perfusion is more challenging to assess in reptiles compared to mammals. Noninvasive blood pressure methods that are commonly used in mammals, such as a Doppler probe with a sphygmomanometer and oscillometric monitors, are often difficult or impossible to obtain with consistent accuracy in reptiles.[22,23]

The pH of reptile blood is variable and has been shown to be inversely related to environmental temperature.[26] General anesthesia can also lead to increases in blood pH. At temperatures between 23°C to 25°C, the normal blood pH of most reptiles ranges between 7.5–7.7.[27] It is postulated that the buffering systems of reptiles are similar to mammals, which would make the bicarbonate-carbonic acid buffer system the most important. Normal total CO_2 values for most reptiles are thought to be 20–30 mmol/L.[28] The most common causes for metabolic acidosis include renal failure, hypovolemia, and diarrhea.[29] A postprandial decrease of chloride and increase of bicarbonate has been reported in alligators, which will lead to a marked physiological metabolic alkalosis—this may also be true of other species.[28] Additional information regarding acid-base of reptiles in general can be found in Chapter 34 of this text, and acid-base parameters specifically related to rehabilitation of sea turtles can be found in Chapter 176.

Diagnostic Imaging

Radiography (including CT), ultrasonography, and other imaging modalities are important for emergency evaluation. Just as in mammalian patients, it is imperative that orthogonal radiographic views are obtained. This includes dorsoventral and horizontal-beam lateral views for lizards, snakes, and crocodilians (vertical-beam lateral is acceptable for crocodilians due to their unique compartmentalized coelomic anatomy), and dorsoventral, horizontal-beam lateral, and horizontal-beam craniocaudal views for chelonians. Single-view dorsoventral radiographs may be utilized as a screening tool for the presence of shelled eggs, metallic foreign bodies, and uroliths; however, a full image series complete with orthogonal views should always be obtained as part of a minimum database (Fig. 87.3). Larger reptilian species, especially large chelonians, may exceed the capacity of small animal radiographic machines, and a large-animal radiographic unit or computed tomography (CT) may be required. The use of abbreviated ultrasonography, such as *abdominal focused assessment with sonography for trauma* (AFAST),[30–32] is used extensively for emergency evaluation of canine and feline patients in emergency hospitals. There is no published equivalent for this in reptiles; however, ultrasonography still has a purpose for emergency evaluation, including determination of coelomic or pericardial effusions (see Chapters 53 through 59).

Electrocardiography

Electrocardiography (ECG) is not recommended in cold reptiles because of the challenge of identifying ECG wave boundaries.[33] The snake's heart is located in the upper third of the body, and ECG leads can be attached about two heart lengths cranially and caudally to the heart with self-adhering cutaneous skin electrodes.[17] In varanids, such as monitors and tegus, the ECG electrodes should be placed either on the limbs or torso. In other lizards, the cranial ECG electrodes should be placed in the cervical regions (as the heart is located at the level of the front limbs). In chelonians, the ECG leads can be placed on the limbs,

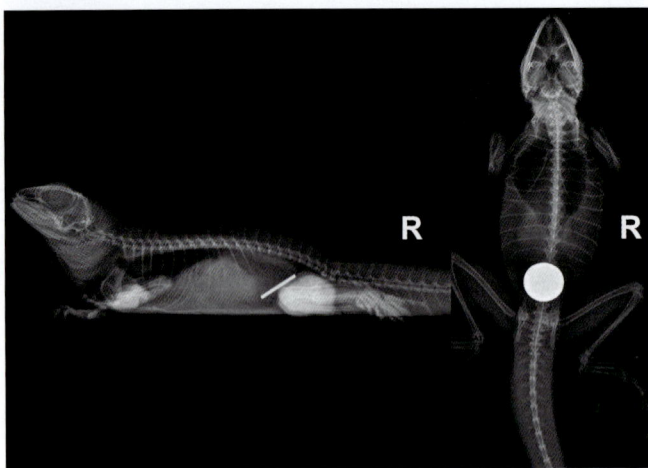

FIG 87.3 Right horizontal beam lateral and dorsoventral whole body radiographs of an adult Chinese water dragon (*Physignathus cocincinus*) that ingested a metallic foreign body (coin). (Courtesy of Karen Schachterle, ACCESS Specialty Animal Hospital.)

although placement of the cranial leads on the skin lateral to the neck and medial to the forelimbs may yield better readings.[17] In smaller species, the alligator clips from the ECG leads can be attached to hypodermic needles that are placed through the skin. See Chapter 68 for more details.

Pulse Oximetry

Pulse oximetry is a modality that is commonly used in emergency medicine for mammals but has limited use in reptiles. It has been shown to underestimate arterial oxygen saturation in green iguanas.[34] In reptiles, pulse oximetry accuracy is influenced by poor tissue perfusion, skin pigmentation, higher levels of methemoglobin, and significant taxa differences in respiratory physiology.[21] Current pulse oximeters are also calibrated to the human oxygen hemoglobin dissociation curve from which the SpO_2 values are calculated, which differs significantly from reptilian oxygen hemoglobin dissociation curves.[21] Therefore pulse oximetry may be used to monitor trends in reptilian species, but specific values should be interpreted with caution.

THERAPY AND INTERVENTION

Oxygen Therapy

In mammals, high carbon dioxide concentrations stimulate respiration; however, in reptiles, respiration is controlled by hypoxia, hypercapnia, and environmental temperature.[35] Many species differences exist, especially between aquatic and terrestrial reptiles. In most species, low oxygen concentrations increase respiration rate, and hypercapnia increases tidal volume. These tenants have been applied to recovery from general anesthesia, and, in a study in green iguanas, prolonged recovery from anesthesia was noted in patients that received 100% oxygen versus room air. This is in contrast to two recent studies in bearded dragons[36] and Dumeril's monitors,[37] both of which found minimal if no statistical difference between animals recovered in room air (approximately 21% oxygen) and 100% oxygen. In cases of true hypoxemia, supplemental oxygen therapy, via facemask or endotracheal tube, is recommended.[17] In fact, it has previously been shown that administration of 100% inspired oxygen resulted in a significant increase in PaO_2 in conscious green iguanas, with no changes in respiratory rate.[34]

Cardiopulmonary Cerebral Resuscitation

Cardiopulmonary arrest is defined as the abrupt cessation of spontaneous and effective ventilation and systemic perfusion. Cardiopulmonary cerebral resuscitation (CPCR) provides artificial ventilation and circulation until advanced life support can be provided and spontaneous circulation and ventilation restored. Basic life support is the cornerstone of CPCR and includes airway management, ventilation, and circulation with external or internal chest compressions. Advanced life support provides more specific interventions based on circumstances of the arrest. The American Heart Association (AHA) publishes updated human guidelines for CPCR, which are often extrapolated for veterinary medicine. There are no established standard guidelines for CPCR in reptiles as there are in humans (AHA) and dogs and cats (RECOVER).[38] Although many of the basic principles of CPCR are applicable, physiological differences among reptile species must be considered.

Airway stabilization via tracheal intubation should be performed with positive pressure ventilation at 6 to 8 breaths per minute and peak positive pressure not to exceed 8 cm water.[17,39] Positive pressure ventilation can be provided via an Ambu bag (Ridge Medical, Lombard, IL) or anesthetic machine. Given that temperature and partial pressure of oxygen are primary stimulators for ventilation in reptiles, in theory, oxygen supplementation may decrease the reptile's own stimulus to breathe. No studies have been performed to assess the role of oxygen therapy in reptile CPCR. Therefore it may be reasonable to initiate CPCR with 100% oxygen when the degree of hypoxemia is unknown, then potentially wean the inspired oxygen gradually to room air to encourage spontaneous breathing.

Cardiovascular monitoring with Doppler scanning and ECG should be performed. If no heart beat is detected, IV or IO epinephrine should be administered at 0.5 mL/kg of the 1:1000 epinephrine concentration.[17] If IV and IO routes are not possible, then the epinephrine should be administered via a catheter through the endotracheal tube at twice the IV dose and diluted with sterile saline at 1 mL/100 g of body weight.[17] Cardiac compressions should be performed when direct cardiac compressions are possible. Atropine can be administered at 0.01 to 0.04 mg/kg IV, IO, or IM, or at 0.2 mg/kg SC or IM.[17] Normal heartbeats can vary from 30 to 100 beats per minute, and IV or IO fluids should be administered to address hypovolemia (see recommendations below). Additional supportive care such as thermal support, blood transfusions, and concurrent treatment for the underlying disease should be provided.

Doxapram has previously been used in cases of severe respiratory distress or cardiopulmonary arrest, but its effect in reptiles has not been as thoroughly evaluated as it has in humans and other mammals.[40] Doxapram is a central nervous system stimulant with various uses in veterinary medicine, such as stimulating respiration in newborns, hastening the awakening from anesthesia, treating respiratory depression, and assisting in diagnosis of laryngeal paralysis in dogs. The use of doxapram is not currently recommended during CPCR in humans, dogs, and cats for reasons such as reducing the cerebral blood flow while increasing myocardial oxygen requirements, resulting in cerebral and myocardial hypoxia.[41,42] Doxapram can also cause transient hypotension before its stimulatory effects.[43] To the authors' knowledge, the effects of doxapram in reptiles during cardiopulmonary arrest have not been studied.

Fluid Therapy

Early goal-directed therapy has demonstrated benefits in outcome in human patients with septic shock and likely increased survival advantage in other patient populations.[44] This treatment strategy has been recommended in veterinary patients as well.[11] This goal-directed strategy directs resuscitation efforts toward restoration of an effective circulating blood volume and adequate end-organ perfusion.[11] The first line of perfusion restoration, and a fundamental component of early goal-directed therapy, is expansion of the intravascular space with fluid therapy. Due to limited veterinary studies, veterinary recommendations have mostly been extrapolated from human studies. The optimal fluid resuscitation plan remains controversial and is still subject to debate.[11,45] Goal-directed therapy in reptiles would also be beneficial, and applicable guidelines should be extrapolated in light of the significant differences and limitations in monitoring and assessing reptiles compared to mammals.

Maintenance fluid rates range from 10 to 15 mL/kg per day in most reptilian patients.[46] The fluid therapy plan should include calculating the patient's maintenance fluid requirements plus dehydration deficits. The fluid deficit volume should be replaced at a rate related to how long the patient may have suffered the fluid loss. Acute fluid losses may be replaced more rapidly than chronic losses. A fluid deficit replacement rate over 72 to 96 hours has been suggested to avoid interstitial overhydration secondary to overly rapid fluid therapy.[47,48] Boluses of crystalloids (5–10 mL/kg) and colloids (3–5 mL/kg) can be given to address perfusion deficits.[17]

Routes for fluid therapy in reptiles include enteral (oral and cloacal), intracoelomic, subcutaneous, intravenous, and intraosseous. Similar to mammals, intravenous or intraosseous fluid therapy is preferred for the critical patient. However, access to these sites are often more challenging in reptilian patients (see Chapter 44). Additional fluid administration routes include subcutaneous and intracoelomic. The authors advise against intracoelomic fluid administration in reptiles due to reduction of space for lung expansion; potential for perforation of lung, intestine, or urinary bladder; and slower rate of absorption.[49] Depending on the species, provision of high environmental humidity can help minimize insensible fluid losses.

Monitoring and reassessment of the patient should be performed regularly during fluid resuscitation. Animals receiving IV or IO fluid therapy should not be left unmonitored over night. Clinical signs of improvement in hydration and perfusion include improvement in mucous membrane moisture and color, skin turgidity, eye position, and mental state. The heart rate, if at their optimal temperature, should also improve. Rechecking blood results can also be performed to monitor progression. Accurate body weight is a useful parameter to monitor in patients receiving fluid therapy, because the amount of weight gain will reflect the amount of fluid gain and correction of the estimated dehydration. Monitoring urination may be useful but one should be aware of the species differences in urination habits. Well-hydrated chelonians should urinate approximately every other day, and the urine volume can range from 0.5% to 3.0% of body weight.[50]

The only visible peripheral vessel in reptile patients is the dorsal buccal vein in snakes, and, due to its location inside the oral cavity, it is not a practical location for indwelling catheter placement in the conscious patient but may be appropriate for a moribund animal.[2] For placement of most intravenous (IV) catheters in reptiles, a cut-down technique is required. In lizards, the cephalic vein can be accessed via cut-down technique, and it is located in a similar location as in mammals, traversing across the antebrachium. The ventral coccygeal vein has also been used for IV catheter placement in lizards (Fig. 87.4). It is accessed blindly, in a similar fashion to venipuncture of this vessel. There have been several reported cases of distal tail necrosis secondary to intravenous placement in this location in several lizard species, and this should be considered. Intraosseous catheters can be used as a substitute for intravenous access, especially in cases of hypovolemia and/or hypotension. The most common placement sites in lizards include the femur, humerus, or tibia (Fig. 87.5). However, possible complications and considerations for this method are leakage, pain and discomfort, and possible

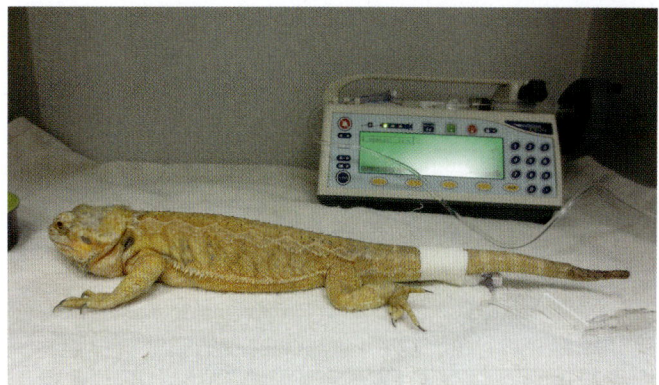

FIG 87.4 An adult female inland bearded dragon (*Pogona vitticeps*) with an intravenous catheter placed in the ventral coccygeal vein. (Courtesy of Olivia A. Petritz, NCSU.)

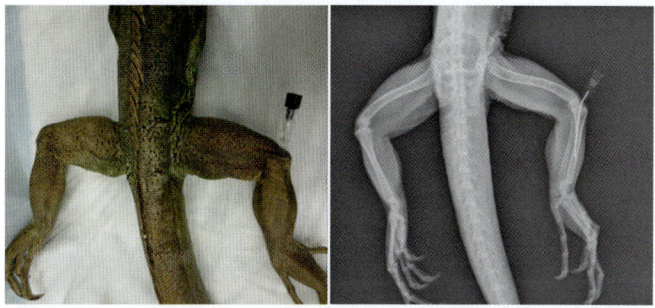

FIG 87.5 A 22-gauge, 1.5-inch spinal needle has been inserted into the right tibia as an intraosseous catheter in this adult green iguana (*Iguana iguana*). (Courtesy of Olivia A. Petritz, NCSU.)

osteomyelitis. Additionally, in reptiles that have nutritional or renal secondary hyperparathyroidism, their compromised bone structure may not support an intraosseous catheter. In snakes, the jugular vein is the most readily accessible, and the right is usually larger than the left. For visualization, a right lateral incision is created 4 to 7 scutes cranial to the heart, at the junction of the ventral scutes and first lateral scale row, or between the first and second lateral scale rows.[17]

The jugular vein of chelonians is the most readily accessible peripheral vessel for IV catheter placement. Long-term jugular catheter placement through a modified Seldinger technique has also been described in chelonians (Fig. 87.6).[51] Intraosseous catheters can be placed in chelonians—the humerus, femur, gular region of the plastron, and the plastrocarapacial junction (bridge) have been described. The humerus and femur are reportedly the most effective in the desert tortoise (*Gopherus agassizii*) when compared with an intravenous jugular catheter.[52] Additionally, a high failure rate for intraosseous fluid administration into the carapacial bridge in the yellow-footed tortoise (*Chelonoidis denticulata*) has been described, and this site was not recommended in this species when they are greater than 3 kg in weight.[53] See Chapter 44 for more details.

Crystalloid Fluids. Crystalloid fluids contain small solutes, mostly electrolytes, that are capable of entering all body fluid compartments and primarily exert their effects on the interstitial and intracellular compartments. Crystalloids have insignificant oncotic (colloidal osmotic) pressure. After infusion of crystalloids, rapid distribution into the extracellular space occurs with 60% to 80% of the administered volume redistributed out of the vascular space and into the interstitium within 30 to 60 minutes in mammals.[45] Only 25% of the infused crystalloid remains in the intravascular space after 30 minutes in mammals.[45] Compared with colloid solutions, larger amounts of crystalloid solutions are required to expand the intravascular space and restore perfusion.

The osmolarity of the commonly available isotonic parenteral crystalloid fluids include Plasma-Lyte A (294 mOsmol/L; Baxter Healthcare, Deerfield, IL), Normosol-R (294 mOsmol/L; Abbott Laboratories, Chicago, IL), lactated Ringer's solution (273 mOsmol/L; LRS; Abbott Laboratories), 5% dextrose (253 mOsmol/L; D_5W), and 0.9% NaCl (308 mOsmol/L) (Table 87.1). Combination fluids can also be made to tailor to a patient's specific needs. Various osmolarity studies in reptiles have shown reptilian osmolarity to be more similar to mammalian osmolarity than previously thought. Further support for the use of the readily available standard crystalloid solutions is given by studies that have shown that reptiles can tolerate severe dehydration as well as a wide range of plasma osmolarity (250 to 400 mOsm/L) and electrolyte concentrations.[46,48]

Diluted crystalloid fluids such as half-strength $LRS/D_{2.5}W$ (262 mOsm/L) or 0.45% $NaCl/D_{2.5}W$ (280 Osmol/L) should be used at the discretion of the clinician. Normal saline is isotonic but is not a physiological buffered solution. It contains a higher concentration of sodium and chloride than other commercially available isotonic fluids and also has a higher osmolarity of 308 mOsm/L. Use of normal saline could be considered for patients with severe hyperkalemia, hypercalcemia, or hypochloremic metabolic alkalosis. Use of large volumes of saline could result in hypernatremia, hyperchloremia, and hyperchloremic metabolic acidosis.[45] Given the potential adverse effects of saline, isotonic crystalloids such as Lactated Ringer's and Normosol-R have been more widely recommended. These solutions are more physiological than saline, contain electrolytes, and contain a buffer such as lactate or acetate.[45] Crystalloid solutions can be classified as "replacement" (e.g., lactated Ringer's, Normosol-R, Plasmalyte 148) or "maintenance" solutions (e.g., Normosol-M, Plasmalyte 56).[54] The composition of replacement fluids resembles that of extracellular fluid and has a similar osmolarity to mammalian plasma (290 to 310 mOsm/L).[54] Maintenance fluids contain less sodium (40 to 60 mEq/L) and more potassium (15 to 30 mEq/L) than replacement fluids and are therefore hypotonic to plasma. Maintenance fluids should never be given as a rapid bolus due to the risk of cerebral edema.[54,55]

Concerns that the use of lactated crystalloids may be harmful to reptiles have not been validated. Reptiles produce lactate and use anaerobic metabolism during shock. Reptiles have been shown to tolerate high blood lactate levels such as 20 mmol/L, most likely making the amount of lactate in commercially available crystalloids clinically irrelevant.[56] Lactate is rapidly converted to bicarbonate by the liver, and use of lactate-containing fluids is not contraindicated

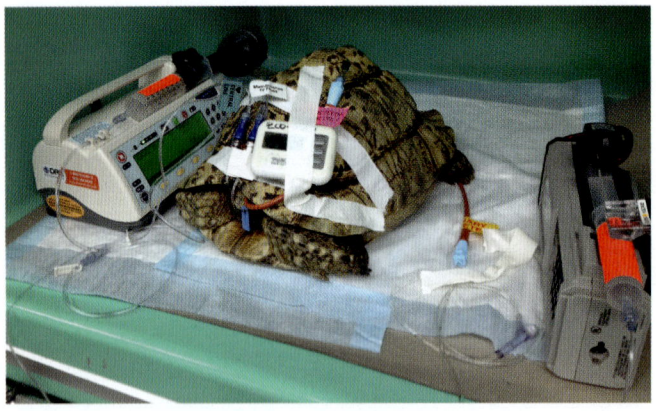

FIG 87.6 An adult leopard tortoise (*Stigmochelys pardalis*) with a central line catheter in the jugular vein, an esophagostomy tube for nutritional support, and an indwelling urinary catheter. (Courtesy of Stephen J. Divers.)

TABLE 87.1	Characteristics of Various Commercial Fluid Therapy Products									
Name	Osmolarity (mOsm/L)	pH	Na⁺ (mEq/L)	Cl⁻ (mEq/L)	K⁺ (mEq/L)	Mg²⁺ (mEq/L)	Ca²⁺ (mEq/L)	Dextrose (g/L)	Buffer	COP (mm Hg)
Crystalloid										
0.9% saline	308 (isotonic)	5	154	154	0	0	0	0	None	0
Lactated Ringer's (LRS)	275 (isotonic)	6.5	130	109	4	0	3	0	Lactate	0
Plasmalyte-A	294 (isotonic)	7.4	140	98	5	3	0	0	Acetate, gluconate	0
Normosol-R	295 (isotonic)	5.5–7	140	98	5	3	0	0	Acetate, gluconate	0
5% dextrose in water	252 (hypotonic)	4	0	0	0	0	0	50	None	0
2.5% dextrose in ½-strength LRS	264 (isotonic)	4.5–7.5	65.5	55	2	0	1.5	25	Lactate	0
Synthetic Colloid										
6% Hetastarch	310 (isotonic)	5.5	154	154	0	0	0	0	None	30
10% Pentastarch	326 (isotonic)	5	154	154	0	0	0	0	None	25
Dextran 40	311 (isotonic)	3.5–7	154	154	0	0	0	0	None	40
Dextran 70	310 (isotonic)	3–7	154	154	0	0	0	None	60	

COP, Colloid oncotic pressure.
Modified from Jarchow J: Hospital care of the reptile patient. In Jacobson ER, Kollias GV, editors: *Exotic Animals.* New York: Churchill Livingstone, 1988.

unless there is concern for hepatic dysfunction.[55] Complications of crystalloid therapy, especially with high volumes, include interstitial fluid gain and expansion of the extracellular space, causing damage to the endothelial surface and impaired capillary exchange. Clinical signs can include interstitial edema, pulmonary edema, cerebral edema, and other organ dysfunction.[45,55] Anemia, hypoproteinemia, electrolyte abnormalities, and hypocoagulability can also occur with large volume crystalloid administration due to hemodilution.[55]

Hypotonic fluids have an osmolarity and sodium concentration much lower than plasma osmolality. Examples of hypotonic fluids include 0.45% saline (154 mOsm/L) and 5% dextrose in free water. Although the 5% dextrose in free water is an isosmotic solution (252 mOsm/L), it has hypotonic effects because the dextrose is rapidly metabolized, leaving behind free water (0 mOsm/L). Hypotonic fluids can be used judiciously to replace free water deficits and treat patients with hypernatremia secondary to hypotonic fluid loss and may also be a safer choice for treating patients with a decreased ability to excrete excess sodium (e.g., renal disease) or decreased tolerance to increased intravascular volume (e.g., heart disease).[57] Hypotonic fluids should never be given as a bolus for intravascular volume resuscitation as they are ineffective at expanding intravascular volume and may also cause life-threatening cerebral and cellular edema.[57] Sterile water (0 mOsml/L) should never be administered intravenously due to the risk of intravascular hemolysis and endothelial damage.[57]

Hypertonic fluid solutions, such as 3% to 7.5% saline, have a higher osmolarity and sodium concentration compared to the patient. Administration of hypertonic solutions causes an osmotic shift of free water from the intracellular space to the extracellular space and can expand the extracellular fluid volume by 3 to 5 times the volume administered.[57] Hypertonic saline may be useful for treatment of hypovolemic shock, intracranial hypertension, and severe hyponatremia (especially given the relatively higher intracellular water content of reptiles). A dose of 3 to 5 ml/kg can be administered as a slow bolus and should be followed with isotonic crystalloids or colloids. Hyperosmotic solutions can cause hemolysis and phlebitis, especially if given repeatedly or through small peripheral veins.[57]

Colloids. Colloid solutions contain larger molecules (>10,000 Da) that tend to remain in the intravascular space after intravenous administration. Natural colloids include whole blood, plasma (fresh, frozen, and thawed), and albumin. Natural colloids such as serum albumin have had controversial effects in dogs, but its use has not been reported in reptiles. To the authors' knowledge, use of plasma administration has also not been reported in reptiles.

Polymerized bovine hemoglobin (Oxyglobin, Biopure, Cambridge, MA) had been commonly used but is currently unavailable. Commonly used synthetic colloid solutions include hydroxyethyl starches such as hetastarch and tetrastarch products. Colloid fluid therapy should be considered in patients that would benefit from intravascular volume resuscitation. Such patients may have severe hypoalbuminemia, hypovolemia, decreased vascular perfusion, or increased capillary permeability. Colloid solutions can be given to reptiles as a 3- to 5-mL/kg bolus over 30 to 60 minutes, and the patient should ideally be reassessed during and after fluid bolus.

Hydroxylethyl starch (HES) solutions are a widely available, cost-effective treatment option for rapid volume expansion. HES solutions are mostly available as an isooncotic 6% formulation. In mammals, synthetic colloidal solutions have been recently associated with adverse effects, including acute kidney injury, coagulopathies, pathologic tissue uptake, pruritus, reticuloendothelial dysfunction, hepatopathies, and anaphylactoid reactions.[45] The coagulopathic effects of HES solutions in mammals are dose dependent.[45] There is much debate on the safety

of HES solutions, and they were recently banned in Europe. Coagulopathic effects have been documented in veterinary medicine, as well as human medicine, although the other adverse effects such acute kidney injury have not been scientifically documented in veterinary medicine at this time. Use in reptiles has not yet been investigated.

Whole Blood. Whole blood transfusions are recommended in cases of acute severe hemorrhage and life-threatening anemia. Ideally a whole blood donor of the same species from the same collection is utilized. Given the thousands of different reptile species, finding a conspecific donor may not always be possible. Heterologous blood transfusions from a different species may be necessary and may still be beneficial (Fig. 87.7). Whole blood transfusion doses of 10 to 15 mL/kg every 24 hours at a rate of 5 to 10 mL/kg per hour has been recommended.[29] The whole blood should be kept cool and warmed to 25° to 30°C prior to administration; the blood should be given within 6 hours of collection.[29] Aseptic technique in collection and handling should always be maintained. Anticoagulants that can be used for blood collection include citrate-phosphate-dextrose adenine (CPDA) in a ratio of 1:9 (CPDA to blood) or heparin at a dose of 5 to 10 units per 1 mL of blood.[29]

Incompatibility reactions such as red blood cell agglutination between both homologous and heterologous donor-recipient pairs have been anecdotally reported; therefore it is advised to perform crossmatches whenever possible. Up to 10% of the total blood volume can safely be removed from a healthy reptile donor.[58] At least 4 weeks should be allowed between blood donations from a given donor.[29] Several case reports have described the successful use of homologous and heterologous blood transfusions.[59] Potential complications of blood transfusions have been infrequently reported. Orange urine post-transfusion in a Hispaniolan slider (*Trachemys decorata*) was noted but was not confirmed to be due to the blood transfusion, because oxyglobin had also been administered.[59] The slider recovered well with no other noted abnormalities. An increased leukocyte response was seen after rapid heterologous blood transfusions in a diamond python (*Morelia spilota*) and a bearded

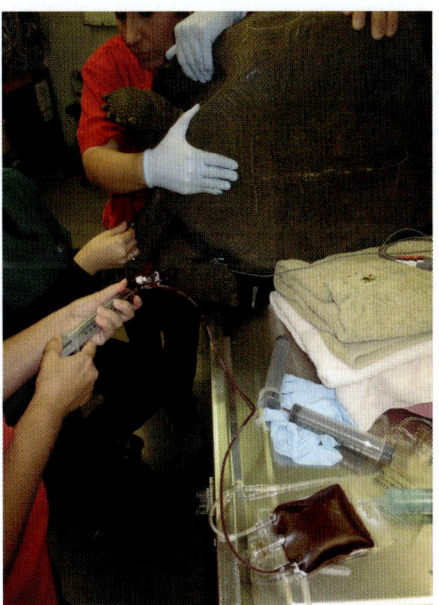

FIG 87.7 Blood collection from an adult Aldabra tortoise (*Aldabrachelys gigantean*) for use in a homogenous whole blood transfusion. (Courtesy of Stephen J. Divers.)

dragon; this leukocyte response was suspected to reflect a possible destructive immune reaction, although no clinical recognizable signs of reactions were observed (McCracken, personal observation).

The use of a blood filter such as the Hemo-Nate18-μ filter (Utah Medical Products, Ltd., Midvale, UT) is standard of care during a blood transfusion to prevent clots and particles from being transferred to the recipient. The 18-μ Hemo-Nate filter resulted in no hemolysis or significant decreases in the packed cell volume in American alligators (*Alligator mississippiensis*) and is recommended for whole blood administration to reptiles.[60]

Analgesics

Many emergency presentations in veterinary medicine involve a pain response, and analgesics are one of the tenants of therapy—reptiles are no exception. Unfortunately, pain has often not been recognized or treated appropriately in reptiles by owners and veterinarians alike. There have been significant advances in the field of reptilian analgesia in the last decade, and any clinician who treats reptiles on a routine or emergency basis should become familiar with these protocols. Although butorphanol used to be the most common analgesic administered to reptiles, it has since been proven to have no analgesic efficacy (determined by use of a thermal noxious stimulus) for a variety of doses in red-eared sliders (*Trachemys scripta elegans*),[61] bearded dragons,[62] and green iguanas.[63] The data on butorphanol usage in snakes is conflicting, with variable analgesic efficacy at high doses in corn snakes[62] but no efficacy on physiological variables in ball pythons when administered at 5 mg/kg IM.[64] Similarly, buprenorphine did not show any analgesic efficacy in green iguanas exposed to an electrical stimulus,[65] nor in red-eared sliders exposed to a noxious thermal stimulus.[66]

Morphine sulfate has been proven to be an effective analgesic in bearded dragons[62] and in turtles.[61,67,68] Significant respiratory depression has occurred at high doses of morphine in certain species, and administration of >5 mg/kg is not recommended.[69] Regardless of the dose, it is recommended to monitor respiratory rates, especially debilitated patients, after parenteral use of μ-opioids. Hydromorphone provided thermal antinociception to healthy red-eared sliders at a dose of 0.5 mg/kg subcutaneously for up to 24 hours, with significantly less respiratory depression.[66] Tramadol, a weak μ-agonist, also has shown analgesic efficacy in red-eared sliders at a dose of 5 to 10 mg/kg[70] and is available for oral administration.

Limited data are available on the use of nonsteroidal antiinflammatory drugs (NSAIDs) in reptiles—particularly their analgesic efficacy and potential negative side effects. No physiological changes indicative of analgesia were noted in ball pythons administered meloxicam at 0.3 mg/kg before a surgical procedure.[64] Pharmacokinetics after intramuscular administration (0.2 mg/kg) of meloxicam has been evaluated in green iguanas,[71] yellow-bellied sliders (*Trachemys scripta scripta*),[72] and red-eared sliders.[73] No significant side effects were noted after these single-dose studies, but clinical efficacy was not assessed. In addition to parenteral administration of meloxicam in yellow-bellied sliders, oral administration was also evaluated, which revealed very low plasma concentrations. Therefore oral administration of this dose could not be recommended in this species. Similar to mammals, the use of NSAIDs in dehydrated patients or those with renal or gastrointestinal disease should be undertaken with caution. For more details on analgesia in reptiles, the reader is referred to Chapter 50.

Antibiotics

Broad-spectrum antibiotic therapy has frequently been recommended in cases of severe integumental (e.g., burns) or gastrointestinal (e.g., intestinal breach and gut-origin sepsis) compromise. However, a systematic review and meta-analysis in human burn victims concluded that antibiotic prophylaxis had no impact on patient survival.[74] In addition, strict criteria and recommendations exist for antibiotic use in cases of gut-origin sepsis.[75] Therefore, given antimicrobial resistance concerns, the essential need for the reptile to be normothermic and hydrated, and the time taken for these drugs to have an appreciable effect, broad spectrum antibiotics are rarely indicated in the reptile emergency room. Specifically, the routine use of advanced cephalosporins and fluoroquinolones should be discouraged, while an antibiotic policy that advocates first-line drugs should be created.[76]

Antibiotic selection would be made based on results of culture and sensitivity testing; however, empirical antibiotic selection may be required before these results are available. In-house cytology and gram stains of potentially infectious exudate may offer some initial direction for antimicrobial therapy. Nevertheless, antibiotics should only be administered after samples have been submitted for microbiological (bacterial and/or fungal) culture, and the patient hydrated with an appropriate body temperature.[76] For a more in-depth review of antibiotic therapy in reptiles, the reader is referred to Chapter 116 in this text.

Other Therapeutics

Reptiles in an acute hypocalcemic crisis will have signs of muscle tremors or seizures, usually as a result of nutritional secondary hyperparathyroidism. Phosphorus, as well as total and ionized calcium, should be evaluated prior to treatment because parenteral calcium may not be required if ionized calcium is acceptable. Calcium gluconate (50–100 mg/kg) should be administered by subcutaneous, intramuscular, or intravenous administration.[77] While calcium chloride contains more elemental calcium in each milliliter of solution, it is extremely irritating to tissues and should only be given intravenously. As in mammals, intravenous administration of calcium should be given slowly, and the heart rate and rhythm should be monitored with an ECG. In cases of concurrent hyperphosphatemia, parenteral calcium supplementation may significantly elevate the solubility index and lead to soft tissue mineralization; therefore phosphate binders and diuresis may be required, along with carefully titrated IV calcium therapy and regular monitoring.

The goal for calcium supplementation, especially in the critical patient, is to alleviate the clinical signs of hypocalcemia rather than to achieve normal plasma calcium concentrations.[78] When the signs of hypocalcemia have resolved, oral calcium supplementation should be initiated with calcium glubionate or calcium carbonate. Severe, chronic hypocalcemia can progress to grand mal seizures, which often require use of midazolam or diazepam in addition to parenteral calcium.[79] Additional information can be found on seizures and nutritional secondary hyperparathyroidism in this text in Chapters 77 and 84, respectively.

Severe hyperuricemia (>25 mg/dL, >1480 μmol/L) can quickly lead to visceral gout and a grave prognosis; therefore administration of allopurinol (25 mg/kg/day) should be considered.[80] Additional information can be found in Chapter 66.

COMMON REPTILE EMERGENCIES

Traumatic Emergencies

As with all species, traumatic injuries often requires emergency evaluation and management. The most common cause of trauma in the authors' practice is predator (another house pet or cagemate) or prey bite wounds (Fig. 87.8). Additionally, hit-by-car injuries, most often in chelonians resulting in shell fractures, are also common emergency presentations. Some owners remain unaware of the severity of the injuries sustained and present the animal for evaluation hours to days after the traumatic event. Specific triage parameters for chelonian shell injuries have been previously published[81] and are discussed in Chapters 113 and 130.

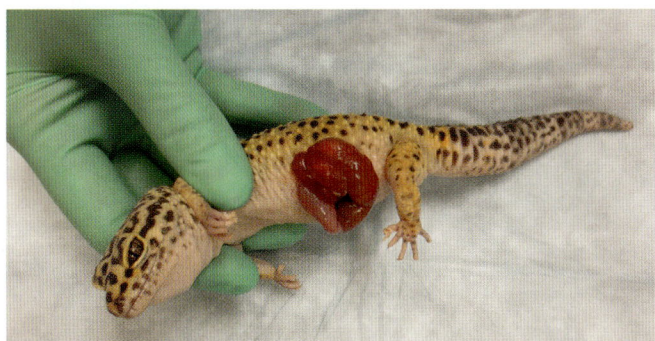

FIG 87.8 A 16-year-old male leopard gecko (*Eublepharis macularius*) who was partially eviscerated secondary to a cat bite. (Courtesy of Olivia A. Petritz, NCSU.)

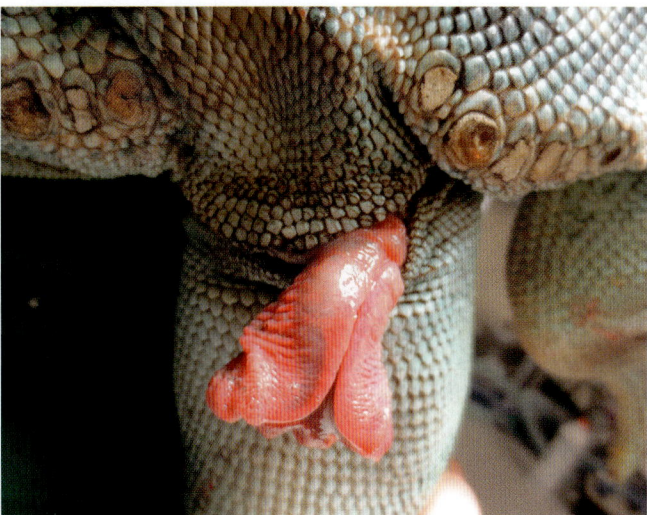

FIG 87.9 A 13-year-old male green iguana (*Iguana iguana*) with a recently prolapsed left hemipenis. (Courtesy of Olivia A. Petritz, NCSU.)

Thermal burns, which may not manifest for several days after injury, should also be addressed as quickly as possible so the appropriate analgesics and fluids can be prescribed (see Chapters 69, 70, and 130). Iatrogenic traumatic injuries inadvertently caused by owners have also been reported, including drill-bit trauma in a blood python.[82] Long bone fractures are another cause for emergency presentation, and methods of external coaptation and surgical fixation are described in Chapters 108 and 109. In brief, the initial management of open fractures is very similar to small mammals, and the same principles should be followed.

Respiratory/Cardiac Emergencies

Acute respiratory emergencies are uncommon, and most are a severe manifestation of chronic disease. Accurate localization of the disease to the upper or lower airways is imperative and follows the same principles from domestic mammal emergency medicine. Common causes of respiratory distress in reptiles include obstructions within the oropharynx or trachea (granuloma, foreign body, neoplasia [tracheal chondroma in ball pythons[83]]), pneumonia, and drowning.[35] Coelomic distension secondary to ascites or organomegaly can also lead to respiratory compromise due to the lack of a diaphragm. Trauma, such as hit-by-car injuries in chelonians, may involve the lungs and present with respiratory distress. Drowning is most commonly seen in chelonians, but any reptilian species is susceptible if given access to deep enough water. These animals may be comatose with no deep pain or corneal reflex on presentation.[17] Despite this seemingly grim prognosis, CPCR is recommended, and successful recovery is possible. Intubation and suctioning of the trachea should be performed in cases of respiratory arrest, as well as placing the chelonian in a head-down position to allow for drainage of fluid. Intermittent positive pressure ventilation and maintaining the animal in its POTZ are usually beneficial.

The most common cardiovascular emergency is severe hemorrhage,[17] and the same principles of hemostasis known in mammals also apply to reptiles. Expedited and effective hemostasis is of utmost importance, as reptile erythrocytes have lower total counts, longer life spans, and slower turnover rate when compared with mammals.[84] Another acute presentation for cardiac emergencies is exposure to cardiac glycosides from the ingestion of fireflies and certain butterfly species in bearded dragons. Shortly after ingestion, dragons exhibit gaping behavior, black beard (gular skin pigmentation) lethargy, depression, and death. Treatment is nonspecific and supportive and often not successful (see Chapter 88). Other cardiac diseases (congestive heart failure, endocarditis, pericardial effusion) usually have a slower onset of clinical signs and are uncommonly presented on an emergency basis (see Chapter 68).

Urogenital Emergencies

A cloacal prolapse can involve one (or more) of the three systems that all terminate at the cloaca: the reproductive, urinary, and gastrointestinal tracts. The clinician should determine whether the prolapsed tissue is viable and which structures are involved. The oviduct and gastrointestinal tracts are both tubular structures with a lumen—longitudinal striations can help differentiate the oviduct from other tissues. The bladder, if present, is a thin-walled, fluid-filled structure that is easily ruptured if exposed for prolonged periods. The phallus and hemipenes terminate in a mushroomlike structure, which helps distinguish these male reproductive organs from other possible prolapsed tissues (Fig. 87.9). Regardless of the origin, it is imperative that any viable prolapsed tissue be addressed as soon as possible to prevent devitalization and further compromise. Following replacement, diagnostics should be performed to determine the cause of prolapse. See Chapters 75 and 106 for additional details.

Dystocia (egg binding) is often a result of improper husbandry, including inappropriate temperature, humidity, and lack of proper nesting areas. Reproductive inertia can be divided into preovulatory (unshelled ova) versus postovulatory (shelled eggs or feti), as well as obstructive (an anatomic inability to pass one or more eggs or fetuses) versus nonobstructive dystocia.[85] The clinician must also differentiate between normal gravid and dystocic females—which can be challenging and is often based on historical information (e.g., laid or gave birth to partial clutch/litter), physical examination, and presence of abnormal clinical signs (i.e., tenesmus). Unlike mammals, dystocia in reptiles rarely requires emergency medical or surgical intervention, and medical management is often pursued initially.[17] See Chapters 80 and 105 for more details.

Neurologic Emergencies

Seizures and muscle fasiculations are cause for emergency presentation, and the same differential diagnosis should be considered as in mammalian patients. These include infectious, inflammatory, toxic, neoplastic, traumatic, and metabolic causes.[79] The latter, specifically hypocalcemia due to nutritional secondary hyperparathyroidism, is the most common cause for seizures and tremors. Total and ionized calcium and phosphorus should be determined and a complete neurologic examination

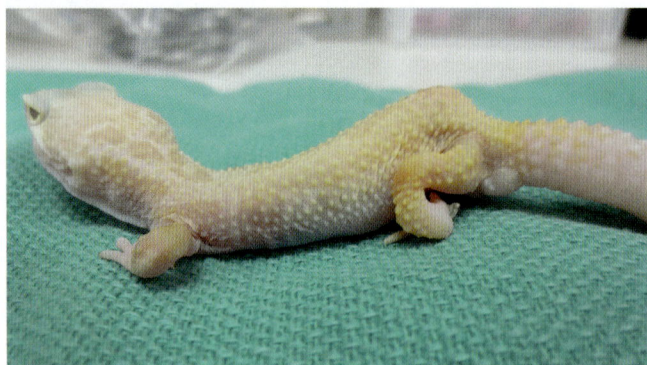

FIG 87.10 A juvenile male leopard gecko (*Eublepharis macularius*) with multiple pathological vertebral and long-bone fractures due to hypocalcemia and nutritional secondary hyperparathyroidism. (Courtesy of Olivia A. Petritz, NCSU.)

undertaken, with additional diagnostics pursued as required for definitive diagnosis (see Chapters 77 and 84). The second most common cause of neurologic presentation includes exposure to toxins such as organophosphates from acariasis treatment or ingestion of heavy metal, and these should be excluded. Vertebral fractures or luxations due to trauma or pathological causes (e.g., nutritional secondary hyperparathyroidism, osteomyelitis) can also result in hind limb paresis or paralysis (Fig. 87.10). Orthogonal views of the skeleton are recommended for assessment of bone quality, fractures, and luxations. Severe nephropathy (uremia and uricemia) and hepatic encephalopathy can also result in neurologic depression (see Chapters 66 and 67).

Gastrointestinal Emergencies

Gastrointestinal foreign bodies, usually secondary to lithophagy or pica, are often a result of a mineral-deficient diet (Fig. 87.11). Animals may present with nonspecific signs, such as anorexia and lethargy, but regurgitation or vomiting is sometimes seen. Depending on the stability of the patient and the size of the foreign object, medical management may be attempted in cases of partial obstructions with laxatives (e.g., mineral oil), fluid therapy, and assist feeding.[17] Cases of obvious complete obstruction, or those where medical management fails, are candidates for surgical intervention. Depending on the size of the patient and the foreign body, gastroscopy may be preferred as a less invasive option. Other differentials

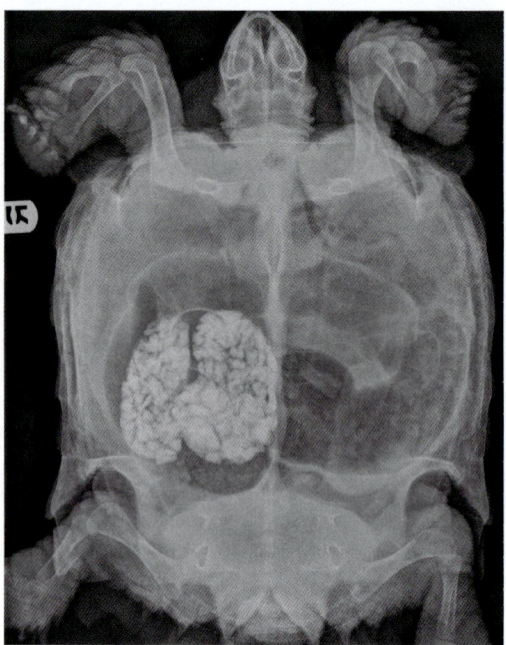

FIG 87.11 A dorsoventral radiograph of an 8-year-old male African spur thigh tortoise (*Centrochelys sulcata*) that presented for acute onset of vomiting. Note the large accumulation of mineral in the small intestine with proximal gaseous distension extending to the stomach, characteristic of an obstruction. (Courtesy of Olivia A. Petritz, NCSU.)

for regurgitation or vomiting in reptiles include inappropriate diet size/amount, postprandial handling, gastroenteritis (parasitic, viral, bacterial, fungal), gastrointestinal stasis, and rarely, secondary to metabolic disease. For additional information on regurgitation, vomiting, and gastrointestinal diseases, the reader is referred to Chapters 73 and 74. Ingestion of certain toxins can also be a considered a gastrointestinal emergency, and the reader is referred to Chapter 88 for additional information on common toxicities and their treatments.

REFERENCES

See www.expertconsult.com for a complete list of references.

88

Toxicology

Kevin T. Fitzgerald and Albert Martínez-Silvestre

Each year, novel industrial molecules, new herbicides and pesticides, over-the-counter and prescription drugs, and even human diets generate a constantly expanding number of potentially toxic substances. Not just humans, but wild species, domestic livestock, companion species, and animals kept in zoological collections are all susceptible to this increasing body of hazardous molecules.

In the last two decades, increasing numbers of more nontraditional "exotic" species have become popular worldwide as household pets. This phenomenon is particularly apparent in the widening number of reptile species being presented to veterinary hospitals. A large and growing number of poisons have been found to be toxic to lizards, snakes, turtles, and crocodilians. Our knowledge of intoxication in reptiles, once an almost anecdotal domain, has grown tremendously in recent years due to more published accounts of reptilian poisonings and more in-depth pharmacologic studies. Thousands of different molecules are capable of poisoning living reptiles. Practitioners cannot be expected to be familiar with every hazardous substance or new poison, but clinicians must understand that toxicology is an essential part of emergency medicine, and they must recognize the most commonly presented toxidromes (toxic syndromes) in exotic species. It is a privilege to practice veterinary medicine, and practitioners must remain duty-bound to keep current both about new species and new toxins. This index of poisons, though not complete, focuses on the most common poisonings of reptiles, their mechanism of action, and potential treatments.

EMERGENCY TREATMENT

Many reptile owners know little about the exotic animals they keep. Coupling this with many veterinarians being unfamiliar with the anatomy, physiology, natural history, and vital signs of captive reptile species creates a recipe for potential disaster. The problem is further compounded since, like many wild species, captive reptiles tend to mask outward signs of disease. As a result, emergencies in reptiles are not always obvious to veterinarians and certainly not to the average reptile owner. Clinicians must remember that the basic tenets of emergency medicine remain the same regardless of species.

Veterinarians can do much to set themselves up for success when dealing with poisoned reptiles. To maximize treatment success, cases of intoxication must be managed swiftly and intensively. Early, aggressive therapy becomes critical in the management of poisoning. For many cases, the telephone is the first line of defense. Often overlooked, receptionists, technicians, and hospital phone staff must be trained in dealing with toxicologic emergencies. Teaching staff to recognize what is deadly and what is harmless can be the difference between life and death.

Emergency care of reptiles begins with a sound history. Often embarrassed by how their animal was housed, how haphazardly toxins were stored, and how long the illness has been going on, owners may be purposely evasive and not give a true history. Nevertheless, treatment starts with a thorough history and husbandry review (see Section 3 for more information).

Required questions in taking a thorough history from a reptile owner include:
- What is the origin of the animal?
- How long has it been with the owner?
- What type of cage setup is employed?
- How long a photoperiod?
- What type of heating system and what are the temperature ranges?
- What food source and how often fed?
- Are cage mates present?

Many reptile emergencies are secondary to inappropriate husbandry, poor diet, and owner inexperience. It is important to obtain information on the diet and how often an animal is being fed and watered, as well as how frequently and with what products are the cage and environment being cleaned. Establishing a consistent and formal pattern of questioning can help reptile clinicians focus on the cause of the problem. Also, species-specific susceptibility to certain poisons must be remembered. Substances that are toxic to birds and mammals may not be toxic to reptiles. Conversely, molecules extremely hazardous to reptiles may not affect birds and mammals.

A complete physical examination is always required. Heart rate, respiration, hydration, neurologic status, and mentation are all critical cues both for diagnosis and for eventual prognosis. In addition to the history, physical examination, vital and clinical signs, and laboratory findings can also help to determine necessary treatment choices. Practitioners must be mindful of the animal's overall condition and treat the patient *not* the poison. Likewise, laboratory results may take days or weeks to return, so one must treat the patient *not* the lab information. Obtaining a diagnosis and patient information through imaging (radiographs, ultrasonography), clinicopathology, biopsy, and gastric lavage are similar in approach to those utilized with small animals. However, since we are limited by the challenges involved in making reptiles vomit, endoscopy may need to be used to obtain stomach samples or to retrieve toxic objects or remove ingested tablets, capsules, pills, or other substances.

Owing to a variety of constraints, intravenous therapy is not always practical for many reptiles. Nevertheless, several viable alternative routes for fluid administration are available. Many desert reptilian species can tolerate remarkable degrees of dehydration, and chelonians, lizards, snakes, and crocodilians can display varying signs of dehydration; however, for most reptiles, sunken eyes, hanging skin, and dry mouths are consistent changes. If intravenous pathways are not practical, intraosseous, intracoelemic, subcutaneous, and enteral routes of fluid administration may be legitimate alternatives depending on the critical nature of the patient. See Chapters 44-46 for guidelines.

Reptilian species have specific preferred body temperatures and optimal thermal zones. For most temperate species, a range of 72°F to 82°F is safe. Caution must be employed since debilitated reptiles may be too weak to thermoregulate. Rigorous, intensive nursing care can do much to help and revive even severely poisoned reptiles. Diets, dietary supplements, and feeding techniques are available to support animals as they are recovering. (See Chapters 44–46 and 87.)

Next follows a discussion, by no means complete, focusing on the most common poisonings of reptiles, their mechanism of actions, and any potential treatments.

PARENTERAL ANTIPARASITIC DRUGS

Ivermectin

Ivermectin is an antiparasitic from a family of chemicals called avermectins. These are marocylic lactones made from fermentation broth of the fungus *Streptomyces avermitilis*.[1] The macrolide ivermectin is available as an injectable, a spray, and an oral formulation. It has activity against a variety of parasites, including nematodes, arthropods, and arachnids.

Avermectins work by potentiating the effects of the inhibitory neurotransmitter gamma-aminobutyric acid (GABA).[1] They stimulate release of GABA by presynaptic sites and increase GABA binding to postsynaptic receptors, which causes neuromuscular blockage. Avermectins also open chloride channels in membranes of the nervous system and further depress neuronal function. These actions cause paralysis and death of susceptible parasites. Ivermectin is absorbed systemically by host tissues. When parasites bite the host, they then absorb the ivermectin. Ivermectin is active against intestinal parasites, mites, microfilariae, and developing larvae.[1] Concurrent treatment with diazepam, which also works through GABA potentiation, may heighten deleterious effects.

Ivermectin can cause depression, paralysis, coma, and death in chelonians.[2] Species susceptible to ivermectin toxicosis may have a blood-brain barrier more permeable than nonsensitive species. This greater permeability may be the result of p-glycoprotein mutation in membranes of the central nervous system (CNS). Another, currently unproven, theory postulates the existence of a specific protein only present in the brains of ivermectin-sensitive species. Ivermectin toxicity has also been reported in several species of lizards and snakes.[3,4] Toxic reaction has been described in terrestrial tortoises, Central American skinks (genus *Mabuya*), Parson's chameleons (*Calumma parsonii*), Panther chameleons (*Furcifer pardalis*), Solomon island skinks (*Corucia zebrata*), and Nile crocodiles (*Crocodylus niloticus*) (Dumonceaux et al, Proc ARAV, 2004, pp 155-157).[5] In the authors' experience, coma and death occurred after 3 days in young Nile crocodiles (*Crocodylus niloticus*) with a single subcutaneous injection.

For many snakes such as common garter snakes (*Thamnophis sirtalis*) or Boelen's python (*Python boeleni*), ivermectin seems to have no adverse effects. However, ball pythons (*Python regius*) in particular may occasionally show mild neurologic signs when treated (Baier, Proc ARAV, 2004, pp 125-127).

Although reported to be safely used in the treatment of *Foleyella* in chameleons (*Furcifer pardalis*) and internal parasites in monitors (*Varanus exanthematicus*) and green iguanas (*Iguana iguana*), ivermectin should always be used with caution.[8–11]

Diagnosis is confirmed by a history of ivermectin exposure and clinical signs. For postmortem testing, samples recommended for submission include frozen brain, liver, and fat. Ivermectin can also be detected in serum.[2] No known antidote or physiological antagonist exists for ivermectin. Treatment is supportive and should include decontamination of any topical sprays with soap and water, fluid therapy,

nutritional support, monitoring of electrolytes, and respiratory (ventilator) support. Recovery may take days to weeks. In the authors' experience, two box turtles (*Terrapene* sp.) and one Hermann's tortoise (*Testudo hermanni*) completely recovered after 4 weeks, and another debilitated box turtle recovered in 6 weeks.

Ivermectin should never be given to chelonians, gravid animals, or neonates. Also, for particularly small species, other therapies should be considered. If any question exists about potential toxicity, ivermectin should only be used topically. The aqueous dilution of ivermectin for injection is problematic. The ivermectin precipitates, thereby making dosing erratic. Alternatively, the mixture of imidacloprid with moxidectin seems to have better tolerance in reptiles.[12]

Fenbendazole

Fenbendazole is a benzimidazole type of antiparasiticide.[12,13] It is safe and effective against many helminth parasites in animals. Fenbendazole and its metabolite, oxfendazole, inhibits glucose uptake in parasites.[12,13] Because of its wide range of activity, its high degree of efficacy, and its broad margin of safety, this antihelminthic is frequently prescribed. Fenbendazole has a high margin of safety and has been reported to be well tolerated even at six times the recommended dosage and three times the recommended duration.[13] Fenbendazole is the drug of choice for treating nematode infections in reptiles. It can be administered orally or per cloaca as a liquid, or the powdered form can be placed on food.

It has been extensively used as an anthelminthic in reptiles at 50 to 100 mg/kg orally (PO) once (repeated in 2 weeks) or 50 mg/kg PO every 24 hours for 3 to 5 days.[14,15] Toxic effects have been reported in birds, rats, cats, and dogs.[16–20] Recently, evidence of fenbendazole overdose has been reported in individuals of a small species of snake given exceedingly large doses of the drug (Alvardo et al, Proc ARAV, 1997, pp 35-36.). Four adult Fea's vipers (*Azemiops feae*) died after administration of single dosages of fenbendazole ranging from 428 mg/kg to 1064 mg/kg. Necropsy findings were suggestive of intestinal changes consistent with fenbendazole toxicity. This study documents adverse effects at doses higher than what is recommended. In Hermann's tortoises (*Testudo hermanni*), fenbendazole has been described as possibly causing heteropenia, leucopenia, and generalized lymphopenia, as well as increases in uric acid, phosphorus, and total proteins or decreased glucose with intensive regimes.[22] Fenbendazole and mebendazole have been shown to cause agranulocytosis in mammals in extremely high dosages and also have been implicated in liver toxicities.[17,20,22] Bone marrow toxicity has also been documented with fenbendazole administration.[23-26]

No antidote exists for this poisoning and treatment is supportive and symptomatic. In long-term treatment, the use of fenbendazole is best indicated in combination with frequent blood tests and vigilant health status evaluation. Additional investigation is needed to determine the effects of antiparasitics such as fipronil and neonicotinoids.

Metronidazole

Metronidazole is used as an antibacterial, antiprotozoal, and appetite stimulant in reptiles. It is formulated as a suspension, as an injectable, and as a tablet. Strict attention must be paid to the dosage, the frequency, and the size of the animal.

The activity of metronidazole is specific for anaerobic bacteria and protozoa.[27] It is specific particularly for *Giardia* and other protozoal organisms. Metronidazole disrupts DNA in target microbes through reaction with intracellular metabolites.

The most severe side effect of metronidazole is dose-related CNS toxicity. Moreover, this drug is hepatotoxic and carcinogenic. High dosages can cause ataxia, inability to walk, nystagmus, opisthotonos, tremors of the lumbar muscles and hind limbs, seizures, and death.[28–30]

Treatment is symptomatic and supportive and involves administration of fluids and both thermal and respiratory support. With supportive care, most patients recover. In severe cases, the patient may need to be placed on a ventilator. Recovery time is dependent on the extent of the toxicity, taking anywhere from 1 to several days.

PARENTERAL ANTIMICROBIAL DRUGS

Antifungal Toxicity

A variety of fungal infections have been documented in reptiles. Ranging from dermatophytes to systemic mycotic infections, these conditions are treated with a variety of antifungal medications. Based on the often small size of the reptilian patient, the mechanism of action of these drugs, and the idiosyncrasies of reptilian physiology, improper dosing can lead to serious intoxications.

Amphotericin B.
Amphotericin B is a macrolide class of antimicrobial that inhibits ergosterol synthesis.[31] Ergosterol is a component of the cell membrane unique to fungal organisms. Amphotericin is a potent nephrotoxin. It produces signs of renal toxicity in 80% of patients that receive it intravenously.[31] Its action causes renal vasoconstriction, reduces glomerular filtration rate, and has direct toxic effects on the membranes of the renal tubule cells.[32] Through these mechanisms, amphotericin B causes acute tubular necrosis. Almost 35% of human patients treated with systemic amphotericin develop hypokalemia sufficient to warrant potassium supplementation.[31]

Clinical signs mimic acute renal failure, anorexia, lethargy, weight loss, etc. Elevated blood urea nitrogen (BUN) and creatinine levels, with decreased potassium and sodium levels, are commonly seen in mammals.[33] In reptiles, uric acid and/or BUN and electrolytes should be monitored. Renal function tests including glomerular filtration rate (GFR) determination by iohexol excretion should be considered.[34]

Treatment includes discontinuation of the drug, aggressive fluid therapy to prevent further kidney damage, and diminishment of renal effects with sodium chloride-containing fluids. Treatment with mannitol may help increase the elimination of amphotericin B.[33]

Prognosis after amphotericin B toxicity depends on the severity of the renal damage. Amphotericin B is still listed as a treatment for aspergillosis in reptiles (1 mg/kg intracoelomically once daily for 2 to 4 weeks).[35] Safer medical and surgical options are available. A less toxic, new formulation of amphotericin B is available for humans and may soon be available for veterinary use. Amphotericin B should not be used for animals with preexisting renal disease.

Griseofulvin.
This antifungal works by inhibiting fungal spindle activity and leads to distorted weakened fungal hyphae.[34,36] It has also been shown to cause bone marrow suppression in mammals, although the mechanism of action is unknown.[36]

Anorexia, lethargy, diarrhea, and anemia have been reported with intoxication.[33] Griseofulvin has been shown to be teratogenic in pregnant animals of many species.[37,38] In reptiles, the recommended dosage for fungal dermatitis is 20 to 48 mg/kg PO every third day for five treatments.[38] It is available as a tablet and a topical ointment.

Treatment includes discontinuation of the drug and symptomatic support. No specific antidote exists. Topical treatments can be removed with tepid water and gentle hand soap. Antifungal overdoses can be best avoided by prevention of fungal infection through good husbandry.

Imidazoles (Ketoconazole) and Triazoles (Fluconazole and Itraconazole).
These antifungal drugs inhibit fungal replication by interfering with ergosterol synthesis. Ketoconazole also has direct effects on the fungal membrane.[38] These fungistatic drugs are metabolized by the liver. Itraconazole is more potent than ketoconazole and is better tolerated with less hepatotoxicity. Clinical signs of intoxication include anorexia, lethargy, weight loss, and diarrhea. Elevated liver enzymes may be present in intoxicated animals.[39] Dosages recommended for reptiles include 2 to 5 mg/kg PO daily for 5 days for fluconazole, 25 mg/kg PO daily for 3 weeks for ketoconazole, and 23.5 mg/kg PO once daily for itraconazole.[38] Minimal side effects seem to occur when using miconazole preparation applied topically. No specific antidote exists for toxicity by these antifungals. Treatment involves stopping the drug, decontaminating any topicals, and supportive therapy (fluids, warmth). For ketoconazole, treatment includes countering hepatotoxicity. Mild intoxications usually improve with simple cessation of the drug.

The safest and most effective drug should be selected for use in the treatment of fungal infections in reptiles. Considerations include the severity of the infection, the size of the animal, and the condition of the animal before treatment. Dosages must be meticulously checked, particularly for systemics and dips to be used on reptiles. Voriconazol has been tested in slider turtles (*Trachemys scripta*) and in bearded dragons (*Pogona vitticeps*) with "yellow fungal disease" or *Nannizziopsis* spp. This drug may be more effective, safer, and less toxic, but requires a longer duration of treatment.[40,41] (See Chapter 117.) Many treatments are best administered by veterinarians and not clients. Finally, reptiles must never be left alone in any bath or medicated dip.

Antibiotic Toxicity

Selection of antibiotics should be made judiciously. Selection depends on experience of the clinician, empirical considerations, the type of infection present based on culture and sensitivity and Gram stains, and most importantly, the size, age, species, and condition of the reptilian patient. No antibiotic can be relied on to be effective for all situations. Many antibiotics have hepatotoxic or nephrotoxic effects. They can prevent or decrease the expected effects of drugs normally used in reptiles such as ketamine, tiletamine, halothane, acepromazine, or pentoxifylline. In addition, antibiotics are no substitute for good wound management, nursing care, nutrition, or husbandry. Ceftazidine causes the least kidney damage and, if indicated by sensitivity testing, is recommended in cases where kidney disease is present.[42]

Gentamicin.
Gentamicin is an aminoglycoside antibiotic. Other aminoglycosides include amikacin, tobramycin, neomycin, streptomycin, and kanamycin. Gentamicin is bacteriocidal and is broad spectrum, except for streptococci and anaerobic bacteria.[42] Its mechanism of action inhibits bacterial protein synthesis by binding to 30S ribosomes. Historically, gentamicin has been used for acute serious infection, such as those caused by gram-negative bacteria. Nephrotoxicity and ototoxicity of gentamicin in reptiles is well documented.[42–45] Recommended dosing for gentamicin varies from 1.5 to 2.5 mg/kg given no sooner than every third day.[46]

Amikacin.
Amikacin is also an aminoglycoside, is bacteriocidal, is broad spectrum in activity, and has the same mechanism of action on bacteria as gentamicin.[47,48] It is indicated particularly against gram-negative organisms, where it may have greater activity than gentamicin.[48,49]

Like gentamicin, nephrotoxicity is the primary toxic effect of amikacin. Patients must remain hydrated during therapy. Ototoxicity has also been reported. If used together with anesthetic agents, aminoglycosides may show neuromuscular blockade in mammals.[47] Dosages for amikacin vary. (See Chapters 116, 127, and 128 for drug dosages).

Chloramphenicol. Chloramphenicol is an antibacterial with a broad spectrum of activity against gram-positive bacteria, gram-negative bacteria, and Rickettsia. Its mechanism of action is by inhibition of bacterial protein synthesis by binding with ribosomes.[50]

The major toxicity of chloramphenicol is hemorrhage.[49,51] In all vertebrates studied, toxicity produces direct, dose-dependent bone marrow suppression that results in reduction in red blood cells, white blood cells, and platelets in mammals.[51] This manifestation is aggravated by inappropriate dosages, extended treatments, and repeated use of the drug. Treatment of chloramphenicol intoxication is supportive and may require blood transfusions. The drug has also been reported to be appetite suppressive. Like gentamicin, chloramphenicol is used less frequently as safer antibiotics appear.[46] The recommended dosage for chloramphenicol is 50 mg/kg administered once daily or every other day.[46]

Enrofloxacin. Enrofloxacin is a fluoroquinolone antibacterial drug. It is bacteriocidal with a broad spectrum of activity. Its mechanism of action inhibits DNA gyrase, thus inhibiting both DNA and RNA synthesis. Sensitive bacteria include *Staphylococcus*, *Escherichia coli*, *Proteus*, *Klebsiella*, and *Pasteurella*.[52] *Pseudomonas* is moderately susceptible but requires higher dosages. In some species, enrofloxacin doses range from 2.5 to 5 mg/kg.[46] Enrofloxacin can cause severe muscle and skin necrosis if administered SC or IM (Fig. 88.1). Only a single IM injection is recommended, followed by oral therapy. Necrosis is caused by its high pH, and dilution is ineffective for practical applications. At a pH of 10 it would be necessary to dilute 1 mL of Baytril with 1000 mL to get close to a pH of 7.

MISCELLANEOUS DRUGS AND PRODUCTS

Chlorhexidine Versus Iodine Toxicity

Chlorhexidine and iodine are antiseptic antibacterial agents used as skin cleansing and wound care agents. Chlorhexidine solution is not impaired by organic material, has broad-spectrum activity with minimal systemic absorption, and maintains residual activity up to 2 days after application. Povidone iodine has broad-spectrum activity against bacteria, fungi, viruses, and yeast but is inactivated by the presence of organic material and has little residual activity.

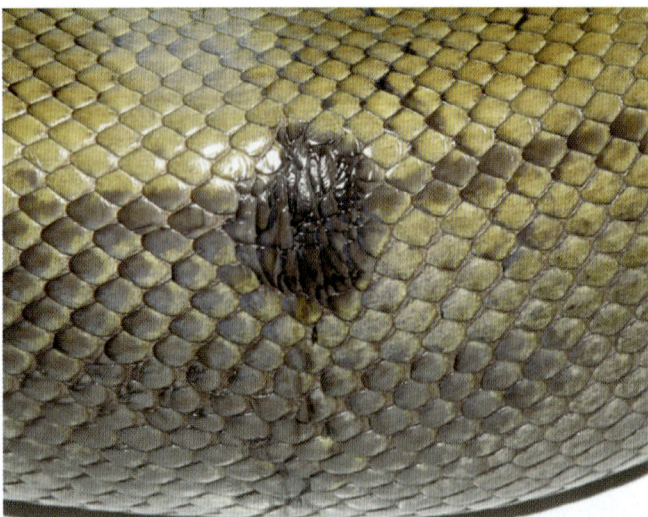

FIG 88.1 Black pigmented scar and skin necrosis following intramuscular administration of several doses of enrofloxacin in an olive Burmese python *(Python bivittatus)*. (Courtesy of Albert Martínez-Silvestre.)

In both cases, caution should be observed with more concentrated formulations, as they are cytotoxic, may slow granulation tissue formation, and ultimately impair or delay wound healing.[53]

Soaking living animals in any solution can be potentially life threatening. Recently, turtles soaked for 1 hour in chlorhexidine scrub have been shown to become intoxicated.[54] Cutaneous absorption of the solution and possible oral and cloacal ingestion of the soaks has been postulated as the cause of the problem. Before any substances are used as a soak, the literature should be checked for preferred usage, dosage, and duration of the soak. Affected animals should be removed from the soak, rinsed, and supported with warmth and fluids. Remember to never leave any reptile unattended in a bath. Animals can drown much faster than anticipated. Also, particular attention must be paid to the depth of fluids in which reptiles are bathed and soaked.

Bleach

Various hypochlorite bleach solutions can be found in most households. Typically, these are 3% to 6% hypochlorite solutions in water.[31,55] Bleaches are moderately irritating. If contact with skin is prolonged, the damage is worsened. Bleaches can be effective in treatment of cage parasites of reptiles but should *never* be applied to live animals. Bleach can cause alkali-type burns if splashed in the eyes of lizards and turtles. Immediate and copious irrigation of the eye minimizes damage. Skin exposed to bleach should be washed with a mild soap and lukewarm water. Animals should be kept out of recently bleached cages for a minimum of 24 hours to prevent respiratory tract irritation. In addition, residual disinfectant can be removed by wiping with a clean cloth or towel and exposing the area to direct sunlight for a few hours.

Dioctyl Sodium Sulfosuccinate (DSS)

DSS is an anionic surfactant substance that traditionally has been recommended as a laxative and stool softener for a variety of vertebrates ranging from humans to rodents.[56] Likewise, DSS has been advocated for the same use in reptiles.[57]

It is generally regarded as a relatively safe pharmaceutical agent with a low toxicity. However, reports of toxic effects exist in the literature for horses, dogs, monkeys, rats, rabbits, guinea pigs, and mice after both oral and topical administration.[58–64] Furthermore, fatalities in reptiles after oral use of DSS have been reported (Paul-Murphy et al, Proc 1st Conference of Zoological and Avian Medicine, 1987). One study documents severe changes in gastric and esophageal mucosa in gopher snakes *(Pituophis melanoleucus)* given oral DSS at a dosage of 250 mg/kg.

A specific dose of DSS has not been established for reptiles, but dosages for other species range from 15 to 40 mg/kg for dogs and cats to 200 mg/kg for horses.[56,63] Concentrations (dilutions) of 1:30 have been recommended for reptiles.[57]

The study in gopher snakes and reports in other species indicate that DSS may not be as innocuous as once believed. These studies demonstrate that DSS can have adverse effects, and, in reptiles, levels greater than 250 mg/kg can result in caustic changes to epithelial surfaces. Additionally, the potential for overzealous oral administration of DSS with resulting aspiration pneumonia exists. Care must be employed if DSS and other laxatives, stool softeners, and enhancers of gastric motility should be considered.

Vitamin Toxicity

For water-soluble vitamins, in which excesses can be excreted into the urine, the margin of safety is large. For fat-soluble vitamins like A and D, this is not the case. Owners, breeders, and veterinarians often over-supplement captive reptiles with these fat-soluble vitamins with deleterious results.

Vitamin A Toxicity. Vitamin A is necessary for normal skin and periocular tissue health, particularly in chelonians and saurians. Turtles and lizards with hypovitaminosis A typically show ocular discharge, palpebral edema, blindness, hyperkeratosis of skin and mouthparts, and aural abscesses. Patients can be treated with oral vitamin A supplementation (2000 IU/kg every 7 days) and an improved diet.[66]

Unfortunately, excessive iatrogenic administration of vitamin A can cause its own issues, including inappetence, full-thickness skin sloughing, secondary bacterial infection, discoloration of the skin, and extreme lethargy. These results usually happen at dosages of 10,000 IU/kg or higher given IM as a single injection.[67] Treatment involves ceasing vitamin A administration, fluid therapy, and nutritional support. The skin lesions may heal slowly, but animals managed supportively can completely recover. Prognosis varies depending on the severity of the lesions.

Vitamin D Toxicity. Dosages of 50 to 1000 times the minimum daily requirement of vitamin D are often given for weeks to months. The use of commercial oral D₃ supplements (Solar Drops Liquid UVB, T-Rex) to avoid the expense and/or substitute for broad-spectrum (UVB) lighting should be actively discouraged. Intoxication can be insidious; particularly when the minimum daily requirement of most mammalian vertebrates for vitamin D is only 10 to 20 IU/kg body weight.[68] Minimum daily requirements have not been established for reptiles. Sometimes a corrective but miscalculated treatment for secondary nutritional hyperparathyroidism may cause iatrogenic vitamin D overdosing. The mechanism of action for toxicity of vitamin D is related to hypercalcemia. This prolonged hypercalcemia causes dystrophic calcification of the gastrointestinal, renal, pulmonary, cardiovascular, and synovial tissues (Fig. 88.2). Definitive and accurate diagnosis is possible by submission of blood for 25(OH)D₃ levels measured by high-performance liquid chromatography or liquid chromatography–mass spectrometry (e.g., Heartland Assays, Ames, IA).[69] Complete

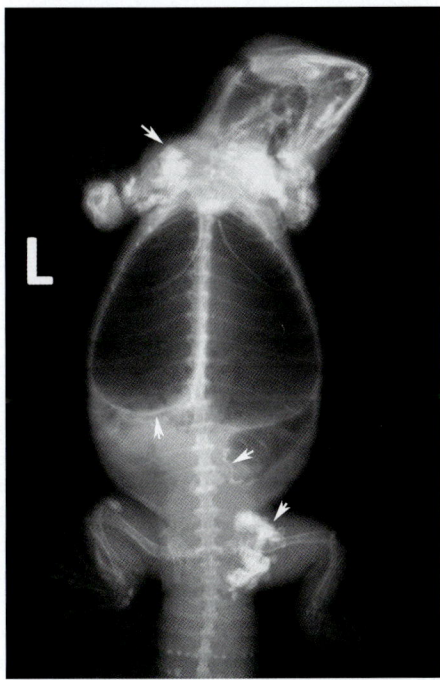

FIG 88.2 Radiographic evidence of soft tissue mineralization (arrows) associated with the pectoral and pelvic musculature, lungs, and gastrointestinal tract in a *Uromastyx* lizard. This animal was supplemented with oral vitamin D₃ and elevated plasma 25(OH)D₃ levels confirmed hypervitaminosis D₃. (Courtesy of Stephen J. Divers.)

removal of vitamin D–containing supplements, diuresis, and cortisone may help control hypercalcemia, but resolution of soft-tissue calcification may not be successful.[69] Calcitonin has historically been recommended for the treatment of vitamin D–induced hypercalcemia, although controlled studies on the efficacy of calcitonin in vitamin D toxicosis are lacking.[69] Pamidronate disodium (a bisphosphonate [Aredia]) has been recommended in dogs to counter hypercalcemia, with 1 to 2 mg/kg given slowly over 2 hours.

In light of the inherent calcium metabolism problems of captive reptiles, veterinarians must counsel clients about proper husbandry, nutrition, and dietary requirements and ensure that no supplements are given to animals without veterinary approval. (See Chapters 27, 84, and 122.)

Organophosphates and Carbamates

Organophosphates are the most commonly used insecticides worldwide.[70] They are the active ingredient in a long list of products. For animal use as insecticides, they are formulated as dips, sprays, topical medications, systemic antiparasitic agents, and flea collars. This group of insecticides includes chlorpyrifos (Dursban), dichlorvos, diazinon, cythioate (Proban), fenthion (ProSpot), malathion, ronnel, parathion, trichlorfon, and vaponna. Their cousins the carbamates include carbaryl (Sevin), bendiocarb, methiocarb, propoxur, and cabofuran. As newer, safer insecticides are marketed, this group is involved in fewer accidental poisonings but still accounts for a large number of intoxications.

Their toxicity in reptiles is well known and even some pesticides are used regularly in different parts of the world to control unwanted populations of iguanas, snakes, and geckos. High concentrations of organochlorine have been proposed as adjuvants to the occurrence of ophthalmic and otic pathologies in the box turtle (*Terrapene carolina*).[71]

Organophosphates and carbamates interfere with metabolism and breakdown of acetylcholine at synaptic junctions.[72] Acetylcholinesterase is the enzyme responsible for breaking down the neurotransmitter at these sites. Acetylcholinesterase is inhibited by organophosphates and carbamates at these cholinergic sites. As a result, acetylcholine accumulates at the synapses, which at first excites and then paralyzes transmission in these synapses, giving it the characteristic "nerve gas" signs associated with organophosphate toxicity. This inhibition of the synapse is irreversible with organophosphates and reversible with carbamates. Organophosphates are readily absorbed by all routes—dermal, respiratory, gastrointestinal, and conjunctival. Overdose with organophosphates may happen more readily if given together with imidothiazoles, such as levamisole.

Clinical signs seen in reptiles include salivation, ataxia, muscle fasciculations, inability to right themselves, coma, and respiratory arrest.[73] Death results from massive respiratory secretions, bronchiolar constriction, and effects on respiratory centers in the medulla, leading to the cessation of breathing.

Blood levels of acetylcholinesterase are variable and poorly diagnostic unless paired. Brain acetylcholinesterase levels are considered definitive. Animals with dermal exposure should be washed with a mild dishwashing detergent and copious amounts of water. Animals should be dried after rinsing to prevent further uptake of the insecticide. The need for fluid therapy to counter dehydration and electrolyte imbalances should be considered. The specific physiological antidote, the muscarinic antagonist atropine, should be given (0.4 mg/kg intramuscularly [IM]) and may help displace the toxin from receptors; however, the more modern poisons tend to bind irreversibly. Atropine should help with salivation, bronchospasm, and dyspnea. Diazepam may be given as needed for seizures. Use of antihistamines as a treatment for insecticide poisonings is controversial and most likely not effective. Prognosis is dependent on dosage, duration of exposure, and size of the animal. It should be noted that, to promote slow absorption and avoid direct contact with reptile skin, some insecticides can be applied to a piece of tape and adhered to the scales for 2 to 3 days (personal observation).

Therapies both effective and safer than organophosphates exist for treatment of parasites in captive reptiles. (See Chapter 120.)

Pyrethrins and Pyrethroids

Pyrethrin is the oldest used botanic insecticide. It is made from the dried and ground flowers of *Chrysanthemum cineriifolium*.[74] Pyrethroids are synthetic derivatives of pyrethrin and are widely available. Pyrethroid insecticides have enhanced stability, potency, and half-life compared with the parent molecule. A variety of dilute pyrethrin-containing and pyrethroid-containing sprays have been recommended for reptiles.[75,76] In fact, the only licensed product for use in reptile parasites is a pyrethroid (Permethrin – Provent-a-mite; ProProducts, Mahopec, NY).[77,78]

These molecules affect parasites by altering the activity of the sodium ion channels of nerves. These poisons prolong the period of sodium conductance and increase the length of the depolarizing action potential.[74] This results in repetitive nerve firing and death. With the right conditions or at higher dosages, these compounds can intoxicate host animals. Because of the potential for transcutaneous absorption, pyrethrin and pyrethroid sprays must be used with caution. As with ivermectin, organophosphates, carbamates, pyrethrin, and pyrethroids should never be given concurrently with other cholinesterase-inhibiting compounds.

Clinical signs have been reported for pyrethrins and pyrethroids, particularly if sprays used also contain insect growth regulators (suc as methoprene). Animals can have signs develop within 15 minutes of application. Signs include salivation, ataxia, inability to right themselves, and muscle fasiculations.[74] Idiosyncratic reactions to pyrethrins can happen at much lower doses than expected. A small percentage of animals appear to be extremely sensitive to pyrethrins and pyrethroids.

No known antidote exists for these molecules. If caught early enough, treatment for pyrethrin/pyrethroid toxicity involves dermal decontamination, isotonic fluids, atropine, and diazepam for seizures. No good antemortem test exists for detection and pyrethrins and pyrethroids produce no identifiable lesions postmortem.[74] Care must be taken to keep pyrethrin/pyrethroid sprays away from reptiles' eyes and mouth to prevent intoxication. Prognosis depends on the strength of the agent used, the duration of the exposure, and the size of the animal involved.

Rodenticides

Each year, rodents destroy crops in the field, eat and contaminate food in storage, serve as vectors for human diseases, bite people, and cause material damage by gnawing. As a result, a variety of rodenticides are ubiquitously used in an attempt to control populations of these animals. These substances prove to be nearly as dangerous to humans and nontarget animals as they are to rodents. Rodenticide intoxication has been documented in a variety of species, including reptiles.[79,80] The original container housing the poison should be provided on presentation so that active ingredients can be positively identified and appropriate treatment initiated. Reptile clinicians are often presented with tortoises that are attacked by rats. Owners often put out rodenticides to control rodents. Great care must be taken to avoid tortoises coming in contact with rodenticide bait.

Anticoagulants. The long-acting anticoagulants are responsible for 80% of rodenticide poisoning in humans and animals in the United States.[81] These long-acting agents have the same action as warfarin; however, they are more potent and their half-life is longer. They are effective after single or limited feedings when compared with other rodenticides. They act by decreasing the activity of the vitamin K–dependent blood-clotting factors (II, VII, IX, X). When clotting factors are sufficiently reduced, bleeding occurs. Currently in the United States, the anticoagulant rodenticides have been taken off the market due to

a dramatic increase in children and nontarget species intoxication, and the only rodenticides available to consumers are bromethalin and cholocalciferol. The most common and most toxic second-generation anticoagulants in use were brodifacoum and bromadilone.

Clinical signs depend on the site and extent of hemorrhage. Most intoxicated animals show anorexia, weakness, and lethargy. The most common clinical sign is dyspnea.[79] Typically, animals bleed into body cavities, abdomen, thorax, joints, and so on. Most of these poisons are packaged as molasses-soaked grain laced with the anticoagulant. These various plant materials can attract herbivorous or omnivorous reptiles. Newer formulations of these baits are dyed turquoise.

Reptiles ingesting toxic levels of anticoagulant rodenticides do not always display hemorrhagic signs. Although hemorrhage was not observed, lethal effects of warfarin and difenacoum after oral ingestion has been demonstrated in brown tree snakes (*Boiga irregularis*).[82] Round Island (Mauritius) was exposed to large amounts of brodifacoum released into the environment (500 kg/ha).[83] Skinks observed eating pellets softened by rain died with high levels of brodifacoum. None showed internal bleeding, and it was postulated the poison interfered with the animals' thermoregulation, causing overheating. Despite these findings, other studies examining lacertids found no evidence of mortality after exposure to brodifacoum at 50 ppm. Balearic lizards (*Podarcis lifordi*), known to be generalist feeders, have demonstrated avoidance of cereal paraffin baits mixed with 50 ppm of difenacoum.[84] Nevertheless, the big-scaled least gecko of Puerto Rico (*Sphaerodactylus macrolepis*) in one experiment showed mortality rates of 15% when exposed to pelleted grains mixed with brodifacoum (50 ppm).[84] Reptiles appear to have a varied response to the effects of anticoagulant rodenticides.

The authors have seen one green iguana (*Iguana iguana*) and two box turtles intoxicated by anticoagulant bait ingestion. Baseline determinations of one-stage prothrombin time (PT) are helpful in animals suspected of consuming anticoagulant poisons in mammals. Comparison PT can be measured in known healthy animals or reptiles. The antidote for anticoagulant poisoning, vitamin K_1, should be administered in animals if PT is increased. Daily dosage recommendations in mammals for vitamin K_1 are 2.5 mg/kg.[79] Therapy with this antidote must be maintained until toxic amounts of the poison are no longer present in the animal. Length of treatment depends on the dose and type of anticoagulant ingested but may be up to 3 to 4 weeks. A PT test should be run 48 hours after cessation of vitamin K_1 treatment. If clotting time is normal, therapy is discontinued. If clotting time is increased, therapy is continued for another week. Vitamin K_1 treatment can be given with subcutaneous injection or orally. Intravenous injections have a high incidence of anaphylactic reaction in mammals.[79] This has not been reported in reptiles. Treatment includes vitamin K_1 and possible oxygen support and plasma transfusion.

Bromethalin. Bromethalin is one of the newer rodenticides that has not been reported to cause poisoning in reptiles, but, because of increasing use, the possibility for intoxication exists. It is formulated in baits of pelleted grain and dyed green or turquoise. Bromethalin is a neurotoxin, but because of its name, it can be confused with the long-acting anticoagulants bromadilone and brodifacoum. Again, one should encourage clients to bring in original containers to obtain valuable label information concerning ingredients.

The mechanism of action of bromethalin is to uncouple oxidative phosphorylation. The brain is the primary target for bromethalin because of its unique dependence on oxidative phosphorylation. The drug causes brain electrolyte disturbances and results in the development of cerebral edema.[81]

Clinical signs include hind limb paralysis, abnormal postures, fine muscle tremors, and seizures. Severely poisoned animals are comatose. Clinical signs are usually seen within 24 hours of ingestion.[85]

Bromethalin is a nonselective vertebrate poison. Antemortem diagnosis of bromethalin poisoning depends on exposure history and subsequent development of appropriate clinical signs. Postmortem diagnosis can be confirmed by the presence of bromethalin residues in frozen fat, liver, kidney, and brain tissues.[81] No antidote exists, and treatment is initially directed at reducing gastrointestinal absorption and providing symptomatic and supportive care. Treatment must also aim at control of cerebral edema seen in severe poisonings. Administration of dexamethasone and mannitol have been recommended to control bromethalin-induced cerebral edema in mammals.[85] Unfortunately, the efficacy of these diuretic agents in controlling bromethalin-poisoned animals is rarely successful. Animals with severe signs such as seizures, paralysis, or coma generally have a grave prognosis.

Cholecalciferol. Cholecalciferol (vitamin D_3), a newer rodenticide, exploits the fact that rodents are extremely sensitive to small percentage changes in the calcium balance in their blood. Cholecalciferol causes hypercalcemia through mobilization of the body stores of calcium predominantly found in bone.[81] This dystrophic hypercalcemia results in calcification of blood vessels, organs, and soft tissues. It leads to nerve and muscle dysfunction and cardiac arrythmias.[69,86] Diagnosis is possible by submission of serum for $25(OH)D_3$ levels measured by chromatography (Heartland Assays, Ames, IA). Prednisone (6 mg/kg) and furosemide (1 to 4 mg/kg) have been recommended in intoxicated mammals.[69] Favorable results have been obtained in several species using these drugs.[69,86,87] Supportive fluids are essential. Calcitonin therapy has been recommended (1.5 UI/kg SID 7 d), but its efficacy is questionable. Pamidronate disodium (Aredia), a biphosphate, has been recommended in dogs, with 1 to 2 mg/kg given slowly over 2 hours.[69,87] Prognosis is poor in animals in which dystrophic mineralization has already occurred.

Metaldehyde. Metaldehyde is the active ingredient in most slug and snail baits.[88] It is formulated in granules, powder, pellets, and liquid. Protein-rich material such as bran or grain is usually added to the bait to make it more attractive to snails. Unfortunately, other animals find it more palatable as well. Metaldehyde poisoning has been reported in a wide range of species, from dogs to livestock.[88] This is not a common intoxication for reptiles; however, the authors did observe one captive tortoise fatality after the poison was encountered in a household backyard garden.

The mechanism of action of metaldehyde poisoning was once thought to be a result of the degradation of the compound to acetaldehyde. Recent studies suggest metaldehyde itself may be the agent that affects the CNS.[89] GABA levels are decreased by metaldehyde, and this decrease can lead to depression, seizures, and coma.

Clinical signs include ataxia, incoordination and locomotor signs, muscle spasms, abnormal postures, and convulsions.[88] The tortoise seen by the author was comatose and nonresponsive and had its head and legs rigidly extended. Clinical signs develop within a few hours of ingestion. Chemical analysis for metaldehyde confirmation is best obtained from antemortem specimens of stomach contents, serum, and urine, and postmortem from frozen liver samples. Bait material can also be tested.

No specific antidote exists for metaldehyde poisoning. Instead, animals are treated supportively. Fluids should be given and oxygen administered to counter respiratory depression. Mammals display the "shake and bake" syndrome and are treated with diazepam or other appropriate anticonvulsants, and steps are taken to counter the hyperthermia. Prognosis is generally better if the animal survives the first 36 hours.[88] The public is strangely unaware of the hazards of this potent poison.

Repticides

Repticides are products used in some parts of the world exclusively to control reptiles as pests.

Alpha-Chloralose. Alpha-chloralose is a humane poison that produces a hypnotic effect by interfering with the body temperature control mechanism of the reptile.[90] Chloralose is both an avicide and a rodenticide used to kill mice at temperatures below 15°C, but its toxic effects also have been widely demonstrated in reptiles. It is part of the composition of a commercial repticide used in Africa, Madagascar, and along the Indian Ocean (Margoillator, Kit Antilezard, La Reunion). The toxic component is mixed with strawberries and dyed pink to attract geckos and other reptiles. It has also been investigated in neuroscience and veterinary medicine for use as an anesthetic and sedative. Affected reptiles become stunned within a few minutes after ingestion and do not move more than 2 m away from the initial feeding point (Fig. 88.3).

Acetaminophen. Acetaminophen (also known as the generic form of *paracetamol*) is a medication used to treat pain and fever. It is typically used for mild to moderate pain in human medicine. Although there is little risk of accidental ingestion in reptiles, it should be avoided as an analgesic by well-intentioned reptile keepers. In fact, this drug is very toxic to reptiles and is even used to control herpetologic pests in different parts of the world. Acetaminophen was registered for use to control brown tree snakes in Guam by the U.S. Environmental Protection Agency.

The acetaminophen dose of 40 mg and 80 mg results in total or near-total lethality for monitors, pythons, and tree snakes. Its toxicity has been described in the Nile monitor (*Varanus niloticus*) and Burmese python (*Python bivittatus*). It has been used as a poison in invasive reptile eradication projects like the lizard *Ctenasaurus similis* and the brown tree snake (*Boiga irregularis*) in Guam.[91–94] In these projects, mice previously injected with acetaminophen are provided to the wild snakes. Snakes die within 48 hours of consumption of poisoned bait.

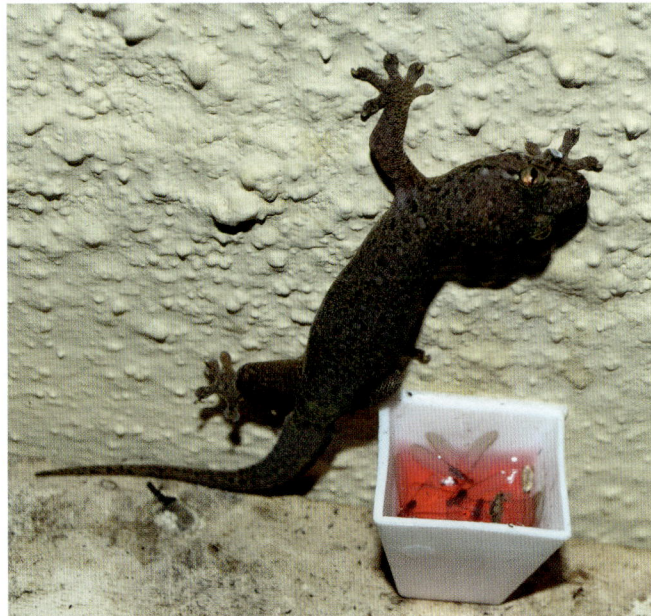

FIG 88.3 Abnormal posture in an Asian house gecko (*Hemidactylus frenatus*) after exposure to a poisonous narcotic used in control of invasive geckos on the island of Mauritius. (Courtesy of Albert Martinez-Silvestre.)

The mechanism of acetaminophen toxicity in reptiles is not known, although it may be due to liver and kidney toxicity, possibly via glutathione depletion, which can lead to hepatic necrosis. Another possibility is the occurrence of methemoglobinemia, which has been observed in cats.[95] Acetaminophen-treated brown tree snakes also displayed severe methemoglobinemia.

Affected animals display no apparent signs of suffering, distress, or discomfort. Only emesis was reported in both monitor lizards and brown tree snakes given the described doses.

Heavy Metal Toxicosis

The risks of heavy metal exposures, such as lead and zinc, is high in free-roaming pets and zoologic collections with public access. However, the occurrence of heavy metal toxicosis among reptiles is not well documented.[96–101] One reason for this is the lack of information regarding reference blood and tissue levels of heavy metals in reptiles. Normal reference ranges have been suggested as a guide to aid in the diagnosis of lead or zinc exposure or toxicity in live iguanas: whole blood lead levels at, 0.06 ± 0.06 mg/mL, and plasma zinc levels at, 2.68 ± 1.66 mg/mL.[102]

Zinc Toxicosis. Zinc is an essential trace element. It is necessary for the synthesis of more than 200 enzymes required for cell division, growth, and gene expression (Cook et al, Proc AAZV, 1989, p 151).[103] Chronic zinc deficiency from improper diet is more commonly seen than acute zinc poisoning from excessive zinc intake. Zinc toxicosis may result from overzealous administration of supplements, ingestion of galvanized metal objects, zinc oxide ointment, or ingestion of pennies. Before 1982, U.S. pennies were more than 90% copper; since that time, they have been 97% zinc (Fig. 88.4). We have seen two iguanas and one snake with gastrointestinal tracts full of pennies that showed signs of

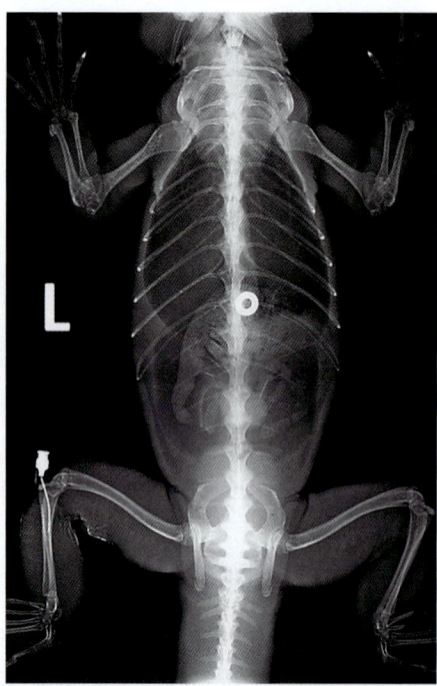

FIG 88.4 Radiographic demonstration of an ingested zinc washer in an iguana that presented with anorexia and lethargy. Plasma zinc levels were significantly elevated confirming the toxicosis. The animal responded to chelation therapy while the washer passed uneventfully. (Courtesy of Stephen J. Divers.)

zinc toxicity. A suspected zinc toxicosis was reported in a Cuban crocodile (*Crocodylus rhombifer*) with a serum zinc concentration of 45.3 ppm (Cook et al, Proc AAZV, 1989, p 151).

The precise mechanism of action of zinc toxicosis is not known. However, the red blood cells, kidneys, pancreas, and liver are most affected. Intravascular hemolysis is the most consistent abnormality seen. Zinc is thought to cause oxidative mechanisms that lyse the red blood cell membrane, leading to anemia.[105]

Clinical signs of zinc toxicosis depend on the amount and form of the zinc ingested. Signs are delayed if coins are the source of the zinc. As few as one or two pennies can cause toxicity. First, the animal may be anorectic and lethargic, and the zinc ingestion may mimic gastrointestinal enteritis. This is followed by intravascular hemolysis, hemoglobinemia, yellow discoloration of the skin and mucous membranes, and weight loss.

Palpation may be positive for coins, but in larger animals, radiographs may be necessary to reveal the pennies (see Fig. 88.4). Elevated zinc levels can be confirmed on a serum/plasma sample antemortem, and in liver, kidney, and pancreas samples postmortem. Treatment consists of removal of the zinc-containing foreign object by endoscopy or surgery. Additional supportive therapy involves fluid treatment to maintain hydration, possible blood transfusion to control anemia, and in severe cases, use of a zinc chelator. However, chelators such as D-penicillamine and calcium-EDTA have been shown to be of questionable value once the source of the exposure has been removed. At our hospital, coins in all three reptiles were successfully removed endoscopically.

Lead Toxicosis. With the prohibition of lead-based paints, lead toxicity is seen less frequently but may still occur. Lead interferes with multiple processes in the body. It affects various cell types, enzymes, tissues, and organ systems. Lead competes with calcium ions, thereby substituting for calcium in bone. Lead mimics and inhibits many cellular actions of calcium and alters calcium flux across membranes.[106] This ultimately increases levels of cytoplasmic calcium in many cell types. Acute calcium-mediated cell death, chronic impairment of neuronal function, diminished energy metabolism by mitochondria result from lead toxicosis, all resulting in apoptosis.

More than 90% of absorbed lead is bound to red blood cells.[101] Lead can be detected antemortem in blood and postmortem in the liver and/or kidney. Care should be taken because blood concentrations do not always correlate with either occurrence or severity of signs.

Clinical signs are similar to those described for zinc, with the addition of neuromuscular dysfunction.[102] In the case of oral ingestion, radiography may show multiple metallic densities in the stomach. Confirmation must be obtained by blood chemical analysis. Published cases of suspected heavy metal toxicosis in reptiles report lead concentrations of 14.7 μg/ml (0.71 μmol/L in a false gharial (*Tomistoma schlegelii*), 3.6 μg/ml (0.17 μmol/L) in a snapping turtle (*Chelydra serpentina*), 4.8 μg/ml (0.23 μmol/L) in a green iguana (*Iguana iguana*), and 8.51 μg/ml (0.41 μmol/L) in a red-eared slider (*Trachemys scripta*) (Cook et al, Proc AAZV, 1989, p 151).[103,107,108] Intestinal perforation has been described in a snapping turtle with lead intoxication (Cook et al, Proc AAZV, 1989, p 151).[104,107,108] In south Spain, high levels of lead were detected in eggs of chameleons (*Chamaelo chamaeleon*), with an associated higher risk of complication of normal incubation or resorption.[109] One case of lead poisoning was cited in a red-eared slider after ingestion of a thermometer containing lead pellets.[108] The main problem is determining if the detected values are greater than the reference ranges of the species.[102]

It is interesting to note that crocodilians are more susceptible to lead poisoning than other reptiles due to the presence of stones in their stomachs. These stones help wear down and dissolve ingested metallic pieces (like saturnism in birds), and liberated lead can then enter the blood stream during digestion.[107,110,111]

Chelation therapy can be started with CaEDTA 30 mg/kg IM SID for 5 days, off for 4 days, and repeated for 5 days.[112] In case of accidental ingestion, prokinetics have been shown to have little effect in lead evacuation.[113]

Successful treatment of zinc/lead toxicity involves removal of the metal-containing objects through surgery or endoscopy and supportive care. Prognosis depends on the amount of metal ingested, the duration of the toxic exposure, and the severity of the resulting anemia. Reptiles must be kept in environments free of potential sources of heavy metal ingestion.

VENOMOUS AND POISONOUS ANIMALS

Snake Envenomations

Snake venoms are complex mixtures of enzymatic and nonenzymatic proteins.[114,115] Derived from modified salivary glands, snake venoms immobilize prey and begin to predigest their tissues (Table 88.1). Hyaluronidase is present in most snake venom and works by catalyzing the cleavage of internal glycosides bonds and mucopolysaccharides.[114,115] This action potentiates the activity of many of the other toxic agents. Phospholipase A$_2$, which causes hydrolytic breakdown of membrane phospholipids, is common to many snake venoms. This molecule displays cytotoxic, anticoagulant (prevents activation of clotting factors), and neurotoxic activities.[114,115] Collagenase is also found in snake venom and leads to the digestion of collagen and breaking down of connective tissue.

Snake venoms are approximately 90% water and, in addition to enzymatic and nonenzymatic proteins, can contain lipids, carbohydrates, and biogenic amines.[114,115,116] The actual toxins that compose the "killing fraction" are referred to as venins. The entire mixture is called venom. Not only does much variability exist in venom composition among snake species, tremendous variability is also seen in susceptibility to different snake venoms by potential prey species.

Venomous snakes do appear to be relatively more resistant to their own venom (Fig. 88.5).[114] Neutralizing antibodies have been documented in the serum of many snakes to the toxins of their own venom.[116,117] In our experience, twice in prairie rattlesnakes (*Crotalus viridus*) and once in western diamondback rattlesnakes (*Crotalus atrox*), snakes were seen to die after being bitten by a conspecific. The severity of the response appears to be dependent on the location of the bite, the volume of venom injected, and the size of the recipient. We have also seen bites between conspecifics and self-inflicted bites that were nonfatal.

Certain nonvenomous snake species that prey on other snakes (including venomous ones), such as the king snake (*Lampropeltis getulus*), also appear to have some resistance to venom.[118] Despite evidence that this venom resistance exists, variability in the venom-neutralizing properties of serum of snakes within genus *Lampropeltis* is also apparent and not always protective. Sometimes when these nonvenomous colubrids are bitten by venomous species, they die.[119]

Beginning in the 1930s, resistance to venoms among both conspecifics and congenerics was observed and theorized. For example, in rattlesnakes, bites between conspecifics, bites between congenetic species, and an individual's bite on itself were documented and observed to be nonlethal.[120] Some species of Australian elapids are not only immune to their own venom but also immune to venom of conspecifics and congenerics of the same continent. In contrast, several authors found examples in other venomous snake species where no such immunity was present, where bites between individuals of the same genus or same species has fatal consequences.[121] In these cases, the bitten snakes displayed clear symptoms of envenomation before death. In captivity, most cases between reptiles of the same species occur during feeding or courtship. In the king cobra (*Ophyophagus hannah*), mating season is a particularly delicate period because males have been seen to bite females. It is noted that in most cases, aside from some tissue damage, the bite is nonlethal.[122,123] In the venomous snake *Bothriopsis taeniata*, death of specimens has been observed in conspecific bites. In the author's experience, we have also witnessed a bite of a male *Agkistrodon contortrix* on a same species cage-mate to be nonfatal, only causing inflammation in the region. Another conspecific bite was observed during copulation from a female upon a male *Trimerisurus trigonocephalus*, with almost no effect apart from a small wound. Also, a female prairie rattlesnake (*Crotalus viridus*) found badly tangled in a ball of masking tape was seen to bite itself multiple times while the tape was removed. Despite numerous bites, the snake showed no ill effects and was successfully released 1 week later.

Humans repeatedly bitten by venomous snakes have claimed immunity to their bite. Satisfactory serologic evidence for these claims has not been established. Effective antivenins exist for many venomous snake bites. A vaccine against rattlesnake bites (Rattlesnake Vaccine, Red Rock Biologics, Woodland, CA, http://www.redrockbiologics.com) has recently been marketed for dogs. However, its overall effectiveness has not been determined.

Lizard Envenomations

Of the approximately 3000 species of lizards, only two known poisonous species exist. The Gila monster, *Heloderma suspectum* (with two subspecies), and the Mexican beaded lizard, *H. horridum* (with three subspecies), comprise the venomous lizards and are found only in the Americas. Their venom is only used in defense.[124]

The venom of these lizards is antigenically unrelated to snake venom.[125] The venom glands are in the lower jaw, and the venom is delivered to the gums at the base of the teeth. Delivery of the venom is dependent on intense chewing action.

Heloderma venom consists of multiple enzymatic proteins, including hyaluronidase, phospholipase, arginine hydrolase, and kallikrein-like

TABLE 88.1 **Some Typical Enzymes Found in Pit Viper Venom**	
Phospholipase A	Protease
Phospholipase B	Arginine ester hydrolase
Acetycholinesterase	Collagenase
Phosphodiesterase	Biogenic amines
Hyaluronidase	RNAase, DNAase

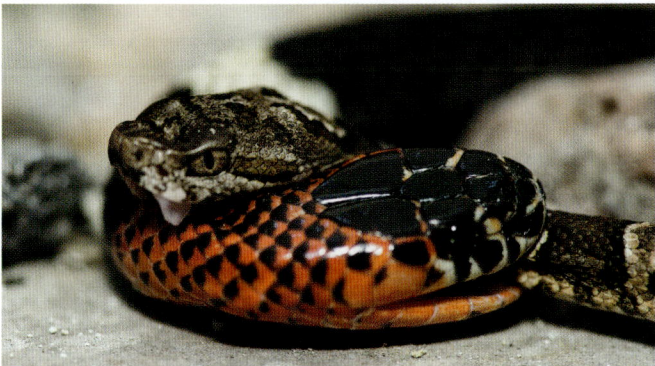

FIG 88.5 Double bite between a coral snake (*Micrurus* sp.) and a South American pit viper (*Bothrops diporus*). (The coral snake, immune to the venom of the pit viper, finished swallowing his foe.) (Courtesy of Fran Brito.)

enzymes.[124] Other proteins have been identified in this venom, including gilatoxin and helothermine.

Hyaluronidase acts as a spreading factor, decreases the viscosity of connective tissue, and catalyzes the cleavage of acid mucoglycosides.[114,115] Arginine hydrolase causes hydrolysis of peptide linkages, and the kallikrein-like enzymes cause vasodilation, increase capillary permeability, lead to edema, and affect the contraction or relaxation of extravascular smooth muscle. Gilatoxin is a neurotoxic protein.[126] Helothermine has been shown to depress the body temperature in mice subjected to this poison.[127] Bites of these lizards to people have been reported as very painful. Currently, no specific antivenom is available for venomous lizard bites, and treatment is supportive. Gila monsters appear to be relatively resistant to the effects of their own venom. The evolution of the venom in these lizards and their primitive delivery system appears to be for defense, for it is not used in the apprehension of prey. This sets it apart from snake and spider venoms, which are used in defense but are primarily designed for immobilization and predigestion of prey.

In lizards, Heloderma bites are common between partners in the same terrarium, either by territoriality, character, or during the breeding season; however, the authors have witnessed no deaths. Conspecific immunity may be because of osteoderms present in their skin that act as a "protective layer," their specific method of envenomation, gender, or a particular immunity to their own venom.[128,129]

Amphibian Toxins

Certain amphibians are poisonous and can cause intoxications. In the United States, two toad species (genus *Bufo*) are the source of most toad poisonings.

The cane or marine toad (*Rhinella* [*Bufo*] *marinus*) and the Colorado River toad (*B. alvarius*) are the two species most implicated.[130]

All *Bufo* species of toads have parotid glands that release toxic substances when the animals are threatened. These are biologically active compounds such as dopamine, norepinephrine, epinephrine, serotonin, bufotenine, bufagenin, bufotoxins, and indolealkylamines.[131] Severe toxicosis has been seen in small animals that bite, masticate, or hold these toads in their mouths. The active compounds secreted from the toad parotid gland are rapidly absorbed by the mucous membranes of the predator and enter the systemic circulation.

Once these compounds have entered the circulation, the greatest effects are seen on the peripheral vascular system, the CNS, and the heart. Bufotenine has pressor effects on blood vessels but may act as a hallucinogen as well.[131] Bufagenin has digitalis-like effects causing alterations in heart rate and rhythm.[130–132] Bufotoxins are vasoconstrictors and add to pressor effects.[131] Indolealkylamines have activity similar to the hallucinogen lysergic acid diethylamide.[126]

Dogs are most commonly affected by amphibian parotid toxins. However, adverse reactions have also been reported in cats and ferrets. Exposure in reptiles has not been documented but anecdotal reports of poisonings do exist. Therefore the assumption is logical that predatory reptiles that include amphibians in their diet might encounter and ingest poisonous toads. No specific antidote is available and treatment is supportive. Therapy includes thorough flushing of the oral cavity. Severely affected animals may need medications to stabilize heart rhythms and control seizures. Supportive care involving fluids may be necessary. Many other toxicoses and conditions can lead to neuropathies, and cardiac arrhythmias can present with signs similar to those of toad poisonings. Differential diagnosis must always be considered and explored.

Fire Ants

In the early 1900s, the imported fire ant reached the United States from South America. The black fire ant (*Solenopsis richteri*) has remained in a small area of central Alabama and Mississippi. The red imported fire ant (*Solenopsis invicta*) has now reached 13 southern states from Texas to North Carolina.[133] In some areas, as many as 60% of local humans report being stung at least once annually.[134] For humans, 1% of stings result in hypersensitivity reactions.[134,135]

These fire ants bite and sting. First, the ant uses powerful mandibles to bite and anchor itself to the skin of the victim, then it uses its abdominal stinger to inject venom in a series of stings rotating in a circle around the head. Unlike the venom of most stinging insects, ant venom is composed primarily of alkaloids, particularly piperadine. Ant venoms have local necrotic and hemolytic effects.[133,134,135]

The authors have seen several small reptiles victimized by these predatory ants in Louisiana and Florida. Neonatal reptiles are especially vulnerable to these aggressive insects.

No antidote therapy exists; however, the use of antihistamines, topical steroid ointments (1% hydrocortisone), topical alcohol, and warm water baths may provide symptomatic relief.

Fire ants generally build mounds in warm sunny areas, places where reptiles typically bask. We can expect more reptile species to fall victim to the bites of these ants as these predatory insects continue to expand their range. Efforts to control the spread of these ants so far have not been effective.

Firefly Toxicosis

Reptile caretakers often supplement the diet of captive animals with freshly caught insects. Fireflies of the genus *Photinus* have been shown to contain steroidal pyrones (lucibufagins) that are poisonous.[136] These pyrones are structurally similar to cardenolides of plants and bufodienolides of toads, both of which are well-studied toxins.[136,137,138] These two compounds cause nausea and vomiting at low concentrations and can be potentially cardiotoxic at higher dosages. If extrapolations from mammals are correct, less than one half of a firefly could be lethal to a 100-g lizard.

Bearded dragons (*Pogona vitticeps*) have shown fatal intoxication after ingestion of fireflies.[139] In both cases documented, the lizards showed signs 30 to 60 minutes after ingestion. Clinical signs included pronounced oral gaping, intense color change in the neck area, and dyspnea. Both animals died within 90 minutes of eating the fireflies. At present, no effective therapy is known.

Lucibufigins protect fireflies from predators. Spiders, birds, and several species of lizard have been shown to avoid fireflies.[140–142] Like many lizards, bearded dragons show indiscriminate eating strategies and may ingest toxic substances. Furthermore, the bearded dragon, an Australian native, has no natural contact with *Photinus* species of fireflies and thus may exhibit no self-protective behavior.

Other lizard species have been shown to eat fireflies without lethal results. In one study, both fence lizards (*Sceloporus undulatus*) and skinks (*Eumeces laticeps*) were fed fireflies.[143] Both species readily attacked and ate the insects but immediately spit them out, wiping their mouths and rubbing their faces on the ground. When offered fireflies a second time (even days later) they refused to eat them and exhibited the same mouth wiping that they displayed after tasting the insects. Next, the authors stuffed five to seven fireflies into live crickets. Both types of lizards ate the crickets but subsequently regurgitated all the crickets they had eaten. No deaths of either species occurred. This study concluded that fireflies were distasteful and could cause regurgitation and vomiting. The conclusion was that the ingestion of fireflies was not always lethal to all lizard species.

Keepers must be advised to feed only safe food items. Any questions should be referred to a veterinarian. Fireflies should not be fed to reptiles nor any insects that sequester cardenolides, such as monarch butterflies (*Donaeus plexxipus*), queen butterflies (*Donaeus gillipus*), and lygaeid bugs (*Oncopeltus fasciatus*).[139] Other lizard species and other captive reptiles may be susceptible to intoxication after firefly ingestion, and they should not be offered as food.

SMOKE INHALATION

Dangerous fires are still a daily occurrence in the new millennium. In the continental United States alone, every 17 seconds a fire department responds to a fire call.[144] Depending on the source, it is estimated that 50% to 80% of fire deaths are the direct result of smoke inhalation rather than injuries from burns or trauma.

When compared to the rest of the world, the United States has one of the highest death rates caused by fire. This may be attributable to wider use of synthetic materials for building and furnishings. These synthetic substances generally produce much more toxic combustion substances. In addition, the nature of our buildings, and the presence of more high rises, skyscrapers, and multifloor dwellings make it much more difficult to escape from the effects of a disastrous fire and much harder to stop the fires once started.

In European countries, forest fires affect mainly Hermann's tortoise (*Testudo hermanni*). If they are not initially killed outright from the fire and burns, they subsequently will succumb to smoke inhalation. In Africa, the species most affected by smoke inhalation due to forest fires are the threatened Malagasy tortoises (*Astrochelys radiata* or *Astrochelys yniphora*). Some species such as gopher tortoises (*Gopherus agasizii*) are said to be more likely to survive fires. This may be a function of their natural history, such as digging burrows or using rabbit burrows as dens.

The pathophysiology of smoke inhalation is complex. Generally, a toxic combustion product (i.e., smoke) exerts its poisonous effects by filling enclosed vital airways with gases other than oxygen and by inducing local chemical reactions in the respiratory tract; chemical asphyxiates elicit toxic changes in tissue distant from the lung.[145] Water solubility of toxic inhalants is the most important factor in determining the level of injury. Injury from water-soluble molecules occurs in the upper airways. Chemical toxicants with low water solubility reach the lungs, where they then exert their damaging effects. In addition, duration of exposure, concentration of the combustion products, and toxin particle size all contribute to the overall severity of the injury. Pathologic changes in the lungs and respiratory tissues may progress over hours to days. Inhalation of super-heated particulate matter in smoke can lead to extensive tissue damage.

In our practice, several captive reptiles have been presented after being exposed to the damaging smoke of house fires. Two young ball pythons arrived after a particularly aggressive apartment fire. Direct laryngoscopy of the animals revealed the accumulation of soot and carbonaceous debris, copious secretions, and edematous laryngeal tissue. Both snakes were in severe respiratory compromise. Their breathing was weak and rapid, and the airways became increasingly edematous. The animals were treated by intubating and administering 100% oxygen and supportive fluids. Despite our aggressive efforts, the smaller snake continued to deteriorate and died. After 2 days of therapy, the larger snake survived. A box turtle presented after a residential fire. The reptile displayed no burns, was nonresponsive, and never regained consciousness despite our efforts, which included supplemental oxygen, fluid therapy, antibiotics, and suctioning the airways. The turtle died roughly 2 hours after exposure. Effective management of smoke inhalation must include establishing airway patency, administration of supplemental oxygen, frequent airway suctioning and removal of both debris and secretions, and cardiovascular support. Early intubation is often more beneficial than waiting for the animal to decompensate. Radiographic evidence of lung damage due to smoke inhalation may not be evident for several hours.

TABLE 88.2	Factors That Affect the Potential Toxicity of Poisonous Plants
Geographic and Seasonal Variables
Plants poisonous in one part of the world may not be as toxic in other areas.
Season.
Plant Part Ingested
Not all parts of poisonous plants are always toxic.
Example: tomato; very edible fruit; stems and leaves contain toxic alkaloids.
Example: apples, peaches, apricots; have cyanide-containing seeds; fruit is edible.
Absorbability of Toxins
Apples, peaches, apricots: cyanide not released unless seeds are broken
Castor bean: poison (ricin) not released unless seeds are chewed
Species That Ingest the Plant
Poisonous plant intoxication often depends directly on the species involved.

Smoke inhalation patients are labor intensive to manage but may result in successful outcomes if animals are treated early and aggressively. Often intoxication from smoke inhalation is seen in wild chelonians after forest fires. It is not uncommon in animals living in areas susceptible to fire. In reptiles, pulmonary edema and congestion is often observed in the respiratory tree during necropsy.[145]

POISONOUS PLANTS

Some plants produce very powerful poisons. For many years, veterinary toxicology largely dealt with livestock suffering from plant poisonings. The last 20 years have seen tremendous growth in our understanding of small and zoologic animal intoxications.

Because many reptiles are either partially or entirely herbivorous, the potential for the accidental ingestion of toxic plants is real (Table 88.2). Although consideration of all plants potentially toxic to reptiles is beyond our present discussion, this section examines the more frequently encountered plant poisonings and those commonly reported in the literature. See Table 88.3 for a list of the most common toxic plants for reptiles.

Heaths (Family: Ericaceae)

The heath family plants (laurel [*Laurus nobilis*], rhodendrons [*Rhododendron*], azaleas [*Rhododendron penthatera* sp., *Rhododendron tusutsusi* sp]) are commonly planted in the United States as ornamental shrubbery. These plants contain grayanotoxins (diterpenoids) that interfere with membrane-based sodium channels.[146,147] The toxin is found in the stem, leaves, flowers, and nectar.[148] Ingestion can lead to bradycardia, gastrointestinal signs, depression, ataxia, and convulsions.[148] No antidote exists; treatment is supportive. We have seen two iguanas poisoned after eating azalea plants, one of which died. Both lizards were recumbent and nonresponsive a few hours after ingestion. Toxic levels in dogs begin at 7 mg/kg.[146,147] The one lizard died shortly after presentation.

Yews (Family: Taxaceae)

Ground hemlock (*Taxus canadensis*), Florida yew (*Taxus floridana*), English yew (*Taxus bacatta*), Pacific yew (*Taxus brevifolia*), and Japanese yew (*Taxus cuspidata*) are all members of a group that contains taxine, a cardiotoxic alkaloid.[146,147] This substance is a sodium channel blocker

TABLE 88.3   List of Plants That Can Be Toxic to Reptiles+

Acokanthera—*Acokanthera* spp. (all parts toxic, except ripe fruit)
Amaryllis—*Amaryllis* spp.
Angel's trumpet—*Datura* spp. (leaves, seeds, flowers)
Apricot—*Prunus armeniaca* (pits, leaves, and bark)
Apple—*Malus* spp., (seeds, leaves, bark)
Avocado—*Persea Americana* (pit, leaves, unripe fruit, stems)
Azalea—*Rhododendron canadenis*
Balsam pear, bitter melon—*Momordica charantia*
Baneberry—*Actaea rubra, A. pachypoda*
Belladonna—*Atropa belladonna*
Bird of paradise—*Poinciana* and related spp. (seed pods and flowers)
Bittersweet—*Celastrus* spp.
Black locust—*Robinia pseudoacacia*
Boxwood—*Boxus* spp.
Bracken Fern—*Pteridium aquilinum*
Buckthorn—*Karwinskia humboldtiana* and related spp.
Burdock—*Arctium* spp.
Buttercup—*Ranunculus* spp.
Caladium—*Caladium* spp.
Calla lily—*Zantedeschia aethiopica*
Catclaw acacia—*Acacia greggii* (twigs and leaves)
Castor bean—*Ricinus communis*
Cherry—*Prunus* spp. (pits, leaves and bark)
Chinaberry—*Melia azadarach*
Clematis—*Clematis montana* and related spp.
Coral plant—*Jatropha mutifida*
Crocus (autumn)—*Cholochicum autumnale*
Cycad or sago cycas—*Cycas revoluta*
Daffodil—*Narcissus tazetta*
Daphne—*Daphne mezerum*
Death camas—*Zigadenus venenosus* and other related species
Delphinium—*Delphinium* spp.
Devil's ivy—*Epipremnum aureum*
Dieffenbachia (dumb cane)—*Dieffenbachia* spp.
Eggplant—*Solonum melongena* (unripe/ripe fruit, leaves)
Elderberry—*Sambucus mexicana* (roots, leaves, stems, bark)
Elephant's ears or taro—*Colocasia* spp.
Euonymus—*Euonymus* spp. (filit, bark, leaves)
European pennyroyal—*Mentha pulegium*
Figs—*Ficus* spp. (sap)
Four o'clock—*Mirabilis jalapa*
Heliotrope—*Heliotropium* spp. (leaves)
Henbane—*Hyoscyamus niger*
Holly—*Ilex aquifolium* and related spp. (leaves, berries)
Horse chestnut—*Aesculus hippocastanum* and related spp.
Horse nettle—*Solanum carolinense*
Hyacinth—*Hyacinthus orientalis*
Hydrangea—*Hydrangea* spp.
Iris—*Iris* spp.
Ivy (Boston, English, and some others)—*Hedera* spp.
Jack-in-the-pulpit—*Arisaema* spp.
Jerusalem cherry—*Solanum pseudocapsicum* and related spp. (leaves, seeds, and flowers)
Jonquil—*Narcissus jonquilla*
Juniper—*Juniperus* spp.
Lantana—*Lantana camara*
Larkspur—*Delphinium* spp.

Laurel—*Kalmia* spp.
Lily-of-the-valley—*Convalleria majalis*
Lobelia—*Lobelia* spp.
Locoweed—*Astragalus* spp. and *Oxytopis* spp.
Lupine—*Lupinus* spp.
Marijuana—*Cannabis sativa*
Milkweed—*Asclepias* spp.
Mistletoe—*Phoradendron villosum*
Mock orange—*Philadelphus* spp.
Moonseed—*Menispermum canadense*
Monkshood—*Aconitum* spp.
Morning glory—*Ipomoea violacea* (seeds)
Mushrooms—*Amanita* spp. and many others, although some species, such as box turtles (*Terrapene* sp.), seem immune to these toxic mushrooms
Narcissus—*Narcissus* spp.
Oak—*Quercus* spp.
Oleander—*Nerium oleander*
Peach—*Prunus persica* (leaves, pit, bark)
Pear—*Pyrus* spp. (leaves, seeds, bark)
Peony—*Paeonia officinalis*
Periwinkle—*Vinca minor, Vinca rosea*
Peyote—*Lophophora williamsii*
Philodendron—*Philodendron* spp. and *Monstera* spp.
Plum—*Prunus* spp. (leaves, pit, bark)
Poison hemlock—*Conium maculatum*
Poison ivy—*Toxicodendron radicans*, includes *T. rydbergii*
Poison oak—*Toxicodendron querciflium* and *T. diversilobum*
Poison sumac—*Rhux vernix*
Poinsettia—*Euphorbia pulcherrima*
Poppy—*Papaver somniferum* and related spp.
Pokeweed—*Phytolacca Americana*
Potato—*Solanum tuberosum* (sprouts, leaves, berries, green tubers)
Pothos—*Eprimemnum aureum*
Primrose—*Prmula* spp.
Privet—*Ligustrum vulgare*
Ragwort—*Senecio jacobea* and related spp.
Red maple—*Acer rubrum*
Rhododendron—*Rhododendron* spp.
Rhubarb—*Rheum rhabarbarum* (leaves)
Rosary pea—*Abrus precatorius*
Sage—*Salvia officinalis*
Shamrock plant—*Medicago lupulina, Trifolium repens, Oxalis acetosella*
Skunk cabbage—*Symplocarpus foetidus*
Snowdrop—*Galanthus nivalis*
Sorrel—*Rumex* spp., *Oxalis* spp.
Spurges—*Euphorbia* spp.
Star of Bethlehem—*Ornithogalum umbellatum*
Sweet pea—*Lathyrus odoratus*
Tobacco—*Nicotiania* spp.
Tomato—*Lycopersicon esculentum* (stems and leaves)
Tulip—*Tulipa* spp.
Virginia creeper—*Panthenocissus quinquefolia*
Vetches—*Vicia* spp.
Water hemlock—*Cicuta* spp.
Waxberry—*Symphoricarpos albus*
Wisteria—*Wisteria* spp.
Yew—*Taxus* spp.

Plant names can vary depending on the source and region. Consult a veterinarian with concerns about plants before feeding them to your reptile or using them in your home or yard.

that can cause both cardiac and neurologic toxicity.[147] The bark, leaves, and seeds are poisonous but not the red fruit surrounding the seeds of these ornamental shrubs.[146,147] Wild birds spread the seeds by eating the fruit (nontoxic) and then excreting the seeds (toxic, but the bird does not chew them). No antidote exists. Poisonings have been reported in livestock, dogs, and caged birds.[149]

Lilies (Family: Liliaceae, Xanthorrhoeaceae, Asparagaceae)

Easter lily (*Lilium longiflorum*), tiger lily (*Lilium lancifolium*), day lily (*Hemerocallis* sp.), Japanese showy lily (*Lilium speciosum*), and Asiatic lily (*Lilium asiàtica*) are known to be poisonous to cats by causing renal toxicosis.[147] All parts of the plant are poisonous.[147] In addition, lily of the valley (*Convallaria majalis*) contains a potent cardiac glycoside.[150] Asparagus contains excess proteins, so as a consequence of it metabolism, excessive uric acid may be produced and the reptile can suffer gout. In our experience, toxic plant ingestion by reptiles is likely possible; captivity exposes animals to all sorts of novel plant exposures. We have administered activated charcoal to an iguana that ingested Easter lilies. The animal survived with supportive therapy, including fluids, warmth, and oxygen.

Fruit Seeds

The seeds of apples, apricots, cherries, peaches, plums, and the jetberry bush contain cyanogenic glycosides.[151] The seeds are dangerous if the seed capsule is broken. In humans, as few as 5 to 25 broken seeds can cause cyanide toxicosis.[152] Cyanide disrupts the ability of cells to use oxidative phosphorylation by poisoning mitochondria. The net effect is tissue hypoxia. The onset of clinical signs may be very rapid, and death can occur suddenly. Treatment for cyanide toxicosis is often not successful but does include 100% oxygen administration, supplemental fluids, and perhaps sodium nitrate or sodium thiosulfate. Attention must be given to what captive reptiles are eating, being fed, or are coming into contact with.

Avocado

Avocado (*Persea americana*) has been shown to be toxic to rabbits, mice, and caged birds.[147,153] All above-ground parts of the plant are toxic.[147] Persin, a compound isolated from the leaves, is believed to be the toxin responsible for avocado toxicity.[153] Intoxicated mammals display cardiac arrhythmias, necrosis of the myocardium, and acute death.[153] Caged birds show respiratory distress.[147,153]

Douglas Mader (personal communication) reports observing green iguanas in the wild eating avocados that have fallen on the ground. However, with all the toxicity reports in other species regarding the ingestion of avocados, they should be avoided in reptile diets.

Ricins (*Ricinus communis*)

Castor bean plants contain ricins, a potent toxin that stops protein synthesis. The poison, present in the whole plant, is most concentrated in seeds.[147] Chewing or breaking of the seed coat is necessary before intoxication can take place. For mice, rats, rabbits, and dogs, one seed can be fatal. In dogs, clinical signs involve the gastrointestinal tract but can include kidney failure and convulsions.[154] No known antidote is available. All ingestions of castor beans should be taken seriously because of the high toxicity. However, seed coats are not always chewed or broken when animals ingest seeds. Often the seeds pass undigested, and animals show no clinical signs.[154]

Cycad (Sago) Palms (*Cycas revoluta*)

These palms are used as house/garden plants and are naturally occurring in tropical and subtropical regions. All parts of the plant are toxic.[147]

The nuts (seeds) are most toxic and only produced by female plants.[147] Toxins induce gastrointestinal, hepatic signs (cycasin), and neurologic signs (B-methylamino-L-alanine).[155] Gastrointestinal signs generally appear within 24 hours of ingestion.[155] No antidote exists; treatment is supportive. Clients should be encouraged to bring in the chewed plant to help identify the species.

Holly (*Ilex* spp.), Mistletoe (*Viscum* spp.), and Poinsettia (*Euphorbia pulcherrima*)

During the holiday season (usually Christmas in the Northern Hemisphere), several potentially toxic plants are often brought into the home.

Mistletoe are evergreen parasitic plants that grow on trees. Human exposures usually involve the berries either eaten by small children or brewed into tea.[156] Attempts to reproduce clinical signs in animals have been unsuccessful. In humans, the most common clinical signs are gastrointestinal. No antidote is available, and treatment is supportive. In children and mammalian companion animals, this intoxication is not lethal.

Holly includes English or Christmas holly (*Ilex aquifolium*), American or white holly (*Ilex opaca*), and winterberry (*Ilex verticillata*). Berries contain the sapponin ilicin, which is a potent gastrointestinal irritant.[147,156] In humans and companion mammalian species, the most common sign is digestive upset. No antidote exists, and treatment is symptomatic. These types of poisonings are not lethal.

Poinsettia (*Euphorbia pulcherrima*) possesses a milky sap rich in diterpenoids.[156] These molecules are fairly irritating to the skin, mucous membranes, and gastrointestinal tract. Reports of toxicity stem from a single account.[157] Poisoning is rare, and treatment is supportive.

Plants Containing Cardiac Glycosides

Several plants contain cardiac glycosides, including oleander (*Nerium oleander*), foxglove (*Digitalis purpurea*), and lily of the valley (*Convallaria majalis*).[147] For oleander, all parts of the leaf are poisonous; a single leaf well-chewed has been reported to be lethal.[158] Foxglove leaves and seeds are toxic. Lily of the valley poisoning comes from leaves, flowers, and roots. The cardiac glycosides are gastrointestinal irritants, may be responsible for a variety of cardiac arrhythmias (irregular pulse, bradycardia, rapid thready pulse, ventricular fibrillation), and can be fatal.

Ivy (*Hedera* spp.)

Ivy is used in greenhouses, as a houseplant, and as a ground cover. English ivy (*Hedera helix*), Atlantic or Irish ivy (*Hederix hibernica*), Persian ivy (*Hedera colchica*), etc., are all potentially toxic.[147] These plants, particularly the berries, contain terpenoids.[147] These molecules can cause salivation, gastrointestinal irritation, and diarrhea. Most ingestions are not serious, and treatment is supportive.

Plants Containing Nicotine

Tobacco products, including pipe tobacco, cigarettes, cigars, chewing tobacco, and snuff, contain the alkaloid nicotine. Nicotine is a stimulant of the CNS and cardiovascular system. It stimulates sympathetic ganglia and increases heart rate and blood pressure. High-dose exposures can cause paralysis of chest muscles and lead to respiratory compromise and cardiac arrest.[159] Cigarettes average from 15 to 25 mg of nicotine depending on the brand. Cigars have four to five times the nicotine of cigarettes. Chewing tobacco is even more palatable to animals because of flavors added (e.g., honey, sugar, molasses, cinnamon, licorice, and various syrups). Aids to stop smoking can also be a source of accidental nicotine ingestion. Nicotine patches usually contain between 7 and 25 mg, and nicotine gum contains 2 to 4 mg per piece. Some garden spray insecticides contain 40% nicotine (Black Leaf 40).

As few as two cigarettes have been shown to cause lethal poisonings in puppies.[159] No data exists for secondary smoke intoxication, but an association between chronic respiratory conditions in captive reptiles and households with one or more smokers have long been suspected by the authors (personal observation). Clinical signs of high-dose nicotine intoxication include excitement followed by depression, diarrhea, seizures, coma, and respiratory or cardiac arrest.[160] No known antidote exists. Treatment includes frequent monitoring of heart rate, and animals may benefit from fluid therapy and oxygen administration. Prognosis is poor for high-dose intoxication.

Captive reptiles may ingest cigar and cigarette butts, pipe tobacco, chewing tobacco, or nicotine patches and gums. We have seen death in one African spurred tortoise (*Centrochelys sulcata*) and one green iguana after eating several cigarette butts.

Treatment includes fluid therapy and oxygen administration. Prognosis is poor for long exposure intoxications. No intoxications have been seen by ingestion of "e-cigarettes" or their nicotine-containing fillers, but the potential for this type of poisoning exists.

Oak (*Quercus* spp.)

Oak trees are found almost worldwide. Acorns, buds, twigs, and leaves have been implicated, but most intoxications involve either immature leaves or freshly fallen acorns in the spring.[161]

Oaks are heterophile plants (leaves of differing ages on the same plant). In several species, the younger trees have leaves that are more pointed than in adult plants and have a different composition, making them less palatable to leaf-eating animals. This may confer a protective advantage to young plants, allowing them to grow and survive.

Toxicosis from oak is produced by high concentrations of tannic acid and its metabolites, gallic acid and pyrogallol. Ingestion of toxic amounts of oak have been shown to cause ulcerative lesions in the upper and lower gastrointestinal tract, liver lesions, and necrosis of renal epithelial cells in the proximal tubules.[147]

A fatal episode of oak intoxication has been reported in a tortoise.[162] An African spurred tortoise was found dead in an outdoor enclosure where numerous oak trees hung over and into the area. On necropsy, the stomach of the tortoise was markedly distended with partially digested oak leaves. Extensive necrosis was found in the oral cavity, esophagus, stomach, and kidneys. The proximal renal tubules showed 45% necrosis.

Reports of this type show the importance for both caretakers and veterinarians to be aware of the potential for toxicity of any plant material ingested either in browsing or as an intentional part of the captive diet. Nutrition of captive reptiles must be carefully considered and continually monitored.

Marijuana (*Cannabis sativa*)

Marijuana continues to be the most used illicit drug in the United States.[163] Due to recent legislation, medical and recreational marijuana has been legalized in some U.S. states. As a result, the potential for companion animals to be exposed to varying forms of marijuana has greatly increased. *Cannabis sativa* has been used for centuries for its hemp fiber, as rope, and for its psychoactive resins. Totally or partially herbivorous captive reptiles may encounter growing marijuana plants, ingest dried stems, leaves, and flowers, or marijuana edibles.

The main active ingredient of marijuana is tetrahydrocannabinol (THC). The highest concentration of this psychoactive constituent is found in the leaves and the flowering tops of plants.[163–165] Hashish is the dried resin of flower tops. The precise mechanism of action of THC is unknown, but the psychoactive effects of this drug are thought to stem from a number of sites within the CNS, including cholinergic, dopaminergic, serotonergic, noradrenergic, and GABA receptors.[163–165] Ingested marijuana shows effects much more slowly than the results of the inhaled smoke; however, the effects of ingested THC last much longer.

Clinical signs after ingestion of marijuana include mydriasis, weakness, ataxia, bradycardia, hypothermia, and stupor.[163] The extent of clinical signs after marijuana ingestion is almost totally dose related.

Treatment for marijuana ingestion is primarily supportive and symptomatic. Marijuana intoxications are rarely fatal because of the wide margin of safety of THC. Activated charcoal administration is recommended to decrease enterohepatic recirculation. For most vertebrates, minimum lethal oral dosage for THC is greater than 3 g/kg.[163] Despite its relative safety margin, recovery after ingestion may be prolonged and take up to 3 to 4 days. Fluids and monitoring of body temperature may be beneficial.

We have treated two reptiles for having ingested large amounts of marijuana. A 4-kg (10 lb) African spurred tortoise showed no effects after eating four marijuana cigarettes. However, a 3-kg (6 lb) male green iguana was stuporous after eating into a "baggie" of marijuana and needed support. Both animals recovered completely. The potential exists for captive reptiles to ingest a variety of illicit drugs. Cannabis intoxication has also been reported in green iguanas.[166]

The herbivorous Steppe or Russian tortoise (*Agryonemis horsfieldii*) has a curious selective diet in the wild. They avoid some plants such as grasses that represent an important component of the plant community. Surprisingly, their preferred food items are the papaveraceae flowers (Opium plants), highly toxic for herbivorous mammals.[167] The tortoise seems resistant to the high concentrations of papaverine. This is an adaptive ecology that avoids sharing the same source of food between different species of herbivorous animals in a harsh environment.

Mushrooms

Confirmed mushroom toxicities are relatively rare, but the potential for such poisonings remain. For humans poisoned by mushrooms in the United States, the exact species is never identified in 95% of cases.[168] Furthermore, for humans known to have ingested toxic mushrooms, the individuals show no symptoms in 50% of the cases. Far and away the most toxic North American mushrooms are members of the *Amanita* species. The next most dangerous are hallucinogenic mushrooms.

The rarity of mushroom poisoning, lack of serious effects, and the inability of most physicians and veterinarians to correctly identify mushroom species involved all contribute to complicating the diagnosis. Nevertheless, a deliberate strategy and treatment plan for suspected mushroom poisoning is necessary. Veterinarians must strive to learn the toxic varieties of mushrooms in their region and their general incidence. Successful diagnosis includes gross identification of the mushroom specimen and a microscopic spore assessment ("spore-prints") by trained mycologists. The authors use mycologists from the Rocky Mountain Poison and Drug Center for mushroom identification in suspected mushroom poisonings. Investigation and confirmation of species by such collaboration is crucial to distinguishing toxic mushrooms from those mistakenly believed to be edible. Veterinarians must establish solid contacts with other local health professionals, such as human toxicologists, university mycologists, and laboratories well versed in toxicologic analysis.

Captive reptiles can be exposed to mushrooms in yards and greenhouses, in household terrariums, and as additives to their diet. Owners witnessing potential toxic mushroom ingestions should present the culprit mushroom for identification. *A. pantherina* occur throughout the United States and usually exists singly.[169] It has a brilliant red cap and is often photographed by naturalists because of its dramatic appearance. These mushrooms contain ibotenic acid and muscicol, its decarboxylated metabolite. Ibotenic acid is related structurally to the stimulatory transmitter agent, glutamic acid. Muscimol is very similar to the neurotransmitter, GABA, and acts as a GABA agonist with typical GABA signs and manifestations. Treatment is supportive. Most GABA manifestations respond solely to supportive care, and the animals completely recover. Benzodiazepines, such as diazepam, may be required for the management of seizures.

We have seen one case where a pet iguana ingested *Amanita pantherina* in a backyard. Within 30 minutes of ingestions, the approximately 1-kg lizard became lethargic and ataxic. The owners brought parts of the remaining mushrooms along with the lizard to facilitate identification and diagnosis. The iguana responded within a few hours to fluids, warmth, and support. No long-lasting effects were noted, and the animal was released after 24 hours. Some tortoises, such as box turtles, have been described as immune to certain toxic mushrooms.[170] Some species of mushrooms eaten by box turtles are quite poisonous to humans. There are cases of nonlethal human poisoning from eating a box turtle.[170]

DIETS TO AVOID

Although some foods may be relished by reptiles, nevertheless, many of these same foods have potentially toxic components and should only be fed in small quantities. Spinach, rhubarb, and beets contain the chelating agent oxalic acid, which binds with calcium ions in the blood to form calcium oxalate crystals. This can lead to a decrease in calcium levels and predispose to bladder stones.[171]

Broccoli, brussels sprouts, and cabbage contain mustard oil glycosides, which have been shown to contribute to the formation of goiter.[171] Fagopyrine found in buckwheat can cause photosensitivity. Iguanas fed buckwheat may develop blepharitis and conjunctivitis when exposed to sunlight. This condition is self-limiting and can be remedied without treatment if animals are kept in the dark and out of the sun for 48 hours.[171]

CONCLUSION

The keeping of any animal is not an inalienable right. Anyone keeping animals is accountable for their well-being and responsible for their treatment. There are 10 million other forms of life on this planet besides human beings. They all share the same life force that we do, thus they deserve our consideration, our respect, and our kindness. Toxins are just one hazard faced by captive reptiles. Exotic animal clinicians must keep current on the ever-expanding number of hazardous molecules that can lead to intoxication in their reptile patients.

ACKNOWLEDGMENTS

To Isabel Verdaguer and Joaquim Soler (CRARC, Spain), Nada Padayatchy and Owen Griffits (Vanille Crocodile Park, Mauritius), Beate Pfau (German Herpetological Society, Germany), Alvaro Camina Vega (Faunia Zoo, Spain), and Jairo Cuevas Lopez (Universidad Complutense de Madrid, Spain), as well as Kristin Newquist for their help and particular comments and suggestions on the manuscript. Additionally, thanks are due to Drs. Doug Mader and Steven Barten for their help and friendship. Finally, we appreciate Drs. Stephen Divers and Scott Stahl for including us in their fine volume.

REFERENCES

See www.expertconsult.com for a complete list of references.

89

Amphibian Medicine

Brent R. Whitaker and Kevin M. Wright†

Our world is changing and so too are our global amphibian populations. In some cases, these changes are in direct response to human activity, such as the development of land for commercial or residential use and the associated creation of transit corridors, all resulting in destruction of habitat and pollution. Similarly, the transition of land to agricultural use has resulted in increased pollution and habitat destruction, which has directly affected terrestrial and aquatic habitats. Other activities, including energy and mining, deforestation, hunting and collecting, and the introduction of invasive species, have all had a significant impact.[1] In other cases, changing climate patterns are known to affect amphibian populations. For example, with the increased frequency of El Nino years resulting in less precipitation in the Cascade Mountains, the western toad has been forced to lay eggs in shallower lakes and pools than they would normally. The lack of depth has increased exposure to ultraviolet light (UVB), causing the eggs to be more susceptible to *Saprolegnia ferax* infection resulting in a greater than 50% mortality.[2]

The emergence of infectious diseases and subsequent extinction of select species will continue, as our environments change along with the biodiversity of organisms that live within them. Amphibian populations exemplify this changing relationship between host and organism (e.g., viruses, bacteria, and parasites). Today we recognize organisms, such as iridoviruses and chytridiomycosis, as pathogens responsible for the global decline of amphibian populations. Veterinarians with a thorough understanding of amphibian medicine are needed to contribute to the care and ultimately to the conservation of these incredible animals.

To accomplish this, the veterinarian must have a thorough understanding of the biology and captive husbandry of amphibians. Amphibians are a unique class of vertebrates that appear in the fossil record during the Upper Mississippian era, more than 300 million years ago. Amphibians were the first vertebrates capable of exploiting terrestrial habitats on a long-term basis, although they still relied on aquatic environments for breeding and the development of young. This class of vertebrates is named Amphibia because of the double life (*amphibios* in Greek) that is characteristic of many of its members: an aquatic larval stage followed by a terrestrial adult stage. The modern-day amphibians have been categorized in three orders: Gymnophiona, the caecilians; Urodela, the salamanders and newts; and Anura, the frogs and toads. (Throughout this chapter the word "salamander" is used to refer collectively to salamanders and newts and the word "anuran" is used to refer to frogs and toads.)

EXAMINATION AND PHYSICAL RESTRAINT

The amphibian examination should be performed in a room that is between 70° and 75°F (21° to 24°C) or is in keeping with the patients preferred body temperature. Rooms suited for housing reptiles kept between 82° and 85°F (27° to 30°C) are unsuitably warm for most amphibians. Unbleached paper towels wetted with chlorine-free water may be used on the examination table. A humidifier in the room may be necessary, especially if the ambient humidity is below 50%. A bottle of clean, dechlorinated water should be in the room to wet down the amphibian as needed. With these precautions, an amphibian may be examined without risking dehydration.

The amphibian's skin is very sensitive to human handling. Soaps, lotions, natural oils, etc. can all irritate or damage the skin. The use of disposable gloves is protective to the animal and to the clinician. It also prevents the spread of pathogens, and for these reasons the authors recommend using them when handling amphibian patients. Several publications, however, caution of potential toxic effects of latex, vinyl, and nitrile gloves when working with amphibian larvae.[3–5] Reactions appear to be species specific. Thoroughly rinsing gloves in fresh water before use with adult or larval amphibians to remove talcum and reduce potential toxins is recommended.

Avoid clutter in the examination room because many amphibians are small and can disappear with surprising alacrity into the instruments and other accoutrements of the typical veterinary practice. For this same reason, close the door to the examination room whenever the amphibian is out of its carrying case.

When setting up the appointment, ask the owner to bring several photographs taken from multiple angles of the animal's normal enclosure, a water sample in a clean container for analysis, and any written records that he or she might have. Upon arrival, peruse the information that the owner has brought as part of the anamnesis. Learn as much about the microhabitat (the vivarium) and the macrohabitat (the environment within which the vivarium is housed) as possible, then proceed with the physical examination of the amphibian patient in a stepwise routine manner to ensure that nothing of importance is overlooked. First, observe the amphibian without handling or removal from its carrying case. Note body stance, responsiveness, and general demeanor, as well as respiratory movements, including gular movements and pulmonary respirations (Figs. 89.1 and 89.2). Body condition, including texture of skin and estimates of hydration status, can often be assessed during this hands-off examination (Fig. 89.3). The nares should be clean and free of debris, and the oropharynx should have no visible lesions. Excessive saliva or the presence of bubbles suggests respiratory complications.

The corneas should be clear, and a blink reflex should be initiated if the ocular globe is approached. Failure to blink mandates further investigation of the eye to determine whether the animal has vision. Slit lamp observation of the cornea and ocular fundus is warranted in any case.[6] Check pupillary reflexes. Note any cutaneous lesions. Erythema may be in response to handling or may signal a more serious underlying cause such as septicemia.

---

†Deceased.

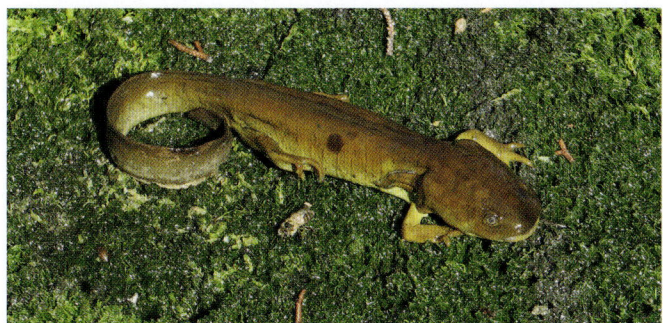

FIG 89.1 The clinician must consider the life stage of the animal being examined. This healthy larval form of the Arizona salamander (*Ambystoma mavortium nebulosum*) will soon absorb the fins on its tail and its gills as it makes its transition to land. Its legs will also become muscular and its broad head will become sleeker, developing eyes that protrude and have eyelids. (Courtesy of Brianna Whitaker.)

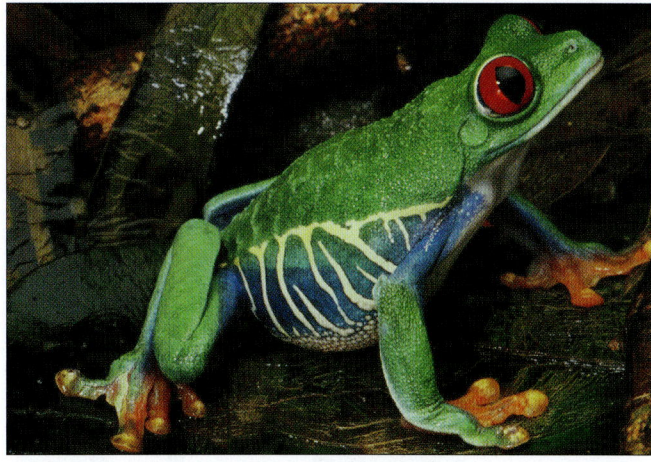

FIG 89.2 This red-eyed leaf frog (*Agalychnis callidryas*) shows the typical body form and posture of a healthy adult anuran: four limbs and a reduced or absent tail. No external neck exists, so the head and body appear unbroken. (Courtesy of National Aquarium.)

As part of the actual physical examination, coelomic palpation should be attempted, but in some species, this is not practical because many amphibians inflate themselves as a defensive maneuver. This defensive bloat appears when the amphibian is upset and can be distinguished from true bloat that remains once the animal has become calm. Edema may also extend down over the legs, especially in anurans. Edema has been associated with renal disease,[7] skin disease, gastrointestinal disease, microbial and parasitic infections, improper environmental conditions, toxins, cardiovascular and lymphatic disease, metabolic imbalances, and liver disease. The stomach may be palpable in recently fed amphibians. Ingested stones and other foreign bodies may be palpated too, as well as the presence of cystic uroliths.

Oral examination is facilitated with the use of a speculum. Use waterproof paper or thin strips of firm plastic, such as a guitar pick, are often used to open the mouth of the anuran. Inserting the paper at the tip of the snout works in some specimens, and inserting at the corner of the mouth works best in others. Large specimens may require a small spatula or thicker piece of plastic, such as a credit card, to pry open the mouth. Care must be taken not to put too much torque on the mouth, because the bones are thin and can easily be fractured if excess force is used. Test and note the withdrawal reflex of the limbs and righting reflex. Auscultation of the pulmonic fields is rarely practical because of the small size of many amphibians.

Proper manual restraint is essential to conduct a safe and informative physical examination, perform clinical diagnostics, and ultimately administer treatment to the amphibian patient. Some species produce toxic secretions, and some, such as the bicolored poison dart frog (*Phyllobates bicolor*), even produce toxins of a potentially lethal nature to humans. Other species (e.g., toads, *Bufo* spp.) produce toxins that irritate mucous membranes and may have lethal effects when absorbed by a human. Some amphibians defend themselves by producing mucilaginous secretions (e.g., slimy salamanders, *Plethodon glutinosus* complex). Wear protective gloves when handling amphibians to eliminate contact with these secretions and take special care not to rub your eyes or nose. Before handling the patient, rinse the gloves under distilled water to remove any talcum powder, which can irritate the amphibian and thereby cause the production of even more defensive secretions. Wearing eye protection is recommended, especially with larger amphibians. When pressure is applied to the parotid gland of a neotropical giant toad (*Bufo marinus*), the gland's secretion may spurt several feet into the air, with unfortunate consequences to the intercepting human.

The bulk of the amphibian's body needs to be supported during manual restraint. Grasp large anurans behind the forelegs.[8] Often the anuran gives a release call, a signal to other anurans that it is either not sexually receptive or is of the wrong sex to be amplexed. The release call may sound similar to a distress call, a vocalization emitted by an anuran in response to predation, but either call may serve to startle a clinician momentarily, resulting in escape.

Many amphibians bite. Some, such as the Argentine horned frog (*Ceratophrys ornata*) (Fig. 89.4), can inflict severe wounds on the human handler. Large anurans often kick violently when first captured, so the handler must be ready to grasp in front of the hind legs immediately after picking up the animal behind the forelegs. Smaller anurans can be encircled with the thumb and index finger, or the hind legs gripped in a firm fist during the examination. For a thorough physical examination, place medium to small specimens inside clear plastic delicatessen cups, or small glass jars, for an unobstructed view of the entire body, including the ventrum.

Grasp medium to large salamanders behind the head and in front of the forelegs and again immediately in front of the back legs. Some salamanders have tail autotomy, so the handler should avoid placing any pressure on the tail. Occasionally, despite the gentlest efforts of the handler, a specimen may drop its tail anyway, so the client should be forewarned that this is a possibility. Small specimens may be examined more closely in a cup or jar as mentioned for anurans. Aquatic salamanders should not be removed from the water except for clinical diagnostics, such as collecting a skin scraping or obtaining the weight, and should be returned to the water as quickly as possible to minimize damage to the skin. Many of the larger salamanders (e.g., Hellbender, *Cryptobranchus alleganiensis*) can inflict painful bites that bleed profusely, so the handler is forewarned to maintain a firm grip when restraining these amphibians and to have owners keep their distance.

Caecilians and some salamanders (e.g., Amphiuma, *Amphiuma* sp.) are somewhat problematic to restrain for examination. An appropriately sized clear plastic tube, such as used for aquarium filtration equipment, or a clear glass jar or clear plastic cup is the most practical way to observe these elongated amphibians. However, to restrain the caecilian for diagnostics such as a skin scrape, without damaging the skin on the rest of the body, can be difficult because many specimens writhe violently when pressure is applied to the body. A soft foam rubber sponge moistened with chlorine-free water can be used to pin the caecilian, and the desired portion of the body can be cautiously exposed for

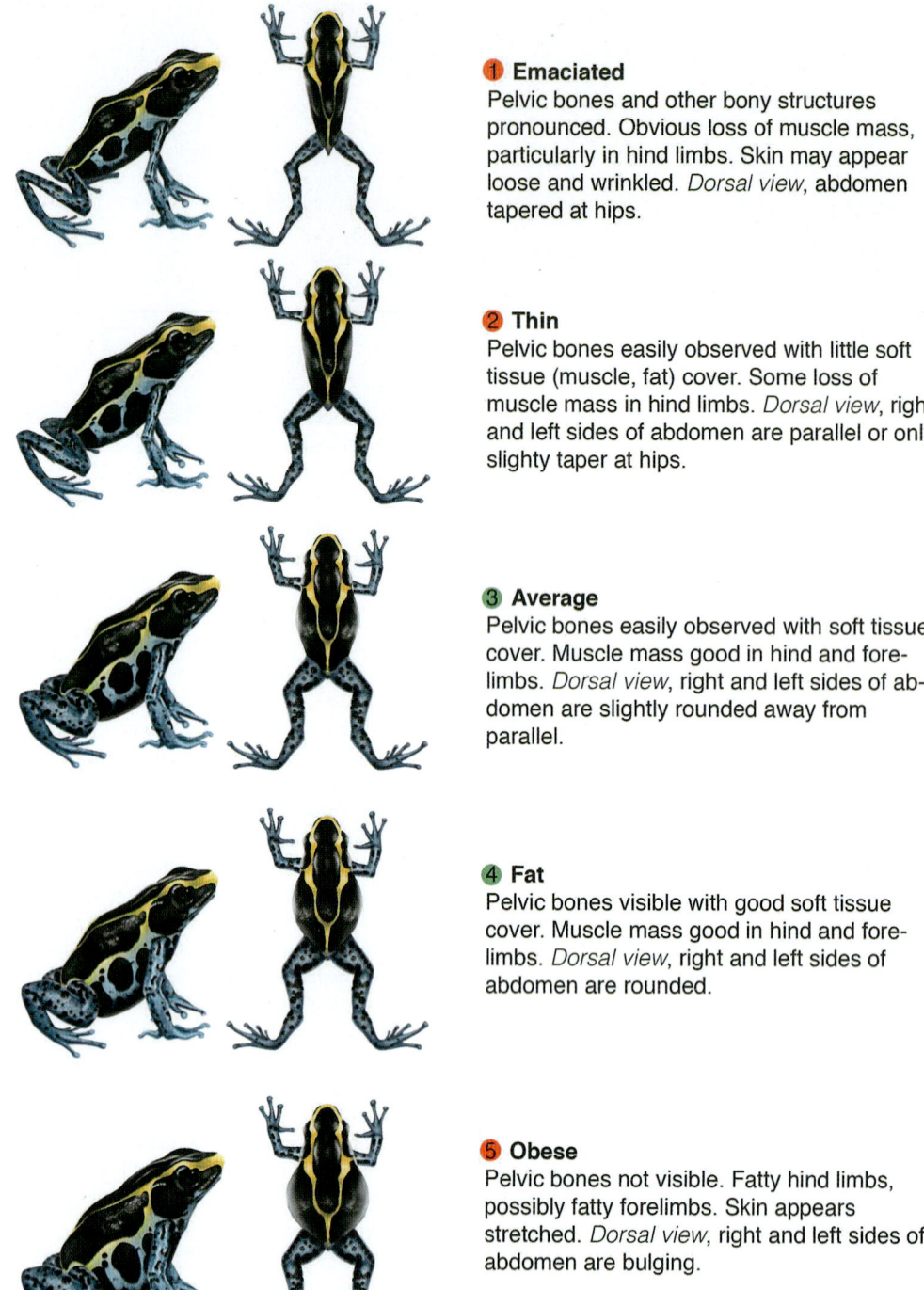

① Emaciated
Pelvic bones and other bony structures pronounced. Obvious loss of muscle mass, particularly in hind limbs. Skin may appear loose and wrinkled. *Dorsal view*, abdomen tapered at hips.

② Thin
Pelvic bones easily observed with little soft tissue (muscle, fat) cover. Some loss of muscle mass in hind limbs. *Dorsal view*, right and left sides of abdomen are parallel or only slighty taper at hips.

③ Average
Pelvic bones easily observed with soft tissue cover. Muscle mass good in hind and fore-limbs. *Dorsal view*, right and left sides of abdomen are slightly rounded away from parallel.

④ Fat
Pelvic bones visible with good soft tissue cover. Muscle mass good in hind and fore-limbs. *Dorsal view*, right and left sides of abdomen are rounded.

⑤ Obese
Pelvic bones not visible. Fatty hind limbs, possibly fatty forelimbs. Skin appears stretched. *Dorsal view*, right and left sides of abdomen are bulging.

● Healthy   ● Unhealthy

© 2013 James Abraham

FIG 89.3 Assessing body condition is important in the clinical evaluation. The body condition scores for the dendrobatid frog, *Dendrobates tinctorius,* is illustrated here. (Courtesy of James Abraham.)

closer examination. Soft damp flannel may also be used. Precoating the "squeeze cage" with water-soluble gel (e.g., K-Y jelly) may be of benefit.

ANESTHESIA AND CHEMICAL RESTRAINT

Physical restraint alone may not yield a thorough examination of certain amphibian patients or may be impractical for other reasons. Chemical restraint is often needed for a thorough evaluation of the amphibian patient. Although familiar veterinary drugs such as sevoflurane, isoflurane, and ketamine hydrochloride may be used for chemical restraint, other drugs, such as tricaine methanesulfonate, isoeugenol, and benzocaine, are the anesthetics of choice for amphibians in most cases. Apnea and cardiac depression are common effects of many anesthetics used in amphibians. Heart rate can be monitored using an ultrasonic Doppler,

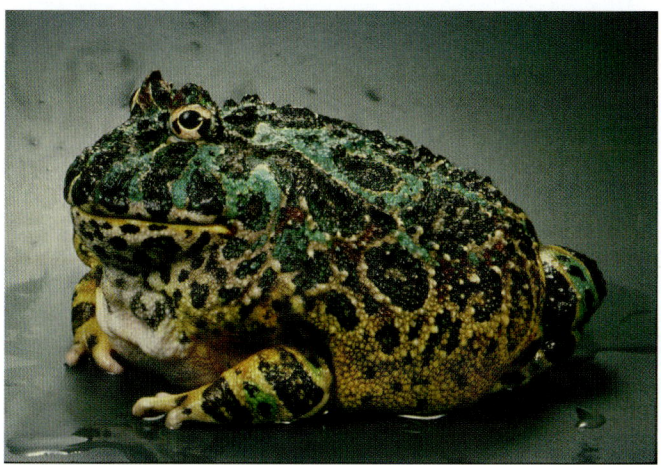

FIG 89.4 Many amphibians bite. Some, such as the Argentine horned frog (*Ceratophrys ornata*), can inflict severe wounds on the human handler. (Courtesy of National Aquarium.)

and gular movements can be visualized to determine apnea in many species.[9]

Immersion anesthetics prepared using water of a neutral pH, and free of ammonia, nitrite, nitrate, chlorine and chloramine, and other contaminants is most effective for amphibian anesthesia. Care must be taken to prevent drowning by keeping the solution below the humero-scapula joint[10] and carefully monitoring the patient.

Tricaine methanesulfonate (e.g., Tricaine-S (MS 222), Syndel USA [formerly Western Chemical], Ferndale, WA) is a water-soluble white powder derivative of benzocaine that can be added to water with the resultant solution used to titrate to the desired anesthetic effect.[11] Because tricaine methanesulfonate is very acidic, buffering the solution using a 1:1 ratio (dry weight) of sodium bicarbonate is recommended in order to reduce the risk of acidosis while increasing the absorbability of the drug. A 0.05% solution of tricaine methanesulfonate (0.5 g/L = 0.5 mg/mL) serves to anesthetize tadpoles and other amphibian larva. A range from 0.1% to 0.2% solution (1 g/L to 2 g/L) is needed for induction of surgical level anesthesia in most frogs and salamanders, but a 0.3% solution (3 g/L) is needed for many toads (*Bufo* spp.). Because the anesthesia is titrated, the final concentration of solution does not have to be precise to be useful; a slightly more dilute or stronger concentration simply increases or decreases the time to induction of the desired plane of anesthesia.

Tricaine solution may be managed simply with premeasured amounts of drugs in a container of known volume. For example, 1 gram of tricaine methanesulfonate in a 2-liter plastic soda bottle yields a 0.05% solution when 2000 mL of water is added. A 0.1% solution requires 2 g of tricaine methanesulfonate in the 2-liter soda bottle, 0.2% requires 4 g, and 0.3% requires 6 g. The concentration does not have to be exact to be effective, as the solution is administered to effect. Precision is only necessary for a controlled study.

A clear plastic bag is an ideal induction chamber for many specimens. Large specimens need correspondingly larger chambers. Plastic sweater boxes and lock-top plastic tubs are inexpensive options. In the case of flighty anurans, the induction tub should be lined with a plastic bag. The loose-fitting plastic serves to cushion the jumps during the excitatory phase of induction. Have readily available a copious supply of well-oxygenated chlorine-free water for the recovery period. If the anesthetic solution is too deep and covers the nostrils, many amphibians drown. This is less important for lungless amphibians and gilled forms that can survive total submergence for varying lengths of time. Nevertheless,

using the shallowest depth of anesthetic solution possible is best to avoid accidents.

Tricaine methanesulfonate may be administered intracoelomically.[12] Aseptic technique must be used to prepare an injection quality solution. Intracoelomic dosages range from 50 to 300 mg/kg.

A surgical plane of anesthesia typically is induced within 20 minutes of immersion into the tricaine solution. Respiratory efforts slow down, and may stop, during tricaine anesthesia, but the cardiac rate is unaffected or even slightly increased except at very deep levels of anesthesia. Renal circulation may become reduced at high concentrations of tricaine methanesulfonate.

Erythema of the ventral skin or other light-colored skin is the first sign of anesthetic induction with tricaine methanesulfonate. The amphibian may appear agitated, and anurans often attempt escape leaps. As mentioned previously, induction of an amphibian inside a plastic bag minimizes the trauma associated with these attempts.

A light plane of anesthesia from tricaine methanesulfonate is characterized by the loss of the righting reflex and corneal reflex, but the withdrawal reflex (deep pain), spontaneous movement, gular respiration, and the cardiac impulse (visible heartbeat) are retained. A deep plane of anesthesia is the stage when only the cardiac impulse is present. The withdrawal reflex is the last reflex to go. An overdose is indicated when the cardiac impulse slows or becomes difficult to detect. Once an amphibian is in a deep plane of anesthesia, place it in tricaine-free water and titrate the level of anesthesia by trickling additional anesthetic solution over the amphibian's body periodically. Once the procedure is complete, anesthesia can be reversed with rinsing the body in well-oxygenated water.

Clove oil (which contains eugenol as its active anesthetic ingredient) and the commercially available pharmaceutical (Aqui-S, http://www.aqui-s.com/) has been used as an anesthetic in adult and larval amphibians.[13–15] One study showed that immersing *Xenopus laevis* in a bath of 350 mg/L of Aqui-S for 15 minutes to be effective in producing short-term surgical anesthesia.[13] Another study concluded that Aqui-S could safely be used to anesthetize southern brown tree frog (*Litoria ewingii*) tadpoles.[15] Researchers implanting passive integrated transponder (PIT) tags found immersing the three-toed amphiuma (*Amphiuma tridactylum*) in diluted clove oil (2 mL/4 L of water) for 5 minutes to be safe and effective whereas surgical implantation of transmitters required at least 10 minutes in the anesthetic.[16]

Propofol has been documented as an anesthetic with intracoelomic injection or intravenous injection in frogs. Intracoelomic injection of 9 to 30 mg/kg resulted in deep anesthesia in White's tree frogs (*Pelodryas caerulea*); a higher dosage was lethal in one specimen.[17] Intravenous injection (10 mg/kg) resulted in sedation or light sedation, but this may reflect perivascular deposition of some of the dose. Topical propofol (100–150 mg/kg) sedated maroon-eyed tree frogs (*Agalychnis litodryas*) of less than 20 g body weight, with the frog rinsed in fresh water once it was sedated (Wright, unpublished data). However, topical or intracoelomic propofol is inconsistent with time of induction, depth of anesthesia, and time to recovery and offers no advantages over topical tricaine methanesulfonate.

Ketamine hydrochloride may be used to immobilize amphibians, but it is less satisfactory than tricaine methanesulfonate or isoeugenol in that a comparatively large volume of drug may be needed, the induction time is extremely variable, the level of anesthesia achieved may vary greatly between species (in fact, many amphibians continue to show spontaneous movement even after the withdrawal reflex is lost), and the recovery time is variable.[18,19] Ketamine may be administered intramuscularly, intravenously, lymphatically via the dorsal lymph sacs in anurans (Fig. 89.5), or subcutaneously, depending on the size of the specimen and the needs of the clinician.

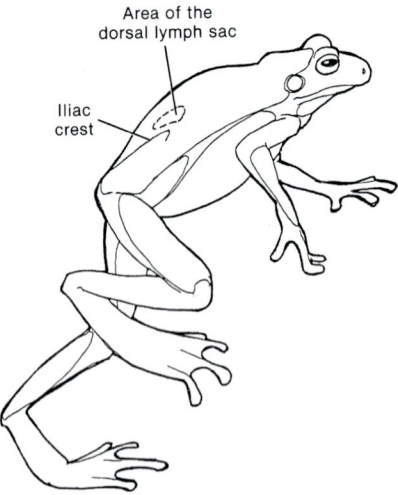

FIG 89.5 In some anurans, a pair of dorsal lymph sacs lies immediately lateral to the base of the sacrum.

Dosages for ketamine are between 75 and 100 mg/kg body weight for most species, although some amphibians may prove extremely sensitive or resistant to ketamine and dosages must be adjusted accordingly. A minimum of 30 minutes should be allowed to pass before the anesthetic stage is evaluated. If a satisfactory level is not achieved, a supplementary dose of ketamine may be administered. If adequate anesthesia is still not achieved, one should consider delaying the effort for 24 hours and starting at a much higher initial dosage. As with tricaine methanesulfonate, anesthetic deaths are rare except in debilitated specimens or through dosage errors of several orders of magnitude. Ketamine (200 mg/kg) combined with diazepam (0.2 mg/kg) administered IM to anesthetize cane toads (*Rhinella marina*) showed minimal activation of the hypothalamic-pituitary-adrenal axis as did tricaine methanesulfonate; however, ketamine-diazepam induction and recovery times were significantly prolonged.[20]

Alfaxalone, a neuroactive steroid and general anesthetic, has recently been made available in the United States and could provide the clinician an alternative option. Although not used extensively, one study using a 5 mg/L immersion bath was successful in anesthetizing a Mexican axolotl undergoing the surgical removal of two gastric foreign bodies.[21] Alfaxalone administered IM to Australian green tree frogs (*Litoria caerulea*) (30 mg/kg) and green and golden bell frogs (*Litoria aurea*) (20 mg/kg) provided sedation within 10 minutes. It also produced a light plane of anesthesia in booroolong frogs (*Litoria booroolongensis*) (20 mg/kg). All doses in this study were insufficient for painful procedures.[22] More work is needed to confirm the benefits and safety of this drug when used in amphibians.

Sevoflurane and isoflurane are inhalant anesthetics that may be used topically in amphibians. Several formulas may be used; a useful ratio is 1 mL isoflurane, 1 mL water, and 3 mL water-soluble gel, stirred to form a viscous liquid. This isoflurane solution is then smeared to the amphibian's ventral surface and rinsed away with fresh water once the animal is in a deep plane of anesthesia. The use of sevoflurane may be preferred. American green tree frogs (*Hyla cinerea*) anesthetized with a mixture of 1.5 parts distilled water, 3.5 parts spermicidal jelly, and 3 parts seroflurane recovered 4.5 times quicker and did not develop the skin lesions that isoflurane-treated animals did.[23] Some amphibians, such as the neotropical giant toad (*Bufo marinus*) or Argentine horned frog, may be anesthetized with directly dripping halothane or isoflurane onto the skin. The problem with either topical technique using inhalant anesthetics is that the induction should be performed under a fume

hood or other system for scavenging waste anesthetic gases as the agent outgases from the solution.

If inhalant anesthetics are used in an induction chamber, a saturation level of 2.5% to 3% is recommended for methoxyflurane,[27] halothane, and isoflurane. The amphibian should be kept in the chamber for 5 to 10 minutes after voluntary movement ceases. A deep plane of anesthesia from a chamber induction usually lasts for 10 to 30 minutes. The chamber should be moistened with fresh water for the amphibian patient's comfort. If an amphibian appears particularly irritated during the process, stop the flow of anesthetic gas and remove the animal from the chamber. Some specimens do not tolerate the volatile anesthetics; epidermal damage may occur if kept in contact with halothane or isoflurane for a prolonged period of time. Large amphibians may be intubated and maintained on gaseous anesthetics, but because of alternate respiratory patterns (e.g., cutaneous, buccopharyngeal routes), maintenance of a steady level of anesthesia via this technique is difficult. An uncuffed endotracheal tube is recommended to avoid damage to the tracheal tissue.

Analgesia should be provided to amphibian patients undergoing potentially painful procedures. The opioid buprenorphine injected into the dorsal lymph sac (37.6 mg/kg) may provide significant analgesia to a common laboratory test of pain and last for up to 4 hours; the alpha-adrenergic agonist dexmedetomidine injected into the dorsal lymph sac (40–120 mg/kg) may provide analgesia up to 8 hours.[25] Alpha-adrenergic agonists appear to be effective in producing analgesia in amphibians. Northern leopard frogs (*Rana pipiens*) administered dexmedetomidine (0.1–3 nmol/g), clonidine (100–1000 nmol/g), epinephrine (1–30 nmol/kg), and norepinephrine (10–300 nmol/g) showed dose-dependent analgesic effects compared with those pretreated with selective alpha-2 receptor antagonists.[26] Meloxicam, a nonsteroidal antiinflammatory drug, has also been used as an antiinflammatory and analgesic in amphibians with apparent success. North American bullfrogs receiving a 4-mm punch biopsy and treated with 0.1 mg/kg IM meloxicam showed a significant decrease in serum PGE2, suggesting that a daily dose of 0.1 mg/kg does provide analgesia.[27] This author has used doses of 0.1 to 0.2 mg/kg SID on a variety of amphibian species. The characteristics of opioid, nonopioid, and partial opioid drugs following systemic administration to *Rana pipiens* in behavioral studies are available[28] and may provide the clinician with alternative options to consider. Further work, however, is needed.

EUTHANASIA

Two agents are noted as methods of sedation and anesthesia in many research articles that are not recommended for the amphibian patient except for euthanasia purposes: ethanol and pentobarbital. An amphibian immersed in 10% ethanol enters a deep plane of anesthesia within 15 minutes. Increasing the concentration of ethanol to 70% kills the animal. An overdose of pentobarbital (>100 mg/kg) can be administered via intracardiac or intracoelomic injection. Evidence exists that amphibians may still feel pain after decapitation for several minutes. If decapitation is necessary for specific reasons, it should follow the induction of deep anesthesia. Other methods of euthanasia have been used, such as immersing small amphibians (<4 g) in liquid nitrogen, but the authors do not consider these to be practical in a clinical setting.

CLINICAL TECHNIQUES

Parasitological diagnostics are similar to those reported for other orders of animals. Direct examinations and flotation concentrations are recommended for detection of most protozoal and helminth parasites. Acid-fast stains of the feces should reveal *Cryptosporidium* spp. if present.

Hematology is an underused tool in the diagnosis and treatment of disease in amphibians. Historically, part of the problem is that large volumes of blood were required to perform relatively simple tests such as hemoglobin analysis. Another problem is that most of the techniques described for amphibian blood collection in the literature were non-survival methods such as decapitation. Thus, most of the data was collected strictly for physiological investigations, and scant attention was paid to the health or survival of the specimens.

Blood collection is relatively simple for total white blood cell counts (WBC), packed cell volume (PCV), total solids (TS), leukocyte differentials, and one or two chemistries on medium-sized amphibians (40–80 g); in larger specimens, one can run complete blood counts and plasma chemistry panels because of the larger volume of sample that can be obtained. Ideally, creating blood smears and evaluating the packed cell volume and total solids is done immediately upon collecting blood from an amphibian. The pretreatment of the syringe and storage of blood using lithium heparin could lead to lower and inconsistent values as observed in one study of blood collected from American alligators.[29] Lithium heparin is the anticoagulant of choice for blood because it does not affect the values of plasma calcium, sodium, or ammonia. One should avoid the use of ammonium heparin when obtaining a sample that is to be analyzed for NH_3 levels or else a falsely elevated reading results. Sodium heparin should be avoided when electrolyte values are desired. Ethylenediamine tetraacetic acid (EDTA) may lyse the erythrocytes of some species of amphibians and is not recommended as an anticoagulant for amphibian blood.

Several options are available for obtaining blood from a frog. A relatively simple procedure is to bleed from the lingual venous plexus that lies immediately beneath the tongue.[30] The authors have used this method on frogs as small as 25 g. Care must be taken to gently pry open the mouth to avoid breaking the thin mandibular bones. A small firm rubber spatula works well, or even a cotton minitip applicator can be used as a mouth speculum. In some animals, working from the lateral edge of the oral commissure is easier, and in other animals, insertion of the speculum into the philtrum, a small divot found just beneath the tip of the nose, is easiest. Once the mouth is opened, a cotton-tipped applicator is used to draw the tongue forward, as if the tongue were flipping out to catch a prey item (Fig. 89.6A). The lingual venous plexus is then visible on the underside of the tongue and the buccal floor. Most frogs have pale-colored tongues, so the purple to red network of veins is readily apparent. One large vein can then be punctured with a 26-gauge or 25-gauge needle, and a heparinized microhematocrit tube can be used to collect the blood that oozes from the vein. Once an adequate sample of blood is obtained, release the tongue. In most cases, this serves to put enough pressure on the vein that it stops bleeding. Occasionally, direct pressure on the venipuncture site with a cotton-tipped applicator is necessary to achieve hemostasis. The disadvantage to this technique is that the samples can be contaminated with saliva and mucus, but this can be minimalized if care is taken to swab the surface of the plexus thoroughly before venipuncture. In the case of a fractious animal, blood collection can be facilitated with sedation or anesthesia.

Large frogs and toads can be bled quite easily from the midline ventral vein on the ventral surface (see Figs. 89–6B and 89–6C). A 26-gauge or 27-gauge needle can be carefully inserted in a craniodorsal direction into this vein and gentle pressure applied to withdraw blood into the syringe. A good insertion site is the point midway between the sternum and the pelvis. Unfortunately, the passage through the bore of these small-gauge needles does tend to distort some blood cells, but a risk of lacerating the midline ventral vein is found with larger-gauge needles.

Salamanders may also be bled from the anterior abdominal vein in the manner described previously, but identification of the venipuncture

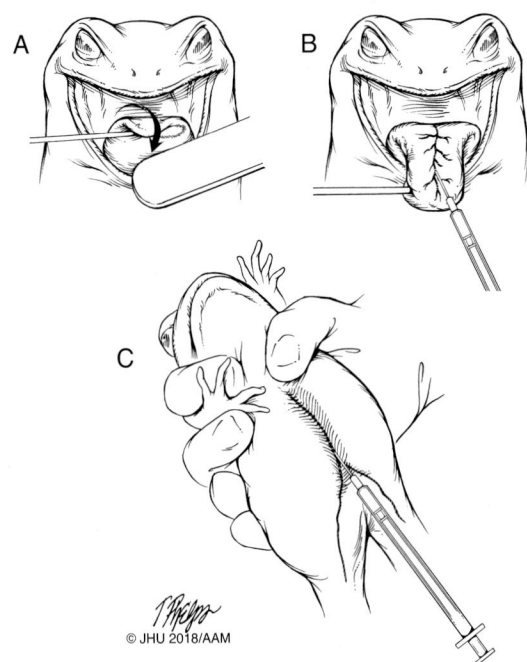

FIG 89.6 (A) Soft smooth speculum can be used to open the mouth and manipulate the tongue of an anuran. (B) The lingual venous plexus is a prominent network of superficial veins that can serve as a phlebotomy site in many anurans. (C) The midline groove on the ventrum lies immediately over the midline abdominal vein and is a good site from which to collect blood. (Courtesy of Tim Phelps, Art as Applied to Medicine, Johns Hopkins University School of Medicine. Copyright 2018.)

site in these amphibians is more difficult. An additional site for venipuncture is the ventral caudal vein, also called the tail vein, which runs immediately ventral to the vertebral bodies. In salamanders weighing less than 80 g, a 27-gauge needle is the most practical choice for venipuncture attempts, but a 26-gauge or 25-gauge needle may be used for larger animals. Some salamanders and newts can perform tail autotomy, and in these species, one should not attempt this method with a conscious animal because it could result in the loss of the specimen's tail during the venipuncture endeavor.

A final choice for the collection of hematologic samples is cardiocentesis. This works equally well for anurans, most salamanders, and even caecilians. If the animal is difficult to restrain, it should be sedated or anesthetized to reduce the risk of pericardial, ventricular, or atrial laceration. Place the amphibian in dorsal recumbency to locate its cardiac impulse (heartbeat). The location of the heart may be quickly determined with a Doppler probe; once located with Doppler, the cardiac impulse is easy to track visually. Once the cardiac impulse is noted, a 25- to 27-gauge needle may be inserted into the central part of the impulse to penetrate the apex of the ventricle. Gentle pressure is applied, and the needle is slowly advanced or withdrawn until a flash of blood is visible in the hub of the syringe. If a clear yellow fluid appears instead, the needle should be withdrawn because the sample is most likely fluid from the pericardial sac. If sufficient pericardial fluid was obtained, it can be submitted for culture (if no anticoagulant was used), have cytological specimens prepared from it, or be analyzed for biochemical parameters. Even a small quantity can be prepared for either wet mount examination or stained slides to determine whether inflammatory cells or other abnormal items are present. A new needle and syringe should be used for a second attempt, but an increased risk exists of a problem arising with each subsequent puncture of pericardial or cardiac tissue.

If a blood flash is detected, pressure should be let off the syringe. A cycle of gentle pressure and release coaxes blood into the syringe with each ventricular beat. Once an adequate sample is obtained, pressure is released, and the needle is withdrawn from the ventricular chamber.

Complete blood counts may be performed in the same manner as described for avian and reptilian species.[31–33] Natt & Herrick's solution allows one to make a direct count of WBCs and red blood cells (RBCs) from the same sample with a hemocytometer. Another option is to use the eosinophil indirect method, such as the Avian Leukopette (VetLab, Palmetto Bay, FL), to count granulocytes and calculate the total WBC/µL by the formula that uses the percent heterophils and eosinophils from the leukocyte differential to correct for the cells not counted in the hemocytometer. Although the eosinophil method may not work in all amphibian species, in the author's experience, it has worked well in axolotls (*Ambystoma mexicanum*), marine toads, smokey jungle frogs (*Leptodactylus pentadactylus*), hellbenders (*Cryptobranchus alleganiensis*), and sirens (*Siren intermedia*) and may be applicable to a wide variety of amphibians.

For each species encountered, the eosinophil technique is not recommended for use until it is verified for that species. This may be done by established guidelines for calculating the allowable total error for the two methods. If the calculated error is ≤ the allowable total error, then the two methods may be considered interchangeable.[34] An advantage to the eosinophil method is that it is much easier to count the stained granulocytes than it is to distinguish leukocytes from similarly sized thrombocytes in the Natt & Herrick's solution. However, the Natt & Herrick's solution allows an accurate WBC independent of the leukocyte differential count. This is important because in amphibians the granulocytes have been poorly described and may vary tremendously in staining characteristics and gross morphology between species.[35–38] Considerable expertise is needed for an accurate leukocyte differential count and interpretation.

Wright-Giemsa solution enhances the detail of the cell's internal morphology and provides consistently richer colors compared with other commonly available stains. It is important to remember that currently granulocytes are described on the basis of their staining characteristics and that the classes of granulocytes generally are not proven to be fully homologous nor analogous to the mammalian granulocytes with similar staining characteristics.[36] Documentation of the disease accompanying the differential leukogram is important to elucidate the role of the various leukocytes seen in amphibians. Few studies report normal blood values for amphibians[32] (e.g., for the American Bullfrog [*Rana catesbeiana*]). (See Chapter 35 for additional hematology and biochemistry values.)

Whenever an amphibian is manually restrained, some damage occurs to the thin epidermis. For this reason, moistened gloves should be worn by the handler to ameliorate the cutaneous injury to the patient. Although the humoral and cell-mediated immunological response in amphibians is poorly delineated, macrophages are responsible for phagocytic removal of cellular debris and bacteria.[36,39] Because of the presence of injured epithelial cells after handling, an amphibian's monocyte count may show a relative and absolute increase on subsequent leukocyte profiles.

Rickettsiae, parasites, and inclusions caused by viruses may be detected on appropriately stained blood smears.[40,41] Trypanosomes and microfilariae are extraerythrocytic parasites. Hemogregarine parasites are common intraerythrocytic inclusions in amphibians. The relative percentage of erythrocytes afflicted with inclusions may be important clinical prognostic indicators. Low levels are probably unimportant or may only be a minor contributing factor to the amphibian's signs. High levels of inclusions may be significant, especially if coupled with signs of anemia such as low PCV or RBC, polychromatic erythrocytes, microcytosis, or hypohemoglobinemia.

With the advent of small inexpensive dry film analyzers (e.g., Heska Element DC, Heska, Loveland, CO; VetScan VS2, VetScan HM5, VetScan I-Stat, Abaxis, Union City, CA; Catalyst Dx Chemistry Analyzer, Catalyst One Chemistry Analyzer, IDEXX Westbrook, ME), plasma chemistry tests on amphibians are now practical to obtain. The small volume of sample needed for analysis by these machines allows even a 0.5 mL sample to yield important results such as total protein/albumin, aspartate aminotransferase (AST, also known as serum glutamic-oxaloacetic transaminase or SGOT), alanine transaminase (ALT, also known as serum glutamate pyruvate transaminase or SGPT), blood urea nitrogen (BUN), ammonia (NH_3), glucose, and electrolytes. For serum samples, the blood should be allowed to clot for a minimum of 20 minutes before centrifugation to minimize the chance of sample coagulation after separation. Plasma samples may be spun down immediately, and then the plasma may be decanted from the cellular component.

Unfortunately, given the paucity of clinicopathologic information about amphibians, even with plasma chemistry data and hematologic values, it is still more of an art than a science to interpret those values in the context of the clinical picture. Interpretation is made more complicated by the fact that normal values may be influenced by environmental conditions, life cycle stage, nutrition, and other variables that directly affect amphibians. Reference values are best generated for a specific species by sampling as many healthy individuals from the population as possible (ideally 60 or more individuals) and analyzing those samples in the same laboratory.[42] If a consistent systematic approach is maintained with evaluation of an amphibian (as is done with evaluation of a domesticated mammal), then each practitioner has the potential to contribute to the development of this field of veterinary medicine.

Coeliocentesis may be performed via the paralumbar region or just off the ventral midline. Obtained fluid should be analyzed for protein content (generally <2 g/dL or <20 g/L), cytological characteristics, and biochemistries and submitted for microbial cultures.

Amphibian bacteria should be cultured at 98°F (35°C) and room temperature. However, most amphibian bacterial isolates can be recovered at 98°F. Although standardized kits may yield useful information as to the identity of the bacterial isolate, more elaborate techniques are often needed to confirm the etiological agent. The laboratory used should be competent in isolating and identifying specimens from other ectotherms (i.e., reptiles and fish), because many human-oriented microbiology laboratories do not have the expertise to identify amphibian pathogens.

Cutaneous lesions should be examined with direct observation of a wet mount, stained samples, biopsy, and microbial culturing. A skin scrape of the lesion may be obtained with the blunt edge of a scalpel blade or a dulled scalpel blade. The scraping should be viewed as a wet mount to determine the presence of fungi and protozoa. A gram stain should be made from the scraping if fungi or bacteria are the suspected etiological agents. A biopsy can be made of epidermal tissue with tenting the skin and removing a small oval of tissue. Tissue glue can be used to oppose the epidermal flaps. Cultures and histopathology of any samples obtained should be submitted if deemed appropriate.

NUTRITIONAL DISEASES

Amphibian nutrition has been a poorly understood aspect of captive husbandry; however, a recent publication on amphibian nutrition and the nutritive value of common feeder insects adds significant information and is recommended reading.[43] Anuran larval forms may be herbivorous, omnivorous, or carnivorous, and caecilian and salamander larvae are entirely carnivorous. Adult amphibians are entirely carnivorous, with the exception of one tree frog (*Hyla truncata*) that includes fruit of the coca tree in its diet.[24] The marine toad has been observed to consume vegetable matter in Florida, but no observations of this are reported in its natural range. Although starvation/emaciation is the most commonly reported nutritional disease, at least two major nutritional diseases are the result of the poor nutritional value of domestically produced insects, primarily crickets and mealworms, which do not provide the proper levels of calcium, phosphorus, vitamin D_3, and vitamin A required. These diseases are preventable in most cases. Vitamin and mineral supplementation through gut-loading or dusting of feeder insects can be effective in correcting the inverse Ca:P ratio and can bring vitamins A and D_3 to appropriate levels.

Nutritional Secondary Hyperparathyroidism (NSHP)

Nutritional secondary hyperparathyroidism (NSHP) is the most common form of metabolic bone disease (MBD) in captive amphibians and is the second most commonly reported nutritional disease in a survey of captive amphibian pathology. An absolute or relative calcium deficiency is likely the underlying cause of most cases of NSPH in amphibians because most of the commonly fed prey items have an inverse calcium-to-phosphorus ratio and a low total calcium. At this point, no descriptions of other forms of MBD have been found in amphibians.

One of the first clinical signs of NSHP in adult anurans is spastic tetany after strenuous movement (e.g., leaping) that subsides during rest. As the disease progresses, swimming may appear uncoordinated, with a lack of direction. Hypocalcemia results in coelomic distension from gastrointestinal stasis and gas buildup, and this may be seen with or without accompanying tetany. With chronic NSHP, amphibians develop spinal deformities, angulation of the long bones, and bowed mandibles that readily bend when manipulated (commonly called "rubber jaw" by herpetologists) (Fig. 89.7).

The clinician may appreciate misalignment of the long bones visually or by gentle palpation. High-resolution radiographs may confirm decreasing bone density in affected individuals and the presence of pathological fractures. The lateral processes of the vertebrae and urostyle become radiolucent early in the course of NSHP in anurans. The long bones typically become radiolucent after the "ghosting" of the lateral processes of the vertebrae and urostyle. If an apparently healthy member of the same species is available, including the healthy animal in the same exposure as the ill animal will assist the clinician in evaluating the skeletal structure. (Be wary in interpretation because the "healthy" animal may simply have subclinical NSHP.) The clinician may wish to retain the humerus, femur, vertebrae, and urostyle of a healthy necropsy specimen to have comparative elements for radiographic studies, in the event that a healthy specimen is not immediately available.

The authors believe that different species of anurans have different calcium and vitamin needs, because one species may develop signs of NSHP when fed the identical diet used to successfully maintain another species. The intake of calcium during the larval stage is especially critical for normal skeletal development and calcium homeostasis of the adult. Calcium absorption is dependent on available UVB, dietary vitamin D_3, and calcium, as well as a healthy gastrointestinal tract, kidneys, integument, and musculoskeletal system.[43] A calcium source such as cuttlebone should be available for the tadpoles of many species; Ramsey Canyon leopard frog (*Rana subaquavocalis*) tadpoles that did not have access to a calcium block developed NSHP as froglets despite being fed a diet used successfully in many other ranid species (Wright, Proc ARAV, 2001, pp 41–42). Thus, any case of NSHP should elicit a thorough dietary review with an examination of the vitamin and mineral supplements administered. Consultation with others who have kept this species may provide essential tips to correct the contributing husbandry (including dietary) problems involved with NSHP.

Amphibians presenting with tetany, spastic movement, muscle fasciculation, bloat, limb paralysis, or rigidity are considered a medical emergency and should be treated immediately for hypocalcemia using

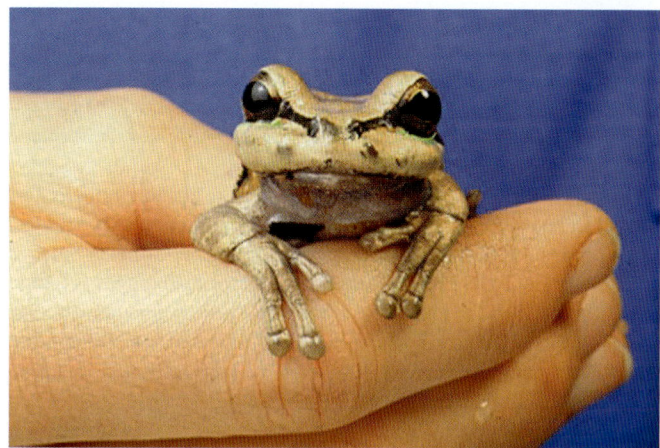

FIG 89.7 Mandibular, skull, and limb deformities as a result of metabolic bone disease of nutritional origin (NSHP) in a New Granada cross-banded frog (*Smiliscus phaeota*). (Courtesy of National Aquarium.)

100 mg/kg calcium gluconate intracoelomically, IM, IV, or SC. Administer treatment a minimum of 1 to 2 times daily (or more frequently if needed) until presenting signs of hypocalcemia resolve. Continue with weekly injections of calcium gluconate until eating, then switch to heavy daily supplementation with calcium carbonate; oral or injectable vitamin D_3 supplements may be required to facilitate calcium utilization. Providing daily baths in 2% to 5% calcium gluconate and 2 to 3 IU/mL vitamin D_3 may allow uptake of the calcium ion in many species but should be used as a supplementary aid and not the single course of corrective efforts. Amphibians with NSHP require several months of treatment for resolution of radiographic lesions and improvement of other abnormalities.

Oral supplementation with Feline Clinical Care Liquid (Pet-Ag, Elgin, IL), Carnivore Care (Oxbow Animal Health, Murdock, NE), or Emeraid Intensive Care (Lafeber, Cornell, IL) may be beneficial. The diet should be corrected so that the amounts of calcium, phosphorus, and vitamin D_3 are balanced. In some instances, the level of calcium may need to be increased over what is considered "normal" for other species—this is especially true for those amphibians that come from hard alkaline environments and those from peat bogs and other weakly acidic environments. Many amphibians are presented too late in the disease to ever regain normal health. Even if calcium homeostasis and normal bone density are achieved, amphibians with deformities of the skull and hyoid bones may not be able to feed on their own. Calcitonin therapy described for reptiles has not proven effective in amphibians because of the major structural differences between amphibian calcitonin and the salmon calcitonin used for the treatment of human osteoporosis.[45]

Hypovitaminosis A

Hypovitaminosis A is a significant disease of captive amphibians, as they are unable to synthesize carotenoids, which includes vitamin A, leading to vision loss, epithelial hyperplasia, squamous metaplasia, and keratinization of mucosal epithelium.[43] This nutritional disorder was first recognized in captive Wyoming toads (*Bufo baxteri*), an endangered species that is the subject of an intense captive propagation program to produce specimens for reintroduction to the wild. An afflicted toad sights and targets a moving cricket and then rocks forward and flicks its tongue out to capture that prey. Often the cricket walks away from this attack, seemingly missed by the tongue flick. Within the Wyoming toad species survival program (SSP), this syndrome became known as "short tongue syndrome" because it looked like the toads were undershooting their targeted prey, as if their tongues were shorter than they should be. The condition appeared to be acquired, with clinical signs usually occurring in subadult to adult animals and slowly worsening over time. Affected toads eventually require assist-feeding as they become completely unable to capture prey.

Pessier determined that the underlying cause of short tongue syndrome was squamous metaplasia of the mucous glands of the tongue rather than an actual shortening of the tongue.[46] These lingual mucous glands were not able to produce mucus. A healthy toad tongue is coated with a sticky layer of mucus that serves to "glue" a prey item to the tongue and hold the prey as the tongue is retracted into the mouth. An afflicted toad was indeed hitting a cricket with its tongue flick, but the tongue lacked the gluey coating necessary to hold the cricket. Squamous metaplasia of the mucous glands is a lesion consistent with hypovitaminosis A in other vertebrates. Since the documentation of this lesion in Wyoming toads, several other amphibians have been reported with lingual squamous metaplasia. Squamous metaplasia has also been noted in the urinary bladder and kidney and may be an underlying etiology for hydrocoelom. Afflicted toads had mean liver retinol levels of 105 ug/kg (range, 44–164 ug/g), whereas the toads with short tongue syndrome had a mean of 1.5 ug/g (range, undetectable to 7.3 ug/g).[46] This finding supported the diagnosis of hypovitaminosis A. Some frogs with conjunctival swellings that were nonresponsive to antibiotic treatments did have resolution after supplementation with vitamin A either orally or topically (Fig. 89.8).

Hypovitaminosis A is associated with an impaired immune system and secondary infections in other vertebrates. It is not clear if hypovitaminosis A impacts the secretions of glands involved in producing and maintaining the cutaneous slime layer, but it does seem likely that at least the mucus production is impaired. This may enhance colonization of the skin by various pathogens and predispose to infection by *Batrachochytrium dendrobatidis*, a fungus that feeds on keratin.

Insects are typically low in vitamin A, so domestic crickets are a poor source of vitamin A, yet crickets are a mainstay of the diets for captive amphibians. One popular commercial supplement lacks vitamin A but has beta-carotene. Frogs that received only this supplement developed conjunctival lesions. Even multivitamin supplements with sufficient vitamin A at the time the container is opened lose their potency if the supplement is stored in areas that have high humidity, warm temperatures, or both. A multivitamin supplement should be used within 6 months of opening the container.

Consideration of vitamin A supplementation in any clinically ill amphibian is reasonable, particularly one with signs similar to short tongue syndrome, swollen eyelids, evidence of infectious dermatitis, hydrocoelom, or simple failure to thrive. Commercially available vitamin A injectable solutions are too concentrated to use in all but the largest amphibians. If a sufficiently low concentration can be made at a compounding pharmacy, an intramuscular dose of 2 IU/g every 72 hours until clinical signs resolve is possible. Another possible treatment route is oral administration at a dose not to exceed 1 IU/g orally daily for 2 weeks or until clinical signs resolve. The oral vitamin A can be expressed from a human-grade vitamin A supplement (liquid gel cap) and diluted with propylene glycol to an appropriate concentration. Propylene glycol may cause irritation in some amphibians, so the client should be advised of possible adverse reactions. Topical treatment with vitamin D₃ is effective in amphibians, so topical administration of vitamin A may be effective.

During a necropsy, the whole tongue should be submitted to rule out hypovitaminosis A. Because the affected glands are more prominent at the rostral tip of the tongue early in the disease, a longitudinal section of the tongue should be examined rather than a cross section. In addition,

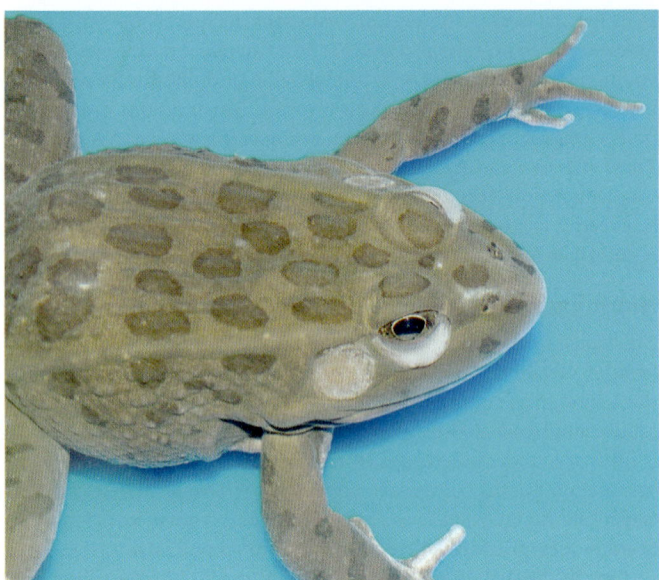

FIG 89.8 An anuran with bilateral conjunctival swelling typical of hypovitaminosis A.

other sensitive structures, such as the bladder, kidneys, and eyelids, should be assessed histologically for evidence of squamous metaplasia. A frozen section of the liver can be submitted for vitamin A analysis. If the levels are below 40 ug/g, and histological evidence of squamous metaplasia is seen in any of the high-risk organs, a diagnosis of hypovitaminosis A is reasonable.

Obesity

Obesity is also a common nutritional disease in captive amphibians, especially in animals that are regularly offered rodents. Some horned frogs (*Ceratophrys* spp.) may reach astounding proportions if fed to satiation on a regular basis. Most of an amphibian's stored fat is in the form of coelomic fat pads; thus, the obese amphibian generally has a grossly distended abdomen and normal-appearing limbs and tail (if present). Although investigations into the long-term effects of obesity in captive amphibians are lacking, obesity in amphibians undoubtedly has a major impact on health. Decreased longevity and poor reproductive performance may be associated with obesity in amphibians.

Gastric Overload or Impaction

Another common syndrome in captive amphibians is gastric overload or impaction (GOI). This potentially lethal condition is generally the result of eating a single overly large prey or consuming too many prey items in a short period of time. South American horned frogs and African bullfrogs (*Pyxicephalus adspersus*) are most likely to be presented with this condition, because many owners take inordinate pride in the gustatory capabilities of their animal. The owner may attempt to see how many prey items (e.g., mice) the anuran can eat in a single setting, unaware of the deleterious consequences this may have. An amphibian is often stimulated to feed when it sees movement. This may cause an amphibian to ingest a smaller cage mate, which is another cause of GOI in captive amphibians. Rocks and other foreign bodies may be ingested incidental to prey capture and swallowing, although pica has been noted in some anurans and aquatic salamanders. Some anurans retch and expel foreign bodies and large meals, but this is not often the case.

Swallowing an overly large meal can decrease respiratory ability. The lung is a simple saclike structure dorsal to the stomach, and when the stomach is distended, the tidal volume and total lung capacity are correspondingly decreased. Another complicating factor is that bacterial decay may outpace enzymatic digestive processes, leading to gastric bloat and endotoxemia. Because the prey often still moves after being swallowed, a distended stomach is prone to perforation, with subsequent contamination of the coelomic cavity with gastric contents. In the case of furred prey, the accumulated mass of undigested hair and bones may cause gastric or intestinal impaction. Gastric washes with hypotonic saline solution may remove ingesta in cases of acute gastric impaction, or if gastric bloating from fermentation is noted. Endoscopic retrieval of items via the esophagus may be possible in some cases. In most cases of GOI, a gastroenterotomy to remove the items is recommended. Pre- and intraoperative antibiotics and fluid therapy are recommended for an amphibian with GOI. The surgeon must determine whether postoperative treatment is needed based on the environment into which the animal will be placed during recovery. The benefit of mucosal protectants such as sucralfate is unknown. If an intestinal impaction from a trichobezoar is suspected, medical therapy (e.g., mineral oil) may be attempted.

Nutritional Support

Liquid formulas designed for the nutritional support of obligate carnivores are generally useful for amphibians, including Feline Clinical Care Liquid (Abbott Laboratory, Chicago, IL), Hill's A/D (Topeka, KS), Waltham Feline Concentration (Leicestershire, UK), Carnivore Care (Oxbow Animal Health, Murdock, NE), Emeraid Intensive Care Carnivore (Lafeber Co, Cornell, IL), or a ReptoMin slurry (Tetra, Blacksburg, VA).

A puree of cricket or mealworm abdomens, earthworms, or pinkie mice supplemented with vitamins and minerals may also serve as a tube-feeding formula, but this may need to be enzymatically digested with pancreatic enzymes to reduce its viscosity enough to flow through small-diameter tubes. Exoskeleton and skin are not digested well by pancreatic enzymes and need to be screened out of the formula to prevent clogs.

A red rubber catheter, polypropylene intravenous catheter, stainless steel gavage tube, or soft silastic tubing may be used as a feeding tube, the choice depending on the size of the amphibian's mouth. Care should be taken to avoid injuring the esophagus or stomach with injudicious use and placement of the tube. The tube only needs to be inserted one-third of the amphibian's snout-vent length to be in the stomach. Begin by diluting the supplement 50/50 with chlorine-free water and giving 1% of the animal's weight daily. This is slowly increased to 2% over a course of days.[47]

Hand-feeding (assist-feeding) may be possible for some debilitated amphibians such as the tiger salamander (*Ambystoma tigrinum*) or the dumpy tree frog (*Pelodryas caerulea*). Even debilitated specimens often swallow a piece of food (e.g., a headless cricket) that is placed in the mouth. Removing the head of the cricket exposes the viscera of the cricket and speeds its digestion. This option is preferred to oral tubing when possible.

INFECTIOUS DISEASES

Viral Diseases

The longest-studied amphibian virus is the herpesvirus, which causes renal adenocarcinomas in the northern leopard frog (*Rana pipiens*).[48] Lucke's renal tumor or ranid herpesvirus (RaHV-)-1 is one of the better-described viral-associated tumors, and its life cycle is generally predictable. Renal tumors grow rapidly during the warm months of the year. Virus replication is greatest at lower temperatures, with viral production occurring in the fall after the tumor has reached maximal size.[49] Viral shedding occurs the following spring, during spawning,

thereby ensuring the infection of the offspring and perpetuation of the disease. Affected frogs become extremely thin and generally die in the months after spawning. Hydrocoelom and hydrops may be noted in the latter stages of renal failure, and coeliocentesis may yield neoplastic cells. At necropsy, either or both of the kidneys may be affected, with a histopathologic diagnosis of papillary adenocarcinoma. Eosinophilic intranuclear inclusions may be detected in the kidneys of infected frogs during the winter months. In many ponds, the entire population of leopard frogs may be infected. A second herpesvirus, frog virus 4 or (RaHV-)-2, has been isolated from the urine of a leopard frog with adenocarcinoma, but the importance of this virus is unclear.[49]

Iridoviruses are DNA-based viruses in the genus Ranavirus that have been associated with die-offs in wild populations of frogs and tiger salamanders (*Ambystoma tigrinum* spp.) globally. A number of factors including persistence in the environment, direct and indirect transmission, the presence of reservoir species including fish and turtles, and changing environmental conditions contribute to the impact of ranaviruses. Ranavirus type III is the iridovirus responsible for tadpole edema syndrome, a disease that is fatal to the tadpole, with adult anurans as asymptomatic carriers.[50,51] Infected tadpoles and metamorphosing froglets have edema and subcutaneous hemorrhage, which may be secondarily contaminated with bacteria. Grossly, the lesions appear consistent with bacterial dermatosepticemia ("red leg disease"). Histopathology reveals intranuclear inclusions within the erythrocyte; a recent finding is that basophilic intracytoplasmic inclusions may also be seen within the glandular cells of the stomach.[52] Bohle iridovirus, implicated in declines of Australian anurans, is closely related to ranavirus III.[53,54] An iridovirus has been associated with mortalities of wild populations of the European common frog (*Rana temporaria*).[55] Gross lesions include erythema, petechiae, ecchymoses, and skin ulcers. Histologically, basophilic and acidophilic intracytoplasmic inclusions may be found within hepatocytes. Secondary bacterial infections are often noted. Frog erythrocytic virus (FEV) appears iridovirus-like and has been found in the erythrocytes of several species of frogs and toads, although the clinical significance of this infection is not known.[49] Ranaviruses can live in aquatic environments for several weeks without a host, emphasizing the need for biosecurity when accepting new amphibians into existing collections. Bleach (3%) and chlorhexidine (0.75%) for 1 minute of contact time are effective disinfectants. In 2016 ranavirus infection in amphibians became a disease listed by the World Organization for Animal Health (OIE) (http://www.oie.int/animal-health-in-the-world/oie-listed-diseases-2017/).

Other viruses have been described from amphibians (e.g., calicivirus, herpesvirus), as have suspected viral-induced lesions, but little effort has gone into the elucidation of disease states associated with viral agents, a fact hampered by the overall paucity of information on normal histology of amphibians. In fact, "poxvirus" lesions originally described from the European common frog (*Rana temporaria*)[56] actually turned out to be normal melanosomes when reviewed with transmission electron microscopy.[55] Nevertheless, viral diseases seem likely to continue to be recognized as a significant source of disease and mortality in captive and wild amphibians.

Bacterial Diseases

Gram-negative bacteria such as *Aeromonas, Pseudomonas, Proteus,* and *Escherichia coli* are part of the bacterial flora that may be routinely cultured from otherwise healthy captive amphibians. Poor husbandry (as exemplified by crowding, poor water quality, inappropriate cage design, spoiled food, exposure to toxins such as pesticides, etc.) may cause immunosupression and allow any one of these organisms to cause disease. Other pathogens, such as iridovirus or *Batrachochytrium dendrobatidis,* may be the primary etiology of disease in many amphibians diagnosed with bacterial infections; the original pathogen may be difficult to detect by the time the amphibian shows clinical signs of illness such as ventral erythema. This clinical sign gave rise to the term "red leg disease" or "red leg syndrome" in early reports of amphibian disease. When this clinical sign is caused by a bacterial pathogen, a more appropriate term for the disease is bacterial dermatosepticemia (Fig. 89.9).

Aeromonas is the most common genus isolated in published cases of clinical bacterial disease in amphibians. *Aeromonas hydrophila*, a common contaminant of water, has historically been associated with bacterial dermatosepticemia.[57-60] However, several other aeromonads and other gram-negative bacteria have been implicated in amphibian disease in addition to *A. hydrophila*. The following discussion is based on what is currently known about bacterial dermatosepticemia in amphibians, with the caveat that appropriate antibacterial therapy ultimately depends on the exact pathogen that has been cultured and definitively identified from the clinical case in question.

Clinical signs of bacterial dermatosepticemia may be brief and extremely rapid in chronology. Dilation of the surface capillaries and petechiation are common clinical signs and cause an erythema that is readily visible against white or pale-colored skin (Fig. 89.10). This condition may progress into ecchymosis and large subcutaneous hemorrhages several hours before death; at this point, the underlying pathogenesis is similar to disseminated intravascular coagulation in mammals. Typically, ecchymosis appears immediately before or during the agonal convulsions.

Bloating from intestinal gas, hydrocoelom, hydrops (Fig. 89.11), anorexia, and lethargy may be noted shortly before the onset of convulsions and sudden death. More than one animal in an enclosure is typically affected as a rule. Postmortem lesions are consistent with disseminated septic thrombi and may also include splenic congestion and areas of hepatic necrosis. Culture of the blood and internal organs of the dead amphibians is recommended to determine the underlying pathogen, and a blood or coelomic fluid (Fig. 89.12) culture of apparently healthy amphibians within the same enclosure is suggested to determine the likelihood of further outbreaks. Some bacteria, such as *Flavobacterium* spp., have as high an epizootic potential as the classic *Aeromonas* spp.[60,61]

Because amphibians commonly have mixed infections by the time they present for clinical examination, the initial therapy for an amphibian with signs of septicemia should target gram-negative bacteria and *Batrachochytrium dendrobatidis*. The patient should be treated immediately with aminoglycosides (5–10 mg/kg intramuscularly [IM] or intracoelomically [ICe] every 48 hours) and then soaked for 10 minutes in 0.01% itraconazole solution or other topical imidazole solutions. Be sure to use solutions that are alcohol-free; note that many of the solutions do not carry this note on the bottle's label and the manufacturer must be contacted to determine whether alcohol is in the solution. If the history suggests possible exposure to sources of *Chlamydophila psittaci*, doxycycline or tetracycline therapy should also be initiated immediately. Immediate evaluation of the husbandry should be performed with the intent of eliminating contributing factors. If possible, isolate, individually monitor, and treat on a case-by-case basis affected and suspect amphibians. Broad-spectrum antibiotics with anaerobic activity (e.g., metronidazole, penicillins) may be warranted, as anaerobic bacteria may be isolated from ill amphibians. Even with appropriate treatment, morbidity and mortality in an outbreak are likely to be high, especially if secondary infections are noted. Soaking the patient in amphibian Ringer's solution, 0.5% to 0.6% sodium chloride, or other electrolyte solution isotonic to amphibian plasma helps combat the metabolic derangement caused by the associated skin pathology.

Chlamydophila species have been reported to cause disease in a number of amphibians.[62] Symptoms may be similar to those observed in animals with dermatosepticemia. Differentiation of this syndrome

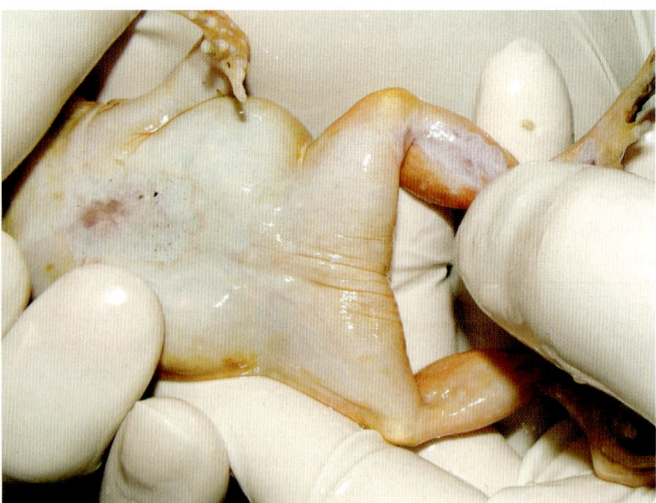

FIG 89.9 Ventral erythema suggestive of "red leg" in this anuran is more appropriately termed bacterial dermatosepticemia.

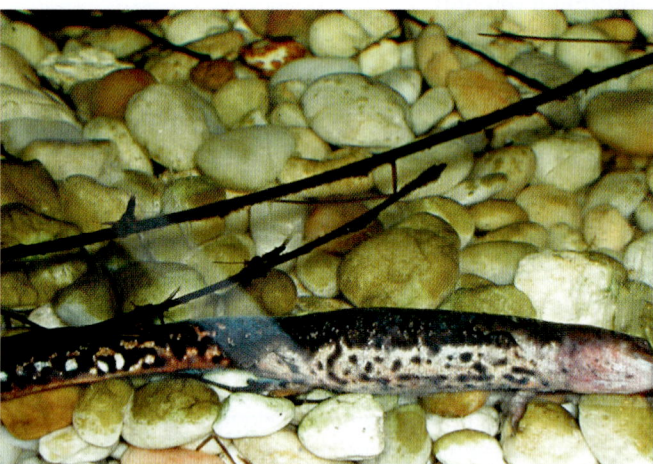

FIG 89.10 A paddle-tailed newt (*Pachytriton brevipes*) dying of bacterial dermatosepticemia. Erythema of the throat region is caused by dilatation and rupture of capillaries during this disease.

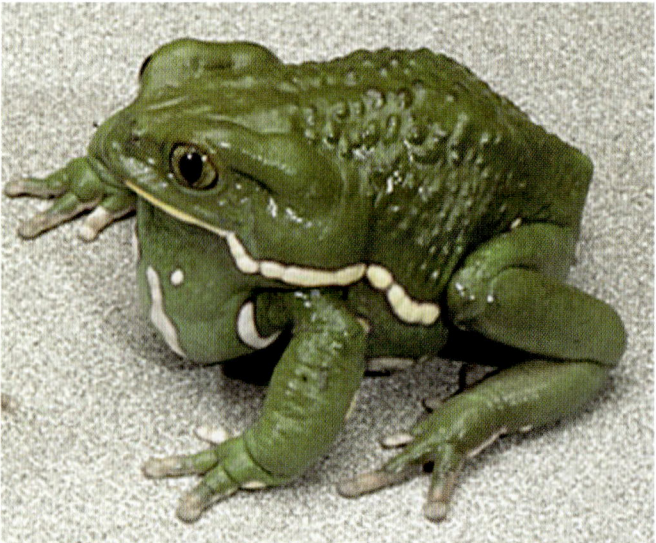

FIG 89.11 A painted-belly monkey frog (*Phyllomedusa savaugii*) with hydrops. Hydrops and hydrocoelom are often associated with septicemia, but in this frog it was caused by renal disease.

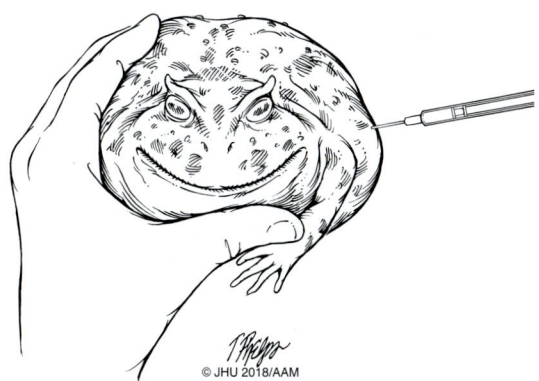

FIG 89.12 Fluid obtained with coeliocentesis may be collected for cytological, microbiologic, and biochemical analyses to help determine the underlying cause of the hydrocoelom. (Courtesy of Tim Phelps, Art as Applied to Medicine, Johns Hopkins University School of Medicine. Copyright 2018.)

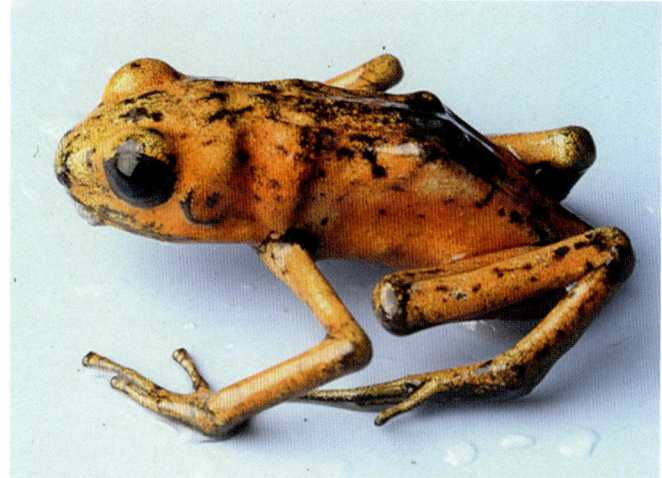

FIG 89.13 An emaciated splendid poison frog (*Oophaga speciosa*). (Courtesy of National Aquarium.)

from classical bacterial dermatosepticemia relies on the absence of bacteria in the cultures obtained and detection of *Chlamydophila* inclusions in the spleen or liver. Distinguishing between chlamydial diseases and rickettsial diseases may be difficult unless antigen or polymerase chain reaction (PCR) tests are used.[63] Doxycycline is the drug of choice for chlamydophilosis,[64] although tetracycline also may be effective.

Chronic bacterial infections are uncommon. Typical presentations include cutaneous ulcers, abscesses, or an amphibian with prolonged lethargy and a poor feeding response. Skin scrapings or cultures of any lesions should be obtained to rule out mycobacterial or fungal involvement. Cutaneous ulcers and abscesses respond quite well to debridement and appropriate antibiotic therapy, both topical and parenteral. The underweight and depressed amphibian likely has internal abscesses or a granulomatous disorder. Internal abscesses are poorly responsive to treatment unless they can be surgically removed. If a granulomatous disease is confirmed, such as mycobacteriosis or chromomycosis (see subsequent), immediate euthanasia is recommended because treatment is ineffective, and the diseases are likely to be zoonotic. A husbandry review is suggested to determine whether any contributing factors are present (e.g., abrasive surfaces, previous occupants that died).

Mycobacterium spp. can cause lesions in amphibians, and the species associated with amphibians are generally waterborne species or those that are soil saprophytes (e.g., *Mycobacterium marinum, M. chelonea, M. ulcerans, M. liflandii, M. ranae, M. xenopi*). Mycobacteria are ubiquitous in the aquatic environment, being found typically in the biofilms coating the animal's aquatic habitat. Infection occurs through direct contact with infected cohorts, consumption of infected organisms, or exposure to contaminated water. Immunologically competent amphibians will remain subclinical for long periods of time, whereas stressed animals typically develop acute and severe disease.[65] Mycobacteriosis must be considered in amphibian colonies, especially those on recirculating systems that are experiencing chronic illness and mortalities. In contrast to the more typical bacterial infections, amphibians with mycobacterial infections generally display weight loss early on despite a good appetite (Fig. 89.13). Clinical signs are typically nonspecific and include weight loss, dermal ulcerations, anorexia, and bloating. If any cutaneous lesions are present, diagnostics should include examination of an aspirate, scraping, or biopsy to determine whether acid-fast bacteria are present. If acid-fast bacteria are detected, samples should be submitted for culture or PCR and identification. The identification of the mycobacterial species does not alter the patient's prognosis but is important because

some species have a higher zoonotic potential than others. If no cutaneous lesions are found, exploratory coelioscopy or coeliotomy may detect internal granulomas consistent with mycobacteriosis. Finding such lesions warrants immediate euthanasia of the amphibian and counseling the client of the zoonotic potential of amphibian *Mycobacterium* spp. In closed, recirculating systems mycobacteriosis can be spread rapidly and infect many of the animals within the colony. Because there is no effective treatment at this time, removal and euthanasia of infected individuals is required to control the spread throughout the colony and prevent the infection of the human handlers.

Fungal and Algal Diseases

Most fungal and algal species that are involved in infectious diseases of amphibians are opportunistic invaders that invade injured or otherwise immunocompromised animals. An important exception is amphibian chytridiomycosis. The causative agent, *Batrachochytrium dendrobatidis* (Bd), was first described in captive amphibians but has since been identified in free-ranging populations and has been implicated in the decline of frogs, toads, salamanders, and newts in seemingly pristine environments.[66] Recently, a second, highly divergent, chytrid pathogen, *Batrachochytrium salamandrivorans* (Bs), has been implicated in the near-extinction of the fire salamander, *Salamandra salamandra*, in the Netherlands.[67]

Chytridiomycosis is typically associated with moist environments where motile zoospores can swim and infect cohorts. Because Bd feeds on keratin, postmetamorphic anurans with keratinized skin are usually affected more than tadpoles, which have only keratinized mouthparts and are usually subclinical. Clinical signs associated with Bd may vary from sudden death with no obvious external signs to progressive lethargy, excessive skin shedding, ventral erythema and petechiation (Fig. 89.14), deformities of the keratin beaks in tadpoles, and cutaneous lesions on the tips of the toes. In contrast, salamanders infected with Bs show multifocal skin erosions all over their body, become ataxic, anorectic, and die within 7 days of being infected.[67] Diagnosis of Bd relies on identification of the agent in skin scrapings or other tissue samples.[68] Biopsies of the drink patch or toe tips are often productive. A commercially available polymerase chain reaction (PCR) test may be used to identify chytrid DNA from skin scrapings and is even more sensitive than histopathology or wet mount examinations (Pisces Molecular, Boulder, CO). Diagnosis of Bs is confirmed using a newly developed PCR. Bd responds to treatment using itraconazole at 0.01% in 0.6%

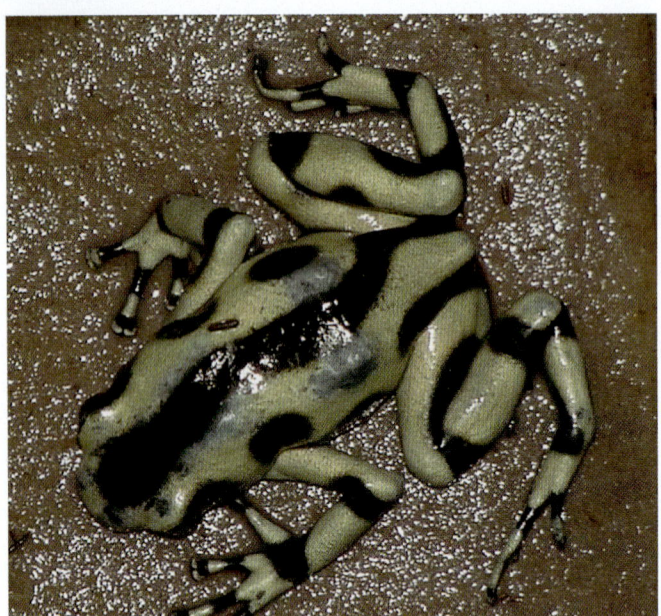

FIG 89.14 Epidermal lesions on the dorsum of a green and black poison frog (*Dendrobates auratus*). Although suggestive of an infectious etiology, these may represent abrasions that have been invaded by bacteria or fungi. A review of the enclosure should accompany the examination of the patient.

saline in a 5-minute bath for 11 consecutive days.[69,70] Spraying animals daily with vorticonazole at 125 mg/L for 7 days may also be effective and much less labor intensive.[71] Elevating environmental temperature to 25°C for 10 days has been effective for Bs.[72] Unfortunately, the fungus appears to persist in wild habitats and may continue to be a proximate cause of the decline of some free-ranging amphibian populations. As of 2016, *Batrachochytrium dendrobatidis* and *Batrachochytrium salamandrivorans* infections in amphibians are diseases listed by the World Organization for Animal Health (OIE) (http://www.oie.int/animal-health-in-the-world/oie-listed-diseases-2017/).

Other than chytridiomycosis, fungal infections are rarely encountered if an amphibian's husbandry is appropriate. Many of these fungi are ubiquitous in aquatic and moist terrestrial environments. An amphibian's covering layer of mucus and other glandular secretions provide protection from invaders, but damage to the slime layer or the epidermis allows fungi to colonize. Cage furnishings may be the source of the amphibian's injury; thus care should be taken to select decorations with nonabrasive surfaces and rounded edges.

Cage-mate aggression may be the source of the traumatic injury, especially if the vivarium is overcrowded. During the breeding season, the vivarium may become functionally smaller, as the inhabitants are more aware of each other and more prone to aggressive displays. In the wild, the subordinate amphibian is able to flee and avoid serious injury, but within the enclosed setting of a vivarium, little chance exists for escape. Reproductive and territorial disputes may culminate in bite wounds. Other sources of cutaneous injury are the nylon nets that are used to transfer fish and amphibians from tank to tank. Care should be taken to use soft netting or a plastic bag when capturing an amphibian to minimize the disruption afforded to the protective slime layer.

Amphibians stressed by other inappropriate husbandry techniques are especially prone to fungal infections. Proper nutrition, sanitation, and water quality are recognized as key elements in prevention of fungal disease in amphibians.

Saprolegniasis is primarily an infection of aquatic amphibians that can be caused by more than 20 different species of aquatic fungi. The characteristic sign of this fungal disease is the presence of a cottonlike material on the surface of the amphibian's skin or gills (Fig. 89.15) or in the oral cavity.[73] This filamentous growth covers an underlying cutaneous ulcer. The fungal mat's color can help the clinician determine the chronicity of the lesion. Acute infections are characterized by a light-colored fungal mat, and more chronic infections often turn green with algae or brown as debris is trapped in the fungal strands. If left unchecked, secondary bacterial infection may occur. A tadpole affected by saprolegniasis may starve as a result of infection of the keratin beak and ulceration of the mouth.[73] Temperature is an important factor in the progress of saprolegniasis, as its incidence rate markedly decreases at water temperatures over 68°F (19°C). Wet mounts of the cottony mat reveal the characteristic fungal hyphae and confirm the lesion as saprolegniasis. Because most cases of diffuse saprolegniasis are eliminated with appropriate use of salt, itraconazole, or benzalkonium baths, it is not necessary to speciate the etiological agent any further. Isolated lesions respond to topical miconazole, dilute benzalkonium chloride, or malachite green.

Chromomycosis is a disease of anurans that is caused by several taxa of pigmented fungi.[74] Cutaneous lesions are usually light-tan or gray to dark raised nodules, and the anuran may show signs of debilitation and weight loss. Presumptive diagnosis is based on finding pigmented fungi in wet mounts of scrapings from a lesion. Etiological diagnosis requires histopathology and fungal isolation. Chromomycosis has a tendency to become systemic, unlike saprolegniasis, which is normally a cutaneous infection, and chromomycotic granulomatous lesions may spread throughout the viscera. The course of this disease may be quite slow, and therapy is usually unrewarding. Cryosurgery may be effective in eliminating individual lesions, but the commonly available antifungal agents and topical antiseptics appear to have little effect on the course of chromomycosis in amphibians. Euthanasia is recommended for infected amphibians due to the zoonotic potential of many of the fungi and the lack of viable treatment modalities to date.

Amphibian eggs often mold if kept in an inappropriate hydric environment. Dendrobatid frog eggs typically need little free water if the humidity is high and the incubation temperature is correct. Salamander eggs often mold if the water is too warm or if the dissolved oxygen is too low. The mold may not kill the embryo but may affect the yolk and kill the tadpole within 48 hours of hatching.

Treatment of fungal disease should be aimed at correcting the underlying cause, so a diagnosis of fungal disease always requires a thorough husbandry review to improve the captive environment of the amphibians.

Mesomycetozoans

Mesomycetozoans are a clade of eukaryotic protists that phylogenetically exist near the animal–fungal boundary. Those known to infect amphibians include *Amyphibiocystidim*, *Amphibiothecu*, and *Ichthyophonus*. Previously reported as *Dermocystidium*, *Dermosporidium*, and *Dermomycoides* ssp., the Dermocystids that infect amphibians are now recognized as two distinct genera, *Amphibiothecum* (previously *Dermosporidium*)[75,76] and *Amphibiocystidium*. Continued molecular characterization of these organisms will likely result in nomenclature changes and taxonomic reorganization. The Dermocystids are spore-forming organisms that appear to be nonlethal, although severe infections may lead to generalized infection and mortality. Infected animals have multifocal nodules and pustules, usually on the ventrum, that resolve in 4 to 8 weeks.

The mesomycetozoan order Ichthyophonida includes the genus *Ichthyophonus*, whose species are pathogenic, causing myositis in pre- and postmetamorphic stages of salamanders and frogs. Clinically, animals

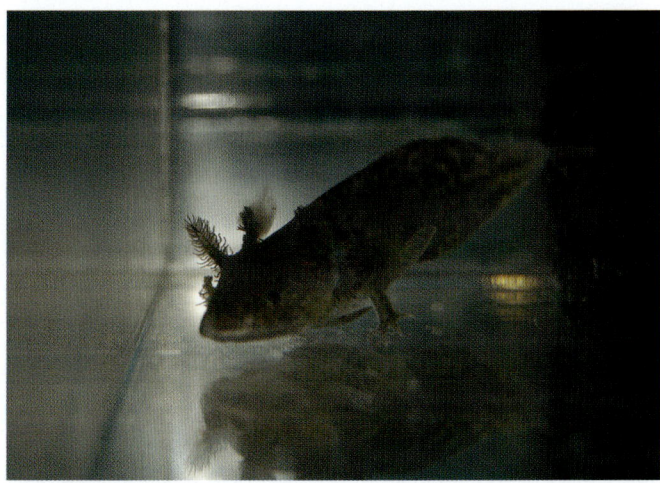

FIG 89.15 An axolotl (*Ambystoma mexicanum*) with saprolegniasis associated with the gills.

show muscle swelling in the thigh, rump, and tail and may appear nodular, especially in tadpoles. Although it may be considered an incidental finding, as in one study that looked at wild amphibians in Quebec, Canada,[77] debilitation may lead to mortality, especially in adults. A similar organism was found infecting the central nervous system of the southern toad (*Anaxyrus terrestris*) in Florida.[78] Diagnosis is based on histopathology or finding characteristic spores in skeletal muscle through microscopic examination of material from the lesions.[79] There is no treatment other than supportive care at this time.

PROTOZOAL DISEASES

Amoebiasis

Entamoeba ranarum is frequently found and has been implicated as a cause of amoebiasis in amphibians. Whether amphibians can recover spontaneously from this disease is questionable. Transmission is accomplished with ingestion of the cysts. The direct life cycle can lead to rapid spread within a collection. Cysts are relatively durable in the environment, and once ingested, the trophozoite stage excysts to mature in the colon. Pathogenic amoebae are most likely to directly attack the colonic mucosa, but the liver and kidneys can also be infected.[80] Certain conditions, such as inappropriate food items, lack of ingesta, or concomitant bacterial or parasitic infections, may predispose amphibians to amoebiasis.

Clinical signs are limited in the early stages of amoebiasis. Anorexia, dehydration, and wasting are common signs of intestinal amoebiasis. Stools change in consistency, becoming liquid and tinged with blood. Failure to pass any stool, as well as regurgitation, may be noted at this point. Hydrocoelom and hydrops may accompany renal or hepatic disease in amphibians. Dehydration is usually associated with renal disease in terrestrial amphibians.

Antemortem diagnosis relies on a combination of clinical signs and accurate identification of the cyst or trophozoite from a fecal sample or a colonic wash. Trophozoites are typical amoeboid forms, generally with a diameter between 16 and 18 μm. Cysts are multinucleate and are between 12 and 20 μm. Direct fecal examination of feces diluted with saline solution reveals the active trophozoite. Cysts are found either with direct smears or with flotation. Detection of the cyst may be enhanced with the use of Lugol's iodine. *Entamoeba ranarum* has very similar morphological characteristics to the familiar mammalian *E. histolytica* but generally has 4 to 16 nuclei. Pathogenic forms are difficult

to distinguish from commensal amoebae, but a preponderance of trophozoites and cysts in the presence of clinical signs such as gastroenteritis, hydrocoelom, hydrops, or dehydration lends support to a clinical diagnosis of amoebiasis. Other stressors are likely present in most cases.

Metronidazole may be used to treat amoebiasis in amphibians, and the preferred dosage and route are 50 mg/kg orally (PO) every 14 days. Aquatic amphibians tolerate a 15-minute to 30-minute bath in metronidazole (500 mg/L), but an oral dose is preferred when practical. If severe signs of intestinal amoebiasis exist, metronidazole may be given at 50 mg/kg PO daily for 3 to 5 days. Fluid therapy may be necessary. If an animal displays signs of neurological disease (e.g., listing, spasticity, lethargy), the dosage of metronidazole should be decreased.

Ciliated Protozoa

Ciliated protozoa are reported from many families of amphibians. At present, ciliated protozoa in the gastrointestinal tract are not clearly shown to have pathogenic effects on the host.[81] Ciliated protozoa are also found in the urinary bladders of some amphibians without apparent pathogenicity.

Finding ciliated protozoa in a gastric wash, colonic wash, or the feces of an amphibian is not unusual. If all other causes for an amphibian's unthriftiness have been ruled out, but a high density of ciliated protozoa is voided in the feces or urine, treatment with metronidazole, tetracyclines, or paromomycin may be warranted. Gastric wash, colonic wash, and fecal parasite examinations usually reveal ciliated protozoa during the direct observation of a sample. Cysts may be found on direct examination and after concentration with flotation. Ciliated protozoa often are found in the lumen of the gastrointestinal tract at necropsy. The absence of signs of an inflammatory process such as heterophilic infiltrates supports the supposition that the ciliated protozoa are commensals. With signs of inflammation, care must be taken to exclude other etiological agents, such as amoebae, coccidia, and bacteria.

Cloudy patches of skin, ulcers, and reddened gills may be related to ciliated protozoal infections in aquatic amphibians. It is most likely to be a problem if water filtration and sanitation are poor and lead to high concentrations of organic debris. Skin scraping and direct observation with a wet-mounted sample usually reveal ciliated protozoa causing cutaneous lesions.

Oral tetracyclines and paromomycin sulfate may be warranted in an ill amphibian (with or without overt gastrointestinal disease) that has a high density of ciliated protozoa in its feces or gastric wash. Dosage is empirical, but a starting level of 10 mg/kg PO once daily (SID) for metronidazole, 50 mg/kg PO twice daily (BID) for tetracycline, or 50 to 75 mg/kg PO SID for paromomycin is suggested. Frequent water changes and improved sanitation and filtration usually eliminate ciliated protozoa in aquatic amphibians. Baths with acriflavin, salt (10–25 g/L), or benzalkonium chloride may be useful in some cases.

Miscellaneous Protozoa

A variety of hemoparasites are found in amphibians, and the description and nomenclature of this group of parasites are beyond the scope of this article. A common finding in amphibian blood films is the presence of trypanosomes. Many trypanosome infections are subclinical and apparently have little effect on the captive amphibian. However, quinidine therapy may be warranted for an amphibian with signs of anemia or debilitation and concomitant trypanosomes. A suggested regimen for quinidine may begin with the method recommended for tropical fish, a 1 hour bath of quinine sulfate (30 mg/L).[82]

Sudden death may occur in amphibians with trypanosome infections. Splenomegaly is a common postmortem finding in these amphibians, and the trypanosome may often be seen in impression smears made of the spleen. Malarial parasites have been found to exert an influence on the performance and reproductive success of certain lizards, and a similar situation likely occurs with amphibians and their trypanosomes.

The introduction of various pathogenic protozoa can occur via feeder fish and via other live aquatic foods (e.g., Tubifex worms) or live aquatic plants placed within a vivarium. A protocol for screening live foods and decorative plants is suggested to minimize the accidental introduction of pathogens into a collection. Dipping the food items and live plants in a hypertonic salt bath (<5 minutes), and following that with chlorinated tap water (<30 minutes) or an acriflavin bath (1–2 hours), helps reduce the possibility of introducing unwanted organisms into the amphibian's enclosure.

METAZOAL DISEASES

Nematodes

Amphibians are host to a staggering variety of nematodes, only a few of which have received intensive study.[83] *Rhabdias* spp. are the best-known lungworms in anurans. Infective larvae penetrate the skin and migrate, with the final molt occurring in the lungs. Little damage may be noted on histopathologic examination of the lungs of an anuran with one or two adult *Rhabdias* present, but heavy infections can result in damage to the pulmonary tissue with associated inflammation and secondary infections. Diagnosis is through fecal parasite or oropharyngeal mucus examination, and the characteristic rhabditiform larvae may be seen. Embryonated ova may be detected in the feces (Fig. 89.16). Some frogs (e.g., glass frogs [*Centrolenella* spp.]) can be transilluminated and thereby reveal large adult worms in the lungs, but this is generally a postmortem finding. Because of the direct life cycle, infected amphibians should be isolated and strict hygiene practiced, preventing spread to other amphibians or superinfection of the original animal.

Strongyloides sp. also have a direct life cycle and may cause severe intestinal lesions. Severe strongyloidiasis may be debilitating and contribute to protein-losing enteropathy and generalized malnutrition.[84] Treatment with anthelmintics may need to be prolonged to eliminate *Strongyloides* sp., as with *Rhabdias* infections, and scrupulous attention to cage sanitation is required. Baths with ivermectin (10 mg/L) or levamisole (100–300 mg/L for 24 hours) weekly for 12 weeks or more may be needed to reduce or eliminate *Rhabdias* spp. Oral fenbendazole (crushed and coated onto crickets for 3 consecutive days) and levamisole (6.5–13.5 mg/kg), applied to the pelvic patch of Houston toads (*Bufo [Anaxyrus] houstonensis*), has been used to effectively decrease the nematode burden of both *Strongyloides* and *Rhabdias* and may offer a practical solution to managing these infections in captive environments.[85]

Filarid nematodes are frequently found free within the coelomic cavity, vasculature, or encysted within various organs.[86] Microfilaria may be noted in some infections, and the presence of microfilaria in the blood of debilitated amphibians does suggest a causal relationship. Treatment with ivermectin may be attempted, but the inflammation associated with the death of the nematode can severely compromise the amphibian.

Some nematodes may cause signs of cutaneous hemorrhage and exfoliation. *Pseudocapillaroides xenopi* has been the causative agent of these signs in the aquatic African clawed frog (*Xenopus laevis*).[87,88] The nematodes and ova can be found in both the mucus and skin scrapings from the lesions. Thiabendazole (50–100 mg/kg PO) and levamisole (5 mg/kg subcutaneously [SQ] followed by 10 mg/kg SQ at day 10 and day 20) was reported as efficacious in eliminating the parasite. Ivermectin baths (10 mg/L) or levamisole baths (100–300 mg/L) for 1 hour weekly are also effective in eliminating cutaneous nematodes.

Signs of gastrointestinal distress may accompany intestinal nematodiasis. Demonstration of parasite ova in feces warrants anthelmintic

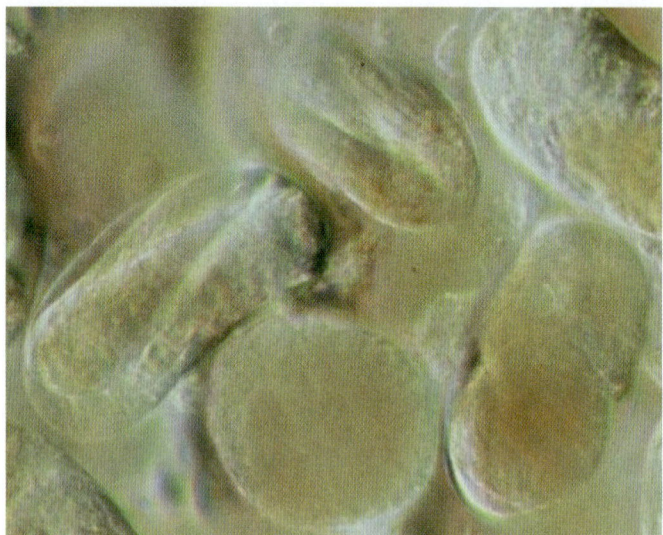

FIG 89.16 Larvated eggs from the lungworm, *Rhabdias*, found in the feces can be difficult to differentiate from other nematode ova. (Courtesy of Sarah Poynton, Johns Hopkins University.)

treatment. Oxfendazole (25 mg/kg PO), fenbendazole (100 mg/kg PO), oxfendazole (5 mg/kg PO), or ivermectin (0.2–0.4 mg/kg PO) is a recommended choice for intestinal nematodiasis. Multiple weekly treatments may be needed to reduce or eliminate some nematodes.

Trematodes and Cestodes

Amphibians may be host to a variety of both trematodes and cestodes, and this situation is further complicated in that the amphibian may serve as the parasite's primary, secondary, or tertiary host, or even as a paratenic host. Larval forms are often found within an amphibian's body with a minimum of associated pathological effects once encysted. However, significant pathology may be associated with migration of the larval forms.[89] Adult trematodes are commonly found in the lung, urinary bladder, kidney, gastrointestinal tract, and skin. One trematode *Ribeiroia ondatrae* has been linked with development of supernumerary limbs in a bufonid *Bufo boreas* and other limb abnormalities.[90]

Antemortem detection is rare unless the trematode is visible, as may be the case for cutaneous infections, or if the trematode is shedding ova in a way that can be detected with routine parasite examinations (e.g., gastrointestinal or urinary tract trematodes). The same may be said for cestodes. The adult cestodes may occasionally reach high enough numbers to cause wasting and anorexia by themselves or in part from obstruction of the gastrointestinal lumen. Therapeutics of trematodiasis and cestodiasis are relatively unexplored. Praziquantel has been used in a number of species of amphibians without ill effect and with some efficacy in eliminating adult and larval trematodes and cestodes.

Other Metazoan Parasites

Microsporidial septicemia with ulcerative dermatitis has been described in the giant tree frog (*Phyllomedusa bicolor*).[91] Microsporidial spores were detected in impression smears from the cutaneous ulcers. Chloramphenicol sodium succinate (5–10 mg/kg ICe) in combination with topical oxytetracycline hydrochloride and polymyxin B sulfate appeared to be an effective treatment.

Myxosporeans are intracellular, obligate parasites that have been found in the gonads, oviducts, kidneys, urinary bladder, ureter, gallbladder, and liver of amphibians.[92] Fatal renal myxosporean infection in Asian horned frogs (*Megophrys nasuta*) has been reported.[93]

Chloramphenicol (70 mg/kg IM every 24 hours) and trimethoprim sulfadiazine (30 mg/kg IM every 24 hours) were not effective.[93] Medicated feed containing 0.1% fumagillin DCH has been helpful in managing *Myxobolus cerebralis* infection in fish.[94] In 2012, the myxozoan parasite *Cystodiscus axonis* was extracted from brain tissue of the critically endangered captive Australian yellow-spotted bell frogs (*Litoria castanea*). Clinical findings included subcutaneous edema, intracoelomic fluid, and swollen kidneys with pale foci. Histological evaluation showed sever tubulonehphropathy and acute encelphalomalacia.[95] *Cystodiscus* was first recognized in 1966.

Acanthocephalans are common gastrointestinal parasites. The ova may be detected on fecal parasite examination. Infection is usually without overt clinical signs, but if the acanthocephalan penetrates the intestinal wall, coelomitis may occur with rapid deterioration of the amphibian's condition. Acanthocephalans require an arthropod host, so the infection is self-limiting within the collection unless the arthropod food supply is contaminated or the amphibian's enclosure is contaminated with ova and suitable arthropods are introduced as prey species and can thereby acquire the parasite before consumption. Treatment is generally unrewarding, although high-dose ivermectin (>0.4 mg/kg ICe) may kill the acanthocephalan.

Leeches are rarely a problem of the established amphibian but may sometimes be seen in freshly imported or otherwise wild-caught specimens. Most leeches are ectoparasites, but one species actually resides within the lymphatic system of anurans. Ectoparasitic leeches are more commonly a problem of aquatic amphibians but have been noted in many nonaquatic species as well. Direct removal is necessary and may be facilitated with exposing the leech to a hypertonic salt bath.

Copepods are occasionally noted on the epidermis of aquatic amphibians. The arthropod can be diagnosed when placed in a wet mount and examined with light microscopy. Antiparasitic hypertonic salt baths as recommended for tropical fish are the suggested therapy for copepod infestation (10–25 g NaCl/L for 5–30 minutes), although ivermectin baths (10 mg/L for 60 minutes) also seem to be effective.

Trombiculid mites are occasionally encountered in terrestrial anurans and salamanders.[96] The suggestive clinical sign is the presence of erythematous vesicles in the amphibian's skin. Scrapings or biopsies of the lesions show the presence of the mites. Topical ivermectin is a suggested therapy in these cases, but hypertonic salt baths may have some effect. Antibiotic therapy may be required in amphibians with extensive cutaneous involvement and secondary bacterial infection. Prevention of this disease in a captive collection is established by heat-treating the soil and leaf litter used in an enclosure before its use.

An uncommonly seen but devastating parasite of terrestrial anurans is the toad fly (*Bufolucilia* spp.). The larvae infest the nasal passage of the anuran and literally eat the host until it can no longer function. Levamisole or ivermectin flushes of the nares and oropharynx may have some efficacy in killing small larvae, and brief exposure (<1 hour) to organophosphates (e.g., no-pest strips) may have some merit. More typical cutaneous and superficial bots may be manually removed.[97] Allergic reactions accompanying the removal of the bot are rare in amphibians. Flushing the wound with an antibiotic solution (e.g., gentamicin in saline solution) and concurrent administration of parenteral antibiotics is recommended in cases of secondary bacterial infection.

TOXICITIES

Amphibians are exquisitely sensitive to many toxins at levels that are tolerated without ill effects by reptiles, birds, and mammals. In part, this is the result of the permeable nature of the amphibian skin, the associated vascular network in those amphibians that rely heavily on it as a respiratory organ, and the high surface area to volume ratio of these generally small animals, all of which enhance the cutaneous absorption and assimilation of many compounds. Clinical signs of toxicosis may be quite vague, and considerable detective sleuthing is necessary to uncover the underlying offending agent. For example, the improper curing of polyvinyl glues used in plumbing vivariums results in the release of methyl-ethyl ketones and tetrahyrofurans, which can be toxic to amphibians, causing the animals to actively try to escape their environment (Whitaker, unpublished data). In some cases, the toxin may be detected with tissue assays of dead amphibians, but the small body size of many amphibians precludes exhaustive analysis in a toxicology laboratory—simply not enough tissue is available for analysis. Environmental samples (e.g., water, soil, food sources) should be obtained for analysis in addition to the samples taken from the amphibian.

A general recommendation for the veterinary clinic is to have a supply of well-aerated chlorine-free water and several clean glass or plastic containers for the treatment of intoxicated amphibians. A gallon of spring water that is aerated using an air pump and stone is an easy and inexpensive solution for clinics seeing the occasional amphibian. Tap water can also be used but may require pretreatment to remove chlorine or chloramine, if present. Chlorine (Cl_2) is easily removed using sodium thiosulfate, sodium hydroxymethanesulfonate (AmQuel, Kordon LLC, Hayward, CA), and/or a carbon filter. Chloramine (NH_2Cl), a combination of chlorine and ammonia, is more difficult to remove. Sodium thiosulfate can be used to break apart the chlorine and ammonia and remove the chlorine, but the ammonia remains at toxic levels and must be removed using zeolite or a biological filter. Sodium hydroxymethanesulfonate, however, effectively splits the chlorine-ammonia bond and neutralizes the resulting ammonia. The chloraminated water is recommended to be adequately aerated for 24 to 48 hours before use. Alternatively, there are water filtration systems now available that use catalytic carbon made from coconut shell to remove chlorine and chloramines that may be effective.

Avoid use of plastic containers that have held anything other than water to minimize the chance that toxic compounds are present (see subsequent iodine toxicity discussion). Rinsing the amphibian with clean water often helps remove some of the more common toxins (e.g., ammonia).

Clinical signs of toxicosis include erythema, petechia, increased mucus production, irritability, agitation, lethargy, dyspnea, convulsions, flaccid paralysis, regurgitation, and diarrhea. Many of the common disinfectants are toxic to amphibians: povidone iodine, chlorhexidine, quaternary ammonium compounds, chlorine, and ammonia. Iodine-based compounds and disinfectants that contain colorizers or perfumes are not recommended for cleaning amphibian enclosures, because the plastic and organic material within the enclosure may retain these compounds and serve as a leach source that subsequently contaminates the captive environment.[98] Stoskopf originally reported an incident of iodine intoxication of poison dart frogs that resulted in agitation and abnormal posturing before death. It was suspected that toxic levels of iodine diffused out of the plastic despite prior rinsing of the enclosure (Proc AAZV 1985, pp 86–88).

Treatment for disinfectant-associated toxicities is aimed at removing the source of the toxin and providing support to the amphibian patient. Rinsing with clean water, parenteral fluids, and nutritional support is indicated. If detected early, most amphibians recover from mild exposure. However, the long-term effects of the exposure may include immunosuppression and resultant secondary infections and other physiological impairments.

High levels of chlorine and ammonia are commonly implicated in the deaths of amphibians. Signs of ammonia toxicity include sudden death, gaping, reddened skin, excess mucus, bright-red gills, disorientation, seizures, failure to gain weight, and dull colors. Diagnosis is difficult, but ammonia intoxication should be suspected if the amphibian has been kept in a vivarium with biologic filtration of the water, and the system has been restarted or otherwise manipulated (e.g., major water change has occurred within the past 2 weeks; antibiotics have been added to tank water). A level above 0.2 parts per million is suspicious for a diagnosis of ammonia toxicosis, and a level above 1 part per million should be considered verification of ammonia as one etiology for the clinical signs. A complete water change is the best therapy for ammonia intoxication. Sodium hydroxymethanesulfonate (e.g., AmQuel) may be used to temporarily bind the ammonia if a water change is not immediately practical. In the event this agent is used, a water change should be done at the earliest opportunity.

Chlorine intoxication is likely if a major water change has occurred within the past 24 hours. Test the source water using a reliable system (e.g., total chlorine checker colorimeter; Hanna Instruments, Woonsocket, RI) to determine whether chlorine is at a dangerous level (i.e., 0.5 parts per million or higher). The affected amphibian should be placed in clean oxygenated water. A bath of 100 mg/mL sodium thiosulfate can be used to manage confirmed chlorine toxicosis. Sodium thiosulfate neutralizes the free chlorine by eliminating its oxidizing properties. After at least 30 minutes in the sodium thiosulfate solution, the amphibian should be placed in well-oxygenated, chlorine-free water.

Heavy metals are often overlooked as a killer of many captive amphibians. Plumbing generally contains copper, lead, or zinc; if tap water is used, the faucet should be allowed to run several minutes before the water is collected. In facilities with galvanized ventilation ducts, zinc toxicosis can occur due to the falling of condensate into the vivarium. Heavy metal toxicoses are far more difficult to diagnose than chlorine or ammonia toxicity unless the clinician is specifically considering it. An amphibian with a heavy metal toxicosis is often beyond the point of effective therapy. The use of chelating agents (calcium versenate, calcium disodium EDTA, dimercaprol) have not been documented but may be of use in managing metallotoxicoses in amphibians.

Salt toxicosis is rare and is generally associated with a marine aquarium near the amphibian enclosure. Amphibian enclosures should be kept well away from a marine tank, and water containers for the marine aquarium should be distinctly labeled to avoid confusion. If the possibility exists within the home, a hydrometer should be used to check the salinity of the enclosure water. Increasing the salinity of the aquarium water has been recommended to prevent ammonia buildup in unfiltered tanks. If significant evaporation occurs, the salinity may reach inappropriately high levels. Therapy for salt intoxication includes the use of hypotonic intracoelomic fluids (see Dehydration section) and rinsing in freshwater baths.

Pesticides are ubiquitous. The amphibian is exposed to these compounds in the wild and within the home. The effects of these compounds in amphibians include immunosuppression, reproductive failure, hepatic disorders, renal disorders, neurological disorders, and developmental abnormalities of larvae. Even a small exposure can have long-term effects in an amphibian—just remember the devastating ecologic effects of the "safe" pesticide, dichloro-diphenyl-trichloroethane (DDT)—and pesticides do not have to be evaluated with regard to their effects on amphibians to be declared safe for the environment. Do not use pesticides around amphibians. If pesticides are used, insect growth regulators are preferred over toxicants. Secondhand tobacco smoke appears to be irritating to amphibians. Amphibia vivaria should be kept in smoke-free rooms.

ENVIRONMENTAL CONDITIONS

Dehydration

Dehydration can quickly progress to desiccation for an amphibian without access to standing water in the absence of appropriately high humidity. Some species (e.g., *Bufo* spp.) are much more tolerant of low humidity than the average amphibian because of their decreased reliance on ammonia as an excretory product. Other amphibians (e.g., *Hyla* spp.) are able to tolerate low humidity by altering body posture to reduce surface area or by excreting protective substances on the epidermal surface. Nevertheless, all species of amphibians are susceptible to dehydration. When water loss exceeds a certain percentage of body weight (dependent on the species, as some species can tolerate over a 30% water loss without lasting ill effect), the excretory system may be irreversibly damaged. Thus, the amphibian may initially respond to therapy, but hydrocoelom and edema may develop within days to weeks due to renal failure.

The severely dehydrated amphibian often has sunken eye sockets, wrinkled and discolored skin, and feels tacky to the touch. Excessive tackiness of the slime coat of an amphibian may be the only sign of mild dehydration. Escapes are not uncommon; placing a shallow water dish on the ground can help support an escaped amphibian until it can be returned to the enclosure.

Rehydration is typically accomplished by placing the dehydrated amphibian in a shallow layer of well-oxygenated, chlorine-free water that is at the species-specific preferred body temperature. Intracoelomic fluids may be necessary and two solutions useful for rehydrating amphibians may be made from intravenous fluids commonly available to the clinician. One solution consists of one part saline (0.9% NaCl) to two Parts 5% dextrose (314 mOsm/L). The second solution consists of seven parts saline to one part sterile water (270 mOsm/L). Do not exceed 25 mL/kg body weight for an initial dose. Avoid use of potassium-containing fluids in the initial therapy, unless hypokalemia has been confirmed. Supplemental doses may be empirically derived based on response to the freshwater baths.

Abrasions

Abrasions are an important route of invasion for secondary pathogens. The environment should be free of coarse-grained woods, sharp rocks, or any other cage furniture that is rough and likely to cause injury to a delicate epidermis. Harsh nylon fishnets are a potential source of injury for aquatic species, so the softer fine-weave nets are preferred. Human hands can be abrasive to some amphibians, so gloves rinsed with aged water should be used when handling smooth-skinned amphibians. Abrasions may require treatment with topicals (e.g., benzalkonium chloride, gentamicin ophthalmic solution) if the wounds appear to be increasing in size, become erythematous, or have an opaque or serosanguineous discharge.

Water Quality

Certain parameters of water quality can cause problems if not within a narrow range: dissolved oxygen, nitrite/nitrate, ammonia, pH, hardness, and turbidity/bacterial blooms. Other parameters, such as tannin concentration, may be important to the animal but difficult to analyze. A sample of the amphibian's tank water should accompany any physical examination for illness, especially if the amphibian is entirely aquatic. Appropriate diagnostic tests should be administered to a sample of the tank water to determine whether any parameters could be contributing to the clinical signs seen. Therapy is aimed at correcting the underlying problem and restoring the tank water to appropriate parameters.

Ammonia and chlorine toxicity can be treated with sodium thiosulfate baths followed with well-oxygenated fresh water, whereas nitrite/nitrate intoxication may respond to treatment with methylene blue baths. Amphibians that have been exposed to a bacterial bloom are at risk of ocular and epidermal infections and systemic disease.

Trauma

Cage-mate aggression is responsible for many of the traumatic injuries in captive amphibians. Some anurans have tusks and sharp dental projections that may be used in territorial battles and may inflict severe lacerations in a fight. Amphibians that lack such armament may still cause injury by badgering the less dominant animals and holding them at bay from food, water, and appropriate niches within the vivarium.

Dendrobatid frogs may drown if maneuvered into deep water by cage mates. Amphibians may try to ingest one another, especially if the group experiences a "feeding frenzy" as has been noted in some anurans and salamanders. This can prove fatal to both animals involved, as frequently the ingested animal is too large (see gastrointestinal overload and impaction). Some larvae are carnivorous and may eat other tank-mates. If cage-mate trauma is the suspected source of any injuries, animals may need to be isolated or set up in a new vivarium with more space and hiding spots. Injuries may necessitate treatment with topical or parenteral antibiotics. Fluid therapy and other therapies may be needed to treat shock in severely injured amphibians.

Clear-sided enclosures are another source of traumatic injury, especially to the rostrum, for many amphibians (Fig. 89.17). This is especially true in active saltatorial anurans that do not recognize the glass as a barrier and may crash into the glass when startled. The clear sides may be covered with an opaque material until an amphibian has grown accustomed to its vivarium. Sudden movements and loud noises startle many amphibians, so a vivarium with these species should be kept in a quiet room with little human or pet traffic.

In addition to acting as a source of heavy metal contamination, metal screen tops can be a source of traumatic injury in anurans and should not be used. Plastic screening or drilled plastic is a preferred ventilation option for the amphibian enclosure.

Hyperthermia

Aquatic amphibians are especially susceptible to hyperthermia. Temperatures should not exceed 80°F to 85°F (27°C–29°C). Hyperthermia typically occurs as seasons change. In the fall, the vivarium that was placed either adjacent to or on the radiator when the heat first comes on can overheat. In the spring and summer, hyperthermia may occur as the vivarium receives more sunlight as the sun shifts in the sky. Malfunctioning thermostats are another source of hyperthermia. For these reasons, questioning the owner about location of the vivarium in the home is essential.

Signs of hyperthermia include frenzied swimming, uncoordinated jumping or walking, lethargy, and death. Autolysis is extremely rapid. If the autolysis is not advanced, histopathology reveals congestion of the cutaneous tissues and gill vasculature. Confirmation of hyperthermia requires skilled anamnesis in the absence of observed temperatures within the enclosure. Therapy is aimed at returning the amphibian's body temperature to normal levels rapidly and can be accomplished with bathing in freshwater ice baths and administering cool intracoelomic fluid therapy. Corticosteroid therapy may be helpful in some cases. If scalding has occurred, parenteral and topical antibiotics may be necessary, especially if there is any tissue manipulation or debridement. Unfortunately, amphibians with even minor burns have a poor prognosis because of the importance of the skin in maintaining water and electrolyte homeostasis. The amphibian may be placed into a continuous bath of full-strength amphibian Ringer's solution to combat fluid and electrolyte imbalances.

Hypothermia

Hypothermia is rarely life threatening in amphibians unless a rapid temperature drop of greater than 15°F (10°C) occurs or the absolute temperature drops below 45°F (5°C). The main clinical sign is lethargy or immobility, although regurgitation of a recently eaten meal or abdominal bloating may be noted. The hypothermic patient should be returned to its preferred body over the course of 12 to 24 hours. Some

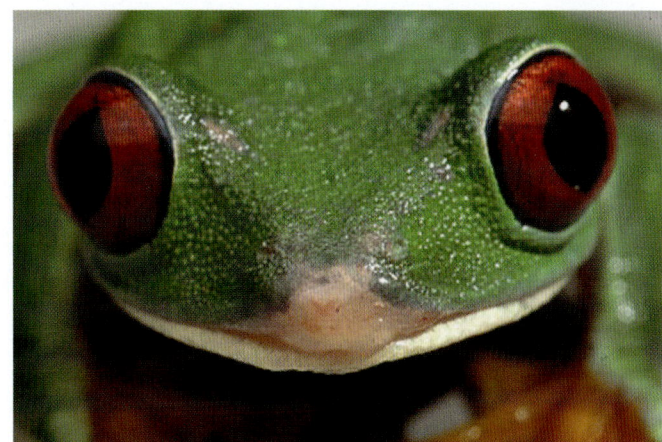

FIG 89.17 Rostral abrasion in a red-eyed tree frog (*Agalychnis callidryas*). (Courtesy of National Aquarium.)

amphibians are immunosuppressed after hypothermia, so the affected animal should be closely monitored for signs of infection over the next 4 to 6 weeks. Antibiotics are warranted if secondary bacterial infection occurs.

Noise and Vibration

Excessive noise and vibration from construction, pumps, and filters can cause stress and resulting health issues in amphibians. In one case, all 175 Xenopus frogs exposed to construction-related vibrations showed excessive gulping at the surface, skin sloughing, and abnormal buoyancy resulting in bloating and the death of seven animals.[99] Whenever possible, relocating animals during construction—creating noise, vibration, or dust—is recommended.

SYNDROMES OF UNCERTAIN ETIOLOGY

Spindly Leg

Spindly leg refers to a group of limb deformities that are associated with metamorphosing tadpoles. The classical sign is a tadpole that starts to develop hind legs normally, but the hind legs do not complete development and are noticeably thin and may show varus or valgus deformation at the time the forelegs emerge (Fig. 89.18). The deformities are not correctable, and the affected animal generally dies. Euthanasia of affected individuals is recommended. This condition has been attributed to various influences: genetic or hereditary, malnutrition, water quality, and enclosure temperature, among others.

Some dendrobatid frog enthusiasts believe the disease is due to improper nutrition of either the mother frog or the tadpoles and have recommended various dietary supplements for the parents and the tadpoles. Iodine solution has been recommended as an addition to the water to prevent development of this syndrome but has been refuted by other hobbyists. The use of water conditioners designed for tropical freshwater fish has been advocated by some. B-vitamin deficiencies and calcium deficiencies have been associated with causing abnormal metamorphosis of amphibian larvae; ensuring larval amphibians have B-vitamin and calcium in their diet or water is recommended. Several factors likely can be involved in the clinical condition called spindly leg. Careful histopathologic analysis of the affected tadpoles and concomitant standardization of the husbandry of the tadpoles and adults may well help elucidate the etiology and pathogenesis of spindly leg and indeed may recategorize this broad syndrome into a number of different diseases. A classification scale has been developed for *Mantella*

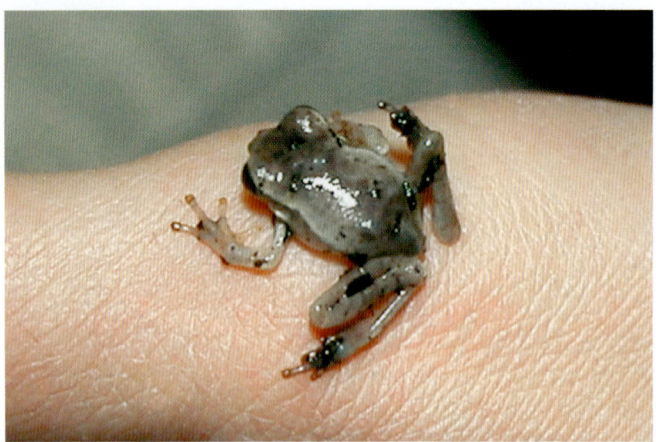

FIG 89.18 Spindly leg in a masked tree frog (*Smilisca phaeota*). Note the poor muscling of all four limbs.

aurantiaca tadpoles and metamorphs (Fig. 89.19A and B).[100] This scheme can be used by the clinician to document and gain a better understanding of the various manifestations of this disease in other species.

Corneal Lipidosis (Lipid Keratosis)

Some anurans have white corneal opacities develop (Fig. 89.20). In many cases, histopathologic analysis of the corneal tissue suggests the presence of cholesterol clefts; this condition is referred to as corneal lipidosis or lipid keratopathy.[101] The actual site of development of the lipid deposits may vary somewhat. It may originate from the scleral margins and advance toward the central cornea, or it may be present as a vertical line across the cornea. The opacities may remain flat or may develop into raised irregular lesions. Most affected anurans have a demonstrable hypercholesterolemia. Typically, the disease is systemic, with cholesterol clefts and inflammation detected in multiple tissues besides the corneas at the time of death.

The diets offered to captive anurans typically consist of pinkie mice and cultured crickets, which have different fatty acid profiles than their wild prey. In a controlled study, corneal lipid deposition was more prevalent in frogs fed a high-cholesterol diet than those receiving a regular diet; however, both groups had higher serum cholesterol than wild frogs.[101] Treatment of corneal lipidosis is generally unrewarding and consists of debulking the lesions and dietary manipulation. Unfortunately, debulking may actually exacerbate the lesion. Dietary management is aimed at the use of wild-caught insects instead of the commonly available monoculture crickets and feeding small amphibians or reptiles in place of mice. Alternatively, sparingly feed high-protein, low-fat foods (e.g., lean chicken heart dusted with vitamins and minerals, earthworms, and crickets that have not fed for 24 hours). The interested clinician may wish to investigate the potential therapeutic use of cholesterol-blocking agents in affected anurans.

Many of the species commonly reported with corneal lipidosis, such as the White's tree frog (*Pelodryas caerulea*), often bask and elevate their temperatures well above 100°F (39°C) in the wild. The opportunity to have these regular high body temperatures is seldom provided to captive specimens. These peak body temperatures may be important for normal fat metabolism. Basking spots should be offered to any amphibian with corneal lipidosis and is an important part of providing proper husbandry to all amphibians.

Gout

Gout has been reported in some anurans. Precipitating causes in amphibians are unknown but probably include dehydration, renal failure,

inappropriate diet, and toxicities. Gout is most likely to occur in those amphibians that commonly excrete a portion of their nitrogenous wastes as uric acid. Waxy tree frogs (*Phyllomedusa sauvagii*) are a commonly kept species that have gout and develop cystic calculi composed of ammonium urate.[102] This is likely due to a number of factors, including the feeding of a high-protein diet together with uricotelism and dehydration. Cystotomy to remove the stones may be required and is readily performed (see Chapter 107).

Gastric and Cloacal Prolapse

Many anurans may evert their stomach and wipe its mucosa clean with their hands. This may help rid the stomach of undigestible or otherwise unpalatable materials. It has also been seen as a sign of toxicosis, anesthesia with clove oil, hypocalcemia, and various other metabolic disorders. It is a nonspecific sign in anurans and may be benign and self-correcting. It usually indicates a serious disorder when noted in salamanders.

Cloacal prolapse is commonly seen. Predisposing conditions include dehydration, hypocalcemia, hypoglycemia, and malnutrition; gastrointestinal foreign bodies; cystic calculi; gastroenteritis; hyperthermia; trauma; and parasitism (Fig. 89.21). Treating an animal with a cloacal prolapse as quickly as possible will improve the likelihood of success. This includes keeping the prolapsed tissue moist and protected before gently massaging it back into place (see Chapter 107). It is important to maintain hydration of the animal, administer antimicrobials if tissue necrosis and infection has occurred, and correct the underlying cause of the prolapse.

NEOPLASTIC DISEASE

Renal, integumentary, hepatic, and gonadal neoplasms are among the most commonly reported tumors of amphibians. Although some anurans appear to have anticancer secretory products and cytoprotective devices, and the urodeles are hypothesized to have reduced tumor susceptibility due to their regenerative capability, neoplasia due to cellular neoplastic transformation occurs. Etiologies may include viral infection, exposure to pollutants, or genetic predisposition.[103] Clinically, examination may reveal the presence of internal or external masses or simply the presence of hydrocoelom and hydrops. Celiocentesis may yield cells with mytotic figures, high nucleus to cytoplasm ratios, and other histopathologic indications of neoplasia. Metastasis appears to be uncommon. Diagnosis of any of these tumors carries a grave prognosis, although some cases may be amenable to surgery (see Chapter 107, Fig. 107.2D).

Fibromas and papillomas are common types of benign tumors encountered. Management attempts may include surgical excision or debulking. Where possible, a surgical margin of at least 0.2 to 1.0 cm is recommended.[103]

A comprehensive review of the literature on amphibian neoplasia that included cases filed in the Registry of Tumors in Lower Animals and a comprehensive overview of amphibian oncology have been published.[103,104]

MEDICAL TREATMENTS

Relatively few studies support the extralabel use of drugs in amphibian species. The formulary in Chapter 128 consists of a variety of drugs that have been published or that the authors have used without ill effect in a variety of amphibian species. So many variables, including environmental temperature, water quality parameters, diet, and health status, affect the absorption and utilization of drugs. Thus no claim can be made to the actual efficacy of a drug for the treatment of a given set of clinical conditions. This formulary is intended solely as a guide for

Stage	Affected Limb	Description
5	R	Rear limbs are extremely stunted or absent despite tadpole body development to metamorphosis. [*]
	F	Forelimbs do not emerge. [*]
4	R	Rear limbs are small, stunted, and stiff. Toes have not developed fully and are not separated. [*]
	F	Forelimbs emerge underdeveloped and are thin. Toes on forelimbs may be underdeveloped or absent. [**]
3	R	Rear limbs are stunted and stiff, and toes have developed. Legs do not bend and may splay outwards. [*]
	F	Forelimbs appear fully developed but thin. One forelimb may fail to emerge or emerge abnormally- i.e. both limbs emerge from the same side of the body. [**]
2	R	Rear limbs are fully developed but thin. Legs splay outwards and may be crossed. [*]
	F	Forelimbs emerge with developed toes but are held abnormally- i.e. parallel against the body. Forelimbs may be thin and weak. [**]
1	R	Rear limbs are fully developed but thin. At rest, tadpole or metamorph does not fully bend legs but legs do not splay outwards. [*]
	F	Forelimbs emerge fully developed and normally positioned, but are thin and weak. Metamorph is able to prop itself up but mobility is compromised. [**]
0	R	Rear limbs and toes fully developed and appear normal. Tadpole may progress through remaining stages as normal, or metamorph may exhibit forelimb abnormalities.
	F	Forelimbs emerge completely and appear normal. Metamorph can hold itself up and move normally, and progresses through remaining stages as normal.

Illustrated SLS Scale

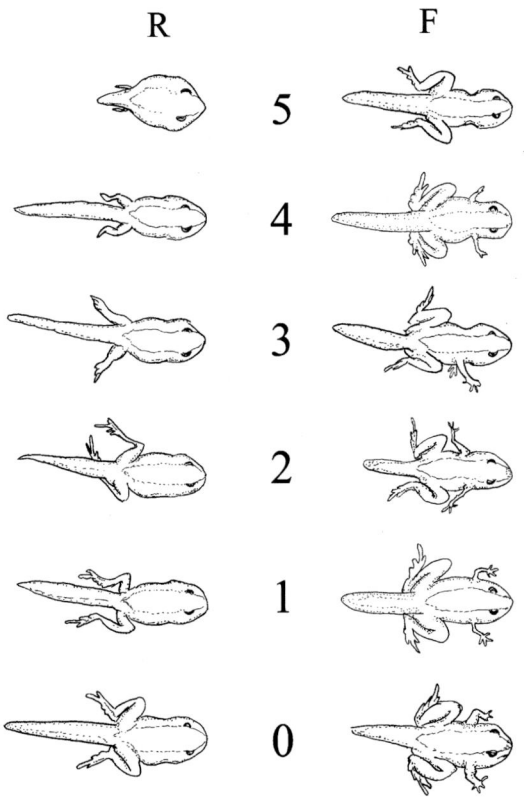

R   F

5

4

3

2

1

0

FIG 89.19 (A) The spindly leg syndrome (SLS) classification scale for tadpoles and metamorphs. A value of 0 represents no clinical signs of SLS whereas a value of 5 represents the earliest detectable developmental stage at which SLS occurs. *Continued development up to tail resorption may occur while limbs remain stunted at this stage, although most will perish before reaching this point. **Most metamorphs are unable or struggle to hold their head above water or climb out of water, and they may not be able to pursue prey. High instances of drowning at this stage. (B) An illustration of the SLS classification scale. (A, Classification scale descriptions modified; B, illustration used with permission).

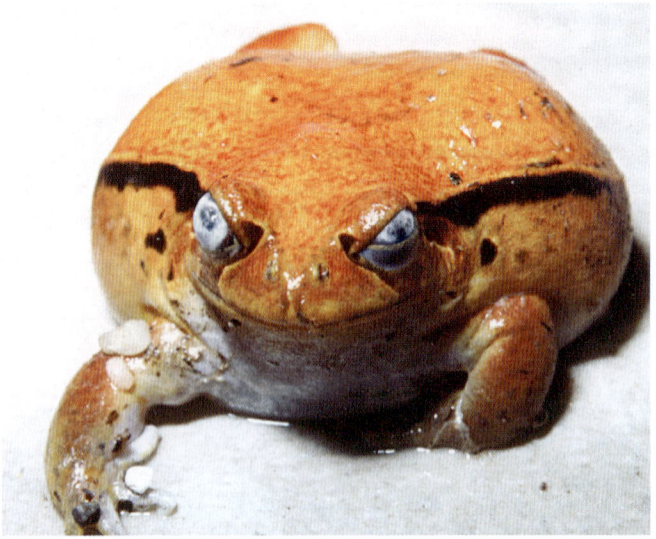

FIG 89.20 A Madagascan tomato frog (*Dyscophus antongilii*) with corneal lipidosis. (Courtesy of Douglas R. Mader.)

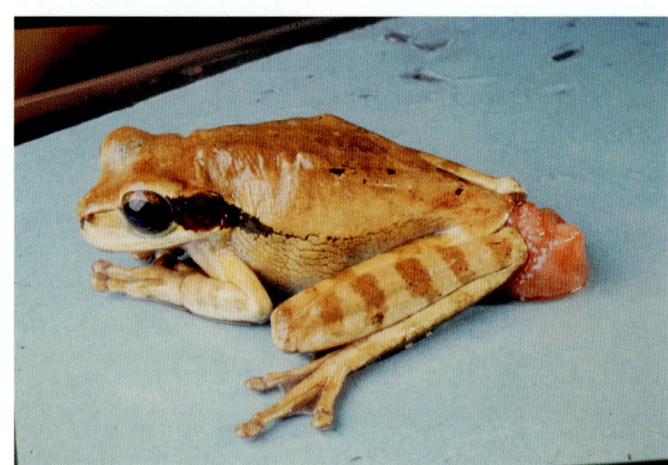

FIG 89.21 Cloacal prolapse in a masked tree frog (*Smilisca phaeota*). Intestinal prolapse is common with nematodiasis, gastroenteritis, or toxicoses. Prolapses of the bladder or other tissues are less common but are more typical of septicemia or toxicoses. (Courtesy of National Aquarium.)

the clinician. Whenever possible, we suggest that referenced papers be reviewed before administering medications to amphibians.

Routes of Delivery

Drug pharmacokinetics are influenced by many factors, including the route of administration. Transcutaneous administration of drugs in the form of a dip, prolonged bath, or topical application is quite effective for cutaneous diseases, such as fungal and protozoal infections. Given the extensive ventral vascularization and thickness of the skin of amphibians, sufficient uptake of the drug may occur to achieve therapeutic levels in the blood and internal organs, and thus antibacterial baths and topical treatments have been successfully used. Other factors that are likely to affect percutaneous absorption include damage and disease to the barrier properties of the skin, appendage density and size, exocrine secretions that coat the skin, and the physiochemical properties of the chemical and its formulation.[105]

Oxytetracycline baths have been advocated in the treatment of aeromoniasis in aquatic larval tanks and adult breeding tanks. Given that many aeromonads are resistant to tetracyclines, the clinician often must use other antibiotics, and many of these antibiotics are not useful for "bath therapy." Gentamicin baths have been an option for management of septicemia, but the drug concentration must exceed 1 mg/mL solution to reach effective blood levels in *Rana pipiens*.[106] Ciprofloxacin 10 mg/L in a 6 to 8 hr bath has been effective in treating many bacterial infections but should be reserved for cases with resistance to more basic drugs.

Ivermectin (0.2–0.4 mg/kg)[107] and praziquantel (8–24 mg/kg) solutions have been applied topically to anurans with subsequent reduction in the numbers of parasitic ova shed via the feces. Given the small body size of many amphibians, such as dendobatid frogs, administration of drugs via oral or parenteral routes may be impractical. When practical, oral or parenteral routes of administration are preferred to ensure adequate uptake and distribution of any given drug. Microliter syringes and pipettes greatly improve accuracy when administering small doses of drugs.

Intracoelomic, subcutaneous, and intramuscular injections are the most common routes of drug delivery used in the treatment of amphibians of sufficient body size. Intracoelomic injections may be given in the paralumbar fossa or just off the ventral midline. The skin over the dorsum, shoulder, or pelvis is usually loose enough to allow tenting of the skin for subcutaneous injections. The epaxial musculature is a useful site for the injection of intramuscular medications in salamanders and caecilians. The maximum drug volume given per site is dependent on the body size/mass of the animal, muscle condition, and irritation/pain associated with the medication administered. The forelimbs are a preferred site for anurans. The ability of the amphibian mesonephric kidney to excrete many of the commonly used drugs and drug metabolites is poorly documented.

Amphibians with hydrocoelom or subcutaneous edema may require baths in electrolyte solutions to reduce fluid volume and correct plasma electrolyte abnormalities. Amphibian Ringer's solution is isotonic to typical amphibian plasma (~230 mOsm/L) and can be created by dissolving 6.6 g NaCl, 0.15 g KCl, 0.15 g $CaCl_2$, and 0.2 g $NaHCO_3$ in 1.0 liter of distilled water (see Chapter 128). A continuous bath in amphibian Ringer's solution is a suggested supplemental therapy for any amphibian with a bacterial or fungal infection. If amphibian Ringer's solution is not available, 0.5% to 0.6% saline solution is an alternative but lacks critical electrolytes. Hypertonic solutions may be needed when the amphibian patient appears grossly distended or edematous from fluid overload. Simple hypertonic solutions are 0.8% to 0.9% saline or the compounds for amphibian Ringer's solution dissolved in 900 mL or less of distilled water. Dextrose (5% or higher concentration) and hetastarch solutions may also be used as short-term hypertonic baths. Monitor the amphibian while it is in the hypertonic solution and remove it if it appears distressed or when it is within 25% of its normal weight. If the amphibian starts to regain fluid when returned to normal water, it should be returned to isotonic or hypertonic solutions for additional therapy. Some amphibians may need to be maintained in isotonic solutions for several days to weeks after recovery from a severe infection.

The intravenous route is largely unused in amphibians, although euthanasia solution may be administered via cardiocentesis.

The oral route is historically how tetracycline has been administered during *Aeromonas* outbreaks. Anthelmintics and nutritional support may be given via this route. An appropriately sized over-the-cuff intravenous catheter is a useful feeding tube for small amphibians. Waterproof paper or a thin wedge of plastic can function as a mouth speculum. Stainless steel rodent feeding tubes work well with larger amphibians.

AKNOWLEDGMENTS

On September 26, 2013, we lost Dr. Kevin Wright, our colleague, our collaborator, and my close friend. Whitaker and Wright were two dreamers alphabetically sitting side-by-side through veterinary school who shared a common interest in everything unusual and who wanted to make an important contribution of some kind. Our original *Amphibian Medicine and Captive Husbandry* book was the result of a mutual interest in these incredible creatures and our ability to study them in our day jobs. This chapter, on amphibian medicine, is likely one of the last works that Dr. Wright and I will write together—at least in this world. Although much of this chapter remains unchanged from that published in Mader's second edition of *Reptile Medicine and Surgery,* new information, illustrations, and references have been added.

To you, the reader, enjoy and discover.

To you, Kevin, farewell my friend. You truly have changed the world. We loved what we did, and we did what we loved. I will carry the bucket with you always.

BRW 2018

REFERENCES

See www.expertconsult.com for a complete list of references.

90

Surgical Equipment, Instrumentation, and General Principles

Stephen J. Divers

In general, performing surgery on a reptile patient should be approached in a similar way to domestic animals, and general surgical principles should not be violated.[1] However, there are some specific anatomical considerations, as well as unique aspects of patient preparation, positioning, and equipment, with which the reptile clinician should be familiar.

WOUND HEALING

Wound healing in reptiles occurs through phases similar to those observed in mammalian species. Initially, proteinaceous fluid and fibrin fill the defect to form a scab. A single layer of epithelial cells migrates beneath the scab. This single layer then proliferates to restore the thickness of the normal epithelium.[2] In addition, macrophages and heterophils migrate into the tissue below the scab to clean up bacteria and debris. A transversely arranged fibrous scar is produced by fibroblasts that migrate into the area. Heterophils are present within the scar tissue matrix until maturation has occurred. This is a slow process in reptiles. Consequently, suture removal is generally recommended 4 to 8 weeks after placement. The activity of the dermis and epidermis during ecdysis appears to promote healing.[2] If suture removal can be delayed until the subsequent ecdysis, wound strength is likely to be better. Peripherally placed sutures may slough off during the first postoperative ecdysis.

Environmental temperature has an effect on wound healing.[2] Maintenance of the patient in the upper end of its optimum range has been shown to promote healing. The orientation of the wound also influences the rate of healing, with cranial- to caudal-oriented wounds healing faster than transverse wounds. With treatment of open wounds, such as those that occur from burns, good environmental hygiene is important. These wounds heal well by second intention with a relatively low incidence of secondary infections.

SURGICAL EQUIPMENT AND SUPPLIES

Instrumentation

Table 90.1 lists some useful manufacturers and distributers of surgical supplies. It can be challenging to maintain a prepackaged "reptile surgery pack" that is applicable for a wide variety of species and procedures (Table 90.2). For truly giant reptiles, including giant tortoises and crocodilians, the use of stronger large-animal instruments is required, but for reptiles between 5 kg and 50 kg, most small-animal instruments are appropriate. However, most patients are less than 5 kg in size, and indeed the majority are typically <500 grams, and for these

animals, small and even microsurgical instruments are often required (see Table 90.2).

Microsurgery instruments are not merely miniaturized versions of standard instruments but rather balanced instruments with fine small tips, which are often the optimal instrumentation for small reptiles (Fig. 90.1). Since microinstruments can be costly, other viable options include ophthalmological instruments, and many practices probably have an "ophtho pack" in their inventory. Standard iris scissors, tenotomy scissors, Castroviejo needle holders, and Colibri forceps can be very useful. Organization of the instrument table is important and aids efficient instrument selection (Fig. 90.2).

One of the most important considerations in surgery is exposure. Plastic self-retaining retractors (e.g., the Lone Star retractor) are sterilizable (by autoclave, gas, or cold immersion), and can be adjusted to fit different sizes and conformations of surgical approaches. These ring-style retractors are lightweight, do not compromise ventilation, and occupy minimal space in the often-limited surgical field (Fig. 90.3). Smaller versions of standard abdominal retractors, such as pediatric Balfour retractors, Haight baby rib spreaders, and so on, can also be utilized but are significantly heavier and more obtrusive. Eyelid retractors can be useful for retracting coelomic incisions in small lizards and snakes.

A variety of surgical drills and saws should also be available. Autoclavable or gas-sterilizable models are preferred. For general orthopedic work of normal bones (which admittedly is rare), the Stryker drill offers excellent control and versatility, even for the smallest of patients (Fig. 90.4A). The oscillating sagittal saw attachment to the air-powered 3M mini-driver provides fine control and reduced tissue trauma compared with rotating saws (see Fig. 90.4B). The VI MiniDriver and MaxiDriver systems appear to be comparable and offer a sagittal saw as well as pin-and-wire driver attachments. A handheld power tool (e.g., Dremel 4000 High Performance Rotary Tool) offers a budget alternative to a dedicated surgical device, and various cutting discs are available (e.g., 22 mm Dremel 545 diamond wheel, 38 mm EZ545 1.5" diamond wheel). Small versions of suction tips, rongeurs, elevators, and bone-holding clamps are also useful.

Epoxy resins (e.g., Enviroset 5-minute epoxy, Environmental Technologies Inc., Fields Landing, CA) or low-temperature veterinary acrylics (e.g., Technovite 8100 MG kit, APEF acrylic packs) may be used for chelonian plastron closures and shell repairs. A two-polymer orthopedic putty is also a very useful aid to external fixation. A selection of intramedullary pins, miniature fixator pins, aluminum/carbon fiber clamps, and titanium/carbon fiber support rods (IMEX Veterinary Inc., Longview, TX) can be used to repair traumatic (nonpathological)

TABLE 90.1	**Sampling of Distributors and Manufacturers of Various Surgical Items**
Veterinary Instrumentation Ltd, Broadfield Road, Sheffield, S8 OXL, UK Tel: +44(0)114 258 8530 Email: clinical@vetinst.com http://www.veterinary-instrumentation.co.uk/	UK distributer of most products mentioned in the text
Jorgensen Laboratories, 1450 Van Buren Avenue, Loveland, CO 80538, USA Tel: +1 9706692500 Email: Info@jorvet.com http://www.jorvet.com	US distributer of most products mentioned in the text
Veterinary Specialty Products, 10504 W 79th Street, Shawnee, KS 66214, USA Tel: +1 8003628138 Email: Info@jorvet.com http://www.vetspecialtyproducts.com	Specialty exotic animal products including adhesive drapes, casting materials, anesthesia masks, Lone Star retractors, and select instruments
General Scientific Corporation, 77 Enterprise Drive, Ann Arbor, MI 48103, USA http://www.surgitel.com See website for international distributors	SurgiTel operating loupes
Ellman International Inc., 400 Karin Lane, Hicksville, NY 11801, USA www.ellman.com/products.html Eickemeyer Veterinary Equipment Ltd, 3 Windmill Business Village, Brooklands Close, Sunbury-on-Thames, Surrey, TW16 7DY, UK Tel.: +44 20 8891 2007 Email: info@eickemeyer.co.uk http://www.eickemeyer.co.uk/	4.0-MHz dual radiofrequency Surgitron
Aesculight, LLC, LuxarCare LLC, 11818 North Creek Parkway N, Suite 100, Bothell, WA 98011, USA Tel: +1 4254879988 http://www.aesculight.com http://www.luxarcare.com	CO_2 lasers
DiodeVet Lasers, 20 Shea Way, Newark, DE 19713, USA Tel: +1 3023687788 Email: info@diodevet.com http://www.diodevet.com	Diode lasers
Mila International Inc., 7984 Tanners Gate Lane, Florence, KY 41042, USA http://www.milainternational.com/index.php/ See website for international distributors	Numerous anesthesia, critical care, and surgical products

fractures in larger reptiles (Fig. 90.5A). A lightweight tubular fixation system, FESSA (Fixateur Externe du Service de Santé des Armées), is small and lightweight and incorporates a pin-clamping mechanism that is preferred for external fixation in smaller animals. The system, available from major distributors, is available in 6- and 8-mm tube diameters, with ranges in length from 31 mm (3.0 g) to 97 mm (12.2 g), and permits the placement of multiple miniature fixator pins close together in small fragments (see Fig. 90.5B). For internal fixation, small locking compression plates are preferred because they facilitate fixed-angle constructs and do not rely on plate-bone compression for stability, which is a frequent cause of cortical fractures when using conventional plates and screws (see Fig. 90.5C).

Lighting and Magnification

Proper lighting is an obvious requirement for surgery. However, it becomes even more important in small patients, and surgical lights should be focused with variable power settings. Modern LED lighting systems are more expensive initially but last longer, are cheaper to run, and produce less heat.

Some degree of magnification is often beneficial if not essential. There are a variety of magnification systems available. Table-mounted operating microscopes are very stable but must be properly positioned to avoid strain and fatigue (Fig. 90.6). Headband- or frame-mounted operating loupes (2× to 4× magnification) with a dedicated LED light source are affordable, versatile, comfortable, and, unlike table-mounted microscopes, have the advantage of allowing the surgeon to adjust surgical perspective (Surgitel, General Scientific Corporation Ann Arbor, MI, USA) (Fig. 90.7). The VITOM (video telescope operating monitor; Karl Storz Veterinary Endoscopy, 1 S Los Carneros Rd, Goleta, CA 93117) system allows practitioners to use their rigid endoscopy tower for operating microscopy.[3] The basic system involves a mechanical arm to hold an exoscope (so called because it is used externally), which is positioned above the surgical field, with the image relayed to the endoscopy monitor (Fig. 90.8). An 11-cm, 0-degree exoscope at 25 cm from the surgical site provides a 7 to 10 cm field of view at 4× to 8× magnification. The standard 2.7-mm telescope (commonly used in exotic animal practice) can also be used in a similar fashion.

TABLE 90.2 Useful Surgical Instruments for Most Procedures Performed in Reptiles Under 5 kg

Items Common to Most Surgeries

Plastic, adhesive drape
LoneStar retractor
Surgitron 4.0 MHz radiosurgery unit
Cotton-tipped applicators
Small scalpel handle and blade (often #15)

Standard Surgical Pack (<5 kg)	Microsurgery Pack
Plain ophthalmic fine thumb forceps	Mini Gelpi retractor
	Eyelid retractor
Adson 1/2 forceps, very fine	Stevens tenotomy scissors
Small scissors (top sharp tip, bottom blunt tip)	Balanced microscissors
	Doolen avian spay hook
Castroviejo retractor	Extra delicate mosquito forceps, straight
Small suture scissors	Extra delicate mosquito forceps, curved
Derf needle holder	Sontec curved tying forceps
Strabismus scissors	Ring-tipped thumb forceps with holes
Four curved ophthalmic mosquito forceps	Castroviejo needle holders
	Two spring bulldog vascular clamps
20 small gauze sponges	
Vetrap 2"	

TABLE 90.3 Comparative Thermal Necrosis Caused by Radiosurgery and CO_2 Laser Devices in Green Iguanas (*Iguana iguana*)[4]

	4.0-MHz Radiosurgery (Filter Cut)	CO_2 Laser (Focused, Superpulse)
Skin	307 ± 94 μm	386 ± 108 μm
Muscle	18 ± 7 μm	91 ± 15 μm

From Hernandez-Divers SJ, Stahl SJ, Rakich PM, Blas-Machado U: Comparison of CO2 laser and 4.0 MHz radiosurgery for making incisions in the skin and muscles of green iguanas (*Iguana iguana*). *Vet Rec.* 164:13–15, 2009.

Hemostasis

A healthy reptile, depending on species, can generally tolerate between 0.4 and 0.8 ml of blood loss per 100 g body weight. Patients in need of surgery are often compromised, and diagnostic blood samples may have been collected prior to surgery. Therefore the amount of intra-operative blood loss that the patient can tolerate may be considerably less. Careful consideration must therefore be given to evaluating, documenting, and reducing hemorrhage intraoperatively.

To allow the surgeon to apply localized pressure to a small vessel and keep track of blood loss, cotton-tipped spears, or applicators, are less traumatic and more manageable in small confined spaces than standard gauze squares. A blood-soaked cotton-tipped applicator typically holds about 0.3 ml of blood. Used applicators should not be discarded out of view but their number recorded to track blood loss.

Vascular clips (e.g., Hemoclips, Weck Closure Systems, Teleflex, Morrisville, NC; Ligaclips, Ethicon Inc., Somerville, NJ) are a convenient and effective way to clamp vessels, which are widely available from distributors (Fig. 90.9). Autoclavable applicators and clips are available in a variety of sizes. Applicators come in a variety of lengths and conformations (straight, angled), and clips come in 10- or 25-clip cartridges. The application of vascular clips is faster than standard suture ligatures, and therefore their use significantly decreases operating time. Any incompletely used cartridge can be cleaned, autoclaved, and reused until empty.

Surgical Lasers and Radiosurgery

A variety of surgical devices are available and most represent major capital investments that warrant careful consideration. A variety of comparative studies have been published and should, in conjunction with a hands-on trial (at a wetlab or in-practice demonstration), help form the basis of an informed purchase decision (Table 90.3).[4–9]

The most commonly used surgical laser (light amplification by the stimulated emission of radiation) in veterinary medicine is probably the CO_2 laser (10,600 nm), although diode devices and Holmium:YAG lasers are also in use and vary in wavelength and tissue absorption characteristics (Fig. 90.10).[10,11] CO_2 lasers offer bloodless dissection comparable to radiosurgery. In contrast, the diode lasers produce more collateral damage but consequently can seal larger vessels, up to 2 mm in diameter. Surgical lasers require enhanced human safety precautions, including a sealed, windowless surgery room and the use of protective glasses specific for the wavelength of lasers being used. Lasers and radiosurgery cause varying degrees of carbonization and produce smoke (which contains DNA, bacteria, and viruses) that should be evacuated with a filtered vacuum (see Fig. 90.10).

CO_2 Laser. There are several companies that sell CO_2 lasers. The CO_2 laser comes in a variety of sizes and power capacities from 2 to 45 W, and all are class IV (Fig. 90.11A). The invisible 10,600 nm beam is beyond the visible wavelength. When laser light is absorbed by a cell, the water within the cell is boiled and the cell essentially explodes. The cell denatures into smoke and the cell remnant, called char (carbonization).

When the laser is used for cutting, cellular destruction is limited to a region only three to four cells away from the target area, thus minimizing tissue devitalization (see Fig. 90.11B). In contrast, tissue destruction can be deliberately maximized for purposes of tissue ablation. Tissue cutting versus ablation can be controlled either by tip size or by "defocusing" the laser's beam. "Focusing" the beam allows the surgeon to use the laser's intensified light beam to "cut" tissue, whereas "defocusing" the beam allows the laser to "ablate" the tissue (Fig. 90.12A). There are three factors that determine the tissue impact of the delivered laser beam: spot size, power, and exposure.

Spot size refers to the diameter of the aperture that contains 86% of the laser's beam. There are several tips that permit precise control of spot (cutting) size (see Fig. 90.12B). The tip sizes range anywhere from 0.25 to 3.0 mm, with the most commonly used tips being 0.25 to 0.8 mm. With focused beam tips, the distance of the tip from the target tissue determines the actual spot size at the target. For most tips the focal distance is typically 1 to 3 mm. Power is measured in watts, which is defined by the amount of energy applied over time (defined as Joules/second). Power is adjusted on the laser by adjusting the wattage. The greater the wattage, the higher the power. Power density is affected by the size of the target area. If the spot size is small, the power is concentrated. If the spot size is large, the power is spread out over a larger area, and the power density is decreased, thus producing a lesser tissue effect. Exposure is also a user-controlled variable and is determined by the duration of the applied laser. The greater the exposure, the greater the tissue impact. Exposure can be delivered as continuous, repeat, or single pulse.

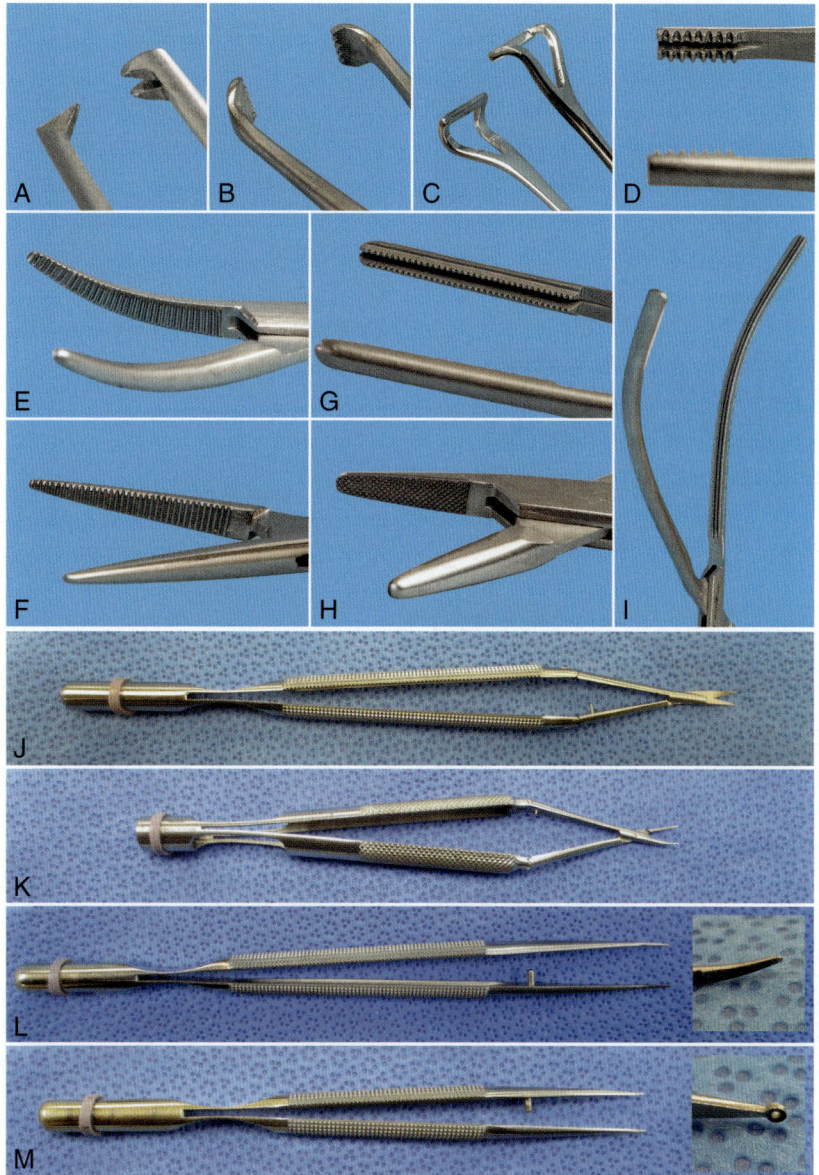

FIG 90.1 A selection of small and microsurgical instruments commonly used in reptile surgery. (A) 1 x 2 Adson forceps are preferred for holding reptile skin. (B) Allis tissue forceps. (C) Babcock forceps. (D) Brown Adson forceps preferred for delicate tissue manipulation. (E) Curved mosquito forceps. (F) Straight mosquito forceps. (G) Debakey forceps are preferred for delicate, especially vascular, tissue manipulation. (H) Mayo Hegar needle holders. (I) Doyen forceps are noncrushing and useful for isolating the intestine. (J) Straight microscissors with round handle and counterbalanced. (K) Micro needle holders with round handle and counterbalanced. (L) Curved micro forceps with platform tips and round handle and counterbalanced. (M) Straight micro forceps with 2-mm ring tips and round handle and counterbalanced. (A–I, Courtesy of Chris Herron, Educational Resources, University of Georgia; J–M, courtesy of Stephen J. Divers.)

Diode Laser. The most common types used in veterinary medicine are the gallium-aluminum-arsenide 810 to 980 nm diode lasers, which are available in varying powers from 15 to 60 W and are all class IV. The laser beam is transmitted from the base unit to surgical site by a solid quartz-core, fiber-optic cable (Fig. 90.13A). A visible light beam is combined with the invisible laser beam to facilitate aiming. Laser fibers come in a variety of sizes (400–1000 μm) and shapes, including flat, conical, orb tips, and air/water cooled. The fibers may be used through the instrument channel of a variety of rigid and flexible endoscopes or in hand-pieces for open surgical use. Unlike the CO_2 fiber, a damaged diode fiber can be trimmed and reused.

The diode laser can be used in direct contact with tissue (contact mode) or at a distance from tissue (noncontact mode) (see Fig. 90.13B). In contact mode the fiber tip is coated with a thin layer of carbon. This is most easily achieved by lightly burning a sterile wooden tongue depressor with the tip of the laser fiber at 10 W. The carbonized tip absorbs virtually 100% of the laser beam, which causes the tip to instantly heat up to ablative tissue temperatures at relatively low power settings, usually just a few watts. The heated tip can then be used to incise, excise, and coagulate tissue, while a 0.3 to 0.6 mm zone of thermocoagulation provides excellent hemostasis of vessels up to 2 mm in diameter (Fig. 90.14). The advantages of carbonized fiber tips are minimized collateral

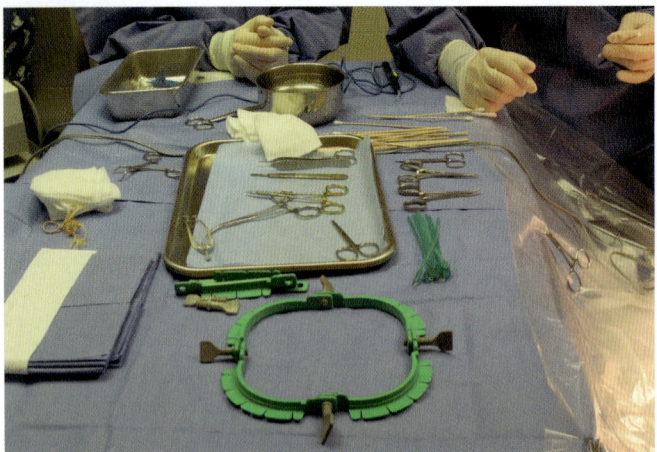

FIG 90.2 Organization of the instrument table is important for efficient instrument use. (Courtesy of Stephen J. Divers.)

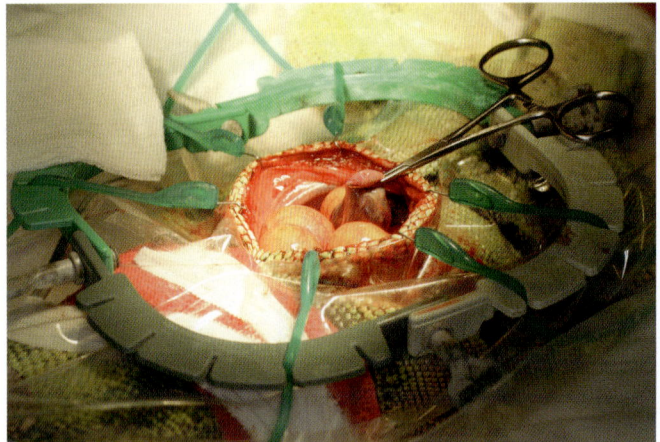

FIG 90.3 The Lonestar retractor incorporates an adjustable plastic ring to which elastic stays where hooks are attached. This retractor is extremely versatile and works well with a variety of species and surgical procedures. (Courtesy of Stephen J. Divers.)

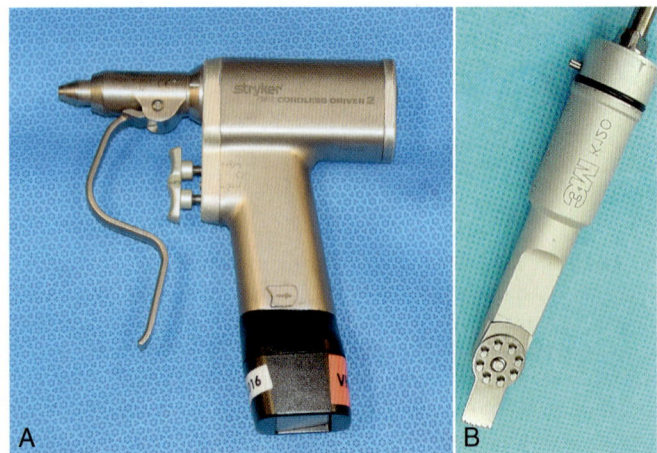

FIG 90.4 Surgical saws. (A) Stryker 4200 Cordless Driver 2 with forward and reverse triggers and a pin/wire collet with finger chuck for quick pin release. (B) Oscillating sagittal saw attachment to the air-powered 3M mini-driver. (Courtesy of Stephen J. Divers.)

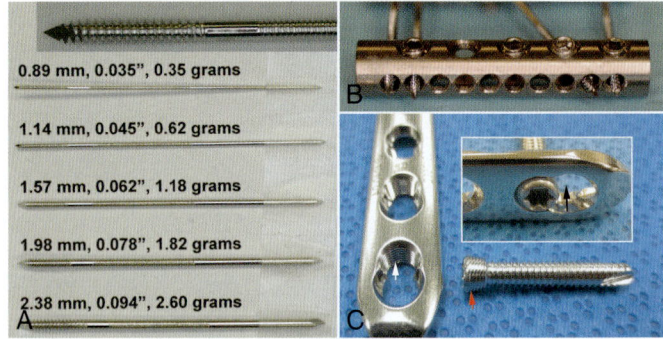

0.89 mm, 0.035", 0.35 grams

1.14 mm, 0.045", 0.62 grams

1.57 mm, 0.062", 1.18 grams

1.98 mm, 0.078", 1.82 grams

2.38 mm, 0.094", 2.60 grams

FIG 90.5 Orthopedic implants. (A) Selection of miniature (mini-IMEX) fixator pins. The top magnified image demonstrates the positive thread profile, which helps resist movement after placement. (B) FESSA bar with four mini-IMEX pins secured using low-profile screws. (C) Small (1.5 mm) locking plate and screw system. The screwhead thread (red arrow) engages the plate (white arrow) as shown in the inset, thereby preventing compression of the bone cortex to the plate. Alternatively, the screw could be inserted through the adjacent aperture (black arrow) to create compression between the plate and bone. (Courtesy of Stephen J. Divers.)

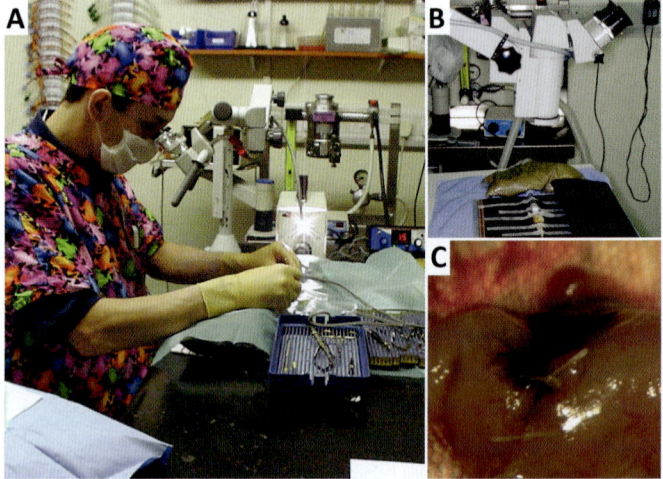

FIG 90.6 (A) Using a Weiss table-top-mounted operating microscope. Notice how the surgeon's back is straight, with the neck slightly tilted and the wrists resting on a support. (B) Operating microscope positioned over a 12-gram *Uromastyx* lizard in preparation for enterotomy. (C) Intraoperative microscopic view of the same *Uromastyx* following enterotomy closure. Note the size of the 6/0 suture used for closure. (Courtesy of Stephen J. Divers.)

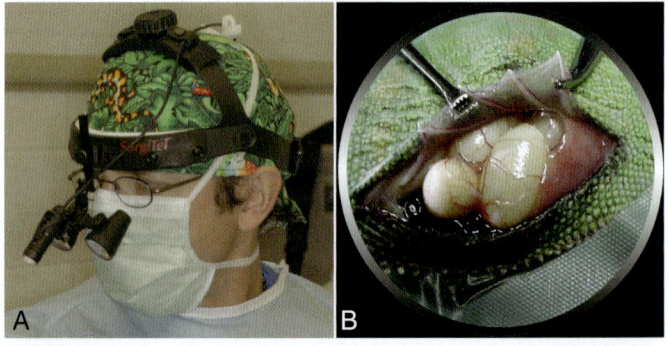

FIG 90.7 (A) SurgiTel headband-mounted 2.5× magnification loupes with integrated light source. (B) Coeliotomy incision in a 120-g chameleon viewed using 2.5× magnification. (Courtesy of Stephen J. Divers.)

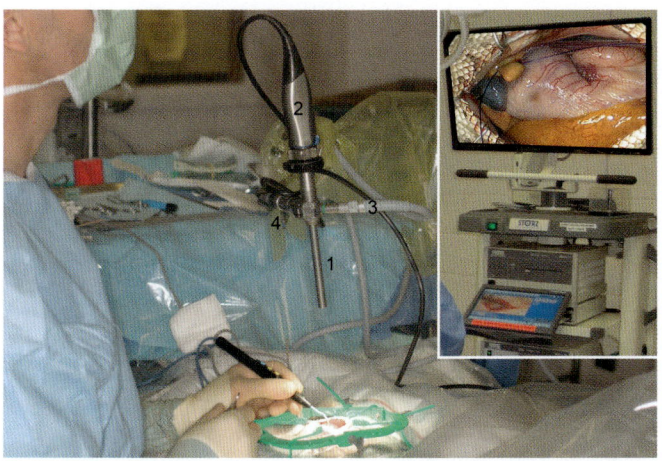

FIG 90.8 Karl Storz video-telescope-operating microscopy. The operating telescope (1) with camera (2) and light cable (3) attached, and supported above the surgical site by a mechanical arm (4), provides a large magnified image on the endoscopy monitor *(inset)*. (Courtesy of Stephen J. Divers.)

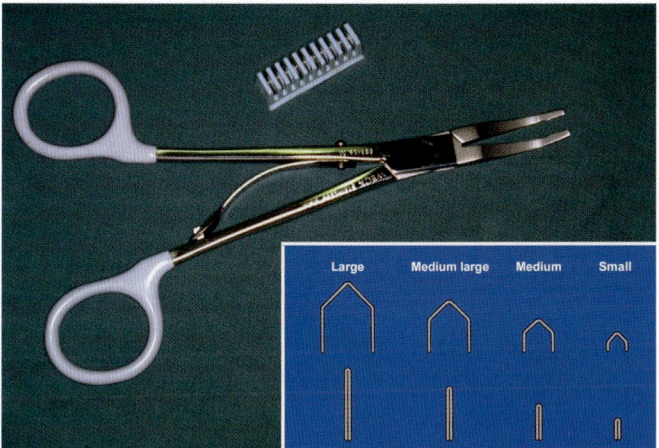

FIG 90.9 Medium vascular clip cartridge containing 10 clips and a medium, straight applicator (Hemoclips, Weck Closure Systems). *(Inset)* Different sizes of vascular clips are available to match surgical conditions. (Courtesy of Stephen J. Divers.)

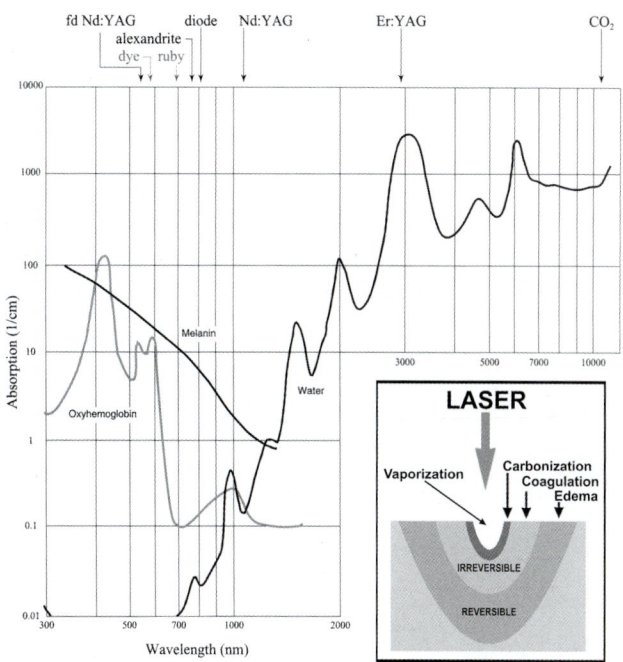

FIG 90.10 The absorption coefficients of hemoglobin, melanin, and water are shown in relation to diode (810 and 980 nm) and CO_2 (10,600 nm) lasers. The diode is more selective for hemoglobin and melanin (pigmentation), whereas the CO_2 has a far greater affinity for water. *(Inset)* The effects of laser on biological tissue. The primary area of vaporized tissue is surrounded by a thin layer of carbonization (char) and then by a zone of thermal necrosis caused by coagulation. The outermost layer is edema and is reversible. (Main illustration, Courtesy of AccuVet Lasers; inset, courtesy of Diomed Ltd.)

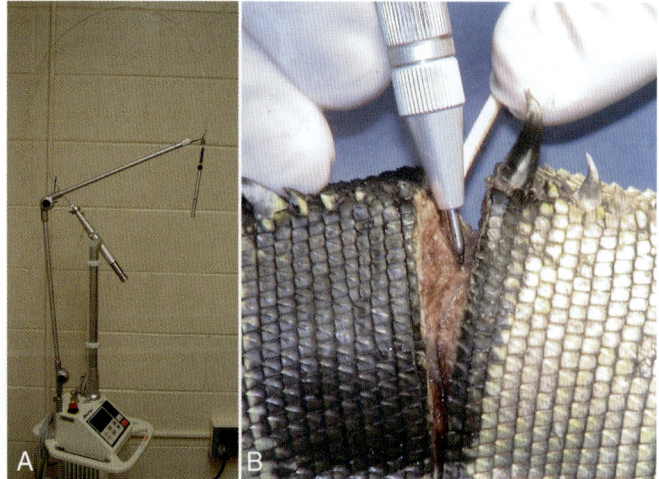

FIG 90.11 NovaPluse CO_2 laser unit with flexible wave-guide to a hand-piece. (B) CO_2 laser incision through the dorsal coccygeal muscles of a large iguanid tail. (Courtesy of Stephen J. Divers.)

damage and reduced tissue penetration (more comparable to those of CO_2 lasers). This is possible because of the dramatic reduction in both laser power and duration required to achieve a given superficial effect.

In noncontact mode the laser is aimed at the tissue from a short distance. The degree of tissue penetration, coagulation, and vaporization depends upon laser type and power setting; duration of exposure; and tissue characteristics, particularly, water content, hemoglobin content, and pigmentation. Generally, diode lasers can penetrate tissue to a greater degree than other lasers (up to 4 mm in nonpigmented tissue) in noncontact mode. Penetration is greatly reduced to around 0.3 mm when carbonized tips are used in contact mode. In practice, contact mode is more accurate and controllable, while noncontact mode is more diffuse with deeper penetration.

For open surgery, the laser fiber is usually housed within a hand-piece that is held much like a pen. The fiber tip is gently stroked across the tissue, either in contact or noncontact modes, until the desired incision or ablative effect is obtained. When used down the operating channel of an endoscope, the fiber is used in contact mode and the entire scope-fiber unit is moved as one. Gentle stroking movements of the scope-fiber unit are used to produce the desired effect, and always under direct visual control.[10] Additionally the diode laser can be utilized in a fluid medium that increases its utility through the endoscopic operating channel, allowing application in the gastrointestinal tract or urogenital system.

Radiosurgery. Radiosurgery utilizes high-frequency radio waves (3.8–4.0 MHz) to cause vaporization of intracellular water, causing the cell to rupture (in a very similar way to CO_2 lasers). Unlike electrocautery, radiosurgery maintains a cooler electrode and offers superior accuracy and reduced collateral damage, comparable with CO_2 laser incisions, at a significantly reduced cost.[4,12] The 3.8 MHz and 4.0 MHz radiofrequency units (Surgitron, Ellman International Inc. Hicksville, NY) offer

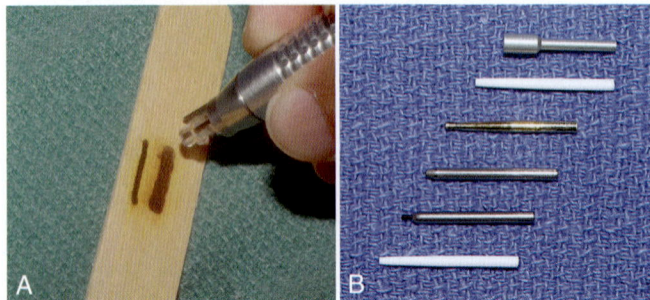

FIG 90.12 (A) The cut on the left is from a 0.4 mm ceramic tip. On the right is a 3-mm scanner tip, used for ablating large tissue areas such as granulomas and surface infections. (B) A variety of tips can be used with the CO_2 laser. Tip size affects spot size, which affects the laser–tissue interaction and power density. The smaller the tip, the more precise the cut. Shown here, top to bottom, are steel 1.4 mm, ceramic 0.8 mm, gold 0.4 mm, steel 0.4 mm, steel 0.3 mm, and ceramic 0.25 mm. (Courtesy of Douglas R. Mader.)

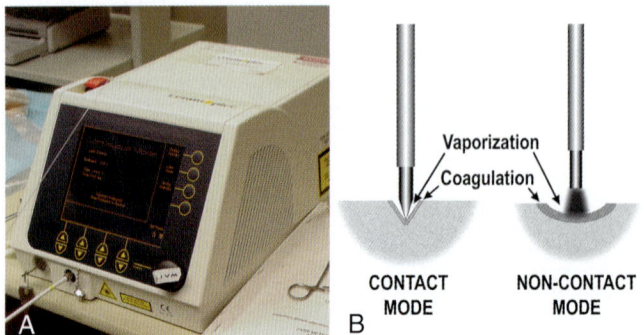

FIG 90.13 (A) 980 nm Ceralas diode laser. (B) Diagrammatic comparison between contact and noncontact modes for the diode laser. Note that the areas of vaporization and coagulation are greatly limited in contact mode. (B, Courtesy of Diomed Ltd.)

monopolar/bipolar applications with foot-pedal/finger-switch control for cut, coagulate, hemostasis, fulgurate, and bipolar modes (Fig. 90.15A).[5,13] Monopolar cutting needles are typically used for dissection, and bipolar forceps for sealing blood vessels (see Fig. 90.15B). A variety of waveforms are possible (Fig. 90.16): (1) A pure filtered waveform utilized for pure microsmooth cutting is used for skin incisions and wire loop excisions, where hemostasis is not expected to be a problem. This waveform gives the least lateral heat and is comparable to focused CO_2 laser incisions (Fig. 90.17A). (2) A fully rectified waveform that blends cutting and coagulation is used where slight bleeding might be expected. It cuts as well as coagulates small blood vessels and gives slight lateral heat to the tissues. (3) A partially rectified waveform is primarily for hemostasis; it cannot be used for cutting but is excellent for coagulation. (4) A fulgurating current that results in spark-gap tissue destruction is very similar to the unipolar diathermy and gives superficial tissue damage by holding the needle electrode close to the tissue and allowing a stream of sparks to burn the tissues. It is suitable for superficial hemostasis and destruction of cysts and superficial neoplasms. (5) Bipolar coagulation allows precise hemostasis obtained by using bipolar forceps (see Fig. 90.17B). Each blade is connected to the radiosurgical unit so that the current passes between the points of the forceps. There are also numerous other radiosurgical attachments for specialized oral, neurological, and endoscopic applications.

Cryosurgery

Cryosurgery is the use of extreme cold (typically liquid nitrogen at −196°C [−321°F]) applied to a tissue to cause cellular freezing and necrosis.[14–16] The technique has been commonly used in the treatment of various dermatological and ocular conditions, especially hyperplastic and neoplastic diseases (Fig. 90.18). However, cryosurgery of visceral lesions is also possible following a traditional or endoscopic surgical approach. A number of cryosurgery systems are commercially available.

Intraoperative Fluoroscopy

A fluoroscopy C-arm (e.g., OEC 9800 Plus Mobile C-arm, GE Medical Systems, Covington, GA, USA) is an expensive but useful device that permits interventional radiographic imaging during surgery. It is particularly useful for the intraoperative assessment of orthopedic repairs and the placement of surgical implants.

Intraoperative Temperature Support

Maintaining patient temperature is essential for similar reasons to mammals. In addition, reduced body temperature in reptiles results in

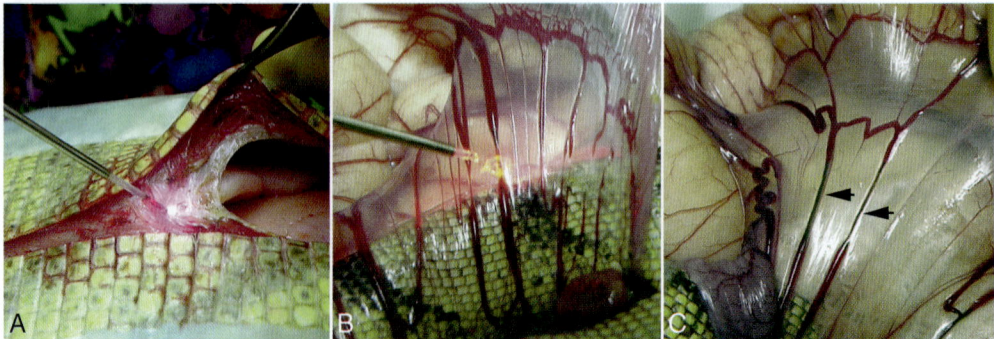

FIG 90.14 (A) 980 nm diode laser incision (contact mode) through the ventral coelomic musculature of a large varanid lizard. (B) Noncontact coagulation of large oviductal vessels in a large iguanid lizard undergoing ovariosalpingectomy. (C) Same iguana demonstrating the ability of the diode to coagulate larger vessels. (Courtesy of Stephen J. Divers.)

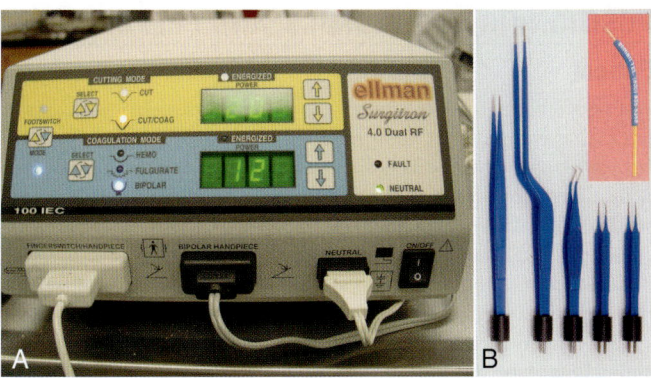

FIG 90.15 (A) 4.0 MHz Surgitron dual-frequency radiosurgery base unit; (B) bipolar forceps and *(inset)* monopolar cutting electrode. (Courtesy of Stephen J. Divers.)

considerable increases in recovery and healing time. Warm-water-circulating blankets and/or forced warm air devices offer the most effective means of maintaining patient temperature (Fig. 90.19).

Suture Materials

In general, the skin of reptiles is strong and acts as the primary holding layer for maintenance of wound closure. For example, with coelomic surgery, the coelomic membrane and body wall are often thin and weak. The success of wound closure relies on strong, well-placed skin sutures. Because the skin is tough, sutures are unlikely to tear through, although tension typically results in necrosis and subsequent dehiscence. Most reptiles do not traumatize their incisions.

Chromic catgut does not appear to be an appropriate suture for use in the reptile patient. In a rhinoceros viper (*Bitis nasicornis*), the material was still present 12 weeks after placement in both the pleuroperitoneum and the subcutaneous tissues.[17] Other absorbable materials not dependent on proteolysis are recommended for deeper tissue closures. Modern rapidly absorbed suture materials (particularly poliglecaprone 25) are recommended for short-term, internal, soft-tissue applications, and antibiotic-impregnated options are now available. Polyglactin 910 has been associated with greater inflammation and less favored.[18] Polydioxanone lasts for several months, but for permanent internal durability nylon is required. Depending upon the expected rate of healing, monofilament nylon, polydioxanone, or poliglecaprone 25 are often preferred for skin suturing, although wire may be necessary for crocodilians and shell repairs. More recently, knotless suture materials (Quill Knotless Closure System, Surgical Specialties Corp Wyomissing, PA; Strarafix, Ethicon Inc.) have become available. When required, suture removal is generally scheduled 6 to 8 weeks after surgery.

Antibiotics

The routine use of broad-spectrum antibiotics following surgery implies a low level of expertise on the part of the clinician. Excessive use of antibiotics has led to widespread drug resistance and is an ongoing major global health hazard for animals and humans. There should be no need to use postoperative antibiotics if appropriate aseptic techniques are employed. However, when performing clean-contaminated procedures (e.g., enterotomy, cystotomy) or procedures where infection would be disastrous (e.g., orthopedics), short-term pre/perioperative (intravenous or intraosseous) antibiotics have been shown to be more effective than several days of postoperative therapy.[19,20] The author does not use postoperative antibiotics routinely, but, when indicated, frequently uses cefazolin at 20 to 25 mg/kg IV or IO, given before moving into the operating room and repeated every 90 to 120 minutes.

Radiosurgery Waveforms Available with the Surgitron

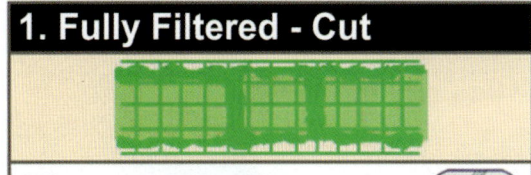

1. Fully Filtered - Cut

Micro-smooth cutting
Minimal lateral heat
Minimal cellular destruction
Preferred for skin incision and biopsy

A

2. Fully Rectified - Cut/Coag

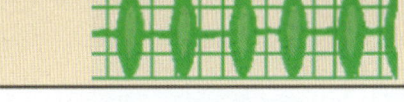

Cutting with hemostasis
Preferred for tissue dissection, esp in vascular areas
Hemostasis with minimal lateral heat and tissue damage

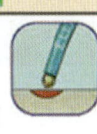

B

3. Partially Rectified - Coag

Coagulation and shrinkage
Preferred for cutting in very vascular tissue with controlled penetration

C

4. Fulgaration

Maximum hemostasis
Preferred for intentional tissue destruction

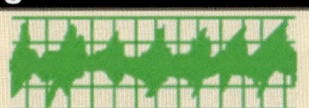

D

5. Bipolar

Pinpoint micro-coagulation
Reduced charring and necrosis
Preferred for hemostasis and coagulation around critical anatomy

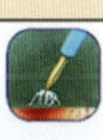

E

FIG 90.16 Different radiosurgery waveforms and their surgical uses. (Courtesy of Ellman International Inc.)

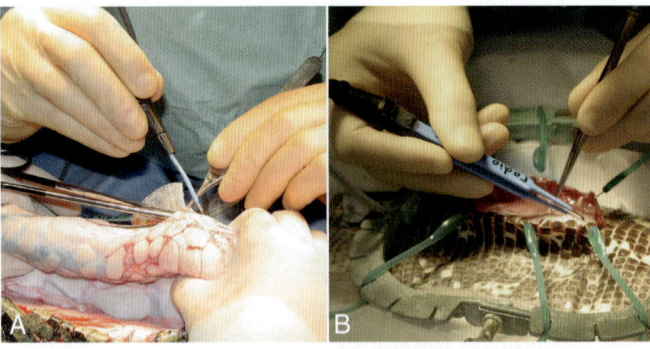

FIG 90.17 (A) Monopolar radiosurgical incision through fascia to access the reproductive tract in a green anaconda (*Eunectes murinus*). (B) Bipolar dissection with hemostasis through the coelomic musculature of a beaded lizard (*Heloderma horridum*).

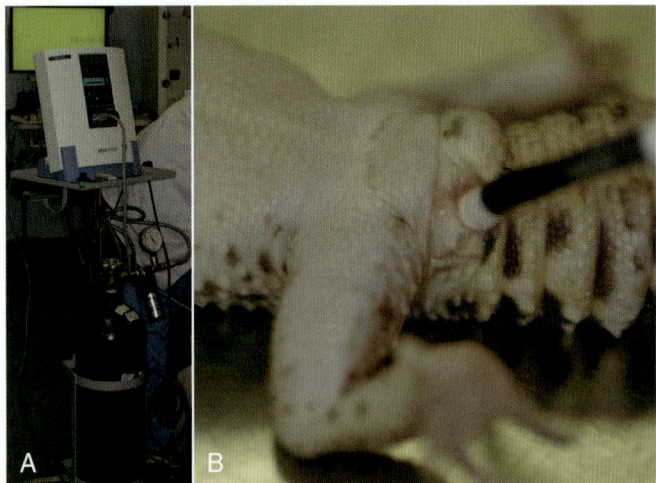

FIG 90.18 (A) Keeler Cryomaster cryosurgery unit with liquid nitrogen tank attached. (B) Cryoprobe being used to treat pericloacal hyperplastic lesion in a leopard gecko (*Eublepharis macularius*). (Courtesy of Stephen J. Divers.)

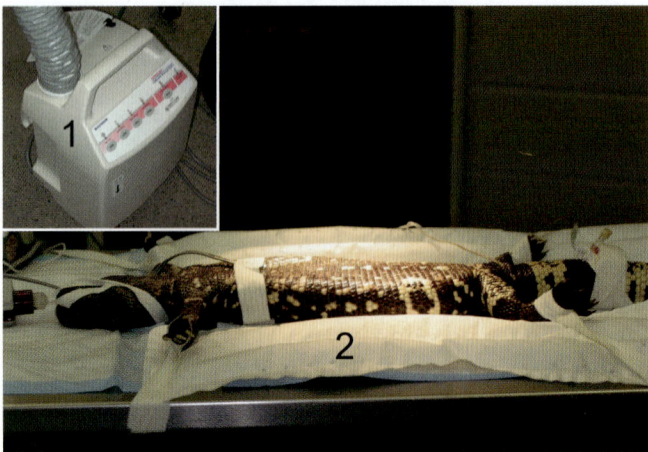

FIG 90.19 The Bair Hugger is a forced-air heating system for maintaining patient temperature. The heat unit (1) is positioned under or adjacent to the table and is connected to an air blanket (2) under this beaded lizard (*Heloderma horridum*). (Courtesy of Stephen J. Divers.)

POSITIONING, ERGONOMICS, AND PREPARATION

Patient

Fasting is often a nonissue, as many diseased reptiles present with days to weeks or even months of anorexia. However, if still feeding, it is wise to fast prior to surgery, especially if a gastrointestinal procedure is planned. A useful rule of thumb is to miss a single feeding cycle. Therefore a small lizard fed every day should be fasted for 24 hours, whereas a large constrictor fed every 2 weeks could be fasted for 2 weeks. Fasting for 24 to 96 hours should result in an empty stomach but is unlikely to have a significant effect on the voluminous large intestine of herbivores.

Prior to surgery a preanesthetic evaluation should be completed and followed by appropriate premedication, induction, intubation, catheterization, and application of intraoperative monitoring devices (see Chapters 48 through 52).

Precise patient positioning will depend upon the species and the nature of the surgery, and specific recommendations are provided in each of the following surgery sections. However, some consideration should be given to maximizing desired surgical access while (1) ensuring that head and neck position does not interfere with ventilation; (2) avoiding excessive compression of the head, limbs, or coelom to prevent pressure necrosis, visceral rupture, or hypoventilation of the lungs; (3) avoiding extreme and prolonged hyperextension or hyperflexion of any joint; (4) ensuring the surgical site is easily accessible and does not require a surgeon to adopt a posture that results in fatigue; and (5) using appropriately sized sandbags, vacuum beanbags, foam supports, and adhesive tape to maintain patient position (Fig. 90.20).

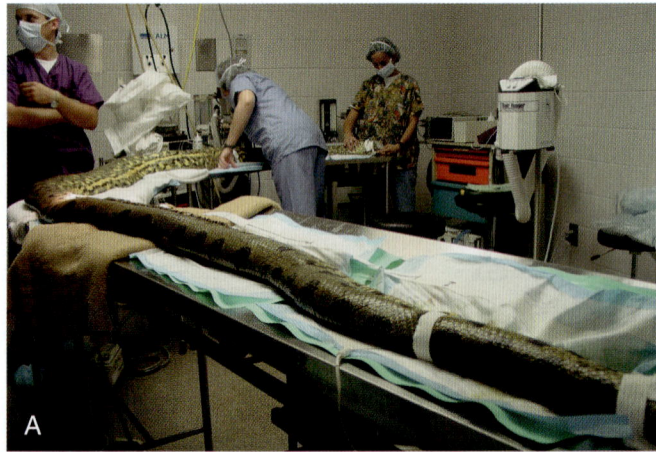

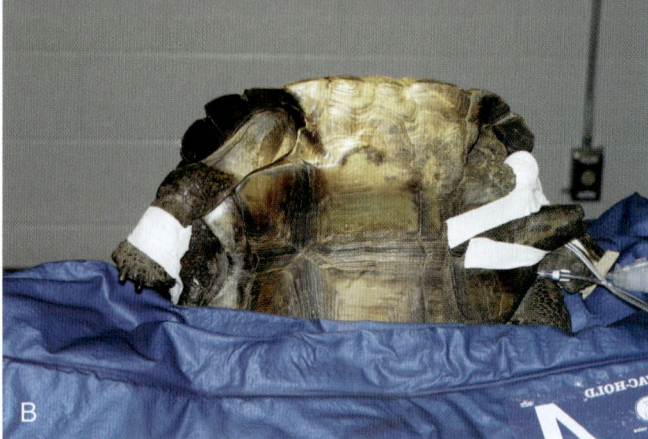

FIG 90.20 Patient positioning. (A) Large green anaconda (*Eunectes murinus*) supported using multiple tables. (B) A tortoise positioned in lateral recumbency using a vacuum positioning bag. (Courtesy of Stephen J. Divers.)

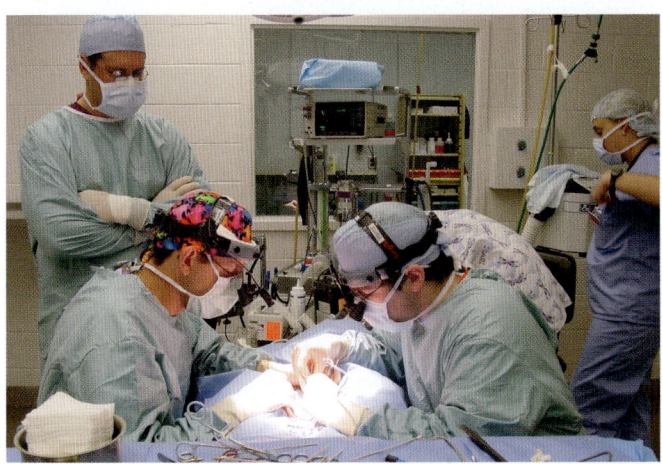

FIG 90.21 Sitting is ergonomically preferred for most procedures, especially when using magnification during microsurgery. This often requires placement of the animal toward one end of the operating table so that the surgeons can sit with their legs under the table, unimpeded by the table pedestal. (Courtesy of Stephen J. Divers.)

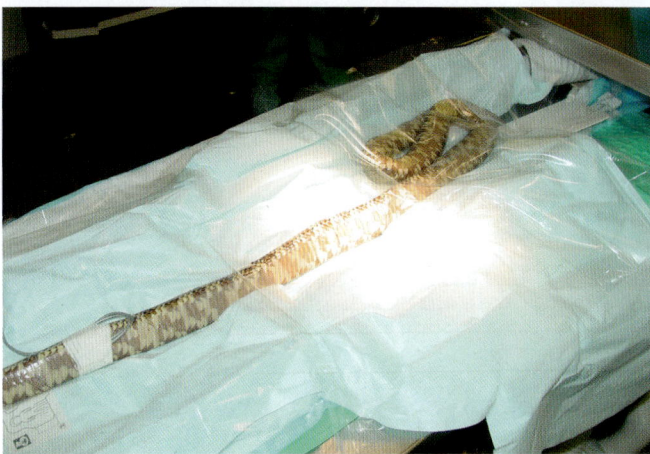

FIG 90.22 This snake has been positioned on a forced-air heater blanket over a water-circulating blanket, and a sterile adhesive drape has been applied. Note the focused illumination of the surgical site. (Courtesy of Stephen J. Divers.)

Surgeon Ergonomics

Rather than assuming contorting positions, the surgeon must dedicate some time to planning factors such as patient positioning and table height if fatigue and musculoskeletal issues are to be avoided.[21] The ideal posture for the surgeon involves sitting (or standing) with a straight back and a slightly flexed neck (see Fig. 90.6).[22] Surgeon posture becomes even more critical during microsurgery, with the surgeon's wrists resting on a padded support on the surgical table (see Fig. 90.6). In most cases, utilizing sandbags or similar objects to support the wrist allows optimal motor control when using microinstruments. Poor positioning will quickly lead to surgeon fatigue, reduced surgical ability, and increased patient morbidity (Fig. 90.21). During microsurgery, surgeons should follow the 20-20-20 rule to reduce fatigue—every 20 minutes look at something 20 feet away for 20 seconds.

Presurgical Preparation and Draping

Aseptic surgery should be performed in an appropriately clean and sterile operating room by surgeons wearing surgical masks, hats, sterile gloves, and gowns. The (non-ocular) surgical site should be aseptically cleaned using standard 0.05% chlorhexidine or 5% povidone–iodine surgical scrub solutions; however, recent studies have indicated that povidone-iodine-alcohol combinations are superior to chlorhexidine-alcohol solutions.[23] A small brush (e.g., toothbrush) is particularly useful for cleaning scaled skin. Dousing with alcohol is not recommended because of increased evaporative heat loss. However, where a surgical solution devoid of alcohol was used for skin preparation, a final alcohol wipe will help ensure a dry grease-free area to which adhesive drapes will readily adhere.

Traditional cloth drapes can be heavy, hinder animal observation for anesthetic monitoring, and are less effective bacterial barriers compared to plastic adhesive drapes.[24] Transparent adhesive drapes have several advantages, including better visualization and monitoring of the patient, maintenance of a waterproof barrier, ability to be secured without towel clamps, and are lightweight with greater aseptic benefits (Fig. 90.22).

POSTOPERATIVE CARE

The two most important points to address postoperatively are thermal support and pain control (see Chapter 50). No excuse exists for not providing postoperative analgesia to patients. During and after anesthetic recovery, the patient should be maintained in a clean, warm, quiet environment. Unless the wound closure is waterproof, incision immersion should be prevented for a period of 5 to 14 days after surgery to allow a scab to form and desiccate. Prevention of brumation (hibernation) for 3–6 months is best to allow complete healing. The fluid and nutritional needs of the patient must be assessed and maintained (see Chapter 87). Fluid therapy is indicated to maintain the hydration status of the patient. Many patients become anorectic after surgery and need nutritional support (see Chapter 122). In some cases, esophagostomy tubes and central jugular lines may be necessary to provide long-term support (see Chapters 44 and 45). It is wise to schedule postoperative examinations after 7 to 10 days (to check for infection/dehiscence) and 6 to 8 weeks (for suture removal).

REFERENCES

See www.expertconsult.com for a complete list of references.

91

Eye

Martin P.C. Lawton

The approach to ophthalmic surgery in reptiles is similar to that used in other species. Many of the techniques utilized for reptiles are modifications of those designed for humans or pet carnivores. An understanding of ophthalmic basics and anatomic differences is essential (see Chapter 71). Most procedures will require general anesthesia. Less often, local anesthesia alone may be adequate, usually with simple procedures, such as a foreign body removal. Sometimes a combination of general anesthesia and either topical, subtenons, or retrobulbar local anesthesia (lidocaine or marcaine) is required.

EQUIPMENT SPECIFIC TO OPHTHALMOLOGIC SURGERY

The size of ocular tissues will make it desirable to use an operating microscope or at the very least a decent loupe system.

Specific ophthalmic instruments should allow atraumatic handling of the delicate tissues. Appropriate suture handling and tying instruments, such as Castroveijos, that will not inadvertently straighten the small swaged on needle or damage the fine suture materials (usually 6/0 to 10/0) should be used. Forceps such as St Martin Forceps (1–2 rat tooth), Bishop Harmans, neurologic forceps, or watchmakers forceps are advantageous.

Aseptic surgery should always be undertaken. Due to the possibility of infection from environmental organisms, it is important to prepare the surgical area with an effective disinfectant/antiseptic, such as 0.5% to 1% chlorhexidine or povidone-iodine (usually diluted 1:4) that has been warmed. Alcohol should be avoided to prevent loss of body heat or damage to the exposed cornea (where there is no spectacle).[1]

There are many disposable drape systems for human ophthalmic surgery that are ideal for reptiles. These drapes are adhesive with a central clear window for keeping the drape in position and for isolating tissues not involved in the surgery. Care should be taken on removing such adhesive drapes as the outer layer of skin may be prematurely avulsed if the reptile is nearing ecdysis.

SPECIFIC OPHTHALMOLOGIC PROCEDURES

Eyelid Repair

Most repairs required are the result of traumatic injuries, including fights, resulting in the loss of the normal integrity of the eyelids. Appropriate perioperative antibiotic therapy may be required. Return to normal conformation and function is the desired effect with minimum scarring or distortion. Where there are substantial damage to the eyelids (e.g., heat lamp burns), a blepharoplasty may be required (Fig. 91.1).[2] In all reptiles with functional eyelids, the lower eyelid is the most important for the protection of the eye and should be the priority in any repair.

Often simple repair to return a normal anatomic apposition using a 6/0 or 7/0 "coated braided suture" such as Vicryl is all that is necessary. The leading edge of the eyelid should be inline to prevent kinks or notches that could later potentially cause corneal irritation or damage. Sutures should be either buried or on the outside of the skin and not on the bulbar conjunctival surface of the eyelid.

Sliding grafts are more difficult to undertake in reptiles than in mammals, but gentle dissection may be able to free up skin for advancement grafts to close any defects.

Spectacle Debridement and Spectaculectomy

The spectacle, being skin, is an ideal area for surgical approaches, such as surgical debridement, repair, or removal of substrate under the surface layer of the spectacle. Any debridement is best performed with the aid of an operating microscope to allow reliable removal of all the foreign material, especially when organic, to prevent the possibility of foreign body reaction or granuloma formation. If the development of scarring should occur during the healing stage, this will usually disappear after

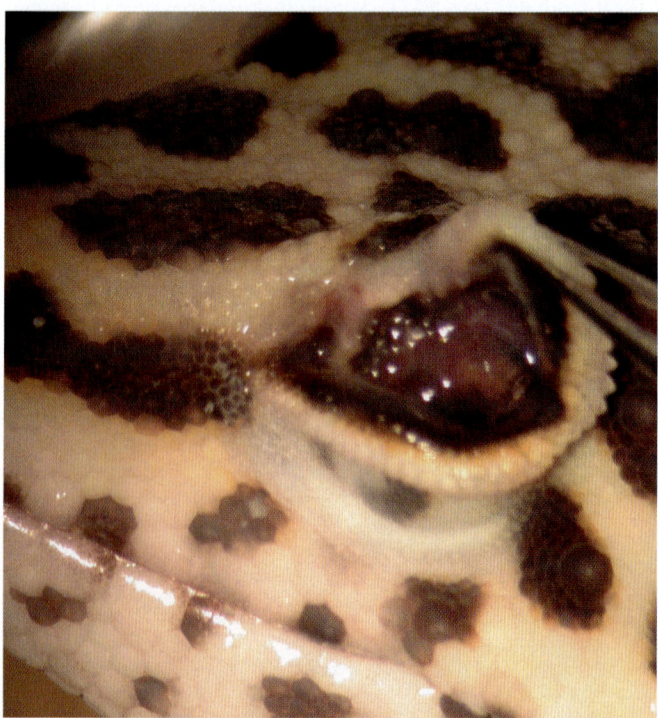

FIG 91.1 Coloboma of upper medial eyelid in a leopard gecko (*Eublepharis macularius*). (Courtesy of Martin P.C. Lawton.)

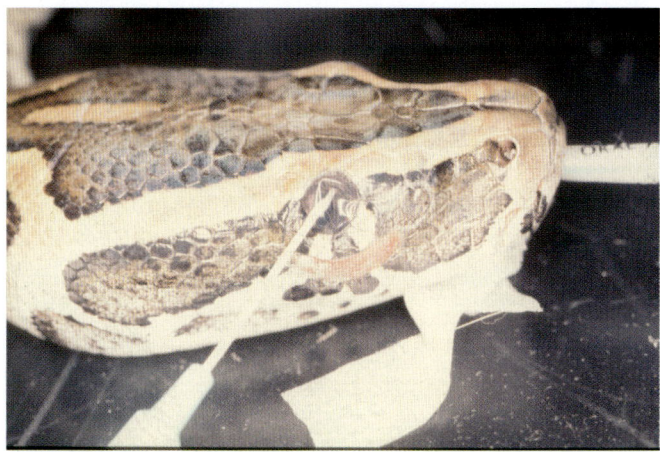

FIG 91.2 Flushing of subspectacular space via the spectaculotomy incision in a Burmese python (*Python bivittatus*). (Courtesy of Martin P.C. Lawton.)

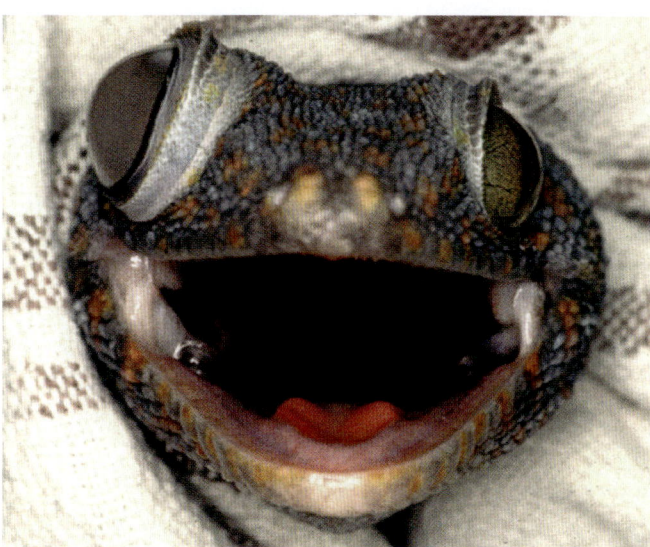

FIG 91.3 Pseudobuphthalmos affecting the right eye of a Tokay gecko (*Gekko gecko*). (Courtesy of Martin P.C. Lawton.)

the next or subsequent slough. Rarely does damage or treatment of abrasions result in permanent opacity to the spectacle.

Treatment and obtaining material for cytology or culture is the ideal approach in dealing with and resolving a subspectacle abscess. The approach requires making a small wedge resection of the spectacle (spectaculotomy), usually at the lateral quadrant. Up to 25% to 30% of the spectacle can be removed by this approach but greater than this could result in excessive loss of the tear film and desiccation of the cornea.[3] If a larger incision is required, then a flap with a temporary suture placement to allow reopening is required. On opening the subspectacular space, a swab should first be taken of any material and submitted for culture and sensitivity; a stained smear may be useful in confirming a bacterial infection. The spectaculotomy wound is left open so that the subspectacular space can be repeatedly flushed out with balanced salt solution (or another suitable solution) (Fig. 91.2) and an appropriate ophthalmic antibiotic solution such as ciprofloxacin or gentamicin once or twice a day. Antibiotics are required if infection is present but are not essential for healing once infection has resolved.[3,4]

Following experimental spectaculectomy in ball pythons, engorgement of the spectacular vessels with edema adjacent to the wound edges is common for several weeks. An amorphous plaque of homogenous proteinaceous material fills the defect and allows reestablishment of the subspectacular space and normal wetting of the corneal surface within 1 week. A variable degree of inflammatory cell infiltration occurs immediately postoperatively and subsides over 4 weeks. Normal wound healing results in regeneration of normal spectacle morphology by 3 months postoperatively. Experimental pythons were not at risk for a higher incidence of ocular or subspectacular infections as a direct result of partial spectaculectomy.[3]

Pseudobuphthalmos

Pseudobuphthalmos is the distension of the subspectacle space with fluid, usually because of a blockage to the normal drainage of the tear film into the mouth (see Chapter 71) (Fig. 91.3). A temporary fistula is required to allow drainage of the fluid and resolution of the distension. There have been descriptions of treating this condition with a small wedge-shaped incision in the ventral spectacle,[5] but recurrence can occur if the wedge is too small.[6] Even with a 30-degree wedge section removed from the inferior quadrant, recurrence was noted and eventually led to the rupture of the lacrimal duct and fluid draining down the face.[7] This author considers that irrespective of the size of the wedge removed, a high risk of recurrence always exists, and, if too big a wedge is removed,

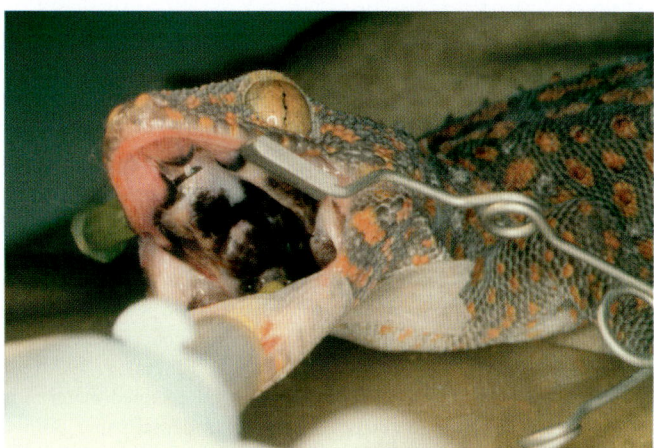

FIG 91.4 Treatment of pseudobuphthalmos by creating a new drainage canal (conjunctivoralostom) in a Tokay Gecko (*Gekko gecko*). (Courtesy of Martin P.C. Lawton.)

problems can develop from exposure keratitis or secondary infection. The critical and essential part of the treatment is to either treat the blocked nasolacrimal duct or create a new drainage canal.[4] A new drainage canal (conjunctivoralostomy) should be formed between the medial aspect of the inferior fornix of the subspectacular space and the mouth, emerging between the palatine and maxillary teeth. This is performed with a 22- to 18-gauge needle (Fig. 91.4); the conjunctivoralostomy should be prevented from closing by placing a 0.625-mm Silastic/silicon tube, sutured in place on the periorbital scales and left in situ for up to 6 weeks.[4,7,8] Any fluid removed from the subspectacular space should always be examined under the microscope (fresh and stained), because flagellates have been found in subspectacular exudates.[7]

Spectacle Avulsion

The total loss of the spectacle will lead to loss of the tear film, desiccation of the cornea, eventual loss of the sight in that eye, and even the loss of the eye. Protection of the cornea is essential by covering the defect until new skin can grow across the defect. This is best done by using mucosal graft, Biosist graft (bovine collagen), or commercially available amniotic membrane.[9] The graft material should be sutured to any

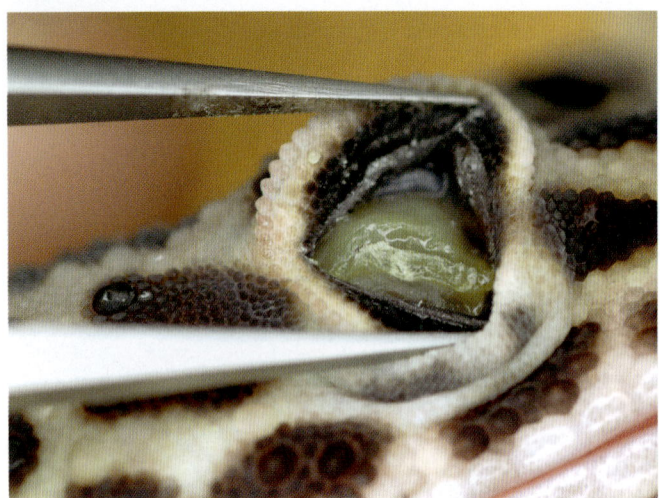

FIG 91.5 Retained eye cap in a leopard gecko (*Eublepharis macularius*). (Courtesy of Martin P.C. Lawton.)

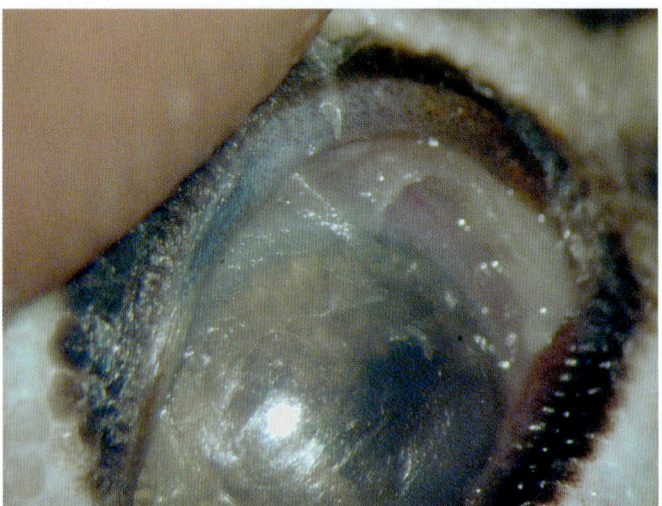

FIG 91.6 Corneal surface in a leopard gecko (*Eublepharis macularius*) after retained eye cap has been removed, prior to removal of remaining material. (Courtesy of Martin P.C. Lawton.)

remnants of the spectacle edge with fine sutures (6/0 to 8/0) to act as a scaffold for the growth of new skin. The transparency of the spectacle is unlikely to be fully regained, and some degree of opacity should be expected.

Gecko Retained "Eye Caps"

This is not a true spectacle condition but a unique syndrome in gecko species with eyelids.[10] A solid mass forms within the palpebral fissure from the retention conjunctival lining and debris under the eyelids, usually with associated secondary infection (Fig. 91.5). Hypovitaminosis A is considered to be a predisposing factor related to this problem, as is low environmental humidity. This procedure may be performed under topical local (proxymetacaine or marcain) or general anesthesia. Magnification is essential to allow removal of all the matter without damaging the cornea (Fig. 91.6). Removal of the retained material is carefully undertaken with forceps or absorbent dental paper points. Lubrication (using balanced salt solution or a viscous tear solution) may be required to soften the material. Repeat surgical intervention, topical antibiotics, and lubrication (e.g., Gentacin – Clincagel, Ceva), and vitamin A supplementation may be required.

Corneal Repair

Superficial corneal damage can typically be treated topically, but deep corneal ulcers should be treated surgically[11] in order to prevent rupture and facilitate healing. A corneal laceration with no loss of tissue can be repaired with simple interrupted sutures of 8/0 or 10/0[12] or the use of a surgical cynoacrylic adhesive (Steribond or Vetbond). Where there is loss of corneal tissue that will not allow direct apposition, the use of a surgical "bandage" is preferred by transposition of a prepared pedicle or bridging graft of conjunctiva that is sutured over the ulcer bed to the edges of healthy cornea with 10/0 Vicryl sutures.

Severe ulcerations in Chelonia and lizards may be treated by performing a third eyelid flap (Fig. 91.7), although Millichamp[11] does not like this approach because it applies pressure to the globe that could potentiate corneal rupture. The placement of the third eyelid flap also has the disadvantage of preventing further examination of the cornea during the healing process.

Corneal Plaque (Keratitis) Removal

Treatment of this condition requires the removal of the plaque from the cornea and appropriate topical antibiotic therapy (Figs. 91.8 and

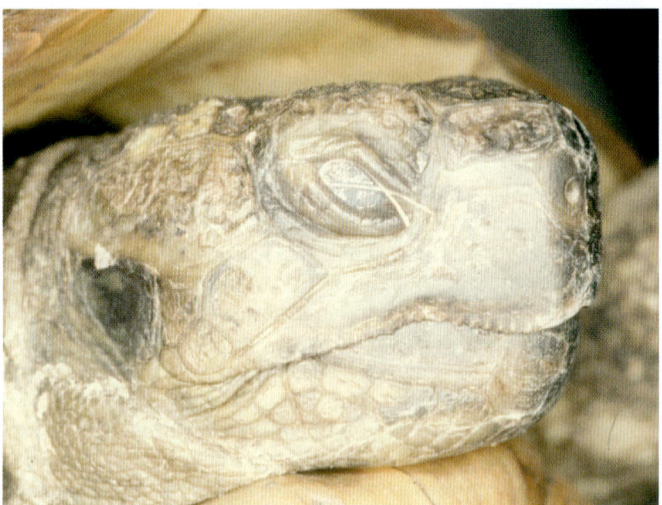

FIG 91.7 Third eyelid flap in a *Testudo* tortoise. (Courtesy of Martin P.C. Lawton.)

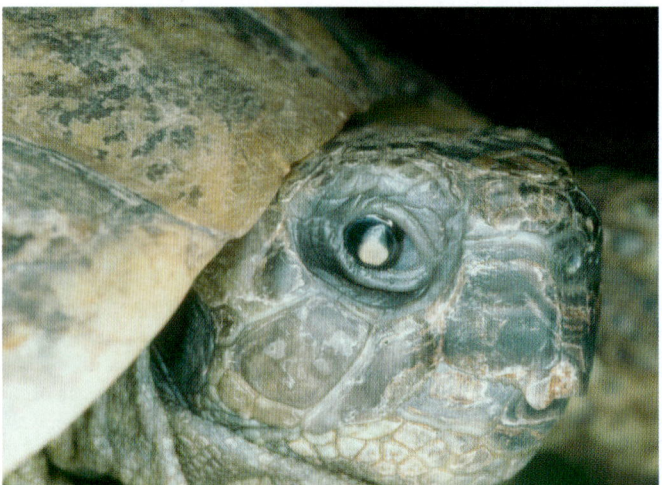

FIG 91.8 Corneal plaque keratitis in a *Testudo* tortoise. (Courtesy of Martin P.C. Lawton.)

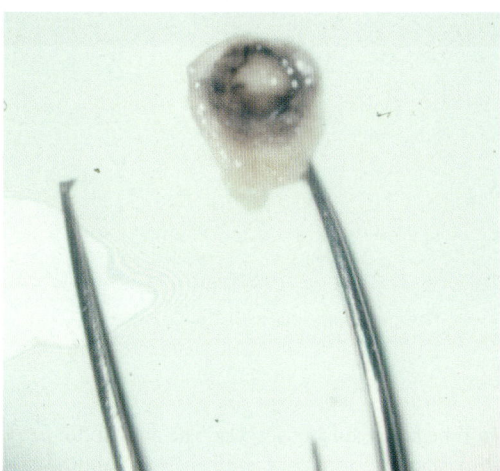

FIG 91.9 Corneal plaque post-removal, showing corneal impression in a tortoise. (Courtesy of Martin P.C. Lawton.)

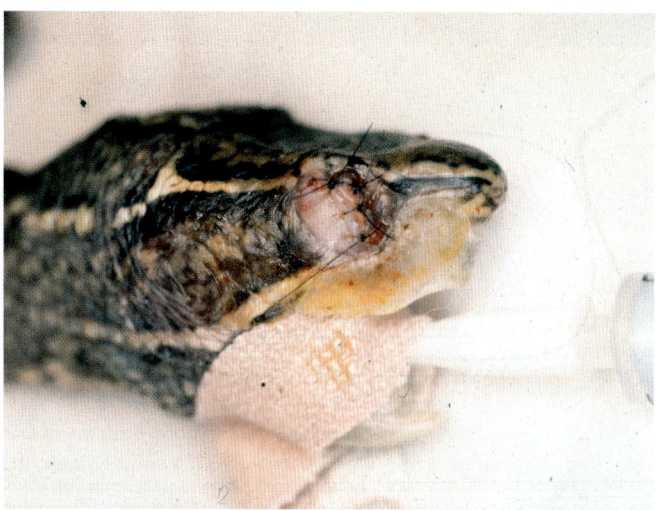

FIG 91.10 Musk turtle (*Sternotherus odoratus*), post-enucleation. (Courtesy of Martin P.C. Lawton.)

91.9). The technique requires the controlled use of a 27-gauge needle to gently lift the mass off the cornea. The plaque can be pretreated with topical antibiotics, often resulting in the mass becoming firmer, which aids removal. Where the mass is very adherent to the damaged corneal surface, superficial keratectomy is performed, and the resulting corneal ulcer treated with appropriate protective products (e.g., hyaluronic drops) and topical antibiotics.

Cataract Surgery

Cataract surgery is indicated in patients whose quality of life is impacted by vision loss. However, the small size of the patient's globe and requirement for specialist equipment (phacoemulsification) renders most reptiles as poor surgical candidates for this procedure.[10]

Cataract surgery in reptiles can be performed in a similar manner to that described for birds. The lens is soft,[13] which means less ultrasound (phacoemulsification) and more irrigation/aspiration is required during removal of the lens nucleus and cortex. Repair of the cornea does not always have to be undertaken, even in aquatic species.[13] Suture materials such as vicryl in the cornea have been reported to cause focal abscesses, which resolved only after the suture was removed.[13] Cataract surgery in reptiles with spectacles is more difficult. Initially the surgeon must incise and flap the spectacle to allow exposure of the cornea before incising into the anterior chamber to deal with the abnormal lens. Visual results can be good, often with reptiles regaining the ability to feed themselves, allowing rehabilitation and a possible return to the wild.[13]

Enucleation

When there is severe infection, inflammation, or trauma of the globe with little chance of recovery, enucleation can be performed. Glaucomatous eyes are particularly good candidates for enucleation,[11] because the prognosis is otherwise poor.

In species with nonfused eyelids, the approach is similar to that described for mammals. Utilizing a lateral canthotomy, the palpebral fissure is enlarged for easier removal of the globe, followed by removal of the eyelid margins and sutured closure to form a permanent tarsorrhaphy (Fig. 91.10). In snakes, the whole of the spectacle and the globe should be removed, the optic blood vessels sealed with hemostatic pressure, and the wound allowed to granulate over a period of 4 weeks.[14]

REFERENCES

See www.expertconsult.com for a complete list of references.

92

Ear

Michelle Kischinovsky and Stephen J. Divers

Generally, the reptilian (and amphibian) ear is not prone to disease requiring major surgical intervention. As with other body systems, the ear can be a site for trauma, dermatologic, and parasitologic insults; however, many are managed medically and supportively. Polyps, neoplasia, abscesses, and other protruding or obstructive growths are likely to need surgical excision to achieve resolution.

Malignant and benign tumors, including nonneoplastic polyps, may develop in or around the aural cavity of the reptilian ear.[1-3] Thorough presurgical assessment of diseased tissue and margin-determination aids in surgical planning and accurate prognosis. This may be done through impression smears, fine-needle aspiration, and/or tissue biopsy. Because the deeper aural regions are difficult to assess, radiography, CT, or MRI may be required.[4] The surgical approach and technique depend on the associated pathology and vascularity of the structure. Conventional surgical techniques can be used, although radiosurgery, laser, or cryosurgery may be favored for speed and improved hemostasis. Magnification (such as operating loupes or microscopy) can be invaluable.

AURAL ABSCESS

Following intubation and the establishment of surgical anesthesia, the oral cavity is packed with moistened gauze to prevent aspiration from eustachian tube lavage during surgery. The animal can be positioned in sternal or lateral recumbency, with the head and neck rotated to position the tympanic area toward the surgeon. Given the close proximity to the ocular structures, aseptic preparation of the tympanic region is best undertaken using dilute povidone-iodine rather than chlorhexidine, and alcohol should be avoided.

A variety of surgical approaches are possible, ranging from a single horizontal incision, cross incisions, partial, and, in severe cases, complete excision of the entire tympanum. For most abscesses, a full-thickness incision made through the tympanum along its ventral border from the 9 o'clock to the 3 o'clock positions and connected horizontally to facilitate removal of the ventral portion (Fig. 92.1). In some cases, it may be necessary to remove the entire tympanic membrane. Inflammatory debris is extracted with small ear loops or curettes, and it is often possible to remove a single caseous plug. Surgical debridement of inflammatory tissue may be required, but care must be taken not to damage the columella during surgery (Figs. 9.21A and 9.22). Because a variety of gram-positive and gram-negative bacteria have been isolated from these lesions, specimens for in-house cytology, Gram stains, culture, and sensitivity should be collected at this time.[5] In addition, acid-fast stains or PCR should be considered if *Cryptospordium* is suspected, and histopathology should be considered if there is granulomatous or other abnormal tissue.[1,2]

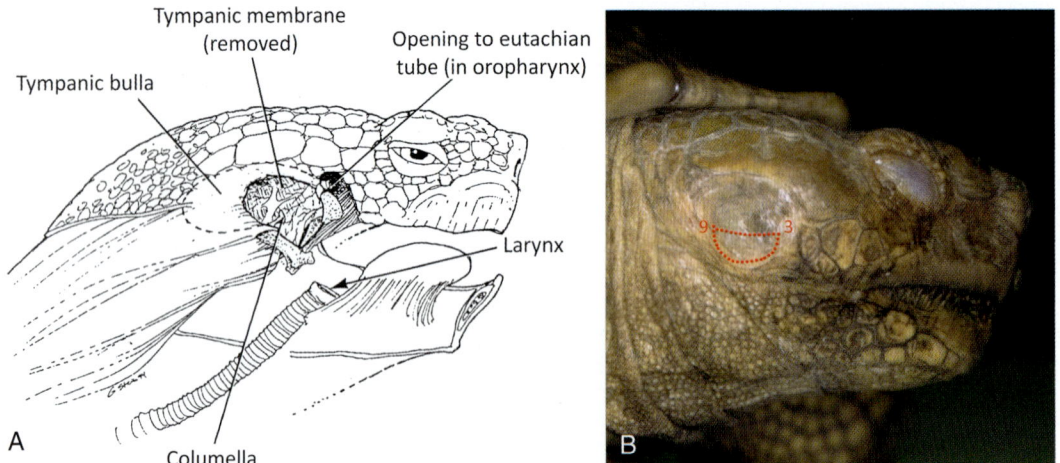

FIG 92.1 (A) Head of a box turtle (*Terrapene* sp.) with the right lower jaw removed. Note the extent of the middle ear cavity demarcated by the dashed line (B) Right lateral view of an African spurred tortoise (*Centrochelys sulcata*) demonstrating the ventral and horizontal tympanic incisions between the 9- and 3-o'clock positions. The excised portion of the tympanic membrane is removed. (A, Adapted from Boyer TH. Common problems of box turtles [*Terrapene* sp] in captivity. *Bull ARAV.* 1992;2[1]:11; B, courtesy of Stephen J. Divers.)

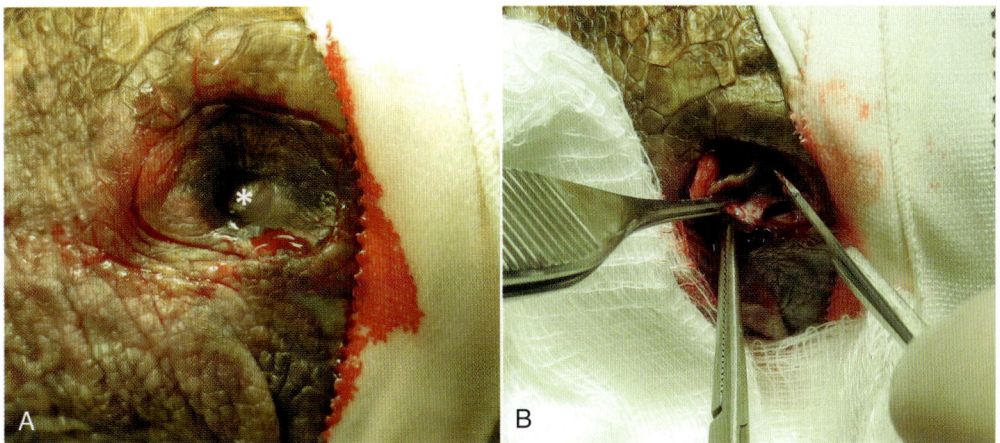

FIG 92.2 (A) Close-up of a right tympanic membrane with a central fistula (*) in a leopard tortoise (*Stigmochelys pardalis*) that presented with chronic otitis. An initial incision has been made around the entire tympanic membrane in preparation for removal. (B) Surgical debridement in the same animal following removal of the tympanic membrane. Chronically infected and inflamed tissue is being removed for histopathology and microbiology. (Courtesy of Stephen J. Divers.)

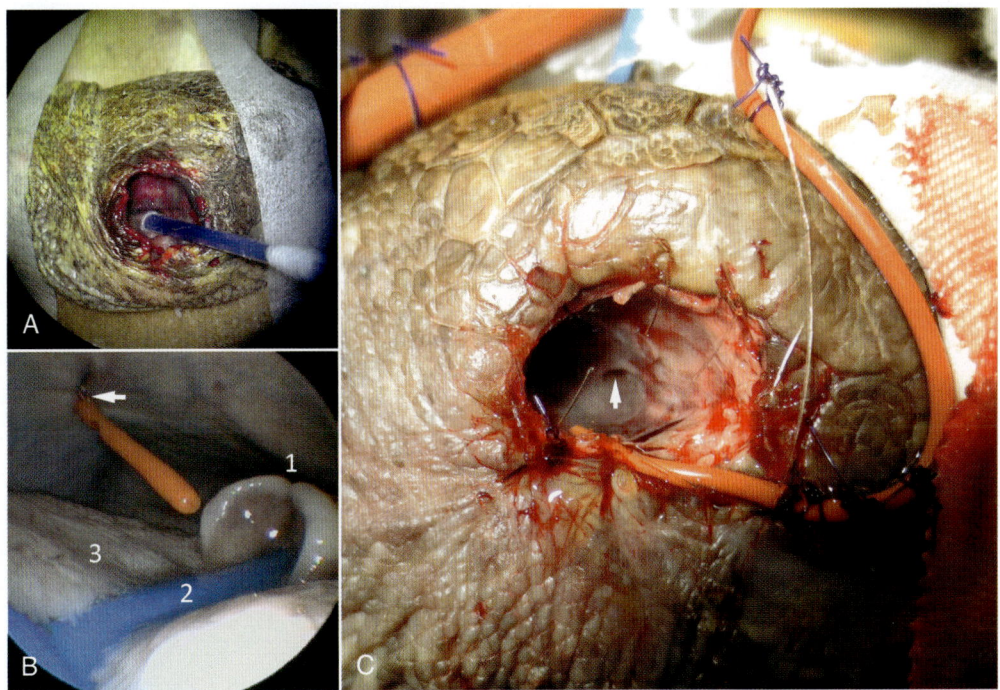

FIG 92.3 (A) Intraoperative view of the tympanic cavity in a tortoise (*Testudo* sp.), with an appropriately sized, cotton-tipped applicator being used to ensure patency of the eustachian tube (cranial to right). In smaller animals a smaller microbrush can be used. (B) Intraoperative, oral view of a leopard tortoise (*Stigmochelys pardalis*) ensuring patency of the right eustachian tube using a red rubber catheter that can be seen exiting the eustachian tube (arrow) into the oropharynx. The larynx (1), endotracheal tube (2), and tongue (3) are also visible. (C) Postoperative view of the same leopard tortoise (cranial to right). The tympanic membrane has been marsupialized to the skin to delay healing until the infection has resolved. A red rubber catheter has been sutured into the tympanic cavity to facilitate flushing and topical therapy in this uncooperative animal. The opening to the eustachian tube is indicated (*arrow*). (Courtesy of Stephen J. Divers.)

The caudomedial aspects of the tympanic cavity are inspected to ensure complete debridement, and patency of the eustachian tube is evaluated (Fig. 92.3A and B). After debridement, the tympanic cavity and eustachian tube are liberally lavaged with sterile saline (with or without an appropriate antimicrobial agent). Indwelling aural irrigation catheters can be used to facilitate twice-daily flushing and topical treatment for uncooperative chelonians (see Fig. 92.3C).

Antibiotics are seldom required following complete surgical removal; however, their use should be governed by established antibiotic policy (i.e., selection of a first-line drug based upon examination of cytology and gram-stained smears, modified by culture and sensitivity results, and preference for local topical therapy over systemic administration). First-line aural antibiotics include trimethoprim-sulfa, amoxicillin, and first- and second-generation cephalosporins. Aminoglycosides should be used with caution given the proximity of neural tissues. Anticoccidial drugs are indicated in cases of cryptosporidiosis. Depending on the degree of surgical manipulation, the routine use of postoperative analgesics for 1 to 3 days is appropriate, with meloxicam and opiates favored by the authors. Aquatic species should be dry-docked for 24 hours and then maintained in shallow water that does not cover the surgical site for the first 10 to 14 days.

Additional support measures including assist feeding may be required based on individual patient response; however, most reptiles recover quickly and are discharged the following day. Clients are instructed to continue daily sterile saline lavage until the wound is closed (often 2–4 weeks) and to make necessary improvements in husbandry (including hygiene) and nutrition (e.g., vitamin A supplementation).[6,7] Reexamination at 1 and 6 to 8 weeks postoperatively is advised to evaluate for infection, assess healing, and remove any sutures.

REFERENCES

See www.expertconsult.com for a complete list of references.

93

Rhinarium

Michelle Kischinovsky and Stephen J. Divers

The rhinarium includes the nostrils, nasal passages, and choana, which open into the oral cavity. The nostrils are often a site of self-induced trauma in captive reptiles, and abscesses involving the maxilla may involve the rhinarium; however, currently there appear to be few indications for rhinotomy.

TRAUMA, ABSCESS, AND OSTEOMYELITIS

Captive reptiles and amphibians are prone to self-trauma from excessive rubbing or striking against enclosure sides. Injuries span from superficial self-limiting abrasions to severe rostral trauma requiring extensive wound management and repeated debridement.

Damage to the rostral area often leads to disruption of air movement through the nares, which results in open-mouth breathing. In turn, this may dry out the oral mucosa, leading to secondary oral and/or respiratory disease as the normal movement of air through the respiratory tract is disrupted. Therefore repairing rhinarial tissue to allow patency

of the nares is critical to long-term success. Husbandry scenarios that result in this damage must also be addressed and resolved for surgical repair, manipulation, or treatment to ultimately be successful.

In severe cases, tissues become secondarily infected, leading to stomatitis, osteomyelitis, or even fractures (Fig. 93.1).[1] If any concerns for bone involvement exist, imaging including radiology, CT, and MRI may be useful in determining a surgical plan and prognosis. Aggressive surgical debridement is usually necessary to remove infected soft tissue and bone to minimize recurrence. Deep, uncontaminated samples should be collected initially for in-house cytology and gram stains, and, if indicated, bacterial and fungal cultures, as well as samples for infectious disease PCR submission (e.g., chlamydia, mycoplasma, ranavirus, herpesvirus, nidovirus) (see Section 4 for more information).

Due to the vascularity of the area, hemorrhage can be a concern because a laryngeal obstruction can result in dyspnea. Use of radiosurgery or laser modalities for hemostasis may be of value when manipulating these vascular tissues. Attention should be paid to protection of the

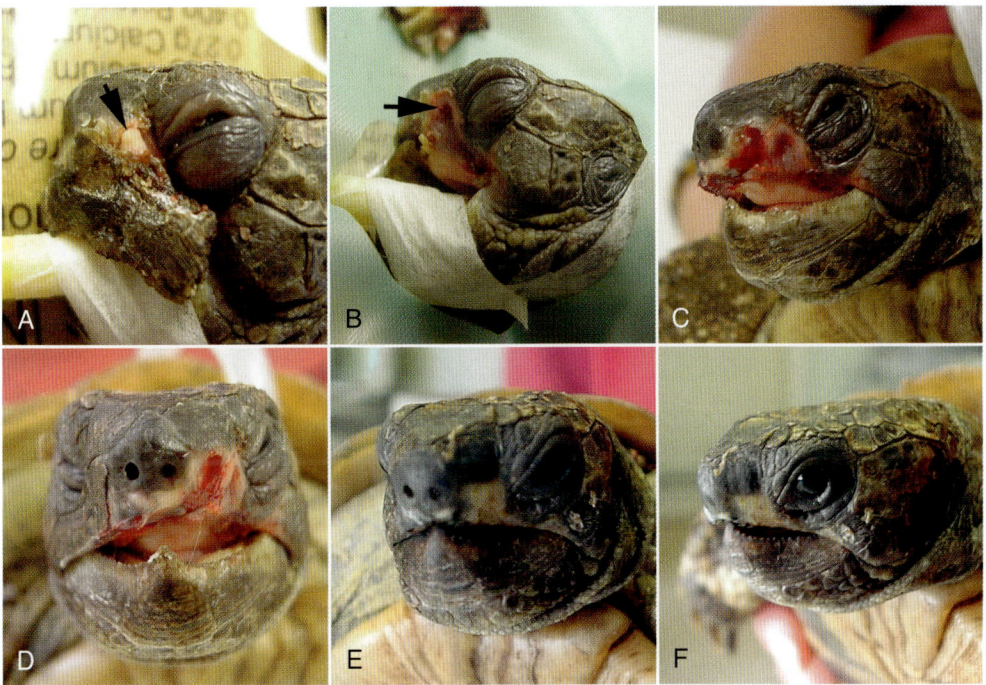

FIG 93.1 (A) Bacterial infection with abscess formation (arrow) associated with a maxillary beak fracture in a Greek tortoise (*Testudo graeca*). The infection has spread to involve the left rhinarium and medial canthus of the eye. (B) Following surgical debridement and removal of the fractured maxillary beak and abscess, a fistula into the left rhinarium is visible (arrow). (C and D) View of the surgical site 4 weeks postoperatively demonstrating healthy granulation tissue. (E and F) View of the surgical site 12 weeks postoperatively showing complete healing with closure of the nasal fistula and maxillary beak regrowth. (Courtesy of Stephen J. Divers.)

larynx itself, especially in procedures where the nares or choana are being flushed, because tissue damage or aspiration can result.

Performing corrective surgery to close wound deficits is difficult, and bandaging any of these areas is generally not possible. Daily or twice-daily flushing using topical antiseptics is essential (e.g., dilute chlorhexidine or betadine, or saline-containing antimicrobials). However, stress to the herptile must be considered when determining frequency of these treatments. In addition, topical treatments may be considered (e.g., manuka honey, silver sulfadiazine, antibiotic ointments). In severe cases where infection is confirmed but topical treatment is ineffective or may require adjunct therapy, systemic antimicrobials are indicated; however, they are no substitute for surgical debridement. Some affected animals may become anorectic, presumably due to interference with olfaction and may need nutritional support (see Chapters 45 and 122). The wounds should be monitored through all phases of second intention healing.

Due to the anatomy and delicate structure of the the rhinarium, and the safety of the surgeon, patients who are fractious or require special attention to internal structures will likely require chemical restraint (see Chapters 48 through 52). To allow safe access to the choana and internal nares, the use of oral speculums, a soft tape roll or other improvised mouth gag device is invaluable. To debride or surgically correct difficult-to-reach areas of the rhinarium, the aid of small and purpose-made (uniquely angled and sized) dental or ophthalmic surgical instruments is useful. Additionally, magnification or video endoscopy, is especially valuable to evaluate the choana and internal nares.

FOREIGN BODIES AND RHINOLITHS

Being an orifice, any foreign object small enough could potentially lodge itself in the cavity. Sea turtles have been described with both a plastic straw and a fork occupying this space.[2,3] In both cases, the object was removed in situ with pliers using forceful retraction and cleaned with a betadine solution before immediate release. In the latter case, it is believed that attempts at regurgitation following ingestion resulted in the foreign body entering the choana and lodging within the nasal turbinates. This highlights the importance of a thorough clinical examination and the use of appropriate imaging modalities (radiography, MRI, CT). It is also a site for fish hook trauma in aquatic and semiaquatic species. Endoscopic evaluation and retrieval may be useful in larger reptiles.

Rhinoliths are seen infrequently, even in burrowing species where dirt could be an obvious nidus. Because the diameter and the angle of the nostrils in most reptilian species usually does not allow great visibility within the nasal cavity, rhinoscopy may aid investigation and removal.

REFERENCES

See www.expertconsult.com for a complete list of references.

94

Oral Cavity, Mandible, Maxilla, and Beak

Michelle Kischinovsky and Stephen J. Divers

This chapter discusses surgical aspects of the oral cavity (teeth, tongue, mucosa), hard palate, mandible, maxilla, and beak (rhamphothecae). Oral cavity pathology requiring surgery is usually the result of trauma. Predisposing conditions and circumstances resulting in injury, such as poor enclosure design and other husbandry-related issues, including nutritional deficiencies, are often contributing factors. A thorough history, clinical assessment, and diagnostic investigation will help to differentiate between a primary injury and one caused by an underlying disease process, and it will help determine a management plan and prognosis.

Neoplastic processes and other growths have been described and are managed similarly to other species with regard to malignancy determination, chemotherapy, radiation therapy, or surgical decisions.[1] Care should be taken when examining the oral cavity to prevent iatrogenic trauma to bone and teeth, as well as soft tissues. Venomous species require particular care and should be examined under general anesthesia (see Chapter 22).

GLOSSITIS AND GLOSSAL PROLAPSE

It is not uncommon for chameleons to prolapse and, in some cases, subsequently "swallow" their tongue. The condition should be treated as an emergency. A full clinical assessment should be made before advising surgical solutions, as the condition is often related to nutritional deficiencies (especially nutritional secondary hyperparathyroidism), and the patient may need stabilization before anesthesia and surgical intervention. In more severe cases where there are concerns related to sepsis, multiple disease processes, and client compliance, euthanasia should be considered. The tissues should be evaluated for viability. A prolapsed or "swallowed" tongue can be replaced to its normal anatomic position using an atraumatic spay hook or similar. If necrosis is evident, then amputation is advised. Bacterial and fungal glossal infections occur in snakes, lizards, and chelonians. Such processes may be diffuse (often acute) or well demarcated (often more chronic). Given the critical roles that the tongue can play in olfaction (snakes and lizards), food prehension (anurans, chameleons), and swallowing (lizards and chelonians), complete amputation can lead to significant postsurgical feeding problems. Although permanent hand feeding is rare, a protracted postoperative recovery period necessitating nutritional support may be required. In general, attempts should be made to retain as much glossal anatomy and function as possible.

Glossal Repair

A novel alternative surgical technique to amputation has been suggested where tissues are viable. In one case involving a Malagasy giant chameleon (*Furcifer oustaleti*), the tongue was brought back into its normal anatomic position after swallowing, then sutured in place with modified cruciate sutures on both sides of the tongue (K. Mathes, personal communication, 2018). Sutures were removed after 5 days, and the patient regained full tongue functionality. Hand feeding was necessary for 3 weeks.

Partial and Complete Glossectomy

The patient is given appropriate preemptive analgesia, induced, intubated, and maintained at a surgical plane of anesthesia. Positioning in sternal or lateral recumbency with the head and neck extended, and rostrally facing the surgeon, is appropriate. Mouth gags can help maintain visualization. Aseptic preparation should be attempted using povidone-iodine rather than chlorhexidine, though with caution because tissues may easily slough. The oropharynx can be gently packed with cotton-tipped applicators or gauze to reduce the chances of aspiration.

In cases of focal, well-encapsulated, or demarcated disease, often involving the fleshy chelonian tongue, gentle dissection along a plane of healthy tissue may enable an abscess or granuloma to be removed (Fig. 94.1). Hemorrhage often occurs, and the judicious use of radiosurgery, pressure, local epinephrine, and hemostatic sponges are effective. Careful consideration should be given to closure because there can be no tension on the glossal epithelium. Fine (4/0–5/0), monofilament, absorbable suture should be used in a simple interrupted pattern, and antibiotic-impregnated poliglecaprone 25 (Monocryl-Plus, Ethicon, Athens, GA) is preferred.

For complete glossectomy in lizards and snakes with a long narrow tongue, a transfixing circumferential ligature is placed on healthy tissue a few millimeters from the nonviable border, and the proximal tissues are amputated using a scalpel, scissors, or radiosurgery (Fig. 94.2). In chelonians and lizards with larger fleshy tongues, multiple mattress sutures may be required. Care should be taken to ligate veins and to avoid damage to the entoglossal process of chameleons, which should be adequately covered by epithelium. Minimal bleeding is expected. Any suture ends should be as short as possible as not to provoke the oral mucosa, although proximal glossectomy usually results in the surgical site retracted within the lingual sheath (see Fig. 94.2C) in species with this structure. The needs, duration, and practicality of nutritional support are important, and placement of an esophagostomy tube should be considered. (See Chapter 45.)

Healing should be monitored closely but is usually rapid for oral tissues, with the patient reevaluated at 1 and 4 weeks postoperatively to assess for possible infection and healing. Prolonged hand feeding may be required, potentially lifelong; however, most patients eventually adapt.

ORAL MASSES AND STOMATITIS

Stomatitis can present as localized or diffuse inflammation and/or infection. In addition, soft tissue swellings or projections may represent abscesses, cysts, papillomas, granulomas, and neoplastic or benign growths

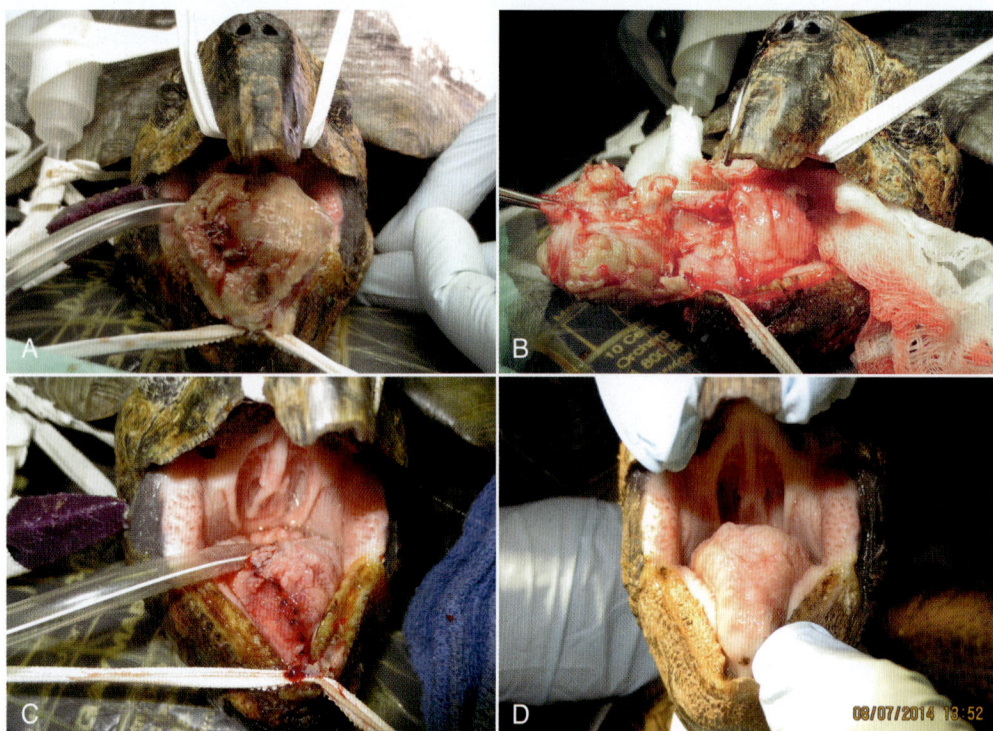

FIG 94.1 Mycotic granuloma and partial glossectomy in a Galapagos tortoise (*Chelonoides nigra*). (A) Gross appearance of the necrotic and inflamed tongue. (B) Surgical resection of diseased tissue by partial glossectomy. (C) Sutured closure of the tongue epithelium using fine simple interrupted sutures of antibiotic-impregnated, poliglecaprone 25. (D) View of the tongue 10 months later during routine examination. (Courtesy of Stephen J. Divers.)

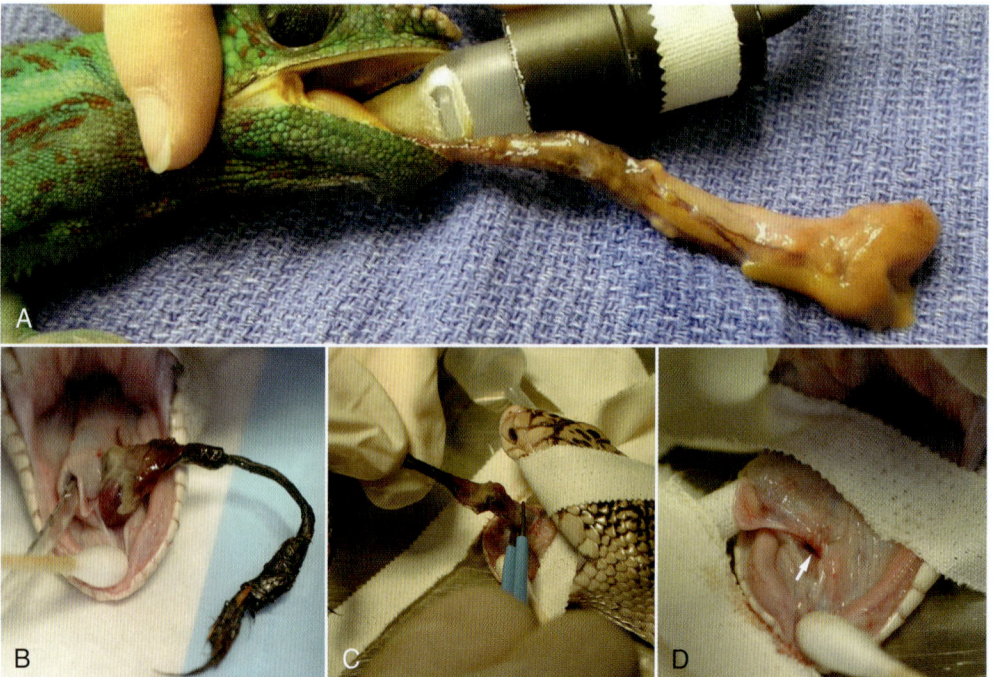

FIG 94.2 (A) Glossal prolapse and abscess in a panther chameleon (*Furcifer pardalis*). (B) Glossal prolapse and necrosis in a northern pine snake (*Pituophis melanoleucus*). (C) Bipolar forceps (not activated) being used to crush the proximal tongue in preparation for a transfixing circumferential suture. Complete glossectomy is then performed distal to the suture with radiosurgical hemostasis. (D) Immediate postoperative view with the glossal stump retracted into the lingual sheath (arrow). (A, Courtesy of Scott J. Stahl, Stahl Exotic Animal Veterinary Services; B–D, courtesy of Stephen J. Divers.)

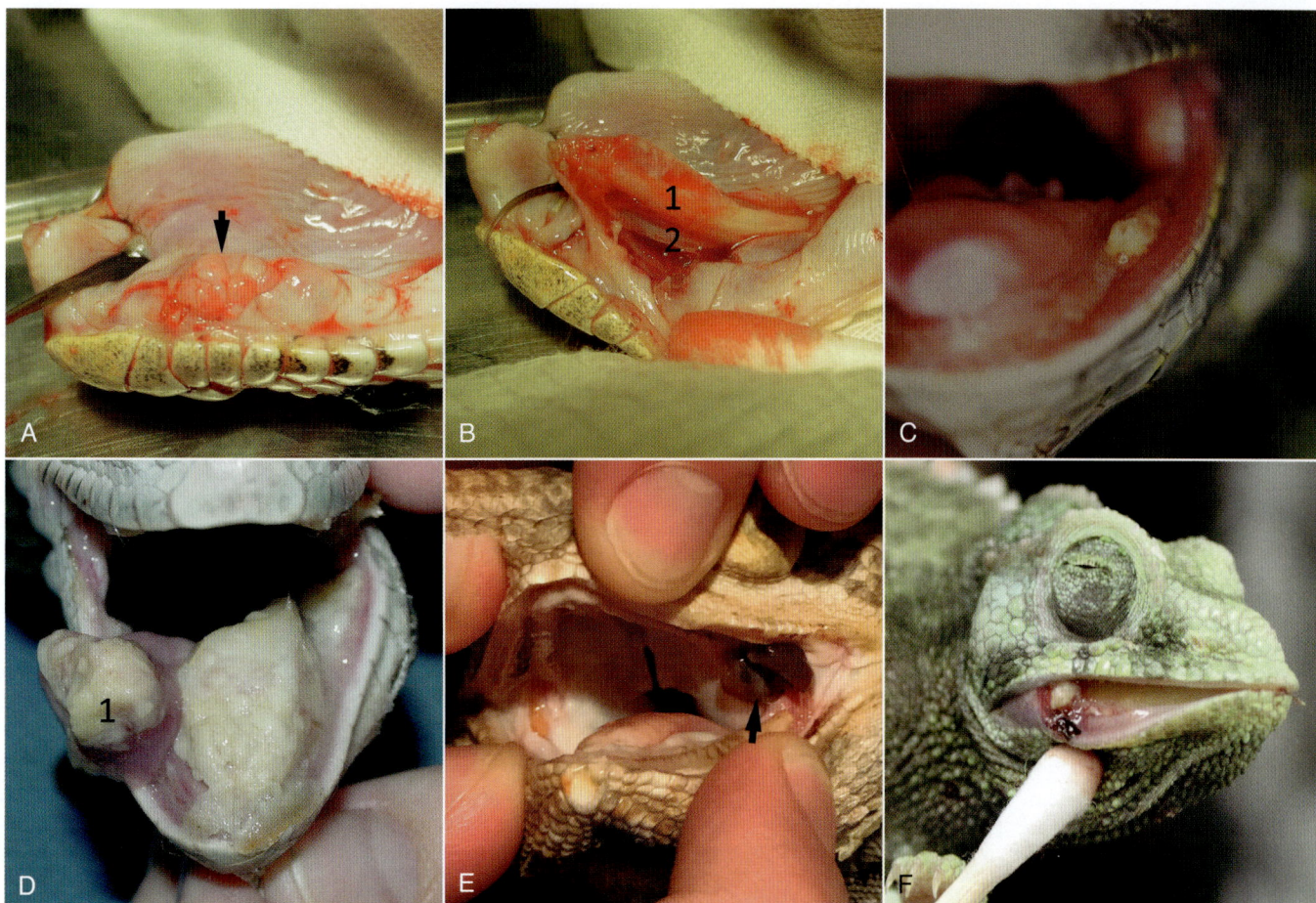

FIG 94.3 (A) Focal soft tissue swelling (arrow) associated with the buccal aspect of the left mandible of a rattlesnake (*Crotalus* sp). (B) Cytology revealed granulomatous inflammation, and the mass was resected. With the lingual gingiva exposed, note the underlying left mandible (1), and the remains of the superficial external adductor muscle (2). The mucosa was closed with fine antibiotic-impregnated, poliglecaprone 25 sutures. (C) Focal gingival abscess of dental origin in a green iguana (*Iguana iguana*). Focal curettage with removal of infected soft tissue and pleurodont teeth is straightforward. (D) Large sublingual and lingual abscesses in a green iguana, which has caused right lateral displacement of the tongue (1). (E) Bearded dragon (*Pogona vitticeps*) with progressive enlargement of granulation tissue at oral commissure. (F) Female Jackson's chameleon (*Trioceros jacksonii*) with temporal gland abscess. (A–D, Courtesy of Stephen J. Divers; E, courtesy of John Stevens; F, courtesy of Scott J. Stahl, Stahl Exotic Animal Veterinary Services.)

(Fig. 94.3). Temporal glands, located at the commissures of the mouth in some old-world chameleons, often present swollen and may be asymmetrical and filled with inspissated material. This is particularly common in Jackson's chameleons (*Trioceros jacksonii*), where green exudate often cultures *Pseudomonas* (see Fig. 94.3).[1] Superficial cytology may be useful but is often poorly diagnostic due to chronicity and oral contamination. Radiography and CT are useful for determining whether there is boney involvement and to plan surgical approaches. Surgical biopsy is often required for a histologic and microbiologic diagnosis to direct treatment. As with the treatment of other abscesses in reptiles these affected glands need to be surgically explored and marsupialized to allow flushing and topical treatment. If bone is involved debridement may be necessary. For such invasive procedures (e.g., debulking, debriding) involving the small and complex nature of most oral structures, magnification, microsurgery, and radiosurgery are often beneficial (Fig. 94.4A).

FACIAL MASSES AND OSTEOMYELITIS

Facial abscesses and granulomas, like their intraoral counterparts, rarely if ever resolve after mere lancing and flushing. Typically, surgical removal *in toto* is required; however, unlike other areas of the body, there is rarely sufficient skin and subcutaneous tissue to ensure closure, and marsupialization or grafting techniques may be required. Although most discrete facial swellings are infectious, aspiration cytology and gram staining can help identify neoplastic or inflammatory masses that may need biopsy for a histologic diagnosis and treatment plan (Fig. 94.4B). Bilateral mandibular swellings, typically due to nutritional secondary hyperparathyroidism, are especially common in lizards and represent a medical, not surgical, condition. Additionally, periodontal disease is a significant cause of oral pathology in captive lizards and is caused by bacterial or fungal invasion of the unique periodontal tissues of lizard species with acrodont dentition, including agamids (e.g., bearded dragons,

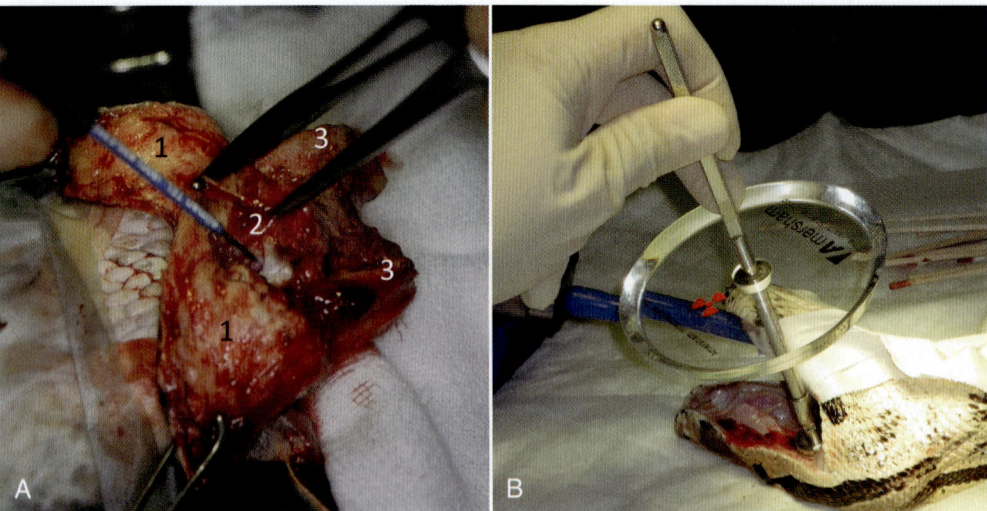

FIG 94.4 (A) Undifferentiated intermandibular sarcoma resection in a Burmese python (*Python bivittatus*). The skin of the ventral mandible (1) has been reflected caudal to expose the sarcoma (2) and facilitate resection from between the mandibles (3). (B) Strontium radiation therapy following resection and debulking of a carcinoma of the right lingual surface in a boa constrictor (*Boa constrictor*). (Courtesy of Stephen J. Divers.)

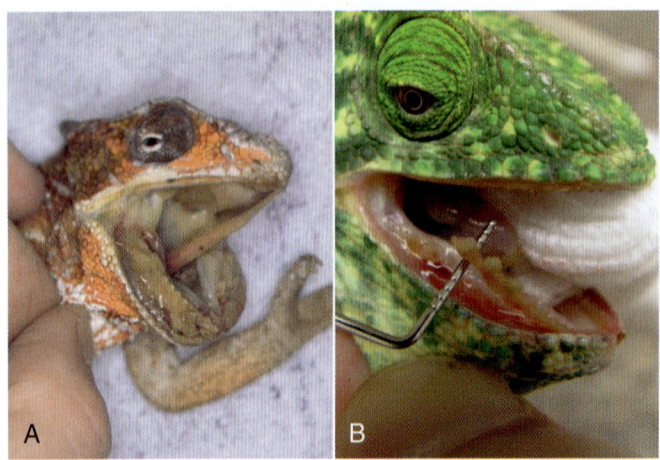

FIG 94.5 (A) Panther chameleon (*Furcifer pardalis*) with severe stomatitis, mandible bone exposure with osteomyelitis, and tongue necrosis that required euthanasia. (B) Parsons chameleon (*Calumma parsonii*) with severe periodontal disease of mandible with associated osteomyelitis and fracture. (A, Courtesy of Stephen J. Divers; B, courtesy of Scott J. Stahl, Stahl Exotic Animal Veterinary Services.)

Pogona vitticeps, and Asian water dragons, *Physignathus cocincinus*) and old-world chameleons.[2] These lizards typically present with asymmetrical swellings and discoloration along mandibular and maxillary bones and improper closure of the mouth. Often osteomyelitis is associated with these lesions, and aggressive therapy to identify and surgically explore these lesions is indicated (Fig. 94.5). (See Chapters 73 and 161.)

Asymmetrical swellings in the region of the maxillae or mandibles should be evaluated radiographically because osteomyelitis is common and does not respond well to medical therapy alone (Fig. 94.6). Typically, surgical exposure, thorough debridement, and marsupialization are required with prolonged antimicrobial therapy, based on culture and sensitivity testing, for 6 weeks or more. Radiographic reevaluation is recommended because disease progression is common.

OVERGROWN BEAK (RHAMPHOTHECA)

Beak disorders are commonly encountered in chelonians. A thorough history and physical examination should be performed, because this is often a multifactorial issue that can be associated with husbandry, nutrition, trauma, infection, and congenital deformity.

Overgrowth of the keratin rhamphotheca (rhinotheca of the maxilla and gnathotheca of the mandible) is especially common and has been controversially associated with nutritional secondary hyperparathyroidism, elevated dietary protein, and soft, easily prehended food items (Fig. 94.7). In severe cases the upper beak becomes compressed, resulting in the rhinarium tissues and the outer nares becoming occluded. Depending on the strength and tenacity of the patient, sedation or anesthesia may be required, and the head and neck are extended and held in place using two fingers behind the jaw. A dremel with a small rounded head is used to correct minor abnormalities, but a cutting disc may be necessary if there are large overgrown sections to remove. Care should be taken as friction heat is created; intermittent tool use and cold saline-soaked gauze or cotton-tipped applicators can be used for cooling. Corrective treatment may only provide temporary relief, as the beak is likely to continue abnormal growth unless underlying causes are identified and corrected.

FRACTURES (BEAK, MAXILLA, AND MANDIBLE)

Fractures of the keratinized beak are not uncommon after severe trauma, especially in free-ranging chelonians. The fractures may be superficial and only include the keratinized structures, or they may involve the underlying maxilla and mandibular bones. Multiple radiographic planes are typically required, although CT is often preferred for identifying skull fractures (Fig. 94.8).[3,4] It is important to appreciate normal radiographic anatomy because the temporomandibular joint is relatively ventral and should not be mistaken for a fracture. If there is no instability or displacement, then preventing beak use by esophagostomy feeding should be sufficient. Distracted or unstable fractures should be reduced and anchored. A variety of techniques can be used as long as the basic principles of fracture stabilization are maintained. Unless the fracture

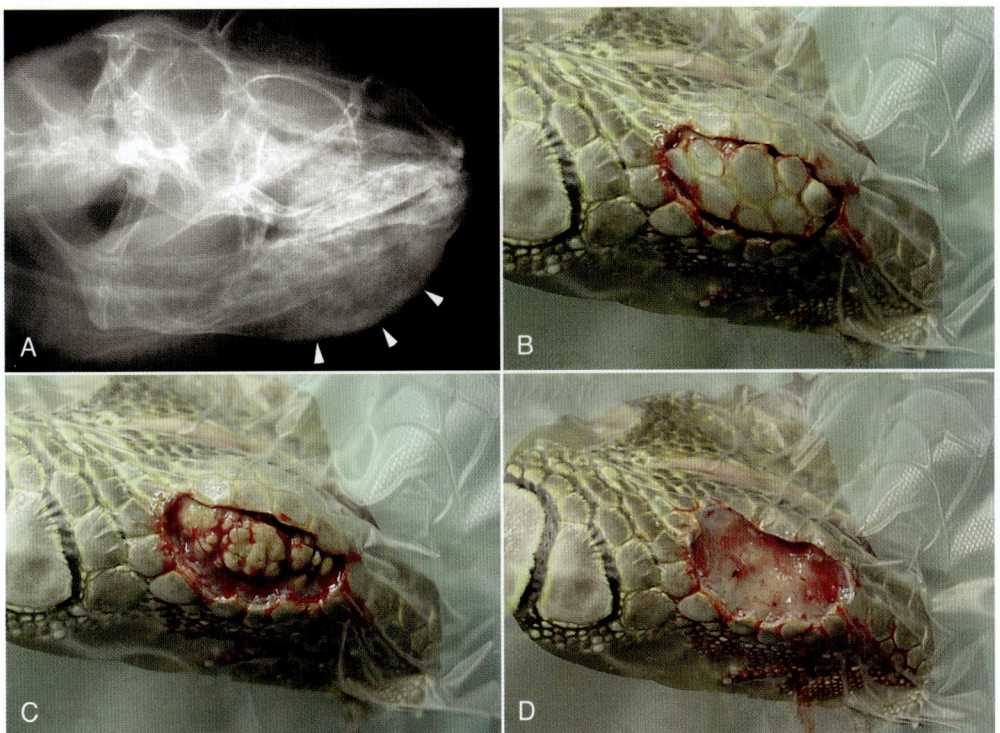

FIG 94.6 Right mandibular abscess with mandibular osteomyelitis in a green iguana (*Iguana iguana*). (A) Skyline (lateral oblique) radiograph demonstrating the proliferative and osteolytic changes associated with the right mandible (arrows). (B) Surgical view of the mandibular swelling following scalpel incision around the prominence. (C) The skin has been removed to reveal the abscess and infected bone. (D) Following debridement and removal of all infected tissue, the surgical site is left open to facilitate twice-daily wound management and healing by second intention. (Courtesy of Stephen J. Divers.)

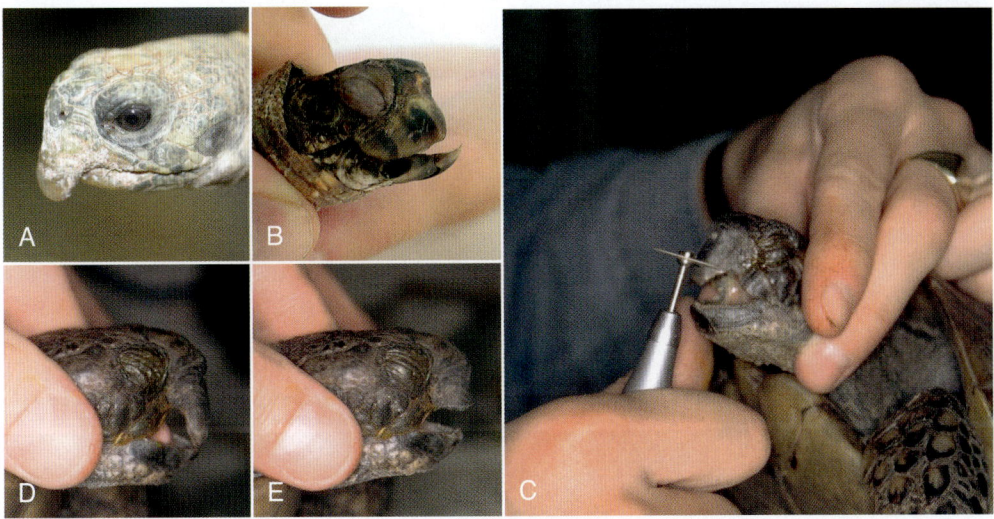

FIG 94.7 (A) Overgrowth of the rhinotheca (Bell's hinge-back tortoise, *Kinixys belliana*). (B) Overgrowth of the rhinotheca and gnathotheca (*Testudo* sp.). (C) Trimming the excessive rhinotheca of a spur-thighed tortoise (*Testudo graeca*) using a rotary tool and cutting disc. Views of the same tortoise preoperatively (D) and after cutting and reshaping using a rotary tool (E). (Courtesy of Stephen J. Divers.)

is <12 hours old, the wound edges should be freshened with a scalpel blade before reduction. Internal fixator pins, tension band wires, and external fixators are commonly used, often in combination with polymethylmethacrylate to provide greater protection and support (Figs. 94.9 and 94.10).[2–5] External fixator pins should not enter the oral cavity,

because contamination and infection of the pin sites becomes likely. Any exposed pin entry sites should be cleaned twice daily. Chronic fractures often become infected, requiring more aggressive debridement and second intention healing (see Fig. 93.1). Implants should not be placed into an infected site or to reduce a pathologic fracture (e.g., in

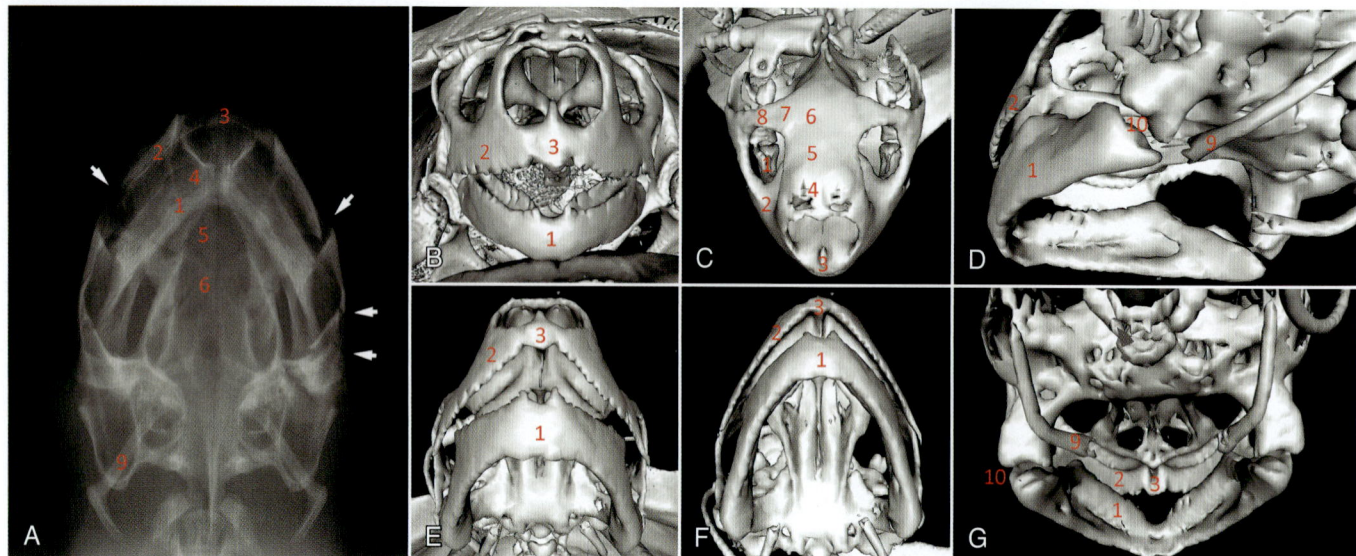

FIG 94.8 (A) Dorsoventral skull radiograph of a *Testudo* tortoise demonstrating multiple, bilateral fractures (*arrows*) of the maxilla. (B–G) 3D surface-rendering reconstructions of the skull CT of a desert tortoise (*Gopherus agassizii*). Mandible (1), maxilla (2), premaxilla (3), nasal (4), frontal (5), parietal (6), postorbital (7), jugal (8), ceratobrachial of hyoid apparatus (9), and temporomandibular joint (10). (Courtesy of Stephen J. Divers.)

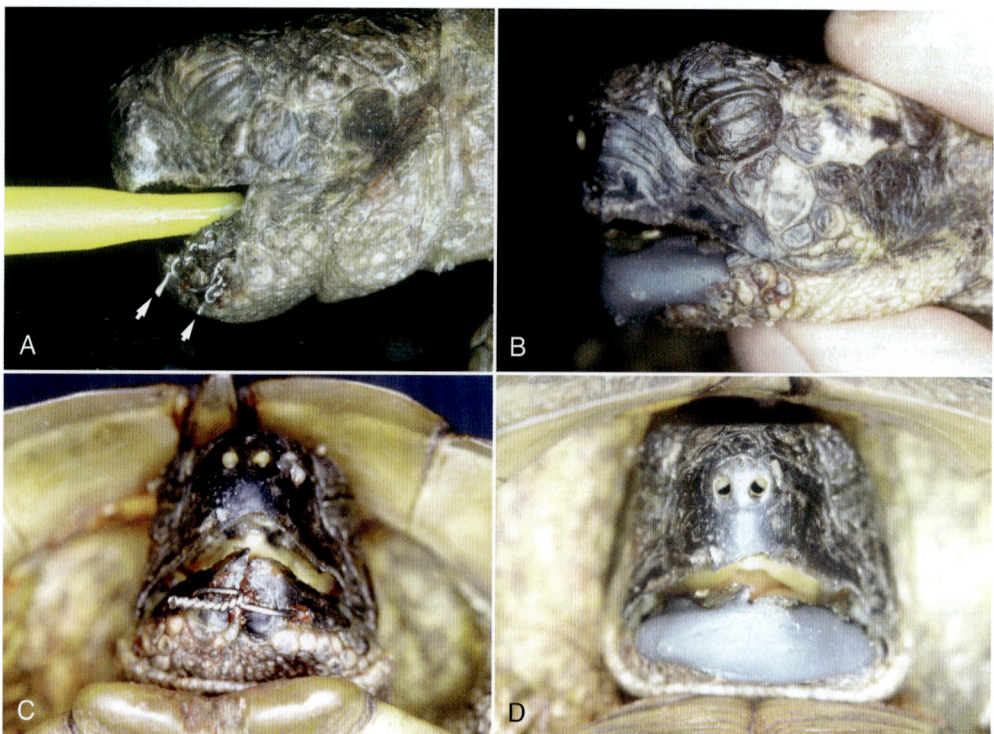

FIG 94.9 Mandibular and gnathotheca fractures in *Testudo* tortoises. (A and B) Lateral fractures of the left mandible and gnathotheca reduced using two wire sutures and covered with polymethylmethacrylate. (C and D) Mandibular symphyseal and gnathotheca fractures reduced using a single cerclage wire and covered with polymethylmethacrylate. (Courtesy of Stephen J. Divers.)

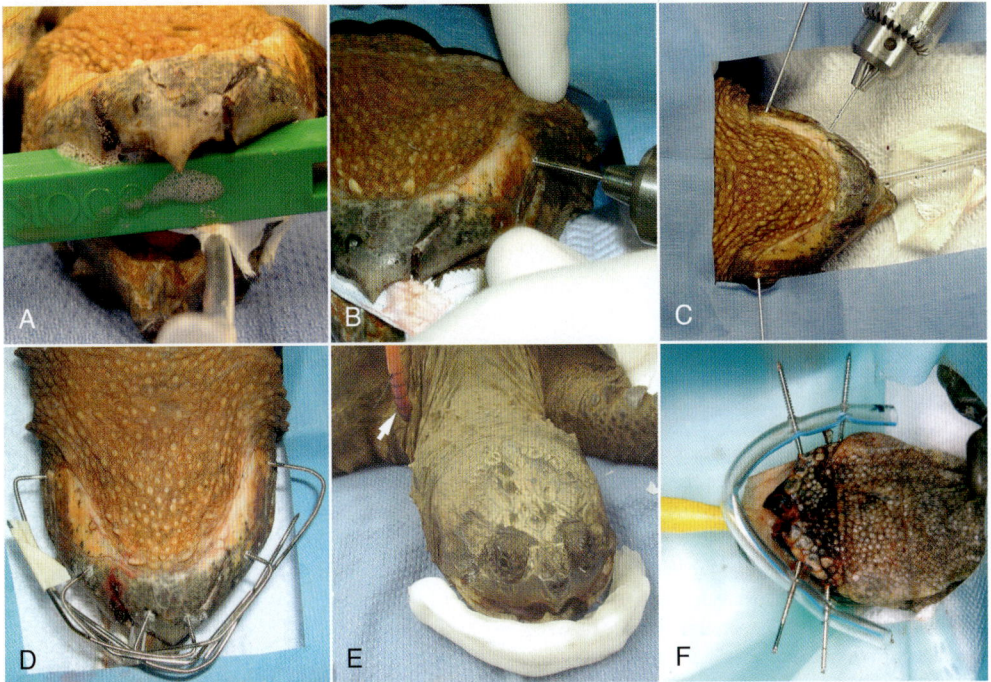

FIG 94.10 (A–E) Multiple mandibular fractures in a common snapping turtle (*Chelydra serpentina*) repaired using six mini-IMEX external fixator pins and covered with polymethylmethacrylate. Note the presence of an esophagostomy feeding tube (E, arrow) to provide nutritional support until healed. (F) Fractured mandible in a *Testudo* tortoise repaired using four mini-IMEX external fixator pins. The tubing pushed over the pins was subsequently filled with polymethylmethacrylate to provide support. (Courtesy of Stephen J. Divers.)

animals with nutritional secondary hyperparathyroidism). Postoperative complications include trauma to any external fixator, pin loosening, and infection. Placement of an esophagostomy tube is recommended to reduce pressures being applied to the beak during prehension. Radiographs should be repeated, often at 4 and 12 weeks, to monitor healing and evaluate for any signs of osteolysis that might indicate infection. Fracture implants are typically left in place for 12 weeks, although radiographic evidence of complete healing is often delayed and can take 12 to 28 weeks.[3–5] However, external fixator removal should not be solely based on radiographic evaluation, but also on clinical evaluation and palpation because a persistent radiolucent line may persist for many months if not years.

A novel, nonsurgical technique has been described in a blue-tongued skink (*Tiliqua scincoides*) that utilized an intraoral plate (U-shaped plastic, 2 mm thick), which was secured in position using a tape muzzle (Köchli et al, ExoticDVM, 2008, 10:25–28). An esophagostomy tube was placed for nutritional support. The plate was removed after 36 days because of damage and loss of teeth, but the lizard resumed eating by day 44 and made a complete recovery.

REFERENCES

See www.expertconsult.com for a complete list of references.

95

Venomoid Surgery

Richard S. Funk

Venomoid surgery is a surgical technique developed to render a venomous snake or lizard nonvenomous by altering the venom production and delivery systems. In some countries, such a procedure is considered a mutilation and is not legally permitted. Additionally, veterinarians who legally perform this procedure should be aware of the liability associated with subsequent envenomation from an imperfect surgery. In the author's experience, an important indication for this procedure is to reduce risk for less-experienced keepers/curators in zoological collections. Additionally, the procedure has been performed on reptiles used in "sting" operations to reduce the risks to all handlers, including the would-be poachers. This procedure is not recommended for those that simply have a desire to keep a venomous reptile.

SNAKES

An early (1937) description of this surgery discussed a crude intraoral approach without surgical hemostasis and "closure" utilizing rubber bands around the patients' heads (excluding lower jaws) for 10 to 48 hours.[1] Another technique utilized in the 1970s involved an approach to the venom apparatus via an incision on the side of the snake's head. Double ligation and transection of a segment of the venom duct was then performed and the venom gland was left intact.[2] A lateral approach for venom duct ligation and resection results in a facial scar on each side, which owners may find cosmetically unappealing, and some snakes (especially elapids) developed a granulomatous response at the surgical site, resulting in a disfiguring swelling. A further modification of this lateral approach was to remove the venom gland and its duct, but a facial scar may still persist. A recent study involving venom duct ligation and resection in four venomous snakes (puff adder [*Bitis arietans*], western diamondback rattlesnake [*Crotalus atrox*], painted saw-scaled viper [*Echis coloratus*], and red spitting cobra [*Naja pallida*]) concluded that scars were virtually invisible after the second postoperative skin shed.[3]

In the 1980s the author developed an intraoral technique that leaves no visible scars and involves the complete removal of the venom gland and the venom duct. Following induction of general anesthesia, the snake is surgically prepped in dorsal recumbency with the mouth opened widely to give full exposure to the buccal surfaces of the maxillae. Care is taken to avoid envenomation of the surgeon. The oral mucosa of the maxillary areas are aseptically prepared. An incision is then made between the palatine-fang axis and the lip margin with radiosurgery, a CO_2 laser, or a no. 15 scalpel blade. Careful dissection with small (preferably ophthalmic) instruments exposes the venom gland and its duct. The venom duct in elapids may be thicker and more difficult to handle. Several small vessels are associated with the gland and the duct, with the largest being encountered dorsomedially; these can be cauterized with the laser or with radiosurgery or, in the case of larger snakes, ligated with absorbable suture and then transected. Good hemostasis is important.

The venom duct is transected at its entrance into the base of the maxillary bone, and the entire duct and venom gland are then elevated and dissected out of the incision as a unit and safely discarded (Fig. 95.1A). To help preserve the cosmetic postoperative appearance of the head, a sterilized silicone prosthesis is cut to a size approximating the

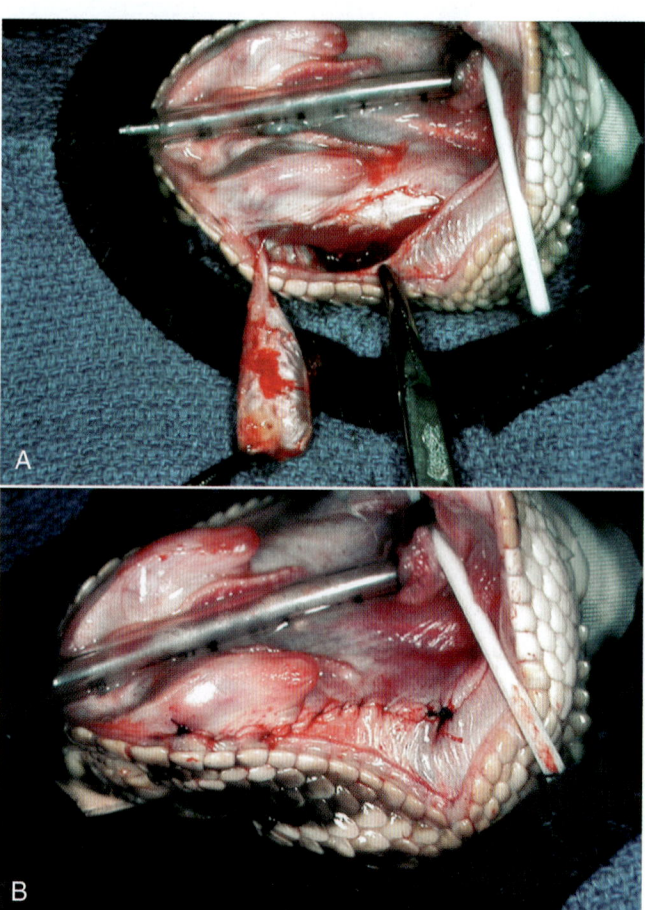

FIG 95.1 Venomoid surgery in an adult eastern diamondback rattlesnake (*Crotalus adamanteus*), with the snake in dorsal recumbency. (A) The right venom gland has been elevated through an intraoral incision, but the venom duct is still attached to the base of the right maxillary fang. The duct will be separated at its attachment, and the venom gland and duct will thereby be removed. (B) The venom gland and its duct have been removed; a silicone prosthesis has been placed into the space formerly occupied by the gland, and the incision has been closed with absorbable monofilament suture in a simple continuous pattern.

size of the gland that was removed, and then placed into the surgical site from which the gland was removed (Silicone Elastomer Block, Implantable Restoration Material, Soft White; McGhan Medical Corp., Santa Barbara, CA). To facilitate future identification, a segment of surgical stainless steel suture may be placed within the silicone prosthesis so that it is visible radiographically, or better still, a microchip transponder may be placed into the prosthesis. The mucosal incision is closed with absorbable monofilament suture in a simple continuous pattern (see Fig. 95.1B). Follow-up suture removal is therefore unnecessary. A broad-spectrum antibiotic is administered perioperatively (e.g., IV cephalosporins).

Following surgery, the snake is not fed for 2 to 3 weeks to help facilitate the healing process and minimize the chances of infection from the oral cavity or from prey abrading the surgical site. The cage is kept clean, and the drinking water is changed daily. Thereafter the snake should be fed only dead prey. No complications have been noted from the uses of these prostheses.

Snakes that this author has rendered venomoid have lived well and even bred subsequently (unpublished data). Legally, most jurisdictions still classify a snake from which the venom glands and ducts have been removed as a venomous species even though it is functionally no longer venomous. In two adult *Crotalus*, one *atrox* and one *pyrrhus*, that underwent this surgery, the snakes were surgically reinvestigated 12 and 14 months later (respectively), and the previous surgical sites from which the venom glands were removed were explored. No trace of gland or duct regeneration was found. Subsequently, test prey envenomation was negative for both snakes (unpublished observations).

GILA MONSTER VENOMOID SURGERY

Venomoid surgery for heloderms, Gila monsters (*Heloderma suspectum*) and beaded lizards (*Heloderma horridum*), is performed differently than venomous snakes because of the anatomic location of the venom glands in the ventrolateral regions on the lower jaws. The location of each gland is indicated by a prominent swelling or bulge along the anterior and middle region of each lower jaw laterally (Fig. 95.2). Under general anesthesia, the skin at the surgical site is aseptically prepared, and a ventrolateral skin incision is made with a scalpel blade, CO_2 laser, or

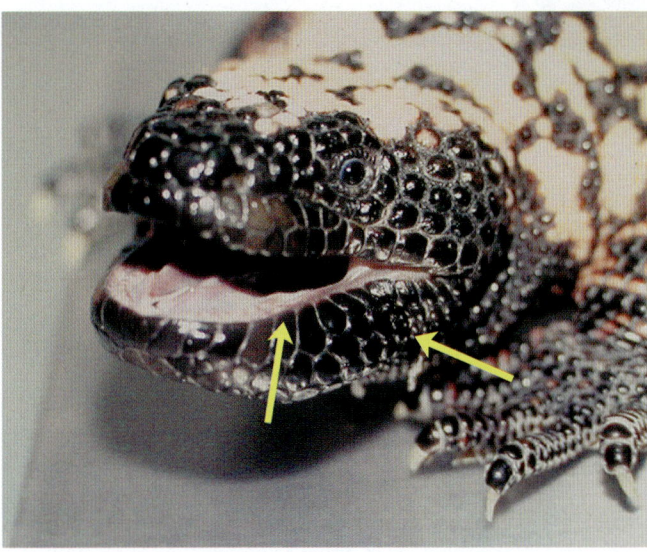

FIG 95.2 The location of the venom gland in the Gila monster (*Heloderma suspectum*) can be noted as swelling or bulge along the anterior and middle portions of the lower jaw (arrows). The gland on each side has a series of tiny ducts leading to the oral cavity.

radiosurgery. The helodermid venom gland differs from snakes in that a single duct is lacking; instead, a number of tiny ducts lead from the lobulated gland to the bases of several teeth. The lightly pinkish venom gland is carefully elevated from the mandible and removed by a combination of sharp and blunt dissection. Hemorrhage is typically minimal. No prosthesis is placed into the venom gland site. The skin is closed with a nonabsorbable monofilament suture in a simple interrupted (noneverting) pattern. Feeding may be resumed in 7 to 10 days. Sutures are removed in 5 to 6 weeks.

REFERENCES

See www.expertconsult.com for a complete list of references.

96

Integument

T. Franciscus Scheelings and Tom Hellebuyck

Surgery of the reptilian integument is frequently warranted for management of wounds, collection of skin biopsies for disease characterization, removal of abscesses and neoplasms, and as a first step in many invasive surgical procedures. Depending on the nature of the pathology and the temperament of the patient, these procedures can either be performed under general anesthesia or by using a combination of sedation and local nerve blocks. Other chapters within this text cover the principles of anesthesia, analgesia, and administration of other therapeutics such as antimicrobials and fluids.

SURGICAL SITE PREPARATION

Established aseptic surgical techniques should be followed for reptile patients. The intended surgical site should be prepared using chlorhexidine or povidone iodine. A sterile toothbrush or a hand brush may be beneficial when trying to adequately scrub uneven, scaled skin. Excessive use of alcohol may lead to patient hypothermia due to evaporative heat loss,[1] but a light, final wipe with alcohol-moistened gauze is still recommended and helps with plastic drape adhesion. There are a range of options available for veterinarians to create a sterile surgical field. Clear, adhesive plastic drapes are particularly useful because they allow for better visualization of the patient, are waterproof, and do not require the use of towel clamps.[1] These are preferred in small to medium-sized animals. For larger reptiles, traditional cloth or paper drapes may be required.

SKIN INCISIONS AND WOUND CLOSURE

Reptilian skin is often heavily keratinized and may be difficult to incise. In addition, many species have enlarged scales or osteoderms, which need to be avoided. Similar to small-animal surgery, the clinician should consider tension lines and incision orientation when planning their approach. To make the initial incision, it is sometimes helpful to tent the skin with a pair of toothed forceps and then stab into the skin with a small scalpel blade. A pair of sharp scissors or a guarded, upturned scalpel can then be used to extend the incision. Radiosurgery and laser units can also be used to make skin incisions in reptiles, although their use should be avoided if histological evaluation of skin margins is required.[2–5] No matter the technique used, the surgeon should avoid cutting directly into scales, which means that many incisions will require a scalloped technique, especially in snakes.

Incised reptile skin tends to invert, therefore an everting suture pattern (e.g., horizontal mattress) is often preferred over simple interrupted patterns for primary closure (Fig. 96.1).[1,6,7] A number of materials are suitable for closing surgical wounds in reptiles, including nonabsorbable (e.g., monofilament nylon, Ethilon; Ethicon, Inc., Piscataway, New Jersey) or absorbable suture (e.g., poliglecaprone 25, Monocryl, Piscataway, NJ).[8] However, braided materials that allow wicking or chromic catgut that causes intense inflammation should not be used.[8] Suture removal is generally 6 to 8 weeks postoperatively, but ecdysis during this time may lead

to premature loss of sutures placed too close to incision margins. Clients should be advised that some degree of dysecdysis may be experienced at the site of the wound, necessitating minor management, but this usually resolves after 1 to 3 shedding cycles (Fig. 96.2). Alternatives to

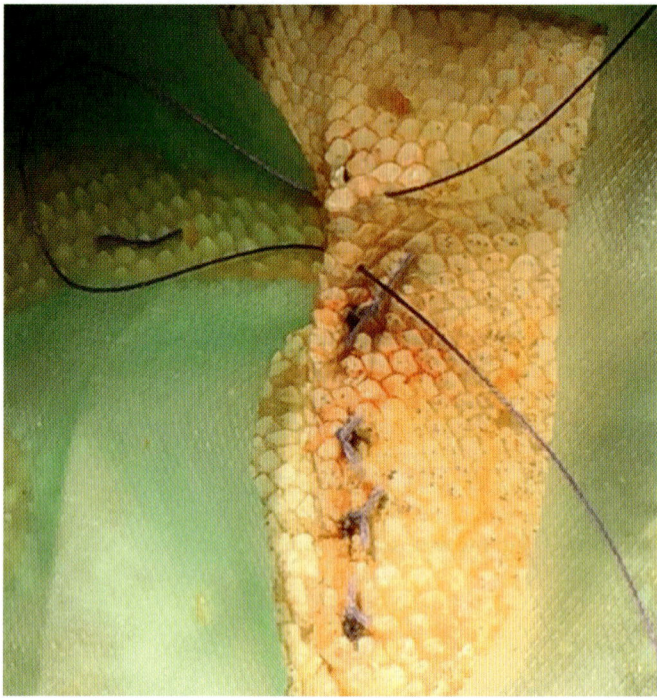

FIG 96.1 Incised reptile skin has a tendency to invert, so an everting pattern should be used. (Courtesy of Tom Hellebuyck.)

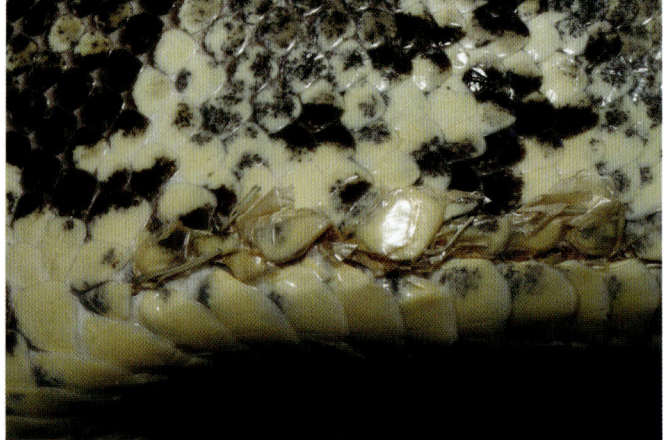

FIG 96.2 As surgical wounds heal, there may be some areas of dysecdysis associated with the incision. (Courtesy of Tom Hellebuyck.)

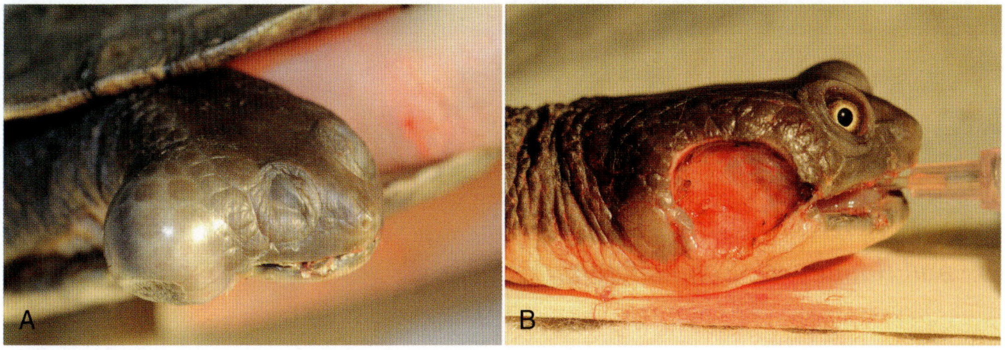

FIG 96.3 (A) Abscesses are commonly encountered in reptile practice, as seen in this chelonian. (B) If wounds cannot be closed, they can be left to heal by secondary intention. (Courtesy of T.F. Scheelings.)

suture material that can be used to close wounds include skin stables, or, in small incisions, cyanoacrylic tissue adhesives (Nexaband Veterinary Products Laboratories, Phoenix, Arizona).

SUBCUTANEOUS MASSES (ABSCESSES, PARASITIC CYSTS, AND NEOPLASMS)

Subcutaneous abscesses are frequently encountered (Fig. 96.3A). They may present as either single or multiple disseminated firm masses entrenched within the skin. Reptile abscesses are typically hard and rarely liquid, so they must be removed completely; lancing and drainage are rarely, if ever, effective. If the surgeon is confident that all the abscess material has been completely removed, then the wound can be closed as previously described. Where there is any suspicion that some contamination may remain, the affected site should be managed as an open wound and allowed to heal by second intention (see Fig. 96.3B). Antibiotics are rarely indicated following abscess removal but, if required, should be based upon fungal and bacterial culture of a portion of the capsule. Differential diagnoses for cutaneous masses include neoplasia and parasitic granulomas, and thus it may be prudent to submit samples of excised tissue for histopathological examination.

OPEN WOUND MANAGEMENT

In some instances, primary closure of wounds is not possible, necessitating second intention healing and delayed closure. Fortunately, reptiles tolerate this well, and it is particularly useful for contaminated wounds or where large deficits exist. Most importantly, the wound needs to be thoroughly debrided and lavaged so that only a healthy bed of granulation tissue remains. Sterile saline is best for wound irrigation, as the addition of antiseptics has not been shown to be beneficial.[9]

Furthermore, these compounds can be cytotoxic and may inhibit wound healing. Surgical debridement may be preferred when anesthesia can be performed. Mechanical debridement (wet-to-dry bandages) is less selective.[10] If clinicians deem mechanical debridement important to wound healing, then it should only be performed during the initial inflammatory phase and should be preceded by administration of adequate analgesia.[10]

Once the wound has been debrided and lavaged, it needs to be covered to prevent it from desiccating and to promote healing. Topical wound coverings such as hydroscopic gels, antibiotic ointments, silver cream, and honey can be utilized to promote wound healing and decrease the risks of post-debridement infection. These, in turn, should be covered by a layer of bandage to provide further protection from mechanical damage. The choice of bandage material used is dependent on the nature of the wound. Products commonly used for small animals translate well to herpetologic medicine. An important sequela of second intention healing is the possibility of significant scar formation and future dysecdysis (see Chapters 69 and 130 for more details). A useful adjunct treatment in managing open wounds is application of low-level laser therapy (biophotomodulation). This can be helpful in the resolution of intractable wounds that are unresponsive to other modalities of treatment (see Chapter 129). The exact method by which lasers promote wound healing is not yet well understood, but they seem to act at molecular, cellular, and tissue levels to promote ingression of inflammatory cells, modulate cytokines, growth factors, and inflammatory mediators, as well as increasing tissue oxygenation.[11]

REFERENCES

See www.expertconsult.com for a complete list of references.

97

Snake Coeliotomy

Richard S. Funk and Rodney W. Schnellbacher

Coeliotomy in snakes is relatively easy for an experienced surgeon to perform. The body cavity is linear, and so the surgical approach involves a linear incision generally over the organ or structure being addressed. But unlike lizards, one short incision will not expose the contents of the entire coelomic cavity. The basic principles of anesthesia and surgical preparation of the patient apply. If possible, try to avoid incising snake skin when the patient is nearing a shed cycle, because the skin is softer and more difficult to handle surgically. Fasting is also recommended to minimize the diameter of the gastrointestinal tract.

When the surgical area is localized, place the anesthetized snake in lateral recumbency and mark the exact surgical site (Fig. 97.1). It is advisable to prep a larger area of the body than originally intended in case it proves necessary to either lengthen the incision or make an additional incision. (Fig. 97.2). The patient may be draped with paper or cloth drapes and affixed with towel clamps, but the authors prefer sterile transparent plastic drapes that adhere to the patient for all but the largest snakes.

An incision should be made, not through the ventral scales, but laterally between the first two or the second and third rows of dorsal scales. If possible, these scale rows are gently spread and the skin incised linearly between the scale rows, trying not to incise any scales (Fig. 97.3A). Make the incision long enough to provide good exposure. Longer incisions take more time to close and may result in a larger scar but may be unavoidable to ensure adequate exposure. After incising the skin, the subcutaneous tissue is incised, exposing the ventral portions of the rib cage (see Figs. 97.3B and 97.4). Hemorrhage is generally minimal and can typically be controlled with gentle pressure, ligation, or with radiosurgery. Continue the incision deeper, just ventral to the rib cage border, incising fascial planes and muscle, and enter the body cavity. Sharp or blunt dissection, radiosurgery, or CO_2 laser may be

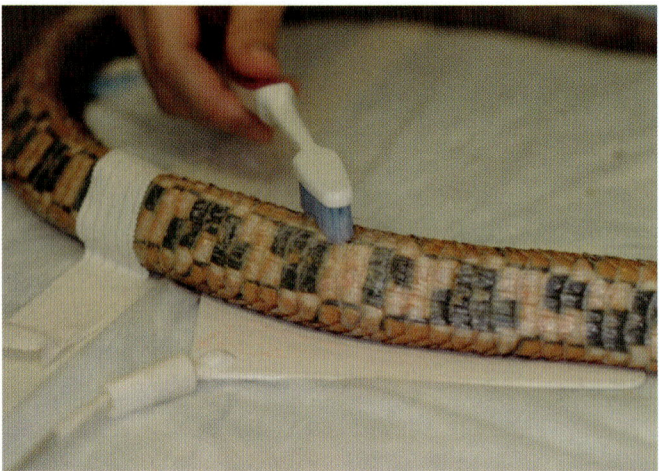

FIG 97.2 A toothbrush can be used to sterilely scrub and prepare the coeliotomy surgery site (in this case the head is oriented to the right). (Courtesy of Stephen J. Divers.)

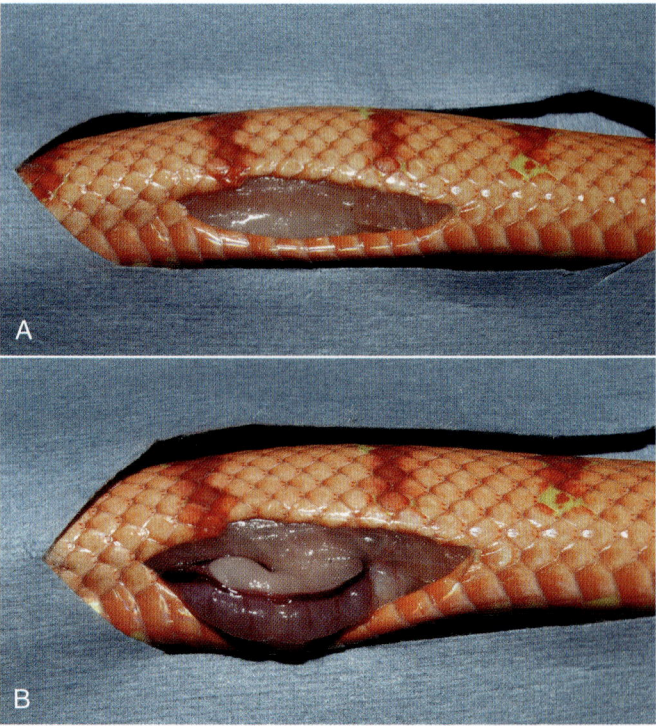

FIG 97.3 (A) A linear incision is made between the first and second dorsal rows of scales, (B) exposing the lower margin of the rib cage. (Courtesy of Richard S. Funk.)

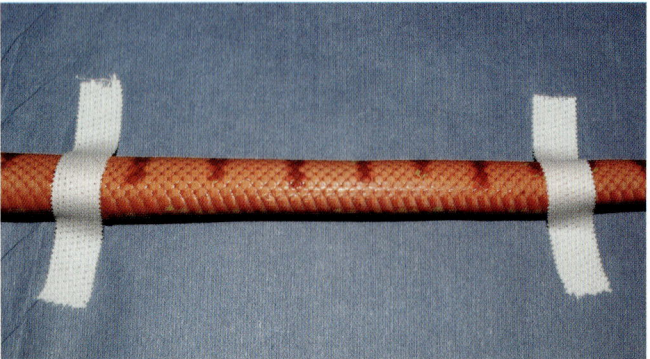

FIG 97.1 The anesthetized snake is placed in lateral recumbency (in this case the head is oriented to the left), and the body is taped to the underlying surgical drape to prevent rotation. (Courtesy of Richard S. Funk.)

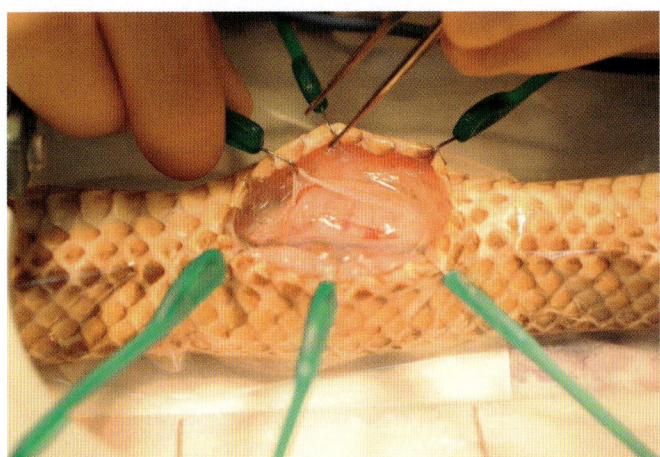

FIG 97.4 Sharp or blunt dissection of the subcutaneous tissues and muscular layers are performed. A (Lone Star) retractor is placed to provide suitable exposure of the coelomic cavity. The coelomic membrane near the ventrolateral body wall is picked up with atraumatic forceps and incised with a scalpel blade. (Courtesy of Stephen J. Divers.)

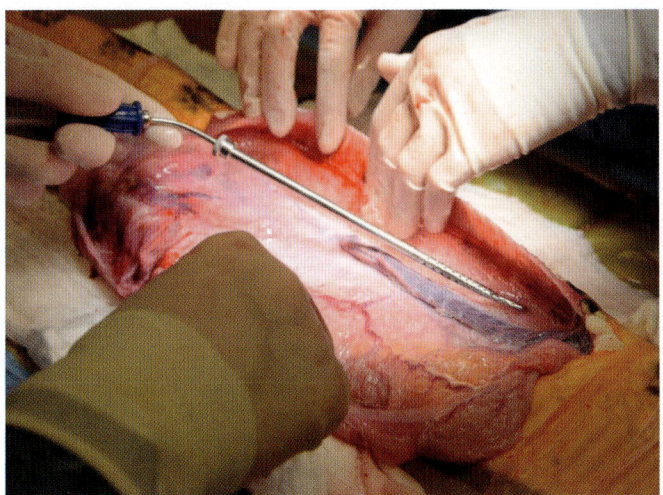

FIG 97.5 The midline ventral abdominal vein seen near the pediatric Poole suction tip in this figure should be avoided. (Courtesy of Stephen J. Divers.)

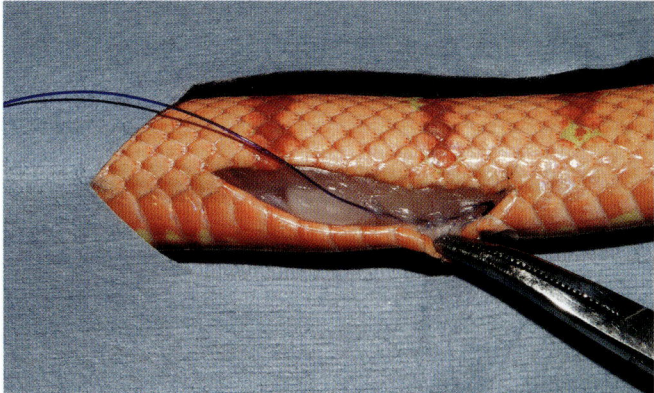

FIG 97.6 The body wall is closed utilizing an absorbable monofilament suture in a simple continuous pattern. (Courtesy of Richard S. Funk.)

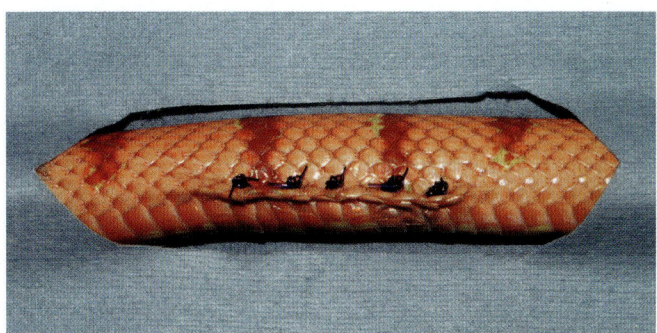

FIG 97.7 The skin incision is closed with a nonabsorbable monofilament suture in a horizontal mattress pattern, with the knots facing dorsally. (Courtesy of Richard S. Funk.)

used in the subcutaneous tissues and muscular layer. To enter the body cavity, gently pick up and tent the coelomic membrane near the ventrolateral body wall with atraumatic forceps and incise it with the scalpel blade's cutting edge facing the surgeon, then advance the incision carefully. This technique will help to avoid cutting any internal structures.

Alternatively, scissors, radiosurgery, or a CO_2 laser can be used based on the surgeon's preference. Authors frequently utilize radiosurgery. The coelomic membranes are thin and tend to be relatively transparent. After transecting these membranes, stay sutures can be utilized to help the surgeon find these delicate tissues at closure. There generally is a midline ventral abdominal vein that should be avoided (Fig. 97.5). The fat bodies (one row on each side within the body cavity) will need to be moved aside to explore the body cavity further; this can be more time-consuming and difficult in very large or obese snakes. At this point the surgeon will locate the structure of interest and follow applicable internal soft tissue surgery principles detailed elsewhere in this volume.

With gastrointestinal foreign body surgery and an enterotomy, it is usually possible to exteriorize that portion of the intestinal tract, which will help to minimize the chances of contamination. With dystocias, an incision at the center of the group of eggs or fetuses often allows you to move the anterior eggs or fetuses caudally into that incision and move the more posterior ones anteriorly, one at a time, for removal. But if these cannot safely be moved, it will be necessary to either extend the incision or create a second or third one. Appropriately sized retractors (e.g., Lone Star retractor) may be useful in providing suitable exposure to the coelomic cavity in larger snakes (see Fig. 97.4). If surgical contamination is suspected, coelomic cavity should be flushed appropriately with sterile fluids before closure (see Fig. 97.5).

During closure, it may be difficult to suture the coelomic membrane, which often doesn't hold sutures well. If the membrane can be closed, it is recommended to do so, using a simple continuous suture of absorbable monofilament material. The body wall is closed with a simple continuous monofilament absorbable suture (Fig. 97.6). The skin is closed using an everting pattern with horizontal mattress sutures of a nonabsorbable monofilament suture. An everting pattern is recommended due to the keratinized skin's tendency to invert, resulting in reduced contact of cut surfaces resulting in poor healing. It is best to orient the knots dorsally to help minimize the adhesion of substrate debris to the knots (Fig. 97.7). In general, and specifically in aquatic species, no or limited access to complete submersion of the incision in water is recommended for 14 days postsurgery. The use of tissue glue around the incision site may also reduce contamination during the healing process in aquatic species. In most cases sutures are removed in about 6 weeks.

Surgery may accelerate a shed cycle, and a snake may shed the sutures intact while shedding its skin. Postoperative management may include appropriate antibiotics if infection is present, or other medications depending on the case. Postoperative pain management should be routinely considered with injectable NSAID medications and/or opioids (see Chapter 50). Changes in husbandry, such as use of a paper substrate to increase cleanliness, postoperative fasting, or a reduction in prey size to reduce the incidence of dehiscence, and increases in temperature within the animal's preferred optimal temperature zone to accelerate healing are recommended.

98

Lizard Coeliotomy

Scott J. Stahl

Surgical coeliotomy in lizards provides important access to most major organs of the coelom and can be an effective diagnostic tool, allowing organ evaluation and potential biopsy. Once the coelom is entered, soft-tissue surgeries, including reproductive procedures, gastrotomy, enterotomy, cystotomy, and other procedures, are performed similar to mammals. However, there are important and unique anatomical considerations that surgeons must appreciate to operate safely. Fasting is recommended to minimize the size of the gastrointestinal tract (especially in species such as monitors that eat large prey items) at surgery. Generally, there are two basic approaches to the coelom in lizards. The most common is the ventral coeliotomy (midline and paramedian) and is the preferred approach for most species. The second approach is a lateral (flank) coeliotomy and is used primarily for laterally compressed lizards such as old-world chameleons.

POSITIONING AND PREPARATION

For ventral coeliotomy the lizard is positioned in standard dorsal recumbency and, for the lateral approach, contralateral recumbency. For ventral and lateral positioning the use of tape, bean-bag supports, or rolled towels is helpful (Fig. 98.1). Standard aseptic preparation is performed before draping, and adhesive clear plastic drapes are generally preferred for better contour and visibility of the patient (Fig. 98.2). One important consideration when using clear plastic drapes involves the adhesive portion, which, when removed after the procedure, can damage the fragile skin of some gecko species such as leopard geckos (*Eublepharis macularius*), African fat-tailed geckos (*Hemitheconyx caudicinctus*), and crested geckos (*Correlophus ciliatus*). Using the nonadhesive portions of the drape or applying a small amount of mineral oil to gently release the adhesive from the skin postoperatively is useful.

VENTRAL COELIOTOMY

There are two different techniques to a ventral coeliotomy, a paramedian and a midline approach. The paramedian approach has been used for many years and involves making a surgical incision in the skin, parallel and lateral to the midline (Fig. 98.3).[1] Following skin incision the thin coelomic musculature is bluntly dissected to avoid hemorrhage (Fig. 98.4). This traditional technique is utilized to completely avoid the ventral abdominal vein (VAV) on approach and allows the surgeon to safely identify the vessel early in the coelomic approach. This procedure is preferred by the author and has been used to safely enter the coelom, avoiding the VAV, in hundreds of lizards of many different species.[2,3] This is the recommended approach for the novice surgeon.

Mader et al. have described a midline coeliotomy technique that also allows safe entry into the coelom by avoiding the VAV.[4] Following an initial ventral midline skin incision, the linea alba is sharply dissected,

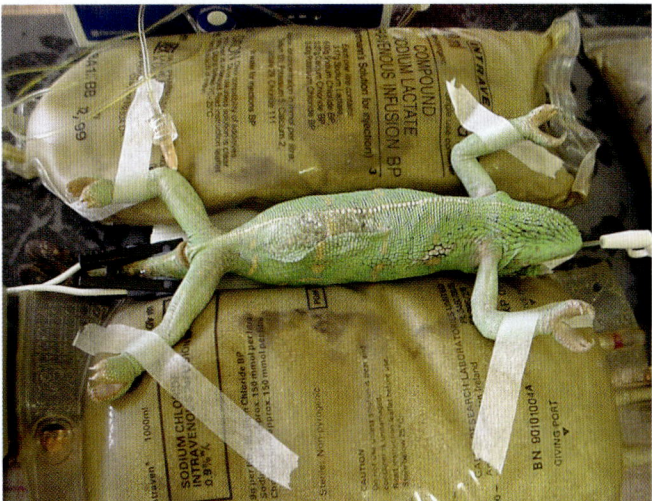

FIG 98.1 A veiled chameleon (*Chameleo calyptratus*) positioned in dorsal recumbency for a paramedian coeliotomy. Sand bags are used to help position and support the lizard. The chameleon is intubated, has an intraosseous catheter placed in the right femur, and a pulse oximetry monitor attached to the tail. (Courtesy of Stephen J. Divers.)

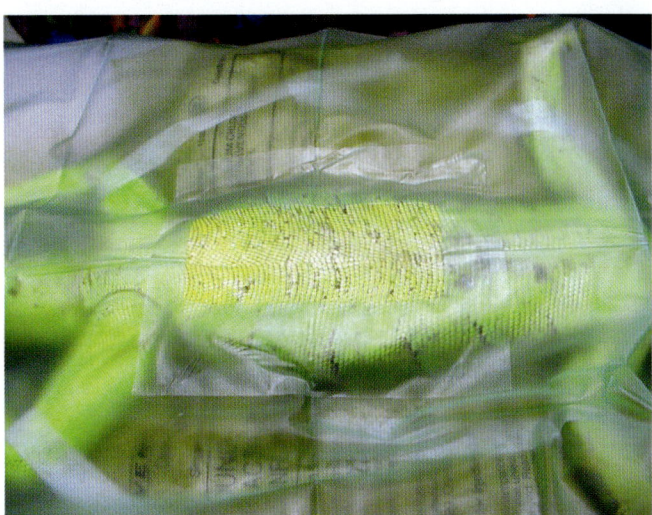

FIG 98.2 A green iguana (*Iguana iguana*) placed in dorsal recumbency and aseptically prepared for a ventral coeliotomy. A clear plastic adhesive drape has been placed and is appropriately cut for ventral coeliotomy. (Courtesy of Stephen J. Divers.)

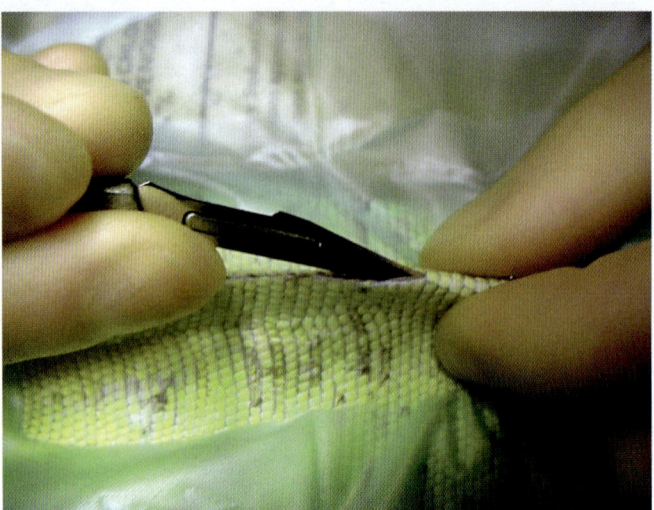

FIG 98.3 An initial paramedian skin stab incision is made in a green iguana (*Iguana iguana*). Often for the initial skin incision the scalpel blade is positioned with the blade upright to allow precise control. (Courtesy of Stephen J. Divers.)

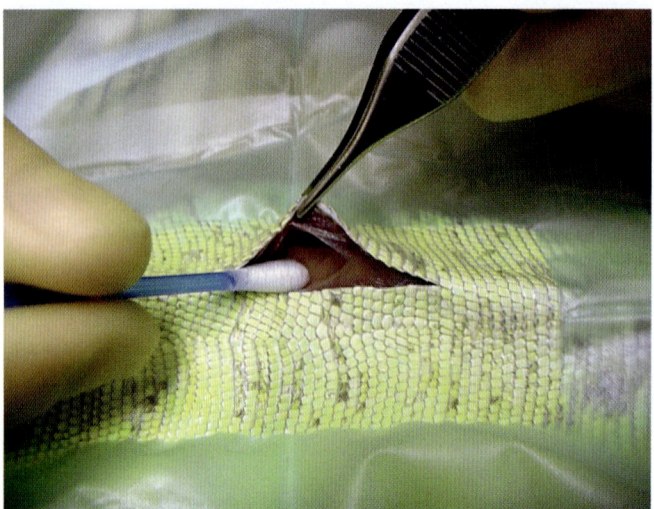

FIG 98.4 After the initial paramedian skin incision in this green iguana (*Iguana iguana*) the thin coelomic musculature is bluntly dissected to avoid hemorrhage and expose the coelom wall. (Courtesy of Stephen J. Divers.)

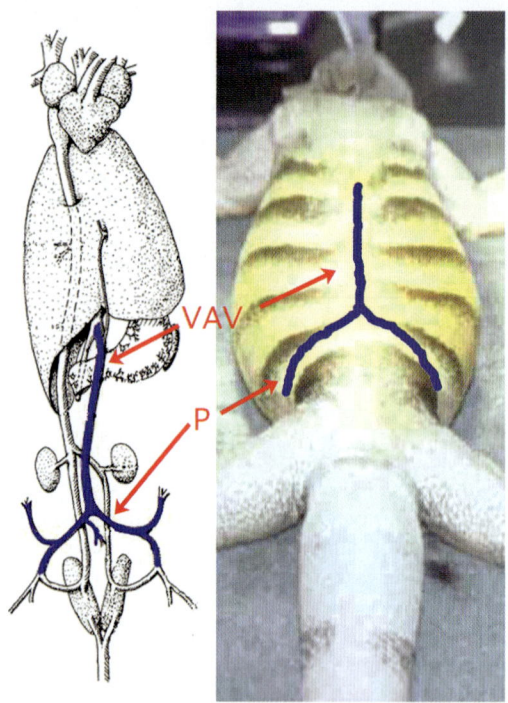

FIG 98.5 The ventral abdominal vein (VAV) is a confluence of the bilateral pelvic veins (P) that are joined bilaterally by the hypogastric veins and the single ventral pubic vein and can be found along the ventral midline, deep to the abdominal muscles. (Courtesy of Douglas R. Mader.)

being careful to avoid the vein. The main advantage of this technique is the presumed reduction in pain associated with an incision through the linea alba (as in most mammals), instead of through the thin coelomic muscles. Regardless of which coeliotomy procedure utilized, a good understanding of the anatomy of the VAV will reduce the likelihood of damage and serious hemorrhage, which if it occurs requires prompt ligation.

The VAV is a confluence of the bilateral pelvic veins, which are joined bilaterally by the hypogastric veins and the single ventral pubic vein. It is located along the ventral midline of the patient, just axial to the abdominal muscles (Fig. 98.5).[4,5] The distance from the pubis to the caudal origin of the abdominal vein varies by species and patient size but is approximately one-fourth the distance between the cranial pubic bone and the umbilicus.[4]

The abdominal vein then courses along the inside of the coelomic wall until it reaches the level of the umbilicus, where it turns dorsad and joins the hepatic vein. Thus the region between the cranial margin of the pubis and extending one-fourth of the distance toward the umbilicus, and the region cranial to the umbilicus progressing to the xiphoid, will have no significant ventral vessels present.[4]

With this anatomical knowledge, the initial surgical incision can occur in either of these anatomical locations without contact with the VAV (Fig. 98.6A and B).[4] As the surgeon proceeds with the incision, the VAV can be gently moved to avoid damage.

Another surgical consideration for the VAV is its variable location within the mesovasorum, which is actually an extension of the ventral coelomic membrane. The mesovasorum varies in size from a couple of millimeters to nearly 1 cm in larger specimens.[4] Although the origin of the mesovasorum is from the ventral midline, the actual location of the vein at surgery depends on the animal's state of repletion and other space-occupying coelomic structures (e.g., bladder calculi, eggs).[4] Thus the vessel may lie on the centerline, or it may be several millimeters off center in either direction (Fig. 98.7). Therefore the surgeon must use caution even when making a paramedian incision as the vessel may be off center.

However, if the VAV is accidently cut and quickly ligated, it is unlikely to be life threatening, as blood will be redirected back through the pelvic veins, into the bilateral renal veins, and directly into the vena cava.[4]

Once exposure is adequate, the linea alba or coelomic aponeurosis (formed by the external abdominal oblique muscle) is gently lifted with forceps to elevate it away from any underlying coelomic structures and carefully incised with a scalpel blade or radiosurgery (Fig. 98.8). After the initial incision, whether using a paramedian or midline approach, the VAV is identified and avoided as the incision is extended to provide adequate exposure for the intended coelomic procedure (Fig. 98.9A–D).

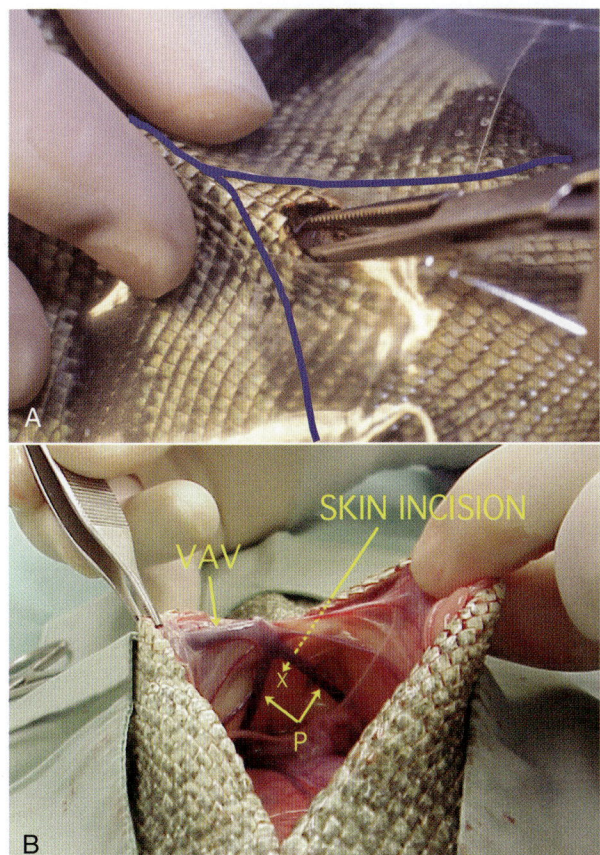

FIG 98.6 (A) The initial surgical stab incision is made between the pubis and the umbilical scar (x) to avoid the ventral abdominal vein (VAV) in lizards. (B) By starting the incision in this location, the blade will not contact the VAV. P, Pelvic veins. (Courtesy of Douglas R. Mader.)

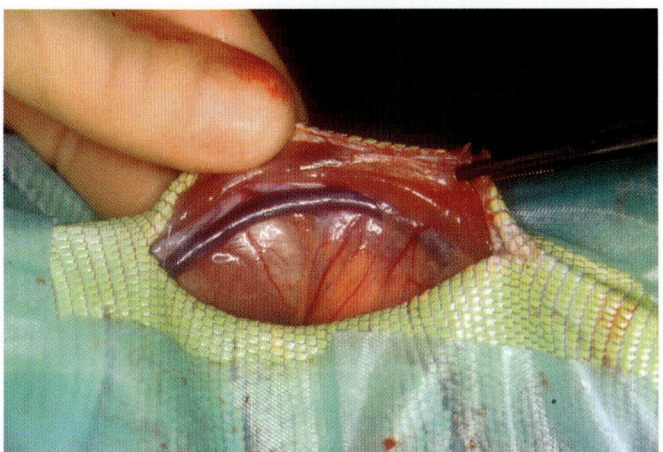

FIG 98.7 The ventral abdominal vein (VAV) of a green iguana undergoing a coeliotomy. The VAV is identified early in the coeliotomy approach to avoid any damage to the vessel. (Courtesy of Stephen J. Divers.)

Caudally the presence of the paired ventral coelomic fat bodies may inhibit the ability to extend the coelomic wall incision to the pubis (Fig. 98.10). These structures are quite vascular and potentially friable, and the surgeon must be careful handling them. If the fat bodies are large they may need to be gently exteriorized (depending on the procedure and species) to allow access to deeper structures. While out of the

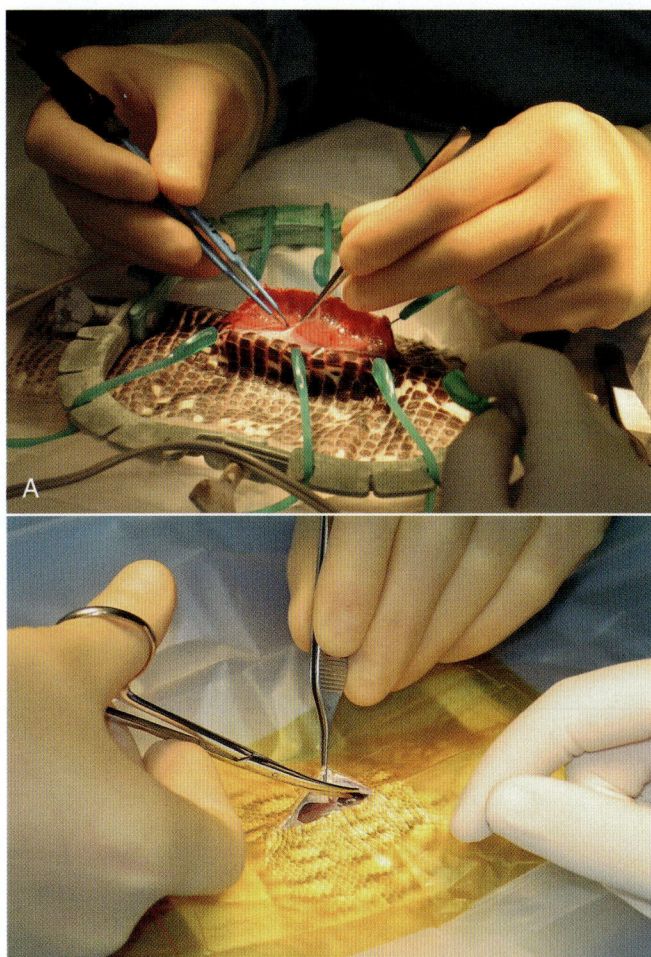

FIG 98.8 (A) Ventral paramedian coeliotomy approach in a Guatemalan beaded lizard (*Heloderma horridum charlesbogerti*). The initial skin incision has been made, a Lone Star retractor is utilized to allow better exposure, and the initial incision into the coelom is made with radiosurgery. (B) Iris scissors are used to carefully extend the initial coelom entry in this bearded dragon (*Pogona vitticeps*). (Courtesy of Stephen J. Divers.)

coelom, they must be protected with moistened lap sponges or gauze. A small amount of "clear" free fluid is not uncommon in healthy lizards. Larger amounts of discolored or flocculent fluid is abnormal and likely an indication of ascites or coelomitis. The use of retractors such as the Lone Star retractor (Fig. 98.11) for larger, deep-bodied lizards or ophthalmic retractors and magnification for smaller lizards can be helpful to allow better coelomic visibility. At this point the surgeon will locate the structure of interest and follow applicable internal soft-tissue surgery principles detailed elsewhere in Section 10.

LATERAL (FLANK) COELIOTOMY

This approach is primarily used for old-world chameleons because of their laterally compressed bodies. The ventral coeliotomy procedure (midline or paramedian) can be used in these species, but the ribs extend caudally and ventrally to the midline, and several ribs may have to be transected to allow access to the coelom (see Fig. 98.9A–D). The paramedian coeliotomy approach is still the author's preferred technique

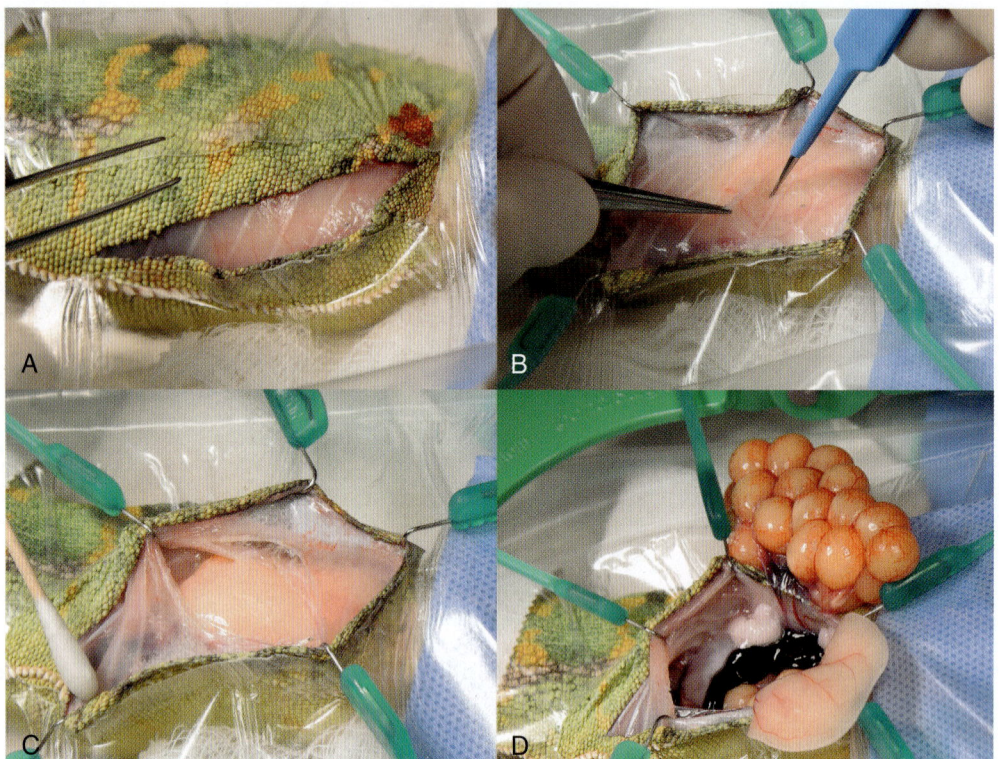

FIG 98.9 Left paramedian approach to the coelom in a veiled chameleon (*Chameleo calyptratus*) with preovulatory follicular stasis. (A) A curvilinear, cranioventral to caudodorsal skin incision has been made using a scalpel. (B) A LoneStar retractor has been applied to retract the skin and expose the lateral flank. Bipolar radiosurgical forceps are used to incise through the intercostal muscles between two ribs. (C) The most cranial and caudal retractor hooks are repositioned first to retract the ribs before adjusting the other hooks. The large fat body can be seen within the coelom. (D) Following the adjustment of all retractor hooks to expose the coelom, the fat body has been reflected caudoventral, and the enlarged left ovary has been exteriorized. (Courtesy of Stephen J. Divers.)

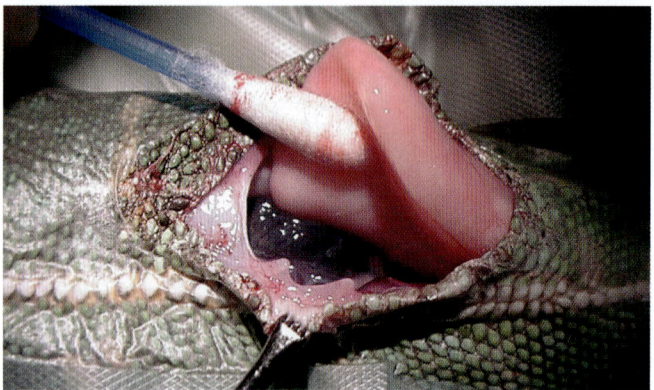

FIG 98.10 A fat body present caudally (to the right in the figure) in a paramedian coeliotomy incision in a veiled chameleon (*Chameleo calyptratus*). The presence of the paired ventral coelomic fat bodies caudally may inhibit the ability to extend the coelomic wall incision to the pubis. (Courtesy of Stephen J. Divers.)

FIG 98.11 Retractors such as this Lone Star retractor system utilized in this bearded dragon (*Pogona vitticeps*) for an exploratory coeliotomy can help the surgeon with coelomic visibility and access. (Courtesy of Greg Costanzo, Stahl Exotic Animal Veterinary Services.)

in chameleons, because it allows greater access to explore the entire coelom. Additionally, compared with the lateral approach, the incision and subsequent scar are not readily visible once healed. Transected ribs heal readily, and complications after paramedian coeliotomy in chameleons are rare. The lateral approach, however, is an effective approach for reproductive procedures such as ovariosalpingectomy, ovariectomy, salpingotomy, and castration.[6] Both sides of the reproductive tract can usually be accessed from a unilateral approach. The incision is made

below the lumbar spine in the paralumbar space, often at an angle (caudal to or between the last ribs) to allow the largest possible incision without involving ribs (Fig. 98.12A and B). Unlike the ventral coeliotomy approach there are no major vessels on entry into the coelom. The initial skin incision is made with a scalpel and carefully extended with iris scissors or a scalpel blade, and the coelomic aponeurosis is incised with iris scissors or radiosurgery to avoid damage to coelomic organs (see Fig. 98.12C). Besides the advantages of avoiding ribs and the VAV, this

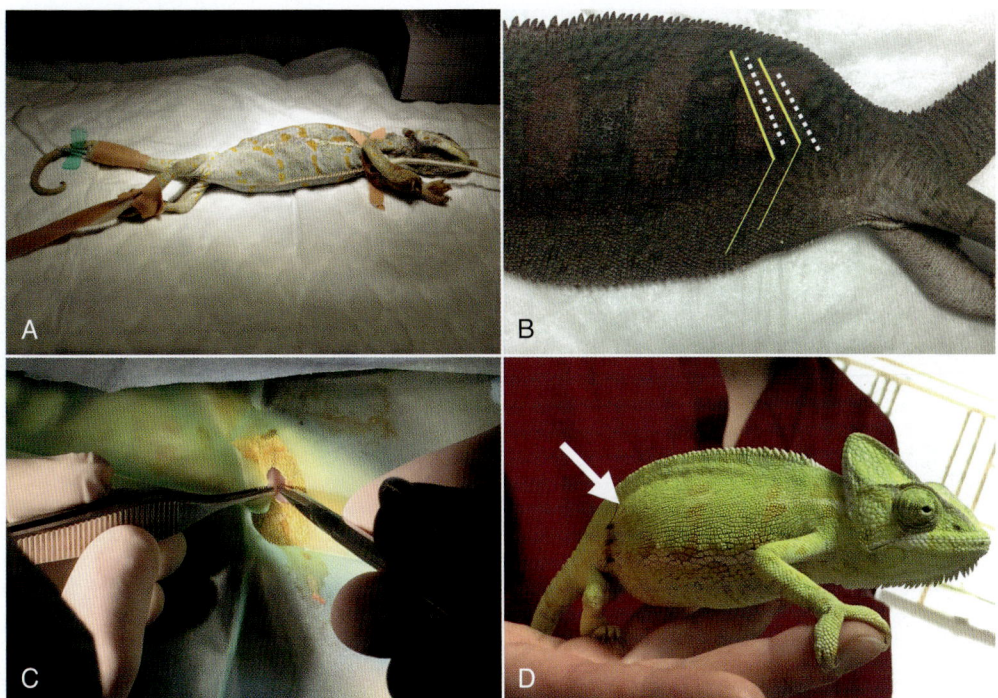

FIG 98.12 Lateral (flank) approach for coeliotomy in old-world chameleons. (A) Proper positioning of the patient for flank approach. Note limb positioning, Doppler placement over heart, and IV catheter placed in coccygeal vein. (B) Potential sites for surgical incision are represented with dotted lines and are caudal to the last rib or between the last and the preceding rib (*yellow lines*). (C) For access to the coelom an initial skin incision is made with a scalpel or radiosurgery followed by iris scissors to incise muscles and coelomic wall. Scissors are preferred to a scalpel to avoid damage to underlying coelomic organs. (D) Appearance of flank approach closure site (*arrow*) in a veiled chameleon (*Chameleo calyptratus*). (Courtesy of Nicola Di Girolamo.)

technique also reduces interference by the paired coelomic fat bodies. One other consideration during old-world chameleon coeliotomy (whether ventral or flank approach) is the presence of air-sac–like extensions of the lungs, which appear as clear finger-like projections often present in the surgical field (Fig. 98.13). These delicate structures must be kept moistened and protected during the coeliotomy procedure.

Before closing the coelom, warm (27°C–29°C, 80°F–85°F) sterile saline irrigation and gentle suction should be performed, especially in cases of coelomitis or following clean-contaminated procedures (e.g., enterotomy, cystotomy). Coeliotomy closure in lizards involves gentle apposition of the coelomic aponeurosis. The muscle and linea tissues are quite fragile and can easily tear with rough manipulation or tension. The goal is to gently bring the wound edges together to create a coelomic "seal," because this closure is not considered a holding layer as in mammals. Absorbable monofilament suture in 3.0 to 5.0 size depending on the patient size, in a simple continuous pattern with minimal tension, is recommended (Fig. 98.14). One exception to this simple continuous closure exists with some gecko species (such as leopard geckos, African fat-tailed geckos, and crested geckos). In these species, the skin is delicate and fragile and does not have the same "holding" strength that more typical keratinized lizard skin does. In these species a simple interrupted suture pattern is recommended to close the coelomic wall, followed by a typical horizontal mattress suture pattern in the skin to increase the strength and integrity of closure (Fig. 98.15).[2,3]

The skin in lizards is closed routinely using nylon (or absorbable monofilament suture if suture removal is unlikely to be possible) with a horizontal mattress suture pattern (Fig. 98.16). An everting pattern

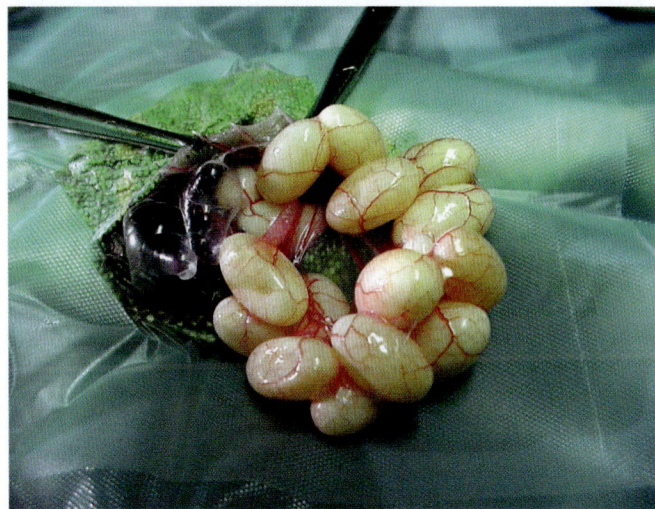

FIG 98.13 A paramedian coeliotomy approach in a veiled chameleon (*Chameleo calyptratus*) with dystocia. One oviduct is filled with retained eggs and is evident on the right. On the left several of the finger-like air sac extensions of the lungs are present in the surgical field. These delicate structures must be kept moistened and protected during coeliotomy procedures in old-world chameleons. (Courtesy of Stephen J. Divers.)

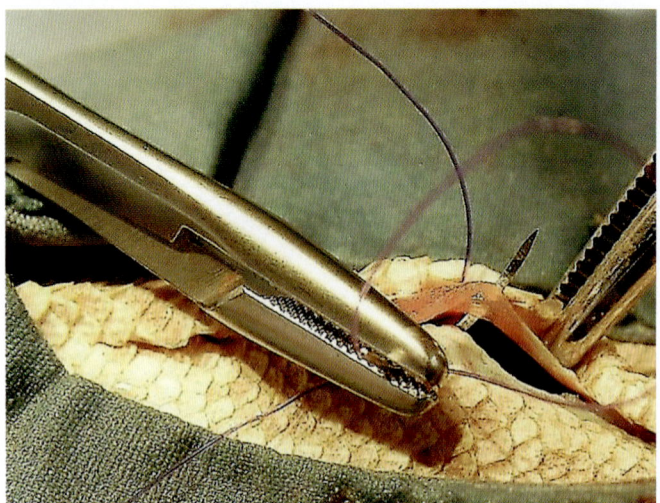

FIG 98.14 The first layer of the coeliotomy closure in lizards involves apposition of the coelomic aponeurosis. The goal is to gently bring the wound edges together to create a coelomic "seal" as this closure is not considered a holding layer (except geckos). A simple continuous pattern with minimal tension is recommended, as utilized here closing the coelomic wall in this bearded dragon (*Pogona vitticeps*). (Courtesy of Scott J. Stahl, Stahl Exotic Animal Veterinary Services.)

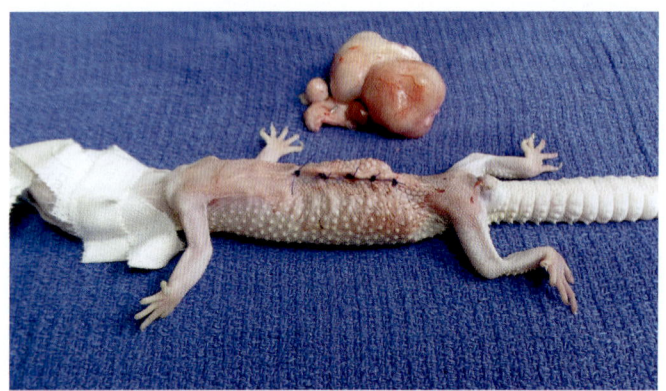

FIG 98.15 A leopard gecko (*Eublepharis macularius*) recovering from a coeliotomy to remove an ovarian neoplasm (present at the top of the figure). The skin is closed with nylon in a horizontal mattress (everting) pattern. In this species (and other geckos) the skin is fragile and does not have the "holding" strength typical for keratinized lizard skin. Therefore, in these species, a simple interrupted suture pattern, instead of continuous (as in Fig. 98.14), is used to close the coelom followed by a horizontal mattress skin closure to increase the strength of the coeliotomy closure. (Courtesy of Scott J. Stahl, Stahl Exotic Animal Veterinary Services.)

is necessary because of the keratinized skin's tendency to invert, resulting in reduced contact of cut surfaces and poor healing (Figs. 98.12D, 98.15, and 98.17). Surgery may accelerate ecdysis, and sutures placed too close to the wound edges may be prematurely shed.

Tissue adhesive can also be placed along the incision line to help with waterproofing and protection. However, when possible, complete submersion of the incision in water is not recommended for 10 to 14 days postsurgery. Lizards that are routinely soaked can be misted or sprayed to encourage drinking and hydration during this period. Postoperative management may include appropriate antibiotics if

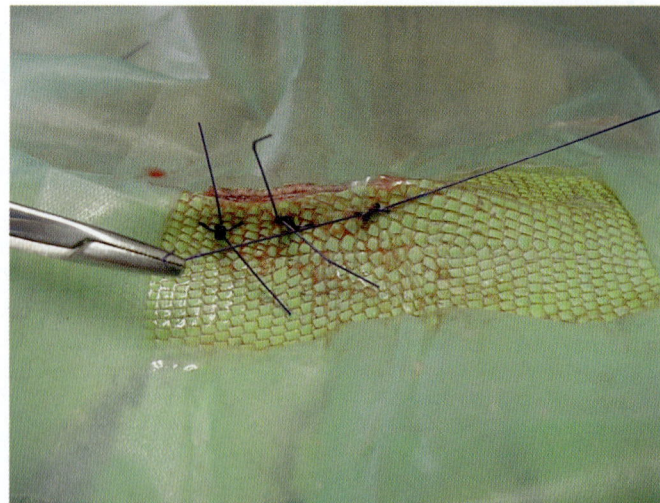

FIG 98.16 The skin in lizards is routinely closed using a horizontal mattress suture pattern as in this ventral coeliotomy skin closure in a green iguana (*Iguana iguana*). (Courtesy of Stephen J. Divers.)

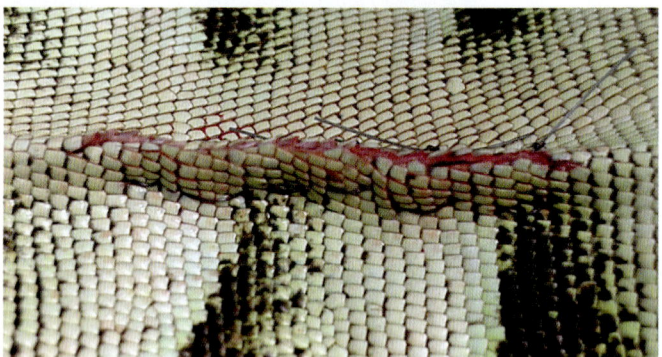

FIG 98.17 An everting suture pattern, such as the horizontal mattress pattern used in this green iguana (*Iguana iguana*) for a ventral coeliotomy skin closure, is necessary in lizards because of the keratinized skin's tendency to invert, resulting in reduced contact of cut surfaces and poor skin healing. (Courtesy of Stephen J. Divers.)

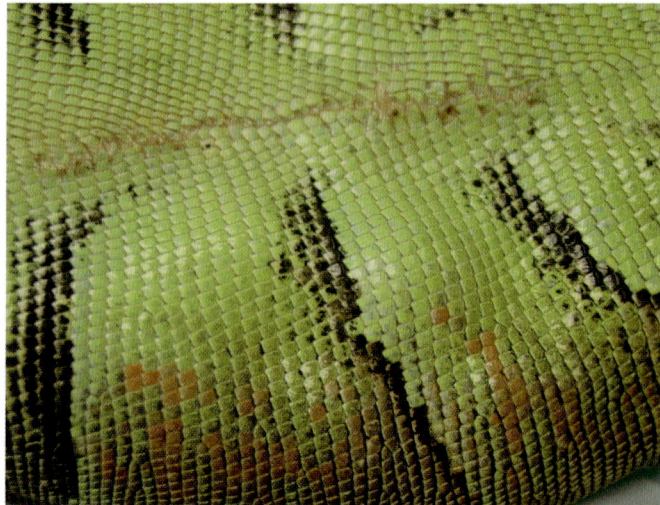

FIG 98.18 A coeliotomy scar on a green iguana (*Iguana iguana*) approximately 1 year after a paramedian coeliotomy. (Courtesy of Stephen J. Divers.)

infection is present and pain management with injectable nonsteroidal autoinflammatory drugs and/or opioids (see Chapter 50). Changes in husbandry, such as using a paper substrate for cleanliness, a short period of postoperative fasting or a reduction in food size or quantity, and increasing temperature to the higher end of the preferred optimal temperature zone (POTZ) to accelerate healing are recommended. In most cases sutures are removed (if still present) 6 to 8 weeks postoperatively (Fig. 98.18).

REFERENCES

See www.expertconsult.com for a complete list of references.

99

Chelonian Prefemoral Coeliotomy

Elisa Wüst and Stephen J. Divers

Surgical coeliotomy provides access to most of the major internal organs of chelonians and thus is useful for a range of surgical procedures, including exploration and biopsy. However, because of the variable anatomy and boney makeup of the chelonian shell, surgical access to the coelom is often challenging. Depending on the species and the surgical site or organ of interest, there are two major approaches to the coelom of chelonians: transplastron and prefemoral. The traditional transplastron coeliotomy approach requires a temporary osteotomy through the plastron, whereas the prefemoral approach is a soft-tissue technique that involves entry into the coelom in front of a pelvic limb (Table 99.1).

Approaching the coelom through the prefemoral fossa is less invasive and can provide unilateral surgical access to the caudal lung, liver, small and large intestine, reproductive tract, kidney, and bladder.[1] This approach is most commonly used for surgery involving the reproductive tract.[1–9] In some species (especially aquatic chelonians such as red-eared sliders, *Trachemys scripta elegans*), it is possible to perform bilateral reproductive surgery with a unilateral approach.[3] In others (including terrestrial tortoises like the Hermann's tortoise, *Testudo hermanni*, and desert tortoise, *Gopherus agassizii*), the suspensory ligaments may be short, the bladder large and obstructive, and/or the prefemoral window small. These factors can complicate access and necessitate a bilateral approach.[2,9] The prefemoral access to the coelom can also be used for organ biopsies, coelomic and gastrointestinal foreign body removal, and urinary bladder stone removal.[10,11] However, when dealing with large cystic calculi or masses, transplastron access to the coelom may be preferable.[12,13]

PATIENT POSITIONING AND PREPARATION

The patient is usually positioned in lateral recumbency, although dorsal recumbency can be more practical for some procedures. Unless anatomic asymmetry or diagnostic imaging dictate otherwise, a left prefemoral approach is often preferred by right-handed surgeons (with a right approach easier for those who are left-handed). Positioning can be achieved using troughs, tape, bean-bag supports, or rolled towels (Fig. 99.1). Tilting the animal into a 30- to 40-degree

TABLE 99.1 Comparison Between Transplastron and Prefemoral Coeliotomy in Chelonians

Transplastron Procedure	Prefemoral Procedure
Technically more demanding, requiring shell-cutting equipment	Technically easier to perform with standard surgical instrumentation
Longer operational times	Shorter operational times
Provides extensive surgical access to all major organs	Provides more limited, and generally unilateral, surgical access; better in species with large prefemoral fossae
Probably more painful postoperatively (involves bone incisions)	Probably less painful postoperatively (only involves soft tissues)
Longer healing times of 12+ weeks	Shorter healing times of 6–8 weeks

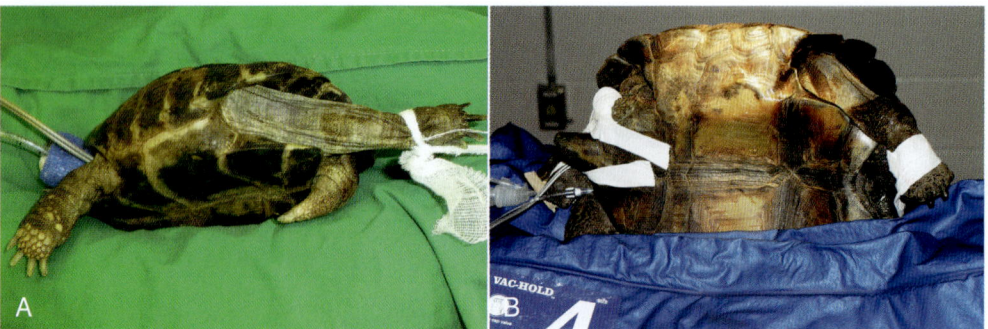

FIG 99.1 (A) Right lateral positioning of a *Testudo* tortoise for left prefemoral coeliotomy using tightly rolled and taped towels. (B) Right lateral positioning of a *Gopherus* tortoise using a vacuum support bag. (A, Courtesy of the Clinic for Birds, Reptiles, Amphibians and Fish, JLU-Giessen; B, courtesy of Stephen J. Divers.)

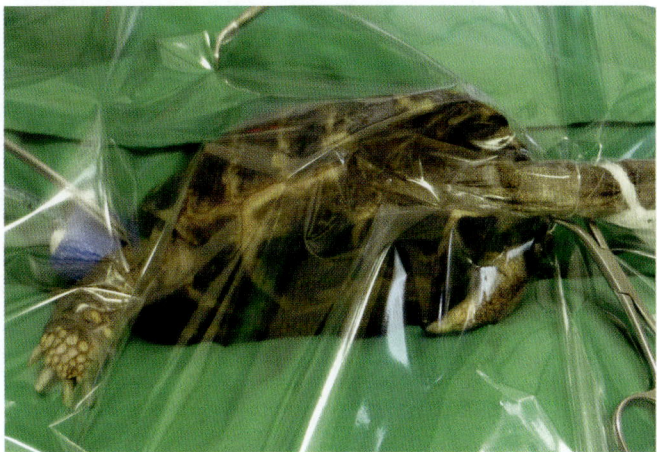

FIG 99.2 Surgical positioning and draping of a male Hermann's tortoise (*Testudo hermanni*) for left prefemoral coeliotomy. The left pelvic limb is extended caudad to maximize exposure. (Courtesy of the Clinic for Birds, Reptiles, Amphibians and Fish, JLU-Giessen.)

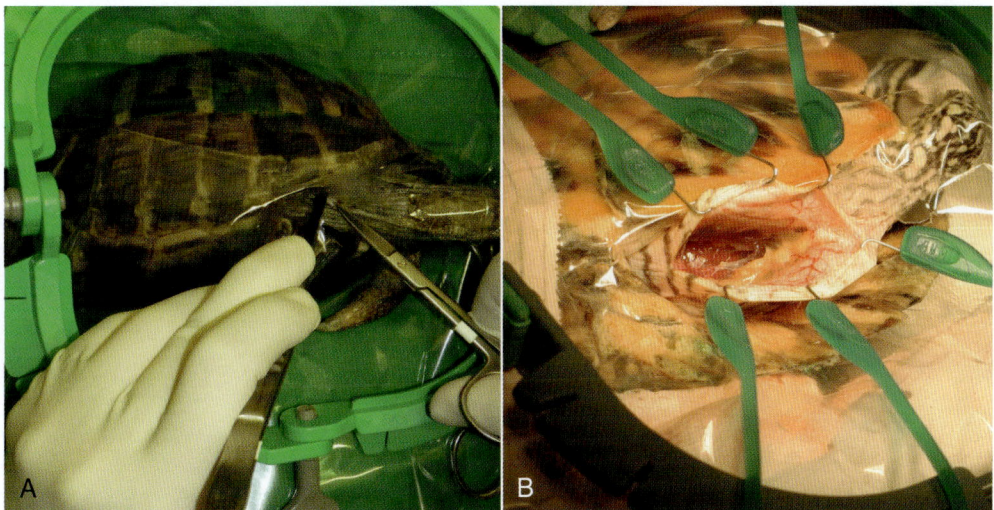

FIG 99.3 (A) Craniocaudal skin incision in the left prefemoral fossa of a male Hermann's tortoise *(Testudo hermanni)*. In this species the incision should be located in the mid to lower ventral third of the fossa. (B) Following skin incision, the coelomic musculature and aponeurosis can be seen in this red-eared slider (*Trachemys scripta elegans*) undergoing a right prefemoral coeliotomy in dorsal recumbency. (A, Courtesy of the Clinic for Birds, Reptiles, Amphibians and Fish, JLU-Giessen; B, courtesy of Stephen J. Divers.)

head-down position can also be helpful.[3] To gain access to the prefemoral fossa, the ipsilateral pelvic limb is maximally extended and secured caudad often by taping to the other pelvic limb, caudal shell, or table. Standard aseptic preparation precedes draping, and adhesive plastic drapes are preferred and can be better contoured to the fossa (Fig. 99.2).

SURGICAL TECHNIQUE

The skin incision is made cranial to the extended limb and in a cranial-to-caudal direction, in the middle of the prefemoral fossa, starting close to the skin insertion at the plastrocarapacial (bridge) junction and ending just cranial to the musculature of the limb (Fig. 99.3A). Blunt dissection cranial to the sartorius and ventral to the iliacus muscles exposes the pale coelomic aponeurosis formed by the external abdominal oblique muscle (see Fig. 99.3B). Gentle perforation of this aponeurosis can then be extended with forceps, scissors, or radiosurgery to gain access to the coelom. Stay sutures or a ring retractor and a focused light source provide significant improvements in visualization (Fig. 99.4). Endoscope-assisted procedures are common and are detailed in Chapter 65.[3–5]

Following clean-contaminated procedures involving the bladder, intestinal tract, or other non-sterile sites, the coelom should be thoroughly lavaged prior to closure. The coelomic membrane, musculature,

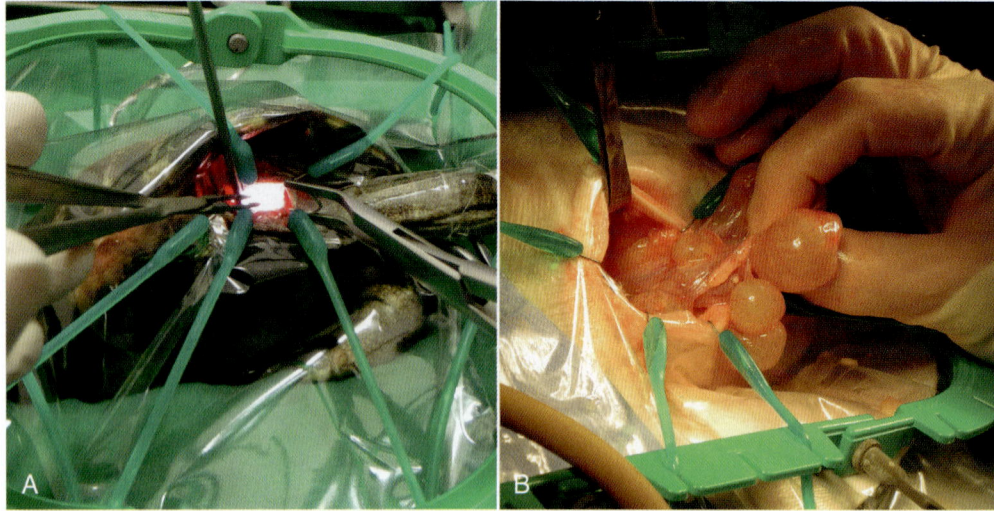

FIG 99.4 Use of a ring retractor and elastic stays to improve visualization in (A) *Testudo* tortoise and (B) *Apalone* turtle. (A, Courtesy of the Clinic for Birds, Reptiles, Amphibians and Fish, JLU-Giessen; B, courtesy of Stephen J. Divers.)

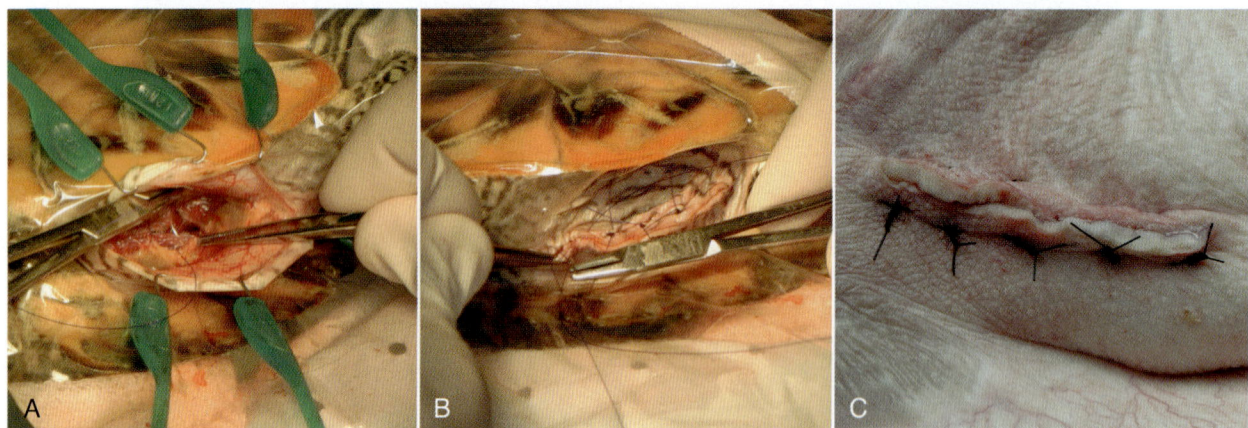

FIG 99.5 (A) Closure of the coelomic musculature and aponeurosis using poliglecaprone-25 suture in a continuous pattern (red-eared slider, *Trachemys scripta elegans*). (B) Routine closure of the skin using polydioxanone in a simple everting horizontal mattress pattern (red-eared slider). (C) Completed skin closure in a soft-shelled turtle (*Apalone*). (Courtesy of Stephen J. Divers.)

and, if necessary, the subcutaneous tissues are closed with a simple continuous pattern using absorbable sutures (e.g., poliglecaprone 25, polyglyconate, or polydioxanone) (Fig. 99.5A). The skin is closed routinely using nylon or polydioxanone and simple, horizontal mattress sutures, which should be removed (if still present) 8 weeks postoperatively (see Fig. 99.5B and C).

REFERENCES

See www.expertconsult.com for a complete list of references.

100

Chelonian Transplastron Coeliotomy

Stephen J. Divers and Elisa Wüst

For decades this approach has been the traditional coeliotomy technique used in chelonians. However, concerns regarding increased surgical trauma, pain and discomfort, and prolonged bone healing have resulted in a shift in preference to the prefemoral approach (with or without endoscope assistance) whenever possible (see Table 99.1). Nevertheless, when extensive exposure (e.g., for large cystic calculus, foreign body, or mass removal) or exploration is required, the transplastron may be preferable, especially in patients with small prefemoral fossae.[1-6]

PATIENT POSITIONING AND PREPARATION

The chelonian is supported in dorsal recumbency using beanbags, towels, and tape, taking care to support the head, neck, and anesthetic attachments. Following aseptic preparation of the ventral plastron (using a brush to remove all debris from the scute interfaces and any plastron hinges), a sterile, adhesive, transparent drape is applied (Fig. 100.1).

SURGICAL TECHNIQUE

Surgical planning must take into account the primary organ/area of interest, the size of any structure(s) to be removed, location of any plastron hinge, shell thickness, and regional subplastron anatomy. Therefore the locations of the heart (usually at the midline intersection of the pectoral and abdominal scutes), paired abdominal veins (running caudocranially within the ventral abdominal musculature), hinges (e.g., between the abdominal and femoral scutes in *Testudo*, and between the pectoral and abdominal scutes in *Terrapene*), and plastron thickness (including its expansion toward the plastrocarapacial bridge) have to be considered before surgery (Fig. 100.2). Careful consideration

must also be given to the degree of access required to perform the procedure (e.g., cystic calculus, mass, or foreign body removal), and, because access cannot be easily enlarged, ensure that the initial cuts are sufficient.

In neonates and young juveniles with poorly mineralized shells, a scalpel blade can be used to incise the plastron (Fig. 100.3A). In most cases, an oscillating sagittal saw couples accuracy with reduced collateral damage and minimal soft-tissue trauma (see Fig. 100.3B), whereas thinner incisions can often be obtained using a fine blade rotary saw (e.g., Dremel) (see Fig. 100.3C). However, rotating saws are less forgiving on soft tissues, and over-scoring at the corners occurs with larger-blade diameters. The saw is held at 45 to 60 degrees to bevel the lateral shell incisions, which are made first (Fig. 100.4A). A fine hypodermic needle or scalpel blade can be used to gauge depth and ensure that the cuts are full-shell thickness (see Fig. 100.4B). The caudal cut and, finally, the cranial cut are made in a similar fashion, but bevelling is not necessary. Penetration of the shell over the heart is generally made last. The caudal or cranial cut can be incomplete, with a few millimeters bone thickness left. While lifting the segment using a periosteal elevator or scalpel handle, the thin bone breaks that will later help to stabilize the loose bone fragment during closure. In addition, blood supply may be maintained, increasing the chances of primary healing. While elevating the cranial or caudal margin of the bony segment, the soft tissues are bluntly dissected free, staying as close to the shell as possible (Fig. 100.5). The paired abdominal veins are closely associated with the plastron. The soft-tissue attachments at the fractured bone line can also be left intact, because the plastron flap is reflected caudal and covered with moistened, sterile gauze. Alternatively, the plastron flap can be reflected cranial, leaving the cranial attachments intact.

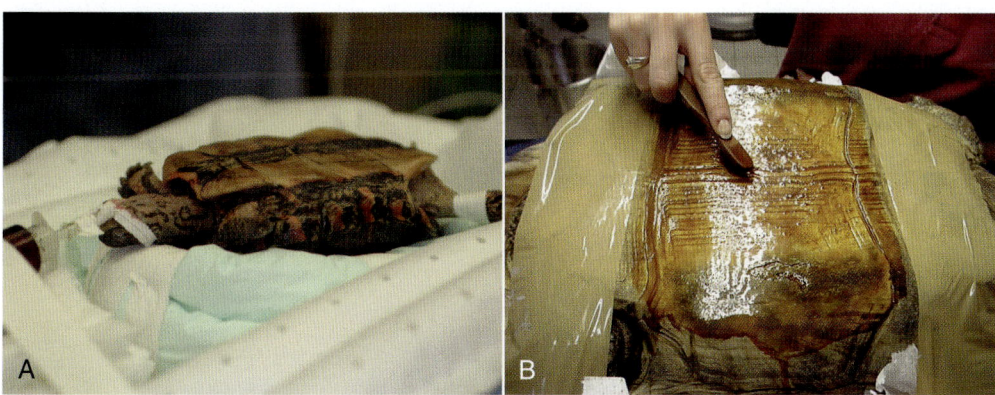

FIG 100.1 (A) Dorsal positioning of a chelonian for transplastron coeliotomy. The animal has been supported on coiled pads. Note the gauze support for the terminal anesthesia circuit. (B) This large tortoise has been positioned on towels with strong tape securing the plastron cranial and caudal. Povidone iodine and a toothbrush are being used to scrub the plastron. (Courtesy of Stephen J. Divers.)

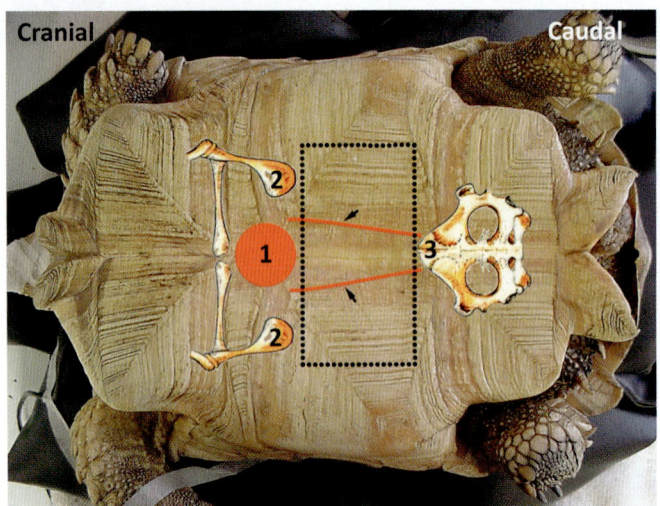

Cranial   **Caudal**

FIG 100.2 Ventral view of a chelonian demonstrating the regional anatomy, including the heart (1), paired abdominal veins (arrows), coracoids (2), and pelvic rim (3). The dotted line indicates the preferred coeliotomy incision lines. (Courtesy of Stephen J. Divers.)

Depending on circumstances, several variations are possible regarding entry into the coelom, including (1) midline incision, between the abdominal veins, through the poorly defined linea alba; (2) unilateral or bilateral paramedian incision(s) lateral to the abdominal veins; and (3) even ligation and transection of one abdominal vein to permit an L-shaped flap for removing large structures (Fig. 100.6). Ligation of both abdominal veins is not recommended, because severe circulatory disturbance would likely ensue. An elastic ring retractor often improves exposure (Fig. 100.7A).

Following clean-contaminated procedures, thorough lavage of the coelom should be performed before a routine two-layer closure (see Fig. 100.7B). The coelomic membrane is closed in a simple continuous pattern using absorbable suture material (Fig. 100.8A). Poliglecaprone 25 or polyglyconate can be used for closure of paramedian incisions, but polydioxanone is preferred for the linea alba. Three or four stabilizing sutures (usually polydioxanone, but wire can be used for large species) can be placed through drilled holes to anchor the bony section to the plastron (see Fig. 100.8B and C). The shell incision line can be filled with sterile antibiotic, absorbable bone wax, or absorbable collagen (Fig. 100.9). The closure is completed using epoxy resin or acrylic (e.g., polymethylmethacrylate), either at four

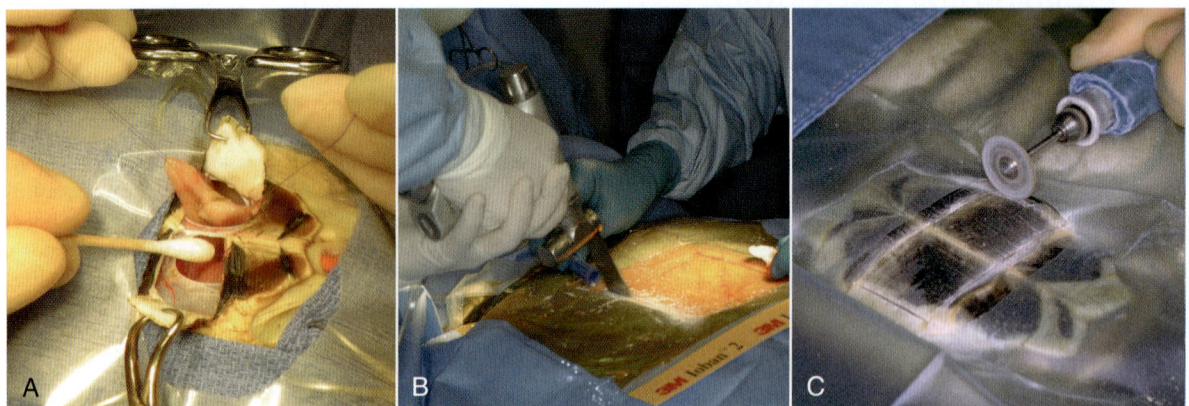

FIG 100.3 (A) In this neonate *Centrochelys* tortoise, the poorly calcified plastron has been incised in the midline, craniad, and caudad, with lateral retraction of the two flaps secured using towel clamps. (B) Use of an oscillating saw to incise the plastron of a *Gopherus* tortoise. (C) Use of a rotary Dremel tool to incise the plastron of a *Testudo* tortoise. (Courtesy of Stephen J. Divers.)

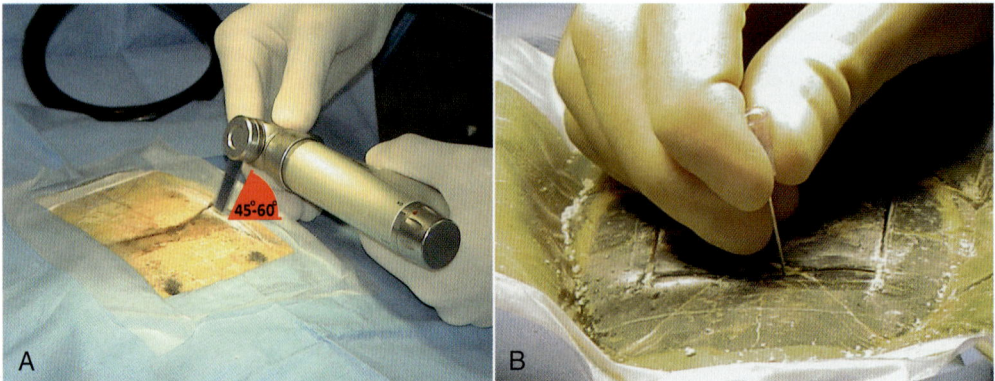

FIG 100.4 (A) The lateral incisions are made first because there are no vital structures or vessels typically below, and they should be beveled at 45 to 60 degrees to prevent the flap from falling under the plastron. (B) A hypodermic needle is used to gauge the depth and ensure full-thickness bone incision. (Courtesy of Stephen J. Divers.)

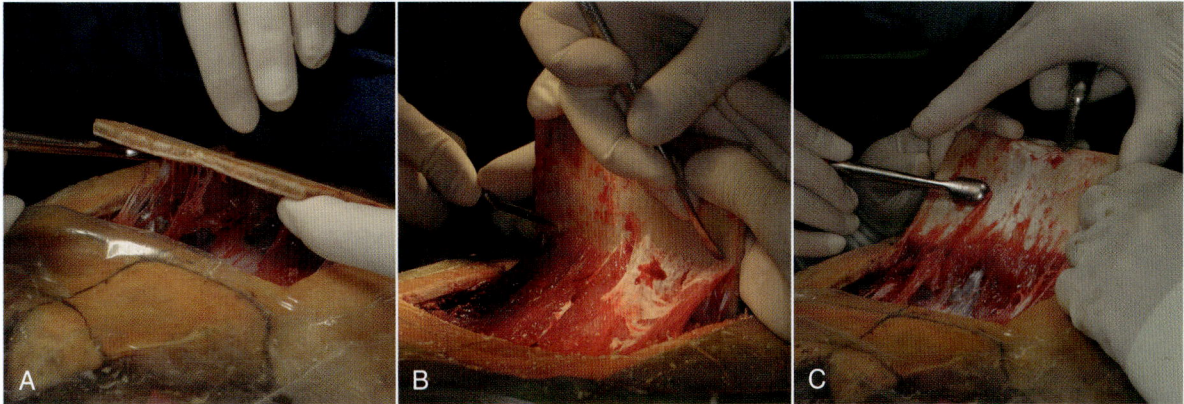

FIG 100.5 (A) Elevation of the cranial margin of the bony flap reveals the musculature attachments below. (B) These muscular attachments are bluntly dissected close to the bony flap. (C) The caudal attachments are left in place and the flap reflected caudad. (Courtesy of Stephen J. Divers.)

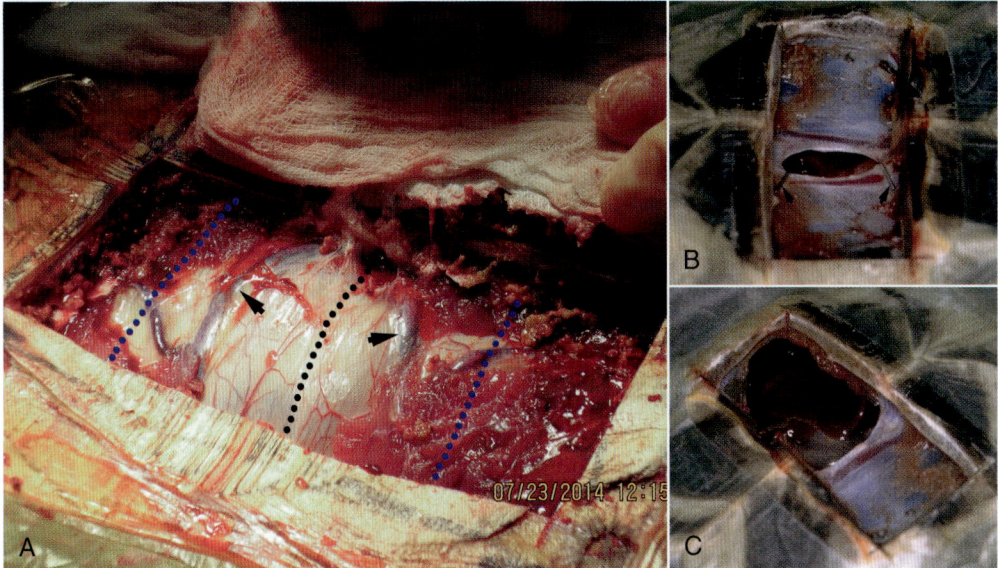

FIG 100.6 (A) Following caudal reflection of the bony flap, the paired abdominal veins can be seen (arrows). Midline, linea alba (black dotted line), or paramedian (blue dotted lines) incisions to the coelom are practical. Laterally, there is often more muscle, and improved hemostasis is required. (B and C) Ligation of one abdominal vein using vascular clips (arrows) to permit a larger access window can be performed when greater exposure is required. (Courtesy of Stephen J. Divers.)

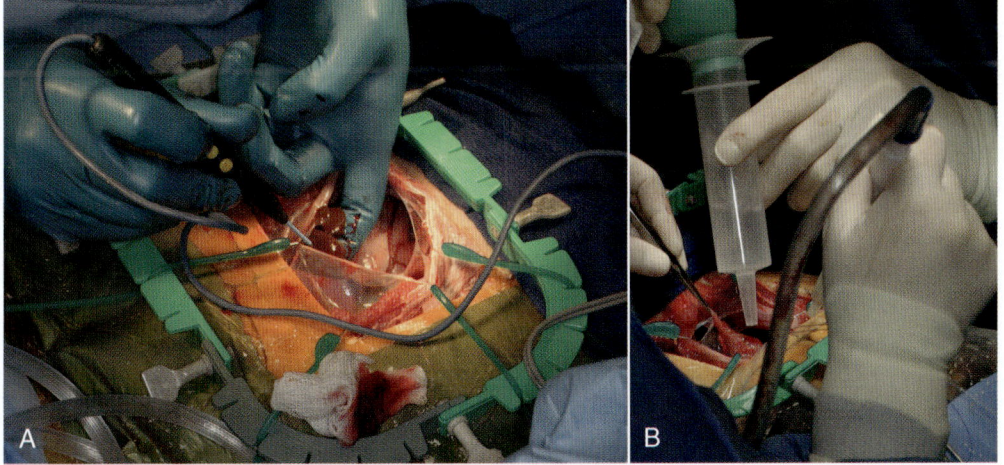

FIG 100.7 (A) Use of a ring retractor and elastic stays (LoneStar) to improve visualization. (B) Copious irrigation and lavage should be performed following clean-contaminated procedures (e.g., cystotomy, enterotomy). (Courtesy of Stephen J. Divers.)

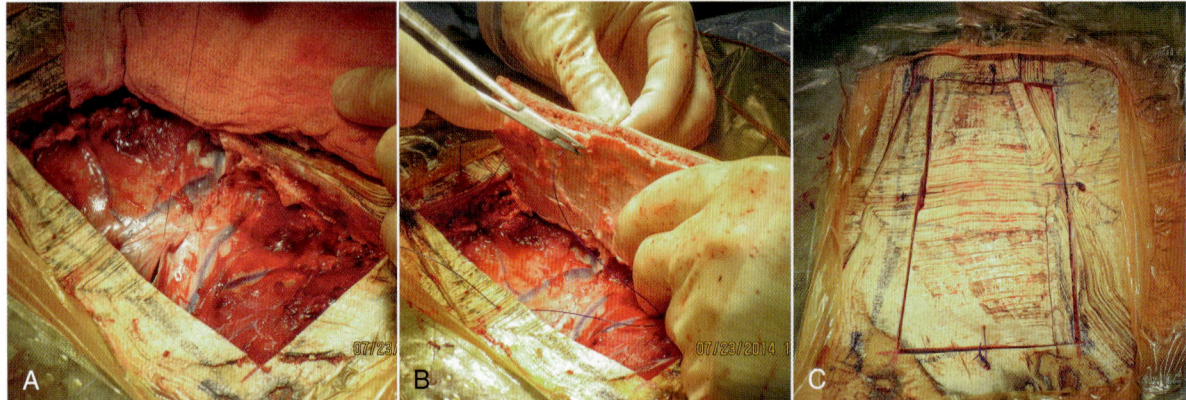

FIG 100.8 (A) Closing the linea alba using absorbable monofilament suture (polydioxanone) in a continuous pattern. (B and C) Placing absorbable monofilament suture (polydioxanone) through predrilled holes to secure the bony flap to the plastron. Anchoring the bony flap results in less movement during epoxy or acrylic application and a more secure bond. (Courtesy of Stephen J. Divers.)

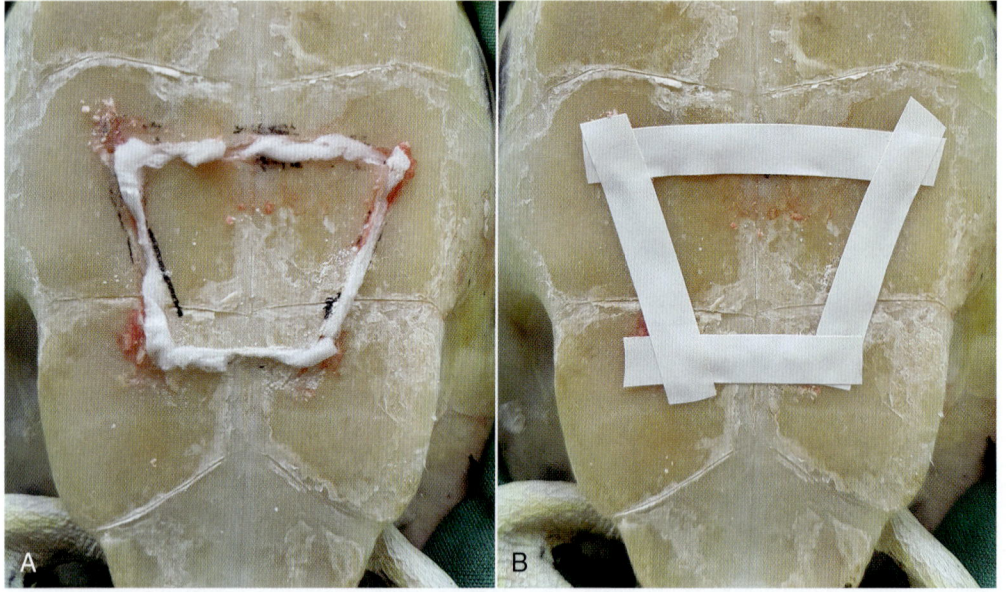

FIG 100.9 Absorbable collagen inserted along the boney incision lines (A) and covered with surgical tape (B) in an aquatic turtle, prior to epoxy covering. (Courtesy of Clinic for Birds, Reptiles, Amphibians and Fish, JLU-Giessen.)

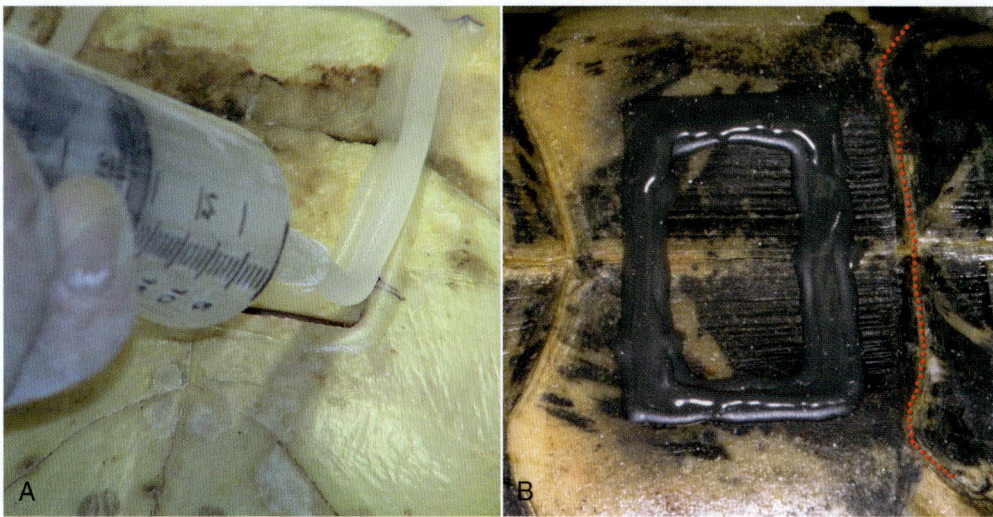

FIG 100.10 (A) Veterinary acrylic (Technovit Jorgensen Labs, Loveland, CO) was mixed in a 60-mL syringe and then applied to either side of the incision and finally over the incision. (B) Completed closure using veterinary acrylic. Note that the caudal hinge of this *Testudo* tortoise (red dotted line) has not been compromised. (Courtesy of Stephen J. Divers.)

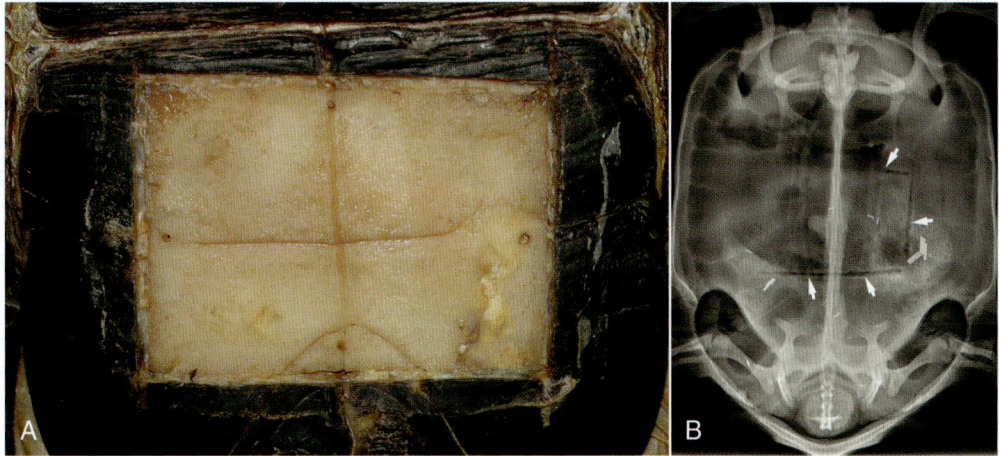

FIG 100.11 (A) Ventral view of the surgical site 12 weeks following surgery and immediately following removal of the bony sequestrum (box turtle, *Terrapene*). An odor was noticed from the bony flap and was promptly removed. No infection was present, but the flap had become a sequestrum with new bone growth below. (B) Dorsoventral radiograph of a *Gopherus* tortoise 12 years following transplastron coeliotomy. Note the persistence of radiolucent lines (arrows) associated with three of the four incisions. The metallic densities are vascular clips. (Courtesy of Stephen J. Divers.)

points or around the entire bony incision. In aquatic species it can be helpful to score or roughen the shell to improve adhesion. The shell is carefully cleaned with an alcohol swab to remove any debris, before epoxy resin or an acrylic is applied (Fig. 100.10A). Temporary masking tape can be used to protect adjacent areas, particularly hinges, before applying the repair material. Any excess, uncured material can then be easily removed along with the tape, thereby creating a clean finish (see Fig. 100.10B). Exothermic materials can cause thermal necrosis, and cold saline drips or cold saline-soaked gauze should be used to control heating.

The healing process depends directly on the size of the bony gap and the quality of the repair. Maintenance of soft-tissue attachments, accurate reduction and immobility of the bony section, aseptic technique, and attention to postoperative hygiene to prevent infection will improve the chances of first or second intention healing. However, it is common for the plastron flap to become a sequestrum that provides temporary protection for new bone growth beneath (Fig. 100.11A). The plastron typically heals within 12 weeks but can take longer, and therefore the covering is usually left in place for 6 to 12 months. Radiography is seldom helpful in the assessment of healing because radiolucent lines tend to persist long after healing is complete (see Fig. 100.11B). However, osteolysis may suggest osteomyelitis, which warrants surgical investigation, debridement and samples for histopathology, and cultures (aerobic, anaerobic, and fungal).

REFERENCES

See www.expertconsult.com for a complete list of references.

101

Crocodilian Coeliotomy

Javier G. Nevarez

Some indications for coelomic surgery in crocodilians may include gastrotomy for removal of foreign body after unsuccessful gastroscopy, enterotomy, follicular stasis, organ or tissue biopsy, and exploratory coeliotomy. However, unlike snakes and lizards, coelomic surgery in crocodilians is far more challenging due to their anatomy, which must be appreciated for successful surgery. There is a limited window for accessing the coelomic cavity. The ventral skin is thicker than on the flanks and can be quite challenging to suture together, especially in older animals and those that have ventral osteoderms (e.g., caiman). Good apposition of the ventral skin is often not possible, leading to delayed healing, and, because of low skin elasticity in this area, stainless steel sutures may be required. For these reasons, a lateral flank approach may be preferred. Nonetheless, some have successfully performed coeliotomy via a ventral midline or paramedian incision.

Within the ventral body wall are free-floating ribs called gastralia, which are found immediately caudal to the sternum (Fig. 101.1). The right and left gastralia are joined by a cartilage at midline. An incision into the ventral coelom requires cutting through the gastralia, which may become more fibrotic or calcified as the animal ages. Though seemingly invasive, cutting through the gastralia generally has no detrimental impact on the animal. The coelomic cavity of crocodilians has two grossly distinct features from other reptile taxa, the presence of a diaphragmaticus muscle (Fig. 101.2) and a distinct mesentery surrounding the intestines (Fig. 101.3). In addition there are eight serosal cavities. The diaphragmaticus muscle originates from the ischia and last gastralia and inserts on connective tissue on the caudal aspect of the liver (see Fig. 101.2).[1] It is incomplete and more horizontally oriented, so it does not create a true separation of the cavity. This thin muscle is thought to

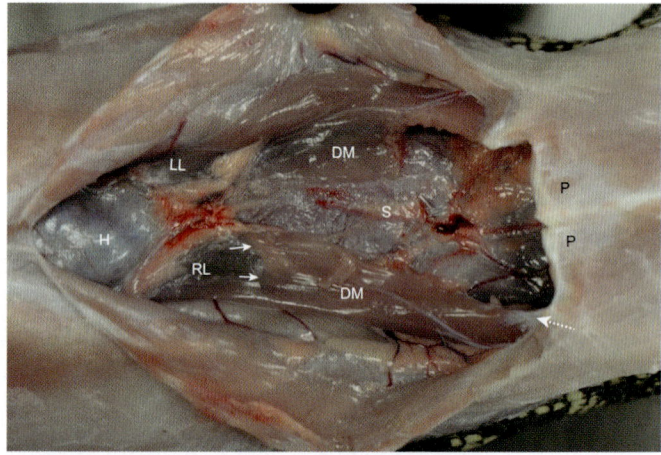

FIG 101.2 American alligator (*Alligator mississippiensis*) with exposed coelomic cavity after ventral midline incision through the gastralia. The diaphragmaticus muscle (*DM*) originates from the ischia and last gastralia (dotted arrow) and inserts on connective tissue on the caudal aspect of the liver (solid arrows). In this image, part of the diaphragmaticus has been transected where the gastralia were incised. H, Heart; LL, left liver lobe; P, pubic bones; RL, right liver lobe; S, stomach. Cranial is to the left of the image. (Courtesy of Javier G. Nevarez.)

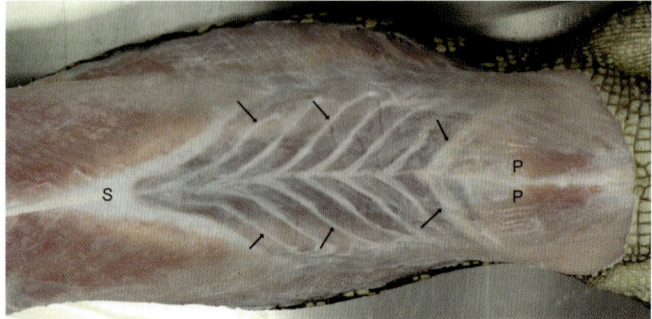

FIG 101.1 Ventral aspect of an American alligator (*Alligator mississippiensis*) with the skin removed. The gastralia (free-floating ribs) are identified with black arrows. They lie caudal to the sternum (S) and cranial to the pubic bones (P). As crocodilians age, these become fibrotic and may calcify. Cranial is to the left of the image. (Courtesy of Javier G. Nevarez.)

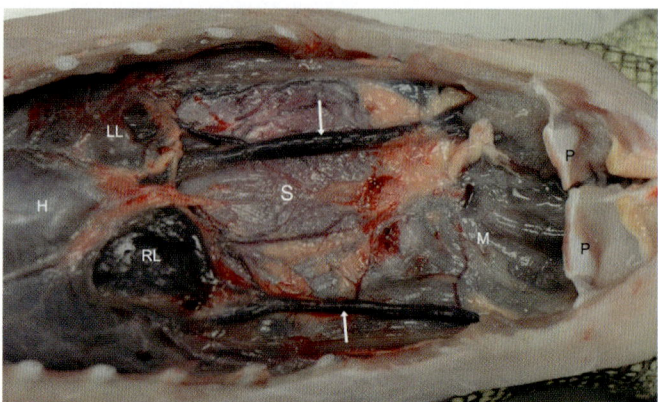

FIG 101.3 Dissection of an American alligator (*Alligator mississippiensis*) showing the lateral abdominal veins (*arrows*). The diaphragmaticus muscle has been removed to allow visualization of the abdominal veins. The pubic bones (P) have been cut to allow better visualization of the coelomic cavity and the mesenteric "sac" (M). H, Heart; LL, left liver lobe; RL, right liver lobe; S, stomach. Cranial is to the left of the image. (Courtesy of Javier G. Nevarez.)

assist with respiration but more likely plays an active role in buoyancy.[1,2] Uriona et al. revealed that transection of the diaphragmaticus muscle can lead to decreased submersion times in *Alligator mississipiensis*.[3] Therefore care must be taken to not transect this muscle during surgery. Crocodilians have a rather unique mesentery that encloses the majority of the small intestine and all of the large intestine, essentially creating a mesenteric "sac" (see Fig. 101.3). This arrangement creates a true separation between the intestines and the rest of the viscera, preventing any direct contact with the stomach, duodenum, liver, lungs, or heart. The duodenum lies in close association with the stomach, right liver lobe, and the gallbladder. To access the spleen, gonads, adrenals, and small and large intestines, an incision has to be made through this mesenteric sac (Figs. 101.4 and 101.5). Suturing this mesentery is challenging, and herniation of the intestines through the incision is a possible complication. The clinical effects of this are unknown. This also makes coelioscopy of crocodilians quite challenging.

Unlike lizards, crocodilians do not have a centrally located ventral abdominal vein but rather two lateral abdominal veins (see Fig. 101.3). These are usually large in size and found deeper within the cavity, dorsal to the diaphragmaticus muscle. On the caudoventral aspect of the coelom, crocodilians have prominent pubic bones that extend ventrocranially from the pelvis and have articulation with the ischium (see Figs. 101.2 and 101.6). The pubic bones obscure visualization of the mesenteric "sac" (see Fig. 101.2) and must be transected to access the small and large intestines (see Figs. 101.3 and 101.4); therefore, incision over this area is not recommended.

An additional consideration before performing a ventral coelomic incision in crocodilians is the postoperative care. Animals will have to be maintained dry to semidry for at least 10 days or until the incision has sealed. The use of a liquid bandage material may help provide additional protection. When maintained outside of water, the weight of their bodies and viscera will place additional strain on the ventral skin incision, affecting its integrity and cleanliness. This could lead to dehiscence and infection of the site. If stainless steel suture was utilized, it will need to be removed once healing is complete.

The numerous, aforementioned issues regarding a ventral incision suggest that a lateral incision through the flank is a better approach to the coelomic cavity (Figs. 101.7 and 101.8). The skin on the lateral aspect of the body is thinner and more pliable and will hold sutures better. There is also less pressure from the body weight and viscera, and the suture line can be maintained dry if the animal is kept in shallow water. In the craniolateral aspect there are still ribs that have to be incised to access the stomach and liver. However, in larger crocodilians these organs may be accessed caudal to the ribs. A flank incision can be made caudal to the last rib and cranial to the pelvis (see Fig. 101.7). The muscle layers must then be incised before entering the coelomic cavity (see Fig. 101.7). Upon entering the cavity, the mesenteric sac can be visualized and must be incised before the intestines can be accessed (see Fig. 101.8). The mesentery sac can be maintained in a taut position by use of a retractor (see Fig. 101.8). Via this approach, most of the small intestines can be exteriorized. It also allows access to the cranial colon (see Fig. 101.8). The caudal aspect of the stomach is

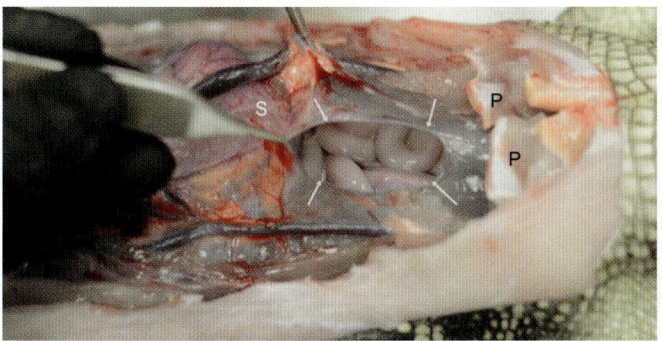

FIG 101.4 An incision through the mesenteric "sac" (arrows) of an American alligator (*Alligator mississippiensis*) reveals the small intestines. The mesentery must be incised to access the intestines and other organs. P, Pubic bones; S, stomach. Cranial is to the left of the image. (Courtesy of Javier G. Nevarez.)

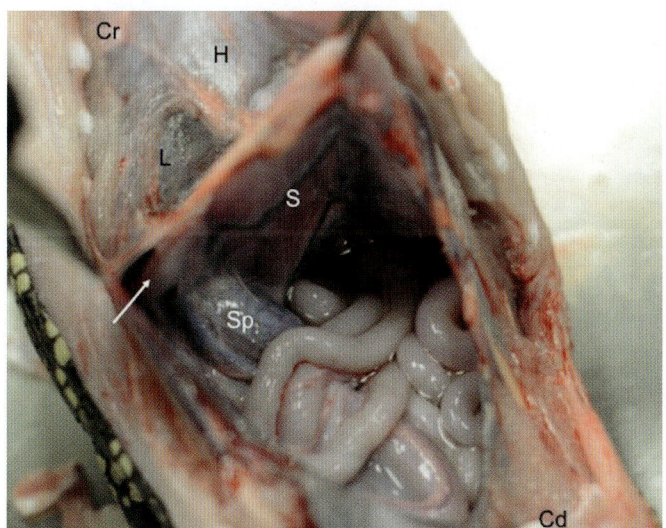

FIG 101.5 View inside the mesenteric "sac" of an American alligator (*Alligator mississippiensis*) showing the duodenm (arrow), spleen (Sp), intestines, and caudal aspect of the stomach (S). This creates a true separation between the lungs, heart (H), liver (L), and the rest of the viscera. Cd, Caudal; Cr, cranial. (Courtesy of Javier G. Nevarez.)

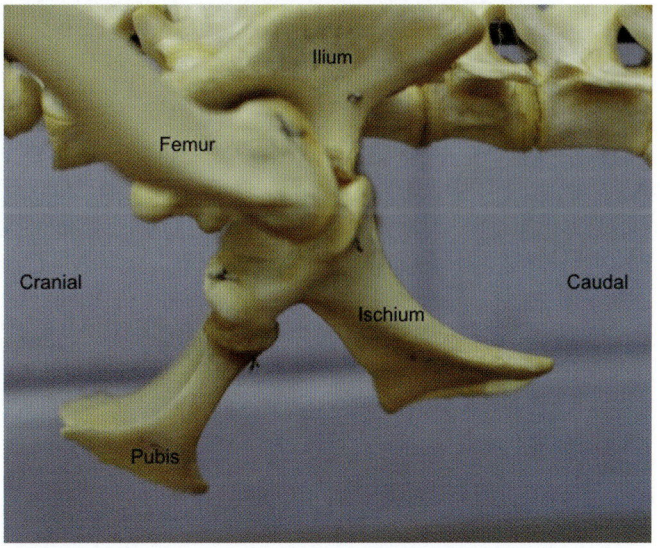

FIG 101.6 Pelvis of an American alligator (*Alligator mississippiensis*) showing the prominent pubic bones that extend cranioventrally into the coelom. The pubic bones articulate with the ischium and are part of the locomotion mechanism of crocodilians. (Courtesy of Javier G. Nevarez.)

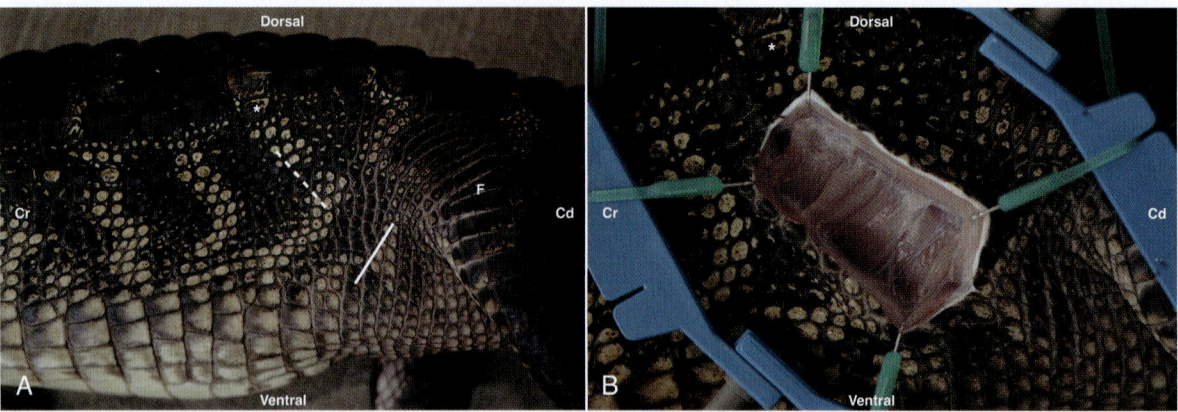

FIG 101.7 Landmarks for a lateral surgical approach in an American alligator (*Alligator mississippiensis*). A lateral incision can be made between the last rib (dotted line) and the pubis (solid line) (A). Incision through the skin reveals various muscle layers that must be incised before gaining access to the coelomic cavity (B). A Lone Star retractor works well to maintain proper exposure (B). CD, Caudal; CR, cranial; F, femur; *, dorsal scute used as fixed reference point for orientation purposes. (Courtesy of Javier G. Nevarez.)

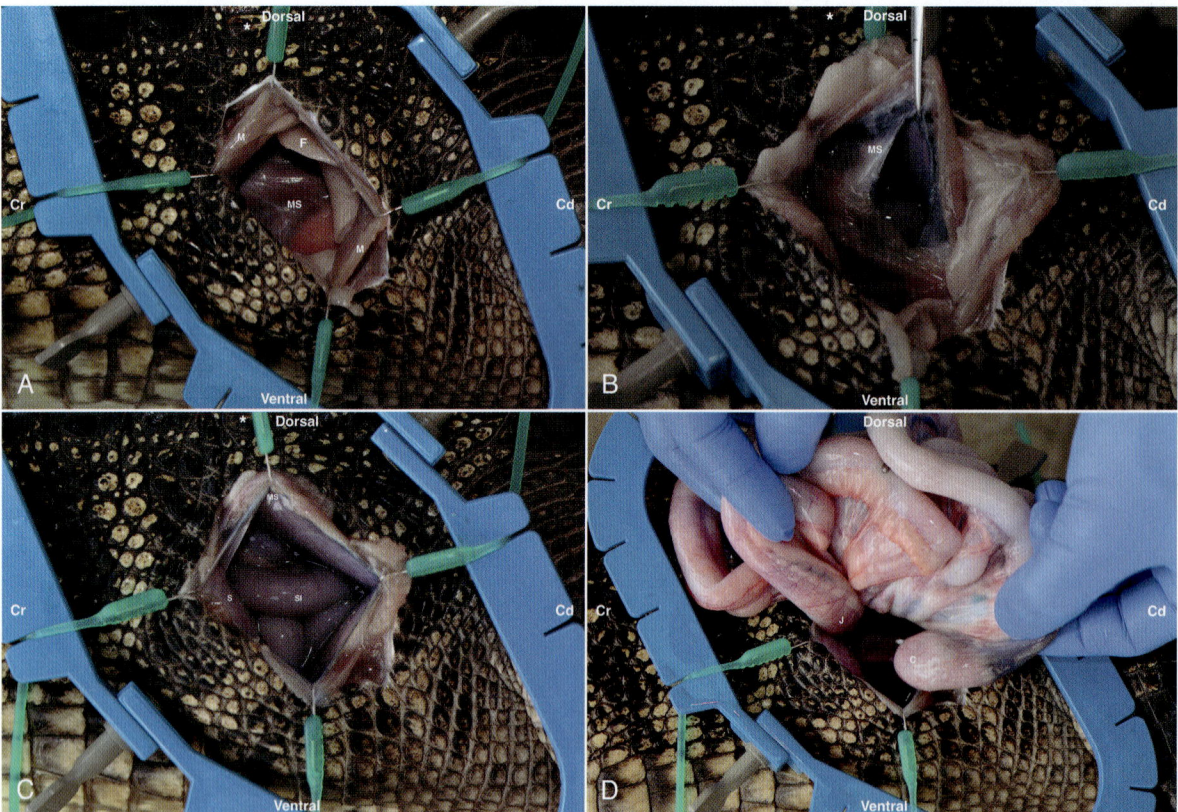

FIG 101.8 View of coelomic cavity through a lateral incision in an American alligator (*Alligator mississippiensis*) (A). A Lone Star retractor is used to maintain tension on the muscle layers (M). Fat (F) and the mesenteric sac (MS) can be visualized in the coelomic cavity. The mesenteric sac must be incised to gain access to the intestines (B). The edges of the mesenteric sac (MS) can be pulled apart with the retractor to allow visualization of the caudal aspect of the stomach (S) and small intestines (SI) (C). Most of the small intestine can be exteriorized (D). This allows easy access all the way from the jejunum (J) to the colon (C and D). CD, Caudal; CR, cranial; *, dorsal scute used as fixed reference point for orientation purposes. (Courtesy of Javier G. Nevarez.)

also accessible, but the duodenum remains fixed inside the coelomic cavity. Access to other organs is limited and may require the aid of an endoscope for visualization.

Based on all these factors, coeliotomy should be considered a last resort in crocodilians. It is certainly possible that a skilled surgeon may successfully perform a specific coelomic surgery. However, the postoperative management of these patients is difficult and results in a more guarded prognosis for successful healing and recovery.

REFERENCES

See www.expertconsult.com for a complete list of references.

102

Lower Respiratory Tract

Stephen J. Divers

By definition the lower respiratory tract encompasses the larynx, trachea, bronchi, and lungs, while the upper respiratory tract is covered in Chapter 93. Primary indications for surgical intervention include surgical or endoscopic biopsy, lung mass removal, and tracheal resection. Endoscopic techniques are covered in Chapters 64 and 65.

There are no specific equipment or instrument items required that are not covered in Chapter 90. However, it is worth noting that it is especially important to appreciate regional anatomy of the neck and coelomic inlet and be particularly diligent regarding vessels, nerves, and other critical structures.

TRACHEAL RESECTION

Tracheal chondroma and lymphoma have been reported in boid snakes, and the author has additionally seen mycotic granulomas in a tortoise (Fig. 102.1). Tracheal resection has been successful in some cases.[1-3] Radiography but especially computed tomography (CT) are required to determine the nature and extent of the tracheal pathology (Fig. 102.2). Before considering resection, endoscopic evaluation and biopsy for definitive diagnosis is important and may dictate the need for nonsurgical therapy (e.g., radiation, chemotherapy, antimicrobials) (see Fig. 102.1A–C). Endoscope-assisted debulking and clinical resolution of a chondroma in a ball python (*Python regius*) utilizing a diode laser has been successful (Stahl S, personal communication, 2018)

Snakes often present with respiratory distress that can be temporarily alleviated by placement of a saccular lung cannula until surgery can be undertaken (Fig. 102.3).[3,4] The temporary cannula should be surgically placed approx. 55% to 70% snout-to-vent to avoid the vascular lung. Maximal ventilation of the anesthetized snake can help identify the caudal lung entry site. A small, lateral coeliotomy incision and intercostal entry

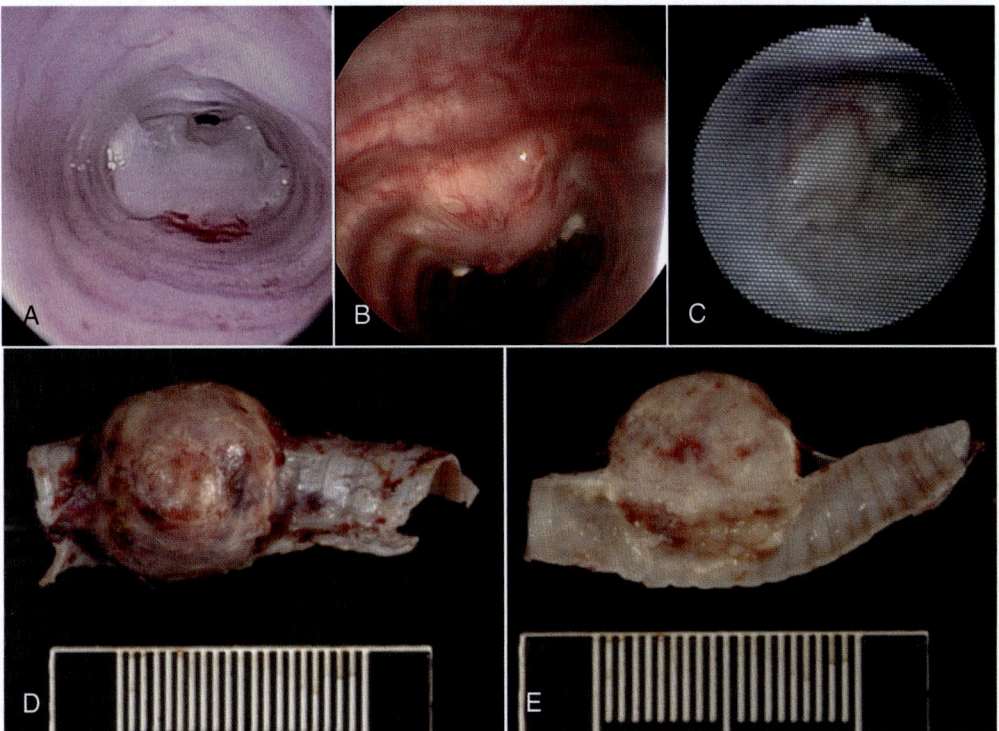

FIG 102.1 (A) Tracheoscopic view of a chondroma in a ball python (*Python regius*) using a 2.7-mm telescope. (B) Tracheoscopic view of a mycotic granuloma in an African spurred tortoise (*Centrochelys sulcata*) using a 2.7-mm telescope. (C) Tracheoscopic view of a lymphoma in a boa constrictor (*Boa constrictor*) using a fiberoptic endoscope. (D and E) Resected portion of the trachea from the same boa constrictor showing an extra- and intramural lymphoma, partially obstructing the tracheal lumen.[3] (A, Courtesy of Scott J. Stahl, Stahl Exotic Animal Veterinary Services; B and C, courtesy of Stephen J. Divers; D and E, from Summa NM, Guzman DS-M, Hawkins MG, et al. Tracheal and colonic resection and anastomosis in a boa constrictor *[Boa constrictor]* with T-cell lymphoma. *J Herp Med Surg.* 2015;25[3–4]:87-99.)

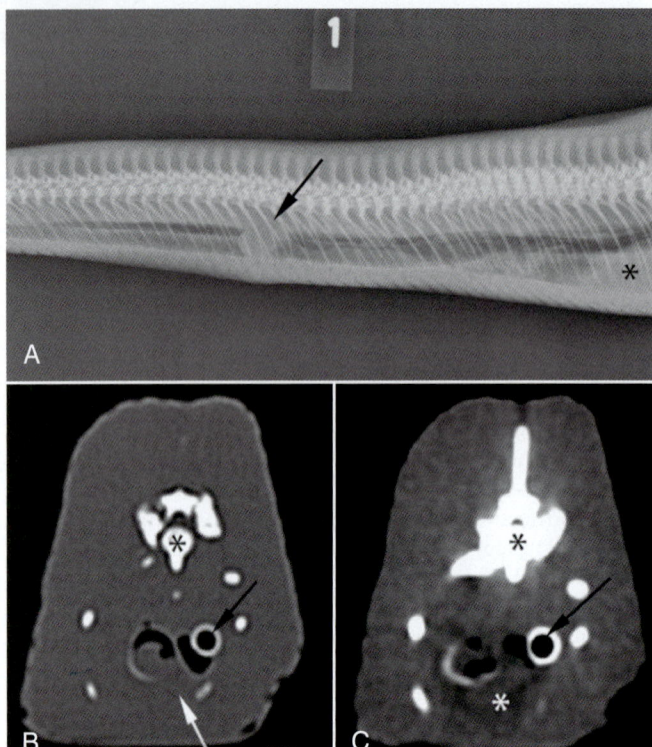

FIG 102.2 (A) Right lateral radiograph of the tracheal region of an 8-year-old boa constrictor (*Boa constrictor*). A round, soft-tissue mass (black arrow) is invading the tracheal lumen at the level of the midtrachea, cranial to the heart (asterisk). (B and C) Transverse computed tomography images of the cervical area of a boa constrictor in a lung algorithm (B) and soft-tissue algorithm (C), which revealed a soft-tissue mass partially obstructing the tracheal lumen (white asterisk). The mass extends ventrally and medially beyond the tracheal wall (white arrow), close to the esophagus (black arrow). A rubber tube has been inserted into the esophagus to delineate this structure during image acquisition (black arrow). The black asterisk indicates the cervical vertebrae.[3] (From Summa NM, Guzman DS-M, Hawkins MG, et al. Tracheal and colonic resection and anastomosis in a boa constrictor *[Boa constrictor]* with T-cell lymphoma. *J Herp Med Surg.* 2015;25[3–4]:87-99.)

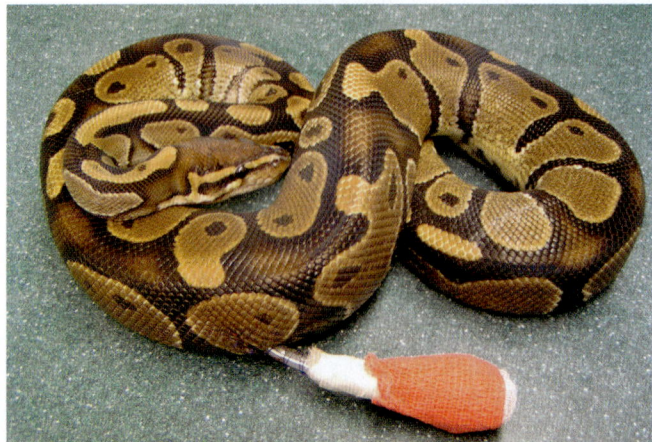

FIG 102.3 A ball python (*Python regius*) with a saccular lung cannula to facilitate breathing. Gauze and bandage material were placed around the tube to prevent debris from entering. (Courtesy of Debra Myers.)

into the coelom permits the placement of a sterile endotracheal tube of equal or greater diameter to that used for tracheal intubation. A cuffed tube is often more secure, but a Chinese finger trap suture is still required, and skin closure can also help maintain tube security. The cannula can be used to maintain anesthesia during tracheal surgery, but a filter should be placed at the entrance of the cannula when not in use to reduce contamination. Nonetheless, a saccular lung cannula should be considered temporary, with removal recommended within 48 hours of placement.

After induction, the anesthetic circuit should be connected to the saccular lung cannula and the trachea occluded using a moistened cotton-tipped applicator or similar. The snake should be positioned in lateral recumbency to afford the best approach to the affected portion of the trachea. The serpentine trachea is often located to the right of midline, making left lateral recumbency preferred and a right approach preferable. After aseptic preparation, a standard craniocaudal coeliotomy skin incision is performed between the first and second or second and third lateral rows of scales. Meticulous dissection and hemostasis is required to avoid the right carotid artery, jugular vein, and smaller vascular supplies to the trachea. The left jugular, left carotid, and esophagus should be deep to the area of interest, but placement of an esophageal catheter may be helpful to aid identification and preservation. If the resection involves the caudal trachea, then appreciation of the thymus and great vessels is required. Placement of stay sutures to elevate the trachea facilitates resection. The tracheal anastomosis is performed using full-thickness, simple interrupted sutures of 4-0 to 5-0 antibiotic-impregnated polydioxanone (PDS-Plus, Ethicon) tied extraluminally. Additional extraluminal tension-relieving sutures on each lateral side encompassing two to three tracheal rings cranial and caudal to the anastomosis site can be considered. The stay sutures are removed and the surgical site carefully inspected for any hemorrhage or esophageal trauma. The subcutaneous tissues are then apposed with a simple continuous suture pattern using 4 to 0 poliglecaprone 25 (Monocryl, Ethicon), followed by routine skin closure. Tracheoscopy 6 to 8 weeks after surgery can confirm healing.

LUNG BIOPSY

There are occasions when a more invasive surgical approach to a lung is required for the purposes of biopsy because appropriate endoscopy equipment is not available, the site of interest is inaccessible (walled off by fibrosis), or small endoscopic biopsies were inconclusive.

Pre- and postcontrast CT images are preferred, but radiography may be acceptable for lesion identification and planning a surgical approach. After aseptic preparation, a 1- to 4-cm craniocaudal skin incision is followed by a 0.5- to 2-cm dorsoventral intercostal approach. Dissection between the ribs is usually blunt or accomplished using radiosurgery to reduce hemorrhage. A ring or eyelid retractor increases intercostal distraction and access to the craniodorsal coelom. An endoscope is valuable for identifying and grasping the affected lung, which can then be exteriorized through the intercostal space. If endoscopy is not available, then holding at maximal inspiration will often facilitate grasping the inflated lung. Abnormal tissue can be sampled or resected. Suturing the lung is problematic, and it is generally more effective to place a transfixing circumferential suture of 4/0 antibiotic impregnated poliglecaprone-25 (Monocryl Plus Antibacterial, Ethicon, Athens, GA, USA) to isolate a small section of lung before sharp distal resection. The lung is replaced and observed for leakage during maximal ventilation. The retractor is removed, and the intercostal incision is closed by placing simple interrupted 4/0 polydioxanone sutures around the adjacent ribs. Skin closure is routine.

In chelonians, a similar lung biopsy procedure as described previously can be used via the prefemoral fossa but is restricted to the caudolateral

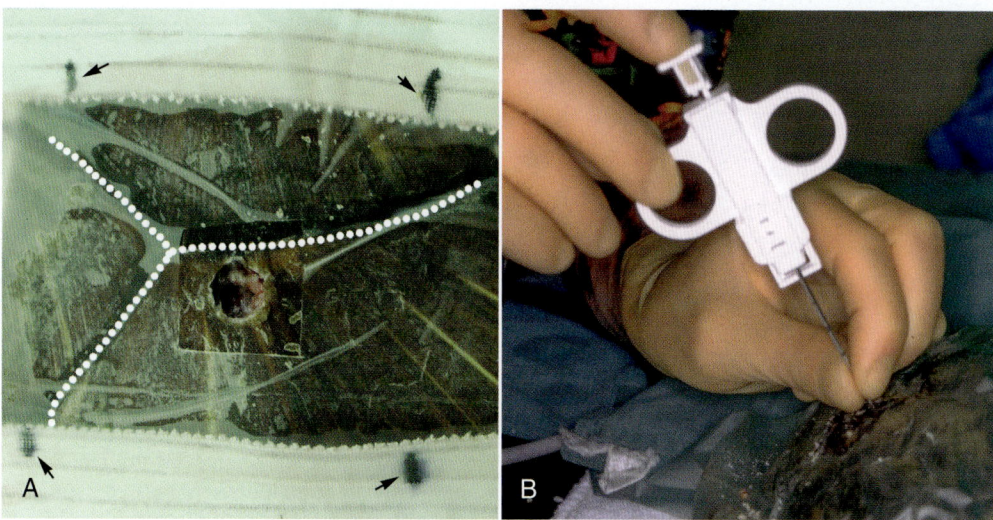

FIG 102.4 Transcarapacial lung biopsy in chelonians. (A) View of the surgical site in a juvenile loggerhead sea turtle (*Caretta caretta*) illustrating the position of the osteotomy through the carapace over the radiographically targeted lesion. The margins of the lesion were marked on tape (arrows). The hole was created close to the intersection of the keratin scutes (white dotted lines) to avoid a bony growth plate. (B) Needle biopsy of the lung of a Greek tortoise (*Testudo graeca*) through a drill osteotomy in the carapace. (Courtesy of Stephen J. Divers.)

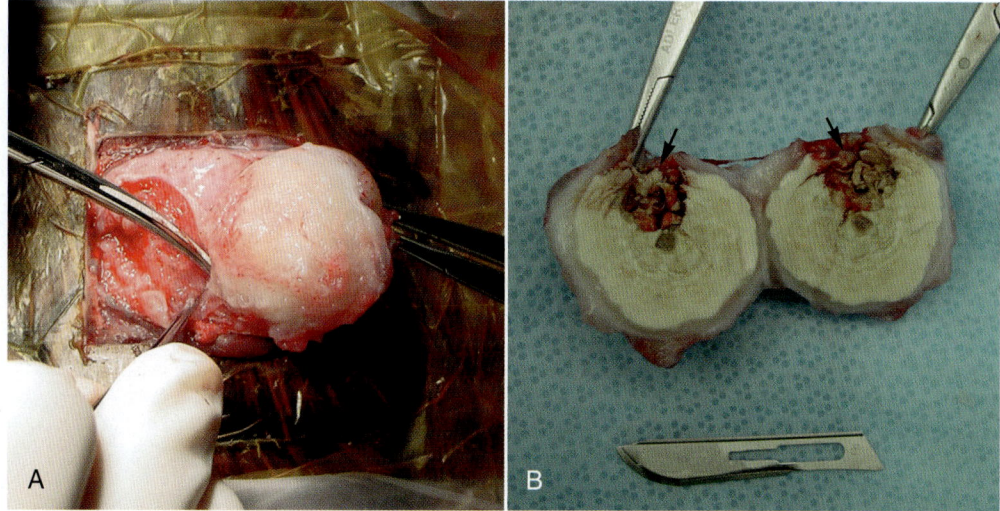

FIG 102.5 (A) Temporary carapacial osteotomy to remove a large fungal granuloma from the lung of a loggerhead sea turtle (*Caretta caretta*). (B) Transection of the granuloma reveals thick encapsulation resistant to drug penetration. Notice the sites of previous endoscopic biopsy (arrows). (Courtesy of Stephen J. Divers.)

aspect of the lung. A 2- to 5-cm craniodorsal prefemoral incision is made, followed by blunt entry into the coelom. An alternative, carapacial approach has also been described (Fig. 102.4).[5] Diagnostic imaging is used to pinpoint a 5-mm drill access hole through the carapace, directly over the pulmonary lesion. While temporarily maintaining maximal inspiration, small hemostats perforate the pleuroperitoneum to allow access for needle biopsy (e.g., Tru-Cut). It is not necessary to close the pleuroperitoneum, but the small osteotomy is closed using epoxy or acrylic. An intrapulmonary catheter can be temporarily secured through the osteotomy to facilitate intrapulmonary therapy.[5]

MASS/ABSCESS/GRANULOMA REMOVAL

When a discrete lung mass (neoplasm, abscess, granuloma) has been identified, a similar, but more extensive, surgical approach to that described previously can be used. In lizards and snakes, a standard ventrolateral coeliotomy provides greater exposure than the intercostal approach. In chelonians, a larger dorsal carapacial flap can be created (Fig. 102.5). Again, the use of a transfixing circumferential suture to isolate the diseased area is often preferred because of the difficulty of suturing lung. This may result in significant loss of pulmonary tissue, which, although well tolerated and unlikely to result in clinically significant respiratory compromise, may result in long-term asymmetrical swimming in aquatic chelonians.

REFERENCES

See www.expertconsult.com for a complete list of references.

103

Gastrointestinal Tract

Ryan De Voe

Surgery of the gastrointestinal tract, including the liver and pancreas, is frequently indicated in reptilian patients. Many of the same procedures that veterinarians are called on to perform in domestic animals can be necessary in reptiles. Indications for performing surgery on the gastrointestinal tract include gastrointestinal foreign bodies, intraluminal impactions, neoplasia, abscesses or granulomas, and intussusceptions, volvulus, or strictures.[1,2] Biopsies of various segments of the gastrointestinal tract and associated organs are often indicated to obtain a diagnosis in disease states or to provide samples for infectious disease screening.[3]

PRINCIPLES OF GASTROINTESTINAL SURGERY IN REPTILES

The same principles of antisepsis and tissue handling used in domestic animal medicine are appropriate for reptiles. A review of literature regarding surgical procedures of the gastrointestinal tract in reptiles does not reveal any unique techniques or procedures that would be unfamiliar to most surgically competent veterinarians.[2,4,5] However, magnification is often beneficial for small species (Fig. 103.1). The phases of wound healing take longer in reptiles but otherwise mirror what is observed in mammals.[1] Longer tissue-healing times may influence decisions regarding antimicrobial, antiinflammatory, and analgesic therapy, as well as nutritional support. It is often beneficial, and indeed is standard practice, to provide intraoperative (IV or IO) antimicrobials prior to entering the nonsterile gastrointestinal tract.[6] Intraoperative antibiotics have been shown to be equal, if not more effective, at reducing postsurgical complications and reducing antibiotic resistance when compared with postoperative therapy.

Prior to entering the gastrointestinal tract of a reptile, the segment of gut should be carefully isolated with saline-soaked gauze or sponges to limit contamination of the coelom. Following closure of the gut, the site should be thoroughly irrigated before removal of the gauze or sponges. With the structures back in normal anatomic position, the coelom should be irrigated thoroughly and then gloves and instruments changed prior to closure.

Surgical incisions into the stomach should be closed in two layers. An initial, full-thickness closure utilizing a simple continuous or simple interrupted pattern followed by an inverting pattern (Cushing or Connell pattern) is preferred. Antemesenteric, longitudinal intestinal incisions closed end to end result in a larger diameter and reduced constriction. Colotomy incisions should also be closed in two layers. The first layer can be appositional or inverting and the second layer inverting. Intestinal closures are often challenging due to the relatively thin wall and small luminal diameter of the intestines of many reptiles. A single layer of accurately placed simple interrupted sutures is usually sufficient to form an adequate seal and encourage normal healing (Fig. 103.2). In all cases, selection of an appropriate suture material and needle is critical for success. Monofilament absorbable suture material, such as polydoxanone or poliglecaprone 25, should be utilized. Those impregnated with antimicrobials (e.g., Monocryl Plus containing triclosan) have been shown to significantly reduce bacterial colonization of suture tracts and reduce infection rates, making them ideally suited for intestinal closure.[7] Fine suture with a tapered, swaged needle is usually indicated,

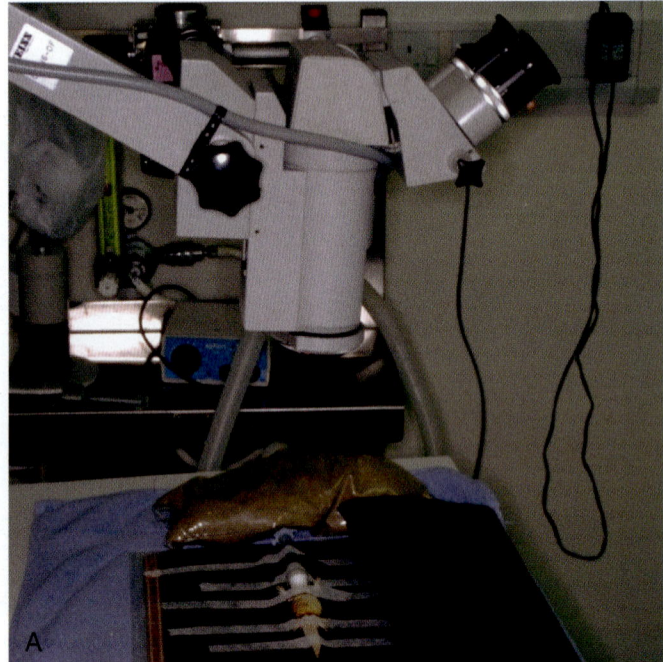

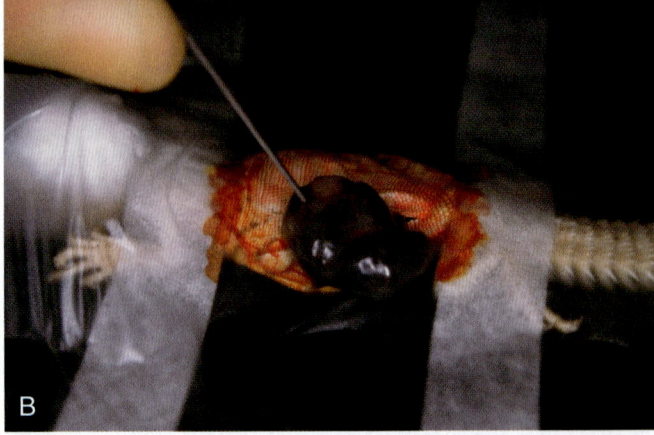

FIG 103.1 (A) Use of an operating microscope to perform an enterotomy in a juvenile spiny-tailed lizard (*Uromastyx* sp.). (B) Exteriorization of the impacted intestinal tract. (Courtesy of Stephen J. Divers.)

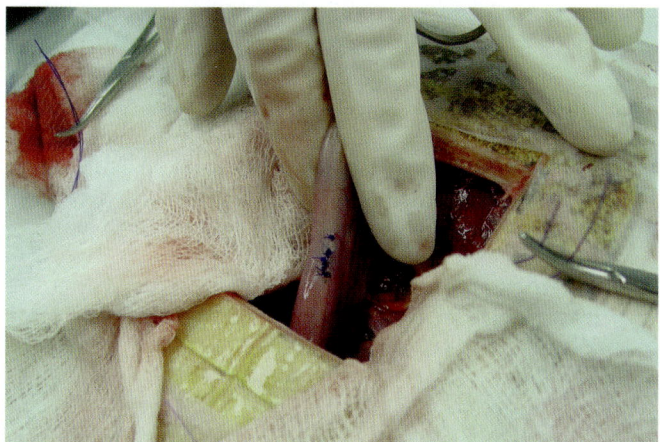

FIG 103.2 Simple interrupted closure of an enterotomy site following foreign body removal in a chelonian. (Courtesy of Stephen J. Divers.)

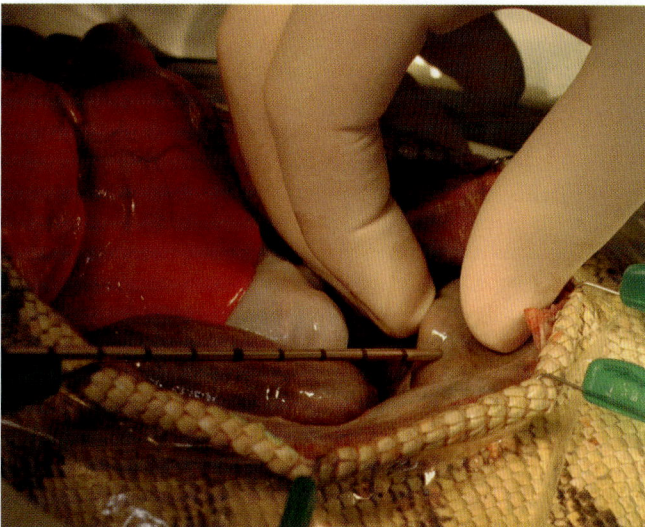

FIG 103.3 Liver biopsy in a green iguana (*Iguana iguana*) utilizing a Tru-Cut biopsy needle. (Courtesy of Stephen J. Divers.)

especially when closing intestinal enterotomies. Even very small cutting needles can create unacceptable trauma in the thin-walled intestines of some species. Gastrotomy incisions in larger species with muscular stomachs may require cutting needles for easy closure. Suturing the serosal surface of an adjacent segment of bowel to the enterotomy site may provide insurance against leakage and dehiscence with questionable closures.[1]

Resection and anastomosis of various segments of the gastrointestinal tract may be indicated due to devitalization of tissue or neoplasia. The technique utilized for anastomosis should be based on size of patient and the segment of gut. Typically, a simple interrupted, appositional pattern is preferred to promote maintenance of luminal patency. Initial placement of sutures at the mesenteric and antimesenteric aspects and closure of the walls in between usually facilitates accurate apposition of tissues and effective anastomosis. Magnification is often required for this procedure when working with smaller species. The prognosis following resection and anastomosis is usually guarded, particularly when resection is necessary due to the presence of abscesses, granulomas, or segments of grossly necrotic gut and/or large lengths of the gastrointestinal tract require resection.

Enterostomy of the lower gastrointestinal tract is possible when the condition of the bowel does not allow for anastomosis following resection of the diseased segment. Enterostomy carries a guarded long-term prognosis[8] Careful case selection is necessary, as aftercare is intensive, both in the immediate postoperative healing and maintenance phases.

PERIOPERATIVE CARE

Due to the slower healing times of reptiles and the potential for contamination, especially with surgeries involving the lower gastrointestinal tract, perioperative antimicrobial therapy is often indicated. IV or IO broad-spectrum antimicrobials (e.g., cefazolin) prior to incision negate the need for postoperative therapy in clean-contaminated procedures, and reduces the chances of favoring antimicrobial resistance.[6] Obviously, if infection is suspected at the time of surgery, samples should be submitted for culture prior to starting therapy, and continued postoperatively.

In most reptile species, postoperative resumption of feeding should not occur for a minimum of 3 to 7 days and even for several weeks in snakes. When feeding is resumed, the composition and volume of the diet should be managed to ensure maximum digestibility and minimize distention of the gastrointestinal tract (and body wall and skin of snakes). The diet should be increased gradually over a period of 3 to 6 feedings until normal intake is resumed.

BIOPSY OF THE GASTROINTESTINAL TRACT

Mucosal biopsies of the esophagus, stomach, and colon may be obtained in most larger species via endoscopic methods. If full-thickness biopsies are required for a diagnosis, celiotomy is necessary. The same techniques that are used in mammals are appropriate in reptiles. Full-thickness wedges of gastric, intestinal, or colonic wall may be collected following isolation of the section of gut with saline-soaked gauze or sponges. Closure of the resultant defect is similar to the technique described following gastrotomy, enterotomy, or colostomy above.

HEPATIC BIOPSY/PARTIAL HEPATECTOMY

Hepatic disease is frequently encountered in reptilian patients and hepatic biopsy may be required to reach a definitive diagnosis. Partial hepatectomy may be indicated to resect hepatic abscesses, granulomas, and parasitic or neoplastic masses. Collection of liver tissue may also be indicated to screen for certain infectious diseases as part of a preventative medicine program. The same methods that are employed in avian and mammalian practice are typically suitable for reptiles. Laparoscopic or percutaneous ultrasound-guided hepatic biopsy is often possible, though the size of the biopsy can limit histologic evaluation depending on available equipment and size of the patient, and gastric perforation and fatal hemorrhage have been reported.[9,10] Laparotomy can facilitate acquisition of larger biopsies via a variety of methods. Intraoperative utilization of various biopsy forceps can be effective. Kevorkian biopsy forceps enable the clinician to obtain relatively small tissue samples without inducing crushing artifact that may inhibit histological evaluation. Skin-punch biopsy tools can also be used intraoperatively with good success. Hemorrhage is the most likely adverse consequence of hepatic biopsy or partial hepatectomy and can result in mortality if not controlled. Hemostasis can be accomplished via strategic application of stainless steel hemostatic clips, sutures, cellulose-based hemostatic agents, or other methods typically employed in avian and mammalian medicine.

Surgery of the biliary system is uncommon in reptiles but occasionally necessary (Fig. 103.3). Surgical removal of choleliths is reported anecdotally in reptiles. There are no special techniques involved in surgery of the reptile biliary system, though taxa-specific knowledge of anatomy is necessary.

PANCREATIC BIOPSY

Pancreatic biopsies are likely underutilized as a diagnostic measure in reptile patients. Derangements of glucose metabolism are frequently encountered in lizards, neoplastic disease of the pancreas is reported and the pancreas may be involved with a variety of infectious diseases. Many of the same methods that are employed with hepatic biopsies can be used to collect pancreatic tissue. There is variation in pancreatic anatomy between reptilian taxa, but the pancreas is typically found adjacent to the duodenum. In some species of snakes (such as members of the family Boidae), the pancreatic tissue contacts the caudal aspect of the spleen forming what can appear to be a single organ referred to as the splenopancreas.[11] This is not the condition in all snakes, however, so normal anatomy should be investigated prior to pursuing a pancreatic biopsy in an unfamiliar species. When performing pancreatic biopsies, care should be taken to avoid causing undue damage to the remaining tissue as iatrogenic exocrine pancreatic insufficiency and diabetes mellitus following resection of masses affecting the organ are reported.[12]

REFERENCES

See www.expertconsult.com for a complete list of references.

104

Urinary Tract

Stephen J. Divers

The urinary system includes the kidneys, ureters, urodeum, and, if present, the urethra and bladder. Surgery of the cloaca is covered elsewhere (see Chapter 106). Following the investigation of urinary tract disease, surgical biopsy or correction may be required (see Chapter 66). The most common urologic surgeries include cystotomy (for the removal of calculi or eggs) and renal biopsy; however, cystectomy and nephrectomy are also possible.[1] Surgical techniques are mirrored from small animal surgery, with adjustments for reptile anatomy and physiology.[2] In many situations, minimally invasive endoscopic options are replacing the more traditional and invasive coeliotomy approaches (see Chapters 64, Diagnostic Endoscopy, and 65, Endosurgery).

CYSTOTOMY AND CYSTECTOMY

Indications for cystotomy include removal of calculi, repair of bladder trauma, biopsy or resection of bladder masses, and biopsy and culture of the bladder wall in cases of severe cystitis. Indications for partial or complete cystectomy include bladder necrosis, neoplasia, or possible management of recurring calculi in some lizard species.[3]

While performing a surgical approach to the coelom, it is important to be cautious of the often full, voluminous, and thinly walled (often transparent) bladder, especially as cystitis and disease may have resulted in greater fragility and tendency to rupture (Fig. 104.1). Bladder (like intestinal) contents should be considered contaminated, non-sterile

sites, and great effort should be made to prevent coelomic contamination and subsequent septic coelomitis. Given the clean-contaminated nature of the surgery intraoperative IV or IO antibiotics should be considered (e.g., cefazolin 20–25 mg/kg IV started 30 minutes prior to first incision and repeated every 90 minutes until closure). However, if bacterial disease (rather than just contamination) is considered likely, then antibiotics should not be started until after the collection of samples for cultures and sensitivity testing.

For lizards, ventral coeliotomy approach is standard; however, for chelonians, a ventral transplastron or prefemoral approach may be used. The decision will depend upon the size, shape, and location of the calculus, and the species of chelonian (because this determines the conformation of the prefemoral fossa). The prefemoral approach is less traumatic but provides reduced surgical access in most terrestrial species. Radiographic evaluation and prefemoral measurements will enable an objective decision to be made regarding preferred approach.

Ideally, the bladder should be gently exteriorized through the coeliotomy incision because this greatly reduces the chances of coelomic contamination (see Fig. 104.1). When this is not possible, the coelomic muscle and skin incisions should be retracted to provide greater exposure and the coelom packed with moistened sterile gauze (Fig. 104.2). The cystotomy incision is made through a less vascular area of the ventral bladder wall (or lateral bladder wall in the case of a prefemoral approach),

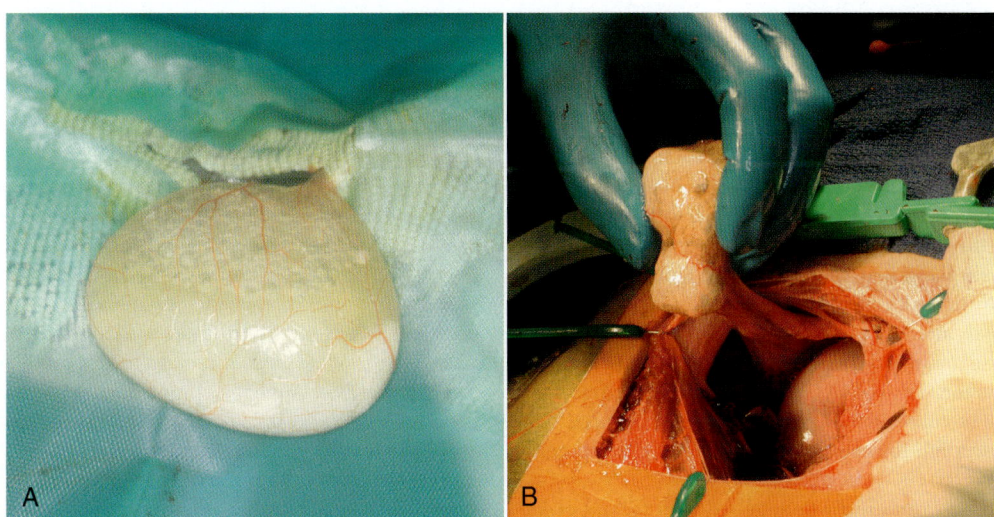

FIG 104.1 (A) View of the exteriorized bladder of an iguanid lizard. Note the very thin, transparent nature and superficial vasculature. (B) Exteriorization of the chelonian bladder via a ventral transplastron coeliotomy. (Courtesy of Stephen J. Divers.)

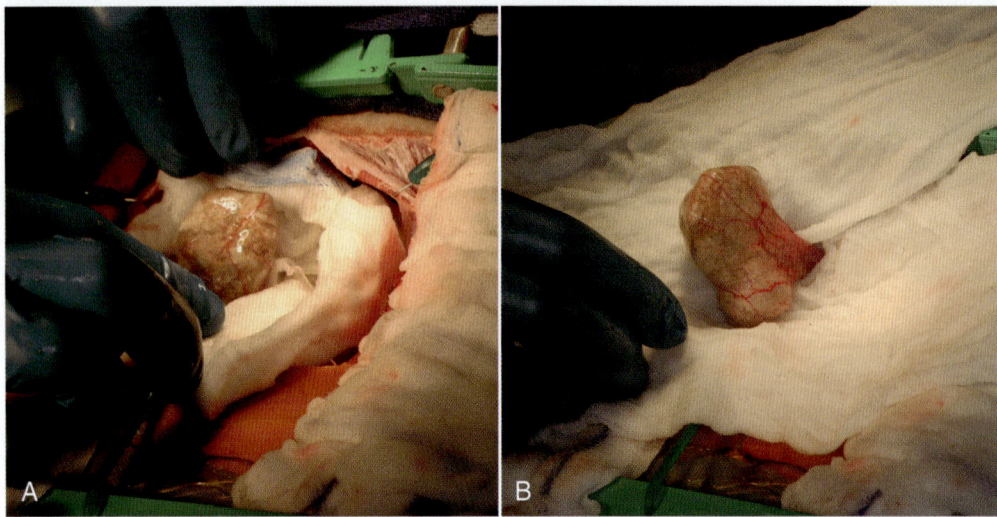

FIG 104.2 (A and B) Packing the coelom of a tortoise with sterile, moistened laparotomy gauze to control any leakage from the bladder. (Courtesy of Stephen J. Divers.)

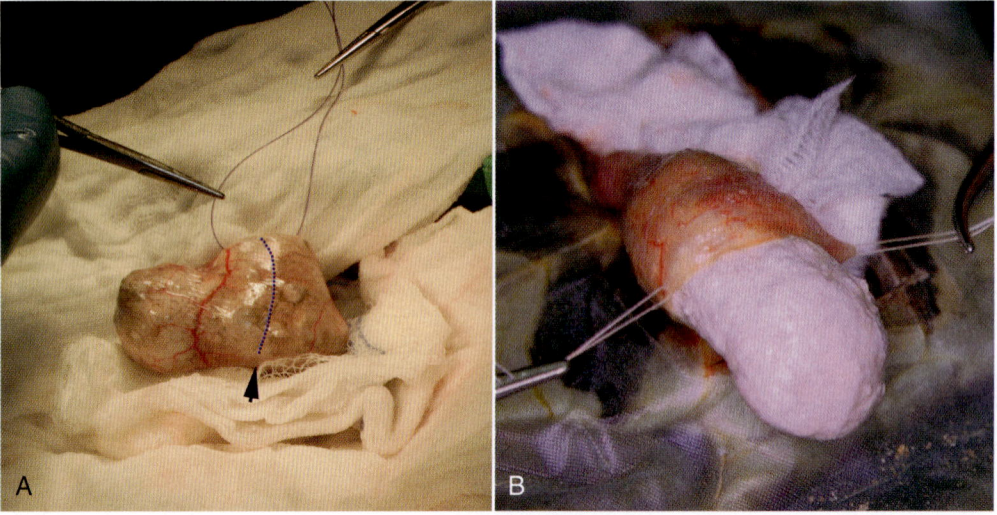

FIG 104.3 (A) The first stay suture has been placed and the position of the second is indicated (*arrow*). The proposed incision is indicated as a dotted blue line. (B) Following incision between the stay sutures, the bladder wall recedes, and the calculus can be removed. Care is required to suction any fluid and prevent contamination of the coelom. (Courtesy of Stephen J. Divers.)

taking care to use suction to remove any fluid from within the bladder (Fig. 104.3A). Stay sutures should be placed and held by hemostats. This will help keep the incision elevated, thereby preventing leakage, and will also maintain incision orientation during suturing (see Fig. 104.3B). When performing a prefemoral cystotomy a lateral incision in the bladder is made, and it is wise to marsupialize the bladder wall to the prefemoral skin incision by using a Lone Star retractor or suture to prevent contamination (Fig. 104.4A). If the bladder wall is abnormal then biopsies should be collected for histopathology and cultures. The easiest place to excise a full-thickness biopsy is along the lateral edge of the cystotomy incision.

Small calculi and eggs can usually be removed with the aid of an angled spoon. It can be difficult to manipulate a large calculus through the incision, and in some cases breaking the calculus in situ may be required; however, excessive fragmentation can create considerable debris

and should be avoided (see Fig. 104.4B). One successful technique to aid in large calculus manipulation and removal is to use large, autoclaved, hardware wood screws (Michael Kiedrowski, personal communication, 2014). Most calculi are relatively soft, and one or two 5-to-8-cm (2″–3″) screws can be placed into the calculus (Fig. 104.5A and B). On rare occasions, when the stone is too hard, a pilot hole may be required. The screws provide greater leverage to facilitate elevation and removal (see Fig. 104.5C). Applying compressive or distractive force between the screws often breaks the stone into two pieces, each with a screw attached for simple removal (see Fig. 104.5D).

Following removal of the calculus or egg(s), the bladder should be inspected, copiously flushed and irrigated with sterile saline, and checked for integrity. Necrotic bladder wall should be debrided and removed. In severe cases of bladder necrosis or neoplasia, most, if not all, of the bladder can be resected without interfering with urine flow; however,

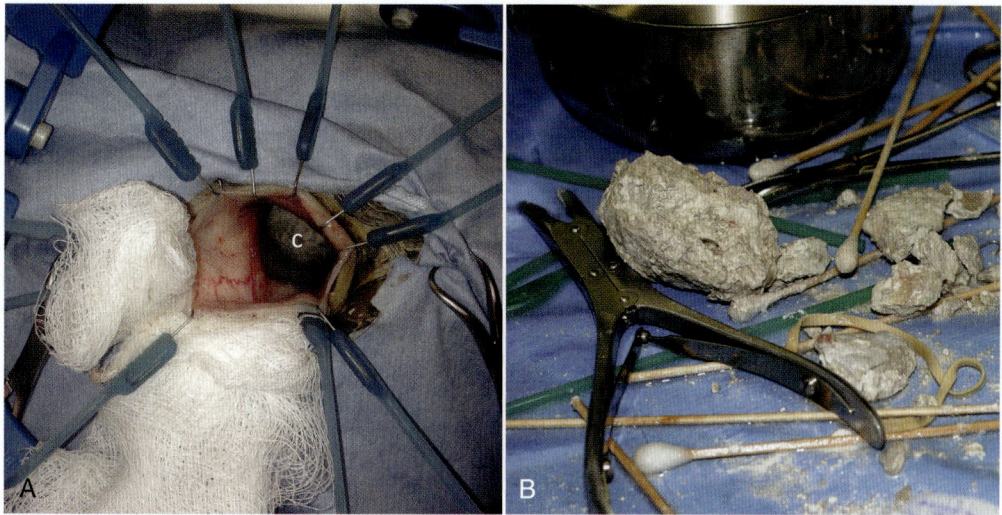

FIG 104.4 (A) Prefemoral approach with the bladder wall temporarily marsupialized to the prefemoral skin incision using a ring retractor and elastic stays. The large calculus (*c*) can be seen within the bladder. (B) Large calculi may require the use of large forceps, ronguers, drills, or saws to break them and facilitate removal; however, severe fragmentation should be avoided. (Courtesy of Stephen J. Divers.)

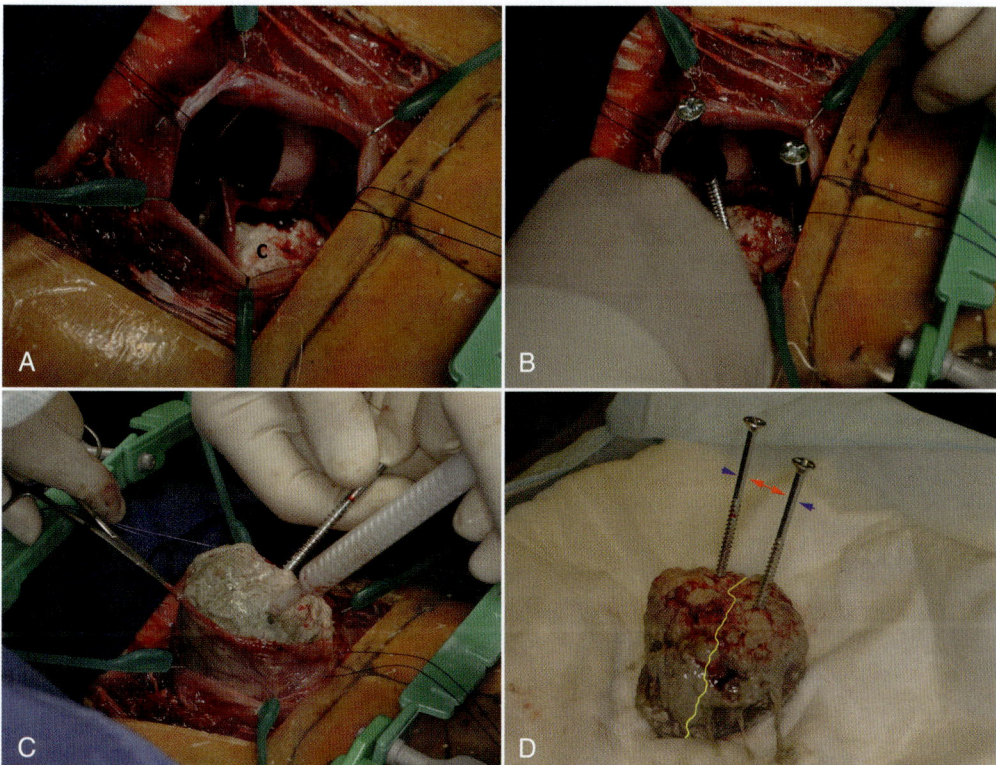

FIG 104.5 (A) Large calculus (*c*) within the bladder supported by stay sutures. (B) Placement of two large screws into the calculus. (C) The screws provide superior leverage and enable the calculus to be lifted out of the bladder and coelom. (D) If necessary, compressive (blue arrows) and distractive forces (red arrows) can be applied to break the calculus in situ, with the fracture generally occurring between the screws (yellow line). (Courtesy of Stephen J. Divers.)

such reptiles will be less tolerant of drought, and therefore wild animals should not be released, although captive reptiles can be adequately managed and thrive.

The bladder wall is closed with fine absorbable monofilament suture, and triclosan-coated poliglecaprone 25 (Monocryl Plus Antibacterial, Ethicon, Athens, GA) is preferred.[4,5] Although a single continuous closure has been shown to be effective with only minimal urine leakage, given the chances of bacterial contamination, a second inverting layer should be routinely performed for added security in reptiles.

RENAL BIOPSY

Histopathologic and microbiologic evaluations of samples from diseased kidneys may be required to determine the underlying pathology causing renal dysfunction. Indications for renal biopsy include neoplasia, nephrotic syndrome, chronic renal disease, and acute progressive renal failure of undetermined etiology.[2] The benefits of a definitive diagnosis should be weighed against the risks of complications and whether the results will change current treatment. The greatest complication is hemorrhage, and consideration should be given to evaluating clotting times prior to surgery.

Endoscopic renal biopsy is safe, effective, minimally invasive, and preferred over open surgical approaches (see Chapters 64 and 66 for more details).[6–8] The advantage of traditional coeliotomy is the ability to collect larger samples, as well as an improved opportunity to more completely evaluate and sample other visceral structures. Access to the dorsal kidneys can be challenging from a ventral coeliotomy approach, and good retraction and packing are often required. In some cases, a lateral coelomic approach directly over the kidney may be easier. Surgical access to the chelonian and intrapelvic iguanid kidneys can be particularly difficult by traditional coeliotomy, and in all cases increased surgical exposure and duration of anesthesia must be considered. Before embarking on renal biopsy in the snake, it is important to appreciate the precise location of both kidneys.[9]

Surgical biopsies collected using a sharp dissection technique with a scalpel blade results in histologic samples with minimal to no artifacts (Fig. 104.6A). However, hemorrhage is often encountered and must be addressed using radiosurgery, laser, or hemostatic materials (e.g., Gelfoam Pfizer, NY). Vascular clips can be used to isolate a small section of kidney prior to sharp dissection, although small biopsy forceps or needle biopsy devices can also be used and typically result in less hemorrhage but greater crush artifact (see Figs. 104.6B and 104.7A). Radiosurgical and laser devices should be avoided when collecting tissue biopsies because they cause significant thermal and histologic artifacts.

A relatively simple technique to biopsy the intrapelvic kidneys of iguanids requires a cranial tail cut-down procedure under local or, more commonly, short-term general anesthesia. A small longitudinal incision is made in the lateral midline just below the lateral processes of the coccygeal vertebrae at the tail base. The incision extends for 1 to 3 cm caudad, starting just behind the hind limb. Blunt dissection between the dorsal and ventral coccygeal muscles permits exposure of the caudolateral aspect of the kidney that can then be sampled (see Fig. 104.7B). This technique is particularly valuable when the kidneys are not enlarged, a surgical approach to the intrapelvic kidneys is difficult, and endoscopy is not available. It is limited to unilateral biopsy unless bilateral cut-down procedures are undertaken. Furthermore, because only a small area of the caudal kidney can be visualized and sampled, this technique is best reserved for diffuse diseases involving the caudal kidney.

NEPHRECTOMY

Indications for nephrectomy include irreparable trauma, persistent infection, renomegaly, obstructive urolithiasis with hydronephrosis, and renal or perirenal masses (due to abscess, granuloma, gout, or neoplasia).[2] Nephrectomy has been performed in a number of colubrids and boids (Divers and Stahl, unpublished data), two cape coral snakes (*Aspidelaps lubricus*), and a monocellate cobra (*Naja kaouthia*).[10,11] Renal neoplasia and localized renal gout were the primary indications. It is critical to evaluate the unaffected kidney and ensure sufficient renal function before considering unilateral nephrectomy. Diagnostic imaging and routine plasma biochemistry, including (depending upon taxa) ammonia, urea, and uric acid, should give some confidence that sufficient renal function remains; however, an iohexol excretion study to measure GFR would be most definitive. Nephrectomy would be more challenging in most lizards and most difficult in iguanids and chelonians.

Prior to serpentine nephrectomy, it is important to appreciate the position and entire length of the affected kidney, as well as the vascular supplies (Fig. 104.8).[9] There are several fascial membranes, including a retroperitoneal membrane, that require transection to expose the kidney (Fig. 104.9A). Once exteriorized, the renal vasculature can be appreciated and ligated using vascular clips or radiosurgery/laser. Starting from the caudal pole of the kidney, the renal portal vein(s) arising from the caudal vein are ligated (see Fig. 104.9B). It is also wise to ligate the

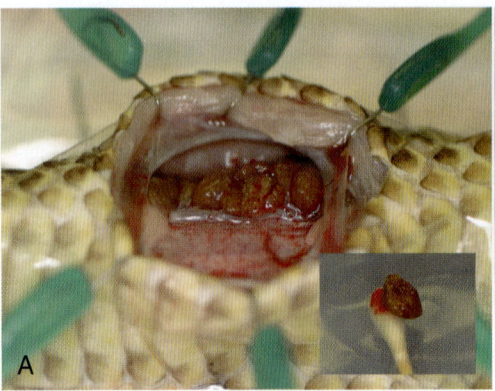
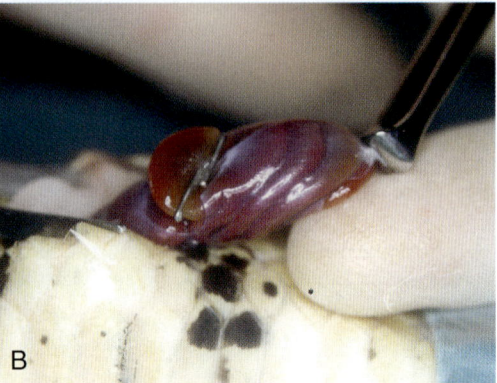

FIG 104.6 (A) View of a diseased kidney in a colubrid snake following sharp biopsy (*insert,* biopsy specimen shown). Although minimal hemorrhage is evident in this case, the surgeon must manage bleeding if it occurs. (B) Vascular clips being used to isolate a renal lobule in a boid snake. (Courtesy of Stephen J. Divers.)

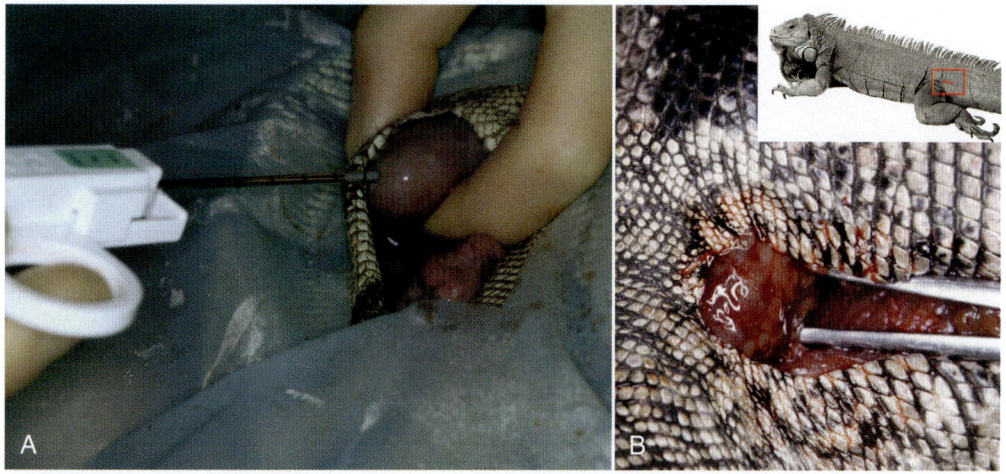

FIG 104.7 (A) Tru-cut needle biopsy of an enlarged iguanid kidney, accessed via ventral coeliotomy. (B) Limited exposure of the caudal pole of the left iguanid kidney following a cranial tail cut-down procedure. (Courtesy of Stephen J. Divers.)

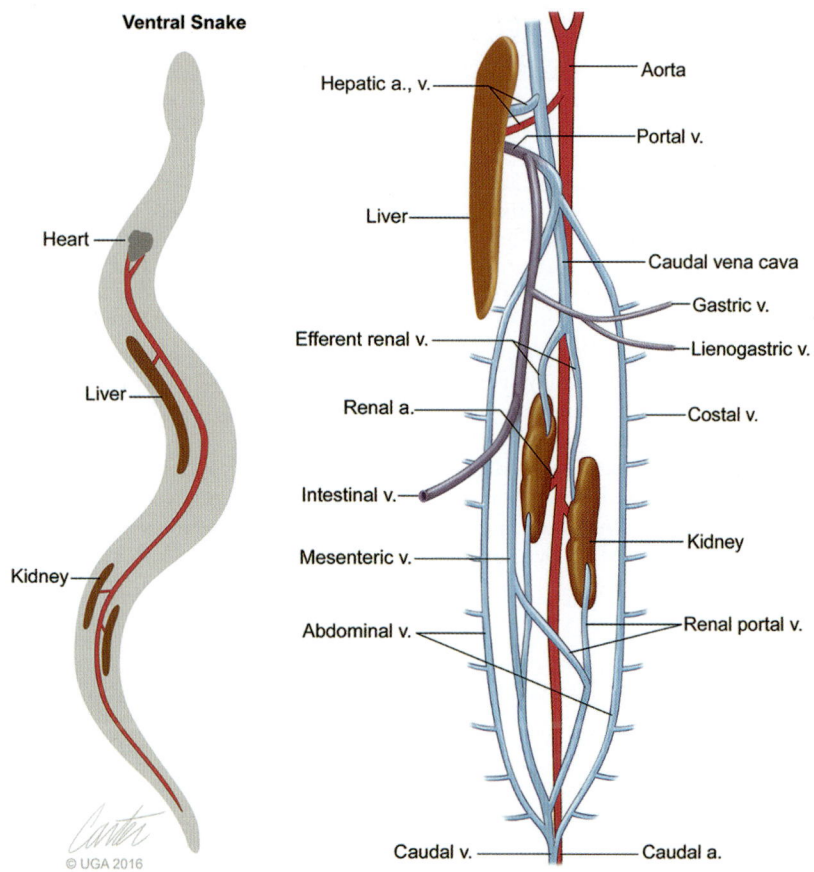

FIG 104.8 Relative position and vascular anatomy of the serpentine kidney. (Courtesy of Kip Carter, Educational Resources, University of Georgia.)

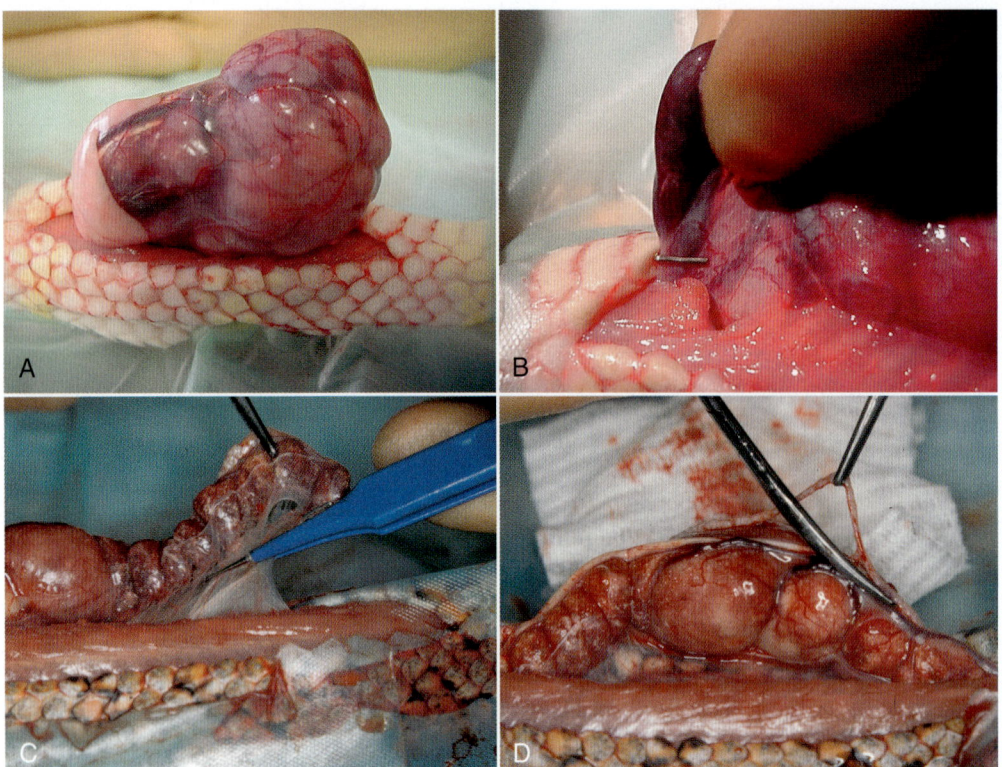

FIG 104.9 Nephrectomy in snakes. (A) Exposure of the right kidney in an albino California king snake (*Lampropeltis getula californiae*) with renal carcinoma. (B) Ligation of the renal portal vein close to the caudal pole of the kidney in the same snake. (C) Dissection of the peritoneal attachments and dorsal arterial vessels of a kidney with severe gout in a corn snake (*Pantherophis guttatus*). (D) Dissecting the closely associated vas deferens away from the kidney is difficult and generally not recommended. (Courtesy of Stephen J. Divers.)

ureter to avoid the retrograde flow and coelomic contamination of urine stored in the terminal ureters. The kidney is then gently dissected free in a cranial direction, taking care to ligate the numerous small renal arteries that arise from the dorsal aorta and enter the dorsal aspect of the kidney (see Fig. 104.9C). The efferent renal veins are then ligated at the cranial margin of the kidney. Care should be taken to avoid damaging the closely associated aorta and vena cava. In males of breeding value, consideration should be given to preserving the closely associated

vas deferens; however, in most cases it is easier to perform a unilateral vasectomy (see Fig. 104.9D). Following nephrectomy, the surgical site should be thoroughly irrigated with sterile saline before routine coeliotomy closure.

REFERENCES

See www.expertconsult.com for a complete list of references.

105

Reproductive Tract

Scott J. Stahl

The reproductive system of reptiles includes the ovaries, testes, salpinges (oviducts), epididymides, vasa deferentia, phallus, and clitoris in chelonians and crocodilians, and hemipenes and hemiclitores in squamates.[1] The urodeum contains the openings of the oviducts and genital papillae (vas deferens termination). A sexual segment of the kidney in squamates is considered part of the reproductive tract.[1] Renal surgery is covered in Chapter 104, and surgical management of the urodeum and cloaca is discussed in Chapter 106. Following a diagnosis of reproductive disease or complication, surgical investigation (including biopsy) or reproductive sterilization may be indicated. Ovariectomy (oophorectomy), ovariosalpingectomy, salpingotomy, orchiectomy, and phallectomy are commonly performed surgical procedures in reptiles. Surgery is often indicated with reproductive disease such as oophoritis, orchitis, salpingitis, paraphimosis, and neoplasia.[2,3] For breeding reptiles, sample collection including surgical biopsies may be performed intraoperatively. Complications from reproductive activity in females (with or without the presence of a mate), including preovulatory follicular stasis, dystocia (postovulatory egg stasis), ectopic eggs, or yolk coelomitis, are common indications for surgery.[2,3] Preventative health measures and behavior management of pet or display reptiles may include elective gonadectomy to eliminate high-risk complications of reproduction in females or to reduce aggression in males.[2–6] When preserving future reproductive capabilities is important, salpingotomy and unilateral ovariosalpingectomy may be indicated.[2,3,7]

In chelonians ovariectomy, orchiectomy, and phallectomies have been utilized to manage population issues in conservation projects.[8–10] Vasectomy was successful in two garter snakes[11] and, although an option for male sterilization, is not commonly performed and not discussed further here. Prolapses involving reproductive organs are common in reptiles and are a frequent indication for surgery.[12] The general equipment and instruments required for surgery are covered in Chapter 90. Many reproductive surgical procedures discussed here can be performed using minimally invasive endoscopic approaches, and the reader is directed to Chapters 64 and 65.[13–17] For a thorough discussion of reproductive diseases and indications for reproductive surgery, see Chapter 80.

MALE REPRODUCTIVE SURGERY

Orchiectomy/Orchidectomy

Indications for castration in lizards and chelonians are to reduce intraspecies and interspecies aggression,[5,6] inhibit the ability to reproduce (population control),[8,9] engage in research,[18] and eliminate testicular pathology such as neoplasia or orchitis (abscess, granuloma).[2,19] Indications for orchiectomy in snakes and crocodilians are less common and are primarily to manage pathological change.

Lizards. For castration in most lizards, a ventral (paramedian or midline) coeliotomy approach is recommended. However, with laterally compressed

species such as old-world chameleons, a lateral (flank) coeliotomy approach can be utilized.[2,19] For details on these approaches, see Chapter 98. Once the coelom is safely entered, the testes are identified. Generally, the testes are paired (right testis slightly more cranial) and found dorsally in the mid to caudal coelom just cranial to the kidneys. The paired coelomic fat pads, bladder (if present), and portions of the gastrointestinal tract may need to be retracted, exteriorized, protected, and kept moist. Exposure of the testes can be improved with the use of retractors such as the lone star retractor. The testes are encased in a fibrous, mesorchium capsule that provides some stability for manipulation; however, if the capsule ruptures, the testis is friable and difficult to manage. When possible, the testis is gently exteriorized through the incision to visualize vessels for ligation. To facilitate elevation of the testis, a suture can be placed through the top of the capsule and gently retracted, or grasped gently with Allis tissue forceps or hemostats (Fig. 105.1). The mesorchium is often tightly adhered to the dorsal coelomic wall, restricting the ability to exteriorize the testis, and the surgeon may have to work within the coelom.

Surgically important anatomical differences exist between the right and left testes in lizards (Fig. 105.2).[1] The right testis is attached directly to the vena cava with short vessels (1–2 mm), and the right adrenal gland is located on the *opposite* side of the vena cava (see Figs. 105.1A and 105.2). Due to its location, accidental damage or removal of the right adrenal gland is unlikely. However, the left testis has its own distinct testicular artery and vein, and the adrenal gland is located *adjacent* to

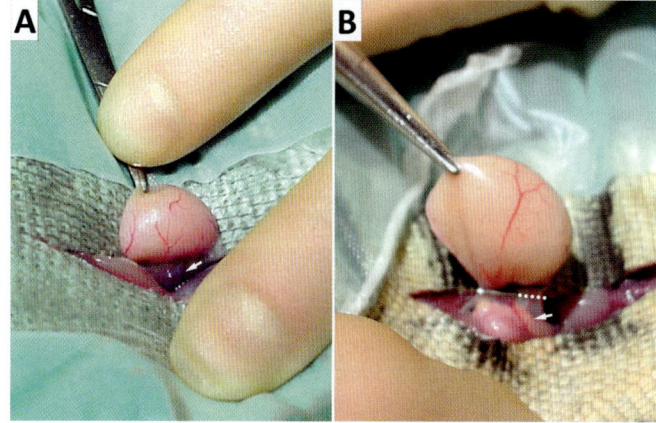

FIG 105.1 Saurian orchiectomy. (A) Hemostats can be used to gently grasp and elevate the testis. The right renal vein (arrow) is located immediately below the testis, and the adrenal gland is below the vein on the right side. (B) A vascular clip has been placed below the left testis and above the left adrenal (arrow); the renal vein is below the adrenal gland on the left side. A second clip is required, as indicated by the dotted line, before the testis can be sharply dissected free. (Courtesy of Stephen J. Divers.)

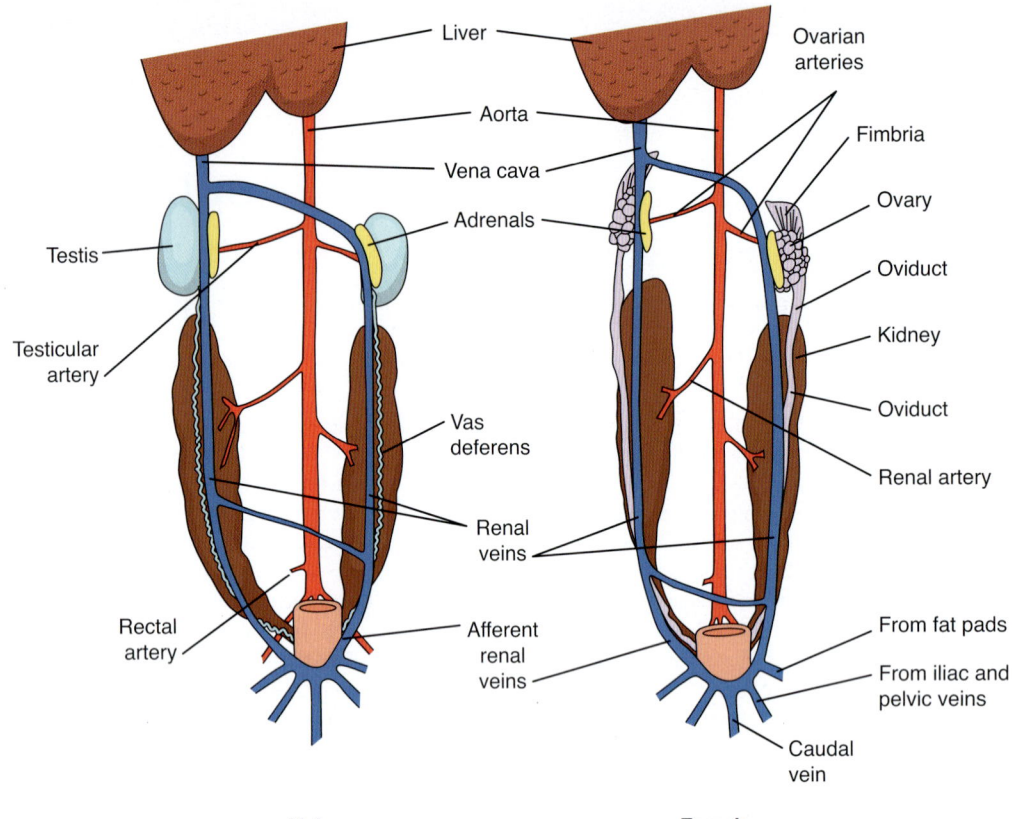

Male   **Female**

FIG 105.2 When performing a gonadectomy in a lizard, it is important to note that the right gonad is anatomically close to the vena cava and the left gonad is attached to the adrenal gland.

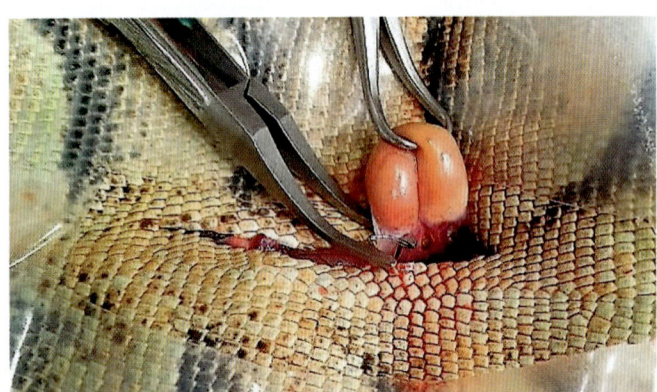

FIG 105.3 Use of vascular clips to ligate the testicular vessels in a green iguana (*Iguana iguana*) orchiectomy. (Courtesy of Scott J. Stahl, Stahl Exotic Animal Veterinary Services.)

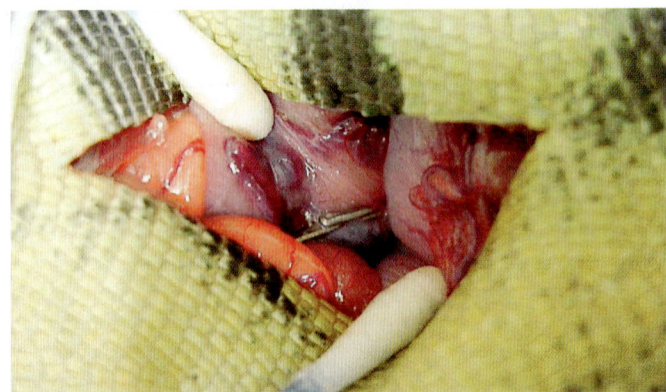

FIG 105.4 After ligation, the mesorchial (or mesovarian) pedicles are observed for bleeding before routine closure. (Courtesy of Stephen J. Divers.)

the left testis utilizing the same vessels. The elongated pink-tan granular adrenal gland should not be accidentally removed or damaged during ligation of the left testis (see Figs. 105.1B and 105.2). Once each testis is isolated, the vascular supply is identified and small windows are made in the mesorchium between the testicular vessels with iris scissors or a scalpel, and the vessels are ligated with vascular clips (Fig. 105.3) or absorbable monofilament suture. In some species (e.g., bearded dragons, *Pogona vitticeps*), the mesorchium is pigmented and the vasculature difficult to visualize. Magnification, focal lighting, and microsurgical instruments can be useful in these situations. After ligation, the mesorchial pedicles are observed for bleeding (Fig. 105.4) before routine closure (see Chapter 98). For laterally compressed lizards such as old world chameleons, a lateral (flank) coeliotomy approach can be utilized. With this lateral coelomic approach the testes are easily identified upon entry,

as they are typically positioned close to the entry site. The same careful ligation of the testicular vessels is performed, and both testes can usually be removed from one incision unless there is associated pathology. Castration of lizards can be performed endoscopically (see Chapter 65 for details).

Chelonians. The least invasive and preferred technique for castration in chelonians is the prefemoral coelomic approach instead of the ventral transplastron coelomic approach.[2,5,11,14,16,17] The testes in most chelonians are accessible from a prefemoral approach (especially with endoscopic assistance), and the trauma of cutting through plastron bone is avoided. However, with testicular pathology or neoplasia, or in some chelonian species, a transplastron coeliotomy may be necessary.[2,13,14,16] For chelonian coeliotomy approaches, see Chapters 99 and 100.

Once the coelom is entered, with either approach, the bladder, intestinal tract, and lungs are gently manipulated to allow access to the testes. The testes of chelonians are paired and found dorsally in the caudal coelom cranial to the kidneys. With the prefemoral approach, the use of retractors such as the lone star retractor can help with exposure (Fig. 105.5). The testis is then identified and grasped with forceps or hemostats and gently manipulated to the level of the prefemoral incision to allow visualization of the mesorchium and the testicular vessels (Fig. 105.6A).[2,18] It is difficult, if not impossible, to exteriorize the testes. With

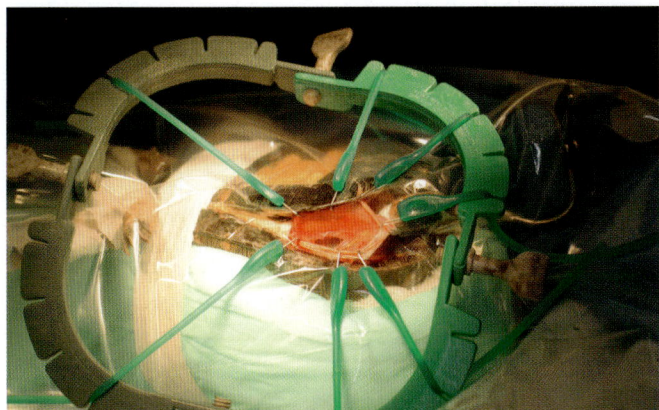

FIG 105.5 With the prefemoral approach to reproductive surgery in chelonians, the use of retractors such as the lone star retractor can help with exposure. (Courtesy of Stephen J. Divers.)

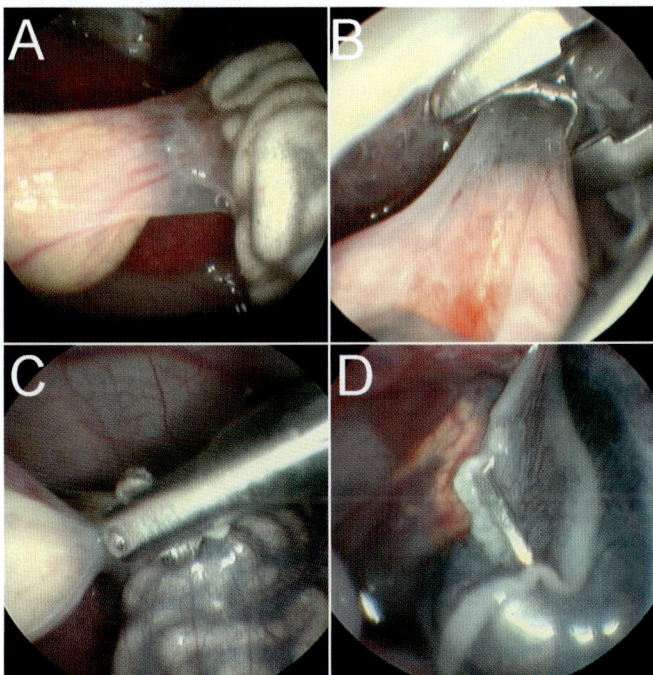

FIG 105.6 Endoscopic-assisted prefemoral orchiectomy in a slider (*Trachemys scripta*). (A) Testis is identified through the prefemoral incision and grasped with forceps or hemostats and gently manipulated up to the level of the prefemoral incision to allow visualization of the mesorchium and the testicular vessels. It is difficult, if not impossible, to exteriorize the testes. (B) The testis and mesorchium are stretched away from the associated epididymis and vascular clamp applied. (C) After ligation the mesorchium is transected with scissors or radiosurgery. (D) The mesorchium pedicle is observed for bleeding before closure. (Courtesy of Stephen J. Divers.)

the transplastron approach the testis is manipulated up toward the ventral plastronotomy incision, but again, the surgeon will generally have to work within the coelom. When the testis is globoid, a single vascular clip may be sufficient, otherwise windows are made in the mesorchium with iris scissors or a scalpel to allow ligation of vessels with multiple vascular clips, suture, or radiosurgery/laser (see Fig. 105.6B and C). Both testes are accessible from a transplastron coeliotomy. However, with a prefemoral approach, the contralateral testis can be difficult to identify and remove from the ipsilateral approach without endoscopy, and a second prefemoral coeliotomy incision is often necessary. The mesorchial pedicles are evaluated for bleeding before routine closure (see Fig. 105.6D and Chapters 99 and 100). Endoscopic-assisted prefemoral castration in chelonians (see Fig. 105.6 A–D) has been found to be effective, minimally invasive, and a preferred technique,[9,13,14,16,17] and complete endosurgery coelioscopic castration can also be performed in many chelonian species.[13,17] For details on these procedures, see Chapter 65.

Testicular Biopsy

In some situations, the collection of histopathologic and microbiologic samples from testes may be required to determine underlying disease or dysfunction/infertility. Indications for testis biopsy include neoplasia, orchitis (abscess, granuloma), and abnormal sperm production (infertility). In most reptiles, endoscopic testis evaluation and biopsy is effective, minimally invasive, and preferred to open surgical approaches (see Chapter 64). However, an open coeliotomy approach may be necessary if endoscopy equipment is unavailable or when evaluating the testes of snakes, which are inherently more challenging patients for coelioscopy.

Phallectomy and Hemipenal Amputation

Phallectomy has been utilized to control reproduction in chelonian conservation projects[10] and in green iguanas (*Iguana iguana*) (Mader DR, personal communication, 2014). It is a less invasive and safer procedure than castration and allows normal (testosterone-driven) social behaviors without insemination of females. Phallectomy (chelonians) and hemipenal amputation (snakes and lizards) are frequently performed procedures, as prolapses are common.[12] One important, unique consideration with reptile phallus surgery is, unlike mammals, amputation does not affect the urinary system, as these structures do not contain a urethra. Additionally, for squamates, the removal of one hemipenis will still allow copulation with the remaining hemipenis. See Chapters 75, 80, and 106 for medical management and indications for removal of the phallus or hemipenis. The anesthetized patient is usually placed in dorsal recumbency, and the phallus or hemipenis is aseptically prepared. Copulatory organs are vascular and transfixing sutures are required. For hemipenal amputation the hemipenis is clamped close to its base with a hemostat, and one or two absorbable monofilament transfixing sutures are placed proximal to the hemostat depending on the patient size (Fig. 105.7). When possible, the remaining tissue should be short enough to allow the sutured stump to recess into the caudal vent/hemipenal sulcus to avoid postoperative exposure trauma.[7,20] In chelonians, the phallus is retracted caudally and clamped at the base with a hemostat or tissue clamp and a minimum of two absorbable monofilament transfixing and encircling sutures are placed, each approximately halfway across the phallus (Fig. 105.8A).[2,3] In larger chelonians, the blood supply to each distinct longitudinal ridge (basically dividing the phallus in half longitudinally) must be identified and each body (corpus cavernosa) and blood supply individually clamped and double ligated with absorbable monofilament sutures.[2,10] Bleeding can be substantial if a vessel is damaged when placing a transfixing suture, and additional sutures may be required. Sutures should be placed close to the base for a good "hold" (but minimize leaving any functional

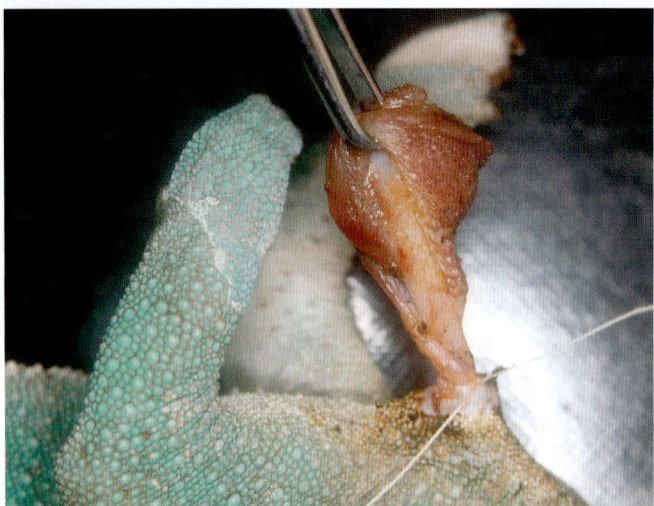

FIG 105.7 Amputation of a hemipenis in a panther chameleon (*Furcifer pardalis*). The hemipenis is ligated close to its base with one or two absorbable monofilament transfixing sutures. (Courtesy of Stephen J. Divers.)

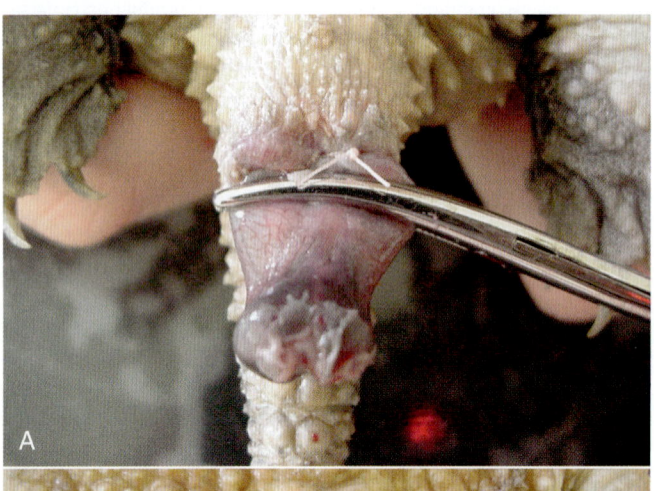

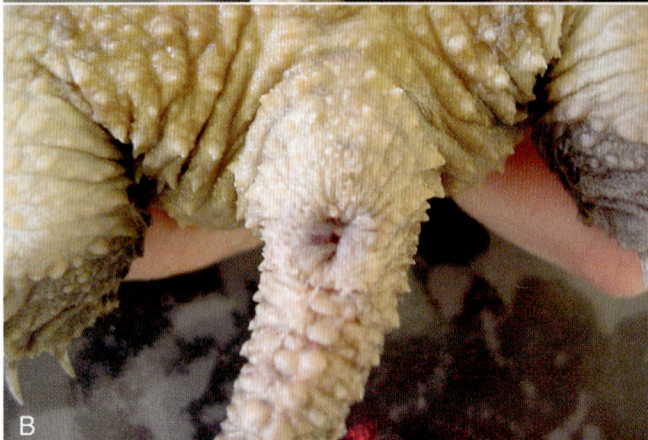

FIG 105.8 Amputation of the phallus in a snapping turtle (*Chelydra serpentina*). (A) The phallus has been retracted caudally and clamped at the base with a hemostat, and the first of two absorbable monofilament-transfixing and encircling sutures has been placed (approximately halfway across the phallus), and the procedure will be repeated on the other half, before phallus transection. (B) The turtle postamputation: the sutures are placed close to the base to ensure any remaining tissue will recess into the cloaca, avoiding postoperative exposure trauma. (Courtesy of Stephen J. Divers.)

phallus) and to ensure any remaining tissue will recess into the cloaca to avoid postoperative exposure trauma (see Fig. 105.8B). The remaining phallus stump can be closed with a simple continuous pattern using absorbable monofilament suture.[2,3,10]

FEMALE REPRODUCTIVE SURGERY

Ovariectomy/Ovariosalpingectomy

The most common indications for ovariectomy and ovariosalpingectomy in lizards, chelonians, and less commonly snakes is to manage reproductive follicular activity and dystocia, although neoplasia is possible.[2,3,14,15,21]

Preventative (elective) ovariectomy can be performed in lizard and chelonian species that are prone to reproductive-related issues.[2,4,5,19]

Lizards

Preventative/Elective and Postovulatory Ovariectomy. For ovariectomy in most lizards, a ventral coeliotomy (midline or paramedian) approach is recommended.[2,19] Once the coelom is entered, the ovaries are identified as paired (right ovary slightly cranial to the left) dorsal structures in the mid to caudal coelom, often just cranial to the kidneys. The paired coelomic fat pads, bladder (if present), and portions of the gastrointestinal tract may need to be retracted, exteriorized, protected, and kept moist. Exposure is improved with the use of retractors such as the lone star retractor. In cases of dystocia, the oviducts are filled with eggs or fetuses and need to be exteriorized and removed first (see Salpingectomy) to allow exposure of the ovaries. With a preventative (immature or seasonally inactive) ovariectomy (Fig. 105.9) or a postovulatory ovariectomy (Fig. 105.10A), the ovaries are generally small and appear as a small cluster of fluid-filled follicles located deep in the coelom. Each ovary is identified and, when possible, gently exteriorized through the incision to visualize the mesovarium and vessels. Often the mesovarium in these inactive ovaries is restrictive, and the ovary is fragile and cannot be exteriorized. The surgeon may have to work within the coelom, and the coeliotomy incision may need to be extended to ensure exposure. Important anatomical differences exist between the right and left ovaries in lizards (see Fig. 105.2).[1] The right ovary is attached directly to the vena cava with short vessels (1–2 mm), and the

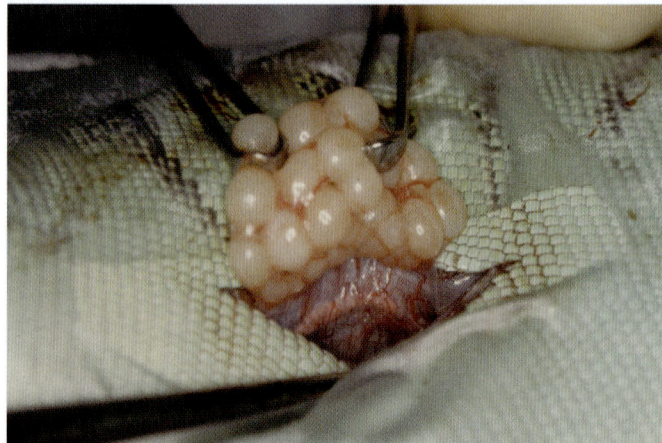

FIG 105.9 A seasonally inactive ovary in a green iguana (*Iguana iguana*); these ovaries are small, located deep in the coelom, and may be more difficult to exteriorize. This is the left ovary, as the adrenal gland (pink-tan elongated structure) is adjacent to the ovary and shares vascularity. Caution must be taken not to damage or accidently remove the adrenal gland when performing the ovariectomy (see Fig. 105.2). (Courtesy of Stephen J. Divers.)

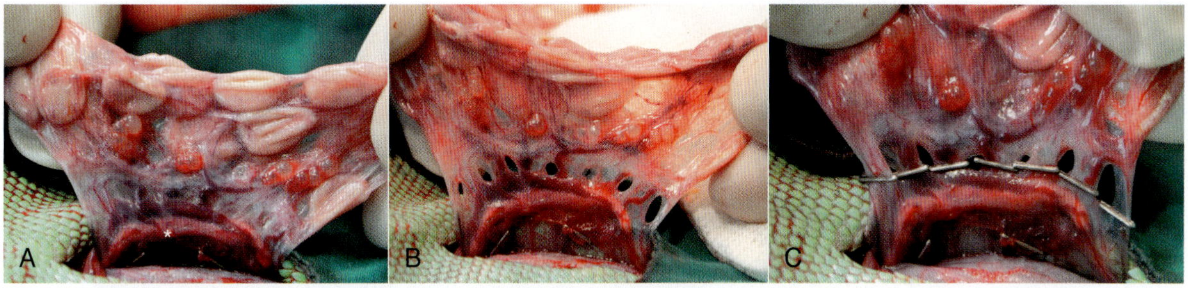

FIG 105.10 A postovulatory right ovary of a green iguana (*Iguana iguana*) exteriorized during ovariosalpingectomy. (A) The adrenal gland (pink-tan elongated structure, indicated by *) is located on the opposite side of the vena cava than the ovary. Note the recent ovulatory change to the ovary and the vascular clips below the adrenal gland, which are ligatures previously placed on the right oviduct vessels, as the oviduct (full of shelled eggs) was removed first to allow access to the ovary. (B) The vascular supply has been identified and small windows are made in the mesovarium between the ovarian vessels with iris scissors. (C) The vessels are ligated with vascular clips, which is easier and preferred; however, absorbable monofilament suture can be used alternatively. (Courtesy of Scott J. Stahl, Stahl Exotic Animal Veterinary Services.)

right adrenal gland is located on the *opposite* side of the vena cava (see Fig. 105.10A) and thus unlikely to be damaged at surgery due to its location. However, the left ovary has its own distinct ovarian artery and vein, and the adrenal gland is located *adjacent* to the left ovary, utilizing the same vessels (Fig. 105.9).[1] The elongated, pink-tan, granular adrenal gland must not be removed or damaged during ligation of the left ovary. Once each ovary is isolated, and proper exposure of the vascular supply is identified, small windows are made in the mesovarium between the ovarian vessels with iris scissors or a scalpel (see Fig. 105.10B), and the vessels are ligated with vascular clips (easier and recommended, see Fig. 105.10C) or absorbable monofilament suture (more difficult).

In some species (e.g., bearded dragons), the mesovarium may be heavily pigmented and the vasculature difficult to visualize for ligation and may obscure the adrenal tissue. Additionally, in bearded dragons the right liver lobe is closely associated with the vasculature of the right ovary, and the surgeon must avoid damaging the liver during ligation of the right ovarian vessels (Fig. 105.11). Magnification and focal lighting, along with microsurgical instruments, can be useful in these situations; however, these anatomical issues make ovariectomy less routine and more challenging in this species. After ligation, the ovarian pedicles are observed for any bleeding before routine closure of the coelom (see Fig. 105.4 and Chapter 98 for details).

For laterally compressed lizards, a lateral (flank) coeliotomy approach can be utilized (see Chapter 98). With this approach the small ovaries are easily identified upon entry, as they are typically positioned near the entry site (Fig. 105.12A and B). However, in cases of dystocia, the oviducts are filled with eggs/fetuses and must first be exteriorized and removed to allow access to the ovaries (see Fig. 105.12E and Salpingectomy). The ovariectomy technique is the same as described previously for the ventral coeliotomy, with careful ligation of the ovarian vessels within the mesovarium (see Fig. 105.12D). Both ovaries can often be removed from a single lateral incision unless there is compounding pathology.[2,19] Preventative ovariectomy (small involuted ovaries) of lizards can be performed endoscopically (see Chapter 65).

Ovariectomy (Preovulatory Follicular Stasis). The same approach is utilized for a preovulatory ovariectomy as described previously, except in these cases large ovulatory follicles are present. Following coelomic entry, the enlarged ovaries, which appear as a "grapelike" cluster of vitellogenic follicles, are obvious (Fig. 105.13A), although in lizards

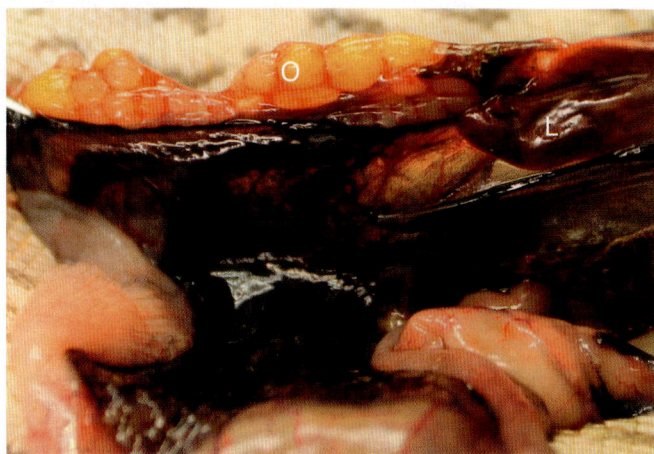

FIG 105.11 The right (inactive) ovary (O) of a bearded dragon (*Pogona vitticeps*). The mesovarium is often heavily pigmented in this species, and the vasculature difficult to visualize for ligation and may obscure the adrenal tissue. Additionally, the right liver (L) lobe is closely associated with the vasculature of the right ovary and must be avoided during ligation of the right ovarian vessels. (Courtesy of Scott J. Stahl, Stahl Exotic Animal Veterinary Services.)

such as geckos, which lay two eggs at a time, only a single static follicle may be present on each ovary (see Fig. 105.13B). The mesovarium is more elastic in these cases and will usually stretch to allow manipulation of the entire ovary out of the incision (see Figs. 105.12C and 105.13A and B). However, the ovary is often larger than the incision, and the follicles may be friable and begin to coalesce (especially if diseased) and can rupture with handling. Gentle manipulation and patience are required, and the coeliotomy incision may need to be extended to allow the entire ovary to be safely manipulated out. Once the ovary is isolated (usually one at a time due to the size), the vascular supply is identified and small windows are made in the mesovarium between the ovarian vessels with iris scissors or a scalpel, and the vessels are ligated with vascular clips or absorbable monofilament suture (Fig. 105.14). Particularly large vessels can be double ligated. The ovary is transected from its mesovarial attachments and removed. The process is repeated for the second ovary. If normal in appearance, the oviducts can be left

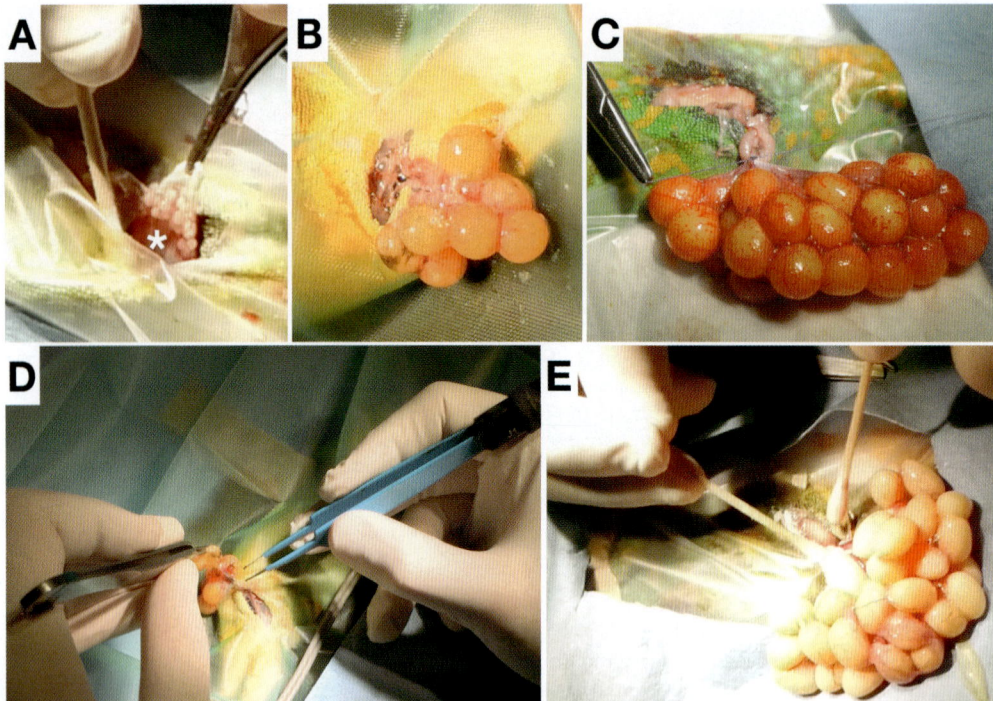

FIG 105.12 Lateral (flank) approach to reproductive surgery in the veiled chameleon (*Chameleo calyptratus*). (A) Identification and exposure of an inactive ovary (preventative ovariectomy) through the lateral approach; the asterisk indicates the mesovarium. These inactive/immature ovaries are more difficult to exteriorize and ligate. (B) A more active ovary with easier exposure through the flank incision. (C) Preovulatory ovary with many large ovulatory ova; the entire ovary is more easily manipulated out of the incision. (D) Use of radiosurgery to transect ovarian vessels after ligation. (E) Postovulatory dystocia surgery with oviduct, filled with shelled ova, manipulated out of lateral incision for removal en bloc, followed by ovariectomy. (Courtesy of Nicola Di Girolamo.)

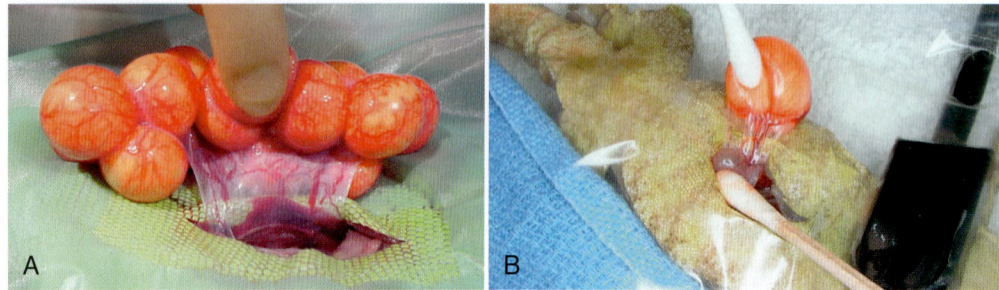

FIG 105.13 A preovulatory ovariectomy involves removing enlarged ovaries with vitellogenic, often static follicles. With this ovarian activity the mesovarium is more elastic and will usually stretch to allow manipulation of the entire ovary out of the incision. (A) A preovulatory ovary in a green iguana (*Iguana iguana*) exteriorized to allow visualization of vessels for ligation. (Courtesy of Stephen J. Divers). (B) A preovulatory ovary in a mossy gecko (*Mniarogekko chahoua*) with one static follicle on the exteriorized ovary. (Courtesy of Scott J. Stahl, Stahl Exotic Animal Veterinary Services.)

in situ. Also, if any ovarian remnant remains, the oviducts can prevent egg yolk coelomitis. This is a legitimate concern, especially in species such as bearded dragons in which the mesovaria are short and pigmented and the liver is closely associated with the right ovarian vasculature. It can be difficult to be certain that all the ovarian tissue is removed in this species, and clients should be warned of this possibility.

Salpingectomy. A salpingectomy is the first procedure performed in cases of surgical dystocia, and upon entry into the coelom the oviducts filled with eggs or fetuses will usually be the first structures identified. The oviducts are paired and found adjacent to the ovaries, and when full of eggs/fetuses, they may occupy most of the saurian coelom. The paired coelomic fat pads, bladder (if present), and portions of the gastrointestinal tract may need to be retracted, exteriorized, protected, and kept moist. Exposure of the oviducts is improved with the use of retractors. Once identified, the oviducts are gently exteriorized from the cranial (fimbria) to caudal (junction with urodeum) to allow visualization of the vascular supply (see Fig. 105.12E). The fimbria is identified, clamped with a hemostat, and ligated with absorbable monofilament suture or vascular clips and transected. In many cases, the fimbria is thin and poorly vascular, and radiosurgical/laser dissection (without ligation) may be all that is required. Starting cranially and

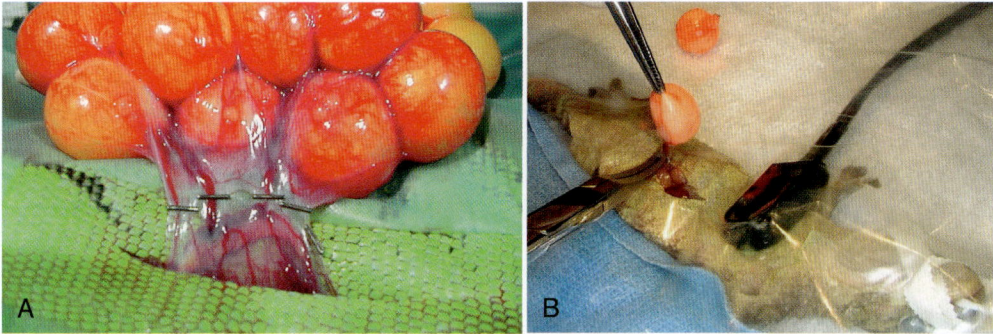

FIG 105.14 (A) In this green iguana (*Iguana iguana*) one ovary has been exteriorized, and small windows have been made in the mesovarium between the ovarian vessels and the vessels ligated with vascular clips. (B) Ligation of ovarian vessels in a mossy gecko (*Mniarogekko chahoua*) with vascular clips. (A, Courtesy of Stephen J. Divers; B, courtesy of Scott J. Stahl, Stahl Exotic Animal Veterinary Services.)

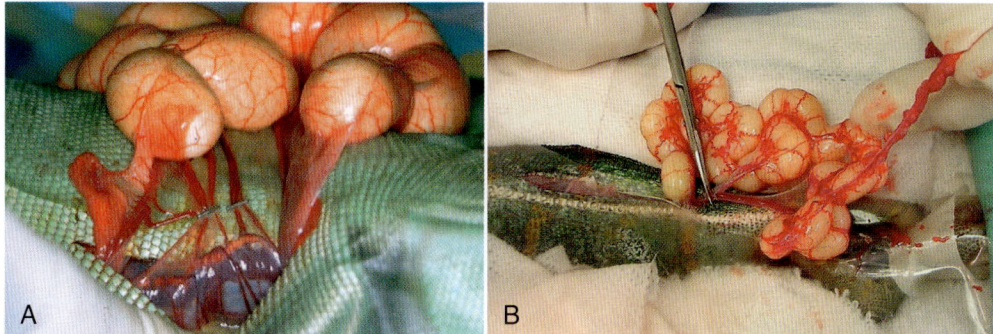

FIG 105.15 Once identified, the oviducts are gently exteriorized from cranial (fimbria) to caudal (junction with urodeum) to allow visualization of the vascular supply. (A) In this green iguana (*Iguana iguana*) small windows have been made in the mesosalpinx (cranial to the left) to ligate vessels in groups using vascular clips prior to transection. (Courtesy of Stephen J. Divers). (B) In this veiled chameleon (*Chameleo calyptratus*), a paramedian approach to the coelom has been performed and the fimbria and vessels of the mesosalpinx (cranial to the left) have been ligated. The distal oviduct is then ligated at its junction with the urodeum with vascular clips before transection. (Courtesy of Scott J. Stahl, Stahl Exotic Animal Veterinary Services.)

working caudally, small windows are made in the fanned out mesosalpinx to ligate vessels individually or in groups using vascular clips, absorbable monofilament suture, or radiosurgery/laser (Fig. 105.15A). Before ligation of the distal oviduct, the pelvic inlet should be checked to ensure no eggs are present. The distal oviduct is then clamped with a hemostat at its juncture with the urodeum, double-ligated with circumferential and transfixing absorbable monofilament sutures or vascular clips (see Fig. 105.15B), and transected, allowing the entire oviduct and contained structures to be removed en bloc (Fig. 105.16). This procedure is repeated on the opposite oviduct. Following the removal of both oviducts, ovariectomy is performed as described previously (see Fig. 105.16). Failure to completely remove both ovaries will result in fatal yolk coelomitis if the lizard ovulates in the future (see Yolk Coelomitis, Ectopic Follicles/Eggs later in this chapter and chapter 80).

Salpingotomy. If a lizard is presented with a dystocia, and maintaining future breeding capability is important, then salpingotomy is recommended. Following identification and exteriorization of the oviducts, the number and location of the retained eggs/fetuses are evaluated and the site for the initial incision can be determined (Fig. 105.17). To improve future reproductive success, trauma to the oviduct must be minimized, and the initial incision is made longitudinally along the

antemesenteric border with a scalpel blade to ensure primary intention healing. The location of the incision should be strategically determined to allow the removal of as many eggs/fetuses as possible through the same incision. Diagnostic samples including oviductal biopsy for histopathology and microbiology can be collected at this time. If necessary, the incision can be extended with a scalpel or iris scissors. Often with dystocia there are fibrin adhesions and secondary inflammation inhibiting the eggs/fetuses from moving freely through the oviduct. If the eggs/fetuses are adhered to the mucosa, the oviduct can be isolated with moistened lap sponges, and warm saline infused into the lumen. The saline, along with gentle manipulation, may allow more eggs/fetuses to be freed and increase the number that can be manipulated out of a single incision.[5] Nevertheless, several incisions may be required to successfully remove all eggs/fetuses. Before closing the oviduct, the pelvic inlet should be checked to ensure no eggs are present. The oviduct incisions are closed with a simple continuous or inverting pattern using fine monofilament absorbable suture. The coelom is lavaged with warm sterile saline and routinely closed (see Chapter 98 for closure).

Snakes
Ovariectomy. Indications for ovariectomy and ovariosalpingectomy are less common in snakes but are often related to damage to the salpinx

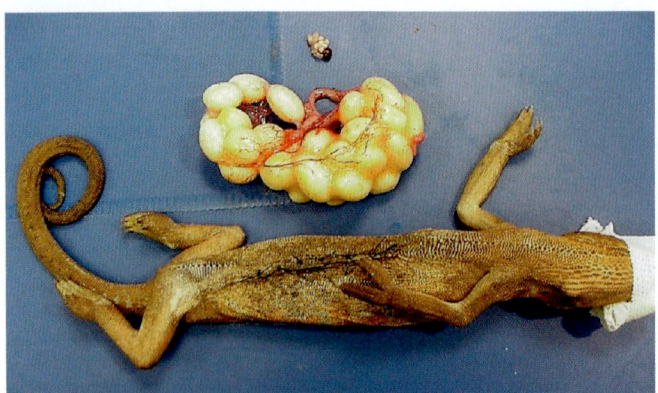

FIG 105.16 A panther chameleon (*Furcifer pardalis*) recovering from ovariosalpingectomy surgery. The chameleon presented with dystocia, and at surgery only one oviduct was involved; a unilateral procedure was performed, as the owner wanted her to remain reproductively viable. Note the abnormal "mass" of retained eggs in the oviduct, which was removed en bloc, and the small (postovulatory) ipsilateral ovary (above oviduct) that was removed as well. (Courtesy of Scott J. Stahl, Stahl Exotic Animal Veterinary Services.)

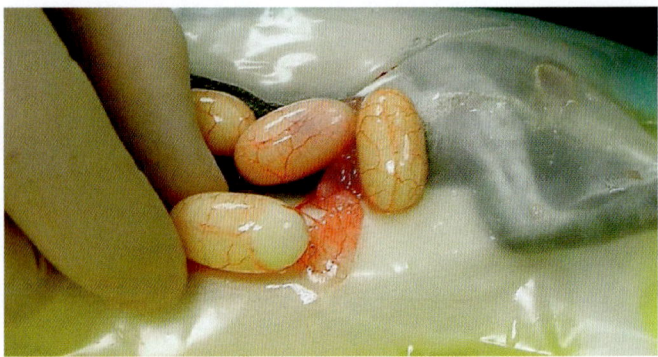

FIG 105.17 Following identification and exteriorization of the oviducts, the number and location of the retained eggs/fetuses are evaluated and the initial incision can be determined. An incision has been made in the oviduct of this panther chameleon (*Furcifer pardalis*), and the eggs are gently manipulated out. (Courtesy of Scott J. Stahl, Stahl Exotic Animal Veterinary Services.)

via prolapse or an obstructive dystocia.[2,7] In these cases, if the oviduct cannot be repaired, the ipsilateral ovary must be removed along with the diseased or damaged oviduct (see Salpingectomy later in this chapter).

For ovariectomy or ovariosalpingectomy in snakes, a ventrolateral coeliotomy approach is recommended (see Chapter 97). McCracken reported the ovaries in most species of snake to be in the 60% to 80% snout-to-vent (SVL) position.[22] However, variation will occur depending on ovarian activity, with folliculogenesis resulting in a larger ovary. Ultrasonography can be useful in locating the ovaries, as follicles are generally easily identified as anechoic to hypoechoic ovoid structures, and this can help determine the incision site. A single long incision or multiple smaller incisions may be necessary to ensure exposure of both ovaries in snakes. Once the coelom has been entered, the ovaries are identified as elongated structures appearing as a string of ovoid, fluid- or yolk-filled structures (follicles) varying in size and color depending on cycle and species of snake. However, there may be several fascial layers to breach in order to obtain direct access to the ovaries. Stay sutures can be used to help identify the layers for eventual closure of the coelom. The staggered, overlapping ovaries (right cranial to left) are found dorsally, with the most cranial portion of the right ovary starting just distal to the gallbladder and the most caudal portion of the left ovary ending just cranial to the kidneys.[1] Unfortunately, because of this elongated morphology and staggered positioning, the surgical exposure necessary to remove both ovaries is extensive. Also, coelomic organs in snakes are more intimately connected by multiple fascial membranes, making exposure challenging. In addition, the saccular lung (air sac) often extends into the reproductive surgical field. Therefore, given these difficulties, ovariectomy is not considered a routine preventative procedure in snakes.

The use of retractors can help with exposure. The ovary is fragile and must be handled gently; however, the mesovarium will usually stretch and allow exteriorization of the ovary (Fig. 105.18A). Once exteriorized and the vascular supply is exposed, small windows are made in the mesovarium between the ovarian vessels with iris scissors or a scalpel blade (see Fig. 105.18B), and the vessels are ligated with vascular clips or absorbable monofilament suture. If the oviducts are unaffected, they can be left in place (see Fig. 105.18C), and closure is routine (see Fig. 105.18D and Chapter 97).

Salpingectomy. Indications for salpingectomy are often related to damage to the salpinx via prolapse or an obstructive dystocia. In these cases, if the diseased or damaged oviduct cannot be repaired and must be removed (Fig. 105.19 A and B), then the ipsilateral ovary must also be removed to avoid ectopic follicles and yolk coelomitis (see Ovariectomy previously).

The coelomic approach is often clearly dictated by coelomic distention. Upon entry into the coelom (see Chapter 97), the oviduct(s) filled with eggs/fetuses are the first structures identified. However, there may be several fascial layers to navigate before achieving direct access to the oviducts. Stay sutures can be used to help identify the layers for eventual closure of the coelom. The oviducts are paired and found adjacent and caudal to their respective ovaries. The affected oviduct should be exteriorized, utilizing the retained eggs/fetuses as a guide. Retractors such as the lone star can help with exposure. It can be challenging to determine which oviduct is involved upon initial entry, which is critical because the ipsilateral ovary must be removed. To expose the entire "affected" oviduct and its ipsilateral ovary, a long incision or multiple smaller incisions may be necessary. Exposed tissues that are to be retained should be protected with moistened lap sponges. Once identified, the affected oviduct is gently exteriorized from cranial (fimbria) to caudal (junction with urodeum) to allow visualization of the vascular supply (see Fig. 105.19A and B). The fimbria is identified and transected as previously described. Working caudally, the mesosalpinx is exposed, vessels ligated, and the mesosalphinx transected, as previously described. The distal oviduct is then clamped with a hemostat, as close to the urodeum as possible, double ligated, and transected. In the case of a prolapsed portion of oviduct, the prolapse may have to be retracted back into the coelom to allow proper ligation and removal. Following removal of the damaged oviduct, the ipsilateral ovary must be removed as described previously (see Fig. 105.19C). The same procedure is performed on the contralateral oviduct and ovary if necessary and is performed through the same incision, although extension may be required. Follicles, eggs and fetuses may be ectopic, and there may be an associated coelomitis from oviduct damage or prolapse. In such cases, warm saline lavage is required before routine closure (see Chapter 97).

Salpingotomy. If a snake is presented with a dystocia involving eggs/fetuses retained in the oviduct(s), and maintaining its ability to

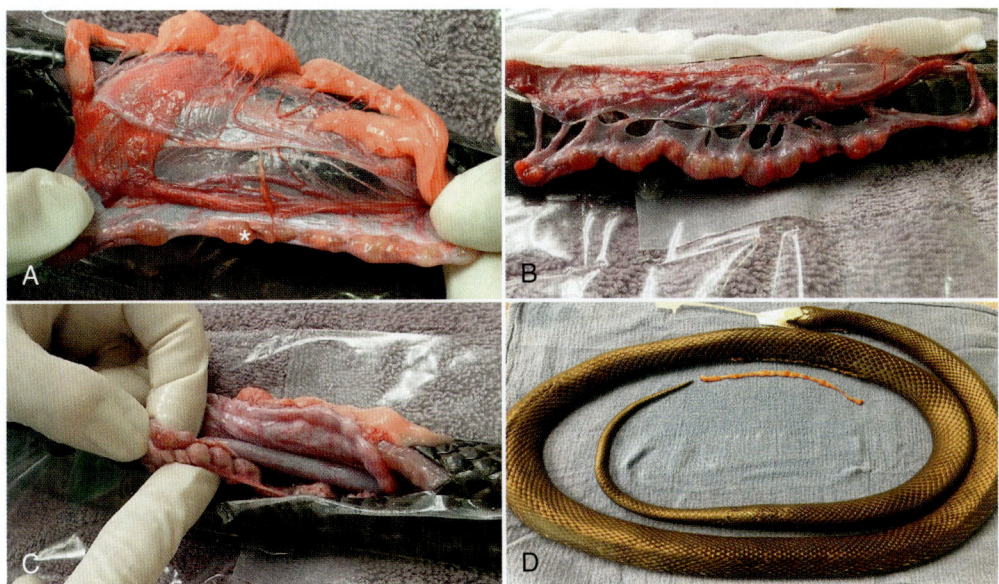

FIG 105.18 Snake ovariectomy. (A) The mesovarium will usually stretch and allow exteriorization of the ovary (*), as with the ovary of this black rat snake (*Pantherophis obsoleta*). (B) Once the ovary was exteriorized (in the same snake), small windows were made in the mesovarium between the ovarian vessels with iris scissors, and the vessels were ligated with vascular clips. In this case one entire oviduct had prolapsed and the ipsilateral ovary was removed. (C) The contralateral ovary (at top) and oviduct (above finger) were inspected and left in place to maintain reproductive potential. (D) The snake on recovery showing unilateral ovariectomy skin incision and removed ovary. This snake went on to lay a clutch of normal eggs from the remaining ovary and oviduct the following year. (Courtesy of Scott J. Stahl, Stahl Exotic Animal Veterinary Services.)

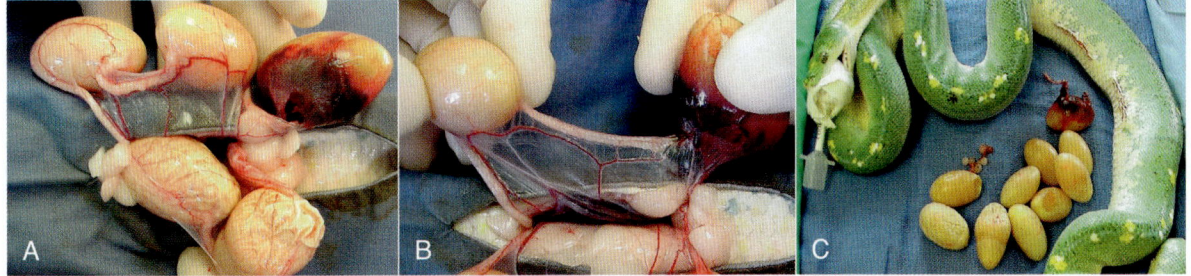

FIG 105.19 Indications for salpingectomy are often related to damage to the salpinx via prolapse or an obstructive dystocia. (A) A green tree python (*Morelia viridis*) presented for a chronic dystocia, and surgery revealed one oviduct had ruptured and was severely damaged. (B) Unfortunately, oxytocin had been inappropriately used in this case and may have contributed to the oviduct torsion and rupture. A unilateral procedure was performed (the other oviduct was empty and normal) to keep the female reproductive. The damaged oviduct, retained eggs, and ipsilateral ovary were removed. (C) The female during recovery; note two incisions necessary to remove the entire ovary and oviduct. (Courtesy of Scott J. Stahl, Stahl Exotic Animal Veterinary Services.)

breed in the future is important, salpingotomy is often recommended (Fig. 105.20).

Upon entry into the coelom (see Chapter 97), the oviduct(s) filled with eggs/fetuses are the first structures identified. However, there may be several layers of coelomic membranes to incise to expose the oviduct. Stay sutures can be used to help identify the layers for eventual closure of the coelom. A portion of the oviduct should be exteriorized utilizing the retained eggs/fetuses as a guide to finding the affected section of oviduct (see Fig. 105.20A). The use of retractors such as the lone star retractor can help with exposure. Once the condition of the oviduct and the number and location of the retained eggs/fetuses are evaluated, the location for

the initial oviduct incision can be determined. To improve future reproductive success, the surgeon's goal is to minimize trauma to the oviduct.

The initial incision is made in a nonvascular area of the oviduct with a scalpel in a strategic location, which allows the removal of as many eggs/fetuses as possible through the same incision. Diagnostic samples including oviductal biopsy, culture and sensitivity, and PCR swabs can be collected at initial entry. The incision is then extended as necessary with iris scissors or scalpel, and the eggs/fetuses are gently manipulated out of the oviduct (see Fig. 105.20B). Often with dystocia there are fibrin adhesions and secondary inflammation that may inhibit the eggs from moving freely in the oviduct.

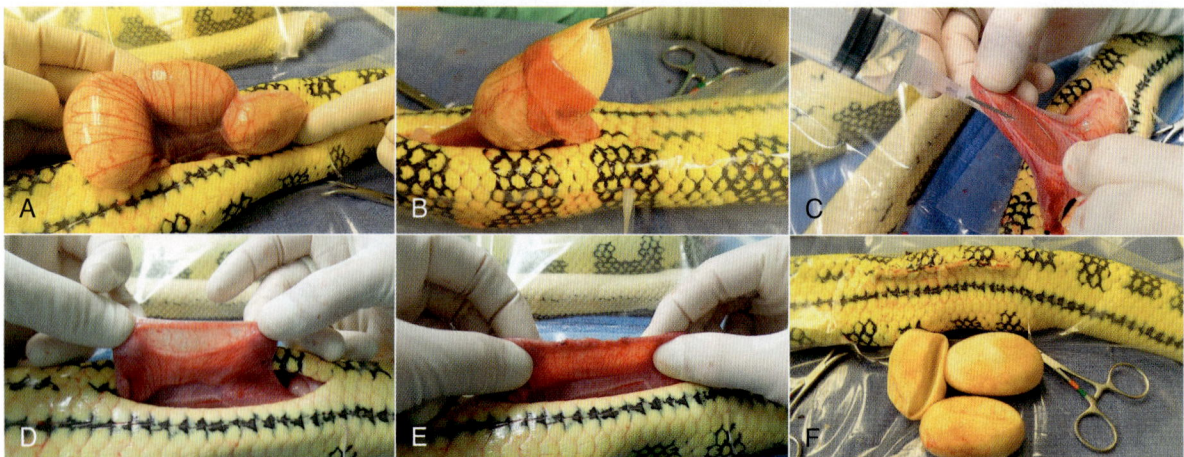

FIG 105.20 If a snake is presented for dystocia, and maintaining its ability to breed in the future is important, salpingotomy is often recommended. A jungle carpet python (*Morelia spilota cheynei*) was presented for dystocia several weeks after laying most of her clutch. (A) Upon surgical entry into the coelom, directed by the presence of retained eggs, one oviduct containing three eggs was identified. (B) The initial incision was made in a nonvascular area of the oviduct, and the first egg was manipulated out. Due to the chronicity of the egg retention, fibrin adhesions were present, and the egg was difficult to detach from the oviduct mucosa (note the thickened, inflamed oviduct). (C) Once the first egg was removed, warm saline was infused into the oviduct lumen, and the saline, along with gentle manipulation, allowed the other two eggs to be manipulated through the same incision. (D) The oviduct after egg removal and (E) after closure with a simple continuous pattern. (F) The coelom was lavaged with warm saline and routinely closed. (Courtesy of Scott J. Stahl, Stahl Exotic Animal Veterinary Services.)

If the eggs/fetuses are adhered to the oviduct mucosa, the oviduct can be isolated with moistened lap sponges and warm saline infused into the lumen (see Fig. 105.20C). The saline, along with gentle manipulation, may allow the eggs/fetuses to move and therefore increase the number that can be manipulated out of the oviduct incision (see Fig. 105.20D).[7] However, often several incisions may need to be made in each oviduct to successfully remove all the eggs/fetuses. The oviduct incisions are closed with a simple continuous or inverting pattern using fine monofilament absorbable suture (see Fig. 105.20E). The coelom is lavaged with warm saline and then routinely closed (see Fig. 105.20F and Chapter 97).

Chelonians

Ovariectomy. The least invasive and thus preferred technique for ovariectomy in chelonians is the prefemoral approach instead of the more traditional ventral transplastron approach.[2,4,8,14–16] The ovaries in most chelonians are accessible from a prefemoral approach (especially with endoscopic assistance), and the trauma of cutting through plastron bone can be avoided. In some species the prefemoral fossa is too restrictive, and there may be situations (such as an obstructive dystocia involving many retained eggs, yolk coelomitis, ovarian neoplasia, cystic calculus) where a transplastron coeliotomy is necessary.[2,3,14] For details on celiotomy approaches in chelonians, see Chapters 99 and 100.

Once the coelom has been safely entered, the bladder, intestinal tract, and lungs may need to be gently manipulated to allow access to the ovaries. The ovaries are paired and found dorsally in the mid to caudal coelom cranial to the kidneys. With the prefemoral approach, the use of retractors such as the lone star retractor can help with exposure (see Fig. 105.5). The ovary is identified, and the interfollicular tissue is grasped with atraumatic forceps and gently manipulated to the prefemoral incision. The ovary is gently teased out of the incision to allow visualization of the mesovarium and ovarian vessels (Fig. 105.21A and B). Vascular clips or absorbable monofilament suture is used to ligate the vessels

before transecting distally and removing the ovary. Once the ipsilateral organ has been removed, the contralateral ovary can often be exteriorized through the same incision. However, if this is not possible, a second prefemoral coeliotomy incision (on the contralateral side) will be necessary.[5,8,14–16] With the transplastron approach, the ovary is manipulated up and out of the plastronotomy whenever possible, or the surgeon may have to work within the coelom.[2,3] Both ovaries are accessible from a transplastron coeliotomy, and each ovary is isolated and removed as described previously (Fig. 105.22). The vascular pedicles are evaluated for bleeding before lavage and routine closure of the coelom (see Chapters 99 and 100 on celiotomy closure in chelonians).

Endoscopic-assisted prefemoral ovariectomy in chelonians is effective, minimally invasive and therefore preferred,[10,13–15] and complete endosurgery coelioscopic ovariectomy can also be performed in many species.[13,14] For details on these procedures, see Chapter 65.

Salpingectomy. Indications for salpingectomy in chelonians are often related to damage to the salpinx via prolapse or an obstructive dystocia. Exploratory surgery is indicated with oviductal prolapse. If attempts to replace and repair the oviduct intracoelomically are not possible, the prolapsed portion is no longer viable, or the salpinx has associated pathology (salpingitis or neoplasia), then salpingectomy with ipsilateral ovariectomy are indicated. A transplastron coeliotomy is recommended with an obstructive dystocia involving many eggs, yolk coelomitis, or with other concurrent coelomic issues (e.g., calculus or egg in the bladder), as this approach allows a more thorough evaluation of the coelom.[2,3] Upon entry into the coelom, the oviduct(s) filled with eggs are often obvious; however, the use of retractors can help with exposure. The oviducts are paired and found adjacent to the ovaries. Once identified, the affected oviduct is gently exteriorized from cranial (fimbria) to the caudal (junction with urodeum) to allow visualization of the vascular supply (Fig. 105.23). The fimbria is identified, clamped with a hemostat, and ligated with absorbable monofilament suture or vascular clips, or,

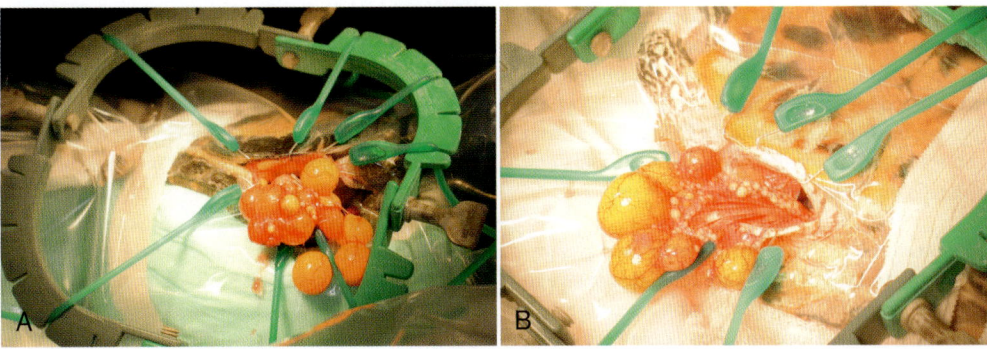

FIG 105.21 The least invasive and thus preferred technique for ovariectomy in chelonians is the prefemoral approach. (A) A lone star retractor was utilized in this tortoise to allow prefemoral access and the ovary identified, the interfollicular tissue grasped with atraumatic forceps, and the ovary gently manipulated out of the incision. (B) In this aquatic turtle the ovary has been gently teased out of the incision to allow visualization of the mesovarium and ovarian vessels. The vessels are then ligated with vascular clips before transecting distally and removing the ovary. (Courtesy of Stephen J. Divers.)

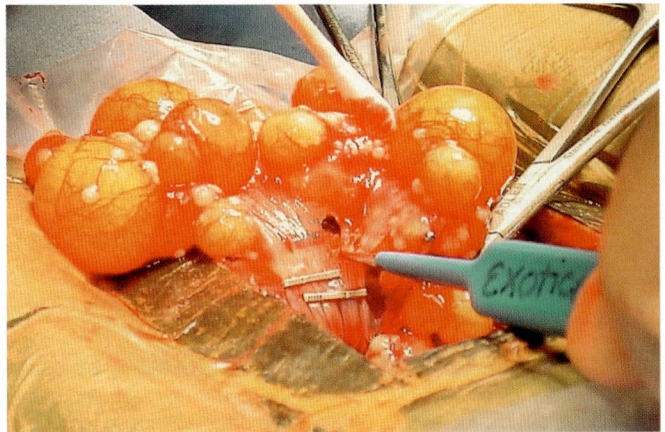

FIG 105.22 With the transplastron approach, the ovary is manipulated up and out of the plastronotomy whenever possible. In this tortoise the ovary has been exteriorized and the ovarian vessels ligated with vascular clips, and the vessels transected with radiosurgery. (Courtesy of Stephen J. Divers.)

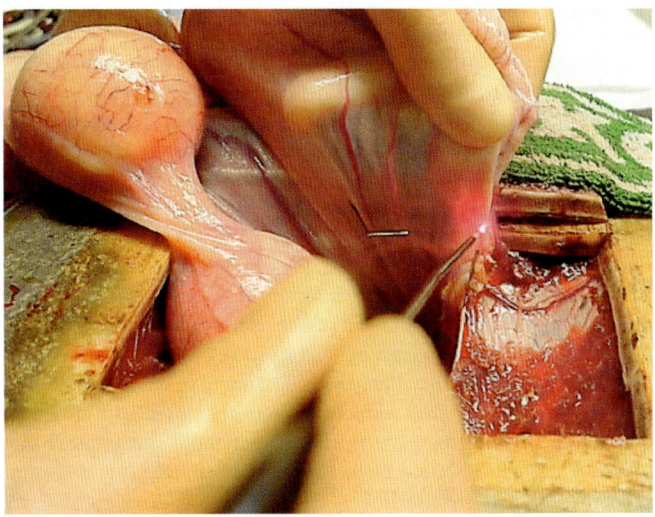

FIG 105.24 A transplastron approach to the coelom in this dystocic tortoise was performed and the mesosalpinx was fanned out to allow windows to be made in the mesosalpinx and vessels were ligated with vascular clips. The vessels were then transected with a diode laser and the oviduct removed en bloc. (Courtesy of Stephen J. Divers.)

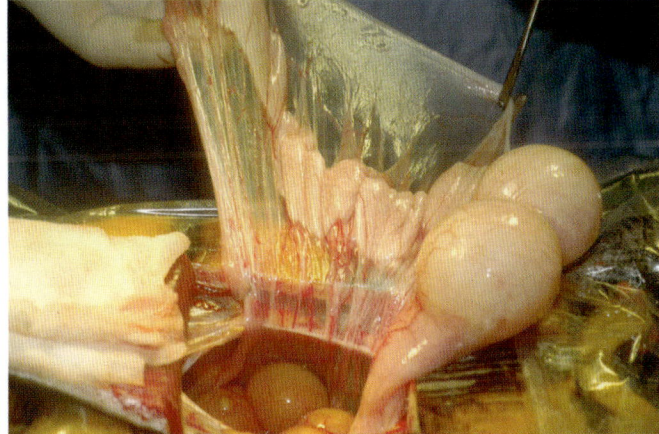

FIG 105.23 A transplastron approach was performed in this dystocic tortoise. The affected oviduct was gently exteriorized, from cranial to the caudal, to allow visualization of the vascular supply for ligation. (Courtesy of Douglas R. Mader.)

if thin and largely avascular, radiosurgery or laser transection is sufficient. Working caudally, the mesosalpinx is fanned out and windows are made in the mesosalpinx to ligate vessels individually or in groups using vascular clips or absorbable suture (Fig. 105.24). Before ligation of the distal oviduct, the pelvic inlet should be checked to ensure no eggs are present. The more substantive distal oviduct is then clamped with a hemostat at its juncture with the urodeum and double ligated with a circumferential and transfixing absorbable suture before being transected to allow en bloc removal. This procedure can be repeated with the opposite oviduct unless unilateral reproductive function is to be maintained. An ovariectomy must be performed on any side where the oviduct is removed or is no longer functional.

In the case of a prolapsed oviduct, the prolapse may have to be "retracted back" into the coelom to allow proper ligation and removal of the oviduct at the level of the urodeum. Following removal of the damaged oviduct, the ipsilateral ovary is removed as previously described.

Often eggs may be ectopic and there may be an associated coelomitis from oviductal damage or prolapse, and warm saline lavage should be considered before routine closure. An endoscopic-assisted prefemoral coeliotomy could be considered for salpingectomy in chelonians where few or no oviductal eggs are involved or the oviduct has prolapsed, and the goal is to perform an ipsilateral (to the damaged oviduct) or bilateral ovariectomy.[3,14,23] For details on these procedures, see Chapter 65.

Salpingotomy.

Salpingotomy procedures are not performed as commonly in chelonians, as unobstructed dystocias are often responsive to medical management with oxytocin.[3] A transplastron coeliotomy is recommended with an obstructive dystocia involving many eggs, yolk coelomitis, ectopic follicles/eggs, or if other concurrent coelomic issues are diagnosed, as this approach allows a more thorough evaluation of the coelom.[2,3]

In addition, unless future reproductive activity is desired, permanent resolution by ovariosalpingectomy is preferred. The coelom is entered, and the oviducts identified and exteriorized as previously described (see Fig. 105.23). Once the condition of the oviduct, and the number and location of the retained eggs have been evaluated, the location for the initial oviduct incision can be determined. To minimize damage and scarring, the initial incision is made longitudinally along the antemesenteric border with a scalpel in a strategic location, which allows the removal of as many eggs as possible through the same incision. Diagnostic samples can be collected, including biopsy following the initial entry. The incision is then extended as necessary with a scalpel or iris scissors (Fig. 105.25), and the eggs are gently manipulated from the oviduct. Often with dystocia there are fibrin adhesions and secondary inflammation inhibiting the eggs from moving freely in the oviduct. If the eggs are adhered to the mucosa, then packing of the oviduct with lap sponges and utilizing saline infusion in the oviduct can help as previously described for lizards and snakes.[7] Nevertheless, several incisions may need to be made in each oviduct to successfully remove all eggs. Before closing the oviduct, the pelvic inlet should be checked to ensure no eggs are present. The oviduct incisions are closed with a simple continuous or inverting pattern using fine monofilament absorbable suture. The coelom should be lavaged with warm saline, and closure is routine (see Chapter 100).

A prefemoral coeliotomy approach (see Chapter 99) could be considered for salpingotomy in chelonians, where just a few eggs are involved (preferably all in one oviduct).[3,13,14,23] This approach may not be possible depending on the female's size and conformation. The use of retractors can help with exposure in the prefemoral area (see Fig. 105.5). An endoscopic-assisted approach is preferred, as the endoscope is used to identify and, with the help of forceps or a spay hook, retrieve the affected oviduct and monitor its manipulation toward the incision. If an endoscope is not available, the use of a spay hook or small spoon in combination with tilting the chelonian patient may allow retrieval of the oviduct.[2,3,23] Once a portion of the oviduct is manipulated out of the incision, it can be used for traction. Stay sutures can be placed in the oviduct, and it is packed off with moistened lap sponges. The portion of the oviduct with retained eggs may be too large to pass through the incision (which is limited by the carapace and plastron).

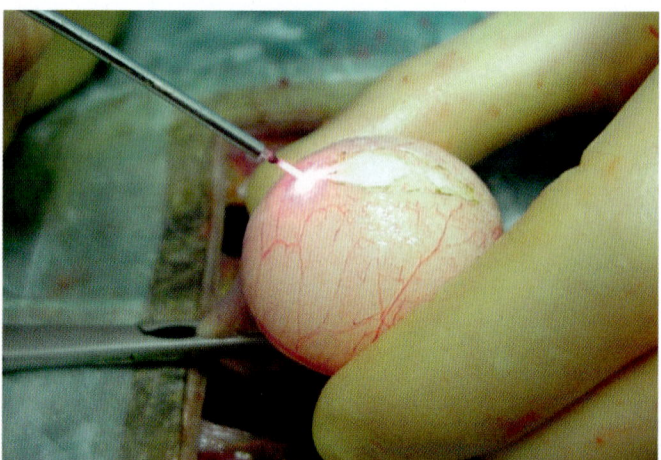

FIG 105.25 Salpingotomy procedures are performed less commonly in chelonians, as dystocias (unobstructed) are often responsive to medical management with oxytocin. After a transplastron coelomic approach in this dystocic tortoise, an incision was made in the oviduct with a diode laser to remove a chronically retained egg. In general, a scalpel salpingotomy incision is preferred over any other surgical device in order to minimize collateral damage and scarring. (Courtesy of Stephen J. Divers.)

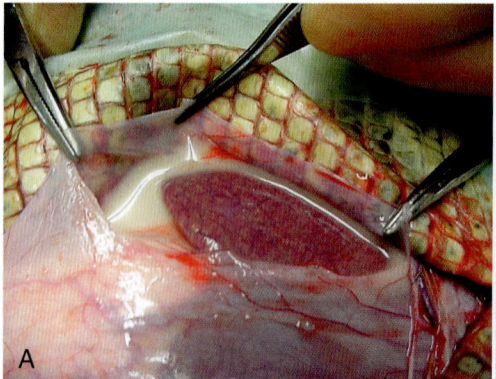 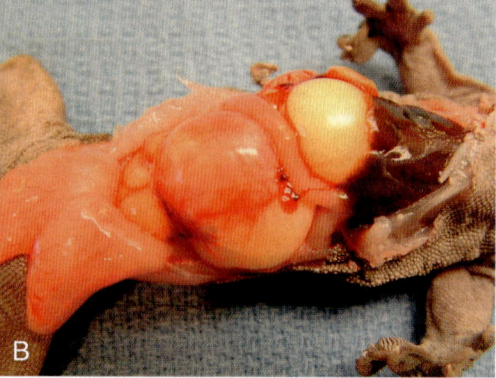

FIG 105.26 (A) A savanna monitor (*Varanus exanthematicus*) with severe yolk coelomitis evident upon entry into the coelom. (B) A crested gecko (*Correlophus cilliatus*) with yolk coelomitis associated with chronic follicular stasis. This species usually only produces one vitellogenic follicle at a time on each ovary, so the change is quite dramatic. The author has seen this condition in several geriatric female crested geckos, and it may be an age-related condition. (A, Courtesy of Stephen J. Divers; B, courtesy of Scott J. Stahl, Stahl Exotic Animal Veterinary Services.)

In such cases, the egg(s) can be aspirated and collapsed following oviductal incision. Again, diagnostic samples can be collected at this initial entry. The process is repeated one by one until all the eggs have been removed. Before closing the oviduct, the pelvic inlet should be checked to ensure no eggs are present. The oviduct is then gently flushed and closed with a simple continuous or inverting suture pattern using fine monofilament absorbable suture. The oviduct is lavaged with sterile saline before being gently returned to the coelom. If the dystocia is bilateral, an endoscope can be used to find and attempt to manipulate the contralateral oviduct toward the same prefemoral incision. If the contralateral oviduct cannot be accessed or manipulated, a second prefemoral approach on the opposite side may be required.[2–4,13,14,23] The coelom is checked for any ectopic eggs or yolk leakage, gently lavaged, and closed routinely (see Chapter 99).

Yolk Coelomitis and Ectopic Follicles/Eggs

Yolk coelomitis is not an uncommon sequela to reproductive disease in females (see Chapter 80 for more details). It is important to thoroughly evaluate the coelom during any reproductive procedure to ensure that such pathology is not missed. Diagnostic samples for histopathology (or cytology) and microbiology should be taken before the coelom is copiously and repeatedly lavaged with warm sterile saline to remove as much yolk material as possible (Fig. 105.26A and B).[5] In more chronic cases, a fibrinlike yolk material may be adhered to serosal surfaces and will require gentle debridement. A gram stain can be performed to help direct immediate antimicrobial treatment and subsequently adjusted based on future sensitivity results.

Ovarian Biopsy

In some situations, the collection of histopathologic and microbiologic samples from ovaries may be required to determine underlying disease or dysfunction/infertility. Indications for ovarian biopsy include neoplasia, oophoritis (abscess, granuloma), and infertility. In most reptiles endoscopic ovarian evaluation and biopsy/aspiration is effective, minimally invasive, and preferred to open surgical approaches (see Chapter 64). However, an open coeliotomy approach may be necessary if endoscopy equipment is unavailable or when evaluating the ovaries of snakes, which are inherently more challenging for coelioscopy.

REFERENCES

See www.expertconsult.com for a complete list of references.

Cloacal Prolapse

Stuart McArthur and Ross A. Machin

Effective treatment of all cloacal prolapses involves a simultaneous balance of medical and surgical interventions. The presentation therefore draws upon many of the techniques described across the clinical disciplines.

Information to assist a clinician faced with a cloacal prolapse in a reptile patient is available in several sections of this book; surgical management is covered here and throughout Section 10. Medical management of a cloacal organ prolapse and associated conditions are also covered in Chapters 75 and 143 and throughout Sections 5 and 9 of this book. We recommend general anesthesia or sedation with additional analgesia, such as opiates and nonsteroidal antiinflammatories, during the surgical resolution of cloacal prolapses, and these techniques and drugs are covered in detail in Chapters 48 through 51 and summarized in Table 75.5 (McArthur S, Machin R, personal observation, 2017).[1-3] See Chapter 16 for further husbandry details and also Chapters 46 and 87.

PHALLUS (CHELONIAN)/HEMIPENIS (SQUAMATE) PROLAPSE

Male reproductive organ prolapse is a common emergency presentation in clinical practice (Figs. 106.1 and 106.2).[4,5] In one UK study that included more than 3000 reptiles, male organ prolapse represented more than 35% of all prolapses and was the most common prolapse type of reptiles and has been reported in chelonians,[4,7-10] lizards,[4,11] snakes,[10,12] and crocodilians.[14] Known causes are covered in more detail in Chapter 75.

Chapter 75 contains a guide to prolapse identification and the conditions predisposing to a prolapse. Prolapse phallus or hemipenis identification is generally straightforward. Only mature male animals will be presented. A phallus prolapse does not contain a lumen and is relatively small and originates within the caudolateral vent in squamates and may be a bilateral presentation as squamates have two (hemipenes). In chelonians, a large single fleshy structure projects out centrally from the cranial cloaca, and this may be a considerable size. In squamates, the main differential diagnoses are hemipenile plugs and infections, which may accompany a hemipenile prolapse. Usually, a reptile can urinate and defecate around this type of prolapse because the male copulatory organ contains no urethra.

A male organ cloacal prolapse can either be reduced or amputated. If a reduction procedure meets significant complications, or is unsuccessful, the clinician can revert to amputation. Amputation affects future reproduction but not the output of the urinary system. In species with hemipenes, the reptile may still be able to successfully copulate and reproduce if only one organ is amputated. Male cloacal organ amputation

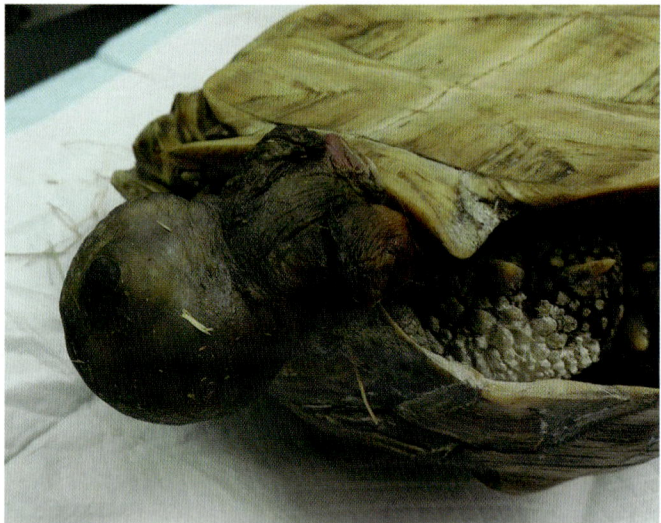

FIG 106.1 Devitalized phallic prolapse in an African spurred tortoise (*Centrochelys sulcata*). Most phallic prolapses can be removed after proximal placement of circumferential transfixion sutures at the prolapse base. (Courtesy of Ross A. Machin.)

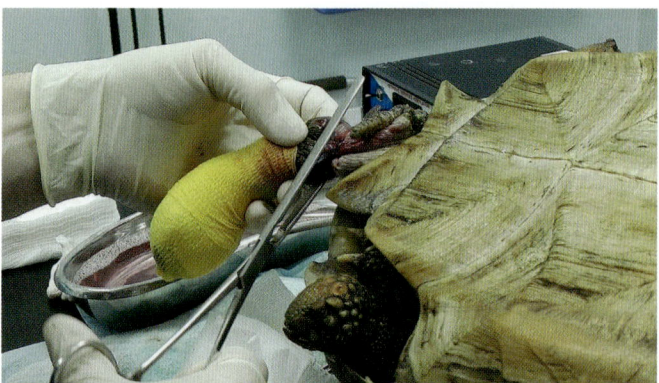

FIG 106.2 Removal of a devitalized phallic prolapse in an African spurred tortoise (*Centrochelys sulcata*). Becaus the ureters empty directly into the urodeum, the phallus does not contain a closed urethra necessary for voiding of urine and so can be removed. (Courtesy of Ross A. Machin.)

carries a favorable prognosis; euthanasia is usually unnecessary. Underlying husbandry and welfare issues must be addressed, as with other presentations.[4-14] Initial stabilization is described in Table 75.3 (see Chapter 75). This includes protection of the prolapsed organ, analgesia, rehydration, and placement in a warm environment.

In an anesthetized reptile with a phallus or hemipenis prolapse, protruding tissue should be assessed for viability, cleaned, lubricated, and gently replaced into the cloaca when possible. A moistened cotton-tipped applicator or tongue depressor may be a helpful tool during prolapse reduction. Application of topical local anesthetic agents (e.g., lidocaine and bupivacaine) mixed with lubricant gels may reduce straining and aid reduction and subsequent retention. Anesthetic agents can be applied topically via infiltration or as an intrathecal block.[1-3] Topical glycerine, dextrose, honey, or concentrated sugar solutions allow osmotic reduction of tissue edema and may be helpful when the organ is profoundly edematous.[21,22] These are often required when managing prolapse of the phallus in chelonians.[8]

Where a prolapse cannot be manually reduced, the vent may be surgically enlarged via a lateral releasing incision, on one or both sides of the vent, with surgical closure after reduction. This allows a swollen prolapse to be reduced and replaced within the cloaca. Once the organ is correctly replaced it rapidly deceases in size. A correctly placed cloacal suture (e.g., 3/0 Polydioxanone), or staples, prevents further prolapse but allows normal urination and defecation.[6,15,16] Sutures or staples are monitored for 1 or 2 days to ensure normal urination and defecation is possible and subsequently removed in 5 to 7 days or longer if necessary to allow a stable reduction to occur.

Where the prolapse is traumatized, severely swollen, or necrotic, amputation is advisable. In both squamates and chelonians, amputation under general anesthesia or sedation is a quick procedure and often simpler than an attempt at reduction. Local anesthetic agents (e.g., lidocaine and bupivacaine) can be infiltrated into tissue at the base of the prolapse, which is then transected distal to a transfixed, circumferential hemostatic suture (e.g., 3/0 Polydioxanone). The amputation stump is replaced within the cloaca where it rapidly reduces in size.

Postoperative complications are unusual and may include hemorrhage or infection. Once the postoperative patient is stable, it can be discharged and managed on an outpatient basis, as long as a suitable recovery environment can be provided. Husbandry should be optimized, and normal perioperative care should be followed, maintaining core body temperature and hydration, and a feeding plan should be established. Provide suitable postoperative analgesia (see Chapter 50) and monitor for urine and fecal production and evidence of straining, discomfort, or pain.[20]

OVIDUCT PROLAPSE

Oviductal prolapses have been reported in female lizards and chelonians (Figs. 106.3 through 106.8). In theory, at least, they may occur in any female reptile. However, reports in snakes appear absent from the literature. In one UK study, only 3% of reptile prolapses were oviducts.[4] Chapter 75 contains information on identification of an oviduct prolapse and conditions predisposing to oviductal prolapse.

Female reptiles with a recent prolapse of an oviduct will present with a tubular prolapsed structure projecting through the vent. The prolapse has a smooth surface with occasional longitudinal striations. A lumen is present. The presence of fecal material is unusual, but surface contamination may occur. Some animals may continue to pass fecal and urinary excretion products around a prolapse. Bilateral prolapses are not reported in the literature and are not known to either the authors or editors. Chronic prolapses quickly become strangulated, necrotic, and traumatized, all of which complicate organ identification.

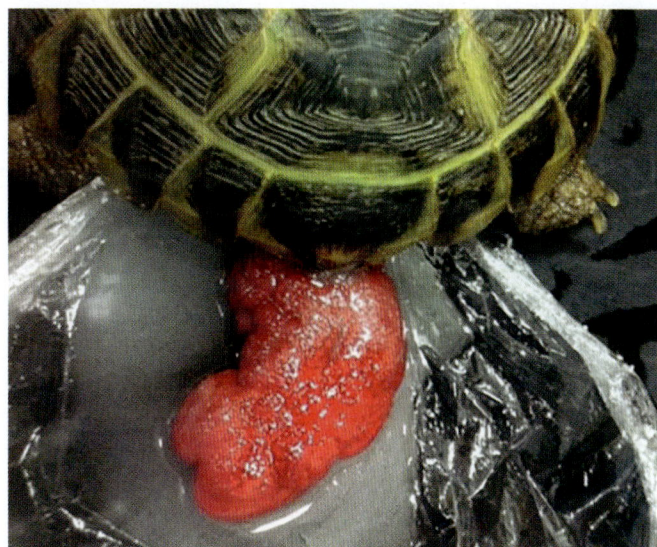

FIG 106.3 Osmotic reduction during stabilization and transportation (*Agrionemys horsfieldii*). An oviduct prolapse is bathed in a concentrated sugar solution and lubricating gel and then wrapped in Clingfilm. This protection is suitable stabilization until a reptile clinician or transportation to a reptile veterinary facility becomes available. (Courtesy of Stuart McArthur.)

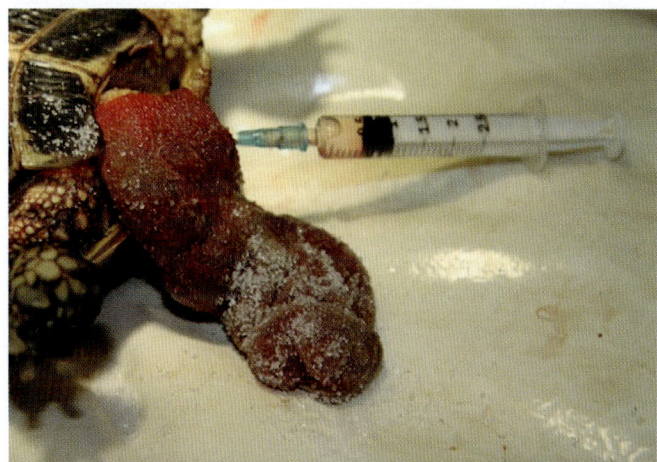

FIG 106.4 Osmotic reduction using sugar (*Agrionemys horsfieldii*). Further reduction is possible under general anesthesia. Here sugar solution is applied in the preoperative period after the prolapse has been cleaned with warm fluid flushing. It is rinsed off and then the prolapse can be reduced. In some cases, oxytocin may reduce the prolapse volume. (Courtesy of Stuart McArthur.)

The primary differential diagnosis of an oviductal prolapse is a prolapse of the colon. Examination of the cloaca with an otoscope or endoscope may be useful and may confirm the presence of a patent colon.

Initial stabilization is described in Table 75.3 (see Chapter 75) and includes protection of the prolapsed organ, analgesia, rehydration, and placement in a warm environment. Suitable analgesia protocols are identified in Table 75.4 (see Chapter 75). Local anesthetic agents can be applied topically, via infiltration or as an intrathecal block.

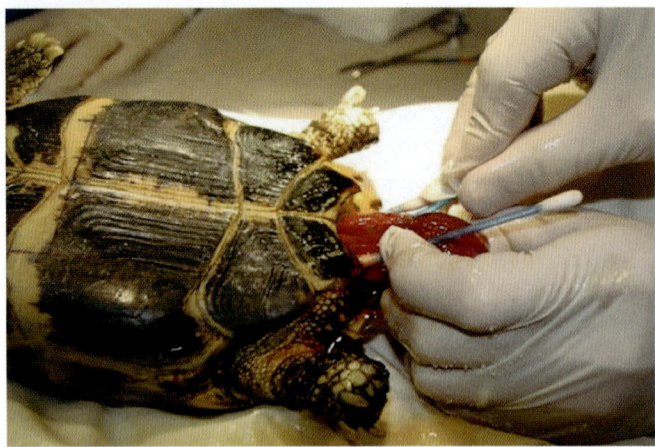

FIG 106.5 Manual reduction following osmotic reduction in the tortoise (*Agrionemys horsfieldii*) in Fig. 106.4. After rinsing off osmotic reduction agents, damp swabs and cotton buds can be used to reduce the prolapse through gentle repetitive compression movements. (Courtesy of Stuart McArthur.)

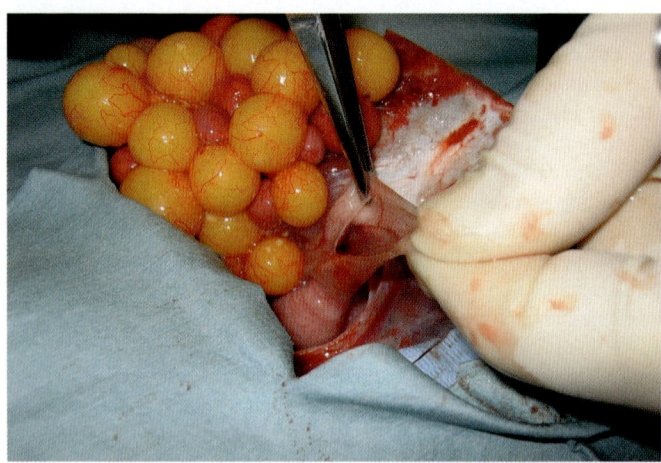

FIG 106.8 Oviduct rupture associated with an oviduct prolapse in a *Testudo hermanni*. (Courtesy of Stuart McArthur.)

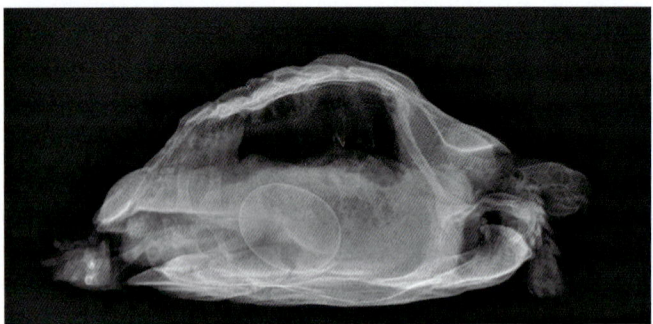

FIG 106.6 Radiographic examination of a reptile with an oviduct prolapse will often reveal a space-occupying mass in the coelom, dystocia (as seen in this *Agrionemys horsfieldii* with a retained egg), or a urolith, or a urolith. Dystocia and relative oversize of eggs accounts for many cases of oviductal prolapse in chelonians that have experienced accelerated growth and early puberty. (Courtesy of Stuart McArthur.)

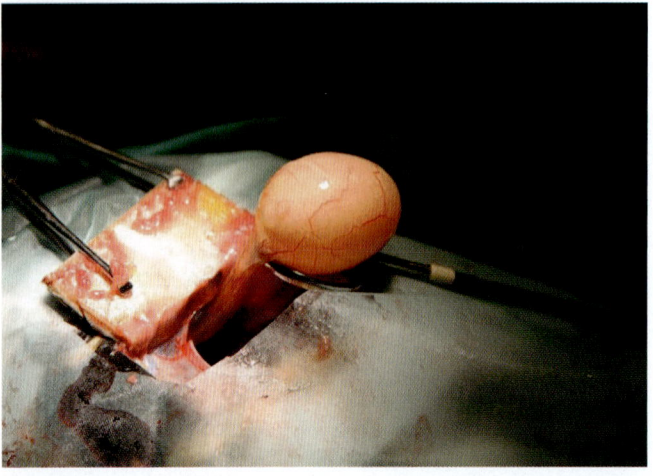

FIG 106.7 Here the oversized egg is removed from the same patient in Fig. 106.6. (Courtesy of Stuart McArthur.)

A coeliotomy (open reduction) with multimodal analgesia is advised as part of the overall management strategy.[1–3] There may be radiographic evidence of dystocia or urinary calculi, which can also be addressed during the coeliotomy. Surgical entry to the coelomic cavity varies with species and is covered in detail in Chapters 97 through 101.

It is rare for a prolapsed oviduct or shell gland to be preserved during treatment. Amputation is usually necessary. Amputation of the externalized prolapse with stump closure is often performed immediately before any coeliotomy, allowing the remaining issues to be addressed, as this ensures only one surgical site is active at a time. Additional coelomic interventions that may be required should be considered, and risks and costs should be carefully and realistically assessed and discussed with the client. Euthanasia may also be considered in severe presentations (e.g., sepsis and collapse) or where there are economic constraints. Closed reduction of an inverted oviduct and temporary retention using staples or purse string sutures is possible; however, it is unusual to simply reduce an oviduct prolapse (e.g., using hydrostatic warm water local irrigation) without persistence of inversion or recurrence.

Exploratory coeliotomy (open reduction) under general anesthesia allows for a comprehensive assessment of the reproductive tract and appropriate management of any dystocia or urolith. Provided the clinician is confident that a prolapse is oviduct and not the colon, then it is acceptable to amputate the prolapse close to the vent before any coeliotomy, closing the residual stump using circumferential transfixion sutures (e.g., 3/0-5/0 polydioxanone or poliglecaprone with triclosan).[6,15,16] Prolapse amputation removes any need to draw necrotic, infected, friable, or traumatized structures back through the vent and cloaca, into the coelomic cavity, during coeliotomy. Where the prolapse has been amputated before coeliotomy, it is usually straightforward to locate the residual oviduct stump, and the subsequent coeliotomy procedure itself is far more straightforward.

Female reptiles all have a bicornuate reproductive system and two ovaries. Removal of the affected portion of the reproductive tract and its accompanying ovary is recommended in most cases of oviduct prolapse, as few reduced prolapses are likely to continue without complication. At coeliotomy, a unilateral prolapse may recover well with removal of just the affected oviduct and its related ovary, leaving the contralateral tract intact.[19] Surgical entry to the coelomic cavity varies with species and is covered in detail in Chapters 97 to 101. Where future reproduction is not a concern, bilateral ovariohysterectomy is preferred to unilateral. This will limit recurrence and additional reproductive tract–related abnormalities. In squamates, the right ovary is anatomically close to the vena cava and care must be taken not to damage this structure. Hemoclips are helpful, although suture material (e.g., 3/0 Polydioxanone) can also be used to ligate ovarian arterial vessels. Irrigate the coelomic cavity with warm saline before closure. Postoperative complications may include infection, hemorrhage, thromboembolism, paresis, or ovarian remnant. Complete removal of ovarian tissue is essential. A bacteriology swab of the coelomic cavity should be taken and culture and sensitivity performed, and then coelomic lavage with warm saline is advised before coeliotomy closure (see Chapter 105).

Husbandry should be optimized, and normal perioperative care should be followed, maintaining core body temperature and hydration, and a feeding plan should be established. Provide suitable postoperative analgesia (see Chapter 50) and monitor for urine and fecal production and evidence of straining, discomfort, or pain.[20]

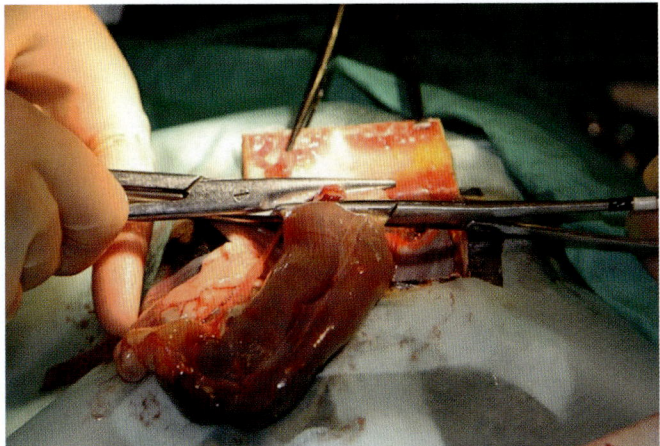

FIG 106.9 After returning the oviduct to the coelomic cavity via gentle traction, it is ligated and removed along with the associated ovary. (Courtesy of Stuart McArthur.)

LARGE INTESTINE (RECTAL/COLONIC) PROLAPSE

Intestinal prolapse has been reported in all reptile classes (Figs. 106.10 through 106.12). Animals may be male or female.[16–18] The main differential diagnosis of a prolapse of the colon in a female reptile is an oviductal prolapse.[16] In one UK study, prolapse of the colon represented one-sixth of the prolapses presented.[4] Chapter 75 contains a guide to prolapse identification and the conditions predisposing to intestinal tract prolapse.

The patient typically presents with a prolapse of a smooth linear structure. There is a lumen. Feces or gas may be present. Because the structure will generally be an intussusception, it may be rigid and inflexible.

Chronic prolapses often become severely swollen or strangulated, and tissues may be necrotic and traumatized, all of which complicate organ identification. Initial stabilization is described in Table 75.3 (see Chapter 75) and includes protection of the prolapsed organ, analgesia, rehydration, and placement in a warm environment. Suitable analgesia protocols are identified in Table 75.4 .

A coeliotomy (open reduction) with multimodal analgesia is advised as part of the overall management strategy of a colon prolapse.[1–3] There may be radiographic evidence of an additional dystocia or urinary calculus that can also be addressed during the coeliotomy. Surgical entry into the coelomic cavity and coelomic closure varies with species and is covered in detail in Chapters 97 through 101. For the patient to remain viable, it is necessary for all (or a significant amount) of the prolapsed colon to be preserved during treatment; therefore a closed amputation is not a realistic option. Euthanasia, or open salvage techniques, described later, may be considered in severe presentations (e.g., sepsis and collapse) or where there are economic constraints.

After lavage of the prolapse, removal of any necrotic tissue, and osmotic reduction as described earlier, coeliotomy (open reduction) allows traction to be applied to the proximal colon during reduction. Milking the intussusceptum slowly and gently out of the intussuscipiens is important. Sustain gentle manual pressure rather than pulling out the intussusceptum to avoid the risk of iatrogenic perforation.[23] After correct reduction, colopexy is performed in an area of healthy viable colon tissue to prevent recurrence. Sutures are placed between the colon

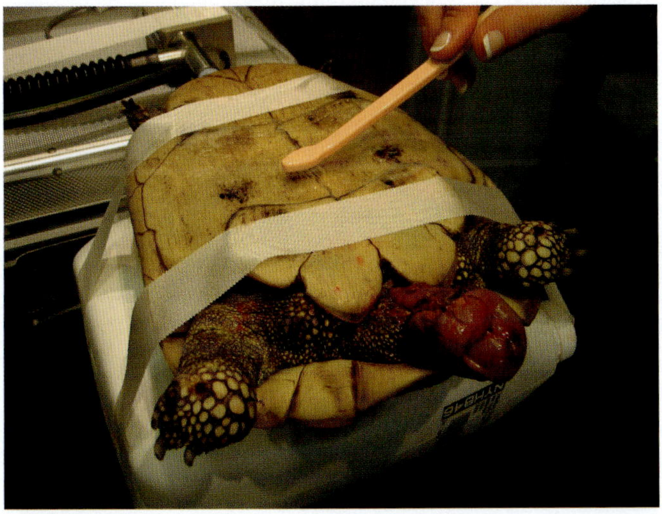

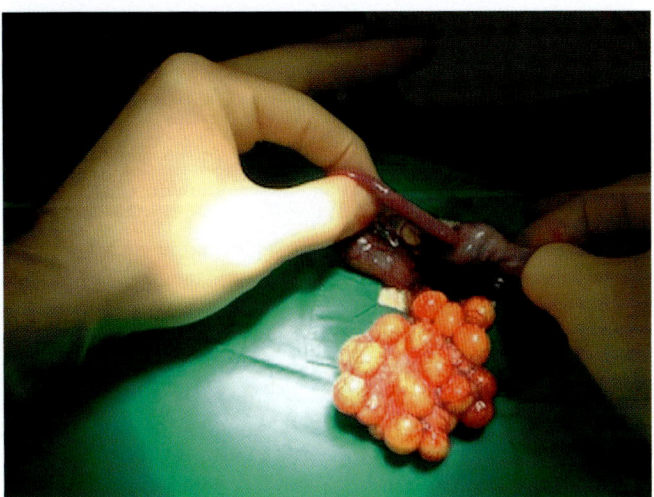

FIG 106.11 The same animal as in Fig. 106.10. Milking the intussusceptum slowly and gently out of the intussuscipiens is important. Sustain gentle manual pressure rather than pulling out the intussusceptum to avoid the risk of iatrogenic perforation. (Courtesy of Stuart McArthur.)

FIG 106.10 Colon prolapse in a female *Testudo hermanni*. This must be differentiated from an oviduct prolapse. (Courtesy of Stuart McArthur.)

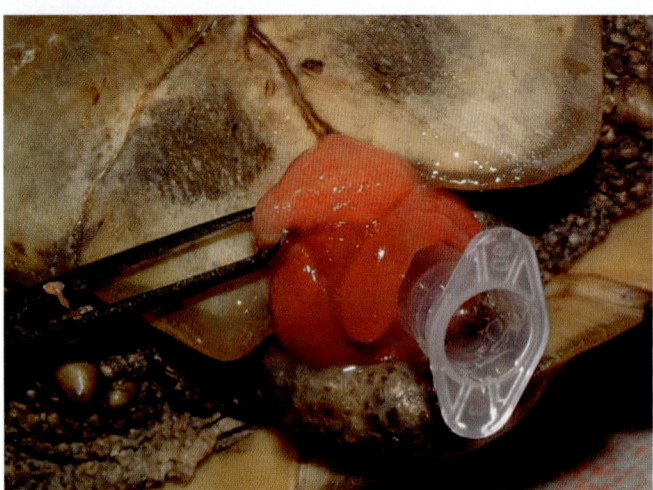

FIG 106.12 Colon resection and anastomosis in a *Testudo* sp. Here, a closed resection is made using a syringe barrel as a stent. This is a salvage procedure where a coeliotomy is not deemed appropriate. (Courtesy of Stuart McArthur.)

and the body wall by using a small atraumatic needle and monofilament absorbable suture material with partial-thickness sutures to minimize potential leakage of colon contents. Alternatively, the colon may be incorporated into the body wall closure. Where exposed tissue is devitalized, a resection and end-to-end anastomosis can be performed. This involves a combination of clean and dirty techniques where an intussusception is retracted back into the coelom during coeliotomy. Resection and anastomosis can be performed with standard soft-tissue techniques. A bacteriology swab of the coelomic cavity should be taken and culture and sensitivity performed, and then coelomic lavage with warm saline is advised before coeliotomy closure.

Provided there is no associated coelomic condition that requires coeliotomy, such as dystocia or urinary calculus, open salvage techniques can be attempted. A fresh nontraumatized prolapse may be hydrostatically reduced using warm water local irrigation after a period of osmotic reduction. Local anesthetic agents can be applied topically, via infiltration or as an intrathecal block and will aid reduction and retention. Contrast radiography, ultrasonography, and endoscopy may be necessary to confirm correct organ replacement. Retention is then achieved via transverse cloacal sutures or staples. However, it is unusual to reduce a colon prolapse without persistence of inversion or recurrence. A pexy between the colon and the body wall may not be necessary. However, if the prolapse remains unstable and recurs, or is likely to recur, then a pexy suture(s) will be required and a coeliotomy (open reduction) necessary to ensure correct reduction.

An anastomosis may also be performed in an unreduced prolapse without coeliotomy, after insertion of a smooth, tubular object (stent) into the lumen of the colon (e.g., a thermometer or clean syringe). The tissue is then transfixed with orthogonal needles, non-viable tissue is excised, and the two remaining layers are anastomosed with monofilament absorbable suture material in a simple interrupted pattern. Alternatively, the sutures can be placed and then the non-viable tissue can be removed.[6,15,16] When the exposed tissue is returned to the coelomic cavity, an inverting end-to-end intestinal anastomosis will have been created. It is essential to monitor these animals postreduction to confirm that they can urinate and defecate and to ensure that no recurrence infection or wound breakdown has occurred. The underlying conditions leading to the prolapse will also require identification and correction.

Systemic or regional postoperative complications should be considered and may include suture breakdown, infection, coelomitis, hemorrhage, thromboembolism, or paresis. Antibiotics in line with local antibiotic policy or based on culture and sensitivity should be considered. Husbandry should be optimized, and normal perioperative care should be followed; maintaining core body temperature, hydration, and a feeding plan should be established. Provide suitable postoperative analgesia (see Chapter 50), and monitor for urine and fecal production and evidence of straining, discomfort, or pain.[20]

BLADDER PROLAPSE

Chelonians and some lizards have bladders that may become prolapsed, and one UK study reported that bladder prolapse represented around 3% of prolapses encountered in a first opinion and referral setting. Chapter 75 contains a guide to prolapse identification and the conditions predisposing to bladder prolapse.

Bladder prolapses present as an amorphous translucent structure protruding from the cloaca, which may or may not contain fluid. There is no lumen. Because the ureters empty into the urodeum without a direct connection to the urinary bladder, it is unusual for them to become damaged during a bladder prolapse. However, their outflow may be temporarily obstructed. The bladder, when present, participates in water and electrolyte reabsorption, and therefore an attempt should be made to salvage as much of the viable tissue as possible.[8]

Initial stabilization is described in Table 75.3 (see Chapter 75) and includes protection of the prolapsed organ, analgesia, rehydration, and placement in a warm environment. A prolapsed bladder should be protected quickly because further trauma is likely due to the thin tissue nature of the organ. Suitable analgesia protocols are identified in Table 75.4. If the animal has been unable to urinate, it is prudent to assess blood potassium and azotemia levels at the start of treatment and take measures to address abnormalities.

When a small viable portion of the urinary bladder is prolapsed, closed reduction in the sedated patient via the cloaca using the hydrostatic pressure of a warm water enema can be attempted. However, if complicating issues such as the presence of urinary calculi or ectopic egg(s) exist a coeliotomy will likely be required. Multimodal analgesia should be used.[1–3] Hydrostatic reduction can be achieved by infusing both the bladder and cloaca with warm fluid via an endoscope sheath or suitably sized crop tube. An appropriate reduction may be confirmed endoscopically or by radiography following infusion of suitable media into the reduced bladder. The patient must be carefully monitored postoperatively for recurrence and ability to urinate and defecate.

Where exposed tissue is not viable, it must be surgically resected and nonviable tissue removed. Using a closed technique, a bowel clamp or set of intestinal forceps is lightly placed across the viable section of tissue, with minimal crushing. A double-layer inverting suture line (e.g., 3/0-5/0 poliglecaprone with triclosan) is placed proximal to the bowel clamp, sealing the urinary bladder.[6,15,16] The nonviable tissue is removed distal to this suture line. The clamp is removed, and the residual bladder is replaced through the cloaca and back into the coelomic cavity. A hydrostatic enema as described earlier can be used to reduce the bladder and return it to a coelomic location, and, if the sheath of a scope is used, endoscopy can confirm the bladder is relocated back where intended.

If a substantial portion of the bladder is damaged, coeliotomy (open reduction) with multimodal analgesia is advised to allow better exposure and excision of the diseased tissue. Local anesthetic agents can be applied topically via infiltration or as an intrathecal block. Surgical entry into the coelomic cavity and coelomic closure varies with species and is covered in detail in Chapters 97 to 101.

During the coelomic exploration, salvage as much of the viable bladder tissue as possible and remove any urolith or ectopic egg. A double-layer inverting suture line (e.g., 3/0-5/0 poliglecaprone with triclosan) is used to close the bladder.[6,15] It will be difficult to avoid contamination of the coelomic cavity with bladder contents. A bacteriology swab of the coelomic cavity should be taken and culture and sensitivity performed, and then coelomic lavage with warm saline is advised before coeliotomy closure.

Husbandry should be optimized, and normal perioperative care should be followed, maintaining core body temperature and hydration, and a feeding plan should be established. Provide suitable postoperative analgesia (see Chapter 50) and monitor for urine and fecal production and evidence of straining, discomfort, or pain.[20] Specifically monitoring blood potassium levels and for azotemia in the postoperative period after this procedure is important.

REFERENCES

See www.expertconsult.com for a complete list of references.

107

Amphibian Soft Tissue Surgery

Brent R. Whitaker and Kevin M. Wright[†]

Amphibian surgery remains poorly documented in the veterinary literature; however, several good references exist.[1–3] Amphibians tolerate anesthesia well when properly used (see Chapter 52), and it is required for the majority of the procedures described here. Our experience is that amphibians make good surgical candidates and that the clinician should consider this therapeutic approach when it is required.

Soft tissue surgical intervention is commonly required to repair wounds and prolapses and perform biopsies, as well as to remove foreign bodies, masses, and damaged eyes. Coeliotomy may be necessary to obtain diagnostic biopsies or remove gastrointestinal foreign bodies, retained eggs, neoplastic masses, or uroliths (Fig. 107.1).

EQUIPMENT

The size of the patient and procedure to be performed must be considered when selecting surgical instruments. Ophthalmic or microsurgical instruments, including scissors, forceps, and hemostats, are often required for delicate surgeries. Ophthalmic knives, for example, come in a variety of sizes, shapes, and angles, making them very useful in smaller patients. Number 11 and 15 scalpel blades also work well. Nonabsorbent clear plastic drapes can be used to create a clean field and minimize desiccation of the patient. Eyelid retractors and plastic ring retractors with elastic stays (e.g., Lone Star retractor) work well to retract coelomic incisions, but care should be taken to ensure that only the minimal amount of pressure needed be applied in order to avoid damage to the skin. Radiosurgery, a laser, or a fine-tipped surgical spear can be used for hemostasis. Magnification and bright but cool illumination are recommended. Many different sutures have been used successfully, including polydioxanone and polyglactin 910; however, one study in the African clawed frog (*Xenopus laevis*) concluded that monofilament nylon showed the least histological reaction and was therefore recommended as the suture of choice in amphibian skin closure. Chromic gut and silk elicited the greatest histological reaction and resulted in a high rate of dehiscence and is not recommended for use in amphibian skin.[4] Polydioxanone, poliglecaprone 25, and polyglactin should be used internally and for muscle closure, although polyglactin is likely to cause greater inflammation.[1] Antibiotic-impregnated sutures may guard against bacterial translocation and are especially useful for GI, bladder closures, and skin closures. Tapered needles with wedged on suture are least traumatic and work best.

Cyanoacrylate tissue glue can also be used in small quantities for skin closure. The glue not only creates a watertight physical barrier but has been shown to have antimicrobial properties, with greatest activity against gram-positive organisms.[5–7] A rigid telescope and carbon dioxide insufflator are useful for minimally invasive coelioscopic and endoscopic examinations (Fig. 107.2).[1,8]

SURGICAL PREPARATION AND POSTOPERATIVE CARE

Maintaining physiological homeostasis for the patient preoperatively, perioperatively, and postoperatively is important for a successful outcome. Temperature of the amphibian's environment must be monitored and maintained within the preferred range. Hypothermia is not an acceptable means to provide surgical restraint or analgesia. Minimal preparation of the surgical site is desired, as amphibian mucus and skin contain antimicrobial peptides produced in granular glands that are protective.[9] Gently cleaning the incision site to ensure that it is free of debris using sterile cotton-tipped applicators dipped in sterile saline or a 2% povidone-iodine in sterile saline solution is all that is needed. The patient should be properly hydrated prior to, throughout, and following surgery. This can make maintaining sterility challenging. Several recipes for balanced solutions exist (see Chapter 89).[1,10,11] Fasting is not required prior to prevent aspiration but may be desirable due to the intended procedure. Gloves should be worn but must be powder free (or powdered gloves must be wiped with saline-moistened sterile gauze). Preoperatively, perioperatively, and postoperatively, the need for antibiotics and pain relief should be evaluated and provided, if necessary. Little information on the clinical effectiveness of analgesics is available; however, the administration of 38–46 mg/kg buprenorphine subcutaneously every

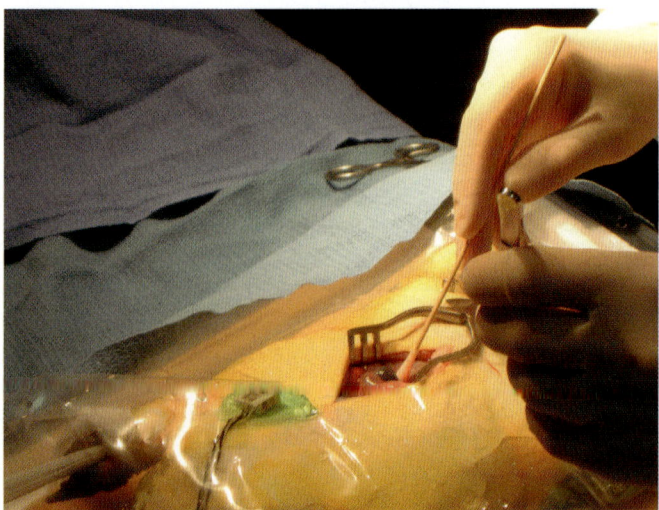

FIG 107.1 Celiotomy in African bullfrog (*Pyxicephalus adspersus*). Note the use of a Doppler to monitor heart rate and the clear plastic drape, which is nonabrasive and helps the animal retain moisture. Eyelid retractors can be used in smaller species as retractors. (Courtesy of National Aquarium.)

[†]Deceased.

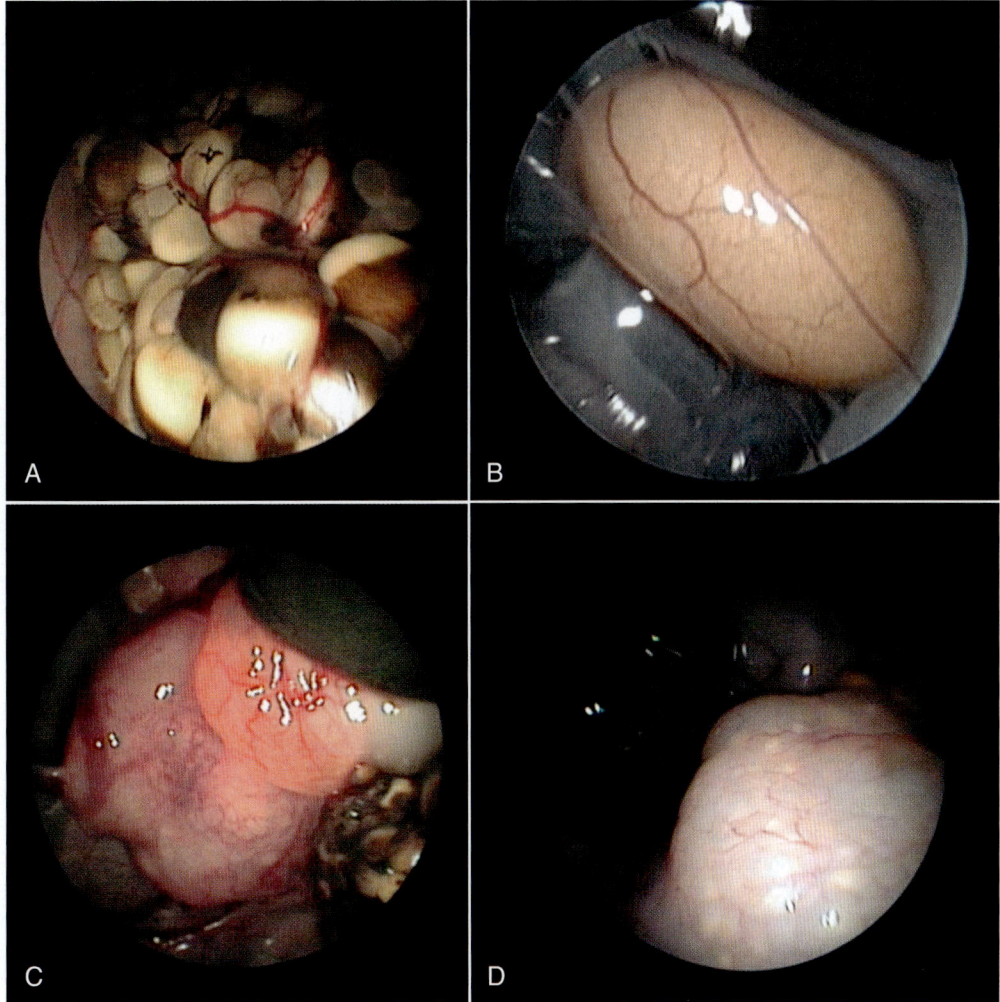

FIG 107.2 Endoscopic images showing (A) a normal ovary in an African clawed frog (*Xenopus laevis*), (B) a normal testis in the American bullfrog (*Lithobates catesbeinanus*), (C) adenocarcinoma in the testes of a White's tree frog (*Litoria caerulea*), and (D) ovarian carcinoma in a giant monkey frog (*Phyllomedusa bicolor*). (Courtesy of Norin Chai.)

4 to 6 hours or dexmedetomidine injected into the dorsal lymph sac (0.6 mg/kg) every 8 hours appears to be effective.[10,11,12] Nutritional supplementation must be provided if the patient is not eating.

TOE CLIP

Toe clipping remains a standard research/institutional method of identification of anurans and urodeles; however, some salamanders will regenerate an amputated digit or limb, limiting the long-term effectiveness of toe clipping as a permanent means of identification in this order.[13] This procedure is not warranted for client-owned pets. For many amphibians, such as poison dart frogs, identification can be achieved using photographs to capture an individual's unique color pattern. Although some field biologists routinely perform this procedure without sedation under research license, ethical and humane concerns exist. Additionally, reports show that toe clipping may have associated complications such as infection, decreased mobility or dexterity, and subsequent increased susceptibility to predation. The rate of return also increases as more toes are removed.[14] When removing a toe from anurans, one should consider that the first three digits of the male's forelimb are important to mounting the female during breeding and that the fourth

hind digit is used by both sexes to remove shed skin and should not be removed. Small anurans can have the toe clipped with iris scissors, and direct pressure is applied to the site until bleeding stops. A small drop of surgical glue adds an additional barrier and can aid in homeostasis. Instruments should be disinfected between individuals. Larger anurans can be toe clipped with stainless steel liga-clips, and the digit distal to the clamp is removed. The clip falls off in 7 to 28 days. Although the regenerated tissue is slightly different in appearance than the original tissue, this can vary.

IMPLANTATION OF TRANSPONDER

A highly successful method of permanent identification of amphibians is the implantation of a transponder chip within the amphibian's body.[15] The procedure is not without risk, as it can cause significant disruption to the skin's bacterial flora and proliferation of resident fungi.[16] Some debate exists about the preferred site of implantation. A subcutaneous site (e.g., underneath the parotid gland of a toad) has been advocated by some instead of an intracoelomic site. The subcutaneous site avoids the chance of abdominal adhesions forming and associated clinical problems arising from migration of the coelomic implant. A subcutaneously placed transponder may be visible and therefore unacceptable for display animals. The intracoelomic implant avoids this problem. The intracoelomic implant may be administered via the paralumbar region or ventrally, lateral to the midline. Long-term studies comparing the advantages and disadvantages of the two site choices are lacking, and choice is currently a matter of clinician preference. Anecdotal reports are found of amphibians shedding their transponders several months after implantation. The transponder likely migrates and is expelled through the bladder, the intestine, or even transcutaneously. Implantation of a second transponder and routine monitoring to ensure both transponders are present and working is recommended for specimens that must have permanent identification.

CLOACAL PROLAPSE

Prolapse of tissue out of the cloaca is a common but life-threatening disorder of amphibians (see Fig. 89.21). Rectum and bladder are among the most commonly seen organ prolapses. Predisposing conditions include metabolic abnormalities such as dehydration, hypocalcemia, hypoglycemia, and malnutrition. Other differentials include gastrointestinal foreign bodies, cystic calculi, gastroenteritis, hyperthermia, trauma, and parasitism. Radiographs to exclude gastrointestinal foreign bodies and cystic calculi are suggested. If the prolapse is detected while the mucosa is viable, the prolapse can be gently replaced using a blunt tool such as the rounded end of an appropriately sized feeding tube. Glycerin gel may be applied to the rectal mucosa to moisten and shrink the tissue before placement. Alternatively, a hyperosmotic saline or sugar solution applied to the prolapsed tissue (not the entire patient) followed in 10 to 20 minutes by a water-soluble lubricant can be effective. If the prolapse appears devitalized, excision of the devitalized intestine and anastomosis of the healthy tissue may be attempted. An antibiotic pessary may be warranted in some cases, as may parenteral antibiotics. A nylon purse-string suture should be used to close the cloaca for 2 to 3 days, and the amphibian should not be fed until after the suture has been removed. Any predisposing conditions should be corrected. Prognosis is guarded, but many anurans respond favorably.

COELIOTOMY

Some of the larger carnivorous frogs, such as the popular Argentine horned frog *(Ceratophrys ornata)*, are well known for pica, or eating abnormal objects, especially rocks. An occasional rock can be manually extracted with long curved Kelly forceps if it is still located in the stomach; however, foreign bodies that have passed the pylorus and entered the small intestine require an enterotomy. Removal of cystic calculi is a common surgery for many phyllomedusine frogs[8,17] because of the number of species that produce uric acid as a nitrogenous waste. Where possible, a two-layer closure of the bladder is ideal, but a one-layer closure is often most practical and works well in our experience. Many of the same techniques used for reptile patients work well for amphibians (see Section 10). Exploratory celiotomy is a useful diagnostic tool and can be used to confirm celioscopic diagnoses, to obtain tissue samples, or for therapeutic procedures such as gastrotomy (Fig. 107.3). Partial ovariectomy is used to harvest ova by exteriorizing a portion of the egg mass through a 3- to 5-mm paramedial incision and excising a sample. Ligation, surgical clips, or radiosurgery of blood vessels may be required if performing a gonadectomy.[1] Closure of a celiotomy site may be problematic because the cutaneous sutures are prone to dehisce. The suture line should be under as little tension as possible. A 3-0 or 5-0 nylon (or antibiotic impregnated absorbable monofilament) in an everting pattern is suggested, with further strength provided with a layer of tissue glue or with internal placement of absorbable sponge material. The patient should be confined in a small

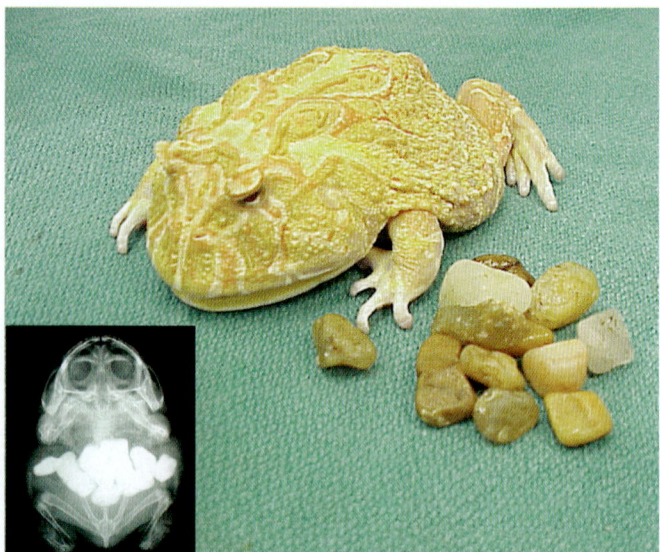

FIG 107.3 Postsurgical photograph of an ornate horned frog *(Ceratophrys ornata)*. Gastrotomy/enterotomy is a common procedure in amphibians. Note the radiograph of the patient showing the multiple ingested rocks *(inset)*. (Courtesy of Douglas R. Mader.)

space and managed with a minimum of handling for at least 10 days after surgery.

OCULAR SURGERY

Corneal biopsies are rarely needed but can be taken. The removal of the lens that had luxated into the anterior chamber of a milk frog *Trachycephalus resinfictrix* was successfully removed using a Snellen loop after making a 180-degree incision at the limbus, decompressing the globe and injecting viscoelastic material into the anterior chamber. After irrigating the globe with saline, the incision was closed with 9-0 nylon suture.[1] Ocular tissue damaged beyond repair due to trauma, infection, or neoplasia can be painful and may require removal. Two critical issues must be managed by the surgeon when performing an enucleation of the eye. The first is that amphibians have a membranous orbit and poorly defined lacrimal bone; caution must therefore be taken not to damage the membrane that separates the globe from the buccal cavity. The second is to control bleeding that can be life threatening in small amphibians. This can be done by first applying pressure with fine-tipped surgical spears and then packing the cavity with an absorbable collagen hemostat or gelatin sponges. If infection is present, placing the patient on an appropriate antibiotic prior to surgery may be helpful.

CELIOSCOPY

Minimally invasive surgical procedures that reduce the size of incision and amount of tissue trauma are preferable. Celioscopy has been used to determine gender in monomorphic species such as giant salamanders *(Andrias* spp.) (Kramer et al. 1983, Proc Am Assoc Zoo Vet, pp 192–194) and goliath frogs *(Gigantorana conrauagoliath)* (Gillespie et al. 1988, Proc Joint Conf Am Assoc Zoo Vet and Am Assoc Wildl Vet, p 62), confirm granulomatous disease, biopsy organs, and biopsy tissue masses (see Fig. 107.2).[1,8,18] A 3-mm incision can be made in the paralumbar region or just lateral to the midline, depending on the purpose of the exam. After inserting the telescope-sheath system into the coelom, carbon dioxide is typically used for insufflation of the cavity.[1] Insufflation pressures of 0.5 to 2 mm Hg with a flow rate of less than 0.5 L/min is recommended.[18] Lateral recumbency may allow the internal organs to fall away from the hypaxial musculature and allow visualization of the testicle and kidneys. A paramedial midline incision allows best access to the liver, and care should be taken to avoid damaging the ventral midline vein. Tissue glue can be used to close the incision. Large incisions may be closed with 3-0 or 5-0 nylon sutures (or antibiotic impregnanted absorbable monofilament), which can be removed in 4 to 8 weeks.[4]

REFERENCES

See www.expertconsult.com for a complete list of references.

108

Orthopedic Principles and External Coaptation

S. Emi Knafo and W. Michael Karlin

Reptiles frequently suffer from fractured bones, either resulting from trauma or pathological processes. Traumatic fractures are most commonly due to inter- and intraspecific aggression, improper handling/restraint, and motor vehicles. Pathological fractures almost always result from any of the various metabolic bone diseases (MBD) that affect reptiles; however, neoplasia, osteomyelitis, or other metabolic diseases may play an underlying role. Many fractures are amenable to treatment with external coaptation, and pathological fractures from MBD are often unsuitable for internal fixation because the bones are unable to support hardware. These fractures are usually best treated with external coaptation (although exceptions exist). In other situations, such as the fracture configuration or size of the reptile, internal fixation may be indicated. In general, if the patient is healthy enough to undergo surgery, internal reduction and fracture fixation will provide superior alignment of fracture fragments, neutralization of fracture forces, and superior healing.[1] In patients with MBD, the underlying cause should be determined and corrected before or concurrent with fracture repair. This requires medical management while treating pathologic fractures. When severe tissue trauma, loss of vascular supply, uncontrolled infection, and inflammation exist, amputation may be required. Reptiles generally function well with partial or complete limb amputations (see Chapter 111).

Most fractures occur as a result of relatively low impact forces, which makes the incidence of comminuted fractures relatively low.[1] Reptiles also have tough inelastic skin, and fractures are often closed. However, open fractures do occur, and any resulting wounds should be thoroughly cleaned, debrided, and sampled for cytology and microbial culture and sensitivity.[2,3] Simple fractures usually carry a fair to good prognosis, whereas contaminated, comminuted fractures or fractures involving a joint can carry a guarded to poor prognosis.[4,5] Limited information is available regarding bone healing in reptiles, though this is discussed in more detail in Chapter 81. Factors that affect bone healing include fracture configuration, age of the animal, nutritional status, and environmental temperature. Bone healing in reptiles tends to occur at a slower rate when compared with birds and mammals, and no secondary cartilage has been demonstrated in the reptilian fracture callus.[6] Healing time for traumatic fractures is generally 6 to 18 months, compared with 4 to 8 weeks in most mammals and 2 to 6 weeks in most avian species.[7] Pathologic fractures that result from MBD seem to heal more rapidly (6 to 8 weeks) if the inciting problem is corrected.

General principles of mammalian fracture fixation apply to reptile patients. Anatomic alignment, stabilization, and neutralization of bending, rotation, compression, and shear forces with minimal disruption of callus and soft tissues should be achieved.[8] Generally, the more forces that must be neutralized by the fixation, the higher the incidence rate of complications and failure. Factors to be considered when deciding on the fixation method to be used include the patient's functional requirements, surgeon's level of experience, the cost of materials/procedure, ease (length of time) of application, and availability of equipment. The patient's size, general health, and metabolic status may preclude a surgical approach to orthopedic repair. Most closed fractures in reptiles may heal without immobilization but will have varying degrees of malunion. However, as the field of zoological medicine continues to advance, it is important to always strive to offer the best treatment options available for the given patient's condition. Even though a given fracture may heal on its own without intervention, it is important to offer hospitalization, (surgical) fracture fixation, multimodal analgesia, and supportive care as part of the initial treatment plan. If financial constraints prohibit such a plan, then modifications to fit the needs of the owner and patient can be made.

PREOPERATIVE AND POSTOPERATIVE CARE

A thorough history, including husbandry details and a physical examination, should be performed before any reptile patient is anesthetized for fracture repair. Anesthetic protocols will vary based on the health of the reptile, species, and size (see Chapter 49). During surgery, all reptiles should be provided thermal support to optimize their anesthetic induction and recovery.[7] The surgical site should be aseptically prepared using 2% to 4% chlorhexidine solution and saline.[9–11] Alcohol can be used, though it exacerbates thermal losses. Aseptic preparation of reptile skin is difficult due to keratinized scales therefore it is recommended to perform a "rough" preparation first. Toothbrushes or commercially available surgical scrub brushes can be used for this initial "rough" scrub to remove debris and clean in between scales. Following a "rough" preparation, an aseptic preparation with contact time of 3 to 5 minutes should be performed.[10,12,13]

EXTERNAL COAPTATION

External coaptation, which involves the use of bandages, splints, or slings to immobilize a fracture, has been successfully used in reptiles of many sizes, including very small lizards, snakes, and giant tortoises. Fractures that are minimally displaced may heal with simple external coaptation. When dealing with pathologic fractures, external coaptation is usually the treatment of choice for initial fracture stabilization. This is because medical management of MBD must be initiated before bone healing can occur, and it is possible for the bones to suffer repeated or additional trauma if not bandaged or splinted. Bone is dynamic, and, during prolonged hypocalcemia (as in MBD), the mineralization process lags behind the deposition of organic bone matrix, resulting in the formation of hypomineralized bone. Reptiles suffering from MBD typically have osteoporosis and weak, thin cortices. Such bones are usually unsuitable (too soft) to support plates, pins, or other orthopedic hardware. If Steinmann pins are inserted, they contact a cortex and then may penetrate rather than being diverted down the medullary canal. Cerclage, hemicerclage, and interfragmentary wires may collapse the soft bone. Bone screws have minimal pull-out resistance when placed in soft bone. Similarly, external skeletal fixation does not function well because the bone purchase of the fixation pins is minimal. In some cases, intramedullary pins can be carefully inserted to provide axial alignment and some bending stability; however, external coaptation should also be applied because cortical purchase may be minimal. Fortunately, once calcium homeostasis has been reestablished, fracture healing progresses rapidly, with a fibrous union providing stability as early as 3 to 4 weeks. Medical therapies for hypocalcemia are discussed in Chapter 122.

Many splinting and casting techniques have been used successfully,[7,14,15] and anesthesia is recommended during application of any external coaptation device. This is to prevent iatrogenic fractures or comminutions and to minimize patient stress and pain. All forms of external coaptation should be monitored closely for evidence of soiling, slippage, vascular compromise, or other problems that may require bandage or splint replacement. Splints and bandages should be changed at weekly intervals (or more frequently if wet/soiled) throughout the healing period to ensure no complications develop and allow the veterinarian to monitor patient progress.

Fractures of digits can be immobilized using ball bandages, in which roll cotton is placed in the palmar or plantar aspect of the foot. Digits are rested in a neutral position over the cotton and wrapped or taped into position. The bandage should include the entire foot and lower limb. If the bandage is at risk of becoming wet or soiled, cotton should be avoided and a nonabsorbent material can be used in its place.[15] Waterproof tape or plastic bags can be used to protect the outer surface of the bandage and reduce the risk of soiling. Owners or caretakers should be instructed to monitor bandages daily for moisture or soiling, which would necessitate a bandage change. Fractures of the forelimb should be bandaged directly to the body to achieve immobilization (Fig. 108.1). The pelvic limbs should be bandaged to the tail (Fig. 108.2). The affected limb should be bandaged to support and pad the fracture site, including joints proximal and distal to the fracture, and then strapped to the body or tail base. For improved rigidity, a small splint can be added between the limb and body or tail. Splints can be made from a piece of wooden tongue depressor covered in tape to protect sharp edges, paper clips, or commercial splint materials such as Hexcelite (Hexcel Medical, Dublin, CA) or other thermal polymer plastic cast material. These lightweight splint materials are ideal in small reptiles

and are particularly useful in cases of metabolic bone disease, where the bones are not strong enough to carry a heavy bandage or splint. In cases of humeral or femoral fractures, similar techniques can be used. However, it is not always possible to adequately immobilize the scapulohumeral or coxofemoral joints, thus providing somewhat suboptimal reduction and immobilization. Depending on the body form of the reptile, some splints can be configured to adequately immobilize these joints by conforming to the affected limb and extending across the body or down the tail base.[15] In lizards, fractures of the humerus or femur can be stabilized with a modified spica splint that crosses over the pelvic or pectoral girdle to the opposite limb, thereby stabilizing the hip or shoulder joint and achieving the goal of immobilizing the joints proximal and distal to the fracture. Most lizards stand relatively low and use lateral abdominal undulation as an aid to locomotion, thus allowing them the ability to ambulate even with this type of device. With fractures of the pelvic limb, the splint should cross midline dorsally to allow normal voiding, and with fractures of the pectoral limb, the splint should cross ventrally (Fig. 108.3A and B). Juveniles that are still growing rapidly are at risk for joint deformity or loss of range of motion if the joints are immobilized for a prolonged period of time.[15]

A tube such as a syringe case of a diameter appropriate to the size of the patient's limb can be padded on one end (proximal end) and used as a splint. Tape stirrups are applied to the limb and secured to the syringe case/tube. Padding should be added to the limb to limit movement and avoid additional strain and fracture within the tube. The tape is then pulled through the tube so that the padded end of the tube is moved into the inguinal or axillary region, and the limb is maintained in traction. The tape is secured to the outside of the tube to maintain the leg in extension and traction.

In chelonians, fractures can be immobilized by restricting limb movement within the shell. The openings between the plastron and carapace (the cervicobrachial and prefemoral fossae) are physically blocked using sturdy tape or other adhesive material (Elastikon elastic tape [Johnson & Johnson], duct tape, etc) to prevent the limb from being extended out from the shell. This provides immobilization but unfortunately does not address fracture alignment and can result in greater fracture displacement. However, the resulting malunion may be acceptable for function (Fig. 108.4).

Snakes are occasionally evaluated because of spinal abnormalities. These spinal changes may be the result of osteoarthritis, osteoarthrosis, vertebral luxation (subluxation), or fracture.[16] In the case of spinal fractures, a body cast has been shown to be effective and easy to apply.[17]

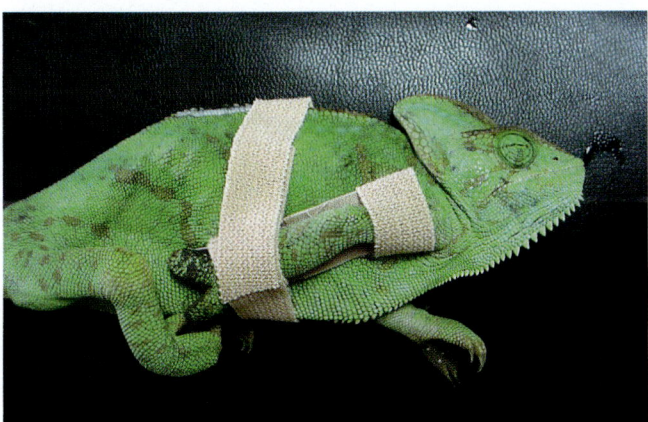

FIG 108.1 Fractures of the humerus, radius, and ulna can be stabilized by pulling the leg caudally to apply traction to aid in reduction and securing forelimb to the body with adhesive tape. Pictured here is a veiled chameleon (*Chamaeleo calyptratus*) with a fractured radius and ulna, with carpus and elbow immobilized using a lightweight splint secured to the body caudally. (Courtesy of Stephen J. Divers.)

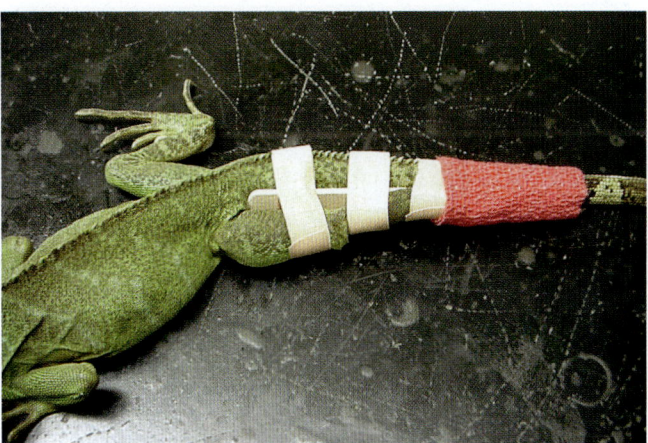

FIG 108.2 Immobilization of the pelvic limb secured to the tail base in a Chinese water dragon (*Physignathus cocincinus*). (Courtesy of Stephen J. Divers.)

The principles of application are to provide an even, continuous layer of cotton padding that conforms to the body and is just thick enough to allow a tube to fit snugly over top. A lightweight, rigid tube (cardboard) is then placed over the affected area. Tube ends should be padded and the tube affixed to the snake using elastic adhesive bandage followed by waterproof tape (Fig. 108.5).[17] It is critical to not add extra cotton padding in areas of depression or to add less over elevated areas, because this will exacerbate the fragment displacement. Snakes in body casts should be fed small food items that will not cause distension of the body wall and can be easily passed.[17]

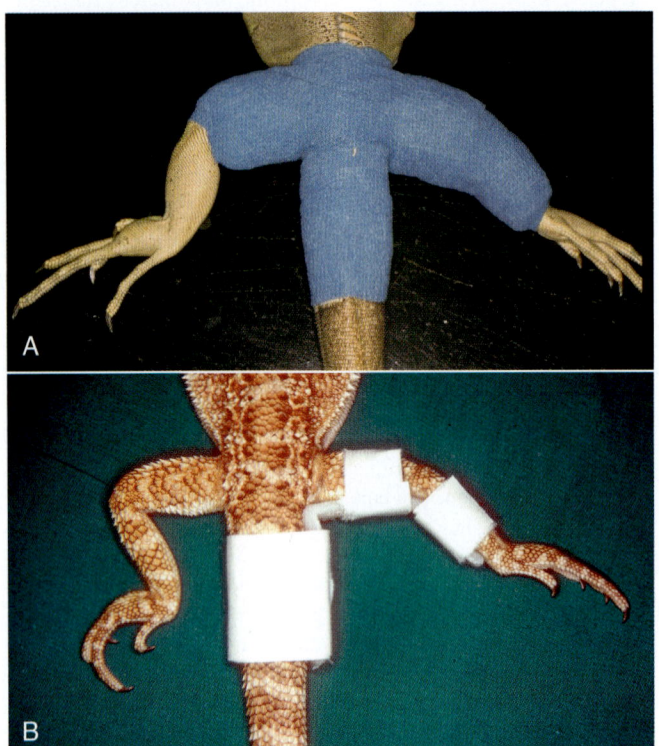

FIG 108.3 (A) A right femoral fracture immobilized using hexalite cast material covered with vetwrap in a green iguana *(Iguana iguana).* The cast extends from the right tarsus, across the dorsal pelvis to the left stifle to immobilize the coxofemoral joints. (B) Fractured right femur in an inland bearded dragon *(Pogona vitticeps).* The stifle and coxofemoral joints are immobilized using a lightweight thermal splint and tape, which extends down the tail base. (Courtesy of Stephen J. Divers.)

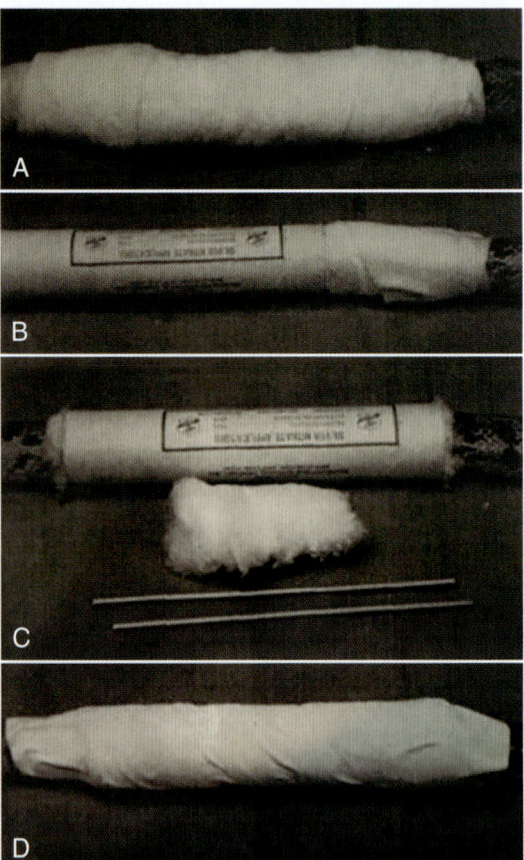

FIG 108.5 Application of a body cast in a snake. (A) Continuous layers of cotton bandage are applied to the affected area, taking care to apply cotton evenly and thick enough for a snug fit of the tube. (B) A rigid tube is fitted over the site. (C) Any openings are filled and padded with additional cotton. (D) The cast is then secured using adhesive bandage, including segments of the body proximal and distal to the tube. Water repellent tape is then applied over top.

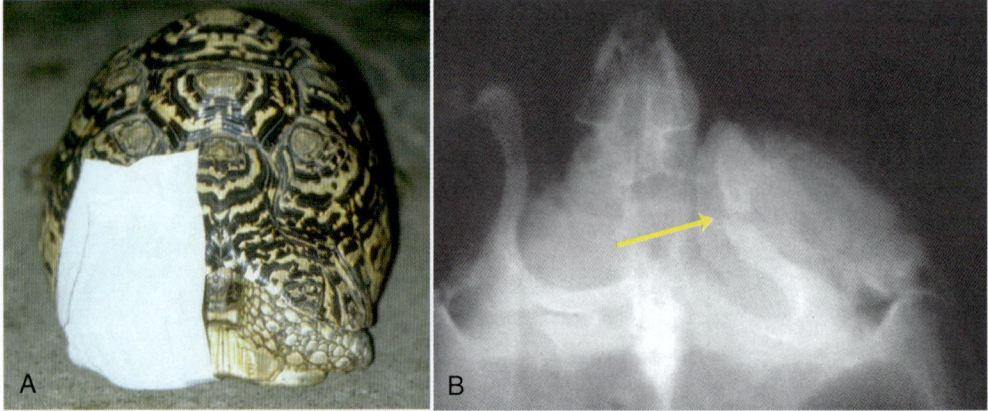

FIG 108.4 (A) In chelonians with a fractured humerus or femur, the limb can be folded into the cavity created between the plastron and the carapace and taped in place to prevent movement, as shown in this leopard tortoise *(Stigmochelys pardalis).* (B) It is recommended to radiograph the limb after it is secured in place to ensure adequate reduction (arrow).

Orthoplast (Johnson & Johnson, New Brunswick, NJ), Hexcelite (Hexcel Medical, Dublin, CA), and veterinary thermoplastic (VTP; Imex Veterinary, Inc., Longview, TX) are rigid at room temperature but when heated in water become malleable. This allows the material to conform closely to the configuration of the limb. Orthoplast is a solid sheet, and Hexcelite is a webbed form available in a roll or sheet. Hexcelite is much easier to conform, but it is not as strong when cool and solid. Veterinary thermoplastic is available in various sizes and thicknesses. It is a solid sheet with a fibermesh reinforcement within the plastic. It is easy to cut to appropriate size, is more malleable than Orthoplast, and is more rigid than Hexcelite, thus making it ideally suited for use as a splint.

Radiography of the limb before and after placement of any bandage or splint is recommended to ensure adequate fracture alignment. If the fracture is not properly reduced, the splint or bandage should be removed, the limb set, and the splint or bandage then reapplied. Sedation or anesthesia is helpful when trying to align the fracture and also decreases patient pain and stress. Fractures splinted in this fashion may take several months to heal. Recheck the patient in approximately 1 to 2 weeks to assess the tolerance of any splints or bandages and the need for adaptations to the coaptation (as swelling reduces). This first recheck also permits assessment of potential complications earlier in the healing process. After the first recheck, the patient should be seen for examination and for radiographs every 4 to 6 weeks until union has occurred. Healing typically takes 6 to 12 weeks (even up to 18 months), and, unlike in mammals, initial healing will be made by fibrous union and may not be radiographically evident for many weeks. Owners should be clearly instructed to remove rocks, branches, or anything else upon which the animal may climb. As a result of enclosure redesign, the heat and light sources may also need to be repositioned to maintain the thermal mosaic within the preferred optimal temperature zone (POTZ) for the species.

ACKNOWLEDGMENTS

The authors would like to acknowledge Avery Bennett and Douglas Mader for their contributions to the previous edition of this chapter.

REFERENCES

See www.expertconsult.com for a complete list of references.

109

Fracture Fixation and Arthrodesis

S. Emi Knafo and W. Michael Karlin

The majority of long bone fractures should ideally be repaired by internal fixation techniques. External coaptation may not be well tolerated by all reptile patients and is not feasible in aquatic and semiaquatic species. However, it is critical to perform a complete physical examination and assess the overall health of the patient, as bones affected by any metabolic bone disease (MBD) are not able to support internal fixation. Most surgical methods for fracture fixation, including bone plates, intramedullary pins, and cerclage wire, have been used successfully in reptiles.[1–7] The surgical approach to the long bones and the principles of application of internal fixation in reptiles are similar to those used in mammalian patients.

Intramedullary Steinmann Pins and orthopedic wires are inexpensive, provide axial alignment bending stability, and require minimal tissue exposure for insertion. Kirschner wires can be used as intramedullary pins and are available in sizes as small as 0.71 mm (0.028 inches). Spinal needles, which are available as small as 25 gauge (0.51 mm) x 8.9 cm (3.5 inches), can also be used as intramedullary pins in small patients.

External skeletal fixation (ESF) can be used for stabilizing a variety of fractures in reptiles. These fixation systems are especially well suited for open, contaminated fractures because they minimize the amount of hardware introduced into the bone through traumatized or contaminated tissues and can be placed without internal or permanent hardware in the surgical site. These devices provide good stability without interfering with joints and may be applied to small patients. ESF devices can include various-size Kirschner wires, Steinmann Pins, or hypodermic needles as fixation pins. Commercially available connecting bars and clamps are now more lightweight (carbon fiber) but can be substituted with acrylic polymer or a penrose drain or small hallow tube filled with acrylic (Table 109.1). In the past, polymethylmethacrylate has been used but presents some concerns for safety risks. Therefore products such as acrylic pin external fixation system (APEFS) or Acrylx from IMEX should be used. ESF is typically not possible in chelonian limbs, as the shell interferes with the external hardware. However, ESF techniques have been used successfully to repair mandibular fractures (see Chapter 110).[8]

In fracture management with ESF, pins must be cleaned daily with antiseptic disinfectant, as ascending infection can lead to pin loosening. It is common practice to provide intra-operative antimicrobial cover starting IV or IO 30 to 60 minutes prior to surgery. However, prevention of infection post-operatively relies heavily on aseptic preparation and appropriate pin management. The routine use of postoperative antibiotics following sterile surgery is inappropriate. Pin loosening is also commonly associated with unthreaded pins, and the components of the fixator should be inspected daily to identify problems early.[9] Highly active or fractious animals should be closely monitored for damage to the ESF or trauma to the affected limb. The success of the repair depends on the ability of the bone to heal before the fixation pins

loosen and the device fails. Because reptile bones heal slowly, the pins are at risk of loosening before the fracture is stable. However, pin purchase can be maximized with positive-profile threaded pins (Fig. 109.1).[10–12] Radiographs should be repeated throughout convalescence to monitor healing. Typically radiographs are rechecked every 2 to 4 weeks, but frequency should be adjusted as needed based on patient progress.

The more heavy-bodied and active the animal is, the more rotational forces will impact fracture reduction and immobilization. Therefore in large patients, bone plating may be the most appropriate fixation technique. Bone plates provide excellent rigid fixation when angular forces may challenge the fixation.[13] However, application of bone plates often requires significant exposure for proper placement, though minimally invasive plate application techniques can be used to improve recovery and outcome.[14] In some instances, closure may be difficult, as reptile skin is less elastic than mammalian skin and may not accommodate the plate easily.[13] Veterinary cuttable plates (Synthes Ltd. USA, Paoli, PA) with screws as small as 1.5 mm in diameter (1.1 mm core diameter) permit plating of bones as small as 3 mm in diameter. Finger plates are also applicable to many long bone fractures in small reptiles. In some reptiles, the long bones are more dramatically curved, and plate contouring will be necessary. The 2.7-mm reconstruction plates may be used to allow the plate to be contoured to such bones. Bone plating requires specific expertise and equipment (Fig. 109.2). Locking plates have also been beneficial in providing a stable internal angle construct, which has the benefit of increased stability compared to traditional systems and is superior in soft bone (Table 109.2).

In most cases, removal of bone plates is not necessary or recommended. As is standard practice in domestic species, the decision to remove intramedullary pins or external skeletal fixators should be based on radiographic evidence of bone healing. However, in reptiles a fibrous union forms before radiographic evidence of healing occurs. This fibrous union may provide adequate stability, allowing fracture healing to proceed to completion if the implants fail or must be removed before the development of radiographic union.

BONE GRAFTING

Due to the nature of most reptilian fractures (e.g., trauma, MBD, hypomineralization, pathological fractures), rigid fixation is often not possible. Compression across the fracture site is paramount to ensure primary bone healing, but this may not always be possible in the reptile patient. Motion at the fracture site is a common reason for fracture repair failure. In many cases, external coaptation holds the limb steady with the fracture fragments in approximation but does not provide the same compression as properly applied bone plates. Incomplete fracture healing may still produce an acceptable outcome for small

TABLE 109.1 External Skeletal Fixator System and Pin Sizes Available

Ex Fix and Pin Size	0.9 mm	1.1 mm	1.6 mm	1.8 mm	2.0 mm	2.4 mm	2.5 mm	3.0 mm	3.2 mm	3.5 mm	4.0 mm	4.3 mm	4.8 mm
Securos Small TITAN ESF	-	-	+	-	-	+	-	-	-	-	-	-	-
Securos Large TITAN ESF	-	-	-	-	-	-	-	-	-	+	-	+	-
Mini SK	+	+	+	-	+	-	+	-	-	-	-	-	-
Small SK	-	-	-	-	+	+	-	+	+	+	+	-	-
Large SK	-	-	-	-	-	-	-	+	+	+	+	+	+
FESSA Ex-Fix 6 mm Tube	+	-	-	+	-	-	-	-	-	-	-	-	-
FESSA Ex-Fix 8 mm Tube	-	-	+	-	-	-	-	-	+	-	-	-	-

For small patients, tiny k-wires or hypodermic needles can be used and acrylic connecting bars can be custom-made to fit the pin configuration. Acrylic Pin External Fixator System, Innovative Animal Products, Rochester, MN; Acrylx ESF Acrylic, IMEX Veterinary, Inc, Longview, TX. Securos Surgical, Fiskdale, MA, connecting rods available: small TITAN system, 6.3 mm; large TITAN, 9.5 mm. FESSA IMEX Veterinary Inc., Longview, TX, SK-connecting rods available in various sizes: for mini SK, 3.2 mm stainless steel; small SK, 6.3 mm in titanium and carbon fiber; large SK, 9.5 mm stainless steel and carbon fiber.
Fixateur Externe du Service de Sante des Armees (FESSA) (Jorgensen Labs, Loveland, CO) external fixatory system connecting tubes (6 mm and 8 mm) available in stainless steel and titanium.

TABLE 109.2 Implant Type and Sizes Available

Implant Type and Sizes Available	1.5 mm	2.0 mm	2.4 mm	2.7 mm	3.5 mm	3.5 mm Broad	4.5 mm	4.5 mm Broad
Dynamic Compression Plate (DCP)	-	+	-	+	+	+	+	+
Limited Contact–Dynamic Compression Plate (LC-DCP)	+	+	+	+	+	+	+	+
Locking Compression Plate (LCP)	+	+	+	+	+	+	+	+
Recon Plates	-	+	+	+	+	-	-	-
Cuttable Plates	+	+	-	+	-	-	-	-
Specialty Plates	+	+	+	+	+	+	+	+

DCP, Dynamic compression plate; *LCP*, locking compression plate; *LC-DCP*, limited contact dynamic compression.

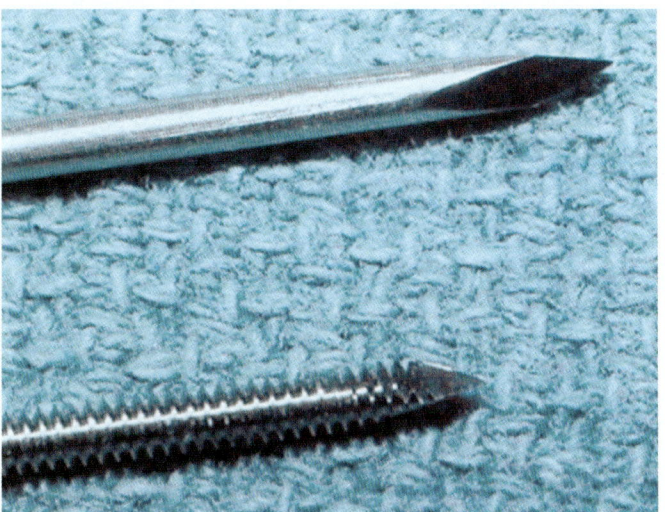

FIG 109.1 Pin purchase can be maximized by using threaded pins, preferably using positive profile pins versus negative profile pins. (Courtesy of Douglas R. Mader.)

terrestrial reptiles and those kept as pets. However, large reptiles, aquatic species, and wild individuals may not do well if their limbs are not completely functional.

As is commonly performed in mammalian patients with complicated fracture repairs, corticocancellous bone grafts may be necessary.[15] Bone grafts can be classified as osteogenic, osteoinductive, and osteoconductive. Osteogenic bone grafts supply and promote bone-forming cells. An osteoinductive bone graft has the ability to induce bone formation when placed into an area where no bone formation will occur. Osteoconductive grafts provide a scaffold for bone formation. In larger reptiles, bone grafts can be harvested from the proximal humerus or femur. A section of rib can be collected, morselized, and used as a corticocancellous graft. In smaller animals, the wing of the ilium is readily accessible. An incision is made over either wing, and a rongeur is used to harvest pieces of bone. These bone chips can be carefully crushed to increase the surface area of the graft and placed in a saline-soaked gauze until they can be packed within and around the fracture site prior to closure. There has been research that shows safety and benefit to the use of platelet-rich plasma in exotic species to promote healing, including a fracture model.[16,17]

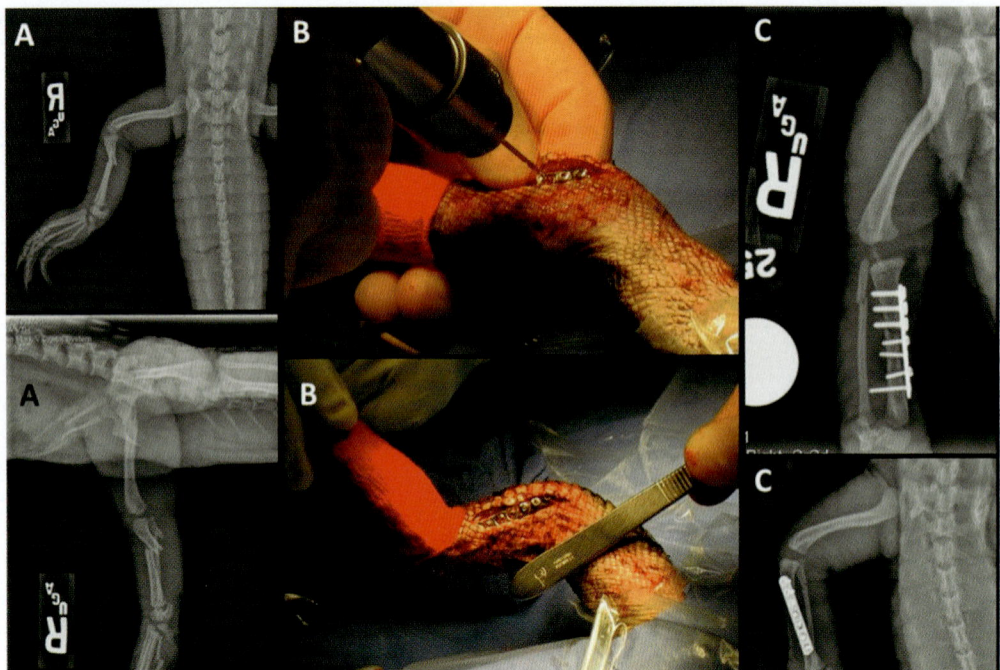

FIG 109.2 (A) Preoperative radiographs demonstrating complete, transverse, mid-diaphyseal right tibia/fibula fracture with moderate angulation (juvenile American alligator, *Alligator mississippiensis*). (B) Intraoperative photographs showing application of a locking bone plate. (C) Postoperative radiographs showing fracture fixation by plating. (Courtesy of Stephen J. Divers.)

Osteogenic bone stimulation can be used as an adjunct therapy to bone graft and external skeletal fixator. Successful use was reported in a Chinese water dragon (*Physignathus cocincinus*) to repair a nonunion fracture of the tibia.[18] A 1.5-volt (DC) battery source provided constant current output (20.5 ma), the IM pin served as the anode, and a subcutaneous implant over the nonunion site acted as the cathode. The fractured tibia was repaired using an IM pin and external skeletal fixator along with a bone graft harvested from the ilium. The osteogenic bone stimulator was left in place for 3 weeks, and the external fixator and IM pin were removed 3 weeks later. Radiographic evidence showed callus formation at the 6-week mark, and the animal recovered well.

COMPLICATIONS OF FRACTURE REPAIR

Implant loosening, migration, bending, and osteomyelitis are all potential complications. Failure of fracture repair should be approached similarly as in domestic mammals. Patient husbandry and nutrition must also be evaluated and optimized. Implants need to be removed from infected sites and cultured for pathogens. Antibiotics should be selected on the basis of culture and sensitivity results. Fistulae should be explored, sequestra removed, affected bone radically debrided, and abscesses treated. Once the patient is stabilized and the infection is controlled, attempts to repair the fracture can be pursued. If owner finances or compliance are concerns, or the limb is not salvageable, then amputation should be considered (see Chapter 111).

Osteomyelitis is a common disease in reptiles, often from hematogenous spread. However, osteomyelitis can also occur secondary to trauma, fractures, and implant infections. Diagnosis is made by hematology, palpation, fine-needle aspirate for cytology and culture, and radiography. Typical signs in mammals, such as swelling, heat, and pain, are not typically appreciated in reptiles.[19] Additionally, radiographically evident periosteal reactions expected in mammals may not be present in reptiles.[13] Implantation of antibiotic-impregnated methylmethacrylate beads has proven successful for the treatment of osteomyelitis. If beads have been placed in a joint, they must be removed once the infection is resolved.

If the beads are placed in soft tissue or in or around bone, the beads do not need to be recovered.

ARTHRODESIS

Techniques used in mammalian orthopedics have been used in reptiles as treatment modalities with varying degrees of success. Coxofemoral luxations are seen frequently in chelonians and lizards. When presented early, these luxations are usually reasonably easy to reduce. Immobilization is achieved by bandaging the limb within the prefemoral fossa of chelonians and maintaining this for approximately 2 weeks. It is important to radiograph post bandaging to ensure that fracture displacement has not been aggravated. If coxofemoral luxations are presented in a chronic condition, reduction can be more challenging. In severe cases, femoral head (and neck) excision may be necessary. Successful use of this technique has been reported in chelonians,[2] but less favorable results have been reported in lizards.[20] Stifle luxation and cranial cruciate ligament rupture was successfully repaired using an over-the-top (with lateral vastus autograft) technique in a tortoise.[21]

In certain cases, arthrodesis may be necessary. Arthrodesis of the elbow was successfully performed in a green iguana (Mader D, unpublished data) with deep soft tissue injuries and osteomyelitis (Fig. 109.3). In this individual, the opposite forelimb had been previously amputated. Therefore amputation of the newly affected limb was not possible, though it likely would have been the treatment of choice. A cubital arthrotomy was performed, and the joint surface was debrided. The remaining space was packed with a cancellous bone graft, and a type II transarticular external fixator was applied (Fig. 109.4). Postoperative cage rest was instituted, and by 12 weeks sufficient callus was observed radiographically to remove the external skeletal fixator. The patient was mobile and was able to climb slightly inclined branches.

A desert tortoise required a carpal arthrodesis after repeated injections of enrofloxacin in the proximal limb resulted in radial nerve paralysis (Mader D, unpublished data). A mid-diaphyseal hole was drilled through the radius. A 20-guage orthopedic wire was then used to encircle ventral

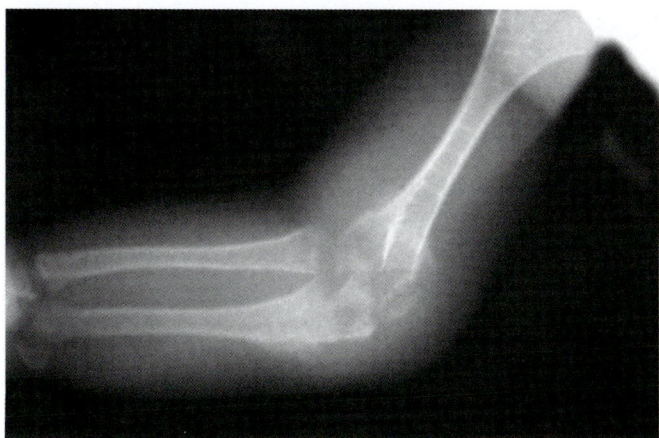

FIG 109.3 Osteomyelitis in the elbow of a green iguana (*Iguana iguana*). (Courtesy of Douglas R. Mader.)

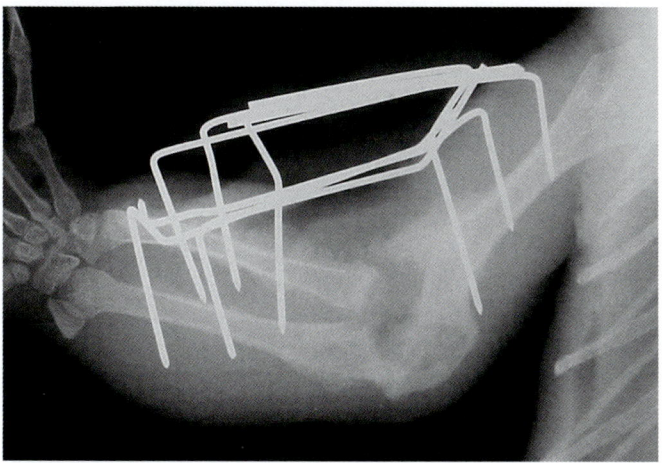

FIG 109.4 An arthrotomy was performed on the elbow joint of the patient in Fig. 109.3. The joint surface was curetted away, and the space was packed with a corticocancellous bone graft. A biplanar external fixator was applied across the joint for stability. Radiographs taken at 6 weeks postsurgery showed initial bridging and callus formation. (Courtesy of Douglas R. Mader.)

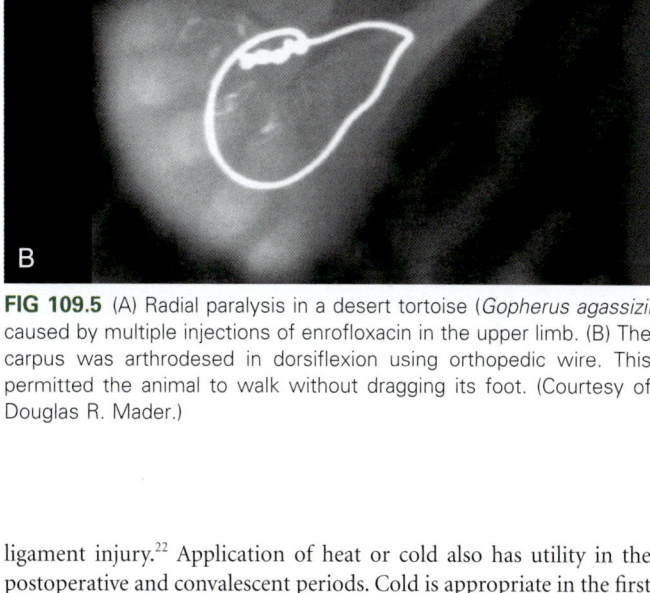

FIG 109.5 (A) Radial paralysis in a desert tortoise (*Gopherus agassizii* caused by multiple injections of enrofloxacin in the upper limb. (B) The carpus was arthrodesed in dorsiflexion using orthopedic wire. This permitted the animal to walk without dragging its foot. (Courtesy of Douglas R. Mader.)

to the digits and connect back to its origin in the radius (Fig. 109.5). With tension on the wire, the carpus was maintained in permanent extension.

PHYSICAL THERAPY

Physical therapy aims to restore full use of an injured body part through increasing blood and lymphatic flow through affected tissues. Such increased perfusion helps resolve inflammation, minimize muscle atrophy, and reduce the incidence of fracture callus entrapment of soft tissues. Range of motion (ROM) is preserved or regained through active and passive ROM exercises. Joint angles should be measured objectively at the start of PT and periodically throughout the course of treatment. Each joint should be moved through 10 flexions and extensions, and then the entire limb moved through full ROM.[22] Massage softens and lengthens tendons and muscles and improves circulation. It also serves to separate abnormally adhered, inflamed soft tissue structures. Other therapies include ultrasound, which produces deep physiological heat and is best used in cases of muscle spasm, adhesions, and tendon/

ligament injury.[22] Application of heat or cold also has utility in the postoperative and convalescent periods. Cold is appropriate in the first 24 to 72 hours after surgery to induce vasoconstriction, and as a result reduces edema and inflammation and decreases pain perception by slowing nerve-conduction velocity. Heat produces vasodilation, which increases local perfusion and aids in drainage of edema. Pain relief is achieved by softening muscles and soft tissues that may be in spasm.[22] Please see Chapter 129 for additional information on low-level therapeutic laser therapy.

Physical therapy (PT) in reptiles is not well described in the literature. Several case reports describe the use of specific techniques in individual animals with varied success. However, postoperative PT is likely an important yet underappreciated tool in aiding recovery in reptile species (see Chapter 131).

A recent case report describes the use of the Wolfe Kinetic Technique to treat severe osteoarthritis in a 20-year-old Komodo dragon (*Varanus komodoensis*).[23] This animal had failed to respond significantly to oral analgesics and suffered from chronic, progressive lameness with decreased mobility. The Wolfe Kinetic Technique (WKT), which uses gentle manual manipulation, aims to change movement patterns to spread the workload of the body as the animal moves. The WKT focuses on the spine, ribs, and pelvis, because the central tenet is that spine and core must move normally in order for the extremities to function normally.[23] This Komodo dragon underwent weekly sessions with a physical therapist that focused on the thoracic spine, scapular stabilizers, lumbar spine, and pelvis. Within the first month, a noticeable improvement in mobility was reported. By 9 weeks, the animal was seen running, and by 12 weeks the animal was able to successfully negotiate a 12-inch step, which had not been witnessed in several years. The animal's gait, comfort, and mobility improved dramatically, and the sessions with the physical therapist were decreased to every other week. Eventually, the animal was taken off all but one oral analgesic, and the dose of that remaining medication was reduced with no adverse effects.[23]

ACKNOWLEDGMENTS

The authors would like to acknowledge Avery Bennett and Douglas Mader for their contributions to the previous edition of this chapter.

REFERENCES

See www.expertconsult.com for a complete list of references.

110

Skull and Spinal Fracture Repair

S. Emi Knafo and W. Michael Karlin

Skull and spinal fractures can occur as a result of traumatic or metabolic causes. Skull fractures are more commonly seen in reptile species with rigid skulls. However, species with cranial kinesis, specifically snakes, still suffer from skull fractures in spite of their relatively malleable skulls. Fractures of the calvarium, mandible, and separation of the symphysis are the most common injuries seen.[1-3] Pathological fractures are associated with metabolic bone disease (MBD), and iatrogenic mandibular fractures (and dental trauma) can occur during attempts to open the mouth in an animal concurrently suffering from MBD or other pathology (especially osteomyelitis).

SKULL FRACTURES

Chinese water dragons (*Physignathus cocincinus*), sail-fin lizards (*Hydrosaurus pustulatus*), and other high-energy, nervous lizards may cause trauma to the mandible by repeated concussive force against enclosure walls. Similarly, snakes may strike glass enclosure walls while attempting to capture prey and injure their jaws. Because their skulls are normally distensible, fractures may initially go unnoticed; however, mandibular fractures are frequently open, which makes the traumatic event more evident to caretakers.[4] The open nature of mandibular fractures also increases the risk of secondary infection.[4-7] Symphyseal fractures in lizards can result in malalignment of dentition if not repaired.[4-7] Circumferential wiring of the mandibular symphysis (Fig. 110.1) creates a stable enough repair to allow healing, as long as the remainder of the jaw is intact. When oral fractures are more severe, interdental wiring with splinting, external fixator, or plating may be necessary.[4-7]

Diagnostic imaging should be performed to completely evaluate fracture configuration. Radiography should be performed before and after fixation. Alternatively, computed tomography or other advanced imaging can help yield greater detail and has been shown to aid in guiding diagnosis and repair in several species.[1,8] External fixation is commonly used to stabilize mandibular fractures in reptiles. Small pins or even hypodermic needles can be used as cross pins to create an external skeletal fixator. Intramedullary pins and cerclage wires can be used depending on the configuration of the fracture and size of the patient (see Fig. 110.1). The use of external or internal fixation

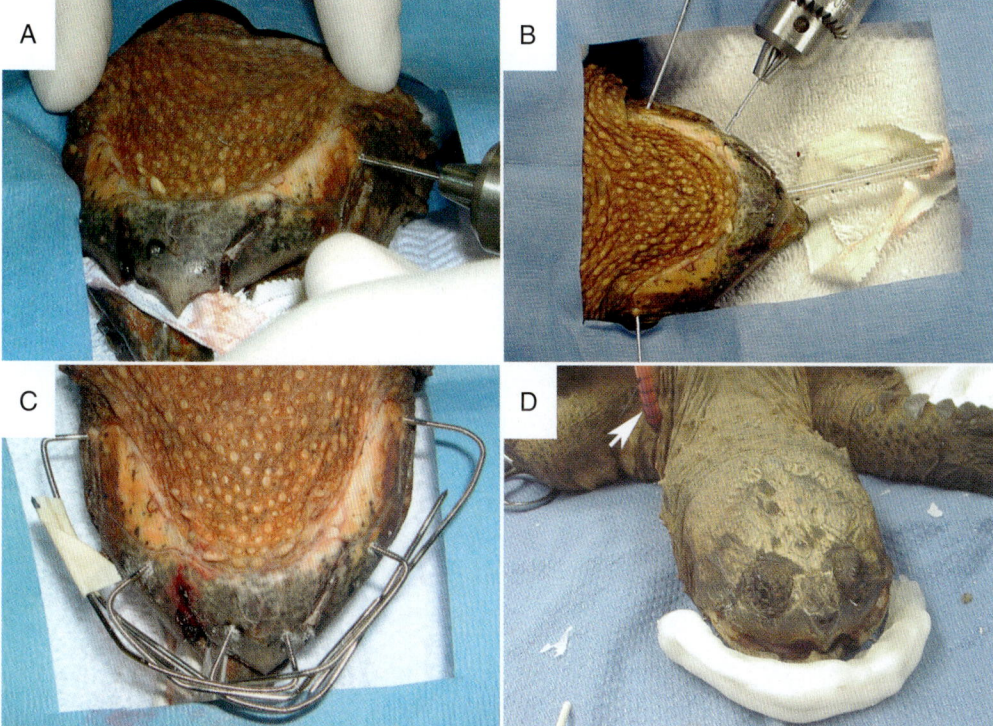

FIG 110.1 (A and B) Placement of cross pins using hand chuck in an anesthetized snapping turtle (*Chelydra serpentine*) with mandibular fractures. (C) Bent cross pins to form a tie-in external skeletal fixator connecting bar. (D) Application of polymethylmethacrylate to strengthen and cover connecting bar. An esophagostomy tube (*arrow*) was placed to permit feeding during the 12-week healing process. (Courtesy of Stephen J. Divers.)

allows the animal to continue eating. However, external coaptation in the form of bandaging the mouth closed can also be used to stabilize jaw fractures.[4–7] In these cases, an esophagostomy tube must be placed to allow nutritional support during healing.[4] Typically, this technique is used in patients with suboptimal bone health, such as in cases of MBD. Traumatic, perforating fractures extending into the nasal cavities and paranasal sinuses in an alligator were successfully treated using methyl methacrylate to create an airtight seal over the perforations during healing.[3]

SPINAL FRACTURES

Pathological fractures of the spine are seen commonly in chelonians and lizards suffering from metabolic bone disease. Snakes have been reported to suffer from bacterial infection of the vertebrae manifesting as segmental, proliferative osteoarthritis and osteoarthrosis of the spine.[9] Most commonly, gram-negative bacteria are isolated, but gram-positive isolates have been reported.[9] Trauma from improper handling can also be a cause of spinal fracture in reptiles. When surgical stabilization of spinal column injury is pursued, it is important to focus on neutralizing the forces that result in bending, compression, shear, and torsion on the affected vertebra.[10–13] Severe injury can potentially occur to the spinal cord or nerve roots with fractures and luxation of the spinal column.[10–13] Stabilization of the spinal column and possible decompression of the cord or both should be explored to mitigate further damage.[10–13] It is important to perform a thorough physical and neurological examination to determine if any concurrent injury may be present. The decision on how to treat luxations and fractures of the spine depends largely on the fracture and the neurological status of the patient. Patients that have an unstable or compressive lesion should be surgically treated.[10–13] Radiographic or CT evaluation is important to determine displacement, but nondisplaced or minimally displaced injuries should be approached cautiously because they can be unstable.[13] Treatment of spinal fractures and luxations can be addressed with conservative or surgical management, used alone or in combination.

The application of a body cast for nonsurgical treatment of spinal fractures is described in Chapter 108. Given that most cases of spinal fracture in reptiles are due to pathological processes (MBD or bacterial infection), surgical repair may not be recommended in all cases. If there is concern for a possible pathological process, then the underlying disease should be addressed. Nonsurgical fracture management techniques may be applied until the patient is more stable and a better surgical candidate. If surgery is to be pursued, the same principles of spinal surgery in mammals apply. In cases where severe neurological deficits are present, the animal's quality of life should be evaluated and euthanasia considered.

Cervical spondylomyelopathy (CSM) is a disease often seen in large- and giant-breed dogs characterized by compression of the cervical spinal cord and/or nerve roots. This is a very complex disease and is not fully understood. Treatment is focused on stabilization and decompression of the cervical spinal cord. Pathophysiology of cervical spondylomyelopathy involves both static (cervical canal stenosis) and dynamic factors. A similar disease of compressive myelopathy of the cervical spine has been seen in four captive Komodo dragons (*Varanus komodoensis*), with three presumptively induced by trauma.[14] Clinical signs and disease progression were similar to what has been seen in small animals; however, the onset of clinical signs is not often associated with a known trauma (in small animals), as was the case in three of the four affected Komodo dragons.[14] The outcome in the case series of Komodo dragons resulted in all dragons being euthanized (range 4 days to 12 months). Komodo dragons have a single occipital condyle (as in all reptiles), single intervertebral articular surface, and ligamentous differences compared to mammals.[1] The difference in anatomy between the Komodo dragon and small animals may be a reason for the poor outcomes noted. Further investigation is needed to ascertain the best way to manage compressive myelopathy in Komodo dragons.

REFERENCES

See www.expertconsult.com for a complete list of references.

111

Limb Amputation

S. Emi Knafo and W. Michael Karlin

Digits and limbs frequently require amputation as a result of trauma or infection.[1,2] Chronic dysecdysis around a toe, or wire/string around a limb, can quickly result in ischemic injury. In cases where infection or pain is not sufficiently controlled, or if there is evidence of osteomyelitis, amputation is appropriate.[1,2] Highly comminuted fractures where blood supply is compromised and cases of nonunion and limb neoplasia may also necessitate amputation.[1,2] Lesions confined to the phalanges are typically amputated at the level of the metacarpus or metatarsus. When disease has progressed more proximally to include the carpus or tarsus, then partial or complete limb amputation is indicated.[1,2] Before amputation is pursued, it is important to assess the animal to determine if any other systemic, orthopedic, or neurological issues are present that may affect outcome once a limb is amputated. In some cases, slinging the affected leg can help determine how the animal will adapt to amputation and get them accustomed to ambulating without the limb. It is important to note that occasionally this can be misleading in dogs, where an individual dog will not adapt well to the sling but does well after amputation.[3] This could also be the case in some reptiles and should be kept in mind when assessing patients and advising owners.

In small animal limb amputations, there are several options for removal of the forelimb and hind limb. In forelimb amputations, techniques include disarticulation of the scapulohumeral joint or removal of the scapula. In hind limb amputations, techniques include osteotomy at the mid-diaphysis of the femur, disarticulation of the coxofemoral joint, and acetabulectomy. These different methods all have their proposed advantages and disadvantages depending on the disease process that is occurring to necessitate amputation.[4] Complications associated with amputations in small animals have been reported to include permanent gait changes, seroma formation, neuroma, phantom pain, and cervical disc herniation.[4]

Partial limb amputation will leave a stump that can be used to aid ambulation. However, such stumps can also become traumatized and (chronically) secondarily infected. The keratinized skin of most reptiles may reduce the risk of ulceration; however, as body weight increases, this complication becomes more common. Therefore partial limb amputation should be reserved for small lizards and chelonians.[1,2] When performing a partial limb amputation, the skin should be incised distal to the intended amputation site to preserve ample soft tissues to create tension-free closures. If possible, the incision should be oriented in

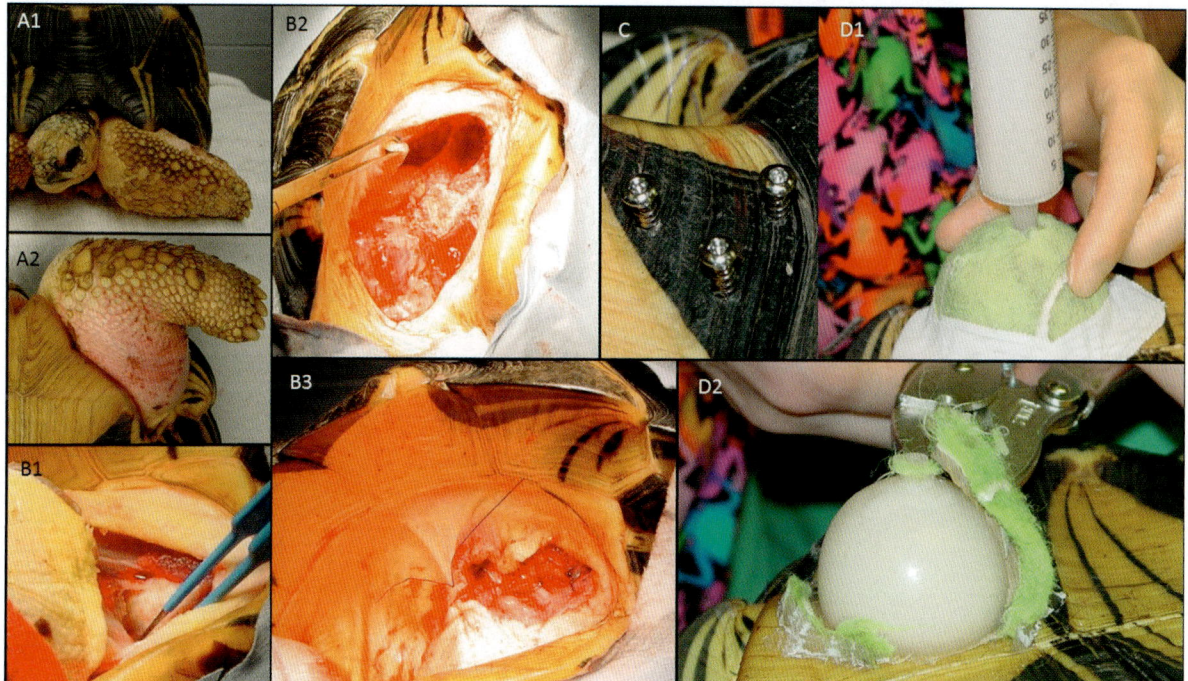

FIG 111.1 (A1 and A2) Sarcoma in the left forelimb of a radiated tortoise (*Astrochelys radiata*). (B1–B3) Amputation of the left forelimb at the scapulohumeral joint. (C) Three screws secured to the plastron. (D1–D2) Half a tennis ball placed over screws from panel (C), used as a mold for polymethylmethacrylate cement, with the tennis ball removed once set. (Courtesy of Stephen J. Divers.)

order to create a flap from the dorsal surface that is placed over the end of the amputated bone and sutured ventrally. This places healthy, keratinized skin on the weight-bearing surface in contact with the substrate. Muscle bellies should be transected at their distal insertions (or as distally as possible) and dissected proximally to allow for adequate soft tissue coverage (padding) over the amputation site. Soft tissues should ideally be transected using radiosurgery or laser to reduce hemorrhage.[2] Major vessels should be identified and ligated with suture, a vessel-sealing device, or vascular clips. A proximal tourniquet may provide additional aid in reducing surgical hemorrhage.

In large lizards, small lizards with proximal lesions, crocodilians, and large chelonians, the entire limb should be removed. This requires disarticulation of the limb at the scapulohumeral or coxofemoral joint.[1,2] A similar surgical approach should be made in these cases, with attention paid to preservation of adequate skin and muscle to allow tension-free closure. The muscles should be elevated proximally from the periosteum until the articulation is exposed. Smooth transection of the nerves with a scalpel, laser, or radiosurgery is recommended. The nerves may be injected with lidocaine or bupivicaine to minimize postoperative pain and help decrease anesthetic requirements. Chelonians undergoing hind limb amputation may benefit from intrathecal anesthesia as described in Chapter 51. In chelonians, prostheses may be provided by securing a furniture caster, wheel, or other appropriate object (tennis or billiard ball cut in half, toy skateboard, etc.) on the plastron ventral to the shoulder or hip joint with an acrylic cement (Fig. 111.1).[2,5] This helps elevate the affected corner of the shell and aids mobility with the remaining limbs. Use of prostheses also prevents dragging and secondary erosion of the plastron. In general, wheeled devices work best on firm level ground, while half-balls work better on natural ground. Postoperatively, bandages should be placed to offer, at minimum, protection of the incision and often compression when indicated. Cage rest and modifications of the enclosure are important during convalescence as the patient adapts to ambulating with three limbs.

REFERENCES

See www.expertconsult.com for a complete list of references.

112

Tail Amputation

Richard S. Funk

It is sometimes necessary to amputate a reptile's tail. Damage to the tail from trauma, including bite wounds, infection, or neoplasia, may leave the tail compromised such that amputation becomes the best treatment. The surgeon should strive to perform the amputation proximally enough to ensure all affected tissue is removed but distally enough to leave as much functional tail as possible. In male snakes and lizards, it is advisable to appreciate the location of and avoid the hemipenes. Along with a thorough physical examination, radiography or CT may be useful to determine bone involvement and help define the best site for amputation.

There is considerable taxonomic variation in the ability of lizards to perform autotomy, and many exceptions exist.[1] Most, if not all, members of the Dibamidae, Anelytropsidae, Lacertidae, Cordylidae, Xantusiidae, Scincidae, Teiidae, Anguidae, and Anniellidae possess postpygal vertebrae and can perform autotomy along the length of the tail. Most members of the Gekkonidae (including Eublepharinae and Diplodactylinae) can perform autotomy, but functional autotomy planes are restricted to the most basal postpygal vertebrae close to the tail base. All agamids that have been examined lack autotomy planes in their caudal vertebrae, but intervertebral breakage takes place in many forms. Vertebral autotomy planes have been reported in many anolines. Vertebral autotomy planes are largely absent or reduced during ontogeny in the iguanids and basiliscines but present in all sceloporines and most tropidurines. No vertebral fracture planes or autotomy have been found in the Varanidae, Lanthanotidae, Helodermatidae, and Chameleonidae. Tail autotomy is rare in snakes but has been reported in some colubrids.[1]

With lizards that are capable of caudal autotomy through an anatomic autotomy plane, it is practical and simple to aseptically scrub the tail and hold the base of the tail with one hand, and then with the other hand bend the tail sharply laterally to effectively amputate through a natural autotomy site (Fig. 112.1). Alternatively, some clinicians may prefer to control the exact location of the amputation (a safe distance above the damage or pathology), and a scalpel blade can be used to completely sever the tail. In either case little hemorrhage occurs, but pressure and styptic powder or solution can be utilized to control bleeding. The tail tip is left unsutured, but a temporary bandage may be applied. The owner can remove the bandage in several days and await the regeneration of a new though modified and shorter tail tip. Sedation or anesthesia is required, and some clinicians prefer to administer a local or ring block using lidocaine or bupivacaine proximal to the projected autotomy site. If the site is closed with sutures, the lizard may not be able to regenerate its tail.[2]

In small lizards, with thin tails, utilizing either a ring block or sedation, the tail is aseptically prepared, and the tail tip may then be cut off with a scalpel blade or with surgical scissors. A styptic powder can be applied, and the exposed tip may be closed with surgical adhesive. Some clinicians may choose to place a small temporary bandage.

With larger lizards that naturally exhibit tail autotomy, such as the green iguana (*Iguana iguana*), once adults and depending on the location of the amputation (if a major portion of the tail is involved) the tail may no longer exhibit autotomy and often requires surgery and closure at the amputation site (Fig. 112.2). Amputation surgery will also be necessary for reptiles that cannot naturally autotomize the tail including some lizards (e.g., helodermatids, varanids) and snakes, chelonians and crocodilians.

The reptile is anesthetized, and local anesthesia can be helpful (e.g., ring block, intrathecal anesthesia) (see Section 6). Squamates and crocodilians are typically placed in ventral recumbency, but dorsal recumbency often affords better visualization around the posterior shell of chelonians. In larger animals a tourniquet may be placed proximal to the surgical site (see Fig. 112.2). It is best to visualize the completed surgical site as a curved stump, either closed dorsoventrally or laterally, before making any incisions. For example, with green iguanas, the author's preference is a laterally closed site, but with bearded dragons, a dorsoventrally closed site is more esthetic (Fig. 112.3). Symmetrical wedge incisons are then made on either side of the tail (or top and bottom). The muscle is then transected, and the tail amputation completed by dissecting between two caudal vertebrae proximal to the tip of the skin where the two wedge tips are, such that closure can be accomplished with minimal tension. If there is too much tension on the skin, additional soft tissue dissection and removal can help. The tail skin is not elastic as it is in mammals. In larger reptiles the individual muscle groups (caudal spinalis, caudal extensor medialis, caudal extensor lateralis, iliocaudalis, caudofemoralis longus, ischiocudalis, and inferior coccygeus) may be identifiable, and the caudal vein or variable vessels may require ligation before skin closure.[3] The muscles should be opposed to cover the exposed vertebrae using absorbable monofilament suture (e.g., polyiglecaprone 25). The skin is trimmed if necessary and closed with eversion utilizing horizontal mattress or simple interrupted sutures.

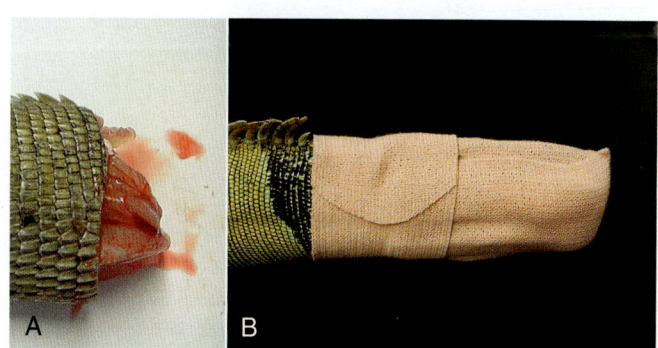

FIG 112.1 Simple tail amputation through a vertebral fracture plane in a green iguana (*Iguana iguana*). (A) Following the snap and twist, the tail separates and the muscle fibers can be trimmed. (B) The tail is not sutured but can be bandaged to prevent gross contamination. (Courtesy of Stephen J. Divers.)

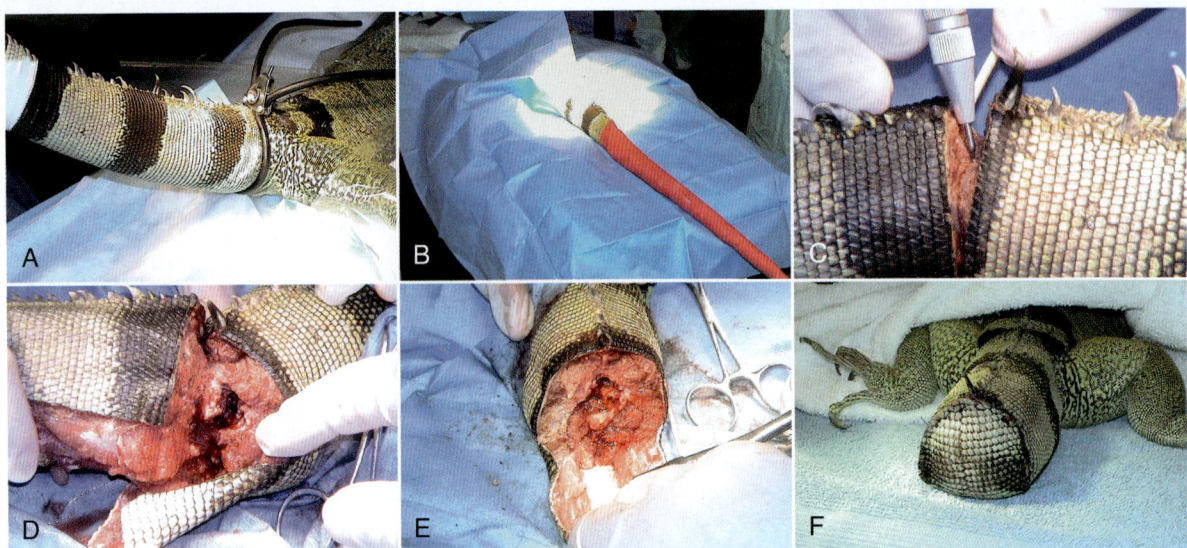

FIG 112.2 Major proximal tail amputation in a green iguana (*Iguana iguana*) by Heather Barron and Michael McBride. (A) Application of a tourniquet to reduce intraoperative hemorrhage. The tail has been suspended to facilitate aseptic preparation. (B) The tail has been placed through a sterile drape and wrapped with sterile bandaging distal to the planned surgical site. (C) Dissection through the dorsal skin and caudal spinalis, caudal extensor medialis, caudal extensor lateralis, and iliocaudalis muscles using a CO_2 laser. (D) Continued dissection through the lateral and ventral muscles, including the caudofemoralis longus, ischiocaudalis, and inferior coccygeus, followed by sharp vertebral separation. A large ventral skin flap is preserved for closure. (E) Following complete dissection of all muscles, ligamentous attachments, and the coccygeal spine, the muscles are sutured over the vertebral stump. (F) The large ventral skin flap is trimmed and sutured closed. (Courtesy of Stephen J. Divers.)

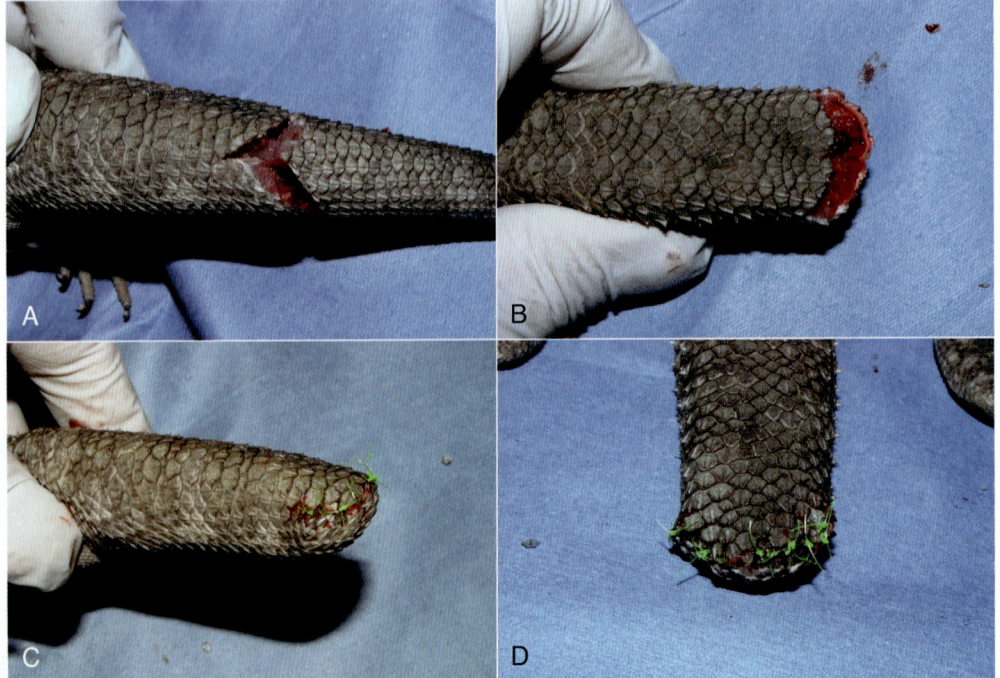

FIG 112.3 (A and B) Symmetrical wedge incisions are made in a top to bottom orientation to amputate the tail in this bearded dragon (*Pogona vitticeps*). (C and D) This wedge incision allows for a dorsoventral closure, which works well in this species. Note that the skin sutures are oriented dorsally to minimize substrate contact. (Courtesy of Richard S. Funk.)

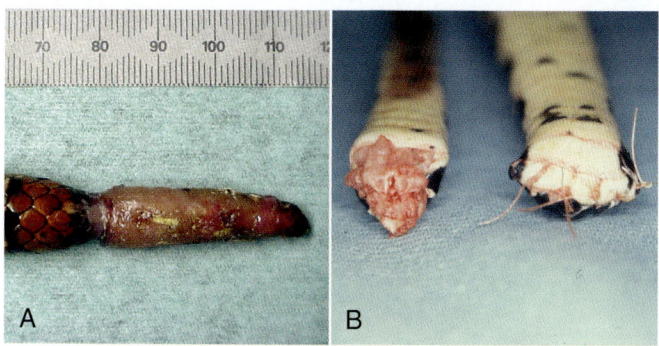

FIG 112.4 (A) Tail necrosis in a corn snake (*Pantherophis guttatus*). (B) View of the distal (amputated) and proximal (sutured) surgical sites following amputation. (Courtesy of Stephen J. Divers.)

Monofilament nonabsorbable (e.g., nylon) or absorbable (e.g., polydiaxanone) sutures may be utilized and removed 6 to 8 weeks later. Sometimes the sutures will be shed during ecdysis. With dorsoventrally flattened tails it is best to place the knots dorsally to minimize substrate contact (see Fig. 112.3).

Snake and chelonian tails may be similarly amputated under general anesthesia, but they tend to be more rounded in cross-section so the approach may be chosen based on esthetics (Fig. 112.4). Depending on access and severity, it may be necessary to resect parts of the posterior chelonian shell. Postoperative pain management is recommended with oral or injectable NSAID medications and/or opioids (see Chapter 50).

REFERENCES

See www.expertconsult.com for a complete list of references.

Shell Surgery and Repair

Terry M. Norton, Gregory J. Fleming,[†] and Jean Meyer

Automobile morbidity and mortality are among the most important conservation issues that affect turtles and other wildlife.[1] Shell trauma is the most common outcome of a turtle being hit by an automobile. These injuries vary in severity and often lead to death or require euthanasia. Other less common causes of shell trauma in turtles include boat strikes in aquatic turtles, lawn mowers and heavy equipment, human malicious behavior, and predation. Shell trauma in captive turtles occurs less frequently but may be caused by dog bites, thermal, crush, and fall injuries.

Although this chapter is focused on triage, repair, and follow-up of shell trauma in chelonians, it is important for veterinarians to be involved and take a lead role in the "bigger picture" mitigation efforts to help reduce the numbers being hit by automobiles. Mitigation efforts are typically applied to areas where large numbers of turtles are affected. Defining hot spots and temporal patterns to target mitigation strategies can be ascertained through active research.[2,3] Mitigation efforts may include placement of converts under roads to allow wildlife to move across the landscape without being hit,[4] static and flashing light signs on the road to alert drivers that turtles may be crossing,[5] active surveillance and moving turtles across road,[2,3,5] nest boxes with predator-proof caging,[6] fencing to prevent the turtle from crossing the road, awareness and education campaigns,[5] egg recovery from injured and dead females, egg incubation, and release of hatchlings or head-starting hatchlings.

With respect to wildlife rehabilitation, if a chelonian can be successfully treated and returned to the wild fully functional, then medical and surgical intervention should be considered. If the chelonian cannot be returned to the wild fully functional, in most cases humane euthanasia is recommended. Occasionally, a nonreleasable chelonian may be used for educational purposes if the appropriate facilities and programs are available and the turtle is comfortable despite its disabilities.

Determining which injuries are not treatable comes with experience, and triaging patients within the first few hours may determine which chelonians can be successfully treated and which cannot. In some situations, the turtle may need to be stabilized and given time to differentiate neurological deficits versus weakness and shock. These decisions are difficult, but with limited time and resources available, it is best to make this decision quickly to save months of work and emotional energy.

TRIAGE OF SHELL TRAUMA

Developing and following a triage system will assist the clinician in formulating a prognosis and implementing a successful treatment course. The following five categories of prognosis have been developed to assist the veterinarian in prognosis and treatment outcomes.[7]

The approximate age of the injury must also be considered when developing a prognosis (e.g., fresh < 6 hours, contaminated 6 to 24 hours, contaminated/infected > 24 hours). The same type of wound will have a very different prognosis depending on if it is recent trauma versus one that occurred a week ago and is now infected.

Excellent Prognosis

Turtles presenting with fresh shell injuries or fractures that are (1) uncontaminated, not infected (< 6 hours old); (2) singular, nondisplaced fracture that does not involve the spine; and (3) with only minor excoriations have the best prognosis for a full recovery. If there are no other associated medical issues, these wounds often heal quickly and may only need a few days to weeks of supportive care before the animal can be released.

Good Prognosis

Chelonians with multiple, unstable and/or open fractures, or dog bites with shallow shell puncture(s), usually have a good prognosis with treatment. Open fractures are characterized by malunion of a fracture with the bone exposed or missing pieces of the bony carapace or plastron. If large pieces of shell are missing or the coelomic membrane is damaged, the prognosis may only be fair to poor depending on the severity of the injury. Injuries in this category that are fresh carry a better prognosis. If the wounds occurred 24 hours or more prior to presentation, they are considered contaminated and are moved to a fair to guarded prognosis depending on the degree of contamination. These animals will usually need supportive care, surgical stabilization, and hospitalization for several months.

Fair Prognosis

Turtles with multiple fractures involving the pectoral or pelvic areas or penetrating punctures of the coelom have a fair prognosis. If the injury is greater than 24 hours, the prognosis becomes worse. Multiple fractures that destabilize the shoulder or pelvis may lead to ambulation difficulties. If the leg cannot be used at all, this would be a grave prognosis for release; the prognosis increases favorably as the ability to move the leg increases. Multiple fractures of the caudal shell narrowing the pelvic canal may lead to dystocia in females entailing a sterilization procedure for a captive animal or euthanasia if the turtle is not to be maintained in captivity.

Guarded Prognosis

Chelonians with open fractures with punctures to the viscera, like fractures of the plastron with concomitant disruption of liver parenchyma (which is lining up to 50% of the ventral coelomic surface, just above the cranial plastron) resulting in substantial blood loss, have a guarded to grave prognosis. In some cases, turtles may be seen with intestines or other organs trailing from the fracture or large amounts of debris,

[†]Deceased.

dirt, and fly larva in the fracture site or fractured limbs. These cases are difficult to treat successfully due to organ damage and infection. A group of high-risk patients are reproductively active females in which depressed fractures may lead to disruption of eggs or follicles, causing severe yolk coelomitis. Further investigation may be warranted, but more severe cases of this type of wound fall into the grave prognosis category, and euthanasia is the best option.

Grave Prognosis

This group includes chelonians with multiple fractures, internal injuries, and head and spinal injuries. Most spinal injuries in chelonians result in neurologic damage affecting the rear legs. In many cases, even though a fracture may proceed across the spine, it may be difficult to visualize this on radiographs. A neurologic examination, including assessment of sensation and deep pain, may assist in making this diagnosis; however, chelonians are capable of spinal walking, which masks spinal injury. Spinal walking consists of reflexive actions rather than conscious movement. Even if the entire spinal cord is severed, spinal walking is still possible. With spinal injuries, a variety of other problems, such as denervation of the bladder and lower gastrointestinal tract, are common. In a few of these cases, a turtle may continue to eat and drink while its urinary bladder and colon enlarges to the point of rupture. If a spinal injury is found, humane euthanasia is recommended. Pelvic fractures may narrow the pelvic canal, which has the potential to cause future dystocia in females. This should be accounted for when developing a prognosis.

Emergency Therapy and Initial Diagnostics

Once the chelonian enters the hospital, it should be evaluated immediately for prognosis, and a decision should be made as to whether to move forward with stabilization or not. An initial diagnostic investigation and emergency care can then be instituted. Emergency care typically includes fluid therapy and pain management.[8,9] If there is obvious infection (or major tissue compromise), broad-spectrum antimicrobials should be started following the collection of material for culture and sensitivity. Sea turtles can usually tolerate phlebotomy whereas most other species will need to wait until stabilized. Serial packed cell volume, total solids, blood glucose, blood gases, and electrolytes will help assess the status of the patient, target the most appropriate therapeutic regimen, and aid in prognostication and evaluation of response to therapy.[8] Radiography and/or CT/MRI, which in addition allow an assessment of internal organs,[10,11] are useful for assessing fractures of long bones, spine, and pectoral and pelvic girdles, and should be performed upon entry to allow for more accurate evaluation. The horizontal beam craniocaudal and lateral views are useful for the assessment of lung fields and can be used to determine carapace uniformity.[7,12] In cases of internal injury, the radiographs may assist in determining the extent of penetration or soft tissue injury.

INITIAL SHELL INJURY AND FRACTURE MANAGEMENT

Shell Wound Care

Wound management techniques used for chelonians are similar to humans and domestic animals. Initially the wound is cleaned and debris removed. Bony shell fragments adhering to the coelomic membrane should not be detached. Copious lavage with warm, sterile saline or lactated ringers, dilute chlorhexidine (0.05%), dilute betadine (0.1% to 1% depending on the degree of contamination and tissue being lavaged), or other commercially available antiseptic irrigation solutions (Octenisept, Schülke & Mayr, GmbH, Norderstedt, Germany; ProntoVet, B. Braun Medical AG, Sempach, Switzerland) is critical. Large quantities

of the irrigating solution should be used under low to moderate pressure.[13] The recommended delivery method to generate the desired pressure (7–8 psi) is a 1-L fluid bag with a cuff pressurized to 300 mmHg with an 18-gauge needle.[13] SilvaKlenz (Molecular Therapeutics, Athens, GA) is a pH-balanced potentiated ionic silver solution that is showing promising results for wound cleansing and flushing in chelonians (Norton T, Ritchie B, unpublished information). Tricide-neomycin (Molecular Therapeutics, Athens, GA) is an antimicrobial that complements the effects of SilvaKlenz. The turtle should be positioned so the flushed solution drains from the fracture/wound site, especially if the coelomic cavity integrity is compromised. One person holds the chelonian and rotates it to direct the opening of the wound ventrally to prevent flushed debris from entering the coelom. Sterile saline or lactated ringers are the preferred solutions to use if the coelomic cavity is compromised. The surround tissue should be thoroughly disinfected prior to lavaging an open coelom.

Regular debridement of dead and infected tissue is critical, especially in the early stages of wound management. For major debridement in a stabilized patient, sedation and analgesia are typically required (see Chapters 48 through 51). Topical lidocaine placed directly on a wound after initial cleaning may provide additional pain relief in some situations. Dental instruments, rongeurs, periosteal elevators, and curettes can be very helpful in removing dead tissue and cleaning out pockets. Fractures of peripheral bones in the shell are often accompanied by soft tissue avulsions creating small defects or pockets. These are prone to infestation with maggots and secondary infection. Affected chelonians are best hospitalized indoors. If the medical management of these dead spaces fails, the overlying bone can be debrided to the point of viable attachment of the coelomic membrane. This enlarges the defect but promotes the healing process.

A variety of topical products for shell wound management are available. The choice of a particular product depends on the wound, stage of healing, and frequency of treatment. Rotating topical antimicrobial products is recommended to avoid resistance. The ultimate goal is to decrease wound-healing time. For relatively minor wounds on the shell, silver-containing products such as silver collasate postoperative dressing (PRN Pharmacal, Pensacola, FL) and silver sulfadiazine cream (SSD, Kings Pharmaceutical, Bristol, TX) mixed with ilex paste (Medcon Biolab Technologies, Grafton, MA) for waterproofing in aquatic species can be applied after cleaning and debridement.[14] Nanocrystalline silver dressings (NSD) are useful because of the extended duration of activity. NSDs have a slower release of silver ions into the wound compared with traditional silver dressings and creams, thus achieving longer bactericidal effects (approximately 3 days). Wound gels (e.g., ProntoVet Gel, B. Braun Medical AG, Sempach, Switzerland; Instrasite Gel, Smith & Nephew, Hamburg, Germany) maintain a moist and antiseptic environment. Commercially available medicinal honey products (Medihoney, Wound Central, Plainfield, IL) come in several forms (gel, liquid, sticky bandages, etc.) that may be used on a variety of wounds. Fresh honey is an alternative. Honeycomb has been used to pack deep wounds. Frequent wound management is usually necessary, and a waterproof bandage is often needed for aquatic species to keep the honey in place. Honey will attract ants, so if the patient is being managed outdoors, an alternative will be needed.

RediHeal (Avalon Medical LTD, St Albans, UK) is a borate-based biological glass wound management product containing factors that promote angiogenesis that can be applied to deep wounds with exposed bone and has proven to be very effective. For deep shell wounds, it can be placed within the wound and then covered with bone cement, impregnated or not with an antibiotic (Figs. 113.1A and 113.2). Doxirobe Gel (Zoetis, Parsippany, NJ) is a topical long-acting doxycycline that allows for very high concentrations at the site of application. Doxirobe

TABLE 113.1 **Wound Care and Other Products Used for Chelonian Shell Fracture Repair**

Topical Medication	Application
1% silver sulfadiazine cream (SSD cream, Kings Pharmaceutical, Bristol, TX) mixed with ilex paste (Medcon Biolab Technologies, Grafton, MA)	Good for most shell and skin wounds. Difficult to remove from some wounds so not the best choice for deep pockets or fractured shell edges. Can mix with Ilex cream (Medcon Biolab Technologies, Grafton, MA), which stays on in aquatic environments better.
SilvaSorb gel (product name: silver antimicrobial wound gel sustained release; Medline, Northfield, IL)	Similar use as SSD cream but does not stick to tissue and is more water soluble so easier to remove. Does not stay on wound long in aquatic environments unless waterproof bandage placed.
Silver collasate postoperative dressing (PRN Pharmacal, Pennsacola, FL)	Collagen-based product with silver. Stays on wound in the water fairly well.
Alginate/CMC dressings with antimicrobial silver (Maxorb Extra Ag+ ReliaMed, Medline, Ft. Worth, TX)	The material is saturated with sterile water and then placed on the wound. Used in a variety of situations from deep pockets to edges of shell fractures/wounds; 72 hrs of antimicrobial activity.
Silverlon Silver Mesh (Webster product name, Silverlon, Nich Marketers, Inc., Gulf Breeze, FL)	This product needs to be saturated with sterile water as well. Use on the surface of the wound for VAC therapy; 72 hours of activity.
SilvaKlenz (Molecular Therapeutics, Athens, GA)	pH-balanced potentiated ionic silver solution for wound cleansing.
Tricide-neomycin (Molecular Therapeutics, Athens, GA)	Antimicrobial used to complement the effects of SilvaKlenz.
Honey and honeycomb	Used on a variety of wounds. Honeycomb is great for packing into wounds and can be impregnated with honey. Honey and honeycomb can be obtained from local beekeepers.
MediHoney products with active leptospermum honey (Derma Sciences, MediHoney Company, Plainsboro, NJ, http://www.dermasciences.com)	Medihoney is expensive but can be cut up into pieces for smaller wounds. Reserve use for open coelomic cavity wounds and deep shell fractures. Comes in several forms (gel, liquid, sticky bandages, etc.).
Doxirobe Gel (Phizer Animal Health, Exton, PA)	Long-acting doxycycline at very high concentrations at the site of application. Useful in treating superficial and deep shell wounds and shell fractures. Provides protection to the wound and stays on very well in an aquatic environment. Does not heat up or smell when mixed.
Bone cement impregnated with gentomycin (Webster product: C-ment 1 J-912 bone cement medium viscosity; Jorgensen Laboratories Inc., Loveland, CO).	Similar benefits as doxirobe. Product heats up and has a strong odor when mixed. Water can get up under the material, so it is important to change weekly or place a waterproof epoxy on the edges.
Rediheal (Avalon Medical LTD, St. Albans, UK)	Borate-based biological glass wound management product containing factors that promote angiogenesis. It can be applied to deep wounds with exposed bone and has proven to be very effective. For deep shell wounds, it can be placed within the wound and then covered with bone cement.
Epoxy cement (Waterweld, J-B Weld Company, Sulphur Springs, TX; AquaStik Epoxy, Two Little Fishies Inc., Miami, FL)	Used to cover screws and wires used in repairing shell fractures. Waterproof and provides further stability.
Equi-Thane Super Fast (Vettec Care, Oxnard, CA)	Quick-drying equine hoof acrylic for attaching bra hooks and zip-tie bases to the shell.
Flexible human sports bandage (NUBandage, West Palm Beach, FL)	Used to cover wounds and hold products in place on shell or limb. Comes in a variety of sizes.

has been useful for treating exposed bone and stays on well in aquatic environments (Fig. 113.3). Cyanoacrylic glue can be used to lightly cover the Doxirobe or bone cement once it is dry to provide further waterproofing. Large carapacial defects may be temporarily covered with either daily adhesive dressings in conjunction with wound gels or a removable prosthesis allowing wound access. An adequate prosthesis can be formed with light curing dental tray material (Henry Schein Inc., Melville, NY) (Fig. 113.4) or generated by 3D printers. Adequately debrided and uninfected, sterile wounds or defects may be filled with glass ionomeres, odontoiatric human bone cement, or dental photopolymerizable nano-hybrid composite.[15] Weekly wound management is usually adequate when using these products in aquatic species.

Shell fractures can be temporarily stabilized with a variety of bandaging materials, including Telfa nonadherent dressing (Medline Industries, Inc., Mundelein, IL) to cover the wound, self-adhering bandaging such as Vetrap (3M, St. Paul, Minnesota) or Elastikon (Johnson and Johnson, New Brunswick, NJ), and Steri-strips (3M, St. Paul, MN) can be used to temporarily hold unstable fractures in alignment or other similar bandaging products. Bone cement, cable ties, and bra hooks can be used to temporarily stabilize fractures and will be described later in this chapter (see Figs. 113.1B and 113.2).

A waterproof bandage for aquatic species consists of placement of petroleum-impregnated gauze over the topical product, Tegaderm (3M, St. Paul, MN) or similar sticky bandaging material with superglue placed around the edges, and finally waterproof tape placed over the entire area with another application of superglue. Dry-docking is an option for freshwater aquatic species that are less water dependent. Rotating between dry-docking and waterproof bandaging may also be an option in some situations. If the injuries are confined to the dorsal aspect of the carapace, the animals may be kept in shallow water after surgical treatment following the same principles as described previously. This allows the turtle to hydrate and feed. With plastral defects or cases of large missing shell areas, the turtle should be dry-docked on moist towels until a primary seal is visible. Another possibility of dry-docking is to place a high plastic grid in a shallow warm water bath, leaving a small freely accessible water surface at one side. This should be narrow enough to prevent the turtle from immerging but on the other hand allow free access to drink and feed. Feces will be passed through the grid, reducing the risk of contamination of plastral injuries. During long-term confinement, careful monitoring for the development of plastral pressure lesions is required. The use of plastic saddle clamps on plastral fractures lifts the animal off the ground, reducing the risk of secondary infections.[16] During the dry-docking period, nutrition and water uptake should be guaranteed by gavage or placement of an esophagostomy tube. A novel technique using a trimmed urine specimen cup, or similar containers with a water-tight lid, glued to the shell with

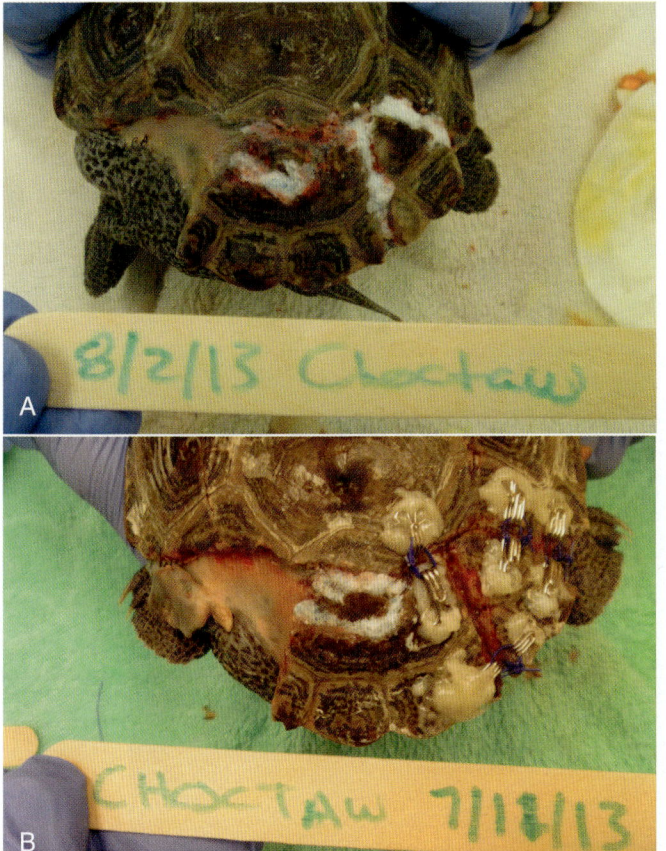

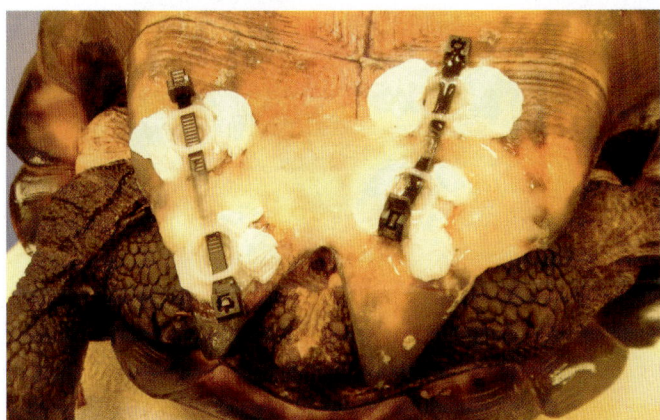

FIG 113.1 (A) RediHeal applied to the open areas of the fracture in a diamondback terrapin (*Malaclemys terrapin*). Bone cement will ultimately cover the RediHeal. (B) Bra hooks with 3.0 PDS II (polydioxanone) Suture (Ethicon US, LLC., Somerville, NJ) material being used to repair a caudal carapace fracture in the same diamondback terrapin. (Courtesy of Terry M. Norton, Georgia Sea Turtle Center.)

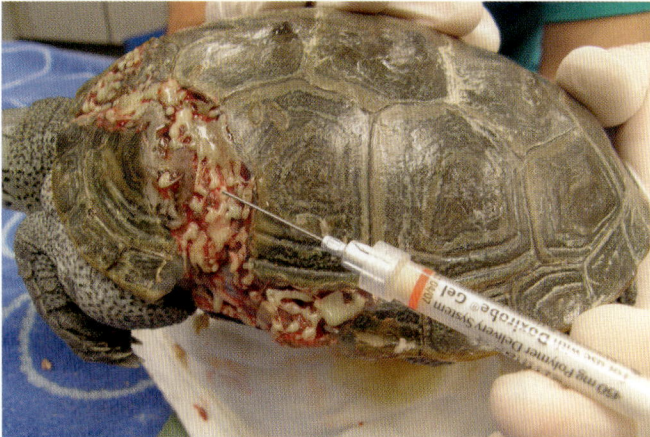

FIG 113.3 Doxirobe applied to a wound post screw and wire removal in a diamondback terrapin (*Malaclemys terrapin*). (Courtesy of Terry M. Norton, Georgia Sea Turtle Center.)

FIG 113.2 Cable ties, RediHeal, and bone cement used to repair a caudal plastron fracture in a gopher tortoise. (*Gopherus polyphemus*). (Courtesy of Terry M. Norton, Georgia Sea Turtle Center.)

underwater epoxy (AquaStik, Two Little Fishies Inc., Miami, FL) can protect the wound from the aquatic environment and allow the turtle to be kept under natural conditions during the healing process[17] (Fig. 113.5). Before gluing the device onto the shell, loose scute material is removed to improve adhesion and guarantee waterproofing. Cleaning and debriding of the wound is achieved through the screw-top lid. After

returning the turtle to the aquatic environment, good water quality has to be assured by frequent water change and high-quality filter systems.

Traumatic injuries that pull the skin away from the shell can be difficult to manage. The authors have used some innovative methods to repair these types of wounds. In an eastern box turtle (*Terrapene c. carolina*) with a severe caudal carapace fracture and skin separation from the shell, bra hooks were adhered to the shell using epoxy cement (WaterWeld, J-B Weld Company, Sulphur Springs, TX), and then the skin was sutured to the hooks (Fig. 113.6). In a green sea turtle (*Chelonia mydas*) with a severe shark-bite injury to the caudal carapace with inguinal fat exposure, plastic hooks were adhered using epoxy cement to the shell, while suture loops and zip ties allowed for a flexible human sports bandage (NUBandage, West Palm Beach, FL) to be attached and hold honey, honeycomb, and petroleum-impregnated gauze on the wound while the turtle was maintained in water (Fig. 113.7A and B).

If single fragments are missing, the prognosis is dependent on the extent of uncovered coelom. There is a reasonable chance that defects involving less than 25% of the shell surface will heal by metaplastic calcification of the coelomic membrane (see also Fig. 70.9A and B) or will be replaced by soft tissue if the defects are peripheral (Fig. 113.8A and B). Detached fragments may be cleaned and fixed in place. Sequestra formation is not uncommon, but they can serve as useful placeholders until new bone forms below.

Vacuum-assisted wound closure (VAC) has been very effective in treating a variety of wounds in chelonians (see Chapter 130 for more details). This technology is often used in patients that have had surgical repair to their shell, or it may be the primary wound-healing modality in some cases. Therapeutic laser therapy has been used for accelerating wound healing in a variety of chelonian species. This type of laser uses two wavelengths of laser light to stimulate cellular energy and increase blood flow (see Chapter 129).

NUTRITIONAL SUPPORT

Many chelonians will start to eat if housed in a semi-naturalistic setting with natural substrate, hide box, appropriate thermogradient, good water quality if aquatic, and outdoor access when appropriate. Short-term tube feeding with a nutritionally complete formula often stimulates the turtle to start eating. Some patients may require tube feeding for long-term oral medication sand nutritional support, thus an esophagostomy tube should be placed. The stomach volume in most chelonian

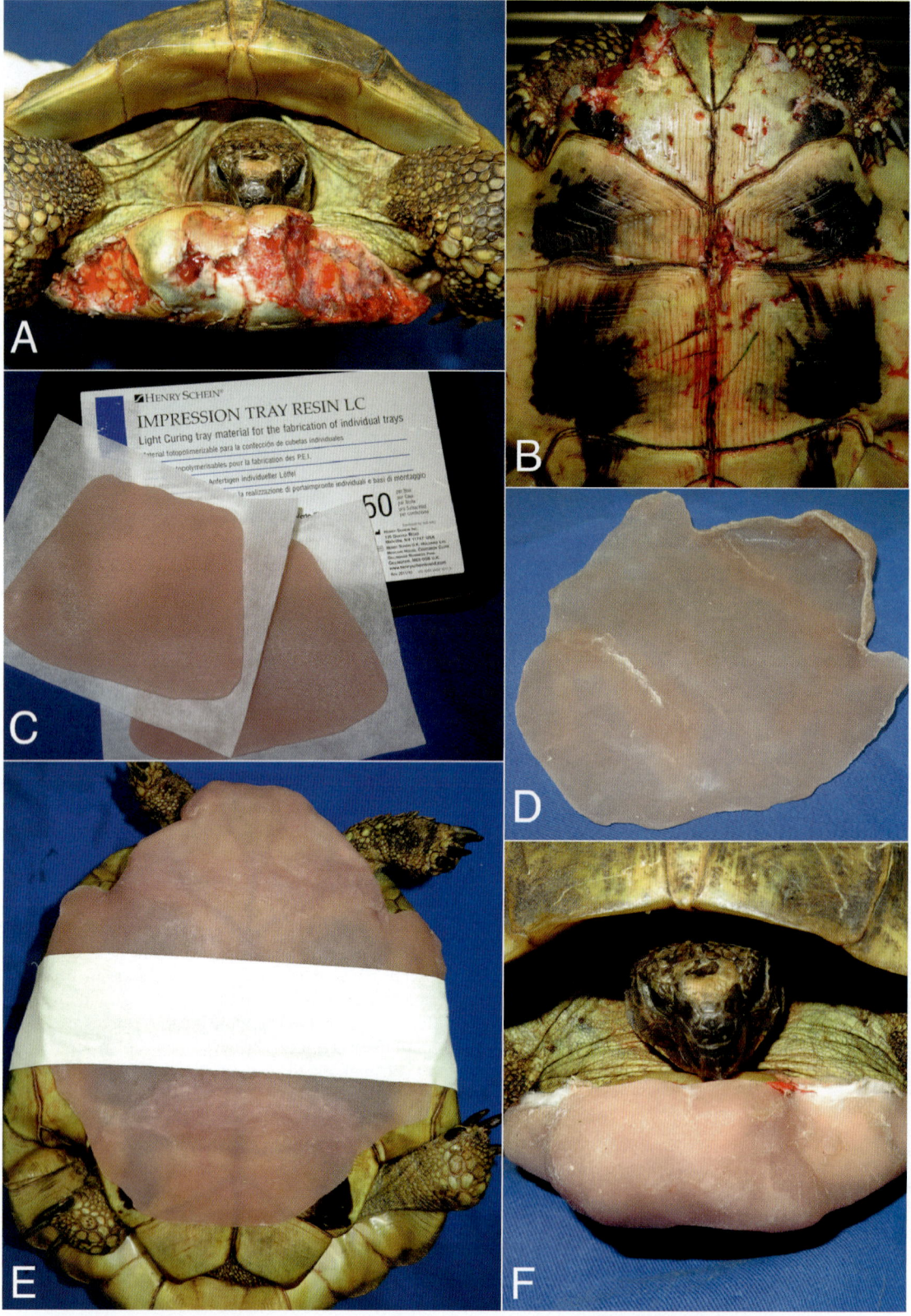

FIG 113.4 (A and B) Severe plastral bite injuries in a *Testudo hermanni*, inflicted by a fox. (C and D) A prosthesis is made out of light curing dental tray material. The tray material comes in plates that can be easily modeled on to the plastron or carapace. Due to the nonstick surface properties of the tray material, the mold can be simply removed after UV light curing. (E and F) The prosthesis is reattached to the shell with a piece of tape. It keeps wound dressings in place, prevents contamination of the wound surfaces by feces or urine, and allows easy changes of wound dressings. (Courtesy of Jean Meyer.)

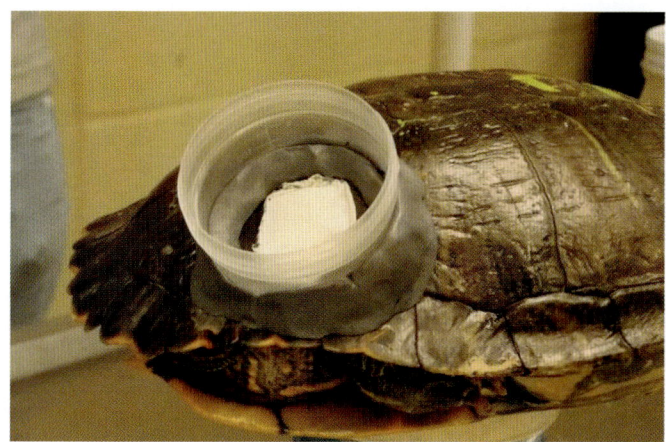

FIG 113.5 Containers with a water-tight lid can be trimmed to size and fixed in place with AquaStik epoxy over perforating shell wounds, as seen in this slider (*Trachemys*) turtle. Wound management is achieved through the open lid. This allows a faster return of the animals into their aquatic environment. (Courtesy of Sypniewski LA, et al: Novel shell wound care in the aquatic turtle. *J Exot Pet Med.* 2016;25[2]:110-114.)

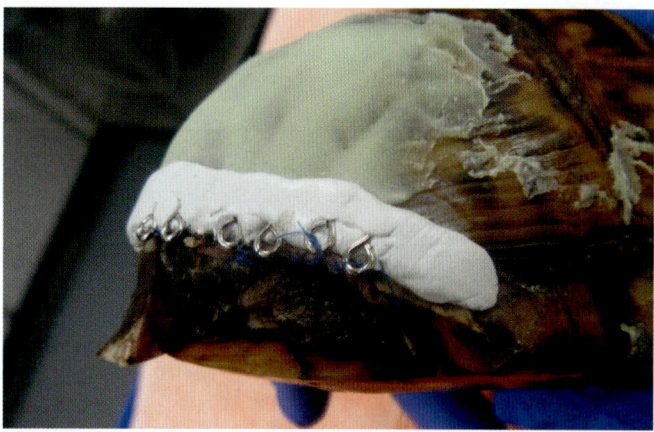

FIG 113.6 An eastern box turtle (*Terrapene carolina carolina*) with a severe caudal carapace fracture and skin separation from the shell; bra hooks were adhered to the shell using epoxy cement and then the skin was sutured to the hooks. (Courtesy of Terry M. Norton, Georgia Sea Turtle Center.)

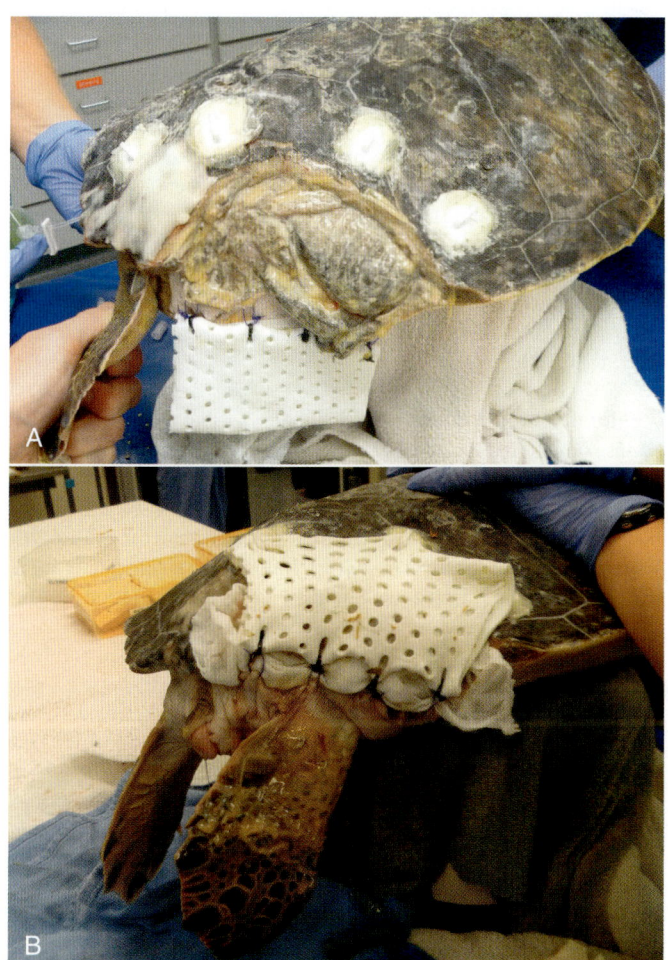

FIG 113.7 (A) Plastic hooks attached using epoxy to the carapace at the edge of the wound with a human sport bandage attached at the other end with suture loops and cable ties used to bandage the wound in a green sea turtle (*Chelonia mydas*) with a severe shark bite. (B) Medihoney gel, honeycomb, and petroleum-impregnated gauze held in place with the sport bandage attached dorsally to the hooks in the same green sea turtle. (Courtesy of Terry M. Norton, Georgia Sea Turtle Center.)

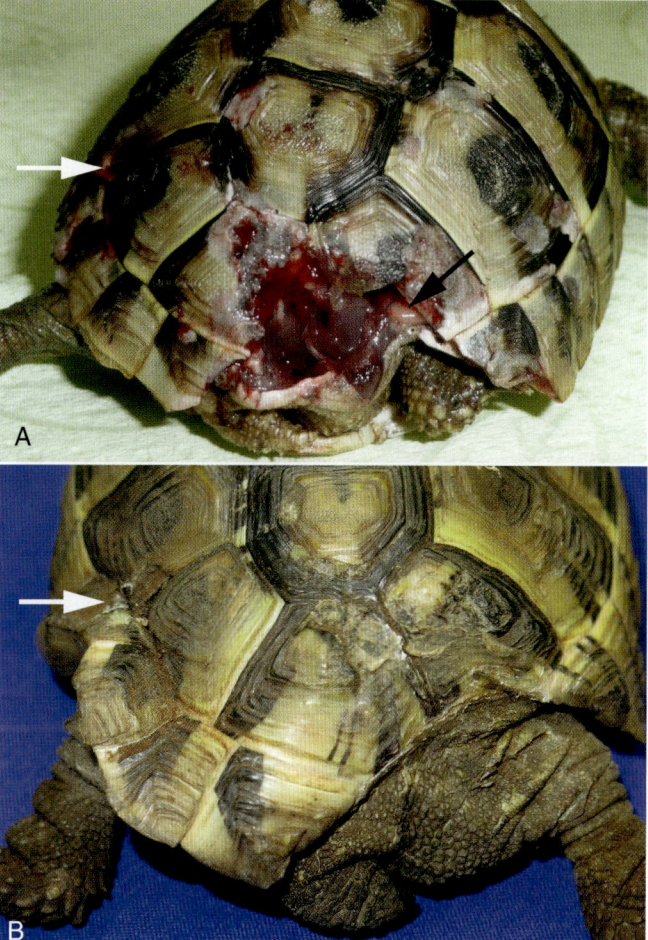

FIG 113.8 (A) Dog bite in a juvenile *Testudo hermanni* with substantial loss of bony carapace, opening of the coelomic cavity, and exposure of the right kidney (black arrow). Deep puncture wound from the canine tooth on the contralateral side (white arrow). (B) Three years after trauma. The skin filling the defect shows physiologic keratinization. The puncture wound on the left side (white arrow) lead to a premature ankylosis of the underlying bony suture with subsequent distorted growth. (Courtesy of Jean Meyer).

patients is about 2% of the body weight or 20 mL/kg.[8] Procedures for placement are described elsewhere in this book (see Chapter 45).[8]

SURGICAL MANAGEMENT

Anesthesia

Anesthetic and analgesic protocols should provide muscle relaxation and pain management when repairing shell injuries. Supplemental heat, consistent with the patient's POTZ, is necessary during an anesthetic procedure to allow normal metabolism of the anesthetics for both induction and recovery. Morphine, tramadol, and meloxicam are used most commonly by the authors for pre- and postoperative pain management. Dissociative anesthetic agents (e.g., ketamine), α-2 agonists (e.g., dexmedetomidine), propofol, alphaxalone, and inhalants, have been found to provide the most reliable results for shell fracture repair (see Chapters 48, 49, and 50 for more details).[18] A combination of injectable drugs are typically used to induce and may be the only anesthesia needed for some fracture repairs.

Fracture Repair and Fixation

Shell repair is a common reason for surgery in rehabilitated chelonians. The general principles for repair in reptiles are similar to other species: apply appropriate wound care principles preoperatively, utilize sterile technique, and provide stability in normal anatomic position for a sufficient time to allow bone healing. Bone healing for the chelonian shell may take 1 to 6 months or even longer depending on the complexity of the fracture repair. This will have an effect on long-term rehabilitation facility housing. The fracture(s) should be described based on the particular anatomical part of the shell that is affected (see Chapter 7, as well as Chapter 70, Fig. 70.3).

If the fracture is nondisplaced and stable, then external bandaging, bra hooks with suture material (see Fig. 113.1B), cable ties (see Fig. 113.2), RediHeal and bone cement with or without an antibiotic (see Fig. 113.2), or a combination of these methods (see Fig. 113.2) may be used as the primary repair. Bandaging should be nonadherent and securely affixed to the shell so as to prevent movement of bone fragments. Regular bandage changes and wound management are required in these situations. If a limb is fractured, then the bandage can splint the limb to the shell to prevent movement. Long bone fracture repair is another option in larger chelonian species and is discussed elsewhere (see Chapters 108 and 109).

Complete shell fractures in rehabilitated turtles should be considered open and typically contaminated, if not infected. Many chelonian shell fracture cases are presented in which where the duration of the injury may be unknown. When reducing shell fractures, strict asepsis should be maintained. Screws and cerclage wires for fracture repairs with regular wound management of the fracture lines and areas missing shell works well for a variety of species. Surgical plates may be used successfully in larger chelonians, such as sea turtles and giant tortoises (Fig. 113.9), and typical principles of repair should be followed.

Many different techniques can be used to repair shell fractures. A combination of techniques may be used initially and throughout the healing process. The use of removable hardware such as screws, bone plates, rods, and wire may be combined with techniques that employ epoxy, hooks, and cable ties. Fragments should be brought as close as possible back into their normal physiologic relationships. A perfect apposition is not mandatory or often even possible. Residual small cracks and voids will be undergrown by granulation tissue and ossifying coelomic membrane.

Adhesives and Epoxy.   The use of epoxy and fiberglass for shell repair has been popular for many years. Epoxy resin with fiberglass is the

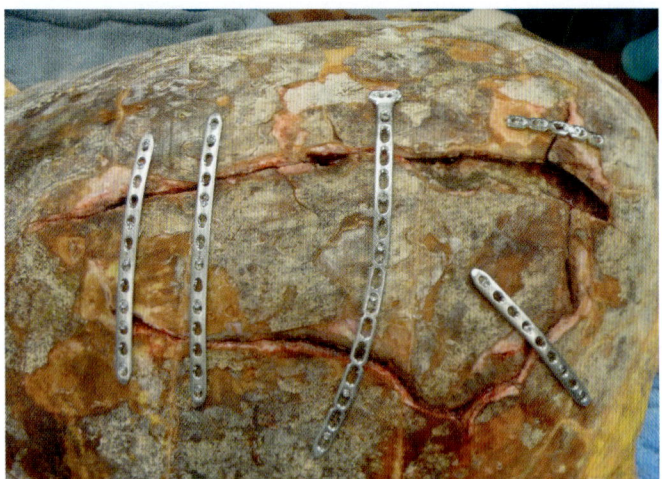

FIG 113.9 A large carapace fracture in a loggerhead sea turtle (*Caretta caretta*) was repaired with small fragment orthopedic plates that had combination holes so the fracture could be fixed in compression with 3.5 mm bicortical screws and also act like an external fixator by placing 3.5 mm locking screws. The plates were bent to fit the curvature of the carapace. The open areas between the plates were filled in with Rediheal and bone cement. The fracture eventually healed and the turtle was released. (Courtesy of Terry M. Norton, Georgia Sea Turtle Center.)

preferred method of closure for plastronotomy. However, for traumatic and infected shell injuries, the use of epoxy and fiberglass is contraindicated, because sealing a contaminated wound will result in infection. Thus, fixation with an open system of wires and screws that allows for wound management is preferred. Epoxy putty, cyanoacrylate glue, and two-part epoxy resin have been used successfully in conjunction with bone plates and cable-tie attachments to stabilize plastron fractures (see Fig. 113.2).

Fixation With Hardware.   For shell fractures that need stabilization, the use of external fixation has provided excellent results. For wildlife cases where finances are often limited, many of the supplies, such as screws, can be purchased from a home improvement store; however, they should be stainless steel because galvanized screws can release zinc systemically and are more likely to rust. If no financial constraints apply, surgical steel–grade implants should be favored. All fixation devices should be sterilized before use.

In most cases, an assistant will be needed to help position and hold the chelonian while the fixator is being placed. The shell and soft tissue around the fixation area should be surgically prepared, debrided, and lavaged. Once the area is prepared and dried, the fixation may take place. If there are missing pieces, the surgeon must try to piece the shell together, leaving an open space where the shell is missing. If the shell cannot be stabilized without the missing pieces, the prognosis is significantly worse. If the shell can be stabilized, applying VAC therapy to such cases may be very helpful.

Screw and Wire Fixation.   The screw and wire method of shell fixation may provide the best stabilization in most shell fracture cases. The first step in fixation is to place sterile orthopedic or stainless steel screws where the fixation wire will be attached. There are two options available, depending on whether the case is client-owned (and approved veterinary orthopedic equipment should be recommended) or wildlife (where finances are limited and hardware supplies may be the only fiscal option available).

Standard orthopedic equipment (plates, screws, and cerclage wire) and techniques can be applied (see Figs. 113.9 and 113.10A–C). A review of available supplies can be found in numerous places, including https://vetimplants.com and https://www.jorvet.com.

For wildlife or financially restricted cases where hardware supplies are utilized, first, select a drill bit that is slightly smaller than the screw. Sterilized, Phillips #6 1/4-inch machine stainless steel screws can be used. Smaller screws are also available. The machine head looks like a mushroom, and the flat aspect of the ventral screw head provides a secure purchase for holding the wire. Screw size needs will vary depending on the size of the turtle and the nature of the fracture to be repaired, thus it is good to have different sizes available.

When drilling into shell fragments, if possible, stay back at least 0.5 cm from the edge of the fracture to provide proper purchase for the screw and to minimize cracking of the shell. When drilling, be careful not to place too much pressure on the drill, as you may sink the bit several centimeters into the coelom and damage the internal organs. Placing a piece of tape around the drill bit at 0.20 cm (⅛ to ¼ inch) of depth will allow for a visual guide to drilling depth. The use of a drill sleeve aids in limiting penetration depth. Two hands on the drill with a slow steady force are recommended when using a power drill. One of the authors (TMN) uses a hand chuck with the appropriate-sized drill bit to make the initial hole (see Fig. 113.10A). Alternatively, the use of a finger clutch, slow-start, forward-reverse electric drill (e.g., Stryker Cordless Driver, https://www.stryker.com) also provides great control.

Fully penetrating the shell thickness should be avoided if possible but should not be a problem as long as trauma to internal organs does not occur. If drilling with a power drill is prolonged, heat may produce tissue necrosis. To avoid this, drip sterile saline on the drill bit when engaged or use a hand chuck to make the initial hole and a handheld screwdriver to place the screws. Once a few screws have been placed, it may be helpful to attach the wire. Each case is different, thus in some cases getting all the screws in place and attaching the wire loosely to start and then tightening to obtain good apposition may be the best option. Fractures of the caudal carapace can be difficult to get aligned, and care must be taken to avoid pulling the fragments upward with too much tension on the wire (see Fig. 113.10B).

To attach the wire, precut a few pieces of wire, 15 cm (6 inches) long (20- to 24-gauge stainless steel wire). It is recommended to have a few sizes of wire available for the different sizes of chelonians and type of fracture that might be encountered. Wrap the wire around one screw head, cross it over between the screws (see Fig. 113.9), wrap one end around the second screw head, and then wrap the two ends around each other. The knot should be between the two screw heads, which allows for the knot to be folded down against the wire but not directly on the shell. At this point, do not tighten the wire with cerclage wire twisters/shear cutters or pliers; only hand-tighten it for two to three twists. If a fractured shell fragment is attached to the underlying tissue but not to the rest of the shell, place screws and wires on all sides and then proceed to hand tighten. Tighten alternate sides to make even contact with the surrounding shell. Some small gaps may not close fully but will heal over time. With more severe cases, the entire shell may not stabilize until the last few wires have been tightened. Once tightened, some of the wires may have become loose and should be removed and retightened. When tightening the wire, the surgeon may need to place five to eight twists on the wire; however, do not over-twist for fear of breakage. In addition, if the wires are too tight, too much pressure may be placed on the tissue margins, causing pressure necrosis. Once the wires are tightened, use cerclage wire twisters/shear cutters or side cutters to remove the twisted knot to the level of four to five twists and use the wire benders or pliers to bend the twist down to be

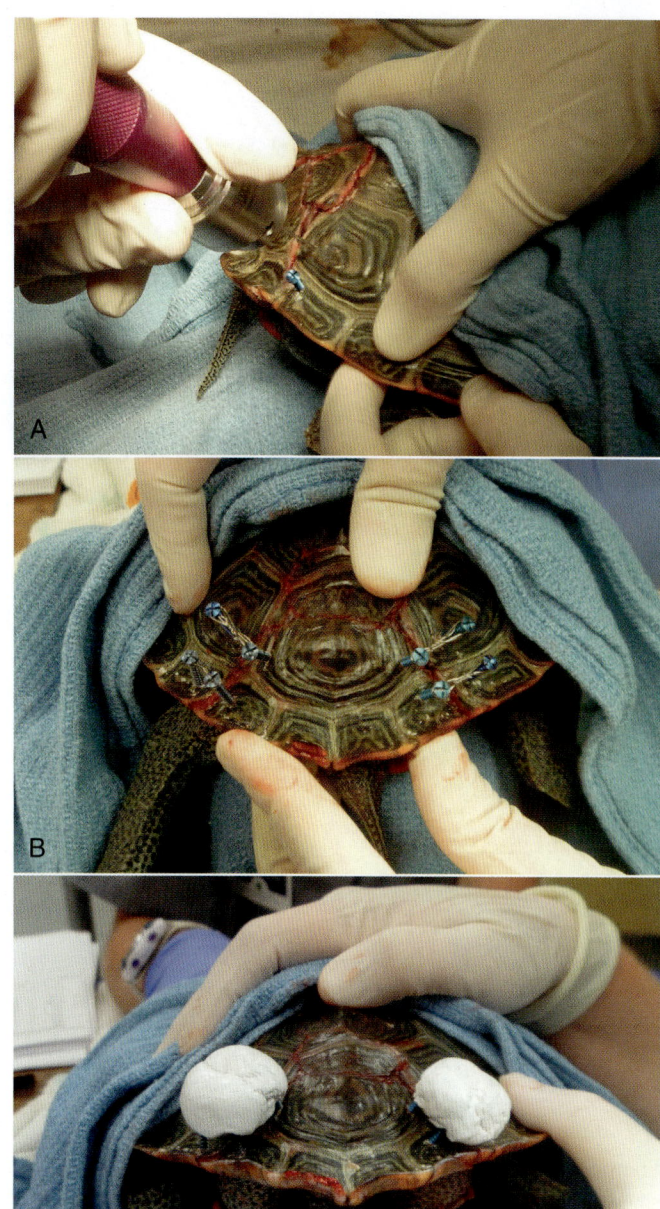

FIG 113.10 (A) Hand orthopedic chuck being used to make a pilot hole with drill bit in a diamondback terrapin (*Malaclemys terrapin*). (B) Sterilized, Phillips #6 1/4-inch machine stainless steel screws and 24-gauge wire placement on caudal carapace fracture. (C) Epoxy putty placed over the screws and wires for added stability, protection, and waterproofing of the fixator. (Courtesy of Terry M. Norton, Georgia Sea Turtle Center.)

parallel with the wire and the shell. Epoxy putty is then placed on the screw head and wire, which allows for further stabilization and waterproofing (see Fig. 113.10C). In some situations, instead of using the wire, the epoxy putty can be used to bridge the screws. This will provide stability but will not put tension on the fracture. One of the authors (TMN) uses RediHeal and bone cement with antibiotics in it along the fracture line. This will need to be changed once a week along with wound cleaning and debridement. This is especially useful in aquatic species.

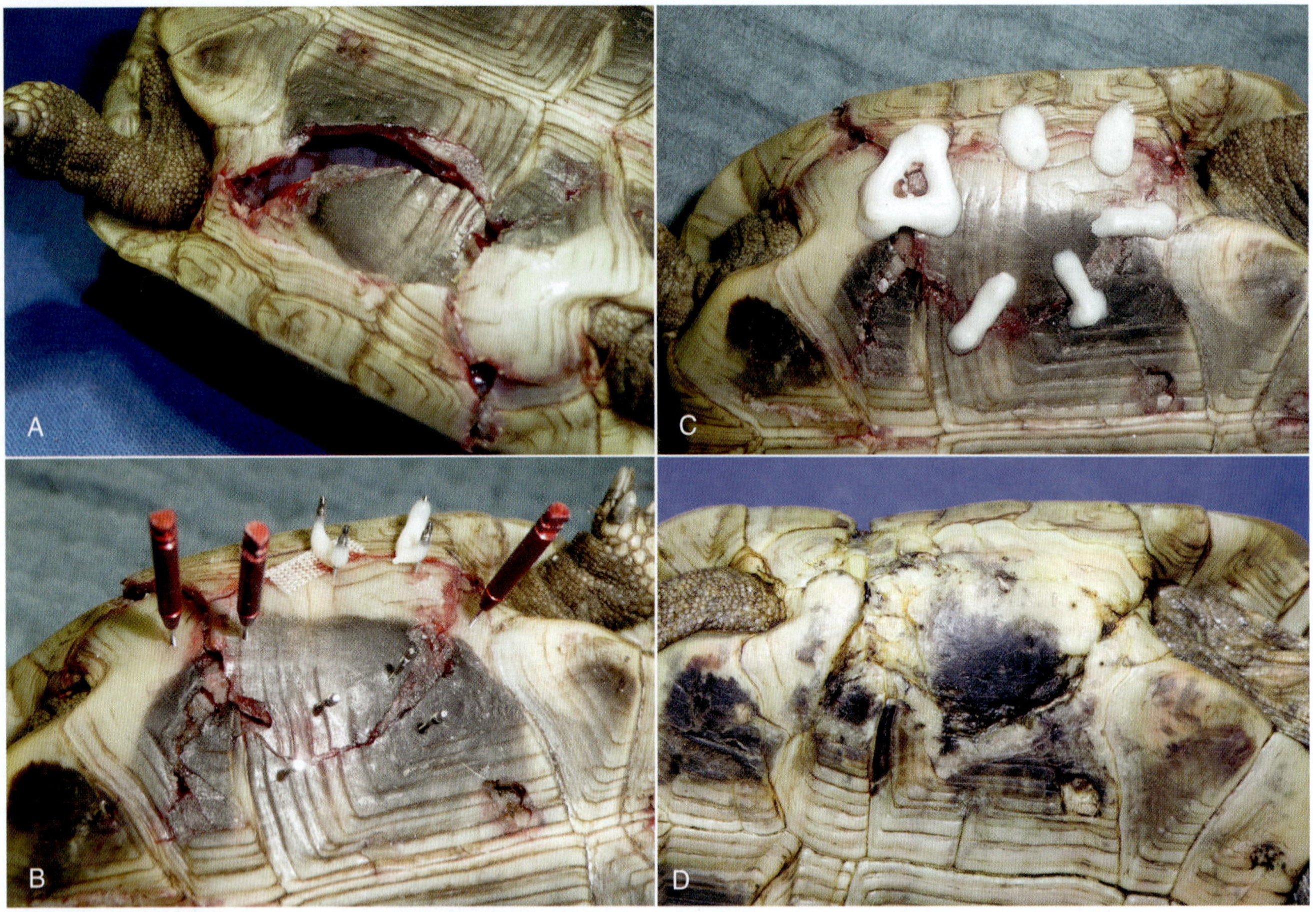

FIG 113.11 (A) An impression fracture of the plastron of a juvenile *Testudo hermanni*. (B) Repositioning of the fragment and fixation with self-threading dental pins in conjunction with UV-activated flowable composite. A small piece of gauze prevents the composite from entering the fracture site (later removed). (C) Finished fixation was left in place for 6 months. (D) Healed fracture 2 years later. (Courtesy of Jean Meyer.)

Fixation Techniques for Young or Small-Sized Chelonians. In small chelonians, self-threading dental pins in conjunction with UV-activated flowable composite (Natural Elegance, Henry Schein Inc., Melville, NY) can be used to bridge over the fracture line (Fig. 113.11A–D). Alternatively, Steri-Strips (3M St. Paul, MN) glued over the fracture site and fixed with a drop of epoxy at each end gives reliable, quick, and inexpensive support (Fig. 113.12). In young, fast-growing animals the time of fixation is kept as short as possible in order to prevent distortions of the shell skeleton during growth.

Cable Tie and Hook Fixation. In some cases of nondisplaced shell fractures where stabilization is needed, alternates to the screw and wire fixation are bra hooks with suture material (see Fig. 113.1B) and cable ties with bases (see Fig. 113.2 and Fig. 113.13). These techniques are less expensive and less invasive but, in general, do not provide as much stabilization as the screw and wire method. Bra hooks and cable tie bases are fastened to the shell with glue or epoxy. Suture material can be used to attach the bra hooks (see Fig. 113.1B) and cable ties are pushed through the bases as shown in Fig. 113.2. The use of a cable tie gun may aid in reducing the fracture. For minor fractures or when anesthesia is not available, this technique may be an option and will save time under anesthesia. These techniques can also be used for temporary fracture stabilization until the patient is more stable. One

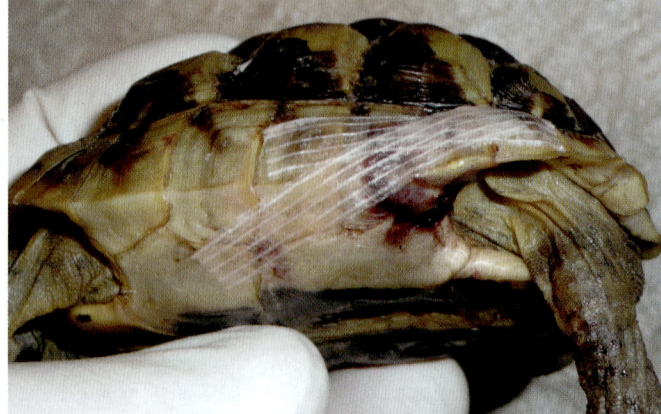

FIG 113.12 Noninvasive fixation of a shell fracture in a juvenile *Testudo hermanni* using Steri-strips. The ends of the strips are secured with a drop of epoxy resin. They can easily be replaced and allow a ventral drainage of the fracture site. (Courtesy of Jean Meyer.)

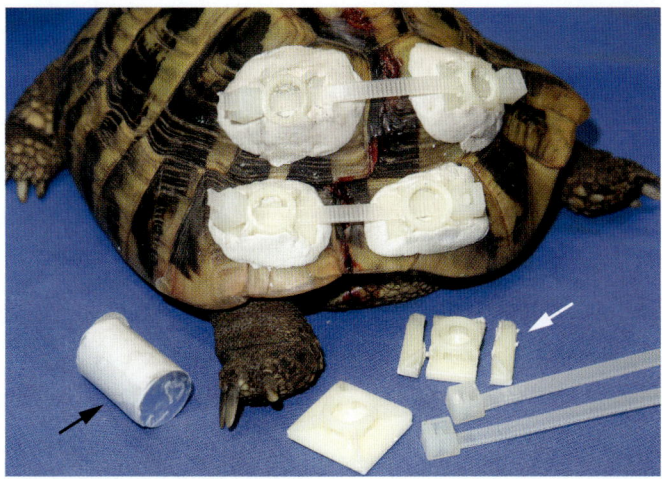

FIG 113.13 Cable tie fracture fixation in a *Testudo* tortoise. Cable tie mounts are cut to size (white arrow) and fixed with epoxy putties (black arrow) to the shell. Putties have the advantage to cling well and smooth the irregularities of the shell surface. After setting, the mounts are connected via cable ties and tightened. This technique allows an open wound treatment. (Courtesy of Jean Meyer.)

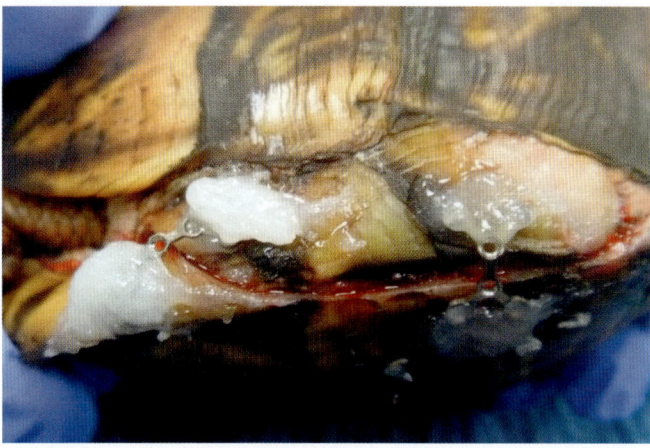

FIG 113.14 Small, phalangeal plates adhered using epoxy to the carapacial and plastron marginal scutes to stabilize a plastrocarapacial bridge fracture in an eastern box turtle. (*Terrapene carolina carolina*). (Courtesy of Terry M. Norton, Georgia Sea Turtle Center.)

of the authors (TMN) uses a quick-drying equine hoof acrylic (Equi-Thane Super Fast, Vettec Hoof Care, Oxnard, CA) for attaching bra hooks and cable tie bases. A tension relief system used in reconstructive surgery (TopClosure, IVT Medical Ltd., Ra'anana, Israel) has proven a durable and inexpensive noninvasive fixation device.[19] Alternatively, saddle clamps might be used to bridge the fracture site.[16] The use of these plastic saddle clamps on plastral fractures lifts the animals off the ground, reducing the risk of secondary infections.

Epoxy and Metal Fixation. Plastron fractures can be stabilized with bone plates, flat pieces of metal, small splints, cable ties, or just RediHeal and bone cement, or a combination thereof (see Figures. 113.2 and 113.5). In many chelonian species, the plastron is relatively flat, and epoxy can be used to attach a bone plate or metal strips across the fracture (Fig. 113.14). The low profile of the bone plate will allow for minimal drag when compared with screws and wire, which may become entangled on rough surfaces. Any open areas will need to be managed with regular wound care as described previously.

Monitoring and Healing Time

The fixation device should be monitored regularly. If the epoxy/screws/wire support becomes loose, they should be removed and replaced, if necessary. Healing time should be approximately 4 to 8 weeks, similar to bone in other species, but some cases may take much longer. This will depend on the severity of the fracture and the stability of the fixation. Simple closed fractures may achieve adequate stabilization in 4 to 8 weeks, whereas more severe cases may take 12 weeks or longer. In more complicated fractures, a staged removal of the screws and wires over 2 to 3 weeks is recommended. Open wound management may be required once the fixation devices have been removed. Radiographs may be helpful but often do not show callus formation. A better guide to a healed fracture is the stability of the fracture on palpation. If in doubt, leave the fixation device on longer.

A common sequel is mold formation on the exposed bony surfaces. Affected areas can be treated daily with terbinafine-containing ointments.

Treatment is discontinued once the open bone surface seals or undergoes demarcation and is sloughed. Chelonians with injuries to the shell should not be hibernated before healing is complete because downregulation of the immune response may predispose to infection.

Removal of External Fixation

The area of the shell should be prepared just as it would for surgery. This procedure may cause some discomfort but does not require general anesthesia; however, analgesia such as meloxicam or tramadol should be used. Screws may be removed with a screwdriver, and then the holes should be lavaged and managed with a preferred topical as discussed earlier. Once screws have been removed, the timeframe to release could be as little as a week to a couple of months, depending on the injury.

MANAGEMENT OF DOG OR PREDATOR BITES

The clinical presentation may be diverse and range from scutal abrasions to cracks, compression fractures, or to the loss of entire parts of the shell. Evaluation and treatment of the injuries should follow the protocol described previously. Fresh bite wounds are generally highly contaminated and should be rinsed with copious amounts of antiseptic solutions and/or sterile saline. Older wounds are generally infected and need debridement and systemic antibiotic treatment based initially on gram stains and subsequently modified by sensitivity results. Dog bites often result in the loss of shell margins, exposing open bone surfaces and significant hemorrhage. The amount of blood loss should be evaluated and monitored by serial PCV measurements. Even if viscera are exposed, these wounds generally have a reasonable prognosis (see Fig. 113.6A–B). Treatment consists of thorough and repeated lavage and appropriate bandaging with local antibacterial ointments or wound gels. Radical debridement is contraindicated, as this may aggravate further hemorrhage. Hemostasis can be achieved by application of sterile surgical bone wax or porcine collagen–based hemostatic absorbable materials (Surgicoll, Medical Biomaterial Products, Germany) or radiosurgery/cautery. All superficial shell wounds will develop dry, yellowish granulation tissue, which should not be mistaken for purulent discharge and should not be debrided. These contaminated/infected wounds should never be simply covered by any kind of epoxy resin, as these materials are cytotoxic and infection is sealed in, leading to osteomyelitis, abscesses, and sequestra.

CONCLUSION

Medical and surgical intervention of chelonian shell fractures can be prolonged but rewarding, because these reptiles often have life spans greater than 50 years. By rehabilitating an adult chelonian, you are assisting with conservation as well as helping individual animals that are often overlooked.

REFERENCES

See www.expertconsult.com for a complete list of references.

Therapeutic Overview and General Approach

Sean M. Perry and Mark A. Mitchell

The class Reptilia is comprised of more than 10,080 species divided into four orders: Squamata (Serpentes, 3567 species; Lacertilia, 6145 species), Chelonia (341 species), Crocodylia (25 species), and Sphenodontida (2 species).[1] Interestingly, since the last publication of this book in 2006, more than 2700 new species have been described. This increase in total species by more than 25% is the direct result of identifying new species and recharacterizing species based on new genotypic information. For the veterinary clinician, this species diversity is a reminder that reptiles presented are not necessarily the same morphologically or physiologically, and that these differences can impact how we manage a case. Veterinarians working with reptiles must develop an understanding of the species-specific requirements of these animals to ensure they make the most informed medical decisions regarding their care.

DEVELOPMENT OF A THERAPEUTIC PLAN

Any good therapeutic plan should focus on treating the underlying disease process while supporting other body systems and optimizing the immune system. Unlike higher vertebrates, reptiles are ectotherms and their metabolic rate and immune response can be impacted by environmental conditions. When considering therapeutic options for the reptile patient, the veterinarian must optimize the environmental conditions to ensure overall treatment success (e.g., drug and fluid absorption) (Fig. 114.1). In this section we will review specific aspects of therapy for reptile patients that may not be prioritized in other taxa.

ENVIRONMENTAL CONSIDERATIONS

Reptiles are ectotherms and depend on environmental temperatures to regulate core body temperature. A number of physiologic factors can be affected by the reptile's body temperature, including metabolic rate, heart rate, immune function, embryologic development, and reproductive activity.[2,3] Reptiles maintain a body temperature similar to their environment; however, exceptions do occur. Strel'nikov found *Lacerta agilis* in a montane environment (13,100 feet) to have body temperatures 29.2°C (84.6°F) above the ambient environmental temperature.[4] The thermal environment is extremely important when establishing a therapeutic plan in reptiles because of a high variability in physiological processes when reptiles are not at their appropriate physiologic state. Whereas the body temperature of a domestic pet mammal is not generally an important consideration in the selection and prescription of a therapeutic, it is an extremely important consideration for veterinarians working with reptiles.

Body temperatures for reptiles are highly variable. Brattsstrom reviewed the literature and published a report summarizing the cloacal and deep groin (chelonians) temperatures for 161 species of reptiles.[5] The range of body temperatures compiled for 13 species of chelonians was 8° to 37.8°C (46.4°–100°F), with a mean of 28.4°C (83°F). The temperature range compiled for 89 species of lizards was 11° to 46°C (51.8°–114.8°F) (mean, 29.1°C, 84.4°F). Overall, the lowest and highest body temperatures recorded were for the tuatara (*Sphenodon* sp.) (range, 6.2°–18°C, 43.2°–64.4°F; mean, 12.5°C, 54.5°F) and American alligator (*Alligator mississippiensis*) (range, 26°–37°C, 78.8°–98.6°F; mean, 32° to 35°C, 89.6°–95°F), respectively. This high degree of variability in body temperatures between reptilian groups and within species reinforces the dramatic physiologic changes that can occur in these animals on a daily basis and the need for an appropriate thermal gradient in captivity.

Veterinarians must be cautious because, despite reptiles' remarkable ability to undergo and survive large fluctuations in temperatures, exposure to excessive temperatures can lead to a fatal hyperthermia. Baldwin[6] showed that *Chrysemys picta* exposed to lethal environmental temperatures (42.2°C, 108°F) die suddenly. Once the animals achieved core temperatures greater than 27°C (80.6°F), they were found to be in

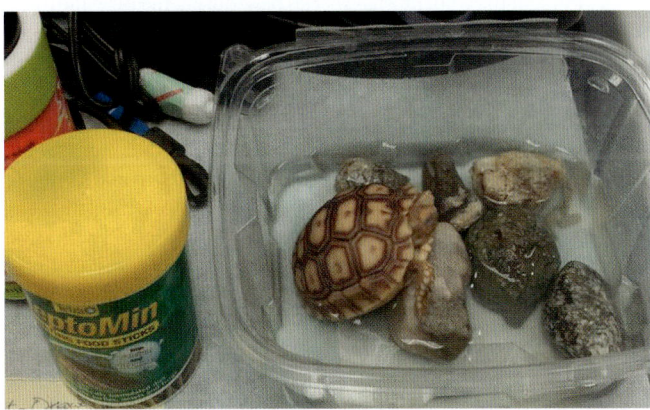

FIG 114.1 A neonatal sulcata tortoise (*Centrochelys sulcata*) set up in a plastic container with an inappropriate substrate (aquatic vs. terrestrial) and diet (carnivorous vs. herbivorous) for this species. Despite the best-developed therapeutic plan, this animal would not recover unless its environment and diet are changed. It is vital to understand each reptile's environmental and husbandry requirements to develop a successful therapeutic plan. (Courtesy of Jonathan Ho.)

obvious discomfort, with tachypnea and frothing at the mouth.[6] A similar series of mortalities was reported in a control group of desert iguanas (*Dipsosaurus dorsalis*) exposed to prolonged elevated environmental temperatures.[7]

Reptiles lack the thermoregulatory function and endogenous thermal set point associated with the hypothalamus in higher vertebrates. In addition, reptiles have been found to self-regulate body temperature and behaviorally stimulate a fever response to control a pathogen. Vaughn found that when a reptile was provided a choice between two different environmental temperatures, the reptile chose the warmer temperature in an attempt to stimulate the immune system to eradicate pathogens. Desert iguanas experimentally inoculated with *Aeromonas hydrophila* sought warmer areas within their environment, whereas no alteration was observed in the behavior of desert iguanas that were given a saline placebo.[7,8]

In contrast to those studies that reported behavioral fever response in reptiles, Warwick has suggested that some reptiles in an advanced state of disease may select lower environmental temperatures rather than higher environmental temperatures. He theorized that these reptiles may undergo a "biological shut down" to reduce the activity level of an inciting pathogen.[9] The theory was based on anecdotal experience with diseased reptiles and was not rigorously tested. However, the authors have had similar experiences with reptiles in advanced disease. Bacterial pathogens are capable of activity at a wide range of temperatures. One of the authors (MAM) has successfully cultured *Salmonella* spp. from reptiles at a range of temperatures (22°–37°C, 71.6°–98.6°F). Although pathogens may remain active, other reasons may exist for why reptiles do not use optimal temperatures, such as general weakness. To ensure the greatest success with these cases, a thermal gradient must be provided that allows the reptile to self-regulate its body temperature. Veterinarians that can provide this specific information to their clients will have greater success with their cases, especially with follow-up to confirm compliance.

REPTILE IMMUNE RESPONSE

The immune system of the reptile is composed of innate, humoral, and cell-mediated arms of the immune system. Although the components of the reptile immune system are similar to those of higher vertebrates, the reptile immune system is more primitive than that described in higher vertebrates. Because reptiles are ectothermic, their immune system is also dependent on the ability to maintain an appropriate core body temperature. In the wild, diurnal species bask during the early morning hours and late afternoon to increase core body temperature. In captivity, reptiles that are not provided an appropriate environmental temperature range may become hypothermic, which can depress immune function.

The humoral component of the reptile immune system functions to produce both specific immunoglobulins (IgY) and nonspecific immunoglobulins (IgM) that interact with foreign antigens and stimulate the cell-mediated immune response. Macrophages phagocytize pathogens or foreign material, process it with a cascade of enzymatic pathways, and present specific antigens to the B-cell lymphocytes for globulin production. IgM is produced first and is a large nonspecific antibody; it is commonly produced in response to gram-negative bacteria and is a lytic antibody that has a half-life of about 10 days.[10] IgY is a smaller antigen-specific antibody that may appear weeks after the initial encounter; it has a longer half-life compared to IgM.[10] IgY is produced in greater quantities than IgM and provides the major defense against infections. It is also passed from the mother to the embryo via the yolk.[11] Recently, an IgA-like antibody has been found in the intestines of the leopard gecko (*Eublepharis macularius*).[12] It is hypothesized that this antibody originated from a recombination between IgM and IgY.[12] Evidence exists that reptiles may also produce the immunoglobulin

IgD. The function of IgD is not entirely understood, but it is expressed on the surface of mature B-cells along with IgM and may play a role in modulating B-cell development.[13] Two IgD immunoglobulin genes, IgD and IgD2, have been sequenced in the leopard gecko.[14] IgD has been detected in tissues from the stomach, intestine, cloaca, liver, kidney, lung, spleen, and blood cells at the same concentrations as IgM. IgD2 was also found in these tissues but at low levels.[14] An IgD gene was also found in the anole lizard (*Anolis carolinensis*).[15] Relative to mammals, reptiles can have a prolonged IgM response before switching to IgY production.[16] Hyperglobulinemia is a common finding with an inflammatory leukogram. Antibody production can be influenced by temperature, antigen type and concentration, and route of inoculation.[13]

The cell-mediated component of the immune system uses T-cell lymphocytes to seek out and phagocytize foreign antigens. Killer T-cells probably have some influence on the destruction of viruses. Functional T-cells have been found in all reptiles tested, including snakes, lizards, turtles, and tuatara.[17] T-cell proliferation is strongly affected by the seasonal cycle in reptiles. Farag and El Ridi found that lymphocytes from the striped sand snake (*Psammophis sibilans*) had the highest proliferation in a mixed leukocyte reaction during the spring and autumn.[18]

Our current understanding of the reptilian immune system is in its infancy, and thus there is a need for us to invest additional resources into evidence-based research to unlock how we can use a reptile's functional immune system to help manage disease processes. For the time being, ensuring optimal environmental conditions is an important start.

NUTRITIONAL STATUS

The nutritional status of the reptile is an important consideration in the development of a therapeutic plan. Reptiles that are fed an inappropriate diet or provided insufficient calories may have multiple concurrent disease processes occurring. Dehydration, cachexia (muscle wasting), myopathies, gastrointestinal senescence, hepatic disease, and renal compromise may all be sequelae from an inappropriate diet. Alterations to hepatic and renal function due to nutritional stress can severely alter the pharmacokinetics of chemotherapeutics that are metabolized and excreted by the liver and kidney. Decreased hepatic function, decreased gastrointestinal function, and renal impairment can all lead to hypoproteinemia, which reduces oncotic pressure within the blood and can alter fluid balance between the intra- and extracellular spaces. This ultimately can affect the success of a fluid rehydration plan.

Reptiles in a negative energy balance can be expected to have physiological disturbances that can affect case management. In severe cases, nutritional deficiency can lead to refeeding syndrome, which is characterized by electrolyte disturbances such as hypophosphatemia and hypokalemia. These electrolyte imbalances can lead to hemolytic anemia or cardiac arrhythmias, and sudden death. Likewise, calcium deficiencies and metabolic alkalosis can lead to severe fluctuations in bound and ionized calcium concentrations, which can also be fatal.

Veterinarians should familiarize themselves with the specific dietary requirements for those species routinely in their care. Reptiles with a negative energy balance should be rehydrated and provided caloric replacement. However, reptiles should be gradually brought up to their resting energy (caloric) requirement over several days or weeks to prevent refeeding syndrome. See Chapter 122 for further discussion on the specific dietary needs of reptiles.

HYDRATION STATUS

Hydration status should always be considered in any reptile when developing a therapeutic plan and a basic understanding of fluid balance in reptiles is important. Reptile total body water content is generally similar to or slightly higher than that found in mammals.[19,20] The primary difference observed between these two groups is where the fluids are located, with higher intracellular (48%–80%) and lower extracellular (20%–52%) fluid volumes in reptiles compared with mammals.[20] In addition, terrestrial reptiles generally have a higher percentage of extracellular fluid compared with aquatic species.[20] Overall, plasma accounts for approximately 3.3% to 7% of the total body weight.[20,21] A high degree of variability exists in the electrolytes important to osmoregulation in reptiles, especially sodium, which represents the primary contributor to osmolality, and while it has been suggested that terrestrial species generally have higher sodium concentrations in the extracellular space than freshwater aquatic reptiles, this is not always true.[19] For example, sodium concentrations can be as low as 120 to 130 mEq/L in terrestrial chelonians.[22] This large variation in sodium, as much as 40%, suggests that osmolalities between species of reptiles may vary significantly, and thus the fluid balance between the extra- and intravascular spaces too. This difference in osmolality should be considered when selecting fluids for rehydration. Although limited, recent studies affirm the variability in plasma osmolalities in different reptiles, with healthy bearded dragons having a mean osmolality of 295 mEq/L and healthy male corn snakes of 344.5 mEq/L.[23,24] It is expected that in unhealthy animals these values would be different. Determining plasma osmolality is best done using freezing-point osmometry. Unfortunately, this is not always available, and thus the authors desired to determine if an algorithm could be used to estimate plasma osmolality. The calculations found to have the best level of agreement for the corn snakes and bearded dragons were 2(Na) and 1.85 (Na +K), respectively. These calculations may be used for these species and as a general rule for other reptiles, but variation dictates determining species-specific calculations, similar to those for cats and dogs. Additional information regarding fluid therapy in reptiles can be found in Chapter 87.

REFERENCES

See www.expertconsult.com for a complete list of references.

115

Routes of Administration

Sean M. Perry and Mark A. Mitchell

Reptiles possess significant diversity in their morphology, and these structural differences need to be taken into consideration when administering drugs or fluids. For example, venomous reptiles can be difficult to handle and present an increased risk to humans who must repeatedly treat them. In these cases, alternative drug delivery methods (e.g., osmotic pumps) can be used to minimize handling and personnel risks. This chapter will review the different methods and routes for administering drugs and fluids to reptile patients.

ROUTES OF DRUG AND FLUID ADMINISTRATION

Enteral Routes of Administration

Gastrointestinal (GI) tract anatomy and motility can affect the absorption and delivery of drugs and fluids in a reptile. Therefore it is important to ensure that every reptile patient is maintained at an appropriate environmental temperature so that the GI tract functions effectively and metabolism is maximized. Medicating per os (PO) can be challenging, especially in chelonians; thus, it is important to understand the different options available for delivering oral medications, including via the diet, directly PO, or through a feeding tube.

Medications can be easily hidden (injected) into food items, or gel diets can be prepared that are combined with the enteral medications. A gel diet can be offered as an exclusive diet during treatment or can be combined with the patient's primary diet. Target feeding or limiting the amount of food offered when treating a reptile with a medication will increase the likelihood of patient compliance; however, if there is any concern that the full dose is not received, then oral dosing must be done to ensure treatment success. Although reptiles have relatively few taste buds, they will avoid distasteful medications. If hidden in food, reptiles will often avoid the area in which the medication is present. To counter this, medications can be flavored too. Many compounding pharmacies can provide a variety of flavors, from fruit (e.g., cherry, grape) to meat flavors (e.g., liver), although any effects on bioavailability are often unknown. Although these different methods for enticing a reptile to eat can be successful, if there is any concern that the reptile is not receiving its full dose, direct oral dosing is recommended.

Fluid replacement should only be done PO for cases with mild dehydration (<5%) and when the GI tract is functioning normally (i.e., no vomiting or diarrhea). This route of administration is often underused in veterinary medicine because of our desire to administer fluids via the parenteral routes; however, since the GI tract is the natural physiological route of fluid absorption, it is appropriate to use when an animal needs mild replenishment. The advantages of administering fluids PO include non-invasiveness, stimulation of GI motility, and the relative ease by which non-veterinary professionals can be trained to perform. The PO route should not be used when the fluid type is a hypertonic fluid, as this can incite an osmotic diarrhea. Additionally,

the PO route should not be used when large volumes of fluids are required, as this can lead to regurgitation or vomiting, and aspiration. The maximum fluid volume that the stomach can hold is 5% to 8% of the reptile's body weight. The authors do not recommend replacing more than 2% to 3% of the animal's body weight PO at a single time to prevent gastric atony and vomitting.

PO fluids or drugs can be administered either via a syringe directly into the mouth or with an esophageal or stomach tube (Fig. 115.1). The authors prefer to administer fluids via an esophageal or stomach tube, because a large bolus can be administered quickly. The tube should be premeasured from the mouth to the midpoint of the coelom, which is the approximate level of the stomach in most species.

Chelonians are more difficult to medicate PO. When a chelonian withdraws into its shell, gaining access to the oral cavity can be extremely difficult. Attempts to extract the head should be done with caution. The caudal cervical vertebrae of a chelonian are fused to the carapace, and aggressive manipulation of the head and neck can result in a cervical spinal injury. Sedation or anesthesia may be necessary to fully withdraw the head and neck. A soft pliable speculum, such as a rubber spatula, or a plastic-coated paper clip may be used to gently pry open the beak. Aggressive manipulation of the oral cavity can lead to fractures of the tomia. Either a soft pliable feeding tube or rigid stainless steel ball-tipped feeding tube can be used to deliver medication or fluids (Fig. 115.2). These tubes are preferred over direct placement of a drug or fluids into the back of the oral cavity because they decrease the likelihood of aspiration or drug loss. The dosing tube should be premeasured to deliver the drug directly into the stomach (approximately midbody to the left of center). When passing a stomach tube, the glottis must be avoided. The glottis is located at the base of the tongue. Passage of the stomach tube may be simplified with lubrication of the tube; however, care should be taken to avoid introducing lubricant into the glottis. Chelonians that need frequent oral treatments should have an esophagostomy tube placed to simplify treatment (see Chapter 45).

Parenteral Routes of Administration

Parenteral routes for administering drugs and fluids are preferred in those cases of severe dehydration and when the GI tract is not working appropriately. Because there are several different parenteral routes for delivering drugs, the patient's response to treatment route can vary. It is important to select the route that considers the size and health status of the patient, any known pharmacokinetic or pharmacodynamic data associated with a treatment, the ease of administration, and any potential adverse effects associated with the route of administration. Parenteral routes for fluid administration should also consider these factors, as well as the type of fluid used, any fluid additives that may be affected by route of administration (e.g., glucose concentration), and desired rate of absorption.

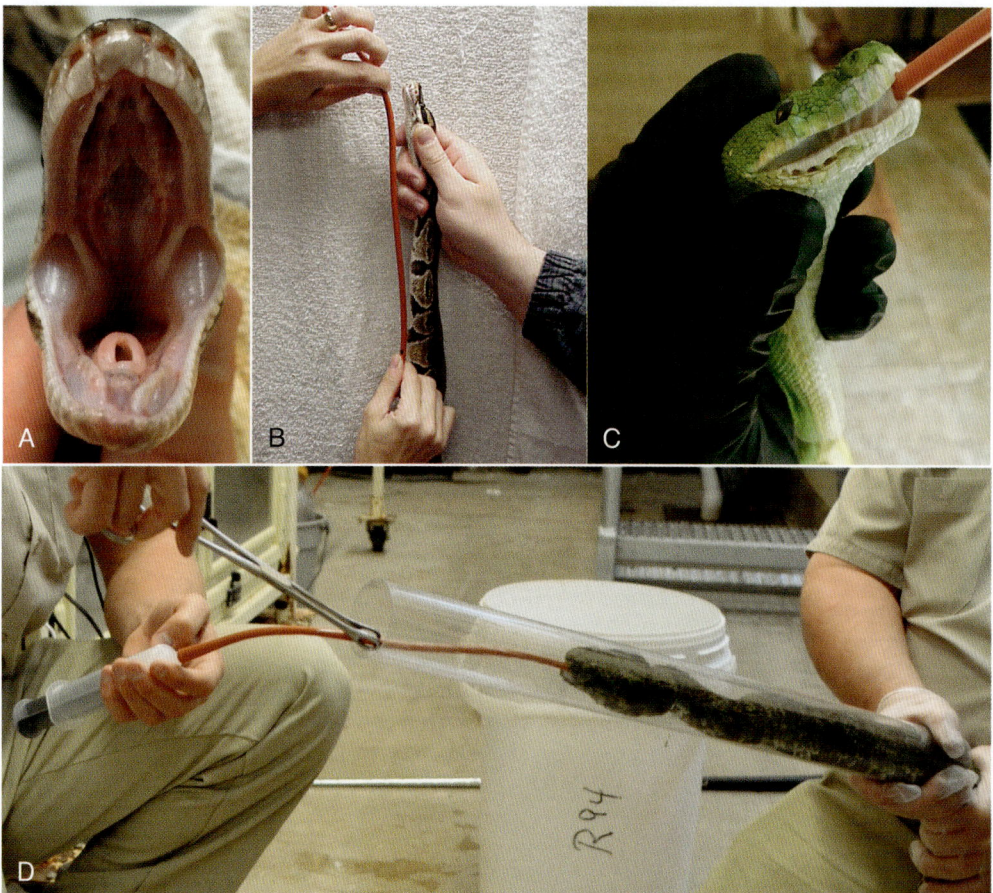

FIG 115.1 (A) Oral administration of medication can be performed utilizing a red rubber tube that is placed into the distal esophagus or stomach in snakes. Ensure that the tube is not passed into the glottis. (B) Tubes should be premeasured before administering medications as demonstrated in this ball python (*Python regius*). (C) In many snake species passing a red rubber tube ventral to the philtrum and between palatine and mandibular rows of teeth allows for easy placement of a distal esophageal or gastric tube, as seen in this green tree python (*Morelia viridis*). (D) Additional equipment may be needed when administering oral medications to venomous reptiles, such as restraint tubes and elongated forceps, as shown here with this Mangshan viper (*Protobothrops mangshanensis*) (A, C, and D, Courtesy of Sean M. Perry.)

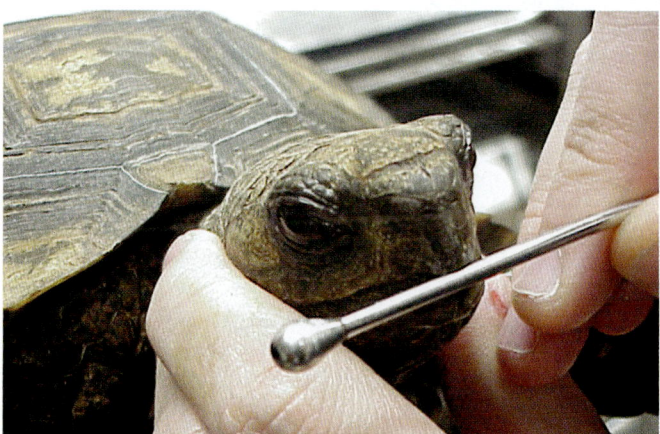

FIG 115.2 A metal gavage tube can be used in assist feeding or administering medications in chelonian species.

Subcutaneous. In reptiles, the subcutaneous (SC) space is small and poorly vascularized compared with mammals. The limited blood supply to the SC space can lead to variable absorption rates, depending on the physiological status. In squamates, the preferred site for administering SC fluids or medications is over the lateral body wall (Fig. 115.3A). In chelonians, SC injections can be given in the axillary and inguinal regions (see Fig. 115.3B). Additionally, in some lizard species small volumes of medications can be administered in the axillary region (see Fig. 115.3C). SC injections in crocodilians are rarely employed but can be given over the lateral body wall. Drugs with pH <7 or >8 (e.g., enrofloxacin), or irritating adjuvants, should not be administered SC because they can cause localized inflammation, tissue necrosis, and skin discoloration or depigmentation (Fig. 115.4). Fluid replacement within the SC space can be used for reptiles but should be limited to those cases where the reptile is <6% dehydrated. Critically dehydrated reptiles should be rehydrated using the intracoelomic (ICo), intravenous (IV), or intraosseous (IO) routes. Hyperosmotic solutions, such as dextrose (concentrations greater than 5%), should be administered IV rather than SC, because there is a chance to induce sterile abscesses, skin necrosis, cellulitis, and sloughing, although in human medicine utilizing subcutaneous dextrose has shown comparable effects to administration IV.[1,2]

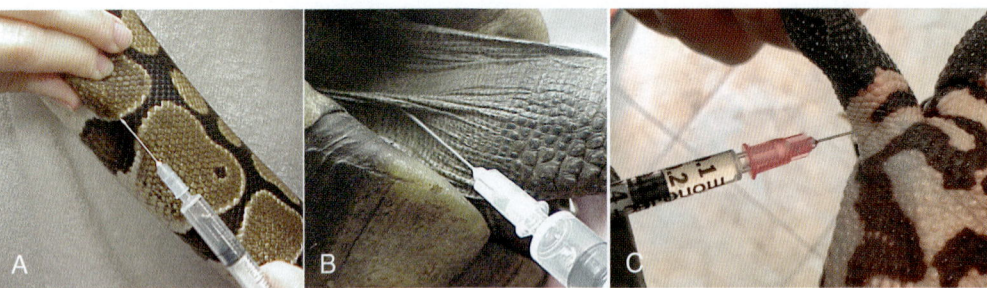

FIG 115.3 (A) The lateral body wall in snakes, such as this ball python (*Python regius*), provides an excellent location for administering subcutaneous fluids or medications; often a pocket at this location allows for subcutaneous fluid to track cranially and caudally. (B) Subcutaneous administration location in the inguinal region of a Burmese mountain tortoise (*Manouria emys emys*). (C) In lizards, small volumes of medications can be administered in subcutaneous space in the caudal axillary region, as in this Gila monster (*Heloderma suspectum*). (C, Courtesy of Sean M. Perry.)

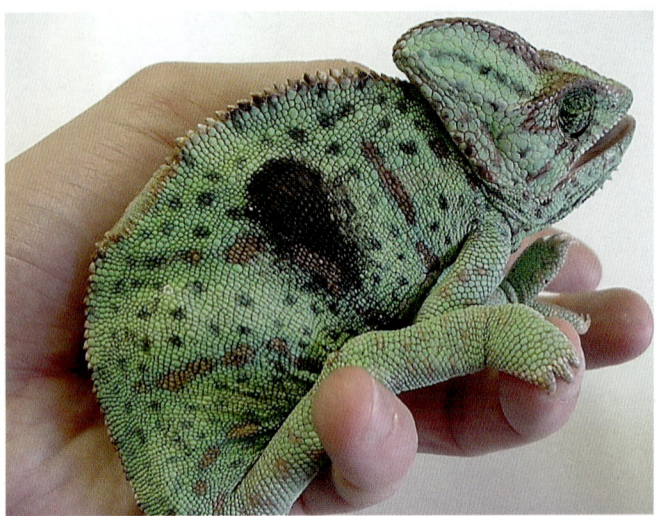

FIG 115.4 Some species such as chameleons often will discolor their skin immediately after any type of injection; the site of subcutaneous injection is obvious in this veiled chameleon (*Chamaeleo calyptratus*). (Courtesy of Stephen J. Divers.)

Administering parenteral drugs via the SC route has become more common in reptile practice. This route of administration is thought to be a less painful route and likely causes less trauma to the surrounding tissue compared with intramuscular (IM) injections. Studies evaluating anesthetics and analgesics have demonstrated that utilizing the SC route was equally as efficacious as the IM route.[3,4,5] Ceftiofur crystaline free acid (CCFA) pharmacokinetics were evaluated utilizing both IM and SC routes in bearded dragons (*Pogona vitticeps*), and there was no observed benefit to the IM CCFA pharmacokinetic profile compared with the SC route of administration.[6] Similar pharmacokinetic profiles showed no clinical differences between these two routes of administration for danofloxacin in loggerhead sea turtles (*Caretta caretta*).[7] More research needs to be performed evaluating more medications and their absorption via the SC route.

Intracoelomic. The coelomic cavity is a large space that is lined with a highly absorptive coelomic membrane. In addition to the coelomic membrane, the serosal surfaces of the viscera are also highly absorptive. Squamates and chelonians do not have a diaphragm, whereas crocodilians only have a pseudodiaphragm. It is important to limit the quantity of fluids placed into the coelomic cavity, as excessive fluids can cause lung compression. Irritating and/or hyperosmolar compounds should not be administered ICo, as they can injure the viscera or lead to fluid accumulation in the coelomic cavity. Care is also required to avoid needle trauma to visceral structures, and some authors no longer recommend this route unless absolutely necessary. ICo fluids should be administered in the ventrocaudal third of the coelomic cavity to avoid the lungs or air sac. Lizard lungs are located dorsally and can extend the length of the coelomic cavity. Placement of the lizard in dorsal recumbency allows for gravity to pull the viscera away from the ventral injection site (Figure 115.5A). The injection site should be disinfected with a topical antiseptic. The hypodermic needle (22–25 gauge) or butterfly catheter (22–25 gauge) should be inserted paramedian at a <15 degree angle to avoid the ventral abdominal vein and viscera, respectively. Once inserted, the syringe should be aspirated to ensure that the needle was not inserted into lung, air sac, or bladder. If air or urine or blood is aspirated into the syringe, then the needle/catheter should be removed and replaced before reinsertion. The same technique can be used to administer fluids to a snake. In chelonians, the authors prefer to administer ICo fluids at the prefemoral fossa where the skin is attached to the shell at the ventral aspect of the bridge. With placement of the chelonian in lateral recumbency, gravity can be used to draw the viscera away from the needle (see Figure 115.5B).

Intramuscular. IM injections are commonly used for administering drugs because of injection site access and rapid uptake and distribution. Physiologic status can have a significant influence on drug absorption via the IM route, as dehydration, hypothermia, and physiological shunting during times of illness or stress can affect muscle perfusion. Adequate hydration and body temperature are required before IM administration of any treatments. Fluids should never be administered via the IM route, because the infusion of a large volume can induce muscle damage and extreme pain. Common locations for IM injections include the triceps and epaxial muscles (Fig. 115.6). In some situations, repeated IM injections are not recommended, such as with irritating compounds or in reptiles with limited muscle mass. Multiple IM injections into a small muscle mass can cause myositis, myopathies, paresis, and changes in ambulation. Over an extended period of treatment, this could cause debilitation. SQ injections can be utilized as an alternative to IM injections for many non-irritating parenteral medications. The SC route is especially useful in small and debilitated reptiles to avoid trauma to muscles.

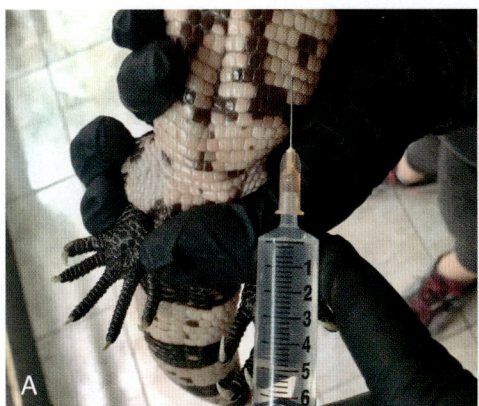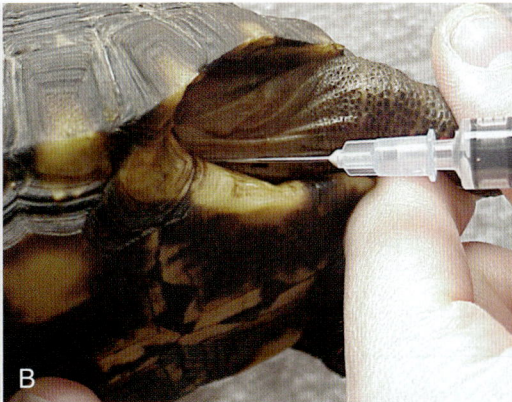

FIG 115.5 (A) Administration of intracoelomic fluids can performed with a lizard in dorsal recumbency and in the ventral third of the body as shown in this Gila monster (*Heloderma suspectum*). (B) Location of intracoelomic fluids within the ventral caudal coelomic cavity of the chelonian to avoid the lungs. This red-footed tortoise (*Chelonoidis carbonaria*) is placed in lateral recumbency. (A, Courtesy of Sean M. Perry.)

Intravenous. The IV route of administration is the most effective and rapid method for delivering drugs and fluids. Fortunately, IV administration has become more routine when performing surgery, providing intensive care, and administering certain therapeutics. Common sites for IV catheters or injections in squamates and chelonians are the jugular (Fig. 115.7A and B) and ventral coccygeal veins, and jugular and dorsal coccygeal veins, respectively (see Chapter 44). The cephalic vein can be used to obtain IV access in large lizards. Most IV catheters require surgical cut-down for placement (Fig. 115.8). The subcarapacial sinus of chelonians is also commonly used for delivering IV drugs; however, irritants or high volumes can lead to temporary or permanent paralysis or death due to presumed intrathecal administration (Fig. 115.9). Central venous catheterization has been recently reported in critical chelonians.[8–10] Arterial catheterization of the carotid artery has also been described in green iguanas for blood pressure monitoring; however, surgery is required to obtain access to this vessel.[11]

Intraosseous. IO catheters can be used when rapid absorption of the fluids is required but IV access is limited or not (see Chapter 44). The proximal tibia is the preferred IO site for lizards. Because the catheter is placed through the periosteum, a local anesthetic and aseptic technique should be used. Spinal needles with a stylet are preferred to prevent bone coring; however, 18 to 25 gauge needles can be used too. The needle may need to be replaced with another if it is obstructed with a bone core, although the second needle must be reintroduced into the same IO site. The authors' preference for hypodermic needles is based on their shorter length. The tibial crest should be used as the primary landmark for insertion. The stifle should be flexed and the needle inserted on the tibial plateau anterior to the joint capsule (Fig. 115.10A). A gentle twisting force should be applied to the needle to ensure proper purchase into the medullary cavity. The catheter can be secured with suture or tape (see Fig. 115.10B). Radiography is recommended to confirm placement (see Fig. 115.10C). Large boluses of fluids are difficult to infuse through an IO catheter because of the small medullary cavity in the tibia. In chelonians, IO catheters can be placed in the distal femur or proximal tibia; however, they can be challenging to place in the femur because of the sigmoid shape of the femur. In addition, if the patient withdraws into its shell, the IO catheter may interfere or be displaced. The cranial and caudal limits of the bony bridge between the carapace and plastron of chelonians have also been suggested as a site for fluid

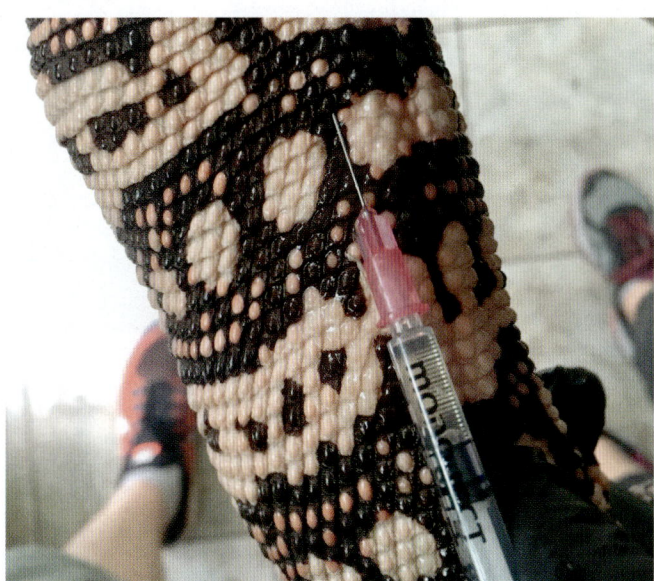

FIG 115.6 Cranial epaxial muscles, as shown in this Gila monster (*Heloderma suspectum*), can be utilized for intramuscular injections without influencing the muscles required for ambulation. (Courtesy of Sean M. Perry.)

administration (Fig. 115.11A–C). This site is considered analogous to the placement of an IO catheter in other species. However, this site can only be accessed via drilling a hole into the shell. It can also be technically difficult to place these catheters, because the size of the medullary cavity in these bridges varies from species to species. Because of the limited accessibility of this site and the invasiveness of the procedure, this site should only be used in rare instances in which other routes of parenteral fluid administration are not possible. In addition to the bridge, the authors have found the gular scute to serve as an acceptable site for IO catheterization in chelonians, especially juvenile animals. Placement of the catheter in these young animals is straightforward and does not require a drill, as the bone is softer. Delivery of fluids through this site

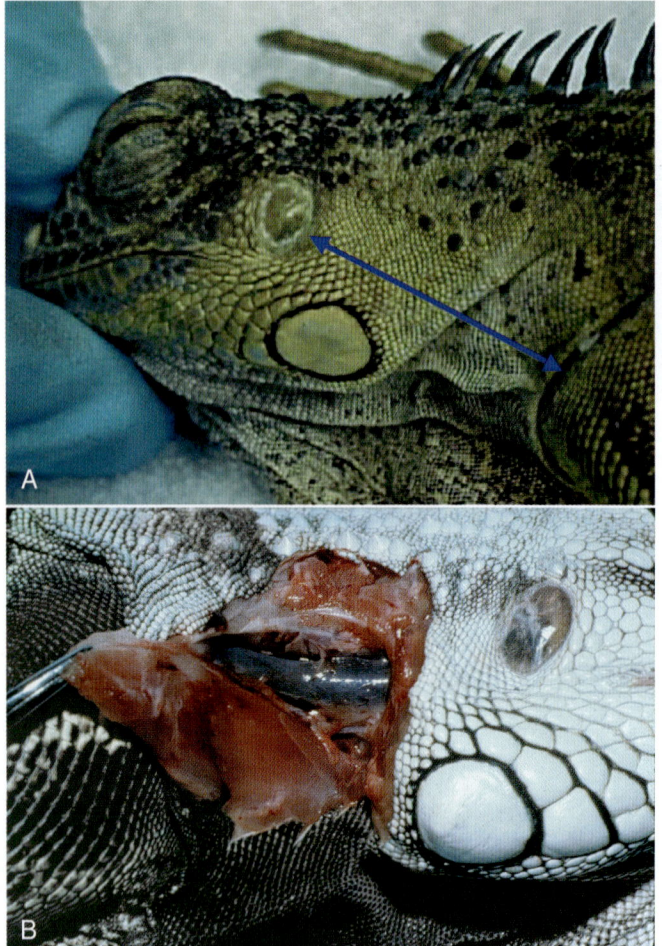

FIG 115.7 (A) The jugular vein in most species of lizards is located in the lateral cervical region. This figure shows the approximate location of the jugular vein in the green iguana (*Iguana iguana*). (B) Postmortem dissection of the jugular vein of an adult green iguana. The large jugular vein is located on the lateral neck caudal to and slightly below the tympanum. This site can be used for venipuncture or intravenous catheterization by drawing an imaginary line from the ear to the point of the shoulder, as seen in (A).

should be done with a syringe pump to limit any potential chance for pressure necrosis and damage to the scute.

Intrathecal Administration. Intrathecal injections have been demonstrated to be a viable option for parenterally administering drugs to chelonians, especially analgesics and anesthetics.[13] Intrathecal injections deliver the drug directly into the subarachnoid space, the location of cerebrospinal fluid (CSF) in reptiles. The dorsal tail of the chelonian should be aseptically prepared for the injection. Palpate the tail and, if possible, locate an intervertebral space as an insertion site. Insert a hypodermic needle (22–25 gauge, 1–1.5") fastened to a syringe into the intervertebral space. Adjustments to the insertion angle should be made to assist in correct placement. Begin insertion with a 45-degree angle once the neural arch is penetrated, then advance the needle into the spinal canal at a 20-degree angle. As the needle is advanced, maintain slight negative pressure. Upon penetration, clear to straw-colored CSF should enter the needle. If unsuccessful, the needle should be redirected

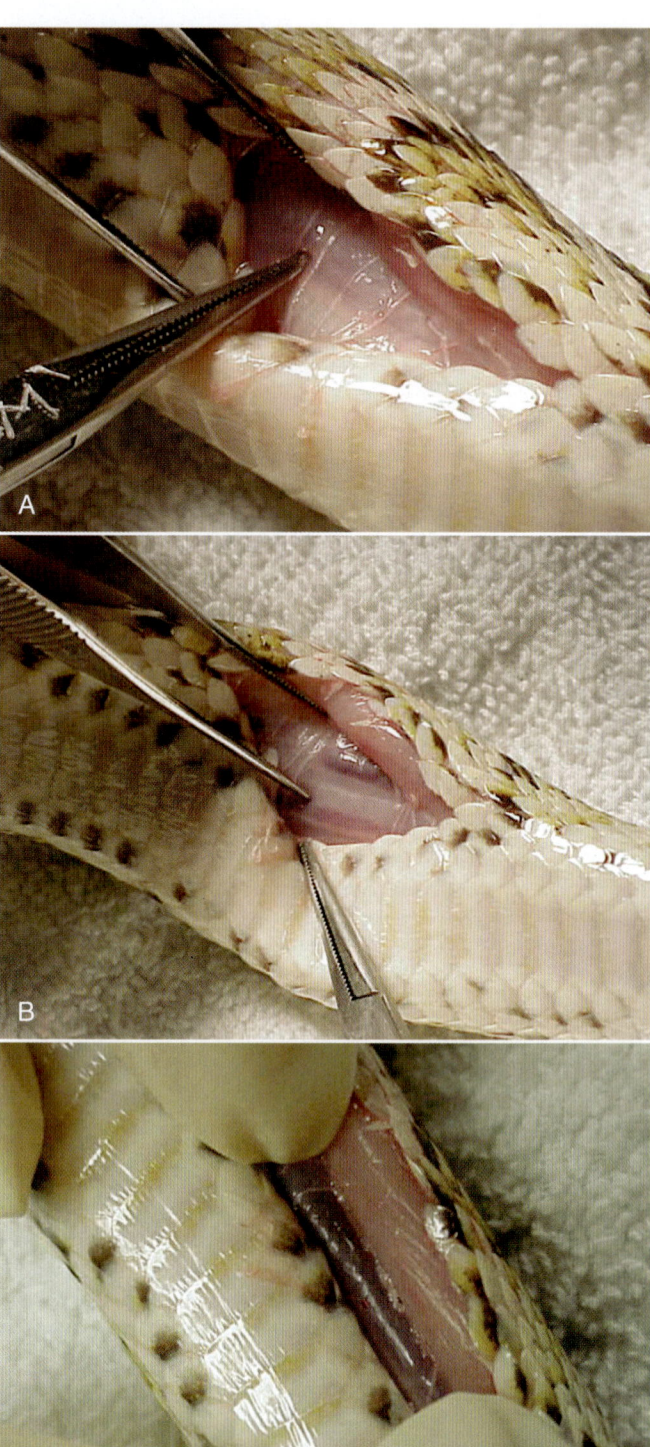

FIG 115.8 (A) The jugular vein of a snake can be located approximately nine scales cranial to the heart. The initial incision should be made between the first and second row of dorsal scales. (B) Blunt dissection of the rectus abdominius is necessary to identify the jugular vein. (C) The jugular vein is a sizable vessel in the snake. Here is an example of a right jugular vein in a reticulated python (*Malayopython reticulatus*).

until CSF is aspirated into the syringe. It is common to aspirate blood from the dorsal coccygeal vessel. If this happens, obtain a fresh needle and start again. Lidocaine (1 mg/kg) has been evaluated as an anesthetic for this procedure in the Galapagos tortoise (*Chelonoidis nigra*) and provides sufficient anesthesia for undergoing a phalectomy with minimal adverse effects.[12]

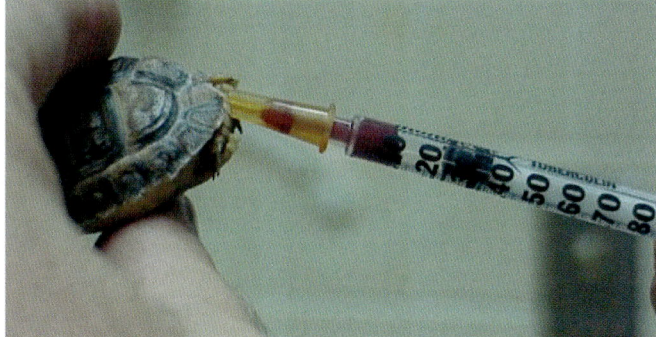

FIG 115.9 Subcarapacial sinus can be used to administer intravenous drugs in chelonians, even in the smallest patients; however, care is required as intrathecal injection is possible. (Courtesy of Mark A. Mitchell.)

Intracardiac Administration. Intracardiac venipuncture is routinely used to collect blood samples and deliver medications to snakes.[13,14] Recent studies in ball pythons *(Python regius)* found that serial cardiac venipuncture was not found to be associated with significant myocardial pathology, and propofol infusion directly into the heart showed minimal microscopic changes to the myocardium.[13,14] The authors have also administered radiographic contrast intracardially without obvious complications (Fig. 115.12). Injecting drugs into the heart is not without potential complications, including laceration of the great vessels or cardiac muscle, and arrhythmias. Although the likelihood of these complications appears to be low for experienced clinicians, they should be discussed with clients before hand.

Additional Routes of Administration

Nebulization. Reptiles have a primitive respiratory tract compared with mammals. Mammals have a well-developed ciliated epithelial lining and mucociliary escalator, whereas the reptile respiratory tract has very few epithelial cilia. Since reptiles lack this component of the immune system, they have a diminished ability to remove foreign material from this system; this can lead to the accumulation of mucous and microbes. Consequently, infections of the respiratory tract can be difficult to manage, and systemic antimicrobials may not be sufficient to control disease.

Nebulization therapy using antimicrobials is routinely done for mammals and birds with equivocal results. To date, only one study

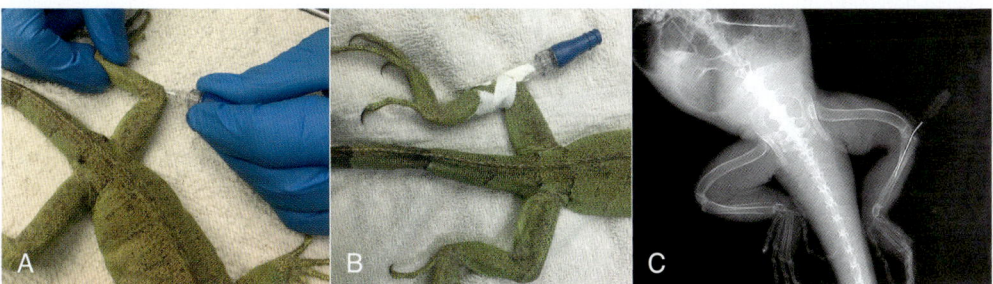

FIG 115.10 (A) Placement of an intraosseous catheter in a green iguana (*Iguana iguana*) in the cranial tibia. (B) Intraosseous catheters can be placed temporarily with tape as shown here in emergency situations while they can be sutured in for long-term placement. (C) Radiographs should be performed after placement to confirm placement within the medullary cavity for appropriate fluid or medication administration. (A and B, Courtesy of Sean M. Perry.)

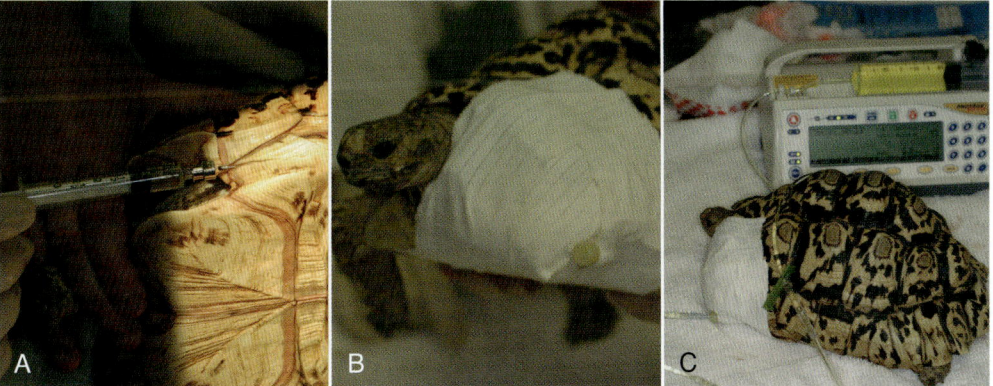

FIG 115.11 (A) Placement of an intraosseous catheter into the right cranial plastrocarapacial bridge in a leopard tortoise (*Stigmochelys pardalis*). (B) Bandaging the right forelimb in flexion to reduce the risk of catheter interference. (C) Tortoise receiving intraosseous fluid therapy using a syringe driver. (Courtesy of Stephen J. Divers.)

exists evaluating the pharmacokinetics of an antifungal medication using nebulization therapy. Kane et al. reported that nebulization therapy using terbinafine in cottonmouths (*Agkistrodon piscivorus*) reached levels higher than in vitro susceptibility concentration (15 ng/mL) for *Ophidiomyces ophiodiicola*. The absorption of the terbinafine is thought to be both via the respiratory tract and cutaneous absorption[15] (Fig. 115.13). Other drugs have been used successfully via nebulization by the authors, such as amikacin and gentamicin. Success with nebulization depends on the drug being used and the particle size of the vapor generated (<5 μm). Larger particles may not penetrate the distal lung and air sac spaces. The use of oxygen as a carrier gas can be associated with suppression of ventilation, and therefore air is recommended for reptiles. The duration of treatment is another important consideration to ensure sufficient penetration (see Chapter 76 for more details).

Reptiles can be nebulized with a variety of antibacterial or antifungal agents, sterile water, or a combination of these compounds. In addition, a mucolytic may be considered. Acetylcysteine 20% can be used to facilitate the breakdown of mucous, increasing the likelihood that the therapeutic is distributed throughout the respiratory tract and maximizing epithelial contact. When using acetylcysteine, exposure time should be limited to 30 minutes because it can be irritating to the tissues.

Intralesional Therapy. Intralesional therapy is a method of administering therapeutics directly to an area of concern either by direct injection of a chemotherapeutic or by implanting chemotherapeutic-impregnated beads. The beads then slowly release the drug into the local tissue to treat either infection or neoplasia for a period of time.

Antibiotic-impregnated polymethylmethacrylate beads can be used to treat osteomyelitis and local infections by providing long-acting, slow-release antibiotics to a specific area.[16] Only heat-stable antibiotics can be used to make the polymethylmethacrylate beads; the authors have had success with aminoglycoside agents (particularly gentamicin and amikacin) and clindamycin. The aminoglycoside antibiotics usually have good efficacy against gram-negative opportunistic pathogens, whereas clindamycin is often effective against anaerobic bacteria. Selecting the appropriate antibiotic-impregnated polymethylmethacrylate beads should be based on microbiologic culture and antibiotic sensitivity testing.

Intrapulmonary administration of amphotericin B has been used to successfully treat pulmonary candidiasis in a tortoise.[17] In reptiles, few case reports exist of intralesional therapy to administer adjuvant chemotherapy to control neoplasia. Squamous cell carcinoma was successfully treated in a yellow-belly slider (*Trachemys scripta scripta*) using a combination of surgery and electrochemotherapy with intratumoral injections of bleomycin.[18]

Transdermal Therapy. Transdermal therapy has become a common method for administering drugs in both human and veterinary medicine. This type of therapy is achieved by placing ointment or a patch delivery apparatus on the skin. In reptiles, the use of transdermal therapeutics is in its infancy. One study tested a loading dose of fentanyl in ethanol and cellulose gel that was enclosed by a plastic barrier with a permeable adhesive membrane on prehensile-tailed skinks (*Corucia zebrata*).[19] All of the animals within the study had measurable plasma concentrations of fentanyl within 24 hours of patch application and concentrations reached the human analgesic range within 36 hours. Another study evaluated the fentanyl transdermal therapeutic system in ball pythons.[20] In these snakes, a fentanyl transdermal patch (12 μg/h) was applied to the dorsum (cranial 1/3) of ball pythons with adhesive and staples. The investigators found detectable concentrations of fentanyl in the blood after 4 hours and human analgesic concentrations (1 ng/mL) starting at 8 hours and continuing for the remainder of the study (216 hours).[20] Both of these studies demonstrated that the scaled skin of a reptile does

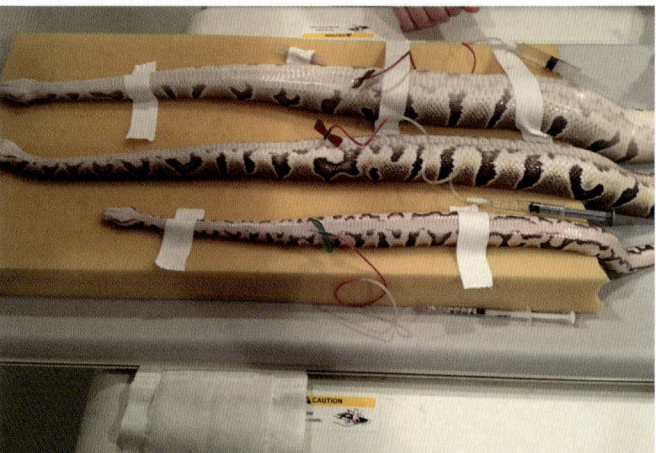

FIG 115.12 Intracardiac administration of medications can be employed in snake species; butterfly catheters are utilized in these ball pythons (*Python regius*) to administer intravenous iohexol before contrast CT. Sedation or anesthesia is recommended to ensure safe venipuncture. (Courtesy of Sean M. Perry.)

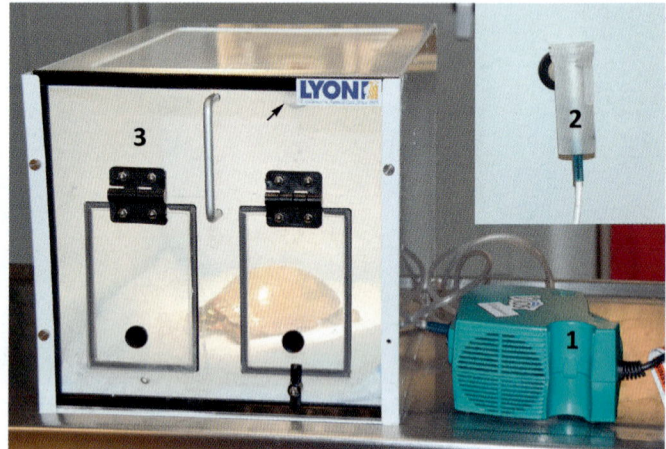

FIG 115.13 Nebulization setup suitable for reptiles. The compressor (1) forces air through the drug reservoir (2), located on external rear wall, to form a fine mist, which is delivered through a port (arrow) into the nebulization chamber (3), which has rubber seals around the front access door to reduce drug vapor escape. (Courtesy of Stephen J. Divers.)

not present an insurmountable barrier to systemic absorption of fentanyl delivered by a transdermal patch and suggest that additional studies are needed in other species.[19,20]

Osmotic Pumps. Alzet osmotic pumps (Durect Corp., Cupertino, CA) are implanted, miniature infusion pumps that provide continuous infusion of therapeutic agents to unrestrained animals. The "pumps" operate via an osmotic pressure difference between the tissue environment and a salt osmotic sleeve. The high osmotic pull of the salt within the pump causes water to diffuse into the pump across a semipermeable membrane and into the sleeve; this increases the pressure within the medication reservoir and initiates the release of the therapeutic agent via a flow moderator at a predetermined, continuous rate that is not dependent on the therapeutic agent's chemical properties.[21] Variable dosing rates can be achieved by altering the concentration of the therapeutic loaded into the pump. In reptiles, osmotic pumps have been used in green iguanas (*Iguana iguana*), corn snakes (*Pantherophis guttatus*), and Mojave rattlesnakes (*Crotalus scutulatus*) to deliver gonadotropin-releasing hormone, amikacin, and florfenicol, respectively.[22–24]

Programmable Infusion Pumps. iPRECIO programmable infusion pumps (Durect Corp., Cupertino, CA) are implanted advanced infusion devices that are miniaturized, fully programmable pumps. These pumps provide the user the ability to program different dosing protocols while maintaining access to a reservoir that can be refilled percutaneously. These pumps utilize wireless data communication and management software that directs dosing and infusion rates. Battery life of these devices varies based on infusion type and model; however, they can last from 47 days to 6 months. There are no reports of these pumps being used in reptiles, although they could certainly have clinical value.[25]

Long-Acting (Depot) Formulations. There has been a movement in veterinary medicine to produce long-acting (depot) formulations to reduce patient stress associated with daily treatment and to increase owner compliance. These same depots would be welcome in herpetological medicine if they provided the same results. Examples of long-acting formulations that have been used to treat reptiles include leuprolide acetate, cefovecin, oxytetracycline, doxycycline, and ivermectin.[6,7, 26–34] A pharmacokinetic study evaluating long-acting oxytetracycline in American alligators (*Alligator mississippiensis*) found it was useful for treating mycoplasmosis;[28] however, cefovecin has been thoroughly investigated and shows no efficacy in green iguanas because it is highly protein bound and has an extremely short half-life.[32–34] These results reinforce the importance of pursuing hypothesis-driven research to generate evidence-based information to ensure treatments will be optimized.

Vascular Access Ports. Vascular access ports are used to repeatedly collect blood samples or administer intravenous medications over time. They are useful in pharmacokinetic studies and for cancer chemotherapy. In a study evaluating these ports in tortoises, a sterile rubber stopper from an evacuated blood collection vial was inserted into a round plastrostomy site created at the location of the cardiac ventricle. This port was used to collect multiple blood samples over time; however, it is important to recognize that multiple injections into the heart can lead to myocardial fibrosis.[35,36] Vascular access ports have also been placed into the common carotid artery of green iguanas to evaluate serial blood gases. The ports remained functional in the green iguanas over several weeks.[37] In another case report, a vascular access port was placed into the ventral abdominal vein of a green iguana with lymphoma to deliver chemotherapy. This port needed to be replaced after 28 days due to dermal necrosis over the port; however, a second port was successfully placed and lasted 6 months without complications.[38]

Topical Administration. Many topical medications are used in reptiles to treat skin disease. Antiparasitics, disinfectants, ophthalmic solutions, creams, ointments, and lavage solutions can all be applied topically to reptiles. These types of drugs are intended to deliver local therapy to an affected area without unwanted systemic uptake and adverse effects.

Topical administration of antiparasitic agents has been evaluated in reptiles, because oral administration of antiparasitics can be challenging in some lizards and chelonians. In the United States the only USDA- and EPA-licensed topical antiparasitic medication for reptiles is Provent-a-Mite; its active ingredient is permethrin. This has been shown to be effective as an acaricide in Komodo dragons (*Varanus komodensis*) and leopard tortoises (*Stigmochelys pardalis*).[39,40] A commercially available topical treatment for intestinal parasites containing imidacloprid and moxidectin (Advantage multi/Advocate, Bayer, Shawnee Mission, KS) is available for companion animals. Frilled dragons (*Chlamydosurus kingii*) and bearded dragons (*Pogona vitticeps*) given a single topical dose of this drug were cleared of *Kalicephalus* sp. and oxyurid ova.[41] Another commercially available topical antiparasitic preparation containing emodepside and praziquantel (Profender, Bayer HealthCare, Shawnee Mission, KS) has been tested for absorption, elimination time, and efficacy in several lizards, snakes, and chelonians.[42–44] Both drugs were absorbed via the skin, except in one case; emodepside was not absorbed in a single red-eared slider (*Trachemys scripta elegans*) that was returned to the water within 1 hour of treatment. [42,43] Treatment with emodepside/praziquantel at doses higher than those used in mammals was followed by a significant decrease in the number of nematode ova in the feces within 48 hours. No adverse effects were observed, and fecal nematode egg counts decreased after treatment in a relatively large (n = 417), uncontrolled clinical trial of emodepside/praziquantel in species from four different reptilian families.[42] Despite these results, a clinical trial with the Texas tortoise (*Gopherus berlandieri*) showed no efficacy when using emodepside/praziquantel to treat pinworms; animals that were treated with topical emodepside/praziquantel had higher egg counts per gram of feces compared with the untreated groups (J. Jill Heatly: Pers. comm., 2016). Additionally, in four Hermann's tortoises (*Testudo hermani*), twenty-two spur thigh tortoises (*Testudo gracea*), two Russian tortoises (*Agrionemys horsfieldii*), and a leopard tortoise, after treatment with topical emodepside/praziquantel, the oxyurid egg count was slightly increased on day 14, although it declined significantly by day 33, which may have indicated a therapeutic effect and moderate efficacy 33 days posttreatment. Topical application of emodepside and praziquantel was well tolerated in our tortoise population.[44] The results of these studies reinforce the importance of pursuing hypothesis-driven research to evaluate species dosing, route of administration, location of treatment, and so on. When faced with a clinical case and no relevant evidence-based science, it is important to thoroughly document protocols used and share them with others to initiate a discussion and, hopefully, an interest in pursuing research.

Topical therapy to aid in wound healing has also been briefly explored in reptiles. Becaplermin, a topical platelet-derived growth factor, was investigated to determine whether it altered the rate of wound closure in bearded dragons. Becaplermin did not have a significant effect on wound closure rates in this species.[45]

Implications of the Renal Portal System and Administration Route

The renal portal system is a unique component of the circulatory system of lower vertebrates. Historically, parenteral drug administration into the tail or caudal extremities was not recommended because of the potential adverse effect (nephrotoxicosis) associated with drug passage through the renal portal system. Although reports exist of nephrotoxicosis associated with the administration of aminoglycosides in reptiles, a review of these cases suggests that the toxicosis was attributed to high doses of gentamicin rather than the route of administration.[46,47]

Research has suggested that parenteral administration of drugs into the caudal extremities may not pose as great a risk as once thought. Holz et al.[48] evaluated renal perfusion in red-eared sliders with radioangiography. The research suggested that intravenous injections of a radiopaque dye into the dorsal coccygeal vein or femoral vein do not necessarily perfuse the kidneys via the renal portal system. The renal portal system most likely serves to perfuse the kidneys, more specifically the tubules, during times of water conservation. During times of water conservation, arginine vasotocin increases water resorption at the level of the tubules while reducing glomerular filtration.[49] Prolactin is the antagonist for this system.[50] Holtz et al.[49] proposed that a valve located between the abdominal and femoral veins might regulate blood flow through the kidneys. At times of water conservation, a valve in the abdominal vein closes, redirecting blood through the iliac veins and into the kidneys. Holz et al.[51] tested the practicality of this concept by performing two antibiotic pharmacokinetic studies in the red-eared slider. Gentamicin and carbenicillin were selected for the study because they are excreted via glomerular filtration and tubular secretion, respectively. The bioavailability of gentamicin was not affected by injection site. However, this was not unexpected because the renal portal system provides blood to the tubules and should not affect glomerular filtration.[48] The area under the curve for carbenicillin plasma concentrations was significantly lower for the hind limb injections at 1, 4, and 8 hours after injection. Although the plasma concentrations were lower for the hind limb injections, the levels recorded remained above the minimum inhibitory concentration (MIC) required for susceptible bacterial pathogens.

The renal portal system of the iguana may behave differently than that described in chelonians. When three green iguanas were given a radiopaque dye intravenously into the ventral caudal vein, the contrast entered the caudal renal parenchyma and moved cranially into the caudal vena cava.[52] When the radiopaque dye was intraosseously delivered into the femur of three green iguanas, the dye entered the common iliac, pelvic, and ventral abdominal veins. The contrast eventually extended into the renal parenchyma. Variation, however, did exist in the movement of the dye in the iguanas, which may be attributed to individual variation or the small sample size.

To determine whether the renal portal system has any effect on drug pharmacokinetics in snakes, Holz et al.[53] evaluated the injection site on the pharmacokinetics of carbenicillin in carpet pythons (*Morelia spilotes variegata*). Seven carpet pythons were used for the study, and each received a 200 mg/kg intramuscular dose of carbenicillin in either the cranial or caudal epaxial musculature. Five months after the injection, the snakes again received a 200 mg/kg intramuscular injection of carbenicillin; however, the site of the injection was reversed from the previous example. No significant difference was seen in the pharmacokinetics between injection sites. Although the concentrations of drugs given in the cranial half of the snakes were higher over the first 6 to 8 hours, the difference was not significant. However, the range of concentrations was quite varied for each time point, suggesting variability within the sample population. A larger sample population may have led to different results. Regardless of the difference, Holz et al.[53] found that the plasma concentrations were sufficient to control susceptible bacterial pathogens.

Research to investigate the pharmacokinetics and the pathological effects of drugs given in the caudal extremities is limited to a few species, and generalization of these results to all 10,000+ species of reptiles could be dangerous. Additional research to elaborate the effects of different drugs on the renal portal system should be pursued.

Treatment of Eggs

In 1975, attempts to reduce or eliminate *Salmonella* in chelonians with antimicrobials led the US Food and Drug Administration (FDA) to ban the sale of turtle hatchlings. Treatment of the freshly laid eggs with oxytetracycline or chloramphenicol with a temperature differential egg dip method was successful at eliminating *Salmonella* in eggs less than 1 day old but did not clear eggs greater than 2 days old.[54,55] However, because of the development and persistence of antimicrobial-resistant strains of *Salmonella*, antibiotic treatment of reptiles or their eggs is not recommended.[56] Alternative techniques have been developed to suppress or eliminate *Salmonella* in red-eared slider eggs. Mitchell et al. demonstrated that two nonantibiotic microbicide compounds (sodium hypochlorite [NaOCl] and polyhexamethylene biguanide [PHMB]) could be used as a bath and pressure-differential dip to successfully suppress or eliminate *Salmonella*.[57]

REFERENCES

See www.expertconsult.com for a complete list of references.

116

Antibiotic Therapy

Sean M. Perry and Mark A. Mitchell

Historic recommendations for dosing and delivering (route of administration) antibiotics have been based on empirical suggestions derived from evidence gained through domestic mammal research or "positive results" derived from case reports. These historic limitations can be attributed to the lack of pharmacokinetic and pharmacodynamic studies specifically evaluating antibiotics in reptiles, although since the last publication of this text, some progress has been made.

ANTIBIOTIC SELECTION

Specific factors that should be considered when selecting an antibiotic for a case include the intrinsic antimicrobial spectrum of that drug (e.g., gram positive vs. gram negative, aerobic vs. anaerobic), acquired antimicrobial resistance, mechanism of action, tissue distribution, potential side effects, metabolic and excretory pathways, dose and volume required, and route and frequency of administration. The antibiotic with the narrowest spectrum of activity should be selected to treat the pathogen to limit collateral damage to the patient's microbiota.

An antibiotic should be administered after confirming the existence of an infection. Ideally, culture and sensitivity profile (or MIC testing) should be done to determine the preferred antibiotic. While pending microbiologic culture and sensitivity testing, the veterinarian must select an antibiotic based on gram stains, cytology, past experience, and best practices. Although limited in sensitivity, cytological examination of a lesion may be used to determine whether the microflora associated with a lesion is homogeneous or heterogeneous. If the bacteria appear homogeneous (all gram positive or all gram negative), then this information may be used to guide antibiotic selection. Most bacterial pathogens isolated from reptiles are gram negative, although gram-positive bacterial infections do occur. Of 141 bacterial cultures and sensitivity panels from clinical reptile cases that were evaluated by a large accredited laboratory, 28% were gram negative and 72% gram positive (Tang et al, Proc ExoticsCon, 2018, p 963).

INDISCRIMINANT ANTIBIOTIC USE IN HERPETOLOGICAL MEDICINE

In both human and veterinary medicine, our management of bacterial infections remains primitive. Currently, our process of isolating and treating a pathogen using an antibiotic suggests a specificity that does not exist. When a reptile, or any vertebrate, is given an antibiotic, the drug can have broad and impactful effects on the individual's microbiota and, more concerning, environmental and human health issues. *Salmonella*-positive green iguanas (*Iguana iguana*) treated with enrofloxacin were cleared of not only the enrofloxacin-sensitive *Salmonella* but *Pseudomonas aeruginosa* and *Citrobacter freundii* as well (Mitchell

M, unpublished data). These latter two microbes were not isolated from cultures collected from the iguanas over 2 to 3 weeks posttreatment. Eventually, these organisms recolonized the gastrointestinal tract; the source was most likely the diet, which was always positive for these two organisms. However, a far greater concern with our current method of treating infections is that it creates a selection pressure that results in the emergence of antimicrobial resistance.[1] Until techniques are found to deliver a treatment that does not affect the commensal microbiota, the risk of creating antimicrobial-resistant organisms will exist, and continued efforts are required to minimize these risks.[2]

In herpetological medicine, it is not uncommon for veterinarians to have cases presented that have been treated empirically with antibiotics previously. Many veterinarians have the mentality that in exotic species, especially reptiles, enrofloxacin is a panacea. The routine use of advanced, broad spectrum antibiotics implies a low level of skill on the part of the clinician. It is our duty to develop appropriate antimicrobial stewardship. Widespread use of antibiotics has led to increases in the reports of antimicrobial-resistant pathogens. Veterinarians should limit antibiotic use to those cases in which their use is warranted. Antibiotic prescription should be limited to one of two reasons: (1) prevent infection (i.e., if an animal is immunocompromised, has severe trauma or wounds, or requires perioperative antibiotics) or (2) treatment of a documented bacterial infection.

MINIMIZING INDISCRIMINATE ANTIBIOTIC USE IN HERPETOLOGICAL MEDICINE

Not all animals that are ill have bacterial infections, and not all bacterial infections require treatment. Worsening of a disease state in critically ill animals does not always warrant escalation of antimicrobial treatments. Viral infections, immune-mediated conditions, and inflammatory conditions can cause signs that can often be attributed to bacterial infections. Early diagnostic testing rather than empirical antibiotic usage can help resolve if an animal needs antimicrobials. Even when bacterial infections are present, systemic antimicrobial therapy may not be optimal. Local therapy with biocidal or antimicrobial drugs may be equally or even more efficacious in some cases. Overall, there needs to be a reduction on the reliance of antimicrobials in veterinary medicine, not just in herpetological medicine. Unfortunately, despite clear efforts in this regard by some areas of the profession (especially small animal and agriculture), herpetological (and exotic pet) medicine is lagging behind. It behooves all of us to critically evaluate our prescribing practices and create appropriate antibiotic stewardship policies within our practices (Table 116.1). For further information on this specific topic we recommend reading the American College of Veterinary Internal Medicine consensus statement published in the *Journal of Veterinary Internal Medicine*.[2]

TABLE 116.1	**Zoological Medicine Service Antibiotic Policy From University of Georgia**	
Tier 1 drugs	Indications: 1. Infection prevention in severely compromised animals. 2. Intraoperative IO or IV administration to prevent infection (e.g., orthopedics). 3. First-line antimicrobial to treat infections, while awaiting culture and sensitivity or MIC results.	Trimethoprim, sulfonamides, or combinations Tetracyclines (e.g., oxytetracycline, doxycycline) Basic/potentiated penicillins (e.g., ampicillin, penicillin, amoxicillin/clavulanic acid) Metronidazole Basic macrolides and lincosamides (e.g., erythromycin, lincomycin, clindamycin) Aminoglycosides 1st- and 2nd-generation cephalosporins (incl intraop ceftiofur) 1st-generation quinolones (e.g., oxolinic acid, nalidixic acid)
Tier 2 drugs	Indications: 1. Only to be used if culture and sensitivity or MIC testing indicate tier 1 drugs are ineffective.	3rd-generation cephalosporins (ceftazidime, ceftiofur) Penicillinase-resistant penicillins (e.g., methicillin) Advanced penicillins (eg piperacillin, cerbenicillin, ticarcillin) Advanced macrolides (e.g., azithromycin, clarithromycin) 2nd-generation fluoroquinolones (e.g. enrofloxacin, orbifloxacin, ciprofloxacin, marbofloxacin) Florfenicol, Chloramphenicol
Tier 3 drugs	Indications: 1. Restricted or prohibited use antimicrobial agents for multidrug resistant infections. Generally, not to be used in veterinary medicine.	Glycopeptides (e.g., vancomycin) Carbapenems (e.g., imipenem) Oxazolidonones (e.g., linezolid) 4th generation and above cephalosporins (e.g., defepine) Ketolides (e.g., telithromycin) Lipopeptides (e.g., daptomycin) Ansamycins (e.g., geldanamycin) 3rd generation and above fluoroquinolones (e.g., levofloxacin)

ANTIBIOTIC DRUGS

Aminoglycosides

Aminoglycosides (Table 116.2) used in herpetological medicine include gentamicin, amikacin, kanamycin, neomycin, paromomycin, streptomycin, and tobramycin. These compounds irreversibly bind to one or more receptor protein of the 30S subunit of the bacterial ribosome, interfering with mRNA translation.[3–5] They are polycations that are minimally bound to protein and poorly absorbed from the gastrointestinal tract. Aminoglycosides are primarily excreted unchanged through the kidneys. This group of antibiotics has a narrow therapeutic index and should be used cautiously. The primary adverse effects associated with aminoglycosides in mammals are ototoxicity and nephrotoxicity. Aminoglycoside toxicity can vary with the specific drug, peak concentration, and hydration and renal status of the patient. Gentamicin is more nephrotoxic than amikacin.[3–5] Veterinarians should evaluate a reptile's renal function and hydration status before initiating treatment with an aminoglycoside. In reptiles, calcium, phosphorous, potassium, total solids, and nitrogenous waste (uric acid, urea, ammonia) concentrations can provide some insight into reptile renal function. An inverse calcium:phosphorous ratio is a strong indication of reduced renal function in lizards.

Aminoglycosides are considered standard of care for gram-negative sepsis and are generally indicated for gram-negative bacterial infections, including *E. coli, Klebsiella* spp., *Enterobacter* spp., *Pseudomonas* spp., *Proteus* spp., *Providencia* spp., *Salmonella* spp., and *Serratia* spp.[6] Aminoglycosides can be used in combination with penicillins to treat gram-positive infections. The MIC required to control gram-negative aerobes with aminoglycosides is dependent on the drug used, with gentamicin having lower MIC concentrations, 3 to 5 μm/mL, than amikacin, 5 to 10 μg/ml.[5] In general, up to three to five times the MIC may be needed to eradicate certain pathogens.[5] Aminoglycosides were one of the first antibiotics used to treat bacterial infections in reptiles. They were also the first class of antibiotics to have pharmacokinetic data that

could be used to determine appropriate dosing intervals. Aminoglycosides should be considered a first-line antimicrobial drug choice.

Amikacin. The absorption, metabolism, and excretion of an antibiotic might be expected to differ when a reptile is maintained at different temperatures. However, no difference was reported in the absorption or elimination rates of amikacin in the gopher snakes (*Pituophis catenifer*) housed at different temperatures.[7] Snakes housed at the higher temperature did have an increased volume of distribution and body clearance compared with those housed at the cooler temperature. In addition, bacterial isolates were more susceptible to amikacin at higher temperatures.[6]

Johnson et al. performed a similar pharmacokinetic study with ball pythons (*Python regius*).[8] Whereas the drug half-lives were substantially higher than those reported in the gopher snakes, however, the dose used was also higher. The increased environmental temperature did not significantly affect the rate of elimination in these snakes. Drug bioavailability following intramuscular injection, which is rarely recorded in reptile pharmacokinetic studies, was substantially less (74%–77%) than that reported in mammals (>90%).[9]

The effect of environmental temperature on amikacin pharmacokinetics has also been evaluated in a chelonian species, the gopher tortoise (*Gopherus polyphemus*).[10] Clearance rates, mean residence times, and area under the curve were significantly different between the two treatment groups. The results of the study strongly suggested that environmental temperature could affect metabolic rate in this species, which in turn can affect drug pharmacokinetics.

Recently amikacin has been successfully delivered in snakes via an osmotic pump. Osmotic pumps were implanted in both corn snakes (*Pantherophis guttatus*) and a Taylor's cantil (*Agkistrodon bilineatus taylori*) to deliver amikacin as a constant rate infusion.[11,12] The results of the study suggested that the osmotic pump could be used for treating bacterial infections in snakes, because the pump delivered the drug at a predictable rate and plasma concentrations were found to reach

TABLE 116.2 Peer-Reviewed Antibiotic Pharmacokinetic Data in Reptile Species to Utilize in Clinical Practice

Aminoglycoside	Species	Dose	Route of Administration	Recommended Frequency of Administration	Half-Life: $T_{1/2}$ (hrs)	Plasma Concentration: C_{Max} (µg/ml) or C_{mean} (µg/ml)	Target Plasma Concentration: µg/ml	Volume of Distribution: V_d (L/kg)
Amikacin	Gopher snake (*Pituophus catenifer*)[7]	5 mg/kg	IM	5 mg/kg loading, 2.5 mg/kg q 72 hrs	25°C—71.9 37°C—75.4	≈18	25°C—1-6 37°C—0.5-6	25°C—0.289 37°C—0.627
	Ball python (*Python regius*)[8]	11 mg/kg (3.5 mg/kg recommended dose)	IC	Once	37°C—110 25°C—126	— —	48	37°C—0.410 25°C—0.465
			IM		37°C and 25°C—109	37°C C_{Max}: 13.87 25°C C_{Max}: 11.93		
	Gopher tortoise (*Gopherus polyphemus*)[10]	5 mg/kg	IM	48 hrs	30°C—30 20°C—176	30°C—C_{mean}: 54.13 20°C—C_{mean}: 0.22	5-25	30°C—0.24 20°C—0.22
	Corn snake (*Pantherophis guttatus*)[11]	2.5 mg/kg	IM		44.8	10.4	8	0.21
		1.7 mg/kg loading—0.026 mg/kg/hr*	IM/Osmo		141	7.62	8	—
		5 mg/kg loading, then 2.5 mg/kg*	IM	72 hrs	121	25.14	8	—
	American alligator (*Alligator mississippiensis*)[21]	1.75 mg/kg	IM	NR	49.4	10.9	12	0.25
		2.25 mg/kg	IM	NR	52.8	13.2	12	0.22
	Red eared slider (*Trachemys scripta elegans*)[16]	10 mg/kg	IM	NR	56.8	25.0	–	–
		6 mg/kg	IM	2-5 days	31.3	14.5	1-5	–
	Box turtle (*Terrapene carolina carolina*)[17]	3 mg/kg	IM	96 hrs	44.3	19.5	2	–
Gentamicin	Blood python (*Python curtus*)[15]	3.0 mg/kg loading, 1.5 mg/kg	IM	96 hrs	100	8.59	6-8	1.1-1.6
	American alligator (*Alligator mississippiensis*)[21]	1.25 mg/kg	IM	NR	37.8	6.2	<6	0.38
		1.75 mg/kg	IM		75.4	9.5	<6	0.28

IC, Intracardiac; *IClo*, intracloacal; *IM*, intramuscular; *IV*, intravenous; *Neb*, nebulization; *NR*, not reported; *Osmo*, intracoelomic osmotic pump (Azlet).

*Some animals became hypercalcemic, these data include those animals in the analysis.

appropriate levels.[11] An osmotic pump has also been used in a clinical case to combat *Salmonella enterica houtenae* osteomyelitis in a Taylor's cantil. Progression of the osteomyelitis was controlled using amikacin (0.026 mg/kg/hour) via the subcutaneous osmotic pump for a total of 10 months. The pump was replaced every 4 weeks and no adverse effects were reported during the treatment period. Unfortunately, 5 months after therapy, the bony lesions progressed and abscesses were observed at the implant site. Euthanasia was elected for this animal.[12]

Gentamicin. Bush et al. was the first group to evaluate gentamicin in chelonians. The average biologic half-life for gentamicin was 32 hours ± 15 hours, with a range of 8 to 76 hours. The large variation in the half-lives can be attributed to the small sample size. Ultimately, the authors concluded that 10 mg/kg every 48 hours for less than 14 days was an appropriate dose (Bush, unpublished data).

Bush et al. were also the first to evaluate gentamicin in snakes, and the average biologic half-life of gentamicin was 82 hours.[13] The half-lives reported in chelonians and snakes were 10 to 40 times longer than those reported for mammalian species.[14] A second study was performed to evaluate serial doses of gentamicin over approximately 14 days. A stairstep increase in serum concentrations of gentamicin was recorded for all groups. The highest concentrations occurred in the groups receiving daily injections. The authors suggested that this might have occurred because the snakes could not excrete the drug in a timely manner. Although serum concentrations were not as high in the groups receiving the antibiotic every 72 hours, they did achieve therapeutic levels and are less likely to produce negative side effects.

Hilf et al. also evaluated gentamicin kinetics in two additional species of snakes, a Burmese python (*Python bivittatus*) and blood pythons (*Python curtus*).[15] The snakes received a single dose of gentamicin (2.5 mg/kg IM). On the basis of the results from the pilot study, and the authors' desire to achieve peak serum concentrations between 6 and 8 µg/mL, the blood pythons (n = 4) were given one of four dosing regimens: 2.5 mg/kg IM followed by 1.5 mg/kg after 72 hours, 2.5 mg/kg IM followed by 1.5 mg/kg after 96 hours, 3 mg/kg IM followed by 1.5 mg/kg after 72 hours, and 3 mg/kg IM followed by 1.5 mg/kg after 96 hours. Peak serum concentration was achieved within 10 hours; however, the biologic half-life varied between 32 and 110 hours. No apparent side effects were seen, although the author used blood uric acid levels to evaluate renal function. Uric acid is not a sensitive assay for renal function in reptiles, and GFR evaluation, renal biopsy, and histology would be more appropriate. Gentamicin accumulation was observed in these snakes, which suggests that multiple dosing could lead to negative side effects. To avoid these potential side effects, the authors suggested medicating pythons with a loading dose of 2.5 to 3 mg/kg and 1.5 mg/kg every 96 hours thereafter.

Raphael et al. also performed a study to determine the pharmacokinetics of gentamicin in red-eared sliders.[16] Differences in the pharmacokinetics of gentamicin between the turtles studied in the Raphael et al. and Bush et al.[13] papers may have been attributed to injection site or temperature variation. The turtles in Raphael et al. were housed at cooler temperatures than those in Bush et al. In addition, the red-eared sliders in Raphael et al. were given the injection in the musculature of the forelimb. This information was not provided by Bush et al., and injection site may have led to alterations in the disposition of gentamicin in these chelonians. On the basis of MIC values for susceptible species, the 6 mg/kg IM dose every 48 to 72 hours was considered appropriate for treatment of susceptible pathogens.

Beck et al. determined the pharmacokinetics for gentamicin in box turtles (*Terrapene carolina carolina*).[17] In addition, the authors also evaluated the role of injection site, forelimb versus hind limb, on the

pharmacokinetics of the drug. No difference was seen in the plasma concentrations of gentamicin between the two treatment groups. Plasma concentrations remained above 2 µg/mL throughout the study, which should be adequate to achieve MIC for most pathogens, although it may be insufficient to achieve the levels suggested by Hoperich.[6] Because gentamicin is excreted via glomerular filtration, these findings were not unexpected. Evaluation of an antibiotic that is excreted via tubular secretion, such as a synthetic penicillin, may be more appropriate for evaluation of the role of the renal portal system in drug pharmacokinetics. Side effects associated with gentamicin have been well documented. The first report in a lizard was associated with the toxic effects on the basilar papilla of *Calotes versicolor*.[18] Gentamicin toxicity was also reported in two boid snakes that received 4.4 mg/kg (2 mg/lb) twice a day for 2 days, and then the same dose once a day for 5 additional days.[19] Both snakes had visceral gout develop, which was attributed to gentamicin-induced renal failure.

Many of the problems encountered with this class of antibiotics have been associated with the use of mammalian drug dosages. Montali et al. evaluated the pathological effects of giving a mammalian dose of gentamicin to two snakes.[20] In the study, two bull snakes (*Pituophis [melanoleucas] catenifer*) were given gentamicin at 5 mg/kg once every 72 hours, and another two bull snakes were given 5 mg/kg once a day for 14 days. Renal biopsy results from the second group of snakes revealed mild to moderate swelling in the proximal tubular cells. One snake from each of the two treatment groups was given an additional dose of 50 mg/kg once a day for 14 days. Again, swelling was noted in the proximal tubules; however, it advanced to tubular necrosis. Variability in the pharmacokinetics of aminoglycosides in reptiles suggests that veterinarians should be cautious and use lower doses when working with an untested species.

Jacobson et al. investigated the disposition kinetics of IM gentamicin and amikacin in juvenile American alligators (*Alligator mississippiensis*).[21] Gentamicin and amikacin were both rapidly absorbed in the alligators. The distribution of both compounds was biphasic. On the basis of MIC values for pathogenic microbes in crocodilians, such as *Aeromonas hydrophila*, 1.75 mg/kg gentamicin and 2.25 mg/kg amikacin were considered appropriate.[21]

Tobramyacin. A single case report of using tobramyacin in a reptile exists in the literature. One Kemp's ridley sea turtle (*Lepidocheyles kempii*) was treated with 5 mg/kg tobramycin (Tobramycin 40 mg/mL, Hospira Inc., Lake Forest, IL) IM every 3 days for 58 days. (Innis C, unpublished data).

β-Lactam Antibiotics

Penicillins. The primary action of the penicillins is against cell wall synthesis; however, this class of drug is susceptible to beta-lactamase. Variable amounts of the semisynthetic penicillins are bound to protein. Distribution of these drugs is greater via the parenteral route. The drugs are excreted primarily via tubular secretion and glomerular filtration. Semisynthetic penicillins cross the placenta in mammals but are not known to have teratogenic effects. Whether these drugs could affect embryos in reptiles is unknown.

There has been no pharmacokinetic investigations into the use of natural penicillins or aminopenicillins, with or without β-lactamase inhibitors. However, these drugs are often effective and are generally recommended as first-line antimicrobials. Of bacterial isolates from clinical reptile cases seen at the University of Georgia, all gram-positive isolates and 65% of gram-negative isolates were sensitive to ampicillin (Divers S, unpublished data).

Carbenicillin and piperacillin are semisynthetic penicillins with extended spectrum against gram-negative bacteria. These drugs were originally found to have antipseudomonal activity; however, increased resistance is reported with increased usage. Lawrence et al. reported pseudomonal resistance to carbenicillin in multiple beta-lactamase-producing pseudomonal species in the early 1980s.[22] The semisynthetic penicillins also have some effect against anaerobes but are generally not recommended as a first-line antimicrobial, but rather when indicated by culture and sensitivity testing.

Studies evaluating the efficacy of the semisynthetic penicillins in reptiles are limited. Hilf et al. determined the pharmacokinetics of piperacillin in blood pythons. The half-life of piperacillin between the snakes used in the study was similar.[23] However, the distribution of the drug was variable after IM injection.

Lawrence et al. determined plasma concentrations of a single IM injection of carbenicillin in four different species of snakes.[22] Blood samples were collected on two different time schedules from the snake subjects, limiting the authors' ability to perform a pharmacokinetic study. Despite its limitations, this study demonstrated a C_{Max} ranging from 177 to 270 µg/mL was achieved 1 hour after injection. Therapeutic concentrations, 50 to 60 µg/mL, were maintained for 12 hours in three snakes. Although a full pharmacokinetic study was not performed, Lawrence et al. recommended 400 mg/kg IM every 24 hours would provide therapeutic levels of carbenicillin for snakes.[22] Holtz et al. reported that carbenicillin at 200 mg/kg IM every 24 hours was appropriate for carpet pythons (*Morelia spilota*).[24]

Lawrence et al. also evaluated the disposition kinetics of carbenicillin in two species of chelonians, *Testudo graeca* and *Testudo hermanni*.[25] A secondary drug peak was reported, which may represent secondary resorption of excreted drug across the bladder wall. Although limited by the numbers of tortoises used in this study, the authors did report that tortoises that evacuated urine during the study did have lower carbenicillin concentrations than those that did not micturate, suggesting that the bladder could serve in some capacity in the reabsorption of this antibiotic. The authors concluded that 400 mg/kg every 48 hours is likely sufficient to provide therapeutic concentrations in these tortoises. Manire et al. evaluated ticarcillin in three captive loggerhead sea turtles and concluded that 50 mg/kg every 24 hours or 100 mg/kg every 48 hours may be appropriate, but that liver enzymes should be monitored.[25a]

Cephalosporins

Cephalosporins were developed from a natural product of *Cephalosporium acreminium*. These antibacterials (Table 116.3) are related structurally to benzyl-penicillin and have a β-lactam ring. They act by inhibiting cell wall synthesis by preventing cross-linking of peptidoglycans. Cephalosporins are divided into five different generations. Unfortunately, there has been little research into the first-line, first- and second-generation cephalosporins, although they are frequently used intraoperatively.

In reptile medicine, third-generation cephalosporins have been evaluated most frequently, but their use should be restricted to infections resistant to more basic β-lactam drugs. Data from the University of Georgia demonstrates only marginally better sensitivity of third-generation (74%) compared with first- and second-generation drugs (57%) for gram-negative isolates, and no difference (75%) regarding gram-positive isolates (Tang et al, Proc ExoticsCon, 2018, p 963). Examples of third-generation cephalsporins used in reptile medicine include ceftiofur, ceftazidime, and cefoperazone.[26] Overall, third-generation cephalosporins have decreased gram-positive activity but increased gram-negative activity. Gram-negative bacteria typically found to be sensitive to these antibiotics include *Escherichia coli*, *Klebsiella* spp., *Pseudomonas* spp., *Proteus* spp., *Pasteurella* spp., *Haemophilus* spp., *Actinobacillus* spp., and *Salmonella* spp. Cephalosporins may be effective against some anaerobes, such as *Clostridium* spp. and *Fusobacterium* spp., but may be limited against others, such as *Bacteroides* spp.[26]

Ceftazidime. Ceftazidime is widely, and perhaps inappropriately, prescribed to numerous species of reptiles because it is broad spectrum, has a low-administration volume (when diluted to 100 mg/mL), and a prolonged dosing interval of 48 to 72 hours. However, clinicians should use caution in using this drug as a first-line antimicrobial to avoid creating resistant organisms and because dosing with ceftazidime has not been evaluated in boids, lizards, tortoises, or freshwater turtles. Lawrence et al. were the first to evaluate the effects of a ceftazidime in eight different snakes, representing five different species, maintained at 30°C.[27] Ceftazidime was selected because of its enhanced activity against gram-negative microbes. This compound also has excellent spectrum against *Pseudomonas aeruginosa*, although given the increased resistance with the continued use of this drug in veterinary medicine, culture and sensitivity testing is important. Peak plasma concentrations for ceftazidime were variable (26–70 µg/mL) and occurred between 1 and 8 hours. The high degree of variability in peak plasma drug levels (26–70 µg/mL between 1 and 8 hours) may have been associated with species differences but could not be evaluated further because of a limited sample size. The half-life of the drug was 24 hours, which is almost 12 times longer than that reported in humans.[28,29] No negative side effects were reported in any of the snakes. The dose administered might be expected to vary with a different environmental temperature. Studies have also been done to determine the pharmacokinetics of ceftazidime in loggerhead sea turtles (*Caretta caretta*), and there appears to be little difference in the plasma concentrations and half-lives following IV or IM routes.[29] In cold-stunned Kemp's ridley sea turtles (*Lepidochelys kempii*) the maximum concentration (C_{max}) was similar to that found in loggerheads, but the half-life in Kemp's ridley turtles was more than double that of loggerheads.[29,30] Further research is needed to determine appropriate dosing recommendations for more species.

Cefoperazone. Cefoperazone, another third-generation cephalosporin, has also been evaluated in reptiles. Although cephalosporins within the same generation typically have similar mechanisms of action, activity, and distribution within vertebrate hosts, some differences do exist. For instance, cefoperazome is more liposoluble than ceftazidime, which can increase its distribution to certain tissues. In addition, cefoperazome is excreted primarily via hepatic pathways, unlike most other cephalosporins, which are excreted via glomerular filtration or tubular secretion. Therefore excretion of this drug may be delayed or negative side effects might be expected in vertebrates with hepatic dysfunction. This may also make it a more appropriate antibiotic than ceftazidime when treating an animal with renal disease.

Cefoperazone pharmacokinetics have been evaluated in a single snake (*Hydrodynastes gigas*) and lizard (*Tupinambis teguixin*) (Speroni, unpublished data). Peak concentrations of cefoperazone were achieved much faster in the tegu (4 hours) than the false water cobra (8 hours). In addition, therapeutic concentrations remained higher in the snake for a longer period of time (96 hours) than in the lizard (<24 hours). From these results, the authors concluded that the snake should be given a dose of 100 mg/kg every 96 hours, and the lizard should be given a dose of 125 mg/kg every 24 hours. However, in the absence of additional animals, these recommendations should be interpreted with caution. The differences found in these animals could have been associated with individual and not species variations because of the limited sample size (n = 1); however, the stark differences between the lizard and snake for this antibiotic do warrant further study with larger numbers of study subjects.

TABLE 116.3 Peer-Reviewed Cephalosporins Pharmacokinetic Data in Reptile Species to Utilize in Clinical Practice

Cephalosporin	Species	Dose	Route of Administration	Recommended Frequency of Administration	Half-Life: $T_{1/2}$ (hrs)	Peak Plasma Concentration: C_{Max} (µg/ml)	Target Plasma Concentration: µg/ml	Volume of Distribution: V_d (L/kg)
Ceftazidime	Loggerhead sea turtle (Caretta caretta)[29]	20 mg/kg	IV	72 hrs	20	69.74	4	0.42
			IM	72 hrs	19	69.9	4	
	Kemp's ridley sea turtle (Lepidochelys kempii)*[30]	22 mg/kg	IM	72 hrs	43	61.31	–	0.3
Ceftiofur sodium	Green iguana (Iguana iguana)[31]	5 mg/kg	IM	24 hrs	15.5	28.6	>2	–
			SC	24 hrs	17.5	18.9	>2	–
Ceftiofur crystalline free acid	Bearded dragon (Pogona vitticeps)[33]	15 mg/kg	SC	10-12 days	89.3	3.14	>1	–
		30 mg/kg	SC	10-12 days	70.8	10.4	>1	–
	Ball python (Python regius)[32]	15 mg/kg	IM		64	14.1	>1	–
			IM	5 days		7.096	0.1	1.98
Cefovecin	Hermann's tortoise (Testudo hermanni)[35]	8 mg/kg	SC	No recommendation	20.7	27.3	Not reported	Not reported
Cefquinome	Green iguana (Iguana iguana)[36]	10 mg/kg	SC	12 hrs–2 days	3.9	35	Not reported	0.30
	Red eared slider (Trachemys scripta elegans)[37]	2 mg/kg	IV	No recommendation	21	8.42	Not reported	0.37
			IM	No recommendation	26.9	3.94	Not reported	–

IC, Intracardiac; IClo, intracloacal; IV, intravenous; Neb, nebulization; SC, subcutaneous.
*Cold stunned animals.

Ceftiofur

Ceftiofur sodium. Pharmacokinetics have been evaluated in green iguanas after IM and SC injections. The mean maximum plasma concentration was significantly higher in iguanas receiving the antibiotic IM versus SC. There was no difference in the terminal half-life or area under the curve by route of administration. Ceftiour sodium maintained concentrations ≥2 µg/mL for more than 24 hours after both IM and SC injections. These results suggested that ceftiour sodium administered at 5 mg/kg IM or SC every 24 hours would be effective against bacteria susceptible at >2 µg/mL.[31]

Ceftiofur crystalline-free acid. Ceftiour is available as a long-acting, large-animal formulation: ceftiour crystalline free acid (CCFA) (Excede; Zoetis, Parsippany, NJ). Adkesson et al. determined the pharmacokinetics of CCFA in ball pythons and confirmed that at 15 mg/kg, the drug is well tolerated and could be effective for bacteria with MIC values of ≤0.1 µg/mL at a dosing interval of at least 5 days.[32] The authors noted that if the bacteria's MIC is ≥0.5 µg/mL, more frequent dosing or a higher dose of CCFA may be required.[32]

CCFA has only been evaluated in a single species of lizard, the bearded dragons (*Pogona vitticeps*).[33] An initial pilot study determined a preferred dose of 30 mg/kg. MIC concentrations ≥1 µg/mL were achieved within 4 hours and remained >1 µg/mL for 12 days via both IM and SC injections. The authors did note that there was less variability with the SC route, which was recommended because of ease of adminsitration.[33]

Cefovecin.

Cefovecin is a relatively new third-generation cephalosporin that has been used extensively in small animal practice due to its long half-life and need for a single injection. However, the first-line use of this drug is discouraged.[34] Pharmacokinetics for this antibiotic have been determined in Hermann's tortoises and green iguanas after SC injection.[35,36] In the Hermann's tortoise, cefovecin at 8 mg/kg was rapidly absorbed, reaching maximum plasma concentrations between 35 minutes and 2 hours postinjection. The C_{max} of cefovecin was considerably lower than that reported in dogs and cats. Cefovecin was detectable at measurable concentrations for 3 days in some of the tortoises but below the level of quantification for all of the tortoises after 1 week. Compared with small animals, the $T_{1/2\lambda}$ mean was much shorter and was attributed to poor protein binding in the tortoises (41.3%–47.5%), compared with dogs and cats (99.5%–99.8%). The authors concluded that administration every 14 days, as with cats and dogs, would not be suitable for Hermann's tortoises.[35]

Green iguanas given a single dose of cefovecin 10 mg/kg SC were found to rapidly absorb the drug, but again, the authors concluded that the 14-day dosing interval used for dogs and cats was not suitable for iguanas. Instead, the authors suggested a dosing interval of 12 hours to 2 days would be more appropriate.[36]

Cefquinome.

Cefquinome is a fourth-generation cephalosporin for use in veterinary medicine. Compared with other cephalosporins, cefquinome has a quaternary ammonium side chain that increases penicillin- binding proteins and penetration into the periplasmatic space of gram-negative bacilli. It has a high antibacterial activity against most gram-positive and gram-negative bacteria, including *Streptococcus spp.*, *Actinobacillus spp.*, Pasturellaceae, Enterobacteriaceae, and *Staphlococcus aureus*. In other species, cefquinome has good absorption, high bioavalibility, and is eliminated by the renal system. See Table 116.3. for dosing and pharmokinectic data for cefquinome. This cephalosporin should be reserved for resistant infections following culture and sensitivity profiles.[37]

Carbapenems and Glycopeptides.

The carbapenems and glycopeptides typically used in veterinary medicine include imipenem, meropenem, and vancomycin. However, the use of these antibiotics should be restricted to limit the likelihood of developing multidrug-resistant infections that can lead to issues in humans. Therefore, these drugs cannot be recommended for reptiles at this time.[2,3]

Tetracyclines.

The tetracyclines represent one of the oldest classes of antibiotics available in human or veterinary medicine and a first-line drug choice (Table 116.4). Tetracyclines available to the clinician include doxycycline, chlortetracycline, minocycline, oxytetracycline, and tetracycline; however, limited, controlled studies exist that evaluate their specific use in reptile medicine. Tetracycline was originally isolated from *Streptomyces aureofaciens*. Tetracyclines are bacteriostatic and act by inhibiting protein synthesis by reversibly binding to the 30S ribosome. At high doses, these compounds can also affect eukaryotic cells. Although these compounds are generally reserved for aerobic bacteria, they have been found (in vitro) to be effective against anaerobes isolated from reptiles. Stewart found that 18 anaerobic isolates, representing 95% of the anaerobes isolated from clinical samples in snakes, were sensitive to tetracyclines.[39]

Tetracyclines are variably bound to protein and have good distribution to most tissues in the body. Tetracyclines are not metabolized but are excreted primarily through the gastrointestinal tract or kidneys. These compounds can be chelated by fecal material, thus reducing their effectiveness. In mammals, food can also diminish the absorption by chelating tetracyclines.[9] Because these compounds are excreted via glomerular filtration, reptiles with renal dysfunction may accumulate the compound over time. Although these compounds are generally broad spectrum, widespread use of these compounds in human and veterinary medicine has led to increased resistance. Of 34 gram-negative and 21 gram-positive isolates tested at a large accredited laboratory, 79% and 67% respectively were sensitive to tetracycline (Tang et al, Proc ExoticsCon, 2018, p 963). These compounds, especially doxycycline, have excellent spectrum against *Chlamydia* spp., *Mycoplasma* spp., and rickettsial organisms.[9,29]

No peer-reviewed studies of doxycycline exist in reptiles; however, one report determined a doxycycline therapeutic regimen to treat sensitive microbes in Hermann's tortoises. In the study, the authors isolated *Staphylococcus* sp. and *Klebsiella* sp. with MIC values of 8.9 µg/mL and 5.6 µg/mL, respectively. Other microbes, including *Salmonella* and *Pseudomonas aeruginosa,* were found to be resistant. The finding of resistance in these microbes should not be considered unusual, because they are highly adapted to the tetracyclines. The authors determined that a loading dose of 50 mg/kg IM once, followed by 25 mg/kg IM every 72 hours, was appropriate for managing sensitive pathogens in this species of chelonian (Sporle, unpublished data).

The emergence of mycoplasmosis in captive crocodilians has led to research to determine the pharmacokinetics of oxytetracycline in American alligators.[39a] The authors concluded that 10 mg/kg every 5 days should maintain appropriate plasma concentrations for susceptible organisms. Oxytetracyclines are also routinely used to manage infections in loggerhead and Kemp's ridley sea turtles. Harms et al. measured the pharmacokinetics of oxytetracycline in loggerhead sea turtles. Based on their data from 25 mg/kg pharmacokinetics and simulations they recommended IM doses of 41 mg/kg as a loading dose and 21 mg/kg every 72 hours to reach a plasma concentration of 1 µg/mL or 82 mg/kg as a loading dose and 42 mg/kg every 72 hours thereafter to reach a plasma concentration 2 µg/mL.[40]

Chloramphenicol.

Chloramphenicol (Table 116.5) is a broad-spectrum bacteriostatic to bacteriocidal drug (depending on concentration and bacterial susceptibility) that was originally isolated from *Streptomyces venezuelae*.[9] This antibiotic has been found to have activity against

TABLE 116.4 Peer-Reviewed Tetracyclines Pharmacokinetic Data in Reptile Species to Utilize in Clinical Practice

Tetracycline	Species	Dose	Route of Administration	Recommended Frequency of Administration	Half-Life: T$_{1/2}$ (hrs)	Peak Plasma Concentration: C$_{Max}$ (µg/ml)	Target Plasma Concentration: µg/ml	Volume of Distribution: V$_d$ (L/kg)
Oxytetracycline	Loggerhead sea turtle (*Caretta caretta*)[40]	25 mg/kg—Dose not recommender; see text for dosing	IM	See text	61	5.5	—	30.7
			IV	See text	64	1.57	—	18.4
	American alligator (*Alligator mississippinenes*)[39a]	10 mg/kg	IV	Every 5 days	—	98	1	—

IM, Intramuscular; *IV*, intravenous.

TABLE 116.5 Peer-Reviewed Miscellaneous Antibiotic Pharmacokinetic Data in Reptile Species to Utilize in Clinical Practice

Miscellaneous Antibiotic	Species	Dose	Route of Administration	Recommended Frequency of Administration	Half-Life: $T_{1/2}$ (hrs)	Peak Plasma Concentration: C_{Max} (µg/ml)	Target Plasma Concentration: µg/ml	Volume of Distribution: V_d (L/kg)
Metronidazole	Red eared slider (Tracheyms scripta elegans)[86]	20 mg/kg	ICoe	48–72 hrs	27	25	–	–
	Colubrid (Elaphe spp.)[87,88]	20 mg/kg	PO	48 hrs	14.8 single dose, 23.1 multi-dose	14.2	2-4	–
							2-4	–
		100 mg/kg	PO		-	7.6	-	-
		150 mg/kg	PO	24 hrs	26	2039	-	-
	Green iguana (Iguana iguana)[89]	20 mg/kg	PO	48 hrs	12.7	1st day—7.6 3rd day—22.8	4	Not reported
Clindamycin	Loggerhead sea turtle (Caretta caretta)[52]	10 mg/kg	IV	Frequency not recommended	17.3	9.83	0.5	6.1
			IM	Frequency not recommended	1.16	6.13	0.5	1.9
			PO	Not a recommended route				
Chloramphenicol	Gopher snake (Pituophus catenifer) (Bush, unpublished data)	40 mg/kg	SC	24 hrs	5.5	26	–	–
		12 mg/kg	PO	Not a recommended route	–	–	–	–
	Water snake (Nerodia sp)[43]	50 mg/kg	SC	48–72 hrs	–	–	5	–
	Crotalus spp.[43]	50 mg/kg	SC	48 hrs	–	–	5	–
	Burmese python (Python bivittatus)[43]	50 mg/kg	SC	24 hrs	–	–	5	–
	Most colubrids[43]	50 mg/kg	SC	12 hrs	–	–	5	–
Florfenicol	Loggerhead sea turtle (Caretta caretta)[44]	30 mg/kg	IV	Not recommended	2-7.8	0.38–8.79	1	10.46–60
			IM	Not recommended	3.2–4.3	0.53–0.79	1	33.56–56.54

ICoe, Intracoelomic; *IM*, intramuscular; *IV*, intravenous; *PO*, oral administration; *SC*, subcutaneous.

aerobic and anaerobic gram-positive and gram-negative bacteria. Stewart found that 18 anaerobic isolates from reptiles, representing 95% of the anaerobes isolated from clinical samples, were sensitive to chloramphenicol.[38] In addition, 100% of gram-positive and 93% of gram-negative isolates evaluated at the University of Georgia were sensitive to chloramphenicol (Tang et al, Proc ExoticsCon, 2018, p 963).

Chloramphenicol inhibits protein synthesis by binding to the 50S ribosomal subunit of the bacteria and possibly mammalian cells. The binding to mammalian cells is the cause of the aplastic anemia reported in humans. Chloramphenicol is widely distributed throughout the tissues in mammals. The drug is primarily excreted via the liver, and a small quantity is excreted unchanged via the kidneys. Clients should be made aware of the potential side effects associated with handling chloramphenicol, and humans with hepatic disease and nonregenerative anemias should never handle the drug.[41]

Chloramphenicol, in combination with ampicillin, has been used to treat *Salmonella* spp. in both lizards and chelonians.[42] Although only 87% of the reptiles were considered *Salmonella*-free after a 5-day course of the two antibiotics, the remaining animals were "cleared" of *Salmonella* after an additional 5 days of treatment. However, one should be cautious with the interpretation of these results, because these animals could have become latent and not actively shed *Salmonella*, or the microbes were shed in such low numbers they were below the sensitivity threshold of the assay. Antibiotics should not be used in an attempt to control enteric *Salmonella* in reptiles.

Pharmacokinetic studies for chloramphenicol in reptiles is still limited to snakes. Bush determined the plasma concentrations of chloramphenicol sodium succinate in gopher snakes after a single 40 mg/kg SC dose. An oral dose of chloramphenicol palmitate (12 mg/kg) only achieved peak plasma levels of 10 μg/mL at approximately 12 hours and was not considered sufficient to provide therapeutic levels against reptilian pathogens. However, the oral dose was considerably less than that given parenterally (Bush, unpublished data).

Clark et al. determined the plasma concentrations of chloramphenicol in 16 different species of snakes.[43] Two different dosing regimens were evaluated, including 25 and 50 mg/kg SC. The 25 mg/kg SC dose was found to produce low plasma concentrations and was discontinued. The plasma concentrations from the 50 mg/kg dose were found to be highly variable between species. Differences in plasma concentrations were also observed between different injectable preparations, with Tevcocin (International Multifoods, Minneapolis, MN) maintaining higher concentrations than Mychel-Vet (Rachelle Laboratories, Long Beach, CA). This difference was attributed to an edematous reaction at the site of injection, which was more common with the Mychel-Vet preparation. One Midland water snake (*Nerodia sipedon*) developed anemia after receiving 6 injections of chloramphenicol every 72 hours; however, no further investigation, such as rib marrow evaluation, was pursued to determine whether the chloramphenicol had a direct effect on blood cell production. Because of the large variation in plasma concentration between species, the authors concluded that chloramphenicol could be given at 50 mg/kg SC every 12 to 72 hours depending on the species. The dosing frequency should also be based on the environmental temperature because it could affect drug metabolism.[43]

Florfenicol. Florfenicol, a fluorinated analog of thiamphenicol, is structurally similar to chloramphenicol, although it lacks the paranitro group that is associated with aplastic anemia in humans.[41] This compound is approved for cattle, poultry, and aquaculture and has also been used to treat other domestic and nontraditional species. Florfenicol is a broad-spectrum bacteriocidal antibiotic that acts against the 50S ribosome of bacteria. In cattle, the drug is moderately bioavailable (79%) after intramuscular injection.[9,41] The drug has good distribution into various tissues, including the central nervous system. Relatively few adverse effects have been reported in mammals and are primarily associated with the gastrointestinal tract. However, these side effects can be significant in horses, and the drug is not generally recommended for equids. Similar considerations may need to be taken into account for reptiles that use hindgut fermentation.

A single published study has been performed to determine the pharmacokinetics of florfenicol in a reptile.[44] In loggerhead sea turtles the plasma half-lives for both the IV and IM routes were short (2–7.8 hours), and florfenicol could not be measured in any of the turtles 12 hours postinjection. The plasma concentrations in both groups were lower than the acceptable MIC for most pathogens. From this study, the authors concluded that 30 mg/kg florfenicol either IM or IV in loggerhead sea turtles was insufficient to manage bacterial infections.[44]

Macrolides

Azithromycin. Azithromycin is an azalide, a subclass of macrolide antibiotics (Table 116.6) that are bacteriostatic and inhibit protein synthesis by binding to the 50S ribosome.[9,41,45] It concentrates in phagocytes and fibroblasts, which may increase its distribution to inflamed tissues. In human tissues, azithromycin is widely distributed but does not pass the blood-brain barrier. Its antimicrobial activity is pH-dependent and is reduced with decreasing pH. In humans, azithromycin is eliminated and excreted unchanged via the biliary and urinary tracts. Renal impairment has a minor effect on elimination. Drug-to-drug interactions are minor and not sufficient to warrant altered dosing. Its antimicrobial spectrum includes many gram-positive and gram-negative aerobes, including *Staphylococcus* spp., *Streptococcus* spp., *Haemophilus* spp., *Bordetella* spp., *Neisseria* spp., and *Moraxella* spp.; anaerobes, including *Peptostreptococcus* spp. and *Prevotella bivia;* and other notable bacteria, including *Legionella pneumophila, Chlamydia* spp., and *Mycoplasma* spp. Hepatotoxicity has been reported in humans, and azithromycin could cause reversible nonregenerative anemia in reptiles. It can contribute to dysbiosis and overgrowth of enteropathogens. Oral preparations should not be given concurrently with aluminum-containing or magnesium-containing antacids or phosphate binders.[45] Azithromycin is available as an oral suspension, tablet, or an intravenous injection and, as a dihydrate, is soluble in water.[45,46] In a single-dose pharmacokinetic study in ball pythons, the authors determined that azithromycin is distributed and excreted similar to humans.[47] The dose used in the study, 10 mg/kg PO, can be given at different frequencies based on the location of the infection. For skin infections, dosing should occur every 3 days, whereas for respiratory and liver/kidney infections, dosing should be every 5 or 7 days, respectively.[47]

Clarithromycin. Clarithromycin is a semisynthetic, bacteriostatic, macrolide antibiotic that inhibits protein synthesis by binding to the 50S ribosome.[48] It is soluble in acetone, slightly soluble in methanol, ethanol, and acetonitrile, and practically insoluble in water. It is available as immediate-release tablets, extended-release tablets, and granules for oral suspension. It is rapidly absorbed from the gastrointestinal tract in humans, with approximately 50% bioavailability, and it is metabolized by the liver into 14-hydroxy clarithromycin, which is also microbiologically active. Clarithromycin and the 14-hydroxy metabolite distribute readily into human tissues and fluids; intracellular concentrations were greater than serum concentrations, but cerebrospinal fluid was not tested.[48] Both clarithromycin and the 14-hydroxy metabolite are excreted primarily in urine. The antimicrobial spectrum of this antibiotic includes a variety of gram-positive and gram-negative bacteria as well as *Mycobacterium avium* complex bacteria, *Mycoplasma* spp., and *Chlamydia* spp. Adverse effects include hepatotoxicity. Hepatic enzymes should be tested before and monitored during therapy. This antibiotic should not be used in gravid or pregnant animals.

TABLE 116.6 Peer-Reviewed Macrolides Pharmacokinetic Data in Reptile Species to Utilize in Clinical Practice

Macrolide	Species	Dose	Route of Administration	Recommended Frequency of Administration	Half-Life: $T_{1/2}$ (hrs)	Peak Plasma Concentration: C_{Max} (µg/ml)	Target Plasma Concentration: µg/ml	Volume of Distribution: V_d (L/kg)
Azithromycin	Ball python (*Python regius*)[47]	10 mg/kg	PO	2-7 days, depending on tissue of interest	51	1.04	4	–
			IV		17	>8	4	5.69
Clarithromycin	Desert tortoise (*Gopherus agassizii*)[50]	7.5 mg/kg	PO	–	–	0.88	–	–
		15 mg/kg	PO	24 hrs	11.69	1.37	≥1	5.3
				2-3 days	30.52	2-7.5		
			IClo	Not recommended (inconsistent absorption)		0.22-1		
Tulathromycin	Desert tortoise (*Gopherus agassizii*)[51]	5 mg/kg	IM	Not recommended	77 hrs	36.2	MIC not established for *M agassizii*	0.53

IC, Intracardiac; *IClo,* intracloacal; *IM,* intramuscular; *IV,* intravenous; *SC,* subcutaneous.

Clarithromycin may be used to treat severe cases of mycoplasmosis in tortoises.[49,50] A recent long-term study showed that clarithromycin can be safe and effective (at resolving clinical signs but not eliminating the organism) in desert tortoises (*Gopherus agassizii*) when 15 mg/kg clarithromycin oral suspension (50 mg/mL Biaxin oral suspension, Abbott Labs, Abbott Park, IL) is administered by gavage every 3.5 days (every 84 hours).[50] The same study also showed that per rectum administration did not achieve target plasma levels.[50] Three Kemp's ridley sea turtles were treated with 15 to 20 mg/kg clarithromycin (Clarithromycin 250 mg tablets, Mylan Pharmaceuticals, Morgantown, WV) PO q72 hr (duration 59–62 days) as part of a treatment regimen. However, plasma levels were low to undetectable suggesting that clarithromycin may not be effective in this species (Innis, unpublished data).

Tulathromycin. Tulathromycin is a long-acting macrolide that has demonstrated efficacy against a variety of respiratory pathogens. A pharmacokinetic study was performed to evaluate the clinical applicability of tulathromycin in desert tortoises after a single IM dose of 5 mg/kg (resulted in a C_{max} of 36.2 ± 29.7 µg/mL and a long elimination half-life of 77.1 h).[51] This study represents a preliminary step in evaluating the utility of tulathromycin in chelonians and demonstrates that population modeling offers advantages for estimating pharmacokinetic parameters when sparse sampling occurs, and there is substantial variability in the data.

Lincosamides

Clindamycin. Clindamycin is a lincosamide (see Table 116.5) that is used to treat infections caused by gram-positive aerobic and anaerobic bacteria in multiple species.[41] One study determined the pharmacokinetics of this antibiotic in loggerhead sea turtles after a single IV, IM, and PO dose. Clearance was rapid and variable with IV dosing, and plasma concentrations persisted above 0.5 µg/mL for only 4 hours. Intramuscular administration revealed inconsistent absorption with a 1.0-hour median half-life and plasma concentrations above 0.5 µg/mL for <4 hours.[52] Oral clindamycin produced low concentrations that were insufficient to calculate pharmacokinetic values. The authors believed this could be attributed to the oral administration technique (in squid). The results of this study indicate that because of rapid clearance, clindamycin administration at 10 mg/kg q 24 hours did not achieve plasma concentrations needed for effective therapy in loggerhead sea turtles. More research is needed to determine whether higher doses and more frequent administration should be considered.[52]

Sulfonamides.

The potentiated sulfas (e.g., trimethoprim sulfadimethoxine) are broad-spectrum antibiotics that are routinely used to treat bacterial and protozoal pathogens in reptiles. Sulfa drugs are generally bacteriostatic; however, the synergism with trimethoprim creates a bactericidal compound. These compounds affect folic acid synthesis. Oral doses are well absorbed in monogastric mammals. This compound has widespread tissue distribution, including the CNS when the meninges are inflamed. Potentiated sulfas are metabolized by the liver and excreted by the kidneys via both glomerular filtration and tubular secretion.[9,53] The primary adverse effects associated with this drug are attributed to hypersensitivity and the potential for crystallization in the urine. These compounds are generally delivered via an oral suspension, although compounding pharmacies can create parenteral forms. Of 141 clinical reptile cultures evaluated at the University of Georgia, 100% of gram-positive and 91% of gram-negative isolates were sensitive to trimethoprim-sulfas (Tang et al, Proc ExoticsCon, 2018, p 963), making these drugs a first-line antibacterial choice.

To date, there have been no pharmacokinetic studies done to evaluate these antibiotics in reptiles. However, Vree and Vree have determined that red-eared sliders can acetylate sulphamethoxazole.[54] Current dosing recommendations are varied, including 15 to 25 mg/kg every 24 hours, 20 to 30 mg/kg every 24 to 48 hours, and 30 mg/kg once a day for 2 days then 30 mg/kg every 48 hours. One should remember that these doses are anecdotal and to consider the general health status (e.g., hydration status) of the patient before selecting a dose. Given the in vitro efficacy against clinical reptile isolates, there is an obvious need for future pharmacokinetic research.

Fluoroquinolones.

Fluoroquinolones (Table 116.7) are synthetic antibacterial agents derived from the 4-quinolone molecule that was first synthesized in the 1960s. Fluoroquinolones specifically inhibit topoisomerase II (DNA gyrase) that controls supercoiling of bacterial DNA. This is the major action of fluoroquinolones in gram-negative bacteria. This disruption of DNA gyrase results in rapid cell death. Their reduced effectiveness against gram-positives is poorly understood; however, it is thought to target topoisomerase IV. They are inactive against obligate anaerobic bacteria. The bactericidal action of fluoroquinolones is fast and concentration dependent. Fluoroquinolones are rapidly absorbed after oral administration in monogastric animals, although administration with food may delay the time to peak plasma concentration. Administration with compounds that contain metal ions will adversely affect plasma fluoroquinolone concentrations. Low protein binding, low ionization, and high lipid solubility result in large volumes of distribution and good penetration into CSF, bronchial secretions, bone, and cartilage. In mammals, concentrations achieved in respiratory and genitourinary tract secretions are higher than plasma concentrations. The major metabolite of enrofloxacin is ciprofloxacin, but the amount of ciprofloxacin produced varies with taxa. Depending on the drug, elimination may be renal, hepatic, or both. For example, enrofloxacin undergoes renal elimination, whereas difloxacin is fecal and marbofloxacin is excreted in both urine and feces. Fluoroquinolones, like enrofloxacin, can achieve a high concentration in the urine, because the kidneys are the primary route of excretion. Urinary drug concentrations are often in excess of MIC values for susceptible pathogens. Because the fluoroquinolones have low solubility in water, they crystallize in acidic urine.[55–57] Crystalluria could be a problem in carnivorous animals fed a high-protein diet. The adverse gastrointestinal effects associated with the fluoroquinolones include nausea, vomiting, and abdominal cramping.[55–57] The descriptions of adverse effects associated with the CNS have been documented in human patients.[57]

Enrofloxacin. Enrofloxacin has been largely abused in the treatment of bacterial infections in reptiles because it is active against most of the gram-positive and gram-negative bacteria that affect these species. Fluoroquinolones should not be considered first-line antimicrobials. At the University of Georgia, sensitivity to enrofloxacin was documented at 89% for gram-negatives and 38% for gram-positives (Tang et al, Proc ExoticsCon, 2018, p 963).

Enrofloxacin administered at a dose of 10 mg/kg IM or 5 mg/kg PO in savannah monitors (*Varanus exanthematicus*) resulted in minimal conversion to ciprofloxacin. The peak serum concentrations recorded in the monitor lizard are adequate to treat susceptible bacteria (Hungerford, unpublished data). Maxwell and Jacobson determined the pharmacokinetics of single-dose PO and IM enrofloxacin in green iguanas. A high degree of variability was found in the plasma concentrations in the iguanas receiving the oral dose, leading the authors to suggest the parenteral route for critical cases. Because ciprofloxacin was not readily detected, the authors suggested that it is not created in appreciable amounts from the metabolism of enrofloxacin in the green iguana (Maxwell, unpublished data).

Pharmacokinetic studies for fluoroquinolones in snakes are scarce. Young et al. were the first to determine the disposition of enrofloxacin in a snake.[58] Burmese pythons given a single dose of enrofloxacin resulted

TABLE 116.7 Peer-Reviewed Fluoroquinolones Pharmacokinetic Data in Reptile Species to Utilize in Clinical Practice

Fluoroquinolone	Species	Dose	Administration Route	Recommended Frequency of Administration	Half-Life: $T_{1/2}$ (hrs)	Peak Plasma Concentration: C_{Max} (µg/ml)	Target Plasma Concentration: µg/ml	Volume of Distribution: V_d (L/kg)
Enrofloxacin	Savannah monitor (Varanus exanthematicus) (Hungerford, unpublished data)	10 mg/kg	PO	NR	36	3.6	–	–
			IM		24	10.5	–	–
		5 mg/kg	PO	NR	40	–	–	–
			IM		40	–	–	–
	Green iguana (Iguana iguana) (Maxwell unpublished data)	5 mg/kg	PO	NR	–	1.16	>0.2	–
			IM		–	2	>0.2	–
	Burmese python (Python bivittaus)[58]	10 mg/kg	IM	48 hrs	6.37	1.66	0.5	–
		10 mg/kg	IM	10 mg/kg loading dose, then 5 mg/kg q48 hrs	27—E	4.81—E: 1 dose / 0.35—C: 1 dose / 2.78—E: >1 dose / 1.1—C: >1 dose	<1—E	–
		5 mg/kg	IM					
	Urutu pit viper (Bothrops alternatus)[59]	10 mg/kg	IM	48–72 hrs	27	4.8—E / 0.39—C	0.53	3.56—E
	South American rattlesnake (Crotalus durisus terrificus)[60]	10 mg/kg	IM	NR	20—E / 33—C	5.49—E / 1.5—C	<1—E	2.12—E
	Gopher tortoise (Gopherus polyphemus)[61]	5 mg/kg	IM	24-48 hrs	23	2.4	<0.25	–
	Indian star tortoise (Geochelone elegars)[62]	5 mg/kg	IM	12-24 hrs	5.1	3.6	0.2	–
	Red eared slider (Trachemys scripta elegans)[63]	5 mg/kg	IM	NR	18-E / 28-C	6.3-E / 0.42-C	0.25	–
		10 mg/kg	PO	NR	33-E / 60-C	3.4-E / 0.35-C	0.25	–
	Yellow bellied slider (Trachemys scripta scripta)[64]	10 mg/kg	ICoe	6-7 days	47-E / 37-C	10.3-E / 3.01-C	<0.5	2.48-E
	Herman's tortoise (Testudo hermanii)[65]	10 mg/kg	ICoe	NR	37-E / 49-C	8.6-E / 0.6-C	0.5	5.2-E / 55.1-C
	Loggerhead sea turtle (Caretta caretta)[65]	10 mg/kg	PO	-	37.8	4.1	1	2.1
		20 mg/kg	PO	7 days	54.4	21.3	1	0.93
	American alligator (Alligator mississippiensis)[67]	5 mg/kg	PO	Not recommended	77	0.50	0.5	–
			PO	72 hrs	21	1.41	0.5	3.39
			IV	72 hrs	40.48	179.5	0.5	0.16
	Saltwater crocodile (Crocodylus porosus)[68]	5 mg/kg	IM	72 hrs	19.02	8.9	0.5	0.41
			PO	NR	64.98	21.04	0.5	0.21

Continued

TABLE 116.7   **Peer-Reviewed Fluoroquinolones Pharmacokinetic Data in Reptile Species to Utilize in Clinical Practice—cont'd**

Fluoroquinolone	Species	Dose	Administration Route	Recommended Frequency of Administration	Half-Life: $T_{1/2}$ (hrs)	Peak Plasma Concentration: C_{Max} (µg/ml)	Target Plasma Concentration: µg/ml	Volume of Distribution: V_d (L/kg)
Marbofloxacin	Ball python (Python regius)[74,75]	10 mg/kg	PO	48 hrs	Not determined	9.4	Not reported	Not reported
			IV			–		Not reported
	Loggerhead sea turtle (Caretta caretta)[71,72]	2 mg/kg	PO	24 hrs	13.3	11.7	2.08	1.6
			IM	24 hrs	19	8.9	≤0.5	.41
			IV	24 hrs	14.9	16.48	≥1	.34
	Red eared slider (Trachemys scripta elegans)[73]	2 mg/kg	IV	24 hrs	–	–	≤1	–
			IM	24 hrs	–	–	≤0.25	–
	Yellow belly slider (Trachemys scripta scripta)[76]	0.4 mg/kg	ICoe	NR	30.6 hrs	.235	–	1.59
		2 mg/kg	ICoe		24.9 hrs	1.04	Not reported	1.5
		10 mg/kg	ICoe		16.1 hrs	7.2	Not reported	.46
	Freshwater crocodile (Crocodylus siamensis)[77]	2 mg/kg	IV	NR	57 hrs	–	0.016-0.56	1.44
			IM		57 hrs	2.7	0.016-0.56	–
Danofloxacin	Loggerhead sea turtle (Caretta caretta)[80]	6 mg/kg	IV		15.4	–	≤1.28	1.02
			IM	48 hrs	14.7	10.25	≤1.28	–
			SC	48 hrs	18.71	10.35	≤1.28	–

C, Ciprofloxacin; *E*, enrofloxacin; *ICoe*, intracoelomic; *IM*, intramuscular; *IV*, intravenous; *NR*, no recommended frequency; *PO*, oral administration; *SC*, subcutaneous.

BOX 116.1 Pharmacokinetically Derived Drug Doses and the Clinical Application of Minimum Inhibitory Concentration (MIC)

Patient Drug Dose (PDD)

1. Obtain cultured bacteria MIC for specific antibacterial medication
2. The host's MIC breakpoint
3. Drug volume of distribution (V_d) in species being treated*
4. Therapeutic factor[†]
5. Target tissue drug concentration = MIC × TF (therapeutic factor)
6. Patient drug dose = PDD × V_d × % bioavailability (unless given IV)

*Known V_d for some reptiles is presented in Tables 116.2–116.7. V_d is limited due to the number of drugs and reptile species numbers. Health status may alter true V_d.

[†]Therapeutic factor is often between 4 to 10; systemic infections: peak plasma levels 2 to 4× MIC (μg/mL); urinary tract (bladder levels): 10× MIC (μg/mL); biofilms 1000× to 1500× MIC (μg/mL).

Adapted from Visser M, Oster SC. The educated guess: determining drug doses in exotic animals using evidence-based medicine. *Vet Clin North Am Exotic Animal Practice.* 2018;21:183–194.

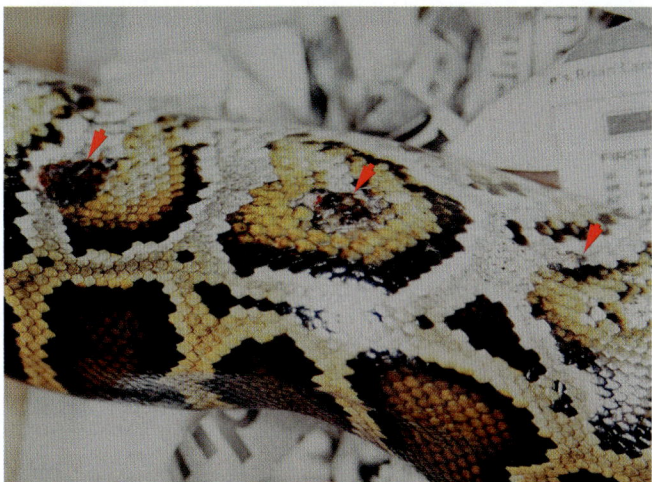

FIG 116.1 Burmese python (*Python bivittatus*) that received repeated injections of enrofloxacin (2.5%) every 3 days. Note the cutaneous necrotic lesions (arrows) at the injection sites. (Courtesy of Stephen J. Divers.)

in a significant conversion to ciprofloxacin; however, the half-life of ciprofloxacin could not be determined. The multiple-dose study revealed that the plasma half-life for ciprofloxacin might be longer than enrofloxacin as a result of the regular conversion of enrofloxacin to ciprofloxacin.

Recently pharmacokinetic parameters for 10 mg/kg enrofloxacin were investigated in seven urutu pit vipers (*Bothrops alternatus*).[59] The drug was slowly absorbed and had a long half-life during the terminal elimination phase, suggesting slow elimination and/or slow absorption in urutu pit vipers.[59]

The pharmacokinetics of enrofloxacin have been evaluated in several species of tortoises. Sporle et al. evaluated the drug in Hermann's tortoises. A dose of 10 mg/kg IM every 24 hours was sufficient to control susceptible bacterial pathogens (Sporle, unpublished data). Prezant et al. evaluated the drug in gopher tortoises (*Gopherus polyphemus*) at a lower dose, 5 mg/kg IM, and found it could be given every 24 to 48 hours to achieve MIC levels for common pathogens.[61] The terminal half-life for enrofloxacin in the gopher tortoise (23.1 hours) was significantly longer than other mammals, birds, and reptiles. Raphael et al. evaluated a similar dose of 5 mg/kg IM in Indian star tortoises (*Geochelone elegans*).[62] In the star tortoises, peak plasma concentrations were approximately 3.6 μg/mL, and the plasma half-life was 5.1 hours. Ciprofloxacin was identified after injection, suggesting that these tortoises can convert enrofloxacin to ciprofloxacin. Enrofloxacin pharmacokinetic studies have also been done with aquatic chelonians. In a study using red-eared sliders, both intramuscular (5 mg/kg) and oral (10 mg/kg) doses of enrofloxacin were evaluated.[63] Ciprofloxacin was measured in the turtles, confirming conversion to this metabolite. No negative side effects were detected in these turtles.

Intracoelomic administration of enrofloxacin was recently evaluated in yellow-bellied slider turtles (*Trachemys scripta scripta*) using a dose of 10 mg/kg and a 10 mg/mL solution.[64] Using the intracoelomic route, the authors were able to obtain therapeutic concentrations with a C_{max} of 10.3 μg/mL. Based on the data presented, 10 mg/kg every 6 days was recommended. The only adverse effects noted were that the animals demonstrated rapid, uncoordinated movements for several seconds postinjection suggestive of pain or discomfort; however, these reactions quickly subsided. Injection site histopathology was not performed in this study.[64] Intracoelomic administration of enrofloxacin has also recently been investigated in Herman's tortoises.[65] Plasma concentrations

of enrofloxacin were detectable in all subjects for up to 240 hours, whereas ciprofloxacin was detectable in all subjects for up to 120 hours.[65]

The emergence of mycoplasmosis in alligators led Helmick et al. to evaluate the pharmacokinetics of 5 mg/kg (oral and IV) enrofloxacin in American alligators.[67] The peak plasma concentration of enrofloxacin (6 μg/mL) was much higher than the MIC (1 μg/mL) determined for the *Mycoplasma lacerti* isolated from the alligators. Additionally, the pharmacokinetics of enrofloxacin have been evaluated in the saltwater crocodile (*Crocodylus porosus*) at 5 mg/kg intravenously, intramuscularly, and orally.[68]

Although adverse effects have been associated with enrofloxacin in mammals, they are rare in reptiles. The most common side effects associated with this antibiotic are pain, inflammation, and necrosis at the injection site (Fig. 116.1). Affected reptiles may withdraw the limb where an injection is given, attempt to escape, or experience skin discoloration or twitching at the site of injection. One report of a more severe reaction was recorded in a Galapagos tortoise (*Chelonoidis nigra*). The tortoise was empirically treated with 1000 mg of enrofloxacin (Baytril, 10% solution, Bayer AG, Leverkusen, Germany) for a suspected pneumonia. The tortoise became hyperexcitable, uncoordinated, and had a profuse diarrhea develop approximately 1 hour after injection. A second, lower dose (500 mg, 5% solution) was given approximately 48 hours later. The tortoise again had a negative reaction postinjection. Because of the similarity in side effects recorded after the enrofloxacin injections, the authors concluded that the tortoise had a hypersensitivity reaction to the enrofloxacin. The adverse effects associated with this case may have been a direct hypersensitivity to the enrofloxacin or could have been the result of a reaction to the carrier associated with the antibiotic (Casares, unpublished data). The authors have used the 2.27% small animal injectable in a number of tortoises, including giant tortoises, without negative side effects. However, the manufacturers do not recommend more than a single IM injection, which should be followed by oral therapy. In addition, when dealing with large animals, the volume should not exceed 20 mL in any site.[69] Other adverse effects such as vomiting, regurgitation, and salivation have been observed in red-footed tortoises (*Chelonoidis carbonaria*) and yellow-footed tortoises (*Chelonoidis denticulata*) and may be seen in other reptiles after intramuscular or subcutaneous injections (Stahl S, unpublished data).

Marbofloxacin. Marbofloxacin is a synthetic, broad-spectrum, bactericidal fluoroquinolone approved by the FDA for skin and soft tissue infections in dogs and cats and for urinary tract infections in dogs.[70] It is available in the United States as an oral tablet and in Europe as both a tablet and injectable. Marbofloxacin is soluble in water, but its solubility decreases in alkaline conditions. This fluoroquinolone is rapidly and almost completely absorbed from the gastrointestinal tract after oral administration in fasted dogs and cats, with a bioavailability in dogs of 94%.[70] In dogs, a small percentage (10%–15%) is metabolized by the liver.[70] Approximately 40% of the oral dose is excreted unchanged in the urine of dogs, and 70% of the drug (85%) and its metabolites (15%) are excreted in the urine of cats.[70] The remainder is eliminated in feces via biliary excretion. Marbofloxacin is bactericidal against a broad range of gram-negative and gram-positive organisms. Marbofloxacin, like other quinolones, is contraindicated in immature animals because it can cause articular chondropathy, and it should be avoided in animals with known central nervous system disorders. Marbofloxacin pharmacokinetic studies have been performed in ball pythons, loggerhead sea turtles, red-eared sliders, and freshwater crocodiles (*Crocodylus siamensis*), and its metabolites have been studied in ball pythons[71–77] (see Table 116.7 for pharmacokinetic data and recommended doses).

Danofloxacin. Danofloxacin mesylate is a synthetic fluoroquinolone approved for SC injection in cattle.[78] The US Food and Drug Administration approved label dose is 8 mg/kg once or 6 mg/kg repeated in 48 hours for bovine respiratory disease associated with *Mannheimia* (*Pasteurella*) *haemolytica* and *Pasteurella multocida*.[78] It is rapidly absorbed, highly bioavailable, and widely distributed in tissues. Danofloxacin has a half-life in cattle of 3 to 6 hours, with negligible accumulation. It is active against gram-negative and gram-positive bacteria.[78,79] A single-dose danofloxacin pharmacokinetic study has been done to evaluate 6 mg/kg dosing via IM and SC routes in loggerhead sea turtles.[80] Danofloxacin has also been administered at 6 mg/kg SC every 48 hours for 30 days to treat chronic mycoplasmosis in *Gopherus* tortoises.[81]

Metronidazole. Metronidazole (see Table 116.5) is a synthetic, nitroimidazole antiprotozoal and antibacterial agent that comes in oral and injectable formulations. It is bactericidal against obligate anaerobes (MIC ranging from 0.25–8 μg/mL) and is protozoacidal against numerous protozoa with an in vitro MIC of ≤1 μg/mL.[82] Metronidazole's antimicrobial action targets DNA synthesis by acting as an electron acceptor in the phosphoroclastic reaction and causes breaks in the adenine–thymine base pairing.[83] Metronidazole is a basic compound with a pKa value of 2.62 and is moderately soluble in water (approximately 10 mg/mL at 25°C) at pH 2.5 to 8.0; the pH of the IV infusion is 5.8.[82–84] Metronidazole is available as an IV infusion (metronidazole HCl), oral tablet (metronidazole base), and oral suspension (Metronidazole benzoate) in many countries; however, the commercial oral suspension is not available in the United States.[85] Oral suspensions using pH-appropriate suspending agents can be procured from licensed compounding pharmacies, and although these are generally the most appropriate formulation for accurate dosing in reptile patients, bioavailability and pharmacokinetics may vary. Metronidazole is well-absorbed after oral administration and is widely distributed to most body tissues and fluids. The major route of elimination of metronidazole and its metabolites is via the urine

(60%–80% in humans), and fecal excretion accounts for 6% to 15% of the dose.[82–84] Metabolism to the 2-hydroxymethyl metabolite occurs, and decreased plasma clearance occurs in patients with decreased liver function but not in patients with renal insufficiency. In humans, adverse effects are typically associated with the gastrointestinal, nervous, hepatic, and hematopoietic systems. Elevated plasma liver enzyme activities have been reported in reptiles after metronidazole treatment.[83] Serious toxic side effects in reptiles can occur at doses between 40 and 100 mg/kg.[19,83] The most common adverse effect observed in reptiles are associated with neurotoxicity, including ataxia, nystagmus, opisthotonos, tremors, seizures, and death. Gastrointestinal toxicity may also occur, including regurgitation and diarrhea. Reported deaths from metronidazole include indigo snakes (*Drymarchon corais couperi*), California mountain king snakes (*Lampropeltis zonata*), and Arizona mountain king snakes (*L. pyromelena*) when doses of more than 100 mg/kg are used (see Chapters 88 and 127). In addition, Jacobson has reported that side effects in Uracoan rattlesnakes may occur with doses >40 mg/kg.[19]

Metronidazole pharmacokinetic studies in red-eared sliders, colubrid snakes (*Pantherophis guttata* and *Pantherophis obsoleta*), and green iguanas have been published.[86–89] In red-eared sliders, side effects were noted, and the authors suggest caution.[86] In colubrid snakes, single doses of 20, 50, 100, and 150 mg/kg PO have been studied, and multiple 20 mg/kg doses have also been studied.[87] No clinically significant adverse behavioral, hematologic, or biochemical effects were observed other than mildly elevated plasma lactate dehydrogenase activity after the last 20 mg/kg dose and mildly decreased glucose after the 50 and 150 mg/kg single doses.[87,88] Taken together, the results support a dosage of 20 mg/kg every 48 hours in *Pantherophis* spp. Higher doses should be reserved for less sensitive infections so that the risk of adverse effects is avoided. A pharmacokinetic study of a single 20 mg/kg dose followed by 20 mg/kg every 24 hours for 10 days in green iguanas identified no adverse hematologic, biochemical, or behavioral changes.[89] The authors concluded that 20 mg/kg every 48 hours would be sufficient for "most" infections and that the dosing frequency could be increased to every 24 hours for more resistant strains.[89]

CONCLUSION

Despite the new information presented in this chapter since the last edition, more research is still needed to determine how we should be using these drugs in reptiles. As some of the results show, not only do we need to better understand how these drugs work across different orders of reptiles, but we also need to further clarify how these compounds affect closely related species and better characterize the effects of temperature and route of administration on these animals. In addition, concerns related to antimicrobial resistance have only increased, and the time has come to challenge the regular first-line use of advanced antimicrobial drugs in herpetological medicine.

REFERENCES

See www.expertconsult.com for a complete list of references.

117

Antifungal Therapy

Sean M. Perry and Mark A. Mitchell

Traditionally, fungal infections in reptiles have been thought of as secondary or opportunistic infections; however, there has been a recent emergence of obligate fungal infections (e.g., *Chrysosporium* spp., *Paranannizopsis* spp., *Ophidiomyces ophiodiicola*) being identified in both wild and captive reptiles. Ultimately, isolation, differentiation, and confirmation of pathogenicity using histopathological (or cytological) examination and culture are necessary to confirm fungal disease. Because fungal infections remain a common and growing concern in both wild and captive reptiles, it is important for clinician scientists to understand the different antifungal drugs available to them to manage these cases and to use evidence-based information when selecting from different antifungals.

Pharmacokinetic studies are most commonly done in healthy animals. Although we assume that the results of these studies can be directly transferred to our clinical patients, that may not be the case. Clinicians need to be cognizant of the physiological disturbances that occur in reptiles affected by disease; by relying on the results of pharmacokinetic studies, we may assume a treatment is working when it is not. The best way to ensure treatment success is to closely monitor our patients during treatment. Another important point to consider from these studies is that the results obtained for one species may not be directly applicable to another closely related species (e.g., two species of sea turtles).

In vitro sensitivity testing is not as routinely performed for fungal isolates as it is for bacteria; however, such testing is often of great value. Although disc sensitivity can be performed, MIC testing is preferred because it not only helps identify the antifungal drug choice but, in combination with pharmacokinetic data (e.g., volume of distribution), can be used to calculate the required patient dose.[1] Evaluation of therapy is important, and checking plasma drug levels should be considered given the lack of pharmacokinetic drug doses available. Just as with antibiotics, antifungal stewardship is often lacking, and the use of the broadest, most modern drugs implies a low level of skill on the part of the practitioner. Drug selection should be based on demonstration of a fungal disease and the use of basic first-tier medications, unless resistance indicates the need for therapeutic change.[2,3]

SYSTEMIC ANTIFUNGAL THERAPY

Amphotericin B

Amphotericin B is a polyene antifungal produced from a strain of *Streptomyces nodosus*.[4] This antifungal agent increases membrane permeability by binding to ergosterol in the fungal cell membrane, leading to depolarization and increased membrane permeability, leakage of the cell contents, and cell death. Amphotericin B has a much stronger affinity for ergosterol in the fungal cell membrane than other sterols, such as cholesterol; however, because it does bind to other sterols, it can cause some toxicity in animals and humans. In addition to fungicidal activity, there is evidence that amphotericin B has immunomodulatory effects. Several drugs are known to interact with amphotericin B when used concurrently. These include antineoplastic chemotherapeutics, corticosteroids, cyclosporin A, digitalis glycosides, flucytosine, imidazole antifungal agents (e.g., ketoconazole, clotrimazole, and fluconazole), other nephrotoxic agents, tubocurarine, and zidovudine.[4]

Amphotericin B is available in two forms: Amphotericin B deoxycholate (Fungizone) and Amphotericin B lipid complex (Albecet).[4] In mammals, the primary benefits associated with amphotericin B lipid complex are that it can reduce toxic side effects (e.g., nephrotoxicity) and improve organ-specific delivery when given intravenously. In addition to reduced toxicity, the lipid complex formulation also has an increased peak concentration, clearance time, volume of distribution, and terminal elimination half-life compared with amphotericin B desoxycholate.[4] It is important to monitor patients closely when using amphotericin B systemically because it can lead to increased concentrations of blood urea nitrogen, uric acid, aspartate aminotransferase, alanine aminotransferase, alkaline phosphatase, lactate dehydrogenase, and amylase. Amphotericin B can also lead to a reduction in phosphorus concentrations and an increase or decrease in blood glucose concentrations. One of the primary concerns when using amphotericin B is that it can be nephrotoxic, causing a reduction in the glomerular filtration rate and direct toxicity at the distal tubules.[4] Animals that are treated systemically with amphotericin B should be well hydrated to limit any potential side effects.[5] Amphotericin B should not be used in a reptile patient with renal disease. The toxicity of systemic amphotericin B is largely mitigated when the drug is used within the respiratory tract (e.g., nebulization, intrapulmonary injection), as it appears to be very poorly absorbed across the respiratory epithelium.[6,7] In addition, studies have demonstrated efficacy against mycotic pneumonia in a number of mammals, birds, and reptiles.[7–10]

In mammals, amphotericin B has been found to be active against *Aspergillus* spp., *Blastomyces* spp., *Candida* spp., *Coccidioides* spp., *Cryptococcus* spp., and *Histoplasma* spp. Antifungal resistance can occur with this drug, particularly with prolonged therapy; therefore treatment should be limited to cases with a confirmed diagnosis, and MIC testing should be considered, especially if clinical response is poor.

Evidence-based research specific to amphotericin B use in reptiles is limited. The minimum inhibitory concentration of amphotericin B against the *Chrysosporium* anamorph of *Nannizziopsis vriesii* (now reclassified, *Nannizziopsis* spp. and *Paranannizopsis* spp.) (Fig. 117.1) cultured from captive lizards was 2 µg/mL.[11] The only other reports of its use are clinical case reports testing nebulization, intratracheal, and intrapulmonary therapy in reptiles.[7–9] Amphotericin B should not be selected as a first-line systemic antifungal agent; instead it should

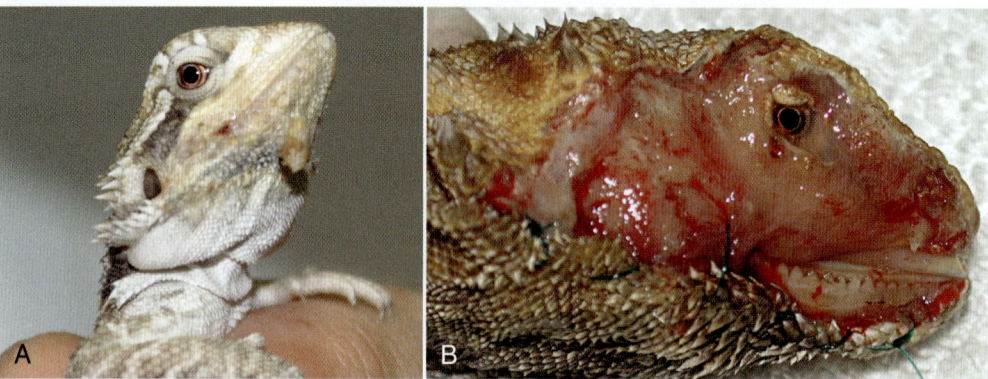

FIG 117.1 Chrysosporium anamorph of *Nannizziopsis vriesii* (CANV) (current characterization: *Nannizziopsis guarroi*) commonly effects bearded dragons (*Pogona vitticeps*) and can range in presentation from (A) small yellow plaques on the skin to (B) severe erosive dermatitis.

only be considered when treatment has failed with other antifungal agents. However, it should be considered as a first-line therapeutic for respiratory infections when administered directly to the respiratory tract.

Azole Antifungals

Azole antifungals are classified into two categories: imidazoles (e.g., miconazole, clotrimazole, and ketoconazole) and triazoles (e.g., fluconazole, itraconazole, and voriconazole). Azoles are often used as first-line systemic therapeutics to treat fungal infections, and a major advantage to azole antifungals is that there are many different oral formulations available. Azoles act by inhibiting ergosterol biosynthesis and thus interfere with fungal cell membrane function. Depletion of ergosterol, along with the accumulation of lanosterol and other 14-methylated sterols, results in destabilization of the cell membrane. This is accomplished by inhibiting P450-dependent 14 sterol demethylase.[5] In mammals, imidazoles are much more potent inhibitors of cell cytochrome P450 than triazoles; however, although largely unknown in reptiles, ketoconazole has been associated with elevated hepatocellular enzymes in a tortoise.[15] Additionally, azole antifungal drugs, such as ketoconazole and itraconazole, are potent immunosuppressive agents, with the ability to suppress T-lymphocyte proliferation in vitro.[5]

Imidazoles

Ketoconazole. The pharmacokinetics of a single oral dose of ketoconazole has been evaluated in gopher tortoises (*Gopherus polyphemus*), resulting in a suggested dose of 30 mg/kg once daily. The only adverse effects noted after a single oral dose of ketoconazole were elevated creatinine kinase (CK), aspartate aminotransferase (AST), and lactate dehydrogenase (LH) concentrations; however, the authors attributed the enzymatic changes to the anesthesia (succinylcholine) used to immobilize the tortoises for catheter placement and blood sampling.[12] The same authors performed a second study at different doses with peak plasma concentrations of 2.2 µg/mL and 4.4 µg/mL at 15 mg/kg and 30 mg/kg, respectively.[13] In mammals, plasma concentrations >1 µg/mL have been found to be effective at clearing approximately 80% of mycotic infections.[14] Based on the results, the authors suggested a single oral dose of 15 mg/kg/day was adequate to manage most mycoses encountered in chelonians. However, because the effectiveness of ketoconazole may be dose dependent, higher doses (30 mg/kg) may be necessary for more resilient fungal infections. Similar

changes in the plasma enzymes, including elevated CK, AST, and LH, were reported in this study. The authors again suggested that the succinylcholine and frequent blood draws were responsible for the enzymatic changes.

Oral ketoconazole (20 mg/kg) has been used in conjunction with topical chlorhexidine solution and terbinafine to successfully treat the fungus formerly characterized as *Chrysosporium* Anamorph of *Nannizziopsis vriesii* (CANV) (current characterization: *Nannizziopsis guarroi*) in a bearded dragon (*Pogona vitticeps*).[15] A similar treatment protocol was also used to successfully treat cutaneous hyalohyphomycosis in two green iguanas (*Iguana iguana*).[16]

Triazoles

Fluconazole. Pharmacokinetic studies evaluating fluconazole in reptiles have been done; however, they are limited to sea turtles.[17,18] A loading dose of 21 mg/kg, followed by additional 10 mg/kg doses every 5 days, were sufficient to treat mycotic infections in loggerhead sea turtles (*Caretta caretta*). In cold-stunned Kemp's ridley turtles (*Lepidochelys kempii*), subcutaneous fluconazole (21 mg/kg loading dose followed by 10 mg/kg every 5 days) failed to attain therapeutic targets for filamentous fungi.[18]

Itraconazole. Itraconazole has become an invaluable antifungal treatment in veterinary medicine and is the most studied antifungal in reptiles. In the spiny lizard (*Sceloporus* sp.), 23.5 mg/kg itraconazole once daily in food for 3 days was considered sufficient to control fungal pathogens for 6 days beyond the peak concentrations.[19]

Manire et al. determined steady-state plasma concentrations of itraconazole in cold-stunned Kemp's ridley sea turtles treated with itraconazole, and in some cases antibiotics, for a minimum of 30 days before having their plasma itraconazole concentrations measured.[20] The plasma concentrations of itraconazole and its primary metabolite, hydroxyl-itraconazole, were comparable, whereas in humans the metabolite concentrations are often twice that of the parent drug.[21] This difference may be attributed to the slower metabolism of reptiles. The itraconazole was well tolerated by these turtles, with no ill effects reported. Based on the study results, a dose of 5 mg/kg per os every 24 hours or 15 mg/kg per os every 72 hours should provide the steady-state concentrations required to kill susceptible fungal pathogens.[20]

Itraconazole is known to cause side effects in mammals and birds and has also been associated with side effects in reptiles too. Anorexia and weight loss are common sequellae in reptiles treated with itraconazole. Additionally, a study evaluating itraconazole in bearded dragons found that an oral 5 mg/kg dose of a commercial suspension (Sporanox, Janssen-Cilag, Berchem, Belgium) was associated with the multiple deaths.[11,22,23] As is common with other species that suffer similar fates, there was no histopathologic evidence of hepatotoxicity in any of the dragons. Itraconazole has been found to accumulate over time in CANV-infected bearded dragons, reaching steady-state plasma concentrations of 4 to 8 µg/mL after 10 days.[11] In vitro MIC$_{90}$ of itraconazole for CANV cultured from infected bearded dragons was 0.25 µg/mL.[11] Fungal organisms could no longer be cultured from CANV lesions after 4 weeks of treatment. In a different treatment trial, seven bearded dragons were successfully treated for CANV with itraconazole (and clotrimazole), but six were euthanized.[23] Although the authors have used itraconazole to treat fungal infections in many different bearded dragon cases, it is important to inform clients about the potential adverse effects, including death, associated with this treatment. Additional work is needed to determine the reason these animals can appear to be healing and die abruptly during treatment.

Itraconazole (10 mg/kg) has also been evaluated in green anacondas (*Eunectes murinus murinus*) infected with CANV.[24] Findings were similar to those reported in bearded dragons and should be therapeutic.[11] Additional work is needed to see if itraconazole produces similar results in other snake families.

Girling and Fraser evaluated the effectiveness of metabolically scaled itraconazole dosing in individual patients (two snake species and two lizard species).[25] These doses (0.5–1.7 mg/kg per os every 53–75 hours for 148–184 days) were found to be effective in treating *Aspergillus* spp. without adverse effects. Although limited in scope, this data does provide some insight into the use of itraconazole and raises the importance of considering the role of metabolic scaling in treating species with a potentially hepatotoxic drug.[25]

It is important to consider novel routes of treatment in cases where oral dosing is not possible or a safety issue. To minimize risk of injury, cloacal itraconazole administration (10 mg/kg) has been attempted in cottonmouths (*Agkistrodon piscivorus*), but plasma levels were low and not considered therapeutic.[26] Itraconazole appears to be well absorbed after oral administration in the few species in which it has been tested, but not after cloacal administration. Higher doses may be necessary, or additional considerations to improve absorption, such as clearing the cloaca and increasing mucous membrane contact time, should be considered.

Itraconazole is effective against fungal pathogens; however, its safety margin may be narrower than other antifungals. Further pharmacokinetic studies in normal healthy and debilitated animals are warranted.

Voriconazole. Voriconazole is a triazole antifungal agent that inhibits fungal cytochrome P450-mediated 14 alphalanosterol demethylation, which is necessary for ergosterol inhibition. Voriconazole has a much higher predilection for fungal cytochrome P450 enzymes than mammalian enzymes.[5,27] It is available as a lyophilized powder for intravenous infusion, film-coated tablets for oral administration, and as a powder for oral suspension.

In humans, the pharmacokinetics of voriconazole via oral and intravenous routes are similar, with maximum plasma concentrations being achieved 1 to 2 hours after dosing.[5,27] Voriconazole is widely distributed into tissues and is metabolized by cytochrome P450 enzymes into multiple metabolites, including N-oxide voriconazole; this metabolite has minimal antifungal activity but accounts for 72% of the circulating metabolites.[5,27] In humans, voriconazole is primarily eliminated via hepatic metabolism; however, more than 80% of the metabolites are recovered in the urine and <2% of the oral dose is excreted unchanged in the urine. Because voriconazole is excreted via the liver, doses in patients with liver disease should be adjusted according to drug plasma concentrations to minimize side effects. No dosing adjustment is necessary in patients with renal insufficiency after oral administration, but intravenous administration should be avoided because the vehicle (sulfobutyl ether beta-cyclodextrin sodium) in the intravenous form can accumulate. The terminal elimination half-life of voriconazole is dose dependent, because the pharmacokinetics are nonlinear. Serious drug interactions can occur with concomitantly administered agents that are also metabolized via the cytochrome P450 enzyme system. Side effects in humans include visual disturbances, gastrointestinal disturbances, hepatic toxicity, fetal toxicity in pregnant women, and electrocardiac disturbances. Voriconazole is effective against multiple genera of fungi, including *Aspergillus*, *Candida*, *Fusarium* (except *Fusarium solani*), and *Scedosporium*. Drug resistance has not been studied thoroughly, but strains that are resistant to fluconazole or itraconazole may also show reduced sensitivity to voriconazole.[5,27] In humans, voriconazole is not a first-line antifungal but is reserved for invasive aspergillosis, candidaemia, disseminated infections, and in patients with mycosis refractory to other antifungal therapy.[28] Consequently, it should not be considered a first-line antifungal in veterinary medicine but reserved for severe or resistant infections.

To date, there have been several studies evaluating the clinical and pharmacological responses of voriconazole in captive reptiles. In vitro voriconazole sensitivity (MIC$_{90}$) against CANV isolated from captive lizards was 0.0625 µg/mL.[11] When voriconazole was used to treat CANV in bearded dragons, only 1/7 (14%) animals died compared with 5/7 (71%) treated with itraconazole; in those that survived, the disease was cleared when treated with voriconazole (Vfend, Pfizer, Ixelles, Belgium) 10 mg/kg per os every 24 hours for 4 to 9 weeks.[11]

A giant girdled lizard (*Cordylus giganteus*) was treated for CANV with voriconazole tablets (Vfend, Pfizer, Ltd, Sandwich, England) suspended in water; the dosing schedule was 10 mg/kg per os every 24 hours for 10 weeks.[8] In vitro MIC of the cultured CANV was 0.25 µg/mL for voriconazole. Weekly fungal cultures from the skin wounds were negative during weeks 7 to 10 of treatment and for 3 weeks after treatment.[8]

Pharmacokinetics of voriconazole have been determined for single and multiple subcutaneous injections in red-eared sliders (*Trachemys scripta elegans*).[29] The results showed that 5 mg/kg achieved target therapeutic concentrations of 1 µg/mL for at most 8 hours, whereas single doses of 10 mg/kg and 20 mg/kg achieved this target for 24 hours. All peak concentrations were above the therapeutic target, whereas the trough concentrations were below the therapeutic target. Using voriconazole at 10 mg/kg subcutaneously twice daily for 7 days is likely to be an effective therapy for fungal infections when the MIC is ≤0.125 µg/mL.[29] Side effects noted in the study included hind-limb paraplegia in two turtles from the multidose study; however, the authors attributed this to repeated subcarapacial sinus venipuncture rather than adverse effects associated with the voriconazole.[29]

There is limited data available regarding voriconazole use in snakes, but preliminary results suggest side effects are common. A single subcutaneous voriconazole dose of 5 mg/kg administered to healthy cottonmouths resulted in the deaths of 3/4 (75%) of the animals within 12 hours of the injection. Necropsy results showed that these animals died from acute degenerative myopathy with a pigmentary nephropathy, suggestive of an acute rhabdomyolysis.[26] Additionally, voriconazole was administered to 2 massasaugas (*Sistrurus catenatus*) and a timber rattlesnake (*Crotalus horridus*) via an osmotically driven pump. Neither massasaugas snake achieved therapeutic voriconazole concentrations for *Ophidiomyces* sp., and one of the snakes died; however, this animal's death was attributed to a concurrent *Ophidiomyces* sp. infection.[26] The timber rattlesnake reached therapeutic concentrations and was able to suppress the infection; however, it was unable to clear the infection based on PCR. This animal died after being released into the wild. Future studies are needed across different families of snakes to determine whether voriconazole can be used to treat susceptible fungal infections without negative side effects.

Posaconazole. To date, there are no clinical reports in the literature for its use in reptiles. In humans this drug is used for invasive or systemic mycosis refractory to itraconazole and/or fluconazole therapy and should not be considered a first-line antifungal.[30]

OTHER SYSTEMIC ANTIFUNGALS

Terbinafine

Terbinafine hydrochloride is an allylamine antifungal agent. In vitro testing suggests it can be fungicidal based on dose/concentration and fungal sensitivity.[5,31] Terbinafine exerts its antifungal action by inhibiting the biosynthesis of ergosterol via inhibition of the squalene epoxidase enzyme; fungi die as a result of the increased membrane permeability from high concentrations of squalene and not ergosterol deficiency.[5,31] It is freely soluble in methanol and methylene, soluble in ethanol, and slightly soluble in water. Oral pharmacokinetics of terbinafine have not been studied in reptiles, but it is well absorbed in mammals after oral administration; peak plasma concentrations generally occur within 2 hours of administration.[32] Terbinafine is lipophilic and rapidly concentrates in the stratum corneum. It has a terminal half-life of 200 to 400 hours in tissues such as adipose and skin, making it well suited for treating fungal dermatoses.[27] Terbinafine is metabolized in the liver via several CYP isoenzymes, not including cytochrome P450, but its metabolites have little antifungal activity.[5] It is primarily excreted in urine; therefore, dosing should be adjusted in patients with renal insufficiency. Terbinafine has been found to have activity against *Trichophyton* spp., *Candida* spp., *Epidermophyton* spp., and *Scopulariopsis* spp. CANV isolated from the skin of bearded dragons has also been found to be sensitive to terbinafine, with an MIC_{90} of 2 μg/mL.[11]

Pharmacokinetics of nebulized and implanted terbinafine has been evaluated in cottonmouths (Fig. 117.3).[33] Snakes provided terbinafine via nebulization were exposed to 0.47 mg/L (18 mg/animal in a 10-gallon tank using 2 mg/mL solution) for more than 30 minutes. Drug absorption was thought to occur by either skin absorption or through pulmonary absorption. Subcutaneous implants of terbinafine (Melatek Implants, MELATEK L.L.C., Middleton, WI) were dosed at 75 to 190 mg/kg. *Ophidiomyces* sp. (Fig. 117.2) from two infected massasaugas showed an in vitro MIC of 0.015 μg/mL, which was determined to be the target. Plasma concentrations from both the nebulization treatment and implants remained above MIC (15 ng/mL) for at least 12 hours in 4/7 (57%) nebulized snakes and for 7 weeks in implanted snakes. However, if conventional antibiotic predictive methods were used, the required therapeutic concentrations were not achieved with either approach. All of the animals in this study tolerated terbinafine well and showed no adverse effects to the medication.[33]

Terbinafine has been used to successfully treat *Exophiala oligosperma* phaeohyphomycosis on the carapace of an Aldabra giant tortoise (*Aldabrachelys gigantea*). Initially, it was used topically in combination with oral itraconazole; however, because the authors did not observe a clinical response, they initiated oral terbinafine (Lamisil, Norvartis Pharmaceuticals, East Hanover, NJ) 3.4 mg/kg per os every 24 hours for 15 months.[34] Plasma concentrations of terbinafine were not measured during treatment.

Terbinafine has also been used to treat veiled chameleons (*Chamaeleo calyptratus*) with systemic *Chamaeleomyces granulomatis*. Unfortunately, both individuals treated with terbinafine died 2 days after initiating therapy. The deaths of these animals were attributed to systemic mycosis rather than the terbinafine.[35]

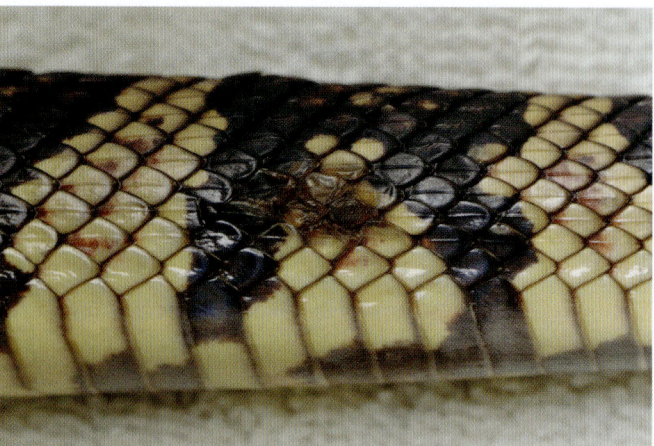

FIG 117.2 Fungal dermatitis caused by *Ophidiomyces ophidiocola* in a Louisiana pine snake (*Pituophis ruthveni*); this animal had other cutaneous lesions that were successfully treated with terbinafine nebulization therapy. (Courtesy of Sean M. Perry.)

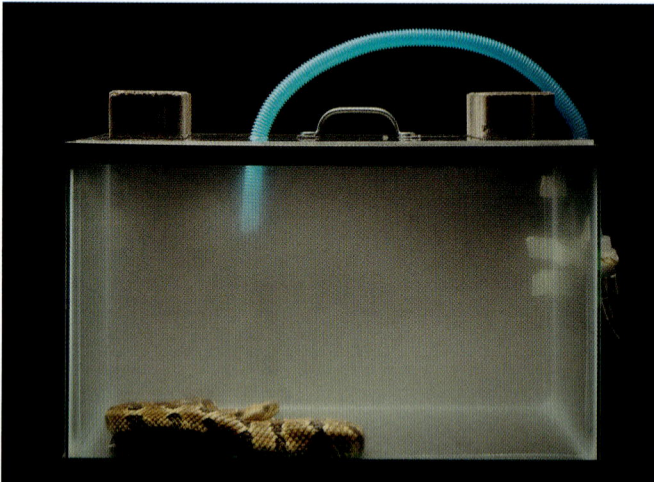

FIG 117.3 A timber rattlesnake undergoing nebulization therapy with terbinafine for snake fungal disease (*Ophidiomyces ophiodiicola*); the one study evaluating pharmacokinetic values of terbinafine used the nebulization setup pictured here in a 10-gallon aquarium. (Courtesy of L. Brian Stauffer and Matt Allender.)

TOPICAL ANTIFUNGAL THERAPY

Ketoconazole

A single case report exists in the literature detailing the use of topical ketoconazole for treating *Fusarium solani* in a loggerhead sea turtle (*Caretta caretta*). In this case the ketoconazole was used in conjunction with a 10% topical iodine solution; therefore its value as a standalone treatment cannot be determined.[36]

Miconazole

Topical miconazole therapy has been used as an adjunct therapy to systemic antifungals in cases of CANV with deep granulomatous dermatomycosis. Additionally, miconazole has been reported to successfully treat fungal keratitis in a gopher tortoise (*Gopherus polyphemus*).[37] However, no studies have evaluated miconazole's efficacy when applied topically to skin and the eye.

Nystatin

Nystatin has been used as a topical adjunct therapy to treat fungal dermatitis; however, no controlled studies have been performed to evaluate its efficacy and absorption as a topical antifungal.[38] *Chamaeleomyces granulomatis* was determined to be sensitive to nystatin based on fungal culture and sensitivity testing from organisms isolated from veiled chameleons.[35]

Clotrimazole

Clotrimazole has been used topically in conjunction with itraconazole to treat necrotizing fungal dermatitis secondary to CANV in a group of 13 bearded dragons. A majority (7/13, or 54%) of the dragons were successfully treated with these topical drugs; however, the remaining 6 dragons (46%) were euthanized.[23]

Terbinafine

As mentioned previously, terbinafine nebulization is thought to act topically and may be absorbed through the skin (Fig. 117.3). Topical administration of terbinafine (Lamisil AT, Novatris Pharmaceuticals, East Hanover, NJ), in conjunction with nebulization therapy, has been used to successfully treat *Ophidomyces* sp. in a Louisiana pine snake (*Pituophis ruthveni*) (SMP and MAM, unpublished data). Topically applied terbinafine (Lamisil, Novartis Farmaceutica, S.A., Barcelona, Spain) has also been used in conjunction with topical chlorhexidine (Cristalmina solucion cutanea, Laboratorios Salvat A.A., Esplugues de Llobregat, Barcelona, Spain) and oral ketoconazole (Panfungol suspension, Doctor Esteve S.A., Barcelona, Spain) to treat CANV in a bearded dragon and two green iguanas.[15,16] Complete resolution of the disease was reported in these animals; however, it was unclear what role terbinafine played in the successful treatment because of the three-drug combination used.

REFERENCES

See www.expertconsult.com for a complete list of references.

118

Antiviral Therapy

Rachel E. Marschang

While the discovery of novel viruses in reptiles and the development of diagnostic methods have progressed rapidly in recent years, methods for treating viral infections have been slower to develop. Therefore, treatment options available to clinicians for managing viral diseases remain frustratingly limited. Many viral infections in reptiles appear to be able to persist for extended periods of time. Thus treatment of clinical disease caused by a viral pathogen may not lead to freedom from infection. Quarantine, barrier nursing, and disinfection are therefore all-important considerations for dealing with viral infections. In large collections, or if an animal is suffering, euthanasia may also be an important consideration. In many cases, viral disease develops because of multiple factors in addition to the virus, including husbandry issues and infections with other agents (e.g., other viruses, bacteria, fungi, and parasites). Optimization of husbandry and treatment of concurrent infections may therefore strongly affect outcome. Specific options for influencing the course of viral infections and the viruses against which each has been used are discussed.

ACYCLOVIR, VALACYCLOVIR, FAMCICLOVIR, AND CIDOFOVIR

Acyclovir, a synthetic nucleoside analogue, is probably the best known antiviral agent in reptile medicine, and it has been used mostly against herpesvirus (HV) infections in tortoises. This class of antiviral drugs competitively inhibits viral DNA polymerases, preventing further viral DNA synthesis. Acyclovir (and various related drugs) has been shown to inhibit the growth of a testudinid HV 3 (teHV3) in vitro with concentrations of 25 and 50 μg/mL inhibiting virus replication in cell culture.[1]

In marginated tortoises (*Testudo marginata*), the oral administration of 80 mg/kg acyclovir (Zovirax suspension, Glaxo Smithkline spa, Verona, Italy) led to a maximum serum concentration of 1.4 ± 0.45 μg/mL for up to 12 hours, with an elimination half-life of 8.85 ± 3.84 hours.[2] In box turtles (*Terrapene* sp.), oral administration of 40 and 80 mg/kg of acyclovir led to similarly low serum concentrations. Valacyclovir, a related substance with higher oral bioavailability, at 40 mg/kg PO, led to serum plasma concentrations similar to those measured for 80 mg/kg acyclovir, although anorexia and lethargy were observed in some treated animals.[3] Administration of higher dosages at more frequent intervals (2–3 times daily) has been suggested. Topical acyclovir on oral lesions of affected chelonians has also been associated with clinical improvement.[4]

Acyclovir and cidofovir have been shown to be ineffective against ranaviruses in vitro (Ferguson SD, Wellehan JFX, unpublished data). Cidofovir and related substances have been used for the treatment of adenovirus infections, although not in reptiles.[5] In a study on erythrocytic iridoviruses in Australian bearded dragons (*Pogona barbata*), an infected and anemic animal was treated with acyclovir (80 mg/kg PO SID) and died within 1 week. Other similarly affected animals that were treated with famciclovir (20 mg/kg PO q48h) had reduced numbers of intraerythrocytic inclusions and did not show overt signs of drug toxicity (Hyndman T, Personal communication, May 2016). Studies in mammals have shown that famciclovir can be a safer alternative to acyclovir.[6,7]

LYSINE

Lysine has been used to treat HV infections in humans and other mammals and has been suggested for use in tortoises with HV infections, although its efficacy in cats has been questioned.[8,9] In tortoises, a dose of approximately 250 mg/kg Viralyse (Vétoquinol, Fort Worth, TX) PO once daily has been described (Wright KM, unpublished observations), but controlled studies investigating the efficacy of this drug do not exist.

DISINFECTANTS

Local application of disinfectants on topical lesions has been suggested, especially for the treatment of stomatitis and glossitis in herpesvirus-infected tortoises (e.g., 0.5% chlorhexidine solution). This could theoretically also help with similar lesions caused by ranaviruses or nidoviruses in snakes, although this has not been investigated in controlled studies. The disinfectant F10 (containing benzalkonium chloride and polyhexanide) has been suggested for treating upper respiratory tract disease of bacterial and/or viral origin in reptiles. It has been used as a nasal wash and for nebulization at a recommended concentration of 0.22 mg benzalkonium chloride and 0.02 mg polyhexanide per ml solution. Although there are no controlled studies evaluating efficacy, this concentration appears to be safe in many species.[10]

MISCELLANEOUS DRUGS

There are a number of other substances that have been used to treat various viral infections in humans and other mammals, such as ribavirin for the treatment of infections with both DNA and RNA viruses, including paramyxo-, corona-, and arenaviruses.[11–13] A wide range of substances targeted against specific viruses, virus receptors, viral proteins, or viral genomes have been developed and tested;[12,14] however, cost and limited commercial interest has resulted in a lack of efficacy, pharmacokinetics, safety, and clinical trials in reptiles. Considering the poor prognoses associated with many reptilian viral infections, the clinician is encouraged to consider antiviral therapy in situations where the owner has provided informed consent, where intervention points and actions (e.g., euthanasia and/or analgesia) have been clearly defined, and where the health of in-contact animals will not be compromised. If therapy is pursued, these experiences, positive and negative, should be shared with the profession to facilitate progress.

TEMPERATURE REGULATION

Adjustment of environmental temperatures has been shown to influence the course of viral infections, with anecdotal and in vitro evidence indicating that this may be true for a wide range of viruses. In most cases, viruses that are specific to reptiles, or to ectotherms in general, tend to replicate better at relatively low temperatures (below 30°C/86°F), and increasing ambient temperature may help slow viral replication. Conversely, reptiles kept at suboptimal temperatures may be more susceptible to viral infection and disease due to increased viral replication or immunosuppression. When adjusting a reptile's thermal environment, it is important to keep them within their preferred optimal temperature zone (POTZ) for that species because changes may affect welfare. Examples for viruses in which temperature has been demonstrated to play a role in the development of disease include gray patch disease (HV) in sea turtles, in which more rapid and severe disease was observed in animals when the water temperature was changed suddenly rather than gradually.[15] Viral replication and disease may also be reduced at higher temperatures for HVs of tortoises. Iridoviruses are temperature limited in cell culture and cannot grow at temperatures above 32°C/90°F. In transmission studies with ranaviruses, temperature has been found to play an important role in the development of disease, with higher mortality in red-eared sliders (*Trachemys scripta elegans*) kept at 22°C (71.6°F), compared with 28°C (82.4°F).[16] Transmission studies with another iridovirus, erythrocytic necrosis virus, in lizards (*Iberolacerta* [*Lacerta*] *monticola* and *Lacerta schreiberi*) showed that infection with these agents can become systemic and may lead to death if the animals are kept at suboptimal temperatures.[17] Temperature regulation may also be helpful in controlling other viral diseases, including ferlaviral, adenoviral, reoviral, and picornaviral disease.

In the case of viruses that can also infect mammals and/or birds (e.g., rhabdo-, bunya-, toga-, and flaviviruses), relatively high temperatures may not be helpful in combating disease development, and high temperatures in captive crocodilians may lead to increased disease and spread of West Nile virus.[18]

IMMUNOMODULATORS

The use of immunomodulators (e.g., Zylexis, which contains inactivated parapox ovis virus; Pfizer AG, Zurich, Switzerland) may be beneficial for treating viral disease in reptiles, particularly for HV-infected tortoises. This is largely speculative, and data on its efficacy are lacking. No adverse effects were reported following IM injection in a large group of mixed reptiles, and subjectively, injected animals appeared to have a higher survival rate than untreated animals (Brames H, unpublished observations).

TREATING SECONDARY INFECTIONS

The majority of viral diseases in reptiles are complicated by other agents, including other viruses, bacteria, fungi, and parasites, which likely play a role in disease progression and outcome. It is important to recognize and treat these concomitant infections appropriately. This has been well-documented for adeno- and reovirus infections in reptiles (see Chapter 30), and evidence suggests that the same is true for other viral infections (e.g., ferlaviruses).

VACCINATION

Vaccination has proven effective in treating poxvirus infections and in preventing West Nile virus infections in crocodilians. An autogenous poxvirus vaccine produced from skin lesions has shown some success in accelerating healing and reducing scarring.[19] West Nile virus can cause serious disease and death in infected crocodilians and is zoonotic. A commercial vaccine is available in the United States (Beohringer Ingelheim, St. Joseph, MO). It is an inactivated vaccine that has been conditionally licensed for use in alligators of age 1 month or older. Uninfected animals that have been vaccinated can be PCR-positive using certain PCR tests, which makes it difficult to differentiate them from infected animals that have not been vaccinated. Efficacy and safety trials are ongoing (Nevarez J, personal communication, 2016).

Vaccination of snakes against a ferlavirus has been attempted using an inactivated cell culture isolate. Western diamondback rattlesnakes (*Crotalus atrox*) were inoculated IM with the inactivated virus with and without the addition of an adjuvant. While no adverse effects of vaccination were noted in any of the snakes, antibody responses to vaccination were variable and transient,[20] and this vaccination method is not currently recommended for the prevention of ferlavirus infection and/or disease.

In the case of HV infections in chelonians, vaccination with an inactivated cell culture isolate has been attempted in a group of HV-infected Mediterranean tortoises (*Testudo* spp.). Inactivated virus with and without adjuvant was injected SC subcutaneously (s.c.) three times. Serology showed no increase in antibody titers against the homologous virus in the vaccinated animals.[21] Anecdotal reports exist on the use of autogenous vaccines made from inactivated material from fibropapillomas to vaccinate sea turtles infected with fibropapilloma-associated turtle HV (FPTHV), but no scientific reports on the effect of such vaccines are available.

REFERENCES

See www.expertconsult.com for a complete list of references.

119

Antiinflammatory Therapy

Kelly Rockwell and Mark A. Mitchell

Antiinflammatories represent one group of pharmaceuticals that are commonly used in veterinary medicine to treat a variety of maladies, and while it was once common to suggest that "no animal should perish without the benefits of steroids," a new mantra has been established that replaces steroids with nonsteroidal antiinflammatories (NSAIDs). Antiinflammatories can impact many different physiological functions in a patient, although much of the current focus on their usage is directed toward their "analgesic effects."

NONSTEROIDAL ANTIINFLAMMATORY DRUGS

Nonsteroidal Antiinflammatories are widely used in reptile clinical practice, even though their effects are still largely unknown. Although not as potent an analgesic as opioids, NSAIDs are commonly used to manage many chronic painful conditions in reptiles, such as pododermatitis, periodontal inflammation, arthritis, spondylitis, osteomyelitis, and articular gout, as well as cases of acute pain or trauma, including surgically induced pain (Fig. 119.1).[1]

The inhibition of the cyclooxygenase (COX) enzyme isoforms is the primary source of the analgesic and antiinflammatory effects seen with NSAID administration. In mammals, NSAIDs block the binding of arachidonic acid to COX, preventing the conversion of thromboxane A_2 to thromboxane B_2 and therefore preventing the formation of the prostaglandins (PG) that serve as potent mediators of inflammation.[2] Studies have shown that NSAIDs act on both peripheral tissue injury sites and at the level of the central nervous system due to the distribution of COX isomers. The COX-1 isomer is considered the constitutive form of COX and is thought to be part of normal homeostasis in many tissues of vertebrates. This isomer is found in tissues throughout the body, including the stomach, kidney, platelets, and reproductive tract. COX-2 is thought of as the induced isomer form, because it can be found at sites of inflammation and is upregulated in response to traumatic injury. However, in skin and muscle biopsies from ball pythons (*Python regius*), production of COX-1 rather than COX-2 was significantly greater at sites of inflammation.[3] In eastern box turtles (*Terrapene carolina carolina*), traumatized muscle also had significantly higher concentrations of COX-1 compared with grossly normal muscle, although both COX-1 and COX-2 were found in liver, kidney, normal muscle, and traumatized muscle samples.[4] As more research is published, it is becoming evident that complete COX-2 inhibition can be detrimental to many normal physiological functions, making COX selectivity an important consideration when prescribing NSAID therapies, as each NSAID may vary in its degree of specificity and subsequent side effects.[2,5]

Because of our limited understanding regarding the impact of long-term NSAID administration in reptiles, the same precautions used in small mammals should be implemented for these species. The primary NSAID side effects observed in mammals are associated with the excretory and gastrointestinal systems. Because most reptiles are uricotelic and their kidneys typically consist of only a few thousand nephrons, compared with the million nephrons found in mammalian kidneys, they are hypothetically more susceptible to nephrotoxic injury than mammals and less able to recover. Additionally, reptiles tend to eat less frequently than mammals and birds, increasing the likelihood that reptiles are receiving regular dosages of NSAIDs on an empty stomach. This can lead to adverse gastrointestinal effects, such of mucosal bleeding and gastrointestinal ulceration.[6] To limit these potential complications, NSAIDs should only be used in well-hydrated patients and preferably after the animal has eaten. Additionally, reptiles prescribed long-term NSAIDs should have their liver and kidney function monitored.

Meloxicam

Meloxicam preferentially inhibits COX-2 and spares COX-1, although at higher dosages its COX-2 specificity is diminished. It is often indicated in both acute and chronic musculoskeletal disorders and to reduce postoperative pain and inflammation following orthopedic and soft tissue surgeries. It is contraindicated in animals with hypotension and should be used with caution in patients with impaired hepatic, cardiac, or renal function, or those with hemorrhagic disorders.[7] In mammals, meloxicam is regarded as relatively safe, with gastrointestinal distress the most commonly reported side effect. Renal toxicity is relatively uncommon in animals with normal renal blood flow.

Carprofen

Carprofen is a COX-1-sparing NSAID, specifically inhibiting COX-2 activity and providing analgesic, antiinflammatory, and antipyretic

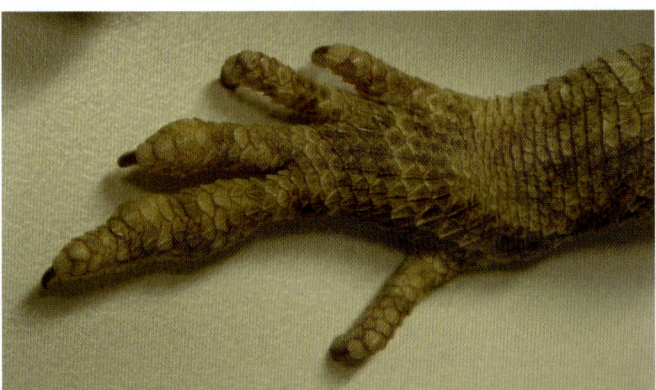

FIG 119.1 A bearded dragon (*Pogona vitticeps*) with swollen toes. A diagnosis of gout was confirmed in this case, and the pain and inflammation associated with this chronic condition were managed with NSAIDs. Monitoring renal function in these cases is valuable, because NSAIDs can contribute to renal disease. (Courtesy of Mark A. Mitchell.)

effects. However, COX-2 specificity appears to be species, dose, and tissue dependent.[7] Carprofen is used to control postoperative pain and acute inflammation, as well as reduce chronic inflammation in cases of degenerative joint disease and osteoarthritis. It is also being investigated as an adjunct therapy for some types of cancer with COX-2 overexpression. Similar to other NSAIDs, it is contraindicated in patients with liver or renal impairment and bleeding disorders. Regular monitoring of hepatic and renal function should be done in patients being treated long term with this NSAID. Because the COX-2 inhibition activity of carprofen may adversely affect renal perfusion, periods of hypotension in patients may exacerbate this effect.[7] Mild gastrointestinal signs (e.g., melena) are the most common side effects in mammals but are very rare in occurrence. Carprofen is currently available in both injectable and oral tablet formulations.

The effects of repeated administration of carprofen for 10 days on blood parameters in green iguanas has been evaluated and showed that IM injections of 2.0 mg/kg had no significant impact on hematologic parameters compared with saline injections.[1] Hemoglobin and packed cell volumes were found to decrease, and the percentage of azurophils increase during the study, but these effects were found in both the carprofen-treated and saline-treated groups. Alanine aminotrasnferase was also found to be increased in the iguanas that received carprofen, but the elevated values were within the physiological reference range for green iguanas.[1]

Ketoprofen

Ketoprofen is a nonselective inhibitor of the COX enzymes, producing both analgesic and antiinflammatory effects. It is commonly used in reptiles for the treatment of musculoskeletal pain and to reduce inflammation. The adverse effects reported with the other NSAIDs have also been reported with ketoprofen, often in more frequency and severity, including surgical site bleeding, gastric ulceration, acute renal failure, and pruritis.[8] Ketoprofen is available in topical, oral, and injectable formulations.

Flunixin Meglumine

Flunixin meglumine is a potent inhibitor of COX enzymes; however, the direct mechanism of action for this NSAID is still unknown. This NSAID can provide analgesic, antiinflammatory, and antipyretic effects; however, its safety threshold is not as wide as the COX-2 inhibitors mentioned previously. For example, if an animal does not respond to an initial dose of flunixin meglumine, additional doses are unlikely to be effective and may increase the chance of toxicity. Adverse effects and contraindications are species specific, and there are currently no warnings regarding its use in reptiles due to lack of experimental studies.[7] It is important for clinicians to pay specific attention to dosing schedules

due to the wide dosage range. Flunixin meglumine is available in both oral and injectable formulations.

Flurbiprofen

Flurbiprofen is a commonly used ophthalmic NSAID that nonselectively inhibits COX enzymes to produce both antiinflammatory and analgesic effects. It is indicated in patients before cataract surgery, as well as for anterior uveitis and ulcerative keratitis when topical corticosteroids are contraindicated. It has been known to cause local irritation and may delay epithelial healing. Flurbiprofen is currently available as a 0.3% ophthalmic solution. Reptiles with intact spectacles, such as snakes and certain geckos, may not gain any benefit from topical flurbiprofen.

GLUCOCORTICOIDS

Glucocorticoids have historically been used to treat a variety of disease processes and trauma-related injuries. They reduce neutrophil/heterophil migration by decreasing the expression of adhesion molecules for these cells in the vascular epithelium, thereby reducing their movement from the blood into tissues. Prostaglandin and leukotriene production is also reduced through the arachidonic acid pathway via inhibition of phospholipase A_2 and, possibly, COX-2 as well.[9]

Antiinflammatory dosages of corticosteroids are commonly administered for conditions such as atopy, angioedema, and urticaria in mammals.[9] Because no pharmacokinetic studies have been done to assess glucocorticoids in reptiles, dosages are empirical. Routine physical examinations and hematologic and biochemistry data should be collected to monitor reptile patients on long-term corticosteroid treatment to manage dosing regimens and screen patients for side effects.

Dexamethasone

In mammals, dexamethasone is 8 to 10 times more potent than prednisone and has a duration of effect that is 48 hours longer.[7] Dexamethasone is available as both an injectable and a 0.1% ophthalmic solution. Though often suggested as a treatment for CNS injury, corticosteroids have not proven to be effective in humans and may actually exacerbate injury. Again, because these drugs have not been fully evaluated in reptiles, they should be used with caution and the patient monitored closely.

Prednisolone

Prednisolone has approximately four times the antiinflammatory potency and half the relative mineralocorticoid potency of hydrocortisone.[7] Like methylprednisolone, it is considered to have an intermediate duration of activity and is suitable for alternate-day use. Prednisolone is available as an injectable, oral, topical, and 0.5% ophthalmic solution.

TABLE 119.1	Dosage Recommendations for Antiinflammatories Used for Reptiles			
Class	Drug	Dosage	Source	Comments
Nonsteroidal antiinflammatories	Meloxicam	0.2–0.4 mg/kg IM, IV, PO q24–48 h	Experimental[6,10,11]	
	Carprofen	1–4 mg/kg IM, IV, PO, SC q24 h	Empirical[11–13]	Following initial dosage, decrease to half dose every 24–72 h[17]
	Ketoprofen	2 mg/kg IM, SC q24–48 h	Experimental[8,11]	
	Flunixin meglumine	0.1–2 mg/kg IM q24–48 h	Empirical[14]	
	Flurbiprofen	1 drop topically q6–12 h	Empirical[15]	
Glucocorticoids	Dexamethasone	0.2 mg/kg IM, IV q24 h for 3 days	Empirical[16]	
		2–4 mg/kg IM, IV q24 h for 3 days	Empirical[15]	
	Prednisolone	2–5 mg/kg PO q24–48 h	Empirical[15]	
		5–10 mg/kg IV as needed for shock	Empirical[17]	

Methylprednisolone

Methylprednisolone is used as an antiinflammatory agent and is authorized for the management of shock in mammals. It has five times the antiinflammatory potency of hydrocortisone and is 20% more potent than prednisolone. In mammals, methylprednisolone has been associated with severe side effects, including thrombocytopenia, increased susceptibility to infections, and gastrointestinal signs. Because of the long-acting duration of this drug, and our limited understanding of its value in reptiles, the authors do not recommend treating reptiles with this drug currently.

CONCLUSION

Antiinflammatory drugs have been and will continue to be an important component of the treatment plans for reptiles. Currently, we do not have strong evidence to support the dosages, routes of administration, and dosing frequencies for these drugs in reptiles. It is important for all veterinarians to document and share their clinical experiences when using antiinflammatories so that we can develop some basic guidelines regarding these important drugs. Additionally, continued pursuit of experimental studies and research to further refine the use of these compounds in reptile species is important. Dosage recommendations for antiinflammatories currently used in reptiles can be found in Table 119.1.

REFERENCES

See www.expertconsult.com for a complete list of references.

Antiparasitic Therapy

Kelly Rockwell and Mark A. Mitchell

Parasites have spent eons creating niches in which to take advantage of their reptilian hosts. In the majority of these cases, the reptile and parasite are in balance; however, in captivity, reduced resources (nutritional, thermal, lighting), immunosuppression, and direct life cycles can often lead to clinical disease. Therefore antiparasitic medications are important tools to minimize the impact of parasitism on captive reptiles.

ENDOPARASITICIDES

Antiprotozoals

Ciliated and flagellated protozoans are common inhabitants of the intestinal tracts of reptiles, especially herbivores. It is important for veterinarians to recognize that most of these organisms are commensals or symbionts of the intestinal tract, and they play vital roles in the digestion of nutrients and the maintenance of the intestinal microbiome. Because of the importance of these organisms in the general health of the intestinal tract, treatment should only be initiated when clinical disease is present.

Metronidazole is the most common antiprotozoal agent used to treat reptiles, and one of the few antiparasitic drugs supported by evidence-based pharmacokinetic studies.[1–4] Metronidazole primarily acts as an amebicide against trophozoites, with limited activity against encysted forms of protozoa.[5] The pharmacokinetic studies performed in reptiles have shown that there is variability in the rate of absorption from the gastrointestinal tract between and within species, suggesting that patients should be monitored closely for a response to treatment as well as adverse reactions to the drug. One of the reasons clinical side effects are common relates to the wide dosing recommendations for this drug (Table 120.1). It is important to utilize evidence-based data first when selecting a dose. Side effects associated with metronidazole toxicity in vertebrates are typically associated with the central nervous system (CNS), including ataxia, an inability to locomote, nystagmus, opisthotonous, tremors of the lumbar muscles and hind limbs, seizures, and death, but may vary with different reptile species.[6] A corn snake (*Pantherophis guttatus*) treated with metronidazole at 250 mg/kg developed severe CNS signs within 24 hours but improved with supportive care over 72 hours (Mitchell M, personal observation). Plasma biochemistry testing showed elevated bile acids suggestive of hepatic dysfunction, whereas the CNS signs were presumably associated with hepatic encephalopathy. Several red-eared sliders (*Trachemys scripta elegans*) experimentally dosed with a single 20-mg/kg intracoelomic injection of metronidazole died 2 to 5 months after the completion of the study.[5] Although it was unclear whether their deaths were due to adverse effects, caution should be exercised when using intracoelomic administration. When using this antiparasitic medication, it is best to follow the guidelines established from the few pharmacokinetic studies reported (see Table 120.1).

Because metronidazole is ineffective at killing protozoal cyst stages, it is often used in combination with iodoquinol, paromomycin, and/or diloxamide furoate (not currently available in the United States) to effectively control both trophozoite and cyst stages in the gastrointestinal tract. The use of paromomycin alone in juvenile bearded dragons (*Pogona vitticeps*)[7] and Gila monsters (*Heloderma suspectum*) was found to be effective at higher doses and decreased dosing intervals, but in leopard geckos (*Eublepharis macularius*) an unknown dosage was only able to clear *Cryptosporidium* infections in two of four animals.[8] When using paromomycin in patients, caution should be used, because systemic absorption can occur in animals with ulcerative gastroenteritis, which can lead to nephrotoxicity, ototoxicity, and pancreatitis.

Other treatments, such as atovaquone-proguanil and halofuginone hydrobromide, were not effective at treating cryptosporidiosis in Boettger's lizards (*Gallotia caesaris*)[9] or snakes,[10] respectively. No adverse effects were reported in the lizards administered atovaquone-proguanil; however, snakes administered halofuginone had hepatotoxic and nephrotoxic changes, including severe, acute liver necrosis, liver hemosiderosis, and cortical and tubular necrosis with iron deposition. Postprandial regurgitation was also observed in several snakes treated with halofuginone and spiramycin.[10] In Boettger's lizard, 10 mg/kg of oral chloroquine for 7 days was also ineffective at decreasing *Plasmodium* sp., but no adverse effects were noted.

Coccidial infections are a common finding in captive reptiles, with most of these infections being perpetuated because of poor hygiene and biosecurity. Coccidial infections are typically self-limiting; however, autoinfection appears common in captive reptiles. Historically, sulfadimethoxine and trimethoprim-sulfamethoxazole (coccidiostats) have been recommended for treating coccidial infections in reptiles (see Table 120.1). Unfortunately, these recommendations were based on empirical data, although later research done by Walden and Mitchell did show that long-term treatment with sulfadimethoxine reduced *Isospora amphiboluri* in bearded dragons.[11] Attempts to control coccidia in reptiles using nutraceuticals (Oregano, *Origanum vulgare*), and probiotics have also been reported and found to be largely ineffective.[11,12] Ponazuril, an antiprotozoal commonly used to treat equine protozoal myeloencephalitis, is recommended for treatment, as it can impact all life stages of the coccidia. Walden[13] performed an experimental study testing the efficacy of ponazuril in bearded dragons and showed that doses of 15 to 40 mg/kg PO once daily for 21 days were effective against coccidia.

Anthelminthics

Nematodes. Nematodes are a common finding in captive reptiles, representing one of the most diverse groups of endoparasites found in these animals. They can travel subcutaneously and, if found in patients, should be surgically removed.[14] Anthelminthics are generally recommended for the treatment of disease, or strategically to control prevalence

TABLE 120.1	Treatment Recommendations for Protozoal Infections in Reptiles		
Treatment/Species	**Dosage**	**Source**	**Comments**
Metronidazole			
All reptiles	100–220 mg/kg PO repeated in 2 weeks	Empirical[5,26,41]	Caution with intracoelomic administration[5]
	50 mg/kg PO q 24 h for 3–5 days	Empirical[5]	
Red rat snakes	50 mg/kg PO q 48 h	Experimental[1]	
Yellow rat snakes	20 mg/kg PO q 48 h	Experimental[3]	
Green iguanas	20 mg/kg PO q 48 h	Experimental[3]	May dose at q 24 h if lack of response
Colubrid snakes	40–50 mg/kg PO	Empirical[26]	
Small chelonians	100–150 mg/kg PO every 10–14 days	Empirical[42]	
Larger chelonians	25 mg/kg PO q 24 h for 5 days, repeated in 10 days	Empirical[42]	
Metronidazole and Iodoquinol			
Aquatic and semiaquatic chelonians	Five days of metronidazole (25–50 mg/kg) and iodoquinol (25 mg/0.75–1 kg), followed by 5 days of iodoquinol alone, then 5 days of both, and a final 5 days of iodoquinol	Empirical[43]	
Terrestrial chelonians	Three days of metronidazole (25–50 mg/kg) and iodoquinol (25 mg/0.75–1 kg), followed by 14 days of iodoquinol alone, and a final 3 days of both	Empirical[43]	
Chelonians	Metronidazole (20 mg/kg) PO q 48 h and iodoquinol (50 mg/kg) PO q 24 h for 3 weeks	Empirical[43]	
Paromomycin			
All reptiles	300–800 mg/kg PO q 24–48 h for 7–14 days, or as needed	Empirical[1,43]	Caution with use—systemic absorption through damaged gastrointestinal tract may lead to nephrotoxicity, ototoxicity, or pancreatitis
Bearded dragons	100 mg/kg q 24 h for 7 days, then twice a week for 6 days, and 360 mg/kg q 48 h for a final 10 days	Experimental[7]	
Gila monsters	300–360 mg/kg q 2 days for 14 days	Experimental[44]	
Chloroquine			
All reptiles	50 mg/kg IM once weekly for three doses, in combination with iodoquinol and metronidazole	Empirical[43]	
Sulfadiazine, Sulfamerazine, and Sulfamethazine			
Lizards	25 mg/kg PO q 24 h for 21 days	Empirical[41]	
Sulfadimethoxine			
All reptiles	90 mg/kg PO once, then 45 mg/kg PO q 24 h for 5–7 days	Empirical[26]	
Bearded dragons	50 mg/kg PO q 24 h for 21 days	Experimental[11]	
Trimethoprim/Sulfamerazine			
Lizards	30 mg/kg PO combined q 24 h for two doses, then q 2 days PO for 21 days	Empirical[41]	
Ponazuril			
All reptiles	30 mg/kg PO q 48 h for two doses	Empirical[5]	
Bearded dragons	15–40 mg/kg PO q 24 h for 21 days	Experimental[13]	All treatments effective; no reinfection 40 days posttreatment

and burden, though caution should be used with these drugs because adverse effects have been reported. Most notably, ivermectin has been found to cause significant side effects in reptiles, especially chelonians, in numerous safety studies[15–19] because of its mechanism of action. Based on most of these reports, its use is contraindicated in chelonians. See Chapter 88 for more information. Ivermectin kills nematodes by causing paralysis with high-affinity binding to the glutamate-gated chloride channels in the invertebrate nerve and muscle cells. It has been used successfully in a variety of reptiles, with snakes apparently tolerating a higher dosage range than other groups without apparent side effects.[19] To date, there are no published pharmacokinetic studies assessing ivermectin in reptiles; however, other than chelonians, skinks, and indigo

snakes (*Drymarchon couperi*), empirical dosing appears relatively safe. Current empirical dosing recommendations for ivermectin can be found in Table 120.2.

Milbemycin oxime analogs are insecticidal and provide anthelmintic activity at very low concentrations by opening glutamate-sensitive chloride channels in neurons and myocytes of invertebrates, leading to hyperpolarization of these cells and blocking of signal transfer. The efficacy and safety of this drug has been compared with ivermectin in several chelonian species using a suspended form of the commercial tablet in propylene glycol (2.5 mg/mL).[16] In the study, red-eared sliders, Gulf Coast box turtles (*Terrapene carolina major*), and ornate box turtles (*Terrapene ornata ornata*) showed no adverse effects to PO or SQ

TABLE 120.2   Treatment Recommendations for Nematode Infections in Reptiles

Treatment/Species	Dosage	Source	Comments
Ivermectin			
Snakes and lizards	0.2 mg/kg PO or SQ repeated in 2 weeks	Empirical[41,45]	Caution in chelonians, skinks, and indigo snakes, fatal
	0.2 mg/kg PO, SQ, or IM repeated in 2 weeks	Empirical[1,46]	toxicity possible; mild side effects (anorexia, depression)
	0.2–0.4 mg/kg SQ or IM	Empirical[26]	in a Senegalese chameleon administered a single 0.2 mg/kg SQ dose[23]
Solomon island skink	0.2 mg/kg IM repeated in 14 days (up to six doses)	Empirical[23]	Fatality reported in one case 24 h after a dosage of 0.2 mg/kg PO
Corn snakes	0.4–1 mg/kg	Empirical[15]	
Dumeril's monitor	0.4 mg/kg	Empirical[15]	
Milbemycin Oxime			
Ornate box turtles	0.25 mg/kg SQ repeated in 8 days	Experimental[16]	
Fenbendazole			
All reptiles	50–100 mg/kg PO repeated in 2 weeks	Empirical[1,41,42,45]	
	50 mg/kg PO repeated in 3 weeks	Empirical[47]	
Snakes	100 mg/kg PO	Empirical[26]	For treatment of snake lungworms, *Rhabdias* and *Strongyloides*
Hermann's tortoise	Single administration of 100 mg/kg PO	Experimental[20]	
Boettger's lizard	Single administration of 0.4 mL/kg active ingredient	Experimental[9]	
Oxfendazole			
All reptiles	Single administration of 66 mg/kg PO	Empirical[20]	Does not require biotransformation and less toxic than fenbendazole
Hermann's tortoises	Single administration of 66 mg/kg PO	Experimental[20]	
Thiabendazole			
Rat snake	110 mg/kg PO repeated weekly for three dosages	Empirical[47]	
Praziquantel			
All reptiles	10 mg/kg PO	Empirical[26]	Caution for anaphylactic-like reactions in ball pythons
Levamisole			
Iguanas	10 mg/kg intracoelomically repeated in 2 weeks	Empirical[41]	
Vercom Paste (34 mg/mL Febantel and 3.4 mg/mL Praziquantel)			
Solomon island skink	0.5–1 mg/kg repeated in 2 weeks	Empirical[23]	
Emodepside + Praziquantel (*Profender*)			
All reptiles	4 drops/100 g body weight	Experimental[45,48,49]	

treatment. Ornate box turtles that received milbemycin SQ were found to have negative fecal screens, although acanthocephalans did pass throughout the course of the study.

The pharmacokinetics of fenbendazole has yet to be assessed in reptiles and, to date, few efficacy studies have been performed. In Hermann's tortoises (*Testudo hermanni*), oxfendazole was more effective at reducing oxyurid fecal egg counts.[20] Recent studies have indicated that a single dose of oxfendazole (25 mg/kg) was able to clear nematodes from green iguanas (*Iguana iguana*) (Kehoe, Divers, unpublished data). Oxfendazole is the active metabolite of fenbendazole responsible for most anthelminthic activity, and thus improved efficacy over fenbendazole is not surprising; oxfendazole has also been shown to be less toxic.[21] In Hermann's tortoises treated with oral fenbendazole, hematologic and plasma chemistry sampling showed marked changes associated with the treatment, although they remained clinically healthy. Their blood results indicated an extended heteropenia with transient hypoglycemia, hyperuricemia, hyperphosphatemia, and equivocal hyperproteinemia/hyperglobulinemia.[22] Such changes should be considered when treating ill tortoises with fenbendazole because these could have significant consequences on recovery. Current recommendations for these drugs are listed in Table 120.2.

Other therapies for the treatment of nematodes in reptiles include the empirical use of levamisole in iguanas, as well as vercom paste (Vercom Paste Anthelmintic, Miles Inc, Shawnee Mission, KS) (34 mg/mL febantel and 3.4 mg/mL praziquantel) in the Solomon island skink (*Corucia zebrata*); in the latter case there were no adverse effects and seemingly better results than ivermectin in eliminating fecal shedding of nematode ova.[23] An experimental application of a combination therapy of emodepside and praziquantel (Profender; Bayer HealthCare, Shawnee Mission, KS) in different reptile species found that both active ingredients penetrate the skin and can be found in serum when given topically, although effective doses may vary with the type and thickness of the integument.

Cestodes and Trematodes.   Praziquantel is commonly used to treat cestodes and trematodes in reptiles. However, the few studies that have assessed the efficacy or pharmacokinetics of this drug have been limited

TABLE 120.3	Treatment Recommendations for Cestode and Trematode Infections in Reptiles		
Treatment/Species	**Dosage**	**Source**	**Comments**
Praziquantel			
All reptiles	10 mg/kg PO or IM, up to 30 mg/kg PO for trematodes	Empirical[26]	Caution for anaphylactic-like reactions in ball pythons
Green sea turtles	50 mg/kg PO three times over a 9h period for 1 day	Experimental[24]	
Loggerhead sea turtles	25 mg/kg PO three times at 3-hour intervals	Experimental[25]	
Emodepside + Praziquantel (_Profender_)			
All reptiles	4 drops/100 g body weight	Experimental[48,49]	

to sea turtles. Green sea turtles (*Chelonia mydas*) orally dosed were successfully cleared of trematode infections.[24] Although no adverse effects were reported in the turtles, treated animals did exhibit elevated alanine aminotransferase and aspartate aminotransferase levels after 3 days of treatment; no notable morphologic changes were noted in the livers of these animals at necropsy. This same finding is reported in humans and mice following praziquantel treatment and may be due to the movement of dead flukes from the mesenteric arteries and bile ducts into the liver, causing the release of hepatocellular enzymes into the plasma. In loggerhead sea turtles (*Caretta caretta*), plasma concentrations of praziquantel were found to be measurable in animals that received a multidose regimen compared with the nonquantifiable concentrations in those animals that received a single dose.[25] The multidose animals had concentrations that persisted for up to 48 hours, though there was some degree of individual variation. One of the turtles that received a single high dose also developed necrotizing skin lesions that resembled toxic epidermal necrolysis 48 hours after administration; the lesions resolved 11 days later. Although praziquantel appears relatively safe, it has been shown to cause anaphylactic-like reactions in ball pythons (*Python regius*) and should be used cautiously in this species.[26] Current recommendations for these drugs are listed in Table 120.3.

ECTOPARASITICIDES

Ticks

The need for tick control in reptiles has grown over the past several decades as more wild-caught animals have been imported with tick infestations. Ideally, external parasites should be removed manually whenever possible, but, with severe infestations, chemical intervention may be necessary for both the animal and the environment. Permethrin has become a common therapy for tick control in reptiles; however, several different commercial formulations contain ingredients that have been found to be toxic to reptiles. For example, piperonyl butoxide, which is added to some formulations as a synergist, has been associated with snake mortalities.[27] Currently, Provent-a-mite spray (Pro Products, Mahopac, NY), which contains 0.5% permethrin, is the only patented United States Environmental Protection Agency– and United States Department of Agriculture–approved acaricide product for use on reptiles and does not contain additives that pose a severe risk to most animals.

Juvenile African spurred tortoises (*Centrochelys sulcata*), juvenile green iguanas, and adult rosy boas (*Lichanura trivirgata*) given 6 applications of Provent-a-mite topically or on their substrate per label directions, but at 10 times the recommended dosage at each application, showed no signs of permethrin toxicosis.[28] One tortoise developed a thick, foamy covering over the skin, but no other signs of ill health were reported. Necropsy of 1 treated snake that had refused food before the study and then exhibited a kinked appearance showed no histologic evidence of an underlying disease process or toxicity. In leopard tortoises (*Stigmochelys pardalis*), permethrin and several other acaricides were

assessed for toxic effects, as well as efficacy against the African tortoise tick (*Amblyomma marmoreum*).[29] Amitraz, cyfluthrin, and permethrin produced transient side effects, including decreased food consumption, reduced defecation frequency, diarrhea, and skin and eye irritation, that lasted for less than an hour after treatment, whereas carbaryl and chlorpyrifos produced prolonged effects lasting several hours. Chlorpyrifos, cyfluthrin, lindane, and permethrin treatment led to 100% mortality of ticks within 24 hours of application; cyfluthrin and permethrin continued to cause 100% mortality when diluted to as low as 1:10,000. Cyfluthrin and permethrin were therefore considered the safest and most effective acaricides for treating leopard tortoises. Comparatively, an additional study in leopard tortoises found that amitraz was successful in detaching and killing ticks without any adverse effects.[30]

A single injection of ivermectin was found to remove ticks on rat snakes, Indian cobras (*Naja naja*), and Indian pythons (*Python molurus*) without any side effects.[31] However, other studies have shown that ticks can recover from ivermectin-induced paralysis with time,[32] so good sanitation and concurrent use of acaricidal sprays may be necessary. Caution should always be used when administering ivermectin to reptiles, because fatal side effects can occur, especially in chelonians, skinks, and indigo snakes. See Chapter 139 for more discussion on treatment options. Current recommendations for these drugs are listed in Table 120.4.

Mites

Severe infestations of the snake mite (*Ophionyssus natricis*) can cause serious health problems for snakes, including skin damage, blood loss and severe anemia, and the spread of bacterial and viral pathogens. If a snake is infested, the parasite will also be present in its habitat, and environmental control, in and out of the enclosure, will be required. Current recommendations for medical therapies to control and eradicate snake mites (or other reptile mites) can be found in Table 120.5.

Currently, the only licensed product for treatment of mites in reptiles is Provent-a-mite spray (Pro Products, Mahopac, NY), though other therapies, such as natural pyrethrin and synthetic pyrethroid, have been empirically used. Pyrethroids tend to be more potent and have a longer half-life than pyrethrins. Both products are applied topically, therefore it is important to remove any residual product by thorough rinsing to prevent systemic absorption and toxicity.[33] Permectrin II (Bayer HealthCare, Shawnee Mission, KS), which contains 10% permethrin, was diluted to a 1% solution (0.1% active ingredient) and applied to several snake species and a blue-tongued skink (*Tiliqua scincoides*), as well as their enclosures topically via spray bottle over an 18-month period. Only one toxic reaction was observed in an adult green tree python (*Morelia viridis*); the animal exhibited convulsions, ataxia, and open-mouth breathing within 30 minutes of spraying but recovered with supportive care. The author suggested that the toxicity was most likely due to an exposure to 2% trichlorfon solution 10 days prior, prompting a recommendation that permethrin should not be used

TABLE 120.4 Treatment Recommendations for Tick Infestations in Reptiles

Treatment/Species	Dosage	Source	Comments
Pyrethrin and Pyrethroids			
All reptiles	1% topically as a spray, remove excess; repeat in 10 days	Experimental[1,28,29]	Do not use with organophosphate insecticides—convulsions, ataxia, and dyspnea can occur. Rinse off as much as possible after application in snakes to prevent absorption and systemic toxicity
Cyfluthrin			
Leopard tortoises	As directed on label	Experimental[29]	Associated with toxicity in snakes and lizards at low doses
Ivermectin			
Rat snakes, Indian cobras, Indian pythons	Single 0.75 mg/kg injection SQ	Empirical[31]	Caution in chelonians, skinks, and indigo snakes; fatal toxicity possible
Lizards	Single dose of 0.2 mg/kg PO or SQ, repeat in 2 weeks	Empirical[41]	

TABLE 120.5 Treatment Recommendations for Mite Infestations in Reptiles

Treatment/Species	Dosage	Source	Comments
Pyrethroid			
Snakes and blue-tongued skink	1% topically as a spray, remove excess; repeat in 10 days	Empirical[33]	Do not use with organophosphate insecticides—convulsions, ataxia, and dyspnea can occur. Rinse off as much as possible after application in snakes to prevent absorption and systemic toxicity
Fipronil Spray			
All reptiles	0.29% topically, remove excess, allow to air dry; repeat weekly or every other week for 6–8 weeks	Empirical (Stahl S, personal communication, 2017)	Use caution when applying to smaller or juvenile reptiles
Ivermectin			
Snakes	5 mg (10 mg/mL) in 1 quart or liter water as a spray; shake vigorously before each use, maintain in an opaque container	Empirical[36]	Use with caution for chelonians, skinks, and indigo snakes; fatal toxicity possible
	0.2 mg/kg SQ once a week for three doses	Empirical[6,37]	
Lizards	Single dose of 0.2 mg/kg PO or SQ, repeat in 2 weeks	Empirical[41]	
Snakes and lizards	0.2 mg/kg IM once a week for up to 3 weeks	Empirical[37]	
	5 mg in 1 liter water sprayed topically once a week for up to 3 weeks	Empirical[33]	
Carbaryl Powder			
Lizards	5% powder topically once a week, rinse off with water after 1–5 minutes	Empirical[41]	Keep out of the lizard's mouth
Predatory Mites			
Stratiolaelaps scimitus mites	1 L, approximately 15,000 mites	Case report[39]	Controlled lizard mites in 5 days
Cheyletus eruditus (taurrus) mites	Predatory mites	Experimental[40]	

concurrently with an organophosphate insecticide.[34] In brown tree snakes (*Boiga irregularis*), pyrethrin applied topically produced mortalities, whereas permethrin showed no toxicity. Oral pyrethrin at both high and low dosages produced mortalities in reptiles too. Affected animals became disoriented and developed muscle tremors and mydriasis; death occurred within a few hours of administration.[35]

One important precaution with the use of natural pyrethrin and synthetic pyrethroid compounds is the increased toxicity associated with

exposure to the fumes of the products. If applied directly to the reptile, it must not be placed in a bag or air-tight container directly afterward, as the product quickly becomes toxic with restricted air flow. If applied to the cage or substrate, they must be allowed to air out and dry before placing the reptile back in the enclosure. Removal of the water bowl for 24 hours to avoid the possibility of the reptile soaking in the bowl right after application and ingesting the water is an important precaution. Additionally, neonate and juvenile reptiles may be more sensitive to these

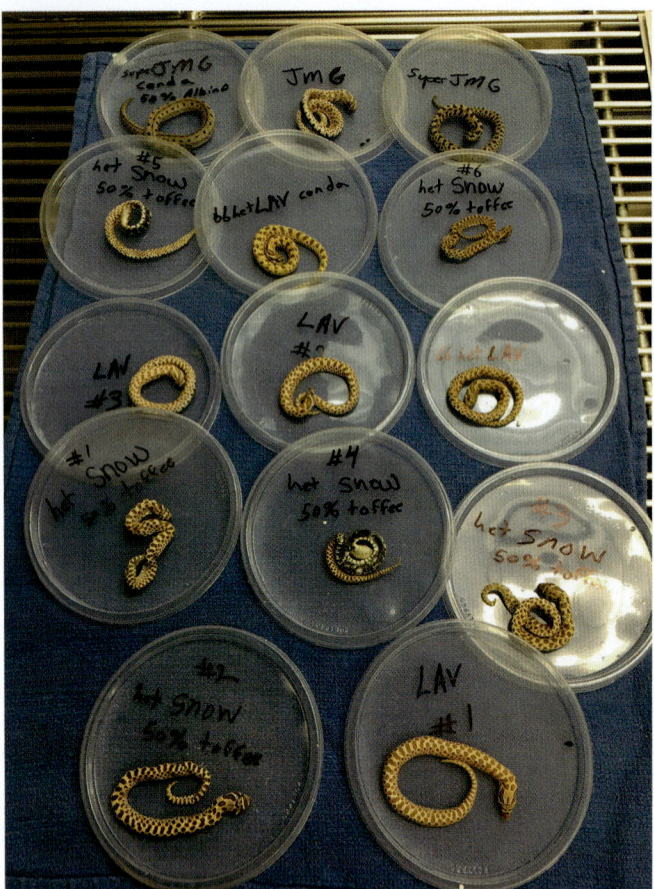

FIG 120.1 A group of juvenile western hognose snakes (*Heterodon nasicus*) that died shortly after being treated for snake mites using the same topical permethrin product and protocol that was used on adult hognose snakes with no adverse effects. Caution must be used in neonates, juveniles, and smaller species of snakes (many colubrids), as they seem more sensitive to these drugs. (Courtesy of Scott J. Stahl, Stahl Exotic Animal Veterinary Services.)

products than adult reptiles. Juvenile colubrids have died following the same directions safely used for adult animals (Fig. 120.1).

Fipronil spray 0.29% (Frontline Fipronil Spray Treatment, Merial, Duluth, GA) belongs to the phenylpyrazole chemical family and is an insect neurotoxin that has been successfully used to treat mites in reptiles. Because the spray is lipid based, it is not water-soluble and is thought to have a residual effect once applied. Stahl (personal communication, 2017) has used fipronil spray extensively to successfully treat snakes for mites. Larger snakes are sprayed directly, avoiding the eyes and mouth, or the spray is applied using latex gloves (spray gloves then rub gloves over reptile) to disperse. Once fipronil is applied, the snake is allowed to air dry before being placed back in its enclosure, or it can be wiped off after 5 to 10 minutes. Caution should be used with topical application of fipronil on smaller or juvenile snakes (apply with sprayed paper towel or cotton-tipped applicators) or use fipronil only in the environment for these more-sensitive reptiles. In these cases when the fipronil is not used directly on the animal, a warm water bath with a pinch of soap added to drown/remove mites from the reptile can be used in combination with environmental treatment with fipronil. Environmentally, fipronil can be liberally sprayed on all surfaces in the cage; however, it is important to allow the fipronil to fully dry before replacing the snake. During the treatment period any particulate substrate and wooden cage furnishings should be removed as they provide places for female mites to lay eggs and make treatment more challenging (this is true for all mite treatments discussed). The water bowl is removed during environment treatment and for 24 hours after fipronil spray has been applied to the snake. The snake and environment can be treated weekly or every other week for 6 to 8 weeks.

Ivermectin therapy has been used for mite treatment, both as an injection and a topical spray. Because ivermectin has a long half-life, it has been suggested that it may make treating the animal's environment unnecessary; however, not treating the environment can lead to reinfection. When using ivermectin spray follow a similar protocol described for fipronil spray, with treatment revolving around application to both the reptile and environment. Stahl (personal communication) has found weekly treatments (with a freshly made "batch" of ivermectin spray solution and by shaking the solution regularly to mix the oil-based ivermectin and water) to the reptile and liberally in the environment for 6 to 8 weeks may be necessary for successful eradication of mites. Recommended injectable doses of 0.2 mg/kg have been shown to be high enough to kill mites, but experimental work with fowl mites (*Dermanyssus gallinae*), which are closely related to the snake mite, require a dose of 0.4 to 0.5 mg/kg to be effective in mice.[4] Further work on ivermectin's effectiveness against *Ophionyssus natricis* and other reptile mites (e.g., lizard mites, *Hirstiella* spp.), as well as its safety in reptiles, needs to be done before dosages can be routinely recommended.[32,36,37] As previously mentioned, caution should always be used when administering ivermectin to reptiles, as fatal side effects can occur, especially in chelonians, skinks, and indigo snakes.

Dichlorvos-containing strips were once recommended for managing mites; however, due to their toxicity to both animals and humans, they should now be avoided. Formulations containing oils, synergistic compounds, or insect growth inhibitors should also be avoided as they can be toxic.[5] The organophosphate trichlorphon was shown to be highly effective against snake mites when applied as a 0.15% spray to both the animal and its cage for 24 hours.[38] It is recommended to remove the animal's water bowl before application and for 24 hours after treatment to prevent accidental ingestion and poisoning. Organophosphates should not be used concurrently with other cholinesterase-inhibiting insecticides, such as other organophosphates or carbamates. When used, animals should be closely monitored for signs of toxicity, including excessive salivation, abnormal posturing, or muscle twitching. Snakes exhibiting any of these signs should be thoroughly rinsed with water and promptly treated with atropine (0.4 mg/kg IM) and fluids.[5]

More recently, predatory mites have been investigated as a nonchemical, biological control method for snake and lizard mites. A recent report found that a 1-L culture of approximately 15,000 predatory soil mites (*Stratiolaelaps scimitus*) was sufficient to eliminate lizard mites (likely *Hirstiella* sp.) from bearded dragons and their enclosure in 5 days.[39] The mites, advertised as *Hypoaspis miles,* are commercially available. *Cheyletus eruditus,* another predatory mite, has also been evaluated as a biological control method for *O. natricis.*[40] When the two species of mites were placed in a tube together, only 6% of the snake mites survived for 48 hours in comparison to a 92% survival rate for snake mites housed alone in a control tube. A follow-up study using *O. natricis*–infested ball pythons found that after 15 days of treatment with the predatory mites, an average of two mites per snake remained, compared with 48 mites per snake in a control group. These predatory mites appear to be a promising nonchemical method of eliminating reptile mites without the potential side effects of some of the chemical treatments.

REFERENCES

See www.expertconsult.com for a complete list of references.

121

Mental Health Treatment (Psychopharmacology and Behavior Therapy)

Leticia Mattos de Souza Dantas and Teresa Bradley Bays

WELFARE AND PSYCHOLOGICAL WELL-BEING

Clinical Significance and Known Etiological Cause(s)

Similar to mammals and birds, reptiles have a wide range of sensory and cognitive abilities that facilitate awareness of their surroundings but can also experience distress related to aversive emotional states.[1] The ability to achieve different forms of learning, including recognition of visual, chemical, seismic, social cues, and special-object arrangement are a few examples of the wide range of cognitive capacities in reptiles.[2] The reptilian neuroendocrine system is comparable to other vertebrates, and many behavioral indicators of stress are often analogous to those of birds and mammals. However, it is important to keep in mind that reptiles not showing recognizable, physiological, or behavioral indicators of stress could still be experiencing distress.[3] Due to the evolutionary gap, some of the most reliable clinical signs in the diagnosis of fear- and anxiety-based problems in mammals, facial expressions and body language, are not always evident in reptiles.[1] Studies to investigate the correlation between behavioral change and the neuroendocrine processes related to distress and specific emotional states in reptiles and amphibians are still lacking.

Clinical Presentation and Diagnostic Confirmation

Behavioral pathologies are diagnoses of exclusion in veterinary medicine. A detailed history that includes behavioral and environmental information, an interview with the client for further clarification, a physical examination, and basic laboratory tests are all necessary to exclude medical causes not related to mental health. See various applicable chapters in this book for detailed information on disease diagnosis.

The most common behavioral symptoms presented by reptiles are aggression, stereotypical or repetitive behaviors (including self-injurious behaviors), and stress/fear-based behaviors.[1,4–6] All of these clinical presentations can be caused by several disease processes. Once a reptile becomes ill, regardless of the cause, it might become fearful or defensive, resistant, and even aggressive toward handling and being touched. Stressors that were previously tolerated will likely lead to distress as a consequence of lowered stress tolerance due to the patient experiencing discomfort.

Preferred Medical Therapy

Mental health treatment in veterinary medicine often includes a combination of recommendations and treatments, including environmental management and enrichment, behavior therapy, and medication. In mammals and birds, this multimodal approach has proven to lead to more effective and quicker results when compared to monotherapy. Studies in these areas are lacking for reptiles, and most interventions are based on environmental management and enrichment. Working with these patients, clinicians and caretakers must strive to avoid fear and aggression-inducing triggers.

When treating a patient that is experiencing psychological distress, all techniques used should target decreasing or avoiding the neuroendocrine stress response. In many cases, simply changing how the animal is handled and the setup of the cage (providing a sense of safety and control, e.g., multiple retreats or hide-outs) can be the most beneficial intervention.[4–6]

One of the most important pillars of behavioral medicine is client education. For any intervention to be effective, the caregiver must learn to recognize behavioral signs of stress for the particular species in hand. Then putting this knowledge into practice by providing safety and management instructions to clients will help them perceive signs of distress in their pet and be educated about what to do next. The same applies for the application of behavior therapy.

Behavior therapy, behavior modification, and cognitive behavior therapy are terms often used interchangeably; however, behavior modification generally refers to any procedure that modifies behavior (including brain surgery and shock therapy), and cognitive behavior therapy specifically applies to treatments that change cognitions. Therefore, behavior therapy (the systematic use of learning procedures to treat psychological problems and change behavior) is the more appropriate term to refer to the interventions prescribed in veterinary behavioral medicine.

Many behaviors develop, evolve, and are maintained through learning processes. The brain is molded by experience as every sensory and cognitive process impacts specific neural circuits, changing how future stimuli will be registered. Behavior therapy aims to affect neural plasticity and lead to behavioral change. Besides helping patients with aversive or distressing emotional states and dysfunctional behaviors, behavior therapy improves daily functioning and can decrease social stress. Data demonstrating the efficacy of specific techniques commonly used for birds and mammals is not available for reptiles. See Chapter 14 for examples of the use of operant conditioning–based therapy techniques to modify behavior.

Desensitization and Counterconditioning Therapy

Based on classical conditioning learning theory, human and nonhuman animals constantly learn through association between stimuli. In the classic example demonstrated by Pavlov, an unlearned response to a stimulus, such as drooling at the sight of food, is paired with a neutral stimulus, such as ringing a bell. Through repetition of ringing a bell every time food is offered, a dog will begin to associate the sound with the physiologic response of drooling in anticipation of a meal. Eventually one can ring a bell without the food present and the dog will begin to salivate. This principle of learning has many applications for veterinary patients, and detailed explanations of learning theory are available.[7]

Classical conditioning learning is commonly how fears are learned and how phobias develop. This process can lead to sustained distress or anxiety if the fear-inducing stimulus is constantly present or is presented repeatedly. A single experience can also be enough for some individuals prone to develop fear- and anxiety-based problems. However, learning via classical conditioning is also an effective therapeutic tool.

In desensitization therapy, the protocol should plan for gradual exposure of the patient to the fear-inducing stimulus. For example, the stimulus should be far enough away or in a reduced amount/time to not elicit the behavioral response. From there, it is slowly moved closer or increased incrementally so that the animal does not show signs of fear or other unwanted emotional or behavioral responses. Each incremental increase should only occur if the animal is showing no signs of stress (or the behavior that needs to be modified) at the current level. If the animal does begin to show signs of stress or aggression, they are becoming sensitized and the exercise must be stopped and restarted from the previous step.

Desensitization should be paired with counterconditioning therapy, which aims to create a positive or pleasant association with the stimulus. A naïve animal can also be *conditioned*, in other words, taught to tolerate and even enjoy a stimulus, interaction, individual, etc., by the same principle. Tools for counterconditioning or conditioning therapy can be as simple as the reptile's preferred foods. This principle is very effective in teaching an animal to tolerate handling and different medical procedures.[8]

Differential reinforcement of alternative behaviors is another type of therapy methodology that attempts to replace unwanted behaviors with actions that are more appropriate for a situation and less harmful for the individual. It is frequently used in conjunction with desensitization and counterconditioning therapy, especially when treating a problem that is a result of stress and fear.

In operant conditioning–based therapy, there are two paradigms: reinforcement (positive and negative) and punishment (positive and negative). Whereas both may lead to behavior change, punishment and negative reinforcement are counterproductive to mental health treatment since they will increase the animal's stress levels and cause fear and many times frustration. Treatments for animals should focus on removing the reinforcements for unwanted behaviors (when possible or applicable), teaching acceptable alternative behaviors in the same context, and using positive reinforcement to maintain these desired behaviors long term.[9] Similar to desensitization and counterconditioning, these principles can be applied to teach reptiles to feel safe and to accept different types of handling.[8]

Environmental Enrichment and Management

Environmental enrichment and management are covered in detail in other chapters of this textbook, but it is worth mentioning that enrichment and proper cage setup are crucial for captive reptile welfare. Most problem behaviors (not related to reproduction or other nonenvironmental-related physiological or endocrinologic changes) reported in the literature stem from a plethora of issues related to poor adaption to confinement, unacceptable physical environments, or inappropriate social interactions. It is also fundamental that the client is instructed to provide a home/cage environment that promotes predictability and consistency to the reptile, which significantly helps in decreasing stress levels.[4–6,10]

Pyschopharmacology and Endocrine Therapy

There are no safety or efficacy studies on the use of any psychoactive drugs for behavioral medicine treatments in reptiles. Most information published to date discusses the use of certain psychoactive drugs for chemical restraint, sedation, anesthesia, and pain management.[11]

A series of studies by Deckel,[12–14] Deckel and Jevitts,[15] and Deckel and Fuqua[16] evaluated behavioral changes in territorial behavior of *Anolis carolinensis* after injection of fluoxetine and other serotoninergic agents, injection of alcohol, and with exposure to mild stress. While these studies have started to shed a light into the interaction of antidepressants and the brain of *Anolis* lizards, controlled studies and clinical applications for veterinary practice are lacking.

Studies on the use of the antidepressant fluoxetine in newts[17] and fish[18] have been published, likewise with no follow-up controlled studies or clinical applications so far. In a study by Larson & Summers, setraline (dissolved in DMSO, resulting in a final sertraline concentration of 10 mg/kg and final DMSO concentration of 1%) was administered in *Anolis carolinensis* with the goal of decreasing aggressive behavior in five pairs of captive males. The animals were separated and treated with sertraline or placebo. Sertraline was given in food to both males or neither male in each pair for 1 week. The pairs were reintroduced, and behavior and social status was recorded. Latency to eyespot darkening was significantly retarded in "dominant" males treated with sertraline, and aggressive displays and attacks were reduced.[19] The role of monoamine neurotransmitters (among other neurotransmitters, neuropeptides, and hormones, such as the melanophore-stimulating hormone) in emotional processes and behavior responses is still unclear for reptiles, making it difficult to make a case for the use of psychoactive medication for the class Reptilia at this time.[20] The author recommends caution when extrapolating doses and treatment regimens from birds and mammals to reptiles because of the significant differences with regard to neurophysiology, neuroendocrinology, general metabolism, and the current lack of knowledge on how these drugs interact in the brain of different reptile species.

Hormone treatments may be used to treat problem behaviors related to the reproductive cycle or that are influenced by reproductive hormones. Castration might be effective in reducing territorial- and breeding-related aggression in some species,[21] but it has no effect on aggression caused by fear or pain. The use of hormones is beyond the scope of this chapter (see Chapters 79, 80 and 125).

Finally, a patient in pain will also be in psychological distress and is more prone to become aggressive and show behaviors that are consistent with distress.[4–6] However, pain management is also beyond the realm of this chapter (see Chapter 50), but it is worth noting that pain prevention and management are paramount for reptile mental health and welfare.[10]

Patient Follow-Up

After treatment is prescribed, close follow-up is advised until the problem behavior is resolved. The frequency of communications with clients may depend on the severity and welfare impact of the problem.

REFERENCES

See www.expertconsult.com for a complete list of references.

122

Nutritional Therapy

Thomas H. Boyer and Peter W. Scott

Warm reptiles to their preferred optimal temperature zone and ensure appropriate hydration before starting nutritional support. A dedicated room kept between 27°C to 29°C (80°F to 85°F) for reptiles with spot heating in cages helps and is better than providing just focal heat. Spot heat can be provided with under-tank heaters or overhead heat sources; be aware that both can burn reptiles. Overhead heat sources can be a fire hazard. Incubators are another excellent means of heat support, but can be too small for larger patients. Use indoor/outdoor thermometers to carefully monitor temperatures; overheating (>41°C, 105°F) kills reptiles quickly (see Chapter 46 for further details).

METABOLIC SCALING

Much has been written on metabolic scaling in reptiles, where metabolic rate (P_{met}) = mass constant × body mass (M_b)$^{mass\ exponent}$. Jacobson cautioned that when considering metabolic scaling for antibiotic dosing there are a host of variables to consider, and many of these apply equally to metabolic scaling of nutritional requirements.[1] For instance, the mass constant, typically quoted as 10 actually varies between reptiles (from 1–5 in snakes, 6–10 in lizards, and unknown for chelonians and crocodilians). The mass exponent also varies within groups (for instance, P_{met} = 4.390 $M_b^{0.98}$ in colubrids, P_{met} = 1.788 $M_b^{1.09}$ in boids, and P_{met} = 3.102 $M_b^{0.86}$ for colubrids and boids combined) and both may be compromised if multiple taxa are combined.[1] In the previous example, mass constant is too low for colubrids, too high for boids, and the mass exponent is too low for both.[1] Furthermore, variable health status (healthy vs. sick will change mass constant), activity level (studies based on active, wild reptiles vs. sedentary captives), body temperature, and physiology of over 10,000 reptile species, makes it hard to derive any universal equation, as even extrapolation between species within groups can be inaccurate.[1] Equations based upon a single species that cover all ages and sizes from neonate to adult would provide the most biologic significance, but only for that species, and few of these complete equations exist.[1] Therefore the best advice is to consider any such equation as a guide and to adjust based on careful monitoring and individual patient response.

DEHYDRATION AND ORAL FLUID THERAPY

Most reptiles are capable of recovering from levels of dehydration that would kill most mammals. Dehydration is difficult to estimate visually in reptiles. Dehydration greater than 8% to 10% results in loss of moisture in the retro-orbital fat pads and sunken eyes. Reptiles have limited skin elasticity, thus skin turgor is of limited value. Hypertonic (hypernatremic, hyperosmolar) dehydration occurs when proportionally more water

than sodium is lost from the body.[2–4] This results in an increased concentration of sodium in the extracellular fluid, which becomes hypertonic regarding the intracellular fluid, and therefore attracts water from the body cells. Hypertonic dehydration is common in reptiles that are not drinking or are hibernating, have end-stage renal disease, or heat stroke (hyperthermia). Isotonic (isonatremic, iso-osmolar) dehydration occurs when proportionally the same amount of water and sodium is lost from the body, so the sodium concentration of the extracellular fluid and hence its tonicity do not change.[2,3] Isotonic dehydration generally occurs as a result of hemorrhage, diarrhea, and short-term anorexia or vomiting. Hypotonic (hyponatremic, hypoosmolar) dehydration occurs when proportionally more sodium than water is lost from the body. This results in a decreased concentration of the extracellular fluid, which becomes hypotonic in comparison to intracellular fluid, which attracts water from the extracellular fluid. Hypotonic dehydration is common with prolonged anorexia and undernutrition.[2,3]

In green iguanas (*Iguana iguana*) subjected to water deprivation, elevations of sodium and potassium increased from baseline (118.5 mmol/L [mEq/L] and 4.2 mmol/L [mEq/l] respectively) to 135.5 mmoL and 4.9 mmol/L by day 3 and 150 mmol/L and 5.3 mmol/L by day 7, respectively. In addition, overt activity was almost nonexistent by day 5.[5] Other parameters that would be expected to elevate with hypertonic dehydration include packed cell volume, total protein, albumin, and chloride. Decreases in sodium and osmolality are good indicators of hypotonic dehydration but must be referenced to species normal or previously unremarkable panels from the same individual.

Maintenance fluid requirements have been determined for some species and range from 10 to 30 mL/kg/day. Daily water budgets for the waxy tree (*Phyllomedusa sauvagei*) and Mexican leaf frogs (*Pachymedusa dacnicolor*) have been documented as 8.6 mL/kg/day; Mojave fringe-toed lizard (*Uma scoparia*) as 11.3 mL/kg/day; diadem snakes (*Spalerosophis diadema*) as 16.7 mL/kg/day; African spurred tortoise (*Centrochelys sulcata*) as 27.6 mL/kg/day; common chuckwalla (*Sauromalus ater*) as 24.5 mL/kg/day; and desert iguana (*Dipsosaurus dorsalis*) as 30.5 mL/kg/day.[6,7] Rehydration typically involves giving maintenance (see Section 11) plus 25% to 33% of the fluid deficit/day. Fluid deficits should be made up over 72 to 96 hours, and rehydration rates of 3× maintenance or greater may be associated with fluid overload and should be avoided. Fluid type has been heavily debated in reptiles due to their larger intracellular fluid volume with presumed lower osmolality relative to mammals, but recent studies have shown reptiles' osmolality similar to mammals for freshwater turtles and crocodilians and sometimes higher than mammals in terrestrial and marine reptiles.[5,8,9] Formulas estimating osmolality in reptiles have been shown to be inaccurate in bearded dragons (*Pogona vitticeps*) and alligators (*Alligator mississippiensis*) but accurate in corn snakes (*Pantherophis guttatus*).[8–10] Recommended fluids include any warmed, balanced, isotonic crystalloid (see Chapter 87, Emergency and Critical Care, for further details). Lactated Ringer's solution, Normosol-R, and Plasmalyte-A are commonly used in reptiles.[11] Dextrose (5%) is isosmotic during administration, but metabolism of the sugar produces net water, which moves into the intracellular space. Consequently, dextrose is indicated where there is profound water deficiency with hypernatremia. Isotonic fluids will not have a severe negative impact on electrolyte imbalances and will benefit the patient until more specific fluid therapy can be determined from clinicopathologic results. LRS does not exacerbate lactic acidosis in mammals, even with liver disease, and reptiles are more tolerant of lactic acidosis than mammals.[12] Dextrose solutions should generally not be administered subcutaneously, but some (e.g., half-strength saline 5% glucose, 5% dextrose, and 4 g/L sodium chloride; two-thirds 5% glucose and one-third normal saline) have been successfully utilized by this route in humans.[12,13]

Fluids can be given by soaking, enterally via stomach tube (Fig. 122.1A–C), subcutaneously, intravenously, intraosseously, or coelomically (or by combination of routes). The authors no longer recommend coelomic fluid administration in reptiles because of the risks of visceral trauma and compression and other variables that may adversely affect absorption and assimilation (e.g., coelomitis, hypoalbuminemia, ascites, etc).[14] If the patient will drink, soaking is typically used for maintenance and mild dehydration. Use 24°C to 27°C (75°F–80°F) shallow, chin-deep water for several hours to overnight. All reptiles can drown in deep

water; if they attempt to swim, the water is too deep. Accurately monitoring of body weight will determine whether they are taking in water. Enteral fluids can be given at 5 to 10 mL/kg every 8 to 24 hours via stomach tube with mild to moderate dehydration (<5%). Close monitoring of body weight, plasma osmolality, PCV, and urination helps evaluate response to hydration; however, monitoring PCV was considered inaccurate for evaluating hydration status in at least one species of avian reptile but has not been evaluated in nonavian reptiles.[15] For details on catheterization and parenteral fluid therapy, see Chapter 44 and Section 11.

NUTRITIONAL SUPPORT

Refeeding Syndrome

Refeeding syndrome is a syndrome consisting of metabolic disturbances that occur as a result of reinstitution of nutrition to patients who are starved, severely malnourished, or metabolically stressed due to severe, sometimes acute illness.[16,17] During prolonged fasting (>4–5 days in cats and >2–5 days in humans but unknown in reptiles), the body maintains extracellular electrolytes by depleting intracellular electrolytes, especially potassium (K), calcium, phosphate (P), and magnesium (Mg). Thiamine is also depleted.[18] Once refeeding starts, blood glucose rises and insulin secretion resumes and pumps glucose and K into cells, which may result in hypokalemia, accompanied by hypophosphatemia, hypomagnesemia, and thiamine deficiency. Electrolyte imbalances may

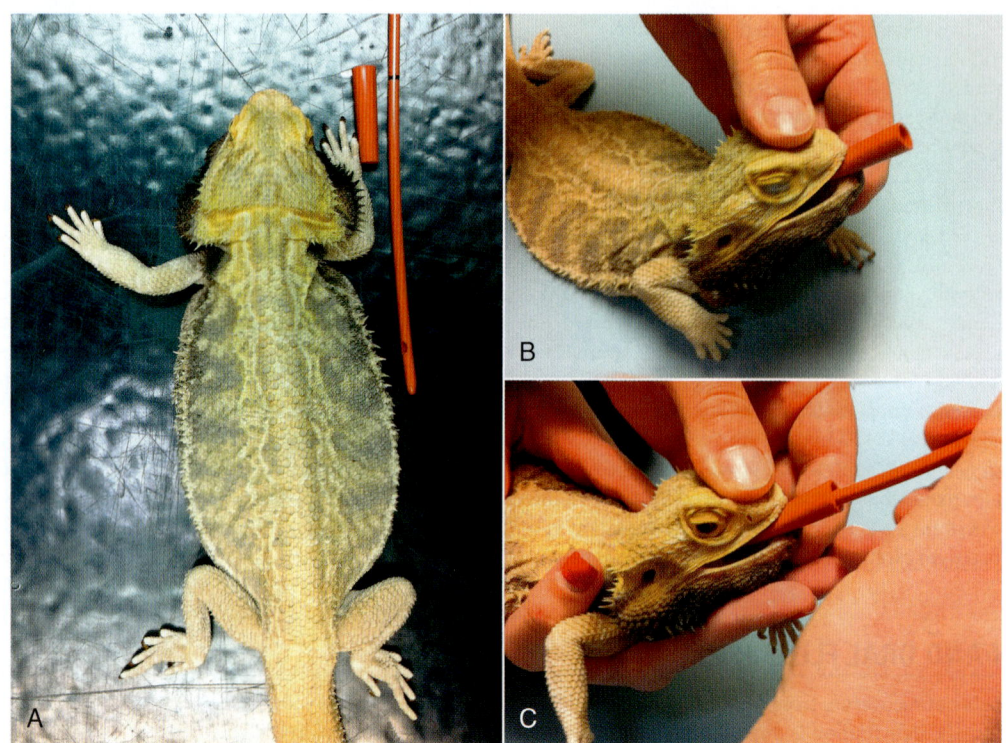

FIG 122.1 (A) To stomach-tube a lizard, here demonstrated in a bearded dragon (*Pogona vitticeps*), measure distal tube placement at one-third to one-half of the distance between front and rear legs. (B) Insert soft mouth speculum, and hold mouth shut on speculum. (C) Pass lubricated premeasured tube and give food slowly.

lead to widespread cellular dysfunction, cardiac arrhythmias/arrest, hemolysis, pulmonary edema, convulsions, and coma.[18]

When nursing a reptile that has been anorectic for a long period, initially focus on rehydration for 2 to 5 days. Supplementation with water-soluble vitamins may be beneficial. When starting nutritional support, limit intake to 10% to 25% of calculated requirements and increase slowly over several days or even weeks. Monitor plasma levels of P, K, Mg (if normal values are available), and glucose as frequently as feasible (ideally every 1-2 days). Watch for the aforementioned worsening clinical signs, or increased lethargy, suggestive of refeeding syndrome and reduce nutritional support if present. Severe hypophosphatemia (≥30% drop from baseline), in particular, is an early warning sign of refeeding syndrome, so monitor closely.[18] Slow reintroduction of food over days to weeks may be required and additional oral supplementation of K, P, and Mg may be indicated if below normal. If the patient remains stable, increasing nutritional supplementation can commence after several days.

Stomach Tubing

Oral feeding of liquid products is generally poorly accepted by most reptiles, and aspiration pneumonia is a significant risk. Stomach tubing is faster, safer, and can be taught to almost all caregivers. Soft, pliable tubes and oral speculums are better than metal or hard plastic to avoid dental or mandibular trauma. For small lizards, use the flared, catheter tip connector end of a red rubber catheter as an oral speculum, and run the cut red rubber catheter through it. In larger lizards speculums can be improvised from 3 mL cut syringes, or syringe cases, generously wrapped with elastic adhesive tape (Elastikon Bandage Tape, Johnson & Johnson, or Veterinary Elastic Adhesive Tape, 3M). Have one person vertically restrain the lizard with one hand behind the head, and with their other hand they can pull down on the dewlap while the feeder holds the maxillae. As soon as the mouth is open, insert the mouth speculum, which the lizard will typically bite down on. Immediately the restrainer should hold the mouth firmly closed so the lizard does not push the speculum out with its tongue. The feeder can then insert the well-lubricated, premeasured feeding tube through the speculum, down the esophagus, and into the stomach, which lies on the left, in the first third to half of the coelom.

Snakes do not require a speculum for stomach tubing and can be fed in the stomach or as far distally in the esophagus as feasible. Stomach location is typically midbody. After feeding, keep the snake's head elevated and gently digitally occlude the esophagus as the kinked tube is withdrawn to prevent regurgitation. Milking food material deposited into the esophagus down to the stomach may help prevent regurgitation.

Chelonians can be stomach tubed, especially if small or weak, but repeated forceful head and neck extension can be traumatic and is not recommended. It is preferable to place an esophagostomy tube if multiple feedings are anticipated (see Chapter 45). For single feedings, it is easiest to pass a stomach tube with the head extended, although a flexible, well-lubricated, small-gauge tube can be passed with the head retracted. Sedation or anesthesia may be required to extract the head. Premeasure and mark the tube from the tip of the mouth, down the extended esophagus, to the mid left pectoral scute. Restrain the head from above, just behind the skull laterally, so that as the chelonian head retracts, the restrainer's thumb and forefinger stop at the cranial carapace (which may need to be padded). Do not let go, as subsequent attempts to extend the head and neck become more difficult. If the mouth opens, immediately block one side with a speculum, but do not place behind the rhamphotheca. If the mouth is not open, with the restrainer's other thumb and forefinger, apply slow, steady downward traction to the mandible until the mouth opens. If this is unsuccessful, the feeder can insert a dull right-angle dental probe into the mouth and direct it ventrally, gently, into the floor of the mouth, until the chelonian opens its mouth and a side speculum can be placed. Many aquatic species can deliver a powerful bite, and caution is required. The lubricated, premeasured stomach tube can be passed down the esophagus—slight resistance may be felt as it passes through the gastroesophageal sphincter—to the level of the left midpectoral scute. Administer liquid diet slowly over a minute, with the chelonian held vertical, and discontinue if any regurgitation is noted in the esophagus or mouth.

Stomach Volume

The maximum gastric volume of most reptiles has not been determined. One study in the viviparous lizard (*Zootoca vivipara*) determined a calculation for stomach volume, where $V = 0.048W^{0.99}$ (V is volume in mL, and W is weight in grams).[19] This equation would give stomach volume of 0.24 mL in a 5 g lacertid lizard (48 mL/kg), but its accuracy in other species has not been determined. In red-eared sliders (*Trachemys scripta elegans*), regurgitation was observed in 43% of the turtles following rapid administration into the stomach of 8 mL/kg of dilute barium, but not when administered slowly over 20 seconds.[20] A dose of 25 mL/kg dilute barium was associated with regurgitation in 22% (4/18) of ball pythons (*Python regius*) and 60% (3/5) of green iguanas (*Iguana iguana*).[21,22] In bearded dragons, a dose of 15 mL/kg dilute barium in the distal esophagus resulted in excellent distention of the stomach for the barium series, yet more than half the dragons showed barium in the cranial esophagus. It was unclear if this represented reflux or tracking of the contrast material as the tube was withdrawn from the caudal thoracic esophagus.[23] Given that reptiles needing nutritional support have often been anorexic for extended periods, stomach volume may be reduced, so the authors often start with 5 mL/kg/feeding and slowly increase the volume over several days or weeks. Too large a volume, or too rapid administration, especially early in treatment, will cause regurgitation, whereas overfeeding can overwhelm the alimentary tract and cause stasis. Multiple small feedings are better than a single large feeding. Regurgitation should be avoided, as it often leads to aspiration pneumonia, which can be fatal.

Esophagostomy Tubes

Esophagostomy tubes can be essential for managing chronic nutritional disease in chelonians and are covered in detail in Chapter 45 (Fig. 122.2A and B). Soft silicon tubes are better tolerated, especially for long-term use, than red rubber tubes. Typically 14 to 24 Fr are used, depending on the reptile's size, whereas intravenous tubing also works for smaller reptiles. Stylets are often needed for softer, more flexible tubes. It is wise to perform a radiographic tube check, flush tubes after each feeding with water, and keep capped when not in use. If the patient regurgitates, check tube placement with radiography or endoscopy, make sure environmental temperature is adequate, and reduce feeding for several days. Tubes can be unblocked by placing a small amount of carbonated cola in the tube until it dissolves the clog.

Critical Care Nutritional Foods

Several commercially available products have worked well for nutritional support of reptiles, including Emeraid Carnivore, Omnivore, or Herbivore (LaFeber Co., Cornell, IL); Critical Care, Critical Care Fine Grind, or Carnivore Care (Oxbow Animal Health, Murdock, NE); and Critical Care Formula (Vetark Professional, Winchester, UK) (Table 122.1 for nutritional information). Low-fat elemental or semielemental diets are typically used for the first week or two. Once the patient is stable, there should be a gradual transition to a more complete maintenance diet.

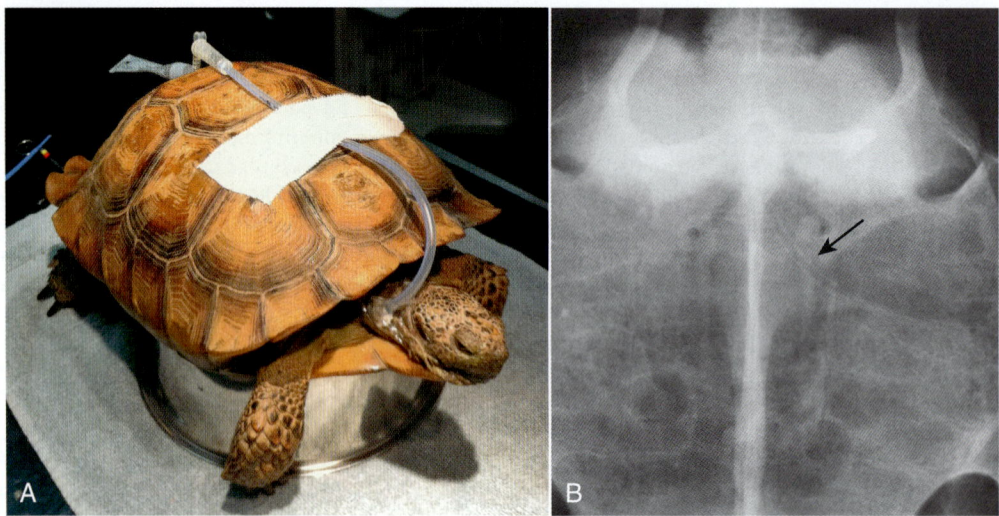

FIG 122.2 (A) Esophagostomy tubes are indicated for long-term administration of fluids, food, or medications to chelonians. (B) Always check tube placement (arrow) with radiography; distal tube should be located within the cranial left quadrant.

TABLE 122.1 **Nutrient Profiles of Commercial Diets Used to Feed Reptiles (% of Dry Matter Basis)**

Diet	Protein	Fat	Ash	CHO	Fiber	Ca	P	Ca:P
Emeraid Intensive Care Herbivore	19.0	9.5	5.3	63.0	32.0	1.00	0.39	2.5:1
Emeraid Intensive Care Omnivore	20.0	9.5	4.8	62.3	2.5	1.00	0.60	1.6:1
Emeraid Intensive Care Carnivore	37.8	33.9	5.9	14.6	4.5	1.00	0.67	1.5:1
Oxbow Critical Care, Normal or Fine Grind	16.0	3.0	10.0	26.1	21.0–26.0	0.40–0.60	0.20	2.0–3.0:1
Oxbow Carnivore Care	45.0	32.0	8.0	5.6	3.0	1.40–1.80	1.20	1.1–1.5:1
Vet Ark Critical Care Formula	14.5	0.3	6.2	79.0	0	0.41	0.22	1.9:1

Ca, Calcium; *CHO,* carbohydrate; *P,* phosphorus.
Thanks to Kelsey Carter for data collection.

Emeraid and Oxbow recommend various diet mixtures for different reptiles; see the manufacturer guidelines: Emeraid, Life Saving Nutrition, a Division of Lafeber, *Emeraid intensive care basic use guide for critically ill exotic animals,* https://emeraid.com/emeraid-intensive-care-basic-use-guide/; and Oxbow Animal Health website, http://www.oxbowanimalhealth.com/our-products/professional-line/. The goal is to maintain body weight and reverse the decline until the patient can eat on their own.

REFERENCES

See www.expertconsult.com for a complete list of references.

123

Cancer Chemotherapy

Antony S. Moore, Joerg Mayer, and Tara M. Harrison

Chemotherapy is the principal modality used to treat systemic cancers such as hematologic malignancies (lymphoma, leukemia) and metastatic carcinomas or sarcomas. In reptiles there is a high incidence of lymphoid neoplasia,[1] suggesting chemotherapy would have a role in the management of neoplasia. The main obstacles for the use of chemotherapy in reptile medicine are the lack of scientific literature from which to infer doses and scheduling, which may in turn exacerbate the preconceptions and misconceptions of owners and veterinarians regarding the toxicity of chemotherapeutic drugs. The goal of chemotherapy in human oncology is to cure the patient, while in veterinary medicine, palliation or remission is a more appropriate goal and, hence, drug dosages and schedules used are less likely to result in side effects. In palliative treatment the primary goal is to improve quality of life, which in veterinary medicine may result in prolonged survival because euthanasia is delayed. Just as quality of life for humans depends largely on preservation of body image as well as essential organ function, owners interpret their impressions of their pet's well-being in terms of their own expectations and beliefs, and this is likely true in reptiles as well. Therefore, communication between the veterinarian and the owner is essential. Options for treatment should never be limited by the veterinarian's interpretation of the owner's finances or preferences; rather, open and honest dialogue will allow an owner to make an informed decision and will ultimately create a "team" approach to chemotherapeutic treatment of the reptile's cancer.

Although it is tempting to think of chemotherapy protocols as a "recipe" for treating cancer, in fact they should be considered a guide. Just as every patient is an individual, their cancer is also individual, and the patient's metabolism and excretion of the drugs is individual. Complete evaluation of the cancer and the patient is therefore very important before administering the first dose of what are potentially toxic drugs.

In general, chemotherapy drugs are most active against cells that are actively dividing and in a particular phase of the cell cycle. Although most tumor cells are in an active phase of the cell cycle, only a small percentage of normal cells are actively dividing. Normal tissues can be classified as static (nerve, striated muscle) in which the capacity for mitosis is limited; expanding (organs, glands) in which mitosis can be induced; and renewing (hematopoietic cells, mucosa, epidermis, gametes, fetal tissues) in which the proliferating proportion approaches that of tumor tissue. In reptiles, proliferation may not be continuous but rather episodic, such as skin renewal (shedding), which could alter the risks for cutaneous toxicity of chemotherapy at that time. In addition, larger predators may induce mitosis in their gastrointestinal tract around feeding, altering the risk for gastrointestinal toxicity at such times. While it may not be practical to avoid chemotherapy at such times, awareness of these specific risk periods may allow for scheduling of drugs that do not target those organs. Toxicity from chemotherapy is most common in tissues that are renewing and is usually related to the dosage of the drug. This has implications for both the patient (toxicity and efficacy)

and for the owner and veterinary staff's safety in handling the drugs during administration, husbandry, and follow-up care. Because of the slower metabolic rate of reptiles, side effects from any given chemotherapeutic agent might be significantly delayed when compared to the common expected time intervals we are familiar with from mammal oncology.

CALCULATING A DOSE OF CHEMOTHERAPY

By dosing chemotherapy on a metabolic basis, the risk of toxicity to the patient is decreased. Although imperfect, and somewhat controversial, current dosage recommendations for cats and dogs are based on body surface area (BSA, m^2). Many drugs used in chemotherapy are given as mg/M^2 (mg per body surface area) instead of as mg/kg. Not much is known about these formulas for reptiles, and systemic chemotherapy is often based on assumptions about drug metabolism and excretion. Although there are Meeh coefficients specifically for reptiles, the published literature uses mg/kg dosing, and that is what is recommended by the authors of this chapter.[2] Please see Chapter 126 for more details on how BSA relates to body weight.

Additionally, anatomic differences in reptiles may mean that drugs are metabolized or excreted prior to reaching therapeutic concentrations. For example, the "renal portal system" means that reptiles have the capability to bypass the systemic circulation by shunting blood from the caudal extremities directly to the peritubular (not the glomerular) renal circulation. This means that if a drug is excreted by tubular secretion it could experience a significant first-pass effect prior to entering the systemic circulation. For drugs such as cisplatin and its transformation products, renal excretion is a complex process involving glomerular filtration, tubular excretion, and tubular reabsorption. For that reason, pharmacokinetics may be altered in different reptilian patients treated with these drugs using the tail vein. Because of the uncertainty of how the renal portal system affects the pharmacokinetic in any given reptilian patient, the authors recommend to avoid injecting chemotherapeutic agents into the caudal portion of the body.

CHEMOTHERAPEUTIC STRATEGIES

Tumors grow most rapidly when they are small. As they grow larger, the growth rate decreases due to a decrease in the proportion of cells in active phases of the cell cycle, increased loss of cells, and cell death due to poor circulation, nutrition, and hypoxia. Larger tumors may also have a poor blood supply; thus chemotherapy drugs may not be delivered to cancer cells at cytotoxic levels. In addition, resistance to chemotherapy can occur through spontaneous mutations in the tumor cell. The likelihood that mutation has occurred is related to the number of cell divisions that have occurred, and therefore resistance to chemotherapy is more likely in large tumors. In general, therefore, chemotherapy will be most active against small tumors, either following early detection or following a cytoreductive ("debulking") procedure such as surgery or radiation therapy. Chemotherapy is rarely effective or curative for large bulky tumors. An exception to this rule is combination chemotherapy for lymphoid neoplasms (as discussed later).

Combination chemotherapy may overcome drug resistance by affecting different metabolic pathways in cells that are resistant to other drugs in the combination. While combination chemotherapy could potentially be more toxic to normal cells, patterns of toxicity vary between drugs, and judicious scheduling of chemotherapeutic agents so that their toxicities do not overlap appears to improve tumor kill without compounding toxicity. For example, drugs that do not produce significant bone marrow suppression (such as vincristine or L-asparaginase) may be scheduled to be given soon after a myelosuppressive agent (doxorubicin, cyclophosphamide), or even on the same day in combination.

BASIC CHEMOTHERAPY DRUG HANDLING

Most chemotherapeutic agents are both toxic and mutagenic. Alkylating agents have been associated with the highest risks to handlers. Organ damage and increased risk of fetal loss have been reported in persons handling and administering chemotherapy with inadequate attention to personal safety. Precautions should be taken when handling chemotherapy drugs during any phase of preparation, administration, and disposal of drugs or waste produced during reconstitution and administration. Personal protective equipment (PPE)[3] consisting of protective eyewear, a respirator mask, a disposable gown with closed-cuff sleeves, and latex (not vinyl) gloves should be worn during any and all phases of handling chemotherapy. A closed-system transfer device is highly recommended, as this reduces the risk for aerosolization and leakage during administration.

Cleaning of a reptile cage for animal waste after chemotherapy should be done by handling waste products with gloves for a minimum of 1 month after each treatment, but this time period could be longer depending on the medication used and in some reptiles where the gastrointestinal transit time is longer (several weeks in some species). Care should be taken to not have immunocompromised or pregnant women handle reptile waste products during the duration of the chemotherapy treatment.

TOXICITY FOLLOWING CHEMOTHERAPY

Myelosuppression is a general term applied to the toxic effects of chemotherapy on the bone marrow. The most chemosensitive cells in the bone marrow are the proliferating hematopoietic progenitors and precursors, which are starting to commit to a particular lineage but are still immature. The more differentiated cells form a nonproliferating pool of maturing hematopoietic cells that will be unaffected by chemotherapy and can continue to provide mature cells for a number of days. This means that the nadir (or low point) of peripheral cell counts occurs at some time after the treatment. The time at which the nadir occurs also depends on the lifespan of the hematopoietic cell. Neutrophils live only hours in both dogs and cats, and their nadir occurs first at 5 to 10 days postchemotherapy; platelets live for approximately 10 days, and their nadir occurs 1 to 2 weeks after chemotherapy; erythrocytes live for 120 days in the dog and 70 days in the cat, and although anemia may occur over a prolonged course of chemotherapy, it is rarely clinically significant. The survival of hematopoietic cells in reptiles is not as well known;[4,5] however, most veterinarians have assumed similar survival times when assessing the effects of chemotherapy on circulating numbers. Like the mature cells, hematopoietic stem cells are largely nonproliferating and so are relatively resistant to chemotherapy toxicity. However, they are stimulated to divide by the loss of proliferating precursor cells and

rapidly replace the lost cells so that nadirs following chemotherapy rarely last more than several days. This also has implications for the interval between administrations of myelosuppressive drugs. If chemotherapy is given when the stem cell pool is dividing (i.e., soon after the previous administration), then severe prolonged myelosuppression due to stem cell destruction may occur. The usual interval between myelosuppressive drug administrations in mammalian species is every 2 to 3 weeks, and that is the interval used in the very few publications in reptile medicine.[6,7] Some drugs (such as lomustine and carboplatin) may have delayed or prolonged nadirs, and dosing intervals are longer for these drugs. EDTA may cause hemolysis in some species,[5] and so it may be advisable to use heparin as an anticoagulant when collecting samples from such species (especially chelonians). Also, veterinarians should be aware that the blood volume of reptiles is 5% to 8% of body weight, so no more than 0.5 ml/100 g should be collected.[5]

When administering chemotherapy, hematology should be performed at the expected heterophil nadir. While in mammalian species this is usually 7 to 10 days after treatment, in reptiles it may be delayed and hematology should be monitored for longer (2 weeks), at least when using a new chemotherapy drug for the first time in an individual patient. Due to lack of information known about the effect of chemotherapeutic drugs and because many apparently normal reptiles often have low leucocyte and heterophil counts, it is extremely important to compare serial hematology samples for each patient in order to try to establish a pattern. This pattern could then be traced back to a normal fluctuation (e.g., seasonal) or a nadir due to a drug reaction.

In one report, the authors recommended that hematology be performed prior to each chemotherapy, and if the heterophil count was 1.5×10^9 cells/L (1.5×10^{12} cells/μL), the treatment was delayed until the heterophil count exceeded 2×10^9 cells/L (2×10^{12} cells/μL).[6] The reason the heterophil count should be in normal range or above before the next dose of a myelosuppressive agent is administered is that treatment before bone marrow recovery may lead to stem-cell depletion and prolonged, occasionally irreversible myelosuppression. If the heterophil count is too low at the time myelosuppressive chemotherapy is due, it is best to delay administration by 1 week or until the heterophil count is more than 2.0×10^9 cells/L. The absolute heterophil count (not the percentage or the total leukocyte count) should be evaluated. Although many animals have a low heterophil count without clinical signs, a nadir count of less than 0.5×10^9/L is sufficient reason to reduce all subsequent dosages of that myelosuppressive drug. A dosage reduction of 25% is a good rule of thumb.

Thrombocytopenia is rarely severe enough to cause clinical bleeding, and normal ranges are difficult to obtain from the literature;[5] therefore, the authors cannot make firm recommendations about dosage adjustments based on thrombocytopenia in reptiles. Also complicating the issue is the finding that thrombocytopenia may be associated with severe inflammatory disease, which can occur as a concurrent response to the cancer. For drugs known to cause thrombocytopenia in mammals (lomustine [CCNU], carboplatin, cisplatin), the clinician is cautioned to assess trends in thrombocyte counts and discontinue if there is a continued downward trend.

The gastrointestinal mucosa is another site of renewing tissue, and toxicity may occur anywhere in the GI system. Some predatory reptiles increase the turnover of their mucosa during episodic feeding, which could increase the risk for gastrointestinal toxicity during such times.[8] While it may not be practical to avoid chemotherapy altogether, it may be prudent to schedule drugs that do not specifically affect the gastrointestinal tract during these times. Clinical signs include nausea, vomiting, inappetence, anorexia, ulceration, or diarrhea. The management of these toxicities will depend on the severity of signs. Vomiting is common in snakes and a terminal event in turtles and lizards; therefore, the clinician will need to evaluate each patient as to the likelihood that vomiting is caused by progression of the cancer, chemotherapy toxicity, or just normal behavior. Similarly, inappetence may be difficult to assess in patients that eat only intermittently. Diarrhea can increase the risk of subsequent sepsis due to breakdown of the protective mucosal barrier to gram-negative intestinal bacteria at a time when the animal is myelosuppressed. Antibiotics, preferably those that target gram-negative bacteria as the ones most commonly implicated in sepsis, should be administered to these animals (with heterophil counts $<1 \times 10^9$/L) in addition to supportive and symptomatic care.

In veterinary mammalian oncology, cardiotoxicity, nephrotoxicity, and urothelial toxicity (sterile hemorrhagic cystitis) have been associated with specific drugs and in specific species. These toxicities are not common to all species (for example, hemorrhagic cystitis after cyclophosphamide is seen in dogs and not cats; doxorubicin is a clinically relevant cardiotoxin in dogs and not in cats, but doxorubicin is renal toxic in cats and not dogs). The reader can see that predicting toxicities in reptiles generally, and particularly in different genera, is impossible, and careful observation is needed to build a body of knowledge around these treatments. Due to the significantly lower number of nephrons in the reptilian kidney, special attention has to be paid to nephrotoxicity, as this side effect may be more severe in the reptilian patient. Concurrent parenteral fluids may be supportive and renal-protective when administering any drug that could be nephrotoxic.

Extravasation of some chemotherapy agents may cause necrosis when they are administered outside the vein. While some drugs may cause temporary irritation, others are truly vesicant, and those are usually classified as DNA-binding and non-DNA-binding drugs. In general, for non-DNA-binding drugs (such as vinca alkaloids), there may be benefit to diluting the extravasated drug using saline and by application of warm compresses to increase blood flow to the area; also the addition of hyaluronidase to improve absorption of the drug has been shown to be beneficial after vinca alkaloid extravasation. In contrast, those that bind to DNA (such as doxorubicin) should be restricted after extravasation by using cold packs and by not flooding the area with saline. Specific antidotes are few, although the use of systemic dexrazoxane appears to reduce the severity of doxorubicin extravasation reactions in mammals. Especially after extravasation of DNA-binding drugs, the tissue necrosis may be severe and surgical debridement may be needed. Prevention is much preferred, and careful use of a "first-stick" intravenous catheter is always recommended. Vesicant drugs should never be administered subcutaneously, intralesionally, or intracoelomically.

Hypersensitivity reactions may occur due to histamine release. This effect usually occurs with rapid administration of some drugs and may be a consequence of the drug itself or due to the carrier solutions in these formulations (as opposed to the drugs themselves). True anaphylaxis rarely occurs in mammalian species following administration of L-asparaginase, an asparagine-specific enzyme, particularly by the intravenous or the intraperitoneal route. If anaphylaxis occurs, the patient should never receive further treatments with that drug. However, to date no published report of an anaphylactic reaction in a reptile exists in the scientific literature. It is possible that this side effect is not a significant concern in the reptilian patient; however, not enough data on reptiles that have been treated with chemotherapy has been collected.

CHEMOTHERAPY DRUG ADMINISTRATION

Systemic chemotherapy is the most common route used; oral or parenteral administration allows for systemic distribution of the active drug at therapeutic levels sufficient to allow damage to the neoplastic cells but

at a level where significant or prolonged damage to normal cells is unlikely. Intralesional chemotherapy may be used under specific circumstances for local (rather than systemic) cancer control; more information follows at the end of this chapter.

As mentioned previously, the authors recommend against administering chemotherapy in the caudal half of a reptile's body due to the potential effect of the renal portal system. Ongoing venous access can be problematic, especially for small reptiles. A subcutaneously implanted vascular access port (VAP), placed surgically under anesthesia, may be suitable for larger reptiles, as they allow venous access with minimal restraint. The use of vascular access ports (VAP) in an (Iguana iguana) with lymphoma has been reported,[6] as has central line placement in tortoises.[9] As with mammalian species, where approximately 10% of patients experience complications (e.g., permanent loss of VAP patency, catheter breakage, suture breakage, infection, and incision dehiscence), in the iguana, reported difficulties included port disconnection, inability to aspirate blood after a few weeks, and infection.[10] Central lines have been successfully placed in a number of chelonians, which remained in place for many weeks and allowed repeated blood collection and intravenous medication without any complications (see Chapter 44 for instructions on how to place a central line).[10] Doxorubicin, which can cause severe tissue necrosis if administered extravascularly, was administered via a VAP to a corn snake (Pantherophis spp.) with a vertebral body osteosarcoma with no significant toxicities noted from either the port or the chemotherapy.[11] One iguana was treated over a 2-year period for lymphoma using three separate VAPs. The lizard experienced acute necrosis over the first VAP placed, and it was removed; the cause was uncertain, but possibly due to extravasation of vincristine. The second port was placed in the coelomic cavity and remained patent for 6 months, at which time the lizard had grown and a subcutaneous VAP was placed and used for an additional 18 months. Doxorubicin, vincristine, cyclophosphamide, and prednisone were all successfully administered to that patient.[6]

CHEMOTHERAPY DRUG DOSING

Dosing of chemotherapy is often based on metabolic rate, but assumptions used in mammals have been refined by multiple studies, including dosage escalation and pharmacokinetic studies; similar studies have been performed in some birds.[12] Unfortunately, chemotherapy dosages in reptiles remain empirical, usually based on dosages used in mammalian species, especially the dog (Table 123.1). Ideally, for each order and probably species, veterinarians will need to develop dosing strategies that maximize efficacy but result in an acceptable toxicity. One approach (at least for a starting dose) is allometric scaling from dog or human dosages, although that is also imperfect (see Chapter 126).

The difficulties are illustrated by one publication, where a dosage escalation for doxorubicin was performed in an iguana with lymphoma, increasing the dosage from the empirical start of 0.26 mg/kg (based on a dog dose reduced by one-third), to 0.75 mg/kg every 3 weeks.[6] During that escalation, the drug showed improved efficacy against the lymphoma but minimal increase in toxicity. Ideally, such a study could be performed in a number of patients from each species to determine the "maximally tolerated dose," which would allow optimum treatment of reptiles. The authors recognize this is difficult and would take a long time. Until those data are available, we will need to rely on case reports and anecdotal information, but if a general principle of dose escalation and scrupulous monitoring for toxicity is followed, eventually that data will be accumulated. It is not enough to say that a drug was nontoxic and not enough to say it was effective; it needs to be both effective and well tolerated.

TABLE 123.1	**Previously Reported Dosages of Chemotherapy Agents Used in Reptiles**		
Drug	**Dose**	**Route**	**Potential Adverse Effects***
Prednisone[7,8,13]	0.2–2 mg/kg	PO, SC, IM, IV	Gastrointestinal ulceration, polyuria, polydypsia, weight gain
Cyclophosphamide[7]	10 mg/kg	IV, PO	Neutropenia, thrombocytopenia, gastrointestinal toxicity
Chlorambucil[8,13]	0.08–1 mg/kg, 2.0 mg/m^2	PO	Neutropenia, thrombocytopenia
Doxorubicin[7]	1 mg/kg	IV	Tissue vesicant if extravascular, hypersensitivity, myelosuppression, cardiotoxicity, gastrointestinal toxicity
Cisplatin[16]	0.5–1 mg/kg	IV, IC, IL	Cumulative renal toxicity, myelosuppression, hepatopathy, hypersensitivity reactions
Carboplatin[17]	2.5–5 mg/kg	IV, IC, IL	Myelosuppression
Cytosar[13,14]	6 mg/kg–30 mg/kg**	IV, SC	Myelosuppression and gastrointestinal disturbances
L-Asparaginase	400 U/kg	SC, IM, IC	Hypersensitivity reaction
Vincristine[7]	0.025 mg/kg	IV	Tissue vesicant if extravascular
Bleomycin[18]	1 u/cm^3	IV, IL	Pulmonary fibrosis

*Adverse effects primarily reported in domestic animals; not enough information in reptiles at this time.
**Too high and possibly fatal.
The reader is referred to other textbook sources on specific chemotherapy agents used in veterinary medicine.[20,21]

Other examples from the reptile literature follow. The chlorambucil dosage in the publications ranges from 0.08 mg/kg PO once (green tree monitor, *Varanus prasinus*, with chronic lymphoid leukemia, died 4 days later)[7] to 1 mg/kg every 7 days (diamondback terrapin, *Malaclemys terrapin*, with lymphoma,[13] was not apparently toxic but not effective either) to 2.0 mg/m^2 every day (King cobra, *Ophiophagus hannah*, with lymphoma [Willette et al, Proc AAZV, 2001, p 20]), which caused minimal hematologic toxicity and then the patient died 6 weeks after starting chlorambucil (but whether due to disease or drug was uncertain); in this latter case the technique for determining surface area was not reported.

Similarly, cytosine arabinoside varies in reported dosage from 6 mg/kg every 7 days (diamondback terrapin with lymphoma, peripheral decrease in abnormal cell counts but widespread systemic lymphoma),[13] to 30 mg/kg SC (24 hours after which the rhinoceros viper, *Bitis nasicornis*, with lymphoma, was dead; presumably due to drug toxicity).[14] Even the prednisone dosage varies in reports from 0.2 mg/kg every 72 hours (sungazer lizard, *Smaug giganteus*, with acute lymphoid leukemia [Martin et al, Proc AAZV, 2003, p 6]), 0.6 mg/kg every 48 hours (terrapin),[13] 0.8 mg/kg every 48 hours (green tree monitor with chronic lymphoid leukemia [CLL]),[7] 40 mg/m^2 SC every 48 hours (cobra with lymphoma [Willette et al, Proc AAZV, 2001, p 20]), to 2 mg/kg daily for 2 weeks then every 48 hours (iguana with lymphoma).[6]

Currently for chemotherapy agents delivered systemically (see later discussion for intralesional administration), we recommend starting with established dog dosages reduced by one-third and at intervals as used in dogs. This may be a reasonable initial approach (at least in one report, there was efficacy and minimal toxicity with this approach).[6] Consultation with a veterinary oncologist is recommended, and if no toxicities are encountered after each treatment, consideration can be given to cautious escalation of dosages (by 10% for every treatment without toxicity) with careful and ongoing monitoring for hematologic and systemic visceral toxicities. All data should be made available for further studies, preferably in a published form, so that repetitive escalations are not performed.

The use of empirical dosing is often unsuccessful, even for tumor types such as lymphoma and leukemias that respond well in mammalian species. Cutaneous lymphoma in a king cobra was initially treated surgically, with recurrence 5 months later, and a second surgery allowed for another 2 months before a second recurrence (Willette et al, Proc AAZV, 2001, p 20). Chemotherapy with doses used for dogs and cats

with L-asparaginase (10,000 IU/m^2 SC), vincristine (0.5 mg/m^2 IV), and prednisone caused a temporary partial response before progression after 4 weeks; chlorambucil caused stabilization for a further 4 weeks, at which time the masses progressed and treatment was ceased. Survival from diagnosis was 15 months (Willette et al, Proc AAZV, 2001, p 20). A diamondback terrapin with lymphoma treated with cytosine arabinoside, chlorambucil, and prednisone showed a decrease in peripheral abnormal cell counts, but widespread systemic lymphoma progressed with death 6 weeks after diagnosis.[13] Conversely, an iguana with lymphoma, treated with multiagent combination chemotherapy (doses discussed previously), was still in complete remission nearly 3 years after diagnosis.[6]

Partial response in chronic lymphoid leukemia was achieved in a green tree monitor for 7 months using chlorambucil and prednisone.[7] A sungazer lizard treated for acute lymphoid leukemia with whole-body radiation and prednisolone was in remission when it died 11 months after radiation (Martin et al, Proc AAZV, 2003, p 6) (see also Chapter 124). Clearly multimodality combinations of surgery, radiation, and chemotherapy should be considered when deemed appropriate to the individual situation.

In addition to systemic chemotherapy, localized (intralesional) chemotherapy is attractive for smaller reptiles. Intralesional chemotherapy is always administered as a suspension in oil or other vehicle, not as pure drug, and is considered a "local" therapy to treat tumors that have not metastasized. The mixture is injected into a tumor, providing a very high drug concentration to the tumor cells but minimal systemic drug levels, thereby avoiding the risk of systemic toxicity. These mixtures are prepared like any chemotherapy agent, but two Luer-lok syringes, one containing the cytotoxic agent and one containing the vehicle (e.g., sterile medical grade sesame oil),[15] should be prepared. The total dose of chemotherapy drug should not exceed the systemic dosage for that drug. Each agent should be placed into a syringe with sufficient capacity to contain both liquids when combined (i.e., 2.5 ml of drug and 2.5 ml of vehicle, each in a 5–6 ml syringe). The syringes are attached to a three-way stopcock, and the two liquids can then be rapidly mixed between the syringes to create an oily emulsion. PPE, as outlined previously, must be worn. It may be wise to mix inside a sealable plastic bag. The syringe that now contains all of the mixture should be detached after covering the attachment with an alcohol-moistened gauze swab to prevent aerosolization, and a 23-gauge needle should be attached. The remaining syringe and stopcock should be discarded as contaminated waste.

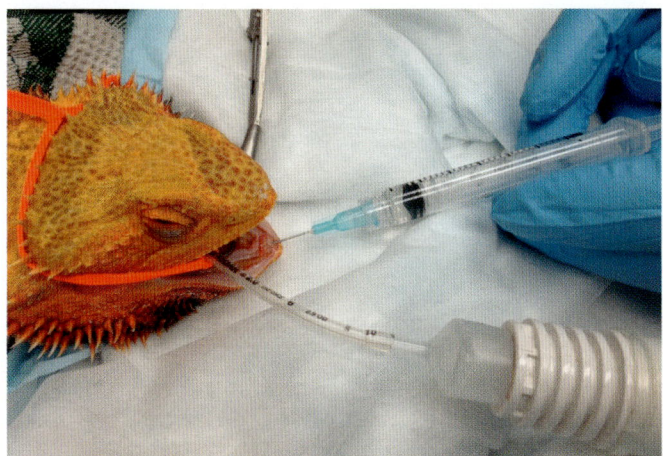

FIG 123.1 A bearded dragon (*Pogona vitticeps*) with mandibular sarcoma, which is being treated with intralesional bleomycin and electrochemotherapy. Note the use of personal protective equipment during administration. (Courtesy of Louis-Philippe de Lorimier.)

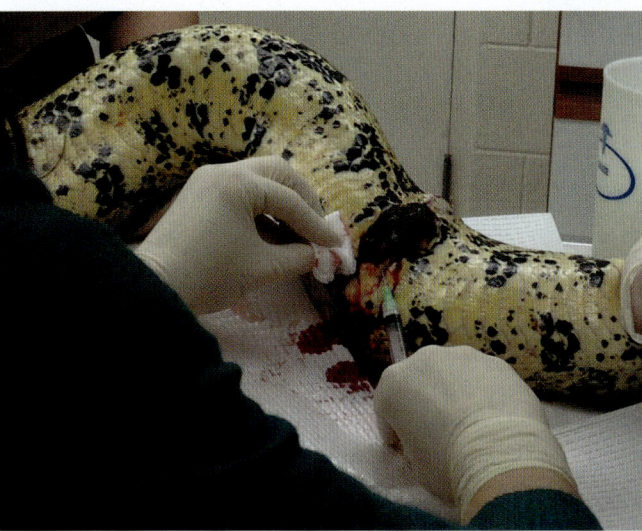

FIG 123.2 Intralesional chemotherapy for a cutaneous metastatic melanoma in a boa (*Boa constrictor* spp.). Note the use of personal protective equipment during administration. (Courtesy of Christine Swanson.)

It is preferable to mix multiple small volumes of drug in this way rather than a single large volume, because separation of drug from vehicle may occur rapidly, thereby reducing the efficacy of the treatment. Likewise, the drug-vehicle mixture should be administered soon after preparation. If a delay is encountered, the drug can be remixed with its vehicle using a new syringe and three-way stopcock. The needles on used syringes should not be recapped. Injection is performed in a grid-pattern to ensure highest possible intratumoral concentration of drug. It is important to use PPE for protection of staff and to watch the area carefully for any leakage of chemotherapeutic agent. If leakage occurs, the area should be swabbed and cleaned with soap and water, and the cleaning materials disposed of as hazardous waste. When removing the needle after intralesional therapy, there is often pressure on the syringe contents that will cause the mixture to leak out when the needle is withdrawn from the tumor. Negative pressure on the syringe when withdrawing will help reduce leakage. The patient should remain anaesthetized until oozing and bleeding stops (Figs. 123.1 and 123.2).

Note that some of the drugs reported for intralesional chemotherapy rely on reconstitution of the lyophilized drug to a higher concentration than would normally be administered systemically. Some of those drugs (e.g., cisplatin and carboplatin) are available as reconstituted drugs, which are too dilute for intralesional use. Drugs that can cause tissue necrosis (such as doxorubicin or vincristine) should never be delivered intralesionally.

The use of intralesional cisplatin has been reported in reptilian species without apparent adverse effect but with unknown efficacy.[16] A 10-year-old female boa constrictor (*Boa constrictor*) with a malignant subcutaneous fibrosarcoma of the body wall was successfully treated with 50 mg (total dose) of intralesional carboplatin in addition to radiation therapy, so the contribution of carboplatin is difficult to assess.[17] Electrochemotherapy uses electrical impulses to improve penetration of chemotherapy into cancer cells and may thereby increase efficacy. Following an incomplete surgical excision, intralesional bleomycin in

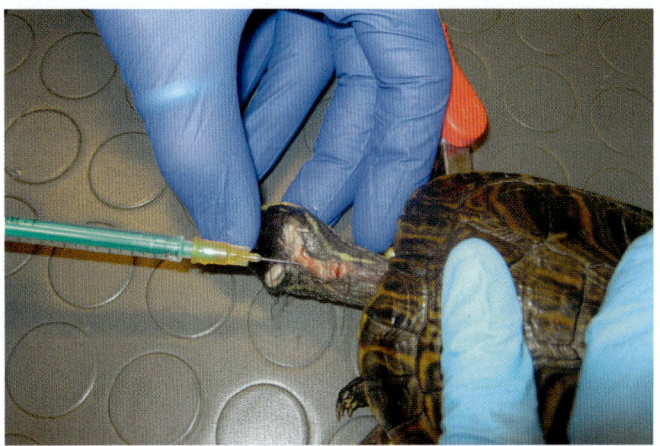

FIG 123.3 An aquatic slider with squamous cell carcinoma treated with electrochemotherapy. This involved intratumoral administration of bleomycin followed by trains of biphasic electric pulses. The treatment was well tolerated, and the turtle was disease-free after 12 months. (Courtesy of Enrico Spugnini.)

combination with electrochemotherapy was used to treat squamous cell carcinoma in a yellow-bellied slider (*Trachemys scripta scripta*). The animal tolerated the treatment and had no evidence of neoplasia 12 months after treatment (Fig. 123.3).[18] Electrochemotherapy and intralesional bleomycin was also used to treat fibropapillomas in a green sea turtle (*Chelonia mydas*). The lesions resolved, and there was no evidence of local recurrence 12 months after treatment.[19]

REFERENCES

See www.expertconsult.com for a complete list of references.

124

Radiation Therapy

Koichi Nagata and Joerg Mayer

Radiation therapy (RT) can be performed in several different ways. The most commonly used RT modality in veterinary medicine is a linear accelerator, which can produce highly penetrating x-rays. Gamma rays are emitted from Cobalt-60 sources or certain radioactive isotopes. X-rays and gamma rays kill the cell mainly by knocking out electrons from the exposed atoms' orbits.[1] The majority of the ejected electrons react with water molecules, which turn into free radicals that damage the DNA and cause double-strand breaks. This is often followed by lethal chromosomal aberrations during the cell division, which results in cell death (mitotic death). Although most cell types die mainly from mitotic death (i.e., cells do not die until they try to divide, which is why the effect or side effects of RT are usually not seen immediately after the treatment), some cells such as lymphocytes and lymphoma cells undergo significant apoptosis (instead of mitotic death), which often results in rapid reduction in tumor size within 24 to 48 hours after RT. Larger tumors are usually more resistant to radiation, partly because the center of the tumor is hypoxic, which makes tumor cells in this zone relatively resistant to the effects of radiation.

SIDE EFFECTS

Radiation side effects are classified into acute effects and late effects. Acute effects typically accompany inflammation and start within days to weeks after starting RT (at least in mammalian species). Late effects usually take months to years after finishing RT before they manifest. Most of the late effects are permanent and nonhealing. A well-known example is a permanent necrosis of the irradiated area.

The risk for radiation side effects may be reduced by careful planning of the radiation field to protect or by reducing the radiation dosage to radiation-sensitive structures. Computer tomography (CT) is the imaging modality of choice for planning, as it can be used directly for computer-based evaluation. In reptile species, achieving vascular access can be challenging, making it more difficult to perform contrast CT studies. In such patients, MRI may be helpful for RT planning in reptiles.[2]

LINEAR ACCELERATOR AND COBALT-60

The following is a summary of various case reports of reptile patients treated by x-ray or gamma-ray radiotherapy.

A 10-year-old Indian Rock python (*Python molurus molurus*) with postsurgical recurrent lymphoma of the ventral oral cavity (approximately $2 \times 2 \times 3$ cm) was treated with 15 Gray (Gy) using a cobalt-60 source.[3] Sixteen days later, tumor regression was observed, at which time the snake was irradiated again with 35 Gy. Approximately 6 months following the first RT, there was no evidence of tumor recurrence. However, the snake became lethargic and died 1 month later. Necropsy revealed lesions in the liver and gastrointestinal tract with the same lymphoma cell type.

The only adverse event from RT was a permanent elimination of dentition at the irradiated site. This indicates that the threshold dose to cause an acute side effect in pythons may be significantly higher compared to the dose tolerated by mammals (in mammals, a single dose of 35 Gy is expected to result in severe acute effects followed by necrosis).

A 2-year-old green iguana (*Iguana iguana*) with a localized lymphoma in the cranial cervical area was treated with a single 10 Gy of radiation.[4] The tumor reduced in size by 90% the next day. Chemotherapy (modified CHOP protocol) was started at that time. The iguana was still in remission when it was rechecked 1008 days after the initiation of treatment. Lymphomas in mammals are known to be very sensitive to RT, and the significant response to RT observed in this iguana may indicate that lymphomas in reptiles also respond similarly to their mammalian counterparts.

It should be noted that when an entire snake is exposed to radiation, the LD50 dose is close to that of humans, which is approximately 300 to 400 Roentgen (2.6–3.6 Gy).[5] Similarly, irradiation of radiosensitive viscera such as lung should be undertaken with caution. A snake treated with 20 Gy to a field that included the lung developed pulmonary vasculitis and was euthanized because of dyspnea.[2] The LD50 in box turtles (*Terrapene* spp.) is reported to be approximately 850 Roentgen [7.5 Gy], indicating that LD50 may vary significantly between taxa. The relatively low LD50 for snakes is surprising, considering that whole body irradiation LD50 for lower vertebrates are higher in general (e.g., 800 Roentgen [7 Gy] in goldfish, 700 Roentgen [6.1 Gy] in frogs, and 1486 Roentgen [13 Gy] in newts) (Fig. 124.1).[5]

Low-dose, whole body radiation may be used for the treatment of lymphomas or lymphoblastic leukemias. An adult sungazer lizard (*Cordylus giganteus*) with acute lymphoblastic leukemia (ALL) and a total white blood cell count (WBC) of $3.1 \times 10^3/\mu L$ was initially treated with 0.2 mg/kg prednisone PO q72 hrs (Janet C. Martin, unpublished observations). However, 3 months after starting the treatment, WBC remained elevated at $34.3 \times 10^3/\mu L$. Two months later, prednisone was discontinued and a single whole body irradiation with 1 Gy was administered. Although WBC was still elevated at 1 month post-irradiation, it decreased at 3 months post-irradiation to $2.9 \times 10^3/\mu L$. Approximately 11 months after RT, the lizard died of femoral pore abscessation, which had been present before starting the treatment for ALL.

Radiation therapy for nonlymphoma tumors have been reported with less success. A 10-year-old boa constrictor (*Boa constrictor ortoni*) with a 4×15 cm subcutaneous fibrosarcoma located 10 cm caudal to the heart was incompletely excised.[6] Three weeks later, cobalt-60 RT (16×3 Gy fractions for a total dose of 48 Gy) was performed over a 21-day period. Hematology following the last radiation fraction revealed leukopenia (2.7×10^3 cells/μL) and severe lymphopenia (likely due to a combination of factors including the neoplasia, multiple coelomic

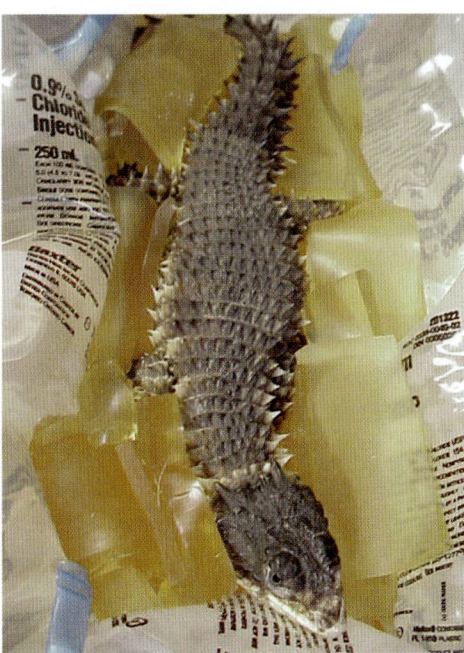

FIG 124.1 A sungazer lizard *(Cordylus giganteus)* receiving whole body irradiation by a linear accelerator. Tissue-equivalent bolus materials (Superflab and saline bags) are placed around the lizard, so that the entire body receives a homogeneous dose of radiation. (Courtesy of Joerg Mayer.)

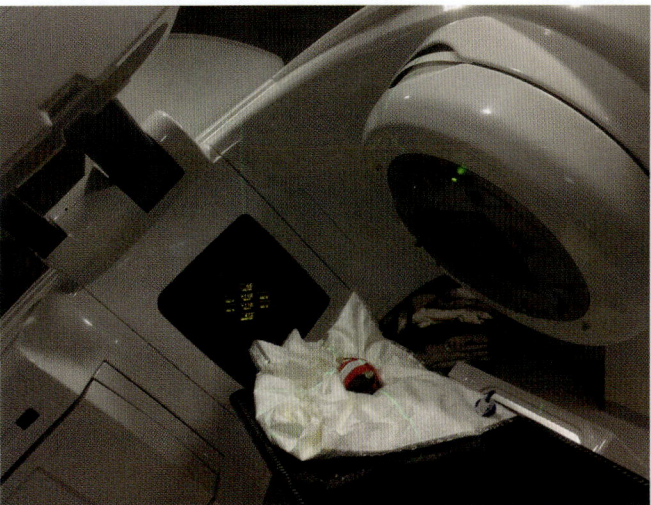

FIG 124.2 Turtle within the linear accelerator (Trilogy, Varian, Palo Alto, CA) at the University of Georgia. The machine is equipped with an on-board imaging system that allows the machine to perform cone-beam CT scans and take radiographs. (Courtesy of Joerg Mayer.)

surgeries, RT, and daily stress of handling). No physical changes to the scales in the radiation field were observed. However, the tumor increased in size during the course of RT. Twenty days after RT, the snake was further treated with intralesional chemotherapy (carboplatin), at which time debulking was also performed. A bacterial culture of the tumor, performed 32 days after RT, revealed *Mycobacterium chelonei*, and the snake was euthanized.

A 15-year-old Madagascar ground boa (*Boa madagascariensis*) with a squamous cell carcinoma was treated with two doses of x-ray radiation (10 Gy per fraction, total 20 Gy) 1 week apart.[2] The tumor increased in size after the first RT. The boa began open-mouth breathing, exhibited dysecdysis, and was euthanized 5 days after the second RT. MRI taken prior to euthanasia revealed streaky hyperintensities dissecting between facial planes surrounding the tumor, which were attributed to RT-induced edema and vasculitis. The electron beams produced by linear accelerators have a limited penetration depth of several (typically 1.5 to 5) centimeters from the skin surface, so electrons can be useful for treating superficial tumors when an underlying organ is to be spared (for example, a skin tumor over the thoracic cavity or the kidneys).

In one report, an adult yellow rat snake (*Pantherophis obsoleta quadrivittata*) with a subcutaneous malignant chromatophoroma in the middle of the body was treated with two surgical procedures.[7] Fifteen days after the second surgery, RT consisting of 4 fractions of 15 Gy (total 60 Gy) was given over 15 days by 6 MeV electron beams (the intervals between the RTs ranged from 3 to 6 days). Dry lackluster scales were noted in the irradiated area, which started 10 days after starting RT. The surgical site healed without a complication. The snake was irritable for several months following RT and anorexic for 20 weeks following the last RT. Ten months after the RT, the snake died with an abscess within the previous site of the tumor. In the caudal coelomic cavity, a lobulated mass was found, which appeared clinically identical to the irradiated subcutaneous tumor, although no histopathologic examination was performed on the new mass. Although the clinical

signs exhibited by this snake could be a result of acute and late radiation side effects, the aggressive radiation protocol used would have resulted in more severe acute effects and necrosis in mammals.

One of the authors (KN) treated a 26-year-old male yellow anaconda (*Eunectes notaeus*) with a 3 × 4 cm squamous cell carcinoma with sebaceous differentiation next to the cloaca. The anaconda was irradiated with 6 weekly doses of 6 Gy of electron beams. By the last fraction of radiation, the lesion had regressed significantly, the patient was noticeably more comfortable, and he had gained weight. At the 6-week follow-up visit, acute radiation effects were noted, including edema and loss of scales. The cutaneous lesions were treated symptomatically with antibiotics and buprenorphine. Despite these treatments, the lesions persisted (but improved) over the next 6 weeks and had almost resolved 16 weeks after therapy. Five months after completion of radiation, a purulent pocket was noted near the vent, which progressed to a nonhealing wound causing pain and bleeding. Fourteen months after treatment, the anaconda was constipated, depressed, had lost weight, and was unable to pass feces. He was euthanized 2 weeks later. Postmortem findings indicated recurrent squamous cell carcinoma of the vent with extensive regional invasion. Although the exact onset of tumor recurrence was unknown, radiation side effects could have contributed to the pericloacal, necrotic lesion seen in this snake.

Stereotactic radiation therapy (SRT) is an emerging method of RT that involves a high dose of radiation (typically x-rays) per treatment (usually 6 to 17 Gy per fraction in mammalian species). The dose used for SRT is significantly higher than the doses usually used for definitive RT (2.5–4 Gy) or for palliative RT (4–8 Gy). SRT is typically delivered in 1, 3, or 5 fractions (instead of 18–20 daily treatments, which is typical for a definitive RT). SRT may be a promising treatment method for reptiles because daily anesthesia episodes may not be feasible in many cases. SRT can be performed by advanced linear accelerators that have an on-board imaging system, which allows a CT scan immediately before each radiation treatment (Fig. 124.2). This technology allows an accurate and conformal beam delivery with a technique called IMRT (intensity modulated radiation therapy), which results in minimal volume of normal tissue exposed to a high dose of radiation. However, the authors are unaware of any documented reports of SRT use in reptiles.

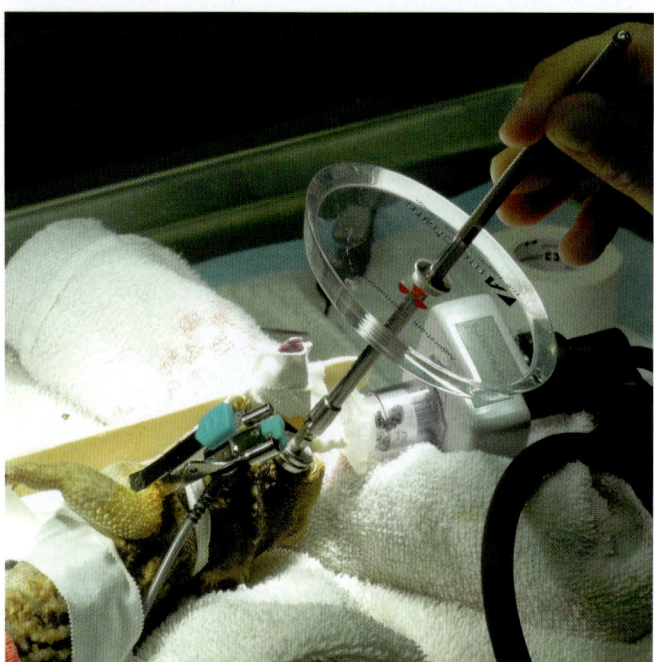

FIG 124.3 A lizard is receiving superficial radiation therapy from a strontium probe. The probe emits electrons that can only penetrate a few millimeters, which makes it suitable for the treatment of small, superficial tumors. (Courtesy of Joerg Mayer.)

STRONTIUM 90

Electrons emitted from a strontium-90 ophthalmic probe, which has an active source diameter of about 8 mm, has very limited penetration (the dose drops to <10% at 3 mm depth), and can deliver a high dose of radiation to the surface of the patient's body (100 Gy or higher) without causing significant side effects in mammals. In the authors' opinion, it should be used with caution if a tumor exceeds 3 to 4 mm in thickness, because the deeper portion of the tumor is likely to be underdosed. Strontium-90 radiation therapy may be an excellent treatment option for small superficial tumors (Fig. 124.3). In one case report, a bearded dragon (*Pogona vitticeps*) with a myxosarcoma on the medial canthus of the right eye was treated with a surgical debulking (all the gross disease was removed with the third eyelid) immediately followed by radiation therapy using strontium-90 ophthalmic probe with 100 Gy.[8] Tumor recurrence was noted 5 months later. Recurrence of the tumor may have been due to the locally infiltrative nature of the myxosarcoma, or the radiation probe may not have been accurately applied to the area of residual tumor tissue. Anecdotally, strontium-90 has resulted in successful treatments in other reptiles (according to the radiation oncologists' ACVR list serve).

RADIOACTIVE IMPLANTS

RT can also be performed by implanting radioactive "seeds" or "straws" directly into the tumor, although this type of RT is far less commonly performed in veterinary medicine. RT by using radioactive seeds was not successful for the treatment of melanoma in a common death adder (*Acanthophis antarcticus*) nor for the treatment of mast cell tumor in an eastern king snake (*Lampropeltis getulus getulus*).[9,10]

CONCLUSION

Given the body of evidence in the literature, radiation therapy may be a good option for some reptilian tumors. Based on some aforementioned case reports, some reptiles may tolerate radiation better than mammals. This may be due to the fact that reptiles are taxonomically closer to birds, which are known to tolerate radiation better than mammals. This may also indicate that radiation therapy should be more aggressively approached for reptiles compared to mammals. However, the greater radiation tolerance of reptiles is not consistently seen in all cases reported here. It is also possible that radiosensitivity may vary among different reptile taxa or even individual patients. Therefore, until more data become available, caution is advised when using aggressive radiation therapy in reptiles.

ACKNOWLEDGMENTS

The authors would like to thank Dr. Lili Duda for her assistance in the preparation of this chapter.

REFERENCES

See www.expertconsult.com for a complete list of references.

Miscellaneous Drug Therapy

Izidora Sladakovic and Rodney W. Schnellbacher

Many reptilian dosages are based on experience, case reports, or extrapolations from other species. Below is an overview of published reports on the use of miscellaneous drug therapies in reptiles for the support of various gastrointestinal, reproductive, renal, and hepatic diseases. Complete reptile and amphibian drug formularies can be found in Chapters 127 and 128.

GASTROINTESTINAL

The effects of cisapride (1 mg/kg PO SID) and metoclopramide (1 mg/kg PO SID) on the gastrointestinal transit time were investigated in desert tortoises (*Gopherus agassizii*) and compared with controls. Neither of these drugs significantly affected transit time.[1] Cisapride (1–4 mg/kg PO SID) has been recommended in bearded dragons (*Pogona vitticeps*) with constipation, in conjunction with correction of underlying conditions.[2] A green turtle (*Chelonia mydas*) received metoclopramide (0.05 mg/kg SC SID) for management of ileus following intestinal resection and anastomosis. After 7 days of therapy, no fecal production was observed. Following a change to cisapride (1 mg/kg PO SID), fecal production was observed after 5 days.[3] Sucralfate (1 g PO SID) was administered to a 23.5-kg loggerhead sea turtle (*Caretta caretta*) with melena, and normal feces were produced within a week.[4] Sucralfate, cimetidine, and activated charcoal suspension were administered to a South American red-footed tortoise (*Chelonoidis carbonaria*) with suspected ibuprofen toxicosis. The patient recovered, and no adverse effects associated with the treatment were observed.[5]

REPRODUCTIVE

A 4.7-mg deslorelin implant was used in a male bearded dragon for aggression. At reevaluation 2 months after implantation, there was significant reduction in aggression and a decline in serum testosterone level.[6] A study investigating the effect of leuprolide acetate on testosterone levels in male green iguanas for 35 days found no significant effect.[7]

In reptiles, arginine vasotocin is the endogenous hormone responsible for oviposition. However, the exogenous form is only available in a research setting; therefore oxytocin is used for nonobstructive dystocia. Oxytocin appears to be most effective in chelonians at relatively low doses and less effective in squamates. There are various treatment protocols and doses published. In general, if no oviposition has occurred after administration of two to three doses, it is unlikely to be effective, and ongoing administration can be detrimental. Concurrent use of prostaglandin $F_{2\alpha}$ or β-blockers may potentiate the effects of oxytocin.[8] See Chapter 80 for more details.

RENAL

Allopurinol (25 mg/kg PO SID) was administered to green iguanas with dietary-induced hyperuricemia, and uric acid concentrations were significantly lower compared with controls.[9] Allopurinol also reduced uric acid concentrations in European tortoises with hyperuricemia (Kolle, unpublished data). Lanthanum carbonate octahydrate reduced phosphorus levels in tortoises with renal disease (P. Kolle, unpublished data).

HEPATIC

Lactulose was used in a green iguana with pseudocarcinomatous biliary hyperplasia and was associated with a reduction in bile acid concentrations.[10]

Additional information on the management of diseases of the abovementioned systems can be found elsewhere in this text. In conclusion, the use of miscellaneous therapies is in its infancy in reptiles and further studies are needed to evaluate the efficacy and safety of these agents.

REFERENCES

See www.expertconsult.com for a complete list of references.

Allometric Scaling

Joerg Mayer

The principles of scaling have been known and used by physiologists for many decades.[1-3] Kleiber first introduced the general formula used in allometric scaling as aM[b], with **a** being the scaling constant, **M** the body mass, and **b** the scaling exponent.[2] The scaling exponent b was considered to be 0.75 for physiological rates (e.g., metabolic rate) and −0.25 for physiological durations (e.g., gestation, elimination). However, a formula that applies to every physiological aspect of every species of reptile is unlikely when dealing in the life sciences. Applying equations to ectothermic animals also brings additional uncertainty with it in regard to providing a predictable outcome. Recently there is also concern expressed that there is no universal 3/4-power law for the body-mass scaling of metabolic rate globally, as the slopes of metabolic scaling vary substantially from approximately 2/3 to 1 depending on the taxonomic group and/or physiological (activity) states.[4] Some studies have shown that a 2/3-power scaling is more accurate within species of mammals and reptiles than is 3/4-power scaling.[5] Gillooly et al. showed that the metabolic rate (the transformation of energy and materials) is governed by two factors: the Boltzman factor (a factor used to describe the temperature dependence of biochemical processes) and the specific allometric relation, used to describe the change of biologic processes with the change in body size.[16] Because the body temperature in reptiles is environmentally dependent and therefore not constant, prediction of the metabolic rates have to be made with the specific temperature optimal for the species. Berner was able to show the significance of this by measuring the oxygen consumption of mitochondria in reptiles at different temperatures.[6] Mader and colleagues were able to show the importance of temperature for pharmacokinetics in the gopher snake (*Pituophis catenifer*) dosed with amikacin.[7] Caligiuri et al. also showed the same effect of temperature on pharmacokinetics in gopher tortoises (*Gopherus polyphemus*) given amikacin.[8] The route of drug excretion is also an important aspect, and this might also complicate calculations just based on bodyweight alone. This phenomenon was observed by authors who examined the allometric basis of enrofloxacin scaling in green iguanas, which showed that enrofloxacin clearance cannot be easily predicted using metabolic scaling.[9]

The advantages of familiarity with certain allometric equations are obvious when dealing with a complex situation such as drug clearance or pharmacokinetic studies. In spite of limitations, these formulas help summarize data and gain information about basic anatomical and physiological facts.

PHYSIOLOGICAL APPLICATION OF SCALING

The fundamental need to apply allometric scaling according to body size has been explicitly published by Kirkwood.[10] The author uses the example of a 1 gm tissue sample from a shrew and a blue whale, pointing out that the tissue sample of the shrew has a 100 times higher metabolic rate than the tissue sample of the whale. With allometric scaling, one

has to keep in mind that all equations are merely descriptive in nature; they should NOT be considered biologic laws. Equations such as these are probably most useful when they are seen as tools to detect general patterns or used for estimations where data on physiological normals or pharmacokinetics are not available.

In the following list, a few reptile-specific formulas are compiled that might be of use to the reptile-oriented practitioner. Knowing physiological rules, such as maximum oxygen consumption (mL/min/kg) in reptiles with varying body temperature, can help monitor anesthetic procedures in controlled (surgery suite) or uncontrolled (field) environments. Growth rate and home range predictions can also be useful in the clinical setting.

Examples (Table 126.1), with **W** as bodyweight in kilograms and **L** as length in centimeters, include:

$13W^{0.8}$ = minimum energy (ME in kcal/d) requirements for free-living existence in lizards[11]
$6.5W^{0.75}$ = ME requirements for maintenance (kcal/d) in snakes[12]
$6W^{0.75}$ = ME requirements for maintenance (kcal/d) in chelonia[13]
$14.6W^{0.23}$ = life span in captivity (years) in reptiles[1]
$W = 0.0003L^{2.85}$ bodyweight in relation to carapace length in *Testudo greaca*[14]
$0.0012W^{0.61}$ = growth rate (g) of reptiles[1]
$4.8W^{0.95}$ = area (ha) home range of lizards[15]

Maximum oxygen consumption (mL/min/kg) in reptiles at varying body temperature[1]:

$3.1W^{0.81}$ lizards at 20°C	$3.3W^{0.83}$ reptiles at 20°C
$6.2W^{0.76}$ lizards at 30°C	$6.1W^{0.77}$ reptiles at 30°C
$9.5W^{0.76}$ lizards at 35°C	$8.1W^{0.71}$ reptiles at 35°C
$8.1W^{0.64}$ lizards at 40°C	$8.1W^{0.64}$ reptiles at 40°C

These calculations can be used to estimate the calorific requirements for hospitalized reptiles, and a calculation form is shown in Table 126.1. It must be remembered that such calculations are merely an estimation and should be modified based upon response and daily weight measurements. In addition there are often physiological variables that must be considered. For instance, when dealing with an emaciated, starving reptile, it is wise to start low (often 10%–20%) of calculated requirements to avoid refeeding syndrome or gastrointestinal overload.

PHARMACOLOGICAL APPLICATION OF SCALING

Allometric scaling can be extremely useful with calculation of a dose for a drug that has not been used in a reptile species before. Allometric data can provide additional information that may help better define and bring a greater level of rationality to the process of attempting to determine a dose that might be effective and not toxic. The formulas used may vary from species to species, between different aged animals

TABLE 126.1 Allometric Food Calculation Examples for Reptiles

Snakes

Species: Ball python	Weight: 0.546 kg
Daily minimum energy requirements = $6.5W^{0.75}$ = 4.13 KCal/day	
Energy factor required:	1
Frequency of feeding:	Every 4 days
Total energy requirement = 4.13 daily = 16.52 KCal every 4 days	
Food make and manufacturer:	Oxbow Carnivore Care
Food energy concentration:	1.6 KCal/mL (2 parts powder to 1 part warm water)
Total feed amount = 10.3 mL every 4 days*	

Lizard

Species: Bearded dragon	Weight: 0.306 kg
Daily minimum energy requirements = $13W^{0.8}$ = 5.04 KCal/day	
Energy factor required:	1
Frequency of feeding:	daily
Total energy requirement = 5.04 KCal daily	
Food make and manufacturer:	Emeraid Omnivore Care
Food energy concentration:	2.39 KCal/mL (3 parts powder to 2 parts hot water)
Total feed amount = 2.1 mL every day*	

Tortoise

Species: Leopard tortoise	Weight: 4.56 kg
Daily minimum energy requirements = $6W^{0.75}$ = 18.72 KCal/day	
Energy factor required:	1
Frequency of feeding:	Daily
Total energy requirement = 18.7 KCal daily	
Food make and manufacturer:	Oxbow Herbivore Care
Food energy concentration:	1.6 KCal/mL (2 parts powder to 1 part warm water)
Total feed amount = 11.7 mL every day*	

*These figures are mere estimates and should be modified based upon clinical situation and patient response. In cachexic reptiles, initial feedings may need to be reduced by 90% to avoid refeeding syndrome or gastrointestinal overload.

TABLE 126.2 Body Weight Conversion Table for Reptiles (K = 10)

BW (kg)	MEC	SMEC	BW (kg)	MEC	SMEC
0.01	0.316	31.623	1.20	11.465	9.554
0.02	0.532	26.591	1.30	12.175	9.365
0.03	0.721	24.028	1.40	12.871	9.193
0.04	0.894	22.361	1.50	13.554	9.036
0.05	1.057	21.147	1.60	14.226	8.891
0.06	1.212	20.205	1.70	14.888	8.758
0.07	1.361	19.441	1.80	15.540	8.633
0.08	1.504	18.803	1.90	16.183	8.517
0.09	1.643	18.257	2.00	16.818	8.409
0.10	1.778	17.783	2.50	19.882	7.953
0.15	2.410	16.069	3.00	22.795	7.598
0.20	2.991	14.953	3.50	25.589	7.311
0.25	3.536	14.142	4.00	28.284	7.071
0.30	4.054	13.512	4.50	30.897	6.866
0.35	4.550	13.001	5.00	33.437	6.687
0.40	5.030	12.574	5.50	35.915	6.530
0.45	5.494	12.209	6.00	38.337	6.389
0.50	5.946	11.892	6.50	40.708	6.263
0.55	6.387	11.612	7.00	43.035	6.148
0.60	6.817	11.362	7.50	45.321	6.043
0.65	7.239	11.137	8.00	47.568	5.946
0.70	7.653	10.933	8.50	49.781	5.857
0.75	8.059	10.746	9.50	54.112	5.696
0.80	8.459	10.574	10.00	56.234	5.623
0.85	8.852	10.415	15.00	76.220	5.081
0.90	9.240	10.267	20.00	94.574	4.729
0.95	9.623	10.129	25.00	111.803	4.472
1.00	10.000	10.000	30.00	128.186	4.273

BW, Body weight; *MEC*, minimum energy cost; *SMEC*, specific minimum energy cost.

$MEC = K \times BW_{kg}^{0.75} = kcal/d$

$SMEC = K \times BW_{kg}^{-0.25}$

K = 10, reptiles
K = 49, marsupial mammals
K = 70, placental mammals
K = 78, nonpasserine birds
K = 129, passerine birds

TABLE 126.3 Allometric Scaling Formulary for Reptiles

Drug	Model	Model Dose	Universal MEC Dose (yields mg/dose)	Frequency Coefficient (yields times/day)	Comments
Allopurinol	Human	300 mg sid	0.18	0.04	
Amikacin	Gopher snake[a]	5 mg/kg IM, then 2.5 mg/kg q 72 h	0.4 (loading) 0.2	0.024	PK dose available for gopher snake, alligator, water turtle
Ampicillin	Dog	22 mg/kg tid	0.665	0.09	
Calcium edetate (CaEDTA)	Avian	35 mg/kg bid	0.333	0.019	Scaled dose used successfully for snapping turtle (Borkowski, personal communication)
Carbenicillin	Dog	15 mg/kg PO, IV tid	0.453	0.091	PK dose available for snake, tortoise
	Snake[b] (1 kg)	400 mg/kg IM q 24 h	40	0.1	
	Tortoise[c] (1 kg)	400 mg/kg q 48 h	40	0.05	
Carprofen	Dog	4 mg/kg IV once	0.12	One time only	
		2.2 mg/kg PO bid	0.07	0.06	

Continued

TABLE 126.3   Allometric Scaling Formulary for Reptiles—cont'd

Drug	Model	Model Dose	Universal MEC Dose (yields mg/dose)	Frequency Coefficient (yields times/day)	Comments
Ceftazadime	Small snake[d]	20 mg/kg q 72 h	2.4	0.04	PK dose available for small snake; scaled dose recommended for large snakes
Cephalexin (Keflex)	Dog	22 mg/kg PO tid	0.665	0.091	
Cephalothin (Keflin)	Dog	15–35 mg/kg IM, SC, IV tid	0.453–1.0	0.091	
Chloramphenicol	Dog	25–50 mg/kg PO IM, IV tid	0.755–1.5	0.091	PK dose available for gopher snake, indigo snake, rat snake, and king snake, boas, rattlesnakes
	Snake[e] (1 kg)	50 mg/kg SC q 12–72 h	10.6	0.063–0.4	
Ciprofloxacin	Human	500 mg bid	0.3	0.08	PK dose available for chicken
Cisapride	Child	0.2 mg/kg qid-tid	0.006	0.1	Used successfully in tortoise (Kaufman, unpublished)
Clindamycin	Dog	10 mg/kg bid	0.271	0.054	
Colchicine	Macaw	0.01 mg/kg bid	0.00013	0.025	Anti-inflammatory for articular gout
Drontal PLUS Small (praziquantel/pyrantel pamoate/febantel)	Dog	1 tab (22.7/22.7/113.4 mg)	0.0064 tab/kcal (0.14/0.14/0.73)	Single treatment	Based on 3 kg dog; manufacturer's dose; successfully used in many herp species (Kaufman, unpublished)
Fenbendazole	Dog	50 mg/kg sid × 3 d	1.5	0.03	Toxicities reported in birds and reptiles; use with CAUTION; many empirical doses available
Fluconazole	Human	200 mg sid	0.12	0.04	
Flunixin meglumine	Horse	1.1 mg/kg sid	0.074	0.068	Used with good effect in reptiles (Kaufman, unpublished)
Gentamicin	Gophersnake[f]	2.5 mg/kg q 72 h	0.25	0.03	MEC dose recommended for large snakes; PK dose available for gopher snake, red-eared slider, alligator, many bird species
Itraconazole	Dog	2.5 mg/kg bid	0.076	0.06	
Ketoprofen	Horse	2.2 mg/kg sid	0.15	0.066	Used IM or IV, follow-up with oral carprofen for long-term therapy; successfully used in many reptile species (Flo Tseng, unpublished)
Metronidazole	Dog	7.5 mg/kg tid	0.2	0.08	Based on canine antibacterial dose; PK dose available for Iguana
	Iguana[g] (1.5 kg)	20 mg/kg PO q 24–48 h	2.2	0.055–0.1	
Praziquantel	Dog	5–10 mg/kg	0.3	Single dose	
Probenicid	Human	250–500 mg bid	0.148	0.08	
Rocuronium	Box turtle[h]	0.3–0.5 mg/kg IM	0.02–0.05	Single dose	For immobilization only, NOT ANALGESIC; reverse with gycopyrrolate/neostigmine
Trimethoprim-Sulfa	Dog	15 mg/kg bid	0.5	0.06	

To calculate a patient's dose:

1. Multiply the universal MEC dose by patient's MEC = mg/treatment
2. Multiply frequency coefficient by patient's SMEC = number of times/day

[a]Mader DR, Conzelman GM, Baggot JD: Effects of ambient temperature on the half-life and dosage regimen of amikacin in the gopher snake, *JAVMA* 187(11):1134–1136, 1985.

[b]Lawrence K, et al.: A preliminary study on the use of carbenicillin in snakes, *J Vet Pharmacol Ther* 7:119–124, 1984.

[c]Lawrence K: Use of carbenicillin in two species of tortoise, *Res Vet Sci* 40:413–415, 1986.

[d]Lawrence K, Muggleton PW, Needham JR: Preliminary study on the use of ceftazadime, a broad spectrum cephalosporin antibiotic, in snakes, *Res Vet Sci* 36:16–20, 1984.

[e]Clark CH, Rogers ED, Milton JL: Plamsa concentrations of chloramphenicol in snakes, *AJVR* 46(12):2654–2657, 1985.

[f]Bush M, et al: Biological half-life of gentamicin in gopher snakes, *AJVR* 39(1):171–173, 1978.

[g]Kolmstetter CM, et al: Pharmacokinetics of metronidazole in the green iguana, *J Herp Med Surg* 8(3):4–7, 1998.

[h]Kaufman GE, et al: Use of rocuronium for endotracheal intubation of North American Gulf Coast box turtles, *JAVMA* 222(8):1111–1115, 2003.
Bid, Twice daily; *IM*, intramuscularly; *IV*, intravenously; *MEC*, minimum energy cost; *PO*, orally; *q*, every; *qid*, four times daily; *sid*, once daily; *SC*, subcutaneously; *tid*, three times a day.

TABLE 126.4   Allometric Scaling Worksheet to Calculate the Universal Minimum Energy (MEC) Cost Dose From Published Dosages in the Literature

Required Data

Drug: _____

Source: _____

Model animal: _____

Body weight (BW; kg):_____

Dose: _____

Model animal MEC = $K \times BW_{kg}^{0.75}$ = _____

Single dose: _____mg (mg/kg × kg)

Universal MEC Dose Calculation

Divide known single dose (mg) by model animal MEC universal MEC
  dose = _____

Frequency Coefficient Calculation

Divide frequency (per 24 hr) by (model animal MEC/BW [kg]) frequency
  coefficient = _____

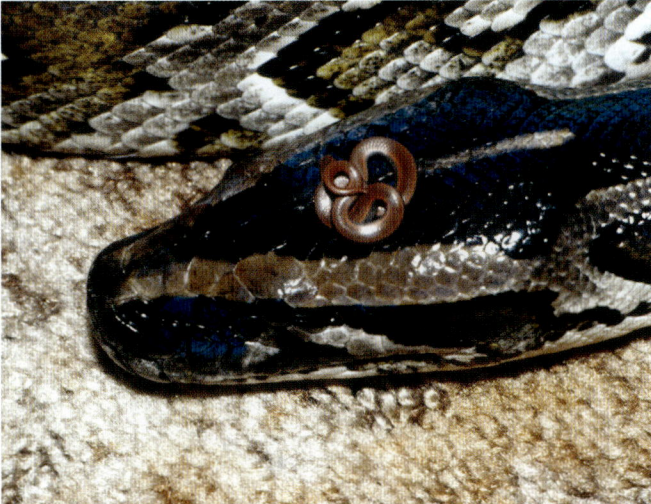

FIG 126.1 Allometric scaling allows extrapolation of dosages between animals of different sizes and between individuals of different species. Here, a full-grown sharp-tailed snake (*Contia tenuis*) has a body mass one one-thousandth of that of an adult Burmese python (*Python bivittatus*). (Courtesy of Douglas R. Mader.)

of the same species, for individuals kept at different environmental temperatures, and between healthy and ill animals.[16] Use of formulas incorporating species-specific data, when available, may help decrease error in prediction, but development of such models is still in the earliest stages. The technique described for drug calculation depends on metabolic rate alone and does not take into account differences in metabolism that may affect the uptake, modification, distribution, elimination, and thus the activity of a drug in a particular individual. This level of uncertainty must be kept in perspective when proceeding with the technique.

Allometric scaling is also extremely useful, and appears to be reliable, when used to calculate a dose from a small to a large animal (and vice versa) within the same or closely related taxonomic group. If a pharmacokinetically derived dose is available for a small snake, this information might be used to extrapolate a more accurate dose for a large snake, instead of merely using the mg/kg dose (Fig. 126.1). This principle is illustrated subsequently with the use of ceftazidime in a large snake.

The practical use of metabolic scaling in large reptiles has recently been illustrated by medetomidine immobilization and atipamezole reversal in large estuarine crocodiles.[17] The authors concluded that medetomidine at a metabolically scaled dosage was effective for immobilizing large estuarine crocodiles. In addition, atipamezole administered at a dosage calculated as a function of surface area effectively reversed immobilization.[17]

REVIEW OF TECHNIQUE

Allometric scaling uses a simple ratio comparing established data from a well-known animal with the unknown patient to derive a logical dose. The energy formula is used as a point of comparison between two subjects to establish predictable data.

Minimum energy cost = $K \times bodyweight_{kg}^{0.75}$

$K = 10$ reptiles

$K = 49$ marsupial mammals

$K = 70$ placental mammals

$K = 78$ nonpasserine birds

$K = 129$ passerine birds

With this formula, the minimum energy cost (MEC) can be predicted for both the well-known animal and the patient. With the addition of the drug dose information for the well-known animal, the drug dose can be predicted for the patient with a ratio:

$$\frac{\text{Well-known animal dose}}{\text{Well-known animal MEC}} = \frac{\text{Patient dose}}{\text{Patient MEC}}$$

The dose derived through this formula gives a suggested one-time or therapeutic dose for a particular drug in a novel patient. Sedgwick suggests a similar manipulation to calculate the periodicity, or frequency of dose administration.[18] This manipulation uses the mass specific minimum energy cost (SMEC).

$$\text{Specific minimum energy cost} = K \times bodyweight_{kg}^{-0.25}$$
$$= MEC/body\ weight_{kg}$$

Again, the ratio is used to develop the frequency of administration on the basis of a well-known animal:

$$\frac{\text{Well-known animal frequency (times per day)}}{\text{Well-known animal SMEC}}$$
$$= \frac{\text{Patient frequency (times per day)}}{\text{Patient SMEC}}$$

Following these two procedures results in a therapeutic dose and a frequency of administration. This dosage regimen may have to be adjusted for practical application. For example, a dose prediction of 4.2 mg to be given 0.4 times per day might be adjusted to 5 mg every 3 days. Adjustments should be made with safety, efficacy, and practicality in mind and must incorporate knowledge of the drug in question. In addition, maintaining careful and detailed records of outcomes after the use of allometrically scaled doses (e.g., measuring plasma drug levels) is prudent. Experience can help build confidence in the safety and efficacy of these estimated doses, which can be valuable in the future.

Choosing a Model

Attempts should be made to minimize metabolic and physiological differences between the well-known animal and the patient by basing comparisons on a pharmacokinetically derived dose of a closely related species as a model. For example, to determine a dose of ceftazidime for a 30 kg snake, an allometrically scaled dose based on the pharmacokinetically derived dose in a 2 kg snake is more accurate than a direct dose from a human or a dog or even the mg/kg dose established in the small snake. The 2 kg snake dose is 40 mg (20 mg/kg) every 3 days.[19] The 30 kg snake dose, based on allometric scaling from the smaller snake, is 307 mg (10.4 mg/kg) every 5 days.

Derivation of a Completely New Application

Considering the first time use of a new drug in a species is a complicated process. Drug discovery is currently moving at a dramatic pace, and newer and better therapies are continuingly being released for humans and domestic animals. Many of these novel antibiotics, antifungal agents, antiprotozoal drugs, and others are proving useful in reptile medicine.

Metabolic scaling continues to be useful in situations where pharmacokinetic information and empirical or experiential data are not available. This occurs most often with the application of new therapies, established in mammals or humans but not yet tried in reptiles. In these situations, a clinician must synthesize knowledge of the particular species involved, the medical condition at hand, and the various options for therapy used in other species with similar conditions.

A recent publication validated the idea of metabolic scaling and acknowledged the complexity of the concept, pointing out that no universal scaling exponent can be obtained for every case.[20] The authors conclude that individual extrapolation models should be built to obtain different scaling exponents specific to the species of interest.[20] At some point, a leap of faith is required to try a particular dosing regimen, hoping that safety is preserved and that efficacy is maintained.

CONCLUSION

Despite the controversies over the accuracy of allometric scaling in reptiles, the clinician dealing with reptiles finds that the methodology of scaling has distinct advantages in that it encourages us to think in detail about our patient's metabolism. As has been pointed out for humans and other mammals, some drugs appear to be scalable and others do not seem to be as predicable with current methods.

It must be restated that the method of allometric scaling should not be regarded as a substitute for pharmacology, but an addition to the problem-solving tool kit that clinicians must use when choosing the proper dosage for extra label pharmaceuticals. In human and veterinary medicine, one of the most common uses of allometric scaling is with the dosing of chemotherapeutic drugs, known to have a narrow margin of safety, by the use of body surface area to derive dosages instead of the standard mg/kg rate. Oncologists have long used body surface area (a rough approximation of metabolism) to derive dosages instead of the standard mg/kg rate.

Despite criticism, the need for allometric scaling is clear. It is of utmost importance when dosing a novel drug, for a novel species, to be conservative for safety reasons and aggressive for efficacy reasons.

The efficacy of antibiotic therapy will become more important as the number of resistant strains of bacteria continue to outstrip the introduction of novel antibiotics to the market. Which method would you use if you had to treat a 1 ton saltwater crocodile with a potentially nephrotoxic antibiotic?

ACKNOWLEDGMENT

The author thanks the coauthors of the previous version of this chapter for their significant contribution that provided the foundation for this updated edition.

REFERENCES

See www.expertconsult.com for a complete list of references.

127

Reptile Formulary

James W. Carpenter, Eric Klaphake, Paul M. Gibbons, and Kurt K. Sladky

This formulary is an updated version of the reptile formulary in the fifth edition of the *Exotic Animal Formulary* (James W. Carpenter, ed. St. Louis: Elsevier; 2018:81–116; 149–166), with permissions by the editor, contributors, and publisher.

For ease of use for the reptile chapter, drug dosages are first listed by "most species," followed by dosages in snakes, lizards, chelonians, and crocodilians; feed and water dosages are generally listed last. Some important considerations with the use of this formulary: Generic (nonproprietary) names of drugs are used in most instances.

Dosages are generally listed in ascending order (hence, dosages for a particular species may not always be listed together). For reptiles, dosages for drugs administered in the drinking water or food, nebulized or administered via nasal flush, are listed last.

Because most of the drugs mentioned in this text are not licensed for use in the species described, in some cases owner consent should be granted before their use. The superscript references include non-peer reviewed sources, including proceedings papers. Authors are encouraged to review the referenced sources and determine their reliability.

See the end of the chapter for a key to the abbreviations used in the formulary.

TABLE 127.1 Antimicrobial Agents[a]

Agent	Dosage	Species/Comments
Amikacin	—	Potentially nephrotoxic; maintain hydration; frequently used with a penicillin or cephalosporin
	26 µg/kg/hr via osmotic infusion pump implant[51,325]	Snakes/PD; consider loading dose at time of implant
	3.48 mg/kg IM once[155]	Pythons/PK (ball pythons)
	5 mg/kg IM, then 2.5 mg/kg q72h[199]	Gopher snakes/PD; house at high end of optimum temperature range during treatment
	5 mg/kg IM, then 2.5 mg/kg q72h[15,316]	Lizards
	5 mg/kg IM q48h[42]	Gopher tortoises/PK; 30°C (86°F)
	2.25 mg/kg IM q72h[146]	Alligators/PD
	50 mg/10 mL saline × 30 min nebulization q12h[99]	Most species/pneumonia; aminophylline at 25 mg/9 mL of sterile saline in nebulizer before antibiotics for bronchodilation[273]
Amoxicillin	22 mg/kg PO q12–24h[70,88]	Most species/use with an aminoglycoside
Ampicillin	—	May use with an aminoglycoside
	10–20 mg/kg SC, IM q12h[148]	Most species, including chameleons
	50 mg/kg SC, IM q12h[297]	Chelonians
	20 mg/kg IM q24h[99]	Tortoises
	50 mg/kg IM q12h[311]	Tortoises/PD
Azithromycin	10 mg/kg PO q2–7d[55]	Ball pythons/PK; single dose study; may cause nonregenerative anemia; *Mycoplasma, Cryptosporidium, Giardia*, and other susceptible organisms; location dictates dosage frequency: skin, q3d; respiratory tract, q5d; liver/kidneys, q7d
Carbenicillin	—	Discontinued; more stable than ampicillin; extended G-spectrum
	200 mg/kg IM q24h[134]	Carpet pythons/PK
	400 mg/kg IM q24h[181]	Snakes/PD; 30°C (86°F)
	400 mg/kg IM q48h[180]	Chelonians/PD (*Testudo* spp.)
Cefazolin	22 mg/kg IM q24h[264]	Chelonians
Cefoperazone (Cefobid, Pfizer)	100 mg/kg IM q96h[90]	Snakes/PD (false water cobras; 24°C [75°F])
	125 mg/kg IM q24h[90]	Lizards/PD (tegus; 24°C [75°F])
Cefotaxime	20–40 mg/kg IM q24h[99]	Most species/may use with an aminoglycoside
	100 mg/10 mL saline × 30 min nebulization q24h[238]	Most species/pneumonia

Continued

TABLE 127.1 Antimicrobial Agents—cont'd

Agent	Dosage	Species/Comments
Cefovecin	—	Short dosing interval is likely for most reptile species[240,329]
	10 mg/kg SC q12h[240]	Green iguanas/PD (25°C [77°F])
	10 mg/kg SC q24h[326]	Red-eared sliders/PK; long-acting cephalosporin; rapid decline in plasma concentrations; not recommended as a long-acting antibiotic; however, adequate to treat select bacteria q24h
Ceftazidime	20–40 mg/kg SC, IM, q48–72h[90,316,338]	Most species/chameleons use q24h
	20 mg/kg SC, IM, IV q72h[15,179]	Snakes/PD; 30°C (86°F); often effective against gram-negative aerobes (i.e., *Pseudomonas*)
	22 mg/kg IM, IV q72h[140,319]	Sea turtles
Ceftiofur	2.2 mg/kg IM q48h[70]	Snakes/ceftiofur sodium
	15 mg/kg IM q24–120h[1]	Snakes/PK; ceftiofur crystalline-free acid; ball pythons; 26.1°C (79°F); dosing interval based on MIC
	5 mg/kg SC, IM q24h[25]	Lizards/PK; ceftiofur sodium; (green iguanas)
	5 mg/kg IM q24h[285]	Green iguanas/PK; ceftiofur crystalline-free acid; no significant adverse affects noted
	30 mg/kg IM, SC[50]	Lizards/PK; ceftiofur crystalline-free acid; bearded dragons 30°C (86°F); interval may be q10–12d
	2.2 mg/kg IM q24h[70]	Turtles/ceftiofur sodium
	4 mg/kg IM q24h[70]	Tortoises/ceftiofur sodium; upper respiratory infection
Cefuroxime	100 mg/kg IM q24h[70]	Most species/30°C (86°F)
Cephalexin	20–40 mg/kg PO q12h[90]	Most species/unknown absorption
Cephalothin	20–40 mg/kg IM q12h[90]	Most species
Chloramphenicol	—	Most species/public health concern; reserve for meningitis or encephalitis caused by susceptible organisms
	40 mg/kg PO, SC, IM q24h, or 20 mg/ kg PO, SC, IM q12h[90]	Most species/20 mg/kg may be given q24h in larger crocodilians
	40 mg/kg SC q24h[40]	Snakes/PD (gopher snakes, 29°C [84°F])
	50 mg/kg SC q12–72h[52]	Snakes/PD; q12h in indigo, rat, king snakes; q24h in boids, moccasin snakes; q48h in rattlesnakes; q72h in red-bellied water snakes
Chlorhexidine (Nolvasan 2%, Fort Dodge)	Topical 0.05% aqueous solution q24h[224]	All species/topical disinfection; dermatitis; infectious stomatitis; periodontal disease in lizards q24h
	Topical 0.07% (1:30 [solution:water])[34,237]	Most species/topical disinfection; infectious stomatitis; abscess lavage; middle ear infection flush in box turtles
Chlortetracycline	200 mg/kg PO q24h[90]	Most species
Ciprofloxacin	10 mg/kg PO q48h[70]	Most species
	11 mg/kg PO q48–72h[167]	Pythons/PD (reticulated pythons)
Ciprofloxacin ophthalmic ointment or drops (Ciloxan, Alcon)	Topical[99]	All species/infectious stomatitis; gingivitis
Clarithromycin	15 mg/kg PO q84h[344]	Tortoises/PD (desert tortoises); upper respiratory tract disease (mycoplasmosis)
Clindamycin	10 mg/kg PO, IM, IV q12h[115]	Loggerhead sea turtles/PK; 29.1–30.3°C (84.4–86.5°F) insufficient to be effective
Danofloxacin	6 mg/kg SC, IM[213]	Loggerhead sea turtles
	6 mg/kg SC q48h × 30 days[99]	Tortoises/upper respiratory tract disease
Dihydrostreptomycin	5 mg/kg IM q12–24h[88,99]	Most species/maintain hydration
Doxycycline (Vibramycin, Pfizer)	5–10 mg/kg PO q24h × 10–45 days[99]	Most species/respiratory infection (i.e., mycoplasmosis)
	50 mg/kg IM, then 25 mg/kg q72h[37,311]	Tortoises/Hermann's tortoise; 27°C (81°F)
Enrofloxacin	5–10 mg/kg q24h PO, SC, IM, ICe[99]	Most species/IM administration is painful and may result in tissue necrosis and sterile abscesses; may cause skin discoloration or tissue necrosis if given SC; to administer SC, dilute with sterile NaCl
	6.6 mg/kg IM q24h, or 11 mg/kg IM q48h[167]	Pythons/PD (reticulated pythons); *Pseudomonas*
	10 mg/kg IM q48h[338,339,351]	Snakes/PK (Burmese pythons, rattlesnakes, pit vipers)
	5 mg/kg PO, IM q24h[218]	Lizards/PD (green iguanas); marked pharmacokinetic variability with PO administration may make IM more suitable in critically ill animals
	10 mg/kg IM q5d[136]	Monitors/PK (savannah monitors); preliminary data
	5 mg/kg IM q24–48h[267]	Chelonians and most other reptiles/PD (gopher tortoises); hyperexcitation, incoordination, diarrhea reported in a Galapagos tortoise[47]

TABLE 127.1 Antimicrobial Agents—cont'd

Agent	Dosage	Species/Comments
	5 mg/kg IM q12–24h[276]	Chelonians/PK (Indian star tortoises); q12h for *Pseudomonas* and *Citrobacter*; q24h for other bacteria
	5 mg/kg IV, IM q48h[176]	Sea turtles/PK (loggerhead sea turtles)
	10 mg/kg ICe q48h[104,286]	Chelonians/PD (Hermann's tortoises; yellow-bellied sliders) dilute with saline to 10 mg/mL
	10 mg/kg IM q24h[311]	Chelonians/PD (Hermann's tortoises)
	5 mg/kg IV q36–72h[125,215]	Crocodilians/PK; PO pharmacokinetics not fully determined; mycoplasmosis
	Nasal flush 50 mg/250 mL sterile water; 1–3 mL/naris q24–48h[99]	Tortoises/URT syndrome; use until no more discharge (5–10 days); may use concurrently with parenteral antibiotics
Gentamicin	—	Nephrotoxicity has been reported,[234] especially in snakes; maintain hydration; use with a penicillin or cephalosporin
	2.5 mg/kg IM q72h[40,41]	Snakes/PD (gopher snakes)
	2.5–3 mg/kg IM, then 1.5 mg/kg q96h[130]	Snakes/PK (blood pythons)
	3 mg/kg IM q > 96h[17]	Turtles/PD (eastern box turtles; 29°C [84°F]); lower dose may be more appropriate
	6 mg/kg IM q72–96h[274]	Turtles/PD (red-eared sliders; 24°C, [75°F])
	1.75–2.25 mg/kg IM q72–96h[146]	Crocodilians/PK (alligators); respiratory infection
Gentamicin ophthalmic ointment or drops	Topical[88]	Most species/superficial ocular infection; lesions in oral cavity
Gentamicin/betamethasone ophthalmic drops (Gentocin Durafilm, Merck)	1–2 drops to eye q12–24h[152]	Tortoises/upper respiratory infections; may also be given as a reverse nasal flush q48–72h or intranasal q12–24h
Kanamycin	10–15 mg/kg IM, IV q24h (or divided doses)[70,88]	Most species/24°C (75°F); give with fluid therapy; avoid in cases of dehydration or renal or hepatic dysfunction
Lincomycin	5 mg/kg IM q12–24h[70]	Most species/wound infection; potentially nephrotoxic; maintain hydration
	10 mg/kg PO q24h[70]	Most species
Marbofloxacin	10 mg/kg PO q48h[56]	Ball pythons/PD
Metronidazole	20 mg/kg PO q48h × ≥ 7 days[99]	Most species/anaerobes
	50 mg/kg PO q24h × 7–14 days[167]	Most species/may be administered concurrently with amikacin for broader spectrum; because of potential side effects at this dose, a lower dose may be prudent
	20 mg/kg PO q48h[31,172]	Snakes/PK (corn and rat snakes)
	20 mg/kg PO q24–48h[173]	Iguanas/PK; use q24h for resistant anaerobes
Oxytetracycline	6–10 mg/kg PO, IM, IV q24h[70,88]	Most species/may produce local inflammation at injection site
	10 mg/kg IM, IV q5d[124]	Crocodilians/PK (alligators; 27°C [81°F]); mycoplasmosis
Penicillin, benzathine	10,000–20,000 U/kg IM q48–96h[90]	Most species/may use with an aminoglycoside
Penicillin G	10,000–20,000 U/kg SC, IM, IV, ICe q8–12h[88]	Most species/infrequently used
Piperacillin	50–100 mg/kg IM q24h[70,88]	Most species/broad-spectrum bactericidal agent; maintain hydration; may use with an aminoglycoside
	50 mg/kg IM, then 25 mg/kg q24h[70,99]	Snakes
	100 mg/kg IM q48h[131]	Snakes/PK (blood pythons)
	100–200 mg/kg SC, IM q24–48h[148]	Chameleons
	100 mg/10 mL saline × 30 min nebulization q12h[238]	Most species/pneumonia
Polymyxin B sulfate, neomycin sulfate, bacitracin zinc ointment	Topical[99]	All species/rostral abrasions, dermal wounds
Povidone-iodine solution (0.05%) or ointment	Topical/lavage[88,256]	All species/fungal dermatitis; dermatophilosis; contaminated wound; can soak in 0.005% aqueous solution ≤ 1 hr q12–24h
Silver sulfadiazine cream (Silvadene, Marion)	Topical q24–72h[197]	All species/broad-spectrum antibacterial for skin (i.e., wounds, burns) or oral cavity; dressing is generally not necessary
Streptomycin	10 mg/kg IM q12–24h[88]	Most species/potentially nephrotoxic; maintain hydration; avoid in cases of dehydration or renal or hepatic dysfunction
Sulfadiazine	25 mg/kg PO q24h[99]	Most species/maintain hydration
Sulfadimethoxine	90 mg/kg IM, then 45 mg/kg q24h[88]	Most species/potentially nephrotoxic; maintain hydration

Continued

TABLE 127.1   Antimicrobial Agents—cont'd

Agent	Dosage	Species/Comments
Ticarcillin (Ticar, SmithKline-Beecham)	50–100 mg/kg IM q24h[88]	Most species/maintain hydration
	50–100 mg/kg IM, IV q24–48h[203]	Loggerhead sea turtles/PK
Tobramycin	—	Potentially nephrotoxic; maintain hydration; potentiated by ß-lactams
	2.5 mg/kg IM q24–72h[70]	Most species
	10 mg/kg IM q24–48h[70]	Chelonians/can be given q48h in tortoises; fluid therapy recommended
Trimethoprim/sulfadiazine or sulfamethoxazole	—	Maintain hydration; parenteral form must be compounded
	10–30 mg/kg PO q24h[99]	Most species/maintain hydration
	30 mg/kg IM q24h × 2 days, then q48h[311]	Tortoises/PD
Tylosin	5 mg/kg IM q24h × 10–60 days[70]	Most species/mycoplasmosis

[a]Because reptiles are ectothermic, pharmacokinetics of drugs are influenced by ambient temperature. Antimicrobial therapy should be conducted at the upper end of the patient's preferred (selected) optimum temperature zone.

TABLE 127.2   Antiviral Agents

Agent	Dosage	Species/Comments
Acyclovir	40–80 mg/kg PO[4]	Box turtles/PK, low maximum plasma concentrations; uncertain efficacy
	≥ 80 mg/kg PO q24h[92]	Tortoises/PK; herpesvirus; poor oral absorption
	80 mg/kg PO q8h, or 240 mg/kg PO q24h[219]	Tortoises/herpesvirus; uncertain efficacy; unlikely to eliminate infection; combine with supportive care
	80 mg/kg PO q24h[255]	Mediterranean tortoises/decreased mortality in those infected with TeHV-3
	80 mg/kg PO q24h[58]	Australian Krefft's river turtles/herpesvirus; uncertain efficacy
	Topical (5% ointment) q12h[88]	All species/antiviral (i.e., herpesvirus-associated dermatitis)
Chlorhexidine solution	0.5% dilution, topical on oral lesions q24h[162]	Tortoises/herpesvirus
Famcyclovir	10–30 mg/kg PO q24h using allometric scaling[302]	Eastern box turtles/treated during outbreak of concurrent TeHV-1 and ranavirus (FV-3); uncertain efficacy
Valacyclovir	40 mg/kg PO q24h[4]	Box turtles/PK, effective plasma concentrations compared with humans; uncertain efficacy or toxicity

TABLE 127.3   Antifungal Agents

Agent	Dosage	Species/Comments
Amphotericin B	0.5 mg/kg IV q48–72h[89]	Most species/nephrotoxic; can use in combination with ketoconazole; administer slowly
	0.5–1 mg/kg IV, ICe q24–72h × 14–28 days[70]	Most species/aspergillosis
	1 mg/kg IT q24h × 14–28 days[147]	Most species/respiratory infection; dilute with water or saline
	0.1 mg/kg intrapulmonary q24h × 28 days[126]	Greek tortoises/pneumonia
	1 mg/kg q24h ICe × 2–4 wk[185]	Crocodilians
	5 mg/150 mL saline × 1 hr nebulization q12h × 7 days[143]	Most species/pneumonia
Chlorhexidine (Nolvasan 2%, Fort Dodge)	20 mL/g water bath[345]	Lizards/dermatophytosis
Clotrimazole (Veltrim, Haver-Lockhart; Otomax, with gentamicin and betamethasone, Schering-Plough)	Topical[281]	Most species/dermatitis; may bathe q12h with dilute organic iodine before use
F10 super concentrate disinfectant (Health and Hygiene, Roodeport, South Africa)	1 : 250 nasal flush, 0.1 mL each nare q24h[49]	Terrestrial chelonians/benzalkonium chloride/polyhexamethylene biguanide HCl
Fluconazole	5 mg/kg PO q24h[345]	Lizards/dermatophytosis
	21 mg/kg SC once, then 10 mg/kg SC 5 days later[116,201]	Loggerhead sea turtles/PK
Griseofulvin	15 mg/kg PO q72h[149–151]	Most species
	20–40 mg/kg PO q72h × 5 treatments[281]	Most species/dermatitis; limited success

TABLE 127.3   Antifungal Agents—cont'd

Agent	Dosage	Species/Comments
Itraconazole	5 mg/kg PO q24h[214]	Most species/some hepatotoxicity noted when used for *Chrysosporium* anamorph of *Nannizziopsis vriesii*; can cause anorexia in bearded dragons without evidence of hepatotoxicity[97]
	5 mg/kg SC[184]	Cottonmouths/deaths in 3 out of 4 animals; not recommended
	10 mg/kg PO q24h[231]	Snakes
	5 mg/kg PO q24h[121]	Panther chameleons
	10 mg/kg PO q48h × 60 days[28]	Chameleons (Parson's)/osteomyelitis
	23.5 mg/kg PO q24h[94]	Lizards/PD (spiny lizards); following a 3-day treatment, a therapeutic plasma concentration persists for 6 days beyond peak concentration; treatment interval was not determined
	5 mg/kg PO q24h, or 15 mg/kg PO q72h[204]	Kemp's ridley sea turtles
Ketoconazole	—	May use antibiotics concomitantly to prevent bacterial overgrowth; may use concurrently with thiabendazole
	15 mg/kg q72h PO[149–151]	Most species
	25 mg/kg PO q24h × 21 days[144]	Snakes, turtles
	15–30 mg/kg PO q24h × 14–28 days[217,260]	Chelonians/PK (gopher tortoises); systemic infection
	50 mg/kg PO q24h × 14–28 days[99]	Crocodilians
Malachite green	0.15 mg/L water × 1 hr bath × 14 days[70]	Dermatitis
Miconazole (Monistat-Derm, Ortho)	Topical[281]	Most species/dermatitis; may bathe q12h with dilute organic iodine before use
Nystatin	100,000 U/kg PO q24h × 10 days[143]	Most species/enteric yeast infections; limited success
Terbinafine	3.4 mg/kg PO q24h × 15 mo[322]	Aldabra tortoises/severe phaeohyphomycosis of carapace; nonresponsive to itraconazole
	Topical[158]	Use in conjunction with oral azoles for *Chrysosporium* anamorph of *Nannizziopsis vriesii*; expect long treatment calendar
Tolnaftate 1% cream (Tinactin, Schering-Plough)	Topical q12h prn[3]	Most species/dermatitis; may bathe q12h with dilute organic iodine before use
Voriconazole	10 mg/kg per cloacal 3/wk × 4 wk[222]	Rattlesnakes/*Ophidiomyces ophiodiicola*; crushed in suspension (Ora-Plus, Paddock Laboratories)
	10 mg/kg PO × 47 days[301,333]	Bearded dragons for *Chrysosporium* anamorph of *Nannizziopsis vriesii*; possible hepatocellular injury
	5 mg/kg SC[138]	Red-eared sliders/exceeded MIC only until 4 hr postinjection; 26°C (78°F)
	10 mg/kg SC q12h × 7 days[142]	Red-eared sliders/resulted in trough concentrations considered subtherapeutic in humans but may reach MIC for some reptile fungal isolates; possible side effects seen
Voriconazole (V)/F10 super concentrate disinfectant (F10, Health and Hygiene, Roodeport, S Africa)	(V) 10 mg/kg PO q24h × 60 days + (F10) 1:250 dilution for 20 min bath q24h × 60 days[289]	Luthega skinks/systemic *Lecanicillium* sp. infection; nonresponsive to oral voriconazole and terbinafine ointment

TABLE 127.4   Antiparasitic Agents

Agent	Dosage	Species/Comments
Albendazole	50 mg/kg PO[99]	Most species/ascarids; most toxic of the benzimidazoles
Carbaryl powder (5%)	Lightly dust animal and environment; rinse after 1 hr; repeat in 7 days[79,90]	Lizards, snakes/mites
Chloroquine	125 mg/kg PO q48h × 3 treatments[99]	Tortoises/hemoprotozoa
Dichlorvos (Vapona No-Pest Strip; United Industries)	6 mm strip/10 ft³ in cage × 3 hr q48h × 2–4 wk[88,347]	Most species/mites; toxicity occurs;[90] prevent contact with animals (e.g., place strip above cage or inside perforated container); avoid in cases of renal or hepatic dysfunction; remove water container; use is discouraged
Dimetridazole (Emtryl, Rhône-Poulenc)	—	Not available in the United States
	100 mg/kg PO once, repeat in 2 wk[99]	Most species/amoebae
	40 mg/kg PO q24h × 5–8 days[143]	Snakes (except milk and indigo)/amoebae; flagellates
	40 mg/kg PO, repeat in 14 days[99]	Milk and indigo snakes/amoebae; flagellates

Continued

TABLE 127.4   **Antiparasitic Agents—cont'd**

Agent	Dosage	Species/Comments
Emodepside (1.98%) + praziquantel (7.94%) (Profender, Bayer)	1.12 mL/kg[225,291]	Many species/PD; nematodes; cestodes; aquatic turtles must be kept dry for 48 hr after application; appears to be safe but need more safety and efficacy data
Fenbendazole	—	Drug of choice for nematodes; least toxic of the benzimidazoles; may have an antiprotozoan effect; overdose may cause leukopenia, avoid in septicemic patients[242]
	25–100 mg/kg PO q14d for up to 4 treatments[37,143,166]	All species/nematodes
	100 mg/kg once[96]	Tortoises/nematodes; shedding of ova continues for 30 days
Fipronil (0.29%; Frontline Spray, Merial)	Wipe on then wash off in 5 min q7–10d prn[76,79]	Most species/mites, ticks; beware of reactions to alcohol carrier; needs safety evaluation[99]
Imidocloprid and moxidectin (Advantage Multi/Advocate, Bayer)	0.2 mg/kg topical q14d × 3 treatments[110]	Lizards/eliminated hookworms and pinworms; needs safety and pharmacokinetic evaluation
Ivermectin	—	Do not use in chelonians,[328] crocodilians, indigo snakes, or skinks[37,99,168]
	0.2 mg/kg PO, SC, IM, repeat in 14 days[80,99]	Snakes (except indigos), lizards (except skinks)[37]/nematodes (including lungworms),[190] mites; can dilute with propylene glycol for oral use; colored animals may have skin discoloration at injection site; rare adverse effects reported in chameleons, possibly associated with breakdown of parasites;[15] do not use within 10 days of diazepam or tiletamine/zolazepam; rare death and occasional nervous system signs, lethargy, or inappetence have been reported;[168] used for pentastomids in monitor lizards (with dexamethasone 0.2 mg/kg q2d)[80]
	5–10 mg/L water topical spray q3–5d up to 28 days[168]	Snakes (except indigos), lizards (except skinks)/mites; less effective than fipronil; spray on skin and in newly cleaned cage, then allow to dry before replacing water dish
Levamisole (Levasole 13.65%, Mallinckrodt)	5–10 mg/kg SC, ICe, repeat in 14 days[15,99,143]	Most species/lungworms; 5 mg/kg in chelonians; 10 mg/kg in lizards, snakes; very narrow range of safety; main advantage is that it can be administered parenterally; avoid concurrent use with chloramphenicol; avoid use in debilitated animals; low dose may stimulate depressed immune system; can be used IM, but less effective
Mebendazole	20–25 mg/kg PO, repeat in 14 days prn[143]	Most species/strongyles, ascarids, effective dosage of 400 mg/kg;[174] may be toxic
Metronidazole	—	Protozoan (i.e., flagellates, amoebae) overgrowth; may stimulate appetite; may cause severe neurological signs at doses > 200 mg/kg;[232] death occurred in indigo and mountain king snakes at 100 mg/kg;[143] injectable form can be administered PO; oral suspension is not available in the United States, but can be compounded
	40–100 mg/kg PO, repeat in 10–14 days[88]	Most species/flagellate overgrowth
	20 mg/kg PO q48h[31]	Corn snakes/PK; 28°C (82°F); protozoa
	40 mg/kg PO, repeat in 14 days[90,143]	Uracoan rattler, milk, tricolor king, and indigo snakes/flagellates
	40–60 mg/kg PO q7d × 2–3 doses[317]	Chameleons/flagellates; amoebae
	40–200 mg/kg PO, repeat in 14 days[228]	Geckos/ocular lesions (40 mg/kg) and subcutaneous lesions (200 mg/kg) caused by *Trichomonas*
	20 mg/kg ICe q48h[137]	Red-eared sliders/PK; ICe administration not recommended; needs further safety evaluation
	25 mg/kg PO q24h × 5 days[99]	Chelonians/amoebiasis
Milbemycin	0.25–0.5 mg/kg SC prn[30]	Chelonians/nematodes; parenteral form is not commercially available in United States; fenbendazole preferred
Nitrofurazone	25.5 mg/kg PO[340]	Most species/coccidia; seldom used
Olive oil	Coat skin q7d[15,79]	Most species, especially small, delicate lizards/mites; wash animal with mild soap (and rinse well) the next day; messy to use; environment must be treated with acaricide
Oxfendazole (Benzelmin, Fort Dodge)	66 mg/kg PO once[96]	Most species/nematodes; may be repeated after 28 days prn
Paromomycin (Humatin, Parke Davis)	35–100 mg/kg PO q24h × ≤ 28 days[88,143]	Most species/amoebae
	100 mg/kg PO q24h × 7 days, then 2×/wk × 3 mo[59]	Snakes/cryptosporidia; reduced clinical signs and oocyte shedding; does not eliminate the organism
	300–360 mg/kg PO q48h × 14 days[261]	Lizards (Gila monsters)/cryptosporidia
	300–800 mg/kg PO q24h prn[54]	Geckos/cryptosporidia; reduced clinical signs; does not eliminate the organism
	360 mg/kg PO q48h × 10 days[109]	Bearded dragons/intestinal cryptosporidia

TABLE 127.4 Antiparasitic Agents—cont'd

Agent	Dosage	Species/Comments
Permethrin (Provent-a-Mite, Pro Products)	Environmental treatment, 1 sec of spray/ft²; wait until dry before returning animal to enclosure[79]	Lizards, snakes/mites; ticks; FDA approved; safe and effective; wash immediately if accidentally applied to skin
	Topical[79]	Tortoises/ticks
Piperazine	40–60 mg/kg PO, repeat in 14 days[174]	Most species/strongyles, ascarids; poor efficacy at < 400 mg/kg[174]
	100–200 mg/kg PO[135]	Crocodilians
Ponazuril	30 mg/kg PO q48h × 2 treatments[32,233]	Bearded dragons/coccidiosis
Praziquantel	—	See also emodepside
	8 mg/kg PO, SC, IM, repeat in 14 days[15,99,148]	Most species/cestodes, trematodes; higher dosages have been administered[90]
Praziquantel (P) and emodepside (E) (Profender, Bayer)	(P) 5.5 mg/kg + (E) 21.5 mg (1 mL/kg) topical[327]	Tortoises/moderate efficacy against oxyurids in 2 of 4 species; efficacy against ascarids was not concluded; well-tolerated
	25–50 mg/kg PO q3h × 3 treatments[2,145]	Sea turtles (green, loggerhead)/PD; spirorchidiasis
Pyrantel pamoate	5 mg/kg PO, repeat in 14 days[168]	Most species/nematodes
	25 mg/kg PO q24h × 3 days; repeat in 3 wk[90]	Most species/ascarids, hookworms, pinworms
Pyrethrin spray (0.09%)	Topical q7d × 2–3 treatments[79]	Most species/use water-based sprays labeled for kittens and puppies; apply with cloth; can also spray cage, wash out after 30 min; use sparingly and with caution; pyrethroids are safer (see permethrin, resmethrin)
Quinacrine (Atabrine, Winthrop)	19–100 mg/kg PO q48h × 14–21 days[340]	Most species/some hematozoa
Quinine sulfate	75 mg/kg PO q48h × 14–28 days[340]	Most species/some hematozoa; toxic at > 100 mg/kg q24h; ineffective against exoerythrocytic forms
Spiramycin (Spirasol, May and Baker)	160 mg/kg PO q24h × 10 days, then 2×/wk × 3 mo[59]	Snakes/cryptosporidia; may reduce clinical signs and oocyte shedding; does not eliminate the organism
Sulfadiazine, sulfamerazine	—	Most species/coccidia; avoid sulfa drugs in cases of dehydration, urinary calculi, or renal dysfunction[232]
	75 mg/kg PO, then 45 mg/kg q24h × 5 days[88,340]	Most species/coccidia
	25 mg/kg PO q24h × 21 days[15,340]	Snakes, lizards/coccidia
Sulfadimethoxine	50 mg/kg PO q24h × 3–5 days, then q48h prn[168]	Most species/coccidia; ensure adequate hydration and renal function
	90 mg/kg PO, IM, IV, then 45 mg/kg q24h × 5–7 days[88,143,340]	Most species/coccidia
	50 mg/kg PO q24h × 21 days[334]	Bearded dragons/coccidia
Sulfadimidine (33% solution)	0.3–0.6 mL/kg PO q24h × 10 days[340]	Most species/coccidia; alternatively, 0.3–0.6 mL/kg, then 0.15–0.3 mL/kg q24h × 10 days
	1 oz/gal drinking water × 10 days[340]	Most species/coccidia
Sulfamethazine	25 mg/kg PO, IM q24h × 21 days[340]	Most species/coccidia
	50 mg/kg PO q24h × 3 days, off 3 days, on 3 days[99]	Most species/coccidia
	75 mg/kg PO, IM, IV, then 40 mg/kg q24h × 5–7 days[143]	Most species/coccidia; ensure adequate hydration and renal function
Sulfaquinoxaline	75 mg/kg PO, then 40 mg/kg q24h × 5–7 days[143]	Most species/coccidia
Thiabendazole	50–100 mg/kg PO, repeat in 14 days[89,143]	Most species/nematodes; fenbendazole preferred
Toltrazuril 5% (Baycox, Bayer)	5–15 mg/kg q24h × 3 days[73]	Bearded dragons/coccidiosis
	15 mg/kg q48h × 30 days[100]	Tortoises/coccidiosis; needs safety, efficacy, and pharmacokinetic study

Continued

TABLE 127.4   Antiparasitic Agents—cont'd

Agent	Dosage	Species/Comments
Trimethoprim/sulfa	—	Most species/coccidia; avoid potentiated sulfa drugs in cases of dehydration or renal dysfunction[232]
	30 mg/kg PO q24h × 2 days, then q48h × 21 days[15,340]	Most species/coccidia
	30 mg/kg IM q24h × 2 days, then 15 mg/kg IM q48h × 10–28 days[340]	Most species/coccidia
	30 mg/kg PO q24h × 14 days, then 1–3 ×/wk × 3–6 mo[59]	Most species/cryptosporidia; can reduce shedding but does not clear infection
Water	Bath × 30 min[79,194]	Snakes, lizards/mites; use lukewarm (29°C [85°F]) water; monitor to avoid drowning; not 100% effective; does not kill mites on head; must treat environment with acaricide

TABLE 127.5   Chemical Restraint/Anesthetic Agents

Agent	Dosage	Species/Comments
Acepromazine	0.05–0.25 mg/kg IM[99]	Most species/can be used as a preanesthetic with ketamine
	0.1–0.5 mg/kg IM[229,259]	Most species/preanesthetic; reduce by 50% if used with barbiturates
Acepromazine (A)/propofol (P)	(A) 0.5 mg/kg IM + (P) 5 mg/kg IV; (A) 0.5 mg/kg IM + (P) 10 mg/kg IV[5]	Giant Amazon pond turtles/sedation with both protocols, longer duration with higher propofol dosage
Alfaxalone(Alfaxan, Jurox)	6–9 mg/kg IV, or 9–15 mg/kg IM[182]	Most species/good muscle relaxation; variable results; drug requires more evaluation; may have violent recovery;[198]don't use within 10 days of DMSO treatment
	6–15 mg/kg IM, IV[298]	Most species
	9 mg/kg IV[290]	Snakes, lizards/induction; not effective for blotched blue-tongued skinks
	12 mg/kg IV[262]	Bearded dragons/effective for induction of anesthesia; respiratory depression noted
	15 mg/kg IM[229]	Lizards, chelonians/induction, 35–40 min; duration, 15–35 min; good muscle relaxation; variable results
	24 mg/kg ICe[111]	Chelonians (red-eared sliders)/surgical anesthesia with good relaxation
	5 mg/kg IV[170]	Turtles, tortoises/induction
	10–20 mg/kg IM[113,164,300]	Horsfield's tortoises (males only)/light to moderate sedation with no to minimal analgesia; red-eared slider turtles/light sedation of short duration; PD turtles administered 10 mg/kg at low temperature more relaxed than warm, and turtles administered 20 mg/kg at warm temperature were most relaxed
	20 mg/kg IM[141]	Red-eared slider turtles, Eastern painted turtles, yellow-spotted Amazon river turtles, other undocumented turtle species/anesthetic induction
	3 mg/kg IV[252]	Crocodilians/induction, but unpredictable results
Alfaxalone (Al)/medetomidine (Me)	(Al) 10 mg/kg + (Me) 0.10 mg/kg IM; (Al) 20 mg/kg + (Me) 0.05 mg/kg IM[113]	Horsfield's tortoises (males only)/deeper sedation than alfaxalone alone with analgesia
Atipamezole (Antisedan, Zoetis)	Give same volume SC, IV, ICe as medetomidine, or dexmedetomidine (5 × medetomidine, or 10 × dexmedetomidine dose in mg)[a,82,309]	Most species/medetomidine and dexmedetomidine reversal; causes severe hypotension in gopher tortoises when given IV[63]
	0.2–0.5 mg/kg IM[81]	Chelonians/shell repair 5–10 min before finished
	0.5–0.75 mg/kg IM,[275] 0.75 mg/kg SC[210]	Chelonians
Atropine	0.01–0.04 mg/kg SC, IM,[33] IV,[89] ICe[295]	Most species/preanesthetic; bradycardia; rarely indicated; generally use only in profound or prolonged bradycardia;[295] may help prevent intracardiac shunting;[149] ineffective at this dose in green iguanas[258]
	0.5 mg/kg IM, IV, IT, IO[232]	Most species/bradycardia, decrease secretions, CPR
Bupivicaine (0.5%)	1 mg/kg intrathecal[206]	Turtles and tortoises/spinal anesthesia
	0.1 mL/10 cm carapace[16]	Green sea turtles/spinal anesthesia
Butorphanol	—	Butorphanol combinations follow; see ketamine for combinations; inadequate for analgesia
	0.4–1 mg/kg SC, IM[295]	Most species/sedation; preanesthetic
	0.5–2 mg/kg IM, or 0.2–0.5 mg/kg IV, IO[23]	Most species/preanesthetic
	1–1.5 mg/kg SC, IM[295]	Lizards/administer 30 min before isoflurane for smoother, shorter induction
	0.2 mg/kg IM[118,275]	Chelonians/minimal sedation

TABLE 127.5   Chemical Restraint/Anesthetic Agents—cont'd

Agent	Dosage	Species/Comments
Butorphanol (B)/medetomidine (Me)[a]	(B) 0.4 mg/kg + (Me) 0.08 mg/kg IM[95]	Green tree monitors/sedation
Butorphanol (B)/midazolam (Mi)	(B) 0.4 mg/kg + (Mi) 2 mg/kg IM[22]	Most species/preanesthetic; administer 20 min before induction
Dexmedetomidine[a] (Dexdomitor, Zoetis)	—	Dexmedetomidine combinations follow; α_2 agonist that has replaced medetomidine;[a] reverse with atipamezole
Dexmedetomidine (De)/ ketamine (K)	(De) 0.03 mg/kg + (K) 6 mg/kg IV[117]	Hatchling leatherback sea turtles/anesthesia; reversal with atipamezole (0.3 mg/kg IM, IV)
	(De) 0.2 mg/kg + (K) 10 mg/kg intracloacally[236]	Yellow-bellied sliders/adequate for light sedation or short clinical procedures
Dexmedetomidine (De)/ midazolam (Mi)/ketamine (K)	(De) 0.1 mg/kg + (Mi) 1 mg/kg + (K) 2 mg/kg SC[211]	Red-eared slider turtles/deep sedation
Dexmedetomidine (De)/ ketamine (K)/morphine (Mo)	(De) 0.075 mg/kg + (K) 8 mg/kg + (Mo) 1 mg/kg IM[223]	Gopher tortoises/anesthesia, reversed with atipamezole
Dextroketamine (DK)	10 mg/kg IV, ICe[132]	Spectacled caiman/mild sedation ICe; PK
Dextroketamine (DK)/ midazolam (Mi)	(Mi) 0.5 mg/kg + (DK) 10 mg/kg IV, ICe[132]	Spectacled caiman/deep sedation IV; PK; no analgesia
Diazepam	—	Diazepam has been replaced by the use of midazolam in many cases; see ketamine for combinations; muscle relaxation; give 20 min before anesthesia; potentially reversible with flumazenil; drug interaction with ivermectin
	0.5 mg/kg IM, IV[232]	All species/seizures
	2.5 mg/kg IM, IV[282]	Most species/seizures
	0.2–0.8 mg/kg IM[295]	Snakes/use in conjunction with ketamine for anesthesia with muscle relaxation
	0.2–2 mg/kg IM, IV[298]	Snakes, lizards
	2.5 mg/kg PO$_2$[95]	Iguanas/reduce anxiety, which often leads to aggression
	0.2–1 mg/kg IM[295,298]	Chelonians/use in conjunction with ketamine for anesthesia with muscle relaxation
Disoprofol	5–15 mg/kg IV to effect[36]	All species/anesthesia; similar characteristics to propofol; not available in United States
Doxapram	4–12 mg/kg IM, IV[295]	Most species/respiratory stimulant
	5 mg/kg IM, IV[22] q10min prn	Most species/respiratory stimulant; reduces recovery time; reported to partially "reverse" effects of dissociatives[183]
	20 mg/kg IM, IV, IO[232]	Most species/respiratory stimulant
	5–10 mg/kg IV[303]	American alligators/immediate dose-dependent increase in breathing frequency
Epinephrine (1 : 1000)	0.5–1 mg/kg IV, IO, IT[232]	Most species/CPR, cardiac arrest
	0.1 mg/kg IM[106]	Snapping turtles/reduction in time to spontaneous respiration after isoflurane anesthesia
Etorphine (M-99, Wildlife Pharmaceuticals)	0.3–0.5 mg/kg IM[229] 0.3–2.75 mg/kg IM[182]	Crocodilians, chelonians/very potent narcotic; crocodilians: induction, 5–30 min; duration, 30–180 min; chelonians: induction, 10–20 min; duration, 40–120 min; not very effective in reptiles other than alligators;[259] poor relaxation; adequate for immobilization and minor procedures; requires an antagonist; limited use because of expense and legal restrictions
Flumazenil (Romazicon, Hoffman-LaRoche)	—	All species/reversal of benzodiazepines, including diazepam and midazolam; seldom indicated
	0.05 mg/kg IM, SC, IV[207]	All species/reversal of midazolam; extrapolated from mammals and birds
	1 mg/20 mg of zolazepam[187] IM, IV[275]	Crocodilians, chelonians/reversal of zolazepam
Fospropofol	25–50 mg/kg ICe[294]	Red-eared slider turtles/muscle relaxation and immobility especially at higher dosage, but prolonged recovery, and profound respiratory depression with resuscitation in 2/8 subjects; use with caution
Gallamine (Flaxedil, American Cyanamid)	0.4–1.25 mg/kg IM[19] 0.6–4 mg/kg IM[288]	Crocodiles/results in flaccid paralysis, but no analgesia; larger animals require lower dosage; reverse with neostigmine;[188] use in alligators questionable; unsafe in alligators at ≥ 1 mg/kg,[259] deaths reported in American alligators and false gharials[185]
	0.7 mg/kg IM[235]	
	1.2–2 mg/kg IM[82]	
	0.5–2 mg/kg IM[177]	Crocodilians

Continued

TABLE 127.5 **Chemical Restraint/Anesthetic Agents—cont'd**

Agent	Dosage	Species/Comments
Glycopyrrolate	0.01 mg/kg SC,[33] IM, IV[22]	Most species/preanesthetic; for excess oral or respiratory mucus; rarely indicated; generally use only in profound or prolonged bradycardia; may be preferable to atropine;[89] does not work at this dose in green iguanas[258]
Haloperidol	0.5–10 mg/kg IM q7–14d[320]	Boids/aggression management
Hyaluronidase (Wydase, Wyeth)	25 U/dose SC[187]	Crocodilians/combine with premedication, anesthetic, or reversal drugs to accelerate SC absorption
Isoflurane	3%–5% induction,[147] 1%–3% maintenance[37]	Most species/inhalation anesthetic of choice in reptiles; induction, 6–20 min; recovery, 30–60 min; not as smooth in reptiles compared with other animals; intubation and intermittent positive pressure ventilation advisable; may preanesthetize with low dose propofol, ketamine, etc.
	3% in 100% O_2 and 21% O_2[248]	Bearded dragons/trend toward shorter induction and recovery with 21% O_2 group compared with use of 100% O_2
	5% via chamber in 5 L/min O_2[129]	Green iguanas/15–35 min loss of righting reflex; mean MAC, 1.62%; pH 7.49
Ketamine	—	Ketamine combinations follow; muscle relaxation and analgesia may be marginal; prolonged recovery with higher doses; larger reptiles require lower dose; painful at injection site; safety is questionable in debilitated patients; avoid use in cases with renal dysfunction; snakes may be permanently aggressive after ketamine anesthesia;[18] generally recommend use only as a preanesthetic before isoflurane for surgical anesthesia
	10 mg/kg SC, IM q30min[33]	Most species/maintenance of anesthesia; recovery, 3–4 hr
	20–60 mg/kg IM, or 5–15 mg/kg IV[99]	Most species/muscle relaxation improved with midazolam or diazepam
	22–44 mg/kg SC, IM[18,19]	Most species/sedation
	55–88 mg/kg SC, IM[19]	Most species/surgical anesthesia; induction, 10–30 min; recovery, 24–96 hr
	10–20 mg/kg IM[231,232]	Snakes, chelonians/sedation
	20–60 mg/kg SC, IM[33,154]	Snakes/sedation; induction, 30 min; recovery, 2–48 hr
	60–80 mg/kg IM[37]	Snakes/light anesthesia; intermittent positive pressure ventilation may be needed at higher doses
	5–10 mg/kg[231,295]	Lizards, snakes/decreases the incidence of breath-holding during chamber induction
	20–30 mg/kg IM[78]	Iguanas/sedation (i.e., facilitates endotracheal intubation); preanesthetic; requires lower dose than other reptiles
	30–50 mg/kg SC, IM[33,154]	Lizards/sedation; variable results
	20–60 mg/kg IM[133,154,259]	Chelonians/sedation; induction, 30 min; recovery, ≥ 24 hr; potentially dangerous in dehydrated and debilitated tortoises
	25 mg/kg IM, IV[99]	Sea turtles/sedation; used at higher doses (50–70 mg/kg); recovery times may be excessively long and unpredictable; combination of ketamine and acepromazine gives a more rapid induction and recovery
	38–71 mg/kg ICe[346]	Green sea turtles/anesthesia; induction, 2–10 min; duration, 2–10 min; recovery, < 30 min
	60–90 mg/kg IM[154,229]	Chelonians/light anesthesia; induction, < 30 min; recovery, hours to days; requires higher doses than most other reptiles
	20–40 mg/kg SC, IM, ICe (sedation), to 40–80 mg/kg (anesthesia)[187]	Crocodilians/induction, < 30–60 min; recovery, hours to days; in larger animals, 12–15 mg/kg may permit tracheal intubation;[295] not recommended alone in Nile crocodiles[177]
	20–100 mg/kg IM[185]	Crocodilians/lower dose for sedation, higher for anesthesia (requires intermittent positive pressure ventilation for hours)
Ketamine (K)/butorphanol (B)	See (K) dosages + (B) ≤ 1.5 mg/kg IM[295]	Snakes/anesthesia with improved muscle relaxation
	(K) 10–30 mg/kg + (B) 0.5–1.5 mg/kg IM[295]	Chelonians/minor surgical procedures (i.e., shell repair)
Ketamine (K)/dexmedetomidine (De)	(K) 5–7 mg/kg + (De) 0.025–0.07 mg/kg IV[141]	Red-eared slider turtles, Eastern painted turtles, yellow-spotted Amazon river turtles, other undocumented turtle species/anesthetic induction
	(K) 10 mg/kg + (De) 0.05 mg/kg IM, IV[268,269]	Desert tortoises/premedication
Ketamine (K)/diazepam (D)	See (K) dosages + (D) 0.2–0.8 mg/kg IM[295]	Snakes/anesthesia with improved muscle relaxation
	(K) 60–80 mg/kg[229] + (D) 0.2–1 mg/kg IM[295]	Chelonians/anesthesia; muscle relaxation
Ketamine (K)/medetomidine (M)[a]	—	Medetomidine is no longer commercially available, but can be compounded;[a] reverse medetomidine with atipamezole
	(K) 10 mg/kg + (M) 0.1–0.3 mg/kg IM[71]	Most species
	(K) 5–10 mg/kg + (M) 0.1–0.15 mg/kg IM, IV[120]	Lizards (iguanas)
	(K) 3–8 mg/kg + (M) 0.025–0.08 mg/kg IV[189]	Giant tortoises (Aldabra)

TABLE 127.5 Chemical Restraint/Anesthetic Agents—cont'd

Agent	Dosage	Species/Comments
	(K) 4 mg/kg + (M) 0.04 mg/kg IM[123]	Green sea turtles
	(K) 4–10 mg/kg + (M) 0.04–0.14 mg/kg IM[81]	Chelonians/sedation and muscle relaxation for shell repair
	(K) 5 mg/kg + (M) 0.05 mg/kg IV[48]	Loggerhead sea turtles/induction of anesthesia for intubation
	(K) 5 mg/kg + (M) 0.05 mg/kg IM[247]	Tortoises (gopher)/light anesthesia; tracheal intubation; inconsistent results
	(K) 5–10 mg/kg IM + (M) 0.1–0.15 mg/kg IM, IV[120]	Tortoises (small-medium)
	(K) 7.5 mg/kg + (M) 0.075 mg/kg IM[247]	Tortoises (gopher)/anesthesia; tracheal intubation
	(K) 10 mg/kg + (M) 0.1 mg/kg IM[169]	Hybrid Galapagos tortoises/sedation
	(K) 10–20 mg/kg IM + (M) 0.15–0.3 mg/kg IM, IV[120]	Turtles (fresh water)
	(K) 5–10 mg/kg + (M) 0.1–0.15 mg/kg IM[122]	Alligators/adults
	(K) 10–15 mg/kg + (M) 0.15–0.25 mg/kg IM[122]	Alligators/juveniles
Ketamine (K)/medetomidine (Me)/midazolam (Mi)	(K) 5 mg/kg + (Me) 0.15 mg/kg + (Mi) 1 mg/kg SC[209]	Leopard tortoises/deep sedation
Ketamine (K)/medetomidine (Me)/morphine (Mo)	(K) 2.5 mg/kg + (Me) 0.15 mg/kg + (Mo) 1 mg/kg SC[210]	African spurred tortoises/deep sedation and analgesia
Ketamine (K)/midazolam (Mi)	(K) 20 mg/kg + (Mi) 2 mg/kg IM, (K) 60 mg/kg + (Mi) 2 mg/kg IM[6]	Giant Amazon river turtles/sedation with both combinations; more rapid and prolonged sedation with higher K dosage
	(K) 20–40 mg/kg + (Mi) ≤ 2 mg/kg IM[29]	Chelonians/sedation; muscle relaxation
	(K) 60–80 mg/kg[229] + (Mi) ≤ 2 mg/kg IM[295]	Chelonians/anesthesia; muscle relaxation
Ketamine (K)/propofol (P)	(K) 25–30 mg/kg IM[229] + (P) 7 mg/kg IV[270]	Chelonians/administer propofol ≈ 70–80 min postketamine; see propofol
Ketamine (K)/xylazine (X)	(K) 30 mg/kg + (X) 1 mg/kg IM[45]	Broad-snouted caiman juveniles/provided mild sedation after either forelimb or hind limb administration
Lidocaine (0.5%–2%)	Local or topical[295]	Most species/local analgesia; infiltrate to effect (e.g., 0.01 mL 2% lidocaine used for local block for IO catheter placement in iguanas);[20] often used in conjunction with chemical immobilization
	0.158 mg/cm intrathecal (combined with epinephrine hemitartrate)[287]	Green iguana/spinal anesthesia
	2 mg/kg intrathecal (IT)[206]	Turtles and tortoises/surgical analgesia/anesthesia of caudal body
	0.038 mL/kg (1 mL/20–25 kg)[277]	Hybrid Galapagos tortoises/surgical analgesia/anesthesia for phallectomy
Medetomidine[a]	—	Medetomidine is no longer commercially available, but can be compounded;[a] reverse with atipamezole; produces poor immobilization alone; see ketamine and butorphanol for combinations
	0.1–0.15 mg/kg IM[22]	Most species
	0.06–0.15 mg/kg[296]	Lizards
	0.15 mg/kg IM[308,309]	Desert tortoises, crocodilians/sedation; incomplete immobilization; generally produces bradycardia and bradypnea
	0.04–0.15 mg/kg IM[185]	Crocodilians/need to reverse
	0.13–0.17 mg/kg IM[250,251]	Crocodilians/moderate sedation/atipamezole (0.1 mg/kg IM) for reversal
	0.5–0.75 mg/kg IM[250,251]	Crocodilians/sedation only when administered in thoracic limb (versus pelvic limb and tail), with atipamezole (2.5 mg/kg) reversal
Meperidine (Mp)/Midazolam (Mi)	(Mp) 1 mg/kg + (Mi) 1 mg/kg IM[16]	Green sea turtles/premedication
Methohexital (Brevital, Lilly)	—	Recovery time of red-sided garter snakes at 21°C (70°F), 125 min; 26°C (79°F), 86 min; 31°C (88°F), 64 min; thinner snakes had longer recovery times; if within 5 wk of parturition, mean recovery time 2 × as long as nongravid; time postfeeding had no effect at 1, 3, 10 days[266]
	5–20 mg/kg SC,[19] IV[89]	Most species/induction, 5–30 min; recovery, 1–5 hr; use at 0.125%–0.5% concentration; much species variability; decrease dose 20%–30% for young animals; avoid use in debilitated animals
	9–10 mg/kg SC,[243] ICe	Colubrids/induction, ≥ 22 min; recovery, 2–5 hr; does not produce soft-tissue irritation seen with other barbiturates; may need to adjust dosage in obese snakes
Metomidate	10 mg/kg IM[71,288]	Snakes/profound sedation; not available in the United States

Continued

TABLE 127.5	**Chemical Restraint/Anesthetic Agents—cont'd**	
Agent	**Dosage**	**Species/Comments**
Midazolam	—	See butorphanol, ketamine for combinations; can be reversed by flumazenil
	0.1–1 mg/kg[11]	Multiple species/mild to moderate sedation
	2 mg/kg IM[18,19]	Most species/preanesthetic; increases the efficacy of ketamine; effective in snapping turtles, not in painted turtles[19]
	0.5–2 mg/kg[296]	Lizards
	1.5 mg/kg IM[254]	Turtles (red-eared sliders)/sedation; onset, 5.5 min; duration, 82 min; recovery, 40 min; much individual variability
	2–3 mg/kg IV[117]	Hatchling leatherback sea turtles/sedation
Naloxone	0.04–2 mg/kg SC[304,305,307,309]	Corn snakes, bearded dragons, red-eared sliders/μ-opioid agonist reversal
	4 mg/kg IM[95]	Green tree monitors/reversal of butorphanol
Neostigmine	0.03–0.25 mg/kg IM[188]	Crocodiles/gallamine reversal; may cause emesis and lacrimation; fast 24–48 hr before use; effects enhanced if combined with 75 mg hyaluronidase per dose when administered SC, IM[188]
	0.063 mg/kg IV[188]	
	0.07–0.14 mg/kg IM[235]	
Pentobarbital	—	Rarely used as an anesthetic agent in reptiles
	15–30 mg/kg ICe[229]	Snakes/induction, 30–60 min; duration, ≥ 2 hr; prolonged recovery (risk of occasional fatalities); venomous snakes require twice as much as nonvenomous snakes;[18] avoid use in lizards
	10–18 mg/kg ICe[229]	Chelonians
	7.5–15 mg/kg ICe, or 8 mg/kg IM[18,229]	Crocodilians
Propofol	—	If administered in supravertebral sinus, be aware for potential submeningeal delivery;[271] see ketamine for combination; anesthesia; rapid, smooth induction; may give 15–25 min anesthesia and restraint in most species; rapid, excitement-free recovery; must be administered IV (slowly; no inflammation if goes perivascularly); may be administered IO; dosages may be reduced by as much as 50% in premedicated (e.g., ketamine) animals; may cause apnea and bradycardia; intubation and assisted ventilation generally required; considered by many to be parenteral agent of choice for inducing anesthesia
	0.3–0.5 mg/kg/min IV, IO constant rate infusion, or 0.5–1 mg/kg IV, IO periodic bolus[298]	Most species/maintenance anesthesia; must provide respiratory and thermal support
	5–10 mg/kg IV, intracardiac[9,288]	Snakes
	10 mg/kg intracardiac[222]	Ball pythons/anesthetic induction for isoflurane maintenance, but prolonged recovery; mild, resolving cardiac lesions
	15 mg/kg IV[27]	South American rattlesnakes/anesthetic induction
	3–5 mg/kg IV, IO[119,120]	Lizards (iguanas)/intubation and minor diagnostic procedures; may need to give an additional dose in 3–5 min; less cardiopulmonary depression than with higher doses
	5–10 mg/kg IV, IO[24]	Iguanas/higher dose is recommended for induction for short-duration procedures or intubation
	10 mg/kg IV, IO[24,71,242]	Lizards, snakes/0.25 mg/kg/min may be given for maintenance;[99] green iguanas/anesthetic induction[242]
	10 mg/kg IV[262]	Bearded dragons/effective for induction of anesthesia; respiratory depression noted; apnea in 2/8 animals
	2 mg/kg IV[22]	Giant tortoises
	3–5 mg/kg IV supravertebral sinus[81]	Chelonians/sedation (i.e., shell repair)
	5 mg/kg IV[106]	Snapping turtles/anesthetic induction
	10 mg/kg IV (supravertebral sinus)[350]	Red-eared sliders/40–85 min anesthesia
	12–15 mg/kg IV[68,318]	Chelonians/lower dosages (5–10 mg/kg IV[295]) may be used; 1 mg/kg/min may be given for maintenance[295]
	20 mg/kg IV (supravertebral sinus)[350]	Red-eared sliders/60–120 min anesthesia
	10–15 mg/kg IV[187]	Crocodilians/duration, 0.5–1.5 hr; maintain on gas anesthetics; experimental IM with hyaluronidase
Rocuronium (Zemuron, Organon)	0.25–0.5 mg/kg IM[157]	Box turtles/neuromuscular blocking agent; no analgesia; for intubation only and small, nonpainful procedures
Sevoflurane	To effect[15,279]	Most species/anesthesia; rapid induction and recovery when intubated

TABLE 127.5 Chemical Restraint/Anesthetic Agents—cont'd

Agent	Dosage	Species/Comments
Succinylcholine	—	No analgesia; narrow margin of safety; generally not recommended, but included for completeness; intermittent positive pressure ventilation generally required; paralysis occurs in 5–30 min; avoid if exposed to organophosphate parasiticides within last 30 days; administer minimal amount required to perform procedure
	0.25–1 mg/kg IM[147]	Most species
	0.75–1 mg/kg IM[33]	Large lizards
	0.25–1.5 mg/kg IM[259]	Chelonians/induction, 15–30 min; recovery, 45–90 min; facilitates intubation
	0.5–1 mg/kg IM[34]	Box turtles/induction, 20–30 min
	0.25 mg/kg IM[177]	Crocodilians
	0.4–1 mg/kg IM[259]	Alligators/rapid onset; 3–5 mg/kg in smaller animals have been used
	0.5–5 mg/kg IM[19,185]	Crocodilians/variable induction and recovery periods
Thiopental	19–31 mg/kg IV[346]	Green sea turtles/anesthesia; induction, 5–10 min; recovery, < 6 hr; erratic anesthesia
Tiletamine/zolazepam (Telazol, Fort Dodge)	—	Sedation, anesthesia; severe respiratory depression possible (may need to ventilate);[37] variable results; may have prolonged recovery; use lower end of dose range in heavier species; good for muscle relaxation before intubation;[83,275] other anesthetic agents may be preferable
	4–5 mg/kg SC, IM[19]	Most species/sedation; induction, 9–15 min; recovery, 1–12 h; adequate for most noninvasive procedures
	5–10 mg/kg IM[22]	Most species
	3 mg/kg IM[120]	Snakes/facilitates handling and intubation of large snakes; induction, 30–45 min; prolongs recovery
	3–5 mg/kg IM[232]	Snakes, lizards/sedation
	10–30 mg/kg IM[229]–20–40 mg/kg IM[147,293]	Snakes, lizards/induction, 8–20 min; recovery, 2–10 hr; variable results; longer sedation and recovery times at 22°C (72°F) than at 30°C (86°F);[321] good sedation in boa constrictors at 25 mg/kg IM;[321] generally need to supplement with inhalation agents for surgical anesthesia; some snakes died at 55 mg/kg
	3.5–14 mg/kg IM[229] (generally 4–8 mg/kg)	Chelonians/sedation; induction, 8–20 min; does not produce satisfactory anesthesia even at 88 mg/kg[259]
	5–10 mg/kg IM, IV[295]	Large tortoises/facilitates intubation; if light, mask with isoflurane rather than redosing
	1–2 mg/kg IM[185]	Crocodilians/recovery takes several hours
	2–10 mg/kg IM[295]	Large crocodilians/may permit intubation
	5–10 mg/kg SC, IM, ICe (sedation), 10–40 mg/kg (anesthesia)[187]	Crocodilians
	15 mg/kg IM[53]	Alligators/induction, >20 min; adequate for minor procedures
Xylazine	—	Infrequently used; variable effects; potentially reversible with yohimbine; preanesthetic for ketamine; see ketamine for combination
	0.1–1.25 mg/kg IM, IV[89]	Most species
	0.1–1 mg/kg IM[185]	Crocodilians/atipamezole better reversal than yohimbine
	1–2 mg/kg IM[187,259]	Nile crocodiles
Yohimbine (Yobine, Lloyd)	—	Xylazine reversal; rarely indicated; atipameazole commonly used to reverse all α_2 agonists

[a]Medetomidine is no longer commercially available in North America, although it can be obtained from select compounding services; dosages are listed here as a guide for possible use with dexmedetomidine, an α_2 agonist that is the active optical enantiomer of racemic compound medetomidine; dexmedetomidine is generally used at half the dose of medetomidine but the same volume due to higher concentration; both compounds tend to have similar effects.

TABLE 127.6 Analgesic Agents

Agent	Dosage	Species/Comments
Bupivacaine	1–2 mg/kg local q4–12h prn[298]	Most species/local anesthesia; 4 mg/kg maximum dose
	1 mg/kg intrathecal[206]	Turtles, tortoises/regional analgesia/anesthesia
Buprenorphine	0.2 mg/kg SC[212]	No evidence of analgesic efficacy in red-eared slider turtles or other reptile species
Butorphanol	—	Recent studies call into question use of particular doses or of this drug in general is providing analgesia in reptiles, including red-eared sliders, ball pythons, corn snakes, bearded dragons, and green iguanas; respiratory depression is a common side effect[292,306,307]
	0.4–1 mg/kg SC, IM[295]	Most species; sedation; preanesthetic; 0.2 mg/kg IM used experimentally in tortoises[98]
	1 mg/kg IM[84]	Green iguanas/ineffective for analgesia; presence of observer may affect iguana response
	20 mg/kg SC[161]	Red-eared slider turtles/ineffective for surgical analgesia
Carprofen	1–4 mg/kg PO, SC, IM, IV q24h,[183] follow with half the dose q24–72h[220]	Most species/nonsteroidal antiinflammatory; no efficacy data in any reptile species
Etodolac	5 mg/kg PO q72h × 30 days[257]	Komodo dragons
Fentanyl	12 μg/hr transdermal patch[61]	Ball pythons/therapeutic plasma concentrations, as defined in mammals, were sustained for the 7-day study, and higher than in mammals; however, efficacy was not determined
	12.5 μg/hr transdermal patch to cranial epaxial muscles[160]	Ball pythons/high plasma concentrations (above analgesic threshold in mammals); analgesic efficacy not proven in any snake species, but anecdotal evidence from certain snake clinical cases demonstrated improved condition after application of patch
	12.5 μg/hr transdermal patch to caudodorsal lumbar region[93]	Prehensile-tailed skinks/no side effects reported after 24 hr when skink blood levels reached human therapeutic levels; environmental temperature can significantly affect absorption
Flunixin meglumine	0.1–0.5 mg/kg IM q12–24h[183]	Most species/nonsteroidal antiinflammatory; use for maximum of 3 days; no evidence of efficacy
	0.5–2 mg/kg IM q12–24h[298]	Most species/nonsteroidal antiinflammatory; no evidence of efficacy
	1–2 mg/kg IM q24h × 2 treatments[36,313]	Lizards/postsurgical nonsteroidal antiinflammatory; no evidence of efficacy
Hydromorphone	0.5–1 mg/kg SC[212]	Red-eared sliders/analgesic efficacy
Ketoprofen	—	Nonsteroidal antiinflammatory
	2 mg/kg PO, SC, IM q24–48h[191,331]	Most species/green iguanas/PK study;[331] loggerhead sea turtles/frequently used due to historical evidence of safety;[191] no efficacy data
Lidocaine (0.5%–2%)	2–5 mg/kg local[298]	Most species/10 mg/kg maximum dosage
	Local or topical[295]	Most species/local analgesia; infiltrate to effect (e.g., 0.01 mL 2% lidocaine used for local block for IO catheter placement in iguanas);[20] often used in conjunction with chemical immobilization
	4 mg/kg intrathecal[206]	Turtles, tortoises/regional analgesia
Lidocaine (L)/morphine (Mo)	2 mg/kg (L) + 0.1 mg/kg (Mo) intrathecal[269]	Desert tortoises/orchiectomy analgesia
Meloxicam	0.1–0.5 mg/kg PO, SC q24–48h[149–151]	Most species
	0.3 mg/kg IM[249]	Ball pythons/physiological changes not consistent with analgesia
	0.2 mg/kg PO, IV q24h[72]	Green iguanas/PD; no evidence of efficacy
	0.1 mg/kg IM, IV[175]	Loggerhead sea turtles/PK; plasma concentrations not consistent with analgesia
	0.1–0.2 mg/kg PO, IM q24h × 4–10 days[81]	Chelonians; no evidence of efficacy
	0.2 mg/kg IM, IV;[332] SC[268,269]	Red-eared slider turtles/PK; plasma concentrations consistent with therapeutic efficacy for 48 hr by IM and IV administration routes;[332] Mojave desert tortoises, postsurgical nonsteroidal antiinflammatory[268,269]
	0.2–0.4 mg/kg IM[141]	Red-eared slider turtles, Eastern painted turtles, yellow-spotted Amazon river turtles, other undocumented turtle species/nonsteroidal antiinflammatory; no evidence of efficacy
	0.5 mg/kg PO, IM, or 0.22 mg/kg IV[278]	Red-eared sliders/PK; found better absorption IM vs PO;[278] after IV administration, plasma levels decreased rapidly and the elimination half-life was 7.57 hr
Meperidine	5–10 mg/kg IM q12–24h[118]	Most species/analgesia; no noticeable effect in snakes even at 200 mg/kg
	20 mg/kg IM q12–24h[183]	Most species/analgesia
	2–4 mg/kg ICe q6–8h[149]	Lizards
	1–5 mg/kg IM[156,306,335]	Turtles, crocodiles/analgesic efficacy of short duration
	2–4 mg/kg ICe[3]	Nile crocodiles/analgesia
Methadone	3–5 mg/kg SC, IM[58,306]	Aquatic turtles/analgesia

TABLE 127.6   Analgesic Agents—cont'd

Agent	Dosage	Species/Comments
Morphine	—	No effective dose for analgesia documented in corn snakes[307]
	10 mg/kg IM[307,341]	Bearded dragons/analgesia; ball pythons/no analgesia
	1.5–6.5 mg/kg SC, IM (Sladky KK, unpublished data)[78,306–307]	Red-eared sliders (long lasting respiratory depression), freshwater crocodiles, *Anolis* lizards/may be effective thermal analgesia
	0.1–0.2 mg/kg intrathecal[206]	Turtles, tortoises/thermal analgesia for 48 hr; regional analgesia caudal body
	2 mg/kg SC[161]	Red-eared slider turtles/surgical analgesia
	1 mg/kg IM[141]	Red-eared slider turtles, Eastern painted turtle, yellow-spotted Amazon river turtle, other undocumented turtle species/analgesia
	0.5–4 mg/kg ICe[309]	Crocodilians/analgesia
Naloxone	0.04–2 mg/kg SC (Sladky KK, unpublished data)[304,307,309]	Red-eared sliders, bearded dragons, corn snakes/μ-opioid agonist reversal
Oxymorphone	0.025–0.1 mg/kg IV[89]	Anecdotal evidence of analgesia in some lizard and turtle species; no efficacy or PK/PD studies; avoid in cases with hepatic or renal dysfunction; no observable effects in snakes even at 1.5 mg/kg
	0.05–0.2 mg/kg SC, IM q12–48h[118]	
	0.5–1.5 mg/kg IM[89]	
Pethidine	—	See meperidine
Prednisolone	2–5 mg/kg PO, IM[183]	Most species/antiinflammatory
Proparacaine (0.5%)	Topical to eye[107,195,284,299]	Iguanas/desensitizes surface of eye; ineffective in animals with spectacles; bearded dragons/IOP by rebound tonometry;[299] Kemp's ridley sea turtles/one drop provided 45 min duration of action;[107] do not exceed toxic dose 2 mg/kg;[99] Yacare caiman/IOP by applanation tonometry[284]
Tapentadol	10 mg/kg IM[102,103]	Red-eared and yellow-bellied slider turtles/analgesia
Tramadol	11 mg/kg PO[108]	Bearded dragons
	5–10 mg/kg PO, SC[13]	Red-eared slider turtles, sea turtles/thermal analgesia, higher doses may affect ventilation
	5–10 mg/kg Po₂[245]	Loggerhead sea turtles/PK; plasma concentrations consistent with efficacy for 48 hr (5 mg/kg PO) or 72 hr (10 mg/kg PO)
	10 mg/kg PO[310]	Turtles, tortoises/analgesia
	10 mg/kg IM[105]	Yellow-bellied slider turtles/PK/PD comparing forelimb and hind limb administration; analgesia; plasma concentrations consistent with analgesia in both forelimb and hind limb

TABLE 127.7   Hormones and Steroids

Agent	Dosage	Species/Comments
Arginine vasotocin (AVT) (Sigma Chemical)	0.01–1 μg/kg IV (preferred), ICe[186] q12–24h × several treatments	Most species/dystocias; administer 30–60 min after Ca lactate/Ca glycerophosphate; more effective in reptiles than oxytocin but not commercially available for use in animals; higher doses have been reported; 0.5 μg/kg commonly recommended
Calcitonin	1.5 U/kg SC q8h × 14–21 days prn[89] 50 U/kg IM, repeat in 14 days[21,99]	Most species (e.g., iguanas)/severe nutritional secondary hyperparathyroidism; administer after Ca supplementation; do not give if hypocalcemic
	50 U/kg q7d × 2–3 doses[102,106]	Green iguanas/salmon calcitonin; do not give if hypocalcemic
Deslorelin acetate	—	No success with use in female reptile reproductive issues
	4.75 mg implant SC[283]	Bearded dragons/abnormal aggression in juveniles; decreased serum testosterone, behavior ceased
Dexamethasone	0.2 mg/kg IM, IV[297]	Most species/laryngeal or pharyngeal edema and inflammation
	0.6–1.25 mg/kg IM, 89	Most species/shock (septic/traumatic)
	0.3–1.5 mg/kg IM, IV, IO[151]	Chelonians/hyperthermia
Dexamethasone sodium phosphate	0.1–0.25 mg/kg SC, IM, IV[99]	Most species/shock (septic/traumatic)
Insulin	1–5 U/kg IM, ICe q24–72h[315]	Snakes, chelonians/doses are empirical and must be adjusted based on response to therapy and serial blood glucose; doses administered ICe may take 24–48 hr before a response is noted
	5–10 U/kg IM, ICe q24–72h[315]	Lizards, crocodilians/see previous
Leuprolide acetate (Lupron Depot 1.875 mg/mL, Abbott)	0.4 mg/kg IM[163]	Iguanas/did not suppress testosterone levels in males
Levothyroxine	0.02 mg/kg PO q48h[112]	Geckos/postthyroidectomy; lifetime management
	0.02 mg/kg PO q48h[246]	Tortoises/hypothyroidism; stimulates feeding in debilitated tortoises
	0.025 mg/kg q24h in AM[86]	Tortoises/monitor T₄ levels

Continued

TABLE 127.7   **Hormones and Steroids—cont'd**

Agent	Dosage	Species/Comments
Methylprednisolone	1 mg/kg IV q24h[151]	Chelonians/ivermectin toxicity
Nandrolone (Deca-Durabolin, Orgamon)	0.5–5 mg/kg IM q7–28d[127]	Most species/hepatic lipidosis
	1 mg/kg IM q7–28d[69]	Lizards/anabolic steroid; reduces protein catabolism; may stimulate erythropoiesis
Oxytocin	—	Dystocias; results are variable; works well in chelonians, less so in snakes and lizards; generally administer 1 hr after Ca administration; use multiple doses with caution
	1–10 U/kg IM[78,99]	Most species/higher end of the range is commonly used; may be repeated up to 3 treatments at 90 min intervals with increasing dosage
	2 U/kg IM q4–6h × 1–3 treatments[10]	Most species
	1–5 U/kg IM,[67] repeat in 1 hr	Lizards/alternatively, 5 U/kg by slow IV or IO over 4–8 hr[67]
	1–2,[35] 2–20,[217] or 10–20[34] U/kg IM	Chelonians
	1–20 U/kg IM q90min × 3 treatments at increased doses, or 50%–100% first dose 1–12 hr later, or IO drip[324]	Chelonians
	2 U/kg IV q2h[65]	Red-eared sliders/faster onset vs IM; fewer animals required second or third doses vs IM route
Prednisolone	2–5 mg/kg PO, IM[183]	Most species/analgesia (chronic pain)
	0.5 mg/kg q24h × 14 days, then q48h until PCV stable[149]	Lizards/autoimmune hemolytic anemia
Prednisolone Na succinate (Solu-Delta Cortef, Pharmacia and Upjohn)	5–10 mg/kg IM, IV,[82] IO[69]	Most species/shock; brain swelling from hyperthermia; may help reduce nephrocalcinosis
Prednisone	0.5–1 mg/kg PO, SC, IM, IV[216]	Most species/lymphoma, leukemia, myeloproliferative disease
	0.8 mg/kg q48h[95]	Most species/chronic T-lymphocytic leukemia; may combine with chlorambucil, but need to monitor uric acid levels
Stanozolol (Winstrol-V, Winthrop)	5 mg/kg IM q7d prn[99]	Most species/anabolic steroid; management of catabolic disease states

TABLE 127.8   **Nutritional/Mineral/Fluid Support**

Agent	Dosage	Species/Comments
Calcium	PO prn[74]	Most species/dietary sources include crushed cuttlebone, oyster shell, egg shell, tablets of Ca salts, or other commercially available products
Calcium carbonate (Rep-Cal, Rep-Cal Labs; Repti Calcium, Zoo Med; Fluker's powdered or liquid forms of calcium)	PO prn[74]	Omnivores, herbivores, insectivores/dietary Ca supplement
Calcium glubionate (Neo-Calglucon, Sandoz; Calciquid, Breckenridge Pharmaceuticals; Calcionate, Rugby)	10 mg/kg PO q12–24h prn[91]	All species/nutritional secondary hyperparathyroidism
	25–50 mg/kg PO q24h prn[208]	All species/nutritional secondary hyperparathyroidism
	360 mg/kg (1 mL/kg) PO q12–24h prn[21,37]	Most species/nutritional secondary hyperparathyroidism; hypocalcemia; dystocia; ensure adequate UVB exposure and proper nutrition
Calcium gluconate	50–100 mg/kg SC, IM, IV[208]	Most species/hypocalcemia (low ionized Ca); hypocalcemic muscle tremors, seizures, dystocia, or flaccid paresis in lizards; when patient is stable, switch to oral Ca; should be diluted in fluids
	100 mg/kg SC, IM, ICe[200,220] q6–24h[21,37]	Most species/hypocalcemia (low ionized Ca); hypocalcemic muscle tremors, seizures, dystocia, or flaccid paresis in lizards; when patient is stable, switch to oral Ca
Calcium gluconate/borogluconate	10–50 mg/kg SC, IM[91]	Most species/hypocalcemia; hypocalcemic dystocia
Calcium glycerophosphate/calcium lactate (Calphosan, Glenwood)	1–5 mg/kg SC, IM[91]	Most species/hypocalcemia; hypocalcemic dystocia
	10 mg/kg SC, IM, ICe q24h × 1–7 days[15,21]	Lizards (iguanas)/hypocalcemia

TABLE 127.8 Nutritional/Mineral/Fluid Support—cont'd

Agent	Dosage	Species/Comments
Carnivore Care (Oxbow Animal Health)	10–20 mL/kg PO or via gavage/esophagostomy q24–48h[98]	Carnivores/short-term nutritional support; anorexia; prepare according to directions; begin after rehydration and stable condition; more dilute in first feeding after anorexia, gradually increase concentration over 3–5 days
	30 mL/kg (3% of body weight) PO or via gavage/esophagostomy q24h;[64] range of 2%–10% body weight PO or via gavage/esophagostomy q24h[208]	Carnivores
Clinicare—feline and canine (Abbott Animal Health)	Gavage prn[348]	Most species/postomphalectomy; use canine formula for herbivores and omnivores, and feline formula for carnivores; initially dilute 1:1 with water and gradually increase to full strength over 48 hr; generally precede nutritional supplementation with 48–96 hr of water or electrolyte solution PO
Critical Care for Herbivores (Oxbow Animal Health)	10–20 mL/kg PO or via gavage/esophagostomy q24–48h[98]	Herbivores/long-term nutritional support; prepare according to directions; begin after rehydration and stable condition
	30 mL/kg (3% of body weight) PO or via gavage/esophagostomy q24h;[64] range of 2%–10% body weight PO or via gavage/esophagostomy q24h[208]	Herbivores
Dextrose in water (2.5%, 5%)	PO, SC, IV, IO, ICe, EpiCe, prn[162]	All species/hyperkalemia;[162] can mix with electrolye solutions
	Calculated water deficit IV, IO[198]	Most species/for intracellular rehydration when mentation is altered and plasma Na > 160 mEq/L; for acute Na toxicosis replace deficit in 12–24 hr; for chronic dehydration slowly replace deficit over 48–72 hr
Electrolyte solutions (Pedialyte, Abbott; Gatorade, S-VC, Inc.)	Voluntary drinking (whole body soak)[98]	All species/oral fluid therapy; early treatment of anorexia; dilute 1:1 with water; caution against drowning
	10–20 mL/kg via gavage or esophagostomy tube q24h[98]	All species/rehydration; when stable; first stage in supplemental nutrition
Emeraid Exotic Carnivore (Lafeber)	5–30 mL/kg gavage or esophagostomy tube q24–72h[99]	Carnivores/nutritional support, severely debilitated, cachectic patients; prepare according to directions; use when hydrated and stable condition; greater dilution in first few feedings
	3% body weight PO or via gavage/esophagostomy q24h;[64] range of 2%–10% body weight PO or via gavage/esophagostomy q24h[208]	Carnivores
Emeraid Herbivore (Lafeber)	5–20 mL/kg gavage or esophagostomy tube q12–48h[99]	Herbivores/nutritional support, severely debilitated, cachectic patients; prepare according to directions; use when hydrated and stable condition; greater dilution in first few feedings
	3% body weight PO or via gavage/esophagostomy q24h;[64] range of 2%–10% body weight PO or via gavage/esophagostomy q24h[208]	Herbivores
Emeraid Omnivore (Lafeber)	5–20 mL/kg gavage or esophagostomy tube q12–48h[98]	Most species/nutritional support, severely debilitated, cachectic patients; prepare according to directions; use when hydrated and stable condition; greater dilution in first few feedings
	3% body weight PO or via gavage/esophagostomy q24h;[64] range of 2%–10% body weight PO or via gavage/esophagostomy q24h[208]	Omnivores
Hydroxyethyl starch (Hetastarch, HES)	3–5 mL/kg slow IV or IO bolus prn[98,198]	All species/hypoalbuminemia; hypovolemic perfusion deficits; increased capillary permeability; use with crystalloids; reduce crystalloid volume 40%–60%; max volume 20 mL/kg[337]
Iodine	2–4 mg/kg PO q24h × 14–21 days, then q7d[99]	Herbivores/iodine deficiency (i.e., goiter); use in species fed a goitrogenic diet; can use a multivitamin-mineral mixture or iodized salt; suggested daily dietary iodine 0.03 mg/kg BW[74]
Iron dextran	12 mg/kg IM 1–2×/wk × 45 days[323]	Crocodilians/iron deficiency; in other species for anemia[99]

Continued

TABLE 127.8   Nutritional/Mineral/Fluid Support—cont'd

Agent	Dosage	Species/Comments
Lactated Ringer's solution (LRS)	15–40 mL/kg SC, IV, IO prn[198]	Land turtles/fluid replacement; use extracoelomically after warming the patient; avoid lactate if hepatic insufficiency
LRS + 0.9% saline (1:1 solution)	20 mL/kg/day ICe[44]	Loggerhead sea turtles/highest percentage of acid-base recovery and electrolyte balance compared with LRS, saline, or 5% dextrose in saline (1:1)
Maintenance crystalloid solution: 1/2-strength LRS and 2.5% dextrose	SC, IV, IO, ICe, EpiCe, prn[198]	All species/maintenance fluid therapy after losses have been replaced
Metronidazole	12.5–50 mg/kg PO[88]	Most species/appetite stimulant (anecdotal; presumably associated with antiprotozoal activity)
	50–100 mg/kg PO[148]	Chameleons/appetite stimulant (anecdotal; presumably associated with antiprotozoal activity)
Multivitamin products (ReptiVite, Zoo Med; Herptivite, RepCal; Repta-Vitamin, Fluker's; Exo-Terra; Nekton)	Dust on vegetables, fruits, or insects q84–168h[312]	Herbivores, omnivores, insectivores/preformed vitamin A; minerals; multivitamin
Polymerized bovine hemoglobin (Oxyglobin, OPK Biotech)	3–5 mL/kg slow IV or IO bolus prn[98,198]	All species/hemoglobin polymer; hypoalbuminemia; hemorrhage; severe anemia; hypovolemic perfusion deficits; increased capillary permeability; use with crystalloids; reduce crystalloid volume 40%–60%; max volume 20 mL/kg;[337] currently under FDA testing by a new manufacturer and unavailable
Replacement crystalloid solutions (Normosol-R, Ceva; Plasma-Lyte, Baxter)	15–25 mL/kg/d PO, SC, IV, IO, ICe, EpiCe prn[36]	All species/replacement fluid therapy; warm to 29°C (84°F)[198]
	10–30 mL/kg q24h, or divided into 2–3 boluses several hours apart[162]	All species/ongoing regurgitation or severe diarrhea
Ringer's solution for reptiles: 1 part Normosol-R + 2 Parts 2.5% dextrose in 0.45% saline [120] or, 1 part Normosol-R + 1 Part 5% dextrose + 1 Part 0.9% saline	10–20 mL/kg q24h[99]	All species/hypertonic dehydration or to prevent nephrotoxicity due to aminoglycosides
	15 (large reptiles) to 25 (small reptiles) mL/kg q24h, or divided into 2 doses per day[36]	All species/hypertonic dehydration; warm fluids to 28°C (82°F)
	20 mL/kg q12h[37]	Chelonians/severe dehydration
Selenium	0.028 mg/kg IM[15]	Lizards/deficiency; myopathy
Sodium chloride (0.45%)	PO, SC, IV, IO, ICe, EpiCe, prn[162]	All species/hypertonic dehydration; correct deficits over 3 days
Sodium chloride (0.9%)	SC, IV, IO, ICe, EpiCe, prn[162,198]	All species/hyperkalemia, hypercalcemia, hypochloremic metabolic alkalosis;[198] can mix with other crystalloid solutions, particularly 5% dextrose; use SC, ICe, EpiCe routes after patient is warm
Vitamin A	—	Overdose causes epidermal sloughing; greater risk with aqueous parenteral formulation; for less severe cases, commercial formulated diets or reptile multivitamin supplements may suffice;[74,230,312] may help infectious stomatitis
	2000 U/kg PO, SC, IM q7–14d × 2–4 treatments[34,37]	Most species/hypovitaminosis A
	2000 U/30 g BW PO once, repeat in 7 days[114,314]	Chameleons/eye swelling, respiratory disease, hemipenile plugs, dysecdysis
	200–300 U/kg[74] SC, IM	Turtles/hypovitaminosis A; give in conjunction with PO vitamin A (2–8 U/g feed DM)
Vitamins A, D₃, E (Vital E + A + D, Stuart Products)	0.15 mL/kg IM, repeat in 21 days[99]	Most species/hypovitaminosis A, D₃, or E; product contains alcohol and may sting when administered; a product without alcohol can be compounded commercially
	0.3 mL/kg PO, then 0.06 mL/kg q7d × 3–4 treatments[34]	Box turtles/hypovitaminosis A; parenteral use may result in hypervitaminosis A and D; given PO may enhance Ca uptake
Vitamin B complex	0.3 mL/kg SC, IM q24h[99]	Most species/anorexia; hypovitaminosis B; use with caution as B₆ toxicity may occur
	25 mg thiamine/kg PO q24h × 3–7 days[10]	Most species/appetite stimulant; hypovitaminosis B
Vitamin B₁ (thiamine)	50–100 mg/kg PO, SC, IM q24h[43]	Piscivores/thiamine deficiency from thawed fish
	30 g/kg feed fish PO[99]	Crocodilians/treat or prevent deficiency
Vitamin B₁₂ (cyanocobalamin)	0.05 mg/kg SC, IM[99]	Snakes, lizards/appetite stimulant
Vitamin C	10–20 mg/kg SC, IM q24h[87,224]	All species/empirical for hypovitaminosis C; stomatitis; skin slough in snakes; supportive therapy for bacterial infections

TABLE 127.8   Nutritional/Mineral/Fluid Support—cont'd

Agent	Dosage	Species/Comments
Vitamin D$_3$	—	Nutritional secondary hyperparathyroidism; hypocalcemia; deficiency and excess may result in soft-tissue calcification
	1000 U/kg IM, repeat in 1 wk[37]	Most species/deficiency; use with oral calcium glubionate and carbonate, general dietary management, and UVB irradiation
	200 U/kg PO, IM q7d[15,21]	Lizards/PO may be safer than IM, but absorption is poor in some species[26,253]
	400 U/kg IM q7d × 3 treatments[196]	Green iguanas/nutritional secondary hyperparathyroidism; use with calcitonin after normocalcemic; also supplement oral calcium
Vitamin E/selenium (L-Se, Schering)	1 U vitamin E/kg[74] IM	Piscivores/hypovitaminosis E; myopathy, anorexia, swollen subcutaneous nodule
	50 U vitamin E/kg + 0.025 mg selenium/kg IM[77]	Lizards/hypovitaminosis E (vitamin E/selenium)
Vitamin K$_1$	0.25–0.5 mg/kg IM[99]	Most species/hypovitaminosis K$_1$; coagulopathies

TABLE 127.9   Miscellaneous Agents

Agent	Dosage	Species/Comments
Activated charcoal-kaolin suspension (ToxiBan, Vet-a-Mix)	5–10 mL/kg PO q24h × 1–3 days[202]	Sea turtles/reduce exposure to brevitoxin
Allopurinol	—	Careful when giving with urine acidifiers and uricosuric drugs (probenecid)[60]
	10–20 mg/kg PO q24h[67,217,272]	Most species/gout; decreases production of uric acid;[193] long-term therapy; tortoises may respond best
	25 mg/kg PO q24h[128]	Green iguanas
	50 mg/kg PO q24h × 30 days, then q72h[171]	Chelonians/hyperuricemia
Aluminum hydroxide (Amphogel, Wyeth-Ayerst)	100 mg/kg PO q12–24h[193]	Most species/hyperphosphatemia (associated with renal disease); decreases intestinal absorption of P; use cautiously in patients with gastric outlet obstruction
Amidotrizoate (Gastrografin, Squibb)	5–7.7 mL/kg PO[205]	Gastrointestinal contrast agent; reported faster transit vs barium; no risk if regurgitation
	7.5 mL/kg PO[227]	Tortoises/gastrointestinal contrast agent; give via gavage; mean transit times: 2.6 hr at 87°F (30.6°C); 6.6 hr at 71°F (21.5°C)
Aminophylline	2–4 mg/kg IM[89]	Most species/bronchodilator
Atropine	0.01–0.04 mg/kg IM, IV q8–24h[226]	Most species/dries up excess mucous secretions with infectious stomatitis
	0.1–0.2 mg/kg IM prn[99]	Most species/organophosphate toxicity
	0.2 mg/kg SC, IM[282]	Most species/respiratory distress associated with excessive secretions
Barium sulfate	5–20 mL/kg PO[46]	Most species/gastrointestinal contrast studies
	25 mL/kg PO, 35% wt:vol concentration[14]	Ball pythons/best gastrointestinal image quality
Bleomycin with high voltage electrical pulses	1 U/cm^3 intralesional, repeat in 33 days[38]	Green sea turtles/fibropapillomas electrochemotherapy; use concurrent local anesthesia
	3.65 mg/kg (1 mg/mL) intralesional, repeat in 2 wk[178]	Yellow-bellied slider turtles/squamous cell carcinoma, postpartial surgical excision
Calcium EDTA	10–40 mg/kg IM q12h[244]	Most species/heavy metal chelation; ensure hydration
Carboplatin	2.5–5 mg/kg IV, intracardiac[216]	Most species/carcinoma, osteosarcoma, mesothelioma, carcinomatosis
Carboplatin 4.6 mg implantable bead (compounded, Wedgewood Pharmacy)	≤ 10 mg/kg total q3wk intralesional or surgical excision sites[153]	Chameleons/squamous cell carcinoma, carcinoma; cut bead into smaller pieces to avoid overdose
Chlorambucil (Leukeran, Glaxo SmithKline)	0.1–0.2 mg/kg PO[216]	Most species/lymphoma, leukemia, myeloproliferative tumors
CHOP Therapy (Modified)	See original paper for full protocol details[85]	Green iguanas/successful management of lymphoma postradiation therapy
Cimetidine	4 mg/kg PO, IM q8–12h[99]	Most species/gastric and duodenal ulceration; esophagitis; gastroesophageal reflux; may use in renal failure to increase phosphate secretion

Continued

TABLE 127.9   Miscellaneous Agents—cont'd

Agent	Dosage	Species/Comments
Cisapride (Propulsid, Janssen)	0.5–2 mg/kg PO q24h[99]	Most species/motility modifier; gastrointestinal stasis; not commercially available in the United States; may be compounded; ineffective in desert tortoises at 1 mg/kg[330]
	1–4 mg/kg PO q24h until defecates[336]	Bearded dragons/constipation
Cisplatin	0.5–1 mg/kg IV (prehydrate), intracardiac, intralesional (in oil)[216]	Most species/carcinoma, osteosarcoma, infiltrative sarcoma (intralesional), mesothelioma, carcinomatosis
Cyclophosphamide	10 mg/kg SC, IM, IV, intracardiac[216]	Most species/lymphoma, leukemia, myeloproliferative tumors
Dioctyl Na sulfosuccinate	1–5 mg/kg PO[101]	Most species/constipation; use 1:20 dilution
Diphenhydramine	2 mg/kg IM q24h[202]	Sea turtles/brevitoxicosis; rapidly reduced conjunctival edema, prevented corneal ulceration
Doxorubicin	1 mg/kg IV q7d × 2 treatments, then q14d × 2 treatments, then q21d × 2 treatments[280]	Snakes/chemotherapy for sarcoma (also lymphoma, carcinoma, etc.); treatment periods variable
Famotidine	0.5 mg/kg SC q3d[342]	Kemp's ridley sea turtles
Furosemide	2–5 mg/kg PO, IM, IV q12–24h[149–151]	Most species/diuretic for edema and pulmonary congestion; while lacking loop of Henle, may affect via other mechanisms
	5 mg/kg IM q24h × 1–3 days[202]	Sea turtles/intentional dehydration with brevitoxicosis, no concurrent fluids given
Hydrochlorothiazide	1 mg/kg q24–72h[69]	Lizards/promotes diuresis; monitor hydration status
Iodine compound (Conray 280, Mallinckrodt)	500 mg/kg IV, IO[69]	Lizards/IV urography; take radiographs 0, 5, 15, 30, and 60 min postinjection
Iohexol (240 mg I/mL; Omnipaque, Sanofi Winthrop)	5–20 mL/kg PO[99]	Most species/gastrointestinal contrast studies; nonionic, organic iodine solution; good alternative to barium;[36] faster transit time than barium; can be diluted 1:1 with water
	75 mg/kg IV[159]	Kemp's ridley turtles (juveniles)/GFR assessment
K-Y Jelly (Johnson & Johnson)	1–3 mL of 50% K-Y jelly and 50% warm water/100 g[8]	Most species/enema
Lactulose	0.5 mL/kg PO q24h[149,150,314]	Lizards, chelonians/hepatic lipidosis
L-asparaginase (Elspar, Merck)	400 U/kg SC, IM, intracardiac[216]	Most species/lymphoma, leukemia, myeloproliferative tumors
Maropitant citrate (Cerenia, Zoetis)	1 mg/kg PO, SC q24h (Klaphake E, personal observation.)	Antiemetic; antinausea; no adverse effects seen; Substance P conserved across classes
Melphalan (Alkeran, Celegene)	0.05–0.1 mg/kg Po[216]	Most species/lymphoma, leukemia, myeloproliferative tumors
Methimazole	2 mg/kg q24h × 30 days[114]	Snakes/excessive shedding from hyperthyroidism; limited effectiveness
Methotrexate	0.25 mg/kg PO, SC, IV[216]	Most species/lymphoma, leukemia, myeloproliferative tumors
Metoclopramide	0.06 mg/kg PO q24h × 7 days[66,99]	Most species/stimulates gastric motility
	0.05 mg/kg PO q24h × 7 days[202]	Sea turtles/intestinal motility stimulant
	0.5 mg/kg IM q24h[75]	Sea turtles/supportive care
	1–10 mg/kg PO q24h[349]	Tortoises/stimulates gastric motility; ineffective in desert tortoises at 1 mg/kg[330]
Milk thistle (*Silybum marianum*)	4–15 mg/kg PO q8–12h[149,151]	Lizards, chelonians/hepatoprotectant
Pentobarbital	60–100 mg/kg IV, ICe[7,39]	Euthanasia
Pimobendan	0.2 mg/kg PO q24h[149]	Lizards
Potassium chloride	2 mEq/kg IV, ICe[21]	Most species/euthanasia; cardioplegic; administer after a euthanasia solution
Probenecid	250 mg/kg PO q12h[265]	Most species/gout; increases uric acid excretion; can be increased prn
S-adenosylmethionine (Denosyl, Nutramax)	30 mg/kg PO q24h[239]	Savannah monitors/liver disease
Sodium bicarbonate	0.5–1 mg/kg IV[99]	Most species/hypoxic acidosis postanesthesia
Sucralfate	500–1000 mg/kg PO q6–8h[89]	Most species/oral, esophageal, gastric, and duodenal ulcers
	200 mg/kg PO q24h[343]	Green iguanas/postduodenoileal anastomosis
Tamoxifen 60-day time-release pellets (Innovative Research of America)	Pellets containing 5 mg tamoxifen implants ICe[62]	Leopard geckos/inhibition of follicular development for 60 days if implanted before vitellogenesis
Terbutaline	0.01–0.02 mg/kg IM[306]	Reduce bronchospasm
	Nebulization, 15–45 min/session q4–12h × 3 + days[263]	Lower respiratory tract particle size should be ≤ 0.5 μm, 2–10 μm for trachea; oxygen flow rates < 10 kg 1–2 L/min, 5 L/min for larger reptiles; use bubble humidifier; possible adverse cardiovascular effects
Tricaine methanesulfonate (MS-222)	250–500 mg/kg ICe 1% solution followed by 0.1–1 mL 50% solution ICe or intracardiac[12,57]	Fence lizards, desert iguanas, garter snakes, house geckos, anole species/euthanasia
Vincristine	0.025 mg/kg IV[216]	Most species/lymphoma, leukemia, myeloproliferative tumors

Abbreviations Used in This Formulary

d	day		MIC	minimum inhibitory concentration
EpiCe	epicoelomic		min	minute
h	hour		mo	month
ICe	intracoelomic		mg	milligram
IM	intramuscular		mL	milliliter
IO	intraosseous		PD	pharmacodynamics/pharmacological data
IT	intratracheal		PK	pharmacokinetic data
IV	intravenous		PO	per os
U (IU)	international unit		prn	as needed
kg	kilogram		q	every
L	liter		SC	subcutaneous
LRS	lactated Ringer's solution		URT	upper respiratory tract
MAC	minimum alveolar concentration		wk	week

REFERENCES

See www.expertconsult.com for a complete list of references.

128

Amphibian Formulary

Brent R. Whitaker and Colin T. McDermott

TABLE 128.1   Antimicrobial Agents Used in Amphibians[a,b]

Agent	Dosage	Species/Comments
Amikacin	5 mg/kg IM q36h[52]	Bullfrogs/PK
	5–10 mg/kg SC, IM, ICe q24–48h[51]	Most species; may be used in combination with piperacillin
Carbenicillin	100 mg/kg SC, IM q72h[52]	
	200 mg/kg SC, IM, ICe q24h[52]	
Ceftazidime	20 mg/kg SC, IM q48–72h[52]	
Chloramphenicol	50 mg/kg SC, IM, ICe q12–24h[52]	Caution: even miniscule exposures carries risk of aplastic anemia in susceptible individuals; wear disposable gloves when handling; aplastic anemia-like findings in Bufo regularis exposed to 125 mg/kg PO q24h × 12 wk[13]
	20 mg/L bath[a] changed daily[52]	
Ciprofloxacin	10 mg/kg PO,[52] ICe[51] q24h	
	500–750 mg/75 L as 6–8 hr bath[a] q24h[52]	May be used for large numbers of animals
Doxycycline (Psittavet, Vetafarm)	50 mg/kg IM q7d[52]	Broad-spectrum antibiotic, part of 4-quadrant therapy; may have anti-inflammatory effect; chlamydiosis
Doxycycline (Vibramycin, Zoetis)	5–10 mg/kg PO q24h[52]	Chlamydiosis
	10–50 mg/kg PO q24h[52]	African clawed frogs/chlamydiosis
Doxycycline 1% topical gel, compounded	Apply topically q8–12h not to exceed 10 mg/kg per day[52]	Useful for localized lesions; may have antiinflammatory effect
Enrofloxacin	5–10 mg/kg PO, SC, IM q24h[52]	Most species/PK (bullfrogs);[52] ICe and topical routes also used but with limited PK data[52]
	10 mg/kg SC, IM[14]	African clawed frogs/PK; high kidney concentrations of enrofloxacin and ciprofloxacin;[14] no significant difference between routes[20]
	10 mg/kg topically[46]	Coqui frogs/detectable tissue concentration for >24 hr, no correlation to plasma concentration
	500 mg/L × 6–8 hr bath[a] q24h[52]	
Enrofloxacin and silver sulfadiazine solution (Baytril Otic, Bayer)	Apply topically to lesions q12h[52]	May have some antifungal effect, but does not appear effective against chytrid
Gentamicin	2–4 mg/kg IM q72h × 4 treatments[52]	
	2.5 mg/kg IM q72h[44]	Coldwater salamanders (i.e., Necturus)/ PD; more frequent dosing may be needed if temperature >4°C (39.2°F)
	3 mg/kg IM q24h at 22.2°C (72°F)[52]	Leopard frogs/PD; at higher temperatures, serum concentrations will be lower
	Topical to eyes[52]	All species/ocular infections; dilute to 2 mg/mL
	Intracameral injection once; not to exceed 4 mg/kg[52]	Panophthalmitis
Metronidazole	10 mg/kg PO q24h × 5–10 days[36]	For chronic diarrhea
	10 mg/kg IV q24h × 2 days[52]	Anaerobic infections
	12 mg/kg topically q24h × 5–10 days[52]	For chronic diarrhea
	20 mg/kg PO q48h × 20 days[52]	Anaerobic infections
	50 mg/kg PO q24h × 3 days[52]	Anaerobic infections
	60 mg/kg topically q24h × 3 days[52]	Anaerobic infections
	50 mg/L × 24 hr bath[a,52]	Anaerobic infections
Ofloxacin 0.3% ophthalmic solution	1 drop q2–4h × 10 days[51]	Keratitis; may also be applied topically to wounds

TABLE 128.1 Antimicrobial Agents Used in Amphibians[a,b]—cont'd

Agent	Dosage	Species/Comments
Oxytetracycline	25 mg/kg SC, IM q24h[52]	Most species
	50 mg/kg PO q12–24h[52]	Most species
	50–100 mg/kg IM q48h[52]	Bullfrogs/PK; especially useful in cases of chlamydiosis (use up to 30 days)[52]
	100 mg/L × 1 hr bath[a,52]	Most species
	1 g/kg feed × 7 days[52]	Most useful with axolotls and Xenopus-fed compounded pelleted diet[52]
Piperacillin	100 mg/kg SC, IM q24h[52]	Anaerobes; may be used in combination with amikacin
Silver sulfadiazine (Silvadine Cream 1%, Marion)	Topical q24h[52]	Antibiotic/antifungal cream
Sulfadiazine	132 mg/kg PO q24h[52]	
Sulfamethazine	1 g/L bath[a] to effect[52]	Change daily
Tetracycline	50 mg/kg PO q12h[52]	
	150 mg/kg PO q24h × 5–7 days[52]	
	167 mg/kg (5 mg/30 g) PO q12h × 7 days[52]	
Trimethoprim/sulfa	3 mg/kg PO, SC, IM q24h[52]	Unspecified sulfa
Trimethoprim/sulfadiazine	15–20 mg/kg IM q48h[52]	Chronic diarrhea[52]
Trimethoprim/sulfamethoxazole	15 mg/kg PO q24h[52]	Chronic diarrhea

[a]Water baths containing antibiotics or topical applications may not provide as consistent distribution as parenteral administration.
[b]SC can be administered in the dorsal lymph sac of anurans.[52]

TABLE 128.2 Antifungal Agents Used in Amphibians[a]

Agent	Dosage	Species/Comments
Amphotericin B	1 mg/kg ICe q24h[52]	Internal mycoses; acutely toxic to *Alytes muletensis* tadpoles at 8 µg/mL bath[28]
Benzalkonium chloride	0.25 mg/L × 72 hr bath[52]	
	2 mg/L × 1 hr bath q24h[52]	Saprolegniasis
Chloramphenicol	20 mg/kg topically (applied as Chlorsig 1% ointment [Sigma], which also contains paraffin and wool fat)[4]	Chytridiomycosis; safe for larvae, recent metamorphs, and adults; confirm negative result by real-time PCR;[4,52] caution: even miniscule exposure carries risk of aplastic anemia in susceptible individuals; wear disposable gloves when handling; aplastic anemia-like findings in Bufo regularis exposed to 125 mg/kg PO q24h × 12 wk[13]
	10–30 mg/L (10–30 ppm) as continuous bath replaced fresh daily for up to 30 days[52]	
	20 mg/L by continuous shallow immersion × 14 days, changed daily[54]	Australian green frog (*Litoria caerulea*); severely ill frogs treated with combination of chloramphenicol, SC fluids q8–12h × 6 days, and temperature increased to 28°C × 14 days[54]
Florfenicol	10 µg/mL topical spray q24h × 14 days[33]	Experimentally infected *Alytes muletensis* adults/reduced zoosporangia numbers but did not eliminate infection; GI and renal toxicity to tadpoles at 100 µg/mL[33]
	30 ppm as continuous bath replaced fresh daily for up to 30 days[52]	Chytridiomycosis; safe for larvae, recent metamorphs, and adults; confirm negative result by realtime PCR[52]
Fluconazole	60 mg/kg PO q24h[52]	
Itraconazole	10 mg/kg PO q24h[52]	Topical route best choice to treat chytridiomycosis; caution with tadpoles[15,52]
	0.01% in 0.6% salt solution x 5 min bath q24h × 11 days[52]	
	0.01% in buffered solution x 5 min bath q24h × 11–14 days[16]	Multiple species/cleared chytridiomycosis by PCR 14 days posttreatment; 6–15 mo posttreatment follow-up yielded positive PCR in some individuals
	0.5–1.5 mg/L × 5 min bath q24h × 7 days[15]	*Alytes muletensis* tadpoles/safe at varying concentrations and duration of 7–28 days; confirmed negative PCR posttreatment; varying levels of depigmentation observed in all individuals[15]
	50 mg/L x 5 min bath q24h × 10 days[22]	Multiple species/cleared chytridiomycosis in subclinical animals; confirmed with PCR
	0.0025% × 5 min bath q24h × 6 days[7]	Australian green tree frog (*Litoria caerulea*), coastal plains toad (*Incillus nebulifer*)/cleared PCR positive juveniles with no clinically apparent side effects

Continued

TABLE 128.2   Antifungal Agents Used in Amphibians[a]—cont'd

Agent	Dosage	Species/Comments
Ketoconazole	10–20 mg/kg PO q24h[52]	
	Topical cream[52]	
Methylene blue	2–4 mg/L bath to effect[52]	Tadpoles/may reduce mortality in newly hatched tadpoles
	4 mg/L × 1 hr bath q24h[52]	Saprolegniasis
Miconazole	5 mg/kg ICe q24h × 14–28 days[52]	Systemic mycoses
	Topical cream or solution[52]	Topical route best choice for chytridiomycosis; solutions containing alcohol may cause irritation; do not use with larvae[52]
Neomycin, polymixin B, bacitracin (Neosporin, Pfizer)	Apply topically to wound q24h[18]	Microsporidian infections; not recommended for bacterial infections, appears to inhibit reepithelialization[52]
Nystatin 1% cream	Topical[52]	Cutaneous mycoses
Potassium permanganate	1:5000 water × 5 min bath q24h[52]	Cutaneous mycoses
Sodium chlorite (NaOCl$_2$)	20 mg/L × 6–8 hr bath[52]	Cutaneous mycoses
Temperature elevation	30°C (86°F) × 10 days[10]	*Lithobates catesbeiana, Acris crepitans*/confirm negative result by realtime PCR[10]
	37°C (98.6°F) for 16 hr[49]	Chytridiomycosis, caution with temperature elevation in sensitive species
Terbinafine HCl (Lamisil AT, Novartis)	0.005%–0.01% in distilled water × 5 min bath q24h × 5 days, or q48h × 6 treatments[6]	Various species/no adverse clinical effects noted with treatment; pH 7.0; confirm negative result by realtime PCR[6]
Voriconazole	1.25 µg/mL q24h topically via spray × 7 days[28]	Poison dart frogs, Iberian midwife toad (*Alytes cisternasii*)/cleared chytridiomycosis in naturally infected individuals in vivo; performed poorly with in vitro assays[28]
Voriconazole (V) + polymixin E (P) + elevated temperature (T)	(V) 12.5 µg/mL q24h topically via spray + (P) 2000 IU/mL × 10 min bath q12h + (T) 20°C (68°F) continuous × 10 days[5]	Fire salamanders/treatment of *Batrachochytrium salamandrivorans*; no effect of medications at 15°C (59°F)[5]

[a]To control the spread of *Batrachochytrium dendrobatidis,* new gloves should be worn after handling each patient. Nitrile gloves are preferred for their ability to kill zoospores on contact. Bare hands are preferred over rinsing the same pair of gloves between patients.[30]

TABLE 128.3   Antiparasitic Agents Used in Amphibians[a]

Agent	Dosage	Species/Comments
Acriflavin	0.025% bath × 5 days[52]	Protozoa
	500 mg/L × 30 min bath[52]	Protozoa
Benzalkonium chloride	2 mg/L × 1 hr bath q24h to effect[52]	Protozoa
Distilled water	3 hr bath[52]	Protozoa
Febantel (in combination with pyrantel pamoate and praziquantel; Drontal Plus, Bayer)	0.01 mL/1 g (10 mL/kg) PO q2–3 wk[34]	Nematodes, cestodes, possibly trematodes
Fenbendazole	—	Fenbendazole combinations follow
	30–50 mg/kg PO[52]	Gastrointestinal nematodes
	50 mg/kg PO q24h × 3–5 days, repeat in 14–21 days[52]	Gastrointestinal nematodes
	50–100 mg/kg PO[36] repeat in 2–3 wk prn	Most species/gastrointestinal nematodes
	100 mg/kg PO,[52] repeat in 14 days	Gastrointestinal nematodes
Fenbendazole (F)/ivermectin (I)	(F) 100 mg/kg PO on day 1, then (I) 0.2 mg/kg PO on days 2,11[52]	Gastrointestinal nematodes
Fenbendazole (F)/metronidazole (M)	(F) 100 mg/kg PO, repeat in 10–14 days + (M) 10 mg/kg PO q24h for 5 days[52]	Concurrent gastrointestinal nematodes and protozoa
Formalin (10%)	—	Do not use if skin is ulcerated; may be toxic to some species
	1.5 mL/L × 10 min bath q48h to effect[52]	Protozoans; may be toxic in some species
	0.5% × 10 min bath once[52]	Monogenic trematodes; may be toxic to some species
Ivermectin	—	See fenbendazole for combination; caution: may cause flaccid paralysis with overdosage; caffeine or physostigmine may ameliorate effects[52]
	0.2–0.4 mg/kg PO, SC, repeat q14d as needed[52]	Nematodes, including lungworms; mites
	2 mg/kg topically, repeat in 2–3 wk[26]	Especially useful for small specimens[52] and Rana spp.[26]
	10 mg/L × 60 min bath, repeat q14d prn[52]	Mites

TABLE 128.3 **Antiparasitic Agents Used in Amphibians[a]—cont'd**

Agent	Dosage	Species/Comments
Levamisole	—	May cause paralysis in some species at suggested dosages;[52] caffeine or physostigmine may ameliorate effects[52]
	6.5–13.5 mg/kg topically to pelvic patch, repeat in 10 days[3]	*Anaxyrus houstonensis*/reduced nematode egg counts
	10 mg/kg IM, ICe, topically,[52] repeat in 2 wk	Nematodes, including lungworms
	12 mg/L bath × 4 days[21]	African clawed frogs/cutaneous nematodes; use ≥4.2 L of tank water/frog
	100 mg/L × ≥72 hr bath[52]	Resistant nematodes
	100–300 mg/L × 24 hr bath, repeat in 1–2 wk[52]	Nematodes, including subcutaneous nematodes in aquatic amphibians; water soluble form is available through aquaculture supply companies
Metronidazole	—	See fenbendazole for combination; toxicity possible at high doses
	10 mg/kg PO q24h × 5–10 days[52]	Protozoa; for unfamiliar or sensitive species
	50 mg/kg PO q24h × 3–5 days[52]	Confirmed cases of amoebiasis and flagellate overload
	100 mg/kg PO q3d[52]	Protozoa
	100–150 mg/kg PO, repeat in 2–3 wk or prn[52]	Protozoa (i.e., Entamoeba, Hexamita, Opalina)
	50 mg/L × 24 hr bath[52]	Aquatic amphibians/protozoa
	500 mg/100 g feed × 3–4 treatments[52]	Ciliates
Moxidectin	200 μg/kg SC q4mo[38]	Nematodes
Oxfendazole	5 mg/kg PO[52]	Gastrointestinal nematodes
Oxytetracycline	25 mg/kg SC, IM q24h[52]	Protozoa
	50 mg/kg PO q12h[52]	Protozoa
	1 g/kg feed × 7 days[52]	Protozoa
Paromomycin	50–75 mg/kg PO q24h[52]	Gastrointestinal protozoa
Piperazine	50 mg/kg PO, repeat in 2 wk[52]	Gastrointestinal nematodes
Ponazuril	30 mg/kg PO q12h × 3 days, repeat in 3 wk; often more effective at 30 mg/kg PO q24h × 30 days; may work with less frequent treatments[52]	Coccidia but not Cryptosporidium; may have some effect on unidentified protozoan cysts
Potassium permanganate	7 mg/L × 5 min bath q24h to effect[52]	Ectoparasitic protozoa
Praziquantel	8–24 mg/kg PO, SC, ICe, topically,[52] repeat q14d	Trematodes, cestodes
	10 mg/L × 3 hr bath,[52] repeat q7–21d	Trematodes, cestodes
Pyrantel pamoate	5 mg/kg PO q14d[34]	Nematodes
Ronidazole	10 mg/kg PO q24h × 10 days[52]	Flagellated protozoa, amoebas
Salt (sodium chloride)	4–6 g/L continuous bath[52]	Ectoparasitic protozoa
	5 g/L bath up to 12h, 10 g/L bath up to 1h (Marcec et al, Proc ARAV, 2011, p 1)	Axolotls, immediate negative clinical effects in baths >20 g/L
	6 g/L × 5–10 min bath q24h × 3–5 days[52]	Ectoparasitic protozoa
	25 g/L × ≤10 min bath[52]	Ectoparasitic protozoa
Selamectin (Revolution, Zoetis)	6 mg/kg topically[11]	Bullfrogs/PK
Sulfadiazine	132 mg/kg PO q24h[52]	Coccidiosis
Sulfamethazine	1 g/L bath[52]	Coccidiosis; change daily to effect
Tetracycline	50 mg/kg PO q12h[52]	Protozoa
Thiabendazole	50–100 mg/kg PO,[52] repeat in 2 wk prn	Gastrointestinal nematodes
	100 mg/L bath, repeat in 2 wk[52]	Verminous dermatitis
Trimethoprim/sulfa	3 mg/kg PO, SC, IM q24h[52]	Coccidiosis; unspecified sulfa

[a]SC can be administered in the dorsal lymph sac of anurans.[52]

Agent	Dosage	Species/Comments
Alfaxalone	5–25 mg/kg IM (Lennox, Proc ARAV, 2013, pp 66–68)	Most species/recommend starting at lower dose (5–10 mg/kg) and titrating up
	10–17.5 mg/kg IM[35]	Bullfrogs/immobilization, respiratory depression, still responsive to noxious stimuli; dose-dependent time to recumbency and time to recovery; no effect by immersion at 2 g/L for 30 min[35]
	18 mg/kg IM, IV, Ice (Hadzima et al, Proc ARAV, 2013, pp 60–64)	African clawed frogs/deep sedation for 1–3 hr (IM, IV), 10–60 min ICe; no effect via immersion at 18 mg/L
	20–30 mg/kg IM[40]	Australian tree frogs/initial effect within 10 min, respiratory depression; insufficient anesthesia as sole agent for painful procedures
	5 mg/L in fresh water bath[29]	Axolotls/single individual; induction of anesthesia, maintained continuous irrigation of gills and skin with additional 0.03 mL drops of alfaxalone for maintenance of anesthesia during surgery[29]
	200 mg/L in fresh water bath[2]	Fire-bellied toads/buffer with sodium bicarbonate to pH 7.2; anesthetic induction in 14 ± 4 min, variable duration of anesthesia up to 30 min; not sufficient for painful procedures
Alfaxalone (A)/morphine (M)	(A) 3 mg/100 mL + (M) 5 mg/100 mL as bath[1]	Fire-bellied toads/provided anesthetic induction and antinociception
Atipamezole (Antisedan, Zoetis)	Titrate to effect IM, IV[27]	Antagonist for dexmedetomidine[27]
Benzocaine (Sigma Chemical)	—	Anesthesia; not sold as fish anesthetic in United States; available from chemical supply companies; do not use topical anesthetic products marketed for mammals; prepare stock solution in ethanol (poorly soluble in water); store in dark bottle at room temperature
	50 mg/L bath to effect[52]	Larvae/dissolve in ethanol first
	200–300 mg/L bath to effect[52]	Frogs, salamanders/dissolve in ethanol first
	200–500 mg/L bath[52]	Dissolve in acetone first
Buprenorphine	38 mg/kg SC[27]	Analgesia & sedation;4 hr; ED₅₀[b] in leopard frogs[27]
	50 mg/kg ICe q24h[23]	Eastern red spotted newts/return to normal behavior after limb amputation; may take >1 hr for onset of clinical effects; postsurgical bath in 0.1% sulfamerazine (w/v; Sigma Chemical Company)[23]
Butorphanol	0.2–0.4 mg/kg IM[52]	Analgesia; efficacy uncertain[52]
	0.5 mg/L continuous immersion for 3 days[23]	Eastern red spotted newts/return to normal behavior after limb amputation; may take >4 hr for onset of clinical effects; postsurgical bath in 0.1% sulfamerazine (w/v; Sigma Chemical Company)[23]
Eugenol (clove oil, 100% eugenol; Aqui-S 20E 10% eugenol)	0.3 mL/L (~310–318 mg/L)[52]	Anesthesia; deep anesthesia after 15 min bath; caused reversible gastric prolapse in 50% of leopard frogs
	0.35 mL in 1 L purified water[17]	African clawed frogs/anesthetic plane for frogs <10 g after 5 min immersion, for frogs ~30 g after 10 min immersion
	0.45 mL/L (~473 mg/L)[32]	Anesthesia; deep anesthesia induced in 80% of tiger salamanders
Codeine	53 mg/kg SC[27]	Analgesia >4 hr; ED₅₀[b] in leopard frogs
Dexmedetomidine	40–120 mg/kg SC[27]	Analgesia >4 hr; ED₅₀[b] in leopard frogs
Diazepam	—	See ketamine for combination
Fentanyl	0.5 mg/kg SC[27]	Analgesia >4 hr; ED₅₀[b] in leopard frogs
Flunixin meglumine	25 mg/kg intralymphatic[9]	African clawed frogs
Isoeugenol (Aqui-S; 50% isoeugenol)	20–50 µL/L[41]	*Litoria ewingii* tadpoles/higher doses resulted in faster induction and longer recovery
Isoflurane	—	Anesthesia; induction chamber
	3%–5% induction, 1%–2% maintenance[52]	Terrestrial species
	5%[52]	Terrestrial species/euthanasia; induction chamber
	Topical application of liquid isoflurane[52]	Bufo spp. (0.015 mL/g BW), African clawed frogs (0.007 mL/g BW)/induce in closed container; once induced, remove excess from animal
	Topical mixture of isoflurane (3 mL), KY jelly (3.5 mL), and water (1.5 mL)[52]	Bufo spp. (0.035 mL/g BW), African clawed frogs (0.025 mL/g BW)/induce in closed container; once induced, remove excess from animal
	Topical mixture of 1.5 parts distilled water, 3.5 parts nonspermicidal jelly, and 1.8 parts isoflurane[55]	American tree frogs/induced in closed container; once induced remove excess from animal; erythematous lesions and signs of systemic illness noted after application[55]
	0.28 mL/100 mL bath[52]	Induce in closed container
	Bubbled into water to effect[52]	Aquatic species

TABLE 128.4 Chemical Restraint/Anesthetic/Analgesic Agents Used in Amphibians[a]

TABLE 128.4   Chemical Restraint/Anesthetic/Analgesic Agents Used in Amphibians[a]—cont'd

Agent	Dosage	Species/Comments
Ketamine	—	May have long induction and recovery times; does not provide good analgesia so may not be suited for major surgical procedures; other agents preferred; ketamine combination follows; see lidocaine
	50–150 mg/kg SC, IM[52]	Most species
Ketamine (K)/diazepam (D)	(K) 20–40 mg/kg + (D) 0.2–0.4 mg/kg IM[52]	Variable results
Lidocaine 1%–2%	Local infiltration[52]	All/local anesthesia; with or without epinephrine; 2% lidocaine in combination with ketamine has been used for minor surgeries;[52] use with caution
Meloxicam	0.1 mg/kg[31]	American bullfrogs/decreased circulating PGE2 levels measured 24 hr post muscle biopsy[31]
	0.4–1 mg/kg PO, SC, ICe q24h[51]	Antiinflammatory; presumptive analgesia; adjunct therapy for septicemia
	0.5% gel topically q24h; do not exceed 0.4 mg/kg[52]	Antiinflammatory for localized wounds
Metomidate hydrochloride	30 mg/L bath[12]	*Rana pipiens*/immersion for 60 min then transferred to amphibian ringer's solution; clinical sedation in 11/11 frogs; surgical anesthesia in 3/11; prolonged recovery; not recommended as sole anesthetic agent
Morphine	38–42 mg/kg SC[27]	Analgesia >4 hr
Nalorphine	122 mg/kg SC[27]	Analgesia >4 hr
Naloxone	10 mg/kg SC;[27] titrate to effect	Antagonist for buprenorphine, butorphanol, codeine, fentanyl, morphine
Naltrexone	1 mg/kg SC;[27] titrate to effect	Antagonist for buprenorphine, butorphanol, codeine, fentanyl, morphine
Pentobarbital sodium	60 mg/kg IV, ICe[52]	Euthanasia; can also be administered in lymph sacs in anurans
Pentobarbital sodium + sodium phenytoin	1100 mg/kg + 141 mg/kg ICe[45]	African clawed frogs/complete cardiac arrest within 3 hr
Propofol	10–30 mg/kg ICe[52]	White's tree frogs/pilot study; use the lower dosage for sedation or light anesthesia; induction within 30 min; recovery in 24 hr
	35 mg/kg ICe[32]	Deep anesthesia in 83% of tiger salamanders[32]
	35 mg/kg ICe[50]	Sonoran desert toads/sedation only; did not achieve surgical plane of anesthesia
	60–100 mg/kg ICe[52]	Euthanasia
	88 mg/L by immersion[19]	African clawed frogs/induced for 15 min, then rinsed; respiratory depression, darkened skin color; death at doses over 175 mg/L
	100–140 mg/kg topically[52]	Maroon-eyed tree frogs (Agalychnis litodryas)/unpublished data; 15–20 min to max effect at 100 mg/kg dose; 10–15 min to max effect at 140 mg/kg;[52] sedation to deep anesthesia; remove and rinse when desired level achieved; recommended only for animals <50 g
Sevoflurane	Topical application	Rapid recovery unless constant reapplication
	Topical mixture of 1.5 parts distilled water, 3.5 parts nonspermicidal jelly, and 3 parts sevoflurane[42,55]	American tree frogs/induced in closed container with 2 mL of sevoflurane jelly per individual; once induced, remove excess from animal; recovery 4.5 times faster than topical isoflurane jelly;[55] in cane toads, reliable loss of righting reflex when 37.5 μg/g sevoflurane in jelly was applied to dorsum[42]
Tiletamine/zolazepam (Telazol, Fort Dodge)	10–20 mg/kg IM[52]	Results variable between species; rapid recovery; not suitable as single anesthetic agent for anurans[25]

Continued

TABLE 128.4   Chemical Restraint/Anesthetic/Analgesic Agents Used in Amphibians[a]—cont'd

Agent	Dosage	Species/Comments
Tricaine methanesulfonate (MS-222) (Finquel, Argent)	—	Anesthesia; buffer the acidity by adding sodium bicarbonate to buffer the solution to a pH of 7.0–7.1; aerate water to prevent hypoxemia; remove from bath on induction or overdosing can readily occur; after bath, place terrestrial amphibians on moist towel or in very shallow water to recovery; some species can be induced at much lower concentrations than listed here; in some cases, anesthesia can be maintained by dripping a dilute solution of this drug (100–200 mg/L) over the skin or by covering animal with a paper towel moistened with the anesthetic[52]
	50–200 mg/kg SC, IM, ICe[52]	Most species/may be irritating administered SC, IM (neutral solution is preferred)[52]
	100–200 mg/kg ICe[43]	Leopard frogs
	100–400 mg/kg ICe[43]	Bullfrogs
	100–200 mg/L bath to effect[52]	Larvae/induction
	200–500 mg/L bath to effect[52]	Tadpoles, newts/induction in 15–30 min
	0.5–2 g/L bath to effect[52]	Frogs, salamanders/induction in 15–30 min
	1 g/L bath to effect[52]	Most gill-less adult species (unless very large)/induction
	1 g/L by immersion, buffered with 1 g/L sodium bicarbonate[50]	Sonoran desert toads/surgical plane of anesthesia
	1–2 g/L by immersion[24]	African clawed frogs/buffered to pH of 7.0 +/- 0.4; 20 min induction then rinsed; respiratory depression; longer duration of surgical anesthesia with higher dosing
	2–3 g/L bath to effect[52]	Toads/induction in 15–30 min
	5 g/L immersion[45]	African clawed frogs/immersion for 1 hr; death within 3 hr
	10 g/L bath[52]	Euthanasia; can be administered ICe or in lymph sacs

[a]SC can be administered in dorsal lymph sac in anurans.[52]
[b]ED50, effective dose for 50% of the population.

TABLE 128.5   Hormones Used in Amphibians[a]

Agent	Dosage	Species/Comments
Gonadotropin-releasing hormone (GnRH)	10 µg SC to female followed by additional 20 µg after 18 hr; 5 µg SC to male[48]	Tomato frogs (Dyscophus guineti)/ovulation and spermiation
	0.1 mg/kg SC, IM, repeat prn[52]	Induction of ovulation in those nonresponsive to PMSG or hCG; administer to females 8–12 hr before males
Human chorionic gonadotropin (hCG)	50–300 U SC, IM[52]	For mating or release of sperm in males; follow with GnRH in 8–24 hr
	250–400 U SC, IM[52]	African clawed frogs, axolotls/induction of ovulation; may be used with PMSG and/or progesterone
Luteinizing hormone–releasing hormone (LHRH)	5 µg ICe per animal[47]	Salamanders (Desmognathus ochrophaeus)/induced oviposition in 94% of animals
	10 µg in 0.05 mL of 40% DMSO applied to ventral drink patch[37]	Bufo americanus, B. valliceps/induced spermiation in 70% of males
Pregnant mare serum gonadotropin (PMSG)	50–200 U SC, IM[52]	African clawed frogs, axolotls/induction of ovulation; administer 600 U hCG SC, IM 72 hr later[52]
Progesterone	1–5 mg SC, IM[52]	African clawed frogs, axolotls/use in addition to PMSG or hCG for induction of ovulation

[a]SC can be administered into the dorsal lymph sac of anurans.[52]

TABLE 128.6   Miscellaneous Agents Used in Amphibians[a]

Agent	Dosage	Species/Comments
Amphibian Ringer's solution (ARS)	6.6 g NaCl, 0.15 g KCl, 0.15 g CaCl$_2$, and 0.2 g NaHCO$_3$ in 1 L water[52]	For treating hydrocoelom and subcutaneous edema; place animal in shallow ARS bath until stabilized (≈24 hr or more); replace with fresh solution daily; may need to wean animal off ARS by placing it in gradually more dilute solutions; hypertonic solution created by using 800–950 mL water instead of 1 L and may be more effective for some cases of hydrocoelom; up to 10 g of glucose may be added per L, but then solution must be made fresh daily[52]
Atropine	0.1 mg/animal SC, IM prn[52]	Organophosphate toxicosis
Caffeine	Use caffeinated tea bag; steep (soak) until solution is "weak tea"; place amphibian in shallow bath, replace q6h[52]	Stimulant; may help reverse ivermectin or levamisole toxicosis, or excessively deep anesthesia[52]
Calcium glubionate (Calcionate, 1.8g/5 mL, Rugby Laboratories)	1 mL/kg PO q24h[52]	Nutritional secondary hyperparathyroidism
Calcium gluconate	100–200 mg/kg SC[52] 2.3% continuous bath (with 2–3 U/mL vitamin D$_3$)[52]	Hypocalcemic tetany Nutritional secondary hyperparathyroidism
Critical care diets	—	Dosages are approximate; may be more appropriate to offer larger volume less frequently for easily stressed animals
• Carnivore Critical Care (Oxbow)	3% bodyweight PO q24–72h[52]	
• Emeraid for Carnivores (Lafeber)	3% body weight PO q24–48h[52]	
• Feline Clinical Care Liquid (Pet-Ag)	1–2 mL/50 g PO q24h[52] 3–6 mL/50 g PO q72h[52]	
• Hill's Feline a/d (Hill's Pet Nutrition)	PO[52]	Nutritional support; mix 1:1 with water; generally gavaged
Cyanoacrylate surgical adhesive (Vet Bond, 3M)	Topical on wounds[52]	Produces a seal for aquatic and semiaquatic species
Dexamethasone	1.5 mg/kg SC, IM[52] 1.5 mg/kg IM, IV[52]	Vascularizing keratitis Shock
Dextrose 5% solution	Bath[52]	For treating hydrocoelom and subcutaneous edema;[52] place animal in shallow bath until stabilized (≈24 hr or more); replace with fresh solution daily; may need to wean animal off dextrose by placing it in gradually more dilute solutions; 7.5–10% solutions may be more effective for some cases of hydrocoelom
	Topically to affected tissues (McDermott et al, Proc ARAV, 2015, p 477)	Small amount can be applied to edematous/inflamed tissue in cases of cloacal prolapse to aid in prolapse reduction
Doxycycline	1.25–2.5 mg/kg PO, SC, ICe q24h[52] 1% gel topically q12h[52]	Antiinflammatory Antiinflammatory
Hetastarch (6% in 0.9% saline)	Bath not to exceed 1 hr without reassessment[52]	May help with initial treatment of hydrocoelom
Hypertonic saline, 5% ophthalmic solution	Topically to affected tissues (McDermott et al, Proc ARAV, 2015, p 477)	Small amount can be applied to edematous/inflamed tissue in cases of cloacal prolapse to aid in prolapse reduction
Laxative (Laxatone, Evsco)	PO[52]	Laxative, especially for intestinal foreign bodies
Methylene blue	2 mg/mL bath to effect[52]	Nitrite and nitrate toxicoses
Oxygen	100% for up to 24 hr[52]	Adjunct treatment for septicemia, toxicoses
Physostigmine (ophthalmic drops)	1 drop/50 g topically q1–2h to effect[52]	May ameliorate flaccid paralysis from ivermectin or levamisole toxicosis
Prednisolone sodium succinate	5–10 mg/kg IM, IV[52]	Shock
Sodium thiosulfate	1% solution as continuous bath to effect[52]	Halogen toxicoses

Continued

TABLE 128.6   Miscellaneous Agents Used in Amphibians[a]—cont'd

Agent	Dosage	Species/Comments
Vitamin A (Aquasol A, 50,000 U/mL, Mayne Pharma)	Dilute 1:9 with sterile water; make fresh weekly; apply 1 drop from a tuberculin syringe with 27-g needle to amphibians under 5 g; 1 drop from tuberculin syringe w/out needle is about 200 U and useful for 15–30 g BW; >30 g, try 1 drop per 10 g BW; topically q24h × 14 days, then q4–7d[52] Dilute 1:10 in sterile water; applied as one drop from 18-g needle; estimated as 50 U/frog q48h to q7d[39] 1 U/g PO daily × 14 days[52]	Hypovitaminosis A; given the plethora of organ systems that hypovitaminosis A may affect, it is reasonable to institute vitamin A supplementation of any clinically ill amphibian, particularly ones with signs similar to "short tongue syndrome," swollen eyelids, evidence of infectious dermatitis, hydrocoelom, or simply "failing to thrive";[52] the use of mixed dietary carotenoids may also be effective in some species[8] African foam–nesting frogs/weight range, 2–7 g; dosing q48h and once weekly significantly increased whole body vitamin A levels over control group and group treated with vitamin A fortified supplement dusted over crickets[39]
Vitamin A gel caps (10,000 U/cap)	Dilute 1:9 with corn oil to yield 1000 U/mL; give 1 U/g PO q24h × 14 days, then q7d[52]	Hypovitaminosis A; given the plethora of organ systems that hypovitaminosis A may affect, it is reasonable to institute vitamin A supplementation of any clinically ill amphibian, particularly ones with signs similar to "short tongue syndrome," swollen eyelids, evidence of infectious dermatitis, hydrocoelom, or simply "failing to thrive;"[52] the use of mixed dietary carotenoids may also be effective in some species[8]
Vitamin B₁	25 mg/kg PO[52] 25–100 mg/kg IM, ICe[53]	Deficiency resulting from thiaminase-containing fish
Vitamin D₃	2–3 U/mL continuous bath (with 2.3% calcium gluconate)[52] 100–400 U/kg PO q24h[52]	Nutritional secondary hyperparathyroidism
Vitamin E (alpha-tocopherol)	1 mg/kg PO, IM q7d[52] 200 U/kg feed[52]	Steatitis

[a]SC can be administered into the dorsal lymph sac of anurans.[52]

Abbreviations Used in This Formulary

d	day		MIC	minimum inhibitory concentration
EpiCe	epicoelomic		min	minute
h	hour		mo	month
ICe	intracoelomic		mg	milligram
IM	intramuscular		mL	milliliter
IO	intraosseous		PD	pharmacodynamics/pharmacological data
IT	intratracheal		PK	pharmacokinetic data
IV	intravenous		PO	per os
U (IU)	international unit		prn	as needed
kg	kilogram		q	every
L	liter		SC	subcutaneous
LRS	lactated Ringer's solution		URT	upper respiratory tract
MAC	minimum alveolar concentration		wk	week

REFERENCES

See www.expertconsult.com for a complete list of references.

129

Photobiomodulation (Low-Level Laser Therapy)

Lara M. Cusack and Stephen J. Divers

Low-level laser therapy (LLLT), or photobiomodulation (PBM), has been used in human and veterinary medicine for decades. More recently, zoological practitioners have begun to utilize LLLT for its anti-inflammatory, analgesic, and wound-healing effects. Though dissent in the level of effectiveness of laser therapy as a treatment modality remains, there exists a growing body of literature around its use as low-risk treatment with potential benefits for a variety of medical conditions. Improved rates of healing for epithelial trauma and musculoskeletal injuries, as well as improvements in chronic pain, have been documented in multiple species, including humans, rats, pigs, and rabbits.[1–7]

Laser light induces a photochemical reaction at the cellular level, which stimulates a biochemical response increasing the production of ATP and results in both local and systemic effects. Photoreceptor cells, such as hemoglobin, cytochrome c oxidase, and melanin, when hit by the laser, absorb the energy, which is stored and used to perform a variety of cellular activities that can have direct effects on healing, including fibroblast proliferation, angiogenesis, and cytokine synthesis.[8–10] An increase in fibroblast proliferation and migration, with subsequent increases in collagen production, contraction of granulation tissue, and improved wound tensile strength, has been attributed to laser therapy treatment and has been documented in multiple wound-healing studies in rats.[12–14] Additional effects, such as analgesia and reduction in edema, have also been documented.[6,7,15–17]

WOUND HEALING

The phases of wound healing in the reptile parallel those in mammals but occur at a slower rate, differ between species, and are affected by a variety of factors such as temperature and restraint-associated stress.[18–20] As infection remains one of the most common complications of wounds, promotion of epitheliogenesis is important both for the primary effects on wound retraction and due to the fact that the epithelial barrier is the primary method of preventing infection.[21] The use of LLLT may be an effective tool in promotion of healing in the reptile patient and may be used for promotion of epitheliogenesis and tissue healing, analgesia, and antiinflammatory effects.

EQUIPMENT AND TECHNIQUES

In a recent survey by *Veterinary Economics*, one in every five veterinarians were using or expanding the use of LLLT in their practices; this availability of equipment greatly increases practical application of this treatment modality for reptile patients.[22] There exists a variety of different veterinary laser units for purchase, each varying in terms of emission mode, power, wavelength, hand pieces, surgical options, and type of delivery system. The emission mode describes the method in which the energy is delivered and is usually described as continuous, chopped, or super-pulse. In general, increasing the pulse duration increases the level of peak power that can be delivered without tissue damage.[22]

The power of the laser is measured in watts (W), which describes the amount of energy (photons) transferred to tissue over time. Increasing wattage coincides with an increase in the number of photons arriving at the tissue. High- and low-power units can deliver an equal number of photons; however, higher-power units will be faster in their delivery.[23] This can be important in a clinical setting, in particular with zoological patients, where minimizing handling times is often desirable. The class of laser is determined by the level of average power, with anything above 500 mW classified as a class IV laser.[23] Due to their increased power, class IV lasers have the ability to damage eyesight and tissue, but they have the advantage of requiring decreased time for treatment.[23] A summary of some of the class IV lasers available for veterinary use is provided in Table 129.1.[22] The wavelength of the laser is measured in nanometers (nm) and is directly correlated to the capability of the laser to penetrate tissue.[22] Detailed information on delivery systems for individual units can be obtained from the specific laser companies.

Penetration of tissues requires the appropriate combination of power, wavelength, and treatment time. The World Association of Laser Therapy suggests that mammalian cells require 4 to 10 J/cm² in order to generate a positive photobiochemical response. Cells closer to the surface require a smaller dose, with deep tissue cells requiring an increased dose.[24] A number of variables of the reptile patient, including pigment, epithelial thickness, stage of ecdysis, and temperature, can make establishment of appropriate dose challenging for the reptile patient, and there are no currently established guidelines for the use of LLLT in any reptile. However, several of the available laser units offer preestablished settings for the exotic patient and for commonly treated conditions such as fractures and wounds, thereby increasing ease of use. The reliability of such presets is unknown, and these settings should be considered a guide at best. Individual animal and species variability can influence the effects of laser therapy, and it is recommended that practitioners maintain a log of settings used for individual patients, conditions, and results.

General recommendations for use of laser on wounds and other tissues involves gentle contact, if using a contact probe, and a continual, sweeping or painting motion of the tissues in order to distribute energy and prevent thermal or photodynamic tissue trauma. Consideration should be given to the level of pigmentation and thickness of the tissue being treated, as the degree of energy penetration will be increased with less pigmented and thinner tissues. Intermittent palpation of the treatment area (or use of a thermal imaging or temperature gun) will allow the operator to ensure that a targeted area is not becoming too warm. Continual visual assessment of the target area during treatment will allow for assessment of any additional signs of tissue trauma. The authors have used laser therapy for a variety of conditions in reptiles, including epithelial wounds, fractures of the carapace and plastron, and joint swelling, and have not noted any negative effects when using the preset

TABLE 129.1   A Summary of Some of the Commercially Available Class IV Laser Units

Company	Emission Mode	Min–Max Power	Wavelength	Handpieces/Probes	Surgery Option
Companion Therapy Laser (LiteCure)	Continuous, pulse	0.25 w–15 w (depending on model)	980, 810, 650 nm (depending on model)	2 deep tissue, 2 superficial treatment	Yes
Cutting Edge Laser Technologies	Continuous, frequenced continuous, super pulse, combined, synchronized	1.2 w (average)	650, 808, 905 nm	Small, large, acupuncture, and intraoral	No
Diowave Laser Systems	Continuous, pulse	1 w–10 w	980 nm, 808/810 nm, 810/980 nm (depending on model)	Multiple	Yes
K-Laser USA	Continuous, pulse, intense super pulse	0.1 w–20 w (depending on model)	660, 800, 905, 970 nm (depending on model)	Quick-release, adjustable for contact and noncontact, optional ear/nose/throat tip	Yes
Pegasus Therapy Lasers (LiteCure)	Continuous, pulse	0.25 w–15 w (depending on model)	980, 810, 650 nm (depending on model)	2 deep tissue, 2 superficial treatment	Yes
Respond Systems Inc.	Continuous, super pulse	1 mw–5 w (depending on model)	660, 810, 850 nm	Small profile with rounded tip, advantage tip, high-power, cluster, acupuncture tip	No

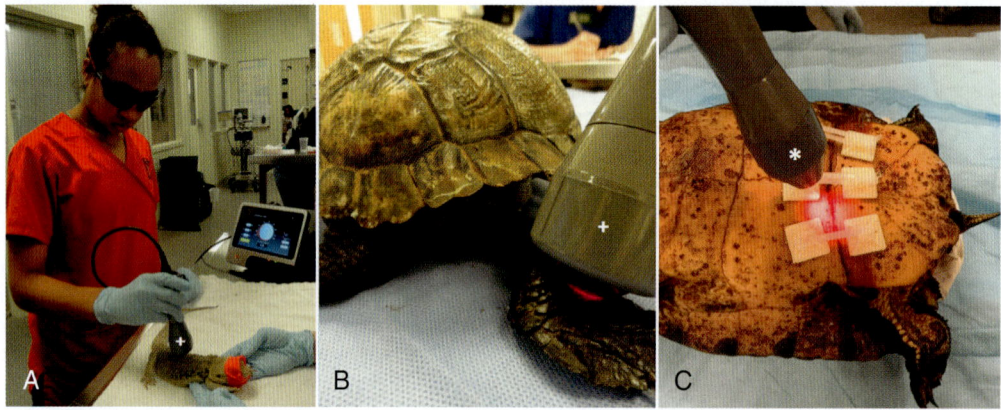

FIG 129.1 The use of different probes, or tissue applicators, can achieve different levels of tissue penetration. (A and B) Deep tissue applicators (+) can be directly applied to the tissue and are useful for deeper wounds and musculoskeletal injuries. (C) Superficial treatment applicators (*) may be used for shell fractures or for injuries where direct contact may be contraindicated. (Courtesy of Lara M. Cusack and Stephen J. Divers.)

reptile treatment protocols as a guideline for therapy. The use of different probes can increase or decrease tissue contact (Fig. 129.1).

Deep tissue applicators allow direct tissue contact and result in much less light being reflected from the skin. The use of such handpieces results in up to 90% more photons reaching the tissue compared to a noncontact hand piece. This may be of particular importance in the reptile patient, as there is a potential for increased reflectivity, or absorption, by the reptilian integument. Handpieces such as the superficial treatment applicators may be more appropriate for injuries such as shell fractures or suture lines, where direct contact may cause iatrogenic tissue trauma or damage to the probe tip.

Additional considerations for the use of laser therapy include the appropriate use of personal protective equipment for both the operator and the patient. Protective eyewear is essential, as high-power laser is known to have negative effects on the eye and should be specific for the wavelength being used (see Fig. 129.1A).

THERAPEUTIC EFFECTS

Despite the growing body of literature supporting the clinical effects of laser therapy in humans, some veterinary studies or reports fail to

document an objective, therapeutic response when compared to controls. The effects of laser therapy vary greatly depending on wavelength, energy, energy density, duration, and the delivery system, and it is likely that the results of wound healing studies are related to these variables, making appropriate dosing important for safe clinical effect. Unfortunately, comparison between studies remains difficult due to variability between treatment protocols, and there is little information on effective and safe laser protocols, especially for exotic species. Therefore, although positive outcomes are possible, the use of nonspecific, unproven regimes may result in no objectively measurable, beneficial effects. Owners should be advised that there are likely no deleterious effects from appropriate LLLT, but clinicians should be cautious regarding unsubstantiated claims of proven efficacy.

Laser therapy has been used for the treatment of skin and shell ulceration in a soft-shelled turtle (*Pelodiscus sinensis*) and for skin wounds in two species of chelonians (*Testudo hermanni* and *Trachemys scripta*); subjective improvement of the lesions was noted in all cases, but results were not verified by histopathology.[25,26] A recent study looking at the effects of therapeutic laser on first-intention incisional wound healing in ball pythons (*Python reguis*) compared rate of healing and histologic wound reaction (reduced inflammation, necrosis, and edema) between wounds treated with therapeutic laser and untreated control incisions. Though there was no significant difference in overall wound healing between treatment groups at the end of the study, the grade of collagen maturity was significantly higher, and gross wound scores were lower for the laser-treated group than for the control group. Treatment in this study consisted of a power output of 0.5 W for 90 seconds once daily for 7 consecutive days, and the dose delivered to each incision was 5 J/cm^2 with a wavelength of 980 nm on a continuous wave sequence. The authors of the study acknowledge that the treatment protocol may have been insufficient because of possible greater reflection or absorption of photons by reptilian scales.[27] A more recent study by the authors investigated the use of laser therapy in the treatment of epithelial trauma in the green iguana (*Iguana iguana*). Epithelial wounds were created and received either topical wound care or laser therapy, at two different doses. The treatment protocol used by the authors in the iguana study used laser therapy at the same dose as the python study for one treatment group and a higher setting (10 J/cm^2), at double the dose, for a second treatment group. Wound measurements were obtained daily for 14 days, and the treatment sites were then evaluated microscopically for ulceration, inflammation, fibrosis, presence of bacteria, and collagen maturity. Subjectively, gross wound scores were less for the wounds treated with 10 J/cm^2 when compared to control wounds or those treated with topical medications or the lower level of laser therapy (5 J/cm^2) (Fig. 129.2). There was no significant difference in histologic evidence of healing between the laser treatment, topical treatment, and control wounds at completion of the study, at which time only 2.4% of wounds had complete epithelialization (Fig. 129.3). Though no significant improvement in histologic evaluation of overall healing was noted with this protocol in this species, there was no obvious damage or disadvantage caused by use of the laser. The low percentage of wounds showing complete epithelialization may support the need for an extended study period.

The effects of treatment with laser therapy have been shown to extend systemically to areas distant from the site of treatment, with one study in rats demonstrating increased healing of wounds that had direct treatment with laser as well as in standardized wounds distant from the site of application. Wounds in the intermediate position had the highest ranks or healing when compared to distant wounds and wounds treated directly.[28] Consideration of tissue characteristics and of the local tissue effects of laser treatment should play a role in the development of appropriate treatment protocols for the reptile patient. Additionally, regular clinical assessment should be performed throughout the course of treatment, allowing for modifications to the treatment protocol.

THERAPEUTIC PLAN

Laser therapy can be used in both acute and chronic conditions and is cumulative in effect. When initiating treatment, laser therapy should be applied in three phases, which include the initial or aggressive treatment phase, a transitional phase, and a maintenance phase. Objective criteria for these three phases in reptiles have not been established; the following are suggestions. During the initial treatment phase, therapy is provided daily or every other day, with clinical evaluation made daily.[29] Dose adjustments can be made during this time, and this period typically is recommended to last for approximately 7 days. Following the initial treatment phase, frequency of therapy is decreased; twice-weekly applications are often recommended (Riegel, 2011, Applications of therapeutic laser in everyday practice. *Veterinary Practice News.*

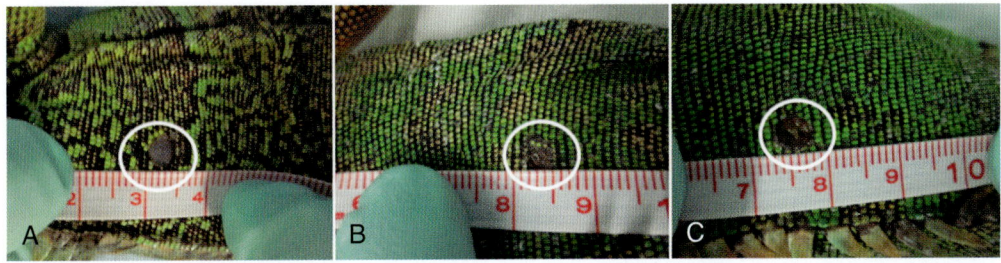

FIG 129.2 (A) Pre-treatment and (B and C) post-treatment epithelial wound in the green iguana (*Iguana iguana*). Post-treatment gross wound scores for (B) wounds treated once daily with laser therapy at 10 J/cm^2 were lower than for (C) control wounds, wounds treated with topical therapy, or wounds treated with laser therapy at 5 J/cm^2. (Courtesy of Lara M. Cusack and Stephen J. Divers.)

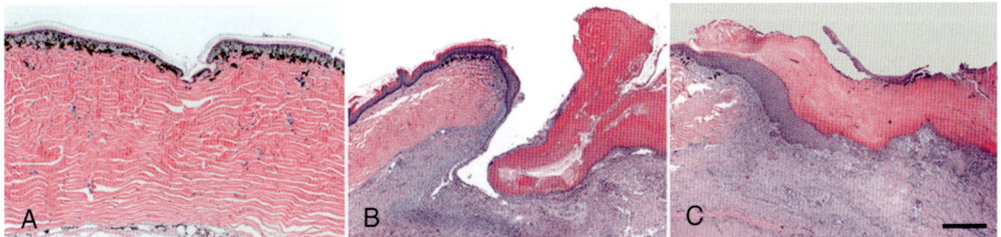

FIG 129.3 Micrograph of pre- and post-treatment epithelium of a green iguana (*Iguana iguana*). Normal, prestudy epidermis and dermis (A). Mild healing was noted when regular epithelial migration was present (B) and partial healing was noted when irregular epithelial migration was present (C). Complete epithelial migration was present in only 2.4% of wounds. Bar = 500 μm. (Reprinted with permission from Cusack LM, Mayer J, Cutler DC, et al. Gross and histologic evaluation of effects of photobiomodulation, silver sulfadiazine, and a topical antimicrobial product on experimentally induced full-thickness skin wounds in green iguanas [*Iguana iguana*]. *Am J Vet Res.* 2018;79[4]:465–473.)

2011;23[8]:26-27). For acute clinical conditions, such as wounds and fractures, the transitional phase lasts until resolution of the condition, whereas in chronic conditions, such as arthritis, this phase often lasts until a clinical goal, such as improved joint mobility, is reached. The maintenance therapy phase can be utilized for ongoing or chronic conditions, and frequency is typically dictated by clinical response. Once- or twice-monthly treatments are often used for maintenance of chronic conditions. In general, the use of laser therapy in the treatment of neoplasia is contraindicated due to the potential for increased growth of tumor cells.

REFERENCES

See www.expertconsult.com for a complete list of references.

130

Wound Management

Maud L. Marin and Terry M. Norton

Reptiles are often presented with different types of wounds on their body. Although their ability to heal wounds is good overall, their healing rate is relatively slow, and significant wounds can take several months and even over a year to fully resolve. It is therefore important to use appropriate techniques in order to minimize healing times. Reptilian wound management follows the general techniques used in small animal and human medicine, but certain products and techniques work better than others in reptiles and will be described below. Wound management is an art, and treatment modalities need to be adapted to each animal, situation, and phase of healing. New products and techniques are constantly discovered, and their application will have to be tested in our reptilian patients.

Wounds commonly seen in reptiles include husbandry-related injuries (dysecdysis, burns, bacterial, fungal, and parasitic dermatitis and shell infections), conspecific- or prey-induced injuries (bites, lacerations, and abscesses), and trauma (fall from perches; lacerations from cage or furnishings; predator attacks; and car, boat or lawn mower accidents). Infected surgical incisions and tumors can also lead to skin wounds.

GENERAL WOUND MANAGEMENT

Husbandry and Management of the Patient

Irrespective of the cause for the wound, providing proper husbandry, nutrition, and a low-stress environment is paramount in optimizing wound healing.[1] The animal should be kept at its preferred optimal temperature zone, with appropriate substrate, excellent water quality (aquatic turtles and crocodilians), and hygiene (see Section 3). Providing nutritional support and a proper diet during the healing phase is also important. When needed, supplemental nutrition can be achieved by assist feeding, tube feeding (snake, lizards, and chelonians) or via an esophagostomy tube (chelonians, lizards, crocodilians). A surgically placed feeding tube also permits long-term administration of fluids and medications in a relatively low-stress manner (see Chapter 45).

Initial Wound Evaluation and Diagnostic Evaluation

Sedation with local analgesia or general anesthesia may be required for initial evaluation and management of serious wounds. It is beneficial to stabilize critical patients prior to anesthesia. Physical and neurologic examinations, and diagnostic investigation (e.g., clinicopathology, diagnostic imaging, and microbiology), are beneficial in establishing an accurate diagnosis and prognosis, which will direct the treatment plan.[2,3] Antimicrobials (following the collection of samples for culture and sensitivity testing) and pain management should be initiated if indicated. Local anesthetics can be injected around the wound prior to debridement to reduce perioperative pain (see Chapters 50, 51, 116, 117, and 119 for further information). Hemorrhage should be controlled and fractures immobilized.

Wound Lavage and Debridement

The initial lavage should be done using a warm, balanced electrolyte solution, sterile saline, 0.05% chlorhexidine solution, or 0.1% to 1.0% povidone-iodine.[4] Surgical debridement should follow if needed, carefully removing all nonviable tissue. Any tissue that has questionable viability can be left in place and reevaluated later or treated with autolytic or enzymatic debridement products (Granulex V, Bertek Pharmaceuticals, Research Triangle Park, NC).[4]

Snakes with generalized dermatitis may be treated with periodic soaking in a medicated water bath (after appropriate diagnostic tests have been performed) containing dilute chlorhexidine or povidone-iodine. It is often beneficial to bathe the snake in water first in case the snake wants to drink. After a 10- to 20-minute antiseptic bath, the animal may be dried off and a thin layer of antimicrobial ointment or cream may be administered topically.

Wound Closure

Reptiles tend to heal well from minor wounds with little intervention. After cleaning/lavage, they may be left to heal by second intention or can be sutured or stapled. Suture materials preferred for use in reptiles include nylon, polypropylene, polydioxanone, poliglecaprone 25, and polyglyconate.[5,6] Apposing and everting suture patterns have been used on reptilian skin, taking care to prevent inversion and subsequent dysecdysis. Although the literature suggests that sutures should be left in place for a minimum of 6 weeks in reptiles, clinically some wounds heal in 2 to 4 weeks with sutures able to be removed at that time.[2,5] Because of the low exudative nature of reptilian wounds, drains are not useful for these patients. The remainder of this chapter will focus on the more challenging wounds that require extensive treatment and bandaging.

Topical Products

Chronic and infected wounds may benefit from topical product application. A wide variety of topical antimicrobials and products that accelerate wound healing are currently available. New products are regularly introduced into the market. It is good to rotate topical antimicrobials over time in order to avoid resistance and to try different products when a wound fails to improve. Topical treatments commonly utilized include silver sulfadiazine cream (Silvadene, Hoeschst Marion Roussel, Kansas City, MO), antibiotic ointments (triple antibiotic ointment; gentamicin sulfate), doxycycline gel (Doxirobe Gel, Pharmacia & Upjohn Company, New York, NY), aluminum spray (AluSpray, Neogen, Lansing, MI), nitrofurazone (Fura-Zone, Squire, Revere, MA), aloe vera gel, sugar, and honey (MediHoney, DermaSciences, Princeton, NJ).[1,7,8] Other wound care products that may help support the healing process include growth factors (Regranex Gel, Ortho-McNeil Pharmaceutical, South Raritan,

NJ), maltodextrin (Intracell, Macleod Pharmaceutical, Fort Collins, CO), chitosan, acemannan hydrogel or the freeze-dried form (CarraVet, Veterinary Products Labs, Phoenix, AZ; Carrasorb Carrington Labs, Irving, TX), and skin protectant cream (ilex Skin Protectant Paste, Medcon Biolab Technologies, Grafton, MA) mixed in with antimicrobial cream. These products can generally be used over an open wound, as well as within the primary layer of a dressing.

BASIC BANDAGING TECHNIQUES

Benefits from applying a bandage include protection from contamination and external mechanical forces, elimination of dead space, immobilization of the injured area, support and comfort, as well as provision of a moist environment.[1,4] Bandaging reptile wounds can be quite challenging. Creativity is required to provide a bandage that is sturdy yet light enough, stays in place, and does not limit the animal's mobility extensively. In aquatic species, some bandages need to be waterproof. Reptile wounds generally produce a thick to hard caseous material rather than a liquid exudate, so light dressings that keep the wound moist are preferred with this group of animals.

A bandage generally consists of three layers. The primary layer consists of a nonadherent dressing placed directly over the wound bed. The most commonly used types of dressings in reptiles are the semiocclusive and occlusive dressings, hydrogels, and hydrocolloids.[1] Examples of semiocclusive dressings include Telfa adhesive pads (Kendall, Mansfield, MA) and Adaptic (Johnson & Johnson nonstick dressings, Arlington, TX). Silver-impregnated dressings have the added benefit of providing a sustained antimicrobial effect on the wound bed (Acticoat burn dressing, Smith and Nephew, Largo, FL; Aquacell Ag hydrofiber dressing with ionic silver, ConvaTec, Greensboro, NC; Silverlon, Argentum Medical, Willowbrook, IL). An example of an occlusive dressing is the Op Site Spray Bandage (Smith and Nephew, Lachine, QC, Canada).[9] Hydrogels come in a flexible sheet or a gel that covers the wound bed and are useful to keep a wound moist. Certain hydrogel sheets also contain silver ions (SilvaSorb, Medline Industries, Mundelein, IL). Hydrocolloids such as DuoDERM (ConvaTec) interact with wound fluid to form a gel.

The secondary bandage layer holds the contact layer in place and can provide support as well as reduction of mobility. Materials commonly used include cast padding and rolled gauze. When needed, a splint can be added into this layer. This layer is not always necessary or useful in reptiles and is often omitted.

The tertiary layer is made with adhesive films (Steri-Drape and Tegaderm, 3M Animal Care Products, St. Paul, MN), bandage wraps (Vetrap, 3M), adhesive tapes (Elastikon, Johnson & Johnson Medical Inc., Arlington, TX) white porous tape or duct tape, and fabrics such as a stockinette. Dressing changes should be tailored to each animal and situation and will vary between daily to once a week. Depending on the patient and the nature of its wounds, the procedure may be performed under manual restraint only, while others will require sedation or general anesthesia.

In snakes, traditional bandages placed around the animal's body do not usually stay in place because of the unique undulating movement they use for locomotion. Adhesive tape and bandages on the skin of snakes can leave a sticky residue, peel off the scales, or even tear the skin. An excellent alternative technique for these wounds is the tie-over bandage technique, which is described later in this chapter.[3,10] Lizards tend to tolerate bandages quite well and are not prone to removing them. Fig. 130.1A through D shows a Komodo dragon (*Varanus komodoensis*) that suffered from severe burns on the ventral skin from a defective ventral heating pad. Wounds on the limbs of chelonians can be challenging to bandage. In certain cases, the affected limb can be kept in place by flexing it into the shell fossa and securing it in this location by placing tape around the shell.

Aquatic animals pose an extra challenge to the clinician when it comes to bandaging. Most conventional bandages are not waterproof and will allow contamination and potential maceration of the wound when they are submersed. Faced with this reality, clinicians may elect to leave the wound unbandaged and unprotected, or periodically dry-dock the animals for wound treatment (more stressful). An alternative is to apply a waterproof bandage. In aquatic chelonians with minor shell wounds, this can be achieved using antibiotic cream covered with an adhesive such as Tegaderm (Fig. 130.2A–C). For more extensive wounds, waterproof tape, Elastikon, silicone, and superglue may be needed to create an adequate water seal. See Chapter 113 for more details on shell bandage waterproofing.

SPECIALIZED BANDAGING TECHNIQUES

Tie-Over Bandage

The tie-over bandage offers an excellent alternative technique for wounds in areas that are mobile or difficult to cover. It is particularly useful in snakes but is also effective in lizards and turtles that have challenging wound locations. The technique has been previously described.[3,10] Briefly, after the wound has been debrided, nonabsorbable suture loops are placed around the wound. A topical medication can be placed over the wound and covered with Telfa pad, hydrogel, or hydrocolloid. Gauze is placed over the primary layer, and umbilical tape is threaded onto the suture loops with the help of a hemostat and tied over the bandage (Fig. 130.3A and B). Bandage changes may be done awake or under anesthesia if further debridement is needed, every 1 to 4 days initially. Later, the schedule should be tailored to the needs and evolution of the wound. In sea turtles, one of the authors (TN) has used a modified technique using metal skin staples instead of suture loops and suture material in lieu of the umbilical tape. In these aquatic animals, Telfa and gauze pads can be replaced with petrolatum gauze. Fig. 130.4A to D show a joint abscess in a Kemp's ridley sea turtle (*Lepidochelys kempi)* that is being treated with a tie-over bandage.

Vacuum-Assisted Closure Therapy

The vacuum-assisted closure therapy (VAC therapy) system (KCI, San Antonio, TX) is an excellent technique used for healing difficult wounds in humans, mammals, and reptiles.[8,11–22] VAC therapy is most beneficial in chelonians when a shell defect is present, usually because of trauma or infection. The reduction of healing time is striking, often saving many months of treatment and hospitalization. The technique is relatively simple to use and can be learned rapidly. The reader is referred to previous publications for a more detailed explanation of the technique.[8,19]

Negative pressure wound therapy (NPWT) promotes wound healing by promoting contraction of wound margins to facilitate closure, encouraging granulation tissue formation, increasing tissue perfusion, removing exudates, and reducing edema.[11–14] In chelonians with an open coelom, NPWT has the added benefit of bringing collapsed lung tissue back into its original location, favoring a more normal anatomic orientation and preservation of the coelomic space.

VAC therapy relies on open-cell foam that is placed into the wound bed, covered by an airtight plastic dressing, and attached to a suction machine by plastic tubing (Fig. 130.5). Additional materials have proven useful for the chelonian patient and are included in Table 130.1. Fig. 130.6A through D shows the use of VAC therapy in a gopher tortoise (*Gopherus polyphemus*), and Fig. 130.7 the use of a waterproof VAC dressing in a Florida cooter (*Pseudemis floridana*).

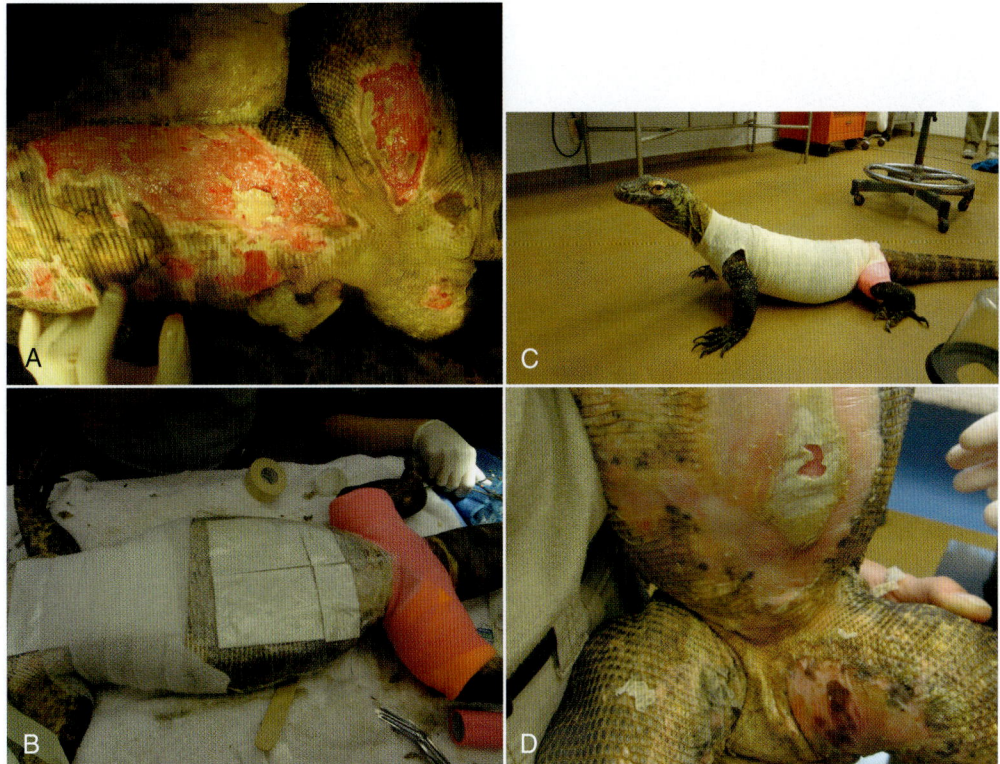

FIG 130.1 (A) Severe burn wounds on the ventral surface of a 4-year-old Komodo dragon (*Varanus komodoensis*) during debridement. This picture was taken 4 weeks after initial presentation. (B) After debridement was performed under anesthesia, primary dressings (Telfa) were placed over the wound. Rolled cotton and Vetrap were used as secondary and tertiary layers. (C) Stockinette was used as a body suit to complete the bandage. (D) Skin wounds 7 months after presentation. The wounds healed after 9 months of intensive therapy. Multiple therapeutic techniques and products were used on this animal, including skin graft, tie-over bandage, and laser therapy. (Courtesy of Maud L. Marin.)

A variety of nonadherent mesh materials (Adaptic, Acticoat, Silverlon) or sterile gauze can be placed on the wound bed with petroleum jelly, saline, or sterile water to keep it moist. Several types of open-cell foam can be used (VAC GranuFoam, GranuFoam Silver, VAC WhiteFoam). Alternatively, inexpensive open-cell foam can be found at home improvement stores (e.g., speaker foam or air conditioning foam with pore size of 400–600 μm) and can be gas sterilized. The open-cell foam is cut to size and placed into/on top of the defect. Multiple foam pieces can be used if needed.

Several types of occlusive plastic adhesive films can be used, including VAC adhesive drape (KCI), Steri-drape, and Tegaderm. If needed, grooves in the scutes can be covered with tape, adhesive materials, or filled in with epoxy. Orthopedic hardware can be covered with adherent bandage material (Elastikon) or epoxy putty before placing the adhesive drape.

Finally, an egress tube (VAC therapy-regulated accurate care [TRAC] pad or red rubber tubing) is placed through the adhesive drape and into the foam, after a quarter size hole is cut at the optimal location. The tube is then hooked to a suction pump. The VAC Freedom suction pump, a surgical suction pump, or a passive suction grenade can be used to generate negative pressure.

When suction is applied, the foam should take on a shrunken appearance beneath the adhesive film. Negative pressure between 100 mm Hg and 175 mm Hg is typically used in chelonians. Continuous suction is generally used, and leaving it on for 24 hours a day is ideal. If during the treatment the airtight seal is lost, it needs to be restored by applying

more clear adhesive dressing. If it cannot be repaired within 2 hours, the whole dressing should be removed and the wound irrigated and left open until a new VAC bandage can be applied. Time off from treatment between bandage changes may be beneficial for the animal to relieve stress and give an opportunity for aquatic turtles to swim freely. Bandages can be changed without sedation or anesthesia, as humans report minimal pain during bandage change or therapy. It is important to monitor fluid loss and hydration status, especially in small patients weighing less than 10 kg. Initially the VAC treatment was used in dry-docked patients, but a waterproof technique was successfully used to treat sea turtles in a hospital treatment pool.[8] VAC treatment time for shell injuries in terrestrial chelonians has been reported to be from 3 to 43 days, whereas in sea turtles, treatment is generally a few weeks to months, depending on the severity of the wound.[19]

SUPPLEMENTAL THERAPIES

Skin grafts (allogenic and porcine small intestinal submucosa [VetBioSIST, Cook, West Lafayette, IN]) have been used successfully in reptiles, with the placement technique being similar to mammals.[5] Proper bandaging techniques, temporary immobilization of the graft, and other protective measures are often necessary for a successful outcome.

Alternative therapies that are suggested to promote wound healing in mammals include low-level cool laser (photomodulation) therapy, electroacupuncture, hyperbaric oxygen therapy, stem cell therapy, and

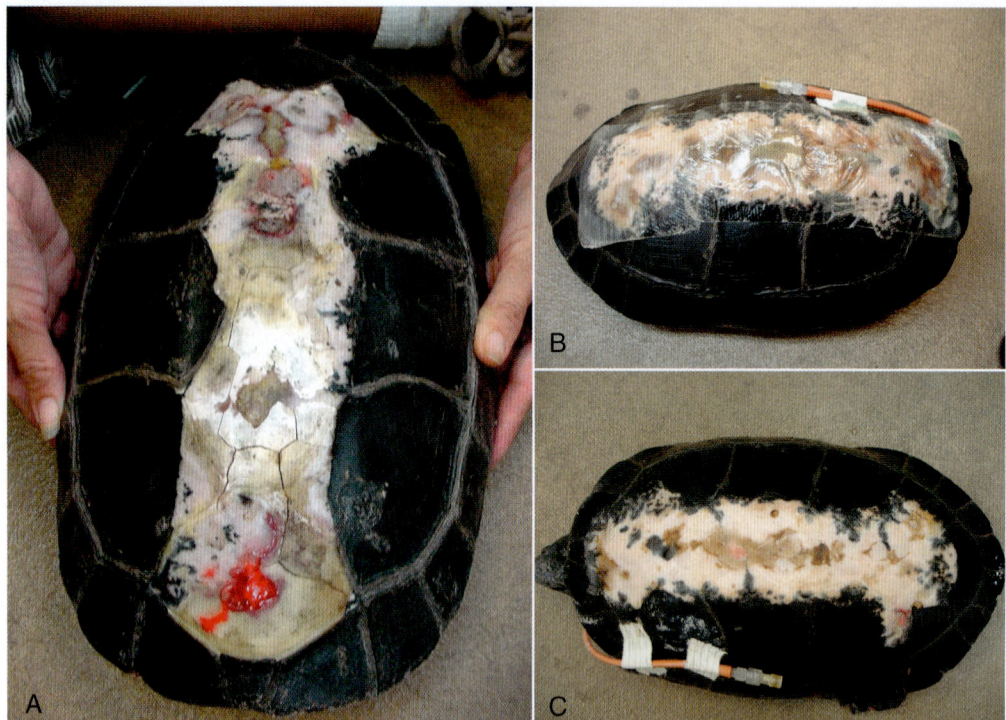

FIG 130.2 (A) Severe wounds on the carapace of a Malaysian giant turtle *(Orlitia borneensis)* because of poor water quality. Note the deep wounds involving the bony plates. (B) After debridement, a small layer of SSD cream was applied to the wound and covered with hydrogel dressing. The dressing was waterproof and the animal was allowed to swim freely. Note the feeding tube placed to help with medical management. (C) Wound(s) progression 40 days post-presentation. Note the healthy granulation tissue and pink epithelium forming over the wound bed. The lesions healed within 60 days, and the dark pigmentation slowly migrated back into the healed tissue. (Courtesy of Maud L. Marin.)

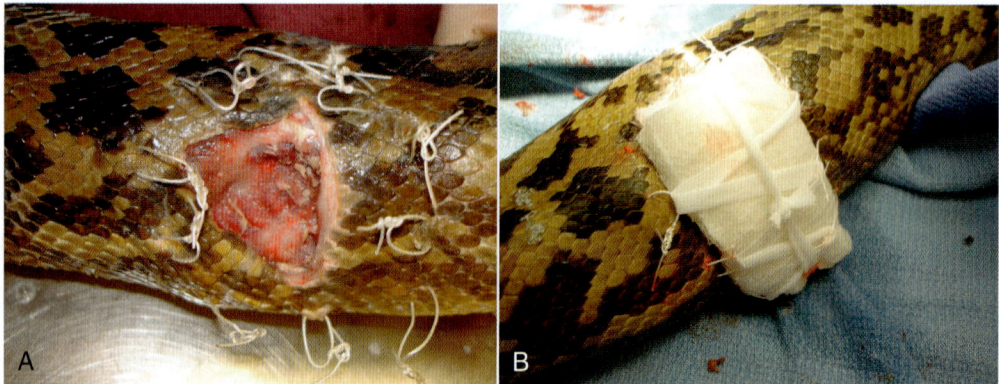

FIG 130.3 (A) Placement of nonabsorbable suture loops around the wound of a 12-year-old Timor python *(Broghammerus timoriensis)* in preparation for a tie-over bandage. (B) A piece of Telfa pad was trimmed to the appropriate size and placed into the wound bed. Dry gauze was added, and umbilical tape was passed through the suture loops and tied over to complete the bandage. The wound closed after 2 months of therapy. (Courtesy of Maud L. Marin.)

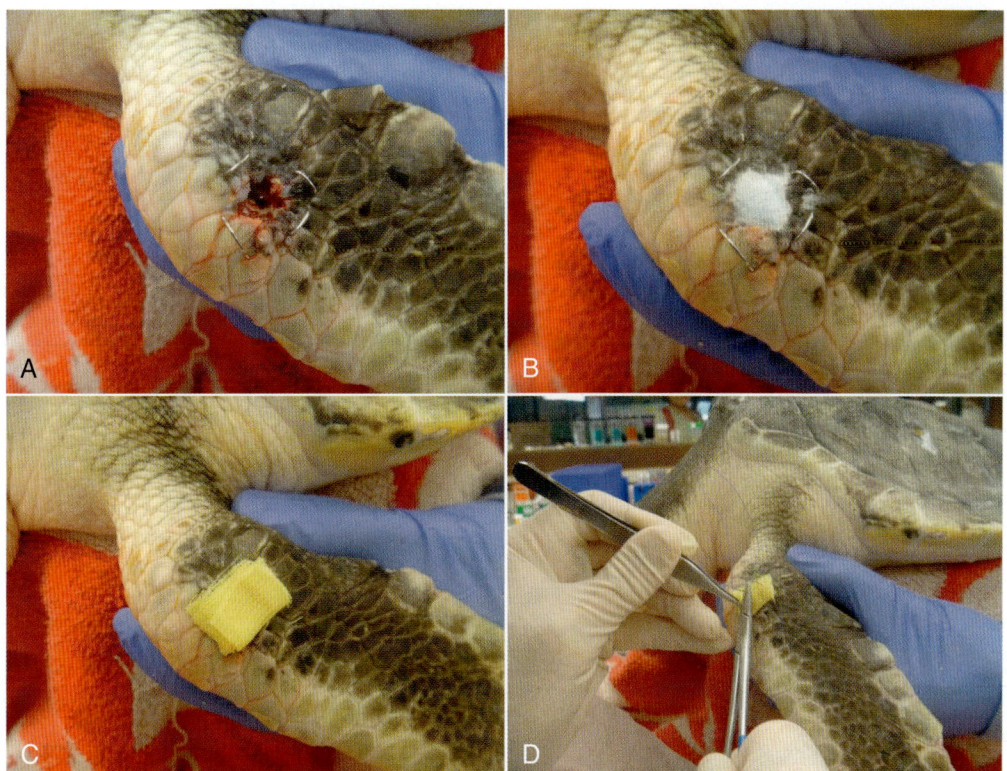

FIG 130.4 (A) Tie-over bandage in a Kemp's ridley turtle, *Lepidochelys kempi*, with a bacterial abscess of the elbow joint. The skin staples were placed around the wound after surgical preparation, flushing, and debridement. (B) Borate-based biological glass (RediHeal, Avalon Medical, Stillwater, MN) was packed into the wound. (C) Vaseline impregnated gauze placed over the wound. (D) Gauze sutured to staples to hold everything in place. (Courtesy of Terry M. Norton, Georgia Sea Turtle Center.)

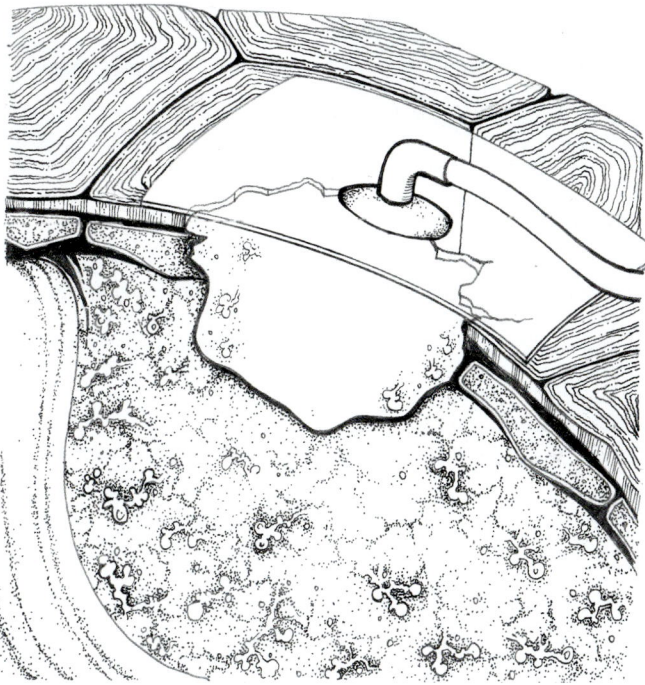

FIG 130.5 VAC therapy on a chelonian patient. The foam is placed into the defect wond covered with a clear dressing. An egress tube is attached and linked to a suction unit (not shown). (Courtesy of Lori E. Lopel.)

TABLE 130.1 Negative Pressure Therapy: Equipment Needed

Components	Best	Good	Adequate
Nonadherent barrier	Silver-impregnated mesh (Acticoat Silverlon) + saline or petroleum jelly	Adaptic+ saline or petroleum jelly	Telfa gauze + saline
Foam	VAC GranuFoam Standard, Silver, or WhiteFoam	Open-cell polyurethane foam (speaker foam at home improvement store)	Loosely placed gauze or laparotomy sponges
Adhesive drape	VAC sterile adhesive drape	Tegaderm, Steri-drape	Food-quality clear plastic wrap with silicone seal on margins
Tubing	Purpose-made pad and tubing (VAC TRAC pad)	Red rubber tube, fenestrated	Any plastic tubing, fenestrated + adaptor
Suction	VAC Freedom or Simplicity Therapy unit	Surgical suction unit	High-volume passive suction grenade

Acticoat burn dressing (Smith and Nephew, Largo, FL); Silverlon (Argentum Medical, Willowbrook, IL); Adaptic (Johnson & Johnson Nonstick dressings, Arlington, TX); VAC products (KCI Animal Health, San Antonio, TX); Steri-drape and Tegaderm (3M, St. Paul, MN).

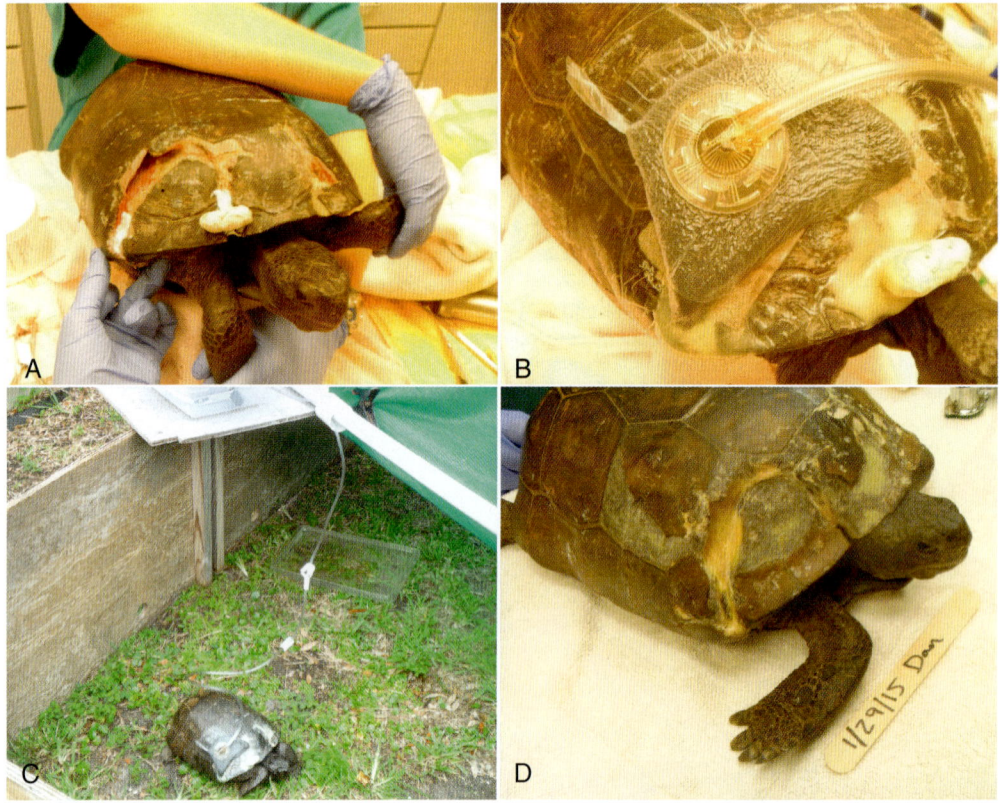

FIG 130.6 (A) Gopher tortoise (*Gopherus polyphemus*) hit by a car with multiple cranial carapace fractures and an exposed coelom and lung on the right side. A set of screws, wires, and epoxy were used to stabilize the fracture. Regular wound management included lavage, debridement, RediHeal and bone cement, and VAC therapy. (B) RediHeal and bone cement were used to manage the wound, seal the coelom, and provide a surface for VAC placement. VAC therapy is being used on this tortoise. (C) The same tortoise in an outdoor pen with VAC unit in place. The tortoise is much more comfortable in an outdoor setting. The VAC unit is protected in a waterproof container. Ice packs are used to keep the VAC unit cool during warmer months of the year. (D) The wound 4 months post initial presentation. (Courtesy of Terry M. Norton, Georgia Sea Turtle Center.)

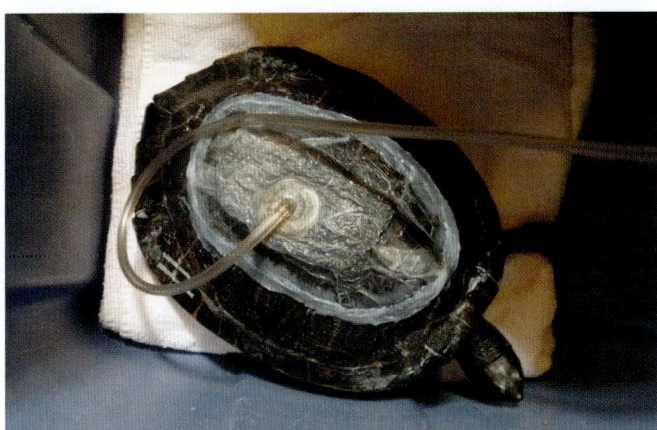

FIG 130.7 VAC therapy was used on this Florida cooter *(Pseudemys floridana)* with an exposed lung and spinal cord. This was alternated with RediHeal and bone cement application to the wound. The turtle continued to feed the entire treatment period and never showed any neurologic deficits. Eventually the turtle was released back to the wild. VAC therapy was critical for the success of this case.

platelet-rich plasma.[23–30] Although few research studies exist on their efficacy in treating reptiles and some refuted efficacy, many clinicians are using them in their reptilian patients with promising results.[28,31] More research is needed on their effects in reptiles.

In conclusion, multiple treatment options exist to treat reptile wounds. Extensive wounds are a challenge to treat, but with proper therapy, as well as husbandry and nutritional support, reptiles have a great ability to heal. Multiple modalities can be used simultaneously, for example, placing a skin graft within a tie-over bandage and using laser therapy on the wound during bandage changes. Finally, the treatment techniques should be reevaluated and modified as needed during the healing period and based on the wound appearance.

REFERENCES

See www.expertconsult.com for a complete list of references.

131

Physical Therapy and Rehabilitation

Albert Martínez-Silvestre and Samuel P. Franklin

The rehabilitation of reptiles encompasses two overlapping disciplines. One involves actual physical rehabilitation, which includes the diagnosis and physical treatment of reptiles with pathologic processes that may hinder their healing or recovery. Application of rehabilitation practices enables these injured reptiles to become as healthy, mobile, and functional as possible. Second, rehabilitation includes habituation of a reptile to a new environment, a new facility, or the preparation of an individual for release into the wild. This chapter describes both aspects of rehabilitation and their application in reptile medicine. Only the rehabilitation of inland reptiles is considered in this chapter. Specific rehabilitation of sea turtles can be found in Chapter 176.

PHYSICAL THERAPY

Response of Musculoskeletal Tissues to Disuse and Remobilization

Fortunately, reptiles spend much of their life in a relative state of inactivity, and their metabolism has a high capacity to adapt to such inactivity. Unlike many other vertebrates, they can quickly change to a state of high energy consumption and high activity such as when hunting, breeding, and avoiding predation, even after days or weeks of inactivity. Some reptiles, such as alligators or lizards, experience a sharp increase in tissue lactate in the pursuit and capture of prey after long periods of inactivity.[1] Resting reptiles have been shown to have blood lactate levels ranging from 4 to 20 mg/dL. Moderate activity results in lactate accumulations of 30 to 80 mg/dL, and prolonged or vigorous activity quickly produces levels exceeding 100 mg/dL. After experiencing such abrupt increases in lactate, reptiles are physiologically exhausted and often unable to appropriately respond to stimuli. Maximum or near-maximum levels of lactate can be produced in only 30 seconds of vigorous struggling in a number of lizard species.

In regard to kinematics and load resistance, generally a reptile's slow walking speed and robust limb bones result in low locomotor forces and limb bone stresses. However, their highly sprawled posture and perpendicular-to-axis femurs and humeri can produce high bending loads. This leads to high limb bone stresses similar to those of avian and mammalian species, as well as high torsion. Turtle limb bones seem considerably "overdesigned" for resisting the loads that they encounter. Additionally, comparisons of bone loading across tetrapod lineages are consistent with the hypothesis that low limb bone loads, elevated torsion, and high safety factors may be primitive features of limb bone design.[2]

Keeping these physiological characteristics in mind, negative side effects associated with extended hospital stays can be overcome by understanding and applying (or minimizing) physical activity specific to each reptile species. Prescribed rehabilitation exercise(s) in tame reptiles are better to be concentrated, not into one long session, but broken up into multiple shorter sessions distributed throughout the day. However, with highly stressed reptiles, it may be more stressful to handle them multiple times. In these cases, once a day rehabilitation is advisable to avoid disrupting their ability to acclimate and feed. Weekly rechecks are recommended to confirm positive progress in the recovery process. In some cases the degree of disuse atrophy can be cumulative and extreme. This is especially true for larger, heavy-bodied reptiles with chronic lameness, as they may be unable to lift their body weight off the ground to allow for normal locomotion. In such cases physical rehabilitation can be used to help them regain strength and enable controlled exercise.

Limb Paresis/Paralysis

Paresis/paralysis of the hind limbs is a common clinical presentation in lizards and turtles. Involvement of all four limbs is less common but may also be seen. Although spinal cord trauma is the most common cause of limb paresis/paralysis, a thorough historical evaluation and physical examination is required to exclude other causes of paresis such as coelomic pain, reproductive activity, neoplasia, renal disease, urolithiasis, neuromuscular disease, metabolic disturbances, and intoxication. A definitive diagnosis for the paretic patient is important, as therapy varies for each of these conditions. Table 131.1 shows the score and the decision-making process in cases of ataxia and postural immobilization.

To diagnose the possible causes of paresis/paralysis, a thorough physical, orthopedic, and neurologic examination are necessary. In cases where coelomic pain is suspected, a pharmacologic review of pain management and analgesia is discussed in Chapter 50. Table 131.1 provides an overview of differential diagnoses for reptile paresia/paralysis and ataxia, the associated etiologies for these conditions, and recommended diagnostic tests including hematology and biochemistry, radiology, cytology, and endoscopy. In cases of suspected vestibular syndrome or nerve injury, magnetic resonance imaging (MRI) is advised, as well as CT for possible vertebral damage.

In addition, we can test the animal's proprioception and mobility using proprioception exercises (see Chapter 77). Generally, land tortoises are scared of heights and they will not jump from a height greater than 30 cm. By placing the tortoise close to the edge of an elevated examination table, we can assess their capacity of vision, proprioception, and ability to escape from danger.

Physical Rehabilitation

Physical rehabilitation can include numerous different approaches to optimize patient function. Manual therapies include the use of mechanical touch, massage, stretching, and joint mobilizations. Physical modalities include treatments such as heat and cryotherapy, vibration therapy,

TABLE 131.1 Functional Scoring System in Reptiles With Possible Spinal Cord Injuries

Five stages of spinal cord injury and related diseases. Each stage is subdivided based on recovery patterns and diagnostic procedures.

0. No pelvic limb movement and no deep pain sensation.
   a. In tortoises, rule out spinal cord trauma, nonspecific coelomic pain, and infection. (Rads, US) (Coe P) (PB) (CT, MRI) (EMG)
1. No pelvic limb movement but voluntary tail movement.
   a. In snakes rule out spinal cord trauma, nonspecific coelomic pain, and infection. (Rads, US) (Coe P) (PB) (CT, MRI) (EMG)
2. No pelvic limb movement with deep pain sensation. Behavioral changes.
   a. In general, rule out end-stage pregnancy, spinal cord trauma, and renal disease. (Rads) (Coe P) (PB) (CT, MRI)
3. Minimal protraction of the pelvic limb(s).
   a. Movement is generally limited to the forelimbs. (Rads) (EMG)
4. Protraction of pelvic limbs >50% of the time. Mild coelomic distension.
   a. Difficulty in urinating and retention of feces. In general, rule out renal disease, pregnancy, obstipation, spinal cord trauma, and metabolic disturbances. (Rads) (Clo T) (PB) (CT, MRI) (EMG)
   b. In the majority of reptiles, rule out ovulation and postovulation pain. (Rads)
5. Protraction of pelvic limbs >50% of the time. Coelomic enlargement.
   a. Chronic urinary retention, azotemia secondary to renal disease, or metabolic disturbances. (Rads, US) (Clo P) (Clo T) (PB)
   b. Rule out acute trauma, spinal cord injury. (Rads) (Clo T) (CT, MRI)

To diagnose all the described diseases in this table, these techniques may need to be performed: *Clo P*, cloacal palpation; *Clo T*, cloacal tone; *Coe P*, coelomic palpation; *CT*, computed tomography; *EMG*, electromyiography; *MRI*, magnetic resonance imaging; *PB*, plasma biochemistry; *Rads*, radiography; *US*, ultrasonography.

electrical stimulation, therapeutic ultrasound, and photobiomodulation. Therapeutic exercise can include aquatic therapy, neuroproprioceptive training, and strength and physical conditioning. Lastly, use of orthoses and prostheses are valuable aspects of physical rehabilitation. Many of the techniques described in the following sections have been assessed for their applicability to reptile rehabilitation in recent years.

Exercise and Joint Mobilization

Ultimately controlled exercise is the greatest tool in physical rehabilitation because it can achieve the objectives of building strength, improving range of motion, and facilitating neuroproprioceptive training. Trained exercises including target training and operant conditioning are widely used in captive crocodiles and large chelonians in zoologic collections and include performing exercises or movements associated with certain commands. Such training can help with completion of therapeutic exercises, improving posture, and allowing diagnostic sampling and feeding control.[3]

It is also important to consider environmental enrichment in physical rehabilitation as is commonly used with sea turtles. Enrichment includes providing food, toys, tactile stimulation, and keeper interaction. Husbandry training is a critical component of this therapy. It elicits the animal's cooperation during treatment, reducing the need for restraint, and provides mental and physical stimulation. Other techniques include conditioning reptiles to feed by tongs, acceptance of tactile manipulation, target training, the following of a trainer, responding to a recall stimulus, and providing a reward for allowing shell scrubbing. These techniques are particularly applicable to land tortoises (*Centrochelys sulcata*,

Stygmochelis pardalis, and *Testudo hermanni*). Initial exercise sessions must be kept short because tortoises can become fatigued after only 10 to 15 minutes of walking, but the sessions can be repeated regularly. In other studies, the use of silhouettes of birds of prey (predators) by artificial models passing over terrariums have been used to induce exercise by encouraging an alert and escape reaction in captive lizards.[4]

In order to help improve muscle mass and strength, and facilitate physical therapy and exercise, anabolic steroids such as stanozolol (5 mg/kg intramuscularly every 7 days) can be used. This hormone also stimulates appetite and reduces protein catabolism and purine degradation and is expected to have a positive effect on erythropoiesis and cellular metabolism in addition to muscle development.[5]

Heat Therapy. Reptiles with chronic pain or old injuries may benefit from superficial heat provided by a hot pack. Indeed, as ectotherms, heat therapy is especially important for reptiles. Superficial heat therapy reduces pain by reducing sympathetic neurologic tone, promoting local circulation, increasing tissue oxygenation, speeding biochemical reactions, and reducing muscle spasms. Heat therapy applied across the coelomic wall can also improve gastrointestinal motility.[6]

If a patient reacts negatively to heat therapy (stops eating, moves less, or otherwise demonstrates results opposite to those expected), the treatment should be discontinued. Caution must be taken to avoid cutaneous burns by excessive contact with heat application in small or young reptiles. Therapeutic ultrasonography or photobiomodulation (low-level laser therapy) are other modalities used for energy application. These therapies may achieve heating of deeper tissues more efficiently and in a shorter period of time than use of heat packs, potentially making them safer and more readily tolerated. Additionally photobiomodulation can be used to promote granulation tissue proliferation, scar formation, and autolytic debridement of necrotic debris in wounds. See Chapters 129 and 130 for more details.

Electrical Stimulation. Use of electrical stimulation for improving strength and muscle mass has not been sufficiently studied in reptiles. However, electrical stimulators have been used in an effort to facilitate tissue regeneration in deep wounds. This treatment may provide advantages over other traditional methods for wound healing. The electrical stimulator device may induce tissue repair without causing severe stress to the patient and could be a potential option for hastening tissue healing in reptiles.[7]

Massage. Massage therapy can be beneficial in many species for pain relief, anxiety reduction, and promotion of the human animal bond. Furthermore, in reptiles massage can generate an increase in temperature locally, making it a useful thermal therapy. Coelomic massage may be helpful in treating posterior paresis by decreasing pain. It can also be an important aid in intestinal transit. Additionally, it may be helpful in removing foreign objects that are in the large intestine or small urinary calculi, although you must use caution not to cause damage to the colon or bladder. Coelomic massage can be performed in lizards by exerting pressure with the thumb in a clockwise direction and at the same time applying digital pressure on the flanks in a dorsoventral and craniocaudal direction. Spinal column massage with pressure points in the cranial coelomic ("thoracic") area prompts inspiration and facilitates lymphatic drainage and blood flow, which allows recovery of spinal movements and improves movement in lizards and snakes. In the authors' experience massage of dorsal column points associated with the lungs, pericardium, and heart stimulates breathing in reptiles in the postanesthetic period and when the patient is suffering from shock. These points are the same that are used in saurian acupuncture (Fig. 131.1) (see Chapter 132).

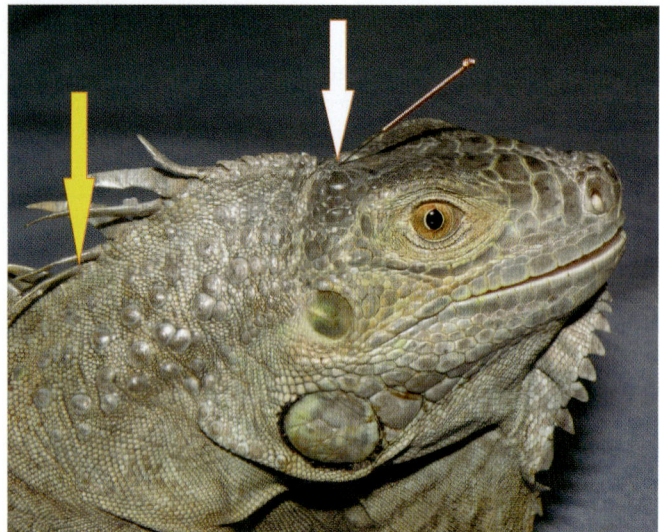

FIG 131.1 Acupuncture/pressure points to stimulate inspiration and breath (yellow arrow) and relax (white arrow) in a green iguana (*Iguana iguana*).

Vibrations. Vibration massagers may be beneficial in the alleviation of gut impactions in tortoises. The vibrator is adhered to the shell for vibrating sessions of several minutes. The vibrator is minimally invasive and well tolerated. A commercial vibrator was used to relieve intestinal constipation in a marginated tortoise (*Testudo marginata*).[8]

Orthopedics

Loss of Limbs. Wild reptiles can lose a limb and still survive; numerous field studies have identified reptiles with limbs that were amputated/removed by predators or other traumatic injuries. Wild turtles often survive the loss of one limb but may not be able to survive in the wild with the loss of multiple limbs. The loss of multiple limbs may affect foraging ability and thus growth in younger animals or reproductive success in mature turtles.

Similarly, in captivity turtles can survive with a loss of up to three limbs, but it is difficult to determine whether they have adequate quality of life. The most common causes of amputation are attacks by rodents (rats and mice), predatory carnivores (e.g., racoons, foxes, weasels, dogs), vehicular accidents, lawn mower damage, or falls from buildings. In cases of limb loss in chelonians, prostheses can be installed (Fig. 131.2).

Loss of forelimbs: Obviously the ability to apply traction using the forelimb is lost and the animal must depend on the propulsive ability of the rear limbs. In these cases the application of wheels or a support that can slide and elevates the plastron such as an acrylic ball cut in half may be useful. In male land tortoises the loss of a forelimb precludes successful mating; therefore, individuals missing a forelimb that are part of a rehabilitation project should not be released into the wild. The loss of a forelimb does not however preclude mating in aquatic turtles.

Loss of rear limbs: Mating is not hindered with the loss of hind limbs. However, in female turtles the loss of hind limbs makes digging a nest for laying eggs more difficult, and the female will need assistance during egg laying. Accordingly, female turtles that are part of rehabilitation projects should not be released into the wild, because they are unlikely to reproduce successfully.

Although wheels can commonly be used to improve mobility in individuals with loss of a limb, wheels are not always the best solution. They are beneficial and function well for tortoises living in terraces,

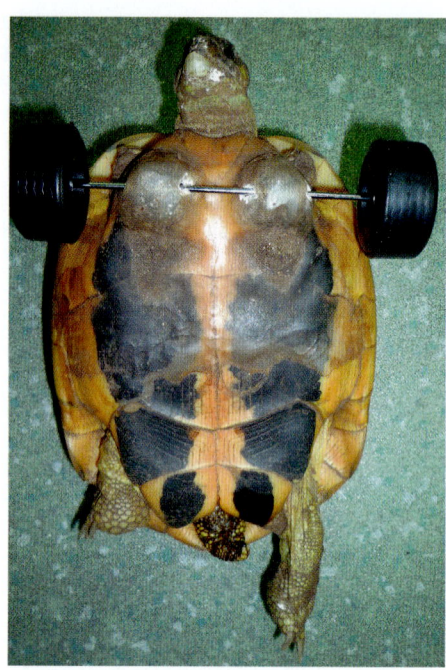

FIG 131.2 Female Herman's tortoise (*Testudo hermanni*) with prosthetic wheels after amputation of front limbs.

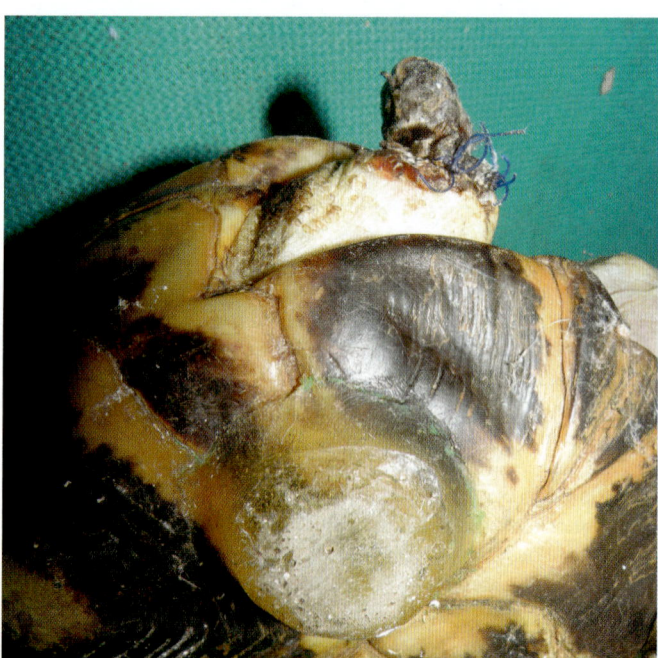

FIG 131.3 Male Russian tortoise (*Agrionemys horsfieldii*) with a nonwheel prosthesis after amputation of right front limb. Prosthesis is glued to the humeral-pectoral scales.

floors, or tiled gardens. However, if wheels are small, or the turtle needs to move through an area of soil, sand, clay, or grass, the wheel may lose the ability to turn and become nonfunctional. In these cases adhering an artificial prosthesis to the plastron that is made of fiberglass, plastic, or wood is a better solution. The prosthesis should be smooth and blunt to allow sliding and minimize adherence of substrate, soil, or plant material (Fig. 131.3).

In unusual cases prostheses are used even when there is no loss of a limb. A red-footed tortoise (*Chelonoidis carbonaria*) with secondary nutritional hyperparathyroidism and a deformed shell was treated with the use of a plastic prosthesis (nonwheel) to enable greater mobility, more involved rehabilitation, and the ability to interact with animals of the same species.[9] In a similar case a radiated tortoise (*Astrochelys radiata*) with a chronic limb lameness was provided with a kind of wheelchair that allowed the limb to move normally so that the animal could exercise and gain strength without having to bear full weight. The wheelchair consisted of an oval platform, made of ½-inch-thick recycled plastic lumber, cut to fit the plastron (Martin, et al. Proc ARAV, 2005, pp 25–26). Session times were gradually increased from 10 minutes to 1 hour daily. After the tortoise had regained sufficient strength, the original castors were replaced with a smaller set that allowed the tortoise to start supporting some of his own body weight. The total duration from initial presentation to complete resolution was approximately 1 year.

Aquatic Therapy. Swimming can be very useful in stimulating spinal movement and improving balance and proprioception. This is especially useful in species that use water periodically in their lives, such as iguanas, monitor lizards, or snakes. It is also useful in making terrestrial reptiles, including lizard species such as Agamidae (*Pogona, Uromastix*), Lacertidae (*Timon, Lacerta*), and Scincidae (skinks), attempt to escape a water bath. As they work to get out of the water they exercise joints and perform repetitive movements. Aquatic therapy in land tortoises consists of daily baths for 1 hour in shallow water to encourage limb movement. A leopard tortoise (*Stigmochelys pardalis*) with a transverse mid-shaft fracture of the right femur was treated with a modified tape bandage combined with aquatic therapy. After 60 days of this treatment and physical therapy the tortoise was ambulating normally (Raiti, Proc ARAV, 2008, pp 59–60).

For muscle building in aquatic turtles, it is necessary to increase the depth of water daily (1 cm daily), encouraging them to exercise to keep afloat. This is especially important in turtles that may lose fitness secondary to inactivity, such as in the softshell turtles (family Tryonichidae) or Fly river turtles (*Carettochelys insculpta*). These patients must be monitored closely to ensure they do not drown.

Rehabilitation Terrariums

The slow metabolism of reptiles necessitates more protracted rehabilitation efforts than generally required for mammal and avian patients. Although it depends on the species and disease, the rehabilitation process is generally no less than a month and can last up to a year or longer. Consequently, reptile rehabilitation facilities must meet certain specific requirements, which may differ from traditional veterinary hospitals. In general, environments and enclosures for rehabilitation should be able to confine the specimens and provide appropriate water, heat, light/photoperiod, temperature, substrate, humidity, ventilation, and visual security and should be easy to clean and disinfect. In many cases it may not be recommended to use elaborate and naturalistic vivaria during this time, as these environments may make it difficult to monitor the patient and eradicate possible contagious pathogens. Sometimes a balance may need to be met as some reptiles may be stressed with such a simplistic environment. In general, plastic, glass, acrylic, or fiberglass enclosures are most useful. For terrestrial species, enclosures can be simply lined with newspaper or paper towels. For aquatic and semiaquatic species, water may be added to the desired depth without substrate (Innis, Turtle and Tortoise Newsletter, 2001;4:14–16).

Reptiles destined for reintroduction to the wild are best maintained in outdoor enclosures. These facilities have to include running and stationary water (in different areas), living spaces consistent with the natural habitat, hibernaculums, surface hiding areas, basking areas, local climate, and predator control (Rossi, Proc ARAV, 1999, pp 59–60). To avoid infectious disease transmission, all tanks, tubs, tools, and other physical features that are used to rehabilitate native reptiles should never be used for exotic species.

Whether endangered species should be on display to the public is debatable. However, it is certainly advisable to prevent human contact or interaction with animals that are attempting to reproduce. However, public exhibition of some animals is essential to helping local human populations learn to value the species. Public education and outreach are important to support conservation efforts. Thus, there should be two types of facilities: those open to the public with educational and cultural themes and those closed to the public with primarily scientific or reproductive aims.

In those facilities in which animals will be displayed to the public, handling and display should be less than 10 minutes at a time to minimize stress. In the turtle (*Clemmys insculpta*), just 1 minute of handling resulted in an increase in heart rate from 28.39 beats/min to 40.2 beats/min (41% increase). This tachycardia persisted several minutes, then the heart rate returned to the baseline value in approximately 10 minutes.[10]

Nutrition During Rehabilitation

Dietary modification is an important aspect of reptile rehabilitation. Diets should be adjusted for age, rehabilitation goals, and disease processes. The diet should be tailored to meet the needs of four vulnerable conditions for the captive reptile: (i) hatchling and juvenile (musculoskeletal growth), (ii) maturity (gestation, ovulation), (iii) coexistence and overcrowding (parasitism, infectious bacterial, viral or fungal disease), and (iv) old age (hepatorenal dysfunction). Consequently, diets must be calculated to meet metabolic requirements, which should initially be based on calculated daily caloric needs (and then modified based upon response, especially accurate body weight). These data can also be used to calculate the total amount of food to be provided by tube feeding (see Chapters 45 and 122). An adequate supply of water is also important. Aquatic turtles absorb water when hunting and eating, and once they stop eating they dehydrate. Water is absorbed from the gut contents, and feces become dry, fluid flow stagnates, and the intestinal contents can produce a blockage. In an animal with gastrointestinal stasis, any new food will build up behind the blockage, and eventually the animal can die. So, solid food must always be mixed with the appropriate amount of water.[11]

In other rehabilitated reptiles, it is possible to produce a condition known as "refeeding syndrome" if too much nutrition is provided too rapidly. In this situation, the animal that has been chronically deprived of nutrition becomes metabolically deranged when calories are suddenly provided. To prevent this, rehydration should precede feeding. Initially, 10% to 20% of calculated caloric requirements should be provided and gradually increased over the first 1 to 3 weeks of rehabilitation (Innis, Turtle and Tortoise Newsletter, 2001;4:14–16) (see Chapter 87). Esophagostomy tube placement and nutritional support in turtles and other reptiles are discussed in Chapters 45 and 122.

Rehabilitation of Wild Reptiles

Successful reptile conservation requires the implementation of both in situ and ex situ programs. Given the current precarious conservation status of many endemic species around the world, it is clear that the captive breeding of reptiles, with the ultimate aim of their possible reintroduction in the wild, is insufficient to preserve a species. The ex situ strategies are needed to help bolster the number of individuals available for reintroduction and maximize genetic diversity. Conversely, the in situ strategies are needed to address the causes of species decline in the wild and focus on conservation of ecosystems that will support wild-born and reintroduced individuals. Both of these approaches are fundamental to preservation of endangered species.[12]

The release of reptiles into the wild must comply with local, national, and international laws (Cooper, et al. Proc iCARE, 2013, pp 242–243). In addition, selection of reptiles to be released should be subject to very strict criteria, including genetic, pathologic, ecological, and behavioral criteria.[13–16] Any individual not meeting these criteria should not be released. Consequently, some animals can never be reintroduced and should ultimately be removed from the rehabilitation program as "unrecoverable" or "unable to be rehabilitated."

Aid to Adaptation

It is important to promote adaptation of newcomers to facilities, including appropriate behavior training for healthy interaction with conspecifics. Reptiles can suffer maladaptation syndrome as a result of transport and changing maintenance conditions and may have difficulty when introduced into a new environment such as a rescue center. Animals that are already present and adapted to local conditions can help with the habituation of recently arrived animals. However, cohabitation of numerous individuals should be done cautiously and with concern for infectious disease transmission. Likewise, caution is required when mixing certain species renowned for intraspecific aggression (e.g., cobras, crocodiles, certain species of iguanas),[17] as well as intermixing of different species that may prey upon one another, such as king snakes due to their known ophiophagus diet and risk of preying upon other snakes and reptiles.

Unrecoverable Reptiles

There are numerous reasons why some reptiles cannot be released into the wild, including that they have spent excessive time in captivity, have suffered maladaptation, pose a risk of communicable diseases to wild individuals, have congenital anomalies or excessive disability (e.g., limb amputation), or are a species/subspecies not appropriate for a specific geographic release site. With this long list of preclusions for release, selection of individuals for release should be done carefully and in accordance with multidisciplinary teams, including ecologists, biologists, veterinarians, and environmentalists. Nonreleasable animals are often relocated to rescue centers or zoologic institutions. However, the role of such animals extends beyond display to the public, and their scientific value should be considered. Unfortunately, unreleasable individuals may need to be euthanized due to poor rehabilitation prognosis, fiscal limitations, or incompatibility within the overall program for species preservation.

Value of Nonreleasable Animals

Blood donors: Blood transfusions are increasingly used in reptile medicine. Hemorrhage secondary to fractures, falls or collisions, severe burns, or hematologic diseases are some of the causes of hemorrhage that warrant a blood transfusion. The possession of healthy nonreleasable animals allows an available pool of blood donors (assuming that appropriate scientific or animal use permits allow such use). When performing a transfusion it is important to perform a matched (homologous) transfusion whenever possible (see Chapter 87).

Mothership effect: Females of some species such as *Python molurus* incubate eggs, provide parental care, or provide protection to offspring other than their own. Eggs of different species of pythons (sick or dead during egg laying, for example) can be incubated by other females in zoos and breeding centers.

Serum bank: It is important for centers that handle endangered species to have a serum bank. This allows for screening of individuals for certain diseases. The ability to detect certain antibodies to disease, and to track trends through time, is important.

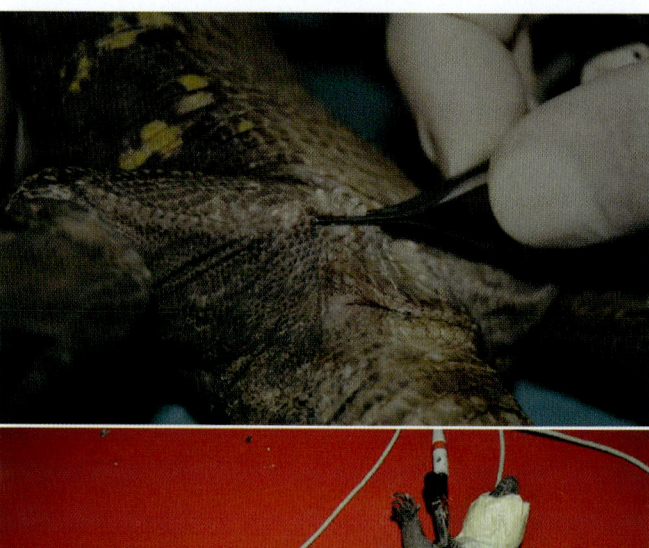
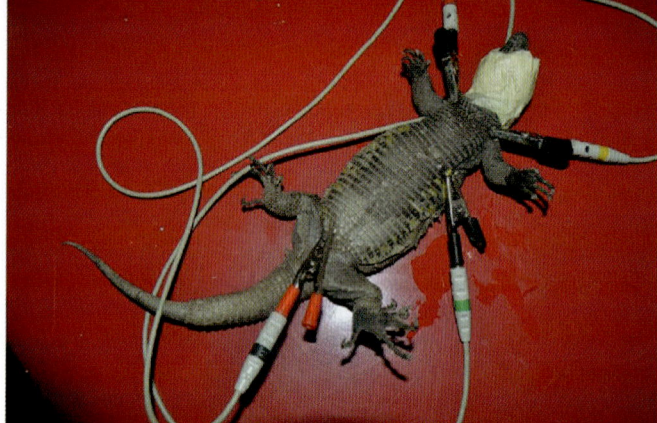
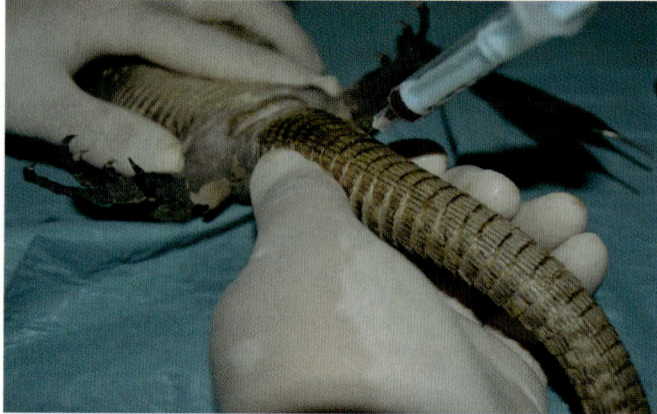

FIG 131.4 Collecting research data including femoral secretions (top), ECG readings (middle), and hematology (bottom) in some nonreleasable El Hierro giant lizards (*Gallotia simonyi*).

Sample size: Nonreleasable animals can help to achieve the ideal number of animals for research, assuming that appropriate scientific animal use permits have been approved.

Physiology research: For all species it is necessary to have established reference values for analytical, diagnostic imaging, or other diagnostic assays.[18] To avoid the risk of extrapolations between species or groups, nonreleasable animals can, with appropriate scientific permit or license, be used to establish reference values for their species (Fig. 131.4).

Semen banks: Nonreleasable reptiles can serve as useful breeders, and their offspring could be released. The collection of semen for artificial insemination is a technique that is beginning to be developed in reptiles[19] (see Chapter 80).

Genome banks: Recent data indicate that within turtle species there is wide geographic variation in genetic variability (not only species but also subspecies, forms, populations, or ecotypes). The safeguarding of some populations may depend on animals that have been maintained in a recovery center. Nonreleasable animals contribute to the protection of viable genes belonging to populations on the brink of extinction.

Environmental education: Education is perhaps one of the most important tools of rehabilitation centers. Showing nonreleasable reptiles is an excellent method to teach visitors. Community education offers a potential to mitigate the impact of human activities that contribute to reptile population decline. Education may also limit the number of healthy animals that are unnecessarily relocated.[20]

Releasable vs Nonreleasable Decision Making

Before the release of any reptile, several factors must be considered, including, but not limited to, structural abnormalities of the animal; infectious disease risks; genetic factors; and national, state, and local laws (Innis, Proc ARAV, 2004, pp 6–8).

Chelonians with repaired shells can be released as long as the repair is inconspicuous to predators. Applying fiberglass and modeling, or 3D-printed shells and subsequent painting, allows released turtles with esthetic prostheses to have high survival rates (Fig. 131.5). However, when considering sealing of shell fractures in turtles, prostheses should only be applied to clean, uninfected wounds that have been managed appropriately. Animals should not be released if infection is present. Many different types of wound sealants and repair materials have been used, including calcium hydroxide pastes, bone cements, and epoxy resins. (For more information, see Chapter 113.)

With regard to hematology, the relative paucity of species-specific reference intervals and use of automated hemacytometers not validated for reptile species mandates a thorough visual examination of blood parameters including smears rather than merely relying upon automated or calculated results. Furthermore, researchers must interpret hematologic results with caution, utilizing the overall picture of an ecological or study population for wildlife monitoring and health assessment.[21] Blood analyses have great potential in ecology, ecotoxicology, and veterinary science, including comparisons between prerelease and postrelease. The major caveat for field researchers, however, is that the established reference intervals derived from captive reptiles may be less appropriate for free-ranging animals. Differences in certain parameters, such as glucose, total proteins, uric acid, and eosinophils may vary in the same animals before and after their release (Martínez-Silvestre, Proc *Congress Mediter-raneend' Herpetologie Marrakesh.* 2007, pp 59–60).

It is important to avoid disruption to wild populations. Reptile translocation can result in a viable increase in the local population. However, augmentation may disrupt existing resident disease or parasitic dynamics and initiate an infectious disease outbreak that could effectively offset any advantages the translocation may have achieved.[15,22] The prevalence of parasites in wild reptiles is often an indicator of the immune status of these animals. In most countries, recovery centers shelter hundreds of animals originating from illegal trade or captive breeding. There are studies that investigate the presence of helminth eggs and worms in feces from free-ranging and captive tortoises and relate the findings to different environmental and host variables. Results show that ascarid infections affect mostly captive animals. Likewise, other diseases such as upper respiratory tract disease are more commonly associated with captive animals. Conversely, in free-ranging populations, oxyurid infections do not appear to be associated with poor health, and their prevalence increases with age. Moreover, in free-living tortoises, the distribution of some ascaris species varies according to habitat and can change significantly with location.[23] Treatment for parasites is recommended; however, in reptiles scheduled for release the goal should

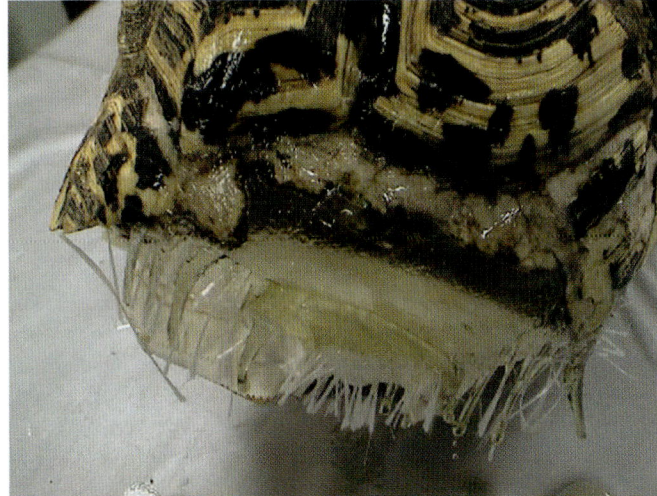
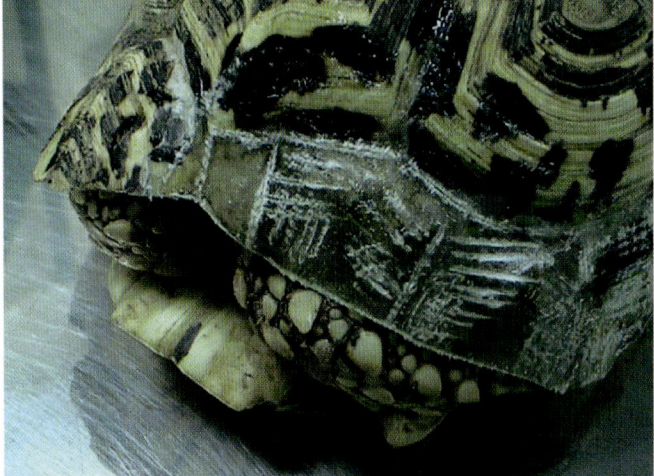
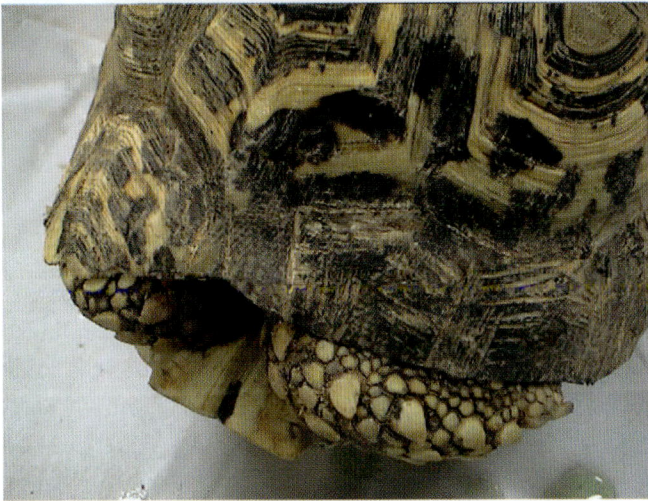

FIG 131.5 Esthetic prosthesis using painted fiber glass in a leopard tortoise (*Stygmochelys pardalis*) bitten by a dog.

be control, not complete elimination, to ensure continued immune recognition.

There is always the concern that asymptomatic carriers of infectious agents released into the wild may spread disease in the environment and to free-ranging populations. There are reports of exposure of wild populations to Ranavirus and Batrachochytrium from released amphibians and herpesviruses and mycoplasmas from released reptiles.

Although mycoplasmas do not usually survive long outside the host unless protected in organic material, numerous other pathogens, viruses in particular, can persist for extended periods in the environment. Rehabilitated animals that are exposed to such infectious diseases in captivity pose a serious threat to wild populations of tortoises (and potentially other reptiles) when they are released. The release of animals with antibiotic-resistant flora is also a concern that should remind the clinician of the importance of appropriate antimicrobial use.

Stress and immune status may affect the presence of pathogens in rehabilitated reptiles. Under stressful conditions, shedding of pathogens, including zoonotic agents, may be enhanced. Occasionally opportunistic pathogens are observed only in hospital conditions such as *Enterococcus* spp. in snakes.[24] In addition, the transmission of *Salmonella* can occur between animals at rehabilitation centers.[25,26] Exotic serotypes of *Salmonella* can be released into the environment with the reintroduction of these rehabilitated animals.[27,28]

Applying diagnostic techniques for isolation or detection of specific microorganisms is important and useful before considering release. These may include bacterial and fungal cultures, polymerase chain reaction (PCR) testing, and antibody testing for chelonian pathogens such as *Mycoplasma* and herpesviruses (Innis, Turtle and Tortoise Newsletter, 2001;4:14–16). Tortoise mycoplasmosis was first reported in desert tortoises from the southwestern United States and California, and has been associated with dramatic population declines. The etiologic agent is *Mycoplasma agassizii*, which has also been isolated from gopher tortoises from Florida. Recently a novel but related *Mycoplasma* species was identified using a PCR assay in box turtles (*Terrapene* sp.) displaying clinical signs consistent with mycoplasmosis. Herpesvirus and *Mycoplasma* have also been isolated from captive and wild moorish tortoises (*Testudo graeca*) in various European and North African countries (Mathes, et al. Proc ARAV 2001, pp 97–99).[29] Infection is usually chronic and can often be subclinical. Clinical signs are often intermittent or cyclical and may be associated with stress. Animals may be chronically infected and should not be released into the wild.

RELEASE STRATEGY

Reptiles can be either "soft released," where acclimation is provided with in situ enclosures, or "hard released" without acclimation, directly into the habitat. Usually, soft releases have resulted in greater survival and site fidelity than hard releases. However, the success of both techniques depends on the species and release habitat (Livoreil, et al. Proc Int Congress on Testudo Genus, 2001, p 32).

Most relocation, repatriation, and translocation projects involving amphibians and reptiles do not have demonstrable benefits for conservation and should not be advocated as acceptable management and mitigation practices.[30] Many reptile translocations fail because the animals are placed in low-quality habitat at the recipient site or dispersed from the release site. Overall success of translocation can be judged by species population viability. For example, the Florida sand skink (*Plestiodon reynoldsi*) is a resilient species that exploits heterogeneous habitats to find suitable microhabitats. Successful translocation of this skink can only be achieved with suitable habitat for this species.[31]

"Head-starting" is a conservation technique for improving survival of individuals from species with high juvenile mortality. This technique is designed to accelerate growth rate and increase body size of captive-born young. Head-started individuals are often kept active year-round to achieve body-size goals and increase survival, omitting or modifying overwintering (brumation). As brumation is part of the life cycle of reptiles, there may be tradeoffs related to temperature response postrelease.[32] This technique has proven useful for the conservation of the West Indian rock iguana (*Cyclura* sp.) (Raphael, Proc ARAV, 2006, pp 32–33).

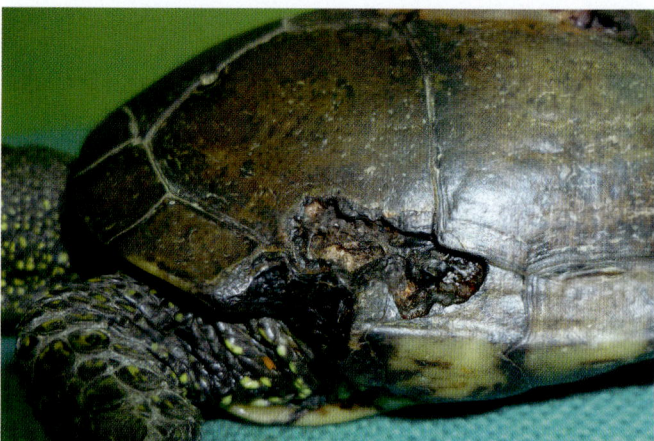

FIG 131.6 Secondary shell infection after marginal scute notching in a reintroduced European pond turtle (*Emys orbicularis*).

There are seldom instances when reinforcement of stable populations with reintroduced animals is recommended. Territoriality of the species and the establishment of hierarchies, especially in turtles, should be considered. Modifications of resident populations may cause stress and compromise their reproductive future. It is important to avoid introducing reptiles in areas where there are already stable and consolidated populations. Instead, the best option is to release individuals into areas previously inhabited by the species, but where the species is currently extinct.[33]

The release of rehabilitated individuals must undergo a detailed sex ratio analysis. Behavioral anomalies have been described in wild Herman's tortoises (*Testudo hermanni*), including the "prison effect," in which the proportion of males and females is highly skewed. In these populations, tortoises exhibit extravagant sexual behaviors, showing homosexual behavior and attempting to copulate with dead conspecifics, empty shells, and stones.[34] The veterinarian plays an important part in reproduction control in both the selection of individuals to breed in captivity and also in postliberation management. In some cases, reptiles have been sterilized to avoid proliferation or genetic contamination in areas in need of sentinel release.[35]

Individual identification techniques in nonmarine reptiles are varied, including microchip (PIT), notches in marginal scutes of chelonian shells, notches in the neck scales or tail of crocodilians and lizards, and colored beads, as well as intracoelomic, subcutaneous, or external transmitters. Peripheral shell/scute notches can become infected and jeopardize the success of the reintroduction (Fig. 131.6). Appropriate technique and prevention of infection is necessary. Techniques that increase animal stress or affect metabolism and/or reproduction should be avoided.[36] A review of marking and tracking techniques in wild and released reptiles can be found in Chapter 175.

When and Where to Release

A conservative approach, maintaining the reptile in captivity for months to allow complete healing, is often preferred before release. Some other authors prefer to release reptiles within weeks of the time of injury if at all possible (Innis, Proc ARAV, 2004, pp 6–8). This philosophy is based on the premise that the patient will heal faster in its native habitat than it will in captivity. As a general rule, reptiles should be released in the evening, avoiding hours of maximum insolation, and in shadowed areas, with water and refuge easily available. Release should also occur during a season of activity for that species (i.e., not during winter) but not during the peak reproductive season (to avoid fights or disturbances). Reptiles may take several days to find refuge and water. When released, reptiles may stay in the same refuge for days or weeks until they feel secure and start to explore their new environment. The habitat chosen should have minimal predators.

Rewilding Programs

Reptile rewilding techniques are mainly restricted to islands. One example includes the rewilding of tortoises on Round and Rodrigues Islands of Mauritius. These islands used to be home to at least two species of giant land tortoises. These endemic species of tortoises were lost from the island ecosystem some 200 years ago due to human hunting. The reestablishment of land tortoises was necessary for restoring ecological function and included extant conspecifics and related taxa. In this case the conspecifics/analogous species chosen for rewilding were Aldabra tortoises (*Dipsochelys elephantina*) from the Aldabra Atoll and Radiated tortoises (*Astrochelys radiata*) from South West Madagascar. In only 5 years, 388 Aldabra and 898 radiated tortoises were naturally hatched in the reserve. Their interaction with vegetation seems to be having the desired ecological effect.[37] The project is transforming these degraded islands of the Indian Ocean into a successful mix of natural biodiversity, along with a popular and sustainable economic and social enterprise (Fig. 131.7). A similar rewilding technique was undertaken using sterilized Galapagos tortoises to engineer a more balanced ecological recovery of Pinta Island in the Galapagos. In this case the released subadult to adult animals were sterilized to avoid interbreeding with future high genetic stock.[35] Animals used in rewilding programs must pass strict health assessments as their role as potential vectors of diseases to the ecosystem must be considered (Martínez-Silvestre, Proc iCARE, 2013, pp 152–155).[38]

ACKNOWLEDGMENTS

To the veterinary team and technicians at the CRARC center (Joaquim Soler, Isabel Verdaguer, Isabel Trimiño, Francisca Claravalls, Anna Saez, Moises Valls, and Adrià Melero); CRT Center (Joan Budo, Xavier Capalleras, Enric Capalleras); Zoologic Badalona Veterinaria (Jordi Grifols, Ferran Bargalló, Simon López); La Vanille Crocodile Park Mauritius (Owen Griffiths, Jim Pether, Gilbert Moutia), and Francois Leguat Rodrigues Tortoise Center (Arnaud Meunier, Aurele Anquetil), as well as Centro de Reproducción del Lagarto de El Hierro (Miguel Angel Rodriguez).

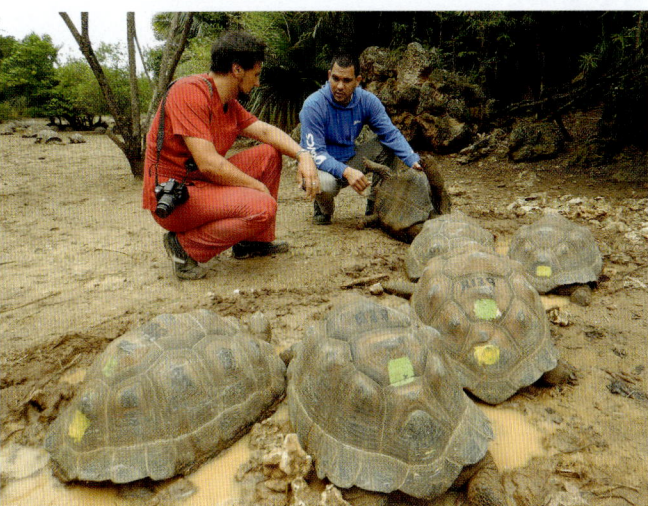

FIG 131.7 Physical examination of Aldabra tortoises introduced in Rodrigues Island (Mauritius).

REFERENCES

See www.expertconsult.com for a complete list of references.

132

Complementary and Integrative Veterinary Therapies

Cynthia L. West and Bruce Ferguson

A number of medical and surgical advances continue to be made in reptile and amphibian health care. Still, many diseases and conditions exist for which conventional medicine is inadequate, impractical, unsafe, or simply not efficacious. In addition, some clients are reluctant to subject their pets to the perceived or real risks of unapproved drugs, anesthesia, and surgery. There may be other methods that we can use to help these animals.

Complementary therapies may be referred to as alternative therapy (or complementary and alternative veterinary medicine [CAVM]) or, less accurately, holistic medicine. They are not generally taught in mainstream veterinary education. Some of these methods have a few thousand years of documented empirical evidence and clinical trials. Others have been developed more recently and have only limited empirical or anecdotal evidence of efficacy with few strictly controlled clinical trials. Traditional Chinese veterinary medicine (TCVM), for example, which incorporates several different disciplines, including acupuncture, herbal medicine, nutrition, massage, and meditation, dates back at least 2500 years, whereas homeopathy has a history of about 200 years.[1] What almost all complementary therapies have in common is that they are targeted to work with the individual animal's natural healing capabilities. They treat the whole individual (thus the term holistic) and support the individual body's healing processes. Much criticism has been aimed at these therapies as being nonscientific and lacking in research, controlled, double-blind studies or other perceived scientific validation. Clinical work is being undertaken worldwide and empirical results are accumulating. The National Institutes of Health's (NIH) website reveals a tremendous amount of ongoing research and has already proven the benefits of CAM for many human diseases.

Available conventional medical treatments can carry serious side effects and can suppress clinical signs while a disease or condition progresses. This is particularly true of chronic diseases like arthritis, asthma, allergies, and dermatologic conditions. In addition, there are few approved pharmaceuticals for use in reptiles and amphibians, and some are potentially harmful. Integrating complementary and alternative therapies into the treatment plan for these species may reduce, eliminate, or shorten the duration of treatment with potentially harmful medications.

Complementary therapies can be used to major benefit in wellness or preventive therapy, particularly for geriatric pets (though also beneficial to young and healthy adult animals) that are more prone to deficiencies, imbalances, and chronic degenerative conditions.

Incorporating these complementary therapies into the treatment plan is not meant to usurp the benefit of proper conventional medical diagnostics. A thorough investigation, including a physical examination, clinicopathology, diagnostic imaging, histopathology and microbiology, and so forth, are still recommended before treatment, along with a detailed history of clinical signs, behavior, husbandry, and nutrition.

This will allow for the most effective integration of conventional and complementary medicine for treatment. However, due to the observational and noninvasive diagnostic tools available to trained practitioners of CAVM disciplines, it is possible to establish a treatment plan for those patients whose caretakers decline to pursue conventional medical testing or for whom invasive diagnostic techniques may prove hazardous or otherwise inadvisable.

Because of the pervasive constraints of time and funding, few of these technologies have been explicitly studied in reptile or amphibian patients. Consequently, little data are available for the use of such methods in these species. Therefore most of the following extrapolates from mammalian data or uses clinical cases from practicing veterinarians.

This chapter is meant to stimulate thought in these emerging therapeutic areas rather than answer all questions. It is a short introduction to some of the integrative and complementary therapies, which may be useful adjuncts in herpetological medicine. Our hope is that the ensuing discussion leads to future applications of the following methods with attendant clinical research. In this fashion, as with all incipient medical systems, a database will begin to accumulate that will enlighten us and benefit our reptile and amphibian patients.

In this section we will briefly introduce some of the more common complementary and alternative therapies found useful by clinical veterinarians, with the primary focus being on traditional Chinese veterinary medicine (TCVM). As stated previously, of the available complementary therapies TCVM is backed by the most clinical and scientific research evidence as well as a 5000-year tradition and approximately 2500-year written history. Many useful and worthwhile complementary therapies, including but not limited to homeopathy, chiropractic, bach flower therapy, aromatherapy, magnetic field therapy and other bioenergetic medicines, Tellington touch, and physical therapy, are omitted from this chapter due to lack of space and the lack of data, especially regarding the multitude of reptile and amphibian species.

Some of these therapies are immediately applicable to most practicing veterinarians (nutraceuticals and some herbs), whereas others require more specialized training (acupuncture, sophisticated herbal medicine, chiropractic, and homeopathy). Readers will find a list of resources for further information, organizations, and, most importantly, further education and training at the end of the chapter. We want the reader to view this introduction to CAVM with the knowledge that this area of herpetologic medicine is in its infancy.

TRADITIONAL CHINESE VETERINARY MEDICINE

TCVM incorporates the disciplines of acupuncture, herbal medicine, nutrition, massage, and meditation. Although some form of meditation is routinely incorporated into the treatment of human beings with traditional Chinese medicine, as veterinarians we normally utilize the first four categories in caring for our animal patients. For the fifth category, we may substitute "lifestyle" changes or improvement in husbandry to complete the balance of holistic care for our patients.

As advocates for our patients, we need to educate owners, to the best of our current knowledge and ability, concerning proper nutrition, housing, environmental enrichment, socialization, and stress reduction. This may be one of the most important aspects for restoring and maintaining health in reptiles and amphibians. Without such knowledge, our ability to offer veterinary care is only sufficient for the acute crisis.

ACUPUNCTURE

The basis and usage of acupuncture may be viewed in either a conventional scientific or TCVM framework. The placement of small needles (usually 30-gauge to 36-gauge) into exact locations in a subject's body may have a number of positive benefits. Western scientific analyses indicate local, immunologic, neuroreflexive, and central nervous system responses to acupuncture.[2] These effects may include shortened healing time in injured tissues and nervous system activation in neurologic trauma. Increased immune surveillance and heightened immune system function along with reflexive changes in organ system function and pain control are also reported as effects of acupuncture. Studies have shown acupuncture results in an increase in endogenous substances such as enkephalins and endorphins, and the analgesic effects of acupuncture can be reversed with naloxone.[3]

Analgesia is not the only measurable effect of acupuncture. Both parasympathetic and sympathetic components of visceral nerves may be stimulated,[4] as well as local changes in cells, nerves, and vessels where the needles are inserted, including mast cell release, vasodilation, and stimulation of neural terminals.[5] Acupuncture can enhance immunity by increasing levels of white blood cells, interferons, antibodies, and immunoglobulins.[6] Hormonal changes, including the release of growth hormone, luteinizing hormone, and thyroid hormones, have also been measured.[7]

In TCVM, health is defined as a state of harmony or balance between the body and its internal and external environment. Illness occurs when the homeostatic mechanisms of the body malfunction, and the resulting imbalance creates a disease condition of excess or deficiency.

Qi is the life force. It is energy and involves the energetic functions of the body, which is the focus of acupuncture. Qi flows through the body and can be accessed through a system of channels or meridians on which we find our acupuncture points. In TCVM, when Qi flows freely, there is balance, health, and the absence of pain. When Qi becomes trapped, obstructed, or stagnant, there is pain; if Qi is decreased, there may be weakness and disease. Acupuncture restores the free flow of Qi and in TCVM may be used to tonify, strengthen, and balance the body's systems.

One using acupuncture for therapy from a strictly western viewpoint would likely choose to treat pain (from trauma, for example) based on local points near the injured area along with a-shi points (Fig. 132.1). A-shi points are points of pain or sensitivity and do not necessarily correspond to known meridian points.[8]

Conversely, a TCVM practitioner might treat an internal medicine case, for example, chronic renal disease, by acupuncturing points that tonify, energize or nourish, and replenish kidney Qi. The TCVM practitioner would also likely use herbs and nutrition to hydrate the body, control and replenish electrolyte problems, and treat clinical signs related to the underlying imbalance. In TCVM, chronic renal disease is not a diagnosis but may present as several different patterns, each with its distinct acupuncture protocol, herbal medicine, and nutritional recommendations.

Most importantly, in modern veterinary medicine, the 2 forms of medical treatment can be successfully and effectively integrated. Chronic renal disease is a common problem in reptiles. An integrated approach might include fluids or diuresis and correction of electrolyte imbalances via conventional medications, along with nutritional and husbandry adjustments. Adding acupuncture to strengthen the kidneys, stimulate appetite, and treat associated problems like constipation and arthritis enhances overall patient support and well-being.

The use of acupuncture on animals transposes traditional Chinese points for humans along 12 major bilaterally distributed meridians, each linked to a specific internal organ, and along 8 extra channels that are not specifically linked to visceral organs. Anatomic differences in species (in comparison with humans), along with uncertain meridian pathways for animals, creates problems with the application of the meridian numbering system. Several studies comparing major points between humans and dogs with various electro point finders, or low skin resistant points (LSR), have revealed a moderately high (79% in one study) correlation between human and canine acupuncture points.[5]

Applying acupuncture to reptiles and amphibians must therefore take anatomic and functional differences into consideration. Meridian points on lizards are easily transposed from canine acupoints, but snakes and turtles are more challenging (Fig. 132.2). Meridians found primarily on the extremities are impossible to directly transpose on a limbless animal. It is likely that many of the points found on legs and digits do exist in some area of the snake's body but have not been discovered or described. Many of the points on the Bladder, Gallbladder Spleen, Liver, Kidney, and Stomach meridians are inaccessible in chelonians (Fig. 132.3). Some species, particularly amphibians and delicate lizards like geckos, may have easily identifiable or accessible points, but handling and stress must be considered when attempting to needle these species. Many of the benefits of acupuncture rely on the release of humoral substances like serotonins and endorphins. Therefore, because corticosteroid and epinephrine release may antagonize many of its positive effects, a highly stressed animal may not receive as much benefit from acupuncture as a calmer, more receptive patient.

Amphibian skin is very delicate and easily subject to damage. Using techniques such as dry needle acupuncture without retention or using the blunt end of the needle handle or moistened, cotton-tipped applicator to briefly stimulate an acupoint may be more appropriate methods for applying acupuncture to delicate amphibian skin.

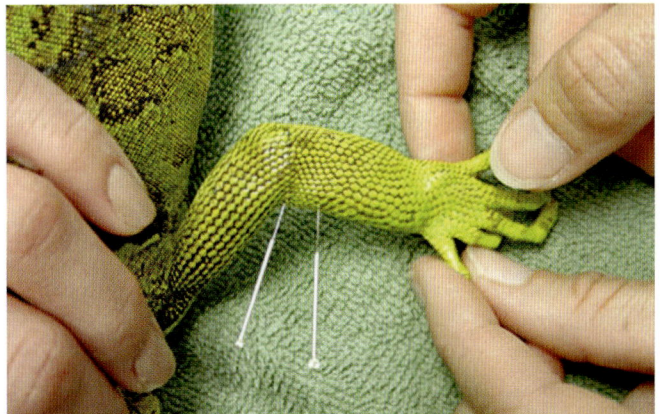

FIG 132.1 For this green iguana *(Iguana iguana)*, a-shi acupuncture points are used to treat pain based on local points near the injured area. A-shi points are points of pain or sensitivity and do not necessarily correspond to known meridian points. (Courtesy of Douglas R. Mader.)

Numerous animal patients have been successfully treated with acupuncture for a wide range of maladies, including, but not limited to, anorexia, constipation, decreased intestinal motility, diarrhea, dystocia, cloacal prolapse, renal failure, respiratory infections, oral inflammation and infection, behavior problems (aggression/anxiety), and musculoskeletal problems such as intervertebral disk disease and resulting neuropathies.

Figs. 132.4 and 132.5 show typical acupuncture points used in lizard and turtle patients. Fig. 132.6 illustrates acupuncture points on an argentine horned frog (*Ceratophrys ornata*). Table 132.1 lists some commonly used acupuncture points, their approximate locations, and a brief description of their primary actions and indications. Specialized techniques such as aqua-acupuncture (Fig. 132.7) and electroacupuncture (Fig. 132.8) can be readily utilized with proper training. To be used safely and effectively, acupuncture requires appropriate training, and we strongly recommend interested veterinarians take a formal course before applying acupuncture to patients.

HERBAL MEDICINE

Herbal medicine encompasses a broad category of uses and applications from various cultures, including traditional Chinese medicine; western herbal medicine, which includes Native American plants; and Ayurveda medicine from India. The components of formulas used in these disciplines may include whole plants or parts of plants, minerals, and even animal parts (Chinese medicine may use all three in their herbal formulas).[9] A practitioner may prescribe a single herb or a combination of herbs (an herbal formula) when treating a patient and has several options for the form used. Herbs can be ordered from professional suppliers as bulk herbs, dried extracts, and liquid extracts (usually extracted in alcohol) and therefore can be administered in several ways, including capsules, powders, drops, teas, and soups. Many Chinese herbal formulas come conveniently concentrated into a pill

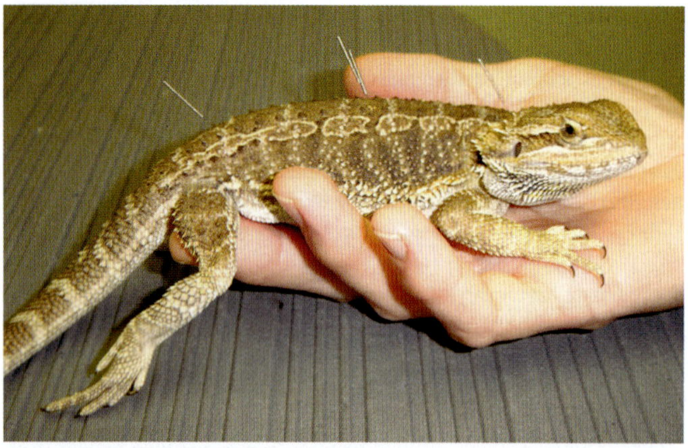

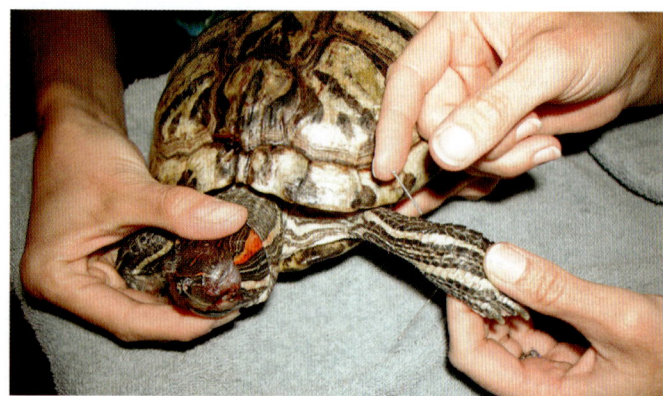

FIG 132.2 Meridian points on lizards (shown here, a bearded dragon [*Pogona vitticeps*]) are easily transposed from canine acupoints; snakes and turtles are more challenging. (Courtesy of Douglas R. Mader.)

FIG 132.3 Most of the bladder and gallbladder meridians and points on spleen, liver, kidney, and stomach meridians are inaccessible on the turtle. Acupuncture (as demonstrated here for a red-eared slider [*Trachemys scripta elegans*]) is limited to the skin of the legs and neck. (Courtesy of Douglas R. Mader.)

TABLE 132.1	Commonly Used Acupuncture Points for Reptiles and Amphibians	
Acupuncture Point	**Actions/Indications**	**Location**
GV 26	Resuscitation	In the philtrum at the level of the ventral limit of the nostrils
GV 1	Diarrhea, constipation, food stasis	On the midline halfway between the vent and the ventral base of the tail
Shan-gen	Appetite stimulation, anorexia	On the dorsal midline on a line just caudal to the caudal aspect of the nostrils
GV 14	Fever, any infection, immune regulation	On the dorsal midline at the space between the last cervical and first thoracic vertebrae
Wei-jian (Tail tip)	Fever, disc injury, spinal injury	At the tip of the tail
ST 36	General weakness and gastrointestinal disorders	On the craniolateral rear limb about 1/5th the distance from the stifle to the hock
LI 10	General weakness and gastrointestinal disorders	On the craniolateral forearm 1/6th the distance from the elbow to the carpus
LIV 3	General pain management, liver disorders, conjunctivitis, and intraocular inflammation	On the dorsum of the rear foot between the first and second metatarsals proximal to the metatarsophalangeal joint
LI 4	General pain management, immune regulation	On the dorsum of the front foot between the first and second metacarpals proximal to the metacarpophalangeal joint
GV 20	Calming, relieves anxiety	On the dorsal midline on top of the head on a line level with the caudal aspects of the orbits
GB 34	Tendon/ligament problems, liver disorders, seizures	On the mid lateral aspect of the rear leg just cranial and distal to the head of the fibula
PC 8	Paresis and paralysis	On the palmar surface of the front foot between metacarpals II and III
KID 1	Paresis and paralysis	On the plantar surface of the rear foot between metatarsals II and III
ST 1	Conjunctivitis, any ocular problem	Just over the orbital rim directly below the center of the pupil

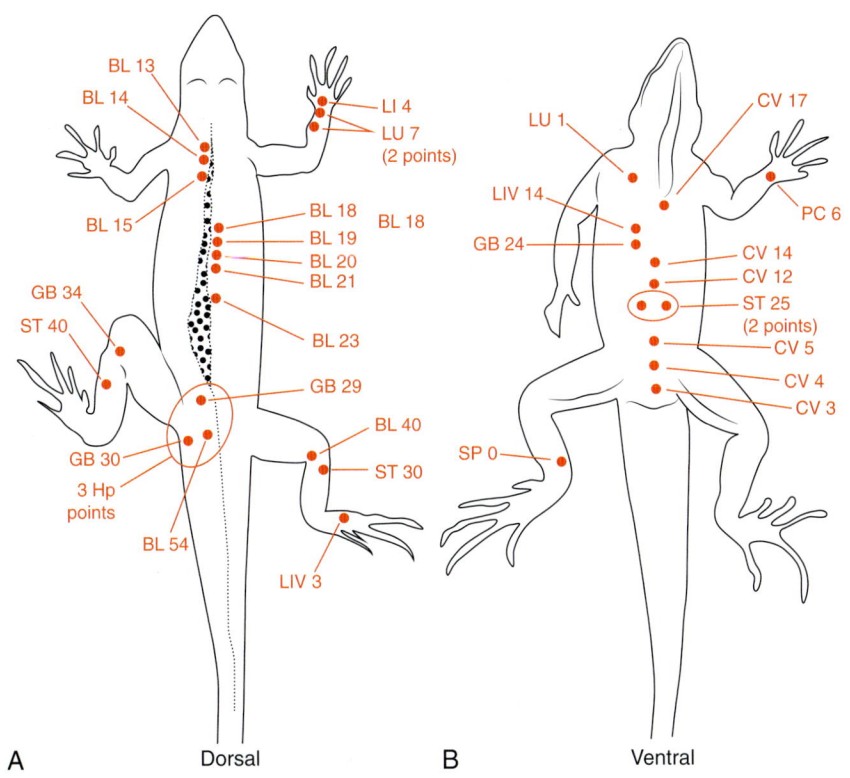

A Dorsal

B Ventral

Lizard Acupuncture (Dorsal View)

Acupuncture Point	Association Point for	Anatomic Location (Bilaterally—1½ Rib Widths Lateral to the Dorsal Midline at the Level of the Intervertebral Space)
BL 13	Lung	3rd intercostal space
BL14	Pericardium	4th intercostal space
BL 15	Heart	5th intercostal space
BL 18	Liver	10th intercostal space
BL 19	Gallbladder	11th intercostal space
BL 20	Spleen	12th intercostal space
BL 21	Stomach	13th intercostal space
BL 23	Kidney	15th intercostal apace

Master Point	Affects
LI 4	Face and mouth
LU 7	Head and neck
BL 40	Back and hips
ST 36	Abdomen and gastrointestinal system

Other Useful Point	Affects/Actions/Indications
LIV 3	Gastrointestinal system, urogenital system, liver, gallbladder, general pain management, conjunctivitis, and intraocular inflammation
GB 34	Tendons
ST 40	Phlegm, ascites, accumulation of damp
GB 29, GB 30, BL 54	Hips, arthritis, paralysis
LU 7	Arteries and respiratory system

Master Point	Affects
PC 6	Chest and cranial abdomen
SP 6	Caudal abdomen and urogenital system

Lizard Acupuncture (Ventral View)

Point	Alarm Point[a] for
LU 1	Lung
CV 17	Pericardium
LIV 14	Liver
GB 24	Gallbladder
CV 14	Heart
CV 12	Stomach
ST 25	Large intestine
CV 5	Triple heater
CV 4	Small intestine
CV 3	Urinary bladder

[a]Pain in these points indicates pain in the corresponding organ.

FIG 132.4 (A and B) Typical acupuncture points for a lizard patient.

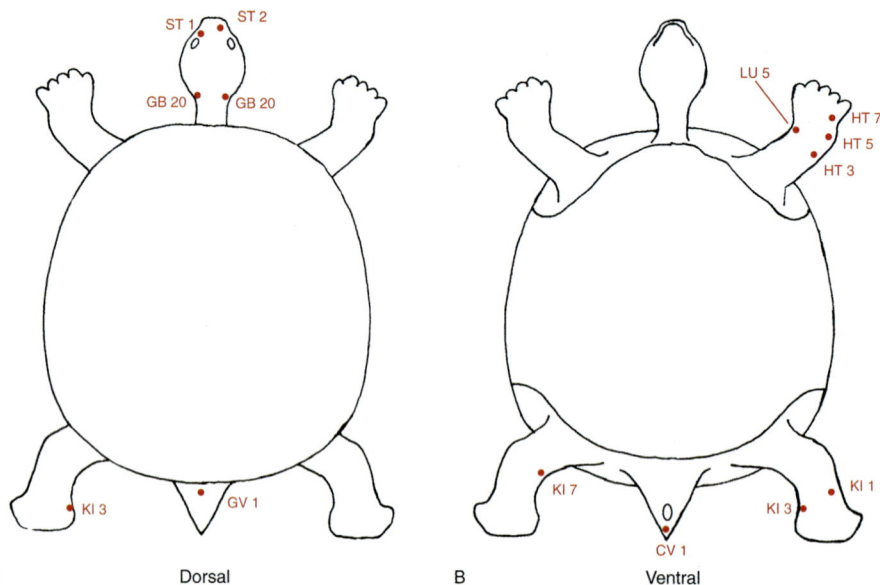

Useful Point	Affects/Actions/Indications	Anatomic Location
GV 1	Diarrhea and rectal/cloacal prolapse	Ventral to tail base and dorsal to vent
CV 1	Constipation and prolapse	Ventral cloacal midline between anus and urinary pore
ST 1	Eye disorders, conjunctivitis	Just over the orbital rim directly below the center of the pupil
ST 2	Eye disorders, conjunctivitis	In the infraorbital foramen rostroventral to ST 1
GB 20	Neurologic disorders and cervical problems	In the shallow depression between the cervicalis and sterno-occipitalis muscles, 1 rib width lateral to the dorsal midline
LU 5	Respiratory disorders and infections	At the elbow immediately lateral to the biceps tendon
HT 7	Sedation, calming, anxiety, and behavioral effects	Immediately proximal to the carpal bone at the lateral carpus
HT 5	Sedation, calming, anxiety, and behavioral effects	Along the same groove as HT 7 but more proximal
KI 1	Revival point, paralysis	Plantar surface of the rear foot between metatarsals II and III
KI 3	Urogenital, cystitis, chronic renal disease	Medial tarsus, caudal to and at the level of the medial malleolus
KI 7	Diarrhea, cystitis, urogenital disorders	Medial rear limb 1/6 of the distance proximal from the medial malleolus to the tibial plateau just cranial to the Achilles tendon

FIG 132.5 (A and B) Typical acupuncture points for a turtle patient. Note: The same points used on the iguana can be used on the turtle *if* accessible. For instance, you cannot access many of the association or alarm points due to the shell.

form as well. When prescribing an herb compared with a conventional western drug, one prescribes a whole plant, substance, or formula where the active constituents may be tempered or enhanced by other parts of the herb or herbal formula. Thus what may be toxic when isolated becomes safer, or absorption may be increased, or effects may otherwise be altered.

Active Constituents and Actions

Some 25% or more of the pharmaceuticals used today are derived from specific substances found in medicinal herbs (Griffith, personal communication). Pharmacognosy has revealed many important biologically active compounds in plants, and one can use this knowledge in prescribing herbal products and incorporating historic uses for dispensing herbal medicines. Some of the more common chemical constituents of herbs and their actions are described in Table 132.2. So, with some understanding of its active constituents and actions, one might prescribe a soothing demulcent such as marshmallow root (*Althea officinalis*) for such diverse conditions as enteritis, colitis, cystitis, and urethritis.

Herbal Energetics

Most indigenous herbal medical systems, including TCVM, are based on the belief that herbs have specific energies or broad therapeutic categories based on their effects in the body. Empirical evidence supports specific effects of herbs, including those that "clear Heat," "drain Damp," "warm," "cool," or "nourish Blood."

For example, a hot pepper is considered to be "warming" and is used to "dispel Cold and clear the exterior." When consumed the pepper elicits sweating, facial redness, and a general warming sensation in the body. Detailed experiments have suggested that these physiological changes are from peripheral vasodilation and increased tissue perfusion and that the flavonoids in the pepper increase neutrophil-killing function and generally increase immune system function.[10] Sweating itself has been shown to have a positive influence on the body's ability to deal with pathogens.

In general, Chinese herbal medicine is heteropathic in nature. Warming herbs are used to treat cold diseases, and cooling herbs treat

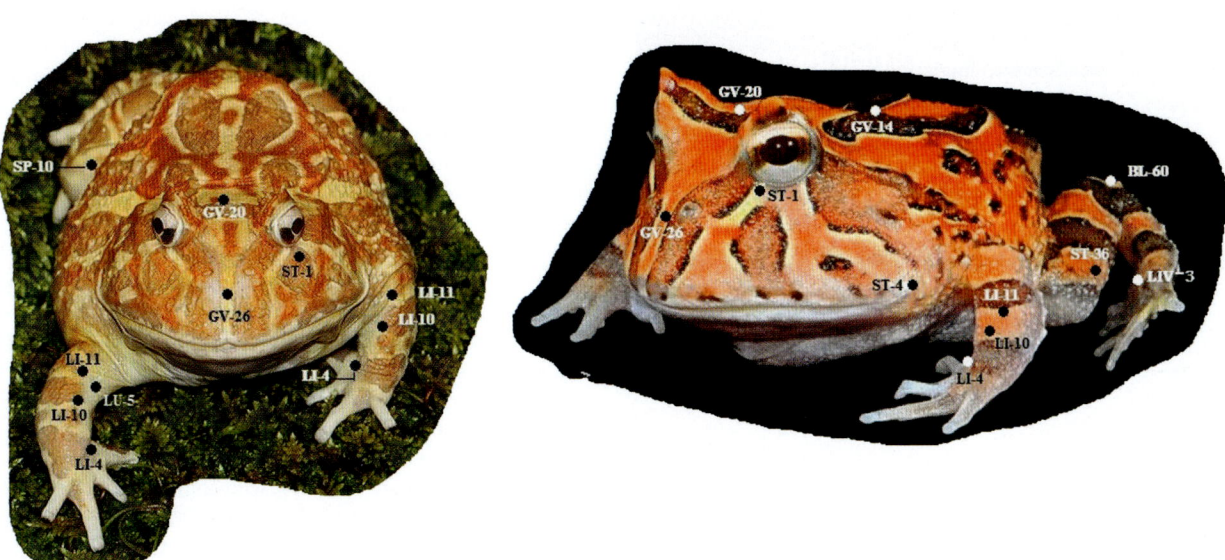

Point	Actions/Indications	Anatomic Location
GV 14	Fever, any infection, immune regulation	On the dorsal midline at the space between the last cervical and first thoracic vertebrae
GV 20	Calming, relieves anxiety	On the dorsal midline on top of the head on a line level with the caudal aspects of the orbits
GV 26	Resuscitation	In the philtrum at the level of the ventral limit of the nostrils
LU 5	Respiratory disorders and infection	At the elbow immediately lateral to the biceps tendon
LI 4	Face and mouth, general pain management, immune regulation	On the dorsum of the front foot between the first and second metacarpals proximal to the metacarpophalangeal joint
LI 10	General weakness and gastrointestinal disorders	On the craniolateral forearm 1/6th the distance from the elbow to the carpus
LI 11	Skin inflammation, diarrhea, constipation, any traumatic injury	At the lateral end of the cubital crease at the lateral elbow
ST 1	Eye disorders, conjunctivitis	Just over the orbital rim directly below the center of the pupil
ST 4	Stomatitis, oral lesions	Just caudal to the mucocutaneous junction at the lateral commissure of the mouth
ST 36	General weakness and gastrointestinal disorders	On the craniolateral rear limb about 1/5th the distance from the stifle to the hock
SP 10	Blood loss, skin inflammation	1½ rib widths proximal and cranial to the medial femoral condyle
BL 60	Back and neck pain, general pain relief	Lateral tarsus, caudal to and at the level of the lateral malleolus
LIV 3	General pain management, liver disorders, conjunctivitis, and intraocular inflammation	On the dorsum of the rear foot between the first and second metatarsals proximal to the metatarsophalangeal joint

FIG 132.6 Acupuncture points of the Argentine horned frog (*Ceratophrys ornata*).

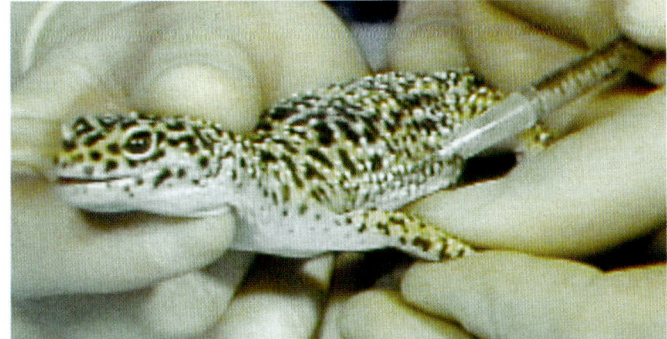

FIG 132.7 Small (such as this leopard gecko [*Eublepharis macularius*]) or easily agitated lizards that do not tolerate needling may benefit from aqua-acupuncture. Aqua-acupuncture is a variance from dry needling where, in this case, vitamin B₁₂, diluted with sterile 0.9% saline, is injected into acupoints instead of using needles. Exercise caution to avoid the renal portal system with any injection into the caudal half of the body (including rear limbs and tail) of reptile and amphibian patients. (Courtesy of Douglas R. Mader.)

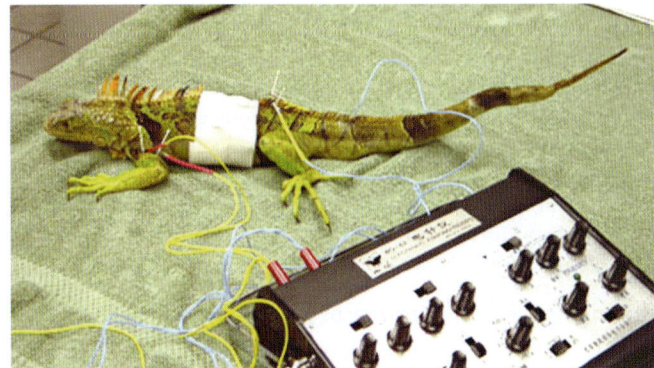

FIG 132.8 As demonstrated in this green iguana (*Iguana iguana*), electroacupuncture, in which dry needles are inserted into specific points and electrical current is applied via an electronic control panel, is a valuable tool for recovery of neural damage. (Courtesy of Douglas R. Mader.)

TABLE 132.2   Common Chemical Constituents of Herbs and Their Actions

Constituent	Actions
Mucilage	Hydrophilic and soothing polysaccharides
Phenols	Broad group of aromatic compounds, astringents (eg, salicylic acid)
Tannins	Coagulate proteins
Coumarins	Anticoagulants, muscle relaxants
Anthraquinones	Irritant or cathartic laxatives
Flavonoids	Complex anti-inflammatory, antioxidant, aromatics
Anthocyanins	Plant pigments that benefit connective tissue
Volatile oils	Ketones, esters, and aldehydes with many effects
Saponins	Steroidal and triterpenoidal compounds
Cardiac glycosides	Digitalis, positive inotrope
Vitamins	Benefit most metabolic processes in body
Bitters	Broad class, stimulates digestion and bile flow
Alkaloids	Broad class (e.g., vincristine, atropine)
Minerals	Support normal metabolic processes (e.g., potassium)

warm or hot diseases. In Chinese medicine, herbs are prescribed based on the individual's TCVM pattern diagnosis and not the specific clinical signs. For example, two patients are seen with chronic diarrhea. One patient has "cow patty" type stools once a day, weak pulses, fatigue, and cool limbs and lower back. The other has bloody, foul-smelling diarrhea; fast, pounding pulses; and hot ears, feet, and groin. The first patient has a deficient and cold-type pattern, and the second has an excess and heat-type condition. The herbal prescriptions for these patients are quite different.

General Use of Herbs in Veterinary Practice

Frequently, the conditions we treat with complementary therapies are chronic problems for which conventional medicine has not been successful, including degenerative joint disease, autoimmune disorders, psychological disturbances, and seizures. Herbal medicine can provide effective treatment choices for these patients when conventional medicines are not adequate or have adverse side effects.

One of the more controversial areas of veterinary medicine is treating behavior disorders with psychotropic drugs. Many perceived "behavior" problems are unacceptable in our homes but natural for the animal in its own habitat. Marking and aggression are frequently seen, and treatment is often sought and administered despite undesirable side effects. Herbal medicine may offer an effective option for calming anxiety while avoiding the adverse consequences of pharmaceuticals such as Depo-Provera, Amitriptyline, Buspirone HCL, and others. An example of this may be incorporating herbal calming preparations for the treatment of farm-raised alligators to reduce skin trauma from heightened agitation when moving the animals to new enclosures. This would not only benefit the animals themselves but also reduce economic loss due to damage to the future harvested hides.

Dosing and Administration of Herbal Medicines

Herbal medicines generally work at a rate somewhere between nutritional therapy and conventional drug therapy. Their actions are generally slower to effect than a pharmaceutical but much faster than nutritional changes or therapies alone.

Metabolic studies conclude that smaller animals generally have a need for relatively higher amounts of herbs than larger individuals due to their higher basal metabolic rates. Herbal components are absorbed, used, and excreted more rapidly, on average, by animals of smaller body size. Our broad recommendation is to calculate herb amounts based on mathematic reduction due to smaller body size and increase that amount to account for increased metabolic rates using metabolic scaling. For example, if an adult 68 kg (150-lb) human dosage of peppermint in an infusion (tea) is 14.8 mL (1 US tablespoon) of herb in 473 mL (US pint) of water, then the dosage for a 34-kg (75-lb) dog is the same, because one increases the amount of peppermint to offset for carnivore inefficiency in using herbal constituents. In other words, a 34-kg (75-lb) dog should take one half of the adult human dose by weight, but this is then increased (doubled) because of the canine gut inefficiency. Note that this increase attempts to consider both body size and natural dietary predilection. These differences may be significant when dealing with herbivorous, omnivorous, or carnivorous herpetological patients.

That said, our reptile and amphibian patients differ drastically in metabolism compared with the small mammalian and avian patients we treat. Dosing should take these species' slower metabolic rate into consideration. As is often the case with conventional pharmaceuticals, this can generally be accomplished by less frequent dosing (q 24 hours vs q 12 hours) for many herbal medicines.

A broad, general dosing recommendation for reptiles and amphibians using oral Chinese herbal medicine is 0.1 to 0.4 g/kg of body weight q 24 to q 12 hours depending on species and herb or formula used. It is best to start with a low dosage of any new substance. If vomiting, diarrhea, or other adverse side effects are seen, discontinue use immediately and restart at a lower dosage or frequency. If the patient has no problems, gradually increase the dosage and monitor efficacy over time. The exact doses of each herb to use in assorted species of animals of dissimilar sizes and metabolism is unknown. Fortunately, however, most herbal medicines lack the dangerous potencies of derived pharmaceutical agents and serious side effects are rare.

Administering herbal medications to animals can be challenging. Many herbs and herbal supplements are given over periods of weeks or months. A significant number of herbal medicines are not particularly palatable for many species. Encapsulating powders and concentrated extracts can provide a more effective means of administration. For some larger species the medicine can be disguised in whole animal foods such as mice or chicks. Some reptiles and amphibians will accept treats such as black soldier fly larvae dusted with herbal powders. Another effective delivery system for herbal medicine is small balls of highly palatable foods. Extracts are generally easy to administer and are believed to have the most rapid gastrointestinal absorption rate (Wynn, personal communication). Alcohol extracts are not very palatable to animal patients, but usually only small amounts are needed. Glycerin extracts are also available and may be more readily accepted but are usually not as concentrated, necessitating a larger volume to be administered. Milk thistle, for example, is available in health food stores in pill, capsule, and both alcohol and glycerin extract forms. We commonly use it for avian hepatic lipidosis, hepatitis, and feline liver diseases and have used it in a green iguana (*Iguana iguana*) with chronic hepatitis.

Topical herbal preparations, such as Yunnan Bai Yao or Coptis powder can be used to good effect for some mild local conditions such as small traumatic wounds and mild local inflammation or infection. It is important, particularly with amphibian patients due to their highly permeable skin, to only choose those preparations that are safe for ingestion to avoid toxicity in these sensitive species. Start with low concentrations and monitor closely for distress or skin irritation. The author has used Yunnan Bai Yao in a free-ranging Southern toad (*Anaxyrus terrestris*) injured by a lawn string trimmer to effectively stop bleeding, prevent infection, and resolve the skin wounds.

In general, herbal medicine is best undertaken by a trained herbalist. Formal training and certification in both western and Chinese veterinary herbal medicine are available both on line and on site from several providers worldwide. However, by careful extrapolation and species consideration, it is possible for new herbal practitioners to provide relief to some patients for chronic and acute conditions when conventional therapies fail or are unavailable.

NUTRITION AND NUTRACEUTICALS

Many chronic health problems in captive reptiles and amphibians are likely secondary to long-term errors in nutrition, husbandry, and the increased stress of confinement. Prior authors have implicated malnutrition in poor performance, disease, and high mortality (see Chapter 27). Micronutrient imbalances are more difficult to discover and are generally inferred from clinical signs or response to treatment. Rarely are all of the important antioxidants, including vitamins C, E, and A, added to manufactured diets for captive reptiles and amphibians. In TCVM, nutritional therapy is based on a heteropathic system of medicine incorporating the ideas of feeding cooling foods for "hot" conditions, warming foods for "cold" conditions, "nourishing" foods to tonify deficiencies, and "clearing" foods to sedate excess conditions. However, to reasonably implement such therapy, we must first understand the nutritional requirements of the particular species being treated. It will do no good to suggest a dietary modification for an animal that incorporates foods inappropriate for that species. Because we are commonly uncertain or unable to reproduce the biologically appropriate diet for each species, investigation of either diverse fresh foods or food additives with nutraceuticals may be prudent.

Many ingested foods have both nutritional and pharmacological effects on the body. Sometimes these two cannot be separated. For example, the US Food and Drug Administration (FDA) defines a food as a substance that provides nutrition, taste, or aroma. By FDA definition, a drug is a substance that is a food or nonfood substance that is used to treat, cure, mitigate, or prevent disease.[11] Nutraceuticals are mostly foods or food derivatives that have known pharmacologic effects. The North American Veterinary Nutraceutical Council defines a nutraceutical as a nondrug substance that is produced in a purified or extracted form and administered orally to provide agents required for normal body structure and function with the intent of improving the health and well-being of animals.[12]

Most veterinarians have some experience with nutraceuticals in the form of supplements for the hair and coat, multivitamin supplements, and joint supplements such as chondroitin sulfate and glycosaminoglycans. Geriatric animals in particular may benefit from these substances because of their decreasing ability to absorb and use nutrients. In these patients nutraceuticals may be used to treat more obvious clinical signs like arthritis, a dry and/or thin skin and coat, and impaired vision.

Nutraceuticals range from macromolecules to simple fatty acids and may act both locally and systemically. For example, numerous species have both quantitative and qualitative fatty acid requirements.[13] Most fats, depending on the natural history and metabolic limits of each reptile, can meet calorific requirements. Some fatty acids may, however, promote inflammation in the body and possibly interfere with normal cytokine production.[14] Furthermore, each bowel segment has an ability to either digest or microbiologically alter fats. Fatty acids that are not biologically appropriate for each species could possibly lead to local bowel inflammation, disharmony, and unbalanced cytokine production and yield less than optimal nutrition to the animal.[15]

Unfortunately, in the still-emerging area of reptile and amphibian complementary medicine we are often left with many uncertainties in the use of nutraceuticals. How to use? When to use? How much to use? Table 132.3 lists some supplements, doses, and possible side effects. We have used joint supplements as recommended on the label but metabolically scaled where warranted.

TABLE 132.3 Common Supplements, Doses, and Possible Side Effects

Supplement	Daily Dose	Possible Adverse Effects
B-complex: B_1, B_2, B_6	5–40 mg	Nontoxic
Folic acid, B_{12}	5–100 mg	Nontoxic
Vitamin C[a]	50–1000 mg	Considered nontoxic
Vitamin E	10–100 IU	Anorexia, increased clotting time
Vitamin A	500–5000 IU	Anorexia, weight loss
Selenium	5–50 µg	Anorexia, ataxia, weakness
Zinc	5–20 mg	Causes calcium/copper deficiency
Omega-3 fatty	25–250 mg	Dyspepsia, diarrhea[b]

[a]Should have mixed bioflavonoids in C:bioflavonoid of 1:1 to 1:2.
[b]Omega-3 fatty acids should be mostly from fish for carnivore supplementation; alpha-lanoline acid from seeds is converted more efficiently to helpful prostaglandins and leukotrienes or eicosanoids in herbivores.

TUI-NA

Our best historic records of the origin of massage as a component of an intact medical system come from China. There, the indigenous manual therapy system Tui-na (literally push-pull) was recorded by the physician Bian Que as being used in 2500 BCE. Regardless of its cultural origin, massage therapy has many proponents and styles.

Known effects of massage therapy include both physiological and psychological changes.[16] Lymphatic drainage and local vascular function are both benefitted by gentle massage and can often be beneficial for reptiles recovering from general anesthesia. Muscle relaxation with attendant reduction in myofascial pain and quicker recovery after exercise are facilitated by massage.

Traumatic fibrosis and sprain or strain injuries respond to deep friction massage techniques and range of motion exercises better than to steroids or surgery. Pain relief is probably the most universally reported effect of massage. Contraindications to massage therapy include avoiding direct massage of cancerous lesions, sites of recent trauma, inflammation, infection, or fracture.

Body work is a superb adjunct to many types of surgery, particularly orthopedic. Physiotherapy technologies in human medicine are advanced compared with veterinary medicine, although a number of universities and referral practices now offer physical therapy and rehabilitation services. For example, after cranial cruciate ligament surgery, the surgical leg should be manipulated daily. In the field of reptile medicine, we may find that soft tissue manipulation techniques can shorten the course of recovery from surgery and trauma.

In some instances, massage may be used instead of surgery. An animal may be a poor surgical candidate, or the owner may not want to pursue surgical options. Massage may contribute to tissue changes that completely relieve the original problem. In an article by Speciale and Fingeroth, the authors conclude, "Persistent use of physical treatment for paralysis that results from conditions affecting the cervical spinal cord may be useful even without concurrent surgical or pharmacologic treatments."[17]

Massage is a valuable addition to acupuncture therapy. Many acupuncture points can be stimulated to good effect with firm finger pressure (acupressure). With proper instruction and the use of selected, gentle techniques, it is possible for clients to extend the effects of acupuncture treatments. Additionally, recalcitrant animals may be treated calmly at home rather than stressfully in the office. Manual therapy courses are available to teach veterinarians Tui-na and massage techniques that they can both apply in their office and show to companion animal caretakers so that the client may treat the animal at home. This empowers and directly includes the caretaker in promoting the healing process for their animal companion. Although unknown, it is likely that such techniques may be of benefit to captive reptiles.

We insert here a word of caution concerning amphibians and all manual therapies. Because of the delicate, sensitive, and highly glandular nature of amphibian skin, all manual therapies must be administered with extreme caution to avoid significant damage and injury to the patient.

Some techniques frequently used with many mammalian species, such as pulling on the tail to relieve pain and stagnation (energy blockage) in the spine, are inappropriate in many lizard species because they may result in inadvertent caudal autotomy.

CHIROPRACTIC

Chiropractic is a separate form of complementary medicine and applies manual spinal manipulation based on the interactions between neurologic mechanisms and the biomechanics of the spine. Treatment is directed at "adjusting" the spine and correcting abnormal positional relationships in the contiguous vertebrae, which, in humans, result in symptoms such as soreness, muscle spasm, tingling, or hard hyperirritable nodular structures called trigger points.[18]

Chiropractic manipulations should only be undertaken by veterinarians with proper training. Great caution must be exercised to avoid further injury when treating small reptiles, where disks are fragile, small, or thin, and when bone integrity is compromised, as with cases of nutritional secondary hyperparathyroidism and osteomyelitis. It is highly questionable whether these techniques are appropriate at all in amphibians because of their delicate and easily damaged skin.

HOMEOPATHY

Homeopathy, a separate discipline from TCVM, is emerging in the field of complementary and integrated veterinary medicine. Homeopathic medicine predates modern medicine by a century or more. Samuel Hahnemann, a German physician, first explored homeopathy in the late 1700s and based his theories and practice on the observation of the body's attempts to heal itself.[19] Homeopathy is said to treat the patient, not the disease, and works on what is called "the law of similars," that is, "like treats like."

Homeopathic practitioners believe that symptoms in humans are an inherent part of the body's defense mechanisms and eliminating them without addressing the source of the problem may suppress the body's ability to heal.[20] In that light, instead of suppressing clinical signs, therapies that augment the body's own defenses may be more appropriate. The homeopathic medicines or remedies used are extremely dilute, so much that there should be no original material left in the solution. Many theories are put forth for the mechanisms of action, including an immunologic basis similar to vaccines. Although research is in its infancy, controlled clinical studies have proven that some homeopathic remedies do work, though mechanisms of action are not yet understood.[19–21]

RESOURCES FOR FURTHER INFORMATION AND STUDY

For those who are interested, the following resources will provide you with opportunities for further education, investigation, and inspiration in applying an integrative approach in your own practices. Organizations and training opportunities in CAVM are listed below.

Academy of Veterinary Homeopathy. James Schacht, DVM, Corresponding Secretary; 6400 E. Independence Boulevard; Charlotte, NC 28212; phone: 704-535-6688.

American Academy of Veterinary Acupuncture. PO Box 419; Hygiene, CO 80433-0419; phone/fax: 303-722-6726; AAVAoffice@aol.com; www.aava.org.

American Holistic Veterinary Medical Association. 2218 Old Enmorton Road; Bel Air, MD 21015; phone: 410-569-0795; fax: 410-569-2346; AHVMA@compuserve.com.

American Veterinarians and Chiropractors Association. 623 Main Street; Hillsdale, IL; 61257; phone: 309-658-2920; fax: 309-658-2622; www.animalchiropractic.org.

Chi Institute. 9791 NW 160th Street; Reddick, FL 32686; phone: 352-591-3165; fax: 352-591-0988; www.chi-institute.com.

International Association for Veterinary Homeopathy. General Secretary: Dr. Andreas Schmidt; Sonnhaldenstr. 18; CH-8370 Sirnach Switzerland; phone: 41 (73) 26 14 24; fax: 41 (73) 26 58 14.

International Veterinary Acupuncture Society. PO Box 271395; Fort Collins, CO 80527; phone: 970-266-0666; fax: 970-266-0777; Ivasoffice@aol.com; www.ivas.org.

REFERENCES

See www.expertconsult.com for a complete list of references.

Differential Diagnoses by Clinical Signs—Snakes

Richard S. Funk and Rodney W. Schnellbacher

The intent of this chapter is to familiarize veterinary clinicians with a brief overview of common clinical signs and differential causes observed in serpents. It is important to be familiar with proper husbandry because many of these clinical signs are related to a poor environment, improper temperature, lack of quarantine, and improper nutrition.

Correct identification of an individual snake is critical to understanding its biology, captive care, and veterinary care. A good reference library therefore is essential. Clients will expect you to be able to identify not only the common pet trade species, but also the snakes native to your area. An individual snake can be identified by photography and the images stored digitally, by making a photocopy of its distinctive pattern or by placing a pit-tag or microchip into the snake.

BEHAVIORAL SIGNS

An increase in activity can be related to a variety of causes, including high environmental temperature, insufficient hiding places, mate-seeking behavior, searching for a nesting site, hunger, thirst, ectoparasites including mites, improper substrate or cage furniture (e.g., no tree branch for an arboreal snake or no burrowing medium for a fossorial snake), odors in the room (e.g., rodents, the family mammalian pets, air fresheners, or incense), or an improper photoperiod (lighting on an irregular cycle or on 24 hours a day).[1] A snake may exhibit defensive behavior if it is a new captive or startled. The authors have observed defensive behavior in an otherwise calm snake in the clinic examination room when a king snake had been the previous patient.

Animals that exhibit signs of lethargy may be ill, gravid, digesting food, being kept too cool, getting ready to shed, or undergoing or preparing for brumation. A snake that is spending increasing amounts of time in its water bowl may be too dry, too warm, nearing ecdysis, have mites, or the water bowl may have been allowed to dry out by the keeper or overturned by the snake.

CARDIOVASCULAR SIGNS

Anemia may originate from blood loss, from neoplasia such as lymphosarcoma, laboratory or clinician error (mishandling or lymph dilution), or possibly hemic parasites, although the latter are generally asymptomatic incidental findings (see Chapter 32). Oral mucus membranes tend to be paler than those of mammals. Oral petechiation is rare but can be associated with stomatitis, septicemia, diffuse intravascular coagulopathy, hyperthermia, intoxication, and only rarely with anemia.

Avascular necrosis of the tail tip has been seen with parasitism, including *Alaria* flukes and microfilariae, or after trauma to the tail. Ischemic tail tip necrosis has been documented in breeding female Burmese pythons *(Python bivittatus)* in association with thromboembolic disease.

Hypovolemic circulatory shock, anemia, or dehydration may cause bradycardia and a weak heartbeat. Snakes that are inactive or at cooler temperatures may naturally have slower heart rates. Infectious diseases have been associated with cardiovascular disease in snakes. Salmonella, Arizona, and *Corynebacterium* sp. have been isolated from a Burmese python with endocarditis.[2] Chlamydiosis also has been associated with myocarditis in snakes.[3] Cardiomegaly has been reported in a variety of captive snakes. Apparent enlargement in the region of the heart (or radiographically the cardiac silhouette) may be caused by cardiomyopathy or pericardial effusion (cardiac tamponade) (Fig. 133.1). Cardiomyopathy has been described in two species of snakes. A mole king snake *(Lampropeltis calligaster rhombomaculata)* presented with lesions characterized by fibroblast proliferation and the replacement of myocardial fibrils with fibrocollagen.[4] A Deckert's rat snake

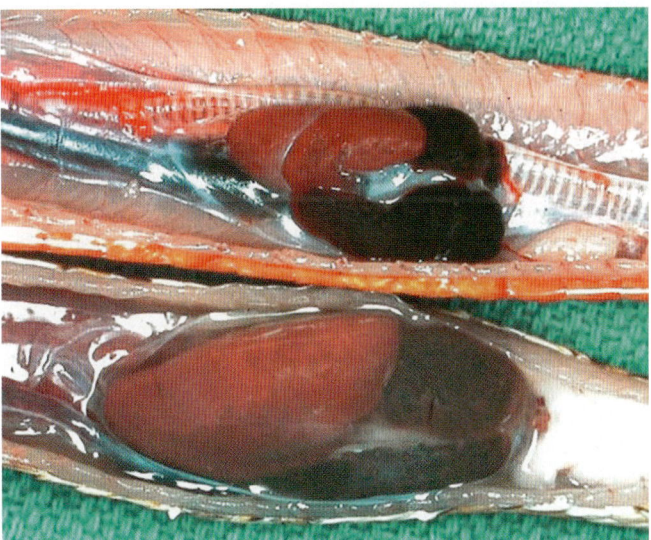

FIG 133.1 Heart comparison of two similar-sized adult corn snakes *(Pantherophis guttatus)*. The heart on the bottom shows significant cardiomegaly from an unidentified cause. (Courtesy of Richard S. Funk.)

(*Elaphe obsoleta deckerti*) presented with necrosis of the myocardial fibers.[5] In both cases, the pathologic changes led to congestive heart failure. Congenital cardiac disease has also been reported (incomplete atrioventricular valve in a neonatal boa constrictor that presented with cardiomegaly).[6] Noncardiac soft tissue mass effects include abscess, granuloma, or tumor.

The presence of mitotic figures in peripheral blood is a normal finding in snakes, although unusually high numbers are suspicious of a disease condition such as lymphosarcoma. Other clinical pathology abnormalities are addressed in the hematology chapter (see Chapter 33).

GASTROINTESTINAL SIGNS

Emesis (Vomiting and Regurgitation)

Emesis is a nonspecific sign and not a discrete disease entity. Vomiting (forceful ejection of the stomach contents) and regurgitation (backflow of undigested food) are difficult to distinguish in reptiles. Snakes possess a poorly developed cardiac sphincter, thus permitting what can appear to be almost effortless regurgitation.[7] Common causes include too large or too many food items, suboptimal temperatures, inappropriate postprandial handling, stress (e.g., no hiding place), or intraspecific interactions. Differential diagnoses must also include gastrointestinal obstruction, functional stasis, gastritis/sepsis (bacterial, fungal, or viral), parasitism (such as *Cryptosporidium*), intramural or extramural masses such as neoplasia, granulomas or abscesses, and exposure to commercial toxins. In a case report of a population of emerald tree boas (*Corallus caninus*), chronic regurgitation was associated with an infection of *Chlamydophila*.[8] Vomitus can be confused with diarrhea when the behavior is not directly observed. Concurrent respiratory disease can be present with any gastrointestinal sign.

Diarrhea

Diarrhea is another nonspecific gastrointestinal sign. First, one must ascertain that the feces is actually abnormal, some species have softer or more liquid stools than others, and in some stools, the quality can vary with prey type. Captive king snakes and rat snakes that are commonly fed rodents may have soft or diarrheic stools after a meal of day-old chicks. The most common causes of diarrhea in captive snakes are inappropriate temperatures (especially too low, inhibiting proper digestion) and gastrointestinal parasites. Foreign bodies, too large a meal, and inappropriate diets (such as dairy products) are also common causes. Bacterial, fungal, or viral intestinal infections can also cause diarrhea (see Chapter 145).

Oral Cavity

A good oral examination should always be performed and may reveal necrotic stomatitis (layterm "mouth rot"), abscessation, foreign objects (e.g., substrate), increased mucus or discharges, respiratory signs, petechiation, tongue abnormalities, icterus, parasites, masses (abscesses, neoplasia), edema, or other problems (see Chapter 167). A mass, broken jaw, or stomatitis can cause a deviation in the opening of the mouth, exposing the gums and leading to an exposure gingivitis.

An inactive tongue can result from a tongue sheath abscess or injury, or rarely the tongue may have been removed by trauma or necrosis. Oral petechiation can be associated with stomatitis, sepsis, hyperthermia, intoxication (as from cedar or organophosphates), or possibly a disseminated intravascular coagulopathy. The oral tissues may also be inflamed from infection, usually bacterial. Edema of the oral membranes has been seen with bacterial cellulitis and uremia secondary to renal failure. Head or intermandibular cellulitis may be bacterial (Fig. 133.2), whereas head edema can result from trauma associated with getting stuck in a hole of a cage or snake bag. Oral discharge or excessive mucus

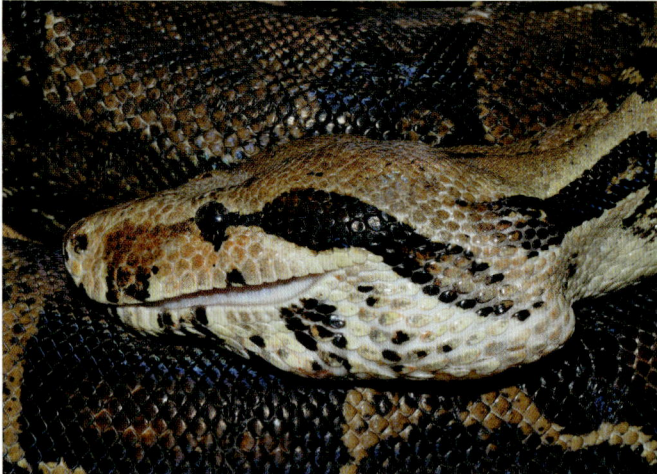

FIG 133.2 Submandibular or pharyngeal edema in a boa constrictor (*Boa constrictor*). (Courtesy of Richard S. Funk.)

may be the result of stomatitis, esophagitis, gastritis, tracheitis, or pneumonia. Dental disease including loose teeth may be seen with stomatitis and osteomyelitis.

Stomatitis (or necrotic stomatitis) is commonly seen in captive snakes and often associated with aerobic and anaerobic bacterial infections. Substandard husbandry and poor hygiene are often predisposing factors. An affected mouth exhibits swelling, exudative material that can be confined to a small area or affect the entire mouth, and increased mucus and may not be able to close properly (Fig. 133.3A and B). Secondary respiratory infection is common due to aspiration of caseous material (see Chapter 167).

Esophagus and Stomach

Emesis or anorexia can occur with stomatitis, which can extend posteriorly down into the esophagus and the stomach. This may not be obvious without endoscopy or being identified at necropsy. Esophageal tonsils may enlarge in boas and pythons with inclusion body (arenavirus) disease. A mass in the precardiac region of the snake could be within the esophagus but might otherwise involve the respiratory system or the rib cage. Cryptosporidiosis can cause marked gastric hypertrophy and is often characterized by a midbody swelling.

Intestines

A mass in the coelomic cavity could be an intestinal granuloma, abscess, neoplasm, foreign body, meal, or cryptosporidiosis, or may be extraintestinal. The snake could be a reproductively active female with enlarged ovaries, retained fetus(es), or eggs that could be mistaken for an intestinal issue. Constipation can be caused by meals that are too large, too frequent, or too heavily furred, or in addition, low environmental temperatures or extraintestinal mass effects (e.g., retained reproductive products, neoplasia, abscess, or granuloma) (see Chapter 145). Such a mass is often palpable but not identifiable as intramural or extramural without contrast radiography or ultrasonography. Advanced imaging, endoscopy, or an exploratory celiotomy may be required for definitive diagnosis. In neonate snakes, a firm midbody intracoelomic mass at the umbilicus may represent a poorly absorbed or infected fetal yolk mass. A prolapse that protrudes from the cloaca may be cloacal, oviductal, hemipenial, or colonic (see Chapter 75).

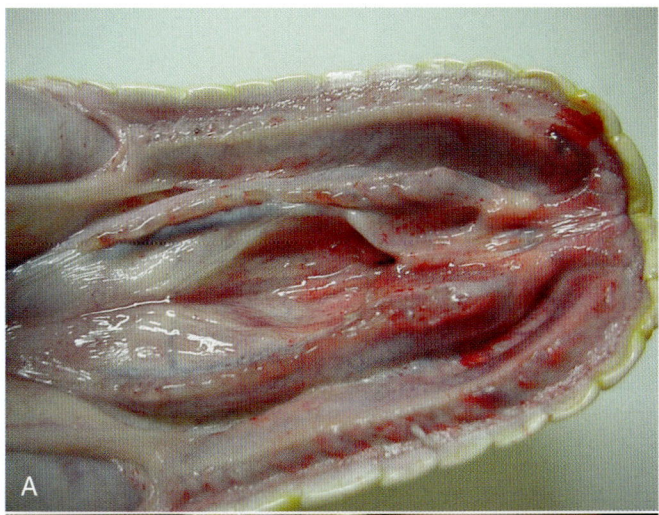

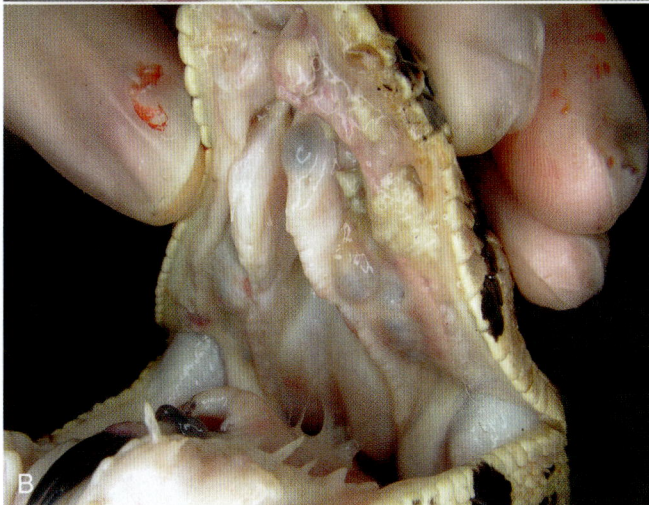

FIG 133.3 Infectious stomatitis, is a common cause of anorexia. Patients that exhibit signs need a thorough physical evaluation, including a discussion of husbandry and management. (A) An acute case of stomatitis with areas of oral petechiation, erythema, and inflammation in a ball python (*Python regius*). (B) A chronic case of stomatitis in common boa constrictor (*Boa constrictor*) with severe inflammation, abscessation, and mucopurulent discharge. (A, Courtesy of Stephen J. Divers; B, courtesy of Scott J. Stahl, Stahl Exotic Animal Veterinary Services.)

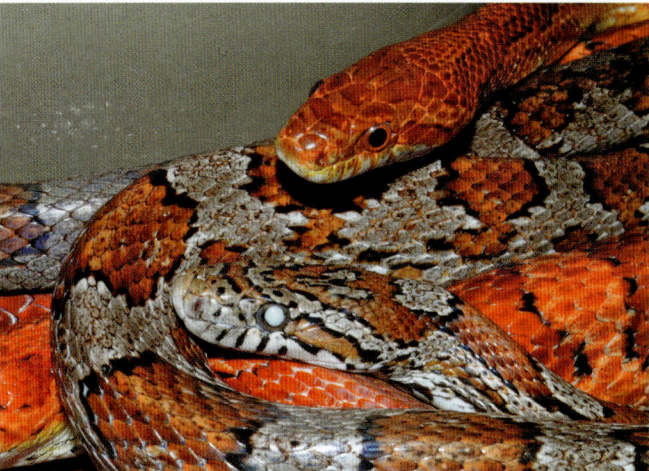

FIG 133.4 Comparison of two similar-sized adult corn snakes (*Pantherophis guttatus*). A mature cataract can be observed in the lower snake. (Courtesy of Richard S. Funk.)

An association with stomatitis and/or respiratory infection must be considered (see Chapter 71).

Microphthalmia may be the result of an infected eye that is becoming phthisical, congenital aplasia, or reduced palpebral fissure partially covering a normal-sized globe. Anophthalmia may occur as a congenital abnormality either unilaterally or bilaterally. Scolecophidians, blind or thread snakes, normally have reduced eyes covered by a head scale.

Cloudy eyes may be normal and indicative of impending ecdysis or associated with a retained/missing spectacle, subspectacular abscess, inflammation of the subspectacular space or cornea, panophthalmitis, or a penetrating wound from a bite or foreign object. The presence of a subspectacular abscess makes examination of the globe very difficult. Occasionally a postbrumation vitreal haziness may develop, which is usually temporary.

Cataracts are occasionally seen in geriatric snakes and as a rare sequela to excessively low brumation temperatures (Fig. 133.4). Any association of cataracts with hyperglycemia, renal disease, hypertension, or increased intraocular pressure as seen in mammals is currently unknown. Blindness can develop with age and cataract formation. Uveitis and hyphemia may also cause a temporary blindness, as can retained spectacles, particularly if more than one is present.

DERMATOLOGICAL SIGNS

Masses and swellings are often abscesses, which are usually bacterial infections and can be fungal or mixed, but granulomas and neoplasms also occur. Myiasis is rare but acariasis is common. Sparganosis may appear as subcutaneous masses, particularly in tropical snakes. A generalized cellulitis may accompany dermatitis or septicemia.

Snout-rubbing abrasions may occur in snakes that need a more secure hiding refuge; are hormonal, especially males trying to escape to breed females; or those kept in cages with a rough edge, or screened top, or that rub and push against a weak or loose area of a cage. Abrasions can become infected, leading to abscessation and or stomatitis. If the inciting cause is eliminated, and the abscess and wounds are properly treated, lesions can heal well after several sheds, although a permanent scar can remain (Fig. 133.5A and B).

Acanthocephalans may also exit the skin and leave small ulcerated wounds.

OCULAR SIGNS

Retention of spectacles may be caused by dysecdysis (often associated with improper humidity), mites in the periorbital space, trauma to the spectacle (and perhaps to the eye as well), ocular abscessation, and husbandry issues including lack of cage furniture to facilitate shedding. Occasionally a normal spectacle may be misidentified as retained, and attempted removal may lead to exposure keratitis of the cornea and often ocular infection (see Chapter 71).

Eyes and periorbital areas may also be infected with the fungus *Ophidiomyces ophiodiicola*, which may cause swelling, cloudiness, and dermatitis. This has been found in wild and captive snakes (see Chapter 31).

Exophthalmia may be the result of an intraocular mass, such as an abscess or granuloma, a retrobulbar mass, subspectacular abscessation, or increased subspectacular fluid due to a blockage of the lacrimal duct.

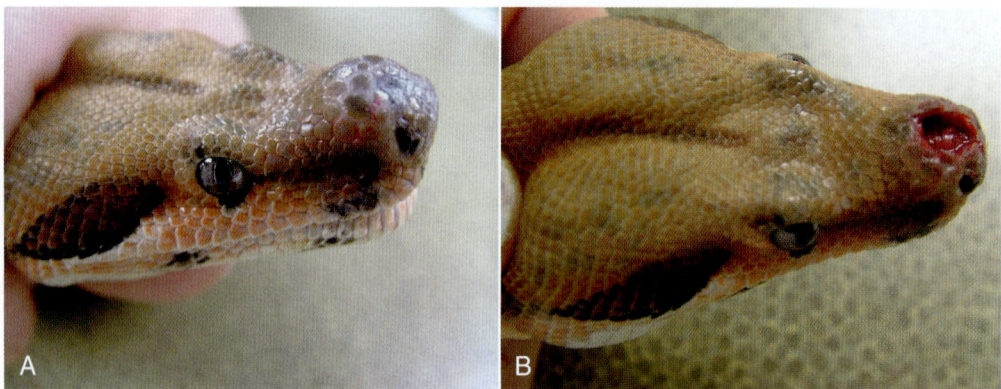

FIG 133.5 (A) This male boa constrictor (*Boa constrictor*) presented with obvious swelling and secondary trauma to the rostrum from attempts to "push out" of its enclosure, as a mature female boa was housed nearby. (B) The same snake after debridement surgery was performed. Note the extent of the abscess and need for aggressive removal of all infected material. In these cases, resolving the underlying condition causing this behavior, such as proximity of female snakes to mature males or the style and type of caging, is critical for success. (Courtesy of Scott J. Stahl, Stahl Exotic Animal Veterinary Services.)

Chemical and thermal burns may result in skin lesions of varying severity, often with fluid-filled vesicles ("blister disease") that may become infected. Poor cage hygiene is a predisposing factor for the development of skin lesions and dermatitis.

Petechiation in the skin may be associated with thermal burns or septicemia. Wrinkling of the skin can be seen with inanition, dehydration, acariasis, dysecdysis, or in postpartum females. Skin damage and bruising can occur secondary to trauma (e.g., tape removal, stuck under a door). A syndrome of skin rupture with separation of the epidermal-dermal layers has been attributed to cachexia and hypovitaminosis C; affected snakes have reduced collagen, but the exact etiology remains obscure. A fungal disease syndrome of the skin of snakes caused by *Ophidiomyces ophiodiicola* has been documented in wild and captive snakes in North America, Europe, and Australia. It can appear as dermal granulomas and crusting dermatitis and can be disfiguring and even fatal (see Chapter 31).

Ectoparasites may be found and are usually *Ophionyssus* mites but occasionally also ticks. Manual removal of ticks is usually possible, but treatments for both, including the use of ivermectin, permethrin, and various acaricides, are discussed in Chapter 32.[9] With mites, the cage and room environments must also be treated. The presence of mites may be suspected if there is dyecdysis, a fine whitish powder on the snake's skin, or if the snake is soaking excessively in its water bowl.

Rodent bite trauma may occur when a snake is offered a live rodent and does not feed immediately, leaving the rodent alive in the snake's vivarium. In addition to any legal and welfare issues, the rodent may cause minor bites to serious wounds that need major surgical repair or even euthanasia (see Chapter 142).

Dysecdysis may occur for numerous reasons, including ectoparasites, malnutrition, dehydration, improper humidity, improper substrate or cage furniture, systemic disease, debilitation, or rough handling during the immediate preshedding phase (Fig. 133.6). The spectacles should normally be shed with the skin as a single piece, but if not, check for mites or husbandry-related problems (see Chapter 149). Snakes with skin wounds, including surgical incisions, may increase their shedding frequency to facilitate healing. Juveniles shed more frequently than adults. A reduction in shedding frequency may accompany reduced feeding and growth.

When wounds heal by second or third intention, scars form and may be depigmented or hyperpigmented, or the scales may be malformed. Pigment-forming neoplasms of the skin, chromatophoromas, appear to be more common in diurnal species.

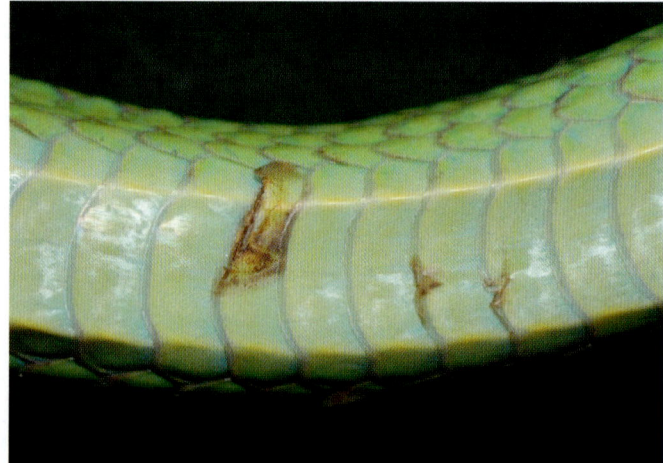

FIG 133.6 Scale dermatitis and necrosis of a rhinoceros rat snake (*Rhynchophis boulengeri*). Cytology and biopsy of scales revealed that dermatitis was caused by a fungal agent. (Courtesy of Rodney W. Schnellbacher.)

A wide variety of captive-bred "morphs" or phenotypes (cultivars) are now available in the commercial pet trade for a growing number of snake species. These include many with patterns and colorations that may differ widely from the wild phenotypes, for example, lacking melanocytes (amelanistic partial albinos), lacking reds and yellows (anerythristic partial albinos), homozygous recessive for both alleles ("snows" and "blizzards"), leucistics (white with blue eyes), piebalds, etc. Occasionally scaleless snakes are seen where the epidermis is keratinized, but scales may be limited to the head and ventrum and/or where mutant scales are rotated.

Subcutaneous and Cutaneous Masses

Masses are usually abscesses until proven otherwise, but granulomas, including those of bacterial or fungal etiology, and tumors may occur. Blisters or vesicles on the skin form from integumentary infections and may (or may not) progress to small abscesses; causes include unsuitably high humidity, excessive moisture, poor hygiene, prey bites, parasitism, and thermal burns. Rib fractures can present as small lumps, as can rib or spinal osteomyelitis and rarely congenital skeletal deformities. Internal

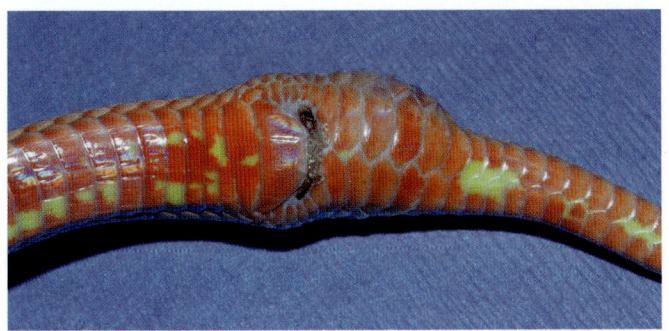

FIG 133.7 Impacted and abscessed scent gland of a king snake *Lampropeltis mexicana leonis*. Abscess was cultured and flushed with saline, and appropriate topical antibiotics were used. (Courtesy of Richard S. Funk.)

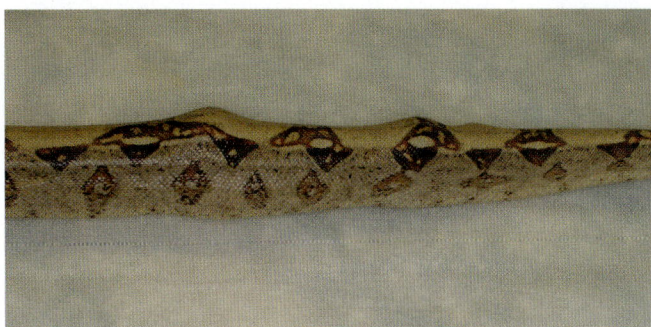

FIG 133.8 A boa constrictor (*Boa constrictor* spp.) presented with an abnormal conformation and limited regional mobility. Radiographs confirmed ossifying spondylosis and areas of scoliosis. (Courtesy of Stephen J. Divers.)

abscesses or granulomas, neoplasia, and organomegaly can cause the appearance of an internal mass. Unabsorbed fetal yolk at the umbilicus may also appear as midbody swelling in neonates. Fecal impactions, fecoliths, and uroliths can appear as caudal coelomic masses. Some snakes nearing shedding may hold feces and urates until ecdysis has been completed. Multiple intracoelomic masses, either visible or palpable, may be present in a reproductively active, gravid, or dystocic female. Unilateral or bilateral impacted or abscessed anal glands or hemipenes in the base of the tail may cause a mass effect (Fig. 133.7) (see Chapter 144). Some, primarily older female snakes, especially corn snakes (*Pantherophis guttatus*), may also develop lipomas on the dorsolateral posterior body.

MUSCULOSKELETAL SIGNS

Musculoskeletal deformities in snakes fed whole prey are rare. Exceptions may be found among snakes that are fed nonsupplemented invertebrates.

Fractures are frequently caused by bites, cage door or lid closures, falling from a perch or branch, unstable cage furniture, and rough handling. Osteomyelitis can weaken a boney area and contribute to a fracture. Rib fractures are common incidental findings on radiographs and, unless they are protruding or penetrating another organ, require no action. One should palpate and look for asymmetry, swelling, and evidence of pain and carefully evaluate skull radiographs or CT scans. Overzealous head-pinning of snakes with snake hooks or tongs may cause iatrogenic head or rib fractures.

Spondylosis, kyphosis, and lordosis, as well as swellings, may be the result of musculoskeletal problems such as abscessation, ossifying spondylosis, osteomyelitis, trauma, fractures, congenital defects, or neurologic disorders (Fig. 133.8).

Many deformities are seen in captive-bred snakes, including shortened jaws or snouts, restricted orbits, domed skulls, arched necks or spines, as well as spondylosis, kyphosis, and lordosis, with some of these conditions attributable to improper incubation or gestation temperatures. A possible role of inbreeding is often invoked but rarely proven. One category of congenital defect that elicits interest from private collectors, including high prices, is two-headed snakes (axial bifurcation).[10]

Tail tips may be damaged by parasites (such as flukes or ticks), prey (e.g., rodent bites) or predators, or accidental trauma (e.g., tail shut or caught in the cage lid or door, or mistakenly tied in the knot of the collecting or transport bag). Thromboembolic disease in Burmese pythons has been shown to cause avascular necrosis of the tail tip.

Paresis and paralysis can occur from musculoskeletal or neurologic abnormalities (see Chapter 77). Spinal lesions are the likely cause of paralysis or paresis in a snake, especially from trauma to the vertebral column but also from spinal infection and abscessation, ossifying spondylosis, or even spinal neoplasia. Affected areas of spine become rigid, and affected snakes have difficulty with locomotion, coiling, and constricting prey. Neurologically related postural abnormalities may be mistaken for musculoskeletal signs.

NEUROLOGICAL SIGNS

Lethargy and depression can be difficult to appreciate and evaluate in snakes. A client may state that a snake is lethargic, and this may not be obvious in the examination room. One should attempt to exclude nonneural causes such as gravidity, ecdysis, low environmental temperature, postprandial behavior, malnutrition, dehydration, or illness (e.g., respiratory or gastrointestinal disease, renal disease, sepsis). In fact, a wide variety of illnesses can cause a snake to be lethargic.

Depression can be the result of head trauma, inappropriately low environmental temperatures, drug reaction, systemic illness, or intoxication (e.g., organophosphates). Some boas and pythons appear to recognize their individual owners and may appear less inactive while their owners are away, only to resume normal activity upon their return.

Paresis and paralysis must be differentiated from musculoskeletal system problems (see Chapter 77). Ataxia may occur from exposure to toxins such as cedar shavings or phenolic cleansers, acaricides and insecticides, over-the-counter medications with questionable ingredients, head or body trauma, hypothermia, spinal osteomyelitis, boid inclusion body disease (arenavirus), meningitis, encephalitis, and thiamine deficiency due to certain fish diets. Ataxia and incoordination may be attributed to hypoglycemia, starvation, general debilitation, hepatic encephalopathy, renal disease, trauma, meningitis, neoplasia, drug intoxication (such as ivermectin), paramyxoviral infection, or boid inclusion body disease (arenavirus).

Inclusion body disease (arenavirus), mostly known to occur in boas and pythons, has now been confirmed in a few colubrid snakes (including *Lampropeltis*), can cause a head tilt, opisthotonos, flaccid paralysis, disorientation, loss of the righting reflex, an inability to prehense or ingest food, and death (Fig. 133.9) (see Chapter 30).

Nutritional deficiencies rarely contribute to neurologic problems in snakes, because most are fed rodents or other whole prey vertebrates. Snakes that are fed invertebrates might be more susceptible to hypocalcemia if the prey are not properly enriched or supplemented. Thiamine and biotin deficiencies have been linked to tremors and convulsions.

Dehydration or aminoglycoside administration can lead to renal disease and gout, which can cause lethargy, incoordination, and death.

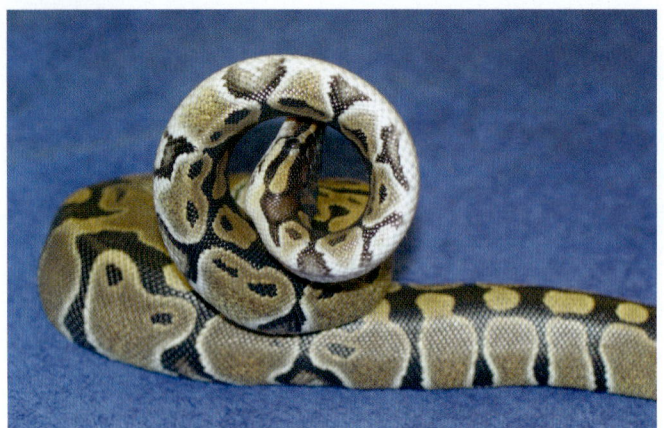

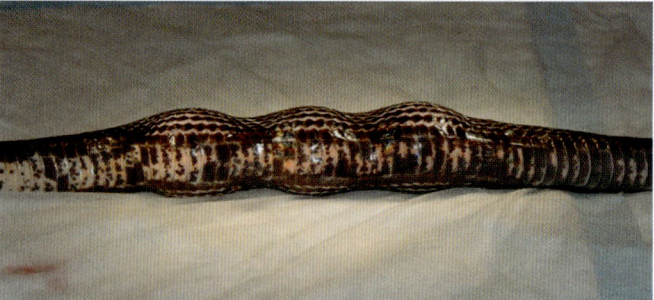

FIG 133.10 Western rat snake (*Pantherophis obsoletus*) with coelomic distension due to egg retention and dystocia. (Courtesy of Stephen J. Divers.)

FIG 133.9 An adult long-term captive ball python (*Python regius*) showing bizarre neurologic behavior. The snake crawled normally, then when stimulated, coiled into a loop. (Courtesy of Stephen J. Divers.)

Hyperactivity may be the result of insecurity (inadequate hiding places), inappropriately high environmental temperature, thirst or hunger, crowding, or mate-seeking behavior, or it may be a naturally active species. None of these are true neurologic disorders.

Central nervous system tumors are quite rare but can cause reduced activity, incoordination, ataxia, convulsions, anorexia, and death. Hepatic encephalopathy, although rarely documented, can be associated with lethargy, inappetence, ataxia, and weakness, and more rarely with opisthotonos. Head tilts are uncommonly seen in snakes but can be the result of head trauma, metabolic disease, unilateral ocular disease, and even sepsis. Central etiologies include encephalitis (due to a variety of infectious agents), abscess, granuloma, or neoplasia. Head trauma can occur from accidents involving cage doors, automobiles, falls, loose cage furniture, or other blunt objects.

Seizures and convulsions can occur from such varied causes as septicemia, including central nervous system abscessation, bacterial encephalitis, viral encephalitis (including paramyxovirus and inclusion body disease), protozoal encephalitis and helminth migration, head trauma, intoxication (including cedar, organophosphates [dichlorvos strips], insecticides, ivermectin over dosage, and paint solvents), heat stroke, metabolic disturbances (e.g., hepatic encephalopathy, uremia), neoplasia, and nutritional deficiencies (e.g., thiamine deficiency).

Unfortunately, many neurologic cases remain undiagnosed following a gross necropsy, and therefore, in addition to submitting tissues in formalin for histopathology, a second set of tissues should be kept frozen for potential toxicology or viral investigations.

REPRODUCTIVE SIGNS

True infertility is difficult to confirm. The failure of a snake to breed necessitates a physical examination to ascertain that the snake's sex has been accurately determined. If the snake was inadequately nourished or improperly cycled, it may not breed. Even if the keeper places the snakes together if not observing them continuously, it can be difficult to know whether courtship and mating has occurred. Infertile eggs may indicate a failure of copulation or sperm transportation, whereas an infection or blockage of the female reproductive tract could lead to failure to produce eggs or offspring.

Snake dystocia occurs when a gravid female does not deliver her brood or clutch or retains a portion of it (Fig. 133.10). This can result from many factors, including obesity, nutrition, dehydration, primipara, "power-feeding" for fast growth but marginal size to carry and deliver a

normal clutch, large or abnormal eggs, improper gestation temperatures, inactivity (restricted cage size), lack of security, lack of a suitable laying or birthing site, oviductal infection or death of a fetus, mass impinging on the oviduct blocking egg/fetus transport, an oviductal torsion or constriction, ectopic egg or fetus, or prolapse of the oviduct. Some snakes will lay their clutch of eggs even without a suitable laying box or substrate, but others will not (for example, female smooth green snakes will die egg bound if no moist site is available for oviposition). Dystocia should always be suspected if a gravid female suddenly becomes anorectic and lethargic, or if there is evidence that the clutch has been retained. Radiography, ultrasonography, and advance imaging may be useful diagnostic tools in assessing reproductive tract, cloaca, and egg and follicle architecture. Medical and surgical treatments for dystocia are addressed in Chapters 80 and 105.

Stillbirth may result from early fetal death or almost any of the factors that contribute to dystocia. Large viviparous snakes that are kept confined to relatively small cages may have a normal delivery but accidentally crush or suffocate neonates because of a lack of floor space.

Cycling female snakes will occasionally produce vitellogenic follicles, then eventually resorb the follicles if are they not ovulated. Follicular stasis or preovulatory stasis is a condition in which follicles neither ovulate nor regress over time and is associated with clinical signs (e.g., lethargy and/or anorexia). Depending on snake size and species, the follicles may be evident as a swelling of the middle to caudal third of the snake. This condition is difficult to diagnose with certainty, mainly because of the interspecific differences in follicular size and development time (see Chapter 80).

Failure of eggs to hatch can be caused by inappropriate incubation temperatures, excessive temperature variation, inappropriate incubation humidity, fetal death, genetic or congenital abnormalities, egg infections, or because of egg infertility. Some neonates will slit the egg and yet fail to emerge and die within the egg when physically they appear normal upon postmortem examination.

A prolapse through the cloacal opening must be carefully evaluated to ascertain whether it is the cloaca, oviduct (in a female), or hemipenis (of a male). The oviduct can prolapse with a retained egg within it. Surgical treatments for prolapses are covered in Chapters 105 and 106).

RESPIRATORY SIGNS

Respiratory signs may include nasal discharge, oral often frothy discharge, dyspnea and open-mouth breathing, abnormal posture (including holding the head and neck elevated), sneezing, wheezes, stridor, and stentor (Fig. 133.11A–C). Respiratory sounds are considered increased

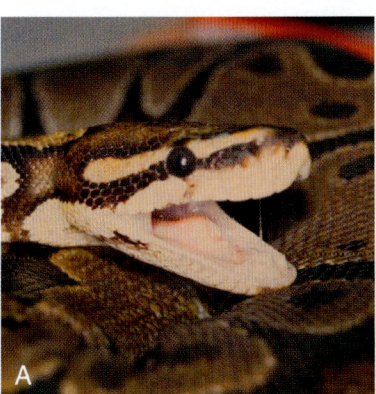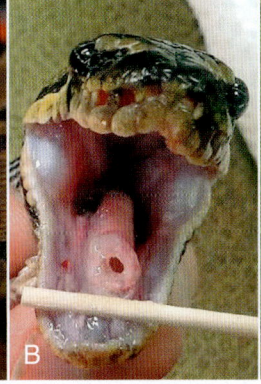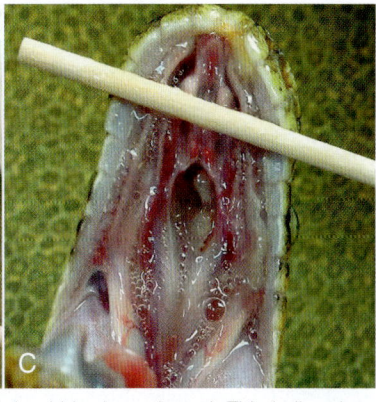

FIG 133.11 (A) Open-mouth breathing is abnormal in snakes and should be investigated. This ball python (*Python regius*) had severe pneumonia, diagnosed via tracheal wash and cytology. (B and C) A ball python on oral examination exhibiting increased fluid in the glottis and oral cavity, and mucopurulent material is present within the choana. Because the glottis resides within the choana with the mouth closed, and increased fluid and material are noted in the glottis with the mouth open, this mucopurulent material is likely coming from the lower respiratory tract. (A, Courtesy of Stephen J Divers; B and C, courtesy of Anibal Armendaris, Stahl Exotic Animal Veterinary Services.)

if audible in the relaxed snake. Abnormal gurgling or wheezing on inspiration, and especially on expiration, should alert the clinician to examine a snake's respiratory system. Some snakes may appear to increase their (normal) respiratory sounds when they become alert. Some snakes may also produce slightly increased breathing sounds when nearing shedding, because the skin lining the external nares thickens in preparation for ecdysis and can narrow the airways. These sounds must be evaluated in comparison with the normal sounds for each particular species, because defensive hissing may be confused with a respiratory problem. For example, *Pituophis* spp. have a cartilaginous structure at the epiglottis that allows the snake to make a loud hissing noise that is normal behavior for these species. Many snakes with respiratory disease are anorectic and lethargic, and sometimes owners may be unaware of the respiratory component to a snake's illness.

Oral and nasal discharges need to be carefully evaluated to ascertain that their origin is from the respiratory system, because gastroenteritis and stomatitis can present with similar discharges. Stomatitis often occurs concurrently with a respiratory infection. Pulmonary neoplasms are rare. Bacterial, mycotic, viral, or parasitic pneumonia may present with dyspnea or with oral or nasal discharges.[11] Snakes lack a diaphragm and have difficulty expelling excessive pulmonary and tracheal mucus. Aspiration pneumonia can also develop following regurgitation, vomiting, or assist-feeding a liquid food.

Dyspnea in snakes can be caused by occluded nostrils, caseous debris or foreign material within the choana, a tongue sheath abscess, an intraoral mass (abscess, granulomas, or neoplasm), a tracheal granuloma or chondroma, hyperthermia, exposure to airborne toxins or irritants (e.g., smoke, incense, or excessive ammonia within the cage), increase in tracheal or pulmonary mucus, or near-drowning events. Any of these conditions can present as open-mouth breathing, either constant or intermittent.

Anatomic snout disfigurements from abscesses, granulomas, cellulitis, or scars may also influence breathing patterns. Epistaxis is rare in snakes but can occur with skull, oral, or body trauma.

Snakes with respiratory disease will commonly inflate their throat region during respiration. Respiratory sounds of snakes can be audible. Abnormal gurgling or wheezing on inspiration, and especially on expiration, should alert the clinician to examine a snake's respiratory

system. Concurrent respiratory disease can be present with severe gastrointestinal enlargement because of lung compression.

Physical examination, collection of hematologic and plasma biochemical parameters, diagnostic samples such as tracheal washes for cytology and culture, imaging modalities, and endoscopic evaluation are essential for respiratory disease diagnosis.[12]

SYSTEMIC SIGNS

Asthenia

Weakness is a nonspecific sign of disease. Disease entities that can be associated with weakness include hypothermia, malnutrition, cachexia, metabolic disease, electrolyte or acid-base abnormalities, anemia, cardiovascular disease, respiratory disease, gastrointestinal disease, dystocia, neuromuscular disease, spinal cord disease, neoplasia, or inflammatory processes including bacterial, fungal, or viral infections. Drug overdoses or intoxications can also be associated with weakness. Pain, including postoperative discomfort, can also manifest as weakness.

Weight Change and Body Condition

It is important to differentiate weight loss and gain from decreases and increases in body condition scores to identify underlying etiologies. Weight gain and obesity are commonly associated with excessive feeding and inadequate activity or exercise (rarely seen in wild snakes). Developing snakes will gain weight as well as length as they grow. Gravid females, constipation, or other causes of coelomic distension commonly can lead to weight gain.

Weight loss has many causes, including underfeeding, malnutrition, increased metabolic rate with inappropriately high environmental temperatures, failure to feed (anorexia) due to any variety of husbandry issues or diseases, maladaptation to captivity, parasites, a postpartum female, cardiac disease, chronic inflammation or infection, dehydration with resultant renal disease, neoplasia, starvation, protein losing nephropathy or hepatopathy, or cancer cachexia.

Coelomic Distension

Coelomic distention can be caused by numerous causes, such as gastrointestinal (GI) disease, organomegaly, neoplasia, and reproductive issues. Knowledge of snake anatomy and topography are important to help rule out specific diseases.

In the gastrointestinal system, coelomic distension can be the result of parasitism, including cryptosporidiosis, a blockage such as a foreign body or fecal impaction, a tumor or granuloma or abscess within the GI tract, intestinal with gas distension, gastrointestinal stasis and putrefaction of ingesta (a result of suboptimal temperatures where digestion cannot proceed effectively), or a normal meal. A fecal impaction or even retained feces yet to be voided may also appear as distension. Retention of large solid uroliths may enlarge the posterior coelom, often with palpable fluid around and anterior to these stones.

Non-GI signs that can cause coelomic distension include extramural organomegaly, such as kidney, liver, or heart. An abscess, granuloma, or neoplasm outside of the GI tract may also cause an abdominal enlargement. General obesity can also cause an enlarged coelom, usually in the posterior coelom because fat bodies are concentrated there.

An owner may not be aware that a snake is gravid, and so developing or retained ova or fetuses may also cause coelomic distension (Fig. 133.10). Reproductive-related distension occurs in the 60% to 70% region of the body from snout-to-vent length in cycling females and is correlated with folliculogenesis and ovulation.

Coelomic transudates (ascites) or exudates (coelomitis) can distend a large portion of a snake's body, and, similar to mammals, this may be attributed to hypoproteinemia, abnormal hepatic function, renal disease, cardiac disease, septicemia, or even neoplasia.[13] Diagnostic tests such as radiographs, gastrointestinal contrast radiographs, ultrasound, and advanced imaging may be useful in diagnosing the cause of coelomic distention.

Anorexia

Anorexia is a nonspecific sign that can be related to husbandry, biology, or disease, or a combination. Husbandry-related issues are very common and include inappropriate temperatures, an improper substrate (e.g., fossorial snake with no appropriate substrate), improper humidity, and excessive or inappropriate handling. A stressed snake with no or too few hiding places or one offered food at the wrong time of day may not feed. Anorexia may be the result of unsuitable caging, for example, in a poor location (high traffic, noisy, domestic pet presence) or inappropriate size.

Almost any disease condition can potentially cause anorexia, including gastrointestinal parasites (nematodes, coccidia including *Cryptosporidium serpentis*, cestodes, amoebas, and flagellated protozoans) and gastroenteritis from bacterial, fungal, or viral infections.[14] Snakes with renal disease or gout commonly stop feeding. Gastrointestinal foreign bodies, constipation, and impactions can lead to anorexia. Oral problems causing anorexia include stomatitis, respiratory disease, occluded nares, bedding trapped in the oral cavity, damage or a bite from a prey item, or a jaw fracture. If the tongue is damaged, missing, or has an abscess within the tongue sheath, the snake may be anorexic. Trauma to the head, oral cavity, or other areas on a snake's body may cause anorexia.

Other causes could be related to improper food items. If the snake has been misidentified, the owner may not be offering it suitable prey,

for example, offering rodents to an insectivorous species such as a smooth green snake (*Opheodrys vernalis*). Freshly imported or newly captured snakes may take a while to acclimate to captivity before feeding. Some may refuse white laboratory mice and feed better on wild-caught native rodents or gray-brown-black domestic rodents. Failure of wild-caught snakes to adjust to captivity is called maladaptation syndrome. Even a newly acquired captive-bred snake may be temporarily anorexic as it adjusts to a new environment. A snake may not eat if the wrong food is offered or if the food is offered incorrectly, for example, on the ground for an arboreal snake or during the day for a nocturnal snake. Juvenile snakes of species with ontogenetic dietary shifts may be problem feeders during the transition, such as from ectothermic to endothermic prey.

Temperate zone snakes may enter a fall anorexia in preparation for brumation, and some new hatchlings that refuse food may feed after a short brumation period. Snakes nearing shedding will typically not feed until after ecdysis.

Reproductive conditions may be associated with anorexia. During the active breeding season, some snakes, especially males, will not feed until the breeding season has ended. Inexperienced owners may not appreciate when a female snake is gravid, and many females will go off feed until after parturition or oviposition.

Acute Mortalities

Often if the snake has been ill and is being treated, the cause may be already known. However, sometimes the owner is convinced it was a "sudden death" scenario without premonitory signs. A good history and full necropsy may be necessary to determine the cause of death or identify factors that could have led to its death. Frequently the death was from a more chronic condition and not sudden.

Husbandry issues can lead to a snake's death, including burns, overheating such as improper use or malfunction of heating devices, drowning, chronic dehydration, chronic malnutrition, trauma from the cage or caging accessories, and trauma from another family pet. Certain medication overdoses could lead to death, for example, gentamicin or environmental insecticides (e.g., dichlorvos strips). Severe parasitism or septicemia can lead to death. Viral infections including paramyxovirus and inclusion body (arenavirus) disease of boas and pythons may also lead to death. Aneurysms have been described in snakes; an aortic aneurysm has been reported in a Burmese python after constricting its meal.[15] Brumation can also be stressful in some snakes and unmask a subclinical condition. Many keepers and owners report an occasional death during brumation or shortly after emergence.

Be careful to correctly diagnose a snake as dead by checking clinical signs, including complete immobility, lack of respirations, absent response to tactile or pain stimuli, and lack of a detectable heartbeat. A snake can be clinically dead and maintain a heartbeat for several hours under some conditions. Use caution when handling deceased venomous snakes because accidental envenomation is possible.

REFERENCES

See www.expertconsult.com for a complete list of references.

134

Differential Diagnoses by Clinical Signs—Lizards

Stephen Barten and Shane Simpson

MUSCULOSKELETAL SIGNS

Lameness and Skeletal and Spinal Abnormalities

Metabolic bone diseases (MBDs), of various origins, are the most common causes of lameness, skeletal, and spinal abnormalities in lizards. MBDs can manifest as fibrous osteodystrophy, osteomalacia, osteoporosis, osteopetrosis, pathologic fractures, and more (see Chapter 158). Swollen or misshapen mandibles, limbs, or vertebral column are common, and lesions may be symmetrical or asymmetrical (Fig. 134.1). Other causes of lameness include fractures or soft tissue injuries from trauma, such as bites from cage mates, neoplasia, cellulitis, abscesses, and osteomyelitis. Joint abnormalities may result in lameness. The affected joints often are swollen and have a limited range of motion. Joint problems may be caused by septic arthritis or degenerative joint disease related to trauma or aging. Articular gout, periarticular gout, and pseudogout have been reported in several lizard species.[1,2] True gout consists of uric acid deposits in the joints. Pseudogout is caused by the accumulation of any crystal other than sodium urate (see Chapters 149 and 161).

Ossifying spondylosis related to age, osteomyelitis, or metabolic abnormalities can cause a lizard's spine and tail to be stiff and unyielding, resulting in an altered gait.

Hypertrophic osteopathy with profound periosteal proliferation of the long bones related to the presence of coelomic space-occupying masses has been reported in the green iguana (*Iguana iguana*).[3]

Tail

Most iguanid lizards as well as many skinks, geckos, and anguid lizards, undergo tail autotomy as a defensive strategy to avoid predation. Each caudal vertebra has a cartilaginous fracture plane through the vertebral body and neural arch. Fracture planes are absent in the cranial part of the tail to protect the hemipenes and fat deposits. In iguanas, the fracture planes are replaced by bone as the lizards grow, so the tail breaks off less easily in adults. The lost tail is regenerated with a cartilaginous rod for support and is covered with smaller, darker scales in an irregular pattern compared with the original tail. One exception is the crested gecko (*Correlophus ciliatus*), which undergoes tail autotomy but does not regenerate the tail once it is lost. Tail autotomy generally does not occur in agamid lizards, monitors, or true chameleons, and these species do not regenerate tails that are lost from trauma or amputation.[4]

Avascular necrosis of the tail is relatively common in green iguanas and central or inland bearded dragons (*Pogona vitticeps*) though is occasionally seen in other species. The distal tail becomes hard, dry, stiff, and discolored. A zone of devitalized tissue characterized by swelling, erythema, and occasional serous discharge often exists between necrotic and healthy tissue at the onset of the problem. Possible etiologies include trauma, hematogenous-borne infection, osteomyelitis of the caudal vertebrae, and iatrogenic damage secondary to blood collection or catheter placement.

Swelling of the ventral tail base, adjacent and caudal to the cloacal opening, in male lizards usually involves the hemipenes. Some male lizards such as green iguanas and various species of chameleons undergo dramatic enlargement of the hemipenes with sexual maturity. Naive keepers occasionally present young adult male lizards to have these normal but newly enlarged hemipenes evaluated. Other species such as blue-tongue lizards (*Tiliqua* spp.) can develop hemipenal sac abscessation (Fig. 134.2). Swelling of the ventral tail base is also caused by

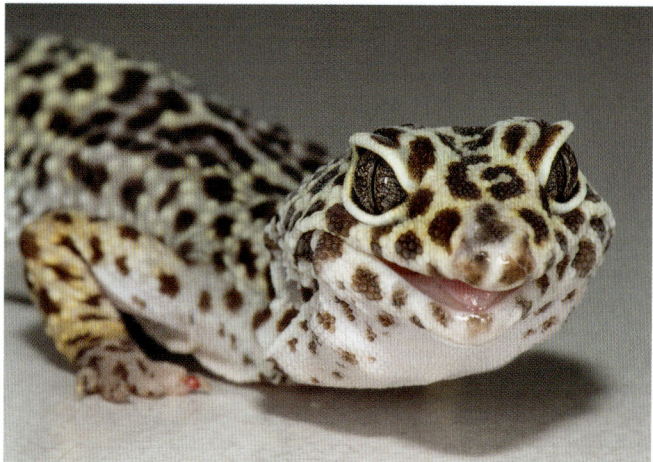

FIG 134.1 Nutritional secondary hyperparathyroidism is the most common of the metabolic bone diseases seen in lizards. Affected animals can present with severe skeletal deformities, such as mandibular deformities as seen in this leopard gecko (*Eublepharis macularius*). (Courtesy of Stephen Barten.)

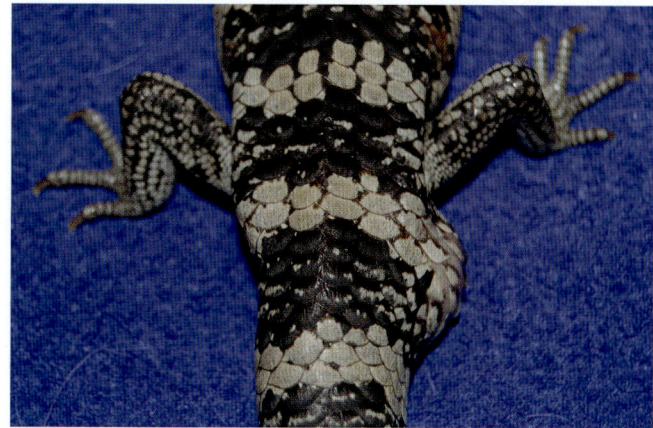

FIG 134.2 Hemipenal sac abscesses present as swellings on either side of the tail base. Abscesses can be bilateral or unilateral as in this eastern blue-tongue skink (*Tiliqua scincoides*). (Courtesy of Shane Simpson.)

so-called seminal plugs. These consist of waxy, caseous debris that collects within the inverted hemipenes and most often are bilateral and symmetrical. The brown dry tips of the seminal plugs often can be seen protruding from the opening of each hemipenis in the caudolateral cloaca. Seminal plugs have been suggested to consist of dried semen and desquamated epithelial cells, but they have been shown to contain no sperm at all.[5] Seminal plugs have been associated with iatrogenic hypovitaminosis A in chameleons and leopard geckos (*Eublepharis macularius*).[6,7]

Deformities

Axial bifurcation, or conjoined (incomplete) twinning, has occasionally been reported in a variety of lizard species.[8,9] Congenital malformations of the head may include foreshortening of the upper jaw, cleft palate, and microphthalmia.[10] Congenitally short, absent, or kinked tails may also be seen.

Kyphosis and scoliosis of the spine occasionally is seen in green iguanas and other lizards. This condition can result from genetic defects, malnutrition, and pathology of the epaxial muscles. Congenital defects may be a result of genetic defects or improper temperatures during incubation. Defects that appear later in life may be genetic or the result of external factors, including infection, trauma, neoplasia, and malnutrition.

DERMATOLOGICAL SIGNS

Dermatitis, Abrasions, Ulcerations, and Open Sores

Rostral abrasions are common in active lizards, such as water dragons (*Physignathus* spp.) and basilisks (*Basiliscus* spp.), and result from repeated trauma with glass or wire cage walls during flight responses to stimuli. Abrasions on the palmar and plantar surfaces of the feet also occur in lizards kept in cages with rough or wire surfaces. Bite wounds from cage mates or live rodent prey or other trauma may result in defects in the skin. (See Chapter 142). Thermal burns result from contact with a heat source or fire and usually involve the ventral or dorsal surface (Fig. 134.3) (see Chapter 69). Chemical burns result from contact with cage disinfectants, such as sodium hypochlorite, that has not been rinsed away adequately. A thorough patient history reveals the cause of the lesion in these cases.

Dermatitis may be ulcerative or necrotizing and result from gram-negative, gram-positive, or anaerobic bacteria and from various fungi and algae.

One significant organism is the fungal pathogen *Nannizziopsis guarroi*.[11–13] This is the causative agent of the syndrome known commonly as "yellow fungus disease" that primarily affects bearded dragons but has been reported in multiple other lizards, including veiled chameleons (*Chameleo calyptratus*) and green iguanas. Affected animals develop severe crusting and ulceration of the skin, particularly around the head, but it can spread to involve all parts of the body (Fig. 134.4) (see Chapter 31).

Dermatitis may also result from mites (*Ophionyssus* sp. and *Hirstiella* sp.). Myiasis may cause one or more open holes in the skin, and the fly larvae are usually visible moving within the hole.

Crusts, Scabs, Flakes, and Dysecdysis

Crusts and scabs may be seen as a result of bacterial dermatitis or burns. Flakes of skin may represent normal shedding. Most lizards shed in pieces, but in some species (e.g., geckos) the old skin comes off in one piece. In addition, some lizards eat their shed skin. Dysecdysis, or difficult shedding, may result in dry, flaking, adherent patches of dead skin (Fig. 134.5). The most common cause of dysecdysis is a lack of humidity. Retained skin surrounding the digits, dorsal spines, or tail tips shrinks as it dries, which compromises the blood flow. This results in necrosis and sloughing of the affected part.

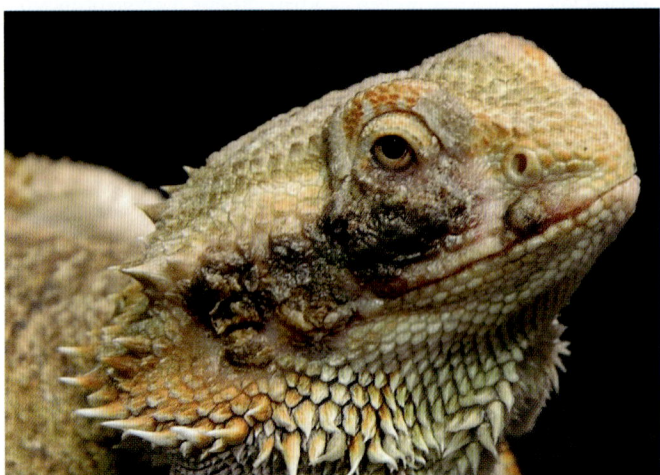

FIG 134.4 *Nannizziopsis guarroi* causes "yellow fungus disease" in central bearded dragons (*Pogona vitticeps*). This fungal infection causes severe ulceration and crust formation predominantly around the head. Treatment may delay its spread and severity, but the infection is usually fatal. (Courtesy of Sue Ciampa.)

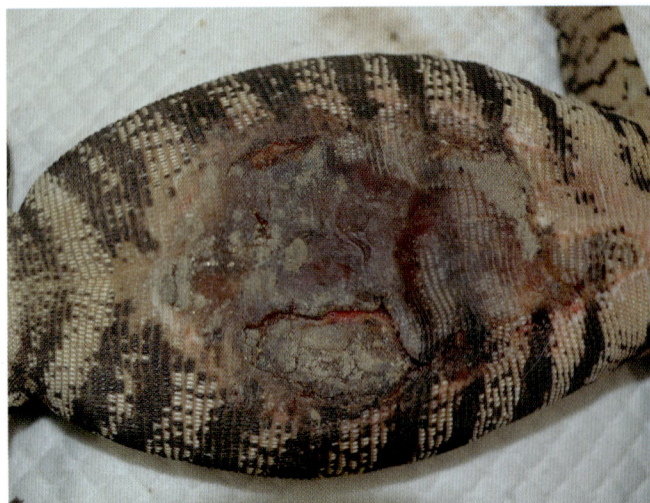

FIG 134.3 A severe, full-thickness burn on the ventrum of a lace monitor (*Varanus varius*) caused by an unprotected heat source with which the lizard was in direct contact. Extensive surgery and prolonged treatment was necessary, but this lizard made a full recovery. (Courtesy of Shane Simpson.)

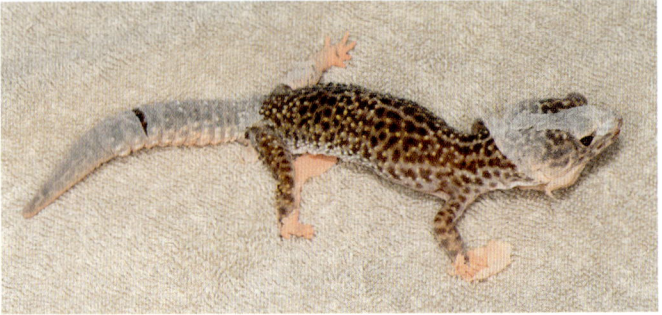

FIG 134.5 Lizards with dysecdysis will retain pieces of shed skin over their bodies, such as in this leopard gecko (*Eublepharis macularius*). (Courtesy of Stephen Barten.)

Dysecdysis has been associated with iatrogenic hypovitaminosis A in chameleons and leopard geckos[7] (see Chapter 147).

Swellings, Nodules, and Blisters

Many lumps in lizards are caused by abscesses, which usually manifest as encapsulated, inspissated pockets of caseous debris. Rarely, reptile abscesses contain mucoid or liquid discharge. Abscesses often are subcutaneous, but they may occur within the coelomic cavity, the middle ear, or under the ocular spectacle. Abscesses usually occur after bacteria, including anaerobes, or fungi enter through a penetrating wound. Cellulitis often precedes the formation of a pocket of debris (see Chapter 138).

Fluid-filled blisters commonly result from conditions of excessive humidity or thermal burns. Cytology should always be done to differentiate between sterile and septic blisters regardless of the cause.

Day geckos (*Phelsuma* spp.) have endolymphatic sacs that are sometimes called calcium or chalk sacs. These appear as bilaterally symmetrical subcutaneous swellings on the lateral and ventrolateral neck. Similar glands occur in crested geckos (*Correlophis cilliatus*) and *Rhacodactylus* spp., such as the gargoyle geckos (*Rhacodactylus auriculatus*), but they are located dorsally in the oral cavity. Their function is to store calcium and thus are radiopaque on radiographs. Anecdotally they are larger in geckos that have been heavily supplemented with calcium and vitamin D. Endolymphatic sacs tend to be larger in females but have been reported in males and, to a lesser extent, juveniles. These are normal structures that might be mistaken for abscesses.

Sebaceous or keratinaceous cysts have been reported in lizards, primarily in the tails of green iguanas and in multiple locations on central bearded dragons. These resemble dry abscesses with a solid core of epidermal debris and can be gently peeled off the underlying skin to leave a shallow crater.[14]

A variety of neoplasms of the integument has been reported in lizards, and these may result in dermal or subcutaneous masses.[15] The types of neoplasias seen include papilloma, squamous cell carcinoma, melanoma, chromatophoroma, fibrosarcoma, and myxosarcoma, among others.

Subcutaneous nematodes and filarid parasites may cause subcutaneous masses. These are especially common in chameleons.[16,17]

Edema may cause swelling of the limbs, pharynx, or coelom.

Cases of pseudoaneurysm or dissecting aneurysm have been observed in the dorsolateral cervical region of captive bearded dragons[18] (Fig. 134.6) (see Chapter 68). Generally adult lizards will present with a large fluctuant to firm swelling on the dorsolateral neck just caudal to the skull. Attempts to aspirate the fluid-filled mass generally yield several milliliters of whole blood. After fluid evacuation, the mass immediately refills with blood, indicating communication with a large or high-pressure blood vessel.

In more chronic cases, the contents of the lesion coagulate and cannot be aspirated. The etiology of this syndrome is unknown. Extensive lesions of smooth muscle in the tunica media of the great vessels have been noted on histopathology and were characterized by distortion and disorientation of the smooth muscle fibers with marked intracellular edema. Hypertension cannot be ruled out as a possible etiology for this syndrome.

Abnormalities in Color, Abnormal Scale Patterns, and Color Change

Abnormalities in color commonly occur in reptiles and are often selected for in captive breeding programs. Red, yellow, and white skin pigments are present in addition to melanin. Amelanosis, hypomelanosis, anerythrism, melanosis, and leucism may be seen. Abnormal scale patterns caused by genetic mutations have also been selected for in breeding

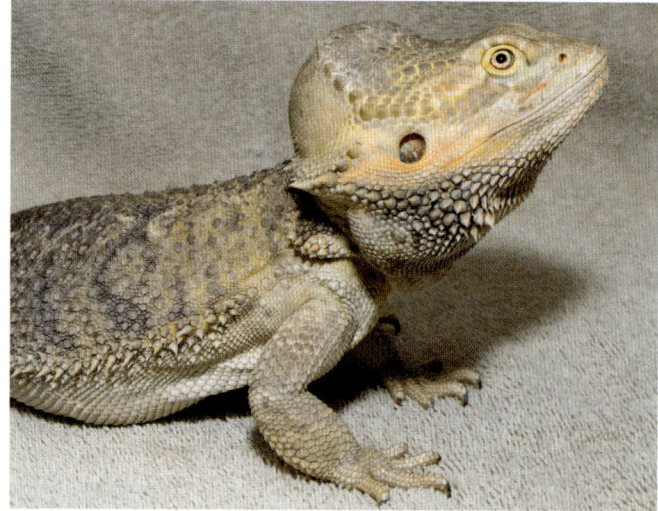

FIG 134.6 Aneurysms have been seen in adult central bearded dragons (*Pogona vitticeps*). When aspirated, frank blood is removed, and the lesion quickly refills. Treatment requires high-risk surgery. (Courtesy of Stephen Barten.)

programs. For instance, popular morphs of the bearded dragon include "leatherbacks," with increased numbers of smaller-sized dorsal scales and fewer spikes, giving the skin a smoother texture, and "silkbacks," with scales so small the skin appears smooth like that of a human. Ontogenetic pattern changes occur in some lizards, for example, the leopard gecko. In this species, the young are banded but become spotted as they mature.

Rapid color change is highly developed in many lizards but most notably among the chameleons (*Chamaeleo* spp.) and anoles (*Anolis* spp.). Control of the chromatophores may be hormonal or neurological or both. Male chameleons confronted with conspecific males or even their own mirror image quickly assume bright "threat" colors as they attack their rival. Chromatophores may react to stimulation from light or changes in temperature; lizards that are cold or in bright sunlight often become noticeably darker. Age, gender, and season may influence color change. Some male green iguanas have a pronounced orange hue develop during the breeding season as a normal condition, and this must be differentiated from the orange discoloration that is sometimes seen with systemic illness. Lizards with systemic disease or malnutrition often become duller or darker than normal. Lizards in an active shed cycle will have a dull appearance to their skin.

Mite infestation may result in color changes to the skin (see Chapter 139).

Scars

Scars from wounds, burns, and other trauma initially are white to pale pink and smooth and lack scales. With each successive shed, the scaleless area becomes smaller as new scales are produced around the periphery of the lesion. The scar does not change appreciably in appearance between sheds but is noticeably smaller immediately after a shed. Once the scarred area has healed, the new scales may be noted to be smaller and darker than the original scales. Also, they usually are arranged haphazardly rather than in even rows.

GASTROINTESTINAL SIGNS

Oral Cavity

Petechiae. Petechiae are uncommon in lizards. Causes include trauma associated with rostral abrasions, running into cage walls during escape attempts, and the forceful use of oral speculums. Focal, early stomatitis can result in petechiae, but this also is rare in lizards. Coagulation disorders are poorly documented in reptiles, but these could result in petechiae. Coagulopathy might also result from the ingestion of warfarin-type rodenticides or prey animals that had ingested rodenticides (see Chapter 88).

Stomatitis, Ulcerations, and Exudates. Stomatitis is much more common in snakes and chelonians than lizards. It is usually the result of poor husbandry conditions, including suboptimal temperatures, malnutrition, and overcrowding. A herpesvirus has been associated with a proliferative stomatitis in green tree monitors (*Varanus prasinus*).[19] However, generally stomatitis occurs secondary to other conditions such as pneumonia and septicemia. Signs can include inflammation, ulceration, abscessation, and caseous deposits (see Chapter 73).

Exposure gingivitis often is mistaken for stomatitis. Lizards that have or have had secondary nutritional hyperparathyroidism (NSHP) commonly have deformed mandibles and maxillae, resulting in the exposure of gingival tissue. This condition also is seen in cases with traumatic defects in the lips. The affected gingiva produces a dry, reddish-brown, scablike material. This condition does not respond to antibiotic therapy. The exposed gingiva should be kept moist with aqueous lubricants and barrier creams, with the discharge periodically removed.

Oral neoplasia has been seen in lizards.[20] Chemical or thermal burns, in theory, could result in oral ulcerations. Lizards with renal failure do not typically develop oral ulcers like those seen in feline patients. Visceral gout can result in inflammation of the oral cavity.

Oral exudates usually result from inflammation of the oral cavity, respiratory tract, or gastrointestinal tract. Stomatitis usually involves exudation. White or mucoid foam may be coughed up in cases of pneumonia. Less commonly, stomach contents may be regurgitated and be present in the oral cavity in cases of gastritis or gastrointestinal obstruction. Septicemia is often present in cases of stomatitis, pneumonia, and gastroenteritis. Inflammation of any tissues is caused by bacterial, viral, fungal, and parasitic agents. Appropriate diagnostic sampling is necessary to differentiate the causative agent. Chameleons (*Chamaeleo* spp.) have temporal glands dorsolateral to the corners of their mouths that sometimes become infected and distended with caseous debris.

Oral Discharge and Ptyalism. Excessive white foam in the oral cavity is occasionally seen in lizards and is associated with septicemia and pneumonia. Affected lizards are usually moribund. Improper husbandry techniques, such as chilling, malnutrition, lack of parasite control, and overcrowding, are often part of the history.

Pharyngeal Edema. Pharyngeal edema has been associated with renal disease in green iguanas and old-world chameleons.[7] Some chameleon species have an accessory lung lobe attached to the trachea in the ventral neck. Swelling in this area can be caused by infection and cellulitis of this structure.

Mucous Membrane Color. Adult bearded dragons and many chameleons normally have yellow-orange mucous membranes that resemble icterus. Many lizards, including various species of chameleons, geckos, and monitors, have melanotic oral cavities. These can vary from jet black to dark purple in color, and the latter must be differentiated from cyanosis.

Icterus is an uncommon sign in lizards. When present, it may be prehepatic or hepatic and result in jaundiced mucous membranes; however, these tend to be a greenish color rather than yellow because of the accumulation of biliverdin rather than bilirubin. Cyanosis may result from respiratory or cardiac compromise but also is rare in reptiles. Erythema and congested mucous membranes may be seen in cases of stomatitis.

Reptile mucous membranes are normally pale pink to white in color and are significantly paler than those of a typical mammal, because the normal packed cell volumes of reptiles are lower than those of mammals.

Tongue. Chameleons (*Chamaeleo* spp.) and monitors (*Varanus* spp.) have long protrusible tongues that retract inside a sheath rostral to the glottis when not in use. Bacterial infection sometimes develops within that sheath. Symptoms include inflammation, discharge, and an inability to protrude the tongue because of adhesions between the tongue and sheath.

In chameleons, hypocalcemia commonly results from malnutrition, lack of ultraviolet B light, or renal disease. One of the first symptoms of hypocalcemia in this group is poor muscle tone manifested as flaccid paralysis of the tongue. The affected chameleons either cannot shoot their tongue at prey in a normal fashion or, if they do, are unable to retract it so that it hangs from their mouth.

The tip of the tongue in the green iguana, leopard gecko, and other lizard species is darker than the rest of the tongue, which may be mistaken for glossitis.

Dental Disease. The teeth of lizards are generally pleurodont (attached to the sides of the mandible without sockets), but in some families, the Agamidae and Chamaeleontidae, they are acrodont (attached to the biting edges of the jaws without sockets). Pleurodont teeth are regularly shed and replaced, and dental disease in these species is rare. Acrodont teeth are not replaced except in very young specimens, although new teeth may be added to the posterior end of the tooth row as the lizard grows. Many agamids have a few pleurodont teeth in the rostral portion of the dental arcade. Periodontal disease has been reported in captive acrodont lizards, including bearded dragons and frilled lizards (*Chlamydosaurus kingii*). Symptoms include gingival erythema, gingival recession, calculus formation, and, in severe cases, osteomyelitis and abscess formation[21-23] (see Chapter 159).

Teeth may fracture as a result of biting or chewing on objects, such as oral speculums. Infected gingiva can result. Teeth may become loosened as a result of NSHP or secondary renal hyperparathyroidism (RSHP).

Anorexia

Anorexia is a common sign among captive reptiles. It is not a disease itself but occurs secondary to other conditions. The causes may be environmental or medical.

Environmental causes of anorexia include low temperature, low humidity, excessive handling of shy specimens, stress from overcrowding, lack of a hide box for visual security, lack of ultraviolet light sources, and presentation of inappropriate or inadequate diets (e.g., carnivorous lizards, such as most monitors, do not accept vegetarian diets). It is therefore important, in the evaluation of the anorexic lizard, that the environmental conditions that *have* been provided and those that *should* be provided are reviewed.

In a few cases anorexia is normal in lizards. Gravid females usually eat less than normal, if at all, because developing eggs or fetuses fill a large percentage of the coelomic cavity and there is no space for expansion of the gastrointestinal tract with food. Assist feeding in this instance is extremely stressful (Fig. 134.7). Likewise, many male lizards become focused on territoriality, fighting with rivals, and searching for a mate during their breeding season, and eating takes on a low priority. Species

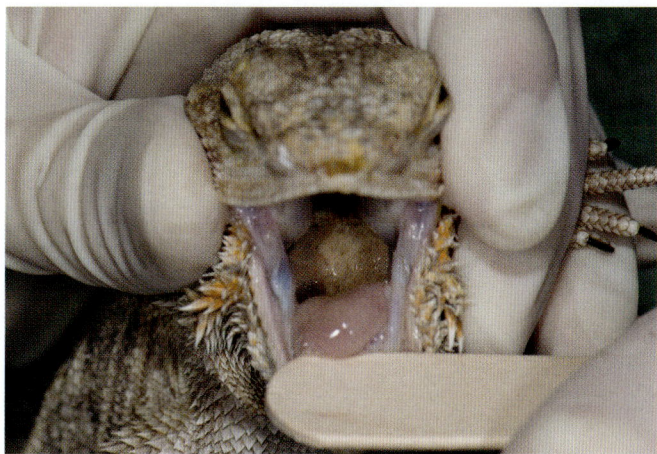

FIG 134.7 A female central bearded dragon (*Pogona vitticeps*) that presented for anorexia and weight loss as a result of postovulatory egg retention. Assist feeding with a semiliquid diet resulted in food remaining in the esophagus and stomach because of the extraluminal pressure of the eggs. Ovariosalpingectomy relieved the dystocia and resulted in a normal return to function. (Courtesy of Stephen Barten.)

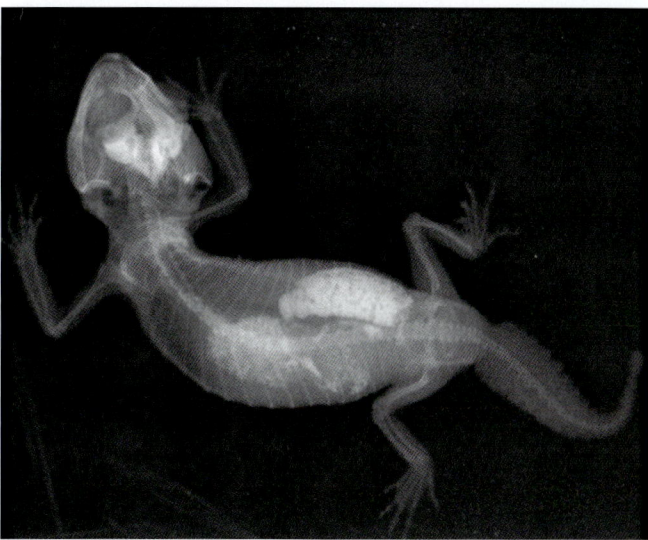

FIG 134.8 Constipation can be the result of many causes, including substrate ingestion such as sand. This radiograph of a smooth knob-tailed gecko (*Nephrurus levis*) clearly shows the large amount of ingested sand. (Courtesy of Shane Simpson.)

that normally brumate, especially wild-caught specimens, may have decreased appetites with decreasing photoperiod in the fall, even when environmental temperatures are kept high.

Medical causes of anorexia are varied. One of the most common signs of any disease is a decreased appetite. Anorexia is common with bacterial or viral infections, parasites, nutritional disorders, foreign body or impaction, stomatitis, and gastroenteritis. Renal disease, liver disease, metabolic disorders, neoplasia, toxemia, and so on all result in anorexia. NSHP often causes soft flexible mandibles and loosened teeth, which can preclude eating, and ileus of the gastrointestinal tract related to hypocalcemia. Tongue lesions or infection can prevent food prehension. A complete history, physical examination, and appropriate laboratory sampling are necessary to establish a diagnosis (see Chapter 42).

Vomiting and Regurgitation

Lizards have a more highly developed cardiac sphincter than snakes and as a result rarely regurgitate. Lizards that are vomiting or regurgitating food are often extremely ill. Causes include septicemia, toxemia, gastroenteritis, parasite burdens, gastrointestinal foreign bodies, and gastrointestinal obstruction caused by intussusception or constipation. Extramural causes of gastrointestinal obstruction include nephritis with renal enlargement, uroliths, the presence of eggs or fetuses, abscesses, neoplasia, and a narrowed pelvic canal from trauma or one of the MBDs. Spoiled food, inappropriate temperatures that prevent normal digestion, and postprandial handling can cause regurgitation. Vomiting may be seen during agonal struggles in terminal cases (see Chapter 73).

Diarrhea

Environmental conditions can result in diarrhea. Low environmental temperatures can cause incomplete digestion, bacterial overgrowth, and diarrhea. Sudden changes in the diet may cause diarrhea in herbivorous lizards, especially when fruits with a high water content are offered. Likewise, lack of fiber in the diet of these lizards can contribute to the formation of loose stools. Feeding chicks, chicken parts, other meat products, or dog food to carnivorous lizards can result in looser and more foul-smelling stool than when rodents are used. Diarrhea is caused by a variety of infectious and parasitic agents. Enteritis results from a number of bacteria, including *Salmonella* spp. Viral diseases are poorly documented in lizards, though agamid atadenovirus infection in bearded dragons is often associated with diarrhea.[24] Parasites that can cause diarrhea include hookworms (*Kalicephalus* sp.), ascarids, strongyles (*Rhabdias* sp. and *Strongyloides* sp.), *Entamoeba* sp., coccidia (*Eimeria* and *Isopora* sp.), flagellates (*Trichomonas* sp., *Monocercomonas* sp., and others), and, less commonly, ciliates (*Nyctotherus* sp.). *Cryptosporidium* spp. is more common in snakes than in lizards, but it has been reported in several species, including leopard geckos,[25] savannah monitors (*Varanus exanthematicus*),[26] and bearded dragons[27] (see Chapter 74).

Constipation

Lack of bowel movements has many potential causes. Associated husbandry issues include inappropriate temperatures, hypocalcemia, and related NSHP from insufficient dietary calcium, dietary vitamin D₃, or UVB lighting; inappropriate or insufficient water sources; lack of activity from a too-small cage; inappropriate food items (long-haired rodent prey, hard-shelled insect prey); and ingestion of indigestible cage substrates such as gravel, rocks, sand, and bark (Fig. 134.8).

Diseases that cause constipation include parasitism and dehydration. Intussusception and cloacitis can cause physical obstruction of the gastrointestinal tract. Extramural causes of gastrointestinal obstruction include nephritis with renal enlargement, uroliths, the presence of eggs or fetuses, abscesses, neoplasia, a narrowed pelvic canal from trauma or NSHP, and neurological deficits related to vertebral lesions such as fracture, scoliosis, kyphosis, and various MBDs.

Constipation is a common presenting sign in bearded dragons. Affected patients have a history of not having defecated for 1 to 2 weeks, anorexia, and lethargy. Examination usually reveals a large mass of urates in the cloaca, preventing the passage of feces.

Prolapse From the Cloaca

Several organs can be prolapsed from the cloacal opening. These include the cloaca itself, the bladder when present, and the colon. Female reptiles can prolapse the shell gland, and males one or both hemipenes. Seminal plugs in males can be mistaken for a prolapsed organ.

A prolapse can occur as a result of anything that causes straining. The most common cause of a prolapsed cloaca in juvenile iguanas is poor muscle tone associated with hypocalcemia and spinal cord deficits from vertebral compression and fracture, usually a consequence of NSHP. Straining may be caused by any cause of gastroenteritis, including bacterial, fungal, viral, or parasitic enteritis; cloacitis; impactions or ingested foreign objects; intussusception; or constipation. Uroliths, bacterial cystitis, or dystocia can result in excessive straining. Extraluminal gastrointestinal blockage caused by renal enlargement, neoplasia, abscesses, or a narrowed pelvic canal from trauma or NSHP all result in straining. Dyspnea can cause straining (see Chapter 75).

REPRODUCTIVE SIGNS

Infertility

Normal courtship and breeding in reptiles is stimulated by seasonal fluctuations in temperature, photoperiod, or rainfall. Many species need a period of brumation to mate successfully. Males and females may fail to produce sperm and eggs, respectively, if they are kept at inappropriate temperatures, humidity levels, or photoperiod. The specific requirements of a species must be researched to avoid exposing them to inappropriate cycling techniques, such as temperatures that are too cold, resulting in illness. Social cues play a role, and for some species successful mating is enhanced by social groups or male-to-male combat, rather than just the introduction of a single male and single female. Some individual pairs may be incompatible with each other. In many of these cases the keeper has misidentified the gender of one or both in the pair. In other cases, the animals are too young to breed. Localized illness, such as infection of the reproductive tract or cloacitis, can prevent breeding, as can systemic illness such as septicemia, malnutrition, or renal failure (see Chapter 80).

Stillbirths and Hatch Failure

Improper environmental conditions for the gravid female or complications with incubating eggs commonly result in stillbirths or failure of eggs to hatch. Low or high environmental temperatures, low or high humidity levels, poor hygiene with mold or fungal contamination of the incubation media, and incubator failure are potential causes. Infection of the cloaca or oviduct, genetic abnormalities, and fetal or egg disease also may be involved (see Chapter 85).

Dystocia

The presence of eggs or fetuses does not indicate the diagnosis of dystocia. Normal gravid females develop distended coelomic cavities and become anorectic. Green iguanas usually refuse food for 4 weeks before they lay eggs.[28] However, they remain bright, alert, and responsive. Gravid lizards with dystocia quickly become depressed and unresponsive and without prompt treatment can die.

Nonobstructive causes of dystocia may include husbandry issues. Lack of a suitable egg-laying site is one of the most common causes leading to postovulatory egg retention. Iguanas need an enclosed egg-laying chamber, and chameleons often lay eggs in the soil of potted plants within their cage if a climbing branch reaches into the pot. Cool temperatures, malnutrition, dehydration, and poor physical condition from lack of exercise can contribute to dystocia. Infection of the reproductive tract can occur, but it can be difficult to differentiate whether the infection has caused the problem or infection is the result of retained ova or fetuses, especially in cases with a delayed presentation.

Obstructive causes of dystocia include anatomic defects that prevent the passage of eggs or young. Oversized, deformed, or fractured eggs

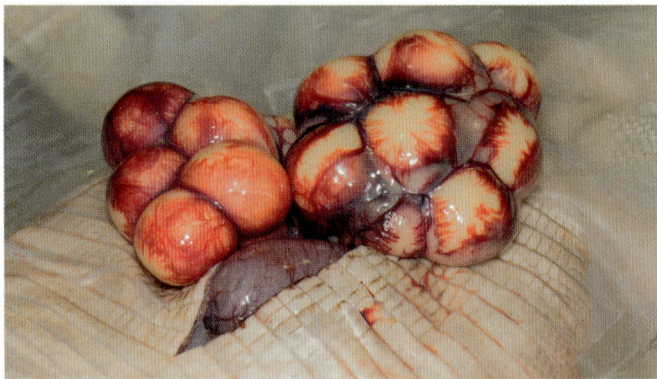

FIG 134.9 Coeliotomy to treat preovulatory follicular stasis in a red tegu (*Tupinambis rufescens*). Marked inflammation and a small amount of free yolk material are visible; these are abnormal and possibly because of trauma from jumping or falling. Without surgical intervention, these patients will succumb to septicemia. (Courtesy of Stephen Barten.)

may be too large to pass through the pelvic canal. The shell gland may have a stricture or torsion. Abscesses, enlarged kidneys, neoplasia, or uroliths may compress and obstruct the oviducts. A narrowed pelvic canal or other spinal deformity caused by one of the MBDs or trauma may prevent passage of eggs.

Preovulatory egg retention occurs when a lizard undergoes vitellogenesis but does not ovulate (Fig. 134.9). The enlarged ova remain on the ovaries but fill the coelomic cavity and cause anorexia. In some cases they are resorbed; in others an ovariectomy is necessary (see Chapters 80, 105, and 148).

RESPIRATORY SIGNS

Dyspnea

Dyspnea may result from upper or lower airway disease. The nostrils can become plugged with unshed skin, normal discharge from the salt excretion glands, or inflammatory discharge from rhinitis and pneumonia. Both the external and internal nares must be examined for discharge, which may be serous, mucoid, or purulent. Pneumonia may be present at the same time as rhinitis. Plugged nostrils result in open-mouth breathing.

Lower respiratory disease with respiratory embarrassment results in dyspnea as the lizard attempts to obtain more oxygen. Pneumonia is caused by a variety of aerobic and anaerobic bacteria. Mycotic pneumonia has been seen in reptiles, including lizards, but is often considered a secondary invader.[29] Verminous pneumonia is usually accompanied by bacterial pneumonia. The helminths *Entomelas* spp. and *Rhabdias* spp. are the common lungworms in lizards.[30] Pentastomes, trematodes, and migrating nematode larvae also may cause verminous pneumonia in reptiles. Among lizards, parasites are most common in chameleons and monitors. Aspiration pneumonia may be a sequela of assist feeding and the oral administration of medication by inexperienced persons.

Untreated chronic respiratory tract disease often spreads to other areas, resulting in abscess formation in the oral cavity, periorbital space, and parenchymatous coelomic organs, notably the liver. Any lesion that compromises the opening of the glottis, such as abscesses or neoplasia of the oral cavity, can cause severe dyspnea.

Drowning and near-drowning injuries are more common in aquatic chelonians but may occur in lizards left soaking unattended or through misadventure.

Primary neoplasms of the respiratory tract are rare in reptiles, but metastasis to the lungs may occur.[15]

Pulmonary edema from cardiac or hepatic disease can result in respiratory signs. Space-occupying coelomic lesions, such as ascites or neoplasia, prevent normal lung expansion and cause dyspnea.

Agonal respiration in terminal patients resembles dyspnea.

Open-mouth panting occurs in some lizards as a cooling mechanism during overheating.

Nasal Discharge

Some lizards have sodium-secreting, potassium-secreting, and chloride-secreting nasal salt glands.[29] These allow the lizard to excrete excess salts without losing significant amounts of water. These secretions appear as a clear, liquid nasal discharge that dries to a fine white powder, which may be observed around the nares or on the sides of the cage.

Sinusitis and rhinitis can produce nasal discharge as well. This material varies from clear with bubbles to thick and mucoid. Because of the position of the internal nares anterior in the oropharynx, stomatitis and pneumonia might also result in nasal discharge. Thorough physical examination helps differentiate between the two groups.

Epistaxis and hemoptysis most commonly occur from metastatic mineralization in green iguanas. Iatrogenic hypervitaminosis D and idiopathic causes are associated with marked hypercalcemia. The resulting mineral deposits commonly occur in the smooth muscle of blood vessels, making them abnormally rigid and prone to fracture with minor trauma, such as a short fall or vigorous restraint. When a mineralized vessel in the lungs fractures, marked epistaxis and hemoptysis result, often with fatal results. Metastatic mineralization is easily demonstrated on radiographs. Other causes of epistaxis are rare in lizards but might include necrotizing rhinitis and sinusitis caused by bacteria, mycoplasma, or fungi, acquired coagulopathy from septicemia, nutritional deficiency or liver insufficiency, rodenticide toxicity, neoplasia, and foreign bodies.

Causes of discharges in the oropharynx are discussed in Chapter 76.

Abnormal Vocalizations

Respiratory sounds may be associated with fluid within the respiratory tract as a result of pneumonia, aspiration, or near-drowning. These must be differentiated from hissing and snorting sounds often used as a defensive gesture in response to a perceived threat. Veiled chameleons will often vibrate their entire body along with hissing and gaping as a normal response to a threat, and this should not be confused with illness. Conversely, a lack of sound might be noted in a fully consolidated lung.

OCULAR SIGNS

Palpebral and Spectacle Abnormalities

Reversible, temporary, bilateral periorbital swelling is occasionally seen in some species of lizard because of venous sinus engorgement. This is particularly obvious when the lizard is restrained behind the head and struggles violently. More permanent venous congestion occurs with systemic and localized infection, cardiac disease, renal disease, and vascular abnormalities such as aneurysm.

Subcutaneous cellulitis, abscesses, and palpebral trauma are common around the eye. These usually result from penetrating wounds secondary to escape attempts, fights with cage mates, and burns from heat lamps.

In species with a spectacle, distention of the subspectacular space with clear lacrimal fluid results in a condition known as pseudobuphthalmos and occurs when the nasolacrimal duct is occluded (Fig. 134.10). Nasolacrimal occlusion can result from infection, pressure

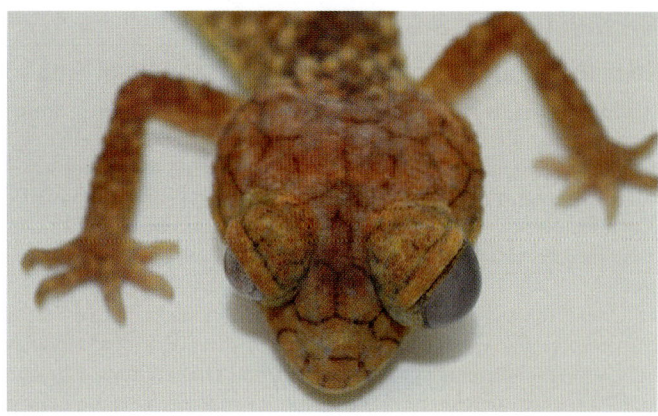

FIG 134.10 Pseudobuphthalmos in a rough knob-tailed gecko (*Nephrurus amyae*). The likely cause of this condition is a blockage of the nasolacrimal structures. (Courtesy of Shane Simpson.)

from surrounding inflamed tissues and mass lesions, fibrosis, or congenital malformation. The subspectacular space also can become distended with caseous debris from a bacterial infection ascending up the nasolacrimal duct or spreading hematogenously. Panophthalmitis must be differentiated from subspectacular abscessation. In the latter condition, the entire globe swells as the interior structures are destroyed by infection originating from wounds or hematogenous spread (see Chapter 71).

Blepharospasm may result from foreign bodies in the eye, such as sand and other particulate bedding materials. Corneal ulcers also cause blepharospasm and may result from foreign bodies, trauma, or infection with bacteria or viruses. Exposure to excessively strong artificial ultraviolet light sources can cause blepharospasm and keratitis.

Palpebral edema, squamous metaplasia, and photophobia have been associated with iatrogenic hypovitaminosis A in many species and commonly chameleons and leopard geckos.[6,7]

Mites and ticks are occasionally found in the ocular adnexa.

Corneal Abnormalities

Keratitis occurs in reptiles as a result of bacterial or fungal infection. Corneal ulcers may result from trauma, foreign bodies, or infection.

In those species with spectacles, exposure keratitis results from iatrogenic avulsion of the spectacle from improper treatment, perhaps related to misdiagnosis, of retained spectacles.

Leopard geckos occasionally develop a plug of caseous debris covering the cornea. Bacterial conjunctivitis, foreign objects such as sand substrate, chronic hyperthermia from excessive use of heat sources, and hypovitaminosis A may be contributing factors in this presentation.[7] The plug usually can be removed in a single piece with flushing and gentle manipulation. Because the inner surface conforms to the round surface of the cornea, the plug is commonly mistaken for a retained spectacle, but of course this species (Eublepharis means "true eyelids") lacks a spectacle.

Arcus lipoides corneae is a white band of material that may partially or completely surround the cornea near the limbus. This condition is associated with aging and requires no treatment.[14]

Lens Abnormalities

Juvenile cataracts with a postulated genetic etiology have been reported in monitor lizards.[31] Senile cataracts may occur in adult animals. Cataracts in brumating reptiles may sometimes be associated with damage from freezing.[31]

NEUROLOGICAL SIGNS

Convulsions, Twitching, Coma, Ataxia, and Head Tilts

Neurological signs in reptiles usually overlap. A condition that causes ataxia frequently progresses through muscle weakness, twitching, convulsions, coma, and death. Muscle fasciculations, tetany, and convulsions sometimes are difficult to separate. Head tilts occasionally accompany other neurological signs; examples include juvenile bearded dragons infected with atadenovirus and idiopathic cases in other species.

One of the most common pathologic conditions in captive lizards is hypocalcemia resulting from unbalanced diets, lack of ultraviolet light sources, and inadequate environmental temperatures. Chronic NSHP cases may develop hypocalcemia with symptoms of tetany, muscle fasciculations, and eventually coma and death (see Chapter 84). Similar signs may also be seen with renal secondary hyperparathyroidism (RSHP) resulting in metabolic disturbances of calcium and phosphorus in particular. Additionally, dehydration and renal pathology can result in gout, causing incoordination and convulsions.

Xanthomatosis (cholesterol clefts) with lesions in the brain resulting in neurological signs have been reported in geckos and water dragons (*Physignathus cocincinus*).[32,33]

Hypoglycemia may result in convulsions, but this condition is rare in reptiles. A heavy parasite burden can result in weakness, lethargy, coma, and death.

Lizards with septicemia may develop brain abscesses with neurological symptoms including convulsions. Tumors involving the central nervous system of lizards are extremely rare.[15]

Neurological lesions may result from physical trauma, such as a blow to the head or damage from freezing.

Toxicity from a variety of substances may result in convulsions. Possible toxins include insecticides; pharmaceuticals such as metronidazole, ivermectin, and aminoglycoside antibiotics; bufotoxins from consumption of certain toads (e.g., the marine toad, *Rhinella marina)*; firefly and Monarch butterfly toxicoses in bearded dragons; and various chemicals such as paint solvents. Toxic plants are occasionally ingested by herbivorous species, the symptoms of which vary with the species of plant (see Chapter 88).

A rare dietary cause of neurological symptoms is vitamin B complex deficiencies. This condition may be seen in carnivorous reptiles that are fed large amounts of frozen fish or in herbivorous lizards fed large amounts of frozen vegetables. Freezing decreases vitamin levels and increases thiaminase activity, resulting in thiamine (B_1) deficiency. Biotin deficiency has been reported in monitors (*Varanus* spp.) fed raw eggs, which contain avidin, a substance with antibiotin activity.[14,34] Symptoms vary with severity but range from weakness and incoordination, through twitching and torticollis, and finally to convulsions and death. The diagnosis is confirmed with response to supplementation with B complex vitamins or histopathology.

Vitamin E and selenium deficiencies are rarely seen in herbivorous lizards with symptoms of muscle weakness, fasciculations, and convulsions. This condition is diagnosed with clinical improvement after the injection of vitamin E and selenium or muscle biopsy.

Paralysis and Paresis

By far the most common cause of paralysis or paresis is spinal cord lesions from the collapse of one or more vertebrae as a sequela to one of the MBDs. Depending on the site of the lesion, paraplegia or quadriplegia may be present. The onset usually is sudden, and a history of trauma may or may not be present. If the lizard is able to defecate and pass urates, the prognosis is fair; if not, the prognosis for recovery is poor. These signs must be differentiated from, but may accompany, muscle weakness, twitching, and fasciculations. Other causes of paralysis and paresis are rare but include spinal cord lesions from trauma such as vertebral fractures, spinal abscesses, and neoplasia.

BEHAVIORAL SIGNS

Aggression

Aggression is generally divided into offensive and defensive aggression. The former involves unprovoked attacks, and the latter is in response to a real or perceived threat or the defense of territory. Some species of lizards are naturally aggressive and pugnacious, for example, many monitor lizards, tegus (*Tupinambis* spp.), and the veiled chameleon. Acquired aggression can coincide with sexual maturation; the onset of breeding season (especially in male green iguanas); stimulation by the presence of conspecifics or mirror images; the display of throat fans, beards, and dewlaps by conspecifics; and exposure to unfiltered sunlight (especially in monitor lizards, Gila monsters, and beaded lizards [*Heloderma* sp.]).

Reproduction

Gravid females may exhibit behavior changes before egg laying that may be mistaken for illness. They often become anorectic and lethargic with distended abdomens. Other individuals become hyperactive, pacing and digging frantically as oviposition nears.

SYSTEMIC SIGNS

Weight Loss

A common cause of weight loss in captive reptiles is an inadequate intake of calories. Some keepers mistakenly offer meals that are too small or too infrequent for the lizard, and nutrition and husbandry must be investigated thoroughly.

Low environmental temperatures can hinder digestion even when adequate diets are eaten. This is especially true in folivorous iguanid lizards that rely on microbial fermentation in their hindgut to break down the cellulose in their high-fiber diet.

Intestinal parasites, renal failure, neoplasia (such as gastric neuroendocrine carcinoma in bearded dragons)[35] (Fig. 134.11), or any systemic disease can result in rapid weight loss.

Anorexia obviously results in weight loss and was discussed in detail earlier.

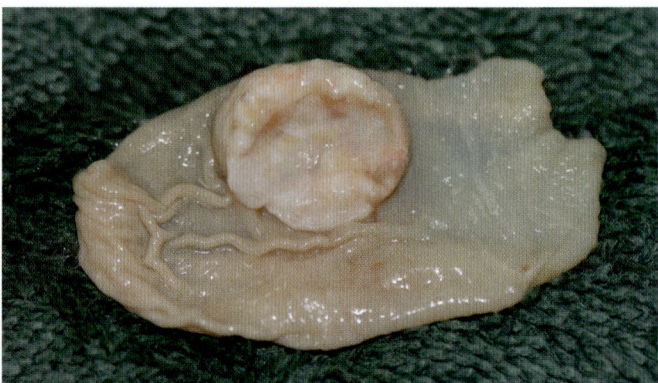

FIG 134.11 Neuroendocrine gastric carcinomas, as shown here attached to the gastric lumen of this dragon at necropsy, have been frequently reported in central bearded dragons (*Pogona vitticeps*). Affected animals often develop a persistent hyperglycemia and profound anemia and present with signs of weight loss and anorexia. (Courtesy of Stephen Barten.)

Distended Coelom

Lizards store fat in paired, symmetrical fat bodies in their caudal coelomic cavity. In obese animals, these may be huge and cause a distended coelom. They appear as fat density on radiographs and often are palpable. Fat bodies may be mistaken for mass lesions.

An apparent distended coelom can result from an enlargement of any of the coelomic viscera. The liver and kidneys may become exaggerated with hepatic lipidosis, granulomatous inflammation, or neoplasia. The gastrointestinal tract can become distended with constipation, foreign objects (notably gravel, sand, or other bedding), obstruction, intussusception, or ileus from a spinal cord lesion or profound hypocalcemia. The bladder often becomes grossly distended with urine when denervated by spinal cord lesions related to trauma or one of the MBDs.

Ascites is caused by similar mechanisms in reptiles as in mammals. Hypoproteinemia, liver failure, renal failure, cardiac disease, septicemia, and neoplasia may cause ascites. Coelomic neoplasia can result in enlargement of the coelom.

Uroliths are occasionally seen in herbivorous lizards with dehydration or unbalanced diets (Fig. 134.12). These tend to be singular and stratified and may be large enough to distend the coelom.

Female lizards that are gravid or have egg retention have an enlarged coelom. The ova can be palpated or visualized with radiology and ultrasound.

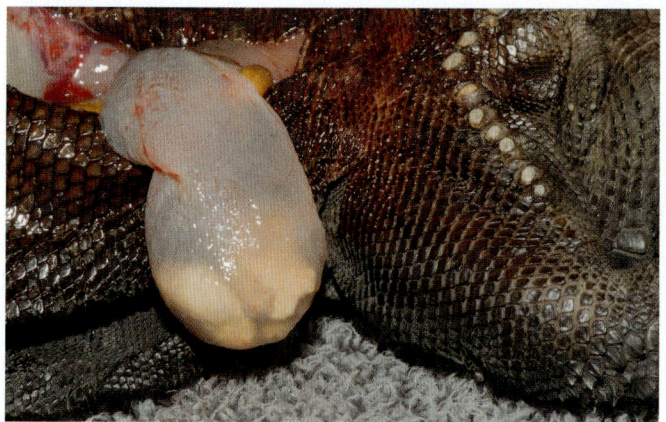

FIG 134.12 Uroliths in the bladder of a *Uromastyx* sp. secondary to chronic urine retention because of paresis from a thoracic spinal lesion. Without intervention and removal these can get quite large resulting in distension of the coelom. (Courtesy of Stephen Barten.)

Lethargy

Environmental conditions, such as low temperatures, lack of ultraviolet light, lack of a hiding place, and social stress, can cause a lizard to be less active than normal. Lizards that are gravid or about to shed commonly have decreased activity. MBDs, nutritional deficiencies, egg retention, renal failure, infections, septicemia, parasite burdens, toxicity, and just about any illness may result in depression and lack of activity.

Often the owners of lizards with lethargy misdiagnose the etiology as attempted brumation, even in cases involving tropical species and the presence of high temperatures. Overly cool temperatures and short photoperiods must be corrected, but other causes should be investigated.

Polydipsia and Polyuria

Polydipsia and polyuria are uncommon signs in lizards, but chronic renal failure is the most common cause. Causes of renal failure include bacterial infection, granulomatous inflammation, chronic dehydration, and excessive use of aminoglycoside antibiotics. Hyperglycemia is uncommon in lizards and has been associated with neoplasia, septicemia, pancreatitis, and metabolic imbalances. True diabetes mellitus (with response to insulin) has not been documented in lizards. Profound hyperglycemia is usually secondary to other causes and not diabetes melitus[36] (see Chapters 79 and 152).

Acute Mortalities

Symptoms of disease in reptiles often are subtle, and owners commonly miss them. Thus many chronic diseases such as septicemia, malnutrition, renal failure, neoplasia, or gastrointestinal obstruction, for example, may present as sudden death when in fact they were chronic in nature. Sudden death often is an acute manifestation of chronic disease.

Heat stroke from exposure to direct sunlight while a reptile is in an enclosed container or thermostatic malfunction in a heating device can result in sudden death. Victims usually are warm to the touch. Drowning causes sudden death, but the history leaves little doubt as to the cause. Ingestion of certain toxic plants results in relatively rapid death. Several reported cases have been seen where the ingestion of a single firefly caused sudden death in bearded dragons.[37] Atadenovirus may cause sudden death with few or no symptoms in juvenile bearded dragons and other species.

REFERENCES

See www.expertconsult.com for a complete list of references.

135

Differential Diagnoses by Clinical Signs—Chelonians

Thomas H. Boyer

ACUTE MORTALITIES

Multiple deaths in a chelonian collection generally indicate infectious disease, environmental failure (e.g., thermostat failure), or intoxication. Common differentials include herpesvirus (Fig. 135.1), intranuclear coccidiosis, adenovirus, entamebiasis,[1] ranavirus, chlamydiosis, reovirus, and paramyxovirus. Indoors, or in a green house, overheating is also a possibility; temperatures above 38° to 43°C (100°–110°F) are rapidly lethal for all chelonians.

DERMATOLOGICAL SIGNS

Cutaneous or Subcutaneous Swelling

Box turtles (*Terrapene* spp.) and occasionally tortoises or aquatic turtles suffer from myiasis caused by *Cistudinomyia (Sarcophaga) cistudinis*. Maggots encyst subcutaneously and breathe through small black-rimmed pores prevalent on the neck, base of the legs, axillary and prefemoral fossae, and sometimes pericloacal area (Fig. 135.2). Swelling associated with joints or feet can indicate articular or periarticular gout; pseudogout or calcinosis circumscripta; joint, bone, or soft tissue infection; foreign bodies; parasites; puncture wounds; fracture; or luxation.[2,3] Aural abscesses are common (Fig. 135.3). Tumors, such as epidermal squamous papillomas, are a rare cause of skin lesions on the feet of aquatic turtles.[2] Bacterial (including mycobacteria) or fungal subcutaneous granulomas are more common. Fibropapillomas, common on green sea turtles (*Chelonia mydas*), are also seen on the other species of sea turtles and are thought to be caused by a herpesvirus (Fig. 135.4). Gas bubble disease can cause large, multifocal, extensive subcutaneous emphysema as a result of supersaturation of water, usually with oxygen.[4,5] Spirochid blood fluke eggs can cause intense granulomatous tissue reactions in many organs, including the skin.[6]

Erythema, petechiae, ecchymoses, purpura, and foul odor of the shell or skin are typically the result of unsanitary conditions (Fig. 135.5). Generally, these signs indicate a bacterial or fungal shell infection. Focal soft areas, palpable under the scutes, may be white to yellow to serosanguinous and indicate osteomyelitis. Shell infections can also result from bite wounds, trauma, calcinosis circumscripta, lack of basking areas, abrasive substrates, or inadequate environmental temperatures. More diffuse shell erythema can also occur with septicemia or starvation. Spirochid blood fluke eggs or granulomas may occlude blood vessels in aquatic turtles and manifest as ulcerative ecchmyotic shell lesions.[6] Chelonians normally have little odor, unless musk glands are expressed under duress.

Erythema

Erythematous skin can indicate septicemia (endotoxins, exotoxins, or hemoprotozoans[2] may cause vascular damage), bacterial dermatitis, burns, or hypervitaminosis A. Many juvenile fresh-water aquatic turtles have reddish aposematic coloration of the plastron, which fades with age and should not be mistaken for erythema (Fig. 135.6).

Aural Abscess (Protrusion of the Tympanic Scale)

Normally the tympanic skin overlying the aural cavity is slightly concave. Aural abscesses cause the skin to bulge outward from solid cellular debris (see Fig. 135.3 and Chapter 92), common in Emydid turtles (especially box turtles and sliders) but less so in tortoises.

Whitish Growth on Skin

Aquatic turtles shed their skin piecemeal, which often remains attached to the turtle, floating around the limbs or body. White growths can also be from scar tissue or fungal, viral, or parasitic infections.

Whitish Areas on Shell

White areas on the shell represent healed shell lesions, exposed healed bone missing scutes, mineral deposits, or ongoing shell infection—bacterial or fungal (see Fig. 7.26A–C versus Fig. 135.5A and B). Chelonian shell is capable of regeneration such that old areas of exposed, devitalized bone and scutes are pushed out by underlying, newly formed scutes and healthy bone. White areas may also be seen in annuli between scutes in rapidly growing turtles and tend to darken with age. Texas tortoises (*Gopherus berlandieri*) are afflicted by superficial whitish scute necrosis that spares the new growth annuli (Fig. 135.7), caused by *Fusarium semitectum*.[7]

Algae Growth on Shell

Green algae often colonize the shell of aquatic turtles, which is generally of little cause for concern. As long as husbandry conditions are adequate, benign neglect or simple periodic scrubbing keeps algae under control. Ultraviolet water filters can eliminate algae in the water.

Sloughing Skin

Chelonians normally shed their skin in a much more piecemeal fashion than squamates, but they still regularly shed. Full-thickness skin sloughing is abnormal and may be associated with iatrogenic hypervitaminosis A (see Chapter 84).[2] Bacterial infection, especially anaerobic bacteria, trauma, starvation, and chemical or thermal burns can also cause skin sloughing. Desert tortoises (*Gopherus agassizii*), kept too damp during hibernation, can develop ulcerative dermatitis from *Aeromonas hydrophila* within deep skin folds.

Sloughing Scutes

Terrestrial chelonians may slough scutes as a result of bacterial or fungal infections brought on by a moist environment or from chronic renal failure.[2] If renal failure is present, bone plates may loosen and ooze azotemic fluid. Ascites may also be present.[2] In tortoises, nutritional deficiencies may cause flaking and sloughing scutes that are secondarily

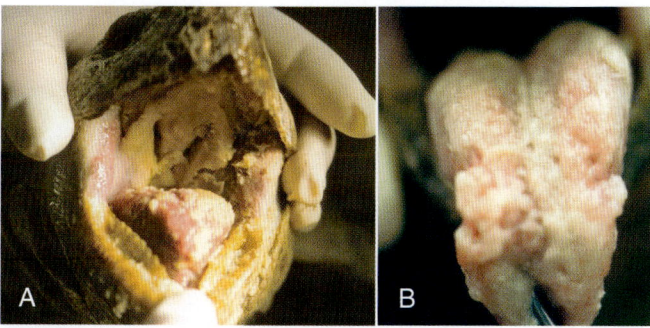

FIG 135.1 (A and B) Multiple deaths in a chelonian collection often indicate viral disease or intranuclear coccidiosis (if husbandry is confirmed as acceptable). This African spurred tortoise (*Centrochelys sulcata*) has classic diptheric plaques due to herpesvirus. (Courtesy of Thomas H. Boyer.)

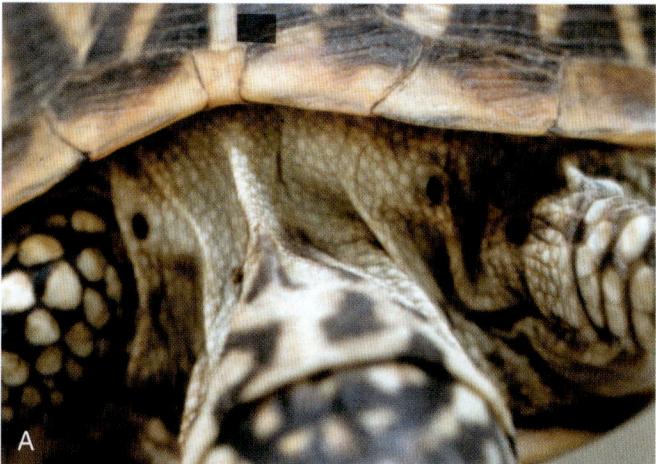

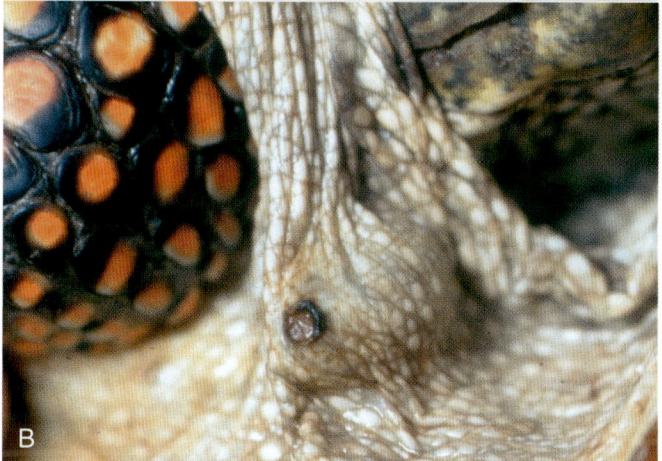

FIG 135.2 (A and B) Several botfly pores are visible around the base of the neck in this ornate box turtle, *Terrapene ornata ornata*. Multiple larvae usually share one portal. (Courtesy of Thomas H. Boyer.)

infected with bacteria or fungi.[8] Aquatic species normally flake off portions of scutes and shed scutes annually.

Shell Ulceration and Necrosis

Traumatic injuries, such as bites from other turtles, or predators, can penetrate the outer keratin layer of the shell. Burns and bacterial or fungal infections can also lead to ulcers on the shell. In terrestrial chelonians, wet shell necrosis tends to be bacterial, and dry shell necrosis tends to be fungal. Ulcerative shell disease or shell necrosis is a chronic

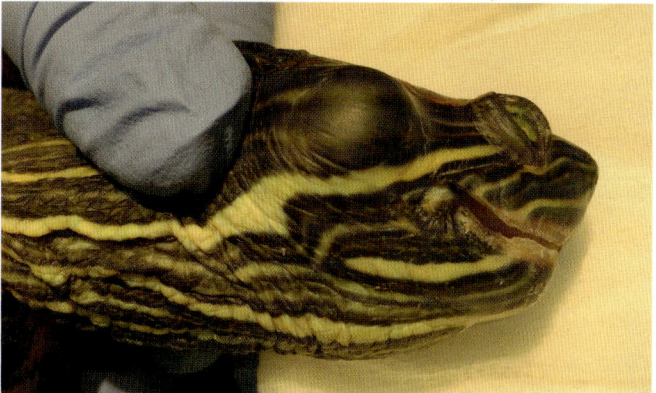

FIG 135.3 Swelling over the tympanic membrane in this slider *(Trachemys)* is generally a sign of an aural abscess; normally the tympanic membrane is slightly concave. (Courtesy of Thomas H. Boyer.)

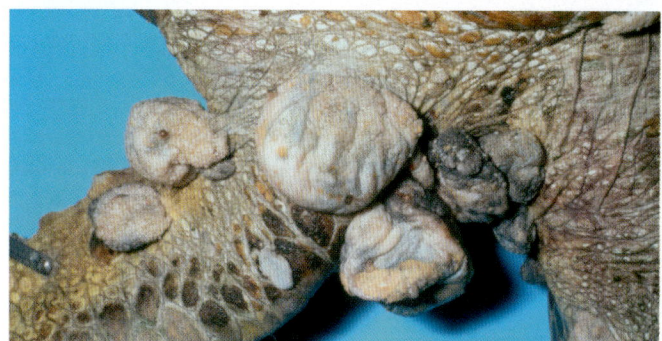

FIG 135.4 Fibropapillomas in sea turtles are thought to be caused by fibropapilloma-associated turtle herpesvirus (FPTHV) spread by marine leeches. (Courtesy of Thomas H. Boyer.)

contagious disease that causes pitting of the shell of aquatic turtles.[9] *Beneckea chitonovora*, a bacteria from shellfish, was thought to be the causative agent.[9] Septicemic cutaneous ulcerative disease causes irregular caseated crateriform ulcers (Fig. 135.8), especially on the ventral surfaces of aquatic turtles such as the softshell turtles.[2] Left untreated, septicemia, hepatic necrosis, paralysis, and death may ensue.[2] The etiologic agent was once thought to be *Citrobacter freundii*, yet poor husbandry and other gram-negative bacteria are undoubtedly involved.[2] Free-ranging desert tortoises can have cutaneous dyskeratosis with a high mortality rate.[10] Lesions commence at the seams and spread toward the middle of the scutes. Lesions are gray-white, sometimes orange, and have a roughened flaky appearance. The plastron is most heavily affected; nutritional deficiency or toxicity is suspected.

Fractures of the Shell

Shell fractures are the result of trauma from dogs, other vertebrate predators, large hoof stock, falls, automobiles, lawnmowers, or boats. Nutritional secondary hyperparathyroidism (NSHP) rarely predisposes to traumatic shell fractures; pathological folding fractures or deformity are more common.

Overgrown Rhamphotheca (Beak) and Toenails

Overgrowth of the rhamphotheca and toenails may indicate an underlying nutritional disease such as NSHP, protein deficiency, or excess. Lack of wear in captivity has been suggested as a cause, yet overgrowth is generally not a problem in captive turtles on balanced diets.[2] Elongated nails (but not rhamphotheca) on the front or rear feet (not both) is a normal secondary sex characteristic in some male chelonians (see Chapter 7).

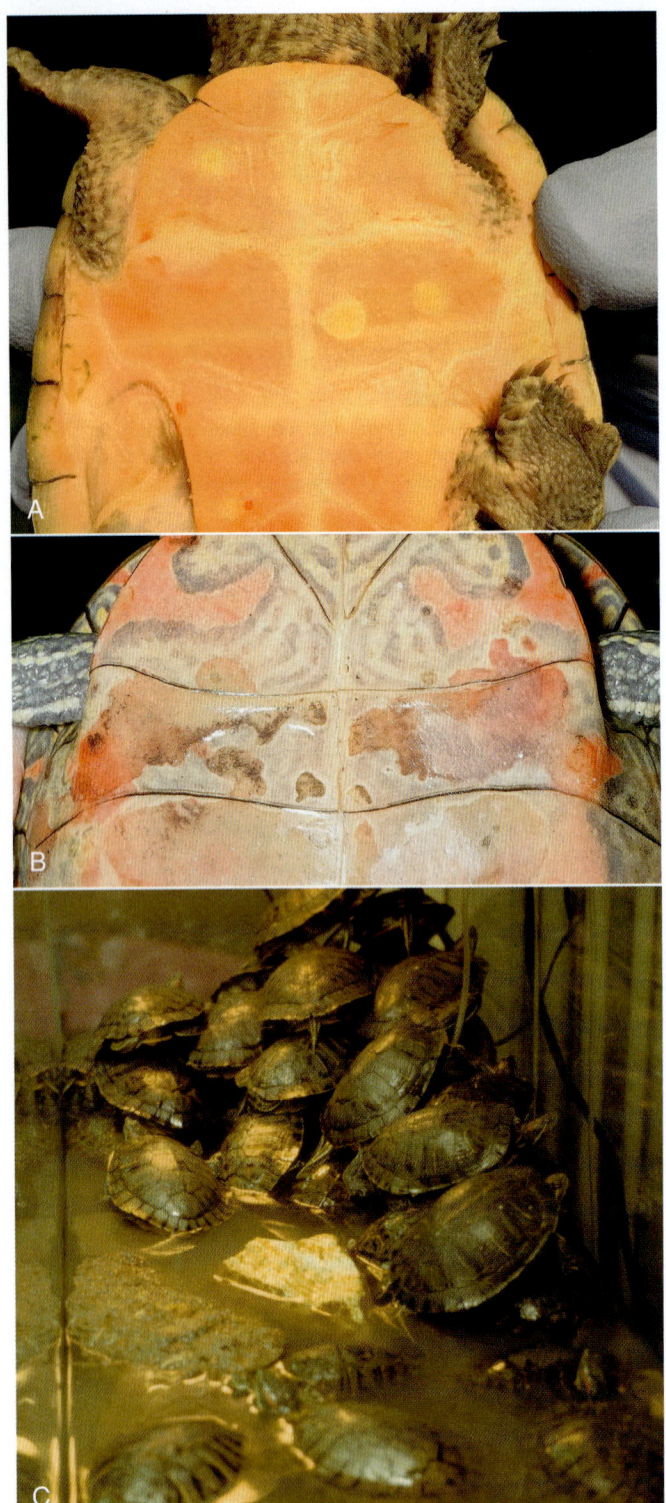

FIG 135.5 Bacterial shell disease (A and B) in aquatic turtles penetrates through the keratin scutes, resulting in osteomyelitis, typically related to unclean water (C). There should be no fluid, discoloration, or soft areas under the scutes of the shell. (Courtesy of Thomas H. Boyer.)

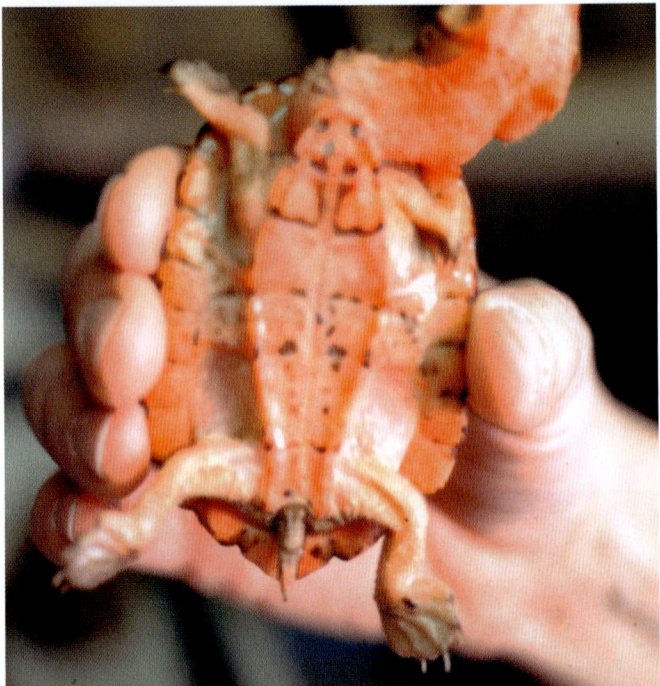

FIG 135.6 Many aquatic turtles have aposematic coloration ventrally, such as this Mata Mata (*Chelus fimbriata*), that fades as they age. This must not be confused with erythema. (Courtesy of Thomas H. Boyer.)

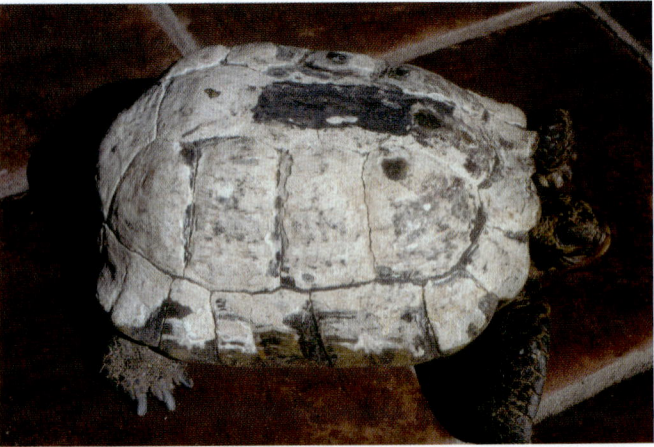

FIG 135.7 Fusarium infection causing superficial scute necrosis in a Texas tortoise (*Gopherus berlandieri*). (Courtesy of Thomas H. Boyer.)

of the few species that normally have soft shells, carapacial fenestrae, or shell kinesis (see Chapter 7).

Distorted Shell

A distorted shell may indicate pathologic fractures and is common with NSHP or healed fractures from previous trauma. NSHP can cause scoliosis of the plastron, lordosis, upturned marginals, increased vertical growth, especially apparent in the bridge area, narrowed or increased shell openings, or lack of shell growth, resulting in a shell that appears too small for the chelonian and often associated penile prolapse. Scute abnormalities can be congenital or the result of various metabolic bone diseases.

Pyramidal Shell Growth

The etiology of pyramidal shell growth remains unknown but is undoubtedly multifactorial. Juvenile tortoises are most often affected.

Soft Shell

A soft shell usually indicates NSHP (see Chapter 84), unless evidence of trauma or bacterial or fungal disease is present. Hatchling chelonians on an adequate ration should have a firm shell within the first few years. Shell should feel like solid bone, much like skull, with the exceptions

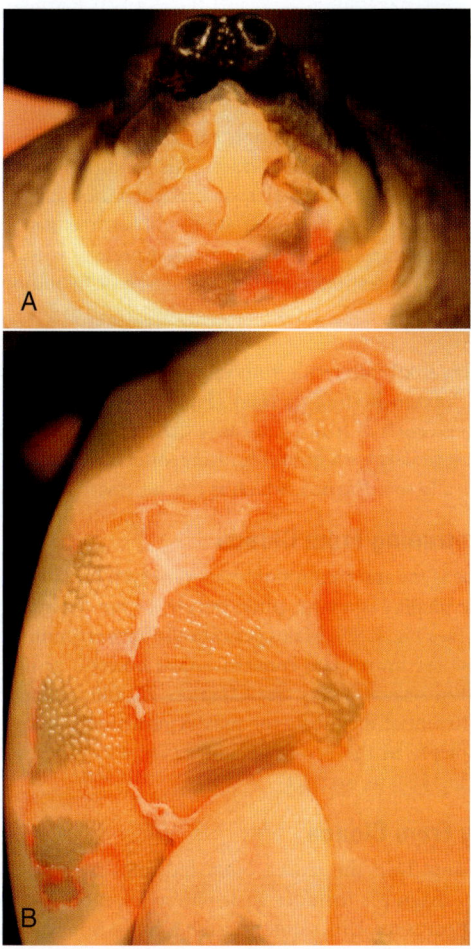

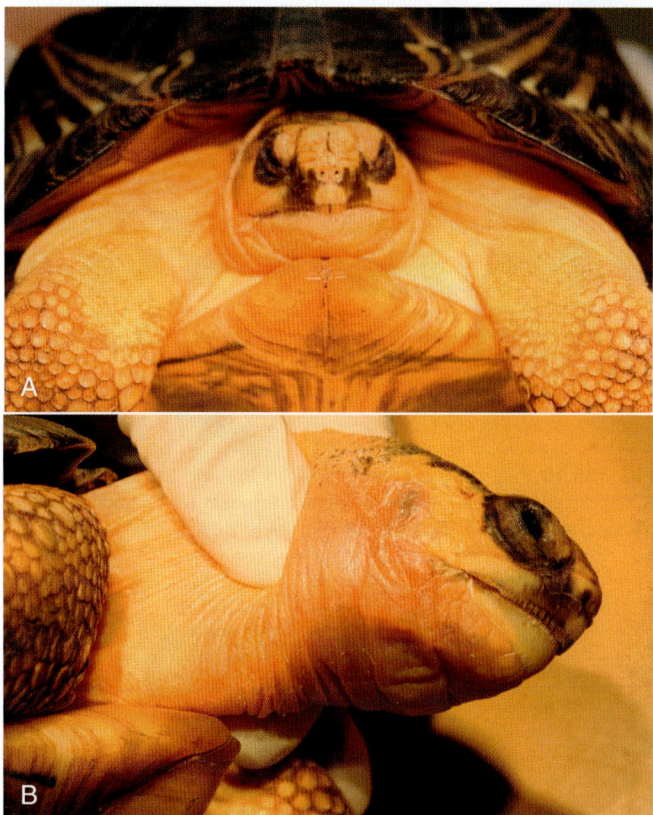

FIG 135.9 Goiter causing myxedema in a radiated tortoise (*Astrochelys radiata*), an unusual manifestation of intranuclear coccidiosis. Goiter is rare in tortoises. (Courtesy of Thomas H. Boyer.)

FIG 135.8 Septicemic cutaneous ulcerative disease in a Fly River turtle (*Carettochelys insculpta*). (Courtesy of Thomas H. Boyer.)

Suggested etiologies include NSHP, too-rapid growth, low humidity, continuous temperature maintenance (no nighttime temperature drop), and species predisposition but not protein excess.[11–13] For more information, see Chapter 27.

Dermal Fistulas

Trauma or myiasis can cause fistulas in the skin (see Cutaneous or Subcutaneous Swelling and Fig. 135.2A and B). Subcutaneous abscesses can also form fistulas.

Edema or Ascites

Edema can result from liver (e.g., hepatic lipidosis), kidney, or cardio-pulmonary disease, from vascular or lymphatic obstruction or hypo-proteinemia.[2] Obese chelonians often have excessive lipid deposition in the axial and prefemoral areas that may be confused with edema. Myxedema has been observed in chelonians (Fig. 135.9) with thyroid/thymus dysfunction (see Chapter 79).[2,14]

GASTROINTESTINAL SIGNS

Anorexia

Anorexia is a nonspecific sign of almost all chelonian illnesses. Some common causes include intestinal or colonic foreign bodies or impaction, NSHP, hepatic lipidosis, hypovitaminosis A, pneumonia, renal failure, low environmental temperature, parasites, and viral infections, especially herpesvirus and intranuclear coccidiosis. Acute bacterial infections can cause anorexia. Most chronic bacterial infections result in reduced

appetite but not complete anorexia. Winter anorexia is common in wild-caught species that normally hibernate.

Poor Body Condition

Emaciation generally indicates starvation from disease, poor husbandry, chronic mycoplasmosis, intranuclear coccidiosis, parasites, neoplasia, or any other debilitating condition.

Pale Tongue and Mucous Membranes

The oral cavity should normally be pale pink, with the tongue even pinker. Pale mucous membranes (Fig. 135.10) are often the result of anemia of chronic disease (especially poor nutrition), poor peripheral circulation in severely debilitated animals, or blood loss. Note that many chelonians normally have lower PCVs than other reptiles or vertebrates. When interpreting blood normal values, always compare them to reference or observed ranges for that species (or closely related species), if previous results from the same animal/cagemate are not available.

Infectious Stomatitis

Herpesvirus can cause necrotic caseous oropharyngeal stomatitis, glossitis, pharyngitis, and tracheitis (see Figs. 135.1A and B and 135.11, as well as Chapters 30 and 169). (e.g., Russian tortoises, *Agrionemys horsfieldii*) may remain latently infected. Herpes has been reported in a variety of tortoises and turtles; all terrestrial chelonians are considered susceptible. Other than herpesvirus, ranavirus, mycobacterial infections, infectious stomatitis is rare in chelonians.

Moisture or Dried Mucus on Rhamphotheca (Beak)

Any accumulation of material on the beak is abnormal and may signify oral infection (herpesvirus, see Fig. 135.10), pneumonia, regurgitation,

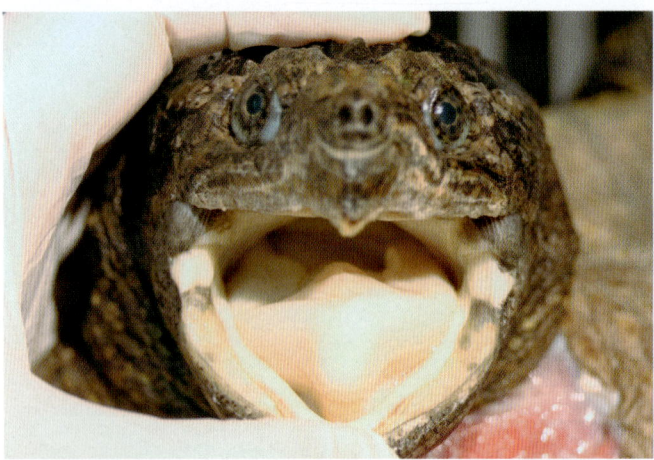

FIG 135.10 Pale mucous membranes in a common snapping turtle (*Chelydra serpentina*). Oral examination is an essential component of the physical examination. (Courtesy of Thomas H. Boyer.)

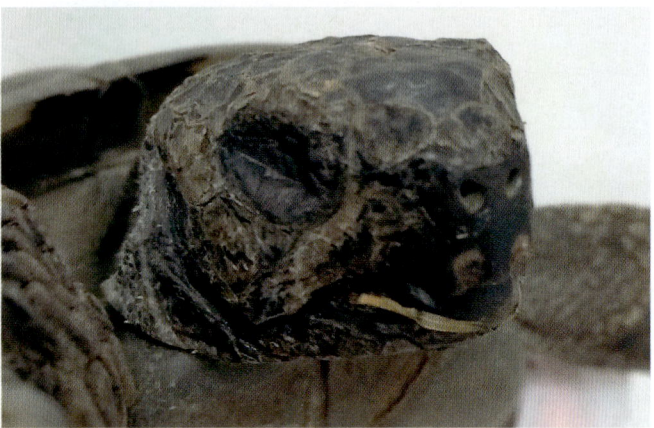

FIG 135.11 Sunken eyes (dehydration) and oral mucus discharge (note the grass stuck to the mandible) are suspicious for herpesvirus infection. *Testudo* tortoises may be carriers of herpesvirus. This long-term captive tortoise developed an active herpesvirus infection during hibernation. (Courtesy of Thomas H. Boyer.)

ulceration, irritation from a foreign body,[15] broken jaw, or a cracked, overgrown, or misshapen rhamphotheca (see Overgrown Rhamphotheca [Beak] and Toenails earlier in this chapter).

Constipation

Chelonians typically defecate daily to every few days. Constipation can arise from small intestinal or, more commonly, colonic impactions, as a result of ingested foreign bodies, such as sand, gravel, rocks, cage litter, or yard debris. Fine sand and crushed gravel are of particular concern. Most tortoises often have a few stones in the gastrointestinal tract that pass uneventfully. Cystic calculi, low environmental temperature, and parasites are less common causes of constipation.

Emesis/Regurgitation

Parasites, foreign bodies, septicemia, and adverse drug reactions can cause regurgitation.[12] The author has seen several chelonians that vomited within 30 minutes of administration of enrofloxacin or vitamin A at normal dosages. Differential diagnoses should include causes of vomiting typical for other animals. Ptyalism, oronasal fluid regurgitation, and vomiting are commonly found in tortoises with intestinal/colonic impactions (Fig. 135.12A).[16] Tortoises may also present for acute and repeated emesis after ingestion of toadstools (species not determined; Jarchow JL, personal communication, 2001).

Bloating

Excessive intestinal gas production can result from fermentation of food within the gastrointestinal tract. This condition can result from an abrupt change to protein-rich or carbohydrate-rich foods; force-feeding sick chelonians inappropriate foods (such as dairy products) or excessive volumes to cachexic animals, especially with suboptimal temperatures; or intestinal/colonic obstruction or hypomotility.[2]

Diarrhea

Loose, watery stools can result from various parasites, bacterial or fungal infections, foreign bodies, or food (Fig. 135.13). Foods with a high water content, such as fruits, can cause diarrhea. For tortoises, lack of roughage, especially with indoor housing, often results in more watery stools, typically semiformed, which is not necessarily abnormal.

Mass Protruding From Cloaca

The phallus is the most common mass observed protruding from the cloaca. The phallus is a large pink, purple, or tan mass with a spade-shaped tip (see Fig. 7.32). Males periodically have erections that should be no cause for immediate concern unless necrotic or if it does not retract within several hours. See Chapters 75, 106, and 143 for more details. Differential diagnosis for masses protruding from the cloaca include prolapse of the urinary bladder (Fig. 135.14A), cloaca, colon (see Fig. 135.14B), or oviduct.[2]

Bleeding From Cloaca

Blood passing from the cloaca often indicates a phallus laceration. Differential diagnosis includes gastrointestinal, urogenital, or cloacal bleeding or parasites. Urocystoliths can be passed from the bladder and lodge in the proctodeum.[17] Cloacaliths have been seen in several tortoise species (Fig. 135.15A and B).

Dilated Cloaca

Urocystoliths can be passed from the bladder and lodge in the proctodeum for extended time and either pass on their own or must be physically broken down and extracted. This extended dilation of the proctodeum may result in a permanently dilated cloaca or slow reduction over many months (see Fig. 135.15C and D).

RESPIRATORY SIGNS

Nasal Discharge

Any nasal discharge, wet or dried, is abnormal in chelonians unless associated with drinking or eating watery foods. Pressure applied on the gular area should not elicit any nasal discharge nor should forcing the head posteriorly into the shell (Fig. 135.16A). Several species of *Mycoplasma* cause upper respiratory tract disease in a variety of chelonians[18] (see Chapter 72). All terrestrial chelonians should be considered susceptible. Clinical signs include clear to white discharge or bubbling from the nares, rhinitis, ocular discharge, conjunctivitis, mild palpebral edema, decreased to no appetite, lethargy, and weight loss, without lesions in the mouth. Nasal discharge may be wiped onto the forelimbs and build up (see Fig. 135.16B).

Several other maladies can cause nasal discharge, including herpesvirus (see Figs. 135.1A and B, 135.10, and 135.12B), ranavirus, adenovirus, intranuclear coccidiosis, chlamydiosis, reovirus, paramyxovirus, foreign bodies (see Fig. 135.12C and D), and oronasal fistulas (see Fig. 135.12E). Multiple deaths are common with viruses and intranuclear coccidiosis but atypical for mycoplasmosis. After mycoplasmosis, herpesvirus is the next most common cause of nasal discharge and almost always also

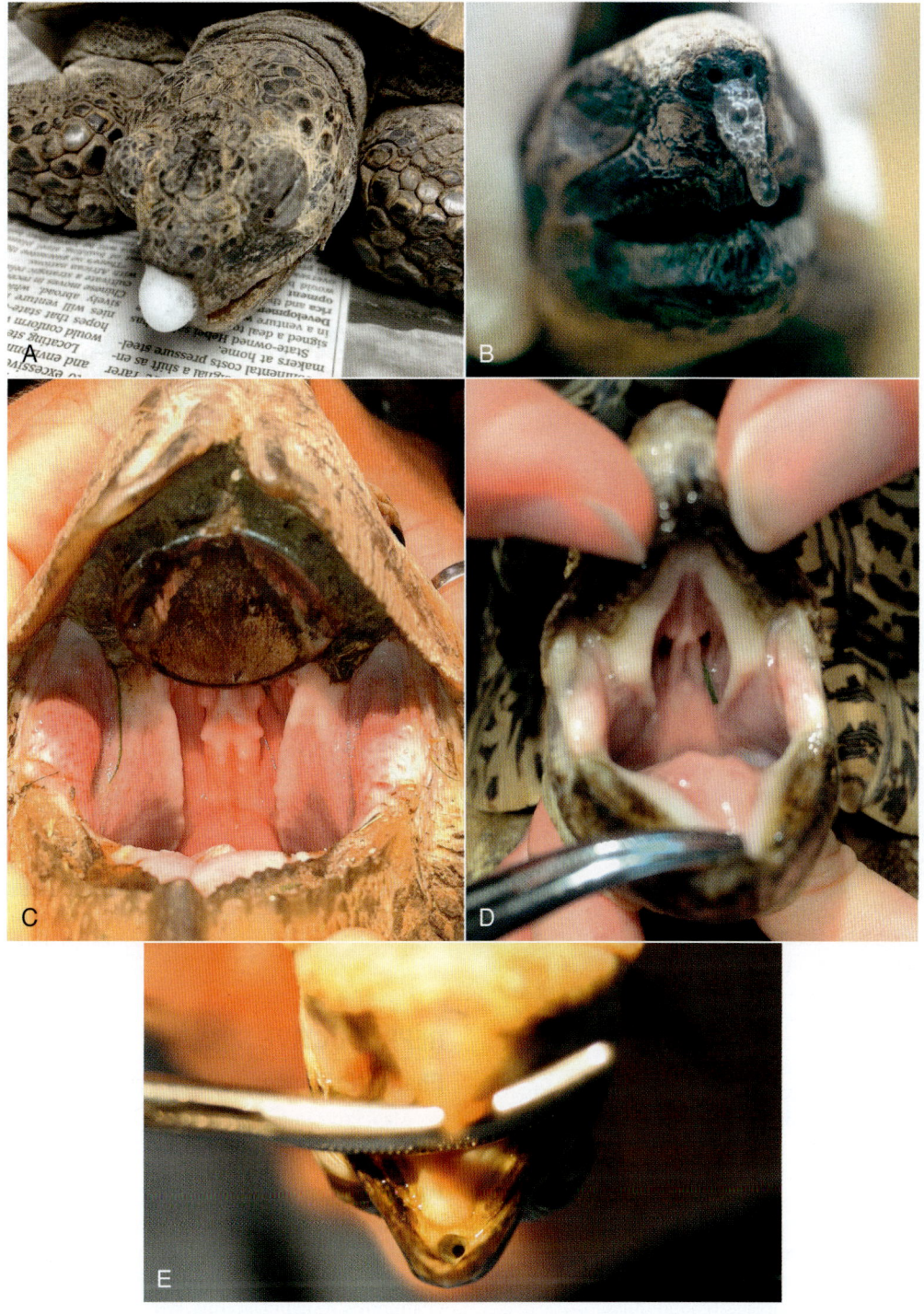

FIG 135.12 Nasal discharge is often the result of mycoplasmosis, but in this case (A) resulted from gastric reflux secondary to colonic foreign body obstruction. The differential diagnoses of nasal discharge also includes herpesvirus (B) (see Fig. 135.1A and B), ranavirus, adenovirus, intranuclear coccidiosis, chlamydiosis, reovirus, paramyxovirus, oral foreign bodies (C, bottle cap; D, blade of grass in choanae), and (E) oronasal fistulas. (Courtesy of Thomas H. Boyer.)

has whitish plaques in the oral cavity (see Chapter 30). Gastric reflux can also cause oronasal discharge (see Fig. 135.12A), and radiography can help exclude colonic obstruction.

Nasal Abnormalities

Chronic upper respiratory tract disease may erode or depigment the nares (Fig. 135.17 and Nasal Discharge section).[15] Chronic upper

respiratory tract disease, NSHP in young growing tortoises, and mycobacteriosis may cause the area around the nares to bulge asymmetrically, much like atrophic rhinitis in swine (see Fig. 135.16B).

Dyspnea and Abnormal Breath Sounds

Dyspneic turtles may stretch the neck and gape their mouth with obvious labored breathing (Fig. 135.18) or pump the head and legs. Movement of

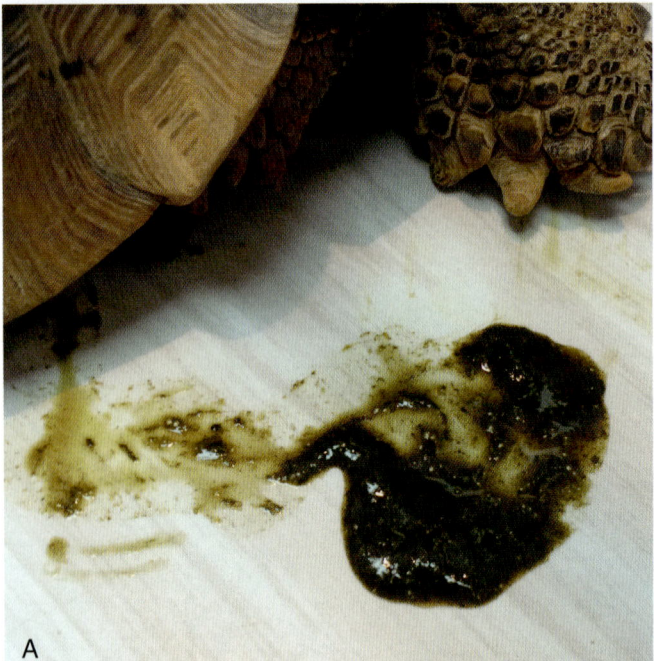

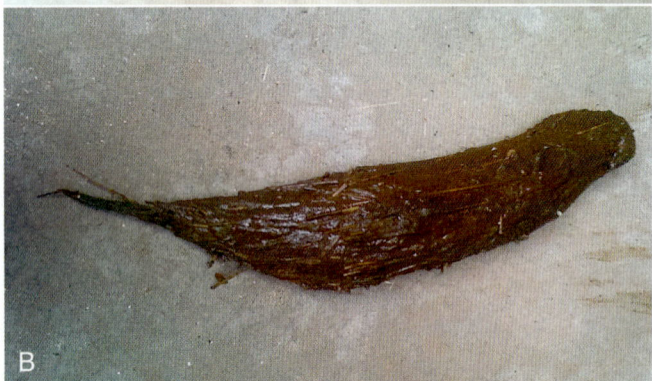

FIG 135.13 Diarrhea in a tortoise (A) compared with a normal stool from a tortoise on a high-fiber grass diet (B). (Courtesy of Thomas H. Boyer.)

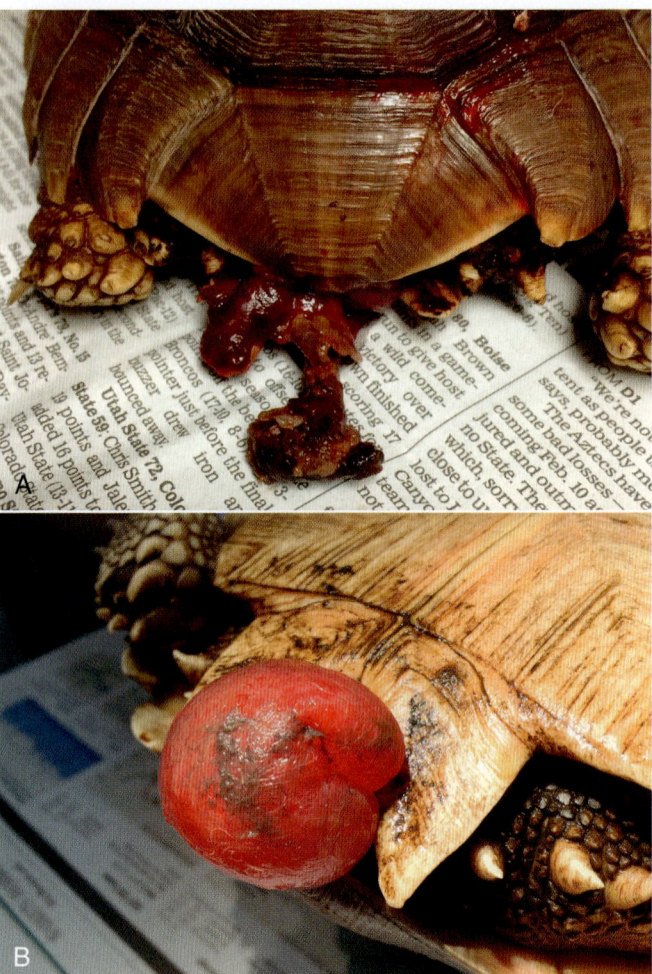

FIG 135.14 Prolapsed bladder (A) and colon (B) in African spurred tortoises (*Centrochelys sulcata*). (Courtesy of Thomas H. Boyer.)

the head and limbs is a normal part of respiration in most chelonians but becomes more pronounced with dyspnea. Gular pumping is associated with olfaction and is not a sign of dyspnea, although some aquatic turtles supplement respiration by buccopharyngeal pumping (bimodal respiration). Dyspnea or abnormal breath sounds, such as a click or slight whistle, usually indicate a lower respiratory tract infection or glottal/tracheal obstruction. Bacteria, particularly gram-negative bacteria, are the most common culprit. Other causes include fungal, viral, or parasitic disease; aspirated tracheal foreign bodies; or neoplasia, such as a tracheal chondromas.

Uneven Floating

Aquatic turtles normally float level from side-to-side but not front-to-back. As material accumulates in a pneumonic lung, the lung becomes heavier and the turtle lists (Fig. 135.19).[2] Any unilateral mass, such as an abscess, tumor, cystourolith, intestinal/colonic foreign bodies, or asymmetrical gas production, as with bloating, can cause similar signs.

Inability to Submerge

Emaciation, pneumonia, tumors, or gas accumulation within the coelom or gastrointestinal tract (from infection, trauma, or obstruction) may cause aquatic turtles to lose the ability to submerge. This is a common problem in sea turtles.

REPRODUCTIVE SIGNS

Phallus Prolapse or Mass Protruding From Cloaca

See Mass Protruding from Cloaca earlier in this chapter (and Chapters 75 and 143).

Failure to Lay Eggs

Nutritional factors or improper husbandry (e.g., stressors, lack of nesting site) should be considered primary to all reproductive failures. Chelonians often fail to lay eggs because of NSHP, hypovitaminosis A, hypocalcemia, dehydration, or lack of an appropriate nesting area. Indoors, females may be reluctant to lay eggs if the substrate is not deep enough (should be twice the length of the carapace). A ruptured, large, or anomalous egg (Fig. 135.20); oviductal rupture; infection; or any mass impinging on the oviduct, such as a urolith, fecalith, or colonic foreign bodies, can also lead to egg retention.[2] Eggs may also become ectopically located in the urinary bladder, coelom, or colon, or lodged in the pelvis. See Chapter 80 for more details.

Mass in Coelom

The differential diagnoses for coelomic masses include ova, eggs, cystic calculi, intestinal or colonic foreign bodies, neoplasia, and abscesses.

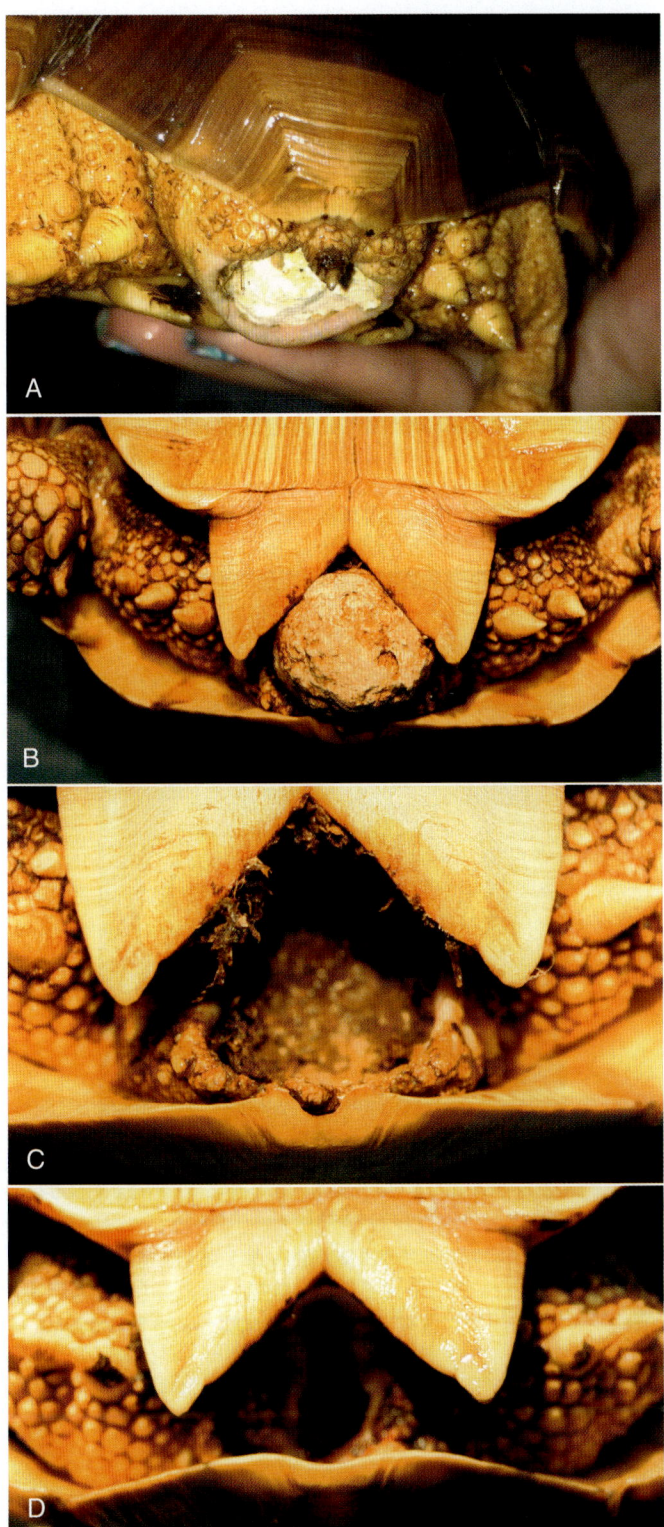

FIG 135.15 Cloacaliths (A and B) can cause constipation and cloacal dilation. In this African spurred tortoise (*Centrochelys sulcata*), note (C) the dilated cloaca and impacted feces immediately after removal and (D) persistent dilation more than a month later. (Courtesy of Thomas H. Boyer.)

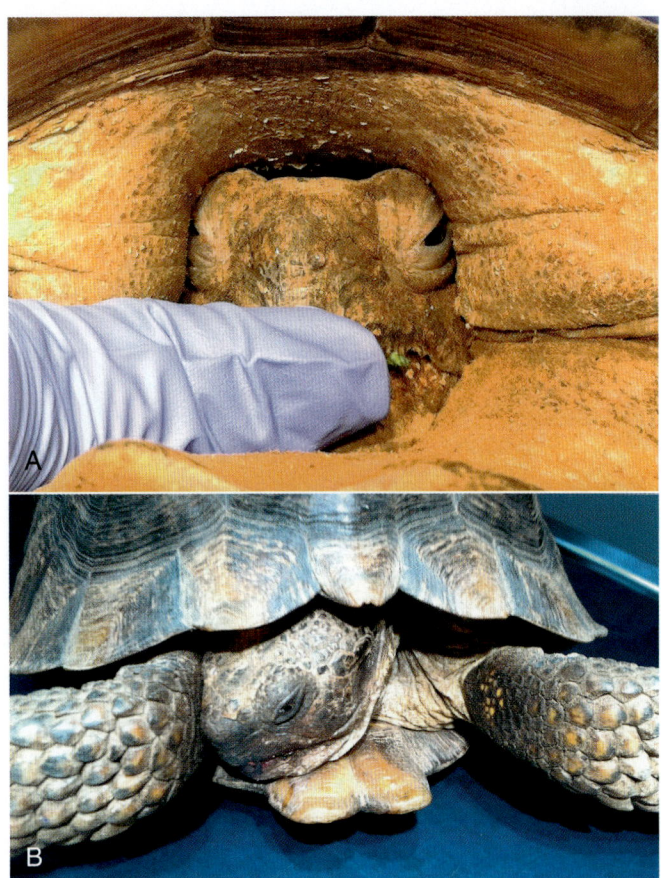

FIG 135.16 Nasal discharge, often a sign of mycoplasmosis, should always be considered abnormal in chelonians (A); note how this tortoise is wiping nasal discharge onto the front right leg (B). (Courtesy of Thomas H. Boyer.)

MUSCULOSKELETAL SIGNS

Lameness

Lameness can result from abscesses, bite wounds, foreign bodies, fractures, osteomyelitis, luxations (Fig. 135.21), trauma, gout, pseudogout, or sepsis and, in females, as a short-term sequela to egg laying and imbalances in calcium homeostasis. Egg retention, cystic calculi, cloacaliths, or constipation can contribute to lameness. One should always consider nutritional or renal secondary hyperparathyroidism as a potential cause of lameness. Large breeding males can traumatize a limb from abruptly dismounting a female.

Asymmetrical Toenail Wear

Uneven wear of the toenails may be associated with lameness in terrestrial species.[15] Be aware of normal secondary sex characteristics (see Sexual Dimorphism in Chapter 7).

Swollen Joints

Joint swelling can result from nutritional disorders, infection, luxation, fracture, articular or periarticular gout, pseudogout, or calcinosis circumscripts.[2,3]

Swollen Long Bones

Long bone swelling can result from healed or healing fractures, neoplasia, osteomyelitis, or fibrous osteodystrophy. Fibrous osteodystrophy, so common in lizards with NSHP, is rare in chelonians.

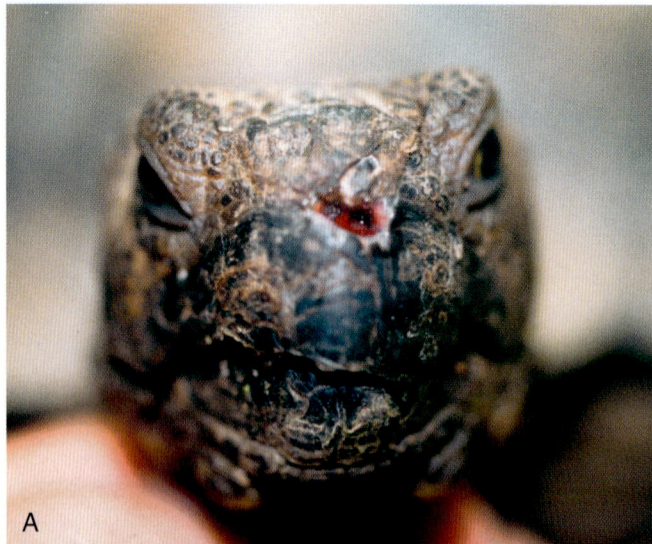

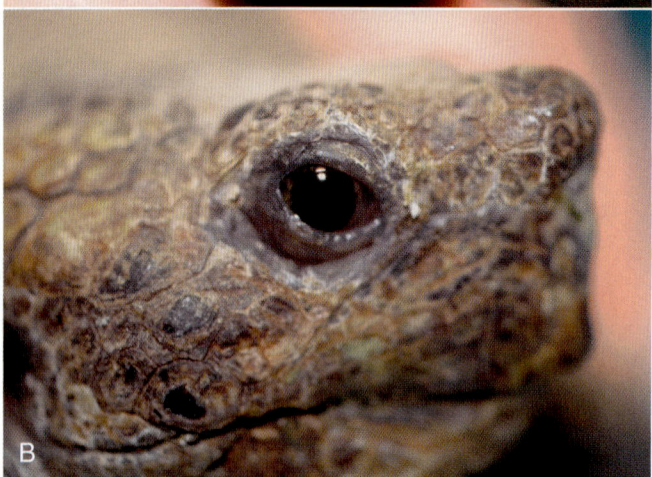

FIG 135.17 Erosion of the nares (A) and bulbous distortion of the nares (B) in desert tortoises (*Gopherus* spp.) with chronic mycoplasmosis. (Courtesy of Thomas H. Boyer.)

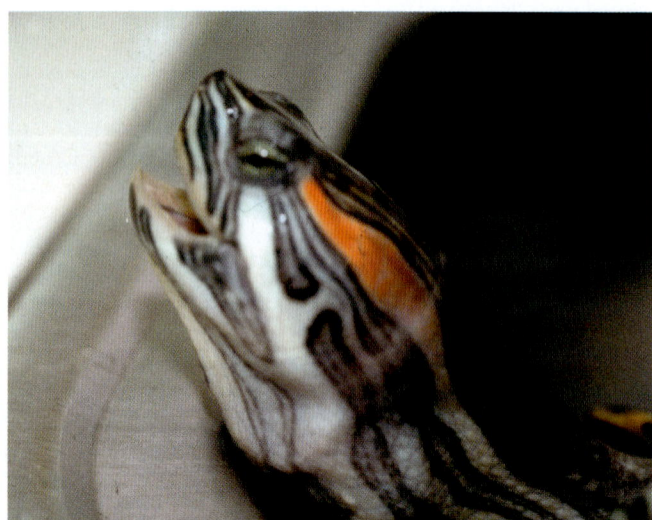

FIG 135.18 Open-mouthed breathing as seen in this red eared slider (*Trachemys scripta elegans*) is abnormal in chelonians and often indicates lower respiratory tract disease if no oronasal symptoms are present. (Courtesy of Thomas H. Boyer.)

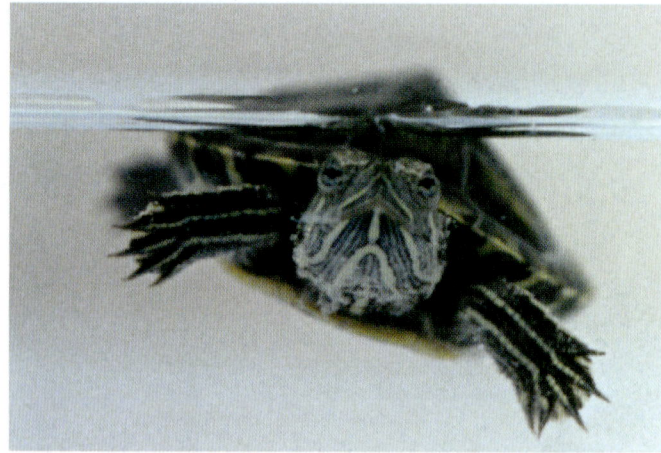

FIG 135.19 Listing laterally is often a sign of pneumonia in aquatic turtles; any unilateral mass or gas production can also cause turtles to list. (Courtesy of Thomas H. Boyer.)

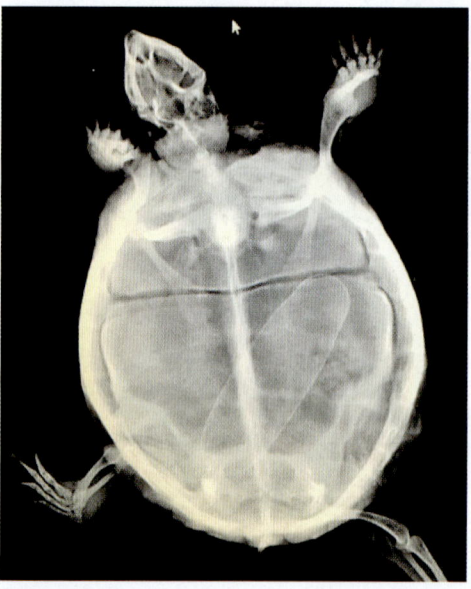

FIG 135.20 Ruptured, or large and anomalous eggs as noted in this radiograph of a box turtle (*Terrapene* sp.) are one of many potential causes of failure to lay. (Courtesy of Brian Loudis.)

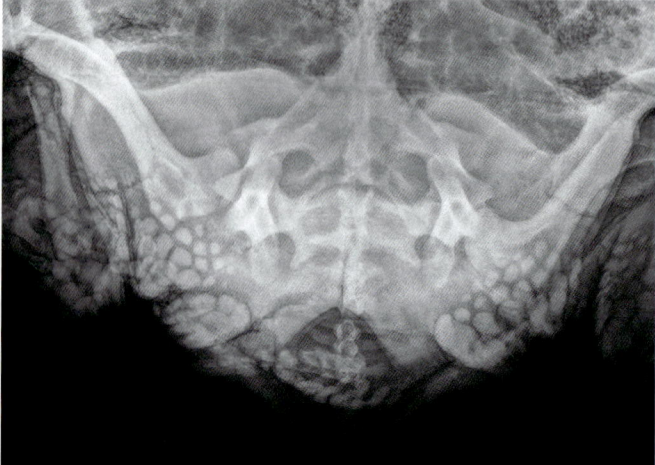

FIG 135.21 Coxofemoral luxation in a Burmese black giant tortoise (*Manouria emys phayrei*), which caused unilateral left rear limb lameness and responded well to femoral head removal. Radiographs, preferably under anesthesia to allow full leg extension, are important to determine the cause of lameness in chelonians. (Courtesy of Thomas H. Boyer.)

Temporal Muscle Atrophy

The temporal muscles are normally prominent with no visible occipital crest. Poor body condition may cause noticeable atrophy of the temporal muscles.[15,19]

NEUROLOGICAL SIGNS

Ataxia/Hypermetric Gait

Severe ataxia and a hypermetic gait have been observed in desert tortoises after episodes of hyperthermia, near-drowning, or joint luxation. Cerebellar injury may be present perhaps as a result of hypoxia, cerebral edema, or encephalitis. Toxin exposure, including the iatrogenic use of ivermectin or organophosphates in mite and tick sprays or the ingestion of toxins such as heavy metals, may also cause neurological signs.

Circling

Circling can be a sequela to freezing during hibernation (see Blindness), toxemia, septicemia, encephalitis, central nervous system damage, or hepatic encephalopathy.[20]

Flaccid Paresis, Paralysis, or Coma

A comatose turtle could have severe systemic illness, such as septicemia, organ failure, end-stage starvation, or be dead. Other less common causes include toxicity to ivermectin, Rhododendrons or other substances, shock, drowning, asphyxiation, hyperthermia, or bloat.[4] If it is uncertain whether the chelonian is still alive, check for a heart beat or pulse with a Doppler ultrasound, echocardiography, or electrocardiogram.

Hind-Limb Paresis

Chelonians can present with hind-limb paresis from the same causes as lameness, as well as from spinal cord damage.

OCULAR SIGNS

Blindness

Blindness has been reported in *Testudo* spp. after freezing and may be associated with hyphema, vitreal haze, lenticular opacities, and retinal damage.[20] Additional symptoms include anorexia, head tilt, circling, or holding the head high. Blindness from other causes is possible but not commonly seen.

Palpebra Edema

Palpebra edema may indicate hypovitaminosis A. Emaciated or dehydrated turtles, such as with herpesvirus infection, also tend to keep their eyes shut, but the globe is more sunken. The differential diagnosis can include trauma, foreign bodies, bacterial or viral infection (often with concurrent respiratory disease), parasites, or metabolic disturbances.[2] Box turtles may hold one eye shut due to aural abscess that may, or may not, be advanced enough to cause tympanic swelling. Ulcers, panophthalmitis, or fire ant stings can also cause blepharospasm.

Exophthalmia

Unilateral exophthalmia may result from retrobulbar abscess, tumor, or injury. Bilateral exophthalmia may result from vascular obstruction or generalized edema.[15] See Palpebra Edema section as well.

Enophthalmia

Bilateral enophthalmia (sunken eyes) can indicate microphthalmia; thiamine deficiency, especially with a diet of frozen fish rich in thiaminases[2]; emaciation or dehydration due to a myriad of chronic conditions, including herpesvirus infection (see Figs. 135.11 and 135.12B); or circulatory collapse (hypotension) in septic or debilitated chelonians. The eyes often sink into the orbit before death. Unilateral enophthalmia may result from orbital injury (particularly automobile trauma) or phthisis bulbi.[15]

Conjunctivitis and Ocular Discharge

Discharge from the eyes can accompany upper respiratory tract disease (see Nasal Discharge section under Respiratory Signs), ocular irritants, and hypovitaminosis A.[2] Sea turtles, red foot (*Chelonoidis carbonaria*), and yellow foot (*C. denticulata*) tortoises normally have a clear ocular discharge because they lack lacrimal ducts.

REFERENCES

See www.expertconsult.com for a complete list of references.

136

Differential Diagnoses by Clinical Signs—Crocodilians

Javier G. Nevarez

STRESS AND IMMUNOSUPPRESSION

Stress and immunosuppression are often underlying factors for many diseases affecting captive crocodilians. Stress has been defined as "a physiological answer to a perceived threat that includes, but is not restricted to, increased adrenal secretion."[1] Stress is also thought of as any event that challenges homeostasis, and likely the response to that challenge involves more than an adrenal response. The autonomic nervous system, the hypothalamic adrenal axis, neuropeptides, neurotransmitters, and neuroimmunologic mediators all have a role in the response of the immune system to stress.[2] Studies in crocodilians have evaluated the stress associated with restraint, long-term corticosterone implants, cold shock, and stocking densities.[3–6] Lance et al. provide an overview of the physiology and endocrinology of stress in crocodilians.[7] Catecholamines, glucocorticoids, glucose, and lactate have been implicated in the stress response of crocodilians. In addition, an argument is made for immunosuppression on the basis of changes observed in the white blood cells.[3–5,7] Factors that influence stress in crocodilian and reptile species are reviewed by Rooney and Guillette.[1] Enough evidence exists to suggest that stress plays an important role in the physiology of crocodilians, and it may indeed predispose them to illness. Overcrowding, handling, excessive noise, diet changes, water and air quality, temperature irregularities, and more should all be considered as predisposing or confounding factors of disease.

SYSTEMIC SIGNS

Anorexia, Lethargy, and Acute Mortalities

The first signs of illness in captive crocodilians are usually nonspecific in nature. These include anorexia, lethargy, and death. In commercial operations, the workers may notice excess food remaining from the day before, which is sometimes followed by a perceived change in the behavior of the animals. One should not underestimate these observations because most workers are well tuned to the daily routine and behavior of the animals. A visit to the ranch or farm should be performed during feeding time to avoid additional stress to the animals. This also allows observation of the feeding and water change practices. At this time, a thorough history and a collection of animals for diagnostics and necropsy can be obtained. In addition to routine samples, tissues should be frozen for possible bacterial, fungal, or viral cultures.

The list of differentials for nonspecific clinical signs must be narrowed after diagnostic results are obtained. However, one must remember that husbandry and disease go hand in hand. Most systemic diseases of captive crocodilians are thought to be secondary in nature. Bacterial and fungal diseases are commonly encountered. The majority of data available on bacterial disease in crocodilians are from studies involving the American alligator (*Alligator mississippiensis*). Table 136.1 presents a large number of isolates from diseased and nondiseased animals, including a survey of fecal coliforms.[8] Huchzermeyer et al. also have extensive data on enteric bacterial and fungal isolates from African Dwarf Crocodiles (Osteolaemus tetraspis).[9] Important bacterial infections reported in crocodilians include *Mycoplasma alligatoris*,[10] *Mycoplasma crocodyli*,[11] and *Chlamydia* spp.

Fungal organisms are often opportunistic invaders of the integument and respiratory system, but primary fungal infections are also reported. Viral diseases are likely underdiagnosed in reptile medicine because of the challenges in diagnostic techniques and scarce information. Poxvirus, West Nile virus (WNV), and herpesvirus have been reported as pathogens in crocodilians. An adenovirus-like infection in captive Nile Crocodiles (*Crocodylus niloticus*) has also been reported.[12] Coronavirus, influenza C virus, and paramyxovirus have been identified with transmission electron microscope in the feces of crocodilians, but their significance remains to be determined. Finally, evidence exists of seroconversion to paramyxovirus and eastern equine encephalitis virus in crocodilians.[13]

Toxicities are not common in captive crocodilians. Lead toxicity is reported from alligators fed lead-shot nutria. Clinical signs include weakness, lethargy, anorexia, and death. Feeding of nutria is no longer common practice.

For privately owned and zoo animals, there are additional differentials to be considered. A faulty or broken heater can lead to sudden death from electrocution. This can also present a risk for humans, therefore, it is important to isolate, protect, and inspect all equipment within the enclosure. A thermostat malfunction can lead to altered water temperatures that can affect the animal's behavior. In colder climates, animals may become lethargic if the heater is not working properly. Conversely, if a thermostat fails, allowing the heater to remain on, the animals' behavior may change because of increased temperatures. At first they may appear agitated but eventually anorexia and lethargy will occur if overheated. Overheating may also occur as a result of inappropriately sized or placed heat lamps.

Foreign bodies should be a differential for anorexic crocodilians, especially those in outdoor exhibits where trash, coins, and other objects may be tossed in by the public. It is also important to pick up and secure all tools such as buckets and hoses, which may also be ingested by animals.

Physiological anorexia can be observed as part of the normal reproductive cycle, in particular during the later stages of egg development. However, dystocia (egg binding) can lead to a more prolonged anorexia that may be the first indication that the animal is ill. Unless the actual mating date is known or the reproductive cycle is monitored by ultrasonography, it can be very difficult to ascertain what constitutes true dystocia. In animals housed outdoors in their natural climate, dystocia should be considered if oviposition has not occurred for 30 days past the expected date. For those housed indoors or outside their

TABLE 136.1   Bacteria Isolated From *Alligator Mississippiensis* With and Without Signs of Disease

Isolate	Tissue	Clinical Signs/ Lesions	Isolate	Tissue	Clinical Signs/ Lesions
Aeromonas hydrophila	Blood[34]	Yes	Klebsiella oxytoca	Skin[55]	Yes
	Lungs, heart, liver, kidneys, intestines, oral cavity[49]	Yes, No		Oral cavity[53]	No
			Klebsiella sp.	Lungs[25]	Yes
	Lungs, blood[50]	Yes	Klebsiella pneumonia	Cloaca[9]	No
	Eye[51, 52]	Yes	Micrococcus kristinae	Blood[34]	Yes
	Oral cavity, water[53]	No	Moraxella sp.	Oral cavity, water[53]	No
	Cloaca[8]	No	Morganella morganii	Blood[55]	Yes
Aeromonas sp.	Lungs[10]	Yes		Oral cavity[53]	No
Acinetobacter calcoaceticus	Oral cavity[53]	No		Lung[10]	Yes
Aerobacter radiobacter	Oral cavity[53]	No		Cloaca[8]	No
Bacteroides asaccharolyticus	Oral cavity[53]	No	Mycoplasma alligatoris	Multiple tissues[34]	Yes
Bacteroides bivius	Oral cavity, water[53]	No	Pantoea spp.	Cloaca[8]	No
Bacteroides loescheii/denticola	Oral cavity, water[53]	No	Pasteurella haemolytica	Oral cavity[53]	No
Bacteroides oralis	Oral cavity[53]	No	Pasteurella multocida	Lungs[56]	Yes
Bacteroides sordellii	Oral cavity[53]	No	Pasteurella pneumotropica	Cloaca[9]	No
Bacteroides thetaiotamicron	Oral cavity[53]	No	Pasteurella sp.	Oral cavity, water[53]	No
Bacteroides vulgatus	Oral cavity[53]	No	Peptococcus magnus	Oral cavity[53]	No
Bacteroides sp.	Water[53]	No	Peptococcus prevotii	Oral cavity[53]	No
Citrobacter freundii	Blood[55]	Yes	Pleisomonas shigelloides	Cloaca[9]	No
	Oral cavity[53]	No	Proteus mirabilis	Blood[34]	Yes
	cloaca[8]	No	Proteus vulgaris	Oral cavity[53]	No
Citrobacter braakii	Cloaca[8]	No		Oviduct[54]	Yes
Clostridium bifermentans	Oral cavity, water[53]	No		Blood[34]	Yes
	Lungs[10]	Yes		Lung[10]	Yes
Clostridium clostridioforme	Oral cavity[53]	No	Proteus sp.	Blood[55]	Yes
Clostridium innoculum	Water[53]	No	Providencia alcalifaciens	Cloaca[9]	No
Clostridium limosum	Oral cavity[53]	No	Providencia rettgeri	Cloaca[8]	No
Clostridium sordellii	Oral cavity, water[53]	No	Pseudomonas cepacia	Oral cavity[53]	No
Clostridium sporogenes	Blood[10]	Yes	Pseudomonas diminuta	Water[53]	No
Clostridium tetani	Oral cavity[53]	No	Pseudomonas fluorescens	Water[53]	No
Clostridium sp.	Blood[10]	Yes	Pseudomonas pickettii	Oral cavity[53]	No
Corynebacterium sp.	Tail abscess[50]	Yes	Pseudomonas vesicularis	Water[53]	No
Diphtheroid sp.	Oral cavity[53]	No	Pseudomonas sp.	Lungs, pharynx[50]	Yes
Edwardsiella tarda	Kidney, feces[54]	Yes		Water[53]	No
	Fat body, pericardial fluid[10]	Yes	Salmonella typhimurium	Gastrointestinal tract[50]	Yes
	Cloaca[9]	No	Salmonella braenderup, anatum Arizona spp.	Cloaca[50]	No
Edwardsiella aerogenes	Cloaca[8]	No	Salmonella sp. (subgroup III)	Lung[57]	Yes
Enterobacter aggiomerans	Blood[55]	Yes	Serratia marcescens	Skin[55]	Yes
Enterobacter cloacae	Oral cavity, water[53]	No		Cloaca[9]	No
	Cloaca[8]	No	Serratia odorifera	Oral cavity[53]	No
Enterobacillus sp.	Lungs[50]	Yes	Staphylococcus aureus	Lungs[56]	Yes
Escherichia coli	Cloaca[8]	No	Staphylococcus cohnii	Blood[34]	Yes
Fusobacterium nucleatum	Oral cavity[53]	No	Streptococcus sp., hemolytic	Lungs[10]	Yes
Fusobacterium varium	Oral cavity[53]	No	Vibrio parahaemolyticus	Blood[34]	Yes
Hafnia alvei	Cloaca[8]	No	Vibrio cholerae, putative	Cloaca[8]	No
			Vibrio fluvialis	Cloaca[8]	No

natural climate, behavior together with plasma biochemistry, hematology, and diagnostic imaging can be used to aid in the diagnosis of dystocia.

Secondary nutritional hyperparathyroidism can also cause animals to be lethargic and anorexic. This is more common in juvenile animals. Older animals may succumb to secondary renal hyperparathyroidism.

Poor Growth and Runting

Another phenomenon seen in captive crocodilian operations is runting, the lack of growth and failure to thrive of some animals within a group. In some operations, animals are separated by size and some buildings contain only the runts. A clear size difference is observed in same-age animals between the runts and the otherwise healthy ones. These animals are not as hardy in the captive environment and are potentially more susceptible to disease. Dominance by other animals, environment, and even incubation factors[14] contribute to the presence of runts.

DERMATOLOGICAL SIGNS

Integumentary disease is often secondary to poor water quality, poor enclosure design, stress, and immunosuppression or a combination of these factors. Lacerations, abscesses, and draining tracts can all be observed in captive and wild crocodilians. Consequently, these open wounds can serve as a nidus for bacteria and fungi. An additional factor in commercial operations or small enclosures is the accumulation of a fatty slime layer on the surface of the water when meat supplements, in particular chicken, are fed in addition to a dry commercial diet. This slime attaches to the skin of the animals and the enclosure, creating an environment for bacterial and fungal growth. The same is true for accumulation of biofilm on the surface of the enclosure. A soap or detergent can be used as a surfactant to help reduce the fatty layer on the water surface. Any product used must be nontoxic, or the animals must be removed from the enclosure while in use. Fungal dermatitis is also common because many fungi thrive in the water column and environment of captive alligators. In most instances, both bacteria and fungi are present in skin lesions. Culture and sensitivity testing can be frustrating in these cases because of the mixed flora found in the lesions. The first step in addressing integumentary abnormalities is to analyze water quality and make improvements as needed. In addition to improvements in water quality, antimicrobial or antifungal therapy may be necessary. Medicating a large group of crocodilians is challenging because it must usually be done orally by mixing the medication with feed. In zoos or private collections, individual crocodilians can be medicated by injecting the prey item or via injection. A pole syringe can be used in large or aggressive animals. There is a lack of pharmacokinetic data for oral antimicrobials in crocodilians, and it has been shown that oral tetracycline is not effectively absorbed in American alligators.[15] These factors pose a challenge for effective treatment and the potential for promoting antimicrobial resistance. Therefore a combination of good hygiene, water treatments with disinfectants, and improved husbandry is recommended.

A number of parasites are known to affect the skin of crocodilians. *Paratrichosoma* spp. are capillaroid parasites that cause a zigzag lesion on the skin. These lesions appear to be purely cosmetic. This parasite is known to affect various crocodile species in the wild and is believed to have a stage of its lifecycle dependent on soil; therefore, it is not observed in captive scenarios where animals are kept on concrete.[13] Regardless of the etiology, good hygiene is essential in the prevention and treatment of integumentary disease in crocodilians. The etiology itself is at times not as important as what conditions predisposed them to the disease. A herpesvirus was identified via TEM from saltwater crocodiles *(Crocodylus porosus)* with concurrent pox virus and bacterial infection of the skin.[46]

Dermatophilosis (Brown Spot Disease)

Dermatophilosis causes brown-red to ulcerative lesions most commonly located between scales on the ventral skin (Fig. 136.1). Most of the cultures appear to resemble *Dermatophilus congolensis*.[16,17] These filamentous bacteria do not respond well to antibiotic therapy; therefore, intensive hygiene practices are necessary to prevent and control outbreaks.

Pox Virus

Parapoxvirus or poxlike viruses have been identified in five different crocodilian species: Spectacled caiman (*Caiman crocodilus fuscus*),[18,19] Brazilian caiman (*Caiman crocodilus yacare*),[20] Nile crocodile,[21,22] saltwater

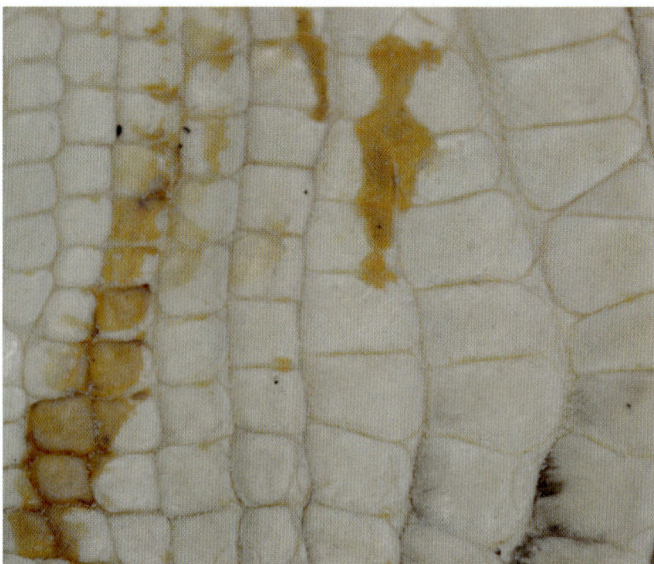

FIG 136.1 Brown lesions typical of dermatophilosis on the ventral skin of an American alligator (*A. mississippiensis*). Lesions usually arise at the junction of the scales and then spread outward. (Courtesy of Javier G. Nevarez.)

crocodile (*Crocodylus porosus*),[23] and freshwater crocodile (*Crocodylus johnstoni*).[23] In caimans, poxvirus is characterized by 1- to 3-mm-diameter, gray to white, coalescing to macular skin lesions. These can be found on the head, palpebrae, maxilla, mandible, limbs, palate, tongue, and gingiva.[18–20] Other signs observed include palpebral and generalized edema. Resolution of clinical signs was observed 6 weeks after improvement of husbandry in one case[19] and after 5 months in another case, with no changes in husbandry.[20]

Lesions in crocodiles are described as 2- to 8-mm-diameter, yellow to brown, wartlike, sometimes firm, and unraised to raised nodules with occasional shallow ulcers. These lesions can be found on the head, palpebrae, nostrils, sides of the mouth, oral cavity, limbs, ventral neck, and coelom and at the root of the tail.[21,22] Resolution of lesions was reported to occur as early as 3 to 4 weeks.[21] Light microscopy reveals epithelial hyperplasia, acanthosis, hyperkeratosis, and necrosis, and at times Borrel and Bollinger's bodies are also visible.[18–22] Secondary bacterial and fungal infections may also be present. Horner reported the use of an autogenous vaccine to treat poxvirus in Nile crocodiles.[21] No specific treatment recommendations exist. Maintaining appropriate husbandry is essential in the prevention and resolution of poxvirus in crocodilian farms.

West Nile Virus

West Nile virus (WNV) has been reported to cause lymphohistiocytic proliferative syndrome of alligators (LPSA).[24,25] LPSA skin lesions are a chronic manifestation of WNV infection and occur in animals that have survived a WNV outbreak.[25] This production problem affects the quality of the hide and consequently decreases profit for alligator ranchers. Gross lesions can be seen as multifocal, 1 mm to 2 mm, gray to red foci on the ventral mandibular, abdominal, and sometimes tail scales (Fig. 136.2). They can be found on any section of a scale and do not appear concave or convex with respect to the scale's surface. Routine microscopic examination reveals dermal nodular lymphoid proliferation with perivascular cuffing. Similar lesions can be found in other tissues besides the skin. Identification of the lesions is complicated by the fact they are sometimes not seen until the hides are removed from the animal. Therefore antemortem identification alone is not very accurate.

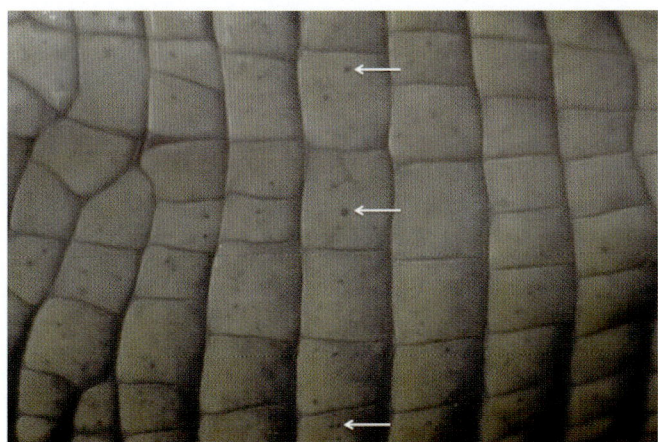

FIG 136.2 Gross lesions (arrows) of lymphohistiocytic proliferative syndrome of alligators on the ventral skin of an American alligator (*A. mississippiensis*). Lesions appear in animals that survived WNV infection. There are over 50 lesions in this image. (Courtesy of Javier G. Nevarez.)

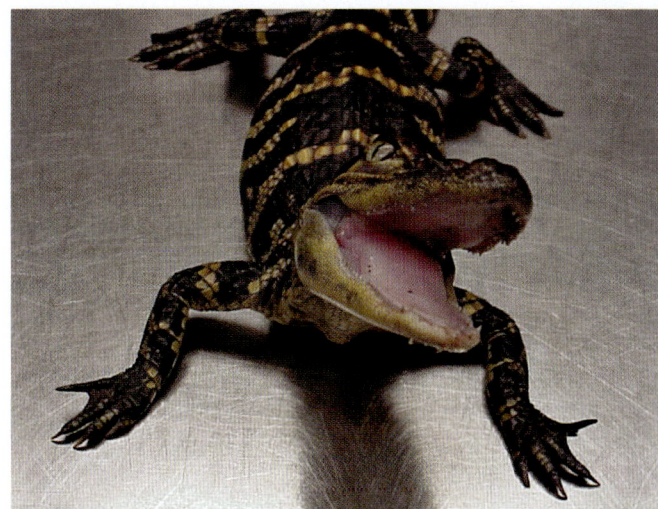

FIG 136.3 Young alligator (*Alligator mississippiensis*) with the head tilt typical of those affected with West Nile virus. Notice that it still maintains an aggressive stand with the mouth open.

NEUROLOGICAL SIGNS

Neurological deficits are not commonly seen in crocodilians and deserve special attention if encountered. Clinical signs may include swimming in circles or on one side of the body, abnormal flotation, lethargy, ataxia, head tilt, and muscle tremors. Anorexia often accompanies the neurological signs. Thiamine deficiencies should be considered in animals fed a frozen fish diet. Signs of thiamine deficiency typically include severe lethargy that leads to coma.

Hypoglycemia has also been reported as a cause of neurological signs in alligators.[26] These animals have muscle tremors, loss of the righting reflex, and mydriasis. Stress seems to be the main contributing factor. The author has also observed neurological signs associated with low oxygen levels inside alligator enclosures. Neurological signs may also be observed after ingestion of metal foreign bodies, including coins, containing lead or zinc.

West Nile Virus

West Nile virus causes neurological signs in captive-reared American alligators raised indoors.[27,28] Presence of antibodies, but no clinical signs, is reported from free-ranging and captive crocodilians housed outdoors.[29,30] WNV in crocodilians is transmitted by mosquitoes and horizontally via fecal shedding. This represents an opportunity for zoonosis in captive operations. Strict building quarantine and hygiene strategies should be implemented to prevent spread to other animals in the facility. WNV is a reportable disease, and one should contact the state veterinarian when diagnosis is confirmed.

WNV can affect an animal of any age, but hatchlings often experience severe per-acute mortalities of up to 50% to 60%.[28] WNV has two disease stages in alligators, acute and chronic. Clinical signs during the acute stage include swimming in circles, head tilt (Fig. 136.3), muscle tremors, weakness, lethargy, anorexia, and death. Animals that survive the acute infection go on to develop LPSA skin lesions, the chronic stage of WNV. There is no treatment. Definitive diagnosis is accomplished with reverse transcriptase polymerase chain reaction (RT-PCR) of liver and brain. However, it must be noted that RT-PCR can detect viral RNA from a commercially available WNV vaccine for alligators (BIVI, St. Joseph, MO). Therefore vaccine status must be known before diagnosis. Maternal transfer of antibodies has also been observed in hatchlings.[31] Veterinarians should take additional precautions during necropsies of suspect animals. Aggressive mosquito control and vaccination have

proven extremely effective at controlling WNV infection in commercial operations.

RESPIRATORY SIGNS

This is one of the most common presentations of captive crocodilians, second only to integumentary disease. Respiratory signs can often be confused with neurological signs, and a clear distinction must be established. However, respiratory disease may accompany neurological disease as a consequence of weakness leading to aspiration. Clinical signs associated with respiratory disease in crocodilians may include dyspnea, tachypnea, nasal discharge, excessive basking, abnormal swimming (either in circles or on one side of the body), and anorexia, among others. As the animals become weak, the basihyoid valve does not function properly and they can aspirate food or water. The pharyngeal anatomy of crocodilians makes aspiration unlikely in healthy animals. Therefore, if aspiration is suspected, evaluation for an underlying illness should be pursued. A number of rhinitis and pharyngitis syndromes have also been described in some crocodilian species.[13] Most respiratory infections are either bacterial or fungal in origin. An early report showed a fungal pneumonia associated with *Beauveria bassiana* in two alligators,[32] and *Fusarium moniliforme* was found in another case.[33]

Mycoplasmosis

One well-documented respiratory pathogen is *Mycoplasma alligatoris.* Clinical signs are nonspecific and include lethargy, weakness, anorexia, white ocular discharge, paresis, and edema (facial, periocular, cervical, limbs).[10] Pneumonia, pericarditis, and polyarthritis are often diagnosed on necropsy. Pathogenicity of *M. alligatoris* has been documented for *A. mississippiensis* and for the broad-nosed caiman (*Caiman latirostris*).[34,35] Other crocodilian species closely related to alligators are also potentially susceptible. Helmick et al. reviewed antimicrobial susceptibility for *M. alligatoris.*[36] A second *Mycoplasma* species, *M. crocodyli,* is known to affect Nile crocodiles.[11] Lesions are similar to those observed with *M. alligatoris.* Some studies have examined the use of an autogenous vaccine for *M. crocodyli,* but work is still needed to determine its true efficacy.[37,38] Currently antemortem diagnosis is difficult and requires a combination of serology and tissue biopsy for PCR. Therefore most cases are confirmed via histopathology and PCR postmortem.

Mycobacteriosis

Although not commonly reported from crocodilians, the author has worked on a number of alligator cases with acid-fast organisms consistent with *Mycobacterium* sp. in the lungs. These animals had evidence of pneumonia on necropsy as shown by multiple white foci, 1 to 4 mm in diameter, on the lung parenchyma. Other cases of pulmonary and enteric mycobacterial infections have been suggested.[39] Difficulties of growing *Mycobacterium* sp. make its definitive diagnosis a challenge.

MUSCULOSKELETAL SIGNS

Musculoskeletal disease can be the result of alterations in the incubation temperature or environment (Fig. 136.4) or trauma from fighting (Figs. 136.5), transport, restraint, neoplasia, or secondary to nutritional disease.

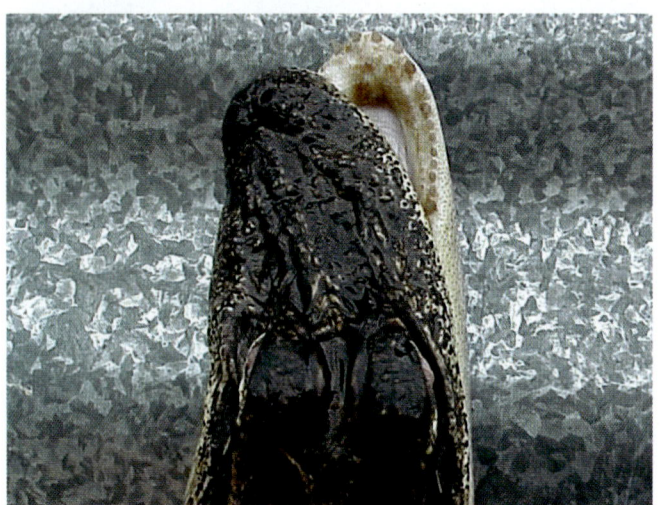

FIG 136.4 Congenital abnormality in an American alligator (*Alligator mississippiensis*). This animal was hatched with this deformity and is able to eat and thrive among others in the group.

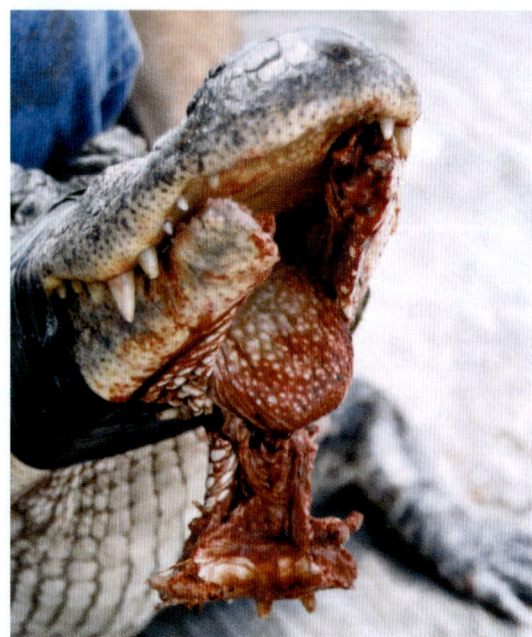

FIG 136.5 Mandibular fracture in a wild alligator (*A. mississippiensis*). This type of lesion is not uncommon in wild animals, particulary in males during breeding season.

Limb fractures and partial amputations can be seen after altercations. It is possible for animals that have lost limbs after a fight to survive to the point of complete healing (Fig. 136.6). These lesions however may also lead to nerve or muscle damage and consequent paresis or paralysis. As mentioned in the respiratory signs section, *M. alligatoris* and *M. crocodyli* cause polyarthritis, which can be evident antemortem.

Nutritional secondary hyperparathyroidism can occur in young crocodilians not being fed whole prey or pelleted diets. Affected animals may also be runts of the group and have concurrent disease. The innate requirement of ultraviolet B light for the production of vitamin D$_3$ in crocodilians is not known. They appear to be able to obtain appropriate levels from their diet, but further research in this area is needed.

Gout also occurs in crocodilians (Figs. 136.7A and B). Clinical signs can be nonspecific in nature, but limb paresis/paralysis and joint enlargement may be observed. A case of gout with concurrent suspected hypovitaminosis A in crocodile hatchlings has been reported.[40]

Deficiencies of vitamins A, B, C, or E can also lead to a variety of musculoskeletal disorders. These are not commonly seen when commercial diets are fed in addition to meat products.

GASTROINTESTINAL SIGNS

Anorexia is likely the most common clinical sign associated with gastrointestinal disease in captive crocodilians. Foreign body ingestion, gastric ulcers, enteritis (Fig. 136.8), and trauma to the oral cavity can be observed in crocodilians. Ingestion of foreign bodies is more common in wild crocodilians. However, it must also be a differential in captive specimens. Malfunction of water pumps, water filters, or construction can lead to the presence of foreign bodies in the enclosures. In outdoor exhibits, the public is often responsible for the presence of foreign objects that are thrown into their enclosures. These can then be ingested by the animals and cause severe problems in the case of nails and other sharp objects (Fig. 136.9).

Infectious enteritis may be difficult to assess grossly because crocodilians have very thick intestinal walls normally. However, crocodilians appear to have a characteristic response to insult of the gastrointestinal tract. Accumulations of fibrous material or necrotizing lesions are commonly seen on necropsy (Fig. 136.10A and B). This reaction is aggressive and can even lead to obstructions caused by the fibrous material. Obstruction can also occur with fecal impactions and torsions. Gastric ulcerations and abnormalities of the gastric mucosa are also routinely observed on necropsy and may be associated with stress and diet. Finally, the intestinal tract contains a large amount of Peyer's

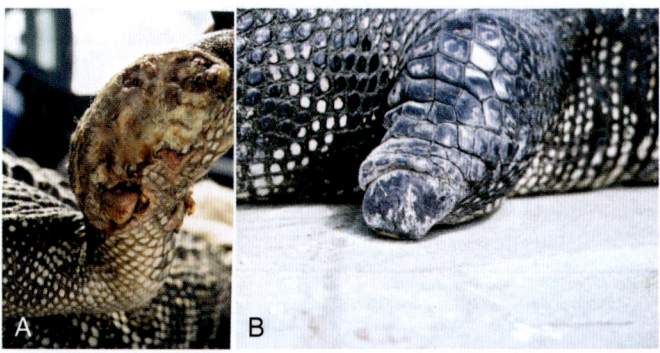

FIG 136.6 (A) Rear limb open fracture with tissue necrosis in a wild alligator (*A. mississippiensis*). Wild animals can recover from these types of lesions, but they can lead to severe septicemia in captive ones. (B) Wild alligator with a healed lesion that resulted in amputation of the distal rear limb.

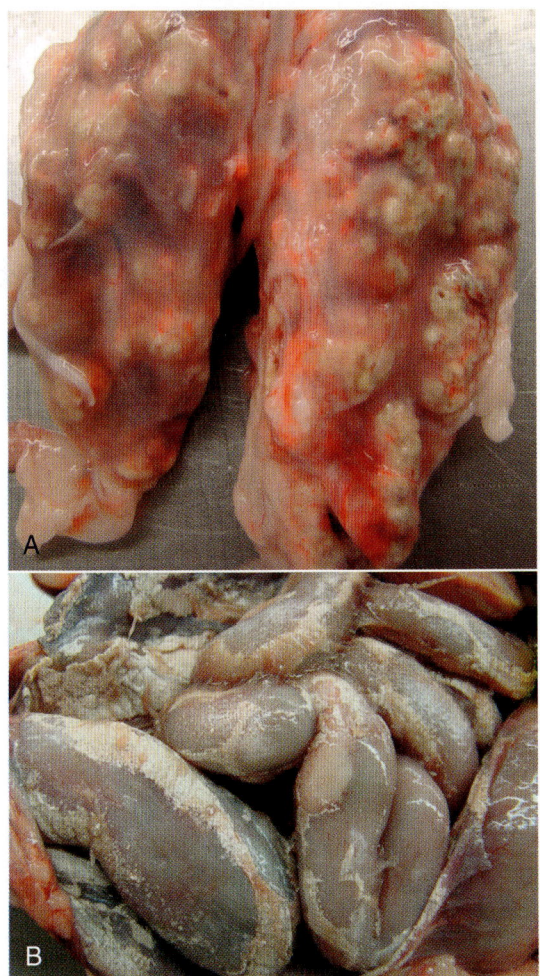

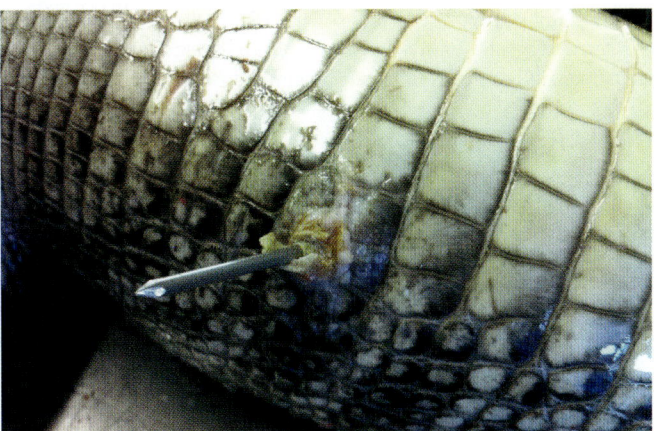

FIG 136.9 Farmed alligator (*A. mississippiensis*) with a nail foreign body that was ingested and perforated its stomach. (Courtesy of Javier G. Nevarez.)

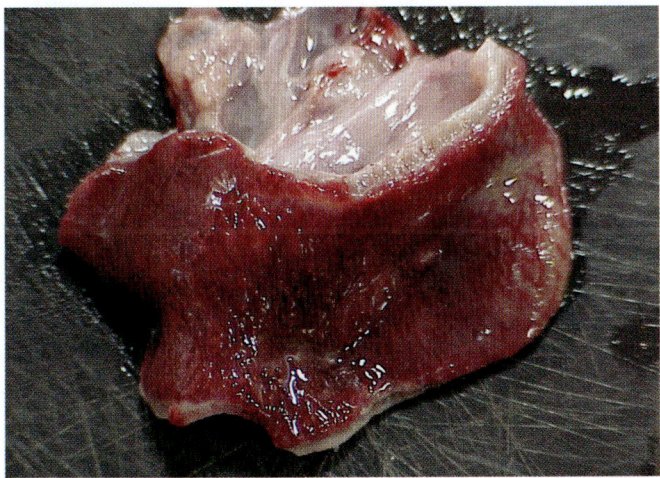

FIG 136.7 (A and B) Renal and visceral gout in an American alligator (*A. mississippiensis*). Oversupplementation with a vitamin and mineral mix was suspected in this case. (Courtesy of Javier G. Nevarez.)

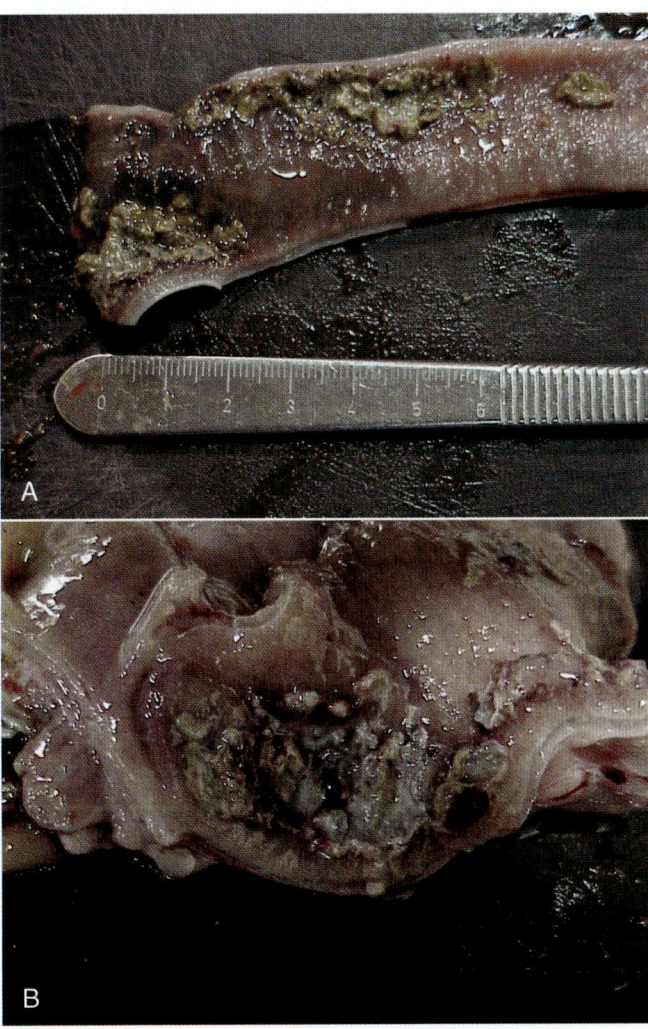

FIG 136.8 Enteritis in a captive-reared alligator (*A. mississippiensis*). Notice the red mucosa.

FIG 136.10 (A and B) Fibrotic membrane on the intestinal mucosa of a captive-reared alligator (*A. mississippiensis*). This was an incidental finding for this animal.

patches and likely represents a site of aggressive inflammatory response to infectious agents. A novel herpesvirus was reported from an American alligator with lymphoid follicular inflammation of the cloaca.[45]

OCULAR SIGNS

Chlamydia

Chlamydiosis has been reported from *C. niloticus* (South Africa and Zimbabwe), *C. porosus* (Papua New Guinea), and *C. siamensis* (Thailand).[41-43] The author has also diagnosed Chlamydiosis in *A. mississippiensis* (United States). Although it has been proposed as a *Chlamydophila psittaci*-like strain in *C. niloticus*,[44] the *Chlamydia* species affecting crocodilians is likely a novel specie(s). Infection usually leads to hepatitis and/or conjunctivitis (Fig. 136.11), but lung and spleen can also be infected. Morbidity and mortality can exceed 50%, resulting in significant economic losses for farmed animals.[42] Treatment with oxytetracycline is anecdotally reported to be effective in crocodiles. This creates significant concerns for possible antimicrobial resistance, zoonosis, and the safety of the meat from these animals.

MISCELLANEOUS

A novel herpesvirus was reported from an American alligator with lymphoid follicular inflammation of the cloaca.[45] A herpesvirus was identified via TEM from saltwater crocodiles (*Crocodylus porosus*) with concurrent pox virus and bacterial infection of the skin.[46] In captive *C. porosus* and freshwater crocodiles (*C. johnstoni*) from Australia, three novel herpesviruses have been identified.[47] *C. porosus* exhibited conjunctivitis-pharyngitis, systemic lymphoid proliferation and encephalitis, or lymphonodular skin lesions.[47,48] *C. johnstoni* had

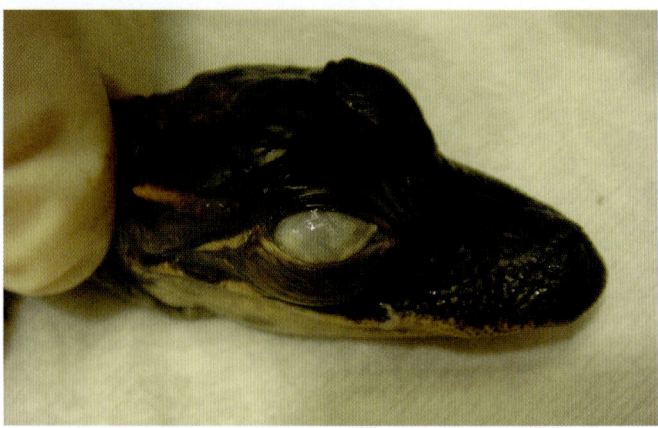

FIG 136.11 Keratitis and conjunctivitis because of chlamydiosis in a hatchling American alligator (*A. mississippiensis*). (Courtesy of Javier G. Nevarez.)

systemic lymphoid proliferation.[47] Chlamydiaceae was also identified from conjunctival and pharyngeal tissues of some of the *C. porosus* cases.[48] Of interest is that these syndromes occur concurrently with other infectious agents and have been associated with significant morbidity and mortality of infected animals.

REFERENCES

See www.expertconsult.com for a complete list of references.

137

Differential Diagnoses by Clinical Signs—Amphibians

Taylor Yaw and Leigh Clayton

This chapter reviews differentials for common presenting conditions in captive amphibians. The primary focus is adult anurans (frogs and toads) and caudates (newts, salamanders, and sirens); larval amphibians and caecilians are not covered in detail. Some guidance is provided for etiologies, diagnostic tests, and management, but readers are referred to other amphibian chapters in this text (see Chapters 12, 28, 52, 89, and 107) for more information on these topics.

ACUTE MORTALITIES

Unexpected deaths of individually housed amphibians and acute mortalities affecting several amphibians in a collection warrant immediate attention by the clinical veterinarian. Acute mortalities are most commonly due to infectious diseases (e.g., chytridiomycosis, ranavirus, lungworm, or bacterial septicemia), sudden environmental changes (e.g., tank flooding or drying, temperature changes), and toxin exposure (e.g., chloramine, chlorine, ammonia, bleach, insecticides). Essential diagnostic evaluations that should be considered include a full history, physical examination of remaining amphibians, water quality testing, skin scrapes, PCR testing (e.g., chytridiomycosis/ranavirus), gill biopsies, full necropsy (including cytology samples and cultures), and tissue submission for histology. Normal blood values for amphibians are largely undefined, but a simple blood smear may help appreciate changes that can be associated with bacterial septicemia. Affected populations should be isolated pending the diagnosis in case of an infectious cause.

Chytridiomycosis, caused by the fungal organism *Batrachochytrium dendrobatidis*, often causes death without premonitory clinical signs and must be considered as a differential in any acute mortality.[1] Nonspecific signs of anorexia, lethargy, ataxia, and cutaneous lesions may be seen before death.[2] Cutaneous lesions include hyperplasia, hyperemia, ulcerations, and brown discoloration of the dermis. This fungal infection has low host specificity and can cause high morbidity and mortality.[3,4] In the authors' experience, outbreaks in larger captive collections may have an insidious onset with increased mortality events over weeks to months. Husbandry parameters, especially temperature, should be reviewed, because outbreaks are often concurrent with environmental stressors. The organism can often be identified on wet mount preparations of shed skin, if the infection is heavy, and PCR of the skin. Chytridiomycosis is reportable to the World Organization for Animal Health (OIE).

Ranaviruses (family *Iridoviridae*) can also cause acute mortality without premonitory clinical signs and have been implicated in mass mortality events in wild amphibian populations.[5] Signs of lethargy, anorexia, buoyancy disorders, edema, coelomic distension, and ventral ecchymoses (especially in the pelvic region) may be observed before death. Internal hemorrhage and hydrocoelom are commonly observed on postmortem necropsy.[6] Several different ranaviruses have been described in amphibians (e.g., frog virus type III, Ambystoma tigrinum virus, Bohle iridovirus, and common midwife toad virus) with varying pathogenicity.[7–10] Susceptibility to the disease varies by species, developmental stage (late larval stage often most severe), and environmental factors.[6] Diagnosis is by histology, PCR, and cell culture; sequencing is needed for definitive identification. Lesions may appear very similar to those of bacterial dermatosepticemia due to secondary bacterial infections, making differentiation difficult without histology, cultures, and PCR. Ranaviruses are also reportable to the OIE.

Lung worms (e.g., *Rhabdias* spp.) can cause acute mortalities in adult amphibians through lung damage and secondary infections.[11] Clinical signs are rarely observed and, if present, are typically nonspecific (e.g., anorexia, poor body condition). The parasites have a direct life cycle and can build up rapidly. Premortem diagnosis may be made by finding ova or worms in oral, nasal, or fecal material. Adult worm burdens are typically obvious on necropsy and histology.

The term "red-leg disease" may still be seen in the literature and is often used interchangeably with bacterial septicemia, particularly *Aeromonas* spp., but is essentially a clinical syndrome that includes erythema and other signs of systemic inflammation.[12] Gram-negative bacteria (e.g., *Aeromonas*, *Pseudomonas*, *Citrobacter*, *Klebsiella*, *Salmonella*, *Proteus*, *Flavobacterium* spp.) are the most commonly reported in septic amphibians. Gram-positive bacteria may also cause disease, particularly atypical *Mycobacterium* and *Chlamydophila* spp., which can cause both acute septicemia and, more commonly, chronic granulomatous disease in amphibians.[5,13–16] Septicemia may be secondary to injury, gastrointestinal inflammation, or immunosuppression and is often correlated with husbandry-related issues.[11]

Abrupt environmental changes, especially changes in water availability and temperature, can lead to acute deaths. A detailed history is essential in identifying inappropriate husbandry (e.g., enclosure type, chemicals utilized for cleaning, diet, supplementation, temperature, humidity, water quality, lighting).[17] Where a visit is not possible, pictures or videos of the primary enclosure and its location in the room can be useful.

COELOMIC DISTENSION

Coelomic distension is one of the most common presenting signs in amphibians. Distension may be due to fluid, soft tissue (often fat or ova), or rarely gas (not covered in this chapter). A full history with water-quality parameters, physical examination, transillumination, radiographs, ultrasound, fine needle aspiration (with fluid evaluation, cytology, and bacterial culture), and PCR (e.g., ranavirus) are commonly utilized to differentiate causes.

Abnormal Fluid Accumulation (Hydrocoelom/Lymphedema)

Fluid may accumulate in focal areas within the lymphatic system but is more commonly generalized to the coelomic cavity (hydrocoelom) or entire lymphatic system (lymphedema) (Fig. 137.1). Hydrocoelom

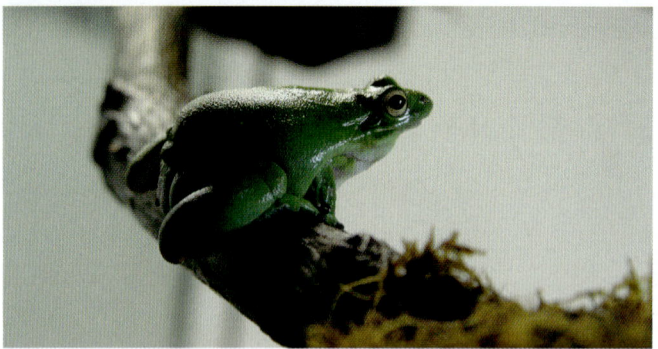

FIG 137.1 A green tree frog (*Hyla cinerea*) with hydrocoelom and lymphedema. These two conditions often present together and are difficult to differentiate in advanced cases. (Courtesy of Amanda Gensemer.)

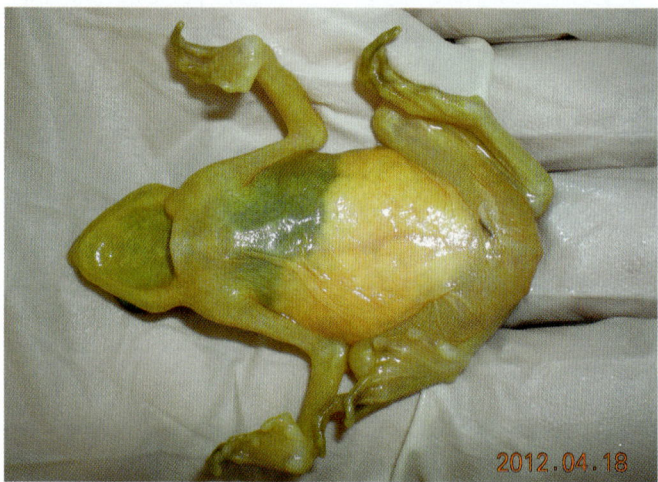

FIG 137.2 A Panamanian golden frog (*Atelopus zeteki*) with coelomic distension due to egg masses. This amphibian also appears to be moderately dehydrated and in poor body condition. (Courtesy of Jessica Nelson.)

is limited to coelomic distension with a rounded coelom. Lymphedema is associated with a rounded appearance over the pelvis and loss of the linea alba, exophthalmos, and limb swelling. Amphibians may show no other clinical signs. Major causes for fluid accumulation include cutaneous lesions, infectious diseases, renal or hepatic diseases, and environmental problems.[14] Cutaneous lesions are covered later in this chapter.

The most common infectious diseases that cause fluid accumulation include chytridiomycosis, ranavirus, and bacterial septicemia. Differentiation of these diseases can be difficult, and further diagnostic assessments are required after initial examination. Secondary bacterial infection can impair diagnosis of underlying viral infections. Skin cytology or histology and PCR are crucial in identifying fungal and viral components. Aspiration of fluid followed by fluid analysis and cytology stains are helpful in identifying signs of infection. Culture and susceptibility of the fluid can guide treatment if a bacterial component is involved.

Renal disease is commonly associated with edema in both terrestrial and aquatic amphibians (Mangus LM, Proc AAZV 2008, p16).[13,14] In the authors' practice, it appears likely that both acute and chronic renal disease can be associated with edema. Infectious diseases capable of causing direct renal damage include local or systemic bacterial, viral, or fungal agents (e.g., mucormycosis, chromomycosis, zygomycosis), as well as myxozoan and microsporidial parasites.[14,18] Noninfectious causes of renal disease include degenerative disease, dehydration, neoplasia (primary and secondary), nutrition (e.g., high oxalates, high protein, hypovitaminosis A), and toxins (e.g., aminoglycosides, heavy metals, polyvinyl chloride glue).[14,19–21] Confirmation is often difficult unless the animal is large enough for renal biopsy for histology and culture.

Hepatic disease can cause edema through the direct effects of hepatocyte necrosis, impaired intrahepatic circulation, or due to low plasma protein levels.[22] Infectious causes of hepatic disease include local or systemic bacterial, viral, or fungal infections as described previously.[23,24] Noninfectious causes of hepatic disease include trauma, neoplasia (primary and secondary), and toxins (e.g., heavy metals, pesticides, herbicides). Tissue biopsy and histology are typically needed for confirmation.

Inappropriate husbandry can predispose amphibians to conditions associated with edema, particularly bacterial and viral infections. Additionally, short-term exposure to cool temperatures (e.g., during transport) has been associated with transient hydrocoelom a few days after exposure that normally resolves without intervention (Clayton, unpublished). Aquatic amphibians housed in water with low dissolved solutes may also accumulate fluid due to low osmotic pressure.[23]

Obesity

Compared with amphibians with edema, obese amphibians retain more definition over the pelvis and linea alba. Obesity is more likely in amphibians fed cholesterol-rich diets (e.g., laboratory rodents, crickets fed on dog food) and sedentary species that readily consume large amounts of food. The coelomic cavity is often firm on physical examination, and fat pads may be visualized via transillumination or ultrasound.

Reproductive Activity

Most amphibians produce large egg masses that may cause coelomic distension (Fig. 137.2). Many also have the ability to retain eggs until suitable environmental cues are received. They may have a pendulous appearance to the body cavity, and there may be focal edema around the upper thighs. Maturing eggs can become lodged in the oviduct, impeding oviposition and eventually forming adhesions requiring surgical attention.[25] Transillumination and ultrasound are often diagnostic, but endoscopy or exploratory coeliotomy may be needed.

Gastrointestinal Impaction/Foreign Bodies

Gastrointestinal impaction with food can cause coelomic distension. In many species, the stomach is distensible and amphibians may consume large food items with no issues. However, maldigestion and gastric stasis due to a primary disease process or husbandry issues can lead to gastric impaction. Gas accumulation can be severe, and the bacterial overgrowth can cause life-threatening complications.[26] In addition, many amphibians have indiscriminate eating habits and will ingest foreign material with food items (Fig. 137.3). Inappropriate feeding locations and ocular disease may predispose consumption of foreign material. Imaging along with endoscopy or exploratory coeliotomy may be indicated for diagnosis and treatment.

Organomegaly (Neoplasia and Granulomatous Disease)

Coelomic neoplasia may present as single or multiple masses in the coelomic cavity. Lymphoma, intestinal and gastric carcinomas, nephroblastomas, sertoli cell tumors, and pancreatic carcinomas have been reported in amphibians.[27,28] Focal granulomatous lesions can cause visceral enlargement and may be observed in one or more locations. Atypical mycobacteriosis, chlamydiosis, and fungal infections are most commonly reported in association with granulomas.[13–16,29] Encysted

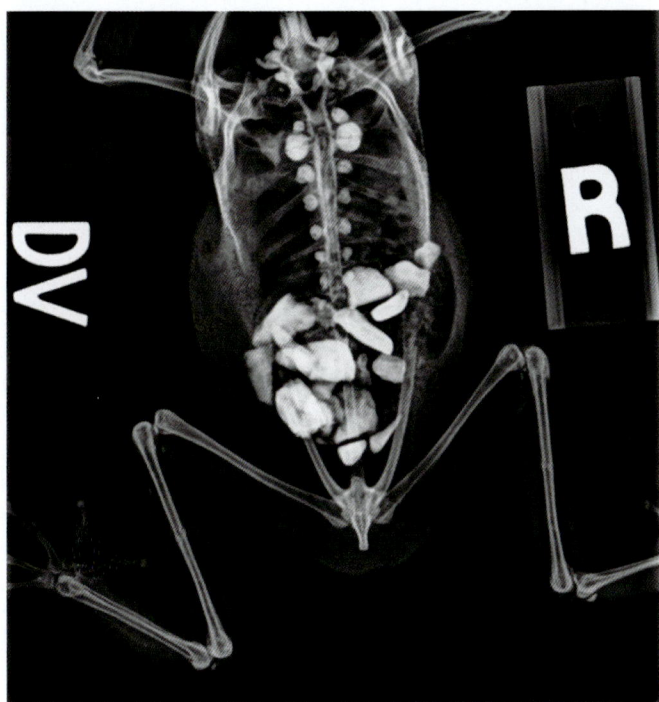

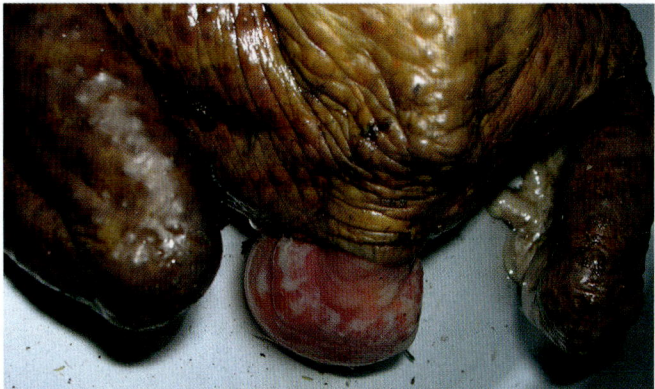

FIG 137.4 A smooth-sided toad (*Rhaebo guttatus*) with a prolapse of the colon and cloaca. (Courtesy of Jessica Nelson.)

FIG 137.3 Dorsoventral radiograph of a giant waxy tree frog (*Phyllomedusa bicolor*) with gastrointestinal foreign bodies.

metazoan parasites can also cause granulomas.[30] Ultrasound-guided fine needle aspirates of affected organs with appropriate cytology preparations (e.g., acid fast, Diff-Quik, and gram stains) and culture can be helpful in identifying infectious agents. Ultimately, biopsy and histology is often indicated for confirmation.

GASTROINTESTINAL SIGNS

Gastrointestinal disease is commonly identified in amphibians, but presenting signs vary. Depending on the number of individuals housed together and the enclosure design (e.g., heavily planted terrariums), caregivers may miss clinical signs such as diarrhea, poor body condition, or reduced appetite. Other signs, such as cloacal prolapse, may be readily appreciated. Standard diagnostics utilized to assess gastrointestinal health include a full history, physical examination, fecal analysis (float, direct preparation, cytology stains), transillumination, ultrasound, and radiographs (with or without positive contrast).

Tissue Prolapse

Prolapsed tissue may be intestinal, urinary, or reproductive (Fig. 137.4). Prolapsed tissue is usually a medical emergency, and owners should be instructed to move amphibians from enclosures with organic substrate into an appropriate medical and/or transport enclosure with high humidity. Definitive identification of the prolapsed tissue is not always possible but should be attempted. Prolapsed cloacal tissue is generally small, smooth, and pink. Prolapsed colon is smooth to ridged, with a tubular appearance. A central lumen and/or feces may be visible grossly on impression smear. Prolapsed urinary bladder is rounded with a thin wall and fluid contents. Prolapsed oviduct includes narrow, coiled tubules that may have longitudinal lines and eggs. In the authors' experience, cloacal and colon prolapses are the most common, followed by the urinary bladder.

Transient, self-limiting prolapses may have no obvious cause and can occur iatrogenically during manual restraint or anesthesia with

tricaine methanesulfonate.[31] These typically resolve within a few hours of presentation. Common causes of prolapses include parasitism, intussusception, gastrointestinal foreign bodies, neoplasia, septicemia, toxemia, dehydration, extraluminal gastrointestinal blockage (e.g., renal neoplasia), toxins, hypoglycemia, hypocalcemia, and malnutrition.[23,24,30] Tissue impression smears and fine needle aspirates of prolapsed tissue may help in identification of tissue and underlying pathology (e.g., parasites).

Gastric prolapses are occasionally reported secondary to other conditions such as terminal disease, toxin exposure, or gastric parasites.[30,32] Iatrogenic gastric prolapse has been reported in leopard frogs (*Lithobates pipiens*) anesthetized with clove oil; prolapses resolved during the recovery phase of an anesthetic event.[33]

Anorexia (Hyporexia)

Anorexia or hyporexia are nonspecific clinical signs that can be associated with most diseases. A thorough history and observation can help distinguish between inappetance and a good appetite but inability to capture or prehend food. As body condition worsens, the amphibian's coelom becomes less distended, the limbs lose muscle, and weight declines (see Fig. 137.2). If the calorie and nutrient imbalance is severe, amphibians may present with neurological signs (e.g., tremors, muscle rigidity, ataxia). Causes of inappetance include inappropriate environmental conditions; musculoskeletal injuries involving the oral cavity; inflammation or infectious diseases (e.g., bacterial septicemia, atypical mycobacteriosis, ranavirus, chytridiomycosis); gastrointestinal, renal, or hepatic disease; neoplasia; and pain.[34] Inability to capture or prehend food is most commonly due to hypovitaminosis A, also known as short tongue syndrome (Pessier AP, Proc ARAV, 2002, p57).[35]

Thin Frog/Emaciation

Weight loss is a nonspecific clinical sign that can be associated with most diseases. Regular weight checks allow for earlier detection of weight loss than just monitoring for changes in body condition. When tracking weight, it is important to look at trends over time, because daily weight ranges can vary dramatically due to urination/defecation. Differentials include those for anorexia as listed previously, malabsorption or maldigestion (e.g., gastrointestinal parasites, inflammation, toxins), and increased metabolic rates (e.g., neoplasia, infectious disease).[17]

Reduced Fecal Production

Normal fecal output varies between species, and long intervals between fecal production are normal in species adapted to more arid conditions (e.g., Hylidae, some Bufonidae). The most common causes of reduced fecal production are anorexia or hyporexia (as stated previously). Other differentials can be divided into mechanical obstructions (e.g., gastric impaction, intraluminal mass, extraluminal mass, severe helminthiasis, intussusception, foreign body, stricture) and functional obstructions (e.g., inappropriate environmental conditions, systemic inflammation or infection, neurological disease, trauma).[30] Amphibians with prolonged anorexia tend to have minimal digesta, and animals with functional or mechanical obstructions tend to have full intestinal tracts that can be observed on palpation, diagnostic imaging, or transillumination.

Diarrhea

Diarrhea must be differentiated from polyuria, which can be difficult. Diarrhea in amphibians has been associated with husbandry related issues such as inappropriate temperature or humidity, or diets high in carbohydrates.[26] Other differentials include gastroenteritis, foreign bodies, and toxins (e.g., heavy metals).[30,32] Amoebiasis, coccidiosis, and some metazoan parasites (e.g., *Strongyloides* spp., *Acanthocephalus ranae*) have been implicated as primary pathogens of the gastrointestinal system.[32,36,37] Ciliates are common in the gastrointestinal tract of a wide variety of amphibians but are typically nonpathogenic.[30] Systemic fungal disease may affect the gastrointestinal tract, whereas *Mucor amphibiorum* can be a primary cause of gastroenteritis.[2,23,38,39] As previously mentioned, ranaviruses can cause intestinal distension with hemorrhage and diarrhea.[24]

DERMATOLOGICAL SIGNS

Amphibians may present with a wide variety of cutaneous disorders. Clinical signs may include coloration changes, erythema, petechiation, ulcerations, abrasions/lacerations, and increased shedding. In many cases, integument changes are due to systemic disease or are related to inappropriate environmental conditions. Differentials should include infectious diseases (e.g., chytridiomycosis, ranavirus, bacterial septicemia), environmental issues (e.g., inappropriate substrate, décor, temperature, water quality, humidity, nutrition), and toxin exposure (e.g., chlorine, ammonia, bleach). Common diagnostic evaluations include a full history, water quality, physical examination, skin scrape (wet mounts and cytology stains), impression smears, bacterial and fungal culture, and biopsy. Necropsy evaluation of the skin should also routinely include skin scrapings as well as histology from multiple sites.

Erythema

Erythema is a common, nonspecific clinical sign, often seen on the limbs and ventral abdomen of amphibians. Erythema can be related to handling, inappropriate environmental conditions, inflammatory or infectious disease, and some neoplastic processes.[4]

Amphibians may develop minor erythema in response to handling, which often dissipates rapidly. Major environmental causes of erythema include rough cage furniture, coarse substrate, use of coarse nets, and poor water quality or environmental irritants (e.g., disinfectants, detergents, chlorine, inappropriate pH). Inappropriate nutrition, in particular hypovitaminosis A, often leads to cutaneous lesions, including erythema. A detailed history with water quality parameters and observation of the enclosure is often diagnostic. Any systemic infection can cause hyperemia, including viral, bacterial, fungal, and parasitic infections. As previously noted, chytridiomycosis, ranavirus, and dermatosepticemia are common infectious processes that must be ruled out (see Acute Mortality section). Other fungal causes of cutaneous erythema not previously mentioned include *Basidiobolus ranarum, Mucor, Saprolegnia*, chromomycosis (e.g., *Cladosporium*), and *Ichthyophonus* spp.[2,4] A variety of cutaneous neoplasms have been described in amphibians. Although these often appear as proliferative masses, neoplasms such as squamous

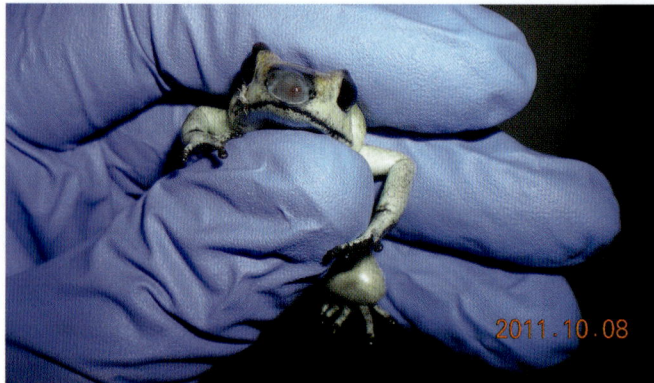

FIG 137.5 A deep rostral abrasion in a terrible poison dart frog (*Phylobates terribilis*). (Courtesy of Jessica Nelson.)

cell carcinomas, adenomas, and adenocarcinomas can exhibit several different characteristics, including erythema and ulcerations.[4]

Abrasions/Lacerations

Abrasions and lacerations commonly occur from traumatic events. Common causes in captive amphibians are tank mate aggression, rostral trauma from enclosure surfaces (Fig. 137.5), entrapment in tank lids or under décor, bites from live prey, inappropriate substrate, and handling with dry hands. If appropriate environmental conditions are provided, most wounds heal well without medical intervention.

Dehydration

Signs of severe dehydration in amphibians include a dry or wrinkled appearance to the skin, dark coloration, sunken eyes, dry stringy mucus in the mouth, or weight loss (see Fig. 137.2). Excessive tackiness of the skin may be a subtle sign of mild dehydration in some species.[4]

Environmental issues, particularly inappropriate water sources, water quality, or temperature, are the most common causes of dehydration. All species of amphibians should have access to water. Other common causes of dehydration are cutaneous disease (e.g., chytridiomycosis, ranavirus, septicemia, thermal burns) and renal disease. Vomiting, diarrhea, and polyuria must also be considered as potential sources of fluid loss but are less common.

Cutaneous Masses

In amphibians, granulomatous inflammation and neoplasia are the most common causes of cutaneous masses. Granulomatous lesions can be due to atypical mycobacteriosis, *Chlamydophila* spp., chromomycosis, mucormycosis, and zygomycosis.[1,2] Cutaneous neoplasia in amphibians include epidermal papillomas, squamous cell carcinomas, cystadenomas, cystadenocarcinomas, melanophoromas, neuroepithelial tumors, and mast cell tumors.[4,28] Of these, epidermal papillomas have shown spontaneous regression. Impression smears, aspirates, and incisional or excisional biopsies for cytology, histology, culture, and PCR can help with diagnosis.

MUSCULOSKELETAL SIGNS

Amphibians showing musculoskeletal signs should be assessed for orthopedic issues, myopathies, and neuropathies. Common diagnostic evaluations include radiography and transillumination. Biopsies and advanced imaging may be indicated.

Ambulation Difficulties

Common musculoskeletal issues include pathologic fractures from secondary nutritional hyperparathyroidism and trauma. Although

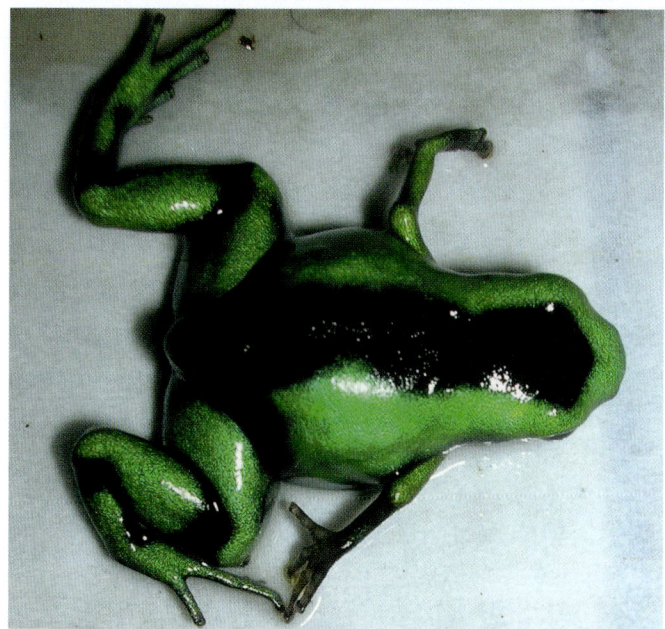

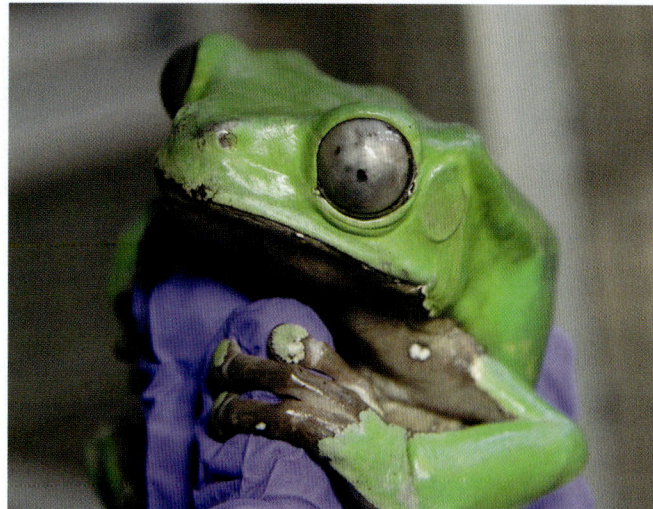

FIG 137.7 Giant waxy tree frog (*Phyllomedusa bicolor*) with advanced corneal lipidosis and stromal melanin deposition. (Courtesy of Jessica Nelson.)

FIG 137.6 Green and black poison dart frog (*Dendrobates auratus*) with thoracic limb malformation (i.e., spindly leg). (Courtesy of Jessica Nelson.)

neuropathies are not reported in the literature, autoimmune diseases, toxins, nutritional deficiencies, trauma, neoplasia, and toxins that could affect the nervous system should be considered as differentials. Secondary nutritional hyperparathyroidism is unfortunately common in amphibians.[11] The most common etiology is an imbalance of calcium, phosphorus, and vitamin D_3 in the diet, but high-fluoride, vitamin A, and oxalates can play a role.[26,40] Primary renal disease can also lead to abnormal bone development due to decreased production of active vitamin D_3. If severe, signs may include spastic tetany after strenuous movement that resolves with rest. If chronic, folding fractures of long bones, spinal changes, and loss of mineral deposition in bones may be present. A detailed history, diet review, and radiographs are often diagnostic.

Developmental Abnormalities (Polymelia and Spindly Leg)

Nutritional and parasitic causes are the most commonly reported etiologies of developmental abnormalities, but traumatic and genetic issues should also be considered. In wild anurans in the United States, polymelia (extra limbs) or amelia (missing limbs) may be due to the digenetic trematode *Ribeiroia ondatrae,* which encysts and disrupts developing limb buds.[41,42] Spindly leg is a developmental disease affecting tadpoles.[26] Classic signs are limited muscling of the limbs, inability to extract the forelimbs during metamorphosis, and a short, round coelom (Fig. 137.6). Enriched parental nutrition can reduce the incidence (Nelson J, Proc Am Assoc Zoo Keepers, 2014, p2).

OCULAR SIGNS

Common ocular presenting signs include increased corneal opacity, ulcers, and cataracts. A full history (including diet and lighting), physical examination, ocular examination with a slit lamp and ophthalmoscope, fluorescein staining, corneal scrapings, cultures, and tonometry are useful diagnostics.

Increased Corneal Opacity

Increased corneal opacity can be caused by edema, vascularization, fibrosis/scarring, pigmentation, or inflammatory cell or lipid infiltrate.

Corneal lipidosis is the most commonly reported ocular disease in amphibians.[43] The disease tends to be bilateral and presents as hazy white or gray corneal opacities starting at the limbus and progressing centrally (Fig. 137.7). Stromal melanin deposition and neovascularization develop in more severe cases.[44] Corneal lipid deposition has been linked to increased lipid in the diet. Female animals may have an increased risk because of egg development. Histology is needed for confirmation of the disease process.

Conjunctivitis, Dacryocystitis, and Uveitis

Inflammation of the conjunctiva, uveal tract, and glandular tissue around the eye presents with redness, discharge, and edema of the affected tissues. If severe enough, increased white blood cells and protein in the anterior chamber may present as flare on ophthalmic examination. Bacterial septicemia is the most common cause, but other causes of systemic inflammation need to be ruled out. Culture and cytologic evaluation can be very helpful for diagnosis and treatment.

Corneal Ulceration

Ulceration can be classified based on depth, onset, and position of the ulceration. Typical signs of corneal ulceration include ocular inflammation, excessive discharge, sensitivity to light, and pain. Although causes of amphibian ulcers are poorly documented, mechanical damage, foreign bodies, inappropriate lighting, humidity, or temperature should all be considered.

Lens Opacity

Cataracts and nuclear sclerosis are common in amphibian lenses. Nuclear sclerosis is always bilateral, spherical, and translucent. Cataracts can be focal or diffuse and are not translucent. Etiologies of cataracts in amphibians are poorly documented, but potential causes include trauma, systemic inflammation, nutritional deficiencies, inappropriate lighting, toxins, and genetics.[44,45] Differentiation of cataracts and nuclear sclerosis can be accomplished by retroillumination.

REFERENCES

See www.expertconsult.com for a complete list of references.

Abscesses/Fibriscesses

Volker Schmidt

DEFINITION

An abscess is defined as a localized collection of purulent material (pus) consiting of degenerate or toxic heterophils, macrophages, lymphocytes, serum, and necrotic tissue in a confined cavity formed by the disintegration of tissues. The reptilian abscess is usually not liquefied but inspissated and surrounded by a fibrous capsule; hence the term fibriscess may be used[1] (Fig. 138.1).

CLINICAL SIGNIFICANCE AND KNOWN ETIOLOGICAL CAUSE(S)

Microorganism (bacteria, fungi, parasites) or foreign bodies embedded in tissue can lead to fibriscess formation with a firm fibrous surrounding wall that is imprenetrable to drug therapy. The portal of entry for pathogenic organisms can be skin, ocular, and periocular tissue and the gastrointestinal or respiratory tracts. Once inside the body,

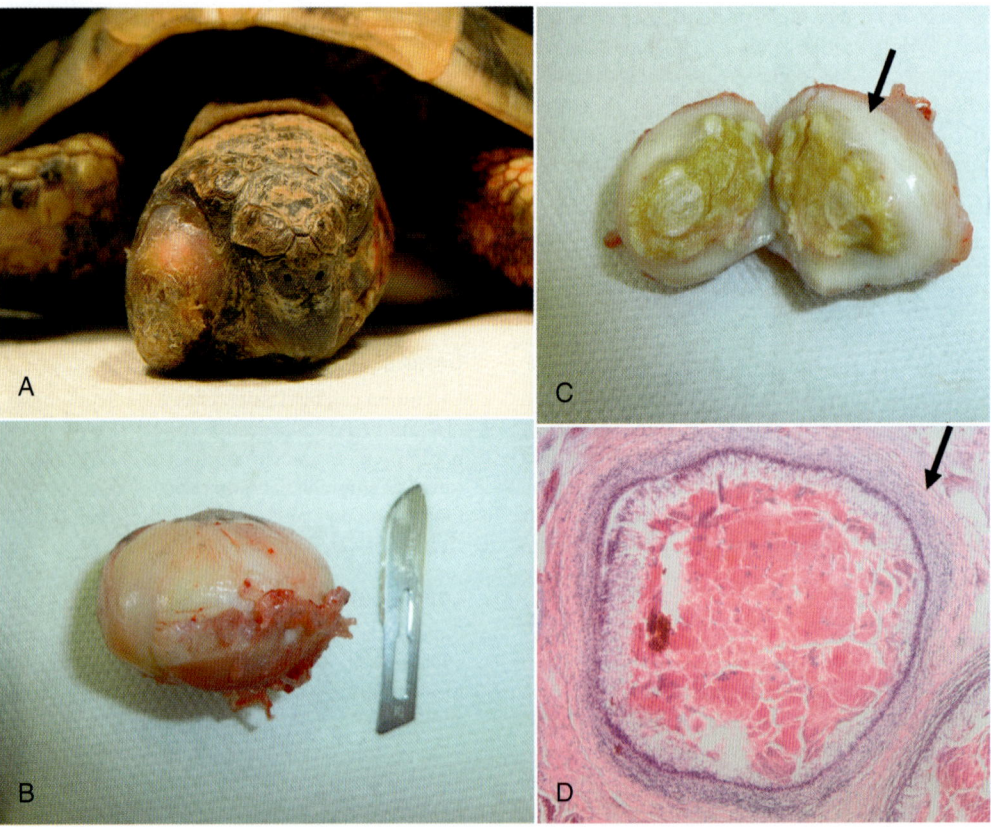

FIG 138.1 Subconjunctival fibriscess in a Hermann's tortoise (*Testudo hermanni*): (A) clinical picture, (B) surgically removed, (C) fibrous capsule (arrow) shown in cross-section, and (D) fibrious capsule (arrow) and central fibrin with bacterial colonies shown in microphotograph, HE stain, 100x. (Courtesy of Volker Schmidt, Department for Birds and Reptiles, University of Leipzig.)

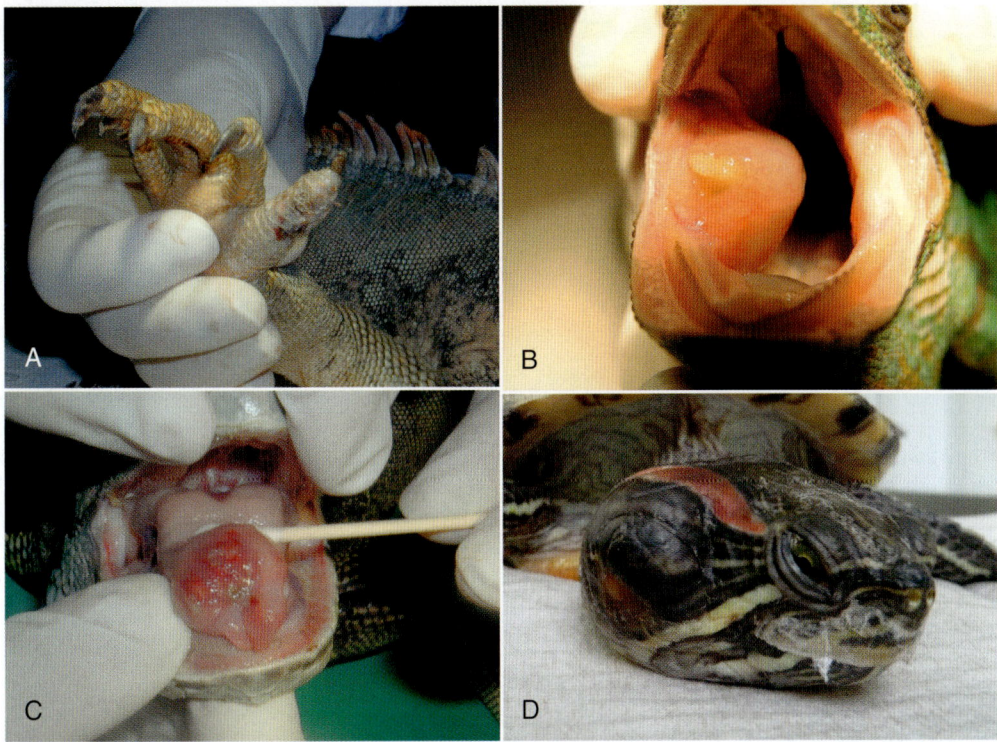

FIG 138.2 Different presentations for abscesses/fibriscesses: (A) cutanous manifestation in a green iguana (*Iguana iguana*) after traumatic injury, (B) glossal manifestation in a green iguana, (C) oral manifestation in a veiled chameleon (*Chamaeleo calyptratus*), and (D) aural manifestation in a red-eared slider (*Trachemys scripta elegans*) often predisposed by hypovitaminosis A. (Courtesy of Volker Schmidt, Department for Birds and Reptiles, University of Leipzig.)

hematogenous spread can disseminate pathogens to other internal organs and tissues. Beside traumatic injuries, which allow infection routes especially for bacteria, hypovitaminosis A results in squamous metaplasia of the epithelium, which often predisposes various reptile species to periocular, perioral, glossal, and aural fibriscesses[2-4] (Fig. 138.2).

CLINICAL SIGNS AND DIAGNOSTIC CONFIRMATION

All reptiles are susceptible to fibriscess formation. Depending on the organ system involved, the clinical signs may vary. Cutaneous or subcutaneous fibriscesses manifest as obvious, generally localized, swellings. Cellulitis, a deep diffuse suppurative infection in areas of low oxygen tension, can have a similar presentation to large fibriscesses but does not have the solid core. The differential diagnoses include any "mass lesions," such as neoplasia, hematomas, scar tissue, gout/pseudogout, and parasitic cysts. Pain on palpation (not always obvious), internal structure (fluid-filled versus solid), and previous history help with evaluation. Because of the solid nature of the fibriscesses, fine needle aspirates and exfoliative cytology are usually nonproductive. Cytology from aspirates usually reveals amorphous debris. Surgical exploration and/or removal of the mass in toto, when possible, followed by tissue cytology/histopathology and bacterial and fungal culture/sensitivity of tissue biopsies are important to confirm a diagnosis. Acid-fast (*Mycobacteria* and *Nocardia*), Gram (bacteria), Grocott (fungi), and periodic acid-schiff (fungi and bacteria) stains/reactions are useful to identify causative pathogens. Samples for microbiology should be collected from the inner lining of the fibrous capsule, not the necrotic center of the lesion, which is often sterile. Radiography, CT, ultrasonography, or MRI can be useful for internal evaluation.

PREFERRED TREATMENT(S)

The key to successful treatment is complete removal of the abscess cavity and surrounding fibrous capsule. Simple lancing and curettage, or removal of the internal caseous material, is not enough to prevent recurrence. Once the capsule has been removed, the wound is generally left open to heal by secondary intention and granulation. Second intention healing ensues, leaving minimal skin scarring in most cases. Healing times vary depending on many factors but in general can take anywhere from 4 to 6 weeks. Thorough surgical debridement is essential and often requires general anesthesia, although local or regional anesthesia may be sufficient in some dermatologic cases. Ablation of the abscess capsule/bed helps sterilize any material left behind after the debridement. Daily lavage and topical treatment of cutaneous lesions is an essential adjunct to initial surgical debridement. Topical antibiotics may be helpful but systemic treatment is seldom indicated following appropriate surgical removal. Incomplete removal often results in recurrence, even if systemic antimicrobials are used. Early in the treatment, weekly reevaluations are recommended.[5,6]

PROGNOSIS AND PREVENTION

Identification and correction of underlying deficiencies in husbandry (e.g., overcrowding, intraspecific agression, poor hygiene, malnutrition, etc.) will help prevent future occurrences. The owner should be given a cautiously optimistic prognosis, with the potential for recurrence or development of new lesions at different locations.

REFERENCES

See www.expertconsult.com for a complete list of references.

139

Acariasis

Kevin T. Fitzgerald

DEFINITION

Infestation with ticks and mites is known as acariasis. Although spiders are the best-known arachnids, ticks and mites are also members of this class. Larval ticks and mites have three pairs of legs, whereas nymphs and adults have four pairs. Head, thorax, and abdomen of ticks and mites are fused; also, they lack antennae and mandibles. These parasites can be difficult to eliminate, expensive to treat, and have a high incidence of recurrence. (See Chapters 32 and 69 for more details.)

CLINICAL SIGNIFICANCE AND KNOWN ETIOLOGICAL CAUSE(S)

Infestation with ticks and mites invariably can be traced to unsanitary conditions, poor husbandry practices, and recent imports of infested animals. Parasitism by ticks and mites occurs in both wild and captive reptiles. Acariasis has been linked to a variety of problems ranging from simple itching and discomfort to dermatitis, anemia, failure to thrive, anemia, and possible transmission of blood-borne diseases. Any level of infestation should be regarded as serious.

Ophionyssus natricis (Parasitiformes, Macronyssidae)—the snake mite—is the most common mite found in reptiles (Fig. 139.1).[1,2] Normally infesting snakes, it can also be found in captive lizards and turtles. *Ophinyssus acertinus*—the lizard mite—is usually red and larger than the black snake mite. More than 250 other mite species can also parasitize reptiles. *Trombiculid* mites—"chigger mites"—affect reptiles but are only parasitic in the larval form. Mites are formidable blood-sucking parasites, and their reptilian hosts often can support up to 10,000 mites.

Seven genera of ticks parasitize reptiles. Both soft- and hard-bodied ticks are found in snakes, lizards, and turtles. Blood-sucking parasites, they can inflict painful bites and under certain conditions result in serious blood loss. Additionally, they may introduce toxins with their bites and have the potential to transmit microbial diseases to hosts and other species.[3] Larger and more conspicuous than mites, they are more likely to be noticed earlier and removed before serious conditions or life-threatening anemia develops.

CLINICAL SIGNS

Anorexia, dermatitis, pruritus, anemia, septicemia, dysecdysis, retained eye caps, dehydration, failure to thrive, and the potential for transmission of blood-borne pathogens have all been documented in tick and mite infestations in captive reptiles. Behavioral changes associated with these ectoparasites can also be observed. Infected snakes may remain coiled in water bowls and soak for extended periods, attempting to rid themselves of these pests. Reptiles may also become hyperactive and will frequently rub against glass or cage furniture in an effort to remove the parasites. Persistent or recurrent dysecdysis in snakes may signal infestation. Even if animals are successful in shedding ectoparasite-infected skin, they quickly become reinfected within the confines of the cage.

Due to the white "dustlike" mite waste material, the skin of mite-infested reptiles may have a dull, lackluster, "dirty" appearance. Skin folds under the chin, under scutes, in the periocular region around the eyes, inside skin folds around the cloaca, and tympanic recesses in lizards are all common regions where mites are found (Fig. 139.2). The host skin at these mites feeding sites becomes hyperemic, edematous, and infiltrated with heterophils, lymphocytes, and plasma cells. Mites vary in color depending on species, gender, and how recently they have fed. Reptiles affected with acarids may be debilitated but remarkably

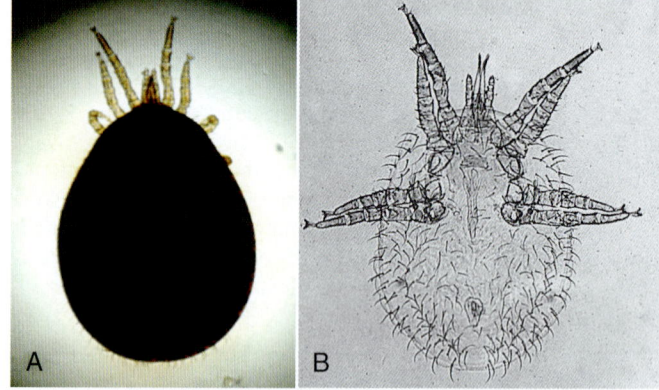

FIG 139.1 A snake mite under magnification. (Courtesy of R. Houston.)

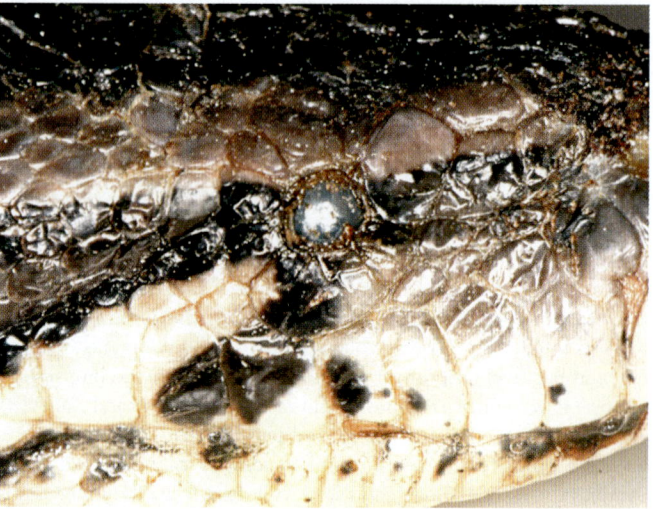

FIG 139.2 A Burmese python (*Python bivittatus*) severely infested with mites. Note the large numbers in the periocular area. (Courtesy of Stephen Barten.)

may still be active, feeding, and seemingly unaffected, even with tremendous parasite loads. Often the most common clinical presentation for reptiles with mites is toxicity from improper and unsafe eradication treatment. These toxicities can be severe, devastating, and often fatal.

CLINICAL PRESENTATION AND DIAGNOSTIC CONFIRMATION

Mites are most readily seen moving on or between scales of the head, around eyes, in axillary folds, or on the trunk of heavily infested lizards. In advanced cases, reptiles may have mites visibly swarming over the body or display conspicuously attached ticks. Casual observation may not be enough to declare animals or cages parasite free. Often mites are not noticed until owners find them on their own skin after handling infested reptiles. Wiping with a wet cotton swab, damp gauze sponge, or a shallow bath may reveal dislodged mites. Ticks are much easier to identify and areas typically targeted should be examined frequently. A regular inspection of captive reptiles and their environments should be performed to identify both free-living and parasite stages. Cages themselves, lids, hide boxes, and cage furniture must be routinely inspected and cleaned. Finally, magnification with a hand lens may help to provide a diagnosis.

TREATMENT

Acaricides—Mites

Preferred Treatment

1. Quarantine: Quarantine of new animals for at least 3 months before introduction into a collection. This may be the **most** important management and control method.
2. Permethrin: 0.5% permethrin spray (Provent-a-Mite, Pro-Products, Mahopec, NY). Lizards, snakes—environment treatment 1 second spray/sq ft.[2] Wait until dry before returning animals to enclosure. Safe, effective—only product licensed as an acaracide for reptiles. **This is the preferred treatment.**
3. Sanitation/cleaning: Mites are killed by hot water >122°F (750°C). Cages, shelves, and lids should be cleaned weekly.

Alternative Therapies

1. Ivermectin topical: 0.5 mL of ivermectin (10 mg/mL) added to 1 quart tap water and applied liberally to the cage and surroundings. Avoid spraying into water bowl. Can be sprayed or wiped on snakes and lizards. Shake solution thoroughly before applying (ivermectin is oil based). Weekly or every other week treatments for 6 to 8 weeks may be necessary in large collections. Ivermectin must never be used on or around chelonians or indigo snakes.[4]
2. Fipronil: 0.29% fipronil spray (Frontline Fipronil Spray Treatment, Merial, Duluth, GA).
3. Resmethrin II: Durakyl -0.35% remethrin (DVM Pharmaceuticals, Miami, FL)
4. Permectin II: 10% permethrin diluted to 1% in tap water used as a spray (Bioceutic Division, Beohringer-Ingelheim Animal Health, Inc., St. Joseph, MO).
5. Dilute pyrethrin: 0.03% dilute pyrethrin (Mite and Lice Bird Spray, 8 in 1 Products, Inc., Itauppage, NY).
6. Imidacloprid plus moxidectin: Commercial Imidacloprid (100 g/L) plus moxidectin (25 g/L)—Advocate Dog (Bayer Corp, Reading, UK) and Advantage Multi (Bayer Corp, Kansas City, MO) has been recommended.
7. Biologic control of mites: Utilization of predatory "cannibal" mites have been recommended as a biologic control for acariasis in lizards.[5]

Treatments No Longer Recommended (Either Unsafe or Ineffective)

- Chlorinated hydrocarbons (DDT)—toxicity
- Organophosphates (Trichlorfon)—toxicity
- 5% Sevin Dust—toxicity
- Dichlorvos strips—toxicity
- Silica gel powder—caustic, toxic
- Olive oil—stressful and not 100% effective
- Drying out cages—ineffective
- Bleach—never apply to animals
- Roccal-D, A-33 Dry—never apply to live animals
- Bathing/soaking—ineffective if done as only treatment
- Insect growth regulators—does not kill mites right away

Acaricides—Ticks

Preferred Treatment

1. Permethrin: Provent-a-Mite (Pro-Products, Mahopac, NY), safe and effective at killing ticks by a spray with a dilution of 0.01% and 0.5%.[6,7] Spray the animal from a few inches away (10 cm). **This is the preferred method.**

Alternative Treatments

1. Cyfluthrin: Cyfluthrin 0.01% (Tempo, Bayer Corp., Kansas City, MO) formulated for premise treatment coupled together with direct permethrin treatment of ticks on chelonians is safe and effective.
2. Ivermectin: Ivermectin has been suggested as a method of tick removal for ticks hiding in nostrils, loreal/labial pits, or other body recesses. Ivermectin must never be given to chelonians or indigo snakes.
3. Permethrin spray: Another permethrin spray (Preventic, Virbac, Ft. Worth, TX) has been suggested for cage, shelving, and room treatment of ticks. This is only for cage environments.
4. Manual removal: Ticks should be removed with delicate forceps. Ticks should be grabbed under the head on the mouth parts and extracted.

PROGNOSIS AND PREVENTION

Success of various therapy protocols for the management of ectoparasites in captive reptiles is dependent on how effective the therapy is in targeting and eradicating the specific life stages of the parasite and how thoroughly the affected housing environment is treated and managed.

In summary, successful treatment of mite infestations generally includes a combination of strategies: a rigorous quarantine system; utilization of the permethrin product Provent-a-mite; and disinfection of the cage, shelving, lids, and associated surfaces, as well as any permanent cage furniture, nondisposable hide-boxes, food, and water dishes. Continued vigilance is essential. Any treatment plan only dealing with the mites on the host and not managing the environment will fail.

Successful tick therapy involves physical removal of the parasite, spray application of the 0.5% permethrin product to affected areas in chelonians, and treatment of the environment and enclosure either with the permethrin product in lizards and snakes or cyfluthrin in chelonians.

Veterinarians treating reptiles must be aware of the zoonotic implications of these parasites and their potential impact on nontarget species.[1,3]

REFERENCES

See www.expertconsult.com for a complete list of references.

140

Amphibian Chytridiomycosis

Norin Chai and Brent R. Whitaker

DEFINITION AND KNOWN ETIOLOGICAL CAUSE(S)

Amphibian chytridiomycosis is a fungal disease caused by *Batracho-chytrium dendrobatidis* (*Bd*) and *Batrachochytrium salamandrivorans* (*Bs*) (Chytridiomycota, Rhizophydiales).

CLINICAL SIGNIFICANCE

Bd has a broad host range and infects at least 520 species of anurans (frogs and toads), urodeles (salamanders and newts), and caecilians. *Bs* seems restricted to salamanders and newts.[1] Horizontal transmission may be direct or indirect, and *Bd* can grow on sterile bird feathers and arthropod exoskeletons. *Bd* can grow on the keratinous paw scales of waterfowl and survive in the gastrointestinal tract of crayfish, which have been suggested as potential nonamphibian vectors for *Bd*.[1] Bd has a global distribution highly linked with international movement of amphibians for research facilities and the pet trade. Asia has most recently been proposed as the origin of Bd. At this time, Bs has been found in Europe and Asia but not in North America. In an effort to prevent the introduction, establishment, and spread of *Bs* in the United States, the US Fish and Wildlife Service recently added all species in 20 genera of salamanders to the list of injurious amphibians (https://www.fws.gov/injuriouswildlife/pdf_files/List-of-Salamander-Species.pdf). This prevents the importation/movement of salamanders into the United States and between states, except by permit for zoologic, educational, medical, or scientific purposes.[2]

CLINICAL PRESENTATION

Gross lesions are generally limited to the skin in postmetamorphic amphibians and to the keratinized mouthparts in larval anurans. Clinical signs are variable and include peracute death, skin lesions (roughness, hyperemia, hyperplasia, small skin ulcers, excessive shedding), necrosis of digits/feet, dehydration, weight loss, loss of righting reflex, lethargy, and abnormal behavior (prolonged periods in the vivarium's water dish, failure to seek shelter, reluctance to flee). In anuran larvae, clinical signs are generally limited to depigmentation of the mouthparts, without morbidity and mortality. Infection due to *Bs* in metamorphosed urodelans is characterized by multifocal superficial erosions and extensive epidermal ulcerations, excessive shedding of the skin, anorexia, apathy, ataxia, and death.

DIAGNOSTIC CONFIRMATION

Cytologic examination of stained or unstained skin smears and skin fragments for the detection of zoosporangia provides rapid diagnosis. PCR or qPCR can be done on skin swabs from mouthparts of live anuran larvae and from the ventral pelvic patch, hind legs, and feet of live postmetamorphic, freshly dead, frozen, or ethanol-preserved postmetamorphic amphibians. Mouthparts of anuran larvae, fragments of shedding skin, multiple skin sections, and toe clips fixed in formalin can be sent for histopathology. Histopathologic changes due to *Bd* include multifocal hyperplastic and hyperkeratotic dermatitis, sloughing of the prominent keratin layer, and numerous fungal zoosporangia. In contrast, *Bs* infection is characterized by erosive skin lesions associated with the presence of numerous intracellular colonial thalli that spread over the epidermis with marked necrosis of the adjacent keratinocytes—hyperplasia and hyperkeratosis are absent.[1] Electronmicroscopy and immunohistochemistry using polyclonal antibodies may be used as an aid in histologic diagnosis.

PREFERRED TREATMENT(S) AND PREVENTION

There is no one treatment against chytridiomycosis that is effective in all species and at all life stages (Table 140.1). There are numerous

TABLE 140.1	Selected Treatments Against Chytridiomycosis	
Treatments	**Dosages—Protocols**	**Comments**
Itraconazole	0.005% (50 mg/L) bath, 5 min/day for 10 days.	Safe and effective treatment in most situations.[3]
	0.01% bath, 5 min/day for 10 days.	Required with higher infection intensities.[3]
	0.0025% bath, 5 min/day for 6 days.	In juvenile *Litoria caerulea* and Gulf Coast toads (*Incilius nebulifer*).[4]
	0.01% bath, 30 min/day for 11 days.	Used in terrestrial African caecilian, *Geotrypetes seraphini*, and aquatic neotropical caecilian, *Potomotyphlus kaupii*.[5]
Voriconazole	Mixed to a concentration of 1.25 µg/mL water and sprayed on to animals daily for 7 days.	Used in Corroboree frog (*Pseudophryne corroboree*), Iberian midwife toad (*Alytes cisternasii*) juveniles, and a few individual poison dart frogs (Dendrobatidae family).[6,7]
Voriconazole and polymyxin E	Polymyxin E submersion baths (2000 IU/mL, 10 minutes) followed by spraying voriconazole (12.5 µg/mL) twice a day for 10 days at an ambient temperature of 20°C.	Effective treatment in *Salamandra salamandra*.[8]

TABLE 140.1 Selected Treatments Against Chytridiomycosis—cont'd

Treatments	Dosages—Protocols	Comments
Chloramphenicol	Combination of continuous shallow immersion (23 of 24 hrs) in 20 mg/L chloramphenicol solution for 14 days, parenteral isotonic electrolyte fluid therapy for 6 days, and increased ambient temperature to 28°C for 14 days.	Effective combination treatment in green tree frogs (*Litoria caerulea*).[9]
Terbinafine	Dissolved in ethanol diluted in distilled water to create solutions of 0.01%–0.005% terbinafine and 1%–0.5% ethanol, respectively. Animals were bathed for 5 minutes daily for 5 consecutive days.	Popular treatment because it is commercially available as an athlete's foot preparation (Lamisil AT Spray, 1% terbinafine hydrochloride, Novartis Consumer Health, Parsippany, NJ).[3,10]
Increased environmental temperature	Environmental temperature is gradually increased over a period of 2 days. Animals are then maintained at this ambient temperature.	Effective treatment at 30°C for 10 consecutive days in *Rana catesbeiana* and *Acris crepitans*.[11] Effective treatment at 25°C for 10 consecutive days in salamanders.[12] Effective treatment at 32.2°C for 72 hrs in aquatic caecilians (*Typhlonectes natans*). Then over a period of 3–4 days the temperature was slowly returned to ambient.[13]

disinfectants that effectively kill *Bd*, including Virkon, a multipurpose disinfectant that contains oxone (potassium peroxymonosulfate), sodium dodecylbenzenesulfonate, sulfamic acid, and inorganic buffers (Antec International, Sudbury, UK) at 2 g/L^{-1} or a solution of 4% bleach.[14] Newly acquired animals should be maintained in quarantine as individuals in separate containers for at least 2 months. Collect skin swabs (or mouthpart swabs from tadpoles) for PCR assay on arrival and 7 weeks later. A thorough necropsy including PCR (ideally qPCR) on the appropriate tissues must be performed on any animals that die.

REFERENCES

See www.expertconsult.com for a complete list of references.

Aural/Tympanic Abscessation

Michelle Kischinovsky and Stephen J. Divers

DEFINITION

Aural abscessation is a condition characterized by an accumulation of caseous material within the middle ear or tympanic cavity, resulting in a protrusion of the tympanum (Fig. 141.1A). The condition exists in both free-ranging and captive reptilian populations and is most commonly seen in chelonians (tortoises and semiaquatic turtles).[1–7]

CLINICAL SIGNIFICANCE AND KNOWN ETIOLOGICAL CAUSE(S)

Aural abscess formation appears to be multifactorial and a result of several predisposing factors. No known cause has been identified; however, it is generally accepted that there exists a correlation between abscess formation and improper husbandry (e.g., suboptimal habitat temperatures, poor hygiene) leading to immunosuppression as well as inadequate nutrition resulting in vitamin A deficiency.[7] Hypovitaminosis A causes hyperplasia and squamous metaplasia of several epithelial tissues, including those of the pharynx, trachea, middle ear, and eustachian tube, leading to an accumulation of exfoliated squamous cells and keratinlike debris within the tympanic cavity, which eventually results in abscess formation.[2,7–9] This assumed relationship is supported by free-ranging Eastern box turtles (*Terrapene carolina carolina*) with pathological aural changes in association with organochloride-containing pesticides known to cause vitamin A metabolism disruption in other species.[8–11] The eustachian tubes, connecting the oropharynx to the middle ear, may provide a pathway for ascending pathogens into the tympanic cavity, which in an immunocompromised animal may contribute to abscess development. However, no consistent bacterial pathogen has been isolated, and most (mainly aerobic gram-negatives) are believed to be opportunistic commensals from the oral cavity.[2,6,12] Though less likely, hematogenous spread and traumatic etiology are possible.

CLINICAL PRESENTATION AND DIAGNOSTIC CONFIRMATION

The tympanic swelling(s) may present as unilateral or bilateral, semifirm to firm, and cause protrusion of the tympanic membrane rather than rupture. Obvious vestibular signs are generally lacking. The absence, in reptiles, of lysozomes (within their granulocytic leukocytes) results in a caseous, inspissated pus. Histologically, cases range from mild squamous metaplasia and hyperplasia to more severe cases involving pronounced inflammation and osteolysis.[2,8,12,13] Diagnosis can often be made solely by visual assessment. Additional tests may add therapeutic or prognostic value and can include fine-needle aspiration cystology (to aid differentiation from neoplasia) as well as hematology and blood chemistry to evaluate systemic disease involvement. Radiography and computed tomography may aid in determination of severity and appropriate management.[13]

PREFERRED TREATMENT(S)

Surgical management is recommended (see Chapter 92 for surgical details). Because of the avascular and inspissated structure of the abscess, it is easily manipulated out of the tympanic cavity in its entirety (see Fig. 141.1B). The deficit is lavaged and dressed daily, and the tympanum is left to heal by second intention. Antibiotics are seldom necessary.

PROGNOSIS AND PREVENTION

Complete excavation of aural debris, appropriate wound and secondary infection management, and correction of any concurrent suboptimal husbandry conditions result in a good prognosis. Recurrence does occur and is typically due to inadequate surgical debridement or failure to address the underlying predisposing factors.[7] Education with regard to appropriate husbandry, sanitation, and nutrition is most beneficial for prevention.

REFERENCES

See www.expertconsult.com for a complete list of references.

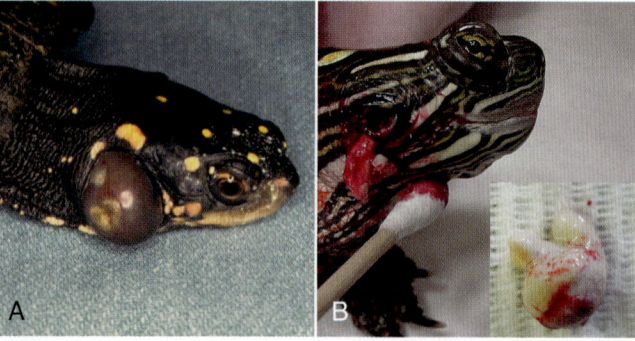

FIG 141.1 (A) Right aural abscess in a Chinese spotted turtle (*Clemmys guttata*). (B) Surgical removal of a right aural abscess from a slider (*Trachemys scripta*). (*Inset*) Removed aural abscess from a tortoise (*Testudo graeca*), demonstrating the caseous, inspissated nature of the infection. (Courtesy of Stephen J. Divers.)

Bite Wounds and Prey-Induced Trauma

Marja J.L. Kik and T. Franciscus Scheelings

DEFINITION

This chapter covers injuries from dogs, cats, predators and rodent/invertebrate prey.

CLINICAL SIGNIFICANCE AND KNOWN ETIOLOGICAL CAUSE(S)

Bite injuries are common in captive and free-ranging reptiles. Injuries may occur as a result of predation, inter- or intraspecies hostility (e.g. dog or cat attack), or from live prey items (especially rodents and crickets).

CLINICAL PRESENTATION AND DIAGNOSTIC CONFIRMATION

Housing sexually mature males together can often lead to serious and violent fighting resulting in extensive wounds (Fig. 142.1A). Conspecific aggression is not limited to sexual rivalry or courtship, as individuals housed in appropriate sex ratios may engage in combat in competition for food or basking resources. Although reptiles housed in mixed exhibits may appear to coexist harmoniously for extended periods, often there is an undercurrent of stress. Reptiles are typically solitary animals that may defend themselves vigorously against rivals. This can

be a difficult conversation for clinicians to have with some keepers as there is a tendency to anthropomorphize the needs of the reptile for companionship.

Bite injuries may also occur from live prey items. Most reptiles will readily accept prekilled prey and the practice of offering live rodents should be discouraged (and may be illegal depending on location). Live rodents left unattended in a cage with an anorectic reptile eventually become hungry, frantic, and may attack or feed on the reptile (see Fig. 142.1B). Rodents may also bite when seized by a hungry reptile, resulting in wounds to the tongue, lips, eyes, or head of the reptile. The bite wounds can be superficial or severe even resulting in death.

Invertebrate prey left in enclosures can bite debilitated reptiles.[1] Although such wounds are typically superficial, they can lead to bacterial infections and even septicemia. Additionally, these nonfeeding interactions with free roaming insects may create stress. Some species of lizards can be fed invertebrates with a pair of forceps avoiding the need to leave them in the enclosure. For others, such as chameleons that utilize their projectile tongues to feed, small but deep containers can be used to localize and contain insects.

Another important source of bite wounds in reptiles comes from dog and cat attacks.[2] This is most common in free-ranging animals but may also occur when reptiles are left unattended in a yard or if they inadvertently escape from an enclosure. These injuries are often severe and commonly result in death or necessitate euthanasia.

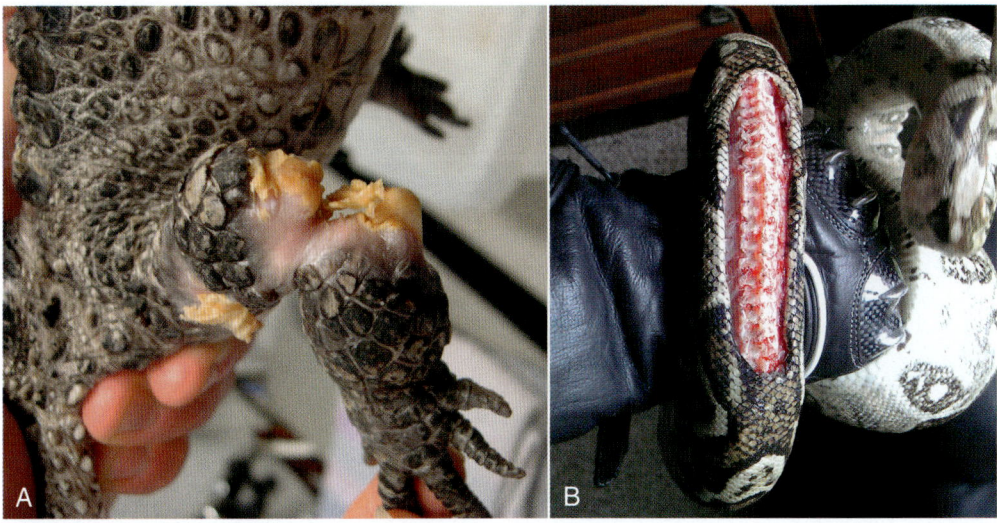

FIG 142.1 (A) Chinese alligator *(Alligator sinensis)* with evidence of severe intraspecific trauma by a cage mate. (B) Boa *(Boa constrictor)* with a bite injury from a rat. (Courtesy of Marja J.L. Kik.)

PREFERRED TREATMENT(S)

Hemorrhage should be addressed. Bite wounds are always contaminated with a variety of microbiota.[3] The wounds should be flushed extensively with sterile saline. Treatment often requires sedation, analgesia and in severe cases general anesthesia (see Chapters 48 through 52).[4] Necrotic tissue should be surgically removed. Defects should only be sutured if wounds are fresh, and not punctures. Amputation should be considered for severely damaged appendages and ruptured globes enucleated. Contaminated, infected, or older (>6–12 hours) wounds should be cultured, not be sutured and be allowed to heal by secondary intention. In some cases, partial closure, still allowing drainage and flushing/treatment may be done. Dressings should be properly applied and changed regularly to keep the wound free from contamination and avoid complications such as myiasis. Topical and systemic antibiotics are often indicated and should be administered based on culture and sensitivity results. Additionally, hematology and diagnostic imaging may be warranted.

For aquatic turtles, wounds should be covered with sterile bandages, including a waterproof adhesive, in order to restore them to an aquatic environment (see Chapter 113 for an extensive discussion on shell treatment and repair). Additional supportive care may include esophageal tube placement for fluid and nutritional support (see Chapter 45). During convalescence animals should be housed under conditions that will not affect wound healing (e.g. unprinted newspaper, paper toweling, and damp towels for aquatic reptiles). See Section 3 husbandry and management, and Chapter 46 hospitalization for more details.

PROGNOSIS AND PREVENTION

Prognosis is varied and depends on the extent of the injury. Superficial wounds involving just the skin have a good prognosis. Deep wounds that result in puncture of the gastrointestinal tract or damage to other internal organs may carry a grave prognosis. In captive situations, these injuries can be avoided by altering husbandry practices and excluding dogs and cats and other predators from reptile areas.

REFERENCES

See www.expertconsult.com for a complete list of references.

Cloacal Prolapse

Stuart McArthur and Ross A. Machin

DEFINITION

A cloacal prolapse is a relatively irreducible, persistent, pathologic protrusion of tissue through the cloaca and vent. A cloacal organ prolapse is a common veterinary emergency seen in both first opinion and referral practice and occurs in all reptile taxa. A cloacal prolapse is a clinical sign, not a diagnosis, because in most cases, a pathologic prolapse is associated with deeper clinical issues and significant debility. The gastrointestinal, reproductive, and urinary systems all terminate at the cloaca, and therefore a wide variety of disorders may manifest as abnormalities around this anatomic structure, especially if obstructive. Prolapses have been described in free-ranging as well as captive reptiles (Machin R, McArthur S, personal observation, 2017).[1–12]

Cloacal anatomy is variable between the orders but is generally divided into three compartments between the caudal colon and the vent.[13–22] The anatomy and physiology of the cloaca is described in Chapter 75.

CLINICAL SIGNIFICANCE

Cloacal organ prolapse is a common reptile veterinary emergency. In one study including more than 3000 captive reptiles, the incidence of reptile prolapses was 1.9%, and they were more common in chelonians and lizards than in snakes. The most common prolapse was the phallus/hemipenes (35.7%). Prolapses were 3.47 times as likely in chelonians and lizards compared with snakes with no statistical differences between males and females, although females were 7.5 times more likely than males to present with a true cloacal prolapse involving no other organs. The authors concluded that species and sex may influence prevalence and type of cases seen.[1]

KNOWN ETIOLOGICAL CAUSE(S)

The presence of a cloacal prolapse is associated with a variety of complex multifactorial causes. These associations are summarized in Table 75.2. They include intestinal (e.g., infections, parasites, constipation, fecoliths, and neoplasia), urinary (e.g., infections and uroliths), reproductive (e.g., male courtship trauma or probing, belanoposthitis, mating injuries, paraphimosis, dystocia, chronic sexual activity, constipation, neurological dysfunction, substrate contamination, hemipenile plugs, hypothermia, neoplasia), metabolic (e.g., hypocalcemia, electrolyte derangements, dehydration, debility, hypothermia, collapse), and coelomic disease (e.g., ascites, coelomitis, neoplasia). In addition, normal tissue (e.g., phallus) may also be intermittently observed by owners during bathing, handling, or urination.[1–12]

CLINICAL PRESENTATION

Left untreated, a cloacal prolapse results in distress and likely pain. The condition must be regarded as a true veterinary emergency, because the prolapsed structure will become rapidly devitalized through ischemic necrosis if not protected and reperfused rapidly. With the possible exclusion of prolapses of the male copulatory organ, untreated prolapses involving the colon, bladder or oviduct are likely to be fatal because of the combined systemic effects of tissue necrosis and compromised body system functions.[1,10]

Treatment of most cloacal prolapses involves a skillful, simultaneous balance of medical and surgical interventions. The presentation therefore draws on many of the techniques described across the clinical disciplines. Information to assist a clinician facing this presentation is located within several sections of this book; surgical management is covered within Chapter 106 and throughout Section 10, whereas medical management is included in Chapter 75 and throughout Sections 5 and 9.

DIAGNOSTIC CONFIRMATION

A detailed history covering husbandry and species understanding is vital in the full diagnosis of a cloacal organ prolapse, because there are many factors that may contribute directly or indirectly to the presenting condition. Features of the history that deserve special attention include the species, age, the suitability of any source of heat or ultraviolet lighting used, the hygiene conditions the reptile has been kept in, whether the reptile was kept alone or in a group, the substrate used, and the humidity and photoperiod used.[11,12]

Organ differentiation may prove challenging due to exposure or trauma. A guide to identification of the organ involved in a cloacal prolapse is given in Table 75.1. It is always important to determine which organ has prolapsed, because this influences both the treatment options and the prognosis. The organ prolapses experienced by each reptile class are summarized in Table 75.1. Prolapsed structures may include hemipenes (snakes and lizards) or phallus (chelonians), cloacal masses or tissue, oviduct, shell gland, colon/rectum, bladder (chelonians), and ovaries (sea turtles).[1,3,4,6,8]

A considered therapeutic plan must have informed client consent. This is occasionally challenging, because many prolapses will require extensive medical management in parallel with surgical reduction or organ removal. Appropriate diagnostic investigations may include clinicopathology (hematology, biochemistry, microbiology, virology), diagnostic imaging (radiography/CT, ultrasonography or endoscopy initially), fecal testing (parasitology, bacteriology), and in some cases exploratory coeliotomy/coelioscopy or advanced imaging techniques may be required.

Following commencement of initial stabilization measures described earlier in Table 75.3, a diagnostic plan should be made and followed, allowing a therapeutic plan suitable to the specific patient.

PREFERRED TREATMENT(S)

It is necessary to treat both the prolapse and the underlying cause. Analgesia, physical manipulation, osmotic reduction, and lubrication

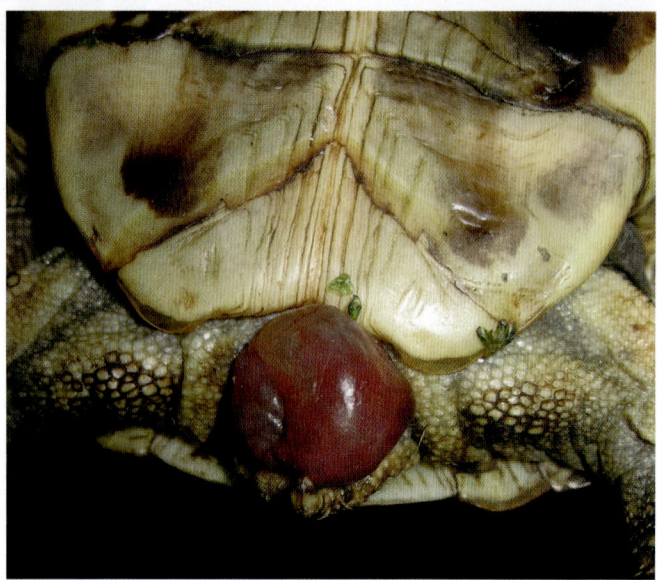

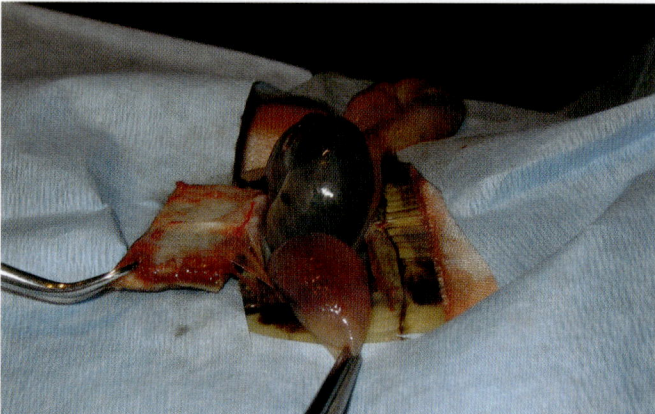

FIG 143.2 The same *Testudo hermanni* as Fig. 143.1. A plastron osteotomy and coeliotomy have been performed. The prolapse has been reduced and the intussusception corrected. The colon will have pexy sutures to the coelomic membrane placed before the osteotomy is closed.

FIG 143.1 Colonic intussusception and prolapse in a Hermann's tortoise (*Testudo hermanni*). The prolapse is fresh and has an obvious lumen.

can sometimes be achieved simply by using materials such as local anesthetic mixed with lubricating gels. However, in many cases, addressing the prolapse may be more complicated. Analgesia options are also covered in Table 75.4.

In the case of a prolapsed phallus or hemipenis, application of lubrication after appropriate lavage often allows a fresh prolapse to then be gently replaced within the cloaca or in the case of a hemipenis inverted back within the ventral tail base. Here it can be retained through a suitable dressing or bandage, or in some cases through a temporary suture. Where the organ has significant devitalized tissue, amputation in a stabilized patient is preferable. Additional conditions behind the prolapse will also require correction; examples include bacterial or parasitic infections, dehydration, and hypocalcemia.

In the case of an oviduct or colon prolapse, a celiotomy is normally required to correctly reduce the prolapse and address factors that lie behind it (Fig. 143.1). If the prolapse is necrotic or devitalized, all or part of the prolapse may require removal during the coeliotomy procedure (Fig. 143.2). Additional conditions behind the prolapse will also require correction, including dystocia, cloacoliths, constipation, and parasitism.

In the case of a bladder prolapse, occasionally these may be reduced without the need for coeliotomy; however, some form of contrast imaging may be required to confirm correct reduction and ensure that that the structure has involuted correctly. It may be necessary to perform a coeliotomy to address any ectopic eggs or calculi within the bladder. Additional conditions behind the prolapse will also require correction.

The longer a prolapse is left vulnerable, with exposure to contaminated substrate, strangulated, engorged, and traumatized, the less likely it is to be viable and the more likely it will require removal.[6] Where organ identity cannot be differentiated because of severe secondary swelling, substrate contamination, avascular necrosis, or an inexperienced clinician, the client should be realistically informed about different options available for managing the patient. These options include referral for diagnostic procedures, surgical options, and possible complications, and they should be issued with a guarded prognosis.[6] For example, in many reptile species it may not be possible to remove a length of necrotic colon and still have a viable patient, and this may not be known until an intraoperative assessment can be made. Surgical procedures and protocols are covered in Chapter 106.

PROGNOSIS AND PREVENTION

The prognosis for a cloacal organ prolapse is dependent on multiple factors; most importantly this includes any underlying cause, the patient's condition, and the prolapse viability and duration of the prolapse. Treatment and prognosis in a young leopard gecko with a hemipenal prolapse that requires amputation following chronic sexual activity will be different than a monitor lizard with severe nutritional secondary hyperparathyroidism and colonic prolapse. Prognosis varies from excellent to grave, and euthanasia should be considered in the most serious cases.

Species understanding and educating owners and caretakers on appropriate husbandry, including stress reduction, environmental enrichment, balanced diet, supplementation, lighting, humidity, and adequate substrate are essential for minimizing or preventing many of these conditions.

REFERENCES

See www.expertconsult.com for a complete list of references.

144

Cloacal Scent Gland Adenitis

Scott J. Stahl

DEFINITION

Paired cloacal scent glands of snakes are uniquely ophidian and are present in all species of snakes.[1] The glands appear in both male and female snakes but are larger in females. These paired glands are located within the tail base (Fig. 144.1A). Cloacal scent glands are specialized exocrine glands that produce a thick semi-liquid material containing pheromones and semiochemicals used to actively mark objects and organisms.[1] See Chapter 80 for more details.

CLINICAL SIGNIFICANCE AND KNOWN ETIOLOGICAL CAUSE(S)

Cloacal scent gland adenitis has been reported in snakes and is not an uncommon presentation.[2] Clinically, scent gland adenitis appears to be more common in older, female, colubrid, and actively breeding snakes.[2] Without release the impacted scent material becomes thick, inspissated, and the gland becomes secondarily infected, swollen, hard, and may rupture.[2] Mineralization and neoplasia are possible and often unilateral. Captive related environmental factors affecting glandular release include humidity, substrate (paper or carpeting versus a natural substrate), poor sanitation, and presence or absence of conspecifics. The author has seen several cases of neoplasia associated with scent glands, and a fibrosarcoma was identified with scent gland adenitis in a colubrid snake (Couture et al, Proc ARAV, 2017, p 352).

CLINICAL PRESENTATION AND DIAGNOSTIC CONFIRMATION

Typically, older and/or actively breeding females are overrepresented. Physical examination is often diagnostic, with snakes presenting with unilateral or bilateral swellings caudal and lateral, and in severe cases craniolateral, to the cloaca (see Fig. 144.1B). In severe cases rupture of the gland may occur. On palpation the gland may be soft to hard depending on changes and duration. Fine-needle aspiration and cytology can confirm gland involvement and may indicate neoplasia. Radiography is less useful except to confirm mineralization. Ultrasonography can help differentiate between neoplastic tissue and impaction. Biopsy for histopathology and microbiological testing at surgery is often necessary for a definitive diagnosis.

PREFERRED TREATMENT(S)

In cases of mild impaction gently massaging the gland (after warm water soak) to move material toward the gland opening may allow release. In larger snakes cannulation of the duct opening (under sedation/anesthesia) can be attempted with a urinary catheter or metal lacrimal duct cannula.[2] Unfortunately, with retention, glandular material becomes thick, grainy, often inspissated, and cannot pass out of the narrow duct opening, necessitating surgery. For surgical resolution, an incision is made between the lateral scale rows over the enlarged gland. The gland

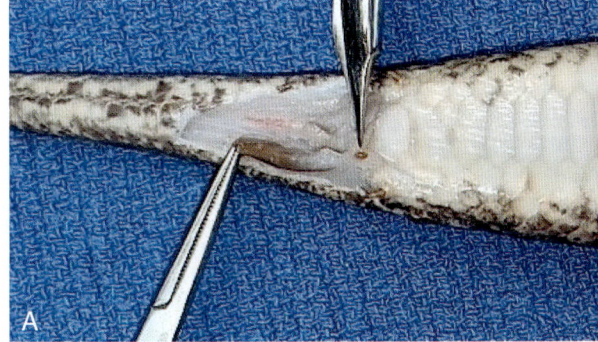
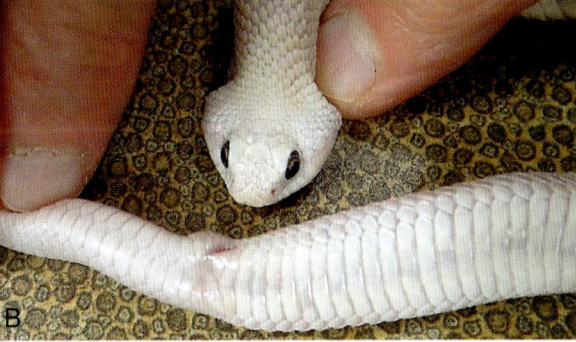

FIG 144.1 (A) A prosection of a female ball python (*Python regius*) showing the location of the paired cloacal scent glands in the tail base. The caudal vent rim, and some subcaudal scales, have been removed to show the location of the left scent gland (grasped by hemostats) and the opening of the scent gland with scent gland material evident (at the tip of the scissors). (B) A leucistic western hognose snake (*Heterodon nasicus*) with cloacal scent gland adenitis in the right gland (at top near snake's head) showing; in severe cases, the gland swelling can be craniolateral to the vent not just caudal. This case was associated with bacterial adenitis. (A, Courtesy of Greg Costanzo, Stahl Exotic Animal Veterinary Services; B, courtesy of Scott J. Stahl, Stahl Exotic Animal Veterinary Services.)

is opened, impacted material is removed, and biopsies of the gland are collected for histopathology and microbiological culture. The gland can then be lavaged and a catheter passed to ensure patency. If the gland was cannulated, it can be closed or marsupialized to allow continued flushing and treatment.[2] Systemic antimicrobials and/or topical antimicrobials may be initiated based on histopathology and microbiological results along with local flushing with antiseptics. Surgical removal of the entire affected gland(s) is often the curative choice in cases that are severe, reoccurring, bilateral, or if neoplasia is suspected/confirmed (Couture et al., 2017, Proc ARAV, p 352).[2] (See Chapter 80 for more details on medical and surgical resolution of scent gland adenitis.)

PROGNOSIS AND PREVENTION

Prognosis is good with complete surgical removal of the gland(s) and if underlying conditions leading to blockage and/or inflammation of the gland are corrected after successful medical treatment. If neoplasia is confirmed, the type of neoplasm determines prognosis. Prevention involves correcting husbandry issues that may be contributing factors.

REFERENCES

See www.expertconsult.com for a complete list of references.

Diarrhea

Kevin Eatwell and Jenna Richardson

DEFINITION

Diarrhea is a clinical sign, not a disease. It can be defined as increased water content in the feces, resulting in soft or liquid feces. Compared with mammals, reptiles have a longer gastrointestinal transit time, and most normal reptile feces are therefore well formed and, in some cases, even desiccated.

CLINICAL SIGNIFICANCE AND KNOWN ETIOLOGICAL CAUSE(S)

Diarrhea can be classified as acute (sudden onset, self-limiting, short duration) or chronic (longer duration, recurrent). Causes of acute episodes include dietary indiscretion, sudden changes in diet, or inadequate temperature provision (see Chapter 74 for more details). Chronic diarrhea is often more concerning due to dehydration and electrolyte imbalances. As with mammals, steatorrhea and melena often indicate a small-bowel problem, whereas fresh blood and mucus are more likely large-bowel related. Potential causes of diarrhea include infectious enterocolitis (e.g., parasitic, bacterial, viral, mycotic), inflammatory or infiltrative diseases of the bowel (e.g., neoplasia), and intestinal malfunction (e.g., partial obstruction).

CLINICAL PRESENTATION AND DIAGNOSTIC CONFIRMATION

Depending on the duration, severity, and underlying cause, the reptile may present bright and active or dull, lethargic, and dehydrated. As diarrhea has many potential causes, a diagnostic investigation is recommended. A full clinical history should be obtained to ascertain any changes in husbandry or diet (e.g., stocking density, hygiene, other reptiles owned, and any concurrent illness). It is also important to appreciate what "normal" feces are for the individual species to avoid misinterpretation based on appearance (Fig. 145.1A). A thorough clinical examination, including detailed palpation of the coelomic cavity and cloacal examination, should be performed. Initial diagnostic tests include fecal parasitology (wet preparation and salt flotation). Speciation of a particular parasite is rarely necessary; however, attempts should be made to place the parasite into a suitable treatment category (e.g., round worm, tape worm, protozoan). Hematology and biochemistry, diagnostic imaging (e.g., radiography, ultrasonography, CT, MRI), and endoscopy (e.g., gastroscopy, cloacoscopy, coelioscopy) may be required. Biopsy may be required for a definitive diagnosis. For more details, see Chapters 32, 74, and 120.

PREFERRED TREATMENT(S)

Treatment is aimed at resolving the underlying cause while providing supportive care to prevent worsening of the clinical condition. Rehydration therapy either parenterally or, if the gastrointestinal tract is functional, orally is recommended. Providing warm water baths may encourage the reptile to drink. Where substandard husbandry is a factor, a full review and correction as necessary will be required (e.g., poor hygiene, inappropriate temperature ranges, dietary items). For parasite burdens, a suitable parasiticide treatment should be selected, with repeat fecal analyses to ensure efficacy. Other therapies will be dependent upon a specific, definitive diagnosis.

PROGNOSIS AND PREVENTION

Prognosis of diarrhea is dependent on the inciting cause and duration of clinical signs. Sensible husbandry and dietary items should be provided. Good hygiene practices, low stocking density, and reducing stressors are all important considerations.

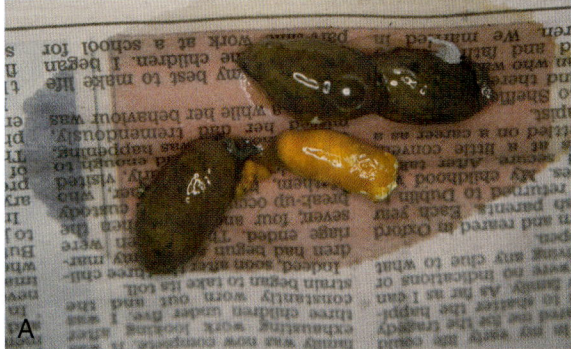 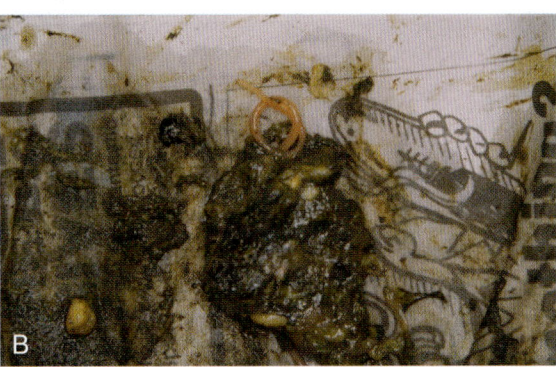

FIG 145.1 (A) Normal feces, urates, and urine from a boa constrictor (*Boa constrictor*). (B) Diarrhea from a spur-thighed tortoise (*Testudo graeca*) containing undigested food, and a large round worm is also visible. (Courtesy of Stephen J. Divers.)

Digit Abnormalities

Geraldine Diethelm

DEFINITION

Digit abnormalities are visible abnormalities of the feet and digits.

CLINICAL SIGNIFICANCE

Foot and digit issues are commonly encountered and often associated with husbandry problems. If ignored they can progress to involve joints and bones, with ascending infections necessitating surgical debridement or even amputation.

ISCHEMIA

Dysecdysis or retained shed (Fig. 146.1) can lead to damage and the loss of toes from strictures formed around the nailbed, disrupting circulation to the appendage. These shedding issues are usually the result of poor husbandry, such as inadequate environmental humidity, or can be the result of generalized illness. Strangulation of digits may also occur from substrate issues such as entrapment with fibers or hair. Additionally, trauma from other environmental issues include digits caught in netting or damaged by screen, attacked by prey, cagemates, or predators (if outside or housepets indoors). Regardless of how damage occurs, infection can ascend and cause inflammation in the remaining digit (Fig. 146.2), joint, and more proximal tissue, ultimately leading to generalized sepsis. Amputation in cases of osteomyelitis, as well as early and aggressive antibiotic therapy, may be necessary to prevent further ascending infection. If infection progresses to involve joints or the spine the prognosis becomes guarded to poor. Husbandry changes, including hygiene, should be discussed with the caretaker in detail. (See Chapter 69 for more details.)

SWOLLEN TOES AND JOINTS

Even with no outward signs of trauma, the differential list should include trauma but also infection, fractures, fibrous osteodystrophy, gout and "pseudogout,"[1,2] and neoplasia. Patients may have nonspecific clinical signs such as anorexia but will often have difficulty ambulating or balancing. Swelling in metatarsal-phalangeal joints often occurs with gout/pseudogout. Diagnostically radiographs can show bone lysis in and around the joints, and needle aspirate cytology or biopsy histopathology will differentiate between infection, neoplasia, and crystal deposits. Whole body radiographs should be taken to exclude other boney involvement (e.g., spine) or calcification of other organ systems. Pain management with nonsteroidal antiinflammatories and/ or opioids should be included. Surgical debridement of any infected or necrotic material is necessary because antimicrobials do not penetrate avascular abscesses. Amputation to prevent spread of disease is a viable alternative to euthanasia. (See Chapter 81 for more details.)

TWITCHING TOES

Tremors or twitching toes are most commonly seen in nutritional or renal secondary hyperparathyroidism and hypocalcemic gravid lizards.

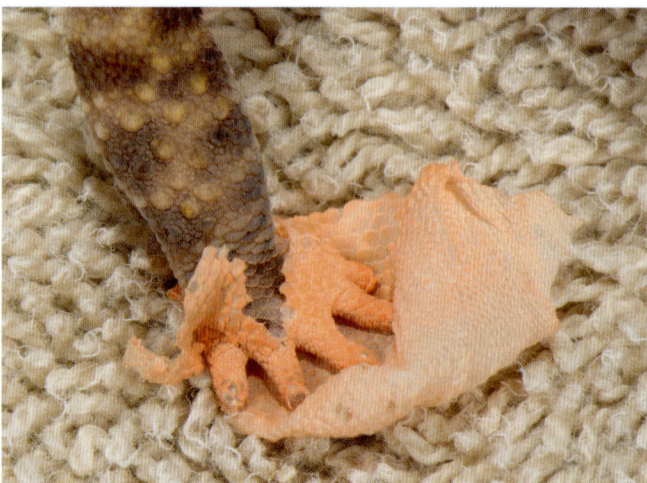

FIG 146.1 Dysecdysis in a leopard gecko (*Eublepharis macularius*). (Courtesy of Stephen Barten.)

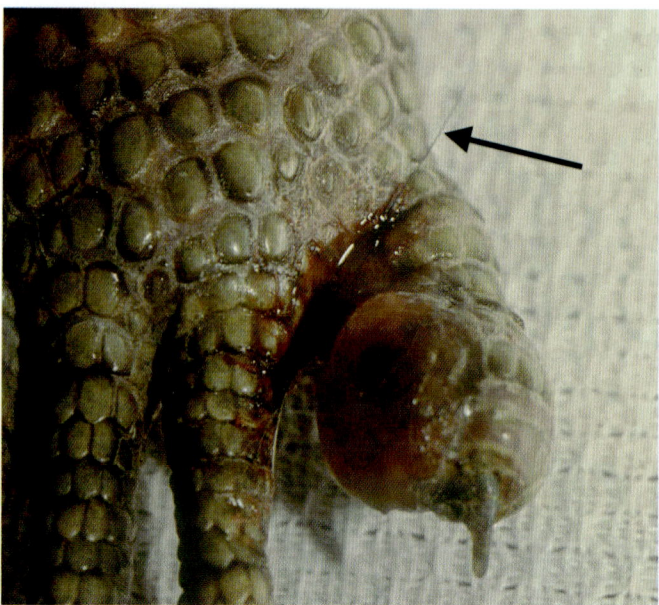

FIG 146.2 Onychitis in a savannah monitor (*Varanus exathematicus*) secondary to fiber (arrow) strangulation. (Courtesy of Douglas R. Mader.)

(See Chapter 84 for more details.) Intermittent, uncontrollable tremors in the toes (and often involving other muscles as well) are typically initiated by excitement and movement. Decreased ionized and total calcium levels result in these clinical signs and, as the conditions worsen, can progress to constant tremoring, seizures, and eventually end in flaccid muscles and paralysis. Differentials should include heavy metal intoxication, hypoglycemia, hypothermia, and sepsis.

SKIN ABNORMALITIES

Necrotic, sloughing, or discolored skin may be caused by burns, trauma, and ectoparasites, as well as poor husbandry, leading to secondary infections.[3] These can result in generalized sepsis. Debridement, topical, and systemic treatment depending on cause, as well as correcting the environment, is necessary. Parasitic reinfestation will occur if the pet is reintroduced into a contaminated habitat. Mites can be detected visually or with a skin scraping. Cytology and culture of material beneath an "uncontaminated" blister or scab can aid in directing effective treatment. (See Chapter 69 for more details.)

REFERENCES

See www.expertconsult.com for a complete list of references.

147

Dysecdysis

Tom Hellebuyck and T. Franciscus Scheelings

DEFINITION

Dysecdysis is the abnormal or impaired shedding of the outer layer of skin of reptiles and amphibians.

CLINICAL SIGNIFICANCE AND KNOWN ETIOLOGICAL CAUSE(S)

Dysecdysis is one of the most commonly observed skin disorders and should be considered a nonspecific clinical finding.[1,2] Knowledge of the normal anatomy and physiology of the reptilian integument is important for recognizing dysecdysis and establishing an appropriate diagnostic and therapeutic approach. Dysecdysis may originate from numerous infectious (e.g., ectoparasites, fungi) (Fig. 147.1) and noninfectious conditions (e.g., low humidity), especially those that interfere with normal skin integrity (see Chapter 69) and disorders resulting in dehydration or hypoproteinemia (Fig. 147.2).[2,3] Dehydration may result in a reduction of fluid necessary at the cleavage zone for normal separation of the old and new epidermal layers. Hypoproteinemia may interfere with the normal enzyme production necessary for the breakdown of the fission layer.[2]

CLINICAL PRESENTATION AND DIAGNOSTIC CONFIRMATION

Retention of sloughed skin may affect the entire integument and adnexa or may be restricted to certain areas (Fig. 147.1). Dysecdysis often presents as constricting bands of old skin, particularly around the digits (Fig. 147.3) and tail in lizards. Failure to recognize and remove incomplete sloughed skin in a timely manner may result in avascular necrosis and loss of distal extremities.[1,2] Retained spectacles in snakes and some geckos may result from the accumulation of several incomplete sloughs. Retained spectacles appear dull and wrinkled compared with normal eyes in nonshedding animals and may occur unilaterally or bilaterally. Discrimination between retained spectacles and other ophthalmologic disorders (e.g., subspectacular abscesses) may be challenging. Clinical evaluation for dysecdysis requires a good understanding of what is normal for the species being evaluated. Additionally, patient age and size, historical details regarding the frequency of past molts and skin issues, and concurrent illnesses should be appreciated. Following a thorough physical examination, additional diagnostic tests may be required to reveal the underlying cause and initiate appropriate therapy. Normal respiratory sounds may increase before and during shedding because of the presence of retained skin around the nostrils.[4] (See Chapter 69 for more details.)

PREFERRED TREATMENT(S)

Aggressively peeling back retained or shed skin should be avoided because these problems are rarely emergent. Premature removal of older epidermal layers before the newer layers have fully developed may result in ulceration or corneal exposure in the case of spectacles and considerable loss of proteinaceous fluids and may permanently damage or scar the skin/eyes (Fig. 147.4). Chronicity often directs the therapeutic approach (see Chapter 69).

Lightly spraying the animal and increasing environmental humidity may be sufficient in minor cases of dysecdysis. Short soaks in lukewarm water are often effective for removing larger portions of retained skin,

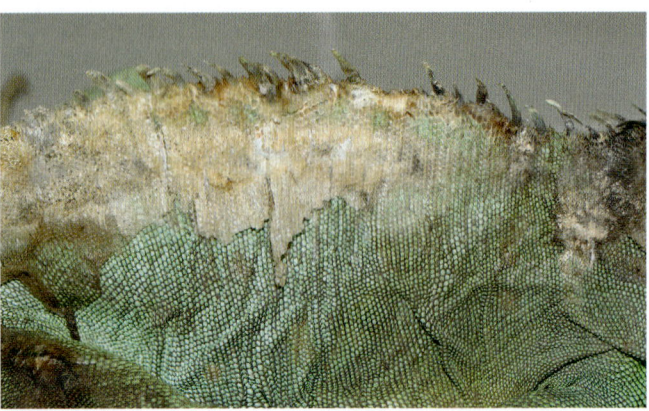

FIG 147.1 This Asian water dragon (*Physignathus concincinus*) shows localized dysecdysis as a consequence of severe dermatomycosis. (Courtesy of Tom Hellebuyck.)

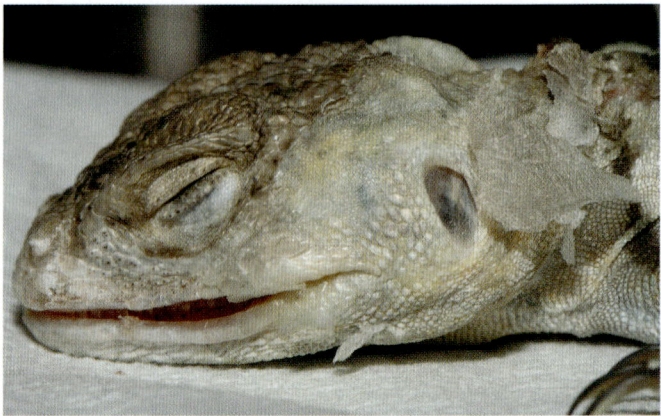

FIG 147.2 In severely debilitated animals such as this collared lizard (*Crotaphytus collaris*), generalized dysecdysis may be observed as a consequence of dehydration and hypoproteinemia. (Courtesy of Tom Hellebuyck.)

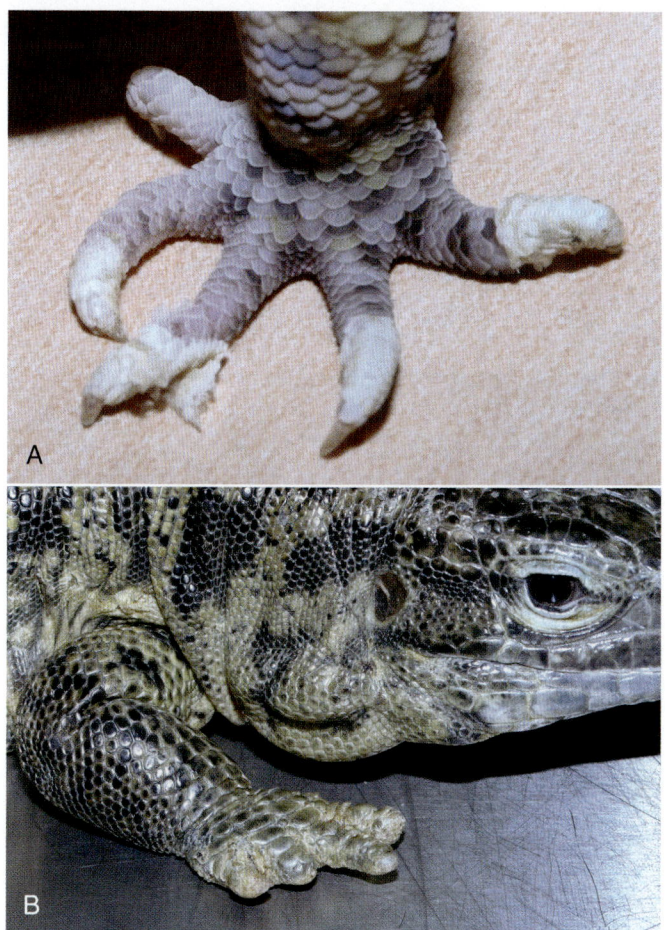

FIG 147.3 Constricting bands of old skin, particularly around the digits in lizards (A) often result in avascular necrosis and dry gangrene with eventual loss of digits, as seen in this tegu (*Tupinambis* sp.) (B). (Courtesy of Tom Hellebuyck.)

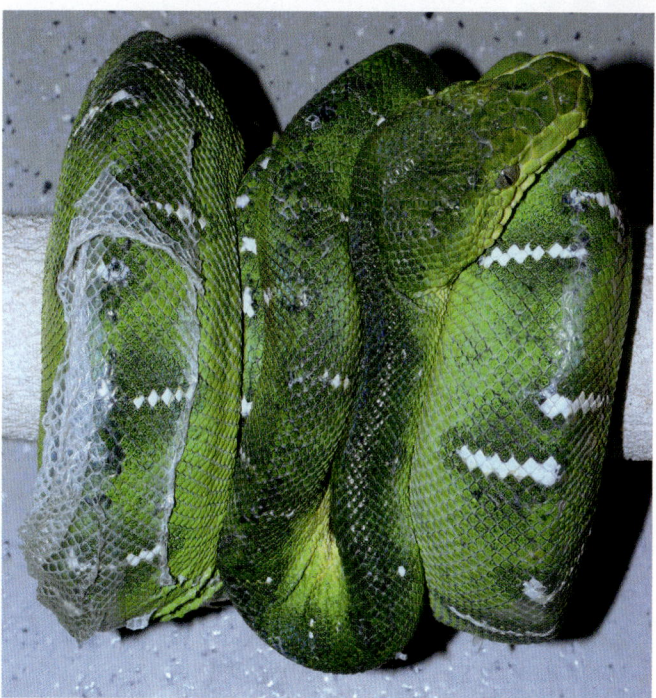

FIG 147.4 Premature removal of older epidermal layers (e.g., during a shed cycle), as depicted in this Emerald tree boa (*Corallus caninus*), due to handling should be avoided, as considerable loss of fluids and proteins and even permanent damage and scarring of the integument may occur. (Courtesy of Tom Hellebuyck.)

especially in snakes. Although various water additions are advocated, plain water is usually sufficient and safest.[2] For many desert-dwelling species, moist/humid retreats often facilitate shedding or resolve shedding disorders. Excessive moisture may result in decreased skin integrity and potentially predispose animals to bacterial and mycotic disease.[1]

PREVENTION

Dysecdysis is typically secondary, and it is effectively prevented by ensuring appropriate, species-specific husbandry. Both clinicians and owners should familiarize themselves with the captive management requirements of commonly kept species. Snakes and certain lizard species should not be handled during sloughing, as the skin is particularly vulnerable to traumatic injury and infection.

REFERENCES

See www.expertconsult.com for a complete list of references.

148

Dystocia and Follicular Stasis

Scott J. Stahl

DEFINITION

Dystocia is the inability to successfully expel term eggs or fetuses from the lower reproductive tract. Preovulatory follicular stasis refers to the inability to ovulate or resorb ova (see Chapter 80 for a more detailed discussion).

CLINICAL SIGNIFICANCE AND KNOWN ETIOLOGICAL CAUSE(S)

Preovulatory follicular stasis occurs commonly in lizards, chelonians, and less often snakes.[1,2] Dystocia is often seasonal, as hormonal cycles, and thus reproductive activity, occur at specific times of the year. The etiologies for dystocia in captive reptiles are often multifactorial and may result from captive stress, inappropriate nesting sites, dehydration, malnutrition, obesity, salpingitis, malformed ova, broken or damaged eggs, obstructive coelomic pathology (e.g., cystic or cloacal calculus), infectious diseases (e.g., boid arenavirus), and abnormal reproductive anatomy.[1,2]

CLINICAL PRESENTATION

Detailed history, thorough husbandry review, and a good understanding of species-specific reproductive strategies are paramount. All chelonians and crocodilians are oviparous (egg-layers), as are most squamates; however, some lizard and snakes are viviparous (live-bearers). Dystocic reptiles may be restless (pacing and climbing), looking for possible mates or nesting sites (Fig. 148.1). Oviparous lizards and chelonians may dig in planters or substrate. Female aquatic turtles may spend extended time out of the water. Coelomic distention with reduced body condition, anorexia, and behavioral changes may be noted. Females may have produced a small clutch or litter but still appear gravid due to several retained eggs/fetuses. Alternatively, the breeder's records may indicate that the female is past her due date. Palpation may confirm enlarged follicles in squamates (not chelonians), but it can sometimes be difficult to differentiate preovulatory from postovulatory ova. Chelonians are more difficult to palpate, but in smaller species digital palpation in the prefemoral area, with the patient held vertically and gently tilted side to side, may allow shelled ova to be detected. It is usually not possible to palpate developing fetuses in viviparous squamates.

DIAGNOSTIC CONFIRMATION

Radiographically squamate preovulatory follicular stasis often appears as a cluster of spherical, dorsal structures that lack a shell. For dystocia cases, radiographs are important to identify the presence and number of shelled eggs and any abnormalities or obstructions (Fig. 148.2). Radiographic demonstration of skeletal structures is only possible late in gestation. Ultrasonography is preferred for identification of preovulatory follicular stasis and to differentiate between preovulatory and postovulatory

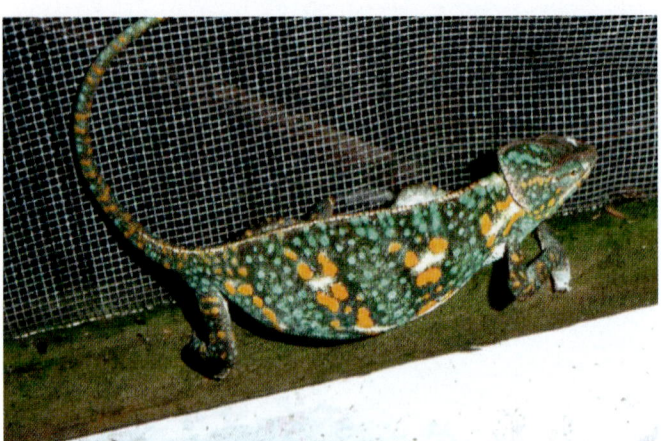

FIG 148.1 Behavior changes may be noted in gravid and dystocic reptiles. This female veiled chameleon (*Chameleo calyptratus*) became restless in her enclosure late in gestation, staying off the tree branches where she typically resided and pacing the cage floor perimeter, looking for an appropriate nesting site. Note the light blue (robin's egg) color spots on her skin, indicative of gravidity in this species. (Courtesy of Bill Love.)

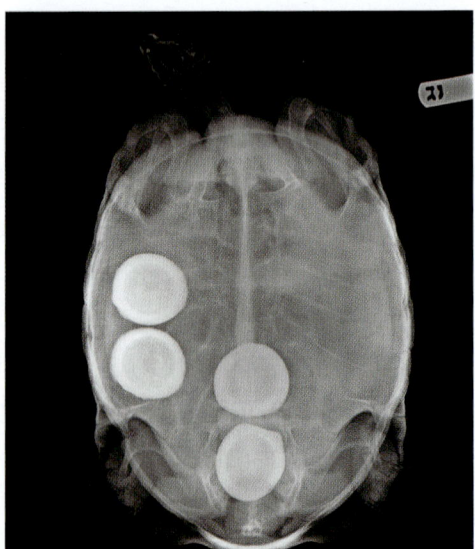

FIG 148.2 A dorsoventral radiograph of a star tortoise (*Geochelone elegans*) presented with chronic dystocia. Multiple treatments by the owner with oxytocin had failed. Chelonians are often responsive to oxytocin; however, before its use, radiographs are important to rule out obstructive dystocias or other concurrent complications such as cystic calculi. In this case note the abnormally thickened calcified shells, usually an indication of chronic retention or ectopic eggs. At surgery all eggs were found to be ectopic, three in the coelom and the most caudal irregularly shaped egg in the bladder. (Courtesy of Shoshana Sommer, Stahl Exotic Animal Veterinary Services.)

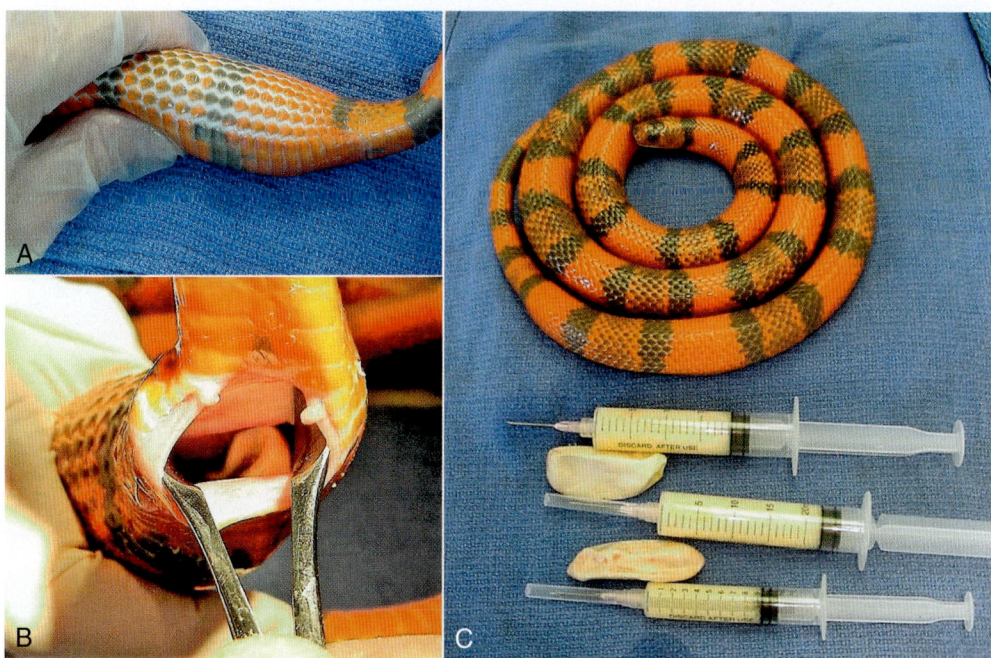

FIG 148.3 (A) A Honduran milk snake (*Lampropeltis triangulum hondurensis*) presented for dystocia after laying a partial clutch of eggs. With general anesthesia and once relaxed, the first egg was found to move freely and was manipulated toward the cloaca. (B) A vaginal speculum was used to dilate the cloaca and allow visualization, an 18-gauge needle was introduced directly into the egg, the liquid contents of the egg aspirated, and the collapsed egg then grasped with hemostats and removed; the procedure was repeated on the second egg. (C) The snake recovering from anesthesia after two eggs were removed through the cloaca. (Courtesy of Scott J. Stahl, Stahl Exotic Animal Veterinary Services.)

ova. Late gestational ultrasonography can determine fetus viability in viviparous species and help differentiate between normal or abnormal presentation. (See Chapter 80 for details on reproductive imaging.) Plasma biochemical changes often include elevations of total calcium but not ionized calcium, which may be low (<1 mmol/L), indicating hypocalcemia with related poor nutrition and husbandry. Complete blood count may show a stress leukocytosis or, in cases of inflammatory/infectious disease, a leukocytosis with left shift.

MEDICAL TREATMENT AND EGG MANIPULATION

Medical treatment may consist of provision of nest box(es) and oral or parenteral calcium supplementation in cases of hypo- to normocalcemia. In cases of unobstructive dystocia, induction using oxytocin, prostaglandins E, and F2a may be effective, with chelonians being more sensitive than squamates (see Chapter 80 for details). NSAIDs and antimicrobials may be indicated. Due to the linear anatomy of snakes, egg manipulation may be possible and is noninvasive.[1,2] However, general anesthesia is required to determine whether the eggs are adhered to the oviduct or if they move freely and can be gently manipulated through the cloaca (Fig. 148.3A). Per cloacal aspiration using a large-gauge needle (16–18g) to collapse can help with removal, per cloaca. (see Fig. 148.3C). Cloacoscopy may be useful in some cases in snakes and chelonians but less so in lizards and is best utilized when only one or several eggs are retained.[1,2] Retained eggs in snakes that are reluctant to move even with the use of anesthesia can be transcutaneously aspirated with a large-gauge

(16–18) needle to collapse and assist with passing. This technique has an increased risk of complications and should only be used when all other options are considered or with economic limitations.

PREFERRED TREATMENT(S)

Surgical management is often the best option for resolving preovulatory follicular stasis (ovariectomy) or dystocia (ovariosalpingectomy), unless the reptile is part of a breeding program. For dystocia cases where future reproduction is important, once the patient is stable and all medical and less invasive management options have been considered, surgery (salpingotomy) may be indicated. (See Chapter 105 for details on performing these procedures.)

PROGNOSIS AND PREVENTION

Prognosis and outcome are generally good for dystocia cases with early diagnosis and intervention. During health examinations of female reptiles clinicians must discuss eventual hormonal influences, familiarize owners with signs of reproductive activity, and offer preventative ovariectomy as an option to avoid future issues.

REFERENCES

See www.expertconsult.com for a complete list of references.

149

Gout

Jorge Orós

DEFINITION

Gout is a metabolic disease characterized by overproduction or underexcretion of uric acid resulting in hyperuricemia and deposition of positively birefringent monosodium urate (MSU) crystals in tissues.[1]

CLINICAL SIGNIFICANCE AND KNOWN ETIOLOGICAL CAUSE(S)

Overproduction of uric acid resulting in hyperuricemia has been associated with high-protein diets (common in herbivorous reptiles fed a diet high in animal protein), whereas underexcretion of uric acid has been associated with dehydration (due to low environmental humidity or inadequate water availability) and/or kidney disease (see Chapter 66). Most cases of gout are the final stage of chronic diseases involving renal failure and/or dehydration.[2] Hypovitaminosis A has also been suggested in producing visceral gout in crocodile hatchlings by the mechanism of reduced renal excretion of uric acid through tubular squamous metaplasia.[3]

CLINICAL PRESENTATION

Articular gout results from the deposition of MSU crystals in the synovial fluid and synovial membranes, resulting in joint inflammation. Deposits of MSU can also be detected around the joints (periarticular gout) (Fig. 149.1). Visceral gout results from deposition of MSU crystals in other soft tissues, such as kidneys (Fig. 149.2), lungs, pericardial sac, serous membranes of liver and spleen, and subcutaneous tissue.[4] Articular gout often precedes visceral gout.[2] Deposits of MSU crystals are called tophi and consist of a complex of MSU crystals surrounded by granulomatous inflammation (see Fig. 149.2, Insert).[4]

DIAGNOSTIC CONFIRMATION

Elevations of plasma uric acid may be suggestive but can be within normal limits, especially for articular gout. Ultrasonography shows MSU crystal deposits as hyperechoic images without posterior acoustic shadowing, which enables their differentiation from calcifications. CT shows crystal aggregates but does not enable specific identification of MSU crystals. Dual-energy CT distinguishes urate crystals from deposits containing calcium.[5] Cytologic examination by phase contrast microscopy of joint aspirates is also useful to identify MSU crystals.[2] Visceral gout can be diagnosed by histopathologic examination of soft tissue biopsy. When using polarized light, the tissues must be fixed in absolute ethanol, because urate crystals tend to degrade and wash out during formalin (aqueous solution) fixation.[6] Determination of the glomerular filtration rate using iohexol excretion can also be useful to evaluate the renal function.[2] Differential diagnoses include hydroxyapatite deposition

disease (HADD) and pseudogout or calcium pyrophosphate dihydrate (CPPD) deposition[6–8] and can be differentiated based on histologic appearance, histochemical staining for calcium, and birefringence under polarized light.

PREFERRED TREATMENT(S)[2,5,9,10]

Treatment consists of fluid therapy to correct dehydration and metabolic disturbances and the judicious use of antiinflammatories (if determined

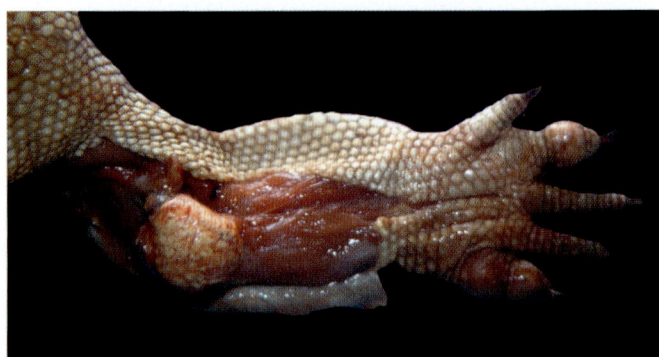

FIG 149.1 Periarticular gout in a savannah monitor (*Varanus exanthematicus*). Note the periarticular accumulation of tophi around the elbow and the swelling of several digits. (Courtesy of Jorge Orós.)

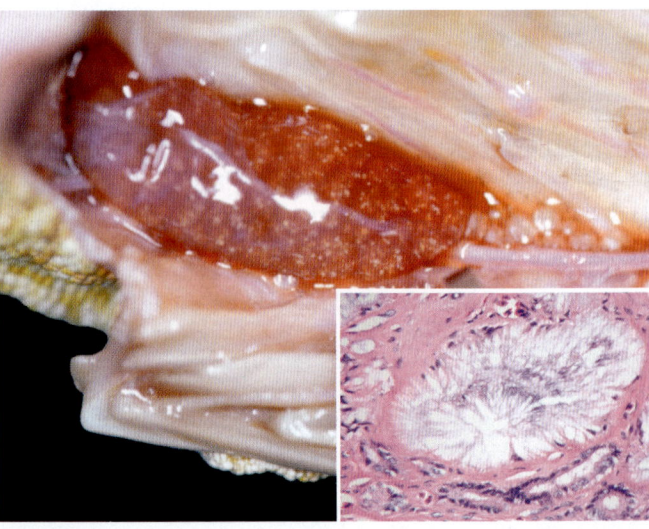

FIG 149.2 Visceral gout in the kidney of a veiled chameleon (*Chamaeleo calyptratus*). (Inset) Histologic appearance of a tophus in the kidney of this animal. HE, ×40. (Courtesy of Jorge Orós.)

safe based on renal evaluation). Surgical removal of isolated articular or periarticular gout, including limb amputation, may be one of the most effective treatment options. Managing pain with appropriate analgesics is important.

Uricostatic drugs may help to reduce uric acid production through competitive inhibition of xanthine oxidase. These drugs include allopurinol (25 mg/kg PO daily in the green iguana, *Iguana iguana*),[2] as well as oxypurinol and febuxostat (used in humans). Uricosuric drugs (e.g., sulphinpyrazone, probenecid, benzbromarone) in human medicine increase urinary uric acid excretion by blocking urate anion reabsorption by proximal renal tubule epithelial cells. Pegylated uricase therapy (pegloticase and pegadricase reserved for selected human patients) reduces urate levels by increasing its metabolism.

PROGNOSIS AND PREVENTION

The prognosis for severe visceral gout is poor to grave. The prognosis for articular gout depends on the extent of the lesions.

REFERENCES

See www.expertconsult.com for a complete list of references.

150

Hemoparasites

Giordano Nardini

DEFINITION

Hemoaparasites are parasitical infections identified within peripheral blood.

CLINICAL SIGNIFICANCE AND ETIOLOGICAL CAUSE(S)

Hemoparasites of reptiles are arguably symbiotes, and most infections are chronic and subclinical. Because they have an indirect life cycle, clinical disease of captive-bred indoor animals is rare.[1,2] The most serious pathogens are *Plasmodium* spp., especially in chelonians and lizards, which can cause anemia, erythroblastosis, and reduced tissue oxygen supply in lizards, and severe hemolytic anemia in chelonians (Fig. 150.1A and B).[1,3,4] *Saurocytozoon* has been reported in lizards, but it is considered harmless;[4] *Haemoproteus* is reported in lizards, turtles, and snakes. It is generally considered nonpathogenic but may cause hemolytic anemia in geckos.[3,4] *Haemogregarina* can be observed in freshwater turtles, tortoises, the tuatara, some lizards, most snakes, and crocodilians. Clinical signs including lethargy, open-mouth breathing, weight loss, and dehydration are uncommon but may be seen in unnatural or aberrant host species, or in immune-compromised patients.[2] In lizards and snakes anemia is possible.[4] *Haemolivia* are encountered in turtles and lizards and are usually nonpathogenic.[5,6] *Hepatozoon* are found primarily in snakes but also in geckos; in snakes, severe consequences on growth and reproduction are reported, including liver necrosis, inflammation, and neurologic signs.[4] *Karyolysus* has been primarily described in squamates

and are rarely pathogenic.[3] *Hemococcidia*, *Lainsonia*, and *Schellackia* have been reported mostly in lizards; *Schellackia* may cause anemia.[3] *Piroplasmids*, *Sauroplasma*, and *Serpentoplasma* have been reported in lizards, chelonians, snakes, and chameleons but are not associated with clinical signs.[7] *Trypanosoma* and *Leishmania* can infect almost all reptile species. *Trypanosoma* can cause severe parasitemia, but infection is often subclinical and lifelong.[7] *Sauroleishmania* may be found primarily in lizards without pathogenicity.[4] *Microfilaria* can be detected in snakes, lizards, chameleons, and crocodilians as incidental findings without clinical signs, even though occlusion of terminal vessels is possible.[3,4]

CLINICAL PRESENTATION AND DIAGNOSTIC CONFIRMATION

Stress (e.g., transport, inadequate captive microclimate, overcrowding, inadequate nutrition) can cause immunosuppression and lead to obvious disease.[1] However, parasite identification in blood smears is frequently an incidental finding. In immunocompromised, geriatric, and young animals, these parasites can cause lethargy, open-mouth breathing, weight loss, hemolytic anemia, splenomegaly, and dehydration.[2,6] Diagnosis is by the microscopic examination of quickly air-dried samples, preferably fixed with absolute methanol and stained with a Romanowsky-type stain or Giemsa/Wright-Giemsa.[1] Light microscopy allows recognition of the parasite genus, whereas morphologic species identification is often difficult and requires molecular analyses, especially for haemogregarines.[1,4] Sporozoites are found in blood cells (erythrocytes, leukocytes, and thrombocytes). Leishmania can be found in macrophages

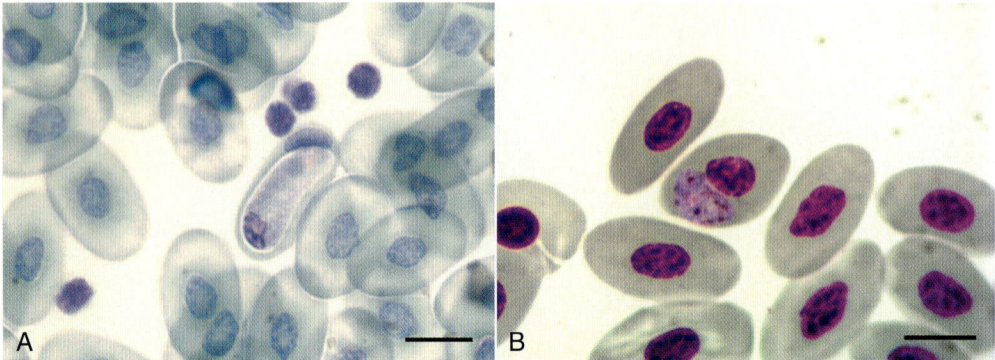

FIG 150.1 (A) *Haemogregarina* in erythrocyte from European pond turtle (*Emys orbicularis*). Giemsa stain; bar = 10 μm. (B) *Plasmodium* sp. in erythrocyte from Mwanza flat-headed rock agama (*Agama mwanzae*). Giemsa stain; bar = 10 μm. (A, Courtesy of M.L. Fioravanti, Department of Veterinary Medical Sciences, University of Bologna, Italy; B, courtesy of M.T. Manfredi and Edoardo Bardi, Department of Veterinary Medicine, University of Milano, Italy.)

and usually is detected by culture techniques. Trypanosoma and microfilaria are found free in the blood film.[1,7]

PREFERRED TREATMENT(S)

No effective treatment is known for reptiles.[8] A decrease in haemogregarine parasitemia, but not clearance, has been noted with atovaquone-proguanil;[9] primaquine and chloroquine have been used against *Plasmodium* in chelonians. In patients with anemia and debilitation, treatment with iron-dextran and quinidine may be helpful.[8,10]

PROGNOSIS AND PREVENTION

Prognosis is generally good. Prevention is by quarantine combined with blood smear examinations, control of potential vectors, and, if necessary, treatment against ectoparasite transmission hosts.[8]

REFERENCES

See www.expertconsult.com for a complete list of references.

151

Hepatic Lipidosis

Stephen J. Divers

DEFINITION

Hepatic lipidosis is abnormal, excessive accumulation of intrahepatic fat. (See Chapter 67 for more detailed information.)

CLINICAL SIGNIFICANCE AND KNOWN ETIOLOGICAL CAUSE(S)

Hepatic lipidosis is a metabolic derangement within the liver that can be associated with many diseases or syndromes. There are a host of factors that have been associated with increased hepatic fat, including high fat diets, reduced activity, nonbreeding females, nonhibernating temperate species, and certain toxins (e.g., ivermectin) (Fig. 151.1A). It is important to appreciate that increased intrahepatic fat is normal in temperate species before hibernation and in females preparing for folliculogenesis.

CLINICAL PRESENTATION AND DIAGNOSTIC CONFIRMATION

Hepatic lipidosis is usually chronic, with gradual reduction in appetite, activity, fecundity and fertility, weight gain (or weight loss late in the course of disease), hibernation problems, and changes in fecal character and color. Plasma biochemical changes including elevations in triglycerides, cholesterol, and lipoproteins are often apparent.[1] Reduced hepatic function can result in elevations of bile acids and hypoalbuminemia. Radiographically, hepatomegaly may be discernible in lizards and snakes but is challenging in chelonians. Ultrasonography and CT are more useful, especially when the hepatic parenchyma is compared with fat bodies. Reptiles with hepatic lipidosis typically exhibit hyperechoic livers and reduced radiographic attenuation (<20 HU).[2] Hepatic biopsy is required for histopathology (and cultures if infection present) in order to reach an antemortem definitive diagnosis.[3,4] Affected livers appear large, friable, and pale tan to yellow in color with a soft fatty "feel" (Fig. 151.1B and C).

PREFERRED TREATMENT(S)

In advanced cases correction of dehydration is the first priority. Vitamin K administration can be considered, especially if coagulopathy has been confirmed. A means of providing long-term fluid and nutritional support (e.g., esophagostomy tube) is typically required. The importance of nutritional support cannot be overemphasized and offers the best therapeutic approach to hepatic lipidosis. When providing nutritional support, it is important to consider (1) the patient's energy and nutritional requirements, (2) the patient's natural dietary preferences, and (3) the use of natural foods for long-term support. The use of artificial, critical care substitutes should only be during initial stabilization. It is important to avoid refeeding syndrome and gastric overload in reptiles that have been anorectic for prolonged periods.

Supplementation with L-carnitine (100 mg/kg/day) may improve hepatic metabolism of fat. Antioxidants such as S-adenosylmethionine (SAMe), which replaces the previous recommendation of methionine, and vitamin E, may also be beneficial. Doses are empirical or derived from allometric calculations from mammal doses.

PROGNOSIS AND PREVENTION

The prognosis is good if diagnosed early before the onset of severe clinical signs. Once hepatic dysfunction is advanced the prognosis is guarded and often requires prolonged nutritional support, medication, and nursing for months or even years. Addressing the following factors

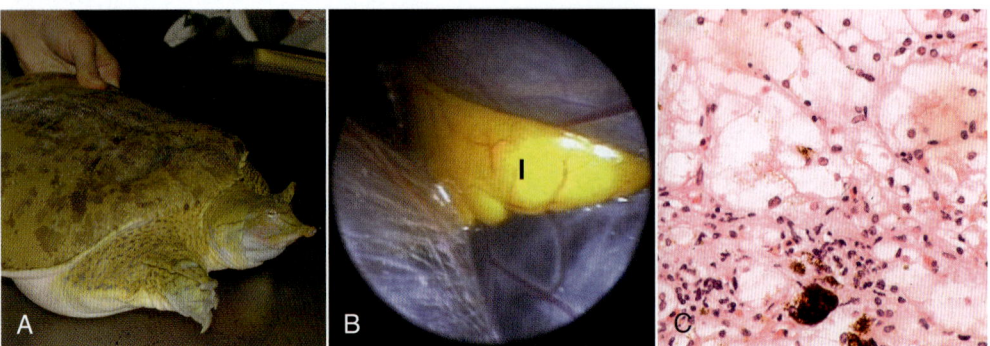

FIG 151.1 (A) Morbidly obese spiny softshell turtle (*Apalone spinifera*). (B) Endoscopic view of a bearded dragon (*Pogona vitticeps*) liver (l) with excessive intrahepatic fat. (C). Histological section of the liver of a Greek tortoise (*Testudo graeca*) shows marked vacuolation of hepatocytes with nuclear margination and pyknosis. H&E, x200. (Courtesy of Stephen J. Divers.)

can often help reduce or prevent occurrence: (1) Provide a suitably large enclosure to facilitate exercise and foraging; (2) avoid excessive feeding (frequency and quantity); (3) facilitate the natural loss of fat from both hepatic and fat body reserve by permitting temperate species to hibernate and intact females the ability to reproduce (or sterilize); (4) keep health logs (including monthly weight and body lengths [straight carapace or snout-to-vent]) and seek annual or biennial health evaluations (including physical examinations and routine blood testing).

REFERENCES

See www.expertconsult.com for a complete list of references.

152

Hyperglycemia

Scott J. Stahl

DEFINITION

Hyperglycemia is defined as a persistent elevation of blood glucose above 300 mg/dL (16.7 mmol/L) and is an uncommon clinical biochemical abnormality in reptiles.[1,2]

CLINICAL SIGNIFICANCE AND KNOWN ETIOLOGICAL CAUSE(S)

Hyperglycemia has not been established as a consistent or specific indicator of pancreatic disease or diabetes mellitus (DM) in reptiles.[1,2] Elevations of blood glucose in reptiles are more often related to physiological variables, metabolic conditions, systemic diseases, stress, and neoplasia.[1–3] Risk factors for hyperglycemia include stress, seasonal variation (especially hibernation and breeding), diving, postprandial response, anorexia/starvation, metabolic disease (liver or renal disease), and neoplasia (pancreatic and nonpancreatic).[1–3] Blood glucose in reptiles appears to be regulated by insulin and glucagon, as in mammals. Generally, DM results from a lack of in insulin (type 1) or an inability of insulin to properly transport glucose into target cells (type 2). Damage to the pancreas from trauma, inflammation, neoplasia, or autoimmune disease resulting in damage or loss of pancreatic neuroendocrine cells can result in elevated blood glucose. Pancreatic pathology, including pancreatitis and primary pancreatic neoplasia, have been reported in reptiles, some associated with hyperglycemia and others not.[1,2] Although several cases of reptile diabetes mellitus have been reported, there is a lack of peer-reviewed publications to support this disease in reptiles.[1,2] Hyperglycemia has not been established as a consistent or specific indicator of pancreatic disease or DM in reptiles; however, there appears to be an association between nonpancreatic neoplasia and persistent hyperglycemia.[1,3] For example, gastric somatostatinoma (neuroendocrine gastric carcinoma) in bearded dragons (*Pogona vitticeps*) usually arise from gastric or pyloric mucosa with aggressive metastasis to multiple organs and are typically associated with severe hyperglycemia (Fig. 152.1).[3] For a review of pancreatic anatomy, physiology, and disease, as well as an overview of reported cases published with persistent hyperglycemia, see Chapter 79.

CLINICAL PRESENTATION AND DIAGNOSTIC CONFIRMATION

Husbandry details related to dietary intake and habits, temperature, humidity, lighting, and other important variables such as hibernation, seasonal cycles, and reproductive activity should be noted. Reptiles with hyperglycemia often present with nonspecific clinical signs (including anorexia, weight loss, and lethargy) and physical examination findings (including loss of muscle mass, weakness, loss of righting reflex, and severe depression). Some reptiles may present overconditioned or obese. Polyuria and polydipsia may be present but are not commonly appreciated.[1] Routine hematology, plasma biochemistry, diagnostic imaging, endoscopy, and exploratory coeliotomy may be required for a definitive diagnosis. In general, fasting blood glucose values for normal reptiles are between 60 to 100 mg/dL (3.0–5.5 mmol/L); however, they can range between 30 and 205 mg/dL (1.6–11.3 mmol/L)[1] (see Chapter 34). A single, fasting blood sample may reveal an elevation in blood glucose but has limited clinical significance. Multiple, serial sampling, or better still continuous (real-time) glucose monitoring is required to confirm persistent hyperglycemia, establish general trends, and determine clinical progression.[1,2] Glucosuria may or may not be noted, whereas the

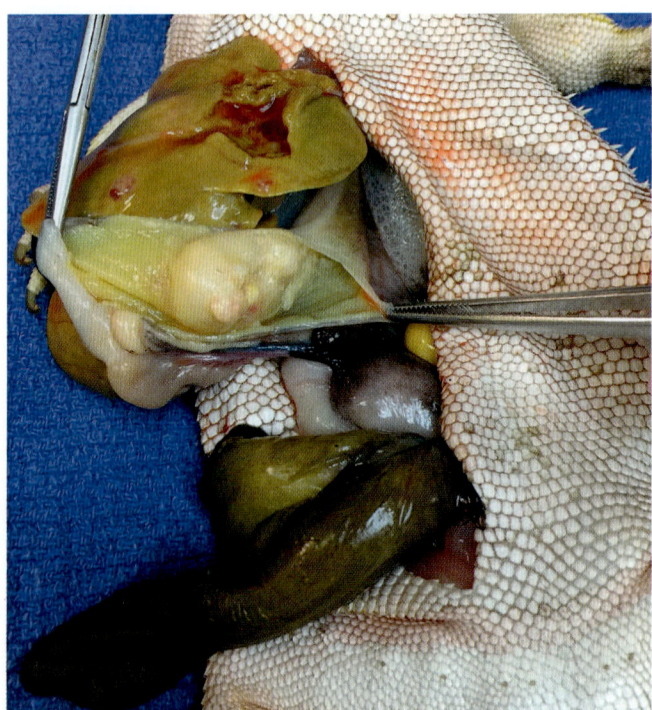

FIG 152.1 A gastric mass (in the gastric lumen between the forceps) was found at necropsy in this bearded dragon (*Pogona vitticeps*), and histopathology identified a gastric somatostatinoma (neuroendocrine gastric carcinoma). These carcinomas arise from gastric or pyloric mucosa and often metastasize to multiple organs. Somatostatin suppresses pancreatic secretions of insulin, lowering insulin receptor sensitivity, likely resulting in the hyperglycemia seen in these cases. (Courtesy of Emily Nielsen, Stahl Exotic Animal Veterinary Services.)

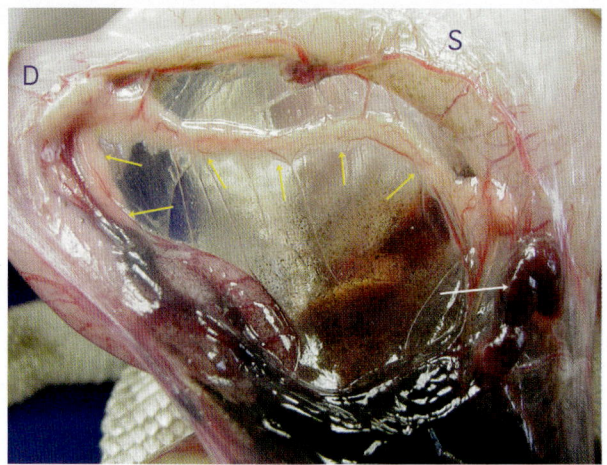

FIG 152.2 The normal pancreas of a bearded dragon (*Pogona vitticeps*) at necropsy. The light-colored pancreas (yellow arrows) is suspended in the mesentery between the stomach (S) and duodenum (D). The spleen (white arrow) is to the right. Note the anatomical complexity of the pancreas with several arms. Unfortunately, biopsy of the reptile pancreas for endocrine evaluation is complicated by high variability in the location of islet cell tissue in the pancreas. (Courtesy of Scott J. Stahl, Stahl Exotic Animal Veterinary Services.)

diagnostic value of insulin, glycated hemoglobin, and fructosamine are largely unknown.[1] Pancreatic biopsy and histopathology may be a valuable tool antemortem, however high variability exists in both the morphology and location of islet cell tissue, both in and outside the pancreas of reptiles (Fig. 152.2).[2] In postmortem cases, it is recommended to submit the entire pancreas, spleen, stomach, and small intestine for histopathologic analysis to avoid missing sites of islet concentration.[1] Metabolic diseases (hepatic and renal), pancreatic disease, and neoplasia should be considered.

PREFERRED TREATMENT(S)

Initial stabilization should include supplemental heat, fluid therapy, liver support, alimentation, and diagnosis-specific therapeutics. Once stable, persistent hyperglycemia should be established and underlying physiological issues, metabolic disease, and neoplasia excluded. If DM is truly determined (a rare diagnosis in reptiles), then insulin therapy (and/or hypoglycemic agents) and close monitoring should be pursued. Compared with mammals and birds, reptiles respond slowly to the administration of mammalian insulin, with lizards and crocodilians less sensitive compared with snakes and turtles.[2]

PREVENTION AND PROGNOSIS

Increasing the fiber in the diet of herbivores and omnivores may prove more effective than glucose-regulating agents. Prognosis for persistent hyperglycemia is guarded. Neoplastic or pancreas-associated hyperglycemia has a poor prognosis. Cases of persistent hyperglycemia related to other intrinsic and extrinsic variables may have a more favorable outcome.

REFERENCES

See www.expertconsult.com for a complete list of references.

153

Hypovitaminosis and Hypervitaminosis A

Thomas H. Boyer

DEFINITION

Hypovitaminosis A is a deficiency often associated with a failure to provide an assimilable form of vitamin A. Hypervitaminosis A relates to excessive vitamin A, which is often iatrogenic and associated with exaggerated dosing in an attempt to prevent or treat a deficiency.

CLINICAL SIGNIFICANCE AND KNOWN ETIOLOGICAL CAUSE(S)

Some omnivores and herbivores synthesize vitamin A from plant carotenoids and are resistant to dietary hypovitaminosis A. Insectivorous amphibians and lizards, as well as emydid turtles, often suffer from hypovitaminosis A, because they may be poor converters of carotenoids to vitamin A, and most insects are vitamin A deficient. Most commercial reptile multivitamin supplements contain β-carotene, which some reptiles cannot convert to vitamin A. Carnivores consuming whole vertebrates rarely suffer deficiency, because the liver is a plentiful source of vitamin A.

Hypervitaminosis A is primarily an iatrogenic disease caused by injections of highly concentrated vitamin A. Before the discovery of mycoplasmosis in tortoises in the early 1990s, it was common practice to give tortoises with upper respiratory tract disease vitamin A injections. This practice is now discouraged because tortoises rarely suffer from hypovitaminosis A because they are herbivores believed capable of converting dietary carotenoids to vitamin A.

CLINICAL PRESENTATION

Clinical signs of hypovitaminosis A manifest by hyperkeratosis and include blockage and swelling of lacrimal and salivary glands, swollen eyelids or lips, and ocular abnormalities (xeropthalmia, corneal keratitis, erosion, ulceration, and keratomalacia) that contribute to blepharospasm and corneal scarring (Fig. 153.1). Blindness can result from corneal scarring and a lack of retinol. Decreased appetite, difficulty catching prey, retained and recurrent hemipenal plugs in lizards, dysecdysis, less vibrant coloration, stomatitis, ear abscesses, pneumonia, or egg retention may also be reported. Farmed crocodiles on a vitamin A–deficient formulated diet had multifocal brown dorsal lingual nodules, as well as renal and visceral gout. In amphibians, especially toads and frogs, vitamin A deficiency causes short tongue syndrome (STS) because of a failure of the mucus-secreting glands in the tongue tip that allows prey to stick to the tongue. Superficially, the rapid-fire tongue appears to fall short of capturing prey.

DIAGNOSTIC CONFIRMATION

Most cases in clinical practice are diagnosed based on dietary history, clinical signs, response to therapy, and sometimes histopathology (hyperkeratosis and squamous metaplasia). Vitamin A levels are not easily measured because most is in the liver, and serum levels do not drop until liver levels are exhausted. Relatively large surgical biopsies or necropsy samples are required to obtain tissue vitamin A levels. Diagnosis of hypervitaminosis A (vitamin A toxicity) in chelonians is made by the clinical presentation of erythema and outer epidermal sloughing. This is usually associated with the recent injection of vitamin A.

PREFERRED TREATMENT(S)

Water-soluble vitamin A palmitate (such as Aquasol A) is more toxic than fat-soluble vitamin A palmitate and is not recommended. Treatment involves dietary improvement. For reptiles, 0.01 mL of fat-soluble vitamin A and D (500,000 IU vitamin A palmitate/mL, 100,000 IU vitamin D/mL) SC or PO, repeated in 2 weeks, reverses clinical signs in 2 to 4 weeks. Remove cellular debris under the eyelids and flush the eyes. Antimicrobials may be required if corneal ulceration or secondary

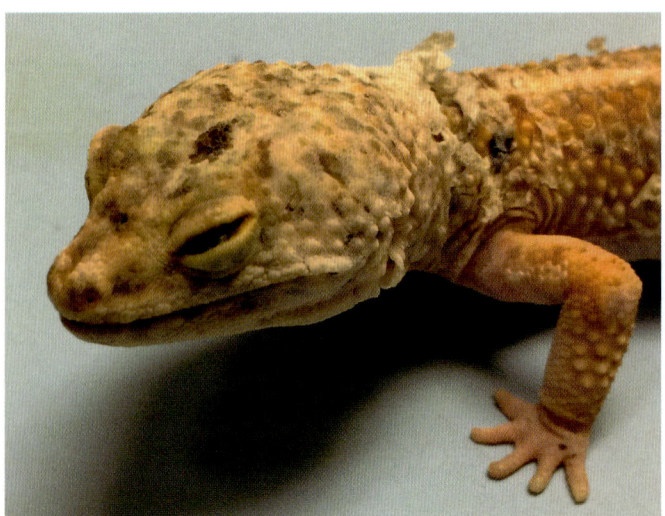

FIG 153.1 Hypovitaminosis A in a leopard gecko *(Eublepharis macularius)* with blepharedema and dysecdysis. Insectivores are prone to vitamin A deficiency because insects are deficient and most reptile multivitamins lack preformed vitamin A.

infection is present and should be based upon culture and sensitivity testing for systemic therapy. Patients do not resume feeding until their eyes open, and therefore nutritional support may be indicated. For STS, 1 drop of vitamin A (vitamin A in oil, 10,000 IU/capsule, Jamieson Natural Sources) can be given PO or transdermally SID for 2 weeks. Treatment for hypervitaminosis A skin sloughing is similar to that for partial thickness thermal burns.

PROGNOSIS AND PREVENTION

Careful attention to the provision of an appropriate and balanced diet will prevent hypovitaminosis A. However, when treatment of a deficiency is required, it is safer to correct the diet and provide oral supplementation than to give injections. (See Chapters 27, 84, and 122 for more details.)

154

Inclusion Body Disease (Reptarenavirus)

Francesco C. Origgi

DEFINITION

Arenaviruses are enveloped RNA viruses and are candidate etiological agents (genus *Reptarenavirus*) for inclusion body disease (IBD).[1–4] IBD is a chronic, multisystemic wasting disease affecting several species of boid snakes worldwide. A similar disease has been documented also in *Colubridae* and *Viperidae*.[2]

CLINICAL SIGNS

The clinical signs are not pathognomonic and may vary, but generally comprise regurgitation, incoordination, disorientation, opistotonus, torticollis, disequilibrium, lack of righting reflex (Fig. 154.1A), flaccid paralysis, and head tremors. Secondary diseases in IBD-affected snakes include pneumonia, stomatitis, and lymphoproliferative and other neoplastic diseases.[2] Affected snakes (e.g., *Python bivittatus*) may die within several weeks or survive for many months (e.g., *Boa constrictor*).[2] Some species differences in clinical signs exist; for example, regurgitation is common in boas but not in pythons.[2] Acutely infected snakes may exhibit leukocytosis, relative lymphocytosis, lower total protein and globulin values, and elevation of aspartate transaminase values, compared with chronically affected animals.[2]

PATHOLOGY

Gross lesions include splenic and pancreatic atrophy with fibrosis and often secondary pneumonia.[2] The histological hallmarks of disease are the intracytoplasmic eosinophilic to amphophilic inclusions (viral nucleoproteins)[1,4] present in multiple tissues in boas and more limited to the CNS in pythons (see Fig. 154.1B).[2] The snake mite (*Ophionissus natricis*) has been implicated as a potential vector of the etiological agent.[2]

DIGNOSTIC CONFIRMATION

Diagnosis of IBD requires laboratory confirmation. Available tests include the following:

1. Reverse transcription polymerase chain reaction (RT-PCR) for the rapid detection of arenavirus RNA from oral and cloacal swabs, whole blood,[5] liver, or esophageal tonsilar biopsies (see Fig. 154.1C).
2. Immunohistochemistry (IHC)[1,3] can be performed on formalin-fixed, paraffin-embedded tissues, including liver, esophageal tonsils (see Fig. 154.1C), pancreas, kidney, and brain (antemortem biopsies when possible or postmortem tissues).[1]

3. Cytological examination of blood smears for detection of inclusions.[6]
4. Histopathology (liver and esophageal tonsilar biopsies [see Fig. 154.1C] or necropsy tissues).
5. Electron microscopy.
6. Virus isolation. Some snakes with inclusion bodies may be RT-PCR negative, and consequently molecular testing should be ideally complemented by histopathology and viral isolation.

PREFERRED TREATMENT(S)

Currently, no specific therapy is available for IBD. Isolation and/or euthanasia of animals within collections is often recommended.

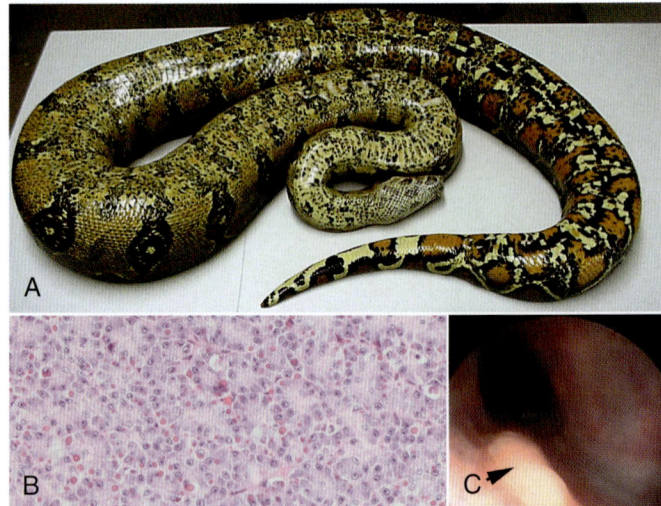

FIG 154.1 Clinical signs, diagnostic "hot spots," and histopathological findings associated with inclusion body disease of boid snakes. (A) A *Boa constrictor* in dorsal recumbency consistent with complete lack of righting reflex is shown in this image. This is a classic, although not pathognomonic, clinical sign observed in snakes with inclusion body disease. (B) Large numbers of glassy eosinophilic intracytoplasmic inclusions are disseminated in this section of pancreas. Histological support of molecular tests for the diagnosis of inclusion body disease is highly recommended. (C) In this endoscopic image of the esophagus of a snake, a prominent esophageal tonsil (arrow) is present. Esophageal tonsils are considered sampling site for antemortem diagnosis of inclusion body disease (A, Courtesy of Scott J. Stahl, Stahl Exotic Animal Veterinary Services; B, courtesy of Francesco C. Origgi; C, courtesy of Stephen J. Divers.)

PROGNOSIS AND PREVENTION

Disease progression in pythons is often rapid and prognosis poor to grave. In boas, the disease can be protracted, and with supportive care, snakes may live for months if not years. However, ultimately the prognosis is poor. Quarantine (at least 6 months), repeat testing, and isolation/removal of positive animals (or those showing consistent signs) are fundamental.[2] Routine testing of a representative set of animals in the collection is recommended. Virus replication is reduced at high temperatures (37°C).[7] Evidence of vertical transmission of co-infecting reptarenaviruses has been recently reported. A juvenile affected snake would develop inclusion bodies from the age of 2 months onward.[8]

REFERENCES

See www.expertconsult.com for a complete list of references.

155

Lizard Cryptosporidiosis

Kevin Eatwell and Jenna Richardson

DEFINITION

Cryptosporidium is a genus of protozoal parasites that are found in wild and captive reptiles. The organism belongs to the suborder Eimeriorina. In lizards, *C. varanii* (*syn C. saurophilum*) has an intestinal predilection, predominantly found in the small intestine mucosa, less commonly in the gastric mucosa, large intestine, and cloaca.

CLINICAL SIGNIFICANCE AND KNOWN ETIOLOGICAL CAUSE(S)

Many lizards infected with *Cryptosporidium* are subclinical with no obvious abnormalities. These individuals can spread infection through collections even if good hygiene is observed. In some individuals, *Cryptosporidium* spp. can lead to clinical disease, which can be highly debilitating for the lizard.

CLINICAL PRESENTATION AND DIAGNOSTIC CONFIRMATION

In asymptomatic cases, oocysts are often detected during routine fecal endoparasite screening. In lizards displaying clinical signs, a chronic enteritis has been reported, with wasting disease seen in geckos (Fig. 155.1).[1,2] Physical examination findings can include loss of muscle mass, reduced appetite, anorexia, lethargy, weakness, diarrhea, and fecal staining may be evident around the cloaca. Cloacal prolapse and cystitis have been reported in a green iguana (*Iguana iguana*).[3] Diagnostic techniques include the identification of oocysts from feces, after modified Ziehl-Neelsen staining (Fig. 155.2). Immunofluorescence antibody tests (IFAT) on fecal samples can also be performed; however, as with the staining technique, the oocyst must be shed in the feces at time of testing for a positive result. As *Cryptosporidium* is intermittently shed; repeat tests for both techniques are required to avoid false negative results. Definitive diagnosis of disease requires intestinal biopsy.

For carnivorous lizards, the presence of *Cryptosporidium* oocysts in the feces may be an incidental finding, ingested with prey items. This can complicate the diagnosis, as the nonpathogenic *C. muris* and *C. parvum* can be difficult to differentiate from *C. varanii* without further testing. Correctly identifying the species can determine clinical outcomes, and this can be confirmed by polymerase chain reaction (PCR).[4]

PREFERRED TREATMENT(S)

Treatment is problematic, as there is no singular agent with proven efficacy. Treatment to eliminate the parasite is a high priority in reptiles because *Cryptosporidium* does not appear to be self-limiting, and chronic shedding occurs.[1] In one study, the burden of *Cryptosporidium* was found to be reduced after treatment using paromomycin (100 mg/kg every 24 hrs for days 1–7, 100 mg/kg twice weekly for days 14–49, 360 mg/kg every 48 hrs for days 50–60).[5] Treatment was effective in green iguanas using halofuginone (110 mg/kg every 7 days for 5 weeks) or a combination of sulfadiazine and trimethoprim (75 mg/kg every

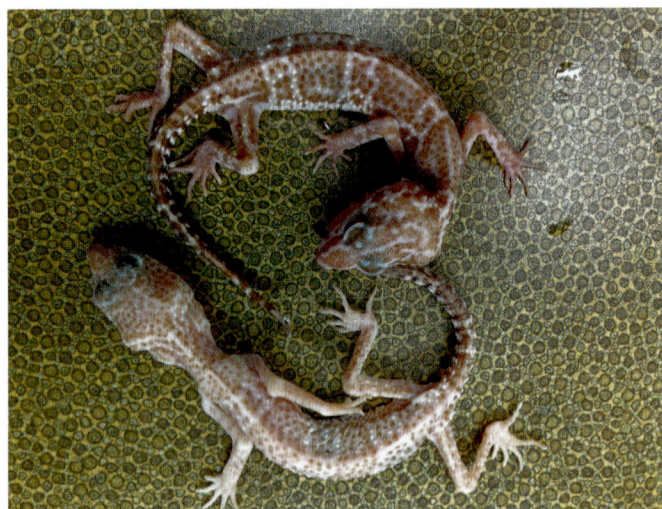

FIG 155.1 Wasting disease is often seen in leopard geckos (*Eublepharis macularius*) infected with cryptosporidium. (Courtesy of Scott J. Stahl, Stahl Exotic Animal Veterinary Services.)

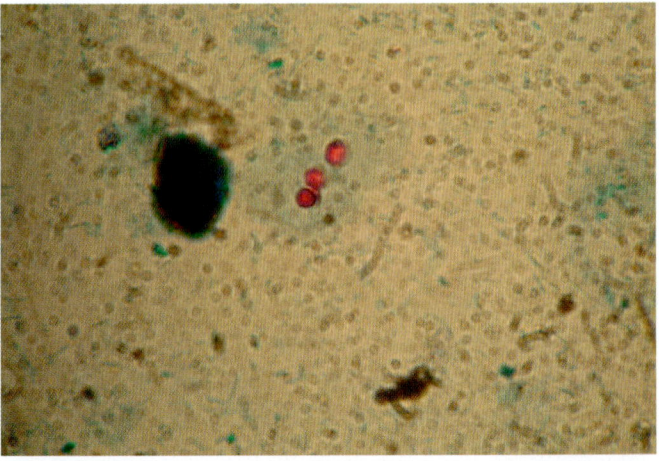

FIG 155.2 *Cryptosporidium* oocysts staining red on a ZN-stained fecal sample from a leopard gecko (*Eublepharis macularius*). The oocysts measure 4 to 8 microns in length. (Courtesy of Kevin Eatwell.)

5 days for 5 weeks) or spiramycin and metronidazole (200 mg/kg every 5 days for 5 weeks) alongside hyperimmune bovine colostrum.[6]

PROGNOSIS AND PREVENTION

Cryptosporidiosis is transmitted via the feco-oral route, either by direct contact between lizards or via contaminated objects or enclosures. Ingestion of sporulated oocytes can then lead to infection. Environmental stressors, high stocking density of animals (particularly in young stock), and reduced health status can all promote the spread of the pathogen. Quarantine and repeat fecal analysis are recommended for all new additions to a collection.

Environmental hygiene is of utmost importance to reduce the environmental contamination by oocysts. Physical removal of all fecal material and contaminated substrate is required. The use of surfactants can aid the removal of organic material on solid surfaces. Specific treatments for the environmental destruction of oocysts include ammonia (5%) and formalin (10%) with a contact time of 18 hours at 4°C. Currently, moist heat (45°–60°C for 5–9 minutes), freezing, or desiccation appears to be the most effective ways to clear the environment after thorough cleaning. More details on protocols can be found in Chapter 18. The zoonotic potential of *Cryptosporidium* is low due to the host-specific nature of the parasite. Sensible hygiene precautions should be performed when both handling and cleaning enclosures.

REFERENCES

See www.expertconsult.com for a complete list of references.

156

Neurological Disorders

Karina A. Mathes and Simon R. Platt

Reptiles with neurological disorders can display a wide variety of neurological signs depending on the species, lesion localization, and underlying cause. The neurological examination should include: evaluation of awareness and alertness, posture, movement and gait, muscle size and tone, assessment of diverse reflexes, evaluation of cranial nerves (I-XII) (see Chapter 77), and response to pain. Evaluating mentation of some reptiles (especially turtles) requires some experience with normal behavior.[1] Reptiles, compared with mammals, may not respond as consistently to certain neurological tests. For example, responses can be quite variable when testing a healthy bearded dragon (*Pogona vitticeps*) for proprioception or a menace response, thus confounding the response (and meaning). Another difficulty encountered when assessing neurological reptiles is the nonspecific nature of clinical signs. Neurological signs are dependent on many factors, including species, lesion localization, and severity of the disease and can include head tilt, circling, buoyancy problems, inability to strike or swallow food, dysphagia, lethargy, blindness, abnormal head and/or body posture (Fig. 156.1), ataxia, loss of reflexes, opisthothonus, seizures, paresis or paralysis, obtundation, stupor, coma, and finally death.

Because of the variety of possible underlying causes, a thorough history and dietary and husbandry evaluation is essential. Neurological or neurological-like signs can be associated with specific neurological disease but also with musculoskeletal or systemic metabolic diseases.

Causes of neurological disease in reptiles include infectious (e.g., viruses, bacteria, fungi, parasites) and noninfectious (e.g., hypoglycemia, hypocalcaemia, metabolic bone diseases, vitamin or mineral deficiencies, intoxication, hypothermia and hyperthermia, trauma (Fig. 156.2), hepatic or renal disease, dystocia, cystic calculi, congenital abnormalities, neoplasia) and vary with reptilian species. Table 156.1 summarizes etiologies for neurological disorders in reptiles. (See Chapter 77 for more details.)

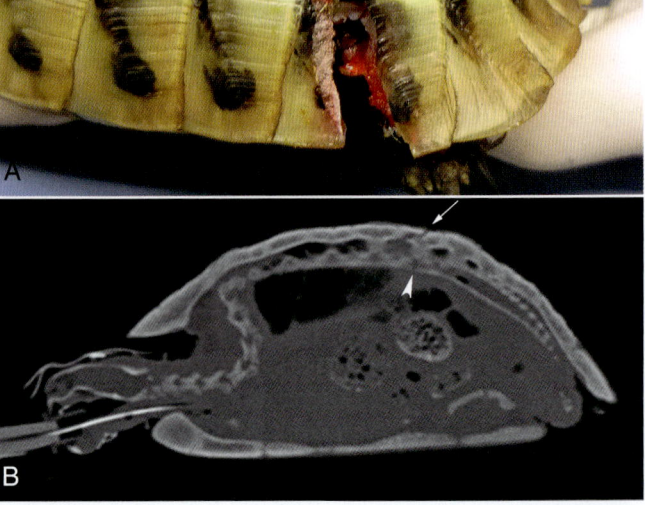

FIG 156.2 Photo (A) and computed tomography (B) of a subadult male Hermann's tortoise (*Testudo hermanni*) with fractures of the carapace (white arrow) and bridge after a car accident, with concurrent trauma of the spinal cord (white arrowhead) leading to paresis of both hind limbs. (Courtesy of Karina A. Mathes.)

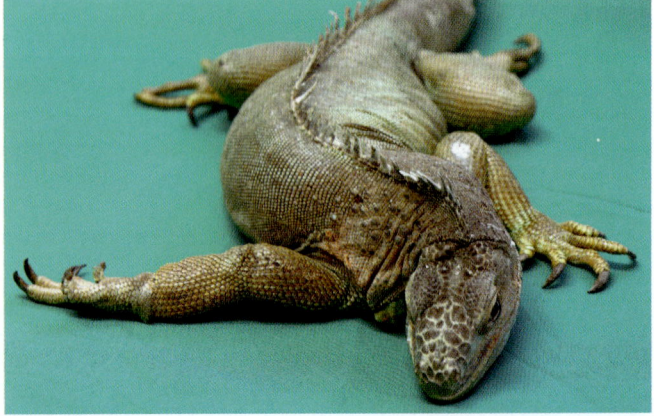

FIG 156.1 Female adult green iguana (*Iguana iguana*) with head tilt and abnormal body posture due to peripheral vestibular disease. (Courtesy of Karina A. Mathes.)

TABLE 156.1   Potential Causes of Neurological Signs and Diseases in Reptiles

Clinical Presentation	Animals Affected	Etiology/Pathogen/Disease	Diagnostic Confirmation	Treatment	Prognosis/Prevention
Infectious Diseases					
Abnormal body position and movement pythons/boas, regurgitation in boas, death in pythons;[2] Torticollis, dysequlibrium, opisthotonus, flaccid paralysis[3]	Snakes	Arenavirus[2,4,5] (previously IBD associated viruses[3,6])	Liver biopsy, blood smears, intracytoplasmic inclusions in multiple tissues; esophageal swabs, whole blood PCR	None specific	Poor prognosis if confirmed, quarantine
Neurorespiratory signs;[7,8] acute meningoencephalitis, flaccid paralysis;[9] head tremor, incoordination, opisthotonus[10]	Snakes Boelen's python Australian pythons	Ophidian paramyxoviruses (including ferlavirus)[7,8] Paramyxovirus infection in a Boelen's python [9] Sunshine virus[10]	Virus isolation from tissue samples, oral and cloacal swabs, electron microscopy, haemagglutination inhibition; virus isolation, PCR	None specific, treatment of secondary bacterial infections	Poor prognosis if confirmed, quarantine
Paresis[11,12] Paralysis[13]	Tortoises	Herpesvirus in tortoises[11,12]	Histopathology, electron microscopy	None specific, symptomatic	Poor prognosis
Meningoencephalitis,[14] circling[14,15]	Tortoises	Herpesvirus in Hermann's tortoises[14,15]	Histopathology, electron microscopy, neutralization test	None specific, symptomatic	Poor prognosis
Head tilt	Snakes	Adenovirus-like infection in a Colombian boa constrictor[16]	Histopathology, electron microscopy	None	Poor prognosis
Intention tremors, swimming abnormalities, opisthotonus	Alligators	West Nile virus in farmed American alligators[17]	Immunohistochemistry of various organs	None	Poor prognosis
Meningoencephalitis, abnormal posture,[18] and blindness[19]	Boa constrictor, reptiles, snakes.	*Staphylococcus aureus,* Salmonella, Mycobacteria[18,19]	Microbiology, fine needle biopsy, Ziehl-Neelsen acid fast stain	Antibiotics	Depending on the severity and location, poor
Vestibular syndrome, sometimes head tilt and circling[18]	Reptiles	Otitis media/interna; due to bacteria or other causes (as vitamin deficiencies, management mistakes)	Microbiology, histopathology	Surgery (removal), antibiotics, optimization of husbandry	Good if treated right
Lytic and proliferative vertebral disease[20]	Reptiles	Osteomyelitis; variety of bacteria and viruses	Microbiology	Antibiotics	Poor prognosis
Ataxia, tremors	Snakes	*Cryptococcus neoformans* in a boa [21]	Histopathology	Chloromycetin, tocopherol	Poor prognosis
Meningoencephalitis, opisthotonus (star gazing) in a boa [22]	Snakes, lizards, rarely chelonians	*Acanthamoeba* spp.[23,22]	Fecal analysis, histopathology	Metronidazole	Poor prognosis, strict quarantine
Seizures (gecko); pseudocysts in the brain (bull snake)[22]	Lizards and snakes	*Toxoplasma* spp. in a Mediterranean gecko[22] and a bullsnake [22]	Fecal analysis, histopathology	None reported in live reptiles[23]	Poor prognosis
Multisystemic infection reported, anorexia	Lizards	*Encephalitozoon* spp. in bearded dragons[24]	Histopathology, transmission electron microscopy	None	Poor prognosis
Varying degrees of paresis	Sea turtles	*Neospirorchis* spp. in wild loggerhead sea turtles[25]	Histopathology	None specific	Poor prognosis
Malnutrition/Deficiencies/Metabolic Diseases					
Muscle tremor, loss of righting reflex, mydriasis	Crocodilians	Hypoglycemia; unknown pathophysiology[26]	Blood glucose levels	Glucose	Depending on the severity
Muscle tremors, fasciculation, tetany	All reptiles	Hypocalcaemia; common in lizards (especially during reproduction)[27]	Measurement of ionized calcium	Calcium administration, correction of underlying causes	Depending on the severity and duration

Continued

TABLE 156.1 **Potential Causes of Neurological Signs and Diseases in Reptiles—cont'd**

Clinical Presentation	Animals Affected	Etiology/Pathogen/Disease	Diagnostic Confirmation	Treatment	Prognosis/Prevention
Variable, nonspecific signs, in case of acute hypocalcaemia: hypocalcemic tetany, loss of balance, loss of righting reflex	Reptiles	Metabolic bone diseases (MBDs); medical disorders that affect integrity and function of bone (i.e., nutritional or renal secondary hyperparathyroidism [NSHP, RSHP])[28]	Measurement of plasma calcium levels	Calcium supplementation, correct diet and housing, vitamin D, calcitonin	Good to grave depending on the etiology and severity
Stargazing, torticollis, seizures	Lizards (*Gecko* spp.)	Xanthomatosis; leaf-tailed geckos with hydrocephalus, encephalopathy[29]	Histopathology	None specific	Poor prognosis
Muscle twitching, incoordination, seizures, torticollis	Snakes (*Thamnophis* spp., *Natrix* spp.)	Thiamine deficiency; feeding frozen and thawed fish to fish-eaters[18,26]	Histopathology, medical history	Thiamine, diet change	Depending on the severity
Muscle tremor, generalized muscle weakness	Egg-eating snakes and lizards (e.g., varanids)	Biotin deficiency; feeding whole raw egg diet[18,26]	Medical history	Vitamin B, biotin, providing of a varied diet	Good prognosis
Muscle tremor, flexion of carpal joints	Green iguanas	Vitamin E/selenium deficiency; tentative diagnosis: nutritional myopathy[30]	Response to medical treatment with selen and vitamin E, elevation of GOT in serum	Selen, vitamin E	Good prognosis
Weakness, muscle tremors	Reptiles	Leaf-tailed geckos with renal encephalopathy (Raiti et al, Proc ARAV, 2000, pp 29–30)	Histopathology	None	Poor prognosis
Ataxia, incoordination, seizures	Reptiles	Gout crystals may form within CNS[27]	Hyperuricemia	Allopurinol, eliminate underlying cause	Poor prognosis if chronic
Intoxication					
Flaccid paralysis, death	Reptiles, especially chelonians	Chlorhexidine toxicosis in red-bellied short-necked turtles[31]	Medical history (immersion in chlorhexidine solution), necropsy	Thorough rinsing with tab water, bath	Poor prognosis
Head tilt, circling, opisthotonus, seizures, convulsions	Reptiles	Organophosphates in snakes[27]	Medical history (dichlorvos strip exposure)	Removal of the toxin, supportive therapy with fluids, sedatives, atropine	Guarded prognosis
Extreme paresis or flaccid paralysis, death	Chelonians, some lizard species	Red-footed tortoises treated with ivermectin[32]	Medical history (ivermectin injection in chelonians), necropsy	Oxygen flow, picrotoxin treatment	Guarded to poor prognosis
Diffuse neurological signs, death	Various snake species, including indigo and king snakes	High doses of metronidazole administration (>100 mg/kg) in indigo snakes[33]	Medical history (metronidazole administration)	Lowering metronidazole dosage down to 40 mg/kg	Guarded to poor prognosis if overdosed
Unusual neurological signs such as walking backward	Reptiles	Lead toxicosis in a Greek tortoise (Chitty, Proc ARAV, 2003, p 101)	Elevated blood lead levels, radiodense object in radiographs	Chelation therapy with sodium calcium edetate	Good prognosis when treated
Facial seizures, head shaking, mouth gaping, death	Bearded dragons	Fireflies containing lucibufagins, may be fatal in bearded dragons (Glor et al, Proc ARAV, 1999, pp 27–29)	Medical history (ingestion), necropsy	Not described	Guarded to poor prognosis
Disorientation, seizures, twitches, death (within hours)	Juvenile European tortoises	Ingestion of branches of English yew (*Taxus baccata*)[34]	Medical history (ingestion), necropsy	None specific, fluids, bath, peroral and cloacal administration of paraffin in surviving animals	Guarded to poor prognosis

TABLE 156.1　Potential Causes of Neurological Signs and Diseases in Reptiles—cont'd

Clinical Presentation	Animals Affected	Etiology/Pathogen/ Disease	Diagnostic Confirmation	Treatment	Prognosis/ Prevention
Seizures, coma, death	Green iguanas	Ingestion of flowers of azalea (rhododendron)[35]	Medical history (ingestion)	Vomitus of the flower, oral fluid supplementation	Good prognosis if removal possible
Trauma					
Opisthotonus, seizures, paresis, paralysis	Reptiles	Traumas causing disorders of the nervous system[27]	Medical history, radiographs	Case depending surgery, supportive fluid therapy, antibiotics, glucocorticoids, mannitol, and where appropriate fracture fixation	Variable good to poor prognosis
Flaccid paralysis hind limbs	Lizards (desert iguana)	Vertebral fracture and spinal cord compression in a desert iguana[19]	Medical history, necropsy, and histopathology	None	Poor prognosis
Miscellaneous Causes					
Relative inability to move and strike prey	Snakes, Burmese python	Spinal osteopathy; *Osteitis deformans* (Paget's disease)[36]	Clinical examination, radiographs, computed tomography, histopathology	None	Poor prognosis
Paraparesis	Chelonians	Chronic dystocia[37]	Radiographs	Treatment of dystocia (conservative or surgically)	Good prognosis
Paraparesis	Reptiles with urinary bladder	Cystic calculi; green iguana with large bladder stone—obstructing pelvic canal[38]	Radiographs	Cystotomy, removal of the cystic calculi	Good prognosis
Head tilt, circling, blindness[27]	Tortoises	Hypothermia; tortoises after hibernation[27]	Medical history	Supportive treatment (including thiamine)	Poor prognosis
Decreased mobility/ inability to move, loss of righting ability	Rattlesnakes	Neoplasia; central nervous system tumor, spinal cord glioma[39]	Clinical examination, histopathology, immunohisto-chemistry	None reported	Poor prognosis
Acute neurological dysfunction, head tilt, obtundation, loss of proprioception and righting reflexes, ataxia, hyperesthesia	Australian water dragons	Unknown etiology; viral or toxic etiology suspected, encephalomalacia, necrosis in the brain[40]	Necropsy, histopathology	Supportive treatment, fluids, antibiotics, antifungals, corticosteroids, atropine—without effect	Poor prognosis

When treating reptiles, clinicians should be aware of their significant ability for tissue regeneration, including the nervous system. Reptiles in general take longer to heal than mammals or birds. Owners should be made aware that progression may be slow and be prepared to allow the time required for regeneration. Preferred medical or surgical treatment depends on the underlying cause. In these patients, it is important to focus on supportive care and environmental management for the necessary time that is required to allow maximal recovery from neurological disease.

REFERENCES

See www.expertconsult.com for a complete list of references.

Nutritional Secondary Hyperparathyroidism

Thomas H. Boyer and Peter W. Scott

DEFINITION

Nutritional secondary hyperparathyroidism (NSHP) occurs when chronic calcium deficiency causes the parathyroid glands to overproduce parathyroid hormone, which stimulates osteoclastic activity, weakens bone, and eventually kills the patient.

CLINICAL SIGNIFICANCE

NSHP, one type of metabolic bone disease, is the most common disease of captive reptiles.

KNOWN ETIOLOGICAL CAUSE(S)

Calcium (Ca) deficiency results from inadequate dietary Ca, a low Ca:P ratio in the diet, and/or lack of vitamin D. Many reptiles and amphibians seem to be more dependent on ultraviolet light (UVB, 290–300 nm) to synthesize vitamin D_3 or cholecalciferol than on dietary vitamin D. As a rule of thumb, UVB is recommended for all reptiles and amphibians, except for a few nocturnal geckos and snakes; however, even these species may benefit from UVB. Bone is the main storage site of Ca within the body; plasma Ca constitutes less than 1% in three main fractions: 45% ionized (free) Ca, 40% total (albumin bound) Ca, and 15% anion bound. When ionized Ca levels drop, parathyroid hormone levels increase, which increases Ca resorption from bone. If bone Ca levels are not replenished, bone weakens, softens, and fractures, and/or fibrous osteodystrophy may develop (lizards) or the shell softens (chelonians). In lizards, life-threatening reductions in ionized Ca can lead to tremors in the digits, limbs, large muscle masses (spasms), seizures, tetany, or flaccid paresis.

Ca is deficient in many vegetables, most fruits, and almost all insects, as well as organ and muscle meats. All whole vertebrates are excellent sources of Ca (because of their bone); hence, Ca deficiency is rarely seen in reptiles and amphibians that eat whole vertebrate prey. Some invertebrates, such as crustaceans, are good sources of Ca, provided the shell is consumed.

CLINICAL PRESENTATION

Signs of NSHP include lethargy, weakness, reluctance to move, declining appetite, and lack of growth or weight gain. Sprawl—and partial to complete lack of truncal and proximal tail, or shell, lifting when ambulating—is common. Lizards are prone to spinal damage from vertebral fractures, which may result in paraparesis or paraplegia of the rear legs and a horizontal flattening of the ribcage and scapula (barrel chested). Both lizards and crocodilians may have bowed, thickened, or fractured long bones or mandibles, pliable mandible and maxillae, overbite, kyphoscoliosis, lordosis or rhoecosis (all three), and walk on the forelimbs rather than plantigrade (Fig. 157.1). Chameleons have a noticeably weakened grip, decreased prehensile ability of their tail, and fall repeatedly. Crocodilians may have teeth that protrude laterally, fall out, or are lucent around their edges. Chelonians have soft shells (normally the shell should feel solid, like skull) (Fig. 157.2) and splay out their legs, but they do not typically have long bone fractures or

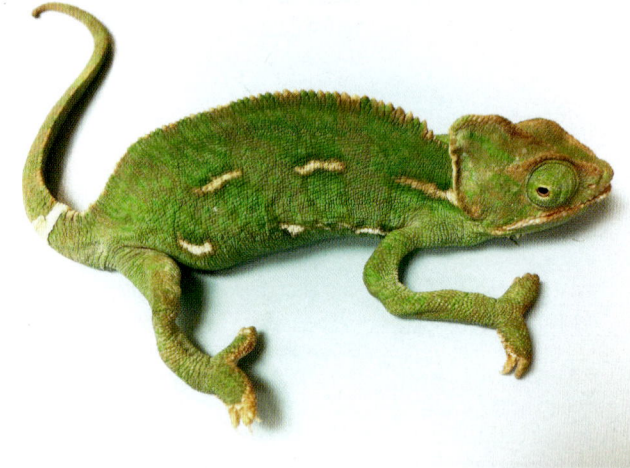

FIG 157.1 Nutritional secondary hyperthyroidism in a veiled chameleon (*Chamaeleo calyptratus*); note the sprawl, bowed legs, mandibular and maxillary malalignment, and uneven spine. This patient made a full recovery.

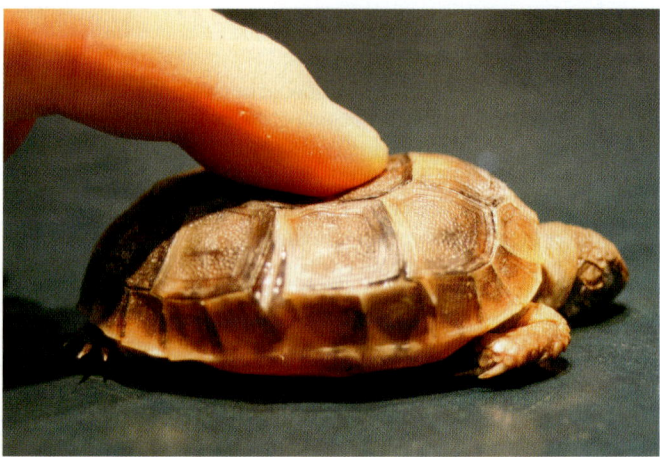

FIG 157.2 Nutritional secondary hyperthyroidism in a desert tortoise (*Gopherus agassizii* or *G. morafkai*). Young anorexic tortoises with soft shells usually die.

fibrous osteodystrophy. In box turtles, the marginal scutes may curl dorsally, the body appears too small for the shell, and the phallus or cloaca may prolapse. Clinical signs in amphibians include lack of truncal lifting, dorsal curling of the toes, vertebral or mandibular deformities, long bone fractures, subcutaneous edema, anasarca, or absence of radio-opaque calcium carbonate in endolymphatic sacs.

DIAGNOSTIC CONFIRMATION

Clinical signs, combined with detailed dietary history, often will suggest a diagnosis. Radiographs are useful to assess fractures and overall bone radiopacity. Radiographs are equivocal in early cases; in mammals 40% to 50% of bone loss must be present to be detected radiographically. Decreased radiographic opacity is more obvious in advanced cases, especially in thin bones. Biochemistry is useful for assessment and excluding kidney involvement, but care must be taken with restraint and venipuncture. Typically, both total and ionized Ca are within normal limits, or low; because bone is such a vast reservoir, reproductively active females may have elevated Ca. With obvious clinical signs diagnostics are often not essential for treatment. More sensitive measures of bone density include quantitative computed tomography and dual energy x-ray absorptiometry.

PREFERRED TREATMENT(S)

Medical treatment includes calcium supplementation, nutritional support, improved husbandry (especially provision of UVB), analgesia, and perhaps calcitonin. Oral calcium supplementation is easiest via calcium-rich syrups, either Ca glubionate (1.8 gm/5 mL or 24 mg/mL elemental Ca) or Ca gluconate (23% w/v or 21 mg/mL elemental Ca), dosed at 1 mL/kg PO bid. Calcium is continued for 1 to 3 months or until the patient is eating calcium-enriched foods well on its own, moving normally and gaining weight. Salmon calcitonin injections have been recommended at 50 IU/kg IM, repeat in 1 week, if normocalcemic, or 1 week after starting calcium supplementation. Do not give calcitonin if hypocalcemic or neurologic signs are present. Patients with hypocalcemic tetany can be treated with 100 mg/kg 10% Ca gluconate IM or intracoelomically q 6 hours until tetany ceases, then switched to oral calcium syrups. Otherwise Ca injections are not recommended. Nutritional support is critical; the patient must start gaining weight and growing, otherwise extensive skeletal damage will not be repaired. Surgical fixation of pathologic fractures is contraindicated.

PROGNOSIS AND PREVENTION

Prognosis is dependent on severity of clinical signs; lizards and crocodilians respond better than chelonians. Early diagnosis and aggressive veterinary treatment is essential; chronic NSHP has a poorer prognosis. Owners must be committed to several months of daily treatment. If no decreased radiopacity of bone is visible, the prognosis is good to excellent. Hypocalcemia and decreasing radiopacity of bone worsens the prognosis. Paresis, paralysis, or obstipation are poor prognostic indicators. Small chelonians with soft shells that are not eating typically die.

Good nutrition with adequate Ca supplementation and UV light is critical; for more information, see Chapters 27, 84, and 122.

Paramyxoviruses (Ferlaviruses)

Francesco C. Origgi

DEFINITION, CLINICAL SIGNIFICANCE, AND KNOWN ETIOLOGICAL CAUSE(S)

With the exception of "Sunshine virus" affecting Australian pythons, all the other partially characterized reptile paramyxoviruses (single-stranded, RNA viruses) are comprised within the genus *Ferlavirus*, subfamily *Paramyxovirinae*, family *Paramyxoviridae*.[1] Lethal infections have been documented mainly in snakes (*Colubridae, Elapidae, Viperidae, Crotalidae, Boidae,* and *Pythonidae*) but also in lizards and chelonians.[1,2]

CLINICAL PRESENTATION

Clinical signs are nonpathognomonic and range from no to severe respiratory disease with or without tracheal exudate.[1–3] Neurologic signs have also been described.[1,2] Snakes (*Antaresia* sp., *Aspidites* sp., and *Morelia* sp.) infected with Sunshine virus showed neurorespiratory signs.[1]

Gross lesions in snakes range from none to caseous-necrotic material in the lung(s), hemorrhages,[1–3] and dermatitis.[4] A characteristic microscopic feature of Ferlavirus infections is a proliferative interstitial pneumonia (Fig. 158.1), with occasional intracytoplasmic eosinophilic

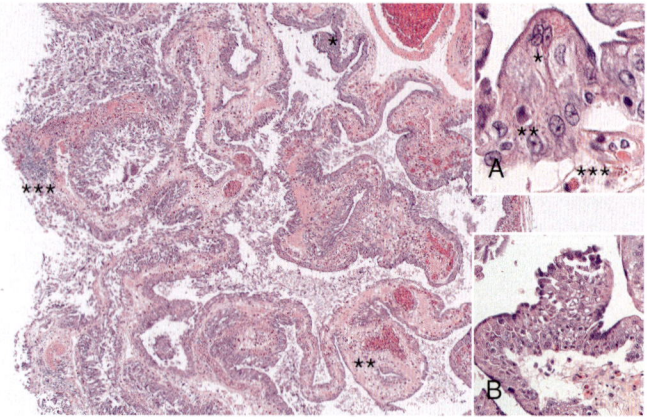

FIG 158.1 Lung of a snake with interstitial proliferative pneumonia. The respiratory epithelium is moderately to markedly thickened (single asterisk), with expansion of the interstitium secondary to edema (double asterisk) and inflammatory infiltration (triple asterisks). *(Inset A)* A classic syncytium is shown (single asterisk). An inflammatory mononuclear cell is infiltrating the epithelium (exocytosis) (double asterisk) and an intact degranulated granulocyte is also present (triple asterisk). *(Inset B)* Marked thickening and proliferation of the respiratory epithelium. (Courtesy of Francesco C. Origgi.)

inclusions in snakes and lizards.[2] Gross findings in snakes infected with Sunshine virus are often unremarkable.[1] The most consistent histologic change is severe spongiosis of the white matter of the hindbrain.[1] Paramyxovirus infections in chelonians may be associated with pneumonia, degenerative liver disease, stomatitis, and dermatitis.[1] Ferlavirus delivered intratracheally causes disease.[3,5] Vertical transmission has also been considered for Sunshine virus.[6]

DIAGNOSTIC CONFIRMATION

Confirmation of clinical suspicion requires laboratory testing (serology, molecular tests, viral isolation, immunohistochemistry, histopathology, and electron microscopy). The most common serologic test is hemagglutination inhibition (HI), whereas the most common molecular test is reverse transcription PCR (RT-PCR) targeting the partial sequence of the L gene.[1,2] A specific RT-PCR is available for Sunshine virus.[1] RT-PCR testing can detect Ferlavirus RNA in the tissues as early as 4 days postinfection (PI), and infected animals remain positive for at least 49 days PI. Lung, small intestine, pancreas, and brain are the tissues of choice for postmortem diagnosis.[3] Overall detection rate (RT-PCR and virus isolation combined) in tissues was shown to be 72%. For antemortem diagnosis, it is best combining RT-PCR and viral isolation on tracheal wash with viral detection as early as 16 days PI. Cloacal swabs may be positive as early as 28 days PI.[3] Detection of HI titers requires a minimum of 16 days and becomes more robust at 28 days.[7] Serologic test results might not be comparable when using different Ferlavirus strains as antigen.[1] Ideal laboratory diagnosis should comprise molecular, serologic, and histopathologic investigations and virus isolation.

PREFERRED TREATMENT(S)

No specific therapies exist against Ferlavirus infection. Supportive therapy has been suggested, with appropriate antimicrobials if secondary infections exist.[1]

PROGNOSIS AND PREVENTION

Quarantine (up to 6 months) while carrying out repeated molecular and serologic tests is critical. Isolation and testing of resident reptiles showing consistent signs is recommended. Prognosis is guarded to poor.

REFERENCES

See www.expertconsult.com for a complete list of references.

Periodontal Disease

Scott J. Stahl

DEFINITION

Periodontal disease involves bacterial or fungal invasion of the unique periodontal tissues of lizard species with acrodont dentition, specifically agamids (bearded dragons, *Pogona vitticeps*; Asian water dragons, *Physignathus cocincinus*; frilled dragons, *Chlamydosaurus kingii*), and all old-world chameleons.[1-4]

CLINICAL SIGNIFICANCE AND KNOWN ETIOLOGICAL CAUSE(S)

Acrodont dentition in lizards appears to predispose to periodontal disease.[1,2] With acrodont teeth only a thin layer of gingival tissue is present along the lateral and medial surfaces of the mandibular and maxillary bones. If this fragile gingival tissue is damaged/abraded, plaque can accumulate, pockets may occur, and microorganisms can colonize, often followed by invasion of deeper tissues and bone. Predisposition for periodontal disease with acrodont dentition may also be related to captive diet and the feeding of less abrasive, cultured insects and soft fruits.[1-3]

Early plaque accumulation with gingivitis is associated with an aerobic, gram-positive cocci bacterial population.[1] With more advanced plaque deposition and increased gingival inflammation, anaerobic organisms, including gram-negative bacteria and spirochetes, invade.[1] *Aspergillosis* spp. was identified in mycotic periodontal disease in a panther chameleon *Furcifer pardalis*.[4]

CLINICAL PRESENTATION AND DIAGNOSTIC CONFIRMATION

Lizards may present with anorexia, soft tissue swellings, or irregular labial closure along mandibular or maxillary bones. Lizards may also have no clinical signs, and oral lesions may be detected during a routine examination using a soft oral speculum to avoid further dental trauma.

Dental probes are useful to assess lesion depth. Early lesions show visible calculus and marginal gingival erythema, with progressive calculus buildup, increased gingival swelling, gingival margin recession, and exposure of underlying mandibular and maxillary bone. In advanced disease, gingival hyperplasia and pockets form with suppurative gingivitis and subcutaneous abscessation. Areas of focal and multifocal osteomyelitis then develop, resulting in loss of bone and teeth and finally pathological fractures and fatal systemic illness. Radiography or CT is useful to assess bone lysis, pathological fractures, bone sequestra, and periosteal proliferation.[1] Culture and sensitivity should be utilized to identify organisms involved and determine appropriate antimicrobial therapy. Because mixed infections are common, both aerobic, anaerobic, and fungal cultures should be submitted, with gram stains used to guide initial drug choices. Biopsy of bone and/or associated soft tissue is the most definitive method for identifying pathogens. Establishing an association between organisms and lesions with histopathology is important, especially in the oral cavity where many opportunistic organisms are present.

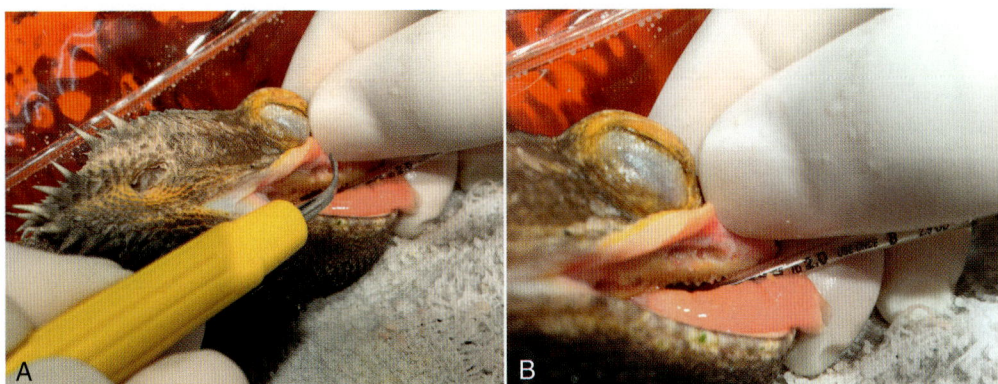

FIG 159.1 (A) An ultrasonic dental scaler is used to gently clean periodontal lesions in this bearded dragon (*Pogona vitticeps*) while under general anesthesia. Once periodontal lesions are present, periodic cleaning under sedation or anesthesia may be necessary to minimize progression of the disease and avoid systemic illness. The patient is intubated to maintain gas anesthesia and to protect the airway during cleaning. (B) The periodontal lesions evident in this same bearded dragon after debridement and cleaning. Notice the significant soft tissue and bone loss and subsequent exposure that will require close monitoring and continued management. (Courtesy of Octavio Romo-Flamand, Stahl Exotic Animal Veterinary Services.)

PREFERRED TREATMENT(S)

Once stable, a thorough oral examination under sedation or general anesthesia is recommended. While under anesthesia, cultures and biopsies may be collected. Removal of calculus is performed, and gingival sulci are cleaned using dental instrumentation and following standard precautions (Fig. 159.1A and B). With deeper lesions, surgical debridement (guided by imaging) and removal of unhealthy tissue and bone is important to expose infected tissue and allow continued topical therapy. Standard wound flushing solutions such as 0.05% chlorhexidine can be used to flush wounds every 1 to 3 days.[1–3]

While awaiting results of culture and sensitivity and/or histopathology, lizards may be started on a first-line, broad-spectrum antibiotic regimen. Due to the high incidence of mixed bacterial infections (aerobic and anaerobic organisms) and the severity of osteomyelitis, combination antimicrobial therapy (gram negative and anaerobic targeting specific drugs) is recommended. With osteomyelitis, systemic antimicrobials may need to be used for 4 to 6 weeks or longer depending on severity.[1,2] Nonsteroidal antiinflammatories, to reduce inflammation and pain, as well as opioids for analgesia are important in the management of these cases (see Chapter 50).

PROGNOSIS AND PREVENTION

Prognosis varies from fair to poor depending on the condition of the lizard at presentation, amount of tissue and bone lost, and the presence of osteomyelitis. Regardless, once initial aggressive treatment is complete, lifetime dental prophylaxis will be required using oral cleansing products (Maxiguard Oragel, Addison Biological Laboratory, Fayette, MO) at home with regular veterinary dental prophylaxis under sedation or general anesthesia.[1–3] Feeding hard-bodied insects (cockroaches, locusts, grasshoppers) and/or (for omnivorous species) more fibrous vegetables (pumpkin, sweet potato, leafy greens) may help to strengthen and keep gingival tissue clean and healthy.[1–3]

REFERENCES

See www.expertconsult.com for a complete list of references.

160

Pneumonia

Stephen J. Divers

DEFINITION

Pneumonia may occur as a primary entity, secondary to stomatitis and aspiration, by hematogenous spread (e.g., endocarditis) or by direct/close anatomical association (e.g., hepatitis, coelomitis). Pneumonia can be focal, multifocal, or diffuse, unilateral or bilateral. Many infections involve commensal or environmental organisms that become pathogenic in an immunocompromised host. Poor captive management, including inappropriate temperatures, ventilation, and humidty, are often intimitely involved with pathogenesis.

CLINICAL SIGNIFICANCE AND KNOWN ETIOLOGICAL CAUSE(S)

Bacterial pneumonia is probably most common and has been associated with aerobic gram-positive and gram-negative species. *Mycoplasma* spp. are important respiratory pathogens of tortoises, crocodilians, and pythons. A number of fungi have been associated with pneumonia in reptiles, including *Aspergillus, Candida, Fusarium, Mucor, Geotrichum, Penicillium, Cladosporium, Rhizopus, Chrysosporium, Paecilomyces*, and *Beauveria*. A variety of viruses have been detected in association with respiratory pathology, including herpesvirus and iridovirus (chelonia), poxvirus (lizards), paramyxovirus, and nidovirus (snakes).

Several genera of digenetic trematodes inhabit the oral cavity, but adults often migrate deeper and can cause focal lesions. Infection of aquatic turtles with digenetic spirorchid trematodes may result in pneumonia. Migrating nematode larvae have caused respiratory signs and/or pulmonary lesions in tortoises (*Angusticaecum*), chameleons (*Hexametra*), and pythons (*Ophidascaris*). Adult lungworms (*Rhabdias*) reside within the lungs of snakes and lizards, whereas migrating larvae (*Strongyloides*) may also be associated with pulmonary lesions. Pentastomid (segmented, wormlike) parasites undergo extensive visecral migrations before locating within the lungs (and less commonly the trachea and nasal passages). Pentastomids can cause localized lesions, and moulting can induce antigenic responses.

CLINICAL PRESENTATION AND DIAGNOSTIC CONFIRMATION

Cases of acute or peracute pneumonia may present as sudden death, although lethargy, anorexia, and respiratory signs, including dyspnea and open-mouth breathing, are common. In aquatic chelonians, asymmetrical position may be evident, with the affected side floating lower than the contralateral side. Although diagnostic imaging may provide convincing evidence of lung disease, a definitive diagnosis relies on the collection of material for histopathology (or cytology) and microbiology (Figs. 160.1 and 160.2). Therefore endoscopic lung

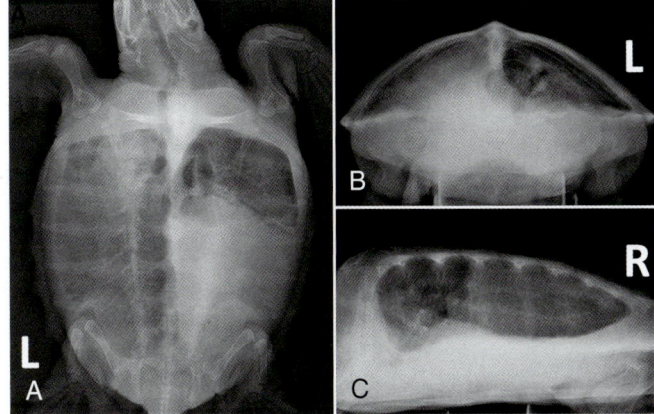

FIG 160.1 Dorsoventral (A), horizontal beam craniocaudal (B), and right lateral (C) radiographic views of a loggerhead sea turtle (*Caretta caretta*) with pronounced consolidation of the mid-to-caudal right lung. (Courtesy of Stephen J. Divers.)

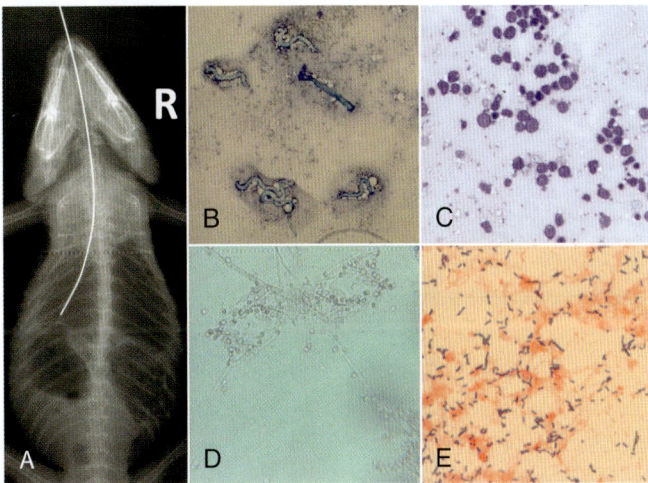

FIG 160.2 (A) Use of a curved stylet to ensure catheterization and lavage of the left lung in a bearded dragon (*Pogona vitticeps*). (B) Lung lavage cytology from a snake with verminous pneumonia demonstrating multiple nematode larvae (Diff Quik, x200). (C) Lung lavage cytology from a tortoise with mycotic pneumonia demonstrating large gram-positive structures consistent with yeast (Diff Quik, x 1000). (D) Lung lavage cytology from a sea turtle with mycotic pneumonia demonstrating fungal hyphae and conidia (wet prep, x1000). (E) Lung lavage from an agamid lizard with bacterial pneumonia demonstrating gram-positive bacilli (gram stain, x1000). (Courtesy of Stephen J. Divers.)

evaluation and biopsy, or lavage, are typically utilized. Verminous cases typically rely on lung lavage and fecal evaluations. Where serological tests exist (e.g., ophidian paramyxovirus), they should be utilized, with paired rising titers differentiating between active infection versus past exposure. PCR testing can be used to confirm the presence of a virus but not necessarily disease.

PREFERRED TREATMENT(S)

High-volume lung lavage and aspiration, or cooperage, have been employed to remove considerable quantities of exudate from the lower respiratory tract of anesthetized or sedated squamates. Systemic and local application of antimicrobials, based upon culture and sensitivity or MIC results, are typically required. Prolonged treatment is often required, along with correction of any predisposing husbandry or nutritional components. Large encapsulated lesions require surgical removal, but even small encapsulated granulomas are often resistant to drug therapy. Pulmonary nematodiasis is often treated with benzimadazoles. Pentastomids can be treated with ivermectin, but parasite death can result in massive antigenic reactions, and physical removal may be necessary.

PROGNOSIS AND PREVENTION

If left untreated most cases progress to generalized sepsis and death, although chronic granulomata or abscesses can develop. Typically the prognosis is poor when dealing with extensive disease. Prevention through strict hygiene and appropriate quarantine practices (including serological testing) is preferable. Improvements in husbandry and nutrition can strongly affect outcome. See Chapter 76 for more details and references.

161

Pseudogout

Jorge Orós

DEFINITION

Pseudogout or calcium pyrophosphate dihydrate (CPPD) is an arthropathy caused by crystal deposits in articular tissues, most commonly fibrocartilage and hyaline cartilage.[1]

CLINICAL SIGNIFICANCE AND KNOWN ETIOLOGICAL CAUSES(S)

There are few confirmed reports of CPPD crystal deposition in reptiles, and they have been presumably associated with chronic renal disease, nutritional imbalance, and joint trauma.[2,3] In humans, risk factors include aging, osteoarthritis, previous joint trauma/injury, familial/hereditary predisposition, and metabolic diseases such as hyperparathyroidism, hemochromatosis, hypomagnesemia, and hypophosphatasia.[4] The key role of local excess of inorganic pyrophosphate (PPi) in cartilage has been demonstrated in humans.[5] PPi is produced endogenously, and crystallization occurs only in the extracellular cartilage matrix, an area of poor vascularity. The passage of crystals to the synovial fluid seems to be required to induce inflammation.[6] CPPD crystals are recognized by innate immune system cells as danger signals, and then activated cells secrete recruiting and activating cytokines, where interleukin-1 plays a central role.[6]

CLINICAL PRESENTATION

Affected reptiles usually exhibit limited and painful mobility.[3] Nodular enlargement of the affected joint may also be noticed.[2] The presentation of both gout and pseudogout in the same animal has also been reported.[3]

DIAGNOSTIC CONFIRMATION

Diagnosis must be based on the identification of CPPD crystals in a synovial fluid sample or from biopsied tissue.[3] CPPD crystals are pleomorphic with rhomboid, rectangular, and rod-shaped forms,[6] and they are variably birefringent under polarized light.[6] Nondecalcified sections of tissue containing CPPD crystals stain positive with Von Kossa or Alizarin Red S stains.[3] In human medicine, chondrocalcinosis on radiographs is considered indicative of CPPD deposition[6] (Fig. 161.1). Ultrasonography shows CPPD crystals as hyperechoic deposits in the depth of hyaline joint cartilage or hyperechoic aggregates in fibrocartilages; their posterior acoustic shadowing enables their differentiation from gout.[6] CT shows calcified deposits but does not enable specific identification of CPPD crystals; in contrast with gout, dual-energy CT has rarely been used in calcium crystal deposition. MRI is relatively insensitive to CPPD deposits.[6]

Differential diagnoses include hydroxyapatite deposition disease (HADD),[7,8] osteoarthritis,[6] and gout.[3] The nonaqueous alcoholic eosin stain is used to allow differentiation of CPPD crystals (exhibiting birefringence) and hydroxyapatite crystals (absence of birefringence) in tissue sections.[9] However, the potential effect of a decalcifier on the birefringence of hydroxyapatite deposits has been reported.[7] By contrast, monosodium urate crystals are needlelike and strongly birefringent, and, in tissue sections, they stain negative with Von Kossa stain.

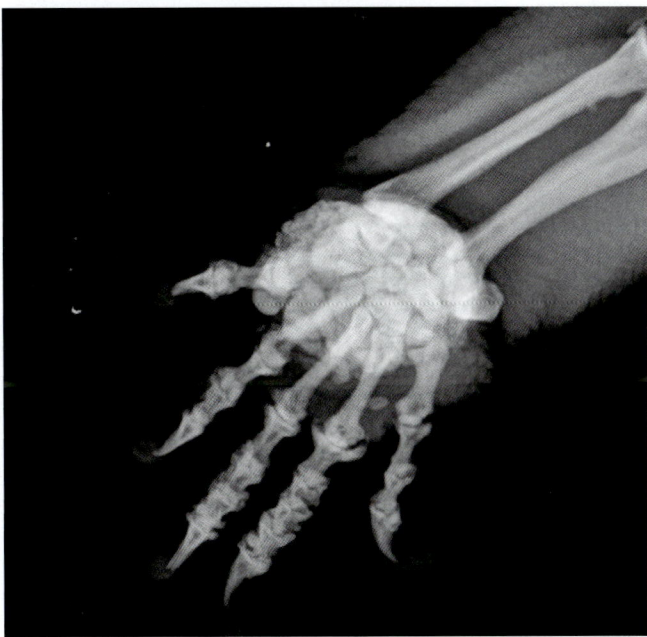

FIG 161.1 Radiograph of the left front foot of a tegu (*Tupinambis teguixin*) showing dramatic soft tissue swelling and mineral deposition. Histopathology on a surgical biopsy of the tissue confirmed a diagnosis of pseudogout with deposition of calcium crystals consistent with calcium pyrophosphate deposition disease. (Courtesy of Gregory Costanzo, Stahl Exotic Animal Veterinary Services.)

PREFERRED TREATMENT(S)[2,10]

No treatment has proven effective in dissolving CPPD crystals; phosphocitrates, pyrophosphatase, and probenecid have failed *in vivo* human testing. Antiinflammatory drugs, including NSAIDs, glucocorticoids (systemic or intra-articular), colchicine, hydroxychloroquine, and methotrexate are used in humans, but their efficacy in reptiles is unknown. Surgical removal may be the most effective treatment, with limb amputation recommended in severe cases. Analgesics for pain management are recommended.

PROGNOSIS AND PREVENTION

Based on the scarce reports, the prognosis for pseudogout in reptiles is guarded to poor.

REFERENCES

See www.expertconsult.com for a complete list of references.

162

Renal Disease

Stephen J. Divers

DEFINITION

Renal dysfunction and disease can be caused by degenerative (most common), inflammatory, infectious, or toxic etiologies, and it frequently results in nitrogenous waste accumulation (e.g., uremia, gout) and electrolyte imbalances.

CLINICAL SIGNIFICANCE AND KNOWN ETIOLOGICAL CAUSE(S)

Degenerative nephrosis represents the most common renal diseases encountered (glomerulonephrosis, tubulonephrosis). Inflammatory conditions are less common but can be associated with bacterial, viral, fungal, and parasitic infections. Severe, acute infections can cause acute renal failure. Therefore, it is important to diagnose these conditions accurately, because prompt and appropriate therapy may result in reclamation of temporarily lost renal function and a complete recovery. Toxic nephropathies have been associated with aminoglycosides and exogenous vitamin D_3 supplementation. Heavy metals, including lead, tend to bioaccumulate in liver and kidney tissues and might be expected to compromise function. When the majority of renal function has been lost, gout and aberrant phosphorus and calcium metabolism (soft tissue mineralization) may result.

High-protein diets are considered a predisposing cause of hyperuricemia, gout, and nephrosis in herbivorous reptiles. The maintenance of high-humidity rainforest species in dry, overheated, captive conditions may result in chronic dehydration and nephropathy. Various bacteria including gram-negative aerobes, *Listeria*, *Leptospira*, *Streptococcus*, *Mycobacteria*, and *Chlamydia* have been isolated from reptile kidneys, either as primary agents of nephritis or secondary to generalized sepsis.

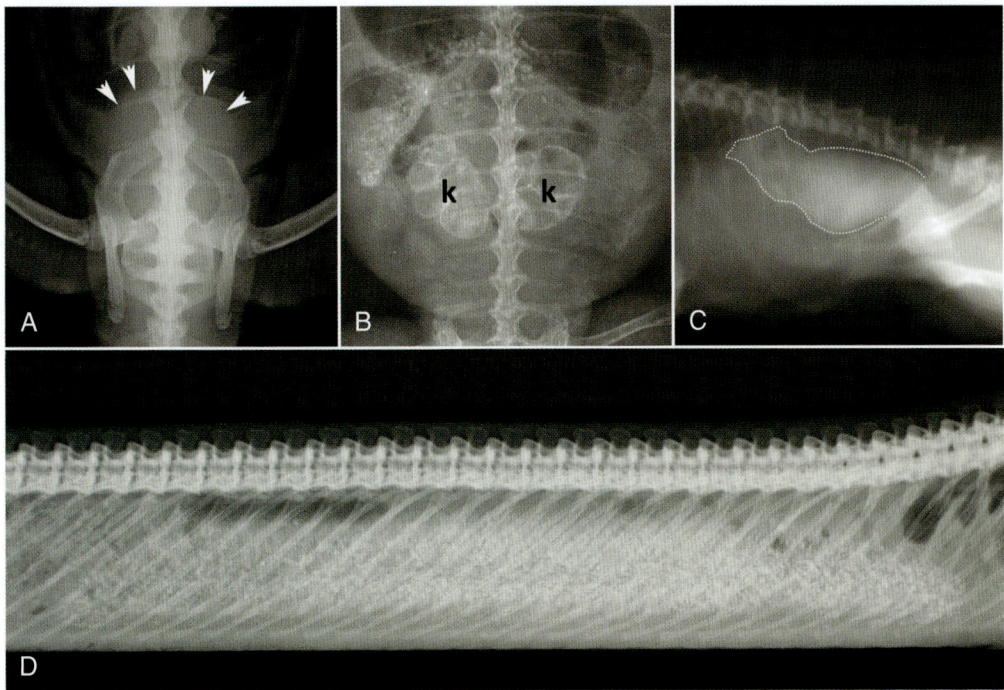

FIG 162.1 (A) Dorsoventral radiograph of the caudal coelom of a green iguana (*Iguana iguana*) demonstrating protrusion of the renal silhouettes (*arrows*) cranial to the pelvic rim, suggestive of renal enlargement. (B) Dorsoventral radiograph of the caudal coelom of a spiny-tailed lizard (*Uromastyx aegyptius*) demonstrating mineralization of both kidneys (*k*). (C) Lateral radiograph (excretory urogram) of a Chinese water dragon (*Physignathus cocincinus*) demonstrating an irregular and enlarged kidney (*dotted line*) following intravenous iohexol administration. (D) Lateral radiograph of a boa constrictor (*Boa constrictor* spp.) with renal gout demonstrating a characteristic starburst pattern along the length of the kidney due to dilation and impaction of the renal tubules. (Courtesy of Stephen J. Divers.)

Renal geotrichosis, phaeohyphomycosis, cryptococcosis, coccidioidomycosis, and candidiasis have also been identified in select individuals with renal pathology. *Entamoeba invadens*, *Hexamita parva*, *Myxidium*, *Klossiella*, and *Caryospora* are documented protozoan causes of nephritis and renal necrosis, whereas *Spirorchis* nematodes have been reported from aquatic chelonians and filarial nematodes from lizards. Herpesviruses, adenoviruses, arenaviruses, and iridoviruses have been associated with inflammatory and/or necrotic renal lesions.

CLINICAL PRESENTATION AND DIAGNOSTIC CONFIRMATION

Typically, chronic nephropathy cases present late in the course of disease when the majority of renal function has been lost, and clinical signs typically include anorexia, weight loss, and poor body condition. Plasma biochemistry may reveal abnormalities associated with electrolytes (Na, K, Ca, P), albumin, and nitrogenous waste excretion (uric acid, urea, and ammonia). Hematology is less specific but may indicate leukocytosis. Radiography, ultrasonography, CT, and MRI may reveal abnormalities in terms of shape, size, mineralization, and blood flow (Fig. 162.1). Iohexol excretion studies are possible to measure glomerular filtration rate and hence determine renal function. Renal biopsy (often endoscopic) is ultimately required for definitive diagnosis, although urinalysis, especially sediment evaluation, can provide valuable clinical insight in cases of parasitic, bacterial, or fungal nephritis (Fig. 162.2). In cases of bacterial or fungal nephritis, culture and sensitivity or, when available, MIC testing is indicated.

PREFERRED TREATMENT(S)

Fluid therapy is used routinely and should be tailored to correct any electrolyte imbalances, with serial biochemistry used to evaluate hydration and progress. Hyperuricemia must be controlled to prevent gout, and allopurinol has been shown to be effective. Other treatments that may be indicated include antimicrobials, intestinal phosphate binders, colchicine, enalapril, calcitriol, or other agents used for management of renal conditions in other species. Antimicrobials should be used only when infection has been demonstrated, with drug selection based on culture and sensitivity or, when available, MIC testing. Protein restriction and selective provision of pyrimidines (thymine and cytosine) over purines (guanine and adenosine) may help reduce uric acid production.

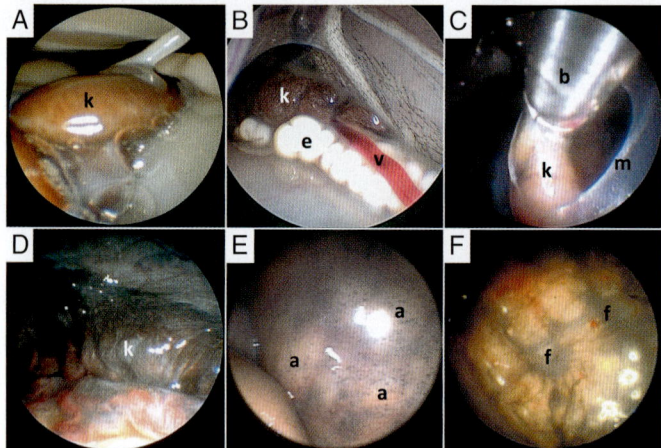

FIG 162.2 Endoscopic views of reptile kidneys using a 2.7 mm telescope. (A) Cranial pole of the left kidney (*k*) of a boa constrictor (*Boa constrictor*). (B) Cranial pole of the right kidney (*k*), right epididymis (*e*), and right renal vein (*v*) of a green iguana (*Iguana iguana*). (C) Biopsy of the left kidney (*k*) of a freshwater turtle (*Trachemys scripta*) using 1.7 mm biopsy forceps (*b*), introduced through an incision in the coelomic membrane (*m*). (D) Enlarged kidney (*k*) protruding into the coelom of a leopard tortoise (*Stigmochelys pardalis*). (E) Kidney of a male red-eared slider (*Trachemys scripta elegans*) exhibiting areas of pallor (*a*) that were confirmed as microabscesses after biopsy. (F) Kidney of a female Greek tortoise (*Testudo graeca*) exhibiting fibrous bands (*f*) across the surface. Biopsy confirmed tubulonephrosis with fibrosis. (Courtesy of Stephen J. Divers.)

PROGNOSIS AND PREVENTION

Prognosis depends on the degree of renal function remaining and the extent of the pathologic change but is generally poor with chronic conditions. Prevention usually centers on good husbandry, including suitable thermal environment, appropriate humidity/temperature, and removal of animal protein from herbivorous diets. (See Chapter 66 for more details and references.)

163

Salmonellosis

Janos Gal and Cathy A. Johnson-Delaney

DEFINITION

Salmonella is a genus of rod-shaped, gram-negative, facultative anaerobic bacteria. They are considered to be a component of the indigenous microflora of reptiles and amphibians, and disease may only manifest after immunosuppressive effects of malnutrition, diet and husbandry errors, stress, concurrent disease, etc.[1-3]

CLINICAL SIGNIFICANCE AND KNOWN ETIOLOGICAL CAUSE(S)

Salmonellae are often found within the gastrointestinal tract of reptiles, spread via the fecal-oral route, and rarely cause disease. Surveys of wild reptiles have shown an incidence of 2.2% to 41% of various *Salmonella* serotypes.[4-6] One zoo population had a 45% infection rate.[7] Although infection and excretion is common, disease is rare, but the zoonotic implications are important.[1,2,8,9] Human salmonellosis often presents with gastrointestinal signs, including acute diarrhea, vomiting, fever, abdominal pain, dehydration, etc.[2] There are known cases in Europe, but overall the numbers appear lower than reported in the United States (see Chapter 174).[9]

CLINICAL PRESENTATION AND DIAGNOSTIC CONFIRMATION

Salmonellae in reptiles usually cause asymptomatic gastrointestinal infections with a lifelong carrier state and intermittent shedding.[1-3,5,7] Onset of clinical disease may be due to predisposing factors such as improper husbandry, transit stress, malnutrition, and concurrent disease. A selected list of serotypes linked with illness in reptiles is listed in

Table 163.1. A wide variety of clinical signs and disease processes may be seen, including anorexia, lethargy, paresis, cachexia, dyspnea, coelomitis, abscesses/granulomas, dermatitis, hypovolemic shock, and death.[3,4,6-8,10-12] Lesions may include necrotic dermatitis; inflammatory, necrotic foci in parenchymal organs; edema in the intestinal submucosa; inflammatory cellular infiltration of the lung; ulcerative enteritis with pseudomembrane formation; spinal osteomyelitis with necrotic lesions; chronic oophoritis; and follicular degeneration (Fig. 163.1), hemorrhages, and pericardial exudates.[3,6,8,10,12] *Salmonella enterica* subsp. *arizonae* serotype 56:Z4,Z23 shows high tropism for bone tissue in different species of reptiles, causing subacute, chronic, progressive, spinal osteomyelitis.[10-12] Due to spinal malformations, affected reptiles have abnormal locomotion.[10,12] Culturing requires selective agar and enrichment.[13] Enzyme-linked immunosorbent assays may have higher sensitivity than cultures. Polymerase chain reaction testing has higher sensitivity and specificity than cultures.[3] Serotyping and pulsed-field

TABLE 163.1 Selected *Salmonella* Serovars Implicated in Reptilian Illness

S. agioboo	S. anatum	S. enterica subsp. arizonae	S. carrau
S. chameleon	S. durham	S. enterica subsp. derby	S. enterica subsp. diarizonae
S. infantis	S. krefeld	S. montivideo	S. muenchen
S. oslo	S. pomona	S. thompson	S. typhimurium
S. saint-paul	S. subgenus II	S. subgenus IV	S. uzaramo

Data from references 3–7 and 9–14.

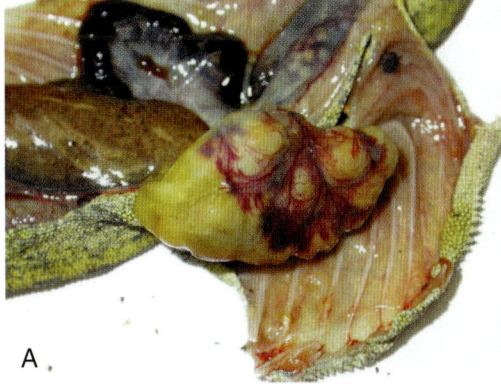
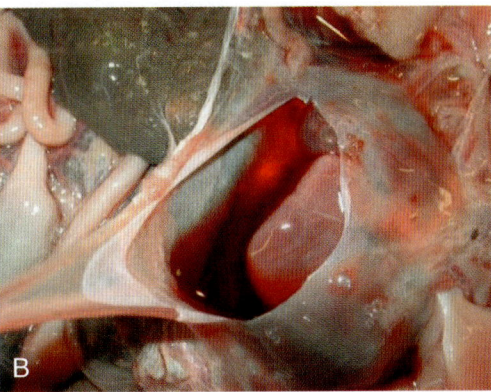

FIG 163.1 Reptile salmonellosis. (A) Follicular degeneration and oophoritis in a Senegal shameleon (*Chamaeleo senegalensis*). (B) Inflammatory-necrotic foci in the liver and pericardial fluid accumulation in a mata mata turtle (*Chelus fimbriatus*).

gel electrophoresis (PFGE) subtyping of *Salmonella* isolates should be performed. In addition to culture, it is important to demonstrate a host pathological response by cytology or histopathology to differentiate between commensal and disease-requiring treatment situations.[12,13] It is not recommended to "test" or "culture" a clinically healthy reptile to attempt to declare it "salmonella free" because of the high likelihood of false negatives due to intermittent shedding.[1,2]

PREFERRED TREATMENT(S)

Attempts to treat reptiles with antibiotics to eliminate *Salmonella* spp. from their intestinal tract have not proven to be effective and cannot be recommended. In clinically asymptomatic animals, antibiotic treatment is contraindicated because it increases the risk of antimicrobial-resistant *Salmonella* strains, which, if transmitted to humans, would complicate their treatment. Attempts to raise "salmonella-free" reptiles have been equally unsuccessful.[1,2]

Supportive care includes fluid therapy, supplemental feeding, and correcting any husbandry deficiencies.[3] In cases of confirmed osteo-myelitis, treatment includes antimicrobial agents selected on *in vitro* sensitivity testing, along with antiinflammatory and analgesic drugs. Surgical debridement and/or amputation/removal of the infected and necrotic bone is indicated where possible. The prognosis depends on the stage and location of the osteomyelitis. Advanced cases or those involving the spine carry a poor prognosis.[14]

PROGNOSIS AND PREVENTION

Appropriate management, stocking densities, and hygiene are helpful. Clinicians must educate owners on the likely prevalence of *Salmonella* in healthy reptiles and amphibians, and how to safely work with them. Updated safety guidelines are available from the Association of Reptilian and Amphibian Veterinarians (ARAV) at their website (arav.org/salmonella-bacteria-reptiles).

REFERENCES

See www.expertconsult.com for a complete list of references.

164

Shell Abnormalities

Jean Meyer and Paolo Selleri

DEFINITION

Shell damage or disease causes disruption of the integrity of the keratin scutes and/or the bony shell.

CLINICAL SIGNIFICANCE AND KNOWN ETIOLOGICAL CAUSE(S)

Infection, trauma (burns, falls, dog or predator bites, car accidents, boat strikes, lawn mowers, crush injuries, persistent courtship/rival behaviors), or neoplasia (e.g., squamous cell carcinoma) lead to cell destruction and/or devitalization with subsequent loss of the epidermal scutes, ulceration, abscess formation, necrosis, and osteolysis (Fig. 164.1A and B). Infections are commonly bacterial (e.g., *Citrobacter freundii*, *Beneckea chitinovora*, *Aeromonas hydrophila*, *Mycobacterium kansasii*, *Clostridium* sp.) and/or fungal (e.g. *Mucor* spp., *Purpureocillium* (*Paecilomyces*) *lilacinus*, *Aphanomyces sinensis*, *Fusarium semitectum*, *Exophiala oligosperma*). Many fungal species may be cultivated from shell lesions but can reflect secondary infection. Viral shell disease is less common but can be associated with herpesviruses (fibropapillomatosis) (primary lesions) and picornaviruses (secondary osteodystrophy). Nutritional or renal secondary hyperparathyroidism may lead to an osteodystrophic softening of the shell.

CLINICAL PRESENTATION AND DIAGNOSTIC CONFIRMATION

Precontrast and postcontrast CT is preferred for evaluating complex fractures or shell disease, although three-view radiography may reveal fracture lines and sequestra (see Chapter 70). Full-thickness shell biopsies should be submitted for histopathology and microbiology and are most reliable. Gram and cytologically stained smears from swabs or tissue impressions may indicate bacterial, fungal, or neoplastic involvement. Aerobic and anaerobic bacterial and fungal cultures from deep swabs or tissue biopsies should be routinely performed. Mycobacterial cultures or PCR should be considered if acid-fast organisms are seen. Antimicrobial selection should be based upon sensitivity testing, with a focus on drugs with known pharmacokinetics.

PREFERRED TREATMENT(S)

Traumatized chelonians should be stabilized with regard to analgesia, supportive fluid therapy, hemostasis, and soft tissue wound care. Eviscerations should be evaluated and replaced after thorough flushing with sterile saline. Surgical stabilization of the fractures should be performed under general anesthesia, after any infection has been resolved. Open wounds necessitate frequent dressing changes every 1 to 3 days. Ulcerated and infected wounds should be initially flushed using antiseptic solutions and sterile saline. Debridement should be performed under sedation with local anesthesia or general anesthesia. Repeated/daily lavage and wet to dry bandages may be required for continued debridement, which can be followed by wound products (e.g., Pronto Vet Gel, Braun, Medical AG, Sempach, Switzerland) and bandaging to promote granulation and healing (Fig. 164.2A and B). Topical antiseptic and antimicrobial products should also be considered.

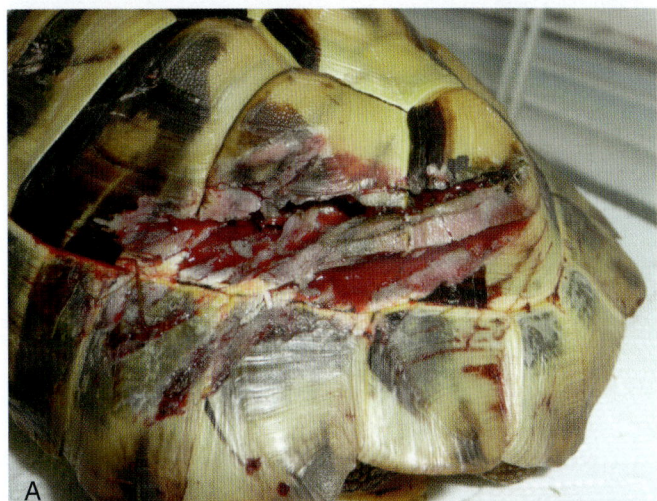

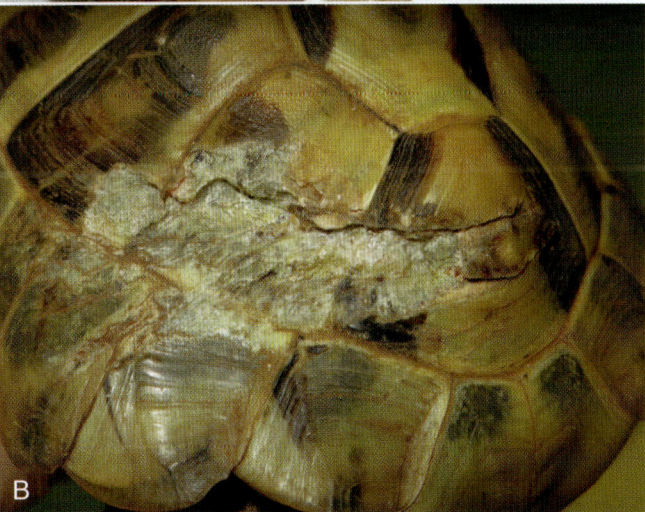

FIG 164.1 Lawn mower injury penetrating the coelomic cavity. (A) Open wound treatment led to sealing of the defect by metaplastic calcification within 5 months (B).

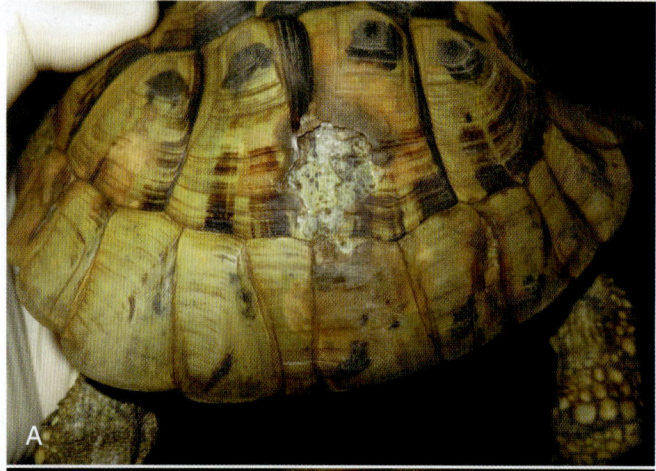

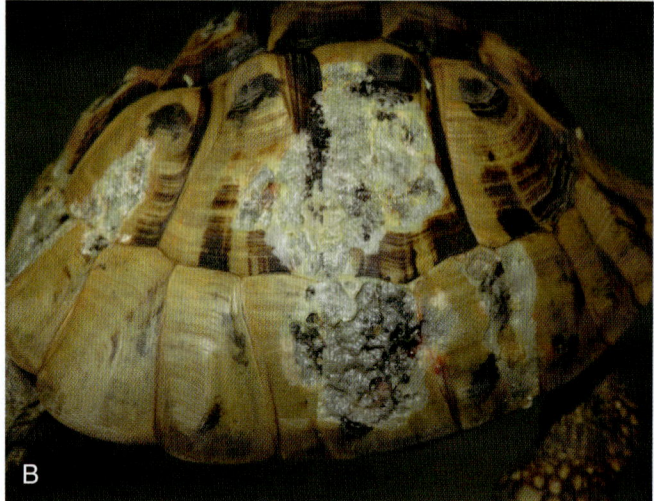

FIG 164.2 Dyskeratosis on the carapace of a Hermann's torotise *(Testudo hermanni)* before (A) and after (B) debridement. Bacterial and fungal infection lead to extensive keratolysis and osteolysis. Defects are sealed with ossified and keratinized granulation tissue.

Vacuum-assisted wound closure with silver impregnated bandaging materials is indicated for extensive lesions. Antimicrobial therapy should be based upon culture and sensitivity testing (see Chapters 70 and 113).

Serious burns require fluid therapy, analgesia, nutritional support, and strict asepsis. Surgical debridement and wound dressing may be required. With the exception of severe burns or integumental loss, antimicrobials should only be used when infection has been confirmed, and narrow spectrum agents effective against the cultured pathogen(s) are preferred. Only where there is significant loss to the integument or severe burns predisposed to infection is the use of broad-spectrum antimicrobials indicated (e.g., 1st- and 2nd-generation cepahlosporins, potentiated sulphonamides, tetracyclines). Metronidazole should be included if anaerobes are present or suspected. Secondary mycotic overgrowth of exposed bone surfaces is effectively treated with local antifungals (e.g., Terbinafine).

PROGNOSIS AND PREVENTION

The prognosis is generally favorable, but complications may result from overlooked visceral trauma, generalized coelomitis/sepsis, or secondary organ failure. Traumatic injuries can often be prevented by taking appropriate precautions (e.g., checking grass before mowing; no unsupervised contact between chelonians and other animals, including children). Appropriate quarantine and housing are required to reduce the incidence of infectious disease and intraspecific trauma.

See Chapter 70 for more details, including references.

165

Snake Cryptosporidiosis

Rodney W. Schnellbacher

DEFINITION

Cryptosporidiosis is caused by coccidian protozoa of the apicomplexan genus. *Cryptosporidium serpentis* infections have been reported in at least 40 species of captive and wild snakes.[1] Although many species are affected, Viperidae (especially rattlesnakes) and amelanotic colubrid snakes appear to be particularly susceptible. *Cryptosporidium varanii* (syn. *C. saurophilum*) has also been identified in a few species of snakes; however, no adverse clinical signs were identified.

CLINICAL SIGNIFICANCE AND KNOWN ETIOLOGICAL CAUSE(S)

Cryptosporidiosis in snakes is a devastating disease that can lead to the loss of valuable animals in a collection. With no effective treatment, it usually results in morbidity and eventually euthanasia. Cryptosporidiosis in snakes is usually characterized by chronic clinical or subclinical infections, leading to primary hypertrophic gastritis. Enteritis, with or without gastritis, as well as a few cases of biliary involvement have also been observed. *Cryptosporidum* spp. is transmitted through the fecal-oral route, by direct contact, or through contaminated fomites. It does not appear to be zoonotic. There is no evidence of infection in snakes from ingestion of avian/mammalian prey infected with *Cryptosporidium.*[2] However, nonreptilian oocytes can be ingested, passed through in stool, and remain infective for mammals and avian species.

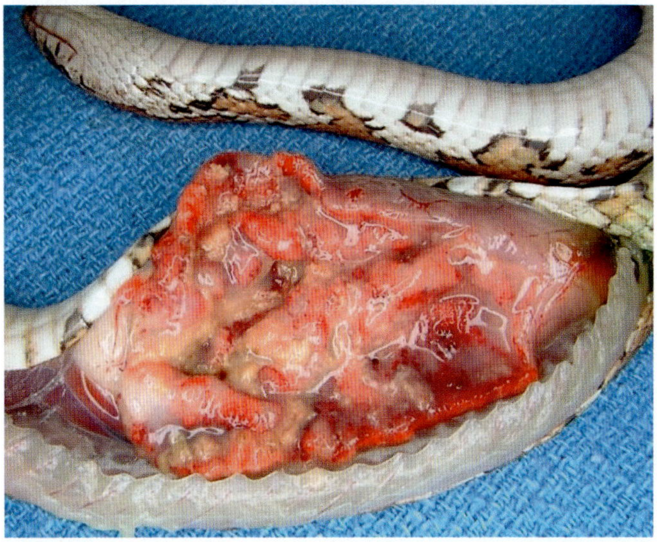

CLINICAL PRESENTATION AND DIAGNOSTIC CONFIRMATION

Clinical signs of cryptosporidiosis are related to gastrointestinal inflammation and hyperplasia (Fig. 165.1). Signs consist of anorexia, weight loss, postprandial vomiting (usually 3–4 days after prey ingestion), lethargy, and midbody swelling of gastric region (Fig. 165.2). Clinically affected snakes may live for days to years. Most snakes that test positive are subclinical, showing no outward signs, and are intermittent fecal shedders, oscillating between no or high levels of oocyte shedding. Differential diagnoses for vomiting and midbody swelling include suboptimal temperatures, inappropriate prey size, stress, obstruction, hibernation-associated necrotizing gastroenteritis, parasitism from other protozoa and nematodes, neoplasia, and infectious gastroenteritis (bacterial, fungal, and viral). Diagnosis can be challenging and is based on clinical signs, physical examination, oocyte analysis, histopathology, and molecular testing. Severely affected snakes often have a firm, thickened, palpable stomach. Ultrasonography or contrast gastric radiography can show gastric mucosal thickening and a delay in gastric emptying (Fig. 165.3). Endoscopically, the stomach rugae can be grossly enlarged, inflamed, or thickened. Diagnosis via oocyte testing can be variable due to intermittent shedding. *Cryptosporidium* sp. oocysts, 4 to 8 μm long, can be detected

FIG 165.1 Gross necropsy of an eastern milk snake (*Lampropeltis Triangulum*) performed after humane euthanasia showing gastric hyperplasia and hyperemia with thickened rugal folds. Histopathology confirmed cryptosporidiosis. (Courtesy of Scott J. Stahl, Stahl Exotic Animal Veterinary Services.)

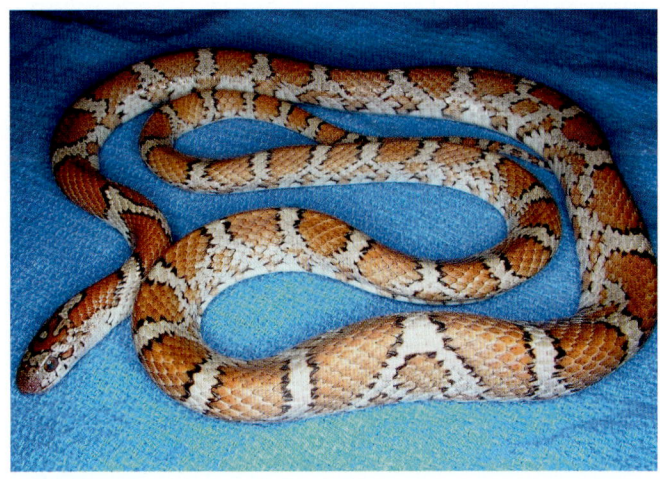

FIG 165.2 The same eastern milk snake (*Lampropeltis triangulum*) as in Fig. 165.1 at presentation with a history of chronic regurgitation, notable weight loss, and midbody swelling evident. (Courtesy of Scott J. Stahl, Stahl Exotic Animal Veterinary Services.)

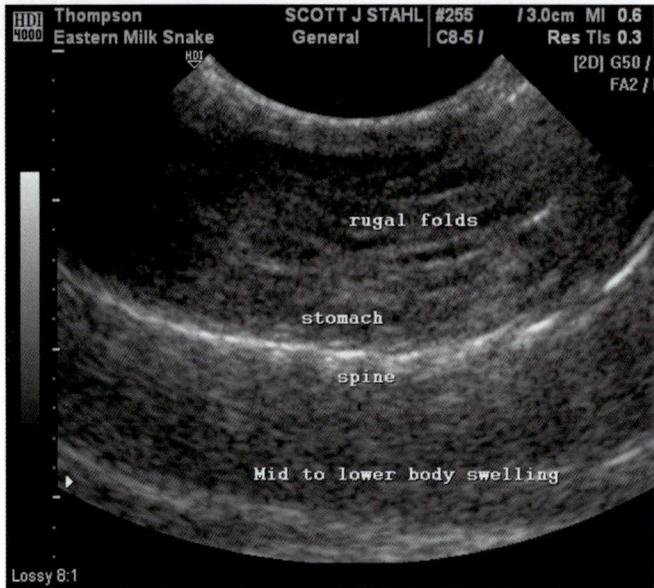

FIG 165.3 Ultrasound image of the same milk snake (*Lampropeltis triangulum*) identifying the midbody swelling as the stomach (located above the spine in the scan; the wording below the spine is a label of the scan itself) with thickened gastric rugal folds, characteristic for cryptosporidiosis in snakes. (Courtesy of Scott J. Stahl, Stahl Exotic Animal Veterinary Services.)

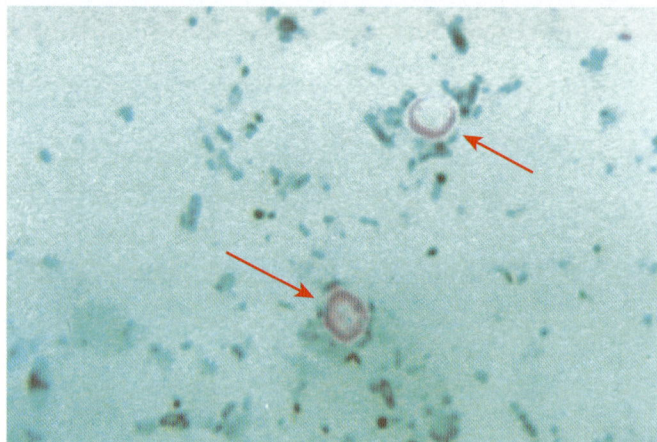

FIG 165.4 *Cryptosporidium serpentis* stained with a modified acid-fast stain (arrows) in a direct wet smear prepared from fecal specimens of a subclinically infected corn snake (*Pantherophis guttatus*). The mean size of *Cryptosporidium serpentis* oocysts is 6.3 × 5.5 μm.

on light microscopy in unstained feces, mucus, or gastric lavage samples, and if detected must be differentiated from mammalian or avian prey *Cryptosporidium* spp. (Fig. 165.4). Sensitivity of fecal testing increases with serial testing, centrifugation concentration techniques, and the use of acid-fast, immunofluorescent staining and PCR (for differentiating mammalian/avian *Cryptosporidium* spp). Gastric lavage (20 mL/kg) is more useful than mucous or feces. Samples are best collected 3 days after feeding. The increased gastric metabolism after feeding is thought to increase *Cryptosporidium* metabolism. Gastric biopsy and histology are the only definitive diagnostic tests (see Chapter 32 for more details).

PREFERRED TREATMENT(S)

Cryptosporidiosis is difficult to treat successfully. Infected and shedding animals should be placed in permanent quarantine or humanely euthanized. Supportive care, including small meals via gavage tube, improvement in environmental conditions, and a reduction of predisposing stressors, may improve health conditions in some individuals. However, animals may become chronic shedders and carriers, with the potential to infect other snakes, and thus should not remain within a collection. Some pharmacological anticoccidial drugs have been shown to reduce the number of organisms or fecal shedding but are ineffective in eliminating all stages of infection; however, treatment with paromo-

mycin was successful in one study in bearded dragons (*Pogona vitticeps*).[3] Hyperimmune bovine colostrum has shown to be efficacious in the treatment of *Cryptosporidium* sp. in a few snakes but is commercially unavailable (see Chapter 32 for more details).[4]

PROGNOSIS AND PREVENTION

Cryptosporidiosis is difficult to manage, and prevention is accomplished through strict hygiene, quarantine, isolation, and diagnostic screening to prevent the introduction of positive snakes into a collection. Reptiles should not be euthanized based on the presence of *Cryptosporidium* in fecal or gastric samples without confirmation of actual disease by biopsy and histopathology. *Cryptosporidium* oocytes are very stable in the environment and may remain infective for 2 to 6 months. Cleanliness and removal of organic matter should be emphasized. Disinfection using 5% ammonia, 10% formalin, or hydrogen peroxide–based products is effective in eliminating oocyst infectivity after 18 hours of contact at 4°C. Exposure to moist heat between 45° and 60°C for 5 to 9 minutes is also effective. Cryptosporidiosis has a poor prognosis and is usually fatal. If supportive therapy is initiated, the animal's quality of life should be considered. Without clinical improvement and/or an unwillingness to eventually eat on its own, euthanasia may be necessary.

REFERENCES

See www.expertconsult.com for a complete list of references.

166

Spinal Osteopathy

Kevin T. Fitzgerald and S. Emi Knafo

DEFINITION

Proliferative spinal osteopathy (PSO) has been described in turtles, lizards, and snakes.[1] Most commonly reported in snakes, these proliferative and progressive spinal lesions have been shown to be associated with chronic bacterial infections. Most frequently, *Salmonella* ssp. are implicated.[2,3] The lesions of spinal osteopathy in reptiles have been compared with osteitis deformans (Paget's disease) in humans.[4] This disease is a localized disorder initially marked by excessive bone resorption followed by deformity and then by excessive bone formation. Affected animals can be dramatically debilitated. See Chapter 81 for more detailed discussion of PSO.

CLINICAL SIGNIFICANCE AND KNOWN ETIOLOGICAL CAUSE(S)

Osteoarthritis is defined as a disorder of moveable joints characterized by deterioration of articular cartilage, osteophyte formation, bone remodeling, and low-grade nonpurulent inflammation.[5] Osteoarthritis can be inflammatory or noninflammatory, caused by trauma, dietary deficiency (hypovitaminosis D, hypervitaminosis A), unknown viral infection, prolonged inactivity due to cage confinement, slow-developing neoplasia, and association with bacterial infection and septicemia. Speculation exists that the spinal lesions may be caused by an immune-mediated reaction from septicemia and triggered by bacterial endotoxins. An association between spinal disease and previous soft tissue bacterial infections has been suggested in various reptiles. *Salmonella*, a bacteria frequently cultured from the gastrointestinal tract of reptiles, but nonpathogenic to the host, has been implicated in vertebral osteomyelitis in snakes.[2,3]

CLINICAL PRESENTATION AND DIAGNOSTIC CONFIRMATION

Clinical signs of PSO in reptiles may vary in severity and location of lesions. Animals with vertebral lesions can show limited movement or no movement at all in affected areas. The affected vertebral regions can be remarkably extensive, sometimes as much as 30 cm (12 in) long. Clinical signs can include vertebral column stiffness and resultant decreased mobility, kyphosis, scoliosis, and occasionally pathologic fractures.

On examination, focal nodular swellings may be visible along the dorsum or bulges on the sides of the body (Fig. 166.1A). Palpation of the spine may reveal variably sized segments of ankylosis, kyphosis, scoliosis, or lordosis. Hyperreflexia or upper motor neuron signs are often seen cranial to the spinal lesion. Caudal to the affected area motor deficits in the somatic musculature, as well as slight or dramatic torsion of the body, may be noted. Additionally torticollis, trembling, and subtle or acute spinal kinking may be exhibited.

Eventually, affected animals cannot move, strike, or swallow prey. If severe luxation and rotation of vertebrae are present, animals may display bizarre corkscrew postures. Affected lizards may show proprioceptive

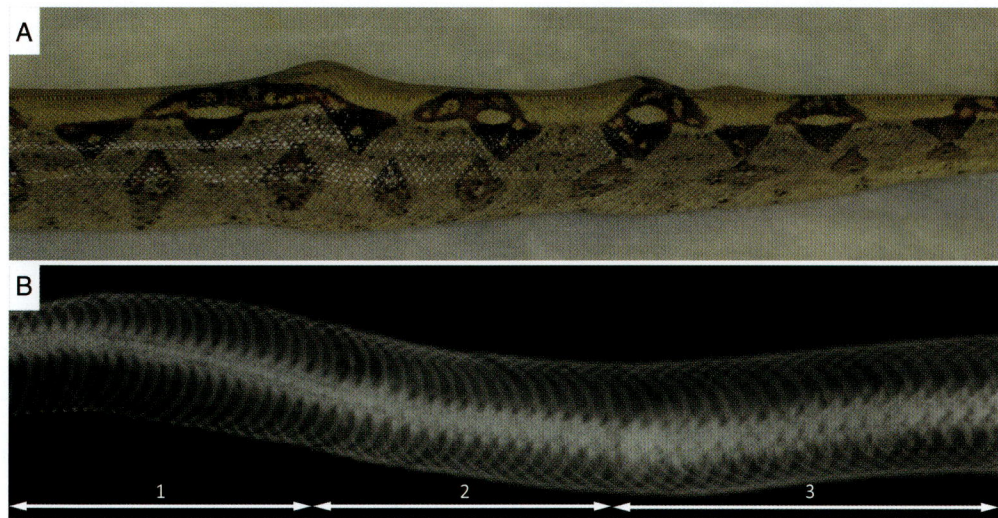

FIG 166.1 Spinal osteopathy in a boa constrictor *(Boa constrictor)*. (A) Clinical presentation demonstrating deformity and swellings associated with the spine. (B) Dorsoventral radiograph of the spine demonstrating normal (1), mildly (2), and severely (2) affected regions. (Courtesy of Stephen J. Divers.)

deficits, severely distorted postures, and partial to total paresis depending on the size and location of the lesion. It is interesting to observe that even severely debilitated animals may continue to eat and drink.

Successful diagnosis of PSO depends on clinical history, physical examination, radiology/CT, bone or blood culture, histopathology, and findings at necropsy. Histopathology is closest to a gold standard for confirming PSO, but it is not always practical or possible. Radiographically, changes associated with PSO typically show evidence of segmented fusion of adjacent affected vertebra (Fig. 166.1B). Vertebrae can be fused dorsally, ventrally, or laterally by foci of irregular proliferative bone, sclerosis of vertebral end plates, and with varying degrees of lysis of vertebral bodies often noted. In advanced stages, periarticular bony proliferation may involve dorsolateral articular facets and costovertebral joints, often resulting in bridging of joint spaces (osseous metaplasia), and ankylosis (Fig. 166.2). Pathologic fractures may be noted and are

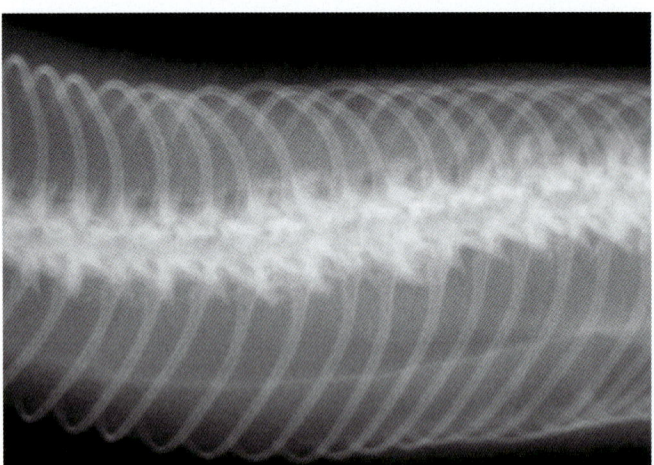

FIG 166.2 Snakes with spinal osteopathy have evidence of segmented fusion of adjacent vertebrae by foci of irregular proliferative bone. Early on, sclerosis is seen on vertebral end plates with or without lysis of the vertebrae. In advanced stages, periarticular bony proliferation involves the dorsolateral articular facets and costovertebral joints. Eventually, osseous metaplasia may bridge adjoining vertebrae (ankylosis). (Courtesy of Douglas R. Mader.)

often associated with proliferative reactive bone exostoses. Radiographs are useful to confirm the presence and severity of spinal disease but cannot identify infection or inflammation. Advanced diagnostics such as nuclear (bone scan) imaging may help identify the site of active disease. Bacterial culture of bone biopsies can be helpful; however, evidence exists that bony lesions of spinal osteopathy may not develop until 22 to 26 months after the initial episode of local infection or septicemia.[6] Animals with radiographic evidence of PSO should have a blood culture. Biopsy of bone in living reptiles is possible, though heavy epaxial muscles over vertebrae make access a challenge. Antemortem rib and vertebral biopsy carries a potential risk of iatrogenic fracture.

PREFERRED TREATMENT(S)

Early diagnosis is essential for successful therapy. Effective treatment can include appropriate antibiotic selection, surgical debridement of granulomatous or lytic areas, use of antiinflammatory medications, and separation of affected and unaffected individuals. Parenteral administration of medication may need to be continued for extended periods. Carprofen and meloxicam have been recommended; although clinical efficacy is difficult to assess. Recently a case report documented establishment of a vascular access port in an iguana for administration of a chemotherapy agent.[7] This may be a reasonable method to deliver therapeutic levels of antibiotics and other drugs in affected reptiles needing long-term therapy.

PROGNOSIS AND PREVENTION

At present, prognosis for reptiles with PSO is poor to grave. Most animals display advanced lesions at the time of presentation. Radiography and CT can be useful to determine severity and monitor progression. Early recognition of this process through implementation of a thorough diagnostic investigation, aggressive long-term antibiotic and analgesic therapy, and/or surgical debridement are the most potentially effective therapies at this time.

REFERENCES

See www.expertconsult.com for a complete list of references.

167

Stomatitis

Ryan De Voe

DEFINITION

Stomatitis is characterized by inflammation and typically infection of the tissues of the oral cavity. Infections can extend from the oral cavity and may result in cellulitis, sinusitis/rhinitis, osteomyelitis, and with aspiration of infectious agents into the lower respiratory tract (pneumonia). More details can be found in Chapter 73.

CLINICAL SIGNIFICANCE AND KNOWN ETIOLOGICAL CAUSE(S)

Although a number of pathogens appear capable of causing primary infections, stomatitis usually occurs secondary to presumed predispositions, such as immunosuppression, poor husbandry conditions, malnutrition, or trauma. Stomatitis is often a sign of systemic disease. Damage to the rostral tissues caused by rubbing on or crashing into barriers, as well as bites from prey items in snakes and carnivorous lizards, can result in stomatitis. Trauma may cause disfigurement, resulting in exposure of the gingiva and associated stomatitis due to desiccation and devitalization of mucous membranes. Lizards with acrodont dentition are susceptible to periodontal disease because of the vulnerable nature of their periodontal tissue. Once this tissue is damaged, invasion of bone from opportunistic organisms (bacterial, fungal) often results and may progress to osteomyelitis (see Chapter 159).[1] Squamous metaplasia of oral mucosa and glandular epithelium due to hypovitaminosis A can create a suitable environment for secondary infections. Nutritional secondary hyperparathyroidism with deformity of the lip margins can cause chronic exposure of the gingiva and stomatitis. The infectious component of stomatitis is caused by a variety of opportunistic bacterial and/or fungal isolates. These bacteria and fungi are often part of the animal's normal oral flora or ubiquitous in the environment. Primarily gram-negative bacteria but also gram-positive and/or anaerobic isolates can cause clinically significant infections. Mycobacterial and mycotic organisms have also occasionally been associated with stomatitis.

Parasitic disease may also result in clinical stomatitis. Nematodes that typically occupy the lower gastrointestinal tract or nasal cavity can occasionally be identified in the oral cavity and may result in pathology.[2] Spirorchid nematodes and their eggs can embolize in small vessels, causing ischemia of oral structures. A number of fluke (monogentic and digentic trematode) species parasitize the oral cavity of various reptile species and can cause or exacerbate existing stomatitis, though usually the presence of these parasites is of little clinical concern to the host.

Certain viral pathogens have a tropism for the oral mucosa and will cause a primary stomatitis. Herpesviruses are well-known causes of stomatitis in chelonians and other reptile taxa.[3-5] Ranavirus infections can also cause stomatitis that can be grossly indistinguishable from herpesvirus infections in some species. Recently nidovirus was found to be associated with stomatitis/pharyngitis in ball pythons (*Python regius*).[6]

CLINICAL PRESENTATION AND DIAGNOSTIC CONFIRMATION

Investigation of reptile stomatitis should focus on defining the pathology in the oral cavity, evaluating overall health, and identifying a predisposing factor or etiology.

Clinical signs may consist of perioral or intraoral swelling/abscessation, pytalism/discharge, disruption of the lip margins, the inability to close the mouth properly, mucosal hyperemia, petechiation and ulceration, mucosal plaques, and dysfunction of the tongue, larynx, and associated structures (Figs. 167.1 and 167.2). Occasionally even with oral pathology there may be no visible abnormalities noted with the mouth closed; therefore, a thorough oral examination is always indicated. Examination of the tongue, especially in snakes, varanid lizards, and chameleons is important to identify glossitis, lingual necrosis, and abscessation of the tongue sheath. Endoscopic evaluation of the oral cavity facilitates access to oral structures and provides magnification. Collection of material from lesions via swabs and scrapes for cytology, culture and sensitivity, virus isolation, and molecular diagnostics should be considered. Radiography or CT is often indicated to identify periodontal disease and osteolysis. Biopsies for histopathology are useful, especially in cases that do not respond as expected to therapy. A minimum database consisting of at minimum a complete blood cell count, differential cell count, and a plasma chemistry panel is recommended in all cases of

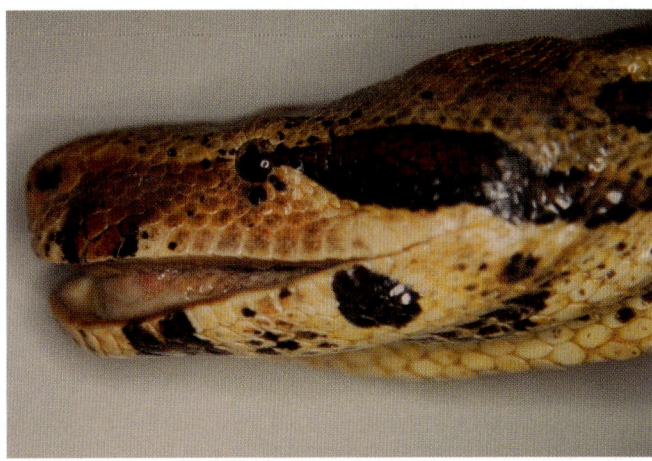

FIG 167.1 Labial deformity in a boa constrictor (*Boa constrictor*), which can result in chronic exposure and damage to gingiva, predisposing to stomatitis. (Courtesy of Stephen J. Divers.)

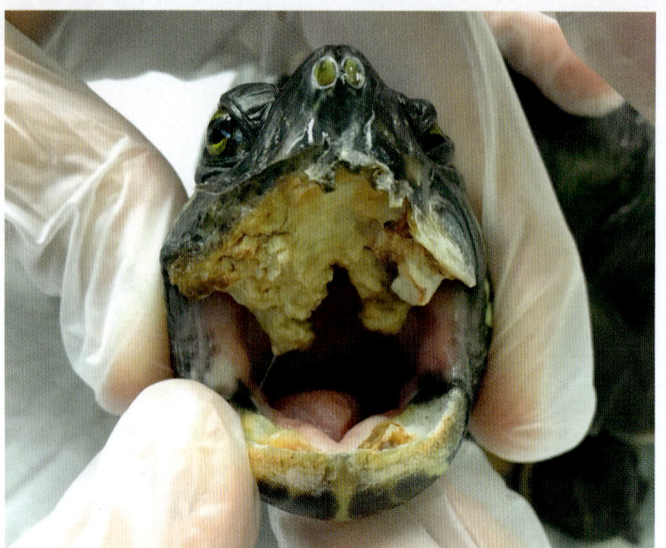

FIG 167.2 Severe, diffuse caseous bacterial stomatitis in a yellow-bellied slider (*Trachemys scripta scripta*). (Courtesy of Scott J. Stahl, Stahl Exotic Animal Veterinary Services.)

stomatitis to help provide insight into the overall condition and health of the animal.

PREFERRED TREATMENT(S)

Animals that are being treated for stomatitis should be kept in optimized husbandry conditions. Appropriate thermal and humidity gradients within their habitat, comfortable hide areas, and adequate lighting are all important in supporting a convalescing reptile (see Section 3 and Chapter 46). Many reptiles with stomatitis will be anorexic or hypophagic

when presented. Gavage feeding, or placement of an esophagostomy tube, may be necessary to bypass a diseased and potentially painful oral cavity (see Chapter 45). Debridement of diseased tissue is required in many cases. Loose teeth that can be removed with little effort should be extracted. Necrotic bone should be debrided. Deep tracts should be marsupialized to facilitate local therapy if there is any question regarding residual diseased tissue following debridement. Systemic therapy with antimicrobial and nonsteroidal antiinflammatory agents may be indicated. Initial antimicrobial therapy should be based on cytology and gram stains and modified by culture/sensitivity results. Local antimicrobial therapy is also usually part of a successful treatment regimen. Cleansing and flushing of affected areas with disinfectants such as dilute chlorhexidine and tris-EDTA solutions can be used effectively. Silver sulfadiazine cream is a commonly used topical therapeutic and has the benefit of being water soluble. When cavities or fistulas are present, sugar or unpasteurized medicinal honey can be effective topically.

PROGNOSIS AND PREVENTION

Prognosis is dependent on cause and severity and can range from good to poor. Mycobacterial or viral etiologies or cases involving bone with associated osteomyelitis have a more guarded prognosis. Prevention of stomatitis in captive reptiles centers on the provision of adequate husbandry, diet, and biosecurity. In cases where there is chronic exposure of gingival tissue, maintenance therapy is often indicated. Periodic cleansing with the aforementioned disinfectants, application of various veterinary oral products such as vitamin C–containing oral cleansing gels, and application of beeswax, petroleum jelly, or other products to protect exposed tissue can be used effectively in maintenance therapy.

REFERENCES

See www.expertconsult.com for a complete list of references.

168

Tail Abnormalities

Richard S. Funk, Robert Johnson, and Stephen J. Divers

DEFINITION

Tail damage results from a variety of causes, including mechanical, traumatic, infectious, and physiological etiologies.

CLINICAL SIGNIFICANCE AND KNOWN ETIOLOGICAL CAUSE(S)

A reptile's tail is a caudal extension of the vertebral column and often used for social signaling, locomotion (counterbalance, swimming), predator avoidance, and even prey luring. In some lizards fat is stored within the tail. Common causes of tail damage and deformity include trauma, autotomy, infection, or a congenital defect. Tail trauma can be caused by cage-mate aggression, the tail being mistaken for a food item and grabbed during feeding, or deliberate or accidental injury inflicted by a human. Caudal autotomy (tail drop) can occur in many lizard species (but not in chameleons, most agamids, monitors, helodermatids, xenosaurids, and lanthanotids), and tuataras but has also been reported in some snakes and amphisbaenids.[1,2] In some lizards the ability to autotomize and regenerate the tail is lost with maturity (including *Ctenosaura, Cyclura, Iguana, Sauromalus,* and some *Tiliqua*). The clinician must be careful in handling susceptible species so as not to cause iatrogenic tail loss (Fig. 168.1A).

CLINICAL PRESENTATION AND DIAGNOSTIC CONFIRMATION

Ascending vascular necrosis of the tail tip is common in the green iguana (*Iguana iguana*), the bearded dragon (*Pogona vitticeps*), monitors (*Varanidae*), tegus (*Teiidae*), and others. Although multifactorial,

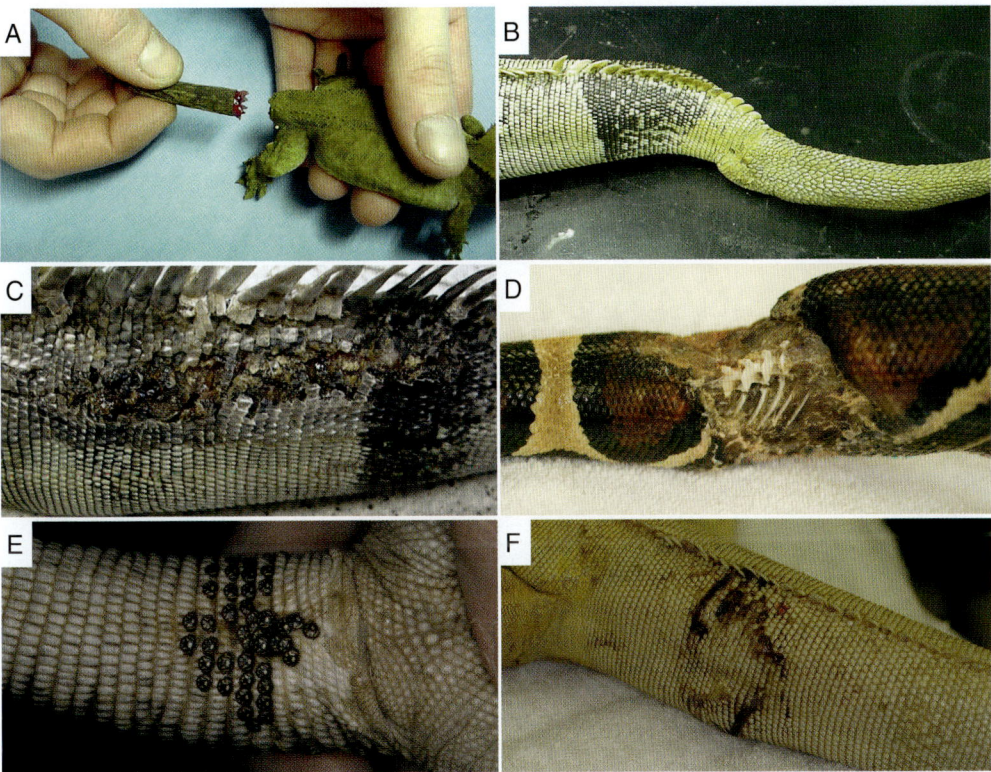

FIG 168.1 (A) Tail autotomy in a *Rhacodactylus* lizard associated with handling. (B) Imperfect tail regeneration in an iguanid lizard. Note the kink at the level of regeneration and the smaller scalation characteristic of regenerated tails in many species. (C) Dorsal tail necrosis and secondary bacterial and fungal infection in a green iguana (*Iguana iguana*) secondary to thermal burn. (D) Rodent-induced tail trauma in a *Boa constrictor*. (E) Ticks feeding along the tail base of a recently imported savannah monitor (*Varanus exanthematicus*). (F) Focal discoloration of the craniolateral tail in an albino green iguana that was associated with osteomyelitis and cellulitis. (Courtesy of Stephen J. Divers.)

a common cause is aggressive or defensive animals slapping their tails against the cage wall or other objects causing injury and necrosis. Vessel calcification, thromboembolism, and reduced peripheral circulation can cause ischemic tail necrosis. A number of different bacteria may be cultured from these necrotic lesions, including *Neisseria iguanae*.[3] Cloacal prolapses and cloacitis may lead to inflammatory lesions on the base of the adjacent tail. Both male and female snakes have paired scent glands located within the base of the tail. These may enlarge as secretions accumulate and may become inspissated or abscessed with a resultant enlargement of the tail base and even ulceration and rupture. The hemipenes of male squamates are located within the tail base, ventral to the scent glands. These may become swollen, impacted, and even abscessed. The condition may be associated with hypovitaminosis A in some species such as geckos and chameleons.[4] Overzealous or improper probing for sex identification, usually in the hands of inexperienced keepers, has been known to cause tail base damage.

Some lizards may develop a forked or deformed tail from an incomplete tail autotomy (see Fig. 168.1B). Tails may also suffer injuries from thermal burns associated with heat lamps and heating pads (see Fig. 168.1C). Occasionally tail skin may be damaged or lost when stuck to tape used in building or decorating an enclosure.

A common cause for tail trauma including tip amputation is trauma from a live rodent bite (see Fig. 168.1D). Damage to the tail skin may result from bacterial or fungal dermatitis/abscesses, contact dermatitis, dysecdysis, ectoparasites (e.g., snake mites, ticks; see Fig. 168.1E), neoplasia, or owner-induced trauma such as forcibly pulling the pet from a refuge or slamming the cage door on the tail. Tail paralysis can be caused by fracture or luxation of one or more caudal vertebrae, a bacterial or protozoal infection that involves the caudal spinal cord, neoplasia, or proliferative ossifying spondylosis or osteomyelitis lesions that usually are bacterial and resistant to resolution (see Fig. 168.1F).

Some terrestrial chelonians (e.g., *Terrapene*), especially juveniles, may lose their tails or tail tips due to retained shed skin when kept in low humidity environments. Wild-caught reptiles commonly exhibit scars or wounds on their tails, presumably from predators or occasionally from prey, other mechanical injuries, or from their human captors.

Iatrogenic tail swelling/infection may result from venipuncture of the caudal (tail) vein. Attention to aseptic technique, proper choice of needle size, limited number of attempts, and mild pressure at the venipuncture site following the procedure should prevent these complications. Tail venipuncture of lizards that can drop their tails should be carefully considered, and sedation/anesthesia may be preferred. Rarely, iatrogenic necrosis of the tail tip may occur after venipuncture.

PREFERRED TREATMENT(S)

Hemipenal plugs can often be removed manually, either by gently grasping and retracting the exposed dried tip, or by a combination of retraction and digital expression with pressure applied in a caudal to cranial direction. Some cases require sedation and sometimes surgical intervention. Many of the conditions discussed previously can be treated with therapeutic agents if indicated; amputation if necessary; surgical removal of abscesses, granulomas, or tumors; or surgical closure of skin defects if possible. Delays in treatment may result in a greater likelihood of infection and permanent scarification.

In the case of surgical amputation of the whole tail, or a portion thereof, the clinician may be able to "assist" natural regeneration by autotomizing it at a natural plane. The wound should be left unsutured so as not to hinder regeneration. In this case conservative treatment, even with a temporary bandage, may be suitable (see Chapter 112).

REFERENCES

See www.expertconsult.com for a complete list of references.

169

Testudinid Herpesviruses

Francesco C. Origgi

DEFINITION

There are at least 20 different chelonian herpesviruses (*Herpesviridae*, subfamily *Alphaherpesvirinae*).[1] Four of them are closely related and have been renamed *Testudinid herpesviruses* (TeHVs) (previously "tortoise herpesviruses").[2] *Testudinid herpesvirus 3* (TeHV3) is considered the most widespread and pathogenic. Any tortoise is considered susceptible, but different species sensitivity exists.[1,2] Highest incidence of disease is seen in early spring and fall.[1] Two distinct genogroups (A, B) of TeHV3 exist and have been associated with lesions of different severity (B > A).[1] The other TeHVs comprise TeHV1 overrepresented in Russian tortoises (*Agrionemys horsfieldii*), TeHV2 in the Agassiz's desert tortoises (*Gopherus agassizii*), and TeHV4 detected in both healthy and diseased African tortoises (Bowsprit tortoise [*Chersinia angulata*] and Leopard tortoise [*Stigmochelys pardalis*]).[3] Transmission is most likely by close contact, although evidence of a likely vertical transmission has been recently reported.[3] Intranasal and intramuscular live virus inoculations cause disease.[2,4]

CLINICAL PRESENTATION

Clinical signs are stomatitis and glossitis with oral and/or nasal discharge, conjunctivitis with ocular discharge, dyspnea, neurological signs, cervical edema, anorexia, and weight loss.[2] Experimentally, stomatitis and glossitis may occur within 12 days postinfection and is detectable for about 2.5 weeks in Greek tortoises (*Testudo graeca*) (see Fig. 169.1). Complete resolution of the clinical signs follows in survivors.[2,4]

Oral diphtheronecrotic plaques are classic (see Fig. 169.1A).[4] TeHV3 is neurotropic;[4] however, the eosinophilic to amphophilic intranuclear inclusions can be seen in virtually any epithelial tissue besides the CNS. Indirect evidence of latency in infected animals exists.[4] Virus reactivation is unpredictable; however, viral shedding in infected tortoises has been reported to occur more commonly after hibernation.[2,3]

DIAGNOSTIC CONFIRMATION

Laboratory confirmation of herpesvirus infection in tortoises is necessary because of the lack of pathognomonic clinical signs and their transitory nature. Differential diagnoses include ranavirus, virus X (Picornavirus) and *Mycoplasma* sp infections.[2] Serological (mainly serum neutralization [SN] and enzyme-linked immunosorbent assay [ELISA]) and molecular tests (mainly PCR) are available together with virus isolation, electron microscopy, and histopathology. SN testing can be applied to any tortoise species as long as the specific herpesvirus strain is available as an isolate, whereas ELISA testing has been validated in Greek and Hermann's (*T. hermanni*) tortoises for TeHV3.[2] Detection of anti-TeHV1 and TeHV2 antibodies in Greek and Hermann's and also other species of tortoises by ELISA is also possible (Origgi F, personal communication). A minimum of two ELISA tests repeated at least 8 weeks apart are necessary to definitively determine infection to TeHV3, and 10 weeks apart are

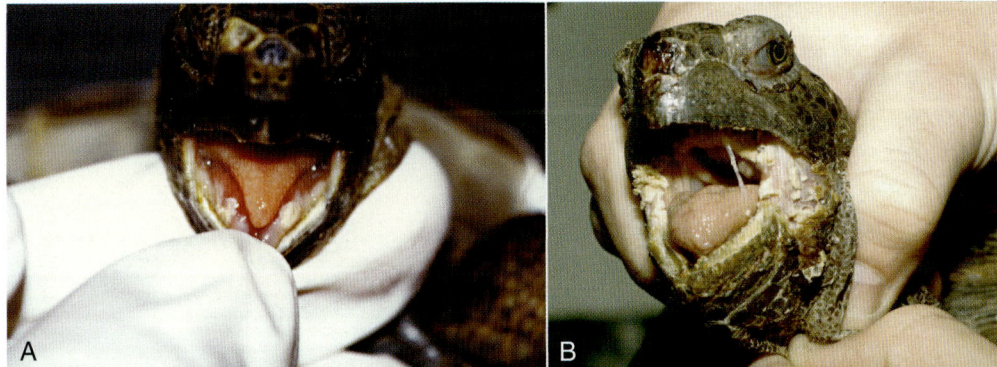

FIG 169.1 (A) Herpesviral stomatitis in a Greek tortoise (*Testudo graeca*). Shown are oral diphtheritic plaques surrounded by hemorrhagic inflammation of the mucosa. Plaques are in the early stage of formation. Notice the perfect symmetry of the lesions. Plaques might not necessarily be symmetrical and may occur also on the tongue. (B) Herpesviral stomatitis and rhinitis in a California desert tortoise (*Gopherus agassizii*). Note the oral plaques and hemorrhagic nasal discharge. (A, Courtesy of Francesco C. Origgi; B, courtesy of Douglas R. Mader.)

suggested for SN.[2] Both tests are equally reliable.[2] Lack of seroconversion may occur.[4] PCR tests include both genotype specific- and pan-herpesvirus protocols.[2] The PCR products need to be sequenced. Virus isolation is the definitive proof of herpesvirus infection. Serology is particularly helpful in chronically infected animals with no clinical disease. Molecular testing is the test of choice during the acute stage of the infection.[2]

PREFERRED TREATMENT(S)

Acyclovir and gancyclovir reduce viral replication *in vitro.*[5] Either 80 mg/kg per os SID or TID of acyclovir have been proposed; however, the effective concentration could not be reached in vivo after a dose of 80 mg/kg.[2] Supportive therapy such as fluid therapy and antimicrobials for secondary infections may also be helpful.[2] Vaccination treatments have been unsuccessful.[2]

PROGNOSIS AND PREVENTION

Herpesvirus infection is for life. Quarantine (6 months or longer) while repeating serological and molecular tests is critical, and separating animals with consistent signs is necessary.[3] Overcrowding and mixing species should be avoided.[2]

REFERENCES

See www.expertconsult.com for a complete list of references.

170

Thermal Burns

Michael Pees and Tom Hellebuyck

DEFINITION

Thermal burns are injuries caused by direct or indirect contact with heated objects or excessive infrared radiation. Burns are generally classified from first up to fourth degree.

CLINICAL SIGNIFICANCE AND KNOWN ETIOLOGICAL CAUSE(S)

Thermal burns are commonly observed in captive reptiles. These injuries can range from mild to life threatening but should always be considered medical emergencies. See Chapter 69 for a more detailed discussion on the treatment, prognosis, and prevention of thermal burns.

The main causes for this condition are the use of inadequate heating equipment or other management faults with respect to environmental temperature maintenance. Common faults are unguarded heat bulbs, hot rocks (Fig. 170.1), or heat mats. The latter are often of poor quality and can reach temperatures that directly lead to thermal damage. It is still not understood why reptiles do not react appropriately to temperatures that will cause immediate burns (e.g., snakes curling around heat bulbs with extreme temperatures), but it is essential that owners are aware of this issue and prepare the reptile's environment appropriately.

CLINICAL PRESENTATION AND DIAGNOSTIC CONFIRMATION

Often historical review of husbandry practices and patient behavior, and a thorough physical examination, will indicate a thermal burn. The classification of thermal burns used in mammals as first-, second-, third-, and fourth-degree burns can also be applied to reptiles (see Chapter 69). Although first-degree burns often appear harmless and might be treated by the owner, clinical monitoring is recommended, because secondary problems (e.g., bacterial infections) may occur. Severity and prognosis depend on several factors, including the kind of heat source (radiant, conductive) and the temperature and time of contact, but also the overall general condition of the reptile, the severity of the skin damage, and the species involved.

Diagnosis and confirmation is based on a combination of clinical signs and investigation into husbandry practices.

PREFERRED TREATMENT(S)

Therapy should be initiated as soon as possible, and proper wound management is essential. Reptiles have a remarkable ability to cope even with extensive wounds, but healing might take several months, and medical treatment should be continued until the wound is closed. Wound cleaning, using mild antiseptics (e.g., chlorhexidine), and a hygienic environment (e.g., paper, towels) are important. Enzyme ointments might be helpful to clean necrotic wounds and stimulate secondary healing. A suitable wet-to-dry bandage may also help with further debridement, whereas iodine gauze can be used to prevent/reduce infection. Systemic antimicrobials should be considered for serious and widespread burns, especially if surgical debridement is planned. The importance of microbiologic examination and susceptibility testing cannot be overemphasized. Fluid and protein loss should be corrected. Analgesia is required for first- and second-degree burns; however, third- and fourth-degree alterations typically result in nerve-ending destruction (Fig. 170.2) and are often less painful.

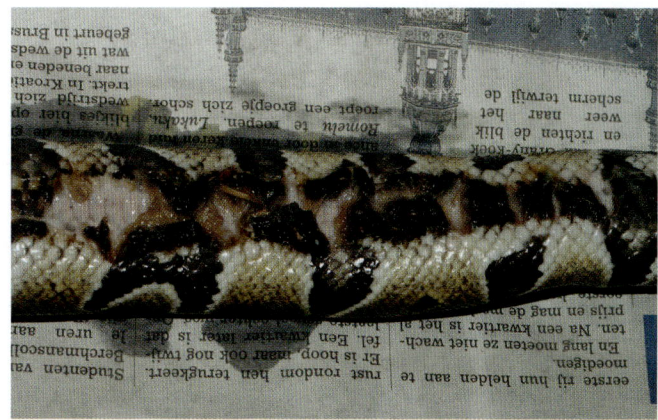

FIG 170.1 Third-degree burn at the ventral body surface in a ball python (*Python regius*) as a consequence of the inappropriate use of a hot rock. (Courtesy of Tom Hellebuyck.)

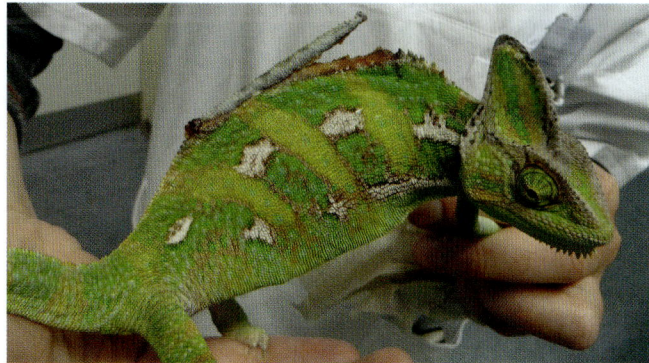

FIG 170.2 Third-degree dorsal burn in a chameleon due to an inappropriately installed heat lamp. The wound healed after several weeks of supportive treatment. (Courtesy of Michael Pees.)

Once reepithelization starts, wound dressings should support healing, and low-level laser therapy (photobiomodulation) may be helpful.[1,2] Scar formation and repigmentation may occur over months and may result in recurrent dysecdysis at the site of damage.

PROGNOSIS AND PREVENTION

Prognosis is dependent on the severity of the condition and an effective therapeutic approach. Appreciation of the natural behavior of reptiles, and establishment of an appropriate and safe thermal environment are necessary. Clinicians should discuss appropriate thermal guidelines with clients.

REFERENCES

See www.expertconsult.com for a complete list of references.

171

Tortoise Mycoplasmosis

Lori D. Wendland and Mary B. Brown

DEFINITION

Mycoplasmosis is an important cause of upper respiratory tract disease (URTD) in tortoises.[1]

CLINICAL SIGNIFICANCE AND KNOWN ETIOLOGICAL CAUSE(S)

Members of the Testudinidae appear to be highly susceptible to *Mycoplasma agassizzi* infection.[1] To date, *M. testudineum* is found only in gopher and desert tortoises (*Gopherus* spp.). In the Emydidae family, a third of *M. agassizii*-like sp. has been identified by PCR.[2] Increased tortoise densities, inappropriate temperature, poor nutrition, and concurrent infections may all exacerbate mycoplasmosis in captive tortoises. Transmission is via direct contact, particularly when animals have nasal discharge. Nasal cavity lesions vary in severity and may include multifocal to focally extensive subepithelial lymphoid aggregates, a mixed inflammatory cell infiltrate, basal cell hyperplasia, mucous and olfactory epithelial metaplasia, and erosion of the ciliated epithelium. *M. testudenium* appears to cause more focal and less severe damage.

CLINICAL PRESENTATION

Clinical signs, alone or in concert, include serous to mucopurulent nasal and ocular discharge, edematous and erythemic conjunctiva, and periocular and palpebral edema (Fig. 171.1A and B). In severe cases, nasal cavities may be completely obstructed with a thick, caseous discharge, and nasal cavity erosion can occur. Once infected, clinical signs may be intermittent or absent, but animals rarely clear mycoplasmal infections. Subclinical animals may have no apparent clinical signs, yet be seropositive, have histopathological lesions, and may shed. Clinical signs intensify and abate cyclically in chronic infections; animals may remain asymptomatic for years before recurrence. In animals that repeatedly exhibit clinical signs, grooves extending ventrally from the nares, eroded nares, and depigmentation around the nares can be observed.

DIAGNOSTIC CONFIRMATION

Optimal diagnostics include both ELISA serology (plasma or serum) and PCR (choanal swabs, nasal discharge, or flushes) coupled with health assessment and observation for clinical signs.[3,4] Western blots are not recommended unless multiple strains or the homologous strain is used as the antigen.[5] ELISA may not detect tortoises in the earliest stages of infection but is the most likely to detect clinically silent, intermittently shedding, as well as chronically infected animals. PCR/qPCR may detect animals in early stages of infection or those currently shedding; however, false negative results can occur in chronically affected, intermittently shedding, or clinically asymptomatic animals or with inadequate sampling of nasal passages. Culture is generally not used,

as *M. agassizii* is fastidious, takes up to 6 weeks for primary isolation, and requires experienced laboratory personnel.

PREFERRED TREATMENT(S)

Treatment recommendations are extralabel, and exact doses may vary for tortoise species.[6] Tetracyclines, fluoroquinolones, lincosamides,

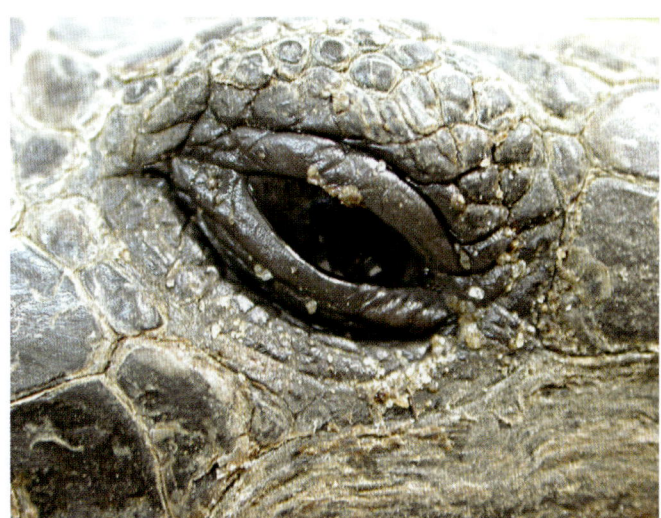

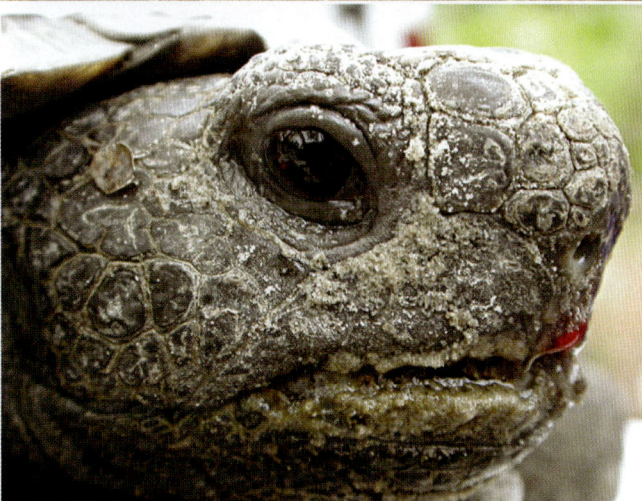

FIG 171.1 (A) Gopher tortoise (*Gopherus polyphemus*) with conjunctivitis, ocular discharge, and severe palpebral edema from mycoplasmosis. (B) Epistaxis, nasal and ocular discharge, and conjunctival hyperemia are seen in this gopher tortoise. These signs may develop as early as 2 weeks after infection.

macrolides, and certain aminoglycocides are effective against *Mycoplasma*; antibiotics targeting cell walls are not effective. Topical (ocular and nasal) antibiotic-corticosteroid combinations used with oral or parenteral antibiotics may minimize the local inflammatory response.[6] Longer treatment may be required in more severely affected animals. Supportive care and housing in the upper ranges of preferred optimal temperature zone will improve response to treatment.

PROGNOSIS AND PREVENTION

Use standard infection control practice for infectious disease, and isolation of ill tortoises for more intensive monitoring and treatment may help contain the flare-ups and decrease frequency of clinical disease. Once diagnosed with URTD, consider that animal as persistently infected and a potential source of infection. Use stringent disinfection and sanitation protocols (e.g., 3%–5% bleach solution). Separate eggs and hatchlings from adults, as hatchlings may develop more acute, fulminant disease. Use adequate husbandry practices to minimize stress and exposure to naive animals. Increased tortoise densities and higher organic load could facilitate environmental persistence. See Chapter 72 for more details.

REFERENCES

See www.expertconsult.com for a complete list of references.

172

Urolithiasis (Cystic Calculi and Cloacal Uroliths)

Krista A. Keller

DEFINITION

Urolithiasis has been reported in chelonians, lizards, and snakes.[1-7] Urolith location may be anywhere along the urinary tract, although cystic calculi are most common.[1-7] Most uroliths are composed of urate salts; however, calcium carbonate, oxalate, and mixed compositions are reported.[1-3,5]

CLINICAL SIGNIFICANCE AND KNOWN ETIOLOGICAL CAUSE(S)

It has been proposed that chronic dehydration and overheating may factor in the etiology of urolithiasis.[3] Urine modification occurs across the bladder epithelium, with water reabsorption along a concentration gradient resulting in further urine concentration approaching that of plasma.[8,9] Thus chronic dehydration and overheating may increase water absorption from the bladder, leading to supersaturation of urate excreta and reduced urination, predisposing to urolith formation. High-protein diets and biological niduses (e.g. parasites, eggs) may also predispose to calculus formation.

CLINICAL PRESENTATION AND DIAGNOSTIC CONFIRMATION

Many cystic calculi have a long subclinical stage where no abnormalities are noted. Physical examination findings suggestive of a cystic or cloacal calculus include cloacal prolapse, egg retention, tenesmus, and lack of production of feces or urine.[3] Physical examination findings that may confirm a cystic calculus include palpation of a hard structure in the prefemoral fossa of chelonians (Fig. 172.1) or the caudal coelom of lizards. Digital cloacal palpation may yield a hard structure within the cloaca. Radiographs are a confirmatory and screening test for uroliths revealing radio-opaque laminar structures in the caudal coelom (Fig. 172.2A) or intrapelvic region (see Fig. 172.2B). Radiolucent uroliths have also been reported but are uncommon.[3] There may be a predisposition in chelonians for cystic calculi location in the left lobe of the urinary bladder.[3] Hematology, plasma biochemistry, and urinalysis do not appear to be routinely beneficial in the diagnosis of urolithiasis in reptiles.[3] However, obstructive uroliths may cause biochemical changes indicative of postrenal obstruction.[1,3,4]

PREFERRED TREATMENT(S)

There are no medical dissolution recommendations for calculi in reptiles, and surgical intervention is recommended. Cystic calculi can be removed during cystotomy (Fig. 172.3), and recurrent cases can be managed with cystectomy.[6] Cloacal calculi can be removed through the cloaca with improved visualization when using cloacoscopy concurrently.[3,4]

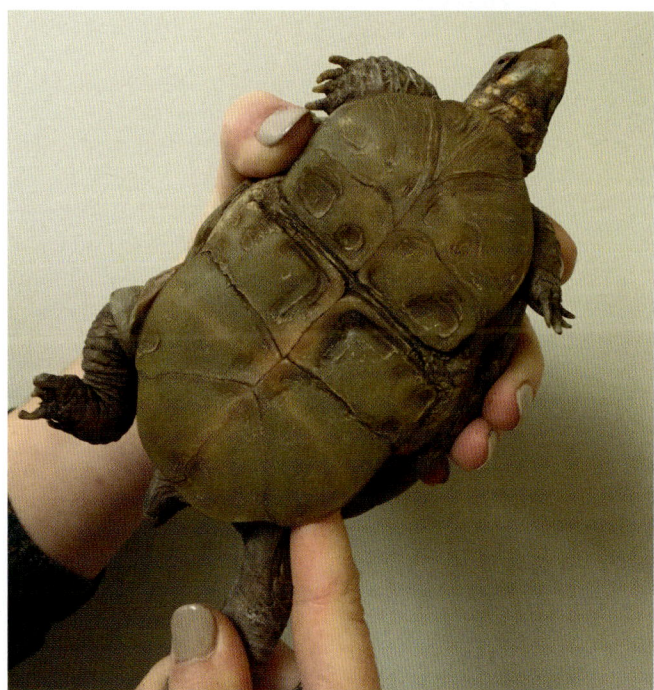

FIG 172.1 Palpation of the prefemoral fossa in a three-toed box turtle (*Terrapene carolina triunguis*) may reveal a hard calculus in the caudal coelom. (Courtesy of Krista A. Keller.)

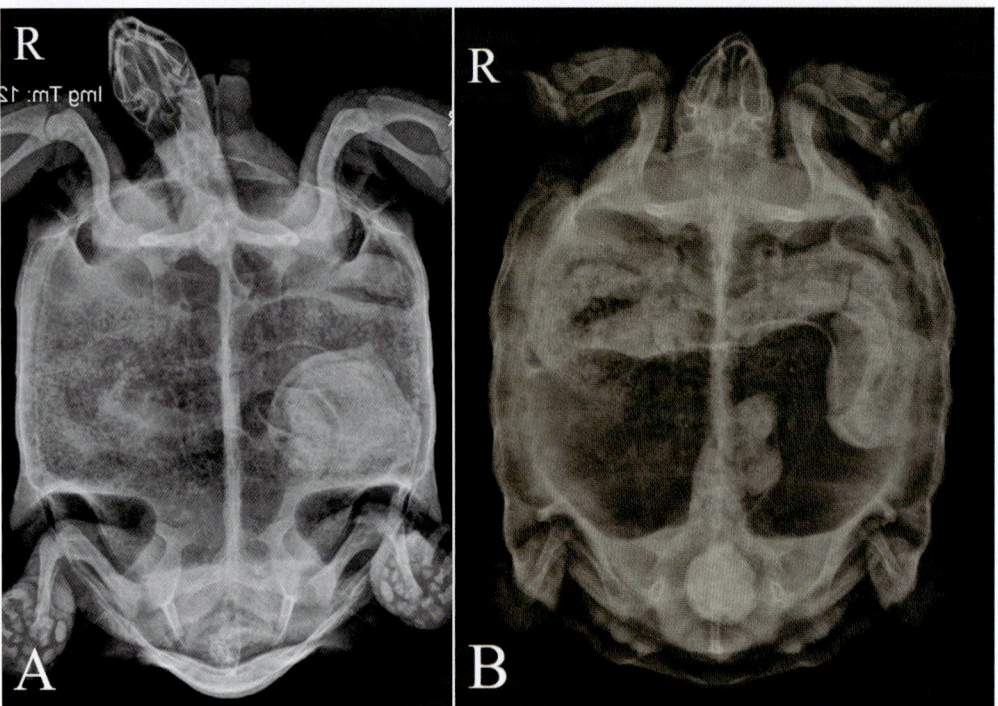

FIG 172.2 Dorsoventral radiographs of desert tortoises (*Gopherus agassizii*) with cystic (A) and cloacal (B) calculi. (Courtesy of Krista A. Keller.)

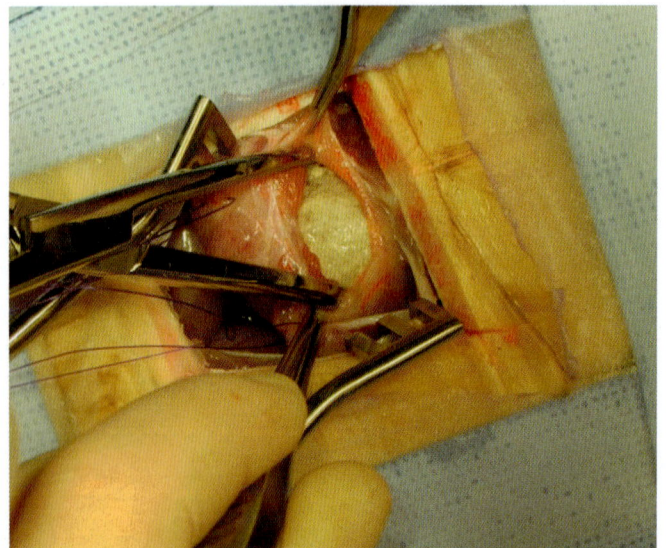

FIG 172.3 Intraoperative photo of cystotomy via plastronotomy approach in a juvenile sulcata tortoise (*Centrochelys sulcata*). Cranial is toward the left side of the image. A Weitlaner rectractor is being used to retract the coelomic membrane, while a curved Kelly hemostat is being used to break down the large cystolith to allow for easier removal. (Courtesy of Krista A. Keller.)

PROGNOSIS AND PREVENTION

The prolonged subclinical stage of cystic calculi has prompted many clinicians not to treat this condition. However, a retrospective study has indicated urolithiasis as a cause of death in 50% of chelonians necropsied with urolithiasis, indicating the need for veterinary intervention.[3] Because of the association of urate urolithiasis with chronic dehydration and overheating, species-specific husbandry recommendations remain the best preventative measure. All species should have access to water and both the high and the low temperatures of their preferred optimum temperature zones at all times.

REFERENCES

See www.expertconsult.com for a complete list of references.

173

Vomiting and Regurgitation

Richard S. Funk and Scott J. Stahl

DEFINITION AND CLINICAL SIGNIFICANCE

Vomiting, or emesis, is defined as a forceful ejection of food from the stomach and anterior intestines. Regurgitation involves the discharge of undigested food immediately, or within a few hours after eating, and is generally passive from the esophagus or pharynx. Both vomiting and regurgitation are clinical signs, not diseases.

CLINICAL PRESENTATION

These two clinical signs can be difficult to differentiate in reptiles. In mammals, testing the pH may help differentiate, with vomitus more acidic (usually pH <3). Often, the vomited or regurgitated material is found in the cage, but unfortunately the history is often incomplete, not allowing differentiation. If the environmental temperature(s) are too cool and food is not properly digested, the material vomited may appear relatively fresh, which adds to the challenge. Turtles and tortoises rarely vomit or regurgitate; consequently, these are serious clinical signs. A thorough history and complete physical examination are important in determining potential causes for vomiting or regurgitation. Behavioral changes, usually related to husbandry issues, are commonplace. For example, nervous snakes that are not provided a secure hiding box may vomit if disturbed or handled after eating a meal. Concurrent diarrhea associated with vomiting often indicates nonspecific gastrointestinal disorders and/or other nongastrointestinal disease. Reptiles with chronic vomiting are likely dehydrated and may have acid-base and electrolyte imbalances. In most reptiles, vomiting, not regurgitation, is occurring and etiologies for vomiting in reptiles are less clearly elucidated than in companion mammals. Consumption of too large a meal, maintenance of the reptile at temperatures not conducive to proper digestion, or the ingestion of partially autolyzed prey items may result in vomiting and diarrhea.

Infectious causes of vomiting include bacterial (including *Chlamydia*) and fungal infections; parasites such as cryptosporidiosis, ascariasis, cestodiasis, and amebiasis; and viral diseases such as adenoviruses and inclusion body disease (reptarenavirus) of boid snakes (see Chapters 30, 32, and 73). In snakes, cryptosporidiosis is a common cause of vomiting and often associated with a midbody (gastric) swelling.

Historically, snakes with cryptosporidiosis usually vomit 2 to 3 days after ingestion the associated gastric pathology inhibits proper digestion, and as the prey item putrefies. Iatrogenic vomiting may also occur after ingestion of oral medications or medicated food; certain specific drugs such as apomorphine, levamisole, xylazine, miticides, and organophosphates; and some species-specific related responses to certain drugs and even the route of administration used (e.g., parenteral enrofloxacin in red-footed tortoises, *Chelonoidis carbonaria*). Poisonings such as the ingestion of toads, resulting in *Bufo* toxicity, and organophosphate or other pesticide intoxication can cause vomiting (see Chapter 88). Inflammatory processes such as pancreatitis, peritonitis (coelomitis), or pyometra, which are commonly associated with gastrointestinal clinical signs in mammals, have not been consistently associated with vomiting in reptiles. Gastrointestinal foreign body (Fig. 173.1 A–C), obstructive neoplasm or granuloma, stricture, intussusception, or congenital defects/atresia may result in vomiting.

Several etiologies exist for regurgitation, with environmental and behavioral causes as described for vomiting being the most common. Other causes include esophageal, pharyngeal, or oral lesions such as stomatitis, esophagitis, neoplasia, esophageal laceration or perforation, strictures, granulomas, and foreign bodies. If regurgitation is chronic, dramatic weight loss and secondary aspiration pneumonia can occur.

DIAGNOSTIC CONFIRMATION

After a detailed history and thorough physical examination, indications for survey and contrast radiography and/or advanced imaging, including CT and MRI, may be recommended. Laboratory analysis and patient evaluation may include complete blood count and chemistry profile. Also, infectious disease–testing, including bacterial and fungal cultures, fecal parasite analysis, PCR testing and acid-fast stains for *Cryptosporidia* in snakes, and samples for virology, may need to be performed. Endoscopy of the esophagus and gastrointestinal system and/or exploratory surgery to obtain appropriate biopsies for histopathology may be required for a definitive diagnosis. For cryptosporidiosis in snakes, a gastric biopsy and histopathology may be required for a definitive diagnosis (see Chapters 73 and 165).

PREFERRED TREATMENT(S)

Correction of dehydration, acid-base imbalances, and mismanagement (such as handling, temperature, provision of shelters, quarantine, and hygiene) is important. Supportive care, including providing appropriate thermal requirements and fluid therapy followed by appropriate chemotherapeutics (e.g., antimicrobials, antiparasitics, gastrointestinal protectants) is critical in managing these cases. Use of antiemetic medications such as metoclopramide may be beneficial. For a review of therapy see Section 11.

Tube- or assist-feeding may be necessary once the underlying problems have been addressed (see Chapter 45).

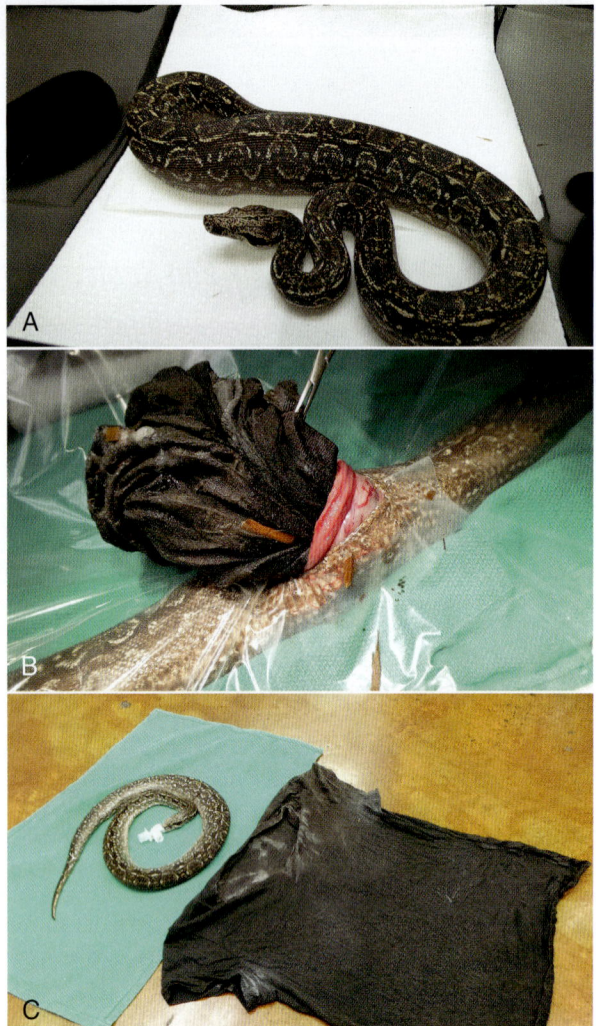

PROGNOSIS AND PREVENTION

Prognosis is dependent on the diagnosis. See Chapter 73 for more information on gastroenterology. If a diagnosis of cryptosporidiosis is confirmed in a snake with clinical signs, the prognosis is poor as no known curative treatment is available. Importantly, these snakes are potentially contagious to other snakes and should be removed from the collection. Vomiting and regurgitation are clinical signs and not specific diseases. If the cause can be identified and corrected, the resulting clinical signs can likely be resolved. Appropriate quarantine, husbandry, and nutrition, with routine health care, can be largely preventative.

FIG 173.1 (A) An Argentine boa (*Boa constrictor occidentalis*) presented for vomiting and midbody swelling. Radiographs revealed a foreign body completely filling the stomach, and on inquiry the owner remembered feeding the snake a frozen thawed rat placed on a t-shirt in the cage, which was missing. (B) At surgery, a gastrotomy was performed, and the t-shirt was manipulated out of the stomach. (C) Snake recovering from anesthesia with t-shirt displayed postop. The snake was fed a small rodent meal 1 month later, vomiting resolved, and the snake made a full recovery. (Courtesy of Scott J. Stahl, Stahl Exotic Animal Veterinary Services.)

Zoonoses and Public Health

Cathy A. Johnson-Delaney and Janos Gal

Most veterinary practitioners working with herpetological species are aware of common zoonoses; however, owners may not be aware of the risks posed by their pets. The veterinarian is often responsible for educating owners. Zoological collections, breeding facilities, wildlife professionals, and research facilities must also be aware of potential risks to their staff and the public. Physicians are often less familiar with reptile zoonoses and with veterinary technology, diagnostics, and treatments used to minimize the risks of zoonoses. The physician rarely seeks consultation with the patient's veterinarian about potential or confirmed problems. Client educational handouts that cover prevention of zoonotic disease from reptiles are helpful; however, veterinarians should be wary of giving advice on human health issues and should always direct an unwell client to their physician.

Humans that are particularly at risk for zoonoses include immunosuppressed or immunocompromised individuals: infants and children under the age of 5 years, the elderly, and those with chronic immunosuppressive disease or who are receiving immunosuppressive therapy.[1–6]

Reptiles have been documented to carry many potential pathogens that, under the right conditions, can cause infections in humans; however, the recovery of such an organism from the reptile does not mandate that the pathogen will be passed to the human and cause disease.[7] Many potential zoonotic pathogens have been isolated from reptiles and amphibians (Table 174.1). Evaluation of the risk potential includes identification of any possible pathogenic organisms, the nature and duration of contact the owner has with the reptile, sources of infection or reinfection by the reptile (i.e., food sources, sanitation measures, housing and husbandry practices), original source of the reptile (e.g., wild caught, domestically bred, exposure to other reptiles), and sources of infection to the reptile during transport and sale (e.g., shipping conditions, pet store housing).

Captive-bred reptiles may be infected with fewer pathogens if the breeders have been careful about screening their wild-caught breeding stock and are meticulous about sanitation. In reality, although some parasitic organisms have been eliminated from the captive-bred reptile, largely because of lack of appropriate intermediate hosts or other determinants in the life cycles, bacterial, fungal, and viral organisms are still found in abundance.[7,8] Bacterial pathogens can originate from contaminated food sources. Risk of transmission may be greater from a live food, such as a chick or a mouse, than from processed food.[7]

Reptiles should not be housed in the kitchen or other areas where food is prepared or eaten. The most important factor to decrease the chance of reptile zoonoses is to always thoroughly wash hands with soap after handling any animal, food/water utensils, or cage furniture

(Table 174.2).[6] Young children should not handle reptiles unless under close supervision, and any oral contact with the reptile or cage furniture must be prevented. Protective gloves should be worn while cleaning the enclosure or utensils (see Chapter 18 for cleaning agents). Water and fecal materials should be drained into the toilet rather than dumped in the sink or bathtub. A splash-guard face shield is recommended to minimize inhalation of potential aerosols or waterborne pathogens coming in contact with mucous membranes during the cleaning process.[7,8] The reptile should have its own soak tub/container rather than the using the owner's sink or bathtub.[6] It is inappropriate to use a children's wading pool outdoors for housing turtles, given the difficulty of preventing children from gaining access (Fig. 174.1).

The risk of transmission can also be minimized by screening the reptile for pathogens as part of a regular preventive health maintenance program.[7] Many reptile veterinarians recommend regular health examinations for pet reptiles, which may include bacterial culturing, particularly for *Salmonella*; however, culture is not recommended because a negative result does not guarantee a reptile is free of *Salmonella* due to intermittent shedding. Owners must be educated that safeguards should always be taken, as any reptile may harbour potentially pathogenic organisms.

BACTERIA

Salmonella

The most recognized reptilian and amphibian zoonosis is salmonellosis.[9] More than 2400 serotypes exist. *Salmonella* is pathogenic to a variety of animals, and although some serotypes are host specific (e.g., *S. java* and *S. urbana* of turtles), all serotypes within *S. enterica* should be considered as potential pathogens for animals and humans.[10,11] *Salmonella* survives well in the environment contaminated by animal feces. There is evidence that amphibians (frogs and toads) in captivity have been associated with *Salmonella* outbreaks.[9]

History. The zoonotic significance of salmonellosis was first reported in 1963 when a 7-month-old child acquired the disease from a pet turtle, although the potential had been recognized since 1946 when *Salmonella* spp. were originally isolated from turtles. In 1968 in response to information about the association of reptile-associated salmonellosis (RAS) and pet turtles, the state of Washington issued a regulation requiring that turtles sold in the state be certified as *Salmonella*-free.[7,8] Because positive results showing that a turtle is free of *Salmonella* spp. is virtually impossible, in large part because of variability in excretion of the organism, this regulation effectively stopped the sale of pet turtles

TABLE 174.1 Selected Potential Bacterial Zoonotic Pathogens Isolated From Reptiles and Amphibians[7,29,35,36,38,39]

Actinobacillus sp.	*Aeromonas* sp.	*Bacteroides* sp.	*Campylobacter* sp.
Chlamydia (Chlamydophila)	*Citrobacter* sp.	*Clostridium* sp.	*Corynebacterium* sp.
Edwardsiella tarda	Enterococci (Vancomycin-resistant)	*Escherichia coli*	*Klebsiella pneumoniae*
Leptospira sp.	*Listeria monocytogenes*	*Mycobacterium* sp.	*Neisseria* sp.
Pasteurella sp.	*Plesiomonas shigelloides*	*Pseudomonas* spp.	*Salmonella* spp.
Serratia marcescens	*Staphylococcus* sp.	*Streptococcus* sp.	*Vibrio fluvialis*
Yersinia enterocolitica; Yersinia ruckeri			

TABLE 174.2 *Salmonella* and Reptiles: Veterinary Guidelines

Veterinarians who treat reptiles should be aware of the following information and recommendations concerning reptiles and *Salmonella* spp:

- *Salmonella* carriage appears to be highly prevalent in reptiles. Reptiles should be considered to be nonclinical carriers of *Salmonella*; the organism is intermittently or continuously shed in their feces and, if ingested by humans, may result in serious illness.
- Veterinarians treating reptiles play an important role in informing reptile-owning clients about salmonellosis and advising them on precautions for reducing the risk of acquiring *Salmonella* infection from reptiles.
- Because *Salmonella* may be shed intermittently in the feces of reptiles, it is not possible to determine whether any individual living reptile is free of *Salmonella*.
- Bacterial culture of fecal specimens from reptiles will not detect all carriers and is not recommended.

Abbreviated information included. Full text posted at http://arav.org, May 2016.

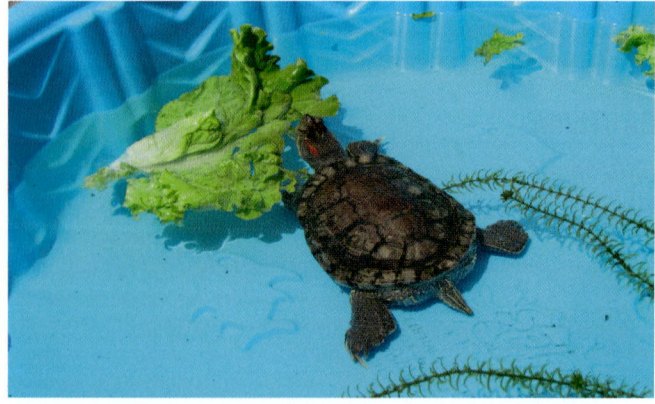

FIG 174.1 This red eared slider (*Trachemys scripta elegans*) is being housed in a children's-style pool, which should be exclusively used for the turtle, and children kept from playing in this pool. (Courtesy of Cathy A. Johnson-Delaney.)

in Washington. Subsequently, other state public health departments conducted detailed surveys of the incidence of turtle-associated salmonellosis.

Epidemiological studies at the time showed that 14% or approximately 280,000 of the estimated 2 million cases of salmonellosis in the United States seen yearly were turtle associated.[12,13] One survey suggested that

at least 22% of cases required hospitalization, which denotes a serious health hazard. A great number of cases probably occur that go unreported, because signs may be nonspecific and self-limiting. RAS in children is most commonly due to contact with turtles (42% of cases in one study), although it is also reported in infants younger than 6 months of age via indirect contact with other species of reptiles that were housed indoors.[13]

In 1972 the Department of Health, Education, and Welfare, United States Food and Drug Administration (FDA), banned the importation of turtles and turtle eggs and interstate shipment of turtles not certified free of *Salmonella* spp. or *Arizona hinshawii* (now classified as *S. arizonae*) by the state of origin.[13,14] In June 1975 the FDA ruled it illegal in the United States to sell viable turtle eggs or live turtles with a carapace length less than 10.2 cm (4 inches), with exceptions made for educational or scientific institutions and marine turtles (families Dermochelidae and Chelonidae). Marine turtles had not been shown to be a reservoir of *Salmonella* spp. and are used to restock coastal waters through the United States conservation programs. Also exempt are turtles sold or held for sale and distribution, turtle eggs not used in connection with a business, and turtles and turtle eggs destined for export only. Carapace length (<4 inches [10.2 cm]) was used as a measure of the potential to transmit *Salmonella* based on the assumption that larger turtles were less likely to be purchased or handled by children under the age of 10 years, the age group most at risk. Any turtle smaller than that carapace size might fit into a child's mouth.[7,13]

After enactment, there was a marked decrease in turtle-associated salmonellosis; however, despite regulations, *Salmonella* colonization of pet turtles continues and cases of human infection from pet turtles and other reptiles continues, especially from lizards.[15–18]

Infection Dynamics. Although more than 2000 recognized serotypes (serovars) of *Salmonella* exist, close to 1000 different serotypes have been isolated from reptiles, many of which have been associated with zoonotic disease in humans.[19–21] All serotypes are considered potentially pathogenic for humans.[7] The variability in excretion of *Salmonella* from reptiles has contributed to the difficulties in isolating the organisms and identifying carriers.[3,22] In one study of RAS in Minnesota during 1996 to 2011, 3.5% of nontypoidal, sporadic salmonellosis cases had reptile exposure; 47% were from lizards, 20% from snakes, and 19% from turtles, whereas 14% reported multiple species of reptile exposure. The three most common serotypes were *typhimurium* (15%), *enteritidis* (7%), and subspecies IV serotypes (7%).[23] A multistate outbreak between 2009 to 2011 of *Salmonella enterica* serovar Typhimurium was traced to contact with water frogs or their habitat.[24] Turtles cultured negative with routine cloacal swabbing and water examination for periods up to 6 months have then later been found to actively excrete the organism. The latent phase of excretion may be interrupted by stress. The organism may be cultured from the feces or cloaca 1 day and not the next.[3,7,22]

Estimates of reptiles harboring *Salmonella* spp. have been reported to be as high as 83.6% to 93.7%, depending on the method of testing. *S.*

enterica subsp. *arizonae* is more prevalent in snakes, estimated at 78.8% harboring the organism. One study utilized polymerase chain reaction (PCR) to demonstrate infection rates of *Salmonella* in hatchling green iguanas (*Iguana iguana*) of 67% to 94%.[25] A retrospective study done at the Bronx Zoo found that *Salmonella enterica* subsp. *enterica* was the most common in cultures (78/175 animals—45%). *Salmonella enterica* subsp. *diarizonae* was common (42/175 animals—24%). It was recovered almost exclusively from snakes, many of which had been clinically ill.[26]

In 1996 the Centers for Disease Control and Prevention (CDC) estimated that approximately 3% to 5% of the 2 to 6 million human salmonellosis cases per year were RAS.[2,3,25] Increasingly reported were human cases associated with iguanas.[2,3,6,22,27,28] In the United States between 2006 and 2014, fifteen multistate *Salmonella* outbreaks were recorded as associated with handling pet turtles.[17]

Although the rate of infection is quite high, most reptiles are asymptomatic. The relationship may be a saprophytic one.[7,29] Reptiles may shed the bacteria intermittently.[29] Isolation of the organism from the reptile does not really elucidate its role in causing disease in the reptile or potential for zoonotic transmission. Strains identified in causing disease in reptiles are listed in Table 166.1.

Reported Human Salmonellosis From Reptiles. Reptiles have been implicated as sources of human salmonellosis as well as livestock and poultry.[7,18] Another risk previously undocumented was from indirect contact from reptiles to children in a zoological exhibit. In one report, children were determined to have become infected from touching the wooden barrier that reptiles (Komodo dragons, *Varanus komodoensis*) had contaminated.[7,30]

Although the public is generally aware of the relationship between turtles and *Salmonella*, they are not as well informed about the connection with other reptiles, including lizards (green iguanas, bearded dragons [*Pogona vitticeps*], crested geckos [*Correlophus ciliatus*], water dragons [*Physignathus cocincinus*]), and snakes. Cases from iguanas were increasingly reported during the years iguanas were popular as pets.[1,3,5–7,11,16,25,28] *Salmonella* I4,[5],12:i:-, Cotham, and Kisarawe have been linked to contact with bearded dragons.[31,32] Pet crested geckos were linked to an outbreak of *Salmonella muenchen*.[33] Other lizards, including chameleons, have been linked with *Salmonella* infections in humans.[7] An infant contracted *Salmonella* serotype Nima carried by a boa that the father routinely handled. The clothing was implicated as the fomite.[11] Reports of RAS from pet turtles continues to dominate the literature and public health recommendations.

In 2008 there was a multistate outbreak of human *Salmonella enterica typhimurium*, with 135 cases in 25 states and the District of Columbia; 45% were in children 5 years of age and younger. In some cases there was contact only with the aquarium rather than the actual turtle. Some involved illegally sized turtles that had been purchased from a street vendor.[34]

The only regulations in effect to deal with the *Salmonella* problem in the United States are the regulations concerning small pet turtles. A client education brochure on *Salmonella* from pet turtles is available from http://www.cdc.gov/healthypets/resources/turtle_brochure.pdf. The Association of Reptilian and Amphibian Veterinarians (ARAV) also has information at http://www.arav.org (Table 174.2).

Attempts to treat reptiles with antibiotics to eliminate *Salmonella* spp. from their intestinal tract have not proven to be effective. Doing so increases the risk of emergence of antimicrobial-resistant *Salmonella* strains, which, if transmitted to humans, would complicate treatment. Attempts to raise "*Salmonella*-free" reptiles have been equally unsuccessful.

With this information in mind, the following guidelines have been developed by the ARAV, in cooperation with the Centers for Disease Control and Prevention (CDC), to help disseminate information to veterinarians and to the general public on how to minimize risks of exposure to *Salmonella* spp. and to help prevent development of reptile-associated salmonellosis in humans.

1. Veterinarians who treat reptiles should educate their clients who own reptiles about *Salmonella* spp. and provide information on the recommended precautions for reducing the risk of transmission of *Salmonella* spp. from reptiles to humans.
2. All veterinarians, staff, and clients who handle reptiles should follow recommended precautions for reducing the risk of transmitting *Salmonella* spp. from reptiles to humans.
3. All reptiles should be presumed to be carrying *Salmonella* spp. in their intestinal tract and to be continuously or intermittently shedding it in their feces. Bacterial culture of fecal specimens from reptiles to determine *Salmonella* infection status is discouraged. If veterinarians are called upon to assist health officials in determining the cause of salmonellosis in a person, bacterial culture of combined fecal and cloacal specimens from reptiles with which that person has had direct or indirect contact are recommended.
4. It is not recommended to treat healthy reptiles with antimicrobial agents with the intention of eliminating *Salmonella* spp. from the intestinal tract. Clients who request treatment of healthy reptiles for *Salmonella* spp. should be discouraged from such treatment and cautioned about the possibility of causing the emergence of antimicrobial-resistant *Salmonella* strains that might pose a greater health risk to humans.

This information was developed by the ARAV in collaboration with the CDC and is intended for information purposes only; please seek advice from your physician and your reptile's veterinarian if questions or problems occur.

Salmonella Bacteria and Reptiles: Information for Owners. This section was adapted from http://arav.org, May 2016.

Most, if not all, reptiles carry *Salmonella* bacteria in their intestinal tract and intermittently or continuously shed these bacteria in their feces. *Salmonella* bacteria usually do not cause any illness in reptiles but can cause serious illness in people.

Salmonella bacteria are easily spread from reptiles to humans. Humans may become infected when they place their hands into their mouths after touching an object, including a food item, that has been in contact with the stool of reptiles. For example, infants have become infected after drinking from bottles of infant formula that became contaminated during preparation. Individuals who prepared the formula had not washed their hands after touching a reptile, or reptiles were allowed to walk on the kitchen counters. For *Salmonella* bacteria to spread from reptiles to humans, the bacteria must be ingested. Therefore simply touching or holding a reptile will not result in the spread of the bacteria unless something contaminated with reptile feces or the reptile itself is placed in the mouth.

Most *Salmonella* infections in humans result in a mild, self-limiting illness characterized by diarrhea, fever, and abdominal cramps. However, the infection can spread to the bloodstream, bone marrow, or nervous system, leading to severe, and sometimes fatal, illness. Such severe infections are more likely to occur in infants and in individuals whose immune system is compromised (e.g., bone marrow transplant recipients, persons with diabetes mellitus, persons infected with the human immunodeficiency virus, and chemotherapy patients).

Unfortunately, *Salmonella* bacteria cannot be eliminated from the intestinal tract of reptiles. Administration of antibiotics to eliminate these bacteria has been unsuccessful and may result in the emergence of *Salmonella* bacteria that are resistant to antibiotics.

Attempts to raise or identify reptiles that do not carry *Salmonella* bacteria have also been unsuccessful; therefore bacterial culture of stool samples in an attempt to identify reptiles that are not carrying *Salmonella* bacteria is not recommended.

Fortunately, the spread of *Salmonella* bacteria from reptiles to humans can be easily prevented by using the following routine precautions:

- Always wash your hands with hot, soapy water after handling reptiles, reptile cages and equipment, and the stool of reptiles.
- Do not allow reptiles to have access to the kitchen, dining room, or any other area in which food is prepared. Also, do not allow reptiles to have access to bathroom sinks and tubs or to any area where infants are bathed. Consider keeping your reptiles caged or limiting the parts of the house where reptiles are allowed to roam free. Always wash your hands after coming into contact with any area where reptiles are allowed or roam free.
- Do not eat, drink, or smoke while handling reptiles, reptile cages, or reptile equipment. Do not kiss reptiles or share food or drink with them.
- Do not use the kitchen sink, kitchen counters, bathroom sinks, or bathtubs to bathe reptiles or to wash reptile cages, dishes, or aquariums. Reptile owners may wish to purchase a plastic basin or tub in which to bathe or swim their reptiles. Waste water and fecal material should be disposed of in the toilet instead of the bathtub or household sink.

The CDC recommends that children less than 5 years of age avoid contact with reptiles and that households with children less than 1 year of age not own reptiles. The ARAV encourages reptile owners with young children to discuss steps to minimize risks associated with owning reptiles with their reptile's veterinarian and their physician. Children should be supervised when they are handling reptiles to ensure that they do not place their hands, or any objects that a reptile has contacted, in their mouths. Reptiles should not be kept in child-care centers.

Aeromonas

Aeromonas spp. have been associated with diseases in fish, amphibians, and reptiles. They are also opportunistic pathogens and have been frequently cultured from clinically healthy reptiles.[35] In one survey of red-eared sliders purchased from 27 different suppliers, *Aeromonas* spp. were isolated from 63%. One survey cultured the oral cavity of 60 pet ball pythons (*Python regius*), and a wide range of gram-negative bacteria was cultured, including *Aeromonas hydrophila*, *Pseudomonas* spp., *Morganella morganii*, *Acinetobacter calcoaceticus*, *Salmonella* spp., *Staphylococcus* spp., and various anaerobic Clostridium species.[35]

Potential infection to humans may occur from contact with the water and open wounds or injuries or from bites or scratches inflicted by reptiles living in aquatic environments.

Plesiomonas

Plesiomonas shigelloides, formerly *Aeromonas shigelloides*, isolated from a boa constrictor with a progressive ulcerative stomatitis was reported to have caused acute gastroenteritis in a healthy young man. This organism may be considered part of the normal commensal flora.[36]

Campylobacter

Campylobacter spp. (*C. jejuni*, *C. fetus*, etc.) are enteric bacteria found in reptiles and mammals. *Campylobacter fetus* has also been isolated from feces of a healthy western hognose snake (*Heterodon nasicus*) and an ill blotched blue-tongue lizard (*Tiliqua nigrolutea*).[37] In one survey of 179 reptiles (human-raised, pet shop, and wild), *C. fetus* was identified in 9.7% in turtles, 1.7% in lizards, and 5.0% in snakes. Only one strain (ST-43) isolated from a red-footed tortoise (*Chelonoidis carbonaria*) was closely related to mammalian strains.[38] In 2004, an isolate from a human with exposure to reptiles was classified as *C. fetus* subsp. *testudinum* subsp. *nov*. Infected humans had a history of eating Asian food

thought to be made from turtles or other reptiles or experienced direct exposure to live reptiles.[37] Pet reptiles should be considered a potential reservoir of *Campylobacter* spp. with zoonotic potential.[39,40]

Other Enteric Bacteria

Many other species of potentially pathogenic bacteria can be isolated from both clinically healthy and diseased reptiles. *Citrobacter* spp., *Enterobacter* spp., *Klebsiella* spp., *Proteus* spp., and *Serratia* spp. were isolated in one study of bacterial flora in red-eared sliders.[41] Clinically asymptomatic lizards and snakes are also known to carry *Klebsiella* spp., *Proteus* spp., and a variety of gram-negative enteric bacteria, which may be transmitted by direct contact.

Yersinia enterocolitica can cause a variety of illnesses in humans, including severe gastroenteritis with abdominal pain that mimics appendicitis. *Y. enterocolitica* and the closely related *Y. intermedia* have been isolated from a number of wildlife species, including snapping turtles (*Chelydra serpentina*).[42] A survey was done of wild European pond turtles (*Emys orbicularis*). Thirty-six bacterial species were isolated, several of which were considered potential zoonotic organisms, including *Salmonella enterica* serovars *newport*, *daytona*, *braenderup*; *Listeria monocytogenes*; *Yersinia enterocolitica*; *Yersinia ruckeri*; *Klebsiella pneumoniae*; *Vibrio fluvialis*; and *Serratia marcescens*. The study concluded that the small number of potential human pathogens isolated indicated that the European pond turtle was of relatively minor importance as a threat to public health.[43]

Pseudomonas spp. gram-negative rods have been cultured from both clinically healthy and diseased reptiles.[35] *Pseudomonas* spp. are common bacteria in oral lesions in snakes.[35] Potentially, humans can contract infection through direct contact with the organism after scratches or bite wounds, inhalation, or ingestion.

Clostridium

Clostridium butyricum producing botulinum type E neurotoxin (BoNT/E) caused disease in two infants. The agent was isolated from water that housed yellow-bellied turtles (*Trachemys scripta scripta*). The turtles were housed in the first infant's home. The second infant was infected after a person had fed the turtle before holding and feeding the infant.[44]

Mycobacterium

Several species of Mycobacterium known to cause infection in humans have been isolated from reptiles, including *M. marinum*, *M. avium*, and *M. tuberculosis*. The majority of *Mycobacterium* spp. isolated from reptiles are classified as atypical forms (e.g., *M. chelonae*).[45] Many of these belong to the Runyon Group IV, which are considered resistant to antibiotics.[45] *M. marinum* has been implicated in cutaneous and subcutaneous nodular disease in humans ("fisherman's finger," swimming pool granuloma).[45] Direct contact with the organism through scratches in the skin, during handling of the animal, or while cleaning its habitat resulted in the human infection.[45] Crocodilians may be used for leather and meat and, if infected, are a potential threat to slaughter staff and tanners.[45] Potential routes of transmission of *Mycobacterium* spp. organisms to humans from infected reptiles include direct contact through defects, scratches, or bites in the skin or with inhalation and contact with oral or respiratory mucosa. The veterinarian, technicians, and staff who handle reptiles with chronic, purulent, or granulomatous lesions should protect themselves by wearing appropriate gloves, mask, face/eye shield (particularly when cleaning cages and tanks), and other garments. Treatment of infected reptiles is not recommended because of the zoonotic potential. The owner should be instructed in proper methods of sanitizing the reptile's environment to minimize exposure and eliminate the organisms.

Coxiella burnetii

In 1978 a cluster of human cases of Q fever caused by the rickettsia *Coxiella burnetii* was diagnosed in employees of an exotic bird and reptile importing company in New York state. These employees had been involved in unpacking and deticking a shipment of ball pythons imported from Ghana. Speculation was that the employees had been infected by inhaling aerosolized particles containing *C. burnetii* during the handling of the pythons or ticks or excreta of the ticks or pythons.[46] It has been identified in snakes, lizards, and turtles during serological surveillance of wildlife, and reptiles may serve as reservoir hosts for the transmission of *C. burnetii* by infected ticks to mammals.[47]

Chlamydia

A study of zoo animals in Japan found that *Chlamydia pneumoniae* DNA was found in 8.1% of reptiles, representing a potential public health risk, as the DNA was close to what had been found in human patients. No human infections directly associated with these reptiles were reported.[7,48]

FUNGI

Zygomycosis, also known as phycomycosis, mucormycosis, or ento-mophthoromycosis, refers to a group of diseases in humans caused by several genera and species of fungi belonging to the class Zygomycetes, orders Entomophthorales and Mucorales. Zygomycetes are ubiquitous saprophytes that produce a large number of spores. Many genera have been found in reptiles that have zoonotic potential. *Entomophthorales* contains members of *Basidiobolus ranarum* (*B. haptosporus*), which, found in anurans, has been documented to cause a granulomatous disease in humans primarily in the subcutaneous tissues.[49,50] *Metarhizium anisopliae* var. *anisopliae* has been found in reptiles. Infections from this fungus in humans are rare and described in an immunocompromised host.[51] *Beauveria bassiana* has caused a fatal granulomatous pulmonary infection in an American alligator and a red-eared slider. Infection of this organism in humans is rarely described.[51] *Purpureocillium lilacinum* has been associated with a number of reptile species. It was the cause of skin lesions in juvenile Chinese soft-shelled turtles (*Apalone sinens*) being raised at large-scale farms for human food and should be considered an important opportunistic pathogen in humans.[51]

Many different mycotic agents have been isolated from diseased reptiles that could also cause infection in humans, including *Aspergillus* spp., *Candida* spp., *Trichosporon* spp., and *Trichophyton* spp. Zoonotic transmission of these fungal agents, although possible, has not appeared in the literature.

VIRUSES

Reptiles may act as reservoir hosts to Western equine encephalitis (WEE; genus: Alphavirus; family: Togaviridae), which causes disease in humans and horses. Infection has been detected in reptile serological surveys, although it does not appear to cause disease. *Culex tarsalis* acts as the vector and can transmit the virus between reptiles. It is thought that reptiles function as reservoir hosts due to their low metabolic rate and reduced immune response during the winter[52] (Fig. 174.2).

Reptiles should not be housed outdoors during an epizootic outbreak in horses in an area. Eastern equine encephalitis virus (EEEV) is also considered zoonotic and may cause fatal encephalitis in humans.[53] In Europe, three species of mosquitoes have been identified that can transmit the virus. Sources for the introduction of the virus have been linked to the exotic pet trade, including reptiles.[53] In the United States, evidence is supporting the role of snakes in the transmission cycle, particularly as overwintering hosts.[54,55]

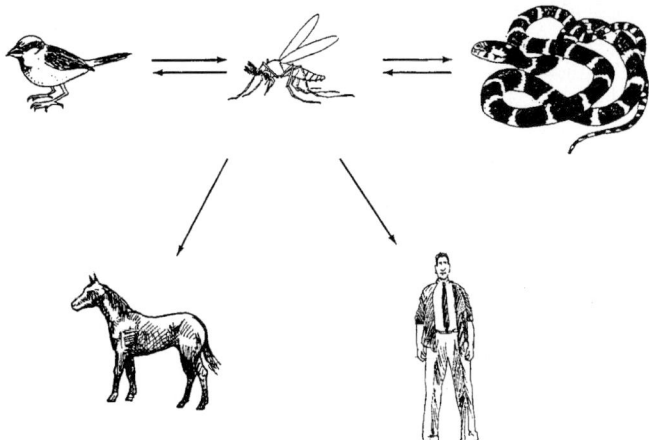

FIG 174.2 Life cycle of western equine encephalitis.

West Nile virus (WNV) is a mosquito-borne flavivirus that is transmitted by various species of *Culex mosquitoes*. WNV is known to have zoonotic potential as a result of infectivity in a wide variety of mammals and birds. Although flaviviruses and arboviruses have been reported to affect ectotherms and in some cases serve as reservoirs, reptiles and amphibians were not initially considered a primary species at risk.[56] The virus emerged in North America in 1999 when it infected and caused deaths in humans, horses, and birds. By 2001, WNV had spread into the southeastern United States and was considered an epizootic, as alligators (*A. mississipiensis*) and a captive crocodile monitor (*Varanus salvadori*) developed neurological signs.[57] The disease had previously been reported in farmed Nile crocodiles (*Crocodylus niloticus*) in Israel.[52,57] WNV has caused substantial losses in farmed American alligators. Eleven different mosquito species can carry the virus. Mosquitoes were probably the most important component of transmission of WNV at alligator farms.[58] WNV has now spread across the western hemisphere.[59] The potential role of reptiles and amphibians in the life cycle and epidemiology of WNV is still not conclusive.[57] If wild and captive species are susceptible, then the range of WNV and zoonotic potential will increase, and captive nonnative herpetological species can serve as reservoirs for the virus.

PROTOZOA

Despite the high numbers of protozoal organisms found in reptiles, most are ectotherm specific. Many varieties are not associated with known disease in the reptile, and their significance as zoonotic pathogens is also unknown. Many may be opportunistic pathogens of the reptile and opportunistic zoonotic pathogens to susceptible humans. Free-living amoebae may also be found in reptile feces. These include *Acanthamoeba, Naegleria,* Hartmanella, *Vahlkampfia,* and *Echinamoeba* sp. There is a potential zoonotic risk.

Cryptospordium

Cryptosporidium is a coccidian protozoan in the family Cryptospori-diidae, suborder Eimeriina. The parasite is not species specific and can easily be transmitted. It has been isolated in many different hosts, including mammals, birds, and reptiles. One study in Italy sampled 120 captive snakes, of which 35% were found to be shedding Cryptosporidium oocysts. Some of the species were considered to have zoonotic potential, although a number were specific for rodents and resulted from the ingestion of the infected prey.[60] The authors concluded that there may be possible public health implications. Another study looked at isolates from captive European tortoises (*Testudo graeca, T. hermanni,* and

T.marginata) in Italy.[61] The zoonotic *Cryptosporidium pestis* (*Cryptosporidium parvum* "bovine genotype") was identified, and the conclusion of the study was that there may be a risk to humans.[61] There have been no documented cases of human cryptosporidiosis from reptile sources.

PENTASTOMIDA

The pentastomes are currently classified in a separate phylum, Pentastomida. Infection by pentastomids may be referred to as pentastomiasis, linguatuliasis or linguatulosis, porocephalosis, or porocephaliasis.[62]

Nine genera have been identified in snakes, three in lizards, four in crocodiles, and two in turtles. *Armillifer* spp. are the most common genera identified from pythonids and viperids, *Kiricephalus* spp. from colubrids, and *Porocephalus* spp. from boids and crotalids. A variety of herbivorous vertebrates may serve as intermediate hosts, including rodents and artiodactylids. Carnivores, nonhuman primates, and humans may serve as incidental hosts[62,63] (Fig. 174.3). Eggs migrate up the respiratory tract, are swallowed, and passed in feces. The life cycle of the pentastomid is considered an oddity in that the intermediate host (rodent, mammal) is higher in the phylogenic scheme than the definitive host (snake, reptile), an uncommon occurrence among parasites.[62,63]

Humans, as aberrant hosts, contract the infection by consuming water or foods contaminated with eggs eliminated in the saliva or feces of snakes by consuming raw or undercooked snake meat or by handling infected reptiles and then placing contaminated hands in the mouth. Other intermediate hosts are infected through ingestion of contaminated water, plants, or the snakes themselves.[64] This may be considered a neglected tropical disease that may become more widespread as tropical species of reptiles are exported for the pet trade.[65] A case has been published of fatal pentastomiasis from *Armillifer armillatus*.[66] The fact that humans can serve as incidental hosts for reptilian pentastomes should alert veterinarians to recognize the zoonotic potential of these parasites. Veterinarians need to educate pet owners about the zoonotic potential of pentastomiasis. Newly acquired wild-caught reptiles should be examined, and, ideally, at least two successive fecal specimens from

the reptile should be examined to reduce the possibility of false-negative results. The need for prompt removal of feces from the reptile's habitat should be stressed. The owner should be instructed on the proper disposal of snake feces (i.e., flush down the toilet versus the family garbage can) and to wear gloves while doing so. Reptile food sources (such as live rodents) should not be allowed to come in contact with the reptile's feces.

HELMINTHS

Reptiles act as the second intermediate hosts for cestodes in the genera *Spirometra* and *Diphyllobothrium*. *Spirometra mansoni*, *S. mansonoides*, *S. erinaceieuropaei* (*D. erinacei*), *S. theileri*, and *S. proliferum* have been associated with sparganosis in humans (i.e., infection with the second-stage larvae called the sparganum or plerocercoid) (Fig. 174.4). Man is generally infected through ingestion of raw or undercooked, infected amphibian, reptile, bird, or mammal meat or through direct contact with infected amphibian or reptile meat used as a poultice for antiphlogistic effects in some Southeast Asian cultures. Use of the poultice has been linked to an ocular form of sparganosis, whereas cerebral

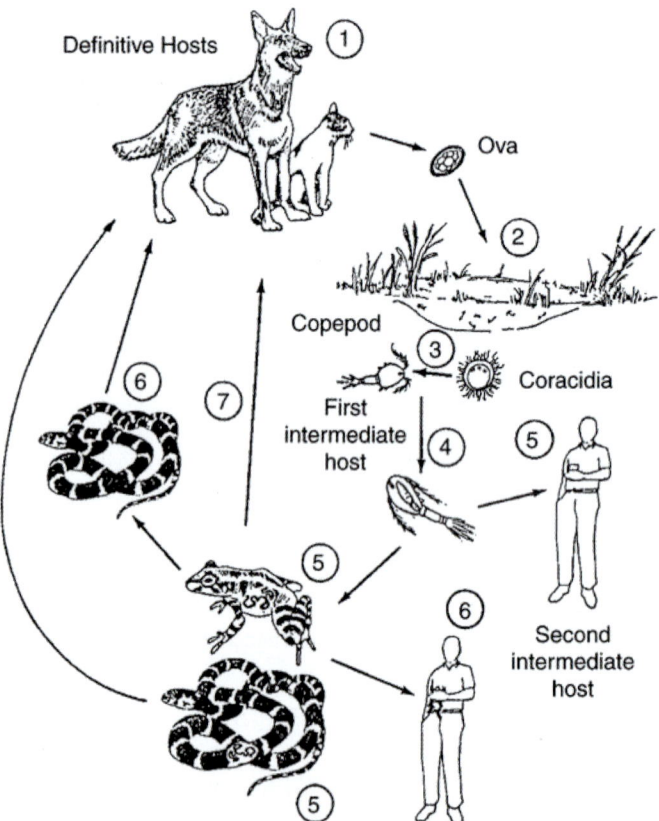

FIG 174.4 Transmission cycle in sparganosis. (1) Definitive host (canids, felids). Plerocercoid attaches to intestinal mucosa, matures in 10 to 30 days, produces eggs. (2) Eggs passed in feces, end up in water containing copepods of the genus *Cyclops*. In the water, eggs become free ciliated embryos called coracidia. (3) Coracidia ingested by first intermediate host (*Cyclops*). (4) Develop into first-stage larvae, "procercoid," in the tissues of *Cyclops*. (5) Ingestion of procercoids in infected *Cyclops* via water by second intermediate host (vertebrates: reptiles, amphibians, birds, small mammals [rodents, insectivores], swine, nonhuman primates, humans). (6) Develop into a "plerocercoid" or "sparganum" in the tissues of the vertebrate host. Plerocercoids in an ingested, infected vertebrate can encyst in new vertebrate host. Humans can be infected with ingestion of either a procercoid or a plerocercoid. (7) Infected vertebrate host with plerocercoids ingested.

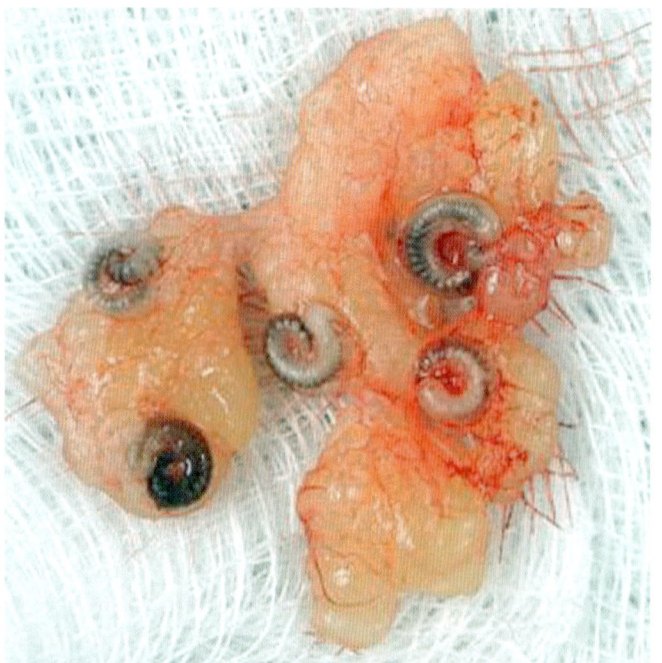

FIG 174.3 Pentastomid parasite from the lung tissue of a macaque monkey.

sparganosis has also been reported.[62] Humans are an incidental host and usually do not play a role in the life cycle of the parasite. Because parasitic life cycles require certain environmental conditions, and most captive reptiles are not intended for human consumption, sparganosis poses a minimal zoonotic risk.

ARTHROPODS

Arthropods that affect reptiles do not pose a direct zoonotic threat. Instead, their importance may be as vectors for viral or bacterial diseases, with the reptile serving as a reservoir or amplification host. The arthropods may cross species, biting reptiles, birds, and mammals, including humans. *Aedes* and *Culex* genera of mosquitoes may feed on reptiles, serving as possible reservoirs for Western equine encephalitis virus, Eastern equine encephalitis, and West Nile virus.[67]

Ornithodoros turicata, also known as the relapsing fever tick, is native to the United States and Mexico and can occasionally be found on reptiles. Heavy infestations have been found on box turtles (*Terrapene* spp.), gopher tortoises (*Gopherus polyphemus*), and rattlesnakes (*Crotalus* spp.). It transmits relapsing fever (also known as tick-borne relapsing fever, borreliosis, or spirochetosis) to humans. The tick may also be a vector of *Leptospira pomona*. All stages readily attack humans.[67]

Immature stages of *Haemaphysalis punctata* have been found on reptiles in Europe, northwestern Africa, and southwestern Asia. This tick may transmit the agent of Siberian (or North Asian) tick typhus (*Rickettsia siberica*). Immature stages of another tick, *H. concinna*, have been found on various reptiles in Europe and northern Asia. This tick transmits the agents of Russian spring-summer encephalitis (a flavivirus) and Siberian tick typhus.[67]

The immature stages of *Ixodes pacificus* are found on garter snakes (*Thamnophis* spp.) and spiny lizards (*Sceloporus* spp.) in the Pacific coastal region of North America. The bite itself causes irritation and trauma in humans and has been implicated in the transmission of tularemia (*Francisella tularensis*). It also may transmit Lyme disease (*Borrelia burgdorferi*). In the United States, *Anaplasma phagocytophilum* was isolated from multiple species of snakes and lizards. This organism causes the potentially fatal tick-borne disease human granulocytic anaplasmosis.[68] In central Europe, *Ixodes ricinus* may occur on European green lizards (*Lacerta viridis*).[69] It has been found to carry Anaplasma, Borrelia, and Rickettsia.[68] However, this tick's bite also causes severe irritation and paralysis in man and may transmit central European tick-borne encephalitis, Lyme disease, and agents of Boutonneuse fever (*R. conorii*).[67]

A study was conducted to look at ticks and the diseases they carried on reptiles and amphibians being imported into Japan for the pet trade.[68] Two species of ticks were identified that are known to bite humans:

Amblyomma dissimile and *Hyalomma aegyptium*. Four human pathogens were found in ticks on reptiles imported from Zambia: *Rickettsia africae*, *Rickettsia raoultii*, *Ehrlichia chaffeensis*, and *Candidatus Neoehrlichia mikurensis*. *E. chaffeensis* causes human monocytic ehrlichiosis, which is an acute febrile systemic illness. *Candidatus Neoehrlichia mikurensis* causes febrile disease in humans.[68] Reptiles and amphibians imported into Japan for the pet trade are not quarantined, so tick-infested animals may go directly into the pet trade.

A study in the Republic of Korea looked at the incidence of reptile-associated ticks and their infection with the severe fever with thrombocytopenia syndrome (SFTS) virus. The study looked at 132 reptiles: 2 species of lizard (49), 1 species of skink (15), and 8 species of snakes (68). Eighty-four ticks were collected in two genera (*Ixodes* and *Amblyomma*). Analysis of the SFTS virus of the ticks collected from two lizards and one snake demonstrated a close relationship with SFTS virus strains found in humans and ticks in Korea, China, and Japan. The study concluded that lizards and snakes may be potential hosts of SFTS virus.[70]

Larvae of trombiculid mites have been found on reptiles caught in the wild or maintained in outdoor enclosures in endemic areas. The most common species in North America is *Eutrombicula alfreddugesi* (also called *Trombicula irritans*), the common chigger. It has been found throughout the western hemisphere on box turtles, various snakes including racers (*Masticophis* spp.), hog-nosed snakes (*Heterodon* spp.), king snakes (*Lampropeltis* spp.), garter snakes (*Thamnophis* spp.), and various lizards. *E. splendens*, common in the southeastern United States, has been found on snakes and lizards. In Europe, *Neotrombicula autumnalis*, the common harvest mite, has been found on lizards and snakes. Only the larvae of these genera are parasitic. The adults are free-living. Control on the reptile includes topical insecticides and cleaning the environment. All of these mites have been reported to cause dermatitis in humans.[67,71,72]

Ophionyssus natricis, a dermanyssid mite of snakes and occasionally lizards, may bite humans. The mite is worldwide in distribution, and heavy infestations can lead to severe anemia, anorexia, lethargy, and death of the host snake. A documented case in humans involved an infested pet python. The family had pruritic papular lesions that had black central dots from skin puncture and bleeding. Some of the lesions appeared vesicular or bullous. They had noticed what they called "small insects" fixed on their skin and large numbers of the same on the snake and in the chair the snake usually occupied. The snake, its cage, and the chair were liberally dusted with a pyrethrum powder. No further bites were noted.[71]

REFERENCES

See www.expertconsult.com for a complete list of references.

175

Working With Free-Ranging Amphibians and Reptiles

Terry M. Norton, Kimberly M. Andrews, and Lora L. Smith

Capturing free-ranging animals for identification purposes, as well as for global positioning systems (GPS) and radio/satellite telemetry applications, is common in amphibian and reptile research and conservation efforts. In the past, these efforts have been predominantly performed by research biologists with minimal veterinary input. Institutional animal care and use committees (IACUC) are now required by most research institutions and for publication of research in the peer-reviewed literature. Veterinarians are being asked more frequently for their input, advice, and expertise in areas of infectious disease prevention, aseptic techniques, pain management, anesthesia, and surgery, all of which are critical in the topics discussed in this chapter. The techniques described here are not all-inclusive but are either commonly used by the authors or represent important techniques used by the scientific community.

AMPHIBIAN AND REPTILE CAPTURE TECHNIQUES

A variety of techniques are available for capturing amphibians and reptiles. Passive capture methods generally do not restrict an animal's movements; thus, they are less likely to result in stress or injury to the animal. Active sampling methods require careful monitoring to prevent morbidity or mortality but can yield valuable data on population size, individual growth rates, health, reproductive state, and survival. A general overview of commonly used passive and active capture methods for amphibians and reptiles is presented in Table 175.1, along with selected references that provide more detail on specific methodologies. Additional information on these methods can be found in Norton et al.[1]

HANDLING

Recommended Precautions to Prevent Disease and Other Health Problems

Infectious diseases can be transmitted within and between amphibian and reptile populations when handled for various procedures by field workers. Some examples of significant infectious and parasitic diseases that may be transmitted when appropriate precautions are not taken include chytrid fungus (*Batrachochytrium dendrobatidis*), snake fungal disease (*Ophidiomyces ophiodiicola*), iridoviruses, *Cryptosporidium serpentis*, paramyxovirus, *Entamoeba invadens*, *Mycoplasma agassizii*, and herpesviruses (see Chapters 29 through 32 for details). The following are some general guidelines for handling and manipulating herpetofauna in the field:

- Avoid using insecticides before handling amphibians and reptiles.
- Wash hands with disinfectant hand wash or wear separate disposable examination gloves after handling each animal.
- Clean any handling equipment with an appropriate disinfectant between each animal.
- Use a separate clean, well-ventilated container or bag for each animal if temporary containment or transport is needed.

- Avoid high or low temperatures during transport of the animal.
- Do not allow contact between animals from different populations when handling or transporting them.
- If wild amphibians or reptiles are held in captivity for various procedures such as surgical placement of radio transmitters, each animal should be isolated in a well-ventilated container that can be easily disinfected. Wood enclosures should be avoided because they cannot be disinfected. Animals should be maintained at their preferred optimal temperature zone with a thermogradient.

MARKING

Recommended Precautions to Prevent Disease and Other Health Problems

Field researchers working with amphibians and reptiles should have some basic aseptic technique and disease prevention protocols established for the field site and species under investigation that are practical but effective. The ultimate goal should be preventing individual animal infections and spreading of disease from one individual to another within a population and, most importantly, preventing population-level disease outbreaks. A risk assessment should be conducted for each project that evaluates the appropriate level of precautions that should be taken for that specific situation.

Amphibians. Because of the permeable nature of the amphibian skin, they are very sensitive to human handling and many toxins at levels that are well tolerated without ill effects by reptiles, birds, and mammals. Soaps, lotions, and natural oils can all irritate or damage the skin. Researchers should wear powderless vinyl or plastic gloves when handling amphibians. Many of the common antiseptics and disinfectants are toxic to amphibians (e.g., surgical scrubs with soaps or detergents, iodine products, chlorhexidine, quaternary ammonium compounds, chlorine, alcohol, and ammonia). For these reasons, surgical, injection, and tag sites should be wiped clean of debris and secretions with sterile saline before the procedure (see Chapter 89).[2]

Reptiles. Depending on the procedure, the area should be cleaned at least once with a surgical scrub (betadine or chlorhexidine), followed by 70% isopropyl alcohol. For invasive surgical procedures, such as internal placement of radio transmitters, surgical preparation that repeats this process four times is recommended. Examination gloves should be worn when minor invasive procedures are performed on reptiles and should be changed between animals. Where feasible, hand washing or an alcohol-based hand disinfectant should be used between animals. Ideally, instruments such as tagging applicators, passive integrated transponder (PIT) tag injectors, and other instruments should be gas-sterilized ahead of time or used with high-level disinfection (2% accelerated hydrogen peroxide, Revital-Ox High Level Disinfectant,

TABLE 175.1   Amphibian and Reptile Capture Techniques

Sampling Method	Description	Target Organisms
Passive		
Cover objects	Untreated lumber, tin roofing, or plastic sheets placed flush with ground offer artificial cover.[84–86]	Terrestrial salamanders, snakes
Leaf litter bags	Bags made from plastic bird netting stocked with leaf litter from a stream offers substrate for aquatic salamander larvae.[87,88]	Salamanders
PVC pipe refugia	Polyvinylchloride pipes (1″–2.5″ diameter) or bamboo placed in the ground or hung vertically on trees offer artificial habitat.[89–93]	Tree frogs
Basking traps	Basking traps consist of either a wire basket anchored to an existing basking log or a floating artificial basking platform to attract turtles. Traps can be checked when the sun is high, and turtles would be expected to be basking.[94,95]	Freshwater turtles
Active		
Netting	Dip nets are effective for capturing amphibian larvae in shallow water. Seine and trammel nets can be used to capture larger amphibians and reptiles in waist-deep water.[96] Foraging sea turtles can be collected by independent fishery trawlers. Twenty-meter, four-seam nets with 20 cm mesh, without turtle excluder devices, are used by one research vessel to capture sea turtles.[97]	Larval amphibians, freshwater turtles, diamond-backed terrapins, sea turtles
Hoop traps	In streams, baited hoop traps are set with the opening pointed downstream, which allows the scent of bait to disperse downstream.[98–100] In ponds or lakes, hoop traps can be set either perpendicular or parallel to the bank, and the top of the trap should be above water to allow turtles to breathe. A fyke net extended from the open end of the trap can guide turtles into the trap.[98]	Freshwater turtles
Funnel traps	These traps come in several forms but rely on inverted funnels to direct animals into the trap. Traps may be handmade from aluminum window screen, plastic trashcans, or be commercially available, e.g., crayfish or minnow traps.[101,102] Funnel traps should be set partially submerged to safely capture air-breathing aquatic organisms.	Larval anurans, aquatic salamanders, and snakes
Pitfall traps	Pitfall (bucket) traps of different sizes can be placed flush with the ground along drift fences (see below) or at the entrance of tortoise burrows.[103] To capture tortoises, the bucket opening must be disguised with newspaper and loose sand. Pitfall traps should be shaded and checked frequently to prevent the animal from overheating.	Small amphibians and reptiles, tortoises
Drift fences	A drift fence is a barrier that directs animals toward traps and may be made from aluminum flashing, hardware cloth, or siltation fence.[104,105] Pitfall, wooden box traps,[106,107] or funnel traps[102] set at the ends or along the fence are effective for small vertebrates. Traps should be well shaded and contain a water source or wetted sponge. Pitfall traps should have drainage holes for rainfall to prevent animals from drowning.	Terrestrial and semiterrestrial amphibians and reptiles
Rod and reel, noose	A rod and reel (treble hook and fishing line) can be used to snag the animal on the osteoderms or bony scutes of the dorsum.[108] A catch pole and noose can be used for further restraint. Spotlights can be used at night to detect eyeshine for nocturnal sampling.	Crocodilians
Cage traps	One-door live cage traps (Havahart; Woodstream Corp., Lititz, PA) can be placed at the entrance of tortoise burrows.[109] The trap should be shaded and checked 2–3 times per day to prevent overheating and stress. Larger versions of these (wire or mesh) can be used to capture crocodilians.[108]	Tortoises, crocodilians
Hand capture	Many amphibians and reptiles can be captured by hand or by using snake sticks/tongs in the instance of venomous snakes. Scuba, snorkeling, and jump/catch/hand grab techniques have been used for freshwater turtles, diamond-backed terrapins, and sea turtles. Nesting female sea turtles can be sighted during nightly beach patrols and processed when she enters a trancelike state without disrupting normal nesting behavior.	Frogs, salamanders, snakes, turtles

See Norton et al.[1] for more detailed descriptions of these techniques.

Steris Corp, Mentor, OH) and sterile water rinsing between animals in the field. A review of the advantages and disadvantages of the available antiseptics and disinfectants can be found in Chapter 18. For true disinfection of instruments, an 8-minute soak time is required before use on the next animal. This precaution may not be practical in every situation; thus, the researcher will need to establish specific protocols depending on the species, potential for disease transmission, and numbers of animals being processed.

Manual Restraint, Analgesia, and Anesthesia

Many of the procedures discussed in this section can be performed with manual restraint alone. Some procedures, depending on the species,

may require local anesthesia, pain management, sedation, or general anesthesia. The research team should consult and collaborate with a veterinarian experienced with amphibians and reptiles when deciding on the implementation of appropriate protocols. Chapters 48 to 52 in this book may be consulted for details in this area.

Marking and Identification Methods

Associated risks and benefits of marking animals for later identification should be carefully considered, and the decision about whether or not to mark individuals should be based on well-conceived research questions. Where research objectives are not long term and permanent marks are not necessary, minimally invasive methods for marking and identifying

TABLE 175.2	Temporary and Semipermanent Marking Methods for Amphibians and Reptiles	
Marking Method	**Description**	**Target Organisms**
Photo identification	High-resolution digital photographs that clearly show natural patterns, anomalies, and injuries of individuals can be taken each time the animal is captured. Photographs of the pineal spot of leatherback sea turtles can be useful for later identification.[110]	Salamanders; snakes; freshwater, marine, and terrestrial turtles
Paint marking	Different color combinations and paint locations can yield numerous individual marks.[18,111–113] Care should be taken to use nontoxic paints, or nail polish, and to apply the minimum amount necessary to identify the animal.	Lizards, snakes, aquatic and terrestrial turtles
Colored beads	Small colored and numbered beads attached to the tail of crocodilians or behind the head of lizards using fishing line[114] or surgical monofilament.[115]	Crocodilians, lizards
Fluorescent polymers and tags	Fluorescent acrylic polymers (also called visible implant elastomers) can be injected into the skin of amphibians. Different injection sites, color combinations, and numbers of marks can allow for large numbers of individuals to be uniquely marked.[116] Small prenumbered fluorescent tags also can be implanted subcutaneously in amphibians.[117]	Frogs, salamanders
Tattoo	Tattooing with a battery-powered tattoo handle has been used to mark the fleshy carapace of softshell turtles as an alternative to shell notching.[118]	Softshell turtles
Claw clipping	Claws of freshwater turtles such as diamond-backed terrapin and softshell turtles may be clipped in a unique sequence to identify individuals.[119]	Freshwater turtles
External tags	Both plastic and metal tags are used to mark crocodilians and sea turtles.[120,121] However, retention of external tags is generally low due to breakage, wear, and entanglement in nets or conspecific encounters. In addition to individual marking codes, contact information can be placed on the back tags to assist with tag recoveries.[121]	Crocodilians, sea turtles

Additional details on these methods are available in Norton et al.[1]

individuals are recommended (Table 175.2). Many of the permanent marking techniques described below are performed by biologists in the field studying large populations of amphibians and reptiles. As this field evolves, veterinarians are becoming more involved and can assist biologists in making decisions about practical but appropriate techniques and where clean and sterile techniques need to be utilized. Apart from zoos and individuals of high value, these techniques are rarely indicated in clinical practice where pet reptiles are involved; however, it is helpful for veterinarians dealing with these species to be familiar with the current marking and identification practices that are performed.

Permanent Marking Methods

Passive integrated transponder tags. Passive radio frequency identification (RFID) tags (or PIT tags) are one of the most widely used and reliable tools for marking amphibians and reptiles.[3,4] A PIT tag is an electronic microchip encased in biocompatible glass that ranges in size from 8 to 22 mm long and about 2 mm in diameter; the smallest tags weigh less than 0.10 g. Tags can be purchased in preloaded sterile syringes or individually and loaded into a sterilized stainless-steel syringe for implantation. All PIT tags should be sterilized before insertion if this has not been done by the commercial source. The preferred technique for sterilization is ethylene oxide gas (STERIS Isomedix Services, Mentor, OH) or hydrogen peroxide plasma sterilization (Sterrad, Advanced Sterilization Products, Irvine, CA). Sterility should be maintained during the loading and insertion of the PIT tag. Infection rates are low provided that appropriate sterilization and site-cleaning techniques are employed.[5]

Tags are dormant until activated by a handheld reader (Fig. 175.1), which generates a close-range electromagnetic field. Each tag contains a unique alphanumeric code that allows an indefinite number of individuals to be marked. The detection range for PIT tags varies with the size of the tag and type of reader. PIT tags can be expensive when large numbers of individuals are marked but have the benefit of small size and a potentially infinite life span. In addition to marking individuals, PIT tags can be used to monitor thermoregulatory behavior and movements of animals. BioMedic Data Systems, Inc. (Seaford, DE) produces

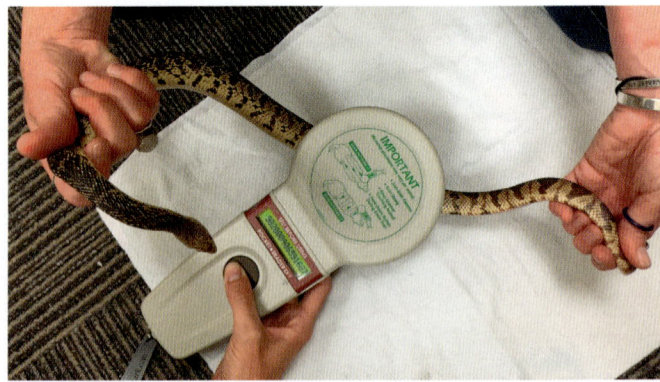

FIG 175.1 The unique alphanumeric code of a passive integrated transponder (PIT) tag is activated when scanned by a manufacturer-specific PIT tag reader. (Courtesy of L. Paden.)

temperature-sensitive PIT tags that have been used to monitor body temperature in snakes.[6,7]

PIT tags are injected most commonly under the skin, into muscle or the body cavity (Fig. 175.2). Application of tissue glue at the insertion site can help with tag retention and can control bleeding. In frogs and toads, PIT tags can be inserted subcutaneously after the area is cleaned as described earlier. For subcutaneous implantation, approximately 4 mm of skin on the ventral surface can be pinched and the tag inserted via syringe.[8] With the advent of smaller tags and insertion needles, PIT tags can now be injected in many amphibian species without the need of a surgical incision. In eastern hellbenders (*Cryptobranchus alleganiensis alleganiensis*), PIT tags were implanted successfully in the dorsal side of the tail approximately 8 cm posterior to the hind leg.[9]

In reptiles, PIT tags are generally implanted subcutaneously, although implantation sites vary by taxa. For example, in crocodilians, PIT tags can be injected subcutaneously at the junction of the ninth and tenth ventral scale rows posterior to the cloaca.[3] In lizards, PIT tags can be

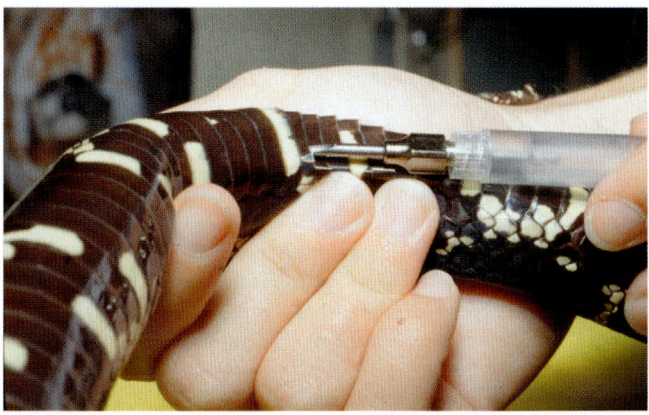

FIG 175.2 Intracoelomic injection of a passive integrated transponder (PIT) tag into an eastern king snake (*Lampropeltis getula*) with the use of a 12-gauge needle. (Courtesy of D.E. Scott.)

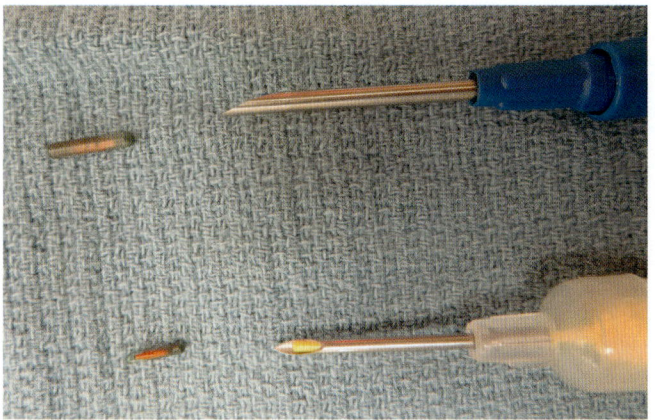

FIG 175.3 Very small passive integrated transponders (PIT) and associated syringe and needle are now available, which allows for easier placement in hatchling and small reptiles. An 8.4 mm PIT tag is shown next to a 12.5 mm PIT tag. (Courtesy of Terry M. Norton, Georgia Sea Turtle Center.)

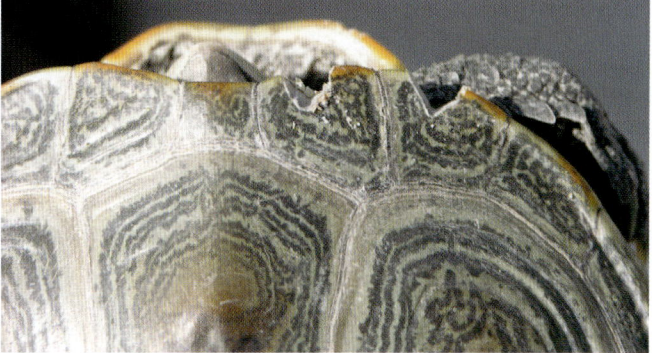

FIG 175.4 Shell marginal notched with a triangular file. (Courtesy of Terry M. Norton, Georgia Sea Turtle Center.)

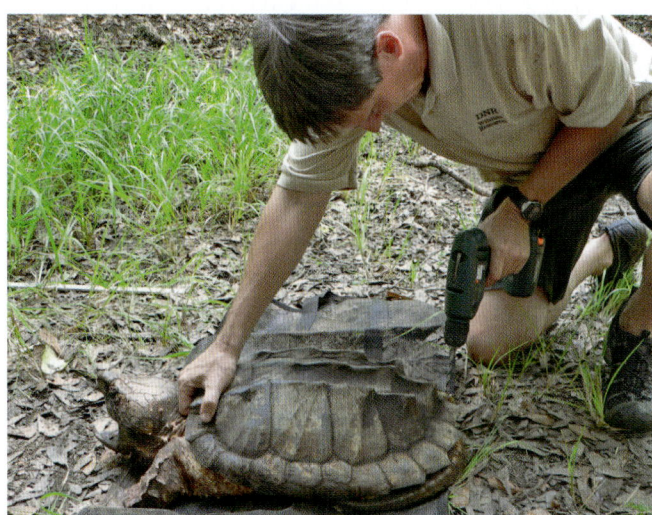

FIG 175.5 Use of a handheld drill to mark marginals on larger freshwater turtles. (Courtesy of Terry M. Norton, Georgia Sea Turtle Center.)

inserted subcutaneously on the side of the animal[10] or anterior to the left hind limb in large lizards or tuatara.[11] In snakes of all sizes, PIT tags can be implanted subcutaneously between the second and third left dorsal scale rows, approximately two-thirds of the way down the body.[4,12] They can also be inserted into the coelom (see Fig. 175.2).

PIT tags in adult freshwater turtles, terrapins, and tortoises can be injected into the loose skin at the shoulder or hind limb on either side of the body. Buhlmann and Tuberville[13] describe a method for implanting PIT tags in small aquatic turtle species such as *Sternotherus* and *Kinosternon* spp. They recommend holding the animal vertically and carefully inserting the needle above a hind limb to implant the tag adjacent and parallel to the bridge of the shell. Before the development of the 8.4 mm PIT tags, researchers had to surgically implant sterile PIT tags in hatchling and small turtles and tortoises by making a small incision into the inguinal skin just in front of the back leg. Local anesthesia or sedation was required.[1] Now the smaller PIT tags can be injected subcutaneously (Fig. 175.3). PIT tags appear to have high retention rates but may migrate from the implantation site;[3] thus, scanning the entire body for tags is recommended.

PIT tags are also commonly used to mark most species of sea turtles. Tags are placed in the left front flipper either in the triceps superficialis muscle (shoulder area) or in the flexor carpi ulnaris (posterior aspect of the flipper, anterior and immediately distal to the second large scale). Tags should not be inserted through fibropapillomas or any abnormal skin. PIT tags are generally used as a secondary marking method in sea turtles, because flipper tags are often lost.[14,15]

Shell notching and drilling. Adult turtles and tortoises can be marked permanently on the 11 to 12 marginal scales of the carapace. Marginal scales at the anterior and posterior portion of the shell are generally flared and have a thin edge that can be carefully notched using a triangular file (Fig. 175.4), cordless Dremel tool,[16] or drilled using a cordless drill with a small bit (Fig. 175.5).[17] The area to be marked should be cleaned with povidone-iodine and alcohol at least once before marking, and the file or bit should be soaked in an appropriate disinfectant between individuals.[16] Lateral marginals on the bridge connecting the carapace and plastron (scales 4–7) should not be marked because they are generally not flared and there is a risk of penetrating the body cavity.

Several different numbering or alphabetical schemes can be derived when scute notching or drilling is used, but in general, scales in each of the four quadrants of the turtle (i.e., front right, front left, rear right, rear left) are assigned a series of numbers (e.g., 1s, 10s, 100s, and 1000s) or letters, such that thousands of individuals can be uniquely marked (see Fig. 175.4).[16] Hatchling turtles can be marked with the same numeric and alphabetical system with the use of fingernail clippers to create a notch in the marginal scutes.

Drilling a hole in a marginal scale can be faster and produce a cleaner, more long-lasting mark than a notch. As a turtle grows, holes migrate toward the edge of the scale, but the mark is generally still visible. In sea turtles, the keratin layer may obscure the hole, so a flashlight can be shined beneath the shell to determine where the keratin layer extends beyond the bone. If so, the same drill pattern can simply be reapplied at the highest part of the keratin. Scale drilling provides an inexpensive alternative to PIT tagging. However, it does not work as well on sea turtles as on freshwater turtles because of their thick shells, extensive growth, and the frequency of marginal shell injury that can obscure marks.

Most chelonians tolerate notching of the shell without analgesia or sedation, but if a drill is used to create a hole in the shell, adequate sedation and analgesia is indicated. Opiates (e.g., hydromorphone, tramadol) in combination with low-dose ketamine and dexmedetomidine are good choices because they are effective, and the alpha-2 is reversible (See section 6).

Toe clipping. Historically, frogs, salamanders, lizards, and juvenile crocodilians were often marked by removal of toes or toe clipping.[18,19] There is some controversy about the level of pain produced by this procedure and whether analgesia or sedation should be used when toe clipping is performed.[2] When large numbers of animals are processed, it may be impractical to provide such intensive care. Researchers using this technique should keep this in mind and consider seeking alternative identification methods when available, and although acceptable if approved under an institutional animal care and use committee, it is never acceptable in clinical practice. The advantage of toe clipping is the low cost and large numbers of unique marks available if individual digits and limbs are assigned a different series of numbers. A single toe can also be removed as a basic cohort mark if unique identification of an individual is not necessary for the research objectives. Excised toes can be preserved in ethanol for genetic analysis or skeletochronology.[20,21]

To facilitate recognition of a toe-clip mark versus a natural injury, researchers can remove multiple toes on different feet. Removal of adjacent toes should be avoided. The thumbs of adult male frogs, which are used in amplexus, should never be removed, nor should more than two digits on any one limb be removed. Stainless steel toenail scissors can be used and toes should be excised at a slight angle. Scissors should be disinfected with an appropriate product before use and between animals. A drop of tissue glue can be used to stop the bleeding. In addition to pain from the procedure, there is concern that toe clipping may affect survival of individuals. Studies have shown that the number of toes clipped may negatively affect frog survival,[22] particularly in arboreal species (e.g., tree frogs, *Hyla* spp.). However, a laboratory study on squirrel tree frogs (*Hyla squirella*) found no difference in growth and survival after toe clipping.[23] Many salamanders and some frogs can regenerate toes quickly; thus, the reliability of the method is further limited. Both toe clips and injectable fluorescent polymers (Table 29.2) have been used to mark individual amphibians;[24] the advantage of using both methods is increased reliability in identifying individuals over time, although the effects of such invasive marking methods on behavior and long-term survival are not known.[25]

Toe clipping is more effective in lizards and juvenile crocodilians than in amphibians because their toes do not regenerate. However, the technique may have negative effects on behavior of arboreal lizards, which have subdigital toe pads for clinging to vegetation.[26] In contrast, a number of studies have demonstrated that toe clipping does not affect sprint speed, which is a measure of fitness in terrestrial lizards.[27–29] The frequency of natural toe loss in lizards has been used as further evidence that toe clipping in lizards is unlikely to influence survival,[30] yet natural toe loss can preclude recognition of toe clips.[31] Although the technique has been used with juvenile American alligators (*Alligator mississippiensis*), natural toe loss from conspecific interactions is frequent and can reduce accuracy and detectability in recaptures. The authors recommend alternative methods for marking juvenile crocodilians and large lizards (see Table 175.2); however, toe clipping (as described previously) is an inexpensive method for marking small amphibians and reptiles (e.g., tree frogs and small lizards) for short-term studies requiring identification of individuals. Again, it is considered unacceptable in clinical practice.

Scale clipping. Scale clipping is an inexpensive technique that is frequently used to mark snakes. Removal of the scale, with small, sharp, sterile scissors, leaves a scar that persists after shedding, and the marks can be accurately read for many years. The method was originally described for subcaudal scales,[32] but Brown and Parker presented a marking system using ventral scales,[33] which are larger and easier to remove than subcaudals.[34] Depending on the numbering system, the entire scale can be removed, or the left or right half of the ventral scale can be removed.[33] Application of tissue glue or New Skin can prevent excessive bleeding. This technique can be used on snakes of all sizes, but fewer scales should be removed and smaller scissors may be required for neonates or small snake species. Local anesthesia with lidocaine (2%; Butler Animal Health Supply, Dublin, OH) or bupivacaine (0.5%, Pfizer, Inc., New York, NY) can provide adequate analgesia for this procedure. A nonsteroidal antiinflammatory drug such as meloxicam may provide postprocedure analgesia.

Scute clipping. Tail scute clipping is one of the more common, affordable, and persistent methods of marking crocodilians. Detectability of clipped tail scutes is reduced slightly with juveniles because of their accelerated growth rates, but overall this technique is the most efficient in terms of ease of application and the ability to identify large numbers of individuals of all age classes.[31] Enumeration systems vary and can consist of numeric or alphabetical ordering. Both left and right sides of dorsal scutes can be incorporated, in addition to tail scutes, to increase the number of potential marks. A sterilized utility knife (X-Acto, Elmer's Products, Inc., Columbus, OH) can be useful for making a clean cut in the least amount of time. Preferably, a fresh, sterile blade will be used on each individual, as dull blades will result in multiple cuts to mark the animal, thereby increasing handling time and stress. The tail scute must be removed down into the muscle; the cut should be made just below where the scales merge with the adjoining scales (Fig. 175.6). If the scute clipping is performed properly, a small amount of bleeding will occur, which indicates that the mark will truly be permanent. Appropriate aseptic technique, as described earlier, should be used. Local anesthesia with lidocaine or bupivacaine will provide appropriate analgesia but is difficult to administer because of the tight skin and lack of subcutaneous tissue.

Branding. Heat branding is a fast, affordable, and straightforward method for marking snakes and is similar mechanically to scale clipping in that it removes the scale tissue. Although the method was originally

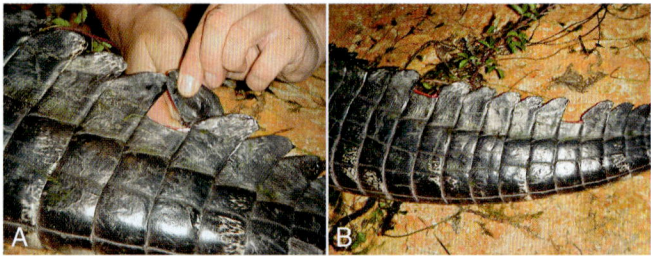

FIG 175.6 (A) Removal of a dorsal scute from the tail of an American alligator (*Alligator mississippiensis*). (B) Completed pattern of a double clip on an American alligator tail. (Courtesy of C. Hagen.)

described as a method to mark amphibians and reptiles,[35] it is most appropriate for use with snakes.[36] Disposable medical cautery units can be used to brand individual scales in patterns similar to those recommended for scale clipping;[37] however, the brands should also be applied to four to five lateral scales that correspond to the marked ventral scales to differentiate between marks and scars from natural injuries (Fig. 175.7). Cautery tips will last longer if overhanging scale material is trimmed off on keeled-scale snakes before branding. High and low temperature settings are available on some cautery units; the low temperature units setting should be used with neonates or small snake species. This technique has been used successfully on a broad array of snake species, both neonates and adults.[37]

Freeze branding, which alters the pigmentation of the scales, has also been used to mark lizards, snakes, and crocodilians. Freeze branding can be achieved with dry ice, ethyl alcohol, or liquid halocarbon (Freon) applied to the skin with a round-tipped copper wire or a synthetic

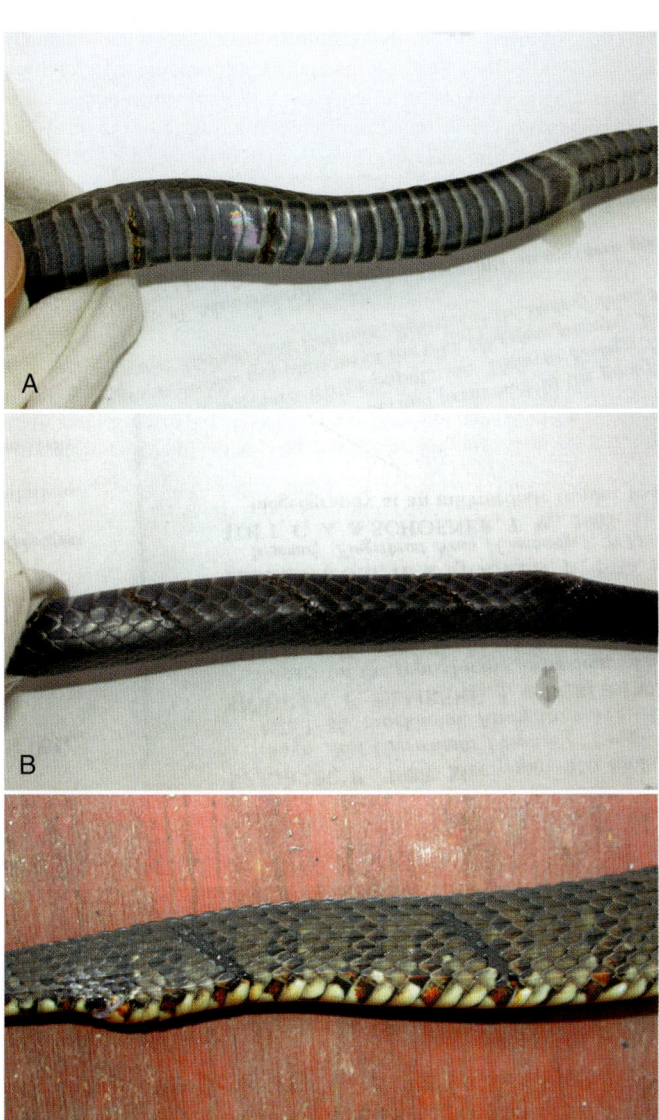

FIG 175.7 (A) Ventral scale pattern after heat branding on a black racer (*Coluber constrictor*). This image displays code 146 (anal plate is skipped). (B) Lateral scale pattern after heat branding for the same individual code as in (A). (C) Image of healed lateral marks from heat branding on a banded water snake (*Nerodia fasciata*). (Courtesy of J.D. Willson.)

sponge-tipped dowel for 20 to 30 seconds.[38] Freeze branding has several shortcomings over heat branding. The marks are more difficult to apply in the field and are variable depending on the original color pattern of the animal and can be difficult to read.

Cohort marks. Magnetized wire tags were used historically to mark large numbers of sea turtles but cannot be used to differentiate individuals unless used in conjunction with another marking technique.[39] Wire tags are typically placed in foreflippers[40] and require a magnetometer for field identification. They are less expensive than PIT tags, have high retention rates (95%–100%),[41] and appear to be effective for the lifetime of the animal.[42] However, the disadvantage of this technique is that magnetometers can be expensive and may detect false-positive animals if there are other magnetic components in the area of the animal,[40] and therefore are no longer a common practice for sea turtles. However, there is potential for this technique to be used for batch marking in other taxa.

Living tags have been used to identify cohorts or year classes of hatchling and juvenile sea turtles[43–45] by applying the mark to different scutes to represent different year classes.[39,46] Living tags are created by autografting a piece of light-colored plastron tissue into a darker scute on the carapace.[40] Grafts can be obtained with the use of a surgical biopsy punch and can be secured with surgical glue.[44] Tags grow with the turtle and appear as spots or streaks in older individuals. It does take a trained eye to identify a mark, particularly on adults that received the tags as hatchlings.

TELEMETRY

The purpose of this section is to introduce some basic principles of telemetry and describe techniques (e.g., VHF, GPS, satellite, biotelemetry, archival data recorders) that have worked well for the authors and other researchers; an exhaustive review of the literature will not be provided due to the rapid rate of change and increased application with these technologies. Amphibians and reptiles are difficult animals to study because they are often cryptic and wary. They can spend considerable periods of time submerged in water or below ground and often live in habitats that are inaccessible to researchers. The ongoing advancement and miniaturization of electronic tagging technology has provided the means to effectively study these animals in the wild with minimal disturbance.[47] In addition, data on physiological function (e.g., heart rate, body temperature, and feeding habits) may be collected. Telemetry refers to an active transmission of data coming from an animal, with the objective of remotely collecting data on an animal's location, behavior and physiology, and characteristics of the environment.[36] Acoustic, electric, magnetic, and electromagnetic (e.g., visible light, radio wave, and microwave) forms of energy can be used to transmit data.[36]

The most commonly used spatial technology for herpetofauna is radio telemetry, which utilizes high-frequency radio waves. The equipment to conduct radio telemetry studies includes a transmitter, a power source (e.g., battery), and a transmitting antenna, all of which must be attached to the animal. Transmitter packages can be externally attached through a variety of methods or surgically implanted internally. Radio signals are detected by receiving antennae, which can be handheld, positioned on land at specific locations, or carried via vehicles, ships, planes, or satellites.[36] Satellite telemetry, including GPS, enables information to be relayed from the transmitter to a receiver via satellites. Biotelemetry refers to the transmission of biological information from sensors on the animal, without direct contact between the transmitter and receiver. Internal physiological data such as heart rate, body temperature, or electrocardiographic results; behavioral data such as diving time and depth; and environmental information such as ambient temperature, light, or salinity can all be relayed. Archival data recorders are self-contained biotelemetric units that collect and archive data for later recovery. This technology allows for researchers to gather information on wide-ranging (e.g., sea turtles) or secretive species that would otherwise be difficult or impossible to study. A wide range of designs, sizes, and methods of application allow for study of a variety of species and are now available for customization through a variety of manufacturers (http://www.telonics.com/wildlife.php, https://atstrack.com/).

Disadvantages and limitations of this technology include (1) high cost and complexity of use, (2) battery capacity and size limitations on transmission longevity and strength, and (3) the physical presence of the device may affect the animal's behavior or that of a conspecific. Internal implantation of transmitter packages requires anesthesia and surgery. Attachment and retention of the transmitter package often presents many challenges. In most instances, transmitting devices should eventually detach from the animal or be removed, which may require recapture and potentially another surgery. Recovery of archival recorders is required to retrieve data, which may also necessitate recapture and even another surgery.

The researcher should select a transmitter package and attachment method appropriate to the animal. The general rule of thumb is that a transmitter package (i.e., battery, transmitter, and antenna) should not exceed 5% of the animal's body mass,[34] and the attachment and placement should not impede the animal's movements, physiology, reproductive success, and survival. Trade-offs between transmitter attachment methods and transmitter weight, transmitter longevity, and transmission range should be determined to optimize performance so that the particular study's objectives can be met.

Radio Telemetry: Nonsurgical Placement

Amphibians. Telemetry placement in amphibians is complicated by their generally small body size and sensitive skin. Most manufacturers can configure a transmitter based on the body size and life history of the focal species. However, projected battery life of the transmitter is limited by battery size, so small transmitters may need to be refurbished with a fresh battery or replaced frequently (every 1–2 weeks to up to 3 months, depending on the size of the transmitter package). Transmitters may be attached externally to frogs with the use of belts or harnesses lined with small beads to prevent abrasion of the skin (Fig. 175.8). The belt must have enough slack to prevent wear on the skin but must be tight enough to prevent the animal from jumping out of the harness or becoming entangled. For external transmitter placement, the antenna is loose and will trail behind the animal (Fig. 175.9). Because of the

body shape and fossorial habit of many salamanders, external attachment of transmitters is generally not used (see the following section on surgical placement of radio transmitters).

Reptiles

Crocodilians. Methods for acquisition and monitoring of behavioral and physiological variables from free-ranging crocodilians through the use of data loggers and via radio, satellite, and acoustic telemetry have been described.[48–51] Radio telemetry has been most widely used to track the movement patterns of crocodilians in addition to body temperatures and heart rates. Measuring body temperature via radio telemetry requires that the transmitter be located internally either via ingestion[52] or by surgical implantation into the coelomic cavity.[53,54] The nuchal shield has been most commonly used as the site for external transmitter attachment. This placement allows the antenna to come out of the water each time the animal surfaces.

In the American alligator, transmitter placement can be conducted in the field at the time of capture in the span of 45 to 60 minutes. The alligator is moved to a shady location to reduce stress and manually restrained. After the alligator is manually restrained, the right forelimb is cleaned with alcohol and an injection of Ketoprofen, a nonsteroidal antiinflammatory drug, is administered at a dosage of 0.2 mL/10 kg (2 mg/kg, 100 mg/mL vial) IM. The body mass of the alligator is estimated based on body length and girth data. The nuchal shield is then cleaned using three alternating applications of povidone-iodine scrub and alcohol. After cleaning, a 22-gauge needle is used to make multiple injections of a local anesthetic, lidocaine, subcutaneously in the area surrounding the nuchal shield at a maximum dose of 2.5 mL/10 kg (5 mg/kg, 20 mg/mL, typically 3 syringes with 1.5 mL of lidocaine and 1.5 mL of sodium bicarbonate will be used). The site is then again prepared with two applications of povidone-iodine scrub and alcohol. At least 10 minutes will be given to allow lidocaine to take effect before drilling. Four small holes are drilled with a sterilized drill bit into the nuchal scutes. Sterilized galvanized steel wire is threaded through the holes and secured to the transmitter through four loops on the side of the transmitter

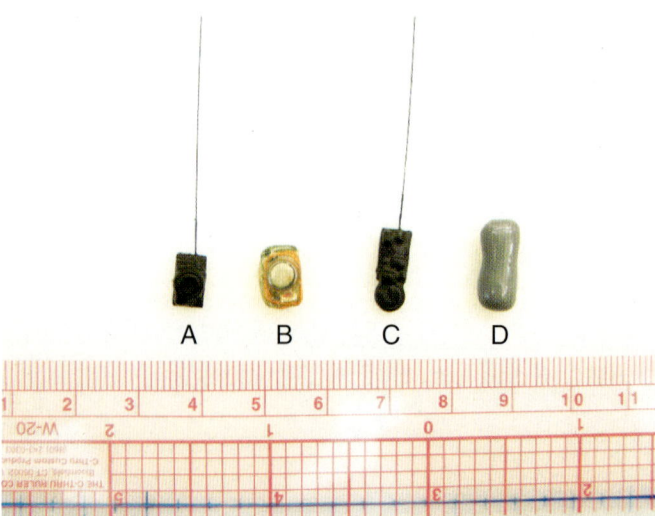

FIG 175.9 Different configurations for small radio transmitters used in amphibians. (A) The transmitter has the battery mounted on top with a free-hanging antenna. (B) The transmitter has the antenna coiled around the battery, and the entire package is encapsulated in acrylic for implantation into the body cavity. (C) The transmitter has the battery mounted at the end of the transmitter, creating a longer but thinner package, also with a free-hanging antenna. (D) A fully encapsulated transmitter with the same configuration as in (C). (Courtesy of Lora Smith.)

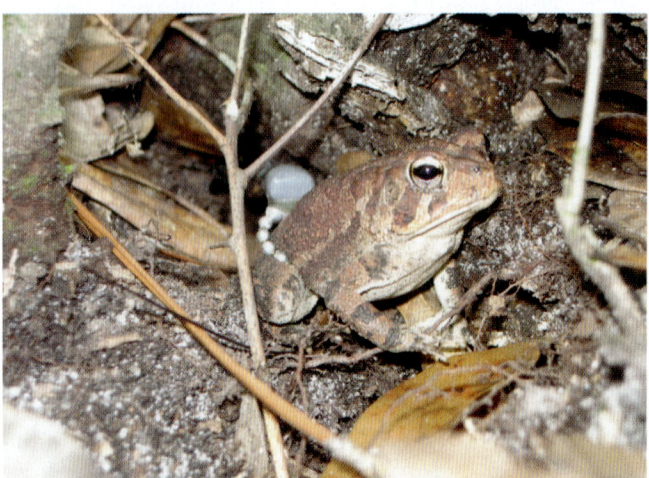

FIG 175.8 Southern toad (*Anaxyrus terrestris*) with belt attachment of a radio transmitter package. (Courtesy of S. Sterrett.)

(Fig. 175.10). Finally, a marine-grade epoxy (J-B Weld WaterWeld Epoxy Putty, Sulfur Springs, TX) is placed around the transmitter to increase transmitter retention time. To camouflage the device, dried epoxy is covered either in dirt or nontoxic paint.

Satellite telemetry has also been used successfully to study long-range movements of estuarine crocodiles (*Crocodylus porosus*).[49] Before attachment of the device, the area around the nuchal shield is surgically prepared after administration of a local anesthetic. Two holes are drilled into each of four scutes in the nuchal shield. A KiwiSat 101 transmitter is attached to the scutes with the use of plastic-coated stainless-steel wire threaded through the drill holes in the scute and then through four steel loops on the sides of the transmitter and fastened with lead crimps (Fig. 175.11). Fifty percent of the animals sent signals for more than 10 months, and four sent signals for more than 15 months.[49]

Archival tags (data loggers) have been used to record diving behaviors, fine-scale movement patterns, and heart rates of crocodilians.[55] Large volumes of data can be stored within these tags and downloaded at a later time. The greatest challenge with this technology is retrieving the tags, which requires additional technologies (e.g., radio telemetry or satellite telemetry) to locate the tag or animal. The tags float and can be designed with a time-release mechanism.[1] Franklin and colleagues describe a technique using a tag and transmitter encased in a neoprene sleeve that incorporated a polystyrene float (Fig. 175.12).[50] Manual restraint and a local anesthetic were used to place the tag. Holes were drilled through the center of four scutes to align with wires from the data package. The wires were threaded through the holes in a manner that minimized any loops of wire being exposed so that the telemetry package would not become snagged. Plastic-coated wire was secured with crimp sleeves.

Lizards. Radio telemetry has been used to study aspects of behavior and spatial ecology in a variety of lizard species, including the beaded lizard (*Heloderma horridum*), Gila monster (*Heloderma suspectum*), Yarrow's spiny lizard (*Sceloporus jarrovi*), lace monitor (*Varanus varius*), southern alligator lizard (*Eligaria multicarinata*), land mullet skink (*Egernia major*), eastern bearded dragon (*Pogona barbata*),[56] and water dragon (*Physignathus lesueurii*).[57] Goodman reviewed a variety of telemetry techniques that have been used in West Indian iguanas (*Cyclura* spp.), including ingested transmitters; transmitters externally applied with duct tape; suture of transmitters to the dorsal crest (Fig. 175.13); transmitter collars, belts, and harnesses (Fig. 175.14); and use of various adhesives to attach transmitters.[56] The signal range did not differ dramatically between most methods but did differ across habitats and among transmitter models, especially in relation to free antenna length.

An additional consideration is the trade-off between signal strength and battery life. Different researchers using the same model of transmitter may select reduced signal strength to increase battery life if the focal species is not wide-ranging; thus, there is substantial variation in signal range and battery life among research projects.[56] Knapp and Owens[58] conducted radio telemetry on hatchling Andros Iguanas (*Cyclura cychlura cychlura*) by placing transmitters on the dorsal side of the pelvic girdle with test monofilament line wrapped around the lizard's body to secure it. This method may also be useful for hatchlings and small lizards of other species.

A harness to attach radio transmitters to water dragons was made by cutting a sheet of nylon mesh or fly screen in the shape of a square with two extending straps.[57] Cutting the square and straps to fit the individual lizard is critical; if they are too large, it may get caught on vegetation, and if too small, it may cause discomfort or abrasions to the skin. The radio transmitter was glued to the harness with adhesive (Super Glue; Super Glue Corp., Rancho Cucamonga, CA) before attaching the harness to the animal. The square part of the harness was placed firmly on the lizard's back above the forearms, while the straps were then pulled over the shoulders, crossed on the chest, and pulled up under the lizard's forearms. After pulling the straps snug, they were adhered to the square with cyanoacylate glue (Super Glue) and to one

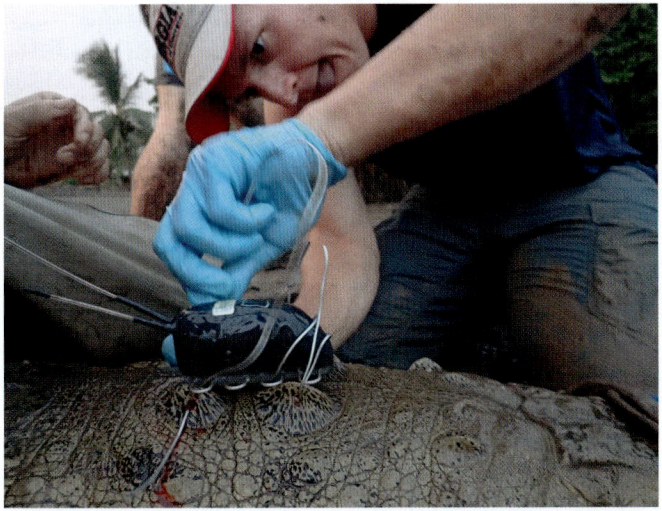

FIG 175.10 Satellite transmitter placed between the nuchal scutes in an American alligator (*Alligator mississippiensis*) using sterilized galvanized steel wire threaded through the holes and secured to the transmitter through four loops on the side of the transmitter. (Courtesy of Kimberly M. Andrews.)

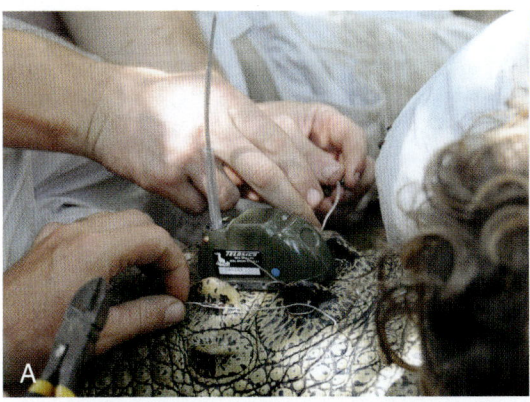
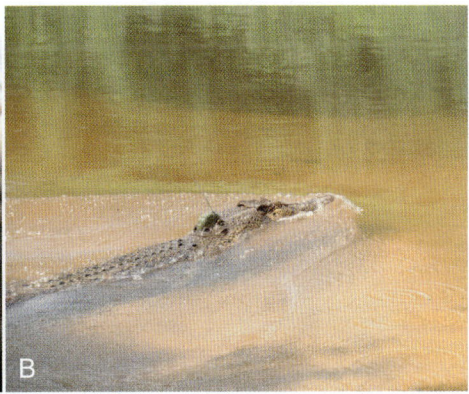

FIG 175.11 (A) Satellite/GPS tag being attached to the nuchal scutes of an estuarine crocodile (*Crocodylus porosus*). (B) Satellite/GPS tag attached to the nuchal scutes of a 2.8-m female saltwater crocodile (*Crocodylus porosus*). (Courtesy of C.E. Franklin.)

another where they crossed on the cranial coelom. The mesh was held together at glue points with forceps. The harness was easily removed by cutting the straps with scissors. Water dragons were monitored for up to 2 months without any harness losses or any noticeable problems for the lizards.

Snakes. Radio or GPS transmitters can be attached externally to snakes to collect short-term movement data.[59,60] The method is ideal for use with juvenile snakes or small-bodied species.[61] Transmitters

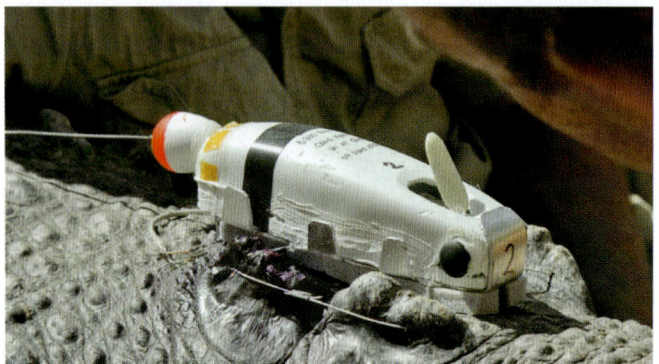

FIG 175.12 Data logger (archival tag) with self-release device attached to the nuchal scutes of an estuarine crocodile (*Crocodylus porosus*). The data logger recorded water depth, acceleration in three dimensions, compass bearing, speed, and body temperature. (Courtesy of C.E. Franklin.)

should be attached dorsolaterally, approximately two-thirds of the snout-to-vent length behind the head with cyanoacylate glue (Fig. 175.15). Transmitters are typically shed during ecdysis and can be retrieved for use on another animal. In rattlesnakes, devices can be attached to the rattle using epoxy and suture material (Fig. 175.16). These transmitters are particularly helpful to use when a snake is waiting for surgical implantation of a radio transmitter. This way the snake can be maintained in a free-ranging state until a surgery can be planned.

Freshwater turtles, terrapins, and tortoises. The predominant way transmitters have been attached to turtles is by mounting the tag onto the carapace. Different techniques have varying levels of success depending on the life history traits, age, and size of the study animals (Fig. 175.17). Boarman and collegues[62] reviewed 113 scientific papers, reports, and semitechnical articles on radio tracking projects regarding turtles with transmitters attached to the carapace by a variety of methods, including epoxy, silicone sealant, dental acrylic, and other types of adhesives. Additionally, there were descriptions of transmitters being strapped on with harnesses or attached via bolts, wire, cable, or nylon ties or with monofilament line, which was passed through holes drilled into the posterior carapace or marginal scutes. In these cases, the transmitter was either attached to the carapace or allowed to trail behind the turtles.

Although there needs to be further research evaluating the effects of transmitters on study animals,[61] there are many possible behavioral (e.g., mating disruptions) and physical problems that can be caused by improper transmitter placement. Shell deformities occurred on hatchling

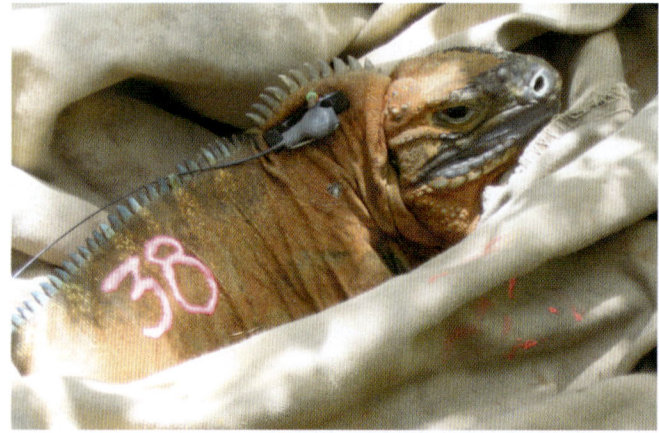

FIG 175.13 A Jamaican iguana (*Cyclura collei*) with radio transmitter sutured to the dorsal crest. (Courtesy of Tandora Grant.)

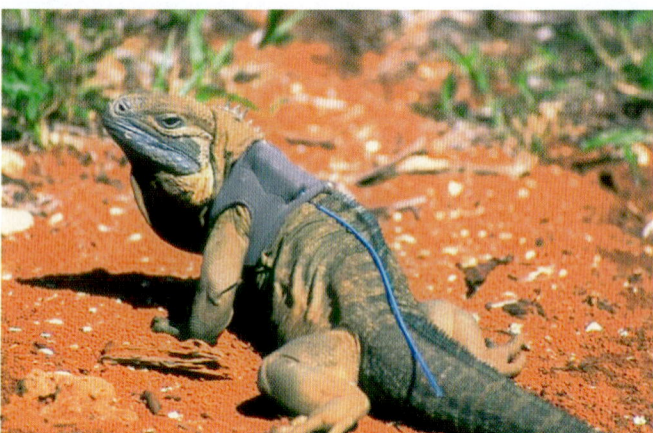

FIG 175.14 A Jamaican iguana (*Cyclura collei*) fitted with a harness transmitter. (Courtesy of Rick Hudson.)

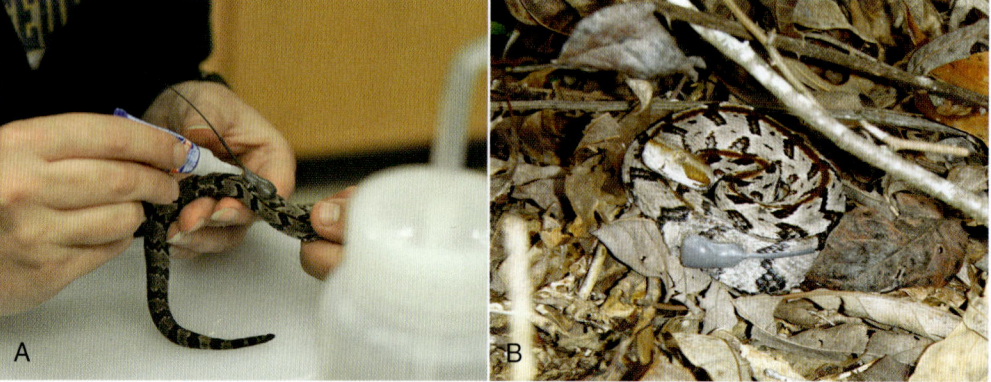

FIG 175.15 (A and B) External attachment of a radio transmitter to a neonate timber rattlesnake (*Crotalus horridus*). (Courtesy of E.M. Schlimm.)

gopher tortoises (*Gopherus polyphemus*) because the epoxy holding transmitters encroached on growth areas,[63] an issue of substantial concern with young, growing animals in particular. Also, transmitters may become entangled in vegetation, usually among gaps between the shell and the transmitter or the antenna. Lastly, transmitters may attract the attention of predators and humans and therefore should be camouflaged in some way (Fig. 175.18). Boarman and colleagues recommended a process for transmitter placement in desert tortoises (*Gopherus agassizii*) that is applicable to other nonmarine turtles:[62]

1. Test the transmitter to confirm that it is functional.
2. Clean dirt off the carapace.
3. Preposition the transmitter to first left or right coastal (pleural) scute and fit as flush to the carapace as possible.
4. To position the antenna, cut short sections of flexible 3 mm plastic tubing and attach each section to the first four vertebral scutes using epoxy. Each section should be cut slightly shorter than its associated scute. Cyanoacrylate glue can be used to hold each section of tubing in place while quick-drying, pliable epoxy putty (nonexothermic that does not heat up) is spread over each section of tubing in a continuous layer from the scute on the side of the tube to the scute surface on the opposite side of the tube. Avoid getting any epoxy on the scute sutures or neighboring scutes to allow for shell growth.
5. Place the antenna through the tube sections leaving approximately 50 to 120 mm hanging loose beyond the posterior of the animal.
6. Attach the transmitter with epoxy putty, using care not to bridge the scute margins and leaving no spaces between the transmitter and the carapace to get caught in vegetation.

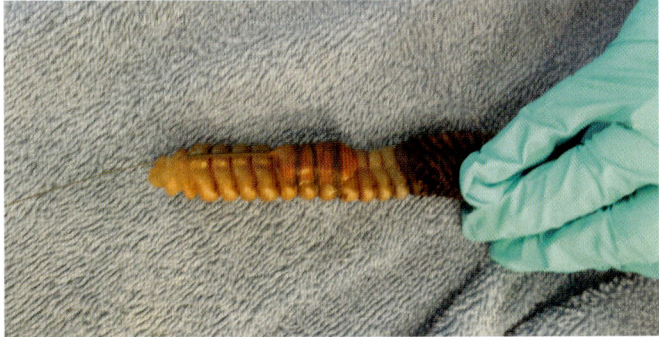

FIG 175.16 A small radiotransmitter is attached to the rattle of an eastern diamondback rattlesnake *(Crotalus adamanteus)* using epoxy and suture material. (Courtesy of Terry M. Norton, Georgia Sea Turtle Center.)

7. Paint the transmitter and putty to reduce reflectivity and contrast and to protect the camouflage capabilities of the animal to reduce predation risk.

In addition to these points, the transmitter placement site should be disinfected, as described earlier in the chapter. The transmitter should not be applied to an abnormal part of the shell (e.g., deformation or site of infection). The carapace can be roughened slightly with sandpaper or a rotary tool (e.g., Dremel) before the epoxy is applied. The authors have had success with using a marine epoxy putty for the initial attachment of the transmitter and then coating it with a liquid epoxy (Power-Fast+, Fast Set Formula; Powers Fasteners, Inc. Brewster, NY). The epoxy putty alone may be successful for securing devices to terrestrial and aquatic turtles and crocodilians, but it is recommended that liquid epoxy be used in most marine turtle species. A digital, distant-laser thermal monitoring device (Raynger ST; Raytek Corporation, Santa Cruz, CA) should be used to make sure exothermic epoxy does not rise above 37.8°C (100°F) during the curing process. If necessary, the area can be sprayed with cool water. In immature growing turtles, it is important not to cross scute suture lines to avoid interfering with the growth of the shell. Hatchling and juvenile tortoises can be radio tracked using small, lightweight radio transmitters attached to the costal scutes with silicon aquarium sealant. This sealant is readily removed without damaging the shell of the tortoise.

Bolts and other fasteners can be used to attach radio transmitters to the carapace of aquatic turtles.[57] A surgical preparation and sterile technique should be used in this procedure, because it requires drilling through the bone of the shell. Transmitter packages with aluminum plates with holes at either end for attachment and whip antennae are available through several manufacturers (e.g., Model A1–2F, Holohil, LTD., Ontario, Canada; Model MOD-125, Telonics, Inc., Mesa, AZ). The preferred site of attachment is on top of the posterior marginal scutes and underlying the peripheral bones of the carapace, typically in a region above one of the hind limbs.[58] Attachment at this site is less likely to create drag or impede movement through substrate or vegetation. The most posterior scute should not be used because it will likely interfere with mating behavior. It is important to preplace the transmitter on the shell to mark the spots to be drilled and to assess how the transmitter fits in relation to the curvature of the shell. If necessary, a small amount of epoxy can be used to create a flat surface for attachment. Holes drilled too close to the outside edge may break down from wear, allowing the fastener to slip, and holes drilled too close to the scute seams often result in excessive bleeding. For pig-nosed turtles (*Carettochelys insculpta*), the epoxy was replaced with neoprene strips cut to the size of the

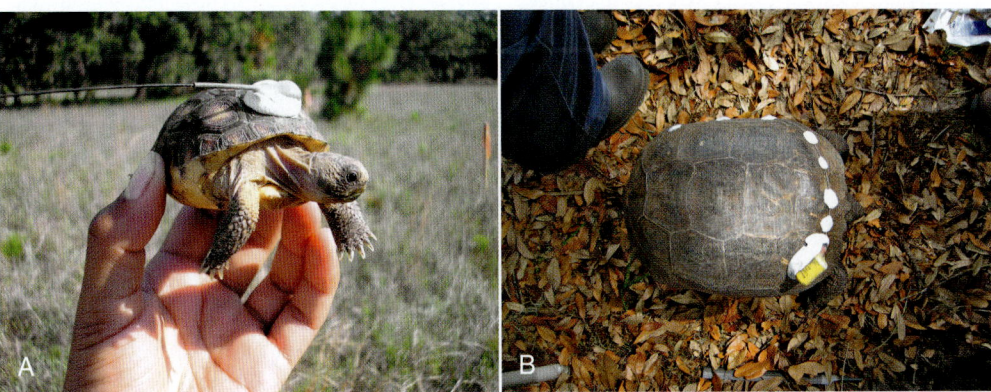

FIG 175.17 (A) Juvenile gopher tortoise (*Gopherus polyphemus*) with radio transmitter on carapace. (B) Adult gopher tortoise with radio transmitter on carapace. (A, Courtesy of T.D. Tuberville, University of Georgia's Savannah River Ecology Laboratory; B, courtesy of Terry M. Norton, Georgia Sea Turtle Center.)

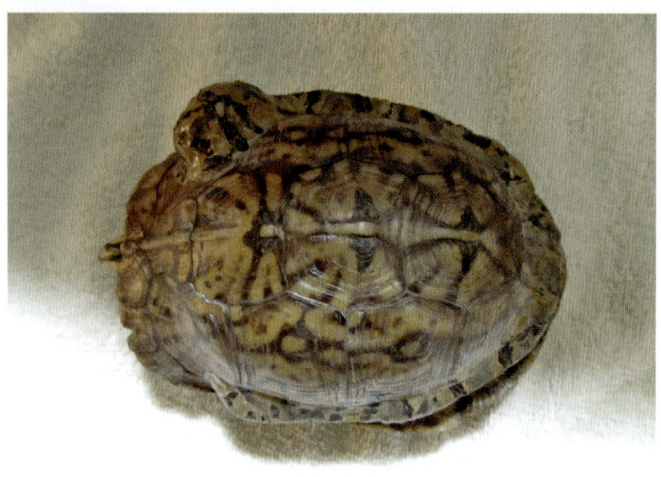

FIG 175.18 Radio transmitter and wrapped antenna that has been painted to camouflage the equipment on an eastern box turtle (*Terrapene carolina*). (Courtesy of J.E. Colbert.)

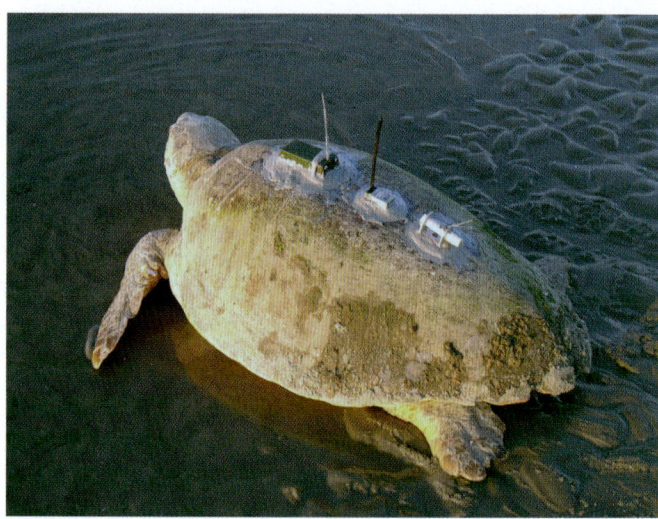

FIG 175.19 Loggerhead sea turtle (*Caretta caretta*) with satellite, sonic, and radio transmitters on carapace. (Courtesy of M. Dodd.)

transmitter, which softened the pressure of the transmitter against the shell. Additionally, pig-nosed turtles have no scutes, so it was critical to ensure that the holes were drilled on or near the seams between the marginal bones, which are clearly visible beneath the skin in this species. Tags were attached with stainless steel bolts and locking nuts threaded with nylon to prevent loosening and corrosion-resistant metal backing plates. The nut should be on top (transmitter side) to allow full leg movement and prevent abrasion of the skin on the legs. Gaps between the tag and the shell were filled with epoxy putty to prevent debris and vegetation from becoming entangled.

Sea turtles. Satellite telemetry has been used most extensively to study long-term, large spatial movements and activities of sea turtles and estuarine crocodiles. This technique is especially important in the marine environment, where very high-frequency (VHF) signals are greatly attenuated and distances to be covered are usually large.[64] The primary disadvantage of this technology is the cost of the transmitters and satellite time.

Most published sea turtle tracking research has focused on postnesting females because of their accessibility. For example, a study was conducted on the Georgia coast to evaluate internesting intervals and postnesting migratory behavior in female loggerhead sea turtles (*Caretta caretta*) (Scott JA, unpublished data, 2006). In this study, a variety of methodologies including acoustic, radio, and satellite telemetry were used to evaluate short- and long-term movement patterns, nest-site fidelity, and interactions with shrimp trawl fishery (Fig. 175.19).

Until recently, very limited information was available on the spatial ecology of male loggerhead sea turtles during the breeding season. Arendt and colleagues evaluated the movement and diving patterns of resident and migrant adult male loggerhead sea turtles during the breeding season in Cape Canaveral, Florida,[65] and after dispersal postbreeding.[66]

A variety of satellite attachment techniques have been used in sea turtles, including tethering of buoyant transmitter housing to the posterior end of the shell, attachment of "backpack-style" transmitters to the anterior vertebral scute with fiberglass cloth and polyester resin, fiberglass filler, two-part epoxy/putty, and combinations of these techniques.[67] Retention time of satellite tags has been and continues to be problematic. Integration of antifouling paints and an alternative adhesive, steel-reinforced epoxy putty (Sonic-Weld, Ed Greene & Co, Tallahassee, FL)[69] has increased retention time.[68]

The GSTC has utilized this technology to track rehabilitated loggerhead sea turtles after release (Fig. 175.20). Satellite placement techniques have been similar to those previously described,[70] except that the transmitter is partially covered with epoxy with only the saltwater switches exposed (Fig. 175.21). A laser temperature gun is used to monitor the temperature of the epoxy; when it reaches 37.8°C (100°F), water is used to reduce temperature. Although these transmitters could theoretically last for 3 years, data collection for more than 1 year has been rare, most likely because of physical damage to the antennae or transmitters and/or biological fouling of the saltwater switch sensor.

Radio Telemetry: Surgical Placement

Only healthy animals should be selected for surgical radio telemetry placement. The signal strength and frequency of the transmitter provided by the manufacturer should be verified with a receiver before placement in the animal to avoid implanting a nonfunctioning transmitter. Surgical procedures should be conducted during the appropriate time of year so that surgical sites can heal adequately. Anesthesia and procedures should be conducted by a veterinarian with extensive surgical experience with herpetofauna. Arrangements can be made with local human hospitals, veterinary schools, or other specialty facilities if this is not available to the researcher. The benefits far outweigh the costs. Although not ideal, individuals without a veterinary degree will likely continue to conduct surgeries following IACUC approval. At a minimum, these individuals should receive specialized training in anesthesia, surgery, and sterile techniques and have close consultation with an experienced veterinarian.

All telemetry devices and data loggers should be sterilized with either ethylene oxide gas or hydrogen peroxide plasma sterilization before surgical implantation, as previously described for PIT tags. High-level (cold) disinfection is inadequate and not recommended.

General Guidelines for Amphibian Surgery. In general, because of their size, many amphibians are not well suited for internal placement of telemetry packages. Internal placement of radio telemetry had been described for large frogs[71,72] and salamanders (e.g., tiger salamanders [*Ambystoma tigrinum*] and spotted salamanders [*Ambystoma maculatum*],[73] and the eastern hellbender[9]). Presurgical preparation of the

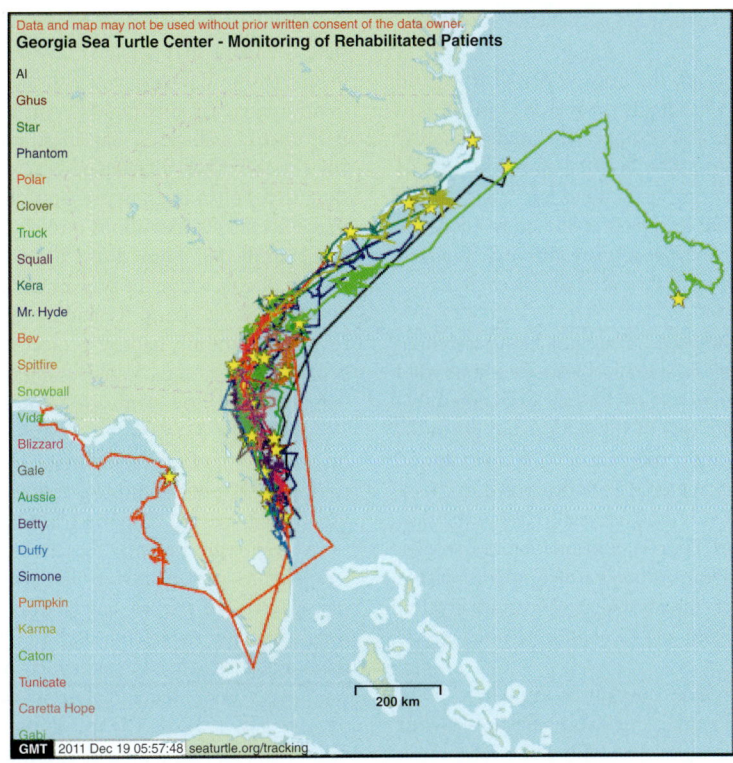

FIG 175.20 Satellite tracks of rehabilitated sea turtles released by the Georgia Sea Turtle Center. (Courtesy of Terry M. Norton, Georgia Sea Turtle Center.)

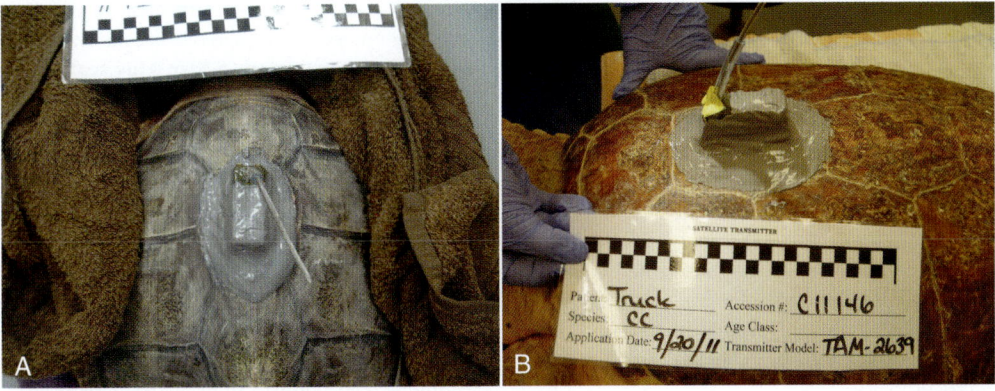

FIG 175.21 (A and B) Satellite transmitter placed on a loggerhead sea turtle (*Caretta caretta*) carapace. (Courtesy of Terry M. Norton, Georgia Sea Turtle Center.)

patient includes ensuring good hydration and electrolyte balance by soaking the animal in a shallow water bath for 60 minutes before surgery. The amphibian can be weighed preoperatively and postoperatively to monitor hydration. The amphibian should be fasted before surgery for a minimum of 4 hours.[74] Appropriate analgesia and anesthesia should be used for internal transmitter placement and other invasive and potentially painful procedures. Although other anesthetic options are available, buffered tricaine methanesulfonate (MS-222; Argent Chemical Laboratories, Inc., Redmond, WA) has been used widely by veterinarians and researchers for anesthesia in amphibians and appears to have a wide margin of safety.[74] After being anesthetized, the amphibian is removed from the anesthetic bath to avoid overdosing or prolonged anesthesia. Well-oxygenated clean water should be provided during anesthesia, and additional anesthetic can be added, if needed.

Although amphibian skin secretions are known to have antimicrobial properties, sterile techniques should be followed. Because of the potential for toxicity from the various available antiseptics, it is recommended that the patient be rinsed with sterile water before placement of sterile drapes. Surgical instruments should be heat or gas sterilized. A small incision is made into the skin, thin muscle layer, and coelomic lining to enter the coelomic cavity. The authors have used transmitters in which the antenna is tightly coiled around the battery, and the entire package is encapsulated in acrylic (see Fig. 175.9D). The transmitter is placed into the coelom, and the incision is closed. The least reactive suture material should be used; polydioxanone (PDS II, Ethicon, Inc., Somerville, NJ) is recommended for internal sutures and skin, and alternatively nylon can be used for skin sutures.[75] Triclosan-impregnated poliglecaprone (Monocryl-plus, Ethicon) suture offers the advantages of faster absorption (4–8 weeks depending on metabolism) and local antimicrobial effects to reduce dehiscence.[76] Internal transmitters will need to be removed or replaced, which is a consideration that researchers should be aware of when working with rare species, those that are difficult to capture, or species that are particularly susceptible to stress.

PIT tags can also be implanted into the body cavity of frogs and salamanders, either by syringe and needle or through a small (2 mm to 3 mm) incision in the skin with the use of surgical methods previously described. In salamanders, the tags can be inserted along the side of the body, approximately 5 mm anterior to the hind leg;[77] tags should be inserted anteriorly, parallel to the long axis of the body. Incisions can be closed with a small amount of cyanoacrylate glue. Anesthetized amphibians should not be released until they are fully recovered.

General Guidelines for Reptile Surgery. Presurgical health screening is recommended. Appropriate analgesia and anesthesia should be used and tailored to each species undergoing surgery. In most cases, injectable sedatives and anesthetics will be followed by intubation and gas anesthesia. Appropriate cardiac and respiratory monitoring equipment should be available. Recommended suture material includes polydioxanone (PDS II),[78] an absorbable suture, that is used internally and in the skin or alternatively nonabsorbable nylon (Ethicon; Ethicon, Inc., Somerville, NJ) can be used for the skin. Triclosan-impregnanted poliglecaprone (Monocryl-plus, Ethicon) suture offers the advantages of faster absorption (4–8 weeks depending on metabolism) and local antimicrobial effects to reduce dehiscence.

Crocodilians. Intracoelomic radio transmitter implantation in crocodilians has been conducted under injectable anesthesia with subsequent intubation and manual ventilation with a bag valve mask (Ambu bag) or Hudson Demand Valve.[48–51] A small skin incision was made between scales in the flank of the abdominal region, just anterior to the right hind limb. Muscle layers beneath the skin were carefully separated to reveal the coelomic lining. Hemostats were used to secure the coelomic lining, and an incision was made to enter the coelom, where the transmitter was inserted. To avoid disturbance when the animals were tracked, the researchers used an automatic and continuous recording station positioned at least 100 m from the waterhole to simultaneously monitor up to 10 individuals. Radio signals from the temperature-sensitive transmitters were received by a four-piece Yagi aerial antenna, mounted 25 m directly above the waterhole that the crocodiles inhabited.[50] Alternatively, using a similar surgical approach, researchers implanted a multichannel radio telemetry system to measure blood flow and pressure, electrocardiographic data, and body temperature in several captive American alligators.[79] The technique has been reported to be promising for free-ranging crocodilians.[50]

The authors (TMN, KMA) developed a technique for surgical implantation of radio transmitters in the muscle of the proximal tail of American alligators. The technique was used on six alligators and is successful on animals that do not occupy estuarine or marine waters that attenuate VHF signals.[80] Following the induction of ketamine-dexmedetomidine-opiate anesthesia, lidocaine was infiltrated into the incision area. Intubation and ventilation with a bag valve mask were performed in all cases. Gas anesthesia can be used to further control anesthesia but has not been necessary with the injectable drug combination used. Following skin preparation, a 3 cm to 5 cm skin incision was made between scales about a third of the way down from the dorsal aspect of the tail. Blunt dissection was used to create a pocket between muscle planes, where the transmitter was inserted (Fig. 175.22). Holohil Systems Ltd. (Ontario, Canada) transmitters (Model SI-2, 50 mm × 11 mm, 36-month battery projected life) developed for snakes have been used. Sterilized copper tubing is threaded caudad subcutaneously before the antenna is threaded through the rigid tubing. A small skin incision at the distal end of the tubing is made to allow the tubing to be removed, leaving the antennae in place. It is difficult to thread the tubing because of the stiffness of the scales; thus, more than one incision was usually needed. The surgical site was closed routinely.

A technique recently described subcutaneous implantation of temperature- or pressure-sensitive acoustic telemetry devices in estuarine crocodiles.[50] The animals ranged from 2 to 5 m in length. The crocodiles were manually restrained, and a local anesthetic was infiltrated into the surgical site. A 2 cm skin incision was made, and a small pocket was formed under the skin along a skinfold, with the use of blunt-ended scissors (Fig. 175.23). The transmitter was then inserted (V16, Vemco-cylindrical, 72 mm long and 15 mm in diameter with rounded ends). The transmitter was positioned so that when the animal surfaced, it remained well below the water. The researchers used fixed receiver stations. The technology has potential to be extremely useful in crocodiles, because the signal transmission occurs through water, and transmission operates irrespective of salinity. Furthermore, the transmitters can be programmed to have a life span of more than 10 years. A variety of sensors are available to measure temperature and pressure (water depth). The signals can be actively tracked or detected by automatic stationary receivers. The authors reported excellent transmission; animals were detected more than 500 m away with the use of a directional hydrophone and active tracking receiver. At the time of the publication, the transmitters had been functioning well for more than 9 months.

Lizards. An effective technique for surgically implanting transmitters in the coelom of anegada ground iguanas (*Cyclura pinguis*) has been reported and has potential for use in other lizard species.[81] With this technique, two-point fixation of the transmitter to the internal body wall was achieved. Antenna placement in the coelom was a critical part of the procedure. Of 23 iguanas, 20 transmitted good signals for at least 10 months after surgery (Fig. 175.24).

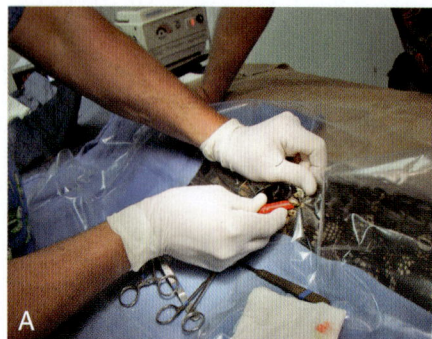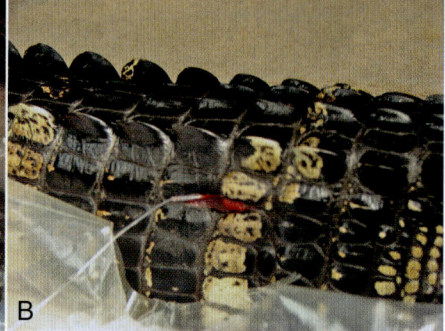

FIG 175.22 (A and B) Surgical placement of a radio transmitter in an American alligator (*Alligator mississippiensis*) tail. (Courtesy of K.M. Andrews, University of Georgia.)

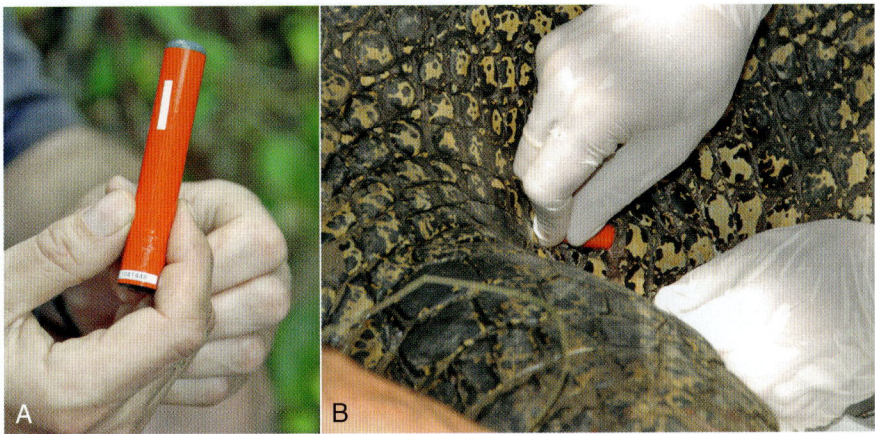

FIG 175.23 (A) Vemco acoustic tag. (B) Surgically implanting a temperature-sensitive or pressure-sensitive acoustic transmitter subcutaneously in a saltwater crocodile (*Crocodylus porosus*). (Courtesy of C.E. Franklin.)

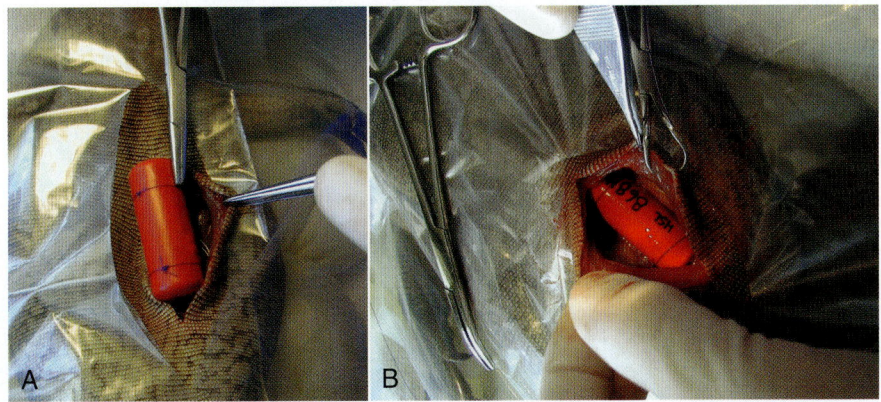

FIG 175.24 (A and B) Surgical intracoelomic placement of radio transmitters in Caribbean iguanas (*Cyclura* spp.) (Courtesy of Fort Worth Zoo Animal Health.)

Another method was described by Doody and colleagues for surgical implantation of radio transmitters in a semiaquatic monitor lizard (*Varanus mertensi*).[57] Gas anesthesia was used. The site was aseptically prepared for implantation. A 2 cm to 3 cm skin incision was made longitudinally on the lateral side of the coelom, approximately 2 to 3 cm anterior from the hind limbs. Muscle was incised to gain access to the coelomic lining, which was then incised. Transmitters (Holohil Systems Ltd, Ontario, Canada, Model 2I-T, 3 g, 2.5 cm × 0.6 cm) with a 10 cm external whip antenna were inserted into the coelom. The transmitter was positioned longitudinally within the coelom. A thin-walled brass tube was threaded subcutaneously from the anterior point of incision along the lateral fold of the animal to just behind the head. The external antenna was positioned inside the tube, and the tube was removed through a small incision made just behind the head, leaving the antenna in place under the skin. No significant adverse effects were noted, according to the authors, over a 2-year study period. Fifty individuals were implanted, and 37 transmitted for more than 16 days; 4 were tracked successfully for 2 years.

Snakes. Radio telemetry devices have been surgically placed in the coelomic cavity of a variety of snake species. Complete healing takes approximately 4 to 8 weeks in reptiles maintained in ideal thermoregulatory conditions. The methodology that follows is a modification of that described previously.[82]

Snout-to-vent and snout-to-tail measurements are taken. The snout-to-vent measurement is divided by three; this distance is measured from the cloaca (vent) anteriorly and used for the incision site for transmitter placement. A permanent marker can be used to mark the skin incision site. The snake is prepared for sterile surgery in a routine fashion. A 3- to 5-cm lateral skin incision is made between the second and third scale rows and then reflected ventrally past the ribs so that an incision can be made in the coelomic lining, which allows access to the coelomic cavity. Care should be taken not to incise the air sac while making the incision in the coelomic lining or accidentally insert the transmitter into the respiratory system.

An appropriately sized transmitter should be selected. Temperature-sensitive transmitters available from select manufacturers or micro-temperature data loggers (iButtons; Maxim Integrated Devices, Sunnyvale, CA) that have been coated in multipurpose rubber coating (PlastiDip; Plasti Dip International, Blaine, MN) and gas sterilized can also be implanted intracoelomically caudal to the transmitter to record body temperatures. Sterilized copper tubing (rigid dog urinary catheter or a similar rigid sterile instrument) is threaded subcutaneously anteriorly. The antenna is threaded into the lumen of the tubing. A small skin incision is made at the level of the anterior end of the tubing. The tubing is removed, leaving the antennae in place. The antenna can be anchored to musculature by one suture (placed approximately 0.5 cm anterior to the transmitter), which reduces the chances of the antennae protruding from the incision site. Care is taken to ensure that the antenna is not crimped (Fig. 175.25). Surgical closure is routine.

Although this technique is expedient and successful in most snake species if proper procedures and sterilization techniques are applied,

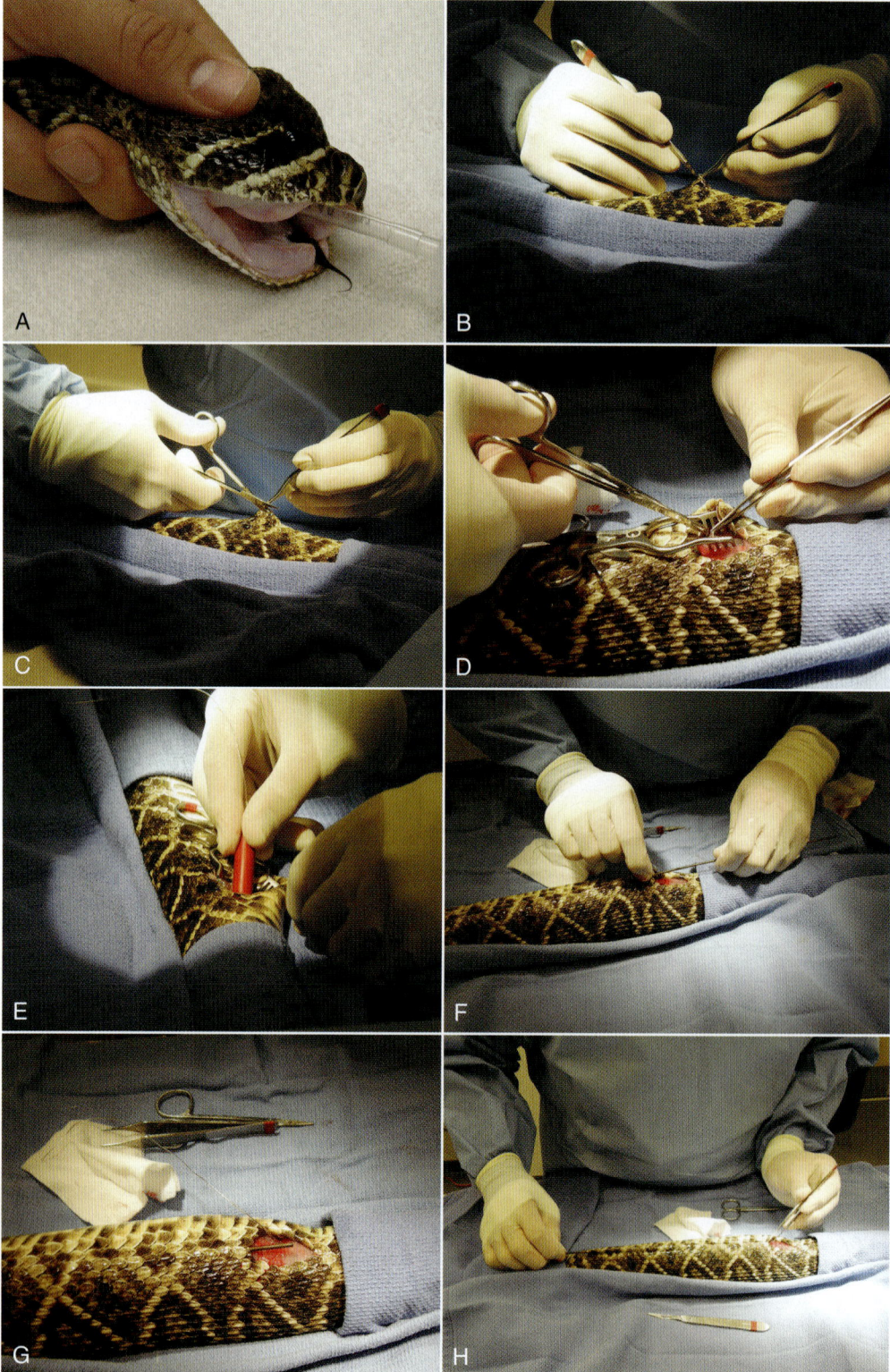

FIG 175.25 Surgical placement of a radio transmitter into the coelom of an eastern diamondback rattlesnake (*Crotalus adamanteus*). (A) Isoflurane anesthesia is administered through an endotracheal tube. (B) Initial stab incision into the skin with a scalpel blade. (C) Skin incision is completed with scissors. (D) Incision of coelomic lining with scissors. Retractors improve exposure. (E) Radio transmitter is being placed into the coelom. (F) Threading copper tubing subcutaneously. (G) Copper tubing in place for threading antenna. (H) Small incision is made to pull out the copper tubing while leaving the antenna in place. (Courtesy of Terry M. Norton, Georgia Sea Turtle Center.)

some species of snakes, such as the eastern indigo snake (*Drymarchon couperi*), are prone to developing bacterial infections at the transmitter site. Recent studies on the eastern Massasauga rattlesnake (*Sisturus catenatus catenatus*) indicate bacterial infections still occur with some frequency, despite proper incorporation of sterile techniques.[83]

CONCLUSION

Capture techniques, marking of individuals for identification purposes, and telemetry placement techniques are used extensively in herpetological research and conservation activities. It is critical that veterinarians and biologists continue to work together to develop sound protocols that provide vital research information while causing minimal negative effects to the individual animals and populations that are being studied and preserved.

REFERENCES

See www.expertconsult.com for a complete list of references.

176

Medical Management and Rehabilitation of Sea Turtles

Charles J. Innis

Fisheries interactions, boat trauma, habitat degradation, poaching, disease, oil spills, and unusual weather events are resulting in increasing numbers of sea turtle injuries, stranding events, mortality, veterinary research, and intervention (Walsh MT et al, Proc ARAV, 2014, p 36).[1–18,20–22] The extensive, but not comprehensive, reference list provided herein reflects numerous recent studies, but the reader is encouraged to explore the many important previous references cited within those studies.

COMMON MEDICAL CONDITIONS

Traumatic injuries may occur due to boat strike, fisheries gear entanglement or hooking, and predator injuries (Fig. 176.1).[1,3] Hook and line or trash ingestion may lead to perforation or obstruction of the digestive tract (Fig. 176.2).[1,6,8,16] Forced submergence by fishing gear may result in near drowning and associated physical and physiological derangements,[3] and decompression sickness may be seen when sea turtles are captured at depth and rapidly brought to the ocean surface (Fig. 176.3).[9]

Sea turtles are susceptible to severe hypothermia or "cold-stunning" in autumn and winter when water temperatures rapidly drop.[4,10–17] Hypothermic turtles are prone to a variety of secondary conditions, including pneumonia, sepsis, and osteomyelitis.[14–16]

Sea turtles are sometimes found stranded in chronically debilitated condition, and various monikers such as "lethargic loggerhead syndrome" and "debilitated turtle syndrome" have been coined.[18] Such turtles are often emaciated, weak, fragile, anemic, and hypoproteinemic.[18] Careful handling may be required to prevent iatrogenic avulsion of skin and bone attachments.

Traumatic injuries or chronic pneumonia may allow air to leak from the lungs into the coelom (pneumocoelom) (Walsh MT et al, Proc ARAV, 2014, p 36). Similarly, any gas-producing coelomic infection or gastrointestinal disease with secondary gas accumulation may cause buoyancy problems. Animals with neurologic damage, especially spinal trauma, may also have buoyancy problems.

Heavy metals and pesticides have been detected in sea turtles, and their presence is sometimes associated with clinicopathologic abnormalities.[20] Brevetoxin, domoic acid, and saxitoxin may also cause toxicity as seen in other marine species.[21] Sea turtles have been exposed to crude oil and petroleum products in small- and large-scale exposure events.[5] Physical, physiological, and postmortem assessments may reveal variably extensive oiling with evidence of oil ingestion and aspiration in some cases. Oiled turtles may be affected by acidosis, electrolyte abnormalities, and presumed physiological stress response, likely caused by combined effects of oiling, hyperthermia, and transport.[5] An experimental study that exposed loggerhead turtles to oil cited possible hemolytic anemia and salt gland dysfunction, but these conditions were not well characterized.[22]

Sea turtles are commonly affected by opportunistic bacterial and fungal infections, often secondary to trauma or hypothermia. It has

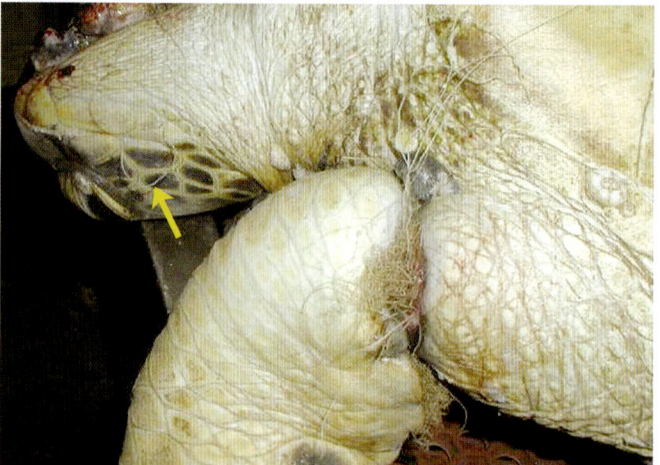

FIG 176.1 Loggerhead turtle (*Caretta caretta*) with nylon fishing line entangling and strangling the flipper. The yellow arrow points to the ingested portion of the line. (Courtesy of Douglas R. Mader.)

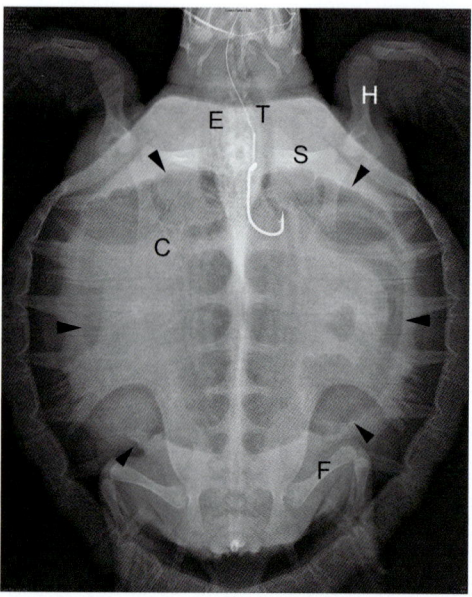

FIG 176.2 Kemp's ridley turtle (*Lepidochelys kempii*) dorsoventral radiograph. There is an ingested fish hook at the tracheal bifurcation. Arrowheads delineate the lung margins. C, Coracoids; E, esophagus; F, femur; H, humerus; S, scapula; T, trachea. (Courtesy of New England Aquarium.)

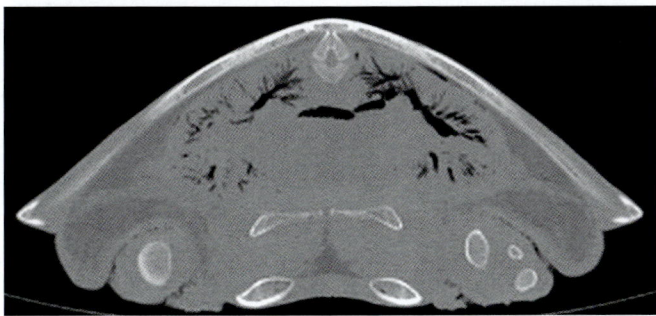

FIG 176.3 Loggerhead turtle (*Caretta caretta*) affected by decompression sickness. Computed tomography at the level of the pelvis demonstrates gas within the renal vasculature. (Courtesy of Daniel García-Párraga.)

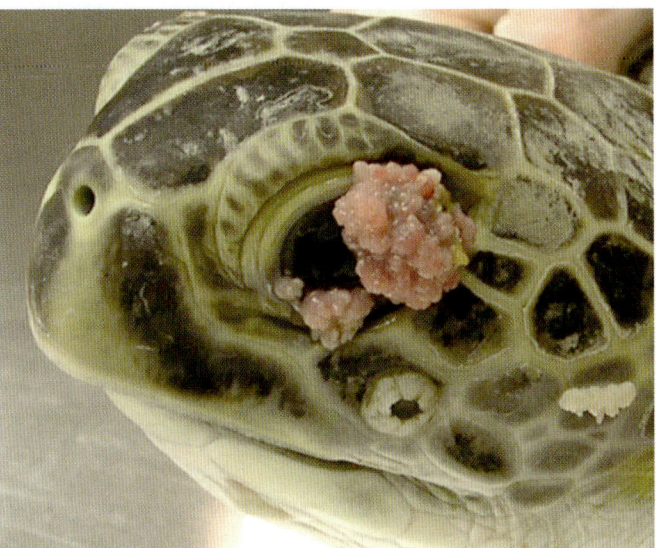

FIG 176.4 Fibropapilloma on the sclera and nictitating membrane of a juvenile green turtle (*Chelonia mydas*). (Courtesy of Douglas R. Mader.)

been shown that hypothermia results in significantly increased plasma corticosterone concentrations, which could contribute to immunocompromise.[14] Most often, infections are caused by bacteria and fungi that are normally present in the environment or associated with the turtle's oral, nasal, cloacal, and digestive tract. Common isolates include various gram-negative aerobic bacteria, *Enterococcus* spp., *Mycobacteria* spp., and *Fusarium* spp.[15,23–26]

Fibropapillomatosis (FP) is common in sea turtles in tropical waters worldwide, especially green turtles (*Chelonia mydas*). It is associated with chelonid fibropapilloma-associated herpesvirus (CFPHV).[26] This debilitating disease is characterized by the proliferation of cutaneous and visceral FP (Fig. 176.4). If FP occurs on or around the eyes, it can lead to visual impairment. Large lesions on the flippers or carapace may affect swimming. Internal FP may develop within the viscera; thus MRI and coelioscopy may be useful for diagnosis.[16] Herpesviruses have also been isolated from cases of "gray patch disease" and "lung-eye-trachea disease" in green sea turtles, and a herpesvirus was described as a cause of cutaneous and mucosal lesions in loggerhead turtles (*Caretta caretta*).[27]

Spirorchid trematodes are common, but they may or may not lead to clinically relevant disease.[7] Adult spirorchids generally reside within the heart or great vessels. When the parasites reproduce, eggs are released into the vasculature, becoming lodged in capillaries and causing granulomas. Spirorchids are among the proposed causes of neurologic syndromes that have been seen in sea turtles.[7]

The coccidian parasite *Caryospora chelonae* may cause fatal enteritis, especially in juvenile green turtles (Pelton CA et al, Proc 44th Annu Conf Internat Assoc Aquat Anim Med, 2012, pp 81–82).[2] Other parasites and epibiota such as nematodes, cestodes, leeches, and barnacles may be seen but are often incidental findings.[29] Sea turtles may be intermediate hosts for some parasite species. Although many debilitated turtles become heavily covered by epibiota, the presence of heavy epibiotia is not always associated with illness, and one study found no clinicopathologic correlates to epibiota coverage.[29]

PHYSICAL EXAMINATION

Sea turtles are relatively easy to examine compared with other turtles, because they cannot withdraw their head and limbs into their shell. Heart rate should be determined using Doppler or ultrasonography, and respiratory rate should be noted visually. Turtles should be weighed and body temperature recorded using a flexible cloacal thermometer gently inserted as deeply as possible, and body measurements should be collected. The mouth is relatively easy to open with gentle traction on the lower jaw or pharyngeal skin. Stranded turtles often have eye injuries caused by scavengers or foreign material (e.g., sand); thus a thorough eye examination, including corneal fluorescent staining, is required. Sea turtle corneas are very sensitive but are desensitized by proparacaine ophthalmic solution.[30] Tonometry data have been reported for loggerhead and Kemp's ridley turtles (*Lepidochelys kempii*), with results of 5 to 12 and 2 to 9 mm Hg (ranges), respectively.[31] A comprehensive neurologic examination should be performed.[32]

CLINICAL PATHOLOGY

There have been more clinical pathology studies published for sea turtles, including data for both healthy and unhealthy turtles, than for any other group of reptiles.[33–49] The number of studies prohibits comprehensive citation, thus the references listed herein have been limited to several of the most recent for each species. Readers are encouraged to explore the many clinicopathologic studies cited within these studies for further insight, taking care to understand the context of the study in which the data were collected (e.g., wild vs captive, adult vs juvenile, postprandial or fasted, injured vs healthy). Recently larger data sets have allowed for the development of mortality prediction indices based on clinicopathologic data.[13,47] Clear trends in improvement of clinicopathologic values during the course of hospitalization have been demonstrated in several studies.[14,15,38,47]

Blood is usually collected from various locations along the external jugular vein. Depending on the site of needle insertion, these sites have also been referred to as the dorsal cervical sinus, postoccipital sinus, or supravertebral sinus.[16] The dorsal coccygeal vein and the interdigital veins may also be used.[49] The subcarapacial sinus can be accessed easily in sea turtles, but serious adverse sequelae have been described for some cases due to its proximity to the cervical spinal cord, including transient paresis and death (Innis CJ et al, Proc ARAV, 2010, pp 8–10). The author reserves use of the subcarapacial sinus for emergency situations when no other vascular access can be obtained.

Blood handling should follow standard reptilian methods, taking care to avoid artifactual influences such as hemolysis, delayed centrifugation, and excessive anticoagulant ratio. Ethylenediamine tetraacetic acid (EDTA) causes lysis of Kemp's ridley turtle blood cells and is generally avoided for all sea turtles, with heparin preferred. No significant differences were found in leatherback turtle (*Dermochelys coriacea*) plasma biochemical values between samples collected in sodium heparin versus lithium heparin, although in general lithium heparin is recommended.[46]

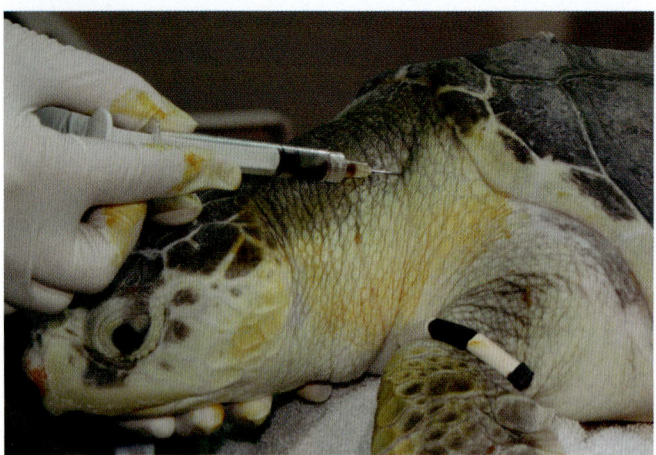

FIG 176.5 Blood collection from a branch of the external jugular vein of a Kemp's ridley turtle (*Lepidochelys kempii*). (Courtesy of New England Aquarium.)

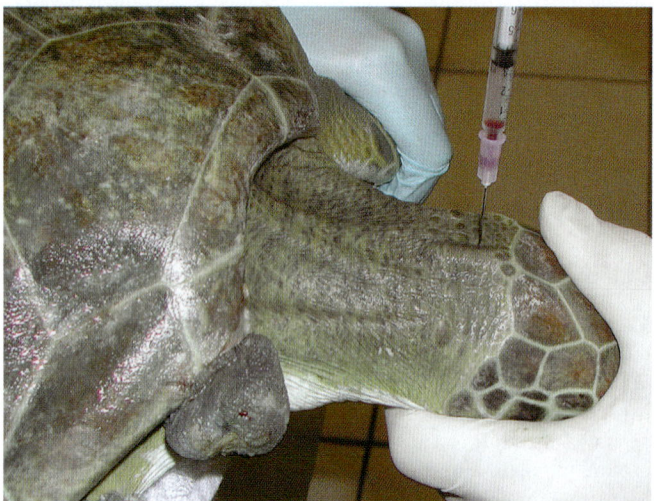

FIG 176.6 Blood collection from supravertebral sinus of a green turtle (*Chelonia mydas*) (Courtesy of Douglas R. Mader.)

For access to the external jugular vein, the head is extended and slightly ventroflexed. The vein is located paravertebrally, lateral to the straplike retractor muscles of the neck (Fig. 176.5). For venipuncture of the supravertebral or postoccipital sinus, the needle is placed to either side of the nuchal crest, caudal to the skull and directed axially toward the dorsal midline of the vertebra (Fig. 176.6).[16] Accidental aspiration of lymph can occur at any venipuncture site, whereas cerebrospinal fluid may be obtained from sites close to the spinal cord.

Healthy carnivorous sea turtles have much higher blood urea nitrogen (BUN) concentrations than terrestrial vertebrates; however, debilitated or nesting sea turtles often have relatively low BUN.[18,44] Interestingly, sea turtles sometimes show increasing BUN values during rehabilitation even though they have not yet accepted food, which suggests that anorexia alone may not explain the reduced BUN seen at admission. Green turtles are more herbivorous than other sea turtle species and have relatively lower BUN values.[10] Plasma uric acid concentrations tend to be quite low in healthy sea turtles (generally <120 μmol/L; 2 mg/dL). Severely elevated uric-acid values are associated with a poor prognosis. Plasma uric acid concentrations are negatively associated with glomerular filtration rate in hypothermic Kemp's ridley turtles.[11]

Both hypoglycemia and hyperglycemia are common in ill sea turtles.[12] In contrast to many other vertebrates, healthy sea turtles often have lower total plasma calcium concentrations and often have an inverse calcium:phosphorus ratio.[18,29] Ionized calcium concentrations in healthy sea turtles are often approximately 1.0 mmol/L.[3,5,12] Hypoproteinemia and hypoalbuminemia are common.[17] Albumin concentrations for turtles are most accurately measured by electrophoresis rather than the bromcresol green method.[51] Protein electrophoresis data have been published for several sea turtle species, but clinical use of these data has not yet become routine.[3,18,43] A variety of plasma enzyme activities are often measured, and the tissues of origin for these enzymes have recently been documented for loggerhead and Kemp's ridley turtles.[35,37] Overall, these enzymes are found in a variety of tissues and thus are nonspecific indicators of cellular injury. Debilitated sea turtles often have elevated sodium, potassium, chloride, magnesium (ionized and total), and ionized calcium concentrations, presumably due to a combination of dehydration, reduced renal and salt gland function, and ingestion or aspiration of sea water.[12] However, a spectrum of derangements is seen, and some individuals may be hypokalemic or hypocalcemic.[12] Severe elevations of sodium and potassium concentrations are associated with mortality.[12] Consistent with observations in other reptiles, creatinine is generally low in sea turtles and considered to be of little clinical importance; however, one study did conclude that creatinine may be of value for prognostication of survival for loggerhead turtles.[47] Sea turtle hematocrit values are generally in the high-20 to mid-30 percentiles. White blood cell counts of healthy sea turtles generally range from 2000 to 25,000 cells/μl (2–25 × 10⁹ cells/L) but are often <10,000 cells/μL (10 × 10⁹ cells/L).

A number of acid-base and blood gas studies have been conducted for sea turtles. Recent studies generally use point-of-care analyzers, which perform analyses at 37°C. The majority of sea turtle physiology and clinical medicine papers utilize mathematical formulae to correct the data for the turtle's body temperature.[3,5,10,12,13,34,38,39] Analyzer-corrected values for pH and PCO₂ may be similar enough to the manually calculated values to be clinically useful.[39] In contrast, analyzer-corrected values for PO₂ do not agree well with manually calculated values.[39] Reptile hematocrit values calculated by automated analyzers are considered inaccurate compared with the manual packed cell volume determinations; however, one study of green turtles reported good correlation of analyzer-generated hematocrit versus manual PCV.[39] Temperature-corrected venous pH in healthy sea turtles at 25°C is generally 7.4 to 7.6, varying somewhat among different studies. Acidosis (both respiratory and metabolic) may be seen in ill, injured, or anesthetized turtles.[5,12,16,34,38] High lactate concentrations have been described in hypothermic sea turtles and anesthetized sea turtles, presumably due to anaerobic metabolism caused by hypoventilation and reduced perfusion.[12,34]

DIAGNOSTIC IMAGING

Radiography, ultrasonography, MRI, CT, scintigraphy, and endoscopy are important tools for the assessment of sea turtles. The reader is referred to a number of primary studies that provide detailed anatomic descriptions using various diagnostic imaging modalities.[52–59] Commonly, imaging is needed for characterization and localization of pneumonia, bone lesions, central nervous system trauma, fish hook or other foreign body ingestion, pneumocoelom, etc. (Figs. 176.2 and 176.7). Unlike some other turtle species, the lung fields of sea turtles are generally well delineated on dorsoventral radiographs (see Figs. 176.2 and 176.7). Gastrointestinal contrast studies may be useful for sea turtles, with due consideration of their normally long gastrointestinal transit time of 2 to 3 weeks.[54] Ultrasound windows are generally limited to the cervical, axillary, and prefemoral spaces. Scintigraphy has been validated as a method for serial monitoring of bone lesions in Kemp's ridley turtles (Fig. 176.8).[59]

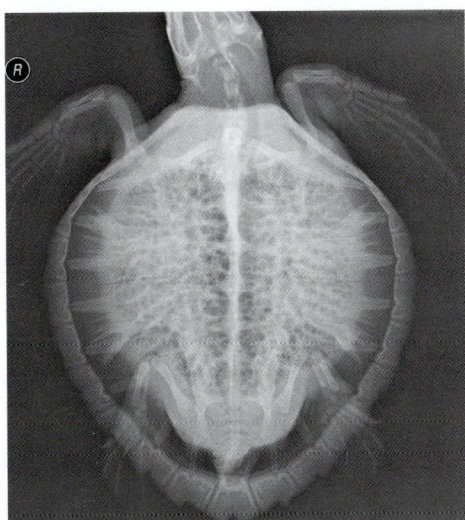

FIG 176.7 Dorsoventral radiograph of a Kemp's ridley turtle (*Lepidochelys kempii*) demonstrating the dramatic edicular lung pattern that is typical of diffuse pneumonia. (Courtesy of New England Aquarium.)

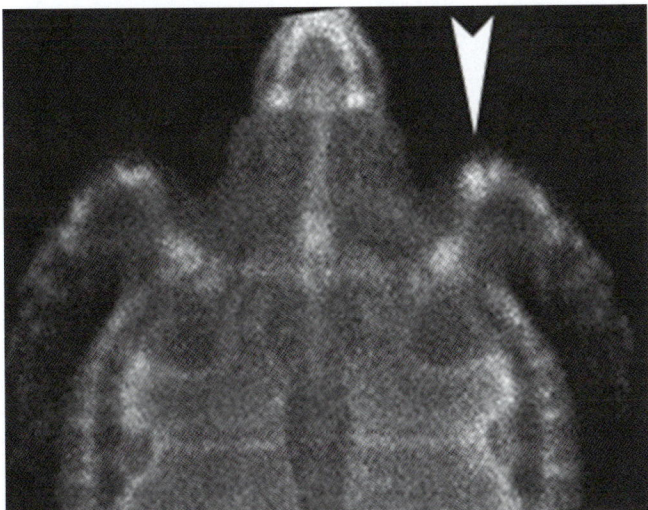

FIG 176.8 Scintigraphy demonstrates an active lesion (arrowhead) in the distal left humerus of a Kemp's ridley turtle (*Lepidochelys kempii*). (Courtesy of New England Aquarium.)

MICROBIOLOGIC AND MOLECULAR DIAGNOSTICS

As for other reptiles, bacterial and fungal cultures and antimicrobial susceptibility are important. When possible, cultures should be incubated at both 37° and 25°C in light of the typically lower than mammalian body temperature of sea turtles. Blood cultures should be considered and are often informative.[14] Molecular methods may be needed for definitive identification of *Mycobacteria* sp., fungi, and chelonian herpesviruses.[23,25–27]

THERAPEUTICS

Principles of therapy for sea turtles follow standard guidelines. Medications are often administered orally. Subcutaneous injections may be given in the lateral cervical and shoulder region or the prefemoral space. Intramuscular injections are most often given in the pectoral muscles. Intracoelomic (ICe) injections are delivered via the prefemoral space but appear to offer little benefit and greater risk compared with SC

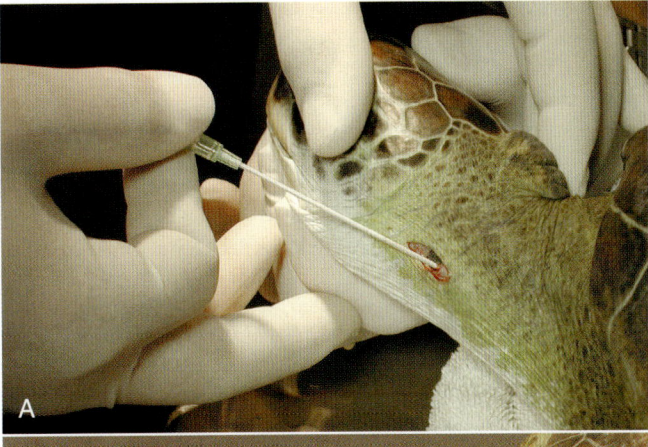

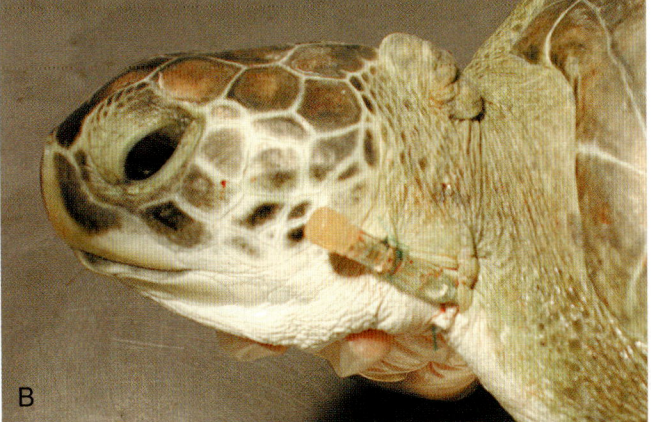

FIG 176.9 (A) A cutdown approach exposes a branch of the external jugular vein to place an IV catheter. (B) Catheter sutured in place. (Courtesy of Douglas R. Mader.)

injection. IV injections can be given in any of the locations discussed for venipuncture, with the jugular vein being preferred, and only with caution using the subcarapacial sinus (Innis CJ et al, Proc ARAV, 2010, pp 8–10). Similarly, given the proximity of the dorsal coccygeal vein and coccygeal spinal cord, caution is warranted. The author accidentally administered contrast media intrathecally, instead of intravenously, via the dorsal coccygeal approach in a Kemp's ridley turtle. Jugular vein catheterization, including central venous catheterization using ultrasound guidance or cut-down techniques, has been effective for sea turtles (Fig. 176.9).[60] Although intraosseous (IO) catheters have been used, they have not become routinely accepted and are unnecessary in most cases.

Bathing sea turtles in fresh water provides a simple form of fluid therapy. However, the author has occasionally observed overhydration, hyponatremia, and even death in several juvenile Kemp's ridley turtles exposed to freshwater. Ortiz et al. experimentally exposed four juvenile Kemp's ridley turtles to freshwater for 4 days and documented decreased plasma sodium, potassium, and chloride concentrations within 48 hours.[61] However, no apparent deleterious effects were noted, and most parameters returned to baseline within 48 hours after return to salt water. Clinical observations suggest that many sea turtle patients are tolerant of freshwater exposure, but close monitoring is essential.

Fluids are generally administered to sea turtles at a maintenance rate of 10 to 20 mL/kg/d SC, PO, ICe, or IV, but higher volumes may be needed for dehydrated patients. Crystalloid fluids commonly used in sea turtles include lactated ringer's solution (LRS), 0.45% saline with 2.5 % dextrose, Normosol-R (Hospira, Inc., Lake Forest, IL), and 0.9% saline. Various cocktails of these fluids are also frequently used. For example, many facilities use reptile ringer's solution made from two parts 0.45% saline with 2.5% dextrose and one part LRS. Camacho et al. reported positive effects in loggerhead turtles treated with a 1:1 ratio of 0.9% saline and LRS.[37] Clinically, LRS appears to be effective and safe for sea turtles.[38] Colloids, blood products, and total parenteral nutrition may be useful for severely hypoalbuminemic, anemic, and hypovolemic patients (Manire CA et al, 2014, Proc 45th Annu Conf Intern Assoc Aquat Anim Med).[62]

Sodium bicarbonate (1 mEq/kg) may be added to fluids to provide increased buffering capacity for acidotic turtles. Dextrose may be added up to concentrations of 2.5% for SC administration to hypoglycemic turtles. Camacho et al. effectively treated hypoglycemic loggerhead turtles and demonstrated significantly increased blood glucose concentration after intracoelomic injection of 0.45% saline and 2.5% dextrose at 20 mL/kg.[38] Calcium gluconate 50 to 100 mg/kg may be added to fluids for turtles with low blood ionized calcium concentrations. Potassium chloride may be added to fluids for hypokalemic turtles (e.g., 20 mEq/L). Severely hypoglycemic turtles may also benefit from IV injection of 50% dextrose (e.g., 0.5 mL/kg). If given as a direct IV bolus, some clinicians prefer to dilute dextrose to a 10% concentration to reduce the likelihood of perivascular tissue reaction. Alternatively, oral glucose supplements such as corn syrup (0.5 mL/kg) or honey may be effective in some cases.

Pharmacokinetic studies are available for ceftazidime, florfenicol, enrofloxacin, danofloxacin, marbofloxacin, oxytetracycline, clindamycin, and ticarcillin, with additional limited data from clinical cases for plasma concentrations of gentamicin, clarithromycin, and tobramycin (Innis C, Proc ARAV, 2014, p 68).[63–64,66–70] Florfenicol, clindamycin, and clarithromycin are expected to lack efficacy in sea turtles based on these studies (Innis C, Proc ARAV, 2014, p 68).[63] Limited clinical investigations indicate that the dosing regimens predicted from single-dose studies may result in unexpected plasma drug concentrations (Innis C, Proc ARAV, 2014, p 68). When possible, plasma drug concentration monitoring is recommended. For gram-positive bacterial infections, ampicillin 30 mg/kg SID appears to be useful.[15] For mycobacterial infections, combination drug therapy including two or three drugs may be needed (e.g., aminoglycoside, tetracycline, and quinolone). Recent positive outcomes and appropriate plasma concentrations have been seen with tobramycin use in Kemp's ridley sea turtles (5 mg/kg IM q3d) (Innis C, Proc ARAV, 2014, p 68).

Fungal infections are common in sea turtles, and deep internal fungal infections such as pneumonia carry a poor prognosis (Fig. 176.10).[24–26,71]

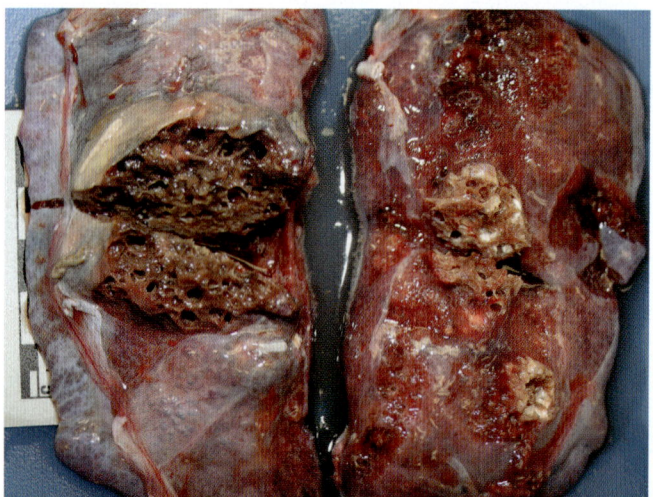

FIG 176.10 Lungs of a Kemp's ridley turtle (*Lepidochelys kempii*) after removal from the body during necropsy. The cut surfaces reveal severe consolidation and white plaques. Histopathologic evaluation revealed severe fungal pneumonia. (Courtesy of New England Aquarium.)

Localized superficial infections such as fungal dermal granulomas may be managed by debridement and topical and systemic therapy.[26] Nebulization of antifungal agents may also be considered. In Kemp's ridley turtles, itraconazole delivered orally at 5 mg/kg SID or 15 mg/kg q3d provided steady-state plasma itraconazole concentrations of approximately 1 µg/mL, which are expected to be efficacious against some filamentous fungi.[71] Pharmacokinetics of fluconazole have been determined in loggerhead turtles and Kemp's ridley turtles; however, comparison of the achieved plasma concentrations to MIC data for many sea turtle fungal isolates suggests that many of these isolates are fluconazole resistant.[24,26] The author has used terbinafine safely for many Kemp's ridley sea turtles at 20 mg/kg PO SID, with treatment durations often lasting several months, although plasma concentrations have not yet been evaluated.

Most clinicians elect to treat sea turtles for parasites only if clinically indicated or if the turtle is to be maintained in permanent captivity. Pharmacokinetic data for oral praziquantel in loggerhead turtles indicate a dosing scheme of 25 mg/kg given three times in 1 day at 3-hour intervals.[72] Anthelminthics such as oxfendazole, fenbendazole, albendazole, thiabendazole, pyrantel, and levamisole may be considered for treatment of nematode infections in sea turtles based on their general safety and efficacy in other reptiles. Metronidazole 50 mg/kg SID × 5 to 7 days may be an effective treatment for *Caryopsora* infections (Manire C, personal communication, 2016). Pelton et al. reported that trimethoprim-sulfa appeared ineffective in eliminating coccidia from a green turtle; however, the turtle was successfully treated with toltrazuril 10 mg/kg PO q7d × 3 (Pelton CA et al, Proc 44th Annu Conf Internat Assoc Aquat Anim Med, 2012, pp 81–82). Another green turtle was successfully treated for coccidia using ponazuril 20 mg/kg PO q7d × 4, but displayed transient anorexia and plasma biochemical abnormalities (Pelton CA et al, Proc 44th Annu Conf Internat Assoc Aquat Anim Med, 2012, pp 81–82).

Topical wound care products, vacuum-assisted wound therapy, acupuncture, and photobiomodulation therapy are routinely used for sea turtles. As for other species, sea turtles likely benefit from therapeutics that target the cardiorespiratory, gastrointestinal, and urinary tract and other organ systems when appropriate. Drugs such as atropine, epinephrine, doxapram, metoclopramide, cisapride, enalapril, furosemide, and others are used with clinical discretion despite a lack of sea turtle–specific data. Furosemide was successfully used for management of brevetoxicosis in loggerhead turtles.[21] Epoetin-α administered at 100 U/kg IM three times weekly in conjunction with iron supplementation increased packed cell volume and shortened treatment time for anemic turtles (Perry SM et al, Proc ExoticsCon, 2015, p 531).

Detailed discussion of analgesia principles and options for reptiles is provided elsewhere (see Chapter 50). Most clinicians utilize nonsteroidal antiinflammatory drugs (NSAIDs) and opiates for sea turtles despite limited pharmacokinetic data and absence of pharmacodynamic data. There is one report of gastrointestinal bleeding in sea turtles that may have been caused by flunixin,[16] but the author has used it short-term without incident in several patients. Meloxicam has become popular for sea turtles, but pharmacokinetic data indicate low plasma concentrations and short half-life.[74] At this time, the choice of NSAID, dose, and dosing interval remain at clinical discretion. Tramadol pharmacokinetics in loggerhead turtles suggest a dosing regimen of 5 to 10 mg/kg PO q48 to 72 hours.[75]

MANAGEMENT OF OILED TURTLES

When treating oiled turtles, human handlers must wear personal protective equipment. External oil can be removed by bathing in dishwashing liquid. Oil is physically removed from the eyes and oral cavity using cotton swabs, gauze, and food-grade oil (e.g., mayonnaise or cod liver oil). Such oils and activated charcoal may also be delivered by tube feeding to facilitate passage and limit absorption of ingested oil.

MANAGEMENT OF BUOYANCY DISORDERS

Treatment and correction of buoyancy problems involves identification of the etiology.[76] Removal of excessive gas by coelomocentesis is successful in some cases. Placement of the animal in freshwater may help because freshwater-specific gravity is lower than that of seawater. Buoyancy problems secondary to spinal trauma carry a poor prognosis, and euthanasia may be warranted. Lung lacerations may be repaired coelioscopically (Walsh MT et al, Proc ARAV, 2014, p 36).

EUTHANASIA

In general, euthanasia of sea turtles is reserved for cases with complete blindness, multiple missing limbs, permanent buoyancy anomalies, paralysis that prevents effective swimming, or to end the suffering of a moribund patient. Due to the endangered status of sea turtles, clinicians must obtain permission from relevant legal authorities. Euthanasia methods should follow modern accepted guidelines for euthanasia methods for reptiles, such as the American Veterinary Medical Association Guidelines for the Euthanasia of Animals. Multimodal euthanasia is recommended (see also Chapter 47).

ANESTHESIA

Anesthesia can be induced with propofol (3–10 mg/kg IV). Dexmedetomidine (0.025–0.1 mg/kg IV) combined with ketamine (2.5–10 mg/kg IV) is also safe and effective, and it is useful for larger turtles due to its relatively low volume of delivery.[34,77–80] Midazolam has been used to sedate leatherback hatchlings at 2 to 3 mg/kg IV and has been used in combination with medetomidine, ketamine, and butorphanol in loggerhead turtles.[79,80] Alfaxalone 3 to 10 mg/kg IV is effective for loggerhead turtles.[81] Tiletamine/zolazepam (3 mg/kg IV or IM) has been recommended in the past, but further observations suggest that recovery times may be unacceptably long (Mader D, personal communication, 2017).[16] Moon and Stabenau reported conscious direct orotracheal intubation and isoflurane induction in Kemp's ridley turtles, and Chittick et al. maintained loggerhead turtles with sevoflurane (0.5%–2.5%) in oxygen.[78,82] Intermittent positive pressure ventilation is required during general anesthesia.

Postanesthetic recovery may take minutes to hours depending on choice of drugs, length of the procedure, body temperature, and individual variation. Sea turtles commonly go through several episodes of apparent recovery before consciousness is completely regained. During prolonged recovery, physiological assessment (e.g., blood gas analysis) is warranted. Reversal drugs should be given if available, and other supportive drugs such as epinephrine, atropine, and doxapram should be considered. Turtles are often kept out of the water and not returned to their tanks for at least 24 hours after anesthetic recovery, although cautious earlier introductions are acceptable for fully recovered individuals.

SURGERY

Common surgical procedures include shell and soft-tissue laceration repair, long bone fracture repair, amputation, enucleation, FP excision, hook removal, and coeliotomy.[83–85] The relatively large prefemoral space allows for effective coeliotomy, exteriorization of portions of the digestive tract, and access to many other viscera, including the reproductive tract, kidneys, liver, bladder, and lungs.[83,85] Access to the esophagus and stomach via a supraplastron approach or axillary approach may be required for hook removal depending on hook location (Fig. 176.11).[84,85] Coelioscopic or coelioscopic-assisted techniques are used routinely (Walsh MT et al, Proc ARAV, 2014, p 36).

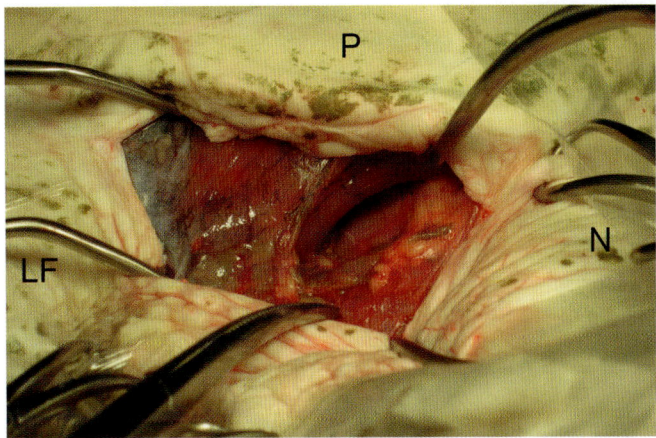

FIG 176.11 Supraplastron approach for access to the distal esophagus during hook removal from a Kemp's ridley turtle (*Lepidochelys kempii*). The patient is in dorsal recumbency, and the incision is held open with retractors. LF, Cranial aspect of left forelimb; N, caudoventral neck; P, plastron (gular scute). (Courtesy of New England Aquarium.)

Hooks and line occasionally pass through a sea turtle's digestive system over time without causing obvious problems, but more commonly they become impaled along the digestive tract warranting surgical removal.[1] Clinicians must use judgment in determining whether conservative monitoring or surgical intervention is warranted. Several approaches to hook removal have been described.[1,53] Hooks located near the heart base are especially dangerous and difficult to remove due to the risk of trauma to the bronchi, great vessels, and heart (see Fig. 174.2). Fatal hemorrhage has sometimes occurred during such surgeries.

Entanglement in fishing lines, nets, and trap lines is common (see Fig. 174.1). The offending material needs to be carefully removed, and the tissue assessed for viability. Sometimes viability is initially unclear, thus patience is needed to monitor healing and viability over time. Amputation is considered as needed. The decision to release a turtle after amputation is dependent on clinical outcome, expected ability to survive in the wild, and discussion with regulatory agencies. In general, release of a turtle with a single amputation is expected, whereas multiple amputations may justify permanent captivity or euthanasia. One exception may be leatherback turtles, for which single forelimb amputation may not be viable but additional study is warranted.

CO_2 laser excision appears to be an effective method for controlling FP.[16] Clinicians should recall herpes latency and understand that surgical excision does not eliminate infection, thus future relapses are possible.

Govett et al. evaluated tissue response to four different absorbable skin sutures in loggerhead turtles.[86] Histologically, polyglactin 910 produced the greatest tissue reaction, whereas poliglecaprone 25 and polyglyconate caused the least tissue reaction. In general, skin sutures need to be left in place for a minimum of 4 to 6 weeks.

MANAGEMENT OF HYPOTHERMIC (COLD-STUNNED) TURTLES

Hypothermic events that affect sea turtles may be classified as acute or chronic. Acute events often occur in winter in the southern United States and are of short duration.[4] These events may involve hundreds or thousands of turtles in a short period of time. Many acutely hypothermic turtles improve quickly with rewarming and supportive care and can be released as soon as appropriate environmental conditions exist.[10] Chronic hypothermic events typically occur in higher latitudes during late autumn and early winter when turtles fail to move to warmer zones. In such events, turtles may be affected by cold for days to weeks before eventual stranding and are thus often in poor physical and physiological condition. Chronically hypothermic turtles are commonly affected by acidosis, respiratory and cardiac failure, decreased renal function, pneumonia, sepsis, and other pathological processes.[12–17,48]

Chronically hypothermic turtles should initially be kept within 2°C to 3°C (3°F–5°F) of their core body temperature.[16] Animals are placed on towels or padding in a climate-controlled space that increases their core temperature to 13°C (55°C) over the first 24 hours. Most animals are treated with fluid therapy. In animals with poor cardiac contractility, as determined by echocardiography and severe bradycardia, atropine (0.05–0.2 mg/kg IV) or epinephrine (0.1 mg/kg IM or IV) may be effective. Although its use has fallen from favor in domestic animal medicine because it increases CNS oxygen demand, doxapram (5 mg/kg) may be effective in stimulating ventilation when administered intravenously in apneic turtles. Cold-stunned turtles that require mechanical ventilation carry a poor prognosis, but if caseload and resources permit, ventilation may save some individuals.[87]

Hypothermic turtles should be provided a shallow freshwater bath adjusted to their core body temperature within the first 24 hours. Stronger turtles may be given access to shallow seawater within 24 to 48 hours, and weaker turtles continue with shallow fresh or brackish water bathing until their hydration and strength have improved.

After the first day of care, patient temperature is raised 3°C (5°F) per day until the temperature reaches 25°C (78°F). Chronically hypothermic turtles may require months of care using the diagnostic and therapeutic methods described previously. Hypothermic turtles are generally not fed until they are able to swim on their own, and their hydration and electrolytes have returned to within normal limits. Body condition, attitude, and activity level should be carefully evaluated before assist-feeding is instituted. In many cases, turtles begin feeding in several weeks voluntarily. Anorectic turtles may be managed with vitamin B complex, tube feeding, thyroxine, or other appetite stimulants (New England Aquarium, unpublished data). The outcome for hypothermic turtles is generally good, with 50% to 80% of turtles successfully rehabilitated and released.[15,16]

LEATHERBACK TURTLE EVALUATION AND CARE

The largest extant species of turtle, the oceanic leatherback turtle, is a unique patient. Adult leatherbacks are often over 150 cm in curved carapace length and can weigh several hundred kilograms. There are approximately eight documented cases of leatherback rehabilitation attempts, some of which are only documented in the popular press and none of which are thoroughly described in the peer-reviewed literature (Fig. 176.12) (Innis CJ et al, Proc 47th Annu Conf Intern Assoc Aquat Anim Med, 2013, pp 77–78).[60] Common reasons for leatherback stranding include boat strike, entanglement, or postentanglement injuries. A body of data has been generated on physical examination, clinicopathologic, microbiologic, toxicologic, parasitologic, and pathologic findings for this species (Innis CJ et al, Proc 47th Annu Conf Intern Assoc Aquat Anim Med, 2013, pp 77–78).[3,34,43,44,46,60,89–91] Entangled and stranded leatherbacks show evidence of physiological stress and negative energy balance.[3,89] Methods for field anesthesia of adult and hatchling leatherbacks have been developed.[34,79] Solitary large intestinal diverticulitis and adrenal coccidiosis are interesting, highly prevalent lesions in this species that

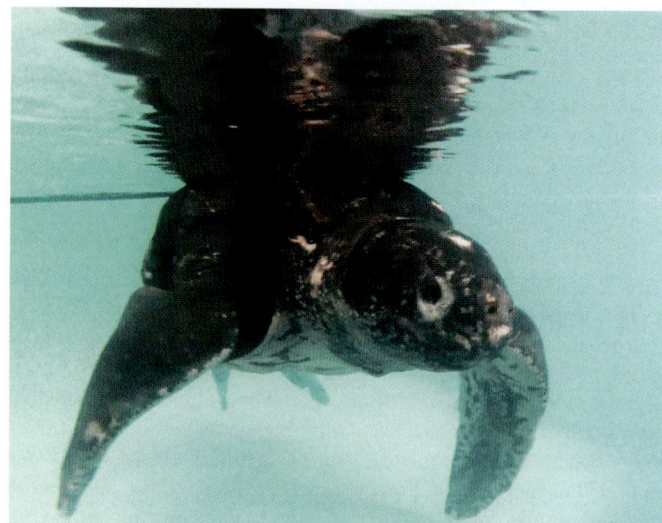

FIG 176.12 A hospitalized adult male leatherback turtle (*Dermochelys coriacea*). A harness loosely surrounds the forelimbs to prevent the turtle from colliding with the tank walls. (Courtesy of New England Aquarium.)

appear to be unrelated to the cause of death (e.g., seen in turtles killed by boat strike or entanglement).[90,91]

Among the few hospitalized leatherbacks, success seems to be greatest when the rehabilitation period is minimized and release is expedited (e.g., several days or less). Supportive care is provided, and as soon as possible the turtle is released at sea. In the only case where postrelease outcome was monitored, a male leatherback traveled 5600 km in 97 days, with diving patterns comparable to healthy leatherbacks tracked in the same region (Innis CJ et al, Proc 47th Annu Conf Intern Assoc Aquat Anim Med, 2013, pp 77–78).

TRANSPORT AND RELEASE

A recent study indicated that Kemp's ridley turtles transported by vehicle for 13 or 26 hours demonstrated a significant physiological stress response, including increased plasma corticosterone and blood glucose proportional to the duration of transport. However, their general physiological status (e.g., heart rate, respiratory rate, electrolytes, blood gases) remained stable.[36] Methods to reduce stress during transport should be employed (e.g., padded, quiet, dark crates) and are worthy of further study. The location at which sea turtles are released is usually determined by governing authorities with assistance from biologists and veterinarians.

ACKNOWLEDGMENTS

The staff and volunteers of Massachusetts Audubon Wellfleet Bay Sanctuary and the New England Aquarium provided access and care for many of the turtles on which this chapter is based.

REFERENCES

See www.expertconsult.com for a complete list of references.

177

Commercial Reptile Farming

Walter Mustin and Javier G. Nevarez

Most people think of cattle, poultry, and swine as agricultural farming, but there is a lesser known agricultural sector, reptile farming. Specifically, this chapter will provide information about commercial reptile farms that produce reptiles as a source of food and textiles. Reptiles are farmed on six continents worldwide and make an appreciable contribution to human well-being through food security and poverty alleviation. In addition, it provides an avenue for the protection of reptile species. Annual production of Chinese softshell turtles alone totaled 344,800 tonnes in 2014.[1] World trade of crocodilian skins exceeded 1.8 million in 2013.[2] The exports of American alligator (*Alligator mississippiensis*) skins from the United States in 2013 numbered 481,341 with an average per skin value of US$241 resulting in an economic value of US$116m.[2] The economic impact of all reptile farms worldwide is not known, but it can be estimated at hundreds of millions of dollars.[2] The benefits of these operations go well beyond the economic impact. These farms also serve as an important source of food in developing countries. In 2013 exports of crocodilian meat were approximately 550 tonnes.[2] These values are only for reported exports and do not take into account local consumption of crocodilian meat, which has a direct impact on the nutrition of local families.

When regulations and enforcement are in place, these farms are also an integral part of creating economic incentives to help protect threatened and endangered reptile species. Engaging local communities is a critical part of the conservation of any species. When those communities benefit economically from conservation, programs are more likely to be successful. Self-sustaining farms maintaining breeding adults and ranching operations where eggs and/or reptiles are collected from the wild and reared in captivity are two systems to commercially farm crocodilians, Caribbean green sea turtles (*Chelonia mydas*), and fresh water chelonians. Many of these species are protected under the Convention on International Trade in Endangered Species of Wild Fauna and Flora (CITES). Therefore their commercial trade across international borders of participating countries is tightly regulated. Captive-bred green sea turtle mariculture and crocodilian farming demonstrate renewable programs with benefits to man and positive conservation implications for endangered and threatened species. Veterinarians working with these species in commercial operations should ensure that animals are maintained according to proper rules and regulations within the country. Furthermore they should strive to improve animal welfare by applying recommendations from the Farm Animal Welfare Committee (e.g., the five freedoms) or the AVMA Animal Welfare Principles.[3,4]

MARICULTURE OF GREEN SEA TURTLES AT THE CAYMAN TURTLE CONSERVATION AND EDUCATION CENTRE

History/Background Information

The Cayman Turtle Conservation and Education Centre Ltd. (CTCEC), first established in 1968 as Mariculture Ltd., and later purchased by the Cayman Islands Government and renamed The Cayman Turtle Farm, Ltd., now operates as a self-sustaining green sea turtle husbandry and research centre where no eggs or adults are removed from the wild. Captive breeders, second-generation offspring from wild stock and eggs legally collected from 1968 to 1978,[5,6] lay their eggs on an artificial beach, part of the 9.3-hectare production, research, and tourist facility. Eggs are collected and incubated in a purpose-built temperature-controlled hatchery for approximately 60 days, after which the hatchlings are transferred to tanks and grown out for eventual release, processing, or for use as breeders. The Centre produces a legal source of turtle meat for widespread local consumption, maintaining cultural culinary practices while providing a deterrent to illegal take.[7] In addition, scientists invited to the facility over a 40-year period have contributed to research on sea turtle health, genetics, sex determination, reproduction, physiology, imprinting, and migratory behavior—all in a unique environment where large numbers of green sea turtles of known ages can be studied in a controlled setting.

From the Centre's inception in 1968, Centre researchers have confronted and solved husbandry problems relating to the reproduction, culture, and health of green sea turtles starting with the initial transfer and successful incubation of eggs obtained from Costa Rica in 1968.[6,8] In 1980 the Centre held and successfully pioneered breeding protocols for the highly endangered Kemp's ridley turtle (*Lepidochelys kempii*) (Wood et al, unpublished data). This research continues to enrich our understanding of sea turtle biology and conservation.

Laws and Regulations

All species of marine turtles are protected under Caymanian law, which includes the *National Conservation Law, 2013,* and the *Marine Conservation (Turtle Protection) Regulations (2008 Revision).* Under this legislation, administered by the Ministry of Tourism, Environment, Development and Commerce, the capture, possession, trade, and export of protected species is prohibited unless authorized by permit. This applies as well to turtles originating from the CTCEC. In 1973 the US *Endangered Species Act* placed the green sea turtle and other sea turtles under protection, making it illegal to catch, sell, import or own any part of the listed species. CITES came into effect in 1977 with green sea turtles listed on Appendix II and later transferred from Appendix II to Appendix I (1977). CITES regulations are implemented by the Cayman Islands through the Cayman *Endangered Species Protection and Propagation Law of 1978* and subsequently through the *Endangered Species (Trade and Transport) Law, 2004.*

Husbandry

Tanks. Turtles are kept in 0.5 to 166 m³ tanks deep enough for them to submerge completely and exhibit normal swimming behavior. Breeders are kept in a 2837 m³ saltwater pond. Tank materials used include concrete and fiberglass with smooth, nonabrasive surfaces that prevent injury to the turtles and allow for easy cleaning.

Water Supply. A continuous flow-through system utilizes high-volume electric axle flow pumps (FPI Pumps, Pompano, FL) to deliver 5000 gpm (18.9 m³pm) of fresh, unfiltered seawater to turtles held in concrete tanks and the breeder pond (Fig. 177.1). Back-up diesel pumps provide redundancy during power outages (see Fig. 177.1)

The water distribution design ensures that fresh seawater flows directly from the ocean to each tank and returns to the ocean without passing through other tanks, preventing the transfer of waste water and minimizing the potential transfer of pathogens between tanks (Fig. 177.2). Depth ranges from 0.7 to 5 meters depending on the size of turtles held. Tank water turnover rates range from 11 to 150 minutes (Table 177.1).

Stocking Density. Specific tank densities are a function of turtle age, size, tank area, depth, volume, water temperature, and flow rates. Tanks full of water allow the turtles, like fish, three-dimensional movement. In contrast, drained tanks confine turtles to a given tank's two-dimensional surface area. Percent coverage (% coverage) is a term the Centre uses to describe the percentage of turtles combined area relative to the tank surface area, where % coverage = (number of turtles × average turtle area/tank area) × 100. Drained tanks where turtles (without stacking or touching each other) completely cover the tank bottom are examples

TABLE 177.1 Tank Size, Volume, and Water Turnover			
Tank	Vol (m³)	Flow Rate (L/min)	Water Turnover (min)
Hatchling tank (102 cm × 165 cm)	0.5	45	11
Hatchling tank (152 cm × 178 cm)	1.4	45	30
Hatchling tank (165 cm × 213 cm)	1.9	45	42
Grow-out tank (9 m × 9 m)	61	757	81
Grow-out tank (15 m × 15 m)	166	1136	146
Breeder pond* (0.2165 ha)	2837	18927	150

*With even slope for 3 meters up to beach.

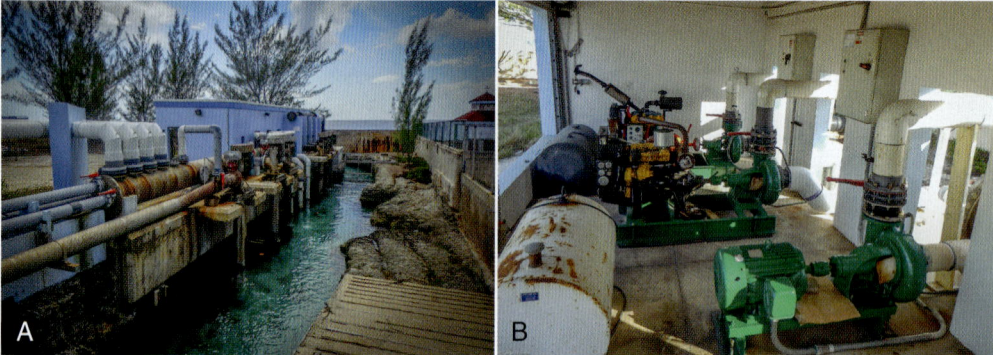

FIG 177.1 (A) Axile flow pumps deliver 5000 gpm (18.9 m³pm) each of fresh, unfiltered seawater to turtles held in concrete tanks and the breeder pond. (B) Back-up diesel pumps provide redundancy during power outages.

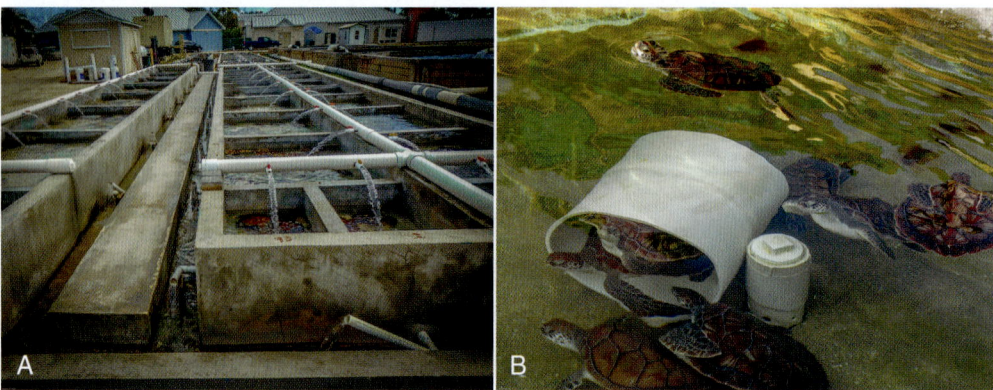

FIG 177.2 (A) The water distribution design ensures that fresh seawater flows directly from the ocean to each tank and returns to the ocean without passing through other tanks. Submerged containers provide enrichment, cover, and shade. (B) Submerged containers such as PVC pipe coupling or plastic flowerpots are effective structures that provide cover, shade, and refuge.

of 100% coverage. The CTCEC hatchling and production tank densities are such that coverage is limited to a maximum of 50%. Turtles are stocked in tanks initially at low percentage coverage. As they grow and their coverage approaches 50%, either their numbers are reduced or they are moved to a larger tank. Table 177.2 shows suggested hatchling tank density schedules that factor in % coverage and other criteria. Table 177.3 shows grow-out tank density schedule for yearling to harvest-size turtles of 5 years.

TABLE 177.2 Grow-Out Tank Density Schedule

Tank Size	Age of Stock	No. of Stock Range
9 m × 9 m (61 m³)	Yearlings	300–800
15 m × 15 m (166 m³)	2 years	500–800
15 m × 15 m (166 m³)	3 years	360–500
15 m × 15 m (166 m³)	4 years	260–360
15 m × 15 m (166 m³)	5 years	200–260

TABLE 177.3 Feed Schedule and Growth Curve for Southfresh and Cargill Feed

Age (mo)	Weight (kg)	Feed
1	0.05	Triton WW 4010 & 3606
6	0.73	Triton WW 4010 & 3606
12	2.36	Triton WW 4010 & 3606
18	4.90	South fresh
24	8.16	South fresh
30	7.44	South fresh
36	16.51	South fresh
42	21.30	South fresh
48	26.30	South fresh
54	31.20	South fresh
60	36.10	South fresh

Diet. A variety of nutritionally complete grain-based commercial extruded floating fish feeds from 0.3 to 1.5 cm diameter are used at CTCEC to grow turtles from hatchlings to breeder size (Table 177.4). Utilizing these diets, sexual maturity of captive green turtles occurs in less than 10 years.

Rations are determined based on a percentage of body weight and age. Early growth is exponential, with 5-year-olds averaging 36 kg (see Table 177.3). Qualitative and quantitative amino acid requirements for hatchling green turtles have been determined.[9] Hatchlings are started on 40% protein diets (Triton 4010 Transition, Cargill, MN). Yearlings and adults receive 36% protein diets (Southfresh Feeds, Demopolis, AL). Decreasing protein levels reflect the natural transition from carnivorous to herbivorous wild diets of green sea turtles. Breeders receive a custom 36% protein diet with added omega-3 fatty acids. Feeding frequency varies from 6 to 7 times/day for hatchlings to 3 times daily for juveniles and adults. Turtles fed too infrequently or an inadequate amount can become aggressive and bite one another. Resulting lesions can become a target for further aggression. However, overfeeding significantly contributes to decreased water quality from uneaten food. Hatchlings are sampled and weighed monthly to adjust rations relative to established growth curves.

Enrichment, Shade, and Cover. Environmental enrichment effectively reduces stereotypic pattern swimming and resting behaviors while increasing random swimming and focused behavior in sea turtles.[10] Floating and submerged enrichment devices are employed at CTCEC to add complexity to the tank environment. Submerged containers such as PVC pipe coupling or plastic flowerpots are effective structures that provide cover, shade, and refuge (see Fig. 177.2). Shade cloths deployed above the tanks provide a refuge from direct sun exposure (Fig. 177.3).

TABLE 177.4 Feed Formulations

Feed	Custom Green Turtle Feed (Southfresh, Demopolis, AL)	Triton WW 4010 (Cargill, Minneapolis, MN)	Triton WW 3606 (Cargill, Minneapolis, MN)
% Protein	36	40	36
% Fat	3.5	10	6
Fiber	6.0	4	3.5

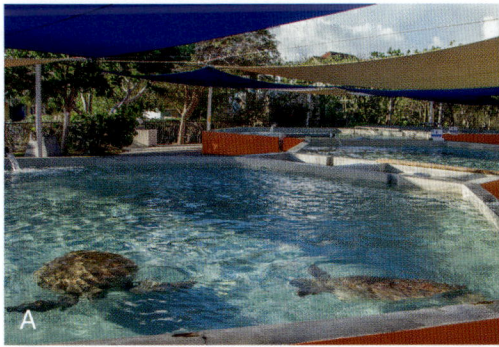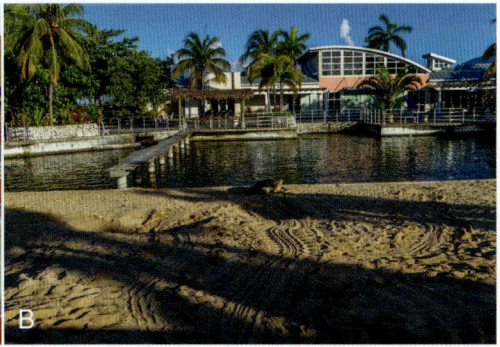

FIG 177.3 (A) Shade cloths deployed above tanks provide a refuge from direct sun exposure. (B) Breeding occurs in a communal breeder pond, and females lay multiple clutches on an artificial beach from April to September.

Hygiene and Preventative Medicine. Successful hatchling husbandry requires regular and sustained removal of uneaten food, feces, and organic material from the water and tank surfaces. Hatchling tanks are drained daily, with the sides and floor scrubbed with a brush, and refilled. Dilute chlorine solutions (100 ppm) are used on tanks weekly after turtles have been temporarily removed from the tanks. Tanks are thoroughly rinsed with fresh seawater before restocking. Excess carapace algal growth can be controlled by scrubbing lightly with 3M Scotch Bright pads (St. Paul, MN) combined with a 15-minute bath in a Halamid Aqua (Chloramine T trihydrate) (Ferndale, WA) solution at 2000 ppm. All turtles 18 months old and older are vaccinated against *Clostridium botulinum* using Botumink (United Vaccines, Inc., Madison, WI), containing *Clostridium botulinum* type C toxoid. A withdrawal period of 60 days precedes harvest. External lesions are routinely treated topically using a 1:1 mixture of petroleum jelly and 1% silver sulfadiazine cream (Dr. Reddy's Laboratories, Shreveport, LA). Necropsies are performed routinely. Animals with clinical signs are isolated in a quarantine area for further tests, observation, and, if needed, treatment. Turtles are randomly sampled for health checks as part of a preventative medicine program.

Breeding Program

Breeding occurs in a communal breeder pond where breeders are housed at a ratio of five females to every male. Females lay multiple clutches on an artificial beach from April to September, with a mean nesting interval of 11 days (see Fig. 177.3). Multiple paternity has been found in 100% of CTCEC clutches.[11] Eggs are transferred from the artificial beach to the hatchery (at or within 12 hours of oviposition) and are packed in (38 × 24 × 30 cm) Styrofoam boxes, sandwiched between layers of sand and light fabric in a way that allow the fabric to be raised for periodic egg inspection (Fig. 177.4). Eggs are incubated an average of 68 days. Upon emergence, hatchlings are transferred to plastic trays (62 cm × 42 cm × 15 cm) until such time that their external yolks are fully absorbed and their plastrons have closed (1–10 days). They are then transferred to outdoor purpose-built concrete hatchery tanks.

Slaughter and Processing

Harvest-sized turtles (mean of 45 kg) are euthanized by captive bolt followed by exsanguination and are processed in a purpose-built, government-inspected abattoir. Dress out of approximately 50% yields a variety of products, including turtle steak, stew, menavalins, and bone, which are sold fresh locally to individuals and restaurants.[7]

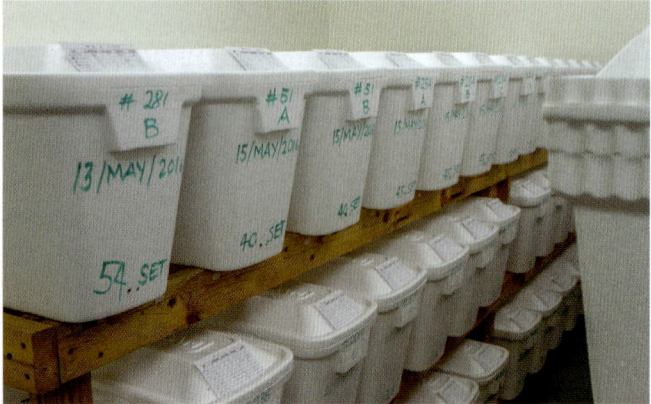

FIG 177.4 Eggs are transferred from the artificial beach to the hatchery (at or within 12 hours of oviposition) and are packed in sand-filled Styrofoam boxes (38 × 24 × 30 cm).

COMMERCIAL REPTILE FARMING OF CROCODILIANS

History and Background

Of the 23 species of crocodilians, the skin and/or meat of 14 species are currently traded internationally (Table 177.5).[12] In the commercial trade, crocodilian skins are traditionally divided as classic (*Alligator mississippiensis, C. porosus, C., novaeguineea, C. niloticus*) and caiman skins.[12] In 2013, there were 878,332 classic skins and 1,010,302 caiman skins in the commercial trade.[2] Although the total commercial value of crocodilian skins is unknown, it can be estimated at over US$200m per year. In addition to skins, crocodilian meat, teeth, and other body parts are also commercially traded, providing additional value.

Twelve species are captive bred in commercial farms (i.e., egg production from captive animals) or ranches, whereas the other two species, *Caiman yacare* in Paraguay and *Melanosuchus niger* in Brazil, are collected through wild harvest only (see Table 177.5).[12] Ranching operations

TABLE 177.5	Worldwide Commercial Trade of Crocodilians	
Species	**Source**	**Country**
Alligator mississippiensis	C, R, W	United States
Alligator sinensis	C	China
Caiman crocodilus	W	Nicaragua, Guyana
Caiman crocodilus	C	Colombia
Caiman crocodilus	C, R*	Brazil
Caiman crocodilus	R, W	Venezuela
Caiman latirostris	R	Argentina
Caiman yacare	R	Argentina
Caiman yacare	C, W, R	Bolivia
Caiman yacare	C, R	Brazil
Caiman yacare	W**	Paraguay
Melanosuchus niger	W	Brazil
Crocodylus acutus	C	Honduras, Colombia
Crocodylus acutus	R, C	Cuba
Crocodylus johnstoni	C, R, W	Australia
Crocodylus moreletii	C, R*	Mexico
Crocodylus niloticus	C, R	Zimbabwe, Kenya, Namibia
Crocodylus niloticus	C, R, W	Madagascar
Crocodylus niloticus	R, W	Tanzania, Mozambique
Crocodylus niloticus	R	Botswana, Malawi, Zambia, Uganda, Ethiopia, Swaziland
Crocodylus niloticus	R*	Egypt
Crocodylus niloticus	C	Mauritius, South Africa, Tunisia
Crocodylus suchus	C	Senegal, Mali
Crocodylus novaeguineae	R, W	Papua New Guinea, Indonesia
Crocodylus porosus	C	China, Singapore, Vietnam, Thailand, Philippines
Crocodylus porosus	C, R, W	Australia, Indonesia, Papua New Guinea
Crocodylus porosus	C, R*, W*	Malaysia
Crocodylus rhombifer	C	Cuba
Crocodylus siamensis	C	Thailand, Cambodia, Vietnam, China

Used with permission from the IUCN-SSC Crocodile Specialist Group.
*, Under development.
**, Program suspended.
C, Captive bred; R, ranching; W, wild harvest.

collect eggs, live hatchlings, or juveniles from the wild with the subsequent growth of the animals in captivity until they reach the market size for the species. All commercially traded species are listed on Appendix I or II of the Convention on International Trade in Endangered Species of Wild Fauna and Flora (CITES). Countries that participate in CITES must demonstrate that commercial trade has no detrimental effect on the wild populations of the species. As part of CITES regulations, all commercial crocodilian skins must be tagged upon skinning of the animal (Fig. 177.5). Some species have different CITES classifications in different countries. Trade of wild-caught CITES I crocodilians is not allowed, but CITES I species are still commercially traded if they are reared in farming or ranching operations only. This sustainable use of crocodilians has contributed to the protection and preservation of various species around the world. In addition it has led to a dominance of legal trade and minimized illegal trade of crocodilian species. In addition to CITES regulations, each country has their own regulatory control over the farming and ranching of their native crocodilian species. In the United States the regulatory control is at the state level whereas in other countries it falls under the federal government or its equivalent. Some countries have produced best management practices documents to assist in the oversight and regulation of their crocodilian operations (Table 177.6).[12–18] Some of these documents also provide specifics as to the welfare and management of the animals.

ALLIGATORS

In the United States, the American alligator is the only crocodilian species in commercial trade. The American alligator population was at critically low levels during the 1960s, but federal and state conservation programs designed to protect wild populations through a 10-year ban on wild harvest brought their population numbers back to sustainable levels. Consequently, captive farming and ranching operations developed.

Farming and ranching operations can be found in Louisiana, Florida, Texas, Georgia, and other southern states where alligators occur naturally. The Louisiana Alligator Industry (LAI) stands as one of the most successful examples of viable, sustainable use of wild species in commercial trade. The Louisiana Department of Wildlife and Fisheries (LDWF) regulates the state's alligator management program. An alligator ranching program was established in 1986. The success of this program can be further documented by an increase in exports in parallel with an increase in the wild populations. In 1986 the United States exported 31,000 alligator skins.[2] This pales in comparison to the 481,304 skins exported in 2013, one of the highest production years for the industry.[2] Today the population of wild alligators is estimated at well over 1 million animals, a 90% increase from the 1960s estimates.

As of 2016 there were 56 alligator ranches that produced approximately 300,000 to 350,000 alligators every year valued at over US $50 million for the hides alone (Elsey R, personal communication, 2016). Under this program, the LDWF granted egg harvest permits to licensed alligator ranchers in the state. Egg collection takes place between June and August. Egg numbers can range from 20 to 60 per nest. Once eggs are collected, they are taken to a private facility for incubation. Eggs collected from the wild are at different stages of incubation, so once in the alligator ranch it may take anywhere from a few weeks to months for the eggs to hatch depending on the time of collection. The total incubation period is approximately 65 days. The majority of alligator ranchers do not attempt to select for a specific sex, which is determined

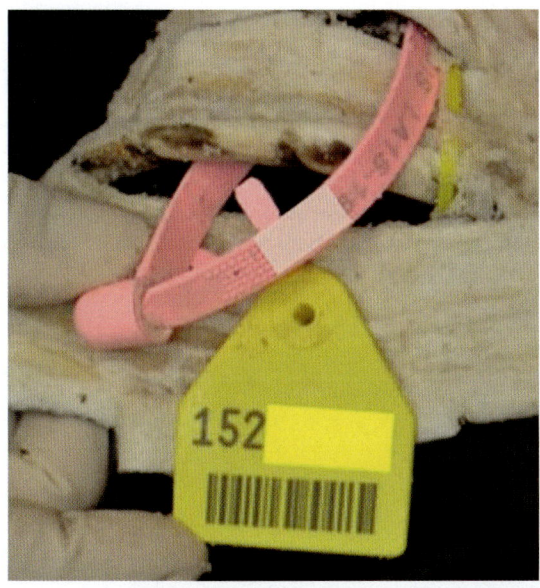

FIG 177.5 Example of identification tags attached through the distal part of the tail skin. The pink tag is a CITES tag and the yellow is attached by the tannery for additional control. The number on each tag has been partially obscured for confidentiality purposes.

TABLE 177.6   Currently Existing Documents That Address Codes of Practice and Best Management Recommendations for Crocodilians

Country	Organization Type	Document	Available Online
Australia	Government	Code of Practice for the Humane Treatment of Wild and Farmed Australian Crocodiles[14]	Yes
Australia	Government	Crocodile Farming Research: Hatching to Harvest[15]	Yes
Australia	IUCN-Crocodile Specialist Group	Best Management Practices for Crocodilian Farming[12]	Yes
United States	Government	Best Management Practices for Louisiana Alligator Farming[13]	No
United States	Government	Alligator Production: Introduction, Breeding and Egg Incubation, Grow-Out and Harvest[17]	Yes
South Africa	Government	South African National Standard: Crocodiles in Captivity[16]	Yes
Thailand	Government	The Agricultural Standard, TAS 7700–2016, Crocodile Farming[18]	Yes
Zambia	Crocodile Farmers Association and Government	Draft Code of Practice (unpublished)	No
Zimbabwe	Crocodile Farmers Association	Codes of Practice	No

by incubation temperature. Once alligators hatch, they are placed in indoor buildings where they are raised until the time of slaughter at 10 to 12 months. Market-size alligators average 36 inches in length (tip of snout to tip of the tail). The alligator hides are then sold to dealers and tanners for further processing. The Louisiana program is the largest supplier of alligator hides in the world. Louisiana alligator hides will eventually end up in high-end retail products such as watch bands, shoes, purses, and other fashion items. These products have the benefit of coming from a natural renewable resource that is environmentally friendly and helps contribute to the wild populations of alligators. In addition to the hide, alligator meat is sold to processing plants and distributed to restaurants, supermarkets, and specialty stores.

The conservation aspect of the Louisiana alligator program comes from the 12% of alligators in each facility (based on the yearly egg hatch) that is destined for release back to their natural habitat each year. This percent of alligators to be released was determined based on an expected survival of the eggs that hatch in the wild and amounts to approximately 40,000 to 50,000 juvenile alligators being released back to the wild every year (LDWF annual report, 2015).[19] Alligators are identified using toe tags and a tail notch before release by personnel from LDWF. Health surveillance of alligators has been performed in alligators destined for release. Veterinary evaluation of disease occurrences in ranches also allows for determination of any potential pathogens of concern for wild populations. This program has been extremely successful and is a model for other crocodilian species around the world.

Husbandry

Housing. Currently the majority of alligators are housed indoors (Fig. 177.6) in fiberglass tubs or concrete pens with a plastic liner to protect their skin. Some facilities have started utilizing custom-built plastic pens similar to those encountered in fish aquaculture. Currently, there are no specific regulations for enclosure size/type or environmental requirements (e.g., air quality, photoperiod) for farmed alligators. Farmers often experiment to evaluate new options for housing of captive alligators.

Water Supply. The water in alligator ranches can be from well, city, or surface sources (i.e., bayous). Facilities have either insulated storage tanks or an on-demand heating system (Fig. 177.7) in order to supply water at the appropriate temperature of 85° to 90°F (29°–32°C). Currently there are no established water quality parameters for alligators similar to what is found in fisheries. Additional research is needed in this area to determine water quality parameters for optimum health and growth.

Stocking Density. Currently there are no specific regulations for enclosure size for alligators. Guidelines for stocking density of alligators are reported as 1 square foot per animal up to 24 inches (61 cm), 3 square feet for those 24 to 48 inches (61–122 cm), and one additional square foot (929 cm^2) for every additional 6 inches (15 cm) beyond 48 inches in length.[18] These recommendations are based on land square footage and do not take into account water volume/depth. Currently most ranches use 18 to 20 inches of water depth within varied pen dimensions. Therefore designing stocking density recommendations based on water volume would be more appropriate. Water levels are increased as the animals grow in order to increase the volume and adjust for their body size. Lower stocking densities have been associated with better growth and lower corticosterone levels.[20] This is an area

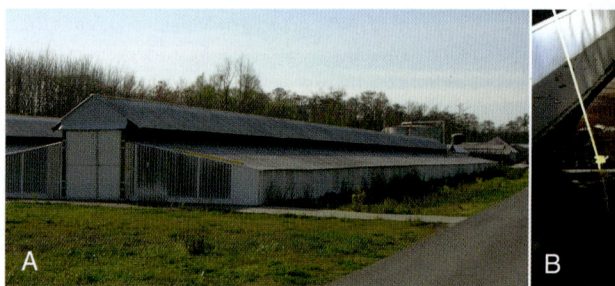
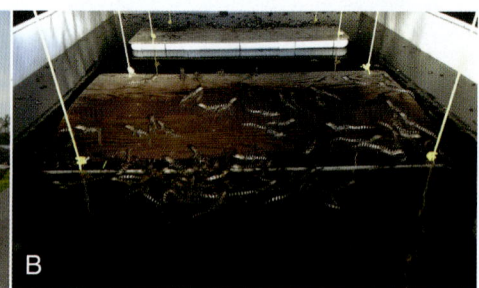

FIG 177.6 (A) Building used in the ranching operation of American alligators (*Alligator mississippiensis*) in Louisiana. (B) Indoor pen housing hatchling alligators. Tables are provided for haul out and feeding area. (A, From Mitchell M, Tully T. *Manual of Exotic Pet Practice.* St. Louis: WB Saunders; 2009, Figure 6.2.; B, courtesy of Javier G. Nevarez.)

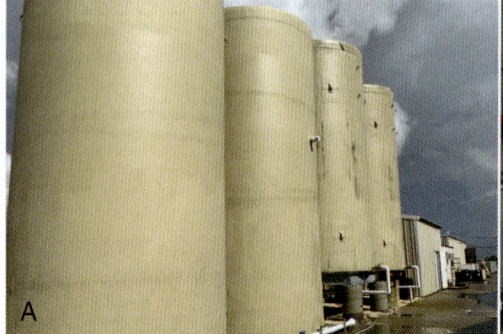
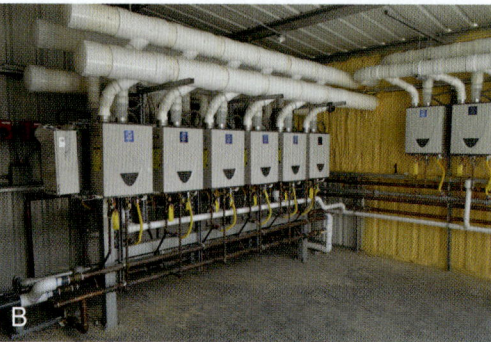

FIG 177.7 (A) Reservoir water tanks in an alligator farm. Tanks are used to hold water after heating and to provide enough pressure for cleaning and washing pens. (B) On-demand water heating system at an alligator farm. This system is highly efficient, does not require storage tanks, and consumes less energy. (Courtesy of Javier G. Nevarez.)

that requires further research to determine what stocking densities provide the ideal combination of efficient growth and optimal health.

Diet. Different feeding regimens and specific nutritional requirements for alligators have been evaluated (Coulson et al, Proc Louisiana Aquaculture Conf, 1992, pp 48–51).[21,22,24,25] Ongoing alligator nutrition research is being performed by the Louisiana State University Agricultural Center. There are commercial, extruded pelletized diets available for alligators. These diets are generally comprised of 45% to 56% protein, less than 11% fat, and fiber content less than 3%. Typically hatchlings are fed the higher protein diet for the first 3 months, and then lower protein diets are used. The majority of the operations will feed a commercial diet exclusively, whereas others mix in fish or chicken. Wooden tables are sometimes placed in the pens and used as a feeding surface, whereas others place the food directly in the water. There is no standardized feeding rate. Some operations feed once per day whereas others feed twice daily. Alligators are typically fed 6 days per week.

Hygiene. There is a wide range of cleaning protocols used across operations. However, in general terms there are two main systems: a fill and flush system and a continuous flow system. In the first system, the pens are drained, flushed, and refilled every 2 to 3 days depending on the age class. In the latter system, there is a continuous but often variable and unknown flow of water into the pens. These pens are only emptied and fully flushed once to twice weekly. When pens are emptied, the walls and floors should be thoroughly scrubbed to reduce the biofilm that forms on the plastic liners. The large amount of organic matter produced by alligators compared with fish precludes the effective use of currently available filtration methods such as bead and sand filters. The development of adequate filtration methods or the use of naturally filtered effluent waters is an area that requires further research. Land application was found to be a viable approach for handling wastewater from alligator farms.[26] Air quality is also an important consideration. Some farms have implemented the use of fans to circulate air through the pens (Fig. 177.8) to improve this aspect, but this is an area that requires further research to determine the best equipment and techniques for this purpose. Finally, implementation of biosecurity protocols such as controlled entry, use of footbaths, and so on, is critical for the control of diseases (Fig. 177.9).

Preventive Medicine. There is currently a WNV vaccine specifically manufactured for use in alligators (Boehringer Ingelheim Vetmedica,

Inc., St. Joseph, MO). It requires two injections administered intramuscularly 3 to 4 weeks apart, with a single yearly booster thereafter. This is the only commercial vaccine available for crocodilians and is strongly recommended for ranches located in areas prone to WNV outbreaks. One of the most effective methods of disease prevention and control is veterinary consultation to evaluate production practices and disease outbreaks. In most instances, necropsy of affected animals is the most comprehensive and effective way to make a definitive diagnosis. Open lines of communication and collaboration between ranchers, veterinarians, and the state agencies are also effective in identifying any potential health issues that may require additional evaluation of animals destined for release to the wild. This helps to ensure the safeguard of wild populations and minimize the introduction of novel disease to the natural habitat.

Breeding Program

Captive breeding programs for American alligators have diminished over the years and represent a minority of the operations. This is not a significant source of animals, but some hatchlings are provided through captive breeding.

Slaughter and Processing

In 2016 the Louisiana Department of Wildlife and Fisheries established a regulation that requires all alligator ranchers and farmers to slaughter the animals according to established guidelines by the AVMA and Swiss Federal Veterinary Office (FVO).[27] Specifically, it includes the use of penetrating and nonpenetrating captive bolt (Fig. 47.2) and spinal cord severance followed immediately by pithing. Decapitation and spinal severance alone are not acceptable methods. This regulation had the

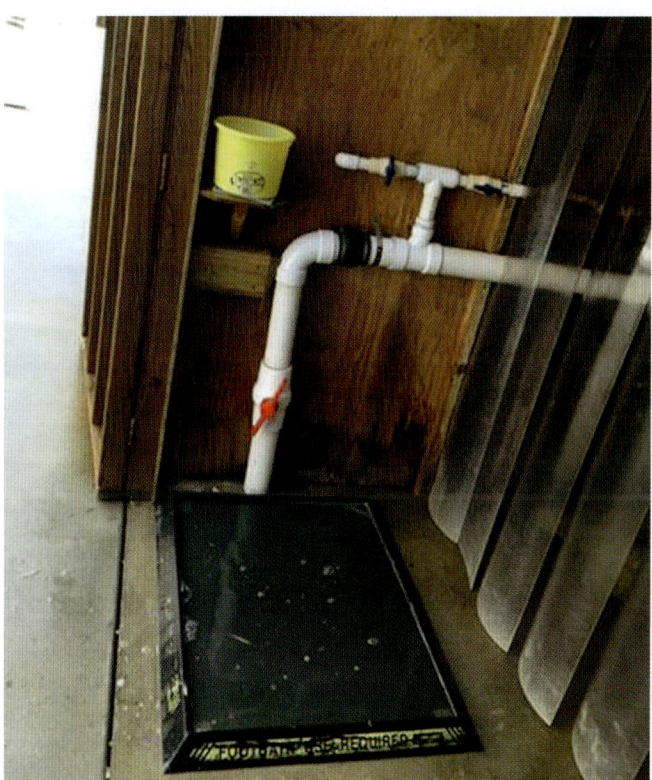

FIG 177.9 Biosecurity measures at an alligator ranch. A foot bath and hand wash station are used before entering the building. Solution is made fresh daily. In addition, doors (shown open) and plastic curtain prevent entry of mosquitoes and other pests into the building. (Courtesy of Javier G. Nevarez.)

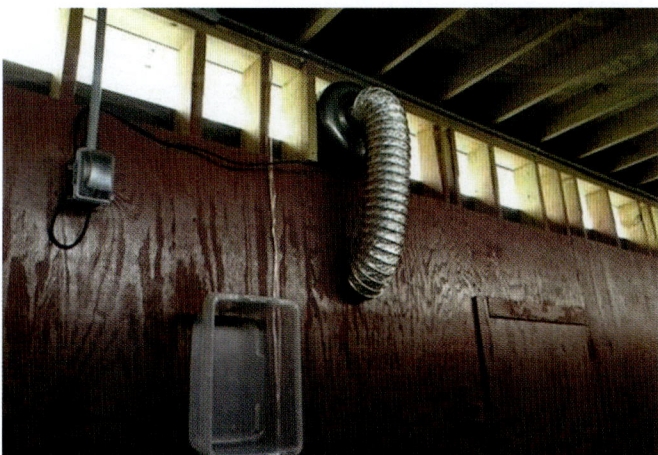

FIG 177.8 Exhaust fan used to promote air exchange in an indoor alligator housing facility. (Courtesy of Javier G. Nevarez.)

full support of the Louisiana Alligators Farmers and Ranchers Association and represents the first instance of regulatory governing of slaughter methods for a commercial reptile species in the United States. These guidelines and regulations also acknowledge that methods may be refined as more research becomes available and strongly encourage consultation with veterinarians to ensure that the methods being used are the most humane possible for each species and circumstance. Further discussion on slaughter can be found in Chapter 47.

CROCODILES AND CAIMANS

There are nine species of crocodiles and three species of caiman in commercial trade (see Table 177.5).[2] In general, crocodiles and caimans are reared in a different manner than alligators. Captive breeding is still an active part of the commercial trade for eight of the crocodile species and two of the caiman species. Ranching is becoming more widespread but still represents a lower proportion of the source for these species. Aspects of their husbandry in commercial operations vary considerably with the wider range of species and countries in which they are reared. Therefore we provide general information about these species and how their captive rearing differs from that of alligators. CITES regulations are in place, but their implementation may vary on a per-country basis.

Husbandry

Housing. In captive breeding operations, the adult animals and often the juveniles are housed in communal outdoor ponds or pens (Fig. 177.10). These can vary from natural earthen ponds to artificial concrete structures. For outdoor rearing, it is also important to provide enough water depth and shade to ensure the animals can seek protection from the sun. Some facilities will keep hatchlings outdoors whereas others maintain them indoors for a period of time. Some facilities are starting to rear animals indoors only, but this practice is not currently widespread.

Water Supply. The water source is more likely to be from well or other natural sources (i.e., lakes, rivers). The use of a water heating system is only necessary where needed as per the local climate and often only used for animals being reared indoors. Animals housed outdoors will experience a more natural variation in temperature because the outdoors ponds and pens are less likely to be heated. Although water temperatures of 85° to 90°F (29°–32°C) will offer maximum growth, the focus in these operations is to ensure the animals have enough water depth to allow for a thermal gradient during the colder times of the year.

Stocking Densities. Stocking densities are a consideration for animal health and husbandry and in the case of crocodiles are also important due to the aggressive nature of some species, such as *C. porosus*. Specific recommendations are available for *C. porosus* and *C. niloticus* (Box 177.1).[12] These recommendations are based on surface area but do not take into account water volume. Because crocodiles and caimans are often housed outdoors, enclosure designs often involve both dry land areas, as well as water areas.

Diet. Diets for crocodiles and caimans vary widely because commercial, extruded pelletized diets are not readily available or not readily accepted by all species. For this reason, whole prey, offal, and animal carcasses from other species (e.g., poultry, swine), with vitamin and mineral supplements, are commonly used.[12] Some farms in South Africa produce their own feed using proprietary formulas. Hatchlings are usually fed daily, and the frequency is decreased to four to five times weekly for juveniles and two to three times weekly for brood stock.[12] The time of the year and season may also influence the type of food and frequency of feeding.

Hygiene. Due to the wide range of species, housing conditions, and countries, hygiene protocols are highly variable. There is little to no treatment of water in natural earthen ponds. Outdoor and indoor pens will have water changes at varying frequencies. Although some farms have biosecurity protocols, this is not widespread.

Preventive Medicine. Crocodile species reared in outdoor earthen ponds are more likely to be exposed to parasites and other diseases due to environmental exposure. In these instances, routine monitoring of fecal examinations and histopathologic evaluation of tissues after slaughter would help establish baseline references for the diseases encountered in a particular facility so that management techniques can

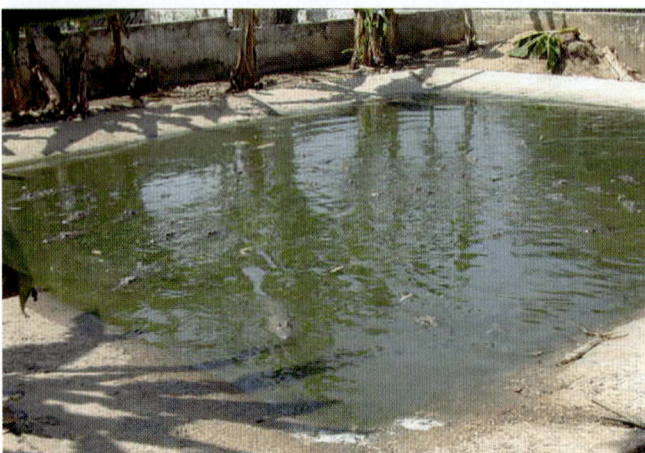

FIG 177.10 Outside enclosure at a Morelet's crocodile (*Crocodylus moreletii*) farm in Mexico. (From Mitchell M, Tully T. *Manual of Exotic Pet Practice.* St. Louis: WB Saunders; 2009, Figure 6.1.)

BOX 177.1   Recommended Stocking Densities for *C. porosus, C. niloticus*, and *A. mississippiensis*

Crocodylus porosus	
Hatchlings	10–15 animals/m²
Animals up to 1 m	2–4 animals/m²
Animals 1–2 m	0.5–1 animals/m²
Crocodylus niloticus	
Hatchlings	<15 animals/m²
Animals 1–1.5 m	2–4 animals/m²
Animals 1.5–2 m	1–2 animals/m²
Alligator mississippiensis	
Animals <0.6 m	<11.1 animals/m²
Animals 0.6–1.2 m	3.7 animals/m²
Animals 1.2–1.35 m	2.8 animals/m²
Animals 1.35–1.5 m	2.2 animals/m²
Animals >1.5 m	Add 0.09 m² per animal for every 0.15 m beyond 1.5 m length

Adapted from the IUCN-SSC Best Management Practices for Crocodilian Farming, with permission.

be applied as needed. Release of animals back to the wild is not as common practice for crocodiles as it is for American alligators. Nonetheless by being reared outdoors, there is still the potential for disease exposure to wild populations via environmental exposure.

Breeding Programs

Captive breeding programs are a common aspect of commercial crocodile and caiman production; however, the specifics of the breeding program will vary according to species and individual farm management. Nonetheless, once the females lay eggs, most facilities will collect them for artificial incubation. Breeding can occur in large communal ponds or in smaller ponds with one male and one to five females.[12]

Slaughter and Processing

The slaughter of crocodiles is carried out by methods recommended within the Analysis of Humane Killing Methods for Reptiles in the Skin Trade published by the Swiss FVO.[28] Further discussion on slaughter can be found in Chapter 47.

GENERAL COMMENTS ON OTHER SPECIES

In addition to sea turtles and crocodilians, freshwater turtles are also widely grown in farms worldwide. These farms supply turtles for laboratory research and educational purposes, the pet trade, and also as food sources. Softshell turtles and sliders (*Trachemys* spp.) are some of the most common species being bred for the food trade. The majority of these farms are closed operations with their own brood stock animals housed in outdoor earthen ponds (Fig. 177.11). Eggs are usually artificially incubated and hatchlings reared in grow-out pens or ponds. Asian countries are one of the largest markets for turtle meat. In Western countries, cultural factors have not allowed reptile meat to become mainstream. Although turtle soup and alligator meat

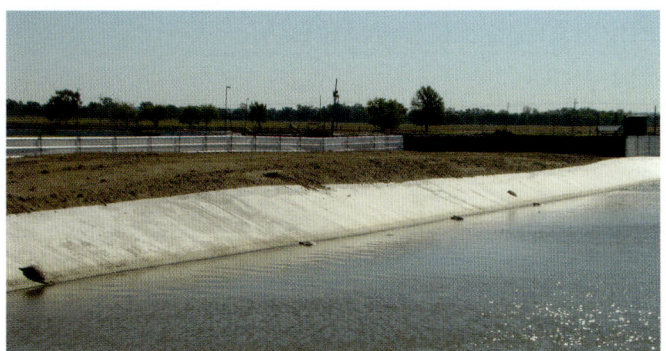

FIG 177.11 Turtle farm pond in Louisiana. This is an earthen pond with a concrete edge and soil area for nesting. (Courtesy of Javier G. Nevarez.)

may be more commonplace in the southeastern United States, meat from other species like green iguanas (*Iguana iguana*) is not welcomed with the same gusto. The availability of farmed turtle meat has curbed some of the illegal trade, but in some countries illegal trade is still very active. One drawback from reptile farms is that like any agriculture endeavor, they can be very labor intensive, and it can take years before a new farm can generate revenue. This of course does not address the immediate economic needs of people and makes it less attractive than traditional farming. When farms are properly managed and regulated by the government, they can have a significant impact on the conservation of the species and the quality of life of the people in local communities.

CONCLUSION

Reptile farming and ranching is a sustainable and profitable agricultural venture in many countries. The benefits are significant for both animal and human populations. A key aspect of the success and sustainability of this trade will be the ability to maintain healthy populations and safeguard the welfare of the animals. This of course is perceived differently across countries but is quickly becoming a critical issue for the long-term survival of farms and ranches. This is an area in which veterinary involvement can have a significant impact. By improving the welfare and health of the animals, farms and ranches can in turn improve productivity. Nonetheless this still remains a challenge in many countries where not even cattle or other traditional agricultural species receive proper veterinary care. The Crocodile Specialist Group has a veterinary group with international members who are actively involved in the care of wild and captive crocodilians. This group serves as a resource for farmers, ranchers, and veterinarians. There is a need for continued research on all aspects of the captive rearing of reptiles in the food trade. This research often has important benefits for the wild populations as well. It is up to current and future generations to ensure that this continues to be a sustainable and renewable industry that benefits the wild population and the communities that share their environment.

ACKNOWLEDGEMENTS

We would like to thank Dr. Ruth Elsey from the Louisiana Department of Wildlife and Fisheries for her guidance and editorial review during preparation of the alligator section of this chapter. Additionally, we thank Mr. Joe Parsons from the Cayman Turtle Conservation and Research Centre for his insight and review of the turtle section of this chapter.

REFERENCES

See www.expertconsult.com for a complete list of references.

178

Large Zoo and Private Collection Management

Paul M. Gibbons

People keep reptiles in large collections for both commercial and noncommercial purposes. Commercial breeding facilities supply the pet trade and produce meat and leather. Noncommercial facilities maintain reptiles for rescue and rehabilitation, for lifetime sanctuary, for pleasure as a hobby, for exhibit and education, and for the conservation of endangered species. Commercial reptile farming is discussed in Chapter 177 and the pet trade is discussed in Chapter 179. This chapter focuses on the management of large collections that are kept for the primary purposes of exhibition, education, and conservation.

Reptile caretakers should provide the five freedoms that all animals need for a life worth living, regardless of the purpose for which they keep them (Table 178.1).[1] To achieve this goal, every captive environment should include species-appropriate physical complexity without potential stressors. Multiple options for heat, humidity, light, water, caging, vegetation, refuge, and substrate must be provided in a manner that allows the reptiles to control how they interact with their environment. Temperature, light, and humidity must cycle daily and seasonally. Provision of feed and water must be based on species-specific natural history. Most reptiles do not feed daily, and some species are adapted to habitats that receive moisture in the absence of rain or experience regular periods without rain or surface moisture. Behavioral enrichment is based on providing varied opportunities for the reptile to select from a mosaic of environmental features and to interact with nonthreatening conspecifics and appropriate prey or browse. Captive reptiles require opportunities to solve the range of problems they might normally face in the wild, with minimal exposure to situations that will induce substantial fight or flight responses. Such enriching care is necessary to achieve the goal of a healthy, reproductively successful, sustainable, large collection.

Large private or public facilities should, at a minimum, meet the standards of regional independent certifying agencies and maintain current certification. Examples of such agencies include the Association of Zoos and Aquariums (AZA) in the United States and the European Association of Zoos and Aquariums. These organizations serve not only to regularly evaluate the operations of member facilities, but they also host the regional authorities for the management of interinstitutional captive populations, studbooks, and species survival plan programs. Current standards for veterinary medical programs and veterinary hospitals at large facilities have been established and are regularly updated by the AZA and the American Association of Zoo Veterinarians.[2]

The International Union for Conservation of Nature (IUCN) is composed of both governmental and nongovernmental organizations. It provides public and private organizations with the knowledge and tools that enable human progress, economic development, and nature conservation to occur together. The Species Survival Commission (IUCN-SSC) is a global network of more than 10,000 scientists working together toward a vision of "a just world that values and conserves nature through positive action to reduce the loss of diversity of life on Earth."[3] Reptile specialist groups include the Anoline Specialist Group, Boa and Python Specialist Group, Chameleon Specialist Group, Crocodile Specialist Group, Iguana Specialist Group, Marine Turtle Specialist Group, Monitor Lizard Specialist Group, Sea Snake Specialist Group, Snake and Lizard Red List Authority, Tortoise and Freshwater Turtle Specialist Group, and Viper Specialist Group. These groups monitor and report on wild population status and conservation programs and maintain the IUCN Red List of Threatened Species for their taxonomic group. The IUCN-SSC Conservation Breeding Specialist Group saves threatened species by increasing the effectiveness of conservation efforts worldwide and provides planning expertise to governments, specialist groups, zoos and aquariums, and other wildlife organizations. Leaders and staff of large private and public collections should actively contribute to these groups and maintain the highest possible level of participation in global species conservation programs.

POPULATION SUSTAINABILITY

Zoologic institutions direct their sustainability efforts toward maintaining healthy, sustainable captive populations, whereas species conservation organizations direct their efforts toward maintaining healthy, self-sustaining wild populations. Both of these directives play an important role in the overall sustainability of reptile metapopulations (*in situ* and *ex situ*), and the differences between them help to explain differences in their activities.

TABLE 178.1 The Five Freedoms of Animal Welfare	
Freedom from hunger and thirst	by ready access to fresh water and a diet to maintain full health and vigor
Freedom from discomfort	by an appropriate environment, including shelter and a comfortable resting area
Freedom from pain, injury, or disease	by prevention or rapid diagnosis and treatment
Freedom to express normal behavior	by providing sufficient space, proper facilities, and company of the animal's own kind
Freedom from fear and distress	by ensuring conditions and treatment that avoid mental suffering

From http://webarchive.nationalarchives.gov.uk/20121010012427/ http://www.fawc.org.uk/freedoms.htm.

Management for Sustainable Captive Populations

The goals of AZA Species Survival Plan (SSP) programs are to maintain self-sustaining zoo and aquarium populations, to maintain or increase the captive populations' genetic diversity, to meet exhibit/education needs, to meet conservation or reintroduction goals, to prevent unnecessary surplus animals, and to minimize inbreeding.[4] In practice, this has led to a focus on creating captive populations that will sustain 90% gene diversity for 100+ years or 10 generations with a positive growth rate so they can survive at least 100 years or 10 generations.[5] This priority is directed toward avoiding the risk of inbreeding depression in the captive population, and it is worth pursuing when the goal of preventing extinction is not compromised by doing so. For some endangered species, the wild population is small, and the captive population cannot be augmented by additional wild founders. In these cases, the priority of the captive breeding program must shift to meet conservation and reintroduction goals to prevent imminent extinction, and inbreeding should be encouraged as needed to increase the size of the remaining global metapopulation. The benefit of preserving the species outweighs the assumed costs associated with inbreeding. The available evidence suggests that many reptile populations, whether naturally occurring or introduced, have become self-sustaining in the face of inbreeding, probably via natural selection and because many species do not naturally outbreed.[6-9] Further research into the normal level of inbreeding in reptile species is warranted.

Captive Management for Sustainable Wild Populations

Conservation breeding is ideally undertaken within the context of a broad conservation action plan that includes a multistakeholder assessment of the conservation status of the species and its habitat and outlines conservation priorities (see Chapter 181). The IUCN provides many tools to support the creation of an action plan, including guidelines on the use of *ex situ* management for species conservation,[10] reintroductions and other conservation translocations,[11] and wildlife disease risk analysis.[12] Effective conservation action plans arise from a formal Population and Habitat Viability Assessment (PHVA) in the form of a workshop that helps people organize and evaluate the available information across a range of disciplines and perspectives. The PHVA can be augmented by an Integrated Collection Assessment and Planning workshop that brings together the stakeholders of the *in situ* and *ex situ* communities to apply the IUCN guidelines for *ex situ* management[10] for regional or global planning. In some cases captive breeding is a primary component of a conservation action plan and in others its importance is superseded by interventions, such as creating a protected area, preventing poaching, eliminating invasive alien species, or otherwise supporting the overall health of the local ecosystem where the species occurs naturally. Ideally, the captive breeding component of the plan is directed toward fulfilling specific objectives to prevent extinction. In many cases, however, substantial new knowledge must be obtained by the reptile caretakers to be successful in keeping the animals alive and then breeding, incubating, hatching, and raising them to an age or size when they can be released in a reintroduction program. These technical limitations can justify the initiation of a captive breeding program in the early stages of a conservation program, many years before the ultimate demographic and genetic needs are defined, the factors leading to the wild population decline have improved, and release sites are secured. Surplus offspring must not be overcrowded and can be transferred into additional assurance colonies, or opportunities should be created for the offspring to participate in creating wild or semiwild populations in locations where they can fulfil the function of an extinct species in an ecological restoration program, a process known as ecological replacement.[13]

For threatened species, a captive assurance population improves the demographic viability of the metapopulation and reduces the risk of extinction in the face of unpredictable threats to the wild population, including disease outbreaks, political instability, catastrophic weather events, and failure of habitat protection efforts. Offspring from captive populations can also be utilized to counteract the challenges faced by small wild populations through head-start programs that address high juvenile mortality and population reinforcement to balance age and sex distribution. The offspring from captive breeding programs can be translocated to recover wild populations when wild stock is not available for translocation.

Every effort should be made to locate *ex situ* breeding colonies as near to the indigenous range of the threatened species as possible. This proximity allows the species to experience the daily and seasonal cycles of light, heat, precipitation, and humidity to which it is adapted. In addition, caretakers can most easily recreate the adapted habitat by providing the feed and environmental features (vegetation, substrate, water, slope, shelter, obstacles, parasites, pathogens, commensal organisms, etc.) present there. After one or more local assurance populations have been established, then additional assurance colonies may be considered in the region and in distant locations. The further from the indigenous range, the greater the risk that captive-raised individuals will lose the traits required for life in the wild, including locomotion, predator avoidance, foraging skills, social interactions, physical fitness, and immunological response.[14] In addition, the risk of exposure to novel pathogens probably also increases with distance from the adapted habitat. This emphasizes the importance of recreating, to the best of a caretaker's ability, a captive environment that matches that of the reptile's native habitat so it can gain the psychological, behavioral, and immunologic competence necessary for longevity and reproduction when captive-raised individuals are repatriated and released.

HUSBANDRY CONSIDERATIONS FOR LARGE COLLECTIONS

Purpose of the Collection and Species to be Housed

Funding, space, labor, and expertise are limited in all facilities, and resources must be directed toward species that best serve the goals of the organization. Zoological institutions select species for their educational value, as representatives of a particular ecosystem, as ambassadors for wild populations, to demonstrate biologic diversity (interesting or unusual features), to inspire people, and to breed for species survival programs. Conservation organizations choose species that require captive breeding to protect them from extinction, particularly when an assurance colony is prescribed in an endangered species recovery plan. On occasion, qualified facilities are called upon to care for reptiles that have been seized from the illegal trade by authorities. A receiving institution may reserve the right to refuse such requests if the species is not among those selected by the facility, and resources are limited to preclude the provision of adequate care.

The first step in planning a captive environment is to gather information about a species' native habitat. A wealth of information exists about the care of common pet species, but such information can be difficult to acquire for rare and endangered species. It may become necessary for the search to expand from electronic resources to printed materials in public and university libraries and even consultation with experienced people and herpetologists. In some cases, it may be important to have multiple visits to the indigenous habitat of the species in question during different seasons to observe and record firsthand how a species interacts with its environment throughout the year. Many rare and endangered species of reptiles require husbandry parameters that differ from the species that are common in captive collections. Commonly kept reptile species have become "common" at least in part because they are particularly hardy and can withstand a range of environmental conditions. The impressed tortoise (*Manouria impressa*) is a good example of a species with specialized needs that was impossible to maintain in captivity before someone observed and reported on its natural history. It is dormant during the dry season and becomes active foraging on the fruiting bodies of fresh mushrooms (Basidiomycota) during the wet season. It lives in dense mountain forests with consistent high humidity, minimal direct sunlight, and moderate temperatures. Even near the native range, creating these features in a captive habitat is difficult for the most experienced reptile caretakers, so conservation efforts for this species must focus on protecting wild populations and their habitat.

Animal Identification and Animal Record Systems

Individual animals in large collections must be uniquely identified to track their signalment, lineage, and medical history, and many identification techniques are available.[15] Photographs can be very helpful because individuals have differences in scalation, scutes, and color patterns, and images that include metadata for identification (e.g., the local identifier and date of the photo) should be captured and stored on accession, at progressing life stages, and at deaccession. Veterinary medical and animal collection records should be electronic, and duplicates should be kept off site in case of fire or a natural disaster. Ideally, all animals should be recorded in Species360 (http://www.species360.org, Bloomington, MN; formerly the International Species Information System), the global, nonprofit, nongovernmental, membership-based organization that systematically gathers and shares information about the animals kept in member facilities. Full participation is evidence that a facility meets modern zoological standards and provides others the opportunity to readily evaluate the collection at a participating facility.

Human Resources

Management of human resources is among the greatest challenges in caring for large collections. Some people who wish to work with reptiles exhibit a set of behavioral traits that interferes with their success. These traits include overconfidence and a reliance on intuitive decision-making that is based on unsystematically recorded personal experience. People who exhibit these and similar traits should be avoided or replaced to achieve the goal of long-term consistent success with species that have highly specialized needs. Skilled, educated, experienced, curious people who are intrinsically motivated to learn about the natural history and husbandry of reptiles may, however, prefer not to perform repetitive tasks, including waste management, cleaning, and feeding. These tasks are necessary to manage large collections and can be assigned to people with limited knowledge, skills, and abilities who are willing to learn, follow protocols, and most importantly, seek assistance when they encounter something that is unfamiliar or outside the protocols.

Staff training and interactions should encourage communication among all levels, and managers should make every effort to be open to and grateful for questioning. Employees who can recognize when a knowledge gap exists, notify their supervisors, seek to learn, and then improve their work using newly acquired knowledge should be acknowledged in public and rewarded. This culture will promote a healthy work environment and maximizes success with the most difficult species.

Senior and supervisory staff must routinely inspect animal enclosures for the regular degradation of habitat quality. Items shift position, plants get trampled or eaten, and substrates become compacted, undergo composting, and lose important compositional features over time. Artificial lighting degrades, and equipment fails. It is ideal for senior staff to perform all of the routine husbandry tasks at regular intervals (e.g., once per week) to identify challenges or impediments to the

execution of protocols. All husbandry staff members should participate in regularly scheduled "morbidity and mortality" rounds to review existing protocols, discuss areas for improvement, and explore new ideas about how to solve difficult problems. Enclosure planning must harmonize ergonomics for the staff, natural history needs of the reptile, provision of environmental parameters, and esthetics.

Building and Enclosure Design Considerations
Indoor Facilities

The interior of large structures such as greenhouses and naturally lighted warehouses with windows and skylights can be managed to provide the background environmental parameters for species from regions with a similar climate. Major climatic zones that are home to reptiles include arid, tropical, mediterranean, montane, and temperate zones. Each indoor facility can be designed to create the daily and seasonal cycles in temperature, humidity, and day length that correspond to a major climatic zone. Individual enclosures within the larger structure are then modified to meet species-specific microclimate needs for vegetation cover, substrate type, shade, basking sites, water, fog, and precipitation. Computerized climate control equipment used in the horticultural industry includes circulating temperature-controlled water systems (Fig. 178.1), centrifugal humidifiers (Fig. 178.2), evaporative coolers, air conditioners, vents, air circulators, and shade systems. It is particularly important to either insulate or heat the flooring of buildings where reptiles are kept in close contact with the floor. Concrete that is not insulated will serve as a heat sink and during cold weather will cause reptiles to exhibit unnatural thermoregulatory behavior that can be life threatening (see Fig. 178.1). Natural sunlight is the best source of background lighting and should be minimally filtered. Mesh screens and ultraviolet-transmitting acrylic panels allow the broadest range of light wavelengths, with or without ventilation as needed. Background

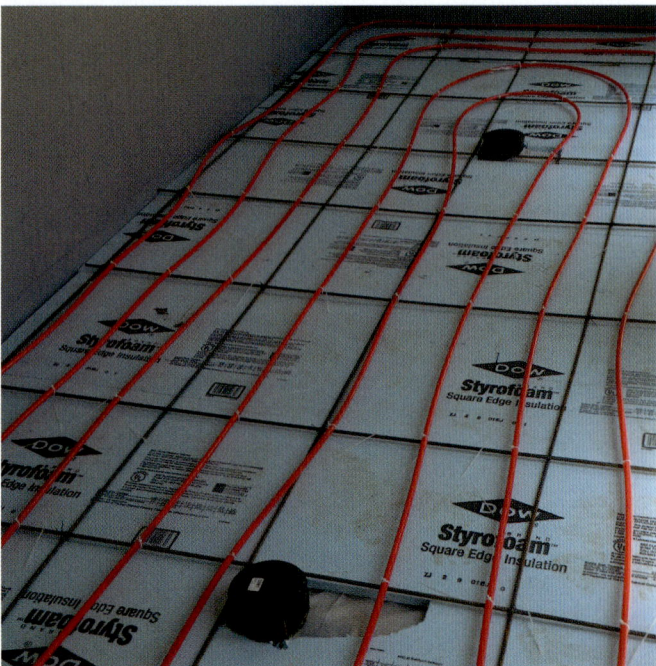

FIG 178.1 Rigid foam board insulation is placed within the load-bearing foundation, and rebar is arranged into a grid on which flexible crosslinked polyethylene (PEX) tubing is secured in place before pouring the concrete slab flooring of a facility that will house reptiles. Warm water is then circulated through the floor by a thermostatically controlled pump. (Courtesy of Paul M. Gibbons, Turtle Conservancy.)

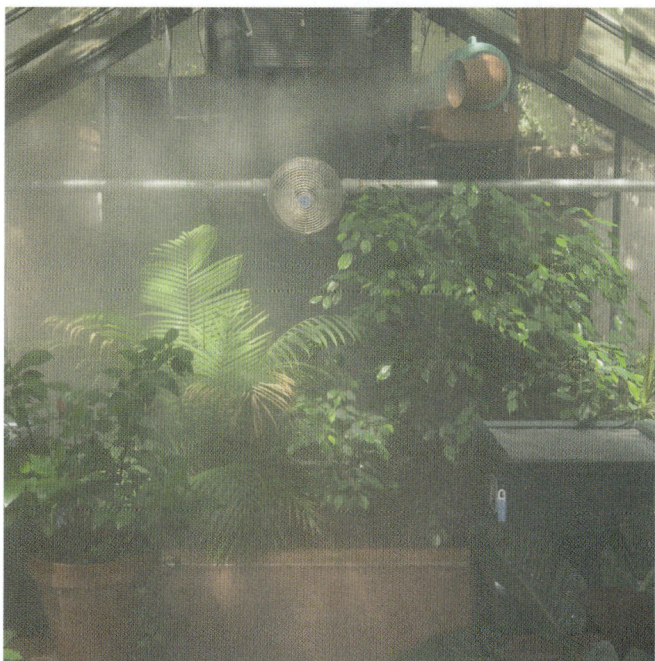

FIG 178.2 A centrifugal humidifier creates a very fine suspended mist similar to that found in cloud forests. (Courtesy of Paul M. Gibbons, Turtle Conservancy.)

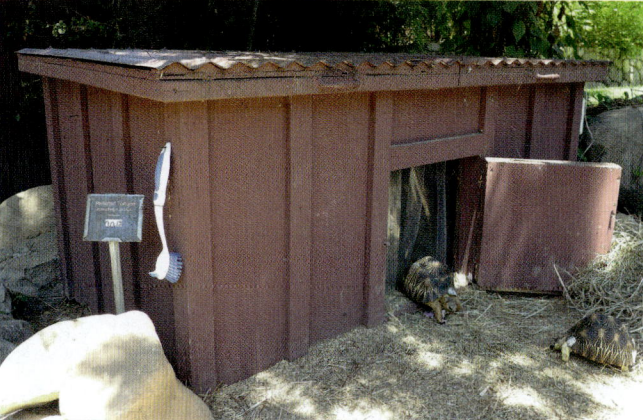

FIG 178.3 Relatively small, well-insulated structures can be used for shelter during brief periods of inclement weather to minimize the need for large structures when maintaining species that can be housed outdoors on most days. (Courtesy of Paul M. Gibbons, Turtle Conservancy.)

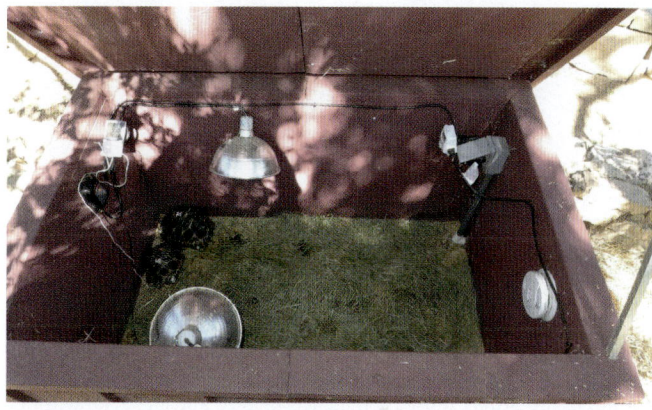

FIG 178.4 The interior of small outdoor structures can be outfitted with thermostatically controlled radiant heaters to blunt nighttime low temperatures and timer-controlled lighting to maintain diurnal light cycles. (Courtesy of Paul M. Gibbons, Turtle Conservancy.)

lighting for day length can be provided with fixed lamps that emit diffuse visible light (incandescent, fluorescent, or LED) if the latitude of the species in the wild differs substantially from that of the facility, and specific needs for infrared and ultraviolet wavelengths can be provided at the microhabitat level.

Outdoor Facilities

Reptiles should be kept outdoors whenever possible. Considerations include potential for escape, the risk of venomous and dangerous species accidentally interacting with people, seasonality, predation, and whether the local environment satisfies the environmental needs of the species. All enclosures for healthy animals at facilities located within the natural range of the species should be outdoors. Judgment is needed to make decisions about daily and seasonal cycles to decide how to optimize the local weather for nonnative species. Relatively small, insulated housing can be constructed for use during brief periods of inclement weather and outfitted with thermostatically controlled radiant heaters to blunt nighttime low temperatures and timer-controlled lighting to maintain diurnal light cycles (Figs. 178.3 and 178.4). A patchwork of shelter from the sun may be all that is necessary for facilities located within the native range of the species (Fig. 178.5). Species that are kept outdoors either within their native range or in a location where the climate closely matches the native range can reproduce (mate, nest, incubate, and hatch) with little to no assistance from caretakers if species-specific social and microhabitat needs are met.

MANAGEMENT OF HUSBANDRY RESOURCES

Large collections of reptiles are often managed by keeping them in groups. To be successful, enclosures that house groups of reptiles must contain replicates of the husbandry resources, including perches, crevices, shelters, basking sites, browse plants, drinking sites, immersion sites, and feeding areas (Fig. 178.6). Multiple visual barriers are necessary,

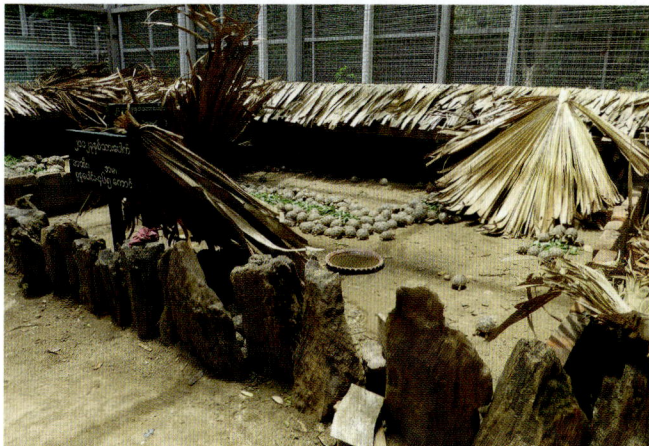

FIG 178.5 Tortoises facilities that are located within the native range of the species may need only to create barriers between groups, feeding slabs, water depressions, and minimal shelter from the sun. Note that this prerelease breeding facility in Bagan, Myanmar, is completely enclosed with heavy-gauge wire mesh to prevent theft. (Courtesy of Paul M. Gibbons, Turtle Conservancy.)

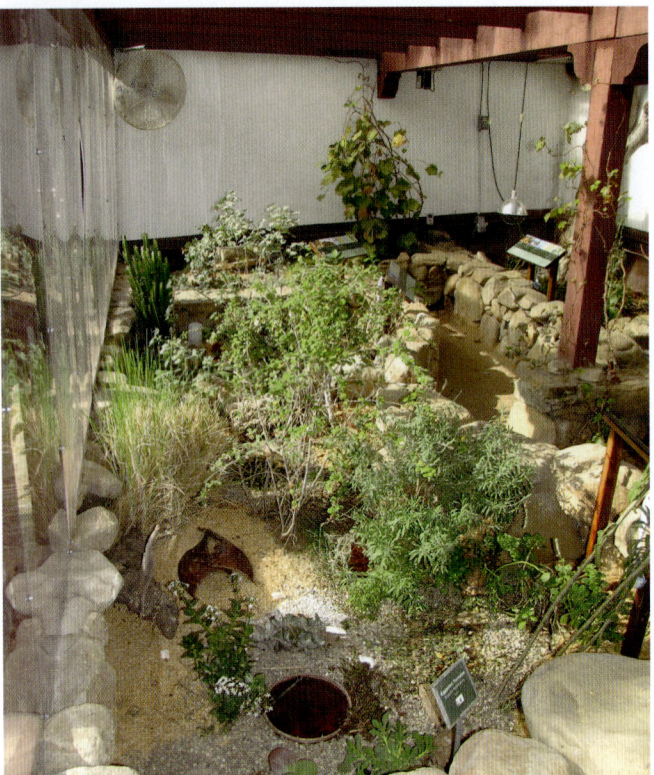

FIG 178.6 A well-appointed enclosure with suitable complexity, shelters, visual barriers, feeding sites, and water dishes to house two male and four female Egyptian tortoises (*Testudo kleinmanni*). (Courtesy of Paul M. Gibbons, Turtle Conservancy.)

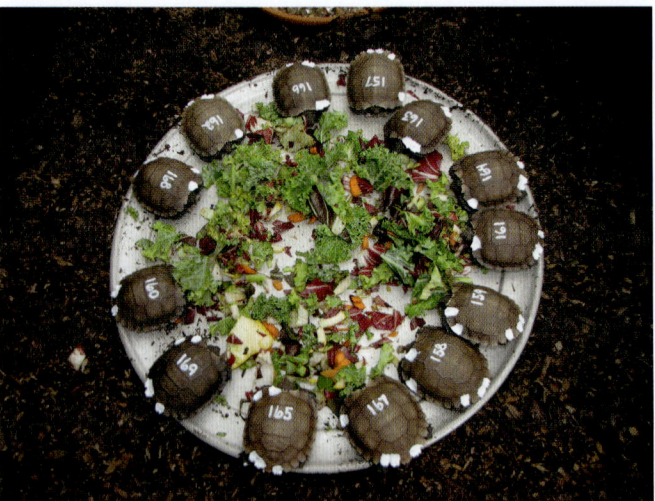

FIG 178.7 When reptiles are housed in groups, the amount of feeding space must be sufficient for all individuals to eat concurrently as shown with this group of hatchling Burmese Black Mountain tortoises (*Manouria emys phayrei*). (Courtesy of Paul M. Gibbons, Turtle Conservancy.)

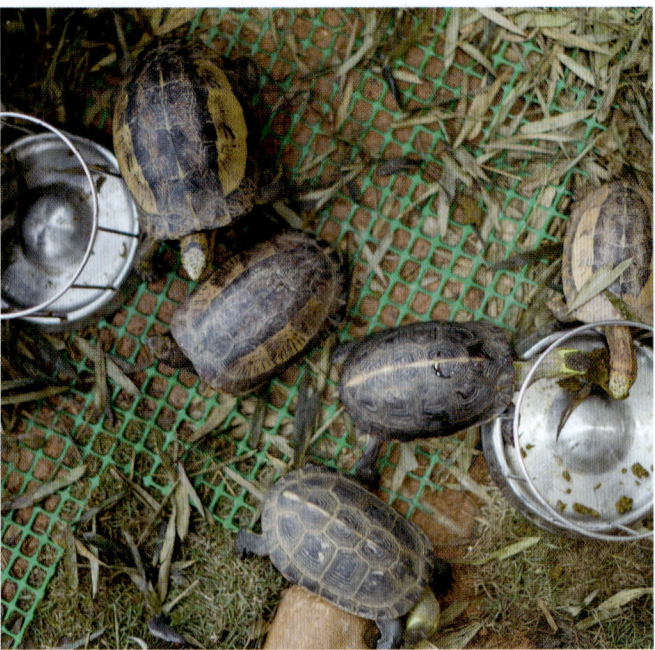

FIG 178.8 Divided feeding plates can improve feeding opportunities for individual reptiles that eat more slowly than others, as shown in this mixed-species group of Asian box turtles (*Cuora* spp.). Similarly divided rectangular troughs can be used to provide food or water to groups of tortoises and larger lizards. (Courtesy of Max Maurer, Turtle Conservancy.)

so individuals need not be in constant visual contact. The animals that comprise the group must be matched by size and behavioral traits. Each individual should be weighed and examined at regular intervals, once every 2 to 4 weeks for most species, to monitor for problems. Some species are predisposed to fighting and cannot be kept in groups, some can be kept in groups until they reach adulthood, and some live peacefully in large groups with only a rare individual that must be separated because it either fights with the others or is not able to fend for itself. The number of individuals in an enclosure must be matched with the individual characteristics of the captive habitat, and social interactions must be managed. There must be sufficient linear space for all of the individuals to eat at the same time (Fig. 178.7). This can be accomplished by creating large or multiple feeding areas or by placing barriers between individuals during feeding. Technology from the food animal agriculture industry, such as divided feeding troughs, can be adapted for reptiles (Fig. 178.8). Heat should be provided in a mosaic with multiple basking sites and multiple areas that are shaded and sheltered from excessive heat. Heat and light from the sun are ideal because they move together in a routine diurnal pattern across an enclosure, providing a thermal environment that varies predictably throughout the day, so the reptiles can choose preferred basking sites as they change.

DISEASE MANAGEMENT

New Acquisitions

The principles of quarantine are described in Chapter 19. It should strengthen the health of new acquisitions in preparation for entry into a large collection. Husbandry in quarantine must not sacrifice any of the essential components of long-term maintenance, including environmental complexity, options, and cycles. Quarantine, both before and after transfer, is a time for the veterinary staff to learn how well the immune competence of a new acquisition matches that of the collection it is to enter. Some microorganisms and parasites that have the potential to cause primary disease or deleterious effects during exposure to poor husbandry can be treated during quarantine. Ideally, quarantine will prevent the introduction of pathogens that do not already exist in the collection with the assumption that immunologically naïve

TABLE 178.2 Common Pathogens of Concern When Introducing New Individuals Into a Collection[16]

Group	Agent	Species	Screening Samples	Recommended Tests
Chelonians				
	Tortoise intranuclear coccidiosis	Tortoises, some turtles	Swab of conjunctiva, oral mucosa, and cloaca	qPCR
	Herpesvirus	Tortoises	Oral swab; plasma	PCR, qPCR; paired PN or ELISA
	Mycoplasmosis	Leopard tortoise, star tortoises, Testudo spp., Gopherus spp.	Swab of conjunctiva, nasal, choanal mucosa; plasma	PCR; paired ELISA
	Systemic amoebiasis	Tortoises and turtles	Feces (fresh and preserved in PVA), cloacal swab	PCR, fecal microscopy direct and trichrome stain
	Iridovirus	Tortoises and turtles	Swab of oral/cloacal mucosa, urine	PCR
Lizards				
	Adenovirus	Bearded dragons	Cloacal swab or wash	qPCR
	Cryptosporidiosis	Leopard geckos, Gila monsters, chameleons, monitors	Gastric lavage, fecal	PCR, IFA, acid-fast stain
Snakes				
	Reptarenavirus (inclusion body disease)	Boas, pythons	Choanal swab	PCR (RNA)
	Paramyxovirus	Viperids, colubrids, less common in pythons/boas	Choanal swab; plasma	PCR (RNA); paired HI
	Nidovirus	Pythons	Choanal/pharyngeal swab	PCR (RNA)
	Cryptosporidiosis	Boas, pythons, colubrids	Gastric lavage, fecal	Acid-fast stain, PCR
Crocodilians				
	Mycoplasmosis	Alligators and crocodiles	Respiratory sample; plasma	PCR; paired ELISA

ELISA, Enzyme-linked immunosorbent assay; *HI*, hemagglutination inhibition; *IFA*, indirect fluorescent antibody immunofluorescent assay; *PCR*, consensus PCR and sequencing; *PN*, plasma neutralization; *PVA*, polyvinyl alcohol; *qPCR*, quantitative PCR.

populations are more susceptible to illness than those that have already been exposed. The collection may experience undesirable morbidity and mortality as it gains herd immunity to a pathogen to which it has previously not been exposed. It may be wise, however, to create a herd that is immunocompetent and prepared for exposure to pathogens that are known to exist in wild populations. Quarantine can be extended for animals undergoing treatment for known diseases, but must be kept as brief as possible. No consensus exists on the minimum duration of reptile quarantine and the logical basis for it. Incubation periods have not been defined for most reptile pathogens. Testing should be based on a risk assessment and directed toward matching immunocompetence among groups (Table 178.2). In situations where there is no evidence of known pathogens, but concerns remain about unknown pathogens and the benefit of introducing a new animal outweighs the risk of losing one or two established individuals, then the new individual can be placed initially with one or two individuals from the established collection. This biological assay can help detect whether a serious yet previously unknown contagious disease is present because it will affect either the newly acquired individual or the test subject(s) without spreading through the entire collection.

Preventive Medicine

The epidemiologic triad considers host, environment, and pathogen factors. Many of the common diseases of captive reptiles can be prevented by providing the necessary environmental parameters to support the health of the reptile and by identifying and eliminating stressors. Many pathogens are opportunistic and can be present in a collection without causing disease unless the environmental parameters change, or a stressor

is introduced. Examples of such diseases include cryptosporidiosis, mycoplasmosis, and amoebiasis. In addition, many nematodes and protozoa that are present in wild reptiles and are directly transmitted can gradually increase over time until they exceed a threshold and then cause disease. The veterinarians who are responsible for managing the health of large collections can use epidemiologic principles to survey for the presence of known, testable, disease-causing organisms and design prophylactic treatment plans accordingly. Similar to large collections of other vertebrates, strategic administration of anthelminthics or antiprotozoal drugs and outdoor enclosure (pasture) management are indicated. Transmission is multifactorial and differs among pathogens; known intermediate hosts should be eliminated when possible. Reptile environments should strike a balance that enhances populations of nonpathogenic microbes and decomposing invertebrates to reduce transmission of pathogens. The combination of environmental features that create this balance may not have been specifically characterized, but general features include sufficient space (not overcrowded), adequate ventilation, live plant communities, circulating water, and good soil drainage. The volume of water and surface area for biologic filtration must be sufficient to maintain nitrogen cycling, and water should be exchanged as needed to prevent the accumulation of nitrogenous wastes. Regular monitoring of environmental quality parameters, including nitrogen cycling and coliform counts, can help to determine whether environmental systems require intervention. Daily spot-cleaning of substrates to remove feces and urine can increase the capacity of an enclosure where biologic systems are not sufficient. Disinfected habitats can be useful when managing reptiles for brief periods of hospitalization, but they present many difficult and unnecessary challenges when used for the long-term maintenance and breeding of reptiles, without providing the intended benefit of reduced disease. In place of disinfection, reptile habitats should be designed to enhance populations of nonpathogenic microorganisms, so pathogens cannot thrive in the environment.

Biosecurity

Biosecurity standards for large collections are directed toward decreasing the risk of disease transmission to susceptible individuals. Written protocols should be regularly reviewed by all of the staff and revised as needed. People must move through the facility with a clear understanding of the likelihood that infectious diseases can be transmitted on hands, shoes, and equipment, in feed, and on free-living animals and pests. Traffic patterns through the facility are orchestrated so that cleaning and feeding routines are accomplished in a specific sequence moving from youngest to oldest animals and working with known sick animals at the end of every day. Feed should be prepared in advance and carried away from the kitchen/food preparation area one time daily without returning. Items used inside of enclosures, including feed plates, should be cleaned in an area that is separate from the kitchen. Disposable gloves should be changed, or hands should be washed with hot, soapy water to remove organic material before feed preparation, between enclosures, after handling animals, and after cleaning equipment. Each enclosure should be entered only once each day, and then only with personal protective equipment including shoe covers and gloves. Enclosures with reptiles that are infected with known pathogens should only be entered with shoe covers, gloves, and designated gowns or coveralls. Equipment is also designated and clearly labeled for each separate area of the facility or group of animals and never transferred to a new area. Small equipment cabinets or boxes help facilitate adherence to the protocols and can be designed to fit into the esthetics of exhibit design (Fig. 178.9). Footbaths may be useful to prevent introduction of pathogens into the hospital or quarantine, and they must be maintained to avoid deactivation of the disinfectant by organic material that is dislodged from the soles of shoes. Regular training sessions for staff members are essential to explain the justification for biosecurity protocols, demonstrate how they are implemented, and identify ways to improve.

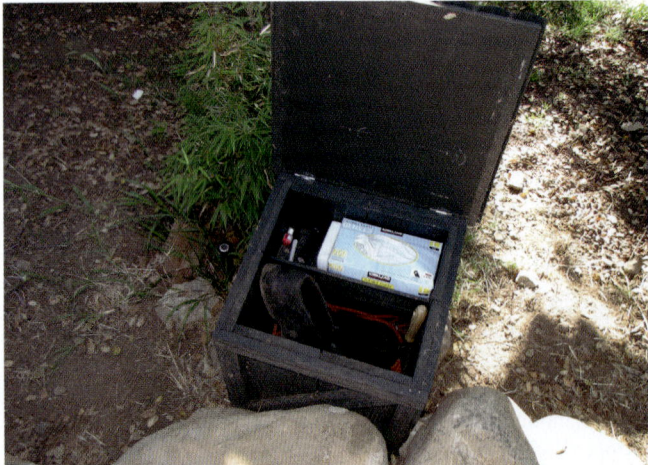

FIG 178.9 A conveniently located biosecurity box that holds gloves, shoe covers, and equipment that has been designated for use only within its adjacent outdoor enclosure is one part of a biosecurity program at the Turtle Conservancy's conservation breeding center. (Courtesy of Paul M. Gibbons, Turtle Conservancy.)

Sick Individuals

Early signs of illness can be difficult to notice in reptiles, especially in large collections or naturalistic exhibits. Animal caretakers must learn each species' normal behavior and routine, and observe all of the individuals in the collection every day. For example, many diurnal reptiles bask in the early morning and eat when their body has reached the optimal temperature for metabolism. They then retreat from the sun and may be observed basking intermittently throughout the afternoon to maintain their body temperature until sunset when they retreat for the night. Accordingly, feed should be provided in the morning and caretakers should take the time to observe each enclosure for sufficient time after feeding to determine which individuals have eaten. Conversely, feed for nocturnal reptiles should be provided in the evening. Not all reptiles will eat every time feed is presented, so individual patterns should be recorded, and any deviation from the normal pattern should be noted and the individual animal identified for observation. One method to identify sick animals is to place a temporary marker, such as a small dab of typing correction fluid or brightly colored nail polish on the skin or shell of the suspect individual. If abnormal behavior continues, then the individual should be separated from the group and placed under observation in an enclosure that is separate from the intake quarantine area and provided with normal husbandry conditions. This offers an opportunity for closer observation and to better determine whether it continues to exhibit abnormal behavior. Body condition is a more useful indicator of chronic nutritional status because absolute body weight can be misleading unless serial measurements over many years are available for review. In general, juvenile reptiles should steadily gain weight over time, and adults should maintain their weight within approximately the 10% to 15% range. It is important to note that body weight normally changes by 10% or more when reptiles nest, defecate, or urinate. In addition, a reptile in poor body condition can retain urine or feces to regain or maintain body weight, and ascites is a common problem that confounds the interpretation of body weight. So rely on body condition, using weight as a logical guide with limitations, to assess nutritional or hydration status. If the observed behavioral concerns and body condition do not improve when the reptile is isolated, then a diagnosis should be obtained and a therapeutic plan instituted. Depending on the relative value of an individual to the goals of the collection (breeder, genetically valuable offspring, or surplus), euthanasia may be considered for individuals with metabolic, degenerative, neoplastic, or other chronic diseases and those that do not respond well to routine treatment. A policy on euthanasia should be clearly defined and implemented to avoid prolonged periods of disease in individuals that will eventually be euthanized.

Necropsy

Chapter 40 describes techniques and protocols for necropsy in reptiles. All animals in a large collection that die spontaneously or are euthanized should undergo gross necropsy. All those in which a cause of death cannot be determined by gross necropsy should be submitted for histopathologic diagnosis. Gross lesions should be photographed. Samples of blood, fluids, and tissue should be collected at the time of gross necropsy and preserved for future testing to determine an etiologic diagnosis based on histopathologic findings. If the facilities and funding permit, tissue samples should be preserved indefinitely for future retrospective disease analyses and genetic banking.

Integrated Pest Management

An integrated pest management program uses regular monitoring to determine what pests are present and then uses the safest approaches to control pest populations while considering environmental concerns.[17]

Pests can consume animal diets, introduce or transmit disease, cause stress, or prey upon susceptible reptiles. The pest management program takes into account the biology of the pests and the effects of the control program on the animal collection and the people involved. A comprehensive program includes a clear definition of the scope and magnitude of the problem, identifies appropriate expertise, outlines a safe and effective plan, implements the program, regularly evaluates the results, and makes improvements when necessary. Indirect suppression methods are the most effective and include modifying enclosures/exhibits, changing human behavior, and educating the staff.[17] Indirect suppression is based on eliminating desirable resources for the pests and is focused on sanitation and cleanliness in animal enclosures and feed storage/preparation areas. Direct suppression or mechanical control of pests differs depending on the pest species and should include a combination of approaches that may include exclusion, baiting, repellants, trapping, removal, euthanasia, and relocation (Fig. 178.10). The most important pests in reptile collections include ants, rodents, procyonids, carnivores, and birds.

CONCLUSION

The principles of managing large reptile collections for educational exhibits or conservation are similar to those of smaller collections, with the added elements of animal identification, recordkeeping, and staff training in husbandry, health, pest management, and biosecurity protocols. The main purpose of breeding endangered species in noncommercial large collections is to prevent extinction, and maintaining genetic diversity is a secondary goal that should be addressed only after the techniques have been refined to keep the species alive and

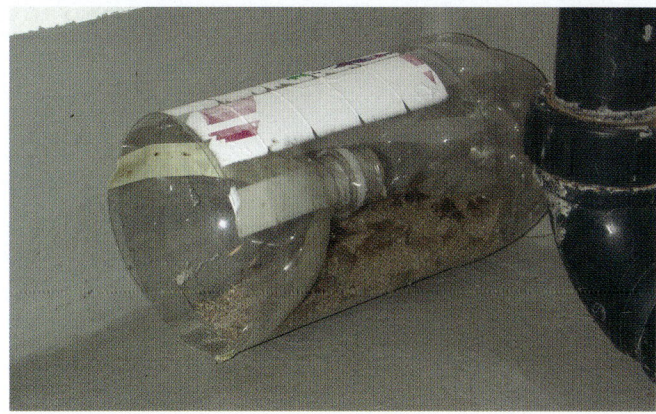

FIG 178.10 Escaped prey can serve as vectors of pathogens. Feral feeder crickets can be captured in a simple trap constructed from a 2-liter plastic bottle with dry feed inside. Masking tape provides a runway for crickets to climb into the inverted opening, which is raised above the substrate to prevent them from climbing out. (Courtesy of Paul M. Gibbons.)

then to breed, nest, incubate, hatch, and raise them to become competent adults that will survive when they are released to restore wild populations.

REFERENCES

See www.expertconsult.com for a complete list of references.

179

Breeders, Wholesalers, and Retailers

Drury R. Reavill and Chris Griffin

Evaluation of recently obtained reptiles from the growing population of captive-bred or wild-caught animals available as pets can be daunting for practitioners. The many different species presented for examination and the dizzying range of requirements for their needs—from husbandry to diet—can overwhelm the time constraints of a veterinary visit. Additionally, the common diseases, parameters of health, and appropriate laboratory tests recommended can vary tremendously.

For collections of reptiles, a herd health approach should be utilized, and a basic knowledge and understanding of reptilian biology, anatomy, and diseases is important. This chapter will present an overview of the species of reptiles currently available in the pet trade, the common husbandry issues and infectious diseases seen, and recommended therapeutic guidelines.

The species of reptiles presented to veterinarians generally fall into two categories: those reptiles that have adapted well to captivity and have been successfully captive bred in large numbers, and those species readily harvested from wild populations. There have been trends in the popularity of reptiles kept as pets. In the 1960s and 1970s, the red-eared slider turtle (*Trachemys scripta elegans*) was a common pet and readily reproduced in commercial ponds. The common green iguana (*Iguana iguana*), though not easily captive bred, was readily imported from farms in South and Central America and thus was popular in the 1990s. Bearded dragons (*Pogona vitticeps*) and a variety of chameleons and geckos are the current popular pets. Large snakes have always had a fan base that seems unchanged over time. Each different species has introduced various disease conditions and challenged reptile veterinarians to provide optimal health care by attempting to understand the natural history of these unique animals. The common reptile species available to the public in the past decade are listed in Table 179.1.[1]

BREEDING COLLECTIONS

Some studies suggest captive-bred animals have better health and survival rates compared with wild-caught specimens.[2,3] These captive-bred animals may be healthier due, in part, to the care of breeding stock and management of disease that can be controlled. There are many diseases presented clinically that can be diagnosed by select antemortem testing. Testing a collection in a systematic manner with a focus on disease prevention may be helpful when dealing with closed breeding collections. A closed collection, characterized by no new animals brought into the collection for breeding or other purposes, is rare; all new breeding animals would be the offspring of the current breeding stock. For breeders, keeping a closed collection is the ideal but is often not adhered to as new morphs or choice individuals of the species being bred become available (Fig. 179.1). In these cases, quarantine is vital, and during the quarantine process testing for the most common pathogens as well as pursuing a diagnosis for any abnormal physical findings is important.

Ideal quarantine facilities should have separate housing and air space from the established breeding population (Fig. 179.2). Biosecurity, especially in terms of isolation of recent acquisitions and separation of species, is important, probably more so with a breeding collection.[2] Disinfectant foot dips are used in some facilities, as well as adequate hand-washing stations. Ideally, quarantined animals are given care last after the breeding population or have different people in charge of each

Table 179.1 **Common Species Available in the Retail Trade**		
Chelonian	**Lizard**	**Snake**
Russian tortoise (*Agrionemys horsfieldii*)	Leopard gecko (*Eublepharis macularius*)	Ball python (*Python regius*)
Red-eared slider (*Trachemys scripta elegans*)	Bearded dragon (*Pogona vitticeps*)	Common boa (*Boa constrictor imperator*)
Malayan box turtle (*Cuora amboinensis*)	Green water dragons (*Physignathus cocincinus*)	Corn snake (*Elaphe guttata*)
Box turtle (*Terrapene* spp.)	Common green iguana (*Iguana iguana*)	Ribbon snake (*Thamnophis sauritus*)
African side-neck turtle (Pelomedusidae family)	Anole (family Polychrotidae)	Milk snake (*Lampropeltis triangulum*)
Marginated tortoise (*Testudo marginata*)	Savannah monitor (*Varanus exanthematicus*)	Garter snake (*Thamnophis* spp.)
Red-footed tortoise (*Chelonoidis carbonaria*)	Emerald swift (*Sceloporus malachiticus*)	Green tree python (*Morelia viridis*)
African-spurred or sulcata tortoise (*Centrochelys sulcata*)	Blue-tongued skink (*Tiliqua* sp.)	King snake species (genus *Lampropeltis*)
Greek tortoise (*Testudo graeca*)	Ameiva (family Teiidae)	Rat snake (genus *Pantherophis*)
	Chameleon species (*Trioceros jacksonii, Furcifer pardalis, Chamaeleo calyptratus*)	
	Uromastyx species (*Uromastyx aegyptia, Uromastyx [dispar] maliensis*)	

population group. Quarantine lengths will depend on the species and can range from 30 to 90 days. The decision when to move animals into the breeding population can be based on assessment of health (eating, drinking, normal behaviors), the source of the animal (wild caught vs. captive bred), results of diagnostic tests and response to any therapies, and vendor/seller reputation (see Chapter 19 for further details).

When assessing breeding collections, it is a good idea to avoid upsetting the routines of breeding animals, so collecting samples and performing examinations is best done before breeding seasons when possible. At a minimum, a review of the records kept by the breeder should be performed once yearly and during every disease outbreak or unexplained cluster of deaths (Table 179.2).[2] Each individual breeding animal should have a calendar log-book entry indicating weights, breeding dates, number of young produced, fecal output, meals offered, meals eaten, shed times, cage cleaning, changes in behavior, and antivenom classification if venomous. Fecal testing, especially in species where parasites are common, can be performed twice yearly, and physical examinations should be done once or twice yearly.

Valuable animals, either as breeders or producers of venom, may warrant more thorough evaluations. These should include (but not be limited to) a detailed history, a thorough physical examination, fecal parasite examinations (e.g., direct, float, and/or special stains), laboratory analysis (complete blood count/chemistry profile), diagnostic imaging, and histology, cytology, and microbiology when indicated (Fig. 179.3).

WHOLESALE AND RETAIL COLLECTIONS

In wholesale and retail situations where individuals are constantly in flux (both in numbers and in species), it becomes quite challenging to

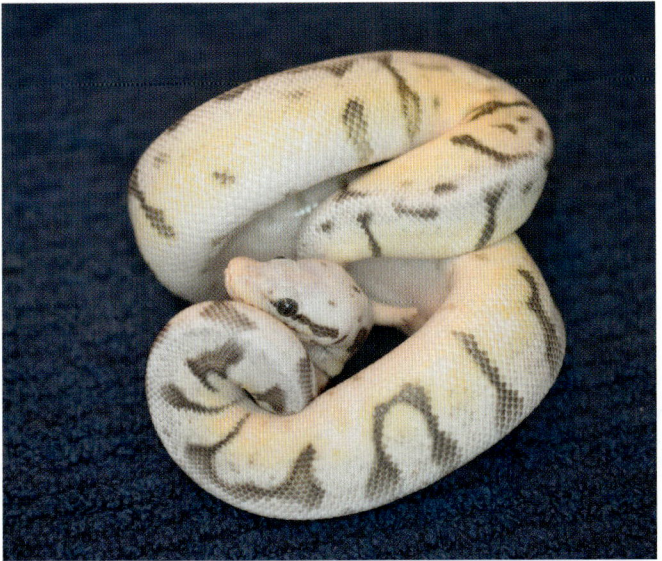

FIG 179.1 Killer bee ball python; genetics: spider (dominant) + homozygous pastel (codominant). (Courtesy of Heather A. Bjornebo.)

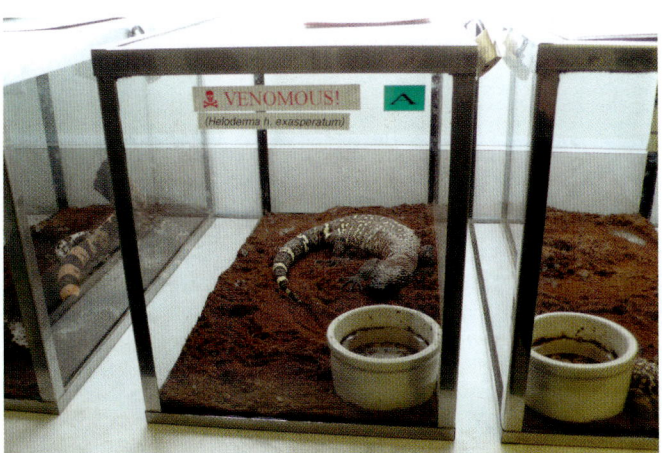

FIG 179.2 Beaded lizard (*Heloderma horridum exasperatum*) maintained in individual display tanks. (Courtesy of Drury R. Reavill.)

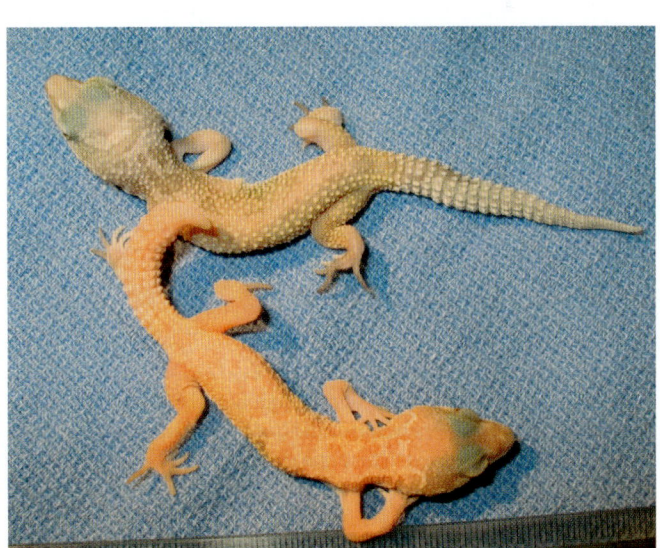

FIG 179.3 The physical examination will be determined by the type and size of animal (leopard geckos, *Eublepharis macularius,* in this figure). Evaluation should include assessment of body condition, color, activity, any swellings/masses, and integrity of the skin. (Courtesy of Chris Griffin.)

TABLE 179.2	Common Infectious Diseases Outbreaks in Reptiles Collections	
Disease	**Species**	**Diagnostic Sampling**
Atadenovirus	Bearded dragons	Biopsy (liver, stomach, esophagus, kidney) and polymerase chain reaction assay (PCR)
Coccidia	Lizards	Fecal analysis
Cryptosporidiosis	Squamates, chelonians	Fecal acid fast, PCR, histology
Herpesvirus	Chelonians	PCR, electron microscopy, and viral isolation
Microsporidia	Bearded dragons	Histology
Mycoplasma	Chelonians, squamates, crocodilians	Culture, enzyme-linked immunosorbent assay (ELISA), and polymerase chain reaction assay
Paramyxovirus	Snake	Hemagglutination inhibition assay (HI), viral isolation, or PCR
Ranavirus	Box turtles, red-eared sliders	Histology, PCR
Reptarenavirus (IBD)	Boas, pythons	PCR, histology

Cage Card _____ Venom:_____ Antivenom clasification: _____

Species (common and Genus species)		
Vendor address	Date in:	
	Date out:	

Band#		Gender	
AVID #		BCS	
Weight		Age	
History			

PE		Location	
DX !		PX	

Caregiver Notes

Date	Initials of Providing		Caregiver Food & Water	Clean Habitat	Notes
	AM	PM			

Medical Notes
Date:

FIG 179.4 Sample of a quarantine cage card. (Courtesy of Drury R. Reavill.)

maintain any sort of continuity of testing or rigid quarantine procedures. Realistically, only animals that appear significantly abnormal will be presented to the veterinary hospital, and basic diagnostics or euthanasia may be all that is allowed. There are financial reasons for this, and although this can be frustrating, a positive impact can still be made for the animals that find themselves part of this pet store experience. Not every case needs advanced imaging or molecular testing, but for unusual cases advanced testing and/or necropsy and histopathology (if the patient dies or is euthanized) should be recommended.

Although a separate room and air space is recommended for quarantine, some physical facilities are not so designed. At a minimum, new arrivals should not be mixed with the current population. Some practical options are grouping neonates or hatchlings together if they originate from the same source. Keeping the same species isolated in the same air space/room is an easy solution, especially if they all came from the same vendor and are moved through as a group before adding new animals. Mixing species and group housing different age groups should be discouraged. Specific quarantine periods need to be determined for each species.

Cage cards can be instrumental in recognizing problems that may arise during quarantine. One of the most important aspects of identifying sick reptiles in the pet store is the proper training of the employees/caretakers. Good observational skills and an understanding of basic health and behavior are paramount to early detection of illness and should then lead to veterinary evaluation. The presentation of a sick reptile 1 to 2 days into an illness often results in a better prognosis than evaluating a reptile 14 to 21 days later. A cage card will help remind employees/caretakers of what needs to be recorded and trigger an early warning of potential problems (Fig. 179.4). This training can also result in better education of customers as to the needs of their new purchase; the public often looks to the sales force as a source of knowledge about the care of exotic animal species.[4]

HUSBANDRY-RELATED CONDITIONS

Deficiencies in husbandry are the most common factor causing illnesses in captive reptiles. For a thorough review of husbandry, see Section 3. Stress, including overcrowding, exposure to sick animals (and their body fluids/excrements), poor nutrition, improper thermal gradients, and many other aspects of care may predispose animals to many of the illnesses that plague reptiles in the pet trade (Fig. 179.5). Many reptiles are shipped to pet stores in containers that are either too small or overcrowded with the same (or different) species and with minimal ability for thermal regulation. Many are shipped from a breeder to a distribution center before being sent to a pet store, and these animals (usually younger ones) may be without food or water for several days during transportation. The basics of thermal support, humidity, feeding opportunities, hiding options, and a reasonable animal-to-space ratio are often not provided, even within a pet store setting.[5,6] These factors may trigger new health conditions or a flare-up of preexisting conditions. Examples include

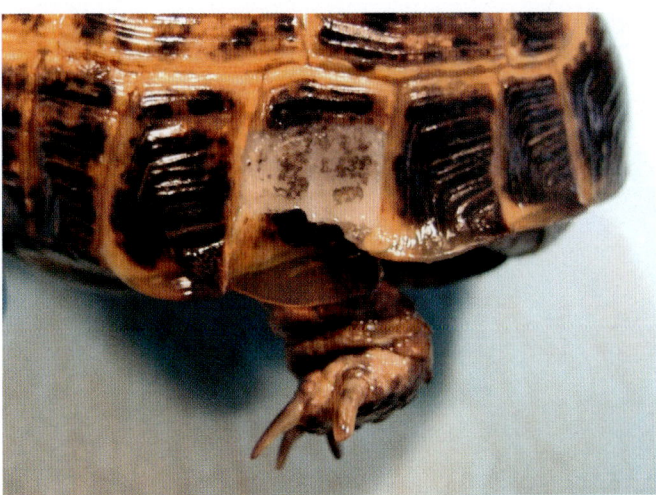

FIG 179.5 Shell damage during shipping of a Russian tortoise (*Agrionemys horsfieldii*). (Courtesy of Drury R. Reavill.)

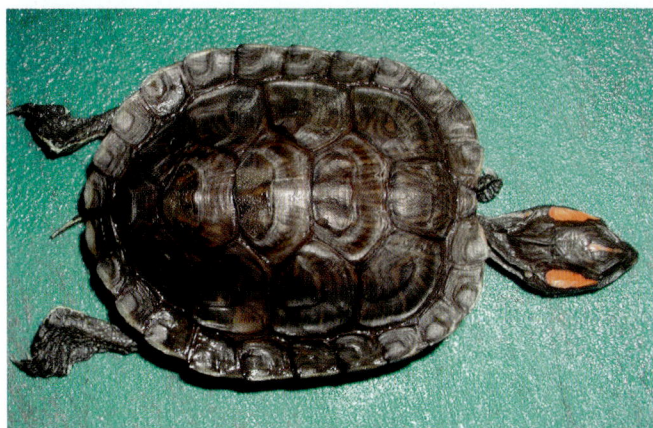

FIG 179.6 A red-eared slider (*Trachemys scripta elegans*) with significant loss of body condition and obvious muscle wasting. (Courtesy of Drury R. Reavill.)

adenoviral or coccidial infections in bearded dragons and cryptosporidial infections in leopard geckos (*Eublepharis macularius*).[7]

Addressing the basic husbandry needs in the store does not need to be complex, and ultimately having healthy animals for sale should result in increased profits/sales. It should be easy to clean enclosures and replace substrate. Visual barriers are important to some species and essential for others. Individual housing may be necessary. Water should be supplied in a manner preferred by the species (e.g., water bowl, tank with a haulout for aquatic species; misting or drip systems for old-world chameleons).

POSTMORTEM EVALUATIONS

In situations where there is increasing morbidity and/or mortality, a complete postmortem evaluation can provide answers. Selecting the most typical presentation of the disease is important in identifying a widespread problem versus a disease condition involving only one animal in a collection. Sometimes necropsies on multiple animals are required to establish the full spectrum of the problem. Indeed, an elective euthanasia and necropsy is often a more rewarding approach, both financially and clinically.

In general, the most recently deceased (or electively euthanized) animal should be considered for necropsy submission during an outbreak of disease or multiple unexplained deaths. Animals that were "found dead in cage" are often not suitable, as heated cages will accelerate autolysis. When possible, paired tissue samples from the same patient (or from multiple patients if more than one is euthanized/dies) should be collected—the first set should be placed in formalin for histopathological evaluation and the second set should be frozen in case future molecular testing (such as PCR) is indicated. Culture swabs should be taken if granulomas or abscesses are observed, and a portion of the affected tissue (if available) can be included in the culture media to increase the chances of isolate recovery (this may be especially true with fungal infections). Intestinal cultures for *Salmonella* may be needed if there are zoonotic concerns.[5] All persons involved with reptiles should be informed and follow the current published guidelines (https://arav.org/salmonella-reptiles-veterinary-guidelines).

Most facilities that will perform a complete postmortem will have procedures in place for body disposal. For animals not submitted for a necropsy (including histopathology), disposal is dictated by local laws. Most locations recommend cremation. Some uncommon species may be held for taxidermy or skeletal preparations. Large species (giant tortoises) in breeding facilities may be buried on-site after consultation with local laws, due to the difficulty in transporting these large specimens.

DISEASE CONDITIONS

The information in the following sections is from case files collected from a large clinical practice and a pathology service.[1] These common disease conditions may not be representative for reptile collections across the world. With increasing awareness of threats to wild populations, additional diagnostic modalities are becoming available that may improve the ability to identify specific disease agents affecting captive populations. A recent example is a Nidovirus that has been associated with a respiratory disease condition in ball pythons (*Python regius*) that had been recognized since the late 1990s as associated with many other etiologies.[8] Another example involves the emergence of highly contagious fungal skin diseases that may result in systemic disease and potentially infect apparently healthy reptiles. The classification scheme for these fungal infections is evolving as more reptile species, both wild and captive populations, are examined and identified. The fungus *Ophidiomyces ophiodiicola* (formerly *Chrysosporium ophiodiicola*) is increasingly being identified in wild rattlesnakes and several species of colubrids, including racers and rat snakes.[9,10] The fungus *Nannizziopsis* is considered a primary pathogen causing dermal infections across different classes of reptiles, most commonly bearded dragons and chameleons; crocodiles; and snakes.[10]

Common Clinical Diseases

Many of the common presentations that are seen in practice are manageable, and most do not necessarily require terminal diagnostic procedures. The most common conditions are discussed here.

In turtles and tortoises, poor nutritional status, failure to thrive, poor/abnormal shell development, and anorexia are common (Fig. 179.6).

In lizards, enteric parasitic infections are common and include coccidia, pinworms, and protozoans in bearded dragons; cryptosporidiosis in leopard geckos; and protozoans in most species (pathogenicity determined by clinical signs and/or histology evidence of associated lesions). Gram-negative enteritis is common in many species. Nutritional secondary hyperparathyroidism (resulting in hypocalcemia and associated changes) remains common in iguanas, uromastyx lizards, bearded dragons, leopard geckos, and chameleons (Fig. 179.7) Ocular issues including conjunctivitis from environmental factors (e.g., reptile bark) or retained sheds (possibly from humidity/hydration issues) and

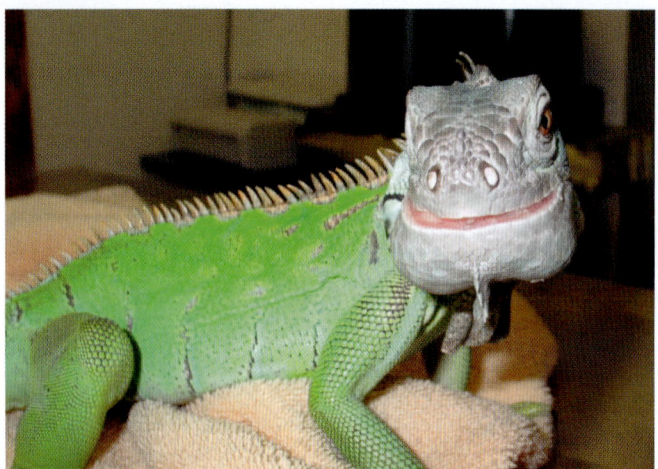

FIG 179.7 The bilateral swelling of the mandible in this green iguana (*Iguana iguana*) is due to fibrous tissue hypertrophy attempting to stabilize soft bones and is a classic sign of nutritional secondary hyperparathyroidism due to poor management. (Courtesy of Chris Griffin.)

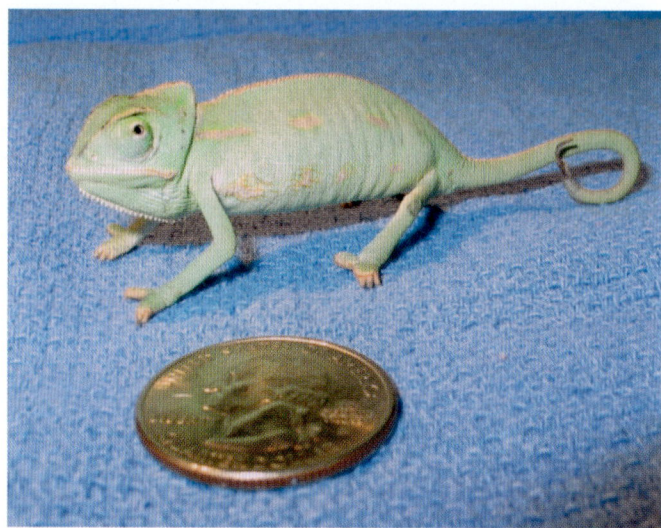

FIG 179.9 A poorly thriving veiled chameleon (*Chameleo calyptratus*) with secondary diseases (including necrosis of the tail tip). (Courtesy of Chris Griffin.)

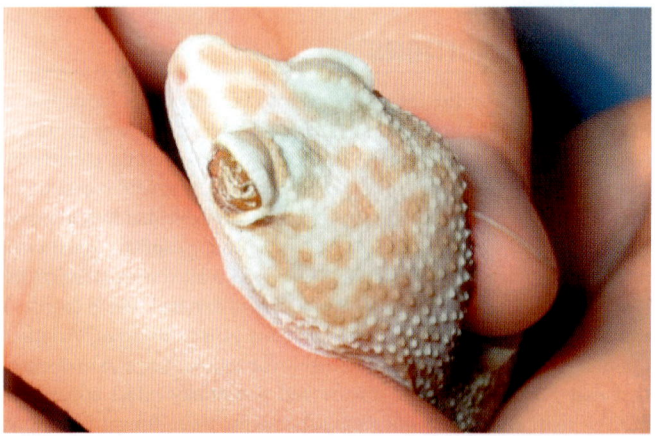

FIG 179.8 In leopard geckos (*Eublepharis macularius*), the skin of the eyelid may be retained following abnormal ecdysis. Failure to shed this skin can result in an accumulation of keratin in the conjunctival sac, subsequent irritation, and infection. (Courtesy of Chris Griffin.)

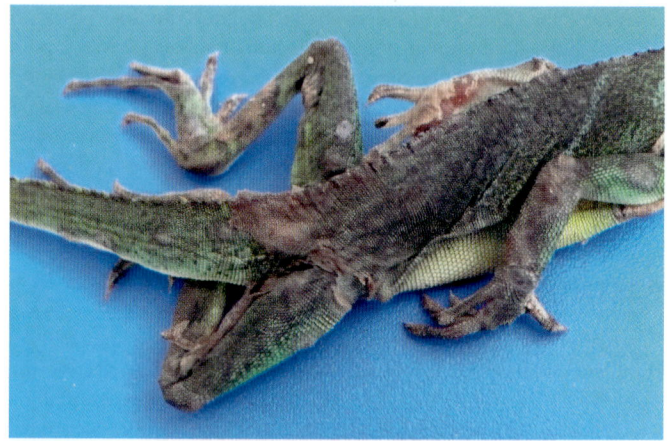

FIG 179.10 Asian water dragon (*Physignathus cocincinus*) with multiple irregular foci of brown-gray hyperkeratotic plaques and dysecdysis due to skin mycosis. (Courtesy of Drury R. Reavill.)

hypovitaminosis A in insectivorous lizards are common (Fig. 179.8). Stomatitis is commonly seen in water dragons, blue-tongued skinks, bearded dragons, and leopard geckos. Atadenovirus in bearded dragons may be more common than reported, and concurrent infections with atadenovirus and parasites (e.g., coccidia and cryptosporidia) can result in more severe signs and a greater chance of mortality.[11] Failure to thrive, a catch-all term used in captive animals to describe illnesses that are not specifically identified but compromise the animal, is seen in more "sensitive" species (e.g., most chameleon species, some geckos, uromastyx, and water dragons) (Fig. 179.9).

Dermal mycoses (formerly classified as Chrysosporium-related dermatitis) are a common skin lesion in anoles, *Ameiva* species, bearded dragons, green iguanas, chameleons, geckos, water dragons, curly-tailed lizards (*Leiocephalus* spp.), and even snakes. Recent molecular analysis has classified these as belonging to the genera Nannizziopsis, Paranannizziopsis, and Ophidiomyces, with a trend to some host specificity.[10] In general, the lesions present as multiple irregular patches of thickened skin supporting a hyperkeratotic exudate (Fig. 179.10). The diagnosis can be made by the fungal morphological and histological features of

the lesions, although confirmation is by culture and PCR. These fungi are a group of keratinophilic fungus that can result in a fatal granulomatous dermatitis[12,13] (Fig. 179.11).

In snakes, mites (*Ophionyssus* spp.), retained shed skin, and dehydration are common in all species. Failure to feed (especially with shy species such as ball pythons) with resulting weight loss and/or failure to thrive is common (Fig. 179.12). Neurological signs (weakness) associated with a generalized debilitated state and/or concurrent ectoparasites or viral infections are also common.

Eye lesions in snakes are usually associated with the spectacle rather than the globe itself. Retained spectacles are common and usually related to a poor shed or mites. Infections of the subspectacular space may be seen in snakes that are under stress while also having difficulty shedding, suffering from stomatitis (and possible nasolacrimal duct involvement as a pathway for pathogens to get to this space), or suffering from a traumatic injury (bite from prey). Primary eye diseases are less common but may result from trauma or developmental issues.[14]

Diagnosis and treatment of the aforementioned conditions can be found in a variety of resources, including other sections of this book.

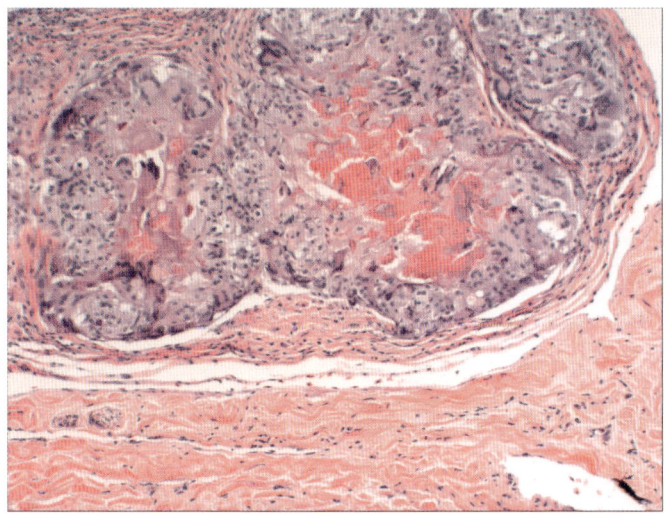

FIG 179.11 Fungal granulomas with a central core of bright eosinophilic debris surrounded by multinucleate giant cells and macrophages. H&E stain; ×10. (Courtesy of Drury R. Reavill.)

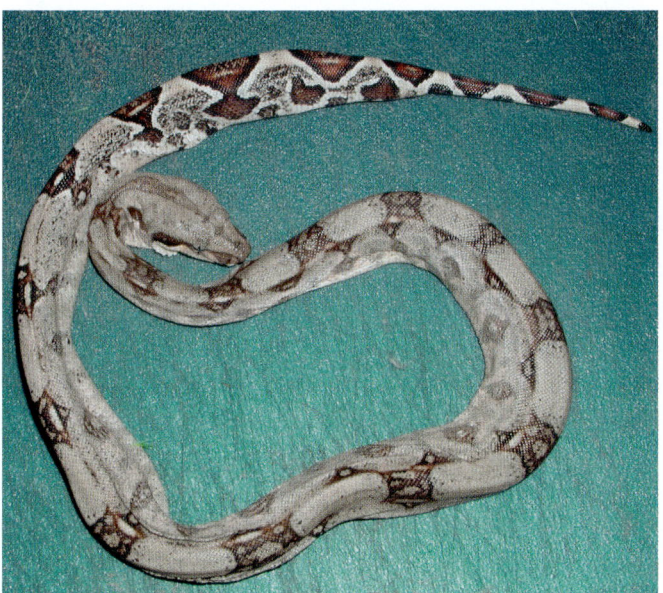

FIG 179.12 Significant loss of muscle mass and severe dehydration are evident in this boa constrictor (*Boa constrictor*). (Courtesy of Drury R. Reavill.)

The reader is referred to the appropriate chapters on specific diagnostic testing and therapeutics for these conditions.

Viral infections are probably more common than previously thought in all species of reptiles. Improved viral identification techniques combined with continued research may shed light on this aspect of reptile disease in the future (see Chapter 30).

Of all the infectious presentations commonly seen, cryptosporidiosis (in any species) may be the most frustrating because the morbidity/mortality rate is close to 100% in diagnosed patients, despite a variety of attempted treatments. Concurrent viral infections (e.g., atadenovirus in bearded dragons) may increase the likelihood of mortality in these cases. Although testing all animals for cryptosporidia and removing chronically infected carriers from the collection may be a consideration for small collections, this may be cost prohibitive in large collections or inappropriate with valuable species. Quarantine, use of proper hygiene, and separation of healthy reptiles from those with obvious clinical signs are viable options. Antemortem tests include fecal acid-fast stain, histological biopsy of the gastric mucosa, or PCR. However, some testing may result in false positives by identifying cryptosporidia from prey items such as rodents.

Diseases Identified Postmortem in Retail Animals

A review of reptiles from several retail facilities submitted to a pathology service identified some disease trends in common pet species (Table 179.3).[1] The majority of the reptiles in the review study were young animals, not older breeding stock. The results of this review are discussed in the following sections. In general, across all reptile groups, the most commonly diseased organ system was the gastrointestinal tract. This suggests that close evaluation of the gastrointestinal system is a priority and also stresses that nutritional support is an essential part of the therapy.

Chelonians. Of the turtles and tortoises examined, the most common finding was chelonid herpesvirus infection of Russian tortoises (*Agrionemys horsfieldii*), which in many cases was from outbreaks involving multiple animals. Herpesvirus-associated rhinitis, stomatitis, glossitis, tracheitis, bronchopneumonia, and, uncommonly, necrotizing hepatitis have been reported in a number of tortoise species: Hermann's tortoises (*Testudo hermanni*); Russian, spur-thighed tortoises (*Testudo graeca*); and marginated tortoises (*Testudo marginata*) (Fig. 179.13). This herpesviral infection is frequently complicated by secondary bacterial infections and generally results in severe debilitation of the tortoise. The transmission is most likely from infected carriers, although the pathogenesis of this viral infection has not been fully described. The early lesions in these Russian tortoises were stomatitis and glossitis. This suggests that specifically testing for herpesvirus in tortoises with this presentation can help separate those animals with this typically fatal disease from those with other potentially treatable conditions.[15]

Nonspecific dermatitis (not involving the shell) was also a commonly recognized postmortem lesion in chelonians, primarily in water turtles such as red-eared sliders (Fig. 179.14). On the basis of the history, these lesions were suspected to be traumatic in origin and were slow to resolve with apparently adequate therapy. Bacterial involvement in cases of dermatitis was based on the presence of bacteria identified in the inflammation and/or bacterial granulomas present within the dermis on histological examination. Fungal dermatitis of chelonians was not identified in this collection of cases.

Sporadic findings of intestinal parasitism were noted. These included nematode, trematode, and cryptosporidial enteropathies.[16] A small number of tortoises and turtles also had a nonspecific enteritis in which a disease etiology was not identified.

Primary pneumonia was uncommon and was usually associated with a variety of systemic diseases.

A small number of the freshwater and box turtles (Emydidae) had intravascular parasites consistent with spirorchid fluke eggs. Adult spirorchid flukes (blood flukes) inhabit the cardiovascular system (heart and blood vessels) of many freshwater and marine turtles. These are analogous to the schistosomes of birds and mammals. Eggs deposited by the adults are carried through the circulatory system and can block small blood vessels in many organs, producing microgranulomas. The eggs then migrate to the lumen of the intestines, which can lead to necrosis and bacteremia. In freshwater turtles, the intermediate host is a snail, of which at least one species has been identified, *Helisoma anceps*.[17] Because antemortem testing is unlikely to identify this infection in the individual animal, a postmortem diagnosis should warrant treatment for all exposed turtles in a collection.[18]

TABLE 179.3 **Summary of Disease Conditions Recognized by Pathological Evaluation***

Lesions/Disease Agents	Chelonians (50/349)	Lizards (108/349)	Snakes (119/349)
Adenovirus† with associated lesions in the liver and/or intestines	—	26 (24%)	3 (2.5%)
Autolyzed sample‡	2 (4%)	3 (2.8%)	1 (0.8%)
Bacteremia	—	1 (1%)	4 (3.4%)
CANV-like† (fungal dermatitis)	—	22 (20.4%)	—
Debilitation, severe§	3 (6%)	12 (11.1%)	49 (41%)
Dermatitis, bacterial†	8 (16%)	9 (8.3%)	1 (0.8%)
Dermatitis, nonspecific‖	2 (4%)	7 (6.5%)	—
Dermatitis, other fungus (not CANV)	—	3 (2.8%)	1 (0.8%)
Encephalitis, nonspecific‖	—	2 (1.8%)	2 (1.7%)
Entamoeba	1 (2%)	1 (1%)	—
Enteritis and/or gastritis, cryptosporidia†	2 (4%)	48 (44.4%)	8 (6.7%)
Enteritis, coccidia	—	7 (6.5%)	—
Enteritis, nematodes	4 (8%)	8 (7.4%)	3 (2.5%)
Enteritis, nonspecific‖	5 (10%)	14 (13%)	52 (43.7%)
Enteritis, protozoal flagellates	—	2 (1.8%)	2 (1.7%)
Enteritis, trematodes	1 (2%)	2 (1.8%)	—
Hepatitis, nonspecific‖	1 (2%)	17 (15.7%)	8 (6.7%)
Herpesvirus† (including necrotizing hepatitis and stomatitis)	19 (38%)	—	—
IBD†	—	—	14 (12.8%)
Kidney, protozoal flagellates	—	5 (4.6%)	—
Mycobacteria†	1 (systemic) (2%)	—	—
Myocarditis, nonspecific‖	1 (2%)	2 (1.8%)	—
Pneumonia, fungal	—	1 (1%)	—
Pneumonia, nonspecific‖	5 (10%)	7 (6.5%)	9 (7.6%)
Renal urate tophi	—	1 (1%)	—
Sarcocyst within skeletal muscle	3 (6%)	—	—
Schistosomes	4 (8%)	—	—
Shell necrosis	2 (4%)	—	—
Skin mites	—	—	5 (4.2%)
Stomatitis, nonspecific‖	2 (4%)	—	—
Trematode, intestines	1 (2%)	—	—
Vacuolar hepatopathy	—	3 (2.8%)	—

CANV, *Chrysosporium* anamorph of *Nannizziopsis vriesii*; IBD, inclusion body disease.

*The numbers will not equal 100%, because animals may have had more than one lesion.

†The etiology, in some cases, was confirmed by further diagnosis with polymerase chain reaction or cultures.

‡The submitted animal was too autolyzed to identify any lesions on histological examination.

§Debilitation was determined by loss of coelomic cavity fat, muscle wasting, and hepatic atrophy.

‖No specific etiological agent was identified.

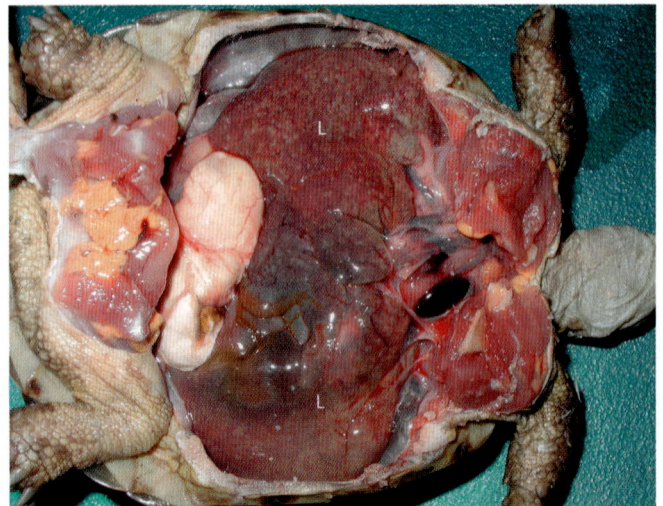

FIG 179.13 Russian tortoise (*Agrionemys horsfieldii*) with multiple foci of hepatic necrosis due to herpesvirus. L, Liver. (Courtesy of Drury R. Reavill.)

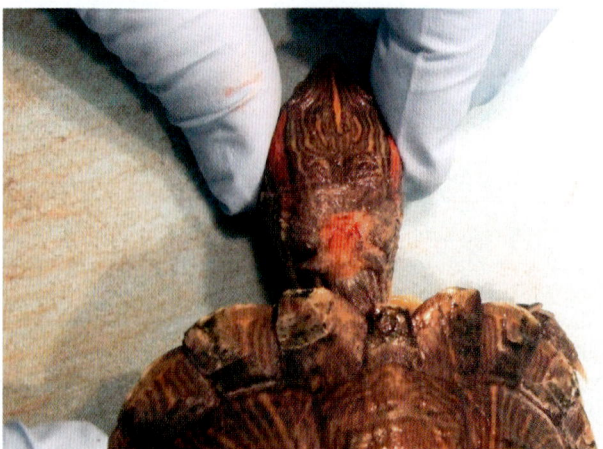

FIG 179.14 Erosive and ulcerative dermatitis on the dorsal neck of a red-eared slider (*Trachemys scripta elegans*), suspected to be caused by trauma. (Courtesy of Drury R. Reavill.)

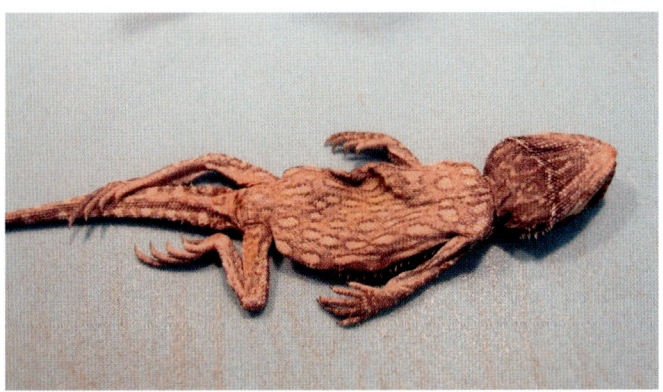

FIG 179.15 A bearded dragon (*Pogona vitticeps*) with enteric cryptosporidiosis. There is loss of body condition with muscle wasting and dehydration. (Courtesy of Drury R. Reavill.)

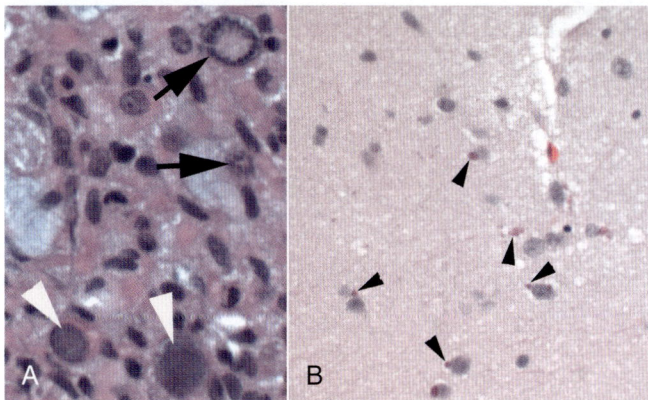

FIG 179.16 (A) Histology of the intestinal mucosa of a bearded dragon (*Pogona vitticeps*) with coccidia (black arrows) and adenovirus (*white arrowheads*). H&E stain, ×40. (B) Round to oval intracytoplasmic viral inclusions (arrowheads) in the brain of a python characteristic of boid inclusion body disease caused by reptarenavirus. H&E stain, ×40. (Courtesy of Drury R. Reavill.)

Lizards. Of the abnormalities reported in lizards, the most common finding was cryptosporidial enteritis and/or gastritis. This is most likely overrepresented because the most common lizards in the pet trade are leopard geckos; and these lizards are frequently infected. Smaller numbers of bearded dragons and water dragons also had cryptosporidial enteropathies. Because these lizards were severely emaciated and dehydrated on postmortem evaluation, the cryptosporidial infections were deemed to be a significant contributor to disease and, ultimately, death (Fig. 179.15).

Atadenovirus infection involving the liver and gastrointestinal tract is common in bearded dragons. This viral infection became established in lizard-breeding colonies in the United States and can result in high mortality rates for immunocompromised animals. The common clinical signs in young bearded dragons are progressive weakness and anorexia. Frequently, these emaciated lizards have concurrent intestinal coccidial infections (Fig. 179.16A).

Dermatitis, including bacterial, fungal, and in some cases with no apparent etiological agent, is commonly seen in young lizards. Additionally nonspecific hepatitis and enteritis are recognized as frequent lesions. The lack of etiological agents for these two conditions could be due to attempts at antemortem therapies. Systemic debilitation, which contributed to decline and death, is characterized by hepatic atrophy and/or atrophy of the coelomic cavity fat pads.

Snakes. Generalized debilitation was a common presentation, especially for young snakes. Almost half of the animals had significant hepatic atrophy, as well as atrophy of the coelomic cavity fat pads. A nonspecific enteritis and/or enterocolitis was also a common finding that could be accounted for by poor husbandry such as inadequate heat and/or humidity.

Inclusion body disease (IBD) of boids, recently associated with the arenavirus, was a frequent finding because the majority of snakes in the pet trade are susceptible to IBD, including the common boa (*Boa constrictor imperator*) (see Fig. 179.16B)[19] (see Chapter 30). Skin mites and gastric cryptosporidiosis were also common, and both diseases are well described in the literature.[20,21]

Diseases Identified Postmortem in Breeding Stock

In general across all reptile groups, tumors, reproductive disorders primarily in females, degenerative lesions of the kidney and liver, and chronic infections such as IBD and mycobacteriosis can develop. These conditions are described in detail in other chapters. Knowing the common diseases in a population of animals and conducting a thorough examination with appropriate diagnostic testing can result in better health of those animals entering the pet trade and improvement in animal welfare.

REFERENCES

See www.expertconsult.com for a complete list of references.

180

Laboratory Management and Medicine

Dorcas P. O'Rourke, Peter Nowlan, and Leslie Retnam

Reptiles and amphibians are encountered in an array of institutional settings, from corporate biomedical research facilities to veterinary colleges and herpetology teaching collections. Some amphibian species, such as the African clawed frog (*Xenopus laevis*), have become so commonplace that entire books are devoted to their husbandry and care in laboratory animal settings.[1] African clawed frogs were originally used for pregnancy assays and toxicology research; more recent biomedical uses include oocyte harvesting for molecular biology research and, along with *Silurana* (*Xenopus*) *tropicalis*, developmental biology studies. In addition to *Xenopus*, commonly used laboratory species of amphibians include axolotls (*Ambystoma mexicanum*), American bullfrogs (*Lithobates catesbeianus*), leopard frogs (*Lithobates pipiens*), tiger salamanders (*Ambystoma tigrinum*), and marine toads (*Rhinella marinum*). Axolotls have long been popular as animal models for limb regeneration studies; research has expanded to include cardiac and central nervous system regeneration. Bullfrogs and leopard frogs are commonly used in physiology laboratory instruction and in endocrinology, nociception, and infectious disease research. Tiger salamanders and marine toads are used as models for studies involving neurology and ophthalmology. Most recently, wild and captive populations of amphibians have been used in environmental toxicology, endocrine disrupter, and chytridiomycosis investigations.

Reptiles are relatively uncommon in biomedical research institutions but are frequently found in universities. Among reptiles, green anoles (*Anolis carolinensis*) and brown anoles (*Anolis sagrei*) are most commonly used for physiology, endocrinology, and behavior research. Parthenogenesis and other reproductive strategies are studied in whiptail lizards (*Aspidoscelis* spp.). Red-eared sliders (*Trachemys scripta elegans*) and related aquatic turtle species are used in physiology laboratories and for infectious disease research. Snakes are typically found in teaching collections and displays and are also used to study behavior, ecology, and evolution. Venom biochemistry and therapeutic use of venom components are specific areas of medical interest. Crocodilians are used commonly in biochemistry, physiology, and environmental toxicology research. Both reptiles and amphibians are extensively studied by herpetologists in laboratories and in the field to better understand their ecology and evolutionary biology and by veterinarians interested in medicine and surgery of these animals.

REGULATORY OVERSIGHT AND ACCREDITATION GUIDELINES

In the United States the USDA requires registration as a research facility if USDA-covered species are used in research and teaching. Registered facilities are subject to at least annual unannounced inspections by veterinary medical officers of the USDA. Significant uncorrected deficiencies in animal care and use programs can ultimately lead to fines and facility closure. At this time, USDA regulations cover only a defined subset of mammals. They are not applicable to reptiles and amphibians and will not be further included in this discussion. The US Government Principles, Public Health Service (PHS) Policy,[2] and *Guide for the Care and Use of Laboratory Animals* (*Guide*)[3] are much broader in scope and cover all vertebrate species. A division of NIH, the Office of Laboratory Animal Welfare (OLAW), is charged with overseeing institutional compliance with the US Government Principles, the PHS Policy, and the *Guide*.[4] This is accomplished through several mechanisms, including reviewing and approving an institution's PHS Assurance and conducting visits to the institution, if warranted. Conducting NIH-funded research activities without approval by an Institutional Animal Care and Use Committee (IACUC) can result in an investigator having to return grant money. In addition to required federal oversight, many universities and research facilities are voluntarily accredited by the AAALAC, International (AAALAC). AAALAC requires adherence to all applicable national, regional, and local legislation and uses the *Guide* as one of its three primary resources.[5] AAALAC conducts triennial site visits to accredited institutions to review animal care and use programs.

US federal wildlife and fisheries agencies require permits to conduct research on certain wildlife species; these will be addressed later. State agencies dealing with natural resources, fisheries, and wildlife may require permits or regulate acquisition and possession of certain species. Local regulations may also apply. When planning research or teaching activities involving reptiles and amphibians, investigators should check federal, state, and local regulatory requirements governing their species of interest.

The Canadian Council on Animal Care (CCAC) is a nonprofit, national organization for setting and overseeing standards of animal care throughout Canada[6]; this is accomplished through peer review assessments and program certification. The *CCAC Guidelines on: The Care and Use of Wildlife* includes amphibians and reptiles.[7]

In Europe, regulatory oversight of research animals involves a number of independent countries and is therefore quite complex. Briefly, there are two overarching regulatory institutions. The Council of Europe,[8] representing 47 independent European states, publishes the European Convention for the Protection of Vertebrate Animals used for Experimental and other Scientific Purposes, Guidelines for Accommodation and Care of Animals (ETS 123, Appendix A), which is relevant to reptile and amphibian research use.[9]

The European Union (EU) has regulatory control over 26 member states and has issued Directive EU 63/2010, which requires each member state to provide an authorization process for the conduct of research using any nonhuman vertebrate animal and cephalopods, and establishment of an oversight agency, the Competent Authority (CA), Directive EU 63/2010 must be implemented by member states. Although there is some flexibility regarding implementation, serious deviations can result in legal action.

EU directive 63/2010 contains a series of appendices that describe requirements relating to animal care and well-being. Annex I lists species that must be acquired from registered breeders and that must be purpose-bred for research, including *Xenopus laevis*, *Silurana tropicalis*, *Rana temporaria*, and *Lithobates pipiens*. Annex III lays down housing conditions for various animals, including reptiles and amphibians.[10] The requirements of Annex III are mandatory, whereas adherence to the more detailed Council of Europe ETS 123 is voluntary. It is important to note that not all members of the Council of Europe are members of the European Union.

Once all appropriate authorizations are in place, parties are subject to regular inspections by inspectors of the Competent Authority (CA). Additionally, each authorized establishment must have an animal welfare body and a compliance officer to monitor study conduct and demonstrate a robust mechanism for ensuring compliance with both the general conditions of the law and the specific conditions of individual authorizations.

Researchers must be trained and competent in theoretical aspects of the law, ethical review 3Rs, and in the practical elements of individual procedures, inclusive of euthanasia; these training programs must be approved by the CA.

In Australia, the eighth edition of the *Australian Code for the Care and Use of Animals for Scientific Purposes* (*Code*) covers all vertebrates and cephalopods and provides an ethical framework and principles for all areas of science using animals, including research, teaching, biologic product production, and environmental studies. The *Code* is endorsed by the National Health and Medical Research Council, Australian Research Council, Commonwealth Scientific Industrial Research Organization, and Universities Australia.[11] States and territories can also require registration and/or licensing to conduct animal research.

In New Zealand, reptiles and amphibians fall under the definition of "animals" under s 2 (1) (a) of the animal welfare legislation. Any research, testing, and teaching (defined in s 5 of the legislation) using such animals can only be done by an institution holding a Code of Ethical Conduct (CEC) approved by the Director General for Primary Industries and following approval by an animal ethics committee properly constituted under the CEC, as required by the Animal Welfare Act. Additionally, native frogs, lizards, and the tuatara are protected, and permits to catch or carry out research on these species are required from the Department of Conservation.[12] The Australian and New Zealand Council for the Care of Animals in Research and Teaching (ANZCCART) provides well-researched, objective information on ethical use of animals in research and teaching.[13]

In Singapore, the Agri-Food and Veterinary Authority (AVA) requires research institutes using vertebrates for scientific purposes (including reptiles and amphibians) to be licensed. Research institutes are subject to at least one annual inspection by inspectors from the AVA.

AAALAC International accredited units can be found in Canada, Singapore, Australia, and throughout Europe.

FUNDING AGENCY REQUIREMENTS

During the 1980s in the United States, several federal agencies formed the Interagency Research Animal Committee (IRAC). Members of this group developed and published the US Government Principles for the Utilization and Care of Vertebrate Animals Used in Testing, Research, and Training (US Government Principles). Agencies that committed to adhere to these principles when conducting and sponsoring research include the Department of Health and Human Services (including the National Institutes of Health [NIH], Centers for Disease Control [CDC],

TABLE 180.1 US Federal Agency Compliance Requirements

Agency	Govt. Principles	PHS Policy	Guide	Other
NIH	X	X	X	
NSF	X	X	X	
DOD	X		X	
NASA		X		NASA Policy
FDA				GLP
EPA				GLP

DOD, Department of Defense; *EPA*, Environmental Protection Agency; *FDA*, Food and Drug Administration; *GLP*, good laboratory practices; *NASA*, National Aeronautics and Space Administration; *NIH*, National Institutes of Health; *NSF*, National Science Foundation.

and Food and Drug Administration [FDA]), the Department of Defense (DoD), Department of Agriculture (USDA), Department of the Interior (DoI), the Environmental Protection Agency (EPA), the National Aeronautics and Space Administration (NASA), and the National Science Foundation (NSF).[14]

Agency compliance requirements are in Table 180.1. Additionally, private granting agencies such as the Morris Animal Foundation require IACUC or equivalent body approval;[15] others may request information on IACUC approval or adherence to animal care guidelines on grant applications.[16,17]

The Natural Sciences and Engineering Research Council of Canada requires all animal research to comply with the CCAC policies and guidelines.[18]

In Australia, the primary federal government funding agency for working with reptiles and amphibians is the Australian Research Council (ARC). The ARC endorses the Australian Code for the Care and Use of Animals for Scientific Purposes.[11] Internally funded university studies are also subject to the Australian Code and state animal research and conservation laws.

In New Zealand, any funding agency would require that all relevant permits (AEC, Department of Conservation [DOC]) have been obtained.

Funding from the Singapore government for biomedical research comes primarily from either the National Research Foundation (NRF), National Medical Research Council (NMRC), or the Biomedical Medical Research Council (BMRC). The application process to obtain funds from the government to conduct research, teaching, and testing on reptiles and amphibians would not be any different from using other live vertebrates.

PUBLICATION REQUIREMENTS

Many professional organizations have standards for ethical conduct of research and criteria for publication in scientific journals.[19–21] The Society for the Study of Amphibians and Reptiles (SSAR), American Society of Ichthyologists and Herpetologists (ASIH), and Herpetologists League (HL) have published *Guidelines for Use of Live Amphibians and Reptiles in Field and Laboratory Research*,[22] which discuss ethical research conduct and expectations for IACUC approval. Other journals have similar requirements (Table 180.2).[23–28]

If an individual wishes to conduct a study and is not affiliated with a university or other institution, she/he may either be able to obtain an adjunct appointment or collaborate with a faculty member of an institution that has a research program and an IACUC in place.

The *Canadian Veterinary Journal* will only consider manuscripts that have obtained IACUC or equivalent approval and have followed CCAC guidelines or equivalent.[29]

European journals broadly adhere to the international guidelines of major journals. Many have implemented the "ARRIVE" guidelines for design of studies using animals[30] and require an ethical review and evidence of compliance with local legislative requirements.

The EU Directive requires project authorization for nonhuman vertebrates or cephalopods to be granted by the CAs of each member state; this process involves an ethical review.

In Australia, each journal's editorial policy delineates specific requirements; however, these increasingly include the ARRIVE guidelines.

The leading journals in New Zealand require ethics approval for publication of research involving the manipulation of animals. The Royal Society of New Zealand's (RSNZ) policy on the ethical use of nonhuman subjects in research states that RSNZ journals endorse the ANZCCART (NZ) policy for the responsible use of animals in science.

The *New Zealand Veterinary Journal* requires conformation with ethical standards described in the Ministry of Agriculture and Forestry (MAF) User's Guide to Part 6 of the New Zealand Animal Welfare Act 1999, the Good Practice Guide for the Use of Animals in Research, Testing and Teaching, published by the National Animal Ethics Advisory Committee (2002), and approval by an accredited animal ethics committee, in accordance with Part 6 of the Animal Welfare Act 1999.

In Singapore, similar to Australia and New Zealand, publications involving amphibians and reptiles for scientific purposes are required to meet specific criteria of the journal.

THE GUIDE FOR THE CARE AND USE OF LABORATORY ANIMALS

The *Guide for the Care and Use of Laboratory Animals* (*Guide*) is used by many institutions within the United States and increasingly internationally when developing and implementing internal policies and procedures for vertebrate animal care and use. Although the term *laboratory animal* appears somewhat misleading, the *Guide* is careful to clearly define laboratory animals as all vertebrates used in research, teaching, and testing. The most recent edition of the *Guide* specifically addresses husbandry and care of aquatic species in research settings. It further explains that even though it does not specifically discuss wildlife and aquatic species in natural settings, it does provide ethical considerations and general principles that are equally relevant to these circumstances.[3]

Performance standards are an integral component of the *Guide*. The *Guide* provides basic standards for animal care and use programs and establishes desired outcomes but allows institutions flexibility in how they achieve those outcomes. For example, air exchange rates in animal rooms must be sufficient to prevent accumulation of excess humidity and ammonia, which is a respiratory irritant. Therefore typical air exchange rates are 10 to 15 air changes per hour. However, species such as reptiles and amphibians with slower metabolic rates and less waste production do not generally require the same rapid turnover of room air; in fact, air exchanges that are too rapid can desiccate species that require high humidity. Consequently, rooms with lower air exchange rates may be preferred for these species and can be appropriately justified through the use of these performance standards. AAALAC-accredited institutions can also refer to recognized reference resources,[31] such as Guidelines for Use of Live Amphibians and Reptiles in Field and Laboratory Research.[22]

In Canada, the *Guide to the Care and Use of Experimental Animals, Vol. 2* (1984), *Guidelines on the Care and Use of Wildlife* (2003), and *CCAC Species-specific Recommendations on: Amphibians and Reptiles* (2004) provide information on reptile and amphibian care and use.[32]

In Europe, the other document that gives more detailed information of best practice and guidelines for reptiles and amphibians is the Council of Europe ETS 123 Appendix A guidelines.

Unlike the *Guide*, which provides a comprehensive overview of all aspects of managing an animal care and research program, there is no single EU document that covers topics such as researcher and staff health and safety, animal transport, captive colony health monitoring, zoonotic disease transmission, and other related components of animal care and use. These subjects are contained in separate documents, and many of them may be national in nature rather than pan-European.

In Australia, the New South Wales animal regulatory body that governs animal research has some useful guidelines on wildlife research that would apply to reptiles and amphibians;[33] other state governments may have similar guidelines. The National Health and Medical Research Council (NHMRC) published guidelines on well-being of animals used in research, and they contain a wildlife section that makes reference to reptiles and amphibians.[34]

New Zealand documents to assist researchers and animal ethics committees on the use of amphibians and reptiles for procedures, such as marking/identification, animal welfare, and practicalities and public perceptions in New Zealand,[35] include the *Guide to the Preparation of Codes of Ethical Conduct*[36] and *Good Practice Guide for the Use of Animals in Research Testing and Teaching.*[37]

In Singapore, the Guidelines for the Care and Use of Animals for Scientific Purposes published by the National Advisory Committee for Laboratory Animal Research (NACLAR) in 2004 is the primary document.[38]

INSTITUTIONAL ANIMAL CARE AND USE COMMITTEE/ANIMAL WELFARE BODY/ETHICS COMMITTEE

The aforementioned US regulations and guidelines require animal care and use program oversight by a body such as an IACUC. For PHS-assured institutions, there must be at least five members on the IACUC. Membership must include a laboratory animal veterinarian, a practicing scientist, a nonscientist, and a community member with no institutional affiliation.[2] Animal care programs with reptiles and amphibians often find it advantageous to appoint IACUC members with experience in these groups of vertebrates. An alternative approach is to utilize consultants with expertise in the species being reviewed; these individuals can often provide valuable information that will enable the IACUC to make sound decisions on proposed animal use.

The IACUC is charged with several important functions, including review of the animal care and use program at least every 6 months.[2] Components of this review include evaluation of the institution's training program for researchers and research staff, animal care personnel, and the IACUC itself; the occupational health and safety program; the veterinary care program; security and disaster plan; deviations from standards in the *Guide;* and mechanisms for reporting concerns about animal welfare.

Collaborations between researchers at institutions are becoming quite common and can create some challenges for IACUCs. Whenever collaborations across institutions occur, there should be a formal written agreement addressing the responsibilities for oversight and IACUC review.[3] These agreements help eliminate ambiguity and reduce redundancy in oversight.

Another IACUC responsibility is inspecting animal facilities and use areas every 6 months. Although inspection of animal housing areas, surgery and procedure areas, and research laboratories is relatively straightforward, accessing remote field stations and research sites can be difficult (Fig. 180.1). Accessibility is further complicated by the seasonality of field work. One solution for evaluating field research is for the IACUC to request videos or photographs of procedures conducted during the field season.

The IACUC must review all proposals for research, teaching, and testing involving vertebrate animals and also must review any proposed changes to approved ongoing activities. No work may begin until protocols and amendments are fully approved by the IACUC. When submitting protocols for consideration by the IACUC, investigators should realize that the content contained in many of the questions is information required by federal regulations and guidelines. This includes rationale and purpose of the animal use; justification of species and animal numbers (statistically justified if appropriate); consideration of the impact on animal well-being and availability of alternatives; assurance that the work is not unnecessarily duplicative; provision of information confirming appropriate training and experience with proposed procedures and species; identification of hazards and methods to minimize risk; description of animal procedures in nontechnical language; provision of information on atypical housing and husbandry; detailed description of anesthesia, analgesia, surgical and other procedures, and postprocedural care; provision of criteria for intervention and rationale for selected endpoints; and description of euthanasia or other disposition of animals.[3] Euthanasia methods must be consistent with the American Veterinary Medical Association (AVMA) Guidelines for the Euthanasia of Animals.[39] The IACUC is required to carefully consider experimental endpoints and humane endpoints and to determine a method of dealing with unexpected outcomes.[3]

Certain procedures demand intense scrutiny by the IACUC, are typically covered in significant detail in protocols, and require rigorous justification. These include prolonged restraint, multiple survival surgery procedures, food and fluid restriction or regulation, and use of non-pharmaceutical–grade substances.[3] Use of hypothermia for anesthesia

in reptiles and amphibians remains controversial and continues to be discouraged.[40,41]

Researchers and instructors submitting protocols involving reptiles and amphibians should be aware of additional items for consideration. Although embryos are not typically covered by the PHS policy, larval forms of amphibians and fish are covered and require a protocol. The use of dead animals or their tissues is not covered unless the animals were killed for the purpose of the collection or if the animals were manipulated before death for the purpose of the study. In those cases, a protocol is required.[42]

Field studies can include a wide range of activities, from capture, identification, and release to invasive sample collection and surgery. Manipulation of animals in the field brings risks and challenges to both animals and personnel, and these must be addressed in the animal care and use protocol. Investigators are encouraged to consult with professional guidelines when planning field studies.[22]

Methods of capture should be described in detail in the protocol. A description of the capture device or method should be provided so that IACUC members unfamiliar with it can clearly understand its operation. Live traps must be checked frequently enough to minimize stress and risk from predators, and any items placed in the trap that increase animal well-being should be included in the description. Site selection should consider protection from the elements and methods to prevent inadvertent capture of nontarget species. Expected mortality rates, adverse effects associated with the capture method, and humane endpoints should also be addressed.

Once reptiles and amphibians are captured, they should be processed as soon as feasible so that stress associated with excess handling is minimized. In some cases, processing requires transportation to a research laboratory, field station, or another site. Animals must be transported in secure containers that prevent escape and injury. During transport, vehicles must have adequate climate control to prevent animals from exposure to temperature extremes. Adequate hydration must also be maintained.

Compared with more traditional laboratory animal species, there are significantly fewer vendors from which to purchase reptiles and amphibians for research and teaching (*Xenopus* is a notable exception). Vendors providing reptiles and amphibians tend to collect from wild or farmed populations, and the condition of animals can be quite variable, depending on the season collected and the holding facilities used (Fig. 180.2). If possible, investigators are encouraged to buy purpose-bred animals from reputable vendors, to ensure healthy research subjects, and to protect wild populations. If reptiles and amphibians are wild-caught, the investigator is responsible for obtaining all appropriate permits; the IACUC will ask for necessary documentation.

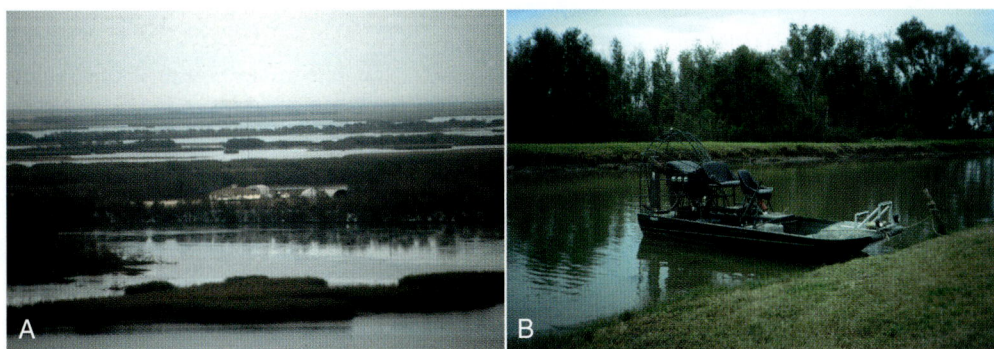

FIG 180.1 (A and B) Field stations are often located at remote sites and require specialized transportation, making them difficult for the Institutional Animal Care and Use Committee (IACUC) to access. (Courtesy of Dorcas P. O'Rourke.)

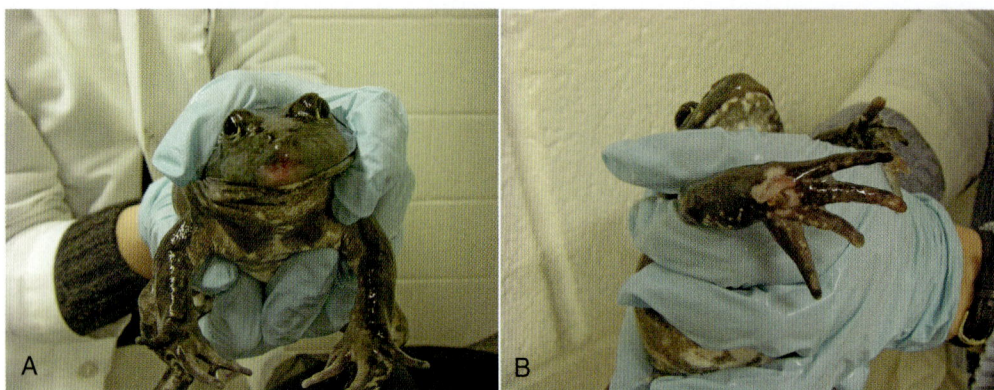

FIG 180.2 (A and B) Wild-caught animals purchased from vendors may have widely variable health status. (Courtesy of Dorcas P. O'Rourke.)

Federal permits may be required for conducting research on reptiles and amphibians. Agencies granting these permits evaluate the risk to the species and population proposed for study and set the criteria for collection, including numbers allowed to be taken. IACUCs may rely on the permitting agency's decision when determining appropriateness of species and numbers. If work is done on federal lands, such as National Park Service land, site-specific permits may be required.[43] Endangered or threatened species of reptiles and amphibians fall under the Endangered Species Act (ESA) and require special permits from the US Fish and Wildlife Service (USFWS); sea turtles require an ESA permit from the National Marine Fisheries Service (NMFS). If endangered species are to be imported or exported, a Convention on International Trade in Endangered Species of Wild Fauna and Flora (CITES) permit is required. CITES permits fall under the authority of the USFWS. State permits may be required in addition to federal permits, and investigators should contact both federal and state agencies for current requirements before protocol preparation and submission.

Occupational health and safety (OHS) concerns must be addressed when research or teaching activities involving reptiles and amphibians is planned. In addition to standard OHS procedures, personnel should be evaluated on the basis of risk and provided appropriate training in relevant zoonoses.[44] They must be instructed in how to correctly use personal protective equipment when required. Written procedures must be in place for dealing with injuries sustained while handling reptiles and amphibians because bites from large lizards, crocodilians, and venomous snakes can be life threatening, and toxins secreted from parotoid glands of some toad species can be problematic. Housing and working with venomous reptiles is especially dangerous, and specific standard operating procedures for handling animals and responding to envenomation must be written and followed. Field studies also require attention to incidental hazards, including extreme heat, water, ticks, venomous species, and plant toxins. Investigators should be prepared to respond to IACUC questions regarding both direct and incidental OHS concerns.

Performing procedures in the field brings additional challenges to the researcher. Methods of individual animal identification are more limited than in the laboratory, and some techniques such as toe clipping remain controversial.[45,46] Identification methods must be described in detail to the IACUC, and justification must be provided in the protocol for proposed methods that cause pain or impact mobility. Survival surgery must be conducted aseptically; this often requires creative approaches and careful planning when the project is designed. Appropriate anesthesia and analgesia must be provided. Inhalant anesthetic vaporizers designed for laboratory rodents are reasonably easy to transport and set up in field stations. Analgesic selection should be species-appropriate and take into consideration potential drug effects

on released animals. Consultation with the institutional veterinarian allows the researcher to plan procedures that address animal welfare in the context of the scientific goals of the study.

Similarly, euthanasia in the field presents a special set of challenges. Drugs typically used for euthanasia, such as sodium pentobarbital, cannot be used in carcasses left for scavengers. If physical methods such as gunshots are used for large crocodilians, the investigator must be prepared to provide evidence of both proficiency and safety in use of that method. In addition to the proposed euthanasia method, the investigator must also provide a proposed method for ensuring death. Any deviations from euthanasia methods approved in the AVMA euthanasia guidelines must be rigorously justified to the IACUC in the protocol (see Chapter 47).

In Canada, Animal Care Committees (ACCs) are required by CCAC guidelines. The structure and function of ACCs is similar to US IACUCs. In Europe, the oversight body in the institute or establishment is the Animal Welfare Body (AWB), which has a mandate to monitor and enforce the conditions of the project authorizations and the housing environment provided by the authorized establishments. The AWB must consist of, at a minimum, the person responsible for the welfare of animals in the establishment, a scientific member, and it shall receive advice from the designated veterinarian. However, in many institutes, the committee will incorporate many more scientists and also include the veterinarian as a member. Tasks to be fulfilled by the AWB include advising staff on matters relating to the welfare of animals in relation to their acquisition, accommodation, care, and use; advising staff on the application of the 3Rs and ensuring they are kept informed on developments in this area; having in place an internal mechanism for monitoring, reporting, and follow-up in relation to the welfare of animals housed in its establishments; following the development and outcome of projects, taking into account the effects on animals and advise with regard to elements that may further contribute to the 3Rs; and advising on rehoming schemes. Many establishments incorporate an animal research ethics committee into the AWB, and it effectively functions as an IACUC, except that the final decision regarding the authorization normally rests with the Competent Authority (CA). The AWB is expected to foster a culture of care. In Singapore, the IACUC system follows the US IACUC system closely.

HOUSING AND CARE OF REPTILES AND AMPHIBIANS IN THE LABORATORY ANIMAL FACILITY

The *Guide* contains few specific criteria for housing and caring for reptiles and amphibians. Rather, it relies on the institution's application of performance standards and IACUC approval of those performance standards. Specific information on reptile and amphibian husbandry and care in laboratory animal facilities is available,[9,47,48] and detailed nutrition and husbandry information is also provided in chapters in this book (see Section 3). Before working with an unfamiliar species, the investigator and veterinarian have a responsibility to learn as much as they can regarding the biology and natural history of that species to develop appropriate guidelines, provide a rationale to justify care standards to the IACUC, and instruct the animal care staff in proper techniques (see Section 2).

Reptiles and amphibians should be housed in enclosures that provide a safe, secure, species-appropriate environment (Fig. 180.3). Cages should be constructed of materials that are nontoxic and can be sanitized. There must be enough room for the animal to engage in species-appropriate behaviors. Hiding places, visual barriers, and substrates conducive to burrowing are essential for most species, and branches or other perches are required for arboreal animals. Group housing may be appropriate for some species of reptiles and amphibians but contraindicated in territorial or cannibalistic species. Provision of an appropriate humidity level is critical to the health and well-being of the animals. The typical range of 30% to 70% relative humidity maintained in animal facilities may be inappropriate for desert species or tropical rainforest species. Although some amphibians do well in warmer temperatures, many species thrive in much cooler temperatures than reptiles; consequently, it may be ill-advised to keep both amphibians and reptiles in the same room. It may be acceptable to house different species of reptiles or different species of amphibians within the same room because of similar environmental requirements; however, careful attention must be paid to the health status of the animals and availability of satisfactory equipment and techniques to prevent cross-contamination. Provision of thermal gradients, basking sites, and full spectrum lighting may be necessary for some species. Aquatic amphibians require water quality analysis as well as chlorine and toxin removal, and husbandry records must reflect this. Feed must be used before expiration dates to ensure

nutritional quality. If used, live vertebrate prey must be covered in the protocol, and attention must also be given to their issues of pain, distress, and humane endpoints. For example, the investigator must discuss why humanely euthanized prey cannot be used. Duration of time that the uneaten prey animal is left in the predator's enclosure should be described, as well as disposition of the prey animal once it is removed from the cage. Sanitation methods and intervals will likely differ from the general recommendations in the *Guide*, and the investigator should be able to provide rationale for these variances. Tanks housing aquatic amphibian species with recirculating life support systems and biofilters may require routine partial water changes and excess debris removal but may not require a complete breakdown and sanitation for prolonged periods, provided that appropriate water quality is maintained. Desert species of reptiles that are singly housed may tolerate less frequent cage changes if enclosures do not become excessively soiled. Territorial species of salamanders that scent mark can become stressed if cage changes occur too frequently. In all cases, it is critical to balance the health requirements with the behavioral needs of the species. In semicaptive or outdoor housing, it is important to consider impacts of environmental factors, such as extreme temperatures, drought, or precipitation. Many environments for semicaptive animals provide limited opportunities for escape from inclement weather, and care must be taken to provide extra protection. Similarly, extra effort should be made to exclude predators.

Institutional veterinarians should have experience with the species housed or must be able to consult specialists who can provide advice and training. There should be appropriate provisions for quarantine of newly arrived animals, isolation of sick animals, routine health surveillance of colonies, and facilities and equipment for anesthesia, surgery, and necropsy. The institutional veterinarian also has responsibility for oversight of other aspects of the program, so researchers should work collaboratively with these individuals when developing and proposing animal care procedures.

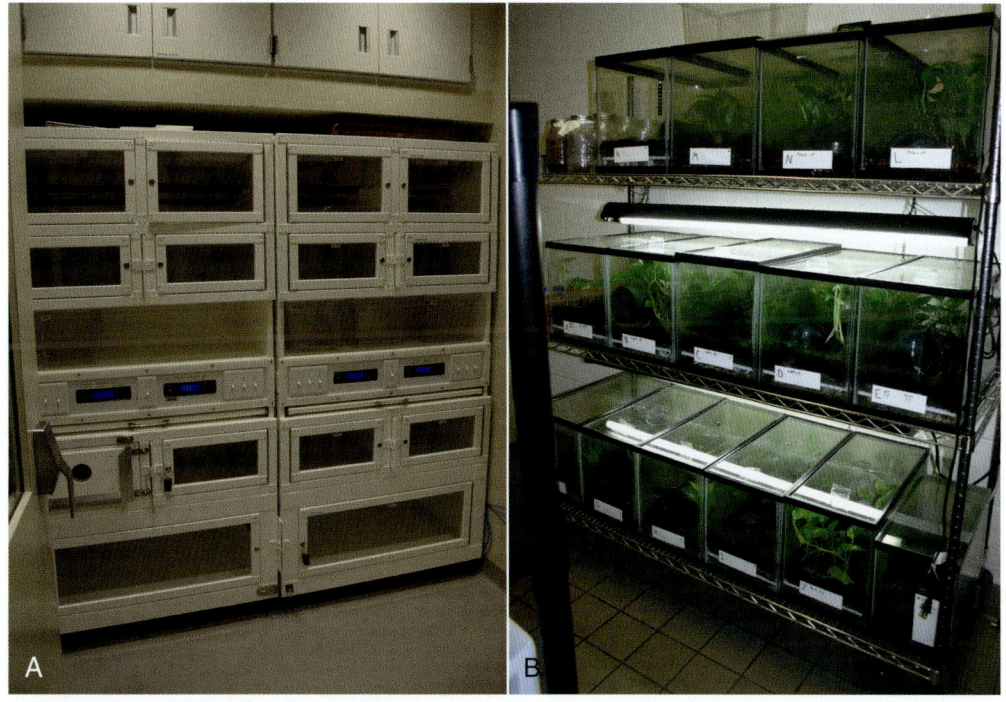

FIG 180.3 (A and B) Reptiles and amphibians should be housed in safe, secure, species-appropriate environments. (B, Courtesy of Dorcas P. O'Rourke.)

CONCLUSION

In summary, investigators interested in submitting proposals for research, teaching, or testing involving reptiles and amphibians should become familiar with national, state, and institutional requirements, as well as those of granting agencies and professional organizations. Collaborative planning with institutional veterinarians and appropriate ethics committees will educate all parties to the species needs and care, as well as the scientific goals, and should facilitate the process of protocol approval.

REFERENCES

See www.expertconsult.com for a complete list of references.

181

Conservation

Shannon T. Ferrell

Conservation can be defined as the protection of a species and its habitat from extinction with the intention of having a viable, sustainable population. Biologists and wildlife managers have typically utilized an assortment of tools to protect a species: habitat preservation/restoration, captive breeding populations, biosecurity from invasive species and predators, economic incentives for the human populace, education, and combating both the illegal trade and the overzealous harvest of animals.[1] The role of this chapter is to briefly examine the conservation of herpetofauna with an emphasis on new philosophies, technologies, and analysis of current programs and methodologies. An excellent review of herpetofauna conservation programs and veterinary involvement is already available.[2]

CURRENT REALITIES—CONSERVATION STATUS

The IUCN (International Union for the Conservation of Nature) Red List provides a global comprehensive inventory of the conservation status of both plants and animals. Assessment of the conservation status of amphibian and reptile species by the IUCN through the Global Amphibian and the Global Reptile Assessments was started in 2004 and 2006, respectively, with continued updates of selected species on an ongoing basis. As of 2016, 26 species of reptiles and 35 species of amphibians are completely extinct, or extinct in the wild, based on conservative estimates from the IUCN.[3] Other estimates place the number of extinct amphibian species at 194.[4] Nineteen percent of 5145 assessed reptile species and 31% of the 6525 assessed amphibian species are also considered threatened (critically to vulnerable).[3] Given the number of reptile species is approximately 9084, the IUCN assessment of reptile species is far from being completed, and it is difficult to fully know how many species are possibly in the threatened category.[5] Assessments of reptile species have mostly relied on regional workshops and the IUCN Species Survival Commissions, which can possibly create geographic and taxonomic bias in the process.[5] For example, North America, Madagascar, and New Caledonia have complete reviews of their reptiles, with more limited evaluations of those species in the Philippines, Europe, and some island groups.[5] Analyses of reptile populations in Asia, Africa, and Latin America are lacking, which can create the task of prioritizing conservation efforts difficult and, likely, biased.[5]

The current rate of amphibian extinction based on losses since 1970 is estimated to be four orders of magnitude (10^4) greater than the normal background level of extinction, whereas another study calculates this same rate to range from 25,039 to 45,474 times the background extinction rate.[4,6] Based on fossil records, five waves of mass animal extinctions have occurred on the planet, with a profound loss of biodiversity during a brief period of time.[7] Considering the reported rate loss of amphibian species in the last century, a sixth mass extinction event is becoming apparent for many species on the planet, but especially amphibians based on their limited geographical distributions in threatened ecosystems.[7]

CAUSATIVE FACTORS—POPULATION DECLINES

The factors associated with amphibian and reptile declines are numerous and varied, with no single factor occurring in isolation but likely working in a synergistic fashion with other factors to extirpate species even in pristine habitats.[8] The most cited factors for herpetofauna declines are (1) habitat alteration, (2) invasive species, (3) climate change, (4) pollution, (5) trade, and (6) infectious diseases.[4,6,9–12]

Habitat Alteration

Habitat loss is intuitively grasped as an obvious cause for animal population declines. Further examination of habitat management practices and policies reveals that even in protected regions, fragmentation of the environment with structures such as roads creates barriers to genetic flow, as animals cannot migrate pass these impediments.[12,13] Moreover, the division of a once-contiguous habitat into smaller, nonassociated sections is highly disruptive even though the surface area of habitat might remain the same by acquiring additional nonadjacent sections.[12,14] With amphibians, the type of habitat to be preserved is highly species-specific and dependent on the life cycle. Some species can be relatively restricted to regions around bodies of water, whereas others can be found in the forest adjacent to a body of water.[14] Research has demonstrated that the uplands forest is critically important when considering protection for wetlands, because many amphibians use the body of water for reproduction, and then the adults and metamorphed progeny will disperse into the forest.[12,14] Furthermore, old-growth forest cover has long been recognized as beneficial to herpetofauna, but human disruption of the landscape has highly fragmented this resource. Because of the financial and political restraints, completely protecting large tracts of forest can be difficult. However, studies in Australia have shown benefit to regrowth of previously cleared forest for maintaining some degree of both reptile population numbers and species biodiversity.[15,16] Overall, habitat fragmentation experiments conducted over the last 35 years on multiple continents and biomes have resulted in a loss of general biodiversity of 13% to 75% in the experimental zones. In addition, significant impacts on ecosystem function were detected in the fragmentation experiments because nutrient cycles were altered and biomass decreased.[17]

Invasive Species

Invasive species can be defined as animals whose presence in a region is attributable to human actions that allowed them to overcome biogeographic barriers and are capable of sustaining a self-replacing population over several life cycles.[18] These species constitute a continued and growing threat to native herpetofauna by direct competition, predation, hybridization, spread of pathogens, and other indirect effects.[18–20] To provide perspective on the breadth of the problem and its etiology, 50,000 nonnative species of animals and plants have been brought into the United States during its history, with the majority of these species introduced for their economic value; however, not all these introductions were permanent or invasive.[21] The most complete review of the costs associated with the prevention and management of nonindigenous species in the United States placed the annual cost to the country at $120 billion.[21] One study evaluating the effects of invasive species on biodiversity determined that the number of reported invasive species (plant or animal) to the Convention on Biological Diversity are underestimated and highly dependent on the level of development and research efforts within a country.[20] Mammalian predators have been the most successful and well-documented invasive taxa, directly causing declines in indigenous reptiles and amphibians, both on the mainland and on islands.[22] A primary factor in the extinctions of at least 14% of all bird, mammal, and reptile species are domestic feral cats (*Felis catus*), who are also the principal threat to at least 8% of the remaining critically endangered birds, mammals, and reptiles.[23] Many reptile species have additionally been impacted by other mammalian predators such as the small Asian mongoose (*Herpestes javanicus*).[21,24,25]

The rise of the exotic animal trade has additionally generated a plethora of reptile and amphibian invasive species that threaten native mammals, birds, reptiles, and amphibians.[26,27] Invasive herpetofauna often have significant impacts on native species, including direct competition for resources, hybridization, inducement of phenotypic change, and species extinction.[26] The prevalent and striking example is the Burmese python (*Python bivittatus*) in the state of Florida, where these large, ambush predators have gained a substantial foothold within the Everglades and surrounding regions due to the hospitable environmental conditions in Florida and the lack of any natural predators.[28] These snakes have attacked humans, pets, large crocodilians, and endangered/threatened species such as the Key Largo woodrat (*Neotoma floridana smalli*) and wood storks (*Mycteria americana*), and they are considered to be responsible for significant declines in wild mammal populations in southern Florida.[27,28] Additional invasive reptile species of particular concern, especially in parts of the United States, are the red-eared slider (*Trachemys scripta*), the brown tree snake (*Boiga irregularis*), the Nile monitor (*Varanus niloticus*), other miscellaneous large constrictors (pythons, boas, and anacondas), and many other lizards such as iguanids and anoles.[27]

Although amphibians are largely thought to be prey items, the cane toad (*Rhinella marina*) serves as a reminder that any species outside of its natural environment can present unique challenges to a naïve ecosystem. These hardy amphibians were introduced throughout the world as biological means to control insects before pesticides, but Australia stands dramatically altered after introducing this amphibian predator into Queensland in 1935.[19] Cane toads are still slowly migrating across Australia while simultaneously reducing numerous animal species through two principal means: consumption of cane toads with resulting fatal intoxication or direct competition for resources such as food during dry seasons and shelters.[19] The ingestion of adult cane toads by native reptilian and mammalian predators has resulted in numerous mortalities from the secreted bufotoxins.[19,29] The affected reptiles in Australia include diverse species of lizards, crocodiles, turtles, and snakes (Fig. 181.1). Finally, the North American bullfrog (*Rana catesbeiana*), the Cuban tree frog (*Osteopilus septentrionalis*), and the Caribbean tree frog (*Eleutherodactylus coqui*) represent other widely dispersed and problematic invasive amphibians (Pitt W et al, Proc 11th Wildlife Damage Management Conf, 2005, pp 112–119).[27,30]

A review of eradication programs found an 86% success rate in targeting and eliminating invasive plants and animals on the mainland

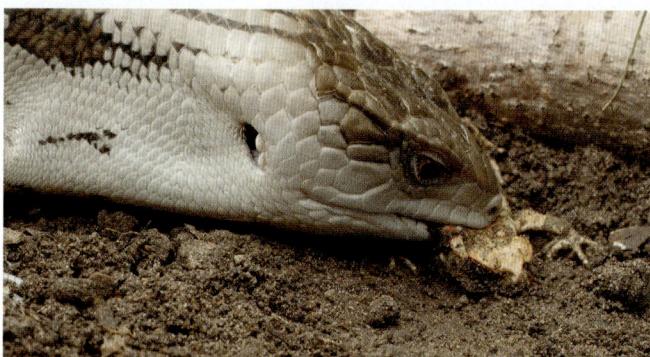

FIG 181.1 A blue-tongued skink (*Tiliqua scincoides*) ingests an invasive cane toad (*Rhinella marina*) that could lead to a fatal intoxication. (Courtesy of Jonathan Webb, University of Technology.)

or islands, with 94.6% of the reported programs targeting vertebrates. However, 97% of the studied eradication programs in the review occurred on islands. The review study could not find any successful, completed, large-scale eradication program on a mainland location with a well-established invasive species.[32] Given these challenges, focus has shifted from the improbable complete eradication of an established invasive species on the mainland to strategies that embrace mitigation and control. Conversely, full-scale eradication of invasive species on islands is being more actively promoted.[33] Islands might only encompass roughly 5.5% of the world's land surface area; however, these fragile habitats hold more than 15% of terrestrial species.[22] Eradication of invasive mammals is a common tool on islands for the conservation of threatened species and has been attempted on more than 700 islands. Rodents, domestic goats, and cats are the three taxa most commonly eradicated from islands.[22] Regardless of the species, removal of invasive animals from islands inhabited by humans is often more difficult and prone to failure than uninhabited islands.[33]

Climate Change

Fluctuations in global temperatures with secondary effects on general weather patterns are slowly being recognized as a biologic crisis as years of meteorologic data are concurrently evaluated with animal movements and extinctions. With the overall trend of global warmth in the last few decades, there has been an evident movement of animals toward the poles and away from the equators, likely to escape abnormally high temperatures.[34] Past extinction rates for reptiles on Aegean islands were found to be greater than for those same species existing on the mainland, when incorporating climatic change into the model, especially for reptiles from cooler environments on isolated, smaller lands.[11] The explanation for the higher extinction rate on islands is the inability to diminish the effects of temperature fluctuations through migration to more appropriate habitats. However, this effect will likely be similar on the mainland as habitat is fragmented through human activities creating similar "islands" of geographic isolation.[11]

Another subtle effect of climate change is the possibility of increasing embryo mortality in reptile eggs and possibly disrupting the adaptive effects of temperature sex determination.[35] Temperature sex determination (TSD) is the environmental, irreversible determination of embryonic sex used by some reptiles during the thermosensitive period of incubation. Some species of turtles use type Ia TSD, where male progeny are produced at the lower range of incubation temperatures. Mixed sex ratios are seen at intermediate temperatures, and female progeny hatch at the higher end of the incubation temperature range. Previous work in painted turtles (*Chrysemys picta*) with type Ia TSD found that increasing the temperature variance around the low mean temperature for male progeny resulted in higher ratios of feminization, leading to a decoupling of the expected effect of the low incubation temperature.[36] A later study in painted turtles demonstrated that greater thermal variance (±5°C) around the respective mean incubation temperatures for each sex (normally 100% male or 100% female) reversed the expected sex ratios of the painted turtles, creating more females at low temperatures and more males at higher temperatures.[35] In addition, either by elevating the mean incubation temperature or by elevating the thermal variance around the female incubation temperature range, the developmental rate of turtle embryos was decreased, and the overall embryonic mortality was increased.[35] These aforementioned effects on sex and embryonic development will have critical impacts on reptile populations as climatic because change conceivably alters both the mean incubation temperatures and temperature variance in reptile nests.[37] Adapting to these climatic challenges, certain turtle species are nesting earlier in the season to take advantage of cooler temperatures that could protect the sex ratios of their progeny.[37] Finally, evidence exists that highly adaptable species, such as certain turtles, might be capable of changing their sex-determining mechanism (conversion from TSD to genetic sex determination) in response to climatic changes.[38]

Pollution

Environmental pollution has repeatedly been listed as another factor in amphibian and reptile declines through direct and indirect toxicologic effects, resulting in severely compromised animals or death.[39–41] Exposure to heavy metals, organophosphates, fertilizers, polychlorinated biphenyls, and other agents have been described as affecting herpetofauna, with the research mostly focused on assessing exposure in wild populations.[40,41] A recent assertion is that amphibians can serve as monitors of environmental quality or "canaries in the coal mine," because their permeable skin, complex biphasic life cycle, and developmental periods in water make them uniquely more susceptible to environmental contaminants.[42] Reptiles are also being investigated as possible bioindicators of environmental pollution due to their longevity and geographic distribution in a variety of different habitats (Fig. 181.2).[43] In reality, with the current, insufficient knowledge base regarding amphibian population sizes and

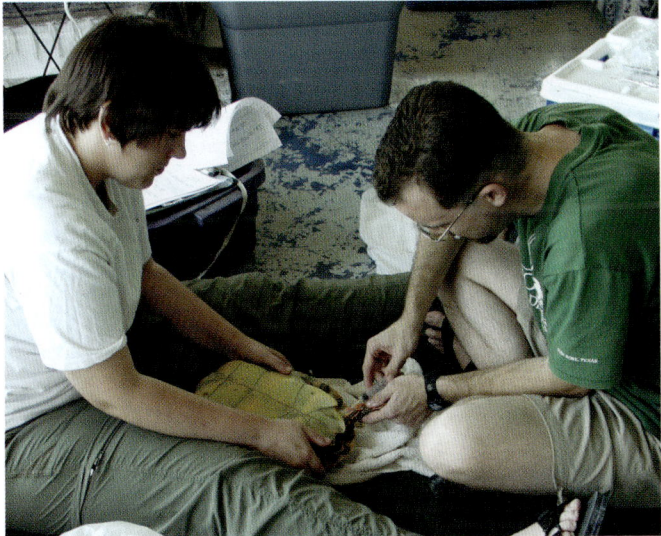

FIG 181.2 Phlebotomy in a Rio Grande cooter (*Pseudemys gorzugi*) for whole-blood, heavy-metal analysis in an environmental health-monitoring study in Texas. (Courtesy of Shannon Ferrell, Zoo de Granby.)

natural population dynamics, amphibians likely are no better than other taxa as indicators of environmental health.[42] One meta-analysis compared the toxicity data regarding numerous water contaminants for amphibians with the same toxicity data for other animal taxa and found that amphibians are more moderate in their responses to a large number of waterborne toxins compared with other animal taxa.[44] However, the authors reiterated that particular amphibians are much more sensitive to certain chemicals than other taxa and that one should review both the species and the information on the chemical agent before drawing conclusions regarding environmental quality.[44] Interestingly, one study, evaluating the use of six different taxa as indicators of biodiversity, found that woody plants and birds were more useful indicators than aquatic or terrestrial herpetofauna in assessing the level of biodiversity in northern Greece.[45]

Whereas the aforementioned environmental contaminants can result in obvious mortality, pollutants known as endocrine-disrupting contaminants (EDCs) can severely affect amphibian and reptile populations through their effects on recruitment for reproduction with little overt effect on immediate individual survival.[46] The WHO and the United Nations define EDCs as exogenous substances or mixtures that alter the functions of the endocrine system and consequently cause adverse health effects in an intact organism, its progeny, or its population.[47] In the past, mostly pesticides or synthetic hormones such as diethylstiberol (DES) were investigated as EDCs in wildlife.[48] The number and types of identified EDCs are growing, as research identifies the various pathways these chemical agents can directly or indirectly affect hormonal systems.[47,48] During the critical periods of organogenesis, minute exposures to EDCs can have significant and permanent effects on the development of certain tissues, especially reproductive organs.[48,49] Numerous studies have highlighted the effects of endocrine disruptors on reproduction in multiple animal species through their estrogenic, androgenic, antiandrogenic, and antithyroid actions.[48] Broad-snouted caiman (*Caiman latirostris*) embryos exposed to bisphenol A, a plasticizer, or endosulfan, an organochlorine pesticide, in ovo demonstrated significant changes in testicular development compared with controls.[49] In three anuran species, exposure to 17α-ethinylestradiol (EE2), a synthetically stabilized estrogen that is the principal ingredient in many female contraceptive pills, at environmentally relevant concentrations during development, resulted in the expression of the female phenotype in genetic males.[50] Inert EE2 is often excreted in human urine, poorly eliminated by sewage plants, and resistant to degradation, accumulating in aquatic sediments.[50] Atrazine is an environmentally persistent, mobile pesticide, with worldwide distribution that can possibly feminize exposed amphibians.[51] In one research study using *Xenopus laevis,* some genetic males exposed to atrazine were capable of producing viable eggs due to testicular oogenesis when bred with normal males. However, the progeny were 100% male as expected, which would obviously impact a population's reproductive fitness.[8,51] Additional contaminants viewed as possible endocrine disruptors of the reproductive system through more indirect pathways are nitrates, chemicals that affect cytochrome activities in the liver, and drugs altering prostaglandin function in the reproductive tract, such as dichlorodiphenyltrichloroethane (DDT).[48]

Trade

Reptiles and amphibians, and/or products produced from their bodies, represent a large amount of the international trade in wildlife. Trade encompasses both legal and illegal transactions, with the majority focusing on commerce for food, leather products, biomedical research, and the pet trade.[52,53] In just evaluating Europe, the trade in reptiles alone accounted for 84% of the value of all European Union (EU) animal imports, reflecting a combination of leather products and skins. Live reptile imports into the EU only represented 22% of the value of animal imports.[53] Amphibians are also imported into the EU in large quantities for meat and the pet trade. About 90 to 230 million individual frog legs are imported annually into the EU, with some estimates placing 84% of these imports being wild caught and supplied from Indonesia.[52] Finally, one examination of the international amphibian trade using species listed by CITES (Convention on International Trade in Endangered Species of Wild Fauna and Flora) and associated country reports for legal import data calculated roughly 480,000 amphibian bodies (live or otherwise) were traded over a 29-year period.[9] The preponderance of live amphibians in international trade consists of three genera in descending order, *Mantella*, *Dendrobates*, and *Ambystoma*, with the vast majority of these live amphibians being wild caught.[9] Based on limited reports of confiscation data, the illegal trade of amphibians is considered to be approximately 10% of the legal trade volume, in part because of the lack of stringent standards and control for amphibian movements.[9,52]

From 2001 to 2012, the trade in live reptiles has declined by about one third based on CITES import data. Importations have declined in animals from both the wild and captive breeding, with the majority of the reductions involving a drop in the trade of the green iguana (*Iguana iguana*).[53] The pet trade likely represents the bulk of the trade in live reptiles, and the survival of animals in the pet trade can have significant effects on the continued demand for replacements. One recent study in the United Kingdom detailed that 3.6% of reptiles acquired as pets in the home died within 1 year of purchase, with captive-bred reptiles having the best chance for long-term survival, which is compatible with other earlier reports.[54]

The demand for live reptiles is still high, with possible sustainable alternatives to harvesting wild populations being captive breeding and ranching. Ranching is defined by CITES as "rearing in a controlled environment of specimens which have been taken as eggs or juveniles from the wild, where they would have a very low probability of survival."[53] Ranching is considered to have a relatively benign impact on wild populations, and possibly a positive one, if some of the ranched juveniles are released back into the wild in their country of origin instead of going into the market.[53] Finally, no matter the decline in the herpetofauna trade as reported by evaluations of the data from CITES, it is imperative to consider much of the trade is not recorded by these entities if the trade is domestic, illegal, or involves a non-CITES–listed species (Fig. 181.3).[53]

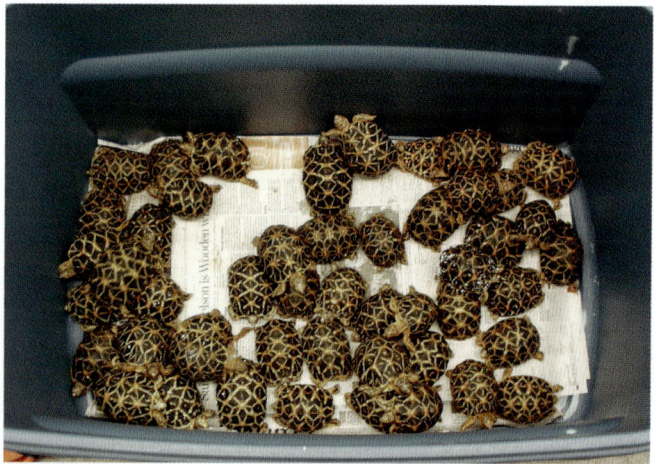

FIG 181.3 Government confiscation of illegally imported Indian star tortoises (*Geochelone elegans*) to undergo a health evaluation before entry into quarantine in a holding facility. (Courtesy of Shannon Ferrell, Zoo de Granby.)

The trade of amphibians internationally has been linked to the transfer of infectious diseases that has put an additional strain on threatened species in their native habitats and contributed to the extinction of species in some habitats.[55] The spread of *Batrachochytrium dendrobatidis* (*Bd*) has been linked to the global amphibian trade, with a growing concern that a more virulent form of this fungal pathogen has emerged through genomic recombination of different variants from multiple geographic regions.[52,56] Poison dart frogs (*Dendrobates* spp.) and western clawed frogs (*Xenopus tropicalis*) are routinely noted as potential vectors of *Bd*. In spite of decades of extensive discussion about this pathogen, methods of limiting its international dissemination are still lacking. For example, a recent surveillance program evaluating the incidence of *Bd* and ranavirus in amphibians leaving Hong Kong in commercial animal shipments found an incidence of 11.7% and 56.8%, respectively, based on skin and cloacal swabs via polymerase chain reaction analysis.[57]

Batrachochytrium salamandrivorans (*Bsal*) emerged in 2013 as a new lethal fungal pathogen restricted to salamanders and newts (Urodela) in Europe, causing lethal skin infections similar to *Bd*.[58] The current hypothesis is that this fungus had evolved with Asian salamanders with little overt pathology in the current native populations; however, the movement in amphibians from Asia to Europe has transferred this fungus to naïve populations of urodeles in western Europe lacking the appropriate resistance.[59] *Bsal* has now been detected in the Netherlands, Germany, and the United Kingdom in both captive and wild populations of salamanders. *Salamandra salamandra* is especially affected and is almost at the point of extinction in the Netherlands.[52,59] Recommendations have been suggested to stop the importation of Asian salamanders to Europe to arrest the distribution of this fungus, but the implementation of these recommendations has been delayed.

Amphibian ranaviruses have been transmitted to novel environments via both the pet trade and the use of amphibians as bait for fishing in the United States.[57,60] The North American bullfrog and tiger salamander (*Ambystoma tigrinum*) have been implicated in the movement of ranavirus throughout the world via international trade.[52] In 2008 the World Organization for Animal Health (OIE) officially recognized both ranavirus and *Bd* as notifiable diseases, but no further actions have been made to limit the movement of either pathogen across the world through biosecurity measures and routine testing of amphibian shipments.[10,52] Finally, *Mycobacterium* has been introduced into different locales through the movement of western clawed frogs and farmed east Asian bullfrogs (*Hoplobatrachus rugulosus*).[61,62] An additional important factor is that water used to house amphibians during shipments is commonly contaminated both with chytrid fungus and ranavirus. The transfer of this water to another country or region and its release into the sanitation system without appropriate disinfection serves as another method to transmit infectious diseases to native amphibians without ever releasing a nonindigenous species into the environment.[57]

Infectious Diseases

Infectious diseases are unlikely to cause an extinction of a species as a sole factor, especially if disease transmission is a density-dependent factor. If density dependent, as the population diminishes below a certain threshold, transmission of the disease drops off rapidly, preserving enough individuals to effectively reproduce.[63] Rather complex interactions between the pathogen, the host, and the environment often dictate the extent and the duration that an infectious disease can spread within a population.[63,64]

Chytridiomycosis and amphibian ranavirus have been implicated in numerous large-scale mortality events in amphibians.[63] However, *Bd* provides a salient example of a population-limiting disease that cannot be simplistically and consistently tied to all amphibian declines. For example, this fungal pathogen has caused numerous losses of amphibian populations in Australia, Central America, and possibly other countries in South America.[4] Conversely, *Bd* has had apparently minor effects on populations in Asia, Europe, and mainland Africa.[4] In addition, in countries with significant amphibian declines such as New Guinea and Madagascar, this pathogen has not been reported as a significant factor.[4] Pertaining to the relationship of host, pathogen, and the environment, exposure of amphibian tadpoles to sublethal levels of ultraviolet B (UV-B) radiation had no effect on leukocyte counts or on their response to an acute antigen challenge. However, the resulting metamorphs did have significant reductions in these aforementioned immune parameters, providing a possible explanation for how environmental changes in UV-B radiation levels could increase the susceptibility of amphibian populations to novel pathogens such as *Bd*.[65]

Ranavirus-induced mortality events in amphibians have been documented on five continents, in varying environmental conditions, and in most taxonomic families of amphibians.[63] The importance of ranavirus to significantly affect amphibian populations is disputed as no clear picture exists as to the distribution, level of virulence, and pathology of these viruses in varying amphibian species.[63,66] It is most likely that the virus functions synergistically with other factors to evoke large-scale mortality events. For example, habitat fragmentation can lead to genetic isolation in some amphibian populations, leading them more likely to suffer from ranavirus epizootics.[63]

CHALLENGES AND HORIZONS

Captive Breeding

Most veterinarians participating in herpetofauna conservation will be involved in translocation projects through the release of conceivably healthy animals to augment the present population (reinforcement) or to reclaim a habitat where the indigenous species has disappeared (reintroduction) (Fig. 181.4).[67] The translocated animals will be either wild-caught specimens that are simply being moved to another location or captive-bred progeny. Important caveats regarding the challenges of these programs should be evaluated, and efforts should be made to reduce any anticipated issues. Captive breeding is a contentious tool for the preservation of species.[68] First, resources, financial and temporal, are shifted from habitat preservation and threat mitigation to the propagation of a species in a captive setting. Many would argue that

these resources are more effective when used for in situ conservation efforts.[68] In situ operations that by definition occur within the range country/region of the species of interest are simpler because of the required climatic factors, light cycles, food items, and more.[66] The release of captive-bred or ranched herpetofauna through conservation translocations has been done for years to combat population declines in native habitats. To be a successful program, these released animals must contribute to the population of reproductively active adults in greater numbers than would naturally occur.[69] Head-start programs have been controversial for many years and will likely continue to be so until more objective evaluations are performed to validate their utility as a conservation tool.[70] The underlying areas of concern are the associated costs of the release programs, the questionable rate of successes, the possibility for disease transmission, and the lack of addressing the underlying problem within the declining population.[71]

Additionally, the progeny of captive-breeding programs suffer from numerous problems associated with a small founder population, such as inbreeding depression, rapid adaptation to captivity, and removal of natural selection.[72] Recent studies have attempted to assess the impacts of captive breeding on the fitness of the prospective progeny to be released. Based on models in fruit flies, adaptation to captivity can be relatively rapid under benign environmental conditions.[72] The predominant concerns in captive progeny are a lack of appropriate response to predators and difficulty in finding food sources. Tadpoles of the Mallorcan midwife toad (*Alytes muletensis*) bred in captivity for successive generations lose their adaptive genetic responses to predators (shallow tail fin depth and rapid growth rate) compared with wild-caught tadpoles.[73] Another study remarked that captive-bred *Rana pipiens* metamorphs exhibited abnormal movement behavior after release, which could affect their ability to locate food sources compared with native *Rana pipiens* in the same area.[74] In conclusion, animal populations can rapidly adapt to captivity within a few generations, and captive-breeding programs should recognize this problem during program design and throughout subsequent monitoring. Recommendations have been made to both preserve genetic diversity but prevent the adaptation to captivity through (1) maintaining a captive environment as close to natural conditions as possible; (2) decreasing the selection pressure from captive environments by reducing mortality rates and ensuring that each individual contributes to reproduction; (3) dividing the captive population into smaller subpopulations that are more fit and diverse than one large population of the same size; (4) increasing the generational interval through delayed matings and cryopreservation techniques as selection and adaptation happen on a generational level; and (5) introducing wild individuals, if possible, into the breeding program.[72]

Further attention also needs to be given to providing a captive situation that helps promote normal physical and mental development of the progeny. Animals are often raised in high-density settings that can lead to disease transmission, stress, and the need for intensive management practices, such as the routine disinfection of the premises, easy-to-clean cages, etc., to reduce disease transmission. This necessity for cleanliness leads to amphibian larvae often being restricted to an aquarium setting with uniform depth and sheer vertical walls. This environment further lacks microclimates, a natural light cycle, appropriate prey variety, and exposure to appropriate microbiota for intestinal flora.[75,76] In addition, prey items are offered, with more emphasis placed on cost and ease. Whether the diet items are truly appropriate for growth based on the ability to ingest and to digest the diet by the larvae or metamorphs is often a secondary concern. The production of healthy progeny capable of surviving after release from captivity to their native environment would likely be improved by deemphasizing a sterile, high-intensive management system with more emphasis given to lower population densities and a more appropriate habitat/diet.[75]

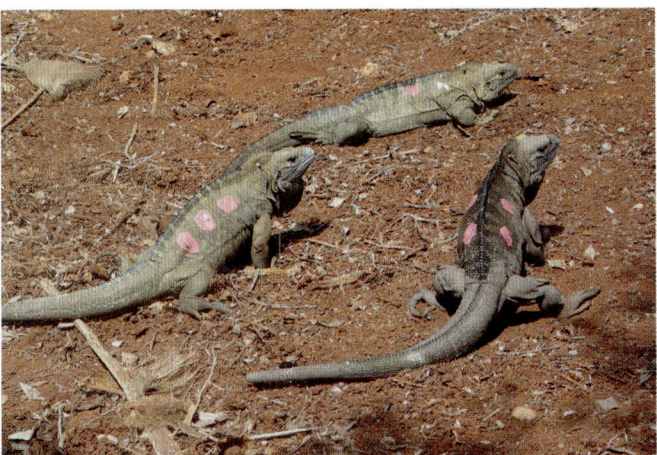

FIG 181.4 Three female Jamaican iguanas (*Cyclura collei*) being released to native habitat after captive rearing in a head-start facility within Jamaica. (Courtesy of Rick Hudson, Fort Worth Zoo.)

Metrics of Evaluation

Evaluating the success of any animal conservation program can be perplexing because of the limited resources available, the cryptic nature of some species making population evaluations difficult, the limited historic data on the population, and in many circumstances, the lack of robust criteria for assessing success of the project.[77,78] Explicitly defining the objectives and providing the data on the observed inputs and outputs can help in this process. Inputs are the resources used in the project, such as monies, equipment, and time. Outputs are the amounts of some specific activity delivered by a project (i.e., progeny released to the environment), which can then help to indicate whether a project has met its specific objectives (i.e., mandated release goal of 500 tadpoles every year).[79] However, assessing the impact or outcomes (the broader consequences of the project for the population and the environment, which are better indicators of long-term success or failure) is essential.[79] Independent evaluators can use a selection of different methods to appraise the actual effects of a project.[78,79]

Many projects simply consider the number of animals translocated as the primary output, but the more salient criteria is the survival of these animals and whether they contribute to the reproduction of the population.[77] Monitoring after release can be considered the most challenging, but likely the most critical, step in any program. However, it is rarely implemented and, if so, in a haphazard fashion.[77,80] Researchers in the Wyoming Toad (*Bufo baxteri*) Project have evaluated a promising methodology for assessing the survival of released metamorphs based on demographic data and a projection model, although the accuracy and reliability with any single year of data is challenging.[77] Monitoring over subsequent years gradually should increase the reliability of demographic estimates and related management inferences, such as the number of metamorphs to release in a year that will survive to become reproductive females.[77]

Genomics

Genomics is considered a discipline of genetics that concerns itself with the study of the genome of organisms through the use of DNA sequencing, bioinformatics, and recombinant DNA to grasp the actual sequences in the genes and their functions. In the past, genetic tools have been extremely useful for (1) estimating the population size of a species where direct estimate data of the population are lacking, (2) protecting genetic diversity in captive-breeding operations, (3) detecting levels of species hybridization, (4) analyzing the frequency and degree of genetic connectivity between adjacent populations, and, finally, (5) using these data to determine important genetic priorities and make informed management decisions.[42,81] Future directions of genomic research are to continue the complete sequencing of various species of reptiles and amphibians to form a bank of genomic data. This databank can then be used to improve retention of genetic diversity in captive-breeding groups through more detailed breeding recommendations and identifying genetic diversity in wild populations that warrant specific conservation efforts. In addition, discussion has been given to analyzing the genome of various animals within a species for factors of disease resistance, which could be useful for evaluating in translocated wild animals or their captive progeny before release into a wild habitat.[81] Of particular merit, by combining genomics with geographical data, conservation biologists can locate specific features in the environment that influence animal movement and genetic movement within a habitat. These features, such as small sections of forest between two habitats or a mature road in a wildlife habitat, can be assessed as having a positive or negative effect on genetic variability within populations. With this information, land managers can demonstrate more objectively the necessity to conserve or to possibly mitigate the damage of specific geographic features.[81]

Finally, genomics can offer a means to assess the success of conservation programs by verifying the genetic diversity after captive animal releases into a threatened population or even just monitoring the viability of a population after conservation of habitat.

Eradication of Invasive Species

Full elimination of any invasive species is difficult on large land masses for many reasons. Hidden environments in the ecosystem, cryptic behavior, high fecundity, lack of predators, incidental species morbidity and mortality with baiting, costs, politics, poor planning and execution, continued reintroductions such as with exotic pets, etc., all work to make invasive eradication close to impossible.[18] As described earlier with the cane toad, the migration of this species has only been slowed, but never halted in Australia.[19] Similar situations have emerged with other introduced species on other continents, despite widespread public and governmental support for eradication measures. In light of these difficulties, conservation biologists have advocated prevention as the primary objective, with an emphasis on information dissemination about the problem to the general public, stringent biosecurity measures, and quarantine procedures.[26,82] The next step in the process if prevention has failed is to have an early detection system with continual surveillance, interception, and immediate removal of a species from a novel ecosystem. Propagule pressure, defined as the frequency with which a species is introduced into a habitat combined with the animal number in each episode, is considered to be the main factor in whether a species becomes established.[82] Therefore decreasing both the introduction frequency and the number of animals introduced can have major benefits in the management of invasive species.[82] The brown tree snake (*Boiga irregularis*) and its possible movement from Guam, where it has extirpated 10 of 13 bird species on the island and bitten thousands of people over a decade, to Hawaii is a case study where prevention and early detection have helped retard the transfer of this aggressive snake.[83] The final step of management through eradication, containment, and control is more commonly studied and practiced because the species of concern has usually already invaded and caused a permanent change in the environment.[26,82] Methods used for eradication (described later) can also be used to simply control both the numbers and distribution of an invasive species if full-scale complete eradication is not feasible.[84] Finally, a detailed system of prevention and early detection that relies on a historic database of exotic animal introductions for a country would be useful for decreasing the frequency and severity of future invasive species incursions as denoted by the successes in New Zealand in dropping this incursion rate since the database's inception.[26,82]

The essential five factors considered critical to a successful eradication effort are (1) early detection of an invasion with abrupt removal efforts, (2) sufficient resources for completion and follow-up surveys, (3) an agency capable of enforcing cooperation, (4) understanding the natural history of the species to target vulnerabilities, and (5) motivated, persistent personnel.[85] The general grouping of eradication methods for invasive species are mechanical, chemical, and biologic.[84] Sponsored hunting, fencing, and trapping are the common examples of mechanical control in which animals are physically removed or excluded from an area.[30,86] Baiting with toxins such as rodenticides as done on islands or the spraying of coqui frogs with citric acid in Hawaii provide examples of chemical control methods.[22,30,86] Finally, many invasive pest species were introduced as predators to control either a native species or an already introduced nonnative species. Obviously, biologic control using predators is highly controversial and fraught with possible unforeseen consequences.[87] A good example of this complexity was the introduction of the mongoose to Jamaica, Puerto Rico, miscellaneous Caribbean islands, and Hawaii to control introduced rats on sugar cane plantations.[21] Sadly, the mongoose did not inhabit the same environmental niche as

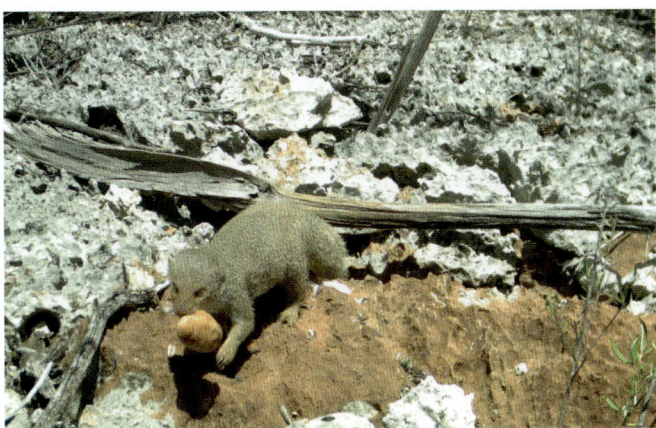

FIG 181.5 One of the primary mammalian invasive species, a small Asiatic mongoose (*Herpestes javanicus*), is removing an egg from an iguana nest. (Courtesy of Rick Hudson and Rick Van Veen, International Iguana Foundation.)

the rats and had questionable benefit on any reduction of the rodent population. However, the mongoose persisted in the ecosystem to plague native lizard species such as the Jamaican iguana (*Cyclura collei*), amphibians, and sea turtles, causing approximately 7 to 12 extinctions of herpetofauna species (Fig. 181.5).[21,25] The success of biologic control methods in some reviews of invasive species eradication only found limited success (<20% achieved complete control and only 41% achieved partial control).[87]

Due to the pressing need to save animal species in light of these precipitous changes, a translocation strategy called assisted colonization has been advocated.[71] In this management technique, species are transported from their native habitat to a region outside their normal physical range (i.e., movement of African reptiles to similar environments in North America) to foster their survival in the face of threats such as climate change. This translocation methodology could have numerous and unforeseen consequences on indigenous animals and their environment in spite of the proposed use of risk assessments to anticipate and mitigate possible impacts. In reality, assisted colonization is viewed by some biologists as another example where an introduced species could become invasive and threaten native populations with extinction.[71]

Enrichment

Enrichment can have three components: environmental, where an environment is provided that offers the animal the chance to pursue normal psychological and physical activity; social, where the opportunities exist for the interaction with other animals; and behavioral, where the animal can demonstrate specific behaviors or behavioral repertoires.[88] Success in captive breeding programs relies on having the necessary species-specific prerequisites for health, reproduction, and development of the progeny. This necessity has largely been recognized in mammals and birds with a gradual application to reptiles and amphibians.[88,89] Beyond simple reproduction, enrichment programs can be used to select for the progeny of amphibians and reptiles who might have the physical and mental attributes to better survive upon release into their native habitat. In addition, researchers question the value of releasing captive-bred progeny into an environment without some basic training in food and predator recognition. Training programs in reptiles have been suggested that could bridge this deficit, while providing both physical and mental stimulation to progeny before their eventual release. Prerelease desert survival training of captive desert tortoises (*Gopherus agassizii*) in California reportedly had significantly improved success with release

trials.[88] Furthermore, blue-tongue skinks (*Tiliqua scincoides intermedia*) were successfully trained with aversive methods to prevent lizards from ingesting toxic cane toads with significant improvements in survival compared with control animals.[90]

However, another study in the common water snake (*Nerodia sipedon sipedon*) found no benefit to prerelease enrichment compared with controls in any measure of postrelease behavior or performance.[70] More importantly, introducing older, larger snakes who had simply undergone a period of simulated winter dormancy resulted in a higher overall survival rate than release of smaller individuals in the previous years, which was similar to the findings in head-started garter snakes.[69,70] In addition, captive-reared snakes that were released into the wild still only grew at a third of the rate of their similarly aged wild conspecifics, pointing to some defect in the ability to hunt in the wild.[70] It is likely that enrichment programs targeting the acquisition of specific associations or skills (i.e., the distaste for cane toad flesh) will be useful if carefully conceived and developed versus merely the introduction of various objects or activities as enrichment that are not directly related to survival.

Prerelease training in amphibians appears to be an important factor for improving survival.[68] Tadpoles produced in a typical laboratory setting have a higher likelihood of predation, and metamorphs are more susceptible to moving in a haphazard direction from a lack of familiarity with normal light cycles and the Y-axis orientation in nature.[75] Using a wire-mesh enclosure placed into the release habitat that incorporates land, land/water interface, and water, tadpoles and metamorphs in this enclosure could remain protected from predators and experience normal light cycles and the Y-axis orientation.[75]

Governance

Although a paucity of independently assessed data was present, a recent study evaluating the outcome success of conservation strategies demonstrated that the allowed use of natural resources (i.e., harvest), the access to markets for those natural resources, and a greater community involvement in the conservation projects were all important factors for successful outcomes.[91] To make these strategies manifest on a regional or national level, conservation institutions such as wildlife and environmental health agencies are looking at internal transformation of their institutional structures.[92] The core guiding principle in the United States has always been the public trust doctrine, where wildlife is owned by the public who entrust wildlife preservation and management to the government at various levels.[92] Because ecologic, political, and economic problems develop in tandem, a set of governance principles are emerging that focus still on the public trust as the foundation with more emphasis on social and economic sciences to foster a greater public participation and personal investment in both habitat and animal conservation.[92,93] Specifically, whether a conservation institution is a zoo, a nongovernmental organization, or a governmental agency, consideration should be given to four key components to create an adaptive and effective entity, if possible: (1) broad-based funding, (2) trustee-based governance, (3) multidisciplinary science as the basis of recommendations from professional staff, and (4) participation of diverse stakeholders and partners.[92]

Relating to governance of habitat management, some biologists argue that conservation targets in the past have been overly precise and narrow in terms of objective goals and methods, leading to outright failure through unintended consequences.[94] Advocates of this view propose that wildlife managers embrace a variety of habitats for a species, even if less than ideal, expanding decision flexibility through less-rigid regulation, and support modifying plans to local circumstances, as needed. In the realm of international wildlife trade, recommendations have been made to create within the current CITES system a new illegal animal trade database to include estimates of illegal trade for all countries and animals, overall world supply of any specific animal product, the demand for these animal products within countries, and their market prices. This information could then be used constructively for more realistically evaluating the utility and efficacy of wildlife trade decisions made by CITES.[95] Finally, CITES trade bans have been implemented for dealing with nontrade threats such as climate change. However, these bans have led to decreased local community support for conservation programs, because the financial benefits to safeguarding the species diminished greatly after the trade restrictions were put into practice. Biologists suggest not using CITES trade bans for nontrade threats and to continue to foster community stakeholders in participatory management with some obvious benefit to community members.[96]

Education

Conservation education is primarily taught through intellectual exercises with varied amounts of visual aids and oral presentations, which appear to have a questionable efficacy and persistent impact on their target audience.[97] In addition, certain groups of animals, such as snakes, are not as highly charismatic as other "flagship" species and might also have been attributed negative stereotypes in various cultures.[97,98] One study found only a modest benefit in changing attitudes regarding snakes after a physical presentation of a snake in a classroom with young children.[98] The children were allowed a brief tactile experience and some didactic lesson material. However, a later study with children found that a field trip in an outdoor setting where the children hunted for and examined nonvenomous snakes had a more significant lasting impact in changing attitudes.[97] The authors point to the necessity for outdoor education with the resulting direct physical and emotional connections to build a better rapport and appreciation for wildlife in young children. These studies highlight the necessity to potentially change how the conservation message is conveyed. Significant strides in conservation might be best obtained by emphasizing less the direct scientific details and more the physical reality of herpetofauna in their native habitats through participatory experiences that might last a lifetime (Fig. 181.6).

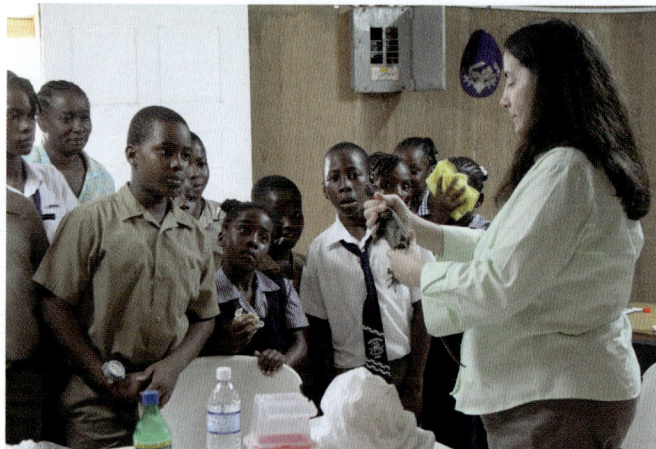

FIG 181.6 A visit by local school children to a reptile head-start program with an opportunity to converse with a veterinarian and participate in a basic health examination. (Courtesy of Rick Hudson, Fort Worth Zoo.)

CONCLUSION

With the physical and political challenges facing conservation issues, facile resignation and apathy can appear to be the logical reactions. However, as veterinarians, biologists, and interested private citizens, our actions, both personal and professional, can serve to affect significant positive changes in herpetofauna conservation. By persevering in the face of this adversity, we create models for our colleagues and future generations to hopefully emulate. Failing at this task is not simply a loss of biologic diversity on the planet but harkens to our own demise.

REFERENCES

See www.expertconsult.com for a complete list of references.

182

Herpetofauna and Ecosystem Health

Scott Connelly

Although often unnoticed in nature, reptiles and amphibians are broadly distributed and represent a great deal of global species-level diversity. Additionally, a disproportionally high level of vertebrate abundance is comprised of herpetofauna in some ecosystems; in humid tropical regions, for example, anurans are often the most abundant vertebrates, and densities of 20,000 frogs per hectare have been recorded at sites within Puerto Rico.[1] As such, reptiles and amphibians can contribute significantly to a wide range of ecological processes, such as energy flow and nutrient regulation, and can strongly influence ecosystem structure. As ectotherms, ingested material is efficiently converted to biomass (rather than mostly lost as heat, as is the case with endotherms) and subsequently may become available energy for upper trophic levels. This energy flux may be especially important with respect to amphibians, as most species have complex life histories that require both aquatic and terrestrial habitats and different food resources dependent on the developmental stage of the individual.

Reptiles and amphibians are similar in many ways regarding their susceptibility to environmental stress, and documenting the causes for, and the magnitude of, their global population declines has received a fair amount of effort during the past two decades.[2,3] This is especially true for amphibians, following the widespread and ongoing species losses due to chytridiomycosis in the late 1980s and other more recent emerging wildlife diseases, such as ranaviruses (Fig. 182.1). However, many reptile populations are imperilled as well, and it has been suggested that reptilian declines are similar in severity, taxonomic breadth, and geographical scale to those currently documented in amphibians.[4] Regional assessments throughout Europe and Africa indicate that between 10% to 20% of reptilian species are threatened with extinction.[5] Like many amphibian declines, losses of reptiles have been attributed to a range of drivers, including habitat degradation, invasive species, pollution, disease, climate change, UV-B radiation, chemical contaminants, commercial exploitation, as well as combinations of these factors.[4,6,7] However, far less focus has been placed on characterizing and quantifying the role that herpetofauna play in supporting overall ecosystem health and, in particular quantifying ecosystem-level responses resulting from their declining abundance and biodiversity.

"Ecosystem health" is a term that encompasses some suite of attributes that can be used to describe the overall condition of a system. These attributes may include the ability of the ecosystem to function within a range of limits and might take into account a measure of system resilience to change, its organization, and vigor. Recently there has been an increased understanding and acknowledgment of the importance of ecosystem services for human well-being. A characterization of ecosystem health may be useful in determining the sustainability of a system, which can be defined as the ability to meet current societal needs from ecosystem services, including provisioning, regulating, and supporting and cultural services, without sacrificing the ability of future

societies to meet their needs.[8,9] Therefore, it has been suggested that an accurate assessment of ecosystem health needs to include a measure of its sustainability; that is, the system's ability to maintain its structure and function through time in spite of external stressors, such as changes in population size. A number of recent studies have demonstrated that biologically diverse ecosystems tend to be more productive, and there has been growing evidence that species extinctions are changing basic processes important to both the productivity and sustainability of global ecosystems,[10] thereby either directly or indirectly influencing the well-being of humans. Unfortunately, we are only beginning to understand the ecosystem-level consequences of changing amphibian and reptile populations on aquatic, riparian, and terrestrial ecosystems,[11] and a complete understanding of the relationships between intact herpetofauna communities and benefits to human populations remains elusive.

INDIRECT ECOSYSTEM SERVICES

Studies investigating the ecological roles of reptiles and amphibians have indicated that their populations, or more specifically declines in their populations, can have measurable effects on ecosystem health, and that in some systems herpetofauna are considered keystone species due to their disproportionally large impact on ecosystem structure and

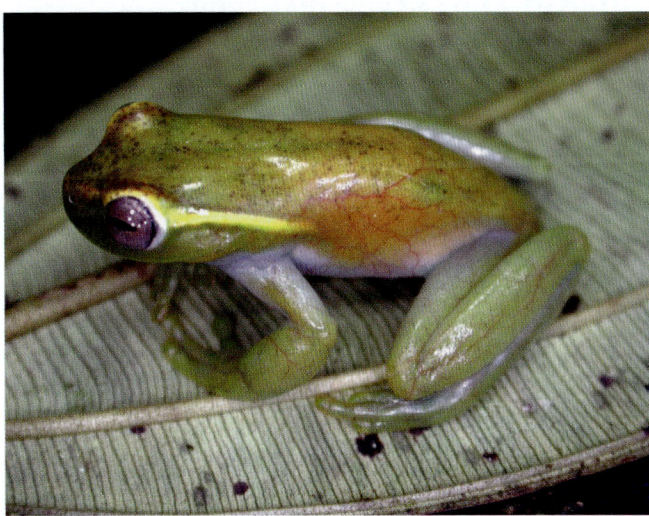

FIG 182.1 Critically endangered *Hyloscirtus colymba* tree frog from Central America, with clear chytridiomycosis symptoms. (Courtesy of Scott Connelly.)

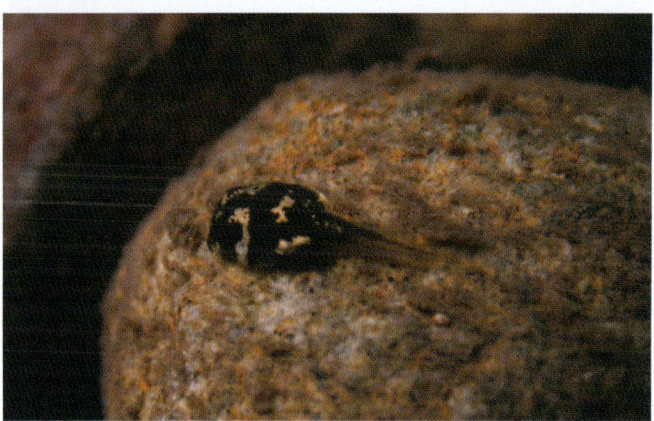

FIG 182.2 Tadpole of *Atelopus zetecki* on a stream bottom, feeding on benthic periphyton and biofilm. (Courtesy of Scott Connelly.)

function. These organisms have been shown to influence a wide range of ecosystem function and processes, such as primary production, decomposition, nutrient cycling, pollination, seed dispersal, and the control of pathogens and pests.

In tropical systems amphibians are often abundant, both as terrestrial adults and as tadpoles, which have been recorded at densities of 1200 tadpoles/m^2. Because frog larvae may play a variety of functional feeding roles, such as carnivore, herbivore, detritivore, filter-feeder, and suspension-feeders,[12] their declining populations should be expected to influence a number of ecological processes. Grazing tadpoles have been found to dramatically decrease primary producer community biomass, both in pond[13] and stream ecosystems,[11] with levels of periphyton biomass often directly related to tadpole densities (Fig. 182.2). Tadpole feeding can also change algal community composition, with studies in tropical streams indicating that tadpole grazing can increase algal species-level biodiversity, and furthermore shift algal assemblages from communities dominated by large upright diatom species to communities characterized by small adnate diatoms when grazed.[14] Additionally, tadpoles have been shown to stimulate algal growth: although algal-grazing tadpoles can significantly reduce algal standing biomass, the algal community that remains after grazing can be more productive, on a per-biomass basis, than algal communities not subjected to grazing.[14]

NUTRIENT AND ENERGY TRANSPORT AND DECOMPOSITION

The potentially important role that amphibians play in the movement of biomass and nutrients through ecosystems has been long recognized, although only a handful of studies have provided reliable estimates of abundance and density of amphibians needed to reveal their true ecological importance. A classic study by Burton and Likens estimated that salamanders within a temperate experimental forest were accountable for ~20% of the energy flow through all bird and mammal populations at the site.[15] More recently, work by Semlitsch et al. found that some previous studies underestimated densities of salamander communities by as much as an order of magnitude, and therefore failed to appreciate the full impact of the roles of salamanders with respect to nutrient and energy flux, and their functional role in regulating invertebrate prey, through ingestion and carbon retention in forests.[16]

Likewise, tadpoles have been shown to influence organic matter dynamics in freshwater systems. The physical disturbance to the aquatic environment, or bioturbation, resulting from larval amphibian feeding activity not only reduces the accumulation of benthic sediments by direct consumption but can also result in the resuspension and transport

of organic matter into the water column. Organic matter transport resulting from aquatic amphibian feeding, in combination with the production and transport of tadpole feces, can be an important source of energy and nutrients (e.g., nitrogen) for downstream communities of aquatic consumers.[11] Additionally, because many anuran species have aquatic larvae that metamorphose to terrestrial adults, they can act as a flux of nutrients from aquatic systems to terrestrial systems. Seale, for example, found that through the ingestion of blue-green algae, and the assimilation of the nitrogen contained within, amphibians moved significant quantities of nitrogen from the aquatic to the terrestrial environment via metamorphosis.[17]

Due in part to their relatively large size, sea turtles may play an important role in the transport of nutrients and energy from marine to terrestrial ecosystems. In a study of nesting loggerhead sea turtles (*Caretta caretta*), it was found that 34% of the energy contained in deposited eggs was transferred to terrestrial dune vegetation, detritivores, and decomposers, and 28% of the energy deposited through oviposition was ingested by predators.[18] Similar trends were documented with respect to the fate of the nitrogen and phosphorus content of the eggs, indicating that where present, these organisms can play a significant role in ecosystem dynamics.[18]

FOOD CHAINS, INVERTEBRATE RESPONSE, AND FUNCTIONAL REDUNDANCY

Herpetological populations have been shown to impact invertebrate communities, both directly and indirectly. Salamanders studied in forested systems, for example, have been found to reduce beetle and fly larvae, adult beetles, ants, and springtails, and increase communities of mites, millipedes, and spiders, presumably indirectly by reducing the competitors and predators of these invertebrates.[19] Insectivorous adult frogs can directly influence prey communities and indirectly alter ecosystem-level processes in terrestrial habitats and have been shown to reduce numbers of aerial insects and rates of plant herbivory.[20] In tropical streams that have experienced catastrophic losses of amphibians due to the pathogenic *Batrachochytrium dendrobatidis* fungus, the dominant larval frog functional group lost was the algal grazers; therefore, subsequent ecosystem responses to their declines might be expected to be most apparent among other invertebrate consumers that also rely on the periphyton food resource. This response was found, as grazing macroinvertebrate communities shifted from generally smaller-bodied to larger-bodied insects.[21] However, even after a number of years of post tadpole declines, no other grazing taxa fully compensated for the role that tadpoles played in the system, suggesting a lack of functional redundancy. Additionally, aquatic macroinvertebrate functional structure differed in unexpected ways, as aquatic insect shredder production significantly decreased after tadpole losses, indicating that less obvious trophic interactions may exist between tadpoles and other taxonomic groups.[21]

Reptilian predators may have significant effects on invertebrate communities as well. Through a manipulative study examining *Anolis* spp. lizards, it was found that the presence of the lizards not only reduced the total number of spider prey and overall prey species richness, but the declines in prey numbers was in large part driven by the resulting loss of rare spider species. Additionally, it was found that the lizards may induce sublethal effects on their prey, as the mean body lengths of a rare spider were larger where the lizard predators were removed.[22]

Because a number of terrestrial turtles and lizards forage on plant foliage, flowers, and fruits, they may exert influence on the biomass and composition of plant communities not only through the direct consumption of biomass but also through the role they may play as pollinators and seed dispersers. In a study examining vegetative consumption by spiny-tailed iguanas (*Ctenosaura hemilopha*), germination trials from ingested and passed seeds indicate that although the lizards may function as seed dispersers of some plant species, especially Cactaceae, the iguanas are poor dispersers for other tree species because they destroy the seeds by ingesting the fruit.[23] However, our understanding of the strength of the herpetofauna on seed dispersal may be underestimated, as the consumption of flowers and fruits by turtles and lizards may influence the terrestrial community composition in other indirect ways and may potentially have measurable economic significance.[24,25]

HUMAN HEALTH, DISEASE, AND MOSQUITOS

Adult mosquitos are a key vector for a suite of wildlife and human diseases,[26] including Zika, malaria, West Nile virus, yellow fever, and others. The World Health Organization estimated yearly costs associated with malaria at nearly $12 billion, which slowed economic growth by 1.3% annually.[27] Indirectly or directly, tadpoles and salamander larvae have been found to affect populations of aquatic grazers or filter feeders, such as dipteran larvae.[28,29] Many *Anopheles* and *Culex* mosquito larvae are filter-feeders, which ingest primarily phytoplankton suspended on the water surface, whereas many larval *Aedes* and *Culiseta* mosquitos feed primarily on periphyton.[30,31] Therefore, feeding by both frog larvae and controphic mosquito larvae can alter algal communities and reduce algal biomass. Competition for limited food resources has the potential for tadpoles to directly lower the growth rates, developmental times, and survivorship of the dipterans. Studies from Papua New Guinea and Australia have suggested that competition with cane toad tadpoles has resulted in smaller female mosquito size and fitness, thereby decreasing the likelihood of mosquito-transmitted disease to humans.[32] Although some tadpole species may increase the ability of aquatic fly larvae to acquire energy by removing sediments from periphyton and thereby exposing additional food resources,[33] most frog/mosquito interactions are generally competitive, and the reduction or removal of larval amphibians will benefit the aquatic mosquito larvae.[34,35] Although adult mosquitos are not likely an important dietetic component of any adult amphibian species, some tadpole species feed on mosquito eggs,[36] and the presence or absence of amphibian larvae has been shown to influence where mosquitos chose to oviposit.[37,38] Direct ingestion of mosquito larvae by the larvae of spadefoot toads[39] and the frog *Hoplobatrachus occipitalis* has been documented, and a significant component of the stomach contents of aquatic tiger salamander (*Ambystoma tigrinum*) larvae have been found to be the larvae and pupae of mosquitos.[40]

WATER QUALITY

A number of studies have characterized how amphibians are impacted by various chemicals, anthropogenically applied nutrients, and other pollutants in the watershed, leading to amphibians often being referred to as "canaries in the coalmine." However, far less research has focused on the influence that amphibians exert on water quality. Many frog larvae are filter-feeders, and as such filter volumes of water equal to their body mass every several minutes; at high tadpole densities their entire aquatic environment can be turned over quickly.[41] Tadpoles have been found to remove bacteria from water bodies and may decrease eutrophication of aquatic systems by ingesting nitrogen-fixing algae.[17]

FOOD AND MATERIALS FROM HERPETOFAUNA

Of the variety of services that intact ecosystems provide to humans, food production is one of the most essential, and the harvesting of

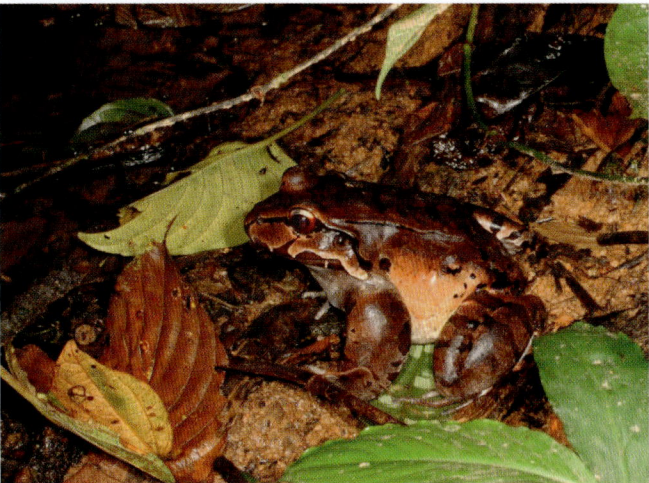

FIG 182.3 An adult tropical *Leptodactylus pentadactylus* (smokey jungle frog), a species commonly harvested for their meat. (Courtesy of Scott Connelly.)

wildlife is an important source of protein in many cultures. In rural areas of Mexico, for example, bushmeat has been estimated to comprise approximately 70% of the protein consumed by humans, with turtles, crocodiles, iguanas, and snakes among the animals hunted.[42] Likewise, in Honduras indigenous people consume several frog, turtle, and lizard species to fulfill basic food needs (Fig. 182.3).[43] Although the widespread harvesting of sea turtles for meat, eggs, and shells has greatly decreased due to overexploitation and resulting species protection efforts, egg harvesting, following stringent conservation guidelines, continues to provide income and protein for some Central American communities.[44] The harvesting of herpetofauna continues to provide food security and significant sources of protein for many local communities throughout much of Latin America, including Argentina, Brazil, Colombia, Peru, Venezuela, and other countries. Apart from the value that herpetofauna provide as a direct food source for humans, their role as consumers of agricultural pests is becoming recognized. Peltzer et al., for example, found that the diets of three frog species found in agricultural soybean fields consisted primarily of herbivore pests of the plants and suggested that the frogs act as important biological control agents in the soybean fields.[45]

In addition to the human value provided as a food source, amphibians and reptiles also provide economic benefits in other consumptive ways. Prestridge et al. reported that the pet trade, for example, was a driver for the importation of 1.48 billion live amphibian and reptiles, including poison dart frogs, boa constrictors, and king snakes, among other species, into Texas alone.[46] Retail prices for these individuals ranged from $30 to over $20,000. Frogs in the genera of *Agalychnis* and *Dendrobates*, and reptiles (*Boa constrictor*, *Basiliscus* spp., and *Sceloporus malachitus*, for example) generated over $1.5 million in revenue for Nicaragua (Figs. 182.4 and 182.5).[47] Products obtained from reptiles, such as hides, have been a significant export for a number of countries; the export of caiman and crocodile hides from the Neotropics to North American and European buyers has been substantial and totaled 300,000 hides from Bolivia and over 11 million from Colombia for the 30-year span between 1950 and 1980.[48] The export of herpetofauna products from countries with especially high levels of biodiversity can create significant revenue. Colombia, for example, generated over $50 million in income between 1929 and 1969 from wildlife exports, with approximately 37% resulting from reptiles.

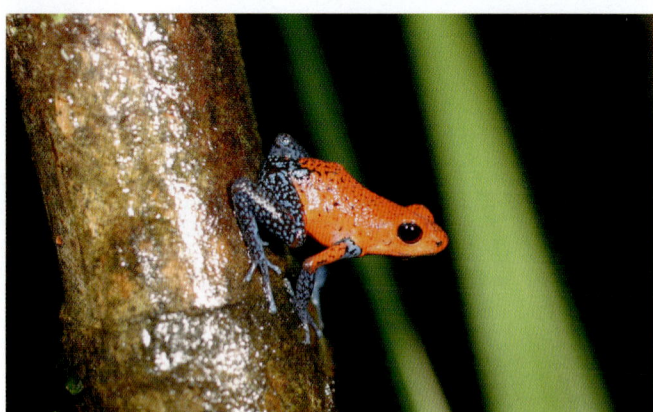

FIG 182.4 Often wild-caught and exported from Central America for the pet trade, an adult *Oophaga pumilio* poison dart frog. (Courtesy of Scott Connelly.)

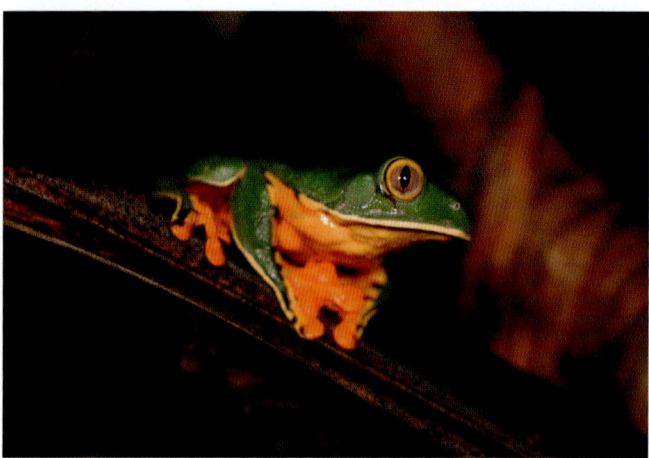

FIG 182.5 Recently offered through the pet trade for several hundred US dollars, an adult *Cruziohyla calcarifer*. (Courtesy of Scott Connelly.)

MEDICINAL, ETHNOBOTANY, AND CULTURAL USES

Amphibians use skin secretions and compounds for a number of biological purposes, including territorial marking, predator defense, and combating microbial infections. Although relatively few chemical properties of amphibians and reptiles have been systematically tested for their potential medicinal properties, humans have recognized for hundreds of years that herpetofauna produce a suite of potentially useful compounds. Amphibians have been used in traditional medicines globally to treat a number of conditions, from warts to heart disease.[49] In the neotropics, more than 60 species of amphibians and reptiles are used in traditional medicine. For example, *Leptodactylus* spp. are sold to treat ailments such as asthma, skin ailments, and tumors.[50] Building on this knowledge, a number of studies have investigated the potential that herpetofauna, particularly anurans, caudates, and snakes, have to contribute to medicine and to the development of novel pharmaceuticals. For example, antimicrobial peptides from frog skin secretions have shown the potential to inhibit infection and transfer of the HIV.[51] A toxin, epibatidine, isolated from the South American poison dart frog *Epipedobates tricolor*, has been shown to be an effective painkiller in rodents,[52] and there has been optimism that synthetic variants of this chemical without side effects can be developed as an alternative to medicinal opiates, such as opioid addiction. In Western culture, ~50% of all manufactured pharmaceutical drugs have been derived from natural sources.[53]

INVASIVES AND ECOSYSTEM STRUCTURE AND FUNCTION

Invasive species are widely recognized as a primary threat to global biodiversity. Although the impact that introduced herpetofauna has on ecosystem structure and function has received relatively little attention, several well-documented case studies indicate that where biological invasions of herpetofauna are successful, dramatic and widespread ecosystem change may follow. For example, the inadvertent introduction of the brown tree snake (*Boiga irregularis*) to Guam has had far-reaching biological consequences, including the extirpations or extinctions of a number of native lizard and bird species.[54] Similarly, declines ranging from 88% to 100% of raccoon, opossum, bobcat, rabbit, fox, and other mammalian species in the Florida Everglades have been attributed to the spread of the invasive Burmese python (*Python bivittatus*).[55] Introductions of amphibians have also driven widespread ecosystem change, with the global spatial expansion of bullfrogs (*Lithobates catesbeianus*) responsible for declines in native species through competition, predation, and habitat displacement.[56] Bullfrogs have also been found to be carriers of pathogens such as the chytrid fungus, and, through their anthropogenic range expansions, have the potential to spread disease, further contributing to species declines.[57] Although the coqui frog (*Eleutherodactylus coqui*), which was introduced to the Hawaiian Islands in the 1980s, has not been found necessarily to compete with native birds for resources, the frogs were associated with ~35% higher abundance of nonnative birds, suggesting that the frogs serve as a food resource for generalist birds that may prey on small vertebrates such as frogs.[58] Due in part to the high densities they may achieve, herpetofauna such as the coqui frog have the potential to alter the concentrations and flow of nutrients; increase overall nutrient availability through their feces, urine, and carcasses; and ultimately stimulate new plant growth.[59]

CONCLUSION

There remains a need to better quantify the ecosystem-level roles of herpetofauna, particularly in light of widespread and ongoing population declines resulting from habitat alteration and loss, overexploitation, disease, and the suite of other stressors that amphibians and reptiles are currently facing.[3,4] How these organisms affect ecosystem structure, function, and overall health is in many ways poorly understood. Quantitative information on basic life history traits (such as growth rates, life spans, and reproductive cycles) and ecosystem roles (such as the part they play in food web dynamics, energy flow, and nutrient cycling) on many taxa is still needed. However, of the studies done, it is apparent that intact amphibian and reptile populations play essential ecological roles in many ecosystems and therefore possess great potential to both directly and indirectly affect human well-being.

REFERENCES

See www.expertconsult.com for a complete list of references.

183

Laws and Regulations—International

Margaret E. Cooper

Reptiles are not the most popular of species. Since time immemorial, reptiles have had bad press in myths and literature. Human beings are often afraid of snakes due to their defense mechanisms of bites, poison, and constriction. People who encounter a snake rarely stop to distinguish between a dangerous or a harmless species and often destroy them before identification. The Crocodilia are also readily recognized as dangerous, and there are countless records of the toll they have taken on people who live and work in their proximity. In parts of Africa contact with chameleons is believed to confer infertility. Only tortoises, turtles, terrapins, and some lizards are widely perceived as being of little or no threat to humans.

Reptile populations that live in the wild are at risk of depletion through habitat decline, persecution, climate change, trade (legitimate and illegal), marine pollution in the case of sea-dwelling species, and inadequate conservation measures, including law enforcement.

The law relating to reptiles has been divided into three parts for this book:
Chapter 183: Laws and Regulations—International
Chapter 184: Laws and Regulations—European
Chapter 185: Laws and Regulations—Americas
In practice, the different levels of law—international, regional, and national—are all interrelated (see Table 184.1). Legislation affects both free-living (free-ranging) and captive reptiles.

This chapter considers the international law affecting reptiles (Box 183.1) and lists the national laws on wildlife and animal welfare of some of the countries not included in the other two chapters (Table 183.1).

ASPECTS OF LEGISLATION AFFECTING REPTILES

For the most part, the international legislation affecting reptiles relates to their conservation. In this field there are a number of international and regional treaties that relate to reptiles or from which reptiles benefit in general terms (see Box 183.1).

The Reptilia are a significant part of the world's biodiversity and worthy of protection. This can be addressed through habitat and species conservation measures and the control of trade. Education has an important role to play in promoting conservation and sustainable use together with changing negative attitudes toward some species. It is essential that these measures are backed by legislation and that the international treaties that address these issues are supported. The law may not always be considered the most successful conservation tool, particularly in locations where there is poor regulatory infrastructure. However, conservationists are beginning to advocate support of better

investigative and judicial powers (coupled with training in skills and the understanding of the importance of species protection) and asking for better legislation and effective enforcement of the law.[1]

Many reptiles are traded for their skins and other parts, and live specimens are supplied to collections, both private and public. They are also in demand for entertainment and display, or they are kept purely out of interest and enthusiasm. Some of this trade is supplied from substantial ranching or captive-breeding enterprises; others are bred on a smaller scale, both commercially or by hobbyists. When endangered species of reptiles are traded across national boundaries permits are likely to be required (as discussed later).

When reptiles are kept in captivity they are dependent on their keepers for their essential needs and general welfare. A keeper should have sufficient knowledge and skills to ensure their well-being and compliance with animal welfare legislation. Such legislation is usually the responsibility of individual countries (see Chapters 184 and 185). The keeping of reptiles in captivity is often regulated at a national or local authority level, and the keeper, be it a private collection, zoological display, or other use, may require a license (see Chapters 184 and 185).

BOX 183.1   International Wildlife Conservation Conventions

Convention on Wetlands of International Importance, Especially as Waterfowl Habitat 1971 (Ramsar Convention)
http://www.ramsar.org/
Convention concerning the Protection of the World Cultural and Natural Heritage 1972 (World Heritage Convention)
http://whc.unesco.org/
Convention on Trade in Endangered Species of Wild Fauna and Flora 1973 (Washington Convention) (CITES)
https://www.cites.org
Convention on the Conservation of Migratory Species of Wild Animals 1979 (Bonn Convention) (CMS)
http://www.cms.int/index.php
Convention on Biological Diversity 1992 (Biodiversity Convention) (CBD)
https://www.cbd.int/

For more details, see Bowman M, Davies P, Redgwel C: *Lyster's international wildlife law*, Cambridge, Cambridge University Press, 2010.

TABLE 183.1 **A Selection of National Wildlife and Welfare Legislation Relevant to Reptiles**

Country	Wildlife	Welfare	Internet Link and References
Legislation			
Albania	Law No. 10253 on Hunting 2010 (as amended)	No specific welfare law Biçoku Y. *Animal Welfare in Albania,* 2013	https://www.ecolex.org/details/legislation/law-no-10253-on-hunting-lex-faoc132101/? http://www.academia.edu/28345042/Animal_Welfare_in_Albania
Australia federal laws	Environment Protection and Biodiversity Conservation Act 1999 (CITES)		
Australia states' legislation (e.g., Western Australia)	Conservation and Land Management Act 1984	Animal Welfare Act 2002 Link

Portal to States' and Territories' legislation | Sankoff P, White S, Black C, eds. *Animal Law in Australasia. Continuing the Dialogue.* Annandale, Australia: The Federation Press; 2013 https://www.agric.wa.gov.au/animalwelfare/other-states-and-territories-animal-welfare-legislation |
China	Law of the People's Republic of China on the Protection of Wildlife 1989 revised 2016		https://eia-international.org/wp-content/uploads/WPL-Final-Law_translation_July-5-2016.pdf
Hong Kong	Wild Animals Protection Ordinance Cap 170; Protection of Endangered Species of Animals and Plants Ordinance, Cap 586	The Prevention of Cruelty to Animals Ordinance Cap 169	https://www.spca.org.hk/en/animal-welfare/welfare-law-development/animal-laws-hong-kong https://www.elegislation.gov.hk/
India	The Wildlife (Protection) Act, 1972, and other laws	Prevention of Cruelty to Animals Act 1960	http://www.envfor.nic.in/legis/wildlife/wildlife1.html https://www.india.gov.in/wildlife-protection-act-1972-3-act-1960
Japan	Law for the Protection of Cultural Properties; Law for the Conservation of Endangered Species of Wild Fauna and Flora 1992	Act on Welfare and Management of Animals (Act No. 105 of October 1, 1973)	http://www.env.go.jp/en/nature/biodiv/law.html https://www.env.go.jp/en/laws/nature/act_wm_animals.pdf
Kenya	Wildlife Conservation and Management Act 2013	Prevention of Cruelty to Animals Act	http://www.kenyalaw.org/lex//actview.xql?actid=No. 47 of 2013 http://www.kenyalaw.org/lex//actview.xql?actid=CAP. 360
Laos	Wild Animals, Fisheries, Hunting and Fishing, Decree on (COM Decree No. 118/CCM, 1989)		http://www.endangeredearth.com/wp-content/uploads/es_laws/Laos_-_Wild_Animals__Fisheries__Hunting_and_Fishing__Decree_on_COM_Decree_No._118_CCM__1989.pdf
Malaysia	Wildlife Conservation Act 2010	Animal Welfare Act 2015	http://www.gunungganang.com.my/pdf/Malaysian-Legislation/National/Wildlife%20Conservation%20Act%202010.pdf https://aaalac.org/resources/Malaysia.pdf
New Zealand	Wildlife Act 1953; Trade in Endangered Species Act 1989; Trade in Endangered Species Regulations 1991	Animal Welfare Act 1999, as amended 2015	Wells N. *Animal Law in New Zealand.* Wellington, New Zealand: Bookers Ltd; 2011. http://www.legislation.govt.nz/act/public/1953/0031/latest/DLM276814.html?search=qs_act%40bill%40regulation%40deemedreg_wildlife+act_resel_25_h&p=1 http://www.legislation.govt.nz/act/public/1999/0142/latest/DLM49664.html http://www.loc.gov/law/foreign-news/article/new-zealand-animal-welfare-legislation-recognizes-animals-as-sentient-bans-cosmetic-testing/
Nigeria federal (state governments also regulate wildlife)	Endangered Species (Control of International Trade and Traffic) Act; Protection of Endangered Species in International Trade) Regulations 2011	Criminal Code 1990, Section 495	http://lawnigeria.com/Laws.php

TABLE 183.1   A Selection of National Wildlife and Welfare Legislation Relevant to Reptiles—cont'd

Country	Wildlife	Welfare	Internet Link and References
Philippines	Republic Act No. 9147, July 30, 2001; an Act providing for the Conservation and Protection of Wildlife Resources and their Habitats		http://www.chanrobles.com/republicacts/republicactno9147.html#.V5fSpY-cGUk
	DENR Administrative Order No. 48, September 13, 1991, Establishment of a National List of Species of Philippine Wild Birds, Mammals, and Reptiles (1991)		http://www.endangeredearth.com/wp-content/uploads/es_laws/Philippines_-_DENR_ADMINISTRATIVE_ORDER_No._48__Pursuant_to_the_provisions_of_Act._No._2590.pdf
	DENR Administrative Order No. 36, of 1991, Guidelines governing the Confiscation, Seizure, and Disposition of Wild Flora and Fauna illegally collected, gathered, acquired, transported, and imported including paraphernalia (1991)		http://sedac.ciesin.columbia.edu/entri/texts/denr.guidelines.florafauna.html
Uganda	Uganda Wildlife Act, Cap 200 of 2000	Animals (Prevention of Cruelty) Act (Cap. 220):	
United Kingdom	Wildlife and Countryside Act 1981 (see Table 80.1)	Animal Welfare Act 2006 and comparable laws for Scotland and Northern Ireland.	http://jncc.defra.gov.uk/page-1376
			https://www.gov.uk/guidance/animal-welfare-legislation-protecting-pets
		Robertson I. *Animals, Welfare and the Law.* Abingdon, UK: Routledge; 2015.	http://www.legislation.gov.uk/ukpga/2006/45/contents
			Cooper ME. Law affecting British wildlife casualties. In: Mullineaux E, Keeble M,eds. *Manual of Wildlife Casualties,* 2nd ed. Cheltenham, UK: British Small Animal Veterinary Association; 2016. Cheltenham

Databases

Country	Wildlife	Welfare	Internet Link and References
European Union N-Lex Portal for national laws of Member States	Including wildlife laws	Including animal welfare laws	http://eur-lex.europa.eu/n-lex/index_en.htm
FAOLEX	Many references to reptile protection in the wild	Numerous animal welfare laws	http://faolex.fao.org/faolex/index.htm
Global Animal Law Project		GAL Matrix: Database of national animal welfare laws	https://www.globalanimallaw.org/index.html
Animal Protection Index	World Animal Protection (formerly World Society for the Protection of Animals)	Assesses quality of animal welfare legislation in individual countries	https://www.worldanimalprotection.org.uk/news/animal-protection-index-api-animal-welfare
Various countries, especially where legislation is not readily available	Individual countries are required from time to time to submit "Country Reports" to the United Nations or to the secretariat of treaties such as CITES or CMS. May contain accounts of current legislation		
Wildlife International website	Lists wildlife laws of 32 countries and the EU		http://www.wildlifeinternational.org/EN/public/agencies/lawdetail.html
			https://theiwrc.org/?s=legislation
Angola, Botswana, Namibia, Zambia, Zimbabwe	Legislation and Policies relating to Protected Areas, Wildlife Conservation, and Community Rights to Natural Resources in partner countries of the Kavango Zambezi Transfrontier Conservation Area		Jones BT. *Legislation and Policies Relating to Protected Areas, Wildlife Conservation, and Community Rights to Natural Resources in Countries Being Partner in the Kavango Zambezi Transfrontier Conservation Area.* Windhoek; 2008
			http://www.tbpa.net/docs/KAZAPolicy%20Review_Dec08.pdf
World Resources Institute	Main wildlife law listed for 49 African countries		http://www.wri.org/resources/maps/rights-to-resources/laws-reviewed
Georgetown Law Library. International and Foreign Animal Law Research Guide		Selection of non-USA national animal welfare laws	http://guides.ll.georgetown.edu/c.php?g=363480&p=2455777

For countries in the Americas, see Chapter 185, Table 185.1.

There is some legislation at the regional level in the European Union (EU) and Council of Europe (COE); this is discussed in Chapter 184.

SOURCES OF INFORMATION ON INTERNATIONAL LEGISLATION

Copies of most international and regional legislation is available on the Internet, and many key treaties also have a website providing the relevant documentation (i.e., the treaty and other legislation and decisions made by the parties subsequent to the treaty, together with detailed information on the implementation of the treaty).

Conservation bodies, such as the International Union for Conservation of Nature (IUCN; https://www.iucn.org/) and the United Nations Environment Programme/UN Environment (UNEP; https://www.unenvironment.org/) have relevant publications, species status reports, guidelines, and other publications.

The IUCN (https://www.iucn.org/) provides ECOLEX, an environmental law resource and library, and the Red List, a definitive authority on the conservation status of animals and plants. The IUCN Species Survival Commission has 10 specialist groups that have experts and resources, in some cases including veterinary expertise relating to particular species, for example, the crocodile, marine turtle, and viper specialist groups (see https://www.iucn.org/ssc-groups-amphibians-reptiles).

TRAFFIC Bulletin (http://www.traffic.org/bulletin/) carries investigations into the trade in endangered species and reports on law enforcement regarding prosecutions of illegal trading. An IUCN publication on wildlife prosecutions reports that among 285 animals of various species, 10 were reptiles (see https://portals.iucn.org/library/sites/library/files/documents/2016-044.pdf).

Special interest NGOs are often very well informed regarding the legislation related to their field of interest and may have useful websites or contacts.

INTERNATIONAL CONSERVATION LEGISLATION

At the international level most of the law regarding reptiles relates to the conservation of species and habitat and comprises international treaties (also called conventions) that are made between countries at diplomatic level and subsequently ratified by national governments. The latter are obliged to put binding agreements such as treaties into effect in their national legislation—thus providing for implementation and enforcement.

The primary conservation treaties are listed in Box 183.1. The two species-orientated conventions, CITES and CMS, are intended to protect listed species, including reptiles, whereas the Ramsar (Wetland Convention) and World Heritage Conventions are aimed at protecting habitat and other significant sites through the designation of protected areas. Although such sites are rarely designated specifically for the benefit of reptiles, species found in such areas will benefit from the protective status accorded to Ramsar and World Heritage sites.

Convention on Biological Diversity

The CBD deals with the conservation and sustainable use of biodiversity in its broadest sense, together with the fair equitable sharing of benefits arising from genetic resources. The latter is supplemented by the Nagoya Protocol on Access and Benefit Sharing (ABS) of 2010, which requires the governments that are party to it to provide a fair and transparent framework for recording and sharing any benefits obtained from genetic resources (by research or commercial development) and ensuring that any benefits are equitably shared with the country from which the genetic resource originated. Any benefit sharing must be on mutually agreed terms. Where new material is collected in a country that is party

to the Protocol, a benefit-sharing agreement should be drawn up. Many resource-rich countries already have existing terms and condition for *in situ* or in-country collection or research. Scientific research institutions, museums, and commercial bodies with existing collections and materials are setting up procedures for assessing and reporting work that produces, or may produce in the future, a benefit to another country. Veterinarians and scientists carrying out research or development with genetic resources, for example, snake venom, should be aware of the new responsibilities if they are working with any of the approximately 100 countries that have joined the Protocol. The European Union and UK already have legislation in place (https://www.gov.uk/guidance/abs).

Convention on International Trade in Endangered Species of Wild Fauna and Flora

CITES is also discussed in Chapters 184 and 185. There are 183 parties to this treaty (as of November 2017); the most recent to join are the EU (2015; the 28 EU states formerly operated as individual parties) and Tajikistan and Tonga (2016). The main purpose of the Treaty it to control the trade in the endangered species listed in Appendices I, II, and III of the Convention. A permit is required to authorize the "trade" of CITES species between countries. The term "trade" in effect means the *movement* for any purpose across national borders. Thus, if a species is listed on an Appendix, a permit is still required even if the purpose is scientific or veterinary rather than commercial. In the case of species listed in Appendix I (as being considered at risk of extinction), permits are not normally given for commercial purposes, whereas a permit may be available for other purposes. A summary of the key provisions is provided in this section.

There are 87 species and 8 subspecies of reptiles in Appendix I, 1278 species and 4 subspecies in Appendix II, and 61 species in Appendix III. As at October 4, 2017, the reptiles listed include alligators; crocodiles and caimans; lizards; geckos; skinks; monitor lizards; many snakes including boas, pythons, and vipers; all sea turtles; and many turtles, terrapins, and tortoises (Table 183.2). Before applying for a CITES permit the current status (the Appendices are updated biannually) of a particular reptile should be ascertained on the CITES website: https://www.cites.org/eng/app/appendices.php. A downloadable list at: https://cites.org/sites/default/files/eng/app/2017/E-Appendices-2017-10-04.pdf.

It is also necessary to check the CITES permit required for a species in the specific countries of import and export, as the status may have been upgraded in the national legislation. This is particularly important with the European Union and UK CITES regulations in which many species have been upgraded.

The essential provisions of the CITES Convention:

- Certain species of reptiles are listed in Appendix I (because they are threatened with extinction), Appendix II (because they may become extinct if trade is not controlled), and Appendix III (when a country asks for cooperation in preventing illegal or unsustainable trade of a species) of the Convention (https://cites.org/eng/app/index.php).
- The CITES provisions apply to live animals, carcasses, and derivatives of listed species (see following section).
- Any international trade of such CITES-listed species must be authorized by a CITES import and export permit issued by the CITES Management Authority of the appropriate country. For a list of these, see CITES website (https://cites.org/eng/cms/index.php/component/cp).
- Trade means international (cross-frontier) movement, whether commercial or not and for whatever purpose (see previous comments).
- In the case of Appendix I species, a permit may be given only for movement that is not of a primarily commercial nature (see previous comments).

Text continued on p. 1444

TABLE 183.2   Reptile Species Listed in Appendices I, II, and III of CITES (as of October 4, 2017)

	Appendix I	Appendix II	Appendix III
Class Reptilia (Reptiles)			
Crocodilia: Alligators, caimans, crocodiles		Crocodilia spp. (except the species included in Appendix I)	

Alligatoridae:
Alligators, caimans
	Alligator sinensis
	Caiman crocodilus apaporiensis
	Caiman latirostris (except the population of Argentina,
	  which is included in Appendix II)
	Melanosuchus niger (except the population of Brazil, which
	  is included in Appendix II, and the population of Ecuador,
	  which is included in Appendix II and is subject to a zero
	  annual export quota until an annual export quota has
	  been approved by the CITES secretariat and the IUCN/
	  SSC Crocodile Specialist Group)		

Crocodylidae:
Crocodiles
	Crocodylus acutus (except the population of the Integrated
	  Management District of Mangroves of the Bay of Cispata,
	  Tinajones, La Balsa, and surrounding areas, Department
	  of Córdoba, Colombia, and the population of Cuba, which
	  are included in Appendix II)
	Crocodylus cataphractus
	Crocodylus intermedius
	Crocodylus mindorensis
	Crocodylus moreletii (except the population of Belize, which
	  is included in Appendix II with a zero quota for wild
	  specimens traded for commercial purposes, and the
	  population of Mexico, which is included in Appendix II)
	Crocodylus niloticus [except the populations of Botswana,
	  Egypt (subject to a zero quota for wild specimens traded
	  for commercial purposes), Ethiopia, Kenya, Madagascar,
	  Malawi, Mozambique, Namibia, South Africa, Uganda, the
	  United Republic of Tanzania (subject to an annual export
	  quota of no more than 1,600 wild specimens including
	  hunting trophies, in addition to ranched specimens),
	  Zambia and Zimbabwe, which are included in Appendix II]
	Crocodylus palustris
	Crocodylus porosus {except the populations of Australia,
	  Indonesia, Malaysia [wild harvest restricted to the state
	  of Sarawak and a zero quota for wild specimens for the
	  other states of Malaysia (Sabah and Peninsular Malaysia),
	  with no change in the zero quota unless approved by the
	  Parties] and Papua New Guinea, which are included in
	  Appendix II}
	Crocodylus rhombifer
	Crocodylus siamensis
	Osteolaemus tetraspis
	Tomistoma schlegelii		

Gavialidae: Gavials	*Gavialis gangeticus*		
Rhynchocephalia			
Sphenodontidae: Tuataras	*Sphenodon* spp.		

Continued

TABLE 183.2	Reptile Species Listed in Appendices I, II, and III of CITES (as of October 4, 2017)—cont'd		
	Appendix I	**Appendix II**	**Appendix III**
Sauria			
Agamidae: Spiny-tailed lizards, agamas		*Saara* spp. *Uromastyx* spp.	
Anguidae: Alligator lizards		*Abronia* spp. [except the species included in Appendix I (zero export quota for wild specimens for *Abronia aurita, A. gaiophantasma, A. montecristoi, A. salvadorensis,* and *A. vasconcelosii*)]	
	Abronia anzuetoi *Abronia campbelli* *Abronia fimbriata* *Abronia frosti* *Abronia meledona*		
Chamaeleonidae: Chameleons		*Archaius* spp. *Bradypodion* spp. *Brookesia* spp. (except the species included in Appendix I)	
	Brookesia perarmata		
		Calumma spp. *Chamaeleo* spp. *Furcifer* spp. *Kinyongia* spp. *Nadzikambia* spp. *Palleon* spp. *Rhampholeon* spp. *Rieppeleon* spp. *Trioceros* spp.	
Cordylidae: Spiny-tailed lizards		*Cordylus* spp. *Hemicordylus* spp. *Karusaurus* spp. *Namazonurus* spp. *Ninurta* spp. *Ouroborus* spp. *Pseudocordylus* spp. *Smaug* spp.	
Gekkonidae: Geckos	*Cnemaspis psychedelica*		
			Dactylocnemis spp. (New Zealand) *Hoplodactylus* spp. (New Zealand)
	Lygodactylus williamsi		
			Mokopirirakau spp. (New Zealand)
		Nactus serpensinsula *Naultinus* spp. *Paroedura masobe* *Phelsuma* spp.	

TABLE 183.2 Reptile Species Listed in Appendices I, II, and III of CITES (as of October 4, 2017)—cont'd

	Appendix I	Appendix II	Appendix III
		Rhoptropella spp.	
			Toropuku spp. (New Zealand)
			Tukutuku spp. (New Zealand)
		Uroplatus spp.	
			Woodworthia spp. (New Zealand)
Helodermatidae: Beaded lizards, Gila monsters		*Heloderma* spp. (except the subspecies included in Appendix I)	
Iguanidae: Iguanas	*Heloderma horridum charlesbogerti*		
		Amblyrhynchus cristatus	
	Brachylophus spp.		
		Conolophus spp.	
		Ctenosaura bakeri	
		Ctenosaura melanosterna	
		Ctenosaura oedirhina	
		Ctenosaura palearis	
	Cyclura spp.		
		Iguana spp.	
		Phrynosoma blainvillii	
		Phrynosoma cerroense	
		Phrynosoma coronatum	
		Phrynosoma wigginsi	
	Sauromalus varius		
Lacertidae: Lizards	*Gallotia simonyi*		
		Podarcis lilfordi	
		Podarcis pityusensis	
Lanthanotidae: Earless monitor lizards			
		Lanthanotidae spp. (zero export quota for wild specimens for commercial purposes)	
Scincidae: Skinks			
		Corucia zebrata	
Teiidae: Caiman lizards, tegu lizards			
		Crocodilurus amazonicus	
		Dracaena spp.	
		Salvator spp.	
		Tupinambis spp.	
Varanidae: Monitor lizards			
		Varanus spp. (except the species included in Appendix I)	
	Varanus bengalensis		
	Varanus flavescens		
	Varanus griseus		
	Varanus komodoensis		
	Varanus nebulosus		
Xenosauridae: Chinese crocodile lizard			
	Shinisaurus crocodilurus		

Continued

TABLE 183.2	Reptile Species Listed in Appendices I, II, and III of CITES (as of October 4, 2017)—cont'd		
	Appendix I	**Appendix II**	**Appendix III**
Serpentes			
Boidae: Boas			
		Boidae spp. (except the species included in Appendix I)	
	Acrantophis spp.		
	Boa constrictor occidentalis		
	Epicrates inornatus		
	Epicrates monensis		
	Epicrates subflavus		
	Sanzinia madagascariensis		
Bolyeriidae: Round Island boas			
		Bolyeriidae spp. (except the species included in Appendix I)	
	Bolyeria multocarinata		
	Casarea dussumieri		
Colubridae: Typical snakes, water snakes, whipsnakes			
			Atretium schistosum (India)
			Cerberus rynchops (India)
		Clelia clelia	
		Cyclagras gigas	
		Elachistodon westermanni	
		Ptyas mucosus	
			Xenochrophis piscator (India)
			Xenochrophis schnurrenbergeri (India)
			Xenochrophis tytleri (India)
Elapidae: Cobras, coral snakes			
		Hoplocephalus bungaroides	
			Micrurus diastema (Honduras)
			Micrurus nigrocinctus (Honduras)
			Micrurus ruatanus (Honduras)
		Naja atra	
		Naja kaouthia	
		Naja mandalayensis	
		Naja naja	
		Naja oxiana	
		Naja philippinensis	
		Naja sagittifera	
		Naja samarensis	
		Naja siamensis	
		Naja sputatrix	
		Naja sumatrana	
		Ophiophagus hannah	
Loxocemidae: Mexican dwarf boas			
		Loxocemidae spp.	
Pythonidae: Pythons			
		Pythonidae spp. (except the subspecies included in Appendix I)	
	Python molurus molurus		

TABLE 183.2 **Reptile Species Listed in Appendices I, II, and III of CITES (as of October 4, 2017)—cont'd**

	Appendix I	Appendix II	Appendix III
Tropidophiidae: Wood boas		Tropidophiidae spp.	
Viperidae: Vipers		Atheris desaixi	
		Bitis worthingtoni	Crotalus durissus (Honduras)
			Daboia russelii (India)
		Trimeresurus mangshanensis	
	Vipera ursinii (only the population of Europe, except the area that formerly constituted the Union of Soviet Socialist Republics; these latter populations are not included in the appendices)		
		Vipera wagneri	
Testudines			
Carettochelyidae: Pig-nosed turtles		Carettochelys insculpta	
Chelidae: Austro American sideneck turtles		Chelodina mccordi (zero export quota for specimens from the wild)	
	Pseudemydura umbrina		
Cheloniidae: Sea turtles	Cheloniidae spp.		
Chelydridae: Snapping turtles			Chelydra serpentina (United States)
			Macrochelys temminckii (United States)
Dermatemydidae: Central American river turtles		Dermatemys mawii	
Dermochelyidae: Leatherback turtles	Dermochelys coriacea		
Emydidae: Box turtles, freshwater turtles		Clemmys guttata	
		Emydoidea blandingii	
		Glyptemys insculpta	
	Glyptemys muhlenbergii		Graptemys spp. (United States of America)
		Malaclemys terrapin	
		Terrapene spp. (except the species included in Appendix I)	
	Terrapene coahuila		

Continued

TABLE 183.2   Reptile Species Listed in Appendices I, II, and III of CITES (as of October 4, 2017)—cont'd

Appendix I	Appendix II	Appendix III
Geoemydidae: Box turtles, freshwater turtles		
Batagur affinis		
Batagur baska		
	Batagur borneoensis (zero quota for wild specimens for commercial purposes)	
	Batagur dhongoka	
	Batagur kachuga	
	Batagur trivittata (zero quota for wild specimens for commercial purposes)	
	Cuora spp. (zero quota for wild specimens for commercial purposes for Cuora aurocapitata, C. bourreti, C. flavomarginata, C. galbinifrons, C. mccordi, C. mouhotii, C. pani, C. picturata, C. trifasciata, C. yunnanensis, and C. zhoui)	
	Cyclemys spp.	
Geoclemys hamiltonii		
	Geoemyda japonica	
	Geoemyda spengleri	
	Hardella thurjii	
	Heosemys annandalii (zero quota for wild specimens for commercial purposes)	
	Heosemys depressa (zero quota for wild specimens for commercial purposes)	
	Heosemys grandis	
	Heosemys spinosa	
	Leucocephalon yuwonoi	
	Malayemys macrocephala	
	Malayemys subtrijuga	
	Mauremys annamensis (zero quota for wild specimens for commercial purposes)	
		Mauremys iversoni (China)
	Mauremys japonica	
		Mauremys megalocephala (China)
	Mauremys mutica	
	Mauremys nigricans	
		Mauremys pritchardi (China)
		Mauremys reevesii (China)
		Mauremys sinensis (China)
Melanochelys tricarinata		
	Melanochelys trijuga	
Morenia ocellata		
	Morenia petersi	
	Notochelys platynota	
		Ocadia glyphistoma (China)
		Ocadia philippeni (China)
	Orlitia borneensis (zero quota for wild specimens for commercial purposes)	
	Pangshura spp. (except the species included in Appendix I)	
Pangshura tecta		
	Sacalia bealei	

TABLE 183.2	**Reptile Species Listed in Appendices I, II, and III of CITES (as of October 4, 2017)—cont'd**	
Appendix I	**Appendix II**	**Appendix III**
		Sacalia pseudocellata (China)
	Sacalia quadriocellata	
	Siebenrockiella crassicollis	
	Siebenrockiella leytensis	
	Vijayachelys silvatica	
Platysternidae: Big-headed turtles		
Platysternidae spp.		
Podocnemididae: Afro American sideneck turtles		
	Erymnochelys madagascariensis	
	Peltocephalus dumerilianus	
	Podocnemis spp.	
Testudinidae: Tortoises		
	Testudinidae spp. (except the species included in Appendix I; a zero annual export quota has been established for *Centrochelys sulcata* for specimens removed from the wild and traded for primarily commercial purposes)	
Astrochelys radiata		
Astrochelys yniphora		
Chelonoidis niger		
Geochelone platynota		
Gopherus flavomarginatus		
Psammobates geometricus		
Pyxis arachnoides		
Pyxis planicauda		
Testudo kleinmanni		
Trionychidae: Softshell turtles		
	Amyda cartilaginea	
		Apalone ferox (United States)
		Apalone mutica (United States)
		Apalone spinifera (except the subspecies included in Appendix I) (United States)
Apalone spinifera atra		
	Chitra spp. (except the species included in Appendix I)	
Chitra chitra		
Chitra vandijki		
	Cyclanorbis elegans	
	Cyclanorbis senegalensis	
	Cycloderma aubryi	
	Cycloderma frenatum	
	Dogania subplana	
	Lissemys ceylonensis	
	Lissemys punctata	
	Lissemys scutata	
	Nilssonia formosa	
Nilssonia gangetica		
Nilssonia hurum		
	Nilssonia leithii	

Continued

TABLE 183.2	Reptile Species Listed in Appendices I, II, and III of CITES (as of October 4, 2017)—cont'd		
Appendix I	**Appendix II**		**Appendix III**
Nilssonia nigricans			
	Palea steindachneri		
	Pelochelys spp.		
	Pelodiscus axenaria		
	Pelodiscus maackii		
	Pelodiscus parviformis		
	Rafetus euphraticus		
	Rafetus swinhoei		
	Trionyx triunguis		

Source: CITES Secretariat.

- Permits are provided for the commercial movement of Appendix II species. Captive-bred specimens of Appendix I species are, subject to certain requirements, treated as if they were listed in Appendix II.
- Special certificates may also be given for the movement of captive-bred animals that are pets or in a traveling exhibition.
- Simplified permit procedures are available in special circumstances such as for the movement of biological and veterinary samples and museum specimens (see later).
- Specific criteria exist for the issue of permits: the trade must not be detrimental to the survival of the species; the animal must have been legally obtained; the animal must be prepared and shipped so as to ensure that it is not at risk of injury, damage to health, or cruel treatment during transportation; the importer must be able to house and care for the animal appropriately (see later).

The detailed provisions of CITES are complex, and further information can be obtained from the CITES Convention website at http://www.cites.org/; and, in view of the extensive additional provisions in the EU law, at the EU website at http://ec.europa.eu/environment/cites/legislation_en.htm and from national resources such as the UK Government CITES website at https://www.gov.uk/guidance/cites-imports-and-exports (also see Chapter 184). For a detailed study of the functioning of CITES, see Wijnstekers.[2]

MATTERS OF PARTICULAR INTEREST TO VETERINARIANS

Derivatives of CITES Specimens

The CITES provisions apply not only to live specimens but also to carcasses, parts, and other derivatives. Originally envisaged to include material such as ivory, traditional medicines, reptile skins, and other artifacts, the provisions also apply to biological and veterinary samples. The CITES permit procedure has often led to the delay of, and damage to, biological and veterinary material essential to the health and management of CITES animals when it is sent to another country for diagnosis, research, or other purposes. CITES now recognizes this problem and provides for a "fast-track," or simplified/partially completed permit procedure in respect of urgent noncommercial samples. See Resolution Conf. 12.3 (Rev. CoP17) permits and certificate (https://cites.org/sites/default/files/document/E-Res-12-03-R17.pdf).[3] This provision may not be well known in many countries, but it is included in Commission Regulation (EC) No 865/2006, Article 18. CITES has also decided that urine and feces are not considered to be derivatives (so do not require CITES permits) under Resolution Conf. 9.6 (Rev. CoP16): Trade in readily recognizable parts and derivatives (https://cites.org/eng/res/09/09-06R16.php).

Transportation

- Animals that are CITES-listed species must be transported in accordance with the CITES "Guidelines for transport and preparation for shipment of live wild animals and plants."[4]
- In the case of air transport, they must be transported in accordance with the most recent airline rules governing the transport of live animals.[5]
- Public road and rail carriers may also have their own requirements.
- International and national postal regulations may forbid the transport by mail of living reptiles. Very precise requirements also exist for the mailing of animal carcasses and pathogens, including special packaging and labeling. These are based on the UN packaging requirements (see, for example, the World Health Organization Guidelines at http://www.who.int/csr/emc97_3.pdf, the relevant national legislation and numerous institutional guidelines).[3]

Captive-Bred Appendix I Specimens

As mentioned previously, such animals may be traded under Appendix II permits. There is an extensive trade in Appendix I reptiles that have been bred in captivity (http://ec.europa.eu/environment/cites/pdf/reports/non_cites_reptiles.pdf). For example, there are many crocodiles, snakes, chameleons, and other reptiles that are also bred for trade in large- or small-scale enterprises.

The criteria set by CITES for captive-bred Appendix I animals to qualify for trade under Appendix II permits is strict, and there is provision for the registration of ranching operations (e.g., crocodile farms) with CITES and identification of the animals and products. There is useful advice and veterinary expertise available from the IUCN specialist groups (as discussed earlier), particularly the Crocodile Specialist Group (http://www.iucncsg.org/).

Many reptiles that are not on CITES are also traded in many parts of the world. The impact on wild populations has been widely studied.[6]

Case Studies

There are various sources of information on law enforcement. CITES infringements and associated prosecutions in many countries are reported in the TRAFFIC Bulletin (http://www.traffic.org/bulletin). Herpetological societies will often note significant cases that have implications for their members, and they will also have information on the impact of relevant legislation, much of which may be available on their websites. Surveys and studies may also provide data on law enforcement.[7,8]

Convention on the Conservation of Migratory Species of Wild Animals

This convention is intended to bring together countries through which certain species routinely pass (range states) in order to provide consistent protection.

There are two appendices. Appendix I requires the parties to the convention to provide full protection to the species listed. Appendix II lists species for which the range states should make agreements regarding measures to take to improve protection within their countries.

The only reptiles listed on Appendices I and II are the yellow-headed side-neck and all marine turtles, as well as the gharial (Appendix I only) and the saltwater crocodile (Appendix II only).

Appendix II agreements that have been made regarding sea turtles follow.

- The Memorandum of Understanding on the Conservation and Management of Marine Turtles and their Habitats of the Indian Ocean and South-East Asia (IOSEA Marine Turtle MOU) and its associated Conservation and Management Plan. (http://www.cms.int/en/legalinstrument/iosea-marine-turtles)
- Memorandum of Understanding concerning Conservation Measures for Marine Turtles of the Atlantic Coast of Africa; see: Conservation Measures for Marine Turtles of the Atlantic Coast of Africa—TS No. 5 (http://www.cms.int/atlantic-turtles/)

Considering how widespread is the habitat of the marine turtle species, such agreements play an important part in developing protection for the various species and in encouraging cooperation between the range states for their protection.

REGIONAL COOPERATION

United Nations Environment (UNEP) Regional Seas Programme

The Regional Seas Programme is designed to bring together countries to conserve the marine environment. This includes not only species and habitat protection but also environmental issues such as marine pollution.

The Programme is divided into 18 regional seas areas, such as the Caribbean, Eastern Africa, the Mediterranean, Black Sea, and the Arctic. There are 143 participating countries and 18 Regional Seas Conventions and numerous Action Plans. This provides a structure whereby nations that have a coastline are encouraged to collaborate and to take responsibility for the marine environment within their territories.

In many cases the culture, politics, economics, and languages of these counties are diverse and may not have marine protection as a priority. The multilateral regional treaties and action plans that address issues of pollution, degradation of coasts and reefs, and the need for legal protection of the marine environment bring the countries together to address marine issues, develop legislation, and arrange cooperation. This is of particular value for marine species such as sea turtles that feed and nest in coastal areas that form part of the territory of a country but migrate through the high seas for which there is no national legal responsibility. For further information, see http://web.unep.org/regionalseas/who-we-are/regional-seas-programmes.

LAW ENFORCEMENT

Implementing legislation and law enforcement are a matter for national law and individual governments. International cooperation in law enforcement is receiving prominence these days. The trade in endangered species is in large part an international matter and the combat of illegal trade requires cooperation and collaboration between governments and enforcing authorities such as the police or wildlife authorities. A number of international or regional cooperative bodies have been set up with such aims, notably the International Consortium on Combating Wildlife Crime, INTERPOL, the Global Partnership on Wildlife Conservation and Crime (World Bank), the Lusaka Agreement Task Force, and the ASEAN Wildlife Enforcement Network. Many nongovernment organizations also contribute support for the enforcement of wildlife conservation legislation (Cooper).[1]

OTHER LEGISLATION

Animal Welfare

Most legislation regarding animal welfare is made at national level, although in Europe there are provisions in EU and COE law (see Chapter 184).

The Organisation Mondiale de la Santé Animale/World Organisation for Animal Health (OIE/WOAH) has taken responsibility for animal welfare standards on the international scene and has drawn up international standards for animal welfare. At the present these are primarily for domesticated species, although the standard on the use of animals in research and education applies to mammals, birds, and reptiles (see http://www.oie.int/index.php?id=169&L=0&htmfile=chapitre_aw_research_education.htm). WOAH is also working on standards for the slaughter of farmed reptiles (http://www.oie.int/infographic/StandardsAW/index.html).

Although legislation on zoos is largely a national matter (see Chapter 184) there are animal welfare standards set on an international basis by the World Association of Zoo Zoos and Aquariums in its animal welfare strategy (see http://www.waza.org/files/webcontent/1.public_site/5.conservation/animal_welfare/WAZA%20Animal%20Welfare%20Strategy%202015_Portrait.pdf).

However, there is considerable concern worldwide regarding the need to encourage animal welfare, because the quality of care for animals varies substantially from country to country. In countries where there is little or no legislation or no interest in enforcing such laws as they exist, it may be possible to develop protocols or standards based on the "five freedoms." These were first put forward in the UK in 1965 in respect of farm livestock and have since been incorporated into legislation for other species and situations, such as zoos and general animal welfare law in a number of countries (see the statement by FAWC[9] at http://webarchive.nationalarchives.gov.uk/20110618120810/http://www.fawc.org.uk/freedoms.htm). The principles are often taught in veterinary schools and provide a widely accepted basis for animal care and management. They are as follows:

1. Freedom from Hunger and Thirst—by ready access to fresh water and a diet to maintain full health and vigor.
2. Freedom from Discomfort—by providing an appropriate environment, including shelter and a comfortable resting area.
3. Freedom from Pain, Injury, or Disease—by prevention or rapid diagnosis and treatment.
4. Freedom to Express Normal Behavior—by providing sufficient space, proper facilities, and company of the animal's own kind.
5. Freedom from Fear and Distress—by ensuring conditions and treatment that avoid mental suffering.

Animal Health

Animal health controls are exercised by most countries when animals, derivatives, or biological samples are imported. While the health controls on domestic and some nondomestic species are strict, reptiles do not always fall within this remit and may be exempt; on the other hand, New Zealand does not allow the importation of reptiles other than for zoos. It is necessary to find out from the animal health authority of the country of importation the documentation and veterinary checks that are required, because requirements may vary from time to time.

Nonnative Species

When planning exportation of reptiles to a country where they constitute an alien species, a permit may be necessary under its nonnative species legislation. Even if importation is allowed, it is likely that it will be illegal to keep or release it without a license to do so.

CONCLUSION

While the veterinarian and others who are working with reptiles may find that national legislation is the normal source of regulation that is likely to affect the management care and treatment of reptiles, it is useful to be aware of the influence that international law has in formulating a country's laws in conservation, animal health and welfare, and other issues. Some of the literature surrounding these topics may be of use, especially to those working in conservation, production, or trade of reptiles.

REFERENCES

See www.expertconsult.com for a complete list of references.

184

Laws and Regulations—Europe

Margaret E. Cooper

The geographic area of Europe extends from the west of Iceland to the east of Russia and from Norway in the Barents Sea above the Arctic Circle to Crete in the Mediterranean Sea and comprises many countries that are diverse in their geography, ecology, history, culture, legal systems, and attitudes toward animals. Not surprisingly, considerable variation exists in the legislation relating to animals, including reptiles, from one country to another not only as to content, form, and stage of development but also in effectiveness and enforcement. Legislation in Europe is heavily influenced by the European Union and the Council of Europe.

SOURCES OF INFORMATION ON LEGISLATION

One can usually obtain printed copies of national legislation from the official government printer, and in some countries (e.g., France, Germany), publishers produce bound volumes of codes of legislation that are to be found in the larger bookshops. International and regional, and in some countries national, legislation is available on the Internet. The laws of individual countries normally are produced in the national language; however, in countries where the language is not widely spoken (such as the Scandinavian counties, the Netherlands, or the newer members of the European Union [EU]); a translation may be available in, for example, English or French. The EU website provides a portal to information on the EU and links to the legislation of member countries (http://europa.eu/index_en.htm). The legislation is available via EUR-Lex at http://eur-lex.europa.eu/homepage.html, a comprehensive website on EU law. The ECOLEX website provides access to a wide range of animal and environmental laws from many countries at http://www.ecolex.org/ecolex/index.php.

Specialist bodies, such as the herpetological societies or wildlife or animal welfare organizations, may have copies of translations of legislation and may also have information or expertise on the application or enforcement of laws relevant to their fields of operation. The newsletter and website of the Federation of Veterinarians of Europe (http://www.fve.org/) is a valuable source of information on recent or forthcoming changes in laws relevant to animal health, animal welfare, veterinary law, and the profession.

Levels of Legislation

Legislation can be found at several levels, ranging from global conventions to city bylaws. These are described in Table 184.1, and examples of the

TABLE 184.1 Levels of Legislation Relating to Reptiles

Level	Description	Type of Legislation	Subjects Relevant to Reptiles
International (or global)	Treaties that all countries may join and that give rise to legal obligations.	International treaties, conventions, agreements.	International conservation conventions (see Box 183.1).
Regional	Multilateral legislation in which countries of a certain region are eligible to participate.	European Union Regulations and Directives. Council of Europe Conventions.	Legislation on conservation, animal health, animal transport, veterinary profession, veterinary medicines, health, and safety.
National (or federal)	Legislation of individual countries. Note: In the United Kingdom, much of the older legislation applies to England, Wales, and Scotland, but since devolution (July 1, 1999), the three countries make some laws separately through the English and Scottish Parliaments and the Welsh Assembly, causing divergence of content. Northern Ireland always has its separate legislation.	Primary laws passed by national parliament. Secondary legislation: orders or regulations made under primary legislation.	Laws on conservation, zoos, research, animal welfare, import/export, veterinary profession, medicinal products, health, and safety.
State	In countries with a federal constitution, each constituent state (e.g., a land in Germany and a canton in Switzerland) may have its own laws (as with states in the United States or Australia and the provinces of Canada).	Laws produced by individual constituent states and effective only within that state.	As for national (see previous), depending on scope given to state by national (federal) law or constitution.
Local	Laws made by local government authorities. Sometimes they also implement national laws.	Laws or bylaws made or implemented by local government authorities under national or state legislation.	Laws on keeping animals for specified purposes (e.g., exhibition). Bylaws regulating, for example, the keeping of animals.

TABLE 184.2   European Wildlife Conservation Legislation Relevant to Reptiles

European Union (EU)	
Habitats and species	Council Directive 92/43/EEC of May 21, 1992, on the conservation of natural habitats and wild fauna and flora (Habitats Directive)
CITES	Council Regulation (EC) No. 338/97/EC of December 9, 1996, on the protection of species of fauna and flora and regulating trade therein
	Commission Regulation (EC) No. 865/2006 of May 4, 2006, laying down rules concerning the implementation of Council Regulation (EC) No 338/97
	Commission Regulation (EU) No 2015/870 of June 15, 2015. Amends Council Regulation (EC) No 338/97
	Commission Implementing Regulation (EU) No. 2015/736 of May 7, 2015, prohibiting the introduction into the Union of specimens of certain species of wild fauna and flora
	Commission Implementing Regulation (EU) 792/2012 of August 23, 2012, laying down rules for the design of certificates and other documents. Amends Regulations 338/97 and 865/2006
	Commission Implementing Regulation (EU) 2015/57 of January 15, 2015, amending Regulation 792/2012
	Commission Regulation (EC) No. 2017/160 of January 20, 2017, amending Council Regulation (EC) No. 338/97 on the protection of species of wild fauna and flora by regulating trade therein
Council of Europe (COE)	Convention on the Conservation of European Wildlife and Natural Habitats 1979 (Berne Convention)
National (and State)	Each country has its own wildlife conservation legislation that is likely to include protection for specified reptiles.
See also Table 183.1	England, Scotland, and Wales share most of this legislation. Northern Ireland has its own very similar laws.
and Table 185.2	EC Regulations on CITES (see previous) have direct application.
	Control of Trade in Endangered Species (Enforcement) Regulations 1997 (SI 1997/1372) (as amended) (COTES)
	Wildlife and Countryside Act 1981 (as amended) (WCA)
	Countryside and Rights of Way Act 2000 (CROW)
	Conservation of Habitats and Species Regulations 2010 (SI 2010/490) (Habitats Regulations)
Useful Websites	
General	https://www.cbd.int/brc/
	http://www.jncc.gov.uk/
	http://www.eu-wildlifetrade.org/pdf/en/2_national_legislation_en.pdf
COE	http://www.coe.int/en/web/conventions/full-list
EU CITES	http://ec.europa.eu/environment/cites/legislation_en.htm
EU CITES	http://ec.europa.eu/environment/cites/pdf/referenceguide_en.pdf
Regulations	
British CITES	http://jncc.defra.gov.uk/page-1376
	https://www.gov.uk/guidance/cites-imports-and-exports

For the international wildlife legislation implemented by the laws in this table, see Box 183.1.
COE, Council of Europe; *EU,* European Union.

legislation relevant to reptiles that has been produced at these levels are shown in Box 183.1 and Table 184.2. Where global or regional legislation on a particular field of law exists, countries that are parties are likely to have some similarity in the content of their relevant national laws.

IMPLEMENTATION AND ENFORCEMENT OF LEGISLATION

Differences also exist in the legal systems as between individual nations. For instance, many have codified legislation (e.g., France) and written constitutions (most nations), whereas Britain has neither of these. Countries may also have fundamentally different judicial systems. For this reason, the implementation (i.e., putting legal obligations into effect, usually with legislation) and enforcement (i.e., ensuring that the legislation is obeyed) of global and regional legislation is the responsibility of individual countries.

EUROPEAN REGIONAL LEGISLATION

The two regional European law-making bodies are the European Union (http://europa.eu/index_en.htm) and the Council of Europe (COE)(http://www.coe.int/en/; http://en.strasbourg-europe.eu/member -states,44987,en.html). Table 184.3 provides some information that may help to clarify their status and the effect of their legislation on reptiles.

FREE-RANGING REPTILES

General

The legal protection of reptiles in the wild includes both species protection and habitat protection. Thus a country's law may specifically afford protection for particular species of reptile, but in addition, reptiles also derive benefit from protection of the habitat in which they can be found.

Substantial wildlife conservation legislation is relevant to reptiles at all levels.[1] See Chapter 183 and Tables 184.2 and 184.4. Most countries have national species and habitat legislation, which is usually a combination of their implementation of global and regional legislation and national provisions. The legislation specifies species and habitats to be protected, methods of protection, offences, penalties, and enforcement powers.

Protected Species

Free-living reptiles have the benefit of protective legislation at a regional and national level. The species covered vary from country to country

TABLE 184.3	European Institutions That Make Regional Wildlife Conservation Legislation			
Institution	Membership	Legislation	Legislation Relevant to Reptiles	Implementation
EU Primary aims of EU: economic, political, and legislative EU aims: also foreign policy and crime prevention	28 member states: Austria, Belgium, Bulgaria, Croatia, Cyprus, Czech Republic, Denmark, Estonia, Finland, France, Germany, Greece, Hungary, Ireland, Italy, Latvia, Lithuania, Luxembourg, Malta, Netherlands, Poland, Portugal, Romania, Slovakia, Slovenia, Spain, Sweden, United Kingdom*.	Regulations have direct application in EU member countries. Directives have to be transposed by each EU country into its national law. Enforcement is responsibility of each EU country. Member countries can be required by the European Court of Justice to implement directives, backed by financial penalty.	†Habitats Directive Transport Directive Scientific Research Directive †CITES Regulations (full titles in text) Professional Directives Medicines Directives	Should be implemented by all member countries.
COE Primary aims: social and cultural, especially democracy, rule of law, and human rights	COE has 47 members and 5 observer countries (including Canada, the Holy See, Japan, Mexico, United States). Nonmembers of COE can join its conventions. 350 NGOs have consultative status.	Conventions must be implemented by member countries that have ratified or acceded to them. Other countries can accede. No specific means to make a country implement a convention.	Relevant conventions: Wildlife conservation (Berne) (ETS 104) Welfare of animals during transport 1968 (ETS 065) Revised 2003 (ETS 193) Scientific research (ETS 123) Pets (ETS 125)	Ratified by: 47 members, 5 other countries and EU 24 countries and Russia 12 countries 21 countries and EC 21 countries

COE, Council of Europe; *ETS*, European Treaty Series; *EU*, European Union; *NGO*, nongovernmental organization.
*In a referendum held on June 23, 2016, the United Kingdom voted to leave the EU. Under the Treaty on European Union (Lisbon Treaty) Article 50, a member state must inform the EU Council of its intention to leave and then, following a maximum of 2 years (unless extended) allowed for negotiation of terms, exit occurs. The United Kingdom will leave the EU on March 29, 2019, and transitional arrangements will apply until the end of 2020.
†See Table 184.2 for the full titles of these laws.

and relate primarily to the species that occur naturally in that country. Table 184.4 shows the listings of protected reptiles for the COE, EU, and by way of an example of national law, English conservation legislation.

Typical Prohibited or Controlled Activities Relating to Reptiles in the Wild

Core offenses likely to be included in a country's species protection legislation are:

- Deliberate killing, taking, or injuring of a protected reptile or its young or eggs.
- Deliberate disturbance of a protected reptile.
- Deliberate disturbance of its breeding or resting place.
- Use of prohibited or nonselective methods (e.g., poison, nets, traps, lights, vehicles) of capture, or killing of protected reptiles that may deplete or disturb local populations or are inhumane.
- Trade (e.g., sale, exchange, barter, transport, or display for sale) in live animals, dead specimens, or derivatives thereof.
- Release of alien (nonnative) species.

Many of these activities can be authorized by license for specified purposes (e.g., conservation, research, education, exhibition, captive breeding, trade in captive-bred specimens, public health, or crop or property protection).

Variation in National Laws

National laws that incorporate some or all of the previous laws may also vary in quantity, quality, and effectiveness, but some uniformity of content does exist within the EU or COE (because the national laws must reflect the regional laws) and among countries that have implemented the global conventions (see Table 184.4 and relevant convention websites). However, the level of protection of a particular species may also vary, because its conservation status can differ from one country to another. This may be so in spite of the listed status of a species at the regional level, because a country can derogate from the main legislation when a species is not at risk, not present, or a country is not willing to protect it; conversely, a country may impose a higher status or stricter regulation than that required by the regional legislation. Likewise, the quality of enforcement is variable, for example, because of the extent of the powers provided or the different degrees of political will or financial resources.

Fieldwork That Involves Reptiles

In addition to the foregoing legislation, those who carry out scientific research in the field using free-living reptiles may need to obtain research authorization or licenses to comply with the species protection laws, or permission to enter the area where the reptiles are studied. If the work involves population management, one should have regard to the IUCN Guidelines on reintroductions, translocation, and other topics.[2-5]

CAPTIVE REPTILES

General

The keeping of animals, including reptiles, is mainly regulated by national or state legislation, although day-to-day control may be the responsibility of local government authorities. The control is likely to depend on the nature of the species and the purpose for which they are kept. Regulation may include provisions for licensing and inspection and require compliance with standards or guidelines.

Reptiles Kept as Pets

The private keeping of reptiles is often controlled, usually at local government authority level, especially if the species (e.g., large or venomous reptiles) represents a risk to the public. Some countries may regulate the keeping of any species of reptile. Others may be selective, as in Britain, where the keeping of specified species is subject to licensing and inspection under the Dangerous Wild Animals Act 1976 (as

TABLE 184.4 **Comparative Table of Protected Reptiles in Europe**

COUNCIL OF EUROPE CONVENTION (APPLIES TO 51 COUNTRIES AND THE EU)	EUROPEAN UNION DIRECTIVE (APPLIES TO 28 COUNTRIES)	AN EXAMPLE OF NATIONAL LEGISLATION: ENGLAND	
Berne Convention (Appendix II)	**EC Habitats Directive Annex IV (a)**	**WCA**	**Habitats Regulations**
Strictly protected species	Animal and plant species of community interest in need of strict protection	Fully or partially protected species listed in WCA	"European protected species" (i.e., those species listed on Annex IV of the Habitats Directive whose natural range includes any area in Britain)
Reptiles			
Testudines			
Testudinidae			
Testudo graeca	*Testudo graeca*		
Testudo hermanni	*Testudo hermanni*		
Testudo marginata	*Testudo marginata*		
Emydidae			
Emys orbicularis	*Emys orbicularis*		
Mauremys caspica	*Mauremyscas pica*		
Mauremys leprosa (*Mauremys caspica leprosa*)	*Mauremys leprosa*		
Dermochelyidae			
Dermochelys coriacea	*Dermochelys coriacea*	*Dermochelys coriacea*	*Dermochelys coriacea*
Cheloniidae			
Caretta caretta	*Caretta caretta*	*Caretta caretta**	*Caretta caretta*
Chelonia mydas	*Chelonia mydas*	*Chelonia mydas**	*Chelonia mydas*
Eretmochelys imbricata	*Eretmochelys imbricata*	*Eretmochelys imbricata**	*Eretmochelys imbricata*
Lepidochelys kempii	*Lepidochelys kempii*	*Lepidochelys kempii**	*Lepidochelys kempii*
		Lepidochelys olivacea	
		Narator depressus	
Trionychidae			
Rafetus euphraticus			
Trionyx triunguis			
Sauria			
Gekkonidae			
Cyrtodactylus kotschyi	*Cyrtopodion kotschyi*		
Phyllodactylus europaeus	*Phyllodactylus europaeus*		
Tarentola angustimentalis	*Tarentola angustimentalis*		
Tarentola boettgeri	*Tarentola boettgeri*		
Tarentola delalandii	*Tarentola delalandii*		
Tarentola gomerensis	*Tarentola gomerensis*		
Agamidae			
Stellio stellio (*Agama stellio*)	*Stellio stellio*		
Chamaeleontidae			
Chamaeleo chamaeleon	*Chamaeleo chamaeleon*		
Lacertidae			
Algyroides fitzingeri	*Algyroides fitzingeri*		
Algyroides marchi	*Algyroides marchi*		
Algyroides moreoticus	*Algyroides moreoticus*		
Algyroides nigropunctatus	*Algyroides nigropunctatus*		
Archaeolacerta bedriaga (*Lacerta bedriagae*)			
Archaeolacerta monticola (*Lacerta monticola*)			
	Gallotia atlantica		
Gallotia galloti	*Gallotia galloti*		
	Gallotia galloti insulanagae		
Gallotia simonyi (*Lacerta simonyi*)	*Gallotia simonyi*		
Gallotia stehlini	*Gallotia stehlini*		
Lacerta agilis	*Lacerta agilis*	*Lacerta agilis**	*Lacerta agilis*
Lacerta clarkorum	*Lacerta bedriagae*		
	Lacerta danfordi		

TABLE 184.4 Comparative Table of Protected Reptiles in Europe—cont'd

COUNCIL OF EUROPE CONVENTION (APPLIES TO 51 COUNTRIES AND THE EU)	EUROPEAN UNION DIRECTIVE (APPLIES TO 28 COUNTRIES)	AN EXAMPLE OF NATIONAL LEGISLATION: ENGLAND	
Berne Convention (Appendix II)	EC Habitats Directive Annex IV (a)	WCA	Habitats Regulations
Lacerta dugesii	Lacerta dugesi		
Lacerta graeca	Lacerta graeca		
Lacerta horvathi	Lacerta horvathi		
Lacerta lepida			
Lacerta parva			
Lacerta princeps			
	Lacerta monticola		
Lacerta schreiberi	Lacerta schreiberi		
Lacerta trilineata	Lacerta trilineata		
Lacerta viridis	Lacerta viridis		
	Lacorta vivipara[†]		
		Lacerta vivipara pannonica	
Ophisops elegans	Ophisops elegans		
Podarcis erhardii	Podarcis erhardii		
Podarcis filfolensis	Podarcis filfolensis		
	Podarcis hispanica atrata		
Podarcis lilfordi	Podarcis lilfordi		
Podarcis melisellensis	Podarcis melisellensis		
Podarcis milensis	Podarcis milensis		
Podarcis muralis	Podarcis muralis		
Podarcis peloponnesiaca	Podarcis peloponnesiaca		
Podarcis pityusensis	Podarcis pityusensis		
Podarcis sicula	Podarcis sicula		
Podarcis taurica	Podarcis taurica		
Podarcis tiliguerta	Podarcis tiliguerta		
Podarcis wagleriana	Podarcis wagleriana		
Anguidae			
Ophisaurus apodus	Ophisaurus apodus		
		Anguis fragilis[†]	
Scincidae			
Ablepharus kitaibelli	Ablepharus kitaibelli		
Chalcides bedriagai	Chalcides bedriagai		
Chalcides occidentalis	Chalcides occidentalis		
Chalcides ocellatus	Chalcides ocellatus		
Chalcides sexlineatus	Chalcides sexlineatus		
Chalcides simonyi (Chalcides occidentalis)	Chalcides simonyi (Chalcides occidentalis)		
Chalcides viridianus	Chalcides viridianus		
Ophiomorus punctatissimus	Ophiomorus punctatissimus		
Ophidia			
Colubridae			
Coluber cypriensis			
Coluber gemonensis			
Coluber hippocrepis	Coluber hippocrepis		
Coluber jugularis	Coluber jugularis		
Coluber caspius (Coluber jugularis caspius)	Coluber caspius		
	Coluber laurenti		
Coluber najadum	Coluber najadum		
Coluber rubriceps (Coluber najadum rubriceps)	Coluber nummifer		
Coluber viridiflavus	Coluber viridiflavus		
Coronella austriaca	Coronella austriaca	Coronella austriaca*	Coronella austriaca
	Eirenis modesta		
Elaphe longissima	Elaphe longissima		

Continued

TABLE 184.4   Comparative Table of Protected Reptiles in Europe—cont'd

COUNCIL OF EUROPE CONVENTION (APPLIES TO 51 COUNTRIES AND THE EU)	EUROPEAN UNION DIRECTIVE (APPLIES TO 28 COUNTRIES)	AN EXAMPLE OF NATIONAL LEGISLATION: ENGLAND	
Berne Convention (Appendix II)	EC Habitats Directive Annex IV (a)	WCA	Habitats Regulations
Elaphe quatuorlineata	Elaphe quatuorlineata		
Elaphe situla	Elaphe situla		
Natrix megalocephala	Natrix natrix cetti		
	Natrix natrix[†]		
		Natrix natrix corsa	
Natrix tessellata	Natrix tessellata		
Telescopus fallax	Telescopus fallax		
Viperidae			
Vipera albizona			
Vipera ammodytes	Vipera ammodytes		
		Vipera berus[†]	
Vipera barani			
Vipera kaznakovi			
Vipera latasti			
Vipera lebetina			
Vipera schweizeri (Vipera lebetina schweizeri)	Vipera schweizeri		
	Vipera seoanni (except Spanish populations)		
Vipera pontica			
Vipera ursinii	Vipera ursinii		
Vipera wagneri			
Vipera xanthina	Vipera xanthina		
Boidae			
	Eryx jaculus		

EU, European Union; *WCA*, Wildlife and Countryside Act.
*Full protection.
[†]Partial protection (killing, injuring, sale).

amended). The animals must be kept in secure and appropriate accommodation, and the keeper must be insured. Reptiles subject to the Act include all crocodilians, some colubrids, all elaphids, front-fanged venomous vipers, and the Helodermatidae (http://www.legislation.gov.uk/uksi/2007/2465/schedule/made).

The COE European Convention for the Protection of Pet Animals 1987 has broad provisions for the responsible keeping of pets, defined as "any animal kept or intended to be kept by man in particular in his household for private enjoyment and companionship." It requires the keeper of a pet animal to adhere to basic principles of animal welfare (see subsequently), and Article 4 provides that a pet should not be caused unnecessary pain, suffering, or distress, nor be abandoned. The keeper of a pet must be responsible for its health and welfare and provide accommodations, care, and attention that take account of the ethologic needs of the animal in accordance with its species and breed. In particular, keepers must give it suitable and sufficient food and water and adequate opportunities for exercise and take reasonable measures to prevent its escape.

Keeping of Protected Species

Restrictions may exist under national wildlife laws (see previous) on the possession of reptiles, particularly if wild caught. A license may be necessary to keep, breed, or trade in native or specified wild-caught or captive-bred reptiles. The keeper of a CITES species may be required to prove that it was imported or obtained legally in accordance with CITES legislation. In the EU, any commercial use of an Annex A CITES species must be authorized (as discussed later).

Exhibition, Display, and Entertainment

Reptiles are used or displayed for purposes such as zoos, circuses, cabarets, or education; such activities are likely to be subject to controls, usually through licensing by a local government authority. Great variation exists in the legislation, enforcement, and actual quality of care provided for exhibited animals in different countries. Countries are required to implement several supranational laws, which are mentioned subsequently.

The COE Pets Convention applies general welfare provisions (see previous) to pets, including reptiles, that are used in exhibitions, entertainment, and competitions and requires that these activities must not interfere with their health and well-being.

The Council Directive 1999/22/EC relating to the keeping of wild animals in zoos applies to collections open to the public and requires EU countries to regulate zoos as briefly summarized:

- The Directive applies to collections of "wild species" that are exhibited to the public on 7 or more days in a year.
- Zoos must be licensed and inspected.
- Accommodation for animals must take into account their biological and conservation needs and provide enrichment; zoos must provide good husbandry, veterinary care, and nutrition.
- Records must be kept; measures must be taken to prevent escapes of animals or the access of pests and to provide for dispersal of animals in the event of closure.
- Zoos must also make a contribution to conservation (e.g., by way of research, training, exchange of information, captive breeding,

reintroduction) and to public education relating to their animals and their habitats.

- The Directive was modeled on the British Zoo Licensing Act 1981 (although the latter has been amended to comply with the Directive).
- British zoos must also comply with the Secretary of State's Standards of Modern Zoo Practice (see https://www.gov.uk/government/uploads/system/uploads/attachment_data/file/69596/standards-of-zoo-practice.pdf).
- The EU has produced an EU Zoos Directive Good Practices Document (see http://ec.europa.eu/environment/nature/pdf/EU_Zoos_Directive_Good_Practices.pdf).
- The EC CITES Regulations[6] (see Table 184.2), in addition to regulating international trade in CITES species (see subsequent), also requires that any use of species listed in Annex A of the Regulation for commercial purposes must be authorized by an Article 10 or, for zoos, an Article 30 certificate. This applies not only to the usual aspects of trade but also to display, which is interpreted to include any exhibit with a commercial element such as zoos, cabarets, and trade shows. Annex A includes all CITES Convention Appendix I animals together with a number of other species that have been upgraded to that status within the EU (http://ec.europa.eu/environment/cites/info_permits_en.htm).

Scientific Research

The COE European Convention for the Protection of Vertebrate Animals used for Experimental and other Scientific Purposes was formed in 1987. The EC Council Directive 86/609/EEC of November 24, 1986, on the approximation of laws, regulations, and administrative provisions of the Member States concerned the protection of animals used for experimental and other scientific purposes has been revised by Directive 2010/63/EU. This legislation relates to experimental or other scientific use of an animal that may cause pain, suffering, distress, or lasting harm and applies to all nonhuman vertebrates, including reptiles, both captive and free-living. Some countries also have detailed regulations or guidance that supplements the main legislation. The controls can include (as in Britain) licensing, inspection, and ethical review; pain controls; veterinary supervision; and the training of researchers. Other countries may or may not have controls of varying content.

TRADE

The trade in endangered species between individual countries is regulated by CITES. This is described in Chapter 183 and the EU CITES Regulations are listed in Table 184.2 and in Cooper.[7]

The essential provisions of EU legislation are summarized later. Other (non-EU) countries in Europe operate CITES by implementing the global Convention on an individual basis. Note that:

- The Regulations implement CITES directly in all EU member countries; they do not have national legislation on CITES.
- Exception: enforcement is the responsibility of individual EU countries (e.g., in Britain by the Control of Trade in Endangered Species [Enforcement] Regulations 1997, as amended).
- Many species (in addition to those in the CITES Appendices) are included in Annexes A to D of the Regulation. The species listed and the status accorded to them may be stricter than the requirements of the CITES Convention. For example, some CITES Convention Appendix II species such as the Mediterranean tortoises have been upgraded to Annex A (equivalent to CITES Convention Appendix I status) and others, not listed on the Convention, have been put onto Annex B (Appendix II status).
- Once legally in the EU, CITES specimens can be moved freely around the EU.

- The importation into the EU of certain Annex B species (including many reptiles) has been suspended (see lists in Commission Regulation (EU) No 888/2014 amended EU 2015/736).
- The "fast track" procedures described in Chapter 183 are incorporated in the Regulations.

For current lists of EU CITES species, see Commission Regulation (EU) No 2017/160 and the list of websites in Table 184.2. The EU CITES provisions are explained in the Reference Guide to the Wildlife Trade Regulations.[6]

EU Trade in CITES Species

Within the EU area and within individual EU countries, the trade of Annex A species (which includes, inter alia, all CITES Appendix I species) is additionally controlled under the CITES Regulations as follows:

- Annex A species may not be used for primarily commercial purposes.
- Annex A species that have been captive-bred from captive-bred parents may be used for commercial purposes if authorized by an Article 10 certificate (or Article 30 for zoos).
- To obtain a certificate, one must produce evidence to show that the animal was legally imported or captive-bred.
- Annex A species in commercial use must be permanently marked with a microchip transponder that conforms to ISO Standards 11784:1996 (E) and 11785:1996 (E) (where this is not physically possible, then with another permanent form of identification). Note: In Britain, although hatchling tortoises are less than 10 centimeters long, they do not need to be marked.
- A CITES animal that has been legally imported or for which an Article 10 certificate has been issued can be traded (in accordance with the terms of the certificate) freely within the EU.
- For an example of these provisions at a national level, see AHVLA[8]
- A thriving trade exists in captive-bred reptiles as pets, among hobbyists, or for other purposes.
- Licensing controls are often imposed on the taking and/or sale of indigenous (and possibly other) reptiles under national wildlife legislation and in conformity with the Habitats Directive and the Berne Convention.
- Local authorities may regulate pet traders and their premises.
- Law enforcement measures are important to deal with illegal trade.

ANIMAL HEALTH CONTROLS

Animal health laws also apply cross-frontier controls, but they operate entirely separately from the CITES provisions described previously.

European Union Directives on Import and Export

Animal health legislation often requires authorization (usually issued by the ministry responsible for agriculture) to import many species of mammal and bird. This legislation also involves veterinary health certification and quarantine for live animals. For such controls to apply to reptiles is unusual. However, permission may be necessary to import pathogenic reptile material, for example, blood or tissues, particularly when the samples are not fixed. Authorization may include conditions relating to packaging, storage, and disposal of the material.[9,10]

National Wildlife Legislation: the Export of Indigenous Species

Some countries forbid the export of indigenous species or derivatives thereof except under license. In addition, national controls may be found on the export and exploitation of genetic materials under legislation implementing the Biodiversity Convention. This might apply to material derived from reptiles and intended for diagnosis, research, or screening for potential value in developing modern medicines.

National Wildlife Legislation: the in-Country Trade in Wildlife

National wildlife legislation usually regulates trade in its indigenous wildlife. The law prohibits the collection and trade in indigenous wildlife, even if the species are not listed on CITES and are not being exported.

Customs and Excise

Animals imported normally are subject to a country's taxes such as customs duty and value added (sales) tax.

REPTILES AND VETERINARY PRACTICE

Veterinary Professional Law

Veterinary practice in most European countries is regulated according to the usual provisions that relate to the registration of veterinarians and control of the profession, together with restrictions on the practice of veterinary medicine by laypersons.

Because the legislation is at national level, the precise provisions and levels of enforcement vary from country to country. To verify whether a reptile must be treated by a veterinarian, one must inquire as to whether reptiles are included in the range of species that must be treated by a registered veterinarian and whether the procedure is one that must be carried out by a veterinarian.

European Union nationals with EU veterinary qualifications are entitled to practice in any EU country. They must register in the given country. Directives 78/1026/EEC and 78/1027/EEC concern the recognition of qualifications and freedom of movement. The nationals may also have to provide a certificate of good standing from the EU country in which they were first or previously registered.

Britain also gives recognition to some (British) Commonwealth degrees from Australia, Canada, New Zealand, and South Africa and also American Veterinary Medical Association (AVMA)–recognized veterinary degrees from the United States (see http://www.rcvs.org.uk/).

Veterinary Medicinal Products

The pharmaceutical legislation that controls the sale, supply, prescription, and administration of veterinary drugs varies from very strict in some countries (with prosecutions and professional conduct [malpractice] proceedings in respect of breaches of the law or for the abuse or mishandling of substances) to lax in other countries. The EU regulates veterinary medicinal products through many regulations and directives. However, the sale, supply, and administration of veterinary medicinal products are controlled by national legislation in accordance with (inter alia) the appropriate directives. Prescription-only medicines for use in animals should normally be prescribed by a veterinarian. In light of the relatively few drugs that are approved for use in reptiles, the veterinarian may have to resort to "off-label" prescribing. In the EU, this must be done with the client's consent, and the drugs must be chosen in accordance with the "cascade" principles. If any patient is eventually to be used for food, then strict withdrawal periods must be observed (see https://www.bsava.com/Resources/BSAVAMedicinesGuide/Prescribingcascade.aspx; http://www.fve.org/uploads/publications/docs/fve_bro_cascade_jan2014.pdf).

OCCUPATIONAL HEALTH AND SAFETY

Occupational health and safety legislation is strong in some countries, including the EU where many directives exist on the subject. In countries in which the legislation is strictly enforced, the management of health and safety is all-pervasive and requires employers use the principles of risk assessment. Thus, in the case of reptiles kept in a zoo or veterinary practice, a risk assessment must be made of the hazards involved, the risks they pose, and the persons affected. Special hazards of reptiles include bites, envenomation, constriction, and salmonellosis. Measures to remove or reduce the risk, written records, and provision for monitoring and reviewing the procedures must be put in place. Legislation may also exist for specific health and safety situations, such as radiography and dangerous substances, fire, and first aid. Information on the EU legislation is available at the website of the European Agency for Safety and Health at Work at https://osha.europa.eu/en/safety-and-health-legislation.

In many other countries, little development may be seen of health and safety so far, and any measures that the veterinarian takes are on a voluntary basis. Any protective measures may help to reduce the risk of compensation claims (on the basis of negligence or employers' liability) that arise from accidents.

WELFARE

European Legislation

There are no international welfare laws relating to the humane treatment of animals, although the OIE (World Organisation for Animal Health, http://www.oie.int/en/) now includes "Recommendations for Animal Welfare" in its Terrestrial Animal Health Code.

Some broad provisions exist in the COE European Convention for the Protection of Pet Animals 1987 (ratified by 13 countries). It covers "any animal kept or intended to be kept by man in particular in his household for private enjoyment and companionship" and therefore includes reptiles kept as pets.

Article 3: Basic principles for animal welfare includes:
1. Nobody shall cause a pet animal unnecessary pain, suffering, or distress.
2. Nobody shall abandon a pet animal.

The article also contains provisions for responsible pet keeping (see previous).

National Legislation

Most countries have national legislation against cruelty to animals, and some may have extensive welfare law. The species covered by animal protection laws vary greatly, so examination of a country's legislation in detail is necessary to find whether it extends to reptiles, captive or free-living.

The provisions vary a great deal, but the forms of animal use or abuse that are addressed may include:
- Specific acts of cruelty
- A general category: causing unnecessary suffering
- The responsibility of the keeper of an animal to provide food, water, and suitable environment
- Poisoning, trapping, and cruel sports
- Mutilations (procedures carried out for nonmedical reasons, e.g., ligation of venom ducts in snakes)
- Use of anesthesia (and analgesics) during surgery
- Specific uses such as research and zoos if separate legislation is not provided
- Transportation (see later)

Some laws include most of the foregoing topics under one law; others have separate provisions, for example, for animals used in scientific research. The English and Welsh legislation is the Animal Welfare Act 2006, and there are comparable laws for Scotland and Northern Ireland. The legislation applies to all domesticated vertebrate species and other vertebrates that are in captivity or under a person's control. The acts include two key provisions: first, the offense of causing unnecessary suffering, and second, the duty of care that is imposed on those who keep animals. This duty requires a person to provide, so far as is reasonable in the circumstances, for the welfare needs of any animal (in accordance with good practice) for which s/he is responsible. The animal must be provided with a suitable environment and diet, be allowed to exhibit normal patterns of behavior, be housed singly or with others as appropriate, and be protected from pain, suffering, injury, and distress. There are also provisions forbidding mutilations, animal fighting, and poisoning.

Welfare During Transportation

European legislation exists on the humane transportation of animals, and this should have been transposed into national legislation. For example, in the English law there are provisions both general and specific that apply to reptiles.

Under the European Convention for the Protection of Animals during International Transport 1968, revised 2003, COE member countries must make provision for the welfare of vertebrate animals (including reptiles) during international transport. The requirements for noncommercial transportation are basic (i.e., that the animal should be fit to travel and that its health and welfare should be safeguarded during the journey). The stipulations for commercial transport are more stringent.

The Council Regulation (EC) No. 1/2005 on the protection of animals during transport and related operations) lays down requirements for the conditions of transport of vertebrate animals within, to, and from the Member States of the EU. It applies to animals that are transported for commercial purposes, for example, reptiles being carried by a commercial breeder or a zoo. It does not apply to transport for noncommercial purposes, transport to and from a veterinary surgery or clinic, or to pets accompanied by their owner on a private journey or when taken to or from a noncommercial event (e.g., as a hobby). Commercial transport requires a transporter authorization, trained handlers and vehicles that meet specified standards. There are conditions relating to journey times, rest times, food, and water for the animals. Animals must be fit to travel.

In England, The Welfare of Animals (Transport) (England) Order 2006 (and comparable legislation in the rest of the UK) implements the European legislation and has some additional requirements that are applicable to animals and circumstances not covered by the EU Regulation, such as reptiles traveling for noncommercial purposes.

Animals of any sort, including invertebrates, must not be transported in any way that causes or is likely to cause them injury or unnecessary suffering. Appropriate transport, containers, and environmental conditions must be provided during transport.

Animals that are CITES-listed species must be transported in accordance with the CITES "Guidelines for transport and preparation for shipment of live wild animals and plants."[11] In the case of air transport, they must be transported in accordance with the most recent airline rules governing the transport of live animals.[12]

Public road and rail carriers may also have their own requirements.

International and national postal regulations may forbid the transport by mail of living reptiles. Very precise requirements also exist for the mailing of animal carcasses and pathogens, including special packaging and labeling. These are based on the UN packaging requirements; see, for example, the World Health Organization Guidelines at http://www.who.int/csr/emc97_3.pdf, the relevant national legislation and numerous institutional guidelines, and Cooper.[9]

CASE STUDIES

There are various sources of reports of law enforcement. CITES infringements and associated prosecutions in many countries are reported in the TRAFFIC Bulletin (http://www.traffic.org/bulletin). Herpetologic societies will often note significant cases that have implications for their members.

CONCLUSION

A wide variety of legislation relates to reptiles either specifically or by way of general application. Although the details of national legislation cannot be included here, this chapter attempts to bring together as many as possible of the relevant principles that may be found in the law of the many countries of Europe. It is also intended to guide the reader toward appropriate sources of further and more specific information on the subject of reptile law.

REFERENCES

See www.expertconsult.com for a complete list of references.

185

Laws and Regulations—Americas

Gregory A. Lewbart and Daniel T. Lewbart

The hobby of captive herpetology is expanding, and more people and herptile (amphibians and reptiles) species are becoming a part of this expanding industry. Although captive breeding is much more popular and successful than it has been in decades past, many wild-caught specimens still find their way into captivity (some illegally) (Fig. 185.1). In some cases, maintenance of cultivated herptiles may also be against certain laws (Fig. 185.2). This chapter focuses on the international, federal, national, state, and local laws regarding herptiles and the authorities that enforce these regulations. Table 185.1 and Box 185.1 highlight information about non-US laws and resources. Several examples of specific regulation enforcement are also included and discussed.

The IUCN Red List of Threatened Species

This excellent resource provides current information for many of the world's plant and animal species at risk. The goal of the IUCN Red List is to "provide information and analyses on the status, trends and threats to species in order to inform and catalyse action for biodiversity conservation." The resource can be accessed via this link: http://www.iucnredlist.org. Following are standard references, one for the loggerhead and one for the hawksbill sea turtle:

Mortimer J.A, Donnelly M. (IUCN SSC Marine Turtle Specialist Group). 2008. *Eretmochelys imbricata*. The IUCN Red List of Threatened Species 2008: e.T8005A12881238.http://dx.doi.org/10.2305/IUCN.UK .2008.RLTS.T8005A12881238.en. Accessed on September 15, 2018.

Ceriani S.A., Meylan A.B. 2015. *Caretta caretta (North West Atlantic subpopulation)*. The IUCN Red List of Threatened Species 2015: e.T84131194A84131608.http://dx.doi.org/10.2305/IUCN.UK.2015-4 .RLTS.T84131194A84131608.en. Accessed on September 15, 2018.

THE CONVENTION ON INTERNATIONAL TRADE IN ENDANGERED SPECIES OF WILD FAUNA AND FLORA (CITES)

Most readers are familiar with the acronym CITES. This multinational agreement was originally written in 1973, was entered into force in 1975, and is meant to protect vulnerable and endangered plants and animals throughout the world from overexploitation. CITES is strictly an international treaty among the participating countries, and enforcement of the CITES provisions is up to the individual member countries (so regulation of CITES is far from consistent beyond the essential requirements of the convention). To date, 183 countries are parties to the CITES Convention. For details about CITES, see the informative website at http://www.cites.org.

Listed CITES animals fall into one of three categories (Appendix I, II, or III), with Appendix I the most protective. However, even Appendix I species can be commercially exploited through a loophole called a "Reservation," which allows participating countries to make exemptions for certain species (e.g., Japan's taking of sea turtles). CITES regulations only apply to the international import and export of listed species, which means legally imported CITES species can be transported, traded, or sold within a given country subject to the legislation of that country (see Chapter 183 for more details).

CITES permits are issued by the management authority for the relevant country; for the United States these and other required permits are available through the US Fish & Wildlife Service Office of

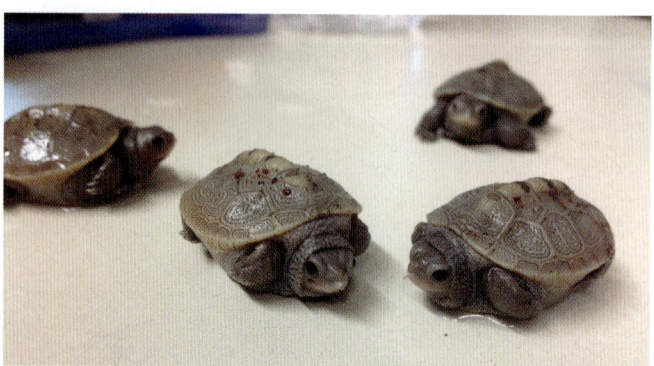

FIG 185.1 These North Carolina diamondback terrapins (*Malaclemys terrapin*) were hatched in captivity. This species is listed as a species of concern at both the state and federal level. (Courtesy of Gregory A. Lewbart.)

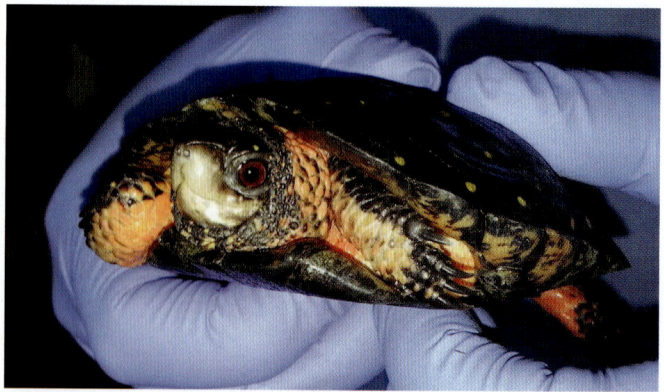

FIG 185.2 This North Carolina spotted turtle (*Clemmys guttata*) was injured by a motor vehicle and is undergoing rehabilitation. This species is listed as federally endangered in Canada, is protected in most US states, is being considered for US federal protection, and is listed as endangered by the IUCN. (Courtesy of Gregory A. Lewbart.)

TABLE 185.1   A Selection of National Wildlife and Welfare Legislation Relevant to Reptiles

Country	Wildlife	Welfare	Internet Link and References
Argentina	Ley Nacional 14.346 -de protección a los animales- Norma Argentina vigente	Law 14346 for the Protection of Animals	http://www.cmc.unl.edu.ar/docs/LEY%2014346.pdf
Bahamas	Wild Animals (Protection) Act (1968)	Animal Protection and Control Act 2010	http://laws.bahamas.gov.bs/cms/images/LEGISLATION/PRINCIPAL/1968/1968–0021/WildAnimalsProtectionAct_1.pdf http://laws.bahamas.gov.bs/cms/images/LEGISLATION/PRINCIPAL/2010/2010–0019/AnimalProtectionandControlAct2010_2.pdf
Brazil	Act No. 9.605 establishing sanctions against environmental illegal activities (1998)	Act No. 9.605 establishing sanctions against environmental illegal activities (1998), Article 32	https://www.animallaw.info/intro/brazil
Canada			
Federal laws	Canada Wildlife Act R.S.C., 1985, c. W-9 Species at Risk Act S.C. 2002, c. 29 Wild Animal and Plant Protection and Regulation of International and Interprovincial Trade Act S.C. 1992, c. 52 (WAPPRIITA) Wild Animal and Plant Trade Regulations 1996	Animal Welfare: Criminal Code RSC 1985 C-45, Sections 445–447	http://laws-lois.justice.gc.ca/eng/acts/W-9/ http://www.ec.gc.ca/alef-ewe/default.asp?lang=en&n=65FDC5E7–1
Provincial laws (provinces having legislation, e.g., British Columbia)	Wildlife Act [RSBC 1996] Cap 488	Prevention of Cruelty to Animals Act [RSBC 1996] CHAPTER 372	Canadian Perspectives on Animals and the Law. (2015) Editors Peter Sankoff, Vaughan Black and Katie Sykes. Irwin Law, Toronto Donihee J. (2000). The Evolution of Wildlife Law in Canada Canadian Institute of Resources Law, University of Canada http://dspace.ucalgary.ca/bitstream/1880/47200/1/OP09Wildlife.pdf
Jamaica	Endangered Species (Protection, Conservation and Regulation of Trade) Act, 2000	Cruelty to Animals Act Cap86	http://moj.gov.jm/sites/default/files/laws/Endangered%20Species%20%28Protection%2C%20etc.%20Act.pdf http://moj.gov.jm/sites/default/files/laws/The%20Cruelty%20to%20Animals%20Act.pdf
Trinidad and Tobago	Conservation of Wild Life Act, Cap 67	Summary Offences Act Ramnath K M (2012). Trinidad Guardian, January 8, 2012	http://rgd.legalaffairs.gov.tt/Laws2/Alphabetical_List/lawspdfs/67.01.pdf http://www.guardian.co.tt/lifestyle/sunday-january-8–2012/address-animal-welfare-legislation
International databases			
FAOLEX	Many references to reptile protection in the wild	Numerous animal welfare laws	http://faolex.fao.org/faolex/index.htm
Global Animal Law Project		GAL Matrix: Database of national animal welfare laws	https://www.globalanimallaw.org/index.html
Various countries, especially where legislation is not readily available	Individual countries are required from time to time to submit "Country Reports" to the United Nations or to the secretariat of treaties such as CITES or CMS May contain accounts of current legislation		
Wildlife International website	Lists wildlife laws of 32 countries and the EU		http://www.wildlifeinternational.org/EN/public/agencies/lawdetail.html
World Resources Institute	Main wildlife law Listed for 49 African countries		http://www.wri.org/resources/maps/rights-to-resources/laws-reviewed
Georgetown Law Library. International and Foreign Animal Law Research Guide		Selection of (non-US) national animal welfare laws	http://guides.ll.georgetown.edu/c.php?g=363480&p=2455777

Data courtesy of Margaret E. Cooper.

BOX 185.1   Wildlife Conservation Legislation Relevant to Reptiles in the Americas

Convention on Wetlands of International Importance, Especially as Waterfowl Habitat 1971 (Ramsar Convention)

Convention Concerning the Protection of the World Cultural and Natural Heritage 1972 (World Heritage Convention)

Convention on Trade in Endangered Species of Wild Fauna and Flora 1973 (CITES) (Washington Convention)

Convention on the Conservation of Migratory Species of Wild Animals 1979 (Bonn Convention)

Convention on Biological Diversity 1992 (Biodiversity Convention)

Courtesy of Margaret E. Cooper.

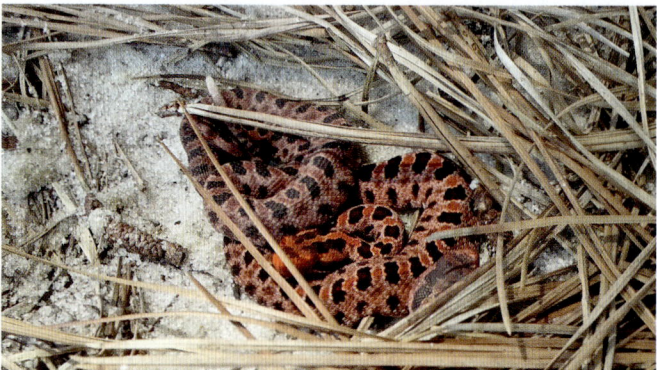

FIG 185.5 These hatchling pigmy rattlesnakes (*Sistrurus miliaris*) were found on a coastal North Carolina island and are protected in this state. (Courtesy of Gregory A. Lewbart.)

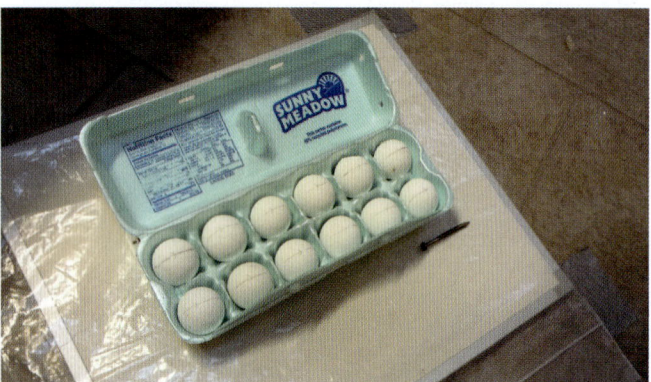

FIG 185.3 This polystyrene carton contains 12 loggerhead turtle (*Caretta caretta*) eggs prepared for radiography as part of a research project. This species is federally protected in the United States and most other countries. (Courtesy of Craig A. Harms.)

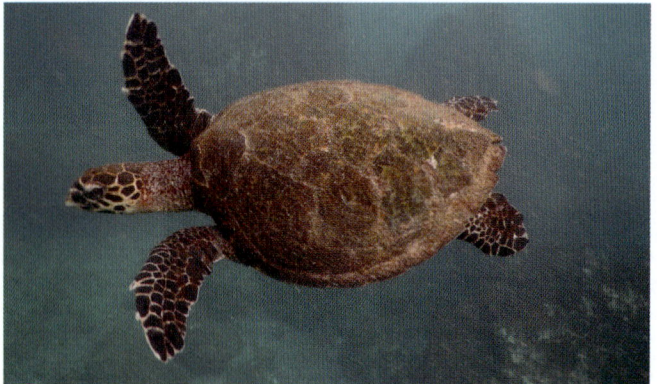

FIG 185.4 This adult wild hawksbill turtle (*Eretmochelys imbricata*) was photographed in the Galápagos Islands. The species is listed as critically endangered throughout its range. (Courtesy of Kelsey Stover.)

Management Authority, 4401 Fairfax Drive, Room 432, Arlington, VA 22203. Visit their website at http://www.fws.gov.

UNITED STATES FEDERAL REGULATIONS

Endangered Species Act

The US Endangered Species Act (ESA) is a federal act that was established in 1973 to protect rare animals and plants, both native and nonnative (see Figs. 185.1 through 185.5). The ESA has also been a model for state endangered species programs and serves as the state regulatory plan in those states without their own legislation. All species of included animals and plants are listed as either threatened or endangered. It also implements CITES in the United States (https://www.fws.gov/). The details of the ESA can be found in title 50, Part 17, of the Code of Federal Regulations (ref: 50 CFR 17). Special permits are required for just about any activity involving a listed species (currently 181 species of herptiles are listed). Some endangered herptiles are the Wyoming toad (*Bufo baxteri*), Shenandoah salamander (*Plethodon shenandoah*), American crocodile (*Crocodylus acutus*), leatherback sea turtle (*Dermochelys coriacea*), Jamaican iguana (*Cyclura collei*), and Puerto Rican boa (*Epicrates inornata*). Some threatened herptiles are goliath frog (*Conraua goliath*), loggerhead sea turtle (*Caretta caretta*), Turks and Caicos iguana (*Cyclura carinata carinata*), and giant garter snake (*Thamnophis gigas*).

Some "special rules" apply to certain situations involving threatened (not endangered) species. These rules eliminate the normal ESA permit requirements. Examples of these special rules include the American alligator (*Alligator mississippiensis*) (state laws apply) and by-catch (accidental capture) of loggerhead, olive ridley (*Lepidochelys olivacea*), and green sea turtles (*Chelonia mydas*).

National Marine Fisheries Service Regulations

The ESA regulations are enforced by both the United States Fish and Wildlife Service (USFWS) and the National Marine Fisheries Service (NMFS); USFWS has jurisdiction only when sea turtles are ashore. Incidental capture permits are required by fishermen who are likely to accidentally take sea turtles. Detailed requirements exist for handling both living and dead-by-catch sea turtles (50 CFR 222.50 and 227.72).

The ESA permits for endangered species are only granted for the following reasons: legitimate scientific research, propagation, species survival, and incidental take. Permits for threatened species may be granted for zoological exhibition, educational purposes, and those listed previously for threatened species. ESA and CITES permits are required for species subject to both documents (in the United States, a single ESA permit fulfills CITES requirements). The ESA only regulates transactions at the interstate level (intrastate commercial activities involving legally obtained species are not regulated by the ESA). Individual states may restrict commercial activity of threatened and endangered species.

Designated United States Ports of Entry

All wildlife entering the United States must do so via one of the following ports of entry unless specified otherwise (50 CFR 14.11 and 14.12):

Atlanta, Baltimore, Boston, Chicago, Dallas/Fort Worth, Honolulu, Los Angeles, Miami, Newark, New Orleans, New York, Portland (Ore), San Francisco, or Seattle. All wildlife shipments are subject to inspection by both the USFWS and the US Customs Service. Specific ports of entry exceptions exist for wildlife (not requiring special permits) originating in Canada and Mexico.

Special Turtle Regulations

The US Food and Drug Administration (FDA) and Public Health Service (PHS) regulate the import of any turtle under 4 inches carapace length and turtle eggs. Restrictions on foreign imports can be found in the PHS regulations (42 CFR 71). Six or fewer turtles and eggs can be imported without a PHS permit for noncommercial purposes. Seven or more turtles/eggs may be authorized with a permit if used for legitimate scientific, educational, or exhibition purposes. Interstate and intrastate transport is governed by the FDA (21 CFR 1240). No turtles of less than 4 inches carapace length, or turtle eggs, may be sold as pets in the United States. Exceptions include legitimate scientific, educational, or exhibition purposes. Confiscated turtles and eggs in violation are subject to humane destruction by the FDA. For more information, go to https://www.fda.gov.

US STATE LAWS

Most US states have their own laws governing the taking and keeping of native reptile species. Some states also regulate the sale and captivity of exotic amphibian and reptile species. See Box 185.2 for a complete listing of state regulatory agencies. Current websites have been included, because laws relating to herptiles are dynamic and the websites allow the interested reader to browse various pertinent web pages.

The Lacey Act (from the USFWS Website)

Passed in 1900, the Lacey Act prohibits import, export, transportation, sale, receipt, acquisition, or purchase of fish, wildlife, or plants that are taken, possessed, transported, or sold in violation of any federal, state, tribal, or foreign law. The 1981 amendments to the Act were designed to strengthen federal laws and improve federal assistance to states and foreign governments in enforcement of fish and wildlife laws. The Act has become a vital tool in efforts to control smuggling and trade in illegally taken fish and wildlife. Another aspect of the Lacey Act regulates the transportation of live wildlife, requiring that animals be transported into the United States under humane and healthful conditions. The Act also allows the interior secretary to designate those wildlife species considered injurious to humans and prohibit their importation into the country.

Individuals convicted of violating the Lacey Act may be fined up to $100,000 and sentenced up to 1 year in jail for misdemeanors and up to $250,000 and 5 years of imprisonment for felony violations. Fines for organizations in violation of the Act are up to $250,000 and $500,000 for misdemeanor and felony violations, respectively. In addition, vehicles, aircraft, and equipment used in the violation, as well as illegal fish, wildlife, and plants, may be subject to forfeiture. Persons who

---

BOX 185.2 United State Agencies That Regulate Herptiles

Alabama Department of Conservation and Natural Resources
Game and Fish Division
Law Enforcement Section
64 North Union Street
Montgomery, AL 36130
http://www.alabamaadministrativecode.state.al.us/docs/con_/index.html

Alaska Department of Fish and Game
PO Box 25526
Juneau, AK 99802-5526
www.adfg.state.ak.us

Arizona Game and Fish Department
Permits Coordinator
2221 West Greenway Road
Phoenix, AZ 85023
www.adfg.state.ak.us

Arkansas Game and Fish Commission
2 Natural Resources Drive
Little Rock, AR 72205
http://www.agfc.com

California Department of Fish and Wildlife
1416 Ninth Street
Sacramento, CA 95814
www.wildlife.ca.gov

Colorado Division of Wildlife
6060 Broadway
Denver, CO, 80216
http://cpw.state.co.us

Connecticut Department of Energy and Environmental Protection
Wildlife Division
79 Elm Street
Hartford, CT 06102
http://www.ct.gov/deep/site/default.asp

Delaware Department of Energy and Environmental Protection
Division of Fish and Wildlife
89 Kings Highway
Dover, DE 19901
www.dnrec.state.de.us/fw/index.htm

Florida Fish and Wildlife Conservation Commission
Bureau of Protected Species Management
620 South Meridian Street OES-BPS
Tallahassee, FL 32399
www.floridaconservation.org/psm

Georgia Department of Natural Resources
Wildlife Resources Division
Law Enforcement Section
2070 US Highway 278, Southeast
Social Circle, GA 30025
http://georgiawildlife.com

Hawaii Division of Forestry and Wildlife
1151 Punchbowl Street, Room 325
Honolulu, HI 96813
www.dofaw.net

Continued

BOX 185.2   United State Agencies That Regulate Herptiles—cont'd

Idaho Department of Fish and Game
600 South Walnut Street
PO Box 25
Boise, ID 83707
https://idfg.idaho.gov

Illinois Department of Natural Resources
Endangered Species Protection Board
524 South Second Street
Springfield, IL 62701
www.dnr.illinois.gov/ESPB/Pages/default.aspx

Indiana Department of Natural Resources
Division of Fish and Wildlife
402 West Washington, Room W273
Indianapolis, IN 46204
www.in.gov/dnr/fishwild

Iowa Department of Natural Resources
Fish and Wildlife Division
Law Enforcement Bureau
Henry A. Wallace Building
502 East 9th Street
Des Moines, IA 50319-0034
www.iowadnr.com

Kansas Wildlife Parks and Tourism
Law Enforcement
512 Southeast 25th Avenue
Pratt, KS 67124-8174
http://ksoutdoors.com

Kentucky Department of Fish and Wildlife Resources
1 Game Farm Road
Frankfort, KY 40601
www.kdfwr.state.ky.us

Louisiana Department of Wildlife and Fisheries
2000 Quail Drive
Baton Rouge, LA 70808
www.wlf.louisiana.gov

Maine Department of Inland Fisheries and Wildlife
284 State Street
41 State House Station
Augusta, ME 04333-0041
www.state.me.us/ifw

Maryland Department of Natural Resources
Wildlife and Heritage Service
Tawes State Office Building
580 Taylor Avenue, E-1
Annapolis, MD 21401
http://dnr.maryland.gov/wildlife/Pages/default.aspx

Massachusetts Division of Fisheries and Wildlife
251 Causeway Street, Suite 400
Boston, MA 02114-2152
www.mass.gov/eea/agencies/dfg/dfw

Michigan Department of Natural Resources
Mason Building
PO Box 30028
Lansing, MI 48909
www.michigan.gov/dnr

Minnesota Department of Natural Resources
500 Lafayette Road
St. Paul, MN 55155-4040
www.dnr.state.mn.us/index.html

Mississippi Department of Wildlife, Fisheries and Parks
1505 Eastover Drive
Jackson, MS 39211-6374
www.mdwfp.com

Missouri Department of Conservation
2901 West Truman Boulevard
PO Box 180
Jefferson City, MO 65102
http://mdc.mo.gov

Montana Department of Fish, Wildlife, and Parks
Law Enforcement Division
1420 East Sixth Avenue
PO Box 200701
Helena, MT 59620-0701
http://fwp.mt.gov

Nebraska Game and Parks Commission
2200 North 33rd Street
Lincoln, NE 68503
http://outdoornebraska.gov

Nevada Department of Wildlife
1100 Valley Road
Reno, NV 89512
www.ndow.org

New Hampshire Fish and Game Department
2 Hazen Drive
Concord, NH 03301
www.wildlife.state.nh.us

New Jersey Department of Environmental Protection
Division of Fish and Wildlife
PO Box 400
Trenton, NJ 08625-0400
www.state.nj.us/dep/fgw

New Mexico Department of Game and Fish
1 Wildlife Way
Santa Fe, NM 87507
www.wildlife.state.nm.us

New York State Department of Environmental Conservation
Division of Fish, Wildlife, and Marine Resources
625 Broadway
Albany, NY 12233-4750
www.dec.ny.gov

BOX 185.2 United State Agencies That Regulate Herptiles—cont'd

North Carolina Wildlife Resources Commission
Division of Wildlife Management
512 North Salisbury Street
Raleigh, NC 27604-1188
www.ncwildlife.org

North Dakota Game and Fish Department
100 North Bismark Expressway
Bismark, ND 58501-5095
https://gf.nd.gov

Ohio Department of Natural Resources
Division of Wildlife
2045 Morse Road
Building G
Columbus, OH 43229-6693
www.ohiodnr.gov

Oklahoma Department of Wildlife Conservation
1801 North Lincoln Boulevard
Oklahoma City, OK 73105
www.wildlifedepartment.com

Oregon Department of Fish and Wildlife
3406 Cherry Avenue NE
Salem, OR 97303
www.dfw.state.or.us

Pennsylvania Department of Conservation and Natural Resources
7th Floor Rachel Carson State Office Building
PO Box 8767
400 Market Street
Harrisburg, PA 17105-8767
www.dcnr.state.pa.us

Rhode Island Department of Environmental Management
Division of Fish and Wildlife
4808 Tower Hill Road
Wakefield, RI 02879
www.dem.ri.gov

South Carolina Department of Natural Resources
Rembert C. Dennis Building
1000 Assembly Street
Columbia, SC 29201
www.dnr.sc.gov

South Dakota Department of Game, Fish and Parks
523 East Capitol Avenue
Pierre, SD 57501
http://gfp.sd.gov

Tennessee Wildlife Resources Agency
Ellington Agricultural Center
PO Box 40747
Nashville, TN 37204
http://tn.gov/twra

Texas Parks and Wildlife Department
4200 Smith School Road
Austin, TX 78744
http://tpwd.texas.gov

Utah Department of Natural Resources
Utah Division of Wildlife Resources
1594 West North Temple
Salt Lake City, UT 84116
http://wildlife.utah.gov

Vermont Fish and Wildlife Department
Law Enforcement Division
103 South Main Street
Waterbury, VT 05671-0501
www.vtfishandwildlife.com

Virginia Department of Game and Inland Fisheries
4010 West Broad Street
Richmond, VA 23230
www.dgif.virginia.gov

Washington Department of Fish and Wildlife
600 Capitol Way North
Olympia, WA 98501-1091
www.wdfw.wa.gov

West Virginia Division of Natural Resources
Capitol Complex, Building 3, Room 663
1900 Kanawaha Boulevard, East
Charleston, WV 25305-0660
www.wvdnr.gov

Wisconsin Department of Natural Resources
101 South Webster Street
PO Box 7921
Madison, WI 53707-7921
http://dnr.wi.gov

Wyoming Game and Fish Department
5400 Bishop Boulevard
Cheyenne, WY 82006
https://wgfd.wyo.gov

Note: The United States Fish and Wildlife Service maintains a web database of state, territorial, and tribal organizations at http://offices.fws.gov/statelinks.html.

provide information on violations of the Lacey Act may be eligible for cash rewards.

CANADIAN FEDERAL REGULATIONS

Canada uses The Wild Animal and Plant Protection and Regulation of International and Interprovincial Trade Act (WAPPRIITA) for regulation and enforcement of its laws regarding both native and nonnative wildlife. The WAPPRIITA web address is http://www.ec.gc.ca/alef-ewe/default.asp?lang=en&n=65FDC5E7-1

Here is a summary of the WAPPRIITA from the website: "The Act applies to the following animal and plant species:
- Species on the Convention on International Trade in Endangered Species of Wild Fauna and Flora (CITES) control list;
- Foreign species whose capture, possession, and export are prohibited or regulated by laws in their country of origin;
- Canadian species whose capture, possession, and transportation are regulated by provincial or territorial laws;
- Species whose introduction into Canadian ecosystems could endanger Canadian species.

The Act forbids the import, export, and interprovincial transportation of these species, unless the specimens are accompanied by the appropriate documents (licences, permits). In all cases, the Act applies to the plant or animal, alive or dead, as well as to its parts and any derived products."

MEXICAN FEDERAL REGULATIONS

The United Mexican States (Mexico) has a rich native herpetofauna with the most reptile species of any country on earth.[1] Over half of the 700-plus species of reptiles are endemic, and along with its nearly 300 species of amphibians, Mexico contains nearly 10% of the earth's herpetofauna diversity.[2] Mexico has been a CITES signatory since 1991 but faces many challenges enforcing illegal trade in wildlife, including herpetofauna. For a thorough review of wildlife conservation in Mexico see Valdez et al. (2006).[2] The National Office of Wildlife, a division of the Ministry of Environment and Natural Resources, oversees wildlife management in Mexico. A copy of the laws pertaining to native wildlife is entitled: "NOM-059-SEMARNAT-2010, Environmental protection – Native species of Mexico forest flora and fauna – Categories of risk and specifications for their inclusion, exclusion or change – List of species at risk." The following link provides information on purchasing a copy of these regulations: http://mexlaws.com/SEMARNAT/NOM-059-SEMARNAT-2010.htm.

CENTRAL AND SOUTH AMERICAN REGULATIONS

There are 27 Caribbean, Central, and South American countries that all have their own laws and regulations regarding wildlife. All of these nations are CITES signatories. For those interested in specific information regarding a particular country, the Latin American Network Information Center provides a starting point: http://www.lanic.utexas.edu/la/region/environment/ (accessed April 15, 2018).

CASE EXAMPLES

Case 1

Facts: A 27-year-old Windsor Ontario man traveled to the United States by car on 6 occasions in 2014 to retrieve illegally taken native US turtles. He used various methods to smuggle the turtles out of Detroit and into China, including taping tutles to his legs and groin, packing them in boots and cereal boxes, and stuffing them into suitcases. The species

of turtles smuggled included the diamondback terrapin (*Malaclemys terrapin*) (see Fig. 185.1) and the spotted turtle (*Clemmys guttata*) (see Fig. 185.2), the latter being listed on the IUCN red list as endangered and the former as threatened. Sometimes the man smuggled the turtles himself and other times he employed a runner. On one occasion he was apprehended with 51 turtles on his person. Each count that the man pleaded guilty to carried a maximun $250,000 fine and 10 years in prison.
Laws violated: CITES, ESA, Lacey Act, and Michigan Wildlife Laws.
Outcome: The defendant was fined $3500 and sentenced to 2 years probation.

Case 2

Facts: In 2012, a 58-year-old Brunswick, Georgia, man was convicted of stealing 156 loggerhead sea turtle eggs (see Fig. 185.3) from nests on Salelo Island, Georgia. The eggs, with a black market value of $15 each, were packed to be sold.
Laws violated: ESA and Lacey Act.
Outcome: The defendant was sentenced to 6 months in jail and required to do 156 hours of community service, one for each egg.

Case 2a

Facts: In 2015, the same man as above (now 61) was convicted of stealing 84 loggerhead sea turtle eggs, again from nests on Salelo Island, Georgia. The eggs, now with a black market value of $25 each, were packed to be sold.
Laws Violated: ESA and Lacey Act.
Outcome: The defendant was sentenced to 21 months in jail, with a comment by the judge that the defendant's next stop would be federal prison.

Case 3

Facts: In 2013, a 28-year-old woman from New York was convicted of conspiring to smuggle 18,000 threatened and endangered reptiles from the United States into Canada.
Laws violated: CITES and ESA.
Outcome: The defendant was sentenced to 18 months in prison and 3 years of supervised release.

Case 4

Facts: In 2015, a 41-year-old man was charged with three counts of purchasing or threatening to purchase threatened turtles illegally captured from the wild. The case involved 100 North American wood turtles with a value of $40,000.
Laws violated: CITES, ESA, United States Postal Laws, and Illinois State Wildlife Laws.
Outcome: The perpetrator was sentenced to 41 months in jail, 3 years of supervised release, $100 special assessment, and was ordered to pay $41,000 restitution.

Case 5

Facts: In 2016, a California development company was convicted of securities fraud and violation of the Endangered Species Act. The company, as required by law, was supposed to mitigate for losses of wildlife and wildlife habitat. In this case it was for a 107-acre development in Contra Costa County. The developer attempted to defraud the city of Dublin with a forged receipt for $3.2 million.
Laws violated: CITES, ESA, and Lacey Act.
Outcome: In January 1999, the Florida businessman pleaded guilty to seven felony counts of conspiracy, smuggling, and violating the Lacey Act and CITES. In April 1999 he was sentenced to 30 months in prison. The conviction of the smuggler was made possible by Operation

Chameleon, a sting operation run by the US Fish and Wildlife Service with cooperation from authorities in Florida, Virginia, Canada, Germany, Mexico, The Netherlands, South Africa, Belize, and Japan.

Case 6

Facts: In 2012 a 63-year-old Tyler, Texas, ecotourism guide smuggled 7 live snakes from Peru into the United States. He purchased the snakes at a market in Lima and smuggled them to Dallas–Fort Worth airport via Lima and Miami. The snakes were illegally obtained and smuggled on his person. He was refused boarding on a Tyler Texas shuttle flight and after taking ground transportation was arrested at his home by Texas game wardens. The perpetrator knew what he did was illegal and was subject to 5 years in federal prison.

Laws violated: Peruvian wildlife laws and Lacey Act.

Outcome: The defendant was sentenced to 3 years probation by a US district judge.

Case 7

Facts: In 2013, eight people were arrested in Puerto Rico for the illegal take, possession, and sale of sea turtle parts intended for human consumption. DNA analysis by the Fish and Wildlife Service Forensic Laboratory identified 15 hawksbill (*Eretmochelys imbricata*) (see Fig. 185.4) and 7 green turtles (*Chelonia mydas*). Enforcement officers from the Puerto Rico Environmental Crimes Task Force, the Puerto Rico Police Department, the Puerto Rico Department of Natural Resources, and the US Marshals Service were all involved in the arrests.

Laws violated: CITES, Lacey Act, and ESA.

Outcome: The defendants faced a maximum 5 years in prison and a $250,000 fine if found guilty.

REFERENCES

See www.expertconsult.com for a complete list of references.

186

Forensics

John E. Cooper, Melinda Merck, and Margaret E. Cooper

This chapter is primarily directed at veterinarians who work with reptiles and amphibians (here referred to as "herpetologic veterinarians") but may also be of use to nonveterinarians, such as field biologists, herpetologists, zoological staff, experienced hobbyists, and lawyers who are asked to advise in this field. Forensic veterinary medicine can be defined as the application of veterinary knowledge to the purpose of the law. Although the use of veterinary forensic medicine is most commonly associated with providing evidence (to the prosecution or to the defense) in court cases relating to the maltreatment of animals or the protection of endangered species, it can also be applied to such matters as environmental impact studies, insurance claims, and allegations of professional misconduct.

Forensic work that involves reptiles and amphibians most often arises from prosecutions for ill-treatment or the smuggling of endangered species. Nevertheless, there are other circumstances in which expert veterinary evidence is required such as theft, keeping reptiles without, or in breach of, an appropriate permit or illegal taking from the wild or unlicensed trade. Public health prosecutions may arise from keeping reptiles and amphibians or from unauthorized importation as bushmeat. Reptiles may be implicated in human abuse situations, for example, the identification of wounds or the cause of injury or death. Civil law claims for compensation for death, personal injury, or damage to property involving reptiles may require an expert veterinary opinion, and likewise in the case of breach of contract, sale of goods, veterinary malpractice, and the verification of insurance claims.

Traditional uses of reptiles or amphibians present particular legal and ethical challenges and at times may lead to investigations and prosecutions under welfare or conservation legislation[1,2] (also see later discussion).

Cooper and Cooper discuss situations in which forensic investigations and evidence are relevant, and Baker provides a brief overview of forensic herpetology.[3-5] Reptiles and amphibians can be the subject of evidence submitted to planning inquiries where their presence on land proposed for development is significant and in cases where human health (especially zoonoses) or environmental pollution is an issue.

A reptile or amphibian may be involved in a potential legal case either as the *victim* or as the causative element (as the *perpetrator* itself or through the *agency* of a person). Investigations are most likely to address questions relating to species identification and origin, cause of death, injury or ill health, and determination of the cause and effects of diseases and wounds sustained by reptiles and amphibians as well as caused by them.

LEGAL CONSIDERATIONS

Some herpetologists and herpetologic veterinarians are aware of legislation that affects their professional activities concerning reptiles and amphibians. It is important that an investigator (expert) understand the particular legal basis of the case for which he/she is to provide evidence. They should also be aware of additional implications for the investigator, such as the welfare of a live animal being examined or the need for authorization to possess animals (particularly endangered species) or their derivatives (including diagnostic specimens) and to transport, store, or dispose of them.

General Legal Principles

Kinds of Law. It is important that the forensic expert is aware of some basic aspects of law such as:

a. Criminal law: Legislation that creates offenses. These are enforced by the state and punished primarily by fines and imprisonment;
b. Civil law: Cases between individuals or legal entities for which the remedies are financial compensation and injunctions;
c. Substantive law: The law upon which a case is based;
d. Procedural law: The rules that dictate how a court or other tribunal deals with a case.

Judicial Systems. In most countries there are separate court systems for different kinds of litigation, particularly civil and criminal. There are a variety of other tribunals for matters such as planning (zoning) and professional discipline. Each system has its own procedural rules, which may include specific instructions for expert witnesses.

The actual procedure regarding evidence varies from country to country. Most "common law" countries (i.e., those that have derived their judicial systems from England [British Commonwealth countries and the United States]) hold adversarial hearings in which either side presents its arguments and its expert evidence to a judge (or equivalent). However, "Roman law" countries (most continental European countries) practice a more inquisitional procedure whereby the presiding lawyer conducts the hearing, which may include expert evidence.

Relevant Law

Legislation is found at international, regional, national/federal, state/provincial, and local levels. For the most part the law that is used to enforce legislation is the national, state, or local laws (see Chapters 183 through 185).

In countries with a federal structure, most of the laws relating to reptiles and amphibians are made at state/provincial level. Consequently there is little uniformity at this level in the provisions, the enforcement powers, and their effectiveness. This is also true of the variability between the laws of different countries. It is therefore necessary to check carefully whether reptiles are included in the definition of "animal" in any piece of legislation. Likewise each law should be examined in detail to determine to what extent it applies to the species and issues in question. An experienced expert can guide a lawyer who is new to the law on animals.

Law relating to reptiles and amphibians is covered in some detail in Chapters 183, 184, and 185, which deal primarily with international, European, and American law, along with some examples of the welfare and conservation laws of other countries. For a more detailed discussion of the various topics with particular reference to forensic evidence, see Cooper.[6–8]

Comments on Aspects Particularly Relevant to Forensics

Conservation. The law generally provides protection for specified species that are at risk, usually in terms of prohibiting or regulating taking, killing, or injuring. Hunting and other harmful sports, trapping, or poisoning are often also controlled. Trade may be prohibited or regulated. All these offenses may require forensic evidence (for example, as to identification, harm caused, time of death, behavior, or ecology) when prosecuted or defended. Reptiles and amphibians dangerous to humans may not be protected in some counties (or even may be classified as vermin), or there may be an exception for self-defense.

Trade. Trade, both legal and illegal, in reptiles and amphibians is widespread. Some species (such as crocodilians) are valuable commercially for their skins or other derivatives or for traditional medicines; other taxa are popular for pets, exhibition, or breeding. Frequent reports of illegal trade are published by TRAFFIC (the wildlife trade monitoring network) and other organizations or governments. Forensic evidence on the identification and origin of confiscated species is required to support prosecutions (and the defense). Animal welfare offenses (including transportation) are often involved as well.

International Trade or Movement. Cross-frontier trade in reptiles and amphibians is common and frequently illegal[9,10]. The Convention on International Trade in Endangered Species of Wild Fauna and Flora (CITES) is a global treaty that regulates the movement of listed species, including many species of reptiles and amphibians (see the Chapters 183 through 185). Most federal countries regulate CITES through national laws, and the EU has regulations that directly apply in all member countries.

Animal Health. Reptiles and amphibians may require a health certification or veterinary check in some countries, and tissue and other diagnostic research or forensic samples might require a permit if they are thought to be pathogenic. Any samples that are being sent for forensic examination or other processes must be packed in accordance with national and international standards as appropriate.

Customs. Customs services may require the services of a forensic expert to verify the identity of imported species against the accompanying documentation. Deliberate misidentification of rare species is common. Dangerous reptiles are also used to disguise consignments of drugs. There are often welfare offenses in illegal consignments, and a veterinary expert may be asked to provide evidence.

Animal Welfare. The need to protect the welfare of captive reptiles and amphibians has long been recognized in Europe. In the UK the classes Reptilia and Amphibia received a level of protection 140 years ago, when they were included in the list of species subject to licensing if they were used for painful experiments in scientific research (Cruelty to Animals Act, 1876). Such protection for them under laboratory and field conditions continues under the UK's Animals (Scientific Procedures) Act 1986 and throughout much of the rest of Europe as a result of (for example) The European Convention for Experimental and Other Scientific Purposes (ETS). Such federal protections are currently lacking

in the United States, as reptiles and amphibians remain excluded from the Animal Welfare Act (1966).

The previous comments regarding the variability of legislation are particularly applicable to animal welfare laws. Many animal welfare laws apply to nondomesticated species that are held in captivity, but this and the specific definition of "animal" must be ascertained for each law. Welfare issues for which forensic evidence is required usually relates to designated forms of cruelty or the broader offense of "unnecessary suffering" such as pain, stress, neglect, or starvation. The modern New Zealand, United Kingdom, and some Australian state laws also impose a duty of care on the keeper of an animal to provide for its essential needs.[11,12,14] These principles are based on the widely used "five freedoms" (see http://webarchive.nationalarchives.gov.uk/20121007104210/http:/www.fawc.org.uk/freedoms.htm). These principles can be used as a benchmark in the assessment of the welfare to support expert evidence.

Animal welfare legislation includes the transport of animals that may apply to reptiles and amphibians. The IATA Regulations and the CITES Guideline for Transport are applicable to reptiles.

Reptiles and amphibians may be used in cultural or traditional activities, which may not meet their welfare needs; if the law does not provide adequate protection, education or public awareness may be considered as an alternative.[2] Information on the assessment of welfare of reptiles in captivity is to be found in Warwick et al.[13] Expert herpetologists and/or veterinarians may be able to provide evidence on needs and optimal environmental requirements of a particular species.[15]

Animals in Captivity. Many countries regulate the keeping of reptiles in captivity. Local authorities may license the keeping of reptiles as private pets or restrict the keeping of dangerous species.

Reptile and Amphibian Collections. The law on keeping reptiles and amphibians in captivity are covered in Chapters 183 through 185 and the literature referred to earlier. Situations that may be regulated include keeping animals as pets, as a hobby, for display or entertainment, and for research. Reptiles and amphibians may also be "hoarded," sometimes as part of a well-meaning but poorly executed rescue program. The standards set by law via zoo associations, both national and international, may provide useful criteria for forensic assessments on welfare and management.

Research. Animal research is regulated in many countries and also extends to work in the field where guidelines apply to work funded by the National Institutes of Health.[16] In the UK, new guidance has been issued regarding wildlife research.[17] Again, this may provide a useful benchmark.

Veterinary Treatment. Increasingly there are veterinarians available who specialize in the treatment of reptiles and amphibians and are able to provide expert evidence in the situations discussed earlier that require forensic evidence. Veterinary law restricts the practice of veterinary medicine to duly qualified persons. The British veterinary law expressly includes the treatment of reptiles as reserved to veterinary surgeons (veterinarians), but it is silent on amphibians. Other countries' veterinary laws may or may not be clear whether treatment of such species is restricted to veterinarians, and in many cases wildlife rescue and rehabilitation is often carried out by nonveterinarians. In the United Kingdom anyone may do this (within the bounds of welfare and other laws), but in some countries rehabilitators must be qualified and authorized.

The law on veterinary medicinal products is discussed in Chapters 183 through 185. Expert evidence might be required in cases where drugs for reptiles or amphibians were wrongly prescribed or illegal products were used.

Health and Safety. In countries where occupational health and safety laws are strict, special risk assessments (regarding handling, envenomation) and precautions may be necessary to protect employees and visitors (for example at zoos or petshops) from the hazards posed by some reptile and amphibian species.[18] Expert evidence may be required regarding the animal's health, welfare, biology, behavior, or management in the event of an accident.

Theft. Some reptiles and amphibians are extremely valuable and at risk of being stolen from private or public premises. Expert evidence may be sought regarding identification and origin of species of stolen animals as well as assessment of the time of theft, death or injury, welfare, or other circumstances.

PROVIDING EXPERT EVIDENCE

Experts on reptiles and amphibians may be needed at various stages of a legal process; in particular, when the investigation of a suspected offense requires herpetologic experts on identification or veterinary care (for example, the examination of the premises where reptiles or amphibians are alleged to be illegally kept). Additionally, experts on identification, handling, behavior, and veterinary care of involved species may be required to manage evidence at the crime scene[19] and to provide reports and oral evidence in the event of a prosecution.

Witnesses

A person may be called as a witness in a court case as either:
a. A witness of fact;
b. A professional witness who gives factual evidence but may also be asked to express an opinion;
c. A person with special expertise, who examines evidence, provides a report, and gives evidence in court that can include an opinion.

Quality of Expert Evidence

In Britain, the judiciary has set high standards for experts and their evidence as to quality, integrity, impartiality, and their duty to the court. In the United States, the "Daubert criteria" must be met before an expert is allowed to give evidence in federal courts and those of many states.[20] These provisions are incorporated in the procedural rules of the courts. Many experts now study, attend training or practical courses, and join schemes that verify their standards.[20–22] For more detailed accounts of forensic work relating to reptiles and amphibians and the provision of expert evidence, see Cooper.[7,20,23]

CONSIDERATIONS IN FORENSIC INVESTIGATION

Although many aspects of forensic work with reptiles and amphibians are very comparable to those that apply to work with domesticated animals, there are certain important differences. Some of these relate to the extent to which reptiles and amphibians are subject to legislation, especially in respect of their welfare and ability to "suffer"; the differences in this respect between (for example) the United Kingdom (UK) and the United States (US) are outlined previously.

Another important difference relates to differences in anatomy and physiology. These can be significant in forensic studies, even within groups of mammals and birds[3,24,62] but are particularly important in reptiles and amphibians, not least because all such species are ectothermic. This will influence such parameters as speed of wound healing and response to insults ranging from pathogens to poisons. This may have to be carefully explained to a judge or jury and outlined in written reports.

In addition there are anatomic variations that may be relevant to forensic examination (both clinical and postmortem) and the

interpretation of the significance of wounds and other lesions. The herpetologic veterinarian will be aware of these variables but others, including clinicians, pathologists, and laboratory-based personnel who are more familiar with domesticated mammals, may need to be reminded of the basic features outlined in Section 2.

Clinical Investigation

A useful compendium of clinical techniques used in herpetologic forensic work was provided by Mitchell and Hernandez-Divers,[25] who emphasized the range and complexity of methods now available. In all investigations—clinical, postmortem, laboratory—as full a history as possible is desirable. Often in forensic work a comprehensive history is not available because the animal (when found or seized) has clinical signs or is dead, and there may (or may not) be an owner or keeper who can provide background information.

Even if history is supplied, it may not be correct and can even be fabricated, so the clinician has to perform an examination on an animal without knowing the true background. The information offered is the initial context for the examination and analysis of findings but may change as the investigation unfolds.

Certain key details should be recorded when the veterinarian is first contacted regarding a case, by telephone, by text/email, or when the animal is first presented. See Box 186.1, an intake form that is adapted from a document designed for suspected cruelty cases but can be modified to suit other forensic investigations, such as those relating to possible breaches of conservation legislation.

The intake form initiates documentation of the case and continues throughout the case (see Documentation of Examination Procedures). The notes made on the form should be factual; they will be used to produce a forensic report. The veterinarian may need to rely upon them if called to testify, and the notes may eventually be requested by lawyers or the court. The date, time, agency (where appropriate—in Europe there may not be an agency involved), case number, name, and contact information of the person who first contacted the veterinarian should be recorded.

As emphasized elsewhere,[28] information should be obtained regarding the type of reptile or amphibian to be examined, how it is being transported, general details of the alleged crime, what is expected of the veterinarian, and a likely time frame to produce findings. The veterinarian should request from the investigator such documents as incident reports, witness statements, photographs, and videos. The number, condition, and quality of these documents should be noted, and each item recorded in the evidence log (see Box 186.2).[29]

The documentation of information is discussed later, as it applies not only to live reptiles and amphibians but also to dead animals and samples. For the same reason, evidence collection and packaging are covered later.

Regardless of species, the animal should initially undergo a full basic clinical examination, similar to that performed during a (diagnostic) veterinary investigation. This means that the animal is examined systematically, even though there may be an obvious presenting wound or lesion of probable importance (Fig. 186.1). Equipment should be available before the examination begins, and the choice may be influenced by the history or allegation.

Use of a clinical record sheet is essential and, like the necropsy sheet (see later), is often best compiled specially for the forensic case rather than relying upon a standard clinical form, which may or may not permit answers to be given to specific questions of forensic importance.

Descriptions for forensic purposes need to be as accurate as possible (they may be checked by someone else). Measurements are important and some "scoring" system is recommended when there is a need to quantify. Color codes are useful and can also be used to help describe

BOX 186.1 Intake Questionnaire for Reptiles/Amphibians

Officer's name: _____ Contact info: _____

Agency (if appropriate): _____ Date and time of arrival: _____

Animal ID/name: _____ Species: _____ Breed: _____ Sex: _____

Status (circle): Stray Abandoned Seized (owned) Seized (relinquished)

Describe cruelty or other offense suspected: _____

_____

Current investigation findings, including any statements (attach officer's report where available): _____

_____

Medical history info: _____

_____

Photos/videos: Copies provided: _____ To be provided: _____ Chain of custody form signed: _____

Date and location animal removed from/found: _____

Animal's demeanor at scene and any changes: _____

Environment description: Indoor/outdoor: _____

Weather/temperature conditions/source of heating/temperature gradient:

_____

Food: _____ Water: _____ Feces/urine: _____

Describe housing conditions, type of shelter, and confinement:

_____

_____

Cleanliness/hygiene: _____

Other animals on premises: _____

Scene description/findings (include physical, biological evidence, weapons, bloodstains):

_____

_____

_____

BOX 186.2 Evidence Log/Chain of Custody (COC) Record for Reptiles/Amphibians

Agency (if appropriate): _____

Case number: _____ Evidence holding location: _____

Item ID: _____ Evidence description: _____

Date: _____ Initials: _____

Purpose of removal/tests performed: _____

Removal date: _____ Receipt date: _____

By _____ By _____

Release Signature: _____ Receipt Signature: _____

feces, urine, and so on. Objectivity is enhanced if reference can be made to colors on a chart (such as those used by purveyors of paint). The consistency of, say, feces can be difficult to describe, and it can be helpful to use a grading system (usually 1–5, liquid–solid) advocated by some of the nutritional companies.

If accurate weights and measurements are to be taken, appropriate equipment will be required.

For reptiles, snout-vent length (SVL) and vent-tail length (VTL) are required. A whole-body length is to be discouraged because of the

possibility of tail damage (see previous). Care must be taken when straightening the animal (putting the animal into a plastic tube will help).

For tail-less species of amphibians (frogs and toads), SVL is required. For tailed amphibians (newts, salamanders, and tadpoles), SVL and VTL are recommended.

A rule with stop is advisable. Take care as discussed previously.

Defining and assessing "condition" is never easy. The definition and determination of "condition" in nondomesticated species can be difficult.

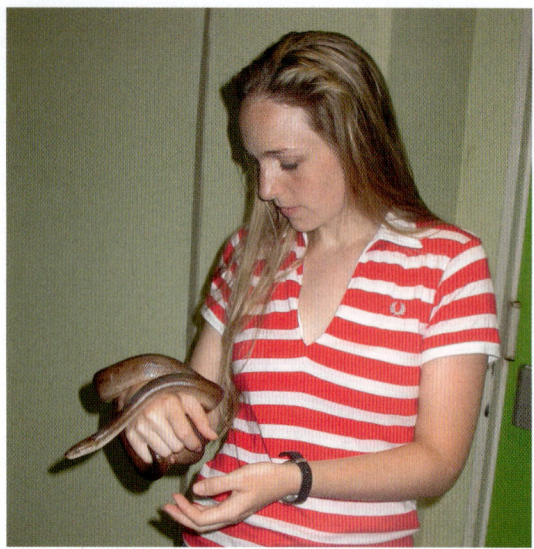

FIG 186.1 Clinical examination should include careful handling. Poor muscle tone may be an indicator of malnutrition or a toxicosis.

"Condition" is an ambiguous term, because it is commonly used both as an indicator of an animal as a whole and also parts of the body (e.g., "condition of the plumage"). Land tortoises and other chelonians present particular problems in terms of assessing "condition" because of the presence of a protective, often hard, carapace and plastron. There are various methods applicable to different taxa of reptiles and amphibians (see, for example, Hailey[31] on Mediterranean tortoises).

Examination of the forensic case brings with it some extra considerations that may not be part of normal clinical investigation. Record-keeping should be meticulous, and contemporaneous notes are essential (hard copies and/or computerized). Investigations or tests may be carried out that would not form part of a normal standard clinical examination; samples should therefore always be taken (see later). With the exception of special issues of *Applied Herpetology* and the *Journal of Herpetology* mentioned in the references, there are relatively few published texts dealing specifically with the forensic clinical examination of reptiles and amphibians. Standard texts on herpetologic diseases are of relevance, and the "expert" appearing in court should not overlook the fact that some excellent texts are published in languages other than English (see, for example, reference 32).

Any veterinary practitioner may be requested to carry out an initial clinical examination of an animal, including a reptile or amphibian, which might be the subject of a legal case. Under such circumstances the veterinarian, who may well not have any specialist postgraduate training, must do his or her best. Some general rules are as follows:

1. Carry out as full and methodical an examination as possible in the time available and with the equipment that is available.
2. Pay particular attention to any organ systems or parts of the body, which may be particularly relevant to the case.
3. Depending on species, certain structures may be particularly relevant to a forensic case (see earlier). Thus for example, when examining a neotenous amphibian, the gills will need careful inspection.
4. If time, facilities, or the veterinarian's lack of experience of the species in question limits a full examination, this should be stated in the report. It is preferable at an early stage to admit that certain examinations were not carried out (or feasible) rather than for this to come to light during cross-examination in a court case or similar hearing.
5. As in all aspects of forensic examinations, detailed contemporaneous notes should be taken together with, as appropriate, tape recordings (audio and/or video) and photographs.

As stressed earlier, reptiles and amphibians are ectothermic, and therefore all metabolic processes are temperature-dependent; see, for example, the earlier work by Smith et al[33] (1988) on the effect of ambient temperature on healing cutaneous wounds in garter snakes. The clinical investigation of an animal cruelty case was extensively covered by Merck et al.,[34] Munro and Munro,[35] and Tiplady,[36] but these authors concentrated on (mainly domesticated) mammals.

Clinical examination alone is usually only one part of forensic investigation. It can be linked with:

- Hematology
- Clinical chemistry
- Parasitology
- Microbiology
- Histology
- Cytology
- Electronmicroscopy
- Radiology and ultrasonography
- Other advanced imaging (e.g. magnetic resonance imaging [MRI], computed tomography [CT] scan)

It is most important that all observations made during a clinical examination are noted and that they, together with verbal comments made by those present during the work, are added to any letter or certificate. Precision is vital.

Veterinarians are increasingly playing an important role in cases involving animal abuse and domestic violence. This followed in the wake of awareness of "battered-pet syndrome,"[37] similar in a number of respects to "battered-child syndrome" and defined by physical abuse characterized by injuries that are nonaccidental—in other words, they have been inflicted intentionally. Suspicion of "nonaccidental injury"(NAI) is often supported by a number of factors, including unusual distribution or appearance of wounds, untreated lesions, an inconsistent history, and suspicious behavior on the part of the owner. Although most of the focus of debate about NAI has been on dogs and cats, they are not the only species that may be abused. Examples of abuse of captive and free-living reptiles and amphibians include:

- *All species:* Physical assaults (e.g., beating with sticks, gouging of eyes), use of fire, (including fireworks), intentional starving, deprivation of water, neglect.
- *Reptiles:* Disemboweling, cutting/pulling off the tail. Predators, for example, crows, may also cause disemboweling. Some lizards shed their tail as a natural defense process (autotomy).
- *Amphibians:* Disemboweling, removal of/damage to limbs by cutting or treading on them, placing toads in a fire to see them "explode."

Reptiles and amphibians that are alleged to have been starved may be examined/seen alive, necessitating clinical examination, or presented dead, necessitating postmortem examination. In view of the particular importance of the subject in respect of animal welfare, starvation is considered here, as a clinical matter, rather than under postmortem examination. It is important to bear in mind that apparent starvation can be due to a variety of causes, not just omitting food. In captive reptiles and amphibians, it can be the result of one or more of the following):

- Failure of the keeper to provide any food or to provide sufficient food in terms of quantity and quality (see later)
- Failure of the animal to accept food, in part or in whole, despite food being offered; failure of the animal to masticate and swallow food, even though food has been offered and, perhaps, taken initially
- Food not remaining within the stomach (on account of regurgitation or vomiting); food not being adequately digested and absorbed in the intestinal tract (because of malabsorption, increased gut transit time, internal parasites, etc)

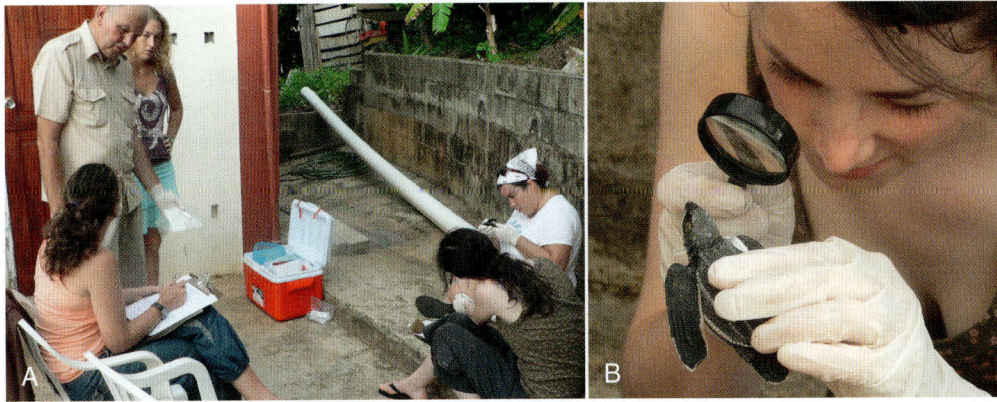

FIG 186.2 (A) Investigation of deaths of hatchlings of leatherback turtles (*Dermochelys coriacea*) in Trinidad and Tobago necessitated immediate action before the bodies began to decompose. This meant recruiting students to help and performing "forensic" examinations in situ, with minimal back-up facilities. (B) A vital initial step in such an investigation is to use a hand lens to examine eyes, skin, and orifices before they dry in the tropical heat.

- Food that has been ingested, digested, and absorbed not being utilized because of metabolic or other disorders

The veterinarian should also remember that reptiles and amphibians, especially the larger species, or those that are maintained at low temperatures, can often go long periods (weeks or months) without feeding, even in the wild.

POSTMORTEM INVESTIGATION

Postmortem examination (necropsy) of reptiles and amphibians plays an important part in certain forensic investigations, especially where there is a need for information about the circumstances of death or whether an animal was in poor health, suffered, or was abused during life (Figs, 186.2 and 186.3). Postmortem examination is an important part of herpetologic forensic work but presents many challenges, not least because of the gaps in our knowledge insofar as interpretation of pathological changes is concerned.[39] This applies also to domesticated mammals.[38] Ideally forensic necropsies should be performed by experienced pathologists, but this is not always possible and the veterinary practitioner must be familiar with proper necropsy procedures.

Necropsies need to follow standard protocols and use appropriate equipment (Fig. 186.4). As emphasized earlier, reptiles and amphibians vary in shape, size, and structure, with great differences exhibited by the diverse species, and thus the person performing the necropsy must have some knowledge of the normal features of these ectothermic species and be familiar with the principles of comparative anatomy (Figs. 186.5, 186.6, and 186.7). Sometimes in legal cases only a portion of a carcass is available, or it consists only of bones plus or minus portions of soft tissues that may have become desiccated and "mummified." Such material requires particularly careful handling and the use of special techniques such as slow rehydration to allow proper examination. Other submissions may essentially be a "soup" of autolyzed material, requiring filtering and sequential drying. No material submitted for necropsy should be considered "unsuitable for examination"; at the very least, it can be radiographed to examine for skeletal trauma, bullets, or implants. On occasion the necropsy will entail careful examination of prey items such as rodents or invertebrates.

Supporting laboratory tests may be required, and it is important that material is maintained, both for production in court and as part of a forensic research and teaching collection. Often a dead reptile or amphibian needs to be investigated, with a view to determining the

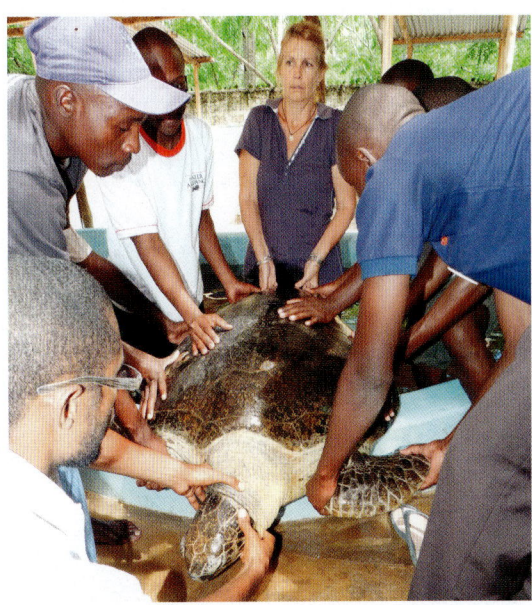

FIG 186.3 "Stranded" sea turtles, such as this green turtle (*Chelonia mydas*) in Kenya, should always be considered potential legal cases. Attention to them must bear this in mind and be performed in a forensic manner.

circumstances—cause, mechanism, and manner—of death. A convenient way of doing so is by trying to answer the following questions about the animal:

- How did it die?
- Why did it die?
- When did it die?
- Where did it die?
- Who might have been involved?

Forensic postmortem examination of wildlife was discussed by Wobeser,[42] and the subject was subsequently reviewed by Cooper and Cooper.[3] There are useful published methods for necropsy (see, for example, Hanley and Hernandez-Divers[43] for reptiles and Pessier[44] for amphibians). Cooper described postmortem techniques for herpetological forensic work,[23] but the diversity in morphology exhibited by diverse species means that the prosecutor must always be innovative

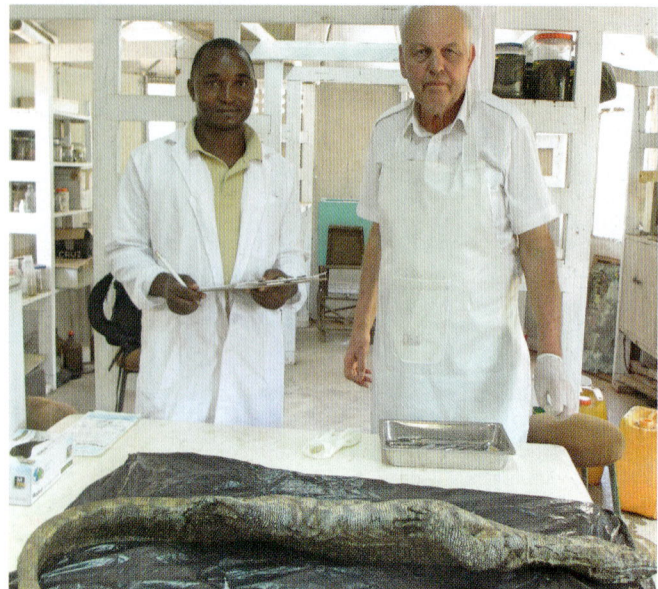

FIG 186.4 A monitor lizard (*Varanus* sp.) is examined postmortem in a simple laboratory in East Africa. One person remains "clean" and serves as scribe.

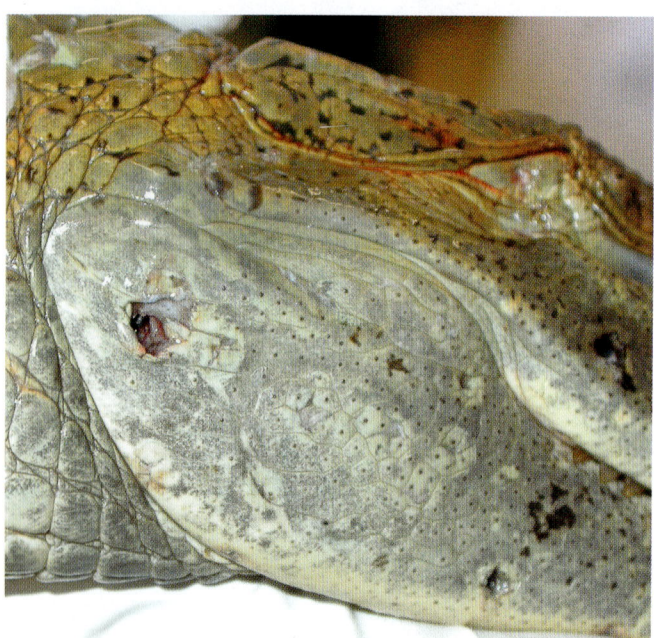

FIG 186.5 Postmortem examination of this spectacled caiman (*Caiman crocodilus*), which died under suspicious circumstances, revealed no significant internal changes, but a small lesion was detected on the side of the head. Probing indicated a deep stab wound and led to investigation of husbandry methods and interrogation of the keeper.

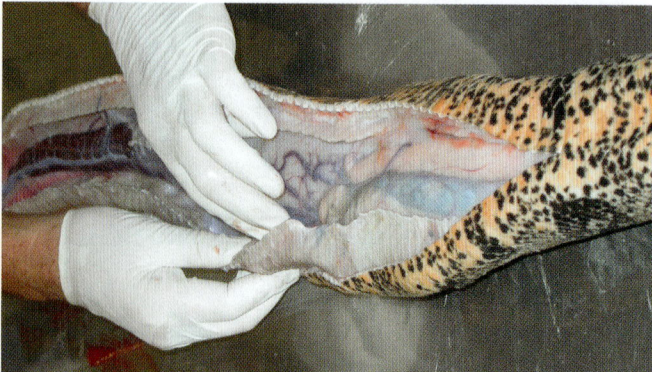

FIG 186.6 Assessment of condition of a reptile at necropsy should include detection, palpation, weighing, and histologic examination of internal fat bodies.

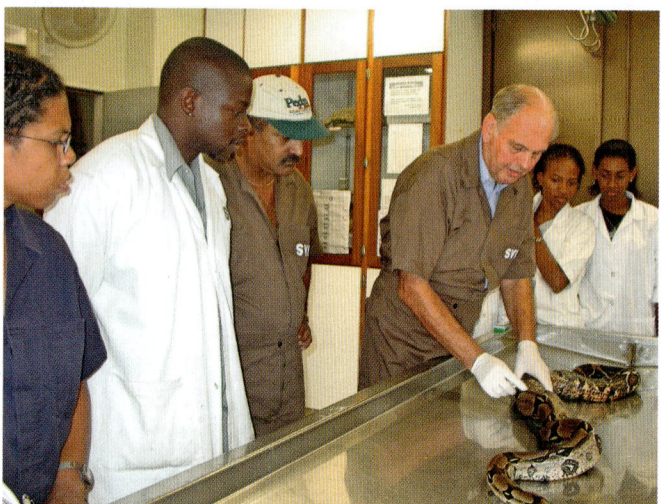

FIG 186.7 A red-tailed boa (*Boa constrictor*) is carefully examined externally. The animal died unexpectedly in a zoo and foul play was suspected. Students attend and learn at first hand routine forensic techniques.

and adaptable. Radiography or other imaging should be carried out whenever possible before postmortem examination.

The forensic necropsy of embryos, eggs, fetuses, and neonates needs special care because of their size (dissection may need to be carried out using microinstruments, such as ophthalmological scissors and forceps, and employing a loupe or magnifying [hand] lens) and some of their unusual features (e.g., osteoderms, gills).

A suggested format for a necropsy examination is provided in Box 186.3. Sometimes different headings and information may be

needed—and can easily be added to the form—for example, when embryos, tadpoles, or eggs (including spawn) are being examined. In herpetologic forensic investigations examination may take place in a purpose-built postmortem room or, especially in "wildlife crime" cases, require the construction of field necropsy area in the bush or by the side of a river. Field necropsies are discussed in Cooper.[9]

The health and safety (H&S) of those performing the necropsy, or likely to be exposed to it or the samples it yields, is of great importance. In many countries this is a legal requirement (see Chapters 184 and 185). All necropsies carry certain standard risks, but reptiles and amphibians may present some extra dangers—for example, venom from snakes/lizards and skin toxins from amphibians. Hazards presented by reptiles and amphibians during necropsy can be broadly divided into (a) infectious, for example, bacteria that may be acquired from the tissues of the dead animal and (b) noninfectious, such as injuries sustained while attempting to cut through the dorsal bony plates (osteoderms) of crocodiles or the bridge between the plastron and carapace in chelonians.

The interpretation of necropsy findings in reptiles and amphibians requires some knowledge of the normal morphology of reptiles and amphibians, for example, the normal presence of two hemipenes in snakes and lizards and the normal black appearance of the liver

BOX 186.3   Forensic Necropsy Examination Form for Reptiles/Amphibians

Submitted by: _____ Species: _____

Reference number: _____ Free-living/captive/captive-bred: _____

Other references: _____ (Amphibians) Juvenile (tadpole)/Immature/Mature: _____ Age: _____ Sex: _____

History (clinical signs, morbidity, mortality, therapy, previous laboratory results, samples sent elsewhere.): Use separate sheet if necessary. _____

_____

_____

_____

Specific request (circle): Cause of death   Cause of ill-health   Background pathology   Other legal/forensic request

Any other special instructions or requests: _____

_____

Date and time of submission to pathology (postmortem) laboratory: _____

Storage before submission: _____

Died/euthanized (date and time of death): _____ Method of euthanasia: _____

Date and time of postmortem examination: _____ Participants, including observers: _____

Gross Postmortem Report

Body weight (g): _____

Measurements: Body length (cm): _____ Snout-vent (SV) (cm) _____ Vent-tail-tip (cm): _____

Other measurements (cm): _____

Condition score (C.S.): _____ Autolysis score (0/1/2/3): _____ Postmortem interval (PMI): _____

External (general): _____

Specific comments on integument: _____

Internal (general): _____

Digestive system: _____

Liver: _____

Cardiovascular system: _____

Spleen/other lymphoid tissues: _____

Necropsy/other nos: _____

Respiratory system lung(s)/gills: _____

Musculoskeletal system: _____

Urinary system: _____

Nervous system: _____

Endocrine system: _____

Reproductive system, including comment on status (gravid, spawn present, etc.): _____

_____

Organs of special senses (including pineal, neuromasts, etc.): _____

_____

Comments on specific organs (e.g., cloaca, paratoid/poison glands): _____

_____

Specimens Selected for

Microbiology: _____ Parasitology: _____

Histopathology: _____ Toxicology: _____

Photography: _____ Radiography: _____

Other, including DNA (specify): _____

Macroscopic findings/gross/preliminary report: _____

_____

Other comments/follow-up work needed: _____

_____

SCRIBE (where appropriate), PATHOLOGIST, and DATE

_____

NA, Not applicable; *NAD*, no abnormalities detected; *NE*, not examined.
1–3 = Minimal, moderate, marked; score changes where appropriate.

in some amphibians and reptiles due to the presence of melanin (easily confused by inexperienced pathologists during postmortem autolysis).

Some changes in organs and tissues can be of particular significance in forensic cases (e.g., traumatic lesions and degenerative changes suggestive of toxicosis). Others, such as bile-staining and pseudomelanosis, are regularly seen features of postmortem autolysis and can be useful in assessing when a reptile or amphibian died or the sort of environment to which it was exposed after death. Skin wounds, contusion, and scarring may provide information about pathologic processes in the animal antemortem. As stressed earlier, reptiles and amphibians are ectothermic, and therefore all such processes are temperature dependent.[33] After the main necropsy and collection of samples, the skeleton of the animal may need to be prepared and examined for further forensic study.

Forensic entomology is important in animal forensic investigations,[3,39] mainly in helping to ascertain how long an animal has been dead. Insects are the prime indicators, as they are in human work, but millipedes, spiders, ticks, and mites can be significant. Any invertebrate found on, in, or in association with a dead reptile or amphibian should be collected and identified and (where appropriate) its stage of development recorded (e.g., a nymphal tick or first-instar maggot). Techniques for sampling invertebrates are to be found in standard texts and described in detail by Barnes[45] and Anderson.[46]

Comparable specialized techniques may also be needed when examining other samples found in association with a dead reptile or amphibian. These include the collection for investigation of (a) plant material, including pollen and seeds (forensic palynology) and (b) mineral deposits, such as dust. Sampling for toxicologic analysis can be challenging; Rotstein provides useful guidance.[48]

Determining when an animal died is often very relevant in forensic work but can be far from easy,[3] especially when dealing with reptiles and amphibians, where published data on postmortem interval (PMI, or time since death estimations) are still scant. Some limited information exists, notably by Frye, who described changes that occur after deaths in reptiles and amphibians (Frye, Proc Association of Reptilian and Amphibian Veterinarians, 1999, pp 23–25), and the paper by Cooper, outlining current knowledge and needs as far as the estimation of PMI in these species.[50]

Reptiles and amphibians present a range of challenges in terms of accurately assessing changes due to autolysis and decomposition, owing to their high variability in morphology and lifestyle; in particular, effects due to ectothermy, the different anatomical features of these two groups of vertebrates, the marked variation in body size of diverse taxa of reptiles and amphibians, and seasonal fluctuations in subcutaneous and internal fat content. Eggs, embryos, fetuses, and larval stages in amphibians present particular challenges.

The postmortem examination of reptiles and amphibians can provide useful information in support of a claim that an animal has been ill-treated but, often this evidence has to be linked with other data on (for example) how the animals have been housed, fed, and handled.

LABORATORY INVESTIGATIONS

Laboratory investigations are an important part of many forensic cases and are applicable to cases involving live or dead reptiles and amphibians. Some of the techniques used are almost entirely laboratory-based—for example, histopathology, toxicology, and DNA technology—but in herpetological work, the investigators are likely to be using a combination of such tests and the evaluation, often in the field, of a live or dead animal or its derivatives. "Derivatives" in a herpetological context include samples that are not a feature of standard mammalian forensic work,

such as urates, frog spawn, and shed (sloughed) skins (Fig. 186.8). Gross and microscopic examination of these materials, including a range of laboratory tests, can be useful and is noninvasive.[51] Techniques of particular value in herpetologic forensics include investigation for ectoparasites, chemical analysis of sloughs for pesticides,[52] and both morphologic and genetic studies for identification purposes.[53]

Molecular techniques have become a feature of forensic investigations concerning reptiles and amphibians in recent years.[54] Various tissues can be sampled, in both live and dead animals. Fetzner[56] described a simplified method for the extraction of high-quality DNA from shed reptile skins. Care must be taken during postmortem examinations not to spread or mix DNA from different sources (see also later discussion).

The two key factors in laboratory forensic work are (a) chain of custody and (b) quality control. The answer to all procedures is to develop and use protocols, whereby the method to be used is clearly defined and followed and will be adhered to in the same way thereafter. Techniques that may be used for samples from live or dead animals or, in some cases, from their environment, were discussed by Cooper and Cooper.[3,39] While many standard procedures are applicable to reptiles and amphibians, some may need modification; for example, microbiological culture may need to be incubated at 24°C.[55] Frye described methods for sampling and standard laboratory techniques in herpetologic forensic work.[56] It is important to use an appropriately accredited laboratory (veterinary/medical/forensic) whenever possible, as results may be challenged. This is sometimes not feasible, however, especially when dealing with wildlife overseas.

Correct sampling will yield reliable results and in turn facilitate accurate interpretation followed by appropriate action. In "forensic" cases such precision is all-important. Mistakes can occur at various stages of sampling (selection, collecting, packing, transportation, reception, processing). An error, inconsistency, or delay at any point can have adverse effects subsequently and thereby prejudice results.

Laboratory techniques cannot be discussed in detail here. Many, but not all, are similar to those used in mammals and birds. The small size of many reptiles and amphibians means that some specimens, such as tiny geckos and tree frogs, may be best embedded, serially or step-sectioned, and then processed for histologic examination.

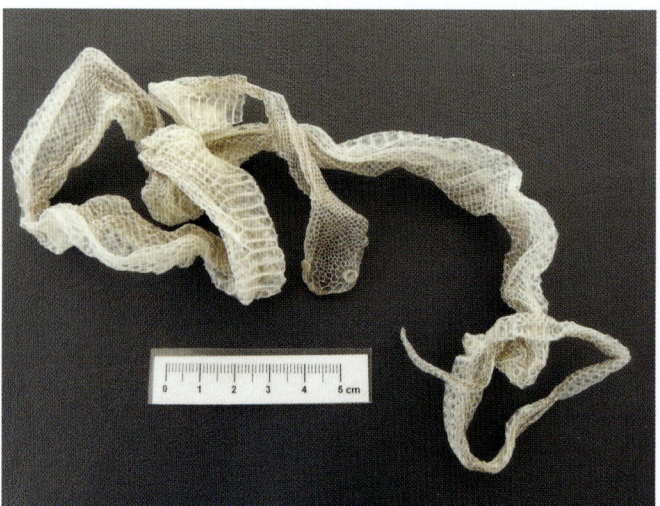

FIG 186.8 The shed skin of reptiles—and to a certain extent of amphibians—can be an important source of information in forensic cases. Such material must be handled with gloves and stored correctly.

CRIME SCENES, FIELDWORK, AND IN SITU COLLECTION OF EVIDENCE

Crime scene investigation in animal forensic cases has been discussed in various veterinary texts, most relating to domesticated species. The particular features of the wildlife crime scene investigation, which is often the norm insofar as reptiles and amphibians are concerned, were detailed by Cooper et al.[57] and by Byrd and Sutton.[58] In such circumstances the "crime scene" may range from just the carcass of an animal—or its parts—to terrain that encompasses topography as varied as coastline, forest, or desert. Often, the location of the wildlife crime scene is isolated, with few facilities for proper investigation and collection of evidence.[59] In poorer parts of the world and in countries that are experiencing social unrest, crime scene investigation may present particular challenges. Equipment, investigative techniques, and scientific technology all need to be appropriate to, and the best available in, the circumstances. Effective investigation under field conditions is likely to require a combination of portable and easy-to-use laboratory equipment, coupled with modern methods of data collection and information transmission.[9]

A whole spectrum of evaluation and interpretation may be needed in wildlife crime scene investigation, and often the veterinarian is working as part of a team. His/her responsibilities may include clinical or postmortem examination of reptiles and amphibians, searching for samples of poisons, correct sampling for toxicologic analysis, and investigation of vegetation, soil, or water. Knowledge of natural history is helpful in wildlife forensic work, as the animals involved may range from terrestrial or arboreal lizards to stranded marine turtles. An interdisciplinary approach is essential. Biologists/naturalists and those experienced in health studies, especially epidemiology, can often usefully complement the role of the police, enforcement officials, and crime scene specialists.[62] Such visits may take the forensic veterinarian to locations as diverse as petshops, zoos, homes of hobbyists, and airports, as well as habitats referred to previously.

RECORD-KEEPING AND COLLATION AND ANALYSIS OF FINDINGS

The forensic examination is a process that requires appropriate, accurate, and full documentation. As stressed by Merck and Mader, everything associated with the case is subject to legal scrutiny that includes all notes, correspondence, photographs, radiographs, examination findings, reports, and the handling of evidence.[28] These are all considered evidence and will be reviewed by the investigator, prosecutor, defense attorney, barrister, and judge. The use of forms is extremely useful in forensic cases to ensure procedures are followed completely and to meet the legal standard for evidence; these include chain of custody/evidence log, photo log, and live and necropsy examination.[28]

CHAIN OF CUSTODY

All evidence must be subjected to a chain of custody (COC). COC refers to a process of documentation in which the evidence is accounted for at all times, and there is a record of any alteration or deviation (for example, when testing is performed) (Appendix 3, Evidence Log/Chain of Custody). Evidence is anything collected or recorded from the animal and includes samples, photographs, radiographs, and the animal itself (Fig. 186.9).

All evidence must be properly collected, packaged, and labeled, and each item must be recorded in the evidence log. Evidence should be kept in a locked cabinet with restricted access. If the evidence is transferred to another person, location, or laboratory, this must be

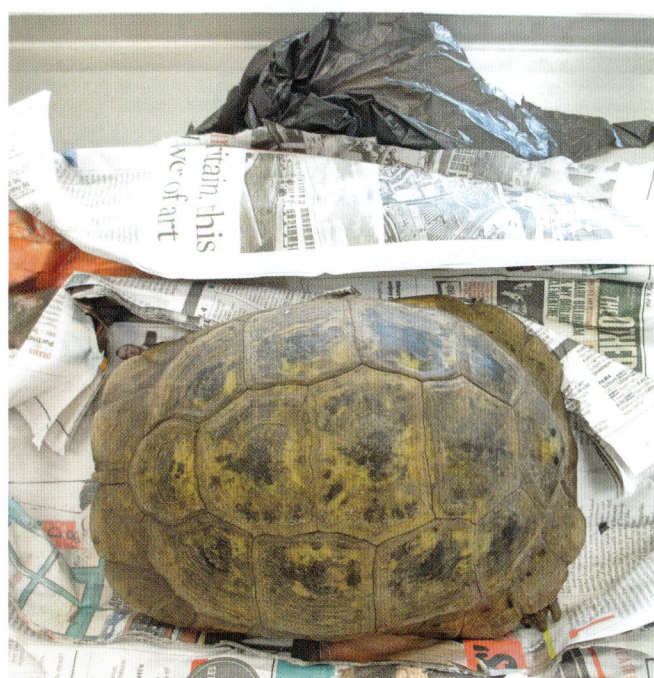

FIG 186.9 In possible legal cases involving necropsy, the packaging material and wrappings must be retained as they may provide forensic evidence and might need to be produced in court.

recorded in the evidence log with the time, date, and a signature from the sender and/or recipient.

Whenever evidence needs to be transferred elsewhere, including the transportation of laboratory samples, COC must again be followed. An evidence receipt form should be sent along with the evidence, containing instructions for the receiving agency/person to complete the COC section and return a copy. It should be recorded on any test request form whether the samples are "evidence," "forensic samples," or involve a "criminal investigation." This information may assist the recipient laboratory to implement appropriate handling protocols and to assign the appropriate person(s) to the analyses.[28]

If evidence is removed from storage, it should be documented in the evidence log, including a note of the purpose, if opened, and of any testing or alteration. Evidence must be held until the court case is over. Because additional legal avenues may be pursued after a case is closed, the prosecuting or other appropriate authority should be consulted before disposing of any evidence.[3,28]

PHOTOGRAPHY AND VIDEOGRAPHY

It is desirable that photographic records, together when appropriate with video documentation, should be kept of all forensic examinations on live or dead animals. This may not always be practicable when investigating free-living reptiles and amphibians under field conditions. The type of camera used is important, and some of the particular precautions that must be taken when photographing cases that are the subject of a legal investigation were described by Merck and Mader.[28] To these can be added the challenges of photography in the field, in cases of wildlife crime. Photographing and examining dead animals and other sensitive material at the crime scene is then best carried out without the attention of on-lookers or the press. Privacy screens may be purchased as such or constructed using canvas or sacking and aluminum poles or strong canes. Camera accessories, including tripods, facilitate the photographing of material that is illuminated with blue light. The use of reflective ultraviolet photography in forensic work is often now standard.

Video documentation is often valuable when examining live reptiles and amphibians, especially when an animal shows difficulty in performing certain functions, such as a snake with neurological or ambulatory signs. In mammals it also helps demonstrate certain types of behavior, such as vocalizing because of pain; these are not usually a feature of herpetological cases, but snakes may hiss or strike or feign death and amphibians secrete excess mucus. Some reptiles and amphibians change color in response to aversive stimuli. If starvation or dehydration is suspected, it is useful to video the animal's response when it is first offered food and water. The same evidence procedures as for photography should be used.[28]

DOCUMENTATION OF EXAMINATION PROCEDURES

When an animal is examined in a forensic case, live or dead, the veterinarian is working on behalf of the court, and there must be full documentation of all the findings, positive and negative. From a legal standpoint, it is likely to be assumed that "it is not documented, it was not done." There should be both written and photographic documentation, but the latter may not always be feasible when investigating free-living reptiles and amphibians under field conditions. It may also be helpful to have a recording device available during examination to permit dictation of findings.

Imaging, including radiography, are important, especially when animal abuse is suspected. Digital radiographs are preferred (although not always possible in poorer countries or under field conditions). If digital radiography is performed, CD copies should be made following the photography protocol advocated by Merck and Mader.[28] Hand-drawn diagrams may be used to document injuries such as bruising and wounds.

Some general considerations should be taken into account for all written documentation.[3] Leaving blank areas on forms should be avoided; *N/A* or a strike through the item should, instead, be used if no entry is required. Editorial remarks on the record should also be avoided. Any errors should be corrected by drawing a single line through the entry, marking it "error," and dating and initialing it.[28]

Details of the headings on the examination form will not be given here as they are featured in Appendix 2, Forensic Necropsy Examination Form for Reptiles/Amphibians.

When a dead animal is received, details of the external and internal packaging are recorded, and photographs should be taken as each layer is removed. Any tears or leakage of the packaging material should be noted, as well as a comment on the degree of decomposition (see PMI). Courier information on the package should be photographed and, if feasible, removed and placed in the case file.[28] All packaging should be retained as possible evidence.

The question of euthanasia is complicated, and the guidelines differ according to the country's laws and veterinary professional regulations.[3] Awareness of the need to relate methods to the specialized features of reptiles and amphibians—for example, the resistance of the nervous tissue of some species to hypoxia—led to guidelines in the UK nearly 30 years ago. Permission for euthanasia may need to be sought. An exception may include a situation in which the animal is in critical condition, and euthanasia is urgently required on humanitarian grounds. These issues, together with the question of the release and disposal of the animal's body, were discussed by Merck and Mader.[28] Specific guidance on forensic record-keeping and the documentation of samples in the context of reptiles and amphibians was given by Hart and Budgen.[60]

THE FORENSIC REPORT

Report-writing has been discussed in various veterinary texts, mainly relating to domesticated species, most recently in the book by Bailey[61] and the chapter by Cooper and Cooper.[62] In the context of reptiles and amphibians it is among topics covered in Chapter 187. Merck and Mader[28] emphasized the importance of the expert's report, stressing that it is written for the whole community: law enforcement agencies, prosecutors, both defense and prosecution lawyers, defendants, judges, and juries.

Merck and Mader stressed that the purpose of the forensic report is to provide a clear understanding of the veterinary evidence.[28] It should include information provided by investigating authorities and/or anyone else involved in the investigation, examination findings, procedures, samples/evidence collected, test submissions and results (medical and forensic), medical diagnoses, treatments and outcomes, and conclusions. Terminology is important in the forensic report, as in the oral presentation of evidence. Some of this relates to medical language, some to the use of words. International differences have to be taken into account, especially in legal cases relating to CITES (see earlier). For example, in most of North America the term "turtle" is used for any chelonian. In Britain, other parts of Europe, Australasia, and some of Africa, a "turtle" is a marine (sea) chelonian, a "terrapin" is a fresh-water chelonian, and a "tortoise" is a terrestrial species.

One issue that deserves further mention here—and which is often a very important point in the forensic report—is the manner or "circumstances" of death.[28] Traditionally, the classifications in humans are homicide, suicide, accident, natural, or undetermined. In animals, the categories often used are nonaccidental, accidental, natural, or undetermined. Alternatively, the questions referred to earlier, under the section Pathology and Postmortem Examinations, can be employed and may prove more intelligible to the court.

THE COLLECTION AND PACKAGING OF EVIDENCE

Appropriate equipment is needed for evidence collection and packaging. Some standard materials are available, such as those in the Animal Cruelty Forensics Kit for veterinarians, available from Tri-Tech Forensics (tritechforensics.com) in the United States. Often, however, especially when investigating possible breaches of conservation or animal welfare law concerning free-living reptiles and amphibians, the veterinarians must fashion their own.[39]

Different types of evidence require different types of packaging and storage. The packaging chosen should be appropriate in size and material for the particular item and should be clean or new to avoid contamination. The goal is to preserve the integrity of the evidence. Clean paper evidence bags and envelopes are preferred over plastic, which may allow moisture to build up over time, thus causing damage. However, plastic storage has been shown not to degrade DNA for up to 3 months (Wilson et al, Proc American Academy of Forensic Sciences, 2010, pp 178–179).

Each item of evidence should be packaged separately. If it is wet or moist, it needs to dry fully. Fragile items should be packed carefully to prevent damage in handling and transport. Gunshot projectiles should be collected with the use of plastic instruments or gloved fingers to prevent damage to any ballistic evidence. They should then be placed in a cardboard box so that damage or marks to the surface are prevented. Small items such as hair or fibers should be placed in coin envelopes or pharmaceutical folds.

Samples from stains of biologic origin may be collected using sterile swabs. For dry stains, a wet–dry technique may be used. Dry swabs may be placed in a paper envelope. If the swab is wet, it should be allowed to air-dry or be placed inside a swab box, which allows the swab to breathe and dry safely. The entire swab box is then placed inside a paper envelope or bag to protect it from contamination while drying.

Arson evidence requires special packaging to prevent vapors from escaping or being absorbed (as occurs when plastic containers are used). Instead, clean unused metal paint cans or special arson packaging containers (available from evidence collection supply companies) should hold the evidence.

Forensic entomology was briefly discussed earlier (see also Barnes[45]). Properly used, it has the greatest potential to provide an accurate time of death. It may also provide information on the time of injury when maggots are found on live animals (myiasis). The documentation, collection, and packaging of insect evidence differs from that of other types of evidence. Collection should include all the different types of insect evidence, including adults (imagines). The oldest life cycles should always be among those collected, because they probably represent the earliest time of insect arrival and colonization. Detailed information about the collection and storage of dipterous larvae and pupae (puparia) is given by Anderson[46] and Barnes.[45]

DNA testing is commonly performed in forensic cases for species determination or when individualization is needed for a match to a questioned sample. The identification of species is especially important in the illegal trade of animals.[3,59] DNA technology and its applications to herpetologic research and forensic investigations involving reptiles and amphibians were described by McDowall.[54] Genetic methodologies in wildlife crime investigations, many of them applicable to reptiles and amphibians, were described in detail by Robinson.[63]

All evidence needs to be properly sealed, not only to protect it but also to indicate readily if its integrity has been maintained.[64] Evidence tape is made to easily tear and is not meant to hold bags closed or boxes together. Packing tape may be used to seal containers, and evidence tape may then be placed over it. The person who packaged the evidence then signs or places his or her initials and the date across the tape.

The package should be properly labeled with the evidence number, case number, date, collection location, description of the item, time collected, collector's name, and signature. If the evidence contains biological fluids or tissue and/or poses a potential hazard to humans, it should be marked with a biohazard label. Each item of evidence is assigned an evidence identification number, and all of it is recorded in the evidence log (see Box 186.2). Chain of custody procedures should be followed, and any transfer, storage, or transport of the evidence must be documented. Reference should be made to documentation, earlier, and to Frye,[56] who described sampling and standard laboratory techniques in herpetologic forensic work.

RETENTION OF FORENSIC EVIDENCE AND OTHER MATERIAL

As emphasized earlier, the retention of material is wise, sometimes essential, because it is likely to constitute evidence. There are three aspects:

1. the storage of everything received, including wrappings, pending a court case where such evidence may need to be produced;
2. the specific selection of relevant specimens for production as evidence (e.g., a piece of damaged carapace);
3. when circumstances, especially legal considerations, permit, the curating and cataloging of appropriate material, after the court case, as "reference" or "voucher" specimens. Cooper et al.[65] discussed the relevance of such reference collections to zoological medicine and conservation biology.

SERVING AS A WITNESS AND APPEARING IN COURT

This important aspect of forensic work is covered in Chapter 187 on Jurisprudence, Expert Reports, Testimony, and Court Appearance by Lawton.

CONCLUSION

Herpetologists and veterinarians who have special knowledge of, and skills with, reptiles and amphibians can make a valuable contribution to forensic evidence. An understanding of the relevant legislation will both enable them to perform their duties more effectively and to comply with necessary legal requirements in preparing and delivering herpetologic forensic evidence.

REFERENCES

See www.expertconsult.com for a complete list of references.

187

Jurisprudence, Expert Reports, Testimony, and Court Appearance

Martin P.C. Lawton

Medical jurisprudence has been defined[1] as the science that applies the principles and practice of the different branches of medicine to the elucidation in judicial proceedings of questions relating to the cause or effect on the legal status of an individual's mental or physical disease or injuries. Despite the age of this definition, it is still pertinent.

Guidance on medical jurisprudence provided to the court is usually by a suitably qualified professional referred to as the "expert witness." Experts were first used in legal matters in the 14th century.[2] The evidence given by medical experts is classed as "opinion" evidence. It consists of the expert providing conclusions (as a scientist) drawn from certain facts, which had been or are supposed to have been proven.[1]

The term "expert" may be misleading, because it means that only by training or experience the witness is qualified to express an opinion, which an ordinary person may not.[2] The acceptance of a witness as an "expert" is ultimately the responsibility of the court (e.g., judge or bench) to decide.

PRINCIPALS OF BEING AN EXPERT WITNESS

A veterinarian may be a witness in a court proceeding in a variety of roles and not always as an expert. A working knowledge and understanding of current regional legislation is advisable when undertaking any potential legal work. Confidence in medical witnesses may be eroded by miscarriages of justice caused by misleading and flawed evidence.[3] Especially true when medical witnesses support conclusions out of synch with their peers or appear to have their own agenda. The roles a veterinarian may be asked to assist with in a court or arbitration include the following:

1. A witness of fact, where the veterinarian may have witnessed an event and be called on to give details of the event. Being a "witness of fact" does not necessarily imply or require the veterinarian to have any special knowledge or experience other than being able to truthfully report events they have witnessed.
2. A professional witness, where a veterinarian is asked to be a witness by virtue of their profession. This does not necessarily require specialist knowledge or experience beyond that expected of a competently qualified veterinarian. The "professional witness" is also a witness of fact and is expected to be able to report on matters experienced but also draw limited conclusions based upon their direct experience only.
3. An expert witness, where a veterinarian may not necessarily have been a witness of fact but by virtue of their qualifications and experience is asked to assess all evidence and draw a conclusion (known as an "opinion") usually in a preprepared report. The expert witness should be prepared to be challenged by the conclusions drawn and be able to defend their assumptions and conclusions under cross-examination.

An expert will most often be called on by either a prosecuting body or, after charges are filed, by the defense team. However, it is important to remember that any expert approached to ultimately assist the court in reaching a decision must remain neutral to either party.[4] Irrespective of what type of witness a veterinarian is when involved in a case, there are a number of golden rules, the most important of which is to not state anything that is not true or is not capable of being supported with argument.

EXPERT REPORTS

The ability to recognize neglect from cruelty can be difficult[5] and will often be the contested issue before the court that requires expert witnesses.

It is standard practice for the expert witness to prepare a detailed report providing information and facts and an "opinion" based on these details to assist the court in understanding scientific facts and to draw a conclusion (verdict). All potential legal cases will require a detailed report, which also acts as a statement of events, findings, and opinions. To prepare a report, further research and consulting with colleagues may be required.[6]

Irrespective of which side calls ("instructs") the expert, they should be nonpartisan[2] and be mindful that they should be working as advisors for the court to help in reaching a fair and correct decision. This is a concept that goes against human nature (not to pick and fight for a side) and must always be forefront in the mind of any expert.[4] Opinions must therefore always be accurate, fair, and, above all, defendable if challenged. A true expert must be able to see matters from both sides and include a weighed opinion in the report, avoiding bias.

All reports prepared by an expert will be subject to legal and critical scrutiny, often with the assistance of another expert ("for the other side"). An important aspect of preparing a report is never to say anything that is either outside of your area of expertise or that you will not be able to later defend and support when challenged.

The most important thing to remember when preparing a report is that it will contain your views and it is what you will be questioned on if the matter comes to court. Your report will be used to establish your "Evidence in Chief." In court you will have access to your reference material, any contemporaneous notes, records, photographs, or other items that you used to formulate your report. This is helpful because it is not unusual for the final court hearing to be many months to years after the original matter or your report was written.

In structuring the expert report, it is standard to include the following:

1. Your full name, qualifications, and details of experience pertinent to the case.
2. A brief curriculum vitae (CV) showing your general experience and supporting why the court should accept you as an expert.
3. Details of the instructions (from the solicitor or attorney), including any specific points on which you have been asked to address or comment or any scenario that you have been asked to consider (especially common when called by the defense).

4. A list of the information (evidence) with which you have been provided (e.g., other witness statements, photographs, videos, laboratory reports, contemporaneous records of interview, etc.).

5. A statement as to whether you have examined the animal(s) involved and details of your involvement and assessments.

6. Conclusions (opinions) drawn from the information provided to you or that can be reasonably drawn from the circumstances of the case.

7. A "statement of truth" and that the conclusion and opinions drawn are within your knowledge. You should also state the facts you have relied on if not already stated.

8. A copy of any references utilized in the making of the report.

The use of technical terms and abbreviations should not be used (unless clearly explained) because the report should be written for a lay audience.[4]

EXAMINATION OF ANIMALS

Although it is not necessary for the expert to have actually examined any of the animals involved in a case, it is always desirable that there be a veterinary report of an examination that can be referred to later. The veterinary examination of live animals should be prompt and as near to the dates of the potential offense as possible. When there is a body(s) involved, a postmortem examination may be delayed or performed at a more convenient time as long as correct storage is maintained to preserve forensic material.

The examination of live or dead reptiles should be thorough and information recorded at the time of evaluation. Recorded information may be written, in a bound notebook (to prevent the accusation of pages being removed or replaced), or digitally recorded (analog is also acceptable) either as a voice recording or a video recording. If the examination is being video recorded, it is important for the clinician to demonstrate what they are doing and point out any abnormalities found so these can be recorded. The video or voice recording may well be presented in court as evidence, and it is import to be mindful that any comments made are appropriate and descriptive and not open to criticism. The recorded examination (in whatever format) will be considered as contemporaneous notes and can be referred to both in the preparation of a report (usually copies are appended to this) and later in court. Any examination records, even if not actually used in court, will need to be provided and disclosed to the other party in case they wish to introduce them as evidence.

In addition to the standard examination covered elsewhere in this book, the veterinarian should always be mindful of the additional requirements necessary in undertaking a forensic examination. For example, it is important to not just record abnormalities but also describe the body systems examined, or not examined, and list any samples taken or additional investigations performed. It is important when recording numerical information, such as lengths, weights, temperatures, and more, to describe with what degree of accuracy this information was collected and detail any equipment used (and if that equipment has been calibrated recently) (Fig. 187.1). If a video recording is not utilized then photographic records of any pertinent findings are important so that reference can be made to this within the report. When taking photographs, it is also important to have identification data such as the case number, specimen number, date, and often a form of measurement in clear view in the images (Figs. 187.2) (especially useful for postmortem examinations or when an abnormality is being recorded).

When samples (blood, feces, swabs, body tissues, etc.) are taken and submitted to an outside laboratory, it is important that there is an effective and unchallengeable "chain of custody." This will start with the veterinarian or technician giving each sample a unique code (usually

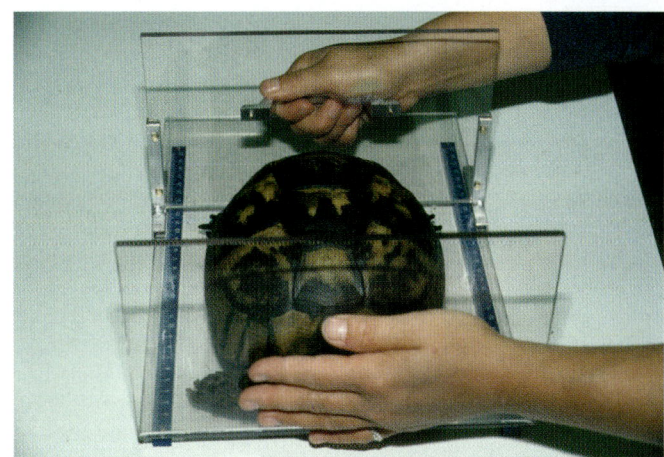

FIG 187.1 Taking an accurate length measurement of a tortoise. (Courtesy of Martin P.C. Lawton.)

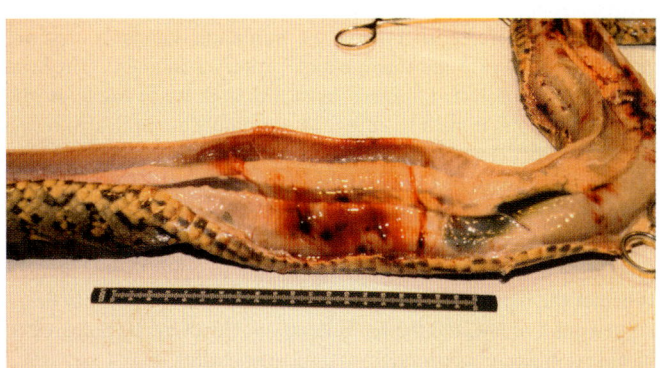

FIG 187.2 Post mortem examination showing "hand-shaped" bruising to a snake caused by rough handling in a cruelty case. (Courtesy of Martin P.C. Lawton.)

the initials of the person taking the sample followed by a number and sometimes the time and date), which is recorded on an "exhibits list" with a description of the sample and method of preservation (if any) that will be appended to the final report. The unique sample number should be used thereafter in any laboratory request form, delivery, and receipt, and should appear on any laboratory report subsequently produced. The method of transporting the sample (courier, in person, or recorded post) should be documented and signatures obtained from all those involved in the process, including the acceptance and processing at the laboratory. It is advised to make contact with a laboratory before the samples are sent to make sure they are aware it is a legal (or potentially legal) case and that they should follow chain of custody protocols.

REPTILE WELFARE AND SUFFERING

A useful summary of many of the laws affecting zoo and wild animals in the United States and elsewhere[7] are given in Chapters 183, 184, and 185.

The involvement of animals in legal situations has been previously considered,[8,9] but a reptile may be either the direct object of the criminal action or the indirect object involved in a nonassociated criminal activity.[4] The direct involvement may be associated with the intrinsic value of the reptile, its rarity (including export or import restrictions and Convention and International Treaty in Endangered Species [of Wild Fauna and Flora] [CITES] requirements), or the potential dangerous nature of the animal and legal restrictions in ownership.[4] However, the largest categories in which a veterinarian as an expert witness will become involved are the welfare and "unnecessary suffering" categories of the various Animal Welfare Acts (where or if they exist).

The use of reptiles and amphibians indirectly in crimes is often encountered when there is a potentially "dangerous" or "fearsome" animal that can be used to reduce the possibility of a certain area (usually the vivaria) being fully searched as part of a criminal investigation (e.g., for stolen goods or drugs).[4] It is rare, but a reptile may also be used as a "dangerous" weapon to cause harm or even death to another human being. The legislation that restricts the ownership of venomous or dangerous reptiles in many countries substantially reduces the risk of the latter being realized, but it is always a possibility.

The welfare categories may not be a deliberate act of neglect or cruelty but have resulted by a lack of understanding the proper care of a reptile; this is known in legal terms as a "failure to meet the needs of that animal." Keeping reptiles or other ectotherms in captivity, compared with mammals and birds, requires an exacting environment and sometimes unusual nutritional requirements often not provided by the owner, leading to suboptimal health and welfare concerns.

Animal welfare legislation set the minimum standards that are expected for the care and treatment of "protected animals."[7] The legal definition of "protected animals" is varied, and, for example, in the United Kingdom, it must be either (1) commonly domesticated in the British Islands; (2) under the control of humans whether on a permanent or temporary basis; or (3) is not living in a wild state.[10] The regional definition of what is a "protected animal" is therefore very important because, in effect, animal welfare legislative requirements (including preventing unnecessary suffering) may not always apply to wild reptiles. Whether the reptile involved is a "protected animal" or not may be an argued point of law, and the veterinarian should always be prepared to be able to make an appropriate argument regarding this.

The welfare categories are linked to the "five freedoms," which are listed as follows:

1. **Freedom from hunger and thirst.** Provided by a ready access to fresh, clean water and a suitable diet appropriate to maintain health and vigor.
2. **Freedom from discomfort.** Provided an appropriate safe environment, including appropriate temperature, humidity, shelter, and a comfortable resting area.
3. **Freedom from pain, injury, or disease.** Provided by frequent checking (ideally daily) and examination of the animal and promptly seeking veterinary advice or treatment as required.
4. **Freedom to express normal behavior.** Provided by appropriate housing, including keeping in suitable and compatible groups such that the animals can act normally or as near to normal as possible.
5. **Freedom from fear and distress.** Provided by appropriate housing away from predators, dominant or noncompatible cage mates and appropriate human/animal interactions.

The unnecessary suffering categories of the various animal welfare legislations are often an important area in which the veterinarian will be asked to define, confirm, and sometimes argue for or against. Questions often posed in courts that the expert may have to answer include whether reptiles do or do not suffer or how they can suffer when they are considered a "lower" vertebrate. Or another argument, less commonly encountered, but just as important: "Do reptiles experience pain?" In both situations, veterinarians typically discuss the scientific literature (e.g., various volumes of *Biology of the Reptilia*) and how these confirm that the nervous pathways of reptiles have been extensively studied and shown to be similar to those of mammals, and thus reptiles can suffer and feel pain. However, the question of what is "pain" may arise and may need to be discussed in court. The accepted definition of pain is "a physiological state caused by any unpleasant sensory or emotional disturbance associated with actual or potential tissue damage." It has been an all too regular defense, especially in chronic neglect cases, that because there may be no pain involved, then there could not be any suffering, thus implying that there cannot be suffering without pain. The legal definition (set by precedent as a ruling in a higher court in the United Kingdom) is that unnecessary suffering "imports the idea of the animal undergoing, for however brief a period, unnecessary pain, distress or tribulation"[11] and clearly sets out that although pain can be part of suffering, suffering can still occur without the involvement of pain. Morton and Griffiths[12] have prepared guidelines on the recognition of pain, distress, and discomfort that may be referred to in support of an expert's argument and conclusions.

The proof of "unnecessary suffering" can sometimes be more difficult to establish, because this requires not only a deliberate act of causing harm to a reptile but the understanding by the perpetrator that such an action will, or would be likely to, result in pain, discomfort, or lasting harm (e.g., suffering). The ability of a person having the understanding of the likelihood of suffering to have occurred or be likely to occur is known in legal terms as malfeasance, and the state of mind of knowing the consequence of particular actions is referred to as "mens rea," which is translated as guilty knowledge or intention to commit a prohibited act. The court often looks to the veterinary expert to qualify any, or the degree of, suffering, and whether it was anticipated or avoidable and thus was unnecessary or not.

COURT APPEARANCE AND TESTIMONY

It is the authors' experience that a court appearance to support the opinions and facts stated in the "expert report" are required in less than 10% of the cases instructed. Once an expert report has been prepared and examined by both parties it may be decided that:

1. there is insufficient evidence for there to be a case (charges) to answer;
2. there is a case to answer but there is an acceptable reason to be offered in mitigation (defense);
3. that the evidence and expert's report is accepted such that the person(s) culpable of the offense (PCO—defendant) offers a plea of guilty ("no contest"); or
4. that charges are laid and the defendant pleads not guilty and a court/tribunal hearing is required.

It is only for the last point (4) that the expert is likely to be called to make a court appearance and give testimony. There are rare situations when even at this point, the expert may not need to attend court, because the expert's report may be "accepted" by both sides and will be put to the court untested (or with agreed redactions). The latter is usually where there are mitigating circumstances raised by the defense that will be argued in court that do not need the involvement of the expert.

Preparation before any court case is required, including taking any pertinent references or text books. The expert may also need to produce secondary or rebuttal reports, depending on any new evidence or other expert reports that are disclosed during the lead-up to the court hearing.

In court, an expert may be asked their opinion on facts established or hypothesized based upon the evidence.[2] It is important for the expert to:

1. Be professional in appearance and during communication at all times.
2. Have a firm opinion and be firm about that opinion.
3. Admit freely if there is room for argument or an alternative opinion.
4. Be concise if possible.
5. Use nontechnical language (without sacrificing accuracy of phrase).
6. Give ground with honesty and good grace.

An unbending expert who is argumentative will often fail to impress the court and carry a lower "weight" in deliberations compared with an expert who is fair and reasonable. However, be wary of the opposing advocate's questions and interruptions. Always listen carefully to the entire question before replying, consider your answer, and then respond. If the question was a series of questions, then state this and that you will deal with each question in turn. Make all replies directly to the judge (or bench) and not to the advocate; the physical movement of your body from facing the advocate to facing the front of the court also reduces the possibility that the advocate will interrupt your reply midflow, as they have lost your attention. It is not unusual for an advocate to ask basically the same question in several different ways. This is known as "testing the evidence" and requires experience to recognize and not be contradictory to answers you have already supplied. Above all else, remember that the expert is there to assist the court in reaching their decision and do not be afraid to reply, "I cannot properly answer that question" or "That matter is beyond my expertise."

REFERENCES

See www.expertconsult.com for a complete list of references.

Page numbers followed by "*f*" indicate figures, "*t*" indicate tables, and "*b*" indicate boxes.

1481